Rockwood and Matsen's

The Shoulder

Rockwood and Matsen's

The Shoulder

FIFTH EDITION

Charles A. Rockwood Jr, MD
Professor and Chairman Emeritus
Department of Orthopaedics
University of Texas Health Science Center at San Antonio
San Antonio, Texas

Frederick A. Matsen III, MD
Douglas T. Harryman II/DuPuy Endowed Professor for Shoulder Surgery
Department of Orthopaedics and Sports Medicine
University of Washington School of Medicine
Seattle, Washington

Michael A. Wirth, MD
Professor
Charles A. Rockwood Jr, MD, Chair, Shoulder Service
Department of Orthopaedics
University of Texas Health Science Center at San Antonio
San Antonio, Texas

Steven B. Lippitt, MD
Professor
Department of Orthopedic Surgery
Northeast Ohio Medical School
Cleveland Clinic Akron General
Akron, Ohio

Edward V. Fehringer, MD
Associate Professor
Department of Orthopaedic Surgery and Rehabilitation
University of Nebraska College of Medicine
Omaha, Nebraska

John W. Sperling, MD, MBA
Professor
Department of Orthopedic Surgery
Mayo Clinic
Rochester, Minnesota

Associate Editors

Samuel Antuña, MD
Shoulder and Elbow Unit
La Paz University Hospital
Madrid, Spain

Aaron J. Bois, MD, MSc
Assistant Professor
Section of Orthopaedic Surgery
Cumming School of Medicine
University of Calgary
Calgary, Alberta, Canada

Frank A. Cordasco, MD, MS
Attending Orthopaedic Surgeon
Sports Medicine and Shoulder Service
Hospital for Special Surgery;
Professor of Orthopaedic Surgery
Weill Cornell Medical College
New York, New York

Jason E. Hsu, MD
Assistant Professor
Department of Orthopaedics and Sports Medicine
University of Washington
Seattle, Washington

ELSEVIER

ELSEVIER

1600 John F. Kennedy Blvd.
Ste 1800
Philadelphia, PA 19103-2899

ROCKWOOD AND MATSEN'S THE SHOULDER, FIFTH EDITION ISBN: 978-0-323-29731-8

Notices

Knowledge and best practice in this field are constantly changing. As new research and experience broaden our understanding, changes in research methods, professional practices, or medical treatment may become necessary.

Practitioners and researchers must always rely on their own experience and knowledge in evaluating and using any information, methods, compounds, or experiments described herein. In using such information or methods they should be mindful of their own safety and the safety of others, including parties for whom they have a professional responsibility.

With respect to any drug or pharmaceutical products identified, readers are advised to check the most current information provided (i) on procedures featured or (ii) by the manufacturer of each product to be administered, to verify the recommended dose or formula, the method and duration of administration, and contraindications. It is the responsibility of practitioners, relying on their own experience and knowledge of their patients, to make diagnoses, to determine dosages and the best treatment for each individual patient, and to take all appropriate safety precautions.

To the fullest extent of the law, neither the Publisher nor the authors, contributors, or editors, assume any liability for any injury and/or damage to persons or property as a matter of products liability, negligence or otherwise, or from any use or operation of any methods, products, instructions, or ideas contained in the material herein.

Library of Congress Cataloging-in-Publication Data

Names: Rockwood, Charles A., Jr., 1936-, author.
Title: Rockwood and Matsen's the shoulder / [edited by] Charles A. Rockwood, Jr., Frederick A. Matsen, III, Michael A. Wirth, Steven B. Lippitt, Edward V. Fehringer, John W. Sperling; associate editors, Samuel Antuna, Aaron J. Bois, Frank A. Cordasco.
Other titles: Shoulder (Rockwood)
Description: Edition 5. | Philadelphia, PA : Elsevier, [2018] | Preceded by: Shoulder / editors, Charles A. Rockwood Jr. ... [et al.]. 4th ed. c2009. | Includes bibliographical references and index.
Identifiers: LCCN 2016008038 | ISBN 9780323297318 (hardcover : alk. paper)
Subjects: | MESH: Shoulder | Shoulder Joint
Classification: LCC RC939 | NLM WE 810 | DDC 617.5/72–dc23 LC record available at http://lccn.loc.gov/2016008038

Executive Content Strategist: Dolores Meloni
Senior Content Development Specialist: Rae Robertson
Publishing Services Manager: Patricia Tannian
Senior Project Manager: Carrie Stetz
Design Direction: Ryan Cook

Printed in China

Last digit is the print number: 9 8 7 6 5 4 3 2 1

We dedicate this fifth edition to the patients worldwide who are faced with disabling conditions of the shoulder. Without question, our patients are our teachers. From them we learn the causes, signs, symptoms, pathoanatomy, diagnosis, natural history, treatment, and prognosis of shoulder disease. They allow us to apply our (at times feeble) efforts to improve their comfort and function. Perhaps most importantly, they are the judges of the merit of these efforts, giving us the sometimes harsh verdict, "I'm not better." Yet we try to learn from these failures so that we and others might avoid them in the future.

We dedicate this edition to our students, those individuals who chose to spend time as apprentices in the practice of shoulder evaluation and management, but who end up being our teachers as well. These aspiring shoulder surgeons are perpetually calling us out, challenging the "generally accepted" beliefs and practices. In many ways they are like the boy in the Hans Christian Andersen tale "The Emperor's New Clothes," who, when everyone else feigns admiration of the imaginary clothes, points out that the Emperor is naked. Through their eyes, sight becomes insight.

Finally, we dedicate this volume to our families, who have given us their fullest support and encouragement during our careers as shoulder surgeons. Without their constant love, we would have accomplished little.

CHARLES A. ROCKWOOD JR
FREDERICK A. MATSEN III

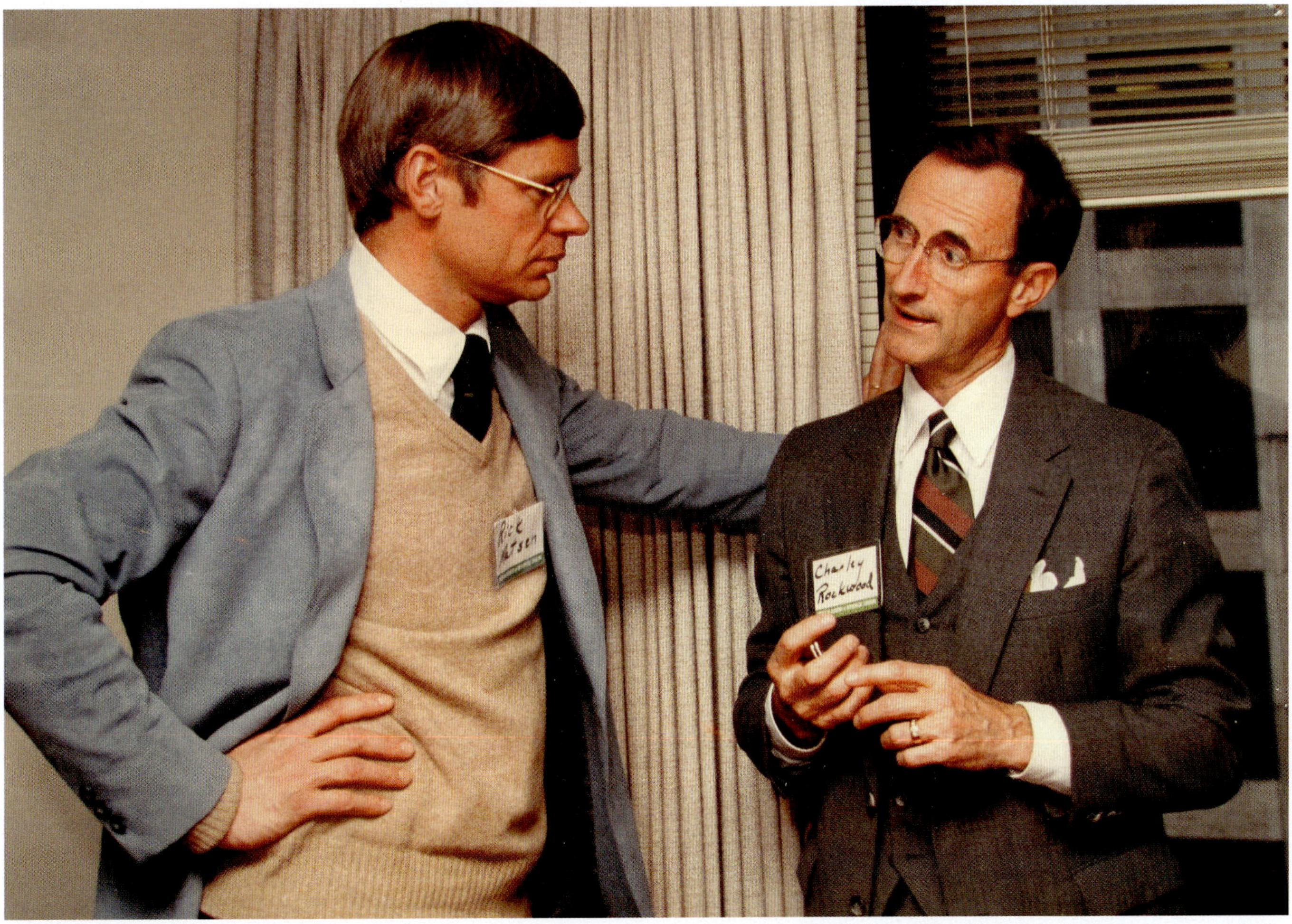

Frederick Matsen *(left)* and Charles Rockwood *(right)* have a 40-year history of close collaboration in advancing the art, science, and teaching of shoulder surgery. (Photo from 1986.)

Preface

It is with great pleasure that we offer our readers an extensively revised fifth edition of *The Shoulder*, a book that has become the definitive resource on the anatomy, mechanics, evaluation, and management of the most interesting joint complex in the human body. We started working on the first edition two decades ago, when we were much younger. Since then we have witnessed a virtual explosion of interest, research, and clinical experience that propelled *The Shoulder* through four highly successful editions.

Since the fourth edition in 2009, the number of articles, surgical techniques, and devices relating to the shoulder has grown almost beyond comprehension. Some of these represent true advances in the field, but others have not been shown to be of value either to the knowledge on which we practice shoulder surgery or to the patients we aspire to help regain the comfort and function of their shoulder. It is time to ask, "Has the increased cost of this new diagnostic tool or implant been justified by an improvement in the clinical results experienced by the patient?" For example, has the increased precision in the measurement of glenoid retroversion using sophisticated three-dimensional reconstruction software translated into a demonstrable improvement in the outcomes for the patient? New methods for imaging and attempting to repair rotator cuff tears continue to emerge, but do these methods lead to higher rates of cuff integrity? We know how to suture the labrum back to the glenoid, but when is this helpful to the patient? Should we be using a coracoid transfer to manage the routine case of recurrent traumatic glenohumeral instability? What should we learn from the historical appearance and subsequent disappearance of laser and radiofrequency techniques or of the intra-articular infusion of local anesthetics via pain pumps? Which patients with proximal humeral fractures are most likely to benefit from nonoperative management, internal fixation, a humeral prosthesis, or a reverse total shoulder? Do resurfacing, stemless, or short-stemmed humeral implants yield better clinical results than the standard type of humeral component that has served patients for half a century?

To help answer these and the many other questions that shoulder surgeons and their patients face daily, we have enlisted the partnership of a magnificent set of authors from around the world—individuals who have spent their lives searching for better ways to serve their patients. These authors have provided us with a fresh new perspective to help guide our practice. But because there are different opinions on every important topic, we have also asked our chapter editors to weigh in at the end of each chapter with their own take on the topic. And, for most chapters, we have asked highly respected international experts or senior editors to provide their thoughts on the subject. In selecting these commentaries our goal was to find surgeons who we knew had a different view so that the reader would be even better informed.

The most engaging feature of shoulder surgery is its dynamism—existing paradigms are constantly being challenged, new approaches to diagnosis and treatment are being evaluated. The published evidence is being continually assessed and reassessed to extract guidance for our practice. Surgeons are holding themselves to increasingly higher standards. We have tried to capture this dynamic by providing the most up-to-date summary of the state of the art today, hoping that this presentation will provide a current framework for practice as well as a foundation for developing what will be an improved state of the art in days to come.

Thank you, our readers, for being a part of this evolution. As we are fond of saying, "Happy shouldering!"

FREDERICK A. MATSEN III, MD

Foreword *to the Fifth Edition*

The first edition of *The Shoulder* was published in 1990 as I was finishing my fellowship with Dr. Rockwood in San Antonio. There were few fellowship-trained shoulder surgeons in the United States, or the world, and even fewer shoulder fellowships. The publication landscape was relatively sparse, with two or three single-author texts and no definitive reference text. Many shoulder conditions that required surgery were managed with traditional open techniques, but arthroscopic management was coming to the forefront. Interest in shoulder surgery was exploding, and the need for additional educational material, especially a reference text, was clear. The first edition was the reference text that this young field needed. It was an outstanding text that was well illustrated and had an extensive reference list. There were two editors, 46 authors, and two volumes.

In the 25 years that have passed since the first edition, the landscape in shoulder surgery has changed dramatically. The number of fellowship-trained shoulder surgeons has increased substantially. It is likely that there are currently more fellowship-trained shoulder surgeons working in New York and Philadelphia than were practicing in the entire United States 25 years ago. Moreover, the number of fellowships offering specialized training in shoulder surgery has exploded, both in the United States and around the world. According to the website of the American Shoulder and Elbow Surgeons, there are 28 fellowships that currently participate in their fellowship match. If one includes sports fellowships and fellowships in Europe and other parts of the world, the total is probably double that number. The need for educational material in shoulder surgery has never been greater.

The fifth edition of *The Shoulder* continues the tradition of excellence that started with the first edition. There are now six editors and three associate editors. The two most senior editors are past presidents of the American Shoulder and Elbow Surgeons and are extremely gifted educators who have dedicated their entire careers to improving the knowledge base of shoulder surgeons. The editorial team has amassed an impressive collection of authors who are nationally and internationally recognized experts in their fields. In addition to chapters on all major shoulder topics and the extensive reference lists expected from this text, there are eight chapters on arthroscopic management of shoulder conditions and a robust accompanying collection of surgical videos. The editorial team and all of the authors should be congratulated on the creation of an outstanding text.

On a more personal note, I would like to address the impressive editorial team that has organized this text. The two most senior editors have had the great foresight to add young leaders and future leaders to their team. The associate editors bring not only a level of energy and enthusiasm that I am sure was helpful, they bring a young perspective that is critical to the success of any educational product today or in the future. Drs. Lippitt, Fehringer, Sperling, and Wirth round out an outstanding editorial team; each is a recognized expert and leader in his own right.

It is hard to overestimate the footprint of Rick Matsen within shoulder surgery specifically and within the field of orthopaedics in general. He and Dr. Rockwood have a very close friendship that has lasted for decades. Together they have impacted all of our careers greatly. I respect Rick immensely; he is a true superstar.

Dr. Rockwood—what can I say. You have had a huge impact on the fields of shoulder surgery and orthopaedic surgery in general throughout the world. Whether it is orthopaedic education, prosthetic design, or leadership, everything and everyone you touch seem to succeed. You have an amazing gift. For me personally, meeting you changed my life forever, both personally and professionally. For this, I will be forever grateful.

GERALD WILLIAMS JR, MD
The John M. Fenlin Jr, MD,
Professor of Shoulder and Elbow Surgery
Orthopaedic Surgery, The Rothman Institute;
The Sidney Kimmel Medical College at
Thomas Jefferson University
Philadelphia, Pennsylvania

Foreword *to the First Edition*

It is a privilege to write the Foreword for *The Shoulder* by Drs. Charles A. Rockwood Jr, and Frederick A. Matsen III. Their objective when they began this work was an all-inclusive text on the shoulder that would also include all references on the subject in the English literature. Forty-six authors have contributed to this text.

The editors of *The Shoulder* are two of the leading shoulder surgeons in the United States. Dr. Rockwood was the fourth President of the American Shoulder and Elbow Surgeons, has organized the Instructional Course Lectures on the Shoulder for the Annual Meeting of the American Academy of Orthopaedic Surgeons for many years, and is a most experienced and dedicated teacher. Dr. Matsen is President-Elect of the American Shoulder and Elbow Surgeons and is an unusually talented teacher and leader. These two men, with their academic know-how and the help of their contributing authors, have organized a monumental text for surgeons in training and in practice, as well as one that can serve as an extensive reference source. They are to be commended for this superior book.

CHARLES S. NEER II, MD
Professor Emeritus, Orthopaedic Surgery
Columbia University
Chief, Shoulder Service
Columbia-Presbyterian Medical Center
New York, New York

Contributors

Joseph A. Abboud, MD
Research Director and Associate Professor
Shoulder and Elbow Division
Rothman Institute
Philadelphia, Pennsylvania

Christopher S. Ahmad, MD
Head Team Physician, New York Yankees
Professor of Orthopaedic Surgery
Center for Shoulder, Elbow, and Sports Medicine
Department of Orthopaedic Surgery
Columbia University
New York, New York

John M. Apostolakos, BS
Medical Student
University of Connecticut
Farmington, Connecticut

Leslie Fink Barnes, MD
Assistant Professor of Orthopaedic Surgery
Department of Orthopaedic Surgery
Temple University School of Medicine
Philadelphia, Pennsylvania

Jan Bartoníček, MD
Professor
Department of Orthopedics
First Faculty of Medicine
Charles University and Central Military Hospital
Prague, Czech Republic

Carl J. Basamania, MD
Orthopaedic Surgeon
Orthopedic Physician Associates
Swedish Orthopedic Institute
Seattle, Washington

Asheesh Bedi, MD
Chief, Sports Medicine and Shoulder Surgery
Gehring Professor of Orthopedic Surgery
University of Michigan Hospitals
Ann Arbor, Michigan

Mohit Bhandari, MD, PhD
Professor of Surgery and Chair
Department of Surgery
McMaster University
Hamilton General Hospital
Hamilton, Ontario, Canada

Kamal I. Bohsali, MD
Shoulder and Elbow Reconstruction
Jacksonville Orthopaedic Institute
Baptist Medical Center-Beaches
Jacksonville Beach, Florida

Pascal Boileau, MD
Professor
Department of Orthopaedics
University Institute of Locomotion and Sports
Pasteur 2 Hospital
Nice, France

Aaron J. Bois, MD, MSc
Assistant Professor
Section of Orthopaedic Surgery
Cumming School of Medicine
University of Calgary
Calgary, Alberta, Canada

John J. Brems, MD
Former Shoulder Fellowship Director
Cleveland Clinic Foundation;
Euclid Orthopaedics
Cleveland, Ohio

Wayne Z. Burkhead Jr, MD
Shoulder and Elbow Fellowship Director
The Carrell Clinic
Clinical Professor of Orthopaedic Surgery
University of Texas Southwestern Medical School
Dallas, Texas

Curtis Bush, MD
Orthopedic Surgeon
Harris Methodist Hospital Fort Worth;
Ben Hogan Sports Medicine
Fort Worth, Texas

Simon Carter, MD
Professor and Director
Orthopaedic Oncology Service
Royal Orthopaedic Hospital
Birmingham, United Kingdom

Michael Codsi, MD
Orthopedic Surgeon
EvergreenHealth Orthopedic & Sports Care
Kirkland, Washington

David N. Collins, MD
Arkansas Specialty Orthopaedics
Little Rock, Arkansas

Ernest U. Conrad III, MD
Seattle Children's Hospital
Seattle, Washington

John Conway, MD
Director, Sports Medicine
Ben Hogan Center
Texas Health Harris Methodist
Fort Worth, Texas

Frank A. Cordasco, MD, MS
Attending Orthopaedic Surgeon
Sports Medicine and Shoulder Service
Hospital for Special Surgery;
Professor of Orthopaedic Surgery
Weill Cornell Medical College
New York, New York

Matthew F. Dilisio, MD
Assistant Professor of Orthopaedic Surgery
Department of Orthopaedic Surgery
Creighton University School of Medicine
CHI Alegent Creighton Clinic
Omaha, Nebraska

Xavier A. Duralde, MD
Associate Adjunct Professor
Department of Orthopaedics
Emory University;
Physician
Peachtree Orthopaedic Clinic
Atlanta, Georgia

Neal S. ElAttrache, MD
Chairman, Kerlan Jobe Orthopaedic Foundation
Director, Kerlan Jobe Sports Medicine Fellowship
Clinical Instructor, Orthopaedic Surgery
Keck School of Medicine of USC
Los Angeles, California

Bassem T. Elhassan, MD
Associate Professor of Orthopedics
Mayo Clinic
Rochester, Minnesota

Nathan Evaniew, MD
Orthopaedic Resident
Department of Surgery
McMaster University
Hamilton General Hospital
Hamilton, Ontario, Canada

Peter D. Fabricant, MD, MPH
Pediatric Orthopaedic Surgery Service
Hospital for Special Surgery
Instructor of Orthopaedic Surgery
Weill Cornell Medical College
New York, New York

Brian T. Feeley, MD
Sports Medicine and Shoulder Service
Department of Orthopaedic Surgery
University of California–San Francisco
San Francisco, California

Evan L. Flatow, MD
Lasker Professor of Orthopaedic Surgery
Icahn School of Medicine at Mount Sinai
President, Mount Sinai West
New York, New York

John M. Flynn, MD
Chief, Division of Orthopedic Surgery
Children's Hospital of Philadelphia;
Professor of Orthopedic Surgery
Perelman School of Medicine
University of Pennsylvania
Philadelphia, Pennsylvania

Albert O. Gee, MD
Assistant Professor
Department of Orthopaedics and Sports Medicine
University of Washington
Seattle, Washington

Guillem Gonzalez-Lomas, MD
Assistant Professor, Department of Orthopaedic Surgery
Hospital for Joint Diseases
NYU Langone Medical Center
New York, New York

Thomas P. Goss, MD
Professor of Orthopaedic Surgery
University of Massachusetts Medical School;
Attending Orthopaedic Surgeon and Chief of Shoulder Surgery
Department of Orthopaedics and Physical Rehabilitation
University of Massachusetts Memorial Health Care
Worcester, Massachusetts

Manny Halpern, PhD
Associate Research Professor
Department of Orthopaedic Surgery
Occupational & Industrial Orthopaedic Center
NYU Langone Medical Center
New York, New York

Richard J. Han, MD
Department of Orthopaedic Surgery and Sports Medicine
Sutter Gould Medical Foundation
Modesto, California

Patrick D.G. Henry, MD
Assistant Professor
Department of Surgery
University of Toronto
Sunnybrook Health Sciences Center
Holland Orthopaedic & Arthritic Center
Toronto, Ontario, Canada

Laurence D. Higgins, MD
Chief, Sports Medicine and Shoulder Service
Department of Orthopedics
Brigham and Women's Hospital
Harvard Medical School
Boston, Massachusetts

John W. Hinchey, MD
Assistant Chief of Orthopaedics
Shoulder and Elbow Fellowship, VA Site Director
South Texas Veterans Health Care System;
Adjunct Associate Professor, Orthopaedic Surgery
University of Texas Health Science Center at San Antonio
San Antonio, Texas

Justin L. Hodgins, MD
Shoulder and Elbow Fellow
Center for Shoulder, Elbow, and Sports Medicine
Department of Orthopaedic Surgery
Columbia University
New York, New York

Jason E. Hsu, MD
Assistant Professor
Department of Orthopaedics and Sports Medicine
University of Washington
Seattle, Washington

Eiji Itoi, MD, PhD
Department of Orthopaedic Surgery
Tohoku University School of Medicine
Sendai, Japan

Kirk L. Jensen, MD
Director
East Bay Shoulder Clinic & Sports Rehabilitation
Lafayette, California

Christopher M. Jobe, MD
Department of Orthopaedic Surgery
Loma Linda University
Loma Linda, California

Herman S. Johal, MD, MPH
Orthopaedic Trauma/Research Fellow
Department of Surgery
McMaster University
Hamilton General Hospital
Hamilton, Ontario, Canada

Natascha Kraus, MD
Center for Musculoskeletal Surgery
Charité-Universitaetsmedizin Berlin
Berlin, Germany

Thomas Lawrence, MD, MSc
Consultant Shoulder and Elbow Surgeon
Trauma and Orthopaedics
University Hospital Coventry and Warwickshire
Coventry, Great Britain

George F. LeBus, MD
Medical Resident
Vanderbilt University Medical Center
Vanderbilt Orthopaedic Institute
Nashville, Tennessee

Mario Lenza, MD, PhD
Orthopaedic Surgeon
Department of Orthopaedics
Hospital Israelita Albert Einstein;
Shoulder and Elbow Surgeon
Department of Orthopaedics
Universidade Federal de Sao Paulo
Sao Paulo, Brazil

Ofer Levy, MD, MCh(Orth)
Reading Shoulder Unit
Royal Berkshire Hospital and Berkshire Independent Hospital
Reading, United Kingdom;
Centre for Sports Medicine and Human Performance
School of Sport and Education
Brunel University London
London, United Kingdom

Steven B. Lippitt, MD
Professor
Department of Orthopedics
Northeast Ohio Medical School
Cleveland Clinic Akron General
Akron, Ohio

C. Benjamin Ma, MD
Professor in Residence
Chief, Sports Medicine and Shoulder Service
University of California–San Francisco
San Francisco, California

Pierre Mansat, MD, PhD
Professor of Orthopedics and Traumatology
Orthopedics and Traumatology
University Hospital of Toulouse
Toulouse, France

Frederick A. Matsen III, MD
Douglas T. Harryman II/DuPuy Endowed Professor for Shoulder Research
Department of Orthopaedics and Sports Medicine
University of Washington School of Medicine
Seattle, Washington

Augustus D. Mazzocca, MD
Professor and Chairman
Department of Orthopedic Surgery
University of Connecticut Health Center
Farmington, Connecticut

Jesse McCarron, MD
Orthopedic Surgeon
Portland VA Medical Center
Portland, Oregon

Ryan A. Mlynarek, MD
Resident, Orthopaedic Surgery
University of Michigan
Ann Arbor, Michigan

Todd C. Moen, MD
Partner
Assistant Director, Shoulder and Elbow Fellowship
W.B. Carrell Memorial Clinic
Dallas, Texas

Brent Mollon, MD
Clinical Fellow, Shoulder and Elbow
Department of Orthopaedic Surgery
Hospital for Joint Diseases
NYU Langone Medical Center
New York, New York

Alexa Narzikul, BA
Medical Student
Sidney Kimmel Medical College
Thomas Jefferson University
Philadelphia, Pennsylvania

Amit Nathani, MD
Resident, Orthopaedic Surgery
University of Michigan
Ann Arbor, Michigan

Stephen J. O'Brien, MD, MBA
Attending Orthopaedic Surgeon
Sports Medicine Department
Hospital for Special Surgery
New York, New York

Bradford O. Parsons, MD
Chief of Shoulder Surgery and Fellowship Director
Associate Professor and Residency Program Director
Icahn School of Medicine at Mount Sinai Medical Center
New York, New York

Scott D. Pennington, MD
Physician
Peachtree Orthopaedic Clinic
Atlanta, Georgia

Djuro Petkovic, MD
Department of Orthopaedic Surgery
Loma Linda University
Loma Linda, California

Wesley P. Phipatanakul, MD
Department of Orthopaedic Surgery
Loma Linda University
Loma Linda, California

Robert H. Quinn, MD
Chair and Professor, Residency Program Director
Department of Orthopaedic Surgery
University of Texas Health Science Center at San Antonio
San Antonio, Texas

Prem N. Ramkumar, MBA
Medical Student
Sports Medicine and Shoulder Service
Hospital for Special Surgery
New York, New York

Robin R. Richards, MD
Professor of Surgery
Department of Surgery
University of Toronto;
Surgeon-in-Chief Emeritus
Sunnybrook Health Sciences Center
Toronto, Ontario, Canada

Daniel S. Robertson, MD
Shoulder and Elbow Surgery
Department of Orthopedic Surgery
Mid-Atlantic Permanente Medical Group
Largo, Maryland

Charles A. Rockwood Jr, MD
Professor and Chairman Emeritus
Department of Orthopaedics
University of Texas Health Science Center at San Antonio
San Antonio, Texas

Markus Scheibel, MD
Center for Musculoskeletal Surgery
Charité-Universitaetsmedizin Berlin
Berlin, Germany

Adam J. Seidl, MD
Assistant Professor
Division of Sports Medicine and Shoulder Surgery
University of Colorado
Aurora, Colorado

Scott P. Steinmann, MD
Professor of Orthopedics
Mayo Clinic
Rochester, Minnesota

Samuel A. Taylor, MD
Assistant Attending Surgeon
Orthopaedic Surgery
Hospital for Special Surgery;
Assistant Professor
Orthopaedic Surgery
Weill Cornell Medical College
New York, New York

Philip Tirman, MD
Medical Director
Renaissance Medical Imaging Associates
Westlake Village, California

I.A. Trail, MD
Professor
Upper Limb Research
Wrightington Hospital
Wigan, United Kingdom

Andreas Voss, MD
Sports Medicine Research Fellow
Department of Orthopaedic Surgery & Department of Orthopaedic Sports Medicine
Technical University of Munich
Munich, Germany;
University of Connecticut
Farmington, Connecticut

Gilles Walch, MD
Centre Orthopédique Santy
Department of Shoulder Surgery
Hôpital Privé Jean Mermoz
Générale de Santé Clinique
Lyon, France

Marie E. Walcott, MD
Department of Orthopedics
University of Massachusetts
Worcester, Massachusetts

Jon J.P. Warner, MD
Chief, MGH Shoulder Service
Department of Orthopaedic Surgery
Massachusetts General Hospital;
Professor of Orthopaedic Surgery
Department of Orthopaedic Surgery
Harvard Medical School
Boston, Massachusetts

Robert W. Westermann, MD
Department of Orthopaedics
University of Iowa
Iowa City, Iowa

Alex E. White, BA
Clinical Research Coordinator
Sports Medicine
Hospital for Special Surgery
New York, New York

Michael A. Wirth, MD
Professor
Charles A. Rockwood Jr, MD, Chair, Shoulder Service
Department of Orthopaedics
University of Texas Health Science Center at San Antonio
San Antonio, Texas

Brian R. Wolf, MD
Congdon Professor and Vice Chairman
Department of Orthopaedics and Rehabilitation
University of Iowa
Iowa City, Iowa

Justin S. Yang, MD
Sports Medicine and Orthopedic Surgery
Kaiser Permanente Los Angeles Medical Center
Los Angeles, California

Joseph D. Zuckerman, MD
Professor and Chairman
Department of Orthopaedic Surgery
Hospital for Joint Diseases
NYU Langone Medical Center
New York, New York

Contents

Video Contents

CHAPTER 1

Developmental Anatomy of the Shoulder and Anatomy of the Glenohumeral Joint

Stephen J. O'Brien, Samuel A. Taylor, Prem N. Ramkumar, Alex E. White

As our human ancestors evolved to become bipedal, the scapulohumeral complex evolved to comply with the specific demands that arise from an orthograde posture and to facilitate prehension. The inherent osseous articular congruity required for weight-bearing activities were sacrificed in the upper extremities for soft tissue stability to afford a greater degree of mobility at the glenohumeral joint.

This chapter focuses on the developmental anatomy of the shoulder girdle and the anatomy of the adult glenohumeral joint. Since the previous edition, several studies and new technologic developments have advanced our understanding of the anatomy and biomechanics of the glenohumeral joint, particularly with regard to the biceps-labral complex and the recently recognized bicipital tunnel.[77]

COMPARATIVE ANATOMY

General Development

The forelimb in humans is a paired appendage whose evolutionary roots can be traced to the longitudinal lateral folds of epidermis in the early fish species *Rhipidistian crossopterygian.*[18] These folds extended caudad from the region just behind the gills to the anus (Fig. 1-1). The pectoral and pelvic fins subsequently developed from the proximal and distal portions of these folds, respectively, and were the predecessors of the human upper and lower limbs (Fig. 1-2).[53]

Over time, muscle buds, along with the ventral rami of spinal nerves, migrated into these pectoral fins to allow for coordinated movement. Peripheral fibers repeatedly divided to form a plexus of nerves, and different regions of muscle tissue often combined or segmented as function evolved.

Cartilage rays called *radials* (Fig. 1-3) developed between the muscle buds to form a support structure, and the proximal portions of these radials coalesced to form basal cartilage, or *basilia.* The radials began to fuse at their base and eventually formed a concrescent central axis, or *pectoral girdle* (Fig. 1-4). These paired basilia eventually migrated ventrally toward the midline anteriorly to form a *ventral bar,* which corresponds to the paired clavicles in some mammals, as well as the *cleitrum,* a membranous bone that attached the pectoral girdle to the skull. The basilia also projected dorsally over the thorax to form the precursor of the scapula. Articulations within the basilia eventually developed at the junction of the ventral and dorsal segments (the glenoid fossa) with the remainder of the pectoral fin, which corresponds to the glenohumeral joint in humans (Fig. 1-5).

As these prehistoric fish evolved into amphibians, their osseous morphology also changed to adapt to gravity out of water. The head was eventually freed from its attachments to the pectoral girdle, and in reptiles, the pectoral girdle migrated a considerable distance caudally.[50] The pelycosaur of the late Paleozoic Era (235 to 255 million years ago) is among the oldest reptiles believed to have been solely land dwellers.[33] These early tetrapods ambulated with the proximal part of their forelimbs held in the horizontal plane and the distal part flexed at a 90-degree angle in the sagittal plane. Locomotion was attained by rotation of the humerus around its longitudinal axis. The cleitrum disappeared entirely during this reptilian stage.

Whereas structural stability was primarily achieved via osseous congruity in these early reptiles, the shoulder evolved to allow greater flexibility and mobility in subsequent species. The basic mammalian pattern developed with articulations arising between a well-developed clavicle and sternum medially and a flat, fairly wide scapula laterally. The coracoid enlarged during this period, and the scapular spine developed in response to new functional demands (Fig. 1-6). Four main variations on this scheme are seen.[8] Mammals adapted for running have lost their clavicle to further mobilize the scapula, and the scapula is relatively narrow. Mammals adapted for swimming also have lost the clavicle, although the scapula is wider and permits more varied function. Shoulder girdles

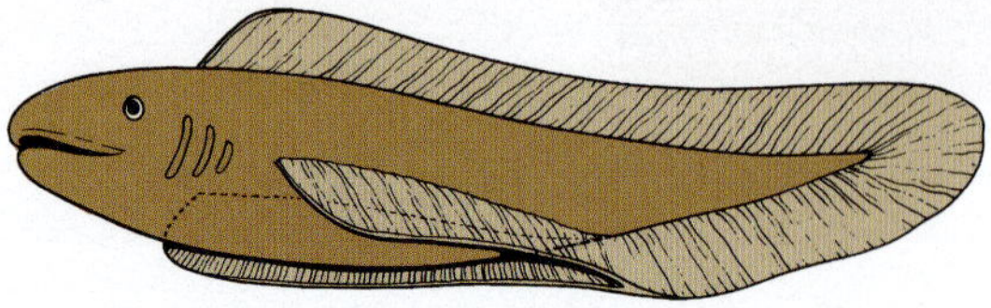

FIGURE 1-1: In the early fish species paired lateral longitudinal folds of epidermis of the fish extended caudad from the region just posterior to the gills to the anus.

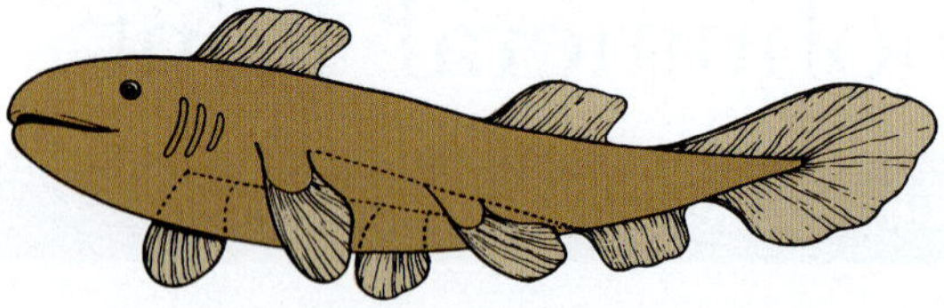

FIGURE 1-2: The pectoral and pelvic fins subsequently developed from the proximal and distal portions of the paired longitudinal lateral folds. These fins were the precursors of the human upper and lower limbs.

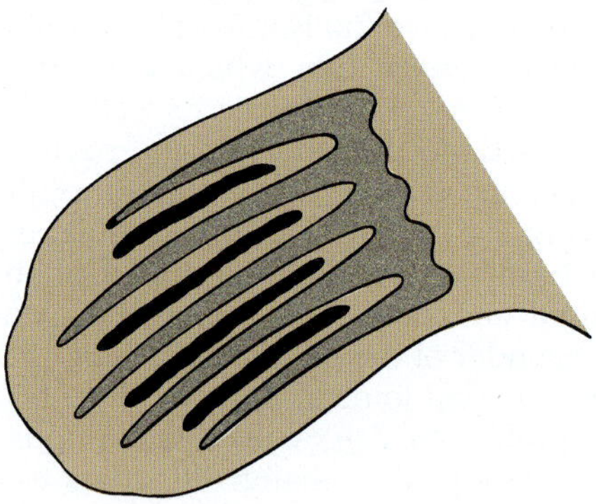

FIGURE 1-3: Cartilage rays called *radials* developed between muscle buds to form a support structure for the limb. The proximal portions of these radials coalesced to form basal cartilage, or basilia.

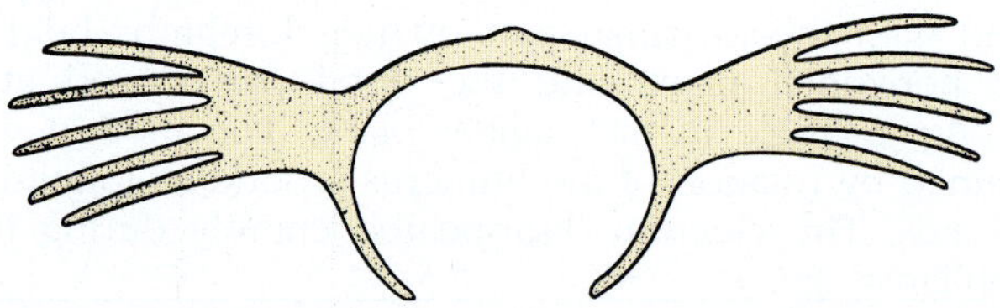

FIGURE 1-4: The paired basilia came together in the midline to form the primitive pectoral girdle. As these basilia migrated, they formed a bar that was the precursor to the paired clavicles.

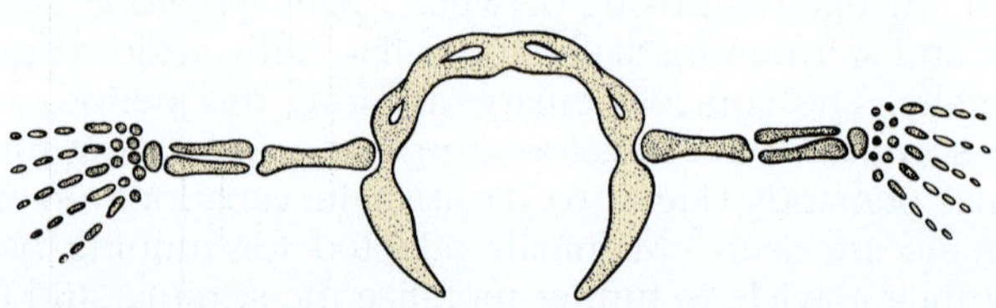

FIGURE 1-5: Articulations within the basilia developed at the junction of the ventral and dorsal segments, which formed the primitive glenoid fossa.

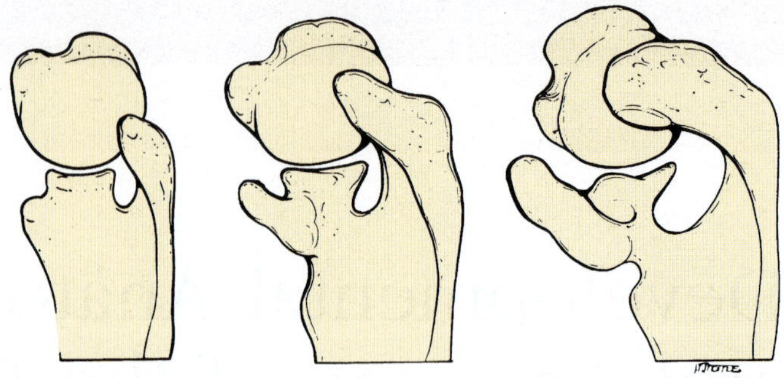

FIGURE 1-6: The coracoid and acromion progressively enlarged in response to the new functional demands of the orthograde posture.

modified for flying have a large, long, well-developed clavicle with a small, narrow, curved scapula. Shoulders modified for brachiating (including those of humans) developed a strong clavicle, a large coracoid, and a widened, strong scapula.

Other adaptations for the erect posture were a relative flattening of the thorax in the anteroposterior dimension, with the scapula left approximately 45 degrees to the midline (Fig. 1-7), and evolution of the pentadactyl limb with a strong, mobile thumb and four ulnar digits. This pentadactyl limb is very similar to the human arm as we know it.

In the following sections, we individually discuss the evolution of the different regions of the shoulder and pectoral girdle as they approach a more human form.

Development of Individual Regions

Scapula

The scapula in humans is suspended by muscles alone and clearly reflects the adaptive development of the shoulder. It has shifted caudally from the cervical position in lower animals; as a result, the shoulder is freed from the head and neck and can serve as a base or platform to facilitate arm movement. The most striking modification in the development of the bone of the scapula itself is in the relationship between the length (measured along the base of the spine) and the breadth (measured from the superior to the inferior angle) of the scapula, or the *scapular index* (Fig. 1-8).[32] This index is extremely high in the pronograde animals with a long, narrow scapula. The scapula is broader in humans and other primates, with the most pronounced differences observed in the infraspinatus fossa, a modification referred to as an increase in the infraspinatus index.

Broadening of the infraspinatus fossa has resulted in a change in the vector of muscle pull from the axillary border of the scapula to the glenoid fossa and has consequently altered the action of the attached musculature. This adaptation allows the infraspinatus and teres minor muscles to be more effective in their roles as depressors and external rotators of the humeral head. Over time, the supraspinatus fossa and muscle have changed little in size or shape, but the acromion, which is an extension

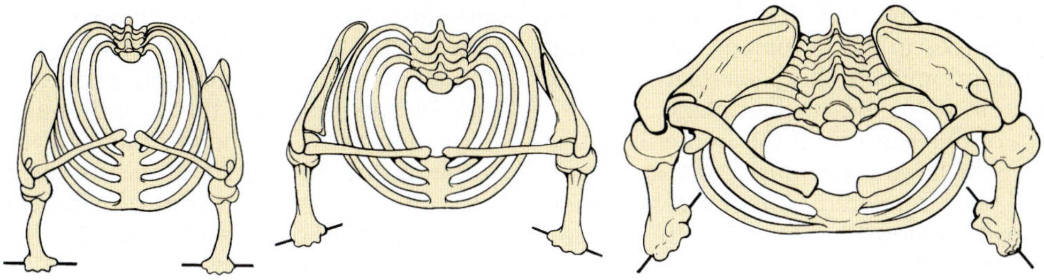

FIGURE 1-7: The anteroposterior dimension of the thoracic cage decreased over time, resulting in the scapula positioned approximately 45 degrees to the midline. The scapula and glenoid fossa assumed a more dorsal position in the thoracic cage, which led to the glenoid fossa being directed laterally. Consequently, a relative external rotation of the humeral head and an internal rotation of the shaft occurred.

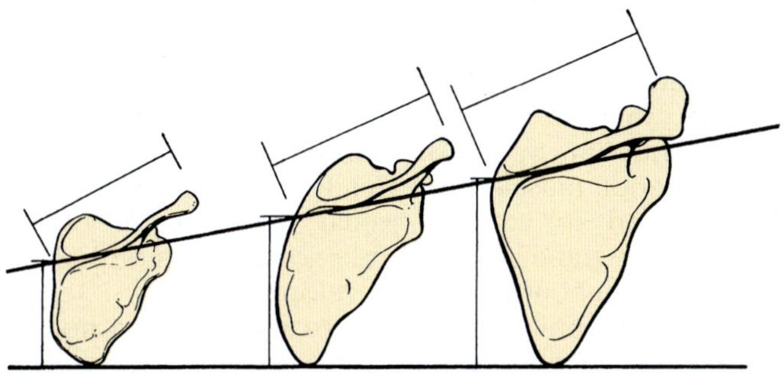

FIGURE 1-8: The size of the infraspinatus fossa gradually enlarged over time relative to the length of the scapular spine. This relative increase has led to a decrease in the scapular index.

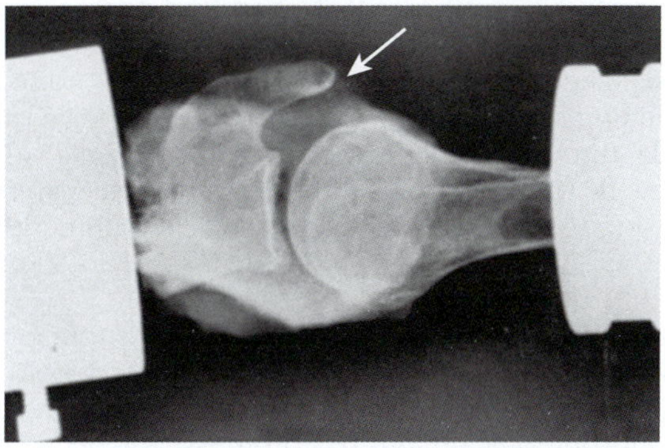

FIGURE 1-9: A radiographic view of an abducted shoulder shows a large overlap (*arrow*) of the coracoid over the glenohumeral joint, which may restrict anterior translation.

of the spine of the scapula, has enlarged (see Fig. 1-6). In pronograde animals, the acromion process is insignificant; however, in humans, it is a massive structure overlying the humeral head. This difference reflects the increasing role of the deltoid muscle in shoulder function. The broader attachment of this muscle on the acromion and its more distal insertion on the humerus have increased its mechanical advantage in shoulder motion.

The coracoid process has also undergone an increase in size over time (see Fig. 1-6).[32] We have performed biomechanical studies showing that with the shoulder in 90 degrees of abduction, the coracoid extension over the glenohumeral joint can mechanically limit anterior translation of the humerus relative to the glenoid. One shoulder tested after sectioning the capsule would not dislocate anteriorly in full abduction until the coracoid process was removed (Fig. 1-9).[59]

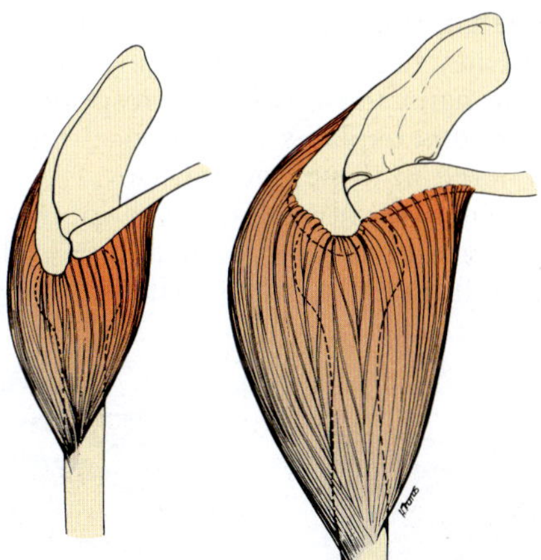

FIGURE 1-10: Over time, the deltoid muscle insertion migrated distally, improving leverage on the humerus.

Humerus

Like the scapula, the humerus has undergone several morphologic changes during its evolution. Over time, the head of the humerus has moved proximally, underneath the torso, as well as from the horizontal plane to a more vertical resting orientation. The insertion site of the deltoid muscle has migrated distally, improving its leverage (Fig. 1-10).[32,37]

In addition, the distal humeral shaft underwent an episode of torsion relative to the proximal end of the humerus, thereby rotating the humeral head internally relative to the epicondyles.[32] As the thoracic cage flattened in the anteroposterior plane, the scapula and glenoid fossa assumed a more dorsal position within it, which led to the glenoid fossa being directed more laterally (see Fig. 1-7). As a consequence, there was external rotation of the humeral head and internal rotation of the shaft relative to it, which led to medial displacement of the intertubercular groove and a decreased size of the lesser tuberosity relative to the greater tuberosity. The resultant retroversion of the humeral head has been reported to be 33 degrees in the dominant shoulder and 29 degrees in the nondominant shoulder relative to the epicondyles of the elbow in the coronal plane.[39]

The other effect of this torsion on the humerus is that the biceps muscle, which was previously a strong elevator of the arm, has been rendered biomechanically ineffective unless the arm is externally rotated. In this fashion it can be used as an abductor, which is often seen in infantile paralysis.

Clavicle

The clavicle is not present in animals, such as horses, that use their forelimbs for standing. In animals that use their upper limbs for holding, grasping, and climbing, however, the clavicle allows the scapula and humerus to be positioned away from the body to help the limb move free of the axial skeleton. In humans, it also provides a means of transmitting the supporting force of the trapezius to the scapula through the coracoclavicular ligaments, a bony framework for muscle attachments, and a mechanism for increasing the range of motion at the glenohumeral joint.

Scapulohumeral Muscles

The scapulohumeral muscles include the supraspinatus, infraspinatus, teres minor, subscapularis, deltoid, and teres major. The supraspinatus has remained relatively static morphologically but has progressively decreased in relative mass (Fig. 1-11).[37] In contrast, the deltoid has more than doubled in its proportional representation and constitutes approximately 41% of the scapulohumeral muscle mass. This increase in size also increases the overall strength of the deltoid. In lower animals, a portion of the deltoid attaches to the inferior angle of the scapula, whereas in humans, these fibers correspond to the teres minor muscle; this explains the identical innervation by the axillary nerve in these two muscles.

The infraspinatus is absent in lower species; however, in humans, it makes up approximately 5% of the mass of the scapulohumeral muscles. The subscapularis has undergone no significant change, except for a slight increase in the number of fasciculi concomitant with elongation of the scapula, and it makes up approximately 20% of the mass of the scapulohumeral group. This adaptation allows the lower part of the muscle to pull in a downward direction and assists the infraspinatus and teres minor to act as a group to function as depressors as well as stabilizers of the head of the humerus against the glenoid during arm elevation.

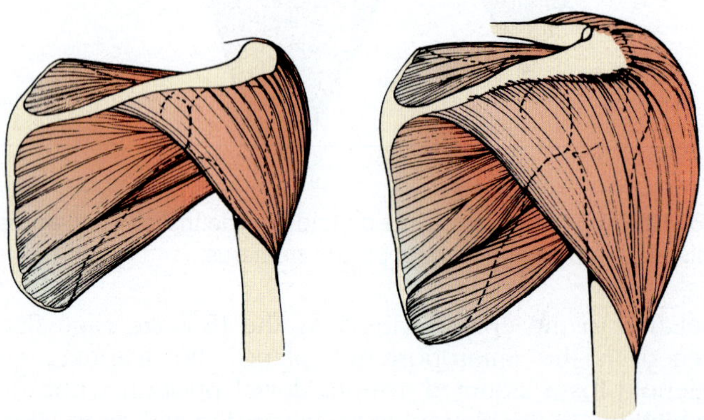

FIGURE 1-11: The supraspinatus muscle has remained relatively static morphologically, but has progressively decreased in mass relative to the infraspinatous muscles, although the enlarged deltoid muscle can be appreciated. The increased importance of the deltoid is evidenced by its increase in relative size.

Axioscapular Muscles

The axioscapular muscles include the serratus anterior, rhomboids, levator scapulae, and trapezius. All these muscles (except the trapezius) originated from one complex of muscle fibers arising from the first eight ribs and the transverse processes of the cervical vertebrae, inserting into the vertebral border of the scapula. As differentiation occurred, the fibers concerned with dorsal scapular motion became the rhomboid muscles, the fibers controlling ventral motion developed into the serratus anterior muscle, and finally, the levator scapulae differentiated to control cranial displacement of the scapula. The trapezius has undergone little morphologic change throughout primate development.

The axioscapular group of muscles acts to anchor the scapula to the thoracic cage while allowing freedom of motion. Most authorities report the ratio between glenohumeral and scapulothoracic motion to be 2:1.[32,28] The serratus anterior provides horizontal stability and prevents winging of the scapula.

Axiohumeral Muscles

The axiohumeral muscles connect the humerus to the trunk and consist of the pectoralis major, pectoralis minor, and latissimus dorsi. The pectoral muscles originate from a single muscle mass that divides into a superficial layer and a deep layer. The superficial layer becomes the pectoralis major, and the deep layer gives rise to the pectoralis minor. The pectoralis minor is attached to the humerus in lower species, whereas in humans it is attached to the coracoid process.

Muscles of the Upper Part of the Arm

The biceps in more primitive animals has a single origin on the supraglenoid tubercle and often assists the supraspinatus in limb elevation. In humans, the biceps has two origins and, because of the torsional changes in the humerus, is ineffective in shoulder elevation unless the arm is fully externally rotated.

The triceps has not undergone significant morphologic change, but the size of the long head of the triceps has been progressively decreasing.

EMBRYOLOGY

Prenatal Development

Three germ layers give rise to all the tissues and organs of the body. The cells of each germ layer divide, migrate, aggregate, and differentiate in rather precise patterns as they form the various organ systems. The three germ layers are the ectoderm, the mesoderm, and the endoderm. The ectoderm gives rise to the central nervous system, peripheral nervous system, epidermis and its appendages, mammary glands, pituitary gland, and subcutaneous glands. The mesoderm gives rise to cartilage, bone, connective tissue, striated and smooth muscle, blood cells, kidneys, gonads, spleen, and the serous membrane lining of the body cavities. The endoderm gives rise to the epithelial lining of the gastrointestinal, respiratory, and urinary tracts; the lining of the auditory canal; and the parenchyma of the tonsils, thyroid gland, parathyroid glands, thymus, liver, and pancreas. The development of the embryo requires a coordinated interaction of these germ layers, orchestrated by genetic and environmental factors under the influence of basic induction and regulatory mechanisms.

Prenatal human embryologic development can be divided into three major periods: the first 2 weeks, the embryonic period, and the fetal period. The first 2 weeks of development are characterized by fertilization, blastocyst formation, implantation, and further development of the embryoblast and trophoblast. The embryonic period comprises weeks 3 through 8 of development, and the fetal period encompasses the remainder of the prenatal period until term.

The embryonic period is important because all the major external and internal organs develop during this time, and by the end of this period, differentiation is practically complete. All the bones and joints have the form and arrangement characteristic of adults. Exposure to teratogens during this period can cause major congenital malformations. During the fetal period, the limbs grow and mature as a result of a continual remodeling and reconstructive process that enables bones to maintain their characteristic shape. In the skeleton in general, increments of growth in individual bones are in precise relationship to those of the skeleton as a whole. Ligaments show an increase in collagen content, bursae develop, tendinous attachments shift to accommodate growth, and epiphyseal cartilage becomes vascularized.

Few studies have focused on the prenatal development of the glenohumeral joint. The contributions by DePalma and Gardner were essential, but did not emphasize clinical correlations between the observed fetal anatomy and the pathology seen in the postnatal shoulder.[16,24,25] Most studies on the developing shoulder have focused primarily on bone maturation, and analysis of the soft tissue structures of the developing shoulder, such as the joint capsule and the labrum, is still incomplete. Studies have not thoroughly evaluated the inferior glenohumeral ligament complex (IGHLC), which has been shown to be an integral component for stability in the adult shoulder.[58] The seminal studies of the fetal glenohumeral joint were completed before the role of the soft tissue structures in shoulder stability was elucidated. There is now a greater appreciation of the anatomy and biomechanics of the static and dynamic stabilizers of the glenohumeral joint and their role in shoulder stability.

Embryonic Period

The limb buds are initially seen as small elevations on the ventrolateral body wall at the end of the fourth week of gestation.[51] The upper limb buds appear during the first few days of the fourth week and maintain a growth advantage over the lower limbs throughout development. Because development of the head and neck occurs in advance of the rest of the embryo, the upper limb buds appear disproportionately low on the embryo's trunk (Fig. 1-12). During the early stages of limb development, the upper and lower extremities develop in a similar fashion, with the upper limb buds developing opposite the lower six cervical and the first and second thoracic segments.

At 4 weeks, the upper limb is a sac of ectoderm filled with mesoderm and is approximately 3 mm long. Each limb bud is delineated dorsally by a sulcus and ventrally by a pit. The pit for the upper limb bud is called the *fossa axillaris*. The mesoderm in the upper limb bud develops from somatic mesoderm and consists of a mass of mesenchyme, which is loosely organized embryonic connective tissue. Mesenchymal cells can differentiate into different types of cells, including fibroblasts, chondroblasts, and osteoblasts (Fig. 1-13). Most bones first appear as a condensation of these mesenchymal cells, from which a core called the *blastema* is formed.[51,76] This development is orchestrated by the apical ectodermal ridge (Fig. 1-14), which exerts an inductive influence on the limb mesenchyme, promoting growth and development.

During the fifth week, a number of developments occur simultaneously. The peripheral nerves grow from the brachial plexus into the mesenchyme of the limb buds. Such growth stimulates development of the limb musculature, where in situ somatic limb mesoderm aggregates and differentiates into myoblasts and discrete

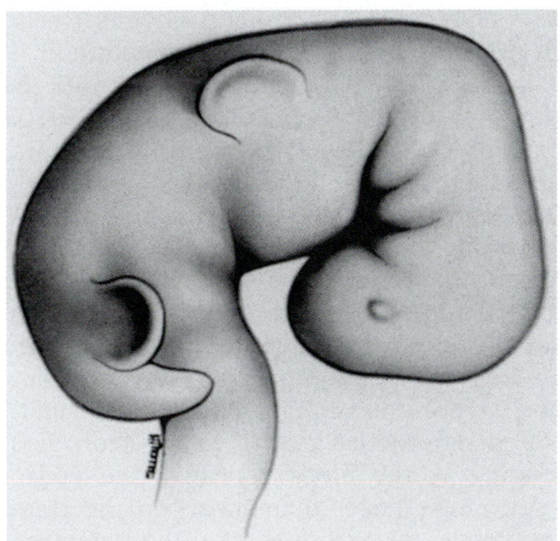

FIGURE 1-12: Because development of the head and neck occurs in advance of the rest of the embryo, the upper and lower limb buds are disproportionately low on the embryo's trunk.

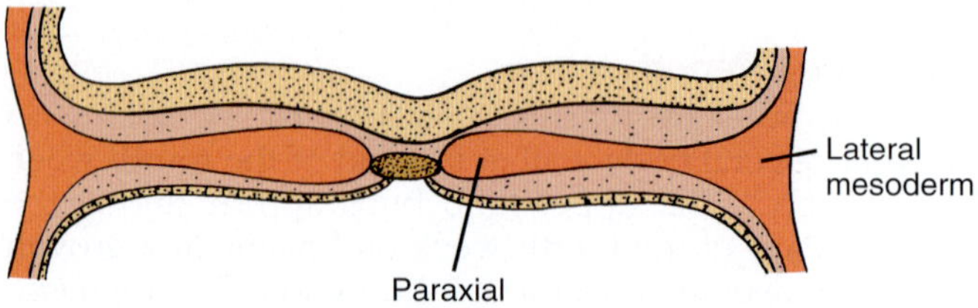

FIGURE 1-13: The mesoderm in the upper limb bud develops from somatic mesoderm and consists of a mass of mesenchyme (loosely organized embryonic connective tissue). It eventually differentiates into fibroblastic, chondroblastic, and osteoblastic tissue.

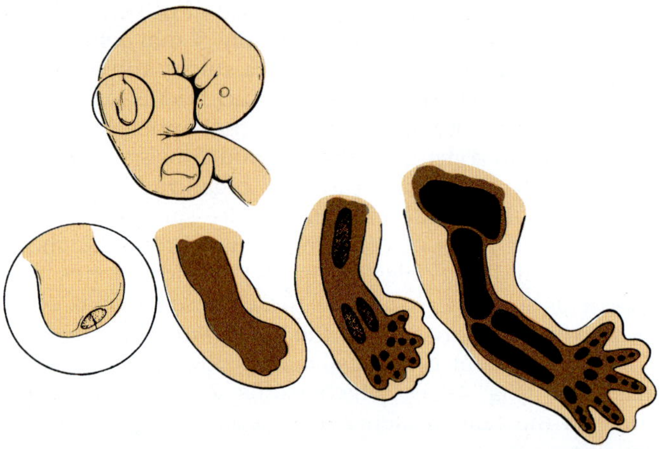

FIGURE 1-14: The apical ectodermal ridge exerts an inductive influence on the development of the upper limb.

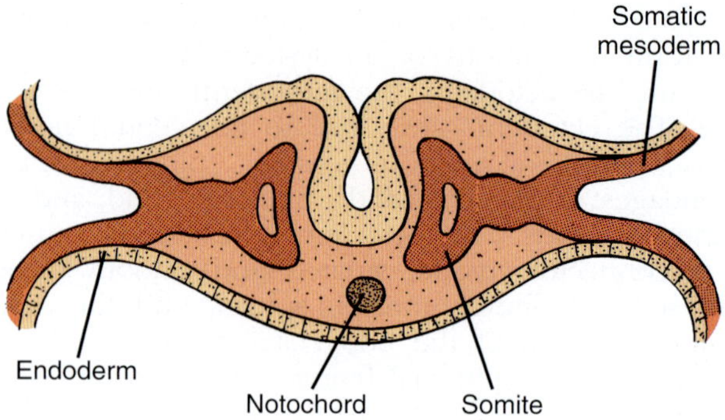

FIGURE 1-15: The axial musculature develops from myotomic regions of somites, which are segments of two longitudinal columns of paraxial mesoderm. This tissue differs from the somatic mesoderm from which the limb develops.

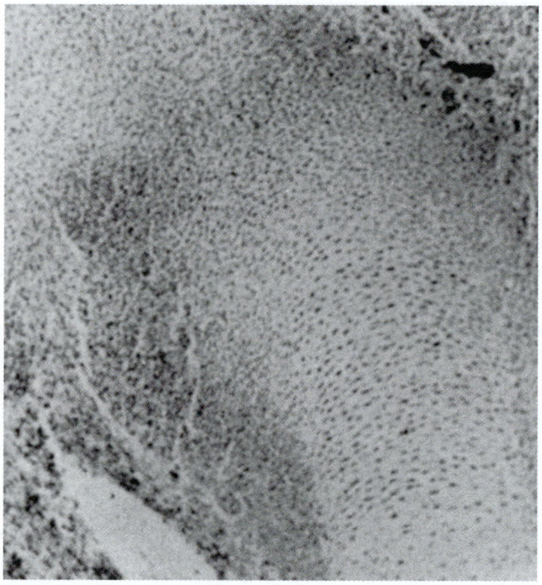

FIGURE 1-16: At 5 weeks of gestation the central core of the humerus begins to chondrify, but a homogeneous interzone remains between the scapula and the humerus. (From Gardner E, Gray DJ. Prenatal development of the human shoulder and acromioclavicular joint. *Am J Anat.* 1953;92:219-276.)

muscle units. This process differs from the development of the axial musculature, which arises from the myotomic regions of segments of two longitudinal columns of paraxial mesoderm known as *somites* (Fig. 1-15). Also at this time, the central core of the humerus begins to chondrify, although the shoulder joint has not yet formed. There is an area in the blastema called the *interzone* that does not undergo chondrification and is the precursor of the shoulder joint (Fig. 1-16). The scapula at this time lies at the level of C4 and C5 (Fig. 1-17),[41] and the clavicle begins to ossify. (Along with the mandible, the clavicle is the first bone to begin to ossify.)

During the sixth week, the mesenchymal tissue in the periphery of the hand plates condenses to form digital rays. The mesodermal cells of the limb bud rearrange to form a deep layer, an intermediate layer, and a superficial layer. This layering is brought on by differential growth rates.[74] Such differential growth in the limb also stimulates bending at the elbow because the cells on the ventral side grow faster than those on the dorsal side, which stretches to accommodate the ventral growth. The muscle groups divide into dorsal extensors and ventral flexors, and the individual muscles migrate caudally as the limb bud develops. In the shoulder joint the interzone assumes a three-layered configuration, with a chondrogenic layer on either side of a loose layer of cells.[27] At this time, the glenoid labrum is discernible (Fig. 1-18), although cavitation or joint formation has not yet occurred. Initial bone formation begins in the primary ossification center of the humerus. The scapula at this time undergoes marked enlargement and extends from C4 to approximately T7.

Early in the seventh week, the limbs extend ventrally and the upper and lower limb buds rotate in opposite directions (Fig. 1-19). The upper limbs rotate laterally through 90 degrees around their longitudinal axes, with the elbow facing posteriorly and the extensor muscles facing laterally and posteriorly.[51] The lower limbs rotate medially through almost 90 degrees, with the knee and

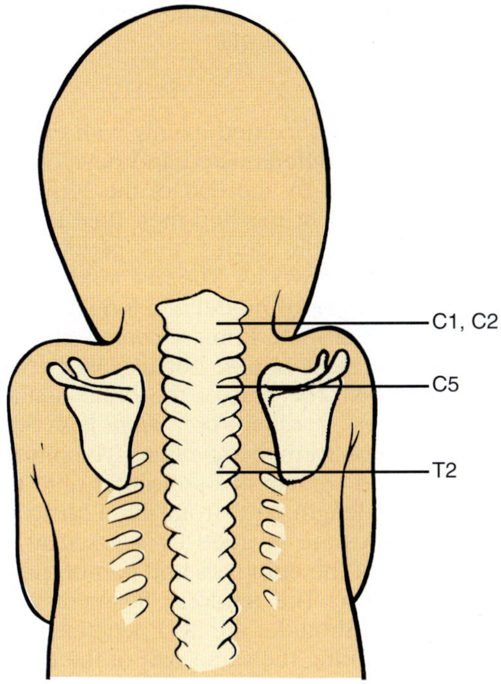

FIGURE 1-17: By the fifth week of gestation the scapula lies at the level of C4 and C5. It gradually descends as it develops. Failure of the scapula to descend is called *Sprengel's deformity.*

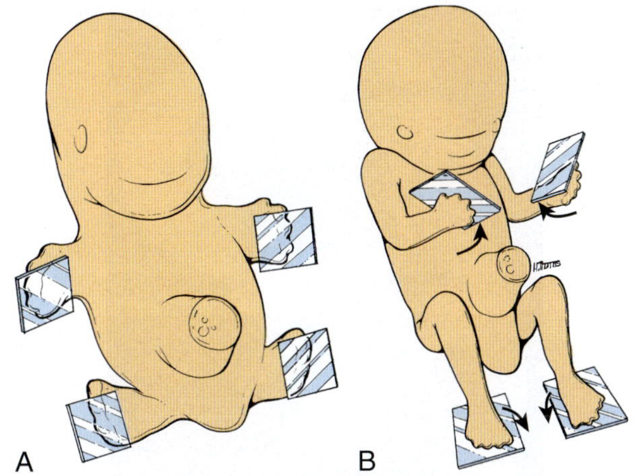

FIGURE 1-19: A, After the seventh week of gestation, the limbs extend ventrally, and the upper and lower limb buds rotate in opposite directions. **B,** As a result, the radius occupies a lateral position in the upper limb, whereas the tibia assumes a medial position in the lower limb, although they are homologous bones.

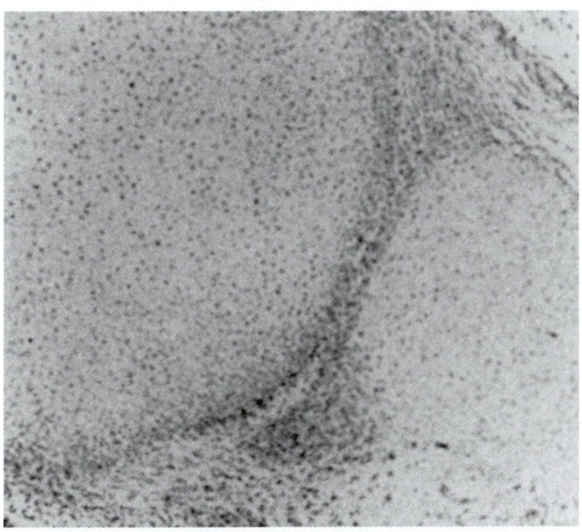

FIGURE 1-18: At 6 weeks of gestation (21 mm), a three-layered interzone is present, and the beginning of the development of the glenoid labrum is evident. (From Gardner E, Gray DJ. Prenatal development of the human shoulder and acromioclavicular joint. *Am J Anat,* 1953;92:219.)

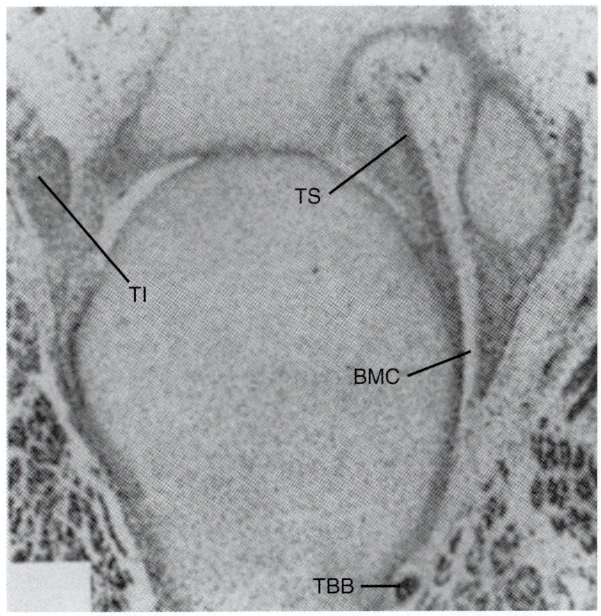

FIGURE 1-20: By the seventh week the glenohumeral joint is well formed, and the middle zone of the three-layered interzone becomes progressively less dense with increasing cavitation. The tendons of the infraspinatus (TI), subscapularis (TS), and biceps (TBB) are clearly seen, as is the bursa of the coracobrachialis (BMC). (From Gardner E, Gray DJ. Prenatal development of the human shoulder and acromioclavicular joint. *Am J Anat.* 1953;92:219-276.)

extensor musculature facing anteriorly. The final result is that the radius is in a lateral position in the upper limb and the tibia is in a medial position in the lower limb, although these are homologous bones. The ulna and fibula are also homologous bones, and the thumb and great toe are homologous digits. The shoulder joint is now well formed, and the middle zone of the three-layered interzone becomes progressively less dense with increasing cavitation (Fig. 1-20). The scapula has now descended and spans from just below the level of the first rib to the level of the fifth rib.[23] The brachial plexus has also migrated caudally and lies over the first rib. The

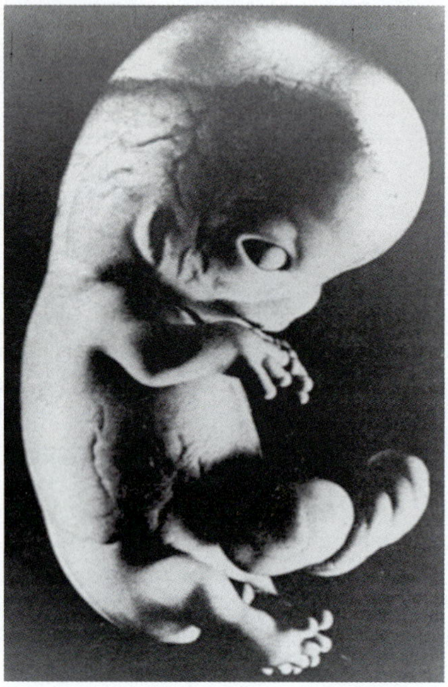

FIGURE 1-21: At the eighth week of gestation the embryo is about 23 mm long. Through the growth of the upper limb, the hands are stretched and the arms are pronated. The firm musculature is now clearly defined.

final few degrees of downward displacement of the scapula occur later when the anterior portion of the rib cage drops obliquely downward.

By the eighth week the embryo is about 25 to 31 mm long, and through the growth of the upper limb, the hands are stretched with the arms pronated (Fig. 1-21). The musculature of the limb is now also clearly defined. The shoulder joint has the form of the adult glenohumeral joint, and the glenohumeral ligaments can now be visualized as thickenings in the shoulder capsule.[51,34]

Although certain toxins and other environmental factors can still cause limb deformities (e.g., by affecting the vascular supply), it is the embryonic period that is most vulnerable to congenital malformations, with the type of abnormality depending on the time at which the orderly sequence of differentiation was interrupted. In gross limb abnormalities, such as amelia, injury to the apical ectodermal ridge is one important factor, which has a strong inductive influence on the limb mesoderm. Matsuoka and colleagues mapped the destinations of embryonic neural crest and mesodermal stem cells in the neck and shoulder region using Cre recombinase–mediated transgenesis[49] and proposed a precise code of connectivity that mesenchymal stem cells of both neural crest and mesodermal origin obey as they form muscle scaffolds. The conclusions suggested that knowledge of these relationships could contribute further to identify the etiology of diseases, such as Klippel-Feil syndrome, Sprengel's deformity, and Arnold-Chiari I/II malformation.[49] Clearly, the timing of embryonic development is critical for understanding anomalies and malformations and is an area of further study.

Fetal Period

Fetal development is concerned mainly with expansion in size of the structures differentiated and developed during the embryonic period. By the end of the 12th week, the upper limbs have almost reached their final length. Ossification proceeds rapidly during this period, especially during the 13th to 16th weeks. The first indication of ossification in the cartilaginous model of a long bone is visible near the center of the shaft. Primary centers appear at different times in different bones, but usually between the 7th and 12th weeks. The part of the bone ossified from the primary center is called the *diaphysis*. Secondary centers of ossification form the *epiphysis*. The physeal plate separates these two centers of ossification until the bone grows to its adult length, and from the 12th to the 16th week, the epiphyses are invaded by a vascular network. In the shoulder joint the epiphysis and part of the metaphysis are intracapsular. The tendons, ligaments, and joint capsule around the shoulder are also penetrated by a rich vascular network during the same part of the fetal period, that is, the third to fourth month of gestation.

A morphologic study of the prenatal developing shoulder joint concluded that the most important changes take place around the 12th week of gestation.[1] At about this time, the glenoid labrum, the biceps tendon, and the glenohumeral ligaments formed a complete ring around the glenoid fossa and led the authors to believe that these structures play a role in stabilizing the joint as well as increasing the concavity of the glenoid fossa. The glenoid labrum consists of dense fibrous tissue and some elastic tissue but no fibrocartilage (as is seen in the meniscus of the knee). The acromioclavicular joint develops in a manner different from that of the shoulder joint. Its development begins well into the fetal period (not the embryonic period), and unlike the glenohumeral joint, a three-layered interzone is not seen (Fig. 1-22). Most of the bursae of the shoulder, including the subdeltoid, subcoracoid, and subscapularis bursae, also develop during this time.

Fealy and colleagues studied 51 fetal glenohumeral joints from 37 specimens to evaluate shoulder morphology on a gross and histologic level and compare it with known postnatal anatomic and clinical findings in fetuses from 9 to 40 weeks of gestation.[21] Specimens were studied under a dissecting microscope, histologically, and with the aid of high-resolution radiographs to evaluate the presence of ossification centers. The fetal gross anatomy and morphology were similar to those of normal postnatal shoulders in all specimens. As noted previously, only the clavicle and spine of the scapula were ossified in the fetal shoulder. The humeral head and glenoid gradually and proportionally increased in size with gestational age. Comparative size ratios were consistent, except for the fetal coracoid process, which was noted to be prominent in all specimens (Fig. 1-23).

In a study by Tena-Arregui and colleagues,[80] frozen human fetuses (40 shoulders) were grossly evaluated

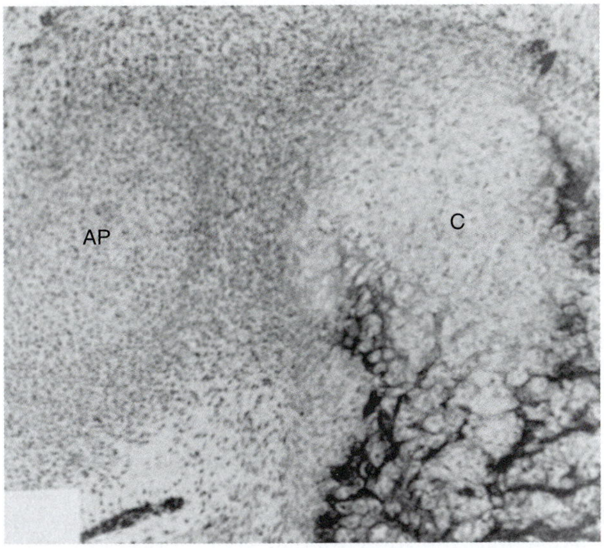

FIGURE 1-22: The acromioclavicular joint develops in a manner different from that of the shoulder joint, and unlike the glenohumeral joint, a three-layered interzone is not seen. *AP,* acromion process; *C,* clavicle.

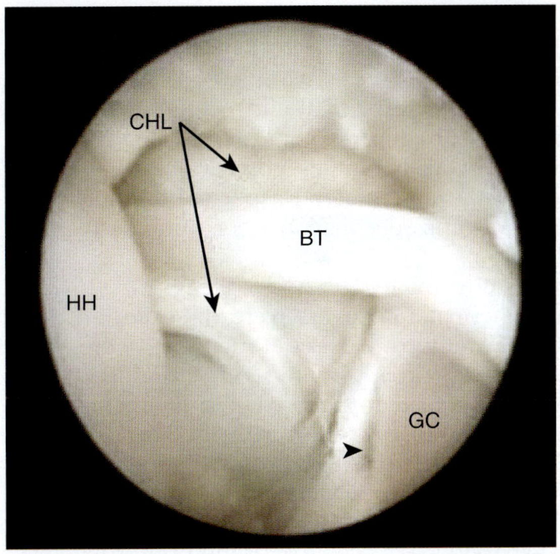

FIGURE 1-24: Arthroscopic view of the left shoulder of a 35-week-old fetus. *CHL,* coracohumeral ligaments; *BT,* biceps tendon; *HH,* humeral head; *GC,* glenoid cavity.

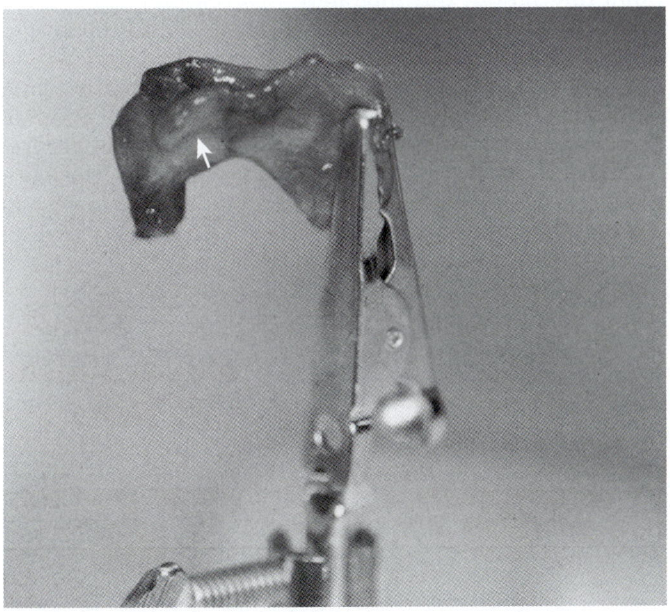

FIGURE 1-23: The fetal shoulder has a proportionally large coracoid process (*arrow*).

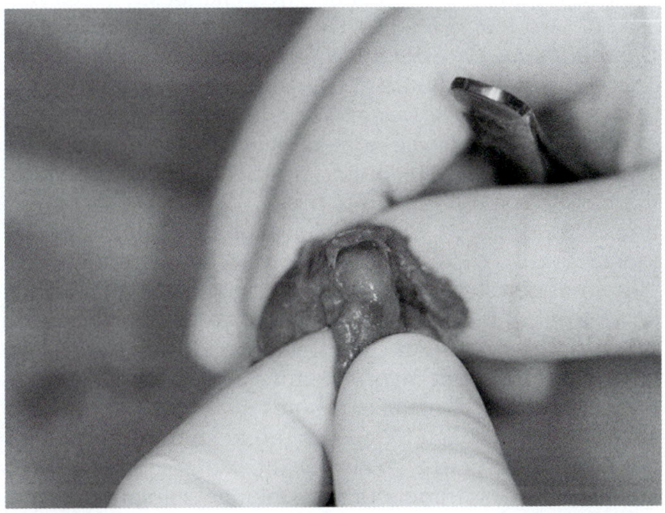

FIGURE 1-25: The fetal acromion process is cartilaginous and adherent to the superior aspect of the humeral head, thus giving the acromion a gentle curve, similar to an adult type II acromion.

arthroscopically, with similar findings. They concluded that the anatomy observed was easier to discern than what is observed in the adult shoulder arthroscopy (Fig. 1-24).[80]

Coracoacromial Arch Anatomy

By 13 weeks of gestation, the rotator cuff tendons, coracoacromial ligament (CAL), and coracohumeral ligament are present. The acromion is cartilaginous and consistently has a gentle curve that conforms to the superior aspect of the humeral head, similar to a type II acromion (Fig. 1-25).[4,10,45] These data suggest that variations in acromial morphology are acquired.

A macroscopic and histologic study conducted by Shah and colleagues analyzed 22 cadaveric shoulders to establish what, if any, developmental changes occur in the differing patterns of acromia.[73] In all the curved and hooked acromia (types II and III), a common pattern of degeneration of collagen, fibrocartilage, and bone was observed, consistent with a traction phenomenon. None of these changes was exhibited by the flat acromion (type I). They therefore supported the conclusion that the different shapes of acromion are acquired in response to traction forces applied via CAL and are not congenital.

In the fetus CAL consists of two distinct fiber bundles that lie in the anterolateral and posteromedial planes, as it does in the mature shoulder.[20] Histologic studies have shown that CAL continues posteriorly along the inferior surface of the anterolateral aspect of the acromion. CAL has well-organized collagen fiber bundles by 36 weeks of gestation.

In a study by Kopuz and colleagues, 110 shoulders from 60 neonatal cadavers were dissected and analyzed for CAL variations.[38] Three CAL types were identified: quadrangular, broad band, and U-shaped. Histologic analysis showed that the U-shaped ligaments had a thin central tissue close to the coracoid. The data suggested that the primordial CAL is broad shaped but assumes a quadrangular shape because of the different growth rates of the coracoid and acromial ends. In addition, broad and U-shaped CALs account for the primordial and quadrangular types, respectively, and Y-shaped ligaments account for the adult types of the single- or double-banded anatomic variants. They concluded that various types of CALs are present during the neonatal period and that the final morphology is determined by developmental factors rather than degenerative changes.

Glenohumeral Capsule and Glenohumeral Ligaments

The anterior glenohumeral capsule has been found to be thicker than the posterior capsule. The fetal shoulder capsule inserts onto the humeral neck in the same fashion as in the mature shoulder and has been found to be confluent with the rotator cuff tendons at their humeral insertion. Superior and middle glenohumeral ligaments are identifiable as capsular thickenings, whereas the inferior glenohumeral ligament is a distinct structure identifiable by 14 weeks of gestation. Anterior and posterior bands are often noticeable in the ligament, consistent with the known IGHLC anatomy in the adult shoulder.[58] The anterior band of the IGHLC contributes more to the formation of the axillary pouch than does the posterior band.

Histologically, the fetal IGHLC consists of several layers of collagen fibers that are highly cellular and have little fibrous tissue during early development. This tissue becomes more fibrous later in gestation. Polarized light microscopy demonstrates that these fibers are only loosely organized, but are more organized than the adjacent capsular tissues. Arthroscopic images of the superior glenohumeral ligament have revealed a defined attachment to the humeral head, forming an intersection of the biceps tendon as it enters the bicipital groove and the attachment of the upper edge of the subscapular muscle tendon.[80]

A rotator interval defect was noted in fetuses by 14 weeks of gestation. This capsular defect was seen consistently in the 1 o'clock position in a right shoulder or the 11 o'clock position in a left shoulder. The interval defect was often covered by a thin layer of capsule that extended from the middle glenohumeral ligament and passed superficially to the defect. Removal of this capsular layer revealed a clear defect between the superior and middle glenohumeral ligaments. Histologic examination of the interval defect in a specimen from the 19th week of gestation revealed a thin surrounding capsule with poorly organized collagen fibers. To our knowledge, this is the first suggestion that the capsular defect is not acquired. Specimens with larger rotator interval defects had greater amounts of inferior glenohumeral laxity. Closure of a large rotator interval defect in adults has been shown to be an effective treatment for inferior glenohumeral instability.[22,29,57]

Biceps Tendon

Although rare, The proximal portion of the long head of the biceps tendon (LHBT) has been reported to develop anomalously. As such, the developmental anatomy of the biceps has been brought to focus in recent studies. Specifically, Audenaert et al. suggested that the proximal LHBT migrates from the glenohumeral capsule and synovial layer into the intraarticular space prior to weeks 20 or 24 of fetal development.[6] Although not widely adopted,[54] this pattern has been observed and reported by others.[84,25,17] Several case reports of anomalous biceps anatomy seen intraoperatively among adults led to the hypothesis that aberrant development can occur at any point throughout this migration.[6] Developmental fusions of the biceps tendon to the supraspinatus, fibrous capsule, and synovial lining have all been observed and would suggest confirmation of this migratory process at varying endpoints. Audenaert et al. proposed a classification of these stages in the embryo, in which the proximal portion of the LHBT originates in the intracapsular position, moves through the synovial layer, and comes to rest in the intraarticular position (Fig. 1-26).[6] Anatomic variation

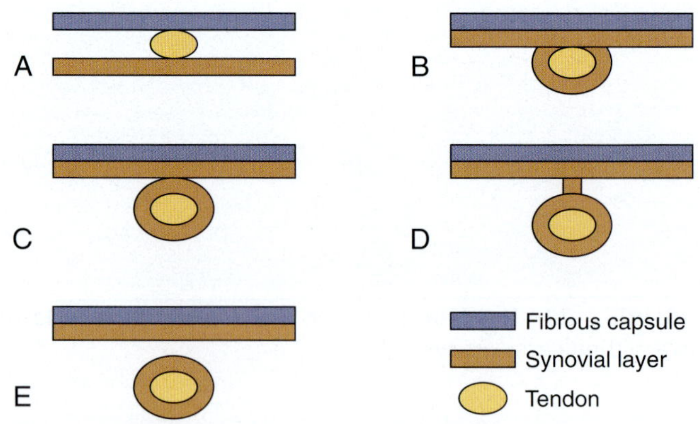

FIGURE 1-26: Schematic representation of embryologic developmental stages and possible positions of the tendon of the long head of the biceps brachii muscle. **A,** Intracapsular position between the fibrous and synovial layers. **B,** Position in a synovial fold. **C,** Intraarticular position, but adherent to the synovial layer. **D,** Intraarticular position, attached by a mesotenon. **E,** Free intraarticular position. (From Audenaert EA, Barbaix EJ, Van Hoonacker P, et al. Extraarticular variants of the long head of the biceps brachii: A reminder of embryology. *J Shoulder Elbow Surg.* 2008;17(1):114S-117S.)

in the long head of the biceps exists as a double structure or insertion within the fibrous capsule.[16] In a recent case, Provencher et al. reported bilateral absence of the intraarticular long head of the biceps in a patient with no history of congenital development abnormalities.[40] Electromyographic analysis of the shoulder motion demonstrates that, despite its presence within the joint, the long head of the biceps is not involved in glenohumeral motion.[7]

Glenoid

The fetal glenoid has a lateral tilt of the superior glenoid rim relative to the inferior rim in the coronal plane; in contrast, the adult shoulder is more vertically oriented. The glenoid labrum has been noted at 13 weeks of gestation. The anterior and posterior aspects of the labrum become confluent with the anterior and posterior bands of the IGHLC, respectively. Detachment of the anterosuperior labrum at the waist of the comma-shaped glenoid has been noted in specimens after 22 weeks of gestation, and such detachment corresponds to an area of variable labral detachment seen in mature shoulders. Gross discoloration of the glenoid hyaline cartilage in the inferior half of the glenoid has been noted in specimens at 30 weeks in approximately the same area as the bare spot that is seen in the mature shoulder. In the embryo no histologic evidence could be found of a bare area of glenoid hyaline cartilage, as seen in the adult glenohumeral joint, suggesting that it may be acquired.

Postnatal Development

Postnatal development of the shoulder is concerned mainly with the appearance and development of the secondary centers of ossification because the soft tissues change only in size after birth. The development of the individual bones is discussed separately.

Clavicle

The clavicle, along with the mandible, is the first bone in the body to ossify, during the fifth week of gestation. Most bones in the body develop by endochondral ossification, in which condensations of mesenchymal tissue become cartilage and then undergo ossification. However, the major portion of the clavicle forms by intramembranous ossification, in which mesenchymal cells are mineralized directly into bone. Two separate ossification centers form during the fifth week, the lateral and the medial. The lateral center is usually more prominent than the medial center, and the two masses form a long mass of bone. The cells at the acromial and sternal ends of the clavicle take on a cartilaginous pattern to form the sternoclavicular and acromioclavicular joints. Therefore the clavicle increases in diameter by intramembranous ossification of the periosteum and grows in length through endochondral activity at the cartilaginous ends. The medial clavicular epiphysis is responsible for the majority of longitudinal growth (Fig. 1-27). It begins to ossify at 18 years of age and fuses with the clavicle between the ages of 22 and 25 years. The lateral epiphysis is less consistent in form; it often appears as a wafer-like edge of the bone just proximal to the acromioclavicular joint and can be confused with a fracture.

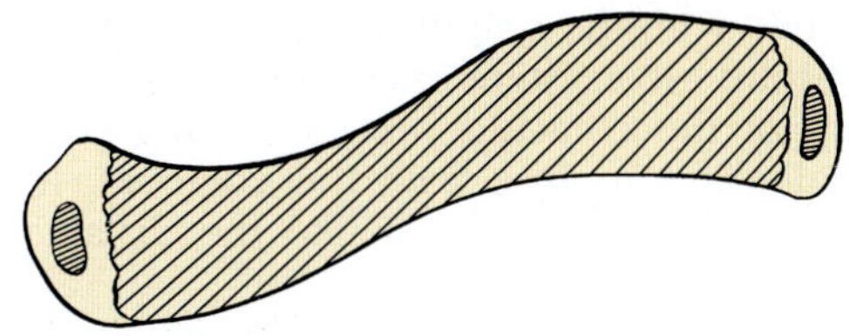

FIGURE 1-27: The medial clavicular epiphysis is responsible for most of the longitudinal growth of the clavicle. It fuses at 22 to 25 years of age. The lateral epiphysis is less consistent in form; it often appears as a wafer-like edge of bone and may be confused with a fracture.

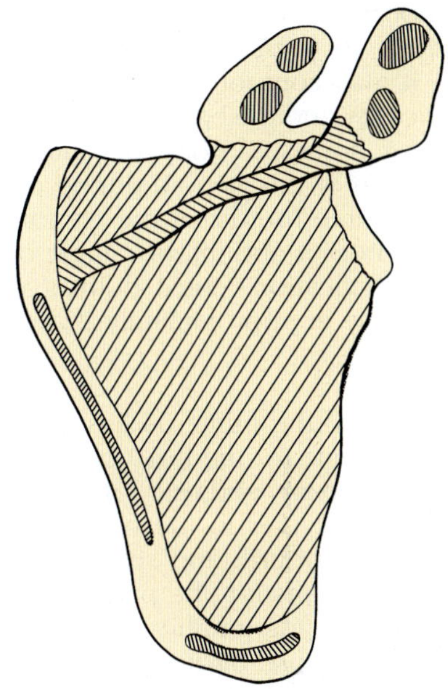

FIGURE 1-28: The coracoid process has two (sometimes three) centers of ossification. A third inconsistent ossification center can appear at the tip of the coracoid process during puberty, and occasionally this center fails to fuse with the coracoid. It may be confused with a fracture. The acromion has two and occasionally three ossification centers as well; an unfused apophysis is not an uncommon finding and often manifests as impingement syndrome.

Scapula

The majority of the scapula forms by intramembranous ossification. At birth, the body and the spine of the scapula have ossified, but not the coracoid process, glenoid, acromion, vertebral border, and inferior angle. The coracoid process has two and occasionally three centers of ossification (Fig. 1-28). The first center appears during the first year of life in the center of the coracoid process. The second center appears at approximately 10 years of age at the base of the coracoid process. The second ossification center also contributes to formation of the superior portion of the glenoid cavity. These two centers unite with the scapula at approximately 15 years of age. A third inconsistent ossification center can appear at the tip of the coracoid process during puberty and occasionally fails to fuse with the coracoid. It is often confused with a fracture, just like the distal clavicular epiphysis.

The acromion has two and occasionally three ossification centers as well. These centers arise during puberty and fuse together at approximately 22 years of age. This may be confused with a fracture when an unfused apophysis, most often a meso-acromion, is visualized on an axillary view. This finding is not uncommon and is often seen in patients with impingement syndrome.

The glenoid fossa has two ossification centers. The first center appears at the base of the coracoid process at approximately 10 years of age and fuses around 15 years of age; it also contributes to the superior portion of the glenoid cavity and the base of the coracoid process. The second is a horseshoe-shaped center arising from the inferior portion of the glenoid during puberty, and it forms the lower three fourths of the glenoid.

The vertebral border and inferior angle of the scapula each have one ossification center, both of which appear at puberty and fuse at approximately 22 years of age.

Proximal Humerus

The proximal end of the humerus has three ossification centers (Fig. 1-29): one for the head of the humerus, one for the greater tuberosity, and one for the lesser tuberosity. The ossification center in the humeral head usually appears between the fourth and sixth months, although *Gray's Anatomy*[85] reports it to be present in 20% of newborns. Without this radiographic landmark, it is often quite difficult to diagnose birth injuries. The ossification center for the greater tuberosity arises during the third year, and the center for the lesser tuberosity appears during the fifth year. The epiphyses for the tuberosities fuse together during the fifth year as well, and they in turn fuse with the center for the humeral head during the seventh year. Union between the head and the shaft usually occurs at approximately 19 years of age.

Adult Glenohumeral Joint

Bony Anatomy

The adult glenohumeral joint is formed by the humeral head and the glenoid surface of the scapula. Their geometric relationship allows a remarkable range of motion. However, this range of motion is achieved with a concurrent loss of biomechanic stability. The large spherical head of the humerus articulates against—and not within—a smaller glenoid fossa, a relationship comparable with a golf ball sitting on a tee. Stability is conferred by the static and dynamic soft tissue restraints acting across the joint.

The head of the humerus is a large, globular bony structure whose articular surface forms one-third of a sphere and is directed medially, superiorly, and posteriorly. The head is inclined 130 to 150 degrees in relation to the shaft (Fig. 1-30).[18,14,61,65] Retroversion of the humeral head can be highly variable among individuals and between sides in the same individual. Pearl and Volk found a mean of 29.8 degrees of retroversion in 21 shoulders they examined, with a range of 10 to 55 degrees.[62] The average vertical dimension of the articular portion of the head is 48 mm, with a 25-mm radius of curvature. The average transverse dimension is 45 mm, with a 22-mm radius of curvature.[31] The bicipital groove is 30 degrees medial to a line passing from the shaft through the center of the head of the humerus (Fig. 1-31). The greater tuberosity forms the lateral wall, and the lesser tuberosity forms the medial wall of this groove.

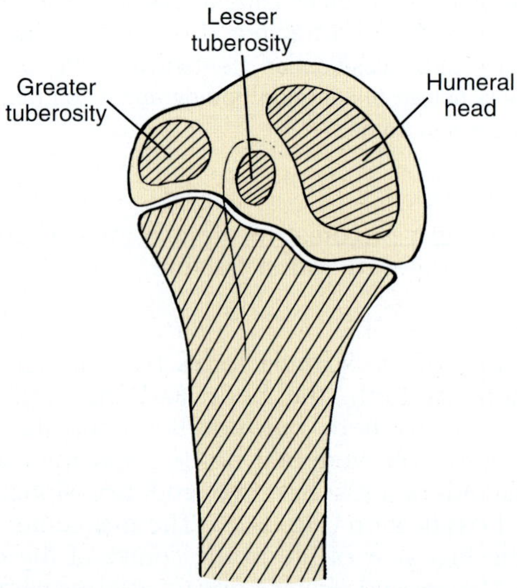

FIGURE 1-29: The proximal end of the humerus has three ossification centers: for the head of the humerus, for the greater tuberosity, and for the lesser tuberosity.

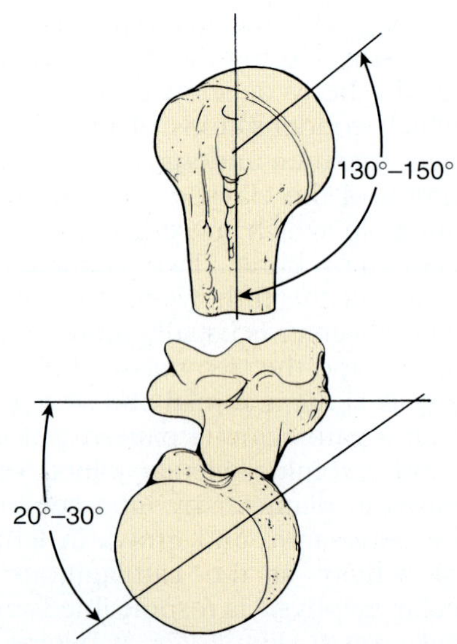

FIGURE 1-30: The neck and head of the humerus are inclined at an angle of 130 to 150 degrees in relation to the shaft (*top*) and have a retrotorsion angle of 20 to 30 degrees (*bottom*).

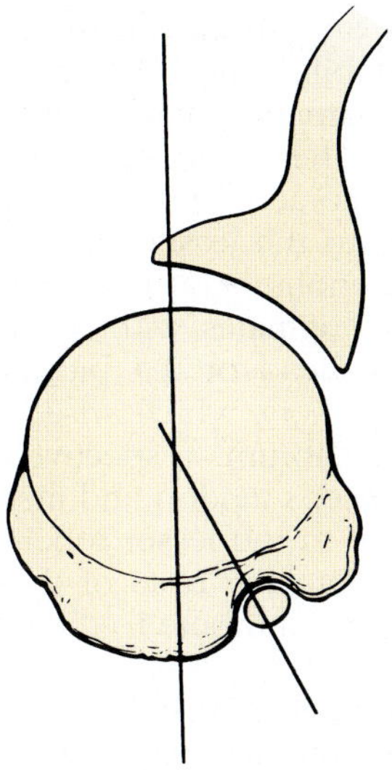

FIGURE 1-31: The bicipital groove is 30 degrees medial to a line that passes from the shaft through the center of the head of the humerus.

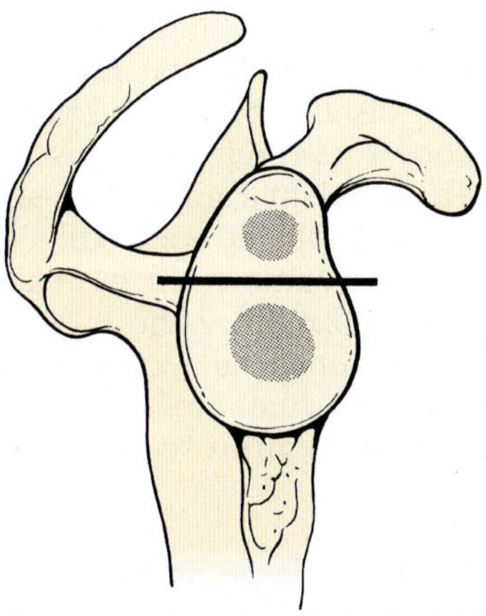

FIGURE 1-32: The glenoid cavity is shaped like an inverted comma. The transverse line corresponds to the epiphyseal line of the glenoid cavity.

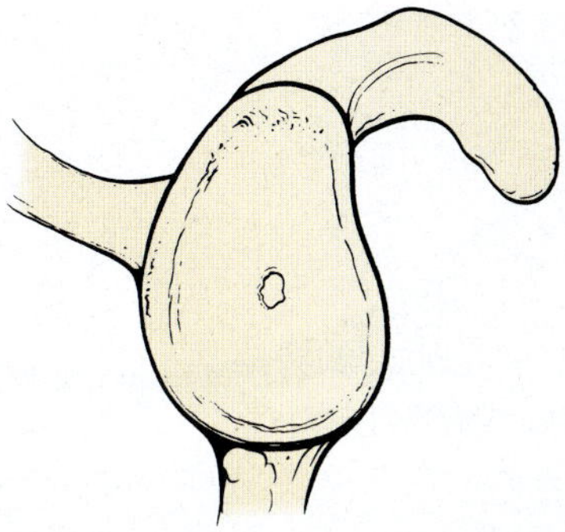

FIGURE 1-33: A bare area is often noted in the center of the glenoid cavity; this area may be related to greater contact pressure and also to age.

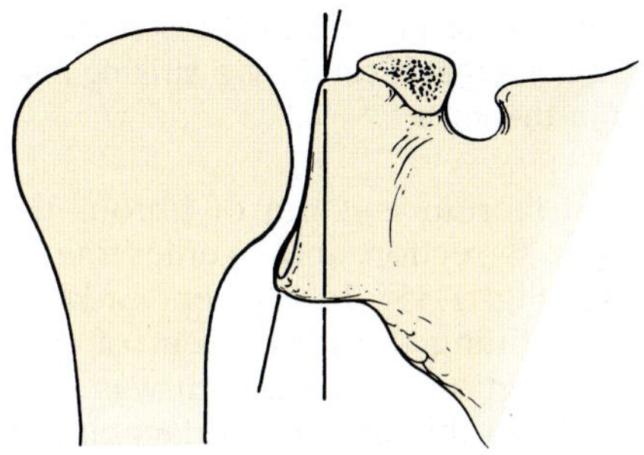

FIGURE 1-34: The superior portion of the superoinferior line of the glenoid is angled at an average of 15 degrees medially relative to the scapular plane.

The glenoid cavity is shaped like an inverted comma (Fig. 1-32). Its superior portion (tail) is narrow and the inferior portion is broad. The transverse line between these two regions roughly corresponds to the epiphyseal line of the glenoid cavity.[16] The glenoid has a concave articular surface covered by hyaline cartilage. In the center of the cavity a distinct circular area of thinning is often noted. This area, according to DePalma and colleagues,[16] is related to the region's greater contact with the humeral head, as well as to age (Fig. 1-33). The average vertical dimension of the glenoid is 35 mm, and the average transverse diameter is 25 mm. In previous studies Saha[68,69,70] noted that the glenoid may be either anteverted or retroverted with respect to the plane of the scapula. He found that approximately 75% of the shoulders he studied had retroverted glenoid surfaces averaging 7.4 degrees of retroversion and that 25% of the glenoid surfaces were anteverted 2 to 10 degrees. Regarding vertical tilt, the superior portion of the superior/inferior line of the glenoid is angled an average of 15 degrees medially relative to the scapular plane, thus making the glenoid surface on which the humeral head lies relatively horizontal (Fig. 1-34).

Based on contact surface studies involving 20 shoulders, Saha[68] originally classified glenohumeral articulations into three types: A, B, and C. In type A, the humeral surface has a radius of curvature smaller than that of the glenoid and has a small circular contact area. In type B, the humeral and glenoid surfaces have similar curvatures and a larger circular contact area. In type C, the humeral surface has a radius of curvature larger than that of the glenoid; the contact is limited to the periphery, and the contact surface is ring shaped. However, Soslowsky and colleagues examined 32 cadaveric shoulders using precise stereophotogrammetry and found that mating glenohumeral joint surfaces had remarkably high congruency, all falling into the type B category. In 88%, the radii of curvature within 2 mm of each other, and all cases were congruent to within 3 mm. Humeral head-to-glenoid ratios were 3.12:1 and 2.9:1 for male and female cadavers, respectively. These authors attributed the relative instability of the shoulder not to a shallow or incongruent glenoid but instead to the small surface area of the glenoid relative to the larger humeral head.[75]

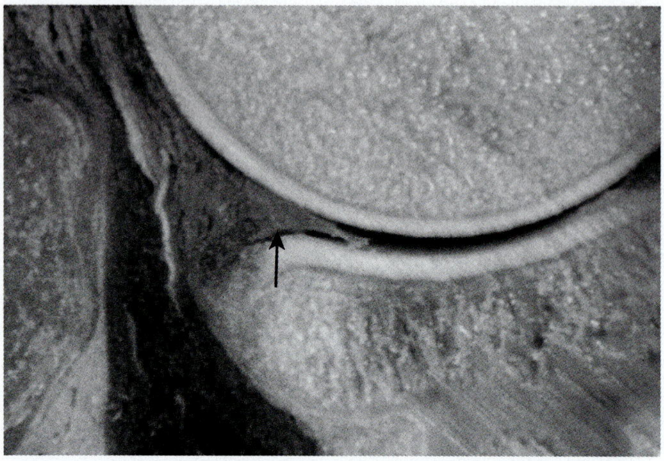

FIGURE 1-35: The glenoid labrum (*arrow*), a rim of fibrous tissue that is triangular in cross section, overlies the glenoid cavity at the rim or edge. It can bear a striking resemblance to the meniscus in the knee.

The glenoid labrum is a rim of fibrous tissue that is triangular in cross section and overlies the edge of the glenoid cavity (Fig. 1-35). In a recent cadaveric analysis quantitatively defining the attachment of the labrum to the fossa, the insertion of the labrum was reported to be consistently at both the articular surface and the neck of the glenoid at the 4 and 6 o'clock positions.[87] It varies in size and thickness, sometimes being a prominent intra-articular structure with a free inner edge and at other times being virtually absent. Previously, the labrum was likened to the fibrocartilaginous meniscus of the knee; however, Moseley and Overgaard showed that it was essentially devoid of fibrocartilage, except in a small transition zone at its osseous attachment.[52] The majority of the labrum is dense fibrous tissue with a few elastic fibers. It is, however, important for maintaining glenohumeral stability.[28,7,9,13,36,43,60] The labrum is responsible for increasing the depth of the glenoid cavity by up to 50% as well as for increasing the surface area in contact with the humeral head.[9,43] It can also act as a fibrous anchor from which the biceps tendon and glenohumeral ligaments can take origin.

Once considered distinct entities, theLHBT and the superior portion of the labrum form a continuous, interdependent functional unit termed the biceps-labral complex. The biceps-labral complex is subdivided into three discrete zones: inside, junctional, and bicipital tunnel.[77] The inside zone refers to the superior labrum and LHBT anchor. Vangsness and colleagues[83] demonstrated four variants that may be present in this zone. The junctional zone refers to the intra-articular portion of the LHBT and its stabilizing pulley. The junctional zone's normal and pathoanatomy can be visualized during standard glenohumeral arthroscopy. The biceps pulley is a capsuloligamentous complex that stabilizes the LHBT within the proximal portion of the groove (bicipital tunnel zone 1). The biceps pulley is formed by a coalescence of fibers from the superior glenohumeral and coracohumeral ligaments, with contributions from the subscapularis and supraspinatus tendons. Together these structures stabilize the LHBT as it rotates 35 to 40 degrees along the articular margin en route to its extra-articular course.[26] The coracohumeral ligament, which stretches from the coracoid process to the greater tuberosity and partially to the lesser tuberosity, is an inferior stabilizer of the glenohumeral joint. The superior glenohumeral ligament originates with or just anterior to the origin of the long head of the biceps and consists of oblique and direct fibers, which arise from the supraglenoid tubercle and labrum, respectively, that course in parallel with the biceps tendon and insert onto the fovea capitis just superior to the lesser tuberosity. Some fibers continue to insert into the base of the bicipital groove, while the remainder contribute to the transverse humeral ligament.[5,35,86]

The bicipital tunnel, which is not technically within the glenohumeral joint, has only recently been described grossly and histologically, by Taylor and O'Brien.[77,78] They defined it as the extra-articular segment of the LHBT and its fibro-osseous enclosure, which extends from the articular margin through the subpectoral region. The bicipital tunnel has been subdivided into three distinct zones. Zone 1 refers to the traditional bicipital groove and is defined proximally by the articular margin and biceps pulley and distally by the inferior margin of the subscapularis. Zone 2, also referred to as "no man's land," extends from the distal margin of the subscapularis to the proximal margin of the pectoralis major tendon (PMPM) and gains its name from its relative invisibility to arthroscopic visualization. Zone 3 is the subpectoral region. The bicipital tunnel is a closed space that commonly harbors lesions that are hidden from standard diagnostic glenohumeral arthroscopy.[77,79]

Shoulder Capsule

The shoulder capsule is large and has twice the surface area of the humeral head. It typically accepts approximately 28 to 35 mL of fluid, with a greater amount in women than in men. However, in pathologic conditions, this amount varies.[55] For example, in patients with adhesive capsulitis, the shoulder capsule accepts only 5 mL or less of fluid, whereas in patients with considerable laxity or instability it can accept larger volumes of fluid.

The capsule is lined by synovium and extends from the glenoid neck (or occasionally the labrum) to the anatomic neck and the proximal shaft of the humerus to varying degrees. The capsule often extends and attaches to the coracoid process superiorly (via the coracohumeral ligament) and on either side of the scapular body (via the anterior and posterior recesses). It can extend down along the biceps tendon for variable lengths and across the intertubercular groove of the humerus. The joint capsule blends with ligamentous structures that arise on nearby bony landmarks and contains within its substance the glenohumeral ligaments, including the inferior glenohumeral complex. All of these structures show great variation in size, shape, thickness, and attachment. A recent cadaveric study demonstrated diminished tensile behavior of the glenohumeral capsule in patients with

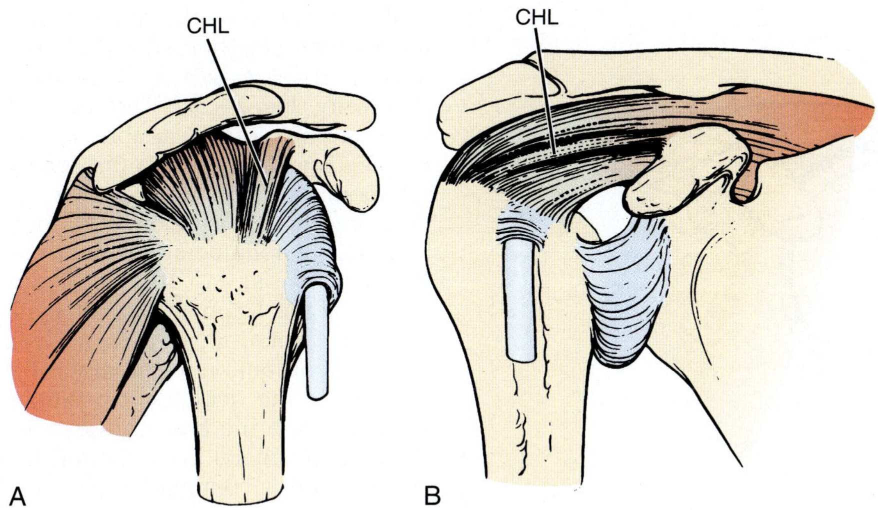

FIGURE 1-36: The coracohumeral ligament (CHL) is a strong band that originates from the base of the lateral border of the coracoid process, just below the coracoacromial ligament, and merges with the capsule laterally to insert on the greater tuberosity. This ligament may be important as a suspensory structure for the adducted arm. **A,** Lateral view. **B,** Anteroposterior view.

anterior instability, highlighting the importance of addressing this capsule with more than plication and suturing in symptom control for this population.[11]

The coracohumeral ligament is a rather strong band that originates from the base and lateral border of the coracoid process just below the origin of the coracoacromial ligament (Fig. 1-36). It is directed transversely and inserts on the greater tuberosity. The anterior border is often distinct medially and merges with the capsule laterally. The posterior border is usually indistinct from the rest of the capsule. Some authors believe that phylogenetically it represents the previous insertion of the pectoralis minor; in 15% of the population, a part of the pectoralis minor crosses the coracoid process to insert on the humeral head.[85] Although the biomechanical contribution of this ligament is not yet fully known, it appears to have a static suspensory function for the humeral head in the glenoid cavity when the arm is in the dependent position. With abduction, the ligament relaxes and loses its ability to support the humerus.

The transverse humeral ligament (Fig. 1-37) consists of a few transverse fibers of capsule that extend between the greater and lesser tuberosities; it helps contain the LHBT in its groove.

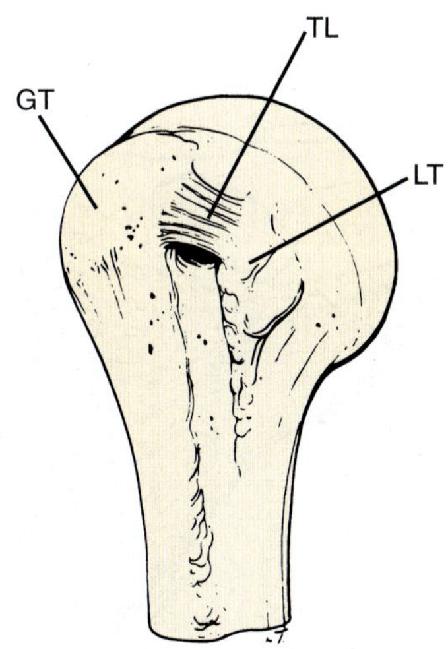

FIGURE 1-37: The transverse humeral ligament (TL) consists of transverse fibers of the capsule that extend between the greater tuberosity (GT) and the lesser tuberosity (LT); it contains the tendon of the long head of the biceps in its groove.

On all sides of the shoulder capsule, except for the inferior portion, the capsule is reinforced and strengthened by the tendons of the rotator cuff muscles, that is, the supraspinatus, infraspinatus, teres minor, and subscapularis (Fig. 1-38). The tendons blend into the capsule over varying lengths and average approximately 2.5 cm. The most prominent of these is the anterior tendinous portion of the subscapularis (Fig. 1-39). Together, they form the musculotendinous or capsulotendinous cuff.

Glenohumeral Ligaments

The glenohumeral ligaments are collagenous reinforcements to the shoulder capsule that are not visible on its external surface. They are best appreciated in situ arthroscopically without distension by air or saline (Fig. 1-40). Their function depends on their collagenous integrity, their attachment sites, and the position of the arm.

Superior Glenohumeral Ligament

The superior glenohumeral ligament is a fairly constant structure present in 97% of shoulders examined in the classic anatomic study by DePalma and in 26% to 90% of specimens in an anatomic study conducted at our institution.[16,60] Three common variations are seen in its glenoid attachment[16]: it can arise from a common origin with the biceps tendon; it can arise from the labrum,

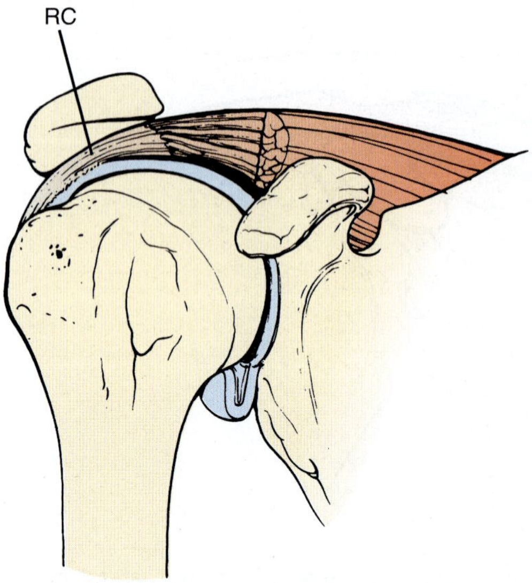

FIGURE 1-38: The rotator cuff (RC) musculature blends into the capsule over varying lengths (on average approximately 2.5 cm) from the insertion site of the rotator cuff on the humerus.

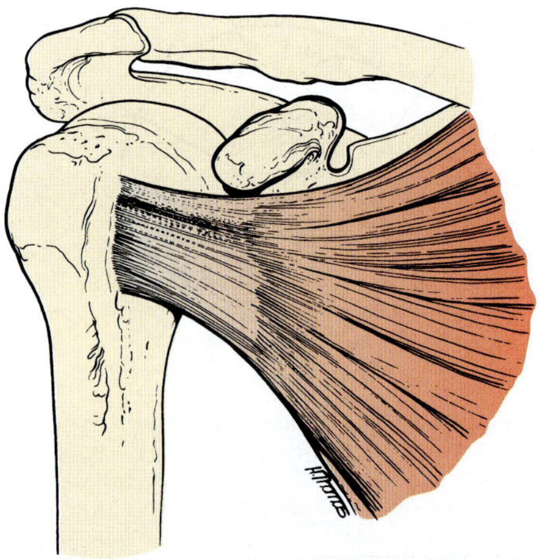

FIGURE 1-39: The subscapularis muscle inserts into the lesser tuberosity with the most superior portion and has a distinct thickening that can resemble a tendon.

slightly anterior to the tendon; or it can originate with the middle glenohumeral ligament (Fig. 1-41). It inserts into the fovea capitis and lies just superior to the lesser tuberosity (Fig. 1-42).[82] The size and integrity of this ligament are also quite variable. It can exist as a thin wisp of capsular tissue or as a thickening similar to the patellofemoral ligaments in the knee.

Biomechanical studies performed by us show that the superior glenohumeral ligament contributes very little to the static stability of the glenohumeral joint.[72] Selective cutting of this ligament did not significantly affect translation either anteriorly or posteriorly in the abducted shoulder. Its contribution to stability is best demonstrated with the arm in the dependent position, where the ligament helps to keep the humeral head suspended (along with the coracohumeral ligament and rotator cuff). Its relative contribution is contingent upon its thickness and collagenous integrity.

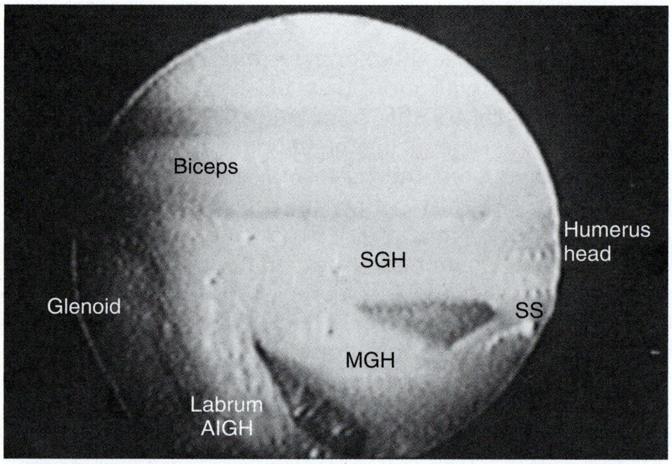

FIGURE 1-40: The glenohumeral ligaments are best appreciated by arthroscopic visualization without distention with air or saline. In this view the various glenohumeral ligaments are seen as they appear from a posterior portal view. *AIGH*, anterior inferior glenohumeral ligament; *MGH*, middle glenohumeral ligament; *SGH*, superior glenohumeral ligament; *SS*, subscapularis.

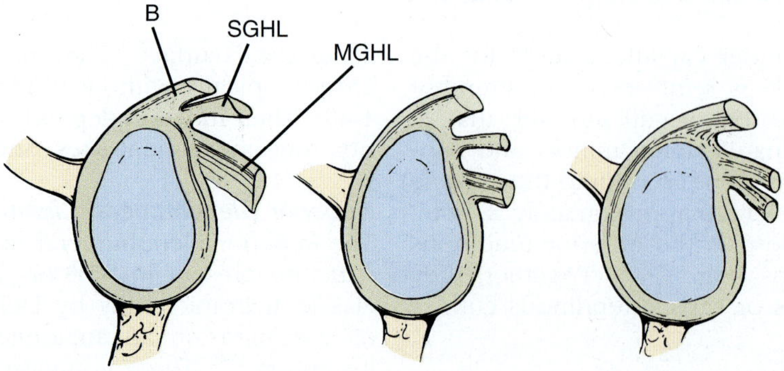

FIGURE 1-41: Three common variations of the origin of the superior glenohumeral ligament (SGHL). *B*, biceps tendon; *MGHL*, middle glenohumeral ligament.

Middle Glenohumeral Ligament

The middle glenohumeral ligament shows the greatest variation in size of all the glenohumeral ligaments and is not present as often as the others. In 96 shoulders studied by DePalma and colleagues,[16] it was a well-formed, distinct structure in 68 cases, poorly defined in 16 cases, and absent in 12 cases. In a subsequent study we found it to be absent in approximately 27% of the studied specimens.[60] In an individual specimen, it may be either quite thin or as thick as the biceps tendon (Fig. 1-43). When present, it arises most commonly from the labrum immediately below the superior glenohumeral ligament or from the adjacent neck of the glenoid. It inserts into the humerus just medial to the lesser tuberosity, under the tendon of the subscapularis to which it adheres (see Fig. 1-42).[82] Other variations are seen in which the middle glenohumeral ligament has no attachment site other than the anterior portion of the capsule, or in which it exists as two parallel thickenings in the anterior capsule. Its contribution to static stability is variable. However, when it is quite thick, it can act as an important secondary restraint to anterior translation if the anterior portion of the inferior glenohumeral ligament is damaged.[72]

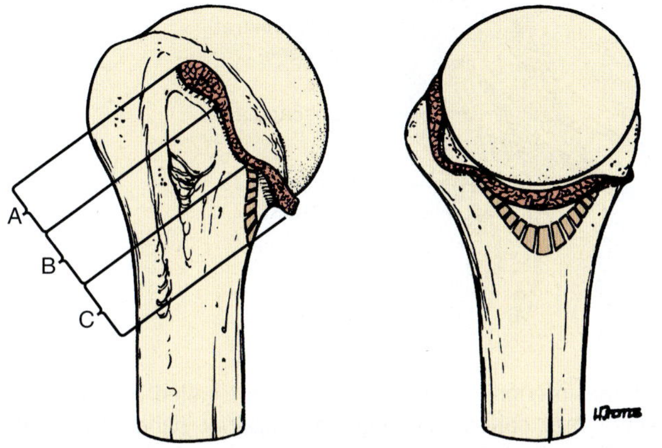

FIGURE 1-42: Attachment sites of the glenohumeral ligaments. *Left*, the superior glenohumeral ligament inserts into the fovea capitis line just superior to the lesser tuberosity (*A*). The middle glenohumeral ligament inserts into the humerus just medial to the lesser tuberosity (*B*). The inferior glenohumeral ligament complex has two common attachment mechanisms (*C*). it can attach in a collar-like fashion (*left*), or it can have a V-shaped attachment to the articular edge (*right*).

Inferior Glenohumeral Ligament

The inferior glenohumeral ligament is a complex structure that is the main static stabilizer of the abducted shoulder. Although it was originally described as triangular, with its apex at the labrum and its base blending with the capsule between the subscapularis and the triceps area, Turkel and colleagues[82] expanded on this anatomic description by calling attention to the especially thickened anterior superior edge of this ligament, which they called the *superior band of the inferior glenohumeral ligament* (Fig. 1-44). In addition, they named the region between the superior band and the middle glenohumeral ligament the *anterior axillary pouch* and called the remainder of the capsule posterior to the superior band the *posterior axillary pouch*.

With the advent of arthroscopy, we have been able to study the joint in situ and to appreciate capsular structures that were disrupted when examination was performed using arthrotomy. By inserting the arthroscope through anterior and superior portals, in addition to the traditional posterior portals, and by observing the joint without distention by air or saline, we have found that the inferior glenohumeral ligament is more complex than originally thought. It is a hammock-like structure originating from the glenoid and inserting into the anatomic neck

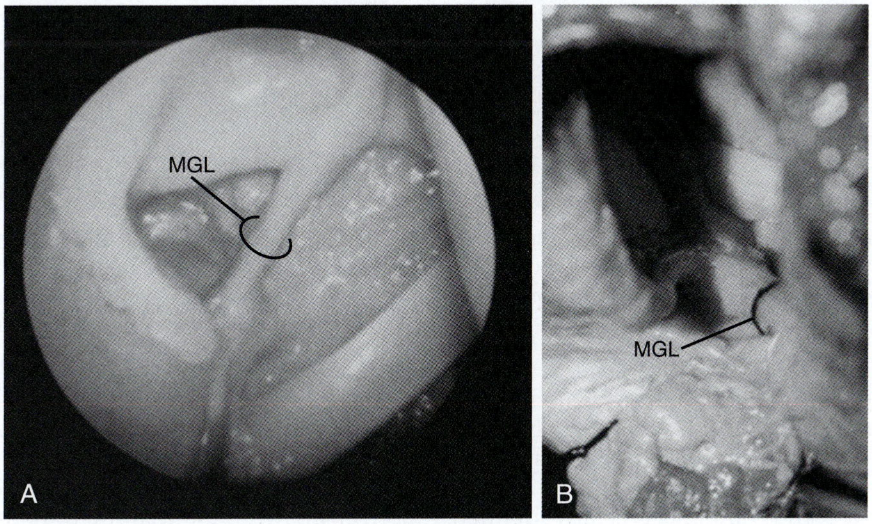

FIGURE 1-43: The middle glenohumeral ligament (MGL) shows great variability. It can exist as a thin wisp of tissue (**A**) or it may be as thick as the biceps tendon (**B**).

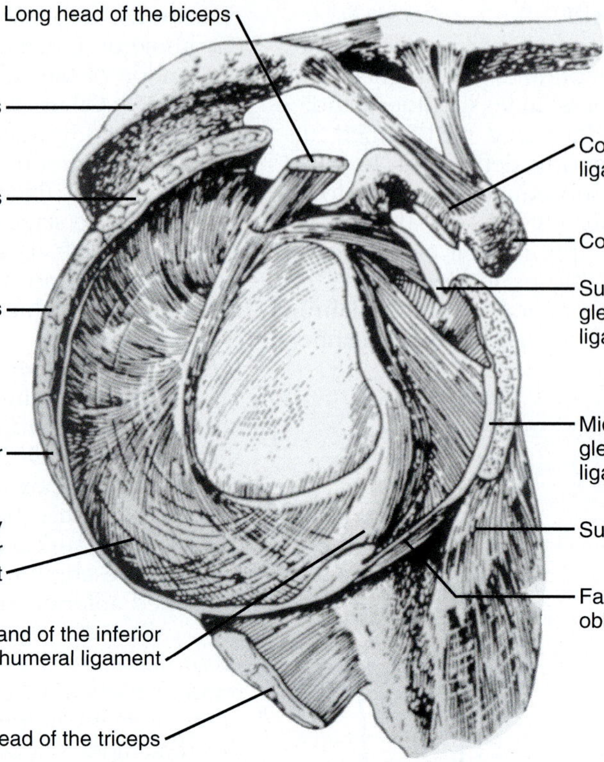

FIGURE 1-44: The anatomic description by Turkel and colleagues of the inferior glenohumeral ligament called attention to the anterior-superior edge of this ligament, which was especially thickened; they called this edge the *superior band of the inferior glenohumeral ligament*. However, no posterior structures were defined. (From Turkel SJ, Panio MW, Marshall JL, Girgis FG. Stabilizing mechanisms preventing anterior dislocation of the glenohumeral joint. *J Bone Joint Surg Am.* 1981;63:1208-1217.)

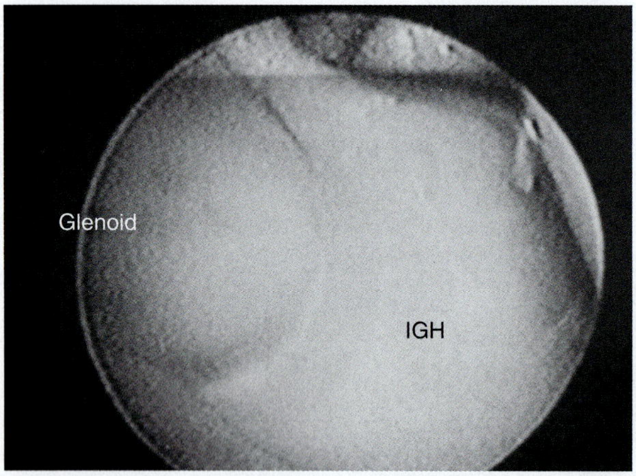

FIGURE 1-45: Posterior arthroscopic view of the inferior glenohumeral (IGH) ligament complex. This hammock-like structure originates from the glenoid and inserts onto the anatomic neck of the humerus.

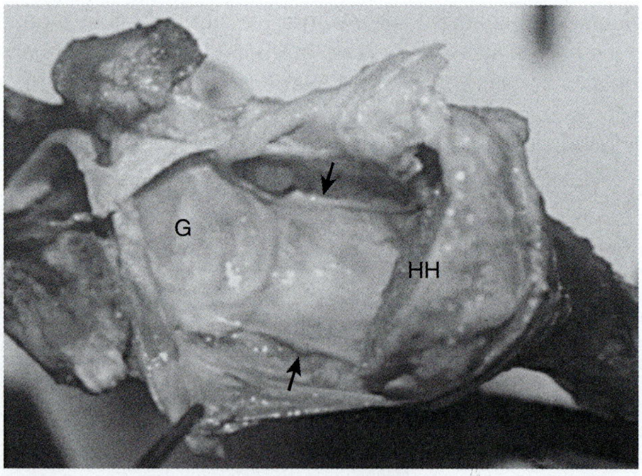

FIGURE 1-46: The anterior and posterior ends of the inferior glenohumeral ligament complex *(arrows)* are clearly defined in this image of an abducted shoulder specimen with the humeral head (HH) partially resected. *G,* glenoid.

of the humerus (Fig. 1-45),[58] and it consists of an anterior band, a posterior band, and an axillary pouch lying in between. We have called this structural arrangement the *inferior glenohumeral ligament complex (IGHLC)*. The anterior and posterior bands are most clearly defined with the arm abducted. In some shoulders, the anterior and posterior bands can only be visualized grossly by internally and externally rotating the arm at 90 degrees of abduction (Fig. 1-46). With abduction and external rotation, the anterior band fans out to support the head, and the posterior band becomes cord-like (Fig. 1-47). Conversely, with internal rotation, the posterior band fans out to support the head, and the anterior band becomes cord-like.

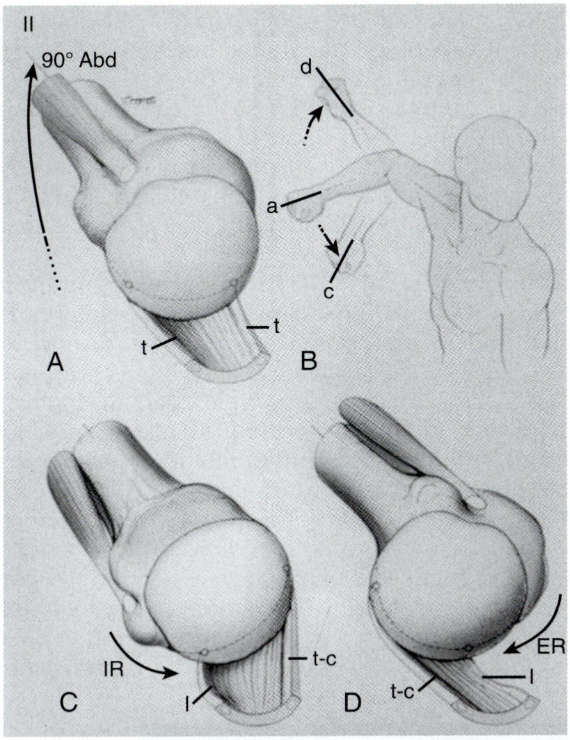

FIGURE 1-47: **A,** The inferior glenohumeral complex is tightened during abduction. **B,** During abduction and internal or external rotation, different parts of the band are tightened. **C,** With internal rotation (IR), the posterior band fans out to support the head, and the anterior band becomes cord-like or relaxed, depending on the degree of horizontal flexion or extension. **D,** On abduction and external rotation (ER), the anterior band fans out to support the head, and the posterior band becomes cord-like or relaxed, depending on the degree of horizontal flexion or extension. *a,* neutral; *Abd,* abduction; *c,* internal rotation; *d,* external rotation; *l,* loose; *t,* anterior and posterior band of the glenohumeral ligament; *t-c,* tight, cord-like.

The IGHLC originates from either the glenoid labrum or the glenoid neck and inserts into the anatomic neck of the humerus. The origins of the anterior and posterior bands on the glenoid can be described in terms of the face of a clock. In our anatomic study of 11 specimens (Fig. 1-48),[58] the anterior band in each specimen originated from between the 2 o'clock and 4 o'clock positions and the posterior band from between the 7 o'clock and 9 o'clock positions. On the humeral head side, the IGHLC attaches in an approximately 90-degree arc just below the articular margin of the humeral head. Two methods of attachment were noted. In some specimens, a collar-like attachment of varying thickness was located just inferior to the articular edge, closer to the articular edge than the remainder of the capsule (Fig. 1-49). In other specimens, the IGHLC was attached in a V-shaped fashion, with the anterior and posterior bands attached close to the articular surface and the axillary pouch attached to the humerus at the apex of the V, farther from the articular edge (Fig. 1-50).

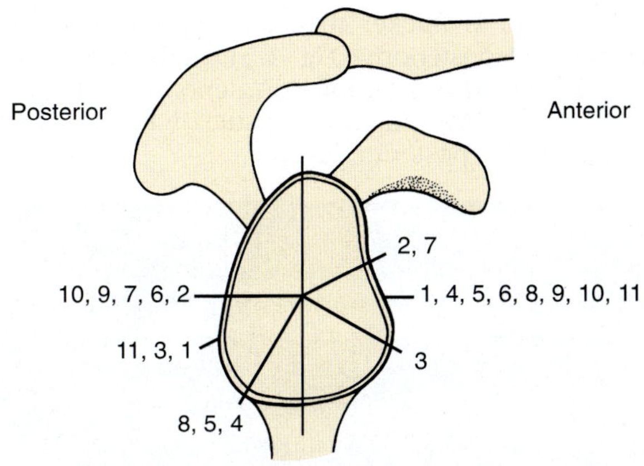

FIGURE 1-48: The glenoid attachment sites of the anterior and posterior bands. In 11 cadaver specimens (indicated by number labels), the anterior band originated from various areas between the 2 o'clock and 4 o'clock positions and the posterior band from areas between the 7 o'clock and 9 o'clock positions.

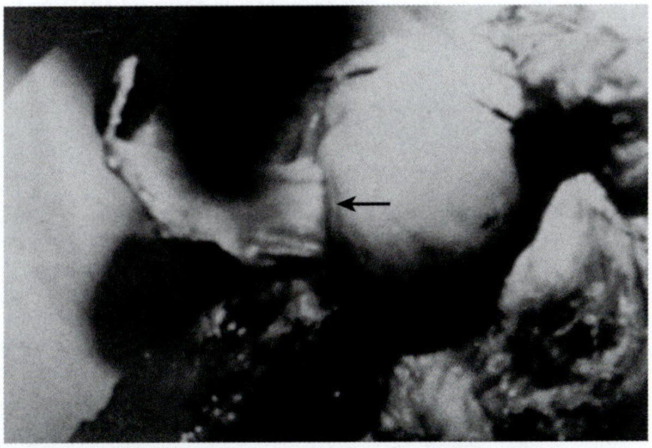

FIGURE 1-49: An example of a collar-like attachment *(arrow)* of the inferior glenohumeral ligament complex just inferior to the articular edge and closer to the articular edge than the remainder of the capsule.

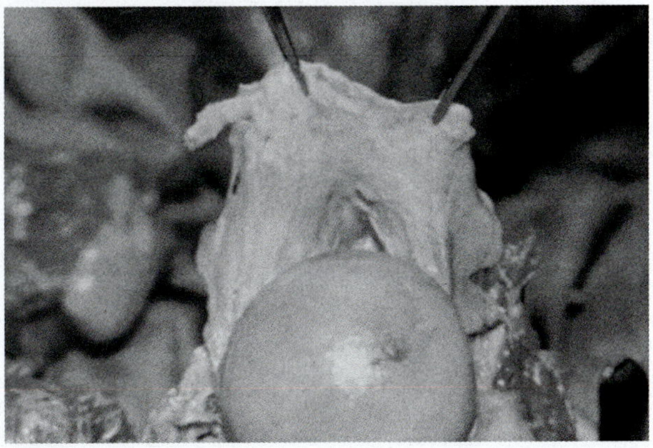

FIGURE 1-50: A V-shaped attachment of the inferior glenohumeral ligament complex of the humerus, with the axillary pouch attaching to the humerus at the apex of the V farther from the articular edge.

The IGHLC is thicker than the capsule adjoining it anteriorly and posteriorly (Fig. 1-51), although considerable variation exists. The inferior glenohumeral ligament is thicker than the anterior capsule, which in turn is thicker than the posterior capsule.

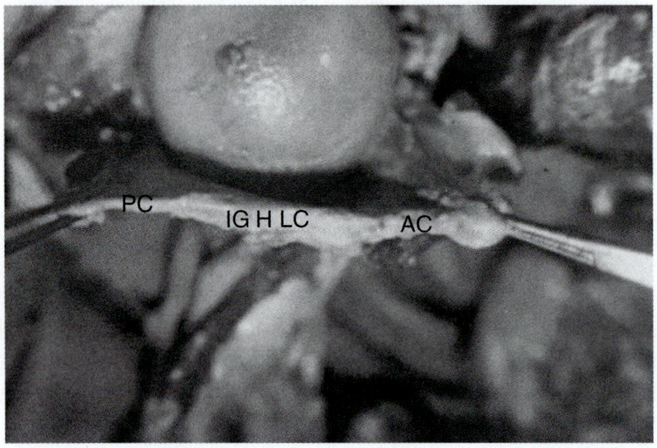

FIGURE 1-51: The inferior glenohumeral ligament complex (IGHLC) is thicker than both the anterior capsule (AC) and the posterior capsule (PC).

The anterior and posterior bands of the IGHLC also show great variation in thickness, but we have been able to identify them in all specimens (Figs. 1-52 and 1-53).[58] Grossly, the anterior band is usually easier to distinguish than the posterior band because it attaches higher on the glenoid and is generally thicker. However, the anterior and posterior bands can be of equal thickness, and occasionally the posterior band is thicker than the anterior band.

Histologically, the IGHLC is distinguishable from the remainder of the shoulder capsule, and the anterior band, axillary pouch, and posterior band are distinct structures.[58] Even in cases in which the bands were poorly defined macroscopically, they were easily distinguishable histologically; in fact, the posterior band is easier to distinguish histologically than the anterior band because of a more abrupt transition from the thin posterior capsule.

The shoulder capsule consists of a synovial lining and three well-defined layers of collagen (Fig. 1-54). The fibers of the inner and outer layers extend in the coronal plane from the glenoid to the humerus. The middle layer of collagen extends in a sagittal direction and crosses the fibers of the other two layers. The relative thickness and

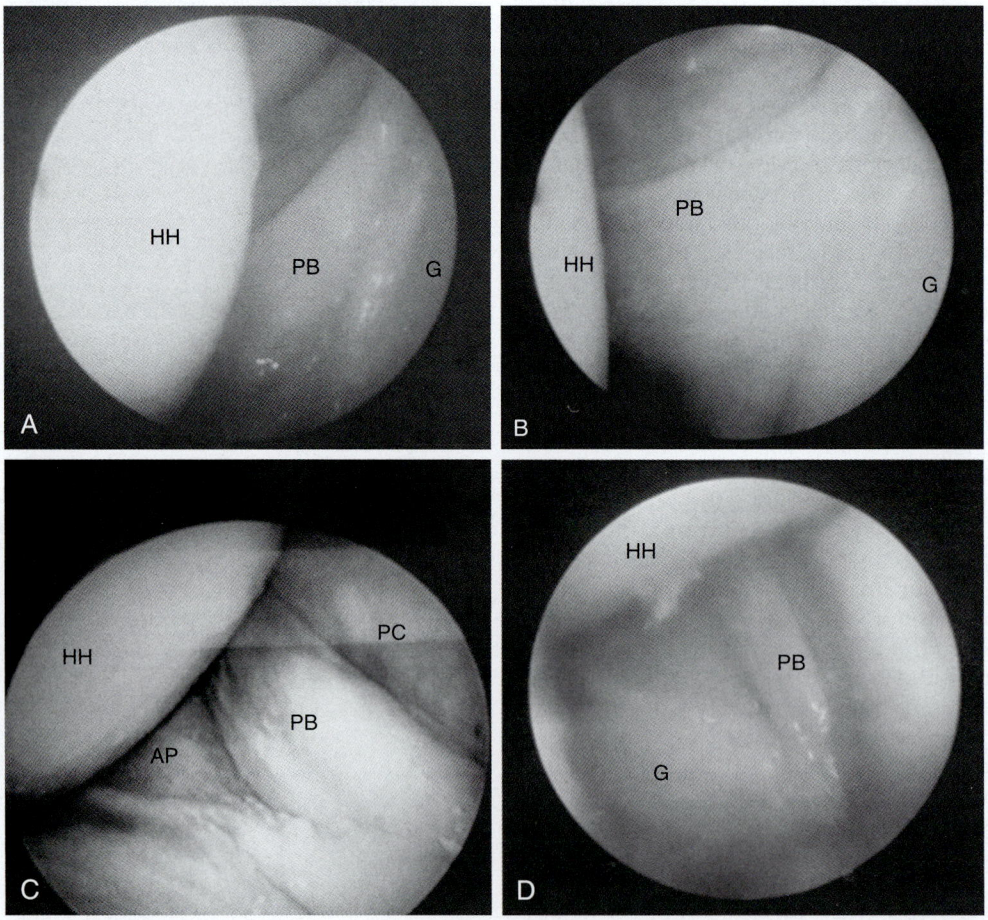

FIGURE 1-52: Various views of the posterior band of the inferior glenohumeral ligament complex as visualized arthroscopically. **A** and **B,** visualized from an anterior portal, show the distinct configuration of the posterior band (PB) with internal and external rotation, respectively. During internal rotation, the posterior band fans out to support the humeral head (HH). **C** and **D** show two superior portal views of the posterior band, the posterior capsule (PC), the axillary pouch (AP), and the glenoid (G).

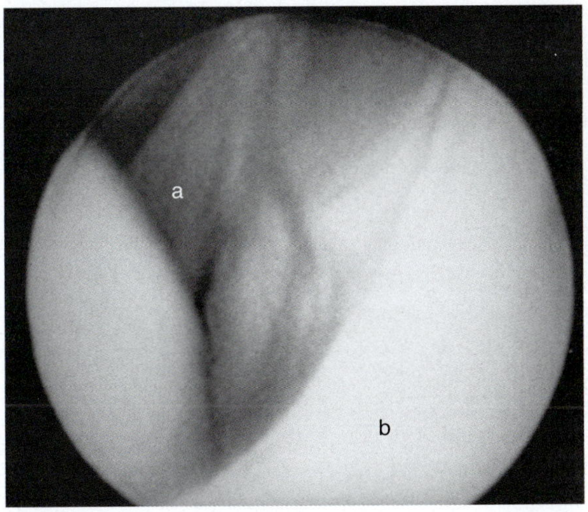

FIGURE 1-53: An anterior arthroscopic view of the inferior glenohumeral ligament complex, showing the anterior and posterior bands (*a* and *b*) and the intervening axillary pouch.

degree of intermingling of collagen fibers of the three layers vary with the different portions of the capsule.

The posterior capsule is quite thin (Fig. 1-55). The three layers of the capsule are easily distinguished, but the outer layer is least prominent and quickly blends into a layer of loose areolar tissue outside the capsule.

The posterior band of the IGHLC exists as an abrupt thickening in the capsule (Fig. 1-56). This thickening is due mostly to the presence of increased, well-organized, coarse collagen bundles in the coronal plane within the inner layer, oriented at 90 degrees to the middle layer. The inner layer is displaced outward at the expense of relative thinning of the outer layer. This finding can be appreciated quite well in coronal views of the posterior band (Fig. 1-57).

The transition from the posterior band to the axillary pouch is less distinct, and the axillary pouch exhibits a gradual intermingling of the coarse longitudinal inner fibers with the sagittal transverse fibers, which are continuous with the transverse fibers of the middle layer

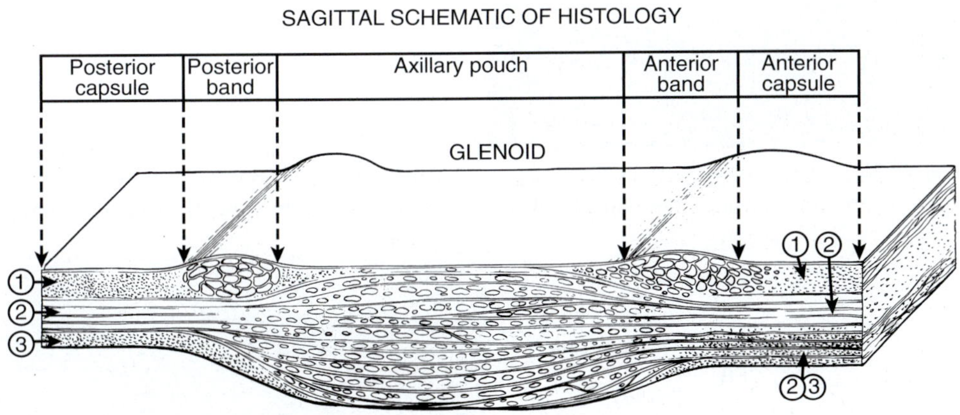

FIGURE 1-54: A schematic representation of the histologic layers of the shoulder capsule. The capsule consists of a thin synovial lining and three well-defined layers of collagen (see text).

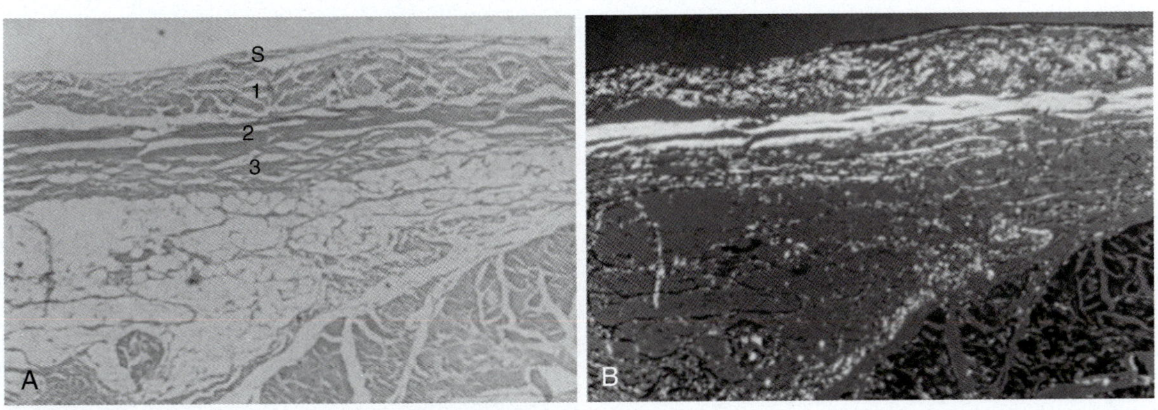

FIGURE 1-55: The posterior capsule is quite thin, and all three layers of the shoulder capsule along with the synovium (S). The posterior capsule quickly blends into a layer of loose areolar tissue outside the capsule. **A,** Hematoxylin and eosin view; **B,** polarized view.

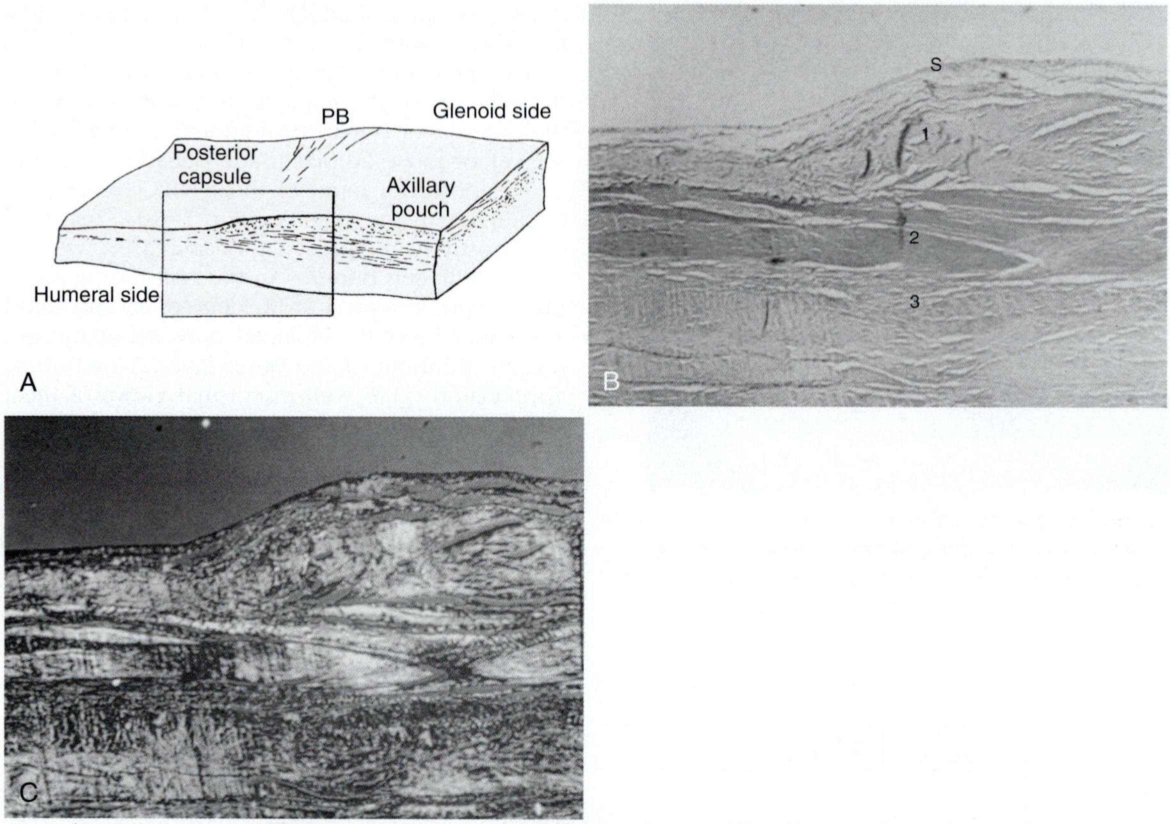

FIGURE 1-56: A, The posterior band (PB) exists as an abrupt thickening in the shoulder capsule. In these sagittal views the thickening can be seen in the inner layer of the capsule. **B,** Hematoxylin and eosin view; **C,** polarized view.

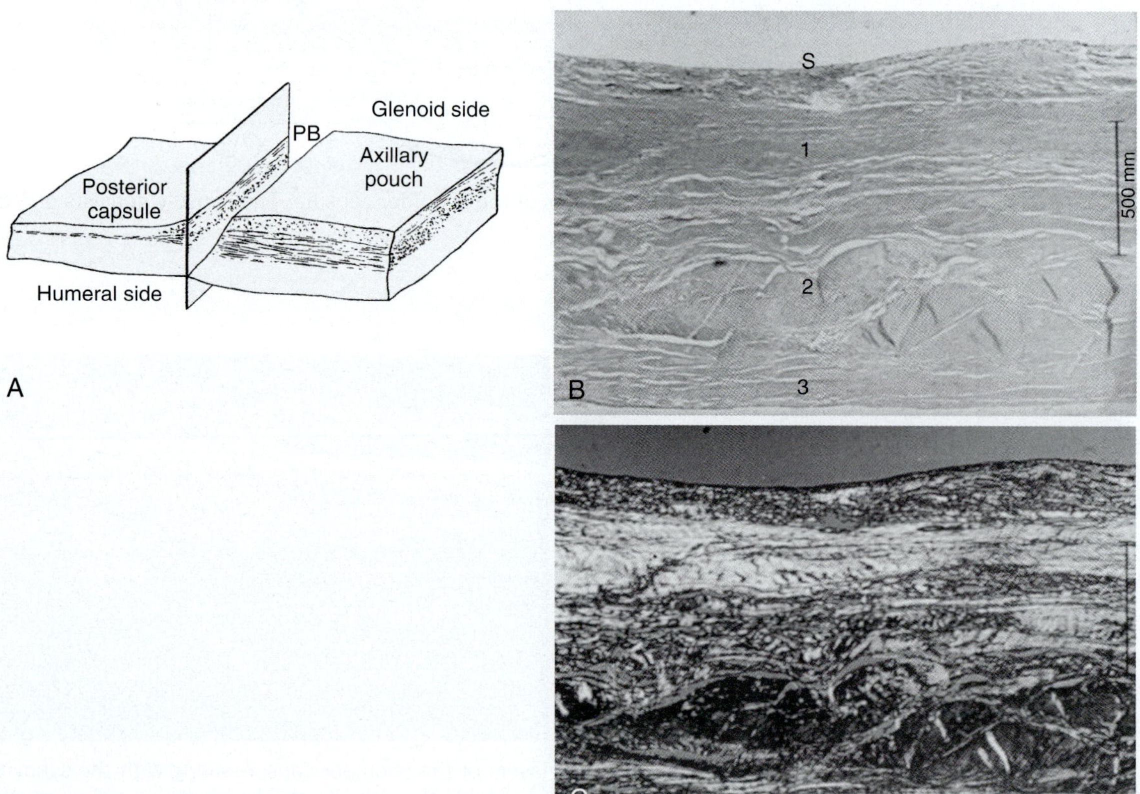

FIGURE 1-57: A, The precise organization of the posterior band (PB) is shown. Coronal views show three well-defined layers (numbered) in this region, along with the synovium (S). **B,** Hematoxylin and eosin view; **C,** polarized view.

(Fig. 1-58). In the axillary pouch region the outer layer is attenuated and virtually disappears.

The anterior band also exists as an abrupt thickening of the inner layer of the anterior capsule, although the distinction is not as marked histologically as the transition between the posterior band and the posterior capsule. The more precise collagen orientation, similar to the posterior band, can be seen, and the coronal view in Figure 1-59 shows a histologic picture virtually identical to that of the posterior band seen in Figure 1-57. Approaching the axillary pouch, these bundles again lose their precise organization and intermingle with the fibers of the middle layer.

The capsule anterior to the IGHLC is qualitatively thicker than the capsule posterior to it, mainly because of the relative increase in the thickness of the middle layer. Extensive intermingling of the middle and outer layers of the capsule takes place in this region (see Figs. 1-51 and 1-54).

Considering the IGHLC as functioning as a hammock-like sling to support the humeral head (Fig. 1-60) provides a unifying foundation for understanding anterior and posterior instability in the human shoulder and explains how damage in one portion of the shoulder capsule can affect the opposite side. This concept has clinical significance for treating instability disorders of the shoulder.

Bicipital Tunnel

As described above, the biceps-labral complex is an intimately associated structure consisting of three anatomic zones: the inside, junctional, and bicipital tunnel zones (Fig. 1-61). The bicipital tunnel is an extra-articular, fibro-osseous structure confining the LHBT that extends from

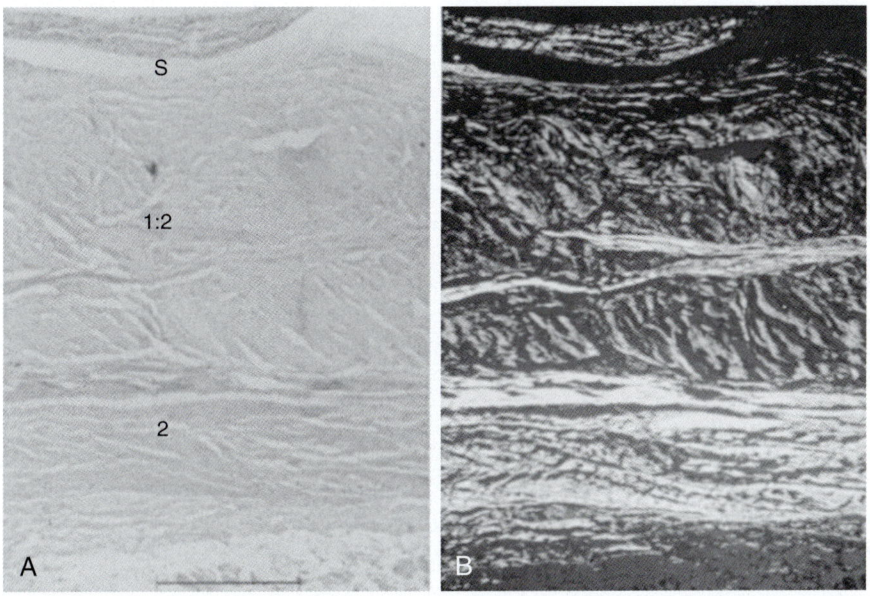

FIGURE 1-58: Sagittal views of the axillary pouch show blending of the inner and middle layers and a continuation of the outermost layer. **A,** Hematoxylin and eosin view; **B,** polarized view. *S,* synovium.

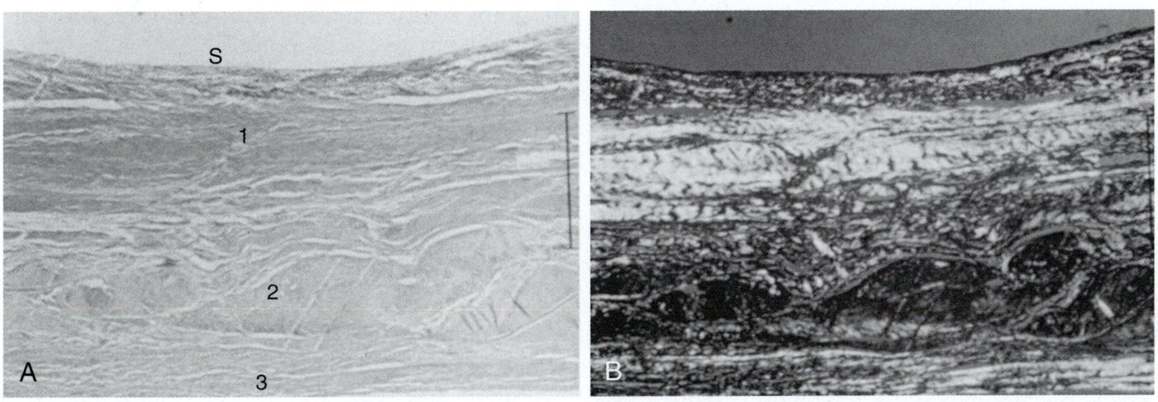

FIGURE 1-59: The more precise collagen orientation returns in the region of the anterior band, as seen in these coronal views. These views are virtually identical with those of the posterior band in Figure 1-57. **A,** Hematoxylin and eosin view; **B,** polarized view, *S,* synovium; *1* to *3,* the three layers.

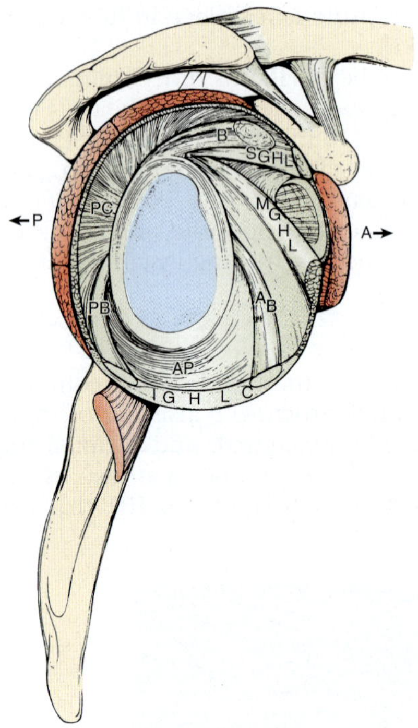

FIGURE 1-60: Anatomic depiction of the glenohumeral ligaments and inferior glenohumeral ligament complex (IGHLC). *A*, anterior; *AB*, anterior band; *AP*, axillary pouch; *B*, biceps tendon; *MGHL*, middle glenohumeral ligament; *P*, posterior; *PB*, posterior band; *PC*, posterior capsule; *SGHL*, superior glenohumeral ligament.

the articular margin through the subpectoralis region. The clinical relevance of this structure was suggested by Sanders et al.,[71] who reported significantly higher failure rate (20.6% vs. 6.8%) for biceps procedures that did not release the structure's extra-articular constraining bicipital sheath.

The anatomy and histology of the bicipital tunnel were described by Taylor et al.[77] in a cadaveric study. They identified three distinct zones. Zone 1 represents the traditional bony bicipital groove and extends from the articular margin to the distal margin of the subscapularis tendon (DMSS). A majority of the LHBT (78%) is visualized under standard diagnostic arthroscopy in this zone.[79] Zone 1 is marked by synovium that circumferentially envelopes the LHBT, a deep osseous groove, and a thick fibrous roof from the subscapularis tendon. Zone 2 extends from the DMSS to the PMPM and represents a "no man's land" since it is hidden from both arthroscopic view and open subpectoralis exposure more distally. In this zone 67% of specimens contained synovium, had a shallow osseous trough along with proximal extension of the latissimus dorsi fibers, and were roofed by axially oriented dense connective tissue fibers and longitudinally oriented fibers of the falciform ligament, which were noted to be distinctly separate structures. Zone 3 is the subpectoralis region, which had a flat osseous floor covered by latissimus dorsi fibers. The roof and lateral constraint of zone 3 comprised the pectoralis major tendon, while the medial constraint came from loose connective tissue or a thin veil of dense connective tissue. Unlike in zones 1 and 2, synovium was rarely found in zone 3. The bicipital tunnel was found to be a closed space with a functional bottleneck between zones 2 and 3 at the level of the PMPM.

Traditionally, lesions of the LHBT have been thought to be a result of proximal abrasion or instability (pulley or subscapularis lesions) and can be readily visualized with arthroscopy. The identification of the bicipital tunnel, however, alters this dogma and suggests hidden lesions as a plausible explanation for suboptimal outcomes during biceps procedures in patients undergoing biceps tenodesis (only 74% reporting good to excellent results and 25% with residual symptoms). A recent study[79] highlighted that 47% of chronically symptomatic patients had hidden extra-articular lesions and 45% of patients with intra-articular lesions had concomitant extra-articular lesions.

Bursae

Several bursae are present in the shoulder region, and a number of recesses are found in the shoulder capsule between the glenohumeral ligaments. Two bursae in particular have clinical importance: the subacromial bursa, which is discussed later, and the subscapular bursa. The subscapular bursa lies between the subscapularis tendon and the neck of the scapula (Fig. 1-62), and it communicates with the joint cavity between the superior and middle glenohumeral ligaments. It protects the tendon of the subscapularis at the point where it passes under the base of the coracoid process and over the neck of the scapula. This bursa is linked to the coracoid process by a suspensory ligament, and in 28% of specimens dissected by Colas and colleagues, the subscapular bursae merged with the subcoracoid bursae, forming a unique wide bursa in this region.[12] The subscapular bursa often houses loose bodies in the shoulder, and it is also a region in which synovitis of the shoulder may be most intense, where small fringes, or villi, can project into the joint cavity.

Although uncommon (and not in communication with the joint cavity), another bursa may be present between the infraspinatus muscle and the capsule. Other synovial recesses are usually located in the anterior portion of the capsule. The number, size, and location of these recesses depend on topographic variations in the glenohumeral ligaments. DePalma and colleagues[16] described six common variations or types of recesses in the anterior capsule (Fig. 1-63), which are really variations in the opening of the subscapularis bursa. Type 1 (30.2%) has one synovial recess above the middle glenohumeral ligament, type 2 (2.0%) has one synovial recess below the middle glenohumeral ligament, type 3 (40.6%) has one recess above and one below the middle glenohumeral ligament, and type 4 (9.0%) has one large recess above the inferior ligament, with the middle glenohumeral ligament being absent. In type 5 (5.1%), the middle glenohumeral ligament is manifested as two small synovial

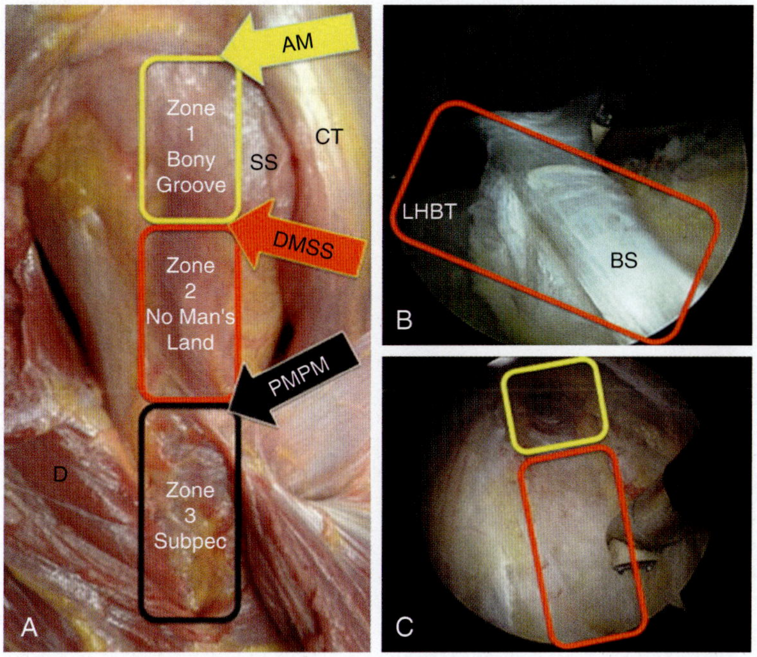

FIGURE 1-61: A soft tissue sheath (**A** and **B**) consistently covers the long head of the biceps tendon (LHBT) to the level of the proximal margin of the pectoralis major tendon (PMPM) and contributes to the roof of the bicipital tunnel. The sheath is clearly visible during open procedures (**A**) and extra-articular arthroscopic procedures within the subdeltoid space (**B** and **C**). The fibro-osseous bicipital tunnel consists of three distinct anatomic zones (**A**). Zone 1 represents the traditional bony bicipital groove (*yellow box*) beginning at the articular margin (AM) and ending at the distal margin of the subscapularis tendon (DMSS). Zone 2 (*red box*) extends from DMSS to PMPM and represents a "no man's land" because it is not viewable from arthroscopy above or from subpectoral exposure below. Zone 3 is distal to PMPM and represents the subpectoral region. The sheath overlying zone 2 can be robust (**B**). *D,* deltoid; *SS,* subscapularis; *CT,* conjoint tendon; *BS,* bicipital sheath.

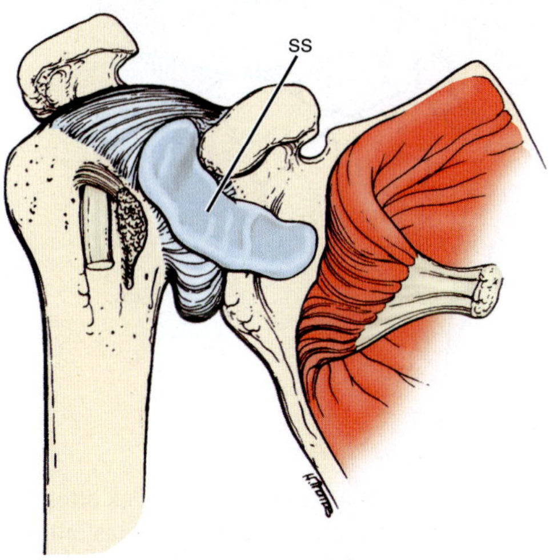

FIGURE 1-62: This subscapular (SS) bursa connects anteriorly and inferiorly under the coracoid process in the anterior portion of the capsule. Loose bodies are often found in this region.

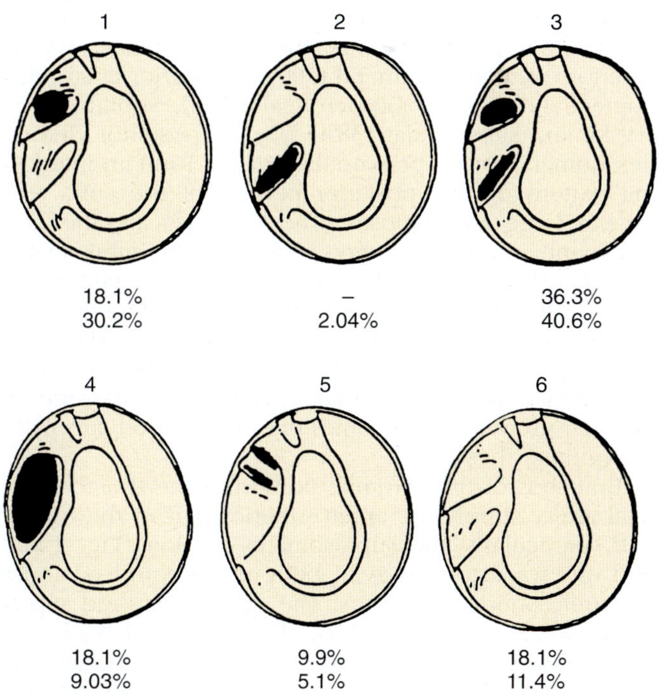

FIGURE 1-63: Variations in the types of recesses in the anterior capsule. The original prevalence percentages of DePalma are listed *(top lines*), along with percentages from more recent anatomic studies (*bottom lines*).

folds, and type 6 (11.4%) has no synovial recesses, although all the ligaments are well defined. Regardless of the arrangement in which they are found, the recesses show extreme variability. DePalma thought that if the capsule arises at the labrum or glenoid border of the scapula, few, if any, recesses would be present. If the capsule begins farther medially on the scapula or glenoid neck, however, the synovial recesses are larger and more numerous. He believed that the end result of such recesses was a thin, weakened anterior capsule that could predispose the shoulder to instability.

Others have referred to this general area of the anterior capsule as the *rotator interval*,[56] which they define as the region between the superior border of the subscapularis and the anterior border of the supraspinatus. The rotator interval includes the region of the superior glenohumeral ligament and coracohumeral ligament, in addition to the middle glenohumeral ligament. Plancher and colleagues[63] found the average area of this region to be 20.96 mm.[53] Some authors believe that enlargement of the interval can cause instability in certain shoulders and that it should be surgically obliterated during stabilization procedures.[56,67] Dynamic testing has shown that the subscapularis and supraspinatus dimensions as well as the total area of the rotator interval decrease significantly with internal rotation and open with external rotation. Imbrication procedures are performed with the arm in a neutral position to avoid loss of motion or insufficient tightening.[63]

Microvasculature

Rotator Cuff

Six arteries regularly contribute to the arterial supply of the rotator cuff tendons: the suprascapular (100%), anterior circumflex humeral (100%), posterior circumflex humeral (100%), thoracoacromial (76%), suprahumeral (59%), and subscapular (38%).[19,66] The posterior circumflex humeral and suprascapular arteries form an interlacing pattern on the posterior portion of the cuff, with several large anastomoses. These vessels are the predominant arteries to the teres minor and the infraspinatus tendons (Fig. 1-64). The anterior humeral circumflex artery supplies the subscapularis muscle and tendon and anastomoses with the posterior humeral circumflex artery over the LHBT (Fig. 1-65). In addition, a large branch of the anterior humeral circumflex artery enters the intertubercular groove and becomes the major blood supply to the humeral head.

Branches of the acromial portion of the thoracoacromial artery supply the anterosuperior part of the rotator cuff, particularly the supraspinatus tendon (Fig. 1-66), and often anastomose with both anterior and posterior circumflex humeral arteries. The subscapular and suprahumeral arteries (named by Rothman and Parke to describe a small vessel from the third portion of the axillary artery to the anterior rotator cuff and lesser tuberosity) make only a minimal contribution.[66] Approximately two thirds of shoulders have a hypovascular zone in the tendinous portion of the supraspinatus just proximal to its insertion. Less commonly, the infraspinatus (in 37% of shoulders) and the subscapularis (7%) also have a poorly perfused area. These areas of hypovascularity correspond to areas where degeneration is common. The hypovascular regions may be present at birth[64]; however, a significant decrease in vascularity can be seen with aging and degeneration.

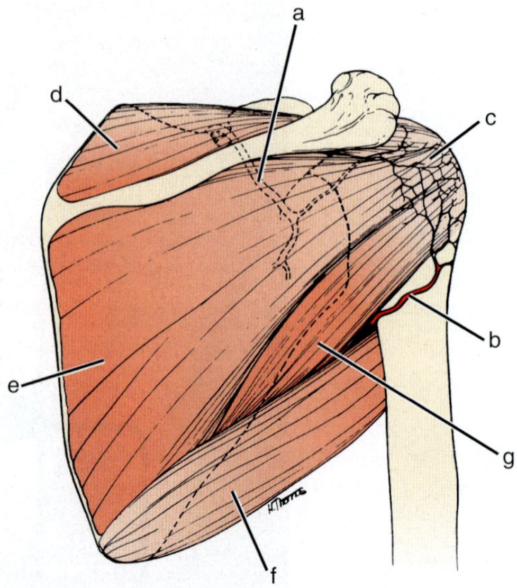

FIGURE 1-64: The suprascapular artery (a) and the posterior circumflex humeral artery (b) form an interlacing pattern on the posterior portion of the rotator cuff (c) with several large anastomoses. Also depicted are the supraspinatus (d), infraspinatus (e), teres major (f), and teres minor (g).

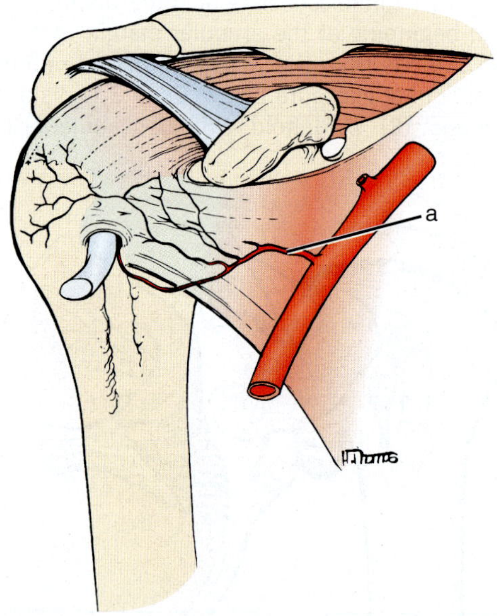

FIGURE 1-65: The anterior humeral circumflex artery (a) supplies the subscapularis muscle and tendon and anastomoses with the posterior humeral circumflex artery over the tendon of the long head of the biceps. In addition, a large branch of the anterior humeral circumflex artery enters the intertubercular groove and becomes the major blood supply to the humeral head.

Rathbun and Macnab[64] demonstrated that in this hypovascular critical zone in the rotator cuff, vascular filling depends on the position of the arm, with less filling noted when the arm is in adduction (Fig. 1-67). Most likely, the filling is also chronically impeded by advanced impingement, with the humeral head and rotator cuff impinging on the acromion, compressing the hypovascular zone, and limiting the potential for repair of small attritional tears in these locations. This mechanism has never been proved, however.

Glenoid Labrum

The glenoid labrum is supplied by small branches of three major vessels supplying the shoulder joint: the suprascapular artery, circumflex scapular artery, and posterior humeral circumflex artery (Fig. 1-68). These vessels supply the peripheral attachment of the labrum through small periosteal and capsular vessels (Fig. 1-69). Although the extent of these microvascular patterns is variable throughout the labrum, they are usually limited to the outermost aspect of the labrum, with the inner rim being devoid of vessels. This arrangement is similar to that observed in the menisci in the knee.[13]

Glenohumeral Capsule and Ligaments

The glenohumeral capsule and ligaments have a predictable blood supply, with contributions from the suprascapular, circumflex scapular, posterior circumflex scapular, and anterior circumflex arteries.

In a study by Andary and Petersen, adult cadaveric shoulders were analyzed to further characterize the vascular patterns to the glenohumeral capsule and

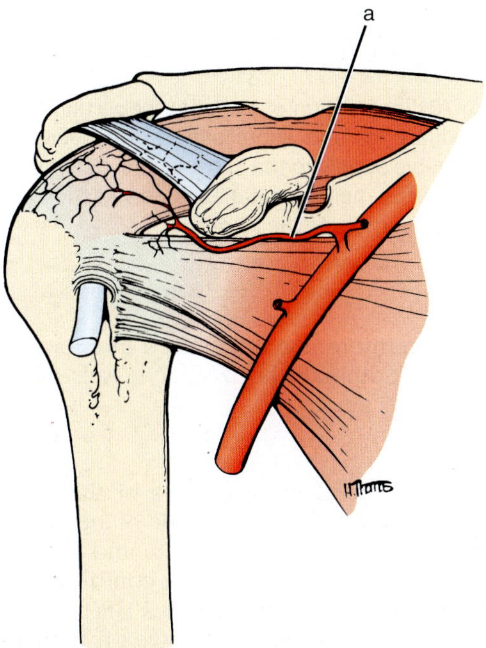

FIGURE 1-66: The acromial branch (a) of the thoracoacromial artery supplies the anterosuperior portion of the rotator cuff, particularly the supraspinatus tendon.

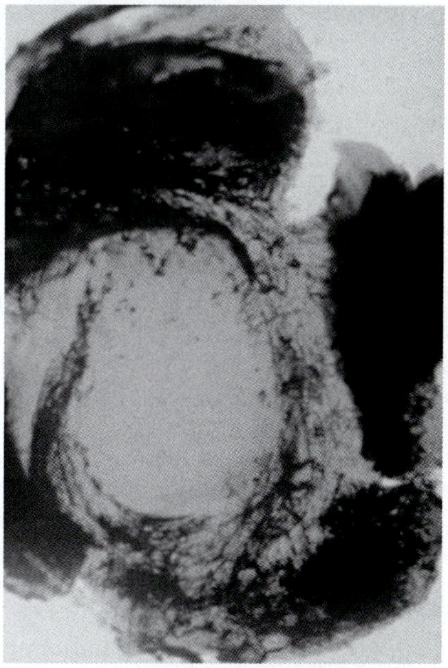

FIGURE 1-68: Microvasculature of the shoulder capsule and labrum. The inferior glenohumeral ligament complex has greater vascularity than the remainder of the posterior capsule, which is relatively devoid of significant vasculature.

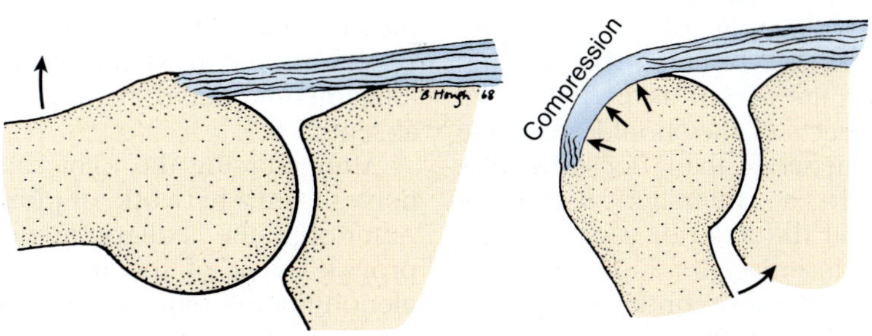

FIGURE 1-67: The hypovascular critical zone in the rotator cuff. **A,** Abduction. **B,** Adduction. Vascular filling depends on the position of the arm, with less filling noted when the arm is in adduction. (From Rathbun JB, Macnab I. The microvascular pattern of the rotator cuff. *J Bone Joint Surg Br.* 1970;52:540-553.)

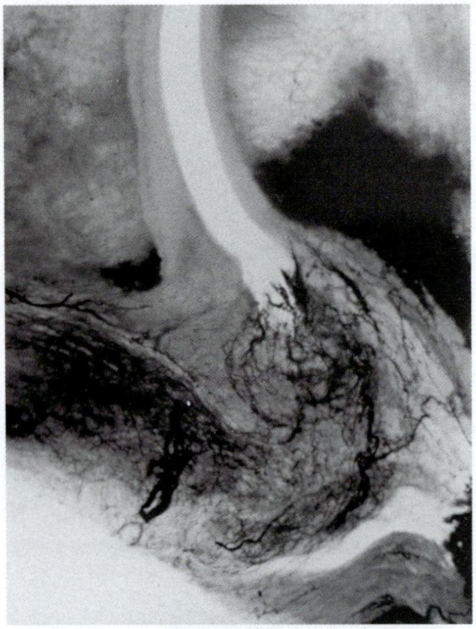

FIGURE 1-69: The vasculature of the labrum's edge is shown. Small periosteal and capsular vessels are visible.

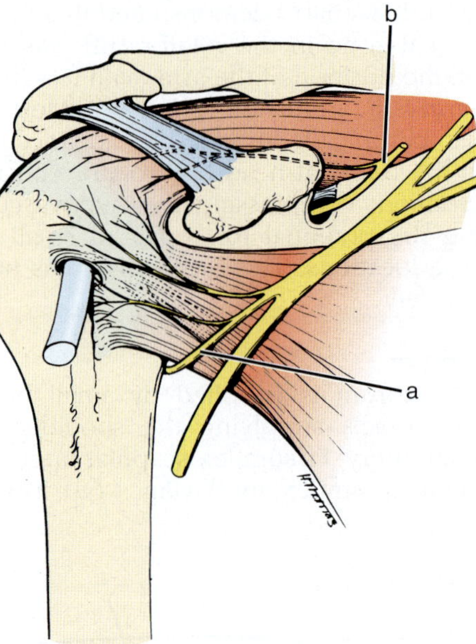

FIGURE 1-70: Innervation of the anterior portion of the shoulder. The axillary (a) and suprascapular (b) nerves constitute most of the nerve supply to the capsule and glenohumeral joint. In some cases the musculocutaneous nerve sends twigs to the anterosuperior portion of the joint.

ligaments.[3] They found that the arterial supply to the capsule is centripetal, entering superficially and then penetrating deeper. Four distinct regions of the capsule receive consistent patterns of vascularity. The anterior and posterior circumflex scapular arteries enter the capsule laterally. The suprascapular and circumflex scapular arteries enter the capsule medially and arborize with the humeral circumflex vessels as they all converge on the middle of the capsule. The anterior humeral circumflex artery supplies the anterior part of the lateral aspect of the capsule, and the posterior part of the lateral capsule is supplied by the posterior humeral circumflex artery. Medially, the periosteal network of the anterior aspect of the scapula supplies the anteromedial capsule, and branches of the circumflex scapular and suprascapular arteries supply the capsule posteriorly. Perforating arteries from the rotator cuff tendons and muscle enter the capsule superficially in the midsubstance and at the humeral insertion, and then penetrate to deeper layers.

The predominant arterial supply of the shoulder capsule is oriented in a horizontal fashion. This orientation is particularly evident in the region of the IGHLC.[58,3] The anterior and inferior aspects of the shoulder capsule exhibit a denser vascular network than does the thin posterior capsule. However, a watershed region of hypovascularity was noted in the anterior aspect of the capsule near the humeral insertion in 5 of 12 specimens.[3] The authors correlated these findings with an associated hypovascular region in the critical zone of the supraspinatus tendon. Based on these results, they warned that surgical approaches to the shoulder that separate the rotator cuff from the underlying capsule could compromise the perforating vascularity to the capsule. Furthermore, laterally based incisions will probably cross the dominant horizontal vessels of the shoulder capsule.

Innervation

The superficial and deep structures of the shoulder are profusely innervated by a network of nerve fibers that are mainly derived from the C5, C6, and C7 nerve roots (the C4 root can also make a minor contribution).[23,15] The innervation of the joint itself follows Hilton's law, which states that nerves crossing a joint give off branches to the joint, providing its innervation. Therefore the nerves supplying the ligaments, capsule, and synovial membrane of the shoulder are medullary and nonmedullary fibers from the axillary, suprascapular, subscapular, and musculocutaneous nerves. Occasional contributions are made from small branches of the posterior cord of the brachial plexus. The relative contributions made by any of these nerves are inconsistent, and the supply from the musculocutaneous nerve may be very small or completely absent.

After piercing the joint capsule, branches from these nerves form a network, or plexus, to supply the synovium. Anteriorly, the axillary nerve and suprascapular nerve provide most of the nerve supply to the capsule and glenohumeral joint. In some instances, the musculocutaneous nerve innervates the anterosuperior portion. In addition, the anterior capsule may be supplied either by the subscapular nerves or by the posterior cord of the brachial plexus after they have pierced the subscapularis (Fig. 1-70).

Superiorly, the nerves making the primary contributions are two branches of the suprascapular nerve, with one branch proceeding anteriorly as far as the coracoid process and coracoacromial ligament, and the other branch reaching the posterior aspect of the joint. Other nerves contributing to this region of the joint are the axillary nerve, musculocutaneous nerve, and branches from the lateral anterior thoracic nerve. Posteriorly, the chief nerves are the suprascapular nerve in the upper region and the axillary nerve in the lower region (Fig. 1-71). Inferiorly, the anterior portion is primarily supplied by the axillary nerve, and the posterior portion is supplied by a combination of the axillary nerve and lower ramifications of the suprascapular nerve.

Alpantaki and colleagues performed an immunohistochemical staining study on cadavers to elucidate the innervation to the LHBT.[2] The authors found that thinly myelinated or unmyelinated sensory neurons provided innervation to this tendon, supporting the concept that the LHBT may be the pain generator in patients with shoulder pathology. This is an area of ongoing study.

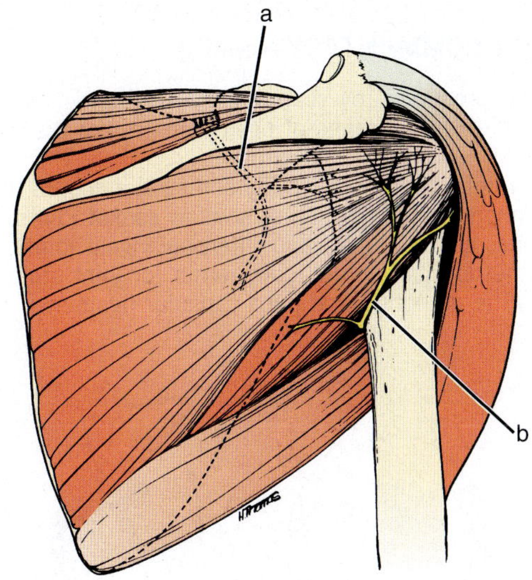

FIGURE 1-71: Posterior innervation of the shoulder joint. The primary nerves are the suprascapular (a) and the axillary (b).

EDITOR COMMENTARY

Steven B. Lippitt

Developmental anatomy of the shoulder, a subject often ignored in shoulder education, is an appropriate first chapter for this extensive fifth edition shoulder reference text. The authors have provided extensive detail relating scapulohumeral anatomy to the unique functional demands of our upper extremity.

In addition to contrasting human shoulder anatomy and development to those of other species, much may be learned by comparison to other human articulations. Our shoulder joint provides a greater range of motion than any other joint in the body and also has the greatest risk of instability. In the hip joint the acetabulum provides a deep socket surrounding much of the femoral head, providing substantial resistance to dislocation. This hip socket limits the extent of femoral motion before acetabular rim impingement occurs. In contrast, the humeral head rests on a relatively small arc of the glenoid and thus is not intrinsically stable, but allows a vast global motion before articular abutment occurs (Fig. 1-72). This large degree of freedom of the glenohumeral

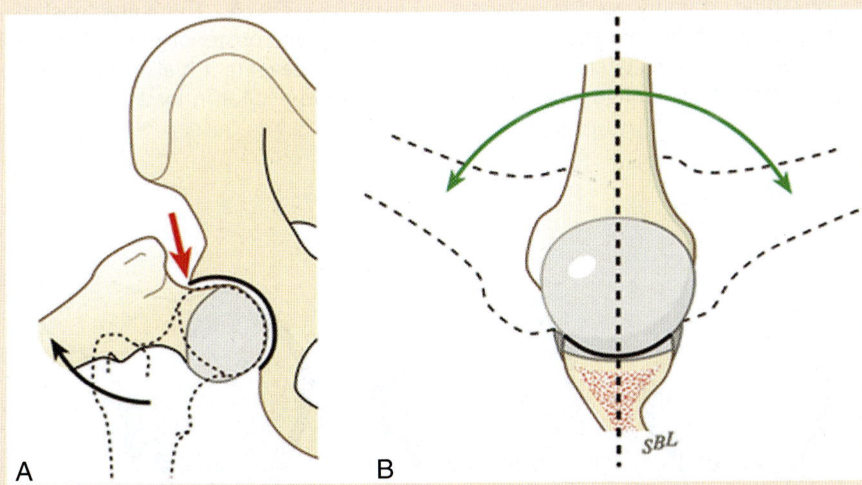

FIGURE 1-72: Hip versus shoulder range of motion. **A,** The hip joint is very stable due to the deep acetabular socket, although femoral motion is relatively limited before rim impingement occurs (*red arrow*). **B,** In contrast, the shallow glenoid of the shoulder joint captures relatively little of the humeral articulation but allows a vast global motion before articular abutment occurs (*green arrow*).

Continued

EDITOR COMMENTARY—cont'd

joint, accompanied by scapulothoracic motion, helps maximize the extensive range of positioning of the distal hand in space.

This unique shoulder mobility comes at a cost to the shoulder's inherent stability. Other shallow socket joints, such as the knee, elbow, ankle, and interphalangeal joints, depend on isometric ligamentous constraints for joint stability (Fig. 1-73). The glenohumeral joint capsular ligaments, however, are lax in mid-range shoulder positions and only provide static constraint when they become taught at the extremes of motion (Fig. 1-74).[43] For example, the inferior glenohumeral ligament provides the principle static constraint to anteroinferior instability when the arm is in extreme abduction, extension, and external rotation, as during the cocking and early acceleration phase of throwing. The knee joint has unique intra-articular cruciate ligaments that prevent anterior or posterior translation of the knee joint throughout its range (Fig. 1-75). The glenohumeral joint differs in allowing humeral translation until the lax capsular ligaments become taught (Fig. 1-76).[30,42] The glenohumeral joint thus requires different mechanisms of stability such as *concavity compression,* the dynamic compression of the humeral head into the shallow glenoid-labral concavity by balanced rotator cuff contraction (Figs. 1-77 and 1-78), and *scapulohumeral balance,* which involves the neuromuscular control of coordinated scapular movement, keeping the glenohumeral joint reaction force positioned

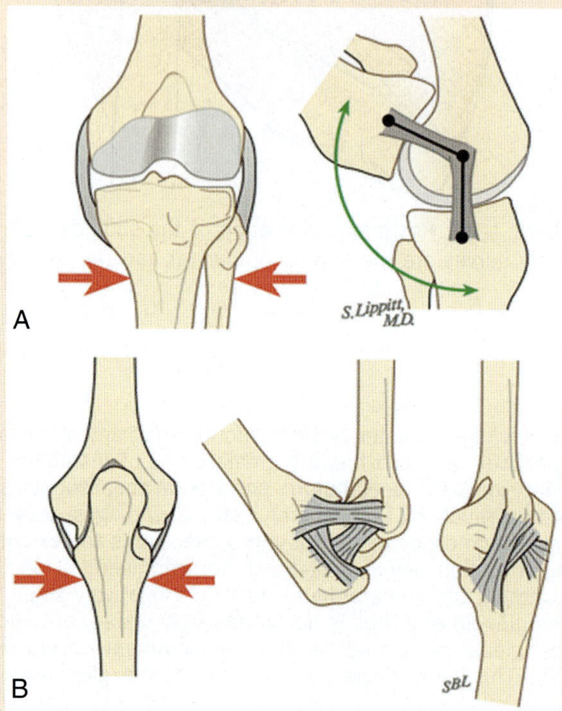

FIGURE 1-73: A, The knee joint collateral ligaments remain in isometric tension, providing stability to varus–valgus stress throughout the full range of flexion and extension motion. **B,** Similarly, the elbow joint collateral ligaments provide stability throughout the elbow's range of motion.

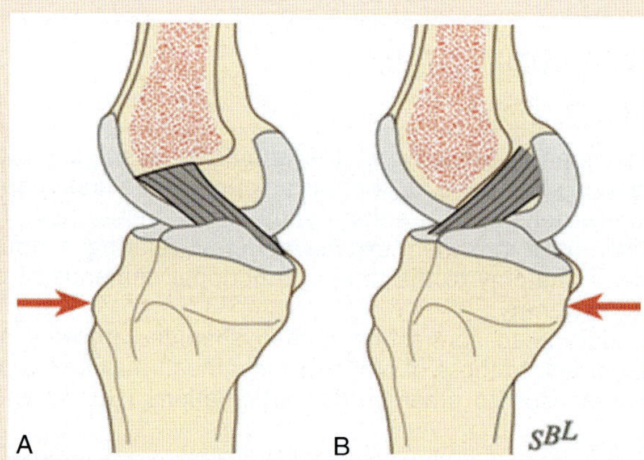

FIGURE 1-75: A, The knee posterior cruciate ligament prevents tibial posterior translation. **B,** The anterior cruciate ligament prevents tibial anterior translation during knee motion and eccentric loads.

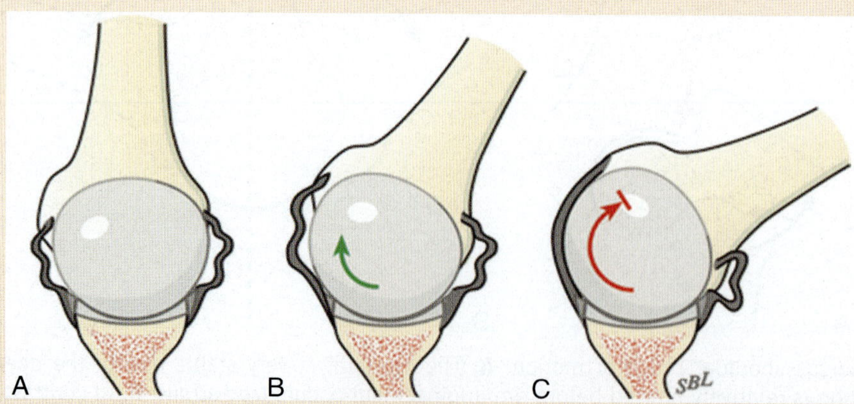

FIGURE 1-74: A and **B,** The glenohumeral joint capsular ligaments are lax in mid-range shoulder positions. **C,** The ligaments only provide static constraint when they become taught at the extreme of the shoulder's range of motion.

EDITOR COMMENTARY—cont'd

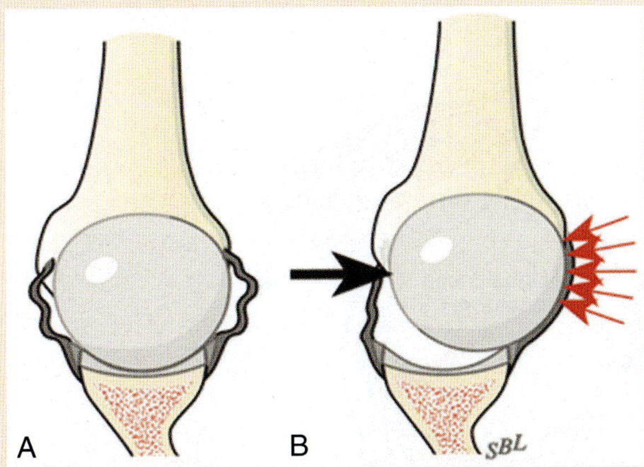

FIGURE 1-76: **A,** The humeral head has lax ligaments when centered in the glenoid in midrange joint positions. **B,** The humeral head translates from the glenoid center with applied external force (*black arrow*) until opposing capsular ligaments become tight (*red arrows*).

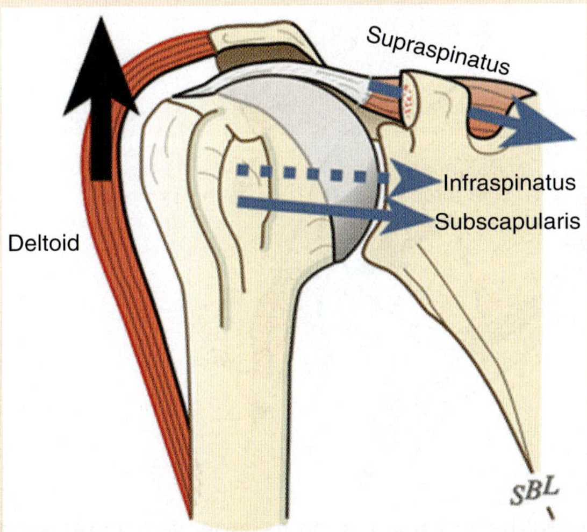

FIGURE 1-77: Stability through concavity compression. The supraspinatus muscle superiorly, the infraspinatus posteriorly, and the subscapularis anteriorly compress the humeral head into the glenoid concavity (*blue arrows*), providing stability.

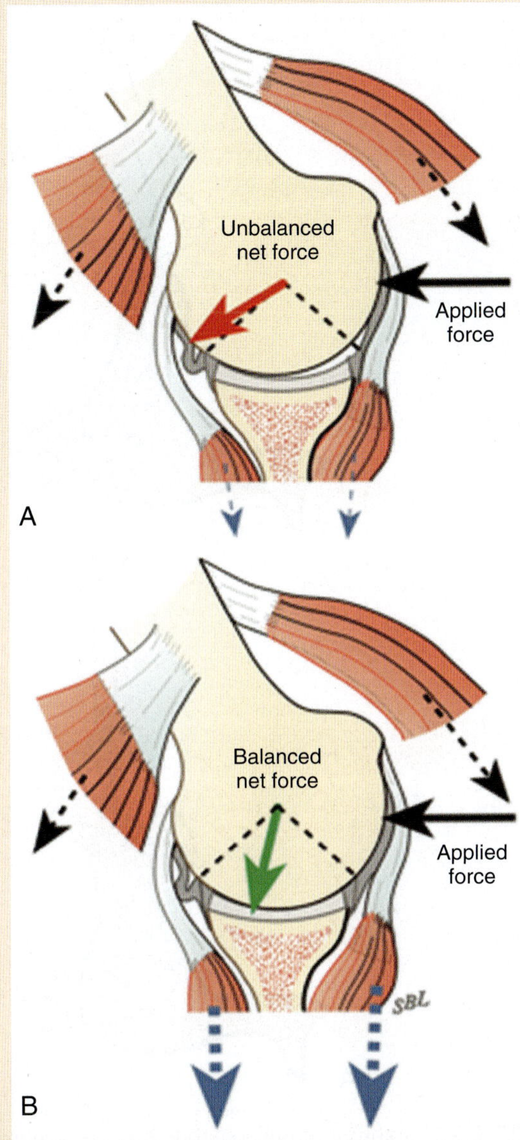

FIGURE 1-78: **A,** Weak contraction of the cuff muscles (*small dotted blue arrows*) does not offset an applied translational force (*solid black arrow*), resulting in an unbalanced net force (*red arrow*) and subsequent humeral translation from the center of the glenoid concavity. **B,** Strong contraction of the rotator cuff (*larger dotted blue arrows*) provides an increased compressive force into the glenoid concavity, balancing the net force (*green arrow*) and centering the humeral head.

Continued

EDITOR COMMENTARY—cont'd

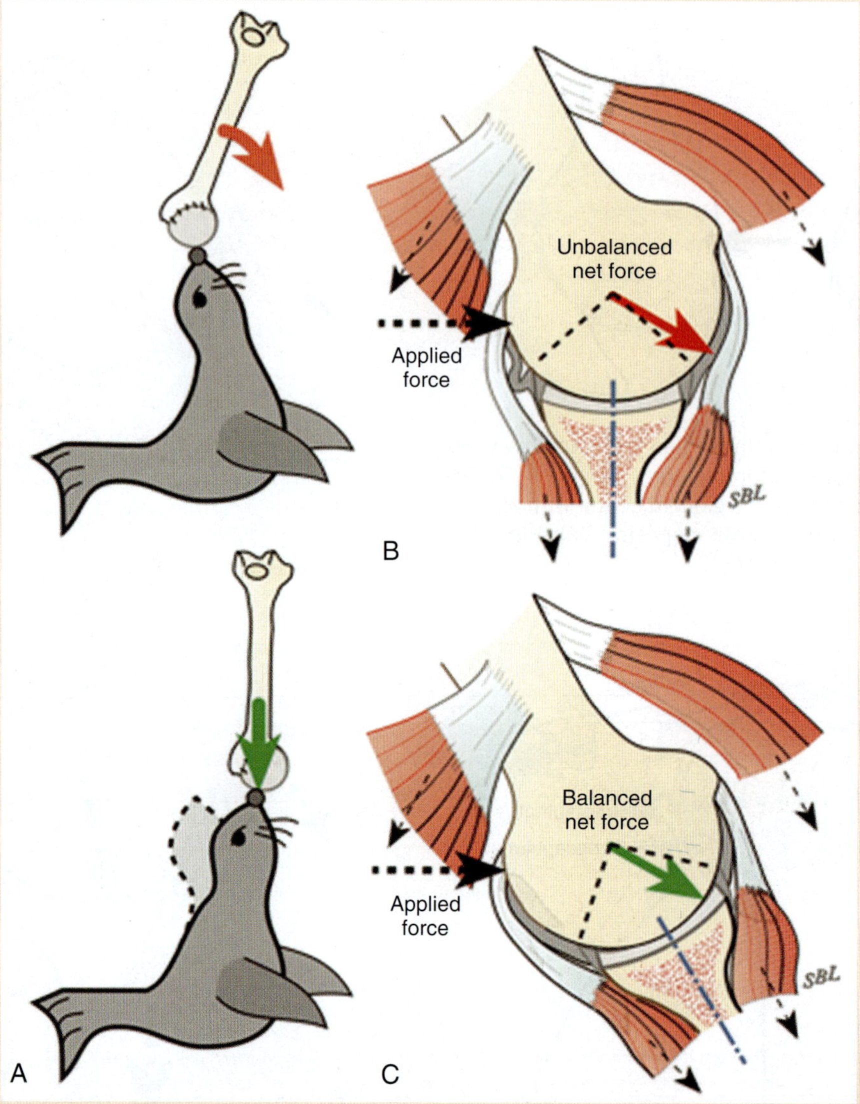

FIGURE 1-79: Stability through scapulohumeral balance. **A,** Like a seal balancing a ball on its nose, varying the scapular position can help balance the humerus in the glenoid. **B,** An applied force results in an unbalanced net force (*red arrow*). **C,** Coordinated scapular movement repositions the glenoid concavity to balance the net humeral force (*green arrow*) within the glenoid concavity.

within the glenoid (Fig. 1-79).[43,44,46,47,48] The shoulder joint is truly an amazing balance of mobility and stability.

This commentary space does not allow detailed discussion of the astounding strength, velocity, and smoothness of various coordinated shoulder joint functions. We can only marvel at a gymnast's iron cross position, a dancer's graceful arm movements, and a baseball pitcher's throw of 100 mph. In absolute awe of the shoulder design, I will personally quote David's Psalm 139:14, "I praise you, for I am fearfully and wonderfully made."[81]

SENIOR EDITOR COMMENTARY

Frederick A. Matsen III

While the anatomy of the human shoulder is evolving at an imperceptible rate, our understanding of this anatomy is continually improving. These authors take us on a fascinating voyage through the current knowledge about our shoulder's evolution and development. As they point out, the scapula of the quadruped lies in the sagittal plane so that the glenoid sits stably on top of the humeral head. The muscles of the rotator cuff are distributed evenly around the humeral head, and the long head tendons of the biceps and triceps anchor the humeral head with their attachments to the superior and inferior aspects of the glenoid lip, respectively. All this adds up to a very stable configuration—a golf ball on top of a golf tee. As we evolved to an erect posture, the humeral loads were delivered in a direction tangential to, rather than directed into, the glenoid fossa—a golf tee driven into the club house door while trying to center a golf ball wanting it to fall to the ground. Attempts of soft tissues to contribute to this stability gave rise to our issues of glenohumeral instability, with deterioration of the glenoid labrum and the rotator cuff. The evolutionary adduction of the arm to the side has placed disproportionate tensile loads on the supraspinatus and long head biceps tendons, resulting in these being some of the most commonly damaged structures in the shoulder. Our use of the upper extremity for lifting objects away from the body (never a part of quadruped shoulder function) further jeopardizes the cuff anatomy by placing large tensile loads on it. Thus evolution has seen the transition from direct loading of the central aspect of the glenoid by the humerus, bone to bone, to the dependency on soft tissues to manage mobility and stability. The golf tee has moved.

These anatomic recognitions provide more than phylogenetic interest. They also suggest methods for injury prevention and rehabilitation. For example, shoulder strengthening exercises are most safely performed in the midrange of glenohumeral motion, where humeral loads are applied perpendicular to the face of the glenoid, rather than in positions at the extreme of motion where soft tissue stabilizers may be excessively challenged. They also advise us to avoid compromising structures such as the coracoacromial arch, which develops as "a gentle curve that conforms to the superior aspect of the humeral head, similar to a type II acromion."

These concepts continue to be refined. We no longer view the cuff muscles as humeral head "depressors," consuming energy in a vain attempt to keep the supraspinatus tendon away from the coracoacromial arch, but rather as "compressors"' that stabilize the humeral head in the glenoid cavity. We are replacing the idea that the inferior glenohumeral ligament is the primary stabilizer of the joint with the recognition that ligaments can only stabilize a joint when they are under tension, losing their effectiveness in most functional positions in which the joint can only be stabilized by concavity compression.

Anatomy is the basic science of shoulder evaluation, rehabilitation, and surgery. The surgeon with a strong foundation in anatomy will recognize and understand the significance of pathoanatomy and its management. Again, thanks to the authors for helping us get there.

CHAPTER 2

Gross Anatomy of the Shoulder

Christopher M. Jobe, Wesley P. Phipatanakul, Djuro Petkovic

We are faced with a paradox in shoulder anatomy. Knowledge regarding the details of shoulder anatomy has increased along with knowledge regarding its clinical significance. However, our exposure is decreasing. The proportion of the medical school curriculum dedicated to anatomy is shrinking, and at the same time, a number of open procedures, where residents and students might observe the anatomy first hand, have been replaced by arthroscopic procedures (Fig. 2-1). This decreased exposure has been offset by new imaging techniques that enable a deeper understanding of the current anatomy, both normal and abnormal, of the patient. Magnetic resonance imaging (MRI) allows a more detailed anatomic study of the patient, and ultrasound adds the ability to dynamically observe some structures.

This chapter details the anatomic structures of the shoulder. According to the concept of a layered portrait, the material is arranged in a layered fashion. The discussion begins with the innermost layer, the bones and joints, which is the most palpable and least deformable structures of the shoulder. They are the easiest to visualize and are the best understood anatomic landmarks. We then reveal the muscle layers that enable motion of the shoulder and the nerves that direct the muscles and provide sensation. We will discuss the vessels that control the internal environment of the tissues of the shoulder and, finally, the skin that encloses the shoulder.

The central theme of the shoulder is motion. The amount of motion in the shoulder sets it apart from all other joints and accounts for the manner in which the shoulder differs from all other regions of the body.

BONES AND JOINTS

The orthopedic surgeon considers bones primarily as rigid links that are moved, secondarily as points of attachment for ligaments, muscles, and tendons, and finally as the base on which important relationships with surrounding soft tissue are maintained. Treatment of fractures has been called the treatment of soft tissues surrounding them.[206] In relation to pathology, bones are three-dimensional objects of the anatomy that must be maintained or restored for joint alignment. Bones exist in a positive sense to protect soft tissue from trauma and provide a framework for muscle activity. In a negative sense, they can act as barriers to dissection for a surgeon trying to reach and repair a certain area of soft tissue and as a barrier to ultrasound visualization. Loss of bone position may endanger soft tissue in an acute sense, and loss of bone alignment may endanger the longevity of adjacent joints.

Joints have two opposing functions: to allow desired motion and to restrict undesirable motion. The stability of joints is the sum of (1) their bony congruity and stability, (2) the stability of ligaments, and (3) the dynamic stability provided by adjacent muscles. The shoulder has the greatest mobility of any joint in the body and has the greatest predisposition to dislocation.

This great range of motion is distributed to three diarthrodial joints: the glenohumeral, acromioclavicular, and sternoclavicular. The last two joints, in combination with the fascial spaces between the scapula and chest, are collectively known as the *scapulothoracic articulation.*[106] Because of the lack of congruence in two diarthrodial joints (the acromioclavicular and sternoclavicular joints), motion of the scapulothoracic articulation is mainly determined by the opposing surfaces of the thorax and scapula. Approximately one-third of the total elevation occurs in this part of the shoulder; the remainder occurs in the glenohumeral cavity. The three diarthrodial joints are constructed with little bony stability and mainly rely on their ligaments and on adjacent muscle at the glenohumeral joint. The large contributions of the scapulothoracic joint and axial body mechanics to the shoulder function have been emphasized over the past decade.

The division of motion over these articulations has two advantages. First, it allows the muscles crossing each of these articulations to operate in the optimal portion of their length-tension curve. Second, the glenohumeral rhythm allows the glenoid to be brought underneath the humerus to bear some weight of the upper limb, which decreases the demand on the shoulder muscles to suspend the arm. Such a division of motion is particularly important when the muscles are operating near the maximal abduction, the point in their length-tension

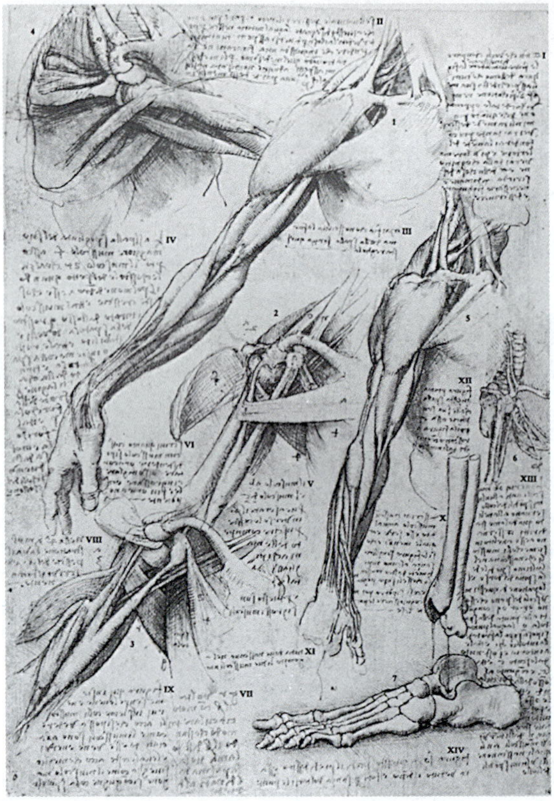

FIGURE 2-1: A page from Leonardo da Vinci's *Notebooks from Anatomical Study.* When compared with other illustrations of the time, the accuracy is striking. This particular dissection is interesting because the acromion is shown as a bone separate from the rest of the scapula. Other illustrations in the *Notebooks from Anatomical Study* show the acromion united. In da Vinci's accompanying notes, neither the fused nor the unfused state is considered normal. (From Windsor Castle, Royal Library. Copyright 1990, Her Majesty Queen Elizabeth II.)

curve at which they produce less force.[139,190] The study of the ultrastructure of ligaments (Fig. 2-2) and tendons concerning the shoulder is in its infancy; however, preliminary studies reveal little difference in terms of collagen biochemistry and fiber structure.[115,194]

Discussion regarding the bones and joints will proceed from the proximal to the distal portion of the shoulder and includes the joint surfaces, ligaments, and special intra-articular structures. Joint stability and the relative importance of each ligament to that stability are elaborated. The morphology of bones and their important muscle and ligament attachments are discussed. Finally, the relationship of bones and joints to other important structures in the shoulder is demonstrated.

Sternoclavicular Joint

The sternoclavicular joint, which is composed of the upper end of the sternum and the proximal end of the clavicle, is the only skeletal articulation between the upper limb and axial skeleton.[95] In both the vertical and anteroposterior dimensions, this portion of the clavicle is larger than the opposing sternum and extends superiorly and posteriorly relative to the sternum.[95,208] The prominence of the clavicle superiorly helps create the suprasternal fossa. The sternoclavicular joint has relatively little bony stability, and the bony surfaces are somewhat flat. The ligamentous structures provide the stability of the joint. The proximal surface of the clavicle is convex in the coronal plane but somewhat concave in the transverse plane. The joint angles from the anteromedial to the posterolateral in the axial plane. In the coronal plane, the joint surface is medially angled towards the superior end; the joint surfaces are covered with hyaline cartilage. In 97% of cadavers, a complete disk is observed to separate the joint into two compartments (Fig. 2-3). The disk is rarely perforated.[56,57] The intra-articular disk is superiorly attached to the first rib below and to the superior surface of the clavicle through the interclavicular ligament. The disk rarely tears or dislocates by itself.[61]

The major ligaments in the joint are the anterior and posterior sternoclavicular or capsular ligaments (Fig. 2-4). The fibers superiorly run from their attachment to the sternum to their superior attachment on the clavicle. The most important ligament of this group, the posterior sternoclavicular ligament, is the strongest stabilizer to the inferior depression of the lateral end of the clavicle.[11] The paired sternoclavicular ligaments are primary restraints so that minimal rotation occurs during depression of the clavicle.

The interclavicular ligament runs from clavicle to clavicle, with attachment to the sternum, and may be absent

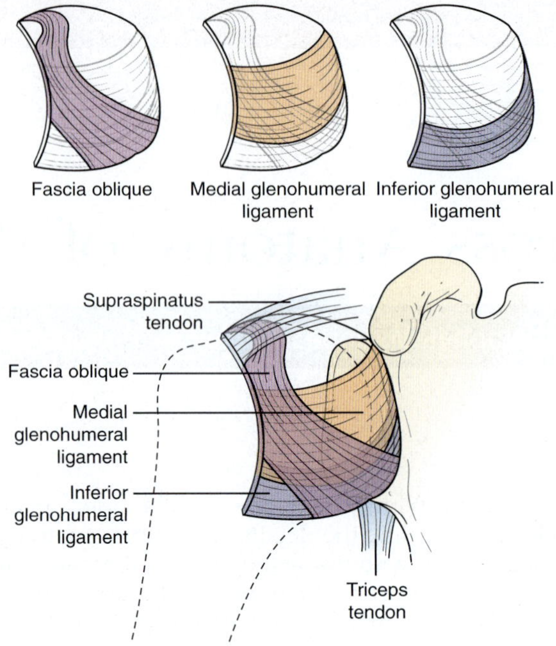

FIGURE 2-2: The dominant orientations of the collagen fibers in the layers of the glenohumeral capsule. (Modified from Gohlke F, et al. The pattern of the collagen fiber bundles of the capsule of the glenohumeral joint. *J Shoulder Elbow Surg.* 1994;3[3]:111-128).

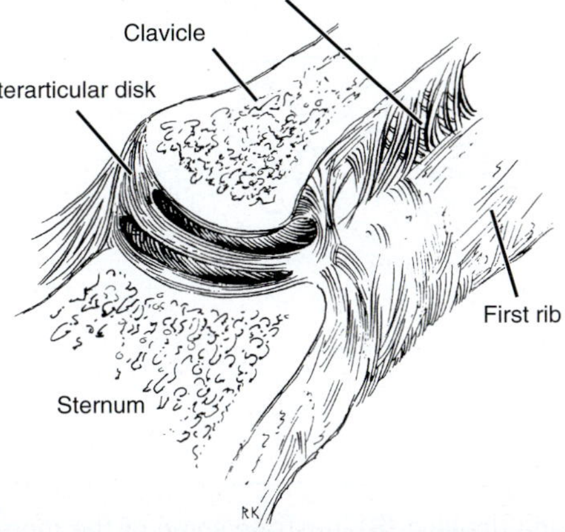

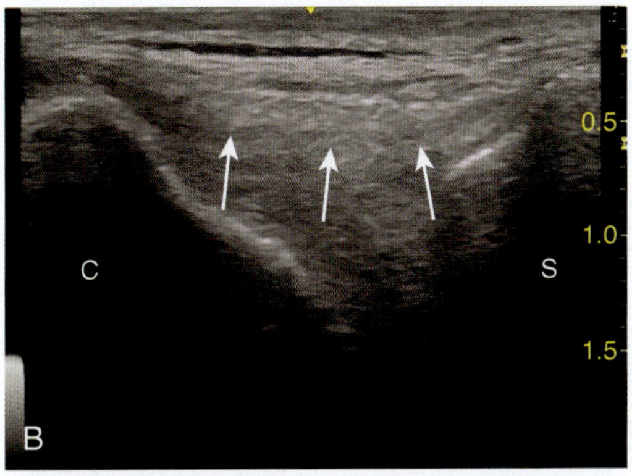

FIGURE 2-3: A, Cross-sectional drawing of the sternoclavicular joint in the coronal plane. A complete disk separates the joint into two compartments. The disk has a firm attachment to the first rib inferiorly and to the ligaments and superior border of the clavicle superiorly. **B,** An oblique axial ultrasound view showing the clavicle (C) on the left and the sternum (S) on the right. The clavicle is somewhat anterior to the sternum. The arrows indicate the anterior sternoclavicular ligament.

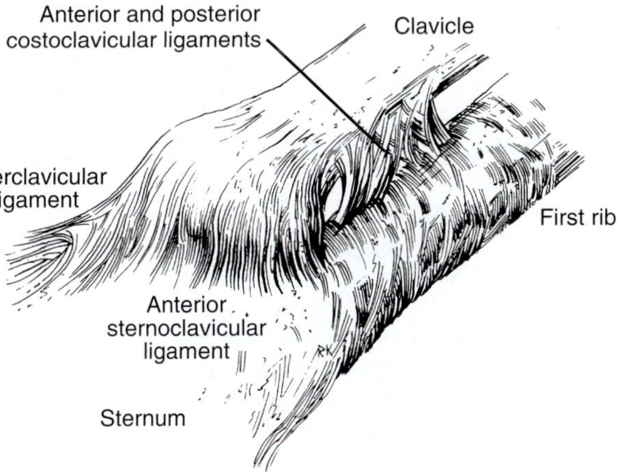

FIGURE 2-4: The exterior of the sternoclavicular joint. This illustration does not show the strongest of the ligaments—the posterior sternoclavicular ligament and the posterior partner of the anterior sternoclavicular ligament. The other important ligaments are shown in their appropriate anatomic relationships.

or nonpalpable in as many as 22% of the population.[115] The ligament tightens as the lateral end of the clavicle is depressed, thereby contributing to joint stability. The anterior and posterior costoclavicular ligaments attach from the first rib to the inferior surface of the clavicle. The anterior costoclavicular ligament resists lateral displacement of the clavicle on the thoracic cage, and the posterior ligament prevents medial displacement of the clavicle relative to the thoracic cage.[4] Cave considered that these ligaments acted as a pivot around which much of the sternoclavicular motion occurs.[32] Bearn found that they were not the fulcrum in depression until after the sternoclavicular ligaments were cut. They are the "principal limiting factor" in passive elevation of the clavicle and are a limitation on protraction and retraction.[11] Perhaps the costoclavicular ligaments enable good results to be reported for proximal clavicle resection.[4]

In the classic study regarding stability of the sternoclavicular joint, Bearn[11] found that the posterior sternoclavicular or capsular ligament contributed most to resisting the depression of the lateral end of the clavicle. He performed serial ligament releases on cadaver specimens and carefully observed the mode of failure and shifting of fulcra. This qualitative observation is a useful addition to computerized assessment of joint stability.

Although reliable electromyographic studies demonstrate that the contribution of the upward rotators of the scapula is minimal in standing posture, permanent trapezius paralysis often leads to an eventual depression of the lateral end of the scapula relative to the other side, although this depression may be only a centimeter or two.[11] Bearn's experiment should be probably replicated using more sophisticated equipment to produce length-tension curves and quantitatively test the response of the joint to rotational and translational loading in the transverse and vertical axes and the anteroposterior axis that Bearn qualitatively tested.[11]

Motion occurs in both the sections of the sternoclavicular joint: elevation and depression occur in the joint between the clavicle and disk,[95] and anteroposterior motion and rotatory motion occur between the disk and sternum. The range of motion in living specimens[106] is approximately 30 degrees to 35 degrees of upward elevation. Movement in the anteroposterior direction is approximately 35 degrees, and rotation along the long axis is 44 degrees to 50 degrees. Most sternoclavicular elevation occurs between 30 degrees and 90 degrees of arm elevation.[106] Rotation occurs after 70 degrees to 80 degrees of elevation. Estimation of the limitation of range of motion as a result of fusion is misleading because of the secondary effects on the length-tension curve of the muscles of the glenohumeral joint and the ability of the glenoid to support the weight of the arm. Fusion of the sternoclavicular joint limits abduction to 90 degrees.[136,183]

The blood supply to the sternoclavicular joint is derived from the clavicular branch of the thoracoacromial artery, with additional contributions from the internal mammary and suprascapular arteries.[95] The nerve supply to the joint arises from the nerve to subclavius, with some contribution from the medial supraclavicular nerve.

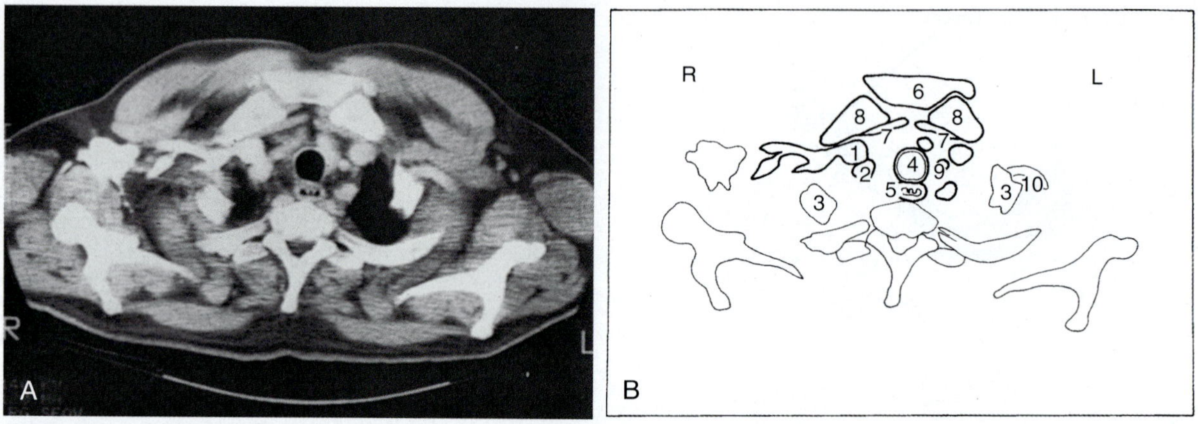

FIGURE 2-5: This contrast-enhanced computed tomographic scan **(A)** and line drawing **(B)** illustrate some of the more important anatomic relationships of the sternoclavicular joint, including the trachea and the great vessels. The structures are labeled as follows: (1) junction of the subclavian and jugular veins, (2) innominate artery, (3) first rib, (4) trachea, (5) esophagus, (6) sternum, (7) sternohyoid muscle origin, (8) clavicle, (9) carotid artery, and (10) axillary artery.

Immediate relationships of the joint are the origins of the sternocleidomastoid in front and the sternohyoid and sternothyroid muscles behind the joint. Of prime importance, however, are the great vessels and trachea (Fig. 2-5), which are endangered during posterior dislocation of the clavicle from the sternum—a rare event that may precipitate a surgical emergency.[118,206,263]

An open epiphysis is a structure not commonly observed in adults. However, the epiphysis of the clavicle does not ossify until the late teens and may not fuse to the remainder of the bone in men until the age of 25 years.[11,263] Therefore the clavicular epiphysis is a relatively normal structure within the age group at greatest risk for major trauma. The epiphysis is very thin and not prominent, which makes differentiation of physeal fractures from dislocations difficult. Instability of the sternoclavicular joint may result from trauma; however, in some individuals, it develops secondary to constitutional laxity.[50]

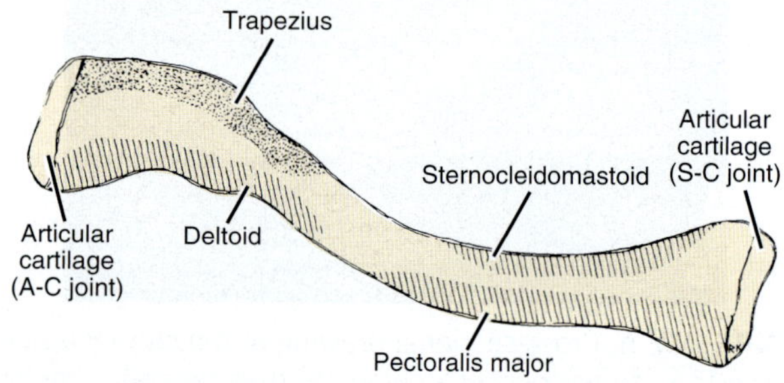

FIGURE 2-6: Superior view of the right clavicle showing its italic S shape; the origins of the deltoid, pectoralis major, and sternocleidomastoid muscles; and the insertion of the trapezius muscle. Note the breadth of the sternocleidomastoid origin. *A-C,* acromioclavicular; *S-C,* sternoclavicular.

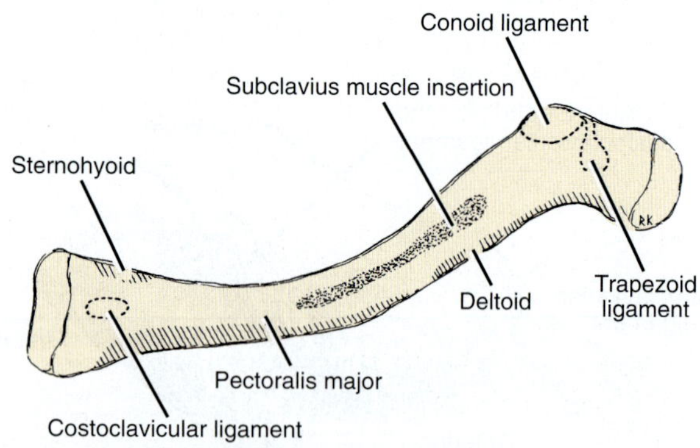

FIGURE 2-7: Inferior view of the right clavicle showing its major ligament insertions and the origins of the deltoid, pectoralis major, and sternohyoid muscles. Also shown is the subclavian groove where the subclavius muscle has its fleshy insertion.

Clavicle

The clavicle is a relatively straight bone when anteriorly viewed, whereas in the transverse plane, it resembles an italic S (Fig. 2-6).[55] The greater radius of curvature occurs at its medial curve, which is anteriorly convex; the smaller lateral curve is posteriorly convex. The bone is somewhat rounded in its midsection and medially and relatively flat laterally. DePalma[9] described an inverse relationship between the degree of downward facing of the lateral portion of the clavicle and radius of curvature of the lateral curve of the clavicle.

The obvious processes of the bone include the lateral and medial articular surfaces. The medial end of the bone has a 30% incidence of a rhomboid fossa on its inferior surface where the costoclavicular ligaments insert and a 2.5% incidence of actual articular surface facing inferiorly toward the first rib. The middle portion of the clavicle contains the subclavian groove where the subclavius muscle has a fleshy insertion (Fig. 2-7). The lateral portion of the clavicle has the coracoclavicular process when present.

The clavicle has three bony impressions for attachment of ligaments. At the medial side is an impression for the costoclavicular ligaments, which at times may be a rhomboid fossa. At the lateral end of the bone is the conoid tubercle and at the posterior portion of the lateral curve of the clavicle and the trapezoid line, which lies in an anteroposterior direction just lateral to the conoid tubercle. The conoid ligament attaches to the clavicle at the conoid tubercle, while the trapezoid ligament attaches at the trapezoid line. The relative position of these ligament insertions is important in their function.[55,95,208] Rios et al.[204] reported that the distance from the lateral edge of the clavicle to the medial edge of the conoid tuberosity in male and female specimens was approximately 45 mm, while the distance to the center of the trapezoid tuberosity was approximately 25 mm. These findings have potential implications in surgical reconstruction of the acromioclavicular joint.[30]

Muscles that insert on the clavicle are the trapezius on the posterosuperior surface of the distal end and subclavius muscle, which has a fleshy insertion on the inferior surface of the middle third of the clavicle. Four muscles originate from the clavicle: the deltoid originates on the anterior portion of the inner surface of the lateral curve; the pectoralis major originates from the anterior portion of the medial two-thirds; the sternocleidomastoid largely originates on the posterior portion of the middle third; and contrary to its name, the sternohyoid to a small extent originates on the clavicle, just medial to the origin of the sternocleidomastoid.

Functionally, the clavicle mainly acts as a point of muscle attachment. Some literatures suggest that with good repair of the muscle, the only functional consequences of surgical removal of the clavicle are limitations in heavy overhead activity,[2,133] and thus its function as a strut[151] is less important. This concept would seem to be supported by the relatively good function of individuals with congenital absence of the clavicle.[239] However, others have found that sudden loss of the clavicle in adulthood has a devastating effect on shoulder function.

Important relationships to the clavicle are the subclavian vein and artery and brachial plexus posteriorly. In fact, the medial anterior curve is often described as an accommodation for these structures and does not form in Sprengel's deformity, a condition wherein the scapula does not descend. Therefore the attached clavicle does not need to accommodate.[23,31,264] The curve is a landmark for finding the subclavian vein.[184] This relationship is more a factor in surgery than in trauma because the bone acts as an obstruction to surgeons in reaching the nerve or vessel tissue that they wish to treat. In trauma, clavicular injury usually does not affect these structures despite their close relationship, and nonunion is rare.[113] Most cases of neurovascular trauma are of the following two groups: injury to the carotid artery from the displaced medial clavicle and compression of structures over the first rib.[101]

Acromioclavicular Joint

The acromioclavicular joint is the only articulation between the clavicle and scapula, although few individuals, as many as 1%, have a coracoclavicular bar or joint.[134,173] Lewis[134] reported in his study that approximately 30% of cadavers had articular cartilage on the opposing coracoid and clavicular surfaces, with no bony process on the clavicle directed toward the coracoid.

The capsule of the acromioclavicular joint contains a diarthrodial joint that is incompletely divided by a disk that, unlike that of the sternoclavicular joint, usually has a large perforation at its center.[56,57] The capsule tends to be thicker on its superior, anterior, and posterior surfaces than on the inferior surface. Upward and downward movement allows rotation of approximately 20 degrees between the acromion and clavicle, which occurs in the first 20 degrees and last 40 degrees of elevation.[106] It is estimated that many individuals have an even narrower range of motion; in some cases, fusion of the acromioclavicular joint does not decrease shoulder motion.[206] DePalma found degenerative changes of both the disk and articular cartilage to be the rule rather than the exception in specimens in the fourth decade or older.[56]

Blood supply to the acromioclavicular joint is mainly derived from the acromial artery, a branch of the deltoid artery of the thoracoacromial axis. Rich anastomoses are present between this artery, the suprascapular artery, and the posterior humeral circumflex artery. The acromial artery comes off the thoracoacromial axis anterior to the clavipectoral fascia and perforates back through the clavipectoral fascia to supply the joint. It also directs branches anteriorly up onto the acromion. Innervation of the joint is supplied by the lateral pectoral, axillary, and suprascapular nerves.[95]

The ligaments about the acromioclavicular articulation and the trapezoid and conoid ligaments have been extensively studied (Fig. 2-8). Traditional and more recent studies have reported that anteroposterior stability of the acromioclavicular joint is controlled by the acromioclavicular ligaments and that vertical stability is controlled by the coracoclavicular ligaments.[206,253] A serial-cutting experiment involving 12 force-displacement measurements was performed using more sophisticated equipment than that used in previous studies.[72] Three anatomic axes of the acromioclavicular joint were used, and translation and rotation on each axis in both directions were measured. The results of the experiment confirmed the previously held views, particularly when displacements were large.

The acromioclavicular ligaments were found to be responsible for controlling posterior translation of the clavicle on the acromion. (In anatomic terms, this motion is really an anterior translation of the scapula on the clavicle.) The acromioclavicular ligaments were responsible for 90% of anteroposterior stability, and 77% of stability for the superior translation of the clavicle (or inferior translation of the scapula) was attributed to the conoid and trapezoid ligaments. Distraction of the acromioclavicular joint was limited by the acromioclavicular ligaments (91%), and compression of the joint was limited by the trapezoid ligament (75%), as discussed later.[72]

The unique findings of the study were the contributions of these ligaments during small displacements. The acromioclavicular ligaments played a much larger role in

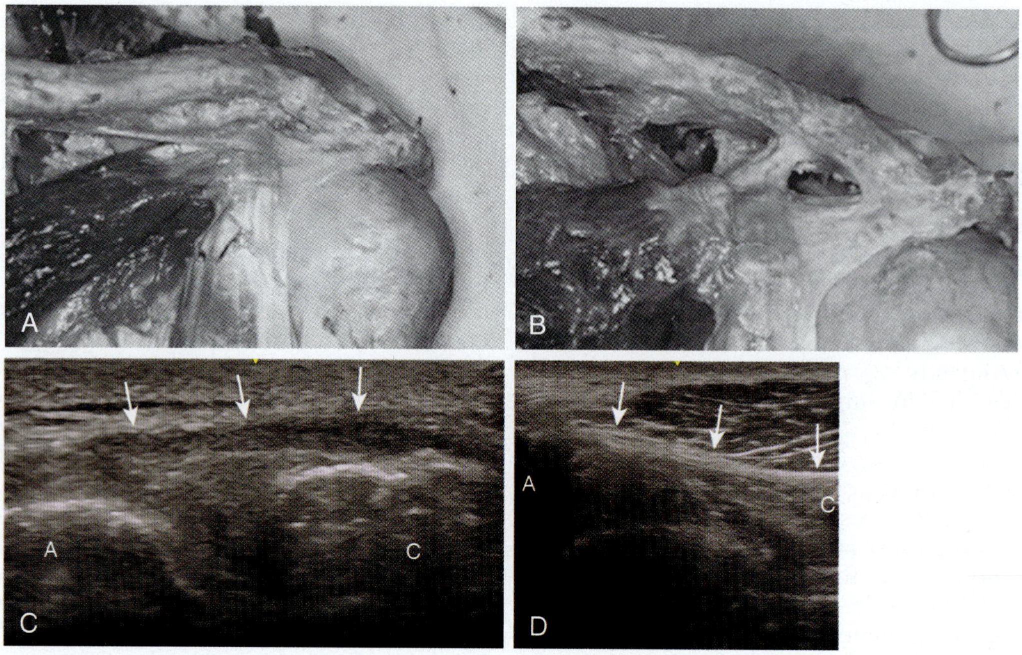

FIGURE 2-8: The acromioclavicular joint complex before **(A)** and after **(B)** excision of the clavipectoral fascia, which was rather prominent in this specimen. Note the thickness of the coracoclavicular ligaments and their lines of orientation, which are consistent with their function. Note also the breadth and thickness of the coracoacromial ligament. **C,** A coronal ultrasound view of the acromioclavicular joint with the clavicle *(C)* on the right, while the acromion *(A)* and the dark acromioclavicular ligaments (*arrows*) bridge the joint. **D,** The coracoacromial ligament (*arrows*), the acromion *(A)* on the left. The coracoid process lies outside the view to the right.

many of these rotations and translations than in larger displacements, which may reflect the shorter lengths of the acromioclavicular ligaments. At shorter displacements, a greater load is applied to the fibers of the acromioclavicular ligaments for the same displacement.

Interpretation of the stability that is attributed to the acromioclavicular ligaments should reflect the additional role that they play in maintaining the integrity of the acromioclavicular joint. Although we would expect the linear arrangement of collagen in the acromioclavicular ligaments to resist distraction, it makes little sense that the acromioclavicular ligaments would resist compression with these fibers; yet in the study, 12% to 16% of compression stability was attributed to the acromioclavicular ligament. Maintaining the integrity of the acromioclavicular joint, particularly the position of the interarticular disk, might explain this discrepancy. We would not expect the acromioclavicular ligament to resist superior translation of the clavicle were it not for the presence of an intact joint below it, creating a fulcrum against which these ligaments can produce a tension-band effect.[72]

These ligaments are seldom called on to resist trauma, and their usual function is to control joint motion. As noted earlier, this joint has relatively little motion, and muscles controlling scapulothoracic motion insert on the scapula. To a large extent, the ligaments function to guide the motion of the clavicle.[73] For example, the conoid ligament produces much of the superior rotation of the clavicle as the shoulder is elevated in flexion.[183]

The distal end of the clavicle does not have a physeal plate. Using microscopic dissection, Todd and D'Errico found a small fleck of bone in some individuals, which appeared to be an epiphysis, but it united within 1 year.[248] We have not observed this structure during surgery or using roentgenogram. The articular cartilage probably functions in longitudinal growth as it does in a physis.

Scapula

The scapula is a thin sheet of bone that mainly functions as a site of muscle attachment (Fig. 2-9). It is thicker at its superior and inferior angles and at its lateral border, where some of the more powerful muscles are attached (Figs. 2-10 and 2-11). The scapula is also thick at the sites of formation of its processes: the coracoid, spine, acromion, and glenoid. The posterior surface of the scapula and the presence of the spine create the supraspinatus and infraspinatus fossae. Three processes, the spine, coracoid, and glenoid, create two notches in the scapula. The suprascapular notch is at the base of the coracoid, and the spinoglenoid or greater scapular notch is at the spine base. The coracoacromial and transverse scapular ligaments are two of the several ligaments that attach to two parts of the same bone. Sometimes an inferior transverse scapular ligament is found in the spinoglenoid notch. This transverse ligament and the ganglia of the labrum may all be factors in suprascapular nerve deficits. The coracoglenoid ligament, which originates on the

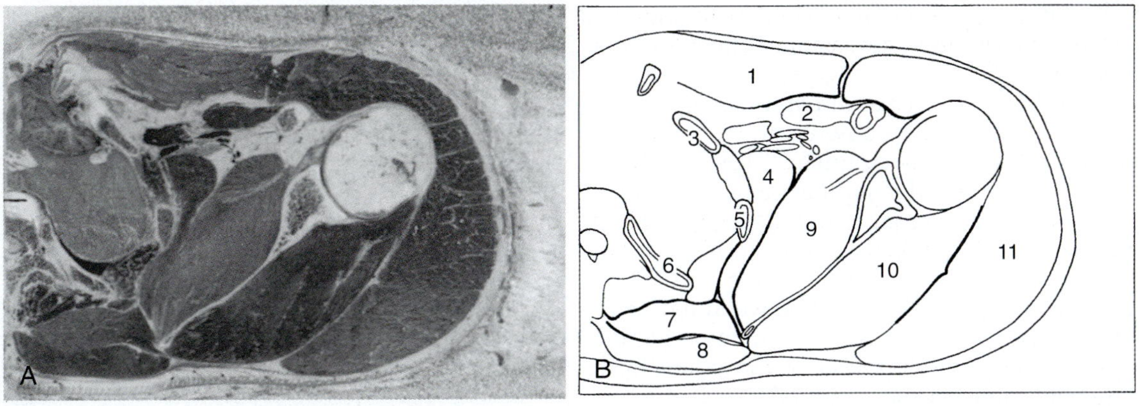

FIGURE 2-9: Image **(A)** and diagram **(B)** of a cross section of the scapula at the midportion of the glenoid. The thinness of most of the scapula and its most important bony process, the glenoid, can be seen, as well as the way in which the muscle and ligaments increase the stability of this inherently unstable joint by circumscribing the humeral head. Hypovascular fascial planes are emphasized. Note that the artist's line is wider than the plane depicted. The labeled structures include (1) pectoralis major, (2) pectoralis minor, (3) first rib, (4) serratus anterior, (5) second rib, (6) third rib, (7) rhomboid, (8) trapezius, (9) subscapularis, (10) infraspinatus, and (11) deltoid.

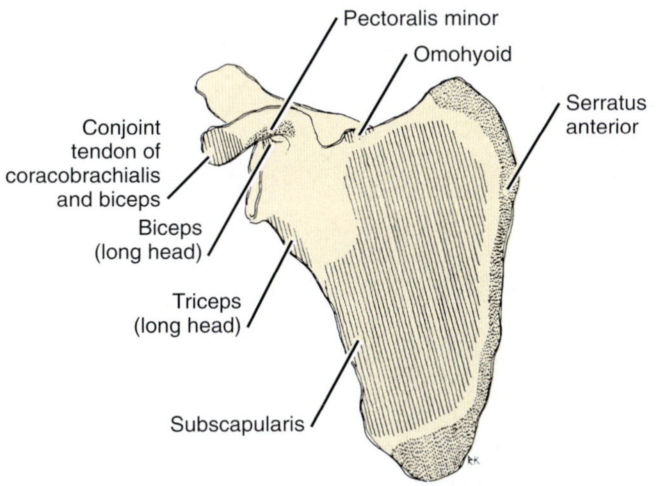

FIGURE 2-10: Anterior view of the scapula showing the muscle origins of the anterior surface (striped pattern) and the muscle insertions (dotted pattern). Ligaments and their origins and insertions are not illustrated.

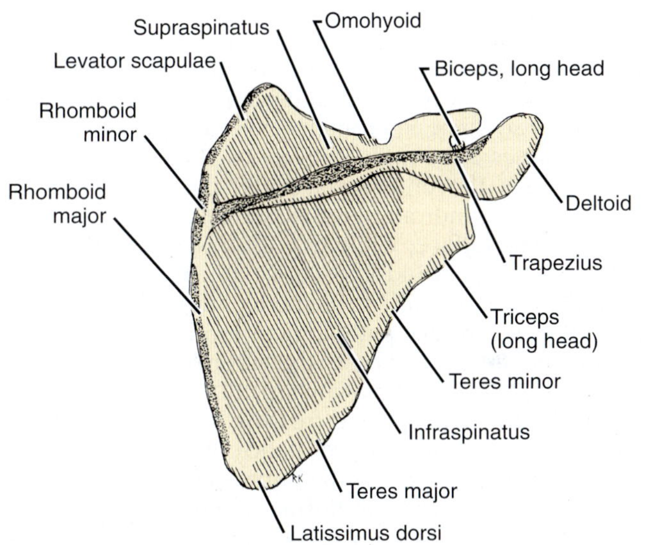

FIGURE 2-11: Posterior view of the scapula illustrating the muscle origins and muscle insertions.

coracoid between the coracoacromial and coracohumeral ligaments and inserts on the glenoid near the origin of the long head of the biceps, is rarely studied.[260] The major ligaments that originate from the scapula are the coracoclavicular, coracoacromial, acromioclavicular, glenohumeral, and coracohumeral.

The coracoid process comes off the scapula at the upper base of the neck of the glenoid and anteriorly passes before hooking to a more lateral position. The coracoid process functions as the origin of the short head of the biceps and coracobrachialis tendons and serves as the insertion of the pectoralis minor muscle and the coracoacromial, coracohumeral, and coracoclavicular ligaments. Several anomalies of the coracoid have been described. As much as 1% of the population has an abnormal connection between the coracoid and clavicle, a bony bar or articulation.[173] Some surgeons have seen impingement in the interval between the head of the humerus and the deep surface of the coracoid.[60,80,81] The coracohumeral interval is smallest in the internal rotation and forward flexion.

The spine of the scapula functions as part of the insertion of the trapezius on the scapula and as the origin of the posterior deltoid. It also suspends the acromion in the lateral and anterior directions and thus serves as a prominent lever arm for the function of the deltoid. The dimensions of the spine of the scapula are regular, with less than 1.5-cm variation from the mean in any dimension. Sacrifice of the entire spine, including the acromion, has a predictably devastating effect on the shoulder function.[149,182]

Because of the high occurrence of pathology involving the acromion and head of the humerus, the acromion is the most studied process of the scapula.[166] Tendinitis and bursitis have been related to the impingement of the head of the humerus and coracoacromial arch in an area called the supraspinatus outlet.[170] When viewed from the front, a 9- to 10-mm gap (6.6 to 13.8 mm in men and 7.1 to 11.9 mm in women) can be observed between the acromion and humerus.[22] Recent advances in radiographic positioning allow better visualization of the outlet from the side or sagittal plane of the scapula.[168]

Several methods of describing the capaciousness of this space or its tendency for mechanical discontinuity have been devised. Aoki et al.[5] used the slope of the ends of the acromion relative to a line connecting the posterior acromion with the tip of the coracoid of the scapula to determine the propensity for impingement problems. Bigliani et al.[15] divided the acromia into three types (or classes) on the basis of their shape and correlated the occurrence of the rotator cuff pathology in cadavers with the shape of the acromion on supraspinatus outlet radiographs. Their classification is generally easy to use; however, the transition between the types is smooth, so some inter-interpreter variability will occur in those cases close to the transitions. Type I acromia are those with a flat undersurface and the lowest risk for impingement syndrome and its sequelae. Type II has a curved undersurface, while type III has a hooked undersurface. As one would expect, a type III acromion with its sudden discontinuity in shape had the highest correlation with subacromial pathology. A report by Banas et al. comments on the position of the acromion in the coronal plane (i.e., the lateral downward tilt). In their series of 100 MRI procedures, an increasing downward tilt was associated with a greater prevalence of cuff disease.[8] The remainder of the roof of the supraspinatus outlet comprises the coracoacromial ligament, which connects two parts of the same bone. It is usually broader at its base on the coracoid, tapers as it approaches the acromion, and has a narrower but still broad insertion on the undersurface of the acromion; it covers a large portion of the anterior undersurface of the acromion and invests the tip and lateral undersurface of the acromion (Fig. 2-12). The ligament may not be wider at its base and often has one or more diaphanous areas at the base.[96] Because of the high incidence of impingement in elevation and internal rotation, the acromia in individuals older than the fifth decade frequently have secondary changes such as spurs or excrescences.

In addition to static deformation of the acromion, one would expect an unfused acromion epiphysis to lead to the deformability of the acromion on an active basis and decrease the space of the supraspinatus outlet.[164] However, Neer found no increased incidence of unfused epiphyses in his series of acromioplasties.[167] Liberson[135] classified the different types of unfused acromia as pre-acromion, meso-acromion, meta-acromion, and basi-acromion centers (Fig. 2-13). In his series, an unfused center was noted on 1.4% of roentgenograms and bilaterally in 62% of cases. The meso-acromion–meta-acromion defect was most frequently found (Fig. 2-14).

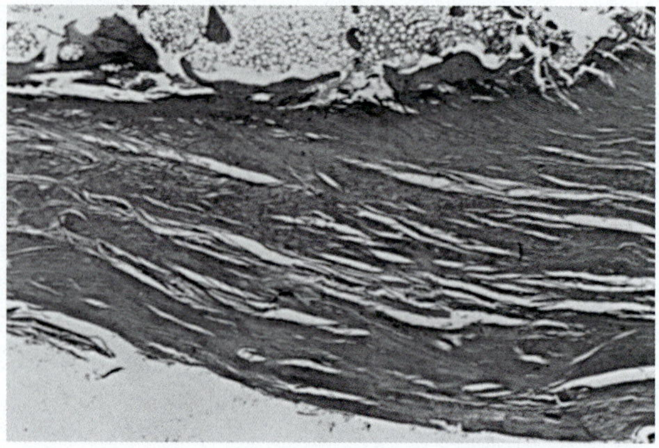

FIGURE 2-12: Photomicrographic view (×12) of the insertion of the coracoacromial ligament into the undersurface of the acromion. The insertion may continue as far as 2 cm in the posterior direction. Note the thickness of the ligament in comparison to the bone.

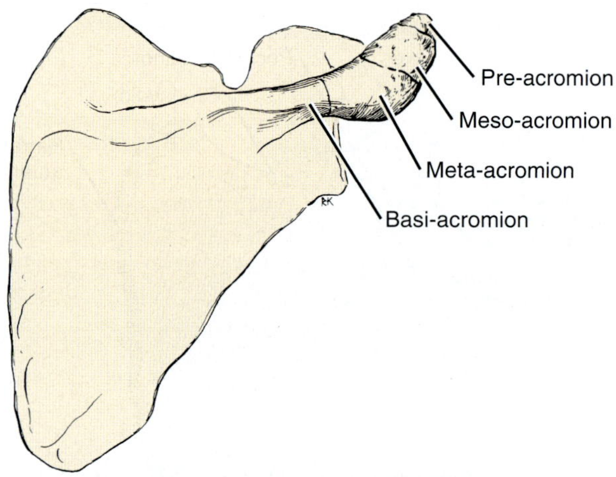

FIGURE 2-13: Different regions of the acromion between which union may fail to occur.

The glenoid articular surface is within 10 degrees of being perpendicular to the blade of the scapula, with the mean being 6 degrees of retroversion in one study.[209] Strauss et al.[226] reviewed multiple studies on various glenoid measurements. The mean glenoid height was found to range between 32.6 mm and 39 mm, with women having smaller glenoid heights. Mean glenoid width ranged from 23.6 mm in females to 28.3 mm in males. The mean glenoid version was found to range from 2 degrees anteversion to 9 degrees retroversion. The glenoid tends to go into more retroversion with osteoarthritis. Churchill et al.[37] found the glenoids of men to be slightly more retroverted than those of women (1.9 degrees vs. 0.9 degrees, respectively) and those of white patients significantly more retroverted than those of black

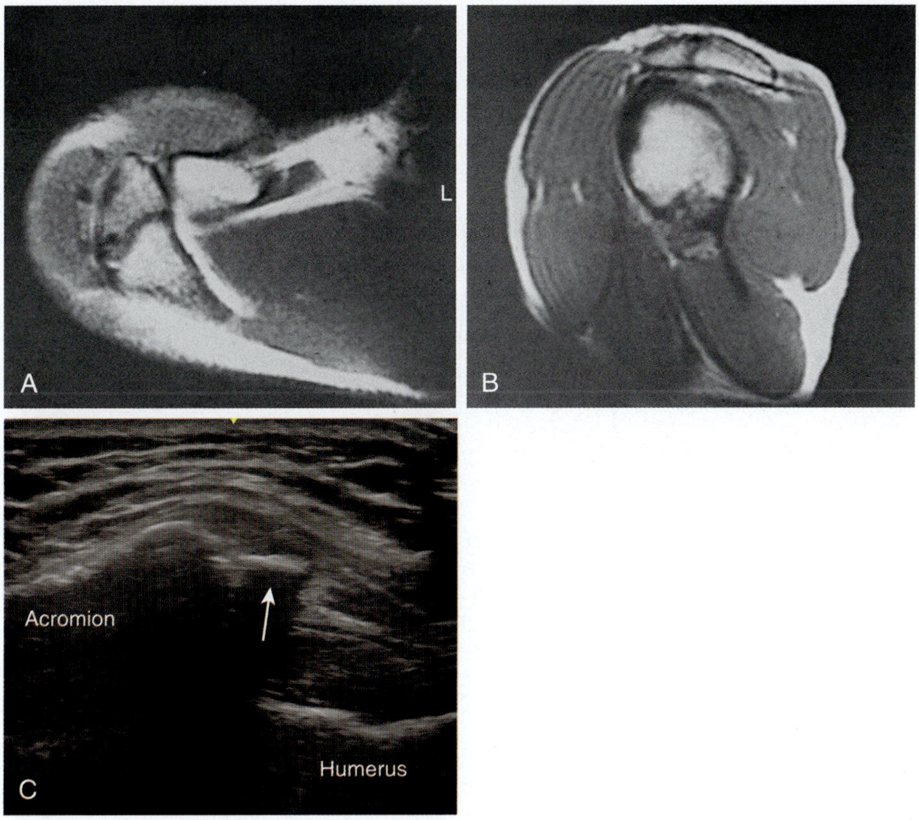

FIGURE 2-14: Transverse (**A**) and sagittal (**B**) magnetic resonance imaging sections of an unfused meso-acromion. **C,** Ultrasound sagittal view of an os acromiale (*arrow*) at the anterolateral tip of the acromion on the right.

patients (2.7 degrees vs. 0.2 degrees, respectively). Churchill et al. also found the inclination to range from 3.6 degrees to 5.3 degrees superior inclination, with no significant difference based on race or gender.

The glenoid articular surface is inferiorly wider in the shape of a pear. The inferior glenoid has also been described as circular.[109] The more caudad portions face more anteriorly than the cephalad portions.[58] This perpendicular relationship, combined with the complementary orientation of the scapula and relationships determined by the ligaments of the scapulohumeral orientation, makes the plane of the scapula the most suitable coronal plane for physical and radiologic examination of the shoulder. The plane of the glenoid defines the sagittal planes, whereas the transverse plane remains the same.[210]

The blood supply to the scapula is derived from vessels in the muscles that take fleshy origin from the scapula (see the "Muscles" section). Vessels cross these indirect insertions and communicate with bony vessels. The circulation of the scapula is metaphyseal in nature; the periosteal vessels are larger than usual, and they freely communicate with the medullary vessels rather than being limited to the outer third of the cortex. Such an anatomy may explain the reason for the subperiosteal dissection being bloodier here than over a diaphyseal bone.[24] The nutrient artery of the scapula enters into the lateral suprascapular fossa[182] or infrascapular fossa.[212] The subscapular, suprascapular, circumflex scapular, and acromial arteries are contributing vessels.

Muscles that were not previously mentioned that originate from the scapula are the rotator cuff muscles: the supraspinatus, infraspinatus, teres minor, and subscapularis. At the superior and inferior poles of the glenoid are two tubercles for tendon origin, the superior for the long head of the biceps and the inferior for the long head of the triceps. At the superior angle of the scapula, immediately posterior to the medial side of the suprascapular notch, is the origin of the omohyoid, a muscle that has little significance for shoulder surgery but is an important landmark for brachial plexus and cervical dissection. The large and powerful teres major originates from the lateral border of the scapula. Inserting on the scapula are all the scapulothoracic muscles: trapezius, serratus anterior, pectoralis minor, levator scapulae, and major and minor rhomboids.

Humerus

The articular surface of the humerus at the shoulder is spheroid, with a radius of curvature of approximately 2.25 cm.[183] As one moves down the humerus in the axis of the spheroid, one encounters a ring of bony attachments for the ligaments and muscles that control joint

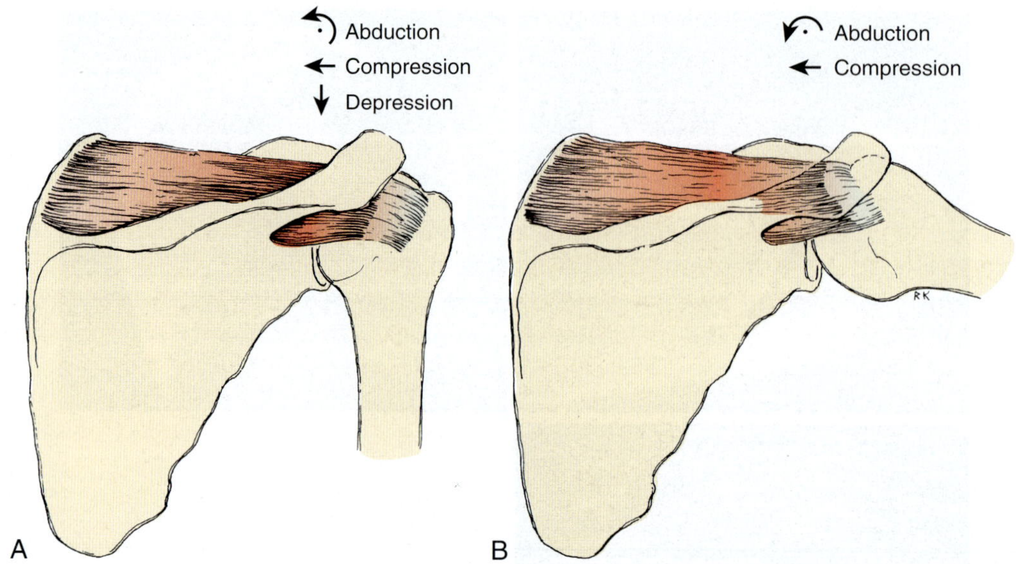

FIGURE 2-15: A, In neutral position, initiation of the use of the supraspinatus muscle produces a compressing force, and because the supraspinatus circumscribes the spheroid of the humeral head, a head depression force is generated. **B,** In the abducted position, when the force of the deltoid muscle does not produce as much vertical shear force, there is loss of the prominence of the spheroid and therefore loss of the head-depressing force of the supraspinatus. An abduction moment and joint compression force remain.

stability. The ring of attachments is constructed of two tuberosities, the intertubercular groove and the medial surface of the neck of the humerus. Ligaments and muscles that maintain glenohumeral stability do so by contouring the humeral head so that the tension in them produces a restraining force toward the center of the joint (Fig. 2-15). In this position, the spheroid is always more prominent than the ligamentous or muscle attachments. For example, when the shoulder is in neutral abduction and the supraspinatus comes into play, the greater tuberosity, which is the attachment of this tendon, is on average 8-mm less prominent than the articular surface, and thus the tendon contours the humeral head.[105] In the abduction and external rotation position, contouring of the supraspinatus is lost. The anterior inferior glenohumeral ligament now maintains the joint stability, and its attachments are less prominent than the articulating surface.

With the arm in the anatomic position (i.e., with the epicondyles of the humerus in the coronal plane), the head of the humerus is retroverted in relation to the transepicondylar axis. In addition, the average retrotorsion is less at birth than at maturity.[107] The degree of retroversion has been a topic of debate. Boileau and Walch[18] used three-dimensional computerized modeling of cadaveric specimens to analyze the geometry of the proximal humerus. They found a wide variation of retroversion ranging from −6.7 degrees to 47.5 degrees. These findings have helped revolutionize shoulder arthroplasty and have brought about the development of the third-generation shoulder prosthesis or the concept of anatomic shoulder replacement. This concept centers on the great range in retroversion that is observed within populations. The surgical goal is to restore the patient's own anatomy. Setting prosthetic replacements at an arbitrary 30 degrees to 40 degrees may not be optimal and does not account for individual anatomic variability.[18] The intertubercular groove lies approximately 1 cm lateral to the midline of the humerus.[49,209] The axis of the humeral head crosses the greater tuberosity at approximately 9 mm posterior to the bicipital groove (Fig. 2-16).[245] The lesser tubercle (or tuberosity) lies directly anterior, and the greater tuberosity lines up on the lateral side. In the coronal plane, the head-shaft angle is approximately 135 degrees.[105] Interestingly, this angle is less for smaller heads and greater for larger ones. The head size (i.e., radius of curvature) most strongly correlates with the patient's height.[105]

The space between the articular cartilage and ligamentous and tendon attachments is referred to as the *anatomic neck of the humerus* (Fig. 2-17). It varies in breadth from approximately 1 cm on the medial, anterior, and posterior sides of the humerus to essentially undetectable over the superior surface where no bone is exposed between the edge of the articular cartilage and the insertion of the rotator cuff. The lesser tuberosity is the insertion for the subscapularis tendon, and the greater tuberosity bears the insertion of the supraspinatus, infraspinatus, and teres minor in a superior to inferior order. Because of its distance from the center of rotation, the greater tuberosity lengthens the lever arm of the supraspinatus as elevation increases above 30 degrees. It also acts as a pulley by increasing the lever arm of the deltoid below 60 degrees.[203] The prominence of the greater

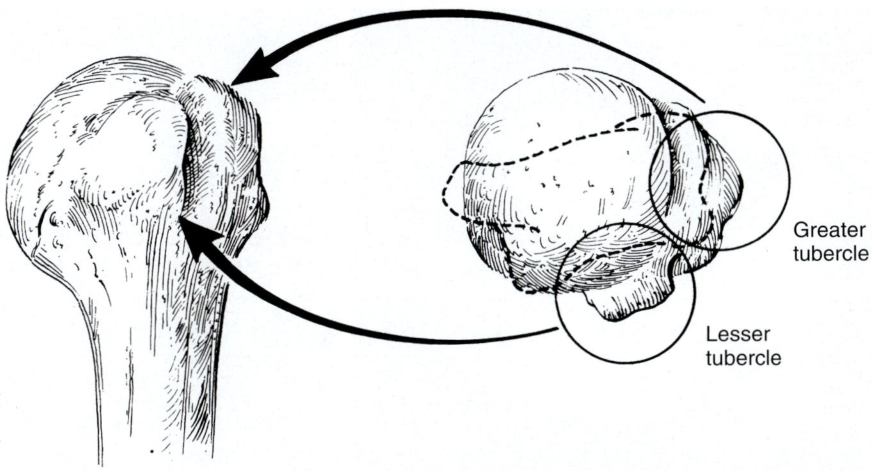

FIGURE 2-16: The head of the humerus is retroverted relative to the long axis of the humerus. The bicipital groove in the neutral position lies approximately 1 cm lateral to the midline of the humerus. Note the posterior offset of the head.

tuberosity can even allow the deltoid to act as a head depressor when the arm is at the side.[74] Below the level of the tuberosities, the humerus narrows in a region that is referred to as the *surgical neck of the humerus* because of the frequent occurrence of fractures at this level.

The greater and lesser tubercles constitute the boundaries of the intertubercular groove through which the long head of the biceps passes from its origin on the superior lip of the glenoid. The intertubercular groove has a peripheral roof that is referred to as the *intertubercular ligament* or *transverse humeral ligament*, which has varying degrees of strength.[81,158] Recent study has demonstrated that the coracohumeral ligament is the primary restraint to tendon dislocation.[180,185,219] The coracohumeral ligament arises from the coracoid as a V-shaped band, the opening of which is posteriorly directed toward the joint. In most cases, the ligament histologically represents only a V-shaped fold of the capsule and has no distinct ligamentous fibers.[43] Tightening this area does affect the shoulder function. The ring of tissue constituting the pulley constraining the biceps tendon comprises the superficial glenohumeral ligament (floor) and the coracohumeral ligament (roof). Because the biceps tendon is a frequent site of shoulder pathology, attempts have been made to correlate the anatomy of its intertubercular groove with a predilection for pathology (Fig. 2-18).[95] Biceps tendinitis was considered to result from dislocation of the tendon secondary to a shallow groove or supratubercular ridge[158] and an incompetent transverse humeral ligament. Meyer[158] attributed the greater number of dislocations of the biceps tendon on the left to activities in which the left arm is in the external rotation, a position that should have been protective. Current opinion is that the dislocation of the tendon is a relatively rare etiology of bicipital tendinitis and that most cases of bicipital tendinitis can be attributed to impingement[186]; dislocation of the tendon is not observed except in the presence of the rotator cuff or "pulley" damage. Walch et al.[256] analyzed long head of biceps dislocations and found that in 70% of cases, the dislocation of the long head of the biceps was associated with massive rotator cuff tears. In particular, the subscapularis was intact in only two of 46 cases. It is possible that the "variable depth of the intertubercular groove" theory may also apply to the impingement syndrome as an etiology. A shallow intertubercular groove makes the tendon of the long head of the biceps and its overlying ligaments more prominent and thus more vulnerable to impingement damage.[167]

The intertubercular groove has a more shallow structure as it distally continues, but its boundaries, referred to as the *lips of the intertubercular groove,* continue to function as sites for muscle insertion. Below the subscapularis muscles, the medial lip of the intertubercular groove is the site of insertion for the latissimus dorsi and teres major, with the latissimus dorsi insertion being anterior, often on the floor of the groove. The pectoralis major has its site of insertion at the same level but on the lateral lip of the bicipital groove. At its upper end, the intertubercular groove also functions as the site of entry of the major blood supply of the humeral head, the ascending branch of the anterior humeral circumflex artery. This artery enters the bone at the top of the intertubercular groove or one of the adjacent tubercles.[79,125]

Two shoulder muscles insert on the humerus near its midpoint. On the lateral surface is the bony prominence of the deltoid tuberosity, over which is located the large tendinous insertion of the deltoid. On the medial surface, at approximately the same level, is the insertion of the coracobrachialis.

The essential relationships to be maintained in surgical reconstruction are the retrograde direction of the articular surface and this surface's prominence relative to the muscle and ligamentous attachments. Longitudinal alignment and the distance from the head to the deltoid insertion should be maintained. In fractures above the insertion

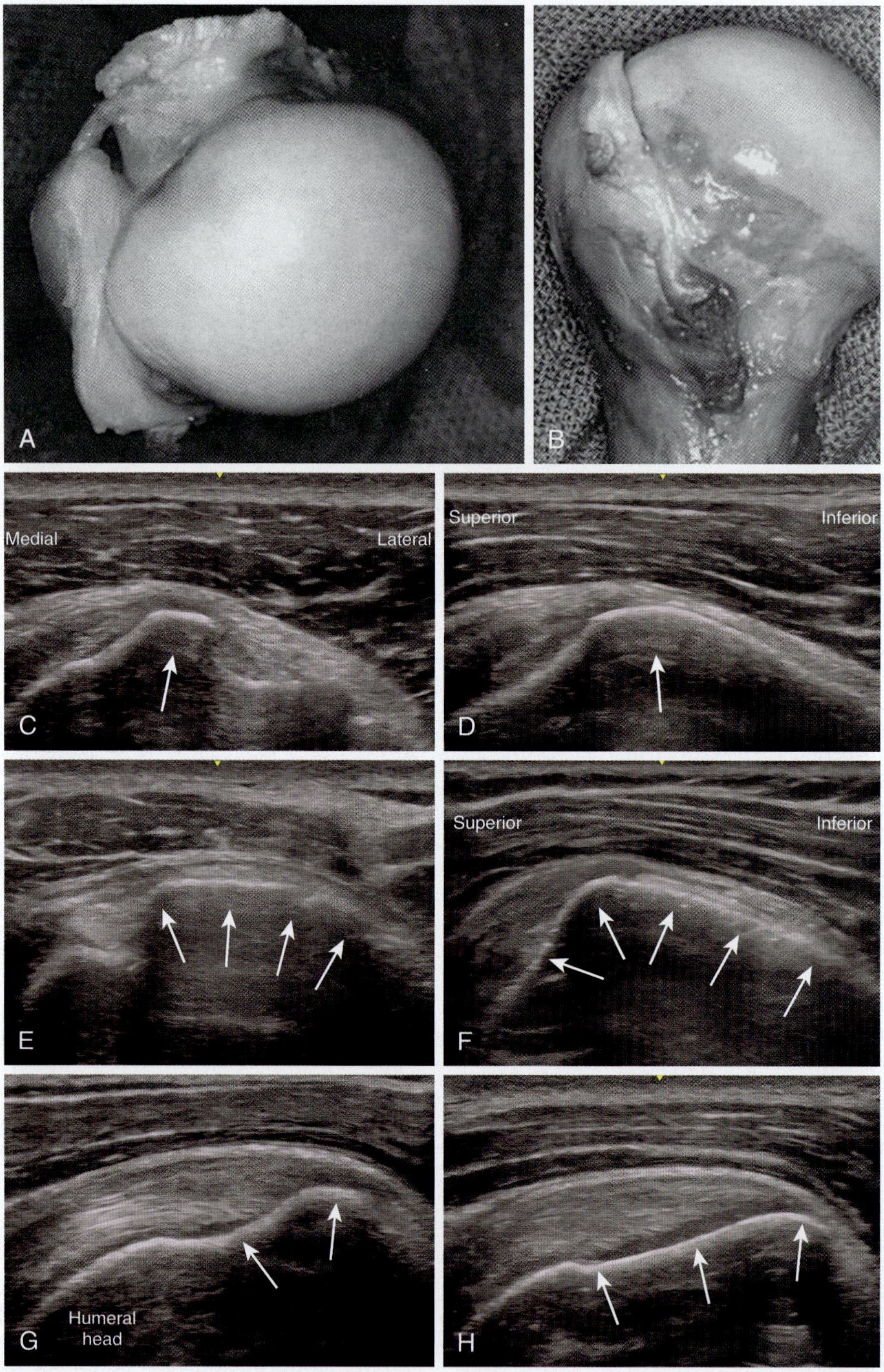

FIGURE 2-17: **A,** Superior surface of the humeral head, where the rotator cuff attaches immediately adjacent to the articular cartilage. The lesser tuberosity is superior and the greater tuberosity is to the left, with the bicipital groove and transverse humeral ligament between them. **B,** Posterior view of the humeral head and the gap between the articular surface and the attachment of the capsule and the tendon. This area is the anatomic neck of the humerus. **C** and **D,** Axial and longitudinal views, respectively, of the lesser tuberosity. Note narrow dimension on the axial view and the pyramidal shape on the longitudinal view. **E** and **F,** Axial and longitudinal views of the greater tuberosity, respectively. Note the broader shape on both views compared to the lesser tuberosity. **G,** Superior facet of the greater tuberosity (*between the arrows*), which is entirely a supraspinatus insertion site. Note the upward curve from the edge of the head. **H,** Middle facet of the greater tuberosity (*arrows*), which has some supraspinatus and infraspinatus inserted into it. Note that this surface is almost tangential to the curve of the surface of the head.

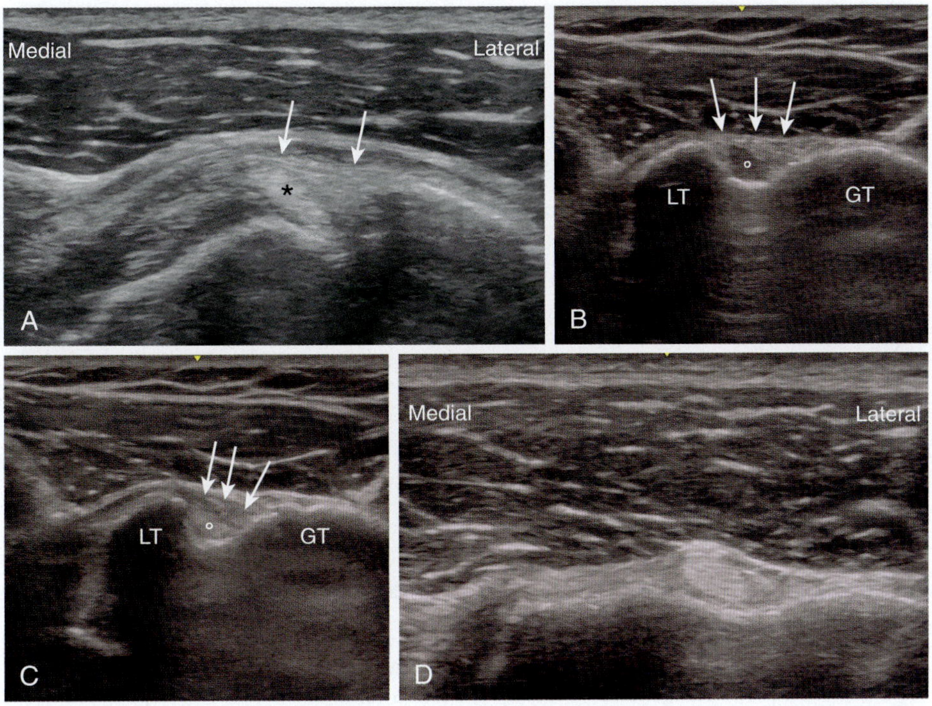

FIGURE 2-18: Superior **(A),** middle **(B),** and inferior **(C)** regions of the bicipital groove. The biceps (*small circle*) lies in the mid portion of each view. The arrows indicate the soft tissue constraints. Note that the upper portion the biceps is mainly stabilized by soft tissues, while in the depth of the groove there is some contribution from the bone. In the upper region, the roof is largely the coracohumeral ligament. In the middle and lower groove, the roof is a continuation of the outer fibers of the subscapularis. **C** and **D** show the tendon in hypoechoic **(B)** and hyperechoic **(C)** anisotropic views.

of the deltoid that heal in the humerus varus or in cases of birth injury that cause humerus varus, the head-depressing effect of the supraspinatus will be ineffective in the neutral position when the shear forces that are produced by the deltoid are maximal.[140] Interestingly, patients with congenital humerus varus rarely complain of pain but have limitation of motion.[235]

MUSCLES

In this section, individual muscles are discussed in terms of origin and insertion, with comments on the type of attachment to bone. The discussion proceeds to the boundaries of muscles and their function that have been described to date. Innervation of muscles is discussed in terms of the nerve or nerves and the most common root representation. The vascular supply and its point or points of entry into the muscle are discussed, with brief mention of anomalies. The muscles are separated into four groups for purposes of discussion. First are the scapulothoracic muscles that control the motion of the scapula. The second group consists of the strictly glenohumeral muscles that work across that joint. Third are muscles that cross two or more joints. Finally, four muscles are reviewed that are not directly involved in shoulder function but are important anatomic landmarks.

For more advanced techniques such as muscle transfers, a functional comparison of the muscles is convenient. To that end, Hezberg et al.[92] have listed the relevant properties of muscles as follows: (1) related groups, (2) internal structure (e.g., pennate vs. longitudinal), (3) excursion, and (4) relative tensions anticipated (Tables 2-1 to 2-3). Muscles are grouped as axial-scapular, scapular-humeral, and axial-humeral. The potential excursion is measured as the resting muscle fiber length in relation to the number of sarcomeres in series without reference to the state of connective tissue restraints. The mass fraction is determined after the fleshy part of each muscle unit is weighed, and the measurements for all shoulder girdle muscles are totaled. The mass fraction is the percentage of the total muscle weight contributed by a given muscle. The relative tension is measured in a physiologic cross-sectional area of muscle fibers and expressed as the percentage of a group of muscles.

Scapulothoracic Muscles

Trapezius

The largest and most superficial of the scapulothoracic muscles is the trapezius (Fig. 2-19). This muscle originates from the spinous processes of the C7 through T12 vertebrae.[12] The lower border can be as high as T8 or as low as L2. The upper portion of the trapezius (above C7) takes its origin off the ligamentum nuchae,

TABLE 2-1 Axial Scapular Muscles

Muscle Unit	Muscle Fiber Arrangement	Potential Muscle Excursion (cm)	Mass Fraction (%)	Relative Tension (%)
Upper trapezius (clavicular)	Longitudinal	13.8	2.9	2.6
Upper trapezius (acromial)	Longitudinal	10.1	2.8	3.5
Middle trapezius	Longitudinal	10.4	2.4	2.9
Lower trapezius	Longitudinal	14.8	3.2	2.7
Levator scapulae	Longitudinal	15.3	2.1	1.7
Rhomboids	Longitudinal	12.5	4.0	4.0
Serratus anterior (upper part)	Longitudinal	11.1	3.5	3.9
Serratus anterior (lower part)	Longitudinal	17.6	7.9	5.6
Pectoralis minor	Longitudinal	13.2	2.3	2.1

TABLE 2-2 Scapulohumeral Muscles

Muscle Unit	Muscle Fiber Arrangement	Potential Muscle Excursion (cm)	Mass Fraction (%)	Relative Tension (%)
Supraspinatus	Pennate	6.7	2.8	5.2
Subscapularis	Multipennate	7.3	8.6	14.5
Infraspinatus	Pennate	8.6	6.7	9.7
Teres major	Longitudinal	8.8	1.8	2.6
Teres minor	Longitudinal	14.9	5.1	4.3
Anterior deltoid	Longitudinal	11.5	3.2	3.4
Middle deltoid (anterior part)	Multipennate	9.2	2.2	3.0
Middle deltoid (posterior part)	Multipennate	9.0	7.8	10.8
Posterior deltoid	Longitudinal	13.9	4.1	3.7

TABLE 2-3 Axial Humeral Muscles

Muscle Unit	Muscle Fiber Arrangement	Potential Muscle Excursion (cm)	Mass Fraction (%)	Relative Tension (%)
Latissimus dorsi	Longitudinal	33.9	15.9	5.9
Pectoralis major (clavicular)	Longitudinal	14.5	2.7	2.3
Pectoralis major (sternal)	Longitudinal	18.8	8.0	5.4

with two-thirds of specimens having an upper limit of origin as high as the external occipital protuberance.[12] Insertion of the upper fibers is over the distal third of the clavicle. The lower cervical and upper thoracic fibers have their insertion over the acromion and the spine of the scapula. The lower portion of the muscle takes insertion at the base of the scapular spine. On the anterior or deep surface, the muscle is bounded by a relatively avascular space between it and other muscles, mostly the rhomboids. Posteriorly, the trapezius muscle is bounded by fat and skin.

As a whole, the muscle acts as a scapular retractor, with the upper fibers used mostly for elevation of the lateral angle.[163] Although some of the other fibers may come into play, only the upper fibers were found by Inman et al. to be consistently active in all upward

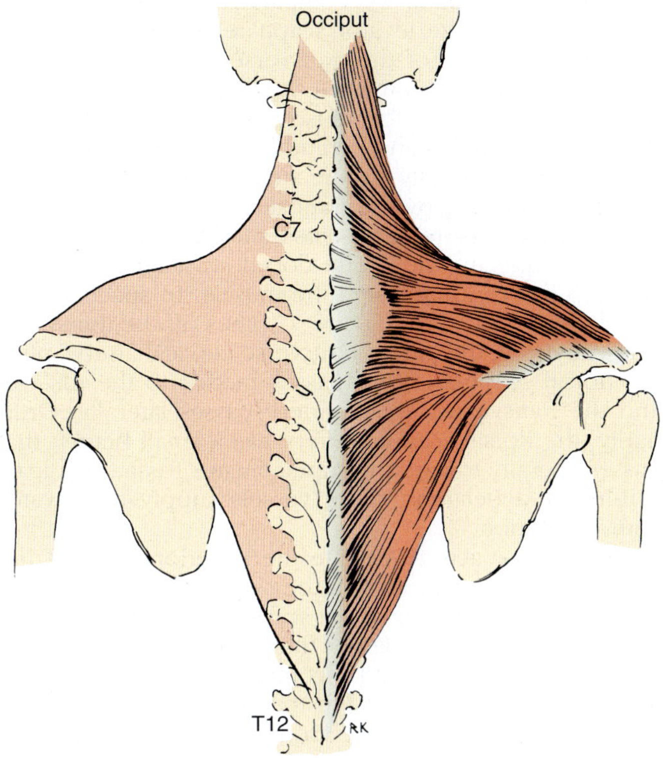

FIGURE 2-19: The arrangement of the trapezius origins and insertions. The muscle takes its origin from the occiput, the nuchal ligament, and the dorsal spines of vertebrae C7 through T12. It inserts on the acromion, the spine of the scapula, and some of the distal part of the clavicle. The trapezius is subdivided functionally into upper, middle, and lower fibers.

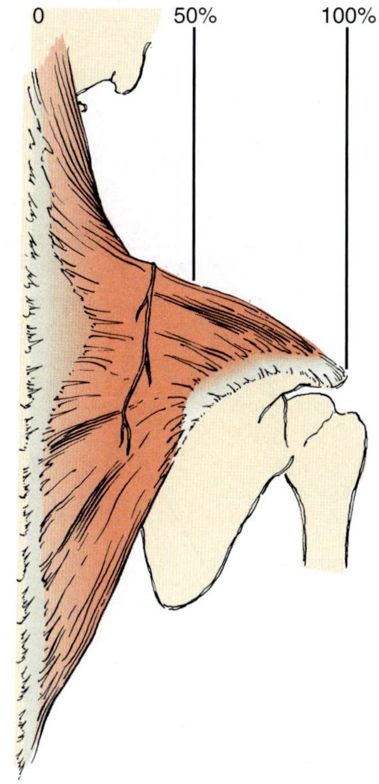

FIGURE 2-20: Course of the spinal accessory nerve relative to the trapezius muscle. If the spinal origins are taken as the "0" point of the muscle length and the acromion as 100% length, the nerve and major branches are all in the medial 50% of the trapezius. The major course is parallel and medial to the vertebral border of the scapula. (From Jobe CM, Kropp WE, Wood VE. The spinal accessory nerve in a trapezius splitting approach. *J Shoulder Elbow Surg*. 1996;5[3]:206-208.)

scapular rotations.[106] The muscle follows a cephalocaudal activation as more flexion or abduction is obtained.[163] In forward flexion, the middle and lower trapezius segments are less active because scapular retraction is less desirable than in abduction.[106] Suspension of the scapula is supposed to be through the sternoclavicular ligaments at rest; electromyographic studies show no activity unless there is a downward tug on the shoulder.[11] The muscle must provide some intermittent relief to the ligaments of the sternoclavicular joint because paralysis of the trapezius produces a slight depression of the clavicle, although not as much as one might expect.[11] The major deformity is protraction and downward rotation of the scapula.[136] The amount of depression may depend on the amount of downward loading of the limb with a paralyzed trapezius.[59] There appears to be a characteristic deficit seen in trapezius paralysis in which the shoulder can be brought up only to 90 degrees in coronal plane abduction but can be brought much higher in forward flexion.[59,98,213] In one case of congenital absence of the trapezius and the rhomboids, the patient compensated by using forward flexion to elevate the arm and lordosis of the lumbar spine to bring the arms up. When his arms had reached the vertical position, he would then release his lumbar lordosis and hold the elevation with the serratus anterior.[216] Acquired loss of trapezius function is less well tolerated.[136,211] A triple muscle transfer of the levator scapulae, rhomboideus major, and rhomboideus minor can be performed to treat trapezius palsy.[240]

The accessory spinal nerve (cranial nerve XI) is the motor supply, with some sensory branches contributed from C2, C3, and C4. The nerve runs parallel and medial to the vertebral border of the scapula, always in the medial 50% of the muscle (Fig. 2-20).[111] The arterial supply is usually derived from the transverse cervical artery, although Salmon found the dorsal scapular artery to be dominant in 75% of his specimens.[212] The blood supply is described as type II,[148] a dominant vascular pedicle with some segmental blood supply at other levels. Huelke[103] reported that the lower third of the trapezius is supplied by a perforator of the dorsal scapular artery and the upper fibers are supplied by arteries in the neck other than the transverse cervical artery. Other authors have attributed the blood supply of the lower pedicle to intercostal vessels.[258] Trapezius muscle transfers are based on supply by the transverse cervical artery.

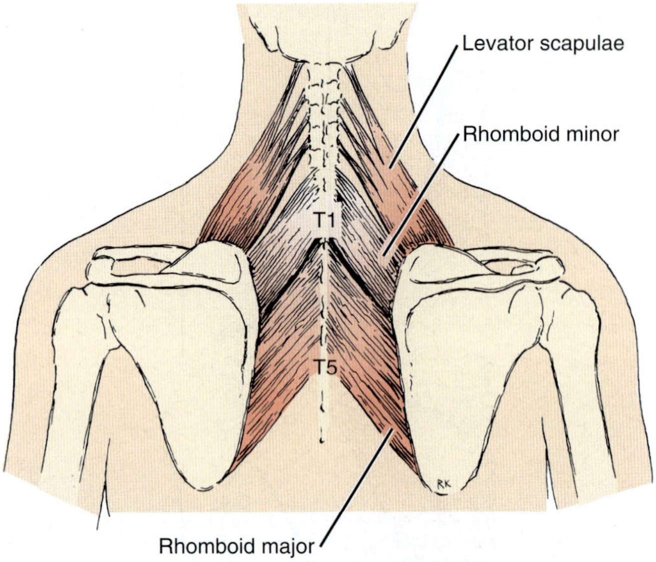

FIGURE 2-21: Rhomboids and the levator scapulae. The dominant orientation of the fibers of these muscles and their relative positions along the medial border of the scapula are shown.

Rhomboids

The rhomboids are similar in function to the midportion of the trapezius,[106] with an origin from the lower ligamentum nuchae at C7 and T1 for the rhomboid minor and T2 through T5 for the rhomboid major (Fig. 2-21). The rhomboid minor inserts on the posterior portion of the medial base of the spine of the scapula. The rhomboid major inserts into the posterior surface of the medial border from the point at which the minor leaves off down to the inferior angle of the scapula. The muscle has, on its posterior surface, an avascular plane between it and the trapezius. The only crossing structure here is the transverse cervical artery superiorly or a perforator from the dorsal scapular artery. On the deep surface is another avascular fascial space that contains only the blood vessel and nerve to the rhomboids. On the muscle's deep surface inferiorly, the rhomboid major is bounded by the latissimus at its origin. Superiorly, the rhomboid minor is bounded by the levator scapulae.

The action of the rhomboids is retraction of the scapula, and because of their oblique course, they also participate in elevation of the scapula. Innervation to the rhomboid muscle is the dorsal scapular nerve (C5), which may arise off the brachial plexus in common with the nerve to the subclavius or with the C5 branch to the long thoracic nerve. The nerve may pass deep to or through the levator scapulae on its way to the rhomboids and may contain some innervation to the levator. The dorsal scapular artery provides the arterial supply to the muscles through their deep surfaces.

Levator Scapulae and Serratus Anterior

Two muscles, the levator scapulae and serratus anterior, are often discussed together because of their close relationship indicated by comparative anatomy studies (see Fig. 2-21). The levator scapulae originate from the posterior tubercles of the transverse processes from C1 through C3 and sometimes C4. It inserts into the superior angle of the scapula. The muscle is bounded in front by the scalenus medius and behind by the splenius cervicis. It is bounded laterally by the sternocleidomastoid in its upper portion and by the trapezius in its lower portion. The spinal accessory nerve crosses laterally in the middle section of the muscle.[95] The dorsal scapular nerve may lie deep to or pass through the muscle. In specimens in which the dorsal scapular artery comes off the transverse cervical artery, the parent transverse cervical artery splits, the dorsal scapular artery passes medial to the muscle, and the transverse cervical artery passes laterally. Ordinarily, the dorsal scapular artery has a small branch that passes laterally toward the supraspinatus fossa. In at least a third of dissections, these vessels supply the levator with circulation.[104]

The levator acts to elevate the superior angle of the scapula. In conjunction with the serratus anterior, it produces upward rotation of the scapula.[183] That the levator (Fig. 2-22) has a mass larger than the upper trapezius is illustrated properly only by comparing the two muscles in cross section; in most illustrations, it is obscured by the overlying musculature.[183] Some authors speculate that this muscle may also act as a downward rotator of the scapula.[95] Innervation is from the deep branches of C3 and C4, and part of the C4 innervation is contributed by the dorsal scapular nerve.

The serratus anterior originates from the ribs on the anterior lateral wall of the thoracic cage. This muscle has three divisions (Fig. 2-23). The first division consists of one slip, which originates from ribs 1 and 2 and the intercostal space and then runs slightly upward and posteriorly to insert on the superior angle of the scapula. The second division consists of three slips from the second, third, and fourth ribs. This division inserts along the anterior surface of the medial border. The lower division consists of the inferior four or five slips, which take origin from ribs 5 to 9. They run posteriorly to insert on the inferior angle of the scapula, thus giving this division the longest lever and most power for scapular rotation.

The serratus anterior is bounded medially by the ribs and intercostal muscles and laterally by the axillary space. Anteriorly, the muscle is bounded by the external oblique muscle with which it interdigitates, where this muscle originates from the same ribs.

The serratus anterior protracts the scapula and participates in upward rotation of the scapula. It is more active in flexion than in abduction because straight abduction requires some retraction of the scapula. Scheving and Pauly found that the muscle was activated by all movements of the humerus.[214] The serratus operates at a higher percentage of its maximal activity than does any other shoulder muscle in unresisted activities.[172,183] Absence of serratus activity, usually because of paralysis, produces a winging of the scapula with forward flexion of the arm and loss of strength in that motion.[124,138] Muscle transfer to replace the inferior slips mainly restores only flexion.[42]

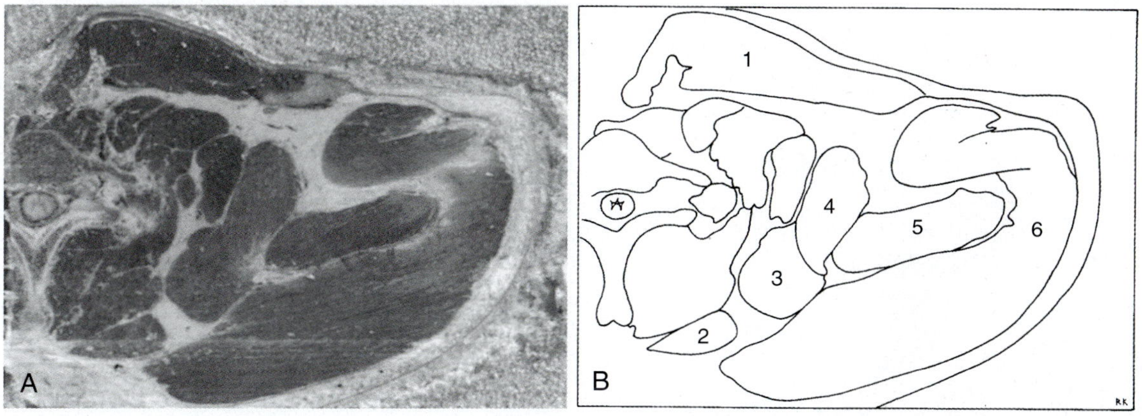

FIGURE 2-22: **A** and **B**, A transverse section at a level slightly higher than the superior angle of the scapula shows the girth of the levator scapulae, seen in cross section. Most of the other muscles noted are shown in their longitudinal section. The structures are as follows: (1) sternocleidomastoid, (2) rhomboid minor, (3) levator scapulae, (4) superior slip of the serratus anterior, (5) supraspinatus, and (6) trapezius.

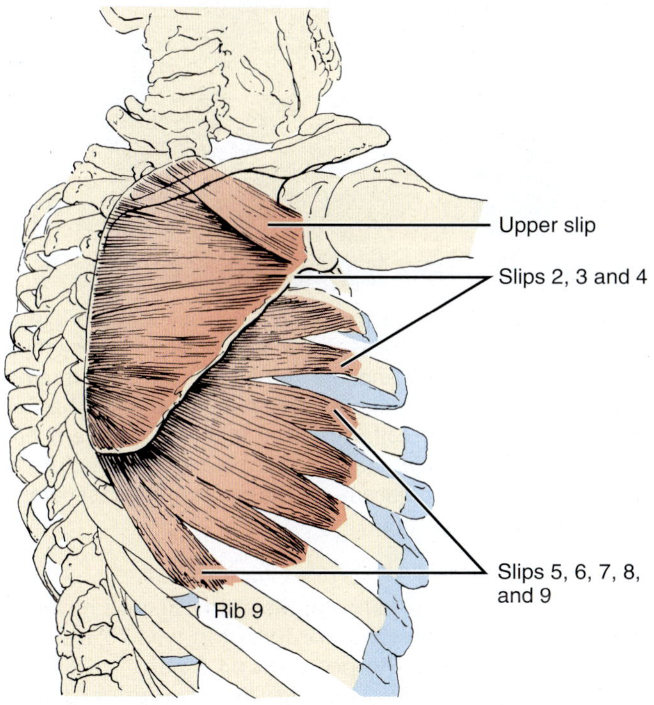

FIGURE 2-23: The three groups of muscles into which the slips of the serratus anterior are divided. The upper slip comes off the first two ribs and the first intercostal space and inserts at the upper edge of the medial border of the scapula. The slips coming off ribs 2, 3, and 4 insert on the broad major portion of the medial border; the slips from ribs 5, 6, 7, 8, and 9 converge on the inferior angle of the scapula.

Innervation is supplied by the long thoracic nerve (C5, C6, and C7). The anatomy of this nerve has been studied intensely because of events in which injury has occurred. The nerve takes an angulated course across the second rib, where it can be stretched by lateral head tilt combined with depression of the shoulder.[100] The blood supply to the serratus is classically stated to be through the lateral thoracic artery.[95] Often, however, the thoracodorsal artery makes a large contribution to the blood supply, especially when the lateral thoracic artery is small or absent. The lateral thoracic artery is the most frequently anomalous artery taking origin from the axillary artery. The thoracodorsal artery may supply up to 50% of the muscle. The upper slips are supplied by the dorsal scapular artery.[212] There, additional contributions from the intercostal and internal mammary arteries take place.

Pectoralis Minor

The pectoralis minor has a fleshy origin anteriorly on the chest wall, from the second through the fifth ribs, and inserts onto the base of the medial side of the coracoid with frequent (15%) aberrant slips to the humerus, glenoid, clavicle, or scapula (Fig. 2-24).[126,138,254] The most common aberrant slip is the continuation across the coracoid to the humerus in the same path as the coracohumeral ligament. The mean width of the pectoralis minor tendon approximates 2 cm with a length of 4 cm.[160] It has been hypothesized that the pectoralis minor is an anatomically feasible option for use inacromioclavicular joint reconstructions.[160] Its function is protraction of the scapula if the scapula is retracted and depression of the lateral angle or downward rotation of the scapula if the scapula is upwardly rotated.

Innervation is from the medial pectoral nerve (C8, T1). Its blood supply is through the pectoral branch of the thoracoacromial artery.[95] Reid and Taylor reported in their injection studies, however, that this vessel does not provide a constant supply to the pectoralis minor; another source is the lateral thoracic artery.[195] Salmon found multiple tiny arteries direct from the axillary that he called the short thoracic arteries.[212] Absence of the muscle does not seem to cause any disability.[261] This muscle was thought to be always present when the entire pectoralis major is present,[95] but Williams reported one case, verified

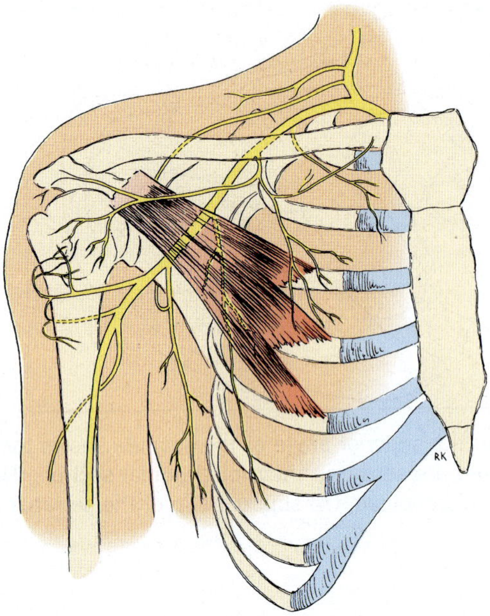

FIGURE 2-24: The pectoralis minor is an important landmark as an anterior border of the axillary space as well as for dividing the axillary space into its proximal, middle, and distal portions. It acts in protraction and depression of the scapula.

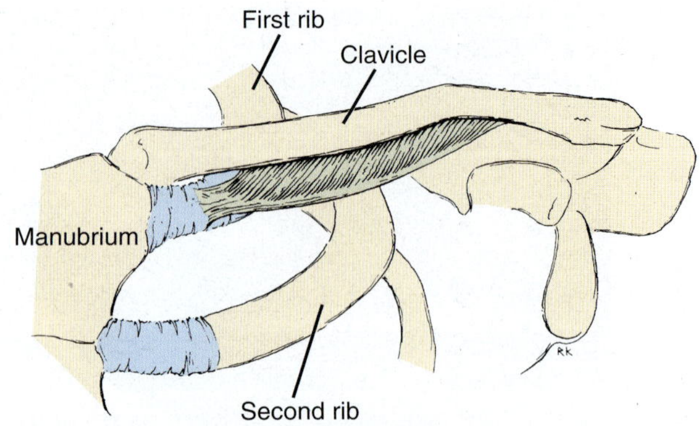

FIGURE 2-25: The subclavius muscle has a pennate structure and a long tendon on its inferior surface.

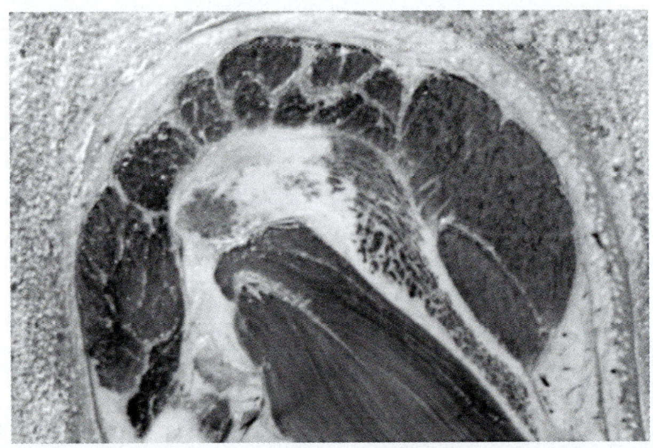

FIGURE 2-26: A cross section taken just below the origin of the right deltoid demonstrates the relative positions of the three divisions of the deltoid and the differences in their internal structure. The middle deltoid, being multipennate, has an abundance of internal collagen. The anterior third (*left*) and the posterior third (*right*) tend to be parallel in structure or partially unipennate adjacent to the septum that separates them from the middle third.

at surgery, in which the pectoralis minor was missing from beneath a normal pectoralis major.[261] Bing reported three other cases in the German literature.[16]

Subclavius

The subclavius muscle is included with the scapulothoracic muscles because it crosses the sternoclavicular joint where most of the scapulothoracic motion takes place (Fig. 2-25). It has a tendinous origin off the first rib and cartilage and a muscular insertion on the inferior surface of the medial third of the clavicle. The tendon has a muscle belly that is pennate in structure. The tendon, 1 to 1.5 inches in length, mainly lies on the inferior surface of the muscle.[33] Its nerve supply is from the nerve to the subclavius. The blood supply is derived from the clavicular branch of the thoracoacromial artery or from the suprascapular artery.[195,212] The action of this muscle is to stabilize the sternoclavicular joint while in motion—particularly with adduction and extension against resistance, such as hanging from a bar (i.e., stabilization in intense activity).[196]

Glenohumeral Muscles

Deltoid

The largest and most important of the glenohumeral muscles is the deltoid, composed of three major sections: the anterior deltoid taking origin off the lateral third of the clavicle, the middle third of the deltoid taking origin off the acromion, and the posterior deltoid taking origin from the spine of the scapula.[1] Typical of broadly based muscles, the origin is collagen-poor throughout its breadth. Insertion is on the deltoid tubercle of the humerus. It is a long and broad insertion. Rispoli reported the mean length of the anterior insertion was 70 mm, the middle 48.4 mm, and the posterior 63.4 mm.[205] Klepps[120] found that the anterior, middle, and posterior deltoid muscle fibers merged into a broad V-shaped tendinous insertion with a broad posterior band and a narrow anterior band. They found that the deltoid insertion in the vast majority of specimens was separated from the pectoralis major insertion by less than 2 mm. The axillary and radial nerves were not very close to the deltoid insertion.[120]

The deltoid muscle's boundary on the external side is subcutaneous fat. Because of the amount of motion involved, the subacromial bursa and fascial spaces bound the deep side. The axillary nerve and posterior humeral circumflex artery, the only nerve and the major blood supply of the muscle, also lie on the deep side.

The three sections of the deltoid differ in internal structure and function (Fig. 2-26). The anterior and posterior deltoid sections have parallel fibers and a longer excursion than the middle third, which is multipennate, is stronger, and has a shorter excursion (1 cm). The middle third of the deltoid takes part in all motions involved in humerus elevation.[183] An abundance of collagen makes it the portion of the muscle most frequently involved in contracture.[13]

Elevation in the scapular plane is the product of the anterior and middle thirds of the deltoid, with some action by the posterior third, especially above 90 degrees.[217] Abduction in the coronal plane decreases the contribution of the anterior third and increases the contribution of the posterior third. Flexion is produced by the anterior and middle thirds of the deltoid and the clavicular portion of the pectoralis major, with some contribution by the biceps (Fig. 2-27). The contribution of the last two muscles is so small that the arm cannot be held against gravity without the deltoid.[41] In summary, the deltoid is active in any form of elevation, and loss of deltoid function is considered a disaster.[86] The deltoid contributes only 12% of horizontal adduction. The lower portion of the posterior deltoid has been suggested to contribute to adduction. However, Shevlin and coworkers attributed this action to providing an external rotation force on the humerus to counteract the internal rotation force of the pectoralis major, teres major, and latissimus dorsi—the major adductors of the shoulder.[217] The deltoid accounts for 60% of strength in horizontal abduction.[38] The deltoid muscle's relationship to the joint is such that it has its shortest leverage for elevation in the first 30 degrees,[183] although in this position leverage is increased by the prominence of the greater tubercle.[203] Gagey and Hue have shown that the deltoid may contribute to head depression at the initiation of elevation.[74]

The anterior third of the deltoid is bounded on its deep surface by the coracoid, the conjoint tendon of the coracobrachialis, and the short head of the biceps and the clavipectoral fascia. The posterior portion of the deltoid is bounded on its deep surface by the infraspinatus and teres minor and by the teres major muscle on the other side of the avascular fascial space. The deltoid has very dense fascia on its deep surface. The axillary nerve and the posterior humeral circumflex vessels run on the muscle side of this fascia.[44]

Innervation of the deltoid is supplied by the axillary nerve (C5 and C6), which enters the posterior portion of the shoulder through the quadrilateral space and innervates the teres minor in this position. The nerve splits in the quadrilateral space, and the nerve or nerves to the posterior third of the deltoid enter the muscle very close to their exit from the quadrilateral space and travel in the deltoid muscle along the medial and inferior borders of the posterior deltoid. Interestingly, the posterior branch extends 6 to 8 cm in length after it leaves the quadrilateral space.[88] The branch of the axillary nerve that supplies the anterior two-thirds of the deltoid ascends superiorly and then travels anteriorly, approximately 2 inches inferior to the rim of the acromion. Paralysis of the axillary nerve produces a 50% loss of strength in elevation,[38] even though the full abduction range is sometimes maintained.[222] The deltoid's vascular supply is largely derived from the posterior humeral circumflex artery, which travels with the axillary nerve through the quadrilateral space to the deep surface of the muscle.[1,95,208,212] The deltoid is also supplied by the deltoid branch of the thoracoacromial artery, with rich anastomoses between the two vessels. The deltoid artery travels in the deltopectoral groove and sends branches to the muscle.[212] Numerous additional arteries are also present. The venous pedicles are identical to the arterial pedicles,[258] except that the cephalic vein is quite dominant, especially for the anterior third of the deltoid.

Rotator Cuff

Before discussing the rotator cuff muscles individually, some remarks regarding the cuff as a whole are in order. Although made up of four separate muscles, the rotator cuff is a complex arrangement. The muscles may appear

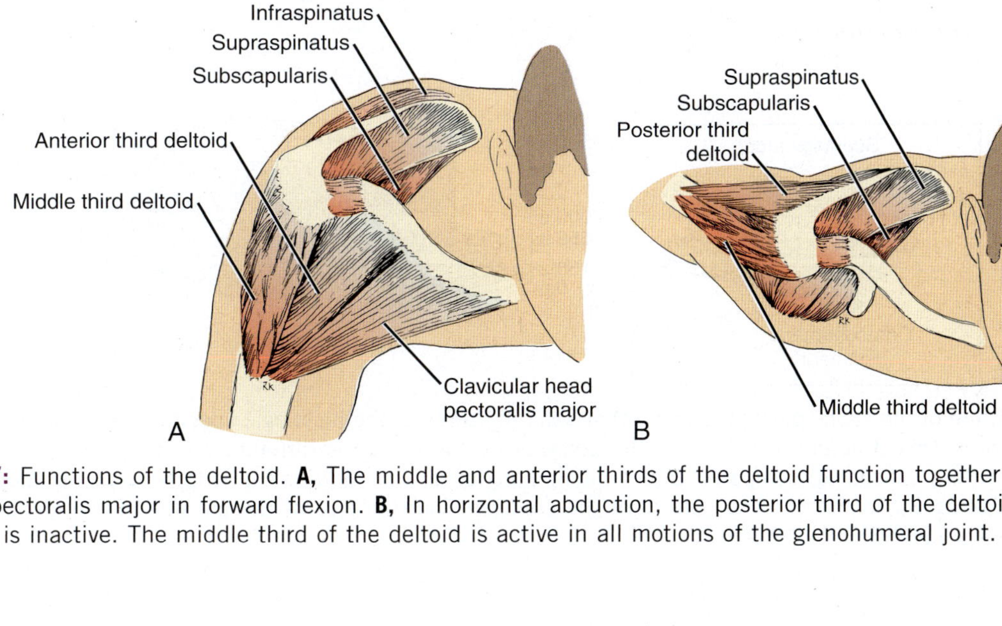

FIGURE 2-27: Functions of the deltoid. **A,** The middle and anterior thirds of the deltoid function together with the clavicular head of the pectoralis major in forward flexion. **B,** In horizontal abduction, the posterior third of the deltoid is active and the anterior third is inactive. The middle third of the deltoid is active in all motions of the glenohumeral joint.

separate superficially, but in their deeper regions they are associated with each other, with the capsule underneath, and with the tendon of the long head of the biceps.[38]

In their deeper regions, the tendons send fascicles into their neighbors. The most complex of this sharing occurs at the bicipital groove, where the fascicles of the supraspinatus destined for the insertion of the subscapularis cross over the groove and create a roof. Conversely, the fascicles of the subscapularis tendon that are headed for the supraspinatus insertion create a floor for the groove by undergoing some chondrometaplasia.[38] Also in their deeper regions, muscles and tendons attach to the capsule. Again, the most complex of these arrangements occurs at the rotator interval. In this region, the coracohumeral ligament contributes fibers that envelope the supraspinatus tendon. This relationship is most apparent on the deep surface, where it is visible to the arthroscopist as a curved cable running from the anterior edge to the back of the supraspinatus tendon and on into the infraspinatus to create a laterally based arch or suspension bridge.[26] This arrangement creates a thicker region of the cuff visible on ultrasound.

Kask et al.[117] described the anatomy of the ligamentum semicirculare humeri (rotator cable) in a cadaveric and MRI study. They divided the rotator cable into three segments—anterior, middle, and posterior. The anterior segment of the rotator cable forms the lateral part of the rotator interval. The segment under the supraspinatus tendon forms the middle portion of the rotator cable. The course of the ligament is perpendicular to the longitudinal axes of the supraspinatus and infraspinatus tendons in this area. The fibers of the rotator cable, covered by the infraspinatus tendon, form the posterior part of the ligament. The descending fibers curve latero-posteriorly and end at the insertion region between the ISP and TM tendons on the posterior side of the greater tuberosity (Fig. 2-28).

Supraspinatus

The supraspinatus muscle lies on the superior portion of the scapula. It takes a fleshy origin from the supraspinatus fossa and overlying fascia and inserts into the greater tuberosity. Its tendinous insertion is in common with the infraspinatus posteriorly and the coracohumeral ligament anteriorly. This complex tendon formation is common to the rotator cuff. The superficial fibers are longitudinal and give the tendon the appearance of a more discrete structure. These more superficial fibers have larger blood vessels than do the deeper fibers. The deeper fibers run obliquely and create a nonlinear pattern that holds sutures more effectively. This tendon sends fibers anteriorly with the coracohumeral ligament over the bicipital groove to the lesser tuberosity. The anterior edge of the tendon is enveloped by the coracohumeral ligament. The

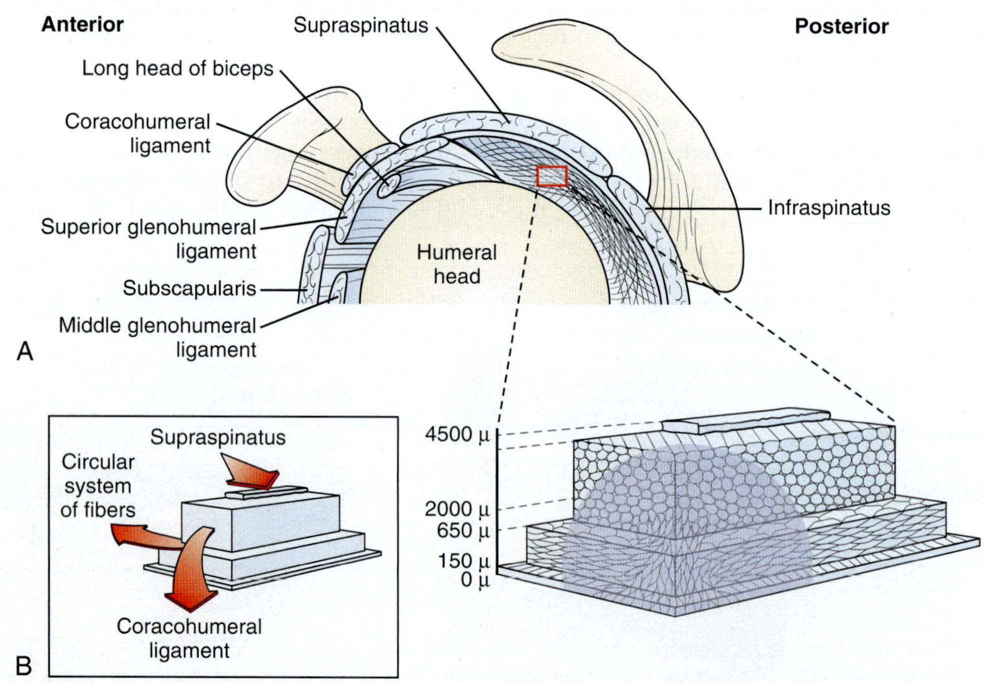

FIGURE 2-28: Structure of the supraspinatus tendon **(A)** shows the source of the histologic specimen; **B** shows the multilayered structure of the tendon. This structure explains why the behavior of this tendon is different with regard to holding suture and reflecting ultrasound (less echogenic) compared with a highly parallel tendon such as the long head of the biceps. (Modified from Gohlke F, Essigkrug B, Schmitz F. The pattern of the collagen fiber bundles of the capsule of the glenohumeral joint. *J Shoulder Elbow Surg.* 1994;3[3]:111-128.)

anterior portion of the supraspinatus is more powerful than the posterior half, with the muscle fibers inserting onto an extension of the tendon within the anterior half of the muscle. This tendon extension can be seen on MRI.[24] Roh et al. found that the physiologic cross section of the anterior muscle belly was much larger than the posterior muscle belly. However, the tendon cross-sectional areas of the anterior tendon were slightly smaller than the posterior tendon. Thus a larger anterior muscle belly pulls through a smaller tendon area.[207]

A portion of the coracohumeral ligament runs on the articular surface of the supraspinatus tendon perpendicular to the orientation of the tendon. This creates a laterally based arch that is visible from within the joint and runs all the way to the infraspinatus insertion. Its tendon may have an asymptomatic calcium deposit in as many as 2.5% of shoulders.[156] Inferiorly, the muscular portion is bounded by its origin off the bone, the rim of the neck of the glenoid, and the capsule itself, which is not divisible from the deep fibers of the tendon (Fig. 2-29).

The function of the supraspinatus muscle is important because it is active in any motion involving elevation.[102] Its length-tension curve exerts maximal effort at approximately 30 degrees of elevation.[6] Above this level, the greater tubercle increases its lever arm.[203] Because the muscle circumscribes the humeral head above and its fibers are oriented directly toward the glenoid, it is important for stabilizing the glenohumeral joint. The supraspinatus, together with the other accessory muscles (the infraspinatus, subscapularis, and biceps), contributes equally with the deltoid to the torque of scapular plane elevation and forward elevation when tested by selective axillary nerve block.[40,41] The supraspinatus has an excursion approximately two-thirds that of the deltoid for the same motion, indicative of a shorter lever arm.[157]

Other muscles of the rotator cuff, especially the infraspinatus and subscapularis, provide further downward force on the humeral head to resist shear forces of the deltoid. If these muscles are intact, even with a small rotator cuff tear, enough stabilization may be present for fairly strong abduction of the shoulder by the deltoid

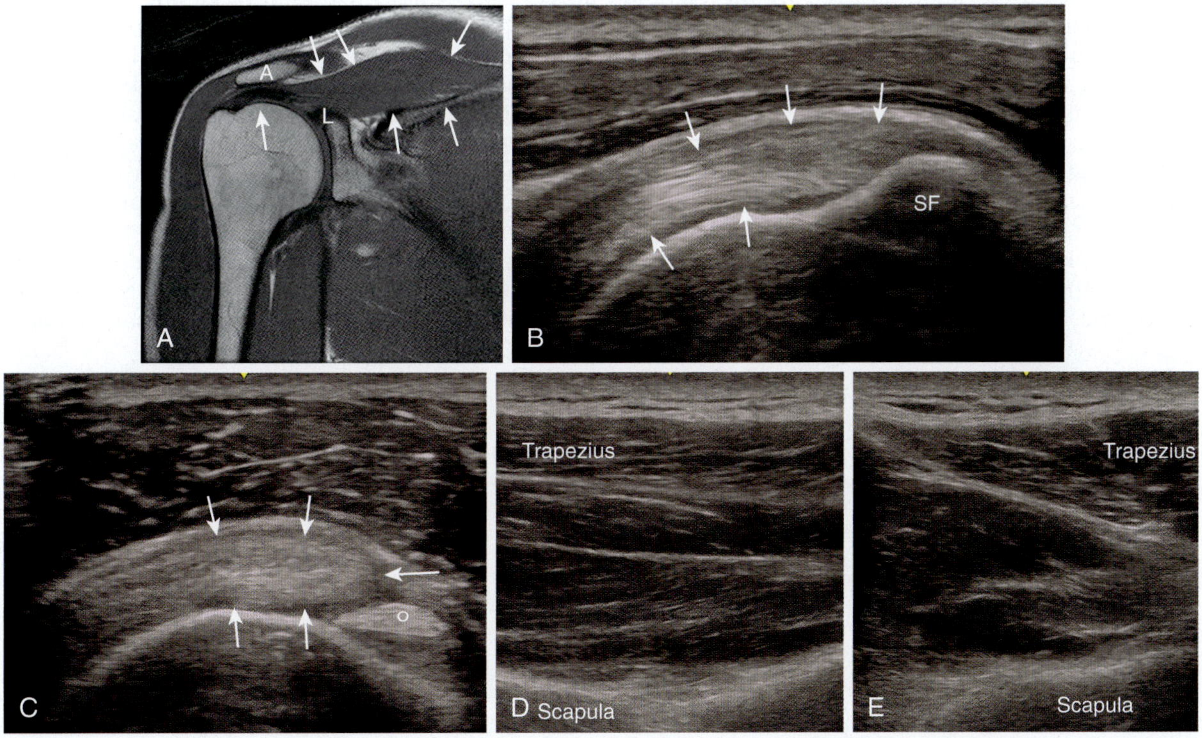

FIGURE 2-29: **A,** Coronal T1 cross section of the scapula in the coronal plane showing the important relationships of the supraspinatus muscle. Among these relationships are the course of the tendon that circumscribes the humeral head—essential to its head-depressing effect—and the tendon's course beneath the acromion, the acromioclavicular joint, and the indiscernible subacromial bursa. Inferiorly, it is inseparable from the capsule of the joint. The subacromial bursa above the tendon, being a potential space, is indiscernible (compare with Fig. 2-60). **B,** Insertion onto the superior facet (SF) of the greater tuberosity, in long axis. The tendon is indicated by the arrows. **C,** Supraspinatus tendon (*arrows*) over the humeral head in short axis with the biceps (*small circle*) on the right marking the anterior border of the supraspinatus tendon. Note how the biceps is more echogenic than the supraspinatus. **D,** Muscle belly in long axis lying between the trapezius and the scapula. **E,** Muscle belly short axis lying between the trapezius and the scapula. Note the central tendon in the anterior supraspinatus on the right. (**A,** Courtesy Allie Blackburn, MD.)

muscle, although the endurance may be shorter.[183] Some patients externally rotate their shoulder so that they can use their biceps for the same activity. Because the supraspinatus is confined above by the subacromial bursa and the acromion and below by the humeral head, the tendon is at risk for compression and attrition. Because of such compression, Grant and Smith's series and others indicate that 50% of cadaver specimens from individuals older than 77 years have rotator cuff tears.[85] A later study by Neer showed a lower incidence.[167]

The boundaries of the path of the supraspinatus tendon are referred to as the *supraspinatus outlet.*[168] This space is decreased by internal rotation and opened by external rotation, thus showing the effect of the greater tubercle.[166] The space is also compromised by use of the shoulder in weight bearing, as when using crutches or doing pushups in a wheelchair.[10] Martin suggested that the external rotation of the arm during elevation is produced by the coracoacromial arch acting as an inclined plane on the greater tubercle.[147] Saha et al. attribute this limitation of rotation during elevation to ligamentous control.[209,210] More recent data suggest that this external rotation is necessary to eliminate the 45-degree angulation of the humerus from the coronal plane, adding 45 degrees to the limited elevation allowed by the glenoid (Fig. 2-30).[110] Innervation of the supraspinatus is supplied by the suprascapular nerve (C5 with some C6). The main arterial supply is the suprascapular artery. These structures enter the muscle near its midpoint at the suprascapular notch at the base of the coracoid process. The nerve goes through the notch and is bounded above by the transverse scapular ligament. The nerve has no motion relative to the notch. The artery travels above this ligament. The suprascapular vessels and nerve supply the deep surface of the muscle. A branch also runs between the bone of the scapular spine and the muscle. The medial portion of the muscle receives vessels from the dorsal scapular artery.[212]

Infraspinatus

The infraspinatus is the second most active rotator cuff muscle (see Fig. 2-30 and Fig. 2-31).[183] It takes a fleshy, collagen-poor origin off the infraspinatus fossa of the scapula, the overlying dense fascia, and the spine of the scapula. Its tendinous insertion is in common with the supraspinatus anterior superiorly and the teres minor inferiorly at the greater tuberosity. On its superficial surface, it is bounded by an avascular fascial space on the deep surface of the deltoid. The infraspinatus is one of the two main external rotators of the humerus and accounts for as much as 60% of the external rotation force.[41] It functions as a depressor of the humeral head.[106] Even in the passive (cadaver) state, the infraspinatus is an important stabilizer against posterior subluxation.[178,179] An interesting aspect of muscle action at the shoulder is that a muscle may have opposing actions in different positions. The infraspinatus muscle stabilizes the shoulder against posterior subluxation in internal rotation by circumscribing the humeral head and creating a forward force. In contradistinction, it has a line of pull posteriorly and stabilizes against anterior subluxation when the shoulder is in abduction–external rotation.[29,183] The infraspinatus is a pennate muscle with a median raphe covered by a fat stripe that can be mistaken at surgery for the gap between the infraspinatus and teres minor muscles. The infraspinatus is innervated by the suprascapular nerve. The nerve tunnels through the spinoglenoid notch, which is not usually spanned by a ligament. Its blood supply is generally described as coming from two large branches of the suprascapular artery.[95] Salmon, however, found in two-thirds of his specimens that the subscapular

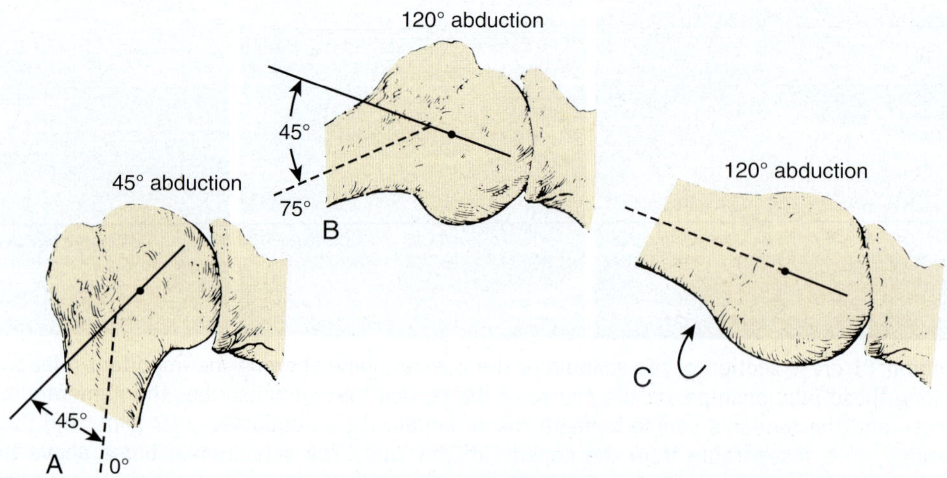

FIGURE 2-30: With some compression of the soft tissues superiorly, this glenohumeral joint allows almost 75 degrees of coronal abduction. Without changing the orientation of the axis of the head to the glenoid, 90 degrees of upward rotation removes the 135-degree neck shaft angle from view, thus making the neck shaft angle appear to be 180 degrees, which adds an additional 45 degrees of apparent elevation in the coronal plane. (From Jobe CM, Iannotti JP. Limits imposed on glenohumeral motion by joint geometry. *J Shoulder Elbow Surg.* 1995;4[4]:281-285.)

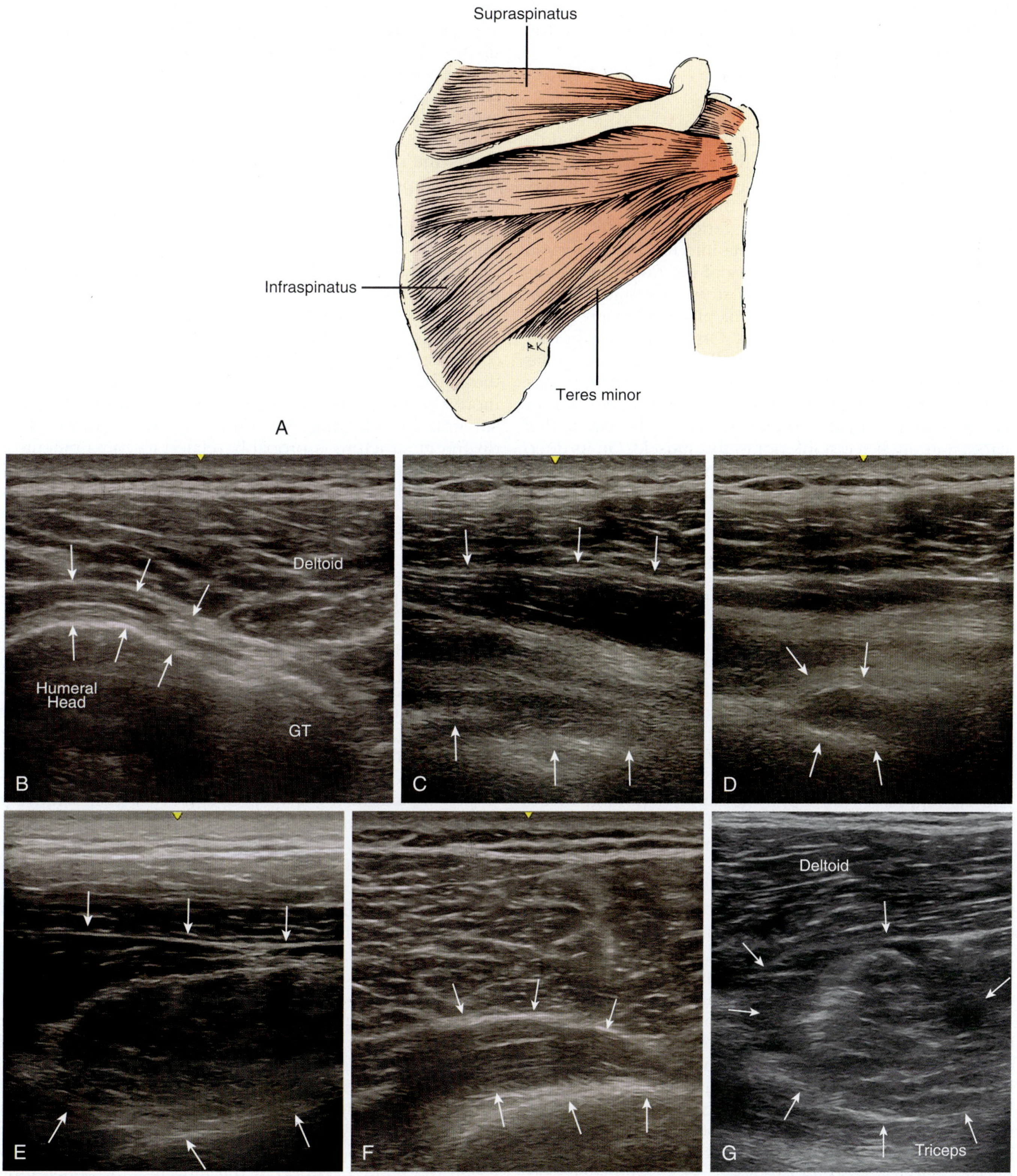

FIGURE 2-31: **A,** The two external rotators of the humerus, the infraspinatus and teres minor muscles, are also the posterior wall of the rotator cuff. Note the median raphe of the infraspinatus, which is often mistaken at surgery for the border between the infraspinatus and the teres minor. **B,** Long axis of infraspinatus (*arrows*) over the head; note the thinness of the structure compared to the thickness of the muscle belly. **C,** Long axis of the infraspinatus muscle belly, between the overlying deltoid and the underlying scapula. **D,** Infraspinatus (the same muscle shown in **C**), in a position that allows the suprascapular vein (*arrows*) to dilate. **E,** Short axis of muscle belly of infraspinatus (*arrows*). The bone of the scapular spine slopes up to the left while the inferior neck of the glenoid lies to the right, marking the lower border of the infraspinatus. The deltoid lies across the top. **F,** Long axis of teres minor near insertion. Note that the tissue is muscle all the way to the bone, without an intervening tendon. **G,** Short axis of teres minor (*arrows*). Teres is Latin for round. The deltoid, which is thicker at this level, lies across the top. The long head of the triceps originates at the right and runs deep to the teres.

artery through its dorsal or circumflex scapular branch supplied the greater portion of the circulation of the infraspinatus muscle.[212]

Teres Minor

The teres minor has a muscular origin from the middle portion of the lateral border of the scapula and the dense fascia of the infraspinatus (see Figs. 2-30 and 2-31). Rarely are individuals found in whom the teres minor overlies the infraspinatus as far as the vertebral border of the scapula.[257] The teres minor inserts into the lower portion of the posterior greater tuberosity of the humerus. On its deep surface is the adherent posterior capsule, and on the superficial surface is a fascial plane between it and the deep surface of the deltoid. On the inferior border lie the quadrilateral space laterally and the triangular space medially. In the quadrilateral space, the posterior humeral circumflex artery and the axillary nerve border the teres minor. In the triangular space, the circumflex scapular artery lies just inferior to this muscle. On its deep surface, in the midportion, lies the long head of the triceps tendon, loose alveolar fat, and the subscapularis. The teres minor is one of the few external rotators of the humerus. It provides up to 45% of the external rotation force and is important in controlling stability in the anterior direction.[29,41] It also likely participates in the short rotator force couple in abduction along with the inferior portion of the subscapularis. The teres minor is innervated by the posterior branch of the axillary nerve (C5 and C6). Its blood supply is derived from several vessels in the area, but the branch from the posterior humeral scapular circumflex artery is the most constant.[212]

Subscapularis

The subscapularis muscle is the anterior portion of the rotator cuff. This muscle takes a fleshy origin from the subscapularis fossa that covers most of the anterior surface of the scapula. It contains multiple interspersed tendinous bands that merge laterally into a flattened tendon in the superior two-thirds of the muscle, while the inferior third of the subscapularis has a muscular attachment almost directly onto the inferior aspect of the lesser tuberosity and the anterior aspect of the humeral metaphysis through a thin membranous structure.[162]

The upper 60% of the subscapularis muscle inserts through a collagen-rich tendon into the lesser tuberosity of the humerus. The lower 40% has a fleshy insertion into the humerus below the lesser tuberosity cupping the head and neck.[93] The internal structure of the muscle is multipennate, and the collagen is so dense in the upper subscapularis that it is considered to be one of the passive stabilizers of the shoulder.[177,234,252] The subscapularis muscle is bounded anteriorly by the axillary space and the coracobrachialis bursa. Superiorly, it passes under the coracoid process and the subscapularis recess, or bursa. The axillary nerve and posterior humeral circumflex artery and veins pass deep below the muscle into the quadrilateral space. The circumflex scapular artery passes into the more medial triangular space. Laterally, the anterior humeral circumflex vessels mark the division between the upper 60% and the lower 40%.[93]

The subscapularis functions as an internal rotator and passive stabilizer to prevent anterior subluxation and, especially in its lower fibers, serves to depress the humeral head (Fig. 2-32).[106] Through this last function, it resists the shear force of the deltoid to help with elevation. Compression of the glenohumeral joint also adds to this function. Another feature of the subscapularis is that its function may vary with the level of training. The function of the subscapularis in acceleration is less in amateur pitchers than in professional throwers, implying that a less-trained thrower is still adjusting the glenohumeral joint for stability, whereas a professional can use the muscle as an internal rotator.[84]

As with the insertions of the other rotator cuff muscles, the subscapularis has parallel collagen superficially and more divergent fascicles deeply. Such anatomy aids the surgeon by allowing the tendon to hold suture. This divergent structure is probably related to containment of the humeral head and upward and downward rotation of the head on the glenoid. One of the more prominent features of this divergence is an upper group of deep fibers that passes on the deep surface of the biceps and inserts into the floor of the bicipital groove all the way to the supraspinatus insertion.

On the deep surface of the upper portion of the subscapularis tendon is the glenohumeral joint. The middle glenohumeral ligament lies beneath the upper portion of the tendon. The anterior inferior glenohumeral ligament lies deep to the mid and lower portions. Innervation is generally supplied by two sources: the upper subscapular nerves (C5), which supply the upper 50%, and the lower subscapular nerves (C5 and C6), which supply the lower 20%. The nerve supply to the intervening 30% varies. The upper subscapular nerves, usually two comparatively short nerves in the axilla, come off the posterior cord. Because of the greater relative motion of the lower portion of the scapula, the lower subscapular nerves, also two in number, are longer in their course.[152]

The blood supply of the subscapularis is usually described as originating from the axillary and subscapular arteries. Bartlett and associates found that 84% of their 50 dissections had no significant vessels off the subscapular artery before the bifurcation into circumflex scapular and thoracodorsal arteries.[9] This finding indicates greater importance of the anterior humeral circumflex artery and the upper subscapular artery named by Huelke.[103] Salmon also described this latter artery as a constant vessel but stated that it is small in caliber. He found that the major supply was derived from branches of the subscapular artery.[212] Small branches from the dorsal scapular artery reach the medial portion of the muscle after penetrating the serratus anterior. Venous drainage is via two veins to the circumflex scapular vein.[258]

Teres Major

The teres major originates from the posterior surface of the scapula along the inferior portion of the lateral border

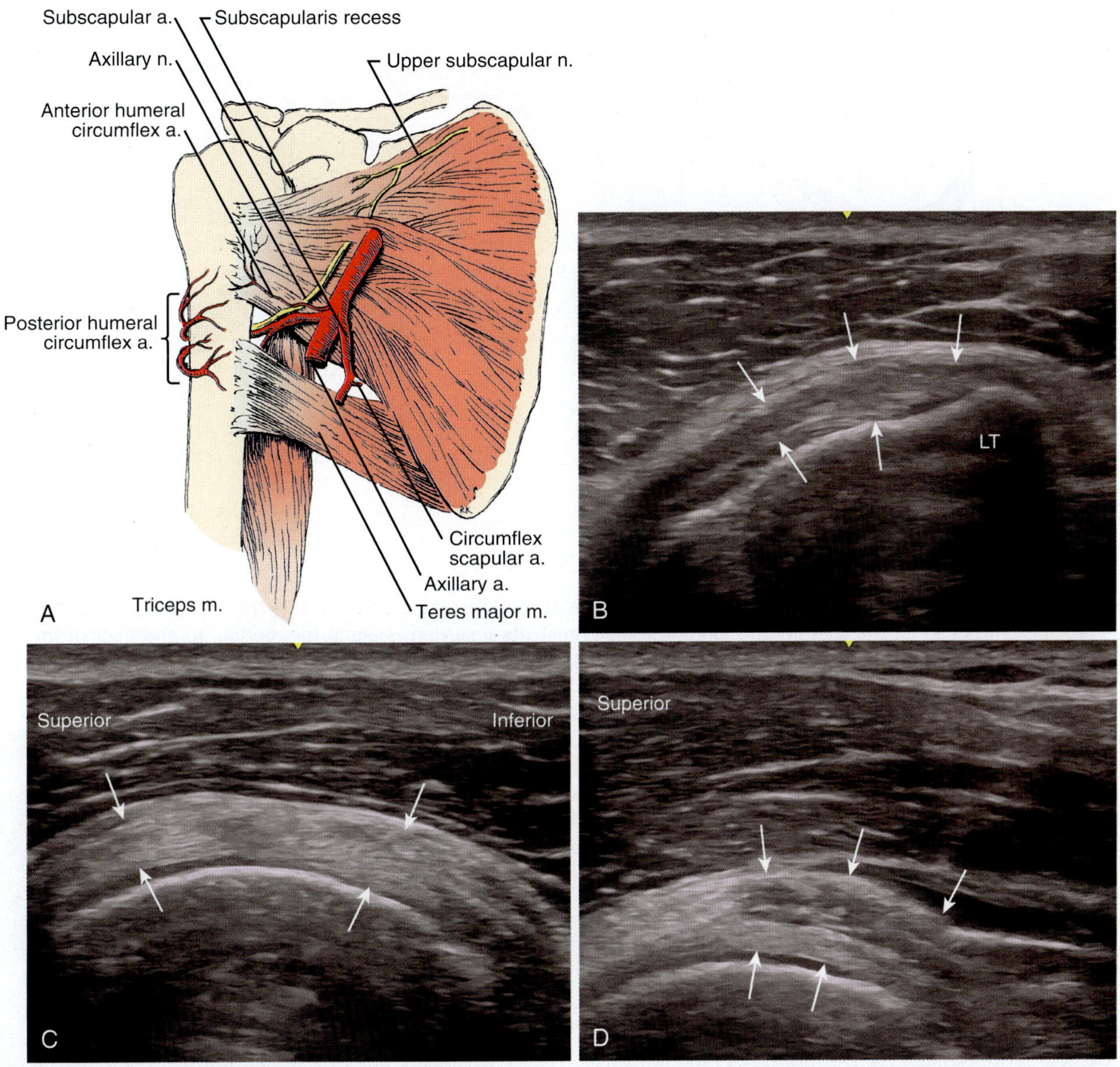

FIGURE 2-32: **A,** The anterior and inferior relationships of the subscapularis muscle. The soft tissues not shown are the axillary space fat and the coracobrachialis bursa. The vulnerable structures within the adipose tissue are the axillary nerve, which crosses the fibers of the subscapularis muscle before entering the quadrilateral space, and the posterior humeral circumflex vessels. The size of the quadrilateral space is enlarged in this drawing for illustrative purposes. The anterior humeral circumflex vessels are also vulnerable anteriorly. The triangular space has been enlarged by the illustrator. **B,** Direct insertion of subscapularis (*arrows*) into the lesser tuberosity (LT). **C,** Short axis view of the subscapularis tendon (*arrows*), over the humeral head. **D,** Short axis view more proximal and medial. The upper left is still tendon. The lower is more muscular at this level. The lower 40% of this muscle, which is not shown on this image, is muscular.

(Fig. 2-33C). It has a muscular origin from the scapula and an insertion into the humerus posterior to the latissimus dorsi along the medial lip of the bicipital groove, a ridge of bone that is a continuation of and posterior to the lesser tuberosity. In their courses, both the latissimus dorsi and teres major undergo a 180-degree spiral; thus the formerly posterior surface of the muscle is represented by fibers on the anterior surface of the tendon. Moreover, the relationship between the teres major and latissimus dorsi becomes rearranged so that the formerly posterior latissimus dorsi becomes anterior to the teres major. In addition to the boundaries of the latissimus dorsi, the teres major is bounded above by the triangular and quadrilateral spaces, posteriorly by the long head of the triceps, and anteriorly in its medial portion by the axillary space. The function of the teres major is internal rotation, adduction, and extension of the arm. This muscle is active in these motions only against resistance.[60] Upward rotation of the scapula may be an additional function of this muscle during activities that involve a

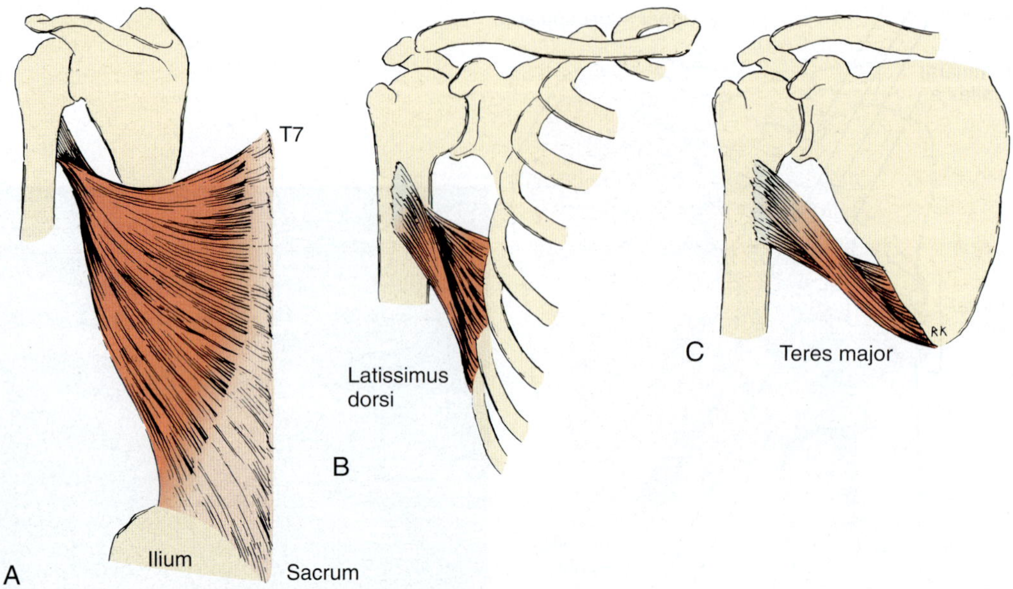

FIGURE 2-33: Posterior **(A)** and anterior **(B)** views of the course of the latissimus dorsi muscle from its origin along the posterior spinous processes from T7 to the sacrum and along the iliac crest. Its insertion is along the medial lip and floor of the bicipital groove. **C,** The accompanying muscle, the teres major, with its similar fiber rotation inserts just medial to the latissimus dorsi.

firmly planted upper limb, such as the iron cross performed by gymnasts. Innervation is supplied by the lower subscapular nerve (C5 and C6), and its blood supply is derived from branches of the subscapular artery, quite regularly a single vessel from the thoracodorsal artery.[212] This branch may originate from the axillary artery directly.

Coracobrachialis

The coracobrachialis has a fleshy and tendinous origin from the coracoid process, in common with and medial to the short head of the biceps, and inserts on the anteromedial surface in the midportion of the humerus. Laterally, the coracobrachialis is bounded by its common origin with the biceps (Fig. 2-34). On the deep surface, the coracobrachialis bursa lies between the two conjoint muscles and the subscapularis. The deltoid, the deltopectoral groove, and the pectoralis major are on the superficial surface. These surfaces tend to be avascular or are crossed by a few small vessels. The action of the coracobrachialis is flexion and adduction of the glenohumeral joint, with innervation supplied by small branches from the lateral cord and the musculocutaneous nerve. Most specimens have a direct nerve to the coracobrachialis from the lateral cord, in addition to the larger musculocutaneous (C5 and C6) nerve. This additional nerve enters the coracobrachialis muscle on its deep surface and provides extra innervation.[71] Because the larger musculocutaneous nerve's entrance to the muscle may be situated as high as 1.5 cm from the tip of the coracoid to as low as 7 to 8 cm, it must be located and protected during certain types of repair. The major blood supply is by a single artery, usually off the axillary. This artery may arise in common with the artery to the biceps.[212]

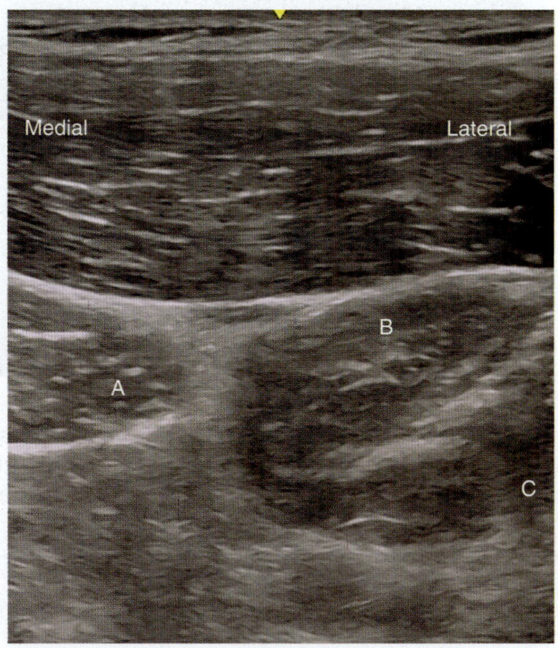

FIGURE 2-34: Short axis ultrasound view of the three muscles attached to the coracoid process: pectoralis minor *(A)*, coracobrachialis *(B)*, and short head of biceps *(C)*.

Multiple Joint Muscles

Multiple joint muscles act on the glenohumeral joint and one other joint, most often the scapulothoracic. When appropriate, the action on both these joints will be mentioned.

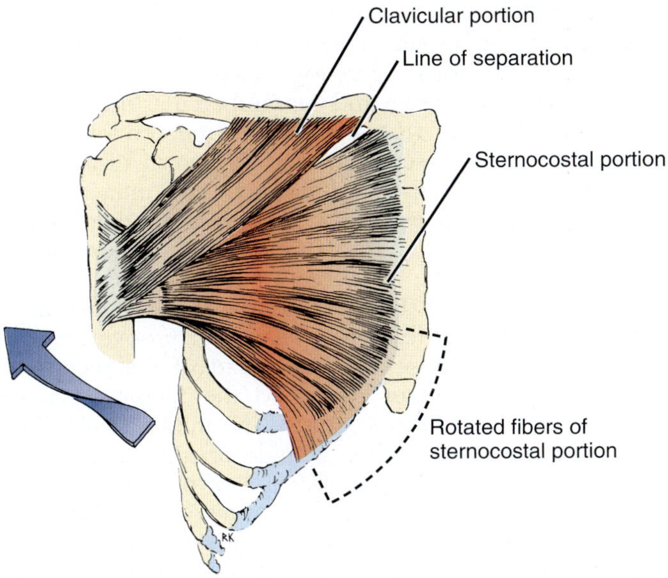

FIGURE 2-35: Two major divisions of the pectoralis major muscle. The separation is often readily discernible. Note the 180-degree rotation of the fibers of the lower portion of the sternocostal division.

Pectoralis Major

The pectoralis major consists of three portions (Fig. 2-35). The upper portion originates from the medial half to two-thirds of the clavicle and inserts along the lateral lip of the bicipital groove. Its fibers maintain a parallel arrangement. The middle portion originates from the manubrium and upper two-thirds of the body of the sternum and ribs 2 to 4. It inserts directly behind the clavicular portion and maintains a parallel fiber arrangement. The inferior portion of the pectoralis major originates from the distal body of the sternum, the fifth and sixth ribs, and the external oblique muscle fascia. It has the same insertion as the other two portions, but the fibers rotate 180 degrees so that the inferior fibers insert superiorly on the humerus. Landry noted that in cases of chondroepitrochlearis muscle anomaly, the twisted insertion is absent.[128] A line of separation is often present between the clavicular portion and the lower two portions. The inferior border is the border of the axillary fold. The superior lateral border is the deltopectoral groove mentioned earlier. On the deep surface superior to the attachment to the ribs lies the pectoralis minor muscle, which is invested by the clavipectoral fascia.

The action of the pectoralis major depends on its starting position. For example, the clavicular portion participates somewhat in flexion with the anterior portion of the deltoid, whereas the lower fibers are antagonistic. Both these effects are lost in the coronal plane. The muscle is active in internal rotation against resistance and will extend the shoulder from flexion until the neutral position is reached.[217] This muscle is also a powerful adductor of the glenohumeral joint and indirectly functions as a depressor of the lateral angle of the scapula. Loss of the sternocostal portion most noticeably affects internal rotation and scapular depression, with some loss of adduction.[146] This loss is significant only for athletics, not daily activities. The clavicular portion is most active in forward flexion and horizontal adduction.[106] Loss of pectoralis major function seems to be well tolerated.[89,261]

Innervation of the muscle is supplied by two sources. The lateral pectoral nerve (C5, C6, and C7) innervates the clavicular portion of the muscle, probably only with C5 to C6 fibers, and the loop contribution from the lateral to the medial pectoral nerve carrying C7 fibers continues through or around the pectoralis minor into the upper sternal portion. The medial pectoral nerve, which carries fibers from C8 and T1, continues through the pectoralis minor into the remaining portion of the pectoralis major. Klepps et al.[121] found that the pectoral nerves innervate the pectoralis major quite medially, far from the humeral insertion. These nerves are safe from surgical dissection as long as one remains lateral to the pectoralis minor and less than 8.5 cm from the humeral insertion point.[121]

The major blood supply is derived from two sources. The deltoid branch of the thoracoacromial artery supplies the clavicular portion, and the pectoral artery supplies the sternocostal portion of the muscle.[195] Additional blood supply is provided via the internal mammary artery, the fourth or fifth intercostal artery, and other anastomoses from the lateral thoracic artery.[195,212] The vessel to the fourth rib area is within an additional deep origin that comes off this rib in the midclavicular line. Venous drainage laterally is through two veins to the axillary vein and medially to the internal mammary system.[195] In a literature review performed in 1902, Bing found that absence of a portion or all of the pectoralis major was the most commonly reported muscle defect, with such defects accounting for 28% of the cases cited.[16]

Latissimus Dorsi

The latissimus dorsi (see Fig. 2-33A and B) originates via the large and broad aponeurosis from the dorsal spines of T7 through L5, a portion of the sacrum, and the crest of the ilium. Frequently, it has origins on the lowest three or four ribs and the inferior angle of the scapula as well.[9] This muscle wraps around the teres major and inserts into the medial crest and floor of the bicipital or intertubercular groove. Given the fascial connections between the latissimus and teres major,[83] these two muscles can be transferred together to provide external rotation.[17]

On its superficial surface, the muscle is bounded by subcutaneous fat and fascia, and along the inferior border, it forms the posterior axillary fold. Anteriorly, it is bounded by the axillary space, and its deep surface is bounded by ribs and the teres major. Actions of the muscle include inward rotation and adduction of the humerus, shoulder extension, and, indirectly through its pull on the humerus, downward rotation of the scapula. Scheving and Pauly found that this muscle is more important than the pectoralis major as an internal rotator.[214] Ekholm et al. found its most powerful action in the oblique motions: extension, adduction, and abduction–internal rotation.[63]

Innervation is through the thoracodorsal nerve (C6 and C7), and its blood supply is derived from the thoracodorsal artery with additional supply from the intercostal and lumbar perforators. The neurovascular hilum is on the inferior anterior surface of the muscle, approximately 2 cm medial to the muscular border.[9] Two investigators have found that this neurovascular pedicle splits inside the muscle fascia into superomedial and inferolateral branches.[9,247] The venous drainage mirrors the arterial supply.[258] They found that such splits are quite predictable and suggested that the muscle could be split into two separate island flaps or free flaps.

Biceps Brachii

The biceps (Fig. 2-36) has its main action at the elbow rather than the shoulder. It is considered primarily an elbow muscle but is listed here with the shoulder muscles because of its frequent involvement in shoulder pathology and its use in substitutional motions. The biceps muscle has two origins in the shoulder, both of which are rich in collagen. The long head originates from the bicipital tubercle at the superior rim of the glenoid and along the posterior superior rim of the glenoid and labrum, and the short head originates from the coracoid tip lateral to and in common with the coracobrachialis. Meyer[44] noted that much of the origin of the long head is via the superior labrum and that the size of the bicipital tubercle does not reflect the size of the biceps tendon. The muscle has two distal tendinous insertions. The lateral insertion is to the posterior part of the tuberosity of the radius, and the medial insertion is aponeurotic and passes medially across and into the deep fascia of the muscles of the volar forearm. Loss of the long head attachment is manifested mainly as loss of supination strength (20%) with a smaller loss (8%) of elbow flexion strength.[145]

The relationships of the biceps tendon are most important in its role in shoulder pathology. The long head of the biceps exits the shoulder through a defect in the capsule between the greater and lesser tuberosities and passes distally in the bicipital groove. This portion of the tendon is that most often involved in pathology. Many studies have attempted to correlate construction of the groove with bicipital pathology (see Fig. 2-18).[94,158] A shallow bicipital groove and supratubercular ridge above the lesser tubercle (the trochlea of the tendon) were thought to predispose the biceps tendon to dislocation, with subsequent tendon pathology. The intra-articular tendon was noted as being broader than that in the groove.[158] Other early authors reported no rupture of the biceps tendon in the absence of supraspinatus rupture. If a correlation exists between bicipital groove morphology and the biceps tendon, a shallower groove may be more likely to expose the long head of the biceps to impingement.[167] Pfahler described the bicipital groove anatomy in a radiographic study. The medial wall of the bicipital groove was higher, with an opening angle of 30 to 40 degrees in the largest fraction of patients.[187]

The bicipital tendon does not move up and down in the groove. Rather, the humerus moves down and up with adduction and abduction relative to the tendon. The bicipital tendon is retained within the groove by a pulley made up of fibers from the coracohumeral and superior glenohumeral ligaments, with some reinforcement from adjacent tendons.[38,255]

Under normal conditions, the action of the biceps is flexion and supination at the elbow. In certain conditions, particularly when paralysis or rupture of the supraspinatus has occurred, the long head of the biceps is hypertrophied, probably because the patient is using the muscle as a depressor of the humeral head by placing the shoulder in external rotation.[183] One patient with a large rotator cuff tear reportedly was employed as a waiter and carried trays on the involved side, a substitution maneuver commonly seen in the days of infantile paralysis.[106,246] Lucas reported a 20% loss of elevation strength in external rotation with rupture of the long head of the biceps.[139] On the other hand, Mariani et al. reported that loss of this head depressor effect is unlikely to worsen impingement.[145] In internal rotation, no loss of strength was evident, and we must remember that impingement occurs in internal rotation.[139] One study

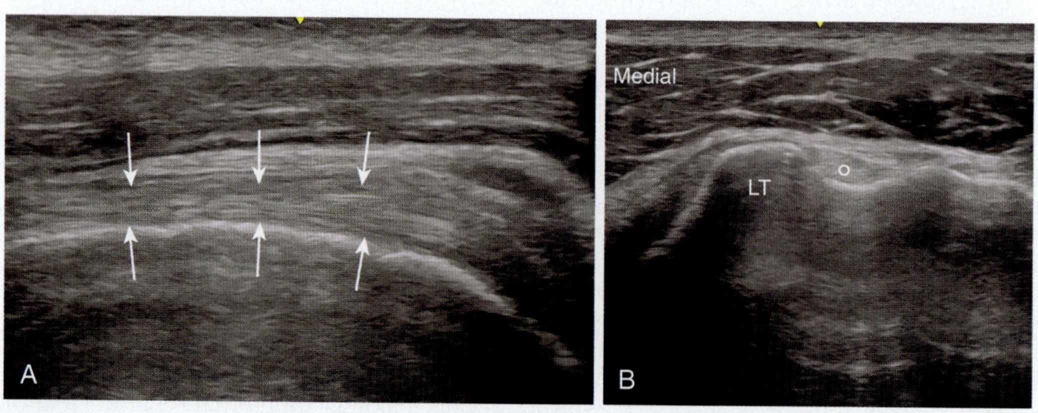

FIGURE 2-36: **A,** Long axis view of the long head of the biceps (*arrows*) in the deep portion of the bicipital groove. **B,** Long head of the biceps (*small circle*) lateral to the lesser tuberosity (LT).

involving cadaver specimens found that the long head could contribute to joint stability and that this stability is increased in external rotation and decreased in internal rotation.[108] It should be emphasized that these are not the usual activities of the biceps in a person without shoulder pathology as determined by electromyography. Innervation of the biceps is supplied by branches of the musculocutaneous nerve (C5 and C6), and the blood supply is derived from a single large bicipital artery from the brachial artery (35%), multiple very small arteries (40%), or a combination of the two types.[212]

Triceps Brachii

The triceps is another muscle that is not usually considered a shoulder muscle but may be involved in shoulder pathology, particularly in the long head. The long head originates from the infraglenoid tubercle. Although this tendon is not intra-articular like the long head of the biceps, the insertion is intimately related to the labrum over a distance of 2 cm centered on the tubercle. The fibers of the tendon adjacent to the capsule radiate into the inferior capsule and reinforce it. The remaining fibers insert into bone. This reinforced capsule, a portion of the inferior glenohumeral ligament, inserts through the labrum and radiates fibers into the circular portion of the labrum.

The origin of the long head is bounded laterally by the quadrilateral space, which contains the axillary nerve and posterior humeral circumflex artery, and medially by the triangular space, which contains the circumflex scapular artery. The teres major muscle passes anteriorly, and the teres minor passes posteriorly. Innervation is supplied by the radial nerve with root innervation through C6 to C8.[95] The arterial supply is derived mainly from the profunda brachii artery and the superior ulnar collateral artery. However, near its origin, the long head receives branches from the brachial and posterior humeral circumflex arteries.

The major action of the muscle is extension at the elbow. In addition, the long head is believed to function in shoulder adduction against resistance to offset the shear forces generated by the primary adductors. In more violent activities such as throwing, the muscle may demonstrate electromyographic activity up to 200% of that generated by a maximal muscle test.[112] A portion of the force would be transmitted to the origin of the scapula.

Landmark Muscles

Some muscles are important to surgeons as landmarks for shoulder dissection, although these muscles are not shoulder muscles in the sense of producing shoulder motion.

Sternocleidomastoid

The most obvious of these landmarks is the sternocleidomastoid muscle, which with the superior fibers of the trapezius, forms the borders of the posterior triangle of the neck. It originates via a tendinous head from the sternum and a broader but thin muscular head from the medial part of the clavicle.[208] The two heads unite and progress superiorly, obliquely posteriorly, and laterally to insert on the mastoid process. This muscle shares the same innervation with the trapezius: the spinal accessory nerve (cranial nerve XI). The blood supply is derived from two vascular pedicles, the superior from the occipital artery and the lower from the superior thyroid artery.

Scalenus Anterior and Scalenus Medius

The anterior scalene muscle originates from the anterior tubercles of vertebrae C3 through C6 and has a tendinous insertion on the first rib. The middle scalene muscle, largest of the scalenes, takes its origin from all of the transverse processes in the cervical spine and also inserts into the first rib. The first rib and the two scalene muscles form a triangle (Fig. 2-37) through which the entire brachial plexus and the subclavian artery pass. The subclavian vein passes anterior to the anterior scalene and posterior to the clavicle. Innervation of these muscles is supplied by deep branches of the cervical nerves. Variations in the muscles and their relationships are believed to predispose an individual to thoracic outlet syndrome.[212]

Omohyoid

The omohyoid muscle is seldom mentioned in a description of surgical procedures, but it divides the posterior cervical triangle into the upper occipital and lower subclavian triangles. It attaches to the superior border of the scapula just medial to the scapular notch and runs anteriorly, medially, and superiorly across the posterior cervical triangle. Deep to the sternocleidomastoid muscle is a tendon in the midportion of the muscle belly. The muscle continues on above to an insertion on the hyoid.

NERVES

The discussion of nerves of the shoulder includes the brachial plexus and its branches, the sympathetic nervous system, the nerves that come off the roots that form the brachial plexus, cranial nerve XI, and the supraclavicular nerves. The brachial plexus is unique in the human nervous system because of the great amount of motion involved relative to the adjacent tissues. By way of introduction, we first discuss the internal anatomy of the nerves. Roots, trunks, and cords of the brachial plexus are also peripheral nerves in their cross-sectional anatomy.[220,230,233] We then discuss the arrangement of the peripheral nervous system relative to other structures of the limbs. As an overview, we note a uniqueness of the brachial plexus in comparison to the rest of the nervous system; this uniqueness is a product of the increased motion of the shoulder.

This section describes the standard brachial plexus and its normal relationships and then discusses nonpathologic variants, variations that do not affect its function but may complicate diagnosis and surgical approaches. Cranial nerve XI, the supraclavicular nerves, and the intercostal brachial nerve are also reviewed.

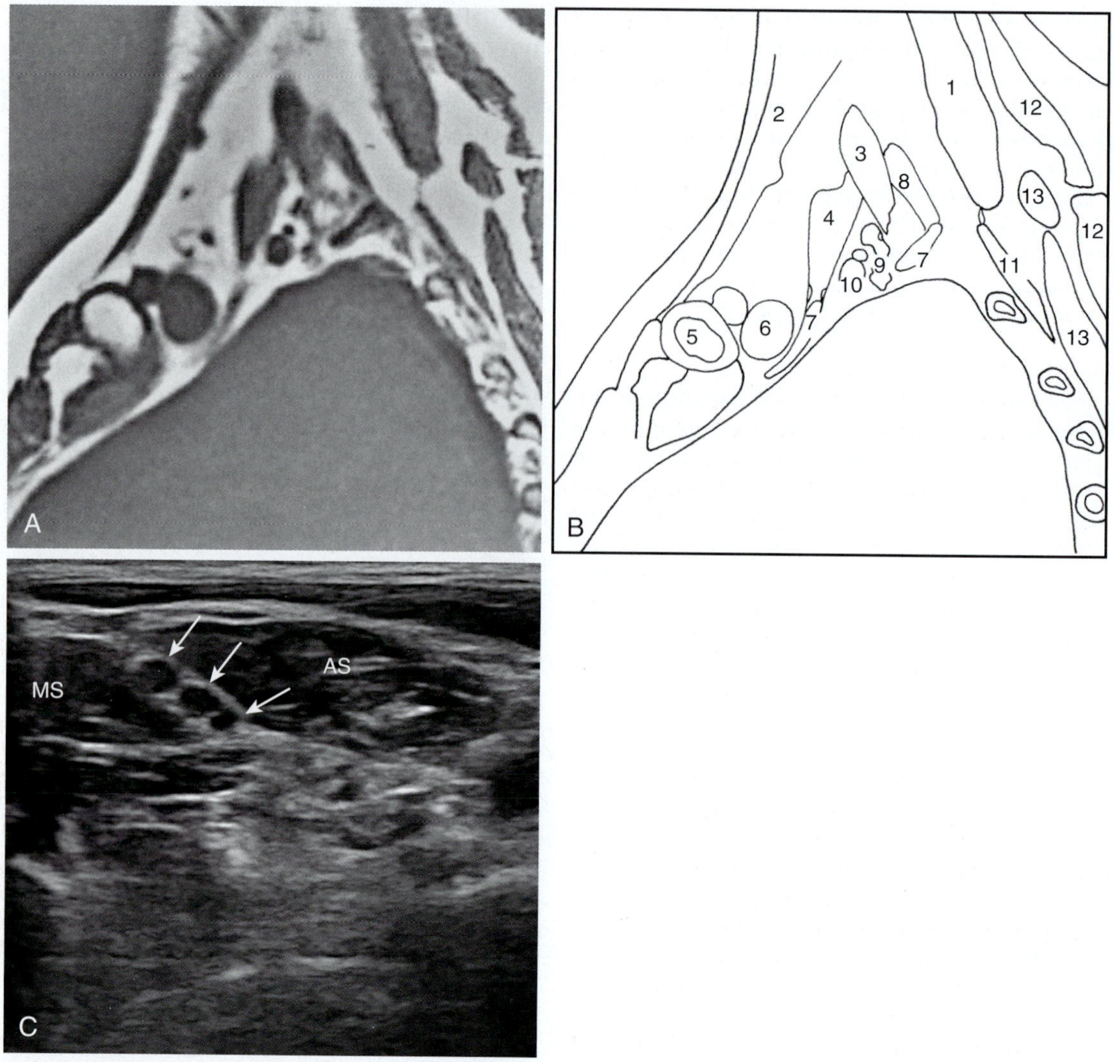

FIGURE 2-37: Magnetic resonance imaging scan **(A)** and diagram **(B)** of the scalene triangle showing its boundaries and the relationship of the important structures. Note that the anterior tilt of the first rib places the more posterior structures at a more caudad level. Note also the greater thickness of the levator scapulae (1) in comparison to the trapezius (12). The labeled structures are as follows: (1) levator scapulae, (2) sternocleidomastoid, (3) middle scalene, (4) anterior scalene, (5) clavicle, (6) subclavian vein, (7) rib 1, (8) posterior scalene, (9) brachial plexus, (10) subclavian artery, (11) serratus posterior superior, (12) trapezius, and (13) rhomboids. **C,** Axial view of the interscalene space with the three upper nerves *(arrows).* C5 lies toward the top, C7 at the bottom.

Nerve Function and Microanatomy

The principal function of nerves is to maintain and support axons of the efferent and afferent nerve cells. Cell bodies of these fibers are located in the dorsal root and autonomic ganglia and in the gray matter of the spinal cord. The axons are maintained somewhat by axoplasmic flow, but conduction of the nerve and its continued function have been found to be dependent on the layers surrounding the axons and their blood supply.[230,231,262] These layers in turn are dependent on an adequate blood supply.[215,236]

The axons in large nerves are contained within Schwann cells either 1:1 or, for smaller nerve fibers, a multiaxon-to-one Schwann cell ratio. These in turn are embedded in the endoneurium. A basal lamina separates the endoneurium from the myelin sheaths and Schwann cells.

Endoneurial tissue is mainly collagen that is closely arranged and contains capillaries and lymphatics.[141,230,262] The next outer tissue, referred to as the *perineurium*, surrounds groups of axons and serves primarily as a diffusion barrier and also maintains intraneural pressure. The integrity of this layer is essential to the function of the nerve and is the tissue most important to the surgeon. The perineurium is divided into multiple layers. The innermost layer has flat cells with tight junctions and appears to maintain the diffusion barrier. The outer layers are lamellated with interspersed collagen. The external layer of perineurium is a proven barrier to infection, whereas the outer layer of the nerve, the epineurium, is not.

The portion of the nerve enclosed in perineurium is referred to as a *fascicle* and is really the functioning portion of the nerve. All axons are contained in fascicles, and fascicles produce the necessary environment for nerve function. The size and number of fascicles vary. Fascicles tend to be larger in size and fewer in number in the spinal nerves and smaller and more numerous around branch points.[220] As a branch point is approached, fascicles bound for the branch nerve are gathered into fascicle groups.[220,262] This variability in fascicle number and size is further complicated by the fact that fascicles travel an average distance of only 5 mm before branching or merging. This arrangement results in a plexiform internal anatomy rather than the cable form that would be more convenient for repair and grafting purposes.[220]

The epineurium is loose alveolar tissue that is richly supplied with blood vessels and lymphatics.[262] It composes from over 80% of the cross-sectional area of the nerve to as little as 25%,[233,262] with an average of approximately 40% to 50% in peripheral nerves and 65% to 70% in the plexus.[220]

The blood supply to the nerves includes extrinsic and intrinsic vessels.[142] Intrinsic vessels are those contained within the epineurium itself, and such vessels constitute the arterial supply of the nerve. Terzis and Breidenbach further classified the nerves and extrinsic circulation according to whether all the extrinsic vessels connect to the same source artery and veins for purposes of free transfer of nerve tissue.[242] The blood vessels within the nerves are redundant and often have a convoluted course. Lundborg found that an average change of 8% in length by stretching had to occur before the development of venous occlusion in the nerves and an average 15% strain for complete cessation of arterial flow. Interestingly, function was normal in laboratory animals in which blood clots and blockage in some of the capillaries persisted even after release of tension on the nerve.[141]

Even the internal arrangement of nerves is designed to accommodate motion (Fig. 2-38). Layers slide past each other and allow almost a laminar motion of the layers relative to their surroundings. The 15% strain limit also has implications for the anatomic relationships of nerves, particularly in the shoulder. The closer a nerve is positioned to a center of joint rotation, the less it will change in length during motion. Two apparent strategies in the design of the brachial plexus protect the nerve against overstretch. First, the location of the nerves directly behind the sternoclavicular joint protects them against stretch during elevation of the clavicle in the coronal plane. The second crucial arrangement is that the brachial plexus in the axilla is not fixed to surrounding structures but, instead, floats freely in a quantity of fat. This design allows the plexus to slide superiorly with elevation of the arm so that it moves closer to the center of rotation and is subject to less strain. The implication of this arrangement is that disruption of the biomechanics of the shoulder may produce neurologic symptoms even though the original trauma or disease may not directly affect the nerves themselves. An additional protective arrangement in a joint that is so highly mobile is that most human motion is conducted forward, thus putting less stretch on most of the plexus. One exception to this tendency is nerves tightly attached to the scapula, which are stretched by scapular protraction.[122]

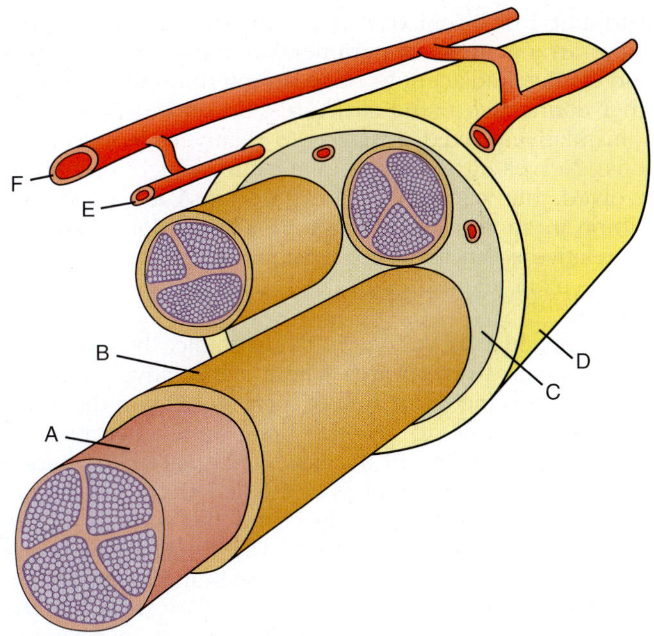

FIGURE 2-38: Internal anatomy of peripheral nerves and how it facilitates motion. *A* and *B* are the inner and outer layers of the perineurium; *C* and *D* are the inner and outer layers of the epineurium. *E* is a blood vessel within the epineurium, and *F* is the blood vessel of the nerve on the outside of the epineurium. Much of the cross section of the nerve is epineurium. The various components of the soft tissue of the nerve accommodate nerve motion. (From Lundborg G. Intraneural microcirculation. *Orthop Clin North Am.* 1988;19:1-12.)

The extrinsic vessels to the nerve tend to have an inverse relationship between their size and number. They reside a short distance (5 to 15 mm) from the adjacent artery. Redundancy of the blood supply is such that a nerve, when stripped of its extrinsic blood supply, will continue to function up to 8 cm from the nearest arteria nervorum.[141,143] This redundancy in blood supply is advantageous to tumor surgeons, who find the epineurium to be an effective boundary in certain tumor dissections. The epineurium is sometimes sacrificed in surgery with good preservation of nerve function. Moreover, radiotherapy can be applied to the axilla without loss of function. The redundancy can be overcome, however, with a combination of epineurial stripping and radiation or an excessive dose of radiotherapy alone, with an adverse effect on nerve function.[66,132]

Brachial Plexus

While studying the circulation of blood to the skin, Taylor and Palmer identified some common elements in the distribution of blood vessels in the body that also apply to the arrangement of peripheral nerves.[238] First, nerves tend to travel adjacent to bone, in intermuscular septa or other connective tissue structures. Second, nerves travel from relatively fixed positions to relatively mobile positions. Nerves rarely cross planes in which motion is involved, but when they do, they cross in an oblique fashion in an area of less motion. This design decreases the relative strain incurred by the nerve while crossing a mobile plane even though the actual total motion is not changed.[238]

The brachial plexus seems to contradict these tendencies. It travels from an area where it is relatively fixed at the cervical spine to an area of high mobility in the axilla and then returns to normal bone and intermuscular septum relationships in the arm. This pattern is unique in the human body and is necessitated by the highly mobile nature of the shoulder and the motion of the brachial plexus nerves on their way to innervate structures in the arm and forearm. This seeming contradiction is understood when we picture the axillary sheath as the connective tissue framework for the nerves and vessels and note that it is the sheath that moves in the axillary space.[76] An excellent review of brachial plexus injury treatment and anatomy was recently published by Shin et al.[218]

Roots

The standard brachial plexus (Fig. 2-39) is made up of the distal distribution of the anterior rami of the spinal nerves or roots C5, C6, C7, C8, and T1. The plexus sometimes has contributions from C4 and T2. A plexus with C4 contributions is called *prefixed*. When contributions from T2 occur, the term is *postfixed*.[218] For C4, this contribution appears in 28% to 62% of specimens,[20] although in terms of neural tissue it contributes very little.[220] The incidence of postfixed plexuses reportedly ranges from 16% to 73%.[119,218] The dorsal root ganglion holds the cell bodies. A preganglionic injury is one in which the roots are avulsed from the spinal cord. An injury distal to the dorsal root ganglion is termed postganglionic. Distinguishing between the two has treatment implications, as there is little recovery potential for a preganglionic injury.[218]

The roots that form the spinal nerves lack a fibrous sheath[66] and obtain a significant amount of soft tissue support only when they exit the intervertebral foramina, at which point they gain a dural sleeve. Herzberg et al. found a posterosuperior semiconic ligament at C5, C6, and C7 that attaches the spinal nerves to the transverse processes.[91] The spinal nerves C8 and T1 lack this additional protection. In most brachial plexus literature, the anterior divisions of these spinal nerves are called the roots of the brachial plexus. Herzberg and coworkers found that the C5 and C6 roots could be followed proximally but failed to find a safe surgical approach to spinal nerves C8 and T1 because dissection involved damage to the osseous structures.[91] Other authors mention the difficulty in exposing the lower two nerves.[144]

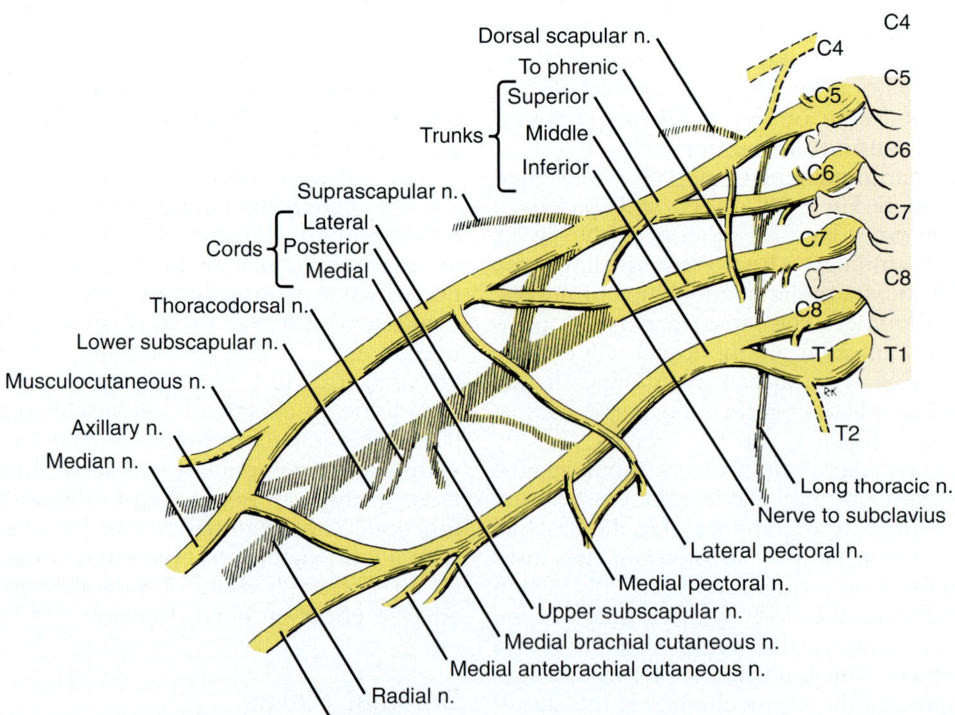

FIGURE 2-39: Standard arrangement of the brachial plexus and its trunks, cords, and terminal branches.

Trunks, Divisions, and Cords

The roots combine to form trunks: C5 and C6 form the upper trunk, C7 the middle trunk, and C8 and T1 the lower trunk.[218] The trunks then separate into anterior and posterior divisions. The posterior divisions combine to form the posterior cord, the anterior division of the lower trunk forms the medial cord, and the anterior divisions of the upper and middle trunks form the lateral cord. These cords give off the remaining and largest number of terminal nerves of the brachial plexus, with branches from the lateral and medial cords coming together to form the median nerve.

The brachial plexus leaves the cervical spine and progresses into the arm through the interval between the anterior and middle scalene muscles (Fig. 2-40). The subclavian artery follows the same course. Because of the inferior tilt of the first rib, the brachial plexus is posterior and superior to the artery at this point; only the lower trunk is directly posterior to the artery on the rib. It is in this triangle made up of the two scalenes that the nerve or vessel can be compromised by any number of abnormalities.[241] The inferior trunk forms high behind the clavicle, directly above the pleura, over a connective tissue layer referred to as *Sibson's fascia*. The upper two roots join to form the upper trunk at Erb's point located 2 to 3 cm above the clavicle, just behind the posterior edge of the sternocleidomastoid muscle. The majority of plexuses are penetrated by a vessel off the subclavian artery, most commonly the dorsal scapular artery, between two of the trunks.[103] The nerves between the scalene muscles become enclosed in the fascia of the scalenes, the prevertebral fascia. This interscalene sheath is important for containing and permitting the dispersal of local anesthetic concerning the nerves.[19]

The plexus splits into cords at or before it passes below the clavicle. As the cords enter the axilla, they become closely related to the axillary artery and attain positions relative to the artery indicated by their names: lateral, posterior, and medial. The prevertebral fascia invests the plexus and vessels and forms the axillary sheath. Two other landmark arteries are the transverse cervical artery, which crosses anterior to the level of the upper two trunks, and the suprascapular artery at the level of the middle trunk and the clavicle.[132]

Terminal Branches

The plexus gives off some terminal branches above the clavicle. The dorsal scapular nerve comes off C5, with some C4 fibers, and penetrates the scalenus medius and levator scapulae, sometimes contributing C4 fibers to the latter.[91] In the remaining cases, the nerve to the levator is a separate nerve. The dorsal scapular nerve accompanies the deep branch of the transverse cervical artery or the dorsal scapular artery on the undersurface of the rhomboids and innervates them.

Rootlets come off nerves C5, C6, and C7 directly adjacent to the intervertebral foramina and contribute to formation of the long thoracic nerve, which immediately passes between the middle and posterior scalenes[20] or penetrates the middle scalene.[99,100] Horwitz and Tocantins

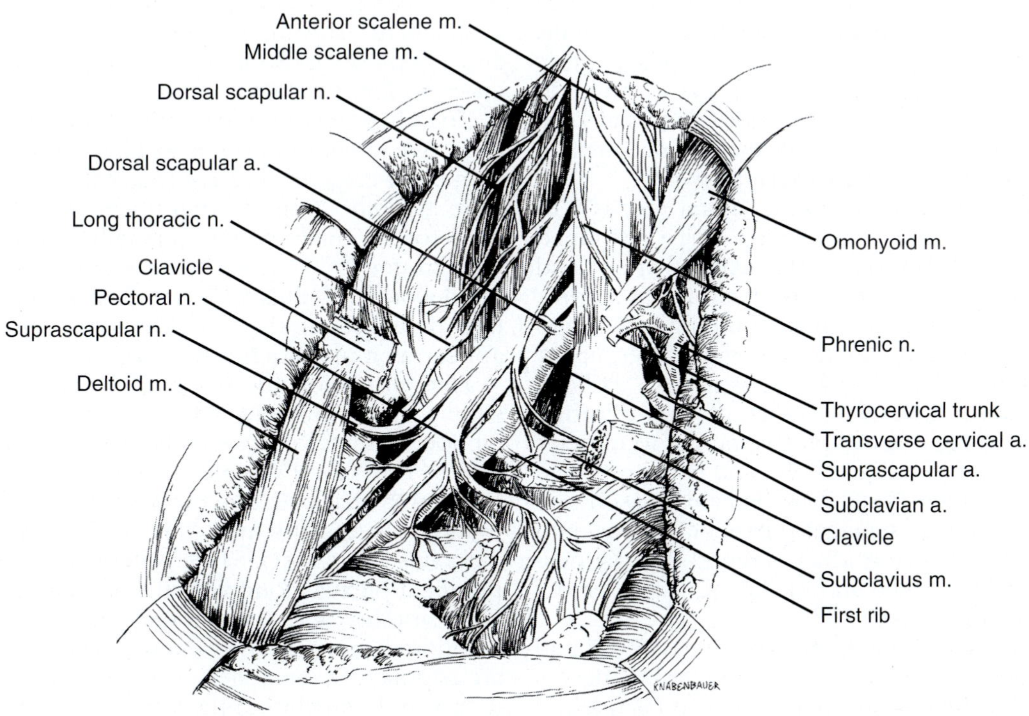

FIGURE 2-40: The more compressed form of the brachial plexus, found at the time of surgery, and its important anatomic relationships. (From Strohm BR, Colachis SC Jr. Shoulder joint dysfunction following injury to the suprascapular nerve. *Phys Ther.* 1965;45:106-111.)

reported that the nerve forms after the rootlets exit the muscle, with the C7 contribution not passing through muscle. They also mentioned that the nerve becomes more tightly fixed to muscle by branches near the distal end of the nerve. This nerve may not receive a contribution from C7, but its composition is fairly regular.[99,100] The nerve passes behind the plexus over the prominence caused by the second rib.[189] This nerve is thought to be stretched by depression of the shoulder with lateral flexion of the neck in the opposite direction. Prescott and Zollinger reported two cases of injury with abduction; several mechanisms of injury may be responsible.[189]

The small nerve to the subclavius also comes off the upper trunk. Kopell and Thompson pointed out an interesting relationship of the suprascapular nerve. Protraction of the scapula increases the distance between the cervical spine and the notch because the scapula must move laterally around the thorax to travel forward.[122] This location also predisposes the suprascapular nerve to injury in scapular fractures.[62]

The lateral cord generally contains fibers of C5, C6, and C7 and gives off three terminal branches: the musculocutaneous, the lateral pectoral, and the lateral root of the median nerve. The first branch coming off the lateral cord is the lateral anterior thoracic or lateral pectoral nerve (C5 to C7), which, after leaving the lateral cord, passes anterior to the first part of the axillary artery. This nerve, 4 cm to 6 cm in length,[88] penetrates the clavipectoral fascia above the pectoralis minor at approximately the midpoint of the clavicle and innervates the clavicular portion and some of the sternal portion of the pectoralis major muscle. The nerve also sends a communication to the medial pectoral nerve, which carries its contribution to the remaining portion of the pectoralis major. This loop usually passes over the axillary artery just proximal to the thoracoacromial trunk.[195] Miller,[159] however, showed the artery to be more proximal. The lateral pectoral nerve also innervates the acromioclavicular joint, along with the suprascapular nerve.[75]

The final lateral cord nerve is the lateral root (C5 to C7) to the median nerve. The median nerve is formed anterior to the third portion of the axillary artery and accompanies the brachial artery and vein into the arm.

The posterior cord supplies most of the innervation to the muscles of the shoulder in the following order: upper subscapular, thoracodorsal, lower subscapular, axillary, and radial. Because of the great range of motion of the muscles relative to the brachial plexus, nerves to muscles in the shoulder tend to be quite long and come off quite high in relation to their destination. For this reason and because nerves tend to segregate in neural tissue into groups of fascicles,[262] several authors report that the posterior cord is poorly formed and may be a discrete structure in only 25% of cadavers.[19,119]

The next distal nerve, the thoracodorsal nerve (C7 and C8), is the longest (12 to 18 cm)[88] of the terminal nerves coming off the brachial plexus in the axilla and is referred to as the *long subscapular nerve*, the *long thoracic nerve*, or the *nerve of Bell*. The nerve follows the subscapular and then the thoracodorsal artery along the posterior wall of the axilla to the latissimus dorsi.[119,132] In the latissimus dorsi muscle, the nerve splits into two branches, as does the blood supply.[9]

The final continuation of the posterior cord is the radial nerve (C5 to C8), which continues posterior to the axillary artery and, shortly after exiting the axilla, disappears into the space deep to the long head of the triceps. The nerves to the long and medial heads of the triceps arise where the nerve is still in the axilla. The posterior cutaneous branch also arises in the axilla. A branch that comes off medially, referred to as the *ulnar collateral nerve* because of its proximity to the ulnar nerve, innervates the medial head of the triceps.

The medial cord has five branches in the following order: medial pectoral nerve, medial brachial cutaneous nerve, medial antebrachial cutaneous nerve, medial root of the median nerve, and ulnar nerve. The medial pectoral nerve (C8 and T1) comes off the medial cord, which at this point has finally attained its position medial to the artery. Anteriorly, it passes between the artery and vein (the vein is the more medial structure) and enters the deep surface of the pectoralis minor. Some fibers come out anterior to the muscle to supply the more caudal portions of the pectoralis major. The nerve length varies from 8 to 14 cm.[111] As mentioned earlier, a communicating branch from the lateral pectoral nerve joins the medial pectoral before it enters the pectoralis minor muscle.

The medial brachial cutaneous nerve contains fibers from T1 and is followed in order by the medial antebrachial cutaneous nerves from T1 and C8. Both are cutaneous nerves that supply the area of skin indicated by their names. The medial brachial cutaneous nerve often receives a communication from the intercostal brachial nerve. The medial root of the median nerve (C8 and T1) passes in front of the third portion of the axillary artery to join the lateral root.

The ulnar nerve is the terminal extension of the medial cord. We would expect it to have fibers of C8 and T1 alone, but researchers have found that 50% of specimens have a contribution carrying fibers of C7 from the lateral cord to the ulnar nerve, generally via a nerve off the median nerve.[20,119] The C7 fibers are usually destined for the flexor carpi ulnaris.[132] The ulnar nerve has no important branches in the shoulder area; its first branches appear as it approaches the elbow.

Like all nerves, the brachial plexus receives its blood supply from adjacent arteries. Because there is little motion relative to the vessels, the arteries are short and direct. The blood supply to the brachial plexus proximally was mapped out by Abdullah and Bowden and found to originate from the subclavian artery and its branches (Fig. 2-41).[3] The vertebral artery supplies the proximal plexus along with the ascending and deep cervical arteries and the superior intercostal artery. The autonomic ganglia lying anterior near the spinal column are supplied by branches of the intercostal vessels in the thorax and branches of the vertebral artery in the cervical area. Distally, adjacent arteries provide contributions. The relationship between the plexus and vessels is abnormal in 8% of shoulders,[159] with nerves penetrated by vessels.

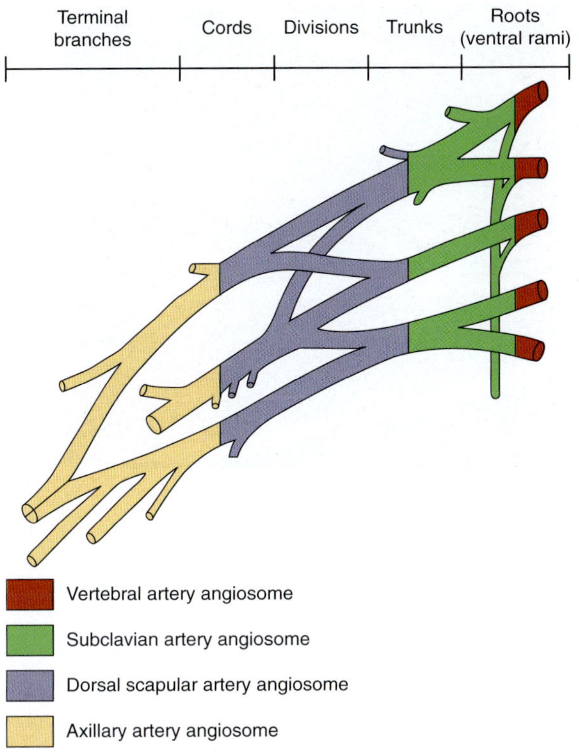

FIGURE 2-41: Blood supply of the proximal brachial plexus and the spinal cord. In the more distal portion of the brachial plexus, the blood supply originates from accompanying arteries and veins. (From Levy SM, Taylor GI, Baudet J, et al. Angiosomes of the brachial plexus: an anatomical study. *Plast Reconstr Surg.* 2003;112[7]:1799-1806.)

SPECIFIC TERMINAL BRANCHES

Because of their importance in surgical dissection in approaches to the shoulder, the following specific terminal nerve branches of the brachial plexus are separately mentioned.

Subscapular Nerves

The upper subscapular nerves (C5) take origin off the posterior cord and enter the subscapularis muscle quite high because there is less relative motion here. These nerves are the shortest of those taking origin from this cord. They supply two-thirds to four-fifths of the upper portion of the subscapularis muscle. The lower subscapular nerves (C5 and C6) follow a long course from their origin before entering the muscles. They innervate the lower portion of the subscapularis muscle and the teres major. Yung, Lazarus, and Harryman[266] specifically dissected out the upper and lower subscapular nerves in relation to their innervation of the subscapularis muscle. They described a safe zone for surgical dissection. They found that the palpable anterior border of the glenoid rim deep to the subscapularis along with the medial border of the conjoint tendon could serve as safe landmarks because all neural branches were at least 1.5 cm medial to the conjoint tendon and all neural branches to the subscapularis were on the anterior surface. Of note, the lower subscapular nerve muscle insertion site is close to the axillary nerve, and the branches are very small. They thus concluded that the location and protection of the axillary nerve could serve as a guide to the insertion point of the lower subscapular nerve.[266] Interestingly, the lower subscapular nerve was recently reported to directly originate from the proximal segment of the axillary nerve in 21% of the cases.[250]

Axillary Nerve

The last branch coming off the posterior cord in the shoulder area is the axillary nerve (C5 and C6). As it disappears into the gap between the subscapularis and teres major, the axillary nerve is accompanied by the posterior circumflex humeral artery. The nerve passes laterally to the inferolateral border of the subscapularis, where it winds 3 to 5 mm medial to the musculotendinous junction. The nerve and artery then pass lateral to the long head of the triceps and are in intimate contact with the capsule.[137] The quadrilateral shape of this space cannot be visualized from the front; when viewed from behind, it is formed by the teres minor superiorly and the teres major inferiorly (Fig. 2-42; see also Fig. 2-32). The medial border is the long head of the triceps, and the lateral border is the shaft of the humerus. Nerve entrapment has also been described in this space.[28]

The axillary nerve divides in the space and sends a posterior branch to the teres minor and the posterior third of the deltoid and an anterior branch to the anterior two-thirds of the deltoid. Ball et al.[7] performed cadaveric dissection of the posterior branch of the axillary nerve and found that the posterior branch divides from the anterior branch just anterior to the origin of the long head of the triceps at the 6 o'clock position. The branch to the teres minor and the superior-lateral brachial cutaneous nerve were observed to arise from the posterior branch of the axillary nerve in all specimens dissected. In most specimens, a branch from the posterior branch was seen to supply the posterior aspect of the deltoid. In all specimens, an additional branch was seen from the anterior branch to the posterior deltoid.[7] The lateral brachial cutaneous nerve supplies the area of skin corresponding in shape to and overlying the deltoid muscle after wrapping around the posterior border of the deltoid.[1] The anterior branch comes to lie approximately 2 inches below the edge of the acromion as the nerve passes anteriorly to innervate the anterior two-thirds of the muscle. One or more small branches attach to the lower border of the posterior deltoid muscle and, unlike the anterior branch, do not proceed vertically toward the spine of the scapula but follow the inferior fibers of the muscle. The axillary nerve also supplies sensory innervation to the lower portion of the glenohumeral joint through two articular branches. The anterior articular branch comes off before the nerve enters the quadrilateral space. The second branch comes off in the space.

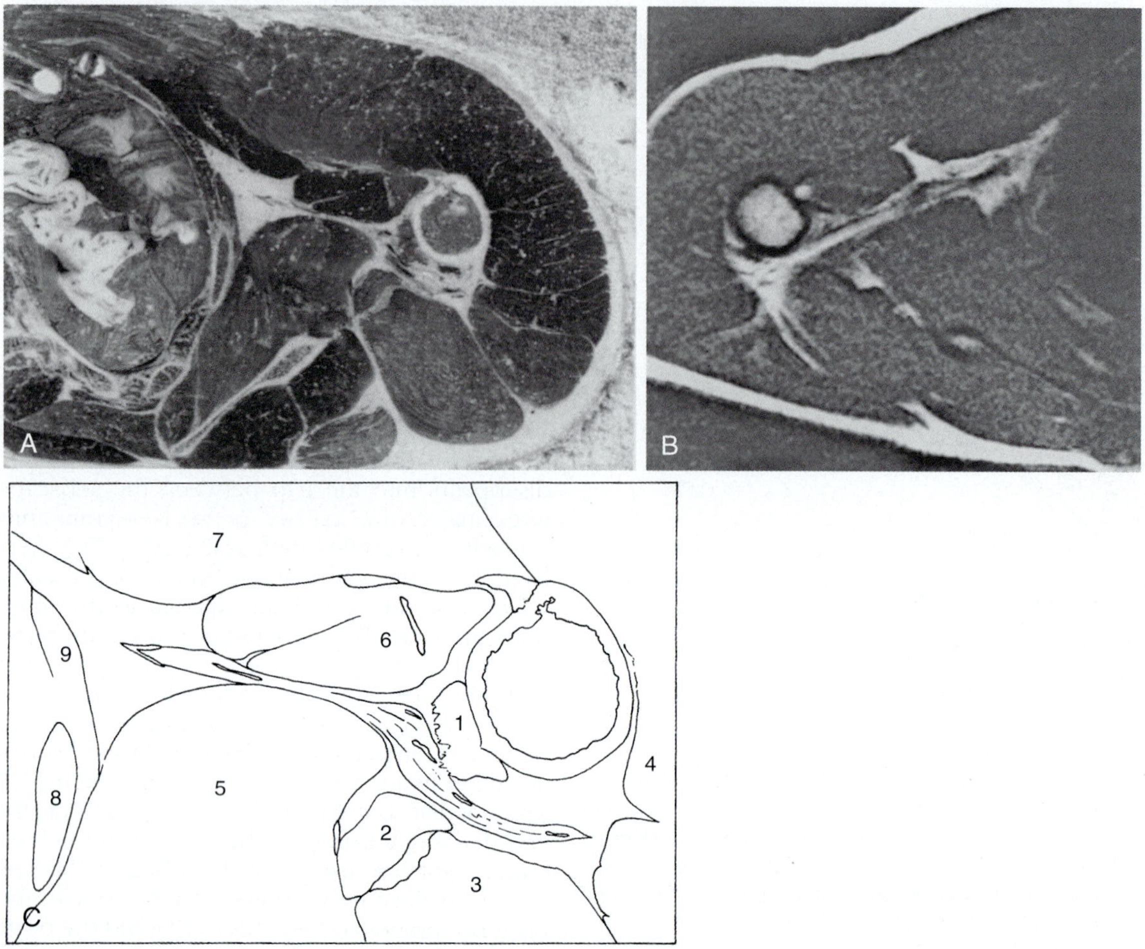

FIGURE 2-42: A, Cross section of a right shoulder showing the quadrilateral space with the nerve and artery coming from the axillary space and passing between the conjoint and subscapularis muscles and then between the triceps and the humerus. Note how small the quadrilateral space is in comparison to the usual representations. **B,** Left shoulder magnetic resonance imaging axial cut showing the quadrilateral space. **C,** Diagram labeling the structures shown in **A:** (1) teres major, (2) teres minor, (3) long head of the triceps, (4) deltoid, (5) infraspinatus, (6) coracobrachialis and short head of the biceps, (7) pectoralis major and minor, (8) rib 3, and (9) serratus anterior.

Together, they are the major nerve supply of the joint.[75] Frequently, another branch accompanies part of the anterior humeral circumflex artery toward the long head of the biceps.

Surgeons worry regarding the axillary nerve safety with deltoid splitting incisions. Cetik et al.[34] performed cadaveric dissection to determine a safe area for the axillary nerve in the deltoid muscle. They found that the average distance from the anterior edge of the acromion to the course of the axillary nerve is an average of 6.08 cm, with 5.2 cm being the closest distance.[34] Stecco et al.[223] looked at the surgical anatomy of the axillary nerve during a transdeltoid approach for proximal humerus locked plating and found the mean distance between the point where the axillary nerve enters into the deltoid muscle and the acromion is 6.8 cm. This coincided with the two distal screws dedicated for the humeral head in their plate, and they recommended avoiding placement of these screws when using a minimally invasive technique. Cheung reported the average distance from the mid-acromion to the superior border of the axillary nerve as 66.6 mm with the shoulder in neutral position. Vertical abduction to 60 degrees moves the superior borders of the axillary nerve significantly, to a distance of 53.9 mm.[36]

Musculocutaneous Nerve

The musculocutaneous nerve (C5 to C7) (Fig. 2-43) originates high in the axilla. The musculocutaneous nerve is commonly thought to enter the coracobrachialis muscle 5 to 8 cm distal to the coracoid process.[97] Flatow et al. found that the nerve did indeed pierce the coracobrachialis at an average of 5.6 cm from the coracoid process.[71] However, they found that the nerve pierces the muscle at a range from 3.1 to 8.2 cm. They also found that small

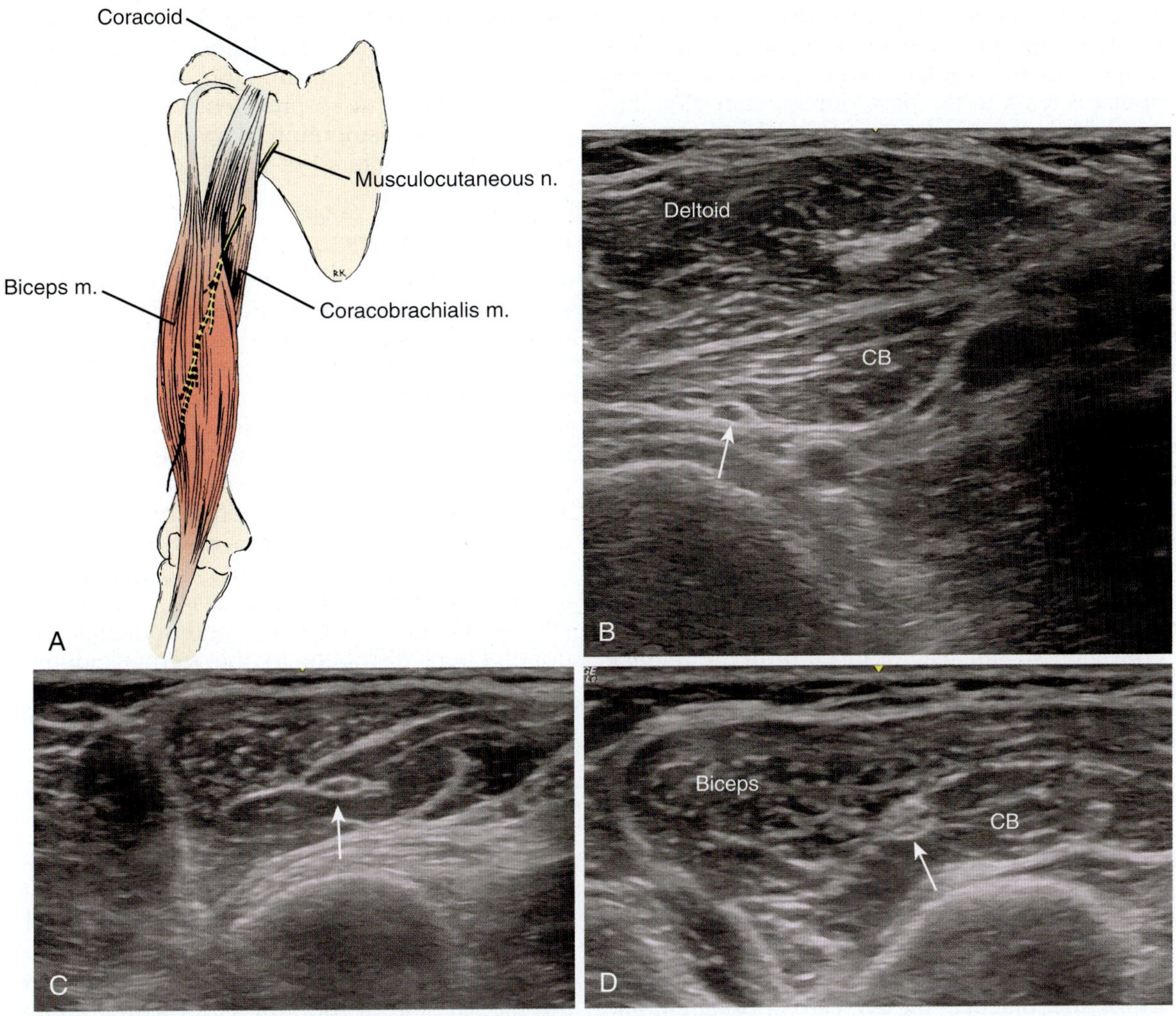

FIGURE 2-43: **A,** Course of the musculocutaneous nerve. This nerve originates from the lateral cord and penetrates the conjoint muscle-tendon on its deep surface. The point of penetration varies; it may be as close as 1.5 cm to the coracoid tip or as far away as 9 cm (average, 5 cm). The nerve continues distally, innervates the long head of the biceps brachii and the brachialis muscle, and appears in the forearm as the lateral antebrachial cutaneous nerve. **B,** Musculocutaneous nerve (*arrow*) at the upper end of coracobrachialis (CB). **C,** Musculocutaneous nerve (*arrow*) in the middle of coracobrachialis. **D,** Musculocutaneous nerve (*arrow*) between coracobrachialis (CB) and biceps.

nerve twigs from the musculocutaneous nerve pierce the coracobrachialis even more proximally, averaging 3.1 cm from the coracoid process, with some as close as 1.7 cm. They concluded that the frequently cited range of 5 to 8 cm could not be relied upon because in 29% of cases, the main nerve entered the muscle proximal to the 5-cm mark. If one includes the smaller branches, 74% of shoulders were found to have one or more nerves entering the muscle in the proximal 5 cm.[71] This entry point is critical because of the number of procedures that may put traction on the nerve. Kerr found nerve branches from the lateral cord or musculocutaneous nerve in slightly more than half of his specimens.[241] The musculocutaneous nerve distally appears in the forearm as the lateral antebrachial cutaneous nerve.

Suprascapular Nerve

The suprascapular nerve arises from the superior lateral aspect of the upper trunk shortly after its formation at Erb's point. This nerve follows a long, oblique course to its next fixed point, the suprascapular notch. This course is parallel to the inferior belly of the omohyoid. The nerve does not move relative to the notch.[197-199] The nerve passes below the transverse scapular or suprascapular ligament and enters the supraspinatus muscle, which it innervates through two branches. Both the origin from the upper trunk and the muscle attachments lie cephalad to the ligament, which forces the nerve to angle around the ligament.[199] This nerve also innervates the infraspinatus muscle through two branches after inferiorly passing around the base of the spine of the scapula.[39]

The suprascapular nerve also provides two articular branches: one in the supraspinatus fossa to the acromioclavicular and superior glenohumeral joints and one in the infraspinatus fossa to the posterior superior glenohumeral joint.[75] The nerve is accompanied by the suprascapular artery, which passes over the transverse scapular ligament. The surrounding bone and ligament form a foramen that may entrap the nerve. Variations in the suprascapular notch anatomy can contribute to nerve entrapment in this area. They include an osseous clavicular tunnel,[175] an ossified transverse scapular ligament, an anterior coracoscapular ligament, and superiorly oriented subscapularis fibers.[174] Paralysis of this nerve has profound effects on shoulder function.[228]

Bigliani et al.[14] performed 90 cadaveric dissections to study the course of the suprascapular nerve, finding that the motor branch to the supraspinatus branches within 1 cm of the suprascapular notch in all specimens. From the base of the scapular spine, the nerve medially curves and innervates the infraspinatus muscle within 1 cm of the base of the scapular spine in nearly 90% of cases. They further found that the nerve courses close to the posterior glenoid rim. The distance from the midline of the posterior glenoid rim to the suprascapular nerve at the base of the scapular spine averages 1.8 cm, with some as close as 1.4 cm.[14] Gumina et al. describe the safe zone to be a distance 2.1 cm from the supraglenoid tubercle to the suprascapular nerve at the scapular notch and 1.1 cm from the midline of the posterior glenoid rim.[87] Compression of the nerve by the spinoglenoid ligament near the base of the spine has been reported.[69,188,244]

Autonomic Supply

All nerves of the brachial plexus carry postganglionic autonomic fibers, with the largest portion (27% to 44%) at C8 and the smallest portion (1% to 9%) at C5.[232] A review of the common structure of the sympathetic nervous system indicates that fibers coming from the spinal cord are myelinated and are collected in what is called the "white" rami communicantes, or type I ramus. Fibers that leave the ganglion (postganglionic fibers) are not myelinated and tend to be collected in the "gray" ramus. Type II rami are gray rami with few myelinated (preganglionic) fibers. Type III rami are mixtures of gray and white fibers. Gray and white rami can also be multiple.[229] The sympathetic supply to C5 and C6 comes through the gray rami from the middle cervical ganglion, the superior cervical ganglion, and the intervening trunks connecting these ganglia. A sympathetic plexus is located on the vertebral artery. Gray rami from the stellate ganglion are received by the C7, C8, and T1 spinal nerves. As mentioned earlier, the autonomic fibers mix immediately with the somatic fibers and do not travel in separate fasciculi.[229] They enter either at the convergence of the roots or proximal to them. Determination of whether a lesion is preganglionic or postganglionic is useful for localizing damage to the brachial plexus. The T2 nerve root is often cited as the cephalad limit of the spinal origin of preganglionic fibers of the sympathetic nervous system, but data indicate that they may arise as high as T1 or C8.[192,229] The caudad limit of preganglionic fibers is T8 or T9.[192] The distribution of sympathetic fibers to vessels is much more prevalent in the hand than in the shoulder. The distribution of sweat and erector pili function probably differs but is still lower in the C5 and C6 areas.[265]

Cranial Nerve XI

The spinal accessory nerve, or 11th cranial nerve, originates from the medulla and upper spinal cord through multiple rootlets. It then ascends back through the foramen magnum and exits in the middle compartment of the jugular foramen. The nerve descends between the internal jugular vein and internal carotid artery for a short distance and then laterally descends as it posteriorly passes to supply the sternocleidomastoid muscle. After exiting the sternocleidomastoid, it continues in an inferior posterior direction across the posterior triangle of the neck and then supplies the trapezius muscle. In the posterior triangle (Fig. 2-44), this nerve receives afferent fibers from C2, C3, and sometimes C4.[45] Some upper fibers distribute to the sternocleidomastoid and the lower fibers to the trapezius. Because the nerve lies so superficially in the posterior triangle, it is at maximal risk for injury.

Intercostal Brachial Nerve

The intercostal brachial nerve is a cutaneous branch of T2 that leaves the thorax from the second intercostal space and crosses over the dome of the axillary fossa. This nerve sends a communication to the medial brachial cutaneous nerve (60%)[119] and may supply sensation on the medial side of the arm as far as the elbow.[19,64] Like many of the cutaneous nerves of the upper part of the arm, it is outside the axillary sheath and is not anesthetized by axillary sheath injection.[19]

Supraclavicular Nerves

The supraclavicular nerves (see Fig. 2-44) originate from the spinal nerves C3 and C4. They are important to the shoulder surgeon because they supply sensation to the shoulder in the area described by their name, the area above the clavicle, in addition to the first two intercostal spaces anteriorly and much of the skin overlying the acromion and deltoid. The ventral rami of C3 to C4 emerge between the longi (colli and capitis) and scalenus medius.[208] The contributions to the supraclavicular nerves join and enter the posterior triangle of the neck around the posterior border of the sternocleidomastoid. They descend on the superficial surface of the platysma in three groups. The medial supraclavicular nerves go to the base of the neck and the medial portion of the first two intercostal spaces. The intermediate supraclavicular nerves go to the middle of the base of the posterior cervical triangle and the upper portion of the thorax in this area. The lateral supraclavicular nerves cross the anterior border of the trapezius muscle and go to the tip

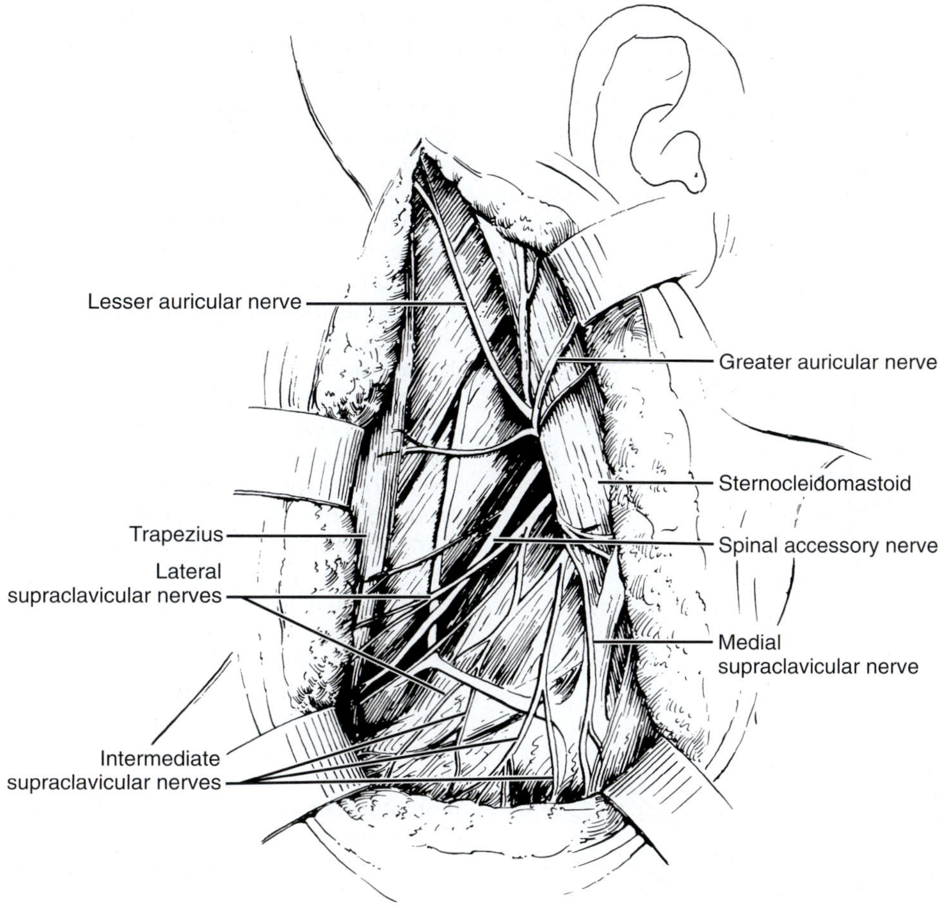

FIGURE 2-44: Spinal accessory nerve and supraclavicular nerves. The supraclavicular nerves in their three groups account for much of the cutaneous innervation of the shoulder. In the posterior triangle, the spinal accessory nerve runs from the sternocleidomastoid to the trapezius, the two superficial muscles of the neck. The spinal accessory nerve lies adjacent to the most superficial layer of deep fascia in the neck.

of the shoulder.[208] The medial nerves may have an anomalous pattern in which they pass through foramina in the clavicle on their way to the anterior of the chest.[78,175,251]

BLOOD VESSELS

Taylor and Palmer,[238] in their extensive studies of circulation of the skin and their literature review, noted basic tendencies in the distribution of blood vessels throughout the body, summarized as follows: (1) blood vessel distribution follows the angiosome concept, the idea that the body is an intricate jigsaw puzzle, each piece of which is supplied by a dominant artery and its accompanying veins; (2) muscles provide a vital anastomotic detour; (3) the arteries link to form a continuous unbroken network; (4) intramuscular watersheds of arteries and veins match; (5) vessels travel with the nerves; (6) vessels follow the connective tissue framework; (7) vessels radiate from fixed to mobile areas; (8) muscle mobility is directly related to the size and density of the supplying vessels (i.e., more mobile muscles will have vessels fewer in number but larger in caliber); (9) the watersheds of vessels are constant, but their origin may be variable; (10) the territory of intramuscular arteries obeys the law of equilibrium (e.g., if a vessel to a structure is larger than the normal surrounding vessels, its neighbors tend to be smaller); (11) vessel size and orientation are the product of tissue differentiation and growth in the area; and (12) muscles are the primary force of venous return.[212,238] We would add here the tendency for vessels to cross joints close to the axis of rotation so that less relative change in length occurs (Fig. 2-45), particularly at the very mobile shoulder. The arteries supplying these blocks of tissue are also responsible for supplying the skin and underlying tissue. These blocks and overlying skin are called angiosomes, in reference to the dominant arterial axes. A fifth tendency reiterated by Taylor and Palmer is an inverse reciprocal relationship between the size of vessels in neighboring contiguous regions, referred to as the *law of equilibrium.*[238]

Elaborating on these themes, they pointed out that vessels rarely cross planes where a great deal of movement takes place.[238] Their illustrations show that when vessels do cross these planes, they have a tendency to cross at the periphery of motion planes or at the ends of muscles, where less relative motion occurs.[238] Moreover, in cases in which the vessel must cross an area of high mobility, it does so in an oblique fashion (Fig. 2-46). Such an oblique crossing is desirable because the strain (strain being deformation expressed as a percentage of the length of the artery) is greatly reduced and yet the absolute motion between the two sides of the plane does not change.

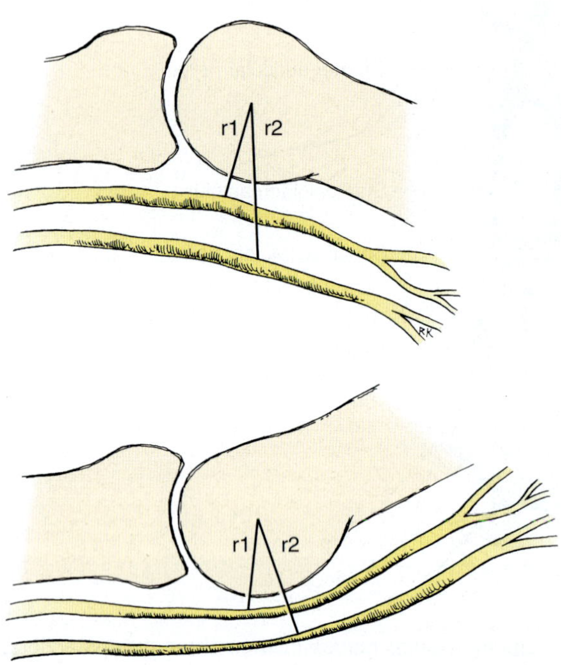

FIGURE 2-45: The strain on a vessel in movement is proportional to its distance from the center of rotation.

The axillary artery and its branches may seem to be an exception to such tendencies. This artery comes from a fixed position adjacent to the first rib and proceeds through a very mobile area within the axilla. The artery returns to another connective tissue framework adjacent to the humerus, where it becomes the brachial artery continuing into the arm. This apparent exception comes about only because of the highly mobile nature of the shoulder. The axillary artery can be thought of as fixed in a connective tissue structure, the axillary sheath, which has some highly mobile adjacent tissue planes, particularly so in relation to the anterior and posterior walls of the axilla. Given this relationship and the tendencies and formation of the vascular system noted earlier, it has been predicted and shown that branches off the axillary artery going to shoulder structures come off more proximal than they would if they followed a direct course to their destination. These branches tend to be long and oblique in the course of their entrance into the muscles and lie outside the axillary sheath. In addition, because structures in the shoulder move relative to each other, one would predict a number of hypovascular fascial planes.[181,212,238] These planes are crossed at the periphery by a few large named vessels rather than directly by a large number of small vessels. These hypovascular planes are frequently found between the pectoralis major and pectoralis minor, between the trapezius and rhomboids, and on the deep surface of the rhomboids (see the section "Bursae, Compartments, and Potential Spaces"). Taylor and Palmer mention the following five angiosomes of the shoulder that have cutaneous representation: the transverse cervical artery, the thoracoacromial

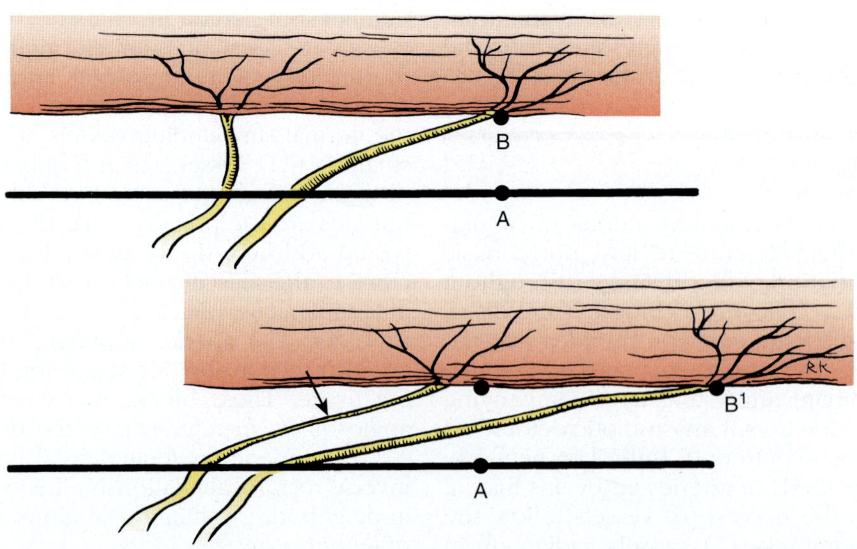

FIGURE 2-46: The oblique course of vessels crossing a motion plane is protective. The vessel that crosses straight across the motion plane is stretched and possibly torn (*arrow*) with the motion that is illustrated, whereas the vessel crossing obliquely has less relative stretch. Crossing at the edge of the plane of motion decreases strain even further.

artery, the suprascapular artery, the posterior humeral circumflex artery, and the circumflex scapular artery.[238]

Arteries and veins are hollow structures with abundant collagen, some elastin, and layers that contain some smooth muscle. They are under control of the autonomic nervous system. Woollard and Weddell found that the distribution of sympathetic nerves to vessels appears to be more abundant in the more distal part of the limb than in the proximal part.[265] In addition, larger arteries and veins have their own blood supply from the base of the vasa vasorum.[95]

Arteries

Arteries (Fig. 2-47) tend to be named by the watershed of the artery rather than the main structure that comes off the axillary or subclavian artery.[249] For example, when the blood supply to the lateral wall of the axillary fossa comes from the pectoral branch of the thoracoacromial artery, it is said that the lateral thoracic artery originates from the pectoral artery rather than the lateral thoracic artery being supplanted by the pectoral artery. Huelke has reported a fairly high occurrence of branches of the axillary artery coming off in common trunks that seem to supplant each other. An interesting exception to the naming rule in the area of the subclavian artery is the dorsal scapular artery. When this artery originates from the thyrocervical trunk, it is called the *deep transverse cervical artery*, although Huelke has tried to correct this nomenclature.[103] *Dorsal scapular artery* is the preferred name.

Subclavian Artery

The blood supply to the limb begins with the subclavian artery, which ends at the lateral border of the first rib. This artery is divided into three portions in relation to the insertion of the scalenus anterior muscle.[52] The vertebral artery originates in the first portion, and the costocervical trunk and thyrocervical trunk take origin in the second portion. Usually, no branches are found in the third portion of the artery. The artery is fairly well protected by the surrounding structures. Rich and Spencer,[202] in their review of the world's literature on vascular injuries, found no large series in which injury to the subclavian artery made up more than 1% of the total arterial injuries. Because the subclavian arteries are protected, injuries affecting them signify more serious trauma than do injuries to other arteries remote to the great vessels.

The first important branch of the subclavian artery, rarely encountered by shoulder surgeons, is the vertebral artery. This branch provides the proximal blood supply to the brachial plexus. The internal mammary artery is always a branch of the vertebral artery.[238] Two vessels encountered more frequently by shoulder surgeons are the transverse cervical artery and the suprascapular artery, which come off the thyrocervical trunk in 70% of cases.[35] In the remaining cases, they come off directly or in common from the subclavian artery. The transverse cervical artery may divide into a superficial branch that supplies the trapezius and a deep branch (when present)

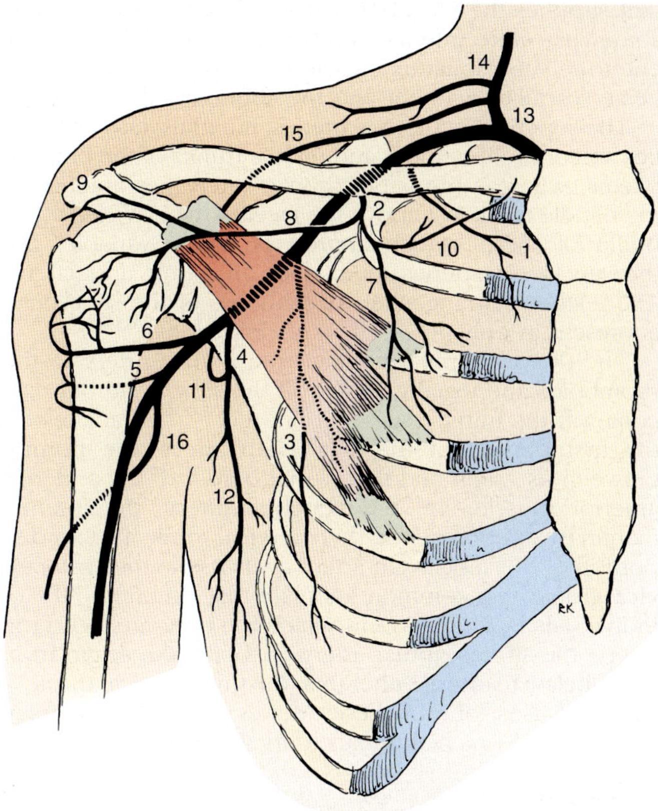

FIGURE 2-47: Major arterial axes of the upper limb. The major arterial axis bears three different names in its course. Medial to the lateral edge of the first rib, it is called the subclavian artery. From the lateral edge of the first rib just proximal to the takeoff of the profunda brachii artery, it is termed the axillary artery, and distal to that it is known as the *brachial artery*. The axillary artery is divided into three portions—superior to the pectoralis minor muscle (as shown), deep to the muscle, and distal to the muscle. This drawing shows the thoracoacromial axis (2) coming off in the first part of the artery, a very common variation. The thoracoacromial axis usually comes off deep to the pectoralis minor. The other variant is the clavicular branch (10), shown as a branch of the pectoral artery. This branch most commonly comes off the thoracoacromial axis as a trifurcation but may arise from any of the branches of the thoracoacromial axis or from the axillary artery itself. Note that most of the branches of the artery are deep to the pectoralis minor and its superior continuation, the clavipectoral fascia. The exception is the thoracoacromial axis and its branches, which lie anterior to the clavipectoral fascia. The labeled branches are as follows: (1) superior thoracic artery, (2) thoracoacromial artery, (3) lateral thoracic artery, (4) subscapular artery, (5) posterior humeral circumflex artery, (6) anterior humeral circumflex artery, (7) pectoral artery, (8) deltoid artery, (9) acromial artery, (10) clavicular artery, (11) circumflex scapular artery, (12) thoracodorsal artery, (13) thyrocervical trunk, (14) transverse cervical artery, (15) suprascapular artery, and (16) profunda brachii artery.

that supplies the rhomboids. The suprascapular artery is somewhat more inferior and traverses the soft tissues to enter the supraspinatus muscle just superior to the transverse scapular ligament and the suprascapular nerve.

The superior of the two arteries, the transverse cervical, lies anterior to the upper and middle trunks of the brachial plexus, whereas the suprascapular artery lies anterior to the middle trunk just above the level of the clavicle.[132] The origin of these branch arteries is highly variable, but the subclavian arteries themselves are rarely anomalous. The textbook arrangement of branches of the subclavian is present in only 46% or less of dissections.[103,191]

The dorsal scapular artery is the normal artery to the rhomboids and usually comes off the subclavian but may come off the transverse cervical artery.[202,208] Branches off the first portion of the subclavian artery, the portion between its origin and the medial border of the scalenus anterior muscle, are the vertebral artery, the internal mammary artery, and the thyrocervical trunk. The second portion of the subclavian artery gives rise to the costocervical trunk.[202] A common anomaly that occurs in 30% of individuals is a variation in which the transverse cervical artery, the suprascapular artery, or both take origin from the subclavian artery rather than the thyrocervical trunk.[193] In most cases, one of these arteries will travel between trunks of the brachial plexus to its destination.[104]

Axillary Artery

The axillary artery is the continuation of the subclavian artery. This artery begins at the lateral border of the first rib and continues to the inferior border of the latissimus dorsi, at which point it becomes the brachial artery. This artery is traditionally divided into three portions. The first portion is above the superior border of the pectoralis minor, the second portion is deep to the pectoralis minor, and the third portion is distal to the lateral border of the pectoralis minor. The usual number of branches for each of the three sections corresponds to the name of the section. The first portion has one branch, the second has two, and the third has three.

First Portion

The first section gives off only the superior thoracic artery, which supplies vessels to the first, second, and sometimes third intercostal spaces.

Second Portion

The first branch given off in the second portion of the artery is the thoracoacromial artery, one of the suppliers of a major angiosome, as defined by Taylor and Palmer.[238] The artery has two very large branches, the deltoid and the pectoral, and two smaller branches, the acromial and clavicular. The acromial branch regularly comes off the deltoid, whereas the clavicular branch has a much more variable origin and can come off any of the other branches, the trunk, or the axillary artery.[195] The thoracoacromial artery pierces the clavipectoral fascia and gives off its four branches.[208] The pectoral branch travels in the space between the pectoralis minor and pectoralis major. In their injection series, Reid and Taylor reported that the pectoral artery supplied the sternocostal portion of the pectoralis major muscles in every case. They found no arterial supply from the pectoral to the pectoralis minor in 46% of dissections and reported that the pectoralis minor received a contribution from the pectoral artery in only 14% of dissections. In 34% of dissections, it appeared that the pectoralis minor received a direct supply from the thoracoacromial trunk.[195]

The arterial supply to the pectoralis major closely coincided with the unique nerve supply of the pectoralis major, with the deltoid artery supplying the clavicular head and the pectoral artery supplying the sternocostal portion.[238] The authors also found that the plane between the pectoralis major and minor is relatively avascular but has a rich layer of anastomoses, with the lateral thoracic artery at the lateral edges of the pectoralis major origin. When the pectoralis major is attached over the fourth and fifth ribs, an anastomotic connection around the fourth rib area is noted. The pectoral branch also supplies most of the skin anterior to the pectoralis major through vessels that come around the lateral edge of the pectoralis major.[238]

The deltoid artery is laterally directed and supplies the clavicular head of the pectoralis major and much of the anterior deltoid. This artery also supplies an area of skin over the deltopectoral groove through vessels that emerge from the deltopectoral groove, usually including one large fasciocutaneous or musculocutaneous perforator.

The acromial artery is generally a branch of the deltoid artery that proceeds up to the acromioclavicular joint. This artery has an anastomotic network with other portions of the deltoid, the suprascapular, and the posterior humeral circumflex arteries and frequently has an important cutaneous branch.[238]

The clavicular artery often comes off the trunk or the pectoral artery and runs up to the sternoclavicular joint. Reid and Taylor noticed that when the clavicular artery was injected, there was staining of the periosteum in the medial half of the clavicle and the skin in this area.[238] The clavicular artery also has anastomotic connections with the superior thoracic artery, the first perforator of the inferior mammary, and the suprascapular artery.

The second artery that comes off the second portion of the axillary artery is the lateral thoracic artery, the most variable of the arteries in the axilla in terms of origin.[104,249] In approximately 25% of specimens it originates from the subscapular artery.[249] At other times, it originates from the pectoral branch of the thoracoacromial artery. The lateral thoracic artery runs deep to the pectoralis minor and supplies blood to the pectoralis minor, serratus anterior, and intercostal spaces 3 to 5. It forms a rich anastomotic pattern with intercostal arteries 2 to 5, the pectoral artery, and the thoracodorsal branch of the subscapular artery. In some cases the thoracodorsal artery gives origin to the vessels of the lateral thoracic distribution. A variation of the second portion of the axillary artery that Huelke found in 86% of cadavers is an upper subscapular artery whose course parallels the upper subscapular nerve.[104] This vessel may prove to be an important artery to the subscapularis because of the absence of important branches off the subscapular artery before the circumflex scapular.[9]

Third Portion

The largest branch of the axillary artery, the subscapular artery, originates in the third part of the axillary artery. This artery caudally runs on the subscapularis muscle, which it reportedly supplies.[95] However, Bartlett et al. found no important branches of the subscapular artery before the origin of the circumflex scapular artery.[9] The subscapular artery gives off a branch to the posterior portion of the shoulder, the circumflex scapular artery, which posteriorly passes under the inferior edge of the subscapularis and then medial to the long head of the triceps through the triangular space, where it supplies a branch to the inferior angle of the scapula and a branch to the infraspinatus fossa.[150] These two branches anastomose with the suprascapular and the transverse cervical arteries. The circumflex scapular artery has an additional large cutaneous branch that is used in an axial free flap.[150]

The continuation of the subscapular is the thoracodorsal artery, which runs with the thoracodorsal nerve toward the latissimus dorsi on the subscapularis, teres major, and latissimus dorsi and has branches to the lateral thoracic wall.

The posterior humeral circumflex comes off posteriorly in the third portion and descends into the quadrilateral space with the axillary nerve. After emerging on the posterior side of the shoulder beneath the teres minor, the artery divides in a fashion similar to the nerve. The anterior branch travels with the axillary nerve, approximately 2 inches below the level of the acromion, and supplies the anterior two-thirds of the deltoid. It has a small communicating branch over the acromion with the acromial branch of the thoracoacromial axis and has a communicating branch posteriorly with the deltoid branch of the profunda brachii. This artery also has small branches to the glenohumeral joint. It supplies an area of skin over the deltoid, particularly the middle third of that muscle, through connecting vessels that directly travel to the overlying skin that is firmly attached to the underlying deltoid. The posterior branch corresponds to and accompanies the posterior axillary nerve.

The next branch is the anterior humeral circumflex artery, which is smaller than the posterior humeral circumflex. It is an important surgical landmark because it laterally travels at the inferior border of the subscapularis tendon, where it marks the border between the upper tendinous insertion of the subscapularis and the lower muscular insertion. The artery has anastomoses deep to the deltoid with a posterior humeral circumflex artery. It supplies some branches to the subscapularis muscle. One branch of the anterior humeral circumflex artery crosses the subscapularis tendon anteriorly, where it is regularly encountered during anterior glenohumeral reconstruction.[106] Another branch superiorly runs with the long head of the biceps and supplies most of the humeral head. Gerber[79] et al. found that the anterolateral ascending branch of the anterior humeral circumflex artery supplies the majority of the humeral head. This branch runs parallel to the lateral aspect of the long head of the biceps tendon and has a constant insertion point where the intertubercular groove meets the greater tuberosity. The terminal end branch is called the arcuate artery. Although the main arterial blood supply to the humeral head is via this terminal branch, Brooks et al.[25] found significant intraosseous anastomsoses between the arcuate artery and posteriormedial vessels from the posterior humeral circumflex. They concluded that some perfusion of the humeral head persists such as in a fracture, the head fragment distally extends below the articular surface. This conclusion has been clinically confirmed in a new proximal humerus fracture classification scheme.[90]

Nonpathologic Anomalies

The function of arteries to deliver blood is related to the cross-sectional area of the delivering artery rather than the particular route the artery takes because arterioles are the resistance vessels.[224,225] Arteries are therefore less dependent on straight line continuity for their function than are nerves. One would expect a higher rate of deviance from the anatomic norm without physiologic consequence among the vessels than nerves, and such turns out to be the case.[144,249] This concept is even more understandable when we recall that contiguous watersheds are connected by choke arteries and that when the vessels in one area are large, those in the adjacent area are small.[181,238] The types of arterial anomalies are similar to those of nerves: a change in the position of origin of the artery, duplication or reduction in the number of stem arteries, and total absence of the artery with its function taken over by another artery.

The oblique route of the arteries as they course to their destination is necessitated by motion in the shoulder. As one might expect, a proximal displacement of arterial origin is more frequent than a distal one. The most common example is proximal displacement of the thoracoacromial axis, which is found in at least a third of cadavers.[104,119,242]

The next most frequently displaced arterial stem is the subscapular artery, which originates in the second part of the axillary artery[54] in 16% to 29% of cases.[104,191] In a small percentage of cases, the superior thoracic artery is proximally moved to take origin off the subscapular artery. Few cases of arteries distally moved have been reported.

Another frequent variation is an increase or decrease in the number of direct branches from the axillary artery.[54,104,191,249] For example, in addition to the branches discussed earlier, Huelke described a seventh branch that he found in 86% of his dissections.[104] This short, direct branch accompanies the short upper subscapular nerve (and is similar in anatomy), thus suggesting the name *upper subscapular artery*.

A change in branch number occurs when a branch of one of the six named arterial stems coming off the axillary artery directly originates from another artery or when two or more are joined in a common stem. In Huelke's series of dissections, he found seven branches in only 26.7% of dissections, six branches in 37%, five branches in 16%, and fewer than five in 11%. De Garis and Swartley reported as many as 11 separate branches from the axillary artery.[54] The most frequent common stems are those of the transverse cervical and suprascapular arteries, which form a common stem off the thyrocervical trunk in as many as 28% of cadavers.[193] The next most common origin is the posterior humeral circumflex artery with the anterior humeral circumflex (11%) or the subscapular artery (15%). The opposite of consolidation can also occur when major branches of these six or seven named branches directly originate from the axillary artery. This anomaly is seen most often in the thoracoacromial axis, where the various branches may come off separately from the axillary artery, although only a small number of cases have been reported.

The final nonpathologic anomaly is total absence of an artery with its function performed by one of the other branches. The lateral thoracic artery is the most commonly absent, and its function is supplanted by branches off the subscapular, the pectoral branch of the thoracoacromial, or both. This variant has been seen in as many as 25% of specimens.[54,104,249]

Collateral Circulation

A number of significant anastomoses contribute to good collateral circulation around the shoulder (Figs. 2-48 and 2-49). The subclavian artery communicates with the third portion of the axillary artery through anastomosis with the transverse cervical, dorsal scapular, and suprascapular arteries and branches of the subscapular artery. Moreover, communications can be found between the posterior humeral circumflex artery and the anterior circumflex, deltoid, suprascapular, and profunda brachii arteries. Communications may also be found between the thoracoacromial artery and the intercostal arteries, particularly the fourth intercostal.

This abundant collateral circulation is both an asset to tissue viability and a disadvantage to assessment of possible arterial injury. Collateral circulation ameliorates some of the effects of an injury or sudden blockage of

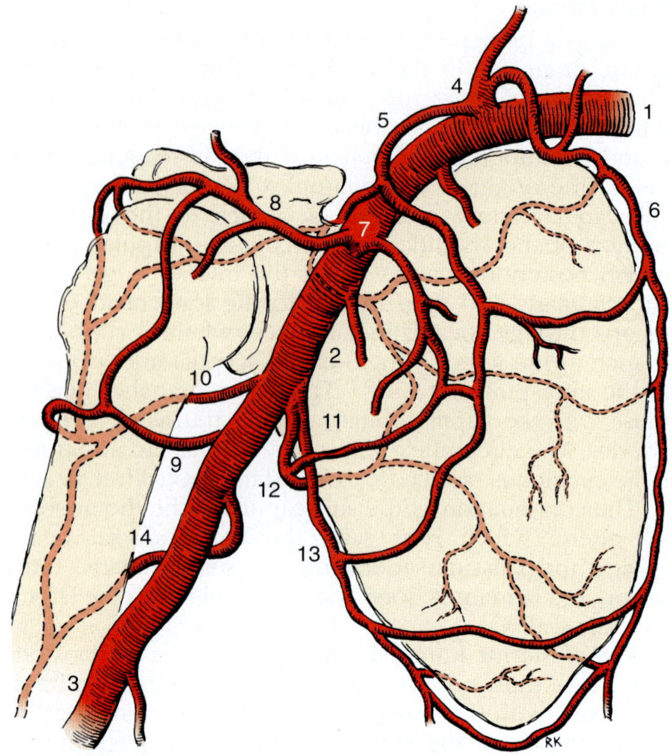

FIGURE 2-48: Diagram demonstrating the large amount of collateral circulation around the shoulder. Some license has been taken in depicting the dorsal scapular and suprascapular collaterals anterior to the major arterial axis. The labeled arteries are as follows: (1) subclavian, (2) axillary, (3) brachial, (4) thyrocervical trunk, (5) suprascapular, (6) dorsal scapular, (7) thoracoacromial trunk, (8) deltoid, (9) anterior humeral circumflex, (10) posterior humeral circumflex, (11) subscapular, (12) circumflex scapular, (13) thoracodorsal, and (14) profunda brachii. (Modified from Rich NM, Spencer F. *Vascular Trauma*. Philadelphia: WB Saunders; 1978.)

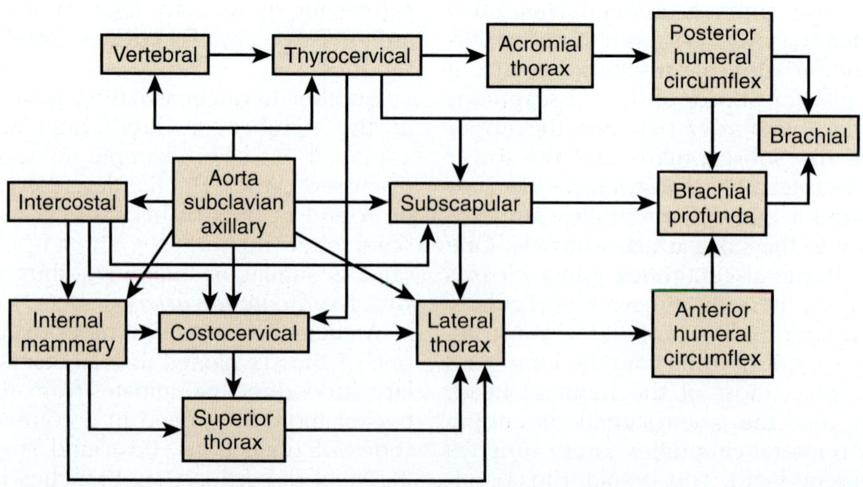

FIGURE 2-49: Diagram of the collateral circulation. The number of collaterals decreases in areas where dense collagenous structures must move adjacent to each other (e.g., near the glenohumeral joint). (Modified from Radke HM. Arterial circulation of the upper extremity. In: Strandness DE Jr, ed. *Collateral Circulation in Clinical Surgery*. Philadelphia: WB Saunders; 1969:294-307.)

the axillary artery. A limb may survive on a flow pressure as low as 20 mm Hg, which would be fatal to the brain or heart.[224] In the Vietnam War, axillary artery injury had the lowest amputation rate of any of the regions of the arterial tree.[200] These anastomoses may on occasion obscure the diagnosis. Although the collateral circulation may transmit a pulse wave (13 to 17 m/sec), it may not be sufficient to allow a flow wave (40 to 50 cm/sec) because flow varies with the fourth power of the radius of the vessels. Even though the collaterals may have a total cross-sectional area close to that of the axillary artery, resistance is greatly increased.[184,224] Furthermore, the same injury that interrupts flow in the axillary or subclavian artery may injure the collateral circulation.[155,202]

The seriousness of a missed diagnosis in injury is demonstrated by reports on arterial ligation. Ferguson and Holt quote Bailey as showing a 9% amputation rate for subclavian artery ligation and a 9% amputation rate for ligation of the axillary artery during World War I.[70] More recent battlefield statistics from DeBakey and Simeon[53] in World War II and Rich et al.[200] in the Vietnam War reveal a much higher amputation rate: approximately 28.6% for subclavian artery injury in Vietnam and 43% for axillary artery injury in World War II.[53] An outstanding exception to this dismal report is the treatment of arteriovenous fistula and false aneurysm, where ligation has very low morbidity, perhaps because of enlarged collateral vessels.[201] Interestingly, in the 10 cases of subclavian artery ligation found in the Vietnam War registry, no subsequent amputations were needed, as opposed to an overall rate of 28% with subclavian wounds. Conversely, both of the two axillary artery ligations ended in amputation.[202] Radke points out that collateral vessels are fewer in number when compact and mobile tissues span the joint.[191]

The percentages of amputations reflect the rate of gangrene necessitating amputation after ligation and ignore the severe nerve pain syndromes that often occur with inadequate circulation.[202] Rich and Spencer believe that the increased gangrene rates among the military in World War II and Vietnam over World War I reflect the increasing severity of war wounds. In any event, neither the old nor the modern gangrene rate is acceptable. Axillary or subclavian artery injuries need repair, if possible, not ligation, and therefore require early diagnosis.[202]

Veins

Axillary

The axillary vein begins at the inferior border of the latissimus dorsi as a continuation of the basilic vein, continues to the lateral border of the first rib, and becomes the subclavian vein.[95,171] This vein is a single structure, in contradistinction to many venae comitantes, which are often double. The subscapular vein is also a single vessel.[9] The axillary and subclavian veins usually have only one valve each,[259] whereas most muscle veins have many valves.[258] Each vein lies anterior to its artery and, especially in its proximal portion, medial or inferior to the artery. Most of the venous drainage is to the axillary vein, except for branches that accompany the thoracoacromial artery, where more than half empty into the cephalic vein rather than continuing all the way to the axillary vein.[195] The relationships of the axillary vein are the artery, which tends to be posterior and lateral, and the brachial plexus. The medial pectoral nerve emerges from the brachial plexus between the artery and the vein. The ulnar nerve comes to lie directly behind the vein as it courses down the arm. The upper limb is similar to the lower limb, which uses a muscle pump action to aid venous return. In the upper limb, the deltoid and triceps muscles receive afferent veins from adjacent muscle and subcutaneous tissue.[258]

Cephalic

The cephalic vein is a superficial vein in the arm that lies deep to the deep fascia after reaching the deltopectoral groove and finally pierces the clavipectoral fascia and empties into the axillary vein.[95] The cephalic vein is absent in 4% of cases. This vein receives no branches from the pectoralis major muscle in the groove[195] and thus drains primarily the deltoid muscle and is often laterally preserved when doing a deltopectoral approach. The cephalic vein is an important landmark in identifying the deltopectoral interval. It is covered by a constant fat stripe in the deltopectoral groove that can be helpful in both identifying the vein and in determining its absence.

The lymph nodes of the axilla lie on the surface of the venous structures. The axillary vein often needs to be excised to obtain adequate node dissection in mastectomy. Lymphatic occlusion, rather than removal of the vein, is believed to be the cause of edema in the arm.[51,116,169] Such a mechanism might mitigate against venous repair, but Rich and associates report that disruption of venous return in the lower extremity results in a higher rate of amputation.[201] Preservation of the cephalic vein, during surgery is thought to potentially reduce postoperative discomfort.

Lymphatic Drainage

Lymph drainage in the limbs is more highly developed superficially, where the lymph channels follow the superficial veins, than in the deep portion of the limb, where the lymph channels follow the arteries.[95,208] Lymphatics in the arm generally flow to the axillary nodes (Fig. 2-50). The more radially located lymphatics in the arm may cross to the ulnar side and hence to the axilla or may consistently drain with the cephalic vein and deltopectoral node, in which case they bypass the axilla and drain into the cervical nodes.[51]

The lymph nodes are named by the area of the axillary fossa in which they lie rather than by the area that they drain. The areas that they drain are rather constant, and each group of nodes receives one to three large afferents.[35] The nodes are richly supplied with arterial blood and seem to have a constant relationship to their arteries.[27] Drainage from the breast area and anterior chest wall passes into the pectoral nodes (thoracic nodes), which lie on the lateral surface of ribs 2 to 6, deep to or

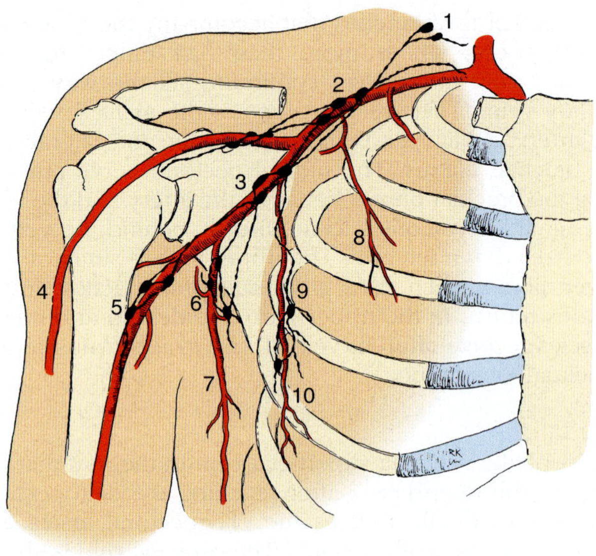

FIGURE 2-50: The location of groups of lymph glands or nodes in the axilla and some of their major interconnections. The main drainage is into the vein, but they also have connections to the deep cervical nodes. Labeled nodes and vessels are as follows: (1) deep cervical, (2) apical, (3) central, (4) cephalic vein, (5) lateral, (6) subscapular, (7) thoracodorsal artery, (8) pectoral artery, (9) pectoral nodes, and (10) lateral thoracic artery.

within the serratus anterior fascia on both sides of the lateral thoracic artery. This group is almost contiguous with the central group. On the posterior wall of the axillary fossa are subscapular nodes that lie on the wall of the subscapularis muscle. They are adjacent to the thoracodorsal artery and nerve and drain lymph from this area, as well as from the posterior surface of the shoulder, back, and neck. These two groups drain into the central, or largest, nodes and higher nodes. The central nodes also receive drainage from the lateral nodes (or brachial nodes) on the medial surface of the great vessels in the axilla and are related to the lateral thoracic and thoracodorsal arteries. All these nodes drain into the apical nodes (subpectoral nodes), which may produce an afferent into the subclavian lymphatic trunk. They then join the thoracic duct on the left side or directly flow into the vein on the right. Some afferents drain into the deep cervical nodes and have a separate entrance into the venous system through the jugular vein.

Relationships

The axillary artery lies in the axillary space, well cushioned by fat, and is relatively well protected from compression damage. As previously mentioned, relatively few injuries occur to the subclavian artery. It is not usually involved in thoracic outlet syndrome. A case in which a normal artery is involved in a compression syndrome is in the quadrilateral space, where the posterior humeral circumflex may become compressed. Although the arteries in the shoulder are arranged around normal mechanics, one would predict that alterations in joint mechanics might endanger the arteries, but such is not often the case. Most indirect arterial damage involves cases of diseased arteries, as occurs in glenohumeral dislocation.[82,114]

BURSAE, COMPARTMENTS, AND POTENTIAL SPACES

With any study of regional anatomy, structures that allow or restrain the spread of substances into or from that part of the body are important considerations. The substances may be local anesthetics, edema from trauma, infection, or tumor. Surgeons are able to extend their surgical exposure or are prevented from doing so by such spaces and barriers. Sufficiency of the barrier is related to the speed with which the substance can spread. For example, we prefer that local anesthetics act within a few minutes. A fascial barrier that prevents such spread may be insufficient to prevent the propagation of postinjury trauma that proliferates over a period of hours. Similarly, a barrier that can contain edema, thus causing a compartment syndrome, may be insufficient to act as a compartment barrier against the propagation of a tumor that enlarges over a period of weeks or months.

Tumor Compartments

Musculoskeletal tumor surgeons have emphasized the concept of anatomic compartments for many years. They point out that tumors centrifugally grow until they encounter a collagen barrier of fascia, tendon, or bone that limits their growth. Tumors tend to more rapidly spread in the direction in which no anatomic barriers are encountered. Therefore a compartment is an anatomic space bounded on all sides by a dense collagen barrier.[67]

Enneking[67] lists four compartments in the shoulder: the scapula and its muscular envelope, the clavicle, the proximal end of the humerus, and the deltoid. The axillary space is a primary example of a space that is, by definition, extracompartmental. It is bounded by fascia posteriorly, medially, and anteriorly and has bone along its lateral border but provides no anatomic barrier to the spread of tumor in the proximal or distal direction.

Infection

Fortunately, infections in the shoulder area are rare in comparison to the hand, probably because of less exposure to trauma and foreign bodies in the shoulder area. Crandon pointed out that a potentiating anatomic feature for the development of infection in the hands is a closed space, which is infrequent in the shoulder.[48] The shoulder has three diarthrodial joints: the sternoclavicular, the acromioclavicular, and the glenohumeral. In the absence of penetrating trauma or osteomyelitis, these areas are the most likely to become infected, especially in individuals who are predisposed by a systemic disease.

Compartment Syndromes

Gelberman reported that shoulder area compartment syndromes are found in the biceps, triceps, and deltoid. These syndromes are most often secondary to drug overdose compression syndromes,[77] which occur when an individual has been lying in one position and does not move to relieve this compression because of a low level of consciousness as a result of a drug overdose. The compression occurs in the most topographically prominent muscles that can be laid upon. Compartment syndromes can also develop after severe trauma in which compression occurs. Gelberman[77] pointed out that the middle deltoid, because of its multipennate nature, actually consists of many small compartments with regard to the containment of edema; however, with the spread of tumor, the deltoid is a single compartment (Fig. 2-51). Therefore decompression of the deltoid requires multiple epimysiotomies in the middle third to adequately release the edema (see Fig. 2-25).

Regional Anesthesia Compartments

The area of the shoulder most closely relevant to anesthesia is the axillary sheath, which begins in the neck as the prevertebral layer of the cervical fascia. This layer of fascia originates in the posterior midline and passes laterally deep to the trapezius. It covers the superficial surfaces of the muscles of the neck and, as it passes forward, forms the floor of the posterior triangle of the neck. It passes lateral to the scalene muscles and lateral to the upper portion of the brachial plexus and then just anterior to the anterior scalene, the longus colli, and the longus capitis muscles. In this anterior position it is truly prevertebral. The axillary sheath laterally and distally continues to surround the brachial plexus and the axillary artery and nerve. The sheath serves the purpose of confining injected material and keeping it in contact with the nerves. In combination with the adjacent brachial fascia, it is also capable of containing the pressure of a postarteriogram hematoma enough to produce nerve compression.[221]

The interscalene position (Fig. 2-52) of the brachial plexus is quite spacious, and the appropriate anesthetic technique requires volume.[68,161] As the sheath laterally proceeds toward the axilla, it is most dense proximally. Thompson and Rorie found septa between the various components in the sheath in anatomic dissections and by tomography (Fig. 2-53).[243] At least three compartments were present, which may account for the need for multiple injections into the axillary sheath to achieve adequate brachial plexus anesthesia and may explain why axillary hematoma does not affect the entire brachial plexus at once. As we continue without pictures of the sheath as a connective tissue structure moving in relation to the adjacent structures, we should not be surprised to learn that the nerves to the shoulder and upper part of the arm already lie outside the sheath in the arm where axillary block is performed, thus necessitating the use of a distal tourniquet to force the proximal migration of anesthetic solutions.

Fascial Spaces and Surgical Planes

Surgical dissection is greatly facilitated by planes or areas of the body that are relatively avascular and without nerves

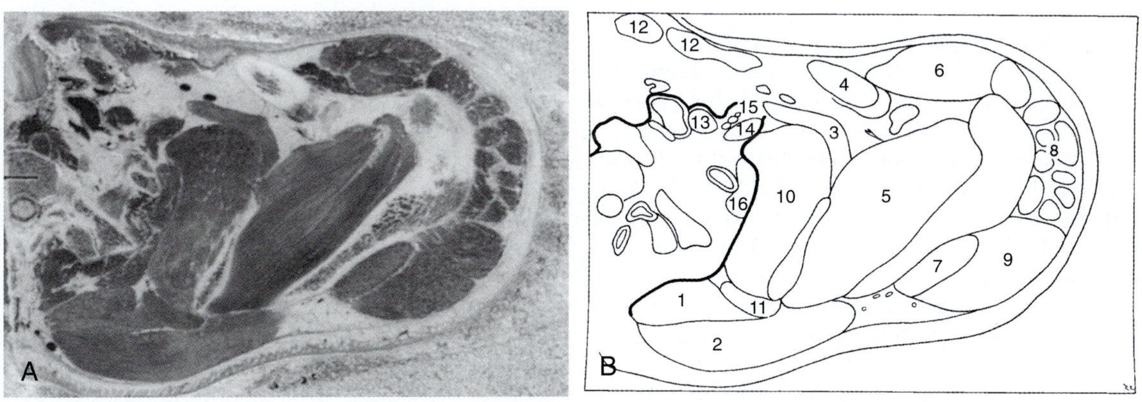

FIGURE 2-51: Image **(A)** and diagram **(B)** of a cross section of the shoulder at the level of the acromion. Several important spaces within the shoulder are demonstrated, beginning with the *heavy line* in B showing the prevertebral fascia, which contributes to formation of the axillary sheath. In the middle portion anteriorly is a deposit of adipose tissue that is the upper end of the axillary space. Posteriorly, at the base of the spine of the scapula, a body of adipose tissue is located between the trapezius and the deltoid, wherein lie the ramifications of the cutaneous branch of the circumflex scapular artery. At the most lateral extent can be seen the multipennate formation of the middle third of the deltoid, which demonstrates why this portion of the muscle should be considered as multiple compartments when treating compartment syndrome. The labeled structures are as follows: (1) rhomboid major, (2) trapezius, (3) omohyoid, (4) clavicle, (5) supraspinatus, (6) anterior third of the deltoid, (7) infraspinatus, (8) middle third of the deltoid, (9) posterior third of the deltoid, (10) serratus anterior, (11) rhomboid minor, (12) sternocleidomastoid, (13) scalenus anterior, (14) scalenus medius, (15) brachial plexus, and (16) scalenus posterior.

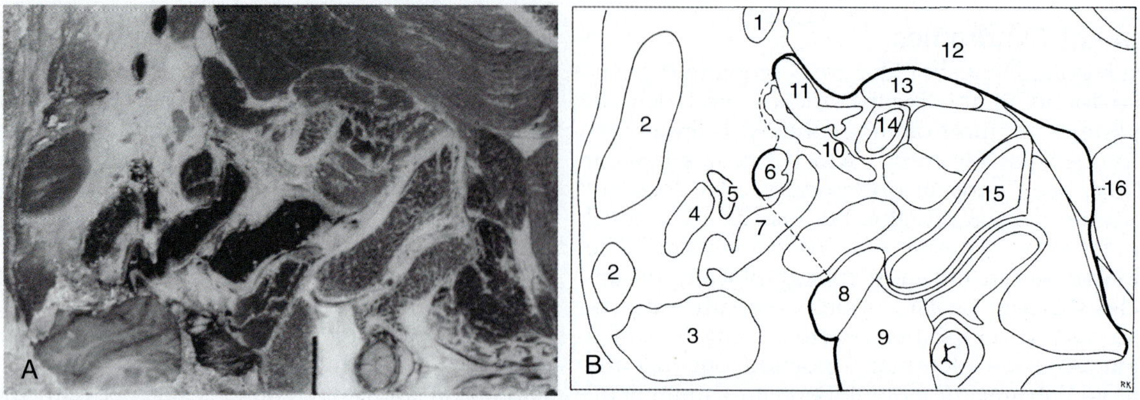

FIGURE 2-52: Image **(A)** and diagram **(B)** of a horizontal cross section of the interscalene interval at the level where the subclavian artery is just beginning to pass behind the scalenus anterior. The heavy line (16) is the prevertebral fascia, which goes on to constitute the proximal axillary sheath at the proximal end. This space is so capacious that anesthesia in this area requires a dose of at least 40 mL. The labeled structures are as follows: (1) omohyoid, (2) sternocleidomastoid, (3) lung, (4) sternohyoid, (5) subclavian vein, (6) scalenus anterior, (7) subclavian artery, (8) longus colli, (9) T2 vertebra, (10) brachial plexus, (11) scalenus medius, (12) serratus anterior, (13) scalenus posterior, (14) rib 1, (15) rib 2, and (16) prevertebral fascia.

(see the sections "Nerves" and "Vessels" for discussion). The crossing of planes by nerve or vessel is greatly discouraged by movement across that plane. This does not mean that no vessels cross such planes, but when these planes are crossed, the vessels tend to be fewer in number and larger in size, are named, and cross in an oblique fashion to accommodate the motion. They tend to enter muscles near the points of origin or insertion and thus decrease the effect of excursion of the muscle. Collateral vessels between adjacent watersheds also cross at the periphery of the planes of motion (Fig. 2-54). The shoulder is the most mobile part of the human body and, as one would expect, contains the greatest number of accommodations for that motion. Three structures specifically allow for motion: bursae, loose alveolar tissue, and adipose tissue.

In loose alveolar tissue, the fibers and cellular elements are widely spaced. The purpose of this type of tissue is to facilitate motion between structures in relation to each other: usually muscle and muscle or muscle and underlying bone. These fascial spaces (Figs. 2-55 to 2-57; see also Fig. 2-54) can be easily penetrated by pus or other unwanted fluid and yet are also useful to surgeons because of the paucity of small vessels and nerves traversing them.[238] Again, this is not to say that no vessels are present. Crossing vessels and nerves tend to be large, are named, and are usually well known and easily avoided. These fascial spaces therefore provide useful passages for dissection. The most commonly observed fascial space is seen deep to the deltopectoral groove, beneath the deltoid and pectoralis major muscles, and superficial to the underlying pectoralis minor muscle and conjoint tendon. This space deep to the pectoralis major and deltoid muscles is crossed by branches of the thoracoacromial artery close to the clavicle, with no other crossing vessels of note.

When a deltoid-splitting incision is used in a posterior approach to the shoulder, a space is encountered between the deep surface of the deltoid and the outer surface of the infraspinatus and teres minor. The crossing structures are the axillary nerve and posterior circumflex artery at the inferior border of the teres minor. Deep on the costal surface of the serratus anterior, posterior to its origins, is a fascial space continuous with the loose alveolar tissue lying deep to the rhomboids. This avascular plane is used by tumor surgeons when performing a forequarter amputation and by pediatric orthopaedists when correcting an elevated scapula in a fashion that results in a less bloody dissection. Note in the illustrations that these spaces are thinner than the ink that the artist used to depict them. Their presence must be borne in mind when interpreting tomograms and planning tumor margins that may be compromised by this loose tissue. This same caveat applies to bursae.

Another way to analyze surgical planes is to think of dissection in layers. Cooper and colleauges[44] found four consistent supporting anatomic layers over the glenohumeral joint. Layer 1 consists of the deltoid and pectoralis major muscles. Layer 2 contains the clavipectoral fascia, coracoid process, conjoint tendon, and the coracoacromial ligament. Posteriorly, the posterior scapular fascia is continuous with the clavicpectoral fascia. Layer 3 contains the rotator cuff muscles. Finally, layer 4 is the glenohumeral capsule.

Adipose Tissue

Adipose tissue provides the double function of cushioning nerves and vessels and allowing the pulsation of arteries and dilation of veins.[238] It also allows movement of tissues in relation to each other. The shoulder has three deposits of adipose tissue that indicate the position of an enclosed nerve or artery. The largest is the axillary space, which contains the brachial plexus and its branches, the axillary artery and vein, and the major

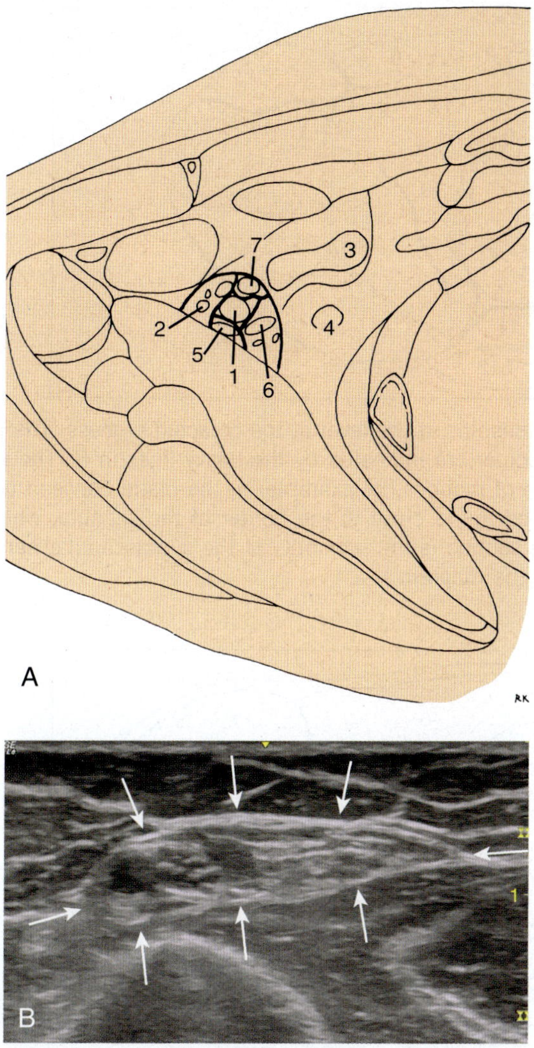

FIGURE 2-53: **A,** Cross-sectional diagram of the axillary sheath demonstrating the septa between the structures contained within the sheath. The labeled structures are as follows: (1) axillary artery, (2) musculocutaneous nerve, (3) vein, (4) lymph node, (5) axillary nerve, and (6) median nerve. **B,** Ultrasound view of the sheath (*arrows*) and the contained nerves and vessels.

lymphatic drainage from the anterior chest wall, upper limb, and back.

The axillary space (Fig. 2-58; see also Figs. 2-51 to 2-56) is bounded posteriorly by a wall of muscle, which from top to bottom are the subscapularis, the teres major, and the latissimus dorsi muscles. The latissimus dorsi forms the muscle undergirding the posterior axillary fold. These three muscles are innervated by the upper and lower subscapular nerve and by the thoracodorsal nerve, formerly referred to as the *middle subscapular nerve.* The anterior boundary of the axillary space is the pectoralis minor muscle and the clavipectoral fascia (see Fig. 2-58). Superior to the pectoralis minor is a dense layer of fascia, referred to as the *clavipectoral fascia,* that continues medially and superiorly from the pectoralis minor. It continues medially to the first rib as the costocoracoid membrane. The pectoralis major muscle and tendon form the more definitive anterior boundary at the inferior extent of the axillary space, although the clavipectoral fascia continues to the axilla. The medial boundary of the space is the serratus anterior muscle and the ribs. The lateral boundary is the portion of the humerus between the insertions of the teres major and latissimus dorsi and the insertion of the pectoralis major, which defines the lower extent of the intertubercular groove. In the anatomic position, the axillary space resembles a warped pyramid; its lateral border actually lies on the anterior surface of the humerus.

The next important body of adipose tissue lies posteriorly, deep to the deep fascia (Fig. 2-59). It is inferomedial to the medial border of the posterior deltoid, lateral to the trapezius, and superior to the latissimus dorsi. This tissue might be considered a continuation of the triangular space because it contains the cutaneous continuations of the circumflex scapular artery, and it is here that the microvascular surgeon seeks the artery and veins of the scapular cutaneous flap.[150]

The third deep deposit of adipose tissue in the shoulder lies between the supraspinatus tendon and the overlying clavicle and acromioclavicular joint (see Fig. 2-29). The tissue cushions and protects the branches of the acromial artery, which is frequently encountered in dissections below the acromioclavicular joint. In summary, for the purpose of dissection, adipose tissue serves to indicate the presence of vessels or nerves.

Bursae

The last structures that facilitate motion are the bursae. Apparently, bursae form during development as a coalescence of fascial spaces.[208] Bursae tend to have incomplete linings in their normal state but may become quite thickened in the pathologic states frequently encountered at surgery. The bursae, being hollow spaces, are totally avascular and can be used as spaces for dissection. Because they are the most complete of the lubricating spaces, they are encountered between the most unyielding tissues: between tendon and bone or skin and bone and occasionally between muscle and bone near a tendon insertion.

The human body has approximately 50 named bursae, and several quite important ones are located in the shoulder.[95,208] The subacromial bursa and the closely related subdeltoid bursa are the most important. These bursae serve to lubricate motion between the rotator cuff and the overlying acromion and acromioclavicular joints. These two bursae are usually coalesced into one (Fig. 2-60). They are the most important bursae in pathologic processes of the shoulder and the ones that cause the most pain when inflamed. Although the subacromial bursa is normally only a potential space and therefore not seen on cross section (see Fig. 2-29) or with imaging

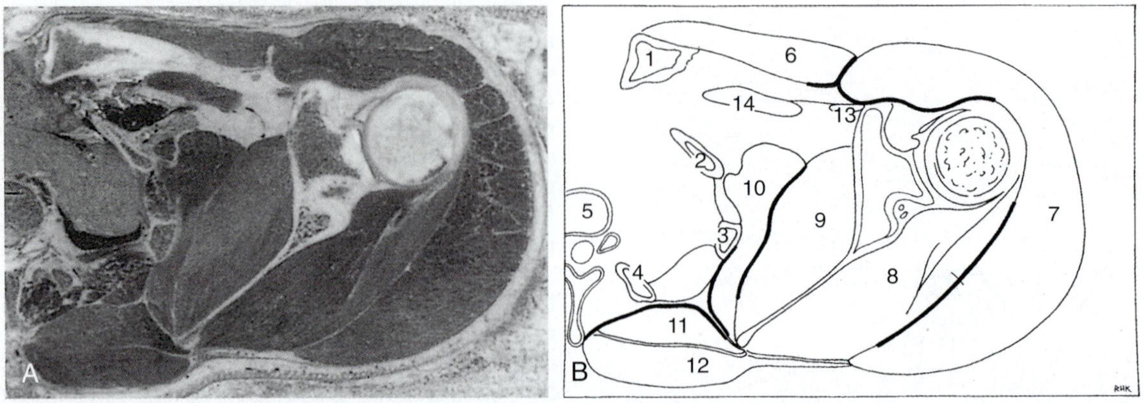

FIGURE 2-54: Transverse section **(A)** and diagram **(B)** showing the relationships at the level of the coracoid process. The planes where most of the motion occurs and that are most likely to be hypovascular are indicated by the heavy lines in B. The vessels that cross these planes are likely to be found at the edges of the planes of motion. For example, in the plane between the serratus anterior and the subscapularis, the vessels crossing are likely to be found close to the border of the scapula, where the relative motion between these two structures is less. Also shown on this section is the proximity of the suprascapular nerve and artery to the posterior rim of the glenoid. (See Fig. 2-57 for the key to the diagram.)

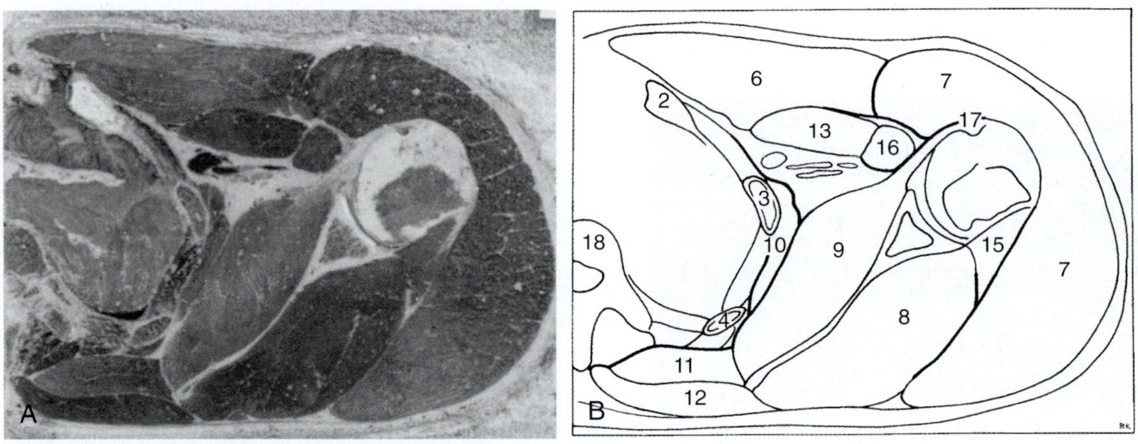

FIGURE 2-55: Cross section **(A)** and diagram **(B)** slightly below the equator of the glenoid. Tissue planes that are likely to be hypovascular are shown by the heavy lines in **B.** (See Fig. 2-57 for the key to the diagram.)

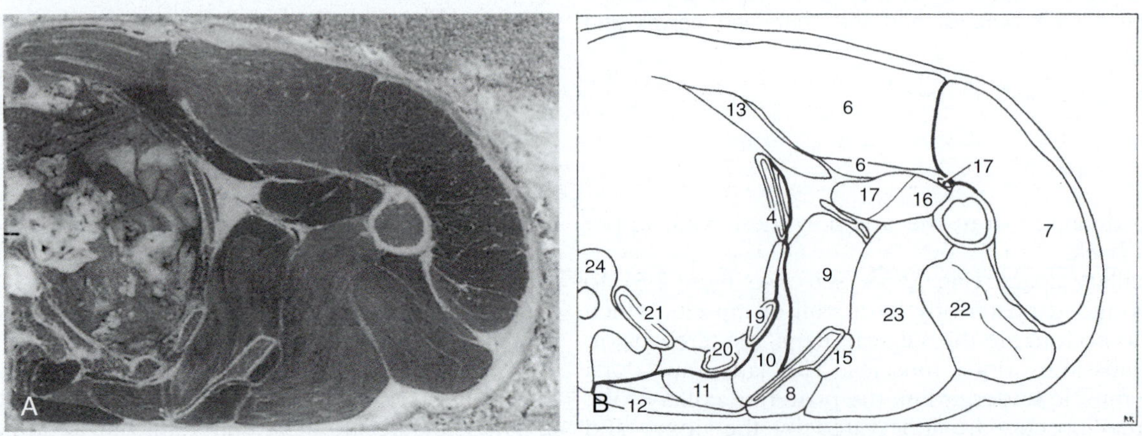

FIGURE 2-56: A lower cross section **(A)** and diagram **(B)** below the level of the quadrilateral space. Careful examination of **A** shows the two layers of the pectoralis major inserting onto the lateral border of the bicipital groove. At the anterior border of the teres major, the fibers of the teres major and the latissimus dorsi can be seen to insert on the medial lip and floor of the bicipital groove. The position of the brachial plexus is well demarcated. (See Figure 2-57 for a key to the diagram.)

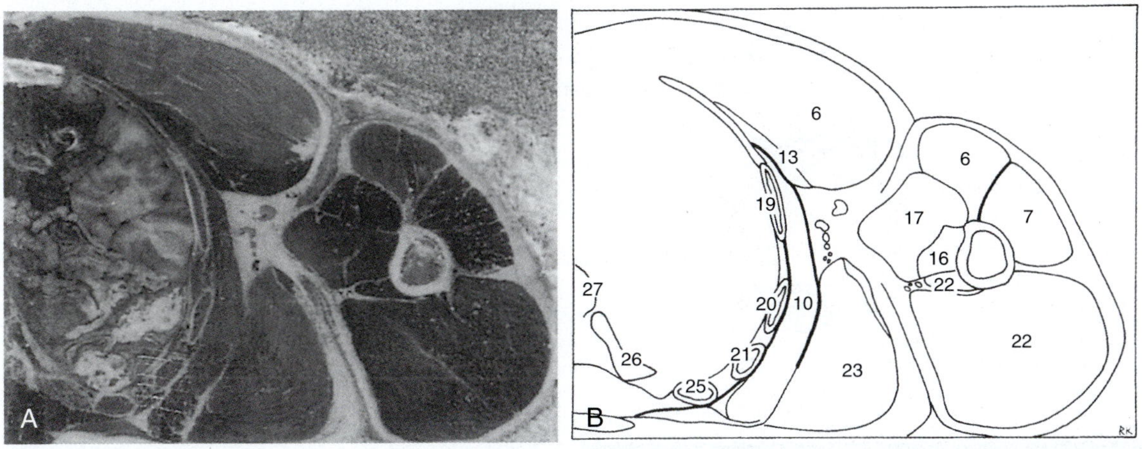

FIGURE 2-57: Cross section **(A)** and diagram **(B)** only a few millimeters superior to the skin of the axillary fossa. The hypovascular planes are again emphasized. Note the large pectoral lymph nodes and the large thoracodorsal vessels. On the lateral side of the teres major, the tendon and a few remaining muscle fibers from the latissimus dorsi can be seen. Labeled structures for Figures 2-63 to 2-66 are as follows: (1) clavicle, (2) rib 1, (3) rib 2, (4) rib 3, (5) T3 vertebra, (6) pectoralis major muscle, (7) deltoid muscle, (8) infraspinatus muscle, (9) subscapularis muscle, (10) serratus anterior muscle, (11) rhomboid muscle, (12) trapezius muscle, (13) pectoralis minor muscle, (14) subclavius muscle, (15) teres minor muscle, (16) coracobrachialis muscle, (17) biceps muscle, (18) T5 vertebra, (19) rib 4, (20) rib 5, (21) rib 6, (22) triceps muscle, (23) teres major and latissimus dorsi, (24) T6 vertebra, (25) rib 7, (26) rib 8, and (27) T8 vertebra.

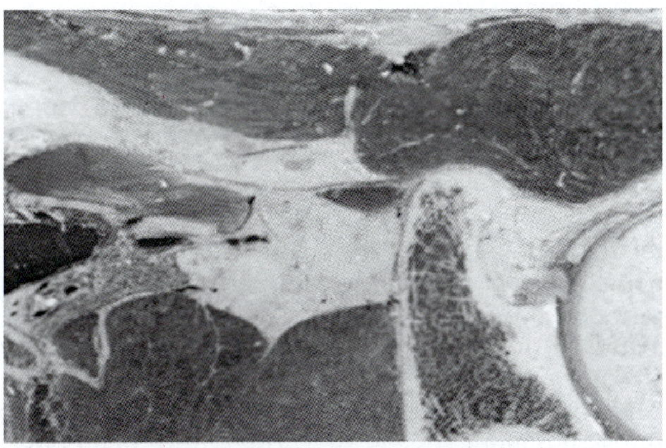

FIGURE 2-58: A magnified view of the axillary space demonstrates a rather prominent clavipectoral fascia starting from the tip of the coracoid and running to the left across the photograph. Just deep to this location and adjacent to the coracoid lies the insertion of the pectoralis minor. The muscle to the left is the subclavius. Immediately posterior to the subclavius can be seen the brachial plexus and axillary vessels.

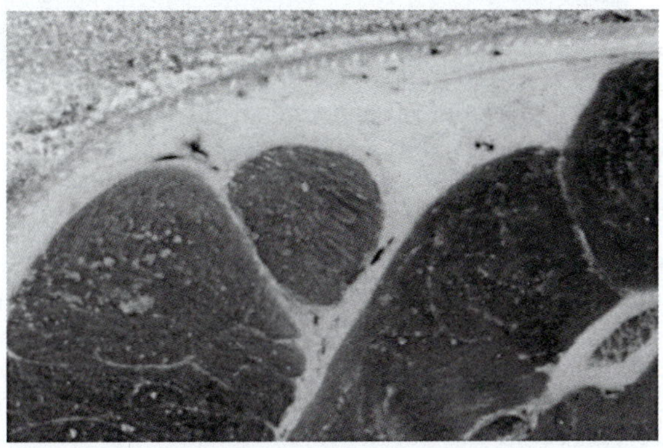

FIGURE 2-59: This cross-sectional view of the back of the shoulder demonstrates the fat pad within which the cutaneous branches of the circumflex scapular artery are located. The muscles on the left are the deltoid and the lateral head of the triceps. The teres minor is anterior, and the infraspinatus is lateral. This adipose tissue might be considered a continuation of the triangular space. Again, the presence of a body of adipose tissue is indicative of an artery or nerve.

techniques, it has a capacity of 5 to 10 mL when not compromised by adhesions or edema.[227] It does not normally communicate with the glenohumeral joint.[65]

Another frequently encountered bursa is the subscapularis bursa, which develops between the upper portion of the subscapularis tendon and neck of the glenoid and, in most cases, actually connects with the glenohumeral joint. Therefore it is usually a recess of the glenohumeral joint rather than a separate bursa. Fairly constant bursae can be found near tendinous insertions as follows: between the muscle and bony insertion of several muscles, including the trapezius, near the base of the scapular spine; the infraspinatus and the teres major near their attachments to the humerus; and an intermuscular bursa between the tendons of the latissimus dorsi and teres major.

A less constant bursa has been found to occur between the coracoid process and the coracobrachialis muscle and the underlying subscapularis muscle. We have seen such bursae inflamed by subcoracoid impingement processes,

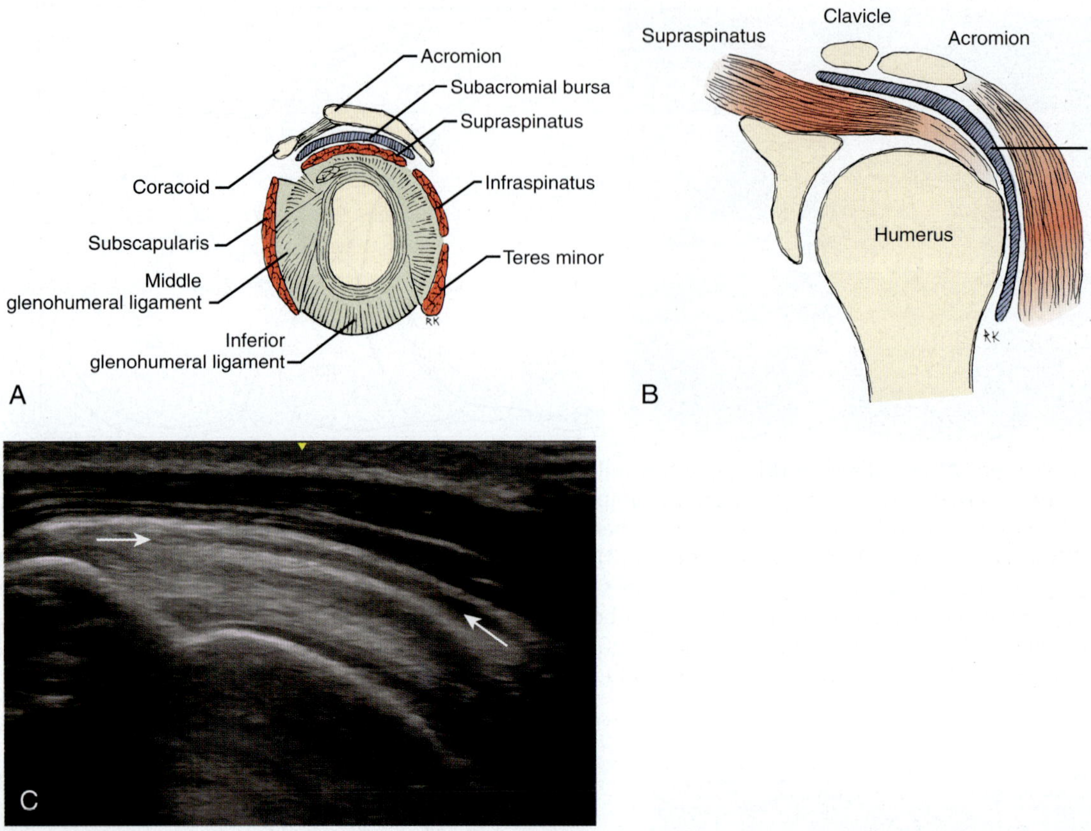

FIGURE 2-60: Sagittal **(A)** and coronal **(B)** views of the distribution of the subacromial bursa. **C,** Subacromial bursa with more fluid than normal.

most often iatrogenic or posttraumatic but have observed two that did not result from antecedent surgery or trauma. The coracobrachialis bursa is often (11% of specimens) an extension of the subacromial bursa.[100] In such cases, the coracoid tip may be visualized through an arthroscope placed in the subacromial bursa.

SKIN

Three requirements with regard to the skin should be considered in surgical planning. The first requirement is continued viability of the skin postoperatively, the second is maintenance of sensibility of the skin, and the last is cosmesis.

Circulation

The skin has several layers of blood vessels. A plexus of interconnecting vessels lies within the dermis itself. The largest dermal vessels lie in the rete cutaneum, a plexus of vessels on the deep surface of the dermis.[131] Another larger layer of vessels is located in the tela subcutanea, or superficial fascia.[95] The blood supply to these layers varies in different areas. Several factors relate to the arrangement of the circulation. The first is the relative growth of the area of the body under consideration. The number of cutaneous arteries that an individual has remains constant throughout life.[238] Growth increases the distance between the skin vessels by placing greater demand on them, which then leads to an increase in the size of the vessels.

The second factor is the path taken by direct vessels to the skin. Direct vessels are those whose main destination is the skin. While indirect vessels are those whose main destination is some other tissue, such as bone or muscle, they also reinforce the cutaneous vessels. The paths of direct vessels are affected by motion among tissues, with a great deal of motion taking place between subcutaneous fat and the deep fascia (Fig. 2-61). With the pectoralis major, for example, the dominant vessels cross at the edge of the plane of motion (i.e., the axilla). Some of these vessels may take direct origin off the axillary artery near its junction with the brachial artery, but they mainly originate from the pectoral area.[238] The vessel travels in the subdermal plexus in the subcutaneous fascia and sends vessels to the rete cutaneum. The plane between deep fascia and subcutaneous fat is an almost bloodless field; dissection can be performed without endangering the primary skin circulation.[238]

When the skin is more fixed, the dominant vessels may lie on the superficial surface of the deep fascia, and vessels to the dermal plexus may run more vertically than obliquely. In these areas, common on the upper part of

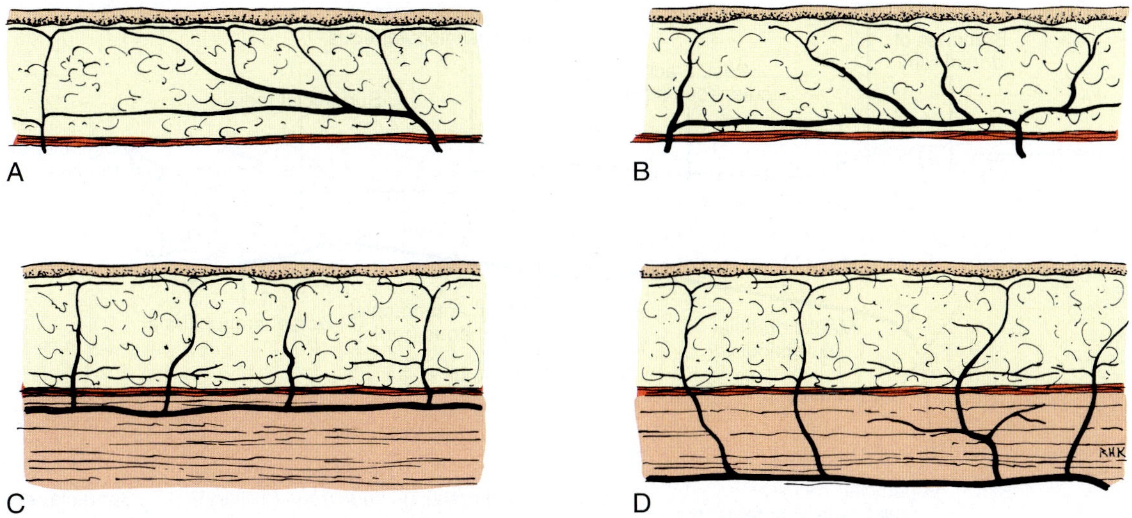

FIGURE 2-61: The four different types of direct circulation to the skin. **A,** Type A is found anterior to the pectoralis major, where considerable motion between the subcutaneous fascia of the skin and the deep fascia of the muscle takes place. The blood supply adapts to this motion by crossing obliquely at the edge of the plane of motion and sending a dominant vessel just deep to the tela subcutanea (subcutaneous fascia). From there, the vessel sends branches to the dermal plexus. **B,** Type B circulation occurs in situations with less motion between the subcutaneous fascia and the deep fascia. In fact, there may be relative motion between the overlying deep fascia and the underlying muscle. Direct vessels branch out on the surface of the deep fascia and subsequently send branches to the dermal plexus. In the shoulder area, such branching occurs over the fascia of the biceps. **C,** In type C, the skin is very tightly attached to the underlying deep fascia, which has an artery running just below it. This specialized situation occurs at the palmar and plantar fascia. **D,** In type D, the dominant vessel supplying this area of skin lies deep to the muscle and sends direct perforators to the dermal plexus. As expected, this type of circulation also occurs in locations with very little motion between the skin and underlying muscle. (Modified from Taylor GI, Palmer JH. The vascular territories [angiosomes] of the body; experimental study and clinical applications. *Br J Plast Surg.* 1930;40[2]:133-137.)

the arm, retaining a layer of deep fascia with skin flaps maintains another layer of circulation.[153] The perforators to this plexus on the deep fascia travel in the intermuscular septa rather than through muscle, where there is motion between muscle and the deep fascia, including muscle in a flap that offers no additional circulation.[101] A number of classifications of fasciocutaneous flaps have been devised on the basis of how the vessels reach the deep fascia.[46,127,154,165]

On the surface, vessels tend to course from concave surfaces of the body toward convexities. Thus they are likely to be found originating in rich supply adjacent to the borders of the axilla and less commonly on convexities such as the breast or outer prominence of the shoulder, which are distal watersheds. As growth increases the length of limbs and the height of convexities, vessels become longer and of greater diameter because of increased demand.[238]

In specialized areas of the body where dominant vessels lie just beneath the deep fascia and the skin is very well fixed, such as the palmar and plantar surfaces, the dermal vessels run vertically straight.

In other areas of the body such as over the middle third of the deltoid, the skin is extremely well fixed to underlying muscle. The dominant vessels, here the posterior humeral circumflex artery and veins,[238] actually course on the deep surface of the muscles, with direct vessels running vertically through the intramuscular septa of the deltoid muscle to the skin. Dissection on either side of the deep fascia will divide these vessels. Only a myocutaneous flap would offer additional vessels to the skin.[176]

These types of skin circulation are not mutually exclusive and may reinforce each other. Over the pectoralis major muscle, for example, direct vessels from the internal mammary vessels reinforce the type A vessels from the axilla.[237] Over the deltopectoral groove, perforator vessels from the deltoid artery reinforce the skin circulation. Much of the deltoid muscle vessels in the tela subcutanea are reinforced by type D vessels from the posterior humeral circumflex. Over the middle third of the deltoid, less overlap is likely, so flap development in this area should be less extensive.

Sensation

Sensation related to shoulder surgery is of less concern to the surgeon and the patient than is sensation in other areas of the body. The incidence of postoperative neuroma of the shoulder is low (Fig. 2-62).

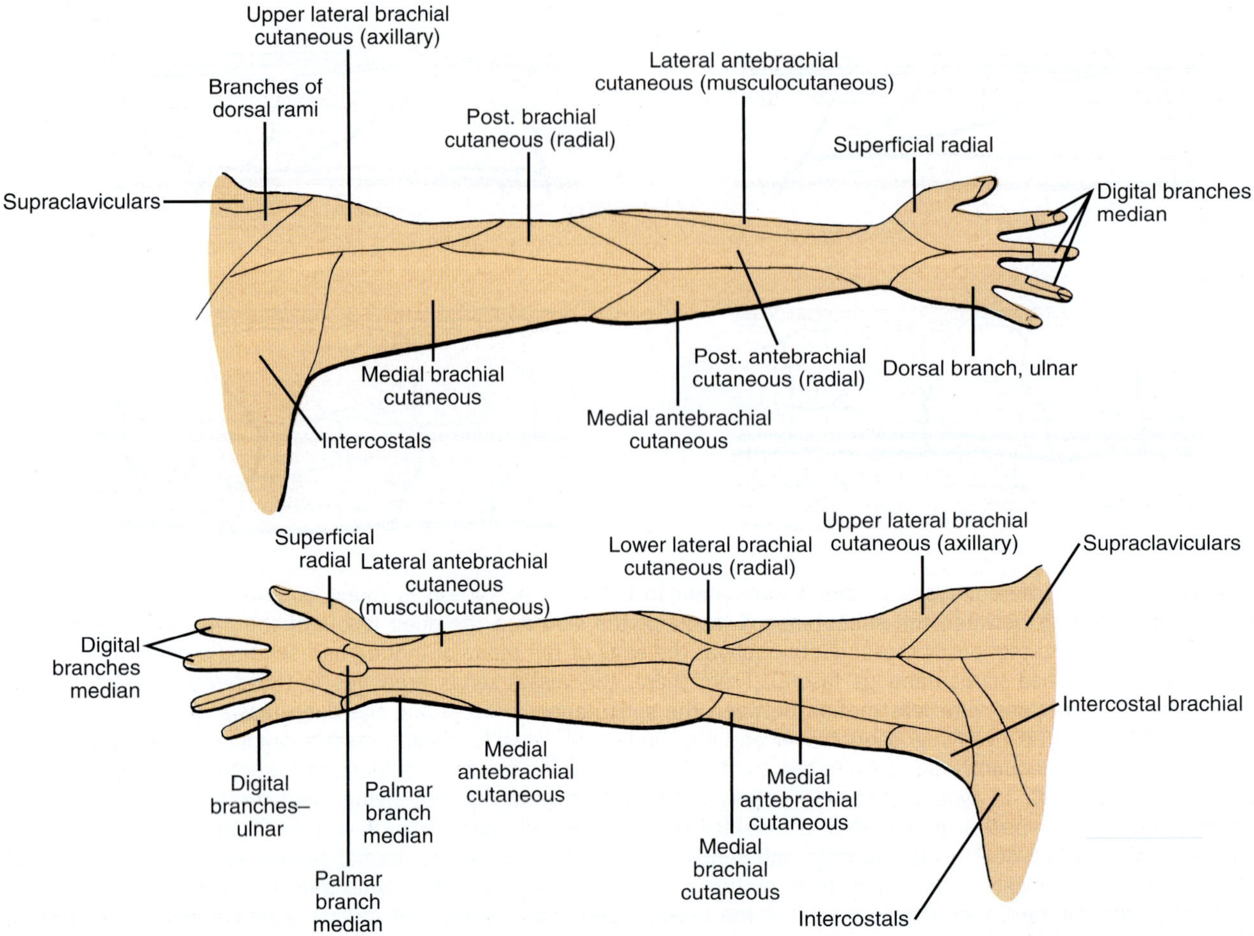

FIGURE 2-62: Representation of the cutaneous sensitivity of the nerves of the upper extremity. Note that of all the nerves to the shoulder, only the axillary nerve has a cutaneous representation. The remainder of the shoulder area is innervated by the supraclavicular nerves and the dorsal rami of the spinal nerves. No sharp demarcation is seen between the area of skin innervated by the intercostal brachial and medial brachial cutaneous nerves because of communication from the former. Intercostal brachial numbness following radical mastectomy is the only cutaneous nerve sensitivity problem common in the shoulder. (Modified from Hollinshead WH. *Anatomy for Surgeons*. 3rd ed. Philadelphia: Harper & Row; 1982.)

The most cephalad of nerves that innervate the skin of the shoulder and lower part of the neck are the supraclavicular nerves. They branch from the third and fourth cervical nerve roots and then descend from the cervical plexus into the posterior triangle of the neck. They penetrate superficial fascia anterior to the platysma, descend over the clavicle, and innervate the skin over the first two intercostal spaces anteriorly.[95] Interestingly, the medial supraclavicular nerves may pass through the clavicle.

The posterior portion of the shoulder and neck is innervated from cutaneous branches off the dorsal rami of the spinal nerves. In the dorsal spine, the area of skin that is innervated is usually caudad to the intervertebral foramen through which the nerve exits. For example, the C8 cutaneous representation is in line with the spine of the scapula, which is at the same height as the third or fourth thoracic vertebra.[95]

Much of the anterior of the chest is innervated by the anterior intercostal nerves. The first branches come forward near the midline adjacent to the sternum and innervate the anterior portion of the chest, somewhat overlapping with the lateral intercostal cutaneous branches. Interestingly, the first intercostal nerve does not have any anterior cutaneous branch.

The lateral cutaneous branches of the intercostal nerve emerge on the lateral aspect of the thorax between the slips of the serratus anterior muscle and innervate the skin in this area. They also supply the larger portion of the chest anteriorly, including the breast.[208]

Only three nerves of the brachial plexus have cutaneous representation in the shoulder, the most proximal of which is the upper lateral brachial cutaneous nerve, a branch of the axillary nerve that innervates the lateral side of the shoulder and the skin overlying the deltoid. The upper medial side of the arm is innervated by the medial brachial cutaneous and the intercostal brachial nerves combined. In the anterior portion of the arm over the biceps muscle, skin is innervated by the medial antebrachial cutaneous nerve.[95]

Relaxed Skin Tension Lines

Although numerous attempts have been made over the past 200 years—and in recent years—to outline the optimal lines for incision, the best description of the basic principles is that of Langer. He found that tension in the skin is determined by the prominence of underlying structures and by motion, with the underlying topography being the predominant influence.[129,130] Langer performed two classic experiments. In the first experiment, he punctured cadavers with a round awl and observed the linear splits that developed because of the orientation of underlying collagen. This he called the *cleavability* of the skin. In the second experiment, he measured skin tension in various ways. In cadavers, he would make circular incisions and observe wound retraction. He would then move the limb to look for changes in retraction. In living patients, such as women in the delivery room who were about to experience a sudden change in underlying topography, he would draw a circle on the skin with ink and observe postpartum changes.

In the twentieth century, cosmetic surgeons have found Langer's lines to be incorrect in certain areas of the body.[47,123] Although the principles outlined by Langer are still held to be valid, newer techniques have been sought to localize the optimal lines in living individuals. These techniques have included further circular incisions, wrinkle patterns, and chemical imprints. All these techniques agree with the incisions empirically found to be best in some regions and not in others.

Contemporary plastic surgeons now speak of relaxed skin tension lines (Figs. 2-63 to 2-65), which refer to their technique of relaxing the tension on the skin between the thumb and the forefinger of the surgeon and observing the pattern of fine lines in the skin. When the relationship is exactly perpendicular to the optimal incision, the fine lines that form are straight and parallel. The skin is then pinched in other directions. The line pattern is rhomboid or obscured.[21,22] This technique allows the surgeon to compensate for individual variability.

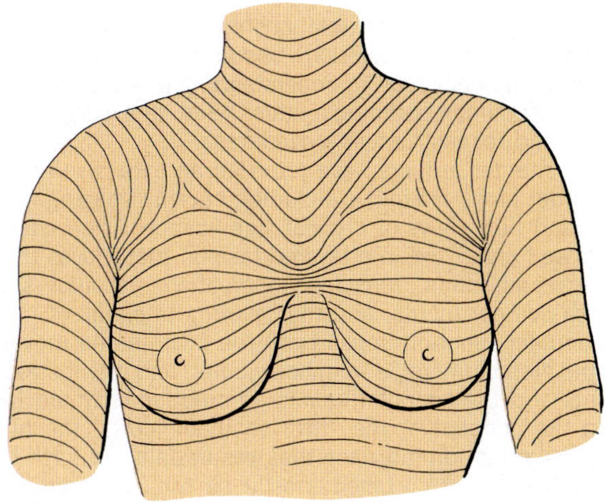

FIGURE 2-64: Because of the different underlying topography, the lines of skin tension in females differ in several respects from those in males. (Modified from Kraissel CJ. Selection of appropriate lines for elective surgical incisions. *Plast Reconstr Surg.* 1951;8[1]:1-28.)

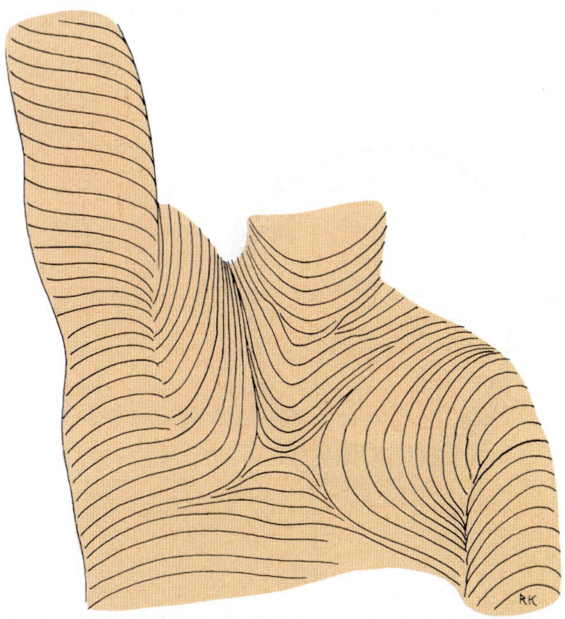

FIGURE 2-63: The usual locations of relaxed skin tension lines in a male. The position of these lines varies among individuals; they should be determined at each operation. (Modified from Kraissel CJ. Selection of appropriate lines for elective surgical incisions. *Plast Reconstr Surg.* 1951;8[1]:1-28.)

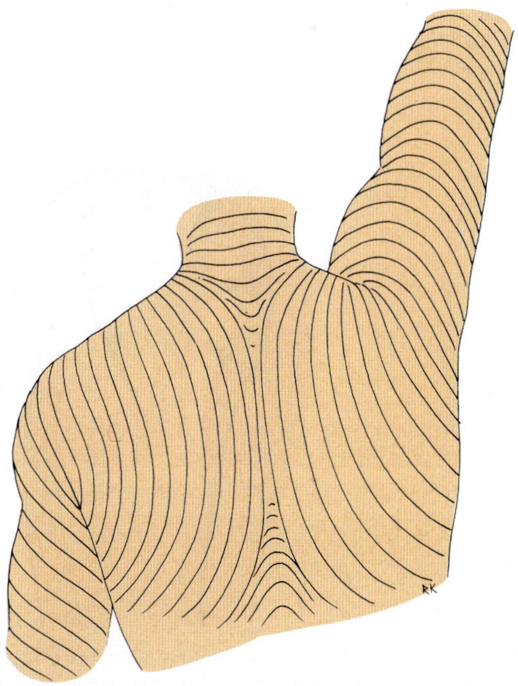

FIGURE 2-65: The usual position of relaxed skin tension lines on the posterior surfaces of the shoulder region. (Modified from Kraissel CJ. Selection of appropriate lines for elective surgical incisions. *Plast Reconstr Surg.* 1951;8[1]:1-28.)

EDITOR COMMENTARY

Steven B. Lippitt

My personal interest in shoulder anatomy was enhanced during orthopedic residency as I proctored upper extremity gross anatomy to medical students during an elective rotation. Current work hour constraints in residency have limited such extracurricular activity. Resident education is potentially more focused on surgical procedures and may miss the overall functional relationship of shoulder anatomy without didactic instruction. Shoulder functional anatomy remains the backbone to understanding physical exam principles, shoulder pathologic states, and safe surgical exposures and reconstructive procedures.

The chapter authors have provided an extensive review of shoulder gross anatomy, including current imaging modalities and new views of clinical significance. The material is very well organized in a layered fashion that moves through bones and joints, muscles, innervation, vascular supply, bursa compartments, and the covering integument.

Shoulder function depends on the coordinated movement of the glenohumeral, acromioclavicular, and sternoclavicular joints and the scapulothoracic articulation. I would like to add the concept of the "fifth shoulder joint," the humeroscapular motion interface that was initially set forth by Dr. Rick Matsen.[155,156] Lined mostly by the subacromial and subdeltoid bursa, this humeroscapular motion interface lies between the inner structures of the proximal humerus, rotator cuff, coracohumeral ligament, and biceps tendon sheath and the superficial layer of the acromion, deltoid, coracoacromial ligament, coracoid process, and the conjoined tendon (Fig. 2-66). Smooth, unrestricted motion at this interface is vital to shoulder mobility as evident when compromised, such as subacromial adhesions in cuff disease and after proximal humerus fracture (Fig. 2-67).

The axillary nerve has an intimate relationship within this humeroscapular motion interface (Fig. 2-68). Because of the primary importance of the innervated deltoid muscle to shoulder function, detailed review of the axillary nerve anatomy is worthwhile. The nerve is a terminal branch coming off the posterior cord of the brachial plexus just proximal to the coracoid process, passing beneath the conjoined tendon anterior to the subscapularis 3 to 5 mm medial to the musculotendinous junction and then lying adjacent to the inferior capsule before entering the quadrilateral space posteriorly. The axillary nerve splits into the anterior and posterior branches within the quadrangular space. The anterior and middle deltoid muscle receives sole innervation from the anterior branch of the axillary nerve. The posterior deltoid muscle innervation varies, with one study showing supply only from the anterior branch in 2.3% of cases, from the posterior branch in 8.5%, and from both branches in 89.1%.[136] The posterior branch of the axillary nerve branches to supply the teres minor muscle and then terminates as the superior lateral brachial cutaneous nerve.

In the anterior deltopectoral approach, the axillary nerve can be palpated by sweeping a finger inferiorly across the subscapularis muscle tendon interface (Fig. 2-69). Nerve palpation can be confirmed by feeling the nerve becoming taught with humeral internal rotation. Prior to transecting the subscapularis tendon, the nerve may be relaxed and the tendon pulled away laterally by humeral external rotation. The anterior motor branch should also be noted on the deltoid undersurface emerging posterior to anterior with the accompanied posterior humeral circumflex artery. Flatow et al. described a "tug test" that helps confirm axillary nerve identity (Fig. 2-70).[73]

In the anterolateral deltoid splitting approach, the axillary nerve crosses approximately 5 cm inferior to the anterolateral acromial corner (Fig. 2-71).[155] However, Burkhead et al. identified that 5 cm does not describe the absolute safe zone for axillary nerve passage and that shoulder abduction

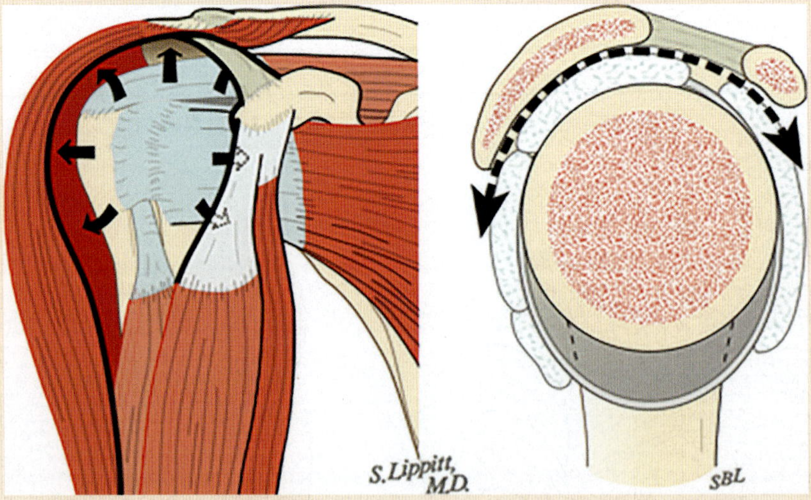

FIGURE 2-66: The humeroscapular motion interface is an important location of gliding movement between the humerus and scapula. The superficial side of this interface consists of the undersurface of the deltoid, acromion, coracoacromial ligament, coracoid process, and conjoined tendons, whereas the deep side consists of the proximal humerus, rotator cuff, and biceps tendon sheath. (Modified from Matsen FA III, Lippitt SE, Sidles JA, et al. *Practical Evaluation and Management of the Shoulder*. Philadelphia: WB Saunders; 1994.)

EDITOR COMMENTARY—cont'd

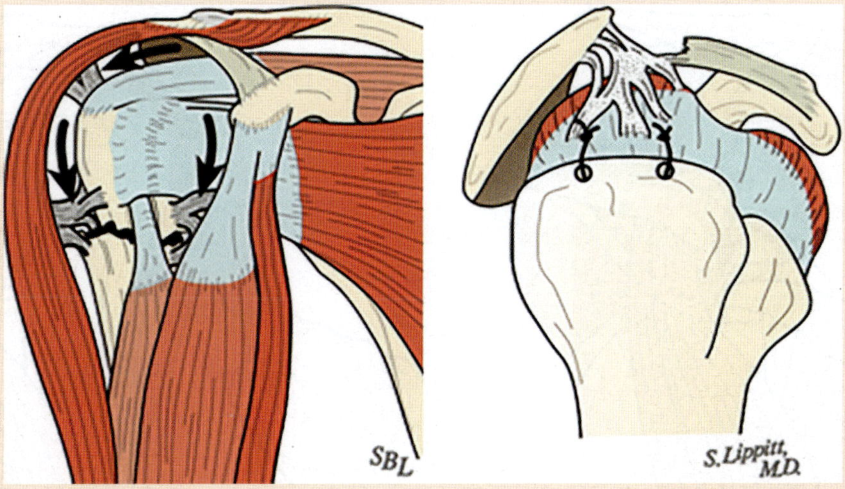

FIGURE 2-67: Adhesions in the humeroscapular motion interface can limit shoulder mobility with examples such as scarring after proximal humerus fracture trauma (*left*) and after acromioplasty and rotator cuff tear repair (*right*).

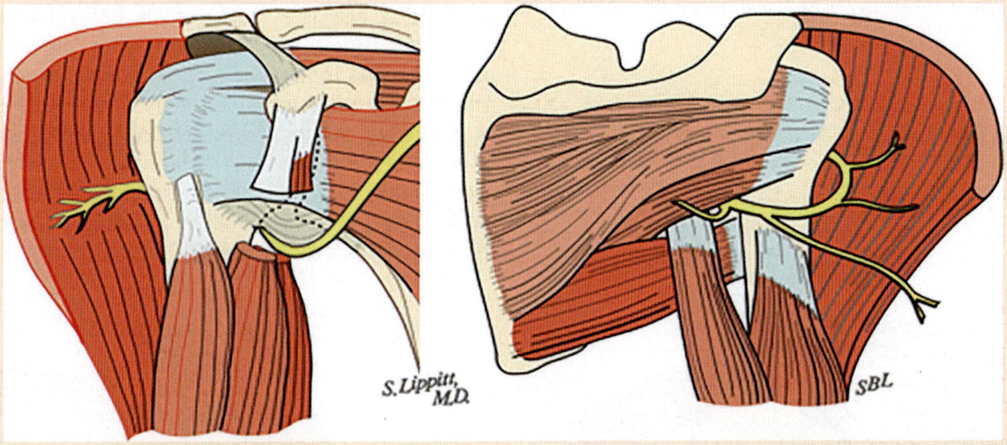

FIGURE 2-68: The axillary nerve in the humeroscapular motion interface between the cuff and the humerus on the inside and the coracoid muscles and the deltoid on the outside.

brings the nerve closer to the acromion landmark.[27] Gardner et al. demonstrated no accessory motor branches to the anterior deltoid crossing the tendinous raphe between the anterior and lateral deltoid, so extending an incision through this raphe after protecting the main motor branch of the axillary nerve does not place the innervation to the anterior deltoid at further risk (Fig. 2-72).[79] This extended anterolateral deltoid approach is more direct to the lateral aspect of the proximal humerus as with plating of a proximal humerus fracture and may decrease the risk to anterior humeral blood supply as compared to the deltopectoral approach.[94,136]

In the posterior deltoid splitting approach, the axillary nerve is approximately 7 cm from the posterior acromial corner (Fig. 2-73).[155] The tendinous raphe between the lateral and posterior deltoid may be split distally to the exiting axillary nerve at the inferior border of the teres minor muscle. The extent of this deltoid splitting approach exceeds that of the similar anterior deltoid splitting approach because the nerve courses more proximal after emerging from the quadrilateral space. The posterior glenohumeral joint can then be exposed safely above the axillary nerve through the internervous plane between the infraspinatus and teres minor.

The axillary nerve course is intimately related to the inferior joint capsule. In a fresh cadaveric dissection study, Uno et al. demonstrated that the axillary nerve is held to the shoulder inferior capsule with loose areolar tissue in the zone between the 5 and 7 o'clock positions relative to the glenoid (Fig. 2-74).[262] The nerve is relatively close to the glenoid in neutral rotation, extension, and internal rotation. With shoulder abduction, external rotation, and lateral joint traction, the capsule becomes taut and the nerve moves away from the glenoid, increasing the safe zone for capsular surgery adjacent to the inferior glenoid labrum.

Continued

EDITOR COMMENTARY—cont'd

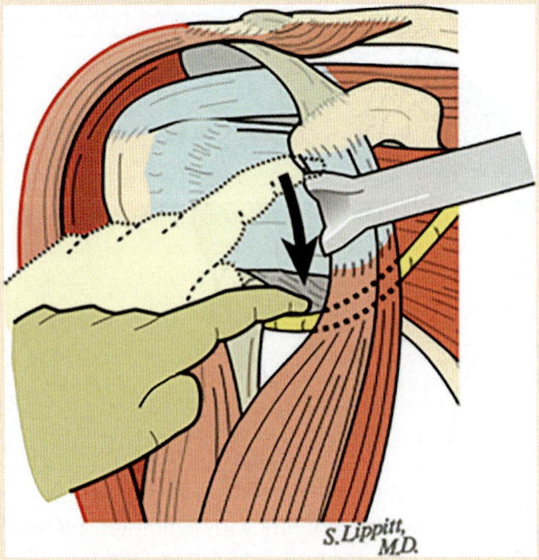

FIGURE 2-69: The axillary nerve may be hooked by sweeping the index finger inferiorly over the anterior subscapularis muscle.

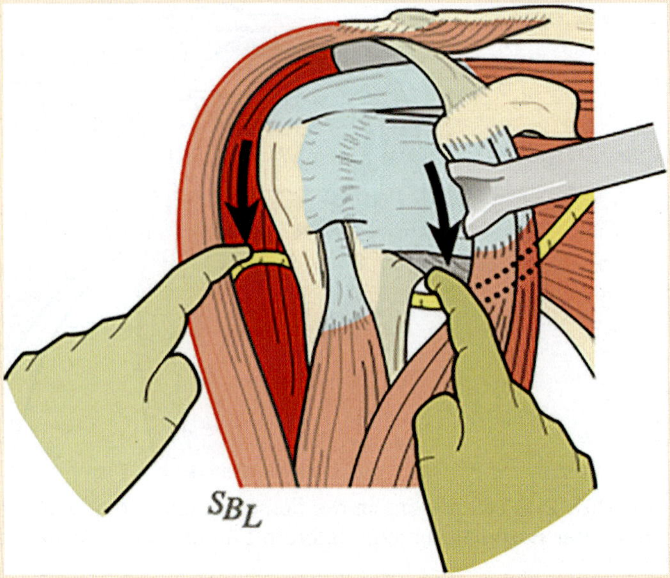

FIGURE 2-70: The "tug test" is performed by simultaneously palpating the axillary nerve inferiorly on the subscapularis with one index finger and the anterior motor branch on the deltoid undersurface laterally with the other index finger. A gentle tug applied by either finger will be palpable to the other and helps confirm axillary nerve identity. (Modified from Flatow EL, Bigliani LU. Tips of the trade. Locating and protecting the axillary nerve in shoulder surgery: the tug test. *Orthop Rev.* 1992;21[4]:503-505.)

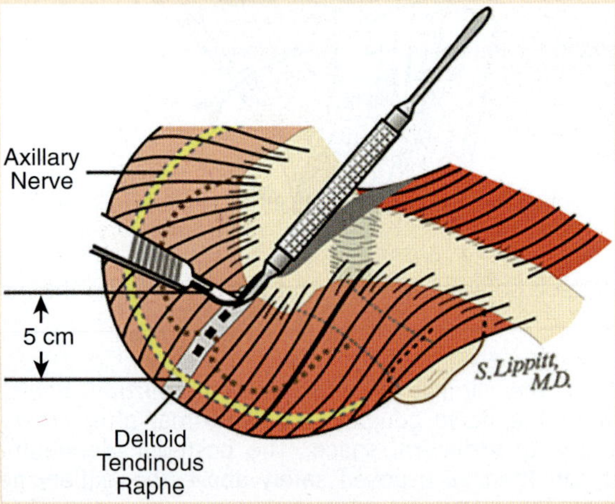

FIGURE 2-71: In the anterolateral deltoid splitting approach, the tendinous raphe between the anterior and lateral deltoid may be split longitudinally from the anterolateral acromial corner to approximately 5 cm distally before encountering the anterior branch of the axillary nerve on the deltoid undersurface.

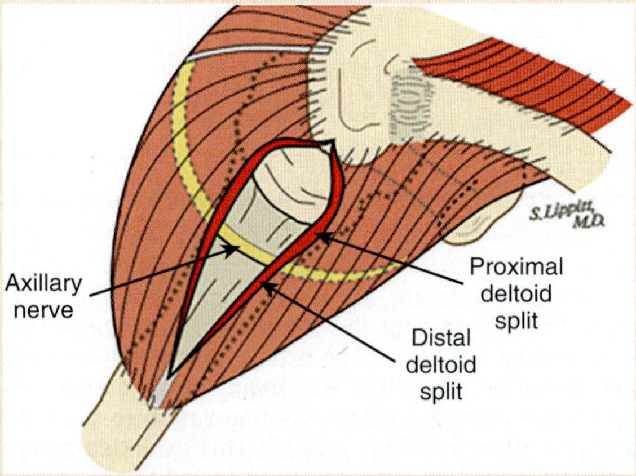

FIGURE 2-72: The extended anterolateral deltoid approach allows splitting of the deltoid distally beyond the identified axillary nerve.

EDITOR COMMENTARY—cont'd

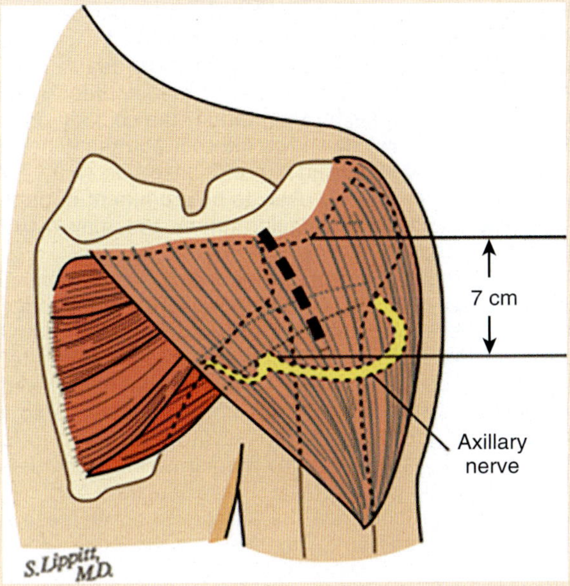

FIGURE 2-73: In the posterior deltoid splitting approach, the tendinous raphe between the lateral and posterior deltoid may be split distally to the exiting axillary nerve at the inferior border of the teres minor muscle.

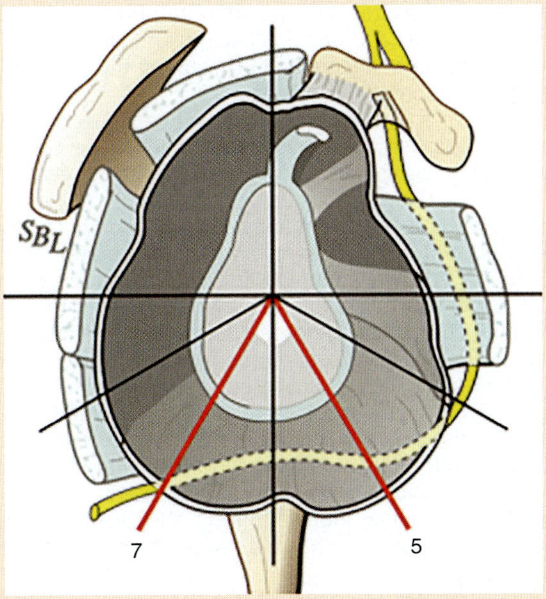

FIGURE 2-74: The axillary nerve has an intimate relationship to the inferior glenohumeral capsule in the zone between the 5 and 7 o'clock positions relative to the glenoid. (Modified from Uno A, Bain G, Mehta J. Arthroscopic relationship of the axillary nerve to the shoulder joint capsule: an anatomic study. *J Shoulder Elbow Surg.* 1999;8(3):226-230.)

Price et al. reported the average distance between the axillary nerve and the inferior glenoid rim as 12.4 mm. The nerve was observed to be closest to the inferior rim at the 6 o'clock position, with the teres minor motor fibers being the closest.[198] Eakin et al. demonstrated a relatively safe margin for arthroscopic suture placement if within 1 cm from the inferior glenoid rim.[63]

Understanding normal anatomy will enhance the surgeon's confidence in protecting such vital structures in shoulder surgery. The surgeon must also recognize this anatomy can become significantly altered by scar tissue, implants, and tendon and bone transfer when patients have had previous procedures.

SENIOR EDITOR COMMENTARY

Frederick A. Matsen III

This chapter elegantly portrays the wonderful complexity of the shoulder's anatomy. It is illustrated by many figures created by Dr. Chris Jobe from his personal ultrasound and cross-sectional studies. Very few, if any, can match this surgeon-anatomist. A few points should be reemphasized in relation to the illustrations in this chapter.

Figures 2-15 and 2-31 demonstrate that the old concept of the cuff muscles as "humeral head depressors" can be laid to rest. The lines of action of the supraspinatus, infraspinatus, and subscapularis do not create any substantial inferiorly directed force; therefore they cannot function as humeral head "depressors." Instead, as demonstrated by Figures 2-9 and 2-55, the rotator cuff embraces the humeral head and compresses it into the glenoid fossa. These two figures, as well as those in Dr. Lippitt's thoughtful commentary, show how the cuff muscles center the humeral head in the glenoid by the mechanism now known as *concavity compression.* Concavity compression can be effective with the arm in any position; this action is in contrast to the stabilizing effect of ligaments, which can only be active in extreme positions where they are under tension.

Figures 2-8A, and 2-32C nicely show the smooth outer surface of the proximal humeral convexity that forms a normal articulation with the coracoacromial arch, as shown in Figure 2-17G. Contact between the proximal humeral convexity and the coracoacromial arch is not "impingement," but rather the way the humeral head is normally stabilized to resist superiorly directed forces.

Figure 2-28 is another important illustration in that it calls attention to the complex intersection of the insertions of the supraspinatus and subscapularis as they join the superior glenohumeral capsule and the transverse humeral ligament. This intersection is the key spot of the shoulder where so

Continued

SENIOR EDITOR COMMENTARY—cont'd

much can happen: tears of the important fibers of the anterior supraspinatus and upper subscapularis, and tears of the transverse humeral ligament with resulting instability of the long head tendon of the biceps.

The vascular anatomy, as shown in Figure 2-48, is useful to remember because these vessels, which can be seen with arteriography, can guide us to the location of the nerves that run along with them. This is particularly useful in cases where the anatomy has been distorted by previous fracture or surgery.

Steve Lippitt has added some additional important illustrations in his editorial commentary. Especially important is Figure 2-66 showing again the two articular surfaces on either side of the humeroscapular motion interface: the proximal humeral convexity on the inside and the coracoacromial arch and deltoid on the outside.

Figure 2-75 shows the cuff hugging the humerus to the glenoid. It also shows how the anterior and posterior glenoid labra deepen the glenoid fossa, further facilitating the concavity compression mechanism that centers the humeral head in the shallow glenoid during the many functional activities performed in the mid-range of shoulder motion. This cross section shows how thin the articular cartilage is that covers the humeral head and glenoid; it is a wonder that it holds up so long in so many individuals. Another image worth including is a section of the shoulder with the arm in abduction and external rotation (the cocking position of the overarm throw). It shows internal abutment between the edge of the glenoid and the cuff insertion (Fig. 2-76). This contact is particularly likely to be prominent in pitchers with a large range of external rotation and may result in deep surface tears of the cuff.

Given that there is so much important and clinically relevant shoulder anatomy, I wish this chapter were longer. I would have loved to learn from the authors regarding the anatomy of the cuff insertion and how it might relate to the pathogenesis of rotator cuff tears. I would have loved to learn how the articular cartilage of the shoulder is so well bonded to the underlying bone. I would have loved to learn the variations in labral anatomy among normal shoulders so that we can avoid calling them "SLAP" tears.

Perhaps we can convince the authors to cover these subjects in the next edition!

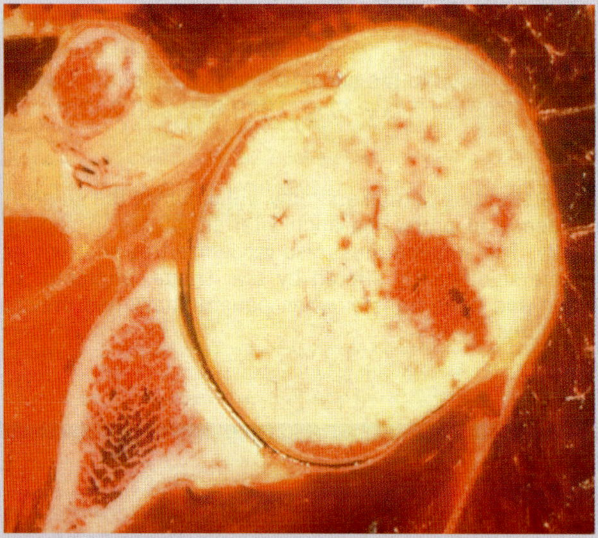

FIGURE 2-75: Shoulder cross section showing the cuff hugging the humerus to the glenoid. (Courtesy Christopher M. Jobe, MD.)

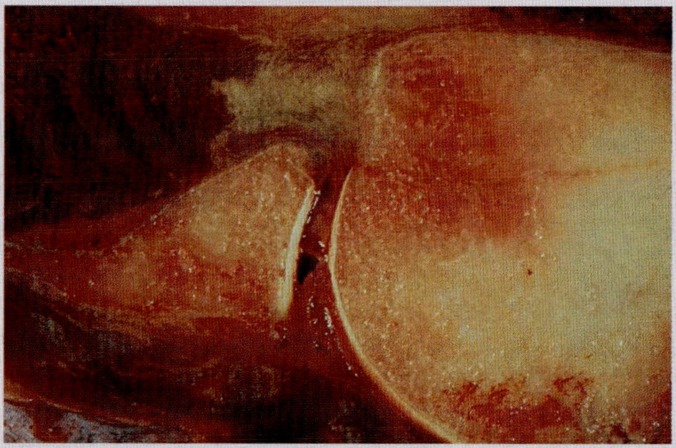

FIGURE 2-76: Section of the shoulder with the arm in abduction and external rotation showing internal abutment between the edge of the glenoid and the cuff insertion. (Courtesy Christopher M. Jobe, MD.)

CHAPTER 3

Clinical Evaluation of Shoulder Problems

Michael Codsi, Jesse McCarron, John W. Hinchey, John J. Brems

From the first days in medical school, physicians are taught that establishing a correct diagnosis depends on obtaining a meaningful and detailed medical history from the patient. This requires the physician to ask specific questions while at the same time actively listening to the responses from the patient. Often physicians formulate their next question without listening to and interpreting the answer to the previous inquiry. Obtaining a good patient history is, in itself, an art that requires experience and patience. One of us (J.J.B.) vividly recalls a mentor stating that all patients come to your office and tell you exactly what is wrong with them when they answer four or five questions. Our task is to decipher their answers to those few questions.

Time is perhaps the most valuable—and least available—commodity in our medical lives in the twenty-first century. We employ physician extenders to help our efficiency and we ask patients to fill out reams of paperwork with numerous questions while we are seeing another patient. We thus lose the advantage of directly listening to our patients, observing their expressions, and interpreting their body language. Each of these facets can offer valuable information to help reach a diagnosis of their shoulder problem. We must recognize that often the answer to one question leads to the formation of the next. This valuable opportunity is lost in the hustle of managing medical care in this era, and it is indeed a lost opportunity. Our duty to our patients is to inquire, listen, examine, test, and then formulate a diagnosis. When performed in this logical fashion, the diagnosis is nearly always straightforward and the treatment then easily rendered.

In evaluating the patient we also must bear in mind that we really are assessing *the patient* not just interpreting radiographic studies or laboratory values. In this increasingly technologic world it is often easy to lose sight of this and to begin treating magnetic resonance imaging (MRI) scans without treating the patient. For example, nearly every MRI of the shoulder we have seen in a patient older than 30 years suggests acromioclavicular joint pathology. Perhaps it is then not surprising that the most overdiagnosed and overtreated condition of the shoulder relates to the acromioclavicular joint.

As clinicians we must evaluate the patient's history and perform a thorough physical examination to establish a strong correlation between the features of each pathologic process. Our confidence rises when the patient's history of the complaint is consistent with the majority of the physical findings. This confidence rises even more when radiographic and laboratory studies are also consistent with the initial diagnosis. When all these features of the patient evaluation point to the same diagnosis, our certainty of the correct diagnosis becomes assured. It is obviously much more disconcerting when a patient's history suggests rotator cuff pathology, the physical examination is more consistent with instability, the radiographs document osteoarthritis, and the laboratory values suggest gout.

We hope the methods described in this chapter for taking a history and performing a physical examination allow every clinician to determine the pathology primarily responsible for the patient's shoulder complaints.

PATIENT HISTORY

Taking a history from a patient is an art. We must ask specific questions, actively listen to the response, and *only then* formulate the next question. The answer to each successive question should ultimately lead the physician to a correct diagnosis. It is important not to develop tunnel vision and lead the patient toward the diagnosis that *you* think is present.

Recall that many widely varying diagnoses manifest with similar symptoms, and differentiation of these diagnoses can only be made after a complete history and examination. For example, if a patient presents complaining of an inability to elevate or externally rotate the arm, the physician might immediately diagnose a frozen shoulder. However, sending that patient, who actually has advanced osteoarthritis, to physical therapy to increase the range of motion (ROM) would ensure a therapeutic failure. A diagnosis is established only after each phase of the evaluation is complete. Anything less in the name of expedience and efficiency does a disservice to our patients.

Age

Most, if not all, disease processes occur in specific patient age ranges. Although malignancies and traumas can occur at any chronologic age, even these processes tend to stratify by age. Surgical neck fractures of the humerus are typical of a postmenopausal woman with osteoporosis rather than an 18-year-old male football player. Osteosarcomas of the proximal humerus are more common in a 20-year-old than in a geriatric patient. The younger, athletic person in the second or third decade of life is more likely to have instability, whereas the 60-year-old golfer with a painful shoulder is more likely to have rotator cuff disease.

Although not fully studied or accurately analyzed, there is a perception that osteoarthritis of the shoulder is occurring at ever-younger ages. Not only is it in the domain of the 70- and 80-year-old patient; often patients in their 50s and younger present with osteoarthritis. Avascular necrosis, infections, and rheumatoid arthritis can occur at any age; thus age is a poor discriminator for these. Spontaneous hematogenous septic arthritis may be slightly more common during youth, but its clinical presentation is usually so specific that the age of the patient need not be considered.

Shoulder instability and its subsets of pathology are much more common during youth and early adulthood. Labral tears, superior labrum anterior and posterior (SLAP) tears, and biceps tendinitis are commonly seen in patients younger than 30 years. However, some activities that span the entire age range, such as downhill skiing, carry a considerable risk of acute shoulder dislocations. Nevertheless, the implications of a traumatic shoulder dislocation are age specific. In a younger patient who sustains a glenohumeral dislocation, the more likely associated injury involves the labrum or biceps anchor. Conversely, in an older patient, an acute glenohumeral dislocation is more commonly associated with a rotator cuff tear. Similarly, trauma to the shoulder can afflict the acromioclavicular joint. In a younger patient disruption of the joint is more common, whereas in older patients, clavicular fracture may be more common.

Some less common conditions afflicting the shoulder still display a predilection for certain age groups. Gout and symptomatic calcific tendinitis usually occur in middle age. Adhesive capsulitis appears in midlife (more commonly in women), and diabetic neuropathic disease is more common in older persons. Cuff tear arthropathy is clearly more common in women in their mid-70s.

Box 3-1 lists common diagnoses associated with typical age ranges. However, it should be borne in mind that any diagnosis can overlap with any age category.

BOX 3-1. Diagnoses Associated with Specific Age Groups

<30 years old: Instability, superior labrum anterior posterior tears, biceps tendinopathy, acromioclavicular joint injury, labral injury
30-60 years old: Rotator cuff disease, adhesive capsulitis, gout, calcific tendinosis
>60 years old: Arthritis, fractures, diabetic neuropathy
>70 years old: Cuff tear arthropathy
No age association: Avascular necrosis, infection, rheumatoid arthritis/inflammatory arthropathy, malignancy

Sex

Most pathologic processes that afflict the shoulder affect both sexes equally. Trauma can occur to anyone; arthritis, infection, cuff tears, avascular necrosis, calcific tendinitis, and gout can likewise occur with equal frequency in male and female patients. However, three conditions, although not exclusive to women, have a significantly higher prevalence in female patients.

Multidirectional shoulder instability is seen much more frequently in female patients between the ages of 15 and 25 years than in male patients of the same age. Why this is the case remains unclear. Male patients might present with clinical evidence of multidirectional laxity, but perhaps because of stronger and better-conditioned muscles, they are better able to compensate for their ligamentous laxity in ways female patients cannot or do not. It remains doubtful that there is a difference between sexes in the pathophysiology of the condition, but the positive biologic response to the condition seems to favor the male patients. A teenage female athlete who presents with shoulder complaints likely has some type of instability pathology. However, the clinician must remain open to other diagnoses and be sure to distinguish patient symptoms from clinical signs. For example, a young person might present with *symptoms* of cuff tendinitis that are caused by underlying shoulder instability.

Female patients also tend to present in far greater numbers than males with adhesive capsulitis.[52] This is in contrast to the idiopathic stiff and painful frozen shoulder, which is equally prevalent among male and female patients and describes restricted shoulder ROM associated with pain. A frozen shoulder can result from any number of pathologic processes, such as posttraumatic stiffness, immobilization, and tendinitis. Adhesive capsulitis is a specific diagnosis most prevalent in women 40 to 60 years of age. It is associated with an idiopathic inflammatory process involving the glenohumeral joint capsule and synovium that results in capsular contraction and adhesion formation.

Although massive rotator cuff tears probably occur in greater numbers in men, it is women, classically older than 70 years, who develop the sequelae of these tears. The diagnosis of cuff tear arthropathy, as defined by painful collapse of the humeral head with superior migration (not iatrogenically provoked by prior release of the coracoacromial ligament), is much more common in geriatric women compared with men, for reasons that are unclear.

Presenting Complaint

When the physician inquires about a patient's chief complaint during the initial visit, pain is the most common response. Subsequent questioning is directed toward better understanding the characteristics of that pain and a presumptive diagnosis follows. Most presenting complaints related to the shoulder are described by patients as pain, stiffness, loss of smooth motion, instability, neurologic symptoms, or combinations of these.

With respect to shoulder pathology, another chief complaint may be one of joint instability. In this case the patient might have no pain and is concerned only by the sense that the shoulder joint is loose, sloppy, or recurrently dislocates. The patient might initially complain of numbness or tingling down the limb, which may be caused by neurologic pathology unrelated to the shoulder. Dissection of this symptom may be more challenging because pathology in the neck might have to be distinguished from shoulder pathology.

Weakness is rarely a sole presenting complaint. Weakness without pain nearly always defines a significant neurologic event or pathologic process. If stiffness of the shoulder is a presenting complaint, it is nearly always accompanied by an element of pain. A patient might present with a complaint of crepitus or popping in and about the shoulder associated with activity or a specific arm motion, but an isolated awareness of crepitus without pain is very rare.

Pain

The discussion of pain is challenging because it is, by definition, a completely subjective complaint. In our vast armamentarium of technology and laboratory analyses, we cannot objectify pain. Pain is a perception of data presenting to our brains. We have all experienced the reality of injuring ourselves with minor scrapes and scratches in our daily lives but have remained fully unaware of this until hours later. Have we all not jumped into a pool of water only to feel cold initially? Within minutes, the initial discomfort fades as we rapidly become conditioned to the water temperature. The water temperature obviously does not change; it is our *perception* of the same data input to our brain that changes.

The same can be the case with other painful stimuli. Psychologists (and perhaps our own experience) suggest that mood can have a dramatic effect on pain perception. People who are depressed or sullen by nature tend to experience greater discomfort and be more disabled for a given level of painful stimuli, and the opposite is likewise true; energetic, optimistic, and happy patients tend to discount even a significant level of otherwise painful stimuli.

Other societal issues are also known to affect a patient's perception and response to pain. Specifically, issues related to material gain can have significant influence on patients' responses to the treatment for the pain. For example, active litigation involving contested remuneration can lead to the perpetuation of a patient's symptoms. Similarly, patients with worker's compensation claims might have little incentive to report improvement in their symptoms. There is no pain meter that can substantiate or dispute such claims.

BOX 3-2. Features of Pain to be Evaluated

Severity (scale of 1-10)
Character (dull, sharp, ache, lancinating)
Onset (acute, chronic, insidious, in a defining moment)
Location (e.g., superior, posterior, anterior, scapular)
Patterns of radiation (neck, arm, below elbow, deltoid insertion)
Aggravating factors (e.g., arm position, time of day)
Alleviating factors (e.g., arm position, medications)
Prior injections (site, response)
Prior treatment

Despite these limitations, obtaining a history related to pain is critically important and valuable. Features of the pain, such as its character, onset, radiating patterns, and aggravating and alleviating factors, nearly always assist the clinician in discerning a diagnosis. Box 3-2 provides an overview of the features of pain that should be evaluated.

Character of the Pain

Despite our inability to *measure* pain, patients use similar adjectives to *describe* their pain. These descriptions can offer much insight into its cause. Pain associated with an acute fracture understandably can be severe and disabling, often remaining minimally responsive to narcotic analgesics for days. In contrast, the pain of impingement and rotator cuff pathology is commonly described as dull, boring, and toothache-like in quality. The pain of a frozen shoulder is typified as all or none: when present at the endpoint of available motion, the pain is truly disabling, whereas when the arm is functioning within its available arcs of motion, pain does not exist. Patients with painful osteoarthritis describe pain that frequently alternates between a sharp stabbing pain under high compressive joint loads and a chronic lower level of pain during less-demanding activities. Patients with severely destructive rheumatoid disease are often so conditioned by the chronicity of their disease that their description of their pain appears to be inconsistent with the degree of joint destruction. These patients tend to be more disabled by their functional loss than by their perceived pain.

Acute calcium deposition in the cuff tendons results in a characteristic type of pain. The pain is so acute and so severe that calcium deposit in the shoulder has been likened to a kidney stone of the shoulder. The pain associated with a kidney stone seems so well understood by the population at large that the pain in the shoulder associated with acute calcific deposit is easily understood as well. Patients with this condition seek a dark, quiet room with minimal competing stimulation. The pain can be so nauseating and disabling that many patients visit an emergency department (ED). The clinical picture is so evident and the radiographs so typical of the condition that the diagnosis is rarely in doubt.

Onset of the Pain

The clinician asks about the onset of the symptoms because this feature has implications in the diagnosis of shoulder pathology. Understandably, with an acute onset of severe pain following a traumatic event, the diagnosis of fracture on a radiograph is not challenging. Other diagnoses may also be discerned by inquiring about the circumstances of the onset of the patient's pain. Impingement and rotator cuff disease more commonly lack a specific date or time of onset; if the patient recalls an insidious onset of the pain, often dating its initiation many weeks or months in the past without a clearly identifiable event, this should make the physician suspicious for cuff-related pathology. Even if the patient presents with a recent onset of pain in the absence of trauma, inquiry needs to be made regarding a history of pain predating the more recent traumatic event.

Radicular pain of cervical origin is likely to have an insidious onset. Patients might acknowledge that turning the head provokes symptoms. Arm pain while driving often indicates a pain of cervical origin. Pain described as sharp and stabbing and occurring intermittently in the scapular muscles and around the top of the shoulder nearly always has its source in the cervical spine.

Location of Pain Perception

Pain is poorly localized around the shoulder girdle. The specific location where the patient perceives the pain is rarely the site of origin of the pain. The most common location for the perception of rotator cuff disease and the associated bursitis is down the arm toward the deltoid muscle insertion. The pain and inflammation associated with bicipital tendinitis is typically perceived down the anterior arm, although the site of pathology is proximal to the intertubercular groove. Pain associated with an acromioclavicular injury usually radiates medially and results in perceived pain along the mid and medial clavicle.

Most intrinsic shoulder pathology has a pattern of pain that radiates down the arm to the level of the elbow, and it is distinctly rare for the pain to be perceived as extending below the elbow joint. Conversely, pain of cervical origin usually radiates from the base of the ipsilateral ear toward the posterior shoulder and into the scapular region. A true cervical radiculopathy, which most commonly involves the fifth and sixth cervical nerve roots, provokes symptoms that are perceived to radiate into the forearm and hand in a dermatomal pattern. In contrast to the pain derived from cervical radiculopathy, pain from adhesive capsulitis does not follow a dermatomal pattern, but often radiates along the trapezius muscle and periscapular muscles. That is because these muscles become strained and fatigued by the excessive scapular rotation that must compensate for the decreased glenohumeral motion.

The pain of an intra-articular infection is not unlike that associated with any joint; it is severe, exquisite, and maximally disabling. The clinical picture is so specific that the suspicion of infection is exceedingly high until a definitive laboratory diagnosis is confirmed.

Aggravating Factors of Pain

As a part of establishing the history of pain, the clinician needs to elicit circumstances that seem to make the pain worse. Often the pain is influenced by arm position, which can provide insight into its cause. Patients might state that the pain is worse or aggravated when the arm is positioned above shoulder level, such as when washing or combing their hair. Activities that result in a long lever arm with the elbow extended, such as reaching across the car seat or reaching out the car window to use an automatic teller machine, increase the pain of a weak or torn rotator cuff. Increasing pain in the shoulder that occurs while pulling bed covers up at night is strongly associated with impingement and cuff disease.

The occurrence of pain at night needs to be elicited, as there appear to be two distinct types of night pain, each associated with a different shoulder condition. The more severe and disabling type of night pain strongly suggests a rotator cuff tear. This pain is described as gnawing, incessant, and unremitting, and it not only awakens patients from sleep but also often precludes any meaningful sleep at all. Patients often relate that the only way they can obtain sleep is to rest semirecumbent in a chair. In a different circumstance patients might acknowledge night pain that is *positional*. They can typically fall asleep but are awakened if they roll onto or away from the affected shoulder.

Patients with positional night pain rarely convey the degree of frustration with sleep interruption that is experienced by those with a cuff tear. Although patients with positional night pain may be annoyed by the sleep interruption, they can generally fall back to sleep easily and do not develop that deep sense of misery associated with persistent sleep deprivation. Positional night pain is most often associated with loss of shoulder internal rotation through muscle stiffness or loss of capsular compliance. Painful arthritis of the acromioclavicular joint can also result in positional night pain and is caused by the compressive loads borne by that joint when lying on the affected side. The pain of these conditions might also be aggravated by lying on the unaffected shoulder; in this position, the weight of the affected arm falling across the chest in adduction also results in acromioclavicular joint compression and posterior capsular stretch.

Patients with adhesive capsulitis describe pain that is characterized by its sudden severity and aggravated by clearly reproducible arm positions. They have no pain until they reach the endpoint of their available motion, when their pain becomes immediate and severe. As their condition progresses they note an increasing inability to perform their activities of daily living, including reaching overhead or reaching behind their back for dressing or personal hygiene.

With an intra-articular process, such as glenohumeral arthritis, patients usually note that aggravation of symptoms comes with activities associated with the repetition of a similar motion. Painting, sweeping, polishing, vacuuming, ironing, and washing a car are activities that predictably aggravate the pain of arthritis and impingement. Loading of the joint and simultaneously performing a repetitious act is particularly aggravating to joint conditions that result from incongruent joint surfaces, such as avascular necrosis, osteoarthritis, and rheumatoid arthritis.

Although inquiry about and analysis of aggravating factors in the assessment of shoulder pain is rarely in itself fully diagnostic, it remains a very important consideration as the history-taking progresses.

Factors That Alleviate Pain

In the same way that analysis of aggravating factors provides insight into the etiology of the shoulder problem, so too does inquiry into the features and factors that alleviate or improve the symptoms. Many times the alleviating factor provides the best information in arriving at the correct diagnosis. Whereas there is much overlap in diagnoses with respect to aggravating factors, it would be unusual to find one alleviating factor that relieves several different problems. For example, if a patient finds that an over-the-counter antiinflammatory truly improves the symptoms, it would logically follow that the patient has an inflammatory condition. Certainly, an antiinflammatory would not solve the apprehension of a shoulder instability problem, nor would it likely manage the pain of an acute fracture. Patients with a frozen shoulder characteristically state that there is absolutely no improvement in their pain with nonsteroidal antiinflammatories. Alleviating factors can include activity modification, positional changes, medications, narcotics, antiinflammatories, injections, or physical therapy. Physical therapy stretching over long time spans usually improves symptoms and needs to be assessed during history taking.

Patients with rotator cuff disease often note that placing the affected arm over their head significantly improves their pain. Often this arm position is the only way they can find meaningful sleep. This is called the *Saha position* (Fig. 3-1), named after the orthopedic surgeon who recognized this phenomenon.

The response to local anesthetic injections in specific anatomic locations around the shoulder can be very instructive and diagnostic. In a patient with chronic subacromial impingement, 5 mL of 1% lidocaine placed in the subacromial space provides immediate and dramatic relief of pain (Fig. 3-2). This response is therefore diagnostic of a subacromial process, and it is especially valuable when trying to discern whether the patient's perceived pain is originating in the shoulder or is referred pain from the neck. A similar local injection test is useful in evaluating the acromioclavicular joint as the source of the patient's pain. Alleviation of pain with arm adduction following an injection of lidocaine directly into the acromioclavicular joint strongly suggests pathology at this joint. Intra-articular and biceps sheath injections can provide similar supporting information regarding the source of a patient's symptoms.

These specific injection tests are valuable in establishing the pathologic process, and, in the case of subacromial impingement, the response to the local anesthetic can predict the response to surgical treatment. Moreover, a negative response to a subacromial local anesthetic can predict a negative response to subacromial surgical treatment.

Response of Symptoms to Self-Prescribed Treatment

With the current advent and ubiquity of the Internet, patients have become more involved in their health care decisions. Countless websites dedicated to patient information help patients self-diagnose, although not always with great clarity or accuracy. There are likely even more websites from which patients can receive a wide variety of treatment recommendations for their self-diagnosed shoulder condition. An Internet search for the term "physical therapy" brings up millions of hits, and searching for "shoulder-specific physical therapy" brings up well more than 1 million websites. No doubt that only few patients arrive at the physician's office these days without some knowledge, opinion, or effort at self-management of their shoulder pain.

It is important to take time to explore which methods, medications, and modalities the patient might have tried

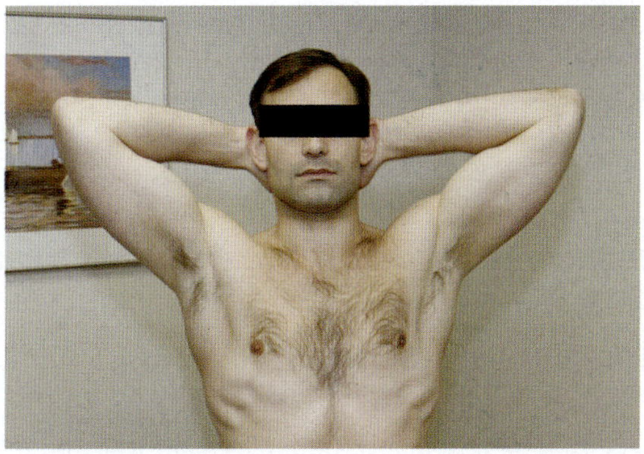

FIGURE 3-1: The Saha position often provides relief from pain related to rotator cuff pathology.

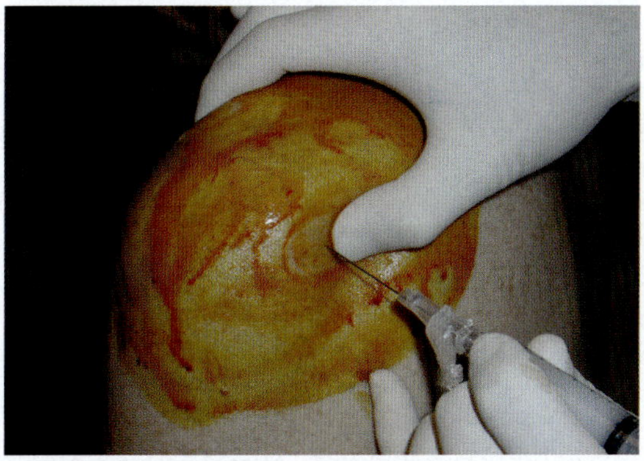

FIGURE 3-2: The subacromial injection technique from the posterior aspect of the shoulder. The physician's thumb is resting on the inferior border of the spine of the scapula.

before coming to the physician. The physician should explore the realm of nutraceuticals and ask specifically about the common ones, including glucosamine, chondroitin, shark cartilage, and methylsulfonylmethane (MSM), because many patients do not consider these to be medicines and do not include them in their medication lists. Many patients consume seemingly countless vitamins and vitamin combinations in their efforts to improve their physical well-being. With the exception of glucosamine and chondroitin, which themselves have not been subjected to the rigors of the scientific method to prove their efficacy, there is little published objective information to make recommendations to patients. Nevertheless, many patients seem certain that some combination of herbs, vitamins, and supplements have affected their medical condition in some way or another. It is important to query and document these treatments during the overall evaluation of the patient with a shoulder problem.

Instability

In this discussion, it is imperative that the concept of instability is understood as referring to a *patient experiencing symptoms* of some shoulder problem. Many asymptomatic shoulders exhibit increased joint translation and are clearly loose during a physical examination. These are defined as *lax*, not unstable. To have shoulder instability means, by definition, that the shoulder is symptomatic for the patient.

In the younger and active age groups, the symptom of shoulder instability may be the patient's presenting complaint. Although there is often a history of acute traumatic event that resulted in an initial, well-defined onset, in many cases there is no history of such traumatic event. Indeed, since the 1980s, genetic factors in ligamentous laxity have been recognized as significant factors in patients' perception of shoulder instability.

The diagnosis of shoulder instability can be very easy when the patient presents with an appropriate history of trauma. Nearly always there has been a trip to ED and radiographs to document the events. However, with the increasing availability of sports trainers at most of the high school, college, and professional competitions, reduction of a dislocation by those personnel results in a history only; there are no ED records or radiographs. Although the history in these situations is still strong, an examination and radiographs even a few days following the event make this a less-than-challenging diagnosis.

A more challenging problem occurs in patients with a sense of slipping and looseness in their shoulder without a history of macrotrauma. More often than not, this more subtle instability pattern is associated with a nondescript level of discomfort and diffuse pain around the shoulder girdle. The discomfort is poorly localized and may be more scapular in location. The association of such symptoms with paresthesia down the arm is nearly always related to shoulder instability. There may be a history of repetitive microtrauma with such activities as frequent swimming, gymnastics, or ballet. Although these activities may not appear to be highly stressful to the joint, they demand muscle function defined by high endurance. Conventional thought suggests that when the ligament quality and integrity do not contribute to joint stability, the surrounding muscle activity and appropriate proprioceptive activity become more important to maintain a functioning joint.

The sense of instability might occur with the arm only in certain positions or it may be present regardless of arm placement or position. True symptomatic multidirectional instability is typically symptomatic in midrange positions before the ligament tension reaches the end of its range. The physician must carefully inquire about which activities and arm positions provoke the symptoms. Patients with this type of instability might have symptoms that are so incapacitating that they tend to avoid extremes of glenohumeral motion. Pain is the more common symptom with a shoulder instability based on ligamentous laxity (AMBRI), whereas apprehension is more common with unidirectional traumatic instability (TUBS). Box 3-3 lists these categories of instability.

The classic patient with traumatic instability is a male athlete who sustained an identifiable traumatic event during the course of a violent activity. Football tackling, a high-speed fall or collision while downhill skiing, or a hyperextension force on an extended arm (such as a basketball blocking shot) are very common scenarios that result in an acute traumatic shoulder dislocation. Conversely, the classic patient with multidirectional shoulder instability is the young, asthenic female ballet dancer, swimmer, or volleyball player with nondescript shoulder pain that also involves the scapula and provokes paresthesia down the arm, occurring in the absence of a defined traumatic event.

Isolated symptomatic posterior shoulder instability is most often associated with a very specific event or process. Although falling on the outstretched arm is a common scenario because the arm is most often placed in the scapular plane to brace the fall and protect the head, and a posterior force is only placed on the hand. As the body continues to fall to the ground, the arm is extended at the shoulder, placing an anterior force on the shoulder. Such circumstances therefore result much more commonly in anterior dislocation; posterior shoulder dislocations are rarely associated with traumatic events that include falls.

Posterior shoulder instability is seen most often in the scenario of electric shocks and epilepsy. It appears that electrical stimulation to the muscles around the shoulder, when provided in a pathologic setting, can

BOX 3-3. Types of Instability

AMBRI: Atraumatic etiology, multidirectional instability, bilateral shoulders, rehabilitation with rotational strengthening, and inferior capsular tightening
TUBS: Traumatic etiology, unidirectional, Bankart ligamentous detachment, surgical repair

BOX 3-4. History Related to Instability

Nature of onset (traumatic or atraumatic)
Perceived direction (anterior, posterior, inferior, or combination)
Degree (subluxation or dislocation)
Method of reduction (spontaneous or manipulative)
Character of symptoms (apprehension, pain, paresthesias)
Frequency (daily or intermittently)
Volition (voluntary, involuntary, or obligatory)
Ease of dislocation (significant energy or minimal energy)
Arm position associated with apprehension

result in posterior shoulder dislocations. Severe electrical discharges, whether from within (major grand mal seizure) or extrinsic (such as an electric shock), appear to result in the posterior shoulder musculature actually *pulling* the shoulder out of joint. Historically, there has also been an increase in posterior dislocations of the shoulder associated with excessive consumption of alcohol and the social activities that can follow. Falling asleep on a park bench with the arms over the back of the bench while inebriated has been associated with posterior shoulder dislocations.

Box 3-4 lists the queries that should accompany a history that suggests instability.

Paresthesia

The most common shoulder-related pathology associated with a perception of numbness, tingling, or paresthesia down the arm is instability. The patient's perception of this neurologic symptom is usually nondermatomal if the process occurs in the shoulder girdle. A patient with multidirectional instability might note a tingling all the way down the arm involving several peripheral nerve dermatomes. In contrast, a cervical root irritation of a herniated cervical disk predictably results in a specific dermatomal pattern of symptoms. An intrinsic shoulder problem, such as a rotator cuff tear, can result in secondary neurologic symptoms. In an effort to support the painful arm, the patient might rest it on an armrest for a prolonged time and develop cubital tunnel syndrome. Similarly, a patient who is protecting the arm and minimizing functional elevation can develop carpal tunnel symptoms from inadequate fluid mobilization and prolonged dependency of the limb.

Weakness

Common causes of weakness include cerebral dysfunction, nerve transmission dysfunction, musculotendinous deficiency, pain, and biochemical causes. With cerebral dysfunction, the patient is not generating the electrical signal (malingering). Nerve transmission dysfunction, such as Parsonage-Turner syndrome, can result from primary neuronal injury. Biochemical problems result from synaptic biochemical pathology, as in myasthenia gravis, polymyalgia rheumatica, and dystrophies.

In a clinical setting, the most common cause of weakness is likely a rotator cuff tear, and although some tears are pain free, most patients experience some pain associated with the weak arm. It is important to ascertain other potential causes of weakness in the complete evaluation of a shoulder-related complaint.

Crepitus

A patient's perception of crepitus around the shoulder is rarely seen without other associated symptoms. Chronic rotator cuff tendinitis and chronic inflammation of the subacromial bursa can result in a crunching sensation and cause the patient to report a noise coming from the shoulder. Because these are inflammatory conditions, they are nearly always associated with some perception and complaint of pain as well. Scapulothoracic bursitis and snapping scapula syndrome can cause a painful crunching sensation in the patient's upper chest posteriorly when the patient elevates the arm. This usually is also associated with some pain.

Following surgery for rotator cuff repair, patients often become aware of painless crepitus in the subacromial space. Although the exact etiology remains unclear, it is likely to be related to the regeneration of the bursa that had been excised as part of the initial surgical procedure. It seems to become most apparent during physical therapy rehabilitation at about the sixth week, and it can linger for several months. Although patients predictably hear the crepitus and perceive the vibration, only rarely is there an accompanying complaint of pain.

Other intra-articular processes can cause noise to be perceived in the shoulder. Minor subluxations may be perceived as a "thunking" sound. Labral tears similarly can cause a low-frequency noise that a patient either hears or feels. Identifying noises and their specific causes can be frustrating and elusive. Fortunately, many other history and physical examination features offer substantive clues to a correct diagnosis.

PHYSICAL EXAMINATION

Cervical Spine (Neck)

The physical examination of the shoulder begins at the neck. Pathology within the cervical spine can manifest with arm pain and nerve symptoms that radiate down the arm. The patient might believe the source of the problem to be somewhere other than the neck. The examiner begins by standing behind the patient and observing the neck and shoulder girdle for symmetry, muscle mass, scars, and deformity. The examiner then assesses the shoulder's ROM, including extension, flexion, rotation, and bending; this is best done while standing behind the patient. Because it is difficult to use a goniometer to make measurements, surface relationships are commonly substituted.

Neck extension is recorded by estimating the angle by which the imaginary line from the occiput to the mentum of the chin extends above the horizontal (Fig. 3-3). Flexion is recorded by noting how many fingerbreadths the chin is from the chest when the patient flexes the neck as much as possible (Fig. 3-4). For lateral flexion, the patient leans the head to the side while looking forward, and the distance from the shoulder to the ear is recorded (Fig. 3-5). Lastly, the patient turns the head from side to side and the examiner notes the degree of rotation (Fig. 3-6). These cervical spine motions are made actively (by the patient) rather than passively (by the examiner).

The Spurling test (Fig. 3-7) is used to assess cervical radiculopathy and has been shown to decrease the foraminal cross-sectional area of all cervical neuroforamina by 70%.[66] This test is performed by placing the

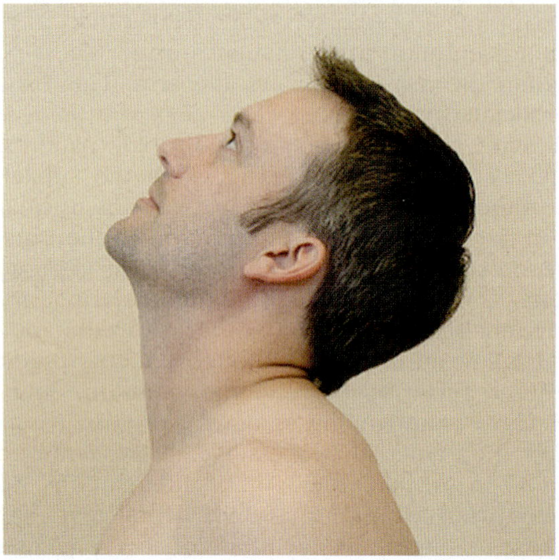

FIGURE 3-3: Neck extension of the cervical spine is assessed by estimating the angle between the horizontal plane and a line connecting the chin and the occiput.

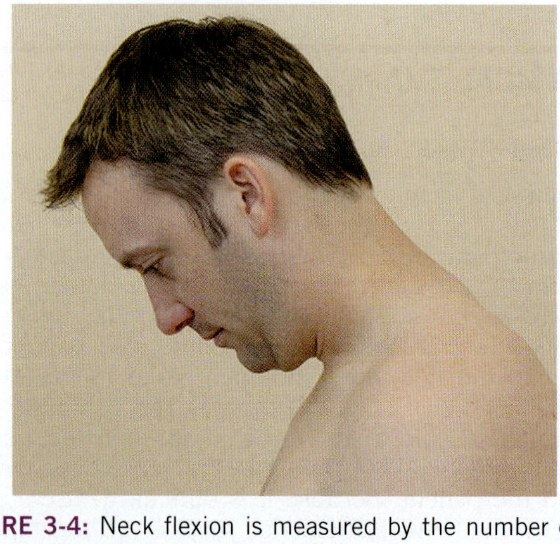

FIGURE 3-4: Neck flexion is measured by the number of fingerbreadths between the chin and the chest.

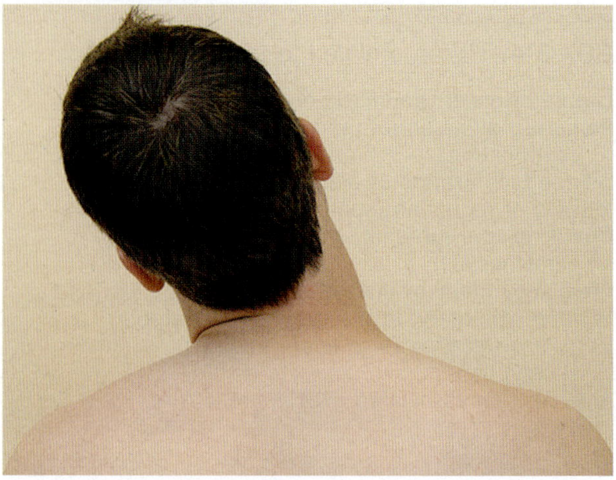

FIGURE 3-5: Lateral flexion is measured by the distance between ear and shoulder. Care should be taken to ensure the patient does not lift the shoulder during testing.

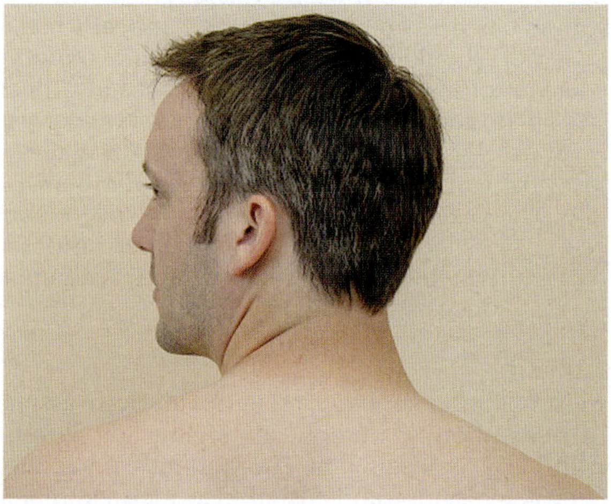

FIGURE 3-6: Lateral rotation is assessed in degrees as the angle through which the patient is able to turn the head from side to side.

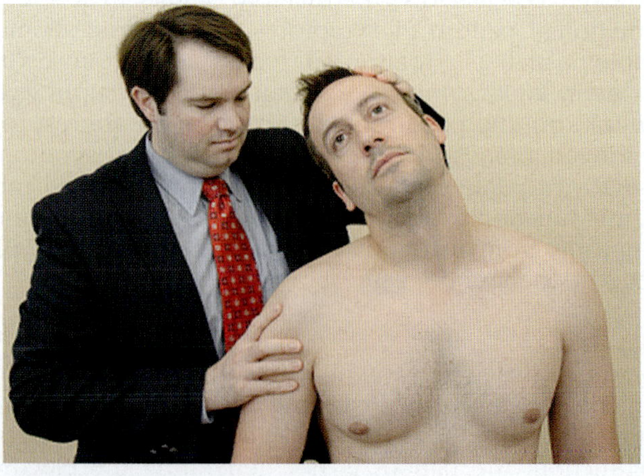

FIGURE 3-7: The Spurling test. An axial load is applied to the top of the head when the cervical spine is extended and rotated toward the affected side.

BOX 3-5. Radicular Patterns of Cervical Nerve Roots

C4: Base of neck pain, trapezial pain
C5: Lateral arm pain (deltoid region)
C6: Lateral forearm pain, along with thumb and index finger pain
C7: Long finger pain
C8: Ring and small finger pain
T1: Medial forearm pain

cervical spine in extension and rotating the head toward the affected shoulder. An axial load is then placed on the spine. Reproduction of the patient's shoulder or arm pain is considered to be a positive response. Conversely, the patient's symptoms may be relieved by flexing and rotating the neck to the contralateral side.[56] Studies have shown a low sensitivity and moderate to high specificity for the Spurling test, ranging from 30% to 50% and 74% to 92%, respectively.[59,69,73] Box 3-5 lists common cervical radiculopathies and their associated upper extremity pain patterns.

Although a detailed neurologic examination is beyond the purview of most shoulder examinations, clinical judgment determines the degree of peripheral nerve assessment necessary to establish a correct and complete diagnosis. Examining the strength of the trapezius, deltoid, spinati, and biceps and triceps muscles suffices for most general shoulder examinations. However, in some situations a more thorough examination needs to be completed, which includes assessment of the motor and sensory distributions of each peripheral nerve of the upper extremity or extremities.

Shoulder

Inspection

Inspection of both shoulders can reveal pathology that would otherwise go unnoticed if the examiner relied solely on the patient history or physical examination (Video 3-1). Both shoulders need to be exposed (Fig. 3-8). First, observe the clavicles for deformity at both the sternoclavicular joint and the acromioclavicular joint. A prominent sternoclavicular joint can be due to an anterior dislocation, inflammation of the synovium, osteoarthritis, infection, or condensing osteitis. A loss of sternoclavicular joint contour is consistent with a posterior dislocation of the medial clavicle, which is worked up urgently to confirm the diagnosis. The acromioclavicular joint is often prominent secondary to osteoarthritis and needs to be compared to that of the opposite side for symmetry.

The relative height of each shoulder is noted as the patient sits with arms by the sides. Small differences in shoulder height are often found in the general population, and such normal differences can be confirmed by asking the patient whether his or her shirt sleeves seem longer on one side than the other. Pathologic causes of a difference in shoulder height can be explained by problems with the articulation of the scapula and thorax or glenohumeral joint. Drooping of the scapula can be caused by trapezius paralysis, scapular winging, scoliosis, pain that results in splinting of the scapula, fractures of the scapula, or disruption of the scapula–clavicular suspensory complex. Deltoid dysfunction can cause the humerus to hang lower on the unaffected side.

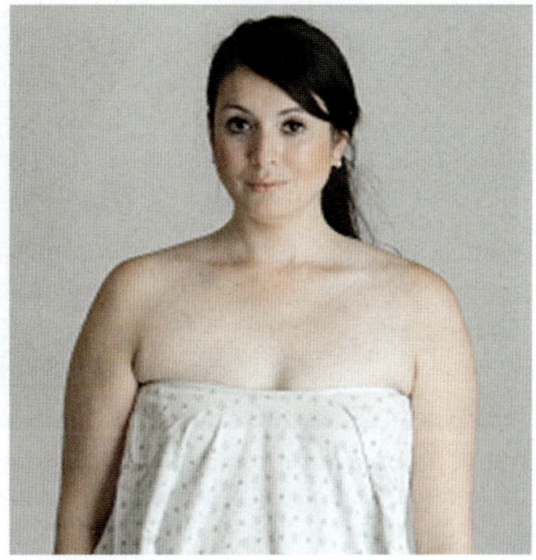

FIGURE 3-8: For female patients, a gown is fashioned such that both shoulders can be visually examined.

Muscle inspection begins with the three portions of the deltoid muscle. Marked atrophy is easy to identify, but deficiencies in the posterior or middle deltoid are more difficult to appreciate until active shoulder motion is initiated (Fig. 3-9). In patients with a large amount of subcutaneous tissue, palpation of the muscle belly may be the only way to distinguish a pathologic muscle contraction from the normal side. Inspection from the back allows assessment of the muscle bulk of the supraspinatus and infraspinatus muscles as well as the trapezius muscle (Fig. 3-10). The anterior and posterior axillary folds are observed for muscle contours of the pectoralis major and latissimus dorsi, respectively.

Once the muscle bulk has been assessed, the static position of the scapulae must be noted. If the soft tissue obscures the view of the medial border or the scapular spine, palpation of these landmarks can help visualize the attitude of the scapula at rest. Excessive lateral rotation of the scapula or an increased distance between the medial border of the scapula and the spine could be caused by trapezius palsy. This can also be accompanied by a prominent inferior tip of the scapula. A laterally prominent inferior scapula tip can also be caused by serratus anterior muscle weakness related to a long thoracic nerve injury, but this might only be recognized during active shoulder motion.

The most common skin manifestations of shoulder pathology are ecchymosis, which occurs after fractures, dislocations, or traumatic tendon ruptures, and erythema,

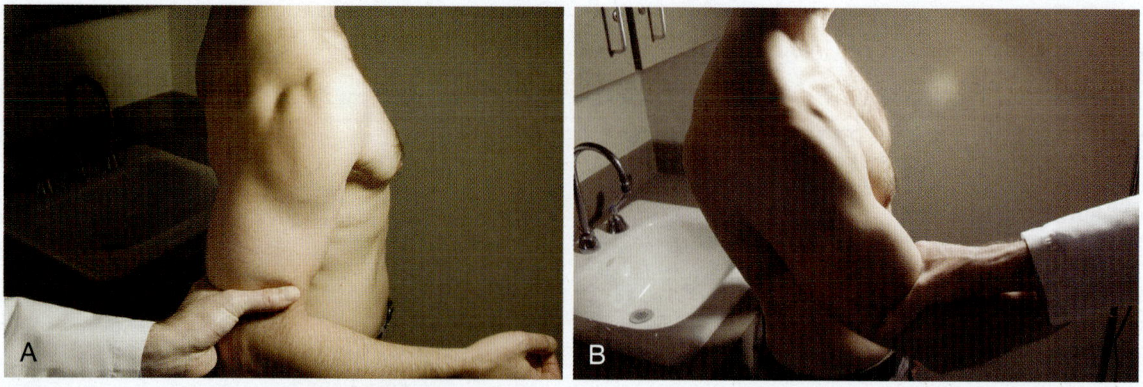

FIGURE 3-9: A, Active muscle contraction against resistance allows the raphe between the middle and posterior bundles of the deltoid muscle to be more easily visualized. **B,** Resisted forward flexion accentuates the raphe between the anterior and middle deltoid muscle bundles.

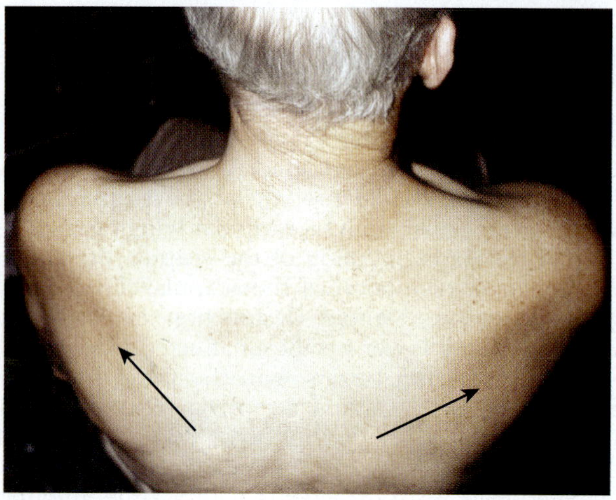

FIGURE 3-10: Bilateral infraspinatus muscle wasting (*arrows*).

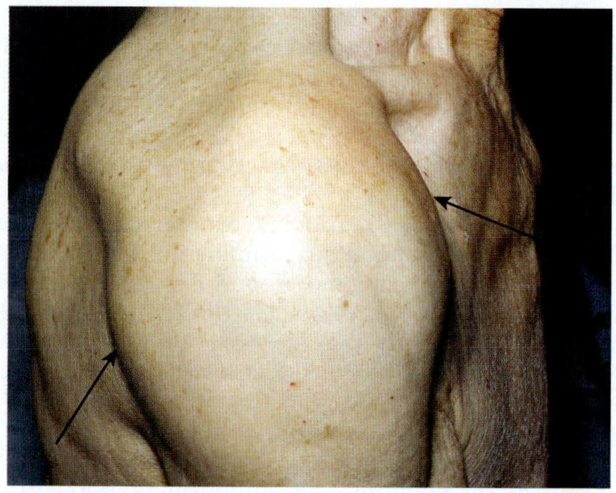

FIGURE 3-11: A fluid bulge (*arrows*) seen here can be an obvious sign of a large or massive rotator cuff tear.

which occurs with infection and systemic inflammatory conditions. Less commonly, the skin around the anterior shoulder is swollen and enlarged due to a subacromial effusion and a chronic rotator cuff tear (Fig. 3-11). The examiner should note the presence of any scars and their location and character. A widened scar can indicate a collagenopathy, often seen in association with shoulder instability.

Palpation

All the joints around the shoulder girdle and any potentially pathologic tissue are palpated for deformity, tenderness, or asymmetry with the normal side (Video 3-2). These locations include the sternoclavicular and acromioclavicular joints, acromion, greater tuberosity, bicipital groove, trapezius, superomedial tip of the scapula, and posterior glenohumeral joint line. The sternoclavicular joint should not be tender and should not move relative to the manubrium.

Localization of the acromioclavicular joint is easy in thin patients, but many patients require the identification of other more easily palpable landmarks. The examiner can start on the medial clavicle and continue laterally until the acromioclavicular joint is felt. In addition, the soft spot where the spine of the scapula meets the clavicle can usually be palpated even in obese patients. Just anterior to the soft spot is the acromioclavicular joint (Fig. 3-12). Lateral to the soft spot is the acromion. The acromioclavicular joint should not be mobile relative to the acromion and should not be tender to palpation. The posterior edge of the acromion can be palpated as an easy landmark to distinguish the lateral edge of the acromion. This is especially useful in obese patients who do not have other easily identifiable landmarks. Knowing where the lateral acromion ends allows palpation of the greater tuberosity and the insertion of the supraspinatus. Any crepitus with passive motion of the shoulder is noted because it can be felt in patients with a rotator cuff tear or calcific tendinitis.

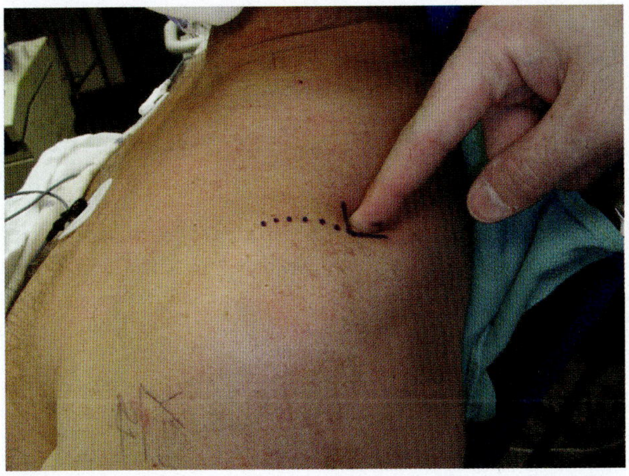

FIGURE 3-12: The soft spot where the spine of the scapula meets the clavicle is easily palpable. Anterior to the soft spot is the acromioclavicular joint (*dotted line*).

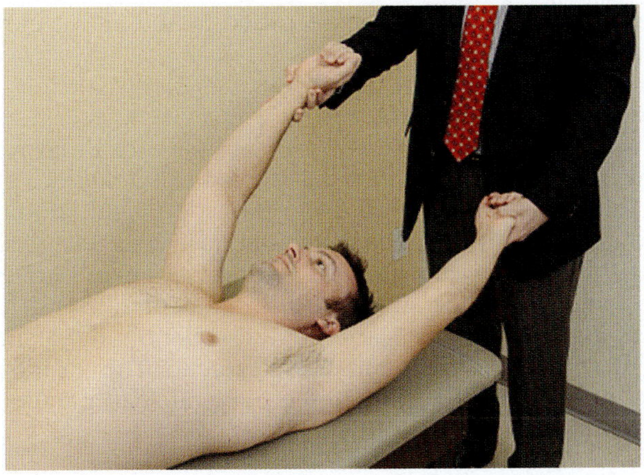

FIGURE 3-13: Supine passive elevation. The patient is placed supine to prevent arching of his or her back during examination. In this case the examination reveals 170 degrees of elevation on the left and 140 degrees on the right.

Crepitus is difficult to palpate during active motion because the contracted deltoid masks this finding.

Palpation of the deltoid muscle may be necessary to ensure that the muscle belly contracts when visualization is obscured by the subcutaneous tissue. Where a fracture is present, small movements in the anterior, lateral, and posterior directions can allow the examiner to quickly assess all three muscle bellies of the deltoid while minimizing patient discomfort.

The bicipital groove is palpated with the forearm rotated in a neutral position or directed straight in front of the patient. The groove is in line with the forearm and approximately 1 cm lateral to the coracoid process when the arm is in neutral rotation. Moving the arm in short arcs of internal and external rotation with the arm at the patient's side allows the examiner to palpate the ridge of the lesser and greater tuberosities, thereby revealing the location of the groove. Many patients have tenderness in this location, especially near the acromion, because of the proximity of the rotator cuff and the subacromial bursa, any of which may be inflamed and tender.

Joint Motion

In measuring and recording ROM it is important that *both* affected and normal shoulders be examined passively and actively (Videos 3-3, 3-4, and 3-5). Furthermore, the active elevation against the force of gravity is recorded both while the patient is supine and while sitting.

Many years ago, the American Shoulder and Elbow Surgeons Society agreed to measure and record the three cardinal planes of motion: elevation in the scapular plane, external rotation with the elbow near the side, and internal rotation using spinal segments as the reference points. Abduction (elevation with the arm in the coronal plane) is not considered a cardinal plane of shoulder motion. However, instability assessment does record both internal and external rotation with the arm in 90 degrees of abduction.

Because shoulder motion is the result of four separate articulations (glenohumeral, scapulothoracic, acromioclavicular, and sternoclavicular), only the *total* motions are recorded, not those occurring at the individual joints. The examination begins by measuring the motion of the unaffected arm initially.

Passive Shoulder Elevation

The patient is placed supine on the examination table without a pillow (unless severe kyphosis or a cervical spine disease necessitates one). The examiner passively lifts the arm over the patient's head and records the highest part of the arc that the *elbow* makes while the axis of the humerus generally points toward the opposite hip (Fig. 3-13). Because the elbow begins at the patient's side (0 degrees), as the arm is passively elevated, the elbow traverses an angle (in the sagittal plane) as the arm is brought overhead. One standard point is the patient's forehead, which typically represents 160 degrees. If the arm can only be brought up so it points to the ceiling, the elbow has traversed 90 degrees. Motion is *not* measured along the axillary crease. The elevation angle is ideally recorded in increments of 10 degrees.

Active Elevation (Supine)

After the passive motion is recorded, the patient elevates the arm under his or her own power in the same fashion as during the passive examination. Once again, the arc of motion recorded is the arc that the elbow makes in the sagittal plane, and the elevation angle is measured to the nearest 10 degrees.

Active Elevation (Standing)

The patient is positioned standing with his or her back against a wall, which prevents hyperextension of the back. The patient lifts the arm toward the ceiling, and the arc of motion is recorded. The patient is observed from the lateral perspective, and the arc of motion that the elbow has traversed is recorded as the active elevation of the arm (Fig. 3-14).

Passive External Rotation

While the patient remains supine, passive external rotation is measured. The elbow is flexed to 90 degrees and the elbow is moved away from the side (slight shoulder abduction) to a distance about the width of the examiner's fist. This establishes an orthogonal angle between the long axis of the humerus and the central axis of the glenoid, which relaxes the superior glenohumeral ligament and the coracohumeral ligament. The examiner cradles the humerus to hold the humeral shaft parallel to the long axis of the spine and prevent the arm from being in relative shoulder extension. The arm is externally rotated by using the forearm as the handle (Fig. 3-15). The arc of motion is recorded from 0 degrees to 90 degrees (or potentially greater with multidirectional instability). The motion is recorded to the nearest 10 degrees.

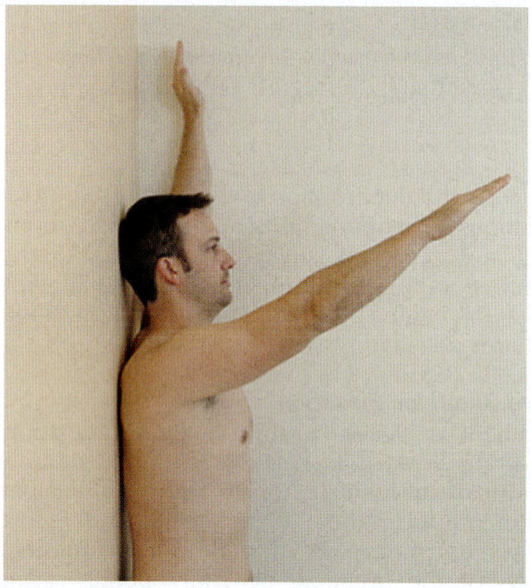

FIGURE 3-14: Active elevation. The patient is positioned standing with the back against the wall, again preventing a perception of increased elevation by arching the back. The patient demonstrates 170 degrees on the left and 120 on the right.

Passive External Rotation in 90 Degrees of Abduction

The patient is positioned supine, with the humerus abducted in the coronal plane to 90 degrees. With the elbow flexed to 90 degrees, the forearm is rotated toward the patient's head and the degree of motion is recorded (Fig. 3-16A). Zero degrees is the starting point with the forearm pointed toward the ceiling. The motion is recorded to the nearest 10 degrees.

Passive Internal Rotation in 90 Degrees of Abduction

With the patient remaining supine, the humerus is abducted in the coronal plane to 90 degrees. The elbow remains flexed to 90 degrees as the forearm is rotated toward the patient's foot, and the degree of motion is recorded (Fig. 3-16B). Zero degrees is the starting point with the patient's forearm pointed toward the ceiling. The motion is recorded to the nearest 10 degrees.

Internal Rotation

The patient reaches behind his or her back and then reaches up between the scapulae (in the fashion of passing a belt or fastening a bra). The examiner pulls the tip of the patient's thumb up the back, and the tip of the thumb determines the level along the spine, which is recorded as the degree of internal rotation (Fig. 3-17). The position of the scapula of the arm that is not being examined provides the proper levels to interpolate. The superior angle of the *nonmeasured side* is opposite T4, and the inferior angle is opposite T7. The iliac crest is at the L4 level. Occasionally the shoulder is so stiff that the patient can only reach the sacrum or greater trochanter of the ipsilateral hip. Severe scoliosis or a stiff elbow on the affected side invalidates these measurements.

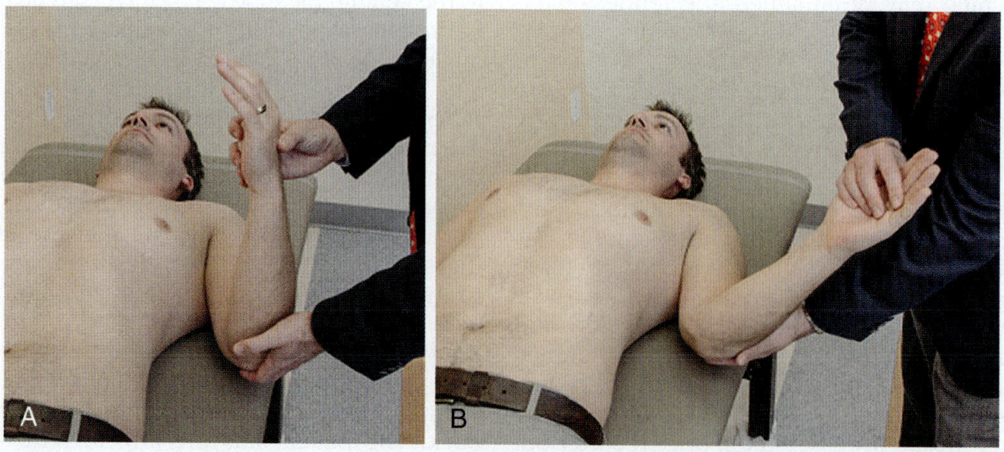

FIGURE 3-15: Supine passive external rotation. **A,** The arm is positioned slightly away from the body and in line with the torso. **B,** The arm is externally rotated, demonstrating 45 degrees of external rotation.

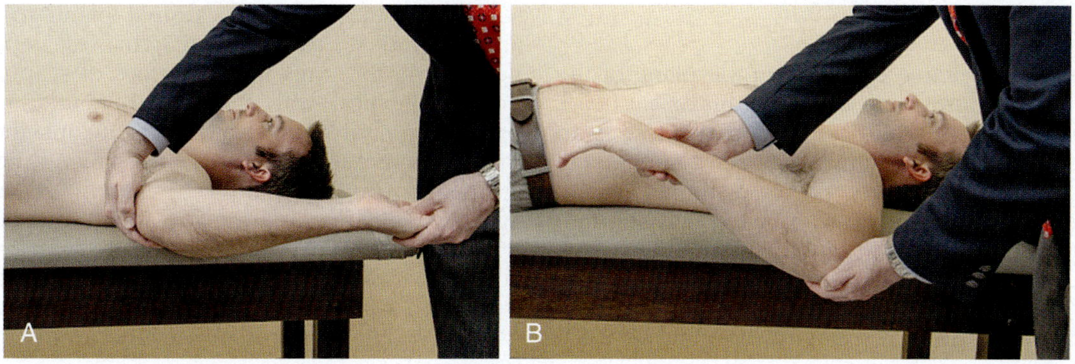

FIGURE 3-16: Supine abducted passive rotation. The arm is abducted 90 degrees and the humerus is kept parallel to the floor. **A,** The arm is passively externally rotated, revealing 90 degrees of rotation. **B,** Internal rotation of the arm, demonstrating 70 degrees of passive motion.

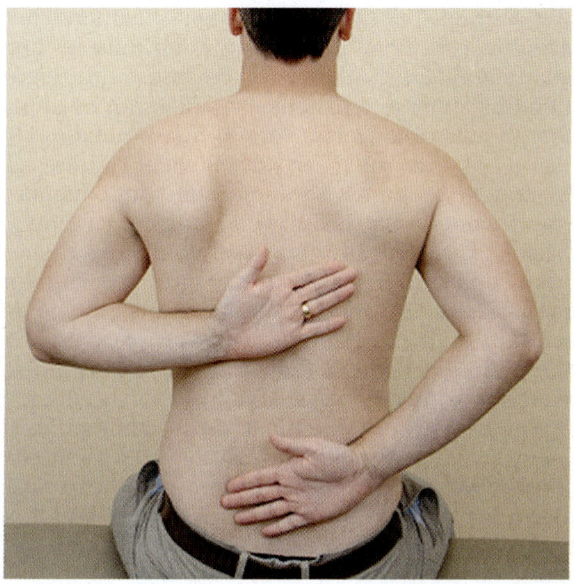

FIGURE 3-17: Internal rotation. This is measured according to the spinal level reached by the tip of the thumb. This patient is able to internally rotate to T7 on the left and L1 on the right.

TABLE 3-1 Strength Grading

Grade	Description
0	Complete muscle paralysis, absence of muscle fasciculation
1	Visible or palpable muscle contraction that is too weak to move the affected joint, even when not working against gravity
2	Muscle contraction that can move the involved joint in the absence of gravity but that is too weak to move the joint through its range against gravity
3	Muscle strength is adequate to move the involved joint through its range against gravity without any added resistance
4	Muscle contraction is adequate to move the joint through its range against gravity with added resistance, but the range is less than full compared to the contralateral side
5	Normal and full range compared to the contralateral side

Active Cross-Body Adduction

Standing or sitting, the patient elevates the arm to the shoulder level, with the upper arm in the scapular plane (0 degrees). The patient then brings the arm across the front of the chest while maintaining it at shoulder level. The arc of motion is recorded.

Functional Strength Testing

General Principles of Functional Strength Testing

Strength testing in the evaluation of a shoulder problem requires a systematic, bilateral assessment of the primary muscles responsible for shoulder ROM. When evaluating patients with more subtle symptoms related to dynamic activities or high levels of athletic performance, a more global assessment of whole-body muscle strength may be needed. This would identify deficits in lower body or core muscle strength, which may be responsible for kinetic chain problems causing overload and injury to the shoulder.

Functional strength testing in the three cardinal planes—elevation in the plane of the scapula, external rotation, and internal rotation—is necessary for understanding a patient's functional limitations and the effect of these on activities of daily living. Assessment of functional strength is often a good place for the orthopedic surgeon to start the strength testing because it can indicate where a more detailed examination of muscle strength should be performed. Isolated muscle strength testing is covered later in the neurologic testing section. Table 3-1 lists the grading system for the assessment of muscle strength.

Functional Strength Assessment

To test strength with active elevation in the plane of the scapula, the patient raises both arms over his or her head. Because most people naturally perform overhead reaching activities by elevating the arm in the plane of the scapula,[26] this simple maneuver usually results in a good demonstration of functional forward elevation strength and allows the assessment of grade 0 to 3 functional strength. Muscle strength of grades 4 or 5 is tested by the patient raising the arms in the scapular plane to shoulder level and then resisting a downward force (Fig. 3-18).

To test functional external rotation strength, the patient keeps the elbows flexed to 90 degrees and at the side while rotating the arms out away from the body. Symmetric external rotation is assessed. Because this movement requires no work against gravity, symmetric motion might indicate only grade 2 strength of the affected shoulder.

Functional internal rotation strength is assessed by placing the patient's arm in neutral rotation at his or her side, with the elbow in 90 degrees of flexion. The patient rotates the arm in toward the abdomen as the examiner applies resistance at the wrist.

Patients who can perform these functional ROM and strength tests should then undergo bilateral isometric strength testing in each cardinal plane to differentiate among grades 3 to 5 strength. This test is performed by positioning the arms in 90 degrees of scapular elevation or in adduction with the arm in neutral rotation. The patient maintains that arm position against the examiner's manual internal or external resistance (Fig. 3-19). An asymmetry in the ability to maintain the arm position against resistance indicates grade 4 functional muscle strength in a given cardinal plane. Symmetrical and full ability to resist the examiner indicates grade 5 muscle strength. Some patients have full and symmetrical strength without being able to maintain the arm position against vigorous force.

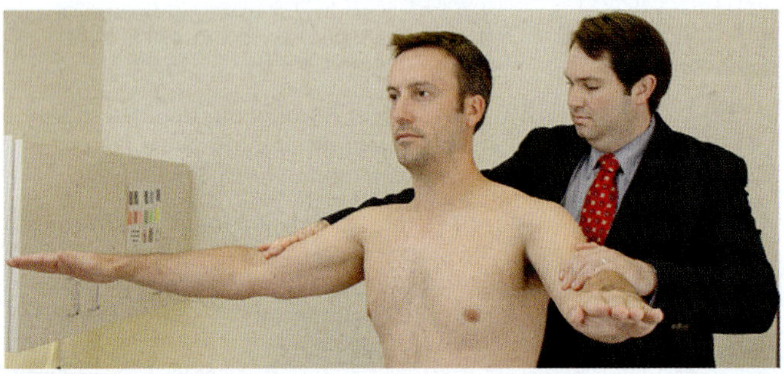

FIGURE 3-18: Functional strength testing of bilateral active elevation.

Stability Assessment

Generalized Laxity Assessment

Stability of the glenohumeral joint is conferred by the passive restraints of the glenohumeral ligaments and by the dynamic restraints of the rotator cuff muscles and the scapular stabilizers (Video 3-6). To assess the degree of ligamentous laxity in a patient's shoulder, an examination of the patient's other joints should first be made. Hyperextension of the metacarpophalangeal joints, elbow joints, and knee joints is often found in patients with general ligamentous laxity (Fig. 3-20). Patients with hyperlaxity can typically flex their thumb to their wrist and place their palms flat on the ground with locked knees. If laxity is found in other joints, it should be expected in both shoulders as well. A history of frequent ankle sprains or patella-femur problems can also be associated with ligamentous laxity of the shoulder. Even if the patient does not exhibit signs of ligamentous laxity in other joints, the shoulders might have excessive laxity. The best way to distinguish between pathologic instability and laxity is to always compare the symptomatic shoulder with the opposite shoulder for all of the following tests.

Sulcus Test

The sulcus test can be performed with the patient sitting or supine (Video 3-7). The examiner pulls the adducted

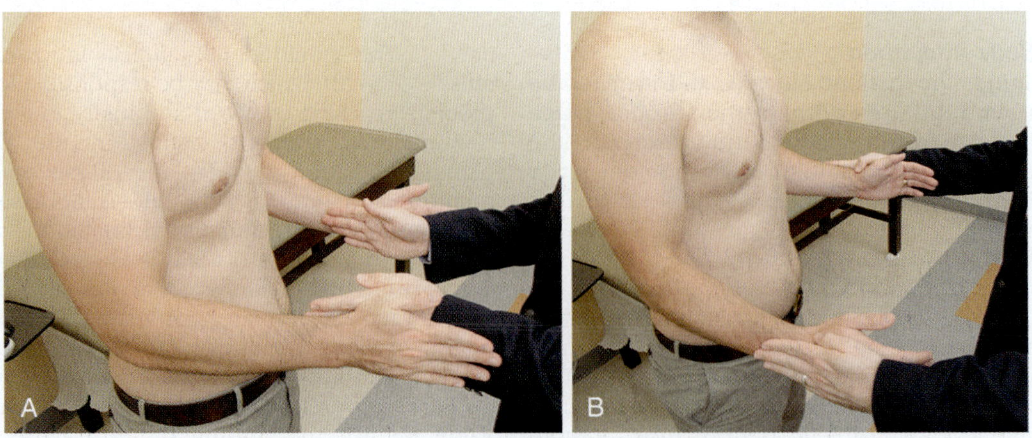

FIGURE 3-19: **A,** Internal rotation and **B,** external rotation strength testing.

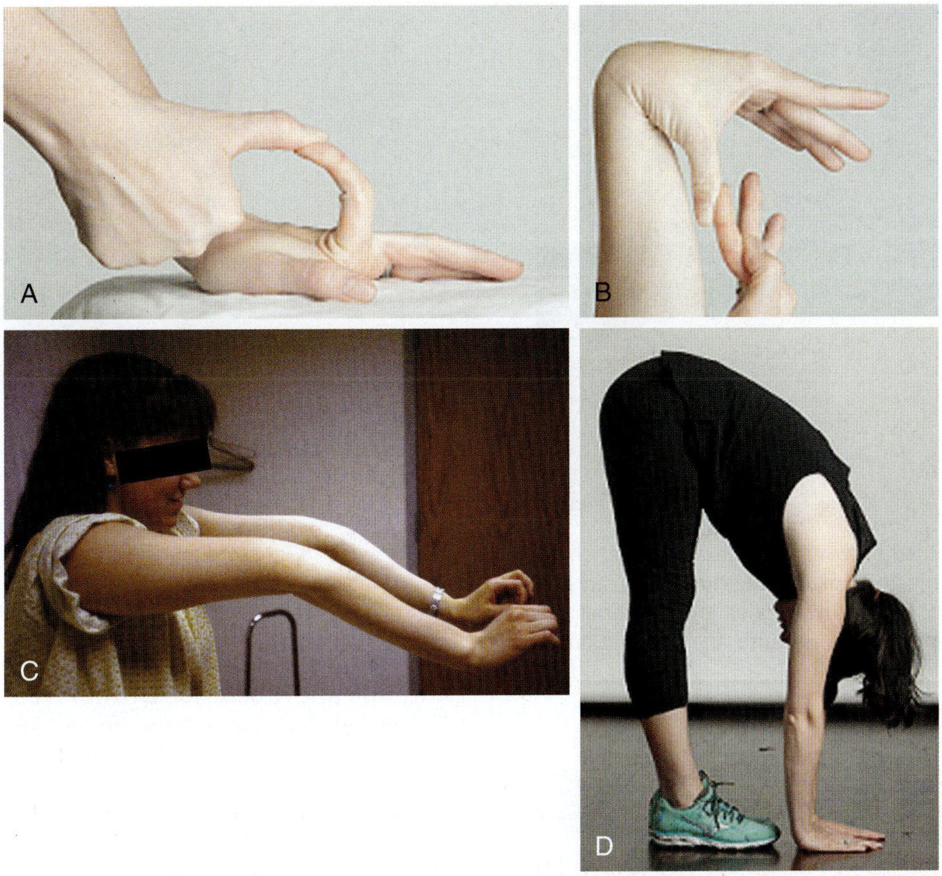

FIGURE 3-20: Generalized hyperlaxity. Hyperlaxity of the metacarpophalangeal joints (**A**), the wrist (**B**), and the elbow joint (**C**). **D,** Patients with ligamentous hyperlaxity can typically place their palms flat on the ground with their knees locked and feet together.

arm at the side toward the foot and measures the amount of translation between the acromion and the humeral head (Fig. 3-21). The translation of the humeral head in centimeters is documented as 1+ for 1 cm and 2+ for 2 cm.[62] The sulcus sign must be correlated with symptoms experienced by the patient. If the patient has a positive sulcus sign, but no symptoms, inferior instability is most likely not a component of their pathology.[3]

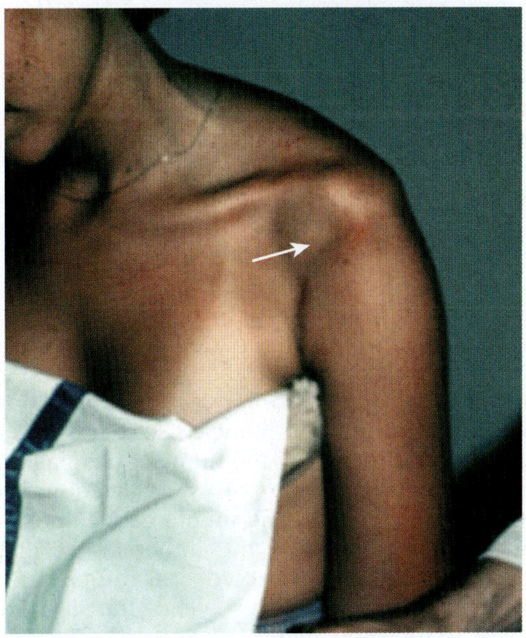

FIGURE 3-21: The sulcus sign *(arrow)*.

Glenohumeral Translation (Load and Shift Test)

Glenohumeral translation can be measured while the patient's arms are resting at his or her side in neutral rotation (Videos 3-8 and 3-9). The examiner stabilizes the scapula with one hand and translates the humeral head with the other hand (Fig. 3-22). The translation of the head is documented as the percentage of the humeral head that can be subluxed anterior to the glenoid rim.[62] The same is done to assess posterior translation. To assess the passive stability conferred by the glenohumeral ligaments, the glenohumeral translation is assessed in varying degrees of internal and external rotation as well as in varying degrees of abduction. The patient is positioned supine and placed at the edge of the table so that

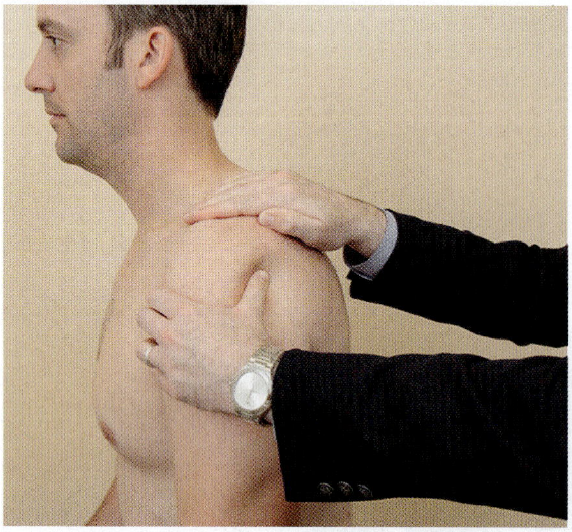

FIGURE 3-22: The load and shift. The examiner stabilizes the ipsilateral scapula and then places the humeral head between their thumb and fingers. Both anterior and posterior translational forces are applied to measure the translation of the humeral head on the glenoid.

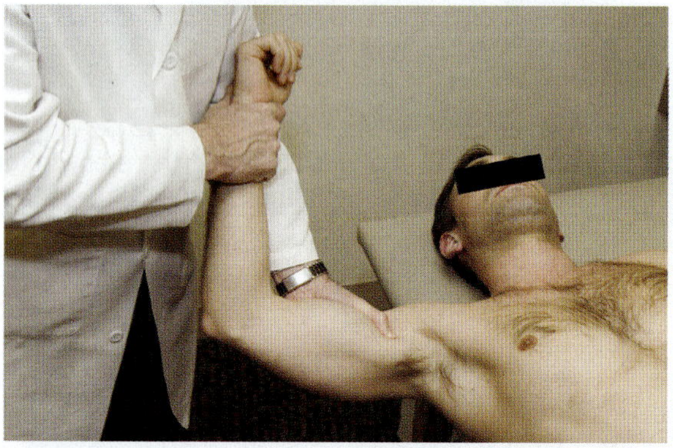

FIGURE 3-23: Assessment of stability conferred by differing aspects of the glenohumeral ligaments. In 90 degrees of abduction and neutral rotation, the inferior glenohumeral ligaments and inferior capsule become taut, providing the majority of ligamentous stability.

the arm can be taken through its full ROM. With one arm, the examiner holds the patient's forearm to control rotation, and the examiner's other hand is placed around the patient's upper arm to control translation. An axial load is placed at the distal humerus so that the examiner can gain a tactile feeling of the humeral head as it articulates with the glenoid. The arm is abducted and rotated into the desired position, and then a gentle anterior shift is made with the hand at the upper arm (Fig. 3-23). Translation of the head is recorded as the percentage of the humeral head that moves out of the glenoid. This maneuver is repeated with a posteriorly directed force. The amount of translation varies with different amounts of arm rotation, so the examiner must repeat the examination on the opposite shoulder using the same arm positions.

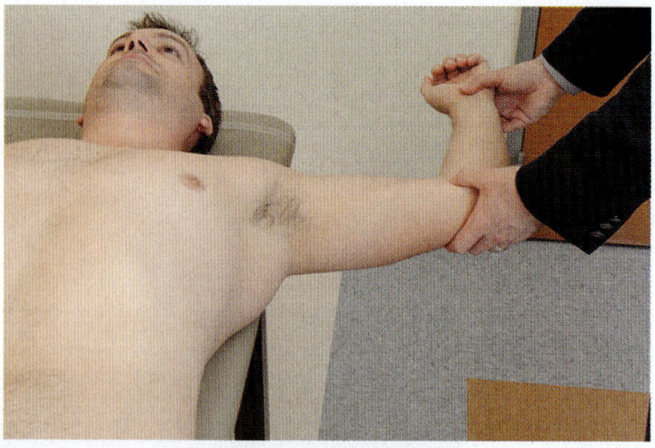

FIGURE 3-24: The apprehension test. The patient is placed in 90 degrees of abduction and 90 degrees of external rotation while supine and assessed for a sense of anterior instability.

Anterior and Posterior Drawer Tests

The anterior and posterior drawer tests as described by Gerber and Ganz[17] are alternative methods for assessing laxity in the shoulder. The patient is placed supine and the arm is abducted 60 degrees. The examiner applies an axial force to the humeral head while holding the arm in neutral rotation. The examiner's other hand is used to translate the humeral head both anteriorly and posteriorly. Translation of the head to the glenoid rim is recorded as grade I, translation over the rim with spontaneous reduction as grade II, and dislocation without spontaneous reduction as grade III.[62]

Apprehension, Relocation, and Surprise Tests

The apprehension test as described by Rowe and Zarins[58] is performed while the patient is supine (Video 3-10). The examiner abducts the patient's arm 90 degrees and then slowly externally rotates the arm to 90 degrees (Fig. 3-24). The patient is asked whether the shoulder feels as if it is about to dislocate. Many patients complain of a vague uncomfortable feeling in the shoulder. Others only show their discomfort with a grimace, or the shoulder muscles involuntarily contract to prevent further shoulder rotation. Any elicitation of apprehension during this maneuver is a positive test. Some patients also complain of pain during this maneuver, and the location of the pain can help the examiner localize the pathology, but pain alone is a poor predictor of traumatic anterior instability. Posterior and superior pain can be caused by posterosuperior labral tears or internal impingement, whereas anterior pain is more likely to be due to an anteroinferior labral tear.

The relocation test as described by Jobe and colleagues[30] is performed in conjunction with the apprehension test. If the patient feels apprehension while the shoulder is externally rotated and abducted 90 degrees, then the examiner applies a posterior force against the proximal arm, which moves the humeral head from an anteriorly subluxed position to a centered position in the glenoid. If the patient no longer has apprehension, but the apprehension returns once the examiner stops applying the posterior force, then the relocation test is positive (Fig. 3-25). Patients with posterosuperior labral tears or internal impingement usually experience an increase in pain during this maneuver because the examiner's posterior force loads the humeral head against the torn labrum.

The surprise test, or anterior release test, is performed at the end of the relocation test, with a sudden removal of the posterior force on the humeral head.[20] The return of an apprehensive sensation is considered a positive test (Fig. 3-26).

The diagnostic accuracy of the apprehension and relocation tests was studied by Farber and colleagues.[15] Physical examinations and subsequent arthroscopies were performed on 363 patients. Of these, 46 had a Bankart tear, Hill-Sachs lesion, humeral avulsion of the glenohumeral ligament on arthroscopy, or radiograph with a documented anterior dislocation; these patients made up the study group, and the rest were used as a comparison group. When apprehension was used as the criterion for a positive test, the sensitivity and specificity of the apprehension test were 72% and 96%, respectively, compared with 50% and 56% when pain was used as the criterion for a positive test. When apprehension was used as the criterion for a positive test, the sensitivity and specificity of the relocation test were 81% and 92%, respectively, compared with 30% and 90% when pain was used as the criterion for a positive test.

In 2013 van Kampen et al. studied the diagnostic value of clinical tests for anterior instability in combination with patient age and history.[72] They found the surprise test to be highly accurate and the relocation and anterior drawer tests to be the most sensitive and specific, respectively. When patient factors and clinical tests were combined, the study revealed that the most important predictors of anterior instability were young age, prior history of dislocation, sudden onset of symptoms, and a positive surprise test. Individual sensitivities and specificities are listed in Table 3-2.

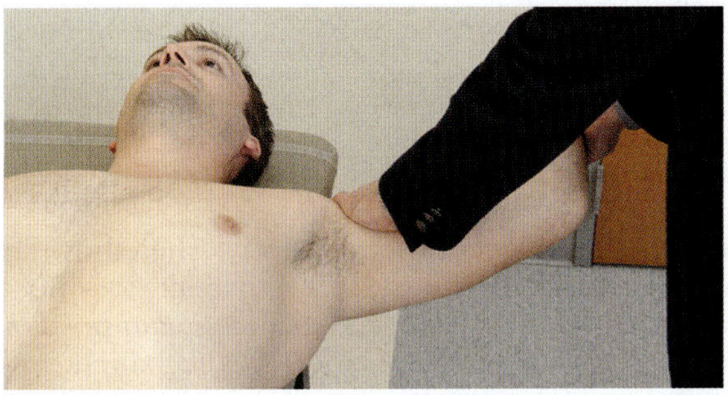

FIGURE 3-25: The relocation test. A posterior directed force is applied to the anterior shoulder while it is in the position causing apprehension. Relief of apprehension symptoms is a positive test.

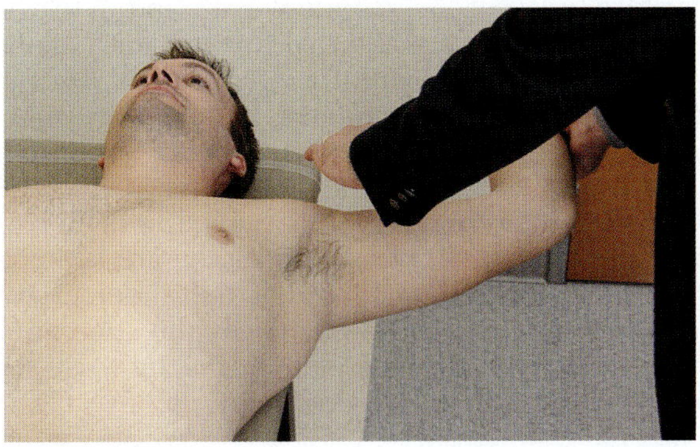

FIGURE 3-26: The surprise test is performed by releasing the posterior directed force and assessing the return of the patient's apprehension.

Posterior Instability Testing

Posterior instability is best tested while the patient is sitting or standing (Videos 3-11 and 3-12). This allows easy visualization of the entire scapula and the posterior muscle contours that often change when the humeral head subluxes or dislocates posteriorly. In patients with severe posterior instability, active forward flexion to 90 degrees, internal rotation, and adduction across the front of the body can cause a posterior dislocation that is easily seen by the examiner. Most patients, however, experience posterior instability only during exertional activities, so the examiner needs to reproduce those conditions to demonstrate posterior instability.

In contrast to anterior instability testing, posterior instability testing begins when the examiner moves the humeral head into a dislocated or subluxated position. This is accomplished by grasping the patient's elbow with one hand and stabilizing the scapula with the other hand. The humerus is brought to 90 degrees of flexion, internally rotated, and adducted across the chest. The examiner then applies a posterior load to the humeral head and maintains that load while slowly abducting the arm (Fig. 3-27). The humerus is kept parallel to the floor and the patient relaxes the shoulder muscles as much as possible. A "clunk" felt when the humeral head relocates into the glenoid indicates a positive test. This test has been

TABLE 3-2 Instability Tests

Test	Sensitivity (%)	Specificity (%)
Apprehension	98	71.6
Relocation	97	78
Surprise	92	84
Anterior drawer	58	93
Load and shift	72	90

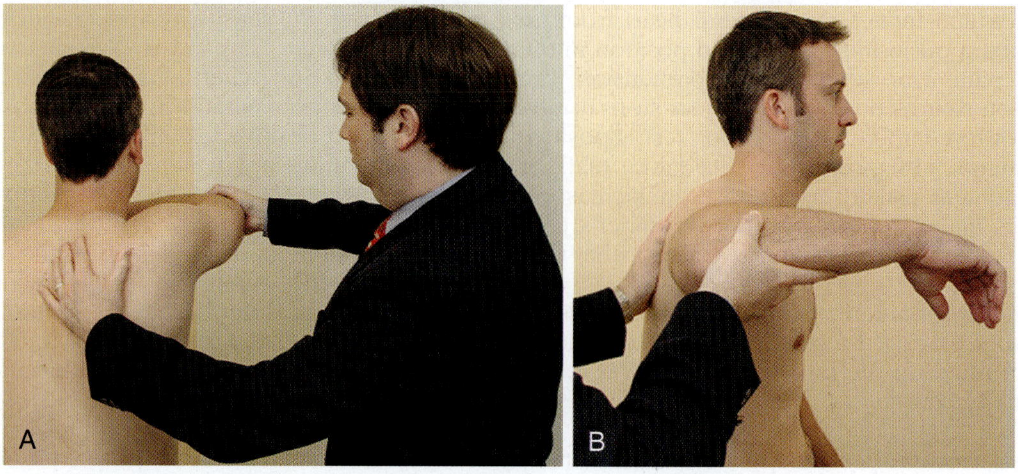

FIGURE 3-27: The jerk test. **A,** The patient's humeral head is subluxated/dislocated posteriorly by placing the arm in 90 degrees of forward flexion and 90 degrees of internal rotation with slight adduction and a posteriorly directed force. **B,** The arm is then abducted while keeping the humerus parallel to the floor. A jerk or clunk is felt when the humeral head reduces.

called the *jerk test* because the shoulder jerks back into the glenoid during a positive test.[39] It has also been called the *Jahnke test* or simply a *posterior load test.*[40]

Rotator Cuff Examination

The rotator cuff examination begins with a visual inspection of the supraspinatus and infraspinatus muscle bulk. Patients with chronic rotator cuff tears often have atrophy of the muscle in the supraspinatus fossa or below the spine of the scapula when compared to the asymptomatic side (see Fig. 3-10). An assessment of the passive and active motion arcs is the second step of the rotator cuff examination, with the expectation that only the active motion is affected in patients with isolated rotator cuff pathology. It is often the case, however, that patients experience a small loss of passive motion secondary to disuse and pain at the extremes of motion.

Subscapularis Muscle

The subscapularis muscle is difficult to isolate with a single specific test because so many other muscles around the shoulder girdle contribute to internal rotation. Tokish et al. found that different arm positions are correlated with the selective activation of different subscapularis muscle regions.[68]

Yoon et al. evaluated several different tests used to evaluate subscapularis deficiency and found the lift-off test to be the most specific for identifying both partial and full thickness tears of the subscapularis.[80] The specificities and sensitivities are listed in Table 3-3.

TABLE 3-3 Tests for the Diagnosis of Subscapularis Tears

Test	Sensitivity (%)	Specificity (%)
Lift-off	12	100
Belly-press	28	99
Bear hug	19	99

Lift-Off Test

The lift-off test can be used if the patient does not have an internal rotation contracture that prevents the patient from passively placing the hand behind his or her back (Videos 3-13 and 3-14). In this test the patient places the hand behind the back at waist level and then, if possible, pushes the hand away from the body. The elbow should not move while doing this.[18] If the patient does not have the strength for this action, the examiner can position the hand away from the waist and ask the patient to hold the hand in that position (Fig. 3-28). If the patient can do this, then the subscapularis muscle is partially functioning. A comparison with the opposite shoulder is always made if the test is abnormal in any way.

Belly-Press Test

Another test specific to the subscapularis muscle is the belly-press test (Fig. 3-29; Videos 3-15 and 3-16).[18] This test requires slightly less internal rotation than the lift-off test and is often less painful to perform for the patient because the hand is not rotated behind the back. The patient must place the hand on his or her belly, keeping the wrist extended so that the elbow is in front of the body. The patient then presses against the belly without flexing the wrist. If the wrist and elbow are locked, this motion can only be performed if the shoulder rotates internally, which is done primarily by the subscapularis. A positive test is when the patient flexes the wrist to push against their belly.

Napoleon Test

A modification of the belly-press test is the Napoleon test (Video 3-17). The patient places the hand on the belly

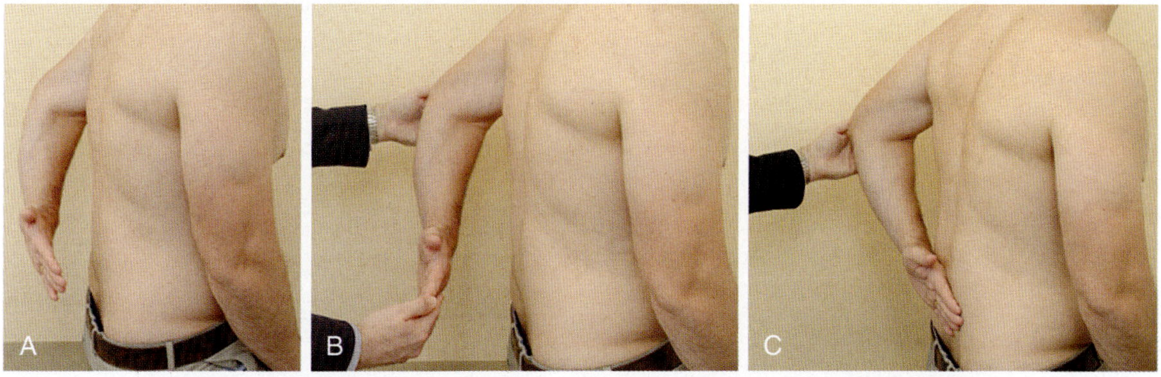

FIGURE 3-28: The lift-off test. **A,** If a patient has the ability to internally rotate and actively hold the hand away from the back, the subscapularis is functional. **B,** A weak subscapularis is suspected if the patient is able to keep the hand off the back only if it is positioned there by the examiner. **C,** An absent subscapularis is suspected if the patient is unable to bring or maintain the hand away from the back.

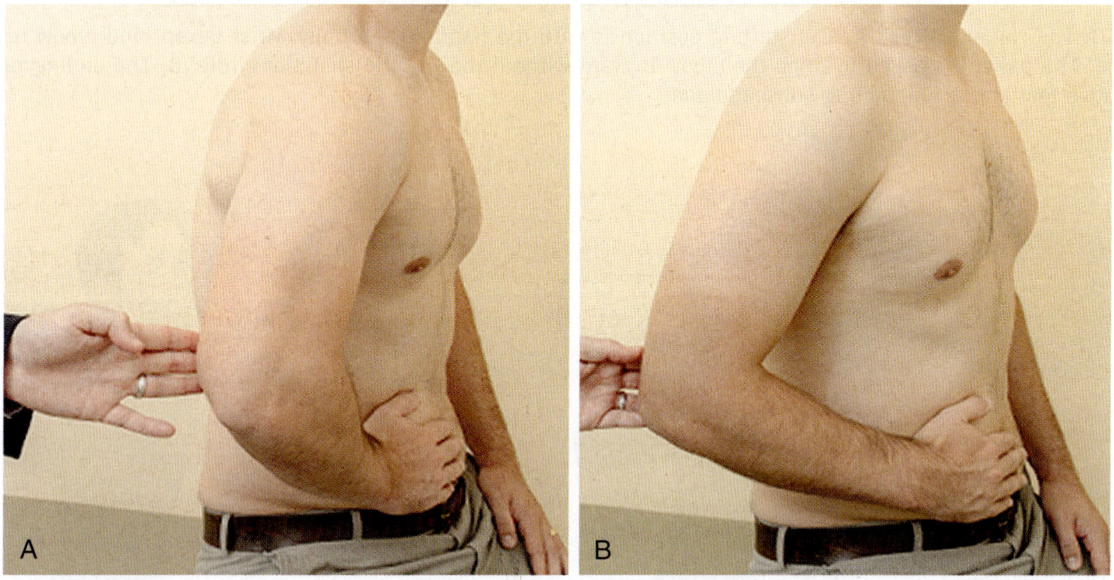

FIGURE 3-29: The belly-press test. **A,** The patient's hand is placed on his or her belly with the wrist straight and elbow in front of the plane of the body. The patient is asked to press against the belly while keeping the wrist straight. **B,** The test is positive, signifying a weak subscapularis, if the patient flexes the wrist to press against the belly.

with the elbow resting at his or her side. While keeping the hand on the belly, the patient pushes the elbow forward (Fig. 3-30). A positive test is recorded when the patient is unable to bring the elbow anteriorly without moving the entire shoulder girdle forward. The examiner can also grade muscle strength by holding resistance against the elbow as the patient attempts to push the elbow forward.

Bear Hug Test

An additional test described is called the bear hug test (Video 3-18).[4] The patient brings the hand over the opposite shoulder. The examiner holds the elbow to prevent elbow flexion during the test, and the patient pushes the hand down against the opposite shoulder or down against the examiner's other hand. Patients with a subscapularis tendon tear or muscle weakness experience pain during this maneuver, or they are unable to push down (Fig. 3-31).

Supraspinatus Muscle

The action of the supraspinatus muscle-tendon unit is difficult to isolate from that of the deltoid because both elevate the humerus (Video 3-19). Rotator cuff muscle testing can also be difficult to perform in patients who experience significant pain that compromises their effort. If the examiner believes pain to be a significant factor in the patient's weakness, then a subacromial lidocaine injection may be used to eliminate pain as a factor.

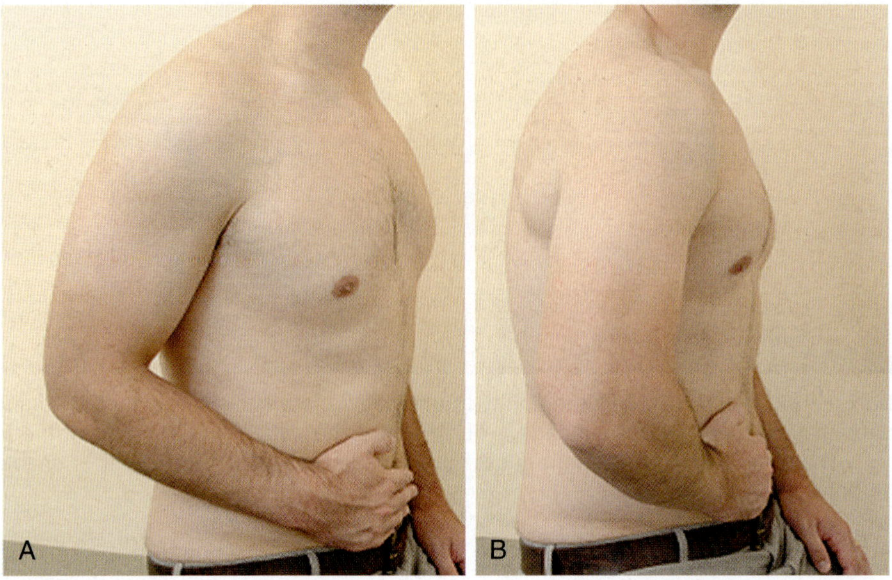

FIGURE 3-30: The Napoleon test. **A,** The starting position is with the hand on the belly, wrist flexed, and elbow resting at the patient's side. The patient is asked to bring the elbow forward without moving the shoulder girdle. **B,** The ending position indicates a negative test and a functioning subscapularis.

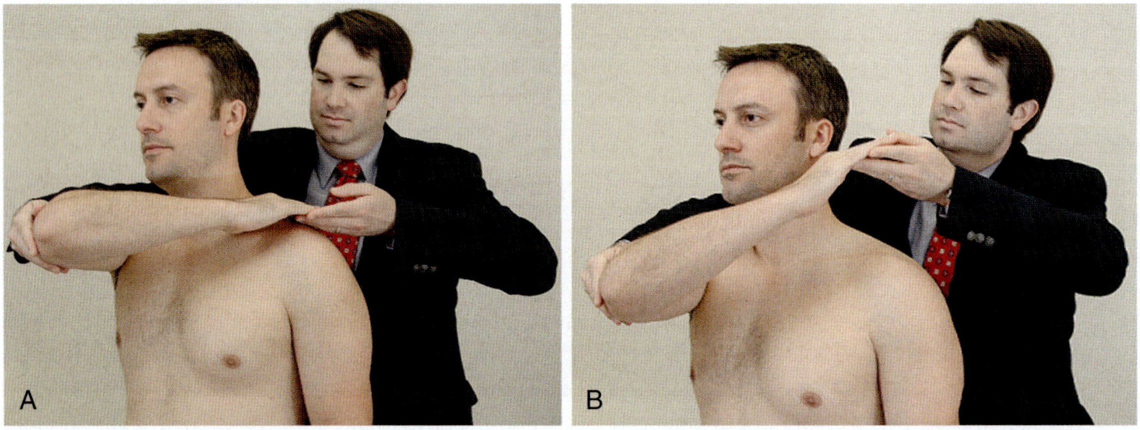

FIGURE 3-31: The bear hug test. **A,** The patient's ability to resist the examiner's attempt to elevate the hand off the contralateral shoulder signifies a functional subscapularis. **B,** A patient with a dysfunctional subscapularis muscle is unable to resist his or her hand being elevated off the contralateral shoulder.

To best isolate the supraspinatus muscle, the arm is internally rotated and elevated 90 degrees so that the muscle-tendon unit is parallel to the floor (Fig. 3-32). Testing both arms simultaneously makes it easy for the examiner to detect subtle differences in strength. The examiner pushes both arms toward the floor while the patient resists. This position has been examined using electromyography to assess supraspinatus activity.[45] The results showed peak supraspinatus activation, but also activation of the anterior and middle deltoid along with the pectoralis major muscle. Any difference in strength can be attributed to the supraspinatus muscle if the deltoid has not been injured. According to a study by Itoi and colleagues, internal or external rotation of the humerus during supraspinatus testing did not improve the accuracy of detecting a torn tendon.[27]

External Rotation

The infraspinatus and teres minor muscles are more easily isolated from the action of the deltoid because the deltoid has very limited ability to externally rotate the humerus. Any loss of strength to external rotation can be attributed to an abnormality in these muscles.

External Rotation Lag Sign

Patients with large or massive rotator cuff tears often have a lag sign (Fig. 3-33), which correlates with disorders of the infraspinatus (Video 3-20).[25,75] This is revealed when the patient holds the arms by his or her sides with the elbows flexed 90 degrees.

The examiner externally rotates the arm as far as it will go passively, and when the examiner releases it, the patient attempts to hold the arm in that position. If the patient's arm internally rotates from where the examiner held it, then the patient has a lag sign that can be documented in degrees. For instance, if a patient has passive external rotation to 45 degrees but can only hold the arm externally rotated to 20 degrees, then the patient has a 25-degree lag sign. In effect the lag sign is simply a way of documenting the difference between the patient's active and passive external rotation.

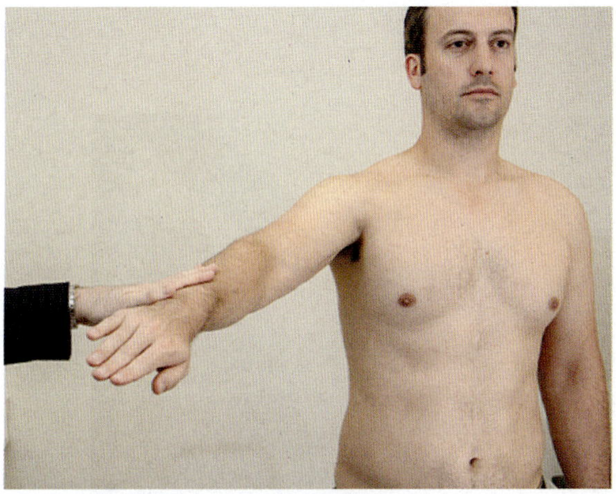

FIGURE 3-32: Supraspinatus strength testing. A downward force is resisted with the arm in 90 degrees of elevation in the scapular plane and internally rotated.

Hornblower's Sign

Originally described in the pediatric obstetric brachial palsy literature, Walch et al. later applied the hornblower's sign to assess teres minor function.[2,75] To perform this test, the examiner abducts the arm 90 degrees in the plane of the scapula, flexes the elbow 90 degrees, and then maximally externally rotates the shoulder (Video 3-21). The patient is asked to hold this position of maximal external rotation. The test is considered positive if the patient is unable to maintain the externally rotated position (Fig. 3-34).

SPECIAL TESTS

Rotator Cuff Tests

Neer Impingement Sign

The Neer impingement sign maneuver, first reported by Neer in 1972 and later fully described by him in 1983,[51] attempts to reproduce compression of the inflamed rotator cuff and subacromial bursa between the humeral head and the undersurface of the acromion and coracoacromial arch. In the classic version of this maneuver, the examiner stands behind the patient and stabilizes the scapula with one hand on the acromion. With the other hand, the examiner elevates the patient's arm in the plane of the scapula. As the arm is brought into full elevation, the examiner holds down the scapula to prevent it from rotating superiorly, bringing the greater tuberosity into contact with the acromion and compressing the potentially inflamed supraspinatus tendon and bursa. In a positive Neer impingement sign, this maneuver reproduces the patient's anterior shoulder pain.

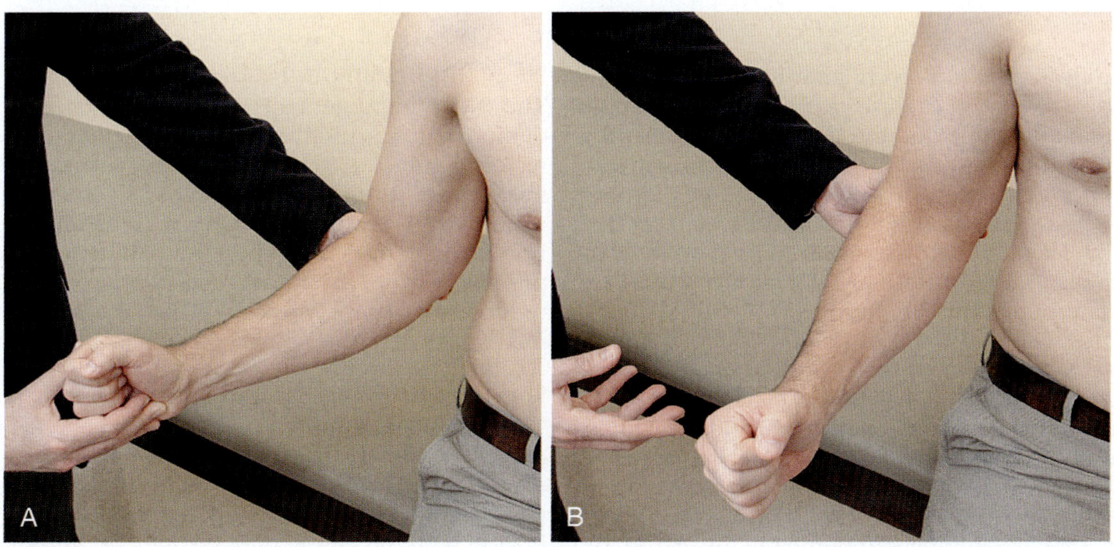

FIGURE 3-33: The external rotation lag sign. **A,** The arm is passively externally rotated to its maximum rotation. **B,** The examiner releases the arm, and the patient attempts to hold the rotated position. Inability to maintain the starting position signifies dysfunctional external rotator muscles and a positive test.

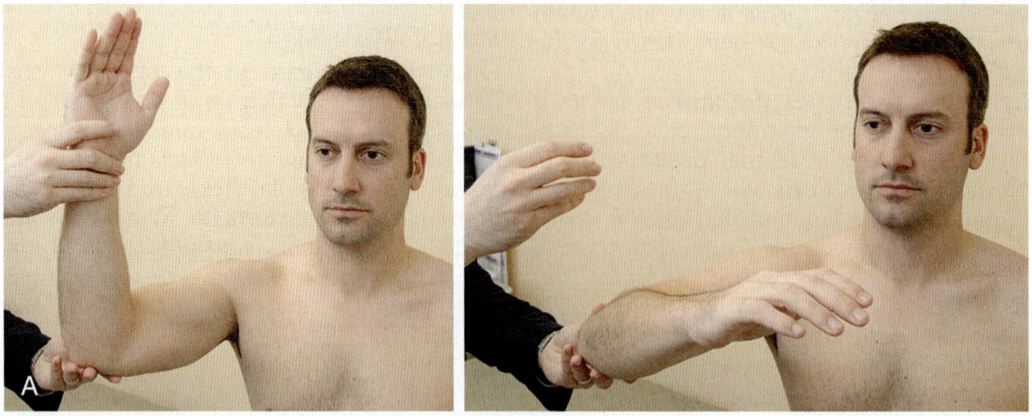

FIGURE 3-34: Hornblower's sign. **A,** The arm is passively positioned in 90 degrees of forward flexion and 90 degrees of external rotation. **B,** A positive test is when the patient is unable to maintain the externally rotated position after the examiner releases the arm, indicating a weak teres minor muscle.

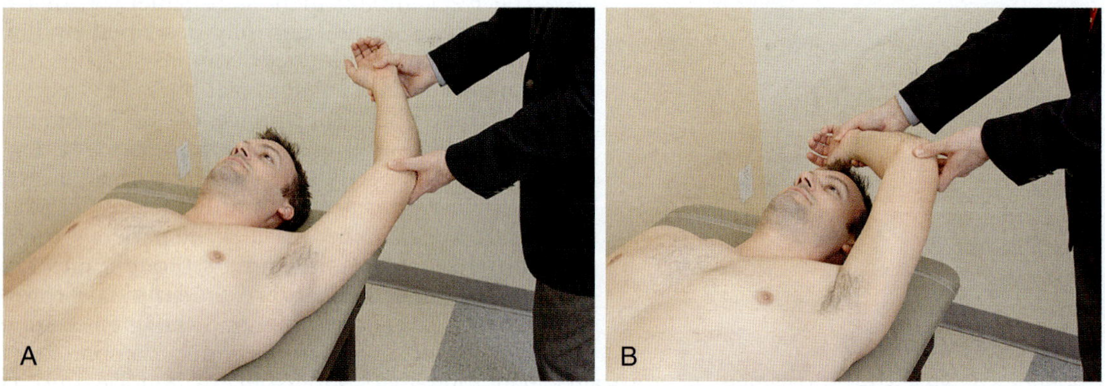

FIGURE 3-35: The modified Neer impingement sign. **A,** The patient is placed supine and the arm brought into full passive flexion in the initial assessment for pain in the anterior shoulder. **B,** A positive test is when this pain is increased by internally rotating the arm.

In a modification of this technique that Dr. Neer has used (personal communication), the patient lies supine on the examination table and the examiner stands at the patient's head. The examiner brings the patient's arm into full elevation and then, with the elbow flexed, applies an internal rotation torque to the arm similar to that described by Hawkins and Kennedy (Fig. 3-35).[22] Performing this maneuver with the patient supine minimizes scapular rotation, eliminating the need for manual stabilization of the scapula by the examiner (Video 3-22).

Neer noted in his original work, and others have confirmed,[44] that other shoulder pathology, especially Bankart lesions, SLAP lesions, and acromioclavicular joint arthritis, often cause pain with this maneuver. Anatomic studies[71] have shown that in addition to rotator cuff and bursal impingement, the greater tuberosity itself or the biceps tendon can directly impinge underneath the acromion when the arm is placed in the Neer position. This likely explains the good sensitivity but limited specificity of the Neer impingement sign.

Neer Impingement Test

The Neer impingement test is performed if a patient demonstrates a positive Neer impingement sign. Approximately 5 mL of 1% lidocaine is injected into the subacromial space. After several minutes the Neer impingement maneuver is again performed. A Neer impingement test is considered positive when the pain associated with the preinjection Neer impingement sign is significantly reduced or absent, indicating that the injected subacromial space was the source of pain.

Hawkins-Kennedy Impingement Test

The Hawkins-Kennedy impingement test was first described by Hawkins and Kennedy in 1980.[22] For this maneuver, the examiner stands at the patient's side, the patient's shoulder is placed in 90 degrees of forward flexion with the elbow bent 90 degrees, and the examiner then forcibly internally rotates the arm (Fig. 3-36; Video 3-23). A positive Hawkins impingement sign is pain as the greater tuberosity rotates under the acromion and

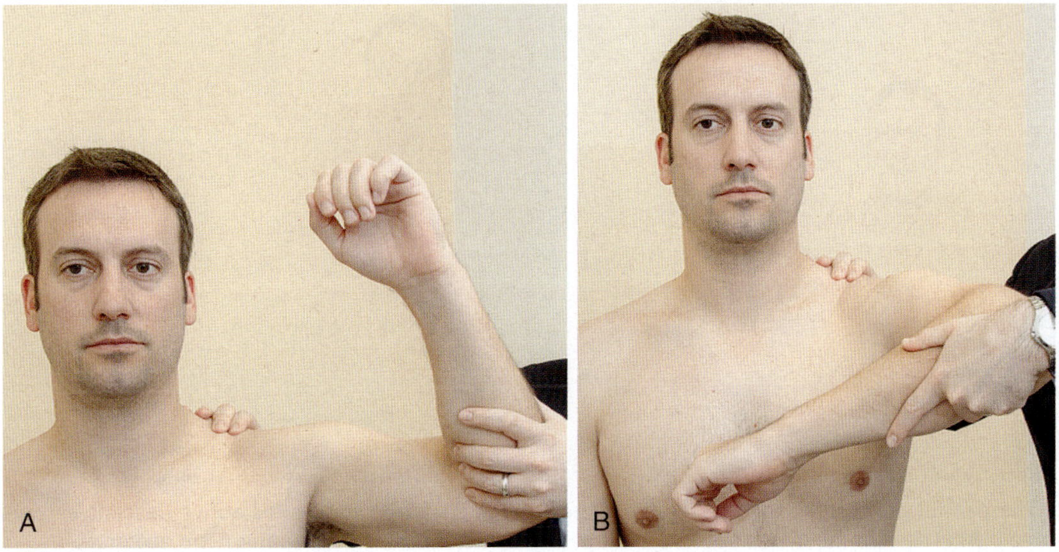

FIGURE 3-36: The Hawkins-Kennedy test. **A,** The arm is initially positioned in 90 degrees of forward flexion. **B,** The examiner then forcibly internally rotates the arm. Reproduction of pain indicates a positive test.

coracoacromial arch, compressing the inflamed bursa and supraspinatus tendon. In one anatomic study[71] all specimens showed direct contact between the coracoacromial ligament and rotator cuff or biceps tendon with this maneuver. As with the Neer impingement sign, this test is sensitive but lacks specificity.

Jobe-Yocum Test

Supraspinatus tendinitis is assessed using the Jobe-Yocum test, first described separately by Jobe and colleagues and by Yocum in 1983.[29,79] Fodor et al. in 2009 demonstrated 90% specificity for supraspinatus pathology with a positive test, but it could not differentiate between tendinosis or tears.[16] With the patient maintaining the arm in 90 degrees of elevation in the plane of the scapula, the arm is placed in internal rotation with the thumb pointing straight down. The patient resists a downward force applied by the examiner to the patient's wrist. The test is positive for supraspinatus pathology if this maneuver is painful. Repeating the same maneuver with the arm in full external rotation should reduce or eliminate the pain (Fig. 3-37). Although a positive test is classically described as pain associated with resistance of the downward force, weakness resulting in the inability to resist the examiner's force may be present as well due to pain-generated muscle inhibition.

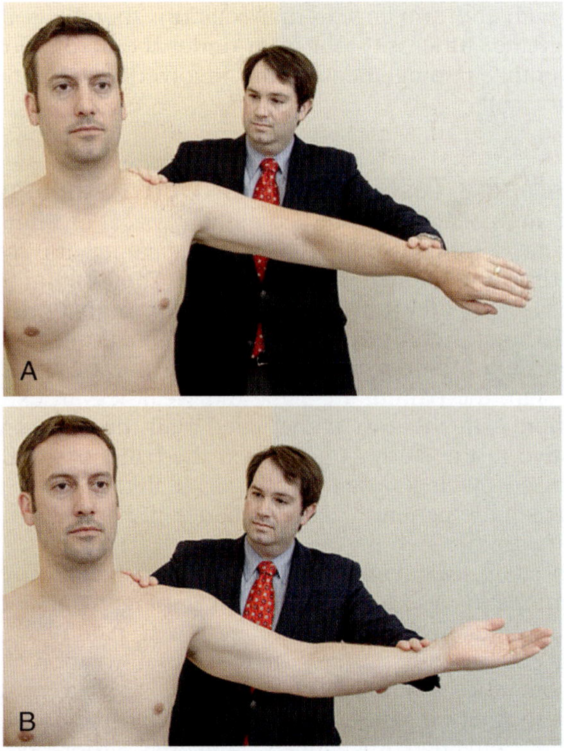

FIGURE 3-37: The Jobe-Yocum test. **A,** This test is used to assess superior cuff and subacromial pathology by asking the patient to resist a downward force with their arm in full internal rotation and in 90 degrees of elevation in the scapular plane. **B,** This is then repeated with the arm in full external rotation. A positive test is when there is pain with the arm in internal rotation, which is relieved with external rotation.

Painful Arc Test

For the painful arc test the patient elevates the arm in the scapular plane with the elbow straight, making sure that the arm is kept in neutral rotation (Video 3-24). Alternatively, the arm can be placed in full elevation and the patient slowly brings the arm down to the side. A

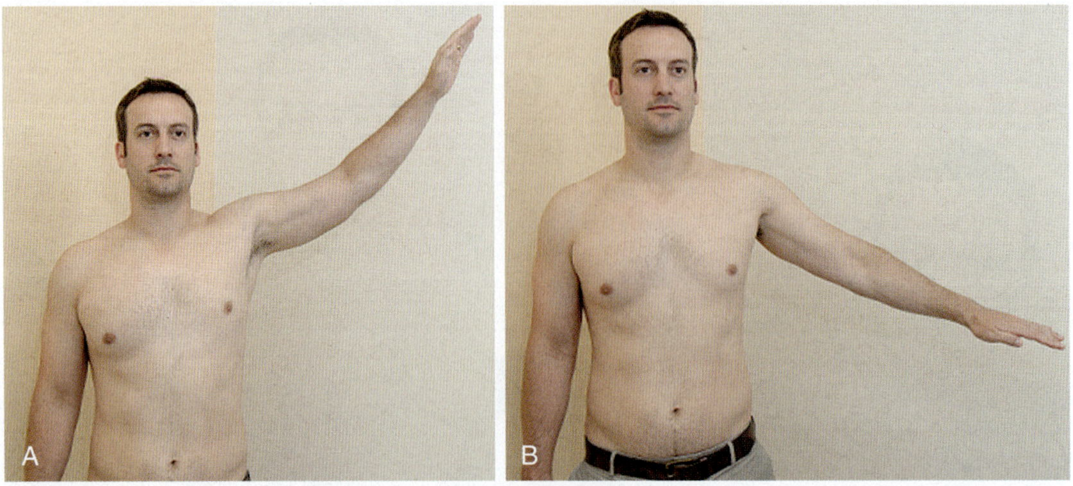

FIGURE 3-38: The painful arc test. A positive test is when there is pain with controlled active descent between 100 degrees (**A**) and 60 degrees (**B**). The arm must be kept in a neutral position to maximize the patient's discomfort.

positive painful arc test is documented when the patient experiences pain between 60 and 100 degrees of abduction during the maneuver (Fig. 3-38). Attention to arm rotation is important when performing this test because patients might minimize or avoid pain by performing the test with the arm in external rotation, thereby rotating the greater tuberosity out from under the acromion and preventing impingement of the involved portion of the rotator cuff.

TABLE 3-4 Rotator Cuff Pathology Tests

Test	Sensitivity (%)	Specificity (%)
Neer impingement sign[23]	72	60
Hawkins-Kennedy[23]	80	56
Painful arc[23]	53	76
Jobe-Yocum[63]	74	30

Combining Tests for Rotator Cuff Pathology

Park and colleagues[55] studied eight physical examination tests to determine their diagnostic accuracy for rotator cuff tears and impingement syndrome. The Neer impingement test was the only test that could predict bursitis or partial rotator cuff tears. The best combination of tests to diagnose a full-thickness rotator cuff tear were the drop-arm sign, the painful arc sign, and weakness in external rotation with the arm at the side. If all three tests were positive in the study cohort, then the patient had a 91% chance of having a rotator cuff tear. If all three tests were negative, the patient had a 9% chance of having a rotator cuff tear.

In 2009, Michener et al. reviewed several physical examination tests for subacromial impingement, including the Neer sign, Hawkins-Kennedy test, painful arc test, Jobe-Yocum test, and resisted external rotation.[47] The authors noted that when three of five tests were positive, the specificity increased to 74%, although the sensitivity of 75% remained unchanged. Similarly, Fodor and colleagues reported on the Neer, Hawkins-Kennedy, Jobe-Yocum, and painful arc tests; with all four tests positive, the specificity was approximately 100% for subacromial pathology, but the sensitivity was low at 40%.[16] Table 3-4 lists the reported sensitivities and specificities of these tests for diagnosing rotator cuff pathology and subacromial impingement.

Internal Impingement

The concept of internal impingement, first introduced by Walch and colleagues in 1992, describes pathologic contact between the articular surface of the posterosuperior rotator cuff and the glenoid and labrum.[74] This typically occurs in the 90-90 position of abduction and external rotation. The following tests are especially helpful in patients involved in throwing activities.

Modified Relocation Test

A modification of Jobe-Yocum's relocation test was reported by Hamner and colleagues in 2000 as a method for testing for internal impingement.[21] To perform this test, the patient lies supine on the examination table with the affected shoulder off the edge of the table. The arm is examined in a position of maximal external rotation and at 90, 110, and 120 degrees of abduction. In each of these three positions an anterior load followed by a posterior load is placed on the shoulder (Fig. 3-39). Pain that is caused by an anteriorly directed force and is alleviated by a posteriorly directed force is considered a positive sign. Contact between the undersurface of the rotator cuff and the posterosuperior labrum was documented arthroscopically in 79% of patients with a positive test. Fraying and undersurface partial thickness cuff tears have been identified in conjunction with a positive test, but the sensitivity and specificity of this test are unknown.

Internal Rotation Resistance Stress Test

The internal rotation resistance stress test was first described by Zaslav[81] to differentiate between intra-articular impingement and subacromial impingement in patients with a positive Neer impingement sign. The test is performed with the patient standing and the arm positioned in 90 degrees of abduction in the coronal plane and 80 degrees of external rotation (Video 3-25). With the examiner standing behind the patient, stabilizing the patient's elbow with one hand and holding the patient's wrist with the other hand, isometric external rotation strength is tested, followed by isometric internal rotation strength (Fig. 3-40). Relative weakness of internal rotation compared to external rotation is considered a positive sign, suggesting internal impingement. Conversely, relative weakness in external rotation suggests rotator cuff or subacromial pathology.

The relative strength of internal versus external rotation in the affected extremity is the important determinant for this examination, and for this reason a comparison with the unaffected contralateral shoulder is not performed with this test. The utility of this test was investigated only in patients who already had an established diagnosis of impingement as defined by a positive Neer impingement sign.

Acromioclavicular Joint Tests

The acromioclavicular (AC) joint is examined initially by direct palpation and application of direct pressure to the joint with the patient's arm relaxed at the side. This is considered positive if pain is elicited at the site of palpation. Walton et al. found this test to be highly sensitive (96%), but not specific (10%).[76]

The acromioclavicular joint is further assessed with the cross-body adduction maneuver. To perform this maneuver, the examiner stands beside or behind the patient. The patient's arm is held forward flexed to 90 degrees, and the examiner adducts the arm across the body toward the opposite shoulder (Fig. 3-41). This maneuver attempts to generate compression across the acromioclavicular joint, causing pain and a positive test.

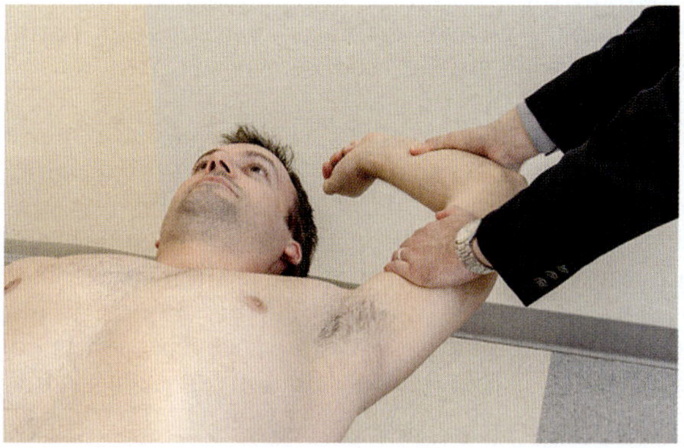

FIGURE 3-39: The modified relocation test. Internal impingement is suspected if pain is relieved with a posteriorly directed force applied to the shoulder in 90, 110, or 120 degrees of abduction.

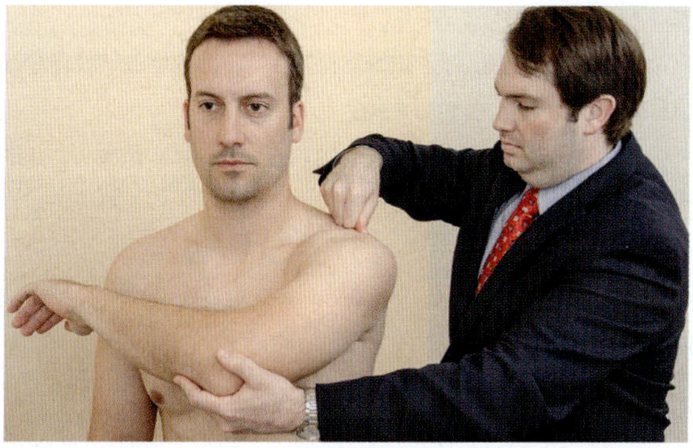

FIGURE 3-41: The cross-body adduction maneuver. The arm is passively flexed to 90 degrees, internally rotated, and then adducted toward the contralateral shoulder. Pathology of the acromioclavicular joint is suspected if there is pain localized over this joint.

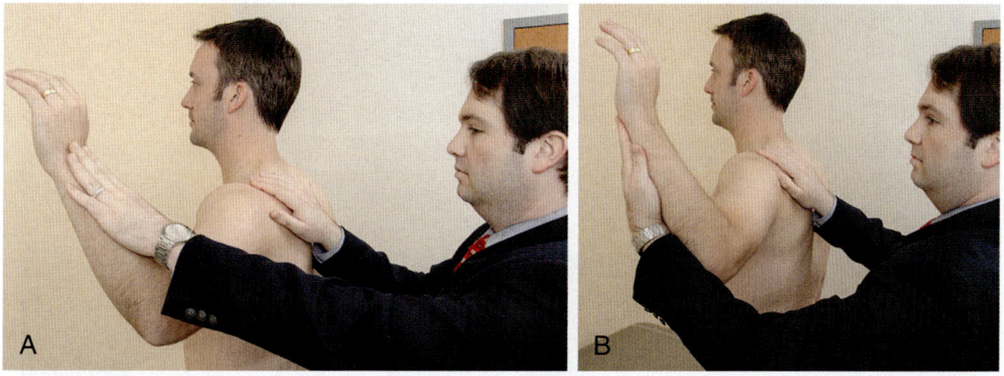

FIGURE 3-40: The internal rotation resistance stress test. **A,** Weakness with resisted external rotation is used to assess subacromial and rotator cuff pathology. **B,** Internal impingement is suspected if there is weakness of internal rotation against resistance.

It is important to establish clearly from the patient the location of any reported pain because this maneuver can produce pain in the posterior shoulder due to posterior capsular tightness or in the anterior shoulder due to subcoracoid impingement. To be considered positive for acromioclavicular joint pathology, this test must reproduce pain located on the top of the shoulder at the acromioclavicular joint.

Further confirmation of primary acromioclavicular joint pathology can be obtained by injecting the acromioclavicular joint with 1% lidocaine after a positive cross-body adduction maneuver. Repeating the maneuver with resolution of pain after the injection establishes the acromioclavicular joint as the source of pain.

Biceps Tendon Tests

Table 3-5 lists an overview of the clinical utility of the following tests for the evaluation of biceps pathology.

Yergason's Test

Yergason's test is performed with the patient's arm at the side, the elbow flexed 90 degrees, and the hand in full pronation. In this position the examiner grasps the patient's hand and asks the patient to attempt to supinate the hand against resistance (Fig. 3-42). Reproduction of pain in the anterior shoulder or bicipital groove is a positive sign suggesting pathology in the long head of the biceps tendon. Chen et al. showed a sensitivity of 32% and a specificity of 78% when this test was correlated with ultrasound findings.[8]

TABLE 3-5 Biceps Tests

Test	Sensitivity (%)	Specificity (%)	PPV (%)	NPV (%)
Speed's[33]	54	87	56	79
Yergason's[8]	32	78	49	64
Upper cut[33]	73	78	63	85

PPV, positive predictive value; NPV, negative predictive value.

Speed's Test

Crenshaw and Kilgore first described Speed's test in 1966.[12] With the elbow extended and the hand in full supination, the arm is placed in 60 to 90 degrees of forward flexion, and the patient resists a downward force at the wrist (Fig. 3-43). A positive test produces anterior shoulder pain or pain in the bicipital groove. Bennett[5] reported a sensitivity of 90%, specificity of 14%, positive predictive value of 23%, and negative predictive value of 83% based on correlations of a positive Speed's test with arthroscopic findings of biceps pathology.

Ludington's Test

For Ludington's test, the patient places both hands on top of the head with palms down and fingers interlocked. The patient then contracts and relaxes the biceps. Pain in the bicipital groove with this test suggests pathology of the long head of the biceps.

Upper Cut Test

The upper cut test for biceps pathology evaluation was described by Kibler et al.[33] To perform this test, the arm is in neutral rotation, the forearm is supinated, and the patient makes a fist. The patient is then asked to bring the fist rapidly to the chin while this motion is resisted at the fist by the examiner (Fig. 3-44). The test is considered positive if the resisted maneuver elicits pain or a

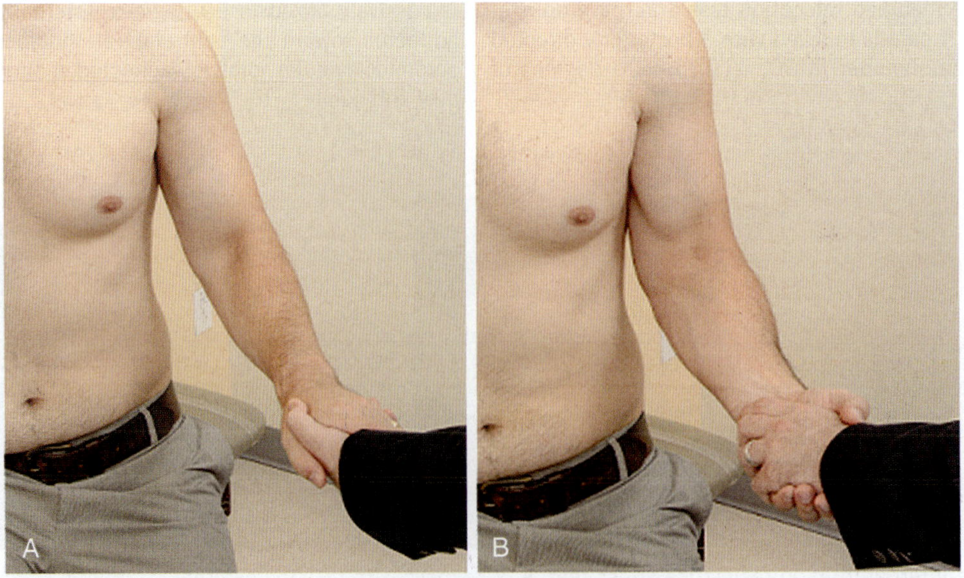

FIGURE 3-42: Yergason's test. **A,** The hand is fully pronated to begin the assessment. **B,** The patient then fully supinates against resistance. This assesses for pathology of the biceps tendon and is positive if there is pain located anteriorly.

painful pop over the anterior portion of the involved shoulder.

Superior Labrum Anterior Posterior Tests

Table 3-6 lists the sensitivities and specificities of SLAP tests.

O'Brien Test (Active Compression Test)

In 1998, O'Brien and colleagues[53] reported on the use of the active compression test to differentiate between acromioclavicular joint pathology and superior labral pathology. The O'Brien test is performed with the examiner standing behind the patient (Videos 3-26 and 3-27). The affected shoulder is flexed forward to 90 degrees and adducted 15 degrees toward the midline. In this position the patient resists a downward force first with the arm internally rotated so that the thumb points to the floor and then with the arm in full supination and external rotation (Fig. 3-45). Anterior shoulder pain relieved with

TABLE 3-6 Tests for Superior Labrum Anterior Posterior Tears

Test	Sensitivity (%)	Specificity (%)	PPV (%)	NPV (%)
O'Brien[11]	85	10	15	78
Anterior slide[33]	48	82	73	60
Crank[54]	9	83	—	—
Biceps load I[37]	91	97	83	98
Biceps load II[11]	67	57	19	90
Modified DLST[11]	92	20	16	93

PPV, positive predictive value; NPV, negative predictive value; DSLT, dynamic labral shear test.

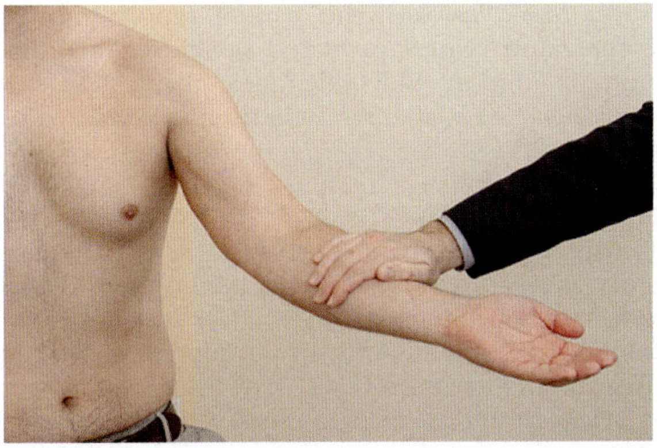

FIGURE 3-43: Speed's test. With the arm in 60 degrees of flexion, the elbow extended, and the hand fully supinated, a downward force is resisted. Recreation of anterior shoulder pain or pain in the biceps groove is a positive test.

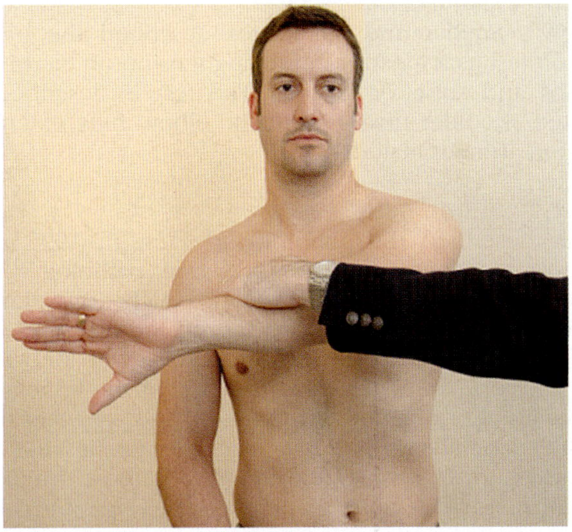

FIGURE 3-45: The active (O'Brien) compression test. This is performed with the arm in 90 degrees of flexion, 15 degrees of abduction, and full internal rotation. Pain over the anterior shoulder when a downward force is resisted indicates superior labral pathology.

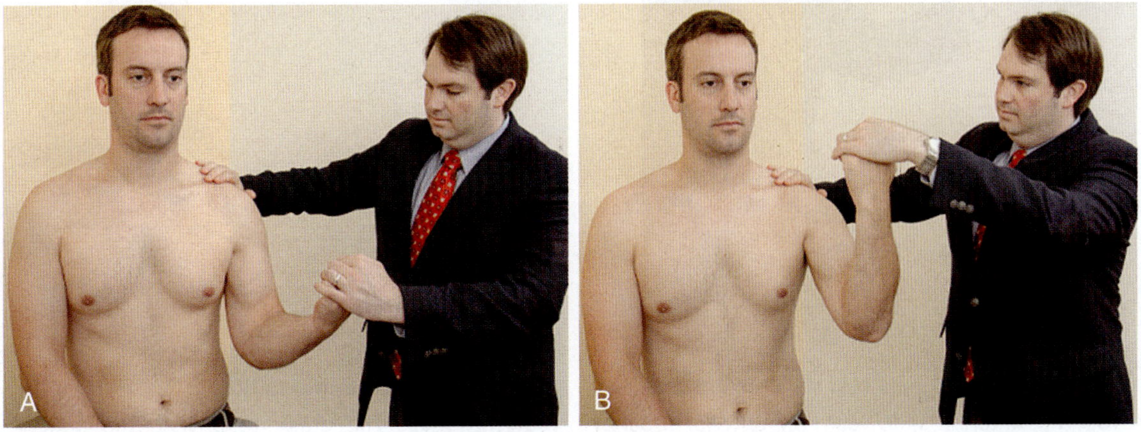

FIGURE 3-44: The upper cut test for biceps pathology. **A,** This is performed with the shoulder in neutral rotation, the forearm supinated with the elbow flexed to 90 degrees, and the hand in a fist. **B,** The patient rapidly moves the hand toward the chin as the examiner applies downward resistance to the fist.

the arm internally rotated, when the maneuver is performed with the arm in full supination and external rotation, is a positive test result indicating superior labral pathology. The location of the pain is also important because pain produced over the top of the shoulder or acromioclavicular joint indicates acromioclavicular joint pathology.

SLAPprehension Test

The SLAPprehension test is a modification of the O'Brien test (Video 3-28). The arm is brought into 45 degrees of adduction instead of 15 degrees, and the same resisted maneuvers are performed as with the O'Brien test. This arm position is thought to place more stress on the biceps origin and superior labrum, but it is also more likely to cause acromioclavicular joint abutment and pain.

Biceps Tension Test

In 1990, Snyder and colleagues described the biceps tension test as a means of applying tension on the biceps anchor and superior labrum. The test is described as resisted shoulder flexion with the elbow fully extended and forearm supinated.[64]

Anterior Slide Test

Kibler described the anterior slide test in 1995 as a method for assessing superior labral pathology.[31] To perform this test, the patient stands with arms akimbo (hands on hips, thumbs along the posterior iliac crests). The examiner stands behind the patient with one hand over the top of the acromion, the tips of the fingers just off the anterior edge of the acromion, and the other hand on the patient's elbow. The examiner pushes the arm forward and slightly superiorly at the elbow while the patient resists this anterosuperior force (Fig. 3-46). Pain or a click over the anterior shoulder is considered a positive sign, indicating a SLAP lesion.

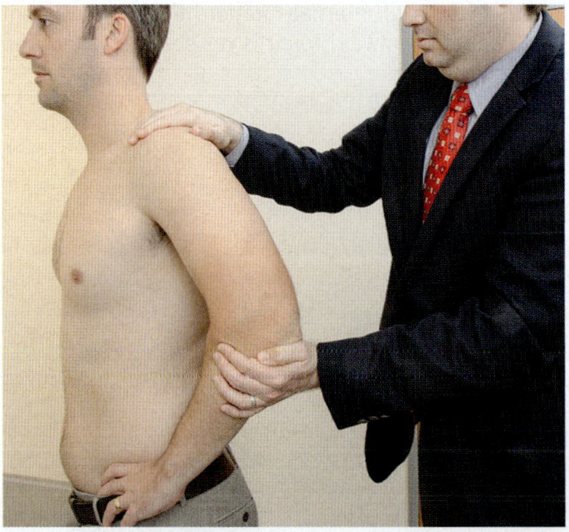

FIGURE 3-46: The anterior slide test. An anterior-superior directed force is applied to the elbow, and a superior labrum anterior and posterior lesion is suspected if there is pain or a click over the anterior shoulder.

Crank Test

The crank test for superior labral pathology is similar to the McMurray test for the knee (Video 3-29). The crank test attempts to detect labrum tears between the two joint surfaces. It is performed in approximately 160 degrees of forward flexion in either the sitting or supine position (Fig. 3-47).[43] Glenohumeral joint compression is created by axial loading through the humeral shaft with the arm in extreme forward flexion and abduction. The arm is then internally and externally rotated. Reproduction of symptoms of pain, catching, or a click indicates a positive test.

Pain Provocation Test

The pain provocation test is performed with the patient sitting and the examiner standing behind the patient. The arm is positioned in 90 degrees of abduction and full external rotation. The patient's hand is then placed in two different positions, first in full supination and then in full pronation[48] (Fig. 3-48). The test is considered positive for a SLAP lesion if the patient reports more pain while the hand is in a pronated position. According to a report by Mimori and colleagues, the test was 100% sensitive and 90% specific when correlated with MR arthrography.[48]

Biceps Load Test I

The biceps load test I for SLAP lesions in patients with a history of recurrent anterior instability was described by Kim and colleagues in 1999.[37] The test is performed by placing the patient's arm in 90 degrees of abduction and full external rotation (as if performing the apprehension test). With the patient's forearm supinated, the examiner externally rotates the patient's arm until the patient begins to feel apprehension. The examiner holds the patient's arm at that position and the patient flexes the elbow against resistance (Fig. 3-49). A decrease in

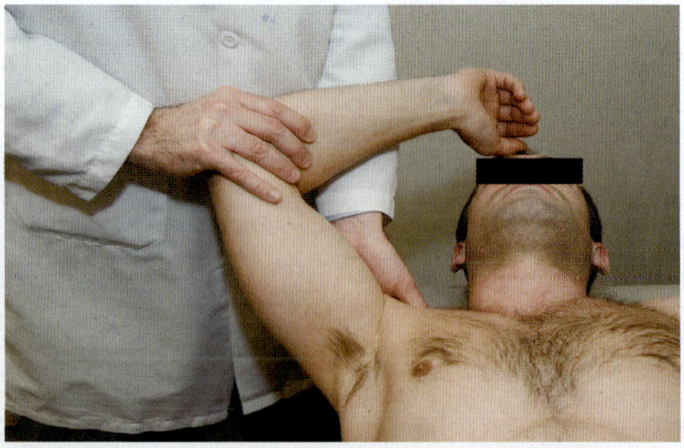

FIGURE 3-47: The crank test. With the patient supine or sitting, the arm is axially loaded in 160 degrees of flexion and then internally and externally rotated with glenohumeral joint compression.

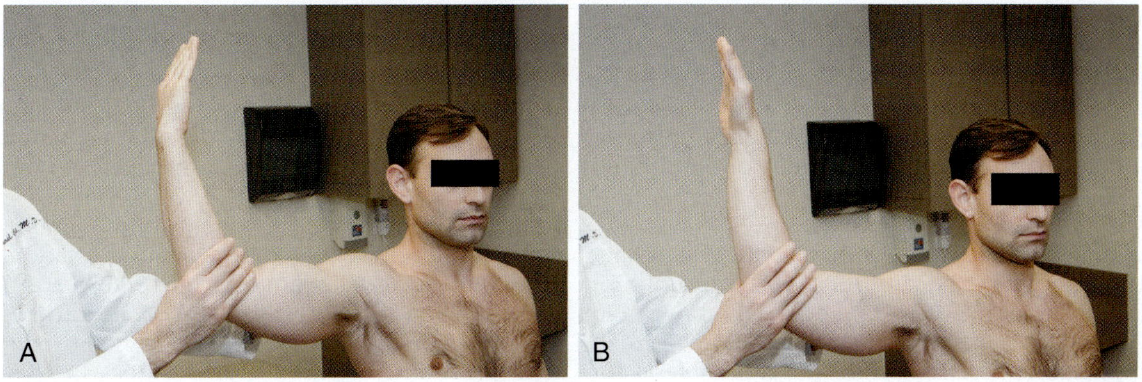

FIGURE 3-48: The pain provocation test. With the arm in 90 degrees of abduction and full external rotation, the hand is placed in full supination (**A**) and then full pronation (**B**). Increased pain in full pronation suggests a superior labrum anterior and posterior lesion.

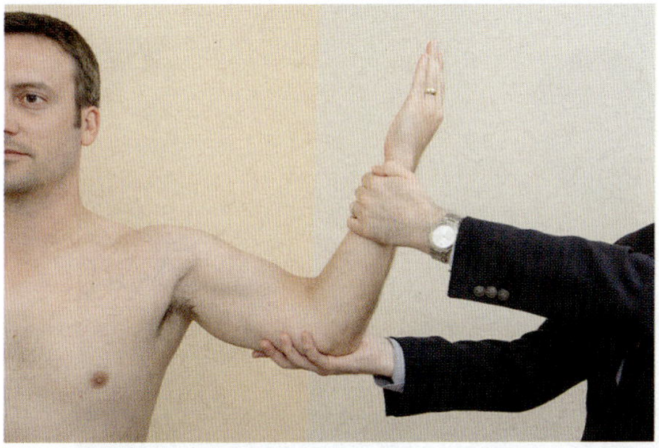

FIGURE 3-49: The biceps load test I. The patient is placed in the position of apprehension with the forearm supinated. The patient then flexes the elbow against resistance. This is used to assess for a superior labrum anterior and posterior lesion in patients with a history of anterior instability.

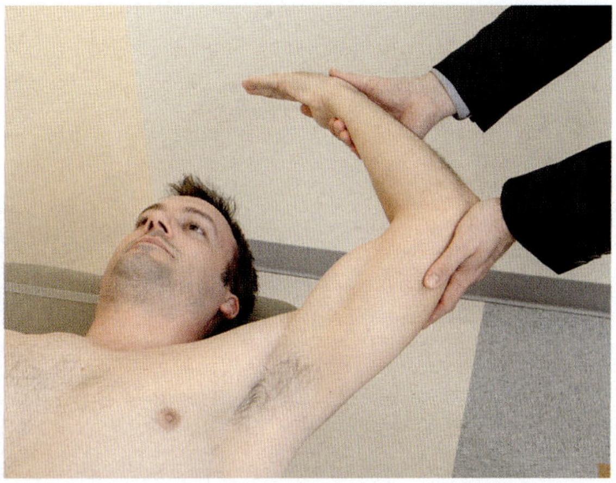

FIGURE 3-50: The biceps load test II. This test is performed in patients without a history of anterior instability. The patient is placed in 120 degrees of elevation and 90 degrees of external rotation, with the elbow flexed to 90 degrees and forearm supinated. The patient then flexes the elbow against resistance. Increased pain indicates a positive test and the suspicion of a superior labrum anterior and posterior lesion.

the patient's apprehension with active biceps contraction indicates a negative test and the absence of a SLAP lesion. No change or worsening of the patient's pain and apprehension indicates a positive test and the presence of a SLAP lesion. This test appears to be highly sensitive (91%) and specific (97%), with a positive predictive value of 83% and negative predictive value of 98%.

Biceps Load Test II

In 2001, Kim and colleagues described a further SLAP test, the biceps load test II, for patients who lack a history of anterior instability.[36] For this maneuver, the patient lies supine and the examiner stands at the patient's side next to the affected shoulder. The patient's arm is placed into 120 degrees of elevation, with full external rotation, the elbow flexed to 90 degrees, and the forearm in full supination. The patient then flexes the elbow against resistance (Fig. 3-50). The test is considered positive if the patient experiences increased pain with the resisted elbow flexion, indicating the presence of a SLAP lesion.

Dynamic Labral Shear Test

The dynamic labral shear test (DLST), described by Cheung and O'Driscoll,[9] is performed with the patient supine. The examiner flexes the elbow to 90 degrees and grasps the olecranon and distal humerus with one hand. This hand is used to maintain 90 degrees of elbow flexion, passively rotate the shoulder externally to its natural limit with only the force of gravity pulling down on the forearm, drop the elbow back into its natural limit of horizontal abduction (toward the floor), and passively elevate the shoulder while maintaining both the horizontal abduction and the external rotation at their natural limits under gravitational force alone. The examiner's other hand is kept on the acromion to stabilize the scapula and to detect a palpable click transmitted through the bony structures. After full overhead elevation, the entire motion is reversed and the arm is brought down to the side while the natural limit of shoulder external rotation and horizontal abduction is maintained. A positive test is indicated by a painful click at the posterior joint line, and/or reproduction of the patient's posterior pain within an arc of 120 and 90 degrees of elevation.[9]

Modified Dynamic Labral Shear Test

Kibler et al. modified the DLST, with the patient standing, instead of supine, and maximal horizontal abduction not being reached until the arm is abducted above 120 degrees (Video 3-30). Otherwise, this test is performed in the same manner as DLST, with the same criteria for a positive test (Fig. 3-51).[33] The principle underlying DLST and modified DLST is to recreate a peel-back lesion and internal impingement.

Posteroinferior Labral Pathology

The Kim test[38] is a provocative maneuver similar to the clunk test used to diagnose posteroinferior labrum tears. With the patient sitting on the examination table, the examiner holds the patient's arm parallel to the floor (90 degrees of forward flexion), with the arm internally rotated 90 degrees. With one of the examiner's hands holding the elbow to control internal rotation, an axial force is directed toward the humeral head. The other hand is used to direct a posterior load on the proximal humerus. The hand on the elbow is then used to forward flex the humerus 45 degrees (Fig. 3-52). Pain in the posterior shoulder is a positive Kim test result. In the only study conducted by the inventor of the test, the sensitivity and specificity for the diagnosis of

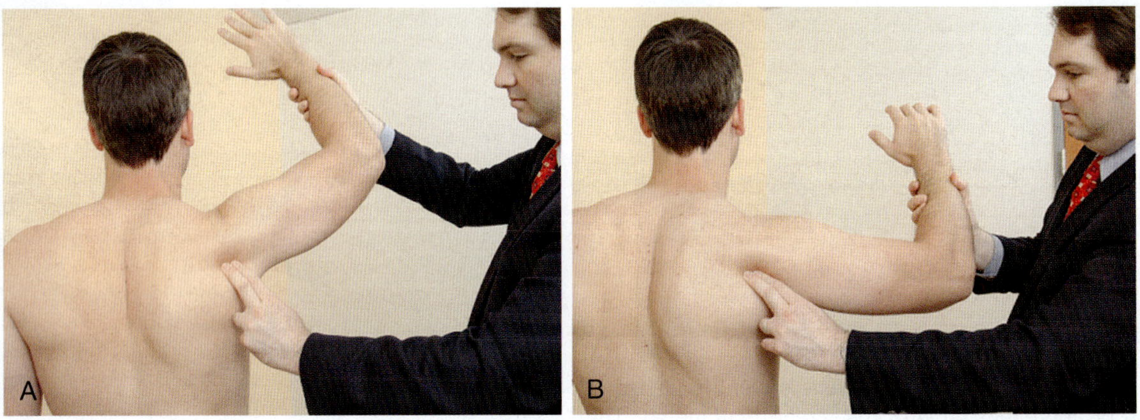

FIGURE 3-51: The modified dynamic labral shear test. **A,** The patient stands with the arm flexed 90 degrees at the elbow, abducted 120 degrees, and fully externally rotated. **B,** The arm is then lowered from 120 to 60 degrees of abduction. The test is positive for a superior labrum anterior and posterior lesion if there is pain, a painful click, or a catch in the joint line between 120 and 90 degrees of abduction.

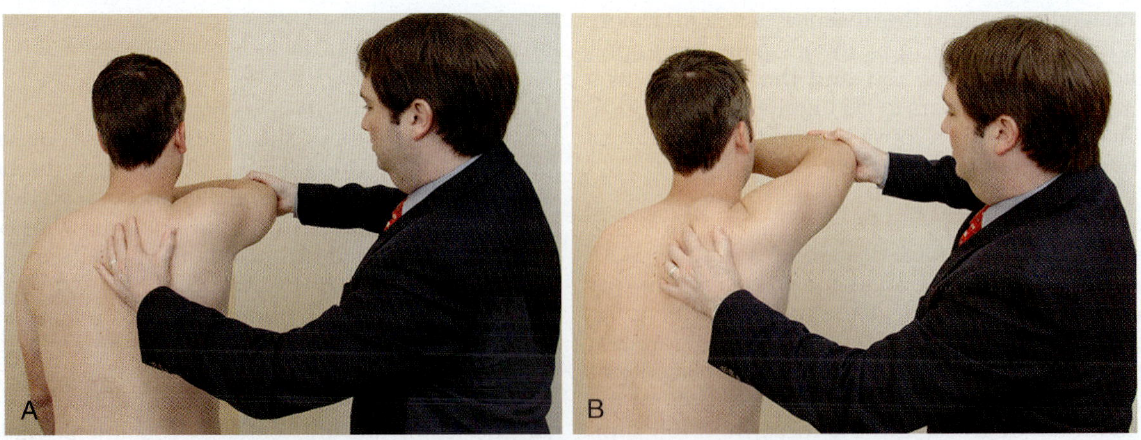

FIGURE 3-52: The Kim test. **A,** The shoulder is forward flexed to 90 degrees and internally rotated to 90 degrees. An axial force is applied to the humeral head, along with a posteriorly directed force on the humerus. **B,** The humerus is then further forward flexed by 45 degrees, attempting to recreate pain in the posterior shoulder that would signify posterior inferior labral pathology.

posteroinferior labral lesions were 80% and 94%, respectively, using arthroscopic evaluation of the posterior labrum as the gold standard. If the test was combined with the results of the jerk test, then the sensitivity increased to 97% for detecting posteroinferior labral lesions.[38]

Subcoracoid Impingement Test

Gerber and colleagues first reported on subcoracoid impingement of the supraspinatus tendon between the coracoid tip and lesser tuberosity in a cohort of postsurgical patients in 1985.[19] This report was subsequently followed by a study by Dines and colleagues,[13] who performed coracoid tip resections in eight shoulders for idiopathic subcoracoid impingement. Through variations in normal anatomy, trauma, or iatrogenic causes, such as proximal humeral osteotomies, there is potential for entrapment of the rotator cuff and other structures between the coracoid and proximal humerus, resulting in pain, weakness, and degenerative tendon injuries.

The subcoracoid impingement test was first described by Gerber and colleagues[19] and consists of two variations designed to reproduce subscapularis impingement between the humeral head and coracoid (Video 3-31). In the first technique the arm is elevated to 90 degrees in the scapular plane combined with medial (internal) rotation of the extremity, reproducing the patient's impingement symptoms and radiation of pain into the upper arm and forearm when the test is positive. The second method involves forward flexion of the arm instead of elevation in the scapular plane, again with medial (internal) rotation of the arm reproducing impingement symptoms and radiation of pain into the arm.

Dines and colleagues described their own version of the subcoracoid impingement test.[13] For this maneuver, the patient's arm is forward flexed to 90 degrees, adducted toward the midline, and internally rotated (Fig. 3-53). The test is positive if it produces anterior shoulder pain or a click in the anterior shoulder.

Tracy et al. showed, using ultrasound, a significant difference for the coracohumeral interval measurements between asymptomatic volunteers and patients with a diagnosis of subcoracoid impingement.[70] The investigators concluded that ultrasound may have a role in assisting the diagnosis of coracoid impingement. In addition, an injection of local anesthetic into the subcoracoid region can be performed if a diagnosis of subcoracoid impingement is suspected based on positive physical examination findings.

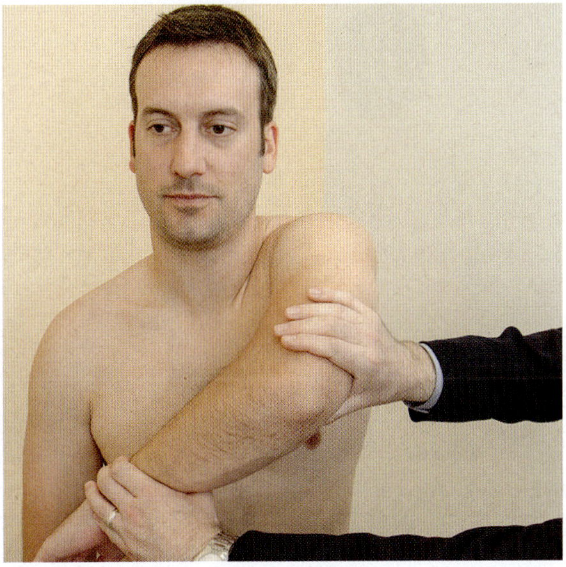

FIGURE 3-53: The coracoid impingement test. Anterior shoulder pain is considered a positive test when the arm is flexed to 90 degrees, adducted, and maximally internally rotated.

Scapular Dyskinesis Tests

Weakness or poorly coordinated muscle activation in the trapezius, levator scapulae, serratus anterior, or rhomboid muscles can lead to malpositioning of the scapula or scapular dyskinesis. The appropriate function of these muscles serves to reduce shoulder load and facilitate effective rotator cuff function. Observing side-to-side differences between the scapulae position at rest and during provocative and stabilization maneuvers can be used to elicit evidence of scapulothoracic dysfunction.

Resting Scapular Positional Measurements

The examiner uses a tape measure to measure the distance between the inferomedial border of the scapulae and the spinous processes in three positions: arms resting at the patient's sides, hands on hips, and arms at 90 degrees of abduction and full internal rotation (Fig. 3-54). Measurement can reveal side-to-side differences due to scapular malposition. A side-to-side difference of 1.5 cm or greater is considered to be a pathologic finding.[7]

Observed Repetitive Forward Elevation

The patient's shoulders and back must be exposed to allow a full view of both scapulae. The examiner stands behind the patient while the patient repetitively elevates and lowers both arms slowly in the planes of the scapulae. The examiner observes any asymmetry along the medial borders of the scapulae or a lack of the normal fluid movement of each scapula as it is protracted and rotated superiorly on the chest wall with arm elevation. Subtle presentations of scapular dyskinesis often manifest during the lowering phase of arm motion as a hitch or jump. This method of evaluation allows assessment of the resting position of the scapulae and the best view of the pattern of motion that occurs with active use of the shoulder girdle. Scapular dyskinesis observed with this method is classified according to the description by Kibler as listed in Table 3-7.[35]

Push-up Test

For most patients, the push-up test is easily carried out by asking the patient to perform a push-up while standing and leaning into a wall. For more muscular,

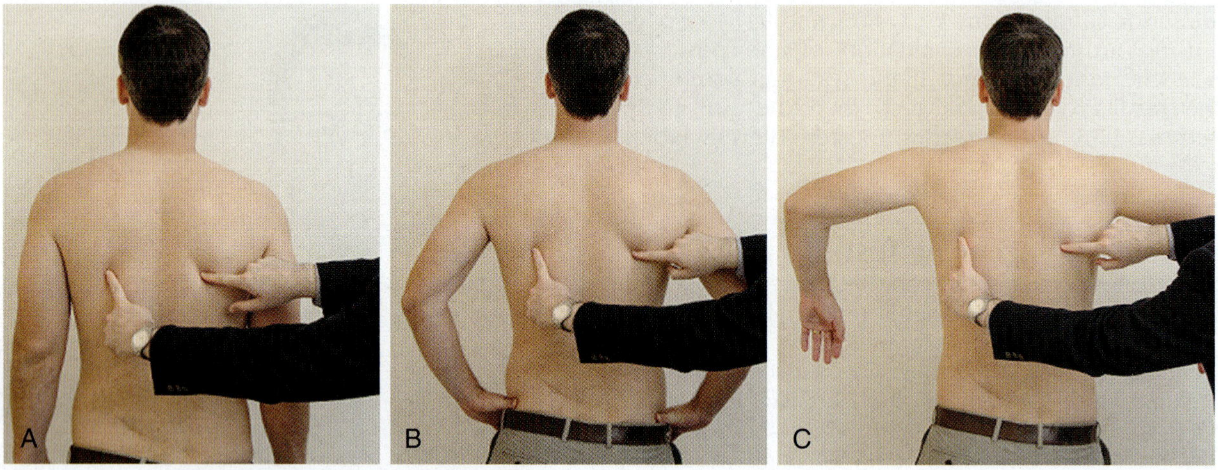

FIGURE 3-54: The resting scapular position test. The static positions of the scapulae are examined with the patient's upper extremities at the sides (**A**), on the hips (**B**), and in 90 degrees of abduction and full internal rotation (**C**).

TABLE 3-7 Patterns of Scapular Dyskinesis

Pattern	Findings
Type I	Prominent inferomedial pole
Type II	Entire medial border prominence
Type III	Prominent superomedial pole
Type IV	Normal symmetric scapular position

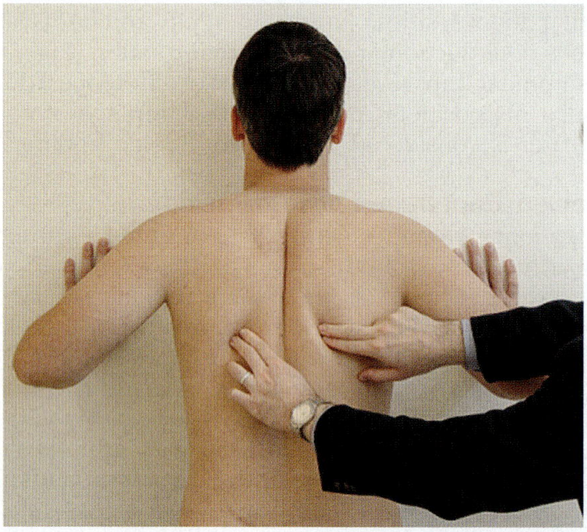

FIGURE 3-55: The push-up test. The scapulae are assessed for symmetric motion or winging as the patient performs a push-up by leaning into the wall.

well-conditioned patients who can do a regular push-up with ease, it is best to have them perform the test in the classic fashion on the floor. As the patient performs the push-up, the examiner observes the exposed scapulae for asymmetry of movement or scapular winging along the medial border of the scapula (Fig. 3-55).

Resisted Forward Elevation

The patient's arms are placed in 30 degrees of forward flexion, and the patient elevates the arms while the examiner applies resistance at the wrist. The examiner looks for winging along the medial border of the scapula.

Scapular Stabilization Test

In patients with shoulder dysfunction and evidence of scapular winging, the scapular stabilization test is used to evaluate the improvement of symptoms and function that can result from stabilization of the scapula. To perform the maneuver, the examiner stands behind the patient and places the palm of one hand on the patient's sternum anteriorly, and the other hand on the medial border of the scapula. With the examiner applying a compressive force to prevent the medial border of the scapula from lifting off the chest wall, the patient elevates the arm in the scapular plane. Improved overhead active ROM or a decrease in symptoms while the scapular border is being stabilized is considered a positive test (Fig. 3-56). A positive test result indicates that the scapular winging is a significant source of the shoulder girdle dysfunction. It also suggests a higher likelihood of improved shoulder function with rehabilitation or surgical stabilization of the scapular winging.

Scapular Assistance Test

As opposed to simply stabilizing the scapula, the scapular assistance test allows the examiner to manually recreate more normal scapular motion by increasing the acromiohumeral space, thereby reducing subacromial impingement during arm elevation and improving dynamic glenohumeral function.[32,61] For this test, the examiner stands behind the patient and manually stabilizes the medial border of the upper part of the scapula with one hand. With the thumb and fingers of the other hand, the examiner assists the inferomedial border of the scapula in superior rotation and protraction around the chest wall as the patient actively elevates the arm (Fig. 3-57).

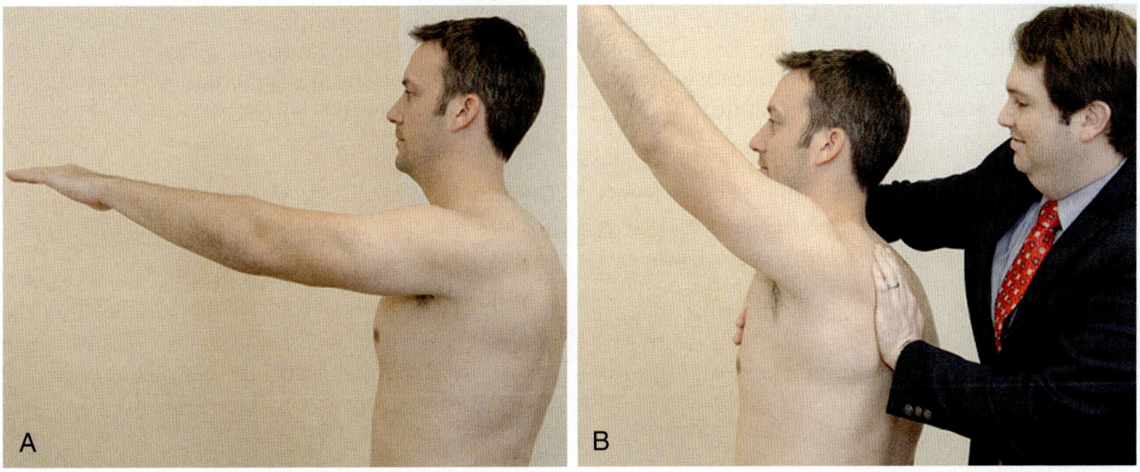

FIGURE 3-56: The scapular stabilization test. **A,** Elevation is limited by medial scapular border winging. **B,** The medial border of the scapula is stabilized by a compressive force applied by the examiner, thereby eliminating the winging. This maneuver improves elevation.

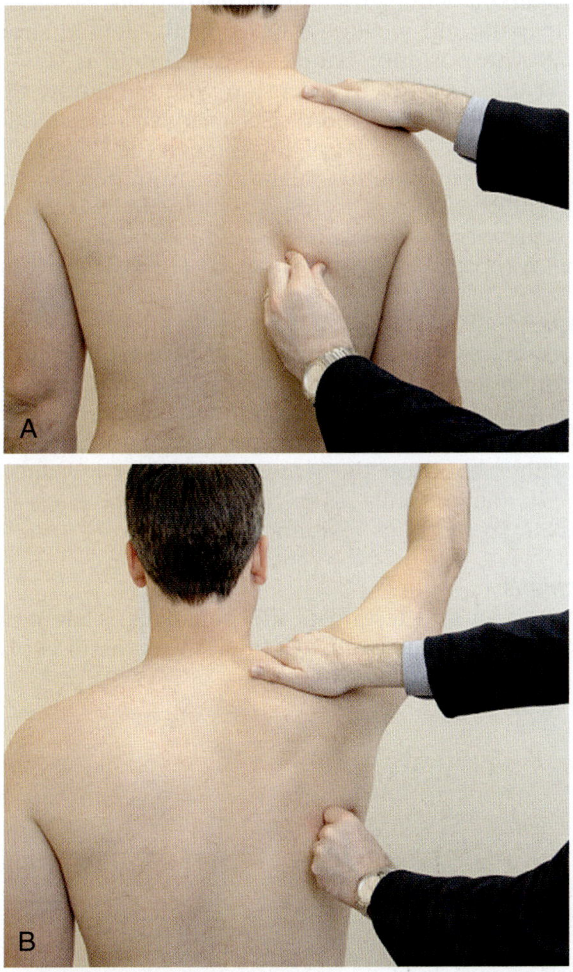

FIGURE 3-57: The scapular assistance test. **A,** The scapula is stabilized with one hand and the inferior pole grasped with the thumb and fingers of the other hand. **B,** The patient actively elevates their arm as the examiner assists the scapula in protraction and rotation.

Reduced pain and weakness with scapular assistance is a positive finding suggesting that abnormal scapular kinematics is contributing to the shoulder dysfunction.

Glenohumeral Internal Rotation Deficit

With the arm in 90 degrees of abduction, the total arc of motion (TAM) is measured by adding the external rotation and the internal rotation together.[77] TAM is then measured, compared, and should be equal within 8 degrees bilaterally. The glenohumeral internal rotation deficit represents the side-to-side differences in internal rotation that can have a negative effect on shoulder girdle mechanics.[7,34]

Crepitus Testing

Crepitus detected on physical examination or reported by a patient can result from bursal pathology or abnormal bone-on-bone contact and can be asymptomatic or associated with pain. Both auscultation and palpation are used to evaluate the location and character of the crepitus.

Subacromial crepitus is best assessed by placing one hand over the top of the shoulder and using the other hand to passively move the glenohumeral joint through its range. Passive ROM is often more effective in reproducing crepitus than active ROM because the rotator cuff is not depressing the humeral head, which allows the humeral head to be brought up into the undersurface of the acromion, where the subacromial bursa can be compressed. In addition, a firm, actively contracting deltoid muscle can prevent palpation of crepitus occurring in the deeper tissues.

Scapulothoracic crepitus usually results from bursitis or bursal scarring at the superomedial, inferomedial, or deep surface of the body of the scapula. The most common location is superomedial.[42] Crepitus involving the scapulothoracic articulation is usually best elicited by active scapular motion performed by the patient, who usually knows how to reliably reproduce the finding. Although more subtle crepitus may only be palpable, scapulothoracic crepitus is often audible because the air-filled thoracic cavity resonates with the crepitus, amplifying the sound.

Glenohumeral crepitus, most often related to articular cartilage loss and bone-on-bone arthritis, is best reproduced by active shoulder ROM against resistance. Assessment with active resisted ROM is better than with passive motion because of the increased compressive contact forces that are generated across the glenohumeral joint with active muscle contraction compared to those during passive joint motion. When palpating over the superior or anterior shoulder, the crepitus produced by bone-on-bone arthritis is usually coarser than that produced by bursal pathology.

Neurologic Testing

Shoulder dysfunction can often be associated with subtle or overt neurologic deficits. Some degree of neurologic testing in the form of isolated muscle strength testing, sensory testing, and reflex testing is therefore needed to fully evaluate most shoulders.

Isolated Muscle Strength Testing

Every assessment of shoulder muscle strength must be performed bilaterally to allow the comparison of the relative strength between the involved and uninvolved shoulders. What might be considered pathologic weakness in one person's shoulder can represent full, normal strength in a less-strong patient. A comprehensive evaluation of muscle strength can identify weakness resulting from pain-related muscle inhibition, reveal weakness not anticipated based on patient history and functional assessments, or demonstrate better strength than expected for a patient's level of functional impairment.

The position of testing also is selected to best isolate the function of each individual muscle group so that groups of muscles are not tested in conjunction with each other. Isometric muscle testing with the involved joint and muscle in a position of optimal mechanical advantage results in the most consistent, reproducible assessment of strength. The exception to this guideline is when testing a muscle group with apparently full strength. Full symmetrical muscle strength is assessed with the involved muscle in its position of maximal shortening because this position accentuates subtle weakness within the muscle that might otherwise go undetected in stronger patients.

Deltoid

Muscle strength testing of the deltoid should independently assess the anterior, middle, and posterior bundles of the deltoid. The anterior bundle is assessed by placing the shoulder in 90 degrees of forward flexion with the elbow extended and the arm in neutral rotation. The patient maintains the arm in this position against a downward force applied by the clinician to the wrist. The middle bundle is assessed by placing the shoulder in 90 degrees of abduction with the elbow extended and the palm of the hand facing up. Again, the patient maintains the arm position against the examiner's downward force applied to the wrist. This position of external rotation in abduction rotates the greater tuberosity out from under the acromion, decreasing the likelihood of supraspinatus impingement within the subacromial space, which can lead to pain and weakness in isometric deltoid strength testing. The posterior bundle of the deltoid is tested by placing the shoulder in extension with the elbow flexed to 90 degrees. The patient resists a forward-directed force applied to the elbow. Applying force at the flexed elbow eliminates confusion that might arise from pushing at the wrist with the elbow extended, which can lead to breaking of the elbow extension and a misperception that the isometric posterior deltoid is weak (Fig. 3-58).

Biceps

The examiner stands in front of the patient and positions the arm with the shoulder in neutral rotation, the elbow flexed fully, and the palm in full supination. The examiner grasps the patient's hand with one hand and places their other hand on the patient's shoulder for stabilization. The patient pulls his or her arm into the chest while the examiner applies resistance.

Brachialis

The position and testing of the brachialis is identical to that used for the biceps except that the forearm is placed

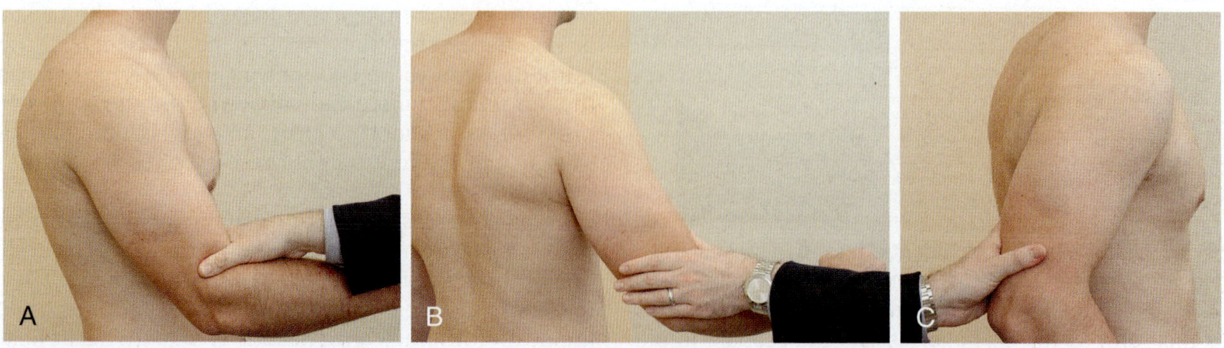

FIGURE 3-58: Deltoid testing. Deltoid muscle testing of the anterior deltoid (**A**), the middle deltoid (**B**), and the posterior deltoid (**C**).

in full pronation to prevent co-contraction of the biceps, which would bring the forearm into supination.

Triceps

The examiner stands beside the patient and positions the arm in 90 degrees of forward elevation with the elbow fully extended and the hand in full supination. The patient resists elbow flexion while the examiner attempts to flex the elbow by stabilizing the arm with one hand on the biceps and applying force at the wrist with the other hand.

Superior Trapezius and Levator Scapulae

The examiner stands behind the patient with both hands on the patient's shoulders. The patient performs a shoulder shrug while the examiner attempts to hold the shoulders in a depressed position.

Middle Trapezius and Rhomboids

The examiner stands behind the patient and places several fingers along the medial border of the scapula. The patient pinches the shoulder blades together. Although absolute strength testing of these muscle groups is not possible with this maneuver, the quality of the contraction can generally be assessed by direct palpation of the involved rhomboids and middle trapezius (Fig. 3-59).

Subscapularis, Supraspinatus, Infraspinatus and Teres Minor Strength Testing

Isolated strength testing of the subscapularis, supraspinatus, infraspinatus, and teres major is covered in the earlier section on rotator cuff testing.

Reflex Testing

Reflexes are tested bilaterally in all patients to allow side-to-side comparison of reflexes. The presence or absence of reflexes is noted, as well as whether they are excessively brisk or sluggish. Table 3-8 lists each reflex, its associated root level, and the peripheral nerve involved. Reflexes are graded as listed in Table 3-9.

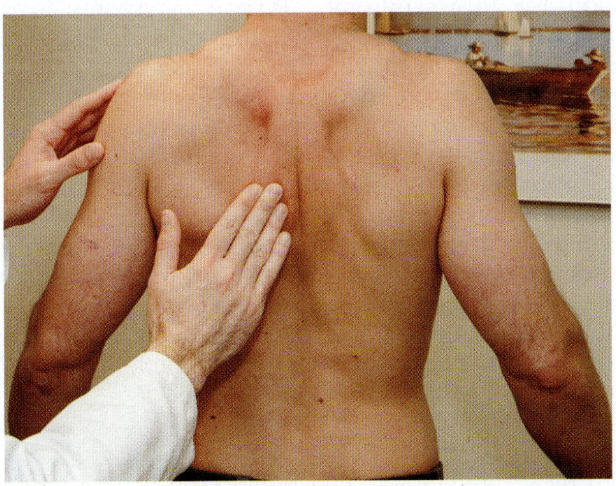

FIGURE 3-59: Assessment of the middle trapezius and rhomboids. The patient pinches the shoulder blades together while the examiner observes and palpates along the medial border of the scapula. The scapular motion and palpable muscle contraction should be symmetric.

Clavicular Reflex

The patient stands with arms hanging at his or her sides, and the examiner taps the lateral aspect of each clavicle with a reflex hammer. This maneuver can produce a reflexive contraction of the trapezius, or, less commonly, other muscles around the shoulder girdle. This reflex does not assess an independent nerve root, but the test can be useful in assessing general irritability of the proximal nerves in the upper extremity.

Scapular Reflex

The patient stands with arms abducted 20 degrees, and the examiner taps the inferior angle of the scapula with a reflex hammer. The reflex response of the rhomboids (dorsal scapular nerve, C5) and middle and lower trapezius (spinal accessory nerve, cranial nerve XI) causes adduction of the arms and medial movement of the scapula.

Pectoralis Reflex

With the patient's arm abducted 20 degrees, the examiner positions a thumb over the pectoralis major tendon

TABLE 3-8 Reflexes

Location	Peripheral Nerve	Nerve Root
Clavicle	Nonspecific	Nonspecific
Scapula	Dorsal scapular	C5
Scapula	Spinal accessory	Cranial nerve XI
Pectoralis	Medial and lateral pectoral	C5-C8, T1
Biceps	Musculocutaneous	C5, C6
Triceps	Radial	C6, C7
Brachioradialis	Musculocutaneous	C5, C6

TABLE 3-9 Grading of Reflexes

Grade	Description
0	No response (always abnormal)
1+	A slight but definitely present response (flicker); may or may not be normal
2+	A brisk response; normal
3+	A very brisk response; may or may not be normal
4+	A tap elicits a repeating reflex (clonus); always abnormal

From Walker HK. Deep tendon reflexes. In: Walker KH, Hall WD, Hurst JW eds. Clinical Methods: The History, Physical and Laboratory Examinations. *3rd ed. Boston: Butterworths; 1990:365-368.*

insertion on the proximal humerus, and taps the thumb with a reflex hammer. Adduction or internal rotation of the arm occurs as a reflex response (medial and lateral pectoralis nerves, C5-C8, T1).

Biceps Reflex

With the patient's elbow supported in 90 degrees of flexion, the examiner places his or her thumb over the distal biceps tendon and taps the thumb. The elbow flexes reflexively (musculocutaneous nerve, C5, C6).

Triceps Reflex

With the patient's elbow supported in 90 degrees of flexion, the examiner uses a reflex hammer to tap the distal triceps tendon just proximal to its insertion on the olecranon. Reflexive elbow extension occurs (radial nerve, C7).

Brachioradialis Reflex

The patient's elbow is supported in 90 degrees of flexion, with the wrist in neutral rotation and neutral flexion/extension. The examiner uses a reflex hammer to tap the brachioradialis tendon approximately 2 cm proximal to its insertion on the radial styloid. A normal reflex response results in elbow flexion (musculocutaneous nerve, C5, C6). The inverted radial reflex is an abnormal reflexive wrist extension that can be seen in response to this test and is a sign of upper motor neuron pathology.

Horner Syndrome

Complete assessment of the upper extremity neurologic status should include observation for Horner syndrome, a constellation of ipsilateral miosis, ptosis, and anhidrosis. This finding is associated with a lesion involving the sympathetic chain at the C6 cervical level. It can be found with very proximal brachial plexus nerve root injuries or with tumors involving the apex of the lung.

Sensory Testing

Evaluation of sensation in the upper extremity can be used to identify focal nerve lesions; regional nerve deficits, such as those caused by syringomyelia; or systemic problems, such as peripheral neuropathy secondary to diabetes. Although dermatomal sensory regions often overlap and are somewhat variable, certain areas on the arm are usually isolated and consistently innervated by a single nerve root level. A light touch or discrimination between sharp and dull can be used to grossly assess sensation in any given area. Sensation is compared bilaterally. Symmetrical alterations in sensation suggest systemic pathology or a more proximal pathology than would be suggested by asymmetric alterations in sensation. Table 3-10 lists the location and dermatome associated with each part of the extremity.

TABLE 3-10 Sensory Testing

Vertebra	Anatomic Location	Peripheral Nerve
C4	Superior aspect of shoulder	—
C5	Lateral aspect of deltoid	Axillary
C6	Lateral forearm and thumb	Musculocutaneous and median
C7	Dorsal tip of the long finger	Median
C8	Medial forearm	Medial antebrachial cutaneous
T1	Medial arm	Medial brachial cutaneous

Vascular Examination

Vascular examination involves the assessment of a wide range of manifestations in the upper extremity. General skin color, texture, temperature, hair growth, and alteration in sensation may relate to changes in the vascular system. An evaluation of all pulses (radial, ulnar, brachial, axillary, and subclavian) and listening for bruits with a stethoscope is indicated, especially when trauma to the extremity has occurred. An evaluation of the autonomic nervous system is important to exclude reflex sympathetic dystrophy (shoulder-hand syndrome). Vascular congestion, especially at the thoracic outlet, can cause shoulder pain. Specific tests can help detect the presence of neurovascular compression in the neck, known as thoracic outlet syndrome (TOS).

Thoracic Outlet Syndrome

TOS is an uncommon condition secondary to compression/irritation of the brachial plexus and/or subclavian vessels. Patients often present with a varied clinical picture and a lack of objective data supporting the diagnosis; the examiners must therefore maintain a high index of suspicion for this syndrome. Typical symptoms involve upper extremity heaviness with above-the-shoulder activities, numbness involving the ulnar aspect of the hand and medial forearm, swelling, and potential cyanosis.[41] Causes of TOS include anterior scalene muscle hypertrophy, cervical ribs, exostosis and malunions of the clavicle, drooping of the shoulder girdle, congenital fibrous bands, and malpositioning of the scapula.[41,57,67]

An inspection of the shoulder girdle for asymmetry may reveal that the affected shoulder is in a more anterior and lower position compared to the unaffected shoulder. The following tests involve provocative maneuvers, which may elicit symptoms in patients with TOS (Table 3-11).

Adson's Maneuver and Modified Adson's Maneuver

With the examiner standing behind the patient and palpating the radial pulse at the wrist, the patient extends the shoulder and arm, turns the head toward the involved side, and takes a deep breath in and holds it (Fig. 3-60). Any decrease or obliteration of the radial pulse suggests subclavian artery compression between the anterior and middle scalene muscles or at the first rib.[1]

The modified Adson's maneuver is performed the same way as the traditional Adson's maneuver except that the patient turns the head away from the involved extremity (Fig. 3-61).[41] Any diminution or loss of the pulse at the wrist is considered a positive test, suggesting thoracic outlet syndrome.

Wright's Maneuver

In Wright's maneuver the arm is hyperabducted and externally rotated, with the patient's head turned in the opposite direction, while the radial pulse is palpated (Fig. 3-62). A decrease or obliteration of the radial pulse is considered a positive test.[78]

Overhead Exercise Test/Roos Test

The patient places both arms in 90 degrees of abduction with the elbows flexed to 90 degrees. The hands are then opened and closed for a 3-minute period (Fig. 3-63).[41]

TABLE 3-11 Thoracic Outlet Syndrome Testing

Test	Sensitivity (%)	Specificity (%)
Adson	79	76
Roos	84	30
Wright	70	53
Adson + Roos	72	82
Adson + Wright	54	94

Data from Gillard J, Pérez-Cousin M, Hachulla E, et al. Diagnosing thoracic outlet syndrome: contribution of provocative tests, ultrasonography, electrophysiology, and helical computed tomography in 48 patients. Joint Bone Spine. *2001;68(5):416-424.*

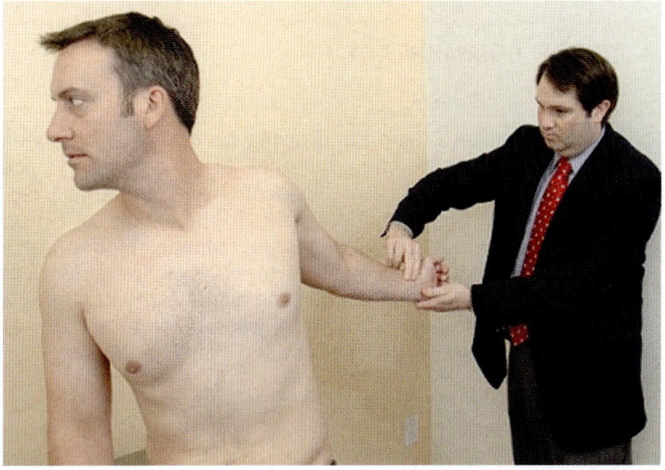

FIGURE 3-61: The modified Adson's maneuver. The head is rotated away from the involved extremity.

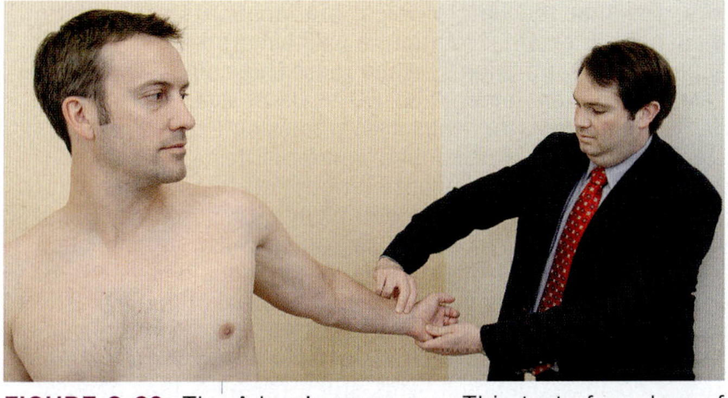

FIGURE 3-60: The Adson's maneuver. This tests for a loss of the radial pulse by hyperextending the patient's arm while rotating his or her head to the ipsilateral side.

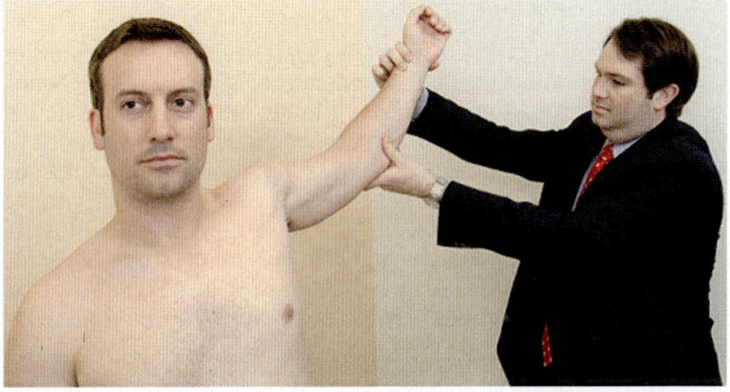

FIGURE 3-62: Wright's maneuver. This assesses for change in the radial pulse as the arm is hyperabducted.

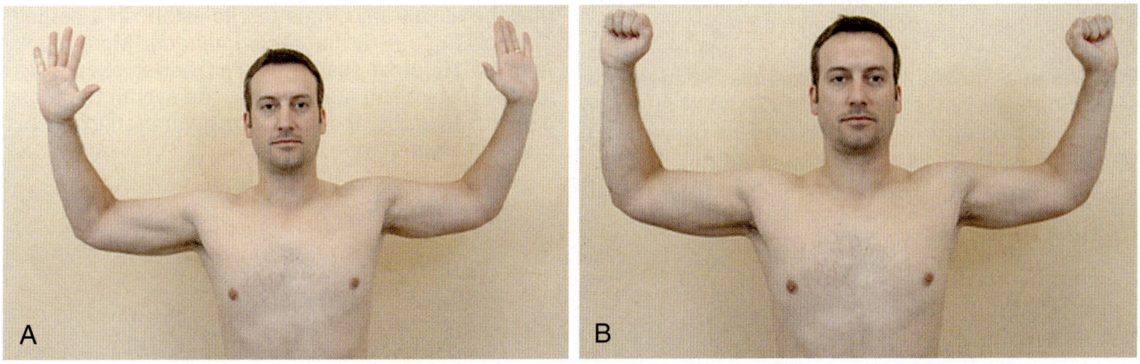

FIGURE 3-63: The overhead exercises test. Both arms are placed in the 90-degree abducted position with the elbows flexed 90 degrees. The patient then opens (**A**) and closes (**B**) his or her fists repeatedly for 3 minutes. Thoracic outlet syndrome is suspected if the symptoms are recreated.

Patients with TOS will experience a recreation of their symptoms, and may not be able to complete the test.

Using pulse oximetry during this test, Braun et al. found a significant drop in oxygen saturation from 98% at rest to 86%.[6] They also noted an increase in heart rate and reproduction of symptoms.

Costoclavicular Maneuver

The costoclavicular maneuver is used to cause compression of the subclavian vessels in the costoclavicular space. As described by Falconer and Weddell in 1943, a backward and downward bracing of the shoulders is performed. Obliteration of the radial pulse is considered a positive test.[14]

EDITOR COMMENTARY

Michael A. Wirth

The art of history taking and laying on of hands has been the a priori cornerstone and bulwark of medicine since antiquity. While the art of diagnosing and directing treatment for the suffering patient dates to the earliest of times, the science of medicine is remarkably recent. In our present era of unprecedented diagnostic technology, the authors of this chapter have reminded us once again of the importance of a thorough history and careful physical examination, as advocated by Dr. William J. Mayo so many years ago:

> *Above all things, let me urge upon you the absolute necessity of careful examinations for the purpose of diagnosis. My own experience has been that the public will forgive you an error in treatment more readily than one in diagnosis, and I fully believe that more than one half of the failures in diagnosis are due to hasty and unmethodic examinations.*[46]

The wisdom of these words is clearly evident in the studies that have noted the high incidence of superior labral tears, bone abnormalities, rotator cuff tears, and acromioclavicular joint arthrosis in asymptomatic shoulders. In a report by Needell and colleagues, dual-echo T2-weighted oblique coronal MRIs were evaluated in 100 asymptomatic patients aged 19 to 88 years, and 75% were diagnosed with acromioclavicular joint arthrosis.[50] In a similar study acromial joint arthrosis was diagnosed using MRI in 41 (82%) of 50 asymptomatic shoulders. Moreover, when the patients were stratified by age, 93% of those in the over-30 age group exhibited arthritic changes.[65] In another report Connor and colleagues utilized detailed MRI scans to evaluate the shoulders of asymptomatic elite overhead athletes. Eight (40%) of 20 shoulders had findings of partial or full-thickness tears of the rotator cuff, but none of the athletes had experienced any subjective symptoms or required any evaluation or treatment for shoulder-related problems during the 5-year study period.[10] More recently, a study presented at the 2015 annual meeting of the American Academy of Orthopaedic Surgeons noted a high rate (72%) of superior glenoid labral tears on MRI in a cohort of 45- to 60-year-old asymptomatic patients.[60] These studies support the premise that imaging studies must be interpreted in light of a thorough history and physical examination and must not be used as a stand-alone method to direct patient care.

The authors of this chapter also remind us that the art and science of clinical evaluation of shoulder problems is a challenge because most physical examination tests are sensitive for a wide range of shoulder conditions, but very few are specific to the presence of a single disorder. A notable exception is anterior shoulder instability, where the specificity of the anterior apprehension test, the relocation test, and the surprise test exceeds 95%.[28] Operationally, these tests are clinically reliable when the reproduction of symptomatic glenohumeral translation (apprehension), and not pain, is used as the sine qua non for diagnosis. In the case of rotator cuff disorders, combining the positive results of several physical examination signs in conjunction with the patient's age has been helpful when diagnosing full-thickness rotator cuff tears. Park and colleagues evaluated the diagnostic accuracy of clinical tests for rotator cuff disorders and reported that the best physical examination signs include weakness in external rotation, a positive drop-arm sign, and a painful arc of motion.[55] When these three signs were positive in a patient older than 60 years of age, there was a 91% chance of a full-thickness rotator cuff tear.[24]

Although specific physical examination tests have demonstrated the ability to diagnose rotator cuff tears and anterior shoulder instability with great facility, this same clinical success has not been generalized to other conditions, such as multidirectional instability of the shoulder or SLAP lesions. In one study by Cook and colleagues, the diagnostic accuracy of five clinical tests for SLAP lesions were evaluated in a prospective, cased-based, and case-control designed investigation.[11] This study revealed that none of the tests provided diagnostic utility to aid decision-making, either as stand-alone examination tools or when used in clusters. Finally, a 2012 systematic review and meta-analysis of shoulder physical examination tests concluded that the use of any single test to establish a pathognomonic diagnosis could not be recommended. Moreover, combinations of shoulder tests provided better accuracy, but only marginally so. Not surprisingly, the overall findings from the data stressed the need for both a comprehensive history and physical examination.[49]

SENIOR EDITOR COMMENTARY

Frederick A. Matsen III

As the authors state at the start of this chapter, the clinical evaluation is the beginning of the doctor-patient relationship. The goal is not so much to come up with a diagnosis that will drive to a specific treatment, but rather to carry out an evaluation of the patient that leads to a reasonable management plan.

I like to emphasize the importance of the four P's that determine the outcome of treatment: the *patient,* the shoulder *problem* the patient is experiencing, the *procedure* used to treat the patient and the problem, and the *physician* rendering the treatment. I place the patient first on this list because as Osler is quoted as saying, "It is more important to know what patient a disease has than what disease the patient has." When introducing myself and shaking the patient's hand I can sense a lot—healthy or frail, positive or negative, smelling of cigarettes or not. To learn a bit more, I ask the patient, "Where are you from and what do you do there?" In an instant I've done a lot to determine if the person might benefit from a surgical approach should one be appropriate for the problem. Next I like to ask, "What can I help you with today?" giving the patient some uninterrupted time to answer. A patient with posterior instability may respond with "I can't do my job," "I need more pain medicine," "My lawyer sent me," or "My shoulder keeps on slipping out when I lift something in front of me"—same diagnosis, but four different problems.

I prefer to avoid dwelling on pain, so rather than asking, "Where does your shoulder hurt?" I ask, "What does your shoulder problem keep you from doing? When does it bother you the most?" I follow this with, "How and when did that problem start?", "How much force was applied to your shoulder in the injury and what position was it in when the force was applied?", and "Tell me about the treatment you've had for it up to now." Trying to learn more about the patient, I ask questions, such as, "How is your overall health?", "How active are you?", "What medications are you on?", and "Have you had prior surgeries and how did they work out?"

My physical exam starts with a "no touch" approach: "Show me which actions are difficult for your shoulder, and what do you feel is happening when you do these things?" To check active motion I ask patients to show me with each shoulder how high they can reach overhead, how far they can externally rotate the shoulder with the arm at the side, how far they can reach across their body, how far they can internally rotate the abducted arm, and how high they can reach up their back. If patients cannot raise their arm actively, I ask them to show how high they can raise it with the help of the opposite arm. At this point, without having touched the patient, I usually have a fairly good understanding of the *problem* and whether the *patient* is likely to be a good candidate for surgical intervention. The remainder of my history, physical examination, and plain radiographs seek to refine this understanding.

The authors have done a marvelous job of cataloging the many tests that have been described for evaluating shoulder problems, but they and Dr. Wirth have also pointed out that these tests are rarely capable of discriminating between these problems. Instead, my exam seeks more tangible findings, such as loss of passive or active ROM, a palpable defect in the rotator cuff, minimal resistance to anterior translation of the humeral head pressed into the glenoid, palpable subacromial crepitus, muscle atrophy, loss of the biceps reflex, or an obvious "clunk" on cross-body adduction.

Bottom line: if the problem is not apparent on history, physical examination, and plain radiographs, or if the patient does not appear to be an excellent surgical candidate, I'm likely to recommend nonoperative management. This remains the case even if MRIs show "acromioclavicular arthrosis," "labral fraying," a "humeral avulsion of the glenohumeral ligament (HAGL)" lesion, or "supraspinatus tendinosis."

CHAPTER 4

Radiographic Evaluation of Shoulder Problems

Kirk L. Jensen, Philip Tirman, Charles A. Rockwood Jr

Radiographic evaluation of the shoulder requires a minimum of two views of the area that are perpendicular to each other. The shoulder is a complicated anatomic unit made up of numerous bony landmarks, projections, and joints. The scapula, which lies on the posterolateral portion of the rib cage, rests at an angle of approximately 45 degrees to the frontal plane of the thorax. Thus the plane of the glenohumeral joint is not the plane of the thorax, and radiographs taken in the anteroposterior plane of the thorax provide oblique views of the shoulder joint (Fig. 4-1). All too commonly, though, a radiographic evaluation of the shoulder consists of two anteroposterior views of the rotated proximal humerus, which are taken perpendicular to the frontal axis of the thorax.

Orthopedists do not diagnose and treat injuries in any other part of the body on the basis of a one-plane radiographic evaluation. With the exception of localizing rotator cuff calcium deposits, the two traditional anteroposterior views of the shoulder in internal and external rotation are, by themselves, inadequate for evaluating injuries and disorders of the shoulder. Rotating the humerus into internal and external rotation does not change the orientation of the scapula to the x-ray beam. Therefore radiographic evaluation of the shoulder should consist of, at minimum, both anteroposterior and lateral views. Specific oblique views may also be required for the further investigation of specific pathologic conditions of the shoulder.

FRACTURES OF THE GLENOHUMERAL JOINT

Recommended Views

The recommended views are the trauma series of radiographs, that is, true anteroposterior radiographs in internal and external rotation and an axillary lateral or a scapulolateral view. Modified axillary laterals or a computed tomography (CT) scan may be required.

Radiographs of the injured shoulder in two planes (anteroposterior and axillary lateral or scapular lateral) are absolutely essential to evaluation of an acutely injured shoulder. McLaughlin,[99] Neer,[110,112] Neviaser,[117] DeSmet,[28] Rockwood and Green,[138] Post,[124] Rowe,[141] Bateman,[6] and many others have recognized the shortcomings of the usual two anteroposterior radiographs of the shoulder and have recommended both anteroposterior and lateral views for a proper assessment of shoulder problems.

The radiographs used to evaluate traumatic shoulder problems are referred to as the *trauma series*. The trauma series can also be used as baseline radiographs to evaluate many chronic shoulder problems.

Following are the recommended radiographs for the trauma series:

- A true anteroposterior view in the plane of the scapula with the arm in internal and external rotation.
- An axillary lateral view. If an axillary radiograph cannot be obtained, one of the following views must be obtained:
  - A scapulolateral view
  - One of the modified axillary views
  - A CT scan

Techniques for Taking the Trauma Series

True Anteroposterior Views

Because the scapula lies on the posterolateral aspect of the thoracic cage, the true anteroposterior view of the glenohumeral joint is obtained by angling the x-ray beam 45 degrees from medial to lateral (Fig. 4-2; see also Fig. 4-1). The patient may be supine or erect, with the arm at the side or in the sling position. An alternative technique is to rotate the patient until the scapula is flat against the x-ray cassette and take the radiograph with the beam perpendicular to the scapula. Sometimes it is difficult for the technician to properly align the patient for the view. A simple technique to assist the technician in positioning the patient correctly consists of using a

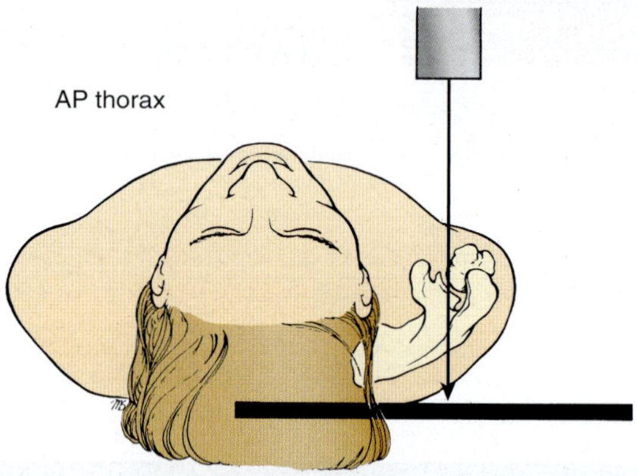

FIGURE 4-1: Anteroposterior (AP) radiograph of the shoulder taken in the plane of the thorax. Note that the film is actually an oblique view of the glenohumeral joint.

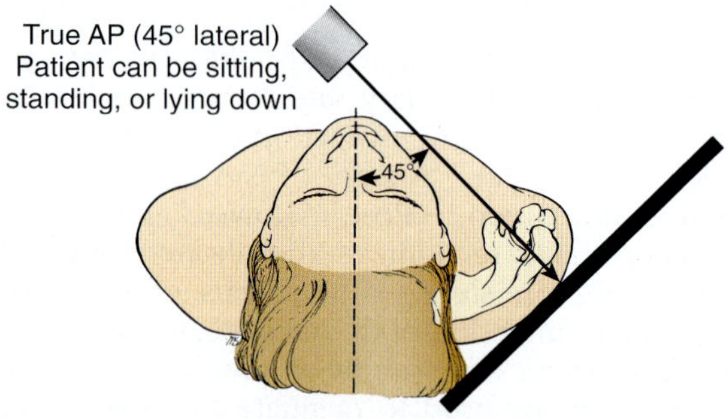

FIGURE 4-2: To obtain a true anteroposterior (AP) view of the glenohumeral joint, the beam must be angled 45 degrees, or the patient can rotate the body until the scapula is parallel to the x-ray cassette.

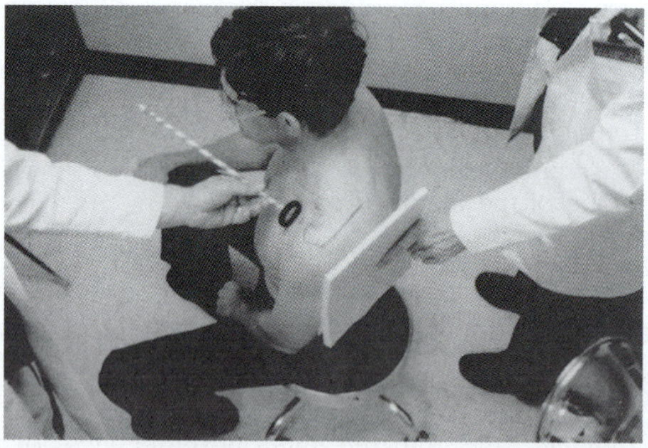

FIGURE 4-3: The position of the patient and the x-ray beam to obtain a true anteroposterior view of the glenohumeral joint.

heavy marking pen to draw a line on the skin along the spine of the scapula. The technician aligns the x-ray beam perpendicular to the line on the skin and directs it at the cassette, which is placed parallel to the line and posterior to the scapula and glenohumeral joint (Fig. 4-3). Although the scapular spine is not exactly parallel to the plane of the scapula, this technique has proved to be effective in clinical practice.

The advantage of the true anteroposterior views of the scapula over traditional anteroposterior views in the plane of the thorax is that the radiograph demonstrates the glenoid in profile rather than obliquely and, in the normal shoulder, clearly separates the glenoid from the humeral head (Fig. 4-4). In the true anteroposterior view, the coracoid process overlaps the glenohumeral joint. If the true anteroposterior view demonstrates the humeral head to be overlapping with the glenoid, the glenohumeral joint is dislocated either anteriorly or posteriorly.

Axillary Lateral View

Initially described by Lawrence[83,84] in 1915, the axillary lateral view can be taken with the patient supine or erect. Ideally, the arm is positioned in 70 to 90 degrees of abduction. The x-ray beam is directed into the axilla from inferior to superior, with the x-ray cassette placed superior to the patient's shoulder (Fig. 4-5). To minimize the amount of abduction required to obtain an axillary lateral view, an alternative technique was devised by Cleaves[19] in 1941. In this technique the patient may be sitting or supine; the arm is abducted only enough to admit a curved x-ray cassette into the axilla. The radiograph is then taken from superior to inferior through the axilla. In situations when abduction is severely limited to only 20 or 30 degrees, a rolled-up cardboard cassette can be substituted for the curved cassette in the axilla (Fig. 4-6).

Axillary lateral radiographs provide excellent visualization of the glenoid and the humeral head and clearly delineate the spatial relationship of the two structures. Loss of glenohumeral cartilage is clearly revealed when the joint space between the glenoid and the humeral head is decreased or absent. Dislocations are easily identified, as are compression fractures of the humeral head and large fractures of the anterior or posterior glenoid rim (see Fig. 4-17 later in chapter). Some fractures of the coracoid and acromion and the spatial relationship of the acromioclavicular joint can also be seen on this view.

If a good-quality axillary lateral radiograph can be obtained, the true scapulolateral view and the modified axillary lateral views are not necessary. However, if because of pain and muscle spasm the patient does not allow enough abduction for a good axillary view, the scapulolateral or the modified axillary lateral views *must* be obtained.

Technique for the Scapulolateral Radiograph

The scapulolateral view is sometimes known as the *transscapular, tangential lateral,* or *Y lateral* view.[140] The position of the injured shoulder, which is usually held in internal rotation (with the arm placed in a sling), is left undisturbed. A marking pen is used to draw a heavy line over the spine of the scapula (Fig. 4-7A). The technician then aligns the x-ray beam parallel to the line on the skin, directed at the cassette, which is placed perpendicular to the line at the anterolateral shoulder. The x-ray beam passes tangentially across the posterolateral chest,

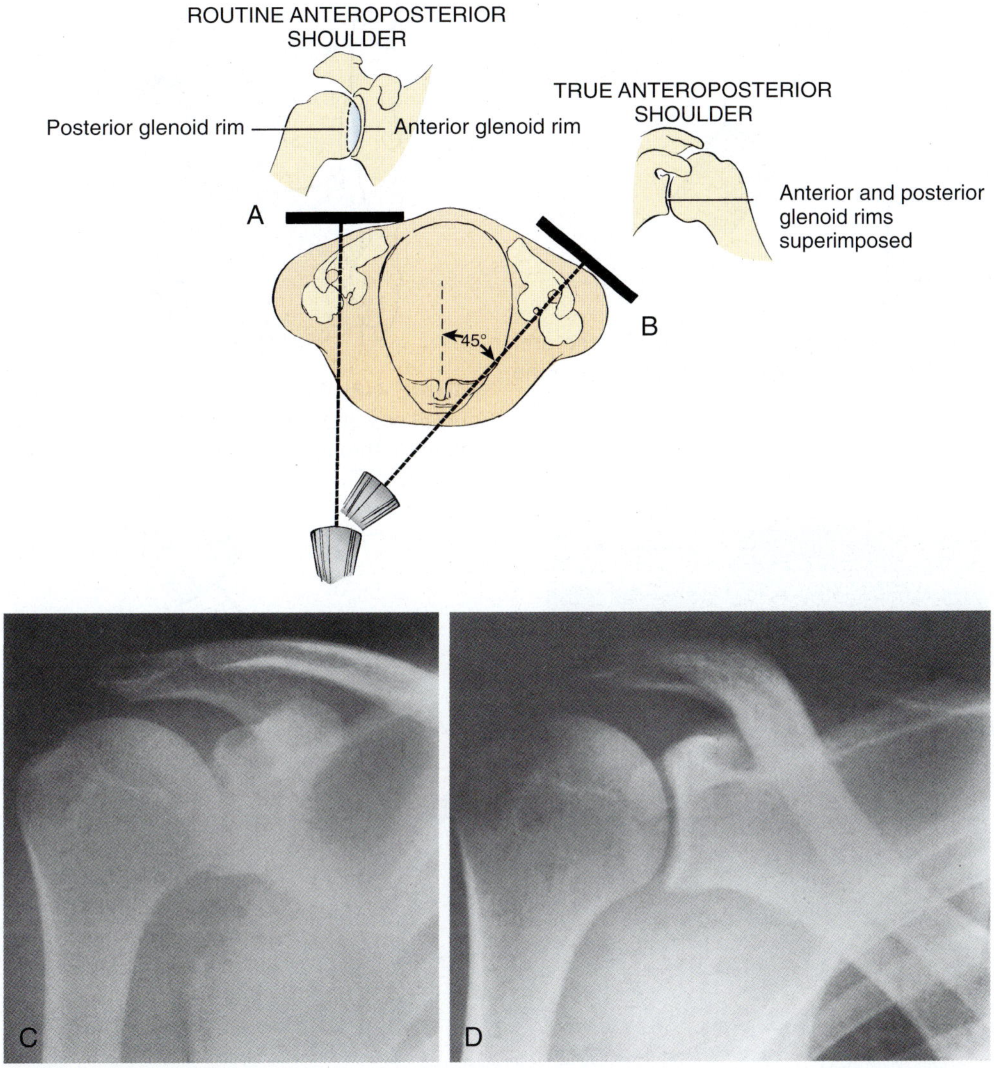

FIGURE 4-4: The difference between the anteroposterior view in the plane of the thorax and true anteroposterior view. **A** and **B,** Note the two angles of the x-ray beam and the placement of the cassettes and the considerable difference between the resulting views of the glenohumeral joint (shown in the schematic drawings and sample radiographs). **C,** A radiograph of the shoulder in the plane of the thorax. **D,** A radiograph of the shoulder taken in the plane of the scapula. (Modified from Rockwood CA, Green DP, eds. *Fractures.* vol. 3. 2nd ed. Philadelphia: JB Lippincott; 1984.)

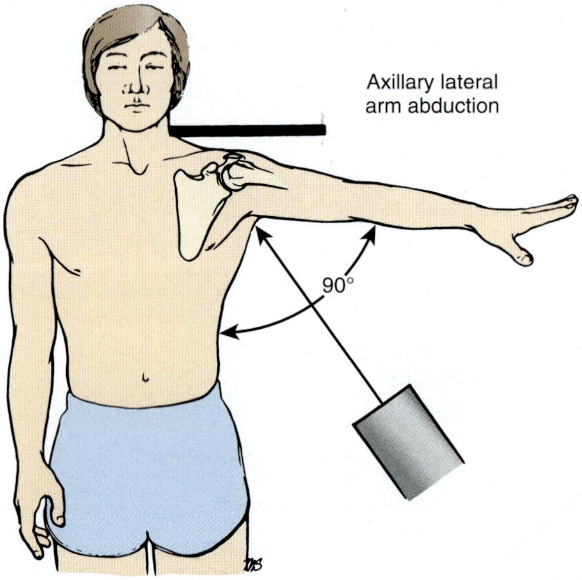

FIGURE 4-5: The axillary lateral radiograph. Ideally, the arm is abducted 70 to 90 degrees and the beam directed up to the x-ray cassette.

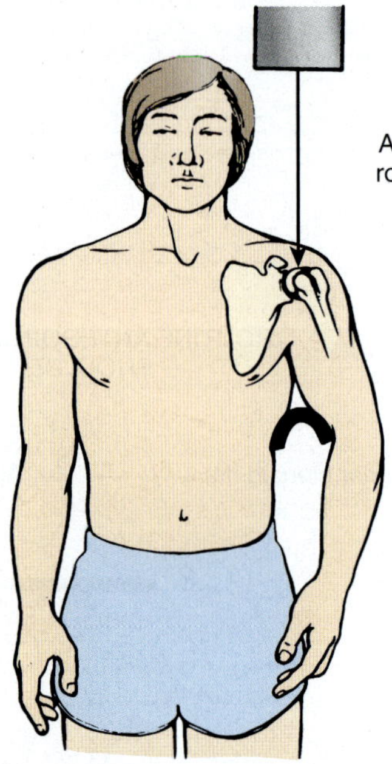

FIGURE 4-6: When the patient cannot fully abduct the arm, a curved cassette can be placed in the axilla and the beam directed inferiorly through the glenohumeral joint onto the cassette.

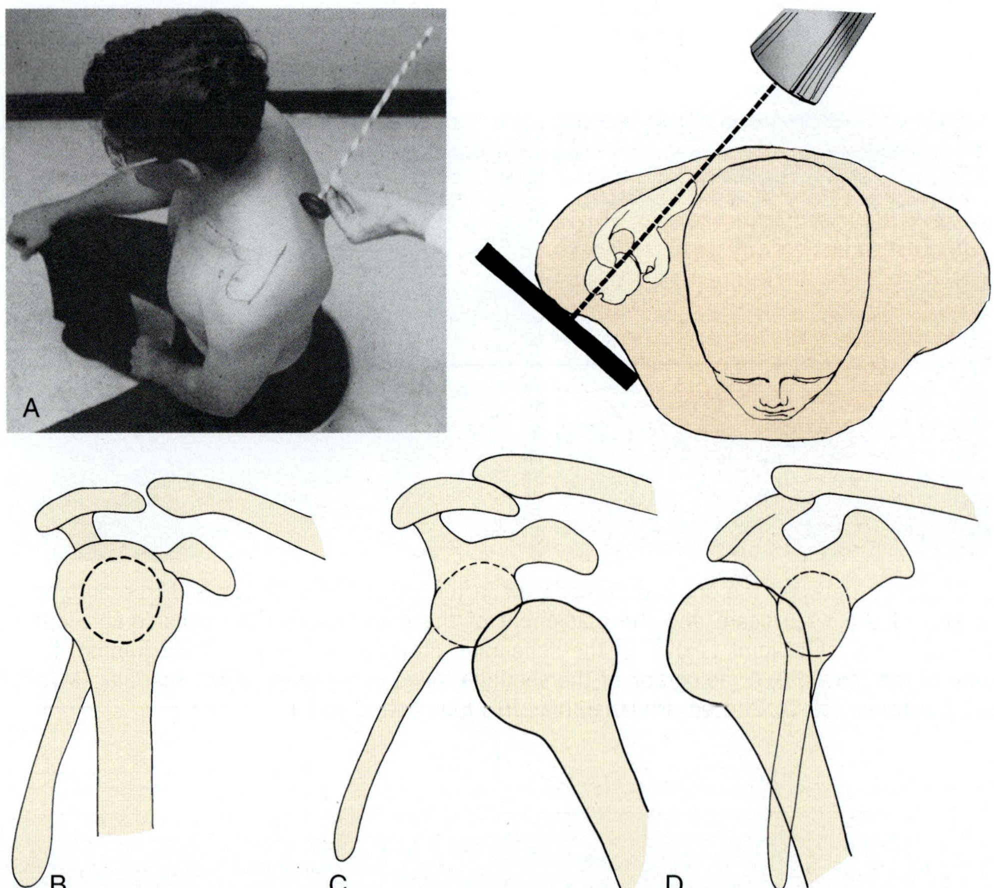

FIGURE 4-7: **A,** A line marked on the skin of the shoulder helps the technician visualize the plane of the x-ray for the true scapulolateral radiograph. **B,** A schematic drawing illustrates how the humeral head on the true scapulolateral radiograph should be centered around the glenoid fossa. **C,** In anterior dislocations of the shoulder, the humeral head is displaced anterior to the glenoid fossa. **D,** In posterior dislocations of the shoulder, the humeral head sits posterior to the glenoid fossa. (**A,** Modified from Rockwood CA, Green DP, eds. *Fractures.* vol. 3. 2nd ed. Philadelphia: JB Lippincott; 1984.)

parallel to and along the spine of the scapula onto the cassette (see Fig. 4-7A and B). The projected image is a true lateral view of the scapula and, hence, of the glenohumeral joint (see Fig. 4-7B).

A lateral projection of the scapula forms a Y shape (Fig. 4-8A to C).[11] The upper arms of the Y are formed by the coracoid process anteriorly and the scapular spine posteriorly. The vertical portion of the Y is formed by the body of the scapula. At the intersection of the three limbs of the Y lies the glenoid fossa. In the normal shoulder, the humeral head is located overlapping the glenoid fossa (see Figs. 4-7B and 4-8D). This view is particularly helpful in determining the anterior or posterior relationship of the humeral head to the glenoid fossa.

In anterior dislocations of the shoulder the humeral head lies anterior to the glenoid fossa (see Figs. 4-7C and 4-8F); in posterior dislocations the humeral head lies posterior to the glenoid fossa (see Figs. 4-7D and 4-8E). The scapulolateral view does not define fractures of the anterior or posterior glenoid rim, but it does reveal displaced fractures of the greater tuberosity. When this view is combined with the true anteroposterior and the axillary lateral views, they together provide three views, all 90 degrees to each other, which maximizes the information available to the clinician for an accurate diagnosis.

Techniques for the Modified Axillary Views

Velpeau Axillary Lateral View

Bloom and Obata's[11] modification of the axillary lateral view of the shoulder is known as the *Velpeau axillary lateral* view because it was intended to be taken with

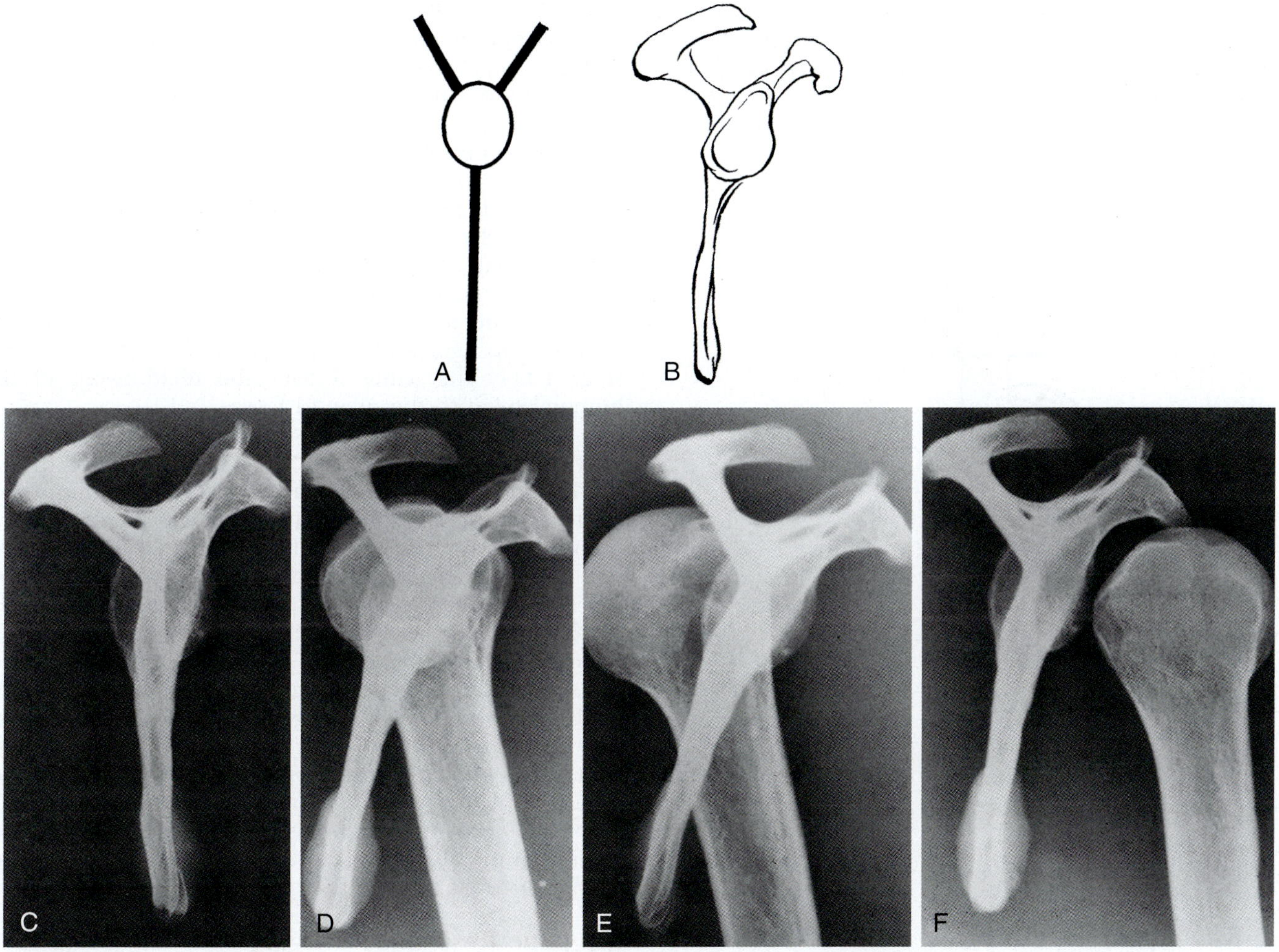

FIGURE 4-8: Interpretation of a true lateral radiograph of the shoulder. **A,** A schematic drawing illustrates how a lateral view of the scapula projects as the letter Y. **B,** Lateral view of the scapula. **C,** A true lateral radiograph of the scapula shows the glenoid fossa located at the junction of the base of the spine and the base of the coracoid with the body of the vertically projecting scapula. **D,** A true lateral view of the glenohumeral joint shows the humeral head well centered around the glenoid fossa. **E,** In a posterior subacromial dislocation of the shoulder, the articular surface of the humeral head is directed posterior to the glenoid fossa. **F,** In an anterior subcoracoid dislocation of the shoulder, the humeral head is anterior to the glenoid fossa. (Modified from Rockwood CA, Green DP, eds. *Fractures.* vol. 3. 2nd ed. Philadelphia: JB Lippincott; 1984.)

the acutely injured shoulder still in a sling without abduction.

With the Velpeau bandage or shoulder sling in place, the patient stands or sits at the end of the radiograph table and leans backwards through 20 to 30 degrees over the table.

The x-ray cassette is placed on the table directly beneath the shoulder, and the x-ray tube is positioned directly over the shoulder so that the beam passes vertically from superior to inferior through the shoulder joint onto the cassette (Fig. 4-9). On this view the humeral shaft appears foreshortened and the glenohumeral joint appears magnified, but otherwise, it demonstrates the relationship of the head of the humerus to the scapula.

Apical Oblique View

Garth, Slappey, and Ochs[40] have described an apical oblique projection that reliably demonstrates the pathology of the glenohumeral joint. The patient may be seated or in a supine position, and the arm may remain in a sling. The x-ray cassette is placed posteriorly, parallel to the spine of the scapula. The x-ray beam is directed through the glenohumeral joint toward the cassette at an angle of 45 degrees to the plane of the thorax and is also tilted 45 degrees caudally (Fig. 4-10A and B).

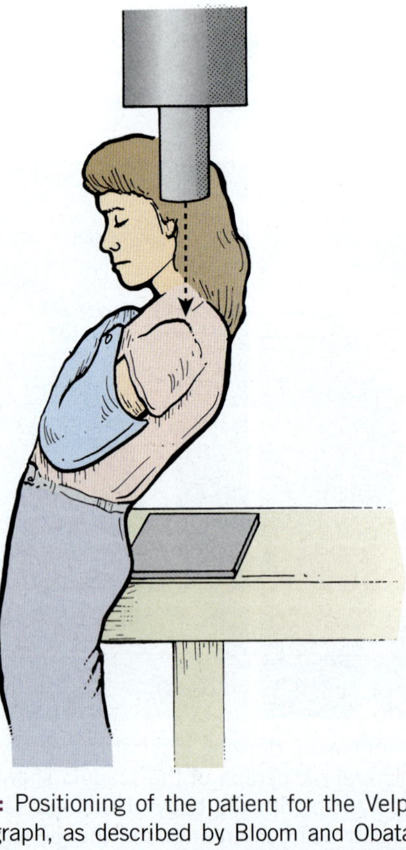

FIGURE 4-9: Positioning of the patient for the Velpeau axillary lateral radiograph, as described by Bloom and Obata. (Modified from Bloom MH, Obata WG. Diagnosis of posterior dislocation of the shoulder with use of the Velpeau axillary and angled up radiographic views. *J Bone Joint Surg Am.* 1967;49(5):943-949.)

The resultant radiograph demonstrates the relationship of the humeral head to the glenoid and therefore identifies the presence and direction of glenohumeral dislocations and subluxations. This view clearly defines the anteroinferior and posterosuperior rims of the glenoid and is useful for detecting calcifications or fractures at the glenoid rim (see Fig. 4-10C and D). Posterolateral and anterior humeral head compression fractures are also revealed.

Kornguth and Salazar[79] reported that this technique is excellent for diagnosis in the acute setting.

Stripp Axial Lateral View

The Stripp axial lateral view, described by Horsfield,[57] is similar to the Velpeau axillary lateral view, except that the beam passes from inferior to superior and the x-ray cassette is positioned above the shoulder.

Trauma Axillary Lateral View

This is another modification of the axillary lateral view and has been described by Teitge and Ciullo.[18,162] The advantage of this view over the Velpeau and Stripp views is that it can be taken while the patient is supine, as is often necessary in patients with multiple trauma. This view can be taken while the injured shoulder is still immobilized in a shoulder-immobilizer dressing. The patient lies supine on the radiograph table, with the involved arm supported in 20 degrees of flexion by placing radiolucent material under the elbow. The x-ray beam is directed up through the axilla to a cassette propped up against the superior aspect of the shoulder (Fig. 4-11). This view defines the relationship of the humeral head to the glenoid fossa.

Computed Tomography Scan

A CT scan reliably demonstrates fractures, the number of fracture fragments, and fracture-dislocations of the glenohumeral joint. However, the addition of a CT scan to the trauma series does not apparently improve the reproducibility of the Neer or Arbeitsgemeinschaft für Osteosynthesefragen (AO) fracture classifications.[151,152] The CT technique should consist of 3-mm-thick contiguous sections with a bone algorithm from the top of the acromion to the inferior pole of the glenoid. It is very important that the scan includes both shoulders so that the physician can compare the anatomy of the injured shoulder with that of the normal shoulder. Three-dimensional CT scans can provide additional information in the acute setting for the evaluation of complex or multiple shoulder girdle fractures.

Magnetic Resonance Imaging

The magnetic resonance imaging (MRI) scan is rarely indicated for managing fractures of the shoulder. However, MRI scans identify the presence of an occult greater tuberosity fracture and associated rotator tendon pathology in a posttraumatic situation[95,97,131] and might also help diagnose the pattern of postfracture avascular necrosis.

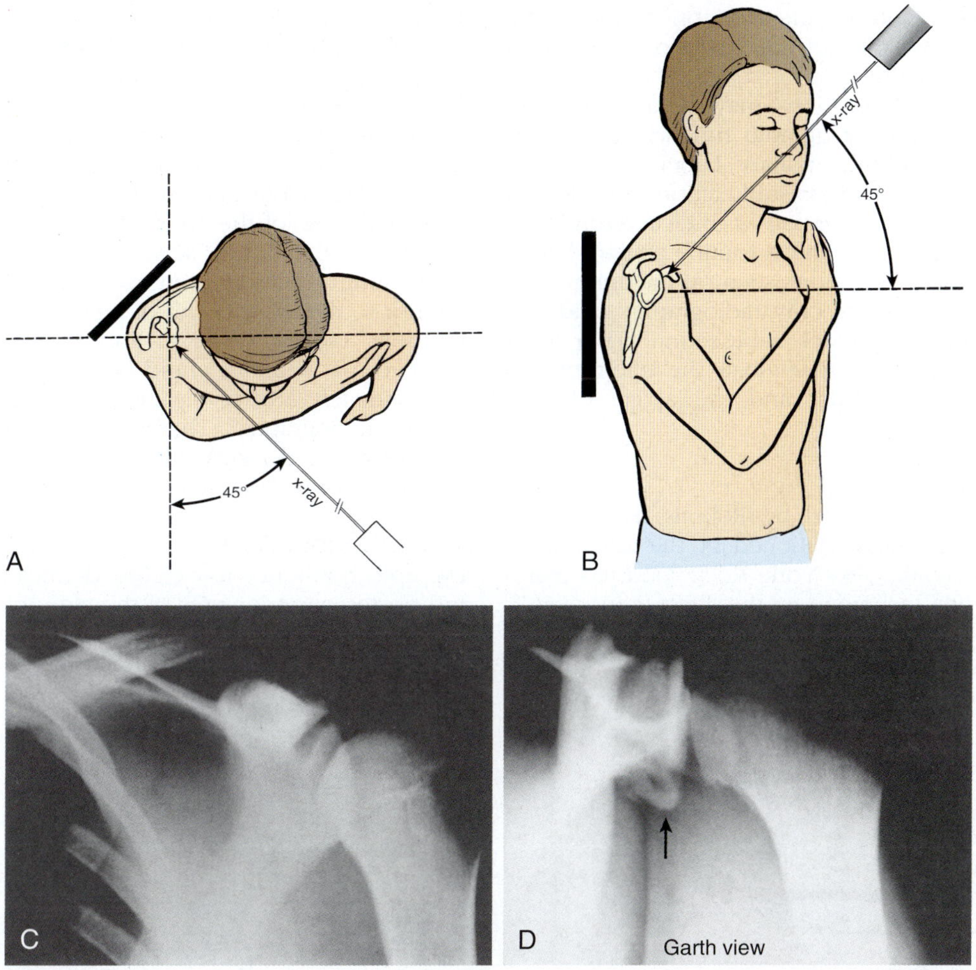

FIGURE 4-10: **A** and **B,** Positioning of the patient to obtain an apical oblique radiograph. This is a true anteroposterior view of the glenohumeral joint with a 45-degree caudal tilt of the x-ray beam. **C,** A radiograph of the left shoulder in the plane of the thorax does not reveal any significant abnormality. **D,** In the apical oblique view, note the calcification on the anteroinferior glenoid rim (*arrow*). (**A** and **B,** Modified from Garth WP Jr, Slappey CE, Ochs CW. Radiographic demonstration of instability of the shoulder: the apical oblique projection, a technical note. *J Bone Joint Surg Am.* 1984;66(9):1450-1453. **C** and **D,** Courtesy William Garth, MD.)

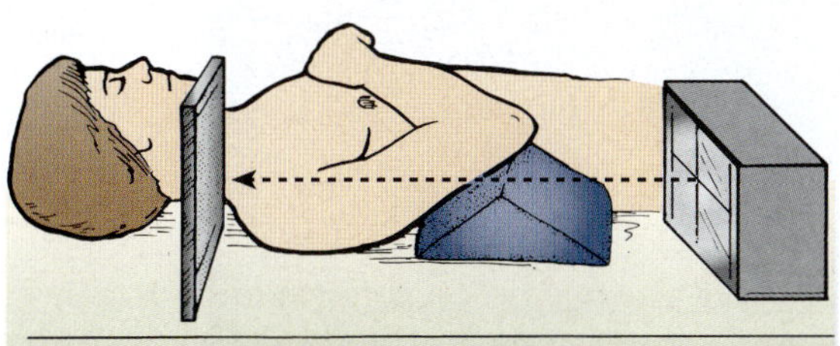

FIGURE 4-11: Positioning of the patient for the trauma axillary lateral radiograph. The patient is supine and the elbow is elevated by a piece of foam rubber to allow the x-ray beam to pass in an inferior direction up through the glenohumeral joint onto the x-ray cassette, placed superior to the shoulder. (Modified from Teitge RA, Ciullo JV. The CAM axillary x-ray. Exhibit at AAOS Meeting. *Orthop Trans.* 1982;6:451.)

ANTERIOR INSTABILITY

Recommended Views

Recommended views for anterior instability are the true anteroposterior views, the West Point axillary lateral, and the apical oblique projection. Arthrograms, arthrotomograms, CT scans, CT arthrography, and MRI scans are discussed in the section "Soft Tissue Evaluation of Shoulder Instability."

With anterior dislocation or subluxation of the glenohumeral joint, there may be bone damage or soft tissue calcification adjacent to the anterior or, particularly, the anteroinferior rim of the glenoid. The true anteroposterior view can demonstrate a fracture of the inferior glenoid that might not be visualized on the anteroposterior views in the plane of the thorax. Although the axillary lateral view may be useful for demonstrating some anterior glenoid abnormalities, the West Point axillary lateral and the apical oblique views provide more information.[133,139]

Anterior shoulder dislocations may be accompanied by fractures of the anterior glenoid rim, which may be demonstrated on a routine axillary lateral radiograph. However, in traumatic anterior subluxation, the glenoid defect almost exclusively involves the anteroinferior glenoid, which cannot be seen on routine axillary lateral views. In many cases the lesions seen on the anteroinferior glenoid rim provide the only radiographic evidence of traumatic anterior shoulder subluxation. Two techniques have been described to evaluate the anteroinferior glenoid rim: the West Point and the apical oblique projections.

West Point Axillary Lateral View

This projection was described by Rokous, Feagin, and Abbott[139] when they were stationed at the US Military Academy at West Point, New York; Rockwood has therefore referred to this technique as the *West Point view.*[138] The patient is positioned prone on the radiograph table, with the involved shoulder on a pad raised approximately 8 cm from the surface of the table. The patient's head and neck are turned away from the involved side. With the cassette held against the superior aspect of the shoulder, the x-ray beam is centered at the axilla with 25 degrees of downward angulation of the beam from the horizontal and 25 degrees of medial angulation of the beam from the midline (Fig. 4-12A and B). The resultant radiograph is a tangential view of the anteroinferior rim of the glenoid.

The usual finding seen in the traumatic anterior-subluxating shoulder is soft tissue calcification located just anterior to the glenoid rim or anteroinferior bony fracture avulsions (see Fig. 4-12C and D). A cadaveric study revealed that a 21% glenoid bony defect appeared to be approximately 18% of the intact glenoid on a West Point axillary radiograph.[60] Therefore the West Point axillary view provides decisive information regarding anteroinferior glenoid rim fractures and their operative treatment.

Apical Oblique View

The apical oblique view clearly defines the anteroinferior and posterosuperior rims of the glenoid. Pathologic findings of the rim associated with recurrent instability, such as displaced malunited rim fractures, glenoid bone loss,

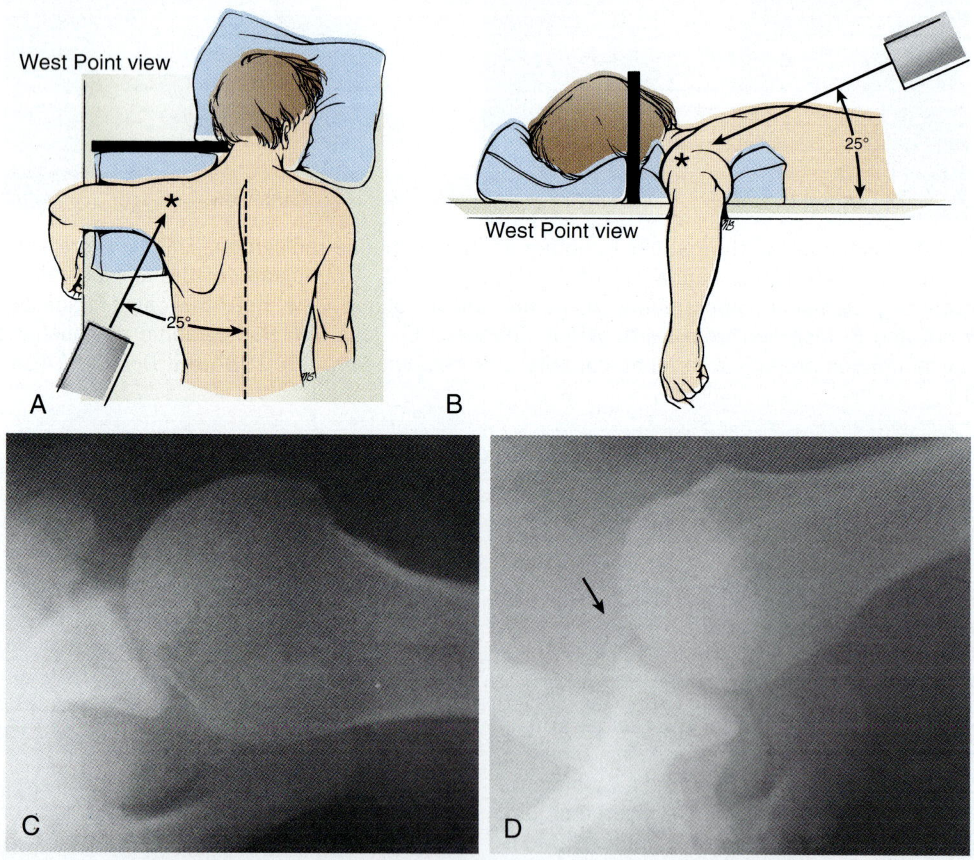

FIGURE 4-12: **A** and **B,** Positioning of the patient for the West Point radiograph to visualize the anteroinferior glenoid rim of the shoulder. *Asterisk,* beam target. **C** and **D,** Examples of calcification on the anteroinferior glenoid rim, as noted on the West Point view. (**A** and **B,** Modified from the work of Rokous JR, Feagin JA, Abbott HG. Modified axillary roentgenogram. *Clin Orthop Relat Res.* 1972;82:84-86. **C** and **D,** Modified from Rockwood CA, Green DP, eds. *Fractures.* vol. 3. 2nd ed. Philadelphia: JB Lippincott; 1984.)

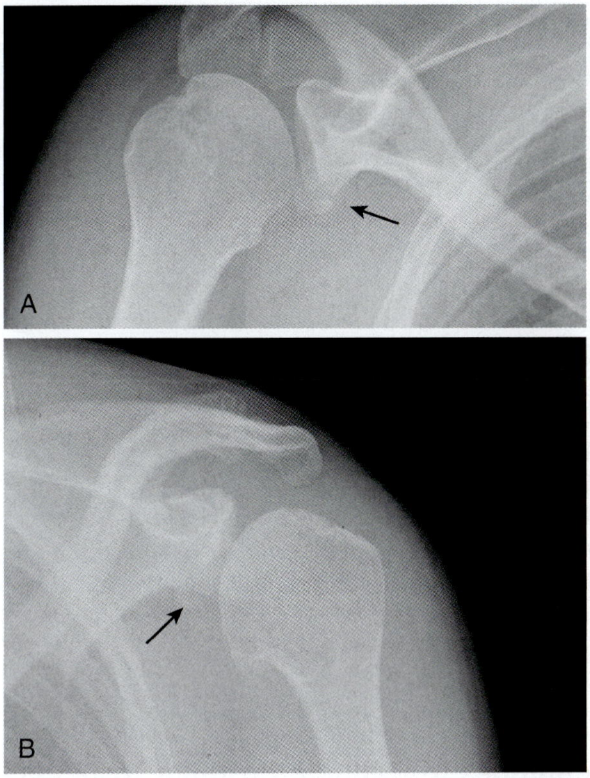

FIGURE 4-13: **A,** Apical oblique radiograph revealing an anterior glenoid rim fracture (*arrow*). **B,** Apical oblique radiograph revealing anteroinferior glenoid cartilage and bone loss (*arrow*).

or anterior inferior cartilage loss, are identified with this view (Fig. 4-13). Posterolateral and anterior humeral head defects are also revealed by this view, although CT is needed to quantify the size of the defect.

Recurrent Anterior Glenohumeral Instability

Radiographic views for recurrent anterior glenohumeral instability include the apical oblique view for anterior glenoid erosion, the Stryker notch view for a posterolateral humeral head defect, and MRI or CT arthrography for detachment of the labrum.

POSTERIOR HUMERAL HEAD COMPRESSION FRACTURES ASSOCIATED WITH ANTERIOR DISLOCATION: THE HILL-SACHS LESION

Recommended Views

The recommended views for posterior humeral head compression fractures are the Stryker notch view, the anteroposterior view with the arm in full internal rotation, and other views.

A commonly encountered sequela of anterior shoulder dislocation is a compression fracture of the posterolateral humeral head. Such a fracture can occur during the first traumatic dislocation or after recurrent anterior dislocations. This is commonly referred to as a *Hill-Sachs lesion* and was reported by Hill and Sachs in 1940 (Fig. 4-14).[53] However, prior to this it had clearly been described by Eve in 1880.[32] In the period between the report by Eve in 1880 and by Hill and Sachs in 1940, it was described by Malgaigne,[96] Kuster,[81] Cramer,[23] Popke,[123] Caird,[17] and Broca and Hartman,[15,16] Perthes,[37] Bankart,[4,5] Eden,[31] Hybbinette,[58] Didiee,[30] and Hermodsson.[52]

The indentation, or compression fracture, may be seen on the anteroposterior view if the arm is in full internal rotation, and it may be seen occasionally on the axillary lateral view. However, we believe that one of the best views for identifying the compression fracture is the technique reported in 1959 by Hall and colleagues[49]; they credited this view to William Stryker, leading Rockwood to call it the *Stryker notch view*.[138]

Stryker Notch View

For the Stryker notch view,[49] the patient is placed supine on the radiograph table with the cassette under the involved shoulder (Fig. 4-15A). The palm of the hand of the involved upper extremity is placed on top of the head, with the fingers toward the back of the head. The x-ray beam is tilted 10 degrees cephalad and centered over the coracoid process. A positive result is a distinct notch in the posterolateral part of the humeral head (Fig. 4-15B).

Anteroposterior View in Internal Rotation

Probably the simplest view, but not the most diagnostic, is the one described by Adams.[1] It is an anteroposterior view of the shoulder with the arm in full internal rotation. This reveals an indentation or compression in the posterolateral portion of the humeral head, a defect that may simply appear as a vertical condensation of bone. Pring and colleagues[125] compared the Stryker view with the internal (60 degrees) rotation view of Adams in 84 patients with anterior dislocation of the shoulder for establishing evidence of a posterolateral defect in the humeral head. The internal rotation view was positive in 48% of patients, whereas the Stryker notch view was positive in 70%.

Other views predating the Stryker notch view have been described by Didiee[30] and Hermodsson[52] and are useful in demonstrating the presence and size of the posterolateral humeral head compression fractures. Although these techniques involve views of the proximal humerus with the arm in internal rotation, they are slightly awkward to obtain. The apical oblique view described by Garth and colleagues[40] also demonstrates the compression fracture. Strauss and colleagues[158] and Danzig and colleagues[25] have independently evaluated the efficacy of the various views in revealing the Hill-Sachs lesion and reported that although none of these views reveals the lesion in every case, the Stryker notch view is probably the most effective. The presence of the

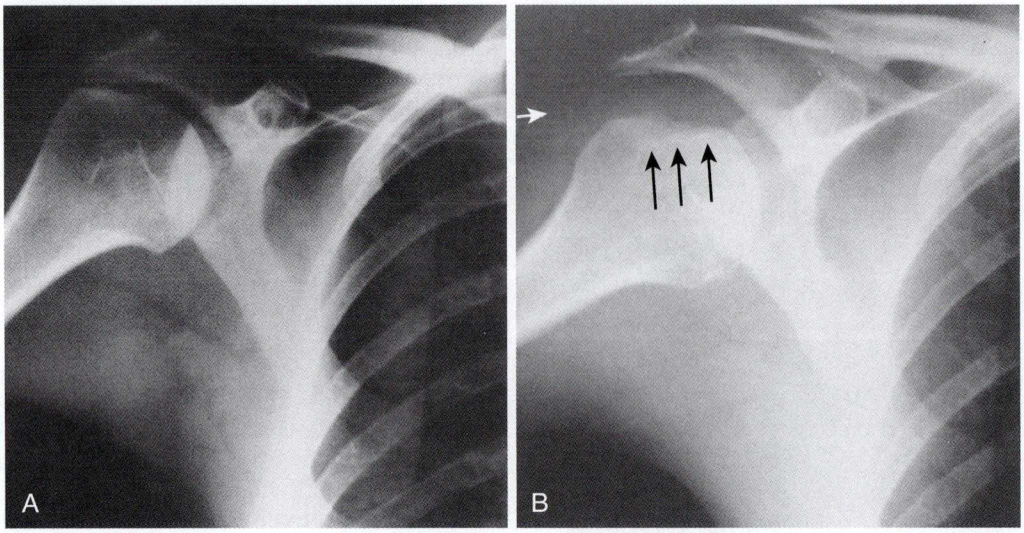

FIGURE 4-14: The Hill-Sachs lesion. **A,** Anteroposterior radiograph of the right shoulder in 45 degrees of abduction and external rotation. Note that some sclerosis is present in the superior aspect of the head of the humerus. **B,** In full internal rotation. Note the defect in the posterolateral aspect of the humeral head (*white arrow*) and the dense line of bone condensation marked by the *black arrows*, the Hill-Sachs lesion.

compression head fracture on the radiograph confirms that the shoulder has been dislocated, whereas its absence suggests that the head may be subluxating rather than frankly dislocating.

After a study of Hill-Sachs lesions created in the posterolateral humeral head, Danzig, Greenway, and Resnick[25] concluded that three views were optimal for defining the lesion: the anteroposterior view with the arm in 45 degrees of internal rotation, the Stryker notch view, and the modified Didiee view.

In a study of 120 patients Strauss and colleagues[157] reported that a specific set of views could confirm the diagnosis of anterior shoulder instability with 95% accuracy; these were the anteroposterior view of the shoulder in internal rotation and the Hermodsson, axillary lateral, Stryker notch, Didiee, and West Point views.

Whereas the Stryker notch view can document the presence of a compression fracture, advanced imaging studies with CT or MRI provide information that affects surgical decision-making. CT, particularly three-dimensional CT, provides images that reveal defect orientation, width and depth, and quantitative information that specifically affects surgical planning (Fig. 4-16).[74,75,100,101,118,126,127]

POSTERIOR INSTABILITY

Recommended Views

Recommended views for posterior instability are the trauma series of radiographs and modified axillary views. Arthrograms, arthrotomograms, CT scans, CT arthrography, and MRI scans are discussed in the section "Soft Tissue Evaluation of Shoulder Instability."

Techniques to Evaluate Posterior Instability

Posterior dislocation of the shoulder is a rare problem, comprising only 1% to 3% of all dislocations of the shoulder, and it is commonly misdiagnosed.[138] There are three reasons for missing the posterior displacement:

1. Inadequate patient history
2. Inadequate physical examination
3. Inadequate radiographic evaluation

All too often, only two anteroposterior views with the arm in internal and external rotation are obtained. Radiographs of the injured shoulder must be made in two planes, 90 degrees to each other. The diagnosis of posterior dislocation of the shoulder can always be made if the anteroposterior view and one of the previously described lateral views are obtained. Usually, the patient does not allow enough abduction to obtain the true axillary view, in which case the scapulolateral or modified axillary view (apical oblique) or a CT scan must be obtained.

Traumatic posterior glenohumeral instability may be accompanied by either damage to the posterior glenoid rim or impaction fractures on the anteromedial surface of the humeral head, the reverse Hill-Sachs lesion (Fig. 4-17). Lesions of the posterior glenoid rim can usually be noted on the axillary view. CT and MRI scans are very helpful in defining the glenoid rim fracture and in determining the size of the compression fracture of the humeral head.

Soft Tissue Evaluation of Shoulder Instability

Patients with recurrent instability often have radiographically occult soft tissue abnormalities. Although their routine

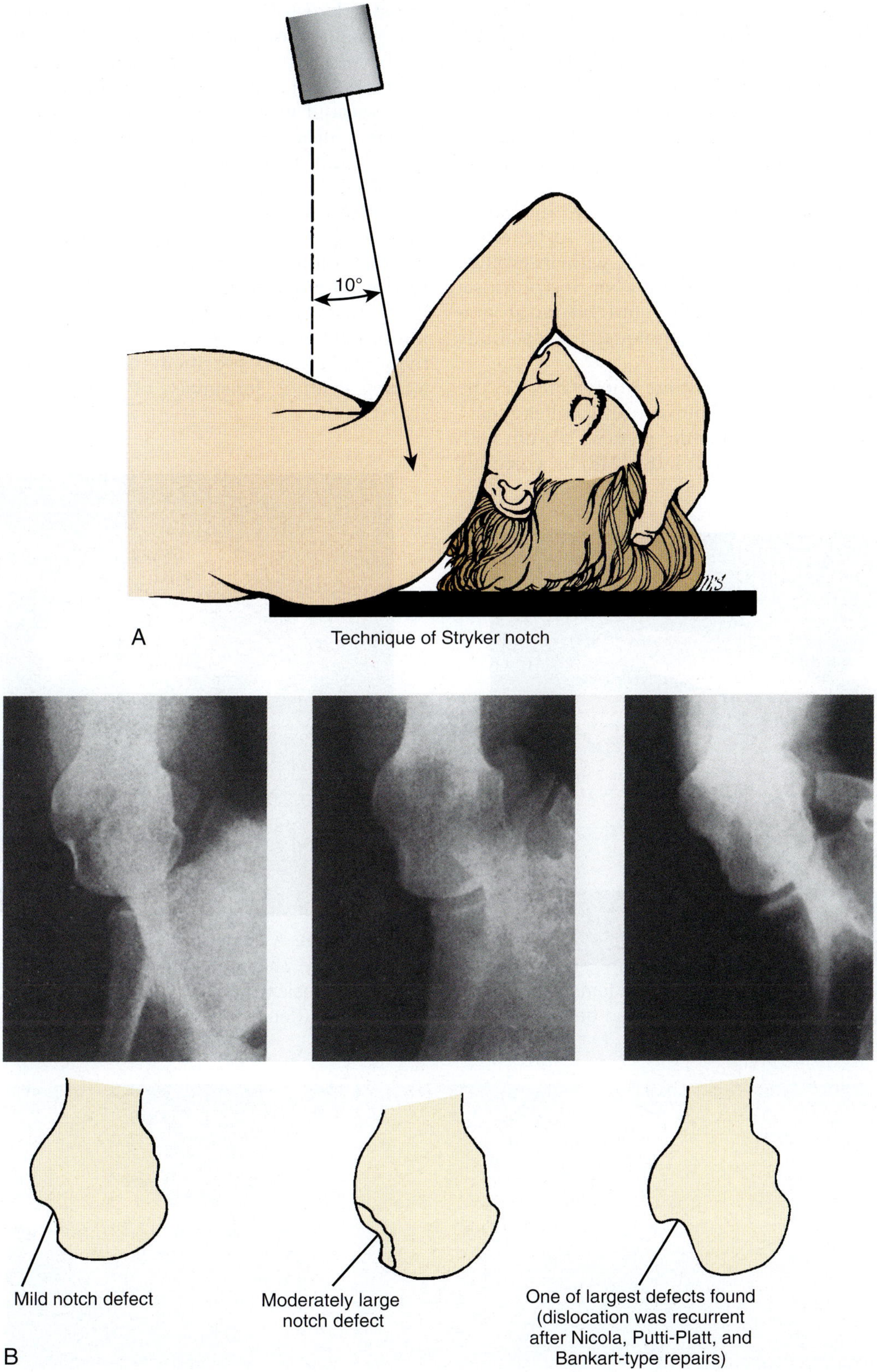

FIGURE 4-15: A, Position of the patient for the Stryker notch view. The patient is supine with the cassette posterior to the shoulder. The humerus is flexed approximately 120 degrees, placing the hand on top of the head. The angle of the x-ray tube is 10 degrees superior. **B,** Defects in the posterolateral aspect of the humeral head seen in three different patients with recurring anterior dislocations of the shoulder. (Modified from Hall RH, Isaac F, Booth CR. Dislocation of the shoulder with special reference to accompanying small fractures. *J Bone Joint Surg Am.* 1959;41-A[3]:489-494.)

radiologic examination may appear normal, a significant injury to the soft tissues is frequently present. In anterior dislocations, the anterior capsule and glenoid labrum may be stripped off the glenoid rim with an intact periosteum forming a pseudo joint-space, as originally described by Perthes[37] in 1906, or a complete avulsion of the labral-ligamentous complex from the glenoid, described by Bankart[4] in 1923.

Plain film arthrography, arthrotomography, and pneumotomography[2,13,76,122] have all been shown to be effective in demonstrating lesions associated with instability, but these are infrequently utilized today for this purpose. CT arthrography,[62,118,127,134,135,150] MRI, and MR arthrography have largely replaced these techniques for instability evaluation.[7,42,45,47,87,106]

CT arthrography can demonstrate the status of the anterior or posterior labrum. Shuman and colleagues[150] used double-contrast CT to study the glenoid labrum with a high degree of accuracy (Fig. 4-18). MRI is currently the standard for imaging a suspected labral and capsular abnormality associated with anterior or posterior instability because it provides anatomic images of soft tissue structures and does not use ionizing radiation.[7,42,45,47,87,143,144] MRI without intra-articular contrast provides only limited specific information regarding glenohumeral instability, and a study that is interpreted as normal—especially by radiologists with limited experience in shoulder instability—does not rule out symptomatic glenohumeral instability. Authors have reported the sensitivity of MRI without intra-articular contrast to detect anterior labral tearing to range from 44% to 100%[8,43,46,86,91] and the specificity from 68% to 95%.[21,36,43,46,71,91,116] Posterior labral abnormalities have been detected with a reported sensitivity of 74% and specificity of 95%[46] and superior labral tearing with a sensitivity of 86% and a specificity of

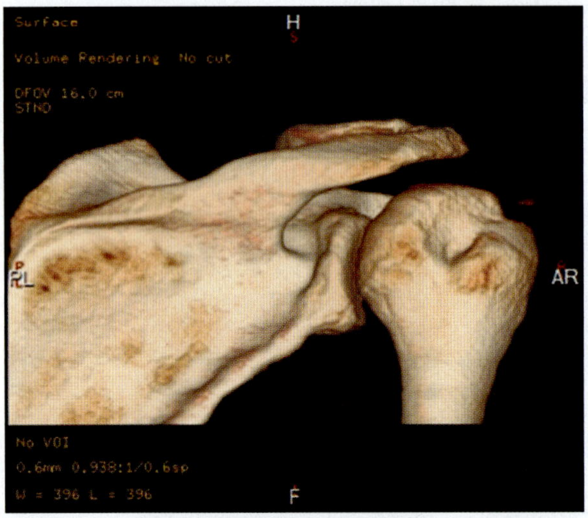

FIGURE 4-16: Three-dimensional computed tomographic scan revealing an engaging posterior humeral head defect.

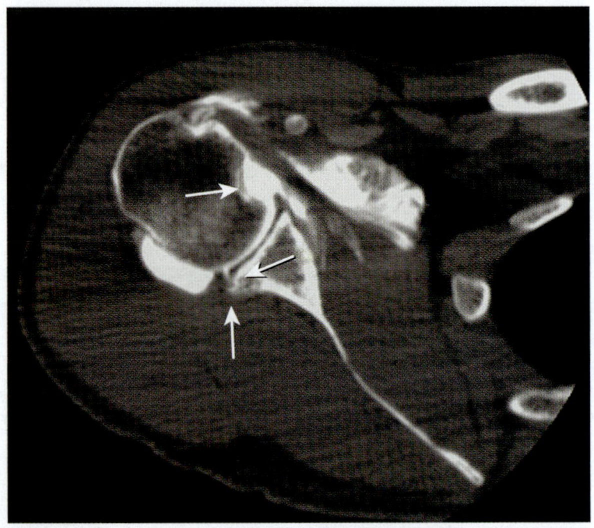

FIGURE 4-18: A computed tomographic arthrogram of posterior instability. The arrows indicate the presence of an impacted Hill-Sachs lesion and traumatic changes to the posterior glenoid rim. (Courtesy Phillip Tirman, MD.)

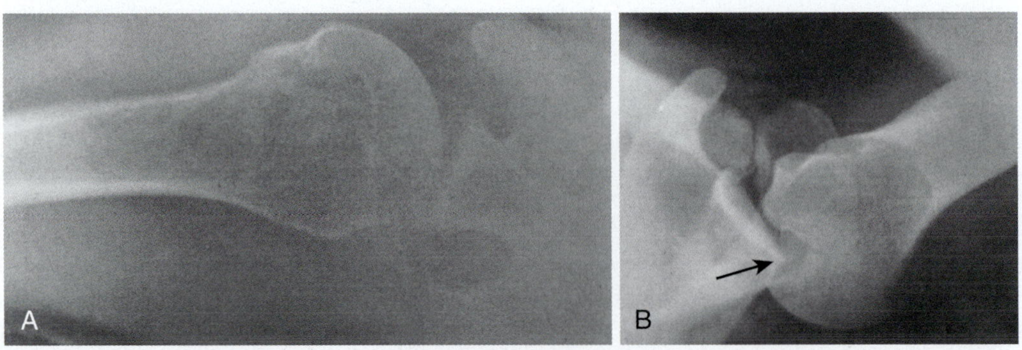

FIGURE 4-17: **A,** An axillary lateral view of a normal left shoulder shows the normal articulation of the humeral head with the glenoid fossa and the normal relationship of the humeral head to the coracoid process and the acromion process. **B,** An axillary lateral view of the injured right shoulder shows a large anteromedial compression fracture of the humeral head, the reverse Hill-Sachs lesion. The *arrow* indicates the posterior glenoid rim that has produced the hatchet-like defect in the humeral head. (From Rockwood CA, Green DP, eds. *Fractures.* vol.3. 2nd ed. Philadelphia: JB Lippincott; 1984.)

100%.[44] Capsular laxity and capsular insertion sites cannot be assessed by MRI without intra-articular contrast.[168] The cost of MRI, initially prohibitive in many cases, is now within the same range as that of CT scans and occasionally even of plain film arthrography. Variability in the accuracy of interpretation of the images has improved, especially with improved communication between the radiologist and orthopedist, and MRI studies for the evaluation of shoulder instability are now commonplace.

MRI combined with intra-articular gadolinium[67] or saline[168] provides images that accurately identify labral and glenohumeral ligament anatomy and injury, associated rotator tendon tearing, biceps abnormalities, and osseous and cartilaginous abnormalities (Figs. 4-19 to 4-21). Intra-articular injection of gadolinium-DTPA (diethylenetriamine pentaacetate) at 2 mmol/L has been shown to have complete passive diffusion from the joint within 6 to 24 hours, and rapid renal elimination has led to almost no systemic side effects.[146] A study evaluating MR arthrography of normal shoulders accurately revealed anatomic variations of the anterior labral signal intensity, form, and size, and the authors concluded that only major tears or detachments of the labrum should be diagnosed.[175] Other studies have shown accurate depiction of labral and capsular abnormalities, especially when accurate history is taken into consideration and there is communication between

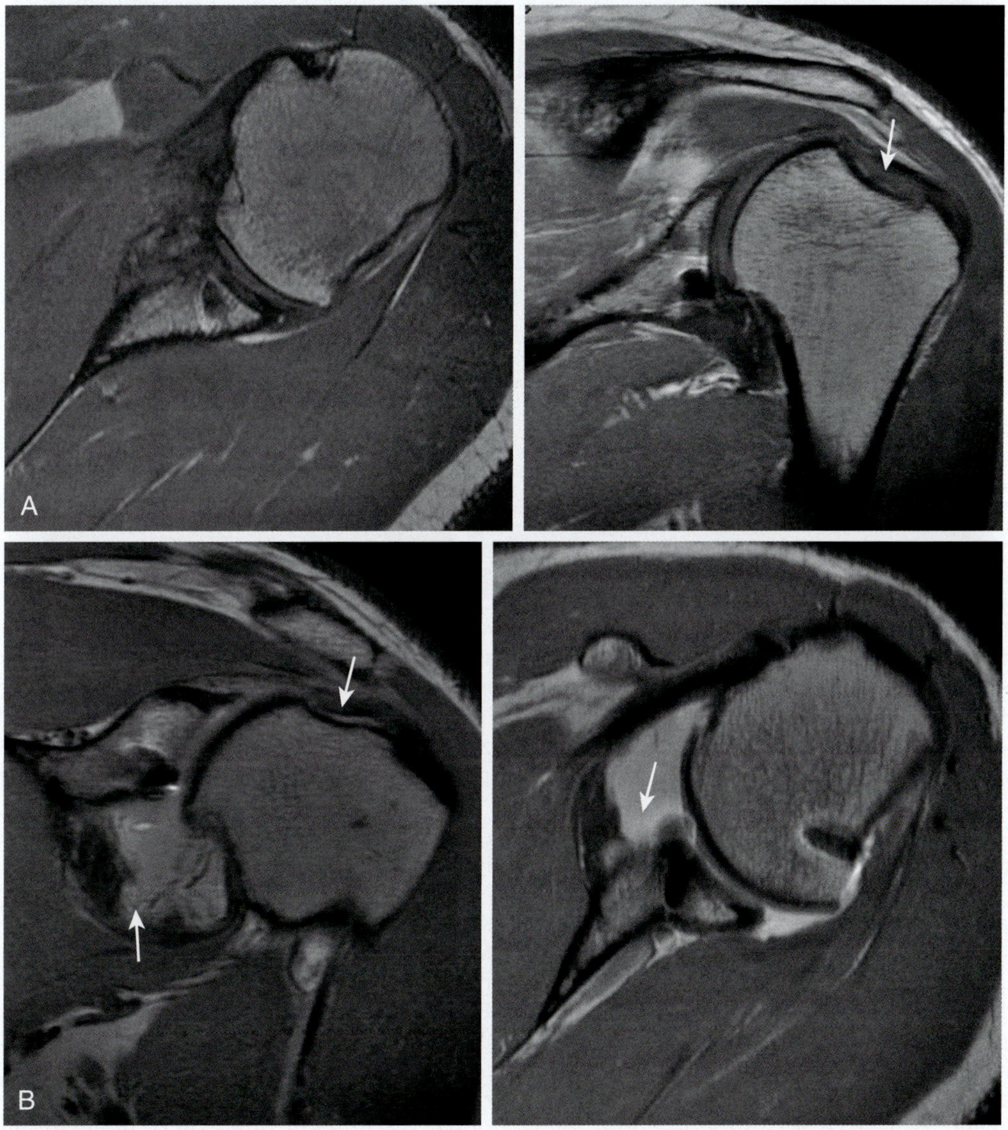

FIGURE 4-19: The benefit of arthrography. **A,** Prearthrographic axial and coronal proton density images demonstrate postoperative changes of a Bankart repair and an impacted Hill-Sachs lesion (*arrow*). This study was initially interpreted as showing expected postoperative findings. However, the patient experienced clinical recurrent instability and therefore arthrography was requested. **B,** After the introduction of intra-articular contrast, the labrum and capsule are lifted away from the glenoid, demonstrating incompetency. The superior arrows in both images point to the Hill-Sachs lesion, and the inferior arrows point to the lesion lifted from its origin by contrast fluid. (Courtesy Phillip Tirman, MD.)

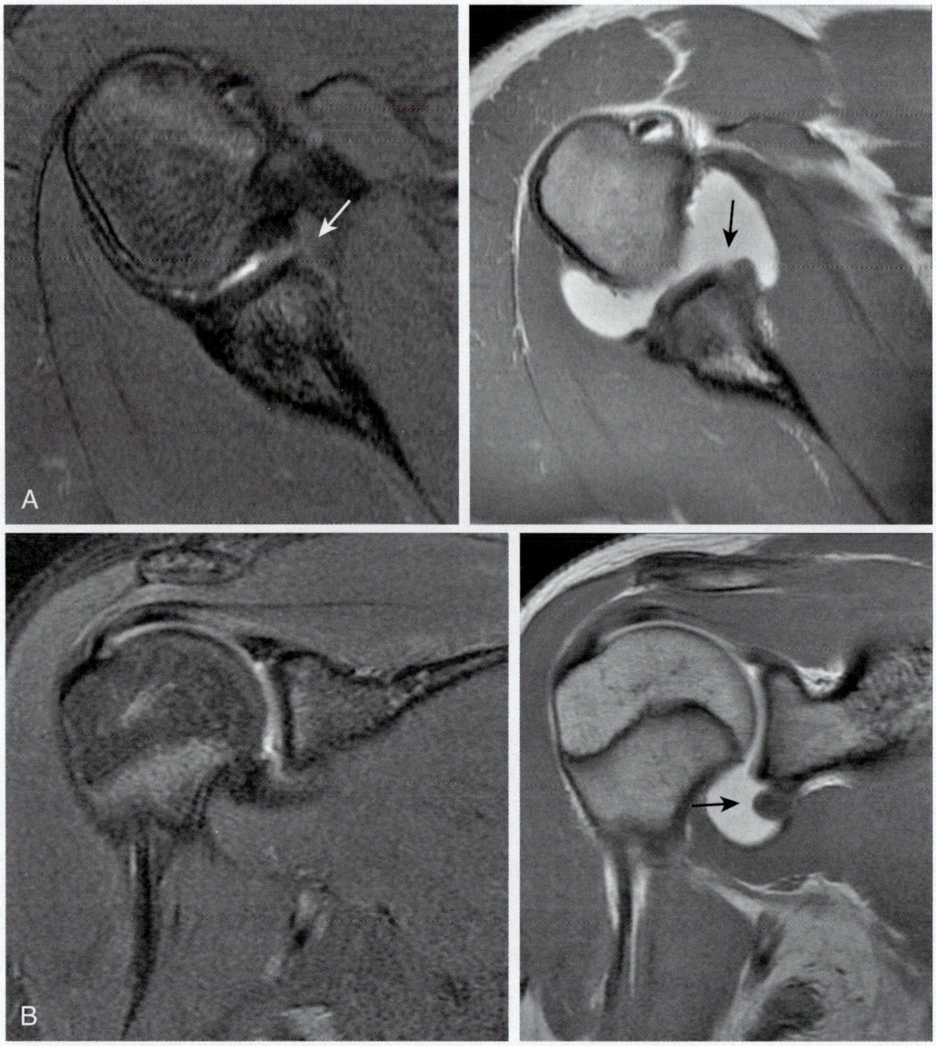

FIGURE 4-20: Arthrogram of an anterior labral periosteal sleeve avulsion lesion before and after the introduction of intra-articular contrast: axial and coronal images. **A,** After the injection of intra-articular contrast, the axial T1 image demonstrates medial displacement of the labral ligamentous attachment site to the anterior inferior glenoid with some overlying fibrotic change and resynovialization. **B,** Before the introduction of intra-articular contrast material, the anteroinferior labrum is shown to be thickened, irregular, and edematous, and there is evidence of healing change. Before contrast the arrow points to the healing tissue. After contrast the arrows reveal displaced labral tissue. The contrast helps delineate the displacement. (Courtesy Phillip Tirman, MD.)

the radiologist and orthopedist.[45,47,106] In a prospective study of 30 patients, surgical correlation was used to show MR arthrography to be superior to CT arthrography in detecting anterior labral pathology.[67] MR arthrography is also useful in evaluating failed anterior instability surgery, with a reported sensitivity of 100% and specificity of 60% in detecting recurrent anterior labral tears.[169] The addition of the abduction and external rotation (ABER) position has been shown to increase the sensitivity of MR arthrography in revealing tears of the anterior glenoid labrum (Fig. 4-22). Cvitanic and colleagues compared conventional axial MR arthrograms to oblique axial MR arthrograms in the ABER position and found the latter to be significantly more sensitive in revealing anterior glenoid labral tears (P =.005; Fig. 4-23).[24]

Capsular laxity remains problematic. In a study of 121 patients undergoing surgery for anterior instability, capsular laxity was missed in all shoulders, and capsular insertion sites were found to have no role in predicting clinical shoulder instability.[121] As MR arthrography can show labral tears and avulsions and the position of the labral ligamentous complex after injury, it is helpful for preoperative planning in distinguishing between regular Bankart lesions, Perthes lesions (which can potentially be deceptively difficult to diagnose in their chronic form), anterior labral periosteal sleeve avulsion (ALPSA) lesions (which can also be deceptively occult with resynovialization), and humeral avulsion of the glenohumeral ligament (HAGL) lesions.[144,164,166,167,172] These lesions can have similar clinical presentations and examination findings and can be difficult to diagnose any other way.

In the past, MRI and MR arthrography were found to be limited in providing diagnostic information important to the patient's surgical management.[26] Close correlation

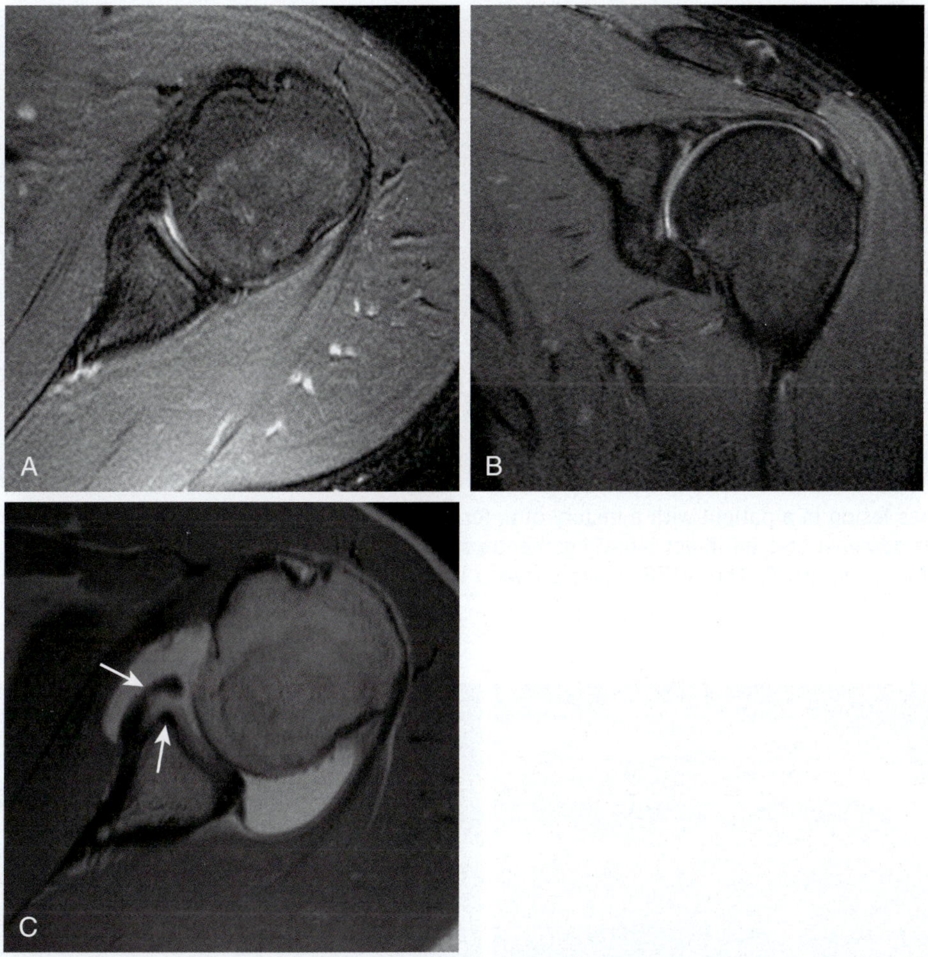

FIGURE 4-21: Arthrogram of Perthes lesion before and after the introduction of contrast. **A,** An axial proton density (PD) fat-saturated image of a patient with a history of multiple dislocations demonstrates slight edema at the base of the anterior labrum. This study was initially interpreted as negative. **B,** A coronal PD fat-saturated image in the same patient demonstrates mild chondral edema with subtle underlying bone marrow edema of the anterior inferior glenoid but no evidence of labral detachment. **C,** An axial T1-weighted image after the introduction of intra-articular contrast material shows stripping of the thickened irregular periosteum and displacement of the anterior labrum at the Perthes lesion site (*arrows*). (Courtesy Phillip Tirman, MD.)

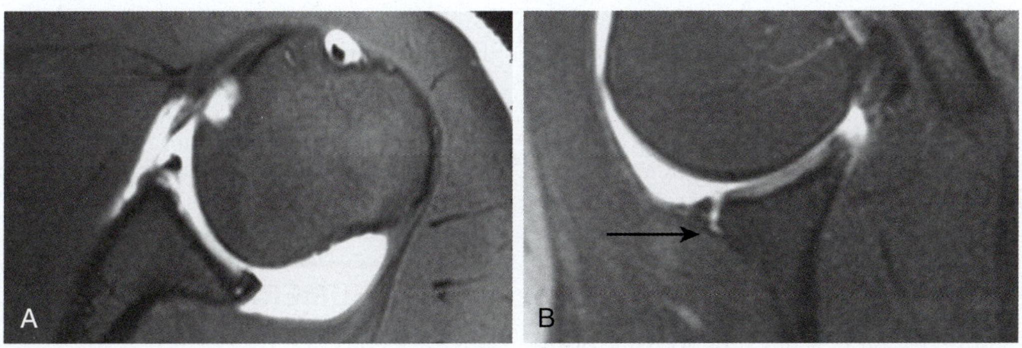

FIGURE 4-22: **A,** An axial, gadolinium-enhanced, magnetic resonance arthrogram that does not identify an anterior labral tear. **B,** Addition of the oblique axial image in the abduction and external rotation position identifies the anterior labral detachment *(arrow)*.

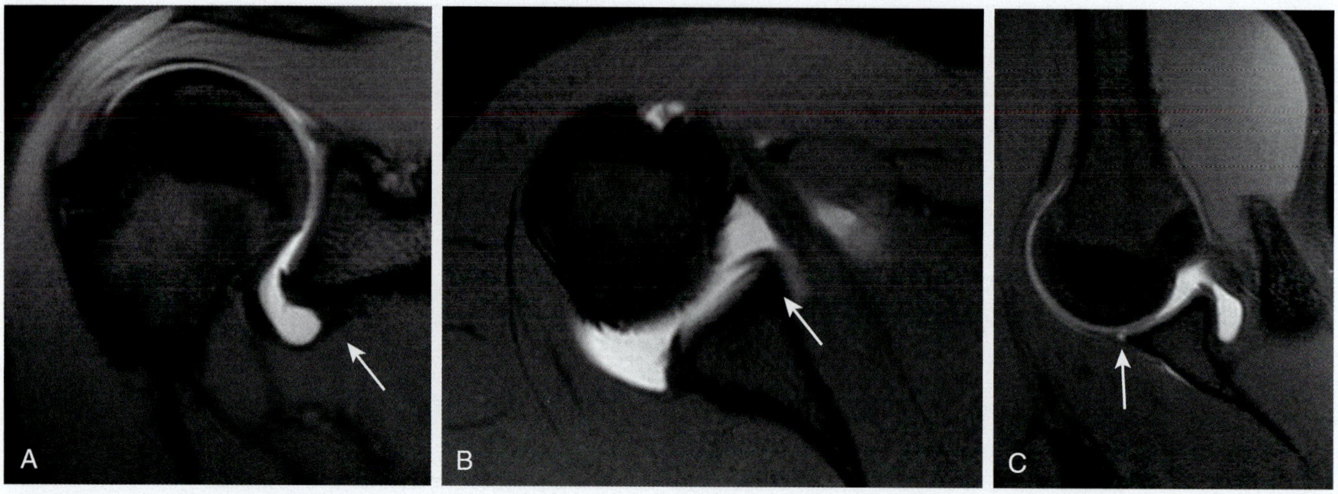

FIGURE 4-23: Perthes lesion in a patient with a history of anterior instability shown on abduction and external rotation (ABER). **A,** The coronal image demonstrates an intact labral ligamentous attachment to the glenoid (*arrow*). **B,** The axial image does not demonstrate detachment (*arrow*). **C,** The ABER image shows a labral tear (*arrow*). (Courtesy Phillip Tirman, MD.)

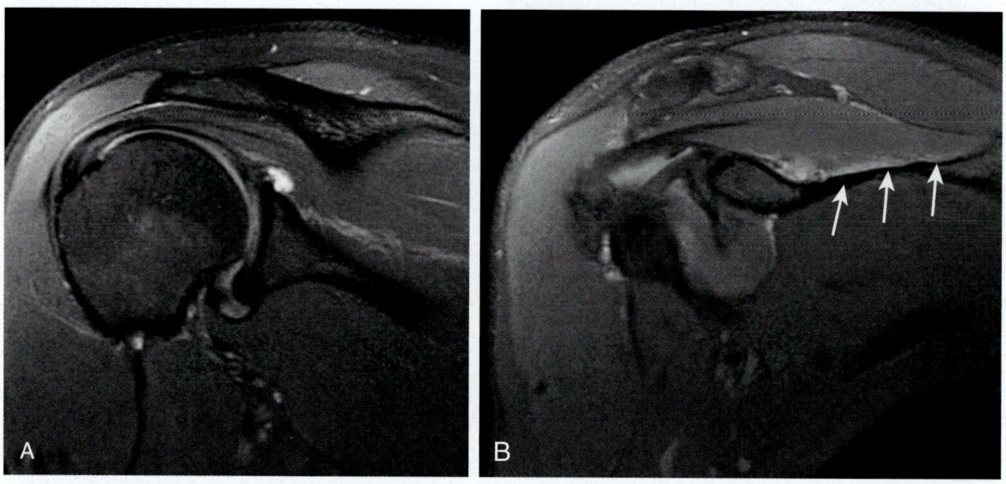

FIGURE 4-24: A superior labrum anterior to posterior lesion with a paralabral cyst. **A,** Coronal proton density fat-saturated image demonstrating a multiloculated cyst adjacent to a torn superior labrum. The cyst extends to the junction between the spinoglenoid notch and the suprascapular notch. **B,** Image anterior to a showing early denervation changes of the origin of the supraspinatus tendon (*arrows*). (Courtesy Phillip Tirman, MD.)

with clinical history, open communication between orthopedists and radiologists, and an increase in the number of musculoskeletal-trained radiologists have led to an improvement in the utility of MRI and MR arthrography in shoulder instability. However, an MR arthrogram study that is interpreted as negative does not rule out symptomatic clinical glenohumeral instability.

Imaging of the superior labrum may be difficult. However, on coronal fat-suppressed proton-density–weighted MRI, a hyperintense linear fluid signal within the superior labrum creating a 5-mm superior shift of the labrum indicates a superior labral tear. Additionally, the presence of a paralabral cyst indicates tearing of the adjacent labrum (Fig. 4-24).[164] Surgical confirmation has shown that MR arthrography reliably and accurately reveals superior labral tears. With a sensitivity of 84% to 92% and specificity of 82% to 91%, along with substantial interobserver agreement, MR arthrography is the gold standard for radiographically evaluating superior labral tears.[9,63]

GLENOHUMERAL ARTHRITIS

Recommended Views

Recommended views for glenohumeral arthritis are the true anteroposterior views in internal and external rotation and an axillary lateral view. A limited CT scan may be required to assess glenoid erosion.

Loss of articular cartilage leads to shoulder pain from glenohumeral arthritis. The radiographic views that demonstrate joint space narrowing or articular cartilage loss are the true anteroposterior, the axillary lateral (Fig. 4-25), and the apical oblique. Osteophyte formation and humeral head deformity are revealed by internal and external rotation anteroposterior radiographs of the shoulder. Posterior glenoid erosion and posterior humeral head subluxation can also be shown by the axillary lateral and apical oblique views. However, the axillary lateral view should not be relied on to determine *glenoid version*, the angle formed by a line between the anterior and posterior rims of the glenoid and a line perpendicular to the axis of the scapular body (Fig. 4-26), because Galinat[39] determined that up to 27 degrees of variation exists, depending on the angle of the x-ray beam and scapular rotation.

Glenohumeral arthritis may be accompanied by various patterns of glenoid erosion (e.g., central or posterior). CT of the glenohumeral joint has been shown to be accurate and reliable in assessing glenoid morphology and version (Fig. 4-27).[37,108] To determine the glenoid version, a limited CT scan of both shoulders should be performed, beginning just inferior to the coracoid process (Box 4-1). The normal glenoid version varies from 0 to 7 degrees of retroversion. The version increases when posterior glenoid erosion is present (Fig. 4-28).[37,65,128]

A preoperative shoulder CT scan to assess glenoid version has been shown to avoid shoulder arthroplasty component malposition and subsequent failure due to unrecognized posterior glenoid wear.[65] A CT scan is recommended before shoulder arthroplasty if the patient has less than 0 degrees of glenohumeral external rotation, has had a previous anterior reconstructive procedure, or has a possible radiographic posterior glenoid erosion or posterior humeral head subluxation. Preoperative three-dimensional CT scans have also been shown to accurately reflect the glenoid vault and surface.[82] This information may be useful in the preoperative evaluation of shoulder arthroplasty patients who have significant glenoid bone loss.

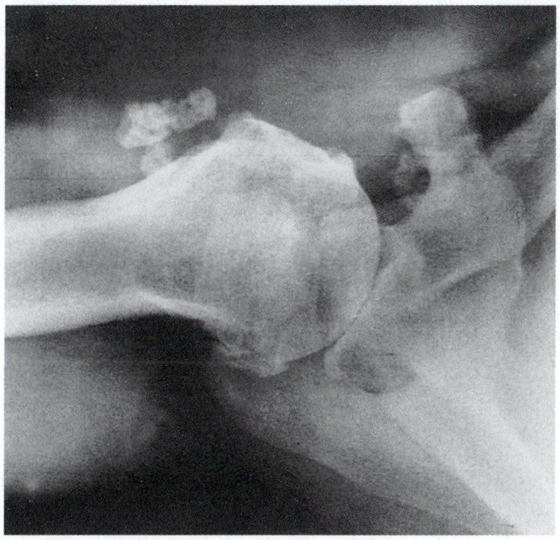

FIGURE 4-25: Axillary lateral radiograph revealing loss of the clear space between the humeral head and glenoid, indicating the loss of cartilage.

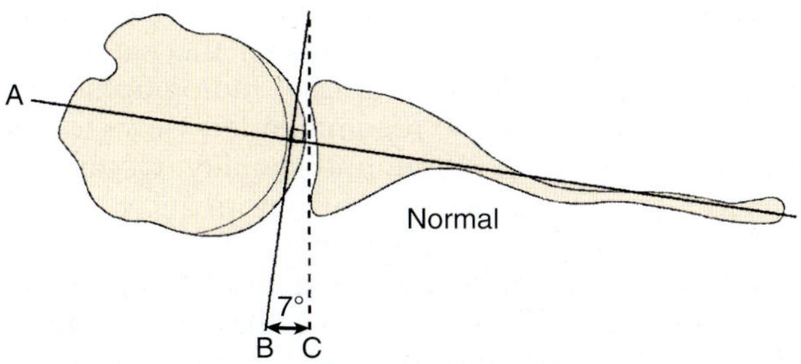

FIGURE 4-26: The normal glenoid version varies from 0 to 7 degrees of retroversion. On a computed tomography scan, measurement of version is accomplished by drawing a line along the axis of the scapular body and then drawing a line perpendicular to it (*B*). A third line is drawn along the anterior and posterior rims of the glenoid (*C*). The angle between *B* and *C* is the glenoid version.

GLENOHUMERAL ARTHROPLASTY

Recommended Views

Recommended views for glenohumeral arthroplasty are the true anteroposterior views in internal and external rotation, and an axillary lateral or apical oblique view.

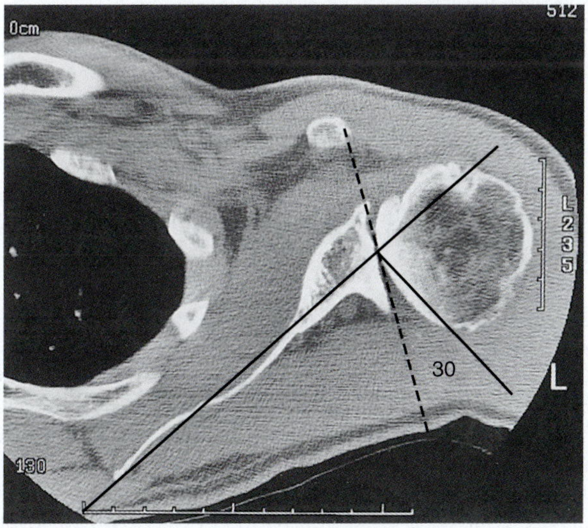

FIGURE 4-27: Computed tomography scan revealing posterior subluxation of the head of the humerus along with posterior glenoid erosion of 30 degrees.

BOX 4-1. Technique for Limited Computed Tomography Scans of the Shoulders

Purpose
To determine the glenoid version of both shoulders

Scout Scans
Bilateral shoulders in a straight line, symmetrically placed across the top of each acromion
Bilateral shoulders with scan lines

Range
No tilt

Filming
Bone windows only (9 on 1, only 1 sheet)
Bilateral shoulders

Intravenous Contrast
None

Display
Bone algorithm

Technique
Arms: Neutral at the sides
Shoulders: Flat, at the *exact* same level or height
kVp: 140 to 160
mAs: 300 or higher
FOV: 28 to 32 cm

Start Location
Inferior tip of the coracoid process

End Location
Six images below the tip

Mode
Axial or helical

Collimation
3 mm

Increments
No gap

FOV, field of view.
Courtesy Becky Laredo, MD, San Antonio, Texas.

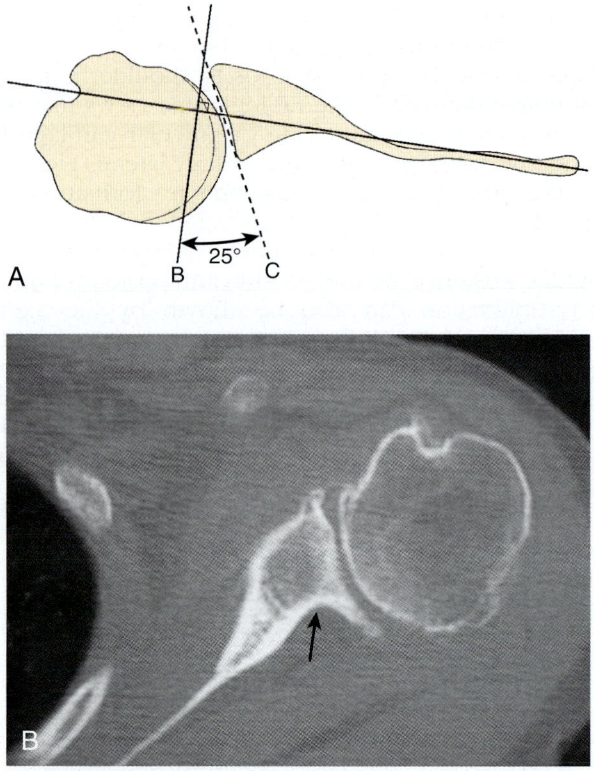

FIGURE 4-28: A, An increase in retroversion to 25 degrees is usually accompanied by posterior subluxation of the head of the humerus. **B,** A computed tomography scan reveals posterior glenoid wear and humeral head posterior subluxation.

Fluoroscopy is helpful for assessing glenoid component fixation. A limited CT scan may be required to assess glenoid erosion.

Evaluation

The routine radiographic evaluation of a glenohumeral arthroplasty should consist of the recommended views for evaluating component position and glenoid articulation. Humeral stem lucencies or migration and humeral head height with respect to the greater tuberosity can easily be followed with anteroposterior views in internal and external rotation.[98] The axillary lateral and apical oblique views can reveal glenoid wear or humeral component instability.

Radiographic evaluation of the glenoid component should routinely consist of a true anteroposterior view of the glenohumeral joint, an axillary lateral view, or an apical oblique view. The presence of lucent lines about a keeled or pegged component should be noted at the first postoperative visit, as well as the seating of the component on the native glenoid.[85] The fluoroscopic positioning of radiographs has been shown to be a more accurate method of identifying glenoid component radiolucent lines,[68] but it exposes the patient to a large amount of radiation and is time-consuming for the patient.

The painful shoulder arthroplasty radiographic evaluation should consist of the recommended views to assess component fixation, position, and stability. Occasionally, a limited CT scan provides useful information regarding glenoid wear or humeral component malposition. CT of a cemented pegged polyethylene glenoid component has been shown to be more sensitive than radiography in identifying the size and number of peg lucencies.[173] MRI[155] and ultrasonography[153,171] have been reported as useful for identifying rotator cuff tendon tears in painful shoulder arthroplasty. MRI with metal-artifact reduction fast spin-echo (FSE) and multiacquisition variable-resonance image combination (MAVRIC) sequencing can reveal synovitis, periprosthetic osteolysis, and supraspinatus tendon tears.[50]

CLAVICLE

Recommended views for the clavicle are an anteroposterior radiograph in the plane of the thorax, a 30-degree cephalic tilt radiograph, a 30-degree caudal tilt radiograph, and occasionally a tomogram or CT scan. These three radiographs are useful for delineating the characteristics of an acute fracture (Fig. 4-29) and are even more helpful in monitoring progress of the fracture toward union. Tomograms or CT scans are required to assess fracture healing and evaluate fractures of the medial portions of the clavicle.

ACROMIOCLAVICULAR JOINT AND DISTAL CLAVICLE

Recommended Views

Recommended views for the acromioclavicular joint and distal clavicle are an anteroposterior view in the plane of the thorax, a 10-degree cephalic tilt view of the acromioclavicular joint, and an axillary lateral view. A scapulothoracic lateral radiograph, stress views, tomograms, a bone scan, CT, or MRI may be required.

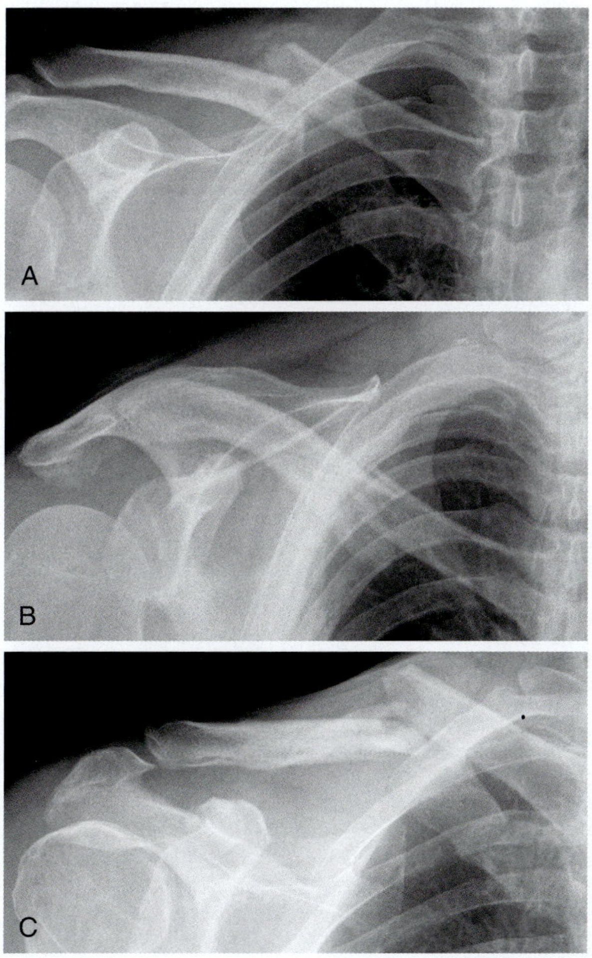

FIGURE 4-29: Clavicle trauma views for delineating fracture pattern and displacement. **A,** A routine anteroposterior view. **B,** Caudal tilt view. **C,** Cephalic tilt view.

Evaluation Techniques

Reduced Voltage

The technician should be specifically requested to take films of the acromioclavicular joint and not of the shoulder because the technique used for the glenohumeral joint produces a dark, overexposed radiograph of the acromioclavicular joint, which can mask traumatic or degenerative changes (Fig. 4-30A). The acromioclavicular joint can be clearly visualized by using 50% of the x-ray voltage that is used to expose an anteroposterior radiograph of the glenohumeral joint (see Fig. 4-30B).

Zanca View

Sometimes, fractures about the distal end of the clavicle or the acromion, osteolysis of the distal end of the clavicle, or arthritis of the acromioclavicular joint is obscured on routine anteroposterior radiographs of the joint because the inferior portion of the distal part of the clavicle is obscured by the overlapping shadow of the spine of the scapula. To obtain the clearest unobstructed view of the acromioclavicular joint and distal portion of the clavicle, Zanca recommended that the x-ray beam be aimed at the acromioclavicular joint with a 10-degree cephalic tilt (Fig. 4-31).[13]

Occasionally, none of the routine radiographs clearly delineate the extent of the pathology in this region, and tomograms, a CT scan, MRI, or a bone scan may be required.

Anteroposterior Views

If the patient has a drooping injured shoulder, it is important to compare radiographs of the injured acromioclavicular joint with those of the normal shoulder. The radiograph may be taken with the patient either standing or sitting and the arms hanging free. If the patient is small, both shoulders may be exposed on a single horizontal 14 × 17 inch x-ray cassette, but for most adults, it is better to use a separate 10 × 10 inch cassette for each shoulder. To interpret injuries to the acromioclavicular joint, the appearance of the acromioclavicular joint and the coracoclavicular distance in the injured shoulder are compared with those in the normal shoulder (Fig. 4-32).[114]

It is important to determine the degree of injury to the acromioclavicular and coracoclavicular ligaments. If both ligaments are disrupted, surgical correction may be indicated. A full description of the various degrees of injury to these ligaments, graded as types I to VI, is given in Chapter 9.

Anteroposterior Stress View

If the original radiographs of a patient with an injury to the acromioclavicular joint demonstrate a complete acromioclavicular dislocation (i.e., type III, IV, V, or VI injuries), stress radiographs are not required. If complete

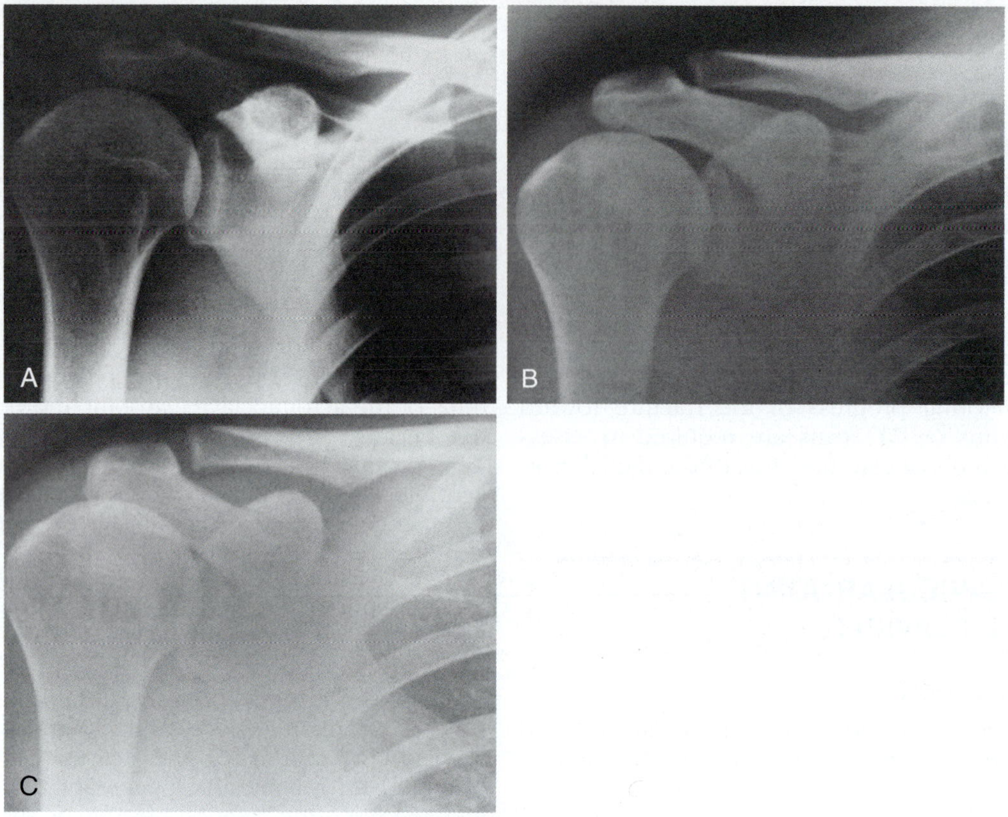

FIGURE 4-30: Routine radiographs of the shoulder often produce a poorly visualized acromioclavicular joint. **A,** A routine anteroposterior view of the shoulder demonstrates good visualization of the glenohumeral joint. However, the acromioclavicular joint is overpenetrated by the radiograph technique. **B,** When the exposure is decreased by 50%, the acromioclavicular joint is much better visualized. However, the inferior aspect of the acromioclavicular joint is superimposed on the spine of the scapula. **C,** With the Zanca view, tilting the tube 10 to 15 degrees superiorly provides a clear view of the acromioclavicular joint. (From Rockwood CA, Green DP, eds. *Fractures.* vol. 3. 2nd ed. Philadelphia: JB Lippincott; 1984.)

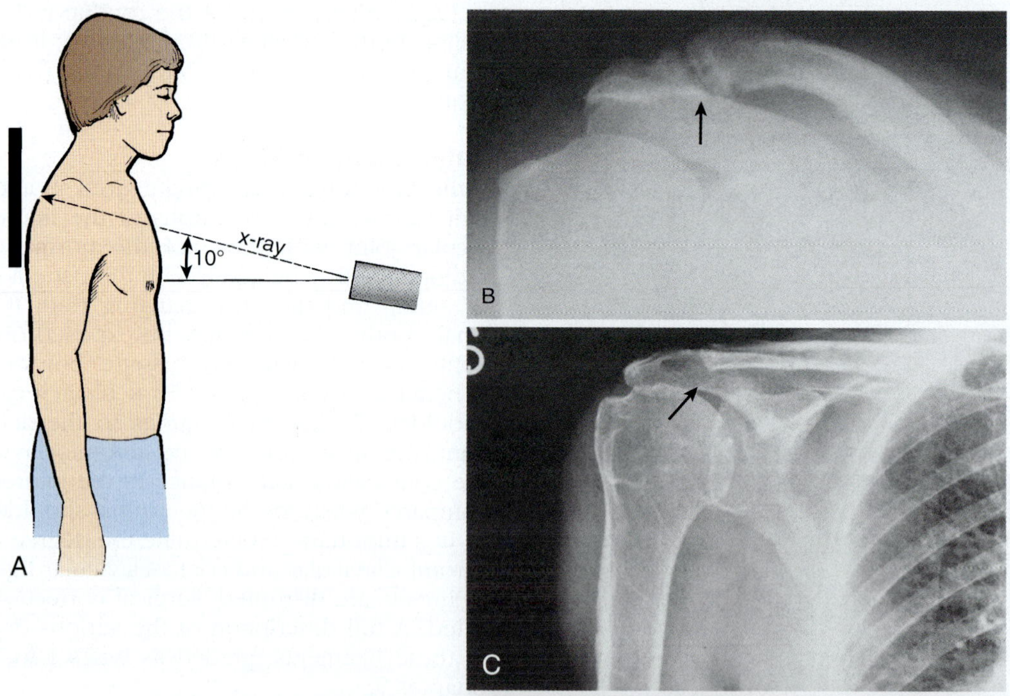

FIGURE 4-31: **A,** Positioning of the patient to obtain a Zanca view of the acromioclavicular joint. **B,** A Zanca view of the joint reveals significant degenerative changes (*arrow*). **C,** An anteroposterior radiograph of good quality fails to reveal any abnormality of the joint. **D,** With the Zanca view, a loose body (*arrow*) is clearly shown within the joint.

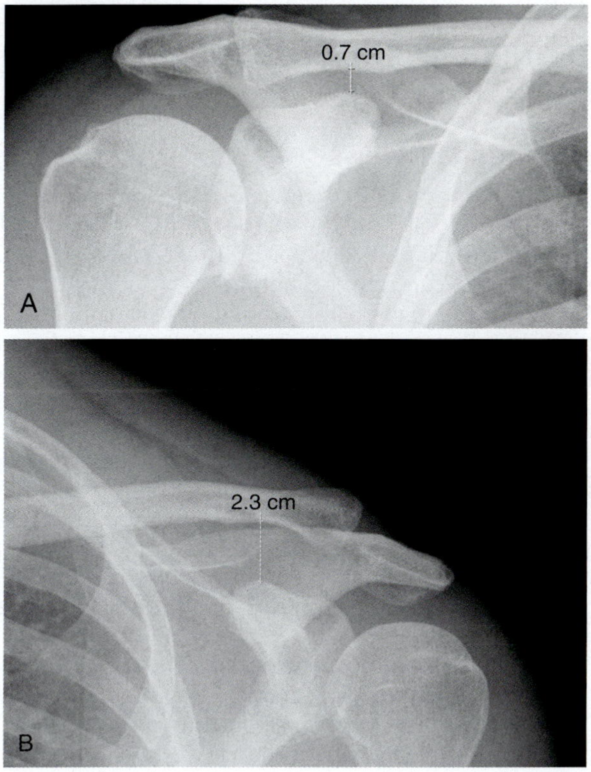

FIGURE 4-32: Comparison of the coracoclavicular distance in the injured and normal shoulders. **A,** In this normal shoulder, the distance between the top of the coracoid and the bottom of the clavicle is 7 mm. **B,** In the injured shoulder, the distance between the top of the coracoid and the bottom of the clavicle is 23 mm, which indicates disruption of not only the acromioclavicular but also the coracoclavicular ligament.

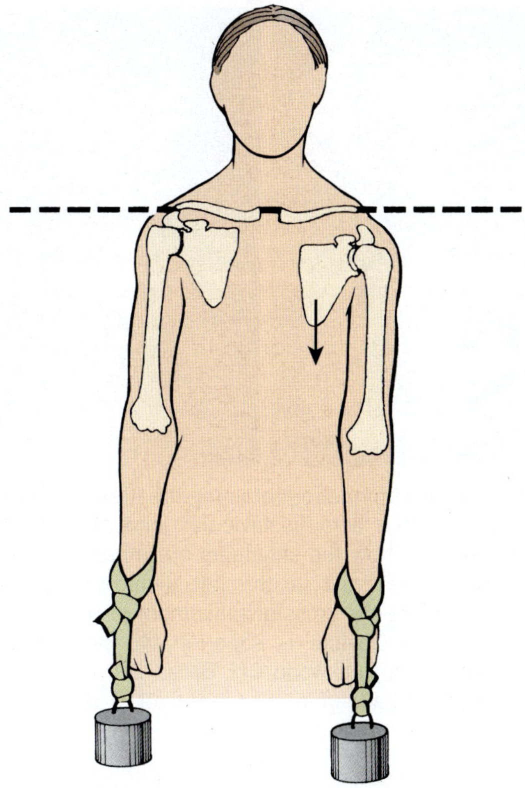

FIGURE 4-33: Technique for obtaining stress radiographs of both acromioclavicular joints with 10 to 15 lb of weight hanging from the patient's wrists. The distance between the superior aspect of the coracoid and the undersurface of the clavicle is measured to determine whether the coracoclavicular ligaments have been disrupted. One large, horizontally placed, 14 × 17 inch cassette can be used in smaller patients to visualize both shoulders. In larger patients, however, it is better to use two horizontally placed smaller cassettes and to take two separate radiographs for the measurements. In disruption of the coracoclavicular ligaments, note that the shoulder is displaced downward rather than the clavicle being displaced upward.

dislocation of the joint is clinically suspected, stress views of both shoulders should be taken. With the patient erect, 10 to 20 lb of weight, depending on the size of the patient, is strapped to each of the patient's wrists while radiographs of both shoulders are taken (Fig. 4-33).[138] Patients should not grip the weights in their hands because the muscle contractions can produce a false-negative radiograph. If stress radiographs demonstrate that the coracoclavicular distance is the same in both shoulders or has a difference of less than 25%, a type III or greater injury can be ruled out.

Axillary Lateral View

With the arm abducted 70 to 90 degrees, the cassette should be placed superior to the shoulder and the x-ray tube placed inferior to the axilla. Obtaining the axillary lateral view is consistent with the basic principle of obtaining at least two views at 90 degrees to one another for evaluation of musculoskeletal trauma. This view can reveal small intra-articular fractures not visualized on the anteroposterior radiograph, and such findings indicate a worse prognosis.[110,111] This view also demonstrates anterior or posterior displacement of the clavicle (as seen in type IV injuries) and the degree of displacement of fractures of the distal end of the clavicle.

Alexander View

Alexander[3,170] described a modification of the true scapulolateral view that he found useful in evaluating injuries to the acromioclavicular joint. This view is a supplemental projection to demonstrate the posterior displacement of the clavicle that occurs with acromioclavicular injuries. The position of the cassette and the x-ray beam is essentially the same as for the true scapulolateral view. While standing or sitting, the patient shrugs the shoulders forward while the true scapulolateral radiograph is taken (Fig. 4-34). If no injury to the acromioclavicular ligament has occurred, no displacement or overlap of the distal

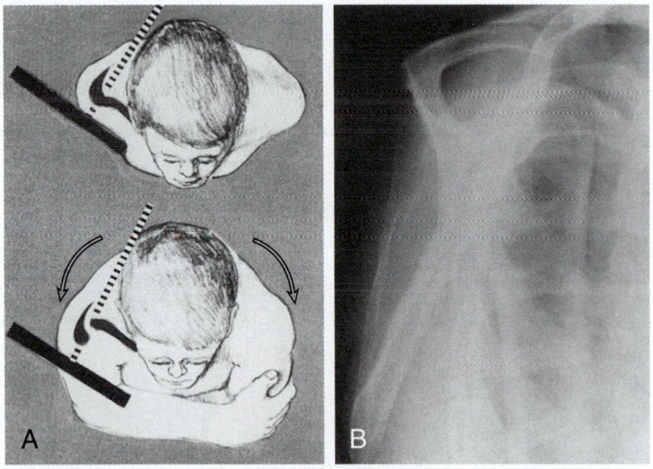

FIGURE 4-34: Technique for obtaining the Alexander or scapulolateral view of the acromioclavicular joint. **A,** A schematic drawing illustrates how the shoulders are thrust forward while the radiograph is taken. **B,** In this left shoulder that has been thrust forward, note the gross displacement of the acromioclavicular joint. The clavicle is superior and posterior to the acromion. (**A,** From Rockwood CA, Green DP, eds. *Fractures.* vol. 3. 2nd ed. Philadelphia: JB Lippincott; 1984.)

end of the clavicle and the acromion will be noted. However, with acromioclavicular ligament disruption, the distal part of the clavicle is superiorly displaced and overlaps the acromion.

Tomogram or Computed Tomography Scan

Occasionally, none of the routine radiographs clearly delineate the extent of the pathology of the distal end of the clavicle or the acromioclavicular joint, and tomograms or a CT scan may be required.

Bone Scan

A bone scan detects early evidence of degenerative arthritis, infection, and traumatic osteolysis of the distal part of the clavicle before changes are noted on a routine radiograph.[136,156,160]

Magnetic Resonance Imaging

MRI of the shoulder can reveal abnormalities of the distal end of the clavicle. An increased T2 signal in the distal part of the clavicle is the most common and conspicuous MRI finding in both posttraumatic and stress-induced osteolysis of the distal clavicle.[27,33,34] However, increased signal is a very common finding, and there appears to be no correlation between the MRI appearance and clinical findings in the acromioclavicular joint.[66] MRI in an asymptomatic population revealed that three-fourths exhibited changes consistent with acromioclavicular joint osteoarthritis that were independent of rotator cuff disease.[109] Therefore an abnormal MRI finding in the acromioclavicular joint is not a reliable indicator that the acromioclavicular joint is a source of pain or is related to associated rotator cuff tendon changes.

STERNOCLAVICULAR JOINT AND MEDIAL CLAVICLE

Recommended Views

A CT scan of both medial clavicles is recommended. An anteroposterior view in the plane of the thorax with a 40-degree cephalic tilt view of both clavicles or a tomogram or bone scan may be helpful.

Although one may be able to diagnose sternoclavicular joint dislocations clinically, appropriate use of radiographs is a critical part of the workup of this condition. Without radiographs, even the most experienced clinicians occasionally misdiagnose injuries to this joint. One cannot rely only on clinical findings to make the proper diagnosis because severe anterior swelling about the sternoclavicular joint, which clinically appears to be a benign anterior sternoclavicular dislocation, can be either a fracture of the medial part of the clavicle or a very serious and dangerous posterior dislocation of the sternoclavicular joint.

Occasionally, routine anteroposterior or posteroanterior chest radiographs demonstrate asymmetry between the sternoclavicular joints, suggesting a dislocation or fracture of the medial part of the clavicle. The ideal view for studying this joint is one taken at 90 degrees to the anteroposterior plane. However, anatomic considerations make it impossible to take a true 90-degree cephalic-to-caudal view. A lateral radiograph of the chest is difficult to interpret because of the density of the chest and the overlap of the medial ends of the clavicles with the first rib and the sternum. As a result, numerous special projections have been devised by Hobbs,[54] Kattan,[67] Kurzbauer,[80] Ritvo and Ritvo,[137] and Rockwood and Green[138] (Fig. 4-35). Although most of these views are very helpful, CT offers the best information for evaluating fractures of the medial part of the clavicle and injuries to the sternoclavicular joint. The *serendipity view* (a 40-degree cephalic tilt view described in 1972) is easy to obtain and reliably demonstrates anterior and posterior subluxations and dislocations of the sternoclavicular joint and some fractures of the medial part of the clavicle.[138] This tomographic view is helpful in making the diagnosis if CT scanning is not available.

Evaluation Techniques

Serendipity View (40-Degree Cephalic Tilt View)

When CT scans and tomograms are not available, the serendipity view[138] can be very helpful in determining the type of injury to the region of the sternoclavicular joint. It can certainly distinguish between a benign anterior dislocation and a dangerous posterior dislocation. The patient is positioned supine on the radiograph table with a nongrid 11 × 14 inch cassette placed under the upper chest, shoulder, and neck region. The x-ray beam is angled 40 degrees off the vertical and centered directly at the sternum (Fig. 4-36). The distance from the tube to the cassette should be 60 inches in adults and 40 inches

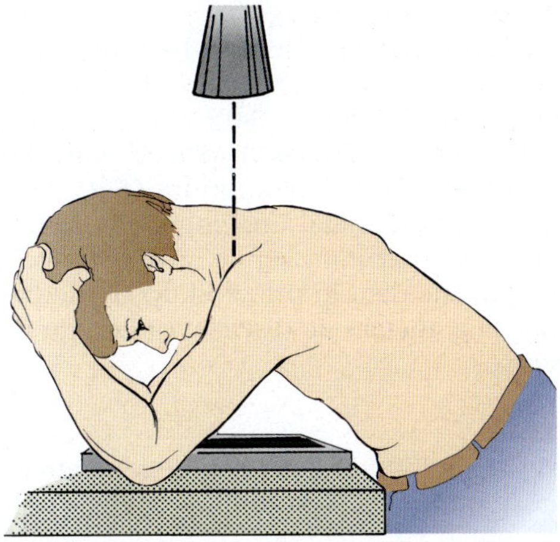

FIGURE 4-35: Positioning of the patient for radiographic evaluation of the sternoclavicular joint, as recommended by Hobbs. (Modified from Hobbs DW. Sternoclavicular joint, a new axial radiographic view. *Radiology.* 1968;90:801. Reproduced with permission from Rockwood CA, Green DP, eds. *Fractures.* vol. 3. 2nd ed. Philadelphia: JB Lippincott; 1984.)

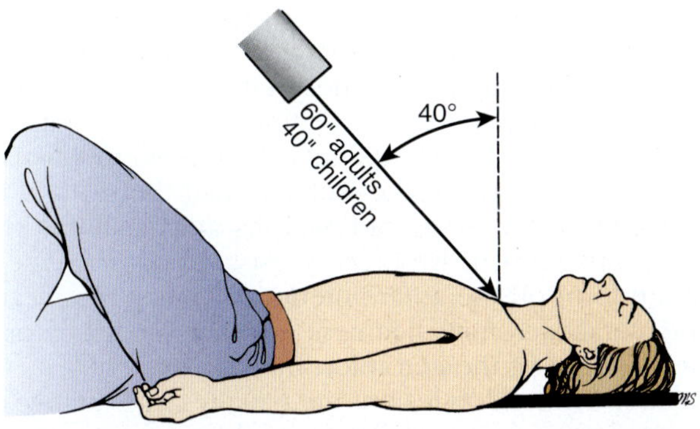

FIGURE 4-36: Positioning of the patient to take the serendipity cephalic tilt radiograph of the sternoclavicular joint. The x-ray tube is tilted 40 degrees from the vertical and aimed directly at the manubrium. The cassette should be large enough to receive the projected images of the medial halves of both clavicles. In children the tube distance should be approximately 40 inches; in an adult with a thicker chest, the distance should be 60 inches.

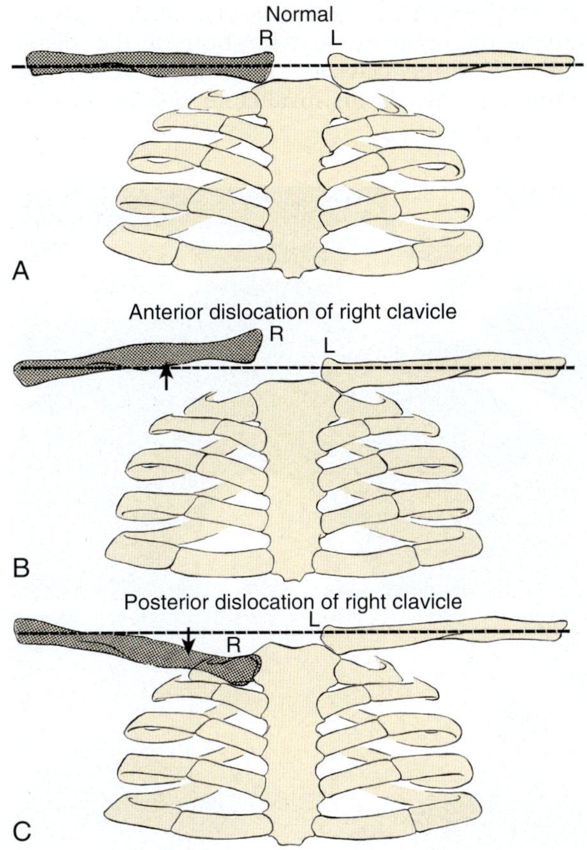

FIGURE 4-37: Interpretation of the cephalic tilt serendipity view of the sternoclavicular joint. **A,** In a normal person, both clavicles appear on the same imaginary line drawn through them. **B,** In a patient with anterior dislocation of the right sternoclavicular joint, the medial end of the right clavicle is projected above an imaginary line drawn through the level of the normal left clavicle. **C,** In a patient with posterior dislocation of the right sternoclavicular joint, the medial end of the right clavicle is displaced below an imaginary line drawn through the normal left clavicle. *L,* left; *R,* right. (Modified from Rockwood CA, Green DP, eds. *Fractures.* vol. 3. 2nd ed. Philadelphia: JB Lippincott; 1984.)

in children. The voltage should be the same as for an anteroposterior chest radiograph. The x-ray beam is adjusted so that it will project *both* clavicles onto the film.

To interpret this radiograph, the relationship of the medial end of the injured clavicle with that of the normal clavicle is compared. In a normal shoulder both clavicles are on the same horizontal plane (Fig. 4-37A). With anterior dislocation, the injured clavicle appears more superior on the radiograph than the normal clavicle (see Fig. 4-37B). In a posterior sternoclavicular joint, the medial end of the dislocated clavicle appears more inferior than that of the normal clavicle (see Fig. 4-37C). Fractures of the medial part of the clavicle can also be noted on this view.

Tomogram

Tomograms can be very helpful in delineating medial clavicular fractures,[1] in distinguishing fractures from dislocations, and in detecting arthritic problems of the sternoclavicular joint.

Computed Tomography

CT scans offer the best information for demonstrating sternoclavicular subluxations, dislocations, fractures extending into the sternoclavicular joint, fractures of the medial part of the clavicle, and arthritis of this joint (Fig. 4-38A)[29,88,92,138] as well as irreducible posterior dislocations. CT scans, especially if enhanced with vascular studies, accurately document the intimate juxtaposition of the displaced medial end of the clavicle to the great vessels of the mediastinum. This is an invaluable preoperative study (see Fig. 4-38B).

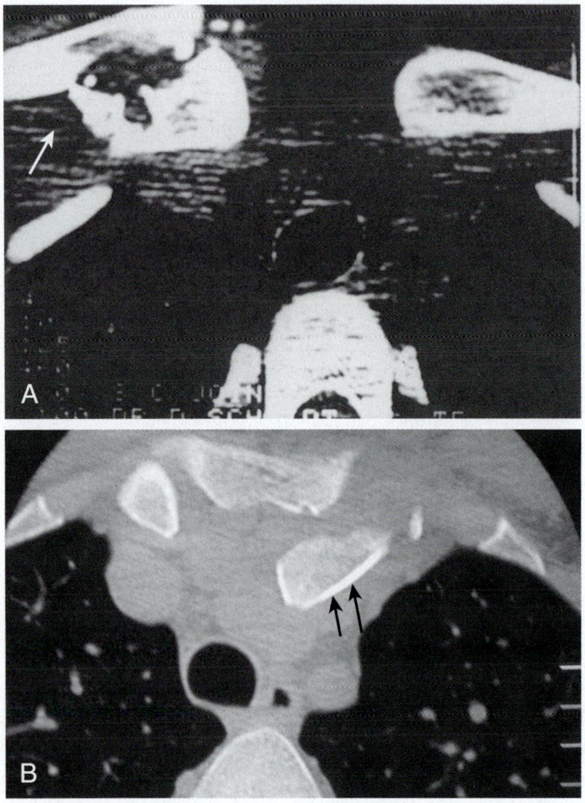

FIGURE 4-38: **A,** A computed tomography (CT) scan clearly demonstrates a fracture of the medial aspect of the clavicle (*arrow*). **B,** A CT scan demonstrates a posterior fracture-dislocation of the left sternoclavicular joint (*arrows*).

Magnetic Resonance Imaging

In children and young adults when the diagnosis is thought to be either dislocation of the sternoclavicular joint or meniscal disk injury, MRI can be used to determine whether the physis has displaced with the clavicle or is still adjacent to the manubrium (Fig. 4-39). MRI is recommended as the initial imaging study in the diagnosis of sternoclavicular joint septic arthritis[12] and provides relevant diagnostic data in the workup of medial clavicular osteomyelitis, metabolic disease, or benign and malignant processes.

Bone Scan

Bone scans are helpful in detecting degenerative changes, inflammatory problems, and tumors of the sternoclavicular joint.[160]

ROTATOR CUFF

Recommended Views

Recommended views for the rotator cuff are the anteroposterior and axillary lateral views, a 30-degree caudal tilt, or the scapular outlet view. Arthrography, CT arthrography, bursography, ultrasonography, or MRI can be used to evaluate the integrity of the rotator cuff.

Impingement syndrome is a common cause of pain and disability in the adult shoulder. It begins with soft tissue compromise involving the subacromial bursa and the rotator cuff; at this stage radiographs are usually normal. As the impingement problem persists and progresses, a spur can form off the anteroinferior acromion, ossification in the coracoacromial ligament may be noted,[113] or an unusual shape of the acromion may be present.[10]

Rotator cuff tendon lesions are usually degenerative and associated with overuse of the shoulder or a progressive

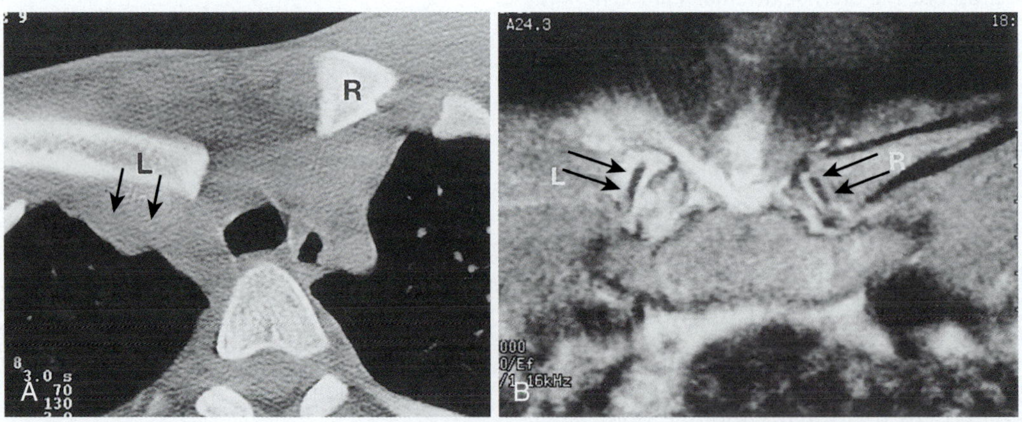

FIGURE 4-39: CT scan of a 15-year-old boy with a posterior dislocation of the left sternoclavicular joint. Usually, in male patients younger than 22 to 24 years apparent dislocation of the sternoclavicular joint is truly a physeal injury to the medial end of the clavicle. **A,** The computed tomographic scan reveals compression of the lung and trachea (*arrows*) by the posteriorly displaced medial left clavicle. **B,** However, magnetic resonance clearly shows that the physis of the left medial clavicle has remained adjacent to the manubrium, just as with the physis of the right medial clavicle (*arrows*). *L,* left; *R,* right. (Courtesy Jesse De Lee, MD, San Antonio, Texas.)

impingement syndrome; only rarely are they traumatic. Radiographic evaluation should include assessment of the coracoacromial arch[178] and, in younger patients, assessment of the anteroinferior glenoid for signs of instability.

Techniques to Evaluate Rotator Cuff Tendinitis

Anteroposterior View

Anteroposterior radiographs of the glenohumeral joint with the arm in internal and external rotation can reveal associated calcific tendinitis in the tendons of the cuff and superior migration of the humeral head under the acromion. Cystic and sclerotic changes may be noted in the greater tuberosity.[38] Degenerative changes may also be seen in the acromioclavicular joint. In addition, sclerotic changes secondary to anterior proliferation of the acromion may be present in the anterior acromion. Narrowing of the acromiohumeral interval has often been noted.

Axillary Lateral View

Routine radiologic evaluation of impingement syndrome should include an axillary lateral view to investigate the presence of underlying glenohumeral arthritis.

Thirty-Degree Caudal Tilt View

Routine anteroposterior radiographs usually do not demonstrate spurs from the acromion, calcification in the coracoacromial ligament, or anteroinferior proliferation of the acromion. However, with the patient in the erect position, an anteroposterior radiograph of the shoulder taken with a 30-degree caudal tilt adequately demonstrates the anterior acromial spur or ossification in the coracoacromial ligament (Fig. 4-40). Anteroinferior subacromial spurs can be noted on the radiographs of patients with either impingement syndrome or rotator cuff problems. Rockwood has used this technique to define spurs since 1979 because this view is easier to accomplish and more reliable for demonstrating spurring of the anterior acromion than is the scapular outlet view (Fig. 4-41). Kitay and colleagues[76] and Ono, Yamamuro, and Rockwood[119] have shown that this technique is highly reliable and that the acromial image correlates significantly with operative acromial spur length.

Scapular Outlet View

For the scapular outlet view, the patient is positioned as for a true scapulolateral radiograph, and the tube is angled caudally 10 degrees. This radiograph offers a view of the outlet of the supraspinatus muscle–tendon unit as it passes under the coracoacromial arch. Deformities of the anteroinferior acromion or the acromioclavicular arch

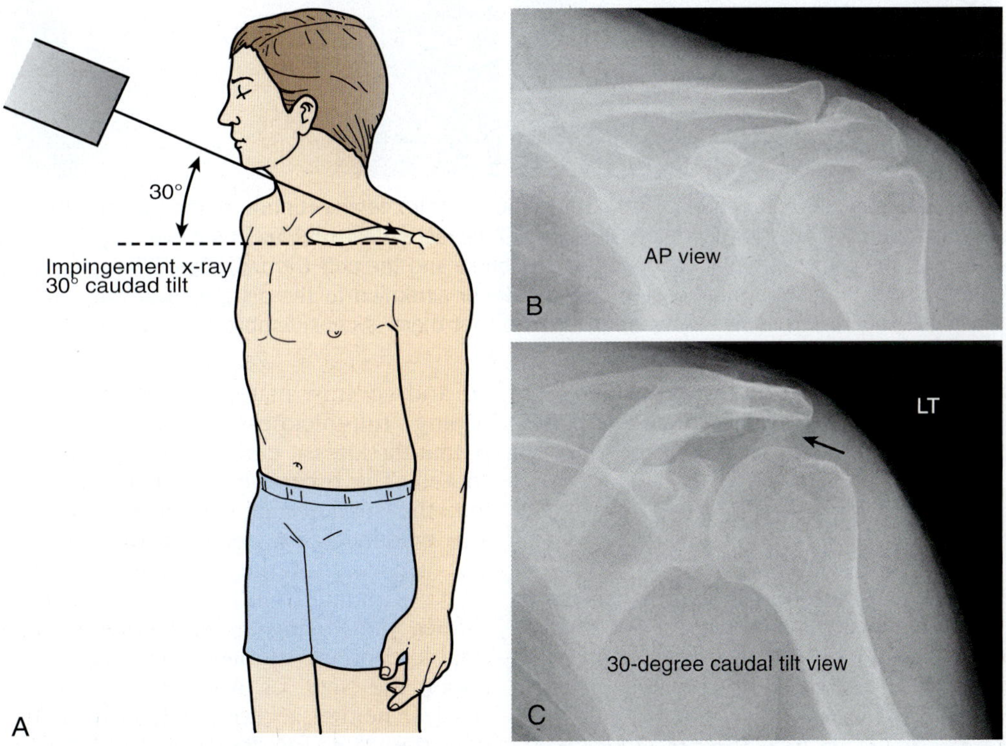

FIGURE 4-40: **A,** Positioning of the patient and the x-ray tube to demonstrate spurring or proliferation of the anteroinferior acromion, which is associated with impingement syndrome and lesions of the rotator cuff. The patient should be erect for this evaluation. **B,** Anteroposterior (AP) radiograph of a 52-year-old patient with impingement syndrome. The acromion does not appear to be abnormal. **C,** However, when the anteroposterior radiograph is taken with a 30-degree caudal tilt of the x-ray tube, the large, prominent, irregular spurring of the anterior acromion (*arrow*) is easily noted. *LT,* left shoulder.

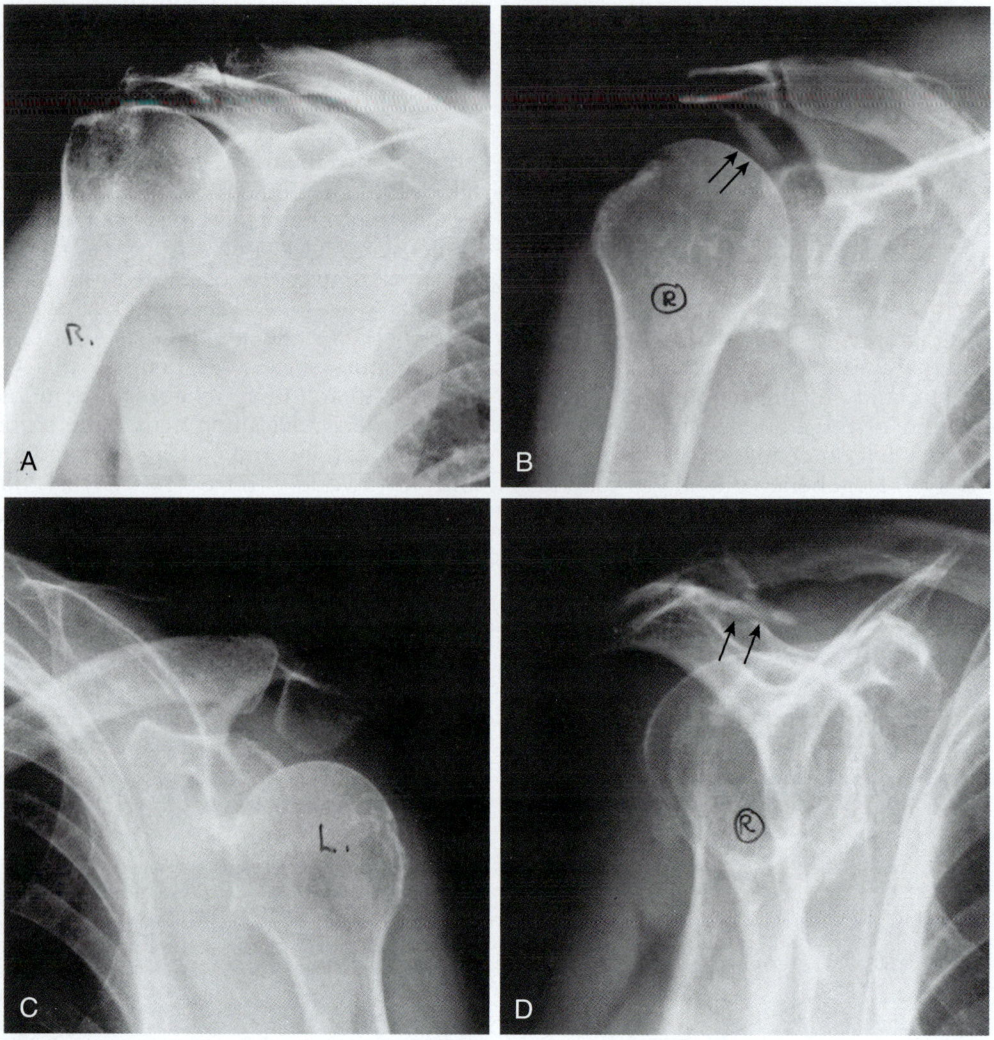

FIGURE 4-41: **A,** Anteroposterior view of a patient with impingement syndrome and rupture of the rotator cuff of the right shoulder. Minimal changes are noted on the anterior acromion. **B,** On a 30-degree caudal tilt view, note the large, irregularly shaped spike of bone that extends down the coracoacromial ligament into the bursa and the cuff (*arrows*). **C,** A 30-degree caudal tilt radiograph of the normal shoulder shows the normal relationship of the anterior acromion to the distal end of the clavicle. **D,** The scapular outlet view of the involved shoulder does reveal the spur (*arrows*), but there is considerable overlap with other structures.

down into the outlet can be noted on this view (see Fig. 4-41D). Bigliani and colleagues[10] identified three distinct acromial shapes on this radiologic view:

Type I: A flat acromion
Type II: A curved acromion
Type III: An anterior downward hook on the acromion

Although this classification of acromial shapes has been shown to have low interobserver reliability,[61,178] the acromial slope measured on the outlet view correlates with acromial thickness.[76]

Techniques to Evaluate Rotator Cuff Integrity

Arthrography, Arthrotomography, and Computed Tomography Arthrography

The shoulder arthrogram, either single contrast with radiopaque material alone or double contrast with both air and contrast material, is extremely accurate in diagnosing full-thickness tears. However, deep surface partial-thickness cuff tears are not always demonstrated. The escape of dye from the glenohumeral joint into the subacromial-subdeltoid bursa provides conclusive evidence of a defect in the rotator cuff (Fig. 4-42). The accuracy of the arthrogram is between 95% and 100%. Goldman and Ghelman favor double-contrast studies (i.e., using air and contrast media).[41] Although double-contrast studies can offer more information about the size of a given tear than single-contrast studies, neither technique is considered more sensitive than the other for detecting tears. Hall and colleagues[48] demonstrated less patient discomfort after arthrography with the water-soluble contrast medium metrizamide. Combining arthrography with tomography or CT scans can help in defining the size of the defect in the rotator cuff.[73,134,174]

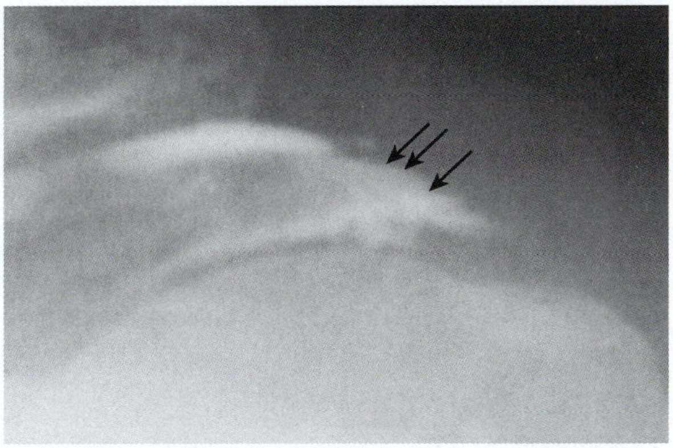

FIGURE 4-42: Positive arthrogram of the left shoulder. The dye is seen not only in the glenohumeral joint but also up into the subacromial-subdeltoid bursa. The size of the tear can also be well visualized (*arrows*).

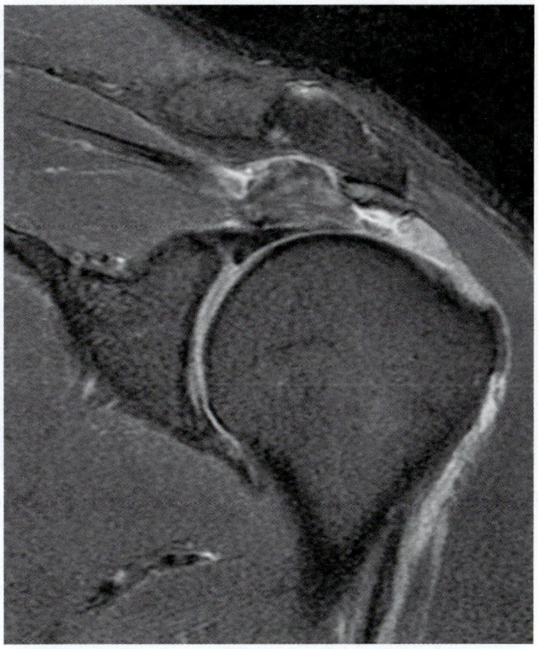

FIGURE 4-43: Supraspinatus tendon tear with retraction to mid humeral head on magnetic resonance imaging. (Courtesy Phillip Tirman, MD.)

Subacromial Bursography

Subacromial bursography has been reported by Lie and Mast,[89] Mikasa,[105] and Strizak and colleagues.[159] In 1982 Strizak and colleagues studied the technique in cadavers and in patients. They reported that normal bursae would accept 5 to 10 mL of contrast medium and that patients with impingement syndrome and thickened walls of the subacromial deltoid bursae would accept only 1 to 2 mL of medium.

Ultrasonography

Reliable demonstration of full-thickness rotator cuff tears with an ultrasound scanner has been reported in 92% to 95% of cases.[22,55,90,93,103,104] It has been shown to be safe, rapid, noninvasive, and inexpensive and has the advantage of imaging and comparing both shoulders. Whereas ultrasonography was previously restricted by equipment limitations and availability, it is now commonly used in the community setting. Sonographic examination is a hands-on experience and allows for a dynamic, reproducible examination that is able to produce recorded images that document normal anatomy and pathologic findings. Ziegler reported surgically confirmed positive and negative predictive values of 96.6% and 93.2%, respectively, for partial-thickness tears and of 92.9% and 96.8%, respectively, for full-thickness tears.[177]

Mack and colleagues have described a real-time ultrasound technique that depends on the absence of motion in the cuff tissue.[93,94] Secondary signs of cuff tear, such as thinning of the cuff or abnormal echoes, are initially more difficult to interpret but become easier to interpret with surgical correlation. These latter findings might not represent a complete cuff tear but may be due to a partial tear, tendinosis, or tendinitis. Kilcoyne and Matsen have proposed that for sonography to offer a useful alternative to arthrography or arthroscopy as a screening procedure, certain criteria should be adhered to: the diagnosis of a complete rotator cuff tear depends on the absence of motion in the cuff tissue when studied sonographically, and if the patient continues to have symptoms suggesting a cuff tear, an arthrogram should be performed to determine whether a small cuff tear is present.[73] Using these criteria Mack and colleagues found that sonography had a sensitivity of 91%, a specificity of 100%, and an overall accuracy of 94%.[94] These results have been duplicated at several other centers.[14,129,161,176] Currently, ultrasonography has become an effective screening tool in the evaluation of subacromial pain.[142]

Magnetic Resonance Imaging

MRI is a commonly used noninvasive technique for investigating lesions of the rotator cuff.[70,72,78,130,132,148,149] It provides information regarding the tendinous attachments of the rotator cuff as well as the condition of the specific rotator cuff muscle belly. MRI has been used to categorize acromial morphology, but interobserver agreement has been shown to be poor[51] because of multiple images revealing a variation in the acromial shape when progressing from lateral to medial.

Various studies have shown MRI to be very sensitive for detecting lesions of the rotator cuff (Fig. 4-43).[59,77,78,147,149] Rotator cuff tendinopathy appears as a thickened, inhomogeneous tendon with increased signal intensity on fat-saturated (FS), proton density-weighted (PD), fast spin echo (FSE) or PD FSE. Partial-thickness tendon tearing can involve the articular side, the bursal side, or the intrasubstance (interstitial) portion of the tendon (Fig. 4-44). Partial-thickness tears can be differentiated from tendinosis by the fluid signal seen on T2-weighted FSE and FS PD FSE images, whereas tendinosis tends to be hyperintense on FS PD FSE only. Unusual tears of the

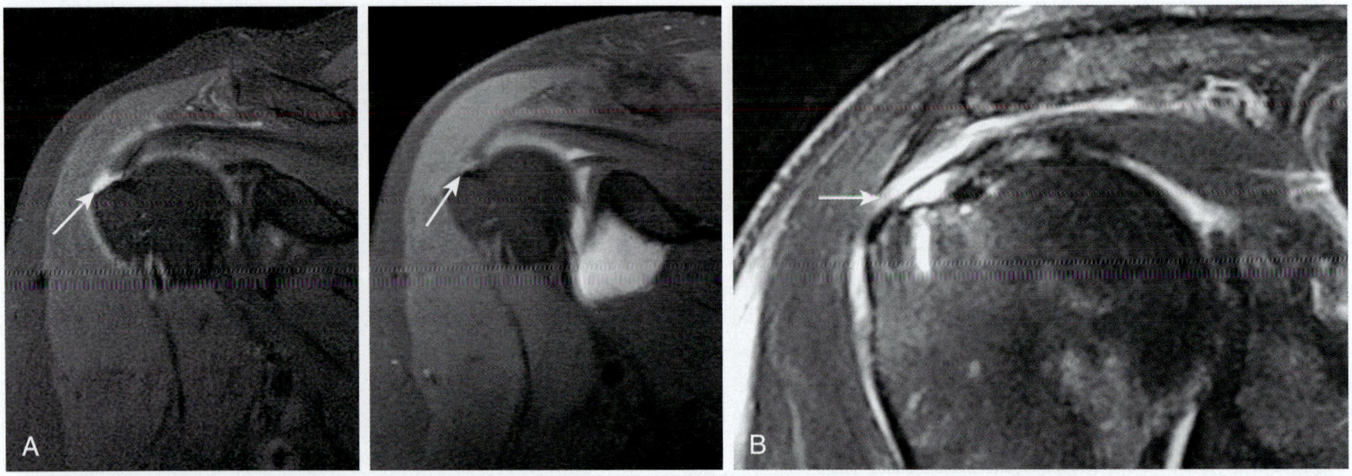

FIGURE 4-44: Articular surface partial tear. **A,** Proton density fat-saturated coronal image demonstrating a deep bursal surface insertional partial tear with a fluid-filled defect identified (*arrow*). **B,** After the introduction of intra-articular contrast, the defect is not enhanced and therefore does not communicate with the joint. (**A,** Courtesy Phillip Tirman, MD.)

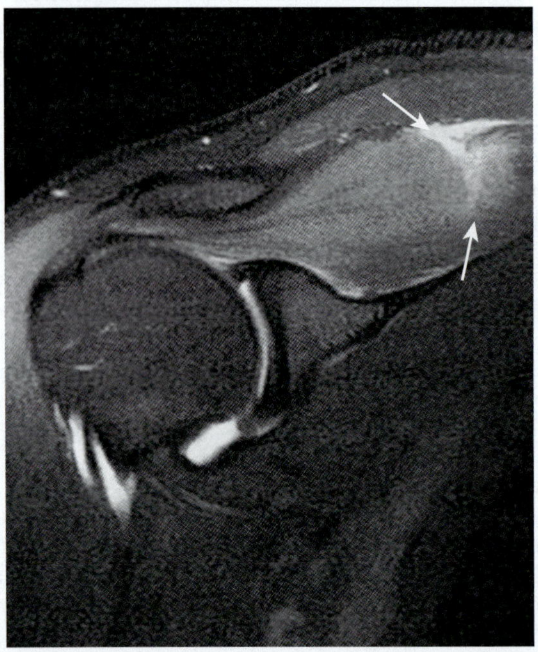

FIGURE 4-45: Supraspinatus muscle tear in a 20-year-old patient after a military press weightlifting injury. Magnetic resonance imaging was ordered to rule out a supraspinatus tendon tear. The coronal proton density fat-saturated image demonstrates a tear of the muscle belly medial to the shoulder joint, with interposed hemorrhage. (Courtesy Phillip Tirman, MD.)

muscle bellies are best shown on FS PD or T2-weighted images (Fig. 4-45).

Surgical correlation studies[56,120] have shown MRI to be accurate in detecting large, full-thickness tears and less accurate in detecting small (<1 cm) tears or in differentiating tendinitis/tendinosis from partial-thickness tears or small full-thickness tears.[64] Rotator cuff tendon tears appear as fluid-filled defects on T2-weighted images, reflecting a discontinuity in the normal tendon signal that is often not evident on the PD scan.[115] Increased signal intensity in the supraspinatus on coronal oblique T1-weighted images has been shown to have no histologic correlation and may be due to the "magic angle" MRI-specific technical artifact.[154] MRI with abduction and external rotation has been shown to be accurate in the assessment of articular surface partial tears of the rotator cuff.[164]

MRI can also be useful in revealing the condition of the muscle belly of a detached rotator cuff tendon.[163] Rotator cuff muscle atrophy is revealed by a reduced cross-sectional area on sagittal images and by the presence of increased signal streaks (fatty infiltrates) within the muscle belly. These are best seen on the coronal oblique images (Fig. 4-46), but can be seen in any plane utilizing T1 or PD images where fatty infiltration appears bright compared to muscle fibers (Fig. 4-47).

Some younger patients with a suspected lesion of the rotator cuff, as suggested by weakness and atrophy, might indeed have a cyst compressing the suprascapular nerve.[165] An MRI can easily detect the cyst, often showing the intra-articular source. Additionally, MRI can show an intratendinous cyst, which has a high correlation with articular-sided tears of the tendons.[143]

The use of MRI to evaluate the integrity of a rotator cuff tendon that has undergone previous surgery can be problematic.[69,145] An artifact from small amounts of ferrous material left in the soft tissues following arthroscopic subacromial burring or shaving causes signal alterations that can obscure the rotator tendon insertion and produce wild-appearing images that suggest infection or other processes. Complete retracted re-tearing is accurately revealed by MRI; however, assessing the size and delineation between partial-thickness or small full-thickness tears is difficult, and clinical assessment is recommended.[107] MRI arthrography is more accurate in

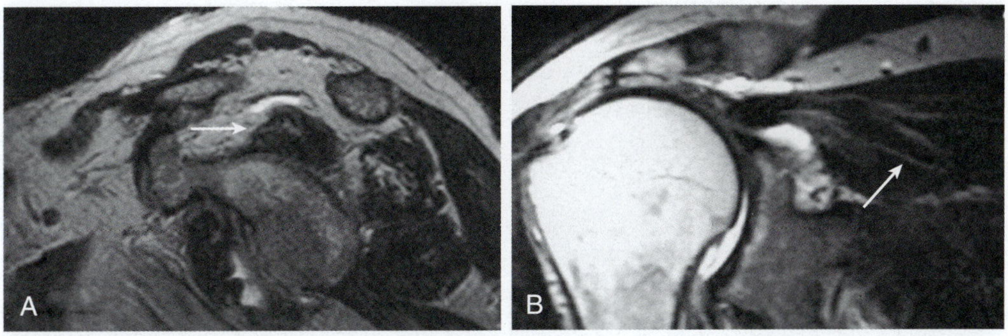

FIGURE 4-46: **A,** Sagittal magnetic resonance image (MRI) revealing supraspinatus muscle atrophy, shown by the diminished cross-sectional area *(arrow)*. **B,** Supraspinatus muscle atrophy demonstrated by coronal oblique MRI, with fat striping (*arrow*) indicating the replacement of muscle by fat deposition. Superior humeral head migration can also be noted.

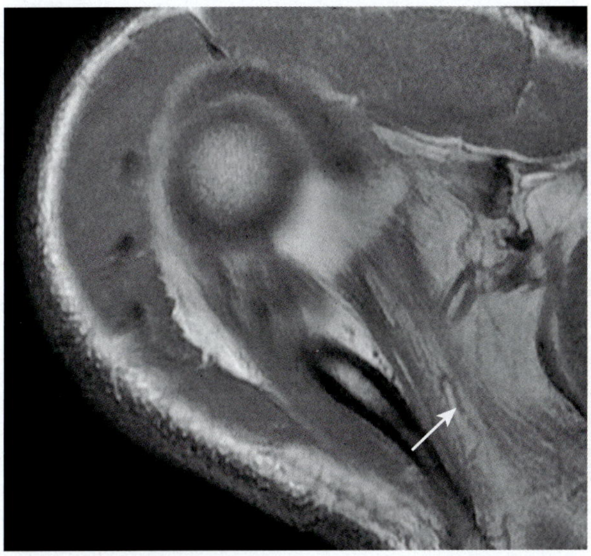

FIGURE 4-47: Muscle belly atrophy. An axial T1-weighted image in the superior aspect of the joint demonstrates fatty atrophy of the supraspinatus muscle belly (*arrow*). (Courtesy Phillip Tirman, MD.)

depicting and characterizing recurrent tears of the rotator cuff as well as other postoperative complications, such as displaced suture anchors (Fig. 4-48). The previous suture repair of a tendon can appear as an increased intermediate signal on T2-weighted images (Fig. 4-49).

SCAPULA

Recommended Views

Recommended views of the scapula include true anteroposterior views and an axillary lateral view. Special views, such as the Stryker notch and West Point views, tomograms, and CT may be required.

The trauma series of radiographs is usually adequate for demonstrating fractures of the scapular body, spine, and neck. Fractures located elsewhere might require other views for optimal visualization. Glenoid rim fractures, although often visualized on the axillary lateral view of the trauma series, may be better visualized on a West Point or apical oblique view of the glenohumeral joint.[40,95] Coracoid fractures may be visible on the axillary lateral view but are much better defined on the Stryker notch view (Fig. 4-50).[49] Acromial fractures can be seen on the axillary lateral view but may be difficult to distinguish from an os acromiale.

A CT scan can be of great value for determining the degree of displacement of fractures of the scapula and for defining the amount of displacement of glenoid fractures (Fig. 4-51).

CALCIFIC TENDINITIS

Calcium deposits in the rotator cuff can be specifically localized in the tendons of the rotator cuff using anteroposterior views of the shoulder in internal and external rotation and an axillary lateral view (Fig. 4-52). MRI is useful in the preoperative evaluation of chronic calcific tendinopathy because it delineates the size of the calcific lesion and can define the amount of rotator cuff tendon involvement (Fig. 4-53).

BICEPS TENDON

Biceps tendinitis is rarely the primary cause of shoulder pain. It is usually secondarily involved as a part of an impingement syndrome or degenerative lesions of the rotator cuff. The anatomy of the bicipital groove can be evaluated by the Fisk view.[35,102] In this view, the x-ray tube is superior to the shoulder. The image of the bicipital groove is projected down onto the cassette, which is held by the patient (Fig. 4-54). Cone and colleagues[20] have extensively studied the radiographic anatomy and pathologic irregularities of the bicipital groove.

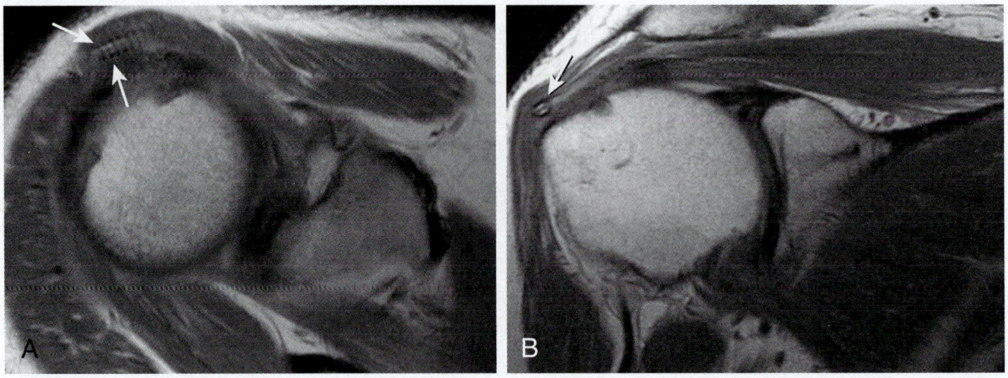

FIGURE 4-48: A displaced fractured suture anchor. **A,** Axial proton density (PD) image showing a fractured displaced suture anchor (*arrows*) in the bursa adjacent to the supraspinatus tendon. **B,** Coronal PD image showing a suture anchor fragment (*arrow*). (Courtesy Phillip Tirman, MD.)

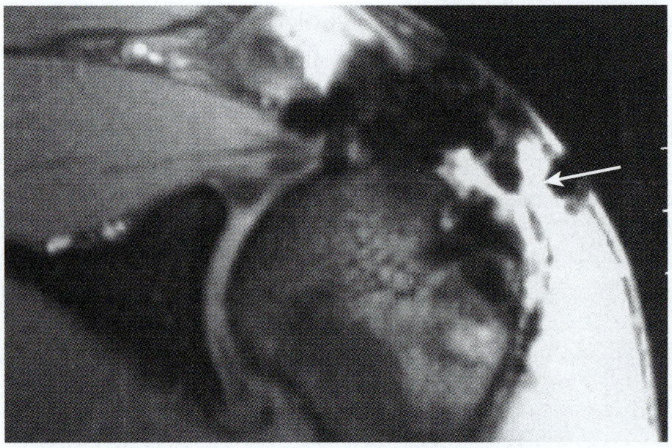

FIGURE 4-49: A T1-weighted coronal oblique magnetic resonance image reveals a low signal artifact from ferrous material; however, retearing of the tendon is apparent (*arrow*).

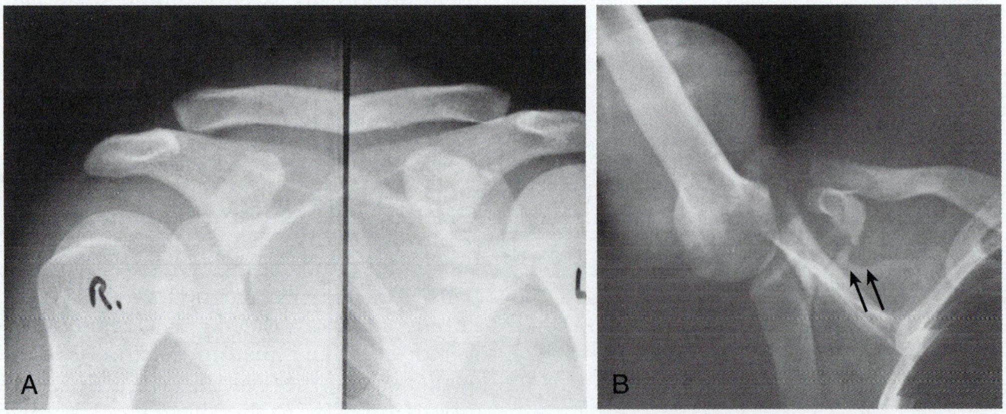

FIGURE 4-50: **A,** A 23-year-old patient with a traumatic injury to his right acromioclavicular joint. Note the superior displacement of the right clavicle from the acromion when compared with the left; also note that the coracoclavicular distance in both shoulders is approximately the same. The fracture at the base of the coracoid is not well visualized. **B,** The Stryker notch view reveals a fracture through the base of the coracoid (*arrows*).

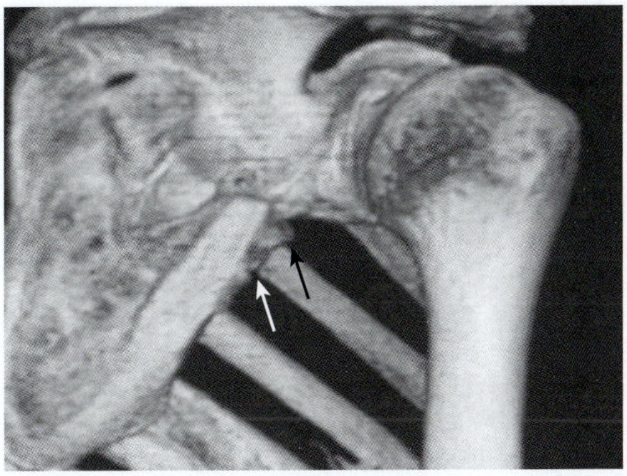

FIGURE 4-51: A three-dimensional computed tomography scan reveals scapular body fractures and lateral border displacement (*arrows*).

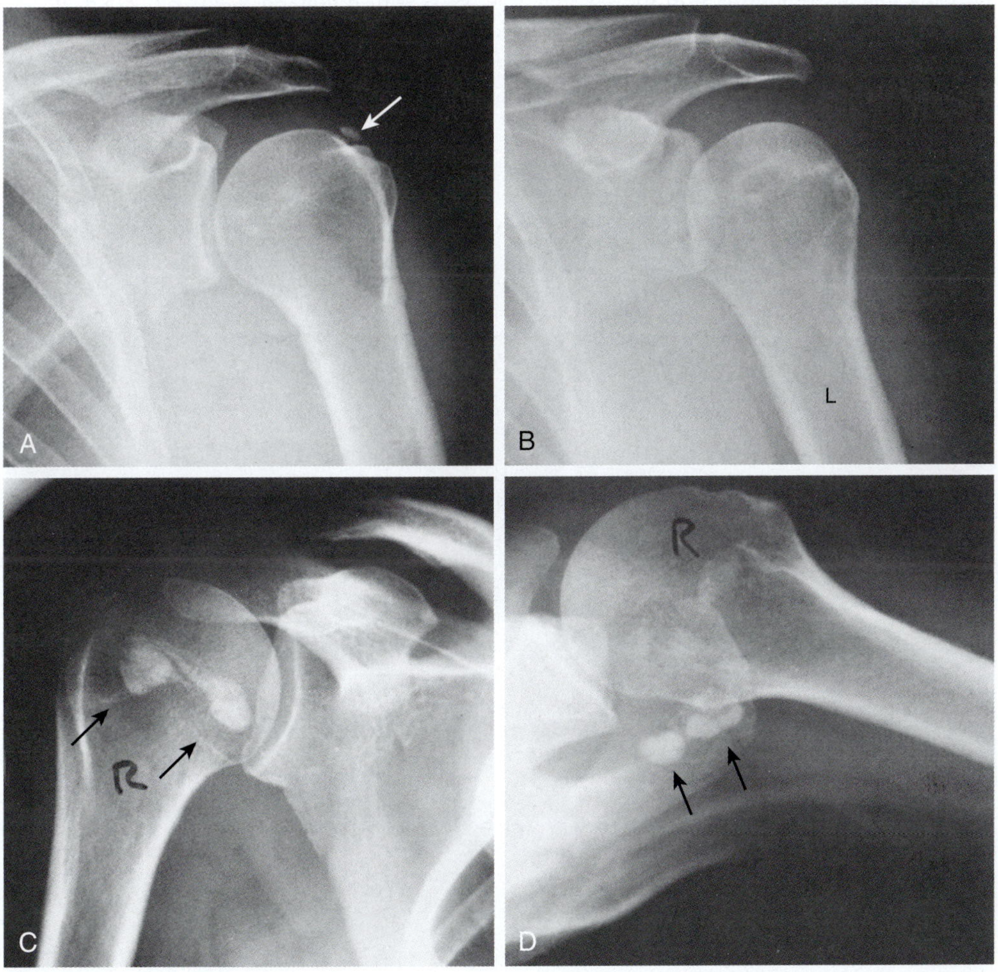

FIGURE 4-52: Calcific tendinitis of the left shoulder. **A,** A calcium deposit is visible with the arm in external rotation (*arrow*). **B,** The calcium deposit is no longer visible with the arm in internal rotation, indicating that the calcium must be in the anterior aspect of the supraspinatus tendon. **C,** A calcium deposit cannot accurately be localized on an anteroposterior radiograph in internal and external rotation, **D,** However, on the axillary view, the calcium deposit is quite distinct and localized in either the infraspinatus tendon or the teres minor tendon.

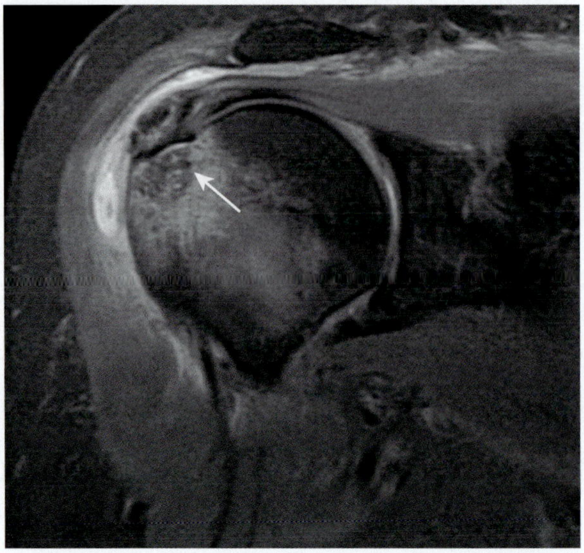

FIGURE 4-53: Calcific tendinitis with intraosseous extension. A coronal proton density fat-saturated image demonstrates calcific tendinitis within the distal supraspinatus tendon, with marked adjacent reactive bursitis. Note that there is intraosseous extension of calcium from the calcific tendinitis into the greater tuberosity, with a marked reactive change. Intraosseous extension tends to elicit a marked reaction. (Courtesy Phillip Tirman, MD.)

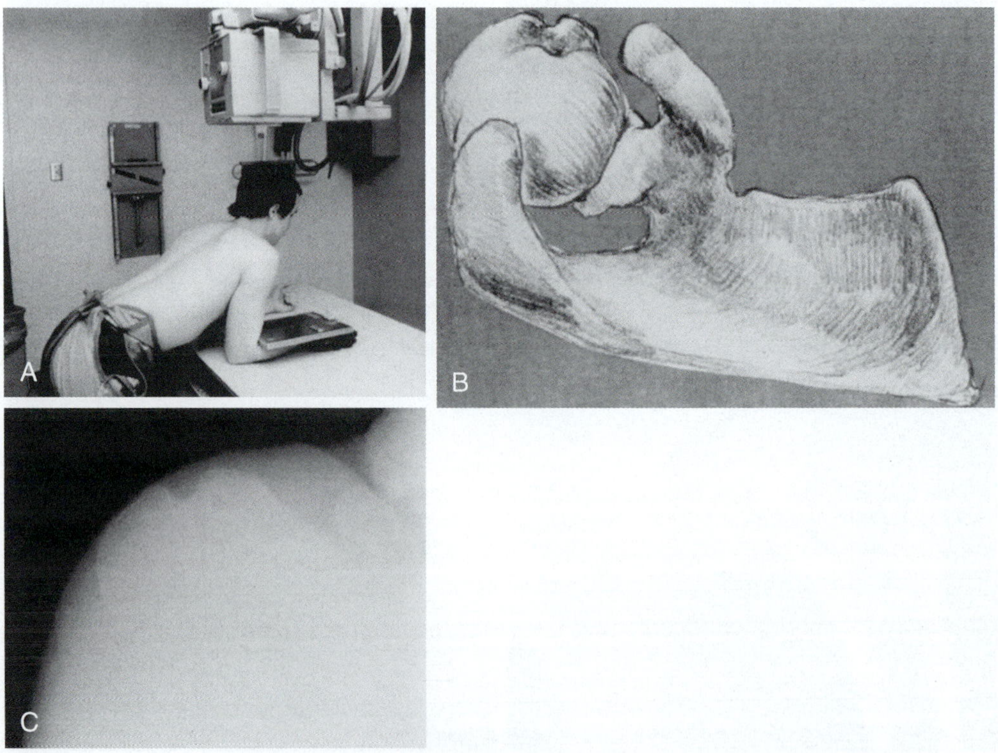

FIGURE 4-54: A, Position of the patient for the Fisk view to visualize the bicipital groove in the proximal end of the humerus. The patient leans forward and holds the cassette so the beam passing down through the bicipital groove will be projected onto the cassette. **B,** Anatomy of the bicipital groove. **C,** Projection of the bicipital groove onto the radiograph film with the Fisk technique. (Modified from Fisk C. Adaptation of the technique for radiography of the bicipital groove. *Radiol Technol.* 1965;37:47-50.)

Bicipital instability is usually associated with rotator interval injury or subscapularis tendon injury, or both. MRI accurately reveals the varying degrees of instability, from a flat long head of the biceps tendon perched on the lesser tuberosity (Fig. 4-55) to dislocation within the glenohumeral joint with complete detachment of the subscapularis tendon (Fig. 4-56).

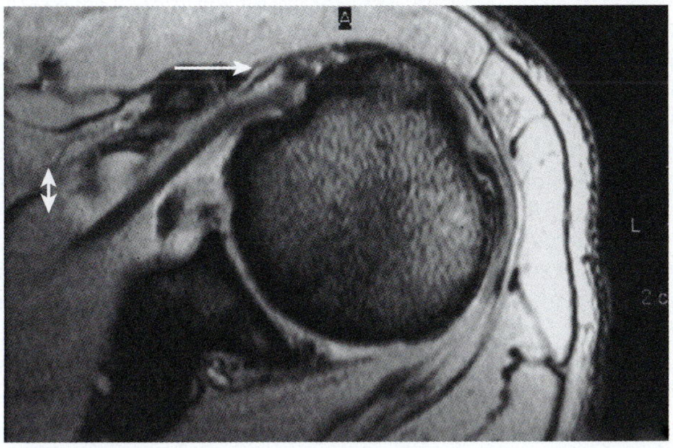

FIGURE 4-55: An axial magnetic resonance image reveals medial subluxation of the long head of the biceps into the substance of the superior part of the subscapularis tendon (*arrow*).

Acknowledgments

We sincerely thank Becky Laredo, MD, musculoskeletal radiologist at the University of Texas Health Science Center in San Antonio, for her contributions involving special radiologic evaluations of the shoulder.

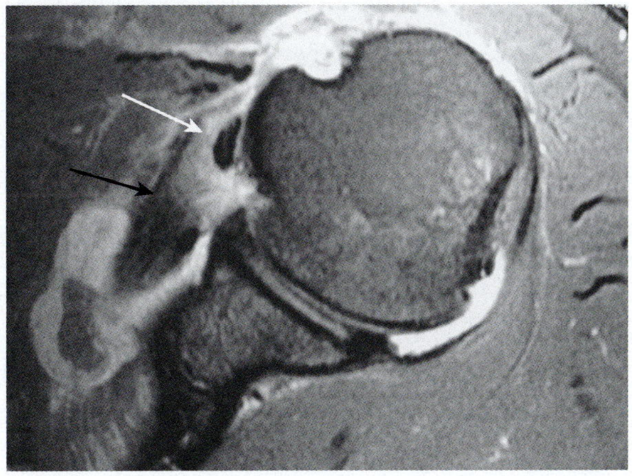

FIGURE 4-56: A magnetic resonance image demonstrates dislocation of the long head of the biceps tendon into the joint (*white arrow*). The dislocation can occur only with rupture of the subscapularis tendon and the capsule. The *black arrow* indicates the stump of the remaining subscapularis tendon.

EDITOR COMMENTARY

Edward V. Fehringer

Dr. Jensen and colleagues have nicely consolidated the work of thousands into a chapter that is easily readable. With the advent and advancement of MRI, it is refreshing to review plain radiographic evaluation and its evolution in the workup of shoulder pathology. While it can be argued that MRI now dominates the radiographic workup of shoulders, all should begin with plain radiographs. If well executed, they often provide what we need to diagnose and treat many shoulder disorders.

While plain radiographs are the workhorse of shoulder workups, the continued development of ultrasound, CT, and MRI allows us to identify more specific diagnoses. As a function of this we use less nonspecific diagnostic terms (i.e., impingement syndrome). Furthermore, we begin to attribute fewer symptoms to plain radiographic spurs, as to do so ignores a constellation of soft tissue and other factors not visualized on plain radiographs.

SENIOR EDITOR COMMENTARY

Frederick A. Matsen III

As shoulder surgeons we use imaging to help establish the diagnosis, plan surgery, and evaluate the change in patients' shoulder anatomy with time. A robust approach to imaging the shoulder needs to recognize that (1) the shoulder is a three-dimensional structure that cannot be represented by a single planar view, (2) critical relationships—such as the degree of centering of the humeral head—change with the position of the arm, (3) shoulder pathology may be found in a large number of different bones and soft tissues, and (4) overlying and superimposed structures as well as metallic implants may complicate imaging the structures of interest. It is possible to spend a lot of time, money, and radiation dosage on imaging; thus surgeons need to develop a judicious approach that yields the information necessary to treat the patient while avoiding the tendency to "over-image." A currently discussed question, for example, is whether three-dimensional reconstructions based on CT scans of the arthritic shoulder help surgeons achieve better outcomes for their patients in comparison to imaging consisting only of two standardized plain films, as discussed in Chapter 16 on the arthritic shoulder, or do complex MRI

Continued

SENIOR EDITOR COMMENTARY—cont'd

analyses of cuff muscle fat content lead to better results in the management of rotator cuff lesions. While more may seem better, we need to ask whether there is an incremental benefit to the patient from the increased cost and time and radiation exposure of more elaborate imaging methods.

The authors of this chapter have done a great job of presenting some of the approaches to imaging. I offer, however, just a few comments.

Regarding the trauma series, in an injured shoulder it may be best to obtain a true anteroposterior view in the plane of the scapula with the arm at the side before abducting the arm to obtain an axillary view. This approach will inform the surgeon of a fracture or a dislocation which could be aggravated by moving the arm. Once the general assessment of the injury is made on the true anteroposterior view, additional imaging can be obtained to further define the pathology.

While the technique of taking an axillary view with a rolled-up cassette may have been useful in the past, currently most imaging is digital and the cassettes cannot be rolled up.

Imaging of the dislocated shoulder is different from that of the unstable shoulder. In the former the displacement is relatively fixed, whereas in the latter the displacement of the humeral head in relation to the glenoid is dynamic. Anterior translation may be more apparent on an axillary view when the arm is extended posteriorly, posterior translation may be more apparent when the arm is adducted across the chest, superior translation may be more apparent when the deltoid is contracted isometrically, and inferior instability may be more apparent when the arm is relaxed at the side. While CT arthrography, MRI, and MR arthrography with the arm at the side may reveal changes in the appearance of the labrum, they cannot reveal dynamic instability. As a result we see patients undergoing repairs for misidentified SLAP, ALPSA, and HAGL or Bankart lesions even though their symptoms were not those of instability.

In imaging the arthritic shoulder, a standardized anteroposterior view in the plane of the scapula and a true axillary view are often all that is necessary for diagnosis and surgical planning. The true axillary view that shows the "eye" or spinoglenoid notch, taken with the arm elevated in the plane of the scapula, is known as the "truth" view because it reveals pathology that would not be expected when imaging (plain film or CT) is performed with the arm at the side. Two important examples are (1) the degree of joint space-narrowing seen when the bald central aspect of the humeral head is opposed to the eroded posterior glenoid and (2) the functional decentering seen when the humeral head drops posteriorly into a pathologic posterior concavity. CT scans may provide a more reproducible measure of glenoid version than standardized axillary views, but it is not clear that CT images lead to any better clinical outcomes in the usual cases of shoulder reconstruction. A final advantage of standardized plain films for arthritic shoulders is that the same radiographic views can be compared preoperatively and as a sequence postoperatively, whereas postoperative CT scans are costly and difficult to interpret because of the metal artifacts.

It is of interest that this chapter continues to use the term "impingement syndrome," which many surgeons consider to be outmoded now that more accurate methods of evaluating the status of the rotator cuff, such as MRI and shoulder sonography, are in common use. It is notable that the ICD-9-CM Diagnosis Code 726.10, which used to refer to "impingement syndrome," is now described as "Disorders of bursae and tendons in shoulder region, unspecified." Variations in the shape of the acromion are no longer commonly believed to be responsible for cuff pathology, and acromioplasty is no longer commonly used as the mainstay of treatment for the damaged rotator cuff.

In closing, we are grateful to these authors for their masterful review of shoulder imaging. My comments are not intended to be critical, but rather to be stimulating the thought regarding how we might apply cost-effective imaging to the complex issues we as shoulder surgeons encounter, as we try to help our patients regain their shoulder comfort and function.

CHAPTER 5

Effectiveness Evaluation of the Shoulder

Patrick D.G. Henry, Robin R. Richards

Evaluating the effectiveness of medical treatment is an important component of the healthcare system. Patients and their families, healthcare providers, administrators, and governments and shareholders within the healthcare system need to be informed as to whether medical treatments are effective. This process is called "effectiveness evaluation," and relies on the accurate assessment of a patient's level of disability that is related to an injury or disease process. Assessing a patient's level of disability before and following treatment provides a means to objectively evaluate the effectiveness of an intervention. Over the last 20 to 30 years, evidence-based medicine has become recognized as an integral part of medical and surgical practice. Accordingly, there has been increased interest in the objective assessment of health outcomes, including those following treatment of shoulder disorders.

The methodology of outcome assessment has evolved in recent decades. However, the ideal outcome instrument for the shoulder remains elusive. A recent review of all shoulder-related publications in the *Journal of Bone and Joint Surgery* (JBJS) between the years 2004 and 2014 concluded the following: "A consensus is needed in shoulder research for more consistent application of validated patient reported outcome measurement tools."[42] This chapter details the history of outcome assessment of the shoulder and the methodology used to assess outcome measures. This chapter also provides a critical analysis of the outcome measures currently available and recommendations regarding the proper use of outcome measures in clinical practice. These concepts are part of the greater field of study known as "psychometrics," which measures the abilities, knowledge, attitudes, and psychological disposition of a patient.

HISTORY

Emery Codman, an orthopedic shoulder surgeon from Boston, is credited for introducing the concept of outcome assessment in the medical community in the early 1900s.[69] He advocated the concept of the "end result idea," wherein the clinician would critically evaluate the surgical results of all cases to identify and understand treatment failures with the goal of improving the care of future patients. This concept was adopted throughout healthcare and is the foundation of evidenced-based medicine. For nearly a century, the effectiveness of intervention was based on the objective clinical assessments such as range-of-motion (ROM), stability, and deformity, combined with the radiographic assessment of other variables such as fracture union and prosthetic position. While initially considered the best method to evaluate a patient's outcome after treatment, such observer-based methodology ignores the patient's perception of his or her condition and fails to address the larger concept of the patient's general health and the role that the shoulder disorder is playing in the well-being of the individual.

Several studies have demonstrated that objective assessment of shoulder function can be inconsistent, with large margins of error. Hayes et al.[47] assessed six different shoulder motions using visual estimation, goniometry, still photography, and reach and found that the standard error of measurement ranged from 14 degrees to 25 degrees between raters and from 11 degrees to 23 degrees for the same rater across different time points. Terwee et al.[105] found that the interobserver agreement was low for assessing active and passive elevations of the shoulder, particularly patients who have severe pain and disability. In a prospective study, Rudiger et al.[95] found a poor correlation between patients and surgeons for objective measurements of shoulder mobility. Dowrick et al.[36] compared self-reported and independently observed disability levels in an orthopedic trauma population. They found that the disability-level ratings greatly varied and that observers consistently rated the disability levels lower than participants (i.e., patients). Furthermore, Hickey et al.[49] found that experienced manipulative physiotherapists had difficulty determining the symptomatic status of patients using observational motion analysis.

As the awareness regarding the limitations of observer-based measurements has increased in the last 20 to 25 years, patient-reported (i.e., self-reported) outcome techniques and tools have emerged.[6] Patient-based general health outcome measures have been used to determine the effect of shoulder conditions on the patient's well-being; more specific instruments (e.g., shoulder specific and those for the entire upper extremity) have also been developed. Cook et al.[28] assessed four patient-based shoulder outcome measures and found them to exhibit good internal consistency across surgical status. In contrast, the observer-based systems assessed in this study revealed inconsistencies across surgical status.

The typical method used for patient-based, self-reported outcomes is a questionnaire. A new method of assessment is emerging, known as Computer Adaptive Testing (CAT). This tool has been used for many types of nonmedical examinations but can also be used for medical questionnaires and functional outcome assessments.[107] This tool involves the use of a computer to ask questions, where each successive question adapts to the responses that have come before it to generate the most relevant next question. This exciting new format enables a shorter and more relevant testing; however, this format is new to modern medicine, and outcome instruments are still in development and yet to be widely implemented.

DEVELOPMENT OF OUTCOME MEASURES AND TOOLS

In the specialty of orthopedic surgery, health-related quality of life (HRQoL) is the main outcome measure of interest because orthopedic interventions for the shoulder are designed to improve the quality of life rather than prolong the lifespan. To understand HRQoL, one must understand the level of disability that a particular condition causes and appreciate the change in disability and function that a treatment renders.

Measuring HRQoL requires asking the right questions and performing the appropriate tests; therefore selecting the appropriate questions and tests is an important and rigorous process. The development of an outcome instrument involves the following steps:

1. Identification of a specific patient population
2. Generation of items (questions)
3. Item (question) reduction
4. Pretesting of the outcome instrument
5. Determination of the instrument's measurement properties (validity, reliability, and responsiveness)

ASSESSING AN OUTCOME MEASURE

Assessing the measurement properties of different instruments is necessary to ensure that the clinical outcome of interest is accurately appraised when using a particular instrument. The properties of an outcome measure that are most important to clinicians include the validity, reliability, and responsiveness; such properties enable the objective assessment of the quality of an outcome measure.[15] Given the plethora of outcome measures available to clinicians, the use of an outcome measure for which data are available is advisable. Background is provided here on the psychometric principles used to compare different outcome instruments published in the literature.

Validity

An instrument is considered valid if it measures what it was intended to measure. Several different terms are used to describe validity. Face validity assumes an instrument is valid if it appears to be measuring what it is intended to measure; this form of validity is the simplest and yet the weakest method of demonstrating validity. Content validity is satisfied when the items that constitute a measure are inclusive of all aspects of the condition of interest. Construct validity is the degree to which a theoretical construct (e.g., shoulder function) is measured by an instrument. For example, because direct measurement of all aspects of shoulder function is not possible, we must also measure other variables associated with shoulder function, such as pain and ROM. Testing construct validity builds confidence in an outcome measure. Validity can be tested by comparing data from a patient-derived assessment with data from a physician-derived assessment of impairment severity, level of pain, ability to perform normal activities of daily living (ADLs), and responses on other contemporary patient-completed questionnaires. Two measures of construct validity are convergent validity and discriminate validity. Convergent validity refers to the extent to which different ways of measuring the same attribute correlate with one another. In other words, convergent validity determines if one outcome measure correlates with another outcome measure that claims to measure the same attribute (e.g., shoulder function). In discriminant (or divergent) validity, a measure does not correlate with dissimilar scales or dimensions of a scale. Furthermore, discriminant validity is the ability of an outcome measure to discriminate across different levels of severity in a patient population. Various statistical measures, including Pearson's product moment correlation coefficient, are used to determine validity.

Reliability

Reliability is the extent to which an instrument yields the same results following repeated administration in a population with stable health status. Shoulder outcome instruments should be sufficiently reliable such that the score derived from the use of an outcome measure does not change, even if the questionnaire is completed on different occasions, provided there has been no change in the patient's clinical status. The term "intrarater reliability" (also known as test-retest reliability and intraobserver reliability) refers to the ability of an instrument to yield the same result (i.e., the agreement between scores) when a single rater or observer repeatedly administers the test to the same patients with stable health conditions. "Interrater reliability" (also known as interobserver reliability) refers to the ability of an instrument to yield the same result when administered to the same patient by two or more raters or observers when no change in the health status of the patient has occurred.

Reliability is assessed in the following manner: (1) recruit a cohort of patients appropriate to the outcome measure being examined, (2) administer the outcome measure, and (3) repeat the process at a predetermined time interval. At the time of the second testing, patients are questioned as to whether their condition has changed since the first test session; if so, they are excluded from the analysis because their score would be expected to change. Reliability is determined using one of the several statistical techniques such as one-way intraclass correlation coefficient, two-way analysis of variance to determine the intraclass correlation coefficient, and Spearman rank correlation coefficients. Furthermore, clinicians can assess the percentage of patients with identical scores and the percentage of patients who have moved between response categories between testing sessions.

Responsiveness

Responsiveness to change is the ability of an instrument to detect true changes in a patient's status (i.e., differences between pretreatment and posttreatment scores) that is beyond random variability. Some authors believe that responsiveness may be the most important property for evaluating a health status instrument. Previous knowledge regarding an instrument's responsiveness aids in the selection of an appropriate outcome measure and also permits estimation of the sample size in clinical studies that use the instrument to ensure that adequate statistical power is achieved.

To determine responsiveness, the difference between the pretreatment and posttreatment scores (i.e., change score) is determined. For example, patients with advanced rotator cuff disease or glenohumeral joint osteoarthritis could be compared before and after rotator cuff repair or total shoulder arthroplasty, respectively. A statistical measure called the *standardized response mean* (mean change score divided by the standard deviation of the change score) can be used to assess the relative responsiveness of an outcome measure. The standardized response mean transforms the change score into a standard unit of measurement, allowing comparison between different instruments. The standardized response mean is frequently used to assess the relative responsiveness of health status instruments used for determining the impact of musculoskeletal conditions. A higher standardized response mean indicates greater sensitivity to clinical change. As previously discussed, the responsiveness of an instrument is an important consideration in research study design because it can serve to minimize the sample size.[56]

The responsiveness of an instrument is related to an important parameter known as the *minimal clinically important difference* (MCID). The MCID of an instrument refers to the smallest change in a test score that a patient would consider clinically relevant or important. For example, the MCID of the Constant score was recently determined to be 10.4 for patients with rotator cuff tears.[59] Two other important parameters related to the responsiveness of an instrument are *ceiling effects* and *floor effects*. A ceiling effect occurs when an instrument cannot reliably differentiate patients who score very high on a scale, while a floor effect occurs when an instrument cannot reliably differentiate patients who score very low on a scale.

APPLICATION OF OUTCOME MEASURES

Clinician Versus Patient Reported Outcomes

Outcome measures are of three main types: patient reported, clinician reported, and performance based. Performance-based outcome measures are typically a subtype of a clinician-reported outcome measure because performance, such as muscle strength or ROM, is usually assessed by a clinician. Clinician-reported and performance-based outcome measures were the mainstay of clinical outcome assessments for the first 75 years of this field. Such measures initially appeared logical because most scientific fields respected the objectivity of observer-based measurement and acknowledged the subjectivity in taking measurements. Performance outcome assessments are important to clinicians and allow the comparison of outcomes between different treatments for the same condition. Therefore, observer-based measurements are still useful to clinicians and patients alike for determining how a particular treatment affects functional outcomes.

Observer-based assessments fail to determine whether patients actually feel better after a given treatment. Patients' perceptions of their disabilities are more relevant than observer-based measurements. However, a clinician's involvement in the administration of a patient-based outcome instrument can be a problem. When an observer (e.g., clinician) questions a patient with regard to function and then records the response, the possibility of observer bias is introduced. Such an effect reduces the validity of the assessment tool.

Patient-reported functional outcomes have been developed and tested using both psychometric and clinometric methods and have several advantages over observer-based assessments: (1) assessment of the patient's perception regarding his or her condition, (2) elimination of bias related to clinician observation, (3) ease of administration by telephone or mail, (4) physical examination not required, (5) cost-effectiveness, and (6) less time required to administer.

Furthermore, recent evidence points to the ability of patients to measure their own performance-based outcomes. In 2014, Yang et al.[122] compared the functional results obtained from patient-reported and clinician-reported outcomes. Patients (n = 120) were mailed instructions explaining how to measure their own ROM using diagram-based questions and strength at home before visiting the clinic 1 year after shoulder arthroplasty. Comparison of these results to clinician-measured values[122] indicated perfect agreement in strength measurements (κ statistic, 0.62 to 0.92); the majority (88%) of patients were within 1 grade of the physician-measured ROM, with patients tending to slightly overestimate their ROM.

Response Methodology

Response methodologies for outcome instruments can be either "yes" or "no" answers, Likert scales, or visual analog scales. Visual analog scales take longer to score than other response methodologies if the value of the patients' responses must be manually determined. Simple responses such as "yes" or "no" limit the number of possible responses and thus may also limit the instrument's responsiveness. Many contemporary outcome instruments use Likert scales; however, the ideal number of response options for a Likert scale has not been determined.

Scoring an Outcome Measure: Categoric Rankings Versus Aggregate Scores

The categoric rankings used to describe outcomes following treatment of a shoulder disorder differ among studies. Most commonly, outcomes are described using terms such as "poor," "fair," "good," or "excellent." The use of categoric ranking may lead to the erroneous assumption that independently designed scoring systems describe similar levels of impairment. The variability in the definition of the terms used for categoric rankings hinders accurate communication between investigators and is an impediment to the objective comparison of results between different studies. For example, different scoring systems have different weights assigned to each domain and different values assigned to each categoric ranking. The outcome measures currently used for the shoulder are based on clinical domains, such as ROM, pain, and ability to perform daily activities; each domain is separately scored. Scores are then aggregated and assigned categoric rankings that range from "poor" to "excellent." Thus a patient with a given raw score may have different categoric rankings depending on which scoring system is used.

The differences between scoring systems are so pervasive that categoric rankings cannot be relied on to provide meaningful comparisons either within or between patient cohorts.[110] Furthermore, study results that use categoric rankings from different scoring systems cannot be combined. Therefore, when reporting categoric rankings for research purposes, the aggregate score should also be included.

Computer Adaptive Testing

CAT is a computerized test administration process that is based on the test-taking philosophy known as *item-response theory,* in contrast to *classical test theory,* in which all subjects must answer the same questions. With CAT, subsequent questions are dependent on the answers provided to previous questions. Apart from the first question, which is identical for all, the test can be tailored to the patient's needs and ability levels by removing redundancy within the test. For example, if a patient cannot lift a pen, the patient will not be asked if he or she can lift a 10-pound weight. The potential benefits of CAT testing include (1) reduced test time and decreased patient response burden, (2) reduced floor and ceiling effects, (3) one-dimensional testing that may clarify the interpretation of results, and (4) the ability to add or subtract questions from the item bank without the need to recreate and validate an entirely new scale.[121]

CAT is the testing platform used by the National Institutes of Health's Patient Reported Outcomes Measurement Information System (PROMIS), which was introduced in 2007.[22] The PROMIS Physical Function score was the first score to be developed, followed by the PROMIS Upper Extremity Score. The PROMIS testing of the upper extremity has been proven to be reliable, with psychometric qualities comparable with other common upper extremity measures (e.g., the DASH score) for various upper extremity conditions. Scoring can be completed by the patient in one-tenth of the time required by other instruments.[35,53,78,83,111] PROMIS and CAT are still in a nascent phase of development and proliferation. The potential of CAT testing is gradually being recognized, and it is likely to become a prominent element of future instruments developed for effective evaluations in the shoulder.

TYPES OF OUTCOME MEASURES

A wide variety of outcome measures are available for use in the shoulder (Box 5-1). In increasing order of specificity, these measurement tools include generic health instruments or health utility measures used to evaluate a patient's overall health, limb-specific instruments used to evaluate upper extremity function, joint-specific instruments used to evaluate shoulder function, and disease-specific instruments used to evaluate patients with a certain disease, such as shoulder instability. The following are examples of instruments used to assess outcomes in patients with shoulder-related pathology.

BOX 5-1. Outcome Instruments Used to Evaluate the Shoulder

Generic
Arthritis Impact Measurement Scale
Duke Health Profile
EuroQol 5-D (EQ5-D)
Index of Well-Being
Nottingham Health Index
Short Form 12 (SF-12)
Short Form 36 (SF-36)
Sickness Impact Profile
Nottingham Health Index

Limb Specific
Disabilities of the Arm, Shoulder, and Hand (DASH)[7]
QuickDASH[11]
Modified American Shoulder and Elbow Surgeons (M-ASES)
Musculoskeletal Functional Assessment[103]
Toronto Extremity Salvage Score[32]
Upper Extremity Function Scale[85]
Upper Limb Functional Index[40]
Functional Impairment Test–Hand and Neck/Shoulder/Arm[67]
Gallon-Jug Shelf-Transfer Test[97]

Shoulder Specific
American Shoulder and Elbow Surgeons Standardized Assessment[87]
Constant-Murley[26]
Abbreviated Constant score[84]
Disability questionnaire[29]
L'Insalata Shoulder Rating Questionnaire
Neer Rating Sheet
Oxford Shoulder Score[4]
Shoulder-Arm Disability Questionnaire[18]
Shoulder Disability Questionnaire[113]
Shoulder Function Assessment Scale[115]
Shoulder Pain and Disability Index[88]
Shoulder Pain Score[120]
Shoulder Questionnaire[33]
Shoulder Rating Scale[60]
Shoulder Severity Index
Simple Shoulder Test[72]
Subjective Shoulder Rating Scale
UCLA End-Result Score[2]
University of Pennsylvania Shoulder Score
Wheelchair User's Shoulder Pain Index[31]

Disease Specific
AC Separation Scoring System
Melbourne Instability Shoulder Scale[118]
Rowe's Rating for Bankart Repair[94]
Rotator Cuff Quality of Life[50]
Western Ontario Rotator Cuff Index[34]
Western Ontario Shoulder Instability Index[57]
Western Ontario Osteoarthritis of the Shoulder Index[65]

Generic Health-Related Quality of Life Instruments

Generic health instruments provide information regarding the impact of a specific condition of interest and any coexisting conditions on a patient's general health. These instruments can be used for almost any type of disorder and can also be used to evaluate a patient's health outcome following treatment of a specific disorder. Such instruments also permit scores to be compared across other orthopedic and nonorthopedic conditions. Therefore the outcomes of different treatments as well as the disability associated with various conditions can be compared using such a score. This type of instrument has important implications for studying health economics in addition to allowing comparative analysis between specialties of the amount of disability that patients perceive themselves to endure. Using this technique, patient-perceived disability due to shoulder conditions was shown to rank similar in severity to five major medical conditions: hypertension, congestive heart failure, acute myocardial infarction, diabetes mellitus, and clinical depression.[41]

Short Form 36 and Short Form 12

The Short Form 36 (SF-36) is the most commonly used tool in orthopedic surgery and clinical medicine to assess general health-related quality of life. This tool measures eight health concepts: physical functioning (10 items), social functioning (two items), role limitations due to physical problems (four items), role limitations due to emotional problems (three items), mental health (five items), energy/fatigue (four items), bodily pain (two items), and general health perception (five items). The reliability, validity, and responsiveness of the SF-36 for conditions of the upper extremity has been demonstrated.[74] An abbreviated version of the SF-36, Short Form 12, has been developed[117] and has been validated to a lesser extent for use in a variety of shoulder conditions, with good correlation to the longer version.[66]

EuroQol 5 Dimensions Questionnaire

The EuroQol group was founded in 1987 and is described as "an international group of researchers dedicated to the measurement of health outcome."[106] Initially a European collaboration, there are now active members worldwide. The evolution of their efforts eventually resulted in the development of the EuroQol 5 Dimensions Questionnaire (EQ-5D), which is an internationally validated general measure of health-related quality of life. The EQ-5D consists of a questionnaire and a self-rated health status assessment using a visual analogue scale (EQ-VAS). The self-assessment questionnaire evaluates the patient's current health in five dimensions: mobility, self-care, usual activities, pain/discomfort, and anxiety/depression. The patient is asked to grade his or her current level of function for each dimension into one of three degrees of disability (severe, moderate, or none). The combination of these grades with the conditions "death" and "unconscious" enables description of 245 different health states. Each health state can be ranked and transformed into a single score (known as the health utility score). The utility score is an expression of the Quality Adjusted Life Years and is commonly used to make evidence-based decisions in analyses of cost effectiveness. Therefore the EQ-5D can be used for health outcomes and economic studies, making it a highly useful and versatile tool for health outcomes and quality improvement research.

The EQ-5D has been used in multiple shoulder studies, and while it is more commonly used in Europe, its use is increasing in North America. One criticism of the EQ-5D is that it may not have high enough responsiveness to detect small but clinically relevant differences in health status.[109]

Limb-Specific Outcome Instruments

Limb-specific (i.e., regional) instruments are based on the presumption that the upper extremity functions as a kinematic chain. According to this paradigm, the shoulder as well as the elbow, forearm, and wrist position the hand for grasping and manipulating objects in the environment. Studies of limb-specific instruments have shown close correlation with joint-specific and disease-specific measures, although they tend not to have the same degree of responsiveness. Nevertheless, a limb-specific instrument may be appropriate when the diagnosis is less certain or when more than one part of the extremity is affected by injury or disease. For example, a condition involving either one of the shoulder, elbow, wrist joint, or the hand can affect one's ability to use a telephone.

DASH and QuickDASH Questionnaires

The Disabilities of the Arm, Shoulder and Hand (DASH) Questionnaire was developed for assessment of single or multiple musculoskeletal disorders affecting the upper limb.[52] The DASH is the third most commonly used upper extremity outcome measure in publications over the last 2 years, after the Constant Murley and the American Shoulder and Elbow Society (ASES) scores.[16] The DASH is a patient-administered, 30-item questionnaire that was designed to quantify physical disability and symptoms in individuals with upper limb disorders. The DASH is divided into three domains: physical function (21 items), symptoms (six items), social/role functions (three items), and two optional modules including sports/music (four items) and work activities (four items). The response to each item is scored on a 5-point Likert scale, and a function/symptom score (from 0 to 100) is calculated; a higher score indicates greater disability. The MCID of the DASH is 10.2 points, with a minimal detectable change of 12 points.[8] The DASH has demonstrated excellent responsiveness compared to joint-specific questionnaires and has been validated for use in both proximal and distal upper limb disorders.[8] It has also been shown to correlate well with the SF-36, but with fewer ceiling and floor effects, supporting its use as a valid measure of health status in patients with a wide variety of upper extremity complaints.[101] This instrument has been validated in many languages including Canadian French,[37] Spanish,[91] Portugeuse,[81] Dutch,[114] Chinese,[62] and Taiwanese.[63]

An abbreviated form of the DASH, the QuickDASH, was developed in 2005.[11] The QuickDASH was developed using three item-reduction techniques on a cross-sectional field of data derived from a study of 407 patients with various upper-limb conditions. This instrument has been found to have similar discriminant ability and test-retest reliability to the DASH.[45,68]

Shoulder-Specific Outcome Instruments

Joint-specific health instruments have been found to be more responsive than generic health status instruments in assessing conditions of the upper extremity. This greater responsiveness is probably because it includes specific items that are relevant to the patient population being studied. The disadvantage of joint-specific instruments is the need for numerous instruments (i.e., for each joint) and the inability to compare outcomes across various conditions, populations, or interventions. A systematic review of 610 articles published between 1992 and 2002 identified 44 different shoulder or upper-limb specific outcome instruments in active use in shoulder surgery research.[46] A more recent review of the literature published in the JBJS (American and British), the *American Journal of Sports Medicine*, and the *Journal of Shoulder and Elbow Surgery* during the years 2013 to 2014 found that the most common shoulder-specific functional outcome instruments used are as follows (from most to least popular): the Constant-Murley score, the ASES, the Simple Shoulder Test, and the University of California–Los Angeles score.[16] Interestingly, another recent review of literature from the past 10 years in JBJS shoulder-related publications found the exact same order of popularity of these instruments.[42]

Constant-Murley Score

The Constant-Murley shoulder score (also known as the Constant score) is a 100-point scoring system (100 points representing the best score) in which 35 points are derived from the patient's reported pain and function and the remaining 65 points are allocated to assessment of ROM and strength. The combination of patient-reported, clinician-reported, and performance outcome measures into a single numerical score make it relatively unique, bestowing a major strength compared to the other outcome measures commonly used. On the other hand, some investigators believe that patient- and observer-based measurements should not be combined into a single score and are best reported separately. The Constant score has been found to be affected by both patient age and sex,[44,116] where the score tends to decrease beginning at age 50 for men and age 30 for women. Age- and sex-matched normative data are available for the Constant score and have permitted the development of an age- and sex-adjusted Constant score. The MCID for the Constant score was recently reported as 10.4 in the rotator cuff tear population[59] and 15 for patients with general subacromial pain.[51]

A major advantage of the Constant score is its popularity, which allows for comparison between various studies. However, despite its popularity, there have been several criticisms of this score, including its only "fair" reliability.[24,89] This lower reliability is likely related to the objective measurements (e.g., strength and ROM components) that make up 65% of the score.[82] In the initial publication, measurement techniques were not described in a standardized format, leading to subsequent publication of guidelines on appropriate techniques for administration of the instrument with specific reference made to the strength measurement component.[25] Compared with patient-recorded outcome measures, the Constant score is also more difficult to administer since a large portion of the score is derived from observer-based measurement[4]; if patients are unable to return for follow-up examination, data collection is considered incomplete as telephone or mail-in questionnaires are not possible. Floor effects for trauma patients[99] and ceiling effects for instability patients[24] have also been noted. Ceiling effects are common with most instability-specific scores due to the unique clinical presentation of shoulder instability compared with other shoulder pathologies.[43]

There is only one pain scale in the Constant score, which likely yields an inadequate representation of a patient's pain since patients often experience different amounts of pain depending on their activities. Improving the accuracy of the Constant score by using the uninjured (i.e., contralateral) shoulder as a reference to yield an "individual relative Constant score" has been suggested; however, this method would be problematic for patients with bilateral shoulder disorders.[39] Due to some of these potential problems with the Constant score, at least two authors have advised against its use in randomized controlled trials.[64,99]

American Shoulder and Elbow Society Score

The ASES Score outcome measure was developed in 1994.[9] This instrument consists of a patient self-assessment section that can be completed independently and a clinician-assessment section regarding the patient's ADLs; however, the final score only includes the patient self-assessment section (100 points total: pain, 50 points; function, 50 points). The MCID has been reported as 12 to 17 points for rotator cuff pathology,[104] while a lower estimate of 6.4 has been reported for general shoulder conditions.[76]

The ASES assessment form has been found to be a valid, reliable, and responsive outcome tool for general shoulder dysfunction[27,76] and for specific shoulder conditions such as instability, rotator cuff disease, and glenohumeral joint arthritis.[1,23,58,61] A major advantage of this instrument is its ease of administration; however, this benefit is slightly outweighed by the requirement to perform calculations afterwards to obtain the final score.[19] The ASES score correlates well with the Constant shoulder score ($r = 0.871$; $P < .01$) and is a highly convenient method of outcome assessment.[98]

One major criticism of the ASES score, as with the Constant score, is that only one pain scale is used. This particular scale asks "What is your pain level today?", which for many patients may not accurately reflect their true pain level because pain level typically varies with the present activity level and time of day. Moreover, three of the 10 questions regarding ADLs pertain to sport or ability level and are not relevant to many patients. Finally, a ceiling effect has been noted in higher-functioning patients.[21]

Simple Shoulder Test

The Simple Shoulder Test (SST) was developed at the University of Washington in 1992 with the belief that outcome instruments could be dramatically simplified yet still retain the same psychometric properties of longer measurement tools. The questionnaire consists of 12 yes/no questions, with two related to pain, seven to function, and three to ROM.

The SST has been shown to have acceptable test-retest reliability, content validity, and construct validity.[43] Responsiveness has been found to be lower in younger patients and in patients with shoulder instability; however, this tool has demonstrated good responsiveness in rotator cuff pathology.[38] Despite this instrument's respectable psychometric properties, the small number of questions and the dichotomous nature of the responses limits its ability to detect small but clinically important changes in patient functionality, both between different patients and for the same patient followed longitudinally. The MCID of the SST is 2 for patients with rotator cuff pathology[104] and 3 for patients undergoing shoulder arthroplasty.[93]

Single Assessment Numerical Evaluation Test

Taking simplicity to the extreme, the Single Assessment Numerical Evaluation (SANE) test attempts to convey everything that the more detailed shoulder scores attempt to accomplish.[119] The SANE test is a one-question test that simply asks the patient, "How would you rate your shoulder today as a percentage of normal (0% to 100% scale with 100% being normal)?"

The SANE test has shown increasing popularity in recent years due to suspicions that the more complicated outcome instruments unnecessarily complicate the assessment process. If the most important element of outcome is patients' perceptions of how they are doing, perhaps we should simply just ask patients this question directly.

This practical approach has resonated with some in the orthopedic community. This test is easily administered and does not require a personal encounter, and patients easily comprehend the question and do not require guidance on how to complete the instrument. The SANE test has been used in several recent shoulder publications to assess patients with rotator cuff pathology, instability, superior labrum anterior to posterior (SLAP) tears, and arthritis[5,54,77,108] and has demonstrated a good correlation with both the ASES and Rowe scores for rotator cuff and SLAP pathology[30,119]; however, this test does not correlate strongly with the QuickDASH or Numeric Pain Rating Scale.[80] The SANE test has not been validated, and the MCID has not been reported.[100]

University of California–Los Angeles End-Result Score

The UCLA end-result score was first described in 1981, making it one of the first published shoulder-specific outcomes measures.[2] This test was developed before the current methodology that applies psychometric principles to develop outcome measures. Although it remains a relatively popular score, there are several criticisms related to the content of this instrument.

The UCLA score is a 35-point scale that evaluates five clinical domains: pain (10 points), function (10 points), active forward elevation (five points), forward flexion strength (five points), and patient satisfaction (five points). The scale has been criticized for its use of descriptive items for pain and function, and one of the items asks whether the patient is "satisfied," which is not a meaningful question for patients who have not yet undergone treatment. Combining patient-based and observer-based items into a single score (similar to the Constant score) may not be appropriate or meaningful. Finally, in the original description, this single score is then reported in terms of a categoric ranking (poor, fair, good, or excellent), which negatively affects the responsiveness of the tool. When using this scale, it is best to report numeric results and avoid reporting categoric rankings. In psychometric testing, the UCLA scale has demonstrated good internal consistency, although the standard error of measurement for the scale was high and factor loading was inconsistent, suggesting that patients may not distinguish between pain and function.[90] The MCID has not been established for this instrument.

Other Shoulder Specific Tests

Many other shoulder-specific instruments are currently in use (see Box 5-1). The popularity of any given test should ideally be based on the qualities of the test for the specific purpose of use; however, other factors such as regional preferences, ease of administration, and other nonpsychometric factors play into this decision. Furthermore, the popularity of a test does not necessarily translate into appropriate use of a test, as several instances have been reported in which a shoulder outcome instrument was used inappropriately.[46]

Disease-Specific Outcome Instruments of the Shoulder

Disease-specific tools, designed to assess specific conditions in a specific joint, are the most specific outcome instruments. The assumption is that a person with a shoulder dislocation has different needs and perceptions of disability than a person with a rotator cuff tear. As a result, such instruments are theoretically more likely to exhibit higher validity, reliability, and sensitivity for a specific disease compared to an instrument with the same psychometric properties that is applied across several different diseases. As a general rule, disease-specific outcome measures are very responsive to small changes in the condition for which they were designed. However, a major limitation of these tools is that a specific tool for each shoulder disorder is required and comparison with other disorders is not possible. The disease-specific instruments most commonly used in shoulder surgery were created by the same working group and include the Western Ontario Shoulder Instability (WOSI) Index for instability, the Western Ontario Rotator Cuff (WORC) Index for rotator cuff disease, and the Western Ontario Osteoarthritis of the Shoulder (WOOS) Index for patients with glenohumeral joint arthritis.[55,57,65]

Western Ontario Shoulder Instability Index

Shoulder instability is a particular diagnosis with features that make it unique to other shoulder conditions. Patients with instability typically have long periods of normal function punctuated by episodes of extreme discomfort related to dislocation events or instability episodes. Instability-specific tools were the first type of disease-specific shoulder tools developed.[92] In 1978, the Rowe score was the first of its kind to be developed.[94] Since then, other scores with better psychometric properties than the Rowe score have been developed, including the WOSI Index, the Oxford Shoulder Instability Score (OSIS), and the Melbourne Instability Shoulder Scale (MISS). Of these, the WOSI Index has demonstrated the greatest validity, reliability, and responsiveness and is currently the recommended disease-specific instrument for shoulder instability.[121] The MCID for the WOSI Index is 220.[121]

Western Ontario Rotator Cuff Index and Western Ontario Osteoarthritis Shoulder Index

The same group that developed the WOSI Index also developed disease-specific outcome instruments for patients with rotator cuff disorders (WORC Index) and glenohumeral joint osteoarthritis (WOOS Index).[55,65] The MCID for the WORC Index is 245 and that of the WOOS Index has not been determined.[34] Both of these scores have demonstrated desirable psychometric properties and are the most frequently used disease-specific instruments for their respective disorders.[34,65,86] However, to date, neither instrument has been used as often as the shoulder-specific instruments described earlier in this chapter.

Rotator Cuff Quality of Life Questionnaire

The Rotator Cuff Quality of Life (RC-QOL) is a 34-item questionnaire developed at the University of Calgary that consists of five domains: physical symptoms, sports/recreation, work-related concerns, lifestyle concerns, and social/emotional concerns.[50] Each item is scored with a

100-point visual analog scale. The sum of all items is divided by 34 to give a final score out of 100, with 100 being the highest and 0 being the lowest functional level. The RC-QOL was recently shown to be predictive of the need for surgery in patients with rotator cuff tears and was found to have similar construct validity to the WORC score.[17] The MCID has not been determined for this instrument.

Outcome Measures That Assess Pain

Pain is a common, subjective, patient-reported measure that is somewhat controversial when included as part of a total score for functional outcome assessment. The amount of pain experienced by patients is certainly one of the most important determinants of outcome for musculoskeletal disorders before and after treatment. However, correlation between self-reported pain and both self-reported disability and observer-based measures of function are sometimes significant but often weak. The measurement of pain often yields much greater treatment effect sizes, or responsiveness, than do physical variables or condition-specific instruments.[70] Furthermore, since the perception of pain is widely variable between patients with the same or similar conditions, some believe that pain scores should not be included in the scoring of functional limitation. This issue can be addressed by scoring and reporting pain and function separately.

Taking these concepts into consideration, the outcome of therapies designed for the treatment of shoulder disease should be described ideally on the basis of a separate assessment of pain, in addition to any generic, region-specific, or condition-specific outcome instruments. Several different scales are available for the measurement of pain intensity, but the most commonly used are the Visual Analog Scale (VAS), Numerical Rating Scales (NRS), and Verbal Rating Scales (VRS).[73]

PUTTING IT ALL TOGETHER: CHOOSING THE RIGHT OUTCOME MEASURE

The choice of an outcome measure(s) should be based on multiple factors, including the disease and treatment being studied, the population involved, the purpose of the assessment (routine clinical assessment vs. clinical research), the personnel available, the time required for administration and scoring, the availability of normative data, and the inherent qualities of the available outcome instruments. Whether the instrument is used to follow individual patients or used in large-scale multicenter trials, most clinicians will use an outcome measure as an initial assessment tool and to determine a patient's progress over time. Therefore the initial selection of an appropriate outcome measure is important. Outcome measurements have varying strengths depending on the population being assessed and the reason for their use. The selection of an instrument for the assessment of outcome must be context specific and should be based on evidence that the instrument has the necessary measurement properties in the population being sampled for purposes of research and/or routine clinical assessment.

The large number of shoulder scoring systems available makes the selection of the ideal instrument challenging. An attempt to compare the Constant score, ASES score, UCLA score, SST, WOSI, and Rowe score found that no score demonstrated superior measurement qualities over the other.[79] A more recent systematic review involving 127 studies applied the EMPRO tool (Evaluating Measures of Patient-Reported Outcome) to 11 shoulder-specific instruments and found that the ASES, SST, and OSS were the highest-rated tools; however, each tool had certain strengths and weaknesses.[96] Another observation is that most of the tested shoulder outcome instruments do not accurately reflect health-related quality of life, and many correlate poorly with each other.[3,79] Thus the outcomes measured using different scoring systems are not typically comparable, and general health is not adequately assessed with more specific scoring instruments. This finding is reflected in other studies comparing shoulder scores to general health quality of life measures.[3] An earlier study comparing the ASES, SST, Severity Score Index (SSI), Shoulder Pain and Disability Index (SPADI), and Subjective Shoulder Rating System (SSRS) found that these instruments performed similarly in describing shoulder function and in discriminating between levels of severity; however, the joint-specific instruments demonstrated lower correlations with generic measures of health than with each other.[10] Therefore inclusion of a general health instrument is recommended as part of any array of outcome assessments. For clinical research purposes, it may be appropriate to use a combination of outcome measures, including a generic health status instrument, joint-specific or limb-specific instrument, a disease-specific outcome instrument, and a pain scale.

FUTURE DEVELOPMENTS

The lack of a universally accepted outcome measure can lead to confusion when attempting to determine shoulder impairment severity. Ideally, a single outcome instrument would be created for the shoulder that has optimal psychometric properties for all conditions, adequately reflects overall health status, is simple to use, and is widely implemented. Through CAT, this ideal instrument may ultimately be developed. However, CAT is still in the early phases of development for health outcomes measurement, and such an instrument would need to be tested extensively.

In the meantime, it may be possible to move towards standardization and widespread use of a combination of current measures that are agreed upon by the shoulder community. Standardization would facilitate communication among investigators, clinicians, healthcare administrators, and the general public. Before standardization of an instrument, more comparative studies are needed to facilitate the recommendation of using one instrument over another. Further work is also required to define the measurement properties for several outcome instruments in specific patient populations.

Senior Author's Current Practice

When assessing a new patient, the senior author (R.R.) currently uses a 20-page survey (Fig. E5-1). The author's practice is oriented toward the assessment and treatment of workers with shoulder and elbow injuries. This survey is presented as an example and is not necessarily applicable to all types of clinical practice. Nevertheless, it is the author's goal that the survey demonstrates the type of evaluation instrument that individual practitioners can develop for their own practices.

Patient consent for the use of data derived from the survey for research purposes is obtained. The survey is configured so that the data can be read by a scanning device. The survey can also be administered using touch screen technology. The importance of answering all the questions is emphasized on the second page of the survey. Page 3 consists of a pain diagram wherein patients are asked to localize their pain and define its severity. Page 4 of the survey asks patients to define the duration of their symptoms and the nature of their onset. Pages 5 and 6 are directed towards defining the severity of the pain, its frequency, and its impact on the patients' normal daily activities and ability to take part in recreational, social, and family activities.

Pages 7 and 8 of the survey are devoted to the Quick-DASH questionnaire. Pages 9 to 15 of the survey are devoted to detailed questions regarding the patients' ability to perform their normal occupational activity, whether they are able to perform modified work, and their attitude towards their work. The author recognizes that most practices would require less emphasis on this area and that practices oriented toward patients who are interested in sports activity would have more emphasis in that area.

Pages 16 to 18 of the survey are devoted to the SF-36 general health outcome measure. Page 19 of the survey is devoted to demographic questions, requesting information regarding the patients' marital status, gender, educational background, height, weight, hand dominance, smoking history, and native language. The final page of the survey is devoted to the documentation of medical comorbidities, if applicable. As noted above, the presence of medical comorbidities can have an impact on patient responses on outcome measures.

The author's current practice uses computer technology to rapidly process the data derived from the survey and have it in a presentable format at the time of the initial patient assessment. The data are presented in a 1-page format that includes normative data and highlights the patient's pain profile and most prominent limitation (Fig. 5-2). Furthermore, such baseline data are very useful in assessing a patient's response to treatment, providing that follow-up data are obtained in a similar fashion. Patients' responses have been observed to change as a function of time and the effects to treatment. Therefore documentation of baseline data is critically important.

CONCLUSION

Ideally, an outcome instrument measures parameters that are directly relevant to the patient and provides a comprehensive assessment of the impact of a condition on a patient's daily life. Additionally, widespread use of such measurement scores facilitates communication among healthcare professionals. Although subjective complaints may be difficult to quantify, pain and disability may be the most valid outcome measures, as these are directly relevant to patients. Self-administered questionnaires have been shown to be more responsive than observer-based physical measures such as ROM, strength, dexterity, and sensation. Self-administered questionnaires are not subject to observer bias. Comparisons between studies that use different scoring systems are generally not valid and the categoric rankings of different instruments are not interchangeable. When categoric rankings are used, the data should also be reported in terms of aggregate scores. In general, both generic and joint-specific measures of health status should be used when assessing shoulder function. The role of limb or joint-specific and disease-specific instruments is evolving at this time. Patient-completed functional questionnaires are the optimal method for assessing the effectiveness of shoulder interventions and encourages the scientific assessment and comparison of treatment outcomes.

Sunnybrook
HOLLAND ORTHOPAEDIC & ARTHRITIC CENTRE
when it matters MOST

3108

Worker-based information

SF-36 health survey scores

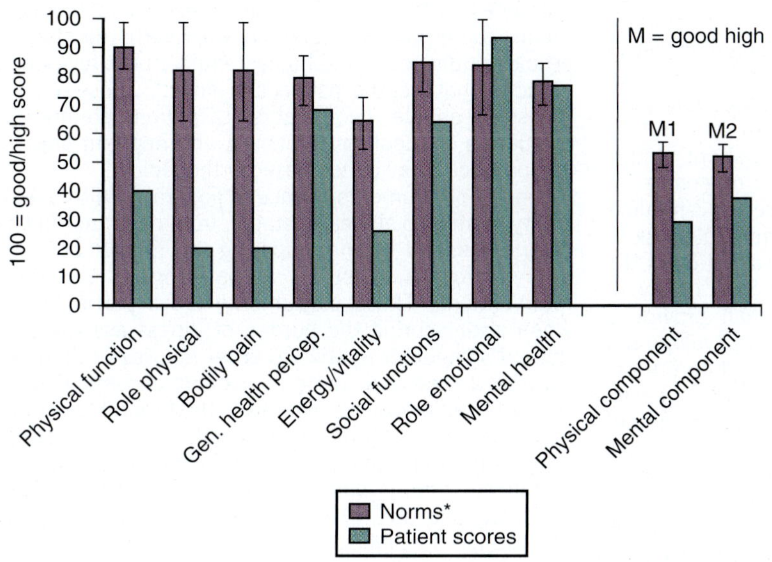

DASH and SPADI scores

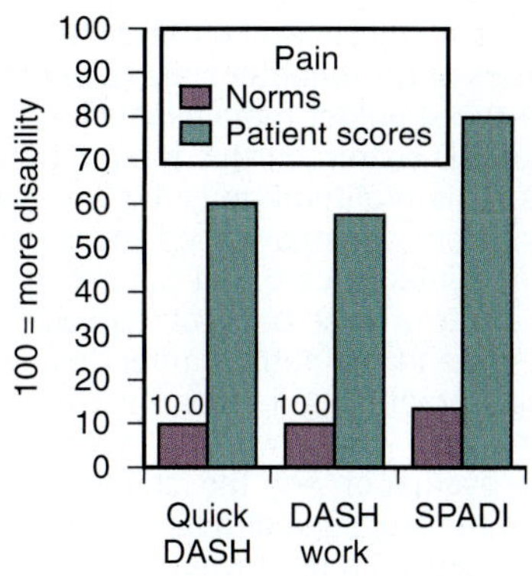

Profile

Age:	35	Sex:	F
		Current occupation:	personal support worker
		Occupation at time of injury:	

Pain scores (greater score = more pain)

von Korff grade (1–4):	Grade 4
Grade 4 = high disability, severely limiting	
Pain intensity scale (/100):	80.0
Days disabled (/180 days):	60
Disability score (0 low-3 high):	2

Cluster score

n/a

Work module

Working?	Yes
Work accomodation underway?	Yes
If 'Yes' what sort?	Modified work because of this

DASH outcome measure scores today

DASH score (0–100, 100 = more disability):	60.0
Open a tight or new jar	2
Place object on overhead shelf	4
Do heavy chores	5
Problem interferes with social activities	3
Difficulty sleeping due to pain	4

Other symptoms

- Arm/shoulder/hand pain
- Arm/shoulder/hand pain on activity

Other health problems Total comorbidities: 1

- Low back pain

FIGURE 5-2: The 1-page summary generated from the survey used by the senior author when new patients are examined. (Courtesy Sunnybrook Holland Orthopaedic & Arthritic Centre, Toronto, Canada. Modified from Hopman WM, Towheed T, Anastassiades T, et al. Canadian normative data for the SF-36 health survey. Canadian Multicentre Osteoporosis Study Research Group. *CMAJ.* 2000;163[3]:265-271.)

INTERNATIONAL EXPERT COMMENTARY

Herman S. Johal, Nathan Evaniew, Mohit Bhandari

Integration of the best available evidence with clinical expertise and patient preferences and values is central to the practice of evidence-based orthopedics.[14] As interventions in shoulder surgery have exponentially increased over the last several decades, so has interest in capturing the full impact of these various techniques and technologies. The authors of this chapter state "the ideal outcomes instrument for the shoulder remains elusive," which is illustrated by a PubMED search on this topic retrieving over 200 publications. This proliferation is likely in part due to a shift in emphasis from clinician-based measures of patient results to patient-centered care and patient-reported outcomes.[99]

There exists a vast body of outcomes used in shoulder surgery,[42,99] and the authors undertook a formidable task in providing a practical guide to effectiveness evaluation of the shoulder. They begin with an overview of the history of outcome evaluation for the shoulder and then provide a primer on the language of outcome instrument development and use. Next, they review features that differentiate clinician-reported, patient-reported, and performance-based outcomes, as well as key concepts related to instrument administration and scoring. The chapter continues with a summary of the most common instruments, including generic health-related quality of life measures and limb-specific, joint-specific, and disease-specific evaluation tools. To navigate the abundance of instruments available, they also provide readers with factors to consider when selecting a shoulder outcome measure.

A thorough understanding of the basis and implementation of shoulder outcome assessment tools is a key component of successful clinical practice and research alike. For clinicians, this chapter provides a set of tools that can be used across an array of shoulder pathologies to define a patient's level of function. This information allows both surgeons and patients to compare treatment results or track the progression of one's disability in a valid, reliable, and responsive manner and to integrate that information into the treatment decision-making process. Such knowledge also allows surgeons to critically appraise outcomes reported in the literature and allows those involved in shoulder research to accurately quantify treatment effects that are observed in experimental settings during the development of new interventions. Overall, effectiveness evaluation methods provide surgeons and researchers with a means to gather, access, interpret, and summarize the functional status of a patient.[13]

When selecting appropriate outcome instruments, clinicians and researchers are faced with a litany of options. Broadly speaking, they can choose performance-based versus patient-reported instruments, and generic versus limb-, joint-, and disease-specific tools. Performance-based measures are typically clinician reported, and these have been the standard tools used to assess effectiveness in the shoulder. Items such as ROM and strength aim to provide useful insight into a patient's overall function. Nonetheless, these observable or physiologic endpoints are only surrogates for shoulder health status, and they may not be as accurate as measuring outcomes from an individual patient's perspective.[20] This realization created a shift to patient-reported outcomes, with over 39 shoulder-specific outcome instruments (both validated and nonvalidated) reported in 167 articles published in the highest impact peer-reviewed orthopedic journal over the last decade alone.[42] These self-reported measures enable incorporation of patient preferences into evaluation of shoulder outcomes, an important step towards the practice of evidence-based orthopedics.

Generic instruments measure general health status and utility relative to all health states, from death to full health.[20] They are useful when comparing the impact of a shoulder injury across a spectrum of pathologies, severities, and interventions. These instruments prove particularly useful when underscoring the burden of illness associated with a patient's shoulder relative to other injuries or illnesses, and provide a means to perform economic comparisons using utility-based measures. However, the broad focus of generic instruments also limits their sensitivity for detecting clinically important changes in shoulder function. In these instances, limb-, joint-, or disease-specific measures are advantageous, as they are designed to inquire about aspects of function specific to the shoulder. These specific instruments are usually more responsive to small but important changes in shoulder health, but they are more difficult to compare across different shoulder pathologies and populations.[20] Comprehensive representations of shoulder health and function can be attained by combining several categories of measurement instruments.[102]

Moving forward, CAT may prove an important initiative for collecting and combining multidimensional information across various shoulder outcome tools in an efficient and user-friendly manner.[48] CAT is still in the developmental phase, but it promises to minimize patient response burden while maximizing evaluation of shoulder function and overall health status.[12,75] In the meantime, surgeons and researchers should select instruments based on the specific purpose of their evaluations. At the end of this chapter, the authors outline their approach to assessing shoulder outcomes, which includes both generic (SF-36) and limb-specific (QuickDASH) measures, with aspects that are both performance based and patient reported. This approach provides an example of how to gain an in-depth understanding of shoulder function and the impact of shoulder pathology on a patient's overall health. As readers progress through the chapter, they should keep in mind that effectiveness evaluation of the shoulder is not an end in itself, but rather a set of principles and tools that help clinicians and researchers ultimately provide better patient care.

EDITOR COMMENTARY

Aaron J. Bois

The authors of this chapter are credited with providing a concise yet thorough summary of the current status of outcome evaluation of the shoulder. The senior author also shares his expertise in this field by providing his current approach to outcome evaluation of a patient presenting with a shoulder complaint that a new surgeon could adopt into his or her clinical practice.

The authors have made clear distinctions regarding the different types of outcome evaluation available to surgeons that range from generic to specific. Generic health-related quality of life instruments (e.g., SF-36) measure physical symptoms, function, and emotional dimensions of health and provide a broad scope of a patient's overall health status. In contrast, limb-specific or regional (e.g., DASH) and disease-specific (e.g., WORC) instruments inquire about specific physical, mental, and social aspects of health affected by the disease; the latter forms of measure can detect small important changes but fail to make comparisons between studies of different diseases because they are so focused and specific. To provide the most comprehensive evaluation of a patient's response to treatment, the inclusion of a combination of measures including a generic health measure, a disease-specific instrument, and a pain scale is recommended.

Surgeons must also understand the fundamental properties of each instrument (i.e., validity, reliability, and responsiveness) before selecting and implementing an outcome measure into clinical practice and/or a clinical trial. Surgeons must be cautious, as some of the available instruments have not been assessed for all such properties. Of equal importance is understanding the differences between clinician- (i.e., observer) and patient-reported instruments; although clinician-based outcomes remain the mainstay of clinical outcome assessment, patient-reported outcomes seem most representative of how a patient is actually doing and helps eliminate observer bias that may be introduced when physician evaluations are performed.

Unfortunately, a universally accepted instrument has not been developed for the shoulder. Some have argued that there are too many joint- or disease-specific measures, preventing comparisons across studies that aim to investigate the treatment effects for the same shoulder condition. Presently, a comprehensive, patient-reported instrument that is widely used and proven valid, reliable, and sensitive to change is needed for clinical and research purposes.

Telling a patient that he or she has "done just fine" following surgery and discharging him or her from your practice is clearly no longer acceptable. To evolve and strive toward providing better care for our patients, we need to obtain outcome data using appropriate instruments to properly evaluate treatment effects and advance orthopedic care.

CHAPTER 6

Fractures of the Proximal Humerus

Kamal I. Bohsali, Aaron J. Bois, Michael A. Wirth

Proximal humerus fractures (PHFs) remain challenging to the treating orthopedist in both their initial diagnosis and classification and in their corresponding management. They account for approximately 5% of all fractures,[61,96,99] and their incidence is expected to increase secondary to an aging population and the associated osteoporosis.[57,101,133,186,196] PHFs are the third most common type of fragility fracture after distal radius and hip fractures in patients aged 65 years and older.[186] In general, PHFs occur more frequently in females than males (3:1 ratio). Nonoperative versus operative management of these injuries depends on the mechanism of injury, the patient's physiologic age, including activity level, and fracture pattern.[155] Although the incidence of PHFs in the elderly did not change from 1999 to 2005, the rate of surgical treatment has increased significantly. In a study evaluating the trends and variance in the incidence and surgical treatment of PHFs in the elderly, Bell et al.[12] noted marked regional variation in the rates of surgical treatment, highlighting the need for better consensus regarding optimal treatment and additional research to determine which fractures are best treated operatively.

Nearly three-fourths of all PHFs occur in patients older than 60 years and are generally the result of low-energy trauma, such as a fall from standing height.[56,155] The majority of these injuries are nondisplaced or minimally displaced and have a good overall prognosis with nonsurgical management despite short-term impairment.[88,99,155,186] Specific risk factors associated with PHFs in the elderly include low bone density, impaired vision and balance, lack of hormone replacement therapy, previous fracture, three or more chronic illnesses, and smoking.[56,118,155]

In contrast, younger patients generally sustain PHFs following high-energy trauma such as motor vehicle collisions, seizures, or electrical shock. These injuries tend to be more severe regarding soft tissue compromise, neurovascular injury, and fracture displacement and often require operative intervention.[99,155]

There remains a wide variation in treatment recommendations for PHFs, with low-quality evidence to support one modality over another. This issue may be partially attributed to the difficulty with radiographic interpretation and the subsequent classification of these injuries.[146]

ANATOMY

To appropriately manage PHFs, it is crucial to understand the complex anatomy of the shoulder girdle. Stability and function of the glenohumeral joint is provided by the interaction of mechanisms that promote a near global range of motion (ROM) and purposeful function. External loads that are transferred to the shoulder girdle are initially offset by joint surface anatomy, joint volume, atmospheric pressure, and joint fluid cohesion and adhesion. Moderate and large loads are counterbalanced by the deltoid and rotator cuff and by the capsulolabral and bone structures, respectively. PHFs alter these complex interactions, resulting in pain, decreased ROM and stiffness, and disability.[96]

The proximal humeral anatomy comprises four main parts: the humeral head, greater tuberosity (GT), lesser tuberosity (LT), and humeral shaft. Following a fracture of the proximal humerus, displacement of each "part" occurs in a predictable manner and is based on the deforming forces created by the tendinous insertions of the pectoralis major, subscapularis, supraspinatus, and infraspinatus (Fig. 6-1).[96]

The normal dimensions and relationships of the bony anatomy of the proximal humerus have been extensively studied. The articular head is spherical and has a diameter of 37 to 57 mm.[30,120] The most superior portion of the articular surface of the humeral head averages 8 mm above the GT,[30] and the humeral version averages 29.8 degrees (range, 10 to 55 degrees).[201] The head is inclined approximately 130 degrees with respect to the humeral shaft.[120]

The bicipital groove lies between GT and LT, and serves as a pathway for the long head of the biceps as it traverses from its intraarticular origin (i.e., superior glenoid–labral complex) into the proximal arm.[96] The distal aspect of the groove is internally rotated with respect to the proximal portion.[123]

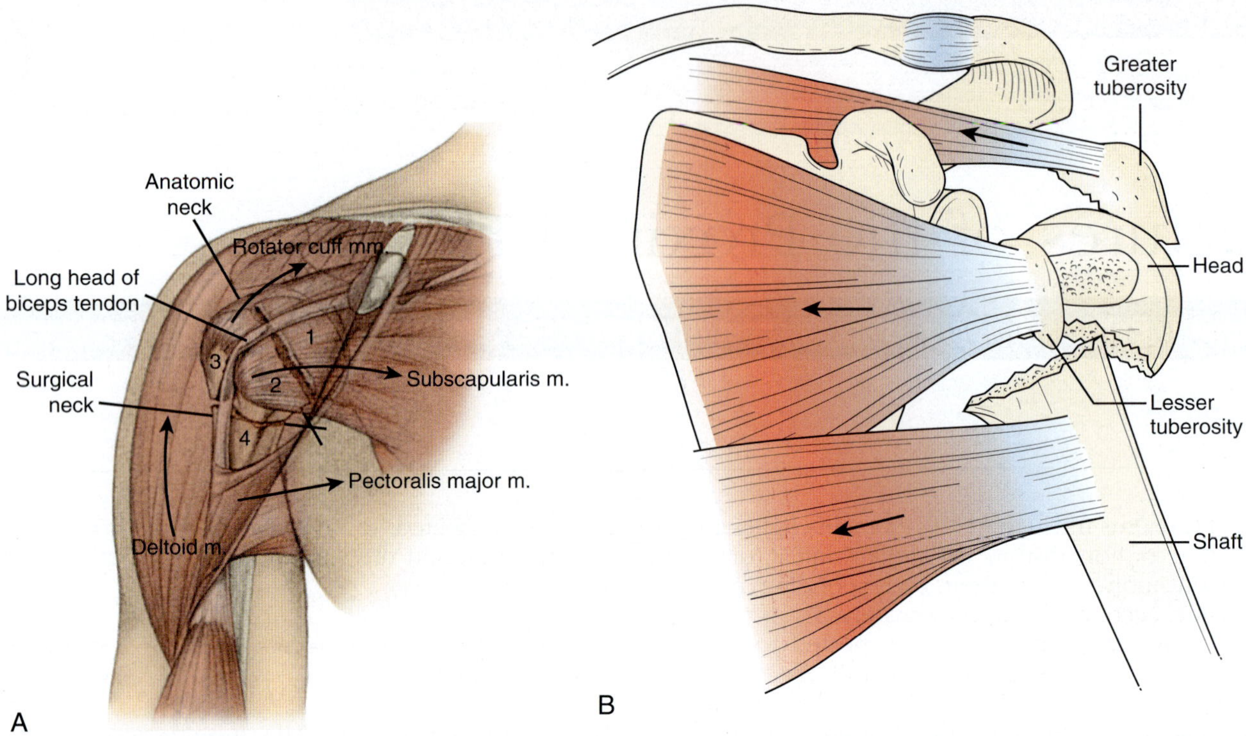

FIGURE 6-1: **A,** The anatomy of the shoulder is complex, and shoulder function depends on proper alignment and interaction of anatomic structures. Displacement of fracture fragments is due to the pull of muscles attaching to the various bony components. The four anatomic components of the proximal part of the humerus are the head (*1*), lesser tuberosity (*2*), greater tuberosity (*3*), and the shaft (*4*). The anatomic neck is at the junction of the head and tuberosities, and the surgical neck is below the greater and lesser tuberosities (metadiaphyseal junction). **B,** The subscapularis inserts on the lesser tuberosity and causes medial displacement, whereas the supraspinatus and infraspinatus insert on the greater tuberosity and cause superior and posterior displacement. The pectoralis major inserts on the humeral shaft and displaces it medially. (**B**, Modified from Neer CS. *Shoulder Reconstruction.* Philadelphia, WB Saunders; 1990:383.)

The anatomic neck of the proximal humerus is located at the junction of the articular surface and the tuberosities. The surgical neck represents an indistinct region (i.e., metadiaphyseal junction) below the tuberosities but above the humeral shaft. There are prognostic implications regarding the precise location of a PHF. For example, a fracture involving the anatomic neck is prognostically worse than fractures involving other regions of the proximal humerus with respect to the potential disruption of the vascular supply to the humeral head and the subsequent development of avascular necrosis (AVN; Fig. 6-2).[93,115,145]

The GT, which is located in a posterior-superior location with respect to the humeral shaft, serves as the attachment site for the supraspinatus, infraspinatus, and teres minor tendons of the rotator cuff. The LT, located on the anterior aspect of the proximal humerus, serves as the attachment site for the subscapularis tendon.

The glenoid is a convex structure of shallow depth shaped like an inverted pear. It articulates with the humeral head, and serves as the attachment for the labrum and joint capsule.[66]

The acromion, the coracoacromial ligament, and the coracoid process form the coracoacromial arch, a rigid bony-ligamentous structure that imparts stability to the shoulder girdle. The rotator cuff, subacromial bursa, and subdeltoid bursa pass underneath the coracoacromial arch. Displaced PHFs can impede normal movement of these structures, causing impingement and disruption of normal glenohumeral motion. In PHFs (displaced and nondisplaced fractures), the subdeltoid and subacromial bursae can become thickened and fibrotic, forming adhesions that can similarly limit normal glenohumeral motion. Early ROM exercises after a fracture have been hypothesized to decrease the formation of such adhesions.[164]

The proximal humerus receives its blood supply from the anterior and posterior humeral circumflex branches from the third division of the axillary artery. The posterior humeral circumflex artery travels with the axillary nerve, enters the quadrilateral space posteriorly, and anastomoses with a branch of the anterior circumflex to supply the posterior cuff. The anterior humeral circumflex artery (AHCA) arises from the axillary artery at the inferior border of the subscapularis, and provides vascular inflow to the humeral head by way of its terminal anterolateral branch known as the *artery of Laing* (also known as the *arcuate artery*).[93,96,145] The ascending branch of the AHCA

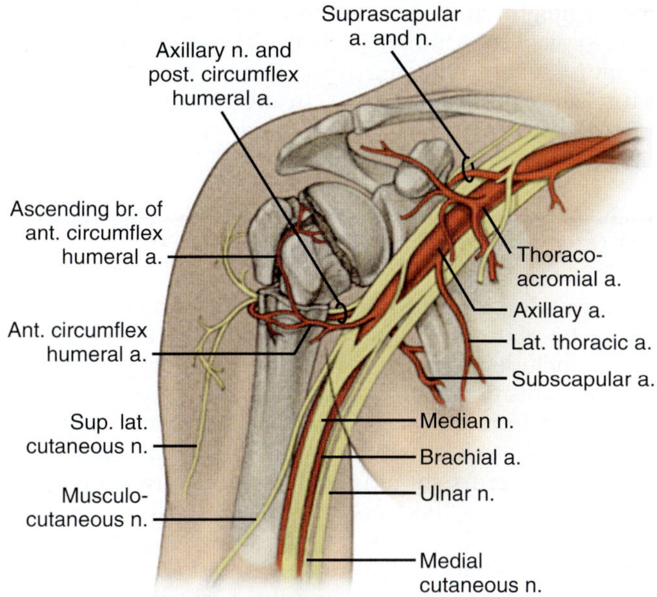

FIGURE 6-2: The brachial plexus and axillary artery lie adjacent to the coracoid process and can be injured with fractures of the proximal end of the humerus. The humeral head receives its blood supply through contributions from the anterior and posterior humeral circumflex arteries. The ascending branch of the anterior humeral circumflex artery penetrates the head at the superior aspect of the bicipital groove and becomes the arcuate artery. Three important nerves are located about the shoulder: the axillary, suprascapular, and musculocutaneous. *ant.*, anterior; *br.*, branch; *lat.*, lateral; *post.*, posterior; *sup.*, superior.

courses parallel to the lateral aspect of the long head biceps tendon, and enters the humeral head at the interface of the bicipital groove and GT (Fig. 6-3A). Injury to the arcuate artery may result in osteonecrosis of the humeral head[93,145]; however, additional extraosseous collateral branches can permit humeral head perfusion despite complete ligation of the arcuate artery.[40] A recent anatomic study has demonstrated that the posterior humeral circumflex artery provides nearly 64% of the blood supply to the humeral head, which may in part explain the relatively low rates of AVN following displaced PHFs (Fig. 6-3B).[115,116]

Vascular injuries following PHFs are uncommon, occurring in 5% to 6% of cases.[22,167] When vascular injuries do occur, they typically involve the axillary artery at the level of the surgical neck just proximal to the trifurcation of the anterior and posterior circumflex and subscapular arteries (i.e., the third part of the axillary artery).[22,167] Most axillary artery injuries occur in patients older than 50 years of age, suggesting that comorbid conditions (e.g., arteriosclerosis) may play a role in this increased incidence.[22,167] A careful neurologic examination must be performed in addition to the vascular assessment secondary to a high correlation between axillary artery and brachial plexus injuries.[22,167]

The brachial plexus (C5-T1 nerve roots, with small contributions from the C3 and C4 nerve roots) provides innervation to the shoulder complex. The most commonly injured nerve following a PHF is the axillary nerve, and it is most susceptible to injury during anterior fracture-dislocations.[255] The axillary nerve arises from the posterior cord of the brachial plexus (C5 and C6 nerve roots), and travels posterior to the surgical neck through

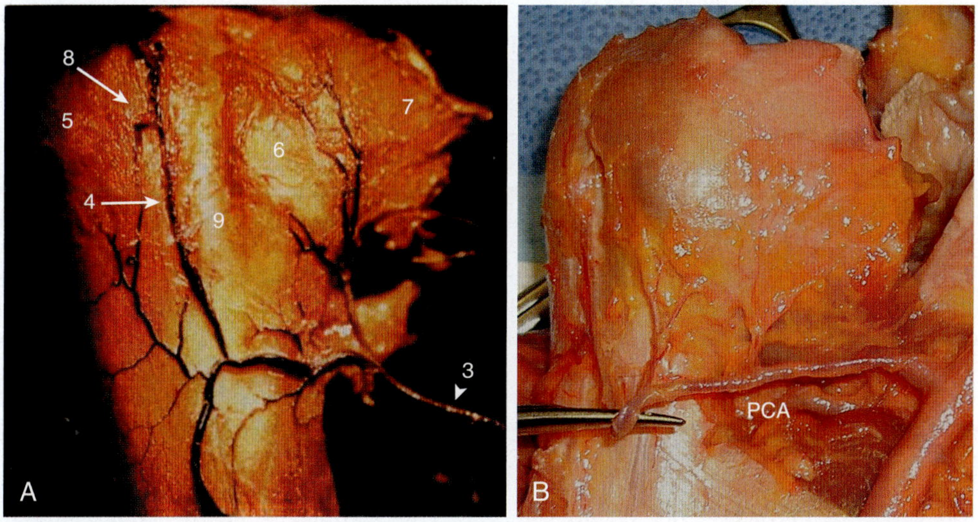

FIGURE 6-3: A, Vascular supply of the anterior humeral head (anterior view). *3,* Anterior humeral circumflex artery; *4,* anterolateral branch of the anterior humeral circumflex artery (arcuate artery); *5,* greater tuberosity; *6,* lesser tuberosity; *7,* insertion of the subscapularis; *8,* site of terminal entry of the arcuate artery into the bone; *9,* bicipital groove. **B,** Vascular supply of the posterior humeral head (posterior view). *PCA,* posterior circumflex artery. (**A,** From Gerber C, Schneeberger AG, Vinh TS. The arterial vascularization of the humeral head: an anatomical study. *J Bone Joint Surg Am.* 1990;72:1486-1494. **B,** From Hettrich CM, Boraiah S, Dyke JP, et al. Quantitative assessment of the vascularity of the proximal part of the humerus. *J Bone Joint Surg Am.* 2010;92:943-948.)

the quadrilateral space along with the posterior humeral circumflex artery. The posterior trunk of the nerve innervates the posterior deltoid and teres minor muscles; a terminal branch of the posterior trunk forms the superior lateral cutaneous nerve of the arm that provides sensation to the overlying deltoid region. The anterior trunk of the nerve continues along the deep surface of the deltoid muscle, and provides branches to the middle and anterior deltoid heads (see Fig. 6-2). Lastly, the axillary nerve supplies an articular branch. Previous anatomic studies documenting the course of the axillary nerve have demonstrated that the mean distance from the proximal aspect of the humerus to the nerve is 6.1 cm (range, 4.5 to 6.9 cm), and the mean distance from the surgical neck of the humerus to the nerve is 1.7 cm (range, 0.7 to 4.0 cm).[34]

The suprascapular nerve, the second most commonly injured nerve, originates from the upper trunk (C5 and C6 nerve roots), and provides motor innervation to the supraspinatus and infraspinatus muscles. This nerve is most susceptible to tractional injury at two locations: the upper trunk where the nerve originates, and the suprascapular notch where the nerve passes below the transverse scapular ligament.[255,256]

The musculocutaneous nerve originates from the lateral cord of the plexus (C5-C7 nerve roots), passes through the conjoint tendon at a variable distance from the coracoid process (3.1 to 8.2 cm), and terminates at the lateral antebrachial cutaneous nerve, supplying sensation to the anterolateral forearm. Injury to the musculocutaneous nerve is a rare event, but can occur with blunt trauma and traction injuries to the shoulder, resulting in the loss of active elbow flexion.[80,81]

Electromyographic studies should be completed between 3 and 6 weeks if clinical recovery is not apparent by physical examination. Documentation of motor denervation without improvement on additional studies may warrant surgical exploration for complete injuries at 3 to 6 months.[155,255,256] Early consultation with a peripheral nerve surgeon is paramount in the proper and timely management of such injuries. Hems and Mahmood retrospectively evaluated 100 patients with injuries to the infraclavicular brachial plexus and noted axillary nerve injury in 15 patients (i.e., 15%) with a PHF due to medial displacement of the humeral shaft. They concluded that specific injury patterns increase the likelihood of nerve injury and that surgical neck fractures require urgent surgical management to decompress the terminal branches of the plexus.[113]

MECHANISM OF INJURY

The most common cause of PHFs is a fall on an outstretched hand from standing height (or less), particularly in patients older than 60 years of age.* Less commonly, high-energy trauma such as a motor vehicle accident, fall from a height, and seizure; these injury mechanisms are more typical in younger patients. These injuries tend to be more severe with regard to the fracture pattern and soft tissue compromise.[67,97,229] In the setting of metastatic bone disease or primary malignancy, a pathologic fracture can occur with minimal trauma.[155]

**References 10, 22, 30, 34, 40, 56, 57, 66, 80, 81, 93, 96, 118, 120, 123, 124, 133, 145, 153, 155, 167, 185, 196, 201, 244, 255, 256.*

CLINICAL EVALUATION

A thorough history and physical examination should always be performed on a patient with a PHF. The history should include patient age, hand dominance, occupation, the mechanism of injury, concomitant injuries, history of malignancy, premorbid level of function, and the ability to participate in a structured rehabilitation program.[225] A review of systems should include queries regarding loss of consciousness, neck pain, ipsilateral elbow or wrist pain, and paresthesias of the hand and upper limb. On physical examination, the surgeon should look for swelling, ecchymosis, soft tissue injuries, and gross deformity. Most patients present with guarding, holding the arm in internal rotation (i.e., forearm overlying the abdomen). Any attempt at active or passive movement elicits significant pain. Palpation of the shoulder reveals crepitus.[155] A careful neurovascular assessment should include evaluation of the brachial plexus, axillary nerve, and axillary artery. Posterior fracture-dislocations can demonstrate flattening of the anterior aspect of the shoulder, with an associated posterior prominence; anterior fracture-dislocations manifest with the opposite findings.[107] The surgeon should assume a vascular injury, even in the presence of a benign examination, in four-part PHFs with axillary dislocation of the humeral head.[40,155,167]

IMAGING

Radiographic evaluation of the shoulder is often difficult due to patient discomfort, but is critical for treatment decision-making. The shoulder trauma series includes a true anteroposterior (AP) of the glenoid (Grashey view), an axillary lateral view, and a scapular Y lateral view (also known as the *transscapular lateral view*).

The true AP view may be taken with the patient's arm in a sling and with the patient standing, seated, or prone (i.e., the most comfortable position). To obtain this view, the unaffected shoulder must be rotated away 30 to 40 degrees, thus allowing the injured side to rest upon the x-ray plate (Fig. 6-4A). Additional AP views (e.g., internal rotation and external rotation AP views) can be obtained to better reveal LT or GT fractures, respectively.[22,155]

The scapular Y lateral (transscapular lateral) view is obtained by placing the anterior aspect of the affected shoulder against the x-ray plate, with the unaffected side rotated out 40 degrees (Fig. 6-4B). This view is essential for assessing associated fractures of the scapular spine and acromion, acromioclavicular (AC) joint injuries (e.g., type IV injuries), and posterior-superior displacement of GT fractures.

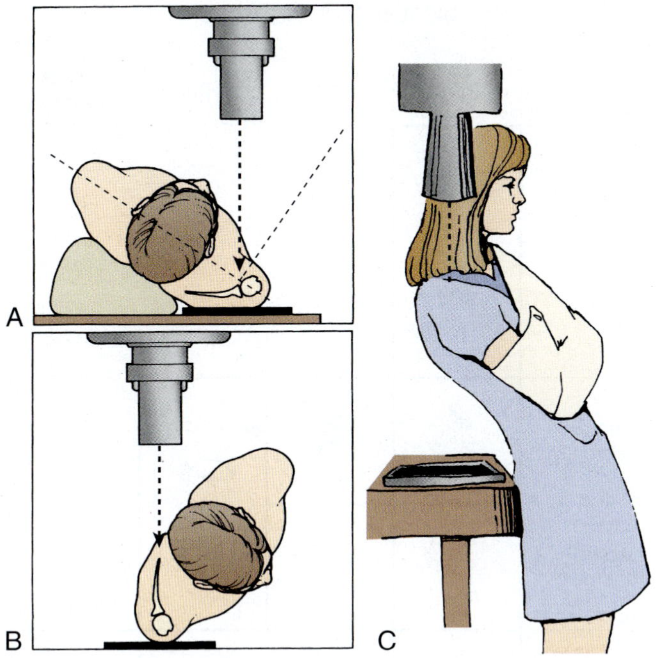

FIGURE 6-4: The trauma series consists of anteroposterior and lateral radiographs in the scapular plane as well as an axillary view. These views may be taken with the patient sitting, standing, or prone. The scapula sits obliquely on the chest wall, and the glenoid surface is tilted approximately 35 to 40 degrees anteriorly. **A,** For the anteroposterior radiograph in the scapular plane (i.e., true AP), the posterior aspect of the affected shoulder is placed up against the x-ray plate, and the opposite shoulder is tilted forward approximately 40 degrees. **B,** For the lateral radiograph in the scapular plane, the anterior aspect of the affected shoulder is placed against the x-ray plate and the other shoulder is tilted forward approximately 40 degrees. The x-ray beam is then placed posteriorly along the scapular spine. **C,** The Velpeau axillary view is preferred after trauma when the patient can be positioned for this view because it allows the shoulder to remain immobilized and avoids further displacement of the fracture fragments. (Modified from Rockwood CA Jr, Green DP, Bucholz RW, Heckman JD. *Fractures in Adults,* 4th ed. Philadelphia: Lippincott-Raven; 1996:1065.)

The axillary view is essential in evaluating the relationship of the humeral head to the glenoid, displacement of the GT, and the glenoid articular surface.[87,170,181] This view can be obtained in the seated, standing, or prone positions. The arm is gently held in 30 degrees of abduction, with an x-ray plate placed on the posterosuperior aspect of the shoulder. The x-ray tube is directed cephalad from a level slightly below the plane of the patient. Due to the nature of the injury, the patient may be unable or unwilling to participate in the abducted axillary view. The Velpeau axillary view is an excellent alternative and is preferred in the trauma setting (Fig. 6-4C; also see Fig. 6-8B). This view is obtained by directing the x-ray beam from superior to inferior as the patient leans backward over the x-ray cassette with his or her arm in a sling.[23]

Magnetic resonance imaging (MRI) is rarely indicated in the setting of an acute injury. If a pathologic fracture is a possibility, then MRI may be useful for staging of the disease. Computed tomography (CT) analysis may be helpful in evaluating tuberosity displacement, the degree of comminution, and glenoid articular surface involvement.[22,107,155] This imaging modality improves the surgeon's ability to make treatment decisions and aids in preoperative surgical planning. A recent review by Berkes et al. did not demonstrate improved interobserver and intraobserver reliability when comparing two- (2D) and three-dimensional (3D) CT imaging with regard to classification and treatment decision-making except among surgeons with limited experience.[15]

CLASSIFICATION

A functional classification scheme should be easy to use, reproducible (i.e., both interobserver and intraobserver reliability), and direct appropriate management. The system must be comprehensive enough to include all variables (patient and fracture variables), but at the same time be specific enough to allow accurate diagnosis and guide treatment.

The most commonly used system is Neer's four-part fracture classification, which was initially reported in 1970.[180] Prior to Neer's system, several others had attempted to classify these injuries according to the fracture location (Kocher [Fig. 6-5]),[136] fracture pattern (Codman [Fig. 6-6], De Anquin and De Anquin, and De Palma and Cautilli),[54,60,65] and injury mechanism (Watson-Jones, Dehne).[259,62]

Jakob and Ganz[127,127a] from the AO (Arbeitsgemeinschaft für Osteosynthesefragen) group proposed a classification scheme involving 27 subgroups based on articular involvement, location, and the degree of comminution and dislocation, with special emphasis on the integrity of the vascular supply. This system helped distinguish valgus-impacted four-part PHFs from other four-part injuries with partial preservation of the vascular inflow to the articular segment through the medial capsule.[96,128,194] The complexity of this system has generally precluded its routine use, despite similar interobserver and intraobserver reliability when compared with Neer's classification system.[237]

The interobserver and intraobserver reliability of the Neer classification system has been previously challenged; however, it remains the most reliable and commonly used system for assessing PHFs.[20,41,182,221,230,239] The classification scheme is based on four segments or parts: the humeral shaft, articular surface, GT, and LT, with emphasis on identifying fracture patterns that are associated with vascular injury to the humeral head (Fig. 6-7). Displacement occurs when a segment or part (articular surface, GT or LT, shaft) has separated more than 1 cm or angulated more than 45 degrees. If this criterion is not met, the fracture is considered minimally displaced, although multiple segments may be involved.[180]

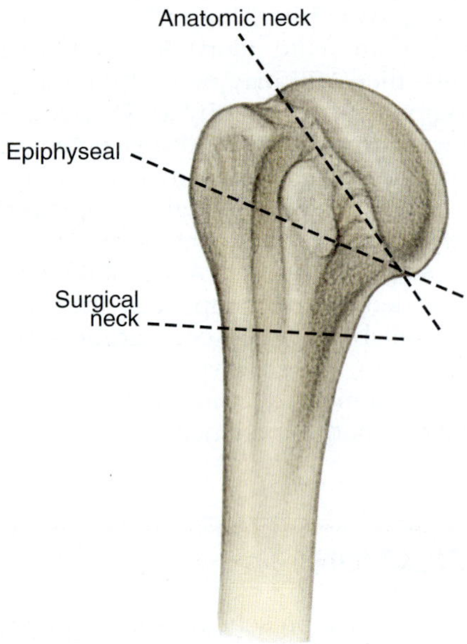

FIGURE 6-5: The Kocher classification is based on three anatomic levels of fractures: anatomic neck, epiphyseal region, and surgical neck. This classification does not allow differentiation of multiple fractures at two different sites, nor does it differentiate between displaced and nondisplaced fractures. (Modified from Kocher T. *Beitrage zur Kenntnis einiger praktisch wichtiger Fracturenformen.* Basel: Carl Sallman Verlag; 1896.)

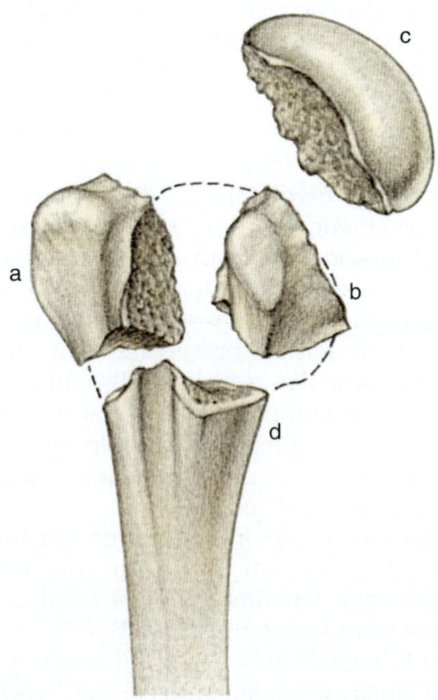

FIGURE 6-6: Codman divided the proximal end of the humerus into four distinct fragments that occur along anatomic lines of epiphyseal union. He differentiated the four major fragments as *a*, greater tuberosity; *b*, lesser tuberosity; *c*, head; and *d*, shaft. (Modified from Codman EA. *The Shoulder: Rupture of the Supraspinatus Tendon and Other Lesions in or About the Subacromial Bursa.* Boston: Thomas Todd; 1934.)

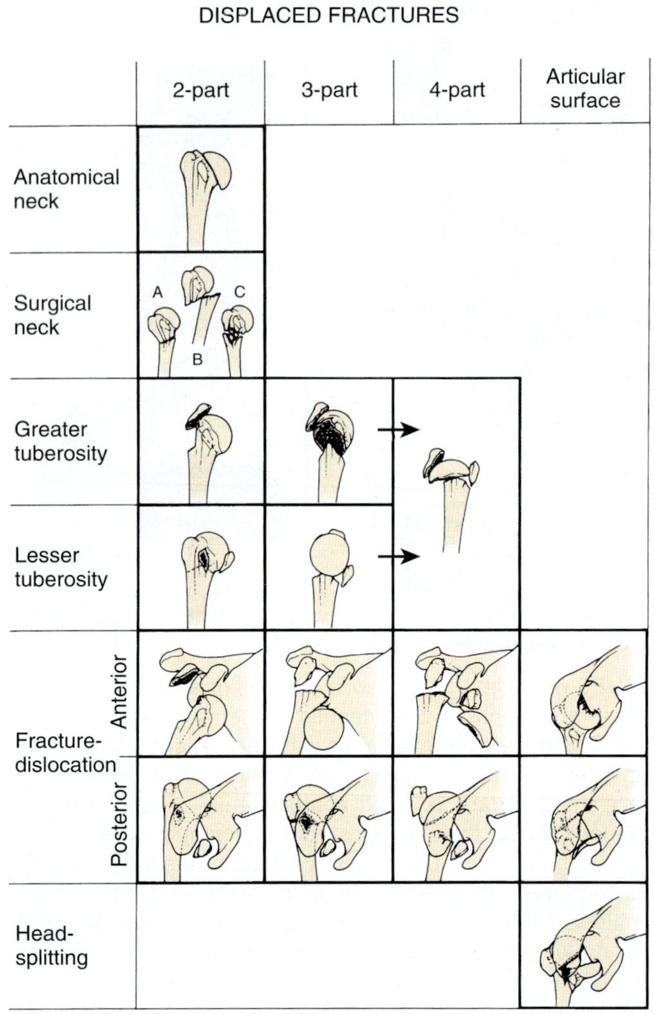

FIGURE 6-7: The Neer classification is a comprehensive system that encompasses anatomy and biomechanical forces that result in the displacement of fracture fragments. A displaced fracture is either two-, three-, or four-part. In addition, fracture-dislocations can be either two-, three-, or four-part. A fragment is considered displaced when it has more than 1 cm of separation or is angulated more than 45 degrees from the other fragments. Impression fractures of the articular surface also occur and are usually associated with an anterior or posterior dislocation. Head-splitting fractures are generally associated with fractures of the tuberosities or surgical neck. (Modified from Neer CS. Displaced proximal humeral fractures. Part I. Classification and evaluation. *J Bone Joint Surg Am.* 1970;52:1077-1089.)

Neer additionally focused on fracture-dislocations of the proximal humerus, head-splitting fractures, and impression fractures of the humeral head. Fracture-dislocations are classified according to the direction of the humeral head dislocation (anterior or posterior) in conjunction with additional displacement of the fracture segments. Head-splitting and impression fractures have specific features of articular surface involvement and have been subdivided according to the percentage of involvement (<20%, 25% to 40%, and >45%) to direct treatment. Classification of these injuries depends on proper radiographs (i.e., shoulder trauma series) and adequate knowledge of the proximal humerus anatomy, including the rotator cuff insertions.

Some authors have attempted to improve the reliability of the Neer classification with CT imaging, but no evidence of decreased variability has been demonstrated with this modality. The same authors have concluded that classification of PHFs remains a difficult task, with reproducibility depending on the surgeon's experience and level of expertise.[16,20,41,182,221,230,238,239] Shrader et al. assert that the problem lies not with an understanding of the classification scheme but with the comprehension of the complex imaging.[236] Similarly, Bruinsma et al.[42] found poor interobserver reliability with the use of 3D CT analysis of PHFs among shoulder and elbow specialists and orthopedic traumatologists.

Hertel et al.[115] modified Codman's original classification to evaluate the predictors of humeral head ischemia after intracapsular fractures of the proximal humerus. According to the authors, the most relevant predictors of ischemia were the length of the dorsomedial metaphyseal extension, integrity of the medial hinge, and basic fracture pattern.[115] The combination of an anatomic neck fracture, short calcar segment (<8 mm of metaphyseal extension), and disrupted medial hinge demonstrated a positive predictive value of 97% when determining humeral head ischemia. Fracture displacement proved less important with regard to humeral head viability. These earlier findings have since been reevaluated by Bastian and Hertel[11] and questioned by Campochiaro et al.[46] Hertel reported on the development of AVN in 51 patients with intracapsular fractures of the proximal humerus. Of the 10 humeral heads that were initially deemed "ischemic," only two developed collapse at the last follow-up, indicating the possibility of revascularization. In contrast, four of the 30 well-perfused humeral heads developed structural changes indicative of AVN. Campochiaro et al.[46] reported a 3.4% rate of AVN in 267 PHFs that were treated with plate and screw fixation, despite "poor quality of reduction" in 50% of cases. The authors concluded that "Hertel's criteria are important in the surgical planning but are not sufficient." These authors also concluded that 3D CT analysis of the medial calcar should be performed to more accurately apply Hertel's criteria.[46]

In a recent study evaluating the reliability of classification systems, Majed et al. determined that the Codman-Hertel classification scheme achieved the highest interobserver score, followed by the Neer and AO/Orthopaedic Trauma Association classification systems.[159] Despite these findings, the Neer classification remains the most commonly used system by orthopedic surgeons for treating PHFs.

METHODS OF TREATMENT

The vast majority of PHFs are minimally displaced or angulated, and do not require surgical intervention.[54,75,155,174,209,216,227] Early protection with gradual mobilization is the guiding principle with nondisplaced injuries. The patient generally wears a sling with an axillary pad for comfort and to prevent skin irritation. The patient is encouraged to perform active finger, hand, wrist, and elbow exercises. The sling is to be used for comfort; most patients are able to wean from the sling between weeks 3 and 6 (often dependent on fracture pattern and patient factors). By 7 to 10 days, gentle passive and active-assisted ROM and pendulum exercises may be initiated as tolerated under the supervision of a physical therapist. Delay of motion beyond 2 weeks has deleterious effects on shoulder ROM, pain, and function.[17,117,141,142] Serial biplanar radiographs should be obtained to monitor possible interval fracture displacement or angulation. ROM gains are generally noted between weeks 3 and 8.[17] By 6 weeks, patients may begin to use the affected arm for activities of daily living (ADLs) as tolerated to improve muscular strength and endurance. Formal strengthening exercises are initiated once there is radiographic evidence of progressive fracture healing and consolidation and when the ROM is approximately 75% to 80% that of the contralateral side.

Approximately 20% of PHFs are comminuted or displaced, and require surgical intervention by means of closed reduction with percutaneous fixation, open reduction and internal fixation (ORIF), or shoulder arthroplasty (i.e., hemiarthroplasty or reverse total shoulder arthroplasty [RTSA]).[65,155] When deciding whether to pursue operative treatment of a PHF, one must collectively consider both the patient (premorbid health status, physiologic age, activity level, and ability to comply with postoperative rehabilitation) and fracture-specific characteristics (severity of the fracture including the degree of displacement and comminution, bone quality, and rotator cuff status).[51] Patients with low demands and significant medical comorbidities (e.g., dementia) should be managed nonoperatively.[117] The ideal goal of treatment, whether operative or nonoperative, is to reestablish a functional pain-free ROM. It is important to note that most of the published treatment algorithms for PHFs are generally based on case series (level IV evidence) in which a single treatment option has been isolated and assessed for efficacy.[240]

Treatment Considerations According to Fracture Subtype

Greater Tuberosity Fractures

Epidemiology

Isolated displaced fractures of GT account for a small percentage of PHFs.[97] Chun et al., in their review of two-part PHFs, reported that 26 of 141 (18%) were displaced GT fractures.[52] As an uncommon event, these injuries may be overlooked or trivialized by orthopedic surgeons and other healthcare providers (Fig. 6-8).

Nature of the Injury

The amount of tuberosity displacement guides the decision-making regarding surgical intervention. In view of Neer's criteria regarding displacement, most authors agree that the shoulder has little tolerance for GT

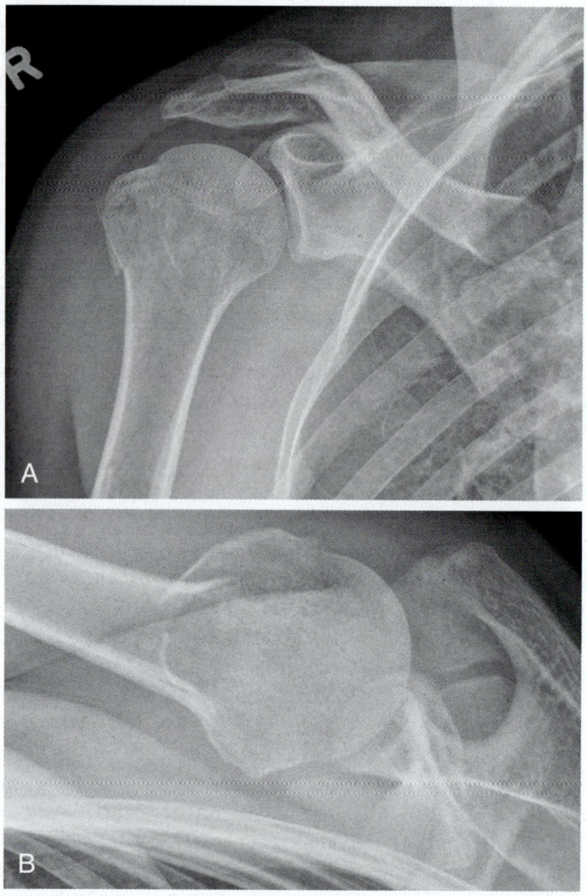

FIGURE 6-8: **A,** True anteroposterior radiograph showing a minimally displaced greater tuberosity fracture in a 36-year-old, right-hand dominant female after a fall onto an outstretched arm. The injury mechanism described by the patient involved hyperabduction of the arm. **B,** Modified axillary radiograph (i.e., Velpeau view) reveals minimal displacement of the fracture. (Courtesy Aaron J. Bois, MD.)

displacement. McLaughlin suggested that displacement of 5 mm or more can cause impingement and rotator cuff dysfunction.[166] Furthermore, Park et al. have suggested that fractures in manual laborers or athletes with as little as 3 mm of displacement should be surgically reduced.[199] The direction of displacement of the tuberosity is just as important as the amount of displacement. Posterior displacement can affect external rotation, but is generally better tolerated than superior displacement, which results in subacromial impingement and weakness with active elevation.

Different mechanisms of injury have been proposed for GT fractures, including impaction (direct fall onto the shoulder or a fall on an outstretched hand forcing the shoulder into hyperabduction, causing compression of GT against the acromion; see Fig. 6-8) or avulsion and shearing (anterior glenohumeral joint dislocation causing the tuberosity to shear across the glenoid rim; Fig. 6-9), although the pathomechanics have not been clearly elucidated.[7]

Peripheral nerve injury is the most commonly associated injury, occurring in nearly 33% of patients following a shoulder fracture-dislocation.[90,148,251] Nearly 50% of patients older than 50 years of age with an anterior shoulder fracture-dislocation have been found to have a peripheral nerve injury. Isolated axillary nerve injuries are the most common nerve injury associated with two-part GT fracture-dislocations.[64,200]

Evaluation

The initial evaluation of a patient with an injured shoulder has been previously discussed including a detailed history and physical examination followed by plain radiographs (i.e., shoulder trauma series). Advanced imaging such as CT and/or MRI are not routinely used; however, 3D CT may be utilized to delineate GT displacement (Fig. 6-10).[97]

Treatment

Nonoperative Management

Nonoperative treatment is reserved for nondisplaced and minimally displaced GT fractures and for low-demand elderly patients. This treatment includes a brief period of sling immobilization for 1 to 2 weeks. Passive ROM exercises are started as early as 7 to 10 days postinjury, starting with pendulum exercises and advancing to stick exercises below the horizontal plane for the first 4 weeks. Passive ROM exercises in all planes as tolerated are encouraged after 4 weeks when there is radiographic evidence of fracture healing and stability without interval displacement. By 6 weeks, patients are permitted to begin active-assisted and active ROM exercises in the form of ADLs, and progressive strengthening exercises may be initiated once there is radiographic evidence of progressive fracture healing and the patient has regained near-normal motion (Fig. 6-11).[97]

In 2013, Rath et al.[210] reported the short-term clinical outcomes of 69 patients following nonoperative treatment of minimally displaced GT fractures (<3 mm). The average Constant score improved from 40 points to 95 points. Of interest, the mean duration of pain relief and improvement in ROM from the time of injury was 8.1 months. Hébert-Davies et al.[112] recently reported a 26% incidence of GT fracture migration in patients younger than 70 years of age when the injury resulted from a fracture-dislocation. Displacement of the GT was 5.6 times more likely with dislocation than without. This reinforces the need for early radiographic surveillance and patient counseling that surgery may be required even when the initial postreduction radiographs reveal a near-anatomic fracture position.[112]

Operative Management

Operative intervention is recommended for GT fractures with more than 5 mm of displacement to prevent fracture malunion and subsequent pain, stiffness, and rotator cuff dysfunction.[166] Patients are placed in the semisitting ("beach chair") position under general anesthesia. An interscalene nerve block may be considered for postoperative pain control, which is performed in the recovery room after a neurovascular examination has been performed on the

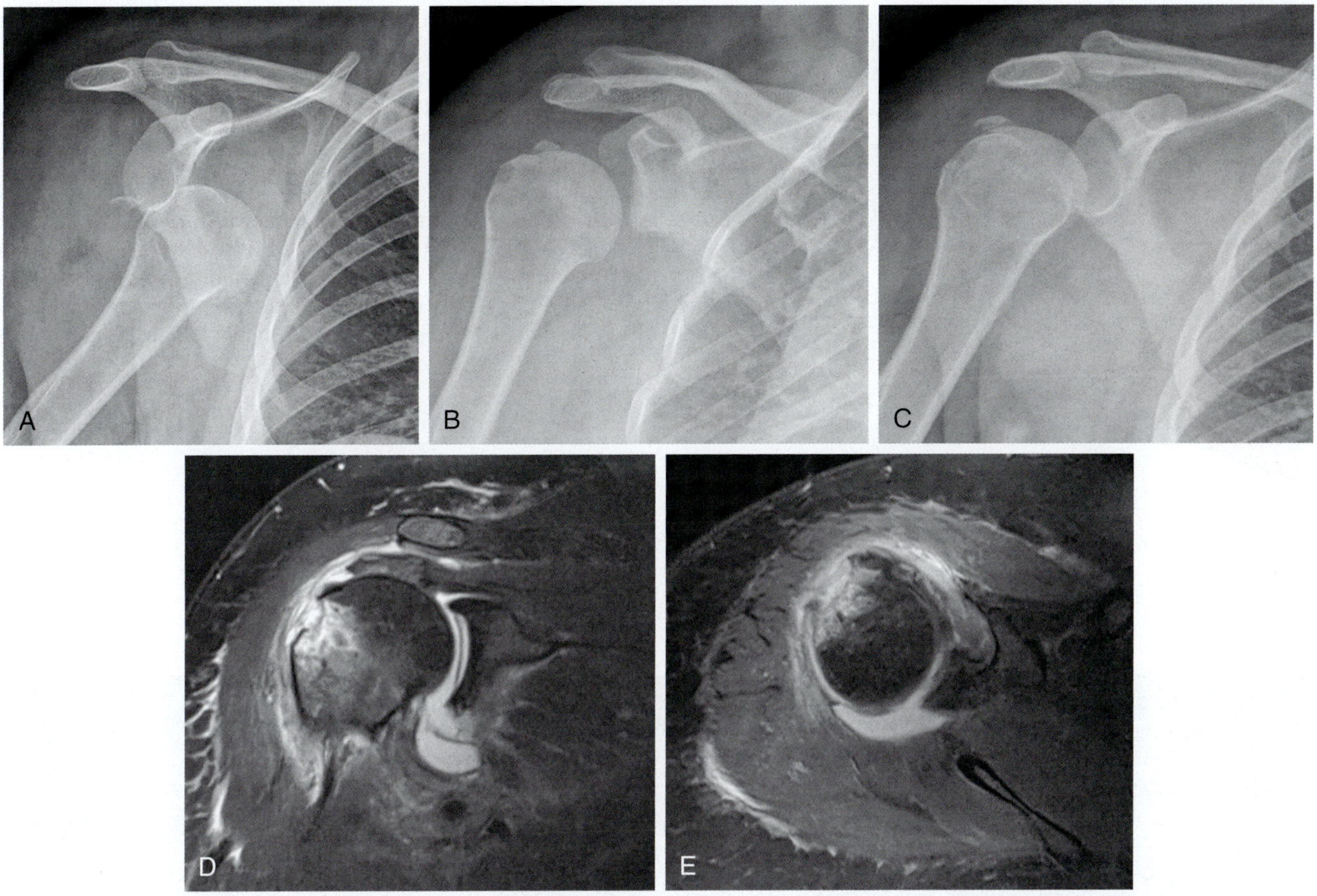

FIGURE 6-9: **A,** Anteroposterior radiograph of a two-part anterior fracture-dislocation with a displaced greater tuberosity (GT) fracture (i.e., avulsion-type fracture fragment). **B** and **C,** True anteroposterior (AP) and AP internal rotation radiographs after closed reduction reveals superior and posterior displacement of the GT fracture fragment(s). **D** and **E,** Coronal and axial magnetic resonance imaging demonstrates medial displacement of the tuberosity fragment(s) with attached rotator cuff tendons. Note the moderate-sized bony defect remaining in the region of the posterolateral wall of the greater tuberosity. (Courtesy Aaron J. Bois, MD.)

operative extremity. An arm-positioning device attached to the beach chair may be used to support the operative limb; alternatively, a padded Mayo stand may be used. A C-arm image intensifier is used to obtain AP and axillary views (Fig. 6-12). The C-arm may be positioned from the head of the bed or from the opposite side of the bed (i.e., surgeon preference) to ensure that proper orthogonal views are obtained.

Surgical fixation of displaced GT fractures may be performed using either open, arthroscopic, or arthroscopic-assisted techniques. Regardless of the surgical technique used, the principles are the same for fracture mobilization and reduction, secure fixation, and repair of concomitant pathology such as rotator cuff tears to provide an environment that will permit early ROM. Surgical exposure for open techniques can proceed by way of a superior deltoid-splitting or deltopectoral approach. Some authors have advocated the use of the deltoid-splitting approach due to the relative ease of visualization of the GT fragment. Fracture displacement must be carefully reviewed on preoperative imaging to ensure that the deltoid split is properly positioned to permit adequate mobilization, reduction, and fixation of the GT fragment. If necessary, an acromioplasty can also be performed with this technique to improve surgical exposure; however, this is rarely required.[81] The deltopectoral approach avoids detachment of the deltoid, and allows exposure of the surgical neck when there is a concomitant proximal humeral shaft fracture; however, this surgical approach should be used with caution in isolated two-part GT fractures, especially when there is posterior fracture displacement.

Multiple open techniques for isolated GT fixation have been described and utilize either all-suture or all-screw and/or plate constructs depending on the degree of comminution present. Traditionally, tension banding and cancellous screw fixation techniques have been used for displaced, noncomminuted GT fractures. Recent biomechanical evidence reveals that tension band constructs provide significantly higher load to failure when

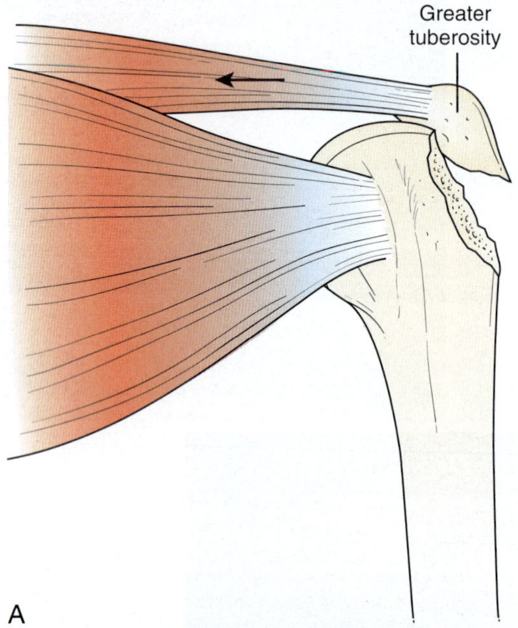

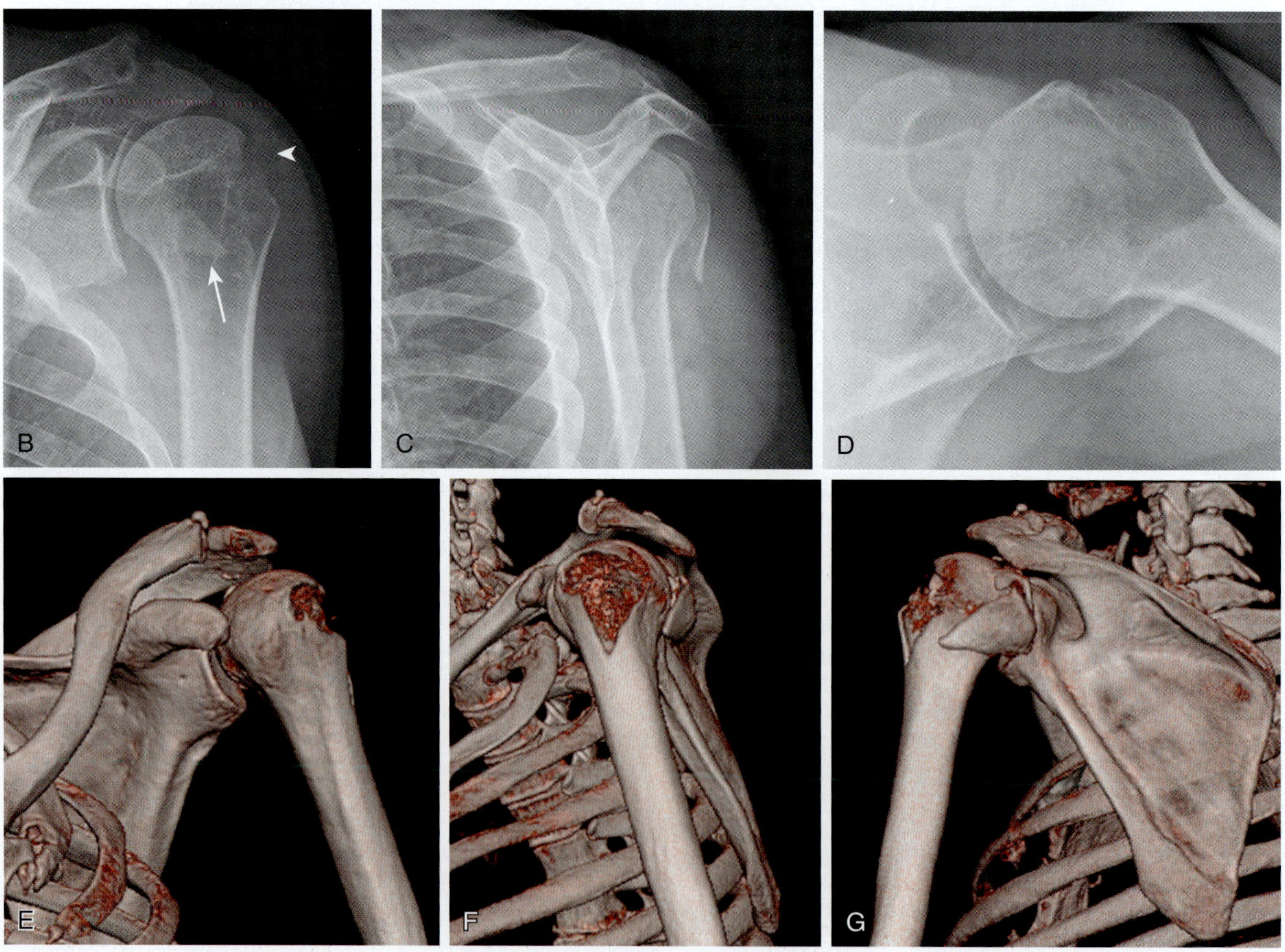

FIGURE 6-10: **A,** Displacement of each "part" occurs in a predictable manner. In cases of two-part fractures involving the greater tuberosity (GT), the supraspinatus and infraspinatus tendons cause superior and posterior displacement of the fracture fragment, respectively. **B,** True anteroposterior radiograph demonstrating a large bony defect and loss of normal contour in the proximal-lateral aspect of the humerus (arrowhead) resulting from a displaced GT fracture (long arrow). **C** and **D,** Transcapular and axillary lateral radiographs reveal a large GT fracture fragment with significant posterior displacement and abutment of the fragment against the posterior glenoid rim. **E** to **G,** Three-dimensional computed tomographic imaging similarly demonstrates a large posteriorly displaced GT fracture fragment. (**A,** Modified from Neer CS. *Shoulder Reconstruction.* Philadelphia: WB Saunders; 1990:377. **B** to **G,** Courtesy Aaron J. Bois, MD.)

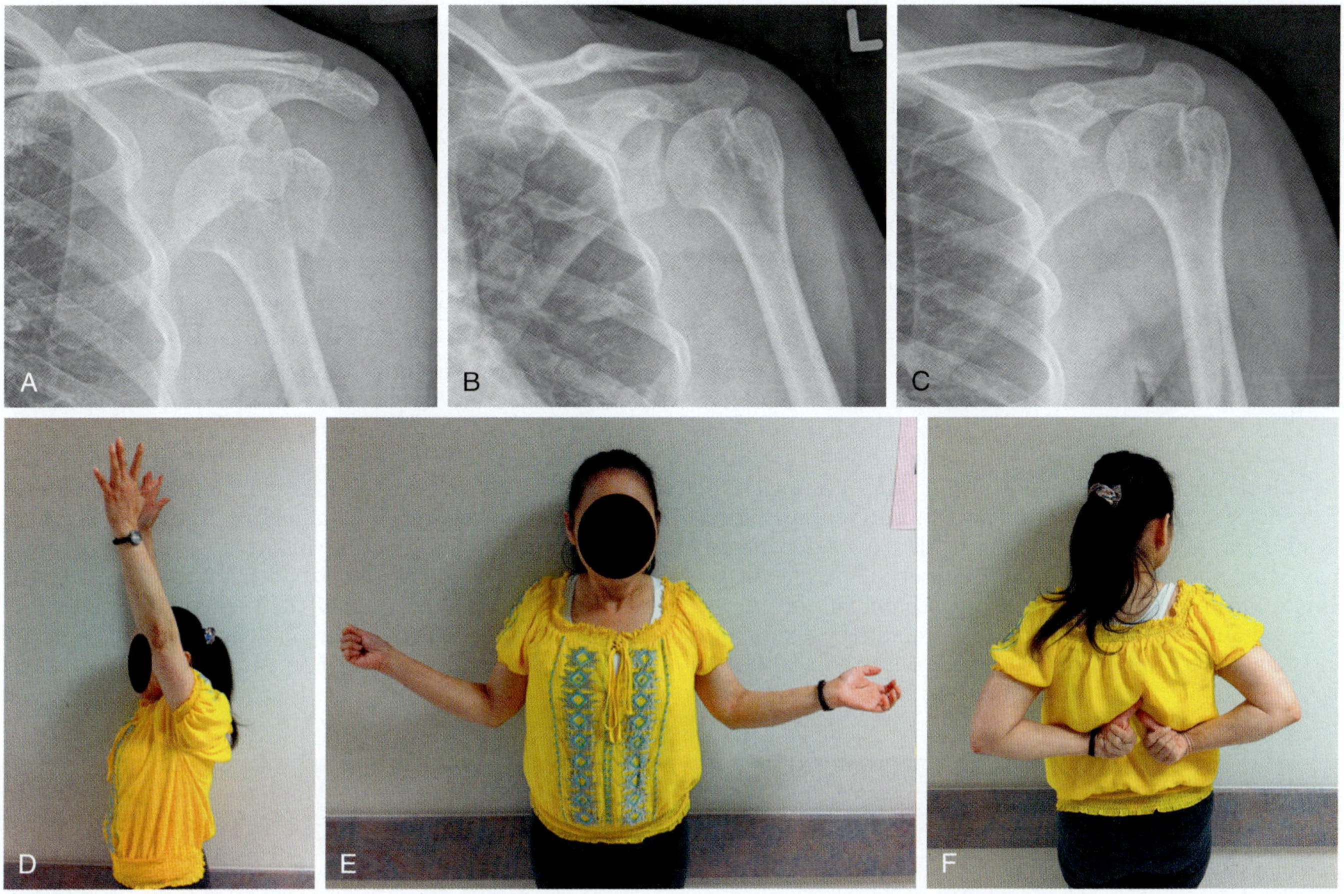

FIGURE 6-11: **A,** Anteroposterior radiograph of a two-part fracture-dislocation with a large displaced greater tuberosity (GT) fracture (left side) in a 53-year-old female following a ground-level fall. **B** and **C,** After closed reduction, the GT fracture reduced and healed without further displacement. **D** to **F,** The patient achieved symmetric range of motion without any further episodes of anterior instability at the 12-month follow-up visit. (Courtesy Aaron J. Bois, MD.)

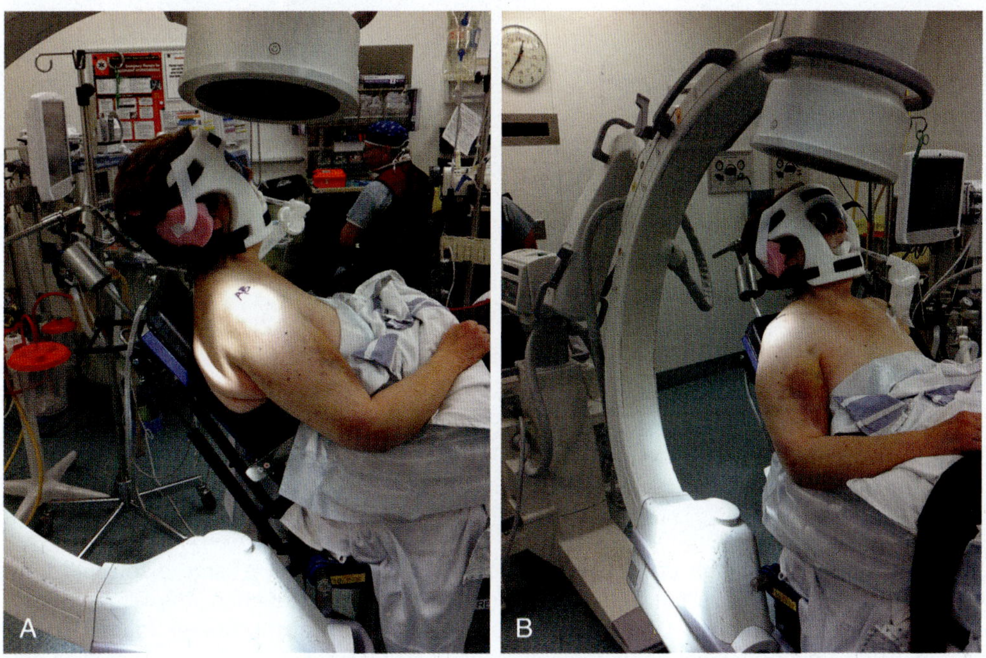

FIGURE 6-12: **A** and **B,** Intraoperative beach chair positioning for concomitant use of C-arm during open reduction and internal fixation of a proximal humerus fracture. The C-arm can either be positioned parallel to the bed and enter from the head of the bed or perpendicular to the bed and enter from the noninjured (contralateral) side. (Courtesy Aaron J. Bois, MD.)

compared with two parallel cancellous screws used alone.[39] Isolated screw fixation is also not recommended because the tuberosity can theoretically fragment or displace around the screw.[97] Screws may be used as a post when placed distal to the fracture when using sutures for tension band fixation. All-suture techniques have also been described using heavy (e.g., No. 5) nonabsorbable sutures placed at the rotator cuff tendon-bone interface, proximally, and through bone tunnels, distally (i.e., transosseous suture construct). Suture constructs used in isolation may fail by suture cutout. More recently, a hybrid fixation construct has been described for noncomminuted and comminuted GT fractures that uses a combination of cancellous screws and suture anchors that are placed distal to the fracture to act as a secondary tension band (Fig. 6-13).[33] Together, each individual construct neutralizes displacing forces created by the other construct and prevents fracture malreduction and subsequent malunion. From a biomechanical standpoint, this hybrid construct may offer fracture stability that theoretically exceeds any single construct and permits early rehabilitation.

Some authors have advocated percutaneous reduction and fixation to minimize soft tissue dissection, although fixation with a single screw or pin remains biomechanically inferior.[91]

Arthroscopic techniques have been described more recently. They have the additional advantage of addressing concomitant pathology such as rotator cuff and labral tears that may be present in patients with an anterior fracture-dislocation. The GT fracture fragment can be visualized and reduced using a grasper device and internally stabilized with pins or screws.[249] Some authors have advocated the use of a suture bridge and double row techniques solely through arthroscopic means with mixed results.[129,242] There are limitations to this technique, specifically in the following settings: (1) subacute presentation and severely displaced GT fractures may preclude reduction due to early fracture healing and soft tissue contracture; (2) large GT fracture fragments may be difficult to visualize and reduce; (3) all-arthroscopic constructs may be technically challenging for those surgeons without specialized training in arthroscopy.[92] Yin et al. have appropriately emphasized that the surgeon must comprehend the "personality" of the fracture pattern, as this often dictates the surgical approach (open vs. arthroscopic) and method of fixation.[267]

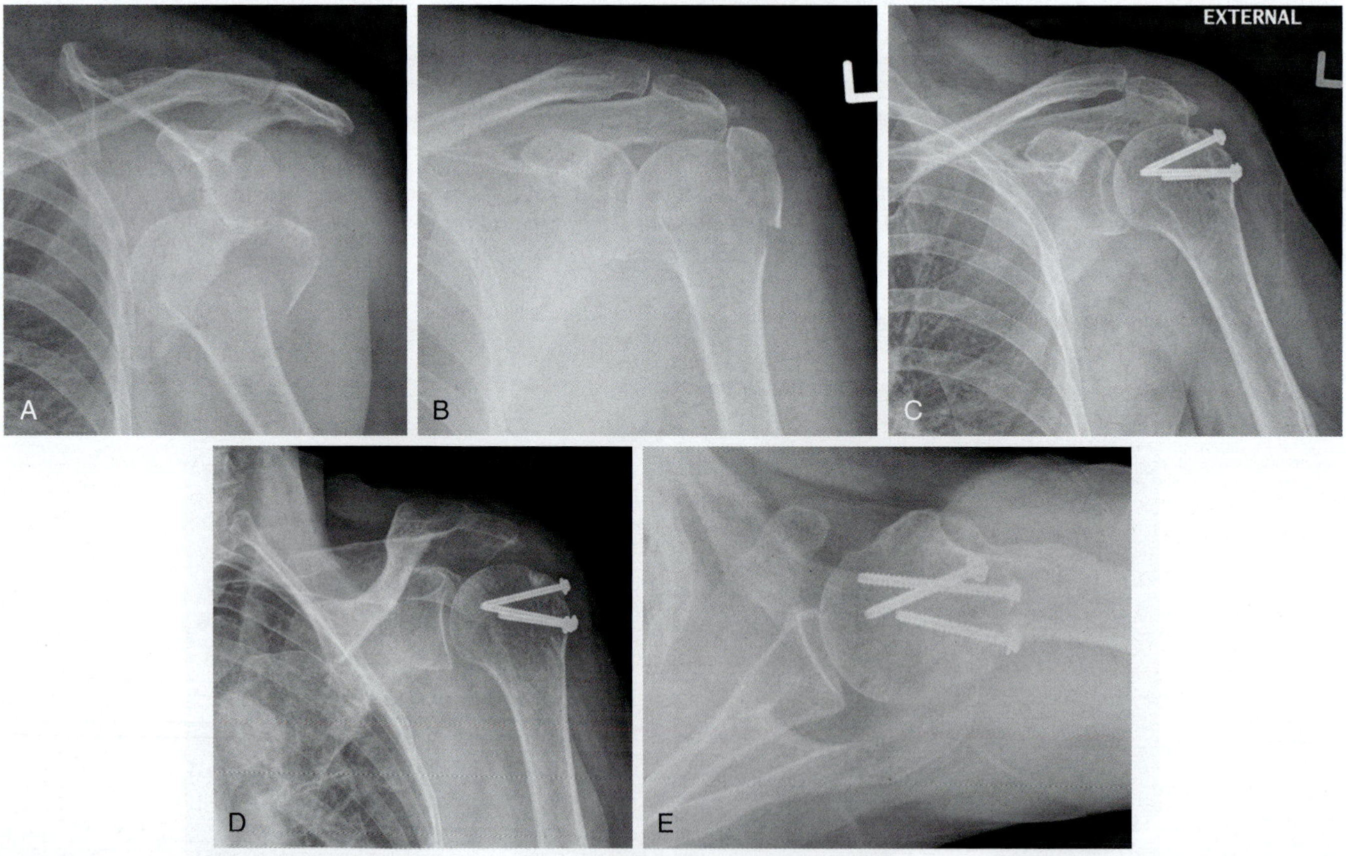

FIGURE 6-13: A, Anteroposterior radiograph of a two-part fracture-dislocation with a large displaced greater tuberosity (GT) fracture in a 61-year-old female following a fall from a height. **B,** After closed reduction, the GT fracture fragment remained displaced in a posterior and superior position. **C** to **E,** Postoperative radiographs at the 8-week follow-up visit after open reduction and internal fixation using a hybrid technique (partially threaded screws and suture anchors [not seen on radiograph] placed distal to the metaphyseal fracture line to act as a secondary tension band).[33] (Courtesy Aaron J. Bois, MD.)

Postoperative Care

Postoperative rehabilitation begins the day after surgery, with pendulum, passive forward elevation to the horizontal plane, and adducted external rotation exercises (i.e., stick exercises). Between 4 and 6 weeks postsurgery, passive ROM exercises are permitted in all planes as tolerated. Internal rotation and adduction maneuvers are avoided until 6 weeks postsurgery. After 6 weeks, active ROM exercises are initiated in the form of ADLs, with concurrent passive stretching exercises in all planes as tolerated. Rotator cuff–strengthening exercises are postponed until 10 to 12 weeks postsurgery when there is radiographic evidence of fracture healing. All patients need to be informed that clinical improvement may not be maximized until 1 year postsurgery.[97]

Outcomes

Stiffness, malunion, and nonunion remain the most common complications that can occur after nonoperative or operative treatment of GT fractures. Shoulder stiffness may be treated early with a dedicated passive stretching program; however, the patient should be informed of the possible need to perform an arthroscopic capsular release with or without an acromioplasty to address concomitant impingement.

Osteotomy and mobilization of a malunited GT fragment has unpredictable results,[4,14,] often requiring a rotator cuff interval slide(s) to reduce the fragment and the rotator cuff. Fixation of the mobilized tuberosity fragment can prove tenuous due to significant osteopenia. In the setting of nonunion, the tuberosity may be markedly displaced, making mobilization and repair difficult secondary to scarring.[14,166,188]

There are limited published studies reporting the surgical results of displaced GT fractures. Paavolainen et al. reported good results in the surgical treatment of six displaced fractures with screw fixation.[195] Chun et al. treated 10 GT fractures with ORIF (eight with screws). At a mean follow-up of 5.1 years, the results were graded as excellent in one patient, good in seven, and fair in three according to Neer's criteria. The mean active forward elevation and external rotation were 118 and 35 degrees, respectively.[52] Flatow et al. reported their experience with surgical fixation of 16 displaced GT fractures using heavy nonabsorbable sutures. At 4.5 years of follow-up, the authors reported six excellent and six good results according to Neer's criteria.[81] Park et al. reported 78% "excellent" and 11% "good" results in 13 fractures treated with suture fixation with a mean follow-up of nearly 4.5 years.[198]

Lesser Tuberosity Fractures

Isolated LT fractures without an associated posterior shoulder dislocation or surgical neck fracture are rare.[217] Because of the subscapularis insertion, the LT fragment will displace medially in the event of a fracture. The mechanisms of injury include sudden resisted abduction and external rotation with eccentric loading of the subscapularis and extension and external rotation of an axially loaded humerus. Diagnosis of these injuries remains challenging, often leading to delayed treatment. Patients may have soft tissue swelling and ecchymosis in the axilla associated with internal rotation weakness, evident with a positive Napoleon sign and modified belly-press test. Plain radiographs may not reveal the LT fracture. Supplementary imaging in the form of a CT scan may confirm the surgeon's clinical suspicion. If the fragment is small, minimally displaced, and does not block internal rotation, a short period of immobilization in slight external rotation (to approximate the fragment to the donor site) followed by early passive and active-assisted ROM exercises is appropriate (Fig. 6-14).[52,68,127,189,217,226] Unfortunately, there are no fracture displacement guidelines as there are for GT fractures to assist the surgeon in treatment decision-making for LT fractures. In 2009, Robinson et al.[220] reported the surgical results of isolated displaced LT fractures in 17 patients. The estimated overall incidence reported in this study was low (0.46 per 100,000). Surgical management routinely resulted in restored shoulder function, with a low rate of complications.

More commonly, isolated LT fractures result from a posterior fracture-dislocation of the shoulder. Surgical intervention is recommended for displaced large tuberosity fragments and for those with articular surface involvement.[127,217,226] The tuberosity may be fixed either anatomically or, if present, into the base of the humeral head defect (reverse Hill-Sachs lesion) if the shoulder is unstable after open reduction (with or without cancellous bone graft to backfill the defect).[226] In 2015, Liu et al. reported their results in 22 of 29 patients available for follow-up who underwent ORIF of an LT fracture associated with a locked posterior dislocation. The mean patient age was 41.7 years, and the majority were male (21 of 22). The length of time until the initial surgery was the only prognostic factor to correlate with an inferior outcome; 9 of 22 patients (41%) in this study were misdiagnosed at the time of their initial presentation, leading to a delay in surgical treatment.[154]

Open reduction may proceed using a deltopectoral approach with the LT fragment stabilized with screws, sutures, and/or suture anchor fixation, or a combination of constructs (i.e., hybrid fixation) (Fig. 6-15).[253] One must assess the medial wall of the bicipital groove and possible associated pathology involving the long head biceps tendon (e.g., tears or medial subluxation of the tendon caused by disruption of the biceps pulley); a biceps tenodesis may be required, and should be discussed with the patient preoperatively. Arthroscopic fixation of a displaced LT fragment has been described by Scheibel et al. utilizing a standard posterior viewing portal, anterior and anterosuperior portals, suture relay, and suture anchor fixation of the tuberosity fragment.[233] Rotator interval closure should be considered in cases of persistent posterior subluxation after the primary fracture fixation is completed; during interval closure, the arm should be held in a neutral position to avoid excessive loss of external rotation postoperatively.

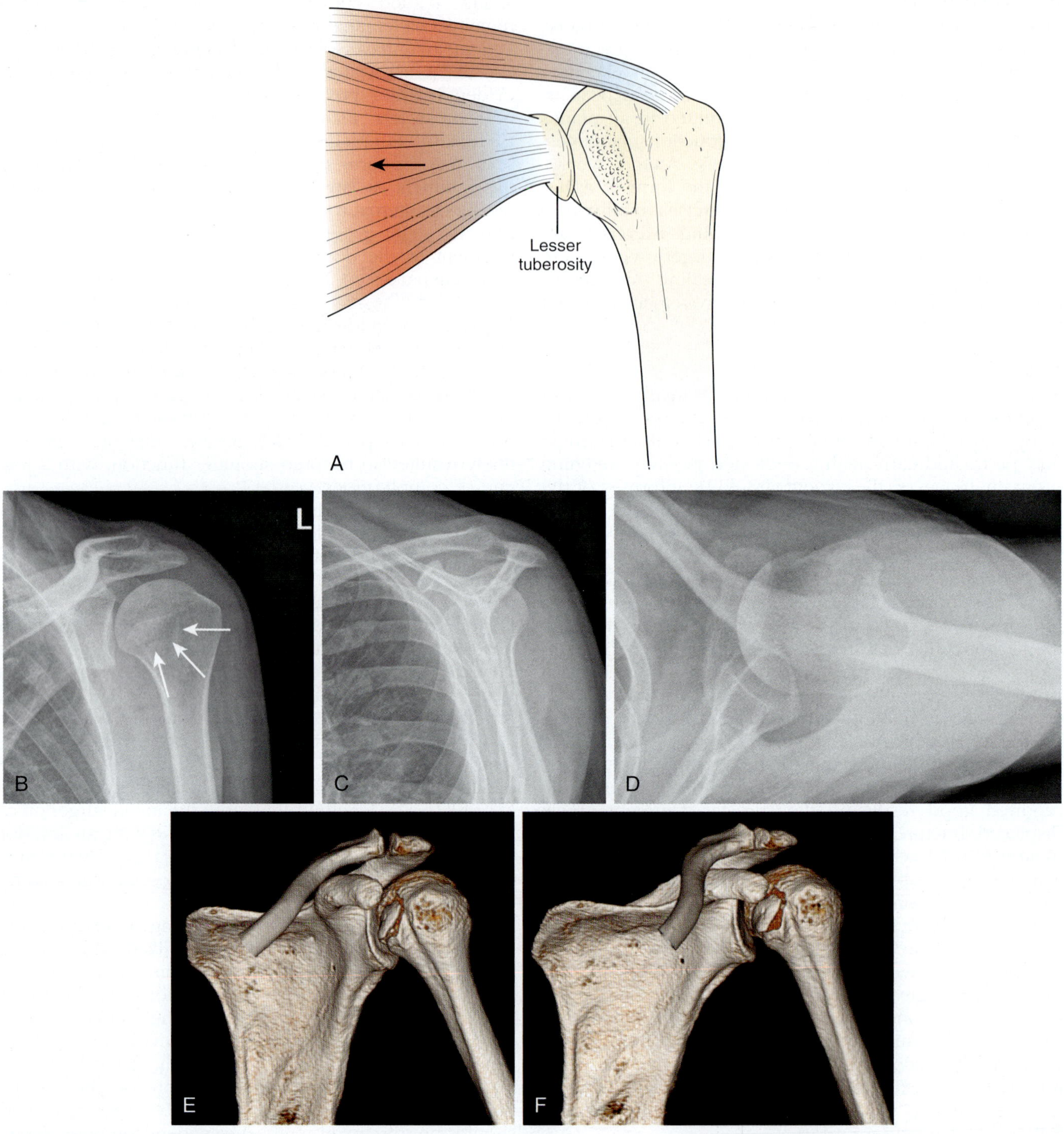

FIGURE 6-14: **A,** Displacement of each "part" occurs in a predictable manner. In cases of two-part fractures involving the lesser tuberosity (LT), the subscapularis tendon causes medial (± inferior) displacement of the fracture fragment. **B,** True anteroposterior radiograph demonstrating a minimally displaced LT fracture in a 46-year-old man following a fall on an outstretched left arm (arrows highlighting fracture lucency). **C** and **D,** Transcapular and axillary lateral radiographs reveal a minimally displaced LT fracture. The fracture is not clearly detected on the transcapular lateral radiograph; however, there is evidence of a small fracture fragment on the axillary radiograph. **E** and **F,** Three-dimensional computed tomographic imaging similarly demonstrates a minimally displaced LT fracture fragment. This injury was treated nonoperatively, with excellent return of function. (**A,** Modified from Neer CS. *Shoulder Reconstruction.* Philadelphia, WB Saunders; 1990:376. **B** to **F,** Courtesy Aaron J. Bois, MD.)

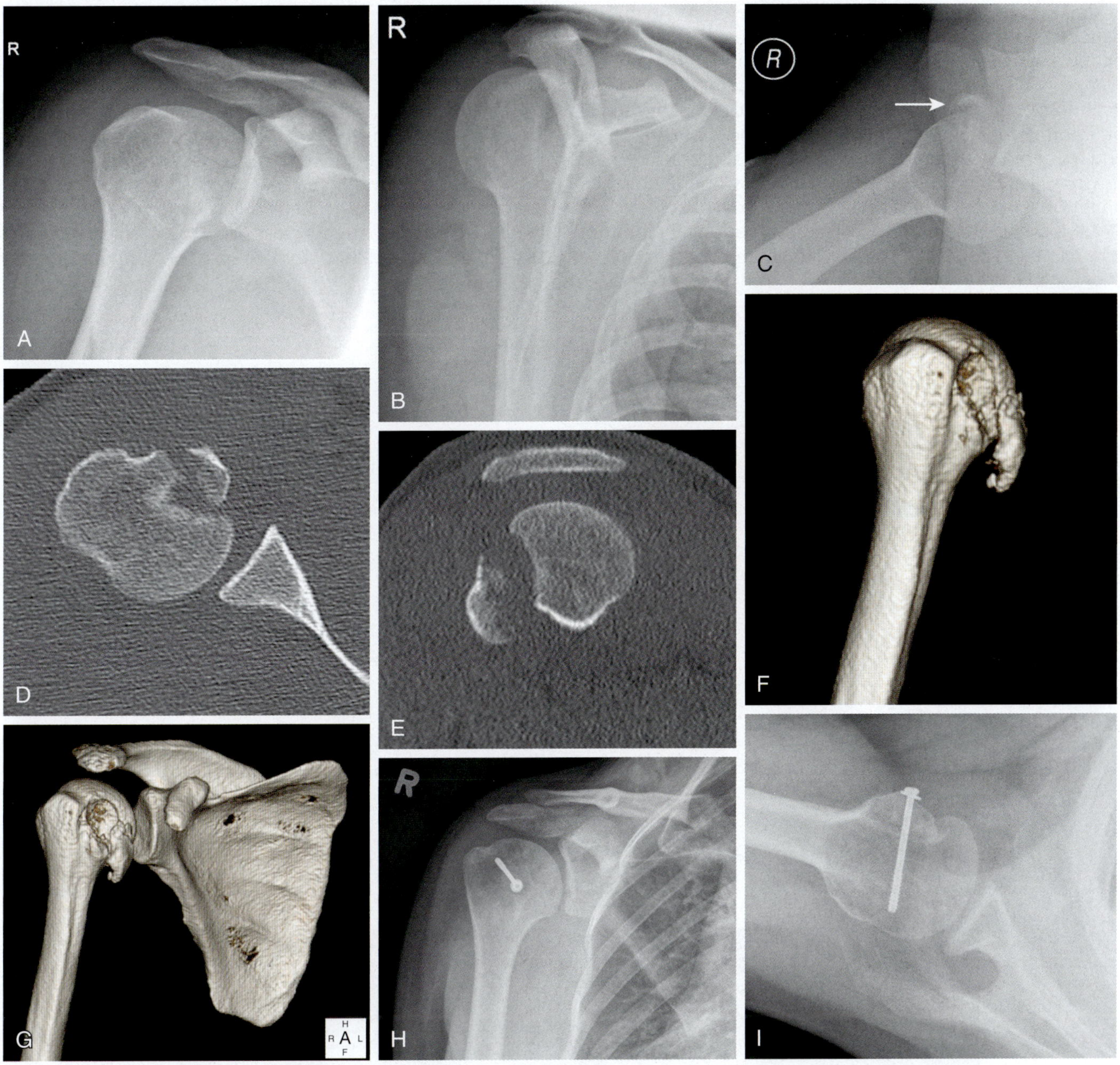

FIGURE 6-15: **A** to **C**, Trauma series demonstrating a two-part fracture-dislocation with a large displaced lesser tuberosity (LT) fracture in a 42-year-old male following a grand mal seizure. Note the displaced LT fracture fragment on the axillary lateral radiograph *(arrow)*. **D** to **G**, Two-dimensional (axial and sagittal cuts) and three-dimensional computed tomographic imaging after closed reduction reveals that the LT fracture fragment remained displaced in an inferior and medial position. **H** and **I**, Postoperative anteroposterior and axillary radiographs at the 12-month follow-up visit following open reduction and internal fixation using a hybrid technique (partially threaded cancellous screw with a washer and transosseous sutures placed from medial to lateral to act as a secondary tension band). (Courtesy Aaron J. Bois, MD.)

Surgical Neck Fractures

Epidemiology

Surgical neck fractures account for the majority (60% to 65%) of PHFs. Nearly 80% of these fractures are minimally displaced and warrant nonoperative management. Surgical indications include fracture displacement, polytrauma, ipsilateral upper extremity injuries, vascular compromise, open fractures, and patient compliance with a postoperative rehabilitation program.[121] Malunion can be tolerated if the tuberosity and articular surface relationships are not distorted.

As Iannotti et al. have suggested, there are two distinct patient populations: young, male patients with high-energy trauma, and elderly, female patients with low-energy trauma. These should be treated differently, even for patients with the same fracture pattern.[121] The young patient typically has good bone quality and can generally comply with postoperative therapy, allowing the surgeon to employ surgical methods such as ORIF with a plate or intramedullary (IM) nail fixation. The elderly patient and patients with dementia may not fully comprehend or appreciate his or her role in the postoperative rehabilitation process. Bone quality in elderly patients tends to be poor, with evidence of comminution after minor trauma; fixation options may be limited, and in some cases of surgical neck nonunion, hemiarthroplasty, or RTSA may be viable options.[121,162]

Evaluation

The amount of displacement is critical when making decisions regarding nonoperative versus operative treatment for surgical neck fractures (Fig. 6-16; also see Fig. 6-32). In the elderly patient, bony contact of fracture segments may be all that is necessary for a functional result. In active patients, less than 50% shaft diameter displacement and less than 45 degrees of angulation may

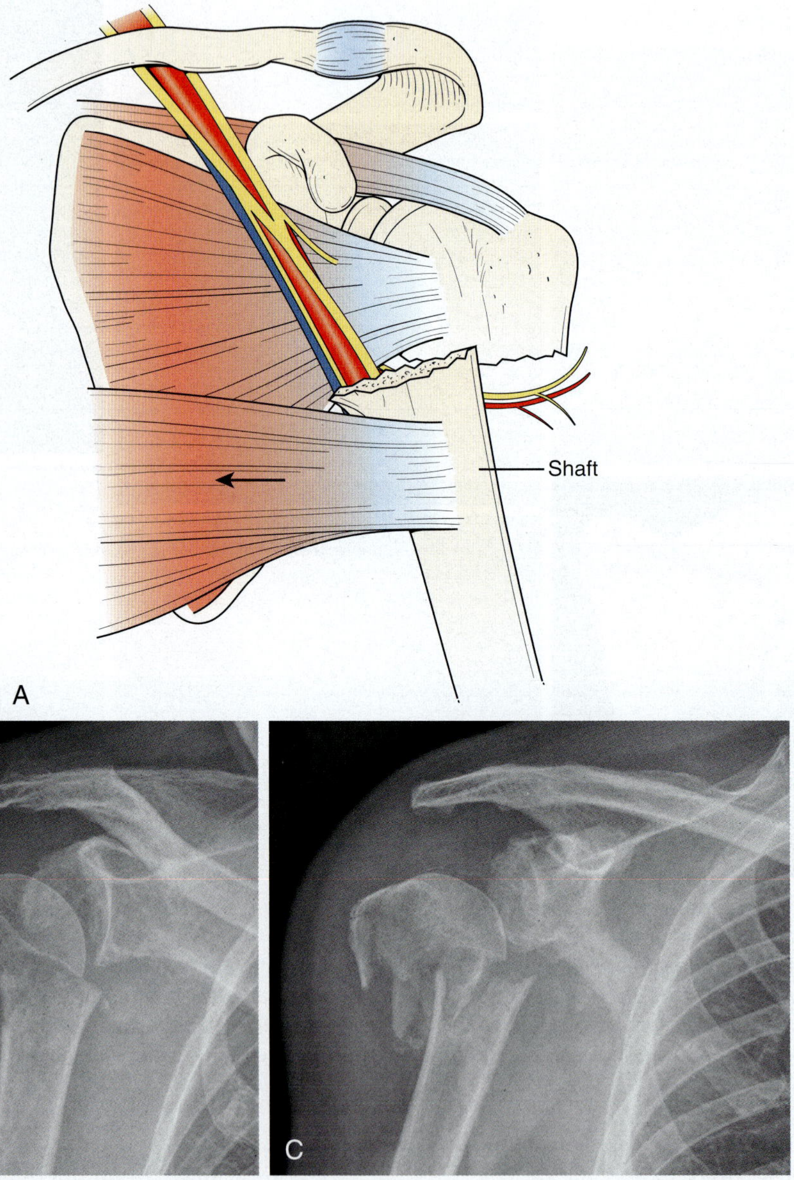

FIGURE 6-16: A, Displacement of each "part" occurs in a predictable manner. In cases of two-part fractures involving the surgical neck, the pectoralis major tendon (and the latissimus dorsi and teres major tendons [not shown]) causes medial displacement of the humeral shaft. Note the close proximity of the neurovascular structures to the proximal-medial aspect of the humeral shaft fragment. **B** and **C,** Anteroposterior radiographs demonstrating a displaced surgical neck fracture in an 81-year-old man following a ground-level fall. (**A,** Modified from Neer CS. *Shoulder Reconstruction.* Philadelphia: WB Saunders; 1990:374. **B** and **C,** Courtesy Aaron J. Bois, MD.)

be tolerated.[22] Varus deformity, valgus deformity, comminution, and 100% displaced surgical neck fractures are considered unstable and require surgical intervention.

Treatment

Management of surgical neck fractures depends on the fracture displacement, bone quality, and the functional demands and mental status of the patient. Nonoperative treatment is generally reserved for patients with minimally displaced or less than 50% displacement who can participate in a rehabilitation program. However, some patients, when treated nonoperatively, do not have good outcomes. Chun et al. reported only 55% good or excellent results in 56 surgical neck fractures treated nonoperatively with a mean forward flexion arc of 104 degrees.[52] Displaced fractures in active patients should undergo ORIF or closed reduction and IM nailing. This latter treatment option works well when the surrounding soft tissue envelope is compromised and concern for postoperative infection exists (Fig. 6-17). In a multicenter retrospective

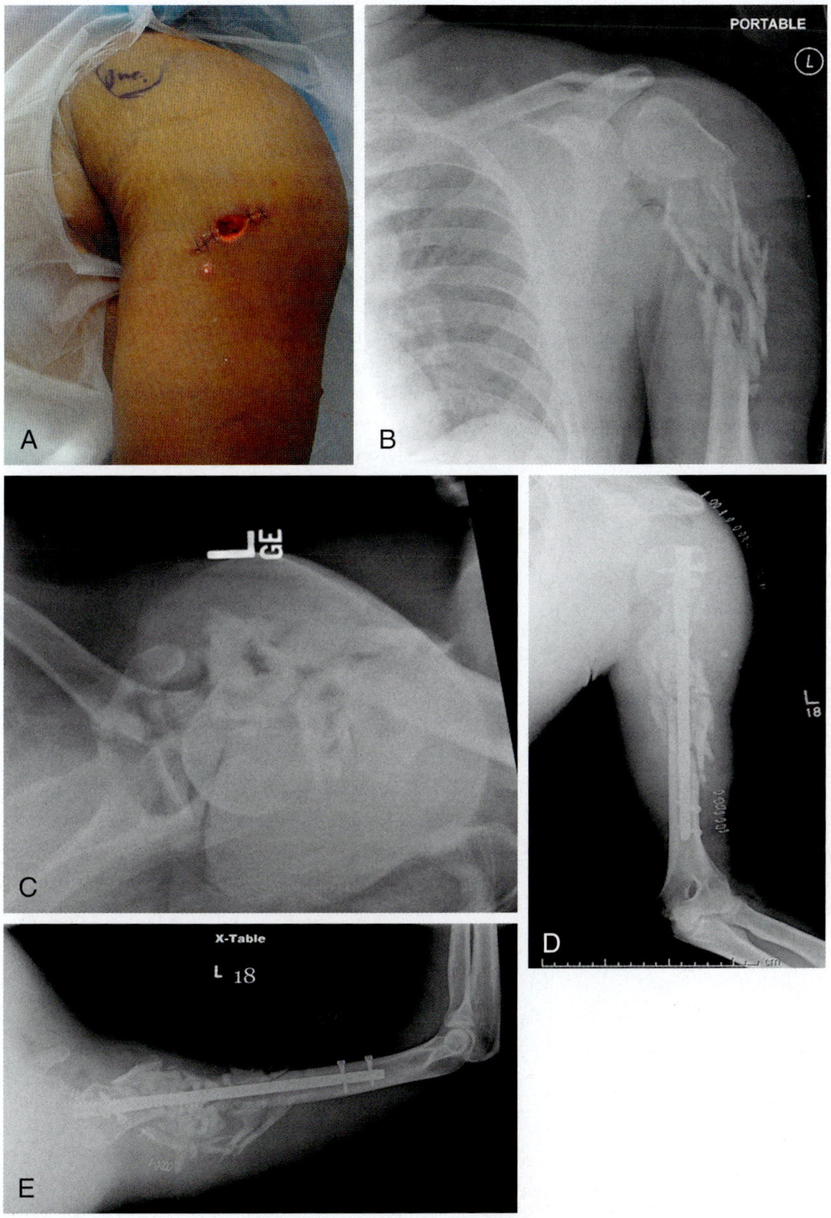

FIGURE 6-17: A, An open wound (i.e., entry wound) in the region of the anterior left shoulder following a gunshot injury with a high-powered rifle. **B** and **C,** Portable anteroposterior (AP) and lateral radiographs of the humerus reveal a comminuted fracture extending from the surgical neck of the proximal humerus to the middle third of the humeral shaft. **D** and **E,** Immediate postoperative AP and lateral radiographs of the humerus following limited irrigation and debridement (with placement of antibiotic beads) and intramedullary nail fixation. This method of fixation was used to bridge the region of fracture comminution and preserve the soft tissue envelope of the arm. (Courtesy Aaron J. Bois, MD.)

observational study, Hatzidakis et al.[109] found that patients with displaced two-part surgical neck fractures that were managed with a locked angular-stable IM had reliable fracture healing, favorable clinical outcomes, and little residual shoulder pain. An alternative option, although technically demanding, involves percutaneous fixation with multiple threaded K-wires after closed reduction. Biomechanical studies have indicated improved fixation rigidity and increased load to failure with a configuration containing parallel descending and ascending pins.[72] The main advantage of this technique is the minimal soft tissue dissection required, which can theoretically minimize the risk of iatrogenic injury to the vascular supply of the articular segment.[121] Disadvantages of this approach include hardware migration, failure of fixation prior to fracture healing, pin tract–related infection, and the necessity for secondary removal of the hardware.[74,169]

Most recently, in 2015, Rangan et al.[208] performed a randomized controlled trial (RCT) comparing operative to nonoperative management of displaced surgical neck fractures. A total of 231 patients (114 operative and 117 nonoperative) were included in the study; the mean age of the patients was 66 years (range, 24 to 92 years). At the final 2-year follow-up, there was no difference in the patient-reported clinical outcomes using the Oxford Shoulder Score (OSS) and the 12-Item Short Form Health Survey. The authors further questioned the growing trend of operative intervention of these injuries in view of these results. However, surgeons should be aware of the limitations that exist with multicenter (and multisurgeon) studies before these data are universally applied to surgical practice.

Three-Part Fractures

In three-part fractures, cleavage lines occur through the surgical neck and GT or LT. The degree of displacement of the segments largely depends on the deforming forces of the rotator cuff muscles. The GT is more commonly involved than the LT, and is usually displaced in a posterior and superior position by the pull of the attached supraspinatus, infraspinatus, and teres minor.[121,178] The humeral head is pulled into internal rotation (i.e., retroversion) secondary to the pull of the subscapularis on the intact LT, while the humeral shaft is displaced anteromedially due to the pull of the pectoralis major. If the fracture involves LT, the subscapularis pulls this segment medially. The intact GT and articular segment are pulled into adduction and external rotation, and the humeral shaft is similarly pulled in an anteromedial direction (Fig. 6-18). Surgical treatment options include closed reduction and percutaneous fixation, ORIF, closed reduction and IM nail fixation with or without suture supplementation, hemiarthroplasty, and RTSA.[131] The latter arthroplasty options are reserved for comminuted osteoporotic fractures that are unsuitable for osteosynthesis in elderly lower-demand, yet physiologically active patients.

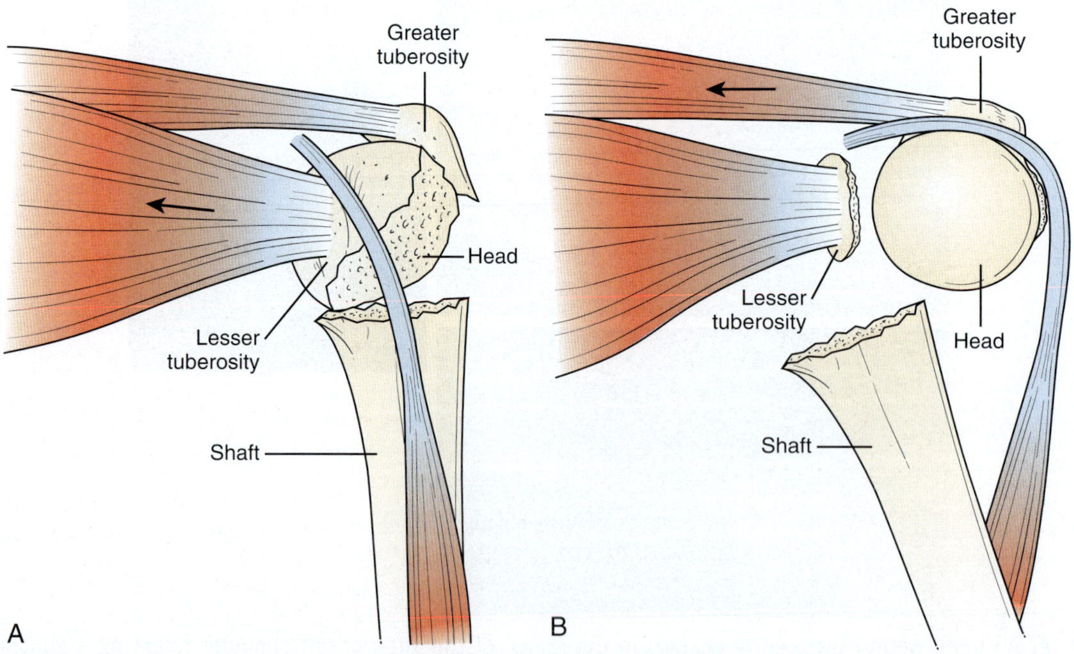

FIGURE 6-18: Three-part fracture displacement patterns. **A,** Greater tuberosity (GT) three-part displacement. The GT fragment is typically displaced superior and/or posterior and the articular surface of the humeral head faces posteriorly by the pull of the subscapularis tendon on LT, which remains intact with the humeral head fragment. **B,** Lesser tuberosity three-part displacement: the LT fragment is displaced medially and the articular surface of the humeral head faces anteriorly by the pull of the intact superior and posterior rotator cuff. (Modified from Neer CS. *Shoulder Reconstruction.* Philadelphia, WB Saunders; 1990:379.)

In 1970, Neer reported his early experience in 39 patients with three-part PHFs treated by closed reduction. Only three patients demonstrated a satisfactory result by his criteria. Poor results were due to malreduction, nonunion, humeral head resorption, and osteonecrosis. He concluded that nonoperative intervention for these injuries was inadequate in active patients.[180] More recent reports by Lill et al.[151] and Zyto et al.[271,272] suggest that good functional outcomes can be achieved after nonoperative management of these injuries. Zyto et al.[272] prospectively evaluated 40 elderly patients (mean age, 74 years) with displaced three- and four-part PHFs randomized to nonoperative management or tension band fixation. At 3 to 5 years of follow-up, they found no differences in functional outcome between the two methods, despite radiographic evidence revealing improved position of the humeral head in the surgical patients.[272] In 2011, Olerud et al. performed a randomized study in 60 patients (mean age, 74 years; range, 56 to 92 years) comparing ORIF using a locking plate to nonoperative management of displaced three-part PHFs. At the final 2-year follow-up, the results for ROM, function, and health-related quality of life (HRQoL) scores were all in favor of the locking plate group; however, critical appraisal of the differences between the groups reveals only marginal improvements in the operative group. Specifically, the mean forward elevation in the locking plate group was 120 degrees (vs. 111 degrees in the nonoperative group) and the mean abduction was 114 degrees (vs. 106 degrees). Functional scores including the Constant score was 61 in the operative group (vs. 58), and the Disabilities of the Arm, Shoulder and Hand (DASH) score was 26 (vs. 35). The small positive results in the operative group were also tempered by a 13% complication rate requiring a "major" revision surgery, and 17% of the patients underwent a "minor" reoperation (total reoperation rate of 30%).[192]

Despite the potential risk for repeat surgery, the majority of displaced three-part PHFs in young adults require operative fixation due to the residual humeral deformity and functional deficits that can prevent the patient from returning to premorbid level of activity.

Four-Part Fractures

Nonoperative management of four-part PHFs should only be employed in the medically unfit and/or low-demand elderly patients. Because of the poor outcomes and high incidence of complications associated with nonoperative treatment (e.g., osteonecrosis, malunion, nonunion, and post-traumatic arthritis), most fractures are treated surgically[151,245]; however, patients should be properly counseled regarding possible risks and complications associated with both forms of treatment.[190] Operative options include percutaneous K-wire fixation,[105,106] ORIF (Fig. 6-19),[9,53,193] hemiarthroplasty,[98,131] and RTSA.[43,59,131,162] Combined or hybrid surgical techniques may be required for complex fracture patterns involving both the proximal humerus and humeral shaft (i.e., segmental fractures) (Fig. 6-20). Closed reduction and percutaneous wire fixation is a viable option for acute injuries (<7 to 10 days) with good bone stock and minimal comminution. Open reduction is generally performed for fractures not amenable to reduction by closed means, for comminuted fractures, and for injuries that are 10 days to 4 months old.

The valgus-impacted four-part fracture is an uncommon but important subtype to identify.[40,127,128,212,214,218] This injury has a more favorable prognosis when compared with other multi-part PHFs secondary to the integrity of the medial capsular blood supply.[40,212] The fracture pattern is characterized by impaction of the lateral aspect of the humeral articular surface due to a fracture of the anatomic neck (Fig. 6-21).[40,212,214,218] The articular surface faces superiorly toward the acromion rather than the glenoid. The tuberosities typically displace into valgus secondary to impaction of the articular surface on the humeral metaphysis, but often do not displace superiorly. The prevalence of osteonecrosis approaches 5% to 10%, much less than that of the corresponding standard four-part PHFs (approximately 20% to 30%).[128,212-214,218]

Jakob et al.[128] achieved a satisfactory outcome in 74% of patients with valgus-impacted fractures who underwent closed reduction or limited ORIF. The major reason for failure was AVN, which occurred in five cases (26%).[128] Resch et al. performed limited ORIF on 22 patients with four-part valgus-impacted fractures, demonstrating no evidence of osteonecrosis at a mean follow-up of 36 months (minimum, 18 months). The results were graded as excellent in 12 patients (54%), particularly in cases in which anatomic reduction was maintained.[212]

Decision-making regarding the appropriate treatment for the aforementioned two-, three-, and four-part fracture subtypes remains challenging, especially in the elderly population (Fig. 6-22). Several studies have attempted to collate the available data through meta-analysis. In 2012, Handoll et al.[105] performed a review of 23 randomized trials involving management of PHFs. Their analysis did not provide fracture-specific management recommendations, except for the early mobilization of nondisplaced fractures.[105] Fjalestad et al.[79] performed an RCT comparing nonoperative treatment and ORIF in 50 elderly patients with displaced three- and four-part fractures. The authors did not find a difference in functional outcome at the 1-year follow-up between the treatment groups.[79] Similarly, Li et al.[150] failed to demonstrate a significant difference in clinical outcomes when comparing operative and nonoperative management of three- and four-part fractures in elderly patients.[150] The authors cautioned against the extrapolation of the results of this study, as the analysis was based on limited data in a specific patient demographic.

Proximal Humerus Fracture-Dislocations

Two-part fracture-dislocations are amenable to ORIF due to the integrity of the vascular supply that is maintained by the soft tissue attachments to one or both tuberosity segments.[22] Three- and four-part fracture-dislocations with or without articular surface involvement similarly require operative intervention (Fig. 6-23). Repeated attempts at closed reduction or delayed ORIF can result in an increased incidence of myositis ossificans.[155] The

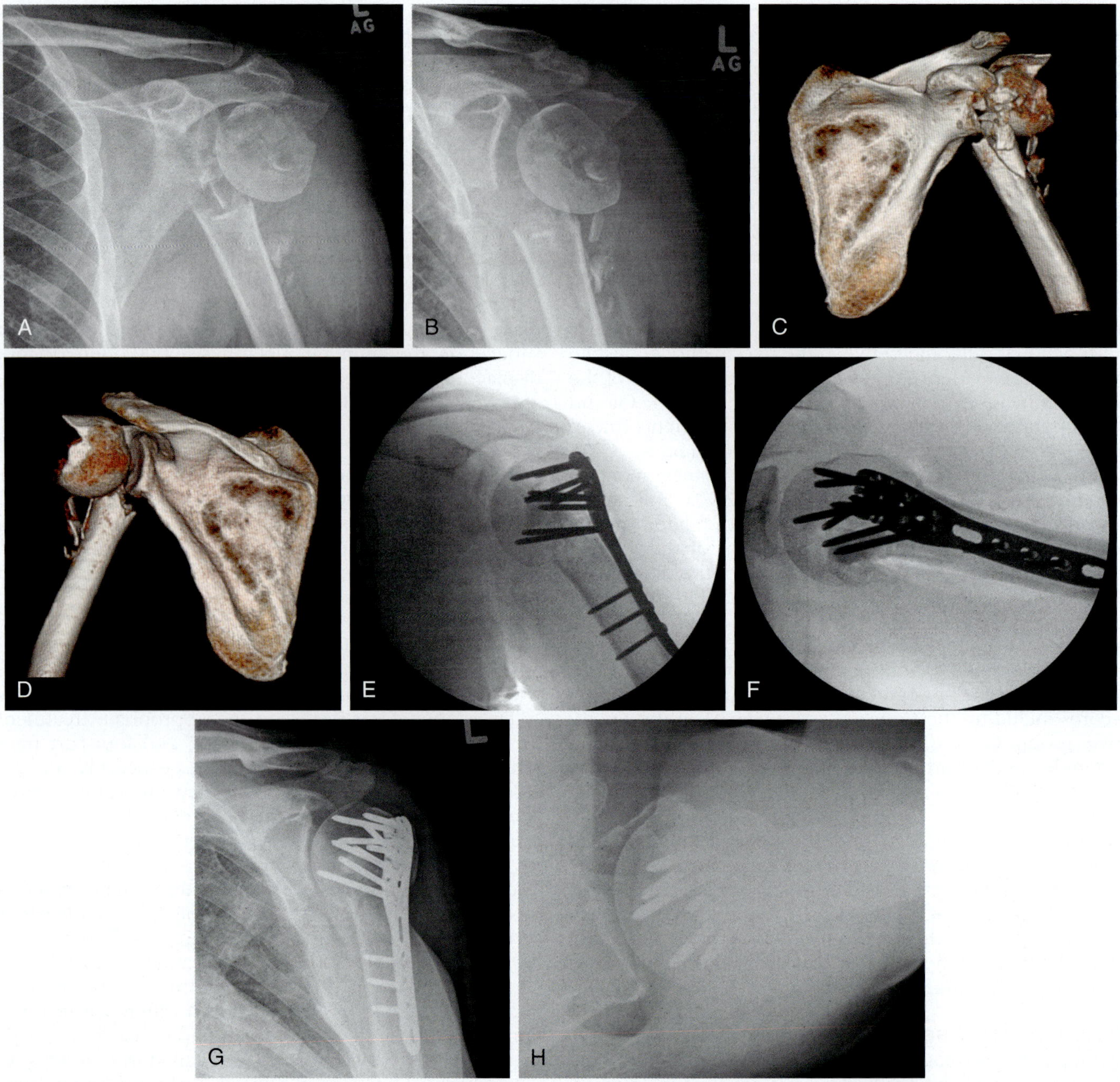

FIGURE 6-19: **A** and **B,** Anteroposterior radiographs demonstrating a comminuted four-part proximal humerus fracture in a 56-year-old man who fell down a stairwell. **C** and **D,** Three-dimensional computed tomographic imaging similarly demonstrating significant fracture displacement. There is a coronal split of greater tuberosity and fracture comminution of the lesser tuberosity and proximal humerus at the level of the surgical neck, with extension into the proximal shaft that was not appreciated on initial radiographs. **E** and **F,** Intraoperative fluoroscopic images following fracture reduction and fixation with a locking plate construct and synthetic bone augmentation of the metaphysis. **G** and **H,** Early postoperative radiographs (anteroposterior and axillary lateral views). (Courtesy Aaron J. Bois, MD.)

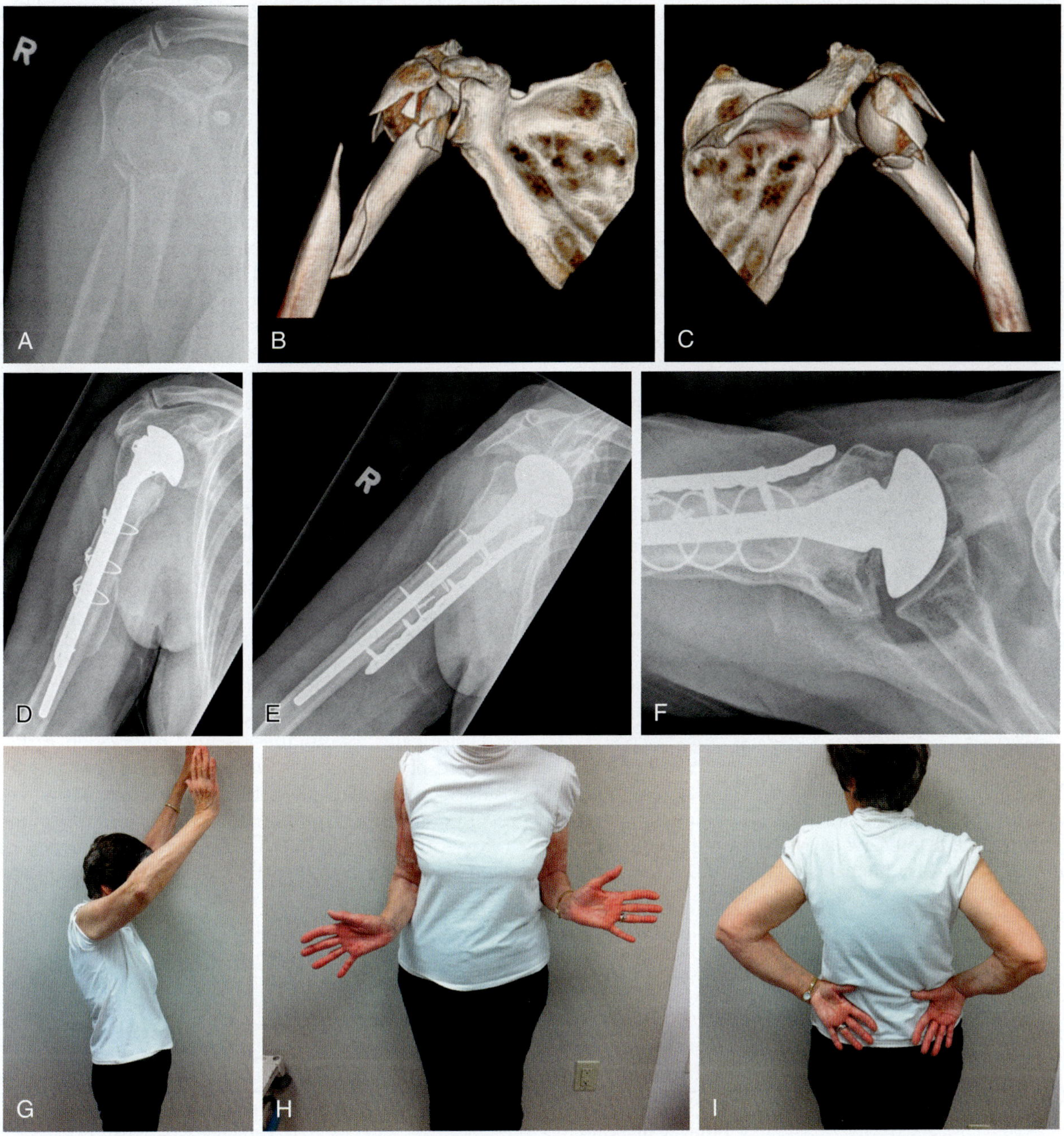

FIGURE 6-20: **A** to **C,** Anteroposterior radiograph and three-dimensional computed tomographic imaging of a complex four-part proximal humerus fracture with extension into the proximal humeral shaft (i.e., segmental fracture) in a 71-year-old female who fell down a stairwell. **D** to **F,** Anterior and lateral humeral radiographs and an axillary radiograph of the shoulder at the 12-month follow-up visit following combined open reduction and internal fixation and hemiarthroplasty. A long-stemmed implant was used to bypass the humeral shaft fracture. A limited cementing technique (i.e., use of proximal cement only) was used to avoid placement of cement down the full length of the medullary canal. Excellent fracture healing was obtained, with near anatomic restoration of the tuberosities in relation to the prosthetic humeral head. **G** to **I,** Active shoulder range of motion at the 12-month follow-up visit. (Courtesy Aaron J. Bois, MD.)

results of ORIF for four-part fracture-dislocations are poor; however, this remains the standard of care in young physically demanding patients. Arthroplasty serves as an appropriate treatment method for such injuries in older patients (i.e., over the age of 65 years) (Fig. 6-24). Closed management should only be considered in the medically unfit patient.

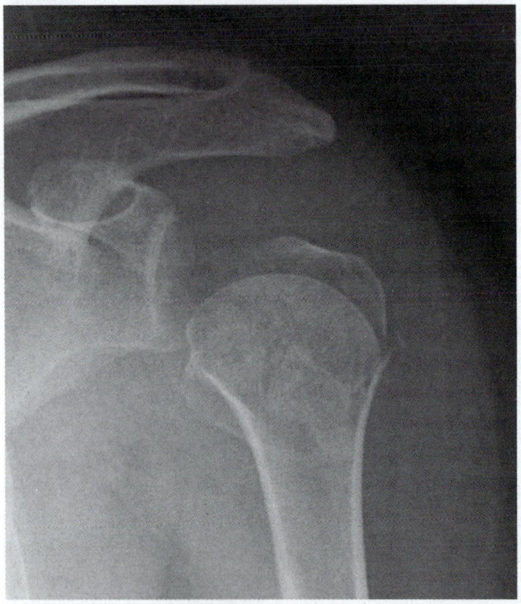

FIGURE 6-21: Anteroposterior radiograph of a valgus-impacted four-part proximal humerus fracture. The medial periosteal hinge remains intact, preserving partial vascular inflow to the humeral head. (Courtesy Michael A. Wirth, MD.)

Operative Techniques: General Considerations

Once faced with the decision for operative management of a PHF, the surgeon must decide to use one of the multiple surgical techniques available, which is dependent on the fracture subtype and surgeon experience.

Percutaneous Treatment of Proximal Humerus Fractures

The goal of surgical fixation of PHFs is twofold: to restore the anatomic relationship between the articular surface and the tuberosities, and to preserve the vascularity of the articular fragment. Closed reduction with percutaneous fixation minimizes soft tissue dissection, and can preserve vascular inflow for anatomic healing. Diminished adhesion formation and improved cosmesis are additional benefits of this approach. The caveat to this technique is that it involves an increased level of technical skill and ancillary support from operating room personnel.[94,171] Percutaneous fixation of PHFs was initially used by Bohler to treat pediatric injuries,[25] and was subsequently applied to adult surgical neck fractures.[125] Because of the growing emphasis on biologic fixation, some authors have advocated percutaneous treatment of three- and four-part fractures.[114,125,213,214] The learning curve is substantial, but proponents of this method cite a decreased incidence of osteonecrosis because the region of the ascending branch of the AHCA is undisturbed (see Fig. 6-3A).[49,73,137,241,262]

Historically, percutaneous and mini-open reduction of PHFs resulted in good outcomes and a low prevalence of osteonecrosis with short-term follow-up. However, more recent data from a multicenter case series with intermediate follow-up demonstrated an increased prevalence of osteonecrosis and posttraumatic osteoarthritis compared with

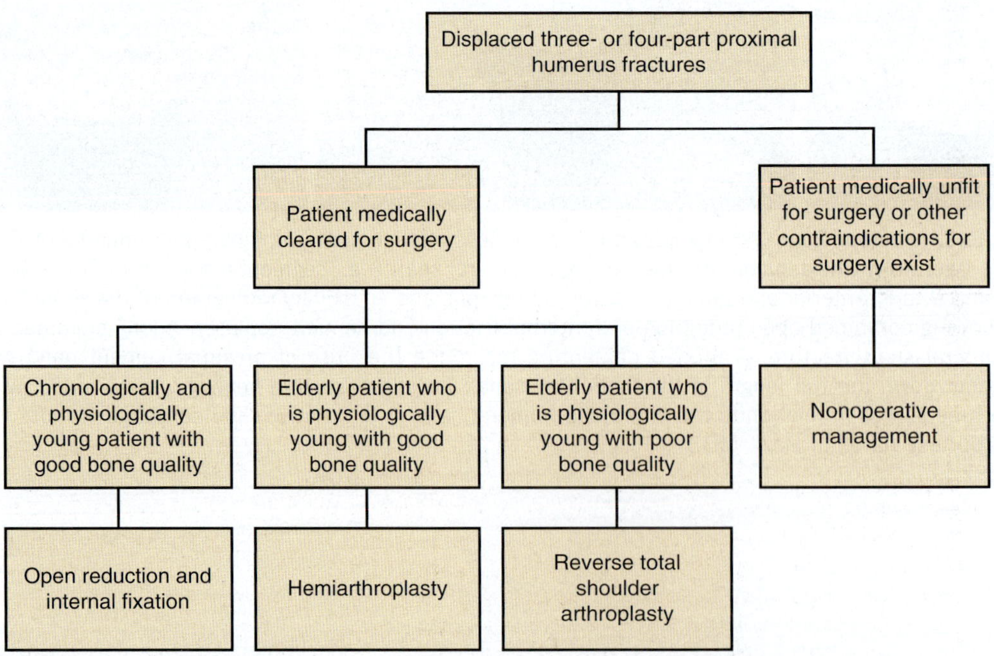

FIGURE 6-22: Treatment algorithm for displaced three- and four-part proximal humerus fractures.

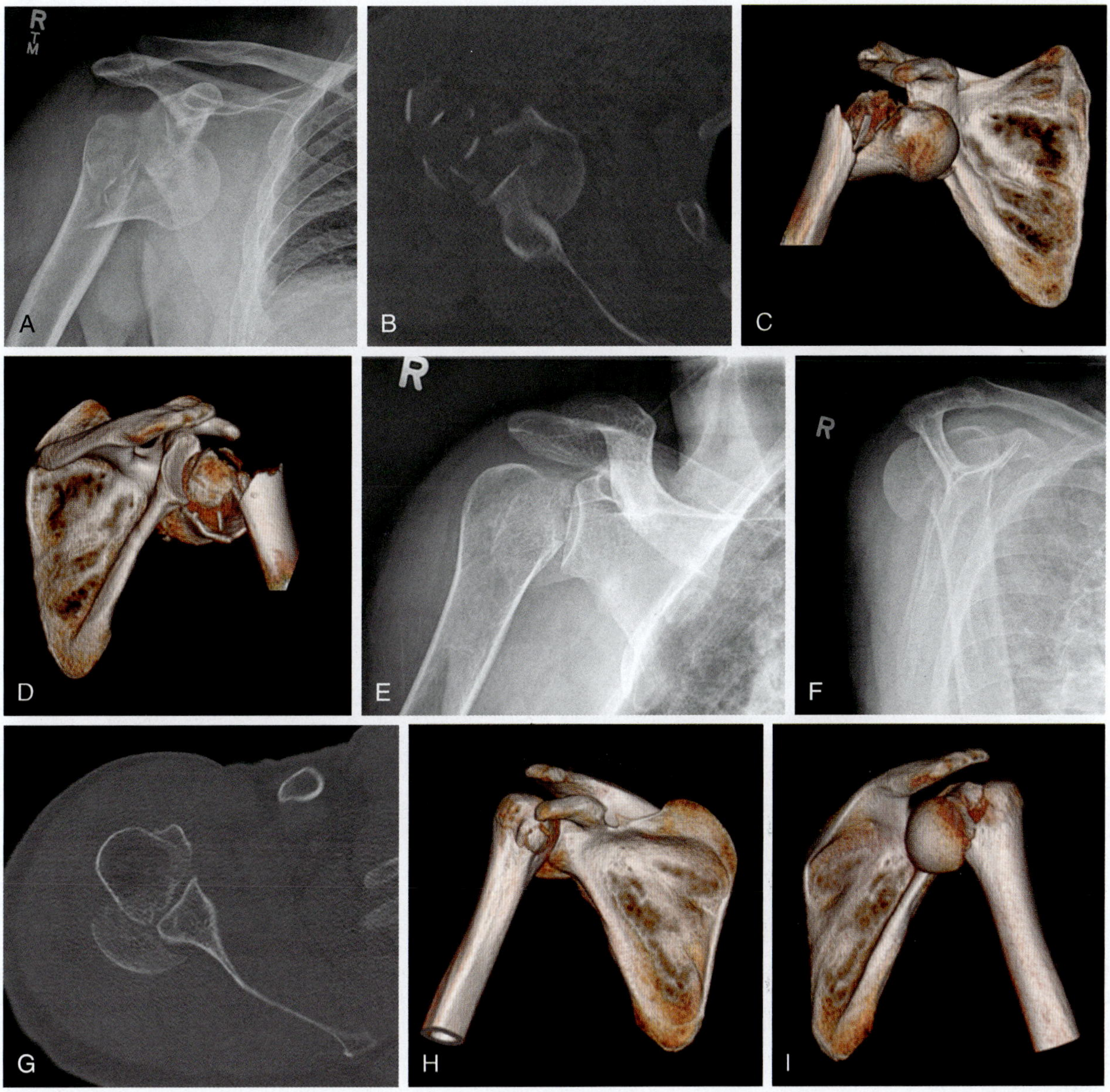

FIGURE 6-23: **A** to **D,** Anteroposterior radiograph and two- and three-dimensional (2D and 3D) computed tomographic (CT) imaging of a comminuted anterior fracture-dislocation in a 49-year-old male who fell from a height. **E** to **I,** Anteroposterior and transcapular lateral radiographs and 2D and 3D CT imaging of a posterior fracture-dislocation in a 53-year-old male after a ground-level fall. (Courtesy Aaron J. Bois, MD.)

that initially proposed. Some patients with these complications presented as late as 8 years postoperatively.[106]

The indications for closed reduction and percutaneous pinning ideally include two-part (e.g., surgical neck), three-part, and valgus-impacted four-part PHFs without comminution in compliant patients with good bone stock. Weekly radiographic evaluation and shoulder immobilization for 4 to 6 weeks are required. Severe comminution and osteopenia are absolute contraindications to this technique. Additionally, numerous attempts to reduce fracture fragments should be avoided; in this situation, the surgeon should be prepared to convert to an open procedure. Fracture-dislocations can prove extremely difficult to manage with this method, and thus it is generally not recommended.[49,73,114,121,125,137,158,171,241,262]

Surgical Technique

Specific technical steps are required to ensure a positive outcome from this intervention. Obtaining good biplanar images after patient positioning and before draping is crucial to the success of this procedure. Neuromuscular relaxation is required in the form of general anesthesia, muscle relaxants, and a regional block (e.g., interscalene block) to facilitate the reduction maneuver.[171] A surgical assistant who can maintain reduction during the fixation process is also recommended.

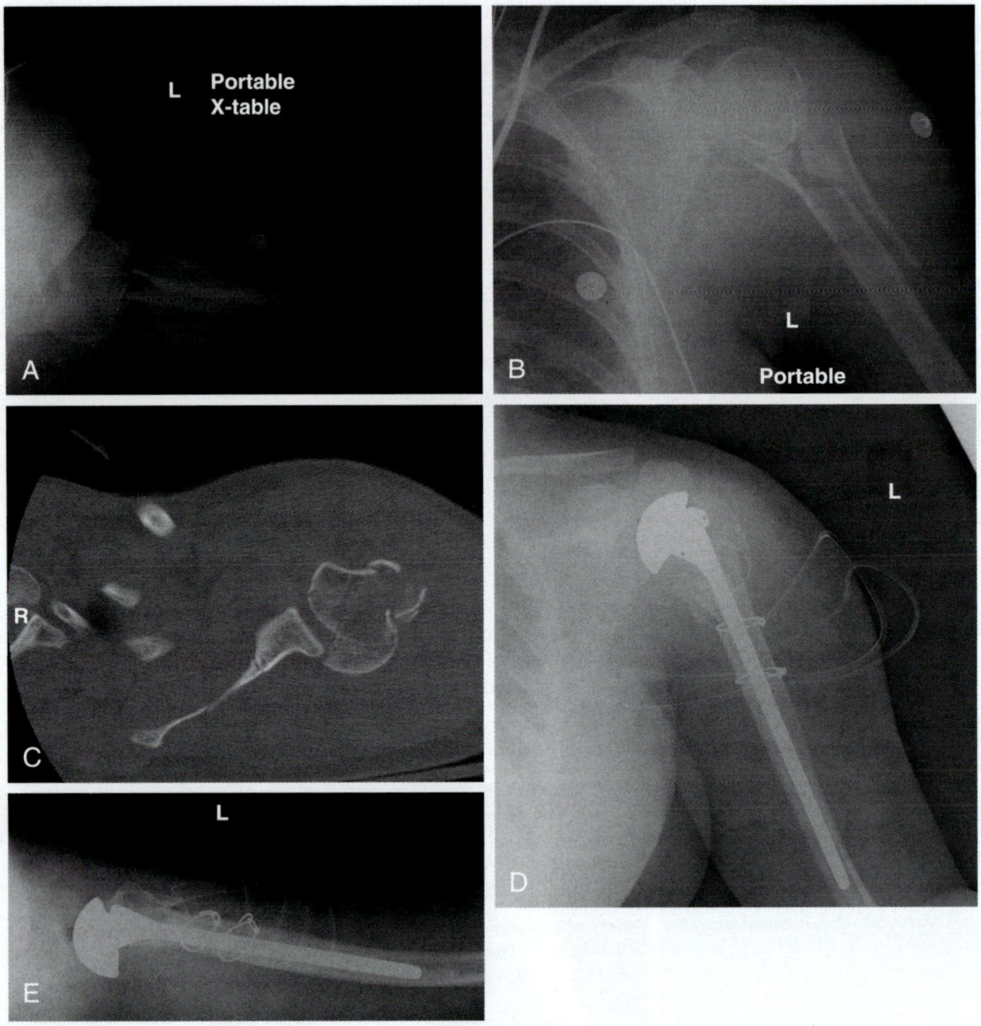

FIGURE 6-24: A, Axillary lateral radiograph of a four-part proximal humerus fracture. **B,** Anteroposterior radiograph of the same fracture with diaphyseal involvement. **C,** Axial computed tomographic image demonstrating articular surface involvement. **D,** Immediate postoperative anteroposterior view demonstrating a modular hemiarthroplasty. **E,** Axillary view of modular implant with reapproximation of lesser tuberosity. *L,* left; *R,* right. (Courtesy Michael A. Wirth, MD.)

Two-Part Fracture

The patient is placed in the beach chair or semi-Fowler's position that allows access to the entire shoulder. Commercially available beach chair positioner attachments and mechanical arm holders will help significantly. Reduction instruments include bone elevators and hooks to manipulate the fragments into position. Terminally threaded 2.5-mm pins and 4.0-mm cannulated screws are commonly used for this technique. The C-arm image intensifier is placed parallel to the table to allow AP and axillary views (see Fig. 6-12).

A provisional reduction maneuver should be performed to determine the feasibility of a closed reduction. With two-part surgical neck fractures, there is apex anterior angulation at the fracture site. The arm should first be placed in 20 to 30 degrees of abduction. Longitudinal traction is then applied to the arm, while the humeral shaft is directed lateral to the humeral head. Concomitant pressure against the anterior surface of the shoulder will help reduce the apex anterior angulation (Fig. 6-25).[121,125]

A single pin is placed on the skin of the anterior shoulder in a distal-to-proximal direction from the lateral humeral cortex to the humeral head. An AP image confirms the inclination, and a skin marker is used to document pin positioning. A 1-cm incision is made on the lateral aspect of the shoulder at the level determined by the C-arm image. Blunt dissection is performed down to the bone with a hemostat. The hemostat is then used to palpate the anterior and posterior cortices of the humerus. The initial pin is then guided under power at the previously determined angle. Initial horizontal pin placement can prevent the pin from sliding across the cortex.

While the assistant maintains the reduction, the pin is advanced under fluoroscopy to engage the humeral head. Because of the approximate 30 degrees of retroversion of the humeral head, fluoroscopy must be used to

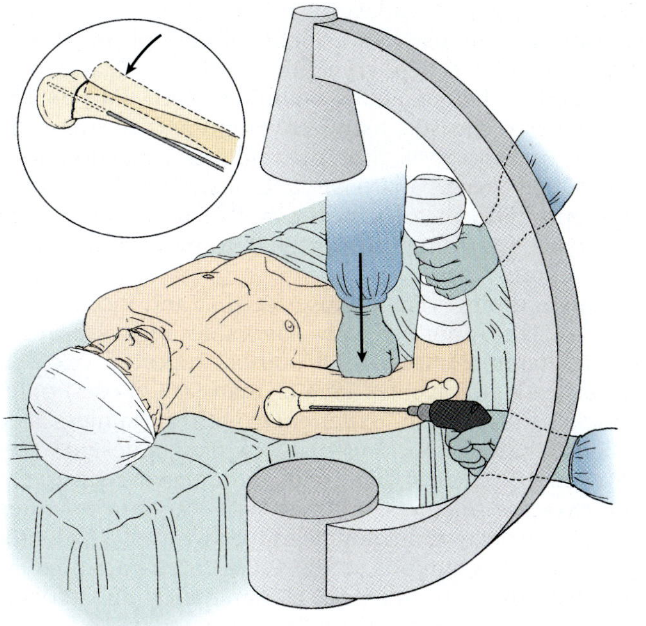

FIGURE 6-25: The reduction maneuver involves slight shoulder abduction, longitudinal traction of the arm, and posterior pressure on the humeral shaft. Anteroposterior and axillary views using C-arm fluoroscopy confirm the reduction. (Modified from Jaberg H, Warner JJ, Jakob RP. Percutaneous stabilization of unstable fractures of the humerus. *J Bone Joint Surg Am.* 1992;74:508-515.)

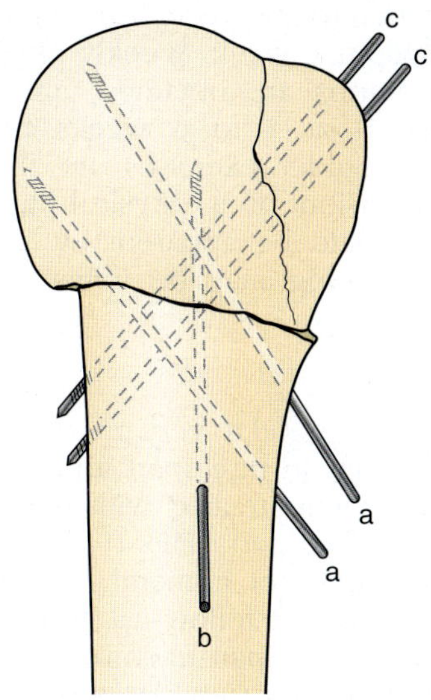

FIGURE 6-26: Two 2.5-mm AO terminally threaded pins are inserted from the lateral shaft, just above the deltoid insertion (*a*). A third pin (*b*) is placed through the anterior cortex and directed posteriorly toward the humeral head. If there is an associated greater tuberosity fracture, it is reduced and held in place with two additional pins (*c*). (Modified from Jaberg H, Warner JJ, Jakob RP. Percutaneous stabilization of unstable fractures of the humerus. *J Bone Joint Surg Am.* 1992;74:508-515.)

confirm appropriate pin placement. A second pin is then advanced parallel to the first with approximately 1.5 to 2 cm of separation. Several authors have demonstrated that parallel pin placement increases torsional stability and rigidity in biomechanical testing when compared with converging pins.[72,130] A third pin is then placed from the anterior humeral shaft into the humeral head. A fourth pin from anterior to posterior may be necessary to augment the fixation (Fig. 6-26).[121,125] An alternative surgical technique involves placement of two K-wires, one in the humeral head and another in the shaft. The K-wires are then utilized as joysticks to achieve fracture reduction, with subsequent placement of terminally threaded pins or cannulated screws.[235]

Three-Part and Four-Part Fractures

Three- and four-part PHFs add a level of complexity that proves difficult to manage with this technique, even in the most experienced hands.[186]

With a three-part valgus-impacted fracture, the humeral head is tilted into valgus while the GT remains at the correct height. After positioning the humeral shaft under the humeral head, a small incision is made laterally to allow placement of an elevator into the fracture site under the humeral head. Under fluoroscopy, the humeral head is then levered upward and into varus alignment. As the humeral head is reduced, the GT will be pulled below the articular surface due to the integrity of the rotator cuff insertion. A 2.5-mm threaded pin or 4.0-mm cannulated screw is then advanced through a separate superior incision to capture the GT and the humeral head. Cannulated screws are usually placed to hold the tuberosity and articular surface reduction, while additional pins or screws are inserted in an antegrade fashion to stabilize the tuberosity to the humeral shaft.[121,125,186]

Four-part fractures, except for the valgus-impacted subtype, generally require open reduction and internal fixation. On the infrequent occasion that percutaneous fixation is attempted, the same steps to reduce the GT, articular surface, and humeral shaft are employed. The LT may be reduced by internally rotating the arm and by placing a hook on the fragment through a laterally based incision. Once reduced, the fragment is held in place with a 4.0-mm cannulated screw. Once satisfied with fracture reduction and fixation, the threaded pins are trimmed below the skin, which is closed. Tenting of the skin from the pin can occur as shoulder swelling diminishes. In some cases, the pin(s) require trimming on an outpatient basis.

Postoperative Care

Most patients are admitted postoperatively for 24-hour observation and continued parenteral antibiotics. The shoulder is placed in a shoulder immobilizer for comfort. Hand, wrist, and elbow active ROM exercises are encouraged immediately. Pendulum exercises may be initiated at 1 week following outpatient radiographs that confirm fracture reduction and hardware stability. Passive forward flexion and external rotation exercises are initiated during the third postoperative week. Weekly physical examination and radiographs are obtained, and the pins are generally removed at 4 to 6 weeks postoperatively. Active-assisted shoulder exercises are then performed under the supervision of a physical therapist. Radiographic union should be apparent by 2 or 3 months. Shoulder strengthening may be initiated by 10 to 12 weeks postoperatively.[74,121,125,171,213,214]

Outcomes

Resch et al. reported good to very good functional results (Constant score, 91% in three-part and 87% in four-part fractures) in 27 patients treated with percutaneous fixation of three- and four-part PHFs (9 three-part, 18 four-part) without evidence of humeral head necrosis at 24 months of follow-up.[214] A follow-up study by Resch et al. on the treatment of four-part fractures indicated good to very good results, with a Constant score of 87% and an osteonecrosis rate of 11% in 18 patients.[213]

Keener et al. reported the results after percutaneous reduction and fixation of two-, three-, and four-part PHFs in 35 patients from three institutions. The mean follow-up was 35 months, with mean visual analog pain, American Shoulder and Elbow Surgeons (ASES), and Constant scores of 1.4, 83.4, and 73.9, respectively. Fracture type, age at presentation, malunion, or osteoarthritis had no significant influence on the measured outcomes. The authors concluded that this technique remained a viable and predictable option in the treatment of PHFs.[134]

Open Reduction and Internal Fixation

Numerous techniques of internal fixation for two-, three-, and four-part PHFs have been described in the literature. These methods include plate and screw fixation, blade plates, tension banding, antegrade or retrograde nailing, or a combination of internal fixation methods with sutures, cables, and metallic implant fixation.[2,24,95,102,121,140,168,178,186,197,223,261] Although the ideal construct for these injuries has not been defined, current advances in locking plate technology have provided surgeons with another viable option in the treatment of multipart PHFs, particularly in patients with suboptimal bone stock.[76,102,223]

The osseous architecture of the humeral head varies with respect to the density of the cancellous bone stock.[250] In elderly patients, this proves particularly problematic when the goal is to achieve rigid internal fixation capable of withstanding a progressive rehabilitation program. Attempts at rigid fixation with prior implants have indicated a high risk of failure due to osteonecrosis, nonunion, malunion, screw cutout, and screw loosening.[95,103,110,143] Blade plate fixation has been used to overcome concerns regarding early hardware failure, but this challenging technique only allows a single point of proximal fixation in the humeral head.[121,122] In addition to the soft tissue dissection required with this technique, some authors have reported unacceptable complication rates related to blade plate protrusion into the glenohumeral joint (eight of 36, or 22% of patients in one study).[168] Using a three-part cadaveric model, Weinstein et al.[260] demonstrated increased torsional stiffness of the locking plate construct when compared with the blade plate construct.[260] Percutaneous pinning and IM fixation can preserve the soft tissue envelope and decrease the risk of osteonecrosis, but the indirect reduction techniques can make anatomic alignment of the fracture fragments difficult to achieve. At this time, there is no consensus regarding the optimal form of fixation for these injuries.[104,105]

Saudan et al.,[232] Frankhauser et al.,[82] and Bjorkenheim et al.[21] have reported early favorable results using a similar titanium implant. All authors reported excellent results, with union rates greater than 90%. Rose et al.[223] reported their 1-year experience with a stainless steel proximal humeral-locking plate of similar design. They followed 16 patients (nine with three-part fractures, five with two-part fractures, and two with four-part fractures) until union or revision at a mean follow-up of 12 months. Of the four nonunions, three were three-part fractures with extensive metaphyseal comminution in smokers. Patients with united fractures demonstrated mean forward elevation and external rotation of 132 degrees and 43 degrees, respectively. The authors were encouraged by the early positive findings, but they emphasized that there are limitations with this method based on the degree of comminution and patient factors (e.g., smoking).[223] Longer term follow-up will be necessary with this surgical technique to better elucidate long-term outcomes and negative sequelae.

Nonlocking and Locking Plate Fixation

Based on a current review of the literature, Nho et al. recommended buttress plate fixation in young patients with diaphyseal cortices greater than 3.5 mm. However, metaphyseal comminution prevented the use of a nonlocking device.[186] The proximal humeral-locking plate has been developed to overcome some of the limitations of conventional plating and to address issues specifically related to osteoporotic bone and metaphyseal comminution. The stability of this implant is based on the fixed-angle relationship between the screws and the plate. The threaded screw heads lock into the corresponding threaded plate holes, preventing toggle, pullout, and sliding. The stability of the fracture-and-plate construct does not depend on any single screw because of the fixed-angle construct.[257] As a single unit, the plate is better able to withstand bending and torsional forces.[102] Precontoured proximal humeral-locking plates provide a mechanical advantage in fractures with metaphyseal comminution (Fig. 6-27). Proximal humeral-locking plates have also evolved to include peripheral holes for rotator cuff fixation and polyaxial screws that allow variable angle screw placement. Both implant traits help mitigate, but unfortunately, have not eliminated, issues related to PHFs with osteoporotic bone.[9,254]

Intramedullary Nail Fixation

Early reports on IM fixation of two- and three-part fractures by Lin et al.,[152] Adedapo et al.,[1] and Rajasekhar

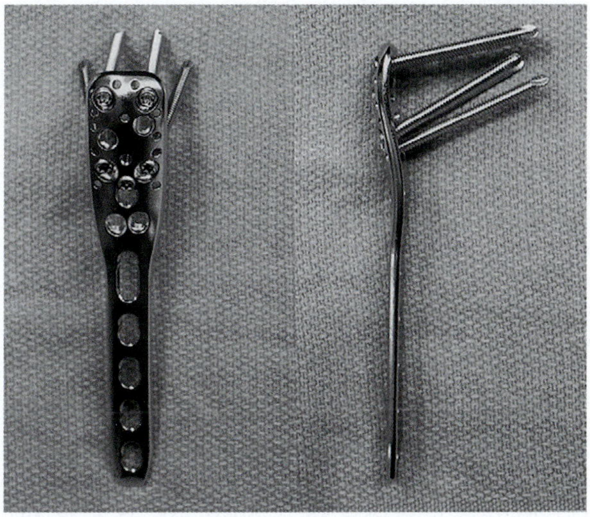

FIGURE 6-27: Photograph of a precontoured proximal humeral-locking plate (Synthes). The proximal screws allow locking fixation into the humeral head. The diaphyseal screws may be conventional or locking. Peripheral holes allow suture or wire augmentation to tuberosity fragments. (From Rose PS, Adams CR, Torchia ME, et al. Locking plate fixation for proximal humerus fractures: Initial results with a new implant. *J Shoulder Elbow Surg.* 2007;16:202-207.)

et al.[207] suggested that this is a reliable technique, with union rates of 100% (21 patients), 97% (29 patients), and 100% (23 patients), respectively. Agel et al.[2] placed emphasis on the appropriate location of nail insertion medial to the GT, and suggested that lateral metaphyseal comminution can contribute to implant failure. Of the 20 fractures treated by these authors, only 65% achieved union at the latest follow-up (range, 4 to 9 months), and 15% (three cases) demonstrated proximal screw loosening. These authors further concluded that IM fixation of PHFs is not effective in the following circumstances: (1) if the insertion site is incorrect, (2) if the insertion site is violated by fracture, or (3) if the fracture contains extensive lateral metaphyseal comminution.[2]

Park et al. performed IM fixation augmented with a tension band and a locking suture technique, and noted fracture union in 25 of 26 patients (95.8%) at a mean of 8.7 weeks (range, 7 to 12 weeks).[197] At a mean follow-up of 39 months (range, 24 to 59 months), ASES scores averaged 85 (range, 40 to 100), with no statistical difference evident when comparing patients younger or older than 65 years of age (range, 27 to 79 years old).[197] The authors concluded that open IM nailing remained a viable technique for PHFs in elderly patients, and good functional outcomes could be expected at midterm follow-up.

Koike et al.[138] reported their results with the use of a commercially available IM nail in 54 patients. Using Neer's criteria, the majority of the injuries were classified as two-part fractures (29 patients or 54%). All surgically managed fractures achieved union, with 43 patients (79%) demonstrating "satisfactory or excellent" results. Residual varus deformity and GT malunion was reported in eight shoulders (15%).[138]

Popescu et al.[204] prospectively evaluated the functional and radiologic outcomes of using an IM nail for fracture fixation in 29 patients (21 proximal and eight humeral shaft fractures). Eighteen patients were older than 70 years of age. All fractures healed at a mean of 2.7 months of follow-up. Complications were limited to a single case of AVN and one case of proximal screw migration. The authors concluded that the proximal locking mechanism of this device reduced the risk of screw failure. There was an additional trend towards better functional results in patients younger than 70 years of age, but this finding did not reach statistical significance.[204]

More recently, Hatzidakis et al.[109] utilized a medial starting point for nail placement to avoid injury to the rotator cuff and reported favorable outcomes in 38 patients with two-part fractures at 1-year follow-up. The study group demonstrated a mean Constant score of 71, a Constant pain score of 13 (range, 0 to 15, with 15 indicating no pain), mean forward flexion of 132 degrees, and a neck shaft angle at union greater than 125 degrees in all but one patient.[109]

Lopiz et al.[156] compared two IM nail constructs in a cohort of 52 prospectively evaluated patients and concluded that an articular entry straight nail resulted in similar outcomes (i.e., union rate) compared to curvilinear implants, with a reduced impact on the rotator cuff and with fewer complications. The authors reported a 42% reoperation rate in the curvilinear nail group (vs. 11% in the straight nail group); 73% of the patients in the curvilinear nail group demonstrated rotator cuff disease–related symptoms (vs. 35% in the straight nail group). Seven of the 11 cases that required revision surgery in the curvilinear nail group were related to screw migration. The remaining four patients required hardware removal, with one case requiring conversion to an RTSA.[156]

Locking Plate Versus Intramedullary Fixation

Kitson et al.[135] investigated the biomechanical behavior of a locking plate versus a locking IM nail for the treatment of three-part PHFs. Paired cadaveric specimens were tested with four directional loads: flexion, extension, varus, and valgus. When cantilever bending loads were below the failure threshold, the nail construct demonstrated significantly higher stiffness results in all directions. The authors also noted different modes of failure for each implant. In all samples, the nail construct failed at the bone-screw interface, whereas all of the plates failed due to bending of the implant at the level of the surgical neck fracture. These authors cautioned extrapolating these data to the clinical setting because the results of controlled osteotomies cannot be equated to PHFs with cortical and metaphyseal comminution.[135]

In contrast, Sanders et al.[231] performed a similar cadaveric evaluation and found that the locking plate construct demonstrated greater stiffness in valgus loading compared with the nail construct (420 vs. 166 N/mm). All other loading vectors showed no statistical differences between the two constructs. Failure in the locking plate occurred in a similar manner through the surgical neck osteotomy site as described by Kitson et al.[135,231] Both studies used similar biomechanical testing techniques; however, it remains unclear whether Sanders et al. performed their testing using a locking version of the IM nail.[135,231] Both studies were limited by sample size, and thus, conclusions must be applied to clinical practice with caution.

Boudard et al.[36] recently performed a retrospective observational study comparing locked plate fixation and IM nail fixation for nonosteoporotic three- and four-part fractures of the proximal humerus. A total of 63 patients (33 with plate and 30 with nail fixation) were available for a 1-year clinical and radiographic follow-up. The mean Oxford, Constant, relative Constant, and Quick-Dash scores did not differ between the groups. Patients with four-part fractures and GT comminution demonstrated statistically significant lower functional scores. Complication rates did not differ between the two surgical groups, although the plate group had three infections. The authors concluded that internal fixation was appropriate for three- and four-part fractures. Although they could not recommend one modality over the other, they suggested that the locking plate technique was “more aggressive.”[36]

In 2016, Gracitelli et al.[273] performed a prospective, single-center, RCT comparing the clinical and radiographic outcomes of PHFs (two- and three-part) treated with either a locking IM nail (third-generation, curved nail with an articular entry point) or locking plate. There were 36 patients randomized to each treatment group; baseline characteristics such as age, smoking status, and fracture pattern and displacement were well balanced between groups. There were no statistically significant differences between treatment groups for the clinical outcome scores (Constant-Murley, DASH, and VAS) at the 12-month follow-up; however, there were significantly more complications in the IM nail group. Specifically, 11 patients (34%) from the nail group and seven (21%) from the plate group had one or more complication. Reoperations were performed in six patients (19%) in the nail group and in one patient (3%) in the plate group.

Arthroplasty

Hemiarthroplasty

In the 1950s, Neer initially developed the technique of humeral head arthroplasty (HA) for treating PHFs.[179] Before this method was developed, these injuries were treated with benign neglect or humeral head resection. By 1970, Neer reported uniformly poor results after ORIF for four-part fractures and fracture-dislocations, and suggested HA for these fractures.[181] Because of the high risk of humeral head osteonecrosis with three- and four-part PHFs, Neer believed that even with anatomic reconstruction with internal fixation, posttraumatic osteoarthritis would develop, resulting in poor outcomes for the patients. Neer reiterated that HA and stable fixation of the tuberosities could provide a reasonable result for the patient.

Clinical studies regarding hemiarthroplasty for PHFs are difficult to directly compare as there remains heterogeneity regarding implant design, surgical technique, rehabilitation, and the outcome instruments used to evaluate patient outcome. In view of these limitations, the literature demonstrates that approximately 90% of patients treated with HA demonstrate minimal pain despite a wide range of function, ROM, and muscle strength. Factors that predict a poor outcome after HA for fractures include tuberosity malposition, tuberosity resorption and associated superior migration of the humeral prosthesis, stiffness, persistent pain, and poor initial positioning of the implant (excessive retroversion, decreased height); women older than 75 years are also at risk for poor outcome.[27,44] Regarding the timing of surgery (i.e., the time between injury and definitive surgery), most authors report poorer outcomes with surgical intervention delayed longer than 2 to 3 weeks, particularly as it relates to functional results.[14,31,175,187,274-276] Robinson et al.[219] reported satisfactory results in patients treated with primary HA with a mean prosthetic survival of 6.3 years. In this study, the majority of patients were pain free at their last follow-up, despite a wide variation in motion, function, and muscle power. Poorer results were noted in elderly patients, especially in the settings of neurologic deficit or instability with retracted tuberosities. Good functional outcomes at 1 year could be anticipated in younger patients who were nonsmokers without postoperative complications or neurologic deficits and with satisfactory radiographs at 6 weeks.[219]

Bicknell et al.[18] performed a pilot study using cadaveric specimens to assess the feasibility of a computer-assisted system in the treatment of four-part fractures. Seven pairs of specimens underwent an HA by way of computer-assisted and traditional methods to anatomically reconstruct the following seven characteristics: humeral head version, humeral head inclination, humeral head offset, humeral length, medial articulation point, GT position, and LT position. The differences between the intact and reconstructed proximal humeral anatomic values were improved in five of seven characteristics, but only humeral head offset demonstrated statistically significant improvement with the computer-assisted method. Although computer-assisted HA is promising, the authors emphasized the need for further investigation and refinement of this technique to allow reproducibility and to facilitate its use in the clinical setting.[18]

Several retrospective and prospective studies have confirmed the viability of HA for the treatment of three- and four-part PHFs that were not amenable to ORIF. Antuña et al.[3] reported their results in 57 patients with a mean age of 66 years and a mean follow-up of 10.3 years (range, 5 to 22 years). Utilizing Neer's criteria, less than 50% of the patients reported satisfactory results (22/57) despite significant pain relief.[3] Fialka et al.[78] demonstrated improved Constant scores at 1 year of follow-up when utilizing a fracture-specific humeral stem; however, nearly 30% of the patients demonstrated tuberosity resorption.[78] Hertel et al.[115] reported their results on 49 patients, with a mean follow-up of 5 years (range, 3.3 to 7.3 years). The mean Constant and Subjective Value Scores were 70 (range, 39 to 84) and 90 (range, 40 to 100), respectively.[115] Boileau et al.[28] demonstrated improved Constant scores in 30 patients at a mean follow-up of 45 months. The absolute mean Constant scores were 68 and 93 when adjusted for age and gender, respectively. Male patients and those individuals under the age of 75 years fared better with regards to functional results after HA. Nearly all patients reported "satisfactory" results after surgery (29 of 30).[28] In 2011, Olerud et al.[191] performed a prospective study of 55 patients (mean age, 77 years; range, 58 to 92 years), who were randomized to either HA or nonoperative treatment for a displaced four-part PHF. At the final 2-year follow-up, the authors concluded that HA resulted in improved quality of life (as per the EQ-5D) and pain relief; however, there were no significant differences regarding the Constant score or ROM. Both groups achieved a mean forward elevation of 90 to 95 degrees despite the use of a fracture-specific stem and reproducible surgical technique. The reoperation rate was low (three patients in the HA group and one patient in the nonoperative group).[191] More recently, Cai et al.[45] randomized 32 patients (mean age, 71.9 years; range, 67 to 86 years) to either HA or internal fixation using a locking plate for a displaced four-part fracture. A control group (i.e., nonoperative treatment) was not included in this study. Twenty-seven patients (84%) were available for the final 2-year follow-up. The functional outcomes (Constant and DASH scores), health-related quality of life, and pain scores favored HA over internal fixation, although most outcomes did not reach statistical significance. ROM parameters were also better for the HA group with regards to forward flexion and abduction.[45]

Reverse Total Shoulder Arthroplasty

Due to growing concerns regarding the potential for poor outcomes following HA related to tuberosity healing or implant malposition, significant interest has developed amongst shoulder surgeons in performing an RTSA for displaced three- and four-part PHFs in the elderly population. The main attraction to this form of arthroplasty is the ability to achieve functional shoulder elevation and abduction regardless of tuberosity healing, position, and degree of comminution; however, the repair and union of the GT fragment(s) during RTSA have been demonstrated to improve functional outcomes including external rotation and patient satisfaction compared to outcomes after tuberosity resection, nonunion, or resorption.[44,139] An additional advantage of an RTSA is that the medial glenoid erosion observed following HA may be prevented through placement of the glenosphere component.

Over the last 10 years, several studies have demonstrated that RTSA is a viable surgical option for acute three- and four-part PHFs and fracture sequelae. Most published studies represent case series (level IV evidence) or systematic reviews; high-level evidence is limited. Boulahia et al.[37] reported their initial results (mean follow-up, 35 months) of a mixed patient population (16 patients) with cuff tear arthropathy and fracture sequelae who underwent RTSA. The mean preoperative-to-postoperative forward elevation increased from 70 to 139 degrees, with a corresponding increase in the Constant score from 31 to 59. The authors did note a revision rate of 12.5%.[37]

Boileau et al.[32] reviewed their results using the Delta III prosthesis (Depuy) in the management of three distinct patient groups: cuff tear arthropathy (21 patients), implant revision (19 patients), and fracture sequelae with associated arthritis (5 patients). Although all groups demonstrated significant increases in forward elevation (55 to 121 degrees) and Constant score (17 to 58), the authors did not observe an improvement in external rotation. More importantly, they reported a 20% (one of five cases) complication rate with the fracture sequelae group (one implant was revised to a hemiarthroplasty due to glenoid fracture). These authors emphasized that functional results are less predictable and complication rates are higher in revision and fracture sequelae cases compared to cuff tear arthropathy cases.[32]

Cazeneuve and Cristofari[47] retrospectively analyzed 23 patients who underwent primary RTSA using the Delta III prosthesis for acute three- and four-part PHFs (18 patients) and fracture-dislocations (five patients). Tuberosity reduction was possible in only five patients. There were 16 patients (70%) available for final clinical and radiographic follow-up; seven patients died prior to the final follow-up. The mean Constant score was 60 (83 for the contralateral, uninjured side) at a mean follow-up of 86 months. Significant gains in forward elevation, abduction, and pain relief were reported. Complications included regional pain syndrome (two patients), infection (one patient, requiring revision), and anterior dislocation (one patient, requiring revision). Based on their results, the authors recommended RTSA for elderly patients with unmanageable tuberosities (e.g., tuberosity comminution or high-risk of tuberosity resorption postoperatively or preexisting rotator cuff pathology) to attain gains in pain relief and forward elevation.[47]

Bufquin et al.[43] reported their results in 41 patients (mean age, 78 years; range, 65 to 97 years) who underwent RTSA for displaced three- and four-part PHFs. The mean follow-up was 22 months (range, 6 to 58 months). The clinical outcome was satisfactory, with a mean active forward elevation of 97 degrees (range, 35 to 160 degrees) and abducted external rotation of 30 degrees (range, 0 to 80 degrees). The Constant and modified Constant scores were 44 and 66%, respectively. Tuberosity displacement occurred in 19 patients (53%) and scapular notching in 10 (25%). The authors concluded that "satisfactory" mobility could be obtained even with tuberosity displacement.[43]

Boyle et al.[38] performed a retrospective case-control study (level III evidence) comparing HA (313 patients) to RTSA (55 patients) for three- and four-part PHFs. Compared with HA, patients who underwent RTSA were significantly older (mean age, 79.6 vs. 71.9 years) and more often women (93% vs. 78%). The 6-month OSS was 28.1 for RTSA and 27.9 for HA. The RTSA group had a significantly better 5-year OSS than the HA group (41.5 vs. 32.3). The authors did not observe a significant difference between the RTSA and HA groups in the revision rate per 100 component years (1.7 vs. 1.1) and in 1-year mortality (3.5% vs. 3.6%). They concluded that patients with acute PHFs who undergo RTSA achieve superior 5-year functional outcomes compared with patients who undergo HA.[38]

Cuff and Pupello[59] performed a prospective cohort (i.e., nonrandomized) study involving 43 patients with three- and four-part PHFs treated with either HA (23 patients) or RTSA (24 patients) with a minimum 2-year follow-up. ASES, Simple Shoulder Test, and patient satisfaction scores were significantly lower in the HA group. Interestingly, tuberosity union rates were higher in the RTSA group (83% vs. 61%). Forward elevation was better in the RTSA group (139 degrees vs. 100 degrees), and three patients from the HA group required revision to RTSA (13% conversion rate). However, analysis of the outcomes relative to tuberosity healing yielded similar results between the HA and RTSA groups. The authors concluded that RTSA resulted in consistently better clinical outcomes and similar complication rates compared with HA for the treatment of comminuted PHFs in the elderly.[59]

In 2013, Mata-Fink et al.[162] performed a systematic review of the literature comparing RTSA to HA. Fifteen studies met the inclusion criteria for the meta-analysis, including 377 patients treated with RTSA and 504 patients treated with HA. The RTSA group had improved forward elevation and functional outcome scores compared with the HA group but diminished external rotation. Complication rates were similar between the two groups. The authors suggested that RTSA is a reasonable alternative for treating older adults (>60 years) with PHFs, but additional research and longer term follow-up are necessary.[162] Sebastia-Forcada et al.[234] performed a prospective study of 62 patients, with equal numbers of patients randomized to either RTSA or HA. RTSA patients had significantly higher Constant scores (56.1 vs. 40.0), forward elevation (120.3 vs. 79.8 degrees), and abduction (112.9 vs. 78.7 degrees), but no difference in internal rotation (2.7 vs. 2.6 degrees). The DASH score was higher in the HA patients (17 vs. 29), denoting greater disability in the HA group. In the HA group, 56.6% of tuberosities healed versus 64.5% in the RTSA cohort. Six patients (19.4%) within the HA group had proximal humeral head migration that required revision to an RTSA. The functional outcome was independent of tuberosity healing in the RTSA group. Scapular notching was observed in one RTSA patient. One patient developed a hematoma, and another developed an infection requiring two-stage revision to another RTSA.[234] Most recently, in 2015, Ferrel et al.[77] performed a systematic review comparing the results of RTSA to HA (30 studies; 1346 patients), and noted improved forward elevation (118 degrees vs. 108 degrees) but inferior external rotation (3 degrees vs. 20 degrees) with RTSA. No significant clinical differences in either the ASES (RTSA 64.7 vs. HA 63) or Constant score (RTSA 54.6 vs. HA 58) were identified. Furthermore, the authors found an increased rate of complications with RTSA (9.6%) but a lower revision rate (0.93%) at the short- to mid-term follow-up.[77]

AUTHORS' PREFERRED METHOD OF TREATMENT

Methods of Treatment

Regardless of the fracture type and surgical intervention selected, a recent Cochrane review of 23 randomized trials involving PHFs failed to demonstrate sufficient evidence to support specific management recommendations (nonoperative vs. operative) with the exception of early physical therapy (PT) for nondisplaced fractures.[105] Despite the lack of evidence to support a preferred treatment method, the goals of intervention include the relief of pain and restoration of function (Fig. 6-28).

Nondisplaced or Minimally Displaced PHFs

Nondisplaced and minimally displaced fractures are treated initially with a sling for comfort. Elbow, wrist, and hand exercises are encouraged during the initial immobilization period. If the fracture is stable, ROM exercises may be started within 10 to 14 days if the pain is tolerable to avoid late sequelae such as stiffness, limited ability to perform ADLs, and an overall poor functional outcome.[142] Serial radiographic evaluation is necessary to evaluate for fracture displacement.[142]

Open Reduction and Internal Fixation of PHFs

The current indications for plate and screw fixation include displaced (with or without comminution) two-, three-, and some four-part PHFs. This method of treatment is also appropriate for fracture-dislocations in young, active adults. The ideal patient is physiologically young with good bone stock, medically capable of undergoing surgery, and compliant with the postoperative rehabilitation program (see Figs. 6-22 and 6-28).[121,186]

Surgical Approach

There are two basic surgical approaches that can be used to treat PHFs. The superior approach to the shoulder involves a skin incision made in Langer's lines just lateral to the anterolateral aspect of the acromion (Fig. 6-29A). The deltoid can be split from the edge of the acromion distally for approximately 5 cm; to protect the axillary nerve, the split should not be extended (Fig. 6-29B). If distal exposure is required, the axillary nerve must be carefully exposed and protected.[22,121,155] The deltoid origin is not removed during exposure of the superior aspect of the proximal humerus. This approach is useful for internal fixation of GT fractures and for IM fixation of two-part surgical neck fractures. Rotation, flexion, or extension of the humerus can allow exposure of the underlying structures for appropriate reduction and internal fixation.[22,121,155]

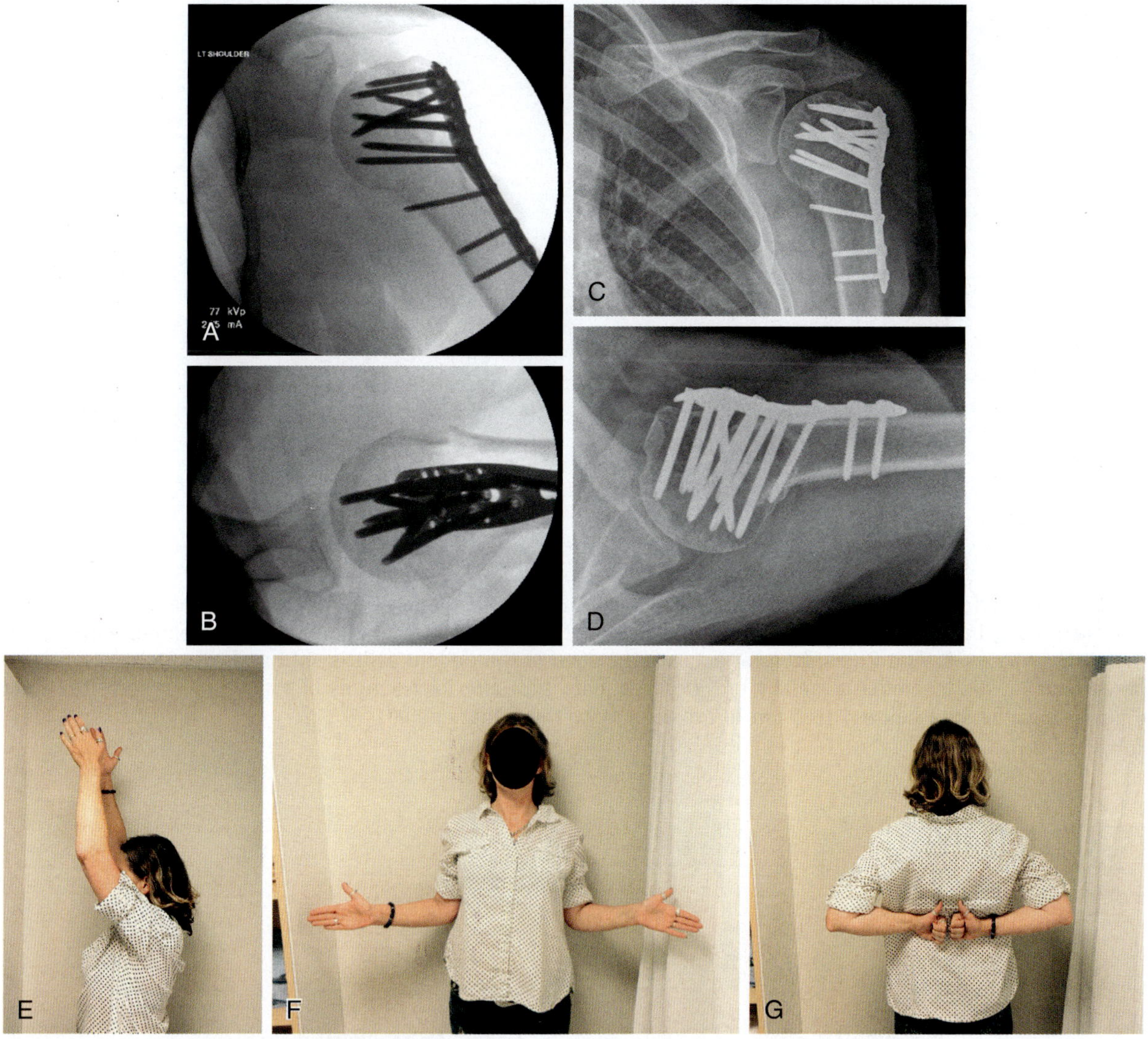

FIGURE 6-28: **A** and **B,** Anteroposterior and modified axillary (Velpeau) fluoroscopic views following open reduction and internal fixation of a displaced three-part proximal humerus fracture in a 49-year-old female (preoperative radiographs not available). **C** and **D,** Postoperative true anteroposterior and axillary radiographs at the 2-year follow-up visit reveal complete healing of the fracture. **E** to **G,** Active shoulder range of motion at the 2-year follow-up visit is nearly symmetric, and muscle strength is normal. The patient has no pain and no limitations with activities of daily living or with recreational sports and activities. (Courtesy Aaron J. Bois, MD.)

The deltopectoral approach remains the workhorse for PHFs (Fig. 6-30A). The skin incision extends from the coracoid process distally toward the deltoid insertion. The cephalic vein should be preserved and is typically retracted laterally with the deltoid. The deltopectoral interval is developed proximally and distally (Fig. 6-30B). If more exposure is needed, the superior 1 to 2 cm of the pectoralis major tendon (PMT) insertion can be divided longitudinally. This approach is useful for internal fixation of two-, three-, and four-part fractures, arthroplasty of three- and four-part fractures, and fracture-dislocations.[22,43,121,155]

Both approaches are useful because they preserve deltoid function, which allows more rapid rehabilitation in the postoperative period. Detachment of the deltoid origin is unnecessary, and if performed, will deleteriously affect shoulder function and prohibit progression during the postoperative rehabilitation program.

Nonlocking and Locking Plate Surgical Technique

The patient may be positioned in the beach chair, lateral decubitus, or supine position on a radiolucent table. We generally prefer the beach chair position and use an extended deltopectoral approach. A commercially available arm-holding device may be used. The anterior third of the deltoid may need to be partially elevated distally from its insertion on the deltoid tuberosity. The displaced

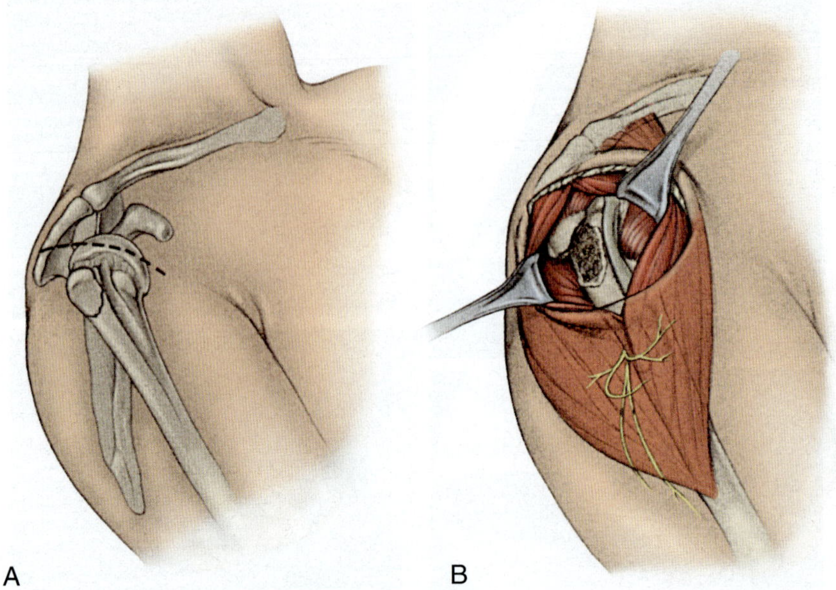

FIGURE 6-29: Superior approach to the shoulder. **A,** The skin incision for the superior approach to the shoulder consists of an oblique incision along Langer's lines beginning on the anterolateral aspect of the acromion and extending down obliquely for approximately 8 to 9 cm. **B,** Two Richardson retractors are placed in the deltoid as it is split approximately 4 to 5 cm from the tip of the acromion. This technique generally provides adequate exposure for fractures of the greater tuberosity. Great care is taken to not extend the split below 4 to 5 cm to avoid injury to the axillary nerve.

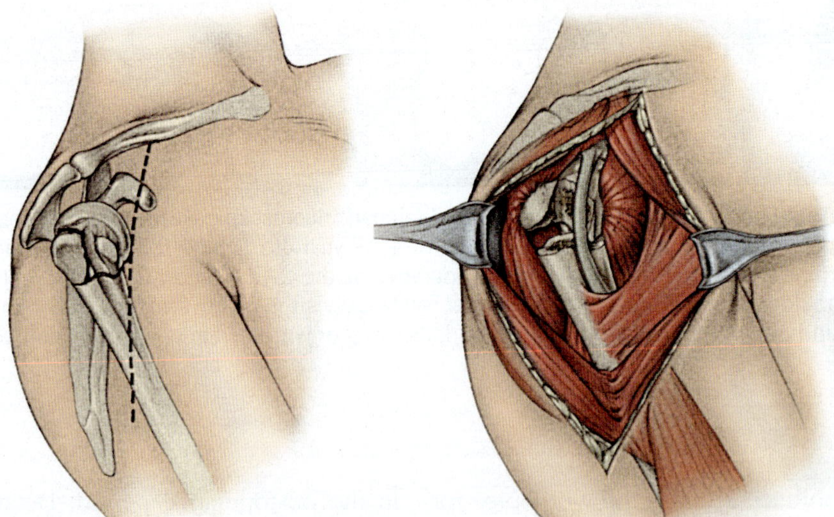

FIGURE 6-30: The extended deltopectoral approach is a utilitarian approach for two-, three-, and four-part fractures. **A,** The incision is made from the clavicle, passes over the coracoid, and extends down to the shaft of the humerus near the deltoid insertion. **B,** The insertion of the pectoralis major can also be released to improve exposure. Care is taken to preserve the deltoid origin on the clavicle. If more exposure is needed, the deltoid insertion can be elevated, although such elevation is rarely necessary.

GT and LT fragments are identified, mobilized, and tagged with multiple No. 5 braided nonabsorbable sutures at the tendon-bone junction for later repair through the peripheral holes in the plate. These sutures can be initially used as traction sutures to facilitate fracture reduction.

For three- and four-part fractures, the tuberosity fragments are initially reduced to the lateral humeral shaft cortex. In valgus-impacted fractures, the medial calcar may be reestablished by using an elevator to disimpact the humeral head. Threaded or smooth 1.6-mm K-wires may be used to provisionally hold the fracture fragments reduced; the wires are initially placed anteriorly from distal to proximal, passing from the anterior humeral shaft into the humeral head. The plate should then be positioned on the anterolateral aspect of the humeral shaft and GT (i.e., lateral to the bicipital groove). Additional wires are then placed through the plate holes into the humeral shaft distally and humeral head proximally to enhance fracture stability. Previously placed sutures from the tuberosity fragment may be delivered through the peripheral holes at this time (Fig. 6-31A). In the AP view, the plate should be placed at a minimum of 8 mm below the superior tip of GT to avoid impingement. Some implant designs require more distal placement of the plate, and the treating surgeon should adjust his or her technique accordingly. Adequate spacing is necessary between the plate and the biceps tendon to prevent injury to the arcuate artery (Fig. 6-31B).

After AP and axillary (or scapular Y lateral) views confirm a satisfactory reduction, an initial compression screw is placed in the elongated hole of the plate. Locked screws are then inserted into the humeral head using the insertion guide. We utilize a sounding technique with the power drill bit to estimate the screw length in the humeral head, which is then confirmed with a depth gauge and lastly with fluoroscopy (in two planes). Typically, we decrease the final screw length by 5 mm in an effort to decrease the incidence of screw penetration; this is especially important in valgus-impacted fractures that have a tendency to "settle" back into valgus over time. Tingart et al. investigated the appropriate positioning of these screws by evaluating the bone mineral density of 18 unpaired cadaveric humeri. They concluded that the pullout strength was least in the anterosuperior portion of the humeral head, and suggested that screws be placed in the regions of the highest bone mineral density that involved all other regions other than the anterosuperior humeral head.[250] At least three distal shaft screws (locking or nonlocking) are inserted (Fig. 6-32). In the event that there is a residual metaphyseal defect, a bone graft or bone graft substitute may be used as an adjuvant to fracture healing (see Fig. 6-19).[186] In this clinical scenario, some authors have recently advocated the use of a fibular strut graft to prevent varus collapse and hardware failure.[6,163,247] A cadaveric study by Bae et al. demonstrated increased load to failure and initial stiffness with the use of a fibular strut allograft in conjunction with a locking plate.[6] Matassi et al.[163] reported promising results with this technique in 17 patients who demonstrated complete union at the latest follow-up, without major complications. Tan et al.[247] demonstrated improved early results in nine patients treated with a proximal humeral-locking plate and IM fibular strut allograft. They believed that the fibular strut graft functioned as a "void filler,"

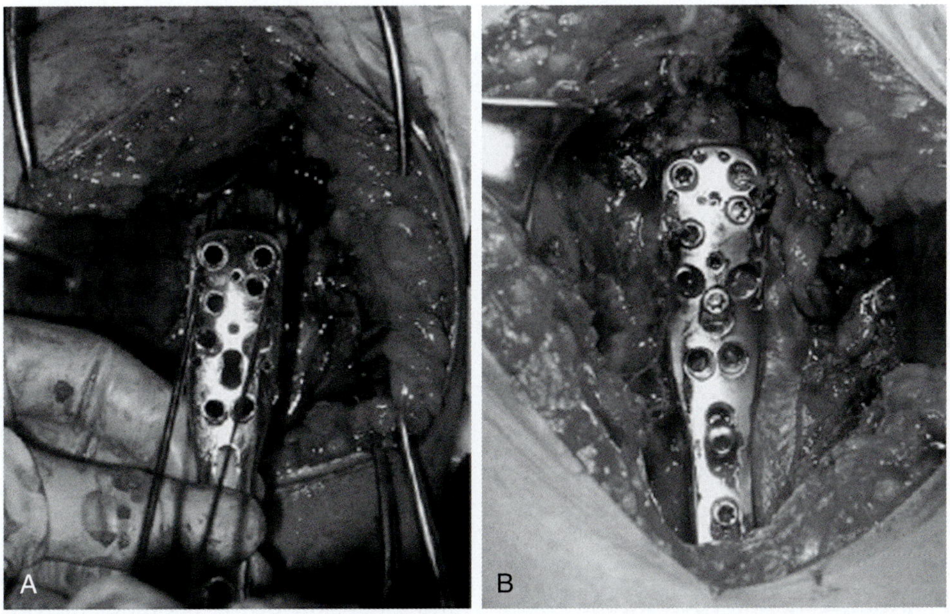

FIGURE 6-31: A, Tagged sutures from the greater tuberosity are placed through the plate. **B,** Locking plate placed in the anterolateral aspect of the greater tuberosity and humeral shaft. (From Nho SJ, Brophy RH, Barker JU, et al. Innovations in the management of displaced proximal humerus fractures. *J Am Acad Orthop Surg.* 2007;15[1]:12-26.)

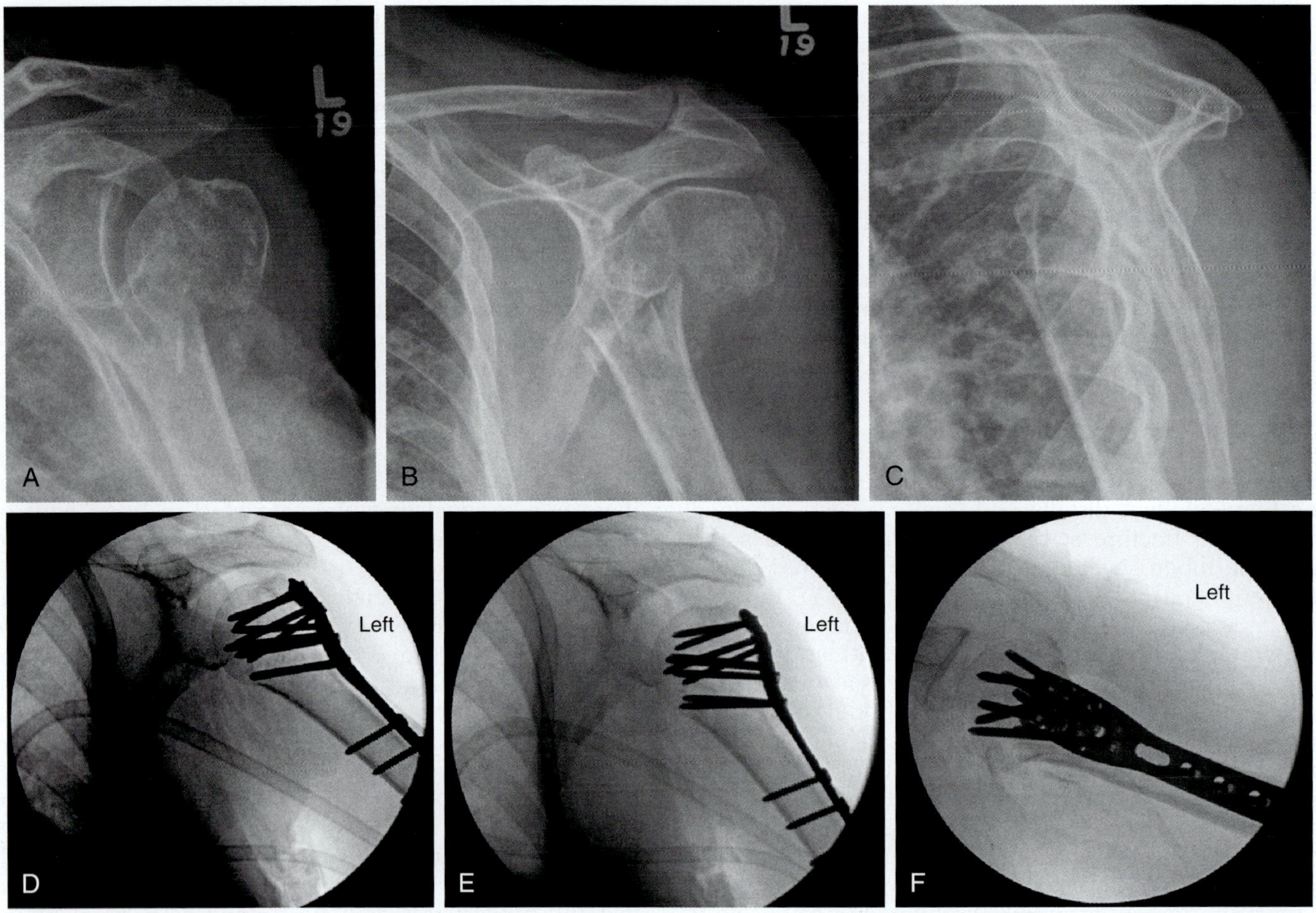

FIGURE 6-32: **A** to **C,** Anteroposterior and transcapular lateral radiographs demonstrating a displaced two-part surgical neck fracture. **D** to **F,** Intraoperative fluoroscopy reveals near anatomic restoration of the proximal humerus and ideal placement of the locking plate and proximal locking and distal nonlocking screws. (Courtesy Aaron J. Bois, MD.)

supported the native humeral head, and provided additional points of cortical fixation to prevent varus collapse and hardware failure in the osteoporotic PHF.[247]

Postoperative Care

The stability of the fixation is evaluated intraoperatively to allow specific tailoring of the postoperative physician-directed rehabilitation regimen. With rigid fixation, patients should begin pendulum and passive ROM exercises on postoperative day 1. Radiographic healing should be apparent by 6 to 8 weeks postoperatively, and active and active-assisted ROM exercises may be performed under the supervision of a physical therapist. By 3 months postoperatively, strengthening exercises should be started. The patient should be made aware that maximal improvement may not be achieved for up to 1 year postsurgery.

Intramedullary Fixation Surgical Technique

Commercially available IM nails have evolved, and now contain design elements that allow for locking screws and/or mechanisms that create a fixed-angle construct. In three-part PHFs with involvement of the GT, the entry point for some commercially available nails is compromised.[2,121,138,207,215] If the LT is involved, the insertion point at the junction of the articular surface and GT is left intact.

The patient is placed in the beach chair position on a radiolucent table. A 3-cm longitudinal incision is made in line with the GT of the humerus. The deltoid is then split in line with its fibers.[215] Under C-arm fluoroscopy, the entry hole of the nail is made with a curved awl or guide pin just medial to the GT and approximately 1.5 cm posterior to the bicipital groove (i.e., if using a curved nail).[207] We prefer to use more modern nail designs that are straight and have fixed-angle locking capabilities for proximal screw fixation (i.e., third-generation nailing); nail entry is through a small split in the rotator cuff and subsequently through the superior articular surface of the humeral head. This helps to reduce damage to the rotator cuff footprint during nail insertion. Adduction of the arm and extension of the shoulder provides adequate clearance from the acromion for the awl and subsequent nail insertion. If closed reduction can be performed (acute cases), it is generally accomplished with longitudinal traction on an adducted arm in neutral rotation.[215] If closed reduction is not possible secondary to soft tissue interposition, adhesions, or early callus formation (subacute or chronic cases), open reduction may be performed before the nail is inserted.[207,215]

A 2-mm guidewire is passed across the fracture and down the IM canal. The nail is inserted and locked proximally and distally. Care must be taken when placing the distal locking screws to avoid injury to the neurovascular structures, including the radial nerve, brachial artery, and median nerve (depending on lateral or anterior screw placement). Gentle blunt soft tissue dissection (nick-and-spread method) and screw placement under C-arm guidance are necessary to avoid iatrogenic injury to these structures.[215] A small longitudinal incision (1 to 2 cm) may be necessary to safely expose the humeral cortex to avoid neurovascular injury during distal locking screw insertion.

Postoperative Care

The arm is placed in a sling or shoulder immobilizer. Gentle pendulum and elbow ROM exercises are initiated on postoperative day 1. Patients are seen at 2 and 6 weeks for clinical and radiographic evaluation. With radiographic union, active and active-assisted ROM exercises may be initiated. By 3 months postsurgery, strengthening exercises can be started.[2,207,215]

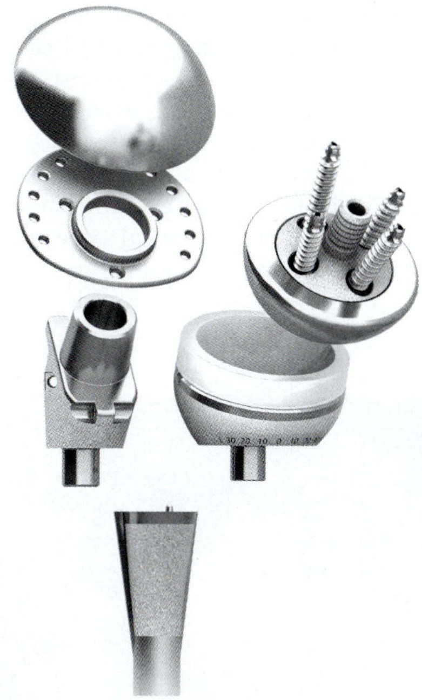

FIGURE 6-33: Modular platform-based stem with a suture collar that allows for hemiarthroplasty reconstruction of proximal humerus fractures with the capability of stem retention and potential conversion to a semi-constrained device. (Courtesy Depuy-Synthes, Warsaw, IN.)

Hemiarthroplasty for Fracture

Patient Selection

The current indications for primary HA include most four-part fractures, some three-part fractures, fracture-dislocations, head-splitting articular segment fractures, and chronic anterior or posterior humeral head dislocations with more than 40% articular surface involvement in elderly patients with osteopenic bone.[181,269] Additional indications include those fractures with greater than 20 degrees of varus precluding internal fixation, associated moderate to severe osteopenia, and sequelae from failed osteosynthesis in a young adult such as AVN of the humeral head.[131]

Iannotti et al. outlined specific anatomic parameters in their cadaveric study that are vital to consider when performing a primary hemiarthroplasty, including humeral head height (8 mm from the GT to the top of the articular surface), radius of curvature (22 to 25 mm), and humeral version (mean, 29.8 degrees; range, 10 to 55 degrees).[120] Initial implant designs were monoblock, and did not offer variations in humeral head sizes. Second- and third-generation "fracture-specific" implants have incorporated modularity and stem body size reduction to match the patient's anatomy while accommodating for tuberosity reduction.[69,172] Additional features of these implants include a recessed proximal body with fins and multiple suture holes to improve tuberosity reduction and fixation. Some implant designs incorporate a central cutout for bone grafting to improve the likelihood of tuberosity healing.[276] "Fourth-generation" platform-based systems (with or without suture collars) may assist the surgeon during the primary reconstruction, with the ability to convert to an RTSA if the initial procedure fails. When using a platform system, the reconstruction begins with stable placement of a diaphyseal component in the desired version and subsequent modular reconstruction of the proximal humerus, including restoration of humeral head height and tuberosity position (Fig. 6-33).

Several studies have indicated that outcomes following primary hemiarthroplasty for acute PHFs are superior to results from late reconstruction.[35,187] Although some studies have recommended urgent intervention (48 hours), most authors suggest preoperative planning with a careful neurovascular assessment of the injured shoulder, medical optimization of the patient, and preoperative templating with standard radiographs of the contralateral uninjured shoulder.[98] A CT scan of the injured shoulder may be useful for surgical planning purposes, especially for complex fracture patterns (A.J.B.) (see Fig. 6-20). As previously outlined, most authors report poorer outcomes when surgical intervention is delayed longer than 2 to 4 weeks, which has also been our experience.[3]

Surgical Technique

The goal of surgery is to anatomically reconstruct the proximal humerus with restoration of humeral height, retroversion, and secure tuberosity fixation. An interscalene block (regional anesthesia) may be used to augment general anesthesia (K.I.B.); however, this is not typically recommended in the trauma setting. Endotracheal intubation is generally recommended to allow intraoperative muscle relaxation.[22,98,107]

The patient is placed on an operative table in the beach chair position (i.e., with the head of the bed elevated approximately 30 to 40 degrees) with the arm positioned in a sterile articulating arm holder or draped free if an appropriate number of assistants are available (Fig. 6-34A).[22,98,107] The surgical preparation site should include the entire upper extremity and shoulder region, including the scapular and pectoral region. Appropriate prophylactic intravenous antibiotics are given to the patient within 30 minutes of skin incision.

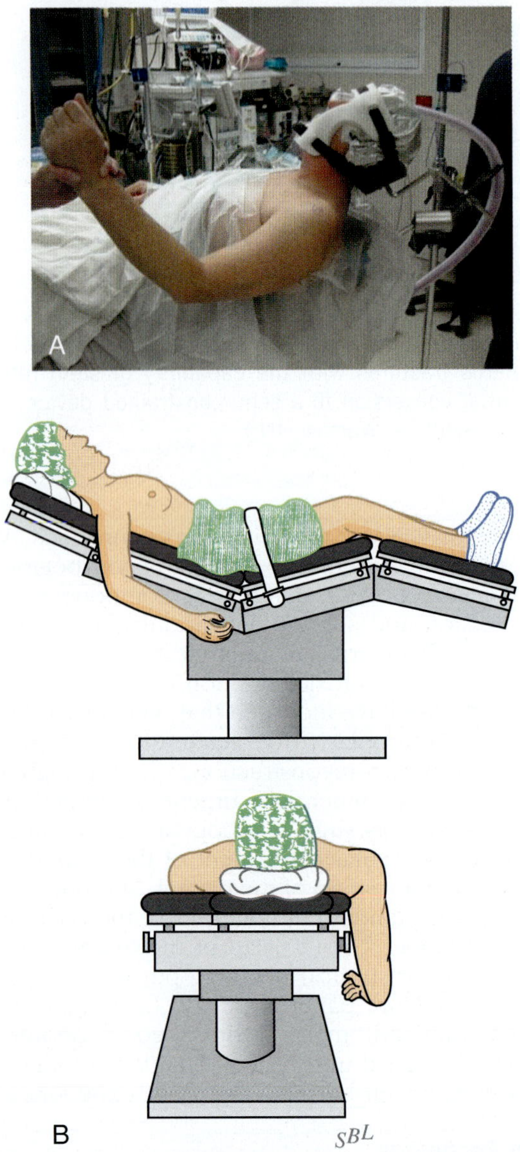

FIGURE 6-34: The "beach chair"/semi-Fowler's position. The patient is placed with the thorax at the end of the table. Commercially available attachments allow for unencumbered access to the medullary canal of the humerus and airway access for anesthesia. A padded Mayo stand or commercially available arm positioner may be used. (**A,** Courtesy Kamal I. Bohsali, MD. **B,** Modified from Matsen FA III, Lippitt SB: *Shoulder Surgery: Principles and Procedures.* Philadelphia, Saunders; 2004:628.)

A standard deltopectoral incision is used. The pectoralis major insertion should be identified and preserved to be used as a guide for restoration of the humeral head height. If additional exposure is necessary, the proximal 1 cm of the pectoralis major insertion may be released (Fig. 6-35). Fracture hematoma is usually encountered once the clavipectoral fascia is incised. Fracture fragments and the rotator cuff musculature become evident.[98,107] The axillary and musculocutaneous nerves may be identified through digital palpation of the anteroinferior aspect of the subscapularis muscle and the posterior aspect of the conjoint tendon, respectively.

External rotation of the humerus results in reduced tension on the axillary nerve.[22,98,107] The tendon of the long head of the biceps is identified as it courses in the bicipital groove toward the rotator interval. The tendon serves as a key landmark when re-establishing the anatomic relationship between the GT and LT. The rotator interval and coracohumeral ligament are both released to allow mobilization of the tuberosities (Fig. 6-36).[22,98,107] An osteotome or saw blade may be used to create a cleavage plane for mobilizing the LT or GT, if the fracture does not involve the bicipital groove. Preservation of the coracoacromial ligament is advisable to maintain the coracoacromial arch and prevent superior migration of the humeral head.

Heavy, nonabsorbable traction sutures are placed through the rotator cuff insertions on the tuberosities at the tendon-bone junction. Two or three sutures should be placed through the subscapularis tendon and three or four spanning through the supraspinatus and infraspinatus tendons. When using a stem with a suture collar, definitive sutures may be placed with a Mayo needle after implantation of the final humeral stem. Tuberosity fragments vary in size, and may require trimming for reduction and repair (Fig. 6-37). With the tuberosities retracted on their tendinous insertions, the humeral head and shaft fragments are easily visualized.[22,98,107] The native articular surface is removed and sized with a template for trial humeral head replacement (Fig. 6-38). All bone fragments, including the cancellous portion of the humeral head, should be saved and morselized for later grafting of the tuberosity and humeral shaft regions. The glenoid must be examined for concomitant pathology. Hematoma, cartilaginous fragments, and loose bone fragments are removed with sterile saline irrigation. Associated glenoid fractures should be stabilized with internal fixation. If the glenoid exhibits significant degenerative wear or irreparable damage, a glenoid component may be required.[22,98,107]

The proximal end of the humeral shaft is delivered into the wound. Loose bone fragments and hematoma are removed from the canal of the humeral shaft. Serial reamers are used to prepare the medullary canal by hand (i.e., without power) for trial implantation. The trial humeral implant is placed with the lateral fin slightly posterior to the bicipital groove and with the medial aspect of the trial head at least at the height of the medial calcar. We currently use a commercially available fracture jig that can maintain the height and retroversion of the

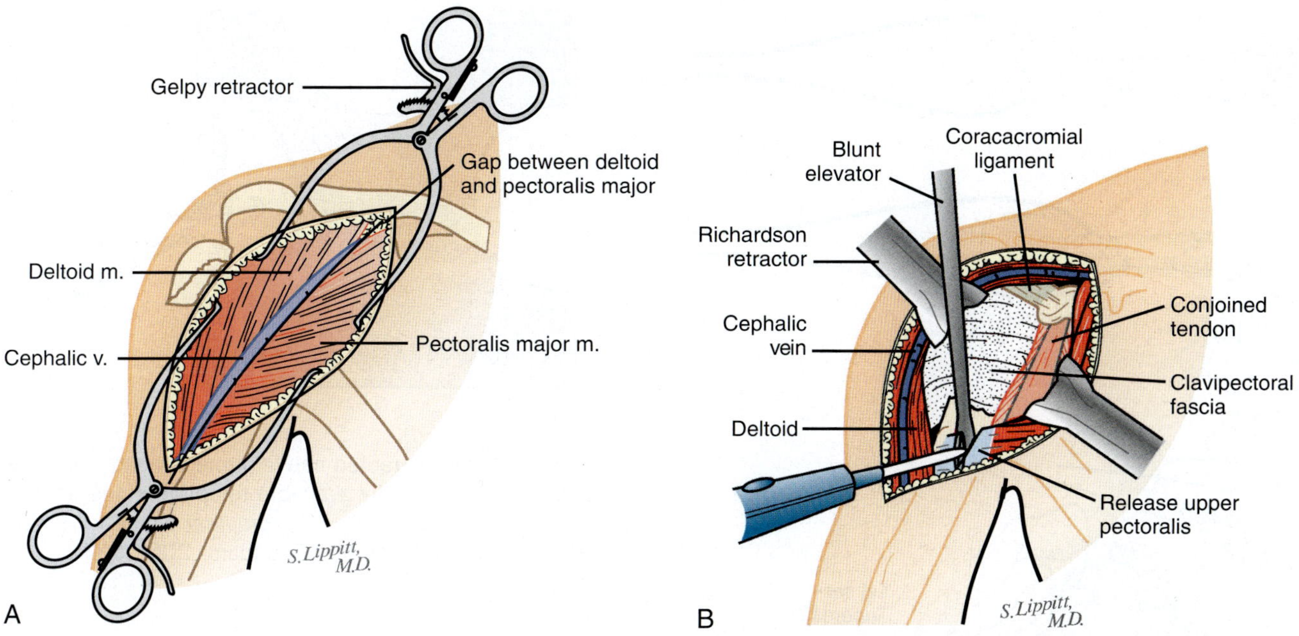

FIGURE 6-35: **A,** The skin incision is centered over the anterior deltoid. The deltopectoral interval is developed with lateral retraction of the cephalic vein. **B,** For more exposure the superior 1 cm of the pectoralis major tendon may be incised. (**A,** Modified from Matsen FA III, Lippitt SB. *Shoulder Surgery: Principles and Procedures,* Philadelphia, Saunders; 2004:629. **B,** Modified from *Global Fx Shoulder Fracture System Surgical Technique.* DePuy Orthopaedics; 1999.)

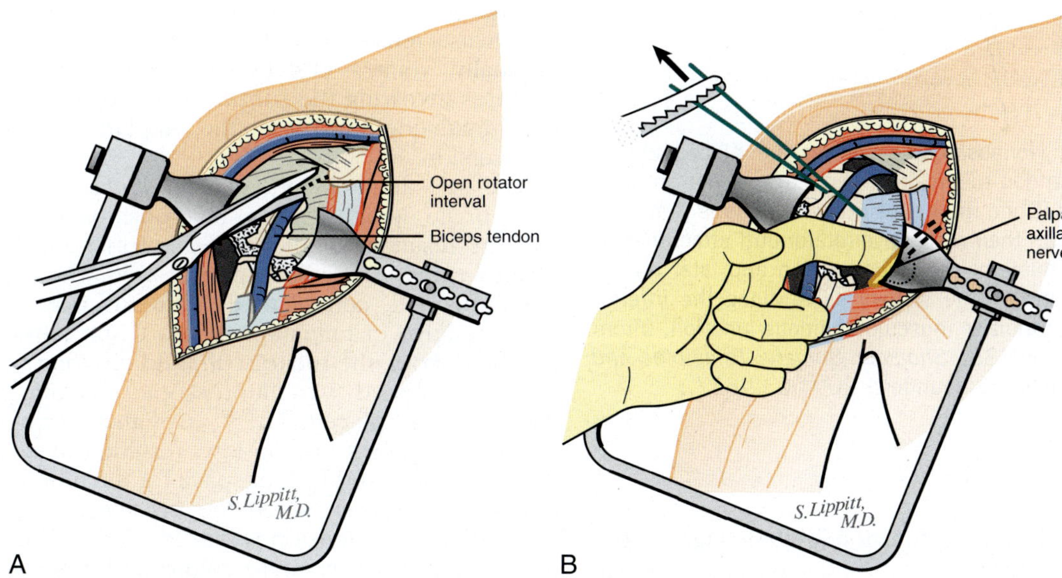

FIGURE 6-36: **A,** The long head of the biceps is identified and traced superiorly to the rotator interval. The tendon serves as a key landmark when reestablishing the anatomic relationship between the greater and lesser tuberosities. **B,** The axillary nerve is identified at the anteroinferior border of the subscapularis. (Modified from *Global Fx Shoulder Fracture System Surgical Technique.* DePuy Orthopaedics; 1999.)

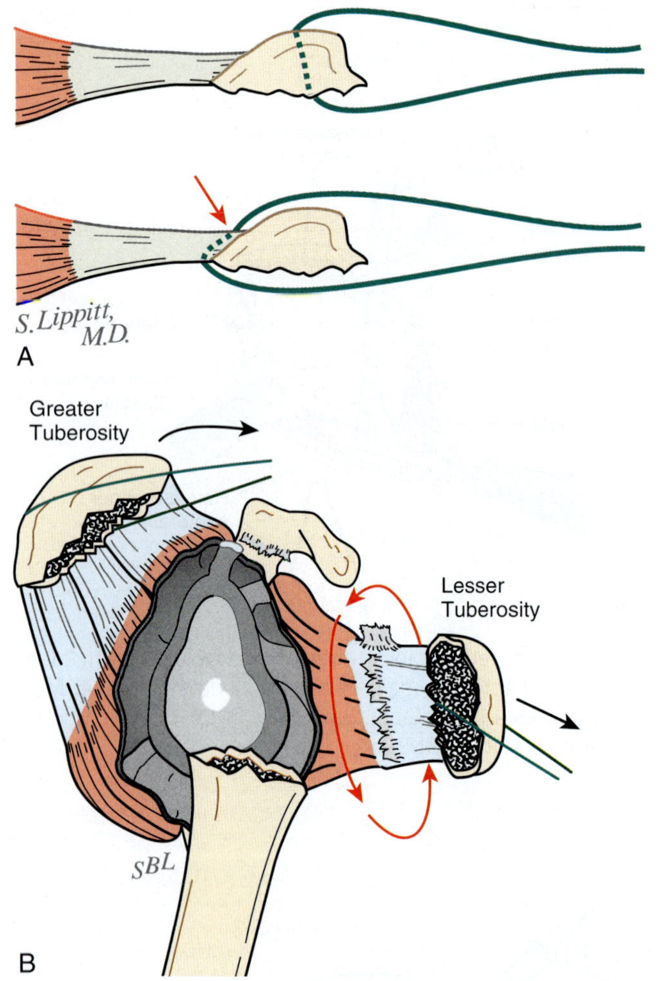

FIGURE 6-37: **A,** Nonabsorbable sutures are placed at the junction of the tendon-tuberosity interface and not through the tuberosities. **B,** Once the native humeral head is removed, the tuberosities, with their respective rotator cuff attachments, are mobilized for humeral canal preparation and later repair. Care is taken to protect the axillary nerve along the inferior aspect of the subscapularis musculotendinous junction. (From Matsen FA III, Lippitt SB. *Shoulder Surgery: Principles and Procedures.* Philadelphia: Saunders; 2004:632-637.)

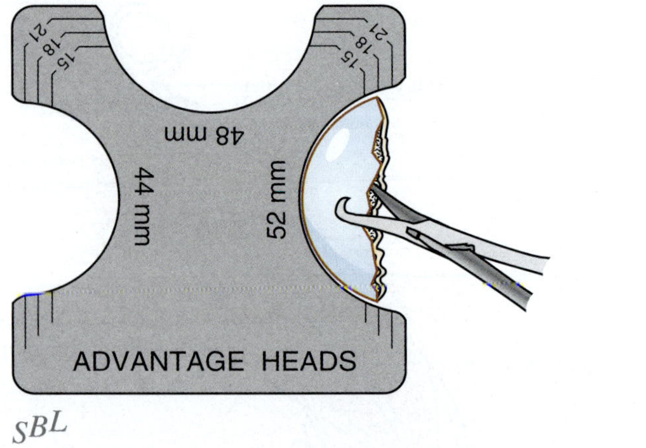

FIGURE 6-38: The extracted native humeral head is sized with the use of a commercially available template guide. (Modified from Matsen FA III, Lippitt SB. *Shoulder Surgery: Principles and Procedures.* Philadelphia: Saunders; 2004:634.)

trial component through a functional ROM (Fig. 6-39).[98] As an alternative, a proximally placed surgical lap sponge may be used to stabilize the stem position during trial maneuvers.

Correct humeral retroversion is critical when recreating the glenohumeral articulation. Most techniques suggest 30 degrees as a guide during reconstruction, although native retroversion varies from 10 to 50 degrees.[120] Several methods are used to gauge this angle:

1. External rotation of the humerus to 30 degrees from the sagittal plane of the body with the humeral head component facing directly medial into the glenoid fossa.
2. An imaginary line from the distal humeral epicondylar axis that bisects the axis of the prosthesis.
3. Positioning of the lateral fin of the prosthesis approximately 8 mm posterior to the bicipital groove (Fig. 6-40).[98,123]

Caution should be utilized when using the bicipital groove as a reference for tuberosity version, as the groove internally rotates distally. In comminuted four-part fractures involving the surgical neck region, the surgeon may inadvertently place the implant into excessive retroversion.[8]

The prosthetic height is also critical to reestablish appropriate length-tension relationships of the rotator cuff and resultant shoulder mechanics. Preoperative templating using AP radiographs of both the injured and uninjured (i.e., contralateral) humerus may be helpful. Intraoperative examination of soft tissue tension including the deltoid, the rotator cuff, and the long head of the biceps combined with fluoroscopic imaging aids prosthetic height placement.[98,107] Common errors involve placing the prosthesis too low, resulting in poor deltoid muscle tension and lack of space for the tuberosities (Fig. 6-39B). In contrast, when the prosthesis is placed too high, inadvertent tension is placed on the tuberosity fixation, leading to premature failure and tuberosity migration (see Fig. 6-51). In the event of significant proximal humerus comminution, Murachovksy et al.[177] have suggested that the pectoralis major insertion be used as a landmark in restoring humeral height. According to their cadaveric study, the distance from the top of the PMT to the superior articular surface of the humeral head averaged 5.6 cm (± 0.5 cm).[177] Ponce et al. have also demonstrated a proportional increase in PMT distance with increasing patient height. The authors reaffirmed the use of the PMT during reconstructive procedures.[203] Drill holes are placed in the proximal humeral shaft medial

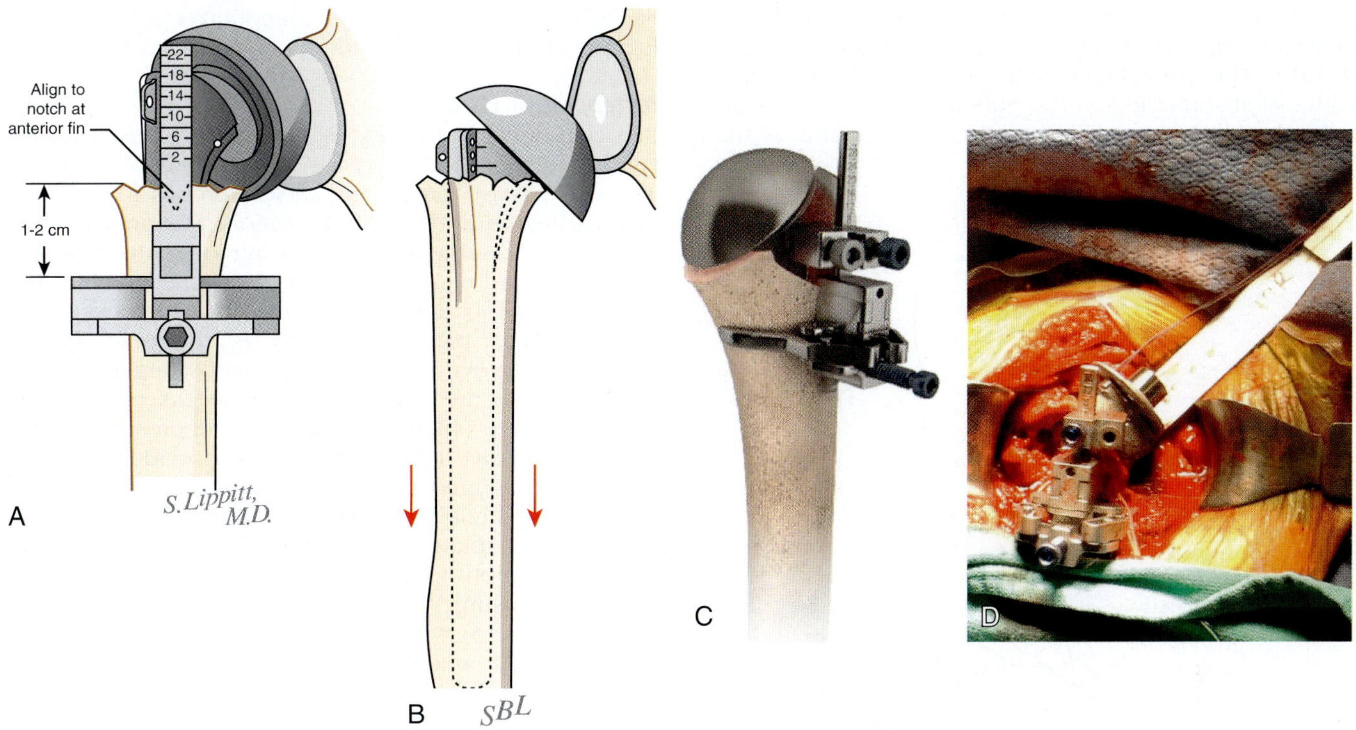

FIGURE 6-39: **A** to **C,** Use of a commercially available fracture jig allows intraoperative assessment of implant height and version. Placing the prosthesis too low results in poor deltoid muscle tension and lack of space for the tuberosities (**B**). **D,** Intraoperative image demonstrating the use of a fracture jig. (**A** and **B,** Modified from *Global Fx Shoulder Fracture System Surgical Technique.* DePuy Orthopaedics; 1999. **C,** Courtesy Depuy-Synthes, Warsaw, IN. **D,** Courtesy Michael A. Wirth, MD.)

and lateral to the bicipital groove approximately 1 to 2 cm distal to the surgical neck, and large nonabsorbable sutures are passed for tuberosity-to-shaft fixation. When using a prosthesis with a suture collar, four drill holes are made through the anterolateral and posterolateral aspects of the proximal humerus, approximately 1 to 2 cm below the fracture line (Fig. 6-41). A trial reduction is then performed, with the mobilized tuberosities placed below the head of the modular prosthesis. A towel clip or GT clamp may be used to hold the tuberosities for fluoroscopic examination and assessment of glenohumeral joint registry and stability (Fig. 6-42; also see Fig. 6-47E). The humeral head should not subluxate anteriorly or posteriorly more than 40% to 50% of the glenoid width or inferiorly more than 25% to 30% of the glenoid height.[98,107]

The final humeral component may be press fit or cemented. When cementing the humeral stem, a cement restrictor is placed to prevent extravasation into the distal humerus. Pulsatile lavage and retrograde injection of cement with suction pressurization is also used (Fig. 6-43).[98,107] Excess cement is removed during the curing phase including around the proximal humeral shaft to facilitate tuberosity healing. A second trial reduction may be performed with a trial head after cement fixation of the humeral stem. The final head may be impacted before the stem is implanted or after the repeat trial reduction.[98,107] When using a suture collar, suture passage may be more feasible without the final humeral head in position. A cerclage suture is placed circumferentially around GT and through the supraspinatus insertion at the tendon-bone junction, medial to the prosthesis, and through the subscapularis insertion at the tendon-bone junction. Several authors have indicated superior fixation with the cerclage sutures when compared to tuberosity-to-tuberosity and tuberosity-to-fin fixation alone.[83-85] Prior to tying sutures, spaces between the tuberosities, prosthesis, and shaft are packed with autogenous cancellous bone graft from the resected humeral head (Fig. 6-44).

Overreduction of the tuberosities should be avoided to prevent limitations in external rotation (LT) and internal rotation (GT).[83-85] The suture configuration and sequence of tying may vary depending on surgeon preference and implant-specific instructions. When using a suture collar, vertical sutures are tied for tuberosity-to-shaft approximation, followed by horizontal tuberosity-to-tuberosity sutures (Fig. 6-45). The lateral portion of the rotator interval is then closed, with the arm in approximately 30 degrees of external rotation using a No. 2 nonabsorbable suture (Fig. 6-46). The deltopectoral interval is generally not closed. Drain suction is recommended in both acute and chronic injuries to prevent hematoma formation. In the event that a regional block was not performed, one of us recommends the use of a commercially available pain pump for postoperative analgesia (K.I.B.). The subcutaneous tissues are reapproximated with 2-0 absorbable sutures. Subcuticular closure is performed with 3-0 monofilament sutures. The arm is then placed in a sling or shoulder immobilizer with 30 to 45 degrees of abduction for comfort (see Fig. 6-47).[98,107]

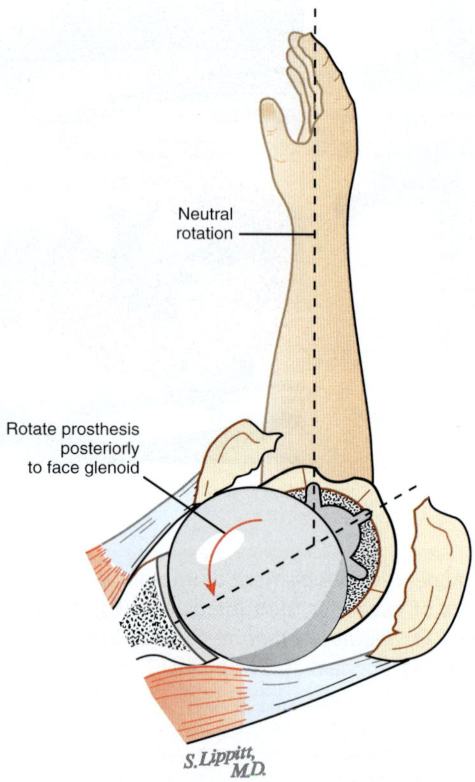

FIGURE 6-40: The anterior fin of the prosthesis is aligned with the forearm in neutral rotation, and the lateral fin is positioned approximately 8 mm posterior to the bicipital groove, establishing a retroversion angle of approximately 30 degrees. (Modified from Matsen FA III, Lippitt SB. *Shoulder Surgery: Principles and Procedures.* Philadelphia, Saunders; 2004:638.)

Postoperative Care

Physician-directed therapy is initiated on postoperative day 1 with gentle, gravity-assisted pendulum exercises and with passive pulley-and-stick exercises to maintain forward flexion and external rotation. Motion limits are placed by the surgeon based on intraoperative stability; passive forward elevation is typically limited to the horizontal plane (90 degrees) for the first 4 weeks. After discharge, the patient's wound is reexamined, and sutures are removed at 10 to 14 days postsurgery. Gentle ROM exercises are continued. At 6 weeks postsurgery, radiographs are obtained to evaluate tuberosity healing. When progressive tuberosity healing is evident, passive ROM exercises are advanced in all planes as tolerated; phase two exercises are initiated with gentle/submaximal isometric rotator and deltoid exercises and active-assisted elevation with a pulley (typically between 8 and 10 weeks postsurgery). At 3 months postsurgery, strength training (phase 3) with graduated rubber bands is implemented. ROM exercises are continued during the strengthening phase of the program. Patients should be aware that maximal motion and function can take approximately 12 months from the date of surgery to achieve.[98,107]

REVERSE SHOULDER ARTHROPLASTY FOR PRIMARY AND SECONDARY MANAGEMENT OF PROXIMAL HUMERUS FRACTURES

Patient Selection

RTSA is now a well-accepted surgical option for complex three- and four-part PHFs in elderly patients. The goals

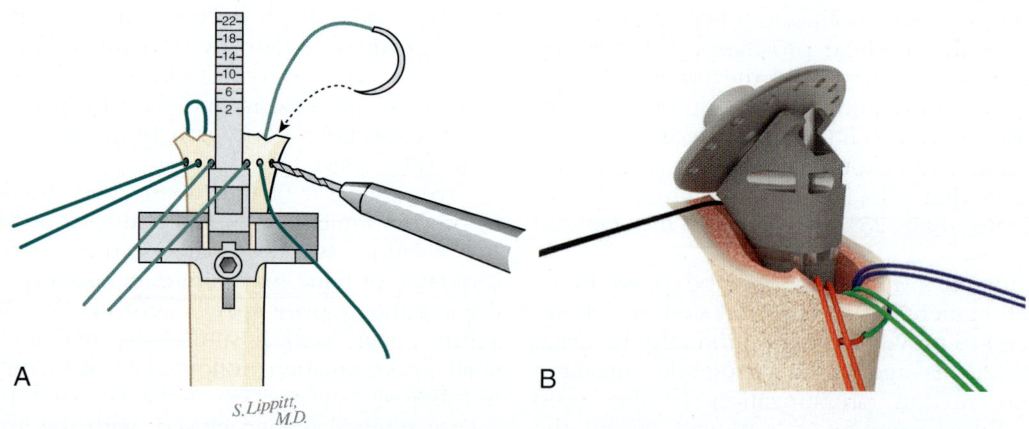

FIGURE 6-41: **A,** Drill holes are placed in the proximal humerus medial and lateral to the bicipital groove with large-caliber nonabsorbable sutures. **B,** Alternatively, with use of a suture collar, four drill holes are made through the anterolateral and posterolateral aspects of the proximal humerus, approximately 1 to 2 cm below the fracture line. (**A,** Modified from *Global Fx Shoulder Fracture System Surgical Technique.* DePuy Orthopaedics; 1999. **B,** Modified from *Global Unite Design Rationale and Surgical Technique.* Warsaw, IN: DePuy-Synthes.)

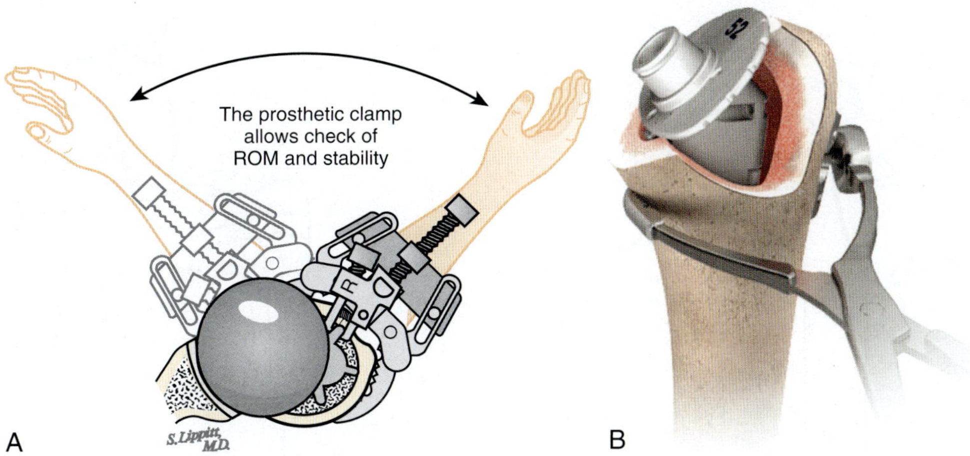

FIGURE 6-42: **A,** A trial reduction may be performed with the fracture jig in place, allowing assessment of the functional range of motion (ROM). **B,** A commercially available tuberosity clamp or large reduction tenaculum may be used for provisional reduction and fluoroscopic assessment. (**A,** Modified from *Global Fx Shoulder Fracture System Surgical Technique.* DePuy Orthopaedics; 1999. **B,** Modified from *Global Unite Design Rationale and Surgical Technique.* Warsaw, IN: DePuy-Synthes.)

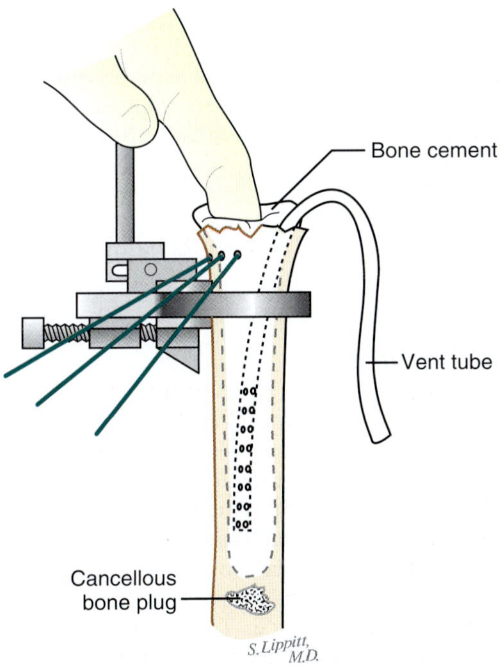

FIGURE 6-43: A cement restrictor is placed to prevent cement extravasation distally. Pulsatile lavage and retrograde injection of cement with suction pressurization is also used. (Modified from *Global Fx Shoulder Fracture System Surgical Technique.* DePuy Orthopaedics; 1999.)

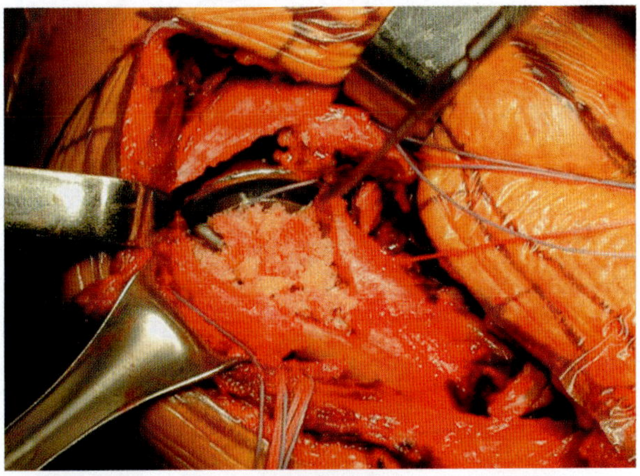

FIGURE 6-44: The technique used for placement of a morselized cancellous bone graft between the tuberosities and humeral shaft. (Courtesy Michael A. Wirth, MD.)

of RTSA for PHFs are nearly identical to those for HA, and involve pain relief and restoration of shoulder function to perform ADLs. Indications for RTSA include elderly patients (ideally over the age of 70 years) in which the fracture pattern, degree of comminution (especially the tuberosities), and bone quality preclude internal fixation or HA. Other factors that favor RTSA over an HA include those with preexisting rotator cuff disease, inflammatory arthritis, heavy smoking, or other metabolic factors (e.g., insulin-dependent diabetes, systemic steroid use) that would negatively affect tuberosity healing. Absolute contraindications for RTSA include axillary nerve injury, significant deltoid muscle dysfunction, and brachial plexopathy. Relative contraindications include open fractures, ipsilateral fractures involving the acromion or scapular spine, and glenoid fracture that prevents stable baseplate fixation. Other relative contraindications include walking aid dependency due to the theoretically increased risk of dislocation or early glenoid component loosening postoperatively with repetitive axial loading of the semi-constrained implant (A.J.B.); however, this remains controversial. It is critical that the

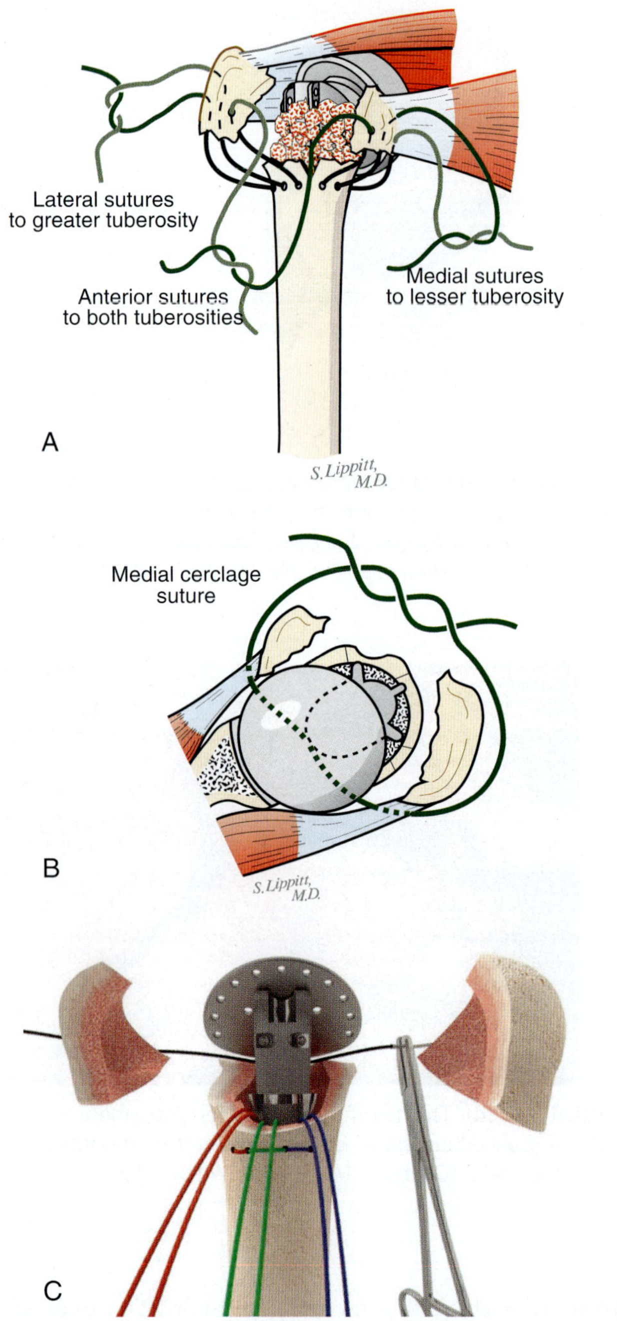

FIGURE 6-45: **A,** Previously placed suture limbs at the tendon-tuberosity interface and shaft are reapproximated. **B** and **C,** Medial cerclage suture is placed circumferentially around the greater tuberosity and through the supraspinatus insertion, and then medial to the prosthesis and through the subscapularis insertion (lesser tuberosity), and tied. (**A** and **B,** Modified from *Global Fx Shoulder Fracture System Surgical Technique.* DePuy Orthopaedics; 1999. **C,** From *Global Unite Design Rationale and Surgical Technique.* Warsaw, IN: DePuy-Synthes.)

patient be able to comply with postoperative restrictions and rehabilitation, as untreated delirium and chronic dementia may negatively affect the surgical outcome. Long-term studies regarding RTSA in this clinical scenario are limited, and as such, caution should be employed when performing an RTSA in certain elderly patient populations.

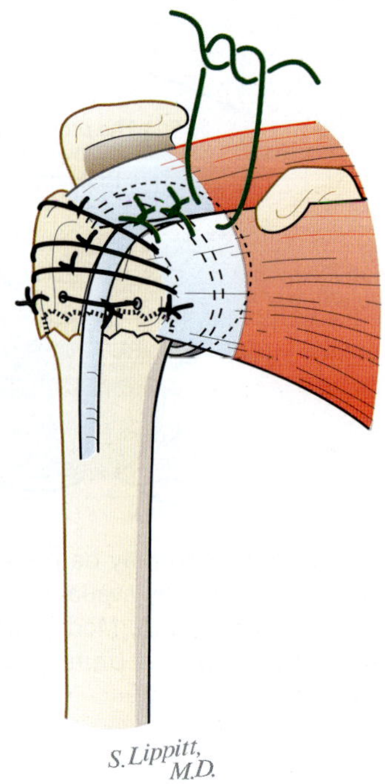

FIGURE 6-46: The lateral aspect of the rotator interval is closed with a No. 2 nonabsorbable suture, with the arm in approximately 30 degrees of external rotation. (Modified from *Global Fx Shoulder Fracture System Surgical Technique.* DePuy Orthopaedics; 1999.)

Surgical Technique

General anesthesia may be performed in conjunction with a regional block (surgeon discretion). We prefer the deltopectoral approach as this exposure is extensile, facilitates tuberosity identification and mobilization, and avoids deltoid detachment. The proximal portion of the PMT may be released to facilitate surgical exposure. The subdeltoid and subacromial spaces are bluntly released of adhesions, taking care to protect the axillary nerve within the subdeltoid space. The clavipectoral fascia, if not already traumatized, may be incised longitudinally in the usual fashion. Effort should be made to identify (i.e., gently palpate) the axillary and musculocutaneous nerves; we do not recommend surgical exploration of neurovascular structures. The long head of the biceps tendon is identified and used to locate the tuberosities. The biceps tendon is tenodesed to the upper border of the PMT. The humeral head is removed and placed on the back table to be later used for bone graft. If feasible, large caliber nonabsorbable sutures are placed through the rotator cuff insertions at the tendon-bone junction (as described for HA) for later repair.

In the fracture scenario, glenoid exposure is typically excellent and unobstructed. Glenoid preparation involves circumferential removal of labral tissue, followed by system-specific steps to implant the baseplate and

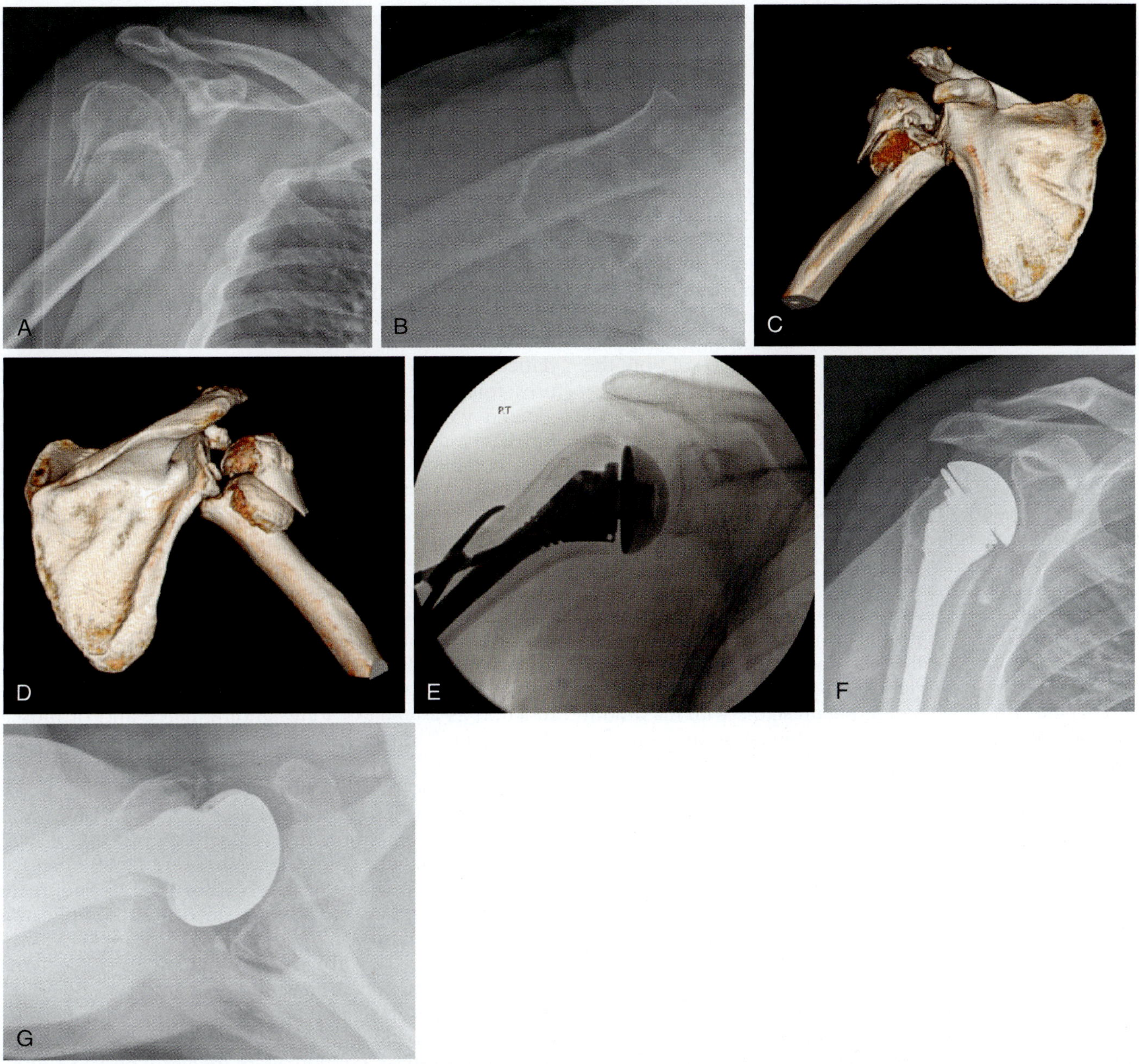

FIGURE 6-47: **A** to **D,** Anteroposterior and axillary radiographs and three-dimensional computed tomographic imaging of a displaced three-part proximal humerus fracture with head-split in a 70-year-old farmer after a ground-level fall. Note the large greater tuberosity fracture fragment. **E,** Fluoroscopic image of the trial implant in place with the tuberosities held in place with a clamp. Note the radiopaque humeral head that permits intraoperative assessment of implant position. **F** and **G,** Postoperative true anteroposterior and axillary radiographs at the 6-month follow-up visit reveal complete healing and anatomic reconstruction of the greater and lesser tuberosities in relation to the prosthetic humeral head. (Courtesy Aaron J. Bois, MD.)

glenosphere. Care should be taken during glenoid reaming to retain subchondral bone for stable fixation of the baseplate. The baseplate should be positioned at the inferior glenoid rim (neutral or slight inferior tilt). Most implant systems allow placement of multiple screws in a nonlocking and locking fashion. Inferior and superior screw placement (lateral pillar of the scapula and coracoid base, respectively) remain the most critical factors with regards to initial baseplate stability. Glenosphere implant size is based on achieving stable and impingement-free ROM.

The humerus is then delivered through the surgical wound with extension and adduction of the upper extremity. Serial reaming of the medullary canal is performed by hand until chatter is encountered. Some implant systems allow press-fit fixation of the humeral stem due to proximal geometry and osteoconductive surfaces such as grit blasting or hydroxyapatite. Fourth-generation platform systems allow for placement of a diaphyseal stem, which is then attached to an epiphyseal component in neutral-to-slight retroversion to allow for improved external rotation prior to mechanical impingement. There are currently no studies that indicate superiority of one design over another. The height and version of the trial implant is judged by the intact medial humeral calcar, tuberosity reduction, and stem version guide. Metaphyseal comminution may preclude the ability of the surgeon to judge stem height; judging implant height and subsequent joint stability remains the most challenging component of this surgical technique. As discussed above, preoperative templating using AP radiographs of both the injured and uninjured (i.e., contralateral) humerus may be helpful for judging humeral component height, especially in cases with significant fracture comminution.

After final stem implantation, a trial humeral cup insert is used to assess stability with the aid of fluoroscopy (surgeon dependent). Implant stability is a qualitative assessment that includes the following: (1) the prosthetic joint should not separate in a neutral position with longitudinal traction ("shuck test"), (2) the conjoint tendon will demonstrate increased tension with digital palpation, (3) external rotation with the arm held in adduction (i.e., arm at side) should allow no more than 2 to 3 mm of gapping between the glenosphere and the humeral liner, and (4) the construct should remain stable with maximum internal and external rotation. If subluxation or instability occurs with any of these steps, stability may be improved by increasing the thickness of the humeral liner, increasing the depth of the liner (i.e., use of a retentive liner), removing soft tissues or osseous structures that cause impingement, and changing to a larger glenosphere.

The GT and LT are grafted with morselized autograft obtained from the native humeral head and repaired in a similar fashion to that described for HA. Most surgeons advocate that the tuberosity-to-implant (i.e., horizontal cerclage) and tuberosity-to-tuberosity sutures be tied prior to tying the vertically oriented sutures (i.e., tuberosity-to-shaft) to prevent overreduction of the tuberosities.[131] In addition, one of us uses the "Nice knot," described by Pascal Boileau, which has excellent loop and knot security to optimize tuberosity-to-implant fixation (A.J.B.). Cancellous autograft is placed into areas of bony deficiency to facilitate tuberosity union. Studies by Bufquin et al.[203] and Gallinet et al.[89] demonstrated improved external rotation strength and function with anatomic union of the GT. The benefits of LT healing are currently unclear. A closed suction drain is placed to decrease the risk of hematoma formation. The surgical wound is then closed in a similar fashion to that described for HA reconstruction.

Postoperative Care

The upper extremity is placed into an abduction sling for 4 weeks. Passive exercises using a pendulum and stick (i.e., adducted external rotation) are delayed until 2 weeks postoperatively to decrease the risk of hematoma formation; however, active ROM exercises of the hand, wrist, and elbow are encouraged during this time. If the tuberosities are repaired at the time of the RTSA, the same protocol as described for HA is followed to protect the tuberosities while they heal due to the improved clinical outcomes observed with tuberosity healing. Deltoid and rotator cuff strengthening may begin at approximately 10 to 12 weeks postoperatively once there is radiographic evidence of tuberosity healing (Figs. 6-48 and 6-49).

Reverse Arthroplasty for Revision of Failed Hemiarthroplasty or Internal Fixation for Proximal Humerus Fractures

Revision of a failed HA or internal fixation is extremely difficult to accomplish, even in experienced hands. Failures following HA might have resulted from excessive glenoid wear, tuberosity malunion, tuberosity nonunion, tuberosity resorption, humeral-stem loosening, infection, or a combination of these factors. Associated soft tissue deficits and contractures, bone loss, and instability all play roles in the loss of glenohumeral joint function. Nerve paralysis may be present and can complicate revision surgery; nerve conduction and electromyography are helpful in the preoperative evaluation of these patients.

Expectations and goals of revision surgery should be realistic and frankly understood by both the patient and the surgeon. Revision surgery is generally indicated for pain relief, as it can be difficult to significantly improve function as a result of longstanding nerve and/or muscle damage and soft tissue contractures.

Levy et al.[149] have suggested that until recently, surgeons have not had a viable option for this clinical scenario. The authors performed an RTSA (with or without proximal humeral allograft) as a salvage procedure in 29 patients (mean age, 69 years; range, 42 to 80 years) to address the issue of failed HA for PHFs. The mean follow-up was 35 months, with an overall complication rate of 28% (eight of 29 patients). The mean ASES score improved from 22.3 to 52.1 postoperatively. The mean active forward elevation improved from 38.1 to 72.7 degrees, and abduction improved from 34.1 to 70.4 degrees. Six patients were dissatisfied with the procedure; four of these patients were treated with RTSA alone (i.e., without allograft reconstruction). The authors found the early postoperative results to be encouraging, and recommended this implant as a salvage solution for failed HA with rotator cuff deficiency or tuberosity failure (Figs. 6-50 and 6-51).[149]

In 2013, Jost et al.[132] reported the revision strategies and outcomes in 121 patients (mean age, 59 years) that were treated for complications related to ORIF of a PHF using a locking plate. A mean of three complications occurred per patient, including malreduction, primary screw cutout, malunion, nonunion, AVN, and infection. Screw penetration into the glenohumeral joint was found in 57% of the patients, leading to secondary glenoid destruction in 33% of patients. Revision arthroplasty (either HA, anatomic total shoulder arthroplasty [TSA], or RTSA) was performed in over 50% of the patients; in six patients, glenoid implantation during revision surgery

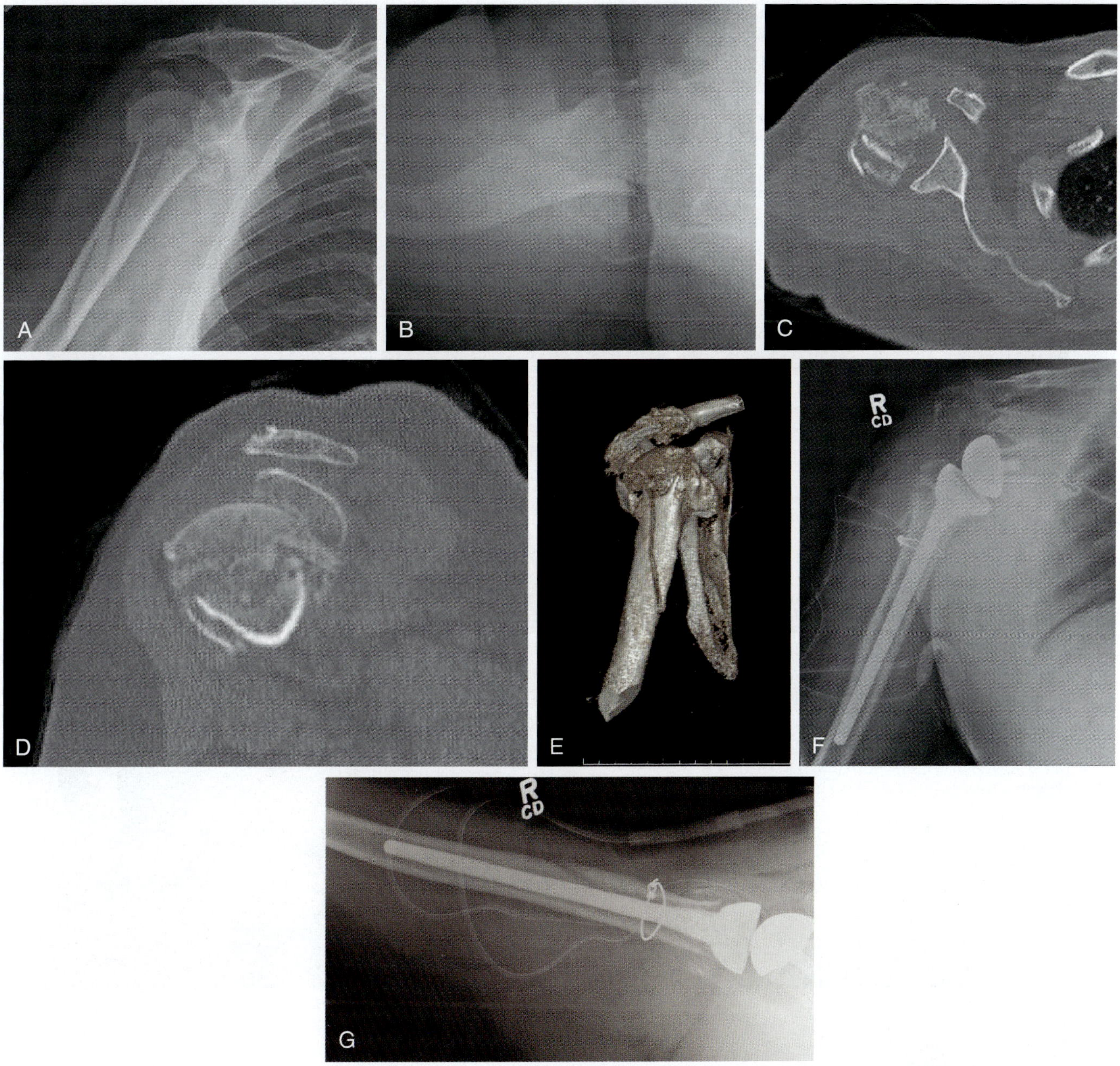

FIGURE 6-48: **A** and **B,** Anteroposterior and axillary radiographs reveal a comminuted four-part proximal humerus fracture with diaphyseal extension. **C** to **E,** Two-dimensional and three-dimensional computed tomographic imaging confirms articular surface and diaphyseal involvement. **F** and **G,** Immediate postoperative radiographs demonstrate a reverse total shoulder arthroplasty reconstruction with press-fit fixation of the humeral stem. (Courtesy Kamal I. Bohsali, MD.)

was not possible due to extensive glenoid destruction. At a mean of 24 months' follow-up, shoulder function improved in all arthroplasty groups; however, overall shoulder function remained substantially restricted.

More recently, in 2015, Hussey et al.[119] evaluated the clinical outcomes in 19 patients (mean age, 66 years; range, 52 to 82 years) with failed internal fixation of a PHF who underwent implant removal and RTSA. The mean follow-up was 36 months (range, 25 to 60 months). Significant improvements were found in all outcome scores; specifically, the ASES score improved from 27.8 to 50.1, the Simple Shoulder Test score improved from 0.7 to 3.2, and the mean visual analog scale for pain score improved from 6.8 to 4.3. Postoperative mean ROM parameters also improved for forward elevation (from 59 to 101 degrees), external rotation (from 11 to 23 degrees), and internal rotation (from buttock to L4). The overall complication rate was 26% (5 of 19 patients). The authors

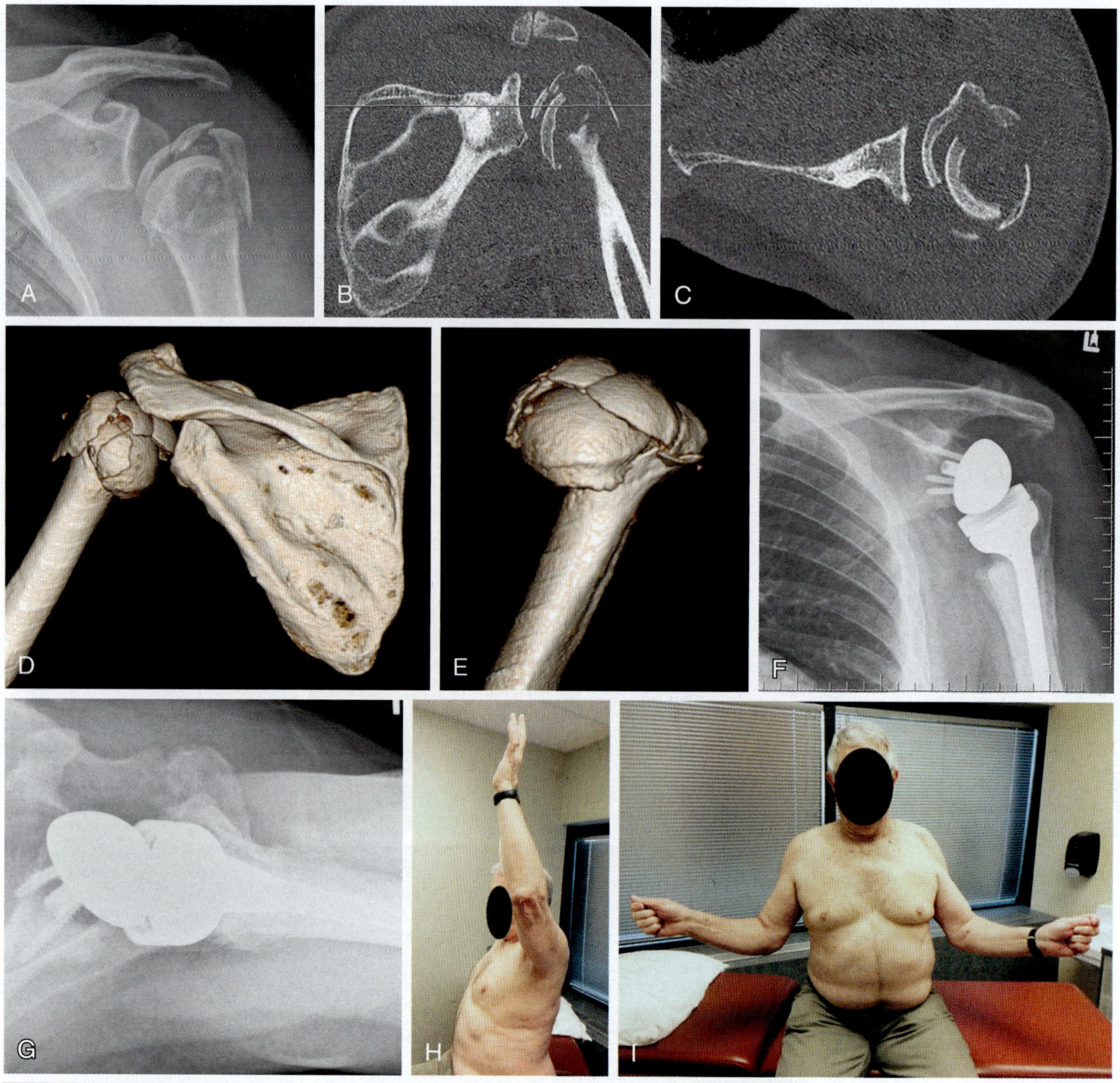

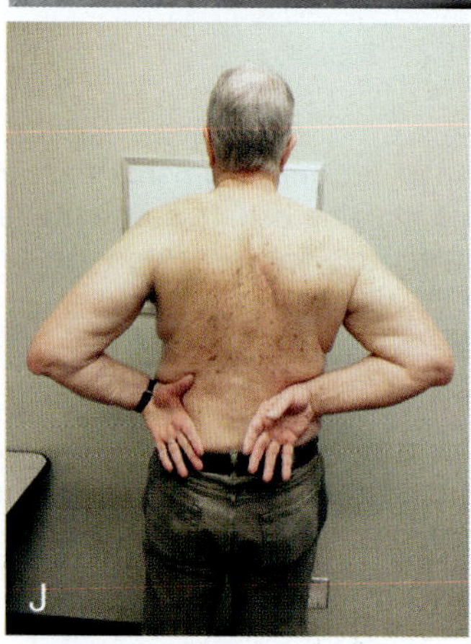

FIGURE 6-49: **A** to **E,** Anteroposterior radiograph and two- and three-dimensional (2D and 3D) computed tomographic imaging reveals a left-sided four-part proximal humerus fracture with head-split in a 69-year-old retired man after a ground-level fall. Note the thin head and tuberosity fragments on 2D CT imaging (**B** and **C**). A scout line is evident on the coronal cut that correlates with the location of the axial cut on 2D CT. **F** and **G,** Postoperative anteroposterior and axillary radiographs at the 12-month follow-up visit reveal complete healing and anatomic reconstruction of the greater and lesser tuberosities following reverse total shoulder arthroplasty. **H** to **J,** Active shoulder range of motion at the 12-month follow-up visit is symmetric. This patient has excellent active external rotation, which is possible secondary to healing of the greater tuberosity. (Courtesy Aaron J. Bois, MD.)

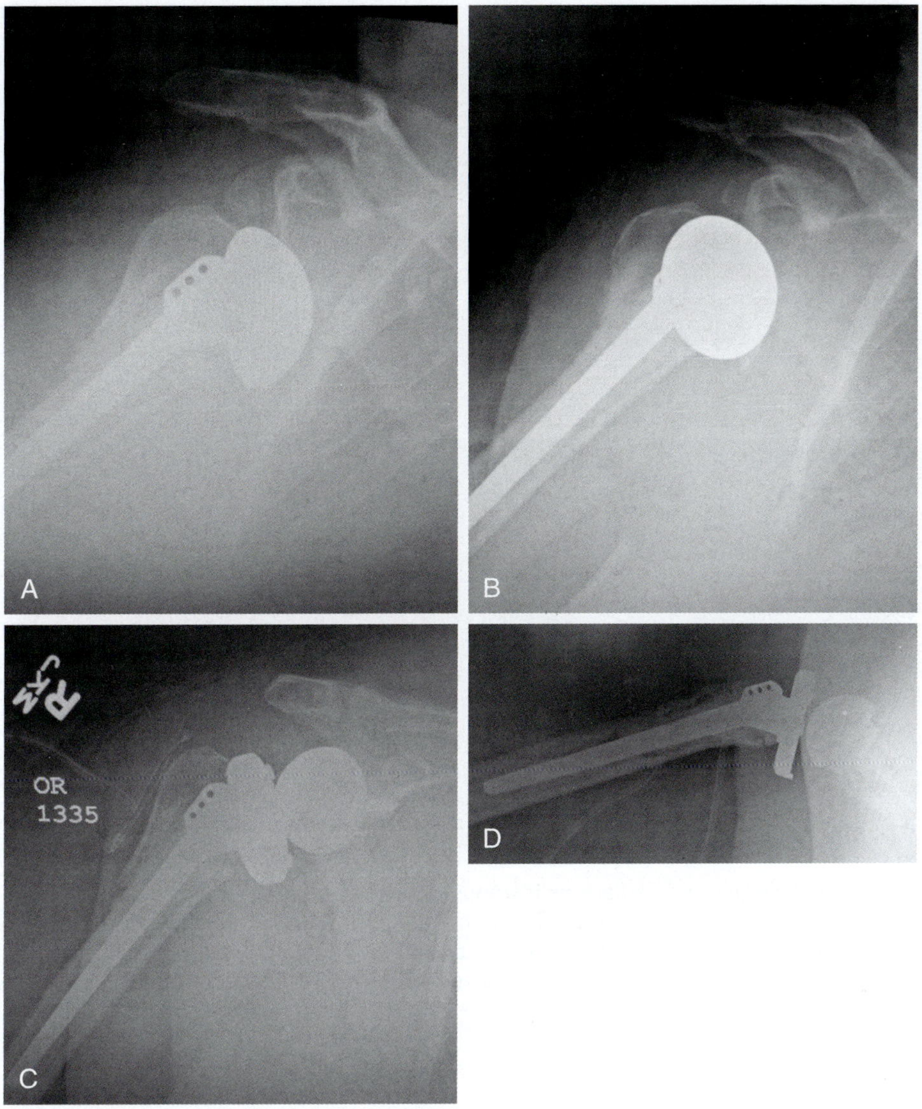

FIGURE 6-50: **A** and **B,** Anteroposterior and scapular Y lateral radiographs reveal anterior subluxation after hemiarthroplasty reconstruction for fracture due to underlying anterior-inferior glenoid bone loss. **C** and **D,** This patient was revised to a reverse total shoulder arthroplasty with stem retention utilizing a platform-based system. (Courtesy Kamal I. Bohsali, MD.)

concluded that an improvement in outcome and pain can be attained following this salvage procedure; however, appropriate patient counseling is required preoperatively to establish realistic patient expectations.[161]

COMPLICATIONS ASSOCIATED WITH TREATMENT OF PROXIMAL HUMERUS FRACTURES

PHFs remain difficult to classify and appropriately manage. Negative consequences can occur as a result of the initial injury or from the surgical treatment itself. Some of these complications include shoulder stiffness, osteonecrosis, malunion, nonunion, and heterotopic bone formation.[22,264] Boileau et al.[29] highlighted some of the challenges when managing the sequelae of PHFs. In a multicenter study involving 71 patients, they identified four complication subtypes of patients who underwent arthroplasty after failure of the initial management (nonoperative and operative): type 1, humeral head collapse or necrosis without tuberosity malunion; type 2, locked dislocations or fracture-dislocations; type 3, nonunions of the surgical neck; and type 4, severe malunions of the tuberosities. The most important factor affecting functional outcome was the need for a GT osteotomy. Positive results were obtained in types 1 and 2, in which osteotomy of GT was not required. All patients in types 3 and 4, who underwent a GT osteotomy, had fair or poor results, with limited active elevation beyond 90 degrees. Petrigliano et al. performed an observational

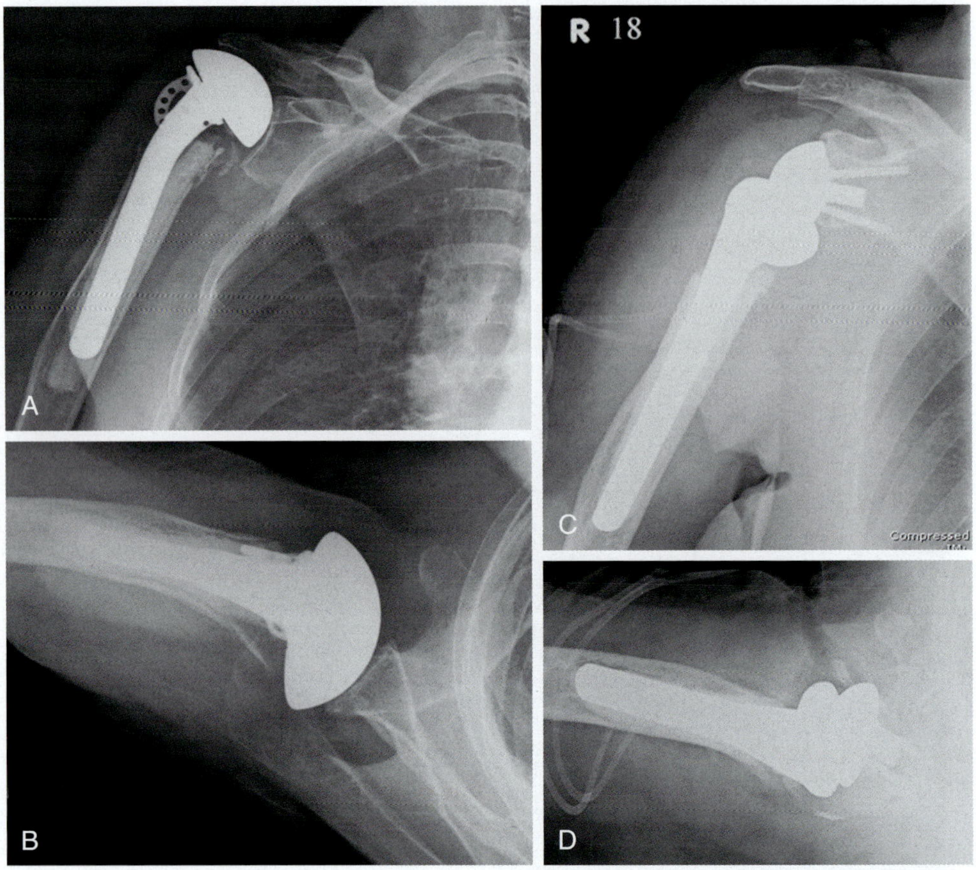

FIGURE 6-51: **A** and **B,** Anteroposterior and axillary radiographs demonstrate a high-riding humeral component relative to the glenoid fossa following a hemiarthroplasty for fracture. The humeral stem is also malpositioned in varus. Both variables (component height and varus angulation) most likely contributed to tuberosity failure and resorption in this case. **C** and **D,** Immediate postoperative radiographs following revision arthroplasty using reverse total shoulder arthroplasty. (Courtesy Aaron J. Bois, MD, and Michael A. Wirth, MD.)

study of 9254 patients who underwent nonprosthetic surgical intervention for a PHF, and found that the following factors were independently predictive of a poor result (i.e., increased risk of short-term complications): age greater than 65 years, male gender, lower socioeconomic status, and coexisting medical comorbidities.[202]

Shoulder Stiffness

Shoulder stiffness remains one of the most common complications after a PHF. Contributing factors include the severity of the initial injury, the duration of the immobilization, articular surface malunion, and patient noncompliance with rehabilitation.[264]

Koval et al.[141] assessed the functional outcome of 104 patients with minimally displaced PHFs treated with a standardized therapy program. At a mean follow-up of 41 months (range, 12 to 117 months), patients who started a therapy program within 2 weeks from the date of injury demonstrated significantly better results (forward elevation, external rotation, pain level) compared with patients who started therapy 2 weeks after injury.[141] Hodgson[117] reaffirmed the necessity for early PT with two-part PHFs, noting prolonged recovery (2 years vs. 1 year) in patients immobilized for longer than 3 weeks.

With regard to hemiarthroplasty, numerous studies have indicated more favorable outcomes with early intervention due to the presence of soft tissue contractures with chronic injuries.[86,183,248] An early physician-directed rehabilitation program should be performed for fractures managed operatively and nonoperatively to minimize stiffness.

Osteonecrosis

The incidence of AVN depends on the severity of the initial injury (e.g., three- and four-part fractures and fracture-dislocations) and surgical technique. Hagg and Lundberg[100] reported an AVN rate of 3% to 14% after closed reduction of displaced three-part fractures and a rate of 13% to 34% after four-part fractures. In addition to fracture severity, exuberant soft tissue dissection has been identified as a major contributing factor.[100] Sturzenegger et al.[246] reported a 34% incidence of AVN in a series of 17 patients treated with ORIF using a T plate.

The early stages of AVN are best detected using MRI. Conventional radiographs will demonstrate later stages of AVN such as humeral head collapse and secondary degenerative changes (Fig. 6-52). The treatment of choice for AVN in the setting of severe pain and functional loss is a hemiarthroplasty or anatomic total shoulder replacement (TSA); the latter method of treatment is considered for end-stage AVN when arthritic changes involve the glenoid fossa.[264]

Prognostic factors and limitations of anatomic TSA for the treatment of posttraumatic AVN were evaluated in a retrospective cohort study by Moineau et al.[173] The study confirmed that the outcomes of TSA are good and predictable when deformation of the proximal humerus does not require a GT osteotomy. Furthermore, the results were negatively affected when there was associated varus deformity of the proximal humerus or fatty infiltration of the rotator cuff on advanced imaging studies.[173]

Malunion

Malunion can occur following nonoperative treatment or failed ORIF (Fig. 6-53). GT malunion (superior, posterior, or both) can lead to impingement against the acromion, resulting in pain, weakness (i.e., from an altered length-tension relationship of the rotator cuff), and diminished ROM (i.e., forward elevation block if superiorly malunited and external rotation block if posteriorly malunited).[22,264] These are extremely difficult problems to manage. If displacement of the malunited GT is greater than 5 mm with functional limitations and pain, this problem is best managed with fragment mobilization, reduction, and internal fixation.[264] For GT malunions that are symptomatic but have lesser degrees of displacement, partial removal of the tuberosity (i.e., tuberoplasty) along with anterior acromioplasty and lysis of adhesions can provide an alternative treatment option.[22] In 2012, Lädermann et al.[144] reported the mid- to long-term results

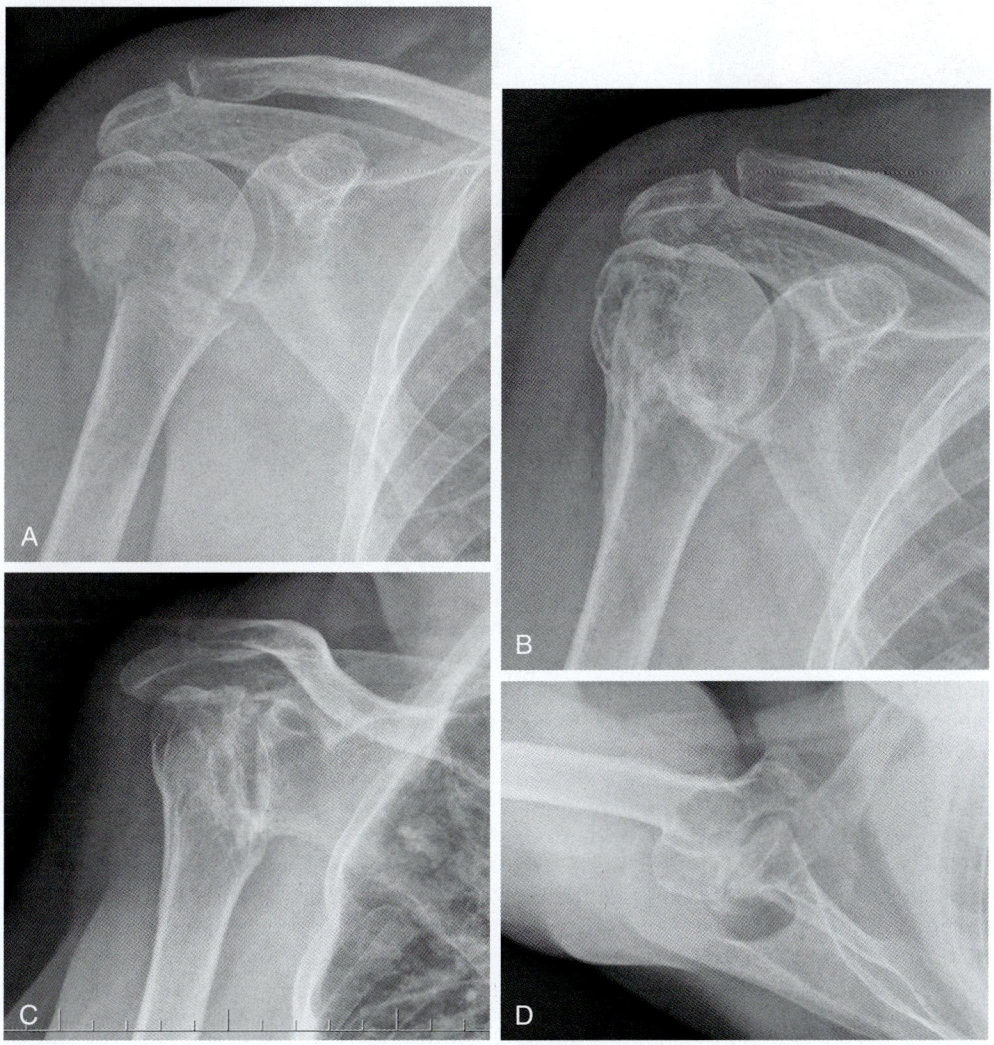

FIGURE 6-52: A, Anteroposterior radiograph demonstrating a minimally displaced three-part proximal humerus fracture in an 81-year-old female. **B,** Radiographic follow-up at 10 months reveals a healed fracture. **C** and **D,** Radiographic follow-up at 3.5 years reveals advanced avascular necrosis with secondary early arthritic changes of the glenoid fossa, including subchondral sclerosis and cysts. (Courtesy Aaron J. Bois, MD.)

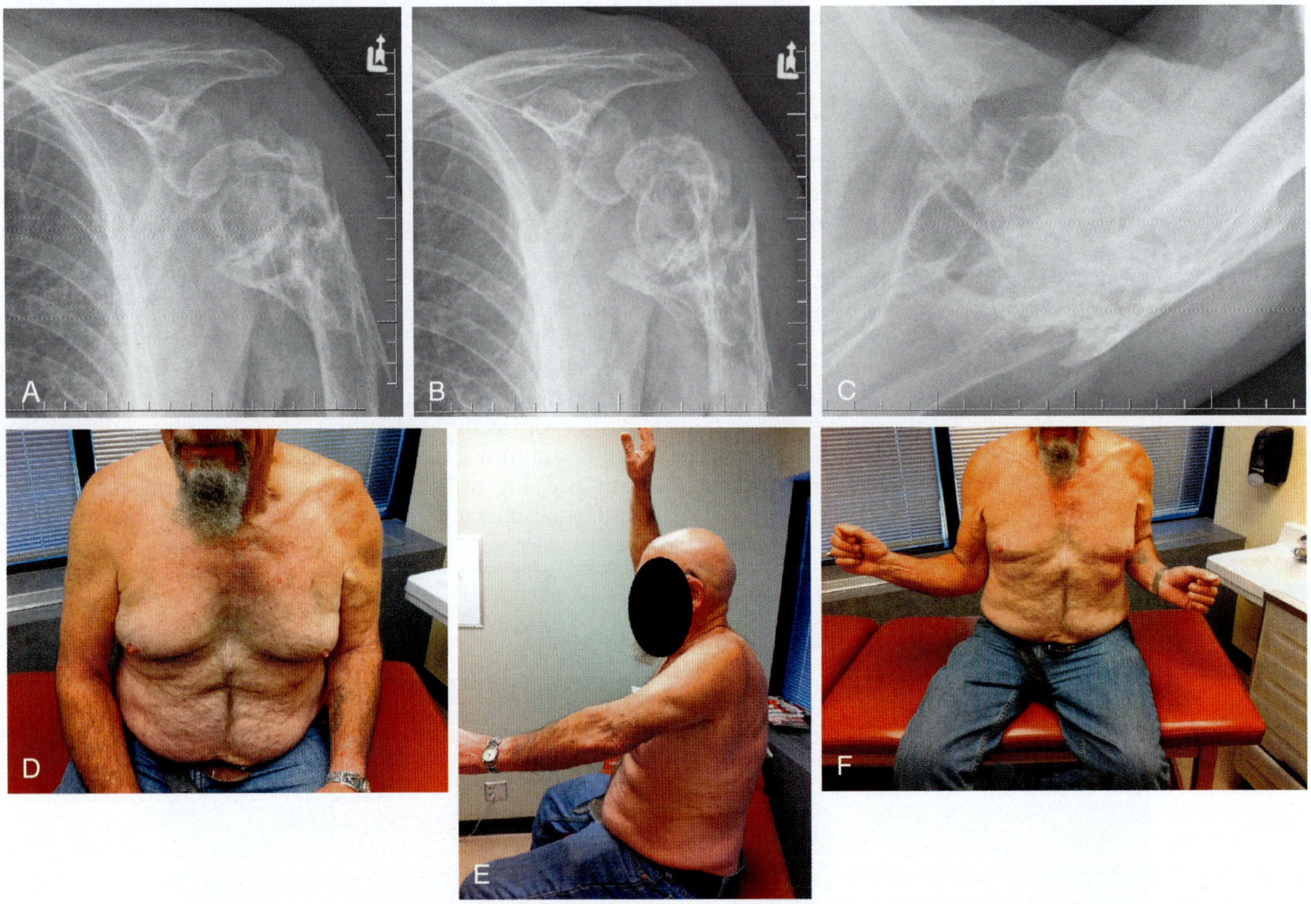

FIGURE 6-53: **A** and **B,** Anteroposterior and axillary radiographs demonstrating a significant deformity of the left proximal humerus following a comminuted fracture involving all "parts," including the humeral head (i.e., head-split, fracture-dislocation subtype) in a 71-year old male following a motor vehicle accident 2 years previously. This patient was referred for persistent shoulder pain and severely limited range of motion. **C,** Clinical appearance of the left shoulder at rest. Note the inferior sulcus sign and deltoid atrophy. **D** and **E,** Active forward elevation and external rotation of the shoulder, respectively. (Courtesy Aaron J. Bois, MD.)

of arthroscopic tuberoplasty and rotator cuff retensioning for proximal humerus malunion in nine patients (mean age, 49 years). Patients showed an improvement in ROM, pain scores, and function; eight patients (89%) were able to return to their previous sports or activities. Care should be taken to avoid GT osteotomy in the setting of hemiarthroplasty due to reported failure rates and poor outcomes.[27]

Two-part surgical neck malunions infrequently cause pain or functional limitations. The occasional varus malunion can result in impingement and require surgical management with arthroscopic acromioplasty or tuberoplasty, or both.[144,264] Osteotomy followed by internal fixation is reserved for severe angulation that prohibits forward flexion (Fig. 6-54).[13] Prosthetic replacement is generally required for three- and four-part malunions with joint incongruity. Tuberosity osteotomies should be avoided when possible as results are adversely affected by this aspect of the reconstruction.[29] Anatomic restoration of the glenohumeral joint must be performed; particular attention to humeral head retroversion and humeral head height is paramount for optimal functional results.[22,264] If significant tuberosity malunion exists necessitating an osteotomy, an RTSA is recommended. Arthroplasty for proximal humeral malunions has demonstrated less favorable outcomes secondary to soft tissue adhesions and displacement of the tuberosities.[22,26,264] Pain relief is usually satisfactory, but it is less predictable than primary arthroplasty.[22,126,264]

Nonunion

Nonunion of PHFs is uncommon, and is usually associated with displaced fractures.[58,147,181,222,243] Nonunion often occurs in elderly, debilitated patients with osteoporotic bone;[180,225] the incidence of nonunion in this patient population is estimated at 23%.[184] Other factors that

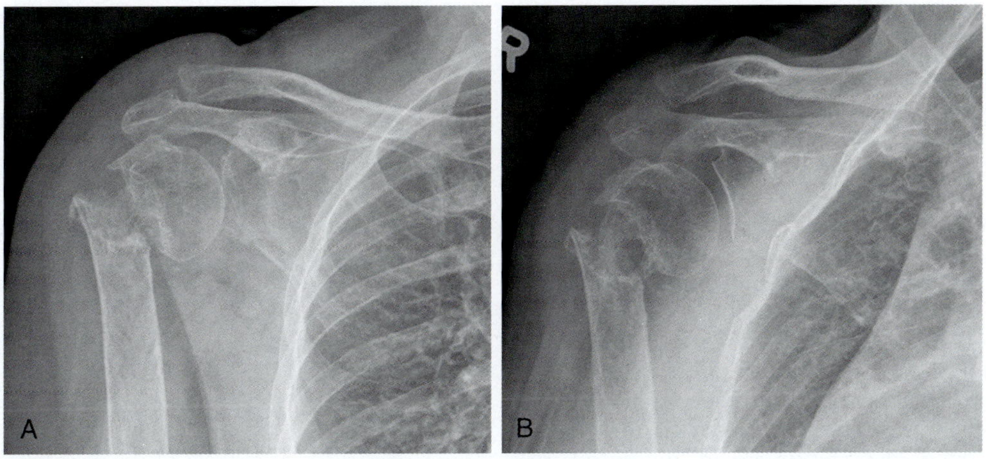

FIGURE 6-54: **A** and **B,** Anteroposterior radiographs demonstrating significant varus malunion of the proximal humerus following a two-part surgical neck fracture in a 63-year-old female who presented with limited shoulder range of motion. (Courtesy Aaron J. Bois, MD.)

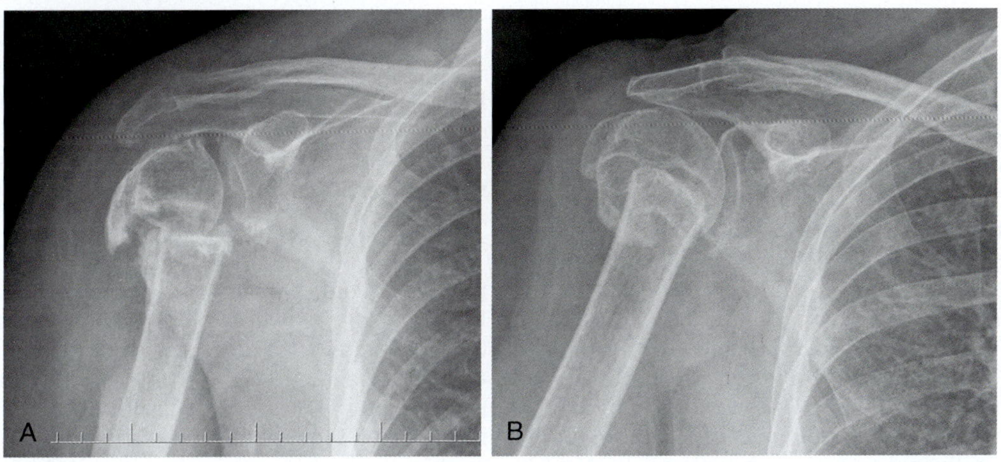

FIGURE 6-55: **A,** Anteroposterior radiograph reveals a surgical neck nonunion following a three-part proximal humerus fracture in a 55-year-old female. **B,** Surgical neck nonunion in a 74-year-old female following a minimally displaced three-part proximal humerus fracture. (Courtesy Aaron J. Bois, MD.)

predispose to nonunion include soft tissue interposition, hanging arm casts, inadequate fixation during ORIF, alcohol abuse, and medical comorbidities such as diabetes mellitus (Fig. 6-55).[58,165,176,211,222]

Indications for surgical treatment are significant pain, deformity, and functional loss. Open reduction and internal fixation using a locking plate construct and the addition of autogenous iliac crest bone graft is the preferred method of treatment if adequate bone stock remains. In cases of surgical neck nonunion, the use of an intercalary strut allograft (e.g., fibular strut) with fixed-angle locked plating provides additional biologic and structural support when the medial calcar is compromised secondary to comminution or osteopenia.[5] In the setting of humeral head resorption and cavitation, a prosthesis (e.g., hemiarthroplasty or RTSA) may be necessary to reconstruct the glenohumeral joint.[264] Surgical reconstruction for surgical neck nonunions results in pain relief in the majority of patients, but the overall results with regard to motion and strength are less predictable.[71,111,224] Reconstruction is often technically challenging and associated with a significant risk of postoperative complications. The risks and benefits of surgical intervention should be discussed in detail with the patient.

In 2012, Duquin et al.[70] reported the results of unconstrained shoulder arthroplasty (i.e., hemiarthroplasty and TSA) for the treatment of proximal humeral nonunions in 67 patients. Thirty-six patients (53.7%) underwent surgical treatment for painful two-part PHFs. Unconstrained arthroplasty was found to decrease pain and improve function in this patient cohort; however, the overall results were "satisfactory" in less than half of the patients. Tuberosity healing about the prosthesis was inconsistent, and had a direct influence on the functional outcome, which is consistent with an earlier report by Boileau et al.[29]

More recently, Raiss et al.[206] analyzed the clinical and radiographic outcomes and complications following semi-constrained RTSA for the treatment of nonunion of the surgical neck. Thirty-two patients with a mean age of 68 years (range, 48 to 83 years) were followed for a mean duration of 4 years (range, 2 to 12 years). Although the clinical outcomes improved significantly, there were 13 complications (41%) leading to nine revisions (28%). The most common complication was a dislocation following RTSA (11 patients or 34%) that was associated with resection of the tuberosities and the attached rotator cuff. These findings are consistent with those of earlier studies, which have also reported an increased risk of dislocation following RTSA treatment for proximal humeral nonunions. Nonoperative treatment may be an option in elderly patients who have minimal symptoms in the nondominant extremity.[206]

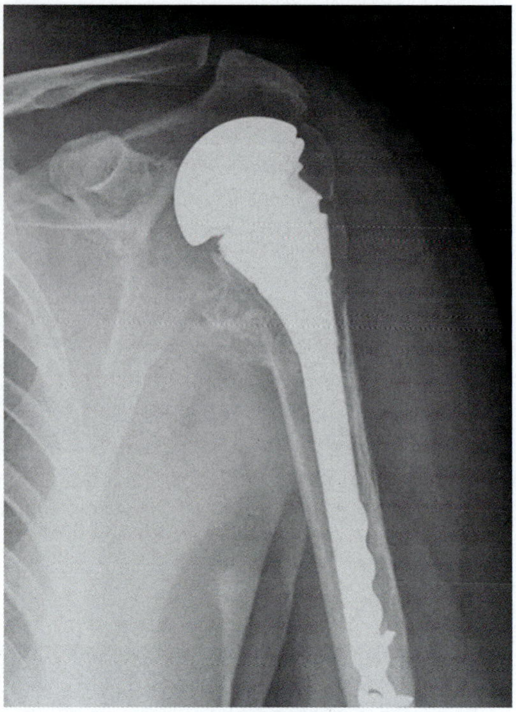

FIGURE 6-56: Heterotopic bone formation noted in the region of the humeral calcar and lesser tuberosity following hemiarthroplasty reconstruction of a four-part valgus-impacted proximal humerus fracture. (Courtesy Michael A. Wirth, MD.)

Heterotopic Bone Formation

Formation of ectopic bone is a common and often incidental finding noted on radiographs in patients with PHFs and fracture-dislocations.[22,181,205,265,266] Neer's report in 1970 on 117 patients treated for three- and four-part fractures and fracture-dislocations indicated an overall rate of 12% of heterotopic bone formation. Factors that increased the likelihood of ectopic bone included the degree of soft tissue injury, repetitive manipulations, and delayed reduction beyond 7 days from the injury (Fig. 6-56).[181] Heterotopic ossification is also commonly associated with neurologic injuries such as traumatic brain or spinal cord injuries (known as *neurogenic heterotopic ossification*) (Fig. 6-57). In the rare situation that ankylosis occurs from heterotopic bone formation, surgical resection is indicated to restore functional ROM.[264]

Complications Specific to Treatment Type

Percutaneous Fixation

Potential complications of this technique include pin migration, infection, AVN, neurovascular injury, and malunion.[72,74,169] The axillary nerve, radial nerve, biceps tendon, and anterior humeral circumflex vessels are all at risk with this method. Soft tissue dissection should proceed carefully down to the bone before pin placement. It is critical to obtain biplanar radiographic views before completing the procedure to confirm correct pin placement.[121,125] To reduce the risk of pin tract infections, pins may be replaced at the time of intervention with partially threaded cannulated screws.

Open Reduction and Internal Fixation

Despite the evidence of positive outcomes using locking plates, postoperative complications may occur (Fig. 6-58; also see the Senior Editor Commentary). Ong et al.[193] reported a complication rate of nearly 21% in 63 patients treated with a locking plate for two-, three-, and four-part fractures. Patients with complications had a significantly lower mean forward elevation when compared with those patients who did not have complications. Similarly, Clavert et al.[53] noted two types of complications: (1) those related to surgical technique, and (2) those intrinsic to the implant. High plate position and inadequate screw length resulted in screw cutout and diminished Constant scores. The authors also observed plate fracture and a nonunion rate of 5.5%, and attributed these findings to the rigidity of the construct.

Intramedullary Nail Fixation

This technique has limitations, particularly when there is significant metaphyseal comminution or humeral head involvement. Nonunions associated with IM nailing appear to be unique to proximal humerus (and humeral shaft) fractures, and tend to be more refractory to secondary intervention (Fig. 6-59).[215] Infection remains a rare event after nailing, occurring in 1% to 2% of cases. More commonly, IM nails are associated with shoulder pain and loss of motion. Subacromial impingement, bursitis, and rotator cuff irritation can occur if the nail is prominent proximally. Iatrogenic fractures have also been reported with vigorous attempts at nail insertion.[215]

Arthroplasty

The most common complications after HA include those related to the greater tuberosity (nonunion, malunion, or resorption), infection, heterotopic bone formation (see

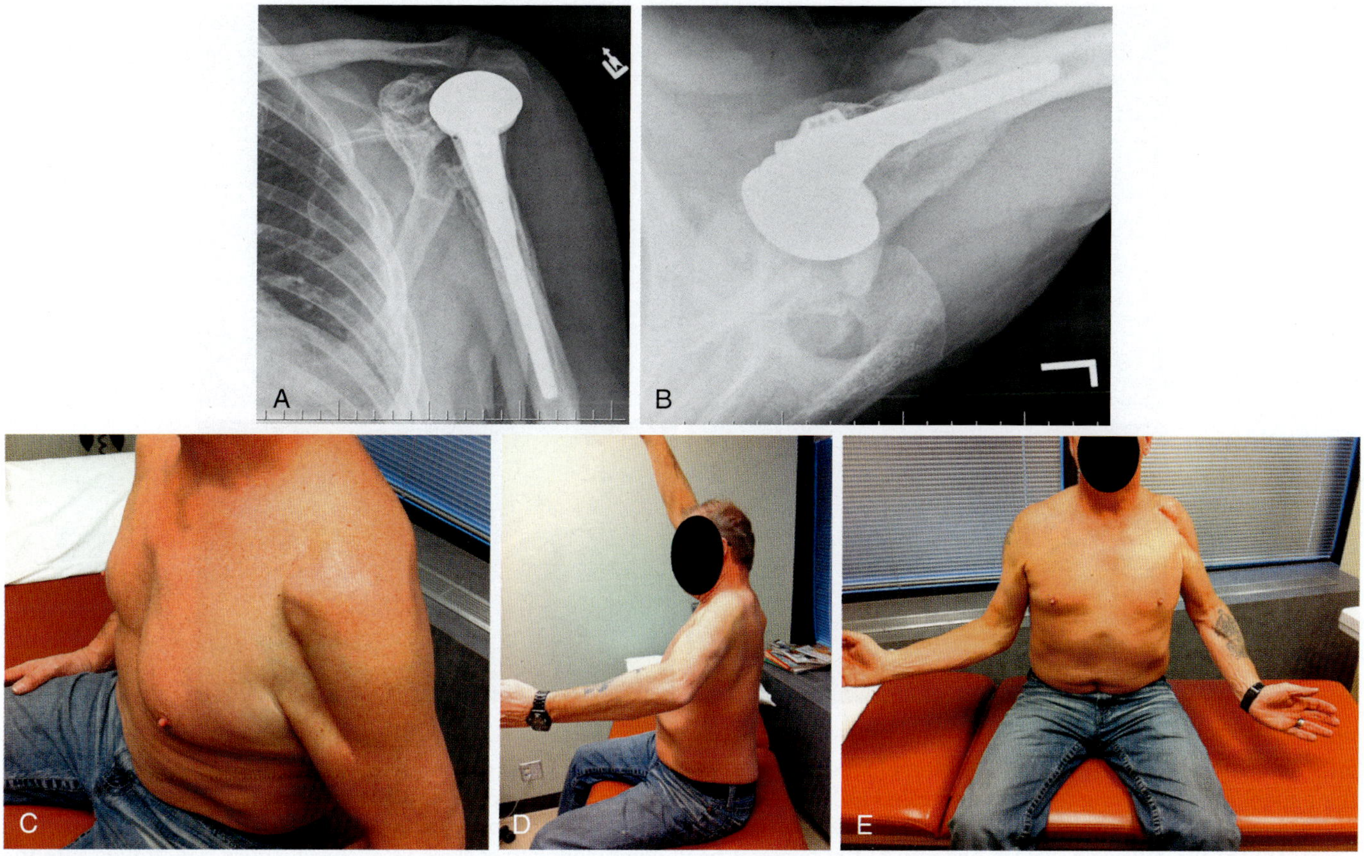

FIGURE 6-57: **A** and **B,** Anteroposterior and axillary radiographs of the left shoulder in a 54-year-old male following hemiarthroplasty (performed 13 years previously for a fracture-dislocation of the proximal humerus) who was referred for shoulder stiffness and weakness. Surprisingly, the patient had minimal shoulder pain. This patient was initially involved in a motor vehicle collision and experienced multiple injuries, including a closed-head injury requiring long-term intensive care unit admission. Note the extensive heterotopic ossification in the subcoracoid region. There is also evidence of component malposition, tuberosity resorption, and superior migration of the implant. **C,** Clinical evidence of anterosuperior escape with humeral head prominence below the skin anteriorly that is accentuated when the patient extends the shoulder. **D** and **E,** Active forward elevation and external rotation of the shoulder, respectively. (Courtesy Aaron J. Bois, MD.)

Fig. 6-55), and proximal humeral head migration (Fig. 6-60).[139] Additional complications include delays in wound healing, nerve injury, humeral fracture, component malposition, instability, rotator cuff tearing, regional pain syndrome, periarticular fibrosis, component loosening, and glenoid arthritis.[26,55,175] Nerve injuries (reported up to 67%) tend to be more common with PHFs and fracture-dislocations than in studies involving HA for nonfracture cases.[63,255,256] In patients with chronic fractures treated with HA, the most common problems encountered are instability, heterotopic ossification, tuberosity malunion or nonunion, and rotator cuff tears.[175] Of all the complications encountered, tuberosity resorption continues to be the most common cause of failure and poor outcomes after HA.[19,59,131,139]

RTSA has proven to be beneficial for the management of certain PHF subtypes. With its increased utilization, surgeons have also encountered negative consequences with its use for treatment of both acute fractures and fracture sequelae. Complications associated with RTSA for fractures vary in incidence from 5% to 40%.[270] Cheung et al. provided a concise summary regarding the potential issues related to this method of surgical treatment. The authors found that the most common complications included neurologic injury (e.g., axillary nerve), periprosthetic fracture, hematoma, and infection, which are similar to those reported for HA, and scapular notching, instability, mechanical baseplate failure, and acromial fracture, which are specific to RTSA.[50] Cazeneuve et al.[48] reported that the most common complications associated with RTSA for fracture were dislocation, reflex sympathetic dystrophy, and infection. The most common reason for revision, much like RTSA for rotator cuff tear arthropathy, was instability. Depending on the type of complication being managed, "salvage options" during the revision surgery include conversion to HA or resection arthroplasty. Options during revision surgery include conversion to HA or resection arthroplasty.[48]

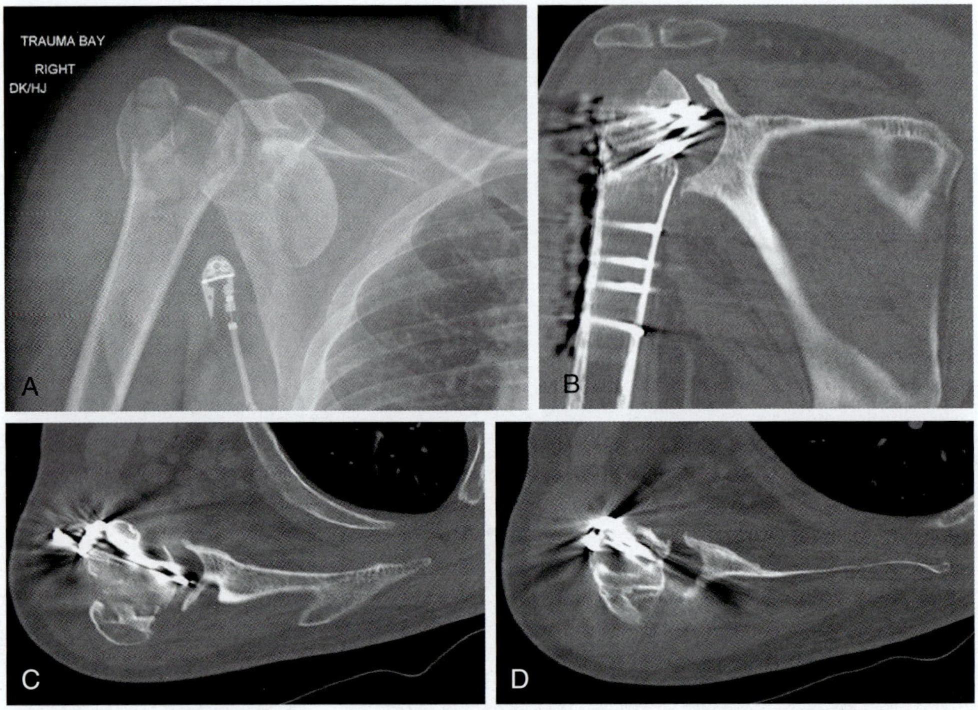

FIGURE 6-58: **A,** Anterior fracture-dislocation of the right shoulder in a 64-year-old male. This patient was referred 1.5 years after an open reduction and internal fixation for persistent shoulder pain and loss of function. At the time of initial presentation, the patient was recovering from an associated axillary nerve injury and was later found to have a deep shoulder infection caused by *Propionibacterium acnes.* **B** to **D,** Coronal and axial two-dimensional computed tomographic imaging in the plane of the scapula demonstrates the following: valgus collapse of the humeral head combined with regions of necrosis, screw penetration into the glenoid vault creating a large contained defect (extending to the base of the coracoid), and posterior malunion of the greater tuberosity. This combination of findings has been referred to as the "unhappy triad" after lock plating by Boileau. (Courtesy Aaron J. Bois, MD.)

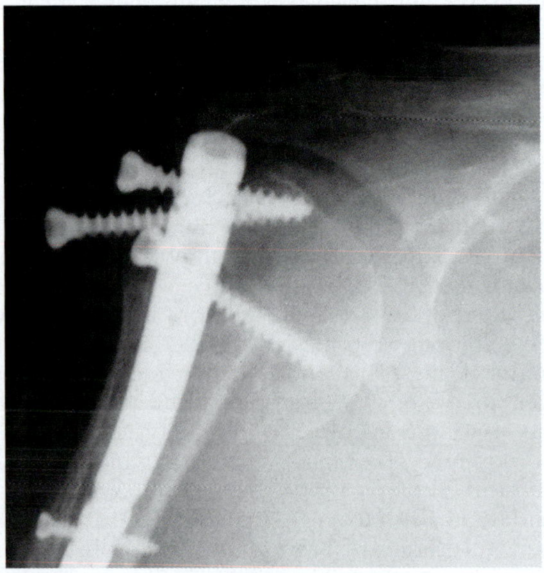

FIGURE 6-59: Intramedullary fixation for a surgical neck nonunion resulting in malunion and hardware prominence in the subacromial space. (From Iannotti JP, Ramsey ML, Warner JJP. Nonprosthetic management of proximal humeral fractures. *J Bone Joint Surg Am.* 2003;85:1578-1593.)

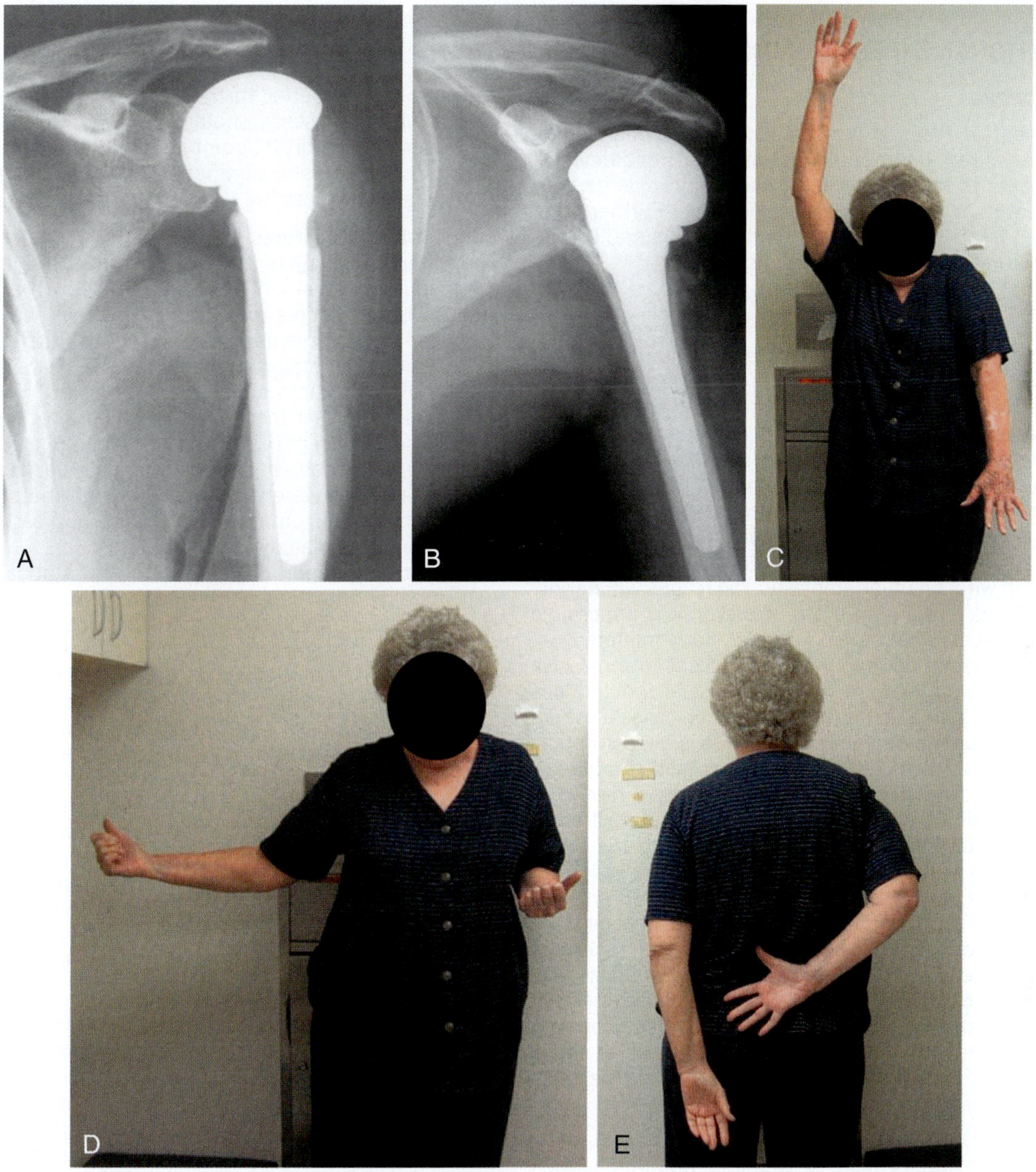

FIGURE 6-60: **A** and **B,** Anteroposterior and axillary radiographs demonstrate tuberosity resorption and increased retroversion of the humeral component. **C** to **E,** This patient presented with poor left shoulder function (i.e., pseudoparalysis) and pain due to tuberosity resorption and component malposition. (Courtesy Michael A. Wirth, MD.)

INTERNATIONAL EXPERT COMMENTARY

Pascal Boileau

The treatment of PHFs is very challenging; so challenging that it has inspired a number of classifications and devices. From implants to rehabilitation, opinions still diverge concerning treatment options and best practice. Furthermore, while a well-treated fracture is forgotten with time, a mistreated fracture may lead to major disability.

Classification and Indications

What is important to remember is the Neer classification. It is our opinion that this is the best classification because it is based on the physiopathology of the muscles and tendons pulling on the GT and LT and the diaphysis. This classification is also very important because it reminds us that 80% of PHFs are undisplaced or minimally displaced, and do not warrant any surgery. In fact, there is some misunderstanding in the treatment of PHFs, mainly because people focus on the humeral head and the possibility of osteonecrosis. While this can be a problem, it is very easy to exchange a necrotic humeral head with a hemiarthroplasty. The results will be very good if the GT is in the right place. However, it is impossible to solve a situation where the GT is posteriorly migrated.

A grossly displaced GT fracture is equivalent to a massive posterosuperior cuff tear, in that the muscle and tendons retract very rapidly and definitively. In revision cases in which the tuberosity was not originally reduced, it is almost impossible to bring the fragment back into place and to obtain a functional shoulder. This is why, for us, the main reason to operate on a PHF is not for the humeral head but for the GT fragment. All efforts should be made to reattach the GT in the right spot so that the cuff will function normally.

Another very important point is that there are two types of PHFs: those that occur in young patients with good bone stock from a very severe trauma and those that occur in elderly patients with osteoporosis from a simple fall. In the first case, there is very good cortical bone, and it is possible to perform fixation well through various forms of osteosynthesis. However, in elderly patients, quite often the bone is too weak to obtain good fixation, and this is why the surgeon should be more inclined to perform arthroplasty in elderly patients.

Imaging

Again, what should be kept in mind is that the correct diagnosis, and therefore the correct treatment, cannot be determined without adequate radiographs. Yet again, the best radiographs to obtain are the Neer series, which includes a true AP view (where you can see the glenohumeral joint line), a true lateral view, and a true axillary view. CT scans can be very helpful in difficult cases, but should not be ordered routinely in my opinion, because sometimes it leads to overtreating the patient.

Greater and Lesser Tuberosity Fractures

Arthroscopic treatment is preferred today with displacement of the tuberosities (>5 mm). If the surgeon does not have the skill to do this under arthroscopy, it can be done open. For LT fractures, it is better to use a deltopectoral approach, while for GT fractures, it is better to use an anterolateral transdeltoid approach.

What should be remembered is that GT fractures are secondary to anterior dislocation or subluxation. Very often, there may be an associated anterior labrum tear (i.e., a Bankart lesion). On the other hand, an LT fracture is very often the consequence of a posterior subluxation or dislocation. Thus in this case there may be a posterior labrum tear, and it is always better to treat them in the same session. This is why arthroscopy should be preferred.

Another very important point is that in tuberosity fractures, the risk of stiffness is significant, and rehabilitation should start as soon as possible.

Surgical Neck Fractures

The pathophysiology of surgical neck fractures is related to the medial displacement of the diaphysis by the force of the latissimus dorsi, teres major, and pectoralis major muscles. The head fragment is undisplaced because the external rotators and internal rotators are still in place. However, the head can be displaced into either varus or valgus. Most surgeons today prefer to treat these fractures with a locked plate. My preference is to treat these fractures through a percutaneous approach with a short, straight, statically locked IM nail. I use either the Neviaser approach (through the trapezius) for varus deformity or an anterior AC joint approach for valgus deformity or translation of the fracture.

Another very important trick is to first statically lock the nail distally, and then perform retrograde hammering (the so-called "back-slap" technique) to place immediate compression on the fracture site. This should be done after positioning the arm in neutral rotation to control the retroversion of the humerus. Then it is easy to finish the procedure by placing one or two proximal screws.

Modern IM nails utilize locking technology to avoid the complications seen in the past, such as screw migration with nonunion or malunion. Additionally, most modern nails are straight and do not damage the footprint of the supraspinatus tendon during nail insertion; therefore they do not lead to the shoulder pain that was seen in the past.

It is my opinion that surgeons should reconsider the use of IM nails in PHFs, especially since the procedure is now carried out with a percutaneous approach.

Three- and Four-Part Fractures

My preferred treatment depends on the patient's age. In patients younger than 60 years, I prefer a locked IM nail. The nail is inserted through a superior transdeltoid approach in the case of GT fracture. It is inserted through a deltopectoral approach in the case of LT fracture and anterior dislocation of the humeral head. In patients younger than 70 years with very severely displaced fractures, I prefer to perform a hemiarthroplasty. In patients older than 70 years with displaced four-part fractures or fracture-dislocations, I prefer to perform a reverse shoulder arthroplasty with GT reattachment.

Complications Associated with the Treatment of Proximal Humerus Fractures

The main and most devastating complication that can be seen after a PHF is posterior migration of the GT. This is the major cause of stiffness and pseudoparalysis of the shoulder. Osteonecrosis can happen, but again, this can be solved easily with a hemiarthroplasty. Glenoid erosion is also a complication of fractures, especially after locking plates or nails. This is also a devastating complication because it leads to revision with a TSA, sometimes in young patients.

Finally, I would like to make surgeons realize that the worst complication that can occur is the combination of the three listed above: proximal/posterior migration of the GT plus osteonecrosis plus glenoid erosion after using a locking plate. I have called this the "unhappy triad after locked plating." There is no way to solve this situation easily. Even a reverse prosthesis will not give a very good result because of the lack of external rotation caused by the posterior migration of the GT.

SENIOR EDITOR COMMENTARY

Frederick Matsen III

I am most grateful to Dr. Pascal Boileau for his thoughtful commentary. Like him, I have been referred so many patients with complications following internal fixation of fractures. Along with some other complications of internal fixation, his "unhappy triad" can be exemplified by the radiographs shown in Figs. 6-61 to 6-70.

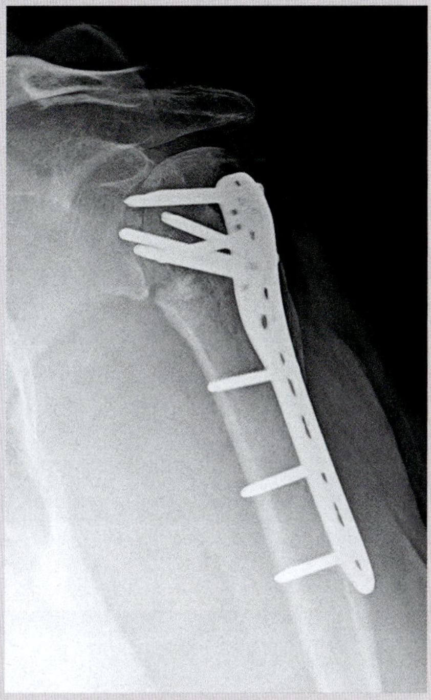

FIGURE 6-61

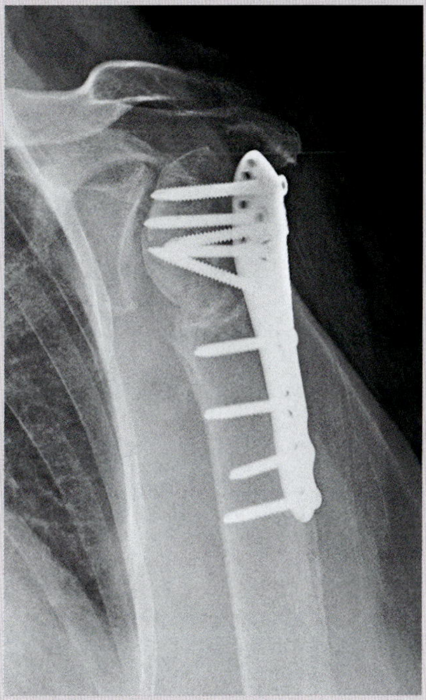

FIGURE 6-62

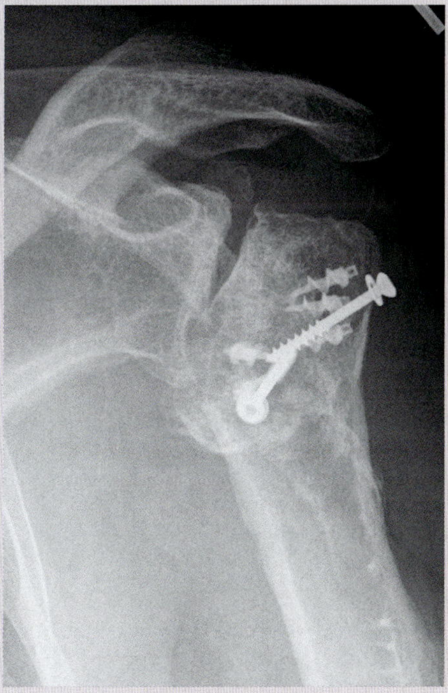

FIGURE 6-63

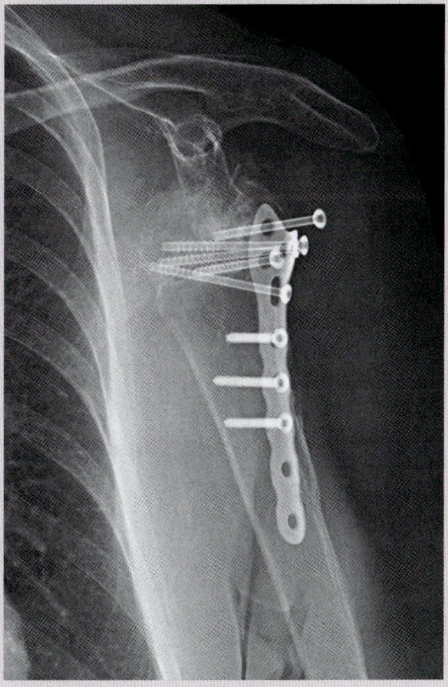

FIGURE 6-64

Continued

SENIOR EDITOR COMMENTARY—cont'd

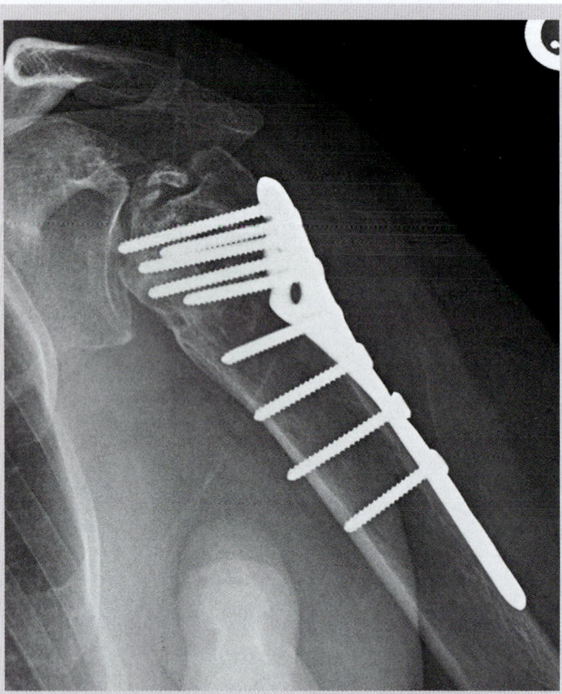

FIGURE 6-65

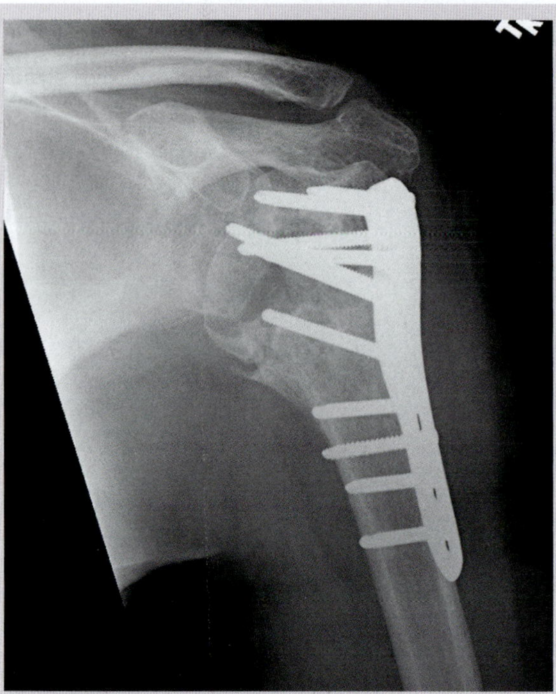

FIGURE 6-66

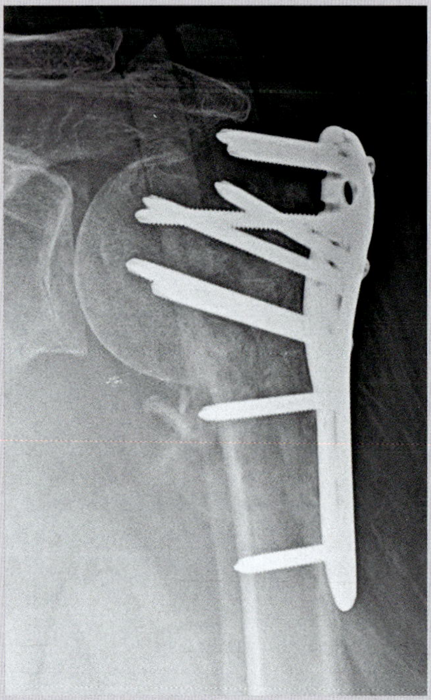

FIGURE 6-67

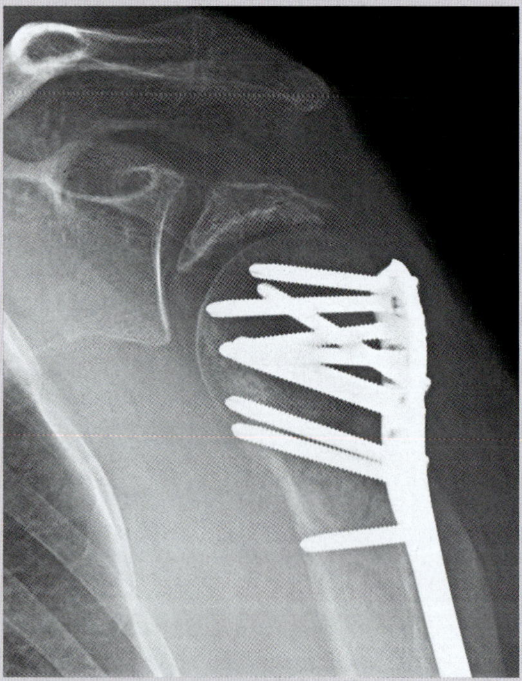

FIGURE 6-68

SENIOR EDITOR COMMENTARY—cont'd

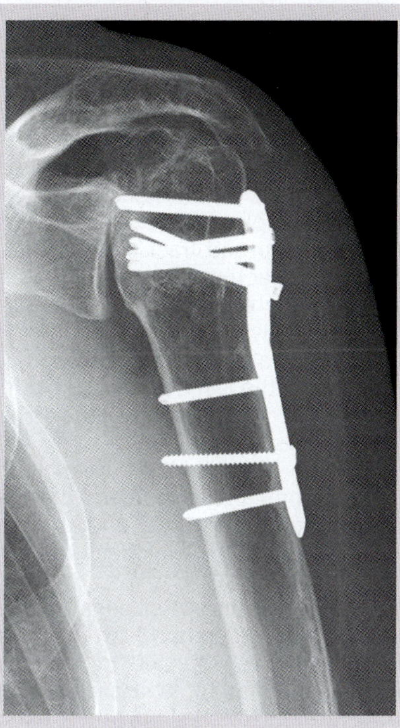

FIGURE 6-69

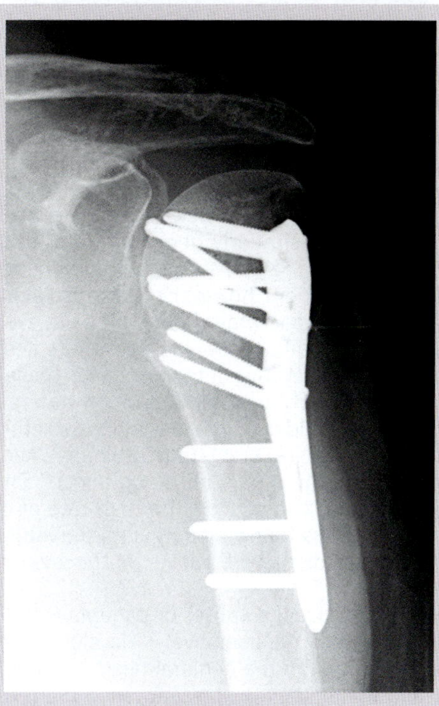

FIGURE 6-70

EDITOR COMMENTARY

Aaron J. Bois

The authors of this chapter are to be commended for their overview and update of the literature of such a diverse and controversial shoulder topic. A review of the recent literature using the PubMed database and the search terms "proximal humerus" and "fracture" revealed several hundred publications in the English literature, most of which represent level IV and V evidence; this highlights both the volume and quality of literature published in recent years and the challenge one faces when trying to use the available literature to assist in the treatment decision-making process.

As previously reported by Charles A. Rockwood (personal communication), and several other experienced shoulder surgeons, there are two distinct patient populations with PHFs: young patients with high-energy trauma and elderly patients with low-energy trauma. These groups should be thought of differently even when they present with the same fracture pattern. In the former group, operative management is often performed in an effort to reconstitute the bony anatomy of the proximal humerus (i.e., the "parts") to reestablish both the registry of the humeral head on the glenoid fossa and the length-tension relationship of the rotator cuff by means of anatomic reduction of the GT; this combination will theoretically restore glenohumeral joint mechanics and shoulder function. The majority of cases in the latter group can (and some argue should) be managed nonoperatively, especially in those patients who are low demand and/or have multiple medical comorbidities precluding them from undergoing surgical intervention, or in patients who clearly lack motivation or are incapable of taking part in a structured postoperative rehabilitation program.

A recent meta-analysis of the available literature on the management of PHFs was published in the Cochrane Database of Systematic Reviews.[105] This review included 23 small RCTs involving 1238 patients. Surprisingly, this analysis concluded the following:

> *There is insufficient evidence to inform the management of these fractures…it remains unclear whether surgery, even for specific fracture types, will produce consistently better long-term outcomes but it is likely to be associated with a higher risk of surgery-related complications and requirement for further surgery. There is insufficient evidence to establish what is the best method of surgical treatment, either in terms of the use of different categories of surgical intervention (such as plate vs. nail fixation, or hemiarthroplasty vs. tension-wire fixation) or different methods of performing an intervention in the same category (such as different methods of plate fixation).*

Continued

EDITOR COMMENTARY—cont'd

This Cochrane Review was recently updated in 2015.[277] Several other important conclusions were made and are worth mentioning: The evidence does not cover the treatment of (1) two-part tuberosity fractures, (2) fractures in young people, (3) high-energy trauma, and (4) less common fractures such as fracture-dislocations and head-splitting fractures.

Since the 2012 Cochrane Review, there have been several other RCTs that have similarly demonstrated no difference in outcome for managing PHFs (operative vs. nonoperative) in the elderly population; however, one must acknowledge some of the methodologic limitations that exist even in level I studies.[79,150,208] Despite these findings, there seems to be a growing trend of operative intervention of these injuries, especially in the elderly population, which has raised concerns by many shoulder surgeons as to whether we as orthopedic surgeons are practicing ethically, keeping our Hippocratic oath in mind of "first do no harm." This should also be kept in mind considering the high rate of complications and reoperations following surgical intervention in this patient cohort (as displayed above in the senior editor's commentary).

In some circumstances, a subset of patients with PHFs that are initially treated nonoperatively develop symptomatic sequelae such as AVN of the humeral head, proximal humeral nonunion, and malunion.[29] At present, such problems cannot always be predicted at the time of the initial fracture, and future reconstructive procedures aimed at reducing shoulder pain and improving shoulder function are technically challenging, with satisfactory outcomes[29,70,108,126,160,161,173,206,263,268] and high complication rates, especially in type III fracture sequelae (i.e., nonunion).[108,161,206,268] In contrast, those patients who are initially managed operatively (e.g., ORIF or HA) are also unpredictably at risk of experiencing postoperative complications. For example, in the HA group, multiple authors have demonstrated a direct relationship between tuberosity healing and patient outcome and satisfaction.[59] This has also been my personal experience. This in turn often leads to a technically demanding salvage-type revision, which also lends itself to a high complication rate (21% to 28%) and modest improvements in ROM and clinical outcomes that must be clearly discussed with patients preoperatively.[119,132,149,252,278]

Despite the results of the highest level of evidence on PHF management, there still remains a role for primary operative intervention in physiologically young and active elderly patients with displaced PHFs, especially in cases of displaced three- and four-part fractures and the corresponding fracture subtypes (fracture-dislocations, head splits, and significant articular impression fractures). Surgical options in this age group typically include one of either HA or RTSA. Although there still remains a role for HA, perhaps the most significant impact over the last decade has been the encouraging results of RTSA in managing acute PHFs; however, more long-term studies are needed.[77,228,258,279,280] Surgeons should also be aware of some of the technical challenges that exist (e.g., obtaining proper humeral component height in cases of comminuted fractures) and the complications associated with using an RTSA for fractures, which vary in incidence from 5% to 40%.[48,50,157,270]

In summary, PHFs remain a challenge to the orthopedic surgeon, especially as it pertains to their management. The incidence of PHFs is expected to increase secondary to an aging population and the associated osteoporosis. With increasing trends towards operative management of such fractures, we must continue to strive toward understanding how to best manage patients with such injuries by means of properly conducted trials with nonheterogeneous patient groups that include nonoperative treatment as part of the study protocol. Recently, efforts have been made to improve the prognostic relevance of how PHFs are classified to help guide the treatment of these complex injuries[281]; however, patient factors remain of utmost importance when deciding between operative and nonoperative management in the elderly population. This stresses the importance of adopting an individualized approach for patient management.

CHAPTER 7

Fractures of the Scapula

Thomas P. Goss, Marie E. Walcott

The scapula is quite important in the functioning of the upper extremity. Lying over the posterior chest wall, it is an integral part of the connection between the upper extremity and axial skeleton via the glenohumeral and acromioclavicular joints and the sternoclavicular articulation. The scapula functions as a semistable, fairly mobile platform for the humeral head and upper extremity to work against. Finally, it serves as a point of attachment for various soft tissue structures (musculotendinous and ligamentous) (Fig. 7-1).

Scapular fractures are usually the result of high-energy trauma (most often direct but occasionally indirect). Avulsion and stress or fatigue fractures can also occur. Numerous fracture patterns have been described.

Fractures of the scapula account for 1% of all fractures, 5% of shoulder fractures, and 3% of injuries to the shoulder girdle (Box 7-1). Such fractures are relatively infrequent for two reasons: (1) the scapula lies over the posterior chest wall and is protected by the rib cage and the thoracic cavity anteriorly and a thick layer of soft tissues posteriorly, and (2) the relative mobility of the scapula allows considerable dissipation of traumatic forces. The vast majority of scapula fractures (>90%) are insignificantly displaced, primarily because of the strong support provided by the surrounding soft tissues, thus making nonoperative management the treatment of choice.[43] As a result, these injuries have received little attention in the literature. However, scapula fractures involve a major articulation, occur in patients with a mean age of 35 to 45 years, and, when significantly displaced, can cause considerable morbidity. Consequently, these injuries deserve more respect and are now receiving increasing consideration in major texts,* general and review articles, and papers dealing with specific issues.†

Because of the significant trauma often involved, patients sustaining a scapula fracture have an 80% to 95% incidence of associated osseous and soft tissue injuries (local and distant) that may be major, multiple, and even life threatening. These patients need to be carefully evaluated when they arrive in the emergency department, and appropriate supportive care must be rendered. As a result, scapula fractures are often diagnosed late, have a delay in definitive treatment, or both. Such delay can compromise the patient's final functional result. In addition, if the associated injuries involve the shoulder complex, the patient's scapula fracture recovery may be even further compromised. Herrera et al.[129] reported on 22 patients with displaced scapula fractures managed operatively 21 to 57 days (mean delay, 30 days) after the acute event. Although technically challenging, they found that the surgery could be safely conducted with good outcomes.

ANATOMY

A thorough knowledge regarding the local bony, soft tissue, and neurovascular anatomy is necessary when evaluating and treating scapula fractures, particularly if operative management is required. The scapula is composed of the scapular body and its four processes: the glenoid, acromial, coracoid, and spinous processes. The glenoid process extends laterally from the scapular body and is composed of the glenoid neck and glenoid cavity which in turn is composed of the glenoid rim and glenoid fossa. The coracoid process extends superiorly from the glenoid process and then anteriorly and laterally. The acromial process extends laterally from the spinous process and eventually anteriorly. The spinous process protrudes posteriorly from the scapular body and extends from the medial scapular border (forming the spinomedial angle) to its junction with the glenoid and acromial processes at the spinoglenoid notch (through which the suprascapular artery and nerve pass from the supraspinatus fossa to infraspinatus fossa). The superior scapular border meets the medial scapular border at the superior angle, and the medial scapular border meets the lateral scapular border at the inferior angle. The scapula takes part in three articulations: the glenohumeral joint, acromioclavicular joint, and scapulothoracic articulation. The

*References 25, 46, 67, 75, 114, 194, 210, 214, 215, 222, 238, 247, 251, 252, 257, 269.

†References 87, 98, 111, 69, 117, 133, 143, 165, 188, 192, 193, 195, 217, 218, 230, 246, 250, 276, 297, 300, 311, 312.

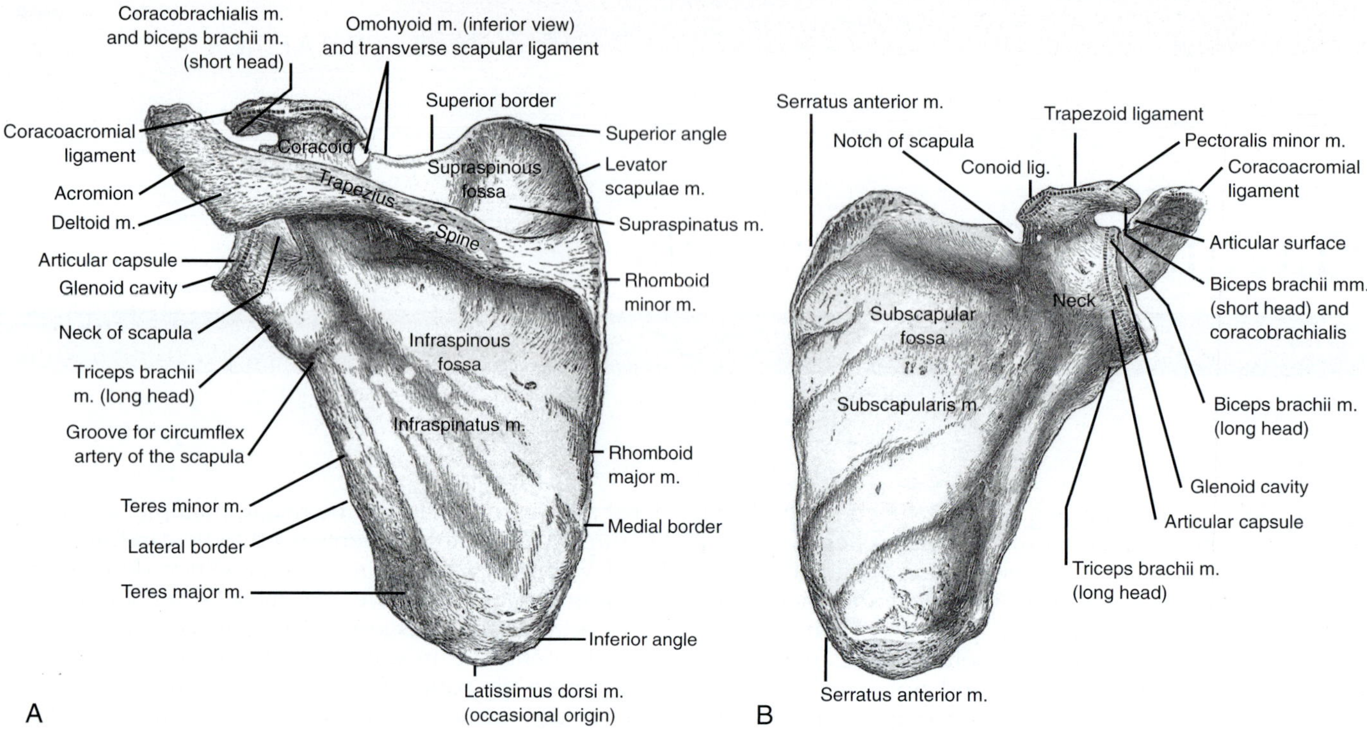

FIGURE 7-1: The many musculotendinous and ligamentous attachment sites on the scapula. **A,** Posterior or dorsal surface of the scapula. **B,** Anterior or costal surface of the scapula. (Modified from Anson B. *Morris' Human Anatomy.* New York: McGraw-Hill; 1966:247-248.)

BOX 7-1. Fractures of the Scapula

1% of all fractures
≥90% insignificantly displaced
Incidence:
- Body and spine: ~70%
- Glenoid process: ~15% (glenoid cavity, ~10%; glenoid neck, ~5%)
- Acromial process: ~8%
- Coracoid process: ~7%

Incidence of associated injuries is 80%-90%, including major, multiple, and life-threatening injuries

scapula serves as a point of attachment for numerous ligaments: the glenohumeral ligaments, coracoacromial ligament, acromioclavicular ligaments, coracohumeral ligament, and coracoclavicular ligament (with its trapezoid and conoid portions). The scapula also serves at a point of attachment for 18 musculotendinous structures. The subscapularis muscle lies over the anterior scapular surface, and the serratus anterior inserts along the inferior angle of the scapula. The supraspinatus and infraspinatus muscles lie posteriorly within the supraspinatus and infraspinatus fossae, respectively. More superficially, the trapezius muscle inserts along the scapular spine, acromion, and clavicle, whereas the deltoid muscle originates from the scapular spine, acromial process, and distal end of the clavicle. The levator scapulae and rhomboids attach along the medial scapular border, while the teres minor and teres major muscles attach along the lateral border. Tendons of the pectoralis minor, short head of the biceps, and coracobrachialis attach on the coracoid process; the latter two form the conjoined tendon. The long head of the biceps originates at the superior glenoid margin, while the long head of the triceps attaches along the inferior glenoid margin. A small slip of latissimus dorsi muscle variably originates at the inferior angle of the scapula, while the omohyoid attaches along the superior scapular border. These muscles are served by nerves arising from the brachial plexus. The brachial plexus and axillary vessels pass medial to the coracoid process and deep to the pectoralis minor tendon. The suprascapular notch is found along the superior scapular border just medial to the base of the coracoid process and is bridged by the transverse scapular ligament. The suprascapular nerve courses through the notch beneath the ligament, while the suprascapular artery passes above the ligament. The scapula is served by two sets of vessels that anastomose with each other. The glenoid process is served by the circumflex scapular artery, which courses inferiorly to superiorly, and the suprascapular artery, which courses superiorly to inferiorly, anastomosing over the posterior glenoid process. The scapular body is served by the thoracodorsal artery, which courses inferiorly to superiorly, and the dorsal scapular artery, which courses superiorly to inferiorly, anastomosing along the medial border of the scapula.

Most shoulder functions involve complex glenohumeral and scapulothoracic movements that occur in a precise sequence. The scapula is capable of six basic movements over the posterior chest wall: elevation, depression, upward rotation, downward rotation, protraction, and retraction. Combinations of these movements allow the positioning of the upper extremity optimally in space. Trauma to the scapular region resulting in fracture nonunion, fracture malunion, soft tissue scarring, muscle damage, and nerve injury can have adverse mechanical and functional consequences.

LOCATION OF FRACTURES OF THE SCAPULA

Quite a number of scapula fracture patterns occur. Typically, they are classified by anatomic area: body and spine, glenoid neck, glenoid cavity, acromial process, and coracoid process. Most scapula fractures involve the body and spine (~70%).[192] The remaining 30% involve its other three processes (Fig. 7-2).

Fractures of the glenoid neck constitute approximately 5% of the total, and fractures of the glenoid cavity (the glenoid rim and glenoid fossa) are approximately 10%. Therefore fractures of the glenoid process account for approximately 15% of all scapula fractures. Approximately 8% of these injuries involve the acromial process and approximately 7% involve the coracoid process.[192]

A group of injuries termed double disruptions of the superior shoulder suspensory complex (SSSC) have also been described and often involve fractures of the coracoid, acromial, and glenoid processes.[107]

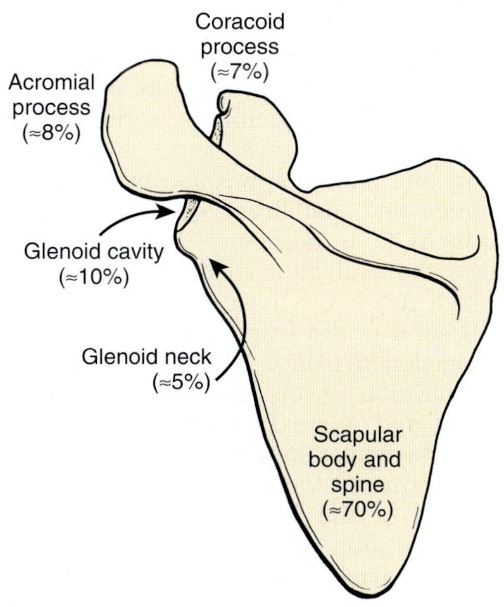

FIGURE 7-2: Incidence of scapular fractures by region.

NEW CLASSIFICATION SCHEME

In 2013 and 2014, the Arbeitsgemeinschaft für Osteosynthesefragen (AO) Foundation and the Orthopaedic Trauma Association (OTA) put forth a new scapular fracture classification system focusing on articular segment and scapular body involvement, respectively. The goal was to describe these injuries in a comprehensive, reliable, reproducible, and accurate manner and to provide a base for further clinical studies. Other variables, such as displacement, were acknowledged as being of equal importance in determining appropriate treatment and predicting outcomes. Fractures of the articular segment are given the designation "F," which includes three groups: F0, F1, and F2. The F1 group has three subgroups, each with three categories and the F2 group has two subgroups. Fractures of the scapular body are given the designation "B," and the involved borders are assigned letters as follows: l, lateral border; m, medial border; and s, superior border. The junction between the articular segment and scapular body is defined by a line parallel to the plane of the glenoid cavity (superior to inferior rim), beginning at the lateral border of the scapular notch and exiting along the lateral scapular margin. Fractures of the acromial and coracoid processes are given the designation "P" and are considered independent systems. While intriguing, this classification system is unfamiliar and somewhat cumbersome and confusing. For example, a Goss-Ideberg type II fracture becomes an $F_1$3a fracture, while a type V_c fracture becomes an $F_1$3b Blms fracture. It remains to be seen whether this system receives wide acceptance.[11,145]

CLINICAL FEATURES

The physician's attention is initially drawn to the scapular region by the patient's complaints of pain. Characteristically, the arm is held adducted, and all movement is resisted, particularly abduction, which is especially painful. Local tenderness is typical. Abnormal physical findings in the area include swelling and crepitus. Ecchymosis is less than what might be expected given the degree of bony injury. However, the specific diagnosis of a scapula fracture is ultimately radiographic. These injuries are often initially missed[123] or detected incidentally on the patient's admission chest radiograph (Fig. 7-3). It cannot be overemphasized that scapula fractures are typically accompanied by associated injuries that often require more urgent management.

ASSOCIATED INJURIES AND COMPLICATIONS

The most significant complications associated with scapula fractures are those that result from accompanying injuries to adjacent and distant osseous and soft

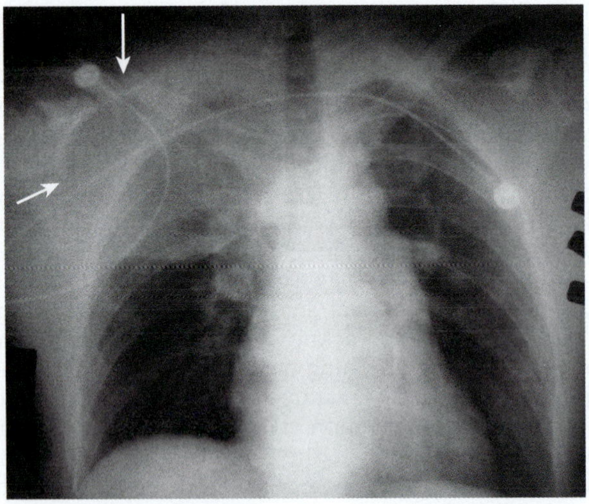

FIGURE 7-3: Anteroposterior chest radiograph of a patient who sustained multiple trauma. The fractured clavicle and scapula (*arrows*) were incidental findings. (From Goss TP. Fractures of the scapula: diagnosis and treatment. In: Iannotti JP, Williams GR Jr, eds. *Disorders of the Shoulder: Diagnosis and Management.* Philadelphia, Lippincott Williams & Wilkins; 1999:600.)

tissue structures.[43,296] Because of the severe traumatic forces involved, these patients have an average of 3.9 additional injuries, with the most common sites being the ipsilateral shoulder girdle,[142] upper extremity, lung, and chest wall.[89] Of these patients, 25% to 45% have accompanying rib fractures, 15% to 40% have fractures of the clavicle, 15% to 55% have pulmonary injuries[196] (e.g., hemopneumothorax, pulmonary contusion), 12% have humeral fractures, and 5% to 10% sustain injuries to the brachial plexus and peripheral nerves.[79,138,277] Fractures of the skull are found in approximately 25% of patients, cerebral contusions in 10% to 40%, central neurologic deficits in 5%, tibia and fibula fractures in 11%,[120,268,277] major vascular injuries in 11%, and injuries that result in splenectomy in 8%. Two percent of these patients die. Landi et al. have described a compartment syndrome associated with a scapula fracture.[167] Various other cardiothoracic, genitourinary, and gastrointestinal injuries have also been reported. Interestingly, Stephens and associates reviewed 173 blunt trauma patients (92 with scapula fractures and 81 controls) and concluded that scapula fractures are not a significant marker for greater mortality or neurovascular morbidity.[270] Veysi et al. also showed no increase in mortality, but they did confirm significantly greater severity scores in trauma patients sustaining scapula fractures.[289]

Complications related to scapula fractures themselves are relatively uncommon. Nonunion, although possible, is quite rare. Malunion can occur in various forms depending on the particular fracture type. Malunion of a scapular body fracture is generally well tolerated; however, painful scapulothoracic crepitus has been described on occasion. Fractures of the glenoid cavity can result in symptomatic glenohumeral degenerative joint disease. Shoulder instability can be associated with significantly displaced fractures of the glenoid neck (angular displacement) and fractures of the glenoid rim. Fractures of the glenoid neck with significant translational displacement can give rise to glenohumeral pain and dysfunction related to altered mechanics of the surrounding tissues.

Complications associated with surgical management are possible and include infection (both superficial and deep), intraoperative neurovascular injury, loss of fixation, and others. A poorly managed postoperative rehabilitation program can lead to unnecessary shoulder stiffness.

Finally, complications related to poor patient compliance can occur. Examples include suboptimal shoulder range of motion caused by unwillingness to follow the postoperative physical therapy program and hardware failure associated with failure to observe postoperative instructions.

RADIOGRAPHIC EVALUATION

A fracture of the scapula is a radiographic diagnosis but precisely defining the injury can be difficult. If a scapula fracture is suspected or noted on other radiographs, a scapula trauma series is indicated, including true anteroposterior (AP) and lateral views of the scapula and a true axillary projection of the glenohumeral joint (Fig. 7-4 and Box 7-2).

The scapula is a complex bony structure. One must be able to visualize and evaluate the scapular body and spine and its three other processes: the glenoid process, acromial process, and coracoid process. The glenoid process is composed of the glenoid neck and glenoid cavity; the glenoid cavity is made up of the glenoid fossa and glenoid rim. The scapula takes part in three articulations (the acromioclavicular joint, glenohumeral joint, and scapulothoracic articulation), each of which must be carefully evaluated. Associated shoulder girdle injuries should also be considered, including those involving the clavicle, proximal part of the humerus, and sternoclavicular joint.

If an injury to SSSC (the linkage system between the clavicle and scapula) is suspected, a weight-bearing AP film is obtained (Fig. 7-4). In some situations, transthoracic lateral and oblique projections of the region may be of value. The scapula trauma series will suffice for many injuries.

If the fracture pattern appears to be complex (multiple fracture lines and significant displacement), computed tomography (CT) is necessary. Images in the superior plane allow the evaluation of the acromioclavicular joint and acromial process, whereas the inferior images allow the visualization of the scapular body and spine and the scapulothoracic articulation (Fig. 7-5). The middle images allow visualization of the glenoid neck, glenoid cavity (glenoid rim and glenoid fossa), coracoid process, and glenohumeral articulation (Fig. 7-6). In certain clinical situations, reconstructed views can be of great value. The proximal part of the humerus can be eliminated for optimal visualization of the glenoid cavity, and other reconstructed images are possible (Fig. 7-7). Three-dimensional (3D) CT can be extremely helpful to an orthopedist trying to evaluate the most complex fracture

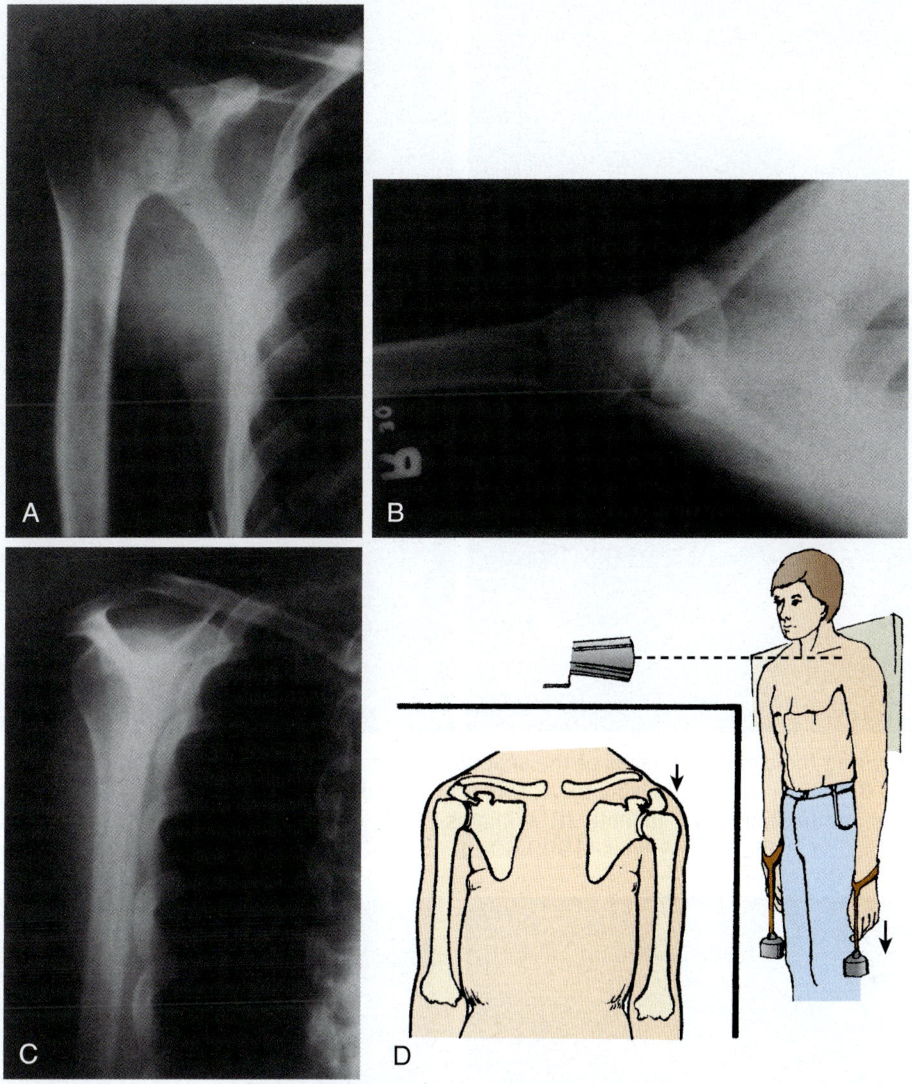

FIGURE 7-4: The scapula trauma series. **A,** True anteroposterior (AP) projection of the scapula. **B,** True axillary projection of the glenohumeral joint and scapula. **C,** True lateral projection of the scapula. **D,** Weight-bearing AP projection of the shoulder complex designed to evaluate the integrity of the clavicular-scapular linkage (optional and depending on the clinical situation). (**A** to **C,** From Goss TP. Fractures of the scapula: diagnosis and treatment. In: Iannotti JP, Williams GR Jr, eds. *Disorders of the Shoulder: Diagnosis and Management*. Philadelphia, Lippincott Williams & Wilkins; 1999:600. **D,** Modified from Rockwood CA. *Fractures*. Philadelphia, JB Lippincott; 1975:733.)

BOX 7-2. Radiographic Evaluation of the Scapula

Fractures often detected incidentally on chest radiograph
Scapula trauma series:
- AP and lateral views of the scapula
- Axillary view of the glenohumeral joint
- Weight-bearing view of the shoulder

CT with and without reconstructions
Three-dimensional CT

AP, *Anteroposterior;* CT, *computed tomography.*

patterns (Fig. 7-8). Images rotated at 15-degree increments in the horizontal, vertical, and oblique planes can be examined and the most useful printed for later reference. McAdams et al. found that CT scanning did not improve the evaluation of glenoid fractures over plain films but did help in identifying associated injuries to SSSC.[187] Finally, it is reasonable to obtain follow-up radiographs at weekly intervals for 2 to 3 weeks after the initial injury to detect inherently unstable fractures that are in acceptable position initially but progressively displace. The clinician must be careful to avoid mistaking nontraumatic radiographic findings (epiphyseal lines, os acromiale, glenoid dysplasia, and scapular foramina) for actual traumatic changes.

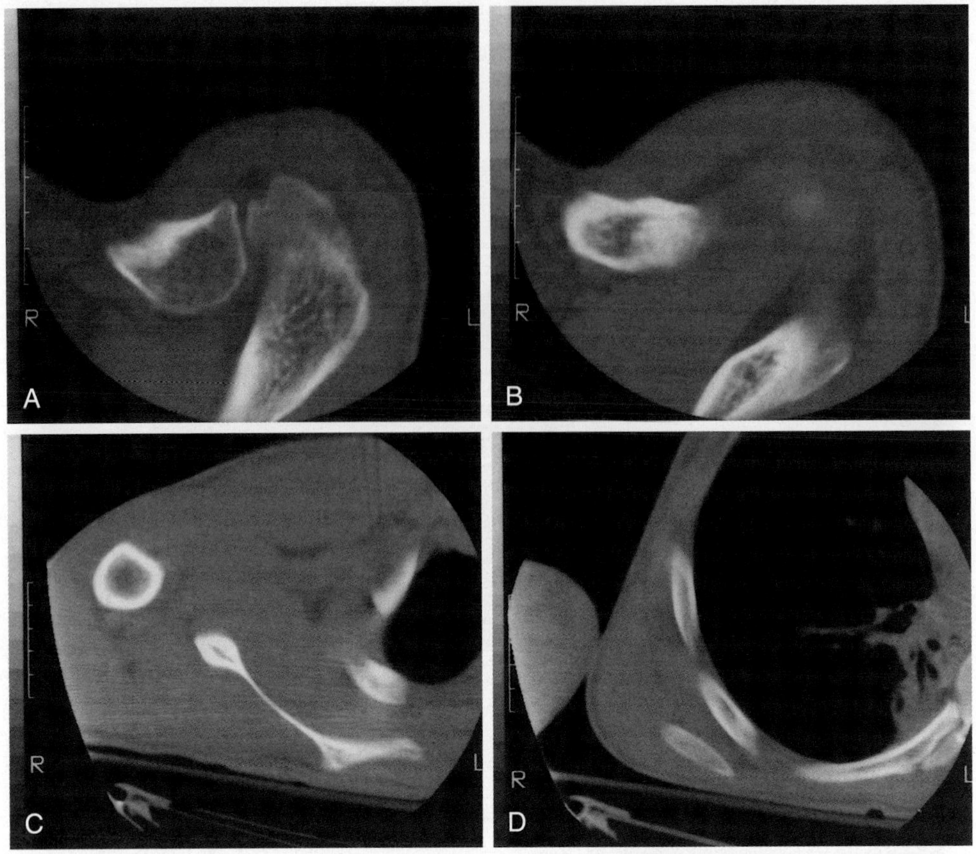

FIGURE 7-5: Axial computed tomographic images of the scapula. **A** and **B,** Superior images showing the acromioclavicular joint and the acromion. **C** and **D,** Inferior images showing the scapular body and scapulothoracic articulation. (From Goss TP. Fractures of the scapula: diagnosis and treatment. In: Iannotti JP, Williams GR Jr, eds. *Disorders of the Shoulder: Diagnosis and Management.* Philadelphia, Lippincott Williams & Wilkins; 1999:601.)

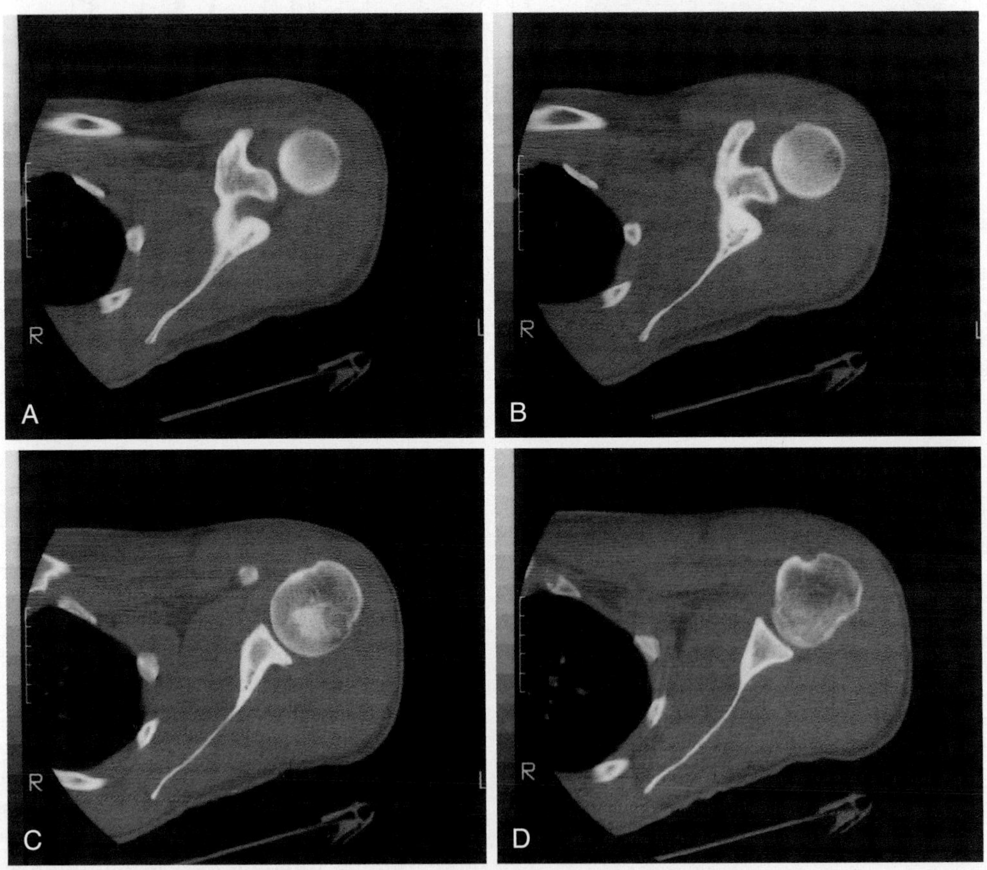

FIGURE 7-6: Axial computed tomographic images through the glenohumeral region of the scapula. **A** and **B,** Most superior. **C** and **D,** Most inferior. (From Goss TP. Fractures of the scapula: diagnosis and treatment. In: Iannotti JP, Williams GR Jr, eds. *Disorders of the Shoulder: Diagnosis and Management.* Philadelphia, Lippincott Williams & Wilkins; 1999:601.)

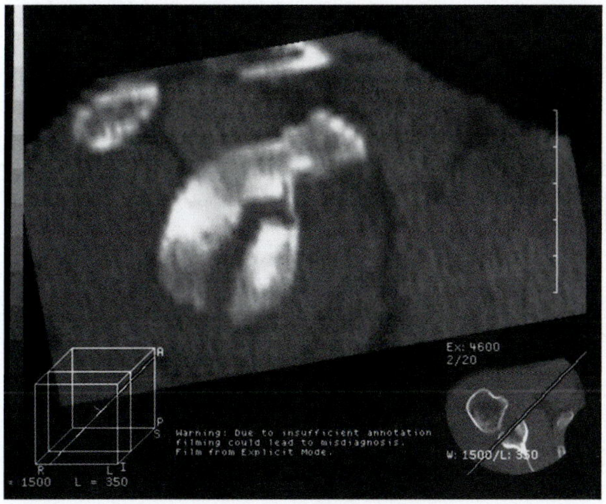

FIGURE 7-7: Reconstructed computed tomographic image showing the glenoid cavity en face with the humeral head eliminated. Note the large anteroinferior glenoid rim fragment with severe separation of the articular surface. (From Goss TP. Fractures of the scapula: diagnosis and treatment. In: Iannotti JP, Williams GR Jr, eds. *Disorders of the Shoulder: Diagnosis and Management*. Philadelphia, Lippincott Williams & Wilkins; 1999:602.)

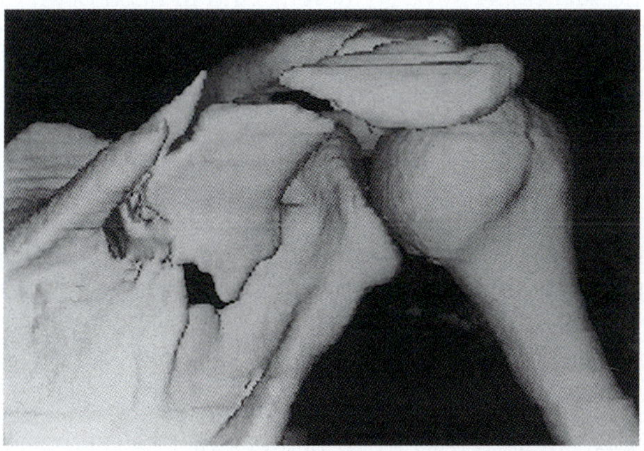

FIGURE 7-8: Three-dimensional computed tomographic image of a patient who sustained a segmental fracture of the acromion. Note the severely displaced intermediate segment. (From Goss TP. Fractures of the scapula: diagnosis and treatment. In: Iannotti JP, Williams GR Jr, eds. Disorders of the Shoulder: Diagnosis and Management. Philadelphia. Lippincott Willims & Wilkins; 1999:602.)

TYPES OF FRACTURES AND METHODS OF TREATMENT

Glenoid Neck (Extra-articular) Fractures

The glenoid neck is that portion of the glenoid process medial to the glenoid cavity and lateral to the scapular body. The coracoid process arises from its superior aspect. The junction between the scapular body and glenoid neck is defined by a line parallel to the glenoid cavity (superior to the inferior rim), running from the lateral border of the scapular notch to the lateral scapular margin. True glenoid neck fractures (which will be discussed here) comprise approximately 5% of all scapular fractures. They exit along the inferior glenoid neck/lateral border of the scapular body, course through the spinoglenoid notch, and exit most often medial to the coracoid process (surgical neck fractures) or, rarely, lateral to the coracoid process (anatomic neck fractures). These injuries are to be distinguished from those far more common disruptions that involve the inferior glenoid neck/lateral border of the scapular body but course through the body to exit through its medial (most common) or superior borders. Such injuries, *termed scapular neck and body fractures,* should simply be termed (and managed as) scapular body fractures to avoid confusion and will be discussed in the section dealing with scapular body fractures.

Glenoid neck fractures may be caused by the following:

1. A direct blow over the anterior or posterior aspect of the shoulder.
2. A fall on the outstretched arm with impaction of the humeral head against the glenoid process.
3. In rare cases, a force applied over the superior aspect of the shoulder complex.

The stability of the glenoid neck is primarily osseous, specifically its junction medially with the scapular body. Secondary support is provided by its attachments superiorly to the clavicular, acromioclavicular joint–acromial strut via the coracoid process, coracoclavicular ligament, and coracoacromial ligament (Fig. 7-9). Tertiary soft tissue support is provided anteriorly by the subscapularis muscle, superiorly by the supraspinatus muscle, and posteriorly by the infraspinatus and teres minor muscles. In a true/complete glenoid neck fracture (a fracture exiting both the superior and lateral scapular margins), displacement may occur (Box 7-3). That these injuries are not more common is somewhat surprising since this portion of the glenoid process is quite narrow. In addition, if its secondary support is compromised (as in a coracoid process fracture, coracoclavicular ligament disruption with or without a coracoacromial ligament injury, clavicle

BOX 7-3. Significantly Displaced Glenoid Neck Fractures

ML translational displacement ≥1 cm
AP angular displacement ≥40 degrees
Decrease in the GPA to ≤20 degrees
Other
Rule out a "false glenoid neck" fracture (i.e., an inferior glenoid neck fracture that does not exit the superior scapular margin)

AP, *Anteroposterior;* ML, *mediolateral.*

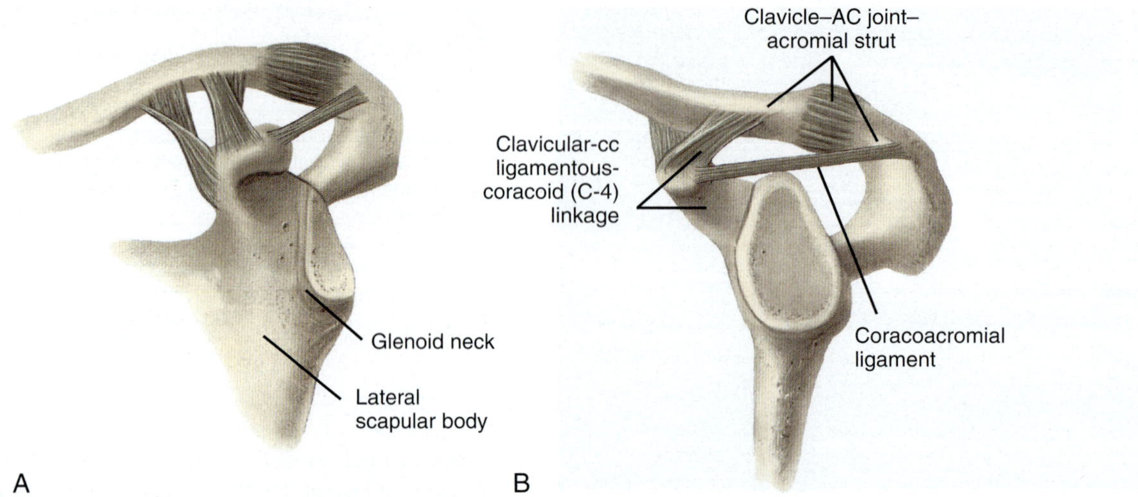

FIGURE 7-9: Structures providing stability to the glenoid process in the region of the glenoid neck. **A,** Lateral aspect of the scapular body. **B,** Clavicle–acromioclavicular (AC) joint–acromial strut via the clavicular–coracoclavicular (cc) ligamentous–coracoid [C-4] linkage and the coracoacromial ligament.

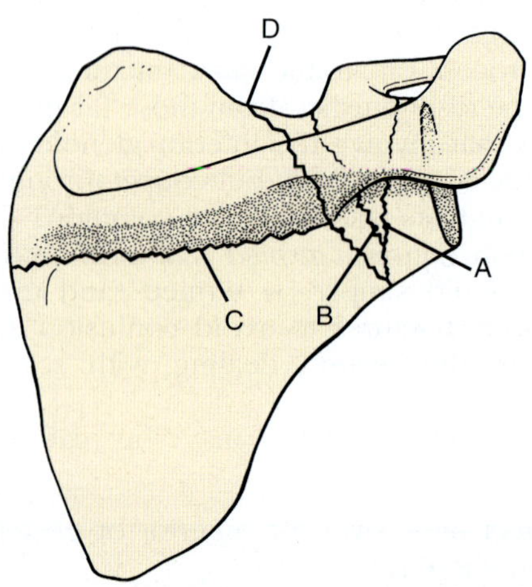

FIGURE 7-10: Four basic fracture patterns involving the glenoid neck. *A,* fracture through the anatomic neck; *B,* fracture through the surgical neck; *C,* fracture involving the inferior glenoid neck that then courses medially to exit through the medial border of the scapular body; and *D,* fracture involving the inferior glenoid neck that then exits through the superior border of the scapular body via the scapular spine (types C and D are managed as scapular body fractures). (From Goss TP. Fractures of the glenoid neck. *J Shoulder Elbow Surg.* 1994;3[1]:42-52.)

fracture, acromioclavicular joint disruption, or acromial fracture), that is, double disruption of SSSC, the fracture has the potential for significant displacement.[104] Hardegger et al.[121] described a rare case wherein the fracture line exited the superior scapular margin lateral to the coracoid process (the anatomic neck) (Fig. 7-10), thereby allowing the glenoid fragment to be displaced laterally and distally by the pull of the long head of the triceps muscle. Arts and Louette[8] described a similar injury. They saw these fractures as inherently unstable (the primary support is completely disrupted and the fracture is lateral to the secondary support system) and in need of an open reduction and internal fixation (ORIF). In contrast, fractures of the surgical neck are only rendered unstable and in need of surgical management when accompanied by associated injuries to the secondary support system. Type I fractures include all insignificantly displaced injuries and constitute more than 90% of the total. Management is nonoperative, and a good to excellent functional result can be expected. Type II fractures include all significantly displaced injuries; "significant displacement" includes medial-lateral (ML) translational displacement of the glenoid fragment relative to the scapular body of 1 cm or more, AP angular displacement of the glenoid fragment of at least 40 degrees, and a decrease in the glenopolar angle (GPA) to 20 degrees or less (Fig. 7-11).[108] Limb and McMurray described the case of a patient with a glenoid neck fracture so severely displaced and inferiorly angulated that the humeral head was articulating with the medial fracture surface and lateral margin of the scapular body.[175] ML translational displacement of 1 cm was chosen by Zdravkovic and Damholt,[307] Nordqvist and Petersson,[220] and Miller and Ada[1,206] as separating major from minor injuries. Bateman[25] stated that this degree of displacement could interfere with abduction. Hardegger and coworkers[121] pointed out that significant ML translational displacement changes the normal relationships between the glenohumeral articulation and the undersurface of the distal end of the clavicle, the acromioclavicular joint, and the acromial process. This displacement alters the mechanics of nearby musculotendinous units, resulting in a functional imbalance of the shoulder complex as a whole (a disorganization of the coracoacromial arch). Miller and Ada[1,206] stated that resultant weakness (especially abductor weakness), decreased

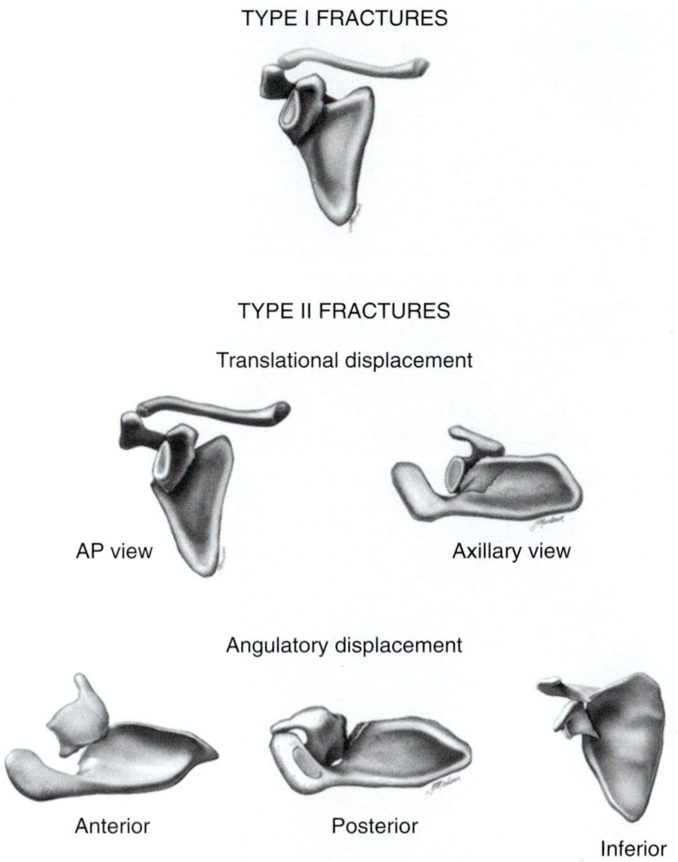

FIGURE 7-11: Classification scheme for fractures of the glenoid neck. *AP*, Anteroposterior.

range of motion, and pain (particularly subacromial pain) were largely due to rotator cuff dysfunction. The premise that significant ML translational displacement of the glenoid process can lead to shoulder discomfort and dysfunction certainly makes sense intuitively. The complex bony relationships in the glenohumeral region are clearly altered, as are the mechanics of the musculotendinous structures that pass from the scapula to the proximal part of the humerus (the deltoid muscle and rotator cuff, in particular). The fracture line usually exits the superior scapular margin medial to the coracoid process (the surgical neck region). The glenoid fragment is then drawn inferiorly by the weight of the arm and either anteromedially or posteromedially by the adjacent muscle forces causing ML transitional displacement. Whether the glenoid fragment displaces medially or the scapular body displaces laterally has been argued but is irrelevant therapeutically (Fig. 7-12).

Bateman[25] and DePalma[74] stated that excessive angulation of the glenoid fragment could result in glenohumeral instability (anterior, posterior, or inferior). Normally, the glenoid cavity faces 5 degrees superiorly and is retroverted 6 degrees relative to the plane of the scapular body. With increasing angulation, the humeral head loses the normal bony support provided by the glenoid cavity (bony instability), which translates into glenohumeral discomfort and dysfunction.[1,25,75,206] Miller and Ada[1,206] stated that AP angular displacement of 40 degrees or more was unacceptable. They saw this degree of displacement as adversely altering not only glenohumeral but also other bony relationships, as well as musculotendinous dynamics, particularly those of the rotator cuff, with resultant pain and overall shoulder dysfunction (diminished range of motion and loss of strength) (Fig. 7-13). Van Noort and van Kampen recommended surgical management for glenoid neck fractures with a decrease in the GPA to 20 degrees or less (5 degrees of superior angulation being the mean in normal individuals).[286] Baroneicek et al. described the management of glenoid neck fractures with various displacements, including those with significant translational displacement in the superior/inferior direction and those with significant superior angular displacement.[22]

Imatani,[143] McGahan and associates,[192] and Lindholm and Leven[176] recommended nonsurgical treatment of all glenoid neck fractures, but their studies give few details to justify this conclusion. Although somewhat ambivalent in their recommendations, two studies do mention surgical management as an option in selected cases. Armstrong and Vanderspuy[6] said that although most of these injuries do well, more aggressive treatment, including ORIF, may be indicated in patients who are young and fit. Wilbur and Evans[297] stated that ORIF might be indicated if the glenoid fragment is markedly displaced or angulated but did not think that they had enough information or experience to warrant definitive surgical indications. Judet,[147] Magerl,[179] Ganz and Noesberger,[93] and Tscherne and Christ[279] reported that operative management of displaced glenoid neck fractures prevents late disability and yields better results. Neer,[214] as well as Rockwood[215] and Butters,[46] presented the recommendations of other investigators, as did a review article by Guttentag and Rechtine.[117] Boerger and Limb[36] reported the case of a patient with a fracture of the glenoid neck, acromial and coracoid fractures, a dislocated acromioclavicular joint, and incomplete paralysis of the infraspinatus muscle treated with ORIF of the acromial and glenoid neck fractures. DeBeer et al. described the operative treatment of a professional cyclist who was able to return to competition after 6 weeks and urged more aggressive management in high-demand patients.[70]

Bozkurt et al. reported on 18 patients treated nonoperatively and found that decreased functional outcome correlated significantly with increased inferior angulation of the fracture and the presence of associated injuries.[41] Van Noort and van Kampen managed 13 patients with neither significant angular displacement, neurologic injury, nor associated ipsilateral shoulder injuries, all of whom had a good to excellent outcome regardless of the degree of translational displacement when treated nonoperatively.[286]

Miller and Ada[1,206] retrospectively reviewed 16 displaced glenoid neck fractures (≥1 cm of ML translational displacement or ≥40 degrees of AP angulation) managed nonoperatively (36-month average follow-up). They found that 20% had decreased range of motion, 50% had

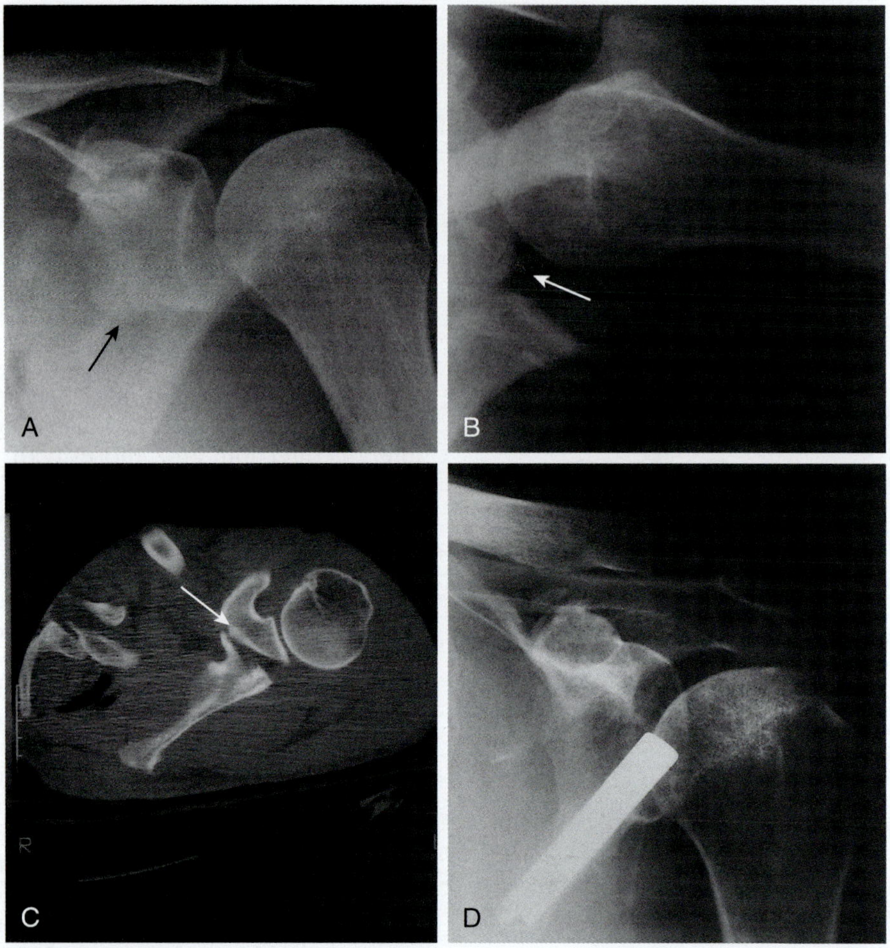

FIGURE 7-12: Radiographs of a patient who sustained a type II fracture of the glenoid neck with significant mediolateral (ML) translational displacement at the fracture site. **A,** Preoperative anteroposterior (AP) radiograph showing the glenoid neck fracture (*arrow*) with significant ML translation. **B,** Preoperative axillary radiograph revealing significant ML translation at the glenoid neck fracture site, probably as a result of an associated disruption of the coracoclavicular ligament (a violation of the C-4 linkage and therefore a double disruption of the superior shoulder suspensory complex) and possibly the coracoacromial ligament. **C,** Preoperative axial computed tomographic image revealing the glenoid neck fracture to be complete and exiting the superior scapular border medial to the intact coracoid process (*arrow*) (a surgical neck fracture). **D,** Postoperative AP radiograph showing anatomic reduction and stabilization of the glenoid neck fracture and glenoid process fragment. (From Goss TP. Fractures of the scapula: diagnosis and treatment. In: Iannotti JP, Williams GR Jr, eds. *Disorders of the Shoulder: Diagnosis and Management.* Philadelphia, Lippincott Williams & Wilkins; 1999:618.)

pain (75% of which was night pain), 40% had weakness with exertion, and 25% noted popping. In particular, these patients often had shoulder abductor weakness and subacromial pain that was due at least in part to rotator cuff dysfunction. They recommended ORIF of glenoid neck fractures with this degree of displacement. Chadwick et al. agreed.[51]

Pace et al. reviewed nine patients with insignificantly displaced fractures and found that the majority had some activity-related pain that was believed to be due to impingement and cuff arthropathy despite 90% good to excellent results.[229] A long-term follow-up study by Zdravkovic and Damholt[307] included 20 to 30 patients (it is difficult to determine the exact number from the text) with displaced glenoid neck fractures and noted that nonoperative treatment yielded satisfactory results. Nordqvist and Petersson[220] evaluated 37 glenoid neck fractures treated without surgery (10- to 20-year follow-up) and found the functional result to be either fair or poor in 32%. They said that for some fractures, early ORIF might have improved the result. Hardegger et al.[121] reported 80% good to excellent results in five displaced glenoid neck fractures treated surgically (6.5-year follow-up). They said that operative management of such injuries prevented late disability and yielded better results. Gagey et al.[92] found a good result in only 1 of 12 displaced

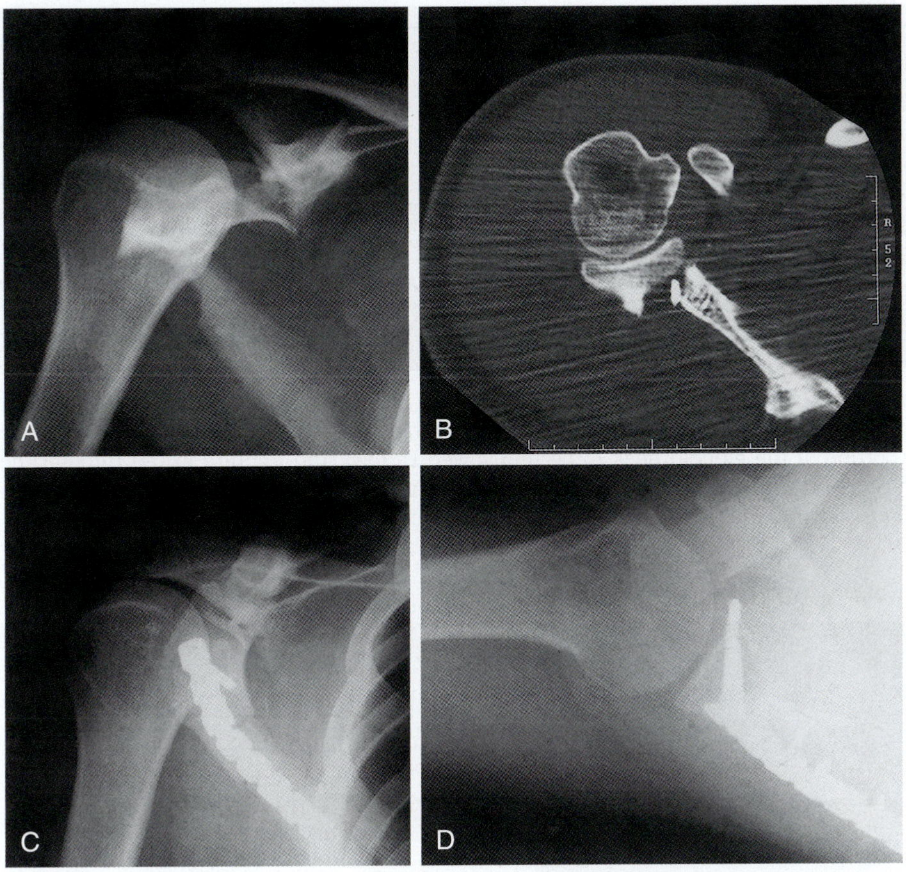

FIGURE 7-13: Type II fracture of the glenoid neck with significant anteroposterior (AP) angular displacement of the glenoid fragment. **A,** Preoperative AP radiograph showing the glenoid neck fracture with severe AP angulation of the glenoid fragment and a fractured coracoid process. Also note the fracture of the scapular body with displacement of the lateral scapular border. **B,** Preoperative axial computed tomographic projection showing the coracoid process fracture (a violation of the clavicular–coracoclavicular ligamentous–coracoid [C-4] linkage), which further destabilized the glenoid fragment and allowed severe angulatory displacement to occur (a double disruption of the superior shoulder suspensory complex). Postoperative AP **(C)** and axillary **(D)** radiographs show the glenoid fragment is reduced and stabilized with a contoured reconstruction plate (the coracoid process was allowed to heal spontaneously).

fractures treated nonoperatively. They stated that such injuries could "disorganize the coracoacromial arch" and recommended ORIF.

Clearly, these investigators agree that the vast majority of glenoid neck fractures can and should be treated without surgery. However, most authors believe that more aggressive treatment, including ORIF, is at least a consideration if not clearly indicated when the glenoid fragment is severely displaced (i.e., type II injuries).

The diagnosis is ultimately radiographic. Plain radiographs are helpful, but because of the complex bony anatomy in the area, CT is generally necessary to decide whether a glenoid neck fracture is indeed complete, to determine the degree of displacement (if any), and to identify injuries to adjacent bony structures and articulations.[187] Again, these injuries should not be confused with the more common fractures that course through the inferior glenoid neck and then exit through the scapular body (see Fig.7-10). CT readily reveals that the latter are not complete disruptions of the glenoid process because the superior aspect of the glenoid neck is intact. These injuries are essentially fractures of the scapular body and are managed as such (Fig. 7-14).[109] Finally, if an injury to SSSC (the clavicular-scapular linkage) is suspected, a weight-bearing AP view of the shoulder is obtained.

Glenoid Cavity (Intra-articular) Fractures

Fractures of the glenoid cavity make up 10% of scapula fractures. The majority (>90%) are insignificantly displaced and are managed nonoperatively (Fig. 7-15 and Box 7-4). Significantly displaced fractures require surgical treatment or at least merit surgical consideration. Ideberg reviewed more than 300 such injuries and proposed the first detailed classification scheme,[140-142] which was subsequently expanded by Goss, who added four varieties (types Ib, Vb, Vc, and VI) to Ideberg's original five. (Fig. 7-16).[105] Type I fractures involve the glenoid rim: type Ia,

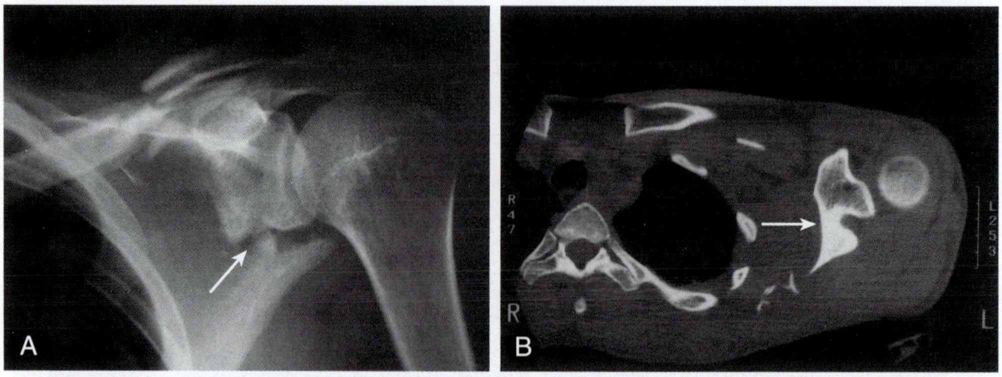

FIGURE 7-14: Radiographs showing what initially, but erroneously, appeared to be a complete fracture of the glenoid neck. **A,** AP radiograph of the shoulder showing a fracture (*arrow*) involving the inferior aspect of the glenoid neck. **B,** Axial CT image showing the superior portion of the glenoid neck to be uninvolved (*arrow*) (the fracture exited through the medial border of the scapular body). (From Goss TP. Fractures of the scapula: Diagnosis and treatment. In: Iannotti JP, Williams GR Jr, eds. *Disorders of the Shoulder: Diagnosis and Management.* Philadelphia, Lippincott Williams & Wilkins; 1999:619.)

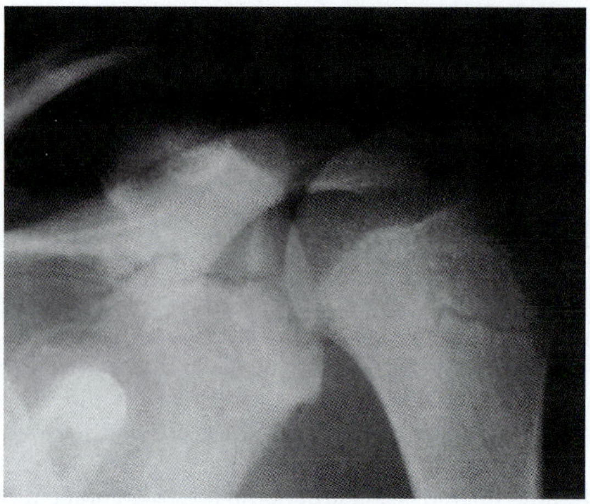

FIGURE 7-15: Anteroposterior radiograph showing an undisplaced fracture of the scapula involving the glenoid process. (From Goss TP. Fractures of the scapula: diagnosis and treatment. In: Iannotti JP, Williams GR Jr, eds. *Disorders of the Shoulder: Diagnosis and Management.* Philadelphia, Lippincott Williams & Wilkins; 1999:603.)

BOX 7-4. Significantly Displaced Glenoid Cavity Fractures

Glenoid Rim Fractures

Unstable glenohumeral articulation:

- Displacement of fragment ≥10 mm
- Involvement of ≥1/4 of glenoid cavity anteriorly
- Involvement of ≥1/3 of glenoid cavity posteriorly

Glenoid Fossa Fractures

Articular step-off ≥5 mm
Unstable glenohumeral articulation
Severe separation of fragments

the anterior rim; and type Ib, the posterior rim. Fractures of the glenoid fossa make up types II to V. Type VI fractures include all comminuted injuries (more than two glenoid cavity fragments).

Fractures of the glenoid rim occur when the humeral head strikes the periphery of the glenoid cavity with considerable violence (Fig. 7-17).[127] These injuries are true fractures, distinct from the small avulsion injuries that occur when a dislocating humeral head applies a tensile force to the periarticular soft tissues.[74] A true axillary view of the glenohumeral joint, CT imaging (routine and reconstructive), and, if necessary, 3D scanning should be used allow one to determine the size and displacement of the rim fragment, whether persistent subluxation of the humeral head is present, and therefore whether stability of the glenohumeral articulation is significantly compromised (Figs. 7-18 and 7-19).

Fractures of the glenoid fossa occur when the humeral head is driven with significant force into the center of the concavity. The fracture generally begins as a transverse disruption (or slightly oblique), for several possible reasons:

1. The glenoid cavity is concave; therefore forces tend to be concentrated over its central region.
2. The subchondral trabeculae are transversely oriented; therefore fractures tend to occur in this plane.
3. The glenoid cavity is formed from two ossification centers; therefore the central region can remain a persistently weak area.
4. The glenoid cavity is narrow superiorly and wide inferiorly, with an indentation along its anterior rim. This anatomy constitutes a stress riser where fractures are particularly prone to originate before coursing over to the posterior rim (Fig. 7-20).

Once a transverse disruption occurs, the fracture can propagate in various directions, depending on the exact

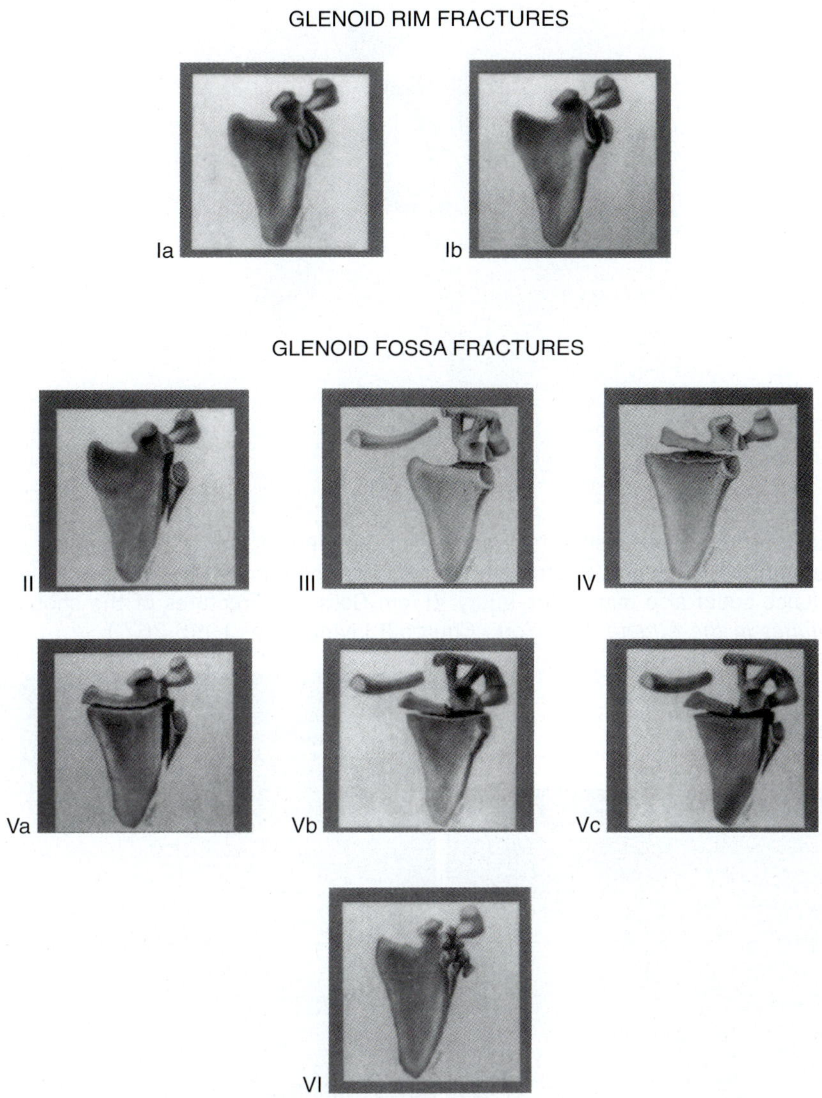

FIGURE 7-16: Goss-Ideberg classification scheme for fractures of the glenoid cavity. (From Goss TP. Fractures of the glenoid cavity [Current Concepts Review]. *J Bone Joint Surg Am.* 1992;74[2]:299-305.)

direction of the humeral head force. An AP projection of the glenohumeral joint, reconstructed CT images, and even 3D CT may be necessary to accurately determine whether and to what degree articular incongruity, separation, or both are present. If an injury to the SSSC (the scapular-clavicular linkage) is suspected, a weight-bearing AP view of the shoulder is obtained.

Type I

Surgical management of fractures of the glenoid rim is indicated if the fracture results in persistent subluxation of the humeral head (failure of the humeral head to lie concentrically within the glenoid cavity) or if the articulation is unstable after reduction. DePalma[74] stated that instability could be expected if the fracture is displaced 10 mm or more and if a quarter or more of the glenoid cavity anteriorly or a third or more of the glenoid cavity posteriorly is involved. Hardegger and coworkers[121] concurred and stated that operative reduction plus fixation of the fragment is indicated to prevent recurrent or permanent dislocation of the shoulder. Guttentag and Rechtine[117] and Butters[46] agreed with these recommendations. Several papers describing the operative management of glenoid rim fractures have appeared in the literature.[10,163,219,262,288] Surgery, if necessary, is designed to restore articular stability and prevent posttraumatic degenerative joint disease (Fig. 7-21).

Type II

With type II glenoid fossa fractures, the humeral head is driven inferiorly, creating an inferior glenoid fragment. Surgery is indicated if an articular step-off of 5 mm or more is present or if the fragment is displaced inferiorly and carries the humeral head with it such that the humeral

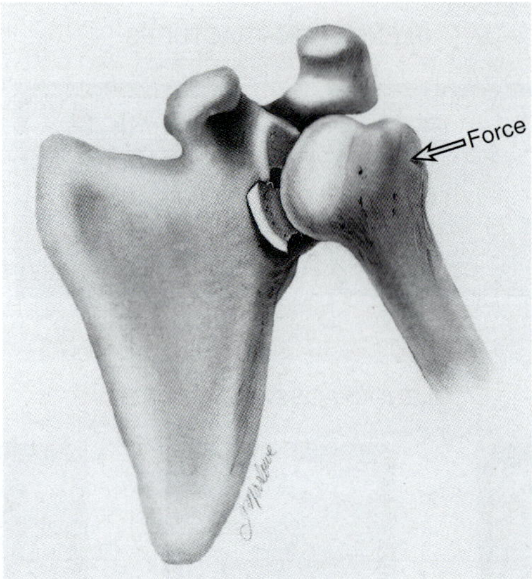

FIGURE 7-17: One mechanism of injury responsible for fractures of the glenoid rim: a force applied over the lateral aspect of the proximal aspect of the humerus. A fall on an outstretched arm driving the humeral head against the periphery of the glenoid cavity with considerable violence could also cause this injury. (From Goss TP. Fractures of the shoulder complex. In: Pappas AM, ed. *Upper Extremity Injuries in the Athlete.* New York, Churchill Livingstone; 1995:267.)

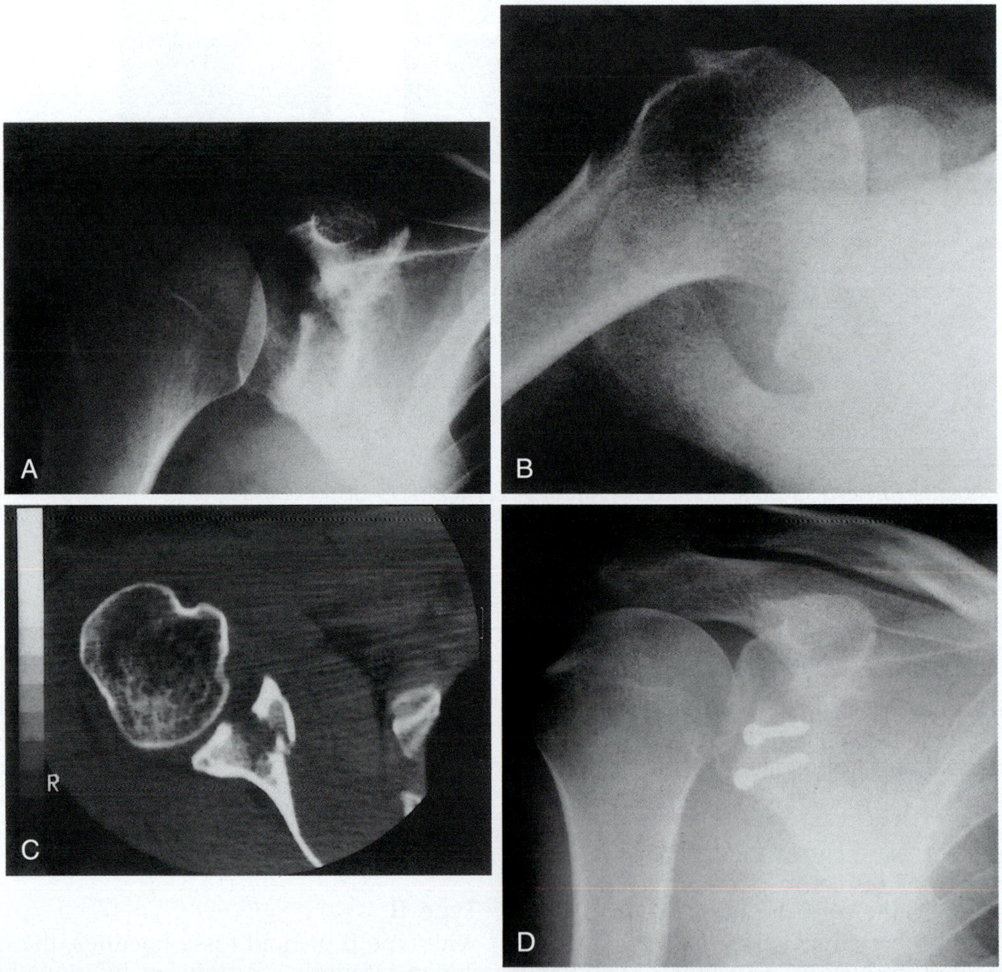

FIGURE 7-18: Radiographs of a patient who sustained a type Ia fracture of the glenoid cavity. **A,** Preoperative anteroposterior (AP) radiograph showing what appears to be a fracture of the anteroinferior glenoid rim. **B,** Preoperative axillary radiograph showing what appears to be a fracture of the anterior glenoid rim with anterior subluxation of the humeral head. **C,** Axial computed tomographic image showing a severely displaced fracture of the anterior glenoid rim. **D,** Postoperative AP radiograph showing reduction and stabilization of the anteroinferior glenoid rim fragment with two cannulated interfragmentary screws. (**A** to **C,** From Goss TP. Fractures of the scapula: diagnosis and treatment. In: Iannotti JP, Williams GR Jr, eds. *Disorders of the Shoulder: Diagnosis and Management.* Philadelphia, Lippincott Williams & Wilkins; 1999:610.)

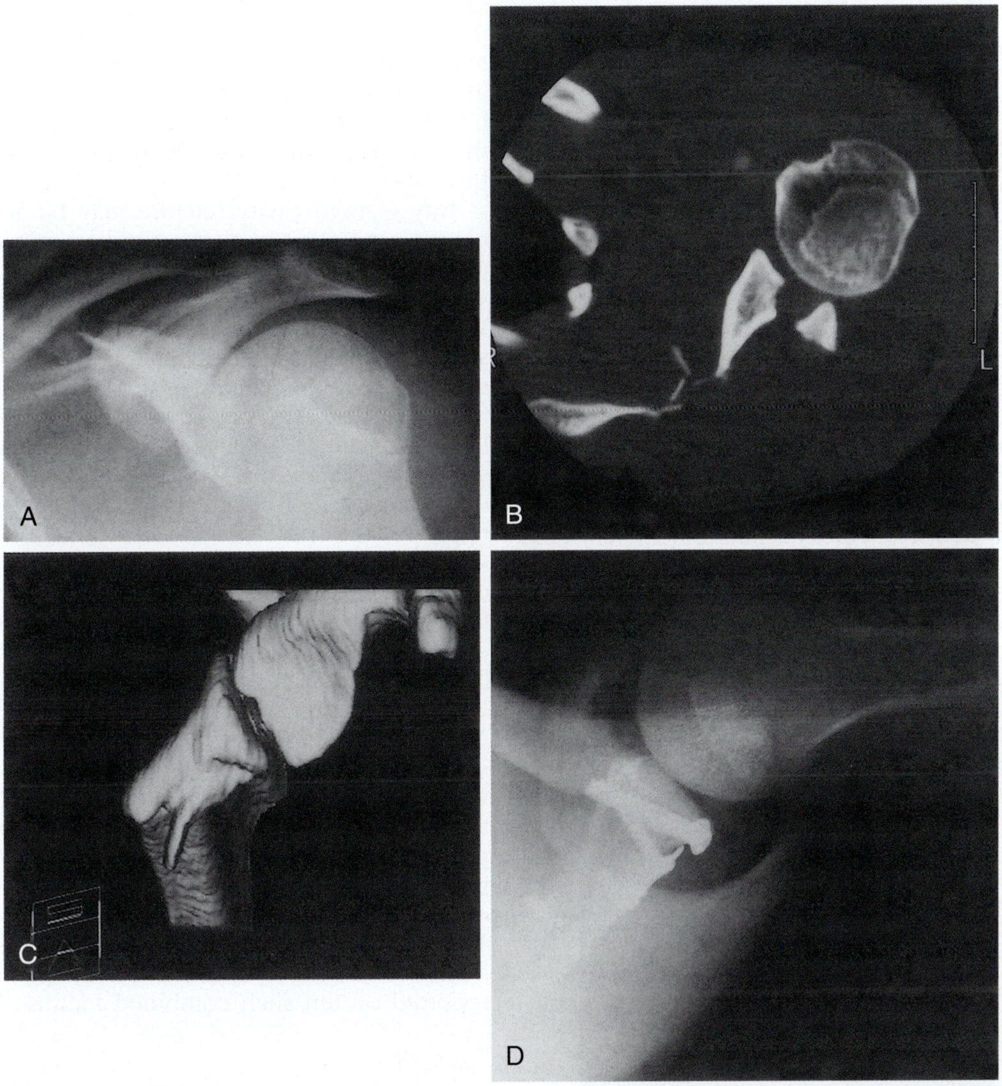

FIGURE 7-19: Radiographs of a patient who sustained a type Ib fracture of the glenoid cavity. **A,** Preoperative radiograph showing what appears to be a fracture of the glenoid cavity with significant posterior involvement. **B,** Axial computed tomographic (CT) image showing a severely displaced fracture of the posterior glenoid rim with posterior subluxation of the humeral head. **C,** Three-dimensional CT image of the glenoid cavity with the humeral head subtracted showing the severely displaced and rotated posteroinferior glenoid rim fragment. **D,** Postoperative axillary radiograph showing anatomic reduction and stabilization of the posterior glenoid rim fragment with restoration of articular congruity. (From Goss TP. Fractures of the scapula: diagnosis and treatment. In: Iannotti JP, Williams GR Jr, eds. *Disorders of the Shoulder: Diagnosis and Management*. Philadelphia, Lippincott Williams & Wilkins; 1999:611.)

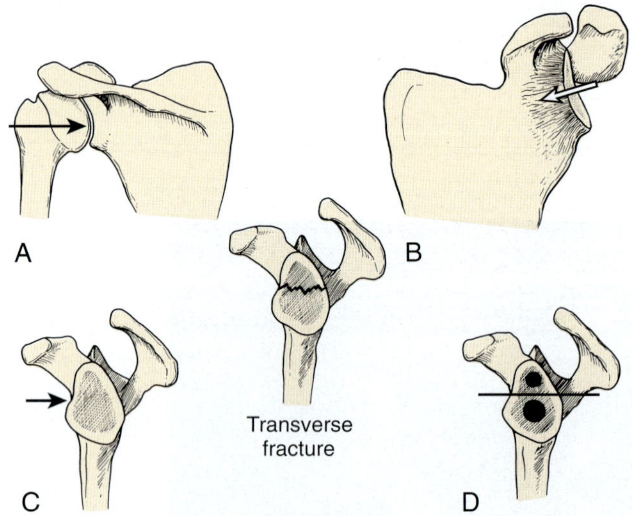

FIGURE 7-20: A transverse disruption of the glenoid cavity and the factors responsible for this orientation. **A,** The concave shape of the glenoid concentrates forces across its central region (*arrow*). **B,** The subchondral trabeculae are oriented in the transverse plane. **C,** A crook along the anterior rim (*arrow*) is a stress riser where fractures tend to originate. **D,** Formed from a superior and an inferior ossification center, the glenoid cavity may have a persistently weak central zone. (From Goss TP. Fractures of the shoulder complex. In: Pappas AM, ed. *Upper Extremity Injuries in the Athlete.* New York, Churchill Livingstone; 1995:268.)

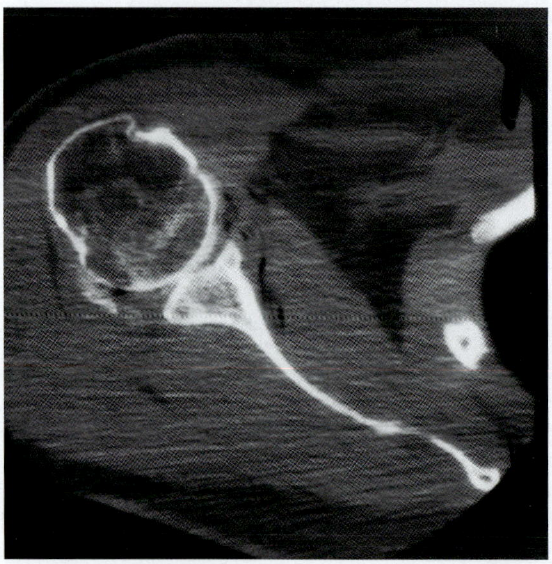

FIGURE 7-21: Axial computed tomographic image of a patient 8 months after a traumatic event. Note the previously undiagnosed displaced type Ia fracture of the glenoid cavity with anterior subluxation of the humeral head and bone-on-bone contact (intraoperatively, the patient was found to have significant posttraumatic degenerative disease of the glenohumeral joint). (From Goss TP. Fractures of the scapula: diagnosis and treatment. In: Iannotti JP, Williams GR Jr, eds. *Disorders of the Shoulder: Diagnosis and Management.* Philadelphia, Lippincott Williams & Wilkins; 1999:610.)

head fails to lie in the center of the glenoid cavity (Fig. 7-22). These injuries can result in posttraumatic degenerative joint disease or glenohumeral instability, or both.[106]

Type III

Type III (glenoid fossa) fractures occur when the force of the humeral head is directed superiorly and causes the transverse disruption to propagate upward, generally exiting through the superior scapular margin in the vicinity of the suprascapular notch.[84,182] Displacement is usually minimal, with the fragment lying medially. Consequently, these injuries are generally treated nonoperatively and heal uneventfully.

Any glenoid cavity fracture may be associated with a neurovascular injury due to the proximity of the brachial plexus and axillary vessels, as well as the considerable violence involved. Type III injuries, as well as type Vb, Vc, and VI injuries, however, are particularly prone to such neurovascular involvement, especially if the superiorly directed force continues further upward and damages SSSC (i.e., if there is an associated disruption of the C-4 linkage or the clavicular–acromioclavicular joint–acromial strut). Neer and Rockwood considered compression of the adjacent neurovascular structures by these and fractures of the coracoid process to be indications for surgery.[215] They and others also described the occurrence of suprascapular nerve paralysis associated with fractures involving the coracoid process and the glenoid neck that extend into the suprascapular notch (electromyographic [EMG] testing was essential to make the diagnosis, and early exploration was recommended).[67,81,265]

Surgical management of type III fractures is indicated if the fracture has an articular step-off of 5 mm or more with lateral displacement of the superior fragment or if a significantly displaced additional disruption of SSSC is present (a double-disruption injury) (Fig. 7-23). Examples include an associated disruption of the C-4 linkage or of the clavicular–acromioclavicular joint–acromial strut.[104] These injuries can result in posttraumatic degenerative joint disease and severe functional impairment. Hui et al. reported on ten such combined injuries.[137]

Type IV

Type IV (glenoid fossa) injuries occur when the humeral head is driven directly into the center of the glenoid cavity.[88] The fracture courses transversely across the entire scapula and exits along its medial border. If there is an unacceptable articular step-off (≥5 mm) with the superior fragment displaced laterally, or if the superior and inferior glenoscapular segments are severely separated, ORIF is indicated to prevent symptomatic degenerative joint disease, nonunion at the fracture site (an extremely rare occurrence but a definite concern in the case shown [Fig. 7-24]), and instability of the glenohumeral joint. Ferraz et al. described a type IV glenoid fossa fracture that progressed to a nonunion. When explored surgically less than 2 years after injury, a 7-mm articular step-off was noted as well as grade III cartilaginous erosion of the humeral head.[85]

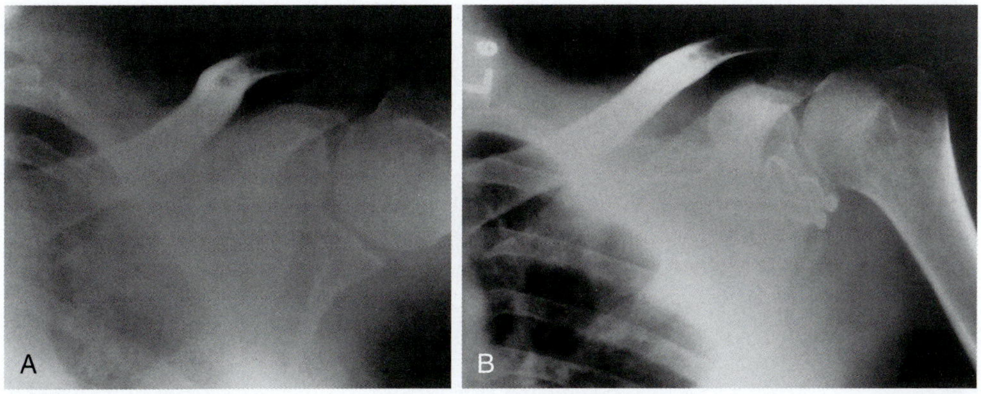

FIGURE 7-22: Radiographs of a patient who sustained a type II fracture of the glenoid cavity. **A,** Preoperative anteroposterior (AP) radiograph showing significant displacement of the inferior glenoid fragment and a severe articular step-off. **B,** Postoperative AP radiograph showing anatomic reduction and stabilization of the inferior glenoid fragment with restoration of articular congruity. (From Goss TP. Fractures of the scapula: diagnosis and treatment. In: Iannotti JP, Williams GR Jr, eds. *Disorders of the Shoulder: Diagnosis and Management*. Philadelphia, Lippincott Williams & Wilkins; 1999:613.)

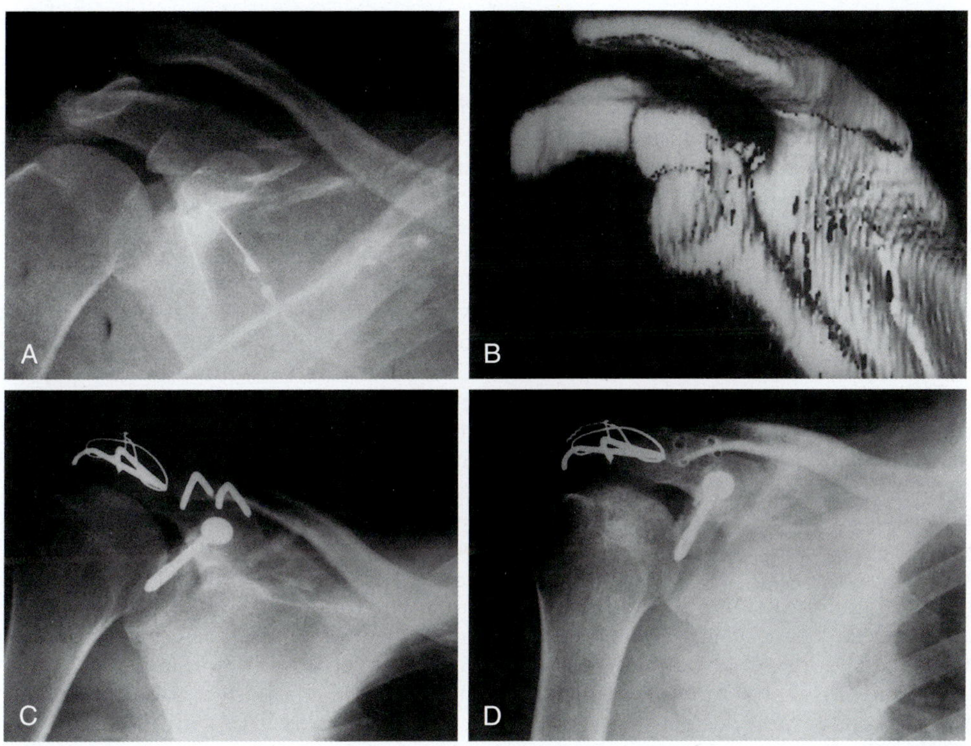

FIGURE 7-23: A patient who sustained a fracture of the acromion, a type III acromioclavicular (AC) joint disruption, and a type III glenoid cavity fracture. **A,** Preoperative anteroposterior (AP) radiograph. **B,** Preoperative three-dimensional computed tomographic image. **C,** Postoperative AP radiograph showing the acromial fracture reduced and stabilized with a tension band construct, the type III glenoid cavity fracture reduced and stabilized with a compression screw, and the AC joint disruption reduced and stabilized with K-wires passed through the clavicle and into the acromial process. **D,** Postoperative AP radiograph showing maintenance of the normal clavicle-scapula relationships after removal of the clavicular-acromial K-wires.

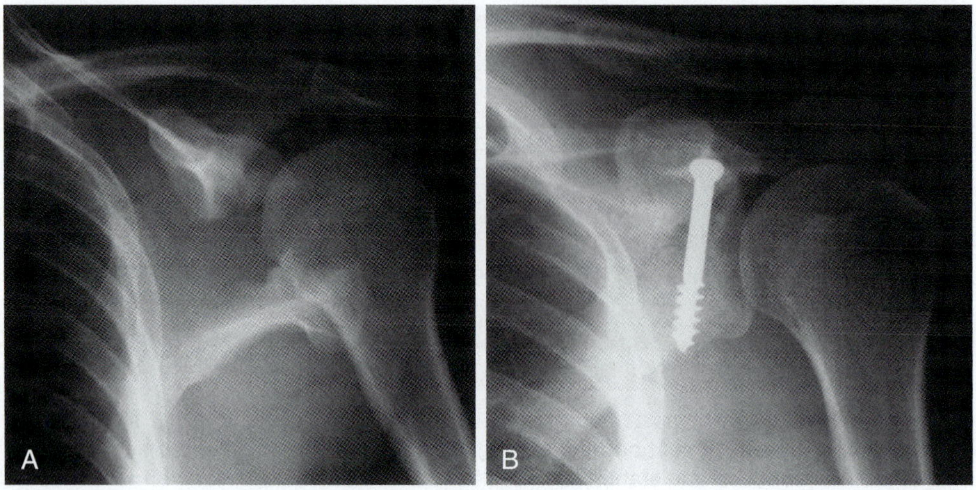

FIGURE 7-24: Radiographs of a patient who sustained a type IV fracture of the glenoid cavity. **A,** Preoperative anteroposterior (AP) radiograph showing severe separation of the superior and inferior portions of the glenoid fossa and scapular body. **B,** Postoperative AP radiograph showing anatomic reduction and stabilization of the superior and inferior portions of the glenoid fossa and scapular body with restoration of articular congruity. (From Goss TP. Fractures of the scapula: diagnosis and treatment. In: Iannotti JP, Williams GR Jr, eds. *Disorders of the Shoulder: Diagnosis and Management.* Philadelphia, Lippincott Williams & Wilkins; 1999:614.)

Type V

These glenoid fossa injuries are combinations of type II, III, and IV injuries and are caused by more violent and complex forces. The same clinical concerns and operative indications detailed for the type II, III, and IV fractures apply to type V fractures (Fig. 7-25). Nork et al. reported on several type IV and type V fractures with associated disruptions of the scapular body that required surgical management of both injuries.[223]

Type VI

Type VI glenoid cavity fractures are caused by the most violent forces and include all disruptions in which more than two articular fragments are present. Operative treatment is contraindicated because exposing these injuries surgically does little more than disrupt whatever soft tissue support remains, rendering the fragments even more unstable and making a bad situation worse.

Reports by Aulicino et al.[12] and Aston and Gregory[10] lend support to the role of surgery in managing significantly displaced glenoid fossa fractures. Lee et al.[170] reported the case of a child who sustained a type II fracture that required ORIF. Ruedi and Chapman[252] stated that "grossly displaced intra-articular fractures of the glenoid that render the joint incongruent and unstable profit from operative reconstruction and internal fixation as incongruities result in osteoarthritic changes." Rowe[251] advocated surgical management of severely displaced injuries. Bauer and coworkers[27] reviewed 20 patients treated surgically for significantly displaced fractures of the scapula (6.1-year average follow-up) and reported greater than 70% good or very good results based on the Constant score. They recommended early ORIF for grossly displaced fractures of the glenoid fossa, glenoid rim, glenoid neck, and coracoid and acromial processes. Hardegger and associates[121] reported that if "there is significant displacement, conservative treatment alone cannot restore congruency," and stiffness and pain can result—"for this reason open reduction and stabilization are indicated."

Kavanagh et al.[151] presented their experience at the Mayo Clinic in which 10 displaced intra-articular fractures of the glenoid cavity were treated with ORIF. They found ORIF to be "a useful and safe technique" that "can restore excellent function of the shoulder." In their series, the major articular fragments were displaced 4 to 8 mm. The authors emphasized that they remained uncertain how much incongruity of the glenoid articular surface can be accepted without risking the long-term sequelae of pain, stiffness, and traumatic osteoarthritis. Soslowsky and coworkers[266] found the maximal depth of the glenoid articular cartilage to be 5 mm. Consequently, if a glenoid fossa fracture is associated with an articular step-off of 5 mm or more, subchondral bone is exposed. Schandelmaier et al.[255] reported a series of 22 fractures of the glenoid fossa treated with ORIF. They stated that "if the postoperative courses are uneventful, excellent to good results can be expected." Leung et al.[173] reviewed 14 displaced intra-articular fractures of the glenoid treated with ORIF (30.5-year average follow-up) and reported nine excellent and five good results. Anavian et al. reported on 33 patients with displaced intraarticular fractures of the glenoid with or without involvement of the scapular body. They noted good functional outcomes postoperatively with a low complication rate.[4] Mayo et al. described their experience with 27 fractures treated operatively for displaced glenoid fossa fractures. They were able to accomplish what they termed *anatomic*

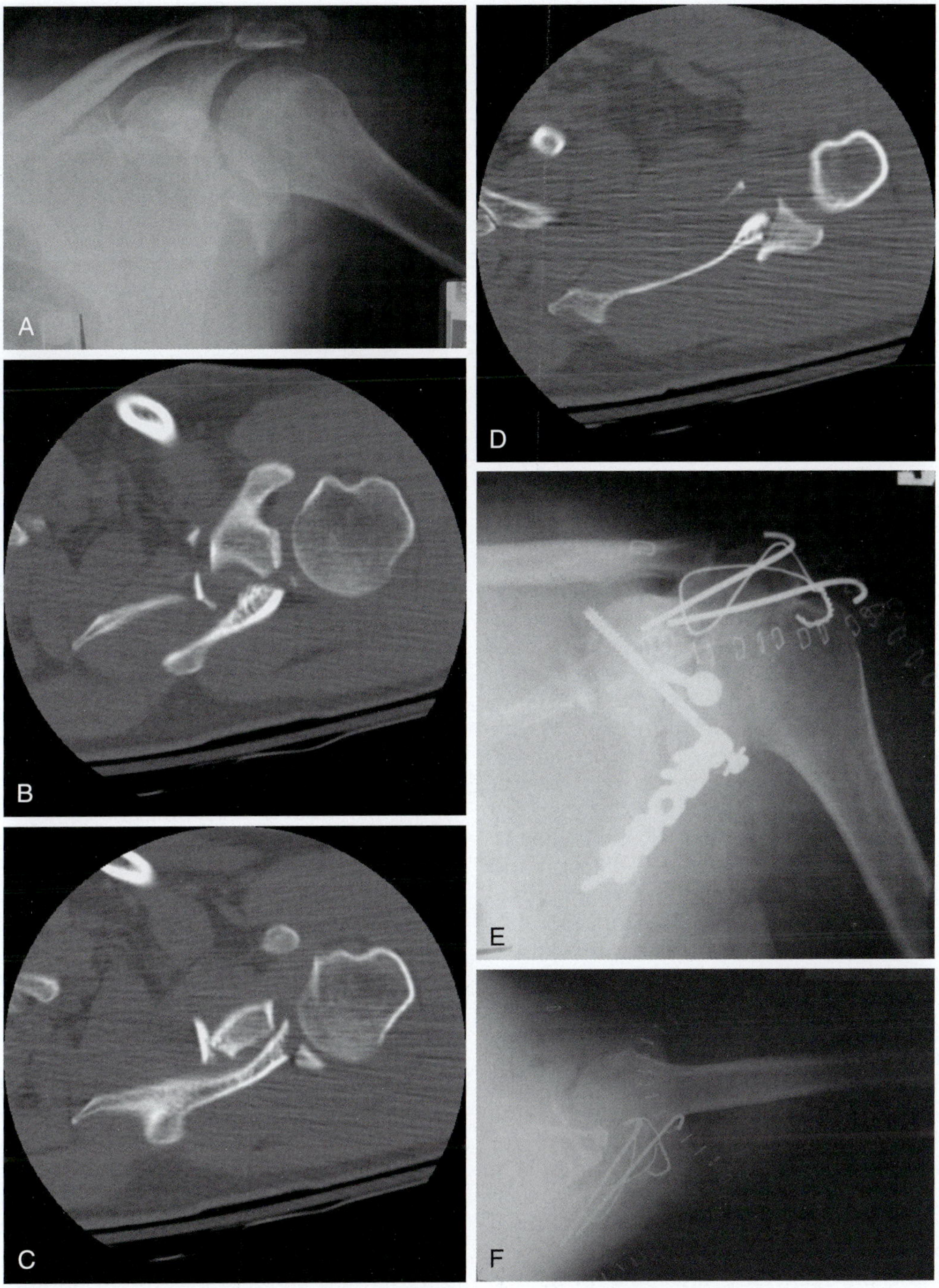

FIGURE 7-25: Radiographs of a patient involved in a motor vehicle accident who sustained a type Vc fracture of the glenoid cavity. **A,** Anteroposterior (AP) radiograph of the glenoid cavity fracture. **B,** Axial computed tomographic (CT) image showing a large anterosuperior glenoid fragment including the coracoid process. **C,** Axial CT image showing the lateral aspect of the scapular body lying between the two glenoid fragments, abutting the humeral head. **D,** Axial CT image showing a large posteroinferior cavity fragment. Postoperative AP **(E)** and axillary **(F)** radiographs, showing the glenoid cavity fragments secured together with cannulated screws and the glenoid unit secured to the scapular body with a malleable reconstruction plate (the acromial fracture was reduced and stabilized with a tension band construct.) (From Goss TP, Owens BD. Fractures of the scapula: diagnosis and treatment. In: Iannotti JP, Williams GR Jr, eds. *Disorders of the Shoulder: Diagnosis and Management.* 2nd ed. Philadelphia, Lippincott Williams & Wilkins; 2007:814.)

reconstruction with a low complication rate and good functional outcomes.[186]

Basis on these reports, it is reasonable to conclude that surgery has a definite role in the treatment of glenoid cavity fractures. Numerous case reports and studies describe arthroscopically assisted fixation of displaced glenoid cavity fractures. The proposed advantages include limited associated soft tissue dissection, preservation of the blood supply to the fracture fragment, direct arthroscopic visualization of the articular reduction, and the possibility of addressing associated capsulolabral and rotator cuff pathology. Sugaya et al. described eight patients with significantly displaced type Ia fractures managed arthroscopically.[272] Yang et al. studied 18 patients with Goss-Ideberg type III glenoid cavity fractures who underwent arthroscopically assisted reduction and fixation with 4.0 mm cannulated screws. At final follow-up (minimum 2 years), they reported excellent range of motion as well as validated patient outcome scores (average Visual Analogue Scale, 0.7; Constant score, 96.8; American Shoulder and Elbow Surgeons, 96.0; and University of California–Los Angeles, 34.3) without complications.[306] Tauber and coworkers reported on ten patients with acute anterior glenoid cavity fractures (Goss-Ideberg type Ia) compromising at least 21% of the glenoid fossa. They used cannulated titanium screws placed percutaneously under arthroscopic visualization. At a 2-year follow-up, nine patients had good/excellent results and one had a fair result. One patient had recurrent instability.[274] Bauer and coworkers reported on five patients with intraarticular fractures of the glenoid cavity who were treated with arthroscopic reduction and suture fixation through drill holes.[26] Multiple case reports have described arthroscopic management using 3.5 mm partially threaded cannulated screws and K-wires.[49,50,96]

Fractures of the Scapular Body and Spine

These injuries are often rather alarming radiographically: extensive comminution and displacement are often present (Fig. 7-26). However, there has been very little enthusiasm in the literature for operative treatment[122] for the following reasons: bone stock for fixation is at a premium, 90+% of these injuries heal quite nicely with nonoperative care,[126] and a good to excellent functional result can be expected.

The reasons for this generally favorable prognosis are as follows: (1) scapular body fractures almost invariably go on to union, and (2) the thick layer of soft tissues within the scapulothoracic interval and the mobility of the scapulothoracic articulation compensate for most residual deformities of the scapular body. The literature does mention a fracture of the scapular body with a lateral spike entering the glenohumeral joint as an indication (albeit extremely uncommon) for surgical management,[121] and a similar recommendation was made in two cases involving patients with fractures of the scapular body and intrathoracic penetration by one of the fragments.[35,256] Bowen et al. reported a case of a significantly angulated greenstick fracture of the scapular body that required a closed reduction.[39] On rare occasions, malunion of a scapular body fracture can result in scapulothoracic pain and crepitus requiring surgical exposure of its ventral surface and removal of the responsible bony prominence(s).[181] Nonunion of a scapular body fracture requiring surgical management has been described.[85,116,150,199]

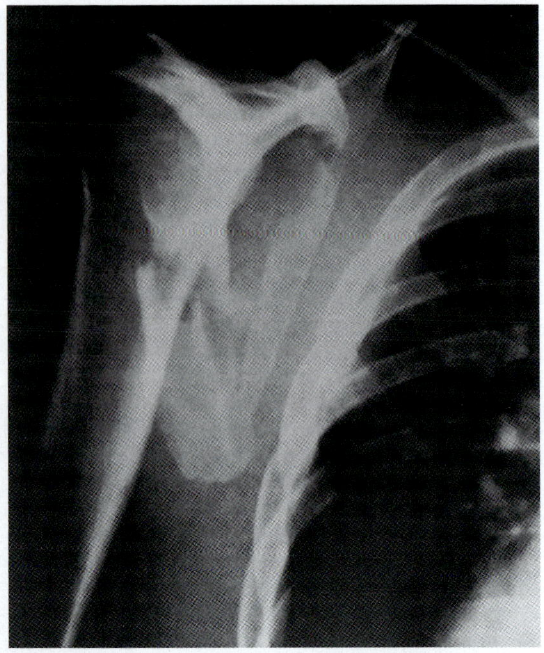

FIGURE 7-26: Anteroposterior radiograph showing a comminuted fracture of the scapular body. (From Neer CS II. Less frequent procedures. In: Neer CS II, ed. *Shoulder Reconstruction*. Philadelphia, WB Saunders; 1990:421-485.)

The vast majority (>90%) of fractures of the scapular body (and insignificantly displaced fractures of the scapula in general) are managed nonoperatively. These patients are initially placed in a sling and swathe binder for comfort. Local ice packs to the affected area are helpful during the first 48 hours, as needed. Absolute immobilization is generally short (48 hours) but can continue for up to 14 days, depending upon the clinical situation. The patient is then permitted to gradually increase use of the upper extremity as symptoms allow, and sling and swathe protection is gradually decreased until the 6-week point.

Physical therapy is prescribed during this period and focuses on maintaining/regaining shoulder range of motion. The program begins with dependent circular and pendulum movements, as well as external rotation to but not past neutral and gradually moves on to progressive stretching techniques in all ranges. Close follow-up is necessary to monitor and guide the patient's recovery, and radiographs are obtained to ensure that unacceptable displacement does not occur at the fracture site(s).

At 6 weeks, osseous union is usually sufficient to discontinue all external protection and encourage full functional use of the upper extremity. However, the rehabilitation program continues until range of motion, strength, and overall function are maximized. Six months to 1 year may be required for a full recovery, but a good to excellent result should be readily obtainable.

Recently, some have recommended dramatic changes in the management of scapular body fractures, and surgical management in certain situations is gaining favor. The group led by Cole has been particularly active in this regard. In 2013, they summarized their approach to the management of scapular body fractures, with an emphasis on surgical indications, approaches, and techniques.[59]

The scapular body is that portion of the scapula medial to a line parallel to the plane of the glenoid fossa (superior to inferior rims), running from the lateral border of the scapular notch (coursing through the spinoglenoid notch) to the junction between the inferior glenoid neck and the lateral scapular border. Its superior, medial, and lateral cortical borders surround a thin central zone. The superior border meets the medial border at the superior angle, while the lateral border meets the medial border at the inferior angle. The scapular spine protrudes posteriorly. It meets the medial border at the spinomedial junction and joins the acromial and glenoid processes at the spinoglenoid notch. The lateral border/glenoid neck pillar is quite important to the overall integrity of the scapula (Fig. 7-27). Fractures of this area if associated with a second scapular body disruption (most often an exit point along the medial border but occasionally at the superior border via the scapular spine) can significantly alter the position of the glenoid process/glenohumeral joint relative to the surrounding bony and soft tissues (destabilizing the overall shoulder complex), with adverse functional consequences. Radiographic findings that indicate significant compromise of the integrity of the lateral border/glenoid neck pillar and the overall integrity of the scapular body include (1) ML translation of the glenoid process relative to the lateral scapular border of greater than or equal to 20 mm as seen on AP radiographs or 3D CT, (2) anteroposterior (AP) angulatory deformity of the lateral border greater than or equal to 45 degrees as seen on a scapular Y view or 3D CT, (3) lateral border/glenoid process ML translation greater than or equal to 15 mm and AP angular deformity of the lateral border greater than or equal to 30 degrees, and (4) a GPA less than or equal to 20 degrees as seen on AP radiographs (Fig. 7-28). In such situations, reestablishing the integrity

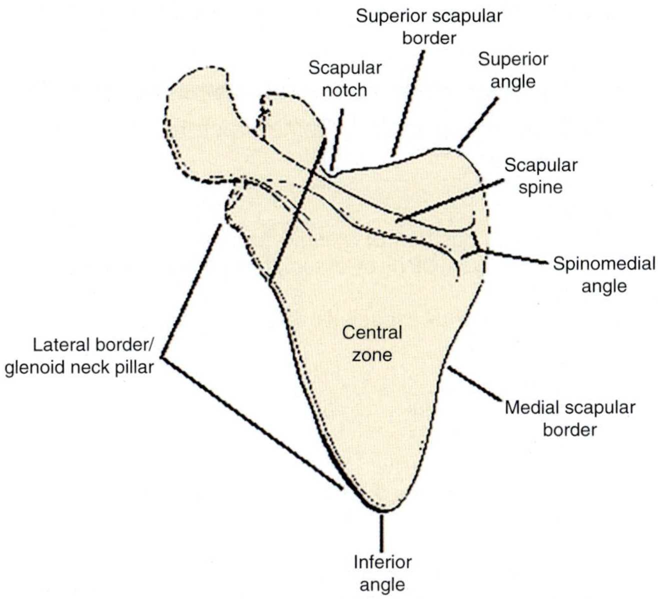

FIGURE 7-27: The scapular body with its various bony landmarks.

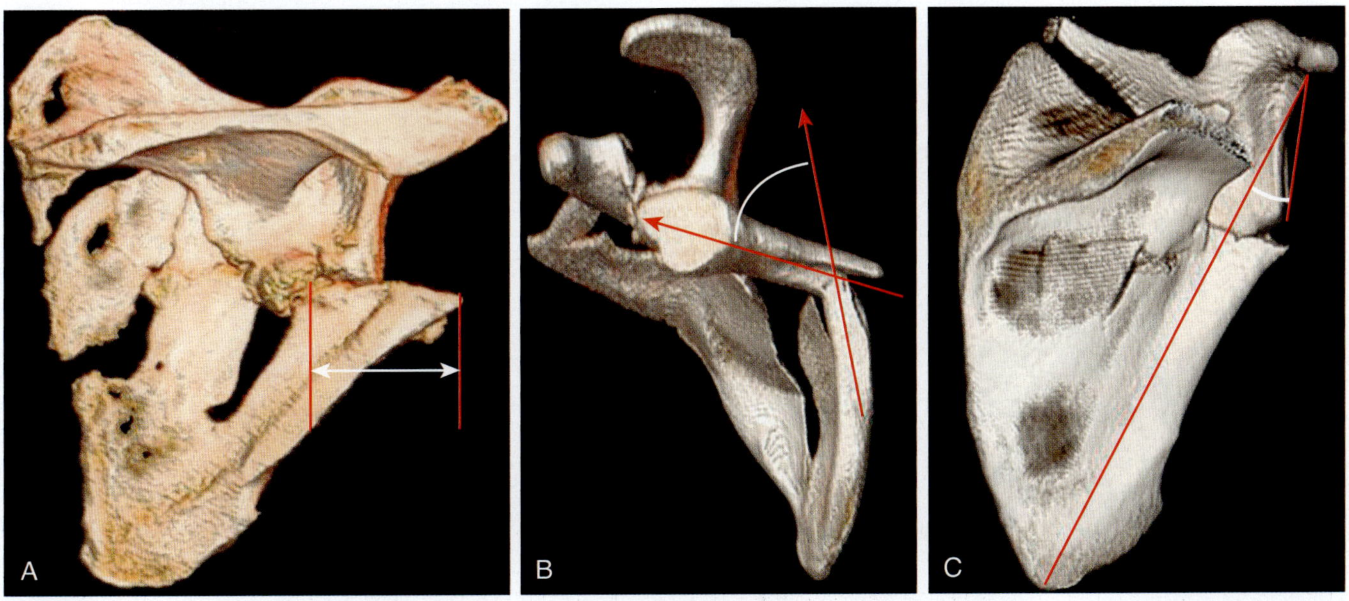

FIGURE 7-28: Computed tomographic images of significantly displaced fractures of the scapular body. **A,** Anteroposterior (AP) view showing significant mediolateral translational displacement. **B,** Lateral scapula Y view showing significant angular displacement. **C,** AP view showing a significant decrease in the glenopolar angle.

of the cortical perimeter of the scapular body (especially the lateral border/glenoid neck pillar but often the medial and/or superior borders as well) has been recommended by several authors in order to restore scapular length, alignment, and rotation and, ultimately, overall shoulder mechanics/function (Box 7-5).

The patient is placed on the operating room table (affected side up), and the scapular body is approached posteriorly. An extensile Judet approach may be used.[148] The posterior deltoid and infraspinatus muscles are detached from their origins and reflected from medial to lateral, allowing access to the lateral and medial scapular borders and the scapular spine. This exposure is limited by the suprascapular neuromuscular bundle, which must be protected. The circumflex scapular artery, if encountered, is tied off (Fig. 7-29). A modified Judet approach with development of the infraspinatus/teres minor interval is used if exposure of the posterior glenoid process and access of the interior of the glenohumeral joint is necessary.[223] Further development of this interval allows access to the lateral scapular border. Access to the scapular spine is gained through the posterior deltoid/trapezius interval. Access to the medial scapular border is gained through the infraspinatus/rhomboids interval. Gauger and Cole described minimally invasive approaches for recent (<10 days old) scapular border fractures with simple patterns (two exit points) in seven patients. They noted outcomes that they described as being comparable to the normal uninjured population without complications.[95]

BOX 7-5. Scapular Body/Spine Fractures: Operative Management

Indications

Unacceptable position of glenoid process
ORIF, which aids ORIF of associated glenoid process fracture
Rare fractures with especially severe displacement

Principles

Approaches:
- Extensile Judet
- Modified Judet
- Minimally invasive

ORIF border disruptions, especially lateral border/glenoid neck pillar
Fixation:
- Dynamic compression plates
- Malleable reconstruction plates
- Locking plates

ORIF, *Open reduction and internal fixation.*

Disruptions of the lateral border, medial border, and superior border/scapular spine are exposed, reduced, and provisionally stabilized. The lateral border/glenoid neck pillar has priority and is managed first, as its reduction reorients the glenohumeral joint and reestablishes an intact post to facilitate reconstruction of the rest of the scapula. Once the scapular perimeter has been reestablished, the borders are definitively stabilized. A dynamic compression plate is used for the lateral border. However, if the inferior aspect of the glenoid neck is involved, a contoured reconstruction plate may be required to gain purchase on the glenoid process. Medial border disruptions are secured with a reconstruction plate contoured appropriately to gain fixation over the medial scapular spine and down the medial border (Fig. 7-30). Disruptions involving the superior border via the scapular spine are stabilized with a dynamic

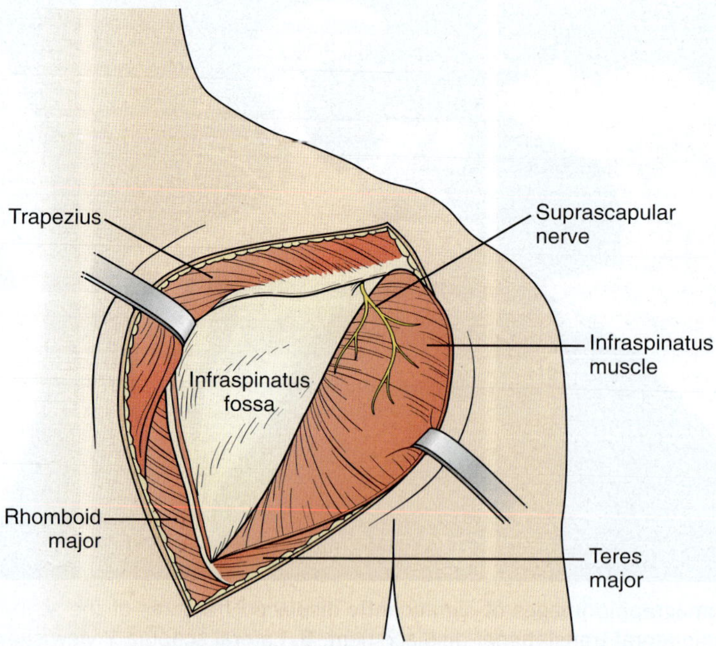

FIGURE 7-29: Extensile Judet approach to the scapular body.

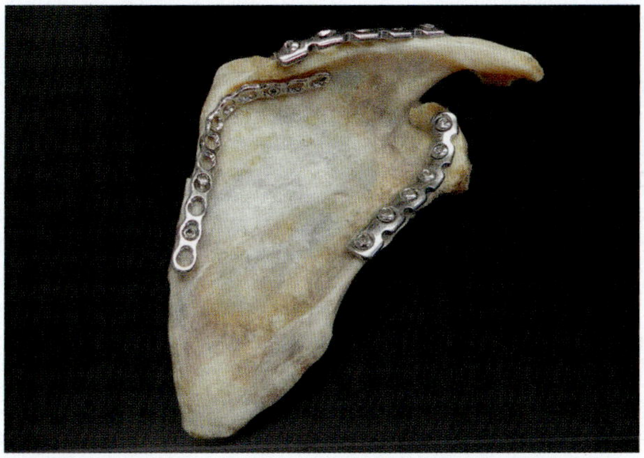

FIGURE 7-30: A scapula with contoured malleable reconstruction plates applied along the medial scapular border/scapular spine, and lateral scapular border/glenoid neck pillar and a dynamic compression plate applied over the scapular spine.

compression plate applied along the scapular spine. Locking plates are used wherever bone stock is deficient. Particularly complex patterns may require other fixation devices (Fig. 7-31). Associated fractures involving the glenoid, acromial, and coracoid processes as well as double disruptions of SSSC are managed according to the principles detailed for those specific injuries.

Nork et al. described 17 patients with displaced Goss-Ideberg IV, V, and VI glenoid cavity fractures with significantly displaced scapular body fractures exiting the medial border. They felt that ORIF of the medial border disruption significantly aided in the ORIF of the glenoid process fracture.[221] Bartonicek and Fric reported on 22 patients with scapular body fractures with or without articular involvement treated surgically (minimal follow-up, 12 months). They stated that in all patients, primary bone union and anatomic restoration between the glenoid process and scapular body were achieved. Congruency and stability of the shoulder was achieved in all, and the average Constant score was 94.[17] Cole et al. described 74 patients with displaced scapular body fractures with or without articular involvement treated surgically. All fractures united in good position. The authors concluded that restoration of normal anatomy was relatively safe and effective, thus affording to the patient the best chance for an optimal functional recovery.[60] Cole et al. reported on five patients who underwent reconstructive surgery for extra-articular scapula malunions. The mean time from injury to surgery was 15 months (range, 8-41 months). All fractures united. All patients were pain free and expressed satisfaction with the result. Four of the five individuals returned to their original occupation and activities.[61]

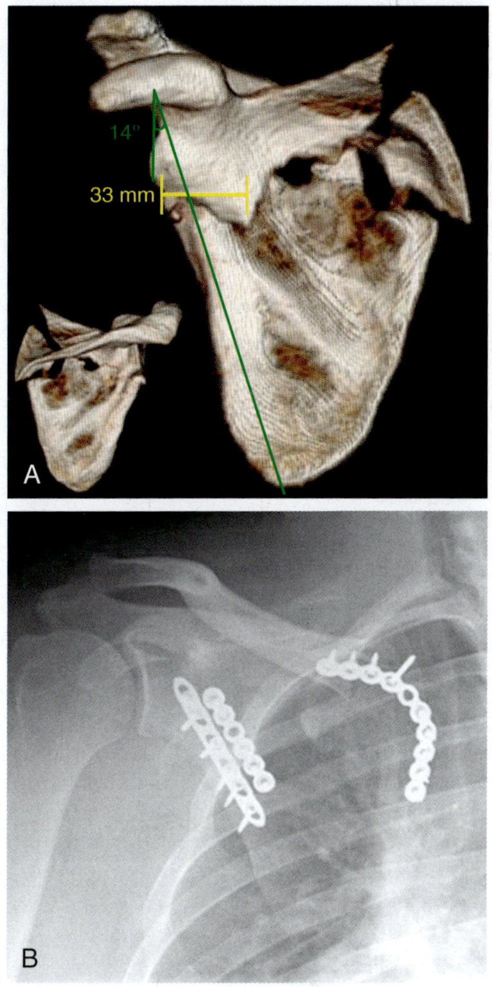

FIGURE 7-31: Images of a patient who sustained a comminuted scapular body fracture. **A,** Preoperative computed tomographic image showing exit points along the superior, medial, and lateral borders with significant mediolateral translational displacement and a significantly decreased glenopolar angle. **B,** Postoperative radiographs showing restoration of the periphery of the scapular body and restoration of the normal position of the glenoid process/glenohumeral joint by means of a reconstruction plate and a dynamic compression plate applied along the lateral border and a reconstruction plate applied along the scapular spine/medial border.

Isolated Acromial Fractures

The acromial process extends laterally from the scapular spine and then anteriorly. Its medial border is defined by a line that courses perpendicular to the surface of the acromial and scapular processes and ends at the deepest point of the spinoglenoid notch. The acromial process is formed from two ossification centers: one for its anterior end and one for its posterolateral tip. The acromial process has four basic functions:

1. Provides one side of the acromioclavicular articulation
2. Serves as a point of attachment for various musculotendinous and ligamentous structures
3. Lends posterosuperior stability to the glenohumeral joint
4. Serves as an important component of SSSC (the scapular-clavicular linkage)

Acromial fractures can be caused by a direct blow from the outside or a force transmitted via the humeral head. Avulsion fractures are the result of purely indirect forces occurring where musculotendinous or ligamentous structures (the deltoid and trapezius muscles as well as the coracoacromial and acromioclavicular ligaments) attach to the acromion. Stress/fatigue fractures have been reported.[119,294] These injuries may be minimally or significantly displaced.[198] Kuhn et al. proposed a classification scheme that prompted some discussion.[160,161,205,275] They emphasized the need for ORIF if an acromial fragment is displaced inferiorly by the pull of the deltoid muscle and is compromising the subacromial space, thereby resulting in impingement symptoms and interference with rotator cuff function.[159]

The diagnosis is radiographic. True AP and lateral views of the scapula and a true axillary projection of the glenohumeral joint detect most acromial fractures. An os acromiale can complicate the evaluation. However, on occasion, CT may be needed to precisely define the injury and disclose involvement of adjacent bony and articular structures. A weight-bearing AP projection is obtained if a disruption of the scapular-clavicular linkage (SSSC) is suspected. Arthrography to evaluate the rotator cuff is considered if an acromial fracture is the result of traumatic superior displacement of the humeral head or chronic superior migration of the proximal humerus, as seen in long-standing rotator cuff disease (e.g., cuff tear arthropathy with a stress fracture of the acromion). Madhavan et al.[178] described a case in which an acromial fracture was associated with an avulsed subscapularis tendon.

Although significantly displaced, isolated, nonavulsion acromial fractures have been described,[100,295] the vast majority are nondisplaced or minimally displaced. Symptomatic nonoperative care will reliably lead to union and a good to excellent functional result. However, significantly displaced injuries require surgical management. Symptomatic acromial nonunion, although uncommon, has been reported in the literature.[77,201] No more than a small fragment should ever be excised.[112] The presence of a large ununited fragment requires surgical stabilization and bone grafting (Fig. 7-32).

Isolated Coracoid Fractures

The coracoid process begins at the superior margin of the glenoid process and extends superiorly, anteriorly, and finally laterally. The coracoid process develops from two constant ossification centers: one at its base that also forms the upper third of the glenoid process, and one that becomes its main body. In addition, the coracoid process has at least two inconstant centers: one at its angle where the coracoclavicular ligament attaches and one at its tip where the conjoined tendon is located. The regions at which the centers finally unite are relatively weak, especially in young adults, thereby making fractures more likely to occur when direct or indirect forces are applied.[208,239]

The coracoid process, which has been called the "lighthouse" of the anterior shoulder, has three basic functions:

1. Serving as a point of attachment for a number of musculotendinous and ligamentous structures (Fig. 7-33)
2. Providing the glenohumeral joint with some anterosuperior stability
3. Serving as an integral part of SSSC (the scapular-clavicular linkage)

Coracoid fractures can be caused by a blow from the outside[64] or contact by a dislocating humeral head or by indirect forces applied through the musculotendinous and ligamentous structures at their attachment sites (avulsion fractures fall into this category).[65,66,86,253] Fatigue/stress fractures have also been described.[38,254] Other causes include fractures associated with coracoclavicular tape fixation used in acromioclavicular joint reconstructions[207] and fractures associated with massive rotator cuff tears. Despite the relative scarcity of isolated coracoid

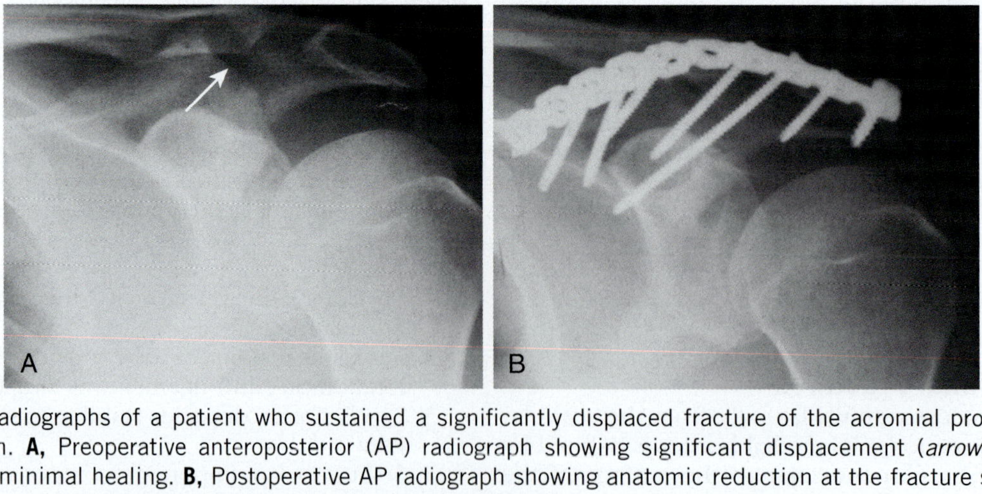

FIGURE 7-32: Radiographs of a patient who sustained a significantly displaced fracture of the acromial process, which went on to a nonunion. **A,** Preoperative anteroposterior (AP) radiograph showing significant displacement (*arrow*) at the acromial fracture site and minimal healing. **B,** Postoperative AP radiograph showing anatomic reduction at the fracture site and stabilization using a plate-and-screw construct (the site was also bone grafted).

fractures, several types have been described.[84,112] These injuries can be anatomically divided into the following categories:

1. Fractures of the tip of the coracoid
2. Fractures of the coracoid between the coracoclavicular and coracoacromial ligaments
3. Fractures at the base of the coracoid process

The diagnosis is ultimately radiographic. True AP and axillary projections of the glenohumeral joint disclose, or at least suggest, the presence of most coracoid fractures. However, because of the complex bony anatomy in the area, oblique views[91,99] or even CT[156] may be necessary to detect and accurately define some fractures and injuries to adjacent bony and articular structures. Accessory ossification centers and epiphyseal lines can complicate the evaluation. A weight-bearing AP view of the shoulder is obtained if the integrity of the scapular-clavicular (SSSC) linkage is a concern.

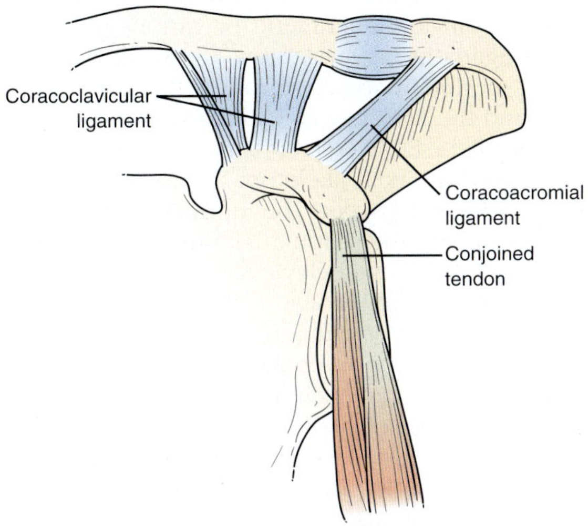

FIGURE 7-33: The coracoid process as the point of attachment for the conjoined tendon, the coracoacromial ligament, and the coracoclavicular ligament. (The coracohumeral ligament and pectoralis minor tendon attach to the coracoid process as well.)

Fractures of the coracoid tip are avulsion injuries—the result of an indirect force applied through the conjoined tendon and concentrated over its attachment to the coracoid process (see Fig. 7-43D). Displacement may be quite marked, but nonsurgical treatment is usually in order.[303,310] Open surgical reduction plus internal fixation has been advocated in athletes, especially those participating in sports that require optimal upper extremity function, and in individuals who perform heavy manual labor. Wong-Chung and Quinlan described a case in which a fractured coracoid tip prevented closed reduction of an anterior glenohumeral dislocation.[302] Late surgical treatment may be necessary if a displaced ununited bone fragment causes irritation of the surrounding soft tissues. Fractures between the coracoclavicular and the coracoacromial ligaments may be the result of either a direct or an indirect force.[72] The distal fragment is usually significantly displaced, drawn distally by the pull of the conjoined tendon and rotated laterally by the tethering effect of the coracoacromial ligament (Fig. 7-34). Treatment may be nonsurgical or surgical, following the same reasoning described for significantly displaced avulsion fractures of the coracoid tip. However, because the fragment is larger, symptomatic irritation of the local soft tissues is more common, and late surgical management is more likely. Fractures at the base of the coracoid process are the most common coracoid fractures. They can be caused by a direct blow from the outside or by a dislocating humeral head.[28] Avulsion fractures caused by strong traction forces are also possible.[9,180,240,249] These injuries are generally

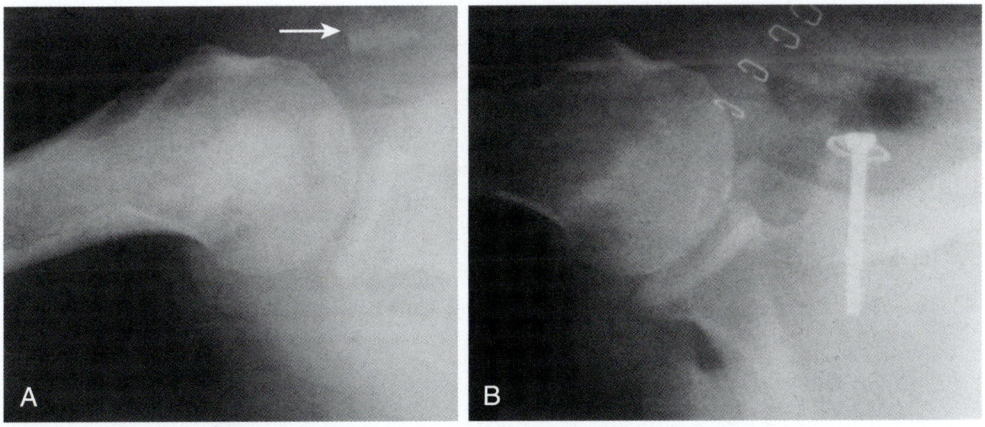

FIGURE 7-34: Images of a patient who sustained a fracture of the distal coracoid process between the coracoclavicular ligament and the coracoacromial ligament. **A,** Preoperative axillary radiograph showing the significantly displaced distal portion of the coracoid process (*arrow*). **B,** Postoperative axillary radiograph showing the bony fragment reduced and stabilized with an interfragmentary screw and a ligament washer. (From Goss TP. Fractures of the scapula: diagnosis and treatment. In: Iannotti JP, Williams GR Jr, eds. *Disorders of the Shoulder: Diagnosis and Management.* Philadelphia, Lippincott Williams & Wilkins; 1999:628.)

minimally displaced due to the stabilizing effect of the surrounding soft tissues, in particular the coracoclavicular ligament (Fig. 7-35). Symptomatic nonsurgical care is usually sufficient, and union occurs within 6 weeks.[97,303,310] McLaughlin felt that fibrous union is not uncommon but is rarely associated with discomfort.[195] If a fibrous union is symptomatic, bone grafting and compression screw fixation must be considered.

Double Disruptions of the Superior Shoulder Suspensory Complex

The SSSC is a bony and soft tissue ring at the end of a superior and an inferior bony strut (Fig. 7-36). The ring is composed of the glenoid process, the coracoid process, the coracoclavicular ligament, the distal end of the clavicle, the acromioclavicular joint, the coracoacromial ligament, and the acromial process. The superior strut is the middle third of the clavicle, and the inferior strut is the junction of the most lateral portion of the scapular body and the most medial portion of the glenoid neck. The complex can be divided into three units: the clavicular–acromioclavicular joint–acromial strut, the three-process–scapular body junction, and the C-4 linkage, with additional support provided by the coracoacromial ligament (Fig. 7-37).

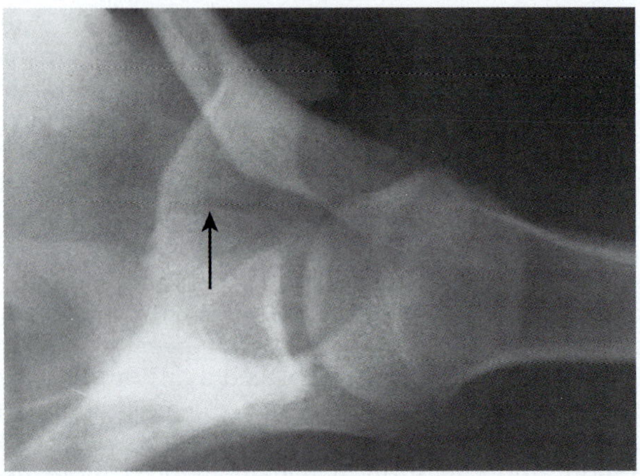

FIGURE 7-35: Axillary radiograph showing an undisplaced fracture of the base of the coracoid process (*arrow*). (From Goss TP. Fractures of the scapula: diagnosis and treatment. In: Iannotti JP, Williams GR Jr, eds. *Disorders of the Shoulder: Diagnosis and Management.* Philadelphia, Lippincott Williams & Wilkins; 1999:630.)

The SSSC is an extremely important structure with regard to the biomechanics of the shoulder complex; each of its components has its own individual function(s). It serves as a point of attachment for various musculotendinous and ligamentous structures, allows limited but very important motion to occur through the coracoclavicular ligament and the acromioclavicular articulation, and maintains a normal stable relationship between the upper extremity and the axial skeleton. The clavicle is the only bony connection between the upper extremity and the axial skeleton, and the scapula is hung or suspended from the clavicle via the coracoclavicular ligament and the acromioclavicular articulation. The SSSC is, in fact, the linkage system between the scapula and the clavicle.

The double-disruption concept (Box 7-6) is a principle that underlies and allows clinicians to understand various difficult-to-treat injuries of the shoulder complex that have previously been described in isolation but are actually united by a single biomechanical theme. The double-disruption concept also has a certain predictive value regarding injuries encountered only rarely.[107]

Single traumatic disruptions of SSSC are common (e.g., type I fracture of the distal end of the clavicle). These situations are anatomically stable because the overall integrity of the complex is not significantly violated, and

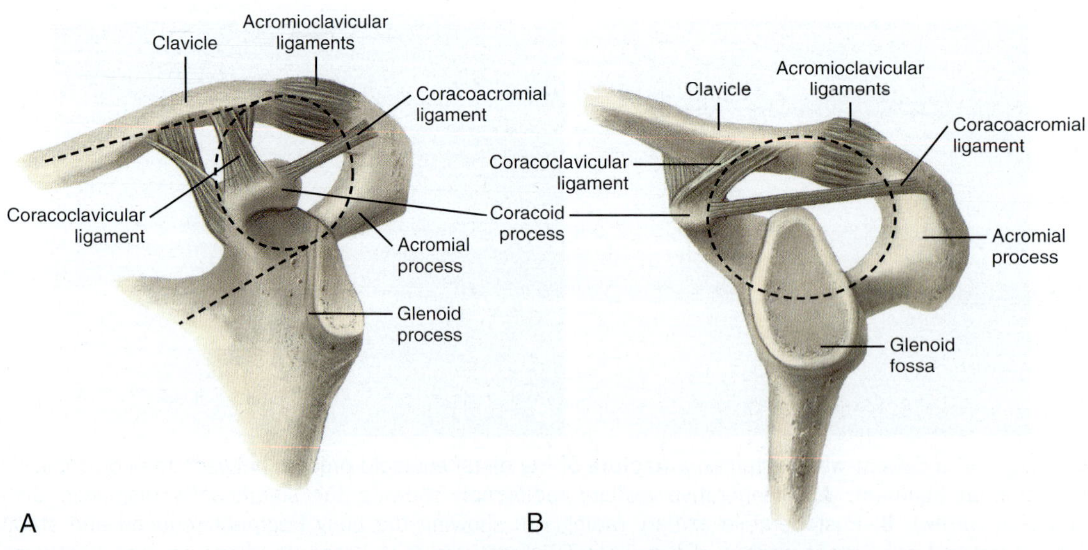

FIGURE 7-36: The superior shoulder suspensory complex. **A,** Anteroposterior view of the bone–soft tissue ring and the superior and inferior bony struts. **B,** Lateral view of the bone–soft tissue ring.

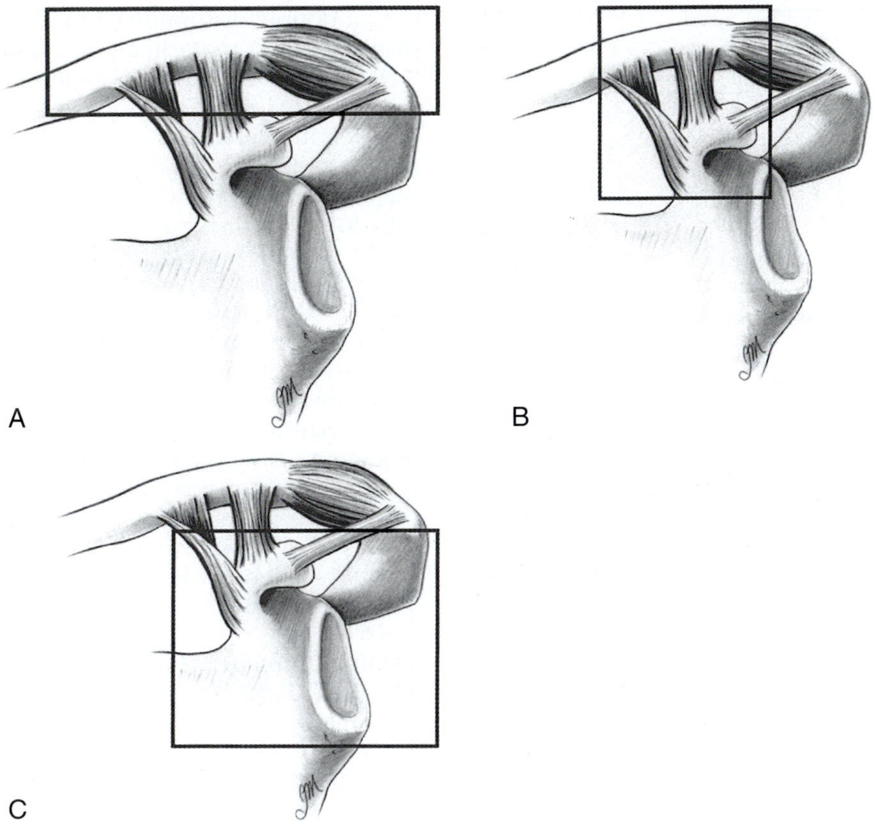

FIGURE 7-37: The three components of the superior shoulder suspensory complex. **A,** The clavicular–acromioclavicular joint–acromial strut. **B,** The clavicular–coracoclavicular ligamentous–coracoid (C-4) linkage. **C,** The three-process–scapular body junction.

BOX 7-6. Double Disruptions of the Superior Shoulder Suspensory Complex

- Principle underlying various injuries to the shoulder complex
- Potentially unstable anatomic situation
- Open reduction and internal fixation required if displacement at one or both sites is unacceptable

nonoperative management generally yields a good to excellent result. However, when the complex is disrupted in two (or more) places (a double disruption), the integrity of SSSC is compromised and a *potentially* unstable anatomic situation is created. Significant displacement can occur at either or both sites and result in bony healing problems (delayed union, malunion, and nonunion[52]), as well as adverse long-term functional difficulties (subacromial impingement, decreased strength, muscle fatigue discomfort, neurovascular compromise from a drooping shoulder, and degenerative joint disease), depending upon the particular injury. Double disruptions can take various forms: two fractures of the bone–soft tissue ring, two ligamentous disruptions of the ring, a fracture and a ligamentous disruption of the ring, fractures of both bony struts, or a fracture of one strut combined with a ring disruption (either a fracture or a ligamentous disruption) (Fig. 7-38). When particularly severe forces are involved, there is the *potential* for complex injury patterns due to multiple ring and strut disruptions. Because the glenoid, acromial, and coracoid processes are all components of SSSC, many double-disruption injuries involve the scapula. In addition, many, if not most, significantly displaced coracoid and acromial fractures are part of a double disruption.

The coracoid process is an integral part of SSSC, serving as one of the bony components of the C-4 linkage that joins the scapula to the clavicular–acromioclavicular joint–acromial strut and a part of the three-process–scapular body junction. Consequently, if a coracoid process fracture is present and associated with another SSSC injury, the potential adverse consequences of a double disruption must be considered and treatment tailored accordingly.[104] Ogawa and coworkers[225] stated that such fractures were usually deep to the coracoclavicular ligament. They classified them as type I fractures and said that they represented a dissociation between the scapula and the clavicle and as such often required ORIF.

The acromial process is one of the components of the clavicular–acromioclavicular joint–acromial strut and part

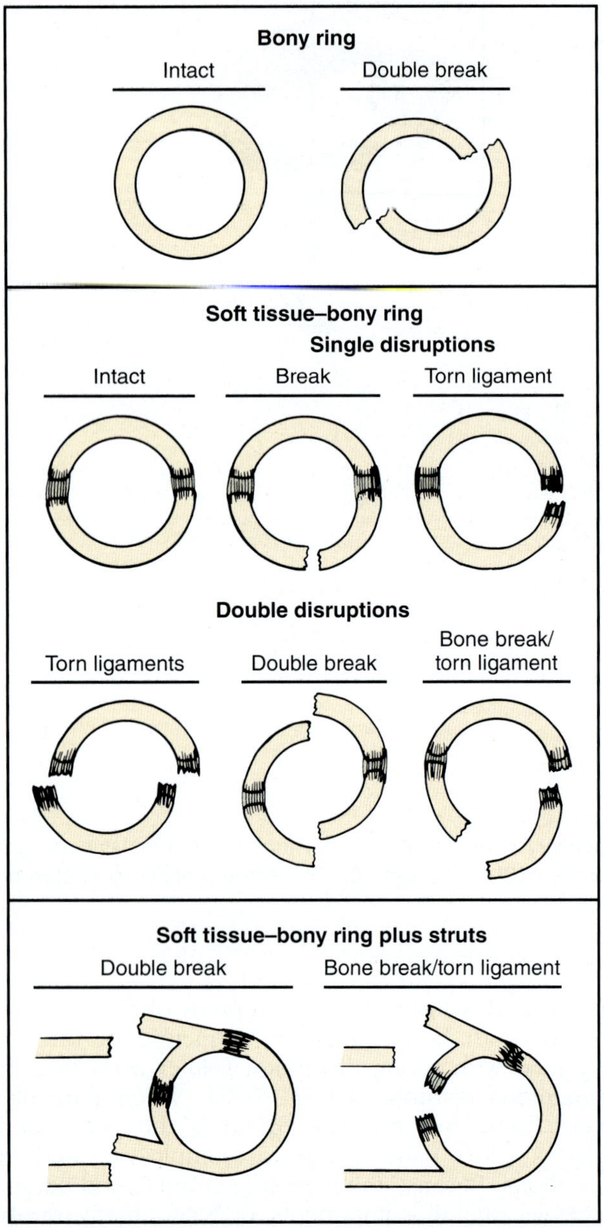

FIGURE 7-38: The many possible traumatic ring-strut disruptions. (From Goss TP. Double disruptions of the superior shoulder suspensory complex. *J Orthop Trauma.* 1993;7(2):99-106.)

of the three-process–scapular body junction. Acromial fractures that are significantly displaced are usually the result of instability created when other fractures or ligamentous disruptions of SSSC are present.[104] These injuries are generally the result of high-energy trauma and often require surgical intervention. Ogawa and Naniwa[224] divided acromial fractures into two types: type I (lateral to the spinoglenoid notch) and type II (descending into the spinoglenoid notch). They said that the mechanism of each was different and that type I injuries were more likely to be associated with other injuries to the SSSC (i.e., a double disruption), more likely to be significantly displaced, and more likely to require ORIF.

If a single disruption is noted on routine radiographs (a true AP view of the shoulder, a true axillary view of the glenohumeral joint, and a weight-bearing AP view of the shoulder to evaluate the integrity of the clavicular-scapular linkage [SSSC]), the clinician needs to look carefully for other disruptions (CT is often necessary because of the complex bony anatomy in the area). If two or more disruptions are present, the clinician must decide whether the displacement at one or both sites is unacceptable ("acceptable" being a relative term, dependent upon the particular clinical situation). If so, surgical management is generally necessary. It cannot be overemphasized that not all double disruptions require surgical treatment—only those in which one or both injury sites is significantly displaced. Finally, in 2013 Lambert et al. offered their perspective on a group of complex injuries to this area which they called "fractures of the lateral scapula suspensory system."[166] Several double disruptions will be described.

Floating Shoulder (Ipsilateral Fractures of the Midshaft Clavicle and the Glenoid Neck)

Importantly, what has been termed a *floating shoulder* represents merely one of many possible double disruptions of SSSC. Thus a floating shoulder is a double disruption, but a double disruption is usually not a floating shoulder. In isolation, each fracture (a glenoid neck fracture and a midshaft clavicle fracture) is generally minimally displaced and managed nonoperatively. However, in combination, each disruption has the *potential* to make the other unstable (the glenoid neck fracture allowing severe displacement to occur at the clavicular site, and vice versa) (Fig. 7-39). The situation is rendered even more unstable if an additional disruption of the clavicular–acromioclavicular joint–acromial strut is present or if the C-4 linkage is violated with or without involvement of the coracoacromial ligament. Hardegger et al.[121] stated that these injuries represent a "functional imbalance" as a result of "altered glenohumeral–acromial relationships." These authors and Butters[46] recommended surgery to reduce and stabilize the injury.

If displacement is unacceptable, surgical reduction and stabilization of the clavicular fracture site (most commonly with plate fixation) is advisable to avoid nonunion, alleviate tensile forces on the brachial plexus, restore normal anatomic relationships, and ensure restoration of normal shoulder function.[131,162] The glenoid neck fracture may reduce satisfactorily with stabilization of the clavicle. However, if significant displacement persists, surgical management may also be required[130,171] (see "Glenoid Neck [Extra-articular] Fractures"). Additional injuries to the clavicular–acromioclavicular joint–acromial strut may require operative treatment, whereas associated injuries involving the C-4 linkage usually heal satisfactorily if the glenoid neck and other disruption sites are treated appropriately.

Leung and Lam reported on 15 patients treated surgically (average follow-up, 25 months).[172] In 14 of the 15

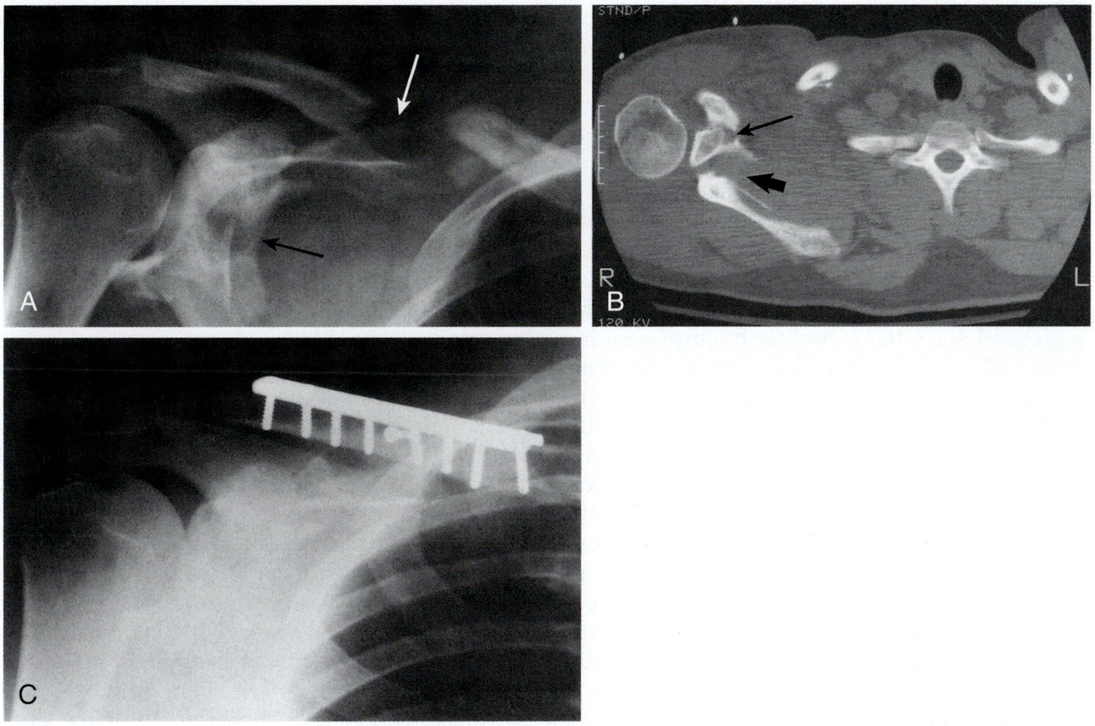

FIGURE 7-39: Radiographs of a patient who sustained a double disruption of the superior shoulder suspensory complex, resulting in a floating shoulder. **A,** Preoperative anteroposterior (AP) radiograph showing a fracture of the glenoid neck with mediolateral (ML) translation (*black arrow*) and a severely displaced fracture of the middle third of the clavicle (*white arrow*). **B,** Preoperative axial computed tomographic image showing the glenoid neck fracture to be complete (*thick black arrow*), with the glenoid fragment and the entire superior shoulder suspensory complex rendered particularly unstable by the associated fracture of the coracoid process (*thin black arrow*). **C,** Postoperative AP radiograph showing anatomic reduction and stabilization of the clavicle fracture. The glenoid neck fracture was managed nonoperatively, although a strong case could be made for open reduction and internal fixation in light of its persistent ML translational displacement (the glenoid fragment remained unstable because of the fractured coracoid process; i.e., a double disruption of the superior shoulder suspensory complex was still present). (From Goss TP. Fractures of the scapula: diagnosis and treatment. In: Iannotti JP, Williams GR Jr, eds. *Disorders of the Shoulder: Diagnosis and Management.* Philadelphia, Lippincott Williams & Wilkins; 1999:624.)

patients, the fractures healed with a good to excellent functional result. Herscovici et al. reported the results of nine patients with ipsilateral clavicular and glenoid neck fractures (average follow-up, 48.5 months.)[132] Seven patients were treated surgically with plate fixation of the clavicular fracture site and achieved excellent results. Two patients were treated without surgery and had decreased range of motion and drooping of the involved shoulder. The authors strongly recommended ORIF of the clavicle to prevent glenoid neck malunion. Simpson and Jupiter in a review article indicated that these injuries often require operative treatment.[261] Rikli and associates expanded this concept somewhat, saying that a fracture of the glenoid neck combined with either a fracture of the clavicle or a disruption of the acromioclavicular or sternoclavicular joint results in an unstable shoulder girdle. They reviewed 13 cases (12 in which the clavicular injury was surgically stabilized) and reported excellent results in nearly all.[245]

There has been continued interest in floating shoulders, including both clinical and basic science studies. Edwards et al. reported excellent results with conservative treatment of consecutive patients with ipsilateral clavicle and scapula fractures; however, in five of 20 patients, the scapula fracture did not involve the glenoid neck.[82] Hashiguchi and Ito reported excellent results in five patients with ipsilateral clavicle and glenoid neck fractures in whom fixation of the clavicle alone was performed.[124] Egol et al. reviewed their results in 19 patients (some treated surgically based upon surgeon preference and some treated nonoperatively) and reported good results with each approach.[83] Ramos and coworkers reported on a series of patients treated nonoperatively who did quite well.[241]

Williams and coworkers conducted a cadaveric study to determine the stability afforded by specific structures. Using a model with ipsilateral glenoid neck and clavicular fractures, they found that instability of the glenoid segment occurred only with subsequent coracoacromial and acromioclavicular ligamentous sectioning. They concluded that floating shoulders only become unstable when there is an associated disruption of those structures.[298]

Van Noort and van der Werken reported on 46 patients with floating shoulder injuries treated operatively or nonoperatively, with mixed results in both groups. They agreed that additional ligamentous disruptions (the coracoacromial, coracoclavicular, or acromioclavicular ligaments) are necessary for significant displacement to occur and concluded that significantly displaced clavicular fractures required ORIF and that glenoid neck fractures with significant persistent inferior angulation also needed to be addressed surgically.[285]

Pasapula et al. stated in a review article that in the presence of a glenoid neck and a clavicle fracture, various combinations of other bony and ligamentous injuries must be present for a true floating shoulder to occur. They also said that due to these associated injuries, ORIF of the clavicular fracture alone might not satisfactorily reduce the glenoid neck fracture.[234] Labler et al. reviewed 17 patients with such injuries and echoed these sentiments.[164] This conclusion would help explain the nature of the injury shown in Figure 7-39. This patient had an associated coracoid process fracture that effectively detached the coracoacromial and coracoclavicular ligaments from the glenoid fragment. These ideas are similar to those expressed for isolated glenoid neck fractures, which usually require damage to their secondary support system to displace significantly.

Other studies by Van Noort and van der Werken[285] and by DeFranco and Patterson[71] concluded that most floating shoulder injuries do well with nonoperative management and that the criterion for operative treatment is not well established, namely, how much displacement at the fracture site(s) is unacceptable. Current experience seems to indicate that the mere presence of a clavicular and a glenoid neck fracture does not demand operative treatment and many do well nonoperatively. However, the more displacement at one or both sites, the greater the need for ORIF, and another disruption of SSSC may be necessary for significant displacement to occur.[228]

Fracture of the Glenoid Neck and Other Non–Midshaft-Clavicle Disruptions of the Superior Shoulder Suspensory Complex

As a component of SSSC and in particular the three process-scapular body junction, the glenoid neck can be a part of other double disruption combinations. One such combination is a fracture of the glenoid neck and a fracture of the base of the coracoid process. As stated earlier, a fracture of the glenoid neck can become displaced only if it is complete (i.e., if the fracture line exits the lateral and superior scapular margins adjacent to the coracoid process). Even so, if the continuity of the glenoid fragment with the clavicular–acromioclavicular joint–acromial strut via the C-4 linkage is intact, displacement is usually minimal. However, if the secondary support system is disrupted with or without involvement of the coracoacromial ligament (e.g. a fracture of the base of the coracoid process), significant displacement of the glenoid fragment (ML translational displacement ≥1 cm, AP angular displacement ≥40 degrees, or a decrease in the GPA to ≤20 degrees) is particularly likely, and surgical management must be considered. Operative treatment consists of ORIF of the glenoid neck fracture, while the coracoid fracture usually heals without direct intervention. Wright and Johnston described a double disruption involving the glenoid neck and the acromial process that allowed significant anteromedial displacement of the glenoid fragment and the glenohumeral joint. Both disruption sites were addressed surgically with a very satisfactory outcome.[304]

Fracture of the Coracoid Process and a Grade III Disruption of the Acromioclavicular Joint

On occasion, especially in young adults, a force that would otherwise cause a grade III sprain of the acromioclavicular joint (a double disruption usually treated nonoperatively with good results) results in an avulsion fracture of the base of the coracoid process or the bony attachment of the coracoclavicular ligament at the angle of the coracoid process instead of a disruption of the coracoclavicular ligament (Fig. 7-43C). A weight-bearing AP projection of the shoulder complex shows displacement of the distal end of the clavicle above the superior border of the acromion, but the coracoclavicular interval remains normal. Treatment of injuries associated with a small bony avulsion fracture of the angle of the coracoid process follows the principles developed for grade III acromioclavicular joint disruptions—specifically, surgical reconstruction of the acromioclavicular joint needs to be considered in young people engaged in athletics or heavy manual labor. Disruptions associated with a fracture of the base of the coracoid process (especially if the fracture is significantly displaced) are considered for surgical ORIF of both sites to avoid the adverse long-term effects of a grade III acromioclavicular separation and nonunion of the coracoid process. Reports in the literature have described both operative and nonoperative management of these injuries.[30,62,84,118,134,162,169,182,208,264,293,309]

Fractures of the Ipsilateral Coracoid and Acromial Processes

Isolated fractures of the coracoid and acromial processes (Fig. 7-40) are usually minimally displaced, and therefore managed nonoperatively. However, when they occur together, they constitute a double disruption of the SSSC, a potentially unstable anatomic situation.[310] If displacement at either or both sites is unacceptable, surgical management is indicated. ORIF of the acromial fracture may be all that is required. This procedure often indirectly reduces and stabilizes the coracoid fracture satisfactorily and is technically less difficult than addressing the coracoid injury. If ORIF of the acromial fracture does not improve the position of the coracoid fracture, the coracoid fracture may need to be reduced and stabilized as well. Lim and coworkers described such an injury managed with ORIF of both sites.[174]

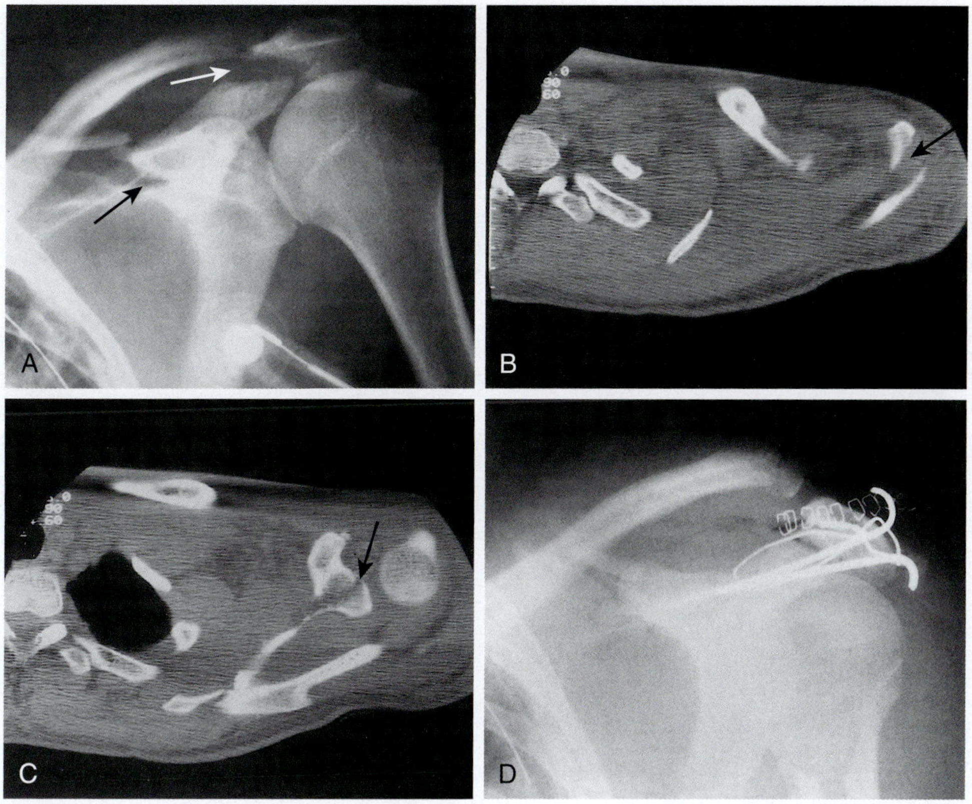

FIGURE 7-40: Ipsilateral fractures of the coracoid and acromial processes and the distal end of the clavicle. **A,** Preoperative anteroposterior (AP) radiograph of the involved area. The *white arrow* indicates the acromial fracture; the *black arrow* indicates the coracoid fracture. **B,** Preoperative axial computed tomographic (CT) image showing wide separation at the acromial fracture site (*arrow*) as a result of the associated coracoid process fracture. **C,** Preoperative axial CT image showing the fractured coracoid process (*arrow*). **D,** Postoperative AP radiograph of the shoulder showing reduction and stabilization of the acromial fracture with a tension band construct. The coracoid process fracture and distal clavicle fracture were not addressed surgically and healed spontaneously. (From Goss TP. Fractures of the scapula: diagnosis and treatment. In: Iannotti JP, Williams GR Jr, eds. *Disorders of the Shoulder: Diagnosis and Management.* Philadelphia, Lippincott Williams & Wilkins; 1999:625.)

Fracture of the Coracoid Process and a Type I Fracture of the Distal Third of the Clavicle (as Well as Type II and V Distal Clavicle Fractures)

Fractures of the distal third of the clavicle can become unacceptably displaced if the continuity of the coracoclavicular ligament between the coracoid process and the proximal clavicular segment is disrupted (type II and type V fractures).[13,32,213,214,232] The same situation can occur with type I fractures if the coracoid process is fractured (Fig. 7-41). Classifying all of these injuries as type II fractures would probably make most sense, expanding this term to include all situations in which the distal third of the clavicle is fractured and the linkage between the proximal/clavicular segment and the scapula (the C-4 linkage) is disrupted.

If displacement at the clavicular fracture site is of such a degree that a delayed union or nonunion is likely, treatment consists of surgical reduction and stabilization of the injury. Associated fractures of the base of the coracoid process may reduce secondarily and heal uneventfully. If not, the coracoid fracture may need to be addressed surgically as well.

Acromial Fracture with Grade III Disruption of the Acromioclavicular Joint

The combination of acromial fracture and a grade III disruption of the acromioclavicular joint creates a free-floating acromial fragment and can lead to a nonunion as well as the well-described adverse long-term functional consequences associated with an acromioclavicular joint disruption. A case report by McGahan and Rab describes a patient with an associated axillary nerve deficit.[191]

If displacement at the acromial fracture site is unacceptable, surgical reduction and stabilization of both the fracture site and the AC joint disruption is indicated. Kurdy and Shah described a patient treated nonoperatively who had "a satisfactory outcome; however, he was 74 years old and an acromial nonunion occurred."[163]

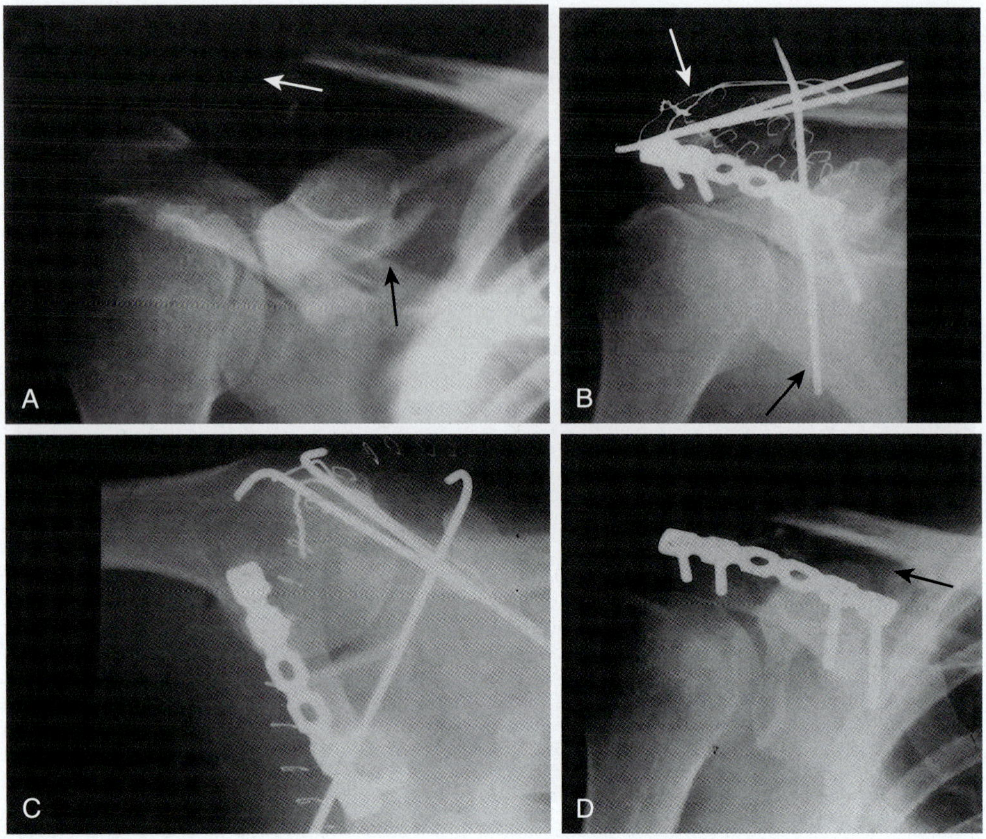

FIGURE 7-41: A patient who sustained a fracture at the base of the coracoid process, a type I fracture of the distal end of the clavicle, and a nondisplaced fracture of the acromion. **A,** Preoperative anteroposterior (AP) radiograph showing severe displacement at the distal clavicular fracture site (*white arrow*) and the coracoid fracture site (*black arrow*). Postoperative AP (**B**) and axillary (**C**) radiographs show reduction and stabilization of the clavicular fracture with a tension band construct (*white arrow*) and reduction and stabilization of the coracoid process fracture by means of a transfixing K-wire passed into the glenoid process (a cannulated interfragmentary screw would now be used). The acromial fracture was plated (*black arrow*). **D,** AP radiograph taken 3 months postoperatively after removal of hardware shows the distal clavicle and coracoid fractures to be healed and the superior shoulder suspensory relationships reestablished (*arrow*). (From Goss TP. Fractures of the scapula: diagnosis and treatment. In: Iannotti JP, Williams GR Jr, eds. Disorders *of the Shoulder: Diagnosis and Management.* Philadelphia, Lippincott Williams & Wilkins; 1999:626.)

Gorczyca et al. described an injury that gradually displaced over time and eventually required surgical ORIF.[101] Torrens et al. described a combined type VI acromioclavicular joint disruption and an acromial fracture requiring ORIF of both injury sites.[278]

Segmental Fracture of the Acromion

As with segmental fractures of other bones, two acromial disruptions create an unstable intermediate segment (Fig. 7-42). If displacement at one or both sites is unacceptable and a nonunion is likely, ORIF with plate fixation or a tension band construct, or both, is performed via a posterolateral approach.

Other Combinations

Type III, Vb, and Vc glenoid cavity fractures associated with another disruption of the SSSC are discussed in the section "Glenoid Cavity (Intra-articular) Fractures" (see Fig. 7-23). Other double-disruption combinations are possible and are treated according to basic therapeutic principles (operative and nonoperative).

Avulsion Fractures of the Scapula

Most of the scapula is formed by intramembranous ossification, but at least six or seven secondary ossification centers are also present. As with other scapula fractures, avulsion injuries are uncommon. By definition, they are caused by indirect forces applied to the surrounding musculotendinous and ligamentous tissues and are concentrated at their scapular attachment sites. Three mechanisms of such injuries are possible: a severe, uncontrolled muscular contraction caused by electroconvulsive treatment, an electric shock, or an epileptic seizure[31,78,128,134,149,153,157,183,236,260,273,296]; a strong, indirect force associated with a single traumatic event[33,73,305,309]; and a gradual bony failure caused by lesser

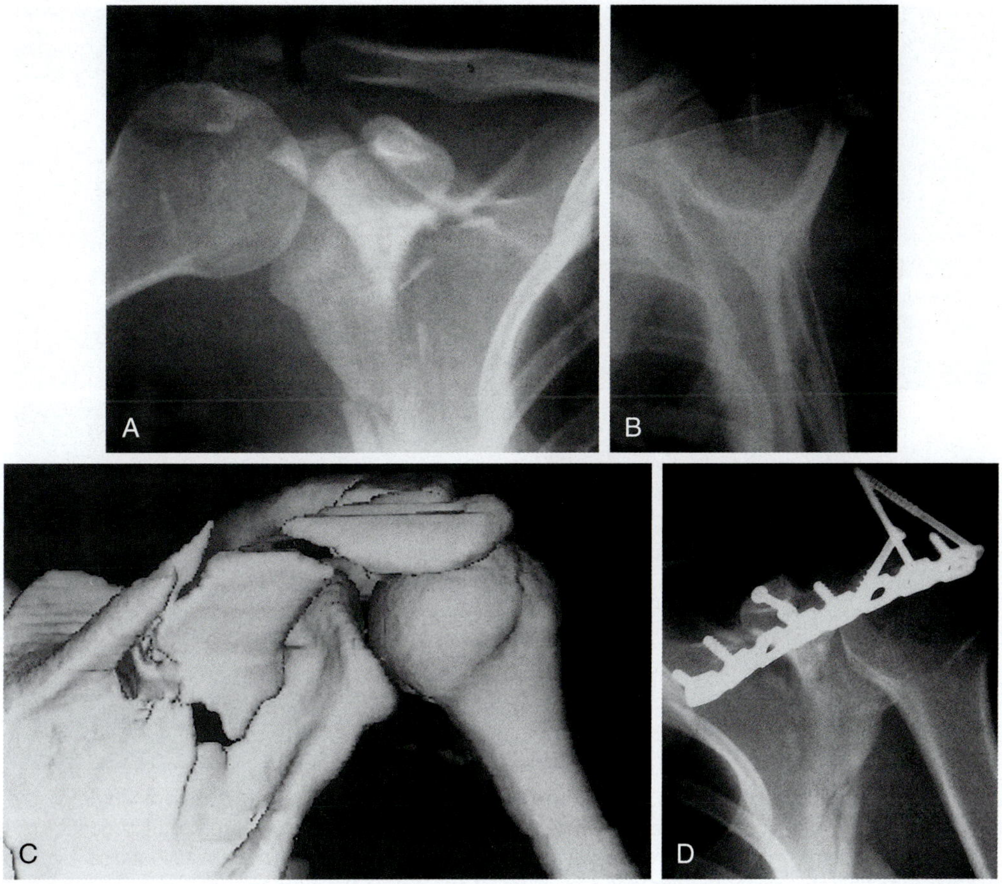

FIGURE 7-42: Segmental fracture of the acromial process and a comminuted fracture of the scapular body. **A,** Preoperative anteroposterior (AP) radiograph. **B,** Preoperative lateral scapula radiograph. **C,** Preoperative three-dimensional computed tomographic radiograph. **D,** Postoperative AP radiograph showing the acromial fractures reduced and stabilized with a malleable reconstruction plate. (From Goss TP. The scapula: Coracoid, acromial, and avulsion fractures. *Am J Orthop.* 1996;25[2]:106-115.)

but repetitive traumatic events (stress[40] or fatigue[294] fractures). The potential varieties are numerous, and many have been described.

Diagnosis and Treatment

True AP and lateral projections of the scapula and a true axillary view of the glenohumeral joint constitute the diagnostic trauma series. The series may be supplemented by a weight-bearing view of the shoulder complex. Treatment is, by and large, symptomatic and nonoperative. However, if the fracture is significantly displaced and of functional importance, ORIF must be considered.[112]

Nonoperative Treatment

Most injuries are managed quite successfully nonoperatively.[12] These include avulsion fractures of the superior angle of the scapula (insertion of the levator scapulae) (Fig. 7-43A)[102]; avulsion fractures through the body of the scapula caused by an accidental electrical shock[76,134,242,273]; avulsion fractures of the infraglenoid tubercle (origin of the long head of the triceps) and the lateral border of the scapula (origin of the teres major and minor muscles)[134]; and avulsion fractures of the infraspinatus fossa (origin of the infraspinatus muscle,[14] which must be differentiated from a developmental anomaly).[241]

An avulsion fracture of the superior border of the scapula can also be managed nonoperatively.[136] This injury is often associated with a fracture of the base of the coracoid process and an acromioclavicular joint disruption.[10,14] Some attribute such fractures to indirect stress applied via the omohyoid muscle,[5,144,299] while others consider it an extension of the coracoid fracture.[301]

Operative Treatment

Some avulsion fractures, such as those of the lateral margin of the acromial process (Fig. 7-43B) (origin of the deltoid muscle), deserve operative consideration at the very least.[134] The deltoid muscle is an important dynamic structure about the glenohumeral joint. Consequently, if this fracture is significantly displaced, surgical reattachment is indicated. Reattachment is simply accomplished using multiple nonabsorbable sutures passed in a horizontal mattress fashion through the deltoid and holes drilled along the periphery of the acromial process.

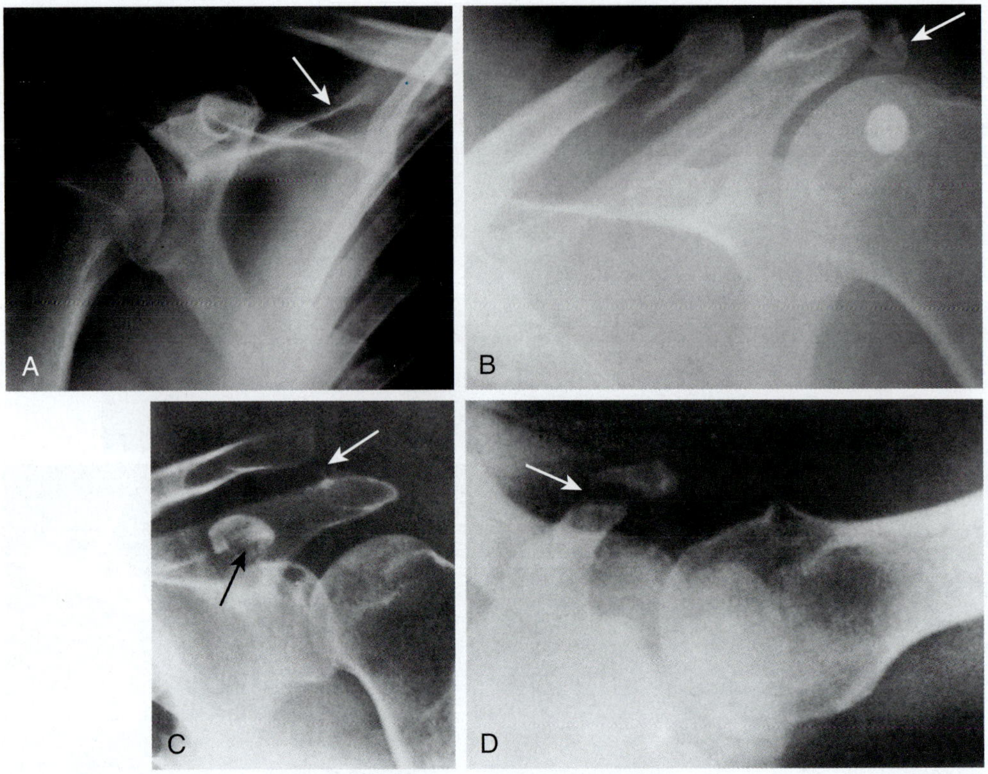

FIGURE 7-43: Various scapula avulsion fractures. **A,** Minimally displaced fracture of the superior angle of the scapula (attachment of the levator scapulae [*arrow*]). **B,** Displaced fracture of the lateral margin of the acromial process (origin of the deltoid muscle [*arrow*]). **C,** Type III disruption of the acromioclavicular joint (*white arrow*) with an associated avulsion fracture at the base of the coracoid process (*black arrow*). **D,** Displaced fracture of the tip of the coracoid process (attachment of the conjoined tendon [*arrow*]). (From Goss TP. Fractures of the scapula: diagnosis and treatment. In: Iannotti JP, Williams GR Jr, eds. *Disorders of the Shoulder: Diagnosis and Management*. Philadelphia, Lippincott Williams & Wilkins; 1999:632.)

Two cases of avulsion fractures through the body of the acromion have been described.[211,243] Both were caused by a significant force transmitted through the surrounding musculature, particularly the deltoid. One was treated nonsurgically, and the second was managed surgically. Bony union and satisfactory return of function were realized in both.

Isolated avulsion fractures of the coracoid process may benefit from surgery (see Fig. 7-34 and "Isolated Coracoid Fractures").

An avulsion fracture of the superior angle of the coracoid process (attachment of the coracoclavicular ligament)[208] or the base of the coracoid process can occur in association with a disruption of the acromioclavicular joint (Fig. 7-43C) (see "Fracture of the Coracoid Process and a Grade III Disruption of the Acromioclavicular Joint").

An avulsion fracture of the inferior angle of the scapula (Fig. 7-44) (insertion of the serratus anterior muscle) is a rare injury.[47] If significantly displaced, this injury causes winging of the scapula and can compromise shoulder function considerably, in which case ORIF is indicated.[125] Such a fracture might be that described by Longabaugh in 1924.[177] Franco et al. described an avulsion fracture of the inferior angle of the scapula presumably caused by prolonged coughing.[90]

An avulsion fracture of the supraglenoid tubercle (origin of the long head of the biceps muscle) indicates a displaced, possibly symptomatic SLAP lesion.[139] It is of interest that the senior author (T.P.G.) published the first report (1982) drawing attention to the fact that labral tears could result in what was termed "functional shoulder instability" as opposed to those tears associated with a subluxing or dislocating shoulder (anatomic instability).[231]

OTHER DISORDERS

Lateral Dislocation of the Scapula (Scapulothoracic Dissociation)

Scapulothoracic dissociation is a rare, traumatic disruption of the scapulothoracic articulation caused by a severe direct force applied over the shoulder accompanied by traction applied to the upper extremity (Box 7-7).[3,79,80,111,135,146,152,168,212,226,251,283] Although the skin remains intact, the scapula is torn away from the posterior chest wall, prompting some to call this injury a closed traumatic forequarter amputation.

Because of the violent forces involved, any of the three bones in the shoulder complex (the clavicle, the

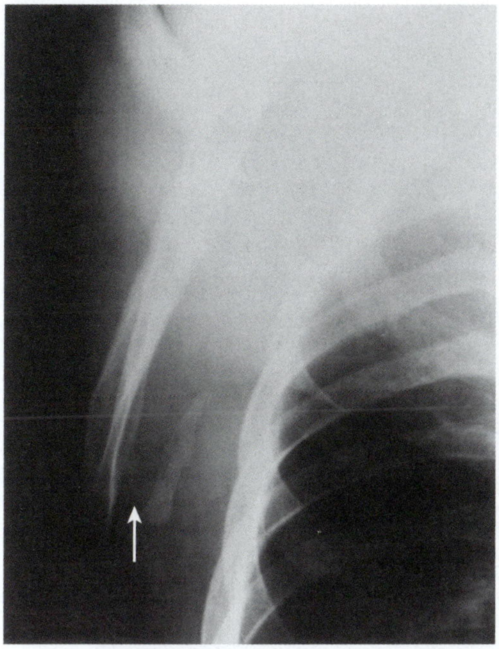

FIGURE 7-44: Lateral radiograph of the scapula showing a severely displaced avulsion fracture of the inferior angle (insertion of the serratus anterior muscle [*arrow*]). (From Goss TP. Fractures of the scapula: diagnosis and treatment. In: Iannotti JP, Williams GR Jr, eds. *Disorders of the Shoulder: Diagnosis and Management*. Philadelphia, Lippincott Williams & Wilkins; 1999:633.)

BOX 7-7. Scapulothoracic Dissociation

Keys to Diagnosis
Violent trauma
Massive swelling
Neurovascular compromise
Lateral displacement on chest radiograph
Awareness of entity

Acute Management
Appropriate treatment of neurovascular injury
Reduce and stabilize the sternal–clavicular–acromial linkage

scapula, and the proximal end of the humerus) may be fractured, and any of the remaining three articulations (the glenohumeral, acromioclavicular, and sternoclavicular joints) may be disrupted. Neurovascular injury is common. Disruption of the subclavian or axillary artery (more commonly the former) and complete or partial disruptions of the brachial plexus are well described. In addition, the soft tissue supportive structures can suffer severe damage, especially those that run from the chest wall to the scapula or from the chest wall to the humerus. Complete or partial tears of the trapezius, levator scapulae, rhomboids, pectoralis minor, and latissimus dorsi have all been reported.

A presumptive diagnosis is based on a history of violent trauma and the presence of massive soft tissue swelling over the shoulder girdle. A pulseless upper extremity, indicating a complete vascular disruption, and a complete or partial neurologic deficit, indicating an injury to the brachial plexus, are quite suggestive. Significant lateral displacement of the scapula seen on a nonrotated chest radiograph confirms the diagnosis. As with all rare injuries, awareness of the clinical entity is critical to making the diagnosis.

Treatment recommendations have focused on the care of the accompanying neurovascular injury. If the vascular integrity of the extremity is in question, an emergency arteriogram is performed, followed by a surgical repair, if necessary. The brachial plexus is explored at the same time. If a neurologic deficit is present, EMG testing is performed 3 weeks after injury to determine the extent of damage and assess the degree of recovery, if any. Cervical myelography can be performed at 6 weeks. If nerve root avulsion(s) or a complete neurologic deficit is present, the prognosis for functional recovery is poor.[44,308] However, partial plexus injuries have a better prognosis, and most patients achieve either a complete recovery or regain functional use of the extremity. If some portions of the plexus are intact and others are disrupted, neurologic repair is a possibility. Late reconstructive efforts are guided by the degree of neurologic return, and musculotendinous transfers are performed as needed.

Care of the surrounding soft tissue supportive structures (musculotendinous and ligamentous) has been nonoperative and consists of protection of the shoulder complex for 6 weeks to allow healing, combined with a closely monitored progressive physical therapy program designed to regain range of motion initially and then strength. Magnetic resonance imaging of the involved area now offers the ability to visualize important disruptions that may be amenable to surgical repair.

Injury to the sternal-clavicular-acromial linkage (a disruption of the sternoclavicular or acromioclavicular joint or a fracture of the clavicle) is usually, if not invariably, present for posterolateral displacement of the scapula to occur. This component of scapulothoracic dissociations has been largely ignored in terms of diagnosis and treatment. Of the three possible disruptions, a fracture of the clavicle seems to be the most common. This anatomic situation is very unstable—the clavicular injury allows maximal displacement of the scapula, and the unstable scapulothoracic articulation often leads to significant displacement at the clavicular fracture site. Consequently, ORIF of the clavicular disruption (screw-and-plate or tension band fixation) is considered in order to avoid delayed union or nonunion, to restore as much stability as possible to the shoulder complex, to avoid adverse long-term functional consequences, and to protect the brachial plexus as well as the subclavian and axillary vessels from further injury caused by tensile forces (Fig. 7-45).[55] Uhl and Hospeder[284] described a lesser injury characterized by progressive subluxation of the scapulothoracic articulation and a clavicle fracture (no neurovascular involvement) requiring ORIF of the clavicle. Similar therapeutic reasoning would

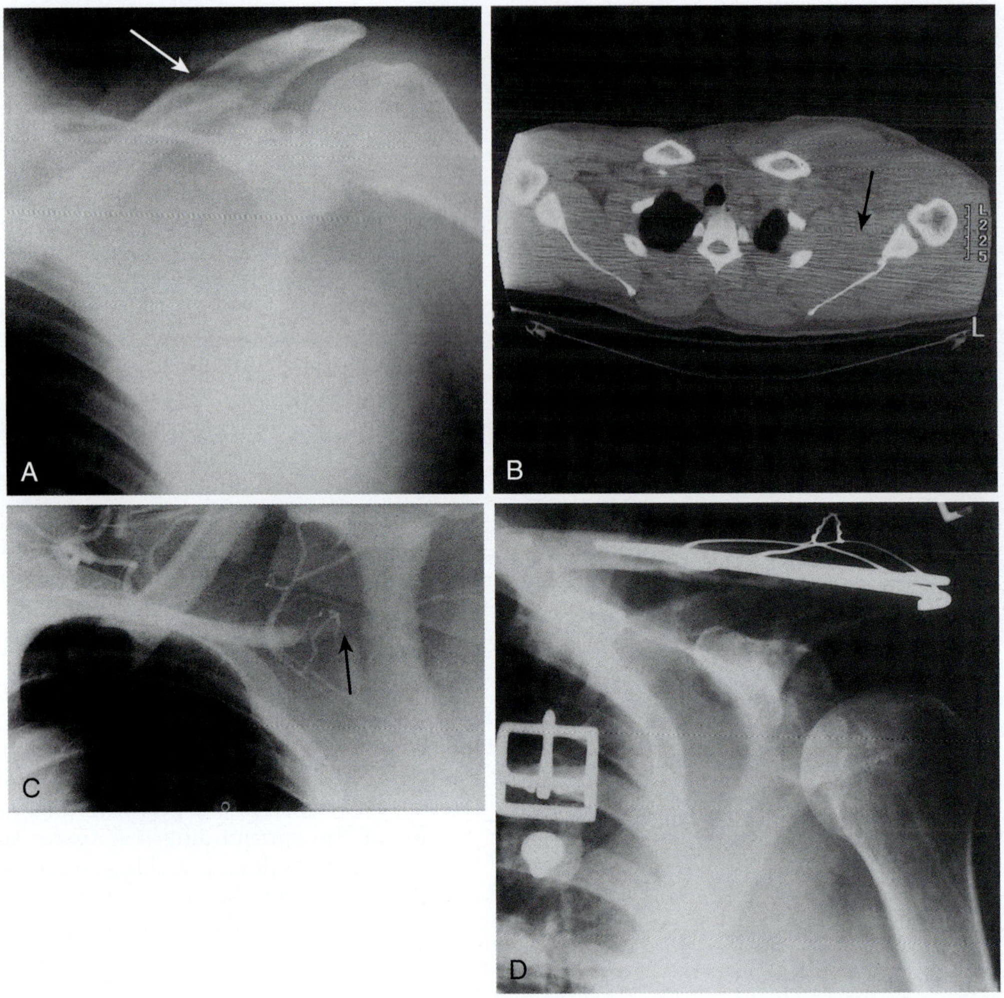

FIGURE 7-45: Radiographs of a patient who sustained a left scapulothoracic dissociation. **A,** Preoperative anteroposterior (AP) radiograph showing significant lateral displacement of the scapula (*arrow*) and a significantly displaced fracture of the distal end of the clavicle. **B,** Computed tomographic image showing significantly increased distance between the left scapula and the rib cage (*arrow*) compared towith the opposite (uninjured) side. **C,** Arteriogram showing disruption of the subclavian artery (*arrow*). **D,** Postoperative AP radiograph showing reduction and stabilization of the distal clavicle fracture (and secondarily the scapulothoracic articulation) by means of a tension band construct. (From Goss TP. Fractures of the scapula: diagnosis and treatment. In: Iannotti JP, Williams GR Jr, eds. *Disorders of the Shoulder: Diagnosis and Management*. Philadelphia, Lippincott Williams & Wilkins; 1999:634.)

apply to scapulothoracic dissociations accompanied by a disruption of the acromioclavicular or the sternoclavicular joint, although with the latter, metallic fixation devices must be avoided.

Intrathoracic Dislocation of the Scapula

Intrathoracic dislocation of the scapula is extremely rare. Cases associated with minimal violence and a preexisting factor (generalized laxity or a locking osteochondroma) have been described.[2] The scapula becomes locked within the posterior aspect of one of the upper intercostal spaces.[216] A second type is caused by more violent trauma, either a direct blow over the posterior aspect of the scapula or a violent outward distractive force applied to the arm. The scapular body is displaced anterolaterally, and its inferior angle becomes lodged between the ribs (Fig. 7-46). The severity of the event usually causes a fracture of the scapula and ribs and a marked disruption of the periscapular soft tissues.[155] Pell and Whipple described a patient who sustained a fracture of the scapular body with the inferior angle locked within the fourth intercostal space that was managed successfully with a closed reduction.[235]

The diagnosis may be missed initially because of associated injuries, inadequate radiographic projections, or both.[216] Displacement of the scapula might not be readily apparent on routine AP chest radiographs. Tangential views (anterior oblique or lateral scapular projections) or a chest CT may be necessary to establish the diagnosis.

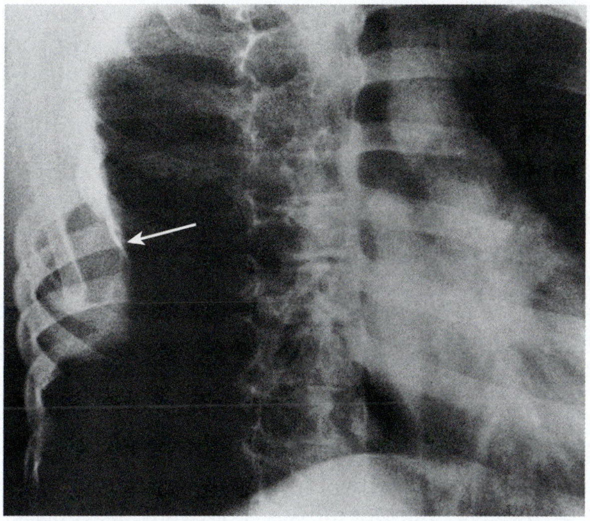

FIGURE 7-46: An anterior oblique radiograph of a patient who sustained an intrathoracic dislocation of his right scapula (*arrow*). (From Nettrour LF, Krufky EL, Mueller RE, Raycroft JF. Locked scapula: Intrathoracic dislocation of the inferior angle. *J Bone Joint Surg Am.* 1972;54:413-416.)

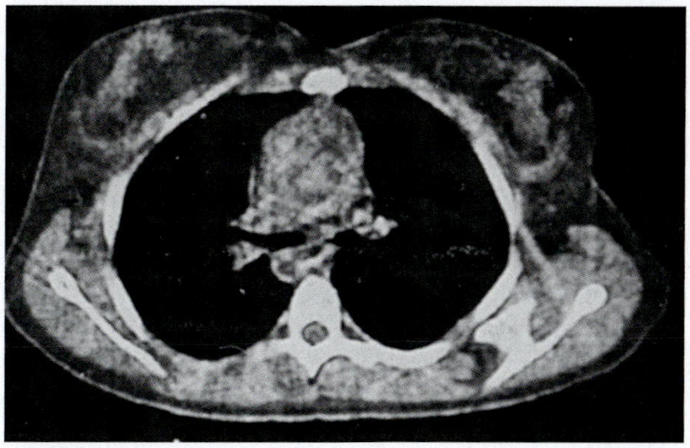

FIGURE 7-47: Computed tomographic image of the scapular body showing a large osteochondroma on the costal surface that caused a snapping scapula.

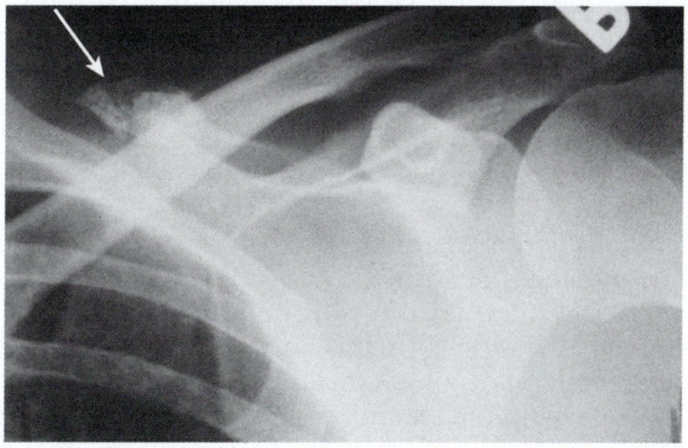

FIGURE 7-48: Radiograph of a patient with pain and crepitus over the superomedial aspect of the scapula (*arrow*). Note the significant exostosis that was subsequently surgically removed, alleviating the patient's discomfort and dysfunction.

Acute injuries are reduced in a closed fashion under anesthesia by hyperabducting the arm and manually manipulating the scapula (rotating the scapula forward and pushing it backward)[75] while steady traction is applied to the arm. The reduction is usually stable, but securing the scapula to the chest wall with adhesive tape or immobilizing the arm in a sling and swathe binder is advisable for comfort and soft-tissue healing.[155] Four to six weeks is generally required for satisfactory healing. Unprotected, progressive functional use of the shoulder and arm is then encouraged. In long-standing cases, open reduction with soft tissue detachment may be necessary, followed by reconstruction of the periscapular soft tissues to reestablish stability.

Scapulothoracic Crepitus

Scapulothoracic crepitus (described under various terms but most often called snapping scapula)[56,58,202,210,214,259] was first described by Boinet[37] in 1867. Mauclaire[185] noted three varieties: *froissemant* (an asymptomatic gentle sound thought to be physiologic); *froittemant* (a louder sound, possibly symptomatic and, if so, most likely due to soft tissue pathology); and *craquemont* (a loud sound, often symptomatic and, if so, most likely to result from bony pathology). These sounds were believed to have two general etiologies: abnormalities within the tissues between the scapula and the chest wall and abnormalities of scapulothoracic congruence.

Etiology

Pathologic conditions affecting the musculature lying within the scapulothoracic interval that can cause crepitus include atrophy,[202,158,246] tears, fibrosis and scarring,[202,203,291] and anomalous muscle insertions.[158,267] Representative cases have been described by Milch,[202-204] Bateman,[25] Strizak and Cowen,[271] and Rockwood.[246]

Bony abnormalities within the scapulothoracic interval that can cause crepitus include osteochondromas over the ventral surface of the scapula (Fig. 7-47),[63,197,203,204,208,233] rib exostoses,[74] Luschka's tubercle[202,292] (a bony prominence at the superomedial angle of the scapula), a hooked superomedial angle of the scapula,[202,244] malunited fractures of the ribs or scapula,[202,203,269] and reactive bony spurs secondary to repeated microtrauma at soft tissue attachment sites (Fig. 7-48).[25,248,271]

Scapulothoracic bursitis can be accompanied by scapulothoracic crepitus.[7,57,58,68,189,190,237,258] The most common sites are at the superomedial angle of the scapula and at the inferior angle of the scapula.[54,154,263]

Other rather rare causes have been described, including Sprengel's deformity (possibly related to the omohyoid bone or an abnormal scapular shape), tuberculous lesions[202] in the region, and syphilitic lues.[202] Finally, scoliosis[103,290] and thoracic kyphosis[56] can cause scapulothoracic incongruence leading to localized crepitus.

Diagnosis

When evaluating such patients, the history, physical examination, and radiologic evaluation can provide numerous clues to the diagnosis. Does the patient have a history of acute trauma involving the scapular body, the ribs, or the scapulothoracic articulation? Does the patient have a history of forceful or repetitive use of the scapulothoracic articulation? Can the patient identify the location of the crepitus or can the physician do the same by palpation or auscultation as the shoulder girdle is put through a range of motion? Visual inspection can disclose fullness or pseudo-winging of the scapula, suggesting a deep surface mass. EMG testing may be indicated to evaluate the neuromuscular status of the shoulder girdle. AP and especially lateral views of the scapula are obtained to visualize the scapulothoracic interval, and a CT and magnetic resonance imaging scan may be indicated in an effort to identify bony or soft tissue pathology (or both) in the region. It must always be kept in mind that the presence of scapulothoracic crepitus may be clinically insignificant, in which case other sources of posterior shoulder discomfort must be considered, including local pathology and referred pain from nearby or distant sources.

Treatment

When considering treatment, the clinician must ultimately decide whether the scapulothoracic crepitus is truly associated with pain, and therefore reflects localized scapulothoracic pathology. In this regard, it is important to remember that scapulothoracic crepitus has been noted in 35% of asymptomatic individuals[115] and that those with hidden agendas or psychiatric conditions can misrepresent its importance. Patients with a well-defined bony prominence within the scapulothoracic interval usually respond quite nicely to surgical removal (Fig. 7-47).[46,209,233]

However, with most patients, the etiology of the painful crepitus is not obvious, making nonoperative care the treatment of choice, at least initially. Such management can include numerous modalities: local application of ice, heat, or both; exercises to strengthen the shoulder girdle musculature[54,202,237]; postural training (a figure-of-eight binder may be used to remind patients to maintain an upright posture)[54,200]; local injections of lidocaine (Xylocaine) and a steroid into particularly symptomatic areas for diagnostic and therapeutic purposes[42,46,56,190,237]; rest or avoidance of aggravating positions and activities; analgesics; nonsteroidal antiinflammatory medications; massage; phonophoresis; ultrasound; and application of ethyl chloride to trigger points. Most patients respond satisfactorily to these measures.

For those in whom nonoperative therapy fails, surgery may be an option if the physician thinks that a definable pathologic lesion is present—the chosen procedure depends upon the nature of the presumed pathology. Procedures have been described wherein a local muscle flap is sutured over the undersurface of the scapula.[185] Rockwood[246] described excision of an avulsed flap of rhomboid muscle with satisfactory relief of pain and crepitus. Partial scapulectomy, including resection of the medial border of the scapula[48] or the superomedial angle,[7,56,158,202,244,271] has been fairly popular when symptoms can be localized to these areas. For symptomatic bursitis associated with crepitus, procedures described have included open bursectomy[155,189,190,216] and arthroscopic bursectomy.[34,54,92,154,184]

AUTHORS' PREFERRED METHODS OF TREATMENT

Scapular Body (and Spine) Fractures

Patients with fractures of the scapular body (and spine) are examined carefully for associated injuries, which are quite common and may be life threatening. The senior author has traditionally (with few exceptions) treated these injuries nonoperatively. Treatment consists of immobilization initially followed by a progressive rehabilitation program focusing on regaining range of motion first and then strength. Six weeks is usually necessary for healing, although continued therapy is often required to achieve an optimal result. A good to excellent outcome can be expected.

However, operative management is gaining acceptance in at least two situations: (1) scapular body/spine fractures with the degree of displacement noted earlier that significantly alters the position of the glenoid process/glenohumeral joint relative to the surrounding soft tissues, potentially resulting in compromised shoulder function and (2) scapular body/spine fractures in which ORIF will significantly improve the reduction and stabilization of associated glenoid process fractures. The surgical approaches and principles are detailed earlier and focus on exposing, reducing, and stabilizing (reestablishing) the cortical perimeter of the scapula, particularly the lateral border/glenoid neck pillar. Surgical indications may change and alterations/improvements in operative management will undoubtedly occur as experience accumulates, but the senior author firmly believes that this more aggressive approach to the treatment of selected scapular body/spine fractures will lead to significantly improved outcomes.

Isolated Coracoid Process Fractures[111]

Fractures of the coracoid tip are generally managed nonoperatively initially. However, late surgical management may be necessary if the displaced bony fragment causes irritation of the surrounding soft tissues.[29] Surgical management (either acute or late) takes two forms[94]: ORIF of the bony fragment if it is sufficiently large and not comminuted, and excision of the fragment if comminuted with suture fixation of the conjoined tendon to the remaining coracoid process (Fig. 7-49). With fractures occurring between the coracoclavicular and coracoacromial ligaments, the fragment is larger and symptomatic irritation of local soft tissues is more common. Consequently, surgical management (acute or late) is more likely. The size of the fragment generally makes it

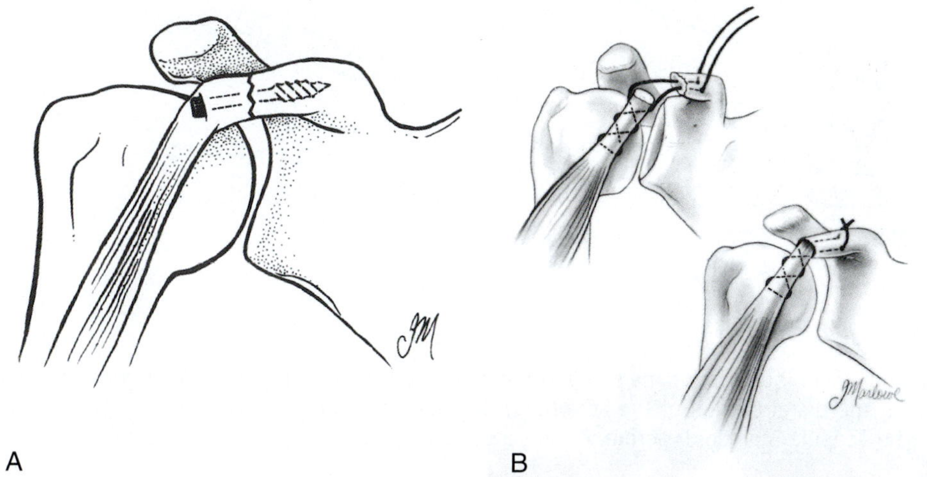

FIGURE 7-49: Two surgical techniques for managing coracoid process fractures. **A,** Interfragmentary screw fixation may be used if the fragment is sufficiently large and not comminuted. **B,** Excision of the distal fragment for small or comminuted fractures and suture fixation of the conjoined tendon to the remaining coracoid process. (Modified from Goss TP. Fractures of the scapula: diagnosis and treatment. In: Iannotti JP, Williams GR Jr, eds. *Disorders of the Shoulder: Diagnosis and Management.* Philadelphia, Lippincott Williams & Wilkins; 1999:628.)

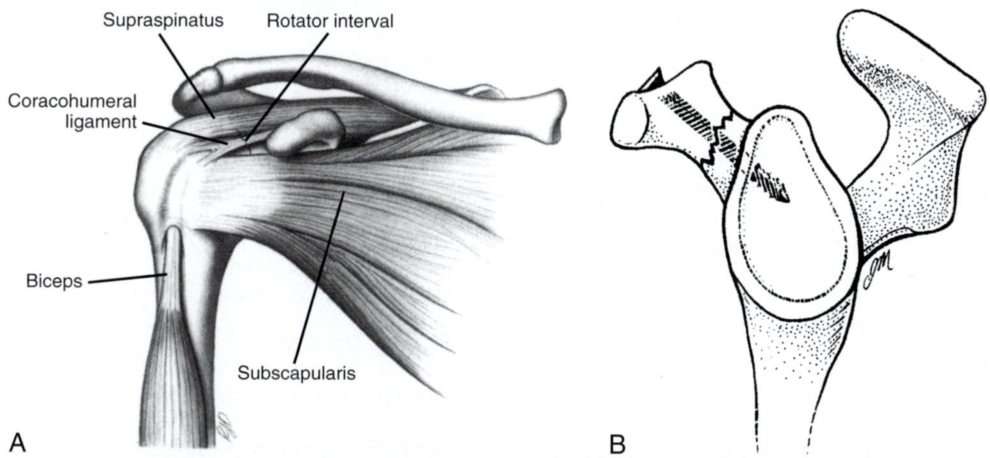

FIGURE 7-50: **A,** The rotator interval and surrounding soft tissues can be opened to expose the coracoid process, including its junction with the glenoid process. **B,** A coracoid process fracture reduced and stabilized with an interfragmentary compression screw.

amenable to interfragmentary screw fixation. Cannulated compression screws are particularly useful. With fractures of the base of the coracoid process, nonoperative care is usually sufficient. However, if significantly displaced or in the event of a symptomatic nonunion, compression screw fixation with or without bone grafting must be considered. As with all coracoid process fractures managed surgically, an anterior deltoid-splitting or a limited deltopectoral approach may be used, and the rotator interval is opened as needed for optimal exposure of the fracture site (Fig. 7-50).

Isolated Acromial Process Fractures

Symptomatic, nonoperative care generally leads to union and a good to excellent functional result. However, if unacceptable displacement is present, surgical reduction and stabilization must be considered.[111] A tension band construct is usually chosen for distal disruptions where the acromial process is quite thin, whereas 3.5-mm malleable reconstruction plates are generally chosen for more proximal injuries (Fig. 7-51).[98]

Double Disruptions of the Superior Shoulder Suspensory Complex

If two (or more) disruptions of the SSSC are present, the clinician must decide whether displacement at one or both sites is unacceptable (unacceptable being a relative term that depends upon the particular clinical situation). If so, surgical management is generally necessary. As emphasized earlier, not all double disruptions require

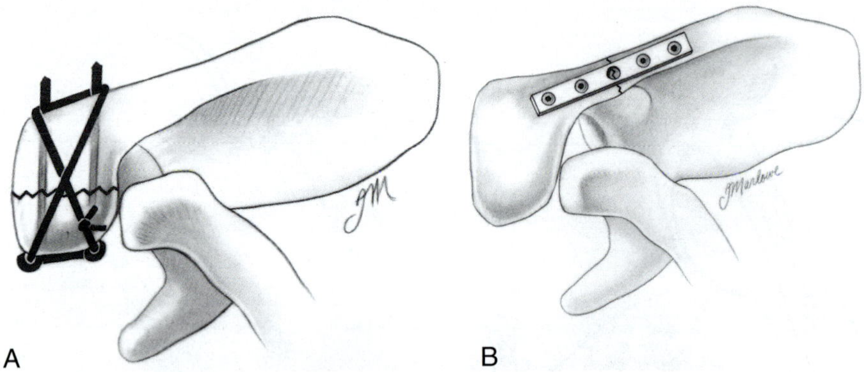

FIGURE 7-51: Two surgical techniques for managing fractures of the acromial process. **A,** A tension band construct (most appropriate for fractures of the distal portion of the acromion). **B,** Plate and screw fixation (most appropriate for proximal fractures). (From Goss TP. The scapula: coracoid, acromial, and avulsion fractures. *Am J Orthop.* 1996;25[2]:106-115.)

surgical management. Reducing and stabilizing one of the disruptions often indirectly reduces and stabilizes the other satisfactorily (whichever injury is easier to manage is chosen). If unsuccessful, both disruptions may need to be addressed. The results, as always, are dependent upon the adequacy of the reduction, the quality of the fixation, and the rigor of the postoperative rehabilitation program.

Avulsion Fractures of the Scapula

The majority of these injuries are managed nonoperatively; however, ORIF is indicated if the fracture is significantly displaced and functionally significant.

Glenoid Process Fractures (General Considerations)

The glenoid process includes the glenoid neck and the glenoid cavity, which includes the glenoid rim and the glenoid fossa. Each of these areas can be fractured in various ways. The vast majority (>90%) of these injuries are managed satisfactorily nonoperatively, and a good to excellent result can be expected. However, most investigators agree that if displacement is significant, surgical management is indicated or should at least be considered.

Principles of Surgery

Several operative principles apply (Box 7-8). The glenoid process may be approached from three directions or combinations thereof, depending upon the clinical situation.[227] The anterior deltopectoral approach is used for fractures of the anterior glenoid rim and at least in part for some fractures involving the superior aspect of the glenoid fossa (Fig. 7-52). Some injuries require only opening the rotator interval (see Fig. 7-50) without detaching the subscapularis tendon. The posterior approach is used for fractures of the posterior rim, most fractures of the glenoid fossa, and fractures of the glenoid neck (Figs. 7-53 and 7-54). The superior approach may be used for fractures of the glenoid fossa that have a difficult-to-control superior fragment (in conjunction with a posterior exposure) and fractures of the glenoid neck that have a difficult-to-control glenoid fragment (in conjunction with a posterior exposure) (Figs. 7-55 and 7-56). Klingman and Roffman described a variation of the posterior approach that allowed ORIF of anterior as well as posterior glenoid fragments.[154] Van Noort et al. described a limited posterior approach,[287] and Ombremsky and Lyman described a modified Judet (posterior) approach for ORIF of glenoid process fractures.[223]

Thick, solid bone for fixation is at a premium because much of the scapula is paper thin. However, four areas are satisfactory: the glenoid neck, the lateral scapular border, the acromial process and scapular spine, and the

BOX 7-8. Glenoid Process Fractures: Surgical Considerations

Surgical Approaches
Anterior
Posterior
Superior
Combinations

Bone Stock
Glenoid process
Acromial process/scapular spine
Coracoid process
Lateral scapular border
Medial scapular border

Fixation Devices
Cannulated screws
Malleable reconstruction plates
K-wires
Dynamic compression plates
Locking plates

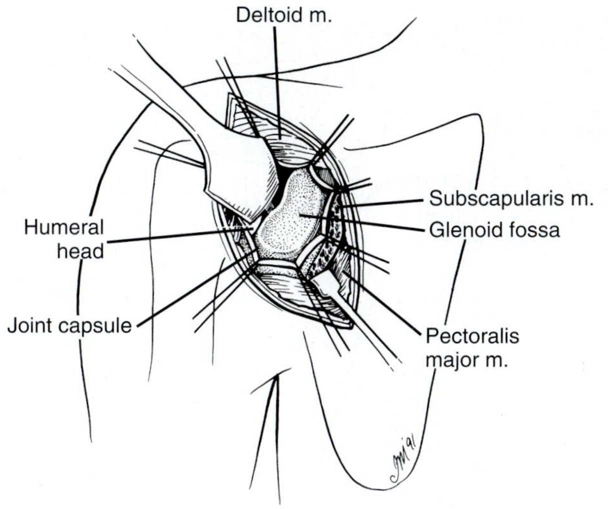

FIGURE 7-52: Anterior surgical approach to the glenoid cavity. (From Goss TP. Fractures of the glenoid cavity: operative principles and techniques. *Tech Orthop*. 1993;8[3]:199-204.)

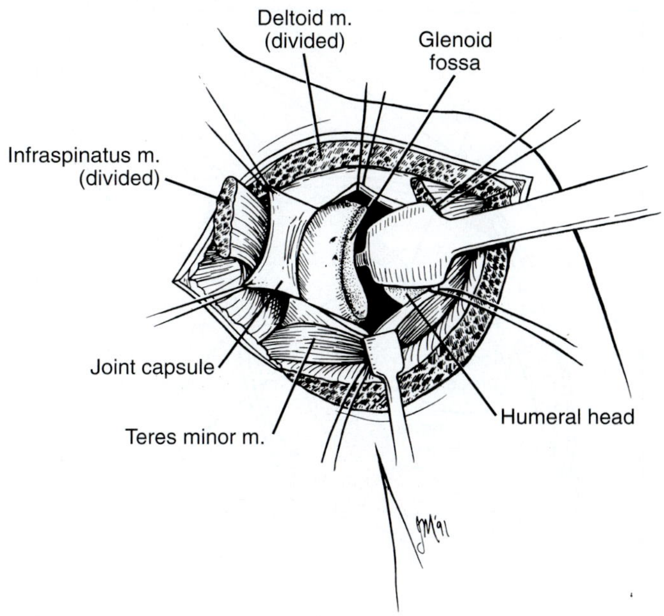

FIGURE 7-53: Posterior surgical approach to the glenoid cavity: standard exposure. (From Goss TP. Fractures of the glenoid cavity: operative principles and techniques. *Tech Orthop*. 1993;8[3]:199-204.)

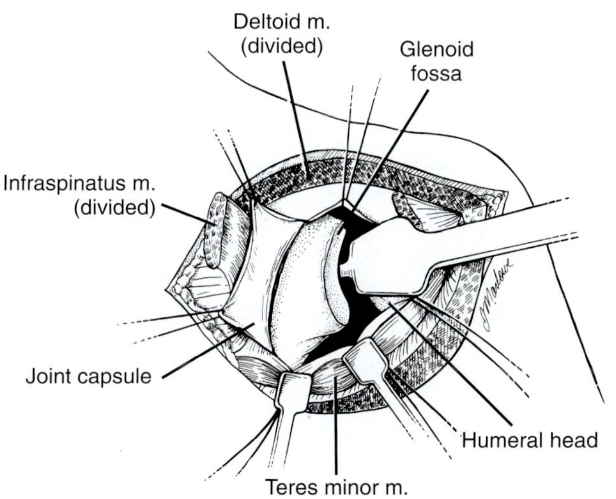

FIGURE 7-54: Posterior surgical approach to the glenoid cavity with development of the infraspinatus–teres minor interval to expose the posteroinferior glenoid cavity and the lateral scapular border. (From Goss TP. Fractures of the glenoid cavity: operative principles and techniques. *Tech Orthop*. 1993;8[3]:199-204.)

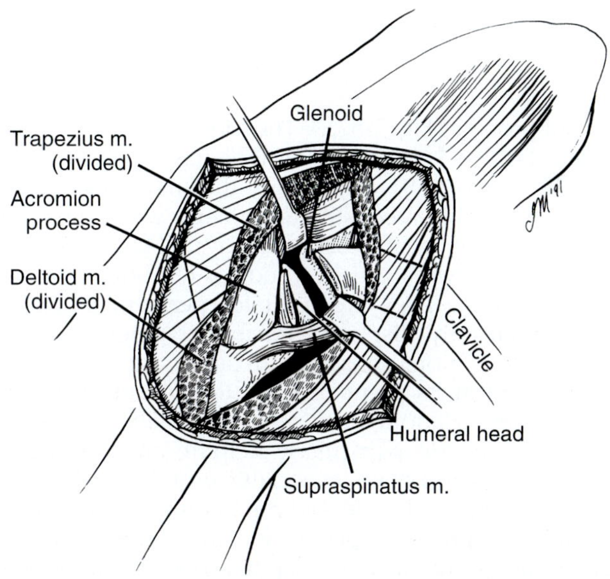

FIGURE 7-55: Superior surgical approach to the glenoid cavity: soft tissue and bony anatomy. (From Goss TP. Fractures of the glenoid cavity: operative principles and techniques. *Tech Orthop*. 1993;8[3]:199-204.)

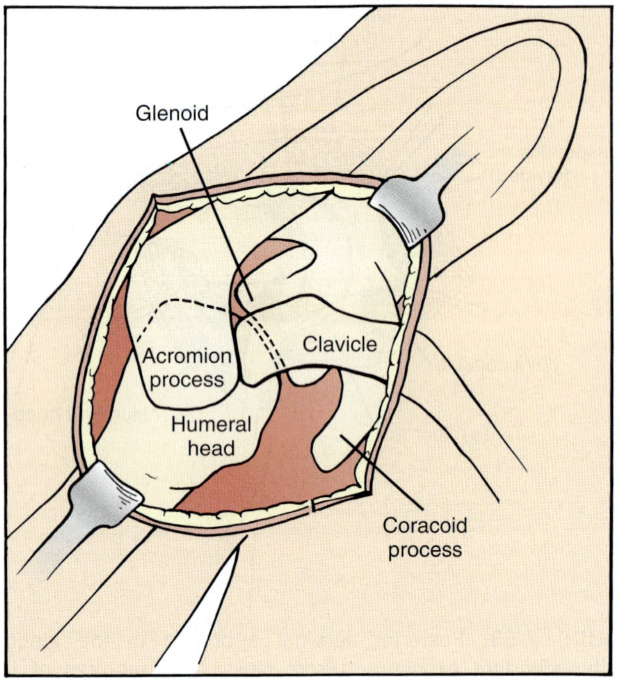

FIGURE 7-56: Superior surgical approach to the glenoid cavity: bony anatomy. (From Goss TP: Fractures of the glenoid cavity: operative principles and techniques. *Tech Orthop.* 1993;8[3]: 199-204.)

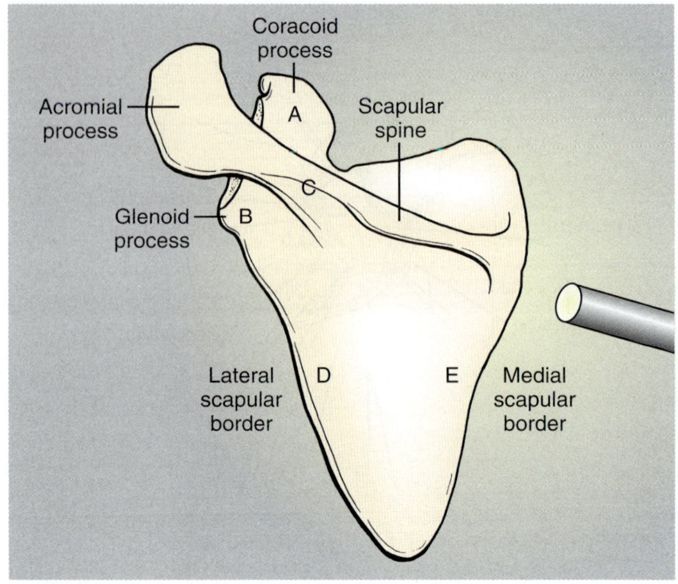

FIGURE 7-57: The scapula and areas of bone stock for internal fixation. *A,* The coracoid process; *B,* the glenoid process; *C,* the scapular spine and acromial process; *D,* the lateral scapular border; and *E,* the medial scapular border (limited bone stock but sufficient for locking plates). (Modified from Goss TP. Fractures of the glenoid cavity: operative principles and techniques. *Tech Orthop.* 1993;8[3]:199-204.)

coracoid process (Fig. 7-57).[45] The medial scapular border cortex is far less substantial. Various fixation devices are available (Fig. 7-58). However, the most useful are K-wires, malleable reconstruction plates, and cannulated interfragmentary compression screws (Figs. 7-59 and 7-60).[105,110,113] K-wires can be used for temporary or permanent fixation. They are used for permanent fixation when significantly displaced fracture fragments are too small to allow more substantial fixation, but the K-wire must be bent at its point of entry to prevent migration. For managing glenoid neck fractures, malleable reconstruction plates are particularly helpful, and cannulated compression screws are especially useful in stabilizing fractures involving the glenoid rim and the glenoid fossa. Dynamic compression plates, locking plates (e.g., for fixation along the medial scapular border), and other fixation devices may be of benefit in specific situations.

These devices may be used alone or in combination depending on the clinical situation and the available bone stock, as well as the surgeon's preference and experience. Rigid fixation is desirable, but inability to achieve this goal does not preclude an excellent anatomic and functional result.

Postoperative Management

Postoperative management of glenoid process fractures depends on the quality of the fixation and stability achieved. Immobilization in a sling and swathe binder is

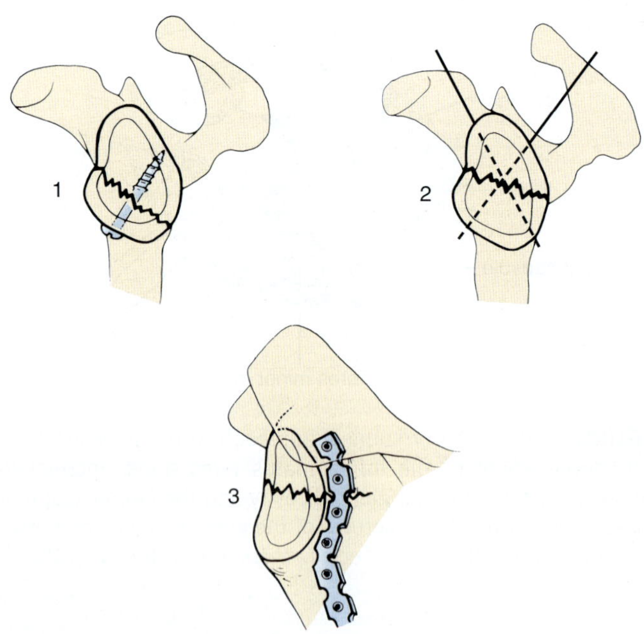

FIGURE 7-58: Fixation techniques available for stabilization of fractures of the glenoid cavity. *1,* An interfragmentary compression screw; *2,* K-wires; and *3,* a contoured malleable reconstruction plate. (From Goss TP. Fractures of the glenoid cavity [Current Concepts Review]. *J Bone Joint Surg Am.* 1992;74[2]: 299-305.)

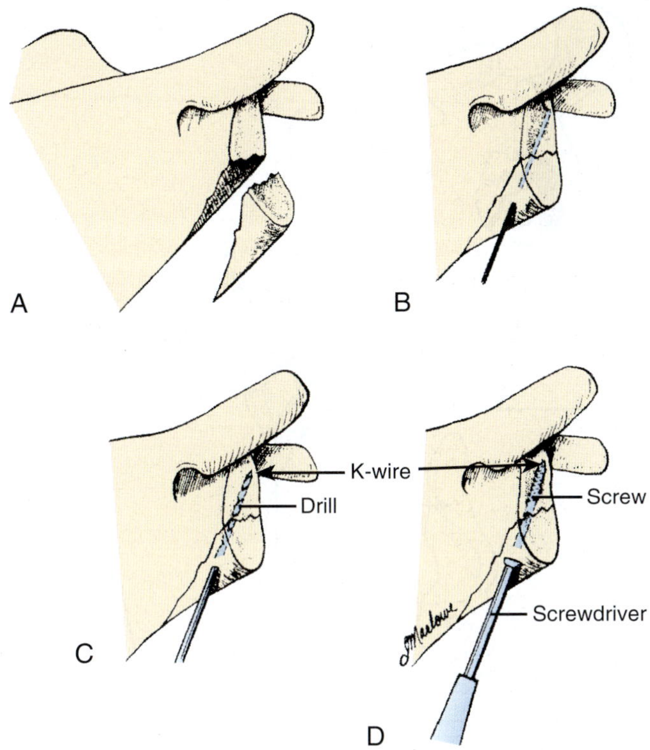

FIGURE 7-59: Reduction and stabilization of a type II fracture of the glenoid cavity with a cannulated interfragmentary compression screw. **A,** Fracture of the glenoid cavity with a significantly displaced inferior glenoid fragment. **B,** Reduction of the glenoid fragment and stabilization with a guidewire. **C,** Use of the guidewire (K-wire) to pass a cannulated drill and eventually a cannulated tap. **D,** Use of the guidewire to place a cannulated interfragmentary compression screw to securely fix the glenoid fragment in position. (From Goss TP. Fractures of the glenoid cavity: operative principles and techniques. *Tech Orthop.* 1993;8[3]:199-204.)

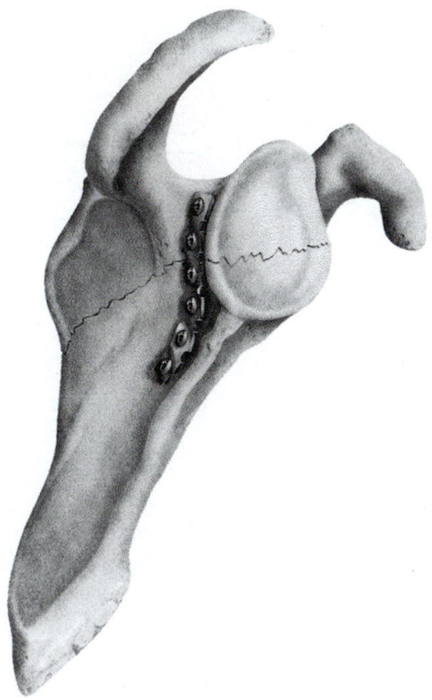

FIGURE 7-60: Reduction and stabilization of a glenoid cavity fracture with a contoured malleable reconstruction plate. (From Goss TP. Glenoid fractures: open reduction internal fixation. In: Wiss DA, ed. *Master Techniques in Orthopaedic Surgery. Fractures.* Philadelphia, Lippincott-Raven; 1998:10.)

prescribed for the first 24 to 48 hours after surgery. If fixation is rigid, dependent circular and pendulum movements are then initiated, as well as external rotation of the shoulder to but not past neutral. During postoperative weeks 3 to 6, progressive range-of-motion exercises in all directions (especially forward flexion, internal rotation up the back, and external rotation) are prescribed with the goal of achieving full range of motion by the end of the 6-week period. The patient is allowed to use the arm actively in a progressive manner within clearly defined limits (moving the weight of the extremity alone when sitting in a protected setting during weeks 3 and 4 and when up and about indoors during weeks 5 and 6).

The patient is evaluated clinically and radiographically every 1 to 2 weeks to make sure that displacement does not occur at the fracture site and to monitor and update the rehabilitation program. At 6 weeks, healing is usually sufficient so as to discontinue all external protection and encourage progressive functional use of the extremity. K-wires spanning bones that move relative to each other are removed at this time, as are those passing through soft tissues (K-wires embedded within a single osseous structure and bent at their entry site to prevent migration may be left in place). Physical therapy continues, focusing on regaining range of motion as progressive strengthening exercises are added.

The patient's rehabilitation program continues until range of motion, strength, and overall function are maximized. Light use of the shoulder is emphasized through postoperative week 12, and heavy physical use of the shoulder, including athletic activities, is prohibited until the 3- to 6-month point. If surgical fixation is less than rigid, the shoulder may need to be protected in a sling and swathe binder, in an abduction brace, or even in overhead olecranon pin traction for 7, 10, or 14 days (depending on the clinical situation) before the physical therapy program is begun. The patient must be encouraged to work diligently on the rehabilitation program because range of motion and strength can improve, and the end result is often not achieved for approximately 6 months to 1 year after injury. Hard work, perseverance, and dedication on the part of the patient, the physician, and the physical therapist are critical to an optimal functional result.

Although the literature remains somewhat deficient because of the rarity of these injuries, increased interest

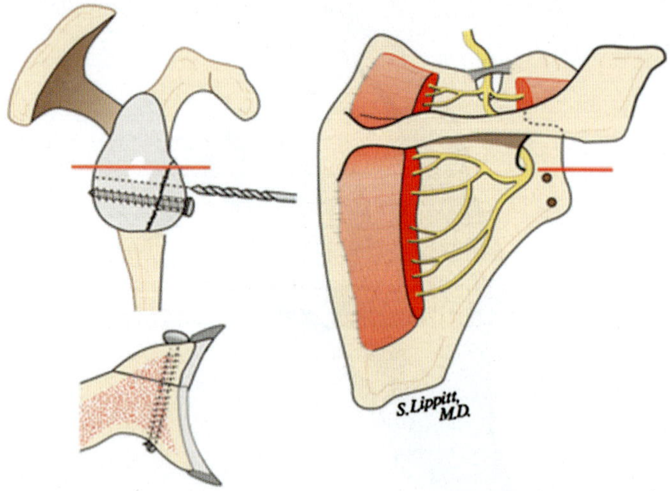

FIGURE 7-61: Recommended placement of two anterior-to-posterior cannulated interfragmentary compression screws below the equator of the glenoid, staying away from the suprascapular nerve. (Courtesy Dr. Steven B. Lippitt.)

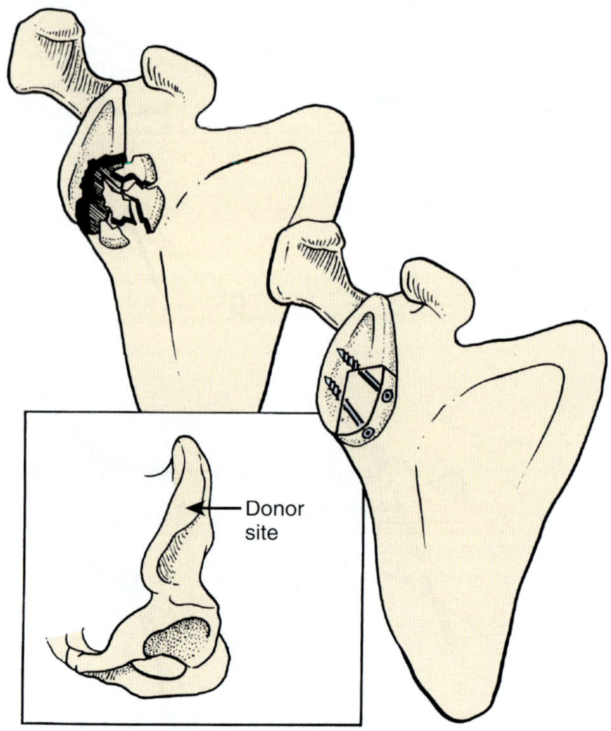

FIGURE 7-62: Use of a tricortical graft harvested from the iliac crest to reestablish bony stability in a patient with a severely comminuted type Ia fracture of the glenoid cavity.

in recent years has resulted in a growing number of case reports and personal series. Although more data are needed, it is reasonable to anticipate a good to excellent functional result if surgical management restores normal or near-normal glenoid anatomy, articular congruity, and glenohumeral stability; if the fixation is secure; and if a well-structured, closely monitored postoperative rehabilitation program is implemented.

Glenoid Cavity Fractures

Type I (glenoid rim)[104-106,108] fractures are managed surgically if the fracture results in persistent subluxation of the humeral head or if the articulation is unstable after reduction. Instability is often the case if the fracture is displaced 10 mm or more and if a quarter or more of the glenoid cavity anteriorly or a third or more of the glenoid cavity posteriorly is involved. Type Ia (anterior rim) fractures are approached anteriorly. The displaced fragment is mobilized, reduced anatomically, and fixed in position with two cannulated interfragmentary compression screws (ideally, two screws are used to provide rotational stability). The screws are placed anterior to posterior below the equator of the glenoid to avoid injury to the suprascapular nerve (see Fig. 7-18, Fig. 7-61). Type Ib (posterior fractures) are approached posteriorly and reduced and stabilized in the same manner (see Fig. 7-19). If the fracture is comminuted, the fragments are excised. A tricortical graft harvested from the iliac crest is then placed intra-articularly to fill the defect (Fig. 7-62). A simple repair of the periarticular soft tissues to the intact glenoid cavity is an option if the bone defect is less than 20% of the articular surface, but restoration of the rim contour is preferable.

Based on available reports, it seems reasonable to conclude that surgery has a definite role in the treatment of glenoid fossa fractures (types II-V). An injury with an articular step-off of 5 mm or more should be considered for surgical intervention to restore articular congruity, and displacement of 10 mm or more is an absolute indication to avoid posttraumatic osteoarthritis. Another indication is such severe separation of the fracture fragment(s) that nonunion at the injury site and/or chronic instability of the glenohumeral joint is likely.

Type II fractures are approached posteriorly. The infraspinatus–teres minor interval is developed to expose the displaced inferior glenoid process fragment and the lateral scapular border. The fragment is reduced as anatomically as possible and stabilized, generally with two cannulated interfragmentary compression screws passed posteroinferiorly to anterosuperiorly (see Fig. 7-22) or with a contoured reconstruction plate placed along the posterior aspect of the glenoid process and the lateral scapular border. Excision of the fracture fragment and placement of a bone graft from the iliac crest is an option if the fragment is severely comminuted. Associated tears of the labral-capsular-ligamentous complex are repaired if possible, as they are with all fractures of the glenoid cavity. Detachments are corrected with nonabsorbable sutures passed through drill holes or with suture anchors. Intrasubstance tears are reapproximated with nonabsorbable sutures passed in a figure-of-eight fashion.

Type III fractures are approached either via a posterosuperior exposure or anteriorly through the rotator interval. A K-wire can be placed into the superior glenoid fragment and used to manipulate it into satisfactory position relative to the remainder of the glenoid process, thereby restoring articular congruity. The K-wire is then driven across the fracture site and used to place a cannulated interfragmentary compression screw. In patients with a significantly displaced additional disruption of the SSSC, reduction and stabilization of the superior glenoid fragment may restore the integrity of the complex satisfactorily. If not, the other injury may need to be addressed as well (see Fig. 7-23). Conversely, if the superior glenoid fragment is severely comminuted and difficult to fix, operative restoration of the additional SSSC disruption can improve glenoid articular congruity indirectly and satisfactorily.

Type IV fractures are approached posterosuperiorly or with a combined posterior-anterior (through the rotator interval) exposure. A K-wire is placed into the superior glenoscapular segment and used to manipulate the fragment into position relative to the inferior segment while directly visualizing the reduction via the posterior exposure. The K-wire is then driven across the fracture site and used to place a cannulated interfragmentary compression screw (see Fig. 7-24). A cerclage wire or cerclage suture passed around the glenoid neck may also be used for fixation, as well as a malleable reconstruction plate. Reduction and stabilization of the fracture at its exit site over the medial border of the scapular body may also be of benefit. As always, care must be taken to avoid injury to adjacent neurovascular structures, in particular the suprascapular nerve and vessels, which pass through the spinoglenoid notch.

Type Va fractures are approached, reduced, and stabilized according to the principles described for significantly displaced type II fractures, although a superior approach may need to be added to gain control over the superior glenoscapular fragment. Type Vb injuries are approached, reduced, and stabilized according to the principles described for significantly displaced type III fractures. If an additional disruption of the SSSC is present, it may require operative reduction and stabilization. Type Vc fractures are exposed via a posterosuperior or a combined posterior–anterior (via the rotator interval) approach. The superior and inferior glenoid fragments are reduced anatomically and rigidly fixed to each other, ideally with a lag screw passed superiorly to inferiorly. The glenoid fragment is then reduced and stabilized relative to the inferior portion of the scapular body using the principles described for ORIF of glenoid neck fractures (see Fig. 7-25). Additional disruptions of the SSSC may require attention as well. Reduction and stabilization of the fracture at its exit site over the medial border of the scapular body may also be of benefit.

Type VI fractures are managed nonoperatively. However, an associated disruption of the SSSC might warrant surgical correction and indirectly improve glenoid articular congruity. The upper extremity is initially protected in a sling and swathe binder, an abduction brace, or even overhead olecranon pin traction—whichever maximizes articular congruity as determined radiographically. Gentle passive rotatory range-of-motion exercises performed by a therapist and the patient are initiated immediately, in hope that movement of the humeral head will mold the articular fragments into a maximally congruous position. By 2 weeks, healing is sufficient to allow protection of such injuries in a sling and swathe binder. Exercises designed to gradually increase range of motion and progressive functional use of the shoulder out of the sling (within clearly defined limits) are prescribed during the subsequent 4 weeks. At 6 weeks, these fractures are sufficiently healed to allow discontinuation of all external protection. Functional use of the shoulder is encouraged and physical therapy continues until range of motion and strength are maximized. These injuries clearly have the highest potential for posttraumatic degenerative joint disease and glenohumeral instability.

Glenoid Neck Fractures

Clearly, the vast majority of true glenoid neck fractures can and should be treated nonoperatively; however, more aggressive management, including ORIF, is indicated when the glenoid fragment is significantly displaced (type II injuries).[109] Some might quarrel with 1 cm of ML translational displacement being an indication for surgery; however, the decision to proceed operatively becomes easier with increasing degrees of displacement. (see Fig. 7-12). Forty degrees (or more, certainly) of AP angular displacement of the glenoid fragment also seems to be a reasonable indication for surgical management as well as a decrease in the GPA to 20 degrees or less. (see Fig. 7-13).

The fracture site is approached posteriorly. The interval between the infraspinatus and teres minor is developed to expose the posteroinferior glenoid neck and lateral scapular border. A superior approach can be added to gain control over the free glenoid fragment. Once a satisfactory reduction has been achieved, temporary fixation can be provided by placing K-wires between the glenoid fragment and the adjacent bony structures (e.g., through the glenoid fragment and into the scapular body or through the acromial process and into the glenoid fragment). Firm fixation is generally achieved by means of a contoured, malleable reconstruction plate applied along the lateral border of the scapula and the posterior aspect of the glenoid process. Supplemental fixation can be provided by K-wires or lag screws. K-wires providing temporary fixation can be retained or used for placing cannulated lag screws (Fig. 7-63).

Conceivably, comminution can be so severe or the size of the glenoid fragment so small that plate fixation is precluded. In these cases, Kirschner-wire or lag-screw fixation of the reduced glenoid fragment to adjacent intact bony structures (e.g., the acromial process, the distal end of the clavicle, or other structures) may be all that is available. If a disruption of the clavicular–acromioclavicular joint–acromial strut is also present, fixation of that injury might indirectly reduce and stabilize the glenoid neck fracture satisfactorily. However, if significant displacement persists, the glenoid neck fracture must also be addressed.[109] Conversely, ORIF of the glenoid neck fracture may satisfactorily reduce and stabilize the second disruption. If not, the associated disruption must be addressed.

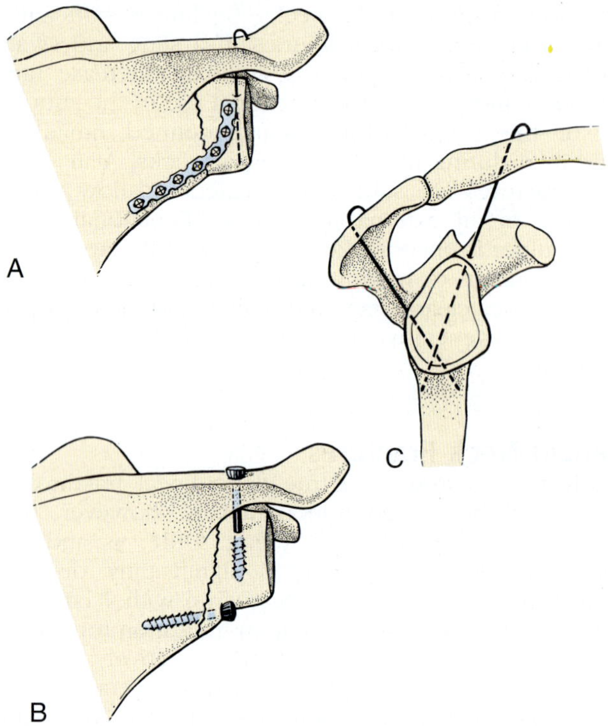

FIGURE 7-63: Fixation techniques available for stabilization of glenoid neck fractures. **A,** Stabilization with a contoured malleable reconstruction plate (note the K-wire running from the acromial process into the glenoid process, which can be used for temporary or permanent fixation). **B,** Stabilization with cannulated interfragmentary compression screws. **C,** Stabilization with K-wires (in this case, K-wires passed from the acromion and clavicle into the glenoid process). (From Goss TP. Fractures of the glenoid neck. *J Shoulder Elbow Surg.* 1994;3[1]:42-52.)

Disruptions of the C-4 linkage with or without a disruption of the coracoacromial ligament are usually managed indirectly by reducing and stabilizing the glenoid neck fracture and any injuries compromising the integrity of the clavicular–acromioclavicular joint–acromial strut. Rarely, if comminution of the glenoid neck and surrounding bony structures is particularly severe, overhead olecranon pin traction must be considered or displacement of the glenoid neck fracture accepted and managed nonoperatively. ORIF of associated scapular body fractures may also aid in the reduction and stabilization of glenoid neck fractures.

Scapulothoracic Dissociation

The senior author has treated five such cases. The key to diagnosis is awareness of the clinical entity. These injuries, although rare, may be more common than previously thought. All the injuries seen have included a disruption of the sternal-clavicular-acromial linkage, most commonly a fracture of the distal third of the clavicle. Every effort is made to reduce and stabilize this component of the injury for the reasons noted earlier.[111] The upper extremity is protected for 6 weeks, during which a progressive rehabilitation program is instituted. Late reconstructive efforts are dictated by the degree of neurologic return.

Intrathoracic Dislocation

We have not encountered this rare injury. Therapeutic principles noted in the literature and detailed earlier are followed.

Scapulothoracic Crepitus

Active management is indicated if scapulothoracic crepitus is truly painful, and thus represents an underlying pathologic condition. Clearly defined bony prominences within the scapulothoracic interval refractory to nonoperative treatment are resected but are rare. Other presumed etiologies are best managed nonoperatively, and the majority respond satisfactorily. Surgery is a consideration in those that do not, especially if symptoms are relatively localized. Exploration of the symptomatic area with judicious bony resection and removal of questionable soft tissue is generally performed, but the results are quite mixed.

AUTHORS' FINAL NOTE

The management of scapular fractures has traditionally been of low priority since they comprise only 1% of all fractures, and the vast majority (≥90%) are treated nonoperatively with highly satisfactory results. However, more recently, significantly displaced fractures of the glenoid process (glenoid rim, glenoid fossa, and glenoid neck) and significantly displaced fractures of the coracoid and acromial processes (frequently part of a double disruption of the SSSC) have drawn the attention of the orthopedic community, resulting in increasing surgical intervention. Papers published by Goss and Ideberg have been particularly important in this regard. Now, disruptions of the scapular body (and scapular spine) requiring operative management are being recognized and treated accordingly. Cole and his group have been especially active in this area. The overall goal is to identify displaced scapular fractures that require surgical reduction and stabilization in an effort to restore the normal bony, intra-articular, and soft tissue relationships within this complex anatomic system and thereby obtain optimal shoulder function. Large series evaluating the results of surgical management have been difficult to obtain since (1) scapular fractures requiring operative intervention are uncommon, (2) a wide variety of disruptions can occur, and (3) follow-up in this patient population is difficult. Nevertheless, series with increasingly significant numbers of operatively managed patients are gradually appearing. As a result, operative indications and surgical techniques are being refined, and functional results are steadily improving.

INTERNATIONAL EXPERT COMMENTARY

Jan Bartoníček

Our commentary on this chapter is based on our experience of a group of 305 scapular fractures, of which 253 were treated with 3D CT reconstruction and 109 were treated operatively. Based on our analysis of this group, we published several articles dealing with the radiodiagnostics of scapular fractures, bilateral scapular fractures, outcomes of the treatment of fractures of the scapular neck, and outcomes of the operative treatment of fractures of the scapular neck. We also published an anatomic study of the internal architecture of the scapula, a clinicoanatomic study of the Judet posterior approach, and a radiologically based anatomic study of the GPA. Two additional studies are in print, namely an epidemiologic study of scapular fractures (250 patients) and a study of the pathoanatomy of fractures of the glenoid fossa (90 glenoid fractures with 3D CT reconstructions).[15,16,18-21,23,24,53,280-282]

Based on these studies, we have developed our own strategy for the treatment of scapular fractures in the following respects.

Anatomy

Based on the study of the internal architecture of the scapula, we have formulated a biomechanical concept of the infraspinous portion of the scapular "biomechanical" body that is formed by two pillars, the spinal and lateral. These pillars transmit compression forces from the glenoid fossa to the scapular body. Therefore our main goal for operative treatment of fractures of the scapular body and neck is to restore the biomechanical continuity of the body.

Diagnostics

A majority of patients in our group sustained an injury caused by medium-energy trauma, such as after fall from bicycle or motorcycle at a relatively slow speed, with the predominance of injuries to the scapula and shoulder girdle, sometimes associated with other injuries. A smaller subset of our group included elderly patients who had sustained scapular fractures after a simple fall onto flat ground or down stairs.

To avoid missing scapular injuries, as is often reported in the literature, we use full-body CT that captures both scapulae. In our view, scapular fractures cannot be reliably classified without 3D CT reconstructions. Therefore, in all patients with scapular fractures, we perform CT examination of the shoulder girdle, including standardized 3D CT reconstructions (anterior, posterior and lateral views) with subtraction of the surrounding bones, particularly the ribs and humeral head (for glenoid fossa fractures).

Classification

Classification into fractures of the scapular body, neck, glenoid, and processes has been generally accepted. Our classification of scapular fractures is based on 3D CT reconstructions and intraoperative findings as described below.

Our classification defines fractures of the scapular neck as extra-articular fractures of the lateral angle of the scapula, that is, fractures of the anatomic and surgical neck and transspinous fractures of the neck. We do not consider the so-called *infraspinous fracture of the scapular neck* as a fracture of the scapular neck but rather as a fracture of the infraspinous portion of the scapular body. This quite frequent fracture does not separate the glenoid fossa from the scapular body but splits the scapular body into two parts. In addition, this fracture is often combined with fracture of the clavicle. Some authors incorrectly classify this combination of fractures as a "floating" shoulder, which causes much confusion and misinterpretation.

With regard to glenoid fractures, we divide them, on the basis of our analysis of 90 fractures with 3D CT reconstructions (52 treated operatively), into fractures of the superior glenoid (intra-articular fracture of the coracoid base), the anterior glenoid rim, the posterior glenoid rim, the inferior glenoid (the most frequent of all glenoid fossa fractures seen in our group and almost always combined with a fracture of the scapular body), and the entire glenoid (all fragments of the glenoid fossa are separated from the scapular neck or body). This division reflects the mechanism of the injury and also dictates the choice of surgical approach.

In our classification, fractures of the processes or borders of the scapula include fractures of the superior angle and superior border of the scapula. These parts serve only for the attachment of muscles and are not involved in the biomechanical function of the scapular body, that is, the transmission of compression forces from the glenoid fossa to the scapular body.

Therapeutic Indications

We treat all nondisplaced or minimally displaced fractures nonoperatively. Intra-articular fractures involving 25% to 30% of the articular surface in the "circular area" (the lower two-thirds of the glenoid fossa), those with a 3- to 4-mm gap or step, and those with instability of the shoulder joint constitute strong indications for operation. Regarding fractures of the superior glenoid, we are more reserved. Regarding extra-articular fractures, we respect Cole's criteria of displacement of fragments of the lateral border of the scapula. Therefore we consider operative treatment in cases involving fractures of the scapular body and neck with a translation of more than 1 cm, with 30% to 40% angulation and mediolateral displacement of more than 1 cm, and with a GPA less than 20 degrees. However, we always consider the patient's general conditions (age, concomitant diseases, level of physical activity), as well as local conditions. We are prepared to operate on selected patients aged 60 to 70 years.

Surgical Approaches

We consider it essential to master the Judet approach and its various modifications. We use this approach in all fractures of the scapular body and neck and fractures of the posterior, inferior, and entire glenoid. Where possible, we prefer a limited approach, without full mobilization of infraspinatus, via the interval between the infraspinatus and the teres minor. If this is not possible, we mobilize partially, or totally, only the infraspinatus and not the teres minor. We use the anterior deltoidopectoral approach in fractures of the superior and anterior glenoid and in coracoid fractures. A superior approach along the scapular spine and acromion is used in fractures of these elements of the scapula.

Internal Fixation Technique

We prefer a stable internal fixation and, where appropriate, we prefer 2.7- to 3.5-mm implants. We do not use K-wires, except for the lost K-wire technique. Locking plates are applied only exceptionally in regions of poor bone stock.

In extra-articular fractures, our aim is to reconstruct both pillars or, where necessary, the circumference of the entire biomechanical body. We usually start on the lateral pillar

Continued

INTERNATIONAL EXPERT COMMENTARY—cont'd

(border). The internal fixation does not need to be massive, depending on the fracture pattern and robustness of the patient. After fixation of the injured pillar(s), we assess the stability of the entire biomechanical body and, if necessary, we add internal fixation in the region of the spinomedial or inferior angle of the scapula.

In intra-articular fractures, the biggest challenge regards those of the inferior glenoid (the most frequently surgically treated fracture pattern in our study group) and the entire glenoid. We have no experience with arthroscopic surgery.

We treat fracture-dislocations of the clavicle and AC joint dislocations after completion of ORIF of the scapula, never before. In our experience, reduction and ORIF of the clavicle alone does not lead to reduction of associated scapular fractures.

Postoperative Rehabilitation

Postoperative rehabilitation is an important part of the treatment regimen. Passive rehabilitation starts on the second postoperative day using continuous passive motion. The start date of active motion exercises depends on the fracture pattern and intraoperative mobilization of the infraspinatus, and is, as a rule, after 3 to 4 weeks postoperatively. According to our experience, mobilization of the infraspinatus increases postoperative pain and so has a negative impact on the course of rehabilitation. In case of a significant limitation in the range of motion in the shoulder joint at the 6-week postoperative follow-up, we seriously consider examination and manipulation of the shoulder joint under general anaesthesia.

Evaluation and Complications

Patients are followed up postoperatively at 6 weeks and 3, 6, and 12 months, with examination including radiographs and, in cases of intra-articular fractures, CT.

We have encountered various complications in scapular fractures. A relatively frequent complication is paresis of the infraspinatus caused by injury to the suprascapular nerve. This complication is most often seen in fractures of the surgical neck of the scapula in which the nerve was entrapped in the fracture line in the spinoglenoid notch. Another possible complication is intraoperative injury during mobilization of the infraspinatus in the Judet approach. We also observed one case of penetration of a screw into the joint cavity. Early postoperative complications included hematoma in the wound (two cases, healed without sequelae after surgical evacuation) and one early deep infection that healed without chronic infection after repeated revisions. Late complications included breakage of the plate (two cases, associated with starting active motion too early and healing without loss of reduction), posttraumatic osteoarthritis of the glenohumeral joint (one case after fracture of the superior glenoid), and a significant limitation in the range of motion of the shoulder (one case of a 70-year-old female patient with a fracture dislocation of the inferior glenoid). Nonunion was not recorded in our group. We operated on one multitrauma patient with a significantly displaced malunion at 4 months after injury involving an open extra-articular fracture of the scapular body. The indication was stiffness of the shoulder joint. Postoperatively, the range of motion improved considerably, and the surgical wound healed uneventfully.

EDITOR COMMENTARY

Steven B. Lippitt

Successful management of scapular trauma requires adequate understanding of relevant anatomy, scapulothoracic and glenohumeral biomechanics, fracture pathology, and appropriate treatment options. Scapular fractures are relatively rare and prove difficult for the casual shoulder surgeon to gain substantial experience in their treatment. Fortunately, the majority of scapular fractures are minimally displaced, often involving the scapular body and lending themselves to nonoperative treatment. Concern is due when presented with complex, displaced, angulated, and comminuted fracture patterns involving the glenoid neck or glenoid fossa.

Given the paucity and diversity of displaced scapula fractures, the literature lacks substantial evidence to guide definitive surgical indications and treatment methods. For example, past recommendations for the so-called "floating shoulder" (ipsilateral glenoid neck fracture and midshaft clavicle fracture) have ranged in treatment from nonoperative management to surgical ORIF of the clavicle, ORIF of the glenoid neck, or both. Classification schemes for scapular fracture (such as the Goss-Ideberg and AO/OTA described in this chapter) vary in defining fracture patterns and relevant displacement, and a reliable system has yet to be uniformly accepted. However, concepts regarding scapular fracture displacement as affecting shoulder girdle function are becoming quite clear. Intra-articular glenoid fractures relate to glenohumeral joint congruity, instability, and the risk of posttraumatic glenohumeral arthrosis. Anterior and posterior glenoid rim fractures with associated humeral subluxation should certainly warrant surgery consideration. Glenoid neck malalignment can contribute to rotator cuff and parascapular muscle dysfunction. Scapular body fracture malunion may lead to painful scapulothoracic crepitance.

Certain aspects of scapular fracture evaluation are worth emphasizing. Many scapular fractures herald significant patient trauma; thorough, serial physical exam is recommended to identify common and often significant associated injuries. Orthogonal radiographs in the scapular plane including AP, lateral Y, and axillary views are important for identifying the scapular fracture pattern. CT and 3D reconstruction better define the extent of fracture comminution and displacement when planning surgical intervention. In addition, the surgeon must understand scapular anatomy, with its limited available bone stock along with potentially unfamiliar extensile exposure, to obtain adequate reduction and fracture fixation. Patient factors such age, activity level, and medical comorbidity must be considered in conjunction with the treating surgeon's expertise when determining final treatment choice.

We are in debt to the esteemed authors, Dr. Thomas Goss and Dr. Marie Walcott, who have provided an exceptional summarization of more recent evidence on this subject of scapular fractures with their preferred treatment guidelines. They have provided in-depth discussion and many pertinent illustrations of glenoid rim, glenoid fossa, glenoid neck, coracoid, and acromial process fractures. The difficult concept of double disruptions of the SSSC is also very well outlined. New to this edition is an international perspective provided by Dr. Jan Bartonicek, of Prague, Czech Republic. His extensive career experience provides a very useful perspective of these complex injuries.

CHAPTER 8

Fractures of the Clavicle

Carl J. Basamania, Charles A. Rockwood Jr

A fracture of the clavicle has been greatly underrated in respect to pain and disability... The "usual or routine treatment" is perhaps far short of satisfying, relieving therapy.[345]

Carter R. Rowe, 1968

Although fractures of the clavicle do not typically pose a significant diagnostic challenge, there have been few injuries with as much controversy with regard to treatment. This clinical relevance is underscored when considering that the clavicle is the most common fracture site in children,[68,389] that an estimated 1 in 20 fractures involves the clavicle,[273] and that fractures of the clavicle constitute as much as 44% of shoulder girdle injuries.[345] Furthermore, it appears that the pattern of these fractures is changing, with fractures of much higher energy now being observed. Possibly as a consequence of this changing pattern, recent studies have shown poorer results with nonoperative treatment than with surgical intervention. There also seems to be a trend to recommend operative treatment for these more displaced fractures.

HISTORICAL REVIEW

The clavicle is entirely subcutaneous and thus is easily accessible for inspection and palpation, thereby possibly accounting for its inclusion in some of the earliest descriptions of injuries of the human skeleton and their treatment. As early as 400 BC, Hippocrates recorded several observations regarding clavicle fractures. With a fractured clavicle, the distal fragment and arm sag, whereas the proximal fragment, held securely by the attachments of the sternoclavicular joint, points upward. It is difficult to reduce the fracture and maintain the reduction:

They act imprudently who think to depress the projecting end of the bone. But it is clear that the underpart ought to be brought to the upper, for the former is the movable part, and that which has been displaced from its natural position.[3]

Union is usual and rapid and produces a prominent callus, and despite the deformity healing usually proceeds uneventfully.

A fractured clavicle, like all other spongy bone, gets speedily united; for all such bone forms callus in a short time. When a fracture has recently occurred, the patients attach much importance to it, as supposing the mischief greater than it really is; but, in a little time, the patients having no pain, nor finding any impediment to their walking or eating, become negligent, and the physician, finding they cannot make the parts look well, take themselves off, and are not sorry at the neglect of the patients, and in the meantime the callus is quickly formed.[3]

The Edwin Smith papyrus provides what is probably the earliest description of the accepted method of fracture reduction; an unknown Egyptian surgeon in 3550 BC recommended the following treatment of fractures of the clavicle[68,273,108]:

Thou shouldst place him prostrate on his back with something folded between his shoulder blades, thou shouldst spread out with his two shoulders in order to stretch apart his collar bone until that break falls into place.

Paul of Aegina, a seventeenth century Byzantine, reported that all that could ever be written about fractures of the clavicle had been written and that treatment included the supine position and the application of potions of olive oil, pigeon dung, snake oil, and other essences.[273]

Some of the earliest documented cases resulted from reports of riding accidents. William III in 1702 died of a fracture of the clavicle 3 days after falling when his horse shied at a molehill. Sir Benjamin Brodie described a "diffuse false venous aneurysm" that complicated a fracture of the clavicle in the case of Sir Robert Peel, who fell from his horse in 1850 on the way to Parliament. As Peel lapsed into unconsciousness, a pulsatile swelling rapidly developed behind the fracture, and his arm was paralyzed. *The Lancet* defended the physician's handling of the case even though many skeptics doubted that death could occur from a clavicle fracture.[71,203,431]

In 1839, Dupuytren, a keen, though controversial anatomist and observer, noted that the cumbersome devices of his day used to hold the reduction were often unnecessary; he advocated simply placing the arm on a pillow until union occurred. Several devices at that time often appeared to aggravate the difficulty created by the fracture or seemed to engender new problems. Dupuytren described a case in which bleeding could not be arrested: "When I was summoned I merely removed the apparatus (the pressure of which was the cause of the mischief) and placed the arm on a pillow. The bleeding immediately ceased."[431,79] He railed against cumbersome and painful treatment methods.

In the late 1860s, the current ambulatory treatment (early mobilization of the patient) was described by Lucas Championniere, who advocated a figure-of-eight dressing, and suggested that recumbency, a popular treatment method of his day, be abandoned.[118] In 1871, Sayre, recognizing the difficulty in maintaining the reduction, advocated a method of ambulatory treatment involving a rigid dressing to maintain the reduction and support the extremity, a method that was echoed and taught in the textbooks of his time and still has many advocates.[354]

In 1859, Malgaigne concluded[229]:

> *But while for a century and a half we see the most celebrated surgeons striving to prefer, or perhaps more strictly to complicate, the contrivances for treating fractured clavicle we may follow parallel to them another series of no less estimable surgeons, who disbelieving in these so-called improvements, return to the simplest means, as to Hippocrates before them. If now we seek to judge of all these contrivances by their results we see that most of them are extolled as producing cures without deformity; but we see also that subsequent experience has always falsified these promises. I therefore regard the thing (absence of deformity) as not impossible, although for my own part I have never seen such an instance.*

This quotation well summarizes the results of most conservative methods of treatment of the fractured clavicle—that is, most fractures unite by various treatment methods. However, many patients are left with residual deformity, some shortening, and a lump. Interference with function, cosmesis, activity level, and satisfaction used to be considered minimal, but more recent studies have suggested that the satisfaction patients achieve after treatment of fractures of the clavicle might not be as high as we previously thought.[91,146,242] In fact, Jupiter probably best summarized these shortcomings when he noted that "we are not meeting our patient expectations with current nonoperative treatment."[177] A study by Nowak showed that nearly 50% of patients still did not consider themselves fully recovered after 9 to 10 years. More specifically, 9% still had pain at rest, 29% had pain during activity, and 27% had cosmetic defects from the fracture.[287]

Although ambulatory treatment of fractures of the clavicle with support of the arm remains the mainstay of care today, there are few other fractures in humans where as much deformity, angulation, and shortening are accepted as the standard of care. Recent studies have shown that nonoperative treatment of clavicle fractures has been associated with chronic pain, weakness, and overall dissatisfaction on the part of the patients.[241,288] In a multicenter, prospective study, patients who were treated nonoperatively did significantly worse in terms of DASH (disabilities of the arm, shoulder, and hand) and Constant scores than those treated operatively.[44] Moreover, the patients treated nonoperatively had a more than threefold increase in the rate of nonunion than the operative patients, and the nonoperative patients had a significant risk of malunion and significantly longer time to radiographic healing.[44] Another study showed significant functional deficits in terms of DASH and Constant scores, with a strength deficit of 20% to 30% at a mean follow-up of 55 months after conservative treatment of a clavicle shaft fracture.[241] Although some of these deficits in patients with malunions and nonunions improved with delayed treatment, there were still significant deficits as compared with patients who were treated acutely.[316] Other studies showed that displacement of more than one bone width was the most significant predictor of poor outcome in nonoperatively treated clavicle fractures,[287] and less than half of the patients returned to their previous recreational and professional activities after a clavicle fracture.[343]

ANATOMY

Development

The embryology of the clavicle is unique in that it is the first bone in the body to ossify (fifth week of fetal life), and is the only long bone to ossify by intramembranous ossification without going through a cartilaginous stage.[112,113,256,257] The ossification center begins in the central portion of the clavicle; this area is responsible for growth of the clavicle until up to about 5 years of age.[68,98] Epiphyseal growth plates develop at both the medial and lateral ends of the clavicle, but only the sternal ossification center is present radiographically.[68,398] This medial growth plate of the clavicle is responsible for the majority of its longitudinal growth, and probably contributes as much as 80% of the length of the clavicle.[291] The sternal ossification center appears and fuses relatively late in life, with ossification occurring between the ages of 12 and 19 years and fusion to the clavicle occurring at 22 to 25 years of age.[169,402] Thus many of the so-called sternoclavicular dislocations in young adults are, in fact, epiphyseal fractures, and are a potential source of confusion unless the late sternoclavicular epiphyseal closure is remembered.

Morphology and Function

The superior surface of the clavicle is essentially subcutaneous over its course, with only the thin platysma providing any muscular coverage and then only to the inner two-thirds of the bone. The supraclavicular nerves, which provide sensation to the overlying skin, are consistently found just deep to the platysma muscle layer.

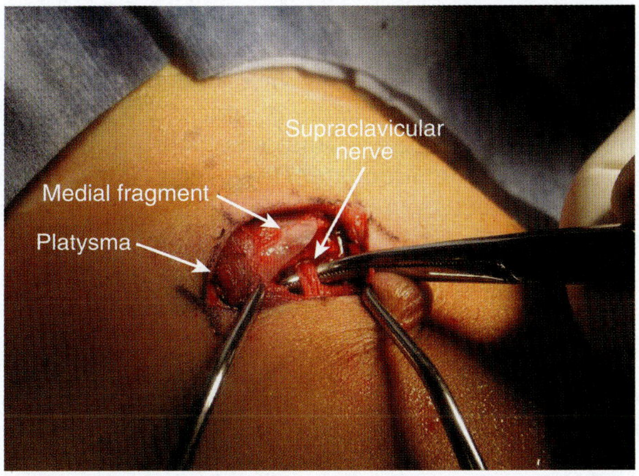

FIGURE 8-1: Surgical view of the middle branch of the supraclavicular nerve entrapped in the fracture site.

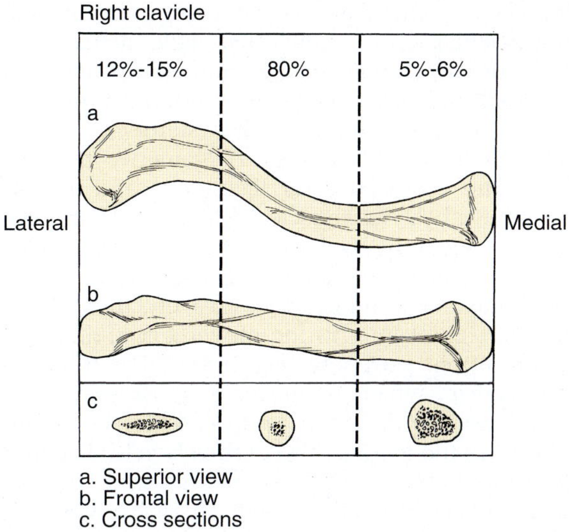

FIGURE 8-2: The clavicle appears as an S-shaped double curve when viewed from above *(a)*. It appears nearly straight when viewed from in front *(b)*. The outer end of the clavicle is flat in cross section, but becomes more tubular in its medial aspect *(c)*.

These nerves have been known to cause painful neuromas when damaged by fracture shards or iatrogenic injury (Fig. 8-1).[245] The clavicle is the sole bone strut connecting the trunk to the shoulder girdle and arm, and it is the only bone of the shoulder girdle that forms a synovial joint with the trunk.[218] Its name is derived from the Latin word *clavis* (key), the diminutive of which is *clavicula,* a reference to the musical symbol of similar shape.[256]

The shape and configuration of the clavicle are not only important for its function but also provide an explanation for the pattern of fractures encountered in this bone. In 1993, Harrington et al.[138] described an image-processing system that was used to evaluate the histomorphometric properties of 15 adult male and female human clavicles. Variations in porosity, cross-sectional area, and anatomic and principal moments of inertia were assessed at 2.5% to 5% increments along the length of the bones. The clavicle's biomechanical behavior (axial, flexural, and proportional rigidity and the critical forceful buckling) was modeled from these data by using beam theory. More than threefold variations in porosity and moments of inertia were found along the length of the S-shaped clavicle, with the greatest porosity and moments of inertia being located in the variably shaped sternal and acromial thirds of the bone as opposed to the denser, smaller, and more circular central third of the bone.

Clavicle orientation, as indicated by the direction of greatest resistance to bending (maximal principal moment of inertia), was found to rotate from a primarily craniocaudal orientation at the sternum to a primarily anteroposterior (AP) orientation at the acromion. Based on cross-sectional geometry, sectional moduli, and estimates of flexural and proportional rigidity, the clavicle was found to be weakest in the central third of its length. These data concur with the fracture location most commonly reported clinically.

An analysis of Euhler buckling predicted a minimal critical force for buckling during axial loading of about two to three body weights for an average adult. Thus buckling, or a combination of axial loading and bending or proportional loading, must be considered as a possible failure mechanism for this commonly injured bone.[138] Although it appears almost straight when viewed from the front, when viewed from above, the clavicle appears as an S-shaped double curve that is concave ventrally on its outer half and convex ventrally on its medial half (Fig. 8-2). Although some reports have noted differences in the shape and size of the clavicle in male and female subjects and in the dominant and nondominant arm, others have not found this to be the case or have discounted their clinical significance.[291,218,75,100]

DePalma found that the outer third of the clavicle exhibited varying degrees of anterior torsion, and suggested that changes in torsion might be responsible for the altered stresses that lead to primary degenerative changes in the acromioclavicular joint.[75] The cross section of the clavicle differs in shape along its length; it varies from flat along its outer third to prismatic along its inner third. The exact curvature of the clavicle and its thickness, to a high degree, vary according to the attachments of muscles and ligaments.[218] The flat outer third is most compatible with pull from muscles and ligaments, whereas the tubular medial third is a shape consistent with axial pressure or pull. The junction between the two cross sections varies with regard to its precise location in the middle third of the clavicle. This junction is a weak spot, particularly with axial loading,[218] which may be one of several reasons why fractures occur so commonly at the middle third. Another reason may be that it is an area not reinforced by muscles and ligaments and that it is just distal to the subclavius insertion.[273,152,160] It is curious that nature has strengthened, through ligaments or muscular reinforcement, every part of the clavicle except the end of the outer part of the middle third, which is the thinnest part of the bone.[31]

The clavicle articulates with the sternum through the sternoclavicular joint, which has little actual articular contact but surprisingly strong ligamentous attachments. The medial end of the clavicle is moored firmly against the first rib by the intra-articular sternoclavicular joint cartilage (which functions as a ligament), the oblique fibers of the costoclavicular ligaments, and to a lesser degree, the subclavius muscle.[75] The scapula and clavicle are bound securely by both the acromioclavicular and coracoclavicular ligaments, the mechanism and function of which have been reported extensively; these ligaments contribute significantly to the movement and stability of the entire upper extremity (Fig. 8-3).[111] The tubular third of the clavicle, which is thicker in cross section, offers protection for the important neurovascular structures that pass beneath the medial third of the clavicle. The intimate relationship between these structures and the clavicle assumes great importance both in acute fractures, in which direct injury can occur, and in the unusual fracture sequelae of malunion, nonunion, or production of excessive callus, in which compression of these structures can lead to late symptoms.

The brachial plexus, at the level at which it crosses beneath the clavicle, consists of three main branches (see Fig. 8-3). Of these branches, two are anterior. One (lateral) branch originates from the fifth, sixth, and seventh cervical roots and forms the musculocutaneous nerve and a branch of the median nerve; the other (medial) originates from the eighth cervical and first thoracic roots, and forms another branch of the median nerve, the entire ulnar nerve, and the medial cutaneous nerve. The posterior branch of the plexus forms the axillary and radial nerves. The cord of the brachial plexus, which contains the first components of the ulnar nerve, crosses the first rib directly under the medial third of the clavicle. The other two cords are farther to the lateral side and posterior. Therefore the ulnar nerve is more often involved in complications arising from fractures of the medial third of the clavicle.

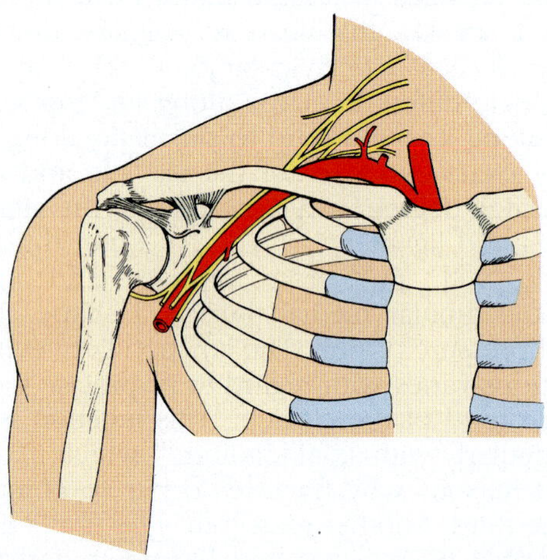

FIGURE 8-3: The clavicle is bound securely by ligaments at both the sternoclavicular and acromioclavicular joints. It is the only bony strut from the torso to the extremity. The brachial plexus and greater vessels are seen posterior to the medial third of the clavicle between the clavicle and the first rib.

The space between the clavicle and the first rib has been called the *costoclavicular space*. This space has been measured in gross anatomic studies and often appears to be quite adequate. However, it is not as large in a living subject as in a cadaver, possibly because in a living subject, the vessels are distended and the dimensions of the cords of the brachial plexus are larger than in a cadaver. In addition, in a living subject, the space is diminished as the first rib elevates because of contraction of the scalenus anticus. Hence when the inner end of the outer fragment of the fractured clavicle is depressed, there is much less space between the first rib and the clavicle; the result is that the vessels (especially the subclavian and axillary vessels) and nerves (especially the ulnar nerve) are potentially subject to injury, pressure, or irritation.[31] The internal jugular, which is adjacent to the sternoclavicular joint (see Fig. 8-3), is not usually injured with middle-third fractures, but has the potential for injury in more medial trauma involving the sternum and sternoclavicular joint. The subclavian vessels, because of their relative proximity to the medial third of the clavicle, can also be injured during operative treatment of clavicle fractures.[172,15,16,372] The clavicle also appears to be unique as a long bone in that it has only a periosteal blood supply and little, if any, intramedullary (IM) or nutrient arterial blood supply. More importantly, the periosteal blood supply has been found to be primarily on the anterior and superior surface of the clavicle. This blood supply, coupled with the poor soft tissue coverage of the clavicle, may be an important consideration in fixation of the clavicle, particularly when significant soft tissue stripping is necessary.[138,194]

Surgical Anatomy

The surgical anatomy relative to the fascial arrangements about the clavicle has been extensively described by Abbott and Lucas.[2] Such knowledge will reduce the risk of damage to neurovascular structures during surgical dissection.[333] It is useful to divide these structures into areas above, below, and behind the clavicle.

Above the Clavicle

At the sternal notch, a layer of cervical fascia splits into two layers, a superficial layer attached to the front and a deep layer attached to the back of the manubrium. The space between these layers contains lymphatics and a communicating vessel between the two anterior jugular veins. The two layers of fascia proceed laterally to enclose the sternocleidomastoid muscle before passing down to the clavicle. For 2.5 cm above the clavicle, they are separated by loose fat. The superficial layer is ill defined and is continuous with the fascia covering the undersurface of the trapezius muscle. A prolongation from the deep layer forms an inverted sling for the posterior belly of the omohyoid muscle, and it continues below to blend with the fascia enclosing the subclavius muscle. Medially, the omohyoid fascia covers the sternohyoid muscle.

Below the Clavicle

Two layers consisting of muscle and fascia form the anterior wall of the axilla. The pectoralis major and pectoral fascia forms the superficial layer; the pectoralis minor and clavipectoral fascia form the deep layer. The pectoral fascia closely envelops the pectoralis major. Above, it is attached to the clavicle, and laterally it forms the roof of the superficial infraclavicular triangle (formed by the pectoralis major, a portion of the anterior deltoid, and the clavicle). The deep layer—the clavipectoral fascia—extends from the clavicle above to the axillary fascia below. At the point where it attaches to the clavicle, it consists of two layers that enclose the subclavius muscle. The subclavius muscle arises from the manubrium and first rib and inserts into the inferior surface of the clavicle.

At the lower border of the subclavius, the two fascial layers join to form the costocoracoid membrane. This membrane fills a space between the subclavius above and the pectoralis minor below and is attached medially to the first costal cartilage and laterally to the coracoid process. Below, it splits into two layers that ensheath the pectoralis minor. The costocoracoid membrane is pierced by the cephalic vein, the lateral pectoral nerve, and the thoracoacromial artery and vein.[2]

Behind the Clavicle

A continuous myofascial layer, which has not been commonly appreciated in surgical anatomy, lies in front of the large vessels and nerves as they pass from the root of the neck to the axilla. From above to below, this layer consists of the omohyoid fascia enclosing the omohyoid muscle and the clavipectoral fascia enclosing the pectoralis minor and subclavius muscles.[2] Behind the medial part of the clavicle and the sternoclavicular joint, the internal jugular and subclavian veins join to form the innominate vein. These veins are covered by the omohyoid fascia and by its extension medially over the sternohyoid and sternothyroid muscles. Behind the clavicle, at the junction between the middle and medial thirds, the junction of the subclavian and axillary veins lies very close to the clavicle and is also protected by this myofascial layer.

Between the omohyoid fascia posteriorly and the investing layer of cervical fascia anteriorly is a space, described by Grant, in which the external jugular vein usually joins the subclavian vein at its confluence with the internal jugular vein.[122] Before this junction, the external jugular is joined on its lateral aspect by the transverse cervical and scapular veins and on its medial aspect by the anterior jugular vein. This anastomosis usually lies just behind the fascial envelope and the angle formed by the posterior border of the sternocleidomastoid muscle and clavicle.[389]

These neurovascular structures are at risk for injury at the time of a clavicle fracture; however, recent studies have shown that these structures, especially the subclavian vein, are at risk for injury during plate fixation of the clavicle, with the subclavian vein being an average of only 4.8 mm from the undersurface of the medial clavicle [372] Furthermore, damage to the subclavian vessels can result in pseudoaneurysms and even death.[15,16]

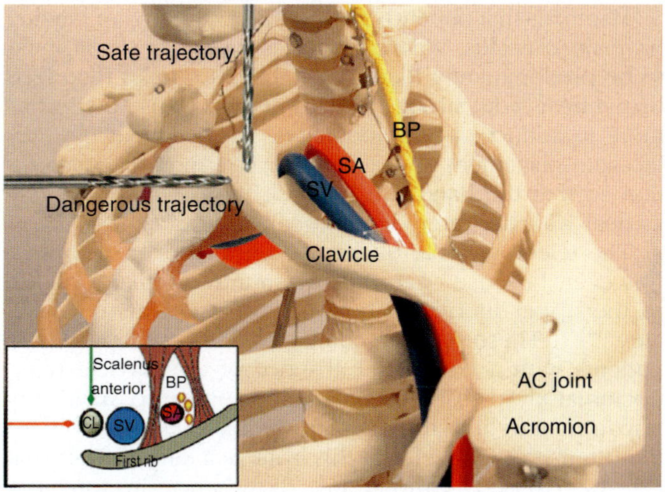

FIGURE 8-4: The relationship of a medial drill relative to the vascular structures below the medial clavicle. The dangerous trajectory is in the central third of the clavicle. BP, Brachial plexus; CL, clavicle; SA, subclavian artery; SV, subclavian vein; AC, acromioclavicular joint. (From Sinha A, Edwin J, Sreeharsha B, et al. A radiological study to define safe zones for drilling during plating of clavicle features. *J Bone Joint Surg Br.* 2011;93[9]:1247-1252.)

On Top of the Clavicle

Aside from the skin, the only two structures that pass over the top of the clavicle are the platysma muscle and the supraclavicular nerves. The platysma muscle is an expression muscle and inserts on the skin and fascia overlying the pectoralis muscle. The cervical branch of the facial nerve innervates it. Although it can be split during IM fixation of the clavicle, it usually has to be transected during plate fixation. We have found that damage to this muscle can cause a painful lump in the neck, and occasionally, changes in facial expression. The supraclavicular nerve usually has at least two major branches, with about 49% of patients having an intermediate branch.[268] This nerve is at risk for injury from a clavicle fracture, but is especially at risk for injury during plate fixation of the clavicle. Studies have shown that up to 83% of patients can have anterior chest wall numbness after plate fixation, with 52% still reporting numbness even 1 year later[53] (Fig. 8-4).

FUNCTION

The function of the clavicle may be inferred, in part, by some study of comparative anatomy. Codman has stated:

> *We are proud that our brains are more developed than the animals: we might also boast of our clavicles. It seems to me that the clavicle is one of man's greatest skeletal inheritances, for he depends to a greater extent than most animals, except the apes and monkeys, on the use of his hands and arms.*[55]

Mammals that depend on swimming, running, or grazing have no clavicles, whereas species with clavicles appear to be predominantly fliers or climbers. Codman theorized that animals with strong clavicles needed to use their arms more in adduction and abduction. The long clavicle may facilitate placement of the shoulder in a more lateral position so that the hand can be positioned more effectively to deal with the three-dimensional environment.[296]

The teleologic role of the clavicle has been disputed, however, because of reports of entirely normal function of the upper limb after complete excision of the clavicle.[62,130,157] These reports, combined with observations in patients with a congenital absence of the clavicle (cleidocranial dysostosis) who do not appear to have any impairment in limb function, are probably responsible for the often-stated belief that this bone is a surplus part that can be excised without any disturbance in function. However, others have noted drooping of the shoulder, weakness, and loss of motion after excision of the clavicle, and have used these observations to attribute the important role of the clavicle in normal function of the extremity (Figs. 8-5 and 8-6).[338,377]

The clavicle does have several important functions, each of which would be expected to be altered not only by excision of the bone but also by fracture, nonunion, or malunion.

Power and Stability of the Arm

The clavicle, by serving as a bony link from the thorax to the shoulder girdle, provides a stable linkage of the arm-trunk mechanism, and contributes significantly to the power and stability of the arm and shoulder girdle, especially in movement above shoulder level.[257] It transmits the support and force of the trapezius muscle to the scapula and arm via the coracoclavicular ligaments.

Although patients with cleidocranial dysostosis and absence of the clavicle do not appear to have significantly decreased range of motion and can, in fact, have an increase in protraction and retraction of the scapula (because of the absence of the clavicle), they can exhibit some weakness in supporting a load overhead. This limitation further suggests that the clavicle adds stability to the extremity under load in extreme ranges of motion.[157]

The clavicle is predominantly supported and stabilized by passive structures,[218] particularly the sternoclavicular ligaments.[28,29] Although evidence of trapezius muscle activity at rest has been demonstrated electromyographically, thus suggesting a role for that muscle in the support of the clavicle,[28] other authors have not been able to demonstrate that muscle activity plays any role in supporting the clavicle.

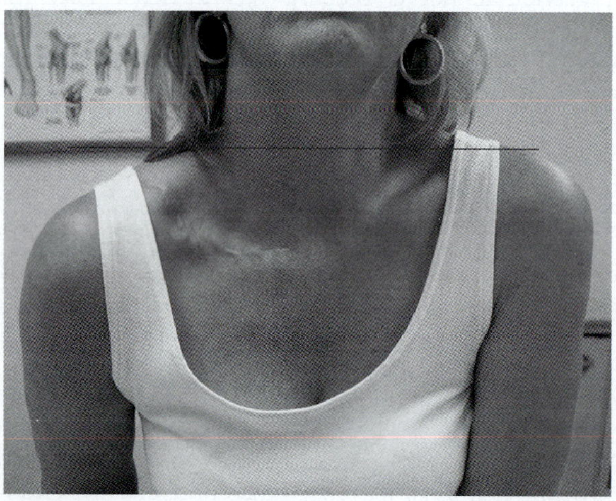

FIGURE 8-5: Appearance of a patient who has had a complete claviculectomy. Note the significant drooping of the right shoulder. The patient complained of chronic pain, hand numbness, and an inability to keep her bra strap on her shoulder.

Motion of the Shoulder Girdle

When the arm is elevated 180 degrees, the clavicle angles upward 30 degrees and backward 35 degrees at the sternoclavicular joint. It also rotates upward on its longitudinal axis approximately 50 degrees. During combined glenohumeral, acromioclavicular, and sternoclavicular movement, the humerus moves approximately 120 degrees at the glenohumeral joint, and the scapula moves along the chest wall approximately 60 degrees. These complex and combined simultaneous movements of the joints and their articulating bony structures (scapula, humerus, and clavicle) seem to imply an important role for the clavicle in the range of motion of the arm. This role is debatable, however, because it has been observed by some that loss of the clavicle does not in fact impair abduction of the arm at all[2,424] and that excision of the clavicle can permit range of motion just as well. However, Rockwood has observed that loss of the clavicle results in disabling loss of function, weakness, drooping of the arm, and pain secondary to irritation of the brachial plexus (see Figs. 8-5 and 8-6).[338]

It has been stated that its contribution to motion may be the most important function of the clavicle, and that this role is related to its curvature, especially its lateral curvature. The 50-degree rotation of the clavicle on its

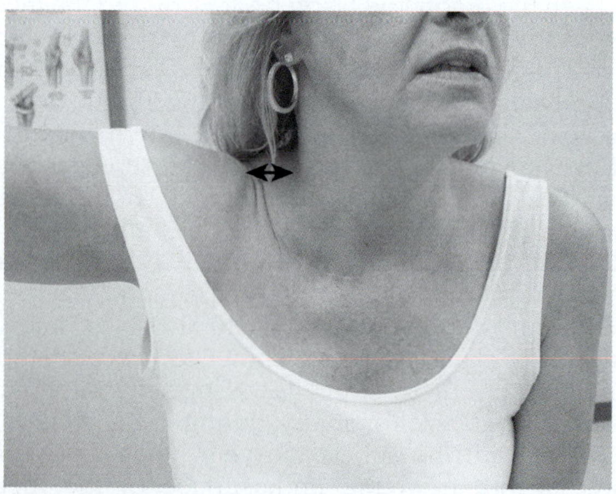

FIGURE 8-6: Note the medial collapse of the shoulder during attempted abduction.

axis appears to be important for free elevation of the extremity. In fact, a direct relationship has been found among the line of attachment of the coracoclavicular ligaments, the amount of clavicular rotation, the extent and relative lengthening of the ligaments, and scapula rotation itself. Of the total 60 degrees of scapular rotation, the first 30 degrees is due to elevation of the clavicle as a whole by movement of the sternoclavicular joint, and the second 30 degrees is permitted through the acromioclavicular joint by clavicular rotation and elongation of the coracoclavicular ligaments. Thus the lateral curvature of the clavicle permits it to act as a crankshaft, effectively allowing half of the scapular movement.[217]

The smooth, rhythmic movement of the shoulder girdle is a complex interaction of muscle groups acting on joints and both the subacromial and scapulothoracic spaces. Although it is difficult to break down all the contributions of the clavicle to the total motion of the shoulder, it appears that its geometric and kinematic design, by permitting rotation, maximizes the stability of the upper limb against the trunk while permitting mobility, particularly of the scapula along the chest wall. The practical result is that the glenoid fossa continually moves, facing and contacting the humeral head as the arm is used overhead.[157]

Nonunion and malunion can cause significant alterations in the orientation of the scapula and glenohumeral joint (Figs. 8-7 and 8-8).[10,83] This altered orientation is typically an anteromedial and inferior rotatory deformity. Malunion represents a fixed or static change in the orientation of the scapula, whereas nonunion is a dynamic deformity, such as would be seen in a significant acromioclavicular separation (Fig. 8-9). This change in the orientation of the scapula results in a change in the resting length of the muscles about the shoulder. Basamania[23] and McKee et al.[242] found significant weakness in the affected limbs of patients with clavicle malunion, regardless of the length of time since their injury. This weakness corrected with the return of the clavicle to its normal length despite no formal physical therapy.

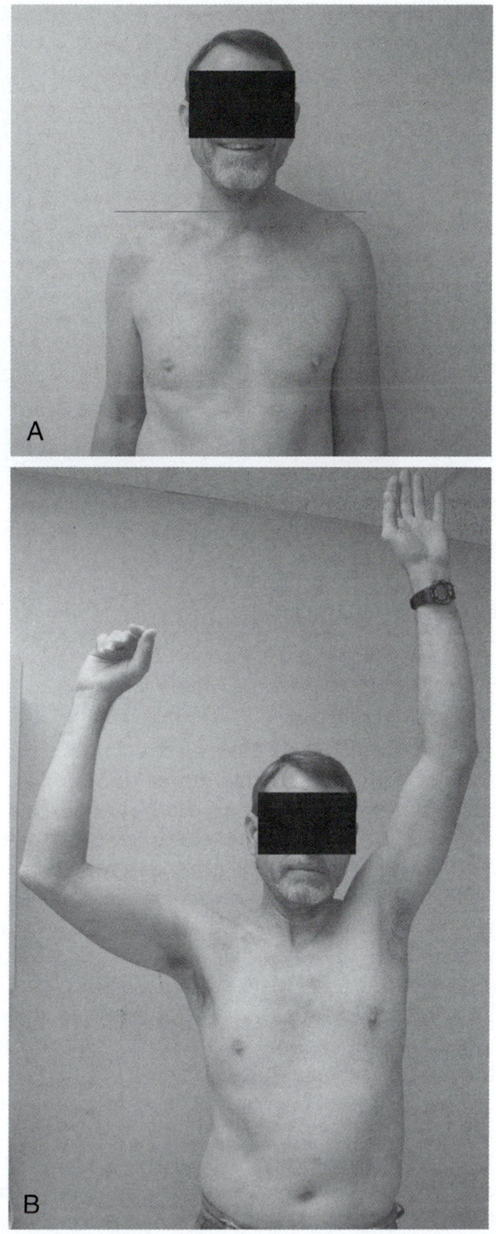

FIGURE 8-7: **A,** Clinical appearance of a patient with clavicle malunion. **B,** Note the drooping of the right shoulder and loss of forward flexion.

Muscle Attachments

The clavicle also acts as a bony framework for muscle origin and insertion. The upper third of the trapezius

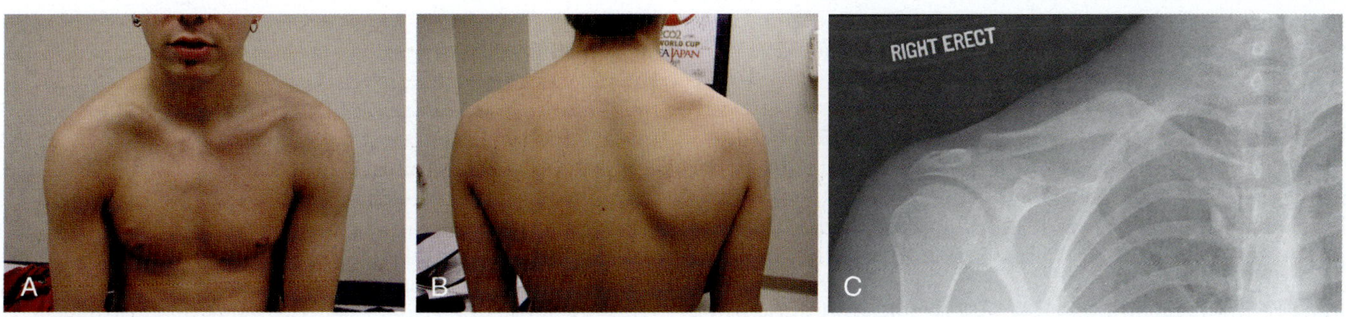

FIGURE 8-8: A patient with a clavicle malunion. **A,** Anterior view. **B,** Posterior view. Note the scapular pseudo-winging. **C,** Anteroposterior radiograph.

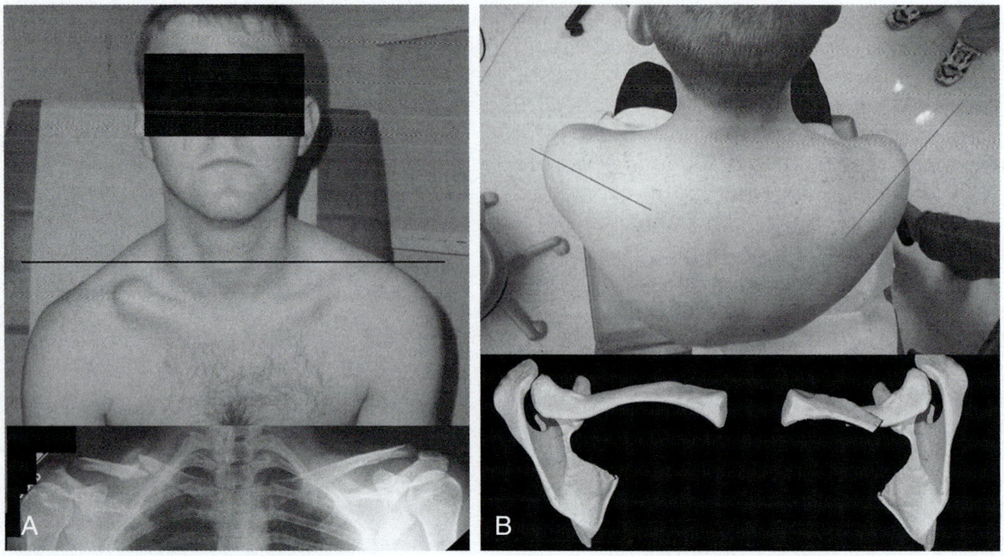

FIGURE 8-9: A, Clinical appearance and anteroposterior radiograph of an acute fracture. Note the inferior displacement of the involved shoulder relative to the normal shoulder. **B,** Same patient viewed from above. Note the anterior rotation of the right shoulder relative to the coronal plane of the body. The changes in orientation of the scapula are shown in the schematic drawing.

inserts on the superior surface of the outer third of the clavicle, opposite the site of origin of the clavicular head of the deltoid along its anterior edge. The clavicular head of the sternocleidomastoid muscle arises from the posterior edge of the inner third of the clavicle. The clavicular head of the pectoralis major muscle arises from the anterior edge of the clavicle. During active elevation of the arm, these muscles contract simultaneously. It has been suggested that in theory, the muscles above the clavicle could be directly attached to the muscles below the clavicle as a continuous muscular layer without an interposed bony attachment,[2] but the stable bony framework clearly provides the advantage of a solid foundation for muscle attachment.

The other muscle that inserts on the clavicle is the subclavius muscle. After it arises from the first rib anteriorly at the costochondral junction, it proceeds obliquely and posteriorly into a groove on the undersurface of the clavicle. This muscle appears to aid in depressing the middle third of the clavicle. Fractures of the clavicle often occur at the distal portion of its insertion. In mid-clavicular fractures, this muscle can offer some protection to the neurovascular structures beneath; however, it can also become entrapped within the fracture site and delay or inhibit healing.

Protection of Neurovascular Structures

The clavicle also provides skeletal protection for adjacent neurovascular structures and the superior aspect of the lung. The subclavian and axillary vessels, the brachial plexus, and the lung are directly behind the medial third of the clavicle. The tubular cross section of the medial third of the clavicle increases its strength and adds to its protective function at this level. The anterior curve of the medial two-thirds of the clavicle provides a rigid arch beneath which the great vessels pass as they move from the mediastinum and thoracic outlet to the axilla. It has been shown that during elevation of the arm, the clavicle, as it rotates upward, also moves backward, with the curvature providing increased clearance for the vessels.[393] Loss of the clavicle eliminates this bony barrier against external trauma.[1] In addition, loss of the clavicle can cause exacerbation of thoracic outlet symptoms because of the drooping of the shoulder and the resultant draping of the brachial plexus over the first rib.

Respiratory Function

Elevation of the lateral part of the clavicle results in increased pull on the costoclavicular ligament and subclavius muscle. Because of the connection between the clavicle and the first rib and between the first rib and the sternum, elevation of the shoulder girdle brings about a cephalad motion of the thorax corresponding to an inspiration. This relationship is used in some breathing exercises and in some forms of artificial respiration.[2]

Cosmesis

By providing a graceful curve to the base of the neck, the smooth, subcutaneous bony clavicle serves a cosmetic function. After surgical excision of the clavicle, the upper limb in some patients falls downward and forward, and gives a foreshortened appearance to this area. Female patients have complained of difficulty keeping their bra strap on their affected shoulder because of this drooping. The cosmetic function of the clavicle is noted by many patients who are concerned by excessive formation of callus after a clavicle fracture or by deformity after clavicular malunion (Fig. 8-10).[1]

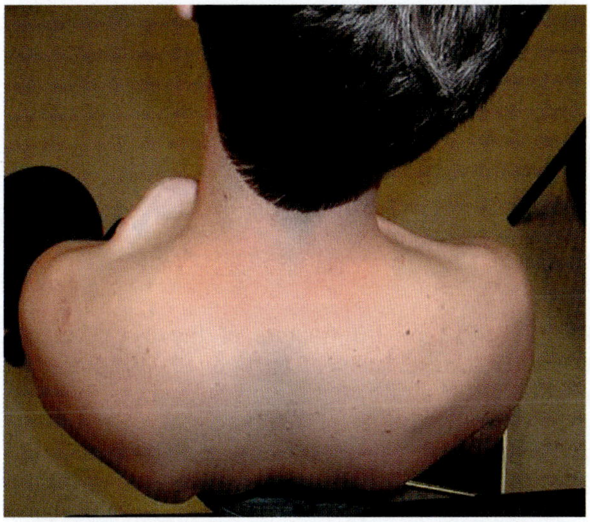

FIGURE 8-10: Significant right clavicle malunion.

CLASSIFICATION OF CLAVICLE FRACTURES

To be effective, a classification system should be accurate in terms of identifying the pathologic anatomy, and it should be able to predict outcome, thereby serving as a basis for deciding on proper treatment. Ideally, a classification system should also be sufficiently straightforward that it is easily reproducible with good intraobserver and interobserver reliability. Unfortunately, most clavicle fracture classification systems are merely descriptive and give no guidance in terms of prognosis. Although clavicle fractures have been classified by fracture configuration (e.g., greenstick, oblique, transverse, comminuted),[392] the usual classification is by the location of the fracture because location appears to better compartmentalize our understanding of fracture anatomy, mechanism of injury, clinical findings, and alternative methods of treatment.[6,86,95,271,299] One of the early classifications of clavicle fractures was Allman's classification. He divided these fractures into three groups[6]:

Group I: Fractures of the middle third
Group II: Fractures of the distal third
Group III: Fractures of the medial third

Neer[273,271,269,270] and Jager and Breitner[164] devised a specific classification for fractures of the distal third of the clavicle.

Craig's Classification

In 1990, Craig[63] introduced a more detailed classification of clavicle fractures that was based on the variable fracture patterns seen within the three broad groups of Allman's clavicle fracture classification (Box 8-1).

BOX 8-1. Craig Classification of Clavicle Fractures

Group I: Fracture of the middle third
Group II: Fracture of the distal third
- Type I: Minimal displacement (interligamentous)
- Type II: Displaced secondary to a fracture medial to the coracoclavicular ligaments
  - A. Conoid and trapezoid attached
  - B. Conoid torn, trapezoid attached
- Type III: Fractures of the articular surface
- Type IV: Ligaments intact to the periosteum (children), with displacement of the proximal fragment
- Type V: Comminuted, with ligaments attached neither proximally nor distally, but to an inferior, comminuted fragment

Group III: Fracture of the proximal third
- Type I: Minimal displacement
- Type II: Displaced (ligaments ruptured)
- Type III: Intra-articular
- Type IV: Epiphyseal separation (children and young adults)
- Type V: Comminuted

Group I Fractures

Group I fractures, or fractures of the middle third, are the most common fractures seen in adults and children. They occur at the point at which the clavicle changes to a flattened cross section from a prismatic cross section. The force of the traumatic impact follows the curve of the clavicle, and disperses on reaching the lateral curve.[276,277,278,376] In addition, the proximal and distal segments of the clavicle are mechanically secured by ligamentous structures and muscular attachments, whereas the central segment is relatively free. This fracture accounts for 80% of clavicle fractures.[273,345]

Group II Fractures

Group II fractures account for 12% to 15% of all clavicle fractures, and are subclassified according to the location of the coracoclavicular ligaments relative to the fracture fragments.[140] Neer first pointed out the importance of this fracture while subdividing it into four types.

Type I fractures are the most common by a ratio of 4:1. In this type of fracture, the ligaments remain intact to hold the fragments together and prevent rotation, tilting, or significant displacement. This fracture is an interligamentous fracture that occurs between the conoid and the trapezoid or between the coracoclavicular and acromioclavicular ligaments (Figs. 8-11 and 8-12).[270]

In type II distal clavicle fractures, the coracoclavicular ligaments are detached from the medial segment. Both the conoid and trapezoid ligaments may be on the distal fragment (IIA) (Fig. 8-13), or the conoid ligament may be ruptured while the trapezoid ligament remains attached to the distal segment (IIB) (Fig. 8-14).[68] There is really no functional difference between these two fractures. The high rate of nonunion in these fractures may be secondary to excessive motion at the fracture site. These fractures are equivalent to a serious acromioclavicular separation in which the normal constraints to anteromedial rotation of the scapula relative to the clavicle are lost.

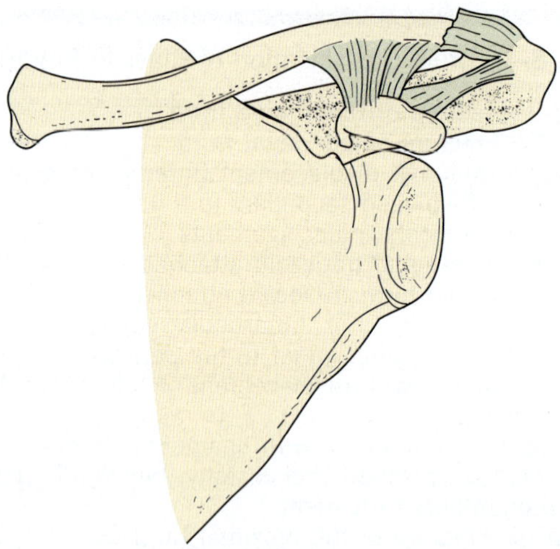

FIGURE 8-11: Type I fracture of the distal end of the clavicle (group II). The intact ligaments hold the fragments in place. (From Rockwood CA, Green DP, eds. *Fractures*, 2nd ed. Philadelphia: JB Lippincott; 1984.)

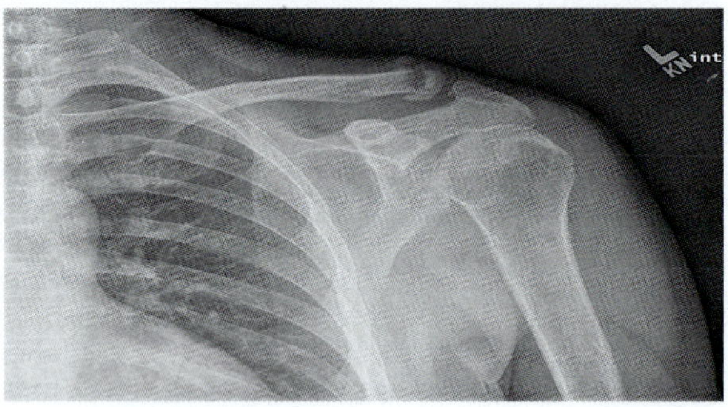

FIGURE 8-12: A type I fracture of the distal end of the clavicle seen radiographically. The fragments are held in place securely by the intact coracoclavicular and acromioclavicular ligaments.

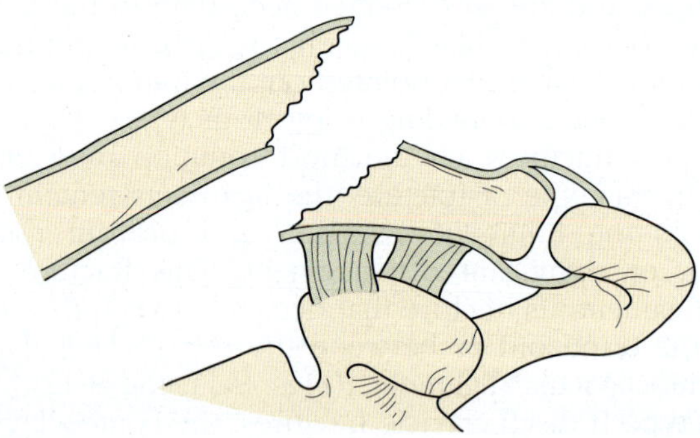

FIGURE 8-13: Type II distal clavicle fracture. In type IIA, both the conoid and trapezoid ligaments are on the distal segment, and the proximal segment, without ligamentous attachments, is displaced. (From Rockwood CA, Green DP, eds. *Fractures*, 2nd ed. Philadelphia: JB Lippincott; 1984.)

Four forces that may impair healing and may be contributing factors to the reported high incidence of nonunion act on this fracture. When the patient is erect, the outer fragment, which retains the attachment of the trapezoid ligament to the scapula through the intact

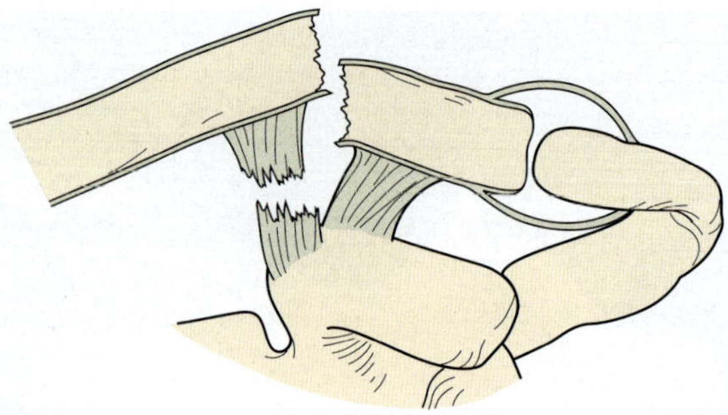

FIGURE 8-14: Type IIB fracture of the distal part of the clavicle. The conoid ligament is ruptured, and the trapezoid ligament remains attached to the distal segment. The proximal fragment is displaced. (From Rockwood CA, Green DP, eds. *Fractures*, 2nd ed. Philadelphia: JB Lippincott; 1984.)

acromioclavicular ligaments, is pulled downward and forward by the weight of the arm; the pectoralis major, pectoralis minor, and latissimus dorsi draw the distal segment downward and medially, thereby causing overriding; the scapula might rotate the distal segment as the arm is moved; and the trapezius muscle attaches to the entire outer two-thirds of the clavicle, whereas the sternocleidomastoid muscle attaches to the medial third, and these muscles act to draw the clavicular segment superiorly and posteriorly, often into the substance of the trapezius muscle.[271]

Type III distal clavicle fractures involve the articular surface of the acromioclavicular joint alone. Although type II fractures can have intra-articular extension, type III fractures are characterized by a break in the articular surface without a ligamentous injury. A type III injury may be subtle, and may be confused with a first-degree acromioclavicular separation, and can require special views to visualize. In fact, it may be manifested as late degenerative joint arthrosis of the acromioclavicular joint. In addition, it has been suggested that weightlifter's clavicle, or resorption of the distal end of the clavicle, might occur from increased vascularity secondary to the microtrauma or microfractures that lead to such resorption.[43,163,273,324]

It appears logical to add a fourth and fifth type of distal clavicle fracture because in a certain series of fractures, bone displacement occurs as a result of deforming muscle forces, but the coracoclavicular ligaments remain attached to bone or periosteum.

Type IV fractures occur in children and may be confused with complete acromioclavicular separation (Fig. 8-15). Known as *pseudodislocation* of the acromioclavicular joint, these fractures typically occur in children younger than 16 years.[336] The distal end of the clavicle is fractured, and the acromioclavicular joint remains intact. In children and young adults, the attachment between the bone and the periosteum is relatively loose. The proximal fragment ruptures through the thin periosteum, and may be displaced upward by muscular forces. The coracoclavicular ligaments remain attached to the periosteum or may be avulsed with a small piece of bone.[86,95,336]

Group III Fractures

Group III fractures, or fractures of the inner third of the clavicle, constitute 5% to 6% of clavicle fractures. As with distal clavicle fractures, they can be subdivided according to the integrity of the ligamentous structures.

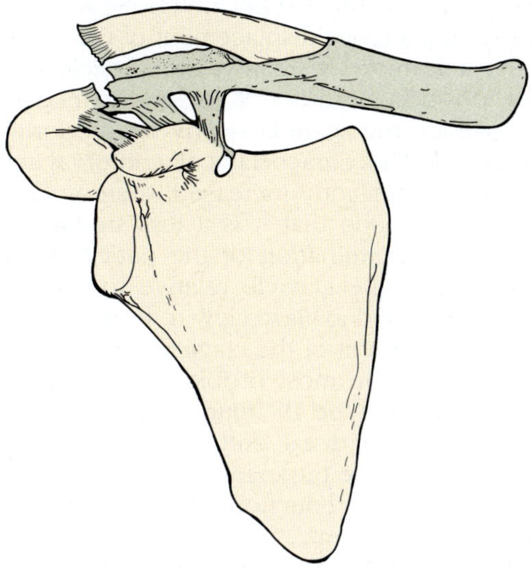

FIGURE 8-15: A type IV fracture occurring in children that has been called a pseudodislocation of the acromioclavicular joint. The coracoclavicular ligaments remain attached to the bone or the periosteum, and the proximal fragment ruptures through the thin superior periosteum and may be displaced upward by muscle forces. (From Rockwood CA, Green DP, eds. *Fractures*, 2nd ed. Philadelphia: JB Lippincott; 1984.)

If the costoclavicular ligaments remain intact and attached to the outer fragment, little or no displacement develops.[6,188] When these lesions occur in children, they are usually epiphyseal fractures.[187] In adults, articular surface injuries can also lead to degenerative changes.[273,425] Based on their observations of 57 medial fractures, Throckmorton and Kuhn classified medial fractures into five different types based on their fracture patterns (Fig. 8-16). It is of interest to note that in their medial clavicle fracture series, 22% of the fractures could only be seen on computed tomography (CT) scan.[395]

Panclavicular dislocation, or a traumatic floating clavicle, is neither a clavicle fracture nor an isolated sternoclavicular or acromioclavicular separation.[30,115,165,223,313] In this injury, both sternoclavicular ligaments and the coracoclavicular and the acromioclavicular ligamentous structures are disrupted.

Rockwood's Classification

Clinically and radiographically, it may be impossible to distinguish between grade III acromioclavicular separations, type II fractures of the distal end of the clavicle, and type IV fractures involving rupture of the periosteum.[270,271,273] Rockwood has classified these fractures in a manner that is roughly analogous to his classification system for acromioclavicular joint injuries in adults (Fig. 8-17). This system is based on the amount of energy imparted to the distal part of the clavicle, which determines the degree of displacement and the direction of the applied force, which determines the direction of the displacement. The subtypes are based on the position of

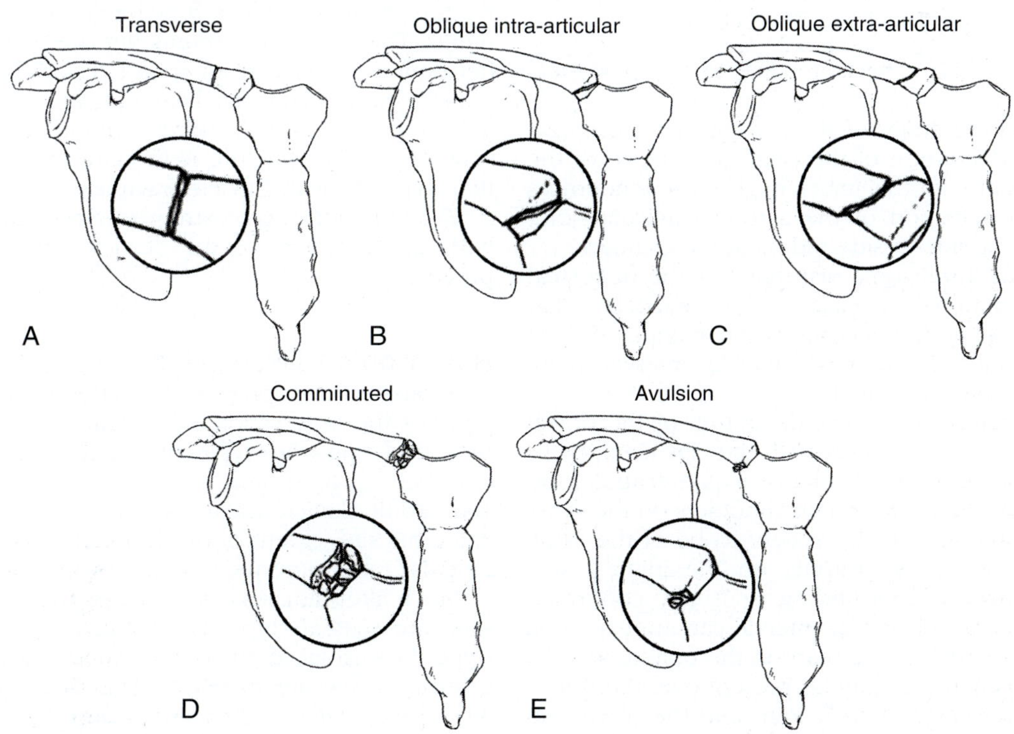

FIGURE 8-16: Classification of medial clavicle fractures. (From Throckmorton T, Kuhn JE. Fractures of the medial end of the clavicle. *J Shoulder Elbow Surg.* 2007;16[1]:49-54.)

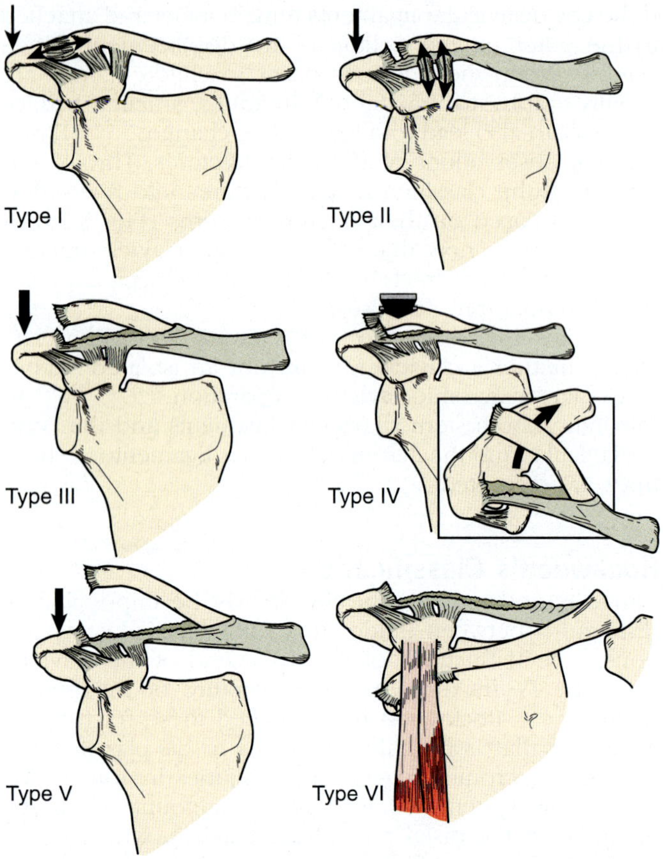

FIGURE 8-17: The Rockwood classification of distal clavicle injuries in children. (From Rockwood CA, Green DP, eds. *Fractures*, 2nd ed. Philadelphia: JB Lippincott; 1984.)

the distal end of the clavicle relative to the periosteal tube.[336]

Type I is a minor strain of the acromioclavicular ligaments without disruption of the periosteal sleeve of the clavicle. A patient with this injury might have tenderness in response to palpation of the acromioclavicular joint but no significant side-to-side radiographic changes.

In a *type II* fracture, some disruption of the periosteal sleeve with a minimal increase in the coracoclavicular interval is noted on radiographs when compared with the uninjured side. The acromioclavicular interval might appear to be slightly widened.

Type III fractures are a gross disruption of the dorsal aspect of the periosteal sleeve, with the clavicle appearing to be displaced upward relative to the scapula. On plain radiographs taken with both shoulders on the same cassette, the clavicles actually appear to be of the same relative height, with the scapula on the injured side drooping downward. This finding is usually confirmed clinically. The coracoclavicular interval can appear to be increased 50% to 100% more than on the uninjured side. Swelling and ecchymosis may be present over the dorsal aspect of the acromioclavicular joint and the distal end of the clavicle in addition to ecchymosis over the posterolateral aspect of the acromion. If the coracoclavicular interval is not widened but the acromioclavicular space is significantly widened, the physician should be suspicious of a coracoid base fracture. With these injuries, the force is dissipated in fracturing the coracoid before the periosteal tube is disrupted. A fracture of the base of the coracoid can sometimes be seen on the axillary view but is best seen on the Stryker notch view.

Type IV is a posterior displacement of the clavicle relative to the acromion. In reality, the clavicle remains in the same position because of its strong medial attachments; however, the scapula is driven anteriorly relative to the clavicle. The coracoclavicular interval might not appear to be significantly increased, thereby leading the physician to conclude that it is a less significant injury. The key to the examination of the patient is palpating the distal part of the clavicle relative to the acromion, and obtaining a good axillary view to look for the relative posterior displacement of the clavicle. In our experience, these injuries are the most problematic in children and adolescents, just as type IV injuries in adults are so disabling, because the distal end of the clavicle can be buttonholed out of the trapezius muscle. Such buttonholing not only prevents reduction but also causes considerable pain for the patient.

Type V is essentially a severe type III injury with complete disruption of the dorsal periosteal tube and significant superior displacement of the distal part of the clavicle relative to the acromion. This injury is presumably due to the additional disruption of the deltotrapezial fascia. Again, the distal end of the clavicle stays in its anatomic position but the scapula drops away. The coracoclavicular interval is typically increased more than 100%. In type V fractures in adults, neither of the main fracture fragments has a functional coracoclavicular ligament. These fracture fragments are displaced by the deforming muscles as in type I distal clavicle fractures, but the coracoclavicular ligaments are intact and remain attached to a small, third comminuted intermediary segment.[299] This fracture is thought to be more unstable than type II distal clavicle fractures.

Type VI injuries are extremely rare, and are associated with displacement of the clavicle under the coracoid process.

Robinson's Classification

The classification proposed by Robinson (Fig. 8-18) is perhaps the only validated classification system in terms of correlating the type of fracture with the typical outcome.[333] His system was based on the observation of 1000 adult clavicle fractures, and takes into account the anatomic site, extent of displacement, comminution, and articular extension and stability of the fracture.

Much like Allman's classification, the primary anatomic sites are medial (type 1), middle (type 2), and lateral (type 3). Displacement further subdivides these primary groups if they are displaced less than 100% (subgroup A) or more than 100% (subgroup B). Type 1 and 3 fractures are subdivided with regard to their articular involvement, with subgroup 1 having no intra-articular

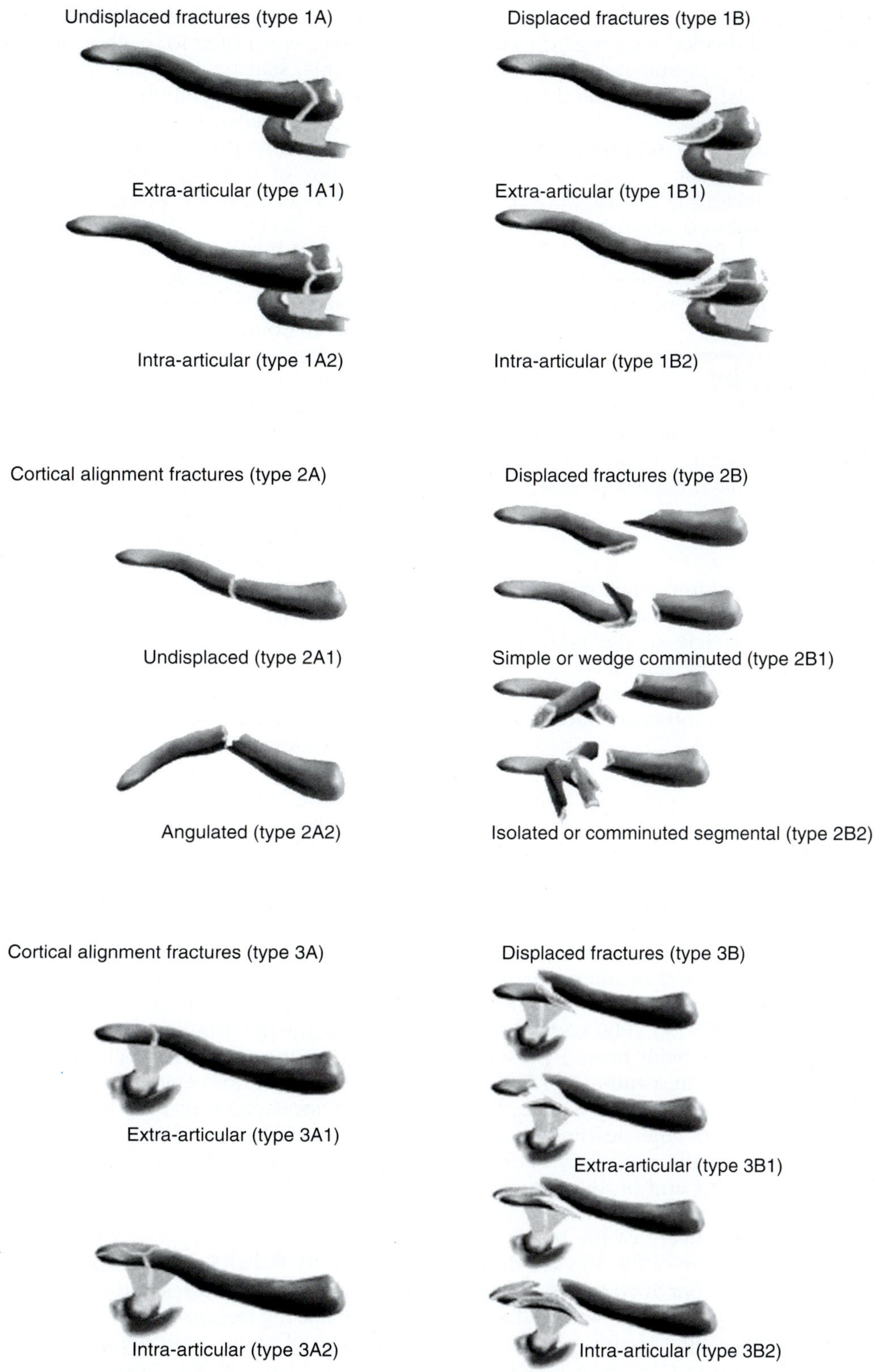

FIGURE 8-18: Robinson classification of clavicle fractures. (From Robinson CM. Fractures of the clavicle in the adult. Epidemiology and classification. *J Bone Joint Surg Br*. 1998;80:476-484.)

involvement and subgroup 2 having intra-articular extension. Type 2 fractures are subdivided with regard to their comminution. Simple or wedge comminution is classified into subgroup 1, and segmental or comminuted fractures are classified into subgroup 2.

By combining these groups and subgroups, virtually all fractures can be described. For example, a comminuted, displaced midshaft fracture is described as a *type 2B2* fracture, and a nondisplaced intra-articular lateral clavicle fracture is a *type 3A2*. Robinson found that both displacement and comminution were associated with an increased risk of delayed union or nonunion.[333]

MECHANISM OF INJURY

Because the clavicle is the bone that is most often fractured, numerous causes of fracture of the clavicle, both traumatic and nontraumatic, have been reported.[88]

Trauma in Children

Fractures of the clavicle in children share many of the same mechanisms of injury as in adults, and can result from a direct blow to the clavicle or the point of the shoulder or from an indirect blow such as a fall on the outstretched hand. However, other features are unusual and unique to children, including obstetric fracture of the clavicle and plastic bowing injury.

Birth Fractures

In 15,000 deliveries from 1954 to 1959, Rubin found that fractures of the clavicle were the most common injury at birth.[347] Although it has been stated that intrapartum traumatic injuries are decreasing as a result of improvements in obstetric care,[111,120,124,173,404] the incidence of clavicle fracture remains quite high, and in infants, it might actually be increasing.[17] Moir and Myerscough found an incidence of clavicle fractures of 5 per 1000 vertex births, which increased to 160 per 1000 with breech presentation.[252] The mechanism of injury in a full-term newborn infant delivered vaginally, when the baby is in a cephalic presentation, is compression of the leading clavicle against the maternal symphysis pubis.[227,391] In a breech delivery, direct traction can occur and produce the same bone injury as the obstetrician tries to depress the shoulders and free the arm during delivery of the head.[184,388]

The overall incidence of fracture of the clavicle during birth is approximately 0.5 to 7.2 per 1000 births. In addition to the presentation of the infant, several factors appear to be involved. Birth weight clearly plays a role because the incidence of fractures of the clavicle increases with increasing birth weight and in larger babies.[48,121] Babies who weigh 3800 to 4000 g or measure 52 cm or longer seem to be at higher risk for fracture. Increased maternal age has likewise been shown to be a risk factor for birth fracture.[27] The experience of the physician is likely also related. Cohen and Otto reported an increased incidence of fractures of the clavicle when babies were delivered by less experienced residents, and a decrease in incidence was noted for each year of obstetrics experience.[56] This statistic certainly merits consideration in obstetrics house staff training. The method of delivery is also important because of an increase in the risk of fracture with midforceps deliveries, which calls into question the wisdom of this obstetric maneuver. On the other hand, Balata et al. noted no fractures in babies delivered by cesarean section.[17]

Fracture of the clavicle does not seem to be related to the type of anesthesia, length of active labor, length of second-stage labor, Apgar score, or parity of the mother. The exact anatomy of fractures that occur during delivery varies, and incomplete, greenstick, and bicortical disruptions with or without displacement have all been reported.[389] In one study, boys were more commonly affected than girls, and the right clavicle was fractured more often than the left clavicle.[17] In 1992, a study suggested a relationship between fractures of the clavicle and mothers who had a second child.[167]

All the literature suggests that more frequent and systematic clinical examination might reduce the incidence or make the diagnosis of clavicle fractures more timely because of what we now know to be risk factors.

Injuries in Infancy and Childhood

Fractures of the clavicle are particularly common in childhood, and almost half occur in children younger than 7 years.[26] Fractures commonly result from a fall on the point of the shoulder or on an outstretched hand. In younger children, such a fall is not uncommonly from a highchair, bed, or changing table. The fracture is occasionally caused by a direct violent force applied from the front of the clavicle; like other fractures of long bones, fractures of the clavicle may be one of several signs of trauma in a physically abused child.

Unlike the situation in adults, direct and indirect trauma to a child's clavicle can result in incomplete or greenstick fractures rather than displaced fractures.[278] In addition, trauma to a child's clavicle can result in plastic bowing alone without evident cortical disruption. Despite an initial appearance of only bowing, on later examination, these fractures usually show evidence of gross healing of complete fractures, with obvious callus visible on radiographs.[37,374]

Trauma in Adults and Adolescents

The incidence of fractures of the clavicle in adults appears to be increasing because of several factors, including the occurrence of many more high-velocity vehicular injuries and the increase in the popularity of contact sports.[315] The mechanism of injury of fractures of the clavicle in adults has been widely reported to consist of either direct or indirect force. It has generally been assumed that the most common mechanism of fractures in adults is a fall onto the outstretched hand.[75] Allman, in dividing fractures of the clavicle into three groups, proposed different mechanisms of injury for each group.[6] He thought that in group I (fractures of the middle third), the most common mechanism of injury is a fall onto an outstretched hand, with the force being transmitted up the arm and across the glenohumeral joint and dispersing along the clavicle. Group II fractures, those distal to the coracoclavicular ligaments, occur from a fall on the lateral aspect of the shoulder that drives the shoulder and scapula downward. Group III fractures, or proximal clavicle fractures, are usually due to direct violence caused by a force applied from the lateral side.

In 1994, Nordqvist and Petersson investigated the incidence of fractures of the clavicle. They reviewed 2035 fractures that occurred between 1952 and 1987.[282] The fractures were classified into three groups according to the Allman system.[6] Each group was further divided into nondisplaced fracture subgroups, with an extra subgroup of comminuted mid-clavicle fractures in group I. Of the fractures, 76% were classified as Allman group I. The median age of the patients in this group was 13 years. Significant differences in age- and gender-specific incidence were noted between the nondisplaced, displaced, and comminuted fracture subgroups. Allman group II accounted for 21% of the fractures. The median age of these patients was 47 years, and no difference in age was found between the subgroups with nondisplaced and displaced fractures. Three percent of the fractures were classified as Allman group III, and the median age of the patients in this group was 59 years. All three groups were characterized by a significant preponderance of male patients.

A study by Nowak in 2000 showed that the incidence of clavicle fractures in Uppsala, Sweden, was 50 per 100,000 population; however, the incidence in male patients was 71 per 100,000, and the incidence in female patients was 30 per 100,000.[286,289] Bicycle accidents were the most common cause of injury, and male patients tended to be younger and to have more comminuted, high-energy injuries. Most (75%) of the injuries were midshaft fractures, and the nonunion rate was 5%.

In 1962, Fowler[105] pointed out that clavicular injuries almost always follow a fall or a blow on the point of the shoulder, whereas a blow on the bone itself is rarely a cause (although a direct blow has certainly been recognized in sports, particularly in stick sports such as lacrosse and hockey[369]). In a large series of fractures of the clavicle (342 patients) studied by Sankarankutty and Turner, 91% sustained a fall or blow to the point of the shoulder, whereas only 1% had a fall onto the outstretched hand.[353]

More recently, Stanley et al. studied a consecutive series of 150 patients with fractures of the clavicle; 81% of the patients described the mechanism of injury.[378] The researchers found that 94% had fractured the clavicle from a direct blow on the shoulder, whereas only 6% had fallen onto an outstretched hand. Further biomechanical analysis of the force involved in the fracture of the clavicle by this group revealed that direct injury produces a critical buckling load that is exceeded at a compression force equivalent to body weight, and thereby results in the fracture of the bone. When force is applied along the axis of the arm, the buckling force is rarely reached in the clavicle. These investigators recorded fractures at every site along the clavicle with a direct injury to the point of the shoulder, and found little support for Allman's concept that fractures at different anatomic sites have different mechanisms of injury. In addition, they theorized that a direct blow to the shoulder might even be the mechanism of injury in those who described a fall on the outstretched hand: as the hand makes contact with the ground, the patient's body weight and falling velocity are such that the fall continues, with the shoulder becoming the upper limb's next point of contact with the ground.

Harnroongroj et al. found that when clavicles were axially loaded, they tended to fracture at the middle third of the clavicle in the region where the curve of the lateral aspect of the clavicle changes to the curve of the medial aspect of the clavicle.[136] The force required to fracture the clavicle was 1526.19 N, and the ratio of the lateral fragment to the total length of the clavicle was 0.49.

Another indirect mechanism of fracture of the clavicle is a direct force applied to the top of the shoulder; the clavicle is forced against the first rib, and a spiral fracture of the middle third is often produced.[75] Another variation of this mechanism is what we refer to as *seatbelt fractures*. The shoulder strap from the seatbelt acts as a fulcrum, typically at the midpoint of the clavicle, and the forward force of the clavicle against this fulcrum causes the clavicle to fracture in a transverse or oblique pattern, with little or no comminution. Although we cannot explain why, it appears that this fracture is more prone to nonunion than more typical fractures (Fig. 8-19). It may be because the amount of energy required to cause a transverse fracture is more than that required to cause the fractures seen with an axial load.

Stress Fractures

Stress fractures of the clavicle have been reported in athletes. They have been seen in a variety of sports, including baseball, diving, gymnastics, and cheerleading.[2,94,344,412,426] It appears that the mechanism of injury is repeated axial loading of the clavicle in all the activities except cheerleading. These fractures tend to be more medial, and should be suspected in patients with chronic clavicular pain associated with overuse. Although plain radiographs can appear normal, bone scintigraphy usually reveals endosteal thickening; however, magnetic resonance imaging can easily detect these injuries and also help rule out pathologic fractures. Most of these fractures occur after changes or an increase in the athlete's training routine, and typically heal uneventfully with rest and activity modification. Stress fractures have also been reported in conjunction with coracoclavicular cerclage fixation of acromioclavicular joint separation.[80]

Nontraumatic Fractures

It is well recognized that the clavicle can be the site of neoplastic or infectious destruction of bone, and a fracture can occur after relatively minor trauma. Certainly,

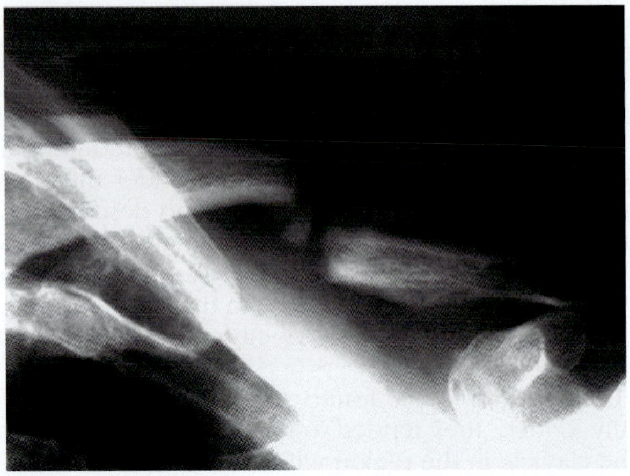

FIGURE 8-19: Atrophic midshaft clavicular nonunion 18 months after a seatbelt injury.

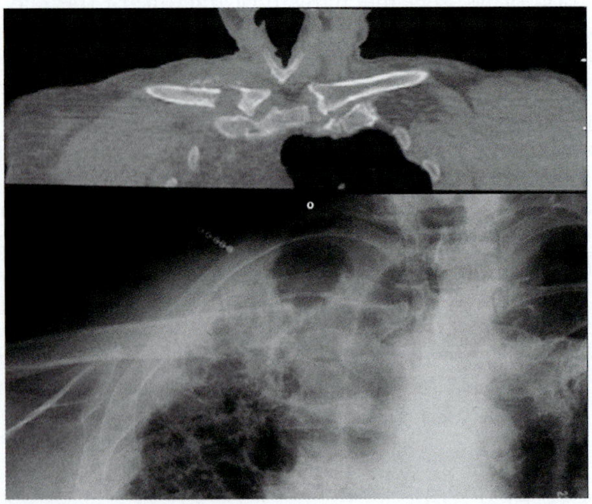

FIGURE 8-20: Medial right clavicular stress fracture 1 year after radical neck dissection for squamous cell carcinoma. Biopsy showed only evidence of a healing fracture with no evidence of tumor.

lack of a traumatic episode should lead the clinician to focus on the possibility that a long bone fracture has occurred in pathologic bone. In addition to both malignant and benign lesions producing pathologic fractures of the clavicle,[377,32] pathologic fracture has also been described in association with arteriovenous malformation, an entity that can mimic a neoplasm.[251]

Atraumatic stress fractures have also been reported in the clavicle.[187] In addition, spontaneous fracture of the medial end of the clavicle has been reported as a pseudotumor after radical neck dissection (Fig. 8-20).[66,101,293,384] Atraumatic clavicular stress fractures have also been reported after reverse total shoulder arthroplasty (Fig. 8-21).[9]

The synthetic material used to treat coracoclavicular disruption has also been reported to produce stress fractures in the clavicle, with subsequent nonunion. Nonunion of the clavicle has occurred after the use of polyester

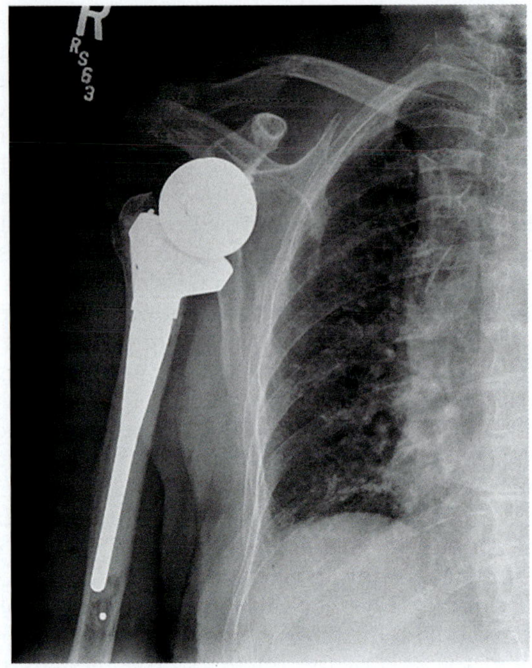

FIGURE 8-21: Clavicle stress fracture seen after a reverse total shoulder arthroplasty. (From Anakwenze OA, Pifer MA, Singh A. Clavicle stress fracture after reverse shoulder arthroplasty. *J Shoulder Elbow Surg.* 2014;23[7]:e170-e172.)

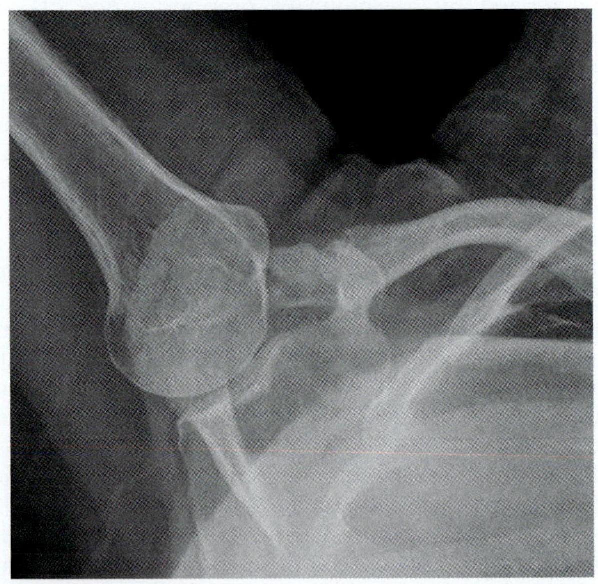

FIGURE 8-22: Erosion of the coracoid and clavicle seen after stabilization of a distal-third fracture using nonabsorbable sutures.

mesh (Mersilene) tape and polyethylene (Dacron) to repair a grade III dislocation of the acromioclavicular joint.[233] Such nonunion is likely the result of the differential motion between the clavicle and the scapula with normal arm motion. When the tape or suture is passed over the clavicle, the differential motion can result in the tape sawing through the clavicle. Figure 8-22 shows an axillary view of a patient who had undergone nonabsorbable suture fixation around the clavicle and coracoid for a distal clavicle fracture.

CLINICAL FINDINGS

Birth Fractures

Two clinical manifestations of birth fractures appear to predominate: clinically unapparent and clinically apparent (pseudoparalysis).

Diagnosis of clinically unapparent fracture may be very difficult because of the presence of few clinical symptoms. A crack heard during the delivery may be the only clue to fracture of the clavicle.[357] Whether the lesion in this group of fractures is truly asymptomatic and is overlooked in the neonatal examination is uncertain, but Farkas and Levine emphasized that many of these fractures are not initially diagnosed. Of the five cases of fracture of the clavicle in 355 newborns in their series, none were suspected after routine physical examination in the delivery room and newborn nursery.[97] On reexamination, however, crepitus could usually be demonstrated at the fracture site. Thus it appears that fractures can easily be overlooked. However, because they are generally unilateral, close examination can reveal asymmetry of clavicular contour or shortening of the neck line. The fracture is often first recognized by the mother after noticing the swelling, which is caused by fracture callus, and typically appears 7 to 11 days after the fracture.[65]

The infant with a clinically apparent fracture is disinclined or unwilling to use the extremity, and clinicians note a unilateral lack of movement of the whole upper limb either spontaneously or during elicitation of the Moro reflex.[106,352] Because these fractures are often complete, local swelling, tenderness, and crepitus can suggest the diagnosis. This injury must be distinguished from other conditions that can make the infant disinclined or unable to use the extremity, such as birth brachial plexus injury, separation of the proximal humeral epiphysis, and acute osteomyelitis of the clavicle or proximal end of the humerus. It is important to remember that a fractured clavicle and a brachial plexus injury can coexist.[389]

Fractures in Children

Almost half of fractures of the clavicle in children occur in those younger than 7 years. Because clavicle fractures in these young children may be incomplete or of the greenstick variety, they might not be obvious, and thus may be overlooked. The mother of the infant might notice that the baby cries after being picked up and appears to be hurt.[26] The baby does not seem to use the arm naturally and cries when the arm is used for any activities or is moved during dressing. On palpation, a tender, uneven upper border of the clavicle may be felt that is asymmetric when compared with the contralateral side. As with a newborn, the mother may take the baby to the pediatrician because of the "sudden" appearance of a lump (Fig. 8-23).[68]

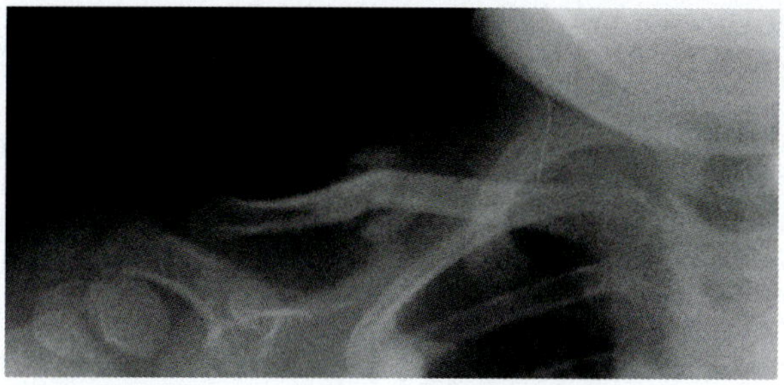

FIGURE 8-23: Clavicle fracture in a 2-year-old child. Prominent callus formation is evident and is manifested clinically as a bump.

However, if the fracture is complete in children who are ambulatory and verbal, the diagnosis is usually obvious. In addition to the child's complaints of pain localized to the clavicle, when these fractures are displaced, a typical deformity caused by muscle displacement of the fracture fragments is apparent. The shoulder on the affected side can appear lower and droop forward and inward. The child splints the involved extremity against the body and supports the affected elbow with the contralateral hand. Because of the pull of the sternocleidomastoid muscle on the proximal fragment, the child tilts the head toward and the chin away from the side of the fracture in an effort to relax the pull of this muscle (Fig. 8-24).[389] Physical examination reveals tenderness, crepitus, and swelling, which are typical for this fracture at any age.

Complete acromioclavicular separations are very unusual in children younger than 16 years. What may be evident clinically as a high-riding clavicle above the acromioclavicular joint and an apparent acromioclavicular separation is often either a transperiosteal distal clavicle fracture or, more commonly, a rupture through the periosteum plus a distal clavicle fracture, with the coracoclavicular ligaments remaining behind attached to the periosteum. This lesion is not often recognized in children younger than 16 years.[86]

Similarly, because the sternal epiphysis is the last epiphysis of the long bones to fuse with the metaphysis (fusion usually occurs from ages 22 to 25 years), the joint may be subject to the usual types of epiphyseal injury. Many misdiagnosed sternoclavicular dislocations are, in fact, separations through the medial clavicular epiphysis. Occasionally, sternoclavicular separations occur with adjacent clavicle fractures in children.[41,207]

It should be pointed out that, although the clavicle is the last bone to stop growing, there is probably very little potential for remodeling after the age of 9 years in females and 12 years in males (Fig. 8-25).[240] Furthermore, although younger patients can remodel an angular deformity, there is little possibility of remodeling shortening. This needs to be taken into account when dealing with these fractures in "little adults."

Fractures in Adults

Because of the characteristic clinical features in adults, displaced fractures of the clavicle present little difficulty with diagnosis if the patient is seen soon after injury. The patient usually provides a clear history of some form of either direct or indirect injury to the shoulder. The clinical deformity is obvious, and may be out of proportion to the amount of discomfort that the patient experiences.[26] The proximal fragment is displaced upward and backward, and may be tenting the skin. Compounding of this fracture is unusual but can occur.[328] The patient is usually splinting the involved extremity at the side because any movement elicits pain. The involved arm droops forward and down because of the weight of the arm and the pull of the pectoralis minor muscle. This drooping further accentuates the posterosuperior angulation seen in most clavicle fractures. Although the initial deformity may be obvious later, acute swelling of the soft tissue and hemorrhage may obscure it. In fractures near the ligamentous structures (acromioclavicular and sternoclavicular joints), the deformity can mimic a purely ligamentous injury.

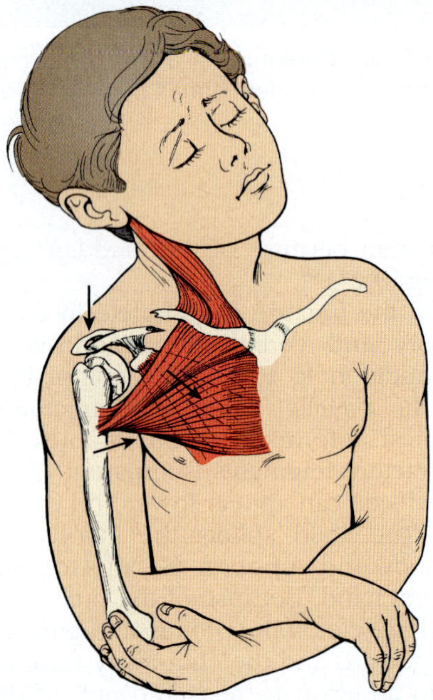

FIGURE 8-24: Clinical manifestation of a displaced clavicle fracture in a child. The shoulder on the affected side appears lower and droops forward and inward. The child splints the involved extremity against the body, supports the affected elbow with the contralateral hand, and tilts the head toward and the chin away from the site of the fracture to relax the pull of the sternocleidomastoid muscle.

Examination of the patient reveals tenderness directly over the fracture site, and any movement of the arm is painful. Ecchymosis may be noted over the fracture site, especially if severe displacement of the bone fragments has produced associated tearing of the soft tissue. Patients might angle the head toward the injury in an attempt to relax the pull of the trapezius muscle on the fragment. As in children, the patient may be more comfortable with the chin tilted to the opposite side. Gentle palpation and manipulation usually produces crepitus and motion, and the site of the fracture is easily palpable because of the subcutaneous position of the bone. The skin over the clavicle, the scapula, or the chest wall might give a clue to the mechanism of injury and might indicate other areas to be evaluated for associated injuries. The lungs must be examined for the presence of symmetrical breath sounds, and the whole extremity must be examined carefully.

Nondisplaced fractures or isolated fractures of the articular surfaces might not cause deformity, and thus may be overlooked unless they are specifically sought radiographically. If the diagnosis is in doubt, special radiographs or a repeat radiograph of the clavicle in 7 to 10 days may be indicated.

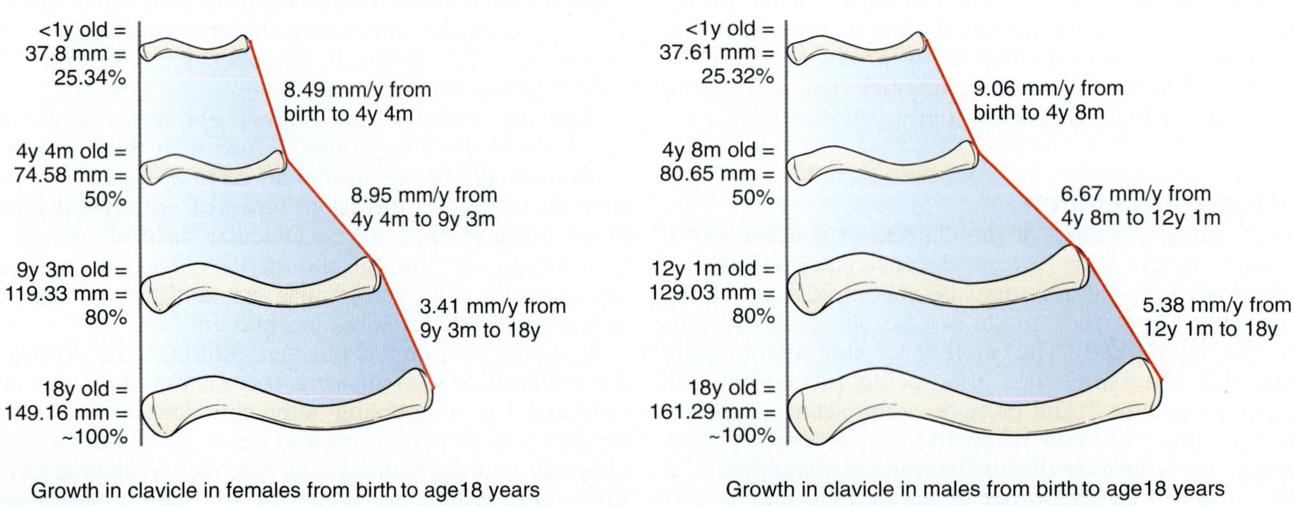

FIGURE 8-25: Growth of the clavicle in females and males from less than 1 to 18 years of age. (From McGraw MA, Mehlman CT, Lindsell CJ, et al. Postnatal growth of the clavicle: birth to 18 years of age. *J Pediatr Orthop.* 2009;29:937-943.)

A panclavicular dislocation is typically produced by extreme and forceful protraction of the shoulder. This injury is usually the result of a major traumatic episode such as a high-speed motor vehicle accident, a fall from a height, or a very heavy object falling on the shoulder,[115] although it has been reported after a minor fall at home.[165] Clinically, patients usually have bruising over the spine of the scapula, and swelling and tenderness at both ends of the clavicle. This injury is associated with anterosuperior sternoclavicular dislocation and either posterosuperior or subjacent displacement of the clavicle. The whole clavicle may be freely mobile and may feel as though it is floating. Radiographs usually confirm this injury.

Associated Injuries

In 1830, Gross reported that "fractures of the clavicle usually assume a mild aspect, being seldom accompanied by any serious accident."[125] Although statistically, most clavicle fractures are relatively innocuous injuries, serious associated injuries can occur, and a delay in treatment may be potentially life-threatening.[203,76] Therefore, in a patient with a clavicle fracture, it is critical that a careful examination of the entire upper extremity be performed, with particular emphasis on neurovascular status, in addition to careful examination of the lungs.[78]

Associated injuries accompanying acute fractures of the clavicle may be divided into associated skeletal injuries, injuries to the lung and pleura, vascular injuries, and brachial plexus injuries.

Associated skeletal injuries can include sternoclavicular or acromioclavicular separations or fracture-dislocations through these joints (Fig. 8-26).[207,42,181,428] As might be anticipated with ipsilateral sternoclavicular or acromioclavicular joint injuries, closed reduction of the ligamentous injury is usually impossible because of the accompanying clavicle fracture.[181] Baccarani et al. reported a fracture of the coracoid process associated with a fracture of the clavicle that they treated by open reduction and internal fixation of the coracoid.[449]

Head and neck injuries may be present,[420] especially with displaced distal clavicle fractures. In one series, 10% of the patients were comatose.[270]

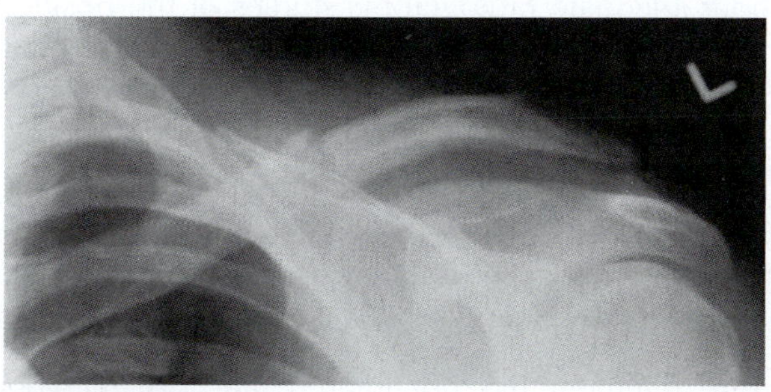

FIGURE 8-26: An unusual case of a fracture of the clavicle associated with complete acromioclavicular separation. The associated clavicle fracture makes treatment of the ligamentous injury very difficult.

Fractures of the first rib are not infrequent and are easily overlooked (Fig. 8-27).[4,417] These rib fractures may be directly responsible for accompanying lung, brachial plexus, or subclavian vein injury. First-rib fractures may be underrecognized because they are not easily seen on standard chest radiographs. Weiner and O'Dell recommended either an AP view of the cervical spine or an AP view of the thoracic spine associated with a lateral view of the thoracic spine to decrease the likelihood that this injury would be overlooked.[417] The location of a first-rib fracture may be either the ipsilateral or contralateral rib to the clavicle fracture.

Weiner and O'Dell have outlined how several of these types of rib fractures occur. The scalenus anticus muscle attaches on a tubercle of the first rib. On either side of this tubercle lies a groove for the subclavian vein anteriorly and the subclavian artery posteriorly. Posterior to the groove for the subclavian artery lies a roughened area for attachment of the scalenus medius muscle. These two muscles elevate the rib during inspiration. The serratus anterior muscle arises from the outer surfaces of the upper eight ribs, and fixes the rib posteriorly during inspiration. These structures can interact to contribute to the occurrence of fractures of the first rib as the clavicle is fractured.

Three basic mechanisms have been theorized to be responsible for this combination of injuries: indirect force transmitted via the manubrium, avulsion fracture at the weakest portion of the rib by the scalenus anticus, and injury to the lateral portion of the clavicle, causing an acromioclavicular separation that leads to indirect force from the subclavius muscle to the costal cartilage and the anterior aspect of the first rib.[417,314] Because of the loss of the suspensory function of the clavicle and splinting

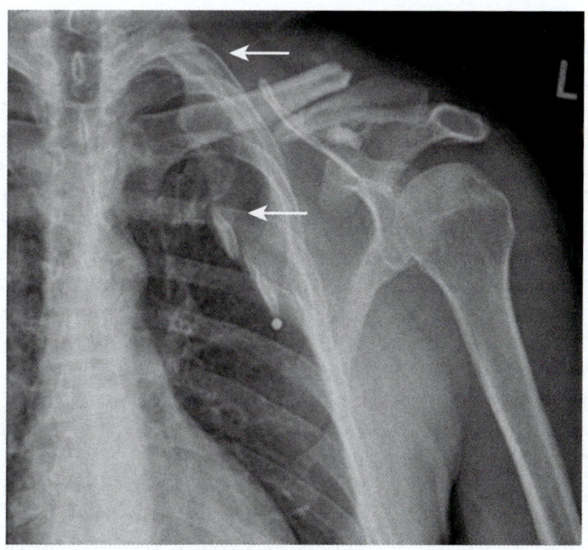

FIGURE 8-27: Fracture of the left clavicle associated with a left pneumothorax (lower arrow). The lung markings are absent on the left side. This patient also had multiple rib fractures including the second rib (upper arrow).

secondary to pain from the clavicle and rib fractures, care should be taken to monitor respiratory function, especially in those with already compromised function, such as patients with chronic obstructive pulmonary disease. These patients can easily decompensate unless given appropriate respiratory and analgesic support.

Fractures of the clavicle may also be associated with dissociation-disruption of the scapulothoracic articulation manifested as swelling of the shoulder, lateral displacement of the clavicle, severe neurovascular injury, and fracture of the clavicle or the acromioclavicular or sternoclavicular joints.[81]

In a combination injury, the floating shoulder consists of fractures of both the clavicle and the scapula, and is associated with an extremely unstable shoulder girdle. In this injury, sequelae such as a drooping shoulder and limited range of motion can develop if this fracture is treated conservatively. Rockwood surveyed members of the American Shoulder and Elbow Surgeons, and concluded that treatment should be directed primarily at stabilization of the clavicle. The primary indication for internal fixation of the scapula is to reduce and internally stabilize a grossly displaced intra-articular fracture of the glenoid fossa.[214,340] Stabilization of the clavicle alone has been shown to produce good and excellent functional results.[222,400] In a case of multiple trauma, Herscovici et al. recommended internal fixation of only the clavicle fracture.[142,143]

Other authors have suggested that although operative fixation does give good results, most cases of floating shoulder are not really unstable, and can be managed with nonoperative treatment.[85,407,422] Williams et al. studied double disruptions of the superior suspensory mechanism, and did not find any significant loss of stability unless the coracoacromial and acromioclavicular ligaments were disrupted in addition to fractures of the clavicle and glenoid neck.[422]

A number of authors have commented on the potentially serious complication of associated pneumothorax or hemothorax with fractures of the clavicle because the apical pleura and upper lung lobes lie adjacent to this bone (see Fig. 8-27).[243] Rowe reported a 3% incidence of pneumothorax in a series of 690 clavicle fractures, but did not comment on how many had associated rib or scapular fractures.[345,346] Although it is easy to see how a severely displaced fracture can puncture the pleura with a sharp shard of bone to produce this lesion, the radiographic appearance may be misleadingly benign, with little evidence to suggest what might have been significant fragment displacement at the time of injury.[78] It is essential that a careful physical examination of the lung be undertaken at the initial evaluation and that the presence and symmetry of breath sounds be identified. In addition, an upright chest film appears to be important in the assessment of all patients with fractures of the clavicle who have decreased breath sounds or other physical findings that suggest pneumothorax, with particularly close attention paid to the outline of the lung.[228] Such assessment is especially necessary in multiply traumatized or unconscious patients who have neither obvious blunt chest trauma nor any external signs of trauma to the chest that might yield a clue to potential lung or pleural complications.[78,162,228,379,381,431]

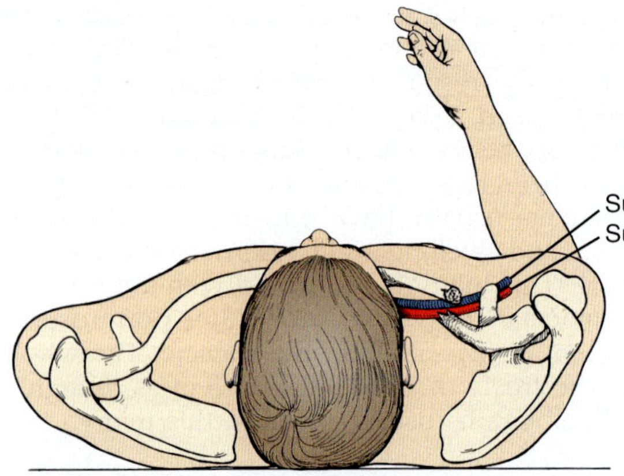

FIGURE 8-28: As the clavicle fractures and displaces, the subclavian vessels immediately posterior to the clavicle may be injured by sharp shards of bone.

Although nerve injuries are rare with clavicle fractures, acute injuries to the brachial plexus do occur.[203] The neurovascular bundle emerges from the thoracic outlet under the clavicle on top of the first rib.[329] As it passes under the clavicle, it is protected to a certain extent by the thick medial clavicular bone; considerable trauma is usually necessary to damage the brachial plexus and break the clavicle at the same time. When the force is severe enough to break the clavicle and injure the brachial plexus, a subclavian vascular injury often occurs concomitantly (Fig. 8-28). The force resulting in nerve injury usually comes in a direction from above downward or from in front downward. As the force is applied, the nerves may be stretched, with the fulcrum of maximal tension being the transverse process of the cervical vertebra. The roots can also be torn above the clavicle, or they may be avulsed from their attachment to the spinal cord.[25] Although the posterior periosteum, subclavius muscles, and bone offer some protection to the underlying plexus, the plexus may be injured directly by the fragments of bone. Such injury is especially worthy of emphasis: Clavicle fragments should not be manipulated without adequate radiographic studies of the position of these fracture fragments.[408]

Direct injury to the brachial plexus usually involves the ulnar nerve because this portion of the plexus lies adjacent to the middle third of the clavicle.

Acute vascular injuries are unusual because of many of the same local anatomic factors that protect the nerves from direct injury. The subclavius muscle and the thick, deep cervical fascia also act as barriers against direct injury to the vessels. If the initial displacement of the fracture fragment has not injured the adjacent vessels, they are unlikely to be injured further, because the distal fragment is pulled downward and forward by the weight of the limb and the proximal fragment is pulled upward and backward by the trapezius muscle. Thus, as with

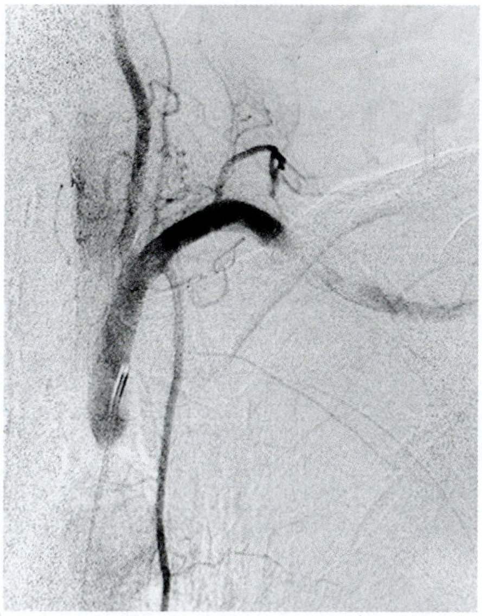

FIGURE 8-29: Subtraction arteriogram showing nearly complete cutoff of the left subclavian artery after a clavicle malunion.

acute nerve injury, a major injury is usually required to produce an acute vascular insult.[303] Nevertheless, injury has been reported even with greenstick fractures.[250] In addition, acute vascular compression resulting from fracture angulation has been described (Fig. 8-29).[67]

When they occur, vascular injuries include laceration, occlusion, spasm, or acute compression; the vessels most commonly injured are the subclavian artery, subclavian vein, and internal jugular vein.[166,193,216,235] The subclavian vein is particularly vulnerable to tearing because it is fixed to the clavicle by a fascial aponeurosis.[129,380] Injuries to the suprascapular and axillary arteries have also been reported.[158,399] Laceration can result in life-threatening hemorrhage, whereas arterial thrombus and occlusion can lead to distal ischemia. Damage to the arterial wall can, in addition, lead to aneurysm formation and late embolic phenomena. Venous thrombosis may be problematic as well; although it does not typically threaten life or limb, it has the potential for pulmonary embolism, which can constitute a threat.[355]

Clinical recognition of an acute vascular injury may be difficult, particularly in an unconscious patient or one in shock. Although a complete laceration can cause life-threatening hemorrhage or result in an extremity that is cold, pulseless, and pale, a partial laceration is more likely to be manifested as uncontrolled bleeding and life-threatening blood loss. The color and temperature of the extremity may be normal, but the absence of a pulse, the presence of a bruit, or a pulsatile hematoma (as the hematoma is walled off or produces a false aneurysm) should make the clinician strongly suspect a major vascular injury.[399] If blood flow is significantly obstructed, the injured limb is usually colder than the uninjured limb, but there might also be a difference in blood pressure between the two.[431] Vascular contusion or spasm can result in thrombotic and, later, thromboembolic phenomena.[416] It is sometimes difficult to recognize the difference between arterial spasm and interruption or occlusion, and it may be reasonable to consider a sympathetic block to help distinguish a spasm from a more serious injury.

If major injury to a vessel is suspected, an arteriogram should be performed.[431] In the rare event of a tear of a large vessel, surgical exploration is mandatory. To gain adequate exposure, as much of the clavicle should be excised as needed to isolate and repair the injured major vessel. Although the vessel may be ligated in some cases, ligation of a major vessel in an elderly patient might well be dangerous because of inadequate remaining circulation to the extremity. In any event, a surgeon skilled in decision-making and in the techniques of vascular repair is essential if a major injury has occurred.

Of particular importance is the association of medial clavicle fractures with the occurrence of almost all of these injuries. Medial clavicle fractures are relatively uncommon in comparison to midshaft and lateral fractures, but they have been associated with a very high incidence of pulmonary problems such as pneumothorax, hemothorax, or hemopneumothorax and pulmonary contusion as well as head, face, and cervical injuries.[395] Most impressive is the very high mortality rate found in association with medial clavicle injuries. Throckmorton and Kuhn found that 20% of patients with medial clavicle fractures die as a result of their associated injuries.[395]

RADIOGRAPHIC EVALUATION

Fractures of the Shaft

With most clavicular shaft fractures, the diagnosis is not in doubt because of the clinical deformity and confirmatory radiographs. Unfortunately, many physicians obtain only an AP radiograph of the shoulder to image clavicle fractures. Because of the multiplanar nature of the clavicle, it is almost impossible to determine displacement and angulation on a single AP radiograph. The primary problem is that the plane of the fracture is oblique to the plane of the x-ray beam. Therefore what is measured as displacement or shortening on an AP radiograph is really equivalent to the base of a triangle, but the true amount of shortening is really the hypotenuse of the triangle (Fig. 8-30). If it is taken into account that the clavicle not only shortens but also becomes angulated inferiorly and rotated medially, the deformity is truly in three planes. Aside from using a three-dimensional Cartesian coordinate system, it is very difficult, if not impossible, to characterize the true deformity on plane radiographs. Furthermore, it is important to obtain standing radiographs of the clavicle because supine radiographs will diminish the effects of gravity on the displacement of the lateral fragment. It is important to note this in regard to CT scans of the clavicle since these are performed in a supine position. It is also important to note that displacement can worsen with time due to the downward

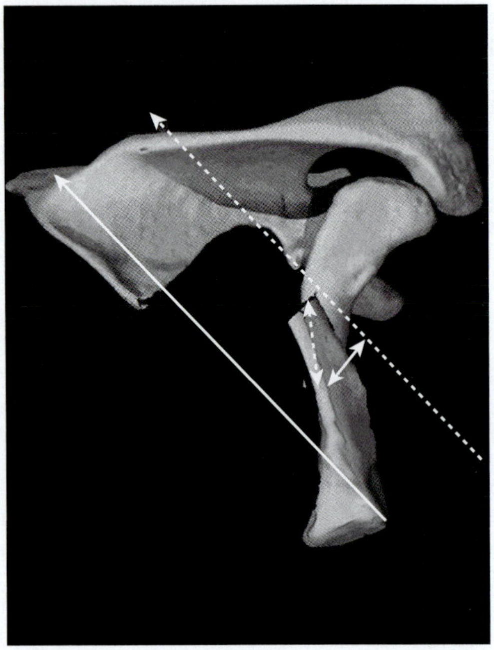

FIGURE 8-30: Shortening cannot be determined on standard radiographs because the deformity is not orthogonal to the x-ray beam. The beam is represented by the long dashed line and the apparent shortening by the short solid line. The true shortening (short dotted line) is really the hypotenuse of the triangle and is longer than the apparent shortening.

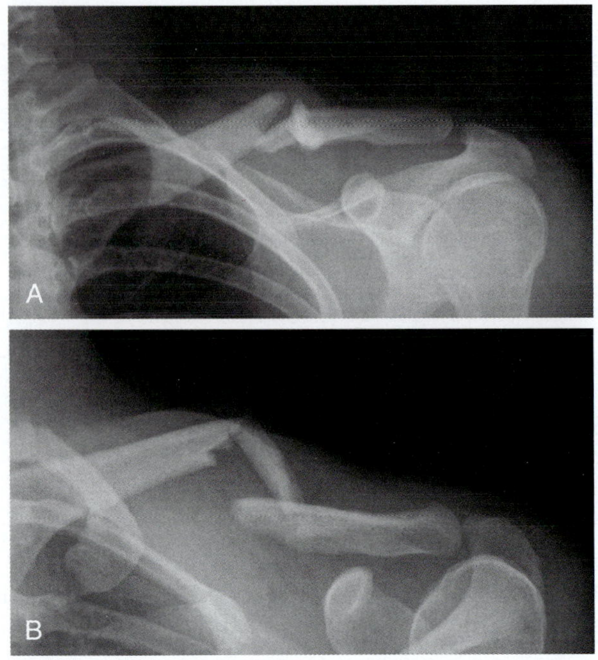

FIGURE 8-31: A, Anteroposterior radiograph of an acute midshaft left clavicle fracture sustained in a mountain bike accident. It appears to be relatively nondisplaced on this view. **B,** A 45-degree cephalic tilt radiograph of the clavicle showing marked displacement and a transversely oriented butterfly fragment.

gravitational pull on the shoulder and also the deforming forces of the muscles about the shoulder. Even if the initial radiographic evaluation suggests minimal deformity, patients treated nonoperatively should receive follow-up radiographs. Significant displacement has been shown to occur in up to 60% of patients initially believed to be nonoperative candidates due to minimal displacement on initial radiographs.[309,331]

To obtain as accurate an evaluation of fragment position as possible, at least two projections of the clavicle should always be obtained: an AP view and a 45-degree cephalic tilt view. In the former, the proximal fragment is typically displaced upward and the distal fragment is displaced downward (Figs. 8-31A and 8-32A). In the latter, the tube is directed from below upward and more accurately assesses the AP relationship of the two fragments (see Figs. 8-31B and 8-32B).[419] Displacement of the fracture is best assessed on the 45-degree cephalic tilt projection. An axillary view with the beam angled slightly cephalad can also help determine fracture displacement, and can be useful in assessing possible nonunion (Figs. 8-33 and 8-34). Quesana recommended two views at right angles to each other, a 45-degree angle superiorly and a 45-degree angle inferiorly, to assess the extent and displacement of fractures of the clavicle.[321] In our practice, we have not really found the 45-degree caudal tilt view to be of benefit.

Rowe has suggested that with an AP radiograph, the film should include the upper third of the humerus, the shoulder girdle, and the upper lung fields so that other

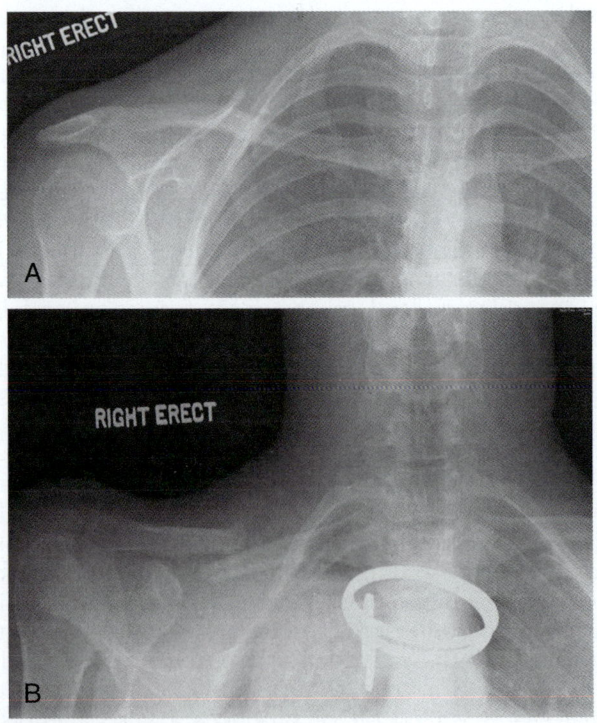

FIGURE 8-32: A, Benign-looking anteroposterior (AP) radiograph of a fracture sustained while the patient was playing Frisbee. **B,** Significant deformity unseen on the AP radiograph. The hint on the AP view of significant deformity is the markedly oblique orientation of the scapula.

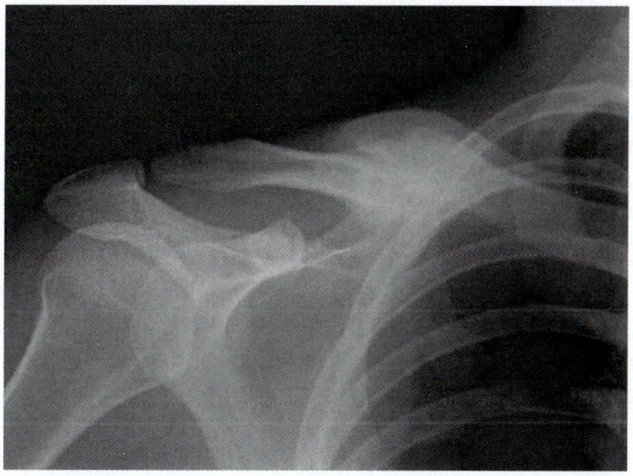

FIGURE 8-33: Anteroposterior radiograph of a clavicle nonunion. On this view, the fracture appears to be healed in acceptable alignment and has adequate callus.

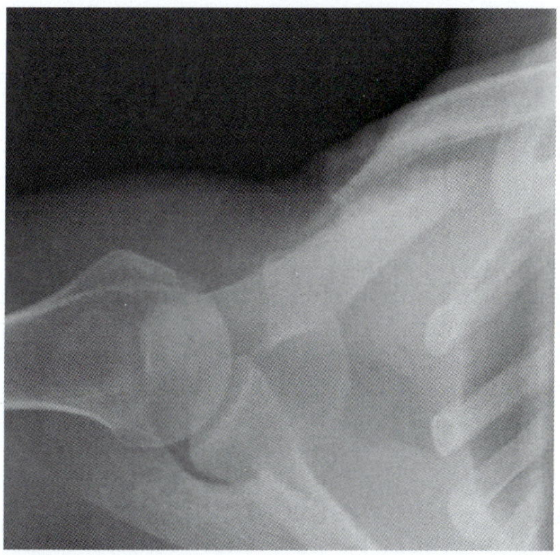

FIGURE 8-34: Axillary radiograph of the same patient in Figure 8-33. The nonunion is obvious, with significant shortening at the fracture site.

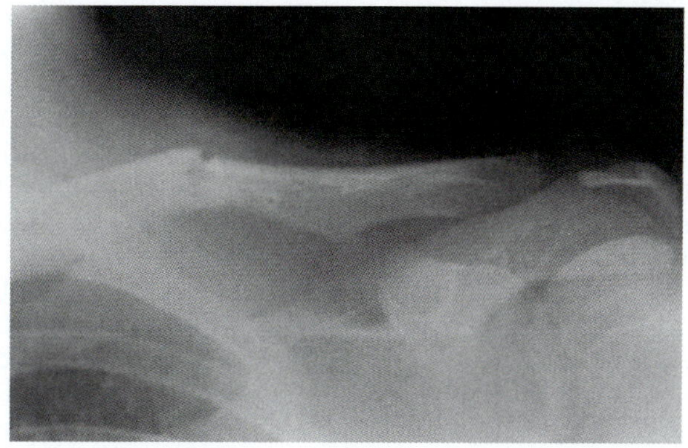

FIGURE 8-35: Greenstick fracture of the left clavicle in a 14-year-old patient. In such a patient, diagnosis may be more difficult.

shoulder girdle fractures and pneumothorax can be identified more speedily.[345] The configuration of the fracture is also important to assess because it can give clues as to the presence of associated injuries. The usual clavicular shaft fracture in adults is slightly oblique; fractures that are more comminuted, and especially if the middle spike is projecting in a superior-to-inferior direction, have generally resulted from a greater force, and can alert the surgeon to the potential for associated neurovascular or pulmonary injuries.

Children's fractures may be greenstick or nondisplaced, or they can appear only as bony bowing, and thus the diagnosis of shaft fractures may be more difficult to make (Fig. 8-35), especially in newborns or infants, in whom the clinical findings may be difficult to assess. Movement by the child or bone overlap can obscure radiographic detail, and an incomplete fracture might not be recognized. However, the surrounding soft tissues of the clavicle are normally displayed as parallel shadows above the body of the clavicle. Although this accompanying shadow might not be seen along the proximal third of the clavicle medial to the crossing of the first rib, it is invariably present on most radiographs. Suspicion of fractures of the clavicle should be aroused by loss of the accompanying shadow unilaterally.[374] If there is any doubt about the presence of a fracture in a child, a repeat radiograph taken 5 to 10 days after the injury will usually reveal callus formation.

In 1988, the technique of ultrasonography was described for the evaluation of clavicular birth fractures.[184] These birth fractures can easily be overlooked and may be confused clinically with birth palsy. In their study, Katz et al. noted no difference in diagnostic accuracy between ultrasonography and plain radiography.[184] In addition, a medial clavicle fracture not seen on plain film was picked up by ultrasonography. In fact, the authors noted that the individual fracture fragments were seen to move up and down with respiration.

With either plain radiography or ultrasonography, it may be difficult to differentiate congenital pseudarthrosis from an acute fracture. However, the radiographic features, the lack of trauma, and the absence of callus usually help distinguish an atraumatic condition such as congenital pseudarthrosis from a birth fracture.

Fractures of the Distal Third

In both children and adults, the usual radiographic views obtained for shaft fractures are inadequate to completely assess distal clavicle fractures. The standard exposure for evaluation of shoulder or shaft fractures overexposes the distal end of the clavicle. The usual exposure for the distal part of the clavicle should be approximately one-third that used for the shoulder joint, especially if it is important to determine articular surface involvement.

Type II distal clavicle fractures can be particularly difficult to diagnose because the usual AP and 45-degree cephalic tilt views typically do not reveal the extent of the injury.[270] If the exposure is appropriate, this distal clavicle fracture may be identified on the AP and lateral views of the trauma series, but to accurately assess the extent of the injury and the presence or absence of associated ligamentous damage, Neer has recommended three views: the AP view, an anterior 45-degree oblique view, and a posterior 45-degree oblique view.

The AP view includes both shoulders on one plate with the patient erect and with 10 lb of weight strapped to each wrist (Figs. 8-36 and 8-37). If the distance between the coracoid and the medial fragment is increased in comparison to the normal side, ligamentous detachment from the medial fragment can be assumed to be present. However, because much of the displacement of the fracture is in the AP plane, two additional views were suggested. An anterior 45-degree oblique view, with the patient erect and the injured shoulder against the plate, gives a lateral view of the scapula and shows the medial fragment posteriorly with the outer fragment displaced anteriorly. A posterior 45-degree oblique view, with the patient erect and the injured shoulder against the plate, also demonstrates the extent of separation of the two fragments. Alternatively, a cross-body adduction AP radiograph can be obtained to assess for ligamentous injury. An AP radiograph is taken with the patient pulling the elbow of the affected shoulder to the midline. If significant ligamentous injury is present, there will be no restraint to anteromedial subluxation of the shoulder relative to the clavicle, and it will appear on the radiograph that the distal fragment is subluxating under the medial fragment.

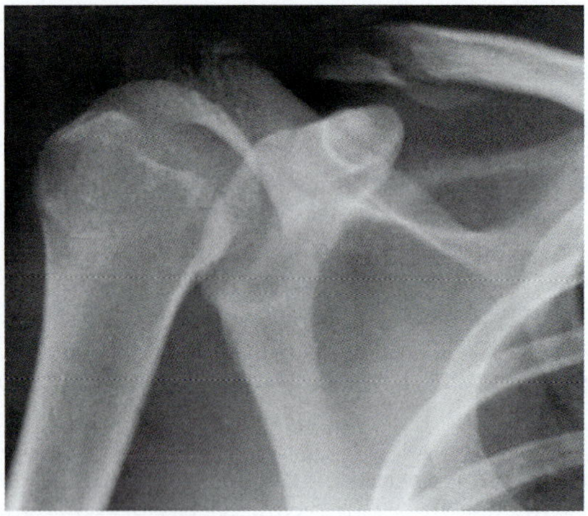

FIGURE 8-36: Fracture of the distal end of the right clavicle. In an anteroposterior view, the location of the fracture suggests ligamentous involvement, with the ligaments attached to the distal fragment.

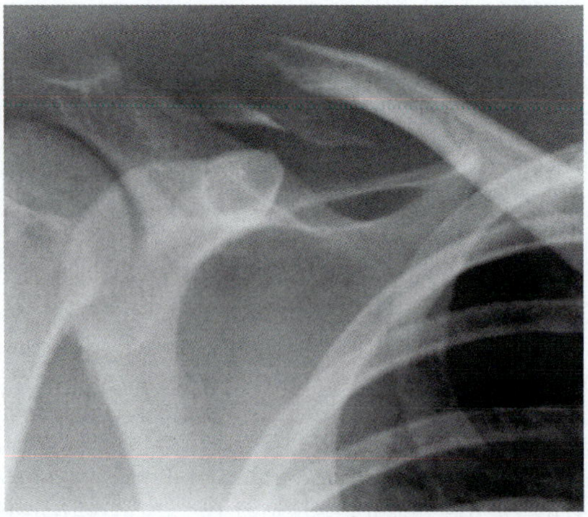

FIGURE 8-37: The extent of ligamentous involvement is confirmed on a weighted view in which separation of the coracoclavicular distance is apparent. The coracoclavicular ligaments are attached to the distal clavicular segment.

In a type II distal clavicle fracture, if radiograph views at right angles to a cephalic tilt view show good bone overlap and proximity of the fragments and if the presence of crepitation confirms contact between the fragments, stress radiographic views with weights are probably not necessary; in fact, the use of weights can further displace otherwise minimally displaced fracture fragments (Fig. 8-38). Posterior displacement of type II distal clavicle fractures is best assessed with an axillary radiograph.

Articular surface fractures of the distal end of the clavicle are easily overlooked unless high-quality radiographs are obtained. A Zanca view with a 15-degree cephalic tilt and soft tissue technique can detect intra-articular fractures much better than standard radiographs can. If the fracture is not seen on a plain radiograph view and clinical suspicion is strong, tomography or a CT scan can reveal the presence and extent of the articular surface injury (Fig. 8-39).

Fractures of the Medial Third

These fractures may be particularly difficult to detect by routine radiographs because of the overlap of ribs, vertebrae, and mediastinal shadows. However, a cephalic tilt view of 40 to 45 degrees or a serendipity view often reveals the fracture, whether in a child or an adult. In children particularly, fractures of the medial end of the clavicle are often misdiagnosed as sternoclavicular dislocations when in fact they are usually epiphyseal injuries. As with distal clavicular injuries, tomography or a CT scan may be useful for demonstrating the intra-articular or epiphyseal nature of the injury in this location.

A study by showed that over 20% of medial-third fractures can be missed on plain radiographs. A high index of suspicion is appropriate, especially in high-energy injuries such as motor vehicle accidents.[395]

Differential Diagnosis

In adults, fractures of the shaft of the clavicle are not usually confused with any other diagnosis, although pathologic fractures are occasionally difficult to recognize as such. However, fractures of the distal or medial end

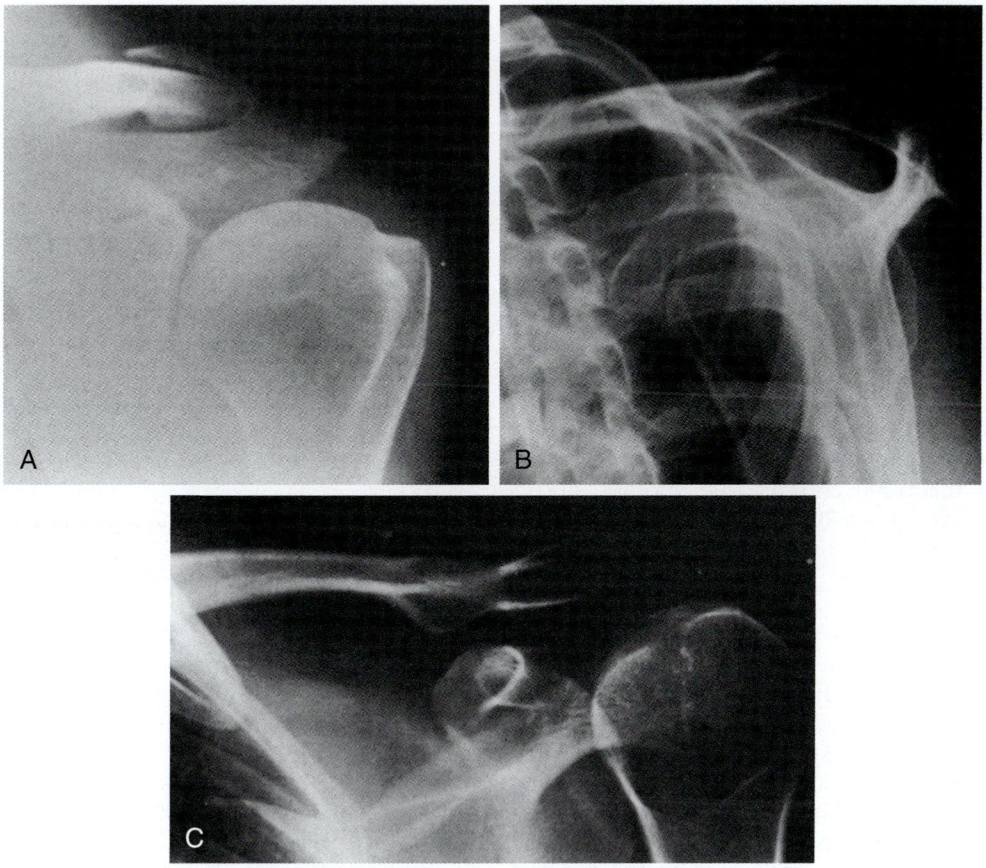

FIGURE 8-38: **A,** Distal clavicle fracture. The proximal fragment has all the coracoclavicular ligaments attached to it, but the segments have good bone contact. **B,** With good bone contact in the perpendicular views, weighted views are not usually necessary and can cause distraction of the fragments. **C,** This distal clavicle fracture healed uneventfully with nonoperative treatment. (From Rockwood CA, Green DP, eds. *Fractures*, 4th ed. Philadelphia: JB Lippincott; 1996.)

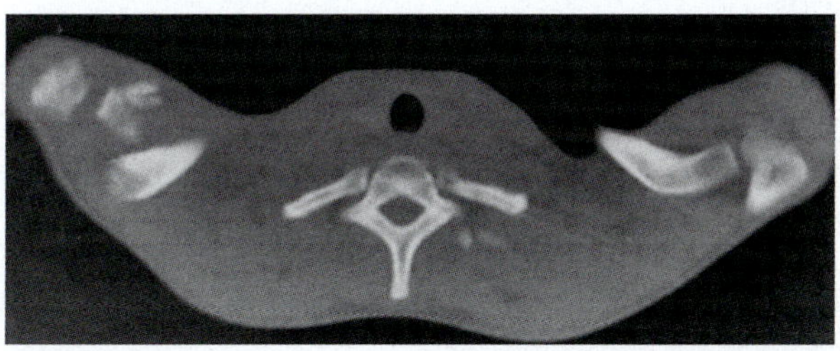

FIGURE 8-39: Computed tomographic scan of a right clavicle fracture. The scan confirms the site of fracture at the distal end of the clavicle and identifies a previously unsuspected intra-articular extension of the distal clavicle fracture.

of the clavicle can clinically appear to be complete acromioclavicular or sternoclavicular separations, although these injuries rarely cause confusion once proper radiographic studies are performed.

In children, it can be easy to confuse injuries to the clavicle with other entities, including congenital disorders and other traumatic conditions.

Congenital Pseudarthrosis

When recognized at birth or shortly thereafter, congenital pseudarthrosis may be confused with either cleidocranial dysostosis or a birth fracture, especially if some trauma has been associated with the delivery. However, birth fractures unite rapidly and leave no disability. The deformity of congenital pseudarthrosis can become more conspicuous as the child grows.[119] Clinically, the lump is painless; the child usually has no history of injury, pain, or disability with this lesion.[192,323] The lump is invariably in the lateral portion of the middle third of the clavicle, and usually affects the right clavicle except in children with dextrocardia, in which case it can occur on the left side.[219,410] Bilateral congenital pseudarthrosis has been reported, particularly in the presence of bilateral cervical ribs.[68]

The cause of this entity is unclear. Although a family history is not typical, some reports have noted a familial incidence, thus raising the question of genetic transmission.[119]

Although there may be a history of trauma with the birth, it is probably incidental; most investigators now agree that congenital pseudarthrosis is not a nonunion of normal bone after trauma.[295] It is probable that abnormal intrauterine development plays the primary role in its appearance, and it has been suggested that pressure from the subclavian artery as it arches over the first rib and under the clavicle may be a primary factor in its development.[219,220] The cervical ribs can also displace the subclavian artery and cause pressure in the same area of the clavicle.[68]

Radiographically, characteristic changes can be noted in congenital pseudarthrosis. The sternal fragment, which consists of the medial third of the clavicle, is larger and protrudes forward and upward, whereas the lateral half is situated below, points upward and backward, and ends in a bulbous mass at the pseudarthrosis site. Other identifying features are an increase in the deformity with age, the proximity of the bone ends to one another, and a large lump palpable clinically. These findings contrast quite markedly with cleidocranial dysostosis.

Cleidocranial Dysostosis

Cleidocranial dysostosis is a hereditary abnormality of membranous bone, such as the skull, and the clavicle is the most commonly involved. The abnormality varies from a central defect in the clavicle to complete absence of the clavicle; the most common manifestation is absence of the distal portion of the clavicle.[68,231] Radiographically, it is distinguished from congenital pseudarthrosis by the larger gap between the bone ends and by the tapered ends of the clavicle rather than the larger bulbous ends.[119] It is more clearly aplastic bone. In addition, multiple membranous bones are involved, and they can each have their own clinical manifestations. Some children have bossing or other skull defects, smallness of the facial bones, scoliosis, abnormal epiphyses of the hands or feet, and deficiencies of the pelvic ring. Usually, a familial history of bone disorders can be elicited.[5,92]

Sternoclavicular Dislocation

Epiphyseal fractures of the medial end of the clavicle can mimic sternoclavicular separations in children because of the late closure of the sternal epiphysis. If it is important to distinguish between these two entities, tomography or CT scanning may be indicated.

Acromioclavicular Separation

Fracture of the lateral aspect of the clavicle in children can also be identical to a complete acromioclavicular separation both clinically and radiographically. If plain radiography does not identify the small fracture fragment, tomography or CT scanning can. However, because the coracoclavicular ligaments remain attached to the periosteal tube in children and healing is uneventful, it is difficult to justify these more elaborate diagnostic modalities in children with this injury.[336]

COMPLICATIONS

Nonunion

One of the greatest fallacies of orthopedics is that "all clavicles heal well." Although many clavicles do heal with nonoperative treatment, the incidence of nonunion is likely much higher than previously thought. Nonunion of nonoperated shaft fractures was thought to be rare, with a reported incidence of 0.9% to 4%.[14,90,171,195,232,269,345,356,370,409] However, more recent research suggests that the actual nonunion rate may be much higher than previously thought, with an incidence of 15% to 25%.[91,146] A review at one of our institutions showed a 10% nonunion rate of fractures that were treated nonoperatively. However, 40% of the fractures in this series were treated acutely with surgery, which means that it could be assumed that the more serious fractures were treated operatively and that this 10% nonunion rate was seen in less severe injuries.

A systematic review also showed that the risk of nonunion was related to fracture displacement (relative risk = 2.3), fracture comminution (relative risk = 1.4), female gender (relative risk = 1.4), and advancing age as shown in Table 8-1.[437]

TABLE 8-1 Probability of Nonunion at 24 Weeks for Diaphyseal Clavicular Fractures

	Displaced (%)		Comminuted (%)		Displaced and Comminuted (%)		Not Displaced, Not Comminuted (%)	
Age (y)	Female	Male	Female	Male	Female	Male	Female	Male
25	19	8	7	3	33	20	3	<1
35	20	11	8	4	35	21	4	<1
45	25	14	10	5	37	25	5	1
55	28	18	12	6	42	29	6	2
65	33	20	18	7	47	33	7	3

From Brinker MR, Edwards TB, O'Connor DP. Estimating the risk of nonunion following nonoperative treatment of a clavicular fracture. J Bone Joint Surg Am. *2005;87(3):676-677.*

Despite some debate in the literature on the definition, most authors consider clavicular nonunion to be defined as failure to show clinical or radiographic progression of healing at 4 to 6 months postinjury,[217,174,350,421] although there is some temporal difference between atrophic and hypertrophic nonunion. Manske and Szabo reported that bone ends that were tapered, sclerotic, and atrophic at 16 weeks were unlikely to unite, whereas they classified other fractures as delayed union at the 16-week point as long as some potential for healing was present.[230] Bilateral posttraumatic pseudarthrosis has been reported in an adult.[134]

Although nonunion of the clavicle is predominantly a problem after fracture in adults, it has been described in children.[281] However, apparent nonunion in a child is likely to be congenital pseudarthrosis. Several factors appear to predispose to nonunion of the clavicle: inadequate immobilization, severity of the trauma, refracture, location of the fracture (outer third), degree of displacement (marked displacement), and primary open reduction.

Predisposing Factors

Inadequate Immobilization

It has long been recognized that the clavicle is one of the most difficult bones to immobilize properly and completely after fracture while providing the patient with the simplicity and comfort that is ideal and practical in fracture treatment. Immobilization, by whatever means, should be continued until union is complete, although it may be difficult to determine this time with certainty. Rowe has provided some guidelines for the usual healing period of fractures of the middle third of the clavicle[345]:

Infants: 2 weeks
Children: 3 weeks
Young adults: 4 to 6 weeks
Adults: 6 weeks or longer

It has been recognized, moreover, that radiographic union can progress more slowly than clinical union, with radiographic evidence of union not appearing for 12 weeks or longer.[279] When in doubt, immobilization should probably be continued. It has been suggested that once clinical union has occurred along with the absence of motion or tenderness at the fracture site, a gradual increase in activity can safely be permitted, even if radiographic union is incomplete.[279]

Severity of Trauma

Up to half of fractures resulting in nonunion follow severe trauma.[24] In their series, Wilkins and Johnston reviewed 33 ununited clavicle fractures.[421] Many of their patients had severe trauma that was manifested by the degree of displacement of the fracture fragments, the amount of soft tissue damage, and associated injuries such as multiple long bone, spine, pelvic, and rib fractures. They pointed out the similarities between the clavicle and another subcutaneous long bone, the tibia, which is also susceptible to nonunion, and emphasized that the subcutaneous position of the clavicle predisposes it to more severe trauma, more severe soft tissue damage, and thus nonunion. As with other bones, open fractures have been implicated as a factor in nonunion of the clavicle.[217] Late perforation of the skin with a free compounding fragment has also been reported.[328]

In a severely traumatic situation, although actual skin defects overlying a clavicle fracture are uncommon, soft tissue coverage appears to be essential to avoid the potential complication of osteomyelitis and nonunion. It may be that most factors associated in some series with clavicular nonunion, such as the degree of displacement, compounding, operative management, poor immobilization, and soft tissue interposition, can simply reflect the cases that have been associated with more severe trauma to the clavicle. The independent statistical importance of some of these associations with nonunion may be questioned.

The increased incidence of nonunion seen in more recent series can reflect more accurate follow-up or the fact that we are seeing more high-energy fractures. Of the patients in the 1968 Rowe study,[345] most were either children or older adults who experienced falls from a standing height. It has been our experience that the fractures we see now are often in bicyclists, particularly mountain bikers.[289,107] In fact, two recent studies showed that the most common injury in bicycle racers is a clavicle fracture. Most of these bikers report flipping over their handlebars at fairly high speeds. Because of the forward momentum in these bikers, they transmit far higher energy to the clavicle when they land on the outer aspect of the shoulder.

We have also seen an increase in what we refer to as *seatbelt fractures* (see Fig. 8-19). These injuries are typically right-sided fractures in passengers and left-sided fractures in drivers. They are generally simple, transverse fractures; however, as a group, they tend to heal very slowly and have a greater propensity for nonunion than lateral impact–type fractures do.

Refracture

A number of studies have identified refracture of a previously healed clavicle fracture as a factor contributing to the development of nonunion.[178,232] In Wilkins and Johnston's series, seven of 31 nonunions occurred in such patients.[421] There appears to be no relationship among the length of time between injuries, the age of the patient, the duration of immobilization of the original fracture, or the severity of the initial or subsequent traumatic injuries and the complication of nonunion after refracture. It has been theorized that because the vascular anatomy of a fractured bone remains altered for a long period even after fracture union,[330] reinjury might in some way prevent this altered blood supply from reacting to the new fracture.[421]

Location of Fracture

Approximately 85% of nonunions of the clavicle occur in the middle third of the bone.[325] Nonetheless, it appears that fractures of the distal third of the clavicle are much more susceptible to nonunion than shaft fractures are. In his series of clavicular nonunions, Neer noted that distal clavicle fractures accounted for more than half of the ununited clavicles after closed treatment.[269] He found the reasons for this increased incidence of nonunion to be multifactorial; the fracture is very unstable, and the muscle forces and weight of the arm tend to displace the fracture fragments.[373] Because these distal clavicular injuries are often the result of severe trauma, local soft tissue injury is extensive and associated injuries may be present and affect generalized biologic and specific fracture healing[270]; it also may be difficult to secure adequate external immobilization.

Even in fractures in which union can occur with closed methods, the union time for distal clavicle fractures is often delayed. This long healing time, combined with the associated degree of soft tissue trauma, can lead to stiffness and prolonged disability from disuse. For these reasons, Neer advocated early open reduction and internal fixation for this injury.[271,270]

Degree of Displacement

In a large series reported by Jupiter and Leffert, the degree of displacement was the most significant factor in nonunion.[178] Wick et al. found that 91% of delayed unions and nonunions had initial shortening of at least 2 cm.[418] However, in many clavicle fractures, marked displacement is often associated with other factors that delay fracture healing, such as severe trauma, soft tissue damage, open fractures, and soft tissue interposition. Manske and Szabo thought that soft tissue interposition alone was a major contributing factor in fractures that failed to heal, and at surgery they often found a fracture fragment impaled in the trapezius muscle.[230] They particularly implicated soft tissue interposition in the development of atrophic nonunion. However, others have reported that muscle interposition is uncommon.[178]

Primary Open Reduction

A number of authors have associated primary open reduction of acute clavicular shaft fractures with an increased incidence of nonunion.[360] Rowe reported an incidence of nonunion of 0.8% in fractures treated nonoperatively, which rose to 3.7% in those treated operatively.[345] Neer had a similar experience, with a nonunion rate of 0.1% in fractures treated nonoperatively and 4.6% when the initial fracture was treated surgically.[269] Schwartz and Leixnering reported a nonunion rate of 13% in patients with clavicle fractures treated by primary open reduction, although they suggested that inadequate internal fixation might have played a prominent role in this high incidence.[360] Poigenfurst et al. reported a complication rate of 10%, with four nonunions in 60 fresh clavicle fractures that were plated.[311]

Poor internal fixation rather than the surgery itself can play the primary role in the increased incidence of nonunion in patients treated by primary surgery. Zenni et al. reported a series of 25 acute clavicle fractures treated by primary open reduction with IM pins or cerclage suture and bone grafting, all of which healed without complication.[436] In some series reporting an increased incidence

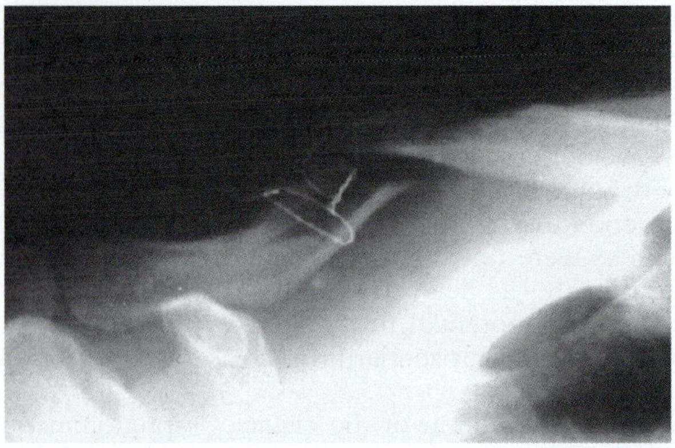

FIGURE 8-40: Failure of fixation in a midshaft clavicle fracture.

of nonunion after open reduction, it is probable that the operative fractures also included many of the more difficult fractures, such as those with more severe trauma, soft tissue damage, and associated injuries, thus contributing to the poor results.

One cannot overlook the fact that most of the surgical complications are related to poor fixation techniques, and it is not the concept of surgical treatment that is the problem, but rather the choice of fixation (Figs. 8-40 and 8-41), possibly because of the tenuous soft tissue coverage about the clavicle and its marginal blood supply. As Wilkins and Johnston have pointed out, the clavicle is very much like the tibia[421] in that it has poor soft tissue coverage. However, very few surgeons, who would never even consider plating a midshaft tibia fracture, see any problem with plating a midshaft clavicle fracture. It may be that the soft tissue injury, combined with the soft tissue stripping that is required for plate fixation, is what contributes to the higher rate of nonunion seen with this popular form of operative fixation.

Diagnosis

Radiographic Evaluation

Although nonunion is often demonstrated clinically by motion at the fracture site, radiographic confirmation is obtained by AP and 45-degree cephalic tilt views. The radiographic signs of nonunion might not always be clear. In patients with minimal displacement of the fracture fragments and no gross motion, tomography or even a bone scan may be useful to demonstrate the presence of nonunion in a symptomatic patient. As with other fractures, nonunion of the clavicle may be manifested as hypertrophic or atrophic bone ends. Patients can have real or apparent bone loss, particularly with comminuted fractures.

Obtaining an AP view of both clavicles on a single large cassette is particularly helpful in evaluating nonunion. In this way the distance from the sternum to the acromion can be measured on the normal side and compared with that on the symptomatic side. Such a comparison can help when deciding whether primary osteosynthesis with bone grafting will be adequate or

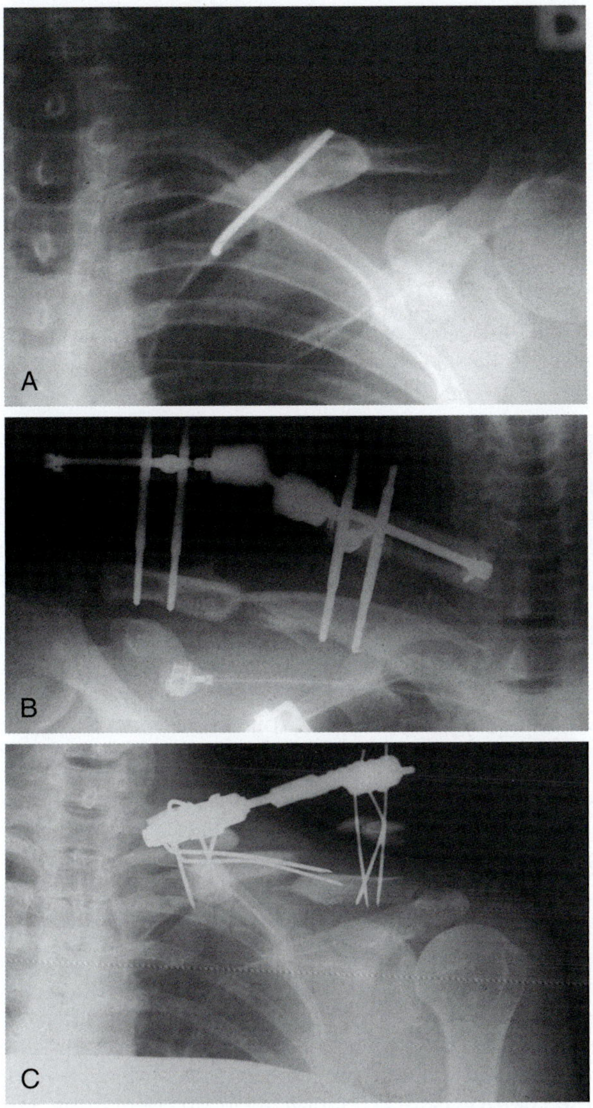

FIGURE 8-41: **A,** Failure of fixation in a midshaft clavicle fracture treated with a single smooth Steinmann pin. **B,** Nonunion and malalignment of a midshaft clavicle fracture treated with an external fixator. **C,** Nonunion and malalignment of a midshaft clavicular malunion that was treated with a fine-wire external fixator.

whether an intercalary segment of bone will be needed to span the area of segmental bone loss. It is very difficult to appreciate the true shortening or deformity of a clavicle on plain radiographs alone.

Symptoms

Approximately 75% of patients with an ununited fracture of the clavicle are symptomatic with moderate to severe pain.[230,178] However, some evidence indicates that patients with atrophic nonunion, although symptomatic initially, may become less symptomatic with time.[421] Pain from nonunion can radiate to the neck, down into the forearm, or even into the hand, especially if nerve irritation is present.[350] The patient might complain of grating or crepitation, which is often palpable. The shoulder can appear to sag forward, inward, and medially, and the apex of the medial fragment may be observed angling upward underneath the trapezius. The rotation of the scapula can also contribute to the posterior medial scapular border pain that can be seen in these patients. Twenty-five percent or more of patients are also affected by neurologic symptoms, which are often caused by compromise of the brachial plexus by overabundant callus.[51,178,221,350] Similarly, chronic vascular symptoms may be present as a result of pressure on the subclavian vein, producing symptoms of thoracic outlet syndrome.[20,58,155,178,197,307]

When considering nonunion as the cause of a patient's painful symptoms, it must be emphasized that nonunion may be an incidental finding. A careful history and physical examination must be obtained because many soft tissue and bone abnormalities around the shoulder, including posttraumatic arthrosis of either the sternoclavicular or acromioclavicular joints, can mimic the symptoms of nonunion. These degenerative changes in the joint can appear several years after the injury.[421]

Physical Examination

Physical examination can reveal motion as the clavicle is manipulated or pain on pressure at a nonunion site. The prominent bone of comminuted fragments may be palpable. Occasionally, patients have limited range of motion at the shoulder joint, but this finding is often associated with soft tissue, subacromial, or glenohumeral joint disease rather than being a direct result of the clavicular nonunion. Loss of motion can occur secondary to malposition of the scapula in the case of significant shortening. If neurologic symptoms are noted, they are often referred to the ulnar nerve distribution, and intrinsic weakness can occur.[350,117]

Malunion

In children with clavicle fractures, foreshortening is common but has not been reported to be a problem, and the angular deformity often remodels. Adults, however, have no remodeling potential, and shortening or angulation can occur. This defect has been described by some authors as a purely cosmetic deformity with little interference with function.[26] However, Eskola et al. reported that patients with shortening of the clavicular segments of more than 15 mm at follow-up examination had significantly more pain than did those without these findings, and they recommended taking care to avoid acceptance of a shortened clavicle.[91] Malunions can also be due to iatrogenic malreduction of the fracture fragments. Although it is less likely with IM fixation, we have seen this with plate fixation where the clavicle was made to match the plate rather than the plate matching the clavicle (Fig. 8-42).

Patients can present with pseudo-winging of the scapula secondary to the fixated anteromedial rotation of the scapula caused by a malunion of the clavicle (see Fig. 8-8B). Although this is not true winging, it represents a static, fixed condition similar to the dynamic

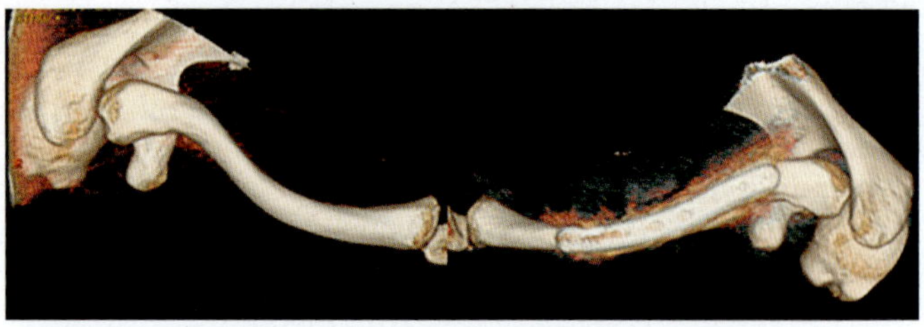

FIGURE 8-42: Iatrogenic malunion of the clavicle caused by making the clavicle match the plate. The clavicle is straighter than a normal clavicle.

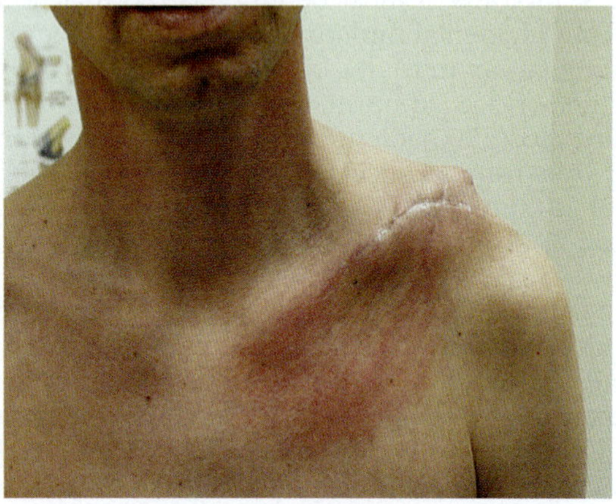

FIGURE 8-43: Clinical appearance of a patient who had undergone plate fixation of a clavicle malunion with an intercalary graft. Loss of distal fixation had occurred.

dysfunction seen with long thoracic nerve injuries. Ledger et al. found that a malunion with shortening of at least 15 mm caused increased upward angulation of the clavicle at the sternoclavicular joint and increased anterior scapular version, and it also caused significant loss of strength in adduction, extension, and internal rotation of the humerus as well as a reduced peak abduction velocity.[205]

If a malunited fracture is a significant cosmetic or functional problem, simply shaving down the bone may be inadequate.[273] This procedure does not correct the primary deformity, which is shortening and angulation, and it can significantly weaken the clavicle. Because of overlapping of the fracture ends, removing the prominence of the deformity can create a unicortical clavicle that is not capable of remodeling. This outcome can predispose the clavicle to refracture and can cause chronic pain. Several authors have recommended osteotomy, internal fixation, and bone grafting.[26,49] The patient must, however, be made aware that nonunion may be a sequela and that the cosmetic appearance of the surgical scar required for plate fixation may be more troublesome than the bump from the malunited bone (Fig. 8-43; see also Fig. 8-53). Furthermore, it must be kept in mind that the deformity is multiplanar, and a single osteotomy can correct only one plane of the deformity.

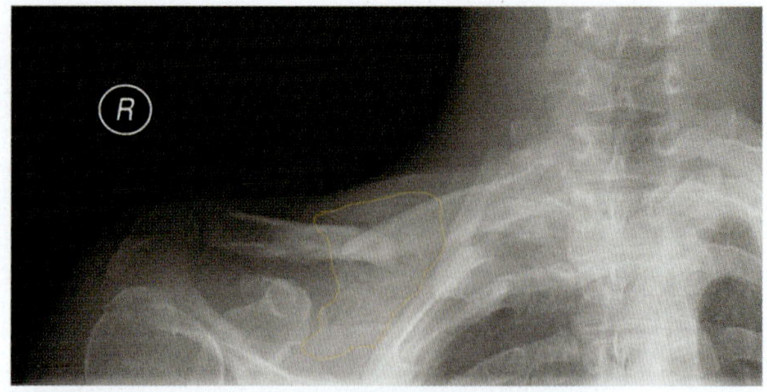

FIGURE 8-44: Massive hypertrophic callus seen 3 months after a midshaft clavicle fracture.

Another approach to this problem is to remove the callus about the fracture site to get down to the original fracture fragments.[22] We have found that even years after the original injury, there is a qualitative difference between the normal cortical bone and the callus. Removal of the callus can be aided through the use of image intensification at the time of surgery to ensure that all of the callus is removed. The fracture fragments are then fixed with an IM pin, which is removed at a later date. The callus is morselized and placed around the fracture site. This procedure can be accomplished through a small cosmetic incision in Langer's lines.

Neurovascular Sequelae

Despite the large amount of callus that follows healing of a fracture in children, the callus mass rarely causes any compression of the costoclavicular space and usually shrinks with time.[68] In adults, however, late neurovascular sequelae can follow both united and ununited fractures.[110,116,260,364,383,397] Figure 8-44 shows a radiograph of a patient with bilateral clavicle fractures who developed severe neurovascular claudication in her right arm 3 months postinjury with no axillary or musculocutaneous nerve function. She was found to have massive callus about the fracture causing compression of the axillary artery and brachial plexus.

Normally, the sternoclavicular angle and anterior bow of the clavicle provide abundant room for the brachial plexus and subclavian vessels in the costoclavicular space. Despite some normal variability in the width and space between the clavicle and the first rib, this room is usually adequate.[151] Occasionally, a congenital anomaly such as a bifid clavicle or a straight clavicle with no medial or anterior angulation can narrow the costoclavicular space and cause neurovascular compression.[342] Thus it is not surprising that abundant callus or significant fracture deformity in some patients can narrow this space sufficiently to cause symptoms that most often involve the subclavian vessels, the carotid artery, or the brachial plexus.[182] These compression phenomena, though uncommon, are important because their clinical manifestation may be confusing to the clinician and problematic for the patient until definitive treatment is instituted. Vascular structures that have been reported to be involved in compression syndromes include the carotid artery, the subclavian vein, and the subclavian artery. Aneurysms and pseudoaneurysms producing brachial plexus compression are also seen.

Vascular Compression Syndromes

Obstruction of the carotid artery can lead to syncope. Such obstruction is associated with fracture deformity or callus at the medial end of the clavicle.

Compression of the subclavian vein between the clavicle and the first rib, with subsequent obstruction, is probably the most common late vascular complication and may be accompanied by plexus and subclavian artery involvement. The point of this obstruction has been shown by Lusskin et al. to be the site where the vein crosses the first rib and passes beneath the subclavius muscle and costoclavicular ligament.[224] A number of authors have emphasized the role of the subclavius muscle and the condensation of the clavipectoral fascia known as the *costocoracoid ligament* in producing venous obstruction and subsequent thrombosis.[93] The syndrome is characterized by dilatation of the veins of the upper extremity and the anterior aspect of the chest on the affected side as a result of congestion of the collateral venous network. This compression is relieved by a downward thrust of the shoulder.[221,93,351,382]

Lusskin et al.[224] reported that this costoclavicular syndrome could be distinguished from the typical anterior scalene, cervical rib, and thoracic outlet compression syndromes, which can also produce arterial and neurologic symptoms but are typically reproduced by Adson's maneuver. The other syndromes are not generally accentuated by shoulder girdle extension.[151,69,128,368] The treatment described by a number of authors has depended on the offending structure. If overabundant callus is causing the problem, addressing the surgery to the clavicle may be indicated. If the clavicle is more normal, however, it might make more sense to resect the first rib. Under no circumstance should the clavicle be removed.[339]

Subclavian artery compression was reported by Guilfoil and Christiansen, who described a case of thrombosis secondary to clavicular nonunion.[128] Although injury to this artery is recognized to occur with acute clavicular injuries,[126,267] it is unusual as a late complication secondary to overabundance of clavicular callus or nonunion (see Figs. 8-29 and 8-44). However, Yates and Guest reported the case of a patient who died as a result of an embolus to the basilar artery that originated from a thrombosis in the subclavian artery after an ununited clavicle fracture.[432]

Traumatic aneurysm[47,73,274] and pseudoaneurysm[365] have been reported after fractures of the clavicle. They may be manifested as pulsatile masses or soft tissue densities in the area of the clavicle fracture or nonunion, and they may be the source of thrombi as well. We have also seen a late vascular injury secondary to a nonunion. Figures 8-45 and 8-46 show an orthopedic surgeon who underwent emergency surgery because of an aneurysm of his subclavian artery that extended into his carotid artery. The aneurysm developed after failed plating of a fracture that progressed to nonunion. Hansky et al. reported a case of aneurysm of the subclavian artery that produced compression of the brachial plexus.[133]

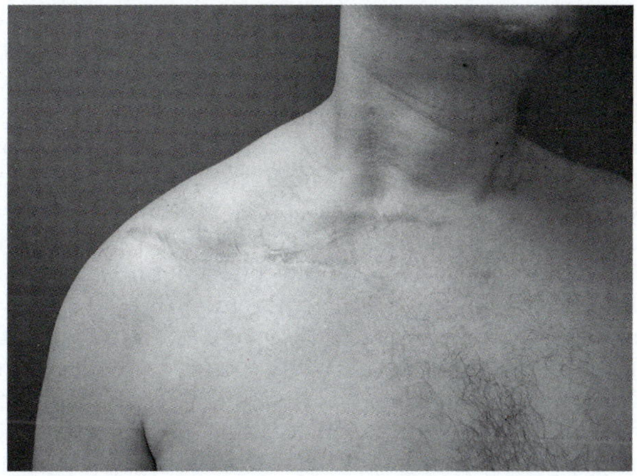

FIGURE 8-45: Clinical appearance of a patient in whom a subclavian artery aneurysm developed and extended into his carotid artery after nonunion of a midshaft clavicle fracture.

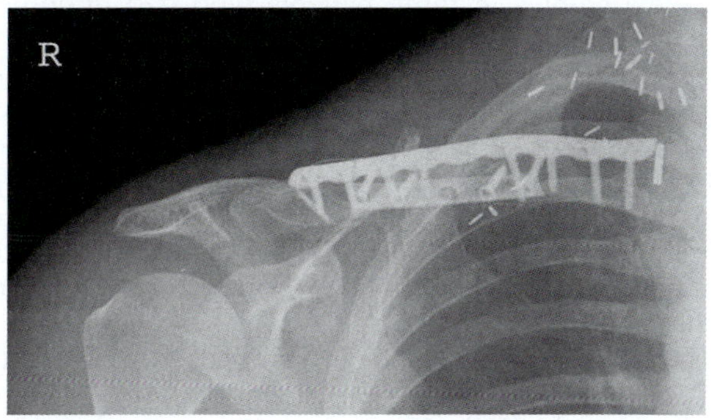

FIGURE 8-46: Anteroposterior radiograph of the patient in Figure 8-45 after successful double plating of the midshaft nonunion.

Neurologic Syndromes

A number of neurologic symptoms have been described as late complications of fractures of the clavicle.[31,89,127,151,186,224,249,277,350] Symptoms can involve the entire brachial plexus or a single nerve. Suso et al. reported an injury to the anterior interosseous nerve secondary to a fracture of the distal end of the clavicle.[387] Bartosh et al. reported an injury to the musculocutaneous nerve after a refracture of the midshaft of the clavicle that occurred 3 weeks after the original injury.[21] Because the onset of symptoms may be variable between the occurrence of a fracture and the establishment of nonunion, the late sequelae can be confused with nerve injuries that occurred at the time of the acute injury. Thus it is particularly important to perform a careful neurologic examination of patients with an acute fracture. Rumball et al.

suggested that a patient with a displaced fracture of the medial part of the clavicle be advised to immediately report the development of any new symptoms.[348]

An early nerve injury is usually a traction neurapraxia, involves the lateral cord, and has a guarded prognosis, but late compression neuropathies typically affect the medial cord, produce ulnar nerve symptoms, and have a more benign prognosis. In this complication, which is typically associated with middle-third fractures, the proximal tip of the distal nonunion fragment is pulled downward and posteriorly, thereby bringing it into contact with the neurovascular bundle, which is squeezed by the nonunion site above and the first and second ribs below. As would be expected, compression neuropathy is more commonly a problem with hypertrophic rather than atrophic nonunion (see Fig. 8-44). Ivey et al. reported a case of reflex sympathetic dystrophy of the anterior chest wall after an injury to the supraclavicular nerve that was associated with a midshaft clavicle fracture.[159]

Ring and Holovacs also reported transient postoperative plexopathies in three patients who had undergone IM fixation of their clavicle fractures. They thought that this might have been due to the force applied to the fragments as they were delivered into the surgical incision and subsequent traction on the plexus.[332]

In addition to compression syndromes, Eilanberger et al. described a patient in whom cardiac arrest occurred after a medial clavicle fracture. They explained the complication as vagus nerve irritation secondary to hematoma of the fracture.[87]

Though seemingly minor in comparison to a brachial plexus injury, we have seen five cases in which the middle branch of the supraclavicular nerve has either formed a neuroma over the fracture site or has become entrapped within the fracture callus itself. This complication may be the source of the chronic superficial pain that can be seen after clavicle fractures (see Fig. 8-1). With midshaft clavicle fractures, the middle branch of the supraclavicular nerve is at highest risk for damage either at the fracture site from the original injury or during an internal fixation procedure, whether an open or closed reduction is carried out.

Diagnosis

The diagnosis of late compression syndrome is usually made by a careful history, physical examination, and electrical studies such as electromyography and nerve conduction velocities.[26,65, 98,117,142,161,192,248] Magnetic resonance imaging may be helpful to outline the relationship between the brachial plexus and hypertrophic callus or clavicular fragments. Dela Santo et al. reported that in 16 cases of clavicle fracture, two patients had early neurovascular complications and 14 had late symptoms of costoclavicular syndrome.[74]

Posttraumatic Arthritis

Posttraumatic arthritis of the joint can follow intra-articular injuries to both the sternoclavicular and acromioclavicular joints, although degenerative disease of the distal end of the clavicle is much more common. Often, this arthritis is a result of the trauma transmitted to these joints at the time of the original injury. It can also be the result of an intra-articular fracture that has gone unrecognized (type III distal clavicle fracture). The patient can have symptoms specifically related to pain at the acromioclavicular joint or symptoms of impingement as a result of extrinsic pressure on the subacromial bursa and rotator cuff by an inferiorly protruding osteophyte of the acromioclavicular joint.[272] Radiographically, cystic changes, spur formation, or narrowing of the acromioclavicular joint may be noted, or resorption of the distal part of the clavicle may be found. Further radiologic studies may be needed to define the lesion, especially in the area of the sternoclavicular joint, and additional tomograms or a CT scan may be indicated. The patient often symptomatically improves after a diagnostic injection of 1% lidocaine (Xylocaine) into the affected joint.

If appropriate nonoperative treatment, including the administration of nonsteroidal medications or a steroid injection, does not provide lasting relief, surgical excision of the joint may be indicated. If the outer portion of the clavicle is to be resected, no more than the distal 10 mm of bone should be removed to prevent injury to the coracoclavicular ligaments, and the deltoid is repaired to the trapezius fascia. If resection of the sternoclavicular joint is indicated, the intra-articular disk can be sutured into the end of the clavicle to help stabilize the medial end, and the clavicular head of the sternocleidomastoid muscle may be used to fill in the area of resection.[242]

TREATMENT

As early as the late 1920s, more than 200 different treatment methods had already been described for fractures of the clavicle.[198,213] In general, excellent results have been reported with nonoperative treatment of these fractures.[283]

The exact method of treatment of a fractured clavicle depends on several factors, including the age and medical condition of the patient, the location of the fracture, and associated injuries. Often overlooked are the functional demands of the patient and the patient's expectations in terms of cosmesis.

Children

Because of their excellent healing potential and the tremendous remodeling that accompanies growth, there is little role for any form of treatment other than nonoperative treatment in children; in fact, it has been stated that operative treatment is contraindicated in children.[389] Occasionally, however—such as for debridement of an open fracture, for neurovascular compromise that does not resolve with closed reduction, or for severe irreducible displacement of the fragments—operative management may be indicated.[160,250,35,215] Although it is generally agreed that closed treatment methods are usually successful, the exact method can vary because children can differ in their comprehension or ability to cooperate with nonoperative treatment regimens.

In a newborn with a birth fracture, little treatment is needed other than measures to keep the baby comfortable. Healing is usually rapid, and occurs within the first 2 weeks with no untoward effects. However, both the nurse and the mother must be instructed in methods of careful, safe, and gentle turning of the infant to minimize discomfort. The arm may be gently bound to the child for a few days to increase comfort level.[68] Direct pressure over the clavicle while dressing the child is avoided.

In children with a greenstick or nondisplaced fracture, treatment often consists of the use of a sling until the symptoms have subsided.[326] In displaced fractures or those requiring reduction, most treatment methods have entailed the use of some form of a figure-of-eight bandage or splint, either alone or reinforced with plaster, to hold the shoulder upward and backward in an attempt to reduce the degree of displacement. Fortunately, in children, these fractures heal rapidly without much morbidity.[312] Treatment of older children and teenagers may be more troublesome, and more often requires plaster reinforcement because of their high level of activity.

Frequent adjustment is often needed by the physician or parent when attempting to treat these young patients with figure-of-eight methods, which can prove frustrating for both patients and surgeons. It has been questioned whether any significant long-term advantage is gained by aggressive attempts at maintaining reduction with these treatment methods.

For adolescent patients, most authors still recommend nonoperative treatment, although there has been a trend toward more aggressive operative intervention in these patients.[359,46]

As noted above, there is less than 20% growth remaining after the age of 9 years in females and 12 years in males. Therefore some authors have recommended more aggressive operative treatment in adolescents.[96,109,150,200,244,265,317,405]

Adults

In adults with clavicle fractures, the goal of treatment (as with other fractures) is to achieve healing of the bone with minimal morbidity, loss of function, and residual deformity. If this objective is kept in mind, reevaluation of some of the traditional, cumbersome methods of immobilization of clavicle fractures might be considered. Historically, the main principles of nonoperative treatment have included bracing of the shoulder girdle to raise the outer fragment upward, outward, and backward; depression of the inner fragment; maintenance of reduction; and the use of the ipsilateral elbow and hand so that associated problems with immobilization can be avoided.

An extensive review of the literature generally leads to the conclusion that immobilization is almost impossible to achieve and that deformity and shortening are usual. Although this shortening was previously not seen as a problem, more recent studies have suggested that shortening alone is probably one of the most significant predictors of dissatisfaction with the outcome of clavicle fractures (see Figs. 8-8 and 8-34).[146,242] The literature is replete with methods of various complexity to immobilize the clavicle, and treatment has ranged from long-term recumbency alone[26,322] to various forms of ambulatory treatment[60] and various internal fixation methods.[38,160,185,206,208,254,263,280,298,322,349,436]

In general, methods of treatment of fractures of the clavicle can be broadly grouped into simple support of the arm, reduction, open or closed reduction with fixation, and primary excision.

Support

With simple support of the arm whether by sling alone, a sling and swathe, a Sayre bandage, or a Velpeau bandage,[213] no attempt is made to maintain a clavicular reduction, provided that the bone appears to be positioned satisfactorily so that union is anticipated.[308] Although sling treatment is certainly the simplest way to treat a fractured clavicular shaft, it is often unsettling to an orthopedic surgeon who wishes to realign the fracture fragments; this mindset likely explains the popularity of the numerous methods of effecting and maintaining a closed reduction. Placing the arm in a sling with the forearm across the abdomen can exaggerate the shortening of the fracture and the anterior medial rotation of the scapula.

Reduction

After reduction, an attempt is made to maintain and hold the reduction by bringing the distal fragment up and back, which may be achieved by a bandage alone (including a figure-of-eight dressing),[33,322] by plaster reinforcement,[61,433] or by full immobilization of the shoulder in various forms of spica casts[191,273,297,345,402] A variety of materials have been used to maintain a closed reduction, including metal, leather, plastic, plaster, and muslin.[273] The position required to reduce the fracture and maintain the reduction (upward, lateral, and backward) is difficult to achieve, is virtually impossible to maintain, may often be uncomfortable for the patient, and has occasionally been reported to cause symptoms of either neurovascular compression or displacement of the fragment[345] if careful attention is not paid to placing the external immobilization precisely. The figure-of-eight dressing can also lie over the apex of the fracture and cause the patient considerable pain and possibly compromise the skin over the fracture (Fig. 8-47).

Few studies have tried to evaluate in a controlled fashion whether a vigorous attempt to effect and maintain a reduction provides a greater chance for a better outcome than does simple arm support for comfort. In two studies directly comparing a figure-of-eight dressing with sling support, it was noted that figure-of-eight dressings were time consuming, required frequent adjustment, might contribute to other problems, and had more complications than simple sling treatment did. The authors

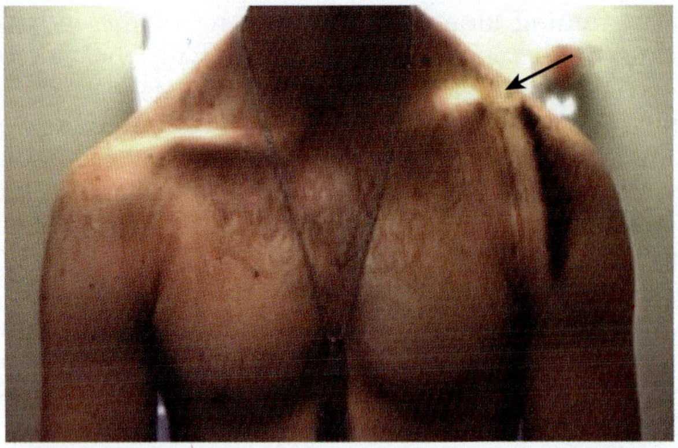

FIGURE 8-47: Clinical appearance of a patient treated with a figure-of-eight harness after a midshaft fracture of the left clavicle. Note that the striations caused by the harness pass directly over the fracture site (arrow).

concluded that the functional and cosmetic sequelae of the two methods of treatment were identical and that alignment of the healed fracture was unchanged from the initial displacement.[11,238]

Another group studied the recovery time after conservative treatment of fractures of the clavicle in 155 patients. No difference was found in the speed of recovery in those treated with a sling and those treated with a figure-of-eight bandage, although the patient's age at the time of fracture did affect the recovery, with 33% of patients older than 20 years still having symptoms 3 months after injury.

Reduction With Fixation

A number of techniques have been described for the treatment of clavicle fractures with open or closed reduction with internal fixation.[131,294,371] These techniques have included cerclage sutures,[402] IM devices (Steinmann pins, K-wires, Knowles pins, Perry pins, modified Hagie pins, Küntscher nails, or Rush pins[367]), or plate fixation.*

Reduction With External Fixation

In some cases, such as open fractures or septic nonunion, open or closed reduction with external fixation can be considered.[358] In one study using the Hoffmann device, the mean length of time for the external fixator to be left on was 51 days; no pleural or vascular complications occurred, and all fractures united.[19] However, this technique is not one with which orthopedists have extensive experience, and this procedure is associated with the potential for serious complications. Xiao reported on a new external fixation device that produced nearly anatomic reduction in 87.4% of his patients.[429] In another report, a small AO (Arbeitsgemeinschaft für Osteosynthesefragen) fixator was used in the treatment of fractures of the clavicle.[19] Although Nowak et al. found no difference in the rate of healing in comparing a reconstruction plate to an external fixator, most patients with an external fixator found the device cumbersome.[290]

In rare instances, primary excision of both ends of the fracture with skin closure and intentional formation of a pseudarthrosis has been advocated.[300]

Nonunion

Asymptomatic clavicular nonunion need not be treated. In addition, nonoperative treatment should probably be considered for nonunion in the elderly. Although nonoperative methods to obtain union have been reported—particularly the use of electrical stimulation and ultrasound—only a few cases of healing of clavicular nonunion by pulsed electromagnetic fields have been documented.[5,10, 39,72] Most authors share the view that electrical stimulation has little role in the treatment of clavicular nonunion, especially because operative methods have shown such a high degree of success.[24,57]

Indications for surgical treatment include pain or aching clearly attributable to the nonunion; shoulder girdle dysfunction, weakness, or fatigue; and neurovascular compromise.[196,298] Although bone drilling has been suggested as a means of stimulating a delayed union to progress,[319] such drilling has little role in established nonunion. Alternatively, some authors have advocated resection of the nonunion. Lateral-third nonunions can occasionally be treated with excision of the distal fragment. Because excision does not address the instability of the remaining medial fragment, some type of ligament reconstruction has to be carried out, such as a Weaver-Dunn type of reconstruction.[275,414]

Partial claviculectomy, with excision of the nonunion site, has been reported by some as a means of treating ununited clavicle fractures. Certainly, in the short term, this procedure can alleviate the crepitus and often eliminates the pain.[230] However, many patients treated in this manner remain mildly to moderately symptomatic,[421,178,339] the stabilizing function of the clavicle is lost, and neurogenic symptoms can be a problem.[217,421] Nonetheless, resection of the nonunion and filling of the defect with cancellous bone chips can stimulate regeneration of the clavicle and, in addition, can decompress the neurovascular structures if the nonunion is accompanied by symptoms of thoracic outlet syndrome.[58,59,155,170] Surgical treatment most commonly consists of an attempt to gain union through some means of internal fixation with bone grafting. The techniques for surgical treatment of nonunion have evolved, as have internal fixation techniques for other long bone fractures and nonunion.

A number of open treatment methods have been detailed. Some authors have used wire sutures through the ends of either clavicular fragment and through an iliac crest graft.[26,117,269] Sutures consisting of other materials, including catgut, braided suture, and even loops of kangaroo tendon, have been used in the past.[273] Simple intrafragmentary screw fixation has been advocated, with fixation of the iliac bone as an onlay graft and cancellous

**References 38, 189, 208, 254, 258, 263, 280, 298, 305, 341, 349, 436.*

bone grafting at either junction.[350,236] However, because of the amount of movement in multiple planes that the clavicle exhibits and because these methods control rotation poorly, neither suture nor screw fixation are secure enough to be reliable when used independently of additional protection. An external cast or brace support is necessary to prevent screw or wire breakage and potential wire fragment migration, which can produce disastrous results.[52,199,225,237,285]

Open reduction plus internal IM fixation with the use of K-wires (with or without screws),[232,273,279,398,403,413,436] Steinmann pins,[189,271,345] Knowles pins,[280] or modified Hagie pins[337] has been a popular method of internal fixation. Although reports have been encouraging with these methods (and they can be successful), rotation is poorly controlled under most circumstances, and the IM fixation can be difficult to insert if the bone ends are atrophic (especially with a flat, curved clavicle). In addition, distraction of the fracture at the nonunion site can occur with the use of threaded pins.[189] If an improper form of IM fixation is chosen, the device can bend or break. Several complications have been reported with pin migration.[199,225,237,285]

However, in 1991, Boehme et al.[34] described a series of 21 patients with nonunion of the clavicle who were treated successfully with an IM pin that was specifically designed for clavicle fixation. It had threads with a differential pitch on either end and a blunt medial tip to prevent penetration of the medial cortex. Furthermore, it had a nut that was secured over the lateral portion of the pin that virtually ensured that the pin would not migrate. The lateral nut and the differential pitch threads also allowed compression of the fragments. These patients underwent open reduction, internal fixation with a modified Hagie IM pin, and autogenous bone grafting. The average duration of follow-up was 35 months (range, 5 months to 11 years). Healing occurred in 20 (95%) of the 21 patients. When compared with other treatment methods, such as fixation with a plate and screws, IM fixation has several advantages. The IM pin can be inserted through a cosmetically acceptable incision in Langer's lines. The pin requires less soft tissue dissection, and after healing, it can be removed through a small incision under local anesthesia (see "Surgical Technique for Intramedullary Fixation").

The application of rigid internal fixation for acute fractures has aided the management of many traditionally difficult fractures, and this concept of rigidly immobilizing fragment ends has had its natural application in the treatment of nonunion as well. Although rigid internal fixation techniques using AO plates without bone grafting have been reported to be just as successful for clavicular nonunion as for nonunion of other long bones,[145,320] the addition of supplemental bone graft to rigid plating has been the most popular treatment of clavicular nonunion. With this method of treatment, reports in the literature have approached a union rate of 100%.[82,84,180,320,327,394,415] Manske and Szabo reported a 100% incidence of union by 10 weeks postoperatively without complications when using open reduction and internal fixation with compression plating and bone grafting.[230] Jupiter and Leffert reported on 23 clavicular nonunions, including two resulting from clavicular osteotomies for surgical access, with an overall success rate of 89% in achieving union. However, 93.7% of those treated with grafting and dynamic compression plating achieved union.[178]

A number of series using an AO reconstruction plate for clavicular nonunion and delayed union have been reported, with results equal to those achieved with the larger dynamic compression plates (DCPs) and semitubular plates.[141] Advantages of the reconstruction plate include its lower profile and its relative ease of contouring to the available clavicular bone. The primary disadvantage of these plates is that they are weaker and do not allow compression at the fracture site.

Eskola et al. reported that 20 of 22 clavicular nonunions healed with rigid plate fixation and bone grafting, but they warned against shortening the clavicle to achieve union.[90] For this reason, if resection of the sclerotic edges of the atrophic margin to achieve primary osteosynthesis would result in significant clavicular shortening, many authors recommend intercalary bone grafting along with plate fixation.[31,217] The reconstruction ratio has been used as an adjunctive means of assessing restoration of clavicular length. A reconstruction ratio of 1 means that the restored length of the clavicle is equal to the length of the contralateral uninjured clavicle. In one series, 16 midclavicular nonunions were treated with a 3.5-mm plate, and 15 of 16 achieved union with a reconstruction ratio of 0.96.[71] Plate fixation with bone grafting is reliable and safe, and has few complications; it has the additional benefit that the rigid internal fixation is usually secure enough that no postoperative external cast immobilization is needed; use of a sling alone is usually adequate. The plate does have the disadvantage of requiring a second operation to remove the hardware if its prominent position irritates the skin. In addition, the screw holes weaken the bone, and protection is thus needed after hardware removal. Some have used this argument to advocate the use of IM fixation if previous plate fixation has failed; they contend that removal of previous hardware and the presence of screw holes from plate fixation make the use of a new plate for rigid internal fixation more difficult.[45]

The advent of low-contact DCPs and precontoured plates has enabled further refinement of well-established principles of plating.[261] The structured undersurface of the plate allows the blood supply to plated bone segments to be preserved, and avoidance of the stress risers produced at plate removal reduces the possibility of refracture after removal of the plate.[310] The excellent biocompatibility of titanium ensures superb tissue tolerance and increases the possibility of leaving plates in situ, thus obviating a second procedure.

Despite apparent success in treating nonunion with rigid internal fixation, a report by Pedersen et al. suggested that care must be taken when choosing the correct plate size.[302] These authors reported on 12 patients with clavicular nonunion treated by plate fixation and bone grafting. Although nine of 12 patients achieved good end results, the primary treatment failed in half of the cases. The authors theorized that a short (four-holed) semitubular plate and insufficient postoperative immobilization were two factors that were significant in the failure of treatment in these patients.

Medial clavicular nonunion, though rare, is particularly troublesome to treat. The proximity to the sternoclavicular joint and vital structures makes IM fixation worrisome, and often, little proximal bone is available to secure a standard DCP. Center plates are often prone to breakage. A postoperative spica cast may be required.

Rehabilitation After Clavicle Fracture

Rehabilitation after a clavicle fracture is started almost immediately, regardless of the treatment modality used. Assuming that no associated injuries have occurred, the patient is allowed to continue lower-body strengthening exercises as before the injury. Aerobic conditioning on an exercise bike or other stationary apparatus is encouraged. The patient is allowed to perform wrist and elbow range-of-motion exercises and grip-strength maintenance exercises immediately. Running is discouraged until the acute pain has resolved. As soon as the acute pain resolves, gentle pendulum exercises and isometric strengthening of the rotator cuff, deltoid, biceps, and triceps are initiated. Normal use of the ipsilateral hand for activities of daily living is also encouraged.

Generally, active range of motion is limited to less than 90 degrees of forward flexion or abduction if any operative fixation has been performed. Such restriction helps limit the initial stress on the hardware. In the absence of hardware, the patient is allowed to advance to active range of motion within the arc of pain tolerance. If no operative fixation is performed, full active range of motion is allowed when the patient is completely pain free, usually after 4 to 6 weeks of healing. When the patient has achieved full pain-free range of motion with radiographic evidence of callus, resistive exercises may be instituted. When the patient has near-normal strength in the injured upper extremity, a plyometrics program may be started.

Return-to-Play Criteria in Athletes

The criteria for return to sport activity are always controversial, and essentially come down to a judgment call by the treating orthopedist. This decision is affected by several factors, including the athlete, the specific fracture, the sport, the position played, the level of sports competition, the level of compensation, and the needs of the team. Occasionally, these factors are in direct opposition to common sense. The treating surgeon must realize that this decision is ultimately a compromise and that all compromises come with inherent risks. The athlete, coaches, and team may be willing to take risks that the orthopedist is unwilling to shoulder. It is our job to protect the athlete from these competing forces just long enough to allow adequate healing of the clavicle fracture. The key word here is *adequate*. We know that fracture remodeling is a long and ongoing process that takes 9 months to 1 year or longer. In theory, the risk of refracture is increased until the bone remodels completely. Stopping sports participation for a year is obviously overkill. We have to make the athlete understand that returning to sports earlier is a compromise and that by doing so, we increase the risk of reinjury. The goal is caution to allow adequate healing without overprotection.

For noncontact athletes, return to sports may be allowed when painless full active range of motion and nearly normal strength have been achieved, as well as evidence of bridging callus, which usually occurs about 6 weeks after fracture. Contact athletes and, in particular, those involved in collision sports are obviously at greater risk for refracture. The position played and the type of fracture also affect this risk. Even if we cannot authorize a return to full participation, we can often permit the athlete to return to practice with the team on a noncontact basis, which allows the athlete to remain at least mentally in sync with the team. We generally permit such participation when the athlete meets the same criteria as those for noncontact athletes. The team trainer can be extremely valuable in keeping the athlete from doing too much, too soon, because the trainer is with the team every day at practice. Generally, the earliest return to contact sports would be between 2 and 3 months. In football, extra protection can at times be afforded by the use of donut pads or, sometimes, fabrication of a fiberglass shoulder shell to dissipate impact forces to the clavicle. If the fracture required operative fixation of any type, the season is generally over for the athlete.

In a study of clavicle fractures in NFL football players, nearly 50% of players with a completely displaced middle-third clavicle fracture were treated successfully with acute surgical fixation without sequela and healed after a mean of 8.8 weeks. Half of these players were able to return to play during the same season. Over half of the players initially treated nonoperatively for a completely displaced middle-third clavicle fracture refractured the clavicle within a 1-year period from the initial injury and missed an average of 1.5 seasons because of the clavicle injury.[255]

Neurovascular Complications

In general, treatment of late neurovascular lesions has depended on the cause of the compromised structure.

If neurovascular compromise is present and due to massive callus formation, and callus debulking is risky, if internal fixation of pseudarthrosis with bone grafting is impractical because of comminution, or if malunion with a severe deformity has occurred and realignment osteotomy cannot be achieved, *resection* of the middle third of the clavicle may be the best choice if the lesion is in this portion. Abbott and Lucas outlined the various areas of the clavicle that can be resected without untoward sequelae and areas that do less well with resection.[2] Although some authors have advocated total claviculectomy, it is probably wiser to perform careful subtotal resections when possible. The primary problem with clavicle excision is that it can exacerbate the symptoms rather than relieve them. The removal of the clavicle can cause drooping of the shoulder and tenting of the brachial plexus and vascular structures over the first rib (see Figs. 8-5 and 8-6).

If excessive callus buildup or malunion of the clavicle has occurred, and the lesion is amenable to bone grafting and plate or IM fixation, removal of the hypertrophic callus and realignment osteotomy with or without segmental interposition of bone graft and cancellous bone grafting often relieves the neurovascular symptoms.

If the clavicle has a satisfactory appearance and is stable, enlargement of the costoclavicular space—and thus neurovascular decompression—can be accomplished by resecting the first rib, with partial excision of the scalene or subclavius muscle.[364,70]

Newborns and Infants

Despite some reports that fracture of the clavicle in newborns may be asymptomatic, we prefer to ensure comfort by treating clavicle birth fractures for a few days. The newborn is supine for many hours in the day; one who is not particularly active may be treated simply by avoiding pressure on the clavicle when dressing the infant and taking care to handle the infant gently and avoid movement of the affected arm during feeding, diapering, and dressing changes. When the newborn is prone, soft padding may be placed under the anterior aspect of the shoulder, with the weight of the body used to help keep the lateral portion of the clavicle back. Avoiding handling of a newborn is neither practical nor desirable.

If pseudoparalysis is present, and the infant avoids using the arm because of pain, we prefer to place a cotton abdominal pad under the infant's arm, flex the elbow fully to 90 degrees, and gently strap the arm to the chest with a padded elastic, Kling, or Kerlix bandage. A sling is difficult to apply and maintain, and is not necessary. Parents may be taught to reapply the bandage for skin care and after bathing. The patient is usually asymptomatic within 7 to 10 days, and healing is generally complete by 2 weeks.

The infant will use the arm normally once symptoms subside. Unrestricted use of the arm is permitted once the wrap is off, and parents may be reassured that the deformity and exuberant callus will remodel in time. After adequate healing, the infant's Moro reflex is retested to ensure that the disinclination to move the arm was, in fact, pseudoparalysis rather than an inability to move the arm secondary to an injury to the brachial plexus.[389]

Children

Ages 2 to 12 Years

Young children are treated symptomatically. In children younger than 6 years, no attempt is made to reduce the fracture because the fracture will remodel and the large lump will be gone in 6 to 9 months.[389] The child is made more comfortable with some type of applied figure-of-eight bandage.

Commercial figure-of-eight bandages are usually too large; the simplest way to construct one is to fill a 2-inch stockinette with cotton wadding, cast padding, or felt. The child is seated, and the dressing is applied as follows: the surgeon, standing behind the patient, passes the stockinette across the front of the uninjured clavicle, through the uninjured axilla and across the back, through the axilla on the fracture side, across the front of the anterior of the shoulder and the clavicle on the fracture side, and across the back behind the neck. To help keep the shoulder up and back, tension is placed on the stockinette, and a safety pin binds both ends of the stockinette together as the tension is maintained. An elastic bandage or 2-inch tape securing the bandage can be placed from one posterior strap to the other to maintain tension and secure the position. Alternatively, the figure-of-eight stockinette may be crisscrossed behind the patient before being applied to the fracture side, and subsequently pinned and tightened. If the 2-inch stockinette appears to irritate the skin, an abdominal cotton pad can be placed beneath the anterior straps.

Parents should be instructed on how to tighten the figure-of-eight bandage to maintain tension by reapplying the anchoring safety pin. Such adjustments should be done in situ without taking the stockinette off. The stockinette can have a tendency to loosen quickly; it should be retightened 2 or 3 days after the initial application and then weekly thereafter. We prefer to see the child weekly to ensure that the bandage is secure and that no skin problems, neurovascular irritation, or any other problems with treatment are occurring. Parents should be made aware of potential circulatory difficulties or skin problems if the bandage is too tight, and we ask them to practice tightening the bandage under our supervision to minimize the anxiety of having to bear the responsibility for handling the bandage adjustment themselves.

In young children, 3 weeks is usually adequate immobilization, but in an older ambulatory child, clinical signs of union, such as absence of tenderness to pressure over the fracture site or movement of the arm, are good signs that can help the physician decide when immobilization may be discontinued. Although union typically occurs in 3 to 6 weeks, symptoms are often dramatically diminished within the first 2 to 3 weeks.

Nondisplaced fractures, incomplete fractures, or plastic bone bowing need not be treated with a figure-of-eight bandage because the position is unlikely to change with ambulatory treatment if activity can be curtailed and reinjury avoided. A simple sling for comfort until clinical union takes place is sufficient. The child should avoid unusually vigorous activity such as gym class until the bone is solid, typically at about 3 months.

Repeat radiographic evaluation is not necessary at each return visit. We typically order a radiograph of the involved shoulder with the immobilization in place, another radiograph to check the progress of healing and the amount of callus, and one final radiograph when union is definite (between 6 and 12 weeks). An additional radiograph showing healing is helpful; in the event of reinjury, radiographic interpretation can be confusing if no radiograph is available that shows union after the first injury.

Ages 12 to 16 Years

This group may be difficult to treat because their activity level often frustrates the most aggressive attempts to maintain reduction and immobilization. Whereas little or no attempt is made to reduce the fracture in very young children, the teenage population has limited remodeling potential, and an attempt can be made to reduce the fracture before applying the immobilization. However, most, if not all, fractures return to their final length within a week after injury.

In cooperative older children, a commercial figure-of-eight clavicular splint—usually an elastic bandage with well-padded areas for the axilla—may be applied. A commercial splint has several advantages, including easy removal for bathing and more resistance to stretching out over time than is the case with a fashioned stockinette. This figure-of-eight bandage does not reduce or rigidly immobilize the fracture, but it may be a reminder to hold the shoulders back when the child wants to slump forward.[68]

Despite reports that there might not be any long-term difference between the use of a sling and a figure-of-eight bandage, we still prefer the latter after an attempt is made to reduce the fracture while maintaining alignment of the clavicle. A figure-of-eight bandage has one advantage that a sling lacks—it leaves both hands and elbows free for use in activities of daily living. In addition, a sling in its usual position holds the arm forward and inward, and the distal clavicular segment is not in position to be lined up with the proximal segment.

In older children, fractures usually heal within 6 weeks. However, we generally maintain the clavicular immobilizer for another 4 weeks after healing to remind the patient to restrict activities. Vigorous athletic activity should be avoided until union is solid, which, in a teenager, should be after 12 to 16 weeks.[68,284]

In a multiply traumatized child, the clavicle fracture may be treated by recumbency if a small pillow is placed between the scapulae to allow the weight of the arm to reduce the fracture. If recumbent treatment is to be instituted, a sling might make the arm more comfortable.

Recent articles have suggested that most bone growth has finished by age 9 years in females and age 12 years in males.[240] This means that there is actually little potential for remodeling after these ages. This has led a number of authors to suggest that a more aggressive approach be taken in treating clavicle fractures in this age group. Although an adolescent may be able to remodel a step off or angulation of a fracture, they cannot remodel shortening. Another study suggested that angulation of a fracture may predispose an adolescent to refracture.[234] Furthermore, the rate of complications from nonoperatively treated clavicles increased with an increase in the age of the patient.[385]

For significantly displaced and shortened fractures in this age group, plate and screw or IM fixation can be used similar to that in adults. The potential for surgical complications must be carefully addressed with the patient and parents.

Medial and Distal Fractures in Children

We prefer to treat both medial and distal clavicle fractures in children with a sling for support and an elastic (Ace) wrap for comfort. Medial clavicle fractures are rare problems, and seldom produce significant displacement. Lateral clavicle fractures, though clinically dramatic (appearing to be a high-grade acromioclavicular separation), are stable because the coracoclavicular and acromioclavicular ligaments remain attached to the periosteal tube and both sides of the joint, respectively. Despite the degree of displacement, the bone will remodel in time (Fig. 8-48). For lateral clavicle fractures, we find that a figure-of-eight bandage is difficult to maintain over the most lateral aspect of the shoulder; the sling and swathe is more practical and quite comfortable, and the healing potential in children negates the need for precise maintenance of reduction.

Adults

Medial-Third Fractures

Medial-third fractures are rare, and account for about 5% of all clavicle fractures in adults. The medial clavicular physis is the last in the body to close, and closure occurs between the ages of 22 and 25 years.[30,64] Many medial clavicle fractures are therefore physeal injuries, which inherently have great healing potential. Physeal arrest is not a concern. Even in cases in which the medial physis has already fused, these fractures heal well. Anterior displacement, even if complete, is not a concern. The great majority of these fractures are best treated nonoperatively with a figure-of-eight bandage or a sling. Healing can be expected to be rapid, with a very low risk of nonunion. This being said, we must emphasize that accurate diagnosis is important for several reasons. These injuries can be misdiagnosed as sternoclavicular joint injuries, which can confound treatment. Medial clavicle fractures that include extension into the sternoclavicular articulation carry some risk of posttraumatic arthrosis, which is something to consider when counseling the patient about the injury.

A medial clavicle fracture that can be very problematic is one with posterior displacement severe enough to impinge on the vital structures at the root of the neck. Patients with complaints of difficulty swallowing or breathing or with any neurovascular compromise require operative reduction of the fracture. Patients without symptoms but with documented CT evidence of impingement of the fragments on vital structures should be considered for operative reduction. Reduction maneuvers or a towel clip reduction should not be performed in the clinic or the emergency department unless the posterior position of the fragment is causing an airway or hemodynamic emergency. This reduction must be performed in the operating room under general anesthesia. The chest must be prepared as for a sternotomy, and a thoracic surgeon must be available in case a vascular problem occurs.

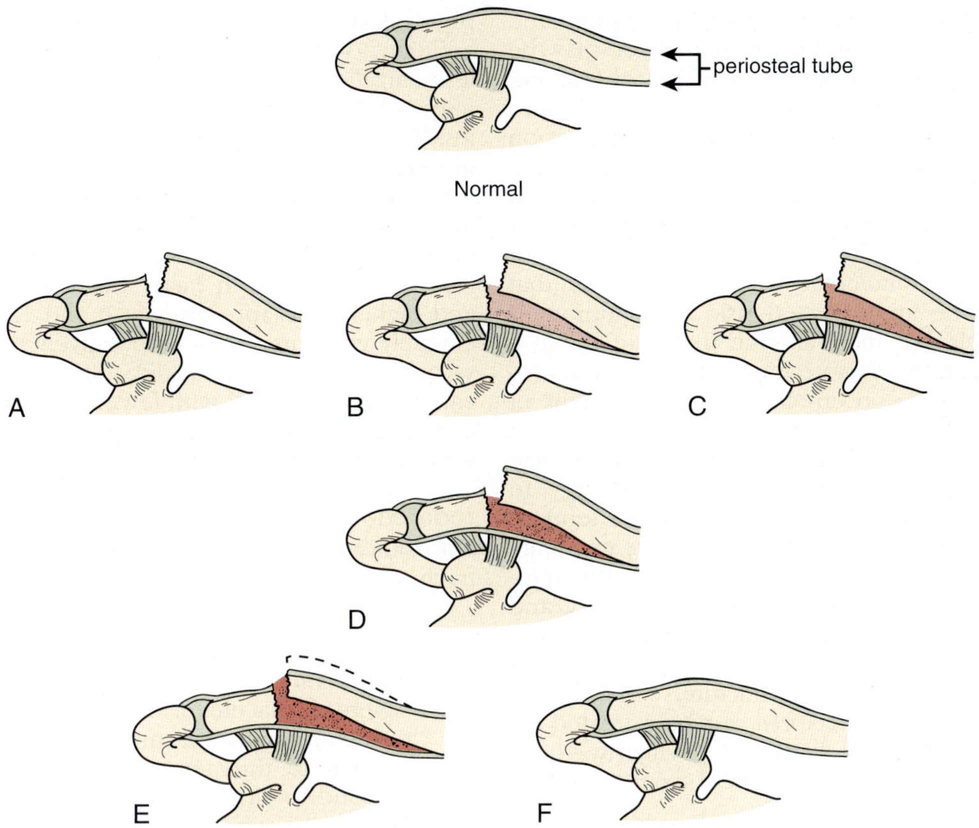

FIGURE 8-48: Sequence of events in a typical type IV distal clavicle fracture in children. **A,** The ligaments have remained attached to the periosteal tube as the medial clavicular fragment ruptures through the superior thin periosteum. This injury can mimic an acromioclavicular separation. **B,** Early filling of the area between the periosteum and the bone is seen. **C,** Further filling in of the bone is apparent. **D,** Bridging callus is seen to reach the top of the medial clavicular segment. **E,** Early remodeling has begun to occur with further consolidation of the fracture. **F,** Remodeling has occurred with complete union. This fracture is best treated nonoperatively, and excellent results can be expected. (From Rockwood CA, Green DP, eds. *Fractures*, 2nd ed. Philadelphia: JB Lippincott; 1984.)

A towel clip can be used to grasp the distal fragment and pull it forward to the proximal fragment. Traction on the upper extremity, or a towel placed between the shoulder blades, might assist in unlocking the fragments and allowing reduction. The reduction is generally stable.

In cases in which the reduction is unstable or cannot be achieved, open reduction is necessary. Removing interposed soft tissue will probably allow reduction, and should stabilize the fracture. Fixation may be obtainable with heavy suture and repair of the soft tissue envelope. In some cases, plate and screw fixation may be necessary. In such cases, the vital structure beneath the clavicle must be protected with a curved Crego or other such retractor to prevent plunging with the drill. You must use all available willpower to resist pinning across the fracture and into the sternum. The literature has many reports of broken hardware that migrated to the mediastinum and neck and even into the great vessels and heart.

There are limited studies reporting open reduction and internal fixation of medial fractures. Sidhu reported on 27 patients undergoing operative fixation of a medial clavicle fracture; 24 had an acute, displaced fracture, and three had fixation for nonunions. Plate and screw fixation was used in 19 cases, and transosseous sutures in eight cases. They reported a 100% union rate with both techniques and excellent DASH scores at 1-year follow-up.[366]

Middle-Third Fractures

Many middle-third fractures or shaft fractures of the clavicle can be managed best by closed means, either with a figure-of-eight splint or a sling. Keep in mind, however, that what you see clinically and on the original injury films is likely to foretell the ultimate result after healing has occurred. Reduction maneuvers and figure-of-eight bandages have not been conclusively shown to hold a reduction or improve cosmesis in these fractures. A fracture that is completely displaced or severely shortened, or both, is likely to stay in this position or revert to this position despite one's best efforts at reduction and the tightest figure-of-eight bandage.

An attempt at reduction can be useful in several circumstances. In extremities with acute neurovascular compromise as a result of a clavicle fracture, an attempt at reduction may be helpful. These cases are rare, but when they occur, a reduction maneuver can turn an emergency into just an urgency and might provide the necessary time for planning or to call in appropriate equipment. Another case in which a reduction maneuver may be useful is in a completely displaced middle-third fracture. This fracture is at greater risk for nonunion according to Thompson and Batten.[394] Crepitus felt with a reduction maneuver suggests that the fracture fragments are less likely to have interposed muscle or other soft tissues. If crepitus is felt and the fracture has no other indications for operative intervention, nonoperative treatment of this fracture could be attempted with the realization that there might still be an increased risk of nonunion. If no crepitus is felt, we must assume that something is interposed between the fracture fragments. Such interposition of tissue raises concern for the development of nonunion.

Problematic fractures of the midshaft of the clavicle are generally those that have absorbed greater energy. In our experience, these higher energy fractures tend to have a remarkably consistent pattern. They are generally shortened and comminuted, and have a butterfly fragment that is consistently inferior. Soft tissue injury and stripping are usually significant, and therefore greater instability is commonly present. All of these problems raise the risk of nonunion in any fractured bone.

We believe that these fractures are best treated by open reduction and internal fixation, for which we have essentially two options: plate and screw fixation and IM fixation.

In the past 2 decades, there has been a significant trend towards operative treatment of clavicle fractures. A landmark article by Hill et al. was one of the first to suggest that patients often do poorly with nonoperative treatment and that the rate of nonunion was considerably higher than previously thought.[146] The Canadian Multicenter study showed a significant decrease in nonunions in patients treated with plate fixation compared to sling; however, there was still a rather troubling complication rate of 31%, with 18% of patients complaining of hardware irritation or pain.[44] Another multicenter study of 1350 patients who underwent midshaft clavicle fixation showed that 24.6% underwent at least one clavicle reoperation.[212]

Because of the high complication and reoperation rate seen with operative treatment of clavicle fractures, some authors, including a recent editorial by the editor of JBJS have suggested that we are possibly over-treating these fractures operatively.[153] It is interesting to note that similar arguments are also being raised in relation to the treatment of distal radius fractures.[423]

There have also been concerns about the significant increase in treatment costs with operative treatment. Some studies have suggested that the number needed to treat to provide financial justification for operative treatment is too high.[301] However, another study showed that despite the cost of operative treatment, the overall cost of nonoperative treatment was over $5000 more than operative treatment. The cost was $12,976.94 for operative patients and $18,068.27 for nonoperative patients. The high cost of nonoperative treatment was due to increased loss of time from work (8.4 days vs. 35.2 days) and increased use of pain medication and need for physical therapy due to prolonged immobilization. In addition to the higher costs, the operative patients had less chronic pain (6.1% vs. 25.3%), less cosmetic deformity (18.2% vs. 32.5%), less weakness (10.6% vs. 33.7%), less loss of motion (15.2% vs. 31.3%), and fewer nonunions (0% vs. 4.8%) than nonoperative patients.[8]

Another study of operative versus nonoperative treatment of clavicle fractures in a worker compensation system found that patients treated operatively returned to work sooner, with faster healing, fewer nonunions, and higher Constant scores at 6 and 12 months postoperatively compared to nonoperatively treated patients in what is typically a very difficult treatment group. The earlier return to work with fewer complications undoubtedly yielded a significant financial benefit, although this was not specifically addressed in this study.[247]

Indications for Primary Open Fixation

Our indications for operative treatment of acute clavicle fractures include the following:

- Neurovascular injury or compromise that is progressive or that fails to reverse with closed reduction of the fracture
- Severe displacement caused by comminution, with resultant angulation and tenting of the skin severe enough to threaten its integrity and that fails to respond to closed reduction
- Shortening of more than 15 to 20 mm and displacement more than the width of the clavicle
- An open fracture that requires operative debridement
- Multiple trauma, when mobility of the patient is desirable and closed methods of immobilization are impractical or impossible
- A floating shoulder with a displaced clavicle fracture and an unstable scapula fracture or with compromise of the acromioclavicular and coracoacromial ligaments[85,142,143,407]
- Type II distal clavicle fractures (see later)
- Factors that render the patient unable to tolerate closed immobilization, such as the neurologic problems of Parkinsonism, seizure disorders, or other neurovascular disorders
- Significant chest trauma such as a flail chest where breathing may be compromised by the drooping of the shoulder onto the damaged area and loss of the support of the clavicle and accessory respiratory muscles
- The occasional patient for whom the cosmetic lump over the healed clavicle is intolerable and who is willing to exchange this bump for a potentially equally noncosmetic surgical scar and the possibility of nonunion.

TREATMENT ALTERNATIVES

There are basically two alternatives in treating this fracture: sling immobilization or surgery. Within the operative treatment alternative, the two choices are plate and screw fixation or IM fixation.

Plate and Screw Fixation

Plate and screw fixation of clavicle fractures is probably the most common method of treatment in use today. Its primary advantages are strong, stable fixation; quick return to function; and basic common internal fixation techniques and relatively easily available and inexpensive fixation hardware, although newer, precontoured plates can be considerably more expensive than older type plates. The primary disadvantages of plate and screw fixation are:

- Large, noncosmetic incision
- Soft tissue stripping
- Stress shielding
- Risk of infection
- Potential for neurovascular injury
- Refracture after plate removal

Plate fixation relies on direct bone healing, which requires very stable, compression fixation. Unfortunately, this can also be a source of bone porosis. Direct bone healing can only be monitored indirectly based on the absence of adverse clinical and radiological symptoms rather than obvious callus. This can cause problems in determining when it is safe to release a patient back to sports.

Although plate fixation provides excellent rotational control, which most IM fixation devices do not, its strength as a tension band is dramatically weakened in cases of comminution. Plate fixation is akin to a cantilever effect in that a dorsally placed plate acts as a tension band. In the case of a perfect transverse fracture, the point of fixation of the cantilever is the sternoclavicular joint, and the plate acts to compress the fracture with bending. Unfortunately, most high-energy clavicle fractures are comminuted, and in this setting, the fixation point of the cantilever moves laterally to the fracture site itself, thereby negating the compression effect at the fracture site and putting significant force on the lateral-most screws (Fig. 8-49). In fact, it has been our experience that when plates fail, they typically do so by pullout of the lateral-most screws (Figs. 8-50 to 8-53). Another problem with plate fixation is that the plate itself sits subcutaneously, and can be the source of irritation and poor cosmesis. If the plate needs to be removed, another involved procedure is required, and the patient is left with multiple stress risers in the clavicle.

If a plate is chosen, it should be a precontoured, low-profile plate or a DCP, preferably a low-contact dynamic compression type of plate such as the AO limited contact dynamic compression plate (LC-DCP). The other choice is a reconstruction plate. The advantage of a reconstruction plate is that it can be easily contoured; however, it provides no compression and is weaker than a DCP in terms of bending (see Fig. 8-51). A one-third tubular plate is not recommended because it does not provide strong enough fixation.

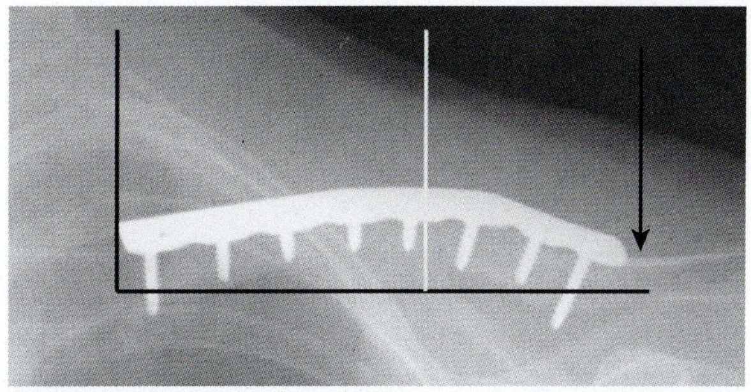

FIGURE 8-49: Cantilever effect when using plate fixation. In the ideal situation, the primary fixation point is at the medial aspect of the plate. With a superiorly placed plate, compression occurs at the fracture site. The arrow points to compression on the distal fragment of the clavicle. However, with comminution, the cantilever point is moved laterally to the fracture site, thereby increasing the force on the distal fixation. This model would predict loss of distal fixation as the primary mode of failure in comminuted fractures.

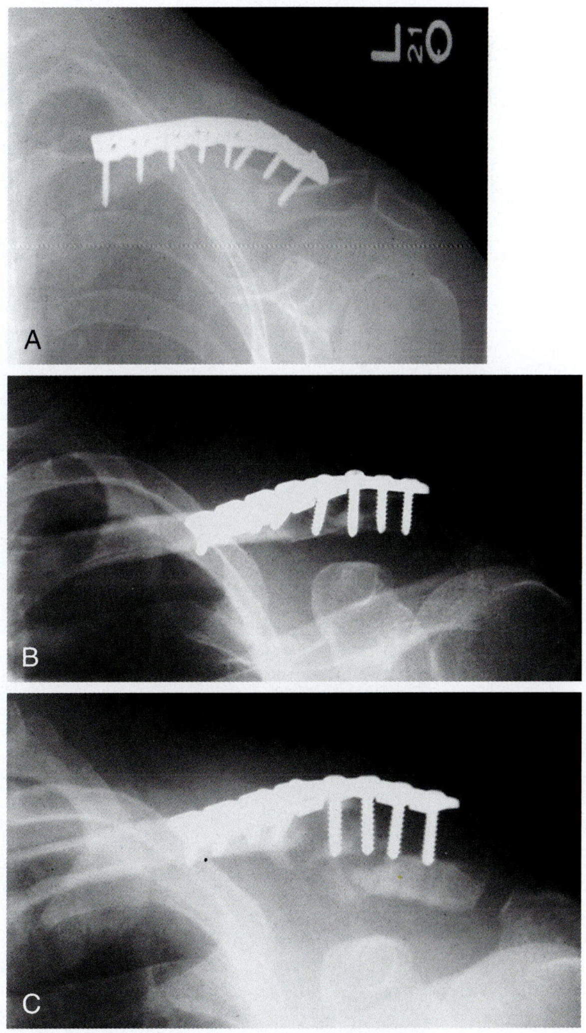

FIGURE 8-50: Loss of distal fixation. **A,** Bending of plate. **B,** Plate on distal clavicle fracture. **C,** Nonunion of distal clavicle previously treated with plate fixation.

Pertinent Anatomy

Plate fixation of the clavicle is complicated because it is an S-shaped bone that is flattened on its lateral end and pyramid-shaped on its medial end. There is considerable variation of the length and curvature of the clavicle; however, the medial arch of curvature always matches the lateral arch. In addition to its S-shaped curve, the clavicle also has a superior bow that has its apex in a variable position on the clavicle.[154] The superior surface tends to be flat medially and laterally; however, the midportion tends to have a convex shape due to the tubular middle clavicle. The anterior medial portion of the clavicle tends to be flat, and the lateral portion tends to be convex and almost angular, making plate fixation laterally more difficult.

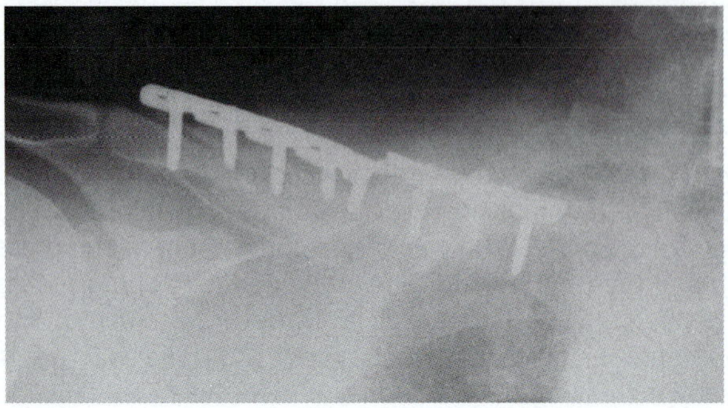

FIGURE 8-51: Loss of distal fixation and plate failure with a locking 3.5-mm reconstruction plate.

Neurovascular structures may be compromised by plate fixation, especially medially. Sinha et al. showed that the average distance between the medial clavicle and the subclavian vein is less than 5 mm.[372] Furthermore, in some patients, the vein is adherent to the underside of the clavicle. A number of reports have shown injury to the subclavian vessels due to screw penetration. It is of upmost importance to prevent plunging with the drill bit or using screws that are more than two to four threads past the inferior cortex. Consideration should also be

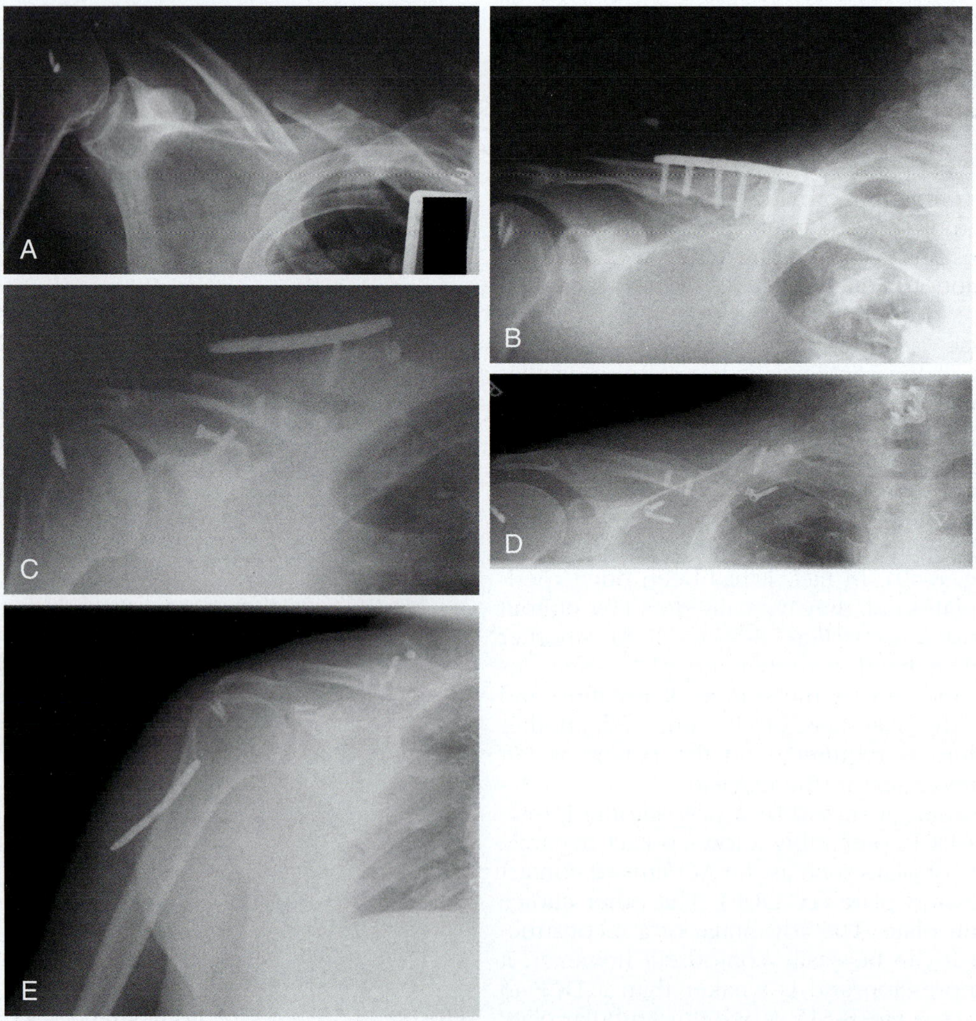

FIGURE 8-52: Significant plating hardware failure. **A,** Injury. **B,** Immediately after surgery with a limited contact dynamic compression plate. **C,** Six months after surgery. **D** and **E,** One year after surgery.

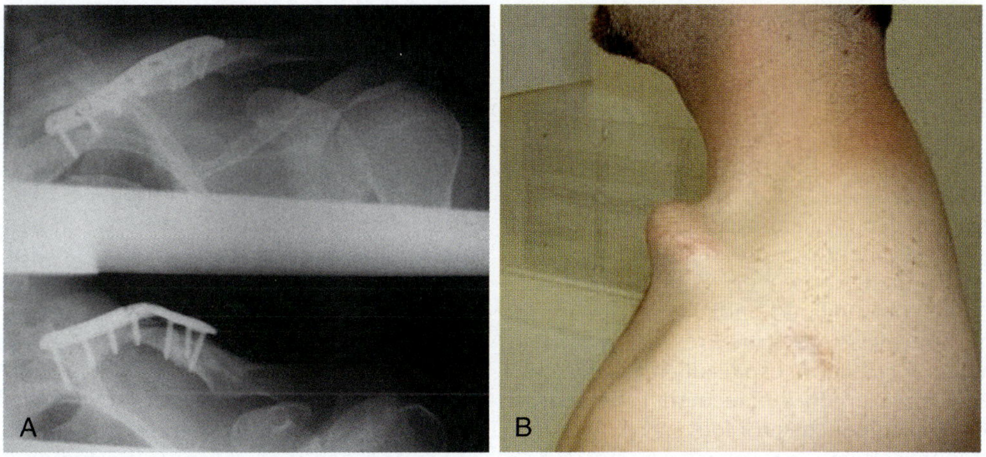

FIGURE 8-53: Loss of distal fixation and plate failure with resultant nonunion of a midshaft clavicle fracture treated with a locking precontoured plate. **A,** Plate fixation that developed failure with angulation of the fracture. **B,** Clinical appearance of angulated clavicle secondary to nonunion of the left clavicle.

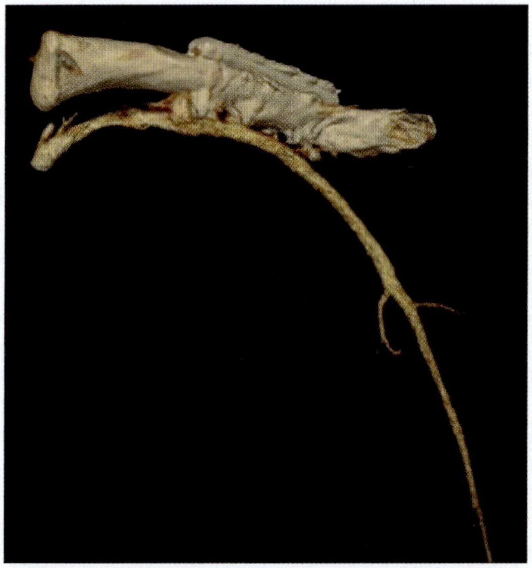

FIGURE 8-54: A pseudoaneurysm of the axillary artery caused by a prominent medial screw. (From Bain GI, Galley IJ, Keogh AR, et al. Axillary artery pseudoaneurysm after plate osteosynthesis for a clavicle nonunion: a case report and literature review. *Int J Shoulder Surg.* 2010;4[3]:79-82.)

given to circumferentially dissecting around the medial clavicle and placing protective instruments such as a Crego elevator under the clavicle to prevent injury to these structures (Fig. 8-54).

Choice of Plate

There are a number of choices in terms of plate fixation. The traditional choices are the 2.7-mm DCP, the 3.5-mm reconstruction plate, and the 3.5-mm LC-DCP. A number of clavicle-specific plates are available, such as the Acumed clavicle plate and the Smith & Nephew Peri-Loc Upper Extremity plate, both of which are precontoured for the clavicle and have locked screw capabilities. However, the Smith & Nephew plate is more of a precontoured 3.5-mm locking reconstruction plate. One of the primary advantages of using precontoured plates versus traditional straight plates is that there is a significant risk of losing the locking screw capabilities of the locking plates when they are contoured. The one-third tubular plate is far too weak to be used in the fixation of clavicle fractures.

There is great variability in the curvature of the clavicle and in the caudal-to-cephalic bow of the clavicle. Huang et al. noted that precontoured plates could fit well on the majority of male clavicles but not female clavicles because of the superior bow, with a poor fit being seen in 38% of specimens from white female donors.[154] Huang et al. also found that precontoured Acumed plates tended to work best with fixation of fractures occurring in the medial three-fifths of the clavicle. Unfortunately, most fractures occur at the junction of the middle and lateral third of the clavicle.

Iannotti et al.[156] found that the LC-DCP provided the most biomechanical stability in terms of fracture rigidity, construct stiffness, and strength. In terms of clinical results, Shahid et al.[363] found that the time to union was faster using a 3.5-mm DCP compared to a 3.5-mm reconstruction plate; however, the hardware had to be removed in half of the patients treated with a DCP because the prominence of the plate caused discomfort.

Although gross motion of fracture fragments can lead to nonunion, a certain amount of micromotion may be a stimulus to bone healing. Because of the considerable forces acting on the clavicle, fracture fixation must be very strong. The paradox in choosing plate fixation for clavicle fractures is that the stiffer the plate, the better able it is to resist these forces but the more likely it is to inhibit healing and allow weakening of the underlying bone because of excessive stress shielding. The stripping of soft tissue about the clavicle to allow placement of a plate can also contribute to osteopenia under the plate, further weakening the bone.

Placement of the Plate

There has been debate about the best position for application of plate fixation, with the primary choices being anterior or superior placement. The advantage of superior placement is that it can be accomplished with minimal soft tissue stripping and there is a broad surface medially for the fixation of the plate; however, there is the inherent problem of plate prominence and the risk of injury to the underlying neurovascular structures when drilling in a superior-to-inferior direction, especially medially.[172,362] The primary advantage of anterior placement is decreased incidence of plate-prominence problems and less risk of damage to the underlying neurovascular structures. However, anterior placement has the problem of more soft tissue stripping for placement of the plate. Furthermore, the anterior surface of the clavicle tends to be more angular compared to the flatter superior surface, making fixation more difficult.

There have been biomechanical studies comparing plate placement. Iannotti et al. found that constructs plated on the superior aspect of the clavicle exhibited significantly greater fracture rigidity and stiffness than the anterior location.[156] It should be noted, however, that the model used in this study was a straight, transverse osteotomy that would have favored a tension-band construct offered by the superior plate position. Unfortunately, this is not the pattern typically seen in real clavicle fractures. In our experience, the vast majority of midshaft clavicle fractures have some element of comminution, usually with an anterior-to-inferior butterfly fragment.

Harnroongroj and Vanadurongwan found that superior plating of a clavicle fracture without an inferior cortical defect provided more stability against the bending moment than anterior plating; however, anterior plating of a fracture with an inferior cortical defect provided more stability than a superior plate.[137]

Some clinical studies have shown no significant difference in outcomes based on plate position, whereas others have.[104,7]

Surgical Technique for Plate and Screw Fixation

As with IM fixation, general anesthesia with intubation is preferred because it allows good muscle relaxation and allows for a postoperative neurological examination in the recovery room.

The patient is placed in either a supine or beach chair position on a radiolucent operating table. The head should be placed in a headrest with the head tilted slightly away from the operative side to allow easier access and drilling of the medial fragment. The arm should be draped out separately to allow movement of the arm to facilitate reduction of the fracture. The clavicle should be exposed from the shoulder to the sternoclavicular joint. There are a number of options for the skin incision. It can be made directly over the clavicle; however, we have found that there is a greater incidence of skin hypersensitivity with this incision. Alternatively, an incision can be made below the clavicle, which minimizes the risk of having the incision directly over the plate. The authors' preference is to make an oblique incision in Langer's lines centered over the distal end of the medial fragment, or in the case of long oblique fractures, it should be centered between the distal end of the medial fragment and the medial end of the lateral fragment. This typically heals more cosmetically than a transverse incision crossing Langer's lines. It can also be extended medially and lateral if necessary in a "Z" fashion. This allows for good exposure to most fractures and minimizes the length of incision directly over the clavicle and plate, and can be used for a minimally invasive approach if so desired. If a minimally invasive technique is used, the plate is slid under the skin, and the screws are placed through small "stab" incisions.

The platysma can be reflected away from the overlying skin and then splint in line with its fibers. Alternatively, it can be left attached to the skin and incised as one layer with the skin. Care should be taken to minimize damage to the branches of the supraclavicular nerves (Fig. 8-55). Unfortunately, this can be a rather daunting task and the patient should be warned that there is a very high probability of anterior chest wall numbness, which can be seen in over 80% of patients, with nearly half still experiencing numbness even 1 year later.

The fragments are exposed, but minimal periosteal stripping should be used to preserve the only blood supply to the clavicle. In most fractures, the medial fragment is superior to the lateral fragment, and the lateral fragment is typically rotated anteriorly due to the pull of the pectoralis muscles. Most butterfly fragments, if present, are anterior and anterior to inferior, and are displaced due to their attachments to the deltoid. Any interposing soft tissue and clots should be removed.

The main fragments can then be reduced with reduction clamps. If the fracture is a long oblique pattern, a 3.5-mm cortical lag screw can be placed across the fracture. Even in significantly comminuted fractures, it is

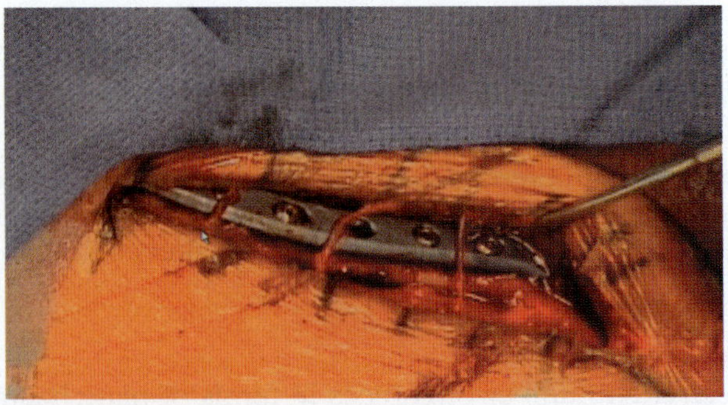

FIGURE 8-55: Branches of the supraclavicular nerve seen overlying a clavicle plate. (From Christensen TJ, Horwitz DS, Kubiak EN. Natural history of anterior chest wall numbness after plating of clavicle fractures: educating patients. *J Orthop Trauma*. 2014;28[11]:642-647.)

usually possible to achieve some bone-to-bone contact between the main fragments.

The senior author prefers to use a superiorly placed precontoured plate for fixation. Anterior plates can be useful in osteoporotic bone and fractures with significant comminution; however, they usually require some take-down of the deltoid and pectoralis muscle attachments. Preoperative radiographs of the uninvolved clavicle can be used to determine the length and shape of the required plate. Care must be taken to ensure that the plate is made to match the clavicle, rather than the clavicle being made to match the plate. Figure 8-42 shows an iatrogenic malunion caused by making the clavicle match the plate.

The plate can then be placed on the fractured clavicle and held there with reduction clamps. The plate should allow a minimum of six cortices purchase both medially and laterally. Although many precontoured plates available now allow for locking screws, we prefer to use a combination of locking and nonlocking screws to decrease the chance of screw pullout, especially laterally.[435] The nonlocking screws should be placed obliquely to decrease the chance of pullout since the deforming forces are usually parallel to the locking screws. Some type of retractor such as a Crego should be placed under the medial aspect of the clavicle to prevent injury to the subclavian vessels.[15,16]

Butterfly fragments should be left attached to their soft tissue and reduced and fixed with interfragmentary screws. If the fragments are too small to allow screw fixation, they can be cerclaged into place with No. 1 absorbable sutures. The platysma is then reapproximated with figure-of-eight sutures of 0 or 2-0 absorbable sutures and the skin closed in a layered fashion with inverted 2-0 or 3-0 absorbable sutures with a running subcuticular absorbable 3-0 suture followed by the use of steri-strips. The skin is then infiltrated with 0.25% or 0.5% bupivacaine with epinephrine. The arm is placed in a sling. If no intraoperative fluoroscopy was used, plain radiographs should be obtained in the recovery room.

Intramedullary Fixation

There are a number of advantages of IM fixation over plate and screw fixation. IM fixation can be performed through a small skin incision in Langer's lines. Studies have also shown that surgical times are typically shorter with IM fixation, with lower blood loss and postoperative pain medication use. It does not disrupt the periosteal blood supply of the clavicle as much as plate fixation, and it requires minimal soft tissue stripping. IM fixation can be removed under local anesthesia. Furthermore, in the setting of comminution, the cantilever effect for a pin extends to the medial-most portion of the pin, thereby providing better fixation in bending loads. It also allows axial compression, which should enhance healing.

One of the primary advantages of IM fixation that is often overlooked is the fact that healing with this type of fixation is callus rather than direct bone healing as is seen with plate and screw fixation. The advantage of this is that healing can be easily evaluated and followed with plain radiographs. Direct bone healing can typically only be inferred on follow-up radiographs because of the lack of complications (i.e., if there is no evidence of loss of fixation or hardware failure/breakage, the bone is assumed to be healed). This may present a problem with a return to sports and other high-demand activities. When bridging callus is seen on postoperative radiographs with IM fixation, there is no question about healing and hence there is more confidence in returning a patient to sports of high-load/demand-type activity.

IM fixation also allows what Perren described as "biologic fixation" of the fracture, utilizing flexible fixation and preservation of the soft tissue envelope with minimal soft tissue stripping and the avoidance of biologic damage caused by overly precise reduction.[304]

The concept of IM fixation of the clavicle is certainly not new. One of the earliest, and more interesting, methods of IM fixation was described in 1930 by Brockway.[40] He described using beef bone inserted into the IM canal for fixation of displaced clavicle fractures. Kuntscher and Maatz beautifully described the anatomy of the clavicle, and suggested that IM fixation should be used in the fixation of clavicle fractures.[201]

Murray also thought that the tubular structure of the clavicle lent itself well to IM fixation.[263] He noted that most clavicle fractures were comminuted, and many had a transversely oriented butterfly fragment that made closed reduction difficult. He used a smooth pin to accomplish reduction, and the pin was passed through the IM canal in a medial-to-lateral direction after drilling a pilot hole through the anterior medial cortex (Fig. 8-56).

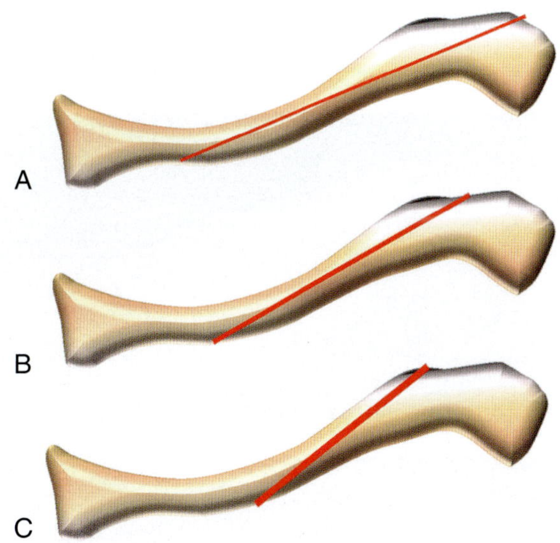

FIGURE 8-56: The length of fixation is determined by the length, diameter, and curvature of the clavicle in addition to the diameter of the pin. As the diameter of the pin increases, it has less fixation because the length of fixation decreases. The larger pin is also forced to exit the lateral fragment more medially than a smaller pin. **A,** Use of small diameter pin in clavicle. **B,** Medium diameter pin. **C,** Larger diameter pin.

He also described the technique similar to the one we prefer for open IM fixation. He made a small incision over the fracture site, passed a pin in an antegrade direction out through the lateral fragment, and then passed the pin in a retrograde fashion into the medial fragment after the fracture was held reduced. Zenni et al. described a similar technique in 1981.[436] Unfortunately, it was not long after this period that Mazet[237] described the migration of smooth wires from the shoulder into the lung.

Types of Intramedullary Fixation

There are basically three types of IM fixation devices (not including beef bone):

1. Smooth
2. Threaded
3. Partially threaded

These can be rigid or flexible and, in the case of hybrid fixation, can have flexible and rigid components.

Pertinent Anatomy

It has been said that IM fixation cannot be used in the clavicle because of its complex shape. Although the clavicle has an S shape with a superior bow, most clavicle fractures occur in its mid-section, where it tends to be relatively straight. If one simply draws a tangent to the straightest portion of the clavicle (see Fig. 8-56), it is easy to see that a fixation device inserted either medially or laterally can traverse this area without difficulty. Use of a hybrid IM device allows even greater length of fixation (Fig. 8-57).

Two important determinants of IM fixation are the diameter of the IM canal and the length of fixation. The IM canal determines the maximum size of the device. The average size of the IM canal at its narrowest point is approximately 6 mm. Although this sounds like a fairly large caliber, one has to keep in mind that the curve of the clavicle makes the effective diameter of the canal much smaller because to span the area of the fracture, the pin has to travel through the isthmus of the clavicle obliquely as shown in Figure 8-56. For the pin to travel the most effective length, it actually makes three-point contact with the walls of the canal: anterolaterally, then posteriorly at the apex of the posterior curve, and then again anteromedially when it makes contact with the anterior medial curve.

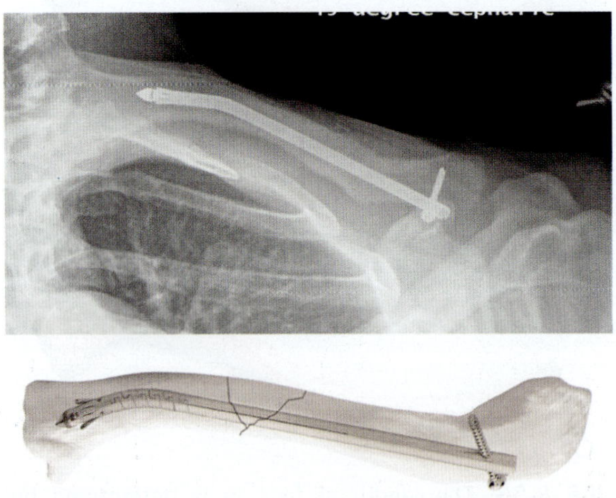

FIGURE 8-57: A "hybrid" intramedullary fixation device with a flexible medial portion to allow greater length of fixation in the medial fragment. It also has "grippers" medially and an interlocking screw laterally to help provide length and rotational control.

The diameter of the device also determines the length of fixation that is possible. Harnroongroj and Jeerathanyasakun found that there was a significant increase in the length of fixation using a 3.2-mm pin as compared to a 4.0-mm pin.[135] Although this seems like a small difference in pin size, they found that the ratio of engagement length to the total length of the clavicle was 0.59 with a 3.2-mm pin and 0.47 with a 4-mm pin, with the smaller pin having almost 2 cm greater fixation length. They also found that the engagement of the 4-mm pin was equivalent to a six-hole reconstruction plate, whereas that of the 3.2-mm pin was equivalent to an eight-hole reconstruction plate. The larger pin had significantly less fixation in the lateral fragment.

Another consideration in the diameter of pin fixation is that the stiffness of the pin is directly proportional to the fourth power of the radius of the pin ($I = \pi r^4/4$); in other words, as the pin becomes larger, its stiffness increases considerably. Just as with plate fixation, some micromotion is preferred to enhance healing. If the pin is too large, it will be excessively stiff, which may actually inhibit healing.

We can now see an important relationship here in that a larger diameter form in IM fixation, whether it be a screw, pin, or smooth wire, will be stiffer and will have potentially less fixation length. Healing can be compromised, and there will also be greater stresses on the short fixation, which could lead to greater risk of loosening, failure of the fixation, and healing. The conclusion from all of this is that the surgeon should pick the smallest pin that has stable fixation within the bone. In our experience, most midshaft clavicle fractures in female patients can be stabilized with a 2.5-mm pin, and most male patients should receive a 3-mm pin. Seldom do we use a larger pin except in very large patients or in older patients who have age-related increases in their canal diameters.

Because the clavicle has very little soft tissue coverage about it, any type of IM fixation that protrudes from the bone can cause soft tissue problems (Fig. 8-58). This was one of the primary factors in the complications in a study by Grassi et al.[123] Although he had a good union rate, he found significant problems with the pin causing irritation to the skin. This was also seen in a study by Strauss et al.[386] It is imperative that the portion of any IM device outside of the bone have the lowest profile possible. The quandary here is that the lower the profile of the device, the harder it is to remove, but the more prominent the hardware, the easier the removal will be.

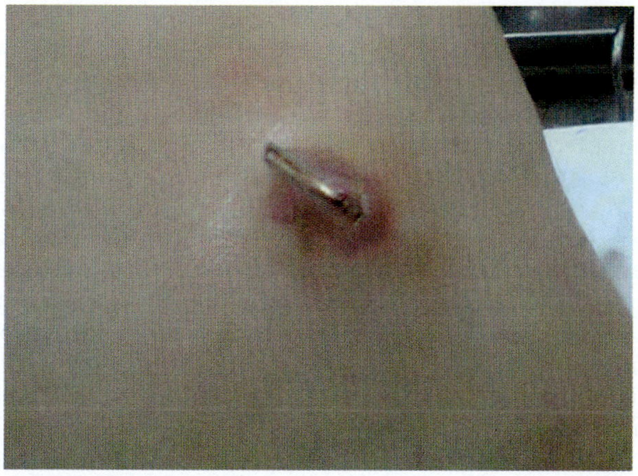

FIGURE 8-58: Skin erosion caused by a prominent intramedullary fixation device.

Choice of Intramedullary Fixation

The primary choices of IM fixation are smooth, threaded, and partially threaded devices. Fully threaded devices are seldom used in the treatment of clavicle fractures because of the risk of gapping at the fracture site. These have far less risk of migration than smooth devices; however, they can prevent compression of the fracture fragments, and thereby impede healing.[123]

There are numerous reports of migration of smooth devices used in clavicle fixation.[225] If these devices are to be used, they need to be followed closely for any radiographic signs of migration. Although smooth pin fixation has declined in popularity, there seems to be new interest in the use of smooth titanium elastic nails (TENs) in treating clavicle fractures.[175-177,188,246,411] One of the primary advantages in using a flexible nail is that it allows considerable length of fixation as compared to a rigid device. The fixation of these devices is said to be facilitated by jamming the end of the device into the lateral fragment. Despite this, there still remains the risk of implant migration, and some studies show a rate of loosening or migration of 5% to 25%.[246,259]

Kettler et al. examined the use of a TEN in 95 midshaft clavicle fractures. They found that an open fracture reduction was required in 53 patients (56%), and they had a nonunion rate of 2%, a malunion rate of 8%, and pin migration in 4%; 5% of patients required a revision surgery.[188] Mueller et al. used a TEN in 32 cases, and they reported a union rate of 100%[259]; however, they also noted that an open reduction was necessary in 50%. They also had shortening greater than 5 mm in 38% and nail migration in eight patients (25%) that required revision shortening of the nail in five of those eight. They also reported breakage of the nail in two patients after the clavicle was healed.[259] It is somewhat difficult to understand how this could have happened after healing unless there was some repetitive micromotion from a subtle nonunion.

One additional problem with TEN fixation is that most studies have relied on insertion of the pin through an anterior medial approach. The dilemma of IM fixation is that unlike plate fixation, the device is intended to be removed once the fracture has healed. The quandary with this is that the device needs to have a low profile so it does not cause skin and soft tissue irritation, but it must be prominent enough to be easily retrieved. In the case of TEN fixation, or any other pin relying on medial insertion, there is very little tissue overlying the medial clavicle, and any prominence can cause significant soft tissue irritation.

Another limitation with IM fixation is that the device length is quite variable, and the surgeon has limited choice of device sizes in terms of length and diameter. There is the risk of compromising fracture fixation. This is particularly true in the case of IM screw fixation, especially cannulated screws where the length of the device is limited by the mechanical properties of the metal used to make the screw. In other words, it is difficult to make a screw of small enough diameter and sufficient length to achieve adequate fixation. For example, studies have suggested using a Herbert cannulated bone screw for midshaft clavicle fractures.[54,148,318] However, the smallest diameter is 4.5 mm, and the longest screw is 100 mm. Low-profile devices do not need to be removed, which is considered an advantage, except in competitive athletes who are at high risk for clavicle refracture.

The recent addition of a hybrid fixation device has alleviated many of the problems associated with IM fixation.[212,435] It has a flexible medial end, which allows it to follow the curvature of the clavicle at its medial end. The device is then activated to become rigid once the desired fracture position is achieved and to deploy grippers at its medial end to lock the device. This gives the device more length and rotation control, which are unachievable with other IM devices. Furthermore, it allows a significantly longer length of fixation than that possible with other rigid IM devices. Laterally, the device is designed to sit flush against the posterolateral cortex of the clavicle, thus minimizing hardware irritation. An interlocking screw is placed through the device and the lateral fragment of the clavicle to further prevent the device from migrating and to stabilize device to give better length and rotation control, thereby reducing the risk of subsequent complications and loss of reduction.

The exposure needed to place an IM pin is significantly smaller than that needed for a formal open reduction and internal fixation with plates and screws. This restricted exposure limits further damage to the already injured soft tissue envelope. The IM pin allows compression at the fracture site and load sharing, which are advantageous in the healing of other long-bone fractures. The IM pin can be removed easily under local anesthesia. IM pins come in different sizes to allow filling of the canal, which again has been shown to be advantageous in other fractures treated with IM devices. Unlike plate and screw fixation, placement of an IM pin does not require drilling perpendicularly through the clavicle. This fact decreases the risk to neurovascular structures and obviates the need to strip the soft tissues to protect these structures.

A number of level I, II, and III studies have shown IM fixation to be equally effective as plate and screw fixation; however, and most importantly, most studies have shown a significantly lower complication rate with IM fixation compared to plate and screw fixation. Thyagarajan et al. found that patients who had undergone pinning had a 100% union rate within 2 to 4 months, with a shorter hospital stay. Plate patients also had a 100% healing rate, but 23.5% also had scar-related pain and 17.5% had discomfort from prominent hardware. The nonoperative group had a 23.5% nonunion rate, 29.4% had cosmetic complaints, and 6% had malunion.[396] Wu et al. examined patients with middle-third clavicular aseptic nonunions treated by plating in 11 patients and IM nailing in 18 patients with supplementary cancellous bone grafting. The time to union was not significantly different between the groups, but the union rate of 81.8% (9 of 11) for plating was significantly lower than the 88.9% (16 of 18) for IM nailing, and the complication rate was 27.3% (3 of 11) for plating and only 11.1% (2 of 18) for IM nailing.[427]

Table 8-2 shows a comparison of plate and IM fixation results.

Surgical Technique for Intramedullary Fixation

Although the following technique is for the hybrid type of fixation, the basic principles can be applied to all types of IM fixation.

All of our IM cases are performed under general anesthesia in an outpatient setting. General anesthesia is preferred for two reasons: coverage of the clavicular regional can be "marginal" with interscalene or regional anesthesia. It also makes postoperative neurovascular examinations difficult in the recovery room. Because of this, we prefer general anesthesia with local anesthesia supplementation. We typically use local infiltration of 0.5% bupivacaine with epinephrine either at the start or at the end of the case. This allows excellent pain control both intraoperatively and postoperatively. Because of the small incision size and minimally invasive nature of IM fixation, virtually all of these procedures are performed in an outpatient setting. Patients are typically given a preoperative dose of antibiotics, with an additional dose in the recovery room.

Rockwood Clavicle Pin

The Rockwood clavicle pin is a smooth pin of different sizes that has fine threads on the lateral segment of the pin and built-up threads on the medial segment to engage the IM canal of the medial canal.

Sonoma CRx Clavicle Pin

Currently, the only type of hybrid fixation device on the market is the Sonoma Orthopedic CRx clavicle pin. It was developed out of concern for the high complication rate due to painful, prominent hardware seen in plate and most types of IM fixation and the problems associated with other types of IM fixation such as poor length and rotational control and poor overall length of fixation with rigid devices due to the S shape of the clavicle. Although the device is manufactured from one piece of metal, the medial 30 mm of the device has a continuous helical laser cut pattern in the cylinder that allows it to be flexible and conform to the curvature of the clavicle, and thereby achieve greater purchase in the medial segment (Fig. 8-59). The remaining rigid portion of the device is the part that transverses the fracture site. Once it is in place, a rod inside the device can be tightened to make the flexible portion rigid by crimping or compressing the helical cuts in the cylinder. As the inner rod is tightened, it also deploys what are referred to as "grippers" or talons that provide further length and rotational control (Fig. 8-60). This not only gives the device better rotational control, it allows for up to 30 mm more length of fixation than could be achieved with a rigid device such as a cancellous screw or a Rockwood pin. The addition of an interlocking screw in the lateral portion of the device also allows for greater length and rotational control, and virtually negates the chances of hardware migration. In addition to the novel concept of the device itself, clavicle specific instrumentation to allow easy insertion of the device was also developed. This included flexible, cannulated reamers, rigid curved and straight awls, and special flexible guide wires that minimize the chance of perforation of the cortical bone. The entire device was

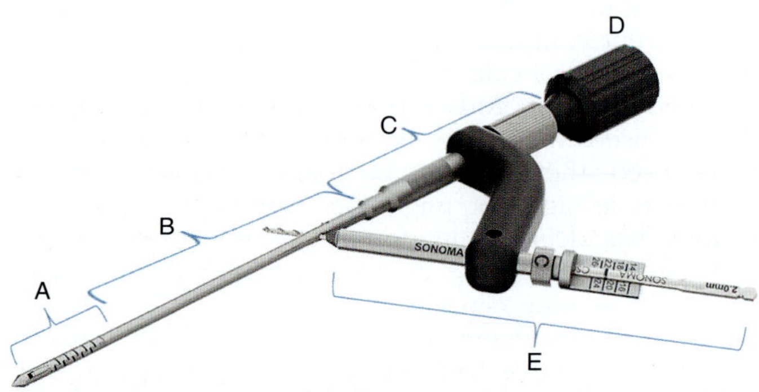

FIGURE 8-59: Diagram of the Sonoma CRx hybrid fixation device with its attached outrigger. *A*, Wavy/flexible body with grippers. *B*, Rigid portion of the device. *C*, Outrigger. *D*, Handle of the torque-limiting screwdriver. ***E***, Interlocking guide and drill. (Courtesy Sonoma Orthopedic Products, Buffalo Grove, IL.)

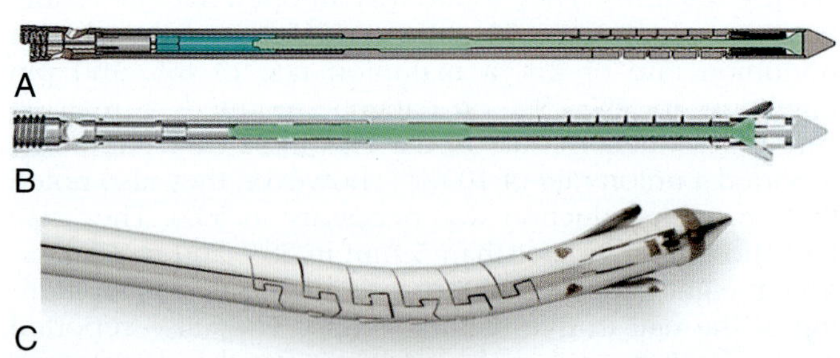

Figure 8-60: Internal mechanism of the Sonoma CRx. **A,** Plunger (represented in green) in the nontightened position. **B,** Plunger in the tightened position crimping the wavy body and deploying the grippers. **C,** The differential cut in the wavy body causes the pin to preferentially curve in one direction when the plunger is tightened. (Courtesy Sonoma Orthopedic Products, Buffalo Grove, IL.)

TABLE 8-2 Comparison of Plate to Intramedullary Fixation Treatment

Author	No. of Patients	Technique Used	Outcomes of Interest	Failure Rate	Complication Rate	Comment	Level of Evidence
Zehir et al.[438]	24 IM 21 MIPPO plate	Sonoma CRx Precontoured plate	Significantly shorter operative times, hospital stay, and time to union and less fluoro use in IM group	4% IM 5% plate	4% IM 5% plate	Cosmetic dissatisfaction higher in plate group; no difference in DASH scores	I
Saha et al.[439]	37 plate 34 IM	TEN Anterosuperior locking plate	Significantly shorter time to union and operative time and lesser blood loss in IM group	0% IM group 3% in plate group	Major: 14% plate vs. 0% IM Minor: 16% plate vs. 38% IM	11% infection rate in plate group; 16% of plate patients rated their scar as "ugly"	I
Assobhi[440]	19 plate 19 IM	TEN 3.5 recon plate	Significantly shorter hospital stay, length of surgery, and scar length and lesser blood loss in IM group	Nonunion: 5.3% plate, 0% IM	Major: 15.8% plate vs. 0% IM Minor: 36.8% plate vs. 21.1% IM	5.3% refracture rate in plate group after hardware removal vs. 0% in IM group	I
Lee et al.[441]	56 IM 32 plate	Knowles pin 3.5 DCP and recon plate	Significantly shorter surgical times and less scar and pain medication use in IM group	Nonunion: 0% 1% plate	0% IM 9.4% plate	Painful hardware: 7.1% IM, 37.5% plate	I
Ferran et al.[442]	17 IM 15 plate	Rockwood screw 3.5 LC-DCP	Mean Constant score of 92.1 IM vs. 88.7 plate	0% both groups	24% IM 80% plate	Hardware removal: 100% planned removal in IM group, 53% due to irritation and infection in plate group	I
Narsaria et al.[266]	32 plate 33 IM	TEN and precontoured plate	No functional differences postoperatively; significantly shorter hospital stay, length of surgery, and scar length and less blood loss in IM group	1 nonunion in IM group 1 revision surgery in IM group, 2 in plate	21.87% wound and scar problems 9.37% refracture in plate group, 0% in IM group	Planned hardware removal in all IM patients, hardware removal in 20 of 32 in plate group	II

Continued

TABLE 8-2 Comparison of Plate to Intramedullary Fixation Treatment—cont'd

Author	No. of Patients	Technique Used	Outcomes of Interest	Failure Rate	Complication Rate	Comment	Level of Evidence
Bohme et al.[443]	20 IM 53 plate 47 nonop	TEN DCP, recon, or LC-DCP	4% infection rate in plate group	0% nonunion in operative groups	15% IM 22% plate	Both operative groups had better pain relief, function, and cosmetic results compared with nonop group	II
Chen et al.[444]	84 plate 57 IM	TEN Reconstruction plates	Significantly shorter time to union, operative time, and less blood loss in IM group	2% IM 4% plate	Infection: 2% IM, 4% plate Hardware failure: 5% IM, 7% plate	43% of plate group rated results as unsatisfactory compared with 14% in IM group	III
Wijdicks et al.[445]	43 plate 47 IM	TEN Reconstruction and locking plates	7% refracture rate in plate group vs. 0% IM	14% implant failure plate vs. 2.1% IM	Major: 26% plate vs. 4% IM	12% major revision plate vs. 2% IM	III
Wenninger et al.[446]	29 plate 33 IM	Rockwood screw 3.5 recon and precontoured plates	Majority of symptoms were from the pressure of the body armor and rucksack wear during training	0% nonunions in both groups	9% IM 31% plate	Active-duty military population	III
Liu et al.[447]	59 plate 51 IM	TEN Straight and contoured superior plates	Significantly shorter operative time, hospital stay, and incision size and less blood loss in IM group	Nonunion: 9.8% IM vs. 10.2% plate Malunion: 7.8% IM vs. 3.4% plate	39% IM 53% plate	Wound complication rate: 5.9% IM, 10.2% plate	III
Kleweno et al.[448]	18 IM 14 plate	Rockwood screw 6 recon, 6 locking, and 2 precontoured plates	Average time to union: 8 months IM vs. 17 months plate	0% IM group vs. 7% plate	28% IM 36% plate	7% delayed union and 14% refracture rate in plate group vs. 0% IM group	III
Thyagarajan et al.[396]	17 IM 17 plate 17 nonop	Rockwood screw LC-DCP plates	IM group had 100% union by 8-12 weeks All IM surgeries outpatient Plate group all had 2- to 3-day hospital stay	IM 0% Plate 6% nonunion Nonop 23.5% nonunion or malunion	IM: 12% superficial wound Plate: 12% implant failure, 35% plate irritation, 24% scar-related pain	All patients in IM group were satisfied with results; 35% of plate group had pain with activity; 12% of IM group had only mild pain	III

DASH, disabilities of the arm, shoulder, and hand; DCP, decompression plate; IM, intramedullary; LC-DCP, low-contact dynamic compression plate; MIPPO, minimally invasive percutaneous plate osteosynthesis; Nonop, nonoperative; recon, reconstruction; TEN, titanium elastic nail.

designed to be entirely IM, with no prominent hardware, as can be seen in Figure 8-56. However, if the device needs to be removed for any reason, it was also designed for easy removal. The medial portion of the pin is made flexible with a torque-limiting screwdriver that loosens the inner rod of the device, thereby allowing the medial portion to become flexible again. A specific extraction device is then secured to the lateral portion of the pin, and it is removed with a slap-hammer type of technique (see Fig. 8-77).

Patient Positioning

The procedure can be performed in a supine or modified "beach chair" position on a radiolucent operating table (Video 8-1). We prefer the modified beach chair position for easier access to the posterior aspect of the shoulder. Clavicle and shoulder access is facilitated by using a radiolucent shoulder-positioning device. The torso of the patient is typically at about 45 degrees relative to the floor. An image intensification device or C-arm greatly facilitates pin placement. The C-arm base can be brought in from the opposite side of the bed from the injured side or it can be brought in from the head of the bed with the C-arm gantry rotated slightly away from the operative shoulder. Drape the C-arm with standard split sheets. It is important to ensure that the entire length of the clavicle including the sternoclavicular joint can be seen and palpated after the draping. The arm should also be draped free to allow movement of the arm to facilitate drilling of the lateral fragment and reduction of the fracture.

The patient's torso should be approximately 45 degrees relative to the floor. The gantry of the C-arm should be situated such that the beam of the x-ray is parallel to the floor (Fig. 8-61).

This gives the equivalent of a 45-degree cephalic tilt view of the medial clavicle, which allows the best view of the anterior curve of the clavicle.

This orientation also gives a cephalic tilt view of the lateral fragment since the placement of any type of retrograde IM fixation in the lateral fragment is crucial to obtaining an anatomic reduction of the fracture. Furthermore, an "AP equivalent" view can be obtained by extending the arm and an "axillary equivalent" view can be obtained by forward flexing the arm (Figs. 8-62 and 8-63).

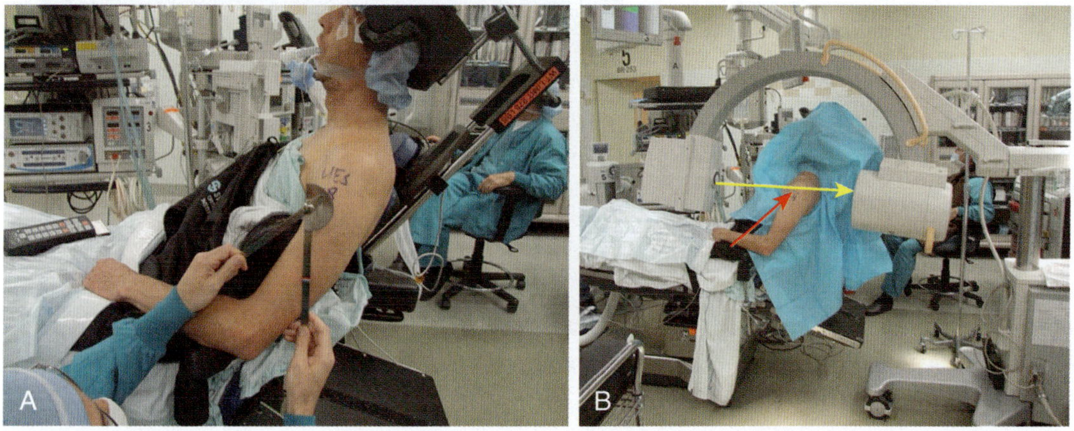

FIGURE 8-61: **A,** The patient is placed in the beach chair position on the operating table with the use of a radiolucent positioner. **B,** The image intensifier is then brought over the top of the patient and draped into the surgical field. The orientation of the imagine intensifier relative to the torso gives the equivalent of a 45-degree cephalic tilt view of the clavicle.

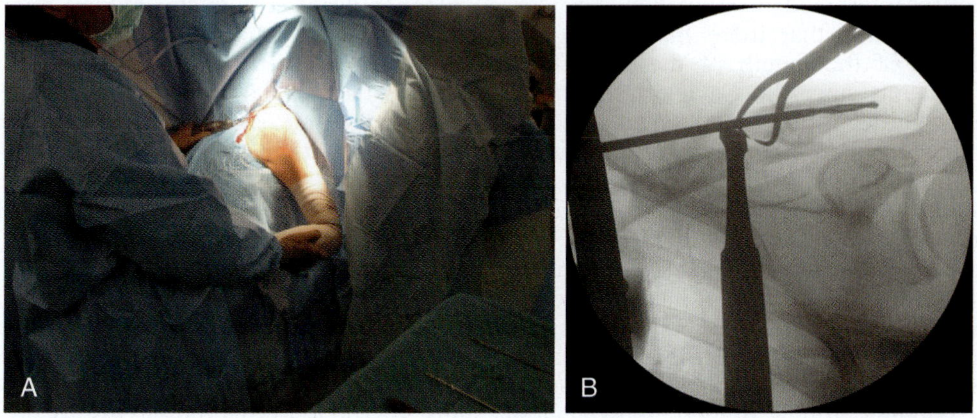

FIGURE 8-62: **A,** Extending the arm of the patient gives the equivalent of an anteroposterior view. **B,** C-arm image. Note the position of the drill bit relative to the equator of the clavicle.

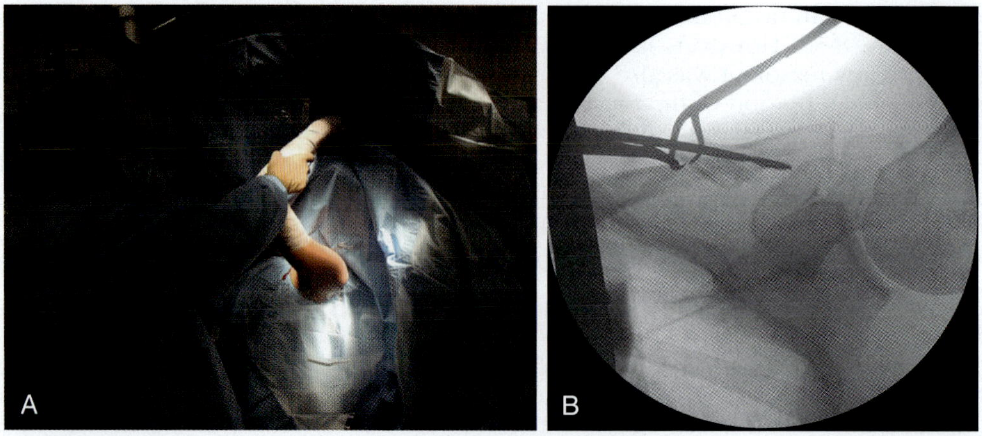

FIGURE 8-63: **A,** Forward flexing the arm gives the equivalent of a "near axillary" view. **B,** Note the exit point of the drill bit halfway between the conoid tubercle and the acromioclavicular joint.

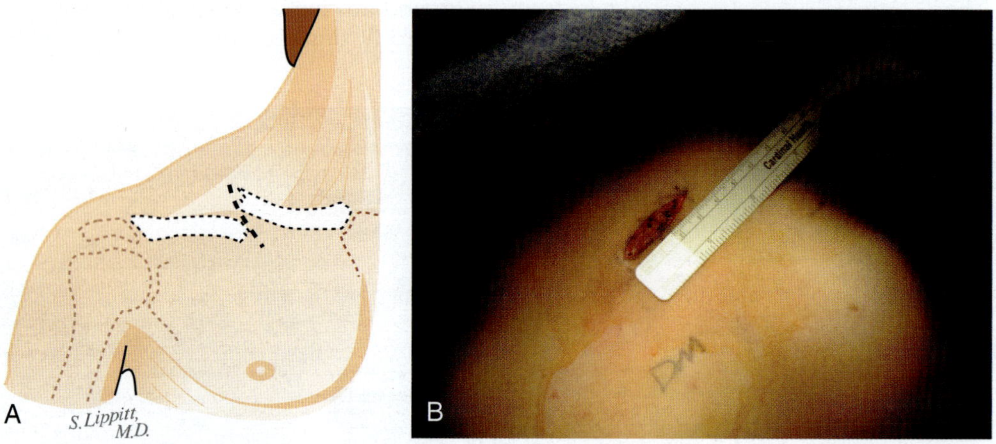

FIGURE 8-64: **A** and **B,** A 3-cm incision is made in the natural skin creases over the distal aspect of the medial fragment. Because of tethering of the skin by the platysma muscle, it is easier to move the skin medially than laterally.

Due to metallic or radiopaque devices on the operative table, the beam of the C-arm may need to be oriented in a posterolateral to anteromedial orientation. The surgeon should be cautioned that there may be significant underestimation of the length of the fracture or overlap of the fragments since the clavicle is obliquely oriented relative to the beam of the x-ray. This underestimation will be exaggerated if the C-arm is oriented in an oblique fashion relative to the torso. If necessary, the patient's shoulder can be brought forward to obtain a better estimation of the true fracture length. It is also important that the entire length of the clavicle can be viewed in one position. Once these points are accomplished, the entire case can be completed with the use of a foot pedal to activate the C-arm, thereby negating the need to have a radiology technician available for the entire case. The patient's arm is draped free to allow movement during the case for better visualization and fracture reduction.

Incision

A 2.5- to 3-cm incision is made in Langer's lines over the palpable distal end of the medial fragment (Fig. 8-64). This technique is used because the clavicle skin is more easily moved medially than laterally (Video 8-2). Most patients have a skin crease in the same area where the incision is made, and placing the incision in this crease typically results in a more cosmetically pleasing scar. In fractures with a long oblique pattern, the incision is made slightly more medially and longer to allow elevation of the medial end of the distal fragment. It should be noted that plain AP radiographs typically underestimate the length of the fracture since the clavicle is oblique to the beam of the x-rays.

Because there is little subcutaneous fat in this region, take care to prevent injury to the underlying platysma muscle. The platysma muscle inserts on the skin near the clavicle, and damage to it may lead to dysfunction of facial expression. Use scissors to free the platysma muscle

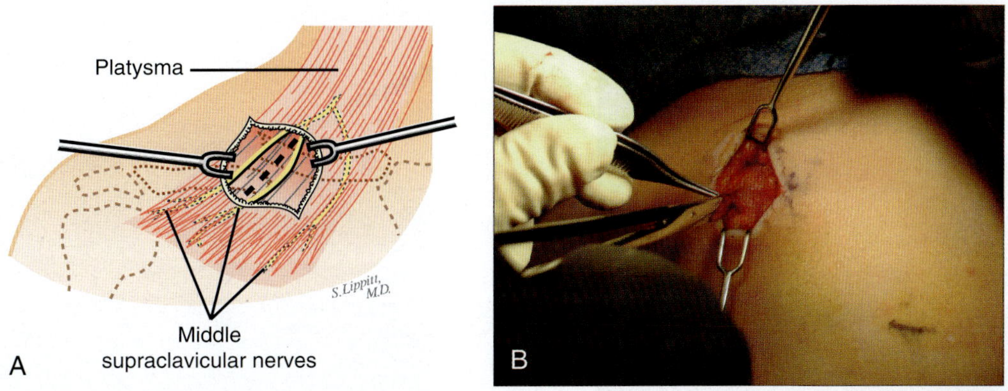

FIGURE 8-65: **A** and **B,** The platysma muscle is typically directly under the skin because there is usually little subcutaneous fat in this region. The middle branches of the supraclavicular nerve are generally found directly under the platysma muscle, and care must be taken to protect them during the surgical exposure, regardless of whether intramedullary or plate fixation is used.

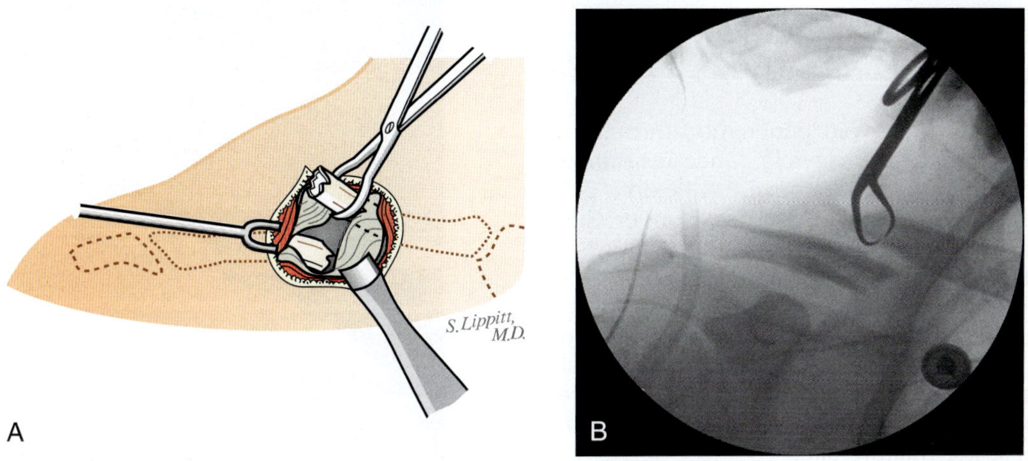

FIGURE 8-66: **A** and **B,** The medial fragment is grasped with a towel clip or bone reduction forceps.

from the overlying skin. Once the platysma muscle has been identified, divide its fibers longitudinally (Fig. 8-65).

Take care to prevent injury to the middle branch of the supraclavicular nerve, which is seen in approximately 50% of patients[268]; it is usually found directly beneath the platysma muscle near the mid-portion of the clavicle. In a number of cases, the nerve has been found in the fracture site (see Fig. 8-1). Injury to this nerve can cause dysesthesia in the anterior shoulder, deltoid, and anterior chest wall in 10% to 29% of cases.[245]

Identify and retract the nerve to prevent injury. With acute fractures, the periosteum over the fracture site is disrupted, and usually requires no further division. In most cases, muscle, typically the subclavius, and/or soft tissue will be interposed in the fracture. On long oblique fractures, we have often found the medial end of the lateral fragment to be embedded in the clavicular head of the pectoralis muscle. Carefully remove them with an elevator or curette. In the case of the medial end of the lateral fragment being in muscle, the fragment can be grasped with a small reduction clamp and with lateral distraction, the medial end can be freed from the muscle with a small key periosteal elevator. Leave small butterfly fragments, usually found anteriorly and inferiorly, attached to their soft tissue envelope. These can be cerclaged after the primary fixation.

Medial Fragment Preparation

The lateral end of the medial fragment is elevated into the incision (Video 8-3). The lateral end of the medial fragment can be grasped with a towel clip to elevate it into the incision. In addition, a half-inch key elevator can be inserted under the lateral aspect of the medial fragment to help elevate it into the incision. Placement of the key elevator under the medial fragment decreases the likelihood of the drill or awl skiving off and going deep to the medial fragment, potentially causing damage to the underlying neurovascular structures (Fig. 8-66). Under fluoroscopic guidance, the medullary canal is identified with a 2-mm drill bit (Fig. 8-67). Palpating the medial aspect of the clavicle can help establish this orientation. Once the orientation is established, the canal can be

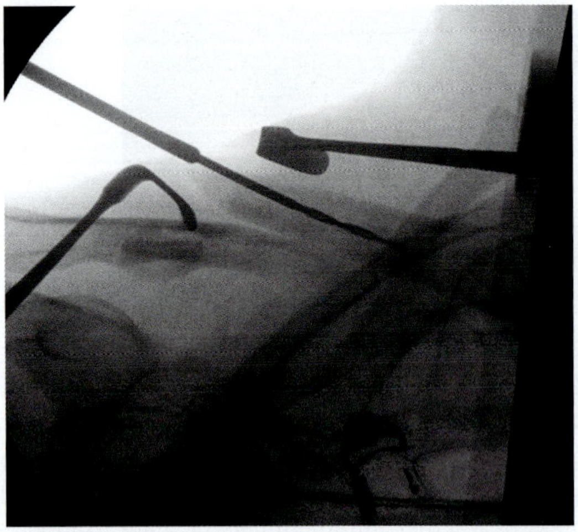

FIGURE 8-67: A 2-mm drill bit is used to localize the intramedullary canal of the medial fragment.

further opened with a 3.5-mm drill bit or a straight or curved 3-mm awl (Fig. 8-68).

Care must be taken to avoid penetration through the anterior medial cortex of the clavicle. Once resistance is met, the straight drill or awl is removed. A flexible guide pin can then be passed into the IM canal under C-arm guidance until it is at least 50 mm past the fracture site. If the bone within the canal is too dense to allow passage of the guide pin, a curved 3-mm awl can be used to further open the canal. Care must be taken to advance the awl using a short back and forth motion. Excessive motion can lead to a windshield wiper effect with eccentric reaming of the canal. The awl should be passed at least 50 mm past the fracture site.

The awl is then removed and replaced with the guide pin. The medial canal can then be reamed with a flexible 4.5-mm reamer (Fig. 8-69). Care must be taken not to pass the reamer too quickly or force the reamer into the canal because the flutes of the reamer can fill with bone, causing a significant increase in friction, with potential thermal necrosis of the bone. If resistance is felt, the reamer should be removed, bone cleared from the flutes, and reaming can then proceed. It is imperative that the medial canal is reamed to at least 50 mm past the medial most extension of the fracture. Failure to do so will place excessive bending forces on the flexible-rigid interface of the hybrid device and may cause early failure. If at least 50 mm of purchase cannot be obtained such as the case with more medial fractures, the hybrid device can be placed in a medial-to-lateral orientation that will be described further below. If changing the orientation still does not give enough purchase, either a different type of IM device such as an elastic titanium nail or a plate should be used. Once the reamer is at least 50 mm past the fracture site, reaming can be continued until resistance is felt; however, in older patients with large diameter canals, the surgeon should be cautioned that when using rigid fixation devices, fixation may be compromised in the broader medial canal rather than improved.

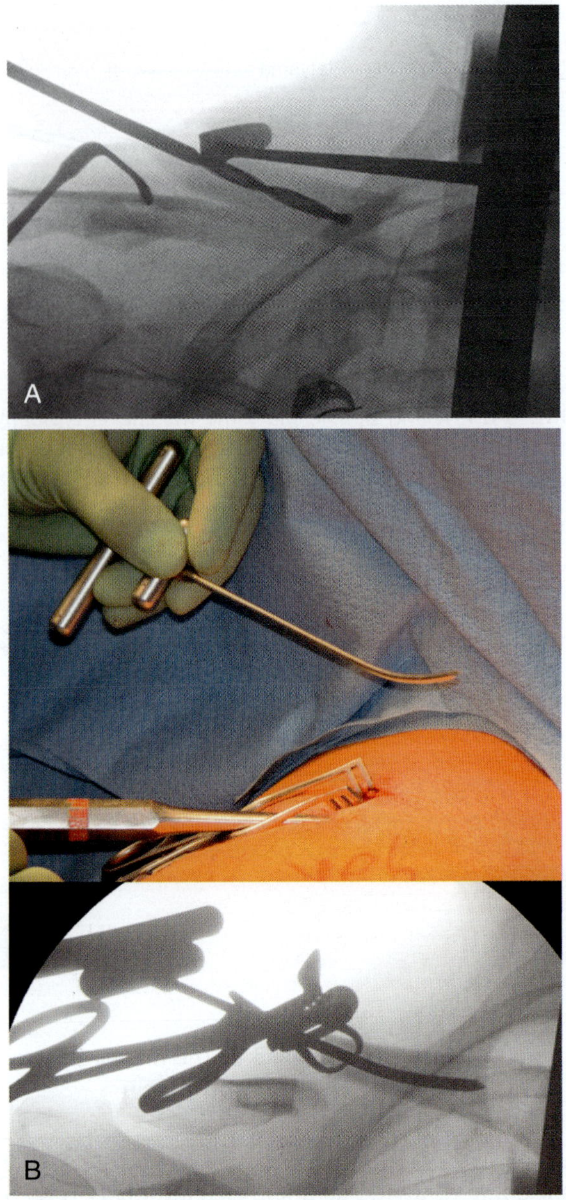

FIGURE 8-68: **A,** Opening of the medial canal with a 3.5-mm drill bit. **B,** A 3-mm straight or curved awl can be used to further open the canal.

If, for some reason, the guide pin penetrates the anteromedial cortex, the tendency for the guide pin is to continue to go out the same perforation. This can be dealt with by using a small curved Frazer-type suction device to "coax" the guide pin past the perforation (Fig. 8-70). The Frazer tip suction device can also be used to help the guide pin past the anterior curve of the clavicle. Once the canal is reamed with the cannulated reamer, the final fixation device will follow the canal since the perforation is too small to allow passage through it.

Lateral Fragment Preparation

The lateral canal preparation can be somewhat more difficult, and proper placement is critical to the technique

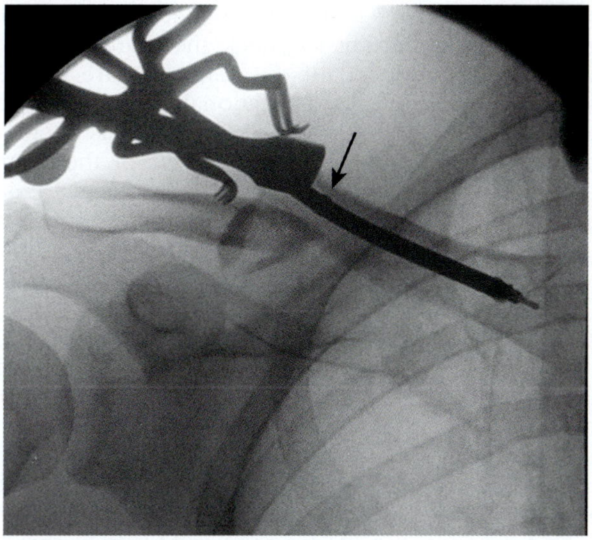

FIGURE 8-69: A flexible 4.5-mm reamer is passed over a flexible guide pin and into the canal until at least 50 mm of purchase is achieved. This is denoted by the band on the reamer (*arrow*).

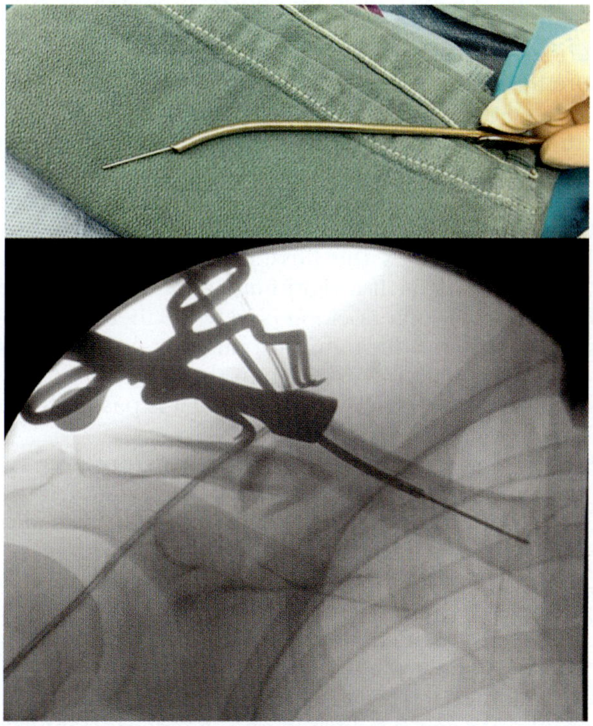

FIGURE 8-70: A small curved Frazer-type suction tube can be used to direct the flexible guide pin into the curve of the medial fragment.

(Video 8-4). The ideal exit point in the posterolateral clavicle is halfway between the conoid tubercle and the distal clavicle and at the equator of the clavicle. Although the exit point is at the equator in most patients, some patients may have an exaggerated downward lateral curve to their clavicle. In these cases, the exit point will be more superior; however, the exit point should never be below the equator of the lateral clavicle as this will cause the distal fragment to be flexed upward relative to the medial fragment and may cause excessive rotation of the distal fragment relative to the medial fragment or problems passing the final fixation device past the spine of the scapula. Although it may seem daunting, it is similar to the importance of the piriformis fossa in femoral nailing, and can easily be achieved with proper drilling and C-arm use.

The medial end of the lateral fragment is usually located posterior and inferior to the distal end of the medial fragment in most cases of lateral impact–type fractures; however, in "seatbelt fractures," the medial end of the lateral fragment may be located anterior to the medial fragment. Once the fragment is identified, it can be grasped with a towel clamp and carefully elevated into the incision. A half-inch key elevator under the tip of the fragment can be used as a "tire iron" to help elevate the fragment. As with the medial fragment, a 2-mm drill is used under fluoroscopic guidance to establish the orientation of the lateral canal. A 2-mm drill bit is used because the orientation can be changed without compromise of the canal. The orientation of the drill bit should be towards the mid-point of the posterior cortex of the lateral fragment. The surgeon can place the tip of his or her index finger at the "V" formed by the junction of the lateral clavicle and the spine of the scapula with the distal interphalangeal joint of his or her finger at the acromioclavicular joint and using this as an "aiming device." This orientation can be checked under fluoroscopy by forward flexing the arm to give more of an axillary view of the distal fragment (see Fig. 8-63). Once this orientation is established, the arm can be extended to allow more of an AP view of the distal fragment (see Fig. 8-62). With this view, the drill bit should be aimed at the "equator" of the clavicle. Once the orientation is verified, the canal is further opened with a 3.5-mm drill bit. Once this is verified to be in a good position, it is passed through the posterolateral cortex. A small incision is then made over the palpable tip of the drill. The 3.5-mm drill bit is then removed and replaced with a rigid Steinmann pin that is brought out through the posterior skin incision. The lateral canal is then "reamed" with a 4.5-mm cannulated drill bit passed in a retrograde fashion over the rigid guide pin. Once the 4.5-mm drill bit reaches the fracture site, the rigid guide pin is removed.

Fracture Reduction

The 4.5-mm drill bit can now be used to help achieve a reduction of the fracture. With downward pressure on the medial fragment and upward force on the elbow to counteract the deformity caused by gravity, the tip of the drill bit can be advanced a short distance into the canal of the medial fragment (Fig. 8-71). This will help temporarily hold the reduction. Once the reduction is verified under fluoroscopy, a flexible guide wire is passed through the 4.5-mm drill bit and advanced until it is seated in the medial-most aspect of the medial fragment.

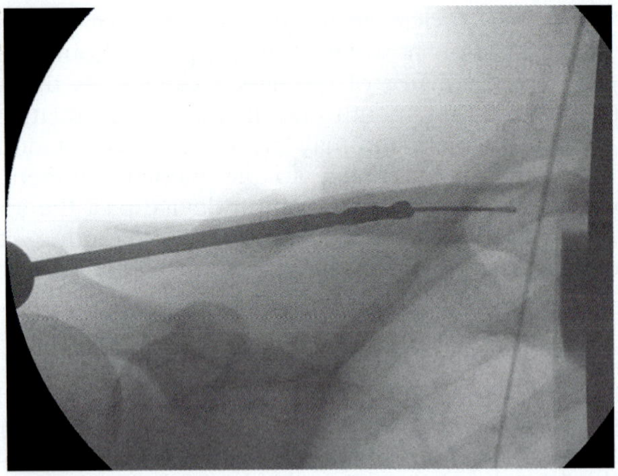

FIGURE 8-71: The 4.5-mm cannulated drill is advanced a short distance into the medial canal to provisionally reduce the fracture. A guide wire can then be passed through this into the medial fragment.

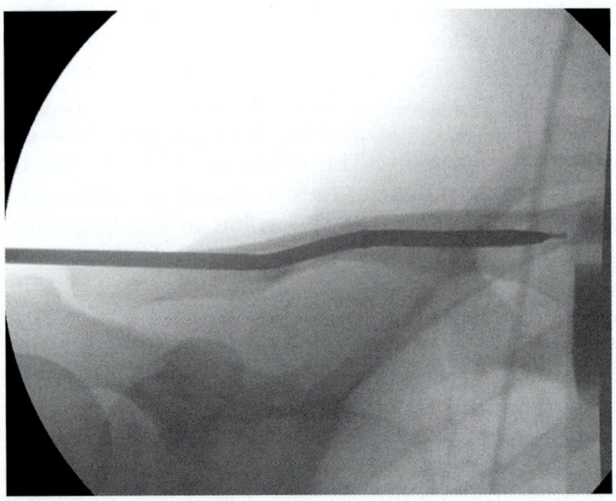

FIGURE 8-72: The entire length of the intramedullary canal is reamed with a 4.5-mm flexible reamer passed over the guide pin.

The 4.5-mm drill bit is then removed, and the entire length of the IM canal is reamed with a 4.5mm flexible reamer passed over the guide wire (Fig. 8-72).

In the case of a long oblique fracture, the fracture can be loosely held reduced with a small bone reduction clamp to prevent shortening of the fracture. In the case of significant comminution, the butterfly fragments can be provisionally fixed by passing No. 1 or 2 sutures around the clavicle and fragments to cerclage them together using a Crego elevator as described below. If a longitudinal fracture is noted in the medial fragment, a cerclaged suture or wire can be passed around the clavicle to prevent propagation of the fracture. Once the flexible reamer has been fully passed, the reduction is checked with fluoroscopy. The fracture should be anatomically reduced. This is not a problem most of the time because if the reamer is IM in both the lateral fragment and medial fragment, it should be anatomically aligned. It is also very important to check the diameters of the fragments once reduced. If the diameters are different, this means that there is a rotational deformity, which needs to be corrected. Once the reduction has been verified, a depth measurement is taken off of the reamer. The reamer is then removed and a guide sleeve passed over the guide pin. The guide pin is then removed and the incisions irrigated with copious amounts of antibiotic fluid.

Final Fixation

An appropriate-sized IM pin is attached to the outrigger, and the tip of the final device is slid along the guide sleeve until it is in the lateral fragment. The sleeve is then removed and the final fixation device advanced until the tip can be seen at the medial end of the lateral fragment. It is very important to advance the pin with direct pressure and not twist the device back and forth, as this may damage the junction between the flexible and rigid portions of the pin. The same reduction maneuver is performed as in the reaming and the pin advanced until it is fully seated. The hole in the device where the locking screw will be placed is visible on the fluoroscopy images, and should be just past the superior cortex to ensure adequate fixation of the locking screw. Once the position is verified with fluoroscopy and the length is checked to ensure that the lateral end of the device is not prominent, the medial end of the pin is "activated" or made rigid by inserting a torque-limiting screwdriver or actuator into the lateral end of the pin and outrigger and turning it until the torque limit is reached and the medial "grippers" or talons deployed (Fig. 8-73).

This also changes the flexible portion of the device into a rigid implant. If a rigid implant is used, please see Video 8-5. The interlocking screw is then placed by passing the guide through the outrigger until it contacts the posterolateral cortex. A 2-mm drill bit is then passed though the distal clavicle and pin until it is passed through the anterior cortex (Fig. 8-74).

Since the drill bit can easily deflect, its position in the pin should be checked by passing the actuator into the pin. If the drill bit is passing through the pin, this should prevent the screwdriver/actuator from fully seating. A depth measurement is then taken and an appropriate length screw is passed through the guide until it is fully seated. Again, the actuator should be used to ensure that the screw actually passes through the pin.

Comminuted fractures should be held out to length before the IM nail is activated and the interlocking screw passed, to ensure that the anatomical length is being restored.

Management of Butterfly Fragments

Once the pin is fully seated and locked into place, the butterfly fragments can now be cerclaged back into place (Video 8-6). A Crego elevator is passed in a posterior-to-anterior direction under the clavicle and fragments. No. 1 or 2 absorbable sutures with a size 1 tapered needle are passed through the soft tissue attached to the butterfly

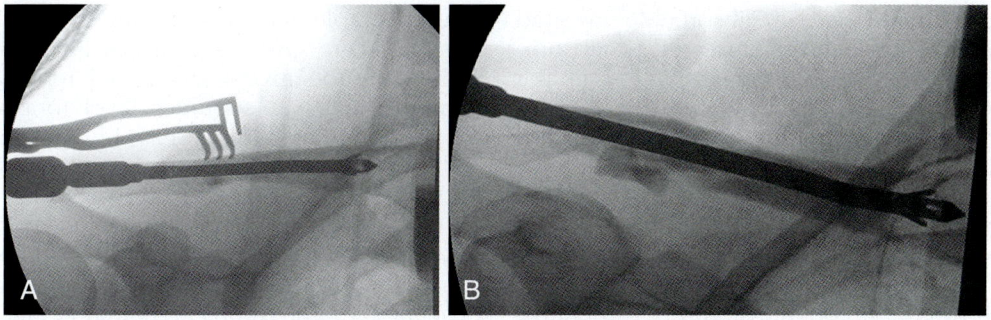

FIGURE 8-73: **A** and **B,** A torque-limiting screwdriver is used to deploy the medial "grippers" and make the flexible portion of the device rigid.

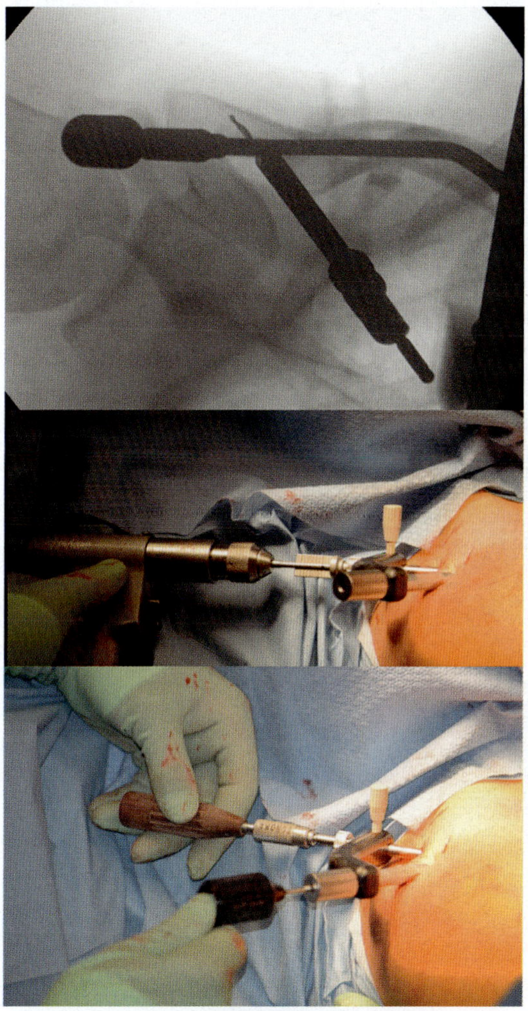

FIGURE 8-74: Drilling and placement of the interlocking screw.

fragments and then under the clavicle. Upward pressure should be kept on the needle to prevent it from going too deep and damaging underlying structures. The needle is then passed until it makes contact with the Crego elevator. Since the curvature of the elevator and size 1

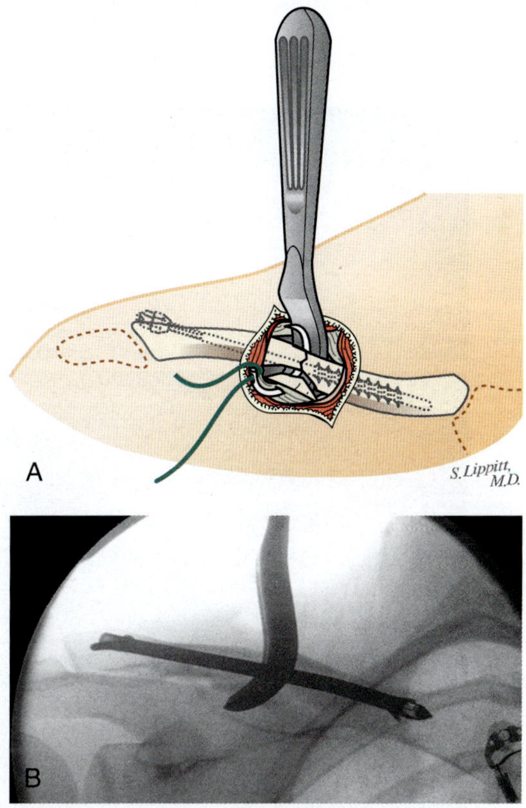

FIGURE 8-75: **A** and **B,** A Crego elevator is placed under the clavicle to protect the underlying neurovascular structures while passing the cerclaged suture or wire.

CT-type needle are essentially the same, the needle should be deflected superiorly until it can be seen and grasped with a needle driver. This is repeated to finish the cerclage (Fig. 8-75). The suture is tied and the wound irrigated again with antibiotic solution.

Final Closure

The periosteum is closed over the fracture with multiple figure-of-eight sutures of size 0 absorbable suture. The platysma is then repaired with size 2-0 absorbable sutures, taking care not to damage the supraclavicular nerve. The skin is then closed with size 3-0 absorbable inverted sutures and running subcuticular sutures of nonabsorbable 3-0 sutures. The posterior incision is closed with the same subcutaneous and subcuticular sutures. The wounds are infiltrated with a long-acting anesthetic and covered with a routine dressing. The arm is placed in a sling for comfort. The patient's neurovascular status is checked and documented when they are alert in the recovery room. An additional dose of IV or IM antibiotics is given in the recovery room.

Figure 8-76 shows the preoperative and postoperative radiographs and incision of a typical case.

Postoperative Care

The patients are placed in a sling for comfort and told they can remove the sling as soon as they want and resume simple activities of daily living. The only restrictions they are given is to avoid lifting more than 10 lb with their operative hand, avoid repeated use of their hand higher than shoulder level to prevent excessive torque on the fixation, and avoid high clavicle risk activities such as contact sports, biking, snowboarding, and horseback riding for 6 weeks. They are instructed to ice the operative site for 20 minutes every 1 to 2 hours as necessary for pain control. They are seen back in the clinic 7 to 10 days postoperatively and AP and 45-degree cephalic tilt radiographs are taken at that time. The same restrictions in terms of upper extremity activity are continued until their 6-week checkup; however, they are allowed to resume stationary bike training and running as tolerated with the obvious advance to avoid falling on the operative side. They are seen again 6 weeks

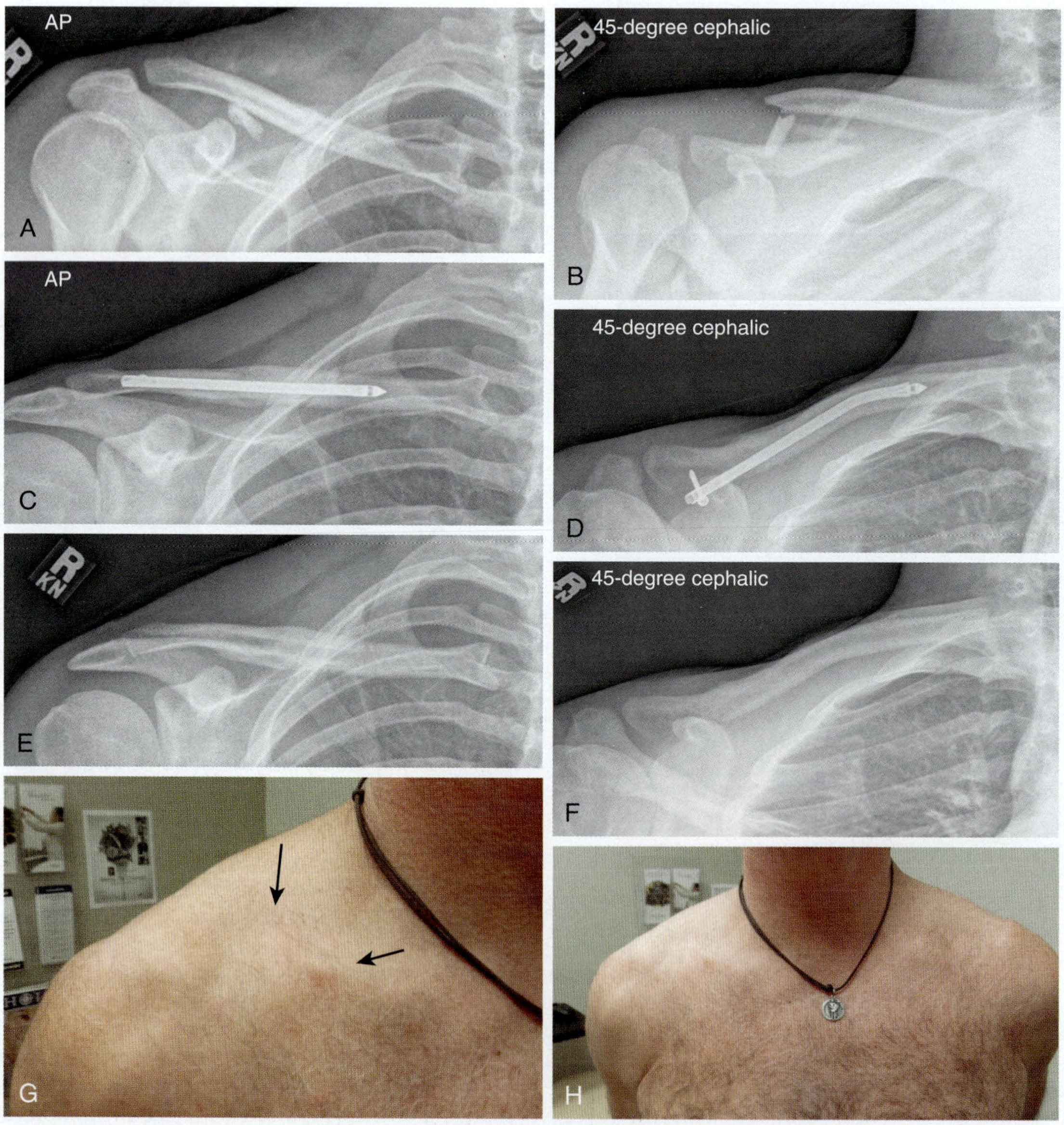

FIGURE 8-76: A to **H,** Before and after radiographs and clinical images. Note the cosmetic "necklace" incision in Langer's lines.

postoperatively, and repeat radiographs are taken. If bridging callus is seen and they are nontender at the fracture site, they are allowed to advance activities as tolerated. If no callus is seen, the weight and motion restrictions are continued. They are then seen again at 12 weeks postoperatively, and repeat radiographs are taken. If the fracture appears to be completely healed, which most are at this follow-up, they are released for unrestricted activities, and they can be scheduled for a routine deep implant removal if they wish.

Implant Removal

Once complete healing has been verified and if the patient desires removal of the implant, they are taken to the ambulatory center. The removal is usually performed with IV sedation and local anesthesia. They are placed in a beach chair position and a fluoroscopy unit is placed over their operative shoulder as in the original procedure. After induction of IV sedation and routine prepping of the shoulder, the area about the posterior incision is infiltrated with a short-acting anesthetic with epinephrine. The old incision is reincised and taken sharply down to the level of the lateral device. The torque-limiting screwdriver/actuator is placed in an extraction adaptor and the tip of the actuator is inserted into the distal end of the implant under fluoroscopic guidance. The extractor is then slid down the actuator and tightened into the lateral end of the implant. The interlocking screw is localized and removed. It is important not to remove the interlocking screw before the extractor is tightened down to the implant because to do otherwise may cause twisting of the rigid portion of the pin relative to the flexible portion, and this could result in shearing of the interface. The actuator is then used to "deactivate" the flexible portion of the implant and release tension on the grippers. A slap hammer is then attached to the extraction adaptor and the device removed. The skin is infiltrated with long-acting anesthetic and closed in the same manner as in the primary surgery (Fig. 8-77).

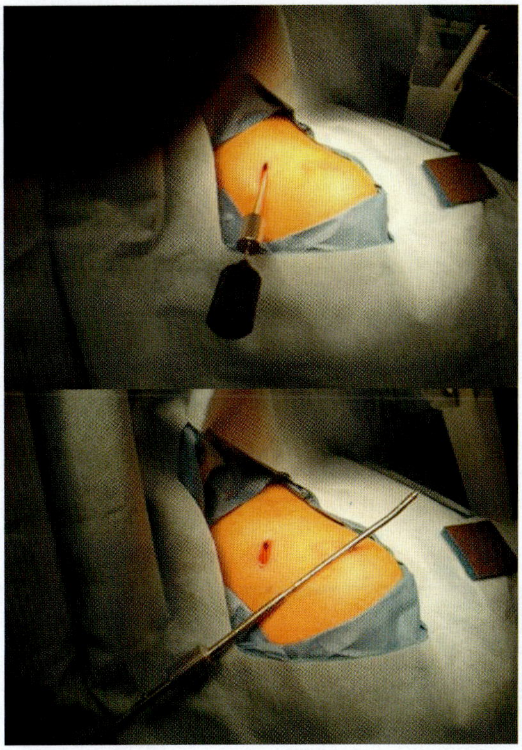

FIGURE 8-77: Removal of the device under local anesthesia.

Postremoval Care

Patients are allowed to resume all activities of daily living with the exception of no contact sports for 4 weeks. They are seen back in the clinic for a wound check at 7 to 10 days postoperatively and seen again 4 to 6 weeks postoperatively, at which time repeat radiographs are taken. Assuming the patient is doing well, they are allowed to return to unrestricted activity as tolerated.

MEDIAL APPROACH

The same IM concept can be used in more medial fractures or if the surgeon prefers a medial approach (Fig. 8-78). The only difference is that the fixation device is brought out through the medial cortex and then antegraded into the lateral fragment without penetration of the lateral posterolateral cortex. The same positioning and fluoroscopy position can be used; however, with the medial approach, the surgery can be performed with the patient in a supine position and the fluoroscopy unit brought in from the injured side of the patient since bringing the pin out through the posterior aspect of the shoulder is unnecessary. If the hybrid device is used and at least 50 mm of fixation at the flexible end cannot be achieved, the surgery must be performed with a medial approach rather than risk compromise of the device by having the junction of the flexible and rigid part of the device too close to the fracture site, where cantilever bending can cause metal fatigue and failure. Although both approaches can be successful, we have found that patients prefer only one anterior incision rather than two as necessitated with the medial approach.

Middle-Third Malunion and Nonunion

Symptomatic nonunion and malunion are treated with the same IM technique as acute fractures. Plate fixation can also be used; however, the IM device allows the procedure to be accomplished through small cosmetic incisions and has all of the advantages noted above in with acute fractures. The primary contraindication to using an IM device, however, is in the presence of bone loss. In these cases, plate fixation and grafting are preferred. These fractures require only minor modifications to the technique noted earlier.

Surgical Technique

For clavicle malunion, incise the periosteum overlying the deformity longitudinally as described earlier. Once

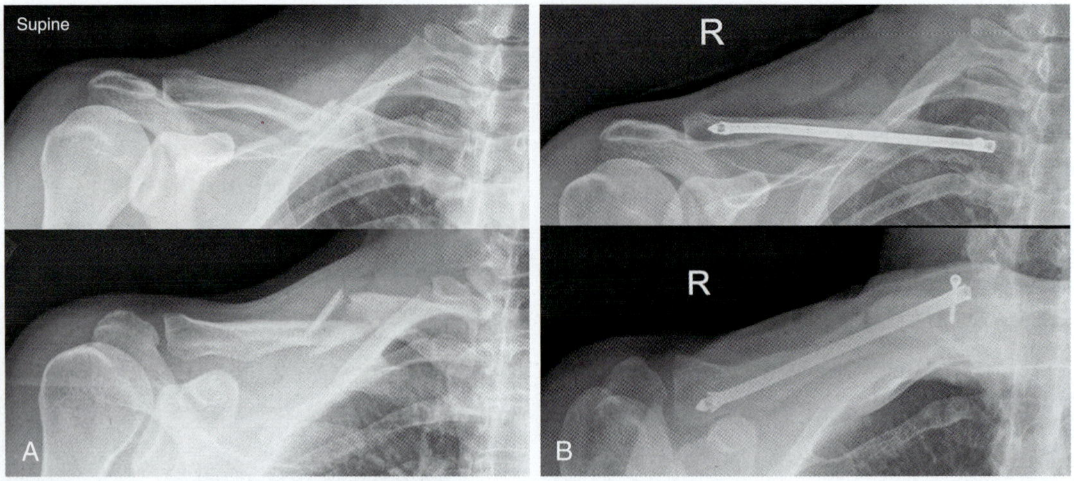

FIGURE 8-78: **A** and **B,** Placement of an intramedullary device in a medial-to-lateral antegrade fashion for a more medially based fracture.

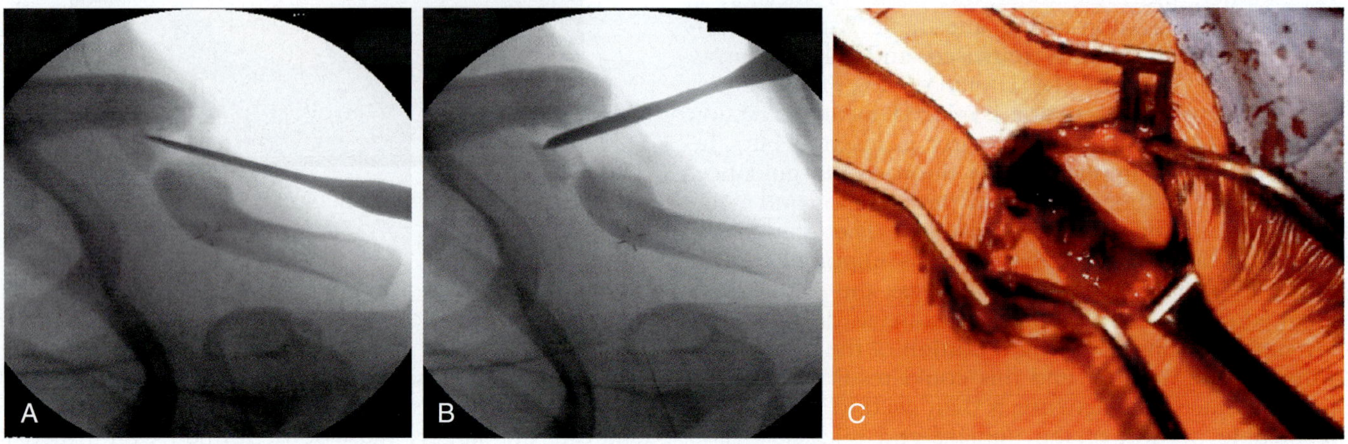

FIGURE 8-79: Resection of callus in a clavicle malunion under image intensifier guidance. **A,** Osteotome identifying callus on the distal end of the medial fragment. **B,** Osteophyte removed to be used for a bone graft. **C,** Intraoperative image showing removal of callus.

the periosteum is circumferentially elevated from the deformity, use a small osteotome to remove the callus from the fracture site. This procedure is best performed under C-arm guidance to ensure adequate removal of the fracture callus (Fig. 8-79).

Use a rongeur to remove the callus from the ends of the medial and lateral fracture fragments. Then find the canal by using the smallest size drill bit, verify its position with a C-arm or radiograph, and drill the canal with the appropriate-sized drill. Pass the clavicle pin as described earlier. A small osteotome can be used to fish scale (rose petal) the cortical bone about the fracture site (Fig. 8-80). Morselize the previously removed callus, and pack it about the fracture site (Fig. 8-81). Autogenous bone graft from the patient should be used when indicated. The periosteum is then carefully closed over the fracture site. Because of the relative loss of mass with debridement of the callus, the periosteum is easily closed. An excellent radiographic and clinical result can be obtained (Fig. 8-82).

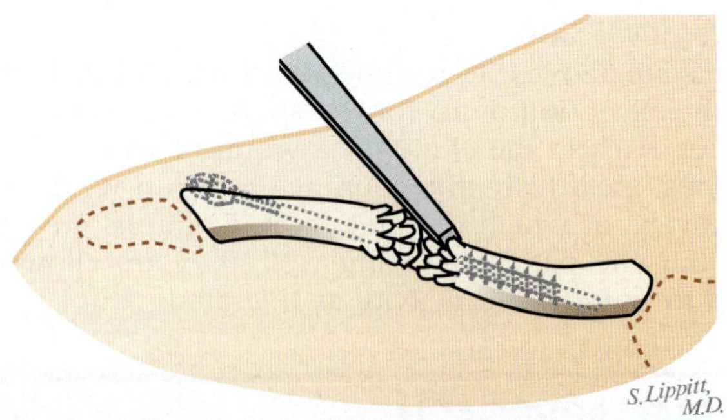

FIGURE 8-80: Fish scaling of the clavicle on both sides of the fracture site.

Hypertrophic nonunion can be treated in the same manner as a clavicle malunion. In the case of atrophic nonunion, remove any tapered ends of the clavicle fragments. Carefully remove the scar tissue with a rongeur. Proceed with treatment as described for clavicle malunion, with the exception of using autologous or autograft bone.

In the case of an atrophic nonunion, the bone ends might have resorbed. It is important to return the clavicle to its normal length (Fig. 8-83), but this can be difficult

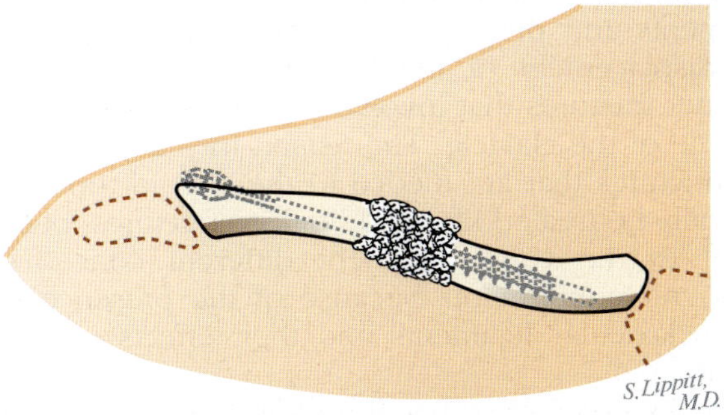

FIGURE 8-81: The bone graft is placed about the fracture site with care taken to not place too much graft on the inferior surface.

to do with IM fixation. In this situation, we remove any nonviable bone from the ends of the fragments. If there is significant loss of clavicular length, a tricortical graft of appropriate length is placed into the defect.[370,361] Because of the difficulty in controlling the intercalary fragment, we prefer to use plate fixation rather than IM fixation. If there is loss of soft tissue coverage in this area, a portion of the clavicular head of the pectoralis major muscle can be swung over the fracture site without difficulty (Fig. 8-84). In the case of severe bone and soft tissue loss, a free vascularized fibular graft can be used in conjunction with an LC-DCP or precontoured plate as shown in Figure 8-84.[253]

Postoperative Care

Postoperative care for malunion and nonunion needs to be modified as required because these fractures typically take longer to heal. On average, the pin is removed in

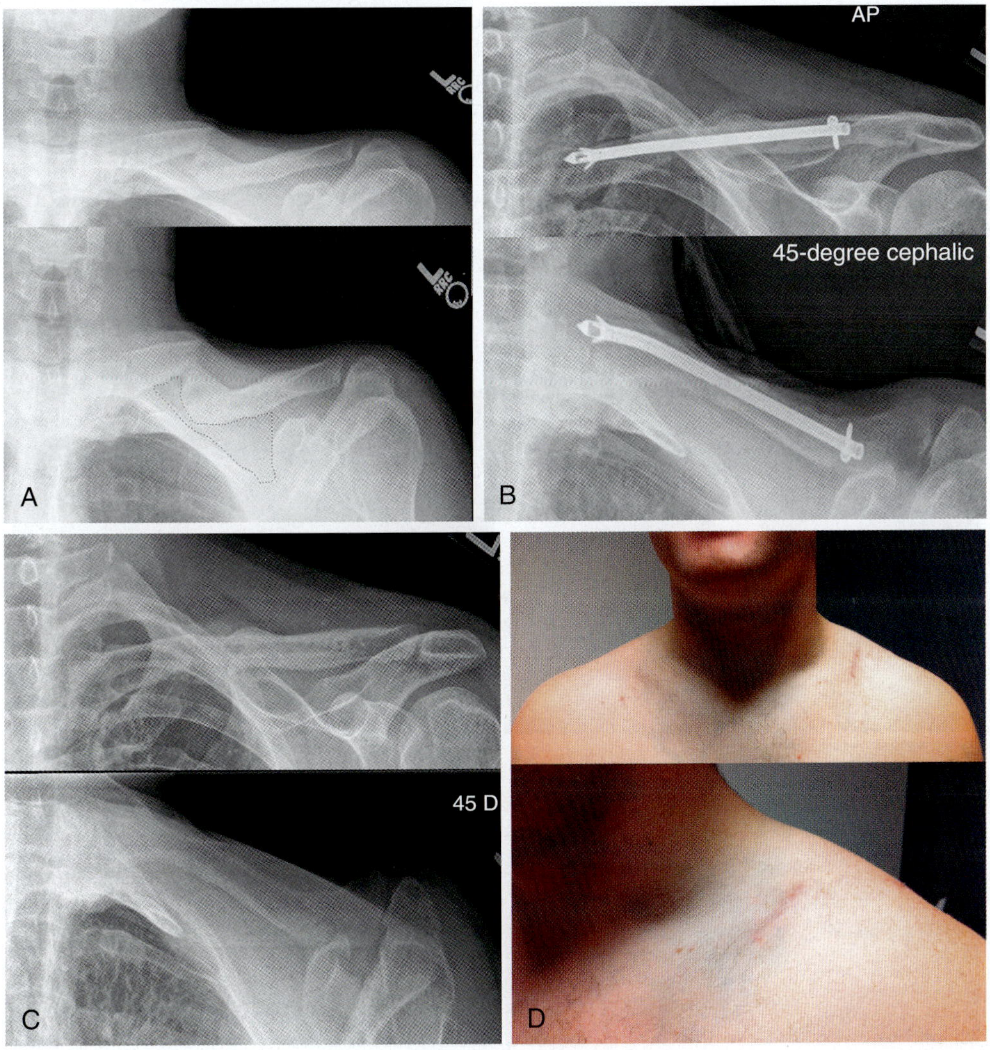

FIGURE 8-82: **A,** Preoperative radiograph of nonunion of a left clavicle fracture through a prior malunion. **B,** Postoperative radiograph with a pin in place. **C,** Postoperative radiograph with the pin removed. **D,** Clinical appearance of a patient with a very small skin incision.

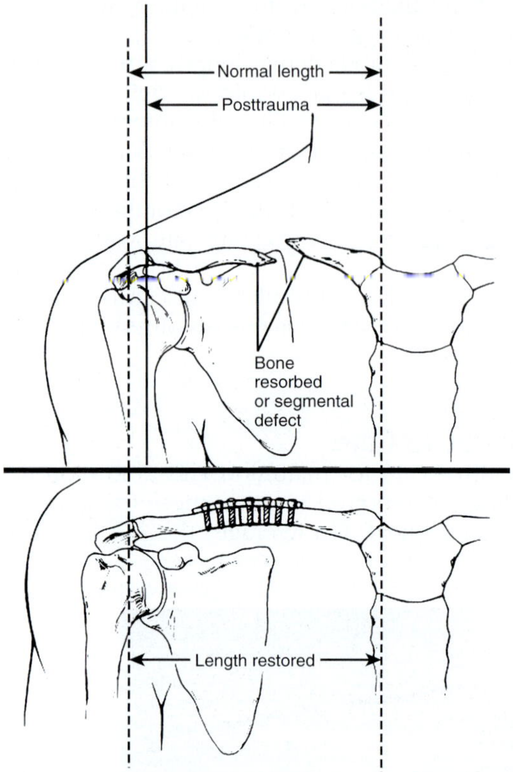

FIGURE 8-83: In cases of nonunion, care must be taken to return the clavicle to its normal length after removal of nonviable bone.

malunion cases at between 12 and 16 weeks, whereas nonunion can take up to 6 months to adequately heal.

Distal Clavicle Fractures

Distal clavicle fractures include fractures with differing treatments and prognoses that depend on the location and displacement of the fracture. In this section, we consider fractures that involve or are distal to the conoid tubercle of the clavicle. The reason for this distinction is that fractures that are medial to the conoid tubercle can generally be treated like middle-third fractures, but those lateral to the conoid present different concerns and treatment requirements because of the presence of the coracoclavicular ligaments and their effects on fracture stability.

Nondisplaced fractures of the distal end of the clavicle are best treated with a sling. As symptoms allow, the patient is weaned from the sling and started on a shoulder rehabilitation program. The earliest return to sports activity is generally around 2 months after the injury. In collision sports, extra padding or a fiberglass shell may be necessary to protect the distal end of the clavicle. The patient must be advised that although he or she feels well, early return to sports is a compromise that involves some risk of refracture or displacement.

Nondisplaced fractures that involve the acromioclavicular joint deserve a special mention. The treatment is the same, but it is important to inform the patient that involvement of the joint increases the likelihood of

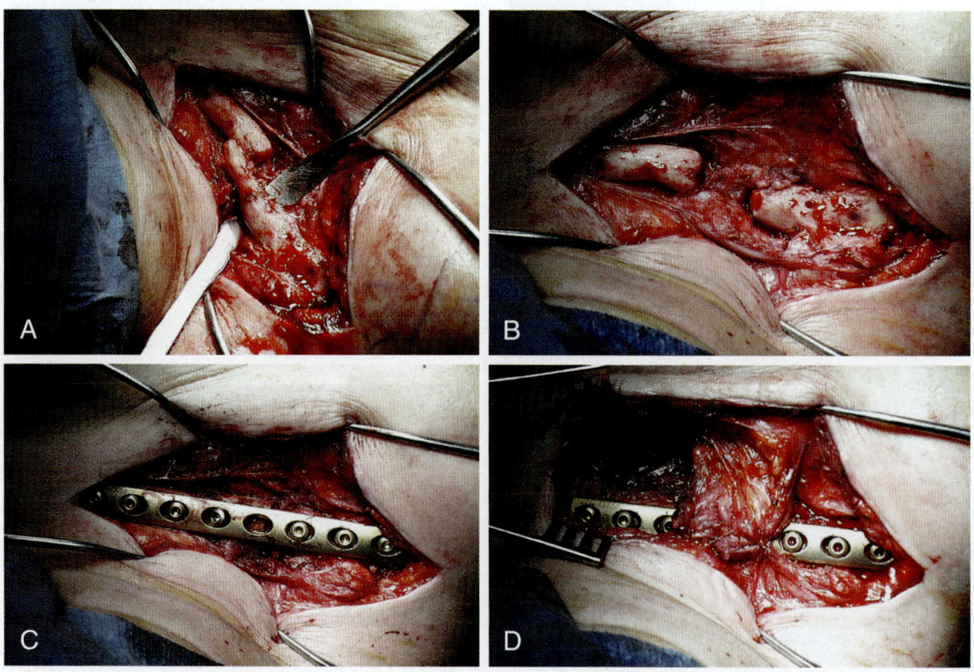

FIGURE 8-84: **A,** Initial appearance of a clavicle nonunion. **B,** After resection of nonviable bone with resultant bone loss. **C,** Limited contact dynamic compression plate incorporating an intercalary tricortical graft. **D,** The lateral position of the clavicular head of the pectoralis major is swung over the fracture site to provide soft tissue coverage.

chronic pain and posttraumatic arthrosis of the acromioclavicular joint. If this complication occurs, a subsequent surgical procedure may be required to alleviate these symptoms, and the patient needs to be aware of this fact.

Treatment of a displaced distal clavicle fracture hinges on the integrity of the coracoclavicular and acromioclavicular ligaments. More precisely, treatment generally depends on whether the conoid portion of the coracoclavicular ligaments is still attached to the medial fragment of the clavicle. If the conoid continues to be attached to the medial fragment, this strong ligament will maintain the coracoclavicular interval, and thereby help prevent large displacement at the fracture site. In fact, it is rare to have a markedly displaced distal clavicle fracture if the conoid ligament remains intact and attached to the medial fragment of the clavicle. The ligamentous stability does not easily allow displacement to occur.

If the conoid ligament is intact, the coracoclavicular interval will be maintained, and the ligamentous and bony anatomy will help prevent the distal clavicular fragment from becoming markedly displaced. The fracture fragments should remain relatively close to one another, and this fracture can be expected to heal with sling treatment. If the conoid ligament is disrupted, the distal clavicular fragment with the attached scapula (through the acromioclavicular and coracoclavicular ligaments) will droop inferiorly and medially under the weight of the attached upper extremity. The medial clavicular fragment, now unencumbered, will elevate away from the distal fragment. Such elevation raises the risk of nonunion and chronic medial rotational instability of the shoulder through the fracture site.

Several clues can be used to ascertain the integrity of the conoid ligament. Often, rupture of the conoid ligament is obvious on radiographs because the fracture is lateral to the conoid tubercle, the coracoclavicular interval is markedly increased, and the fracture is markedly displaced. With fractures occurring at or very near the conoid tubercle, this can sometimes become more difficult. When both coracoclavicular ligaments are attached to the distal fragment, the fracture line is usually oblique, and the coracoclavicular interval is maintained with the lateral fragment. The fracture is typically widely displaced. In equivocal cases, medial rotational instability at the fracture site can be demonstrated by performing a cross-body adduction view of the shoulder (Fig. 8-85). This stress radiograph accentuates conoid ligament detachment from the medial clavicular fragment. An increase in fracture displacement, an increase in the coracoclavicular interval, and marked underriding of the distal fragment beneath the proximal fragment are generally seen. These findings represent medial rotational instability occurring through the fracture site. Failure of these findings to occur suggests that the conoid ligament is still attached to the medial fragment of the clavicle.

Treatment Options

Treatment options for lateral clavicle fractures include coracoclavicular fixation (Fig. 8-86), plate fixation, IM screw fixation, and K-wire fixation.

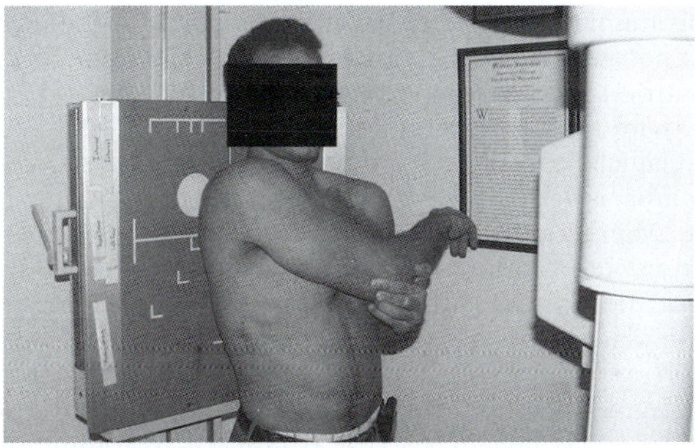

FIGURE 8-85: Method for obtaining a cross-body adduction anteroposterior radiograph. The patient pulls the elbow to the midline while keeping the arm against the chest.

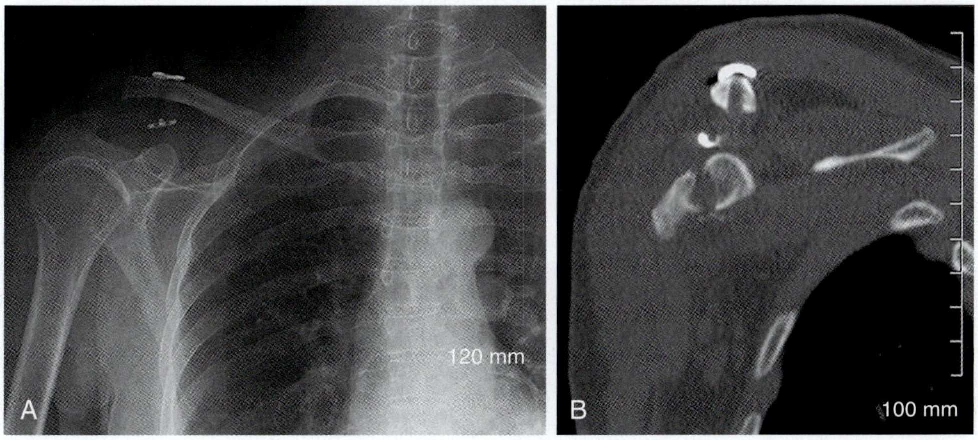

FIGURE 8-86: Fracture through the coracoid of a toggle-type anchor device. (From Gerhardt DC, VanDerWerf JD, Rylander LS, et al. Postoperative coracoid fracture after transcoracoid acromioclavicular joint reconstruction. *J Shoulder Elbow Surg.* 2011;20[5]:e6-e10.)

Plate fixation of this fracture can be problematic. The exposure required is relatively large. The distal fragment is small, and the acromioclavicular joint limits the length of plate that can be used. A small T-plate sometimes allows enough screws in the distal fragment for adequate fixation. Newer specialized plates allow better fit of the plate onto the distal clavicle and the insertion of multiple divergent locking screws to improve fixation strength (see Fig. 8-93).

One significant problem with plate fixation of distal fractures is that there are significant forces on the distal fixation. The distal fragment is softer metaphyseal bone and can be quite small, which makes it hard to get even two or three screws into the distal fragment. Because of this problem, some authors have advocated the use of a hook plate that relies on a fingerlike projection that goes under the acromion to give added stability while still allowing some rotational movement at the acromioclavicular joint.[102,103,131,132,183,262, 264,390] Although in concept this may be better than carrying the fixation out onto the acromion, a number of authors have reported complications such as dislocation of and mechanical failure of the plate, acromial erosion or osteolysis, and impingement (Fig. 8-87).[50,132,183] Muramatsu et al. found evidence of hook migration into the acromion in 87% of patients.[262] This necessitates early removal of the plate, which must be carried out through the same large incision.

K-wire fixation down the IM canal of the distal end of the clavicle can create problems as well. The force on this area is large, and hardware breakage is quite possible. Migration of broken hardware in this region is well documented,[225] and we prefer to avoid this possibility.

For the unstable variety of this fracture, we generally prefer placement of a coracoclavicular screw,[18,99,168,226,401,430] which reduces the coracoclavicular interval and brings the fragments into close proximity to allow healing. Use of the coracoclavicular screw is limited by comminution extending medial to the conoid tubercle. Comminution distal to the conoid tubercle is not a factor. It has been suggested that proper placement of a screw for coracoclavicular fixation is too difficult; however, with proper fluoroscopic technique, it is actually quite easy. The coracoclavicular screw offers several advantages. The exposure required is small, and sometimes we do not even have to open the fracture site. The fixation is solid, with true bicortical fixation in the coracoid giving nearly 750 to 1000 N of strength to failure, which nearly approximates the strength of the native acromioclavicular and coracoclavicular ligament complex,[139] whereas a hook plate has only 460 N load to failure.[239,294] In comparison to a hook plate, a coracoclavicular screw can be inserted with minimal exposure and minimal soft tissue stripping. Under C-arm guidance, this procedure can be performed almost percutaneously. After fracture healing, the screw can be removed easily under local anesthesia, thereby avoiding breakage of the hardware, whereas a hook plate requires significantly greater exposure for removal. Suture and suture anchors have also been used for treatment of distal clavicle fractures either by themselves or in conjunction with plate fixation. The primary advantage of these is that they do not need to be removed. The primary problem, however, is that since they are not removed, they can cause osteolysis of the clavicle and/or coracoid due to the differential motion of the scapular relative to the clavicle, and can also fracture through the clavicle with later trauma (see Figs. 8-22, 8-86, and 8-95).

A meta-analysis of distal clavicle fixation techniques showed that union was achieved and 98% of patients with similar functional outcomes with the above mentioned techniques; however, complications occurred in 22% of the operative group. There was an 11-fold increase in major complications with hook plate fixation compared to IM fixation and a 24-fold increased risk of major complications compared to suture anchor fixation. Complications with the other fixation methods were as follows: K-wire plus tension band wiring (20.0%), coracoclavicular stabilization (4.8%), and IM (2.4%) and interfragmentary fixation (6.3%).[273] Numerous complications have been reported with hook plate fixation especially medial peri-implant fracture, acromial erosion, and dislocation of the fixation device (see Fig. 8-87B). Because of this, it is typically recommended that the device be removed as soon as possible once healing has been achieved.[292]

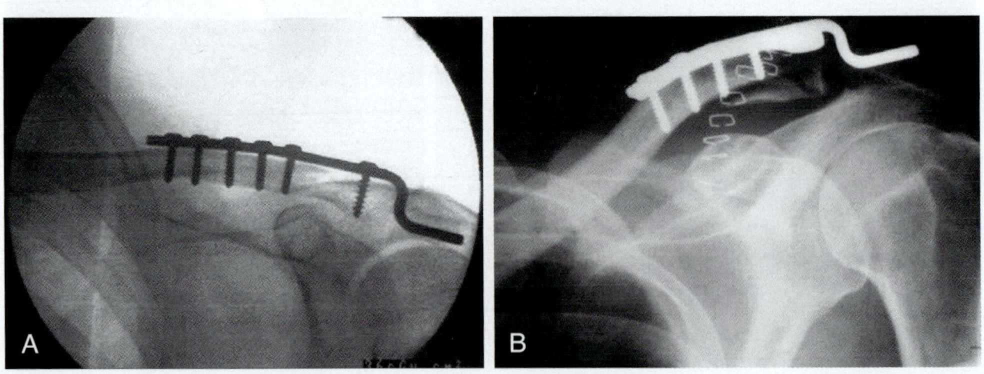

FIGURE 8-87: A, Hook plate for a distal-third clavicle fracture. **B,** Dislocation of the acromial portion of the plate. (From Haidar SG, Krishnan KM, Deshmukh SC. Hook plate fixation for type II fractures of the lateral end of the clavicle. *J Shoulder Elbow Surg.* 2006;15[4]:419-423.)

Coracoclavicular Screw Technique

The patient is positioned much the same as for IM pinning. The primary difference is that the C-arm is oriented in a posteromedial-to-anterolateral direction (Fig. 8-88). This gives what we refer to as a *cortical ring sign* of the coracoid. We have found that when the coracoid is viewed in this position, placement of the coracoclavicular screw into the superior apex of this ring virtually guarantees placement in the center of the base of the coracoid (see Fig. 8-91C).[114]

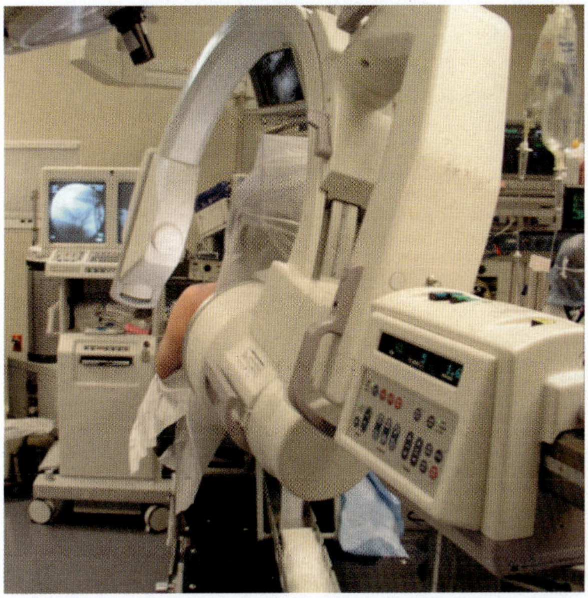

FIGURE 8-88: Position of the C-arm for coracoclavicular screw placement. The posteromedial-to-anterolateral orientation make the coracoid appear as a "ring."

A skin incision that allows exposure of the fracture site is then made in line with the clavicle. The fracture is held reduced with a reduction forceps, and the clavicle is drilled by placing a 4.5-mm drill bit above but slightly angulated relative to the coracoid in the mid-portion of the clavicle (Fig. 8-89). Oblique placement of the screw can improve its pullout strength. A 3.2-mm drill guide is passed through this hole until it makes contact with the coracoid. This allows a collinear placement of the screw holes, which facilitates passage of the screw. This position is verified under C-arm guidance (Fig. 8-90).

Both cortices of the coracoid are drilled with a 3.2-mm drill bit. It is very important to drill both the superior and deep cortex of the coracoid because bicortical fixation has significantly greater resistance to pullout than a unicortical screw. A depth gauge is used to measure the length of the screw, and an appropriate-sized screw with a washer is passed through the clavicle and into the coracoid (Fig. 8-91).

If there is significant comminution, the coracoclavicular screw can be used in conjunction with a small T-plate or specialized distal clavicle plate for what we call *hybrid fixation*. This combination is still significantly stronger than a hook plate and prevents compromise of the acromion (Fig. 8-92). With hybrid fixation, the coracoclavicular screw still needs to be removed due to the differential movement of the scapula and clavicle. Suture anchors with endobuttons have been used in a similar fashion. The primary advantage of these is that they do not need to be removed. Unfortunately, a number of cases have been reported of the devices pulling through the clavicle and/or the coracoid. Since the acromioclavicular ligaments and usually the trapezoid ligaments remain undamaged, it is not necessary to repair or augment the conoid ligament since the acromioclavicular ligaments will provide stabilization once the bone heals.

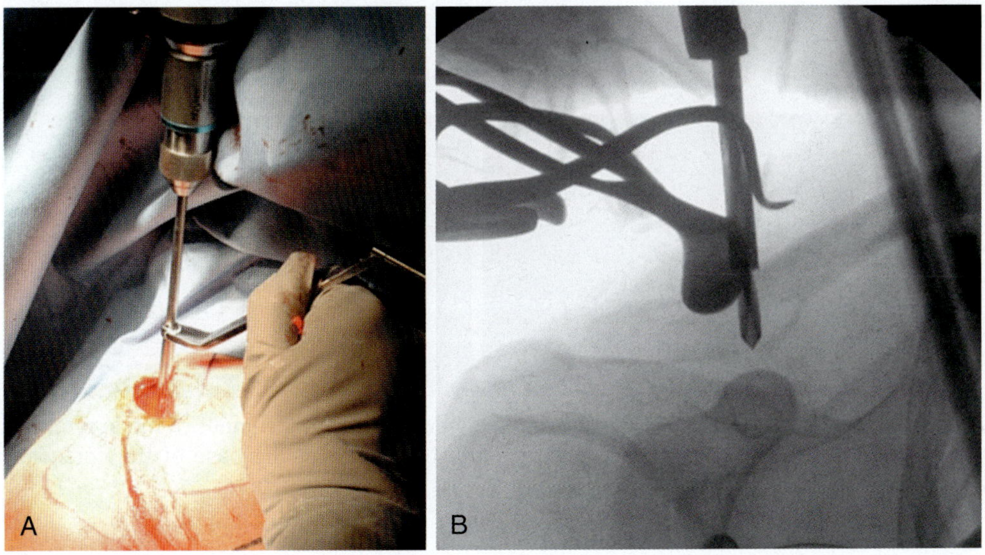

FIGURE 8-89: **A** and **B**, Fracture is held reduced, and a 4.5-mm drill is used to produce the hole through both cortices of the clavicle directly above the ring of the coracoid.

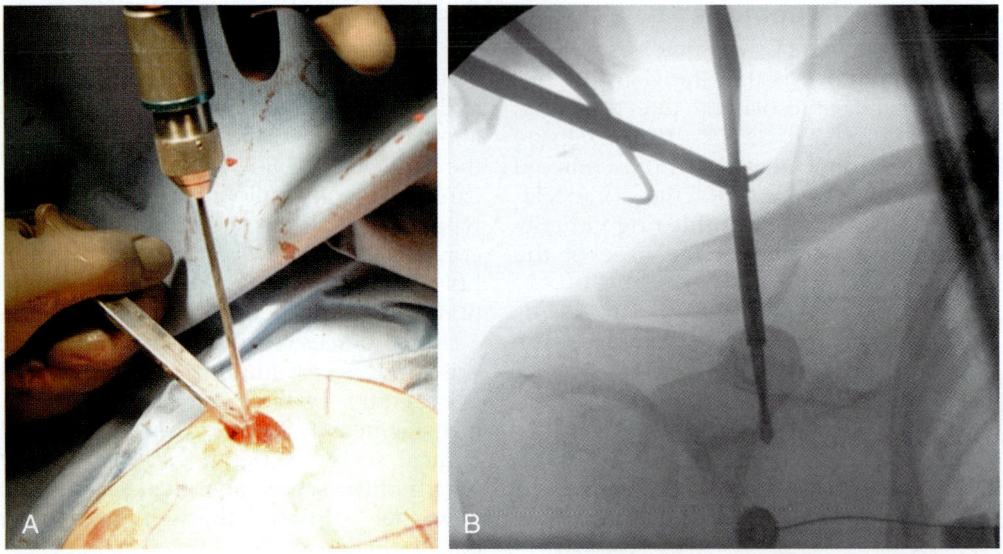

FIGURE 8-90: **A** and **B,** The drill hole in the coracoid is made by passing the drill guide for a 3.2-mm drill through the hole in the clavicle.

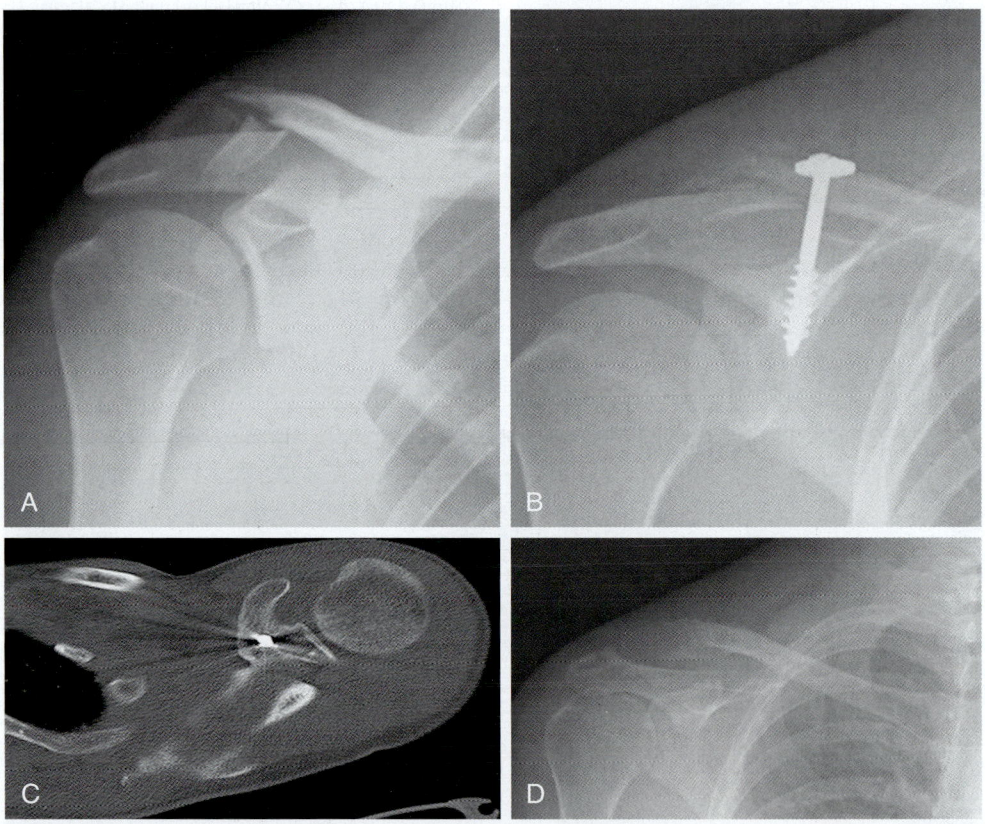

FIGURE 8-91: Preoperative **(A)** and postoperative **(B)** radiographic views showing placement of the appropriate-length screw and washer. **C,** Computed tomographic scan confirming placement into the center of the base of the coracoid. **D,** After hardware removal.

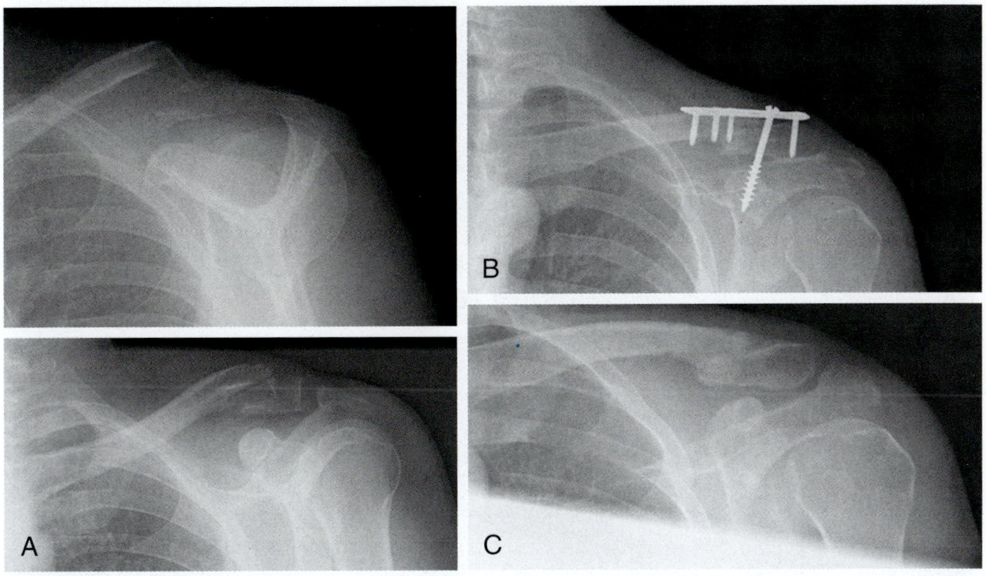

FIGURE 8-92: A hybrid plate and coracoclavicular screw combination may be used when the fracture is significantly comminuted. Preoperative **(A)** and postoperative **(B)** radiographs of a hybrid fixation technique. **C,** After removal of both the plate and screws.

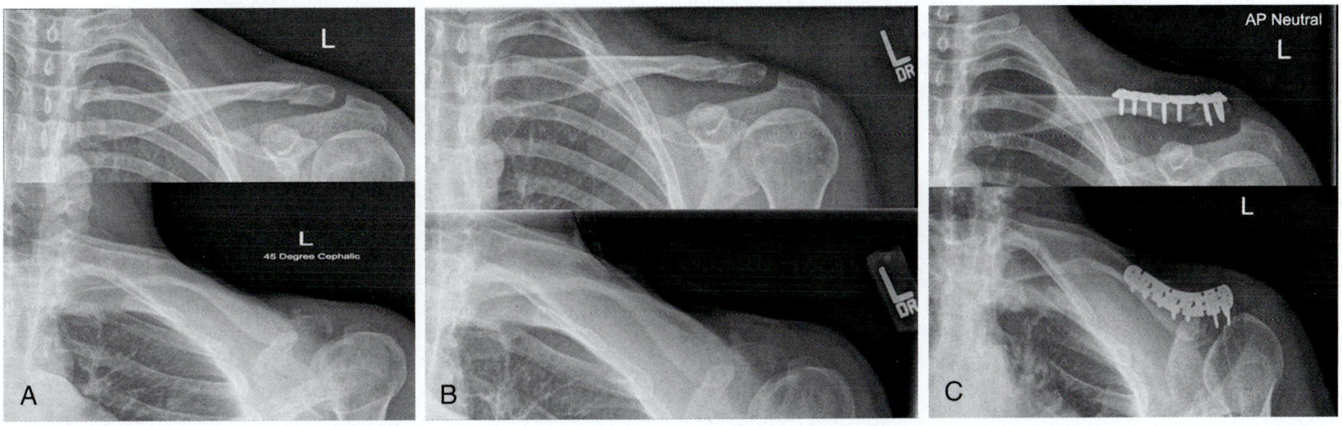

FIGURE 8-93: A, Injury radiographs in a 24-year-old man. **B,** Nine months postoperative radiographs showing no healing. **C,** Postoperative radiographs at 6 months.

Furthermore, reduction of the fracture within the first few weeks after the injury will reapproximate the torn ligaments and allow them to heal much like the healing of the syndesmotic ligaments with syndesmotic screw fixation.

Other alternatives are available for both stronger bone and even weaker bone. Due to the multiple divergent screws, many new precontoured devices can be used with and without supplemental coracoclavicular fixation. An example of an unexpected nonunion after a minimally displaced distal clavicle fracture treated with a clavicle-specific low-profile plate with divergent distal screws is shown in Fig. 8-93. Although it is a rare indication for a fracture in an older patient, new woven polyester devices specifically designed for distal clavicle fixation can be used (Fig. 8-94). This was chosen because of the significant comminution of the distal fragment with compromise of the overlying skin and the relative porosity of the bone due to the patient's age. It was believed that the bone would have been too weak and compromised for plate fixation or coracoclavicular fixation, and the risk of complication of a hook plate was felt to be too high in the patient. The surgeon is cautioned, however, that any device that goes around the coracoid and clavicle can cause erosion of both or either of these bones. Therefore careful postoperative monitoring is necessary. If any evidence of erosion occurs, the devices should be removed immediately (see Fig. 8-22 and Fig. 8-95).

Postoperative Care

The patient is placed in a sling for the first 4 weeks. The patient is allowed out of the sling for hand, wrist, and elbow range of motion exercises. Repeat radiographs are

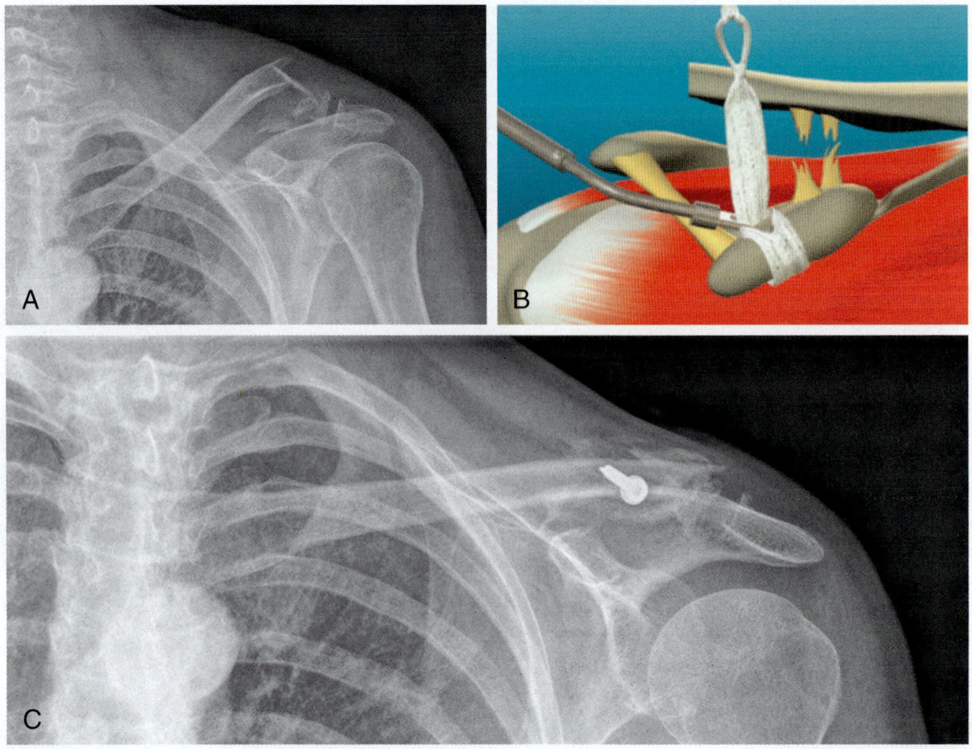

FIGURE 8-94: **A,** An active 79-year-old female fell while skiing. **B,** Polyester weave device. **C,** Clinically healed fracture 3 months postoperatively. (**B,** Courtesy LockDown Medical Ltd, Redditch, UK.)

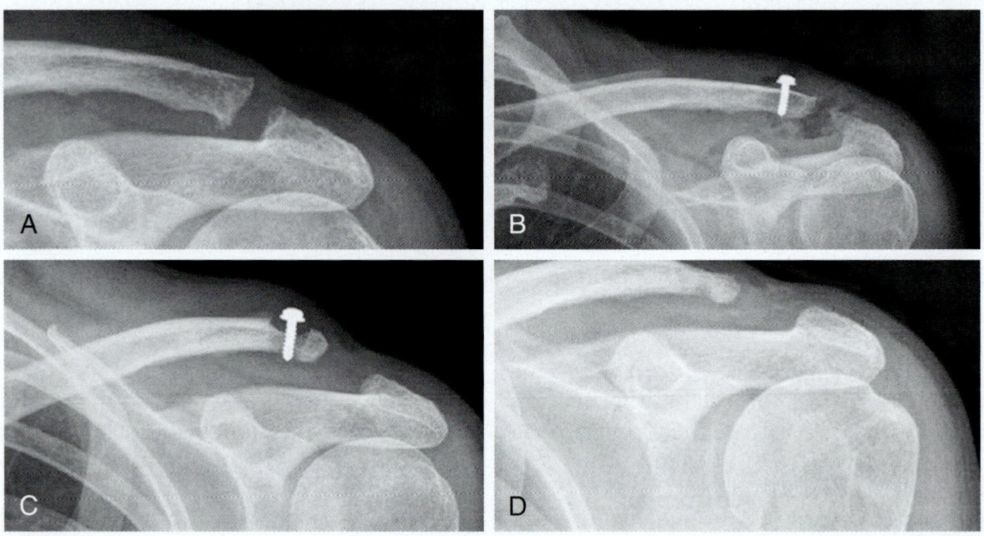

FIGURE 8-95: **A** to **D,** Osteolysis of the distal clavicle after placement of a polyester device. (From Dearden PMC, Ferran NA, Morris EW. Distal clavicle osteolysis following fixation with a synthetic ligament. *Int J Shoulder Surg.* 2011;5[4]:101-104.)

taken at 4 weeks. If there has been no change in the position of the screw fixation, the sling is discontinued and the patient is allowed to perform activities of daily living with a lifting restriction of 5 lb and no repeated use of the operative-side hand above shoulder level. Once healing has been confirmed on follow-up radiographs, the screw is removed under local anesthesia approximately 8 to 12 weeks postoperatively. The patient is instructed to avoid contact sports for 6 weeks and advance activities as tolerated. If a hybrid-type fixation is used, only the coracoclavicular screw needs to be removed, and this can still be done under local anesthesia. There is no need to remove the rest of the plate and screws unless the patient so desires.

What Is the Best Fixation for Fractures of the Clavicle?

Both IM fixation and plate fixation have high rates of union, with significant reductions in the relative risk of nonunion.[437] In terms of choosing which to use, the surgeon has a number of considerations: the fracture pattern, comfort level with the different techniques, the patient's expectations in terms of return to work, and concerns for scarring. The one absolute indication for plate and screw fixation is a clavicle fracture nonunion with bone loss. These typically require an intercalary graft with very stable fixation, and occasionally even double-plate fixation. For other types of fractures, malunions, and nonunions, either technique can be used. Because of the lower risk of major complications with IM fixation, the authors prefer this technique. With complex, comminuted fractures, hybrid fixation is preferred. Although smooth pin fixation can be used, such as a TEN, there is little length and rotational control and a relatively high risk of hardware migration. With the Rockwood pin, there is little risk of hardware migration; however, there has been a relatively high incidence of painful, prominent hardware in some studies with this device.[123,386] Since the hybrid Sonoma CRx device allows for both length and rotational control, it can be used in all types of clavicle fractures, including highly comminuted fractures. Furthermore, unlike other types of IM fixation, the device does not need to be removed routinely as it has been shown to cause little irritation.[190,435] As a result, we recommend this as the preferred treatment for most clavicle fractures.

INTERNATIONAL EXPERT COMMENTARY

Mario Lenza

This chapter provides a very worthwhile review of the literature. Congratulations to the authors for the thoroughly well-written chapter. Treatment of clavicle fractures is an important area of current surgical controversy, and this chapter would certainly be helpful to keep the readers updated. Having read this update as a new reader, my main feeling is that the chapter is full of important information. Overall, this is a very mature report as it includes key updates on treatment interventions.

My commentary emphasizes how my personal approach to treat clavicle fractures is similar or differs from what the authors have presented, with specific reference to (1) how I evaluate the patient, (2) the treatment options I consider and eventually select, (3) the technique I use for surgery, (4) the approach to postsurgical rehabilitation, and (5) the postsurgical evaluation, including potential complications.

How I Evaluate the Patient

I agree with the first point about the diagnosis of clavicle middle-third fractures, which is easily made on the basis of a typical history of trauma and the clinical evaluation, which usually shows bruising and deformity. My practice differs, however, on the imaging protocol. Diagnosis verification may also be made from a single AP chest radiograph, which is commonly available in an urgent trauma setting. Preferably, to evaluate the characteristics of the fracture (e.g., the degree of displacement, angulation, shortening, and comminution), I have two incidence radiographs taken in the upright position: Zanca view[434] (a 10- to 15-degree cephalic tilt of the standard view) and the Velpeau axillary view for clavicle (Fig. 8-96). These two incidences help characterize the fractures; the first one with the angulation and displacements in the coronal plane and the Velpeau axillary view in the axial plane.

Lateral clavicle fractures can also be well visualized with AP radiography using the Zanca view, which helps delineate the fracture by removing the overlap of the thoracic cage. Additional CT scanning is useful for intra-articular fractures.

For medial clavicle fractures, CT scanning is the procedure of choice; however, some radiograph projections could be performed as the initial investigation, such as the serendipity and Hobbs views.[202,147]

Treatment Options I Consider and Select

I agree with the authors that there are mainly three options for treating midshaft clavicle fractures: simple support (sling immobilization), surgery with IM fixation, and surgery with plate and screw fixation.

Middle-third clavicle fractures have traditionally been treated in a conservative fashion given the generally low incidence of nonunion after conservative treatment.[8,123,146,179,204,269,283] Common indications for surgical intervention include open fracture, severe displacement, an imminent lesion of the skin by a sharp edge of the clavicle, neurovascular injuries, and floating shoulder. More recently, other indications have been adopted, including high-energy fractures such as clavicle shortening greater than 20 mm, complete displacement (lack of cortical apposition), and severe comminution.[44,179,204,334]

These findings of high-energy fractures have prompted a recent increase in preference for surgical treatment. When surgical intervention is chosen, there are several techniques of open reduction and internal fixation using a plate and screw or IM fixation. Surgical treatment has the advantage of anatomic reduction of the fracture, with shorter immobilization periods and faster return to full activities. Nevertheless, complications of surgical treatment can occur, which include wound infection or dehiscence, deep infection, and problems with the hardware used for fixation. The rates of infections range from 0% to 18%,[36,310] and the rates of hardware irritation requiring removal of material range from 50% to 100%.[179,44] In addition, there are other adverse events with surgical interventions, such as refracture after hardware removal, hardware migration, hypertrophic and noncosmetic scar, complex regional syndrome, transient brachial plexus symptoms, and nonunion.[36,310,179,44]

Continued

INTERNATIONAL EXPERT COMMENTARY—cont'd

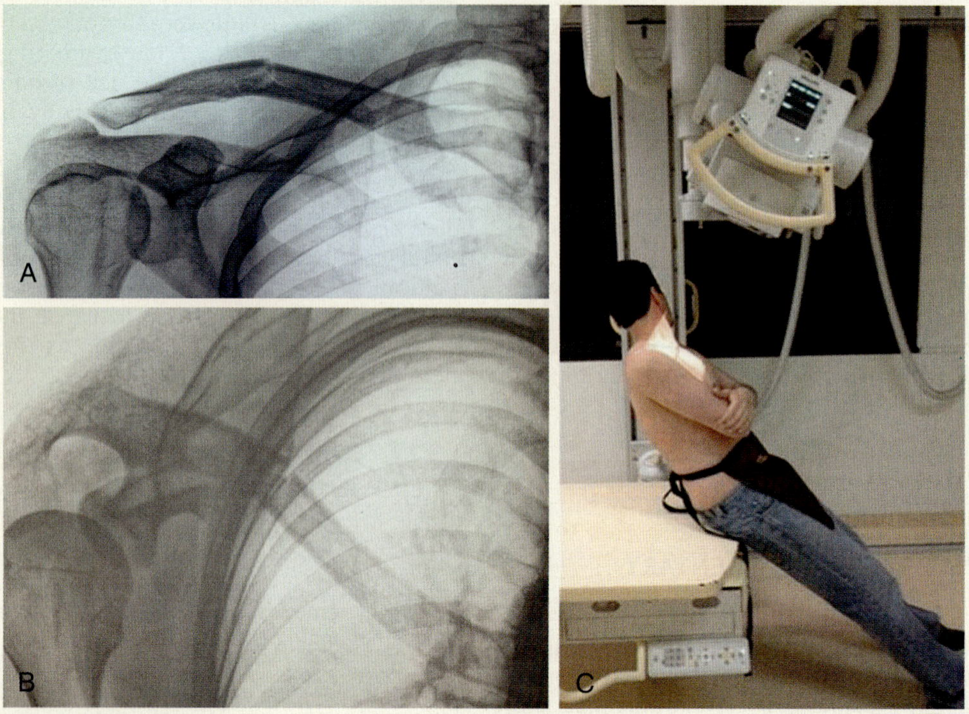

FIGURE 8-96: A, Routine radiographic Zanca view (10- to 15-degree cephalic tilt) shows a nondisplaced middle-third clavicle fracture. This view helps evaluate angulation and displacements in the coronal plane. **B,** Velpeau axillary view radiograph for clavicle—this view helps evaluate angulation and displacements in the coronal plane. **C,** Positioning of the patient for the Velpeau axillary view radiograph.

In contrast to fractures at other skeletal sites, there are few randomized trials that have compared either conservative or surgical approaches to the management of clavicular fracture. There is also limited evidence from single trials only regarding the effectiveness of different methods of surgical and conservative interventions for treating clavicle fractures.[209,211,210]

Lenza et al.[209] concluded that evidence generated by only two clinical trials published in the 1980s[12,149] is insufficient to determine the effects (benefits and harms) of different methods of conservative treatment of acute middle-third clavicle fractures in adults. A search strategy updated in January 2014 did not find any new studies that compared conservative interventions for treating clavicle fractures.

The current literature reinforces that the topic around the best conservative treatment for middle-third clavicle fractures in adults is controversial, and most U.S. surgeons prefer to use a simple sling rather than the figure-of-eight bandage for conservatively treating patients (94% simple sling vs. 6% figure-of-eight bandage) according to a recently published study.[144] However, another Germany survey study on the conservative treatment of clavicle fractures concluded that simple clavicle fractures are treated in a nonsurgical way and orthopedic surgeons prefer the use of a figure-of-eight bandage in 88% of cases.[306]

Lenza et al.,[210] based on evidence from eight trials with a high risk of bias, identified some low-quality evidence that surgical interventions may not result in significant improvement in upper arm function, and chose to evaluate the effects (benefits and harms) of surgical versus conservative interventions for treating midshaft dislocated clavicle fractures in adults. The authors of this review concluded that treatment options must be chosen on an individual patient basis, after careful consideration of the relative benefits and harms of each intervention and of patient preferences.

Three more randomized controlled trials assessing surgical versus conservative interventions were published after the review above. The first one was a multicenter, high-quality, powered, and well-designed randomized clinical trial that evaluated 200 patients with acute dislocated midshaft clavicle fractures treated with primary plate fixation or a collar and cuff for 3 weeks; the results of this study demonstrated better functional outcomes and significant fewer rates of nonunions with surgical interventions, but the authors did not support routine primary surgical treatment for these fractures.[335] The other two randomized controlled trials found similar results in favor of surgical interventions.[77,247]

Considering the current literature, my personal preference to treat acute middle-third clavicle fractures depends on the fracture pattern. (1) For nondisplaced fractures, I prefer simple support with a sling that will be used for between 3 and 4 weeks. Patients are encouraged to discard the sling when the pain has subsided. (2) For completely displaced middle-third clavicle fractures (no cortical contact between

INTERNATIONAL EXPERT COMMENTARY—cont'd

the main proximal and distal fragments), I prefer open reduction and plate fixation. The decision, however, is not limited by the evidence and fracture characteristics only; I also consider patients' expectations of treatment benefits and perceptions on the risk factors for nonunion with conservative treatment and on the potential complications of the surgical intervention. In addition, variables such as activity level and time to return to daily activities should be taken into account when selecting treatment.

Technique I Use for Surgery

Based on evidence from four trials with a high risk of bias, a recent systematic review[211] identified some low-quality evidence of a lack of a clinically important difference in function between IM fixation and plate fixation. On the safety side, the review showed that overall adverse events may be less frequent after IM fixation, but I am very uncertain of the reliability of these findings because of the limited and low-quality evidence on the relative effectiveness. The review also indicated that, where plate fixation is considered appropriate, the use of a reconstruction plate fixed superiorly on the main distal fragment and anteriorly on the main proximal fragments may be more effective than fixation with the plate shaped in the form of an S and fixed on the superior surface. Again, the low- or very-low-quality evidence for these comparisons raises questions over the reliability of these findings.

After the results of Lenza and Faloppa,[211] four additional randomized controlled trials were published. Sohn et al.[375] compared superior plating versus anteroinferior plating using minimally invasive plate osteosynthesis to treat 37 patients with acute displaced clavicular shaft fractures. The authors found no statistical differences between the two methods when assessing the incidence of nonunion and Constant and UCLA scores. Three other randomized controlled trials[13,266,406] compared plate fixation versus IM nailing for treating displaced midshaft clavicle fractures; the authors found no statistical differences between the two methods regarding the functional endpoints and incidence of nonunion at 1-year follow-up.

While there are many benefits of IM fixation, it appears that the results of this method are more unpredictable than the results of plate fixation. From my point of view, the anatomy and biomechanical aspects of fixation appear to be inferior in resisting displacement compared with plate fixation. Figure 8-2 shows that the clavicle is a thin bone mainly in the lateral expansion where it articulates with the acromion.

In my current practice, when surgery is the option of treatment, I perform open reduction and fixation of the fracture with precontoured 3.5-mm clavicular DCP (Fig. 8-97).

Patient positioning. Under general anesthesia and brachial plexus block, patients are placed in the beach chair position. An oblique incision is made over the site of the fracture, and larger branches of the supraclavicular nerves are identified and protected.

Surgical approach. A superior approach and plating is my preferred technique.

Technique. The distal and proximal fragments are reduced with the aid of reduction forceps; they can be held temporarily with a lag screw or a K-wire. A precontoured plate is then applied to the superior surface of the clavicle. If a lag screw is placed, then it is sufficient to insert three bicortical screws (six cortices) proximally and three distally. If it is not possible to place a lag screw, then four screws should be placed proximally and four distally.

Approach to Postsurgical Rehabilitation

There is no sufficient evidence to guide postsurgical rehabilitation; therefore my protocol is based on clinical practice and includes the following procedures: after surgery, a standard arm sling is used for 2 or 3 weeks (patients are encouraged to discard the sling when the pain has subsided); at 7 to 10 days postoperatively, the wound is checked and the stitches are removed. After 3 weeks of surgery, patients are instructed about some simple home stretching exercises such as forward elevation and external rotation stretches and Codman pendulum exercises. I recommend avoiding contact (e.g., football, boxing, hockey) or unpredictable (e.g., soccer, basketball, downhill skiing) sports for up to 12 weeks after surgery.

Postsurgical Evaluation Including Potential Complications

The most common adverse events following conservative treatment are nonunion and malunion. While studies of nondisplaced fractures have reported low rates of nonunion (around 0.03%), studies of displaced fractures have reported high rates of nonunion of up to 15%.[334,335] From my point of view, most of these nonunions are asymptomatic in side of fracture (there is no pain), and the symptoms are related to the disruption of the stable relationship between the upper extremity and the axial skeleton, since the majority of the patients have dysfunction of the scapulothoracic rhythm. Of note, nonunion is the most important predictor of a detrimental/negative functional outcome; it is likely that better functional outcomes are related to the union of fractures.

Most of the complications and need for secondary procedures in patients who undergo open reduction and plate fixation are related to hardware irritation and/or prominence of the plate. In my practice, more than 50% of patients need plate removal. Anteroinferior plating is associated with fewer symptoms of hardware irritation; however, I prefer superior plating due to the ease of technical intervention.

Regarding other topics such as lateral and medial fractures, the brilliant and experienced opinion of the authors is consistent with my current practice.

Continued

INTERNATIONAL EXPERT COMMENTARY—cont'd

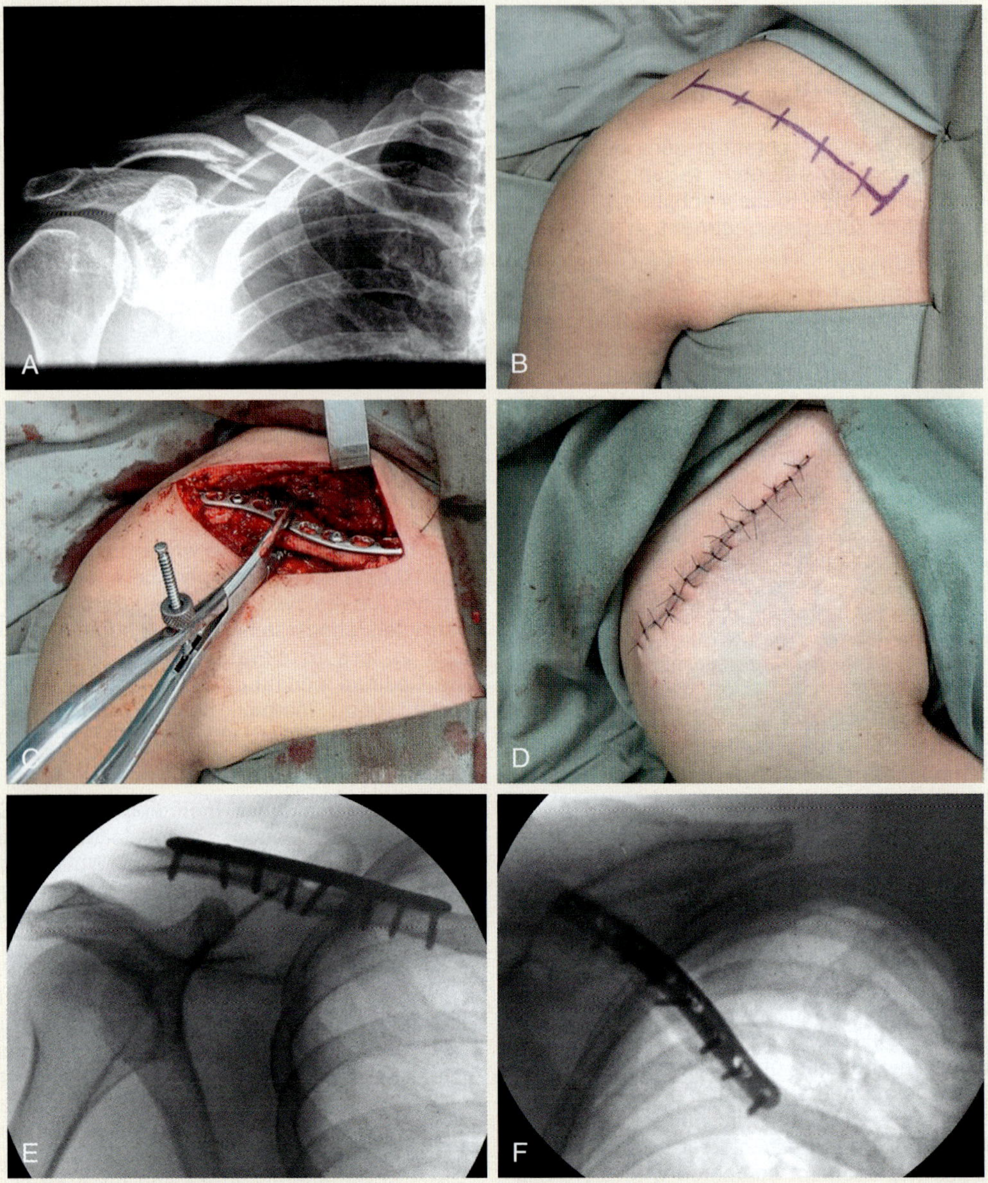

FIGURE 8-97: **A,** Zanca radiographic of an acute displaced middle-third clavicle fracture. **B,** Demarcation of a direct incision over the clavicle along Langer's line. **C,** Intraoperative image of open reduction and internal fixation with a superior contoured small-fragment plate (held with a reduction forceps). **D,** Suture of incision. **E,** Postoperative Zanca view radiograph. **F,** Postoperative axillary view radiograph.

EDITOR COMMENTARY

Edward V. Fehringer

Drs. Basamania and Rockwood have once again very comprehensively and thoughtfully reviewed and updated us on the diagnosis and treatment of a fractured bone that was historically ignored far too often. The understanding of post-fracture difficulties from which many patients suffered has caused several authors to look much closer at these often-perceived innocuous fractures. As it is somewhat difficult to ascertain with upper extremity metrics to provide crisp and objective data, we know now that midshaft fracture nonunion rates are significantly higher than we had previously thought, been taught, and taught to our patients. Moreover, for fractures that have healed in malunited positions, upper extremity function has not necessarily been ideal or without significant consequences for patients.

Proper radiographic evaluation of clavicle fractures is critical to the understanding of the pathoanatomy and its treatment. With its odd shape and position, it is easy to underestimate shortening, displacement, and contour. As a general rule for infants, children, and adolescents, rarely are there operative indications for clavicle fractures. However, with the advent of teenage years and entering of adulthood, we are gaining a better understanding of the fractures for which surgical intervention should be considered. While it is probably inaccurate to state that all completely displaced midshaft clavicle fractures should be addressed surgically, it is also inaccurate to state that all clavicle fractures heal. Due to the great work of many in studying a fracture that was often forgotten, a clearer picture is developing of the fractures at risk for nonunion or malunion from which significant sequelae ensue.

Dr. Basamania favors an IM approach for the majority of midshaft fractures that he deems suitable for surgical repair. I prefer plate-and-screw fixation, as do many who have familiarity with its use in other bones as well as its predictable results in the clavicle. While maybe slightly less cosmetically appealing, I find clavicle plate-and-screw fixation to be predictable, rotationally stable, and applicable in all clavicle cases. Particularly in fractures with extensive comminution, I like to add smaller 2.4-mm plates anteriorly if necessary to augment superiorly placed 3.5-mm main constructs. While precontoured plates help due to their lower profile, I frequently find the need to contour them a bit more intraoperatively to "fit the bone," rather than fitting the bone to the plate, particularly in cases of nonunion. Finally, without a doubt, I have been admittedly influenced, regardless of the data, by how much simpler it is to address acute fractures than it is to address nonunions. The level of complexity is markedly reduced in the acute setting. I am not convinced that this should be the reason alone that I should be surgically addressing more midshaft fractures acutely; however, I look forward to further work that helps delineate the midshaft fractures that should, without a doubt, be addressed acutely with surgical fixation. Simple operative costs alone should not be the argument used to avoid surgery. A number of costs (including lost workdays) are difficult to measure but need to be considered. Nonoperative treatment is not inexpensive.

Fortunately, most medial clavicle fractures heal with simple immobilization. For those with significant displacement or nonunions, T-type locking plates improve the ability to address them. I have successfully used volar distal radius plates (with bends removed) in this area prior to more recent locking T-shaped plates for clavicles.

Surprisingly, on the lateral clavicle end as well, there is often more bone anterior to posterior than first realized. Axillary views confirm this, as do CT scans. "Flooding" the small distal fragment with screws anterior to posterior can be very useful in obtaining fixation in the distal fragment. I do not believe that use of a hook plate is of value, but feel that locking distal clavicle plates and fixation into the coracoid (depending on the fracture pattern and ligamentous injury) have significantly improved our ability to address challenging fractures in this area.

I am equally impressed with Dr. Lenza's commentary. I found it to be a candid and practical approach to diagnosing and treating clavicle fractures. I will incorporate the Velpeau axillary view into my workup, as I am confident that I have often underestimated anterior-posterior displacement. Dr. Lenza's work in systematically evaluating clavicle fractures as well as their nonoperative and operative treatment is commendable. Given the breadth of his clavicle fracture diagnosis and treatment acumen, I was pleased to learn that my nonoperative and operative approaches mirror his. I have also found, as he noted, that each fracture and patient must be evaluated and treated individually. Along those lines, I have found that acutely treating distracted midshaft fractures with early plate/screw constructs makes sense. While they are uncommon and the literature does not contain compelling data to address them surgically, it may be surmised that these fractures and soft tissues have sustained greater trauma and are inherently more unstable. We thank Dr. Lenza for sharing his expertise and images to help refine our understanding of clavicle fracture diagnosis and treatment.

CHAPTER 9

Disorders of the Acromioclavicular Joint

David N. Collins

In those cases where the acromion has been torn off, the bone which is thus separated appears prominent. The bone is the bond of connection between the clavicle and scapula, for in this respect the constitution of man is different from that of other animals.[4]
Hippocrates

DEVELOPMENTAL ANATOMY

The clavicle and scapula are joined together by ligamentous structures existing in two separate locations, one a diarthrodial joint and the other a space, partially occupied by a ligamentous complex.

Clavicle

In the human fetus, as the sixth postconceptional week approaches, the clavicle develops two centers of ossification for its body. They join together approximately 1 week later and become the first bone to ossify in humans.[681] In contrast to the other bones in the body, which form from cartilaginous precursors, clavicle ossification evolves from a mesenchymal or precartilaginous stage, sometimes termed *membranous* or *dermal* bone.[399] Medial and lateral cartilaginous masses develop thereafter, resulting in linear growth of the clavicle, predominantly from the medial mass (Fig. 9-1).[681] A secondary center of ossification not present at birth appears in the medial end of the clavicle at 18 to 20 years, with union to the remaining clavicle before 25 years. A similar ossification center both appearing and uniting in the 20th year at the lateral end of the clavicle was described by Todd and D'Errico.[913] Duplication of the clavicle, especially distally with the formation of two distinct acromioclavicular joints (ACJs), is an extremely rare phenomenon uniquely captured with computed tomography (CT) scan surface reconstruction (Fig. 9-2).[942]

Acromion and Coracoid Processes

The acromion and coracoid processes are cartilaginous at birth. As many as three secondary ossification centers have been reported for the coracoid process, which phylogenetically is a separate bone.[399] These centers and two for the acromion appear between 13 and 16 years and typically unite to form a single bond between 14 and 20 years. Nonunions are possible at all sites but are most commonly seen in the acromion (os acromiale).

ANATOMY AND FUNCTION

Overview

The human torso bears the upper limb by means of suspensory muscles to the scapula, clavicle, and humerus, maximizing the opportunity for movement. The muscles also serve as support for the sternoclavicular joint (SCJ), the limb's only true articulation to the axial skeleton. The clavicle braces the upper limb at a fixed distance from the axial skeleton that permits optimal movement and power (Fig. 9-3). This is possible only through the clavicle's attachment to the scapula at the ACJ and at the coracoid process via the coracoclavicular (CC) ligaments. So linked to the axial skeleton, motion of the scapula on the thorax is possible only through the combined motions occurring via the sternoclavicular (SC) and ACJs.[413,902]

The ACJ is served by sensory branches from the suprascapular, axillary, and pectoral nerves.[401,251] Its blood supply is derived from the acromial branch of the thoracoacromial artery, posterior humeral circumflex artery, and suprascapular (transverse scapular) artery. These vessels converge to form a smaller network (acromial rete) that overlies the acromion and penetrates the joint.[401]

Skin

The innervation of the skin overlying the distal clavicle, ACJ, and acromion process is predominantly via the supraclavicular nerves, deriving from cervical roots C3 and C4.[400] From anterolateral to posterolateral, the coverage can overlap with the upper lateral brachial cutaneous nerve, a branch of the axillary nerve derived from cervical root C5. Branches of the supraclavicular nerve are spared with skin incisions directly over the ACJ, while more medial skin incisions and dissection are likely to encounter the lateral branch consistently and sometimes the intermediate branch, if present.[643]

Muscle Attachments

The anterior head of the deltoid muscle originates from the anterosuperior (AS), anterior, and anteroinferior (AI) aspects of the lateral clavicle; ACJ ligaments; and anterior acromion process. The trapezius inserts onto the posterosuperior (PS) aspect of the lateral clavicle, ACJ ligaments, and medial aspect of the acromion process. The actions of these two muscles contribute to the stability of the ACJ and aid the suspension of the upper limb from the clavicle and the axial skeleton. The coracobrachialis and the short head of the biceps brachii originate from the tip of the coracoid process. Proximal and inferomedial to the tip is the insertion of the pectoralis minor. Although not in its immediate vicinity, other muscles, including the pectoralis major, sternocleidomastoid, levator scapulae, rhomboid major and minor, and serratus anterior, have significant action on the ACJ.

Pertinent Osteology

Distal Clavicle

The S-shaped clavicle tapers from being a cylindrical bone medially to a more flattened bone laterally, where

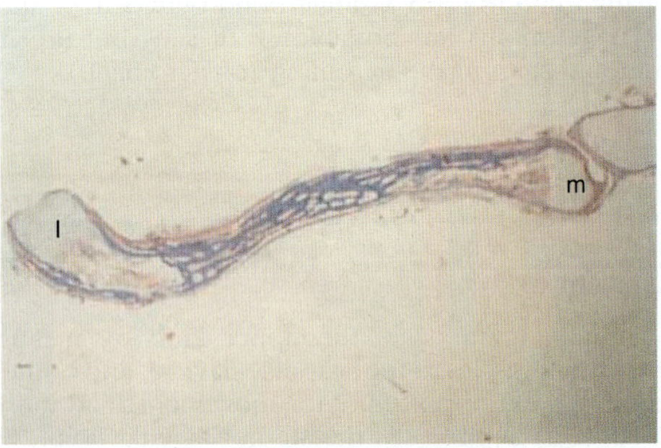

FIGURE 9-1: Transverse section of an 11-week-old human fetus clavicle. Note the developing diaphysis and the lateral (l) and medial (m) cartilaginous masses. The shape at this early stage of development resembles the adult clavicle. (From Ogata S, Uhthoff H. The early development and ossification of the human clavicle: an embryologic study. *Acta Orthop Scand.* 1990;61[4]:330-334.)

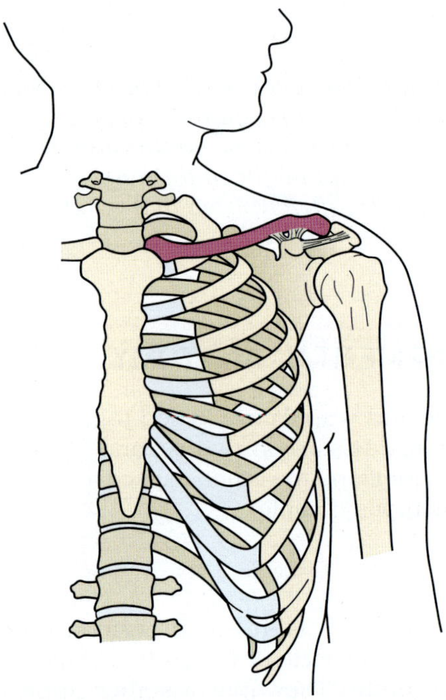

FIGURE 9-3: The clavicle functions as an intercalary strut between the axial skeleton and the upper limb via its interconnecting ligaments with the scapula.

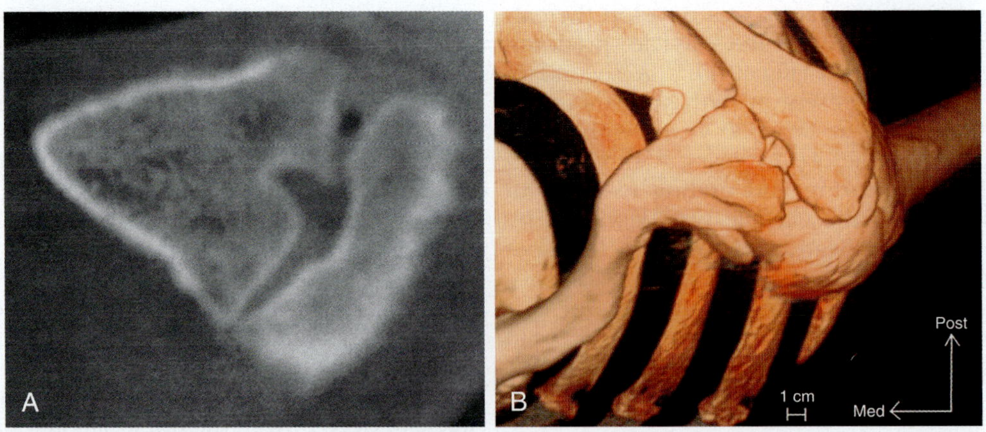

FIGURE 9-2: Computed tomography scan images of duplication of the acromioclavicular joint. (From Viard B, Karp J-S, Tremlet J, et al. Unilateral duplication of the acromioclavicular joint: case report and literature review. *Surg Radiol Anat.* 2013;35[10]: 973-977.)

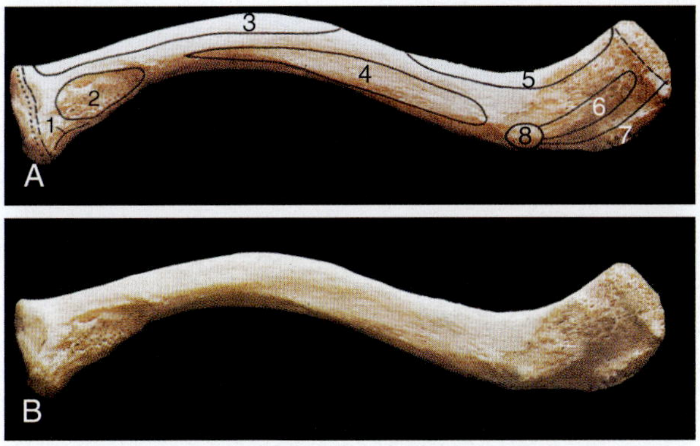

FIGURE 9-4: Osteology of the clavicle, from below. **A,** The attachments for the trapezoid *(6)* and the conoid *(8)* ligaments are outlined. *1,* Sternohyoid; *2,* costal tuberosity; *3,* pectoralis major; *4,* subclavius; *5,* deltoid; *7,* trapezius muscle. **B,** The inferior aspect of the clavicle. (Modified from McMinn RMH, Hutchings RT. *Color Atlas of Human Anatomy.* Chicago, Year-Book Medical Publishers; 1985:93-94.)

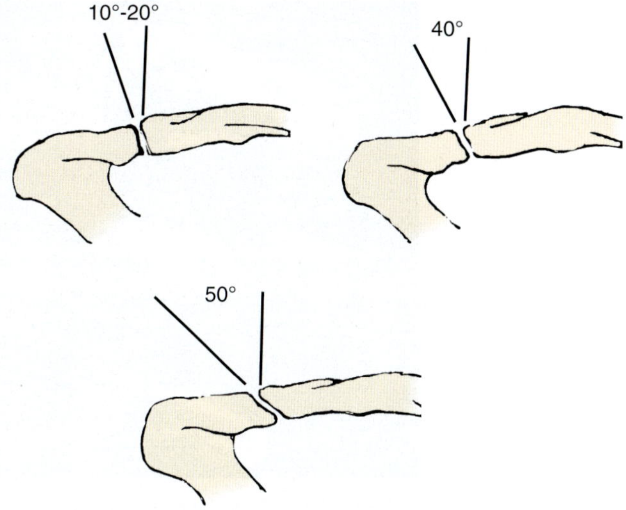

FIGURE 9-5: The sagittal plane orientation of the acromioclavicular joint shows great variability.

superior and inferior surfaces are distinguishable. The anterior portion of the lateral clavicle articulates with the acromion process of the scapula, and hence, the ACJ. On its inferior surface, points of attachment for the CC ligaments are delineated by a slightly prominent tubercle and a more subtle line for the conoid and trapezoid ligaments, respectively (Fig. 9-4). Bone mineral density progressively increases from the most lateral aspect of the clavicle to an area of optimal bone density corresponding to the insertion area of the CC ligaments.[316]

Coracoid Process

Oriented superior, anterior, and lateral to the axis of the scapula, the coracoid process assumes a hooked shape as it projects from the superior body of the scapula. The coracoid attachments of the coracoacromial ligament (CAL) as well as the conoid and the trapezoid ligaments, together sometimes referred to as the CC ligament or CC ligament complex, although relatively constant in location, lack specific identifying osseous prominences. The distance separating the coracoid's superior aspect from the overlying clavicle's inferior aspect ranges from 1.1 to 1.3 cm.[64,110]

Acromion Process

A rather small, facet-like portion of the anterior medial aspect of the acromion process is the articulation area with the lateral clavicle. The acromial attachment of the CAL is without identifying prominence.[257,287]

Acromioclavicular Joint Architecture

Prior to the last 10 to 12 years, investigations of the morphology of the ACJ had been limited.[255,373,752,929] The hyaline cartilage–covered convex lateral clavicle and the concave medial acromion articulate as a true diarthrodial joint. Whether it remains so throughout life is uncertain. Transitional changes of hyaline cartilage to fibrocartilage have been reported to occur on both sides of the joint between the second and third decades of life.[926] In a cadaver study with the mean age at death of 81 years (range, 69 to 91 years), Hatta et al. documented that the articular cartilage in the lower half of both the clavicle and the acromion was significantly thinner than that in the upper half accompanied by more articular cartilage degeneration.[379] From anterior to posterior, the changes were consistent.

The joint normally varies in size and shape with respect to adult age, gender, and skeletal morphology.[110,731,779] Likewise, the orientation of the coronal plane of the joint is variable, ranging from nearly vertical to, less frequently, angulations from superior lateral to inferior medial approaching 50 degrees, a phenomenon that results in increasingly greater overriding of the lateral clavicle on the medial acromion (Fig. 9-5).[224,255,929] Although less common, angulations from superior medial to inferior lateral leading to underriding of the clavicle with respect to the acromion have also been reported.[622] It is not unusual for some degree of vertical incongruence of the ACJ to exist in the complete absence of pathologic events.[929,455] In a cadaver study that utilized dissections and CT scanning, Colegate-Stone et al. identified three main 3D shapes of the ACJ: flat, oblique, and curved (Fig. 9-6).[175] On the basis of the intra-articular disk, Emura et al. identified three primary types of ACJs and their incidence in a cadaver study (mean age, 82.9 years): type I, complete disk (3.8%); type II, incomplete disk (25%); and type III, absent disk (71.2%).[270]

The relatively lax joint capsule enables essential movement while resisting displacement of the acromion over the clavicle.

Intra-Articular Disk

Composed of fibrocartilage superiorly and dense connective tissue inferiorly, a disk of variable shape and size separates the ACJ, either partly (meniscoid) or completely, into two halves.[270,379] Although it is presumed to

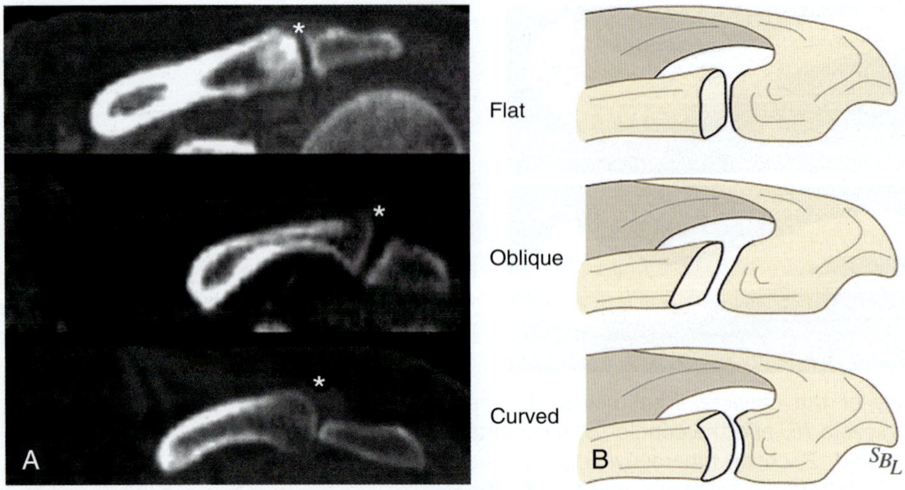

FIGURE 9-6: **A** and **B**, Morphology of the acromioclavicular joint. (**A**, From Colegate-Stone T, Allom R, Singh R, et al. Classification of the morphology of the acromioclavicular joint using cadaveric and radiologic analysis. *J Bone Joint Surg Br.* 2010;92[5]: 743-746. **B**, Courtesy Steven Lippitt, MD.)

function in a manner similar to a meniscus in the knee (contributions to load distribution, joint stability, motion, and articular cartilage nourishment), its actual role is unknown. The articular facets of the lateral clavicle and medial acromion may be intrinsically incongruent, in which case the intra-articular disk morphology is the conforming intercedent structure.[270] In younger patients, it is a structure potentially at risk for an acute injury, including contusion, tearing, or maceration. Structural and functional survival beyond the active years is unlikely as the disk succumbs to age-related degeneration.[223,717,797] In the Hatta et al. cadaver study, disks were absent in 24% of the specimens and meniscoid-like in the remainder.[379]

Ligaments

A relatively weak, thin capsule encloses the ACJ. Distinct acromioclavicular (AC) ligaments, named by their location—anterior, posterior, superior, and inferior—augment the strength of the capsule.

The CC ligament is actually two ligaments, the trapezoid and conoid ligaments (Fig. 9-7). Despite their morphologic differences, the trapezoid and conoid ligaments have similar dimensional, viscoelastic behavioral, and structural properties.[192,373,797]

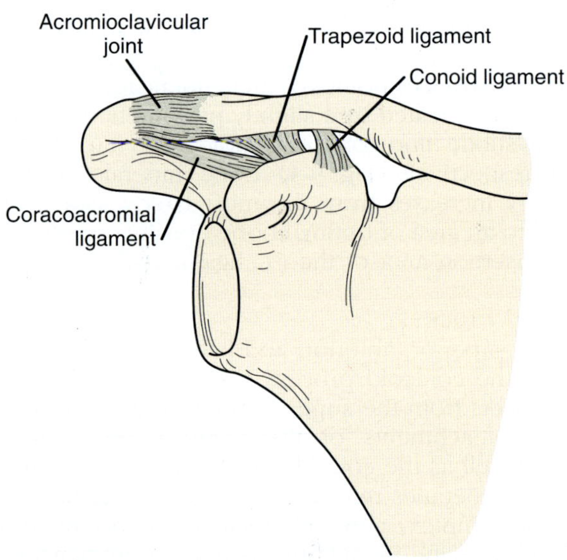

FIGURE 9-7: The ligamentous anatomy around the acromioclavicular joint.

Both ligaments attach to the superior aspect of the angular region of the coracoid process. From a more anterior and lateral site that begins at the angle of the coracoid, courses in the direction of its tip, and ends posterior to the pectoralis minor tendon attachment, the trapezoid ligament is oriented toward the clavicle in a superior, anterior, and slightly lateral direction to attach at the trapezoid line on the inferior clavicle. From a more posterior and medial site on the angle, the conoid ligament expands in circumference as it runs superiorly and slightly medially toward its point of insertion, the conoid tubercle. Here, the lateral one-third and medial two-thirds of the clavicle join to form the posterior curve of the clavicle; at the curve's apex, the conoid tubercle can be identified on the posteroinferior clavicle, just posterior and medial to the most medial aspect of the trapezoid line (see Fig. 9-4).

Distal to the angle, on the lateral aspect of the more horizontal part of the coracoid, is the attachment of the CAL (Fig. 9-8). It joins onto nearly the entire width of the acromion process at its AI edge.

Rios et al. showed that regardless of gender or race, the length of the clavicle can serve as a gauge for the determination of the anatomic attachments of the trapezoid and conoid ligaments.[757] Reliable anatomic points in osteology specimens and fresh specimens were used to measure to the center of the trapezoid ligament and the medial edge of the conoid ligament. The distance from the lateral edge of the clavicle to the respective ligament point of reference was measured and used to express a ratio of the measured distance to the clavicle length. This value was 0.17 for the trapezoid and 0.31 for the conoid. In another cadaver study, Renfree et al. determined that there were no gender differences for the measurement from the center of the articular surface to the lateral-most point of the trapezoid ligament, but the lateral-most point of the conoid ligament was more medial in men than in women.[751] The only significant gender variation identified by Takase was in the coronal dimension of the undersurface of the clavicle and the sagittal dimension of the trapezoid ligament attachment.[889]

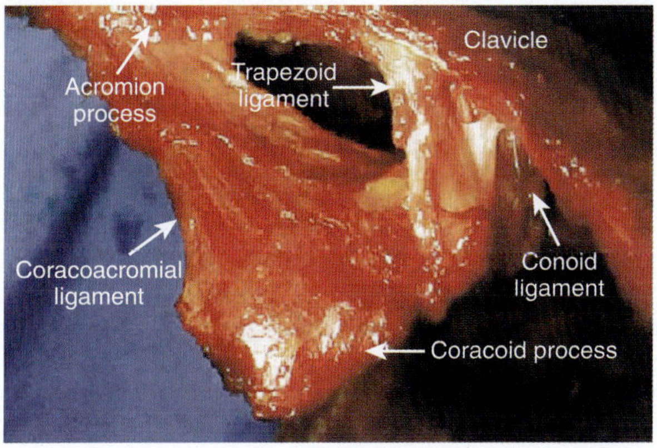

FIGURE 9-8: The coracoacromial ligament attachment to the superolateral aspect of the coracoid process. (Modified from Fealy S, April EW, Khazzam M, et al. The coracoacromial ligament: morphology and study of acromial enthesopathy. *J Shoulder Elbow Surg.* 2005;14[5]:542-548.)

Salzmann et al. demonstrated coracoid anatomic landmarks that facilitated identification of the dimensions and orientation of the insertional footprint of the CC ligaments (Fig. 9-9).[800] In a similar anatomic study, Xue et al. determined that the location of the center points of the footprints could be accurately expressed by the ratios of the conoid and trapezoid centers to the dimensions of the clavicle and coracoid process.[1001] Similarly, Takase precisely defined the anatomic parameters of the two CC ligaments.[889] Knowledge of these landmarks may prove useful intraoperatively when anatomic reconstructions are being considered.

By way of its attachments to the clavicle and scapula, and their respective relationships to the axial skeleton and torso, the CC ligament helps to link scapulohumeral motion and scapulothoracic motion.[173,413,457] These two ligaments create a much stronger union of the clavicle to the scapula than the AC ligaments. This ensures that the clavicle and scapula will move simultaneously as the ligaments reach maximum tension, signifying the limits of the natural excursion of the ACJ. The functional strength of the ACJ increases in the presence of intact CC ligaments.[929,127] Thus the effective suspension of the upper limb from the torso via the SCJ and supporting musculature is assured.

Although it is tempting to simplify the function of the AC and CC ligaments as anterior-to-posterior and superior-to-inferior stabilizers, respectively, displacement resistance of the lateral clavicle is significantly more complex, as borne out in the results of experimental cadaver investigations.[209,215,216,306,471,509,763,764,766] Not only are the ligaments distinguishable as discrete anatomic structures, the individual roles they play biomechanically are becoming more clear. Collectively, in the midst of a wide range of load, displacement, and restraint variables, these studies have shown that anterior restraint is afforded by the inferior AC ligaments and conoid ligament, posterior

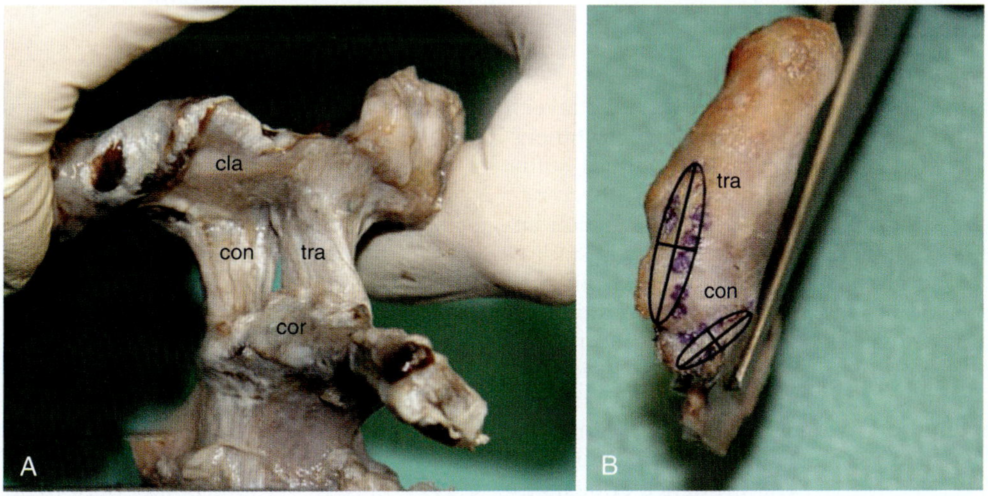

FIGURE 9-9: **A** and **B**, The coracoclavicular ligaments with their footprint on the superior left coracoid process. *cla,* clavicle; *con,* conoid ligament; *cor,* coracoid process; *tra,* trapezoid ligament. (From Salzmann G, Paul J, Sandmann G, et al. The coracoid insertion of the coracoclavicular ligaments: an anatomic study. *Am J Sports Med.* 2008;36[12]:2392-2397.)

restraint predominantly by the superior and posterior AC ligaments and the trapezoid ligament, superior restraint by the conoid ligament, and ACJ, compression restraint by the trapezoid ligament.[374,1009] The results of the in vitro studies of Dawson et al. suggested the importance of the CC ligaments for equally restraining both anterior-posterior (AP) and superior-inferior movements, while the restraint of the AC ligaments was threefold greater in the AP plane than the superior-inferior plane.[209] In their study, joint compression contributed to joint stability in a reverse linear fashion, signifying the importance, at least experimentally, of the distal clavicle articulation with the acromion.[209]

Considerably more attention is being paid to the investigation of horizontal instability of the ACJ. Recent research that has included the serial ligament section and tracking measurement has brought this concept to light by demonstrating serially increased translations of the clavicle posteriorly or the acromion anteriorly with sectioning of the AC ligaments and further translations with sectioning of the CC ligaments.[762] The clinical implications of the resultant excessive translations and altered articulation between the medial clavicle and lateral acromion cannot be overlooked, and may help to explain patterns of pain and dysfunction after such injuries.

Experimental sectioning of either the conoid or trapezoid ligaments had no effect on the overall strength of the C ligament.[374] Complete dislocation of the lateral clavicle superior to the acromion process requires the interruption of the integrity of the conoid and trapezoid ligaments.[127,729,763,764,766,929] In an experimental study loading shoulders to failure, ligament disruptions were more common than fractures.[209,474] In another, the conoid was the first to fail.[585] Age, height, and weight showed no significant relationship with the ligament cross-sectional area or the mechanical properties of the shoulder. It has been shown in finite element analysis based on human CT scan information that during progressive abduction, the conoid ligament progressively lengthens while the trapezoid ligament remains relatively unchanged but ultimately becomes lax at full abduction.[826]

Coracoclavicular Articulation

Although lesser bursae can interdigitate between the layers of the conoid and trapezoid ligaments, a more prominent bursa can exist between the ligaments, sometimes sufficiently expanding to create a CC joint between the coracoid process and the clavicle.[525] Twenty cases of such an articulation were documented by dissection or with radiographs in 1939.[343] The gross and histologic appearance is that of a diarthrodial joint with cartilage-covered articulating surfaces and a synovial-lined capsule, and correlates with its radiographic properties.[152,171,343,525] The incidence of this unusual shoulder articulation is probably around 0.5% but, depending on geographic region, can vary widely from 0.04% to 27%, and it is often bilateral (Fig. 9-10).[159,172,282,358,368,450,530,640,651,677,726] The incidence appears to increase with age.[159] It can develop in response to restricted movement of the scapula caused by variations in the shapes of the scapulae, clavicles, and first ribs.[640]

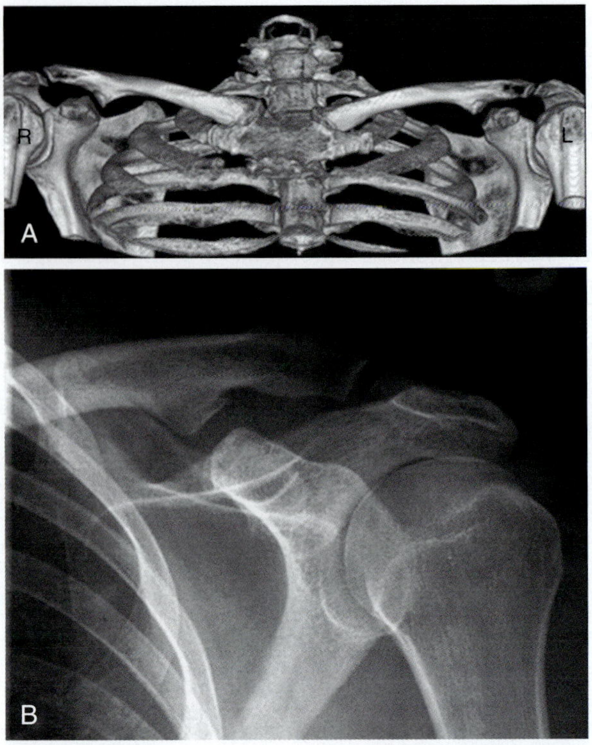

FIGURE 9-10: Coracoclavicular joint. **A,** Three-dimensional computed tomographic scan of shoulder girdles showing bilateral coracoclavicular joints. **B,** Anteroposterior radiograph showing the coracoclavicular joint. (From Cheung TF, Boerboom AL, Wolf RF, Diercks RL. Asymptomatic coracoclavicular joint. *J Bone Joint Surg Br.* 2006;88[11]:1519-1520.)

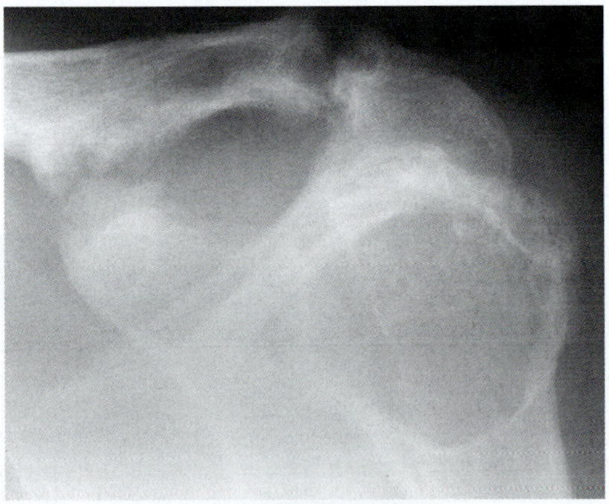

FIGURE 9-11: The coracoclavicular joint in a male patient with ankylosing spondylitis. Note the ipsilateral acromioclavicular joint.

Symptomatic CC joints have been reported in the settings of osteoarthritis (OA) and rheumatoid arthritis (RA), trauma, and thoracic outlet syndrome, but the overall clinical significance of the CC joint is uncertain (Fig. 9-11).[367,513,651,665] Troublesome peripheral ipsilateral limb pain, paresthesias, and weakness may evolve.[366]

Lehtinen et al. recognized resorption of the undersurface of the clavicle and believed it to be an atypical manifestation of RA involvement of the CC joint.[513] Singh et al. conducted an extensive review of the features of the CC joint, leading to a proposed algorithm for treatment.[843] Corticosteroid injection into the joint has been successfully used to treat a painful CC articulation.[665] Surgical excision of the joint to resolve pain has been reported.[282,366,651,976]

Neurovascular Structures

Familiarity with the subcoracoid neurovascular structures is essential when surgical repair or reconstruction of the ACJ is undertaken, as highlighted by Tom et al.[915] They examined the relationship of bony landmarks of the shoulder, including the ACJ and the coracoid tip to the musculocutaneous nerve, posterior cord and lateral cords of the brachial plexus, and the axillary artery. The musculocutaneous nerve was the furthest and the lateral cord the closest structure from both landmarks. A 30-mm safe zone exists around the anteromedial tip to the coracoid process. At a distance of more than 8 cm, the relative safety of these neurovascular structures is virtually assured during surgery about the ACJ.

EXCISION OF THE DISTAL CLAVICLE

Complete Excision

Surgical removal of the lateral clavicle is the definitive treatment for a multitude of disorders of the ACJ. The method of excision initially described was the contemporarily termed "open" technique. Arthroscopic excision of the distal clavicle was first described by Johnson in 1986.[438] Snyder and Esch et al. separately reported arthroscopic excision of the distal clavicle in 1988.[274,855]

Excision of the lateral portion of the clavicle is indicated when the cause of shoulder pain can be attributed solely to the ACJ or a component of a shoulder pain–generating syndrome. The diagnosis is confirmed by the response to intra-articular injection of local anesthetic.[675] Suspicion of additional or alternate diagnoses requires thorough diagnostic investigation, occasionally including arthroscopy of the shoulder performed in conjunction with arthroscopic distal clavicle resection (DCR).[242]

It seems that either Facassini or Morestin first performed excision of the distal clavicle about a century ago.[127,593] In 1941, Gurd and Mumford independently gave the first published accounts of the procedure.[360,631] Subsequently, it has been the subject of many investigations seeking to define the essential yet safe extent of excision. Nearly all recommendations that have been proposed, whether the technique is performed in the traditional open manner or with an arthroscope, take into account the protection of the investing ligamentous support for the ACJ and the CC ligaments. By doing so, postresection instability that might contribute to discomfort and dysfunction is potentially minimized.

The recommended resection length varies from 0.5 to 2.5 cm. Although the precise amount to be excised in each instance is unknown, it would not be erroneous to suggest removing approximately 1 cm of the lateral clavicle.[831,453]

However, this recommendation lacks a high level of evidence support from the literature.[741] Branch et al. suggested that 5 mm is adequate to prevent bony abutment in both rotationally and axially loaded shoulders if the CC and AC ligaments are intact.[112] This recommendation was confirmed in a study by Edwards et al.[261] They further showed that if the resection was 2.5 mm or less, abutment was likely to occur between the acromion and the clavicle, particularly inferiorly and posteriorly, and that joint stiffness diminished with the amount of bone resected. Boehm et al. advised a resection of no greater than 0.8 cm in women and 1.0 cm in men based on cadaver studies using magnification and microcalipers.[99] Exceeding the recommended amount consistently resulted in detachment of some portion of the trapezoid ligament. The anatomic study by Renfree et al. measured the distance from the center of the articular surface of the distal clavicle to the resected edge of the clavicle.[751] They concluded that resection of less than 11.0 mm should never violate any portion of the trapezoid ligament in 98% of men or women, and resection of less than 24.0 mm should never violate any of the conoid ligament. Resection of more than 7.6 mm of the distal clavicle in men and 5.2 mm in women, performed by an arthroscopic approach, can violate the superior AC ligament.[751] Eskola showed that patients with a resection of more than 1.0 cm have more pain than patients with less than 1 cm of resection.[277] The findings of their cadaveric dissections led Stine and Vangsness to advise that to preserve the integrity of the investing AC ligaments and CAL, ACJ resections should be 5 to 7 mm by removing 2 to 3 mm from the medial acromion and 3 to 4 mm from the lateral clavicle.[877] This recommendation is supported by the results of an in vitro biomechanical investigation by Pandhi et al., whose investigation compared peak load to failure of specimens undergoing 1 cm DCR to specimens undergoing mm resection of the medial acromion and distal clavicle, and showed significantly higher resistance to failure with symmetric mm resection of bone from the ACJ.[693]

In a biomechanical cadaver study, Matthews et al. determined no significant differences in residual ACJ stiffness and compressive contact between the acromion and the lateral clavicle when comparing mock 5-mm arthroscopic resection to 10-mm open resection.[576] Beitzel et al., when examining horizontal translations of the clavicle in cadavers undergoing sequential excision of the distal clavicle, documented progressively increasing AP excursions compared with the native joint with inferior capsule excision and 10-mm bone excisions, even when the superior and posterior AC capsular ligaments and the CC ligaments remained intact.[75] Further excursion was observed with complete AC capsule excision, suggesting the significant importance of protection or reconstruction of the joint capsule.

In a cadaver study by Harris et al., 15.3 mm was the mean distance between the end of the clavicle and the most lateral fibers of the trapezoid ligament.[373] Rockwood et al. observed cases with persistent pain after lateral clavicle excision that they attributed to inadequate resection and confirmed radiographically.[768] He recommended excision of at least 2 to 2.5 cm of the clavicle, acknowledging that resection to this extent sacrifices the majority of the trapezoid ligament but spares the conoid ligament so that the lateral clavicle remains stabilized. With open techniques for lateral clavicle excision, meticulous closure of the superior capsule and investing AC ligaments is extremely important.[16]

Under experimental conditions, it was predicted that when the distal clavicle is resected, higher loads may be borne by the adjacent soft tissues.[190] In the same model, the intact surrounding soft tissues exerted a dampening effect, with a reduction in the compressive loads across the ACJ. In another study using cadavers, posterior translation of the clavicle was significantly reduced when the CAL was incorporated as an augment to the capsule repair performed at the time of open excision of the distal 1.0 cm of the distal clavicle.[189]

In an attempt to further spare the investing stabilizing ligaments, the plane of resection should mimic the plane of the angular orientation of the existing joint when possible.[877] To prevent the abutment of the acromion and clavicle during adduction of the arm, Neer advocated the removal of 1.5 to 2.0 cm, resecting more superiorly and posteriorly than inferiorly and anteriorly.[649] Intraoperative ultrasonography has been used for verification of appropriate arthroscopic DCR.[98] On the basis of their investigation and to prevent further supraspinatus outlet–encroaching osteophytes, Roidis et al. recommended DCR at the time of surgery for impingement with or without rotator cuff repair (RCR), even when no symptoms could be attributed to the ACJ.[770]

Partial Excision

Concern exists for the fate of acromial stability at the time of open or arthroscopic subacromial decompression operations, especially when performed with coplaning of the ACJ and distal clavicle. The inferior AC ligament can extend as far as 10 mm lateral to the joint line.[227,489] In addition, the fibers of the medial-most CAL can be found intimate to the inferior AC ligaments and capsule.[797,227,623] It has been shown experimentally that it is impossible to perform standard subacromial decompression without violating the integrity of the inferior AC ligaments on the acromion process.[227] Although the immediate effect in the experimental cadaver model is AP and superior compliance increased as much as 32%, in vivo factors such as ligament healing and muscle recovery can dampen the effect of acromioplasty and coplaning. In a cadaveric study by Edwards, coplaning the lateral clavicle together with acromioplasty contributed to more joint laxity and translations of the lateral clavicle than did acromioplasty alone.[260]

According to studies with 4- to 7-year follow-up data, coplaning of the ACJ at the time of arthroscopic subacromial decompression did not contribute to instability, pain, or further surgery at the ACJ.[50,51,121,460,967] Contrary to these reports, Fischer et al. reported increased OA and instances of symptomatic ACJ instability, some necessitating reoperation, and expressed their concerns with coplaning at the time of arthroscopic subacromial decompression.[295] This experience led to their recommendation for either resection or preservation of the entire lateral clavicle. Other authors have observed that arthroscopic subacromial decompression accompanied by coplaning or partial excision of the lateral clavicle can result in AP laxity and instability symptoms arising from the modified ACJ.[96,383,489,759] Kuster et al. reported that arthroscopic subacromial decompression did not accelerate the development of osteoarthritic changes in the ACJ.[489] In the report by Kharrazi et al. in 2007, nearly 50% of patients who underwent reoperation for ACJ symptoms following arthroscopic subacromial decompression and ACJ surgery had persistent symptoms.[459] Contrary to their earlier report, they identified no reason to perform concomitant coplaning or complete excision of the distal clavicle.[460] The evidence from the literature is conflicting, but suggests that coplaning can create or intensify symptoms arising from the ACJ.[741]

Results of Excision

Rabalais and McCarty performed a systematic review confirming that the best level of evidence for the excision of the lateral clavicle is level III or level IV.[741] From their careful analysis and identification of low levels of evidence, they concluded that the method with the best results or fewest complications could not be determined. That stated, there is little argument that excision of the lateral clavicle successfully addresses the majority of the pathologic entities encountered at the ACJ. However, there are unsatisfactory outcomes because of cosmesis, pain, and dysfunction that have at their root mechanical more so than nonmechanical factors. The factors are often interrelated, and include improper resection, instability, loss of soft tissue integrity, heterotopic ossification, scars, and neuromas. The vast majority of clinical scenarios for which excision of the lateral clavicle is the only reasonable treatment to consider offer absolutely no technical challenges. Therefore it is the execution of the technique that results in unsatisfactory outcomes.

OPEN

In the orthopedic literature, there are abundant citations of the results of DCR performed open.* The report by Rabalais and McCarty indicated 76.8% excellent and good results.[741] Cheung et al., at a mean follow-up of 8.3 years, reported a mean Simple Shoulder Test (SST) score of 10.9 and a mean American Shoulder and Elbow Surgeons (ASES) score of 88.3, with expectedly improved pain and satisfaction.[153] In a systematic review, Pensak et al.

**References 153, 129, 183, 277, 279, 351, 661, 671, 715, 718, 719, 791, 808, 847, 949, 994.*

recognized excellent and good results in 79%.[713] The clinical outcome impact of the associated acromioplasty was insignificant.[153] In the presence of heavy manual labor or worker's compensation or litigation, the results might not be as predictable.[671,715,153] Alford and Bach noted savings of operative time with open DCR.[16]

ARTHROSCOPIC

Numerous publications that describe the techniques and the results have followed the seminal work of Johnson, Snyder, and Esch et al.* The report by Rabalais and McCarty indicated 92.5% excellent and good results with arthroscopic DCR.[741]

In the systemic review by Pensak et al., excellent and good results were achieved in 91%.[713] The trend for excellent and good outcomes continues to be shown in reports that utilize isolated arthroscopic DCR and when performed in conjunction with treatment of lesions of the rotator cuff (RC), biceps tendon, glenohumeral joint (GHJ), and labrum.[90]

Several studies have compared the results of arthroscopic and open excision of the lateral clavicle with confirmation of the benefits of each method.[296,303] Flatow et al. reported earlier recovery of comfort with the arthroscopic method.[296] Freedman et al., using validated outcome measurement tools, showed no significant differences at 1 year, with the exception that the improvement in visual analog scores from before surgery to 1 year postoperatively was significant for their arthroscopic group but not their open group.[303] With the arthroscopic method, there is opportunity to diagnose and treat intra-articular lesions.[115] Elhassan's group validated comparable results in both groups, although 90% of the arthroscopic group had subacromial decompression as well as many other additional procedures compared with the open group.[266] Patient dissatisfaction, regrowth of the distal clavicle, and revision surgery were more frequent in the arthroscopic group, although pain directly over the ACJ was less frequent. In a comparative assessment at the 4- to 5-year follow-up, the only difference between open and arthroscopic DCR was less residual pain in the arthroscopic group.[760]

The ACJ may be approached arthroscopically either directly (superior) or indirectly (bursal or inferior).[35,88,296,297,313,454,914,1015] Although the direct approach can yield results similar to those of the bursal approach, a possible disadvantage is that it places the important superior stabilizing structures at risk.[371,523] Hardeman et al. experimentally compared the effect of soft tissue–sacrificing indirect (inferior) DCR with soft tissue–sparing direct (superior) DCR specifically to determine the effect on residual horizontal stability.[371] They found that for horizontal stability, the ultimate failure strength with the direct approach exceeded the ultimate failure strength of the indirect approach.

Pensak et al. stated that the indirect approach mandates a concomitant subacromial decompression, which imposes additional risks of complications, especially when performed in the absence of impingement.[713] A level I comparative study of both approaches determined that the outcomes were comparable in athletes, with faster improvement and earlier return to sports with the direct approach.[144]

As with open excision, patients with a worker's compensation claim undergoing either isolated excision or excision concomitant to another procedure may be more likely to have an unsatisfactory outcome.[459,547,856,914]

Continued pain and instability in the AP plane have been reported after arthroscopic DCR, sometimes necessitating further reconstruction (Fig. 9-12).[96,295,523,675,683] Inadequate or uneven bone resection has been reported after DCR.[88,296,314,521]

Rabalais and McCarty analyzed level IV evidence reports of lateral clavicle excision performed in conjunction with other procedures (subacromial decompression, RCR, etc.) and reported 94.7% excellent and good results.[203,453,519,521,523,547,571,741,856] This was confirmed in the study by Pensak et al.[713] Razmjou et al. determined that inferior outcomes could be expected in patients with OA of the ACJ (even when determined arthroscopically to be mildly involved) in whom DCR was omitted at the time of RCR.[748] In a level I investigation, Oh et al. showed that better results were not obtained with preventive (asymptomatic) arthroscopic DCR in conjunction with arthroscopic RCR and that it risked the development of iatrogenic symptomatic AC instability.[683] In the presence of an asymptomatic ACJ, Kim et al. advised excision of the distal clavicle at the time of arthroscopic RCR.[464] They determined that pain and functional scores were better at final follow-up when the AC arthritis is advanced and when inferiorly directed osteophytes are observed arthroscopically. Blasiak et al. found similar outcomes in patients undergoing arthroscopic RCR regardless of the presence or absence of symptomatic arthritis of the ACJ.[95] In a level I evidence study, Park et al. identified no outcome differences resulting from the treatment of patients with confirmed symptomatic ACJs and RC tear with RCR with and without excision of the distal clavicle.[697]

Heterotopic ossification and calcification can occur after an ACJ injury or following the excision of the lateral clavicle.[79,129,183,571,856] Symptomatic ossification or calcification are quite uncommon, although it may be an offending lesion when the outcome of DCR by either open or arthroscopic methods is not considered satisfactory (Fig. 9-13).[79,718,856] Patients at high risk for developing heterotopic ossification, such as those with a previous history of the lesion or patients with either hypertrophic pulmonary osteoarthropathy or spondylitic arthropathy, may be candidates for pharmacologic prophylaxis.

Arterial injury with adverse consequences accompanying arthroscopic DCR is a very rare lesion that might occur during routine anterior portal placement for arthroscopic examination of the shoulder.[966]

It appears that DCR, regardless of method, following trauma to the ACJ produces fewer excellent and good

References 34, 35, 68, 76, 88, 140, 274, 296, 297, 313, 314, 427, 432, 438, 453, 454, 518, 521, 523, 571, 675, 825, 831, 855, 856, 914, 1015.

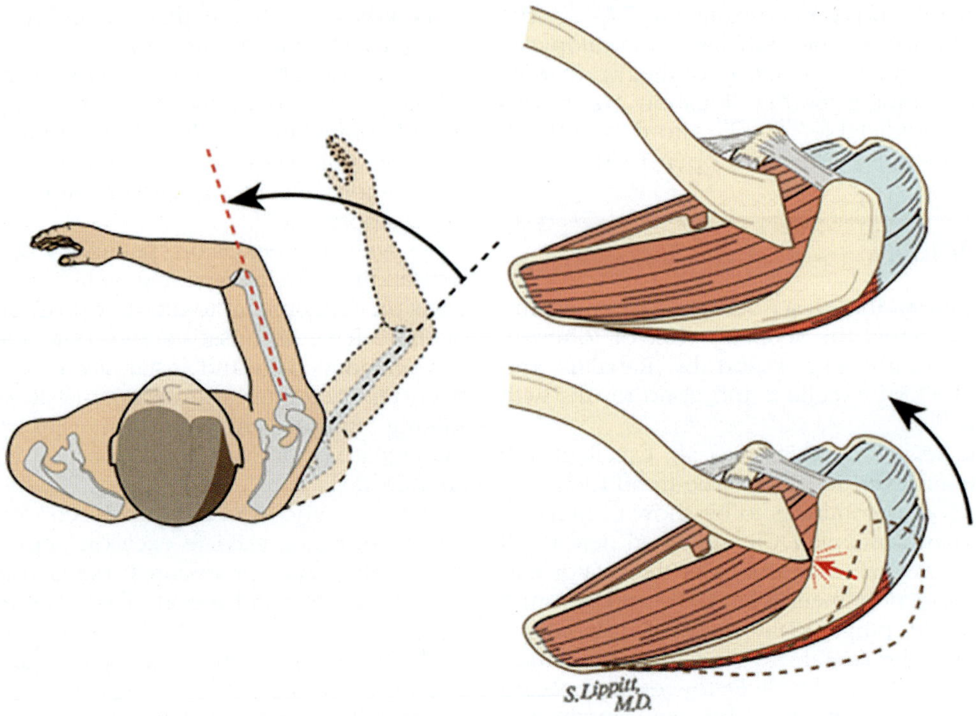

FIGURE 9-12: A proposed mechanism for painful instability after lateral clavicle excision is abutment of the remaining posterolateral clavicle against the posteromedial acromion (*arrow*). (Courtesy Steven Lippitt, MD.)

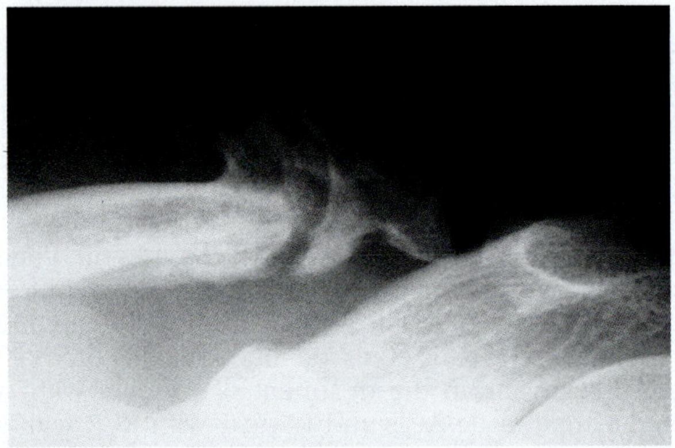

FIGURE 9-13: An extreme example of heterotopic ossification with nearly complete restoration of the lateral clavicle following open excision.

results than when it is performed for nontraumatic conditions.[183,277,571,671,715,718,741,809,1015] Reoperation after arthroscopic DCR was performed three times more often in patients with existing worker's compensation and litigation claims.[459]

COMPLICATIONS OF EXCISION

Open

In the series by Chronopoulos et al., a complication rate of 64% was reported.[163] They found not only the usual complications but also several not reported in the literature such as ACJ tenderness (55%), incisional scar sensitivity (55%), hypertrophic incisional scar (14%), and infection (10%). The incidence of postoperative stiffness is reportedly as high as 29%.[163,277]

Arthroscopic

The incidence of reoperation for inadequate excision ranges from 0% to 6.2%.[144,266] Fracture of the distal clavicle attributable to misidentification of the ACJ was reported by Ghodadra et al.[323] Iatrogenic excision of the CC ligaments can result in a type III AC dislocation.[491] A secondary operation to treat heterotopic ossification has been reported.[144]

MANAGEMENT OF FAILED DISTAL CLAVICLE EXCISIONS

Failure to obtain a successful outcome after DCR may be attributable to technical and nontechnical actions. A classification of complications by Basamania et al. included diagnostic error, inadequate resection, joint instability, and miscellaneous factors.[57] Strauss et al. believed that most complications were related to improper surgical technique.[879]

Failure to resect enough distal clavicle can result in continued, symptomatic abutment of the acromion and the clavicle. The problem is usually secondary to inadequate visualization or underestimation of the amount of resection when DCR is performed arthroscopically. The solution is straightforward in most instances. A secondary operation is performed to address the residual distal clavicle more often openly than arthroscopically, unless concomitant shoulder lesions have been identified or suspected.[879] The results to be expected are potentially excellent.

Overresection, which is most often accompanied by manifestations of instability, is a far more challenging problem, nearly always resulting in more significant pain and dysfunction than underresection. Different degrees of overresection and extent and directions of instability are possible. Exceedingly generous resections, usually radiographically apparent, place the important CC ligaments at risk, especially the most lateral trapezoid. Refractory symptoms usually necessitate a formal reconstructive stabilizing procedure to specifically address the instability pattern. The extent of instability determines the extent of reconstruction.[879] The results to be expected are not always predictable but probably range from fair to good, not always achieving the patient's goals.

Persistent incompetence of the ligaments released at the time of DCR and left inadequately repaired (usually open) or unrepaired (typically arthroscopic) may confound an otherwise successful excision of the distal clavicle. The more subtle but nevertheless disabling symptoms are probably attributable to translational microinstability in the AP plane. Treatment varies from secondary repair with imbrication of the deltotrapezius fascia and the underlying residual AC capsule and ligaments to a more sophisticated reconstruction that utilizes joint-spanning material, either synthetic or biologic.

Motion limitation after an appropriate period of healing is occasionally reported.[163,571,277] Undetected stiffness existing at the time of the index procedure is probably the most common precipitating factor. Identifiable risk factors such as diabetes mellitus should be recognized preoperatively. Satisfactory management may prove difficult but a patient approach is probably best. Alternately, additional surgical treatment could be entertained.[879]

The formation of mechanically significant heterotopic bone at the site of DCR is rare. In its presence, it is wise to look for other causes of shoulder pain after DCR rather than being seduced into a secondary operation that includes its removal.

Miscellaneous conditions reported to confound the results of DCR include preexisting psychiatric illness, suprascapular neuropathy, infection, and osseous bridging of the ACJ.[163,560,879,925]

Author's Preferred Method

The patient is placed in the beach chair position with the head supported on an adjustable well-padded headrest to allow free access to the superior aspect of the shoulder. The skin incision is made in the relaxed skin tension lines approximately 1 cm medial to the ACJ, extending for 3 to 4 cm (Fig. 9-14). A small, straight Gelpi retractor is placed into the subcutaneous tissue, which is gently elevated from the underlying fascia.

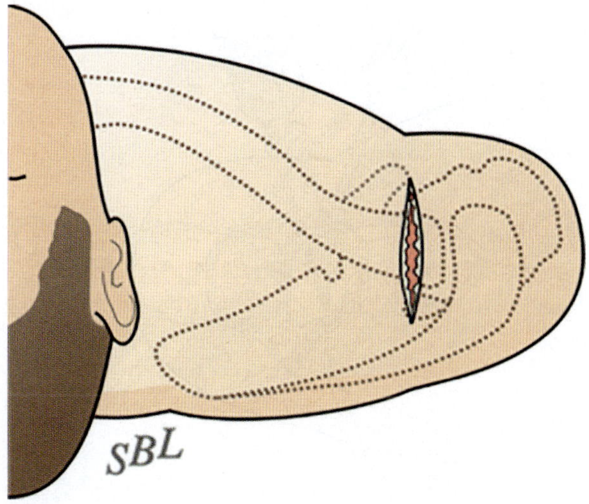

FIGURE 9-14: A superior incision in the relaxed skin tension lines is made slightly medial to the acromioclavicular joint for a distance of 3 to 4 cm. (Courtesy Steven Lippitt, MD.)

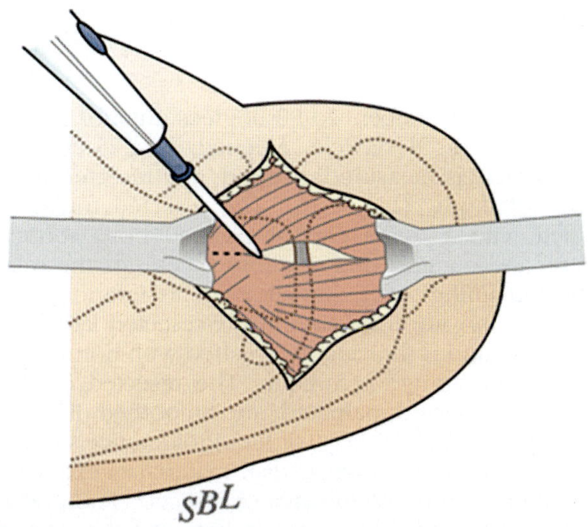

FIGURE 9-15: In line with the clavicle, the deltotrapezius fascia and underlying acromioclavicular joint capsule are divided and reflected from the distal clavicle. (Courtesy Steven Lippitt, MD.)

Beginning 2.0 to 2.5 cm medial to the ACJ, electrocautery is used to incise the soft tissue overlying the superior aspect of the clavicle (Fig. 9-15). The incision should be carefully placed to avoid the trapezius and deltoid muscles from their respective insertions. The incision is continued laterally through the capsule of the ACJ onto the acromion process for a distance of approximately 0.5 to 1 cm. Subperiosteal dissection of the distal clavicle is carried out with electrocautery to create anterior and posterior soft tissue flaps that include the capsule, the superior ligaments of the ACJ, and the adjacent muscles. Complete soft tissue dissection is confirmed with a 0.25-inch key elevator enabling the placement of two small

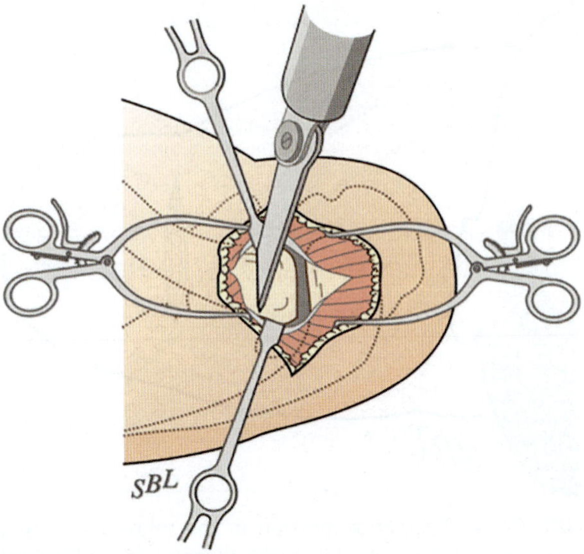

FIGURE 9-16: The surrounding soft tissues are protected as the lateral clavicle is excised with a microsagittal saw. (Courtesy Steven Lippitt, MD.)

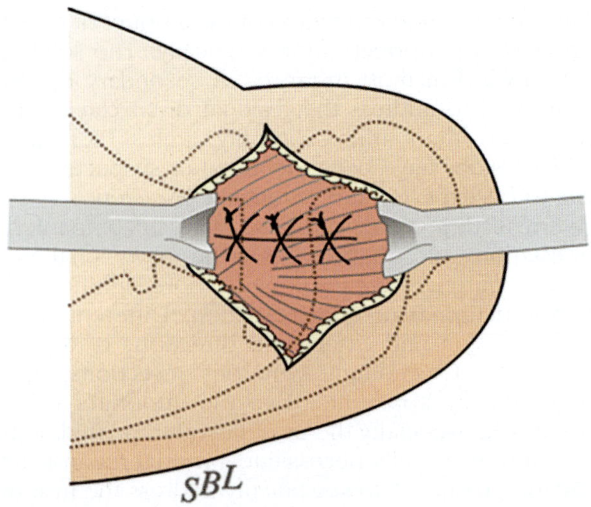

FIGURE 9-17: The residual defect is closed by careful repair of the deltotrapezius fascia and acromioclavicular joint capsule. No more than three sutures placed with a figure-of-eight technique are usually necessary. The sutures are tied with four throws to limit the likelihood of palpable and potentially painful knots beneath the skin at the surgical site. Leaving a small tag further reduces the possibility of palpable suture. (Courtesy Steven Lippitt, MD.)

Chandler retractors bent to 90 degrees anterior and posterior to the distal clavicle. A length of 1.25 cm of the distal clavicle is measured, marked, and resected using a microsagittal saw (Fig. 9-16). The resected fragment is grasped with a towel clip or pointed bone reduction forceps and manipulated to allow access for the release of the remaining soft tissue attachments inferiorly.

Upon removal of the completely resected lateral clavicle, the wound is thoroughly irrigated with normal saline by the bulb syringe technique. The resected clavicular surface is inspected, palpated, and smoothed, if needed, using a pinecone bur, rasp, or file. Proliferative synovium and abnormal intra-articular disk material is excised. By placing a fingertip into the area of resection and performing extremity adduction, contact between the acromion and the residual distal clavicle is recognized and corrected by additional resection.

The surrounding soft tissues are infiltrated with a local anesthetic solution consisting of equal parts of 0.5% Marcaine with epinephrine and 1% lidocaine. With the medial subcutaneous flap retracted with a bent Army Navy retractor, a 6-D Mayo trocar needle delivers No. 2 nonabsorbable sutures through the anterior and posterior soft tissue flaps (Fig. 9-17). No more than three sutures placed with a figure-of-eight technique are usually necessary. The sutures are tied with four rows to limit the likelihood of palpable and potentially painful knots beneath the skin at the surgical site. Leaving a small tag further reduces the possibility of palpable sutures. For extremely thin patients, absorbable sutures are preferred. The subcutaneous tissue is closed with 2-0 absorbable sutures using a buried technique, capturing the dermal layer to ensure excellent superficial soft tissue apposition. Strips of 0.5-inch adhesive-backed paper tape cut in half are applied to the skin. A sterile dressing covers the wound, and the arm is placed in a sling.

Patients are discouraged from active arm elevation without the assistance of the opposite limb for 3 to 4 weeks to protect the deep soft tissue repair. Heavy use of the extremity is not recommended for 6 to 8 weeks to ensure that sufficient preliminary healing of the AC ligaments has taken place and that the residual void created at the time of DCR has been filled with scar. Hydrotherapy to obtain range of motion is suitable as soon as the wound is dry. Return of full strength, range of motion, and full function can be expected in most cases by 12 weeks.

Technical Pearls and Pitfalls

Cosmetically unappealing scars may be avoided by carefully placing the incision in the relaxed skin tension lines.

Placing the skin incision approximately 1 cm medial to the palpable prominence of the distal clavicle enables optimum and safe placement of the saw. The angle of resection favors removing slightly more bone superiorly and posteriorly than inferiorly and anteriorly (Fig. 9-18). This orientation of the plane of resection prevents contact between the remaining clavicle and the acromion when the arm is placed in cross-body adduction. A saw is preferred to the use of either a bur, which creates more bone debris, or an osteotome, which can shatter the bone.

The soft tissue sleeve that includes the ACJ capsule and its supporting ligaments is carefully closed side to side without an attempt to obliterate the dead space formed by

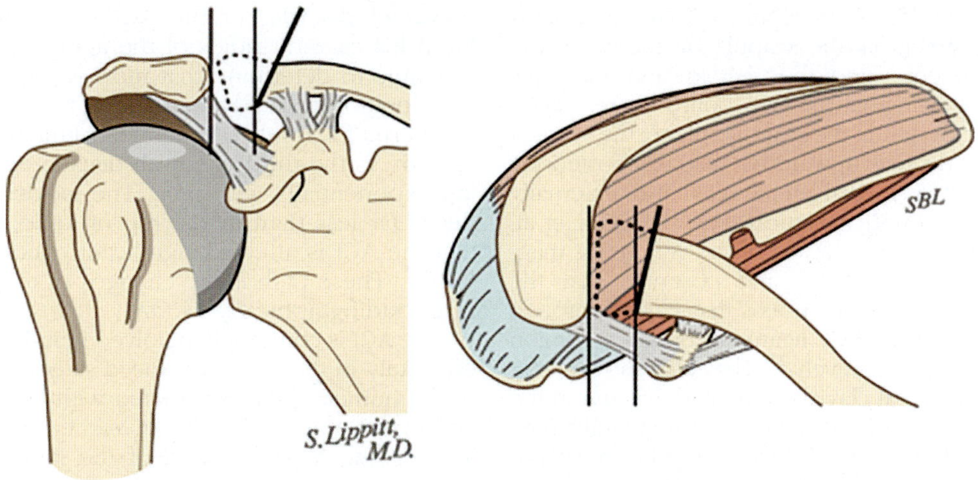

FIGURE 9-18: The plane of resection favors slightly more bone removal superiorly and posteriorly to prevent abutment of the acromion process on the clavicle during extremity adduction. (Courtesy Steven Lippitt, MD.)

the absence of the lateral clavicle. It is important that the repair suture engage the entirety of the reflected soft tissue, not just its most superior portion. This effectively reconstructs the superior AC ligaments and capsule, which reduces the possibility of iatrogenic AC instability. The temptation to create an interposition arthroplasty using the soft tissues adjacent to the joint should be resisted. Their relative immobility risks a closure under tension that can lead to dehiscence of the tissues at the repair site. Overtightening the trapezius or deltoid muscle at the resection site can contribute to focal discomfort. Likewise, an insufficient closure can be painful, cosmetically unappealing, and functionally compromising.

Heterotopic ossification can develop at the surgical site. Preventive measures include subperiosteal dissection with electrocautery rather than sharp or blunt elevation of the soft tissue from the bone, thorough irrigation of the surgical site to remove residual bone debris, and prophylactic administration of pharmacologic agents such as indomethacin.

Summary

Disorders of the distal clavicle that result from internal derangement of the ACJ or irreversible deterioration of its articular surface can be effectively treated with excision of the distal clavicle through a limited open surgical approach. It is very important to carefully preserve the soft tissues contiguous with the joint capsule. Sufficient resection requires removal of no less than 1 cm and no more than 2.5 cm of the distal clavicle.

An anatomic approximation of the soft tissues at the time of closure will safeguard the horizontal stability of the ACJ. Cosmesis is maintained through the use of proper skin incision orientation and by making no attempt to interpose a large volume of the adjacent soft tissues. Technical ease and swiftness of performance predictably resulting in favorable and durable outcomes are the hallmarks of this operation.

BIOMECHANICS OF ACROMIOCLAVICULAR MOTION

Based on observations of patients with ACJ arthrodesis, observations of the movement of pins drilled into the skeleton under certain conditions, and the data from investigational laboratory models, opinions vary with respect to the amounts and types of movement that take place at the ACJ. With upper limb elevation, Inman et al. recognized 20 degrees of ACJ motion and 40 to 50 degrees of clavicle rotation.[413] Codman was the first to suggest that the motion was far less, at around 5 degrees.[173] Caldwell's patients with AC arthrodesis had excellent range of motion.[130] The studies of Kennedy and Cameron provided the initial description of the downward scapular rotation occurring in conjunction with upward rotation of the clavicle during upper limb elevation.[456,457] Codman's opinion was later supported by the investigations of Rockwood, who detected only 5 to 8 degrees of ACJ motion.[173,763,764,766] Rockwood surmised that in the presence of the diminutive amount of motion at the ACJ, full or nearly full elevation of the upper limb was only possible with 40 to 50 degrees of upward rotation of the clavicle and by the simultaneous downward rotation of the scapula. He termed the phenomenon synchronous scapuloclavicular motion, and acknowledged the earliest description by Codman and later by Kennedy and Cameron.[173,456,457] It was recognized that motion limitations between the clavicle and scapula (coracoid process) induced either by natural or surgical phenomena had no significant effect on the range of motion of the upper limb. However, the results of some recent experimental investigations have not lent support to this concept.[826]

Recent studies have enabled a more complete understanding of the complex motion interactions of the upper limb, scapula, clavicle, and thorax, and appear to have validated the conclusions of the pioneering investigators. As the upper limb is raised, the clavicle elevates 11 to 15 degrees and retracts 15 to 29 degrees.[549] This motion is linked to the movement of the scapula by means of the ACJ, the CC ligaments, and the deltoid and trapezius muscles, whose attachments the two bones share. When the upper limb is elevated in the scapular plane, the scapula not only rotates 50 degrees upward but also tilts posteriorly 30 degrees around a medial-lateral axis and externally rotates 24 degrees around a vertical axis.[587] Sahara et al. performed a 3D kinematic analysis of the ACJ using magnetic resonance imaging (MRI), and observed that the scapula rotated 35 degrees on an axis that passed through the insertions of the AC and CC ligaments on the acromion and coracoid process, respectively.[794] They also showed that with abduction, the lateral clavicle translated 3.5 mm in the AP and 1 mm in the superior directions. Subsequently, they demonstrated that during arm abduction, significant scapular multiplanar rotational motion (15 to 20 degrees) with respect to the clavicle occurred through the ACJ.[793] In an electromagnetic surface motion analysis tracking the shoulder girdle, Teece et al. demonstrated coupled motion patterns between the clavicle and the scapula that facilitated clearance of the humeral head beneath the acromion during scapular plane abduction.[902] This resulted from scapula upward rotation, internal rotation, and posterior tilt relative to the clavicle at the ACJ. Ludewig et al. studied limb elevation (flexion, coronal abduction, scapular abduction) in humans with skeletal pins attached to electromagnetic tracking sensors to show multiplanar rotational motion of 8 to 19 degrees.[550] Later, the same investigational center demonstrated small differences in kinematics of the shoulder when painful and painless shoulders were compared.[506] Interruptions of the normal integrity of the AC and CC ligaments unfavorably alter the normal linkage between the scapula and the clavicle, resulting in significant dyskinesis patterns during limb movement in whole cadavers.[684,685] This may lead to the loss of the clavicular strut function, imposing abnormal contact and even overriding of the clavicle on the acromion, especially with abduction of the internally rotated arm.[684] Dyskinetic patterns of the scapula and clavicle are also observed in patients with AC arthrosis with or without RC tear, perhaps compensatory to ameliorate pain.[864]

Changes in the position of the scapula with respect to the clavicle are accompanied by a subtle gliding motion between the articular surfaces of the ACJ and virtually undetectable motion through the CC ligaments. Mazzocca et al. considered the mechanical coupling of the clavicle, the scapula, and upper limb elevation vital to upper limb motion and function.[581] They stated that "the ACJ should not be fixed, either by fusion, joint-spanning hardware (screws, plates, pins) or by CC screws. Motion will be lost, limiting shoulder function, or the hardware can fail." This interpretation and conclusion has been reached by others, derived from their respective results of in vitro investigational studies.[826]

SPECTRUM OF DISORDERS

Nearly one-third of patients with shoulder pain will be identified to have a lesion of the ACJ.[688] The most prevalent disorder of the ACJ is degenerative disease. From his classic studies of the aging shoulder, DePalma was able to determine that most people experience ACJ deterioration with advancing age.[222,225] His work revealed a pattern of age-related changes within the joint emerging as early as the third or fourth decade of life and increasing exponentially with time. The incidence in the shoulder is far less than in the hip or knee, but it is notable that the ACJ is affected significantly more often than the GHJ.[721] These pathologic changes of the joint are recognized radiographically as OA.

The ACJ is commonly involved in inflammatory arthritis, especially in the more advanced stages.[514] Superior ascent of the humeral head associated with cuff-tear arthropathy and massive defects in the RC can erode the ACJ, eventually leading to destruction of the joint, sometimes with the formation of large cysts that can mimic a soft tissue tumor.[618,650,921] Crystal arthropathy with ACJ involvement and other forms of AC arthritis are uncommon. Transient exacerbation of pain arising from the ACJ often accompanies adhesive capsulitis (frozen shoulder syndrome).[23] Infections of the ACJ are uncommon, even when the general health of the patient is compromised.[496] Neoplasms, both benign and malignant, as well as proliferative disorders of the synovium, very rarely affect the ACJ.[544]

It is, however, trauma to the ACJ and its environs that has garnered the greatest attention, as much due to its relative frequency of occurrence as to the quest to optimize recovery from the lesions thus produced. Evidence supporting this fact is found in literally hundreds of clinical and experimental investigations dealing with ACJ trauma. Therefore the bulk of the remaining chapter is devoted to this topic.

Characteristics of the Painful Acromioclavicular Joint Evaluation

This section focuses on the assessment of the atraumatic causes of ACJ pain and dysfunction.

History

Pain is the most common symptom of an ACJ disorder. Without prompting, nearly all patients point directly at the ACJ or its vicinity when they begin to describe their symptoms. However, the expression of ACJ pain may be altogether different as reported in an interesting study by Gerber et al.[319] Hypertonic saline injected into the ACJ of otherwise asymptomatic volunteers resulted in variable pain patterns that included not only the ACJ but also the area of the anterolateral deltoid, the suprascapular region including the trapezius and the supraspinatus, and the anterolateral aspect of the neck. The results of a pain mapping study enabled Bayam et al. to report that the pain resulting from ACJ pathology was predominantly sharp and stabbing, localized to the anterior shoulder, and seldom radiated to the forearm (Fig. 9-19).[63] It was the most focal and the least severe compared with pain arising from other shoulder disorders.

The positive value of pain diagrams for detecting and diagnosing AC disorders was shown by Walton et al.[952]

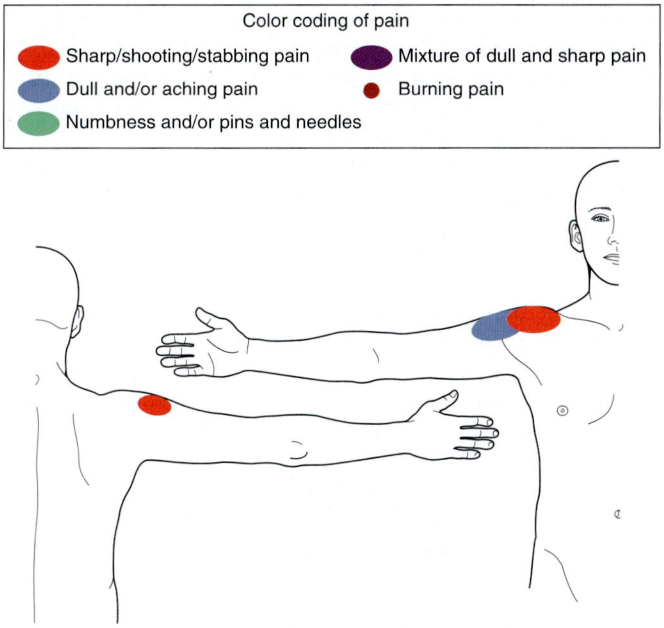

FIGURE 9-19: Mapping for acromioclavicular joint pain. (Modified from Bayam L, Ahmad MA, Naqui SZ, et al. Pain mapping for common shoulder disorders. *Am J Orthop*. 2011;40[7]:353-358. Copyright 2011 The American Journal of Orthopedics.)

For the patient exhibiting shoulder pain between the mid-clavicle and the deltoid insertion with a positive Paxinos test (described under "Physical Examination") and a positive bone scan for uptake at the ACJ, the researchers were convinced that the diagnosis of ACJ pain was "virtually certain." Patients with a problematic ACJ do not commonly mention swelling or crepitus arising in or about the joint.

Physical Examination

With the patient either sitting or standing and the overlying clothing removed from both shoulders, the examiner looks for asymmetry: shoulder posture at rest, skin color, muscle bulk, and surface topography (Fig. 9-20). Both shoulders are examined for active motion, voluntary provocative maneuvers, skin temperature, tenderness, ligamentous laxity, passive motion, sensation, strength, circulation, and discriminatory maneuvers. The depth of examination of the cervical spine, remaining components of the shoulder girdle, and the upper limb is variable and determined individually.

The patient may be asked to identify as precisely as possible, the location of the pain. A positive "one finger test" is recognized when the patient points directly to the ACJ.[591]

Asymmetric tenderness well localized to the ACJ indicts the ACJ as the source of the symptoms, especially if the pain so produced is essentially the same in character as the pain experienced by the patient. It is sometimes very difficult to confidently identify and successfully palpate the ACJ when the patient is obese or very muscular. In these instances, it might prove helpful to reference the triangle formed by the clavicle, scapular spine, and base of the neck. The ACJ is directly anterior to an examining fingertip placed just medial to the acromion process at the lateral apex of the triangle (Fig. 9-21).

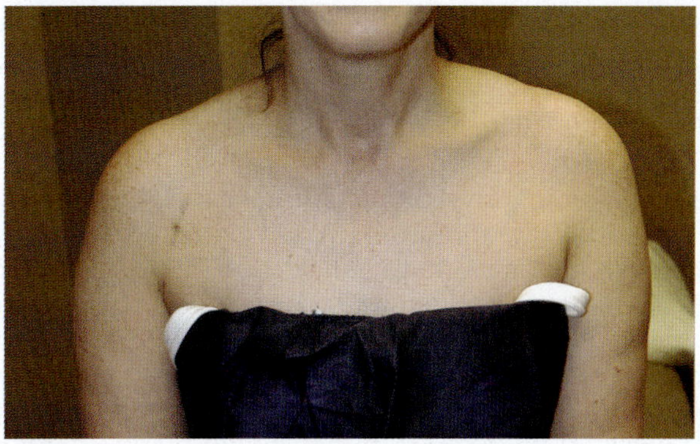

FIGURE 9-20: Patient preparation for physical examination requires unimpeded access to both shoulders.

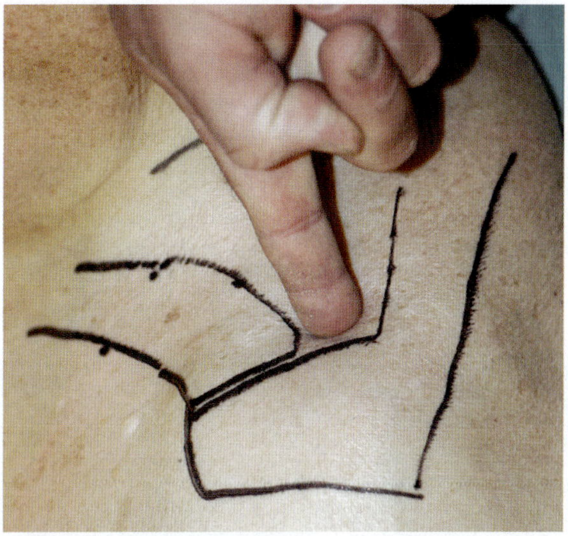

FIGURE 9-21: Surface landmarks helping to identify the acromioclavicular joint, which lies directly anterior to the soft spot at the apex of the isosceles triangle formed by the scapular spine, the clavicle, and the base of the neck.

Provocative Testing

Several pain-exacerbating examination maneuvers that suggest ACJ pathology have been described, including the cross-body adduction stress test, the AC resisted extension test, Buchberger test, the active compression test, and the Paxinos test.[119,420,592,678,952] However, in a systemic review with meta-analysis, Hegedus et al. concluded that the diagnostic accuracy of these orthopedic special tests could not be substantiated.[388] With the cross-body adduction stress test, the examiner passively elevates the upper limb to 90 degrees in the sagittal plane and, with the elbow either extended or flexed slightly, moves the limb medially (Fig. 9-22).[592] The test is considered positive if it reproduces pain in or near the ACJ.

The passive external rotation test uniquely stresses the ACJ compared with more traditional tests such as cross-body and active compression tests. With the arm at the side maintaining the thoracohumeral relationship with the flexed elbow, the arm is passively externally rotated to achieve the maximum range possible. The anterior deltoid muscle is passively stretched, resulting in pressure on the ACJ as the distance between the clavicle and acromion are reduced.[698]

The AC resisted extension test starts with the upper limb elevated 90 degrees in the sagittal plane, the elbow flexed to 90 degrees, and internal rotation to 90 degrees (Fig. 9-23).[420] With the examiner's hand fixed in the space against the posterior elbow, the patient extends the shoulder in the transverse plane, meeting the examiner's resistance. The test is considered positive if pain is experienced in the ACJ.

The Buchberger test combines inferiorly directed force to the lateral clavicle with passive forward elevation of the slightly adducted and externally rotated upper limb.[119] The test is considered positive if pain is invoked or intensified in or near the ACJ. To perform the Paxinos test, the examiner places a thumb over the posterolateral acromion and the ipsilateral or contralateral index or long finger (or both) over the superior aspect of the mid-part of the clavicle.[952] AS pressure is applied by the thumb while inferior pressure is applied to the acromion. The test is considered positive if pain is produced or intensified in the region of the ACJ (Fig. 9-24).

The active compression test is begun by requesting the patient to fully extend the elbow and forward elevate the upper limb 90 degrees in the sagittal plane followed by 10 to 15 degrees medial to the sagittal plane (Fig. 9-25).[678] The thumb is pointed downward by full internal rotation of the shoulder and pronation of the forearm. An inferiorly directed force is applied to the upper limb thus positioned. The force is released, the forearm is fully supinated, and the force is reapplied. The test is considered positive if pain is produced with the first maneuver and reduced or eliminated with the second maneuver. Pain in or near the ACJ indicates a problem of the ACJ.

The Bell–Van Riet (BVR) test, described in 2011, is a variation of a cross-body adduction test. The upper limb is passively elevated to 90 degrees, maximally adducted, and fully internally rotated, with the elbow in full extension and the forearm pronated.[935] The examiner facilitates maintenance of the extreme position—pain is considered a "positive cross-arm adduction sign." A resisted downward force on the forearm that evokes pain and inability to maintain the starting position is considered a positive

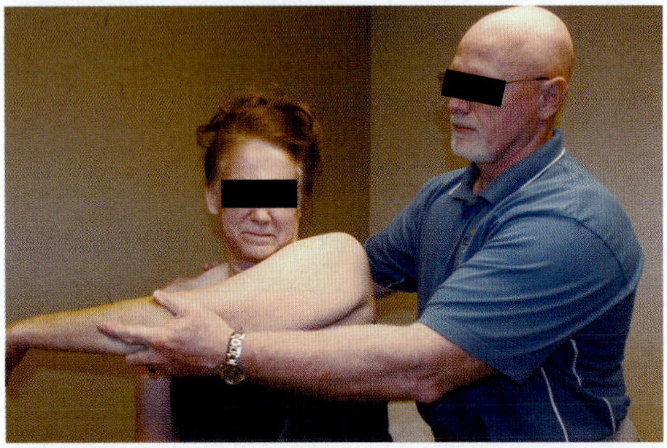

FIGURE 9-22: The cross-body adduction stress test.

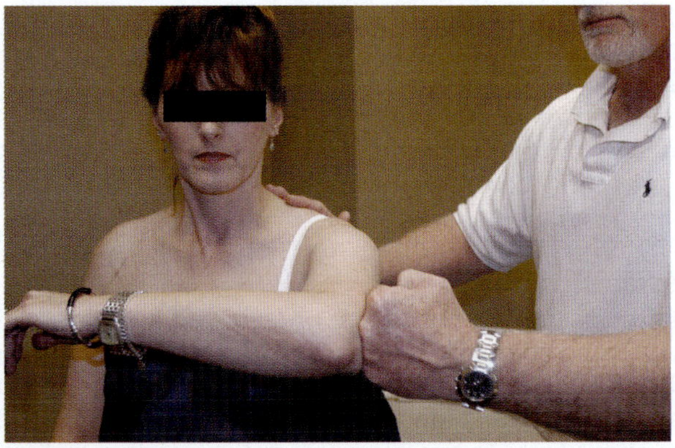

FIGURE 9-23: The acromioclavicular resisted extension test.

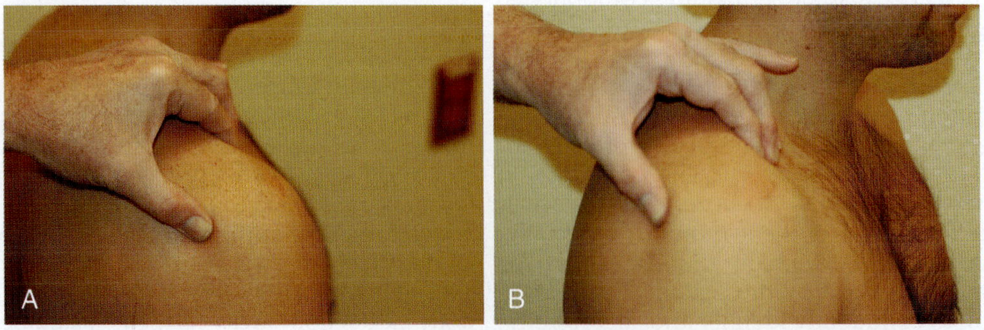

FIGURE 9-24: The Paxinos test. The examiner's thumb and finger are squeezed together. (From Walton J, Mahajan S, Paxinos A, et al. Diagnostic values of tests for acromioclavicular joint pain. *J Bone Joint Surg Am.* 2004;86[4]:807-812.)

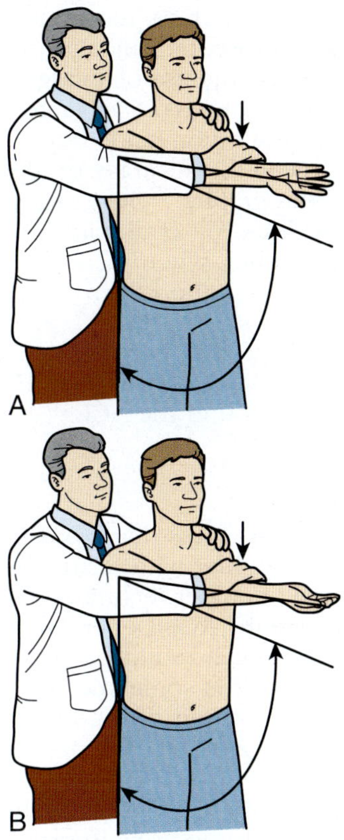

FIGURE 9-25: The active compression test. This two-step maneuver can help to distinguish between acromioclavicular joint and labral lesions. **A,** This maneuver may reproduce pain in the shoulder. Note a downward force being applied to the hyperpronated adducted limb, which has been raised to 90 degrees. **B,** This maneuver may reduce or eliminate shoulder pain. Note the limb in full supination. The test is considered positive if pain produced with maneuver one is reduced or eliminated with maneuver two. Both acromioclavicular joint and labral tears may be discerned by the location of the pain. (Modified from O'Brien SJ, Pagnani MJ, Fealy S, et al. The active compression test: a new and effective test for diagnosing labral tears and acromioclavicular joint abnormality. *Am J Sports Med.* 1998;26:610-613.)

BVR test. The maneuver can be repeated with the limb in external rotation. Essentially the same test was described in a nearly identical publication in 2013 and designated the sac test.[788] To better understand how the BVR test evoked pain, Alta et al. invited healthy volunteers 23 to 60 years of age with no history of shoulder problems to undergo 4D CT scanning of the shoulder with the arm adducted plus resisted elevation, essentially simulating the BVR test.[19] They observed that the clavicle translated posteriorly and superiorly, with some opening of the superior joint space and maintenance of joint width. Reduced translation and increased age were positively correlated.

I learned the hug test from Douglas Harryman and Frederick Matsen as an additional clinical tool for assessing the ACJ (Fig. 9-26).[375] The examiner stands at a right angle

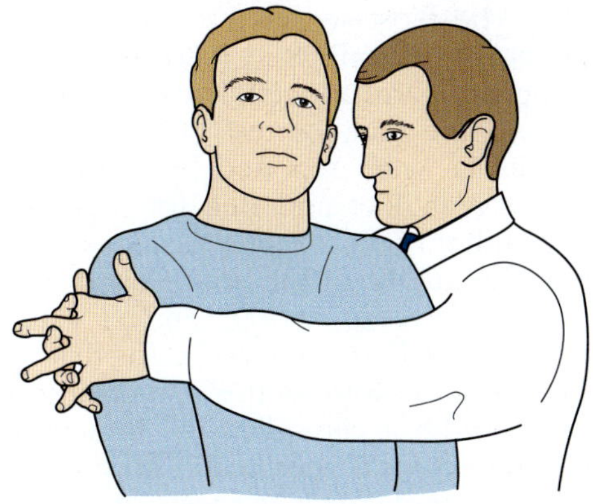

FIGURE 9-26: The hug test elicits pain from the affected acromioclavicular joint.

to the patient's symptomatic side, reaches around the patient's shoulders, and locks both hands together. The hug is then performed, compressing both shoulders in the coronal plane between the examiner's chest and hands. The test is considered positive if pain is produced or aggravated in or near the ACJ closest to the examiner.

Maritz and Oosthuizen showed high sensitivity for ACJ line tenderness and cross-body adduction stress testing.[567] O'Brien et al. determined that the active compression test exhibited a high degree of accuracy (100% sensitive and 96.6% specific) for ACJ lesions.[678]

In a study by Walton et al., ACJ tenderness to direct palpation had the greatest sensitivity for the detection of ACJ disorder in patients with shoulder pain, followed by the Paxinos test.[952] They also reported that the most accurate clinical maneuver for detecting an AC abnormality was the Paxinos test. Chronopoulos et al. analyzed patients with isolated chronic disorders of the ACJ to determine the diagnostic value of physical examination provocative testing techniques.[164] The most sensitive test, the cross-body adduction test, was also the least accurate. The active compression test had the greatest specificity, the least sensitivity, and the most accuracy. The AC resisted extension test was between the other two for all diagnostic values. Interestingly, provocative maneuvers described for other shoulder maladies (Neer impingement sign, Hawkins impingement sign, painful arc sign, drop arm sign, and Speed's test, Jobe's sign, neck tenderness) are capable of inducing pain in patients with chronic lesions of the ACJ.[567,164]

Using dynamic ultrasonography of the ACJ in normal volunteers, Park et al. concluded that the cross-body adduction and active compression tests resulted in more stress to the ACJ than the passive external rotation test, highlighting their utility.[698]

The response to local anesthesia instilled into the ACJ can help identify the cause of shoulder pain.[952,935] This is especially true when provocative testing is performed both before and after the injection. Von Reit and Bell ascertained the sensitivity of provocative clinical tests with local anesthetic and corticosteroid injection testing of the ACJ.[935] The most sensitive test was the BVR performed in internal rotation (98%), followed by the O'Brien test (83%), the cross-arm adduction test (67%), the Jacob's test (41%), and the Paxinos test (12%). Curiously, the exact same results were reported by Saccomanni, who failed to credit Van Riet and Bell for their work.[788] In addition, the author of this chapter has personally spoken with Shaffer, the author of the article cited by Von Riet and Bell and Saccomanni, and Dr. Shaffer stated "… I'm afraid that I did not find a reference for that test in my manuscript, nor am I aware of this particular test or have any experience with it clinically."[78,831] In a primary care setting that utilized local anesthetic injection testing followed by certain traditional ACJ tests, the limited diagnostic value of the tests was realized while combinations of aspects of history and physical examination appeared to provide more diagnostic value for identifying painful ACJ conditions.[128]

Despite the very superficial location of the ACJ, its relative size, variable anatomy, and pathologic changes often confound arthrocentesis. Successful needle entry into the joint often lacks tactile confirmation (Fig. 9-27). Bisbinas et al. reported incorrect placement more than 60% of the time when orientation to the joint was obtained by palpation alone.[89] Accuracy of intra-articular placement confirmed by arthrography was 43.3% in a study by Wasserman et al.[961] In cadaver studies, ACJ injection accuracy by palpation was 57% to 70%.[103,701,725] The use of ultrasound guidance improved the accuracy to 90%.[103] When the accuracy of injection in the clinical setting is deemed critical, some authors recommend using image intensification or fluoroscopic guidance to improve accuracy.[89,725] Others advise the use of sonography, which has been shown to be 98% to 100% accurate compared with the 40% accuracy of injection guided by palpation.[708,785,258] Edelson et al. showed the accuracy of ultrasound-guided injection with arthrography.[258] Reiterating their sources, Daley et al. as well as Aly et al. cited that the injection accuracy rate is higher when performed with image-guided assistance versus the landmark-guided approach (palpation) (93.6% vs. 68.2%).[202,20] Surgical decision-making with respect to the response to injection should take into account all the factors and current data relevant to injections in and around the ACJ.

Imaging

Plain Radiographs

Due to its composition of less-dense bone and its location in a region of the shoulder with relatively less soft tissue coverage, standard shoulder techniques must be altered to properly delineate the ACJ. Depending on the patient's stature or body habitus, a reduction of x-ray kilovoltage by as much as one-half is sometimes necessary in order to gain optimal visualization of the ACJ.[768,1012]

Anteroposterior View

It is preferable to obtain this view with the patient either standing or sitting with the arms unsupported and neutrally positioned in the sagittal plane. Anatomic variations and technical inconsistencies are effectively dealt with by imaging bilateral ACJs simultaneously on a single cassette or on two smaller cassettes for wider patients (Fig. 9-28).

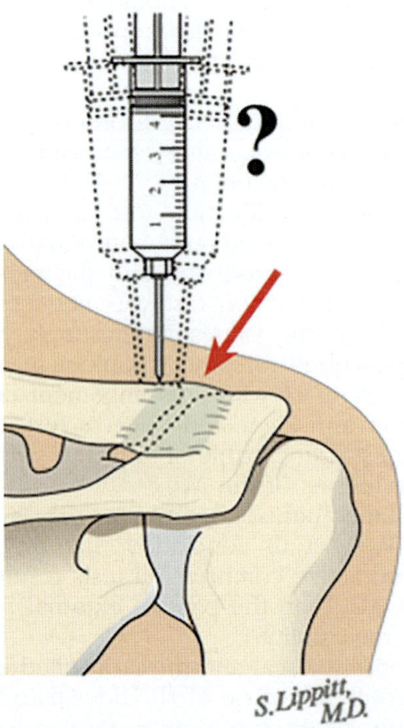

FIGURE 9-27: Even with vast experience, acromioclavicular joint injections are easier said than done. (Courtesy Steven Lippitt, MD.)

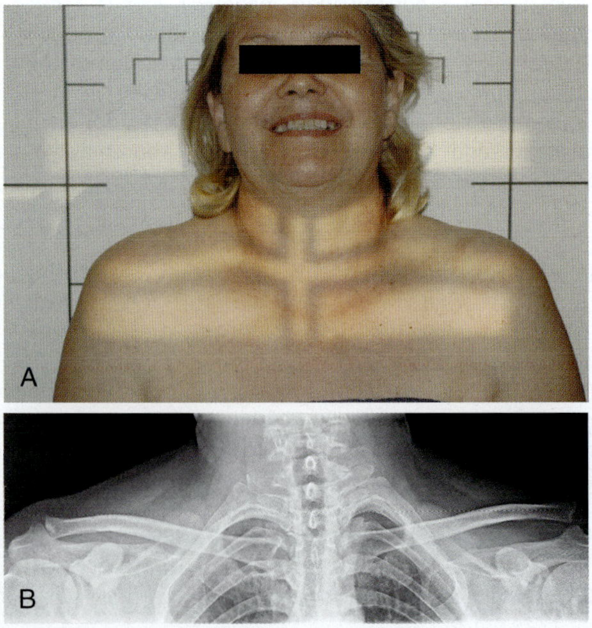

FIGURE 9-28: Positioning and technique for Zanca views. Both shoulders **(A)** are imaged simultaneously on one or two cassettes **(B)**, depending on the width of the shoulders.

A 10- to 15-degree cephalic tilt applied to the x-ray beam optimizes the image of the ACJ by eliminating its superimposition on the posterior acromion and lateral scapular spine (Fig. 9-29).[1012]

Dimensions and configuration are extremely variable, mandating a cautious approach to interpretation in the setting of injury.[446,929] AC width ranges from 0.5 mm to 7 mm,[686,720,1012] and the CC interval ranges from 1.1 cm to 1.3 cm.[64,110]

Lateral Views

One of two views is selected: either an axillary lateral view or a scapular Y view. The axillary view offers an advantage for determining the anterior or, much more commonly, posterior displacement of the clavicle (Fig. 9-30). The scapular Y view highlights superior displacement of the clavicle, although posterior displacement can be demonstrated (Fig. 9-31).

Other Views

The axial and tangential views of the ACJ have been described in normal volunteers.[150] The views are not in widespread usage, and their role in injury assessment and treatment has not been investigated.

Stress Views

It is sometimes possible to subject the acutely injured shoulder to an additional deforming stress as an aid to diagnosis. A radiograph obtained simultaneously with the stress maneuver often captures the critical information sought by the examiner. Stress views can facilitate the diagnosis and characterization of the severity of an AC dislocation, although some question their value.[71,104,166,900,1004] In a survey of members of ASES, which had a 94% response rate, 81% indicated that they did not recommend the routine use of stress radiographs in the emergency department,[1004] and 57% did not use the views. Only 9% changed their treatment plan based on the outcome of the views. The radiographic assessment for nontraumatic conditions of the ACJ does not usually incorporate stress views.

Anteroposterior Stress Views

For standard AP stress views, the technical principles and patient positioning are unchanged from routine AP views of the ACJ. Stress of 10 to 15 pounds is applied to both upper limbs while the patient is invited to relax as much as possible. The method of weight attachment to the upper limb, hand-held versus wrist-suspended, might not be important.[850] It may be possible to ascertain avulsion of the anterior deltoid by other forms of stress application, but the accuracy of a weight-lifting view and its role in the routine assessment of suspected AC dislocations has yet to be determined.[48]

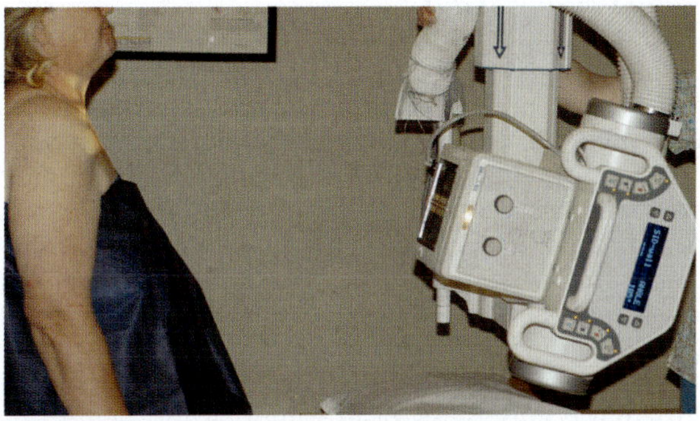

FIGURE 9-29: The Zanca view is taken with the x-ray beam directed 10 to 15 degrees cephalad.

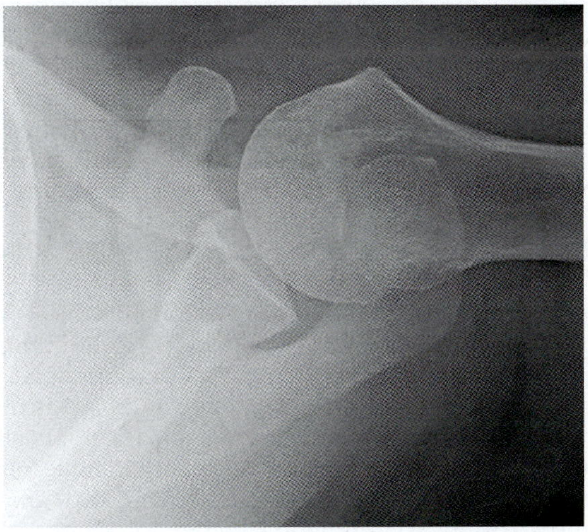

FIGURE 9-30: The axillary lateral view enables assessment for anterior or posterior displacement of the clavicle with respect to the acromion.

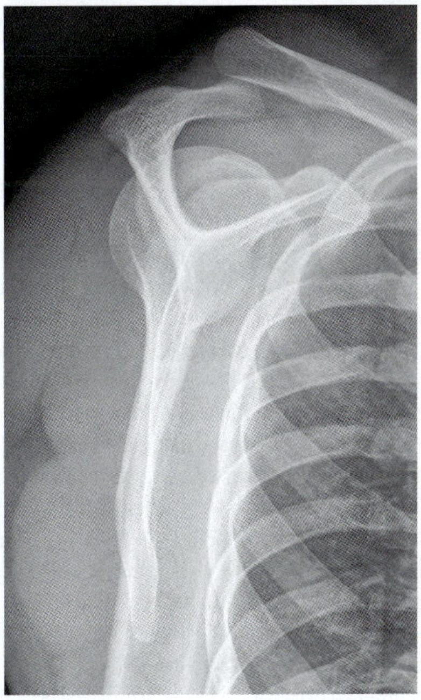

FIGURE 9-31: Scapular Y view showing superior displacement of the clavicle resulting from an injury.

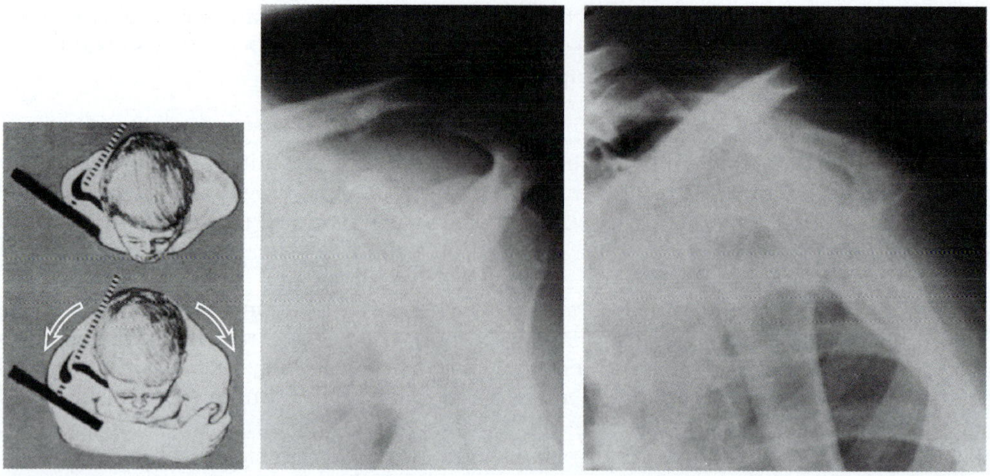

FIGURE 9-32: Lateral stress or Alexander views to assess for injury of the acromioclavicular joint. *Left,* The shoulders are thrust forward while the radiograph is taken. *Center,* Alexander view in the relaxed position. The acromioclavicular joint is only minimally displaced. *Right,* With the shoulders thrust forward, the acromion is displaced anteriorly and inferiorly under the distal end of the clavicle.

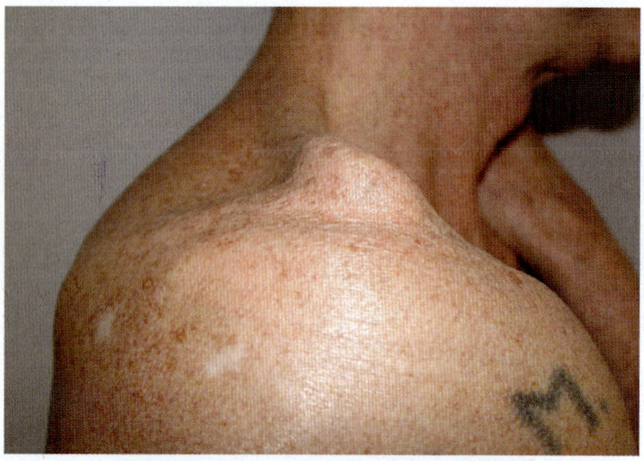

FIGURE 9-33: Clinical appearance of the lateral stress view.

Lateral Stress Views

It is possible to demonstrate pathologic relationships between the acromion and the clavicle by using a shoulder-forward view (Alexander view), obtained like a scapular Y while the patient actively protracts the shoulder (Figs. 9-32 and 9-33).[13-15] Although it is anticipated that this stress will displace the acromion anterior and inferior to the clavicle, more comprehensive imaging may be necessary to properly define the severity of injury.[950] A similar cross-body adduction view was reported and used by Barnes et al. to help identify a stable or unstable ACJ, and was identified by Beitzel et al. as the Basamania view (Fig. 9-34).[71,54] Tauber et al. described the advantages of dynamic axillary views in instances of suspected ACJ injury for determining the presence of horizontal instability.[900] With this view, they introduced the concept of gleno-acromio-clavicular angle as a means to quantify the translations of the distal clavicle observed while the shoulder assumed three specific positions for the axillary radiograph (Fig. 9-35).

Computed Tomography

The primary purpose of CT is to obtain a more accurate assessment of the morphology of the distal clavicle, coracoid process, and acromion process and, to a lesser extent, their relationships with one another. Accounting for differences in patient positioning, reduced gravitational forces may come to bear upon CC and AC relationships. It can aid in the analysis of complex injuries, fractures, neoplastic processes, or infections, especially when postprocessing 3D images are generated (see Fig. 9-10A). Wide view 4D CT scanning (dynamic) has been described, and provides an opportunity to document multiplanar components of ACJ injuries and better understand their significance (Fig. 9-36).[249]

Nuclear Medicine

When there are no other clues to a diagnosis in the presence of vague shoulder pain, bone scintigraphy is helpful to rule out an occult osseous lesion of the shoulder girdle. It is an excellent imaging tool for accessing semiacute injuries to the ACJ and ACJ arthropathy. The scan is positive when it demonstrates focal increased radioactive tracer uptake when compared with the uninjured contralateral side, especially if the plain radiographs demonstrate bilateral symmetrical AC arthrosis (Fig. 9-37). It confirms the ongoing osseous activity in cases of osteolysis. Walton et al. found that bone scanning had a higher degree of accuracy for determining an AC abnormality than did MRI or plain radiographs.[952] In this study, it had a higher predictive value (positive and negative) than did clinical testing or local anesthetic injections. While usually not necessary, single-photon emission computed tomography (SPECT) scan imaging has the capacity to render the active processes at the ACJ in a dramatic manner (Fig. 9-38). Tc-99m leukocyte imaging has proved useful in instances of septic arthritis of the ACJ.[1017]

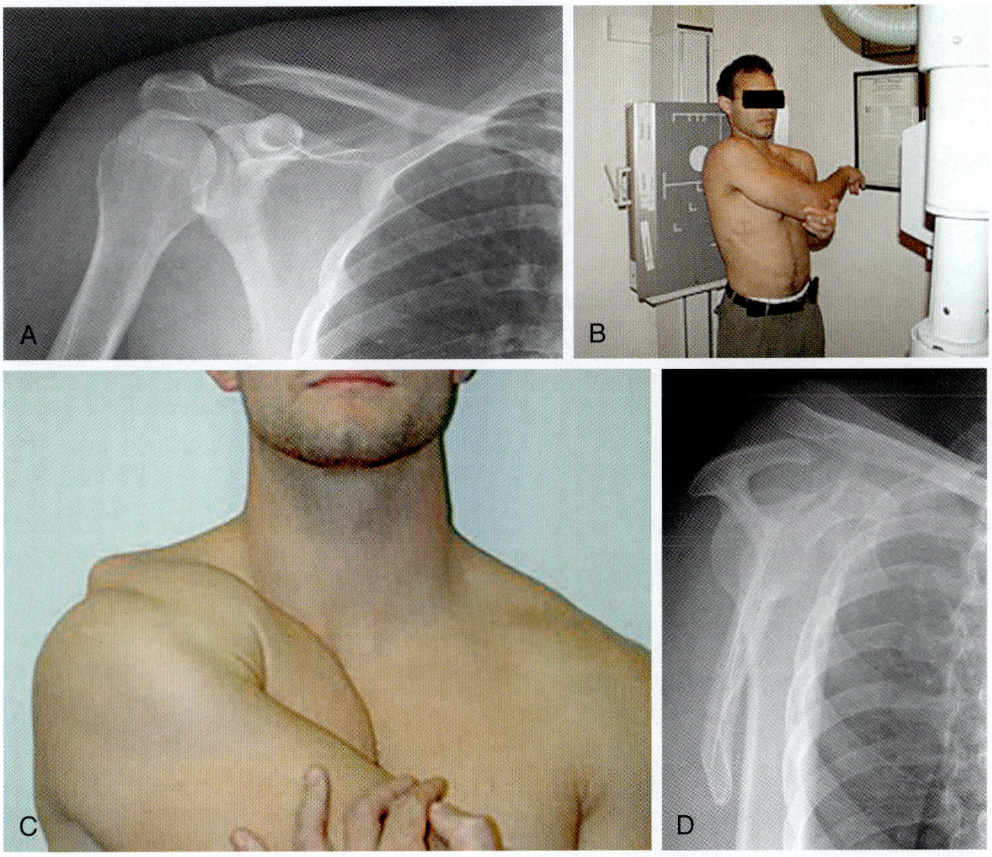

FIGURE 9-34: Basamania view. **A,** Anteroposterior view showing widening of the acromioclavicular joint and the coracoclavicular interval. **B,** The patient pulls the elbow of the affected arm to their midline using the unaffected arm. **C,** Clinical appearance. **D,** The acromion process of the scapula has rotationally translated internally, medially, and inferiorly beneath the distal clavicle, which is indicative of instability. (Courtesy Carl Basamania, MD, The Polyclinic, Seattle, WA.)

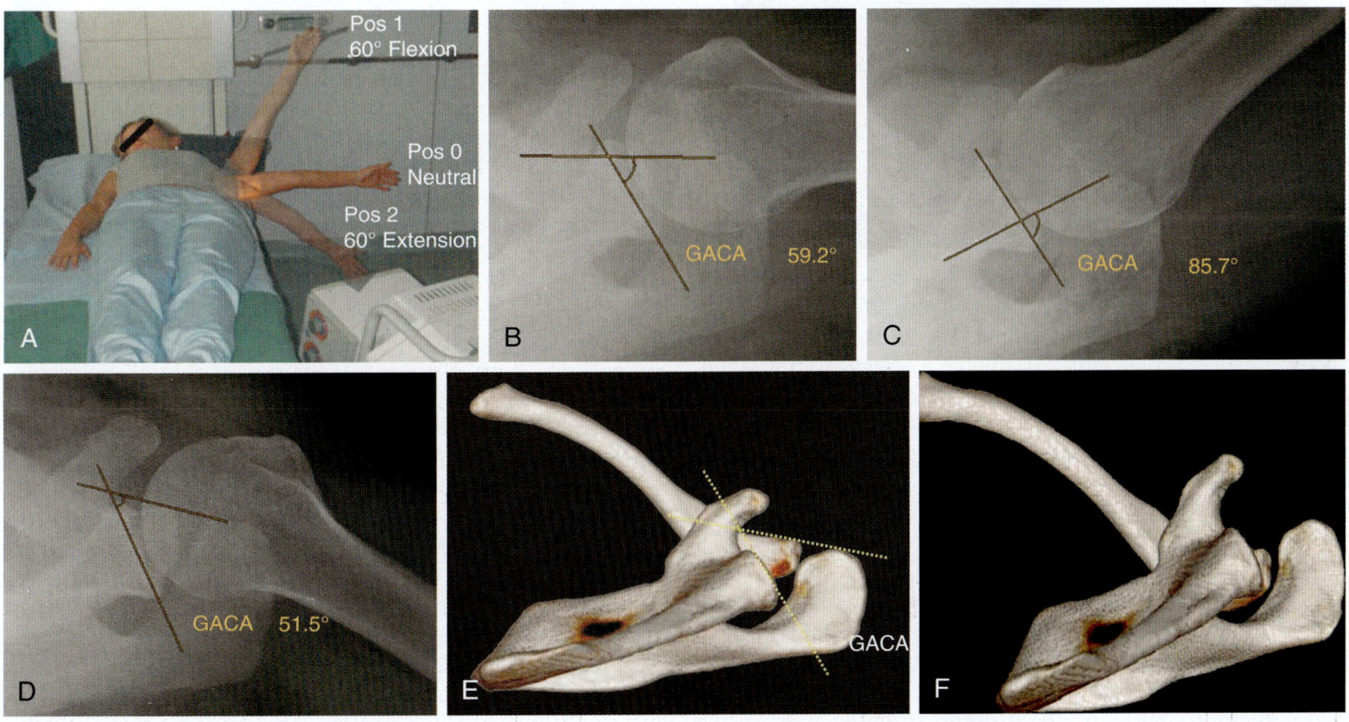

FIGURE 9-35: Functional axillary view used to reveal dynamic horizontal instability. **A,** Patient positioning. **B,** Position 0. **C,** Position 1, detecting posterior dislocation. **D,** Position 2, detecting anterior dislocation. **E,** Surface computed tomography of position 0. **F,** Surface computed tomography of posterior dislocation. GACA, Glenoacromioclavicular angle. (From Tauber M, Koller H, Hitzl W, et al. Dynamic radiologic evaluation of horizontal instability in acute acromioclavicular joint dislocations. *Am J Sports Med.* 2010;38[6]:1188-1195.)

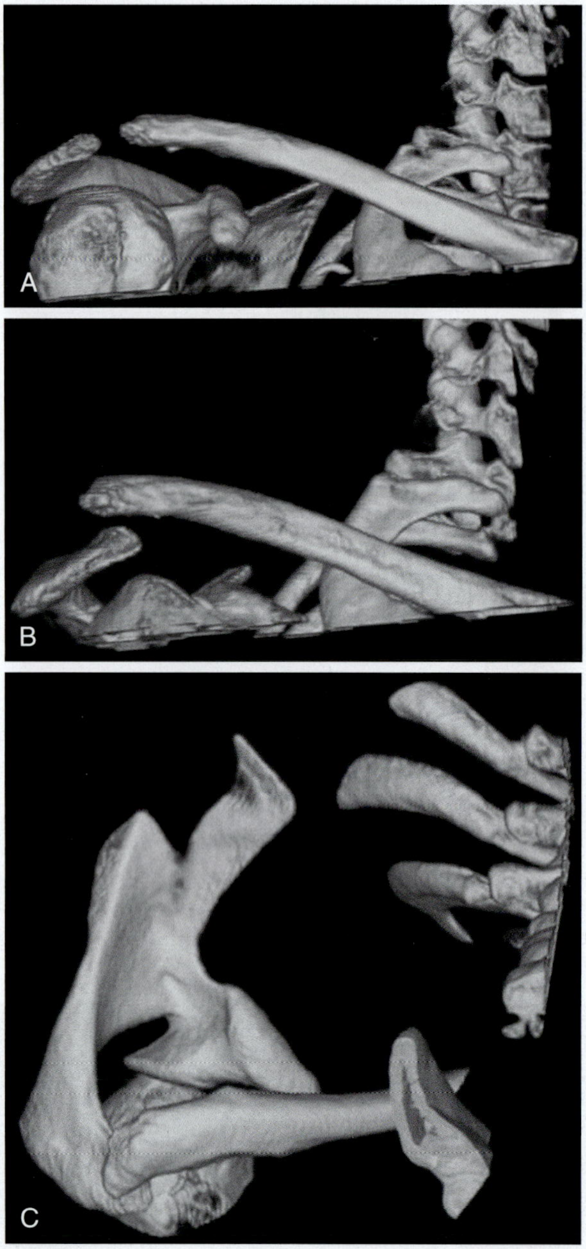

FIGURE 9-36: **A** to **C,** Examples of the type of advanced imaging that may enhance acromioclavicular joint classification schemes. (From Dyer DR, Troupis JM, Kamali MA. Wide field of view CT and acromioclavicular joint instability: a technical innovation. *J Med Imaging Radiat Oncol.* 2015;59[3]:326-330.)

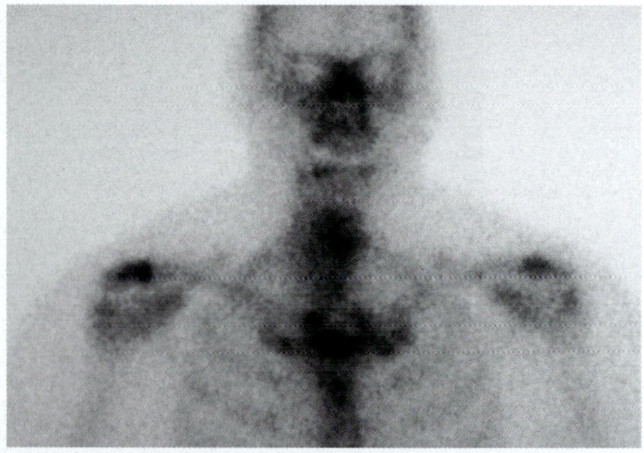

FIGURE 9-37: The 2-hour delayed image technetium-99m bone scan revealing intense uptake in the right acromioclavicular joint.

Magnetic Resonance Imaging

MRI effectively displays the pathologic changes that result from injuries and nontraumatic disorders that involve the ACJ.[21,25,341,654] New MRI scan orientations for the ACJ and specifically to appropriately image the CC ligaments have been described and their utility confirmed in a report by Schaefer et al.[21,25,810] Complete correlation of clinical, plain imaging, MRI and pathologic findings may prove difficult.[54,654,810] While currently not particularly practical, stress MRI has been shown to distinguish partial from complete injuries as well as functional integrity of the ligament.[419] However, plain films usually suffice and do so at significantly less expense.

MRI is the best imaging modality for assessing masses or cysts in the region of the ACJ.[254,496,833] In that setting, it can delineate the internal characteristics, margins, and surrounding tissue response to the mass. Concomitant massive RC tears are identified in many instances.

The value of the routine use of MRI for the diagnosis and management of arthropathy of the ACJ has been questioned.[646] One reason is because it is exceedingly rare that an MRI report for a patient with shoulder pain fails to mention an abnormality of the ACJ due to its high sensitivity for detecting AC abnormalities.[646,871,952] Another is that degenerative findings of the ACJ are just as likely to be present in asymptomatic persons.[871] The importance of the clinical evaluation in the presence of this particular imaging abnormality cannot be overemphasized.

In the study by Walton et al., MRI had a higher predictive value (positive and negative) than did clinical tests or local anesthetic injections.[952] It has been shown to be more sensitive for OA than conventional radiography.[210] Fiorella et al. reported a 12.5% incidence of increased T2 signal in a series of shoulder MRI examinations, and stated that it usually was of no clinical significance except in patients with chronic AC pain and no other imaging abnormalities.[294] Increased T2 signal intensity representing edema is also a common finding in traumatic and arthropathic conditions of the ACJ (Fig. 9-39).[221,294,441] MRIs of patients with symptomatic ACJs are more likely to show edema in the distal clavicle and higher grades of OA than in asymptomatic patients. Reactive bone edema in the distal clavicle, medial acromion, or both is a more reliable predictor of AC pathology than are degenerative changes.[839] Fluid in the ACJ is a common MRI finding in patients with shoulder problems (Fig. 9-40).[822] Advancing age, ACJ osteophytes, and GHJ fluid are notable associated findings that suggest a relationship between ACJ fluid and OA.

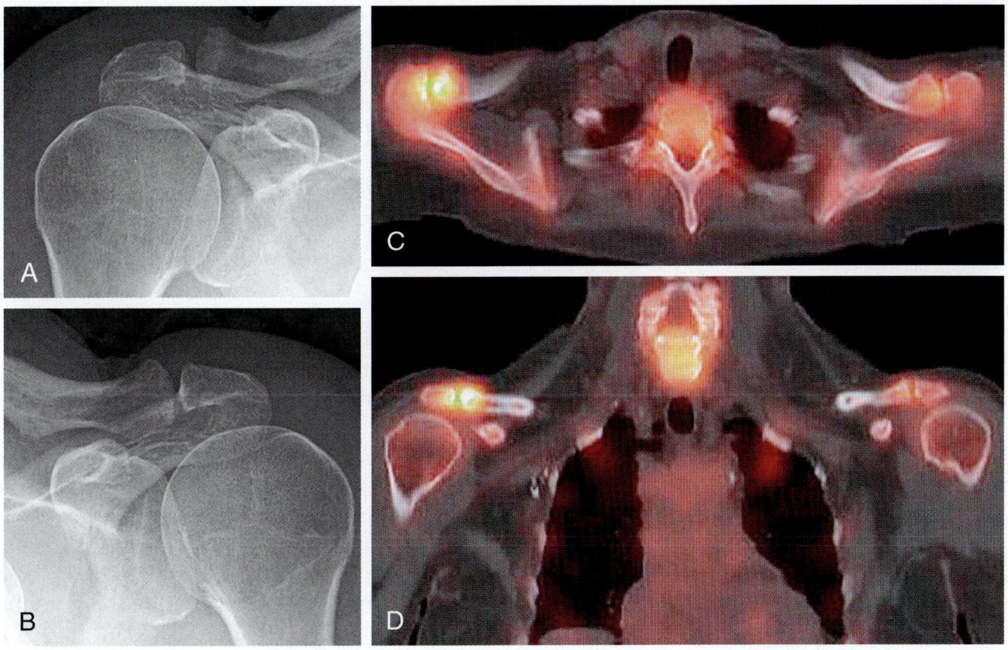

FIGURE 9-38: Single-photon emission computerized tomography images provide remarkable identification of an active process at the acromioclavicular joint on the right. **A,** Symptomatic joint. **B,** Asymptomatic joint. **C,** Axial cut. **D,** Coronal cut.

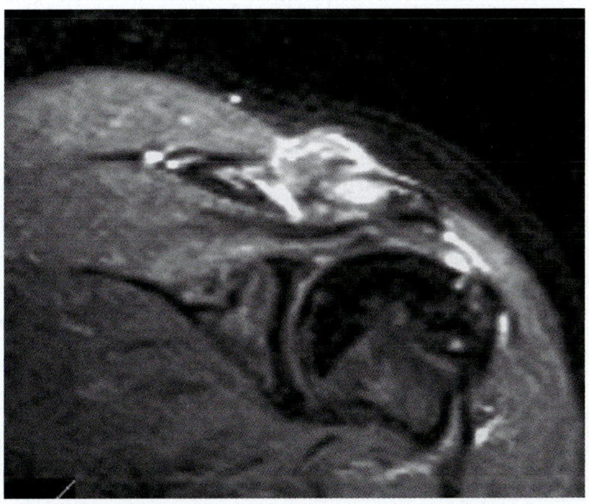

FIGURE 9-39: Magnetic resonance image showing increased T2 signal in the lateral clavicle.

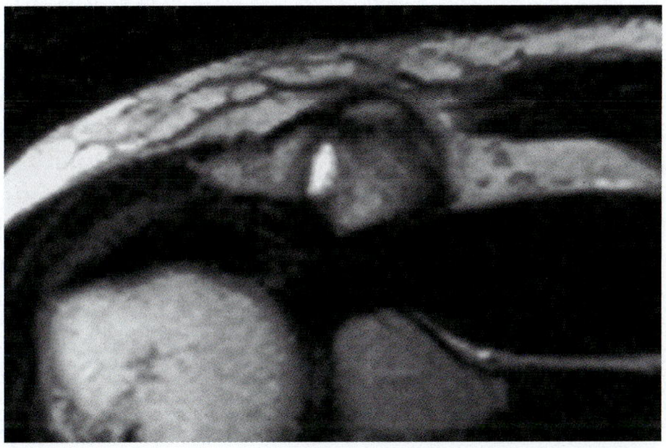

FIGURE 9-40: Magnetic resonance image showing fluid in the acromioclavicular joint.

With special techniques, the intra-articular disk may be distinguishable, when present, from the adjacent articular cartilage.[292]

Ultrasonography

Technologic advancements together with the expanding capabilities of ultrasonography have further stimulated an interest in applying this form of imaging to the ACJ.[290,386,414,574,695] Its reliability for the injured ACJ is well documented.[10,288,475,575,818, 850,851] Heers and Hedtmann have demonstrated the advantages of ultrasonography for determining the extent of injury to the deltoid and trapezius muscles and their common fascia.[387] They expressed concern that conventional sagittal plane radiography might have the limitations of either overestimating or underestimating the extent of soft tissue injury. A simple dynamic provocative maneuver performed with ultrasonography can aid in detecting lesser injuries to the ACJ, such as type I injury.[710]

Blankstein et al. favored ultrasonography for assessing patients presenting with atraumatic anterior shoulder pain, citing less pain, negligible ionizing radiation, and the visualization of degenerative changes that can go undetected by conventional radiography.[94]

Ultrasonography has proven utility for diagnosing septic arthritis of the ACJ.[979]

TRAUMATIC DISORDERS

Overview

As many as 40% of shoulder injuries involve the ACJ.[774] Most injuries to the ACJ and its environment are due to minor episodes of trauma that result in nothing more than contusions, minor strains, and sprains, never coming under the scrutiny of a healthcare provider, and from which full recovery is the norm. However, it is not infrequent that the events that result in injury to the ACJ are of sufficient magnitude to damage adjacent soft tissue structures, especially if the conditions of the sustaining force are considered high energy. Under these circumstances, the AC and CC ligaments and the attachments of the deltoid and trapezius muscles are susceptible to partial or complete tearing or avulsion.

ACJ dislocations represent 12% to 15% of all dislocations of the shoulder girdle and 8% of all joint dislocations in the body.[141,395,754] Emergency department visits for AC dislocation was 1.8 per 10,000 inhabitants in an Italian epidemiologic investigation, and 8.9 per 10,000 in a Scottish review.[156,395] In a Swedish urban population of nearly one-quarter million, taking into account both sexes and all ages, AC dislocations represented 4% of all shoulder injuries.[669] Dislocations were eight times more common in male subjects, and the prevalence was highest in the age group younger than 35 to 39 years, a finding also observed in previous investigations.[156,204,231,777,791,908,965] Shoulder injuries often happen during alpine skiing, and around 20% affect the ACJ.[472,963] In a prospective study of junior hockey players, ACJ injuries were second only to facial lacerations in terms of frequency of injury.[882] A recent study of shoulder injuries in competitive rugby players documented a 32% incidence of ACJ involvement.[384] Injury to the ACJ is the sixth most common among injuries sustained by collegiate-level football players (2.8%).[233] More than 96% are incomplete injuries (see below). The injury is 12 to 14 times more likely to occur during a game than during practice.[233,244] The incidence of ACJ injuries among all shoulder injuries sustained by players in the national football league during a 12-year period was 29.2%.[552] That review also found that quarterbacks sustained the highest rate of injury, with 21 injuries per 100 players.

Associated Injuries

Potentially high forces risk damage to other structures in proximity to the ACJ. Fractures of the ribs, scapula, humerus, and clavicle have occurred.[84,208,442,452,680,737,858,907,993,999,1006] Rarely, a simple avulsion from the clavicle may occur.[996]

Scapulothoracic dissociations have been reported, and add complexity to the management of ACJ injuries.[600,768] Isolated dislocation or sprain of the ACJ is infrequently associated with severe head, great vessel, or thoracic injury.[342] Pulmonary injuries have been reported.[49]

Neurologic injuries that can include the brachial plexus are rarely associated with AC injuries.[309,320,597,884]

Accompanying intra-articular GHJ lesions identified arthroscopically in both acute and chronic dislocations have included partial-thickness and complete-thickness tears of the RC, biceps tendon, and rotator interval; osteochondral humeral head defects; labral tears, especially type 2 SLAP lesions; and GHJ dislocation, sometimes treated concomitantly with the ACJ dislocation.[31,328,705,706,912] Individuals over the age of 45 years are at threefold greater risk of having such a lesion.[31]

Classification

The extent and severity of injury to the interconnecting and surrounding soft tissues of the scapula and the clavicle (the ACJ capsule with its intimate investing AC ligaments and CC ligaments and the deltoid and trapezius muscles) define the current and most widely accepted classification of ACJ injuries. Zaricznyj suggests that the term AC dislocation is an incomplete description of the most severe form of injury to the uniting structures of the two bones and that a complete separation of the two bones should be termed scapuloclavicular dislocation.[1013]

Injuries to the AC and CC ligaments may be distinguished by the preservation or loss of the gross structural integrity of the ligaments. Incomplete injuries result in no or only slight elongation of the ligament fibers, and complete injuries tear the ligament fibers into at least two separate pieces.[127] By virtue of strength alone, the AC ligaments are more vulnerable than the CC ligaments. The lowest energy injuries result in isolated damage to the AC ligaments, and higher energy injuries affect both the AC and CC ligaments. The most severe injuries damage the deltoid and trapezius muscles or attachments. This phenomenon of sequential injury, first mentioned by Cadenat, became the fundamental principle upon which the earliest classification schemes were based, and continues to captivate contemporary investigators with respect to pathoanatomy and mechanism of injury.[18,54,56,127,918]

Incomplete injury to the AC ligaments and no injury to the CC ligaments was termed type I. Complete injury to the AC ligaments with incomplete injury to the CC ligaments was termed type II. Complete injury to both the AC and CC ligaments was termed type III. Bannister et al. and Rockwood astutely recognized that certain injuries with displacement were sufficiently severe to warrant strong consideration for surgery as the preferred method of treatment, and proposed additional classification: type III subcategories A, B, and C by Bannister and separate types IV, V, and VI by Rockwood.[48,766,981] Rockwood's proposal gained widespread acceptance, and together with the original classification, it encompassed injuries to the ACJ in all recognized forms (Fig. 9-41). Type IV injuries are the result of a summation of force vectors that result in the clavicle eventually resting posterior to the acromion, penetrating the trapezius muscle, sometimes completely through its substance. The clavicle in type V injuries is displaced superiorly but because of disruption of the attachments of the deltoid and trapezius muscles, significantly more than in type III. Type VI injuries feature a clavicle displaced inferior to

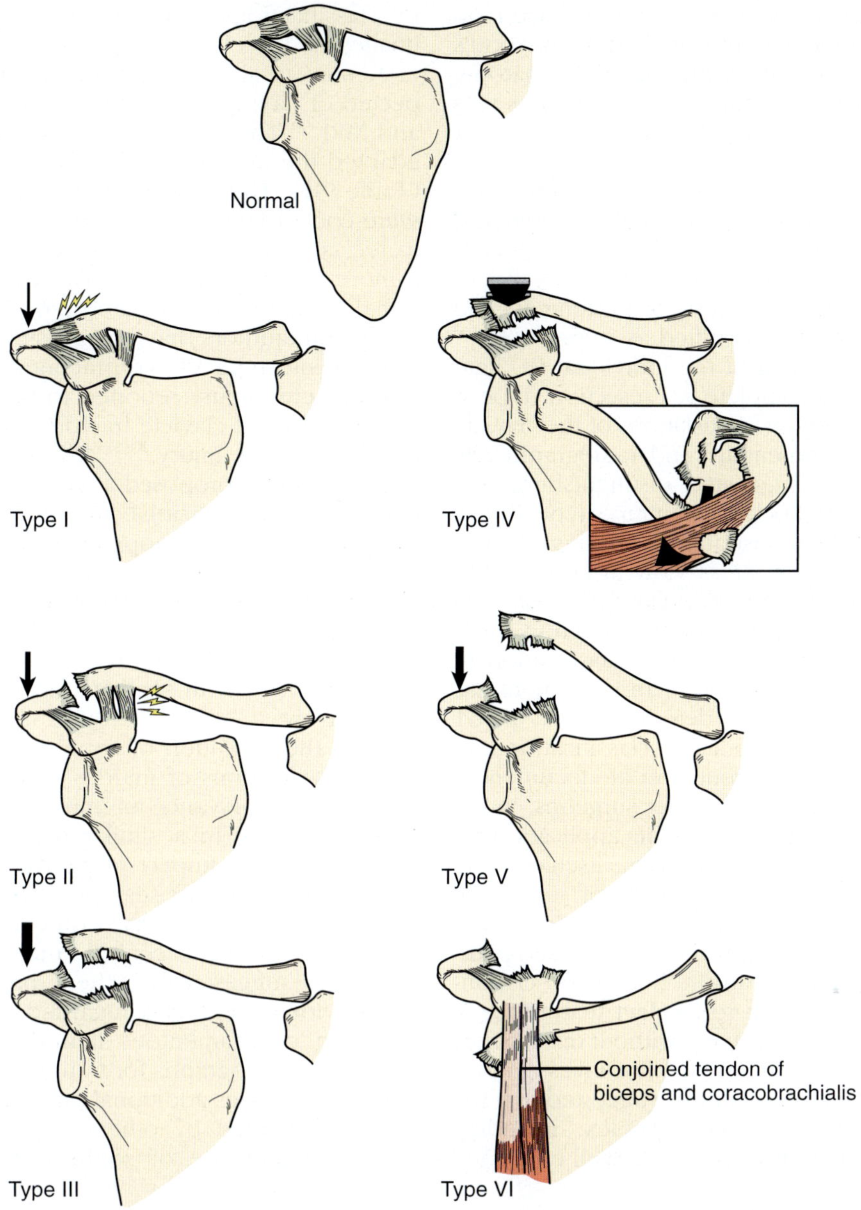

FIGURE 9-41: Classification of ligamentous injuries to the acromioclavicular joint. *Type I,* The acromioclavicular and coracoclavicular ligaments are intact. *Type II,* The acromioclavicular ligaments are completely torn, but the coracoclavicular ligaments remain intact. *Type III,* The acromioclavicular and coracoclavicular ligaments are disrupted. *Type IV,* The acromioclavicular and coracoclavicular ligaments are disrupted, and the distal end of the clavicle is displaced posteriorly into or through the trapezius muscle. *Type V,* The acromioclavicular and coracoclavicular ligaments are completely torn, and due to the severity of injury, the deltoid and trapezius muscles are detached from the distal clavicle. *Type VI,* The acromioclavicular and coracoclavicular ligaments are completely torn, and there is inferior displacement of the clavicle beneath the coracoid process.

the acromion or the coracoid process. An investigation of observer reliability for the diagnosis of ACJ injuries (limited to types III to V) found that consistency of grading was more common individually than it was among the individuals.[481]

Rockwood's classification represents an amalgamation of historical data derived from the analysis of plain and stress radiographs, anatomic dissections, cadaver experiments, and surgical observations infused with extensive, in-depth personal experience. On this basis, and rightly so, the pathoanatomy is often inferred, only to be resolved by direct visualization at the time of operative treatment or by means of more sophisticated imaging such as MRI and ultrasonography.[54,387] The latter concept was applied to four acutely injured patients, two uninjured patients, and one fresh frozen cadaver.[54] In two of the four injured patients, the type of injury based on classic plain radiographic parameters and Rockwood's classification did not correlate with the pathoanatomy detected by MRI. However, confirmation of findings was only possible in one of the four patients who elected for operative treatment.

Differences in ligament attachments and orientations support the notion of individual sprain of the conoid and trapezoid ligaments with ACJ injury.[889] Perhaps this is what Neer astutely recognized decades earlier as a subgroup of injuries resulting in less displacement and healing with stability that he identified as "type II ½."[647] Selective sequential sectioning of the individual CC ligaments in the presence of complete AC resection (type II "plus") documented pathologic translations of the clavicle rendering the joint experimentally and radiographically unstable.[585] Beitzel et al. suggested distinguishing two variations of the type III Rockwood injury: type IIIa, a stable injury without a demonstrable overriding clavicle on the cross-body adduction stress view, and type IIIb, an unstable injury with resistant scapular dyskinesia and an overriding clavicle on the cross-body adduction stress view.[71] The reliability of the Rockwood classification of ACJ dislocations as a tool for diagnosis and treatment has been questioned.[56,158,481] Cho et al. determined that 3D CT did not add further to the reliability of classification and treatment of these injuries.[158] Kraeutler et al. documented the inconsistency, even among shoulder surgeons, in the use of the Rockwood classification and its application for treatment decision making.[481] In cadavers, Eschler et al. investigated the plain radiographic results of sequential sectioning of the AC ligaments and joint capsule and the CC ligaments.[275] Their results confirmed the inferred pathoanatomic changes designated in the Rockwood classification, and also drew attention to the fact that a type V injury could be produced in cadavers without disturbance of the deltoid or trapezius attachments. The investigations and experiences of other authors have suggested that the instability patterns may be more complex, including medial instability, and may not always be well explained by classifications based on static rather than functional images.[44,56]

Nemec et al. prospectively imaged 44 patients suspected of having an acute ACJ injury with plain imaging and MRI.[654] Their findings resulted in a classification that adapted the Rockwood classification to the MRI findings (Table 9-1). The classification on plain imaging and MRI were concordant in 52.2%, and the results of the MRI led to reclassification to a less severe injury in 34.2% and to a more severe injury in 11.4%. The MRI identified additional ligamentous lesions in 25% of the patients.

Several authors have suggested subclassification of type VI into type VIa (supracoracoid or subacromial), a lower energy injury reported to be always accompanied by a diaphyseal clavicle fracture, and VIb (subcoracoid), a higher energy injury.[208,353,442,475]

Elamin et al. proposed a type VII injury based on their experience with a single instance of a locked superior AC dislocation.[265] Intraoperatively, the joint was irreducible and complete tearing of the AC and CC ligament with periosteal stripping of the lateral clavicle was observed. Resisted engagement with the acromion was reconciled by DCR, while CC and AC reconstruction was performed with synthetic ligament and direct repair, respectively.

With the evolution of sophisticated imaging, perhaps new classifications of injuries will emerge that take into account the relevance of multiplanar aspects of injury (see Fig. 9-36). In a similar manner, it is intriguing to contemplate the impact of similar clinical investigations with expanded databases upon the classification of these injuries.[387] Until then, based on current information gathered from relevant clinical and imaging reports, the author, as suggested by others, proposes a modification of the widely and highly regarded classic Rockwood classification of ligamentous injuries of the ACJ obtained from plain radiographs for traumatic disorders of the ACJ, that encompasses additional patterns of injury recognized and documented by others (Fig. 9-42).[71,208,249,265,353,442,475] Perhaps wider use of sophisticated imaging that may

TABLE 9-1 Ligamentous Lesions According to Rockwood Classification Adapted for Magnetic Resonance Imaging

Injury Type	Acromioclavicular Ligament	Coracoclavicular Ligament	Coracoacromial Ligament	Trapezoid and Deltoid Muscles
I	Partial tear	No tear	No tear	No tear
I+	Partial tear	Partial tear	No tear	No tear
II–	Complete tear	No tear	No tear	No tear
II	Complete tear	Partial tear	No tear	No tear
II+	Complete tear	Partial tear	Partial tear	No tear
III	Complete tear	Complete tear	No tear	Detachment from distal part of clavicle
III+	Complete tear	Complete tear	Partial tear	Detachment from distal part of clavicle
IV	Complete tear	Complete tear	Complete tear	Detachment from distal part of clavicle

From Nemec U, Oberleitner G, Nemec SF, et al. MRI versus radiography of acromioclavicular joint dislocation. AJR Am J Roentgenol. *2011;197(4):968-973.*

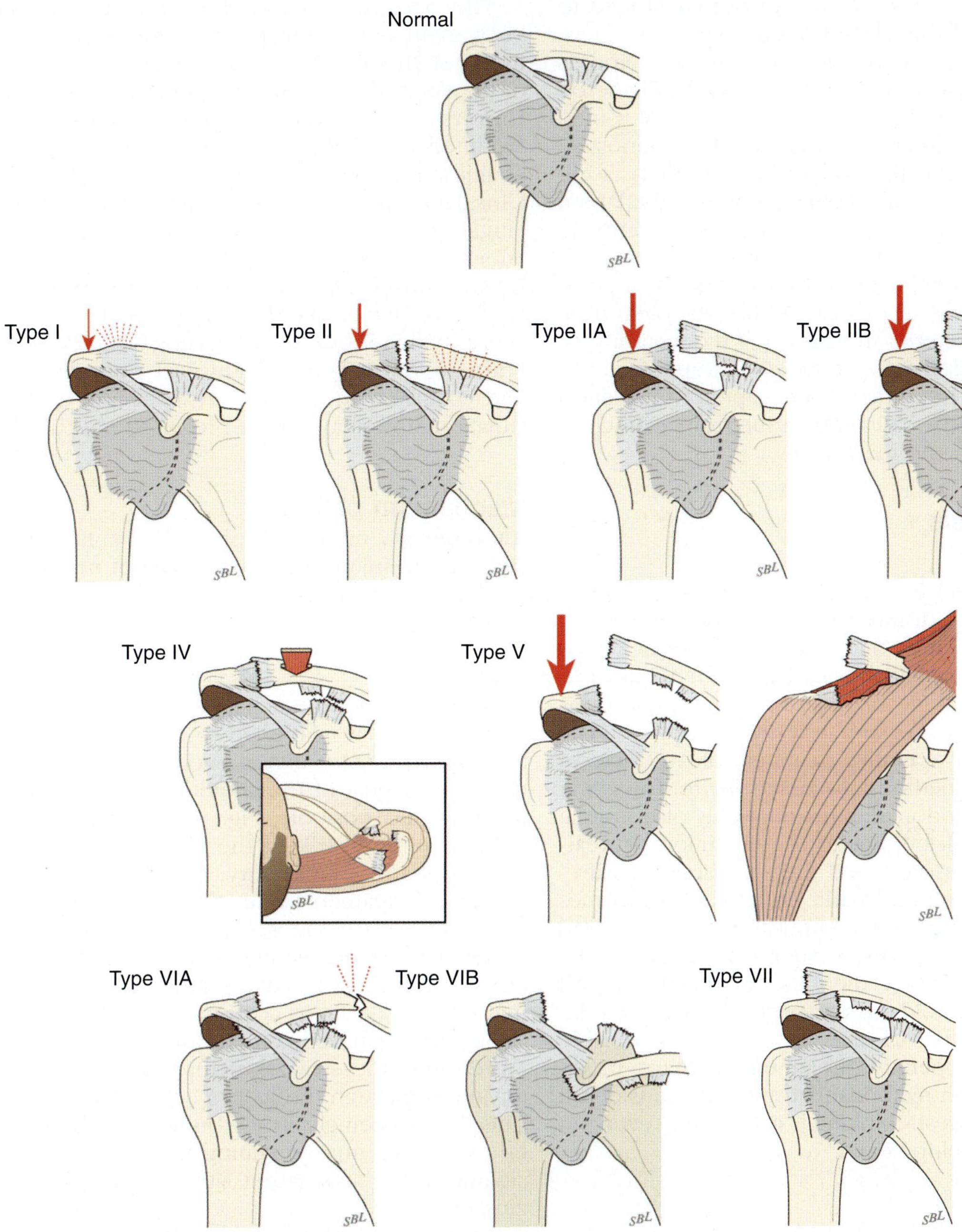

FIGURE 9-42: Author's proposed contemporary modified Rockwood classification of acromioclavicular joint injuries. *Type I,* The acromioclavicular and coracoclavicular ligaments are intact. *Type II,* The acromioclavicular ligaments are completely torn, but the coracoclavicular ligaments remain intact. *Type IIIa,* The acromioclavicular and coracoclavicular ligaments are torn. The extent of tearing of the conoid ligament enables stability with adduction stress testing. *Type IIIb,* The acromioclavicular and coracoclavicular ligaments are torn. The extent of tearing of the conoid ligament prevents stability with adduction stress testing. *Type IV,* The acromioclavicular and coracoclavicular ligaments are disrupted, and the distal end of the clavicle is displaced posteriorly into or through the trapezius muscle. *Type V,* The acromioclavicular and coracoclavicular ligaments are completely torn, and due to the severity of injury, the deltoid and trapezius muscles are detached from the distal clavicle. *Type VIa,* The acromioclavicular and coracoclavicular ligaments are completely torn, and there is inferior displacement of the clavicle beneath the acromion process but above the coracoid process accompanied by a diaphyseal clavicle fracture. *Type VIb,* The acromioclavicular and coracoclavicular ligaments are completely torn, and there is inferior displacement of the clavicle beneath the coracoid process. *Type VII,* The acromioclavicular and coracoclavicular ligaments are completely torn, and there is superior displacement of the clavicle above the acromion process. (Courtesy Steven Lippitt, MD.)

validate the results of in vitro investigations will lead to further refinement of this classification.

Classification of injury in the immature skeleton is similar to that in adults, and has been offered by Dameron and Rockwood.[205] Type I injuries are the result of a mild sprain without compromise of the investing periosteal tube. Type II injuries result from partial disruption of the superior periosteal tube with slight widening of the lateral clavicular physis. Type III injuries result from a complete disruption of the periosteal tube with less than 100% superior translation of the metaphysis. Type IV injuries result from a complete disruption of the periosteal tube with superior and posterior translation of the metaphysis. Type V injuries result from a complete disruption of the periosteal tube with more than 100% superior translation of the metaphysis. Type VI injuries result from a subcoracoid displacement of the metaphysis.

Treatment Analysis

General

According to Tamaoki et al., "… the available evidence for treating acute AC dislocations is of poor quality."[894] Beitzel et al. further stated that "there is lack of evidence to support treatment options for patients with AC dislocations."[70] With the passage of time, operative indications and treatment methods for any lesion come and go. The same can be said for operative treatment of ACJ dislocations. Some of the methods discussed in the following pages have been abandoned, remaining only of historical interest for their contributions to the evolution of treatment. Other methods described may be rarely or infrequently used either for predictable, unfavorable outcomes or unacceptably high rates of complications. General and specialty orthopedic surgeons today remain energetically engaged in the pursuit of the best treatment for ACJ dislocations. What unfolds in the pages ahead is a relatively brief summation of the application of reliable classic methods of operative treatment, perhaps modified, interspersed with methods that might be considered "state of the art," "fresh-thinking," novel, and even, in some instances, developmental.

Results

Comments and citations found in the treatment sections for types III below are generally relevant and applicable to types III, IV, V, and VI because many references include the treatment of more than one type of injury. Some authors have grouped treatment of types IV, V, and VI with the consideration that nonoperative treatment is the method of choice for types I, II, and III. Numerous authors have combined their results for treating type IV and V. Citations that report the results of comparative treatment are very frequent, and may likewise be applicable to more than one type of injury. Many authors report simultaneously the results of treatment of both acute and chronic injuries. The reader is advised to access the specific article as needed for clarification when necessary.

The outcomes of the treatment of ACJ injuries have been expressed in most of the validated scoring systems used for the shoulder. These include the Bother Index of the Short Musculoskeletal Function Assessment (MFA), University of California at Los Angeles (UCLA), UCLA Modified AC Score, SST, ASES, various versions of Disabilities of the Arm, Shoulder, and Hand (DASH) score, L'Insalata Score, Shoulder Pain and Disability Index, Single Assessment Numeric Evaluation (SANE) score, Subjective Shoulder Value (SSV), Constant-Murley (C-M), Japan Orthopaedic Association score, Nottingham Clavicle Score, Oxford Shoulder Score, Neer Score, Poigenfurst Score, Walch Score, Visual Analog Scale (VAS) Pain, Short Form-36, Short Form-12 Physical Component Summary, and cosmesis. In addition, ACJ-specific evaluation tools (Imatani, Taft) have been proposed and used.[410,501,811,887]

Mechanism of Injury

Although any number of physical events may be responsible for an injury, the mechanism of injury is a product of forces characterized by direction, magnitude, and point of application.

Direct

The most common mechanism for injury to the ACJ is a direct force that is applied to the superior aspect of the acromion process such as would occur with a fall onto the outer aspect of the shoulder with the upper limb in an adducted position (Fig. 9-43). A falling object or a deliberate blow striking the superior acromion is a rarer mechanism of direct injury.

The AC ligaments offer the weakest resistance to the forces that push the acromion inferiorly and medially; stronger resistance is afforded by the intact clavicle and SCJ.[65,989] Although isolated injuries are most common, AC injuries that occur in conjunction with clavicle fractures or SCJ injuries have been reported.[27,67,180,253,317,389,423,732,803,999] More often, these two structures are spared as the force advances through the ACJ to act upon the CC ligaments. This is an extremely strong buffer, but should its integrity be overcome, any remaining forces are likely to be dissipated at the attachment sites of the deltoid and trapezius muscle.

An inferiorly directed force acting upon the superior lateral clavicle can cause more damage when the upper limb is abducted and the scapula is retracted, and can result in an inferior dislocation of the clavicle beneath the coracoid process.[594,704]

Indirect

Indirect mechanisms of ACJ injury are exceedingly rare. A fall onto the adducted upper limb is apt to drive the humeral head into the inferior aspect of the acromion, subjecting the ACJ to variable degrees of injury (Fig. 9-44). The integrity of the acromion process and glenohumeral stability is risked when extremely high superiorly directed forces are encountered. The ACJ may be injured by pulling or traction-like forces applied to the upper limb.[530]

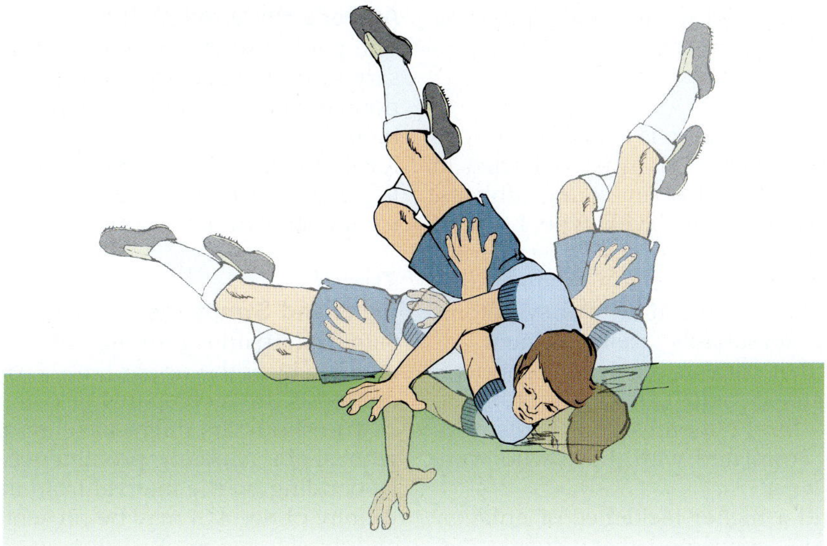

FIGURE 9-43: Acromioclavicular joint injuries most often result from a fall directly onto the point of the shoulder.

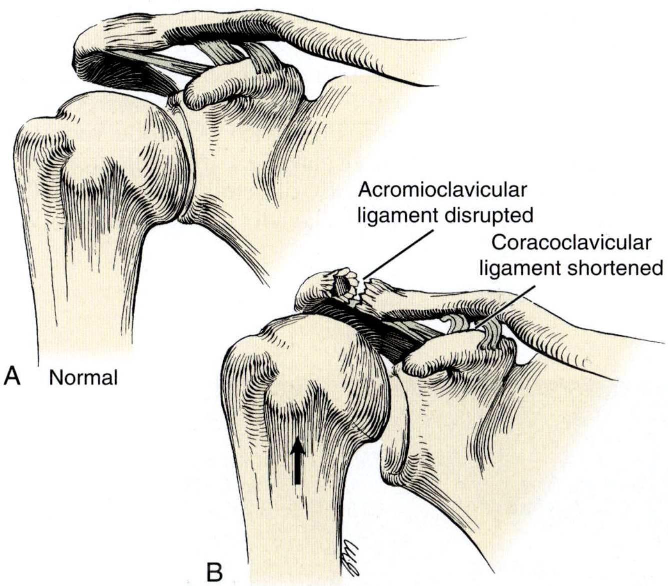

FIGURE 9-44: An indirect mechanism of injury that might occur from a fall onto the adducted upper limb results in complete tearing of the acromioclavicular ligaments while preserving the integrity of the coracoclavicular ligaments. (From Rockwood CA, Green DP, eds. *Fractures*. 2nd ed. Philadelphia: JB Lippincott; 1984.)

Acute Lesions

Type I

Signs and Symptoms

Mild pain is well localized to the ACJ, and may be aggravated by movement or maneuvers that load the upper limb. Although the ACJ may be slightly swollen, the shoulders are not unusually asymmetric in appearance. Active motion through a full range is sometimes hindered due to pain. Tenderness to some degree is appreciated at the ACJ but not overlying the CC ligaments. Palpable deformity of the joint is not present.

Imaging

Sometimes, the plain films demonstrate mild soft tissue swelling that accompanies type I injuries. Otherwise, the ACJ appears normal and exhibits symmetry to the uninjured shoulder.

Pathoanatomy

The AC ligaments sustain a mild-to-moderate sprain, maintaining the ACJ integrity. The CC ligaments and the deltoid and trapezius muscles are normal.

Treatment

Virtually all type I injuries should be treated without surgery.*

Methods

A sling or immobilizer for the upper limb helps to place the shoulder at rest. During the first 24 hours, cryotherapy can help reduce pain and swelling. Nonnarcotic analgesics are usually adequate for successful pain management. As the pain subsides, motion quickly recovers, and external support is discontinued. Although formal physical therapy is usually not necessary, some authors have advised non–pain-provoking gentle range of motion exercises, closed chain exercises, and muscle rehabilitation.[138,193,329] As the symptoms abate, isotonic progressive resistive exercises and open chain exercises are employed.[193] Participation in contact or collision activities is best avoided until motion has fully recovered,

References 18, 43, 47, 70, 91, 244, 516, 527, 628, 673, 674, 724, 747, 767, 768, 887, 918, 969.

tenderness has disappeared, and manual muscle testing is not painful.

Results

Full recovery of comfort and function is expected for type I injuries treated nonoperatively. This was confirmed in a report by Babe et al.[38] Time lost in young athletes, including collegiate football players with type I and II injuries was 10 to 12 days.[244,691] On occasion, symptoms are reported anywhere from 6 months to 5 years following injury.[80] More than 90% of the time, the symptoms remain insignificant or reasonably well tolerated.[80,194] Shaw et al. determined that patients receiving nonoperative care for type I injuries could expect symptoms to resolve, in most cases, by 12 months.[832] Patients with symptoms at 6 months correlated with those who were symptomatic beyond 1 year.

Mouhsine et al. found a higher incidence of unfavorable outcomes, and were concerned that adverse outcomes were underestimated.[628] In their study, operative treatment was necessary in 13% of type I injuries.

Complications

It is possible but quite unlikely that posttraumatic arthrosis would appear following a single type I injury. However, degenerative changes of the ACJ were reported in 56% of patients following a type I injury in the study by Mouhsine et al.[628] In some instances, degeneration was accompanied by pain, and necessitated a reduction in activity. Rarely, osteolysis of the distal clavicle develops as a late phenomenon after this type of injury.[1011]

Author's Preferred Method

The patient wears an upper limb sling as long as necessary to provide comfort and protection. Cryotherapy and nonnarcotic analgesics are preferred for pain management. Motion recovery is accelerated according to the level of pain. Resolution of ACJ tenderness and full, painless range of motion signal complete healing and return to unrestricted activities.

Type II

Signs and Symptoms

Significant pain is present both at rest and with attempted movement of the upper limb. Loss of functional range of motion is an accompanying complaint.

The shoulders might have an asymmetric appearance, with slight superior prominence of the distal clavicle. Depending on the interval from injury, ecchymosis in the vicinity of the ACJ may be present. Pain limits both active and passive range of motion as well as strength. The ACJ may be exquisitely tender, inhibiting reliable instability testing that might otherwise be positive for excessive excursion only in the AP plane. This can be demonstrated with a two-hand maneuver: With the clavicle and the acromion in grasp, opposing forces in the AP plane are applied to each bone, resulting in excessive movement of one with respect to the other when compared with the contralateral shoulder (Fig. 9-45). A subtle rebound phenomenon of the lateral clavicle can result from the application of light inferiorly directed pressure to the superior aspect of the lateral clavicle. CC ligament tenderness is present.

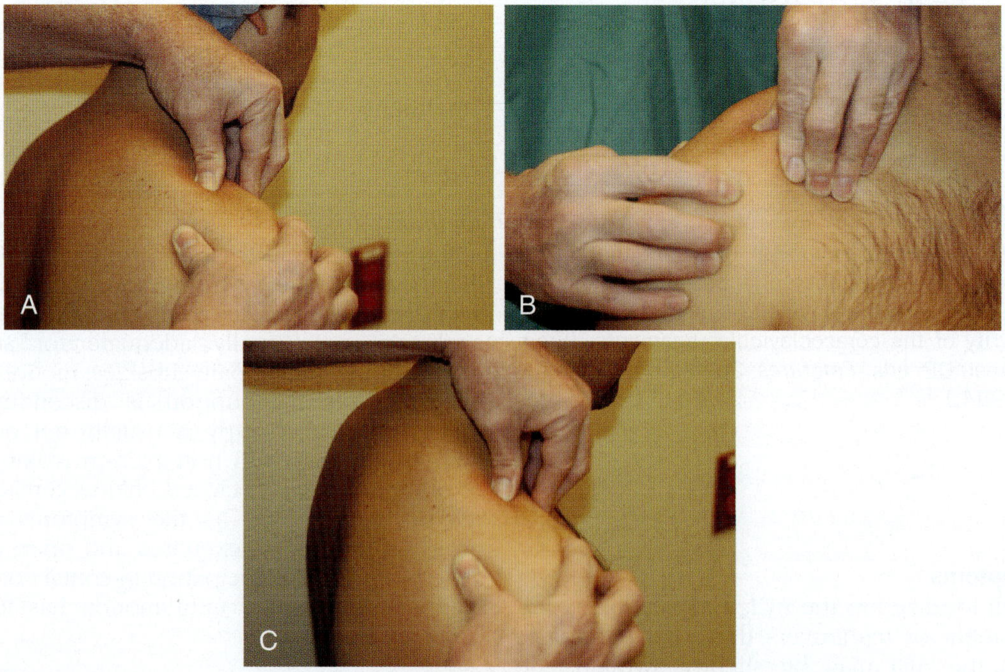

FIGURE 9-45: Anteroposterior stress test of the acromioclavicular joint. The clavicle is held as stationary as possible (**A**) while straight anterior (**B**) and posterior (**C**) stresses are sequentially applied to the acromion process.

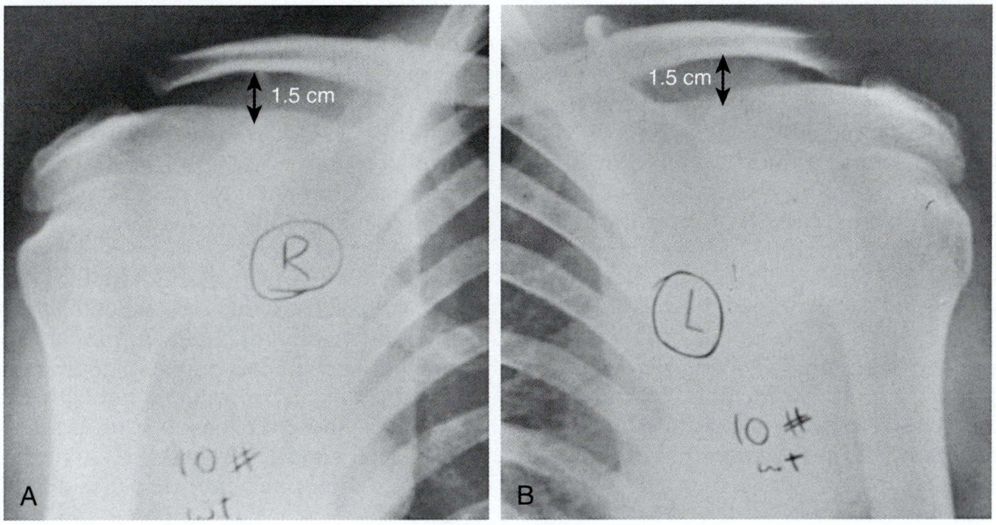

FIGURE 9-46: Radiographic appearance of a type II injury to the right shoulder. With stress radiographs, the coracoclavicular distance in both shoulders (**A** and **B**) measures 1.5 cm. However, the injured right shoulder (**A**) has a widened acromioclavicular joint compared with the normal left shoulder (**B**).

Imaging

Plain films can demonstrate subtle differences from the opposite, uninjured shoulder. The ACJ may be widened and have a slight incongruence resulting from the superior displacement of the lateral clavicle. The CC interval is normal and remains so when stress is applied (Fig. 9-46). The utility of MRI to distinguish type II from type III injuries has been suggested.[21,654]

Pathoanatomy

The AC ligaments are completely torn, resulting in disruption of the ACJ. The joint widens in the transverse and, less often, coronal planes. The CC ligament sustains a mild or moderate sprain that can result in slight widening of the CC interval. The deltoid and trapezius muscles are susceptible to partial detachment from the lateral clavicle. An extremely rare associated finding is fracture of the coracoid process.[239]

Treatment

Nonoperative treatment is preferred for type II injuries.*

Methods

The same fundamental methods for treating a type I injury are used for a type II injury. A sling or immobilizer for the upper limb helps to place the shoulder at rest. During the first 24 hours, cryotherapy can help reduce pain and swelling. Nonnarcotic analgesics are usually adequate for successful pain management. As the pain subsides, motion quickly recovers, and external support is discontinued. Although formal physical therapy is usually not necessary, some authors have advised muscle rehabilitation, particularly of the scapular stabilizers.[138,193,329] Later, as postinjury irritability subsides, more sophisticated exercises are employed.[193] Participation in contact or collision activities is best avoided until motion has fully recovered, tenderness has disappeared, and manual muscle testing is not painful. This is usually a bit longer for type II injuries, and can require 6 weeks or more.

Some authors have been tempted to treat the deformity associated with type II injuries. These methods use the concept of opposing forces applied to the clavicle and the acromion in a manner that theoretically reduces the subluxation and sustains the congruity of the ACJ until healing has been completed. Nearly 40 different methods have been described, all with limitations that include noncompliance, skin breakdown, and loss of reduction.[18,929-931] Most authors have abandoned an active form of nonoperative treatment in favor of a simple sling that is worn for a short time. At the risk of further, more serious injury while the ligaments heal, it is generally recommended that forceful maneuvers with the upper limb as well as contact or collision activities be avoided for up to 12 weeks.

Results

Shaw et al. determined that patients receiving nonoperative care for type II injuries could expect symptoms to resolve, in most cases, by 12 months.[832] Patients with symptoms at 6 months correlated with those who were symptomatic beyond 1 year.

Even with slight degrees of incongruence of the ACJ, full recovery with return to their preinjury status is expected in most cases.[91,696] However, sometimes, despite apparent ligament healing, discomfort and dysfunction linger unexpectedly long after the acute event, which is attributable to residual instability, infolded capsule, articular cartilage injury, meniscal injury, residual joint incongruity, and

**References 43, 70, 91, 194, 516, 527, 628, 673, 674, 724, 747, 754, 767, 768, 969.*

repetitive residual trauma.[59,80,194,385,556,674,861,878,951,982] A theoretical mechanism for such instability has been demonstrated in a cadaveric study.[585] Occasionally, such posttraumatic sequelae may necessitate operative treatment.[561] Mikek reported a mean follow-up of 10.2 years for type I and II injuries, and found that more than half of patients will experience symptoms and obtain noticeably lower functional scores when compared with the uninjured shoulder.[604] In their series, treatment was not necessary for symptoms. While joint dimensional differences were detected by ultrasonography, radiographic degenerative changes were not observed.[604]

Weakness has been reported.[385] Factors that can contribute to persistent symptoms include posttraumatic lateral clavicle osteolysis, intra-articular soft tissue entrapment, free-floating chondral or osteochondral bodies, and an unstable intra-articular disk.[67,878,17]

Complications

Reinjuries that occur before the ligament is completely healed can unexpectedly convert a type II into a type III injury. Skin breakdown beneath immobilizing devices forces abandonment of type II injury treatment while the integument heals.

ACJ incongruence, especially in the setting of extreme use, can precipitate symptomatic arthrosis. Such degenerative changes (arthrosis and osteolysis) of the joint have been reported, with an incidence as high as 70% (Fig. 9-47).[17,749,1011]

Author's Preferred Method

Nonoperative treatment is directed toward effective pain management by means of a sling, cryotherapy, and narcotic analgesics. This can require 1 to 2 weeks. Pool therapy is encouraged, and hastens the recovery of active, pain-free movement. Once motion fully recovers and tenderness abates, strength rehabilitation is initiated. Forceful use and contact and collision activities are avoided for 12 weeks.

Type III

Signs and Symptoms

The patient has moderate to severe shoulder pain. Pain is not only localized to the ACJ but can also emanate from the CC and periscapular regions. Motion, either active or passive, in any direction and to any degree, exacerbates the pain. Neurologic symptoms are very rare.

The patient appears acutely injured, often with the affected upper limb postured in a protective and stress-relieving manner: supported higher than usual by the opposite hand and arm and braced against the torso. The soft tissue overlying the acromion may be abraded or contused. Ecchymosis might or might not be present. The lateral clavicle is prominent beneath the skin, and the remaining shoulder has a drooped appearance (Fig. 9-48). The clavicles remain relatively level, while the weight of the upper limb displaces the clavicle inferiorly (Fig. 9-49).

Motion and strength assessment are unreliable due to pain. Tenderness is more diffuse: ACJ, distal clavicle, and CC region. Pain permitting, global instability of the clavicle is demonstrable. With the clavicle stabilized with one hand, it may be possible to reduce or nearly reduce the dislocated ACJ by placing the other hand beneath the flexed elbow and applying a superiorly directed force sufficient to often completely obliterate the visible deformity. The deformity returns when the force is removed. According to some authors, type III may be distinguished from type V if a well-performed shoulder shrug reduces the AC dislocation, implying intact deltotrapezius fascia.[584]

Imaging

The ACJ is incongruent from widening, and there is at least 50% contact loss between the acromion and the clavicle.[918] In the majority of type III injuries, there is no contact between the articular surfaces of the lateral clavicle and the medial acromion. The CC interval is widened 20% to 100% (Fig. 9-50).[64,768,981] An optimally positioned scapular Y view is particularly helpful (Fig. 9-51). Stress

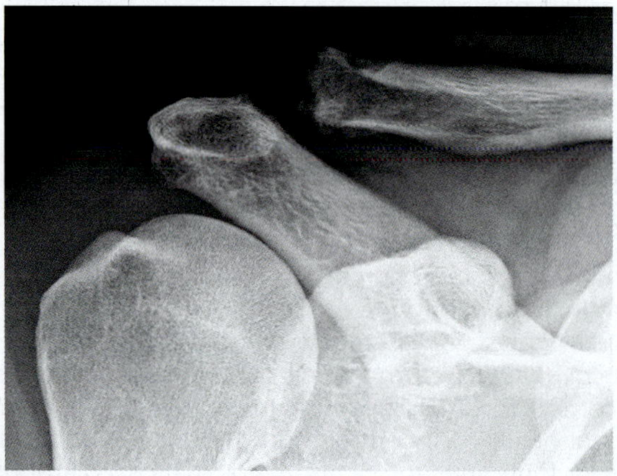

FIGURE 9-47: Traumatic osteolysis and remodeling of the distal end of the clavicle.

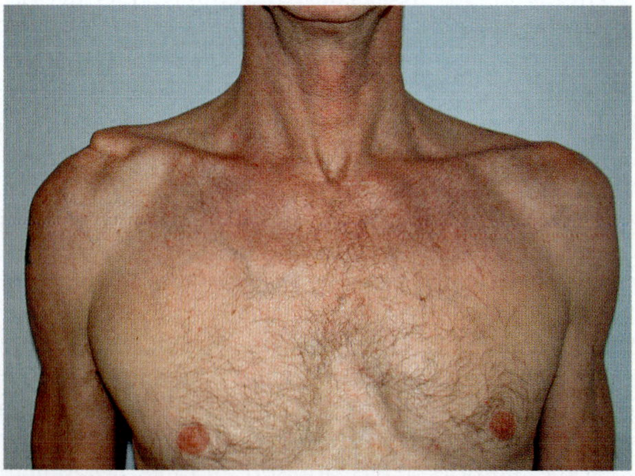

FIGURE 9-48: This type III injury results in an uneven appearance to the shoulders. The injured right shoulder does not droop in this instance secondary to pain that results in splinting by the foreshortened trapezius muscle.

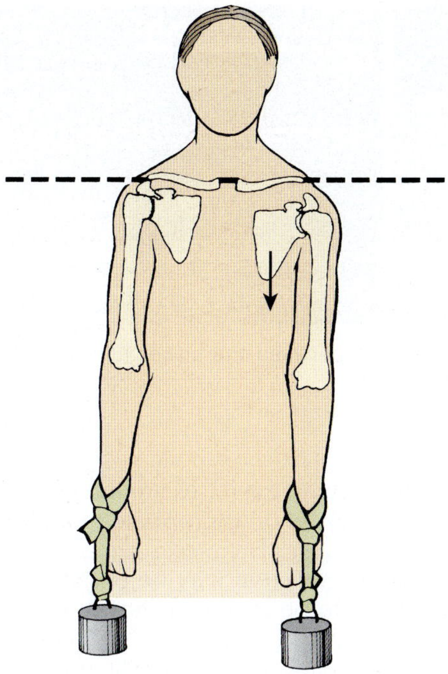

FIGURE 9-49: The type III injury results in deformity because of the downward displacement of the acromion process together with the upper limb, not because of superior displacement of the clavicle.

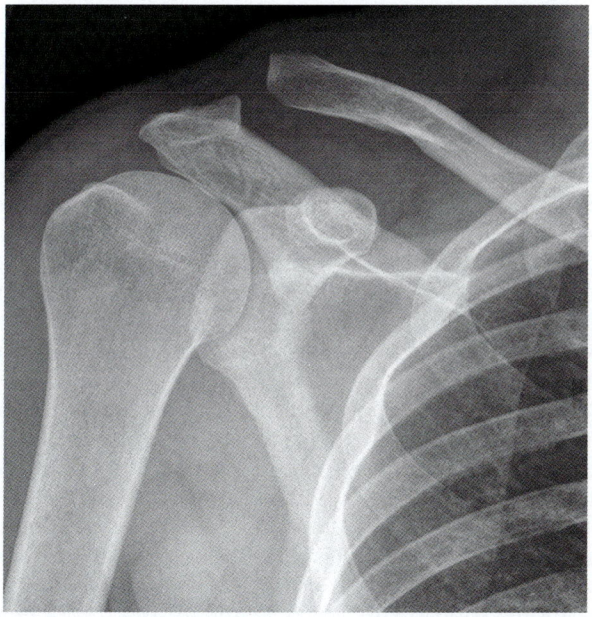

FIGURE 9-50: Anteroposterior view of a type III injury. The articular surfaces of the acromioclavicular joint are widely displaced. The coracoclavicular interval is significantly increased.

views are a consideration, and demonstrate similar findings (Fig. 9-52). The utility of a cross-body adduction view has been cited by some authors as a discriminatory imaging tool to highlight ACJ instability persisting beyond the acute injury period of 3 to 6 weeks.[54,56,71] In addition

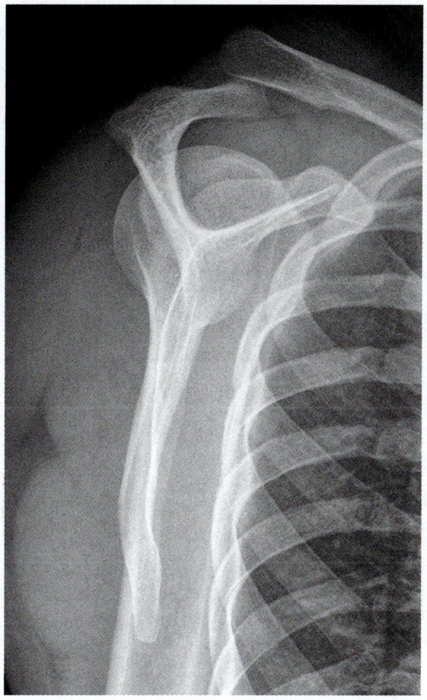

FIGURE 9-51: High-quality scapular Y view.

to ligamentous injury, joint effusion, bone marrow edema (bone bruise), edema, and detachment of the deltoid and trapezius muscles to some degree are often observed on MRI.[654]

Pathoanatomy

The lateral end of the clavicle is exposed as a result of stripping of the periosteal sleeve. The AC and CC ligaments are torn completely, resulting in dislocation of the ACJ. Midsubstance tearing and avulsion from the clavicle occur nearly equally. In comparison to the normal shoulder, the CC interval may be widened by up to 100%. There is a high probability that deltoid and trapezius muscles are detached from the distal clavicle.

Treatment

The treatment of type III injuries has been, is, and will remain in the foreseeable future, a subject of significant controversy. About every 10 to 20 years, certain orthopedic surgeons are compelled to solicit opinions regarding the treatment of type III injuries from other orthopedic surgeons, including academic department chairs, by the distribution of survey material.[195,590,666,734] Although the purpose of these surveys varies, treatment styles emerge as beacons that divinely light the way for practitioners of the period. This was true in 1974, and it remained true in 2007, as expressed by the conclusions of Nissen et al.: Nonoperative symptomatic treatment is preferred, and operative treatment should include resection of the lateral clavicle, reconstruction of at least the CC ligaments with either sutures or local ligament graft, and protection of the reconstruction with rigid fixation between the coracoid and the clavicle.[666] Subsequently, the ever-growing body of pertinent literature has

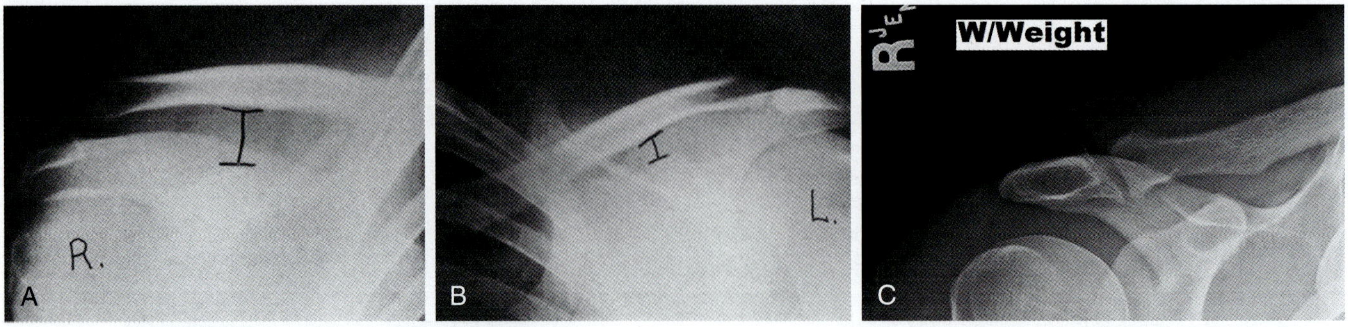

FIGURE 9-52: Anteroposterior stress views demonstrating no appreciable difference between the unweighted and the weighted views. **A,** Contralateral side. **B,** Unweighted. **C,** Weighted.

been exhaustively perused by several authors, from which have emerged current concepts reviews, systematic reviews, meta-analyses, and summaries of evidence-based publications attempting to reveal the best evidence for the treatment of all AC dislocations, and in particular, acute type III injuries.[724,865,142,894,70,613,853,463,477,527]

Nonoperative Treatment

Nonoperative treatment is recommended by many authors, and it is the conclusion of the extensive reviews by Ceccarelli et al., Spencer, and Phillips et al.* Hootman concluded that evidence current at the time did not support operative treatment to achieve better functional outcomes and patient satisfaction.[403] Tamaoki et al. concluded from their review of randomized controlled trials that substantive evidence supporting the decision or timing of surgical treatment did not exist at the time of their review.[894] Beitzel et al. and Modi et al. reached similar conclusions.[70,613] From their review, Korsten et al. stated that for these lesions, there was no conclusive evidence for the treatment.[477] For the majority of patients, nonoperative is the preferred form of treatment for type III injuries. This specifically includes patients such as contact and collision athletes and cyclists, who remain at high risk for repeated injuries to the ACJ. There are no contraindications to nonoperative treatment.

Methods

Taking advantage of the fact that the dislocated joint is easily reducible in the acute setting, some authors have advocated a closed reduction accompanied by external immobilization. Various techniques and methods have been used through decades of experience with the type III injury.[207,217,867,930,938] None has proved any better than another, and each has its own pitfalls.[457,507,734,887,986]

Recognizing the difficulties with maintaining a satisfactory reduction, many authors have recommended symptomatic treatment only with sling support for the upper limb.[329,330,355,663] Motion and strengthening exercises are initiated as the resolution of pain permits. The pace of therapeutic exercise parallels the resolution of symptoms. Closed and open chain exercises are integrated following a 6- to 12-week period of appropriate mobilization. With only minimal scapular dyskinesia remaining, release to activities without restriction may be possible. The role of orthotics to facilitate periscapular muscle rehabilitation is uncertain.[193] Return to higher levels of activity demands enthusiastic participation in a rehabilitation program that emphasizes progressive restoration of strength, function, and sport-specific drills.[138,327,330] An excellent in-depth review of nonoperative care for not only type III but types I and II injuries forms the basis of best practice guidelines.[750,439]

Results

Excellent and good results are obtainable with nonoperative treatment.* An earlier return to work and other activities is often possible.[330,424,555,501,775,217,244,304] Korsten et al. concluded that the price paid for a shorter duration of rehabilitation was a worse cosmetic outcome.[477] Delays to return to sport are sometimes as long as 2 months.[691] At mid- to long-term follow-up, 90% to 100% of patients have very favorable outcomes.[47,91,747,887,734,232,848] At the completion of rehabilitation, strength and endurance approaches that of the opposite upper limb.[986,815]

Overall, satisfactory results obtained with nonoperative treatment derived from a meta-analysis review of the literature was 87%.[724] Calvo et al. demonstrated that there were no differences in the outcome of nonoperative and operative treatment.[131] Spencer searched 469 publications to identify nine studies with level II and level III evidence that compared nonoperative and operative treatment.[865] From this in-depth analysis of what he considered limited low evidence, he concluded that nonoperative treatment was more appropriate because the results of operative treatment "were not clearly better and were associated with higher complication rates, longer convalescence, and longer time away from work and sport." De Carli et al. reached a similar conclusion.[217] They also noted poor satisfaction with the cosmetic results in 50% of the patients.

Many authors have observed that pain, flexibility, range of motion, and strength after nonoperative treatment are

**References 26, 47, 142, 217, 304, 330, 410, 424, 501, 555, 629, 724, 865, 909, 934, 986.*

**References 47, 91, 217, 232, 304, 310, 330, 355, 410, 424, 501, 555, 734, 775, 815, 887.*

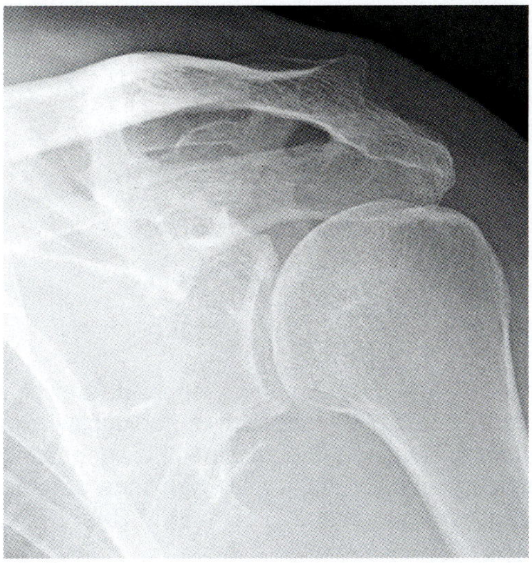

FIGURE 9-53: High-energy shoulder girdle trauma with resultant fractures and apparent type III injury that went on to spontaneously fuse.

at least equal to, if not better than, those after operative treatment.* If differences exist, they are slight or activity specific.[887,815] A higher rate of complications and a slower return to work has been observed with operative treatment.[310,501,217] Although not all authors agree, heavy manual laborers and high-performance overhead athletes such as pitchers might not fare as well with nonoperative treatment because they are less likely to be completely pain-free and have normal function.[766,590,304] Pain and weakness have been reported in up to 50% of patients.[986]

After treatment, the extent of congruity or incongruity, the presence of OA, and the development of heterotopic ossification appear to have no correlation with the outcome, regardless of the treatment method. An exceedingly rare consequence of an apparent type III injury is AC fusion (Fig. 9-53).

Complications

Although not really a complication, the asymmetry of the shoulder becomes obvious after swelling resolves (Fig. 9-54). The extent of deformity may be unexpected and undesirable, perhaps necessitating treatment. Pressure-related skin breakdown is possible with certain types of external immobilization.[18]

Persistent pain and weakness are the most common late sequelae with type III injuries. Ossification is often present in the CC interval at the completion of the period of healing (Fig. 9-55).[17,30,217,355,607,929-931,970] The significance of the ossification is uncertain, but it does not seem to disturb recovery.[17,768,970]

Osteolysis of the distal clavicle has been reported.[1011] The risk of posttraumatic OA has been shown to be lower after nonoperatively treated injuries, as is the incidence of CC ossification.[131]

**References 47, 231, 310, 330, 385, 410, 411, 502, 555, 735, 909, 986.*

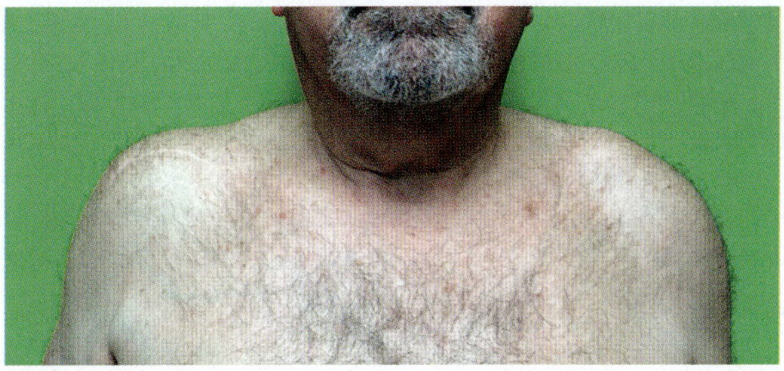

FIGURE 9-54: Shoulder asymmetry resulting from type III injury. Note the prominence of the left distal clavicle and the inferior attitude of the shoulder compared with the contralateral shoulder, which had been previously treated for acromioclavicular injury.

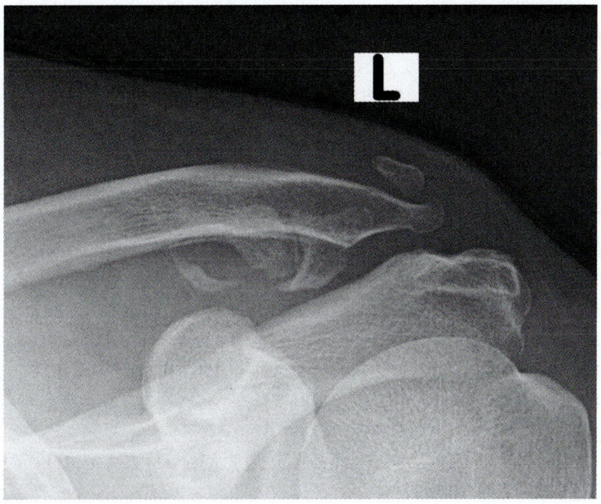

FIGURE 9-55: Abundant heterotopic ossification resulting from a type III dislocation.

Author's Preferred Method

Nonoperative treatment of type III injuries differs only slightly from the treatment of type II injuries. The cornerstone is effective pain management by means of a sling, cryotherapy, and narcotic analgesics. This can require 1 to 2 weeks. Pool therapy is encouraged, and hastens the recovery of active, pain-free movement. Once motion fully recovers and tenderness abates, strength rehabilitation is initiated. Protective measures are more relaxed for type III injuries than for type II injuries.

Operative Treatment

Surgical treatment of ACJ dislocations has been performed since 1861, and appears to continue to play an important role for some clinicians in the care of carefully selected patients with these injuries.* On the basis of the available evidence, firm conclusions are elusive regarding operative versus nonoperative treatment, the timing of surgery, open versus arthroscopic surgery, and choice of surgical procedure with respect to (1) ACJ fixation,

**References 47, 48, 123, 184, 244, 333, 501, 515, 516, 589, 765, 767, 783, 886, 918, 986.*

(2) fixation between the coracoid and the clavicle, and (3) ligament reconstruction.[613,853] A meta-analysis that analyzed operative versus nonoperative treatment recognized that, from the dearth of well-designed investigations, the emergence of the optimum treatment was impossible.[853] From their comparative study, De Carli et al. concluded that "... results cannot support the routine use of surgery to treat type III ACJ dislocations."[217]

Several investigators analyzed their data to compare and distinguish the results of early (acute) versus delayed (chronic) treatments.[247,264,345,444,479,611,772,969] Song et al. performed a systemic review of early versus delayed operative treatment.[862] From their review, they opined that early intervention may have an edge for improved functional outcomes and quality of reduction; however, their opinion was supported only by low-level evidence studies.

Indications

Operative treatment offers the only opportunity for structural and cosmetic restoration. Reserving it for heavy manual laborers, patients 25 years and younger, athletes, and frequent overhead users has been suggested.[501,502,768,919] That said, in one review, there appeared to be no evidence to support the claim that the outcome of operative treatment is better than that of nonoperative treatment.[865] Currently, proof is lacking that special groups of patients mandate consideration for operative treatment. Trainer et al. advocated a 3-month period of nonoperative treatment to optimize the recovery of motion, strength, and shoulder coordination.[919] Patients with persistent symptoms were offered surgical treatment.

Contraindications

Extremely low demand and inactive patients might have nothing to gain with operative treatment. Significant skin abrasions can delay operative treatment.

Methods

Sage and Salvatore reported primary AC ligament repair with joint meniscus reinforcement over 50 years ago.[791] Even recently, direct ligament repair backed up with a temporary CC screw has been described[33] (Fig. 9-56). The ligament could be coapted with repair in 38% and aligned and approximated in 62% with the use of autogenous palmaris longus or in its absence, half of the flexor carpi radialis, along with nonabsorbable suture. Rushton et al. stabilized the ACJ via two pairs of transosseous tunnels.[780] Sandmann et al. reported a triple cerclage technique whereby one trans-ACJ and two CC sutures maintained the joint reduced.[804] Sobhy used a single nylon tape around the coracoid, through the clavicle, and across the ACJ.[857]

The ACJ may be reduced by a closed or open technique and repaired with metallic wires or pins that temporarily transgress the articular surfaces of the acromion and the clavicle.* The importance of supplemental

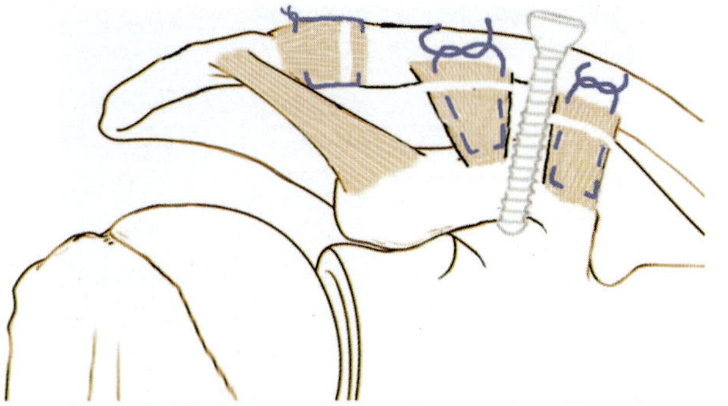

FIGURE 9-56: Acromioclavicular, trapezoid, and conoid ligament suture repair protected with a coracoclavicular screw. (Modified from Assaghir YM. Outcome of exact anatomic repair and coracoclavicular cortical lag screw in acute acromioclavicular dislocations. *J Trauma.* 2011;71[3]:E50-E54.)

techniques performed in conjunction with the method of internal fixations has been emphasized by some authors. These techniques include the additional repair of the AC and CC ligaments, AC and CC ligament repair reinforcement with the intra-articular disk, repair or imbrication of the deltoid and trapezius attachments, adjacent soft tissue transfers (CAL, biceps short head), lateral clavicle excision, autologous fascia lata suspension, CC suture augmentation, and clavicle osteotomy.* The duration of temporary fixation is typically longer than 6 weeks but varies with the technique. Motion restrictions are mandatory to protect the integrity of the pins or wires until their removal. Thereafter, motion and strengthening programs are introduced.

Nearly 40 years ago, Balser published in German the first account of the use of a hooked plate.[46] While the appearance of the plates may vary, the principles since inception of the concept have not wavered. The open reduction and internal fixation method with a precontoured hooked plate affords rigid internal fixation and spares the articular surfaces of the joint (Figs. 9-57 to 9-60).† The device has the advantage of simultaneously stabilizing the CC (superior-inferior) and the AC (anterior-posterior) ligaments. With no other means of fixation augmentation, stability is afforded by scar that accompanies healing of the surrounding soft tissues. Several authors have described the use of supplemental fixation including CC fixation with polydioxanone sulfate (PDS) sutures, direct CC ligament repair, suturing the capsuloligamentous sleeve of the ACJ, additional screw fixation through the plate, and transposition of the CAL as per Weaver and Dunn.[146,283,355,538,796,901,1010] Some authors have advised early range of motion within a day of the operation.[165,535,796,872,901] Others permit a limited range after a brief period of protection.[236,355,422,714,1010] Implant removal

*References 7, 36, 37, 55, 59, 60, 122, 165, 206, 224, 243, 278, 279, 281, 404, 410, 412, 413, 479, 501, 515, 537, 541, 542, 555, 579, 605, 624, 655-660, 679, 723, 736, 742, 777, 690, 929, 791, 842, 854, 875, 887, 932, 940.

*References 7, 33, 36, 59, 122, 206, 404, 479, 537, 541, 542, 579, 624, 655-660, 679, 734, 736, 791, 854, 940.

†References 11, 114, 165, 213, 236, 240, 241, 264, 333, 346, 355, 362, 390, 422, 429, 443, 478, 601, 638, 714, 796, 814, 819, 841, 872, 901, 945, 990, 997, 1010.

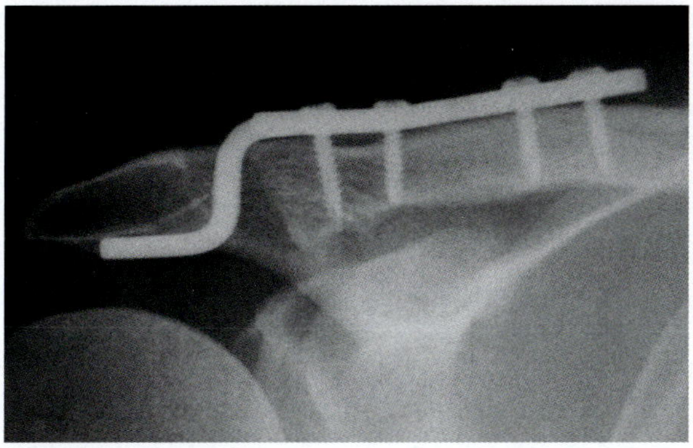

FIGURE 9-57: Hook plate for type III injury enabling excellent restoration of anatomy.

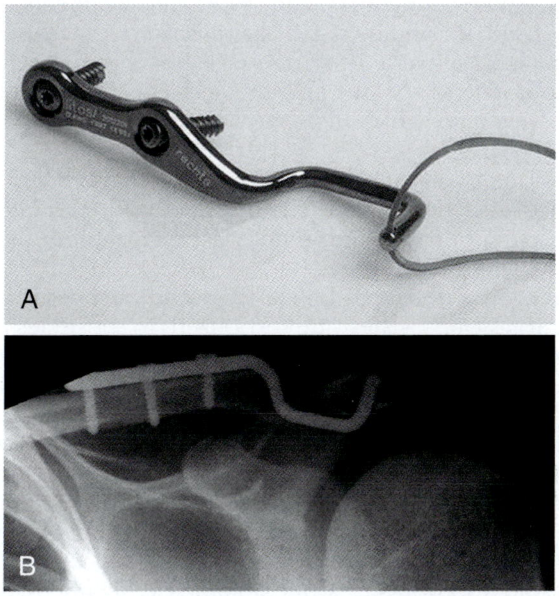

FIGURE 9-58: AC-Hakenplatte tifix plate. (From Kienast B, Thietje R, Queitsch C, et al. Mid-term results after operative treatment of Rockwood grade III-V acromioclavicular joint dislocations with an AC-hook-plate. *Eur J Med Res.* 2011;16[2]: 52-56.)

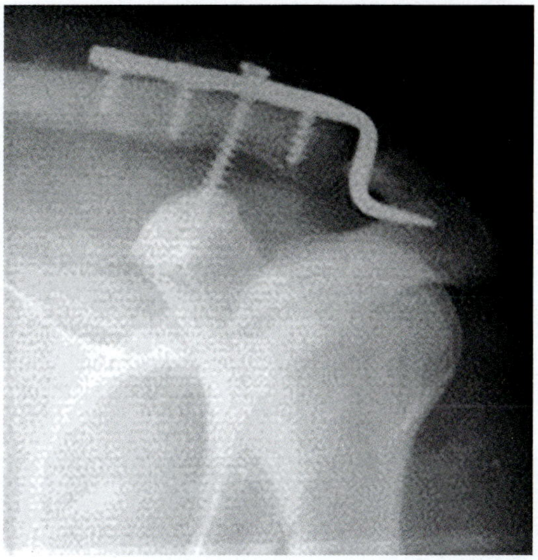

FIGURE 9-59: Hook plate application with a supplemental coracoclavicular screw through the plate. (From Darestani R, Ghaffari A, Hosseinpour M. Acromioclavicular joint fixation using an acroplate combined with a coracoclavicular screw. *Arch Trauma Res.* 2013;2[1]:36-39.)

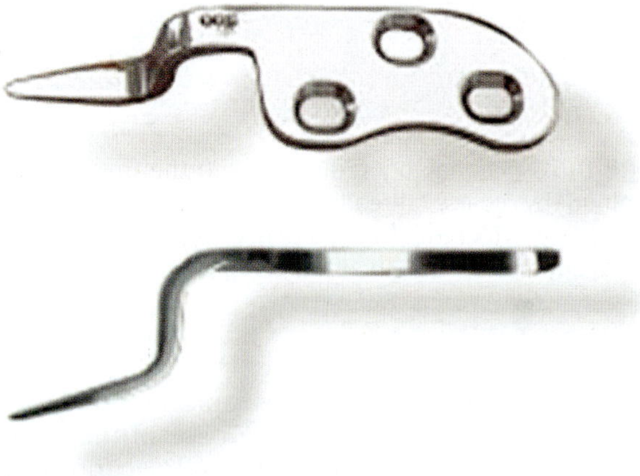

FIGURE 9-60: Acroplate (aap Implantate AG). (From Cîrstoiu C, Rădulescu R, Popescu D, et al. Acroplate—a modern solution for the treatment of acromioclavicular joint dislocation. *J Med Life.* 2009;2[2]:173-175.)

is reported between 4 and 24 weeks. Infrequently, the duration of implant retention is as long as 7 to 13 months.[146,264] Some authors do not routinely remove the device.[213,283,901] Asymptomatic patients may occasionally refuse a secondary operation to remove the plate.[872] Immediately after plate removal, vigorous efforts toward motion and strength recovery are initiated.

Liu et al. designed and utilized the articulated micromovable and anatomic AC plate (MAAP; Fig. 9-61).[540] Ryhanen et al. have described the use of a CC nitinol C-shaped hook implant (AC-Hakenplatte tifix).[782] Insertion with arthroscopic assist has been described.[325]

The clavicle and the coracoid process offer secure points of fixation that can be used to maintain either a closed or open reduction of the ACJ. These stabilization techniques may be used independently or as a supplement to other forms of either temporary or permanent means of fixation. In addition, direct repair of the AC and CC ligaments performed concurrently with the CC stabilization can be considered.

Bosworth was the first to describe the use of a screw between the clavicle and the coracoid process to achieve ACJ stability.[107] Others have used the technique as described by Bosworth or have made modifications in the technique (Figs. 9-62 and 9-63).* Garrigues et al.

*References 29, 47, 276, 310, 410, 456-458, 546, 555, 722, 775, 886, 887, 896, 922, 970.

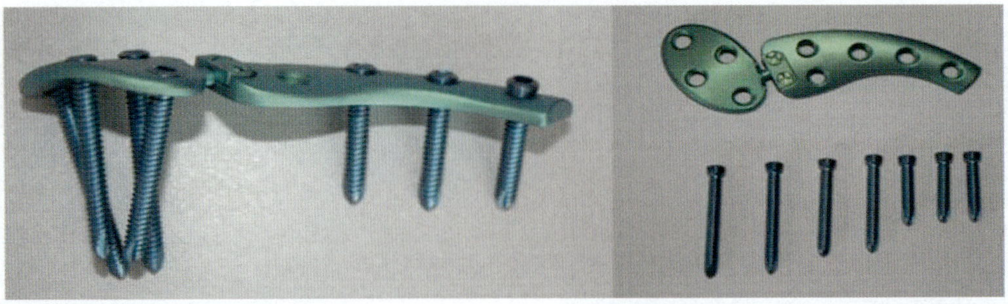

FIGURE 9-61: Articulated hook plate applied across the acromioclavicular joint to permit some joint motion. (From Liu Q, Miao J, Lin B, et al. Clinical effect of acute complete acromioclavicular joint dislocation treated with micromovable and anatomic acromioclavicular plate. *Int J Med Sci.* 2012;9[8]:725-729.)

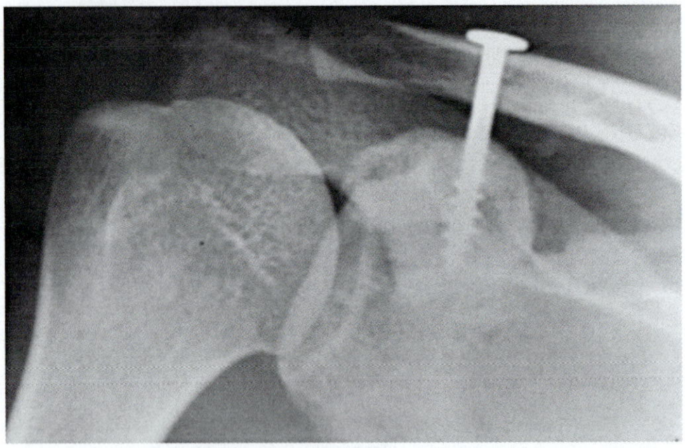

FIGURE 9-62: Satisfactory reduction with the Bosworth screw maintained by coarse threads in the base of the coracoid process. (From Rockwood CA, Green DP, eds. *Fractures.* 2nd ed. Philadelphia: JB Lippincott; 1984.)

described an intraoperative fluoroscopically aided method for the proper identification of the base of the coracoid process to facilitate the placement and security of purchase of a percutaneously placed CC fixation device such as a screw.[312] The method is applicable to more recent CC devices that incorporate cortical suture buttons, described below.

The exploration and debridement of the ACJ has been advocated,[361,456,457,970] but some authors do not consider this an essential component of treatment.[107-110,922] In the setting of CC stabilization, the necessity for the direct repair of the CC ligaments is uncertain. Bosworth and others have elected to leave the ligaments unrepaired.[26,107-110,456,457, 922] Some authors have emphasized the importance of supplemental CC ligament repair at the time of CC stabilization.[361] Repair of the trapezius and deltoid attachments can contribute to the overall strength of the repair and has been emphasized by several authors.[55,361,456,541,970]

There are significant variations in the recommendations for postoperative immobilization, restrictions, rehabilitation, the necessity for implant removal, and the timing of implant removal.[17,64,107,456, 970]

The extraosseous, intraosseous, and transosseous placement of absorbable sutures, nonabsorbable sutures, wires, cables, anchors, and synthetic ligaments have been used for indirect ACJ stabilization (Fig. 9-64).* If the material is passed through drill holes in the clavicle, in the coracoid, or in both, the reduction is potentially more accurate, and the outcome may be improved (Fig. 9-65).[147,217,237,269, 404, 492,548,621,776,1005,1010]

Various types of synthetic ligaments have been used for reconstruction.[324,444,565] The ligament is looped beneath the coracoid process and then passed through tunnels in the clavicle and secured.

Reconstructions that utilize CC suture techniques date back to 1996.[305] They are espoused to pose less risk to adjacent neurovascular structures with comparable strength of the native ligaments, and are minimally invasive.[113,160, 885] Additional advantages are less blood loss, shorter operative time, and no secondary incision or hardware to remove.[160,167,305] The relatively simple suspension method of Huang et al. incorporated subcoracoid and transclavicular passage of large, nonabsorbable sutures through tunnels at the sites of the conoid and trapezoid footprints.[409] Concomitant CC ligament repair can be performed, and is believed by Lu et al. to be one of the most important components of their repair technique.[160,548] The potentially less invasive aspects of some of the newer implants, such as TightRope (Arthrex) has been touted.[404,429]

Concomitant supplemental AC ligament repair has been described. Zhang et al. modified the technique by placing a stabilizing suture anchor across the ACJ.[1016]

Transposing the CAL into the resected distal clavicle was suggested in 1917 by Cadenet, advocated by Nevisier in the early 1950s, and was reported by Weaver and Dunn in 1972, who used the technique for both acute and chronic type III injuries.[127,655,656,964] Other authors used the CAL in the same or a similar manner.[220,247,451,655,656,658,746,837] Modifications of the Weaver-Dunn method were subsequently described by other authors, and were felt to be especially useful for

*References *17, 64, 147, 149, 167, 168, 174, 200, 201, 217, 237, 238, 269, 298, 333-335, 348, 392, 393, 404, 409, 444, 445, 492, 548, 562, 565, 579, 617, 621, 653, 696, 969, 722, 776, 781, 857, 869, 885, 888, 941, 1005, 1007, 1010.*

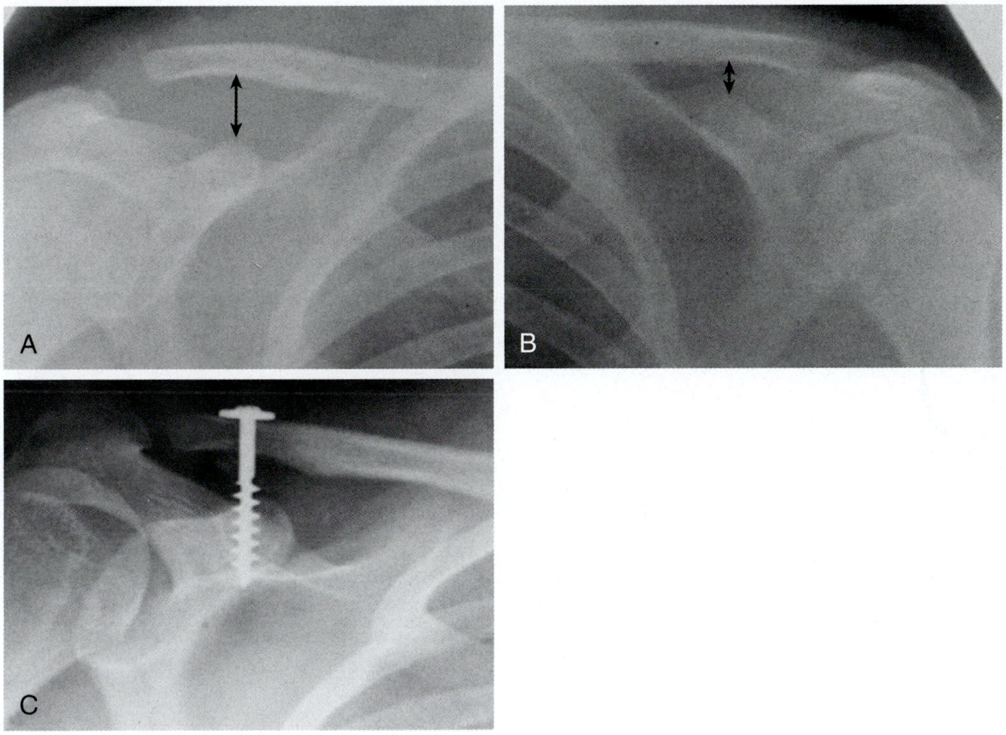

FIGURE 9-63: Excellent reduction with restoration of a normal coracoclavicular interval with a coracoclavicular screw. **A,** Anteroposterior stress radiograph of the right shoulder in a patient with a type III acromioclavicular dislocation. **B,** A stress film of the left shoulder revealed it to be normal. **C,** Postoperative radiograph showing the acromioclavicular joint reduced and held temporarily in place with a special modified coracoclavicular lag screw. (From Rockwood CA, Green DP, eds. *Fractures.* 2nd ed. Philadelphia: JB Lippincott; 1984.)

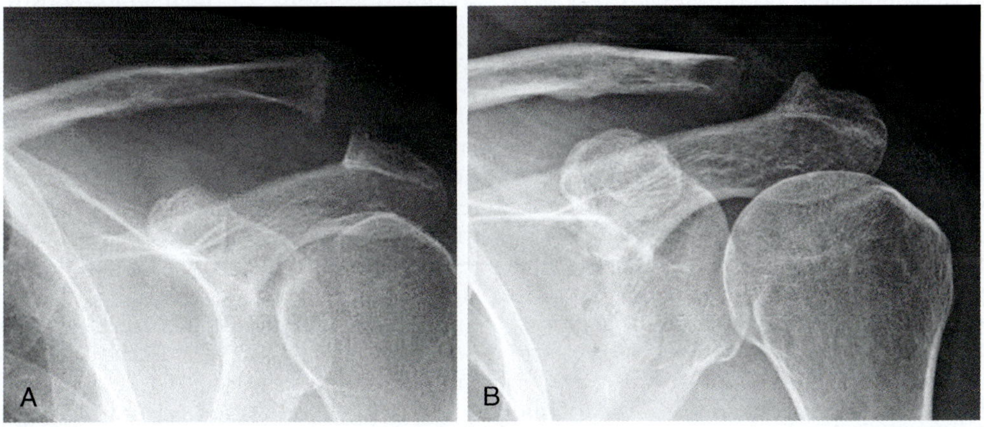

FIGURE 9-64: Acute type III injury. **A,** Preoperative. **B,** Final postoperative treatment using encircling permanent sutures with distal clavicle resection.

a more active population.[516,586,673,730,735,771,911,969] The CAL, with or without an accompanying piece of bone, may be transferred to the clavicle with or without supplementary fixation.[125,187,211,487,490] Such concepts of CC augmentation in conjunction with the Weaver-Dunn operation have been supported by the results of experimental studies.[228]

A Cadenet procedure was described by Cerciello et al. that has been modified by the addition of CC cerclage, CC ligament remnant suturing, and transarticular dual K-wire fixation of the reduced ACJ.[143]

Another method for incorporating the CAL was originally described by Vukov.[947] It differs in that the ligament is left intact, and the reduced distal clavicle, having undergone a limited distal resection, is "elastically" affixed with sutures passed through transosseous tunnels in the clavicle.

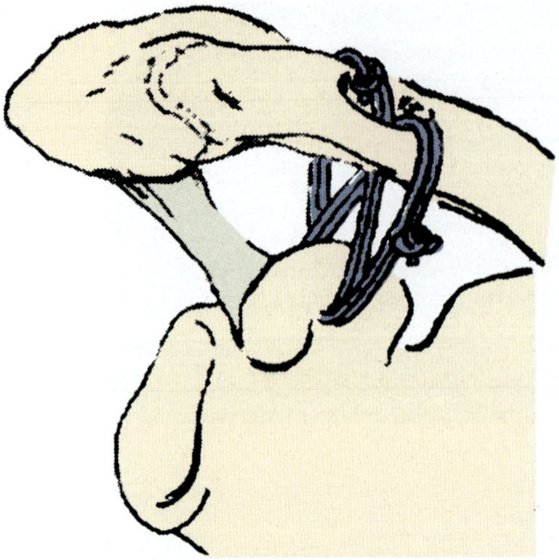

FIGURE 9-65: A method of coracoclavicular reconstruction with loops passing through a prepared hole in the clavicle. (Modified from Dimakopoulos P, Panagopoulos A. Functional coracoclavicular stabilization for acute acromioclavicular joint disruption. *Orthopedics* 2007;30[2]:103-108.)

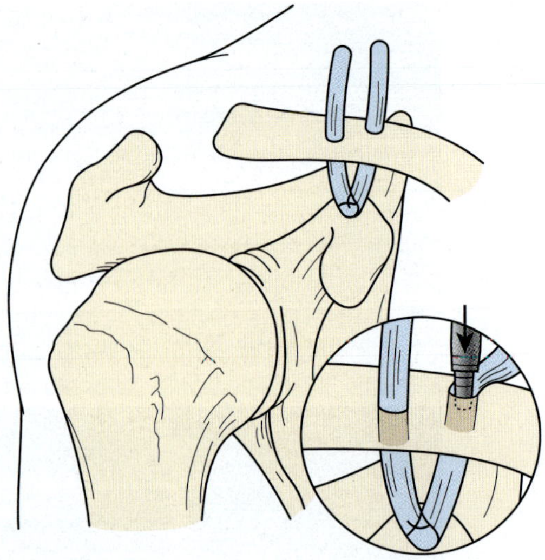

FIGURE 9-66: A coracoclavicular reconstruction that is considered anatomic uses autograft or allograft tendon. (Modified from Mazzocca AD, Conway J, Johnson S, et al. The anatomic coracoclavicular ligament reconstruction. *Oper Tech Sports Med.* 2004;12:56-61.)

In 1941, Gurd described excision of the distal clavicle as a treatment for type III injuries.[360] In the same year, Mumford reported the same operation for type II injuries, and advocated that treatment of symptomatic type III injuries should also include CC ligament reconstruction as well as DCR.[631] The role for excision of the lateral clavicle at the time of surgical treatment of a type III injury is not clear.[969] There were no differences reported between CC ligament fixation alone and CC fixation with excision of the lateral clavicle.[116] Likewise, when the outcome of AC fixation and CC ligament repair with and without lateral clavicle excision were compared, no differences were observed, with the exception of the more frequent appearance of degenerative changes when the lateral clavicle was retained.[852,854]

In 1965, muscle transfers were suggested as a reasonable treatment for type III injuries.[41,230] The tip of the coracoid process, including the coracobrachialis and the short head of the biceps, was osteotomized and attached to the clavicle. Scattered reports appeared later, some with slight modifications of the technique.[42,83,117,196,331,333,954] Transposition of the biceps long head or a slip of the conjoined tendon have been described as substitution methods for the CC ligaments.[120,495,937] Jiang et al. described reconstruction with a proximally base-conjoined tendon transfer supplemented with transclavicular clavicular sutures anchored in the coracoid process.[435,436]

In the last 8 years, there has been an explosive trend to seek a more anatomic and biologic solution for CC ligament reconstruction. The notion is that reliable restoration of function and comfort is dependent on the durable restoration of anatomic parameters, including the congruity and stability of the ACJ. The method often includes substituting synthetic or biologic material for each CC ligament separately entering the clavicle and coracoid as close as possible to the footprints of the native ligaments.

Early biomechanical investigations followed the initial report of Jones et al., who described the surgical technique of using autologous semitendinosus tendon, and applied the method in a revision case.[191,354,374,426,440,512] Mazzocca et al. were among the earliest advocates for so-called anatomic CC ligament reconstruction (ACCR) of the CC ligament complex using autograft or allograft tendon[582] (Fig. 9-66). Additional biomechanical work by Lee et al. led to the first clinical application and report of the use of autologous hamstring tendon by Nicholas et al.[512,662] Subsequently, some form of "anatomic" repair or reconstruction that utilizes autogenous or allogenous tendon is being reported more frequently as a preferred method of treatment.[39,45,138,214,284,337,505,554,610,744,758,834,960] ACJ reconstruction that utilizes the same graft for CC reconstruction has been described.[138,437,524] In 1928, a similar method was eloquently described by Bunnell, who incorporated a fascial graft weave that offered stability between the clavicle and the scapula at both sites (Fig. 9-67).[123]

An arthroscopic method for treating type III injuries was first described by Wolf and Pennington.[988] In this study, either sutures or allograft semitendinosus were used for CC stabilization. Lafosse et al. presented the initial description of an arthroscopic technique that did not require autologous tendon.[494] Since then, other arthroscopic methods using the CAL, various types of sutures, or tendon autograft or allograft have been described.*

Arthroscopic-assisted percutaneous CC screw insertion has been described.[151,773,920] Somers and Van der

**References 39, 62, 151, 214, 581, 611, 712, 773, 859, 916, 920, 960, 987, 1008.*

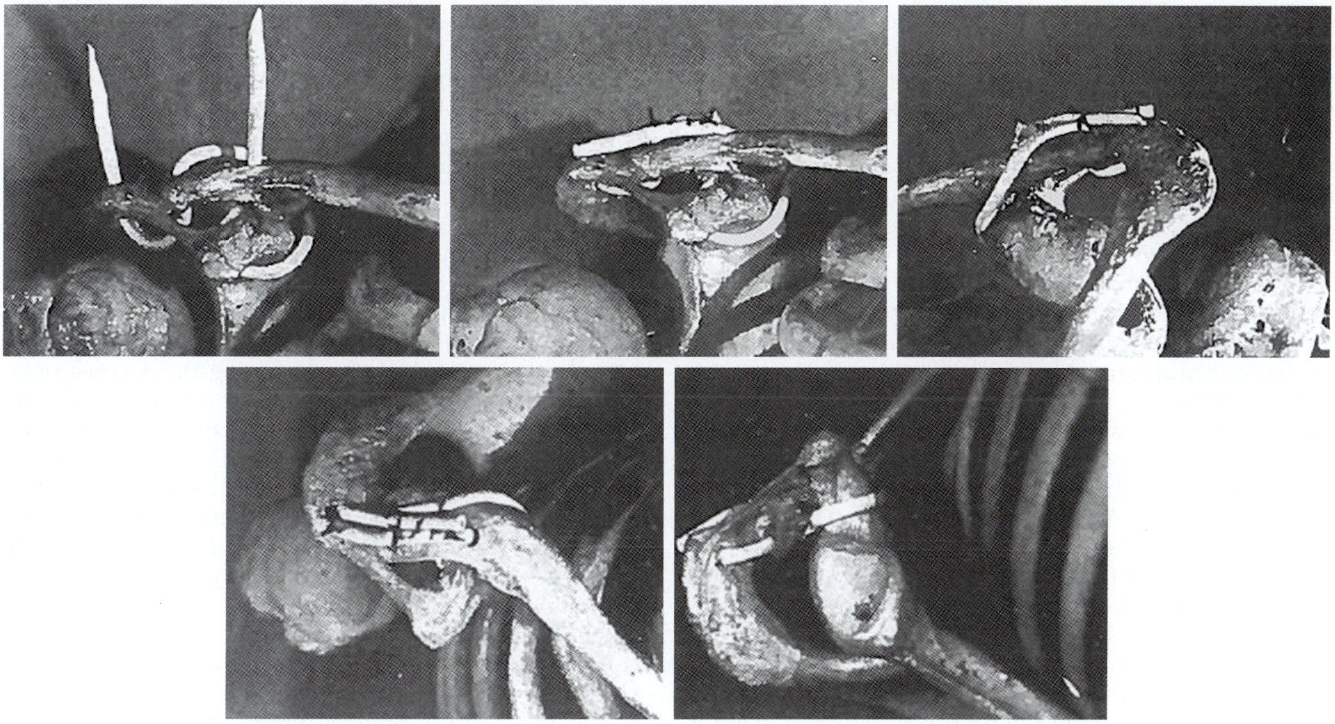

FIGURE 9-67: Various perspectives of a cadaver shoulder with rubber tubing depicting Bunnell's fascial weave technique anatomically stabilizing the clavicle and the acromion. (From Bunnell S. Fascial graft for dislocation of acromioclavicular joint. *Surg Gynecol Obstet.* 1928;46:563-564.)

Linden reported transclavicular sutures with coracoid suture anchors performed arthroscopically.[859] Further arthroscopic techniques have been investigated, recommended, and performed.[974,692,174,444] Appropriate visualization with the arthroscopic method is by one of two ways: an intra-articular approach via the rotator interval and a subacromial approach. In general, arthroscopic CC stabilization may enable the safer and more accurate placement of materials used for stabilization.[635] Perhaps an additional advantage is the finding of coexisting lesions, which often require additional treatment; the incidence ranges as high as 25% to 35.3%.[429,635,868] These include SLAP tears, disorders of the biceps long head, Bankart lesions, glenoid cartilage fissures, humeral head or glenoid minor chondral defects, and partial- and full-thickness RC tears.[610,635,859]

In 2006, the use of a contoured, metallic, buttonlike device designed to rest against the outer cortex of bone and a nonabsorbable reinforced suture system was first described by Hernegger and Kadletz.[392] In 2007, the technique of using such buttons in a flipping manner was presented.[534,881,973] Many authors have since reported on the use of one or more pairs of flipping CC buttons spanned by nonabsorbable sutures, both open and arthroscopic assisted.*

**References 81, 174, 181, 214, 217, 218, 328, 404, 532, 539, 601, 635, 692, 776, 801, 802, 835, 868, 939, 968, 1007.*

Experimental Investigations. Impetus to find an effective way to render the injured ACJ stable has resulted in scores of investigations that have attempted to analyze and compare the multitude of methods, old and new.

Thirty years ago, upon comparing techniques for AC fixation, Kiefer et al. found that the most rigid fixation was provided by the Bosworth screw.[461] Restoration of ACJ congruency using seven different methods of fixation between the clavicle and the coracoid were studied by Jerosch et al.[431] They demonstrated satisfactory vertical stability with all of the techniques. Excessive horizontal translations between the acromion and the clavicle were demonstrated with all of the loop techniques and the Weaver-Dunn reconstruction, whereas the joint anatomy was best restored with the Bosworth screw or bone anchor reconstruction.[431] Harris et al. showed that Bosworth screw placement with bicortical purchase provided strength and stiffness as good as or better than the intact CC ligaments.[374] In a cadaver model comparing the biomechanical function of different surgical procedures for ACJ dislocations, the Rockwood screw resulted in decreased primary and coupled translations, and showed increased stiffness.[426] CC sling and CAL transfer resulted in increased primary and coupled translations. In situ forces increased for all three reconstructions.

Additional experimental screw fixation for CC ligament reconstruction has been investigated.[892] In this study, CC fixation comparing stainless steel and bioabsorbable 4.5-mm screws showed no difference in pullout strength and fixation strength that exceeded the intact CC ligaments. In a study by Motamedi et al., 6.5-mm CC screw fixation with one-cortex purchase was significantly weaker and stiffer than the intact CC ligaments.[625]

In a cadaver model, McConnell et al. performed reconstructions with CC loop (No. 5 polyester fiber [Mersilene]), CC screw, and hook plate fixation, and subjected the specimens to stiffness and failure testing.[588] Hook plates reproduced physiologic stiffness more closely. The CC screw failed at the highest load and was the stiffest reconstruction, and the CC loop was the least stiff. In a comparative investigation, Fialka et al. identified the poor mechanical properties of the Bosworth technique, especially at more than 90 degrees of abduction. While transarticular K-wires were rigid and stable, a high rate of migration was observed. The most favorable mechanical stability was with the ligament augmentation and reconstruction system (LARS) device.[293]

In an in vitro model of the ACJ, Nüchtern et al. not only showed the physiologic stiffness of the hook plate but also showed the relevant role of the ACJ ligaments for restoring physiologic properties about the ACJ at the time of reconstruction for complete dislocations.[676] Kim et al. investigated changes in 3D motion taking place at the ACJ with and without the presence of a hook plate.[467] In patients who had undergone hook plate for distal clavicle fracture, they showed diminished internal rotation (mean, 16 degrees) and increased anterior translation (2 mm) of the clavicle with respect to the medial acromion compared with the nonoperative side.

Wickham et al. compared the maximum tensile strength and resistance to deformation of one or two strands of Ethibond No. 5 suture, one or two strands of polyester (Mersilene) tape, size 0 polydioxanone braid, and size 2 poly(L-lactic acid) suture braid in a CC model, and demonstrated the significantly greater tensile strength of poly(L-lactic acid) sutures.[978] Two strands of polyester tape, polydioxanone braid, and poly(L-lactic acid) braid exhibited similar resistance to deformation with cyclic loading but performed significantly better than the other test samples. Failure loads comparable to the intact CC ligament (725 N) were observed in the experimental reconstructions performed with braided polydioxanone and braided polyethylene passed around or through the clavicle; failure loads of a 6.5-mm screw with single-cortex purchase in the coracoid were around one-half those of the intact CC ligaments. The strength and stiffness properties of the braided polyethylene suggested that it could serve effectively as an augmentation for ACJ repairs and reconstructions. Martetschläger et al. concluded that inferior biomechanical properties of PDS sutures used to reconstruct the AC and CC ligaments were responsible for failure to achieve vertical stability.[569]

In experimental repairs performed by Wellmann et al., loop or button fixation of polydioxanone sutures exhibited significantly higher ultimate loads than did coracoid suture anchor repairs with No. 2 high-strength polyethylene (Ultrabraid) sutures.[974] In a cadaver model, ACJ congruity was not restored by any CC loop fixation through drill holes in the clavicle but was more closely restored when the drill hole was placed more anteriorly in the clavicle.[44]

Different configurations of synthetic suture direction and orientation have been investigated. Abat et al. determined that passage via double tunnels in both the clavicle and the coracoid results in a reconstruction that is biomechanically more like the native state compared with a V configuration, where only one tunnel is in the coracoid.[1] Schliemann et al. compared the coracoid side flip button tendon graft with tendon looping around the coracoid with synthetic suture augmentation, and found the biomechanical properties of the reconstruction to be comparable.[816] The benefit of passing the reconstruction material transosseous as opposed to extraosseous is less abrasive changes observed in the material and the adjacent bone in contact with the material.[468] The use of a transosseous TightRope method rather than fiber mesh cerclage for such augmentation resulted in less translational motion.[1019] Lädermann et al. demonstrated the advantages of AC and CC cerclage over V-shaped orientation synthetic suture (TightRope) CC reconstruction and hooked plate.[493] Their work suggested that CC cerclage might better reproduce the native ligament stiffness.

Tunneling through the bone as opposed to passage around the bone is seen by many as the most effective option to create the so-called "anatomic" reconstruction that hopes to restore normal kinematics and forces for stabilizing the ACJ.[344,354,1009] Various ways of creating tunnels in the clavicle and coracoid for passage of synthetic sutures with or without augmentation biologic grafts and securing different holding sutures over different types of cortex-preserving devices (buttons) have been described.[72,74,169,289,417] Beitzel et al. identified no difference between one and two tunnels in the clavicle.[72-74] As a result of in-depth biomechanical investigations and early clinical experiences, recommendations are coming forth for tunnel sizing, positioning, and spacing in the clavicle and coracoid process.[138,289,923] Rylander et al. showed the benefits of a 4-mm versus a 6-mm tunnel in the clavicle.[784] When loaded to failure, drilled specimens failed by button pullout, and looped, undrilled coracoids failed by fracture. According to Spiegl et al., hamstring through 6-mm tunnels significantly weakened the clavicle compared with cortical button and suture through 2.4-mm tunnels.[866] Dumont et al. determined that clavicle strength or resistance to ultimate failure were not enhanced by the presence of interference screws placed in the tunnel to achieve tenodesis.[246] Ferreira et al. showed that load-to-failure testing of a 6-mm tunnel through the coracoid process was significantly higher when the entry and exit of the tunnel was center and center or medial and center, respectively.[289] The mechanism of failure was predominantly in the repair construct and not a fracture of the coracoid. In a 3D virtual shoulder model, Coale et al. were able to highlight the significant risks when attempting to restore the anatomic footprint of the conoid and trapezoid ligaments.[170] In their model, it was not possible to create reconstruction tunnels that both restored anatomic ligament footprints and maintained, without significant risk of cortical breach and fracture, the integrity of the bone through which the tunnel passes. In a similar model, Xue et al. observed a 90.5% incidence of clavicle or coracoid cortical breach with collinear drilling of a 4-mm tunnel based on anatomic landmarks.[1000,1002] Alternately, noncollinear drilling of the coracoid tunnels determined by the ligament footprint on the superior aspect of the coracoid process directed to the inferior surface to a position that respected an adequate bony bridges and the cortical margins did not result in cortical breach. They also calculated the angulation of the coracoid tunnels. The advantages on non–image-guided navigation over drill guide technique in cadavers for the accuracy of tunnel placement has been demonstrated in a cadaver investigation.[904] In a matched-pairs cadaver study of coracoid tunnels, Campbell et al. determined that cortical button fixation strength was greater with a 4.5-mm tunnel compared with a 6-mm tunnel.[132] In their study, central and proximal fixation was stronger than eccentric and distal fixation. Experimental reconstructions with semitendinosus graft have shown the ability to reproduce peak loads equivalent to that of the native CC ligaments.[870,344] Compared with the native ligaments, stiffness is lower.[870] Walz et al. demonstrated the efficacy of the dual tunnel TightRope technique with buttons in reproducing and exceeding the vertical and horizontal forces of the native CC ligaments.[953]

Reconstructions that incorporated the ACJ restored the biomechanical characteristics of the native ACJ specifically by reducing undesirable AP translations that could not be overcome by isolated CC techniques.[3,795] Nüctern et al. also identified the significant role in joint stiffness contributed by the AC ligaments.[676] Using a constant technique of CC ligament reconstruction while comparing four different AC reconstruction, Beitzel et al. showed the benefit of the additional ACJ reconstruction and the superiority of the stability of the direct wrapping and suturing technique.[72] The utility and efficacy of reconstructing the ACJ with an intramedullary free semitendinosus graft in vitro have been shown.[302,311,603] Garg et al. demonstrated the superiority of intramedullary over various extramedullary ACJ reconstructions.[311] Shu et al. documented the effectiveness of a novel reverse CAL transfer when compared with isolated CC ligament reconstruction and comparable to intramedullary allograft tendon.[838] When AC and CC reconstructions are simultaneously performed, significantly greater horizontal stability has been shown.[338,603] Kowalsky et al. showed that the AC ligaments rather than the articulation of the distal clavicle may have a protective role for a CC reconstruction, hence a supportive rationale for DCR, when necessary.[480] On the other hand, biomechanical testing of the reconstruction may mirror the native state even when the AC ligaments are not included.[75,272,906]

The CAL transposition as used in the Weaver-Dunn reconstruction is, experimentally, one-fifth the ultimate load of the intact CC ligament.[625,512] Deshmukh et al. demonstrated that the Weaver-Dunn method was significantly more lax than the native ligaments.[228] In their model, CC augmentation was less lax than the Weaver-Dunn reconstruction but more lax than the native ligament. Harris et al. showed that CAL transfer in the manner of Weaver-Dunn was the weakest and least stiff experimental reconstruction when compared with the intact CC ligament, CC screw fixation, woven polyester vascular graft slings, and suture anchor technique with No. 5 braided polyester.[374] The Weaver-Dunn procedure, even with modifications, fails to reproduce the load-to-failure durability of the intact AC and CC ligament complex.[354,583] In a cadaver model that assessed the motion between two points fixed respectively on the distal clavicle and acromion process, an unaugmented Weaver-Dunn reconstruction demonstrated significant multiplanar laxity when compared with an intact joint.[984] In the same study, a reconstruction augmented with CC suture with anchor into the coracoid was neither more nor less mobile than the intact joint. In contrast, LaPrade et al. recognized that when the Weaver-Dunn reconstruction was performed with coracoid transclavicular cerclage, motion at the ACJ was restored to near-normal values.[500] In their comparative study, Lee et al. drew similar conclusions, but also documented the superiority of the transclavicular coracoid cerclage that used semitendinosus.[510] From their investigation, Luis et al. concluded that for sufficient resistance to undesirable ACJ motion, the Weaver-Dunn reconstruction should always be accompanied by supplemental stabilization methods.[551] A similar conclusion was reached by Wellman et al., who used only the medial one-half of the CAL together with polyester cord secured with flip buttons.[972] Transfer of the CAL as per Weaver-Dunn at the time of CC hamstring tendon grafts did not yield superior stability or biomechanical strength.[169] Several biomechanical studies have been completed that illustrate that ACCR more closely approximates the stiffness of the CC ligament complex and produces less anterior-to-posterior translation at the ACJ as compared with the Weaver-Dunn procedure.[159,172,191,354,368,450,583,900] Other studies have identified the inferior biomechanical properties of the Weaver-Dunn reconstruction when compared with alternate, more "anatomic" or alternative reconstructions.[73,74,526,906] The stabilizing advantages of additional coracoid reconstruction at the time of the Weaver-Dunn method have been shown.[468,1019]

Portions of the conjoined tendon have been used for experimental CC reconstruction. Sloan et al., in a cadaver model of single load to failure, demonstrated that the strength of the lateral half of the conjoined tendon (265 N) was at least as strong as that of the CAL (246 N) in a simulated reconstruction, although it lacked the strength of the intact CC ligaments (621 N).[849] They cited potential advantages of this technique, including retention of the CAL integrity and significantly longer autologous graft material.

The tendon of the pectoralis minor tendon morphology and tensile strength has been investigated in cadavers and compared with that in the AC ligament.[614] It can offer structural properties that render it as suitable as, or even more suitable than, the CAL. Although it has yet to be evaluated clinically, its use for this purpose circumvents the potential complications that may arise from the sacrifice of a normal and functionally important part of the coracoacromial arch.

The rationale for the use of biologic CC ligament substitutions has been investigated. The requirement for a biologic graft may not depend so much on the strength of the reconstruction, which can be comparably achieved with nonbiologic materials, but rather the necessity of the presence of a biologic substrate.[971] In load-to-failure studies, anatomic allograft reconstructions have been shown to be superior to modified Weaver-Dunn, nonanatomic allograft, anatomic suture, and graft-rope techniques.[906] An experimental anatomic reconstruction with semitendinosus tendon in a cadaver model failed to show significant elongation with cyclic loading in a manner similar to the intact CC ligament complex.[191] In addition, the stiffness and ultimate load of the anatomic reconstruction decreased significantly by 40% and 25%, respectively, compared with the intact CC ligament complex. Comparing reconstructions using semitendinosus supplemented with either hook plate or PDS suture braid in paired cadavers, Dierckman et al. demonstrated superior biomechanical properties with the hook plate, although no difference to maximum load to failure.[235] CC ligament reconstructions with tendon grafts demonstrate greater stability and less translation in vitro when compared with the Weaver-Dunn procedure in its original or modified forms.[354,583] Accurate graft positioning and tensioning are required to reduce the incidence of failure. An in vitro investigation by Stübig et al. demonstrated the superiority of 3D C-arm flat detector navigation compared with freehand arthroscopic technique aided by 2D fluoroscopy for the creation of transosseous tunnels based on anatomic landmarks.[883] In a similar in vitro study, the advantages of electromagnetic navigation compared with standard minimally invasive reconstruction methods in terms of tunnel accuracy and time of preparation were observed.[398] Constraint on the graft has been shown to be reduced experimentally if fixation takes place in the sitting position with the arm in 90 to 120 degrees of abduction.[418] An in vitro CC reconstruction with semitendinosus looped beneath the coracoid and through anatomic clavicular drill holes comparing knot versus interference screw fixation showed no differences in the biomechanical properties except in the mode of failure: graft elongation versus slippage at the screw-tendon interface, respectively.[870] A theoretical advantage is avoidance of additional stress risers in the coracoid process. It has been shown that a CC sling compared with a transcoracoid tunnel results in more pure anterior translation and AP translation of the clavicle under load testing.[1009,344] Comparing graft fixation techniques, Tashjian et al. found that square knotting had superior ultimate strength compared with interference screw fixation but the greatest elongation with cyclic loading versus side-to-side suture fixation and interference screw fixation.[897] The side-to-side construct was the stiffest of the three methods of fixation. The superiority of biointerference screw fixation has been shown, and can be further enhanced with augmentation with nonabsorbable sutures.[272] In cadaver specimens, Breslow et al. identified comparable fixation and stability achieved by a CC fixation method with sutures compared with one with suture anchors.[113]

The concept of surgical recreation of separate CC ligaments has support, both theoretically and from experimental investigations.[826,870,906] Different tendons have been used, and have shown no differences in the mechanical properties of in vitro reconstruction.[272,512] Tunnel placement in the area of the clavicle corresponding to the attachment of the CC ligaments has the best bone density, and correlates with higher loads to failure experimentally.[316] In a virtual shoulder simulated from normal shoulder MRIs, the kinematics of normal CC ligaments could not be restored by three common methods of CC reconstruction, leading the authors to conclude that it may be prudent to select graft fixation techniques most compatible with the type of instability being treated.[417] In addition, the importance of simultaneous AC ligament reconstruction cannot be overlooked.[795]

The direction being taken by investigators with interest in ACJ stabilization is toward the use of stronger materials or methods. There is growing evidence, mostly experimental, that supports a strategy of repair or reconstruction that includes both the AC and CC ligaments.[209] Experimentally, a comparison of retention or excision of the distal clavicle in conjunction with reconstruction of the CC and AC ligaments revealed no significant difference in motion versus the intact state.[66] It is not entirely clear at this time whether rigid or nonrigid fixation is better. The greatest attention has been focused on direct methods to achieve CC stability and, for the most part, indirect methods to achieve AC stability. Therein lies the challenge. It is intuitive that the preservation of the clavicle in its entirety would afford the best opportunity for preserving strength, motion, and function. However, even with maintenance of a congruent ACJ reduction, the necessity for excising the lateral clavicle might not be obviated. Biologically compatible materials as well as grafts are receiving more attention, as are methods considered less invasive.

Results

When compared with nonoperative treatment, operative treatment can result in less pain and better endurance, especially during work.[43,411,696] Operative treatment resulted in improvement with regard to pain and patient satisfaction both in the short term and long term in several studies.[724,735,853] However, from the meta-analysis of Smith et al., no differences were observed in strength, pain, throwing ability, or OA.[853] Better cosmesis and greater duration of sick leave occurred with operative treatment. From their systematic review, Korsten et al. recognized that subjective and objective outcomes were better with operative treatment, although radiographic abnormalities were more common.[477] While subjective and radiographic outcomes were better with operative treatment, objective parameters (UCLA, C-M, ASES, Acromioclavicular Joint Instability [ACJI] scores) were not significantly different. In high-performance overhead athletes, complete pain relief and return to normal was achieved more with operative treatment (92% vs. 80%).[590]

Return to professional football required nearly 60 days.[552] A trend toward earlier return to Australian rules football with a more satisfactory outcome with operative treatment was reported by Cardone et al.[136]

Direct AC and CC ligament repair via transosseous sutures that were protected with a temporary 4.5-mm CC screw for 8 weeks resulted in excellent clinical and radiographic outcomes at a mean follow-up of 72 months.[33] Methods that temporarily transfix the ACJ with pins can produce some excellent and good results.[410,501,515,555,734,887,940] A recent study by Verdano et al. reported a mean C-M score of 92.7, DASH score of 3.2, and SST score of 11.4.[940] Reduction was maintained or there was minimal loss (less than 3 mm) in 85.7% of the patients. Increasingly stable if not improving long-term benefit up to 11 years has been shown.[515] Fair and poor results have been reported to be 50% to 100% as common as excellent and good results.[734,410] Intermediate outcomes, with 60% excellent and good outcomes, were observed.[243] From what might be the report with the longest mean follow-up (24.2 years), by Lizaur et al., the clinical outcomes (Imatani, DASH, UCLA, SST, and VAS satisfaction) were both satisfactory and pain free in 92.1%.[542] Radiographically, reduction was maintained in 86.8%, and the incidence of moderate to severe OA of the ACJ was 16%.

The PDS triple cerclage technique described by Sandmann et al. resulted in 94% excellent and good results, a mean C-M score of 94.3, ASES score of 94.6, and DASH score of 3.46.[804] With respect to the CC distance, they found 85% less than 5 mm, 12% 5 to 10 mm, and one patient with more than 10 mm, none of which affected the clinical outcome. The AC and CC weave with nylon tape resulted in a mean Constant score of 84.9, ASES score of 81.7, and satisfaction in 88.2%, with 94% radiologic reduction.[857] Occasional concomitant direct CC ligament repair did not impact the outcome.

Hook plates have been used extensively in Europe, resulting in reports from various centers as far back as 33 years.* In the earliest reports, the follow-up period was relatively short, with the results mixed and inconsistently reported.† Since then, the clinical and radiographic reliability of the method has been verified in multiple studies, and its use has become more widespread (Fig. 9-68).[236,264,283,429,478,714,872,901,1010] Consistently high mean C-M scores (>92) have been reported.[236,264,422,478, 601,796,1010] In 225 patients with a mean follow-up of 36 months, the mean Taft score in a report by Kienast et al. was very good and good in 84%.[462] Additionally, in their study, both AC and CC intervals were appropriately reduced. Tavakoli et al. reported no redislocations.[901] Minor joint asymmetry may exist at the completion of treatment.[796,901] A poor correlation between clinical and radiographic results is not uncommon.[213,429,796,841,1010] On the contrary, Di Francesco et al. noted a clear correlation between radiographic findings and clinical results. They utilized postreconstruction MRI to assess ligamentous healing and the presence of scar tissue.[236] Healing was present in 37 (88%) (stable) and not present in 5 (12%) (unstable). This correlated with greater than 50% joint subluxation and only fair clinical results. The clinical scores are lower in the infrequent presence of persistent anterior-posterior instability.[429,601] Return to work and sport, often early, is the norm.[236,283,601,714,796,872]

Gstettner et al. performed a comparative study of hook plate versus conservative treatment, and achieved better clinical (Constant 90.4 vs. 80.7, SSV 89.2 vs. 77.6, excellent/good 87.5% vs. 58.8%) and radiographic (CC interval 12.1 mm vs. 15.9 mm, reduction in sports activity 16.4% vs. 23.5%) results in hook plate cases.[355] Ejam et al. observed no significant differences in the outcomes of acute or late operations.[264] Compared with the Phemister method, the Acroplate favored a more complete and rapid recovery without mobility complications.[165]

More recent reports out of Asia have highlighted the ability of the hook plate to produce excellent clinical scores and radiographic parameters.[146,243,1010] Chen et al. reported no loss of reduction and improved clinical outcomes after plate removal.[150] The mean C-M score was 89. Dou and Ren reported 100% excellent and good clinical outcomes.[243]

With the MAAP, Liu et al. reported a mean Constant score of 94, excellent and good results in 94%, and anatomic reductions in 88%.[540]

The outcome of the use of CC screws is generally excellent and good in more than 77% of patients.[29,276,410,546,555,886,887,896] This is the case even when ossification forms between the clavicle and coracoid or is encouraged to form.[456,546] A relatively recent report by Esenyel et al. highlighted a mean Constant score of 98, excellent results in 86.7%, and normal alignment in 96.7%.[276] Percutaneous screw insertion is more difficult, and results in higher rates of complications.[922]

Bone-encircling and bone-engaging fixation with a multitude of flexible materials produce generally favorable clinical outcomes.[160,348,393,409,626,1005,1010] If desired, return to preinjury activity levels can be expeted.[269,305,328,570,565,626] Martetschläger et al. identified an 83% survivorship rate at 2 years using these techniques.[570] Implants specifically designed for initial mechanical and supplemental biologic stabilization demonstrate a favorable immunologic response as well as a histologic response that suggest a functioning implant.[473] In one of the longer term (mean, 70 months) studies using PDS cerclage, Greiner et al. reported favorable clinical outcomes (C-M 91.7, DASH 5, and SSV 92).[348] CC interval increase of more than 5 mm was observed in 20% of the patients; OA was observed in 36%.

Favorable outcomes in the C-M, DASH, and Taft scores can be expected with transclavicular nonabsorbable sutures secured to the coracoid with suture anchors.[160,305] A similar outcome was reported with the addition of supplemental suture anchor fixation across the ACJ.[1016] Somers and Van der Linden reported favorable clinical

*References 11, 114, 213, 236, 240, 241, 264, 283, 333, 346, 362, 390, 429, 443, 601, 638, 714, 814, 819, 841, 872, 945, 990, 997, 1010.

†References 11, 114, 145, 213, 240, 241, 333, 346, 362, 390, 443, 638, 814, 819, 841, 945, 990, 997.

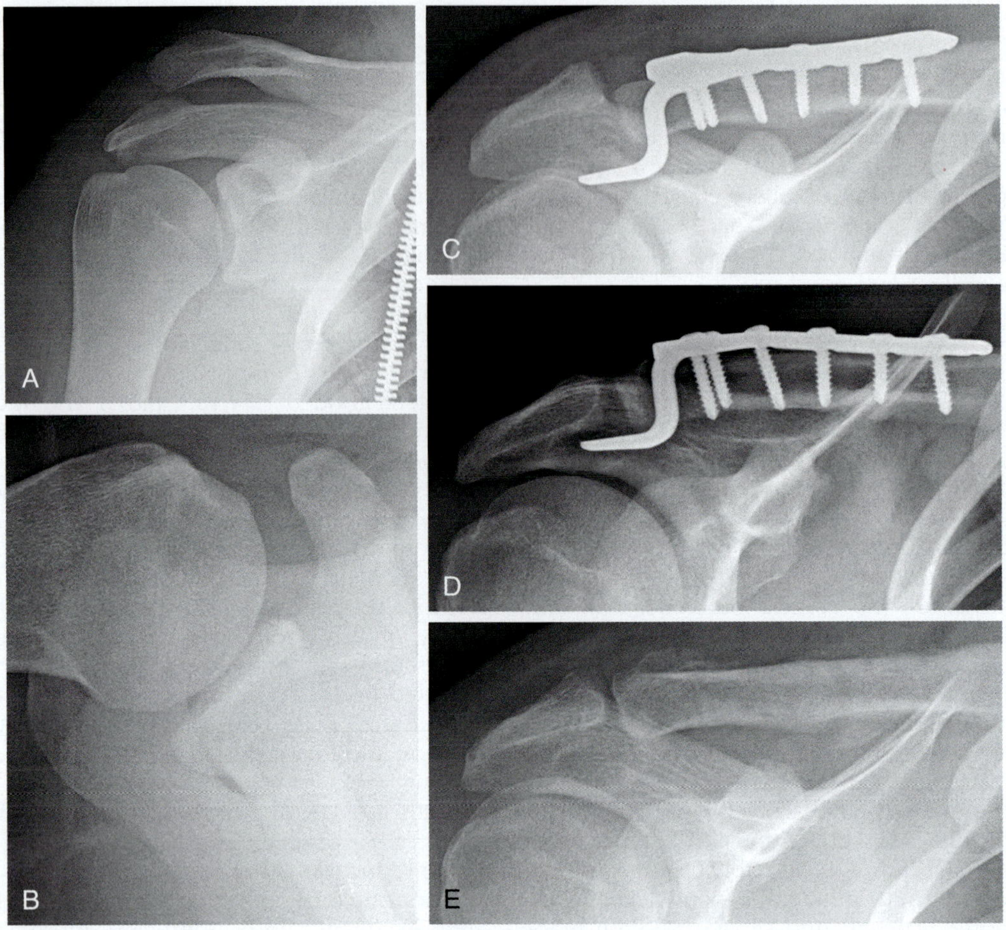

FIGURE 9-68: Treatment with hook plate. **A,** Preoperative anteroposterior (AP) image. **B,** Preoperative axillary lateral image. **C,** First postoperative image (overcorrection). **D,** Preoperative AP removal. Note osteolysis of the acromion at hook. The overreduction was reconciled. **E,** Final image. Note persistent osteolysis, favorable reduction, and remodeling of the screw holes.

and radiologic outcomes with high satisfaction rates using a similar technique performed arthroscopically.[859]

The clinical results of reconstructions using synthetic ligament (Ligastic) indicate a mean C-M score of 82 versus 90 on the healthy side.[565] Despite this score, satisfaction for the postoperative result was high (96%), although some patients complained of residual pain (33%), scar concerns (7%), weakness (1%), work issues (1%), and sport issues (1%). A greater CC distance on the operative side did not adversely affect the outcome. Kany et al., using double braided polyester, reported excellent and good outcomes in 88% of their patients.[444] The efficacy and safety of the LARS device has been shown.[324,626] Motta et al. identified complete and incomplete ossifications in 96% of patients who recovered normal ACJ motion as demonstrated by 90 degrees of abduction and 0 degrees of external rotation against resistance and cross arm test.[626] They showed full clinical recovery, and no correlations were recognized with radiographic or clinical outcomes.

Ye et al. reported a mean C-M score of 95.3 and markedly improved VAS score with transclavicular and subcoracoid passage of titanium cerclage multifilament cables with 82% anatomic reduction.[1005] They recommended removal 6 months after implantation to avert fatigue breakage.

Transosseous sutures spanning the CC interval may be secured through holes in metal buttons held intimately to the bone cortex by knotting the passed suture over the button. With such an open technique, an early (mean, 12 to 18 months) clinical success rate of nearly 90% together with radiographic stability restoration was achieved.[81,217,328,601,968,1007] At a mean follow-up of 24 months, De Carli et al. noted very high outcome scores (mean C-M, 98.2; ASES, 100; ACJI, 87.9), with the only significant difference from nonoperative treatment being for the ACJI score.[217] Subjective and radiographic parameters favor operative treatment. Yi and Kim recognized that when the surgeon controls variables of clavicle and coracoid tunnel alignment, oriented as perpendicularly as possible, both clinical and radiographic improvement are favored.[1007] Shin and Kim reported a mean C-M score of 97.5 at 25.6 months.[835] Loss of reduction did not influence the C-M score significantly. With a slightly longer follow-up (mean, 39 months), Rosslenbroich et al. showed a mean C-M of 94.7 and a mean Taft score of 10.8.[776] An influence of age on outcomes was observed, with younger patients achieving higher outcome values.

Grassbaugh et al. showed an advantage to suture button techniques compared with other techniques, some historical, for the rate of revision and radiographic outcomes.[345] However, in their review of their experience with eight different methods of treatment, they could show no statistically significant differences in clinical function or pain regardless of the treatment method. They observed poorer results for the treatment of chronic injuries and in the presence of DCR.

Some series of arthroscopic suture button techniques show a higher rate of successful clinical versus radiographic outcomes at early-to-intermediate term follow-up.[174,181,218,328,404,482,570,635,801,939] Original buttons with a diameter of 6.5 mm migrated more often than a wider button (10 mm).[174] No significant CC interval differences were observed by Cohen et al. who also obtained a C-M score of 91 despite piano key deformity and superior-inferior mobility in 40%.[174] Pan et al. reported excellent functional recovery, no or minimal pain, and no radiographic failures at a mean of 2 years.[692] The influence of tunnel orientation on the results is inconclusive.[482] Glanzmann et al. emphasized the ability to eliminate pathologic posterior translation radiographically.[328] Cook et al. obtained as many excellent and good results as fair and poor results.[181] If failures were excluded, the mean C-M score reported by Spoliti et al. improved from 89.7 to 92.4.[868]

Open techniques deemed "anatomic" reveal definite improvement in both pain and function, with an ASES score of 92 and Constant score of 94.7.[138] Three failures yielded a success rate of 82%. Similar outcomes with respect to ASES scores as well as favorable SANE scores (89.1), QuickDASH (5.6), and excellent satisfaction were reported by Millett et al.[611] Radiographic reduction was maintained in 82% of the patients. Arthroscopic-assisted techniques with interference screw autograft fixation in bone tunnels in both the clavicle and coracoid yielded a C-M score of 96.6, minimal (<2 mm) to mild (2 to 4 mm) or less displacement, and excellent functional and subjective outcomes.[1008]

Studies that have compared the results of AC and CC fixation report conflicting outcomes.[53,498] Favorable results were reported by Weaver and Dunn and subsequently reiterated by other authors who performed the operation as originally described.[125,746,959,964] Modified Weaver-Dunn operations also produced favorable outcomes.[516,586,673,735,969] With a modification of the Cadenet method, Cerciello et al. reported mean C-M score of 94.3, VAS pain score of 0.91, 92% satisfaction 88%, complete reduction, and no degenerative changes.[143] Sood et al., from their systematic review of the published literature available at the time, concluded that there was a low level of evidence to support the use of CAL transfer.[863] In addition, supplemental fixation did not improve the results secondary to complications of its usage. A high rate of recurrent deformity was expected. Acute and chronic cases fared equally. The outcomes with retention or excision of the distal clavicle did not differ unless the retained clavicle manifested OA, in which case the results were inferior.

Comparing the Vukov and Phemister methods, Radovanovic et al. found similar outcomes but a shorter recovery time with the technique of Vukov.[742]

Mixed results have been reported for the treatment of type III injuries with transposition of the tip of the coracoid process, which includes the short head of the biceps and the coracobrachialis to the clavicle.[782,42,83,846] Skjeldal et al. advised that the procedure not be performed in patients with acute type III injuries.[846] The proximally based conjoined tendon with CC sutures method of Jiang et al. resulted in superior clinical scores (ASES 91.4, C-M 90.6, SST 10.9), with overall excellent or good results in 89% of the patients.[435] The majority returned to the same work and sports.

The early results of using autologous tendon indicate both efficacy and safety when grafts such as gracilis are utilized.[505] A comparison study analyzing the results of reconstruction with Ethibond sutures through tunnels and semitendinosus autograft demonstrated no clinical or radiographic differences.[564] Material costs related to certain newer implants may not completely offset any realized savings gain accompanying their usage.[404]

Several studies report the lack of correlation between clinical outcome and abnormal radiologic findings.[515,776,817,1008] However, in the occasional instances of AP instability, inferior outcome scores are to be expected.[601]

Complications

The systematic review of Korsten et al. determined that complications were more prevalent with operative treatment.[477] Isolated ACJ fixation has a higher complication rate than CC fixation.[53,498,738]

The ability of the stabilization method to maintain the operative reduction is considered the hallmark of the worthiness of the procedure. The incidence of recurrent deformity has been reported to be as high as 80%.[181] The definition of loss of reduction with "anatomic" reconstruction varies from author to author. Anything other than anatomic reduction (referencing the contralateral side) varies from 6% to 100% (Fig. 9-69).[138] It is generally believed that after treatment, the extent of congruity or incongruity as well as the presence of OA and the development of heterotopic ossification appear to have no correlation with the outcome, regardless of the method.

A high failure rate is expected for soft tissue reconstructions if either AC or CC fixation techniques are not incorporated as additional protection from deforming forces.[33] However, a very concerning complication of ACJ repair or reconstruction is hardware failure. Pins and wires used to stabilize the ACJ can break or loosen and subsequently migrate, as reported by Lyons and Rockwood and others (Fig. 9-70).[250,479,515,529,536,553,580,670,928,985] Serious injury and death can result from pin migration.[2,299,347,363,487,529,553,753,828] The materials used for CC loop techniques and foreign body reactions to these materials can result in failures, the majority of which result from

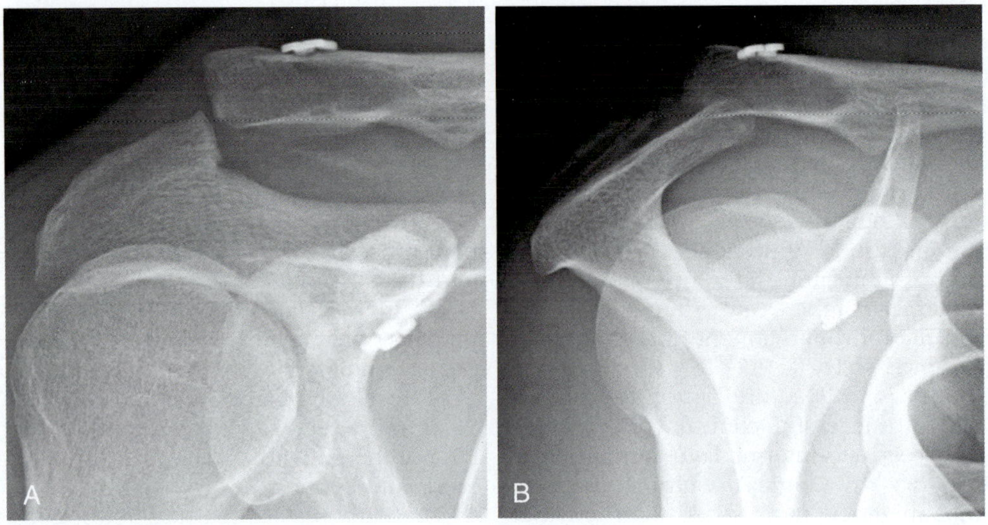

FIGURE 9-69: Early loss of reduction of acute type III dislocation treated with synthetic sutures tied over cortical buttons.

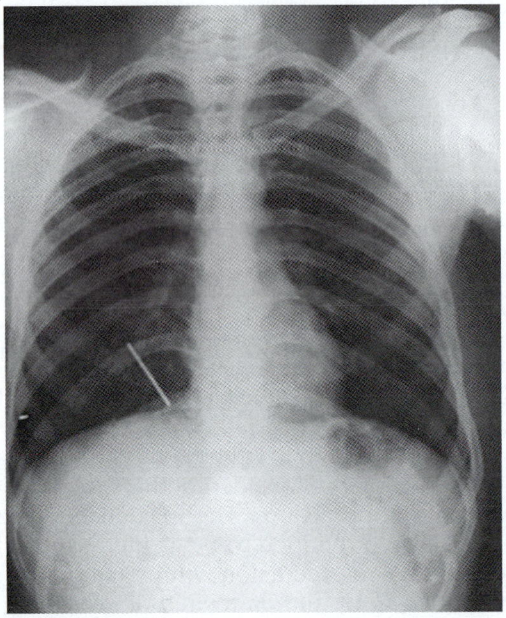

FIGURE 9-70: Steinmann pin fixation was chosen for an acromioclavicular joint repair. After breaking, it migrated to the right lung. (From Rockwood CA, Green DP,eds. *Fractures*. 2nd ed. Philadelphia: JB Lippincott; 1984.)

the erosion or fracture of either the clavicle or the coracoid process (Fig. 9-71).[101,176,201,248,307,334,479,568,616,876,1005] Screws, wires, cables, or nonmetal synthetics can suffer fatigue breakage, leading to recurrence of the deformity (Fig. 9-72). Screws can lose their purchase in the coracoid and pull through (Fig. 9-73).

The propensity for complications related to the engaging hook was realized in the static cadaver investigation by ElMaraghy et al.[267] Hook positioning was unpredictable, especially because of the widely variable acromial and sometimes distal clavicular morphology. In their study, the incidence of subacromial bursa violation was 87%, supraspinatus muscle belly contact was 60%, and the focal contact of the tip of the hook with the undersurface of the acromion was 60%. These phenomena were validated and others recognized including subacromial impingement and RC lesions (partial thickness) in the study by Lin et al., who performed dynamic sonography of the subacromial space and environs after hook plate procedures.[535] The engaging hook of the hook plate can lead to acromial osteolysis or erosions with varying frequency and extent, sometimes progressing to a fracture (Fig. 9-74).[146,155,355,429,467,535,638] No acromial osteolysis secondary to the hook was reported by Metzlaff et al., who removed plates between 10 and 13 weeks from the time of implantation.[601] While the duration of implant retention may yield excellent stability, the price paid in terms of acromial osteolysis and ACJ degeneration has been recognized.[146,422] It can also lose its purchase beneath the acromion process (Fig. 9-75). Loss of reduction can spontaneously occur after removal of the implant, but is infrequent.[213,236,264,478,796,1010] Reports of hardware failure are not unique to the hook plate used by Kienast et al.[462] Other complications related to the hook plate include medial clavicle fracture and screw failure (Fig. 9-76).[283,901] Hypertrophic incisional scars were observed in as many as 63% of patients.[429] Additional complications reported include progressive degeneration of the ACJ, frozen shoulder, hematoma, and wound-healing problems.[146,236,355,390,478,841]

Loss of reduction by suture anchor malpositioning was reported by Choi et al.[160] Other notable factors contributing to loss of reduction include obesity, heavy, muscular limbs, and noncompliance with postoperative protective measures.[305,1016]

Contemporary techniques that promote "anatomic" reconstruction, including bone tunneling performed at the time of transosseous CC reconstruction, are solely responsible for fractures through the clavicle and coracoid, although coracoid looping techniques are not without risk. With the recent explosion of these techniques, the frequency of iatrogenic

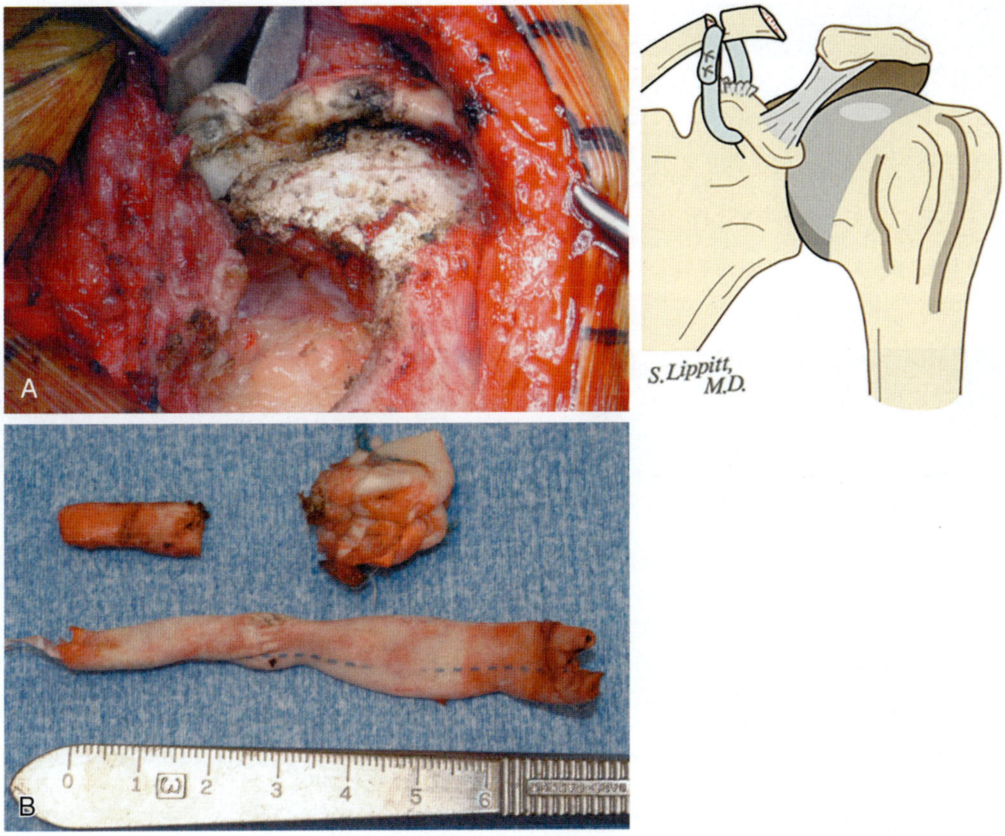

FIGURE 9-71: Coracoclavicular loop fixation with vascular graft. **A,** In situ vascular graft that has eroded into the clavicle. **B,** Bulky vascular graft removed because of painful soft tissue irritation. (Illustration courtesy Steven Lippitt, MD.)

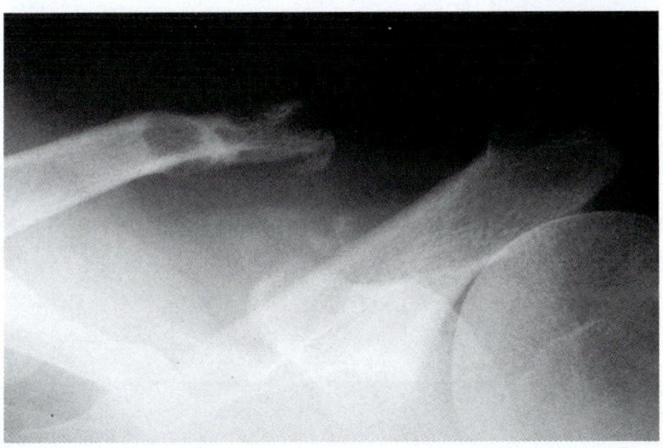

FIGURE 9-72: Failure of nonabsorbable sutures used for a type III injury, with recurrence of deformity and reactive changes within the clavicle.

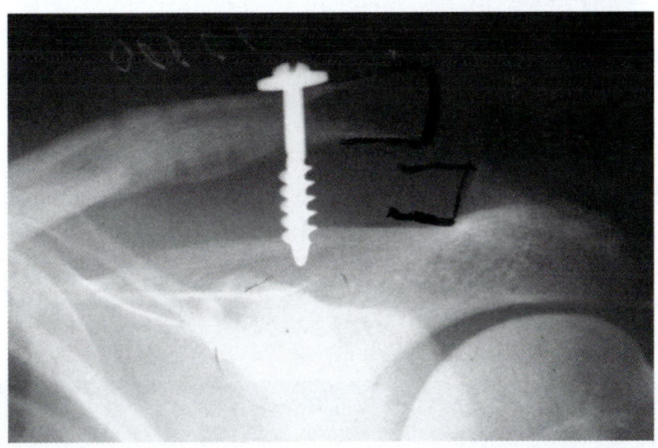

FIGURE 9-73: Loss of fixation of the coracoclavicular screw used for a type III injury, with recurrence of deformity.

fracture is increasing (Fig. 9-77).[321,570,606,611,727,817,900,923,1008] In a series of 27 patients, complications were more common in coracoid tunneling (80%) versus coracoid looping (35%) methods.[606] To avoid iatrogenic clavicle fractures from tunnels, several authors adhere to techniques whereby biologic graft encircles both the clavicle and the coracoid.[583,960] A coracoid fracture with subcoracoid passage of tendon graft was reported by Tomlinson et al.[916] Millett et al. reported a revision and complication in 8 of 31 cases (25.8%).[611]

Many of these techniques employ flipping buttons, sometimes placed arthroscopically, that may migrate with loss of surgical correction in as many as 92% of cases.* Most often, this phenomenon is related to tunnel malpositioning, expansion of the drilled tunnel, and sometimes

---

**References 181, 218, 328, 482, 534, 570, 606, 627, 633, 635, 776, 801, 835, 857, 868.*

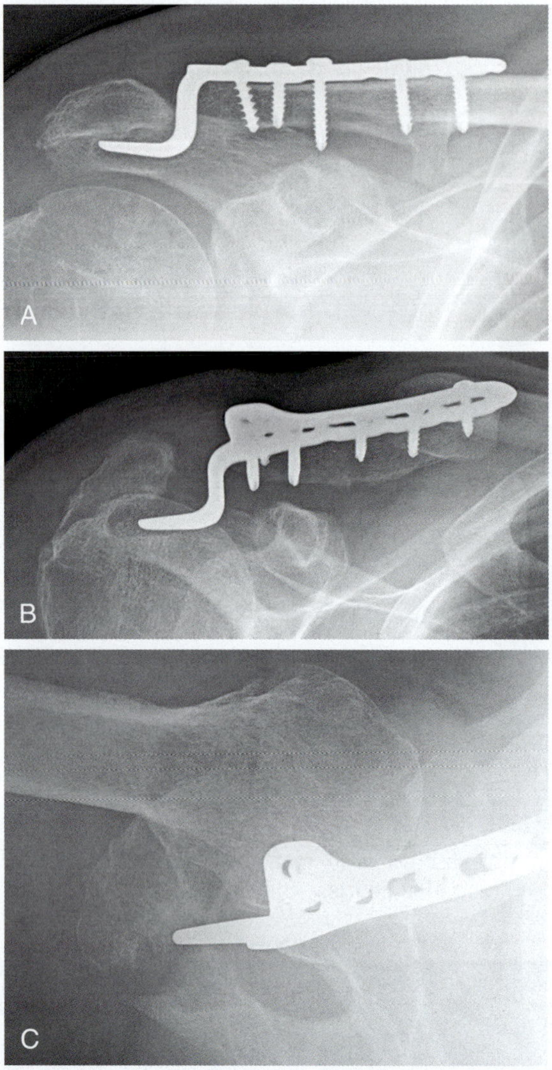

FIGURE 9-74: **A** and **B,** Two examples reveal a large zone of osteolysis around the hook of the plate indicative of substantial motion unwisely performed in the presence of the hook plate. **C,** Fracture of the acromion process as a result of osteolysis.

fracture through the respective bone (Fig. 9-78).[181,321,835] As an exception, Motta et al. identified #5 FiberWire failure in four patients with ligamentous hyperlaxity.[627] Cook et al. showed that medialized tunnels were a significant predictor of early loss of reduction.[182] Carofino and Mazzocca advised minimization of tunnel diameter spaced no closer than 20 to 25 mm with the most lateral tunnel 10 to 15 mm from the lateral edge of the clavicle.[138] This phenomenon was diminished if the conoid tunnel was placed at 25% of the clavicle length from the

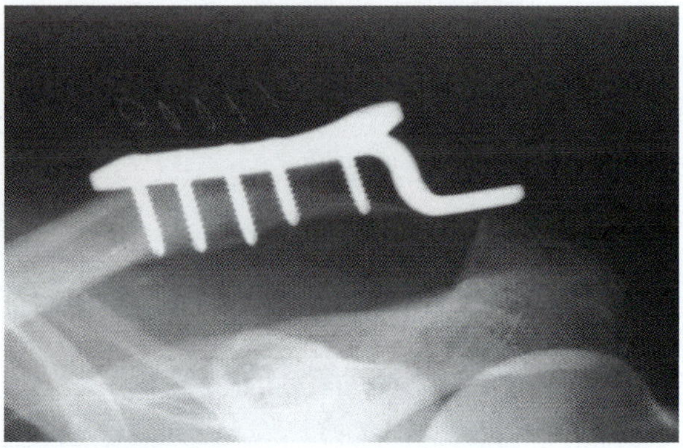

FIGURE 9-75: Hook plate no longer secured beneath the acromion process.

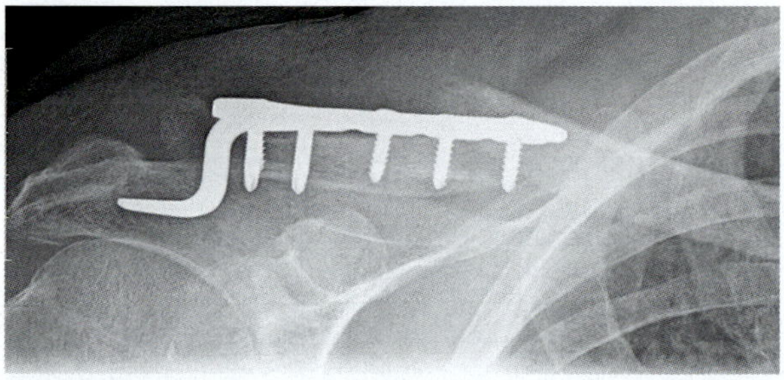

FIGURE 9-76: Fracture of clavicle propagating from the medial screw.

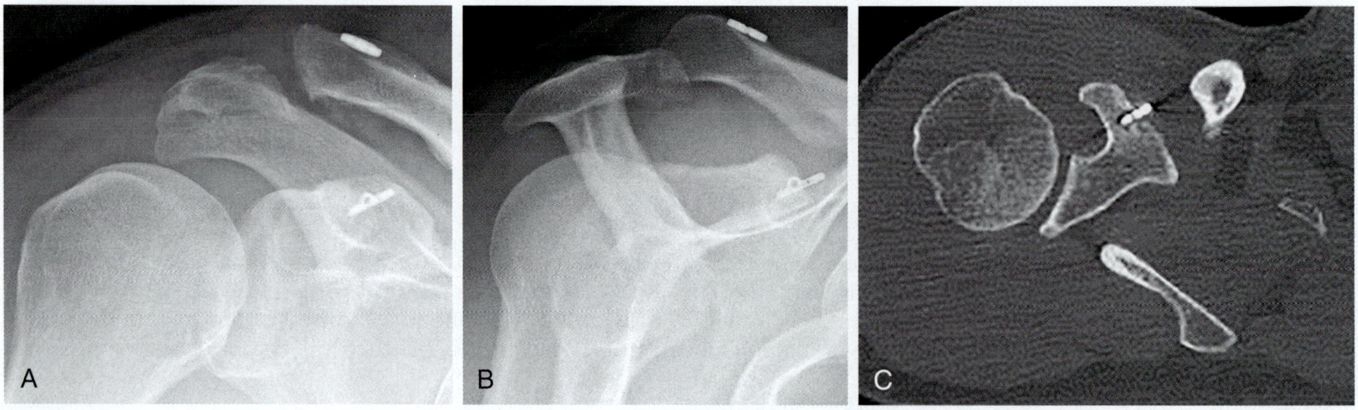

FIGURE 9-77: **A** to **C,** Iatrogenic fracture of the coracoid secondary to malposition of the tunnel created to place the cortical button.

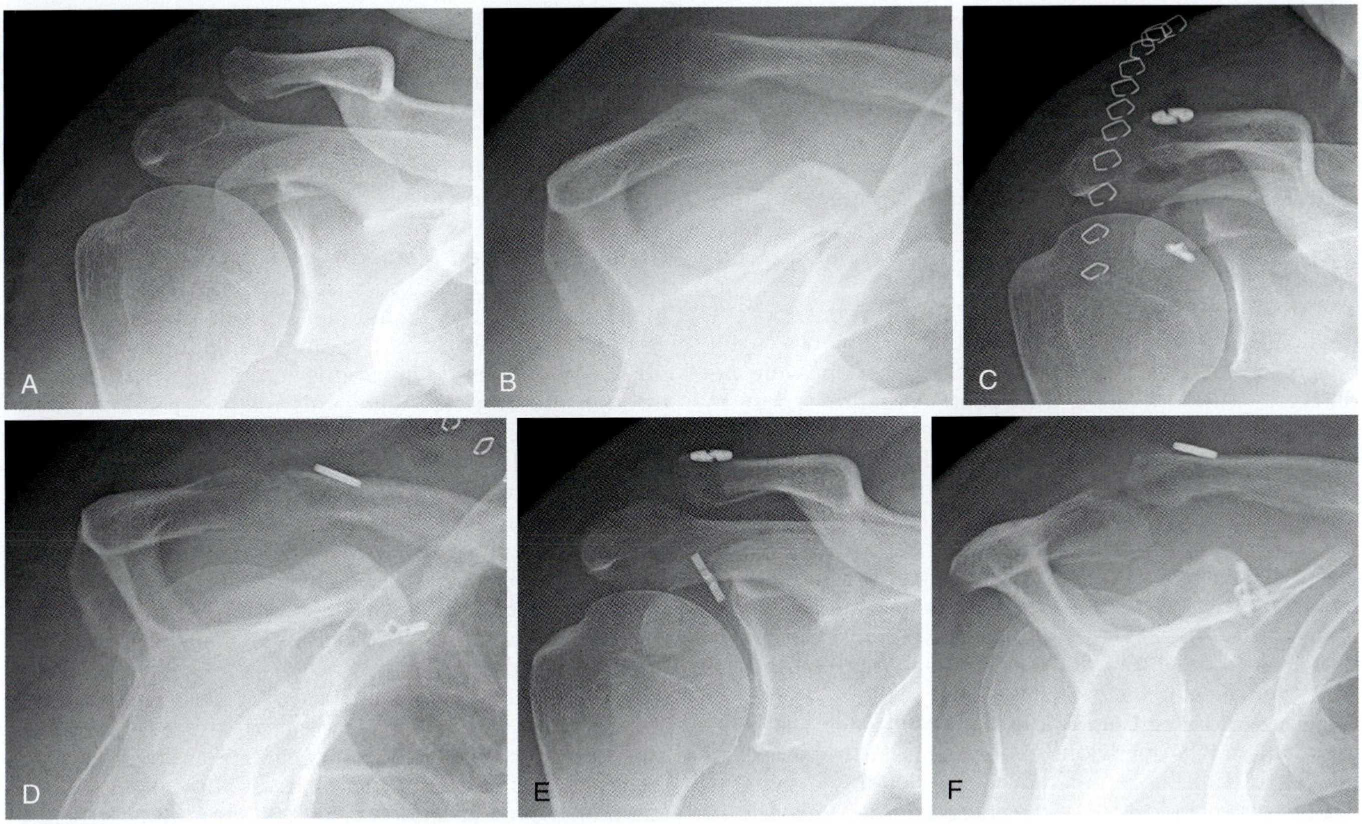

FIGURE 9-78: Tunnel malposition leading to early loss of reduction of an acute type III dislocation treated with synthetic sutures tied over cortical buttons. **A** and **B,** Preoperative images. **C** and **D,** Early postoperative images. **E** and **F,** Images taken 5 weeks later.

lateral edge of the clavicle. The incidence of posterior instability, static or dynamic, may be as high as 53%.[482,817] Instances when clavicular and coracoid buttons were not aligned perpendicular to each other suffered greater loss of reduction.[817] In this study, the authors also observed that younger patients achieved superior clinical and radiographic outcomes. Patients with complications did not fare any different than those without complications, but they were less satisfied with their operation and did not experience good or excellent results.[570] Rosslenbroich et al. identified a 22% loss of reduction (subluxation more than 50%).[776] Shin and Kim reported a complication rate of 44%, including clavicle fracture propagating from a drill hole, fixation failures, clavicular erosion, and ACJ arthrosis.[835] Despite a variable degree of loss of reduction (more than 50% difference in 33%) and complications in 44%, the mean C-M scores in patients with complications and reduction loss were 95.2 and 95.6, respectively. Woodmass et al. performed a systematic review of complications of arthroscopic treatment of AC dislocations.[992] Soft tissue irritability over the clavicular hardware was the most common complication in acute cases.

In a long-term follow-up using PDS cerclage, complete redislocation was observed in 2 of 50 patients (5%).[348] The rate was 9% with the triple cerclage technique in a shorter study by Sandmann et al.[804] One redislocation was observed with nylon suture weave.[857]

Synthetic ligament complication may be unique to the device. Use of Ligastic-type reconstruction was abandoned as a result of progressively increasing osteolysis appearing at the site of ligament passage through the clavicle in 22% of the patients.[565] A 14% incidence of OA or osteolysis was noted as well. Kany et al. observed a 21% loss or reduction and a 12% incidence of night pain and capsulitis.[444] One sleeve migration occurred. One instance of clavicular tunnel enlargement was observed in each of two reports.[162,324]

Infection, usually superficial, at the site of ACJ reconstruction has been reported.* Staged reconstruction may be possible after the removal of all foreign material, rendering the operative site sterile. An aseptic response to braided polyester synthetic ligament, Nottingham Surgilig (Surgicraft), resulting in osteolysis of the distal clavicle was reported by Dearden et al.[212]

Technical overcorrection of the CC interval, while enticing to preempt anticipated superior subluxation after repair, may result in compression of the brachial plexus.[492,301] Entrapment of the brachial plexus with devastating consequences resulting from subcoracoid looping techniques has been documented.[903]

**References 16, 138, 160, 217, 236, 264, 328, 348, 462, 645, 776, 796, 859, 940, 955.*

Inadvertent injury to subclavian neurovascular structures during clavicular drilling associated with placement of a hook plate is a potential complication that can be averted with a keen knowledge of recognized safe drilling angle and depths.[739]

Posttraumatic arthritis has been shown to be more common after operative than after nonoperative treatment.[131] Posttraumatic arthritis can result and is more likely in ACJs that remain incongruent at the completion of their treatment.[887,179]

Calvo et al. have shown that the incidence of CC ossification is higher after operative treatment.[131] Millbourn reported that the incidence and severity were not different with operative treatment.[607] In the report by Greiner et al., one instance of revision operation was necessary secondary to prolific CC calcification.[348] At 10 years of follow-up, posttraumatic arthritis was reported to be more common when AC fixation, as opposed to CC fixation, was used.[887]

Scapular dyskinesis and scapular malposition, inferior medial border prominence, coracoid pain and malposition, and dyskinesis of scapular movement (SICK) syndrome have been reported in 11.7% and 2.9% of patients with type III injuries.[633]

Salvage of Failed Coracoclavicular Stabilization. Depending on the index operation, any number of salvage options may be available as reported by Geaney et al.[315] Confounding factors include loss of the integrity of the clavicle or coracoid due to erosion or fracture, clavicle foreshortening, and tissue exhaustion (CAL, conjoined tendon, deltotrapezius fascia). The optimal conditions for revision exist when the clavicle and the coracoid remain intact, and specific points for materials anchorage are preserved. CC looping techniques or their variations, with supplemental but temporary rigid fixation, would appear to offer the best options. For these extreme cases, there may be advantages to using biologic as opposed to synthetic reconstruction techniques. The first report of the use of autologous tendon between the clavicle and the coracoid was used for this indication.[911] The continued use of autologous semitendinosus tendon is supported by its strength properties and results in a few cases.[370,440,469,499,625,898,899] Deveci et al. incorporated the use of autogenous anterior tibialis tendon through transosseous tunnels with a hook plate to offload the bone tendon interfaces during the healing period and optimize integration of the tendon in the tunnel.[229] They reported lower C-M scores (mean, 77.7) than for index procedures but no loss of reduction. The use of a braided polyester ligament in this setting has been described.[430]

Salvaging iatrogenic fracture of the coracoid process may prove difficult.[606,980] It usually thwarts any opportunity to achieve stabilization for intraosseous fixation between the clavicle and scapula unless substantial, high-quality bone remains available at the intersection of the base of the coracoid process with the body of the scapula and the glenoid neck. The best option may be the use of a hook plate and separate internal fixation of the clavicle fracture if feasible.[452,606,980] Transposition of some or all of the origin of the conjoint tendon with or without bone is another consideration.[435,436,465]

Recurrent deformity resulting from iatrogenic fracture of the clavicle may be reconciled as simply open reduction internal fixation of the fracture.[570] When reconstruction is not deemed possible as a result of deficits of bone and soft tissue, total claviculectomy, reported for other indications, could be considered as the terminal, definitive reconstruction.[483]

Author's Preferred Method

I originally used Dacron vascular CC loops for type III injuries. When the technique fell out of favor due to erosion, nonabsorbable sutures ranging in size and number were passed in various combinations around and through the clavicle. When this method resulted in frequent failures, a more rigid form of fixation was found with the Rockwood screw. Even with the best visualization for optimal screw placement into the coracoid process, failures continued. A combination of Rockwood screw and modern nonabsorbable suture (FiberWire) did not solve the problem of failures with recurrent deformity. Since 2004, I have been using a hook plate in conjunction with nonabsorbable CC sutures (Fig. 9-79).

With the patient in the beach chair position, a skin incision is made in Langer's lines over the clavicle in a line just lateral to the tip of the coracoid process (Figs. 9-80 and 9-81). Generous subcutaneous flaps are raised and the deltotrapezius fascia is incised over the lateral clavicle, extending over its end, where the supporting structures are disrupted and just onto the acromion process (Figs. 9-82 and 9-83). The ACJ is inspected and debrided as needed, preserving the entire length of the clavicle (Fig. 9-84). Sufficient subperiosteal exposure of the clavicle is performed to permit application of the shortest plate. The surgical approach at this location does not jeopardize the

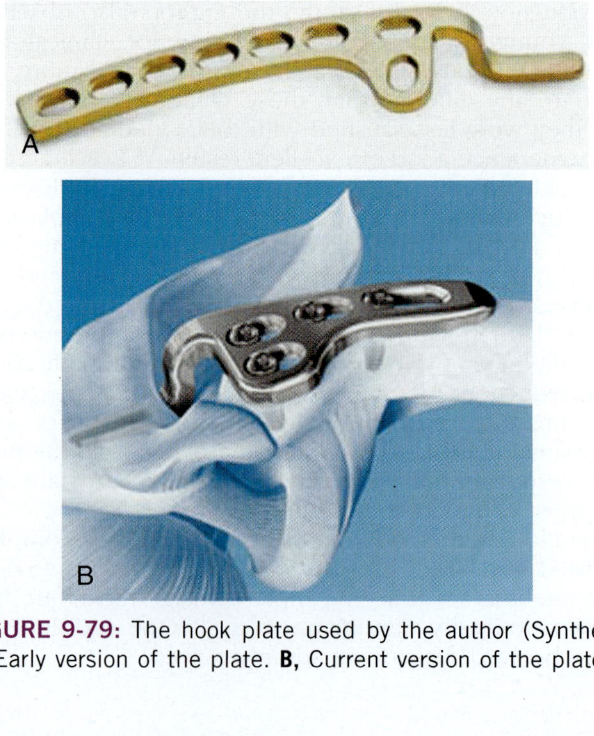

FIGURE 9-79: The hook plate used by the author (Synthes). **A,** Early version of the plate. **B,** Current version of the plate.

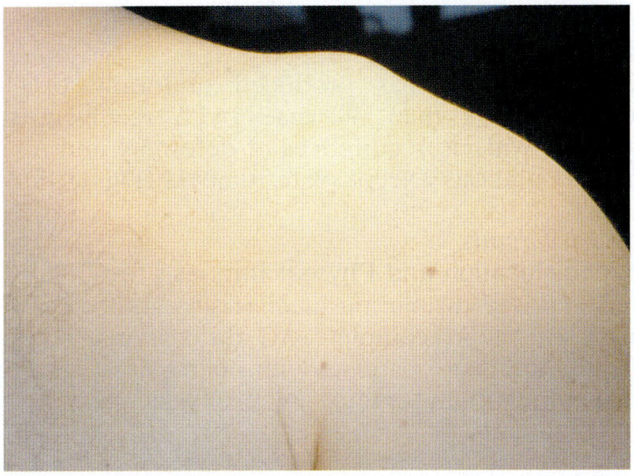

FIGURE 9-80: Acromioclavicular joint deformity apparent at the time of the operation.

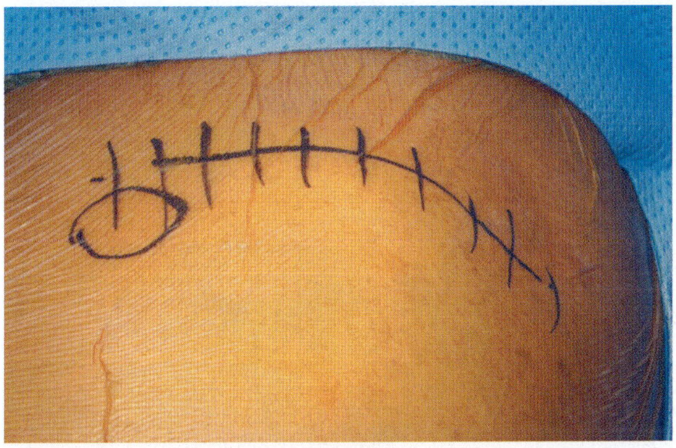

FIGURE 9-81: Skin incision in the relaxed skin tension lines.

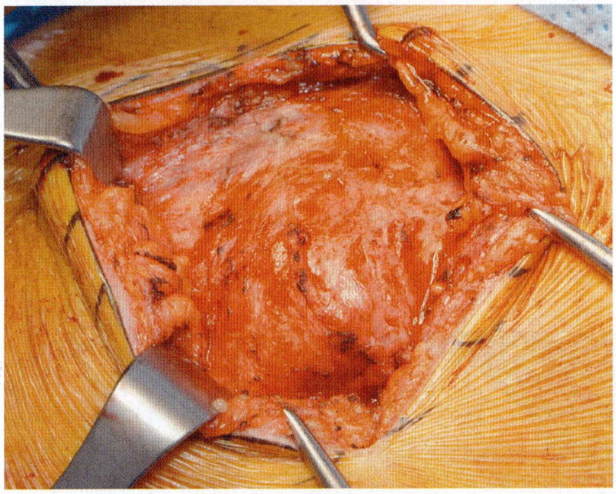

FIGURE 9-82: Superficial dissection to expose the deltoid, trapezius, clavicle, and acromioclavicular joint.

integrity of the major neurovascular structures, which are more than 4.5 cm from the clavicle.[761]

Three 1-mm cotton Dacron sutures are passed beneath the coracoid process as close as possible to its base, then posterior to the clavicle and back toward the coracoid

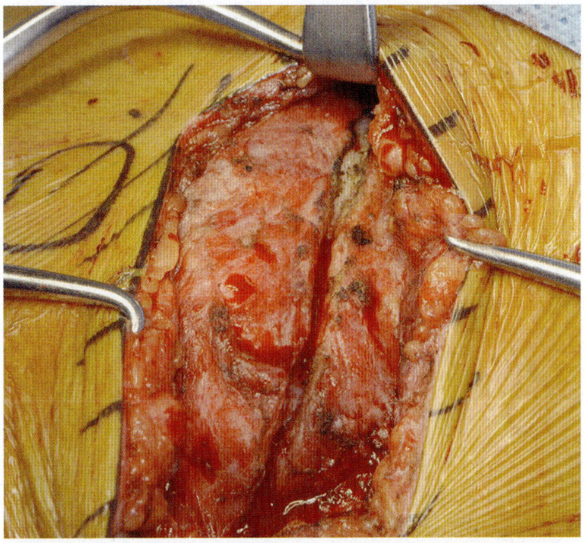

FIGURE 9-83: Deep dissection between the deltoid and the trapezius, with entry into the injured acromioclavicular joint.

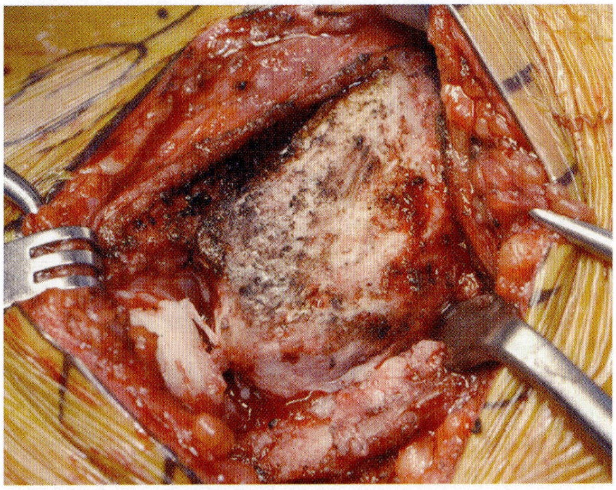

FIGURE 9-84: Exposure of the lateral clavicle. Note the disruption of the intra-articular disk.

(Figs. 9-85 to 9-87). They are not tied at this point. Access for the hook portion of the plate is created by blunt dissection at the junction of the medial acromion and the scapular spine. This important step enables proper placement of the hook beneath the acromion process, advancing it laterally as far as possible (Fig. 9-88). A trial implant is selected based on the estimated height of the joint and the requirements for adequate screw purchase in the clavicle (Fig. 9-89). The joint is reduced by manually stabilizing the plate, which now lies superior to the clavicle, while the acromion is brought into proper relationship with the lateral clavicle by axial force delivered through the upper limb. Occasionally at this point, the plate has to be removed and contoured slightly to optimize the fit to the clavicle. It is then held in the reduced position with a bone-holding forceps (Fig. 9-90). Reduction is confirmed, and then the plate is secured to the clavicle with screws. The sutures, which have come to lie beneath the plate, are tied (Fig. 9-91).

The deltoid, trapezius, and ACJ-supporting structures are closed anatomically or, where necessary, imbricated (Fig. 9-92). The skin is closed with adhesive strips (Fig. 9-93). The upper limb is immobilized for 6 weeks and used to a very limited extent only below the shoulder for another 6 weeks. The plate is routinely removed between the 12th and the 16th week after the operation (Fig. 9-94).

This technique has produced uniformly excellent results in more than 30 cases with relatively short follow-up, with no recurrences of deformity and no secondary operations except plate removal (Fig. 9-95).

Type III Variants

Pseudodislocation and Physeal Injuries

When exposed to injuring mechanisms and forces sufficient to result in complete AC dislocations in adults, skeletally immature patients with open physes and thick periosteum sustain unique injuries generically termed type III variants.[682]

Signs and Symptoms

Although the patient appears acutely injured, pain is usually less than with a similar injury in a skeletally

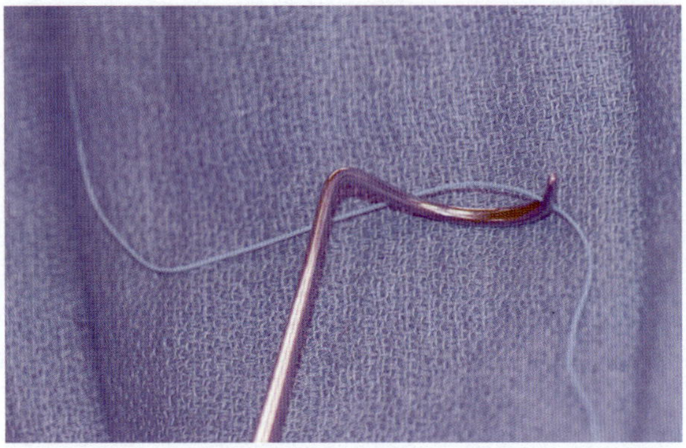

FIGURE 9-85: Curved instrument used to pass the pulling sutures beneath the clavicle.

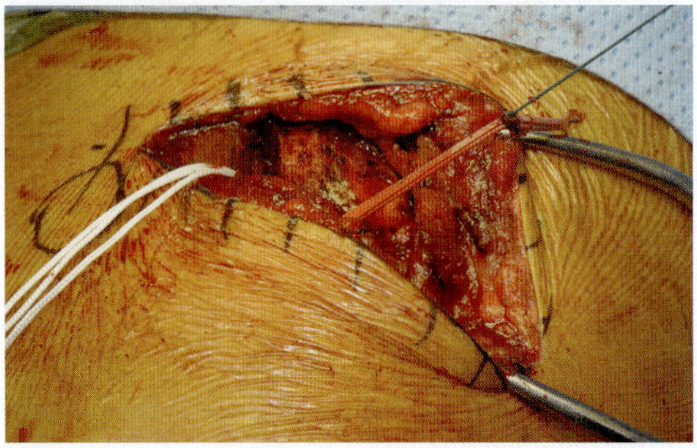

FIGURE 9-86: Three 1-mm cotton Dacron sutures being pulled beneath the coracoid process.

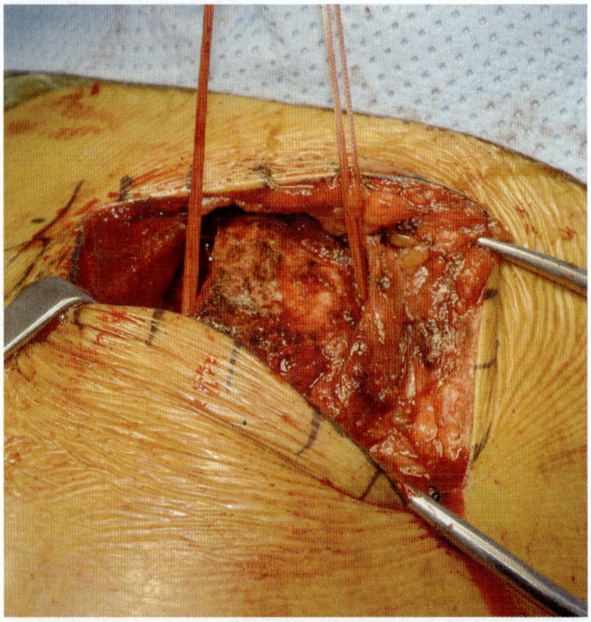

FIGURE 9-87: Sutures passed posterior to the clavicle.

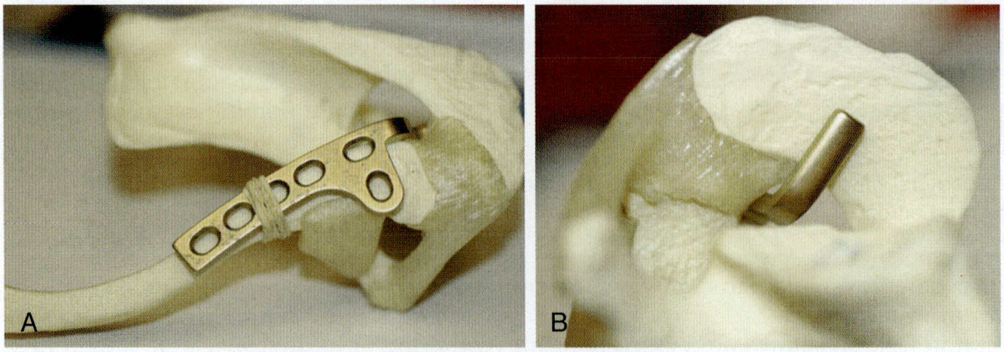

FIGURE 9-88: Positioning the implant. **A** and **B,** Saw bone models demonstrate the proper position of the plate. Note that it is as lateral as possible.

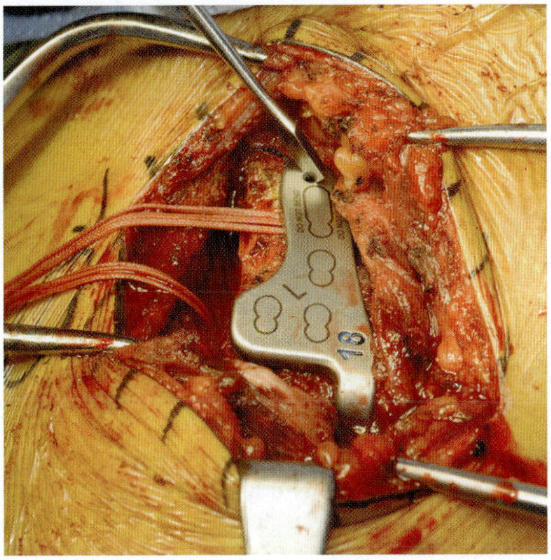

FIGURE 9-89: Implant trial being positioned.

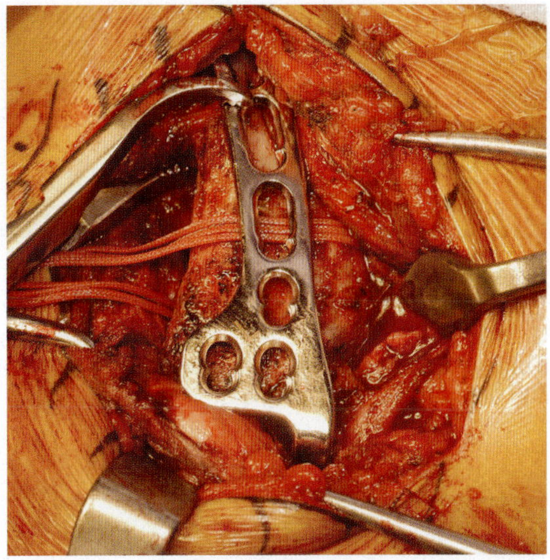

FIGURE 9-90: The definitive implant is provisionally secured.

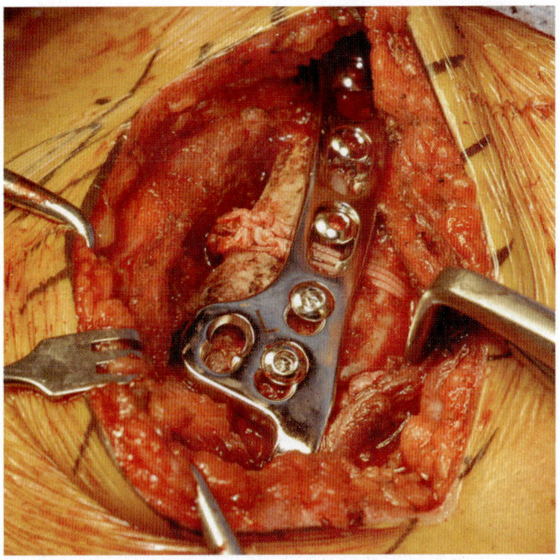

FIGURE 9-91: The definitive implant is secured to the bone with screws, and the sutures are tied.

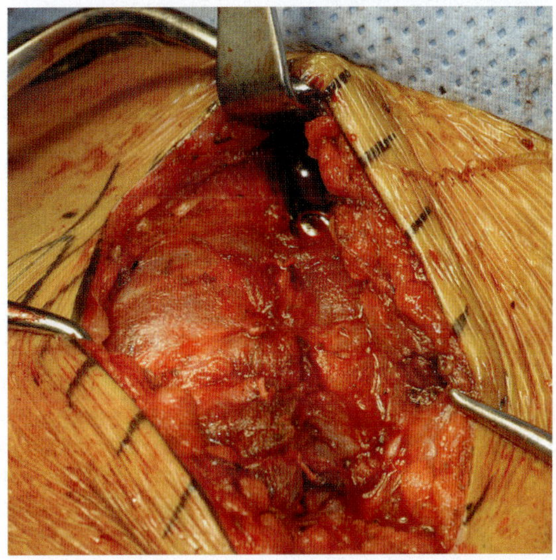

FIGURE 9-92: Deltotrapezius and acromioclavicular joint closure.

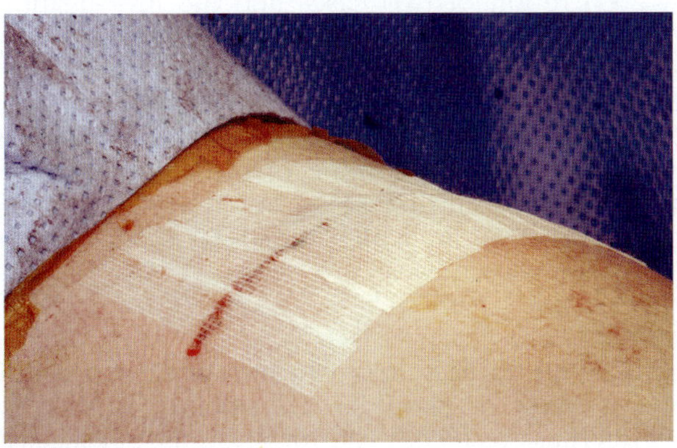

FIGURE 9-93: Skin closure with notable absence of the previous deformity.

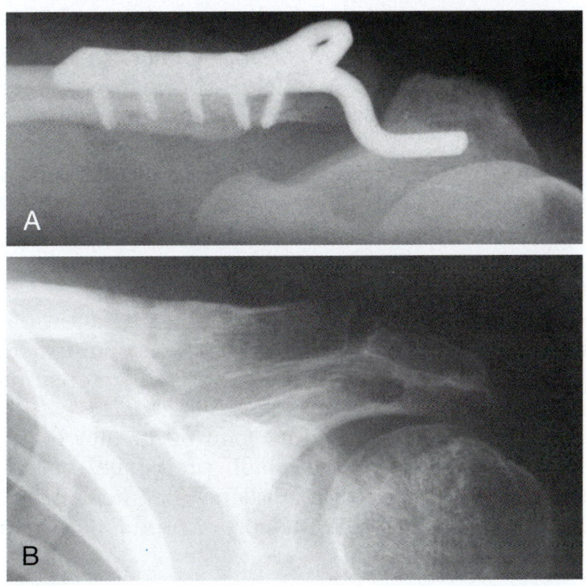

FIGURE 9-94: **A,** Radiograph after the operation. **B,** Radiograph at the final follow-up.

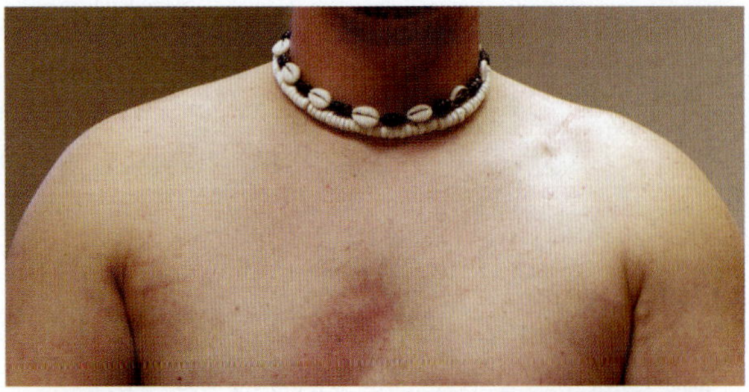

FIGURE 9-95: Clinical appearance after hook plate implantation, healing, and implant removal, with a notable lack of deformity and an aesthetically pleasing scar.

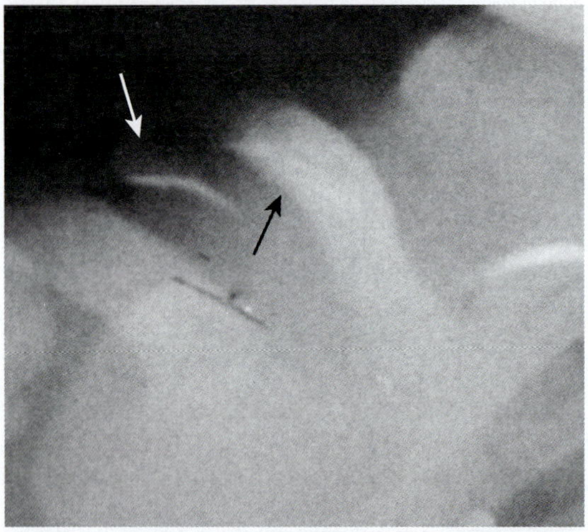

FIGURE 9-96: Type III variant in the immature skeleton. A Thurston Holland fragment *(white arrow)* has resulted from this injury. The *black arrow* shows apparent coracoclavicular interval widening due to clavicular disruption from the periosteal tube. (From Ogden JA. Distal clavicular physeal injury. *Clin Orthop Relat Res.* 1984;188:68-73.)

mature patient. Guarding is not as strict. The injured limb is held in a protective manner adjacent to the torso, less often with the assistance of the opposite upper limb. Superior soft tissue abrasion, bruising, and swelling may be present. Active and passive motion are resisted, inhibiting the accurate assessment of motion and strength. Tenderness is confined mostly to the superior aspect of the lateral clavicle.

Imaging

The most obvious finding is complete separation of the acromion and the lateral clavicle that is accompanied by widening of the CC interval. A vertical CC interval more than 12 mm and 11 mm in skeletally immature males and females, respectively, or more than 50 greater than the contralateral side suggests a high probability of an AC dislocation.[511] A Thurston Holland fragment may be detectable (Fig. 9-96). MRI may prove useful to determine preservation or injury to the CC ligaments and the ACJ capsule.[470]

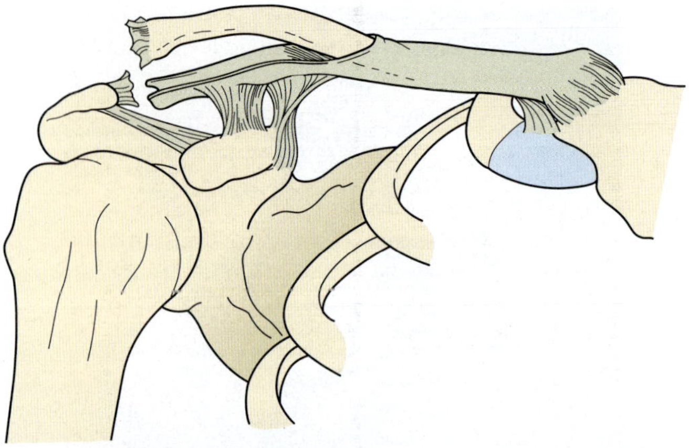

FIGURE 9-97: Type III variant. Shown is the displaced osseous clavicle leaving behind, inferiorly, a periosteal tube attached to the cartilaginous epiphysis that maintains the integrity of the acromioclavicular joint.

Pathoanatomy

The structural properties of the physeal-metaphyseal interface of the lateral clavicle render it the weakest link of the scapuloclavicular composite in a child or adolescent. Therefore the forces of injury result in a fracture through the physis (Salter-Harris type I or type II) without disturbing the integrity of the ACJ and the adjacent epiphysis of the lateral clavicle. The metaphysis of the lateral clavicle rips through the superior periosteal sleeve, which is then peeled away from the lateral clavicle by any remaining inferiorly directed forces and by the weight of the upper limb (Fig. 9-97).[92,199,263,280,381,449,682] The CC ligaments remain securely attached to the periosteal sleeve of the lateral clavicle and the coracoid process.

More rarely in children and adolescents is the instance of injury resulting in fracture of the lateral clavicle (Salter-Harris type II), with complete rupture of the CC ligaments but maintenance of the lateral clavicle (epiphysis) attachment to the acromion.[263,470]

A 2005 report of two cases and the investigation of museum specimens by Edelson et al. was the first to describe an even rarer form of this injury, whereby the lateral clavicle, having sustained a Salter-Harris II injury, is displaced downward and backward into the supraspinatus outlet toward the spine of the scapula.[256] A case similar to this occurring in an adult was described by Yanagisawa et al., in which the distal clavicle impaled the supraspinatus muscle.[1003]

Treatment

Essentially all of these injuries can be treated nonoperatively. A sling or shoulder immobilizer is used until the tenderness resolves. The physeal injury heals within 3 weeks, enabling rapid motion recovery. When the periosteal healing response is mature, the patients are

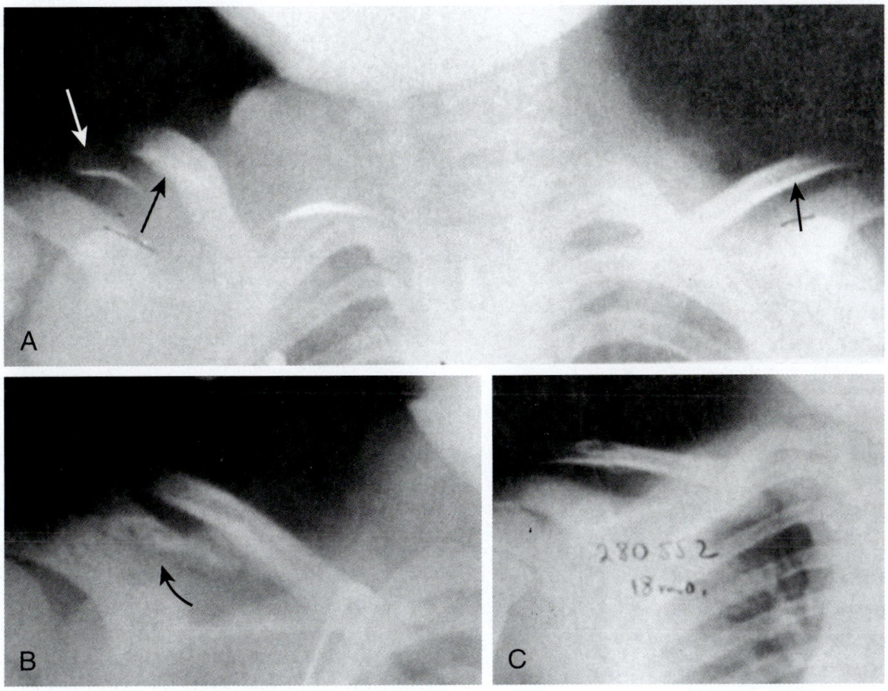

FIGURE 9-98: **A** to **C,** Type III variant. A brisk healing response is usually observed with remodeling, which results in a clavicle that appears normal. **A,** The *white arrow* indicates a Thurston Holland fragment. *Black arrows* show apparent coracoclavicular interval widening due to clavicular disruption from the periosteal tube. **B,** *Curved arrow* indicates a normal coracoclavicular interval now apparent as a result of new bone formation arising from the periosteal sleeve. **C,** Restoration of normal anatomy at the completion of remodeling. (From Ogden JA. Distal clavicular physeal injury. *Clin Orthop Relat Res.* 1984;188:68-73.)

permitted to return to vigorous activities (Fig. 9-98). Rashid et al. recommended surgical treatment in type IV and V injuries to avert potentially annoying cosmetic deformity.[745]

If, based upon extreme displacement, the lateral clavicle is suspected of spearing the trapezius muscle, it would be appropriate to proceed operatively with the intent of repairing the torn superior periosteal sleeve.[263,280,682] Edelson et al. advised operative treatment of the unique injury that they described for children older than 13 years.[256]

In the absence of extenuating circumstances, I prefer nonoperative treatment for this injury.

Results

The results are usually excellent, with no significant complications. A rare phenomenon of duplication of the clavicle by means of intense healing within the periosteal tube, especially in cases with wide displacement, has been observed.[336,924] Types IV and V may result in cosmetic deformity without functional impairment.[682,745]

Fracture of the Coracoid Process

Complete dislocation of the ACJ combined with fracture of the coracoid process is a very rare injury.* A similar lesion has been described in the immature skeleton.[177,433,709]

**References 52, 82, 86, 139, 245, 359, 364, 452, 466, 484, 528, 572, 619, 639, 805, 996.*

Signs and Symptoms

The patient experiences moderate to severe shoulder pain. Pain is not only localized to the ACJ but might also emanate more to the anterior aspect of the shoulder. Motion, either active or passive, in any direction and to any degree, exacerbates the pain.

The patient appears acutely injured, often with the affected upper limb postured in a protective and stress-relieving manner. The soft tissue overlying the acromion may be abraded or contused. Anterior shoulder ecchymosis resulting from the fracture is possible. Motion and strength assessment are unreliable due to pain. Palpation of the coracoid process induces pain.

Imaging

The most obvious finding on the AP view is complete separation of the acromion and the clavicle, with preservation of a normal CC interval. This radiographic feature is most indicative of a fracture at the base of the coracoid, which may be difficult to see unless an axillary view, a Stryker notch view, or a CT scan are obtained (Figs. 9-99 to 9-101).

Pathoanatomy

Although the CC ligaments usually maintain their secure attachment to the clavicle and the coracoid fracture fragment, two instances of their concomitant complete rupture resulting in an extraordinary injury triad, or triple lesion, have been reported.[955,983]

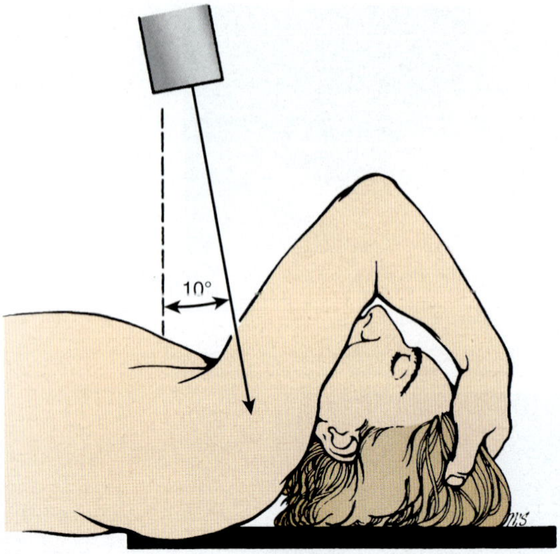

FIGURE 9-99: Fracture of the base of the coracoid process is best seen with the Stryker notch view. The hand is placed on the top of the head, putting the humerus in approximately 120 degrees of flexion as the x-ray beam is directed 10 degrees cephalad.

Treatment

Historically, with little difference reported between the results of operative and nonoperative treatment, the latter is usually preferred.[82,245,364,415,433,484,504,572,709,852,854,955,983] However, it appears that operative treatment has been preferred in recent reports.[245,452] Bhatia described a percutaneous technique.[86]

Type IV

These rare injuries are characterized by the posterior displacement of the distal clavicle into or through the substance of the adjacent trapezius muscle, sometimes with extreme deformity.[49,134,378,508,558,664,792,860] Even more rarely, posterior dislocation of the ACJ is accompanied by anterior SC dislocation, termed bipolar clavicle dislocation.* The association with a middle third clavicle fracture treated with open reduction internal has been described.[910,993] Wade et al. reported a very rare variation of this injury that resulted from medial clavicular epiphyseal fracture.[948]

Signs and Symptoms

The patient experiences moderate to severe shoulder pain. Damage to the trapezius muscle can result in pain that radiates throughout its substance into the neck, superior shoulder, and medial periscapular region. Motion, either active or passive, in any direction and to any degree, exacerbates the pain, which is especially intense if the clavicle has completely penetrated the trapezius.

The patient assumes a guarded posture to ease the significant pain resulting from the acute injury. The affected upper limb is held close to the body with the support of the opposite upper limb. Superior skin abrasions, soft tissue swelling, and ecchymosis are often observed. The ACJ is visibly and palpably deformed by superior and posterior displacement of the clavicle (Fig. 9-102). Extreme posterior displacement occurs if the clavicle penetrates the trapezius completely and comes to lie directly beneath the skin. In this case, it is not likely that the joint is reducible (Fig. 9-103). Like the type III injury, pain inhibits the accurate assessment of motion and strength. The ACJ, distal clavicle, CC ligament, and trapezius muscle are tender to palpation.

Imaging

The lateral clavicle is displaced, to some degree, above the acromion process, and the CC interval is widened. Posterior displacement of the clavicle may be overlooked unless an axillary lateral view is obtained (Fig. 9-104). However, Rahm et al. observed a very high incidence of false-positive axillary views for posterior subluxation of the clavicle in a cadaver study, and cautioned regarding its interpretation.[743] Dynamic horizontal instability may be a component of the injury pattern, which may be best identified with functional axillary radiologic evaluation as described by Tauber et al.[900] It may exist independent of the type of superior instability. Careful assessment of bilateral Zanca views provided Vaisman et al. with sufficient information to describe and validate a radiographic index measurement for the diagnosis of type IV injuries[933] (Fig. 9-105). They determined that a type IV injury could be recognized when the ACJ width index (injured side plus uninjured side divided by injured side) was more than 60%, with a sensitivity of 95.7% and a specificity of 97.5%. When this view is not possible because of pain or body habitus, or the diagnosis is uncertain from plane imaging, a CT scan might prove helpful. 3D scanning is extremely useful for diagnosis (Fig. 9-106).[807]

Pathoanatomy

The AC ligaments are always disrupted. The CC ligaments are usually but not always torn. The clavicle is displaced posterior to the acromion, coming to rest in, or sometimes through, the trapezius muscle. This usually changes the orientation of the CC interval. There is a high probability that the deltoid and trapezius muscles are detached from the distal clavicle.

Nonoperative Treatment

As a result of the extent of displacement and the severity of soft tissue damage, nonoperative treatment is usually not a consideration for type IV injuries.[24,253,378,527,558,664,860] It is such a painful lesion that even the most inactive patient will benefit from operative treatment, even if it is only a closed reduction. Opinions vary with regard to the choice of treatment for bipolar dislocations.[27,77,252,798,803]

Operative Treatment

Indications and Contraindications

With rare exception, all type IV injuries should be considered for operative treatment.[792] Extremely low demand

**References 27, 28, 67, 77, 180, 234, 252, 253, 271, 317, 423, 434, 507, 545, 648, 694, 732, 765, 803, 813.*

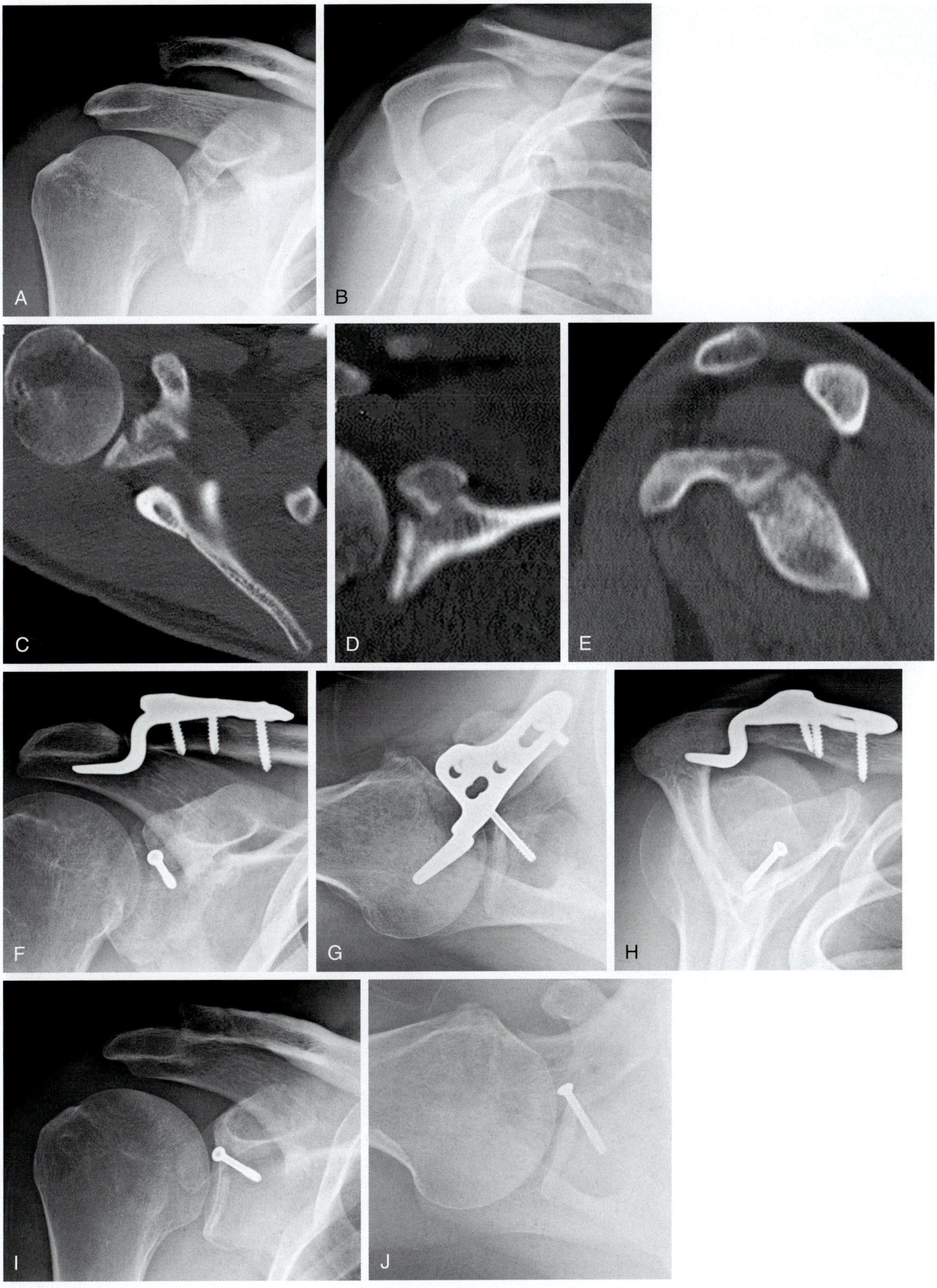

FIGURE 9-100: Coracoid fracture with intra-articular extension managed with open treatment and hook plate acromioclavicular stabilization. **A,** Preoperative anteroposterior (AP) view. **B,** Preoperative scapular Y view. **C** to **E,** Computed tomographic images. **F,** Postoperative AP view. **G,** Postoperative axillary lateral view. **H,** Postoperative scapular Y view. **I,** Final AP view. **J,** Final axillary lateral.

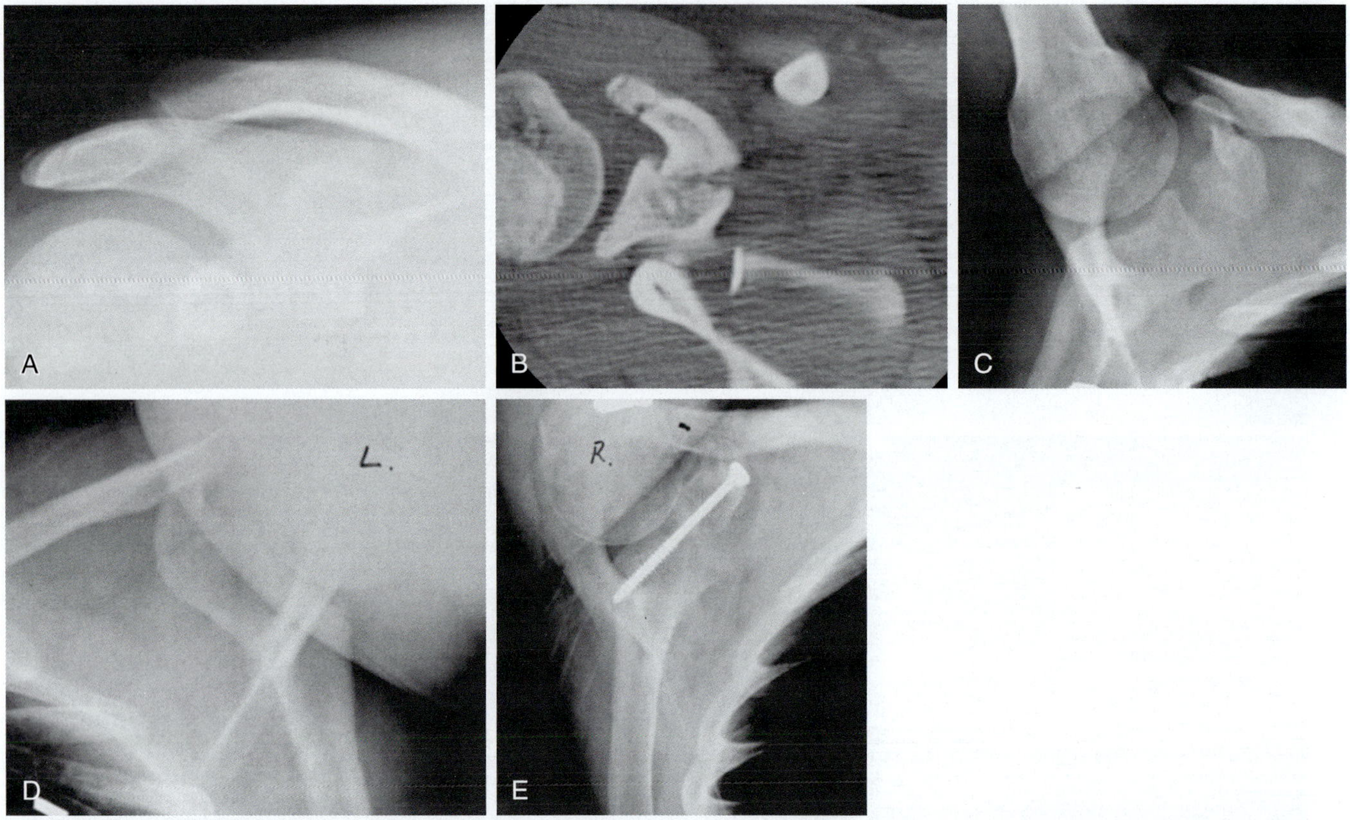

FIGURE 9-101: Nonunion of the base of the coracoid. **A,** The right acromioclavicular joint is unstable. **B,** Computed tomographic image of a fracture of the base of the coracoid process. **C,** Nonunion demonstrated on the Stryker notch view obtained 6 months after the acute injury. **D,** Stryker notch view of the contralateral shoulder. **E,** Nonunion repair with internal fixation and bone graft.

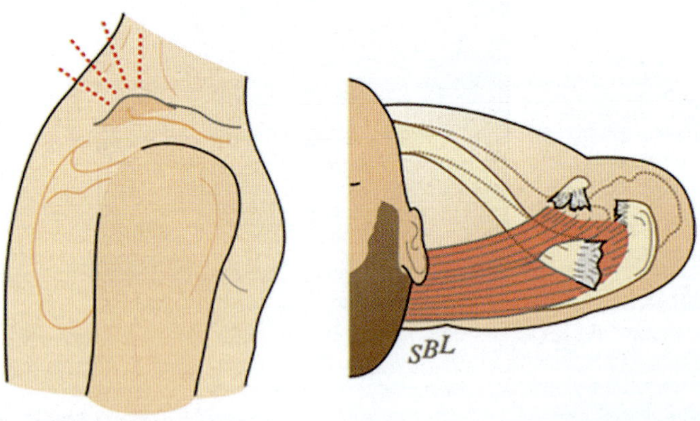

FIGURE 9-102: Patient with a type IV acromioclavicular joint injury. Note that the distal end of the clavicle is displaced posteriorly back into and through the trapezius muscle. (Courtesy Steven Lippit, MD.)

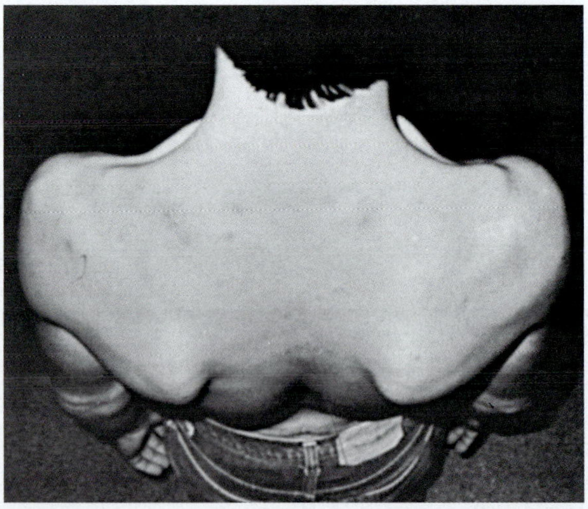

FIGURE 9-103: Type IV injury. The clavicle inclines posteriorly, producing a bump where it penetrates the trapezius muscle. (From Rockwood CA, Green DP, eds. *Fractures,* 4th ed. Philadelphia: JB Lippincott; 1995.)

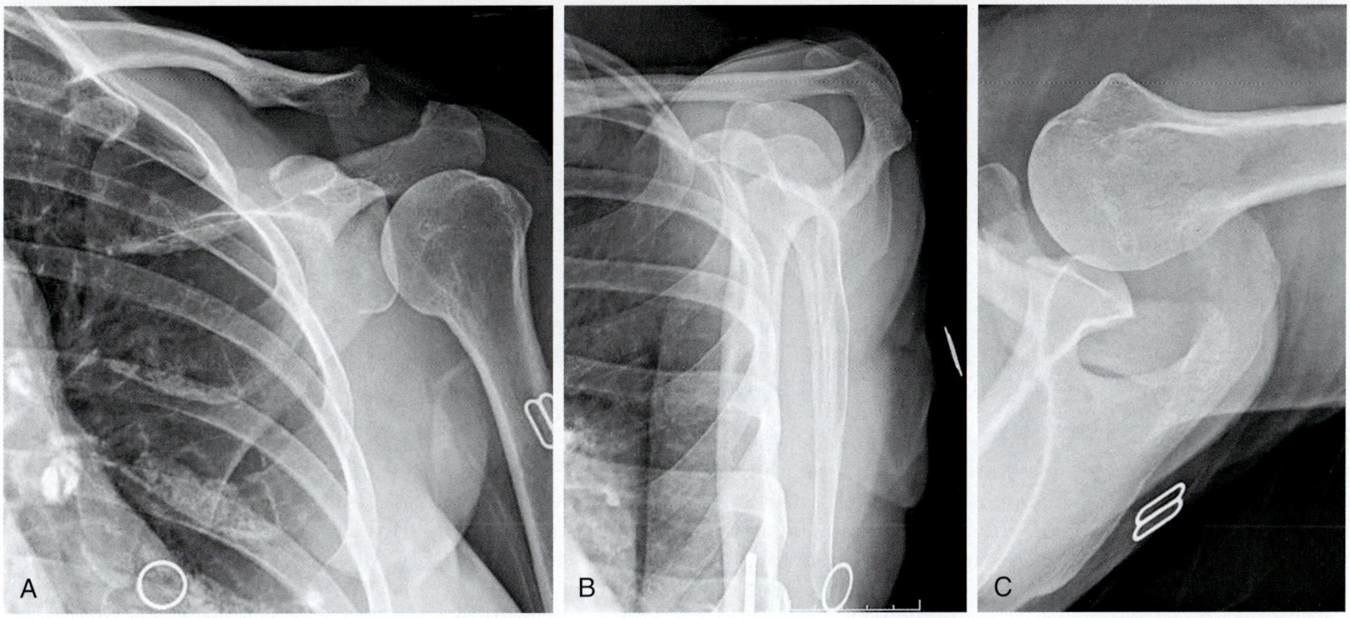

FIGURE 9-104: Acute type IV injury. **A,** Anteroposterior view shows the acromioclavicular joint appearing wider than the coracoclavicular interval. **B,** Scapular Y view and the telling axillary lateral **(C)** view clearly show the posterior dislocation.

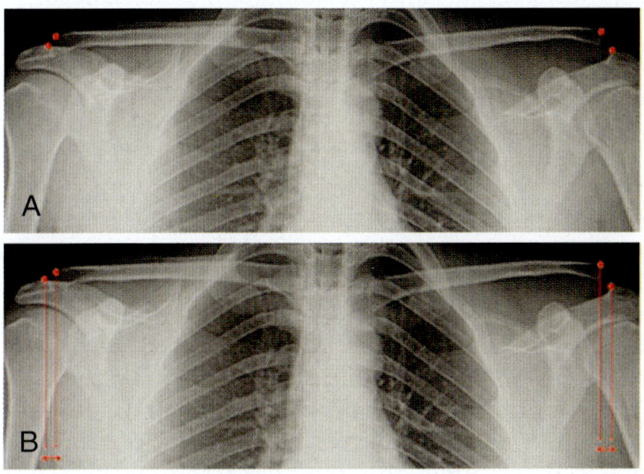

FIGURE 9-105: **A** and **B,** An acromioclavicular joint width of 60% or greater supports the diagnosis of a type IV injury. Obtained from measurements taken from bilateral Zanca views and calculated as width of injured side—width of normal side/width of normal side. (From Vaisman A, Villalón Montenegro IE, Tuca De Diego MJ, et al. A novel radiographic index for the diagnosis of posterior acromioclavicular joint dislocations. *Am J Sports Med.* 2014;42[1]:112-116.)

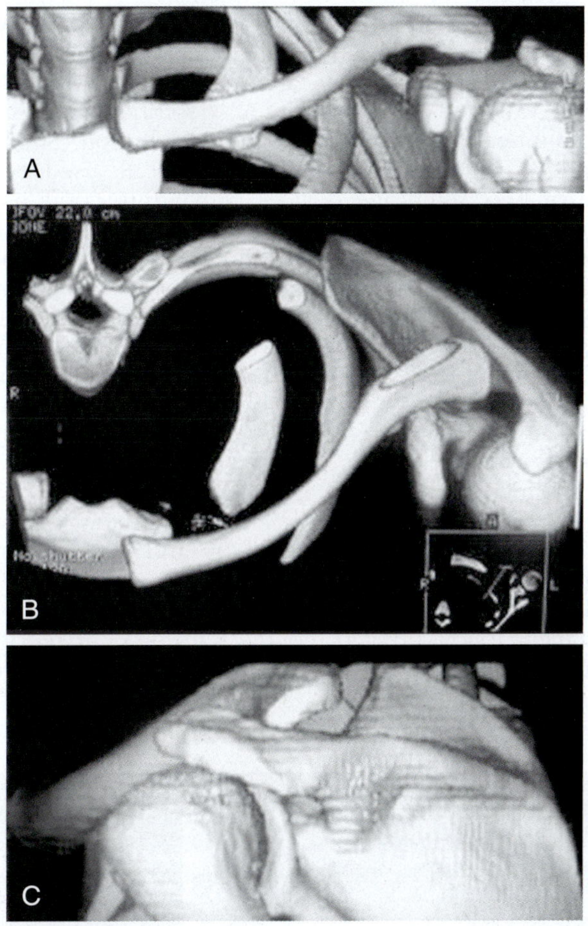

FIGURE 9-106: **A** to **C,** A type IV injury is clearly demonstrated with three-dimensional computed tomography. The sternoclavicular joint is anteriorly dislocated. **A,** Viewed from the anterior, the acromioclavicular joint appears widened, whereas the coracoclavicular interval appears normal. The medial clavicle is anterior to the manubrium. **B,** From above, the abnormal relationships of the acromioclavicular and sternoclavicular joints and the coracoclavicular interval are obvious. **C,** The lateral clavicle is not only posterior but also superior to the articular surface of the acromion. (From Scapinelli R. Bipolar dislocation of the clavicle: 3D CT imaging and delayed surgical correction of a case. *Arch Orthop Trauma Surg.* 2004;124[6]:421-424.)

and inactive patients might have nothing to gain with operative treatment. Significant skin abrasions can delay operative treatment.

Methods

Closed reduction under general anesthesia may be possible and all that is needed for the extremely low demand, frail patient.[673] Otherwise, open treatment is required to disengage the lateral clavicle from the trapezius. It is possible that, immediately after the reduction, the only way to preserve joint congruity is by internal fixation that temporarily transgresses the joint.[378,508,664] Depending on the findings, AC and CC ligament repair or reconstruction is considered.[24,527] Use of the hook plate has been reported, and may have a more significant role in fracture-dislocation.[24,458] Millett et al. described their "docking technique, a variation of the Weaver-Dunn method, which was augmented by nine braided strands of No. 1 PDS.[609] Isolated lateral clavicle excision is reasonable in the presence of intact CC ligaments.[558,860] Chernchujit et al. described an arthroscopic-assisted CC fixation with synthetic sutures spanning dual coracoid suture anchors, the clavicle, and a small titanium plate over which the suture was tied.[151] Katsenis et al. described the use of single-tunnel CC fixation with the Endobutton (Smith & Nephew) (flipptack fixation).[448] Thiel et al. used either one or two TightRope devices with arthroscopic assistance.[905] Basyoni et al. described the use of nonabsorbable sutures with anchors in the coracoid secured over a small button plate on the clavicle, with the hope to reduce the risk of neurovascular complications.[58]

Argintar et al. chose total claviculectomy as the definitive treatment for a case with union between the clavicle and the first rib accompanied by bipolar cartilage loss.[28]

Results

Successful operative and nonoperative treatment have been reported.[28,378,508,527,558,609,664,860] Chernchujit et al. obtained a mean C-M score of 95 and 77% anatomic reduction.[151] Millett et al. showed 94% maintenance of reduction and a mean ASES score of 86 at 29 months.[609] At a mean follow-up of 42 months, Katsenis et al. reported a mean C-M score of 93, mean Short MFA Bother score of 20.88, and CC distance equivalent to the uninjured side.[448] Basyoni et al. achieved a mean C-M score of 92.8, return to work at a mean of 11.2 weeks, and 93% satisfaction.[58] Satisfactory functional results by SST (11/12) were reported by Thiel et al.[905]

Complications

Loss of reduction and superficial infection have been reported in the few published cases. Posttraumatic degenerative changes are likely sequelae (Fig. 9-107).

Author's Preferred Method

Operative treatment is preferred. A closed reduction would suffice in the most inactive patients. Open reduction allows thorough exploration of the ACJ and CC interval. In the rare instance that the CC ligament is only sprained, the trapezius is repaired after ACJ reduction. If instability persists, a hook plate is applied and left in place for 12 to 16 weeks. It is then removed under general anesthesia, and rehabilitation commences.

Type V

Signs and Symptoms

The pain of a type V injury is often more intense than the pain in type III or type IV injuries because the damage to the soft tissues is more severe and includes disruption of the muscle attachments from the lateral part of the clavicle. For this reason, the pain is widespread and exacerbated by motion, either active or passive, in any direction and to any degree. Neurogenic pain is possible due to the effect of the unsupported weight of the upper limb on the brachial plexus.

The patient holds the affected upper limb close to the torso with the help of the opposite upper limb. The lateral clavicle tents the overlying skin as the unsupported upper limb assumes an extreme inferior attitude (Fig. 9-108). Lateral stress testing can create a remarkable deformity of the shoulder. The soft tissue overlying the acromion is likely to be abraded and contused, and more diffuse swelling and ecchymosis, the result of extensive muscle detachment, is observed. Like the other dislocations, pain inhibits the accurate assessment of motion and strength. The shoulder is diffusely tender.

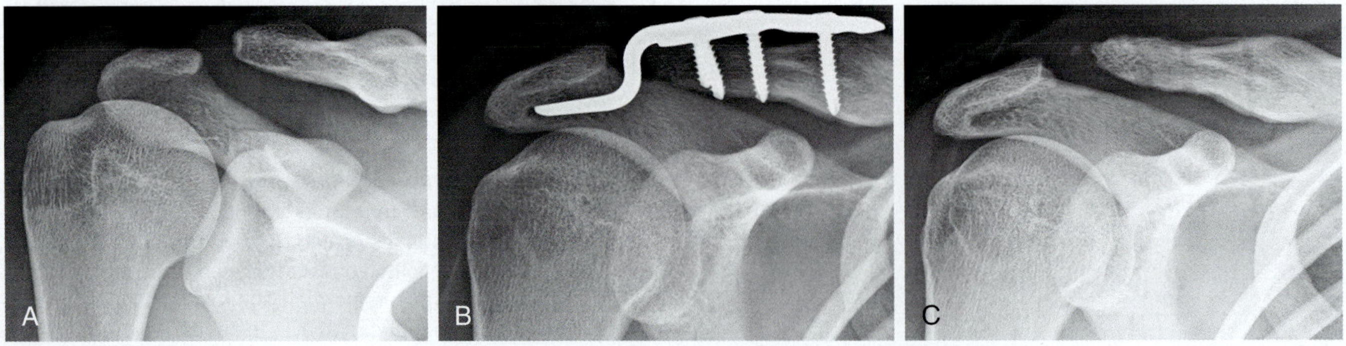

FIGURE 9-107: **A** to **C**, Treatment of a type IV dislocation using a hook plate with resultant degenerative changes of the distal clavicle.

Imaging

There is extreme incongruity between the lateral clavicle and the acromion process as the scapula, no longer adequately suspended by the clavicle, drops away. It is not unusual for the CC interval to widen by as much as 300% (Fig. 9-109).

Pathoanatomy

The AC and CC ligaments are torn completely, resulting in dislocation of the ACJ. In comparison to the normal shoulder, the CC interval may be widened twofold to threefold. There is the highest probability that the periosteal sleeve and the deltoid and trapezius muscles are detached from the lateral half of the clavicle.

Operative Treatment

The extreme displacement and the severity of soft tissue damage preclude nonoperative treatment for type V injuries.

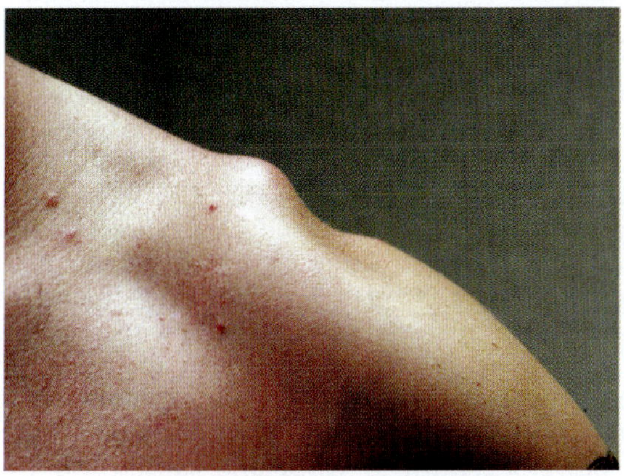

FIGURE 9-108: Type V injury.

Methods

As in type III injuries, open and arthroscopic-assisted CC fixation with synthetic material have been used.[268,811,836,941] The use of autogenous and allogenous tendon with or without additional synthetic suture augmentation has been reported.[45,407,662,891] Both the modified Cadenat procedure and the modified Dewar procedure were compared and reported by Takase et al. and Takase and Yamamota.[890,891] Temporary transacromial K-wire fixation in conjunction with coracoid process transfer (Dewar method) was reported by Wang and Zhang.[957] Temporary fixation while transferring the CAL to the inferior distal clavicle as well as the lateral of the conjoined tendon was reported by Kim et al.[465] Von Heideken et al. reported on the use of the hook plate while analyzing the benefits of acute versus chronic treatment, which included the Weaver-Dunn procedure.[946] Liu et al. described the combined use of the classic Weaver-Dunn procedure and hook plate for types IV, V, and VI (Fig. 9-110).[538] Shin et al. described CAL transfer to the inferior aspect of the distal clavicle together with paired transclavicular sutures secured to the coracoid process with anchors.[836] Temporary fixation spanning the ACJ supplemented with AC and CC ligament repair was reported by Virtanen et al.[943] A similar method was reported by Wang and Wong, who also supplemented the repair with transosseous CC suture.[956] El Sallakh reported the all arthroscopic technique of transosseous flipping buttons with synthetic sutures (Fig. 9-111).[268]

Results

The results of treatment have been mixed. An early report of the use of autogenous semitendinosus resulted in high outcome scores, patient satisfaction, and no loss of reduction.[662] Verhaven et al. reported nearly 30% of patients with fair or poor results.[941] Loss of reduction, OA, ossification, or osteolysis did not correlate with outcome.

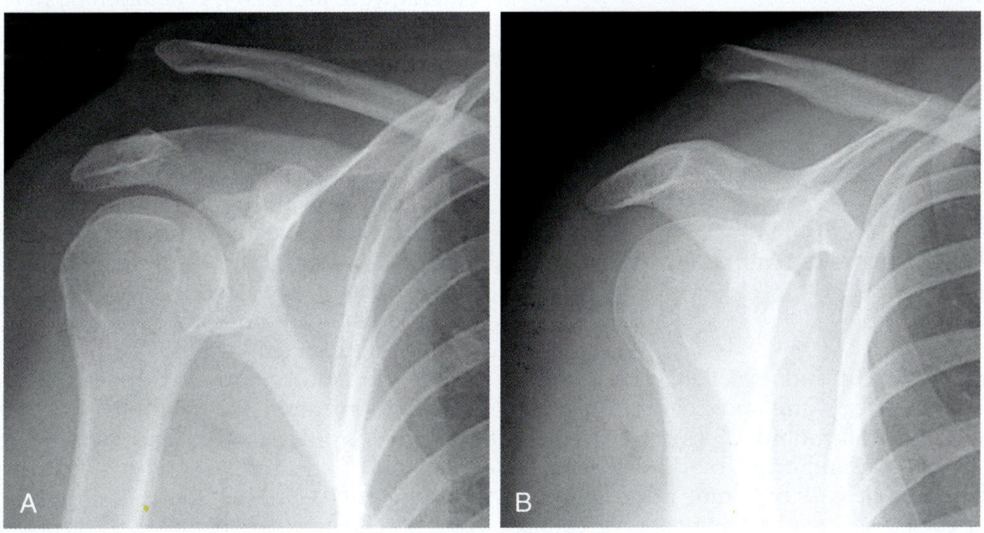

FIGURE 9-109: Type V injury. There is extreme widening of the coracoclavicular interval (**A**) and significant inferior displacement of the acromion on the scapular Y view (**B**).

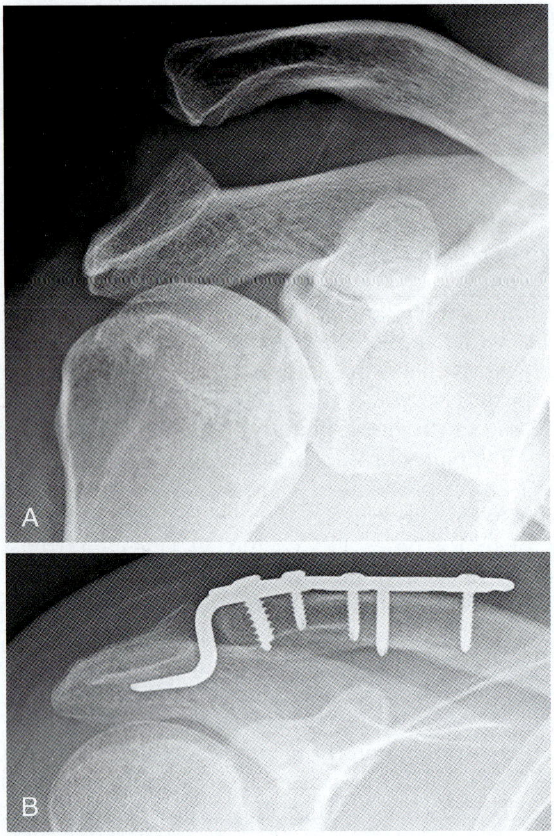

FIGURE 9-110: Type V injury treated with a hook plate.

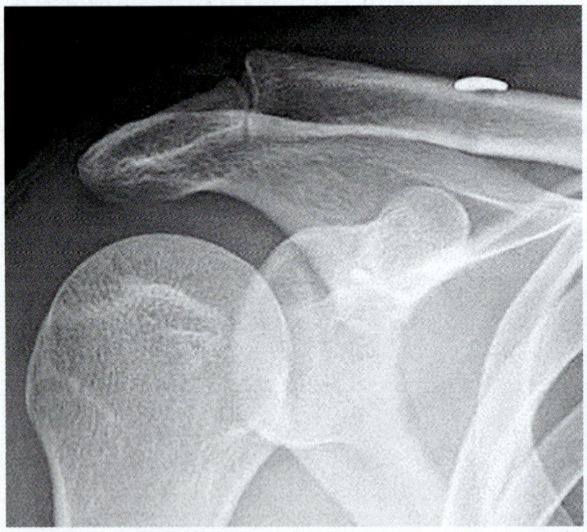

FIGURE 9-111: Type V injury treated with arthroscopic-assisted cortical suture buttons.

Excellent and good clinical and excellent radiographic outcomes were reported by Wang and Zhang.[957] A mean UCLA score excluding satisfaction of 28 (more than 27 of 30 = excellent, good) was reported by Takase et al.[890] Superior subluxation of less than 5 mm and OA were noted in 25% and 12%, respectively. The results of Takase et al. indicated very similar UCLA scores (mean of more than 27 of 30 = excellent/good) but more frequent and significant superior subluxation and OA with the modified Dewar procedure compared with the modified Cadenet procedure.[890] The best radiographic results reported by Takase and Yamamoto were with a double-bundle reconstruction that combined the use of autologous palmaris longus for the conoid and artificial ligament (Dacron) for the trapezoid, with both secured with Endobutton.[891] The UCLA score was not significantly different to that with the Dewar or modified Cadenet procedures. Scheibel et al. reported a very high rate of clinical success as revealed by SSV, C-M, Taft, and ACJI scores.[811] One hundred percent coracoid process healing was observed by Wang and Zhang.[957] A mean modified UCLA score of 18.5 together with no reduction loss was observed by Kim et al.[465] No correlation between functional and radiographic outcomes were reported. Hou et al. reported excellent and good results in 70% and 18% for two- and one-hole techniques, respectively.[407] Augmentation with synthetic sutures did not result in a significant difference. Successful use of a "luggage tag" technique with autogenous or allogenous semitendinosus tendon with a redisplacement rate of 5% was reported by Baldwin et al.[45] Von Heideken et al. reported a Constant score of 91, with 91% of the patients self-rating the results as excellent or good.[946] Radiographically, the CC interval was increased by 39% compared with the uninjured side, and the joint subluxation with weighted radiographs was 38% of the clavicle diameter. No correlation between Constant score and radiographic findings was found. Both clinical and radiographic outcome parameters were better for acute versus chronic treatment.[946] At 3.5 years after treatment, the return to work/activity rate was 96%, with a mean Constant score of 88 for patients treated with a combination of the Weaver-Dunn procedure and hook plate.[538] With the TightRope technique, El Sallakh reported a mean C-M score of 96.3. Return to work and satisfaction with the functional results and cosmesis was the norm.[268] Shin et al. reported a mean C-M score of 96, with return to normal life at a mean of 3.1 months.[836] Anatomic reduction criteria were met in 83%. Virtanen et al. reported excellent functional outcomes (mean C-M score of 90, DASH score of 5.1, SST score of 11).[943] Radiologically, normal ligament was observed in 78%. There were no correlations between the radiographic and functional outcomes. Of interest was the observation that half the patients with redislocation were found to have anatomic reductions during the period of follow-up. Wang and Wong reported a mean C-M score of 94.5, even exceeding the uninjured side with only 0 to 4 mm CC intervals in 62% at follow-up.[956]

Experimental Treatment

Ammon et al. created type V injuries in cadavers, compared the failure load and pullout strengths of fixation, and demonstrated that titanium Bosworth screws were superior to poly(L-lactic acid) screws.[22]

Complications

Loss of reduction, sometimes early, is not infrequent, usually with no effect on shoulder function (Fig. 9-112).[941,811,836,946] Scheibel et al. reported a 43% incidence of radiographic

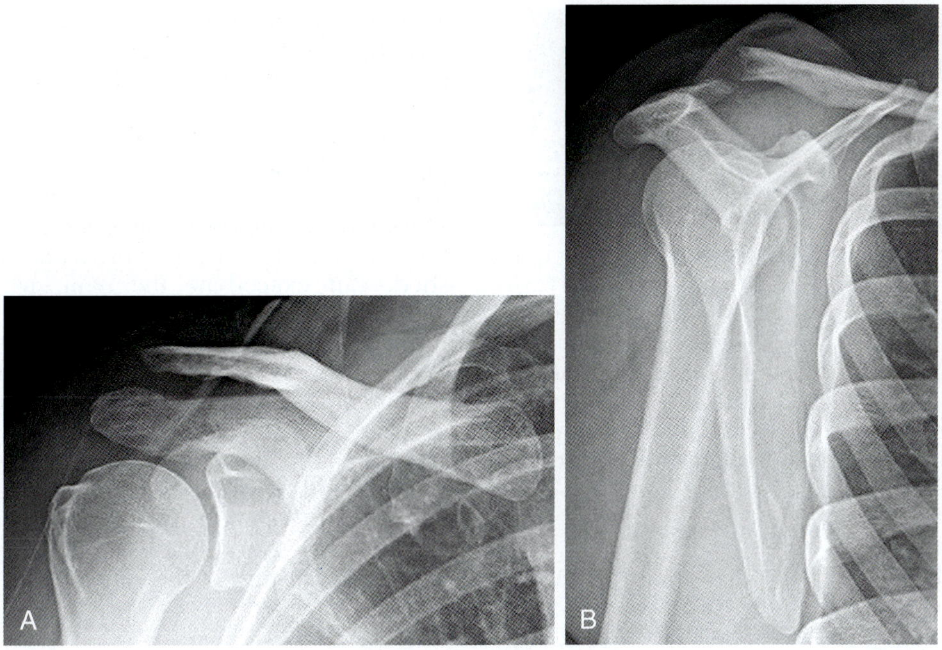

FIGURE 9-112: **A** and **B,** Acute type V dislocation treated with a hook plate shown with loss of reduction after plate removal.

signs of posterior instability following the use of the TightRope.[811] Liu et al., using Weaver-Dunn and hook plate reconstruction, experienced two redislocations without any effect on the functional outcome.[538] Takase and Yamamoto reported three complete dislocations with the Dewar method.[891] They noted permanent motion loss in 62% of patients but only in those undergoing the Dewar procedure. One instance of technical error resulting in coracoid tunnel malposition led to fracture with a loss of reduction.[268] Kim et al. used temporary K-wire fixation across the ACJ and observed 66.7% incidence of radiographic AC arthritis.[465] Virtanen et al. reported no outcome (C-M, DASH, SST, or VAS pain) differences between groups with or without complications.[943] Hoffler and Karas, by their account, reported the first known hook plate erosion through the acromion.[397] Superficial and deep infections are rarely reported.[538,943,946]

Author's Preferred Method

I treat the injury with a hook plate as in type III injuries.

Type VI

Type VI injuries, like type IV, are extremely rare.[24,133,320,376,594,644,704,790,820,917,1003] They are usually produced by high-energy force that results in additional systemic injuries.

Signs and Symptoms

Type VI injuries often occur simultaneously with other musculoskeletal or systemic injuries that affect the overall expression of pain. However, an isolated type VI injury manifests with severe pain localized to the lateral clavicle. The patient typically experiences upper limb paresthesias until the fracture is reduced.[320,594,704]

The patient holds the injured limb in a protective manner adjacent to the torso with the opposite limb, resisting all attempts at movement. With type VI injuries, the normal sloping appearance of the superior shoulder flattens. The acromion becomes unusually prominent, as does the inferiorly distinct coracoid process. However, diffuse swelling and ecchymosis resulting from additional injuries nearby can obscure the deformity of the ACJ. Altered peripheral cutaneous sensation is possible. Vascular perfusion of the upper limb remains stable. As with the other high-grade dislocations, pain inhibits the accurate assessment of motion and strength. Diffuse tenderness is the rule.

Imaging

Subacromial dislocations result in narrowing of the CC interval as the lateral clavicle is displaced inferior to the acromion process. A diaphyseal fracture of the clavicle is usually observed.[208,353] With subcoracoid dislocations, instead of a CC interval superior to the coracoid process, a new CC interval is created inferior to the coracoid process (Fig. 9-113). Inferior dislocation accompanied by glenoid neck fracture and scapulothoracic dissociation has been observed.[376]

Pathoanatomy

The AC ligaments are completely torn. The CC ligament remains intact with the subacromial type but is completely torn with the subcoracoid type. The ACJ is dislocated. The clavicle is displaced inferior to the acromion or the coracoid. The CC interval is decreased (subacromial) or no longer anatomically exists (subcoracoid). The origin of the conjoined tendon has a deformed appearance because the lateral clavicle usually rests directly

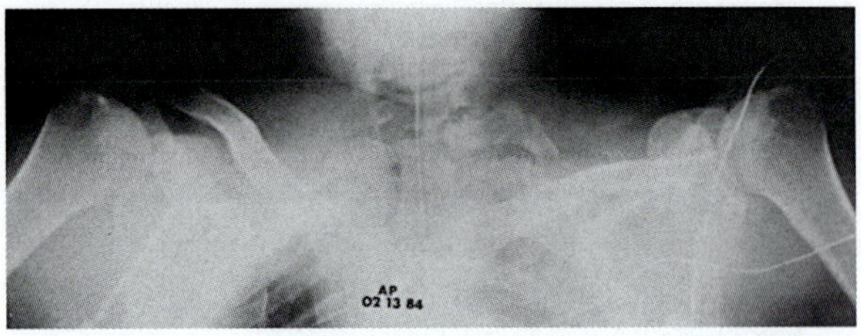

FIGURE 9-113: Type VI injury: subcoracoid dislocation of the left clavicle.

posterior. There is a high probability that the deltoid and trapezius muscles are detached from the distal clavicle, but it depends on the extent of displacement. Vascular injuries have not been documented. Multidirectional instability has been observed.[376]

Operative Treatment

The nature and severity of the injury precludes consideration for nonoperative treatment for type VIa injuries, while a trial of conservative management for type VIb might be a consideration in selective instances.[320,353,442,475,594,641,704,790,917]

Contraindications

There are no specific contraindications to operative treatment. Unstable multisystem injuries and significant skin abrasions might require a temporary delay.

Methods

A consistent method of operative treatment has not emerged due to the relative rarity of type VI injuries. Closed reduction with various combinations of soft tissue repair, CAL transfer, temporary transfixation of the ACJ, CC screw fixation, immobilization, and lateral clavicle excision have been reported (Fig. 9-114).[133,320,353,376,475] Subacromial dislocations remain stable after internal fixation of the ipsilateral clavicle fracture.[208]

Results

The cases reported in the literature have achieved successful outcomes without complications.

Chronic Lesions

Rockwood's classification scheme of types I to VI facilitates the understanding of acute traumatic lesions more so than chronic ones. From the perspective of treatment, the rudimentary classification espoused by Cadenet is, perhaps, more appropriate: incomplete (excision of the lateral clavicle) and complete (stabilization).[127] Incomplete lesions include Rockwood types I and II. Practically speaking, complete lesions include only Rockwood type III injuries. The reason for this is that types IV to VI are recognizable as the most severe forms of complete injury, and as such have been treated acutely in most instances.

Recurrent or habitual forms of complete injury are quite rare. Four cases of recurrent subacromial dislocations of the clavicle that were treated operatively have been reported.[517,644,790] Single cases of bilateral nontraumatic anterior dislocation, one recurrent, were reported separately by Janecki and by Richards et al., and can represent a less severe variant of a type VI injury.[425,755]

Incomplete (Types I and II)

Signs and Symptoms

Mild to moderate pain that is well localized to the ACJ is the most common manifestation of a chronic incomplete injury. Movement, which may be slightly diminished, can exacerbate the pain, which is sometimes sufficiently intense to contribute to weakness of the upper limb.

The physical findings are often subtle. A slightly more prominent distal clavicle can result in the appearance of an enlarged ACJ when compared with the opposite side. The scapula might track abnormally as the upper limb is elevated and lowered. Deficits of internal rotation and cross-body adduction are possible as a result of pain. Crepitus arising from the ACJ is usually not appreciated. Provocative testing of the ACJ may be beneficial.

Imaging

The plain films are occasionally normal or symmetrical to the opposite ACJ. More often, a chronic type I injury cannot be distinguished from OA and is, in fact, a secondary type of OA. Classic findings include eccentric narrowing of the joint space, subchondral cyst formation, densification of the adjacent subchondral bone, and osteophyte formation (Fig. 9-115). One or more loose bodies may be present (Fig. 9-116). At other times, the predominant manifestation is one of osteolysis expressed as a loss of the subchondral bone with radiolucent cysts scattered throughout the epiphysis. Plain films might demonstrate an incongruent ACJ with slight superior displacement of the lateral clavicle. A small increase in the CC interval is possible.

Pathoanatomy

Depending on the extent of injury, scar tissue can form in the vicinity of the ACJ. Slight superior displacement of the lateral clavicle is possible. The findings are those of OA of varying degrees. They include capsular and synovial hypertrophy, joint effusion, thinned or absent articular cartilage, eburnated subchondral bone, and perhaps punctate cysts visible within the subchondral bone. The congruency of the joints varies with the amount of displacement and the extent of arthritis. The lateral clavicle may be tapered with an irregular surface as a result of osteolysis. Copious joint fluid can accumulate, sometimes under pressure.

Nonoperative Treatment

Methods

The mainstays of nonoperative treatment are rest, nonsteroidal antiinflammatory medication, and the liberal use of ice or heat. Judicious use of intra-articular corticosteroid injections is reasonable.

Results

The therapeutic response primarily depends on the severity of the pathologic changes in the ACJ. Symptoms can

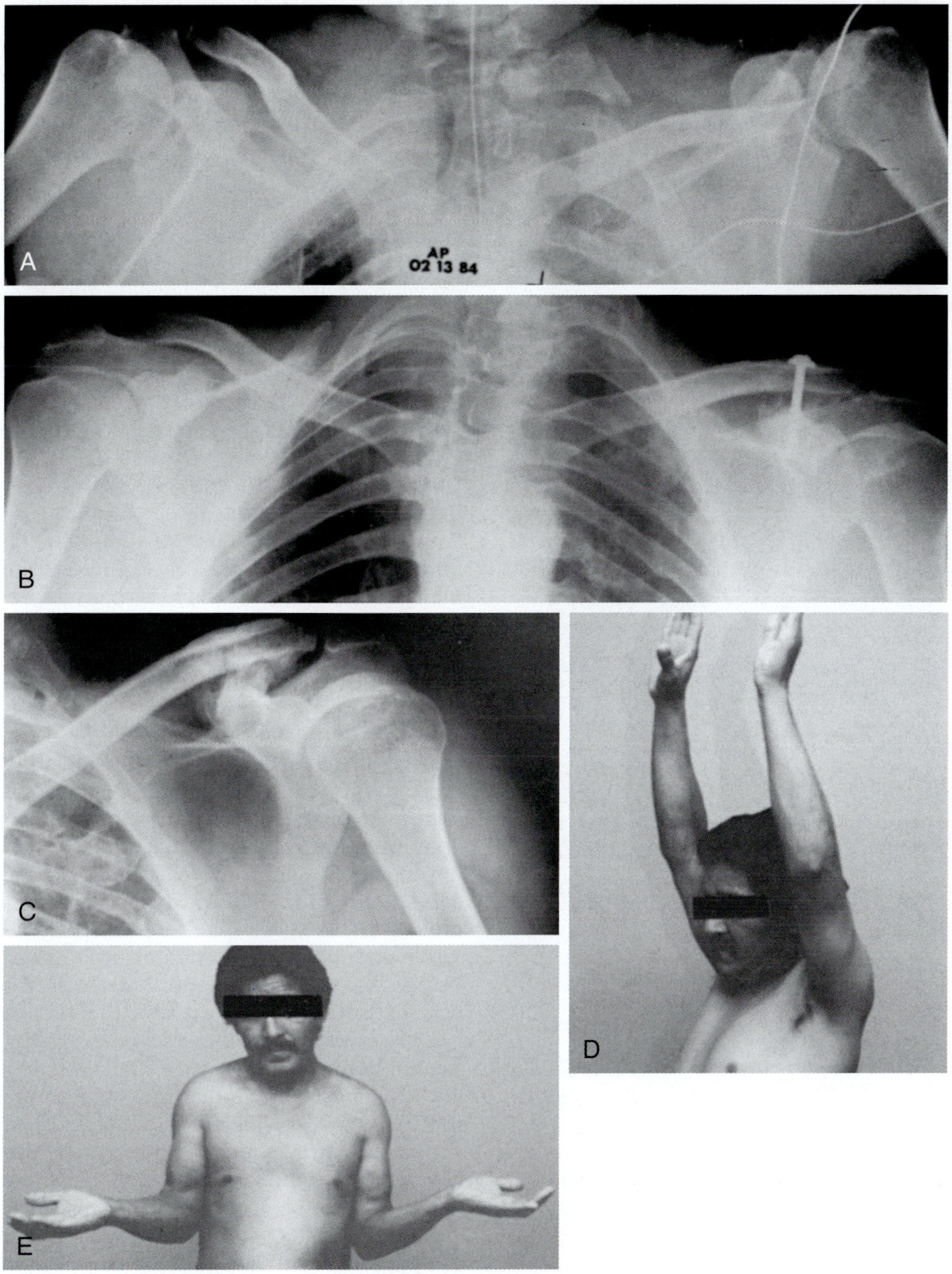

FIGURE 9-114: Type VI injury. **A,** This injury resulted from a train-pedestrian accident. In addition to the type VI subcoracoid dislocation of the clavicle, the patient sustained multiple rib fractures. **B,** Treatment included open reduction and placement of a coracoclavicular screw. **C,** At 6 weeks, the screw was removed. At 13 months, heterotopic ossification has formed in the coracoclavicular interval. **D** and **E,** Even with the coracoclavicular interval heterotopic ossification, full range of motion is essentially possible.

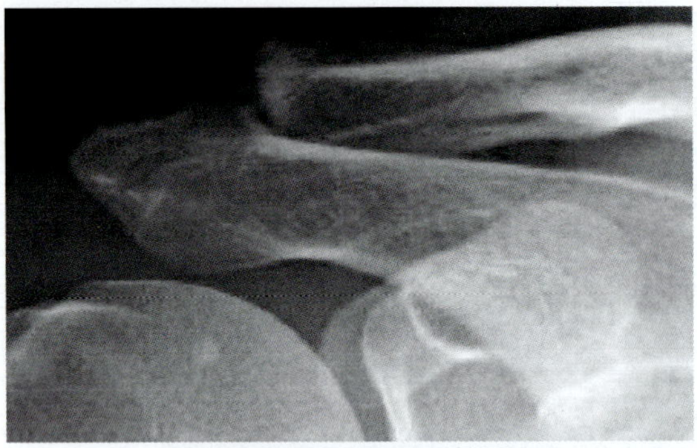

FIGURE 9-115: Secondary osteoarthritis of the acromioclavicular joint, a sequela to a type I injury.

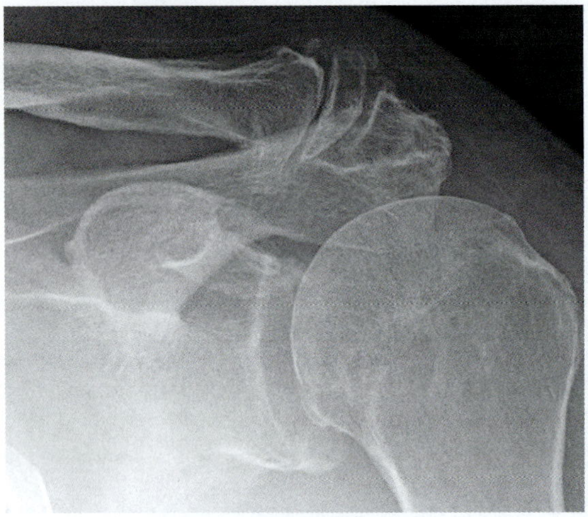

FIGURE 9-116: Osteochondral (loose) body in an acromioclavicular joint with advanced osteoarthritis.

wax and wane or become refractory to all means of treatment.

Complications

The only complications of concern are those related to treatment, including side effects of systemic medication and iatrogenic septic arthritis caused by joint injection.

Operative Treatment

Indications and Contraindications

Intractable pain and dysfunction that has become unresponsive to nonoperative treatment is the indication for operative treatment. There are no specific contraindications to operative treatment.

Methods

The mainstay of operative treatment for chronic type I injuries is excision of the lateral clavicle as described by Mumford in 1941.[631] The techniques have been previously described. There are concerns for its use in occult instability or in patients with generalized ligamentous hypermobility.[88,313]

Results

The results of lateral clavicle resection for chronic type I injuries cannot be discerned from the literature. In theory, the results should not differ from that of lateral clavicle excision for degenerative disease, which means that comfort and function can be reliably restored.

Complications

Complications of lateral clavicle excision have been described. Heterotopic ossification can develop after excision of the lateral clavicle, and is sometimes sufficiently symptomatic to warrant additional operative treatment. Pain can persist because of the excision of too little or too much lateral clavicle. Careless technique can result in the functional loss of the AC ligaments, leading to symptomatic instability in the horizontal (AP) plane.

Complete (Types III and V)

Signs and Symptoms

Pain is the predominant feature of a chronic complete injury. As a result of the effect of more extensive soft tissue injury on shoulder mechanics, pain is present not only in the area of the ACJ but can also be more widespread. With the loss of the scapula's connection with the clavicle, the sturdiest component of upper limb suspension, the periscapular muscles are pressed into a higher state of activity. Both factors can result in the development of periscapular pain and even pain radiating into the upper limb due to excessive traction on the brachial plexus. An increased prevalence of neck pain appears to be attributable to an acquired cervical hypolordosis.[356] A variation of impingement syndrome can result in infra-acromial and subdeltoid pain. Motion is usually normal, although range limitations are possible due to pain. Overall shoulder girdle strength may be diminished on the basis of disuse or because of the mechanical absence of a sturdy articulation between the scapula and the clavicle. Scapular dyskinesis and syndrome (scapular malposition, inferior medial border prominence, coracoid pain and malposition, and dyskinesis of scapular movement) have been reported in 70 and 58% of patients with type III injuries.[357]

Prominence of the lateral end of the clavicle is the most notable physical feature of a chronic complete injury (Fig. 9-117). As with acute complete injuries, the shoulder girdle and upper limb assume a drooped appearance with respect to the opposite side. Mild disuse muscular atrophy is sometimes observed. Range of motion is usually not restricted, but with elevation and lowering of the upper limb, a variation of winging of the scapula, a scapular dyskinesis, is often observed.

Forced internal rotation and cross-body adduction induces ACJ pain. Crepitation at the ACJ may be produced by upper limb movement or with direct palpation. Manual muscle testing for strength exhibits no significant deficits. The ACJ and the periscapular and infra-acromial regions might exhibit tenderness. The joint might or might not be reducible. Due to the disturbance of scapular motion, impingement signs may be positive. The results of ACJ provocative testing may be unreliable or misleading in this setting.

Imaging

Chronic and acute complete injuries have a similar radiographic appearance in that there is no contact between the articular surfaces of the lateral clavicle and the medial acromion, and the CC interval is widened (Fig. 9-118). A wider CC interval in chronic versus acute injuries was reported by von Heideken et al.[946] Heterotopic ossification is sometimes present in the CC interval.

Pathoanatomy

Scarring is present in the region of the ACJ and the lateral clavicle, making it difficult to distinguish the ACJ capsuloligamentous complex from the healed attachments of the trapezius and deltoid muscles. The gap between the acromion and the clavicle may be filled completely with scar tissue or may be a pseudarthrosis. The intra-articular disk is usually undetectable. In the absence of a CC interval that has been obliterated with scar tissue and bone, the CC ligament stumps may be palpable. The hyaline cartilage usually remains on the medial acromion and the lateral clavicle but might not be mechanically sound. Heterotopic ossification in the CC space is often observed, and rarely poses a conflict to joint reduction at the time of reconstruction.[977]

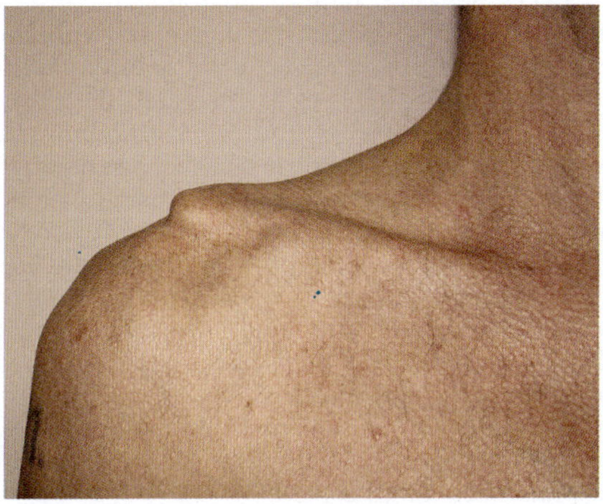

FIGURE 9-117: Clinical appearance of chronic complete acromioclavicular dislocation of the right shoulder.

Nonoperative Treatment

Methods

Overuse can provoke a symptomatic flare of the chronic complete injury, necessitating an initial period of rest. It is appropriate to dispense nonsteroidal antiinflammatory medication or nonnarcotic analgesics along with recommendation for the use of ice or heat. Because there is no longer a true articulation, it is not appropriate to consider a corticosteroid injection. In the presence of scapular dyskinesis, a specific rehabilitation program directed toward the improvement of periscapular muscle strength and flexibility is advised.

Results

The success of nonoperative treatment of chronic complete injuries depends on compliance with activity modification. Simple modifications are sometimes all that are necessary to render the shoulder both comfortable and functional. If aggravating factors are unavoidable, nonoperative treatment will fail. Nearly 80% of patients with disabling scapular dyskinesis may have resolution of their symptoms.[135]

Complications

The only complications of concern are those related to treatment with systemic medication.

Operative Treatment

Indications and Contraindications

Intractable pain and dysfunction that have become unresponsive to nonoperative treatment are the indications for operative treatment. There are no specific contraindications to operative treatment.

Methods

Excision of the lateral clavicle will rarely address the symptoms that result from a chronic complete injury, and

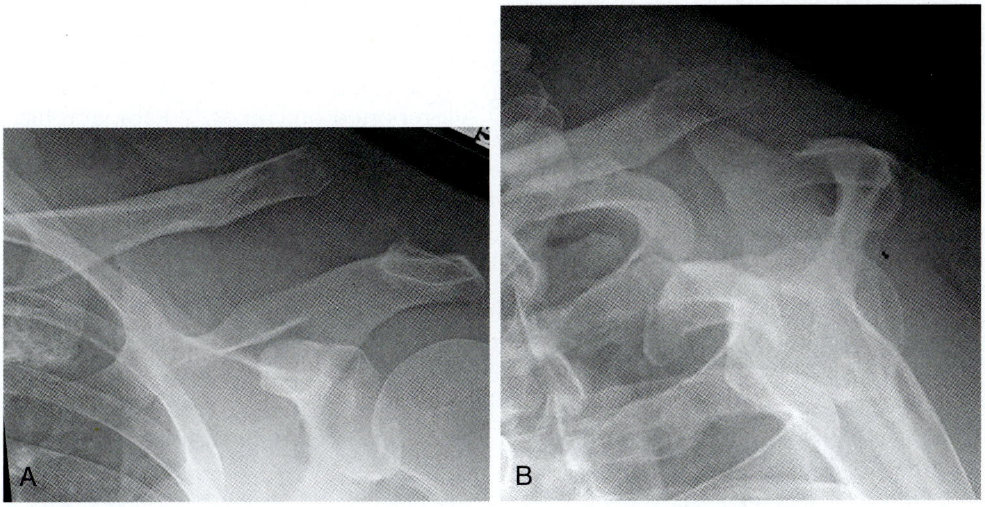

FIGURE 9-118: Chronic type V injury: anteroposterior (**A**) and scapular Y views (**B**).

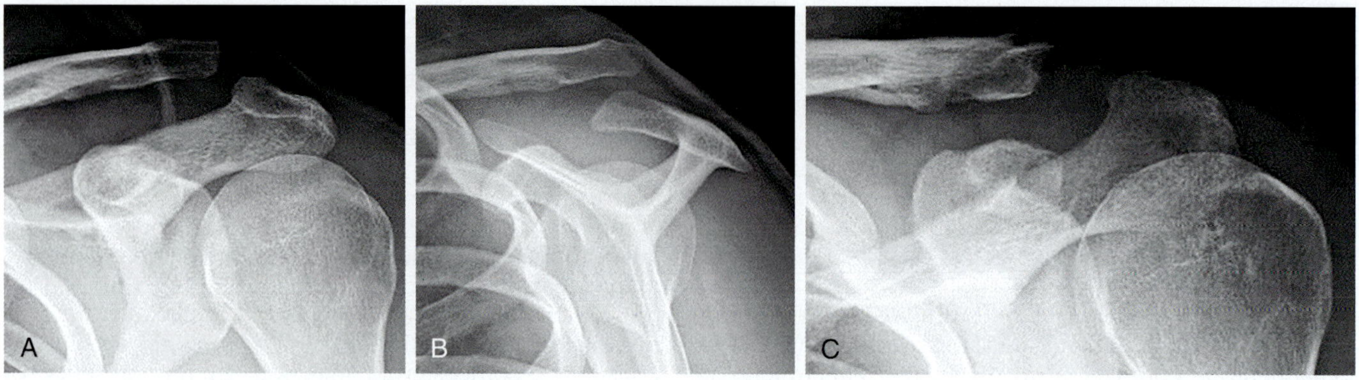

FIGURE 9-119: Chronic type III injury treated with cerclage suture and distal clavicle resection. **A,** Preoperative anteroposterior view. **B,** Preoperative scapular Y view. **C,** Postoperative Zanca view.

is not advised.[768,831] Reconstructions of the ACJ are most successful when the operation incorporates, by some means, fixation between the clavicle and the coracoid process (Fig. 9-119).* Biologic tissue or synthetic materials have been used to reconstruct the AC and CC ligaments simultaneously without excision of the lateral clavicle (Fig. 9-120).[69,298,699,789,1014]

Tauber et al. used subcoracoid and two-tunnel transclavicular passage of autogenous semitendinosus.[899] Saccomanno et al. reconstructed both the AC and CC ligaments with pretensioned autogenous semitendinosus graft without additional fixations.[789] Parnes et al. reported a similar technique performed with arthroscopic assistance with either autograft or allograft.[699] Scheibel et al. utilized an arthroscopic method using autogenous gracilis tendon through bone tunnels in the clavicle and with augmentation of the coracoid using the TightRope technique.[812] A similar prospective investigation by Nordin et al. utilized autogenous gracilis tendon augmented with Graftrope.[668] Natera et al. used semitendinosus allograft through coracoid and clavicular tunnels augmented and protected by a synthetic flip button system (ZipTight, Biomet).[642]

Synthetic materials, including a braided polyester ligament, are an alternative to biologic tissue.[87,430,485,991] Touted advantages are that with early range of motion possible, rotation of the clavicle is not impeded, and the ligament remains well fixed to the clavicle, inhibiting its erosion by a sliding fixation device. The use of LARS has been reported.[162,324,561]

Ejam et al. reported the use of a hook plate with no additional biologic or synthetic augmentation.[264]

Dynamic muscle transfers, as described in the treatment of acute type III injuries, have also been performed in chronic cases, with or without excision of the lateral clavicle.[83,230, 291,958] Some authors have supplemented this method of treatment with the addition of a hook plate.[958]

Transposition of the CAL to the end of the resected clavicle was described by Weaver and Dunn in 1972 and subsequently performed by others as originally described or with subtle technical modifications, sometimes including encircling CC sutures or biologic material or transosseous techniques with synthetic sutures and Endobuttons (Fig. 9-121).* Seeking a more anatomic reconstruction, Payvandi et al. transferred the ligament with a bone wafer to the inferior clavicle with suture anchor CC supplementation.[707] Millett et al described their "docking technique," a variation of the Weaver-Dunn method, which was augmented by nine braided strands of No. 1 PDS.[609] The Cadenat method, modified using a hook plate instead of transacromial K-wires, has been reported.[620] In a study that included only type V injuries, von Heideken et al. reported the use of a hook plate in conjunction with the Weaver-Dunn method.[946] Boström et al. chose to compare this method with one that used CC suture loop (PDS braid) augmentation.[106]

The importance of reconstructing the ligaments of the ACJ as well as the CC ligaments to achieve optimum stability has been emphasized.[944,428]

Results

The transposition of the CAL to the end of the resected clavicle yields excellent or good results in at least 80% of patients.[111,361,479] When used together with a hook plate, von Heideken et al. reported a mean C-M score of 85 and a mean SSV of 80, with 79% excellent and good self-reported outcomes.[946] Radiographically, the CC interval was increased 101% compared with the uninjured side, and the joint subluxation with weighted radiographs was 63% of the clavicle diameter. No correlation was found between the C-M score and radiographic findings. Tauber et al. obtained significantly superior clinical and radiographic outcomes with a semitendinosus graft compared with the modified Weaver-Dunn method.[899] The Weaver-Dunn method supplemented with CC fixation with Mersilene tape resulted in a mean C-M score of 91, with excellent and good outcomes in 93%, and 100% satisfaction yet unfavorable results in 26% due to two

**References 8, 85, 100, 106, 218, 286, 300, 318, 430, 620, 642, 789, 806, 899.*

**References 8, 85, 100, 111, 125, 187, 218, 318, 361, 406, 485, 486, 503, 609, 707, 837, 897, 899, 964, 991.*

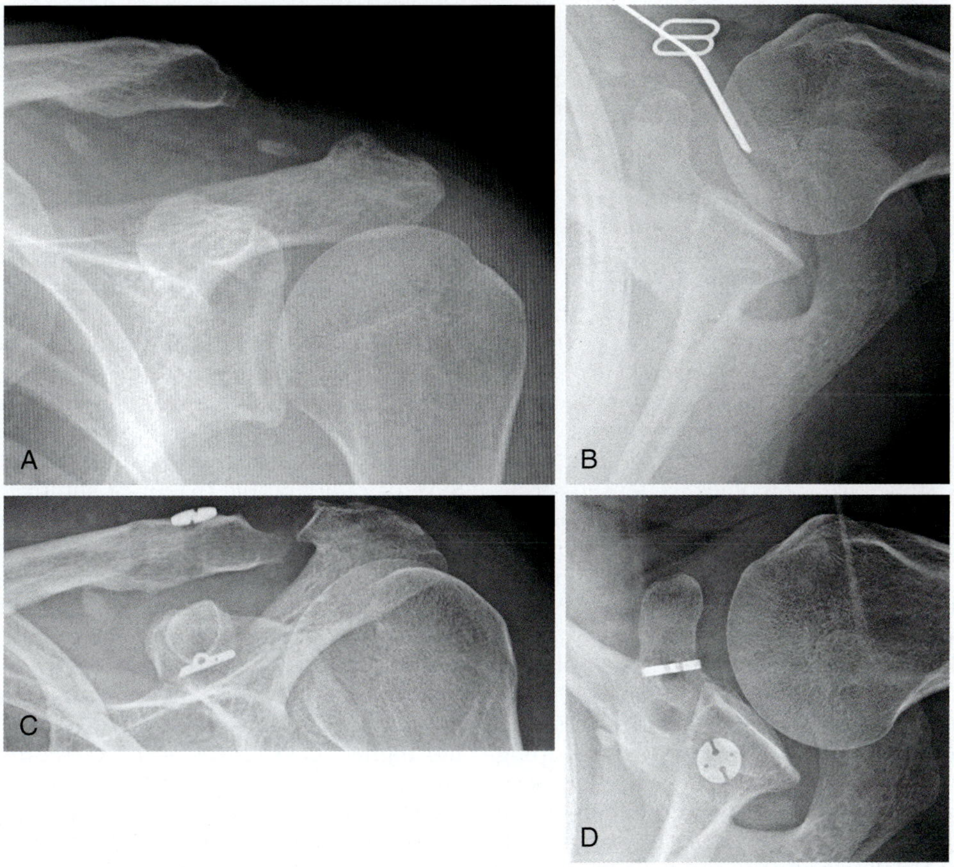

FIGURE 9-120: Chronic type IV injury stabilized with nonabsorbable sutures augmented with allograft fascia spanning the acromioclavicular joint and the coracoclavicular interval. **A** and **B,** Preoperative views. **C** and **D,** Postoperative views. The reduction was never obtained.

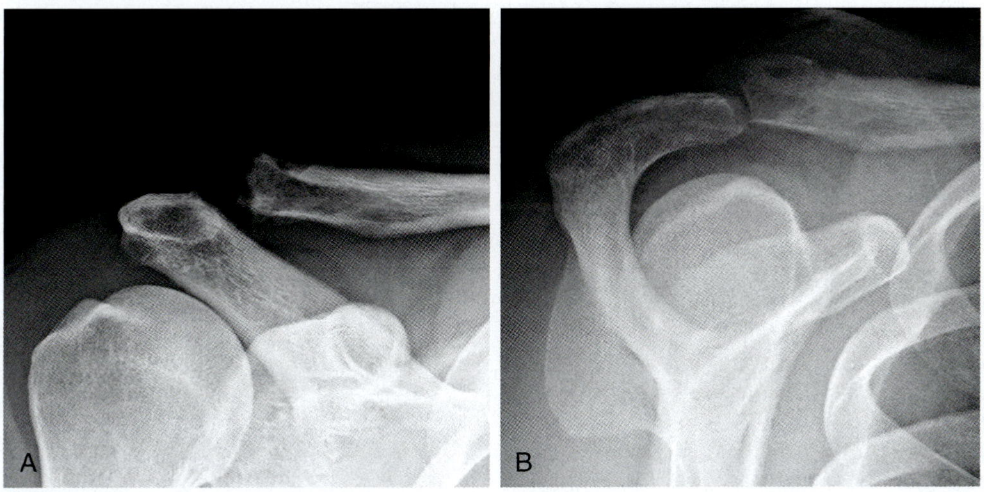

FIGURE 9-121: **A** and **B,** Chronic type III dislocation treated with the Weaver-Dunn method and hamstring coracoclavicular reconstruction.

instances of stiffness that produced pain and two asymptomatic prominent distal clavicles.[486] When performed concomitantly with the Surgilig device, short-term clinical and radiologic outcomes were uniformly successful.[991] With the Weaver-Dunn-Chuinard method augmented with two titanium buttons using heavy nonabsorbable suture, the UCLA modified AC score was 16.5/20 and the SSV was 82% with no losses of reduction.[100] Ejam et al. reported a mean C-M score of 94 and mean L'Insalata score of 93.[264] A modified Cadenet method that uses a hook plate rather than K-wires has shown success.[620] The long-term follow-up (mean, 18 years) reported by Virtanen et al. revealed successful functional results, including a C-M score of 90, DASH score of 5.1, and SST score of 11 out of 12.[943] Radiographic anatomic alignment was maintained in 76% of the patients.

Biologic tissue or synthetic materials have been used to reconstruct the AC and CC ligaments simultaneously without excision of the lateral clavicle.[298,69,1014] Very favorable results and an extremely high satisfaction rate have been reported for reconstructions of the AC and CC ligaments performed simultaneously without excision or limited excision of the lateral clavicle.[298,69,1014,428,789] However, CC ligament reconstruction with autogenous hamstring tendon through tunnels with or without superior AC reinforcement with tendon graft only gave moderately favorable subjective outcomes.[943] Jensen et al. reconstructed the AC and CC ligaments with autogenous gracilis and GraftRope, with better clinical than radiographic outcome parameters, and horizontal instability was effectively addressed in 87% of the patients.[428] Parnes et al. achieved a mean C-M score of 96, SSV of 95%, and SST score of 11/12 at a mean follow-up interval of 30.4 months with no loss of radiographic reduction.[699] A more anatomic reconstruction with the LARS ligament resulted in improved functional outcomes compared with looping Dacron vascular graft, which resulted in fair or poor results in 83% of patients.[300] Better outcomes were achieved with allograft semitendinosus compared with synthetic ligament (LARS) in the study by Fauci et al.[286] Previous attempts at operative stabilization did not have a significant impact on clinical scores or radiographic instability.[286] A 44% incidence of concomitant findings were recognized during the arthroscopic-assisted reconstruction performed by Jensen et al., and included both degenerative (calcifying tendinopathy, biceps long head) and traumatic (partial supraspinatus and subscapularis tears and SLAP lesions).[428] In the absence of complications, 75% excellent results (3/4) were reported by Nordin et al.[668] Utilizing a dynamic transfer with supplemental hook plate, Wang and Zhang reported a mean Constant score of 91 with no loss of anatomic reduction, which was obtained in all instances.[958] Return to work and sport with no change in status was the norm.[958]

Bezer et al. reported a mean Constant score of 90 with reduction maintained in 90% of the patients.[85] Reduction parameters were derived from measurements obtained from models created from 3D CT scans with stress applied to the limb. Inverse correlation for C-M score was present only in the parameter craniocaudal AC distance (CCD): the superior margin of the acromion and the superior margin of the clavicle in the sagittal plane. In addition, increased CCD was observed only in dissatisfied patients unwilling to undergo the operative treatment again. Al-Ahaideb achieved a mean C-M score of 97 with 77% anatomic reductions and return to full activities at 6 months.[8] Lower clinical outcome scores were noted in chronic cases in which the Weaver-Dunn method supplemented the TightRope technique was compared with acute cases in which only the TightRope technique was used.[218] Millett et al. showed 94% maintenance of reduction and a mean ASES score of 86 at 29 months.[609] The use of a synthetic ligament (Surgilig) resulted in a mean C-M score of 92 at an average of 55 months with 10 out of 11 excellent or good results.[430] Using the same device, Bhattacharya et al. reported a mean C-M score of 83.1, Imatani score of 81.2, and Bhattacharya score of 14.1, with satisfaction in 82%.[87] The results of reconstruction with the Surgilig were compared with those of the Weaver-Dunn method in the study by Kumar et al.[485] Better outcome scores and earlier return to work and sport were observed in the patients undergoing the Surgilig method. Comparing the Weaver-Dunn method augmented by PDS sutures versus hook plate, Broström et al. could show no significant differences with respect to C-M score, QUICKDASH, total excellent and good results, SSV, or radiographic extent of subluxation.[106] There was no correlation between the grades of subluxation versus function. They concluded that the hook plate afforded no advantages over suture augmentation at the time of treatment with the Weaver-Dunn method, resulted in more pain at follow-up, and were obligated to a secondary operation. Chouhan et al. reported a mean C-M score of 91 and ASES of 93 with no radiographic complications.[162] Using the same device, Giannotti et al. obtained the highest C-M scores and SST scores possible.[324] Marcheggiani et al. confirmed significant improvement in clinical outcomes using LARS with C-M and Oxford scores of 94 and 45, respectively.[561] An overall 98% success rate was observed. The outcomes of professionals and nonprofessionals were essentially identical.

Complications

Essentially the same complications are encountered whether one is treating an acute or a chronic lesion of this type (Fig. 9-122). Isolated excision of the lateral clavicle is significantly more prone to complications in the setting of chronic complete injuries and is best avoided (Fig. 9-123). Woodmass et al. performed a systematic review of complications of arthroscopic treatment of AC dislocations.[992] Loss of reduction was the most common complication in chronic cases, especially those utilizing graft reconstruction (Fig. 9-124). Saccomanno

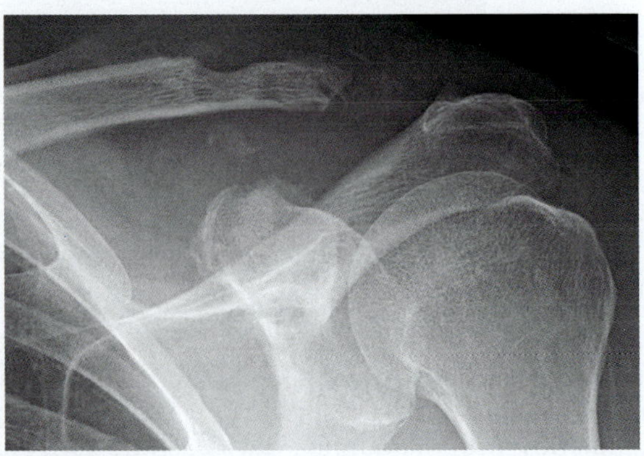

FIGURE 9-122: Loss of anatomic reduction with erosion of the clavicle by encircling nonabsorbable sutures.

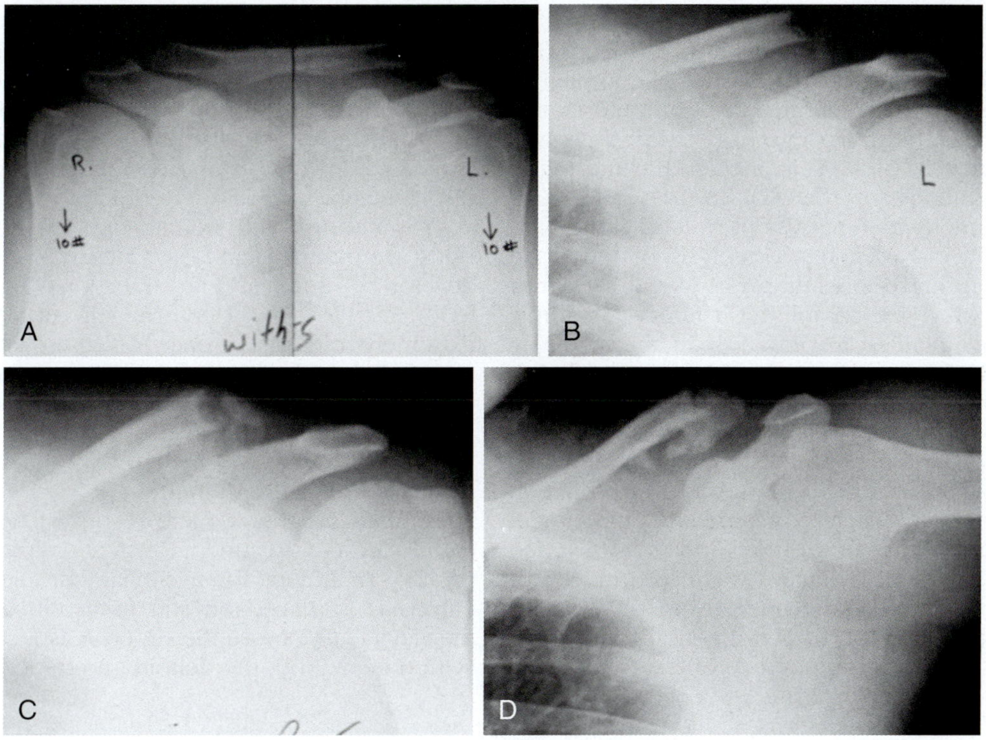

FIGURE 9-123: Complication of instability from lateral clavicle excision for chronic, complete acromioclavicular joint dislocation. **A,** Acute, complete acromioclavicular dislocation on preoperative radiographs. **B,** Six months later, due to continued pain, the lateral clavicle was excised. **C,** Four months after surgical treatment, the patient had increasing pain, heterotopic ossification, and widening of the coracoclavicular interval. **D,** Continued symptoms at 8 months after the index operation. (From Rockwood CA, Green DP, eds. *Fractures.* 2nd ed. Philadelphia: JB Lippincott; 1984.)

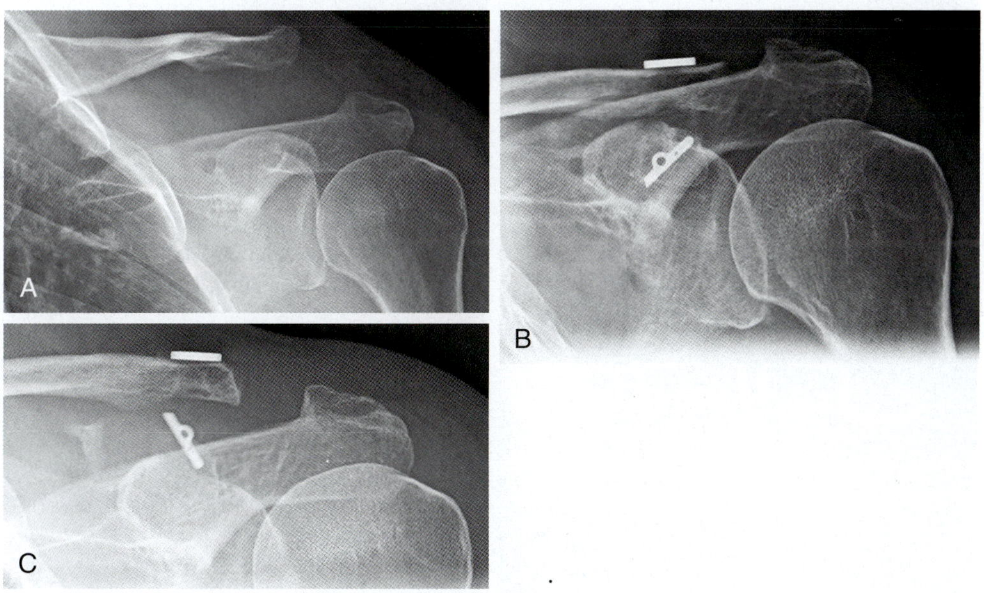

FIGURE 9-124: **A,** Type V injury. **B,** Overcorrection. **C,** Failure on the coracoid side, but reduction is fairly well maintained by the biologic allograft.

et al. observed asymptomatic recurrent deformity in 11% of the patients in their series,[789] with DASH and C-M scores of 6.6 and 90.3, respectively. Issues of compliance and overaggressive rehabilitation may contribute to this phenomenon.[396] A concerning rate of complications was noted by Virtanen et al.[944] This included clinical and radiographic instability of the ACJ in 44% and 56%, respectively. Tunnel widening was prevalent, along with clavicle and coracoid fractures, osteolysis of the distal clavicle, infection, and reoperation (Fig. 9-125). Dacron vascular graft had a 43% complication rate.[300] Anatomic reduction was maintained in only 47% in the study by Jensen et al.[428] They also observed clavicular tunnel widening of 10 mm (initial 6-mm tunnel) (Fig. 9-126). A prospective study utilizing GraftRope with autogenous gracilis tendon with 6-mm tunnels was abandoned by Nordin et al. due to 50% incidence of loss of reduction in the first 6 weeks.[668] They expressed discouragement by the present and future fixation methods that included coracoid tunnels. Loss of reduction was noted in 21% of the patients in the series of Marcheggiani et al.[561] A coracoid fracture due to erosion by a synthetic ligament has been reported.[430] Other reported problems with the device include breakage and fixation screw prominence with loosening.[87] Broström et al. reported two redislocations, each requiring a revision stabilization procedure.[106] Von Heideken et al. reported a superficial infection and an instance of hook dislocation requiring revision reconstruction.[946] Ejam et al. reported superior hook plate displacement with ill-advised activity leading to removal at 3.5 months with no adverse effect on outcome.[264] Both symptomatic and asymptomatic AC arthrosis may develop.[957] Surgical site infections have been reported.[100,106,162,485,561,699] Alentorn-Geli et al. reported the extremely rare occurrence of distal clavicle osteolysis with a slightly modified classic Weaver-Dunn method that did not include the supplemental use of metal or other material spanning the ACJ.[12]

Author's Preferred Method

I prefer to use hook plate reconstruction (as described earlier for the treatment of acute type III injury) as a primary treatment for a similar chronic lesion. Greater emphasis is placed on soft tissue dissection inferior to the clavicle to expose the superior aspect of the coracoid. With this method, the deltoid and trapezius are detached

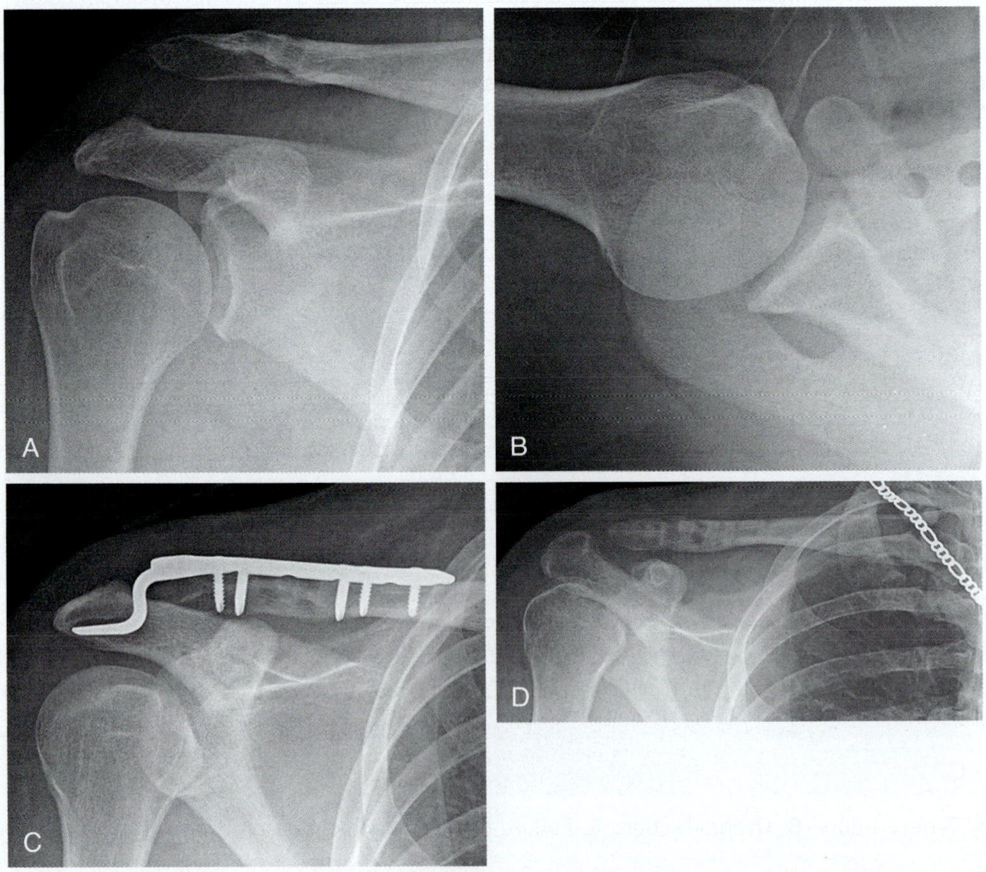

FIGURE 9-125: **A** and **B,** Failed type V injury treatment with subcoracoid allograft tendon passed through the transosseous tunnels and secured to itself using permanent sutures with addition coracoclavicular sutures. **C,** Secondary reconstruction with hook plate, coracoclavicular sutures, and deltotrapezius imbrication. **D,** Three weeks after hook plate removal. Anatomic restoration of the acromioclavicular joint and the coracoclavicular interval.

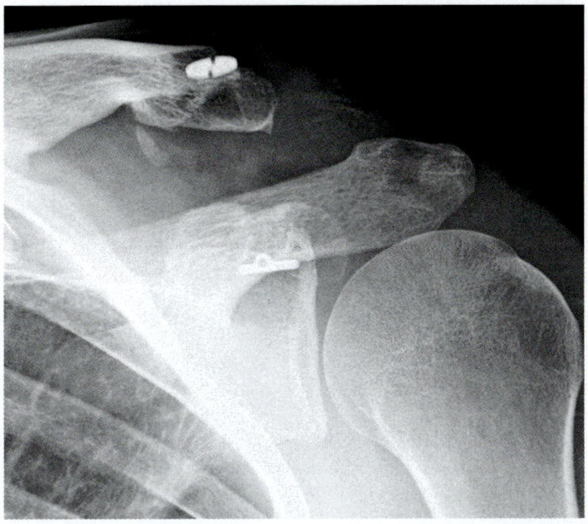

FIGURE 9-126: Result of the case shown in Figure 9-120. Reduction has been lost.

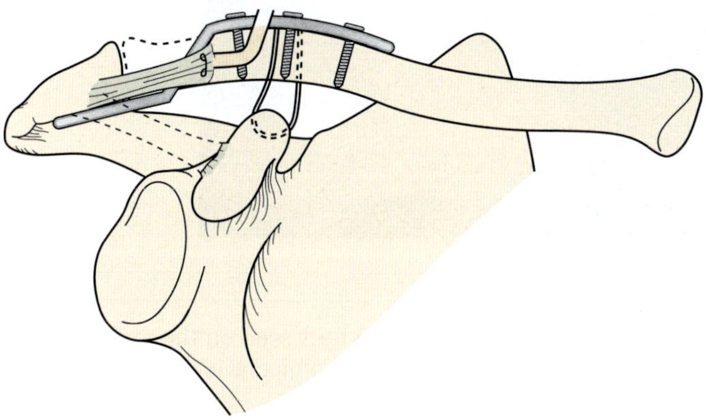

FIGURE 9-127: Chronic complete reconstruction that uses the coracoacromial ligament, detached from the coracoid and attached to the lateral clavicle, spanning the acromioclavicular joint. The hook plate provides rigid internal fixation, and the coracoclavicular interval is spanned with nonabsorbable suture.

more extensively. The end of the clavicle often undergoes attritional changes that do not favor its durability if it is once again opposed to the medial acromion. For this reason, it is unhesitatingly excised even if it has a normal appearance.

Success with this technique depends on the formation of scar tissue in critical locations: between the coracoid process and the clavicle, between the acromion process and the clavicle, and superior to the clavicle. The strength and stiffness of the hook plate maintains the proper osseous relationships during the formation of the stabilizing scar tissue. To avert the possibility of residual AC horizontal or medial instability, there are two options to consider. The first option is to strengthen the linkage between the acromion process and the lateral clavicle, which in nearly all cases, has been resected. The CAL can be detached from the coracoid and attached to the lateral clavicle, spanning the ACJ (Fig. 9-127). The same reconstruction can be performed with tendon graft. The second option is interposition arthroplasty using autografts or allografts or other material that might be considered biologically active. The method has the benefit of a cushioning effect and, to some extent, a stabilizing effect.

LESS COMMON INJURIES

Anterior dislocation (type IV variant) of the distal clavicle is an extremely rare injury, usually sustained in sporting activities as reported by Baek et al.[40] It usually results from a direct injury to the shoulder, typically a fall. Deformity manifests by anterior prominence of the distal clavicle. Ecchymosis, diminished motion, and focal tenderness are the hallmark physical examination findings. Radiographically, while the AP view may not appear normal, the most informative view is the axillary lateral view, which shows the clavicle anterior to the acromion (Fig. 9-128). Surface reconstruction CT scanning is diagnostic as well. Open treatment is required as the distal clavicle skewers the deltoid muscle, which along with the trapezius muscle is stripped from the lateral end of the clavicle. In this case, the CC ligaments were intact. Stability is restored after reduction by means of a suture technique that reconstructs the AC ligaments. With appropriate aftercare and rehabilitation, uneventful recovery is expected.

NONTRAUMATIC DISORDERS

Acromioclavicular Osteolysis

The relationship between osteolysis of the distal clavicle and trauma has been well documented as evidenced in the literature review conducted by Schwarzkopf et al. in 2008.[821] The earliest reports of the condition are found in the non-English literature.[262,330, 975] The strong association with trauma was verified by others.[421,556, 636] The role of repetitive trauma, perhaps best thought of as overuse, or atraumatic, first mentioned by Ehricht more than 5 decades ago, was noted by Seymour in 1977, and subsequently strongly supported by a report by Cahill, who documented an undeniable relationship to weight training.[129,262,829] Other authors have confirmed this relationship with repetitive trauma or overuse, especially weight training.[577,808, 809] It is reported less frequently in female patients, perhaps due to less risk-activity exposure.[577,599,687,769]

Various mechanisms for the development of osteolysis under these conditions have been suggested, including vascular compromise, microfractures, nervous system dysfunction, osteoclastic activation, and synovial hyperplasia.[32,118,129,520,556,636,687,740]

The radiographic findings are variable, depending on the duration of the process, and have been effectively described by all reporting authors. In addition to osteolysis, these can include osteoporosis, irregular or absent subchondral bone, alteration of the distal clavicle morphology such as tapering, cysts of various dimensions,

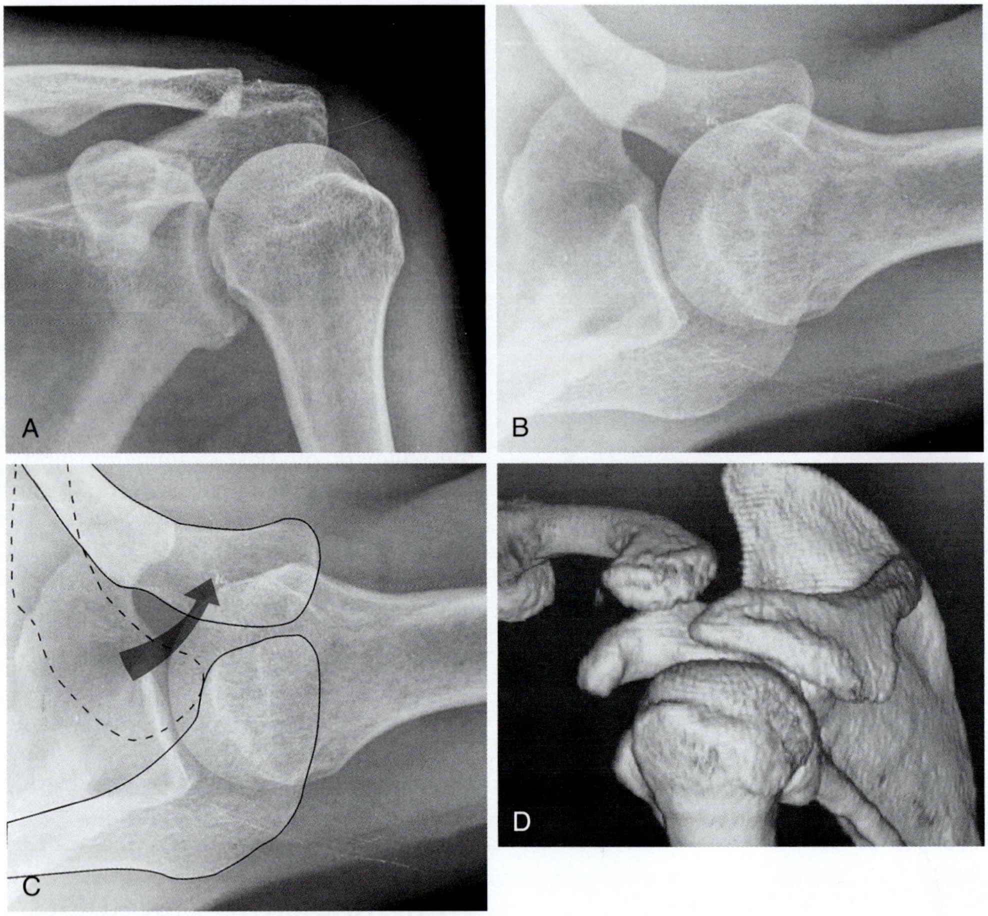

FIGURE 9-128: **A** to **D**, The extremely rare anterior acromioclavicular dislocation (type IV variant) best seen on the axillary lateral view. (From Baek SH, Oh CW, Wallace WA, et al. Anterior clavicle dislocation associated with acromioclavicular dislocation in a soccer player: a case report. *Am J Sports Med.* 2007;35[10]:1752-1755.)

calcification, and osteophytes (Fig. 9-129). Bone scan activity is usually intense and well localized to the ACJ and distal clavicle (Figs. 9-130 and 9-131).[129] MRI, often performed but rarely necessary, might reveal edema within the marrow elements of the distal clavicle, nondisplaced subchondral distal clavicle fracture, cortical erosions, ACJ effusion, focal capsular disruption, and cysts.[221,447,703,1011]

Histologic findings obtained at the time of operative treatment were reported by Asano and others, and may be extensive: synovial hyperplasia, articular cartilage destruction of the distal clavicle, bone necrosis, vascular proliferation, reactive woven bone, fibrous tissue invasion, multinucleated giant cells, inflammatory cells within the bone marrow, and preservation of the intra-articular disk.[32,350,497,556,636,1020] Asano et al. also documented noninvolvement of the acromion process.[32]

Another etiologic category has been proposed by Hawkins et al.—nontraumatic.[382] They described the clinical presentation of three healthy patients without exposure to trauma or overuse and without evidence for metabolic disease or any other known cause of osteolysis.

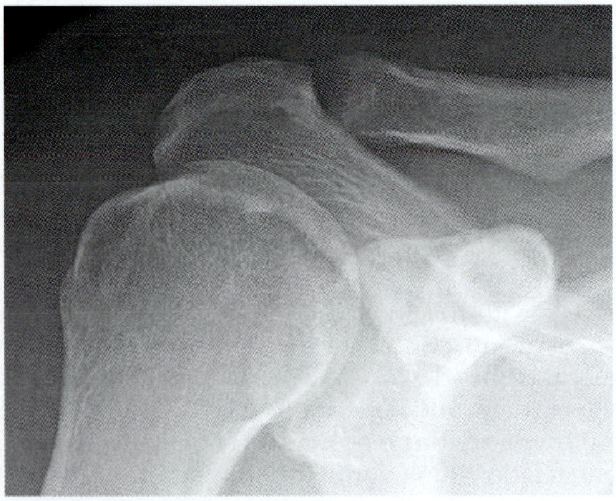

FIGURE 9-129: Posttraumatic osteolysis manifesting loss of subchondral bone, cysts, and osteopenia.

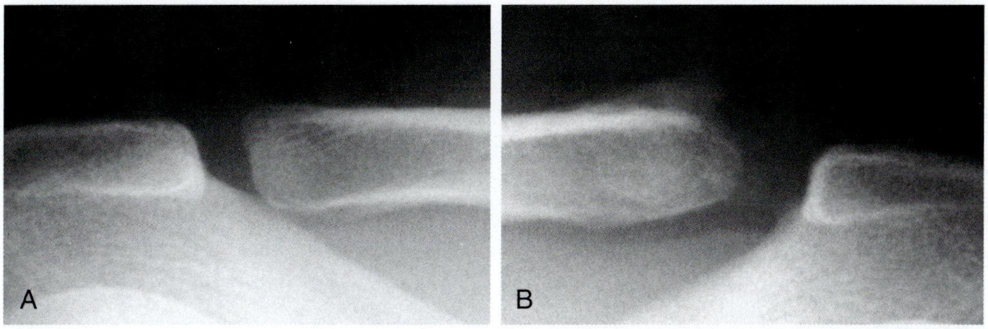

FIGURE 9-130: Osteolysis. **A,** Normal acromioclavicular joint. **B,** Tender, enlarged acromioclavicular joint.

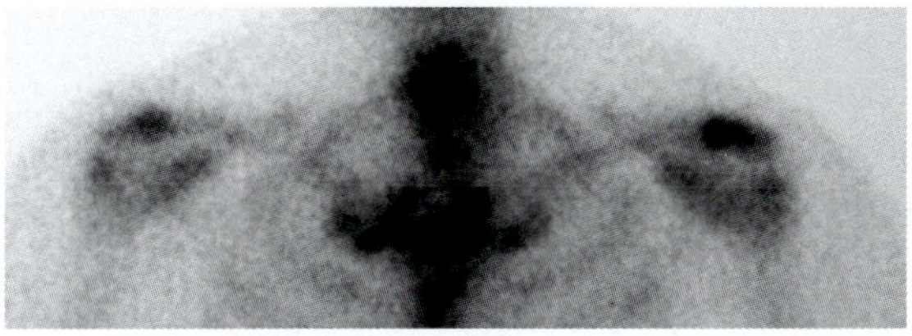

FIGURE 9-131: Bone scan (correlating with plain radiographs in Fig. 9-130) showing intense tracer uptake in the acromioclavicular joint with osteolysis.

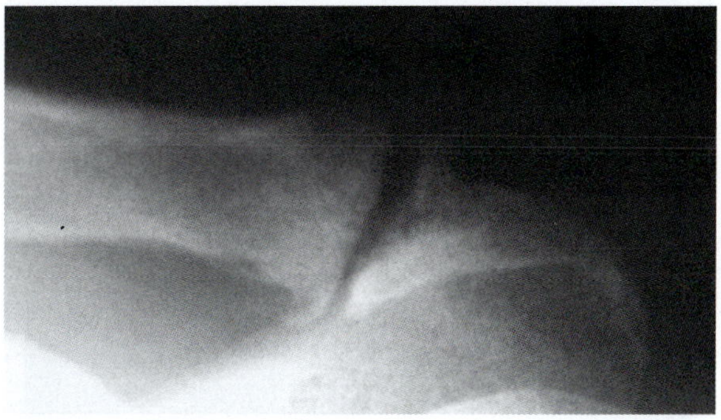

FIGURE 9-132: Osteoarthritis of the acromioclavicular joint seen on the Zanca view. Note eccentric joint space narrowing, osteophytes, and subchondral cysts.

The differential diagnosis of atraumatic occurrence is limited. Systemic diseases such as hyperparathyroidism, RA, and scleroderma should be given consideration, especially with bilateral involvement. Local processes that can resemble classic osteolysis are massive osteolysis (Gorham-Stout disease), infections, metastatic malignancy, primary bone tumors such as multiple myeloma, and crystal arthropathy, especially gout.

Activity-related pain with local tenderness and perhaps slight swelling are the hallmarks of this disorder. Night pain may be present to a variable degree depending on the intensity of the inflammation that is associated with the process.

A conservative plan of care should be undertaken for osteolysis of the distal clavicle, at least initially. The cornerstone of treatment is rest and activity modification, even going so far as to completely discontinue participation in weight-training programs that are undertaken to maximize athletic performance and vigorously encouraged by coaches and trainers. Nonsteroidal anti-inflammatory medication can be prescribed and from time to time, during the course of recovery, it may be reasonable to perform a corticosteroid injection. Although it can require 6 to 12 months, instances of relatively atraumatic osteolysis of the distal clavicle are capable of recovery of comfort, function, and bone integrity with conservative treatment.[118,308,522,769] Frequent findings on MRI at a mean follow-up of 4.3 years included flattening of the distal clavicle from subchondral resorption (79%), abnormal widening of the ACJ space (50%), and secondary OA (71%), which, in more than half of the cases, was moderate and severe, resulting in clinical symptoms.[769]

When nonoperative treatment is deemed a failure, excision of the lateral clavicle will definitively terminate the process and, in nearly all cases, result in an excellent or good outcome.[153,382,808,847]

Acromioclavicular Arthritis

There are more than 100 different types of arthritis that can involve the ACJ. Only three are mentioned here.

Osteoarthritis

Because of the prevalence of OA of the ACJ in the population, it is near certainty that nearly all providers of musculoskeletal care evaluate and treat the disorder at some point (Fig. 9-132).[126,391,596] Recent reviews reinforce this notion.[559,598] However, it may be very difficult to ascertain whether the condition is primary or secondary, although the former is not commonly symptomatic and the latter, especially trauma-related OA, is more prevalent (Fig. 9-133).[80,313,887] An ultrasonographic investigation of asymptomatic males aged 40 to 79 years identified a 65% prevalence of ACJ OA.[326] Extra-articular fractures of the clavicle that result in malunion do not appear to be associated with an increased incidence of OA.[148] Type III acromions and smaller supraspinatus outlets have been observed in the presence of more severe degeneration of the ACJ.[770] Increasingly severe OA is four-fold more common in individuals with spinal cord injuries than in matched, able-bodied persons.[273] Distal clavicle osteophytes (48%) and ACJ space narrowing (13%) are findings identified on plain radiographs in a small sampling of

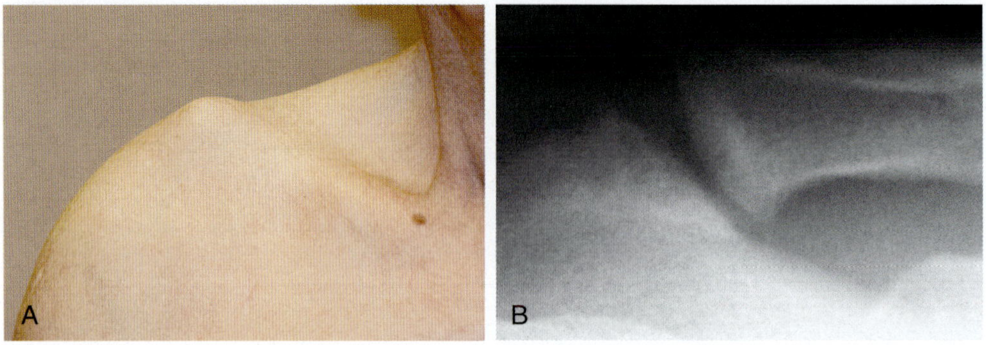

FIGURE 9-133: Osteoarthritis. The patient was asymptomatic. **A,** Clinical appearance. **B,** Radiographic correlation of primary osteoarthritis.

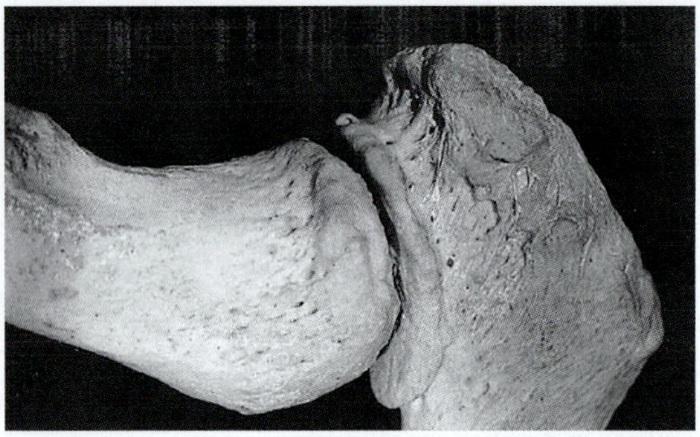

FIGURE 9-134: Archival dried skeleton demonstrating degeneration of the acromioclavicular joint, especially on the acromial side, resulting in a "ball and socket" appearance. (From Edelson JG. Patterns of degenerative change in the acromioclavicular joint. *J Bone Joint Surg Br.* 1996;78[2]:242-243.)

major league baseball pitchers (average age, 29 years) and appear to correlate with innings pitched.[995]

From observations of archival dried skeletons, Edelson recognized patterns of degenerative change that included acromial side elongation in the sagittal plane, principally in the posterior facet[255] (Fig. 9-134). In this setting, SI osteophytes were diminished. Corresponding AP-directed clavicular side broadening and rounding-off resulted in a ball-and-socket–like articulation. In another investigation, Edelson and Taitz observed that AC degeneration was independent of spurring or faceting of the rest of the acromion process.[259]

From their observations of the ACJ space narrowing with age, Petersson and Redlund-Johnell concluded that an interval of 0.5 mm or less between the acromion and the clavicle in a patient older than 60 years might not indicate disease.[720] Bonsell et al. drew attention to a negative correlation between the age-related radiologic findings of OA and symptomatic ACJs.[102] The occurrence of traction osteophytes arising from the lateral articular facets of the clavicle significantly correlates with increasing age.[557] However, it should be recalled that the true incidence of AC OA is underestimated by plain radiography or tomography.[874] As discussed earlier, the sensitivity of MRI and ultrasonography verifies its presence earlier in life as well as an increasing incidence with age. In addition, the widespread use of MRI of the shoulder has led to the recognition of a high prevalence of age-related changes in the ACJ, which are not infrequently found in asymptomatic patients.[646,833,840] Wulff et al. reported a 10-year longitudinal MRI investigation of the ACJs of manual laborers that correlated progressively increasing AC degeneration (33% higher) when engaged in forceful work.[998] Elhassan et al. reported that nearly 50% of patients undergoing DCR for painful ACJ arthritis had normal radiographs but documented eburnation of the distal clavicle.[266]

In cadavers, OA was also age related, and was especially prevalent after 70 years.[717] Besides age, other risk factors for the development of OA are extreme labor and sports participation.[873]

The treatment of OA of the ACJ differs very little from that of other joints in the body, and include activity modification, nonnarcotic analgesics, nonsteroidal anti-inflammatory medication, and the liberal use of ice and heat. The role of manual physical therapy for a select group of patients has been advocated.[372]

Peterson and Holer, in 2010, reported that there were no systematic reviews, meta-analyses, or randomized controlled trials regarding therapeutic injections of the ACJ.[716] The results of intra-articular corticosteroid injections vary but usually result, at the least, in short-term pain relief and improvement in range of motion.[297,420,488,602,785,914,962] The effectiveness of injection would seem to be predicated on the accuracy of delivery of the therapeutic agent into the ACJ. When injecting painful ACJs with clinical and radiographic arthritis, Scillia et al. reported an accuracy of 36.5% for intra-articular confirmed with contrast and fluoroscopic evaluation.[823] However, in the study by van Riet et al., 64% expressed no relief at the 1-month follow-up to injection. The symptoms had resolved in 28%, and the results remained favorable when the patients were followed up to 42 months.[936] Ultrasonography showed no advantages over palpation technique for pain relief and functional recovery.[785] The long-term benefits of steroid injection into the arthritic ACJ was investigated by Hossain et al. in patients with a minimum 5-year follow-up.[405] The C-M score improved significantly at a steady rate, and 25% of patients had symptom reduction for 1 year. Significant deterioration was observed at 5 years compared with 1 year, but patients were still significantly better than preinjection. Other investigations have noted shorter term relief (1 week), with return to baseline pain by 3 weeks.[786,787] A controlled investigation comparing ultrasound guidance intra-articular versus periarticular local anesthetic with steroid injections revealed similar improvement over a 3-week study period in both groups.[787] The recommended dosages of local anesthetic and steroid into the ACJ are often exceeded by orthopedic surgeons.[844] The success of pain relief with intra-articular injection of local anesthetic and corticosteroid is directly related to joint capsule hypertrophy (>3 mm) demonstrated by MRI.[880] A 3-T MRI comparison of asymptomatic with symptomatic ACJs revealed that the only discriminating observation was the degree of superior capsular distension in symptomatic joints.[161]

The disease can be definitively treated by excision of the lateral clavicle with predictably satisfactory outcomes if appropriate surgical guidelines are followed (Fig. 9-135).[242] The prevalence of OA of the ACJ led Pennington et al. to state that "radiological features should only be used as an adjunct in the decision to excise the ACJ."[711] Injection testing may prove useful to discriminate sources of pain and guide treatment in the presence of disorders of the RC.[927]

Rheumatoid Arthritis

The ACJ is affected in at least 50% of patients with RA—even more commonly than the GHJ.[719] Only rarely is operative treatment performed.

Crystal Arthritis

Gout and pseudogout (also termed *calcium pyrophosphate deposition disease*) of the ACJ have been reported.* The crystal deposition is often accompanied by solitary massive tophi, pseudotumors, and pseudocysts with resultant dramatic physical and imaging findings. An instance of gout involvement of the ACJ resulting in cystic swelling has been observed.[578] Bilateral ACJ involvement with gouty arthritis and pseudotumor (saturnine gout) was reported by Podgorski et al.[728] Acute attacks of pseudogout of the ACJ are extremely rare.[185,365,408] The incidence of chondrocalcinosis of the ACJ observed on chest radiographs was 1% and restricted to patients 75 years or older.[700] Associated with knee chondrocalcinosis, its presence suggests the possibility of pseudogout or secondary OA.

**References 97, 185, 226, 322, 352, 365, 408, 563, 578, 608, 637, 728, 921.*

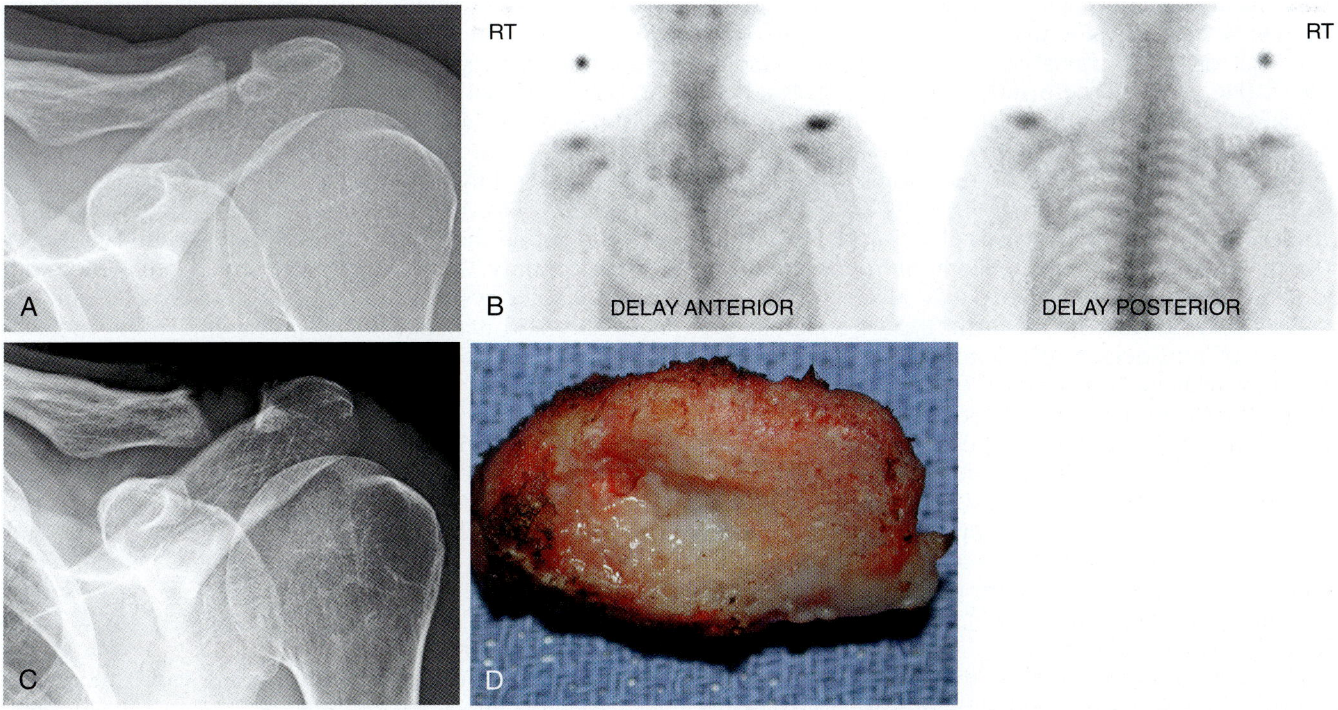

FIGURE 9-135: Painful acromioclavicular joint with imaging confirmation. Appropriately oriented and spaced distal clavicle resection. Erosion, chondrolysis, osteolysis, cyst formation, eburnation of subchondral bone, and to a lesser extent, osteophyte formation, observed in a resected specimen.

Other Diseases Involving the Acromioclavicular Joint

Synovial chondromatosis has been reported.[702,615] One instance of primary hemochromatosis involving the ACJ has been reported.[285] A single occurrence of fibroma of tendon sheath in a 16-year-old female was reported by Glover et al.[332]

Cysts of the Acromioclavicular Joint

The ACJ is a common site for the development of cysts or, more accurately, cyst-like structures that are nearly always the result of insidious, degenerative massive and usually irreparable tears of the RC. Syringomyelia of the cervical cord and Charcot arthropathy of the shoulder have been reported to initiate a cascade of events resulting in the formation of an ACJ cyst.[9] Regardless of the initiating process, the pathogenesis of those related to tears of the RC relates to instability of the humeral head. No longer constrained by sufficient medially directed forces, the humeral head ascends until it makes contact with the fibro-osseous coracoacromial arch. Lacking the protective covering of the RC, the articular cartilage deteriorates and presents a much rougher surface to the overlying arch. The relatively thin inferior ACJ capsule begins to erode, while the unusually large effusion that typically accompanies this condition escapes by way of the path of least resistance into the ACJ. The attachments of the deltoid and trapezius muscles act as reinforcements for the anterior and posterior portions of the capsule, while exposing the relatively weak superior capsule that bridges them to the ebb and flow of joint fluid under pressure. The capsule eventually fails, permitting the fluid to slowly dissect into the overlying soft tissues. In response, a new, flexible pseudocapsule forms and becomes a discrete permanent enclosure that remains in close proximity to the ACJ or, rarely, finds its way into the surrounding muscles (Fig. 9-136). These cystic structures, isolated AC synovial cysts and the rare, isolated true periarticular ganglions are well documented in the literature and should not be confused with infections or neoplasms.* Crystals are sometimes detected in the fluid (Fig. 9-137).

Hiller et al. published an excellent in-depth manuscript that included a complete literature review and four additional cases.[394] They opined two distinct etiologies for cysts in proximity to the ACJ. Type I arises in the presence of nonspecific ACJ degeneration. It communicates only with the subacromial bursa and not the GHJ because the RC is intact (Fig. 9-138). Type II is the classic "cyst" of the ACJ evolving in the presence of a significantly large RC tear, often with degenerative changes of the GHJ (see Fig. 9-138).

Cysts have been observed in the setting of gouty involvement of the ACJ that acquires a characteristic pattern of bony projections from the acromion, giving it the name porcupine shoulder.[226] Detection on a plain radiograph is exceedingly rare.[578]

The cysts present no specific threat unless the overlying, protruding skin is threatened by pressure or excessive friction. The investing, stretched integument can be further compromised by repetitive aspirations, leading to spontaneous drainage and risk of infection.[845] Local pain, cosmesis, and irritable contact with the adjacent tissue during movement may be indications for surgical treatment. Spontaneous resolution has been observed.[219]

*References 124, 157, 198, 339, 361, 394, 476, 556, 618, 630, 689, 733, 778, 824.

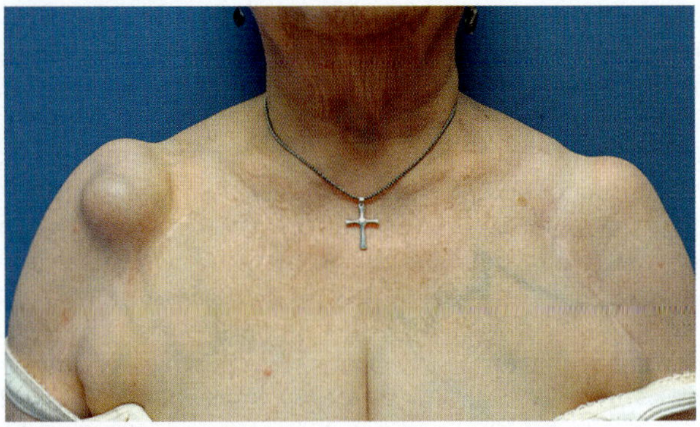

FIGURE 9-136: Acromioclavicular cyst in a patient with a small rotator cuff tear in the presence of anatomic total shoulder arthroplasty.

Ultrasonography or MRI are the best ways to image the cyst, and are sometimes as dramatic as the most extreme form of the geyser sign observed with arthrography (Fig. 9-139).[186,197,921]

Distinction is made between the treatment of type I, which are isolated synovial cysts, and type II, which are those forming in the presence of RC tear. For type II, isolated excision of the cyst mandates a soft tissue repair sturdier than originally present to prevent recurrence or, even worse, an arthrocutaneous fistula.[634] Techniques employed during treatment may include DCR, closure of tracts from the subacromial bursa to the ACJ, RCR, acromioplasty, and special attention to potentially redundant skin (Fig. 9-140).[672] In some instances, another consideration is to interpose synthetic or biologic allograft material into the debrided ACJ to create an effective "seal," thereby eliminating the opportunity for recurrent fluid accumulation.[845,543] On the contrary, Cho, having documented experience with infection after cyst excision, believes that patches are not necessary and may encourage postoperative infections.[157] Mullett et al. reported successful arthroscopic treatment of a massive cyst.[630] Cyst recurrence after excision of the lateral clavicle is rarely observed.[157] The cuff is usually irreparable, and GHJ arthropathy may be present. In these instances, prosthetic arthroplasty contributes to the successful management of the cyst.[352,830] Type I cysts and ganglia can be effectively treated by excision and DCR.[476] Complications of cyst excision only may include recurrence, a draining sinus, and infection.[157]

Infections of the Acromioclavicular Joint

Since the seminal report by Griffith and Boyadjis, more than 30 cases of infectious arthritis of the ACJ have been reported.[349] Most infections of the ACJ are caused by operations or injections intended to treat a disorder of the joint. Blood-borne infections have been recognized.[61,105,340,377,416]

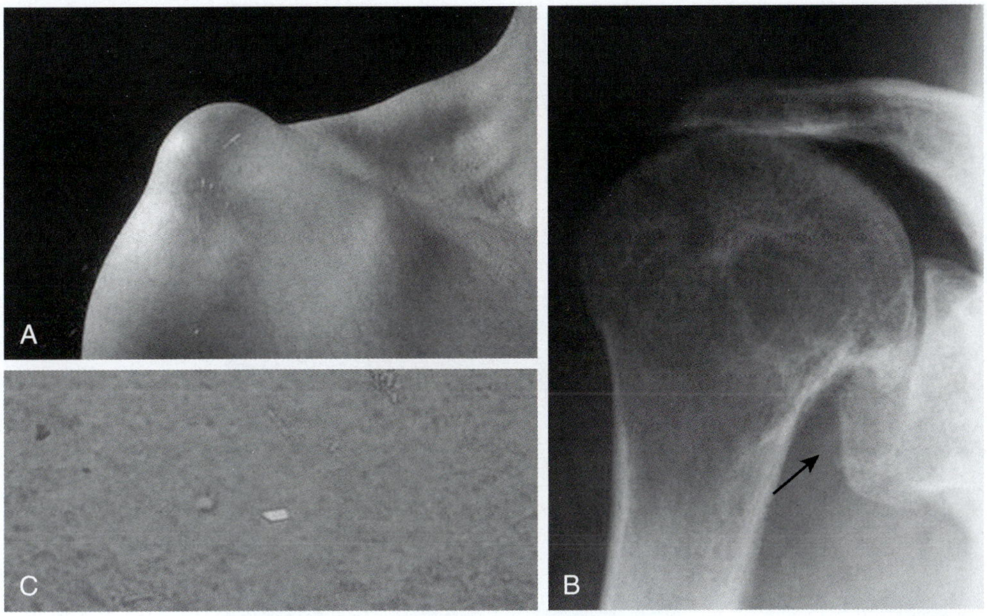

FIGURE 9-137: Acromioclavicular cyst. **A,** Clinical appearance of the cyst. **B,** Accompanying radiograph indicating a massive irreparable rotator cuff tear. Calcific radiodensity within the joint space (*arrow*) indicates crystal deposition within the cyst. **C,** Calcium hydroxyapatite crystals obtained from the fluid-filled cyst.

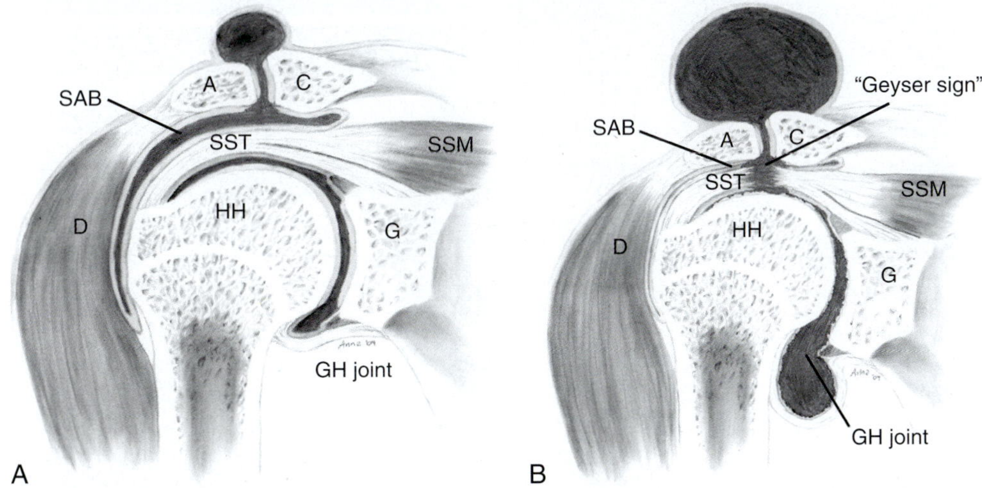

FIGURE 9-138: Acromioclavicular joint cysts. **A,** Type I: arising from the diseased acromioclavicular joint in the presence of an intact rotator cuff. **B,** Arising in the presence of a massive, irreparable rotator cuff tear, often accompanied by arthropathy. *A,* acromion; *C,* clavicle; *D,* deltoid; *G,* glenoid; *GH,* glenohumeral; *HH,* humeral head; *SAB,* subacromial bursa; *SSM,* supraspinatus muscle; *SST,* supraspinatus tendon. (From Hiller AD, Miller JD, Zeller JL. Acromioclavicular joint cyst formation. *Clin Anat.* 2010;23[2]:145-152.)

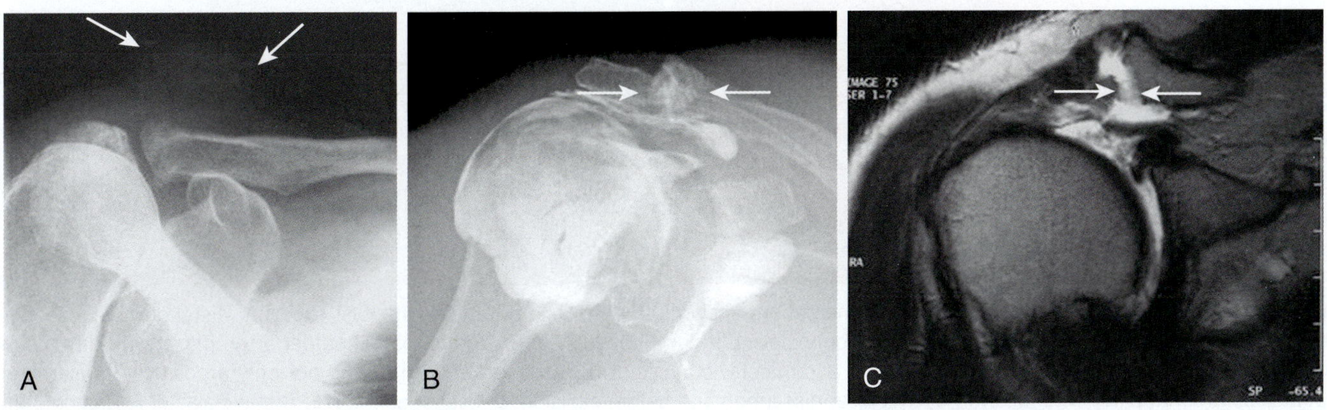

FIGURE 9-139: Acromioclavicular cyst images. **A,** The humeral head abuts the acromioclavicular joint. The soft tissue outline of the cyst is shown by the *arrows*. **B,** Arthrography demonstrates the Geyser sign (*arrows*). **C,** Magnetic resonance imaging shows the rotator cuff tear and the fluid communicating between the acromioclavicular joint and the glenohumeral joint (*arrows*).

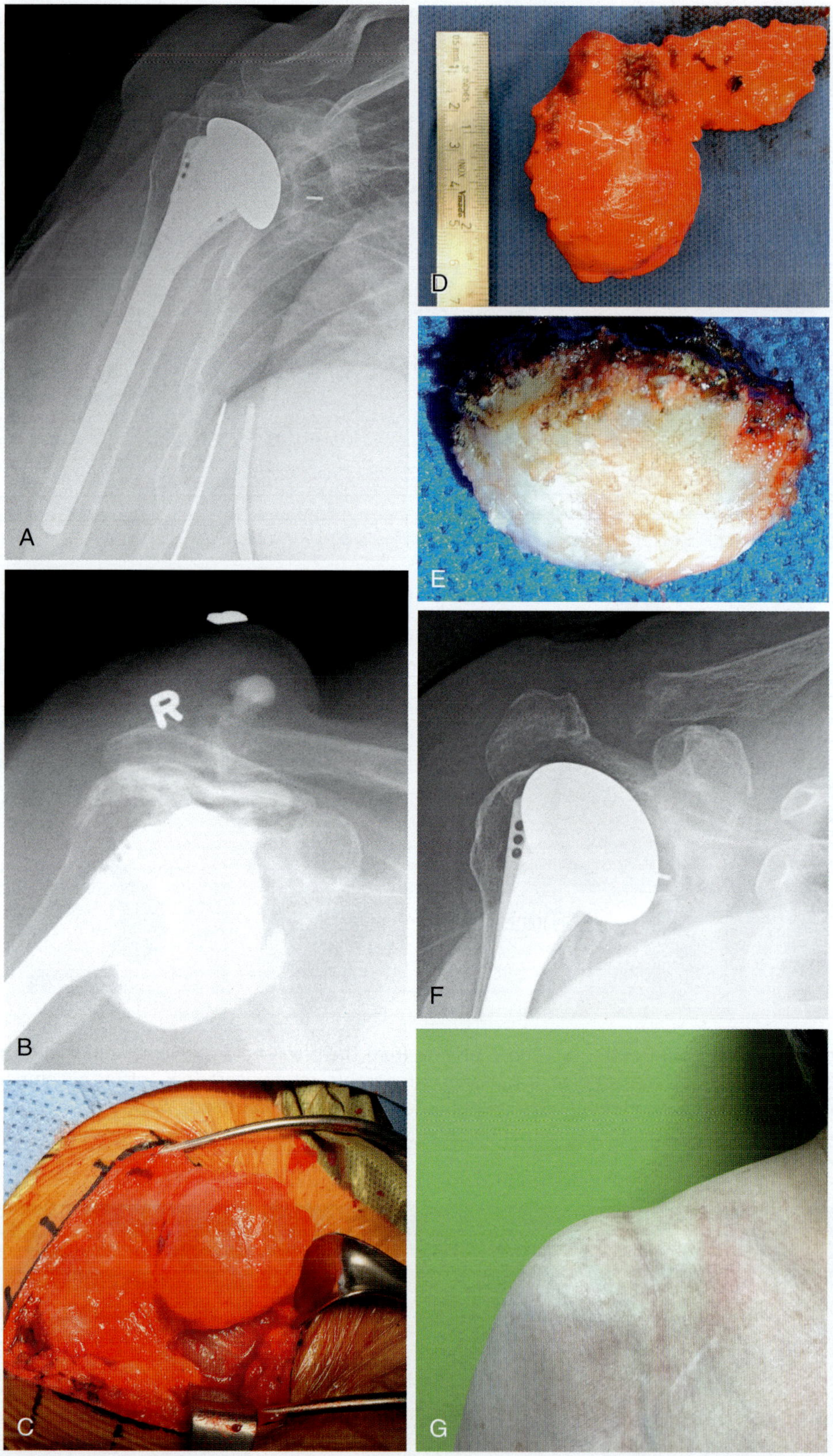

FIGURE 9-140: Acromioclavicular cyst in the same patient shown in Figure 9-136 treated with cyst excision, distal clavicle resection, and soft tissue imbrication to seal the inferior acromioclavicular joint capsule. **A,** Anatomic total shoulder arthroplasty with diminished acromiohumeral interval and osteoarthritis of the acromioclavicular joint. **B,** Arthrography exhibiting not only a positive "geyser sign" but also contrast tracking into the cyst. **C,** Cyst after dissection and before excision. **D,** Cyst specimen. **E,** Distal clavicle. **F,** Radiographic appearance 18 weeks after distal clavicle resection. **G,** Clinical appearance 18 weeks after resection and soft tissue reconstruction.

Rarely is the infecting organism acquired directly from infected tissue in the vicinity of the joint.[105] Primary septic arthritis is exceedingly rare.[416] A few reports of bacterial arthritis in healthy individuals have been published.[61,93,105,137,154,188,349,402,416] Immunocompromised persons are at higher risk.[105,154,178,349,369,496,573,632,667,893,979,1018] Bilateral involvement is extremely rare.[154,340,377] Nonbacterial infections, including *Mycobacterium*, *Candida*, and cryptococcosis have been reported.[5,6,533,632,756,893,895,612] Unless otherwise contraindicated, surgical treatment and systemic antibiotic is preferred and uniformly successful.

Other Disorders of the Acromioclavicular Joint

Osteonecrosis of the lateral clavicle has been reported.[652] Its radiographic, gross, and histologic features allow it to be distinguished from osteolysis. The extraordinarily rare rapid idiopathic osteolysis (Gorham-Stout disease) involving the lateral clavicle was reported by Sestan and Miletic.[827] An inexplicable painful, motion-limiting condition of the ACJ may persist in the shoulder with adhesive capsulitis (frozen shoulder), for which manipulation, with successful outcome, has been described by Lilje et al.[531] Adolescent throwers, particularly older ones, may acquire a shoulder pain syndrome localized to the ACJ associated with superior capsular hypertrophy identified with ultrasonography.[380] Bioabsorbable suture anchors placed for RCR have been found in the ACJ as a result of failed RCR with disengagement of the anchor, leading to migration into the joint.[595] Uneventful retrieval at the time of RCR revision followed.

INTERNATIONAL EXPERT COMMENTARY

Natascha Kraus and Markus Scheibel

How We Evaluate the Patient

Clinical evaluation of ACJ instability includes a thorough examination of ACJ pathologies as well as overall shoulder function. As degenerative or secondary glenohumeral changes may mimic or mask symptomatic chronic ACJ instability, care needs to be taken to distinguish between the two. Evaluation of scapulothoracic rhythm, scapular dysbalance, and SICK scapula syndrome is essential. In addition to a visible vertical instability in acute and chronic situations, an accompanying dynamic posterior translation (DPT) of the clavicle due to AI scapular rotation may be present and tested clinically by fixing the acromion with one hand and moving the clavicle anteroposteriorly. Comparison with the nonaffected side is mandatory, as congenital hyperlaxity may be present.

Radiographic evaluation should include bilateral AP as well as bilateral lateral stress views (Alexander views) in order to visualize vertical and horizontal translation in ACJ instability. A DPT, which is not evaluated in Rockwood's classification, is not restricted to high-grade injuries and has to be considered also in low-grade instabilities. A DPT can be evaluated on dynamic axillary or bilateral Alexander views.[15,900] DPTs can be graded into a nondisplaced situation (Fig. 9-141A) or a partial (see Fig. 9-141B) or complete translation (see Fig. 9-141C). Persisting complete DPT on Alexander views is associated with worse clinical results after surgical stabilization.[811] Our unpublished data show that patients with a complete DPT present with a clinically worse situation in the acute posttraumatic setting (maximum 7 days posttrauma) in comparison to patients with or without a partial DPT. Besides, patients with a CC difference of less than 30% achieved significantly better clinical results in comparison with patients with a higher CC difference of more than 30%, whereas there was no difference between patients with a Rockwood type III (25% to 100%) and those with a type V (>100%) injury. Therefore we use a new classification of ACJ instability (Table 9-2). It remains unknown if a complete DPT with low-grade CC translation necessitates surgical intervention. However, if surgical stabilization is indicated, DPT should be addressed as well.

Treatment Considerations and Selection Decision

As there is currently a lack of level I evidence regarding conservative or surgical treatment of acute and chronic ACJ instabilities, treatment considerations are based on both patient-specific factors such as age or functional and cosmetic demands, and surgeon-specific experience. In the majority of cases, conservative treatment of acute low-grade instabilities (Rockwood type I/II) is chosen, despite the risk of persisting pain and the development of chronic ACJ instability. High-grade injuries with complete rupture of all stabilizing ligamentous structures are usually treated by surgery due to the loss of stability of the shoulder girdle and the subsequent scapula-thoracic imbalance. Accompanying DPT in Rockwood type III injuries should be considered a factor in favoring surgical over conservative treatment.

TABLE 9-2 New Classification of AC Joint Instability

Type I: Partial vertical instability (CCD <30%)	A. None/partial dynamic horizontal translation B. Complete dynamic horizontal translation
Type II: Complete vertical instability (CCD >30%)	A. None/partial dynamic horizontal translation B. Complete dynamic horizontal translation

CCD, craniocaudal acromioclavicular distance.

Continued

INTERNATIONAL EXPERT COMMENTARY—cont'd

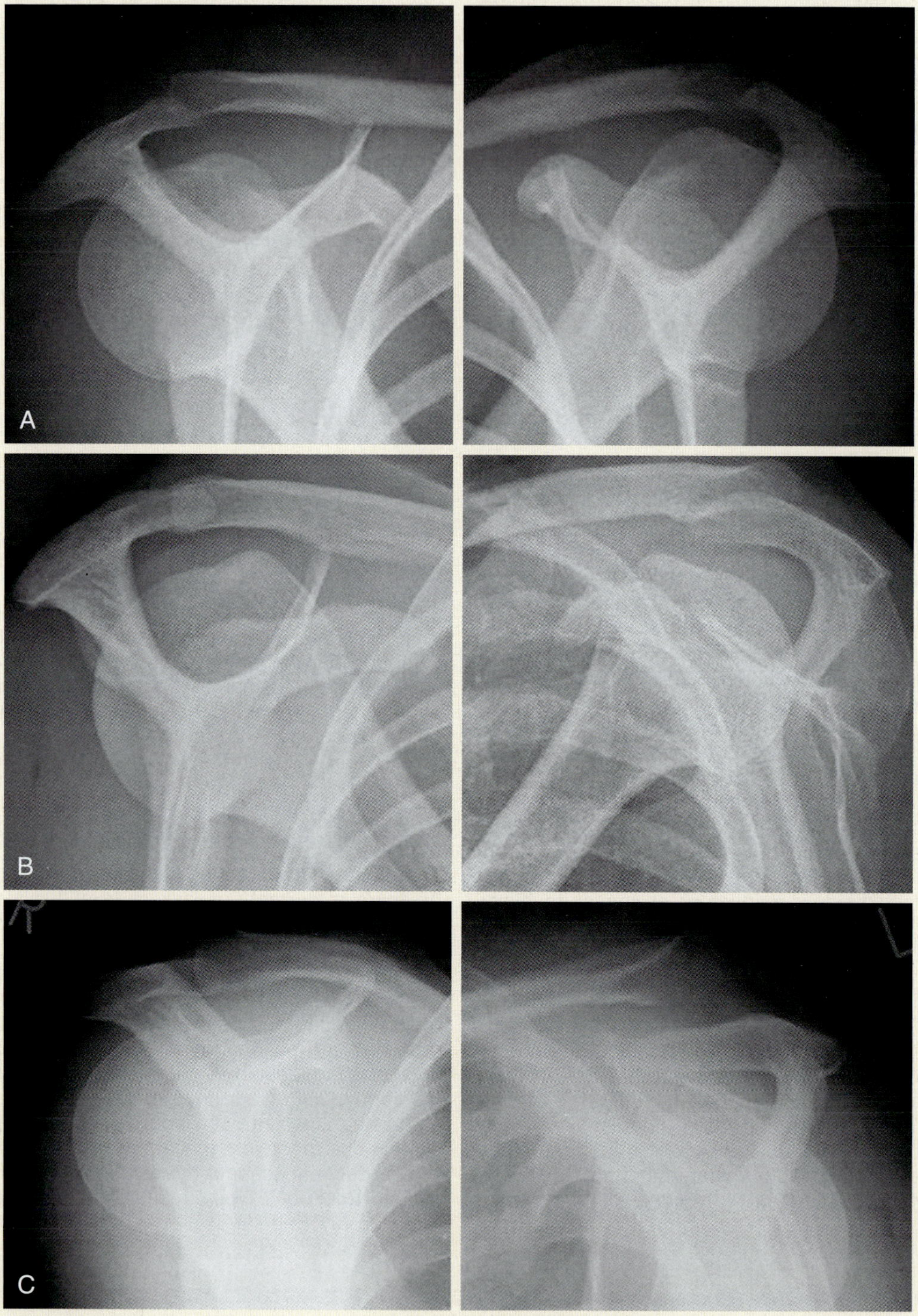

FIGURE 9-141: Evaluation of the severity of dynamic posterior translation (DPT) (left side, healthy; right side, affected side). **A,** Stable situation without DPT. **B,** Partial DPT: enlarged translation of the clavicle with a reduced overlapping of the clavicle and acromion compared with the contralateral side. **C,** Complete DPT: no overlapping of the clavicle and acromion. The clavicle is posterosuperiorly dislocated more than one shaft width.

INTERNATIONAL EXPERT COMMENTARY—cont'd

In chronic ACJ instability, surgery is indicated after failed conservative therapy of 3 to 6 months. If secondary arthritis is the main problem in cases of low-grade instability, a lateral clavicle resection may be sufficient. Biologic augmentation should be considered for chronic high-grade instabilities, accounting for the lack of intrinsic healing and scar-forming potential of the ligamentous tissue in this chronic situation. One-directional vertical high-grade instabilities can be treated in an all-arthroscopic CA ligament transfer. A modification of this technique includes an additional synthetic augmentation with a transclavicular-transcoracoidal stabilization with a TightRope implant. This approach has been shown to provide better results regarding anterior and superior translation of the clavicle.[406] Combined vertical and horizontal high-grade instabilities require a more stable reconstruction method such as a free tendon graft (e.g., gracilis or semitendinosus tendon) and an additional synthetic augmentation with a pulley-like implant to correctly restore the anatomic and biomechanical situation of the native CC ligament complex.[812] A modification of this technique includes an additional AC stabilization to sufficiently treat horizontal instability.

Surgical Technique

Acute AC Joint Instability (Arthroscopic-Assisted Combined CC and AC Stabilization)

The patient is placed in the beach chair position under general anesthesia and perioperative antibiotics (Fig. 9-142). All K-wire and drill hole placements should be carried out under fluoroscopic control in addition to the arthroscopic view to ensure adequate mediolateral placement in the clavicle. After diagnostic arthroscopy via a posterior standard portal, two additional portals (AI and lateral) and a 1.5-cm incision superior to the clavicle and approximately 3 cm medial of the ACJ are created. With the exception of tenodesis of the long head of the biceps, associated glenohumeral lesions are treated after AC stabilization. Hence, the undersurface of the coracoid and the subcoracoidal space are prepared using an electrothermic device via the AI portal. With the aid of an anterior cruciate ligament (ACL) drill guide and with its marking hook introduced beneath the coracoid base via the AI portal, the first oblique drill hole is placed transclavicular-transcoracoidal. First, a 2.0-mm K-wire is placed and overdrilled using a 4.0-mm cannulated drill bit. A nitinol suture passing wire is introduced through the drill bit and retrieved via the AI portal. The second drill hole is established in a similar fashion in line with the trapezoid ligament. Next, the drill holes for the AC cerclage are established in the clavicle and acromion. No additional incisions are needed. Hence, the TightRopes are shuttled via the first two nitinol wires and inserted into the subcoracoid space under arthroscopic control. Next, the clavicle is reduced, and the TightRopes are knotted securely. The AC cerclage is performed by inserting a FiberTape via the last two nitinol wires. The clavicular incision and the arthroscopic portals are closed in a standard fashion.

Chronic AC Joint Instability (Arthroscopic-Assisted Stabilization With Autologous Tendon Graft and Synthetic Augmentation)

After portal placement and preparation as described above, the tendon graft (gracilis/semitendinosus tendon) is harvested from the ipsilateral knee and prepared analogous to ACL surgery (Fig. 9-143). Next, the arthroscope is reintroduced into the joint, and both the transclavicular-transcoracoidal drill holes are created. The third transclavicular drill hole is placed 1 cm lateral to the second drill hole, approximately 2.5 cm from the lateral edge of the clavicle. Next, the TightRope is introduced into the CC space via the second drill hole, the clavicle is reduced under fluoroscopic control, and the sutures are tied, thereby reducing the

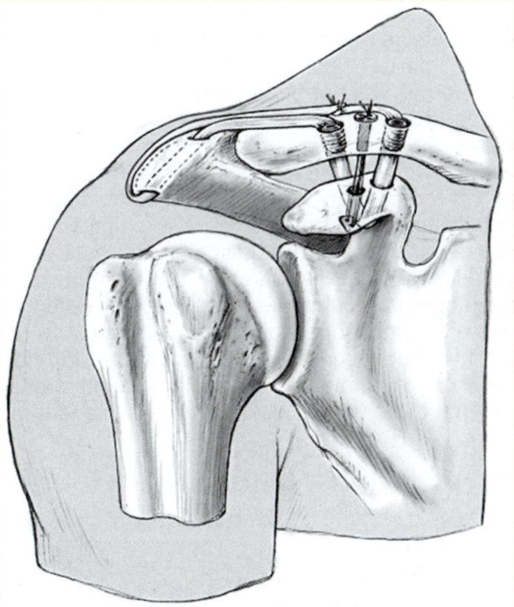

FIGURE 9-142: Arthroscopic-assisted coracoclavicular and acromioclavicular stabilization in a double TightRope technique with additional acromioclavicular cerclage. (From Gerhardt C, Kraus N, Greiner S, et al. Arthroscopic stabilization of acute acromioclavicular joint dislocation. *Orthopade*. 2011;40[1]:61-69.)

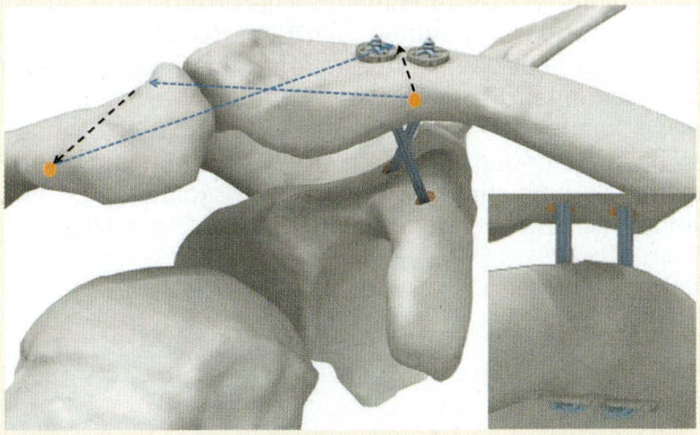

FIGURE 9-143: Arthroscopic-assisted stabilization with a free tendon graft and TightRope augmentation in a combined coracoclavicular and acromioclavicular technique. (From Kraus N, Gerhardt C, Greiner S, et al. Arthroskopische Behandlungsmoeglichkeiten chronischer Schultereckgelenkinstabilitaeten. *Arthroskopie* 2010;23[4]:293-303.)

Continued

INTERNATIONAL EXPERT COMMENTARY—cont'd

clavicle. The tendon graft is now pulled into the first drill hole via the first nitinol wire. Next, the graft is shuttled back via the third transclavicular portal lateral to the coracoid. Each graft end is attached with a PEEK tenodesis screw (Arthrex) while applying tension to both ends. Hence, the AC stabilization is carried out. Therefore a transacromial drill hole is placed via the lateral portal. The long end of the tendon graft is then pulled through the acromion and above the ACJ. With the aid of an arthroscopic knot pusher, the graft is pushed subcutaneously superior of the acromion and returned to the incision above the clavicle. Both graft ends are sutured together. A careful ACJ resection can be added in cases of symptomatic secondary ACJ arthritis. Next, the clavicular incision and the arthroscopic portals are closed in the standard fashion.

Postsurgical Rehabilitation Approach

After arthroscopic-assisted stabilization of acute ACJ instability, the shoulder is protected in a 20- to 30-degree abduction brace for 6 weeks. After free tendon graft augmentation in the chronic situation, this is prolonged for 8 weeks postoperatively. During the first 3 weeks, passive range of motion is restricted to 45 degrees of flexion and abduction. After tendon graft augmentation, the shoulder is immobilized for 2 weeks with mobilization of the hand and elbow only in order to preserve the construct until tendon integration has begun. During the following 3 weeks, passive range of motion is limited to 90-degree flexion and abduction. From the seventh to ninth weeks on, passive range of motion is unlimited, and active movement may be started. Forceful, ACJ straining movements and carrying heavy loads is discouraged for 12 weeks postoperatively. Muscle-strengthening exercises and sport-specific training are delayed up to 10 to 12 weeks.

Outcome Evaluation and Complications

In the majority of cases, good to excellent clinical results after surgical stabilization of acute ACJ stabilization are described in the literature, regardless of the chosen technique.[236,348,799,811] However, as mentioned before, likewise unrelated to the technique, recurrent instabilities are reported in up to 10% to 20% of cases. So far, the reasons remain unknown. The majority of cases remain cosmetically dissatisfying, yet asymptomatic. The arthroscopic-assisted CC stabilization in a double TightRope technique achieved good to excellent clinical results after a mid-term follow-up. Some patients displayed radiographically evident partial vertical recurrent instability without clinical relevance as has been described in various other techniques as well.[811] However, a persisting DPT could be associated with worse clinical results. Therefore we added an AC cerclage to the procedure. So far, patients with an additional AC cerclage have displayed comparable clinical results to isolated CC stabilization with a lower rate of DPT. A partial DPT was not associated with worse clinical results. So far, only a complete DPT seems to influence the clinical midterm outcome.

Surgical treatment of chronic ACJ instability remains a challenge, not least because of the reduced healing potential. CC stabilization with free tendon grafts displayed good clinical results with pain reduction and a radiographically stable situation in the revision setting.[898] However, isolated biologic augmentation may lead to high rates of failure, osteolysis of the lateral clavicle, and drill hole enlargement.[899] Biomechanically, an additional transacromial stabilization provided more horizontal stability compared with an isolated CC stabilization, and was comparable to the native situation.[338] Patients in our own institution achieved on average 86 points in the CS, 91% in the SSV, 10.8 points in the Taft score, and 87 points in the ACJI. Thirteen patients had undergone previous surgery. One patient displayed a visible asymmetry between their clavicles. Radiographically, there was no difference between the CC distance on both sides. However, three patients had a recurrent vertical instability and required revision tendon augmentation. One patient displayed a complete DPT.

Various complications such as implant migration and irritation, CC ossification, drill hole enlargement, recurrent vertical and/or horizontal dislocation, and even coracoid and clavicle fractures have been associated with arthroscopic and open techniques in both acute and chronic situations. Implant migration occurred when using the first generation implant of the TightRope, but was not associated with a major loss of reduction.[811] Since a modification of the device with larger buttons exists, implant migration has become rare. On the other hand, implant irritation because of the suture material above the clavicle may still be a cause of symptoms, and may necessitate partial implant removal. Redislocation after implant removal has not been seen in our cases. Ossification in the area of the former CC ligaments occurs in up to 75% of patients 2 years after surgery.[811] So far, ossification has not lead to worse clinical results or a restricted range of motion. On the contrary, patients with combined CC ossification in both ligaments tended to have a significantly shorter CC distance and less DPT. Clavicular drill hole enlargement has been described in the literature.[482] The influence on clinical or radiographic outcomes has not been noted. Coracoid fractures after TightRope stabilization are rare, but have been reported to occur. In order to avoid eccentric drill hole placement and wrong implant position that might predispose to coracoid fracture, fluoroscopic control is mandatory in this procedure.

EDITOR COMMENTARY

Samuel Antuña

Although the ACJ has since long ago been considered a source of potential shoulder pain, a huge interest on this small joint has risen within the last 10 years. It is really fascinating how novel knowledge on biomechanics and detailed morphology variations has led surgeons into a renewed focus on reproducing the mechanics and anatomy of this joint more precisely. Dr. Collins has written a fantastic review of what we know about the ACJ contemporarily, which is very useful indeed for understanding the pathology and possible treatment options.

It could be considered fair to acknowledge that DCR has been occasionally overused in the past. Often times, resection was performed routinely as part of associated procedures in the subacromial space, even as a prophylactic measures. Today, we should probably only consider joint resection indicated when there is clearly symptomatic ACJ OA that has not been resolved by conservative measures or when there is posttraumatic pathology in the joint with or without joint dislocation. Whether to perform this simple operation open or arthroscopically depends on many factors but mainly on the surgeon's experience and the necessity of addressing associated problems, such as cuff tears or ACJ instability. The most common complications we see after this operation are excessive resection or postoperative instability; both of these complications can be prevented with adequate technique. If well indicated and executed, DCR is a reliable surgical procedure with good predictable results.

Contrary to what has happened with ACJ resection, ACJ stabilization procedures have recently become extremely popular. In fact, their popularity has influenced the decision-making process of many surgeons in an attempt to preserve joint mechanics and anatomy as close to normal as possible after ACJ dislocations. Fortunately, the majority of patients with grade I or II ACJ injuries do very well with observation and early pain relief measures. However, one needs to be aware that a small percentage of these patients may present late with pain over the ACJ. These posttraumatic painful joints may have occult menisci injuries or subtle AP instability, and may require a surgical intervention either to debride or stabilize the joint.

The hot topic is still the best treatment for complete ACJ dislocations. We now recognize the importance of assessing posterior translation of the distal clavicle, as this has been related with a poorer outcome. When facing a complete dislocation of the ACJ, three factors should be considered before the final decision on treatment is made, namely the patient's expectations and requirements, the surgeon's experience, and specific variations in pathology, more importantly the degree of posterior instability associated with superior displacement. The younger and more active the patient is, the more experience the surgeon has in less invasive techniques, and the higher the degree of posterior translation present, more likelihood of pursuing a surgical treatment. However, an honest approach should include a thorough explanation to the patient of the potential benefits of nonsurgical treatment and the fact that the available literature still does not favor operative over conservative treatment.

Stabilizing the ACJ is a fun operation. CC fixation with a screw was a brilliant idea that has evolved over time to more reliable methods of fixation with anchors or cortical fixation and sutures. All of these acute CC fixation methods are successful in the majority of cases and can be performed arthroscopically, with the advantage of preserving the deltoid attachment. If significant posterior translation of the distal clavicle is detected, the surgeon should consider additional AC fixation with transosseous sutures. The hook plate is also a very valuable option with the only disadvantage of requiring later plate removal. Symptomatic chronic instability of the ACJ may be a more challenging problem. Many techniques have proved their efficacy, but if one common thought we could extract from the literature and experience is that adding a biologic CC fixation with tendon allograft or even autograft seems a reasonable thing to do in order to achieve long-term stabilization.

In conclusion, after reading this chapter, I am sure readers have profoundly increased their knowledge on ACJ problems and have probably become more aware of the potential complications related to both conservative and operative treatment. However, knowing more and better technical skills does not mean operating more: we, as surgeons, must offer our patients their best option, and quite often, this is the simplest option.

CHAPTER 10

Disorders of the Sternoclavicular Joint

Aaron J. Bois, Michael A. Wirth, Charles A. Rockwood Jr

The first detailed case report of a sternoclavicular (SC) joint injury appeared as early as 1843,[158] and numerous related articles were published in the late nineteenth century. However, it was not until the 1920s and 1930s that such articles appeared in the U.S. literature.[40,49,116]

Injuries to the SC joint are an uncommon problem, and many authors apologize for reporting only three or four cases. The rarity of these injuries and the lack of standardized methods for treating them, measuring outcomes, and reporting complications increase methodologic flaws in structured literature reviews and often preclude a meaningful meta-analysis. From a literature review and in our combined 50 years of clinical experience, anterior dislocations are best treated nonoperatively, and posterior dislocations, which have accounted for deaths, need to be promptly diagnosed and reduced. Anterior and posterior injuries in adults up to the age of 23 years are usually physeal injuries and heal without specific surgical treatment; however, true posterior dislocations do occur in the skeletally immature population and require similar treatment to their adult counterparts. Special radiographs are usually required to make the diagnosis. In our experience, high-definition computed tomography (CT) images with three-dimensional (3D) reconstructions are the gold standard for evaluating these injuries.

SURGICAL ANATOMY

Because less than half of the medial clavicle articulates with the upper angle of the sternum, the SC joint has the distinction of having the least amount of bony stability of the major joints of the body.

The SC joint is a diarthrodial joint and is the only true articulation between the upper extremity and axial skeleton. The articular surface of the clavicle is much larger than that of the sternum, and both are covered with hyaline cartilage. Articular cartilage covers approximately 67% of the medial end of the clavicle, with coverage only on the anteroinferior aspect of the clavicle and on the underside of the clavicle at its articulation with the manubrial cartilage and first-rib costal cartilage (Fig. 10-1).[110] In 2.5% of patients, there is a small facet on the inferior aspect of the medial clavicle, which articulates with the superior aspect of the first rib at its synchondral junction with the sternum.[30] The enlarged bulbous medial end of the clavicle is concave front to back and convex vertically and thus creates a saddle-type joint with the clavicular notch of the sternum. The clavicular notch of the sternum is curved, and the joint surfaces are not congruent.

Ligaments of the Sternoclavicular Joint

The SC joint has so much incongruity that integrity of the joint must come from its surrounding ligaments; that is, the intra-articular disk ligament, extra-articular costoclavicular ligament (rhomboid ligament), the capsular ligaments, and interclavicular (IC) ligament.

Intra-Articular Disk Ligament

The intra-articular disk ligament is a very dense, fibrous structure that arises from the synchondral junction of the first rib with the sternum and passes through the SC joint. This ligament divides the joint in the sagittal-oblique plane to create two separate joint spaces (medial or sternal and lateral). Anatomic studies have shown that the disk has a robust insertion on the posterosuperior aspect of the clavicle (see Fig. 10-1).[110] Anteriorly and posteriorly, the disk blends into the fibers of the capsular ligaments; inferiorly, the disk has a less robust attachment (Fig. 10-2).[110] The diameter and thickness of the articular disk, on average, are 18 mm and 5.4 mm, respectfully.[110] DePalma[47] has shown that the disk is perforated only rarely; the perforation allows free communication between the two joint compartments (see Fig. 10-2).

The intra-articular disk acts as a checkrein against medial displacement of the medial clavicle. Histologic studies have demonstrated that the sternal side of the disk is composed of fibrocartilage and dense connective tissue, whereas the clavicular side of the disk is composed of only fibrocartilage. Therefore it is likely the clavicular side of the articular disk that has the function of resisting the compressive load to the clavicular surface.[55]

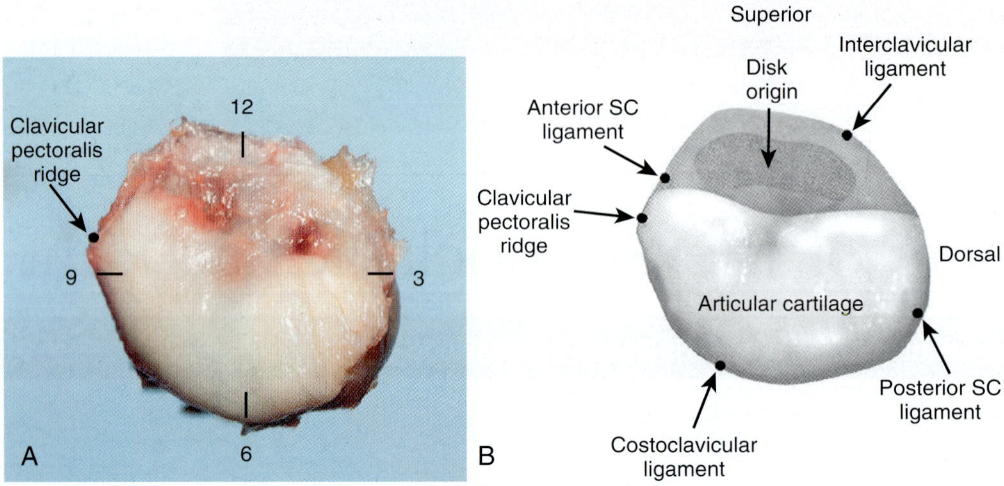

FIGURE 10-1: Anatomy of the medial end of the clavicle (right) with clock face positions indicated (lateral view). **A,** The most anatomically superior point is 12 o'clock, and 9 o'clock faces anteriorly. **B,** Anatomic illustration of the medial end of the clavicle showing the extent of the articular surface and the attachment locations of the sternoclavicular (SC), interclavicular, and costoclavicular ligaments. Note the limited articular cartilage coverage and the large attachment area of the intra-articular disk. (From Lee JT, Campbell KJ, Michalski MP, et al. Surgical anatomy of the sternoclavicular joint: a qualitative and quantitative anatomical study. *J Bone Joint Surg Am.* 2014;96[19]:e166.)

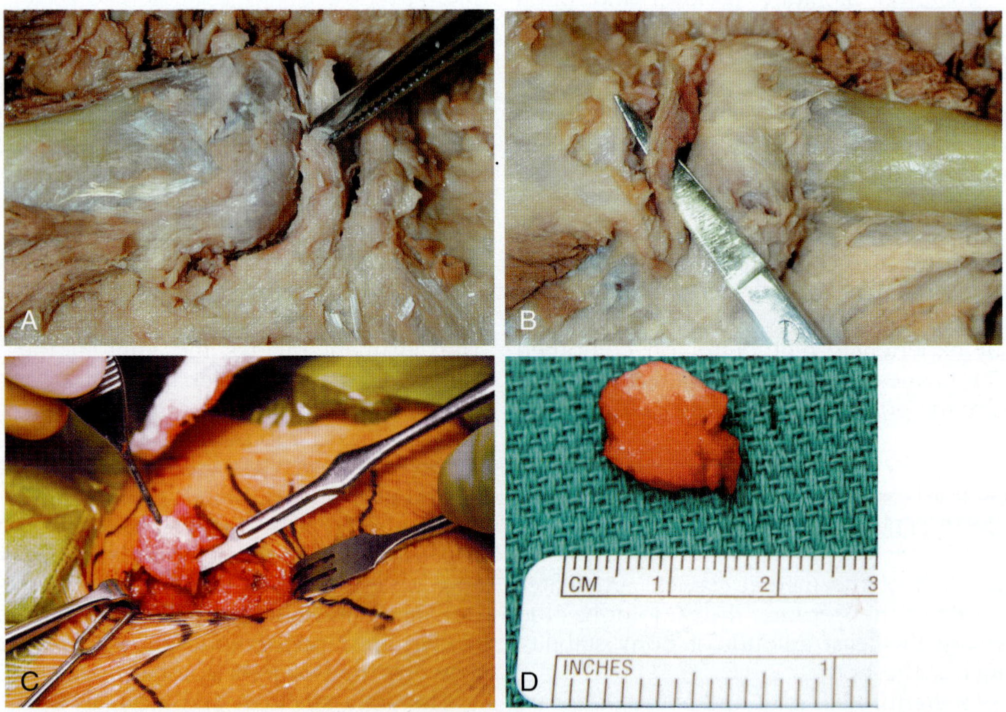

FIGURE 10-2: **A,** Normal-appearing articular disk ligament of the right sternoclavicular joint (held by forceps). **B,** Degenerative articular disk ligament with a central perforation (left sternoclavicular joint). **C,** Intraoperative photograph demonstrating excision of a symptomatic articular disk ligament (held by forceps). **D,** Surgical specimen of excised articular disk ligament.

Costoclavicular Ligament

The costoclavicular ligament, also called the *rhomboid ligament*, is comprised of an anterior and a posterior fasciculus is the largest ligament of the SC joint. The fibers of the anterior fasciculus arise from the anteromedial surface of the first rib and are directed upward and laterally. The fibers of the posterior fasciculus are shorter and arise lateral to the anterior fibers on the rib and are directed upward and medially. The costoclavicular ligament attaches superiorly to the margins of an impression on the inferior surface of the medial end of the clavicle, sometimes referred to as the *rhomboid fossa*.[76,156] Cave showed, in a study of 153 clavicles, that the attachment point of the costoclavicular ligament to the inferior clavicle can be one of three types: (1) a depression, the rhomboid fossa (30%); (2) a flat surface (60%); or (3) an elevation or prominence (10%).[29] More recently, Lee et al.[110] observed that the costoclavicular ligament consistently attached to a palpable tubercle in all of the 11 cadaveric specimens studied, known as the *costoclavicular tubercle*, which likely corresponds to the "elevation" described by Cave in 1961. The anatomy of the costoclavicular ligament is in many ways similar to the structural configuration of the coracoclavicular ligament on the outer end of the clavicle (Fig. 10-3).

The dimensions of the costoclavicular ligament have also been described. Cave reported that the average length is 1.3 cm, maximum width is 1.9 cm, and average thickness is 1.3 cm.[29] Lee et al.[110] found that on the clavicle, the center of the costoclavicular ligament is on an average 13.8 mm lateral to the inferior SC articular margin, while the most medial fibers are 10.3 mm lateral to the same point of reference. On the first rib cartilage, the center of the insertion was 14.8 mm lateral to the inferior manubrial articular cartilage margin, and the most medial fibers of the ligament were 8.3 mm.

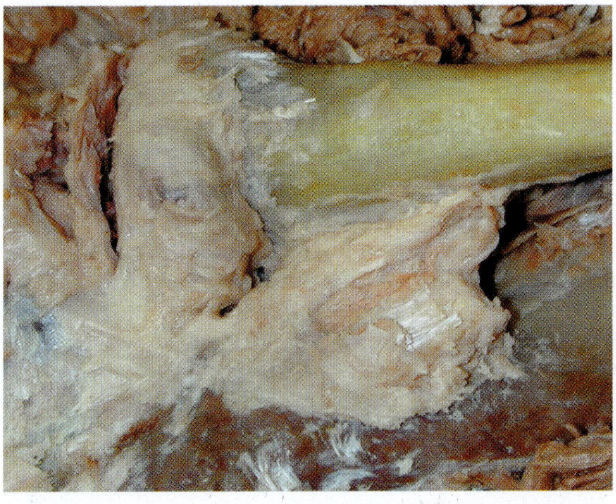

FIGURE 10-3: Left medial clavicle demonstrating the rhomboid appearance of the costoclavicular ligament and the anterior sternoclavicular capsular ligament.

The fibers of the anterior and posterior components cross and allow stability of the joint during rotation and elevation of the clavicle. Bearn[12] has shown experimentally that the anterior fibers resist excessive upward rotation of the clavicle and that the posterior fibers resist excessive downward rotation. In addition, the anterior fibers resist lateral displacement and the posterior fibers resist medial displacement (Fig. 10-4).

Interclavicular Ligament

The IC ligament connects the superomedial aspect of each clavicle with the capsular ligaments and the upper part of the sternum (Fig. 10-5). Lee et al.[110] found that the IC ligament was the "most readily identified of the SC-associated joint ligaments as a discrete ligament between the two clavicle heads." The IC ligament attachment is located at the 1:30 o'clock position on the medial clavicle (i.e., right clavicle) (see Fig. 10-1).

The IC ligament assists the capsular ligaments in producing *shoulder poise*, that is, holding the shoulders up. The function of this ligament can be tested by putting a finger in the superior sternal notch; with elevation of the arm, the ligament is quite lax, but as soon as both arms hang at the sides, the ligament becomes tight. Spencer et al.[185] have shown experimentally that the costoclavicular and IC ligaments have little effect on anterior or posterior translation of the SC joint. In an anatomic study, Tubbs et al. found that the IC ligament prevented superior displacement of the clavicle with shoulder adduction and depression.[199]

Capsular Ligament

The capsular ligament covers the anterosuperior and posterior aspects of the joint and represents thickenings of the joint capsule (see Figs. 10-3 and 10-5). This structure is the strongest of all the SC ligaments and is the first line of defense against the upward displacement of the medial clavicle caused by a downward force on the superior aspect of the shoulder. We have observed that the clavicular attachment of the ligament is primarily on the epiphysis of the medial clavicle, with some secondary blending of the fibers into the metaphysis. In a more recent anatomic study, Lee et al.[110] found that the anterior SC ligament is an oblique capsular thickening running from inferomedial to superolateral, attaching at the 10 o'clock position on the medial clavicle (i.e., right clavicle). In contrast, the posterior SC ligament appears as a diffuse thickening of the posterior joint capsule with no discrete ligament and a broad footprint on the manubrium and clavicle and attaches at the 4:30 o'clock position on the medial end of the right clavicle (see Fig. 10-1).

Although some authors report that the intra-articular disk ligament greatly assists the costoclavicular ligament in preventing upward displacement of the medial clavicle, Bearn[12] has shown that the capsular ligament is the most important structure in preventing upward displacement of the medial clavicle (see Fig. 10-4). In an experimental postmortem study, he determined that after cutting the costoclavicular, intra-articular disk, and IC ligaments, they had no effect on clavicle poise. However,

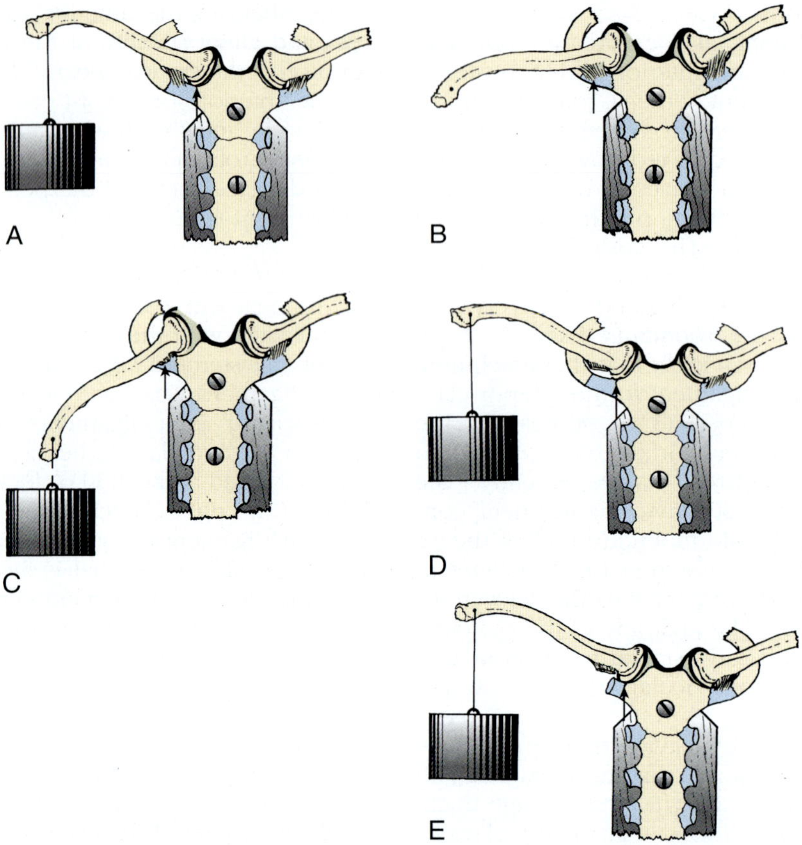

FIGURE 10-4: The importance of the various ligaments around the sternoclavicular joint in maintaining normal shoulder poise. **A,** The lateral end of the clavicle is maintained in an elevated position through the sternoclavicular ligaments. The *arrow* indicates the fulcrum. **B,** When the capsule is divided completely, the lateral end of the clavicle descends under its own weight without any loading. The clavicle seems to be supported by the intra-articular disk ligament. **C,** After division of the capsular ligament, it was determined that a weight less than 5 lb was enough to tear the intra-articular disk ligament from its attachment on the costal cartilage junction of the first rib. The fulcrum was transferred laterally so that the medial end of the clavicle hinged over the first rib in the vicinity of the costoclavicular ligament. **D,** After division of the costoclavicular ligament and the intra-articular disk ligament, the lateral end of the clavicle could not be depressed as long as the capsular ligament was intact. **E,** After resection of the medial first costal cartilage along with the costoclavicular ligament, there was no effect on the poise of the lateral end of the clavicle, as long as the capsular ligament was intact. (From Bearn JG. Direct observation on the function of the capsule of the sternoclavicular joint in clavicular support. *J Anat.* 1967;101:159-170.)

the division of the capsular ligament alone resulted in a downward depression of the distal end of the clavicle. Bearn's findings have many clinical implications for the mechanisms of injury of the SC joint.

Spencer et al.[185] performed a cadaveric study measuring the anterior and posterior translation of the SC joint in both intact specimens and following transection of randomly chosen ligaments about the SC joint. Cutting the posterior capsule resulted in a significant increase in both the anterior and posterior translation. Cutting the anterior capsule produced a significant increase in anterior translation. This study demonstrated that the posterior SC joint capsule is the most important structure for preventing both the anterior and posterior translation of the SC joint, with the anterior capsule acting as an important secondary stabilizer.

Subclavius Muscle

Reis et al.[150] studied the function of the subclavius muscle and found that the basic function of this muscle was to stabilize the SC joint. They also reported that the subclavius could act as a substitute for the ligaments of the SC joint. We believe that this is an important study as it might explain why some people, after loss of the medial clavicle and the supporting SC ligaments, do not have instability of the medial end of the clavicle and provides further support to leave the subclavius muscle intact during operations on the SC joint (Fig. 10-6).

Applied Surgical Anatomy

Surgeons planning an operative procedure on or near the SC joint should be knowledgeable regarding the vast

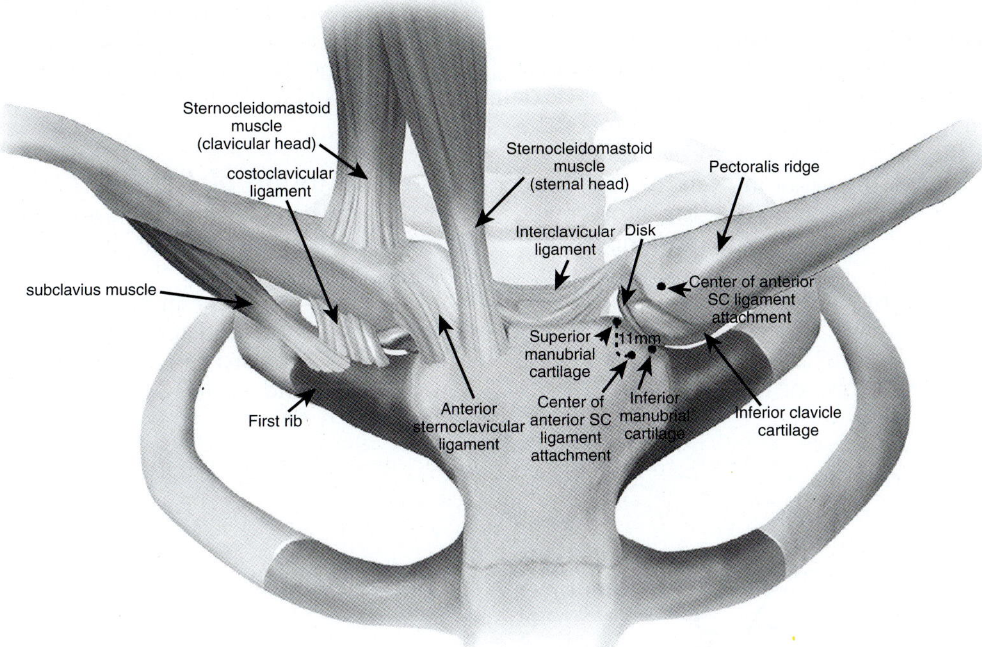

FIGURE 10-5: Anatomic illustration of both sternoclavicular joints (anterior view). Muscle attachments are excluded from the left sternoclavicular (SC) joint to illustrate the intra-articular structures. Cartilage is depicted as darker than the surrounding osseous structures. (From Lee JT, Campbell KJ, Michalski MP, et al. Surgical anatomy of the sternoclavicular joint: a qualitative and quantitative anatomical study. *J Bone Joint Surg Am.* 2014;96[19]:e166.)

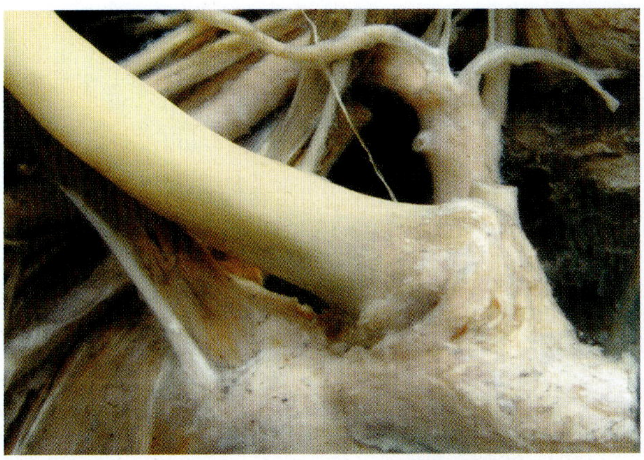

FIGURE 10-6: Normal anatomy around the sternoclavicular joint. Note that the tendon of the subclavius muscle arises in the vicinity of the costoclavicular ligament (from the first rib) and has a long tendon structure.

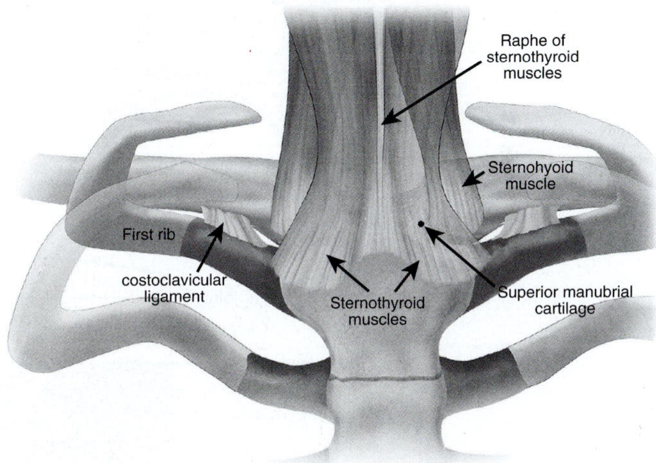

FIGURE 10-7: Anatomic illustration of the sternoclavicular joints (posterior view), showing the topography of the muscles in relation to the joint. Cartilage is depicted as darker than the surrounding osseous structures. (From Lee JT, Campbell KJ, Michalski MP, et al. Surgical anatomy of the sternoclavicular joint: a qualitative and quantitative anatomical study. *J Bone Joint Surg Am.* 2014;96[19]:e166.)

array of anatomic structures immediately posterior to the SC joint. A curtain of muscles—the sternohyoid and sternothyroid—are located posterior to the SC joint and the medial third of the clavicle and block the view of vital structures. The sternohyoid muscle is a thin strap muscle that inserts onto the posterior aspect of the SC joint capsule and medial clavicle. The sternothyroid is located more posterior than the sternohyoid muscle and has a more inferior insertion on the posterior aspect of the sternum and costal cartilage. In addition, there is a fascial attachment between the right and left muscle bellies of both strap muscles with a midline raphe that inserts onto the posterior aspect of the manubrium (Fig. 10-7).[110]

Some of the vital mediastinal structures posterior to the SC joint include the innominate artery (also known as the brachiocephalic trunk), brachiocephalic vein, vagus nerve, phrenic nerve, internal jugular vein, trachea, and esophagus (Fig. 10-8). Ponce et al.[143] used contrast CT in 49 patients without identified injury to the neck or chest to define the proximity of these structures. The mean distance to the nearest anatomic structure deep to the clavicular region of the SC joint was 6.6 mm and was 12.5 mm for the sternal region. The brachiocephalic vein was the closest vital structure to the posterior aspect of both the right (average distance 6.0 ± 2.4 mm) and left (7.0 ± 2.5 mm) SC joint. As a percentage of all the nearest mediastinal structures, 26.0% were within 5 mm, 73.2% were within 10 mm, 87.2% were within 15 mm, and 92.9% were within 20 mm of the posterior SC joint. When operating in the region of the SC joint, it is critical to realize that an avascular plane (i.e., "safe zone") exists anterior to the fascial layer and muscle bellies of the strap muscles (Fig. 10-9).[81,110,143]

Range of Motion of the Sternoclavicular Joint

The SC joint is freely movable and functions almost like a ball-and-socket joint in that the joint has motion in all planes, including rotation. The clavicle, and thus the SC joint in normal shoulder motion, is capable of 30 to 35 degrees of upward elevation, 35 degrees of combined forward and backward movement, and 45 to 50 degrees of rotation around its long axis (Fig. 10-10). It is most

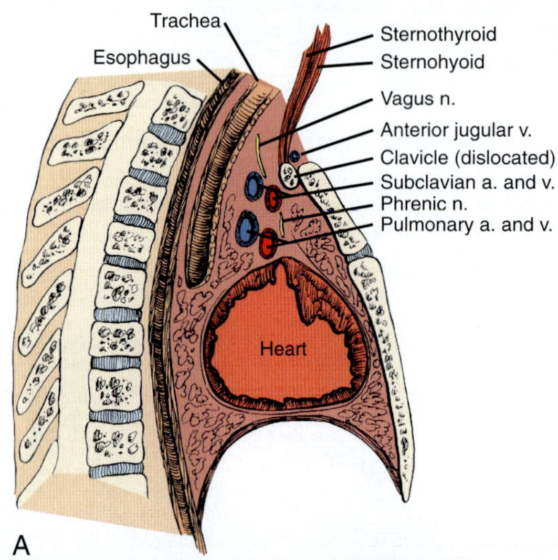

A

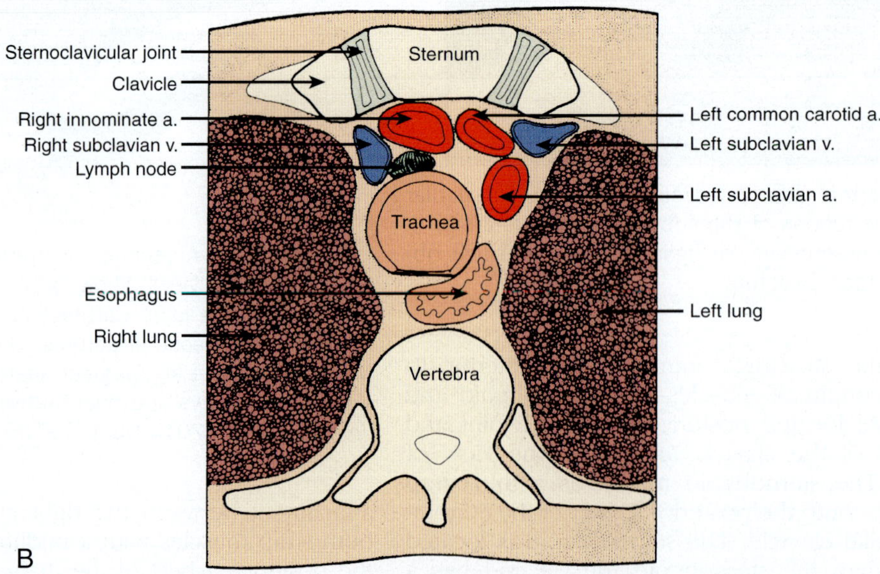

B

FIGURE 10-8: Applied anatomy of the vital structures posterior to the sternoclavicular joint. **A** and **B,** Sagittal view and cross section demonstrating the structures posterior to the sternoclavicular joint.

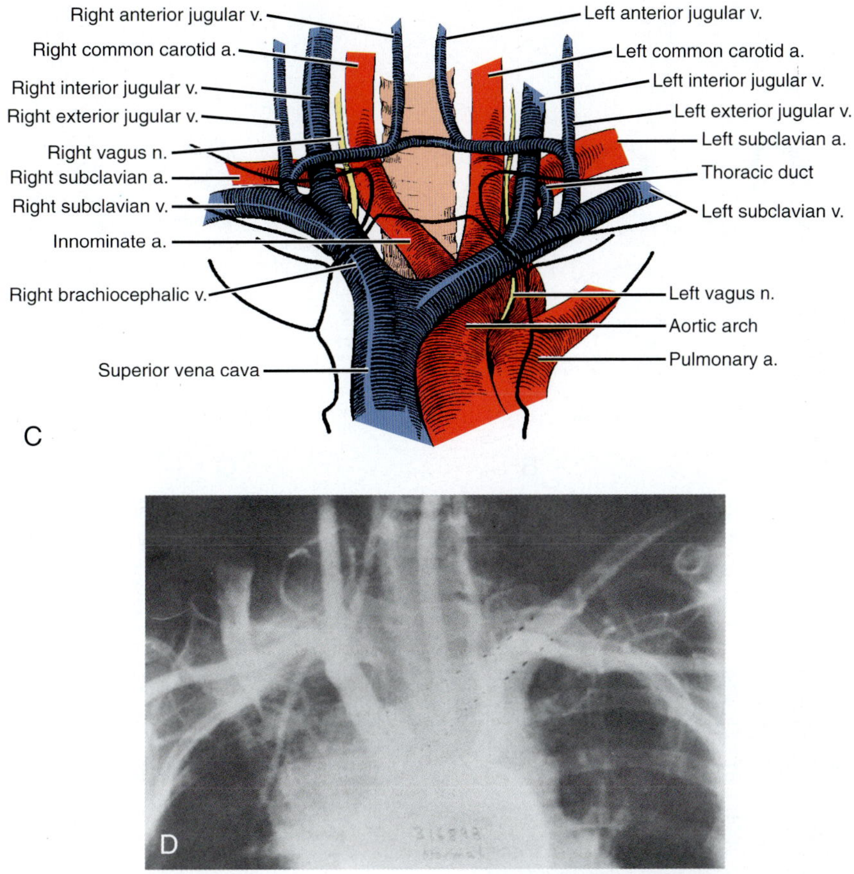

FIGURE 10-8, cont'd C, A diagram demonstrating the close proximity of the major vessels that are posterior to the sternoclavicular joint. **D,** Aortogram showing the relationship of the medial end of the clavicle to the major vessels in the mediastinum. (From Bucholz RW, Heckman JD, eds. *Rockwood and Green's Fractures in Adults.* 5th ed. Philadelphia: Lippincott Williams & Wilkins; 2001: 1260.)

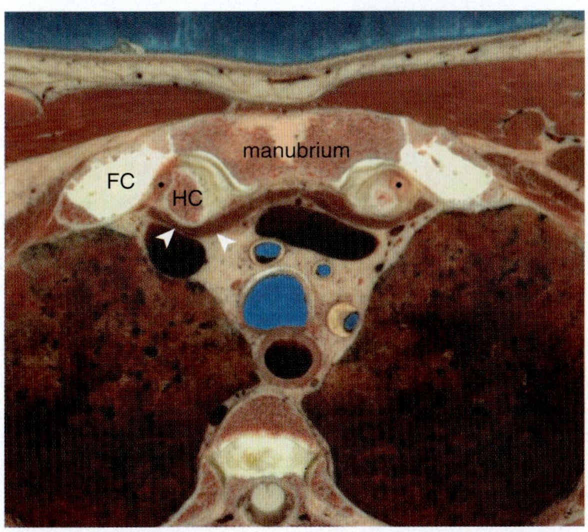

FIGURE 10-9: Axial cryosection image showing a part of the SC joint space (black dots) lateral to the right and left heads of the clavicle (HC). The sternothyroid and sternohyoid muscles (white arrowheads) form a curtain anterior to the vital mediastinal structures. Performing surgery anterior to the strap muscles creates a "safe zone" (i.e., avascular plane). FC, First costal cartilage. (From Han DH, Nam YS, Ahn MI, et al. Underrecognized soft-tissue structures inferior and lateral to the head of the clavicle: anatomy with computed tomography correlation. *Clin Anat.* 2010;23[7]:803-810.)

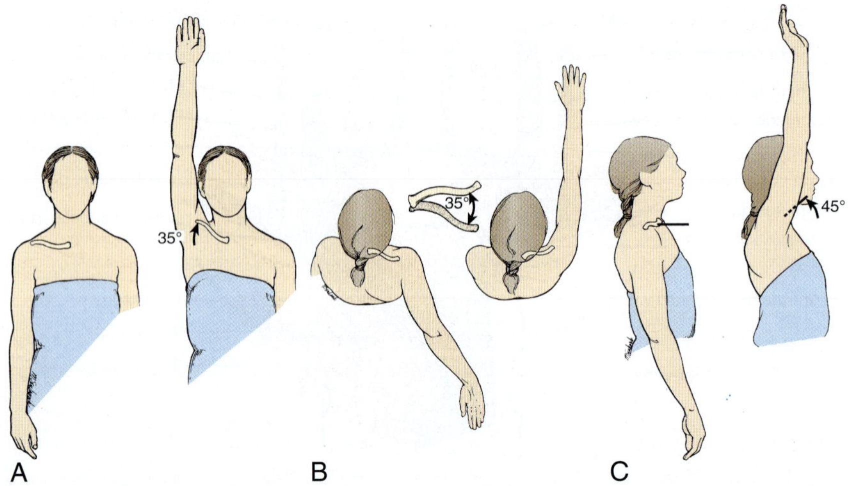

FIGURE 10-10: Motions of the clavicle and the sternoclavicular joint. **A,** With full overhead elevation, the clavicle elevates 35 degrees. **B,** With adduction and extension, the clavicle displaces anteriorly and posteriorly 35 degrees. **C,** The clavicle rotates on its long axis 45 degrees as the arm is elevated to the full overhead position.

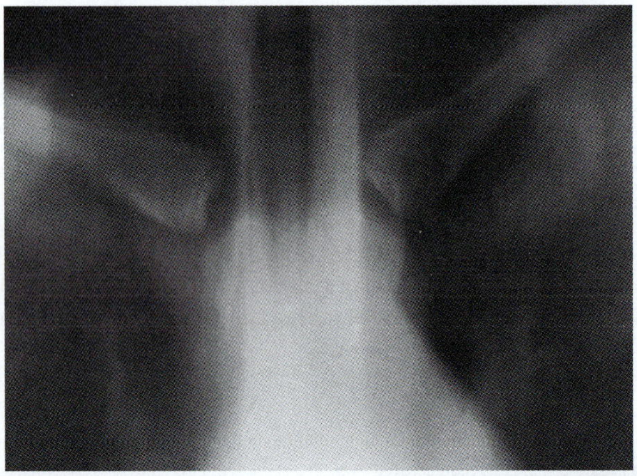

FIGURE 10-11: Tomogram demonstrating the thin, wafer-like disk of the epiphysis of the medial part of the right clavicle. (From Rockwood CA, Green DP, eds. *Fractures.* 2nd ed. Philadelphia: JB Lippincott; 1984.)

likely to be the most frequently moved joint of the long bones in the body because almost any motion of the upper extremity is transferred proximally to the SC joint.

Epiphysis of the Medial Clavicle

Although the clavicle is the first long bone of the body to ossify (intrauterine week 5), the epiphysis at the medial end of the clavicle is the last of the long bones in the body to appear and the last epiphysis to close (Fig. 10-11). The medial clavicular epiphysis does not ossify until the 18th to 20th year, and it fuses with the shaft of the clavicle around the 23rd to 25th year. In an extensive cadaveric study of the medial clavicular physis in 605 males and 254 females, Webb and Suchey[213] reported that complete union might not occur until 31 years of age. This knowledge of the epiphysis is important because we believe that many of the so-called SC dislocations in the younger population are fractures through the physeal plate.

CLASSIFICATION OF STERNOCLAVICULAR JOINT DISORDERS

Classification Based on Etiology

Detailed classifications are confusing and difficult to remember, and the following simple classification and differential diagnosis of SC joint problems is suggested (traumatic versus atraumatic) (Fig. 10-12). This section of the chapter focuses on traumatic injuries to the SC joint.

Traumatic Injury

Traumatic injuries can be further subclassified in terms of severity (sprain, subluxation, dislocation), direction (anterior or posterior), onset (acute or chronic), and age of the patient (skeletally immature or mature). An anterior dislocation is the most common type of SC joint dislocation; the medial end of the clavicle is displaced anteriorly or anterosuperiorly to the anterior margin of the sternum (Fig. 10-13). Posterior SC joint dislocation is uncommon; the medial end of the clavicle is displaced posterior, posteroinferior, or posterosuperior with respect to the sternum.

Because the SC joint is so small and incongruous, one would believe that it would be the most commonly dislocated joint in the body. However, the ligamentous supporting structure is extremely strong and has evolved in such a manner that it is one of the least commonly dislocated joints in the body. Traumatic dislocation of the

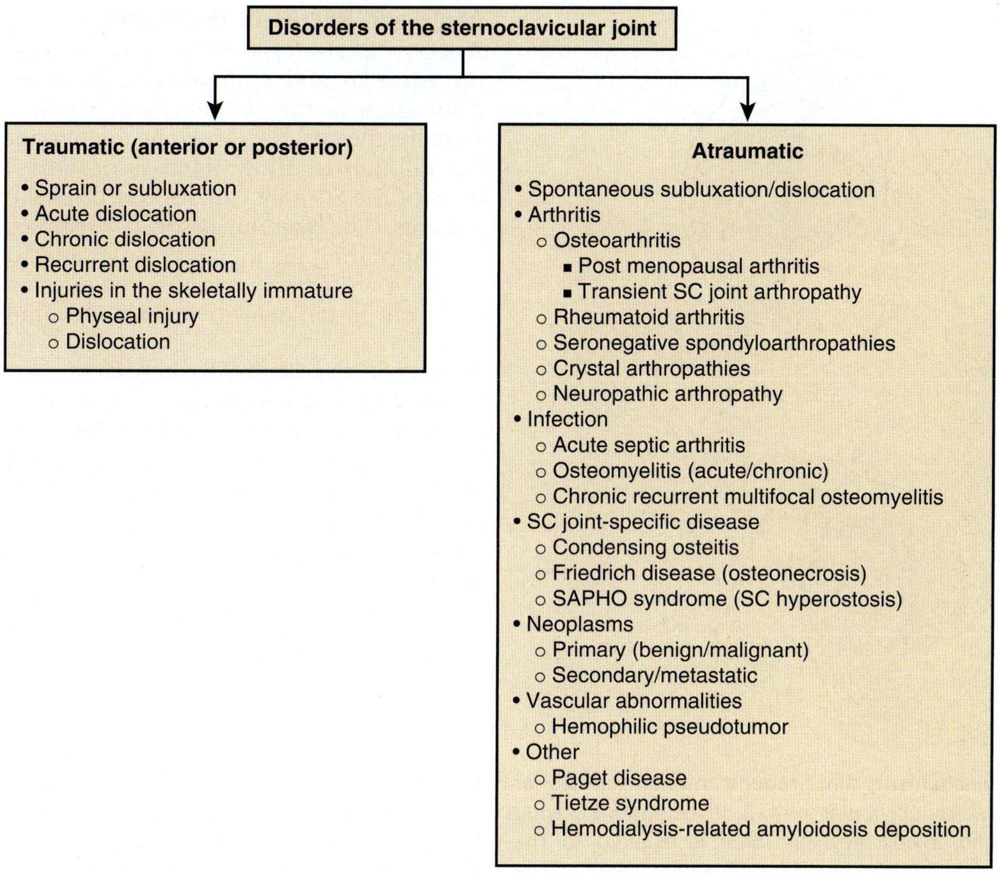

FIGURE 10-12: Classification and differential diagnosis of sternoclavicular joint disorders. *SC,* sternoclavicular; *SAPHO,* synovitis acne pustulosis hyperostosis osteitis.

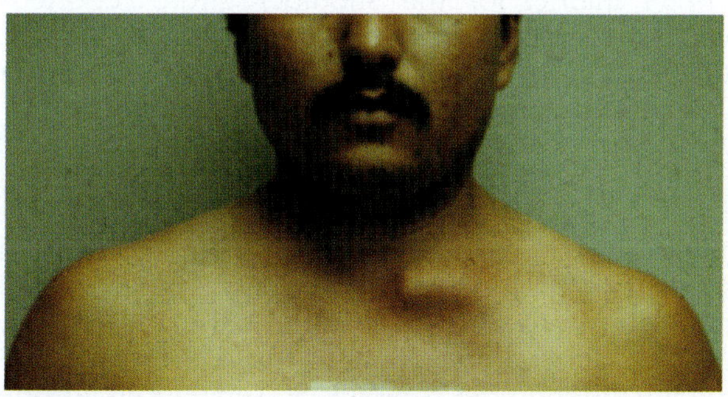

FIGURE 10-13: Clinical view demonstrating anterior dislocation of the left sternoclavicular joint.

SC joint usually occurs only after tremendous force, either direct or indirect, has been applied to the shoulder.

Mechanism of Injury

The most common mechanism of injury to the SC joint is an indirect force applied to the anterolateral or posterolateral aspect of the shoulder. Mehta et al.[123] reported that three of four posterior SC dislocations were produced by indirect force, and Heinig[85] reported that indirect force was responsible for eight of nine cases of posterior SC dislocations. Indirect force was the most common mechanism of injury in our series of 185 patients as well. If the shoulder is compressed and rolled forward, an ipsilateral posterior dislocation results; if the shoulder is compressed and rolled backward, an ipsilateral anterior dislocation results (Fig. 10-14). Posterior SC joint injuries can also occur when a significant force is applied directly to the SC joint or the anteromedial aspect of the clavicle from blunt trauma (Box 10-1).

Most Common Cause of Injury to the Sternoclavicular Joint

The most common cause of dislocation of the SC joint in adults is vehicular accidents; the second is an injury sustained during participation in sports.[129,134,210] Omer,[134] in his review of patients from 14 military hospitals, found 82 cases of SC joint dislocations. He reported that almost 80% of these occurred because of vehicular accidents (47%) and athletics (31%). In contrast, Tepolt et al.[193] performed a recent meta-analysis of posterior SC joint injuries in the adolescent population (comprising both true dislocations and physeal injuries; mean age, 15.2 ± 1.8 years) and found that 71% of injuries occurred during participation in sports (football, rugby, and wrestling).

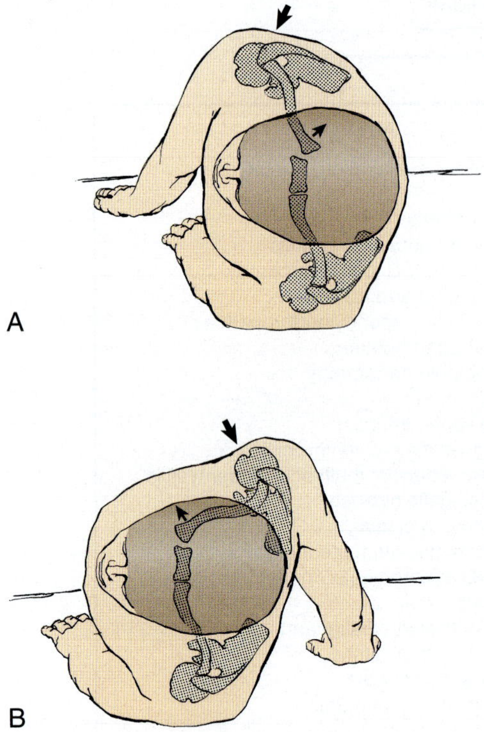

FIGURE 10-14: Mechanisms that produce anterior or posterior dislocation of the sternoclavicular joint. **A,** If the patient is lying on the ground and a compression force is applied to the posterolateral aspect of the shoulder, the medial end of the clavicle will be displaced posteriorly. **B,** When the lateral compression force is directed from the anterior position, the medial end of the clavicle is dislocated posteriorly. (From Bucholz RW, Heckman JD, eds. *Rockwood and Green's Fractures in Adults.* 5th ed. Philadelphia: Lippincott Williams & Wilkins; 2001: 1247.)

BOX 10-1. Direct Injury Mechanisms to the Sternoclavicular Joint

- An athlete lying supine on the ground is jumped on, and the knee of the jumper lands directly on the medial end of the clavicle.
- A kick is delivered to the front of the medial clavicle.
- A person is run over by a vehicle.
- A person is pinned between a vehicle and a wall.

Traumatic Injury Subtypes

Sprain or Subluxation

Acute sprains of the SC joint can be classified as mild, moderate, or severe. In a *mild* sprain (type I), all the ligaments are intact, and the joint is stable. In a *moderate* sprain (type II), the capsular, intra-articular disk, and costoclavicular ligaments may be partially disrupted, resulting in a subluxation of the SC joint (anterior or posterior).

Acute and Recurrent Dislocation

A *severe* sprain (type III) involves complete disruption of the capsular and intra-articular ligaments, resulting in a dislocation of the SC joint (anterior or posterior). Occasionally, the costoclavicular ligament is intact but stretched out enough to allow joint dislocation. Isolated dislocations of the SC joint can also occur in skeletally immature patients (i.e., without associated physeal injury).[111,212] If the supporting ligamentous structures fail to heal following joint reduction, mild-to-moderate force may produce recurrent instability; however, this is rare.

Injuries in the Skeletally Immature

Acute Physeal Fracture. Traditional teaching describes SC injuries in childhood and adolescence as physeal fractures with either anterior or posterior displacement of the medial clavicle, not dislocation of the joint. However, more recent literature has supported the finding that skeletally immature patients may in fact have isolated SC joint dislocation without associated physeal injury,[111,193,212] with one such study reporting that both forms of SC injury occur with equal prevalence.[111]

Chronic Physeal Fracture. Similar to SC dislocations, physeal fractures of the SC joint are at risk for being missed on initial presentation, and unfortunately, a delayed presentation is not uncommon. In the skeletally immature population, posterior SC joint injury may be missed in nearly 25% of patients on initial presentation.[111] Delayed diagnosis affects treatment options because successful closed reduction after 48 hours is rarely reported in the literature.[111,193]

Incidence of Injury to the Sternoclavicular Joint

The incidence of SC dislocation, based on the series of 1,603 injuries of the shoulder girdle reported by Cave et al.,[30] is 3% (specific incidences of dislocation in this study were glenohumeral, 85%; acromioclavicular [AC], 12%; and SC, 3%). In the series by Cave et al., and in our experience, dislocation of the SC joint is not as rare as posterior dislocation of the glenohumeral joint.

In a study of 3,451 injuries during alpine skiing, Kocher and Feagin[106] showed that injuries involving the shoulder complex accounted for 39.1% of upper extremity injuries and 11.4% of all alpine skiing injuries. Of the 393 injuries involving the shoulder complex, SC separations accounted for 0.5%.

The largest published series from a single institution was reported by Nettles and Linscheid,[129] who studied 60 patients with SC dislocations (57 anterior and 3 posterior). However, in our series of 185 traumatic SC injuries, 135 patients had anterior dislocation and 50 patients had posterior dislocation.

Orthopedic Injuries Associated With the Sternoclavicular Joint

Bilateral Dislocations

In 1896, Hotchkiss reported a bilateral traumatic dislocation of the SC joint.[91] The senior author (C.A.R.) has treated four cases of bilateral SC dislocation. Bilateral traumatic anterior SC joint dislocations have also been reported following a motorcycle accident in a 28-year-old male.[36] In 2010, Baumann et al.[11] reported the first case of a bilateral traumatic posterior physeal fracture dislocation in a 15-year-old boy who fell forward on his chest while downhill skiing. Closed reduction under anesthesia with a clamp was initially successful; however, recurrent instability occurred just 2 days later as confirmed on repeat CT, necessitating open reduction and internal fixation with transosseous sutures.

Dislocations of Both Ends of the Clavicle

Dislocation of both ends of the clavicle is a rare, high-energy injury with fewer than 30 cases reported in the literature. In 1990, the senior author[168] reported six patients who sustained a dislocation of both ends of the clavicle (anterior dislocation of the SC joint and posterior dislocation of the AC joint). Two patients who had fewer demands on the shoulder did well with only minor symptoms after nonoperative management. The other four patients had persistent symptoms that were localized to the AC joint. Each of these patients underwent reconstruction of the AC joint that resulted in painless full range of motion and return to normal activity.

Combined Sternoclavicular Joint Injury and Fractures of the Clavicle

Elliott[52] reported on a tripartite injury about the clavicular region in which the patient sustained an anterior subluxation of the right SC joint, a type II injury to the right AC joint, and a fracture of the right midclavicle. Velutini and Tarazona[206] reported a unusual case of posterior dislocation of the left medial clavicle, the first rib, and a section of the manubrium. Others have reported fracture of the clavicle associated with anterior SC joint subluxation, and injury to the long thoracic nerve.[140] All of these combined injuries were associated with severe trauma to the shoulder region (e.g., the involved shoulder struck an immovable object or was severely compressed) (Fig. 10-15).

Combined Sternoclavicular Joint Dislocation and Scapulothoracic Dissociation

Tsai et al.[198] reported a patient with an SC dislocation associated with a scapulothoracic dissociation. The patient had also sustained a transection of the axillary artery, an avulsion of the median nerve, and a complete brachial plexopathy. Surgical management included vascular repair and an above-elbow amputation.

Signs and Symptoms of Injuries to the Sternoclavicular Joint

Traumatic Subluxation

In a mild sprain (type I injury), the patient complains of mild-to-moderate pain, particularly with movement of the upper extremity. The joint may be slightly swollen and tender to palpation, but instability is not noted. A moderate sprain or subluxation of the SC joint (type II injury) often results in swelling, and pain is marked, particularly with any movement of the arm. Anterior or posterior subluxation may not be obvious to the examiner when the injured joint is compared with the normal SC joint.

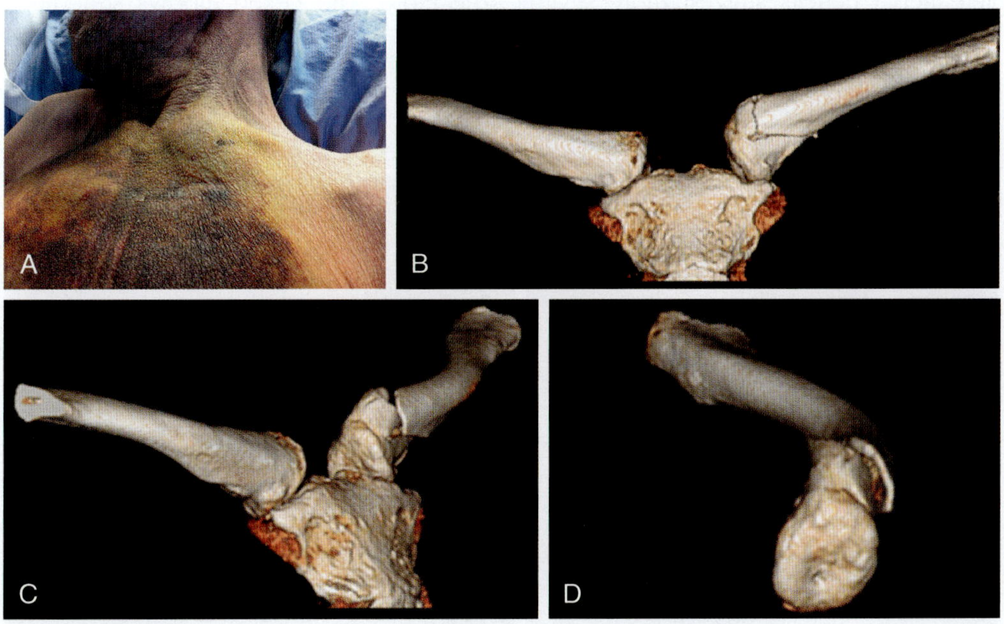

FIGURE 10-15: **A,** Clinical view of an elderly man with an isolated left medial clavicle fracture and anterosuperior subluxation of the sternoclavicular joint after a fall. Note the significant bruising of the anterior chest wall. **B–D,** Three-dimensional computed tomographic views of the ipsilateral injuries to the medial clavicle and sternoclavicular joint with preservation of the medial articular surface.

Signs Common to Anterior and Posterior Dislocations

The patient with an SC dislocation has severe pain that is increased with any movement of the arm, particularly when the shoulders are pressed together by a lateral force. The patient usually supports the injured arm across the trunk with the normal arm. The affected shoulder appears to be shortened and thrust forward when compared with the normal shoulder. The head may be tilted toward the side of the dislocated joint, and discomfort increases when the patient is placed in the supine position.

Signs and Symptoms of Anterior Dislocations

With an anterior dislocation, the medial end of the clavicle is visibly prominent anterior to the sternum and can be palpated anterior to the sternum. The clavicle may be fixed or quite mobile.

Signs and Symptoms of Posterior Dislocations

The patient with a posterior dislocation has more pain than a patient with an anterior dislocation. The anterosuperior fullness of the chest produced by the clavicle is less prominent and visible when compared with the normal side. The medial end of the clavicle is displaced posteriorly, and the corner of the sternum is more prominent but this is usually difficult to appreciate because of swelling. Venous congestion may be present in the neck or in the upper extremity. Symptoms can also include a dry, irritating cough and hoarseness. Breathing difficulties or shortness of breath may be secondary to a pneumothorax. Circulation to the ipsilateral arm may be decreased. The patient might complain of difficulty swallowing, a tight feeling in the throat, or a choking sensation. The distal neurologic examination may reveal diminished sensation or weakness secondary to brachial plexus compression. Complete nerve deficits suggest more severe injury patterns.

RADIOGRAPHIC FINDINGS OF INJURY TO THE STERNOCLAVICULAR JOINT

Anteroposterior Views

Occasionally, routine radiographs of the chest or SC joint suggest that something is wrong with one of the clavicles, because it appears to be displaced compared with the normal side (Fig. 10-16). For example, a difference in the relative craniocaudal position of the medial clavicle greater than 50% of the width of the clavicular head suggests dislocation. It would be ideal to take a view at right angles to the anteroposterior (AP) plane, but because of the complex 3D anatomy, it is impossible to take a true 90-degree cephalic-to-caudal lateral view. Regardless of a clinical impression that suggests an anterior dislocation, a CT scan must be obtained to confirm one's suspicions.

Heinig View

For the Heinig view,[85] with the patient in a supine position, the x-ray tube is placed approximately 30 inches from the involved SC joint and the central ray is directed tangential to the joint and parallel to the opposite clavicle. The cassette is placed against the opposite shoulder and centered on the manubrium (Fig. 10-17).

Hobbs View

For the Hobbs view,[89] the patient is seated at the x-ray table, high enough to lean forward over the table. The cassette is on the table, and the lower anterior rib cage is against the cassette (Fig. 10-18). The patient leans forward so that the base of the neck is almost parallel to the table. The flexed elbows straddle the cassette and support the head and neck. The x-ray source is above

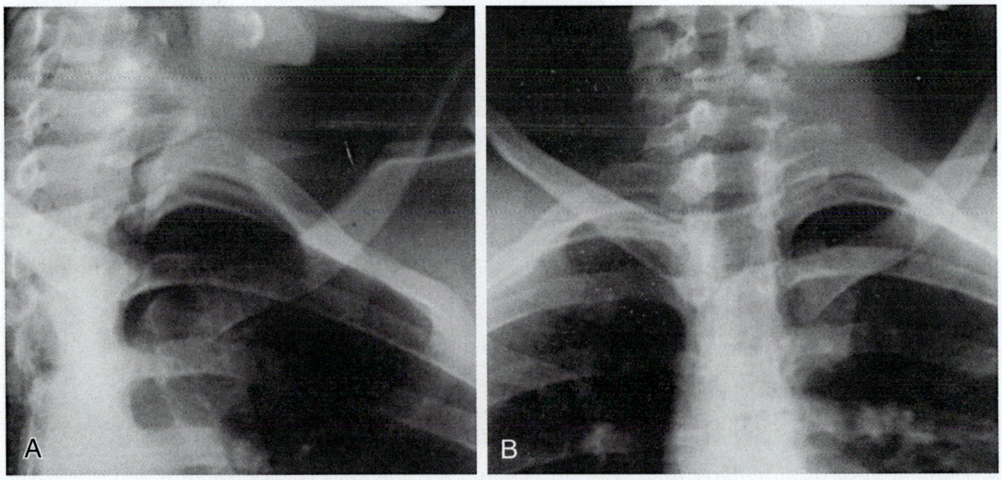

FIGURE 10-16: **A** and **B,** Routine radiographs of the sternoclavicular joint are difficult to interpret, even though this patient has a classic posterior dislocation of the left sternoclavicular joint. (From Rockwood CA, Green DP, eds. *Fractures*. 2nd ed. Philadelphia: JB Lippincott; 1984.)

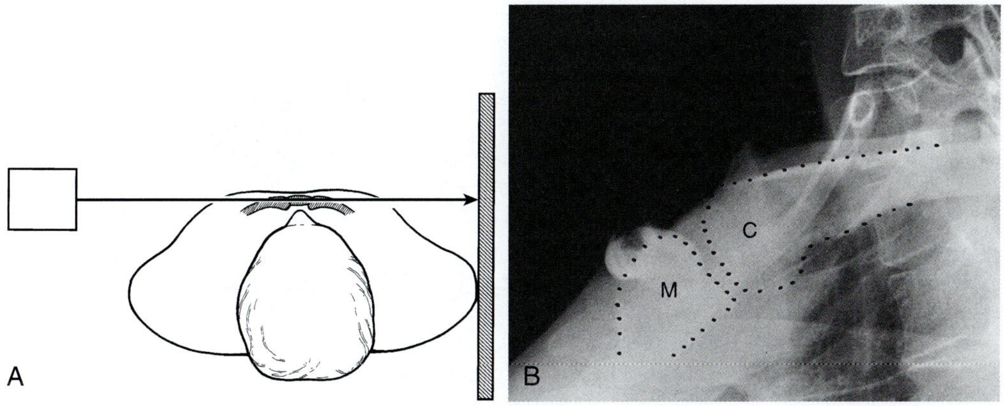

FIGURE 10-17: **A,** Positioning of the patient for radiographic evaluation of the SC joint, as described by Heinig. **B,** Heinig view demonstrating a normal relationship between the medial end of the clavicle (*C*) and the manubrium (*M*). (From Bucholz RW, Heckman JD, eds. *Rockwood and Green's Fractures in Adults.* 5th ed. Philadelphia: Lippincott Williams & Wilkins; 2001: 1250.)

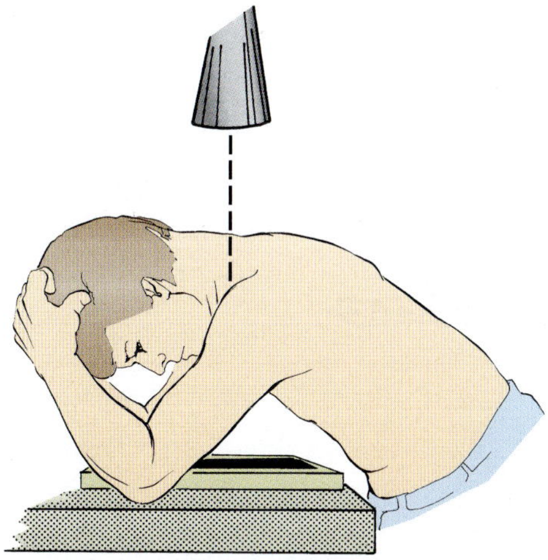

FIGURE 10-18: Positioning of the patient for radiographic evaluation of the sternoclavicular joint, as recommended by Hobbs. (Modified from Hobbs DW, The sternoclavicular joint: a new axial radiographic view. *Radiology.* 1968;90:801-802.)

the nape of the neck, and the beam passes through the cervical spine to project the SC joints onto the cassette.

Serendipity View

The senior author accidentally found that the next best thing to having a true cephalocaudal lateral view of the SC joint was a 40-degree cephalic tilt view; hence, the *serendipity view.* The patient is positioned supine on the x-ray table. The tube is tilted at a 40-degree angle off the vertical, and is centered directly on the sternum (Fig. 10-19).

Computed Tomography Scans

Lucet et al.[117] used CT scans to evaluate the SC joints in 60 healthy subjects homogeneously distributed in terms of gender and decade of life from 20 to 80 years old. They reported that 98% of the subjects had at least one sign of abnormality, such as sclerosis, osteophytes, erosion, cysts, or joint space narrowing. The number of signs increased with age, and the number of signs in the clavicle was greater than those in the sternum. Similarly, Tuscano et al.[200] obtained CT scans from 104 healthy subjects free from SC joint symptoms, and demonstrated that greater than 10% of patients show substantial asymmetry in the SC joints (i.e., SC joint space and distance between the manubrium and anterior margin of clavicular head), which may be interpreted as pathologic. These authors suggest exercising caution in attributing a disease state to asymmetry because of the frequency of this finding in the asymptomatic population. These findings become clinically useful in the setting of chronic subluxation or dislocation of the SC joint.

Magnetic Resonance Imaging

Magnetic resonance imaging (MRI) has been correlated with anatomic sections of SC joints, and is an excellent method for evaluating the anatomy of the SC joint and surrounding soft tissues in great detail. The sagittal plane is useful to assess the integrity of the costoclavicular ligament and the attachments of the intra-articular disk to the SC ligaments. This view is also helpful in assessing the location of the great vessels, trachea, and esophagus. T2-weighted images were superior to T1-weighted images in depicting the intra-articular disk. MR arthrography has the added advantage of delineating perforations in the intra-articular disk and more subtle injuries to the capsular ligaments. In children and young adults, MRI is especially helpful in distinguishing between a dislocation of the SC joint and a physeal injury (Fig. 10-20). MRI is far superior to CT in its ability to detect bone marrow abnormalities, cartilage injury, effusions, and the surrounding soft tissues.

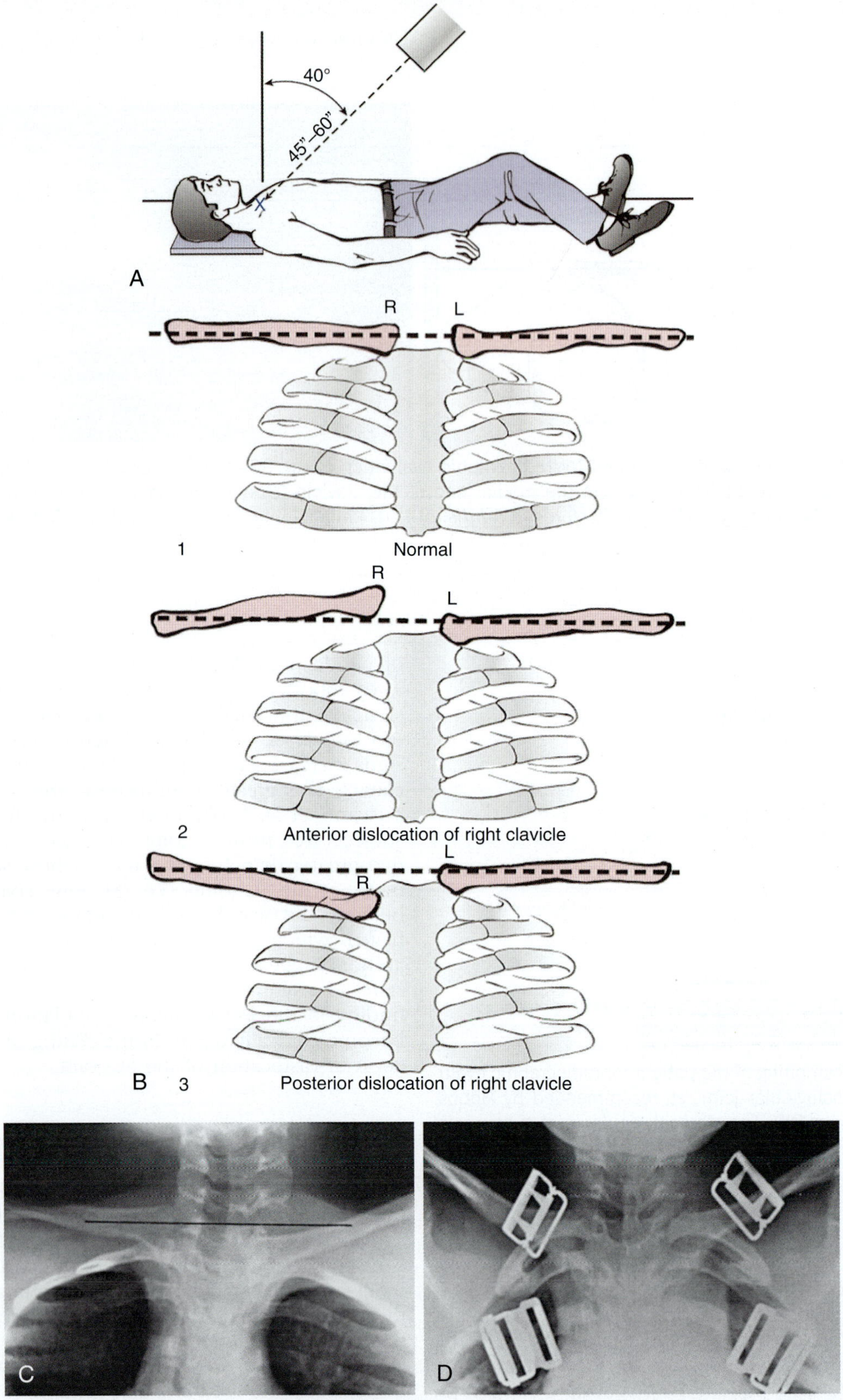

FIGURE 10-19: **A,** Positioning of the patient to obtain a "serendipity view" of the sternoclavicular (SC) joints. The x-ray tube is tilted 40 degrees from the vertical position and aimed directly at the manubrium. **B,** Interpretation of the serendipity view. *1,* In the normal scenario, both clavicles appear on the same imaginary line drawn horizontally across the film. *2,* Anterior dislocation of SC joint. The medial half of the right clavicle is projected above the imaginary line drawn through the level of the normal left clavicle. *3,* Posterior dislocation of the SC joint. The medial half of the right clavicle is displaced below the imaginary line drawn through the normal left clavicle. **C,** Clinical example of a posterior dislocation of the left SC joint as seen on a 40-degree cephalic tilt radiograph in a 12-year-old boy. The left clavicle is displaced inferiorly to a line drawn through the normal right clavicle. **D,** After closed reduction, the medial ends of both clavicles are in the same horizontal position. The buckles are a part of the figure-of-eight clavicular harness that is used to hold the shoulders back after reduction. (**A** and **B,** From Court-Brown CM, Heckman JD, McQueen MM, et al. *Rockwood and Green's Fractures in Adults.* 8th ed. Philadelphia: Lippincott Williams & Wilkins; 2015: 1616. **C** and **D,** From Rockwood CA, Green DP, eds. *Fractures.* 2nd ed. Philadelphia: JB Lippincott; 1984.)

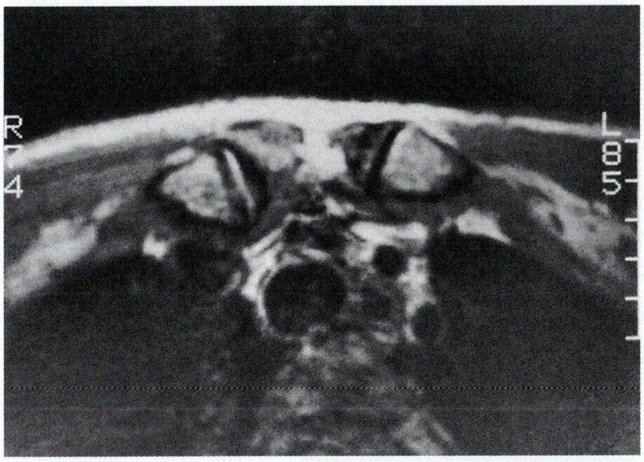

FIGURE 10-20: Magnetic resonance image of the sternoclavicular joints. The epiphysis on the medial aspect of both clavicles is clearly visible. (From Bucholz RW, Heckman JD, eds. *Rockwood and Green's Fractures in Adults.* 5th ed. Philadelphia: Lippincott Williams & Wilkins; 2001: 1253.)

Ultrasound

The role of ultrasound is limited in comparison to CT and MRI except in the case of intraoperative evaluation, where it can be nearly impossible to precisely determine the adequacy of reduction. In this setting, the value of ultrasound is unsurpassed in accurately confirming whether a closed reduction has been successful.[177] However, sonography is dependent on operator experience and knowledge of regional anatomy. In 2012, Sullivan et al.[188] described the use of an O-arm intraoperative CT system to verify reduction in two cases of posterior SC joint dislocation. Lastly, duplex ultrasonography can be helpful for diagnosing thrombosis and vessel occlusion in cases where vascular insult is suspected. However, the role for advanced vascular imaging such as CT angiography cannot be understated and should be performed if vascular injury is present or suspected acutely to define the location and extent of vascular injury. CT angiography should also be considered for all chronic or late presentations of posterior SC joint injury.

ATRAUMATIC DISORDERS OF THE STERNOCLAVICULAR JOINT

Like other diarthrodial joints, the SC joint is also susceptible to the normal spectrum of inflammatory and degenerative diseases, as well as a number of other disorders that are specific to the SC joint (see Fig. 10-13). Such disorders can present either acutely or insidiously with localized pain, swelling, and even subluxation or enlargement of the joint.[86,88,155] A simple algorithm is outlined that reviews the clinical approach to a patient who presents with such complaints without a history of trauma (Fig. 10-21).

Spontaneous Subluxation and Dislocation

This condition typically occurs in women during their late teens or young adult life, and usually occurs in patients who have generalized ligament laxity of other joints. Although both SC joints can be affected, usually the dominant side is more symptomatic (Fig. 10-22). As the patient raises the arm forward, the medial clavicle spontaneously displaces anteriorly and superiorly, and, when the arm is returned to the patient's side, the medial clavicle is reduced. Atraumatic subluxation and dislocation are usually anterior, and are usually not associated with a great deal of pain. In some patients, the anterior subluxation of the SC joint is painful and is associated with mechanical symptoms (e.g., a snap or pop) as the arm is both elevated overhead and again lowered to the patient's side. In middle-aged women, spontaneous anterior or anterosuperior subluxation can be associated with condensing osteitis of the clavicle.[204]

Arthritis

Osteoarthritis

Osteoarthritis represents the most frequent cause of pain and swelling of the SC joint, and is characterized by narrowing of the joint space, osteophytes, subchondral sclerosis, and cysts on both sides of the joint. Because hyaline cartilage covers only the anteroinferior aspect of the medial clavicle, most of degenerative changes occur in this region of the joint. The sometimes discrete degenerative changes are best seen on CT scans (Fig. 10-23). The swelling may be asymptomatic; however, a symptomatic joint is characteristically painful on abduction or forward elevation of the shoulder beyond the horizontal plane. Other findings on clinical examination include prominence at the medial end of the clavicle (caused by osteophytes), a fixed subluxation, or crepitus with range of motion.[86] Most often, there is no history of previous injury to the joint. High-risk groups include postmenopausal women, patients with chronic SC joint instability, and manual laborers. Sternoclavicular joint arthritis and hypertrophy can also develop after radical neck surgery, particularly when the spinal accessory nerve is sacrificed.[25,172] The mechanism for this is believed to be the result of chronic downward and forward position of the shoulder that results after denervation of the trapezius muscle.[88] The incidence of SC joint arthritis in such circumstances is reported to be as high as 54%.[25]

Sadr and Swann[164] reported on 22 patients with *postmenopausal arthritis* involving the SC joint. The majority of cases involved the SC joint of the dominant arm, and were believed to be the result of normal degeneration of a frequently moved joint. The majority of patients are asymptomatic; a lump develops at the SC joint and, occasionally, a vague ache will develop when the joint is stressed. Patients have no previous history of injury or disease. Radiographs reveal sclerosis and enlargement of the medial end of the clavicle, reactive sclerosis of the sternum, and subluxation of the joint. The pathologic changes are those of degenerative arthritis.

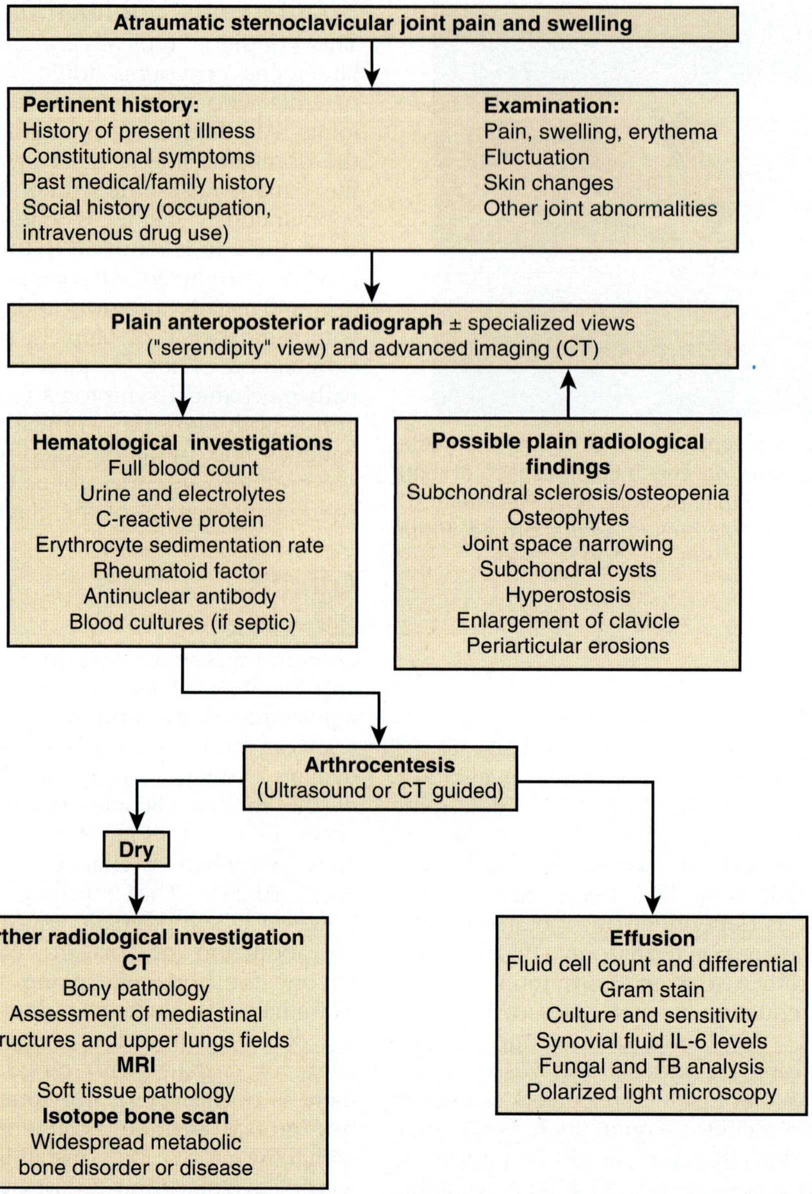

FIGURE 10-21: Diagnostic protocol for the investigation of an atraumatic sternoclavicular joint problem. *CT*, computed tomography; *IL*, interleukin; *MRI*, magnetic resonance imaging; *TB*, tuberculosis. (Modified from Robinson CM, Jenkins PJ, Markham PE, et al. Disorders of the sternoclavicular joint. *J Bone Joint Surg Br*. 2008;90[6]:685-696.)

In a recent report, Sternheim et al.[187] identified a group of 25 female patients (mean age, 59 years; range, 50–71 years) with monoarticular arthritis of the SC joint that had a benign, self-limiting clinical course. The patients presented with complaints of pain (72%), local swelling (88%), and redness (8%) that progressed over a 4-week period. The physical examination revealed tenderness (84%), swelling (88%), and limited range of motion (16%), which persisted for a median of 5 months. All patients underwent blood work to rule out infection and inflammatory arthritis, which was normal. Plain radiographs revealed arthritic changes in only five patients (25%); however, of the six patients who underwent advanced imaging such as CT, five patients (83%) had joint space narrowing, sclerosis, and subchondral cysts. Pain resolved spontaneously in all patients, leaving only swelling in nine patients and tenderness in one patient. The authors described this clinical entity as *transient sternoclavicular joint arthritis.*

Rheumatoid Arthritis

Rheumatoid arthritis (RA) is a chronic, systemic inflammatory disorder of unclear etiology characterized by an erosive, symmetrical polyarthritis of synovial joints.[33] RA is the most common form of inflammatory arthropathy; the estimated prevalence is 1% worldwide, with a female-to-male ratio of

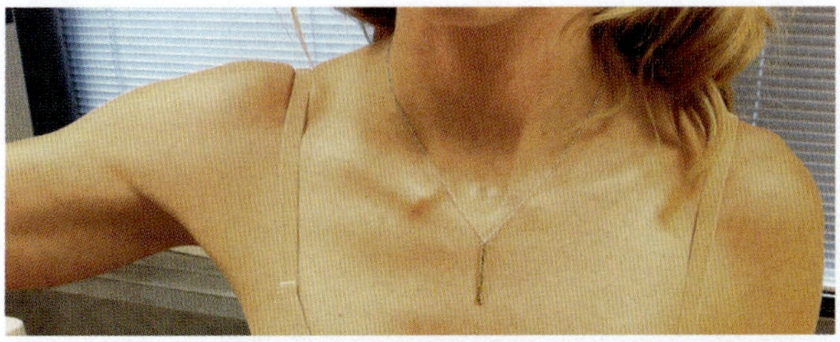

FIGURE 10-22: Spontaneous anterior subluxation of the right sternoclavicular joint in a young adult woman. With the arm in an abducted and extended position, the medial end of the right clavicle spontaneously subluxes anteriorly without any trauma. When the arm is brought back down to the side, the medial end of the clavicle spontaneously reduces. Such subluxation episodes are not usually associated with any significant discomfort.

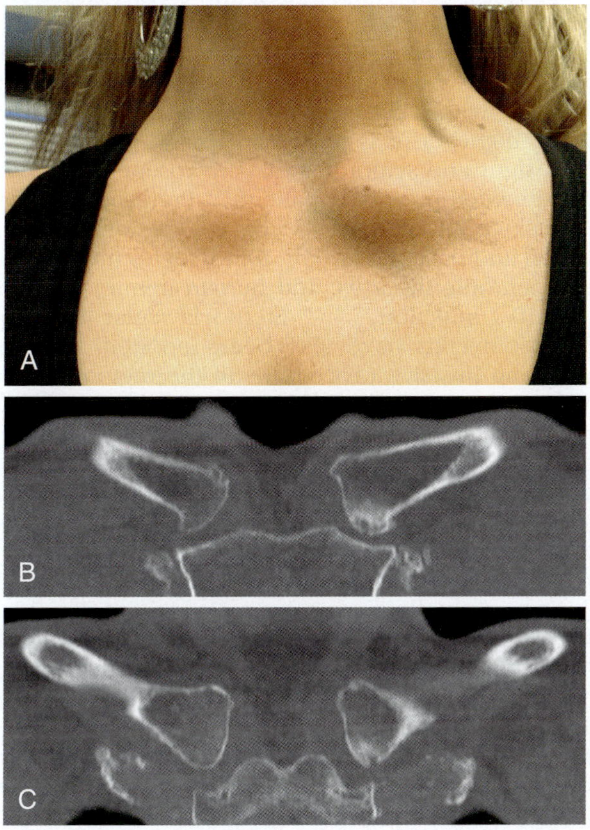

FIGURE 10-23: **A,** Clinical appearance of swelling and deformity of the left sternoclavicular (SC) joint in a 56-year-old postmenopausal patient with degenerative arthritis of the SC joint. **B–C,** Computed tomography (coronal images) of both SC joints reveals the typical findings of osteoarthritis, including joint space narrowing, subchondral sclerosis and cysts, and osteophytes. Similar mild degenerative changes are seen involving the patient's asymptomatic right SC joint.

3:1 that diminishes with age. Approximately 91% of patients with longstanding RA (>5 years' duration) develop glenohumeral joint symptoms[33]; however, symptomatic SC joint involvement is less common, ranging from 19% to 30%.[101,159] Like RA involvement of other joints, RA of the SC joint is characterized by osteopenia, soft tissue swelling and synovitis, and periarticular erosions (Fig. 10-24).

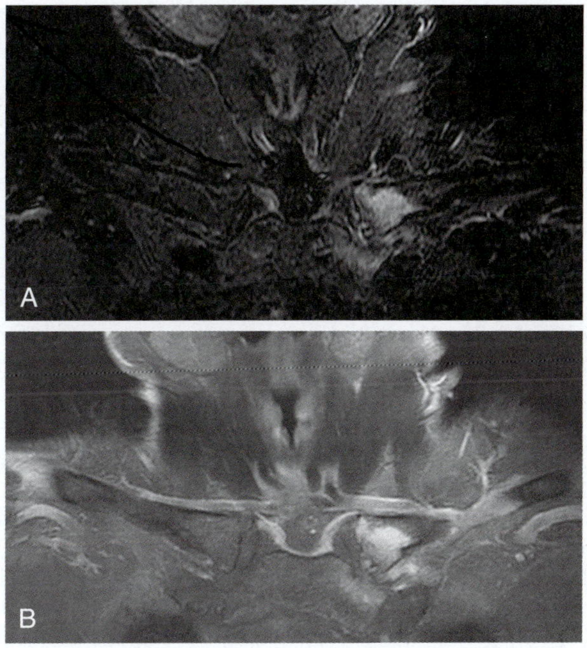

FIGURE 10-24: A 60-year-old male presenting with pain and swelling of the left sternoclavicular joint and fullness within the supraclavicular fossa. **A,** Coronal magnetic resonance image (short tau inversion recovery [STIR] sequence) reveals the characteristic findings of bone marrow edema on both sides of the joint, synovitis, and periarticular erosions (medial clavicle). **B,** Coronal T1 weighted fat-saturated image demonstrating the thickened synovium within the sternoclavicular joint and periarticular erosions.

Seronegative Spondyloarthropathies

These inflammatory arthropathies include a heterogeneous group of diseases characterized by axial spine involvement (e.g., ankylosing spondylitis), asymmetric peripheral arthritis (e.g., psoriatic arthritis), enthesopathy, inflammatory eye (e.g., Reiter syndrome), and bowel (e.g., colitic arthritis) disease occurring in the absence of serum rheumatoid factor and association with HLA-B27. These arthritides may also destroy articular cartilage but characteristically are more destructive toward collagen and fibrocartilage. Limited published studies have assessed the SC joint involvement in this group of arthropathies. Emery et al.[53] reported involvement of the SC joint in only 2 of 52 (4%) patients with ankylosing spondylitis. In contrast, Taccari et al.[189] found that the SC joint was clinically symptomatic in 5 of 10 patients (50%) with severe psoriatic arthritis.

Crystal Arthropathy

Crystal deposition disease has been described in multiple joints, including the SC joint. Identification of calcium pyrophosphate dihydrate (CPPD) crystals or monosodium urate crystals in synovial fluid, articular tissue, and rarely, the periarticular tissue, allows one to differentiate between

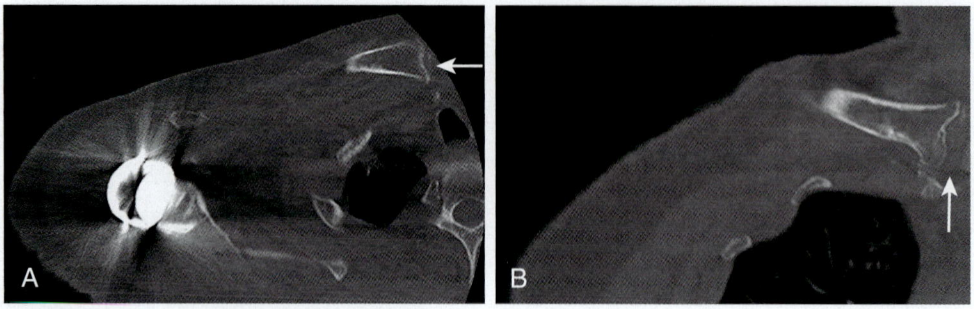

FIGURE 10-25: A and **B,** Axial and coronal computed tomographic images of a patient with calcium pyrophosphate dihydrate deposition syndrome of the right sternoclavicular joint (*arrow*).

crystal deposition disease and other inflammatory and degenerative arthritides. Examination of joint fluid with a polarizing light microscope reveals characteristic positive (pseudogout) or negative (gout) birefringent crystals.[86] CPPD crystal deposition disease may be asymptomatic[175] or may cause an acute, gout-like attack of inflammation and pain, referred to as pseudogout (Fig. 10-25).[46] In a recent study, Shirazian et al.[175] retrospectively evaluated CT studies of the cervical spine in 209 patients that were free of SC joint symptoms; the overall prevalence of CPPD crystal deposition in the SC joint was 17.2% (36 of 209 patients). The rarest manifestation of CPPD deposition is tophaceous pseudogout, which is characterized by a mass containing CPPD crystals arising within or adjacent to the SC joint. Richman et al.[153] have reported a case of tophaceous pseudogout extending posteriorly and inferiorly from the left SC joint, causing a mass effect on the adjacent brachiocephalic vein requiring excision.

Gout is a heterogeneous group of diseases resulting from monosodium urate crystal deposition in tissues or from supersaturation of uric acid in extracellular fluids. The initial episode of acute gout usually follows decades of asymptomatic hyperuricemia, and is predominantly a disease of adult men, with incidence peaking in the fifth decade of life. However, gout involving the SC joint has been described in limited reports and in less predictable clinical circumstances, including a case in an 18-year-old female.[169]

Less Common Forms of Arthritis

Neuropathic arthropathy is a destructive arthritis characterized by fracture, subluxation, and dislocation of articular structures in the setting of neurologic damage to the involved joint. Syringomyelia is the most common cause of neuropathic arthropathy in the upper limb; only two cases of SC joint involvement have been reported in the literature.[34,43] Other uncommon conditions that cause erosive changes to the medial clavicle include the systemic inflammatory syndrome of polymyalgia rheumatica,[130,136] hemophilic pseudotumors,[96] and hyperparathyroidism.[192] Hemodialysis-related deposition of amyloid (β_2-microglobulin) in the SC joint in long-term hemodialysis patients has been described.[222] The clinical and imaging features may be similar to that of infection, warranting synovial biopsy and specific staining for the β_2-microglobulin component of amyloid.[24,223]

Infection

Spontaneous, unilateral, painful, and erythematous swelling of the SC joint with the appearance of joint subluxation should be considered an infectious etiology until proven otherwise. Such clinical presentations may be associated with acute, subacute, or chronic bacterial arthritis; however, it is important to recognize that such clinical signs and symptoms may be absent in the elderly or immunocompromised patient.[155] Predisposing conditions include intravenous (IV) drug addiction, distant site infection and bacteremia,[103,127] RA, diabetes mellitus, alcoholism, chronic diseases, and human immunodeficiency virus (HIV) infection.[41,160,219] Sternoclavicular joint sepsis and osteomyelitis have also been reported in patients undergoing invasive procedures in the region of the SC joint including subclavian vein catheterization,[114,144,151] coronary angiography,[90] tracheostomy tube placement,[83] and other head and neck surgical procedures of the larynx, pharynx, and esophagus.[208] However, one must recognize that SC joint infection can occur in otherwise healthy adults without identifiable risk factors.[8,35,51,160,170] Ancillary investigations such as CT are very helpful in making an early diagnosis of a septic SC joint (Fig. 10-26); however, MRI has been shown to be more sensitive than CT in diagnosing septic arthritis[16] and osteomyelitis of the SC joint (Fig. 10-27). The typical findings on imaging include joint capsular distension of 10 mm or greater over both the clavicle and sternum, and adjacent bone marrow fluid signal on MRI.[98] Regardless of the advanced imaging modality used, definitive diagnosis of SC joint infection requires image-guided aspiration or open biopsy followed by consultation with an infectious disease specialist to ensure that appropriate laboratory evaluation of the specimen is undertaken. The joint fluid should also be analyzed to rule out crystal-induced monoarthritis.

In 2004, Ross and Shamsuddin summarized the findings of 180 cases of septic SC joint arthritis published between 1970 and 2004.[160] The mean age of the patients was 45 years (range, 11–88 years) and the majority were male (73%). Presenting symptoms included chest pain (78%) and shoulder pain (24%); painless swelling was the presenting complaint in only 4% of patients, including 50% of those diagnosed with tuberculous arthritis. Only 65% of the patients were febrile. Laboratory investigations revealed an elevated white blood cell count in only 56%

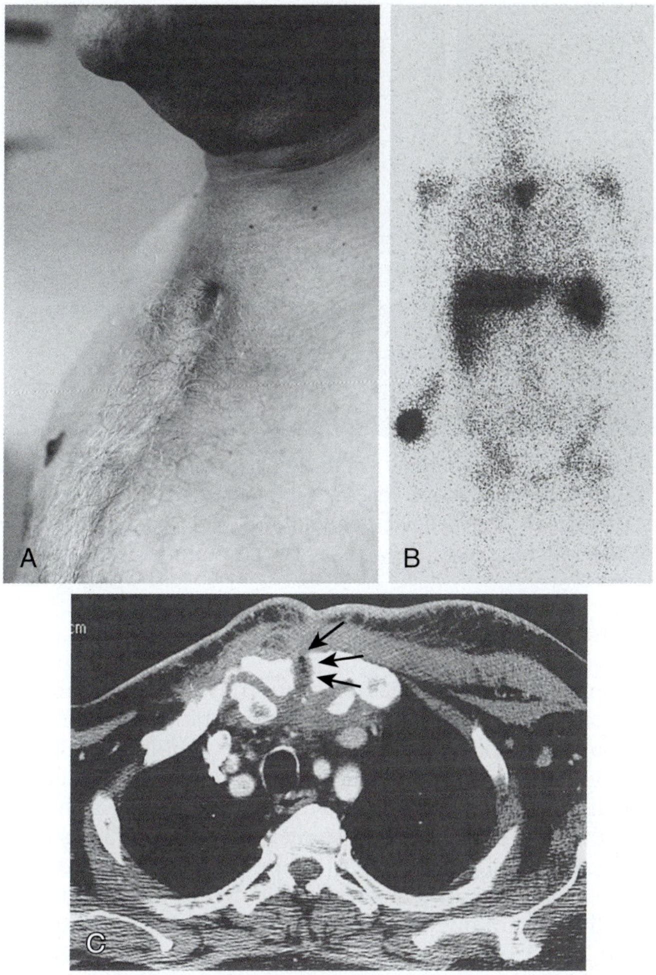

FIGURE 10-26: A, This patient had longstanding insulin-dependent diabetes and underwent a coronary artery bypass procedure that was complicated by a postoperative wound infection. **B,** Indium-enhanced white blood cell scan consistent with infection in the region of the left sternoclavicular joint. **C,** Computed tomographic scan revealing significant soft tissue swelling, interspersed locules of air (*arrows*) within the sternal osteotomy site, and focal irregularity of the posterior aspect of the sternum consistent with an infectious process. (From Rockwood CA, Green DP, Bucholz RW, Heckman JD, eds. *Fractures in the Adult.* Philadelphia: JB Lippincott; 1996.)

of the patients (erythrocyte sedimentation rate and C-reactive protein values were not reported); bacteremia was demonstrated in 62% of the patients. When needle aspiration was performed, cultures were positive in 50 of 65 patients (77%). Eighty-seven of 102 (85%) initial plain radiographs were normal, whereas all 95 patients (100%) who underwent CT scans demonstrated at least one abnormality, including osteomyelitis (69%), chest wall abscess (57%), joint space widening (25%), mediastinitis (20%), and extrapleural abscess (1%). The most common risk factor was IV drug use (21%), followed by infection at a distant site (15%), diabetes mellitus (13%), trauma (12%), and infected central lines (9%). *Staphylococcus aureus* was responsible for 49% of the cases. Other common and uncommon pathogens that have been reported include *Streptococcus pyogenes*,[170] methicillin-resistant *S. aureus*,[127] *Neisseria gonorrhoeae*,[80] and *Salmonella*.[5,35] Atypical infections such as *Pseudomonas aeruginosa* and *Candida albicans* have been previously reported in IV drug users;[73,75] however, in the review by Ross and Shamsuddin[160] and in more recent reports,[72] methicillin-sensitive *S. aureus* was still the most prevalent organism isolated in this patient group.

In developing countries, there have been reports of joint infection from *Mycobacterium tuberculosis*.[31,56,154,160,165] Richter et al.[154] reported on nine patients with infection of the SC joint secondary to tuberculosis. The average time from onset of the disease to diagnosis was 1.4 years. Higoumenakis[87] has stated that unilateral enlargement of the SC joint is a diagnostic sign of congenital syphilis. The enlargement of the SC joint can be mistaken for an anterior dislocation. He reported the sign to be positive in 170 of 197 patients with congenital syphilis. The enlargement is attributed to hyperostosis of the medial aspect of the clavicle occurring in the SC joint of the dominant extremity, which reaches its permanent stage and size at puberty. Joint enlargement has also been seen in leprosy.

Disorders Specific to the Sternoclavicular Joint

Condensing Osteitis of the Medial Clavicle

This condition has also been termed hypertrophic osteitis. In 1974, Brower et al. first described the clinical entity of condensing osteitis of the medial clavicle in two young adult women.[20] Since this original report, there have been fewer than 50 cases of condensing osteitis of the medial clavicle published in the English literature. This rare condition usually affects women in their fourth and fifth decades of life (range, 20–65 years)[71,77,107,180]; only three reports in men have been published.[2,131,180] Most cases involve the medial end of one clavicle; only two cases of bilateral condensing osteitis have been reported.[93,109] The etiology of condensing osteitis is unknown, and is likely to be multifactorial. Brower et al.[20] hypothesized that the histopathologic changes of the medial clavicle (increased number and thickness of trabeculae combined with obliteration of marrow space) was probably a reaction to abnormal repetitive mechanical stress; however, only 2 of 11 cases (18%) reviewed by Outwater and Oates[135] had a history of occupational or athletic-related recurrent stress. Other etiologies have been proposed[2,13] and some investigators believe condensing osteitis represents low-grade osteonecrosis.[77] In children, condensing osteitis most likely represents chronic recurrent multifocal osteomyelitis.[99]

The clinical signs and symptoms consist of intermittent or constant pain of variable intensity that is localized to the medial clavicle that radiates to the supraclavicular fossa and ipsilateral anterior chest and shoulder. By the time patients first seek medical attention, the symptoms usually

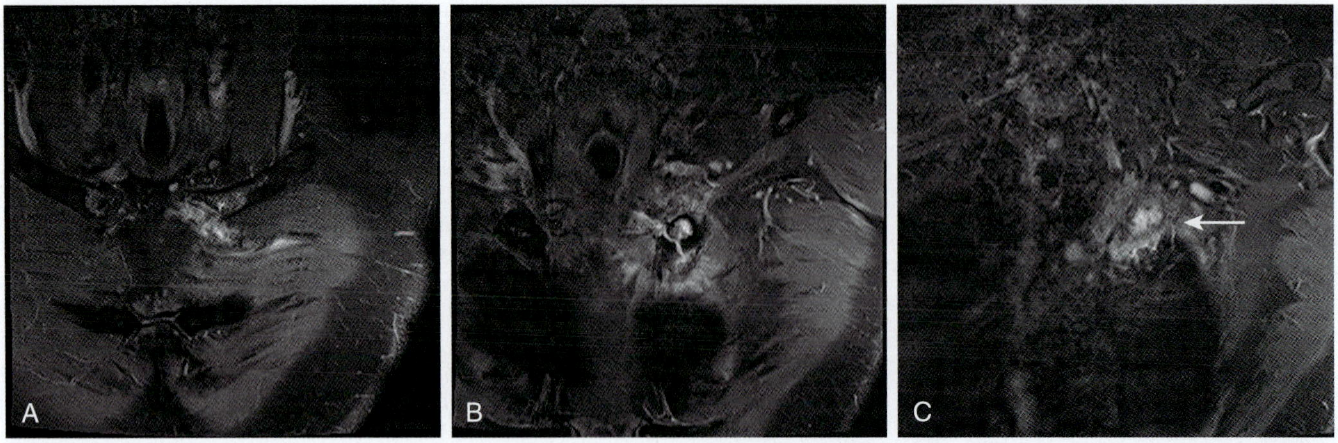

FIGURE 10-27: A 61-year-old male presented with a 3-month history of progressive pain, swelling, and erythema over the left sternoclavicular joint and anterior chest wall. Coronal T2-weighted fat-saturated magnetic resonance imaging demonstrates findings consistent with septic arthritis and destructive osteomyelitis of the left sternoclavicular joint (**A**), contiguous spread of infection into the first costochondral junction (**B**), and empyema of the left lung apex (**C**; *arrow*). Tissue cultures were positive for methicillin-sensitive *Staphylococcus aureus* infection.

will have been present for months to years. There is often swelling and tenderness over the medial clavicle, and pain is reproduced with shoulder abduction or forward elevation; however, the swelling may be painless.[93]

Radiographs show sclerosis and slight expansion of the inferior margin of the medial third of the clavicle. Occasionally, there is an inferior osteophyte present, but the joint space is preserved. The changes in the inferior-medial clavicle are best detected by CT (sclerosis and marrow cavity obliteration).[82] Radionuclide studies reveal increased uptake of the isotope. The differential diagnosis includes Paget disease, SC hyperostosis, Friedrich disease, infection, Tietze syndrome, and osteoarthritis. Several authors have described the use of MRI as an adjunctive method for diagnosing this entity.[190,207] In some cases, a biopsy may be required to differentiate this entity from primary or metastatic bone tumors.

Friedrich Disease

Aseptic osteonecrosis of the medial end of the clavicle, also known as Friedrich disease, was first described in 1924.[61,64] Friedrich wrote that this disease shares some similar characteristics with Perthes disease, Köhler disease, Kienböck disease, and Preiser disease.[64,88] Since this original report, there have been fewer than 25 cases of Friedrich disease published in the English literature; even fewer cases have been confirmed by histopathology with the pathognomonic finding of osteonecrosis (i.e., devitalized bone) surrounded by normal intact bone.[37,102,113,118,174] Some authors believe it is difficult to differentiate cases of condensing osteitis from Friedrich disease, and postulate that both conditions may be one of the same that follow along a spectrum of disease.[100,148]

The majority of reported cases are in female patients, both children and adults, although cases have been reported in men.[37,113] It is usually unilateral; we are aware of only one bilateral case.[113] This condition usually presents with swelling and tenderness over the medial end of the clavicle; however, some patients present with a painless swelling as their primary complaint.[37] Similar to condensing osteitis, laboratory tests for inflammatory and rheumatologic markers are normal. Radiographs and CT reveal irregularity and bony deformity of the sternal end of the clavicle[113]; MRI may demonstrate necrotic islands of bone in the metaphysis.[86] The symptoms are usually self-limiting, and complete resolution with remodeling of the medial end of the clavicle typically occurs over a period of 12 to 18 months.[113,155]

Synovitis Acne Pustulosis Hyperostosis Osteitis (SAPHO) Syndrome

Starting in the 1960s, there have been reports of an association between cutaneous lesions and musculoskeletal manifestations such as peripheral synovitis or aseptic osteitis affecting the anterior chest wall.[214] Since then, more than 50 designations have been used to describe these combinations, including one of the more common terms, sternocostoclavicular hyperostosis (SCCH).[27,182,183,194] In 1987, a group of French researchers who suspected that these disorders might share common characteristics coined the acronym SAPHO.[32] The complete syndrome described by the acronym is not common; the dermatologic manifestations are not frequently concomitant with the joint symptoms.[27] In one of its rarest presentations, Tamai and Saotome described a patient with palmar and plantar lesions associated with bilateral osseous fusion of both the AC and SC joints.[191]

SAPHO syndrome affects predominantly children and adults, and is not common in individuals older than 60 years; chronic recurrent multifocal osteomyelitis is considered the pediatric equivalent of SAPHO syndrome.[27] There is no predilection for gender, except for the male predominance in patients with severe acne.[27] The etiology remains unknown, and its consideration as a variant of the spondyloarthropathies is controversial and not definitively established. Others have theorized that SAPHO may be the result of an autoimmune process following long-term persistence of low-virulence organisms such as *Propionibacterium acnes*; this pathogen has been identified in bone biopsies of the affected chest wall, and in spinal and peripheral lesions.[27] Enthesitis can represent an initial symptom of SAPHO syndrome in some patients. Inflammatory enthesopathies can cause ossification, contributing to the formation of bone bridges; the painful swelling of the anterior chest wall is caused by hyperostosis and osteitis.[27] The anterior chest wall (i.e., sterno-costo-clavicular junction) is involved in 60% to 95% of patients with SAPHO syndrome.[48] The characteristic skin changes include severe acne and palmoplantaris pustulosis, which have been found in approximately 25% and 50% to 75% of patients with SAPHO, respectively (Fig. 10-28).[27] Such dermatologic changes may precede or follow the osteoarticular manifestations. The high variability in the clinical and imaging presentation depends on the stage of the lesions and the imaging method used.[27]

Prior to using the all-inclusive acronym SAPHO, Sonozaki et al. described the condition known as SCCH.[182,183] SCCH involves adults of both genders between 30 and 50 years of age, and is usually bilateral. The process begins at the junction of the medial clavicle, the first rib, and the sternum as an ossification in the ligaments, and later involves the bones. In some cases, the hyperostosis is extensive, and forms a solid block of bone consisting of the sternum, ribs, and clavicle. Patients may have peripheral arthritis. Subperiosteal bone changes have been noted on the radiographs of other bones of the skeleton, specifically, the humerus, pelvis, tibia, ribs, and vertebral bodies. The most common clinical finding is intermittent pain in the upper chest that may radiate to the shoulder and arm. Pain and swelling may increase with exertion. As might be expected with fusion of the SC joint, shoulder motion is severely restricted.[88] SCCH is a seronegative and HLA-B27–negative rheumatic disease; however, a previous retrospective study of 52 patients with SAPHO revealed that 8% of the patients were HLA-B27 positive.[166] Inflammatory markers (i.e., erythrocyte sedimentation rate and C-reactive protein) may be mildly elevated.

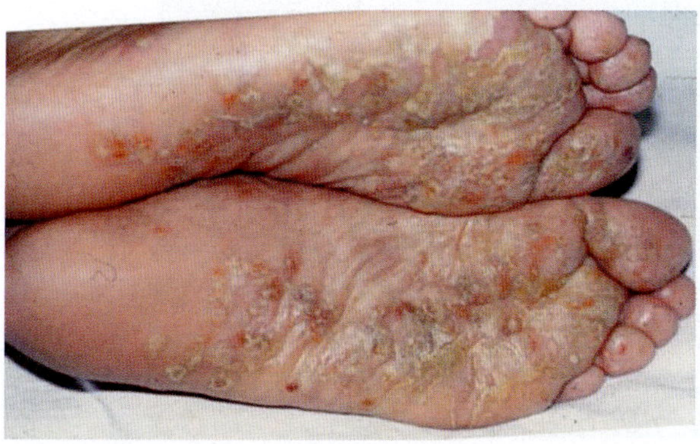

FIGURE 10-28: Palmoplantaris pustulosis is occasionally observed in patients with SAPHO syndrome (synovitis, acne, pustulosis hyperostosis, osteomyelitis). (From Carneiro S, Sampaio-Barros PD. SAPHO syndrome (synovitis, acne, pustulosis hyperostosis, osteomyelitis). *Rheum Dis Clin North Am.* 2013;39[2]:401-418.)

The radiographic appearances of SCCH have been subdivided into three stages (I, II, and III) by Sonozaki et al.[182,183] Stage I comprises mild ossification in the costoclavicular ligaments. Stage II is characterized by an ossific mass between the clavicle and the first rib. In stage III, a bone mass exists between the clavicle, sternum, and first or upper ribs. CT clearly shows the bony changes and any associated soft tissue mass (Fig. 10-29). On radionuclide bone scans, there is an increased uptake of the radioisotope in the affected areas with the characteristic and highly specific "bullhead" sign, even if their radiologic appearance was normal.[63] In this condition, hypostosis can appear in the spine, long bones, sacroiliac joints, and the SC region.

Other Conditions

Tietze Syndrome

Tietze syndrome is a benign, self-limiting condition characterized by tender swelling in the region of the anterior chest wall of unknown etiology. Tietze first described the condition in 1921,[196] and it has also been termed costosternal syndrome, anterior chest wall syndrome, and costochondritis.[88] The condition is usually unilateral, and occurs most frequently in the second through fourth decades of life. The site most involved is the costosternal junction of the second rib; the SC joint and costosternal junction of other upper ribs may be involved. Radiographic studies are of little diagnostic use, and laboratory analysis is usually normal, and thus it is considered a diagnosis of exclusion.[88] The symptoms of pain and tenderness in the anterior chest wall may disappear in weeks, but the swelling may persist for months. Patient reassurance is extremely important; because of the condition's benign course, treatment is aimed at alleviating symptoms.[88]

Other benign causes of SC joint swelling unrelated to Tietze syndrome include ganglion cysts and synovial osteochondromatosis (Fig. 10-30).

TREATMENT

Traumatic Injuries: Anterior

Sprain/Subluxation

The initial treatment of a mild sprain (type I) or subluxation (type II) injury consists of ice, 3 to 4 weeks of rest, and nonsteroidal antiinflammatory drugs (NSAIDs).

Acute Dislocation

There still is some controversy regarding the treatment of acute or chronic anterior dislocation of the SC joint.

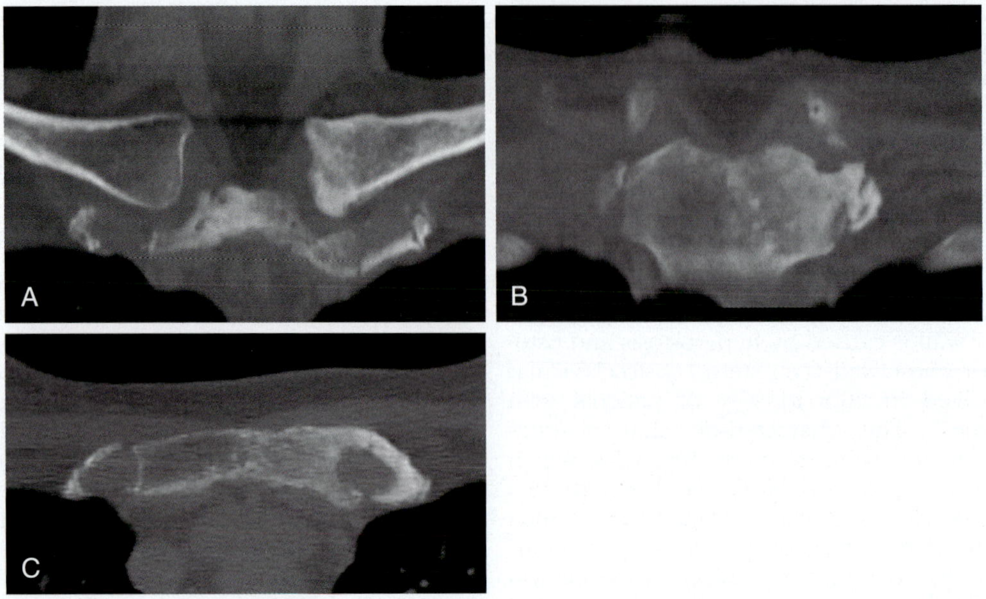

FIGURE 10-29: CT findings in a 52-year-old female with SAPHO syndrome (synovitis, acne, pustulosis hyperostosis, osteomyelitis). **A–C,** Mixed sclerotic and lytic changes involving the medial aspect of the left clavicle and throughout the manubrium. There is periosteal reaction and bony expansion at the medial aspect of the clavicle and ossification at the ligamentous insertions surrounding the sternoclavicular joint. Erosions are present in and around the joint and involve the left and right first costosternal junctions.

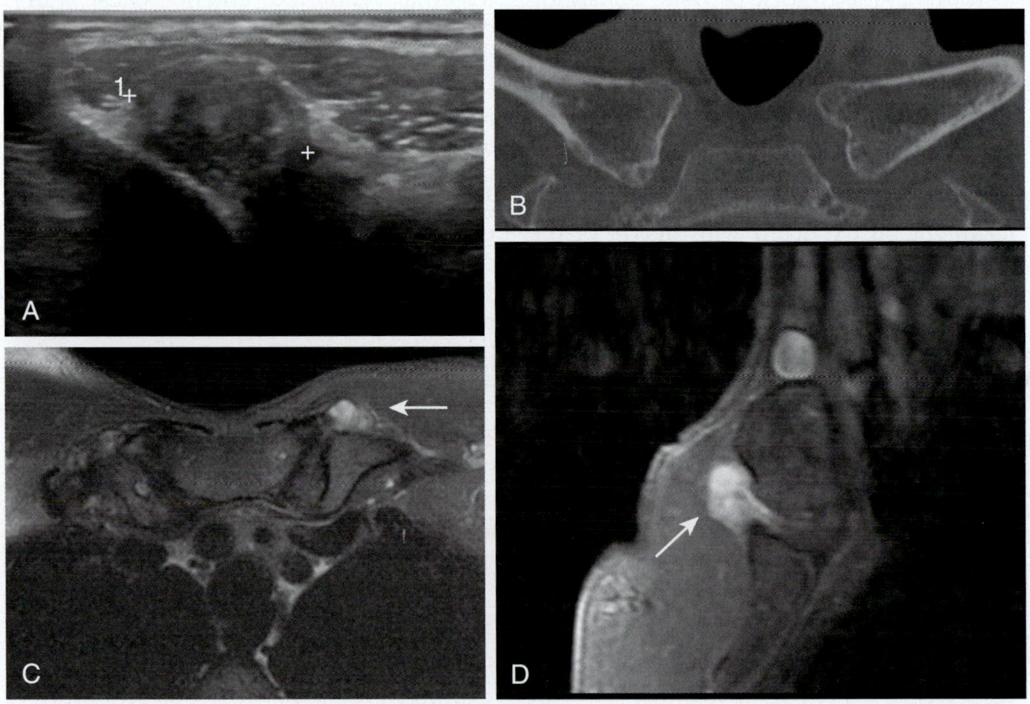

FIGURE 10-30: A 64-year-old female presenting with an acute onset of swelling over the left sternoclavicular joint described by the patient as a "tender lump." **A,** Ultrasound reveals a soft tissue mass ($1.8 \times 1.0 \times 1.8\ cm^3$) arising from the sternoclavicular joint. **B,** Coronal computed tomographic image demonstrates mild degenerative changes in both sternoclavicular joints. **C** and **D,** Axial T2-weighted and sagittal T1-weighted fat-saturated postgadolinium magnetic resonance imaging reveals a small, well-circumscribed enhancing periarticular lesion arising from the anteroinferior aspect of the left sternoclavicular joint that has an appearance most compatible with a complex capsular ganglion cyst with internal synovitis.

In 1988, Fery and Sommelet[60] reported the results of 49 SC dislocations (anterior and posterior) that were treated either operatively or nonoperatively. Only 55% of the patients were available for follow-up assessment at an average of 6.7 years. They had good and excellent results with both closed and operative treatments; however, most of the unsatisfactory results in this series were of patients with unreduced dislocations that were treated nonoperatively. In 1990, de Jong and Sukul[44] reported long-term follow-up results in 10 patients with traumatic anterior SC dislocations. All patients were treated nonoperatively with analgesics and immobilization. The results of treatment were good in seven patients, fair in two patients, and poor in one patient at an average follow-up of 5 years.

Chronic Dislocation

Surgery is considered for the patient who fails conservative treatment with persistent or worsening symptoms of at least 6 months' duration. Removal of the torn or degenerated intra-articular disk along with a capsulorrhaphy can improve pain and eliminate mechanical symptoms of popping and grating.[45,202] Complications are not uncommon when attempting to stabilize an anterior injury, and include recurrent instability,[60] loss of motion, and pain.[57]

Panzica et al.[137] recently reported the long-term operative results of 11 patients with anterior SC joint instability who were managed with either resection arthroplasty (6 patients) or ligament reconstruction (5 patients). Treatment occurred an average of 19.1 months after injury or diagnosis in the resection group and within 2 weeks of injury in the reconstruction group. The results of treatment were evaluated at a mean of 9.9 years using the American Shoulder and Elbow Surgeons, Disabilities of the Arm, Shoulder, and Hand, and Constant-Murley outcome scores. The outcome evaluation and postoperative pain scores did not differ significantly between the two operative groups; however, the overall results were worse in the reconstruction group when the SC joint reconstruction was not performed soon after injury and in the resection arthroplasty group if the costoclavicular ligament was not preserved or reconstructed. Unfortunately, a control group (i.e., nonoperative treatment group) was not available for comparison in this study. In 2013, Guan and Wolf[79] reported good results at a mean follow-up of 40 months after reconstruction of the SC joint using a hamstring autograft in a series of six patients with either traumatic or atraumatic anterior instability (acute or chronic). In this small heterogeneous series, one surgical failure occurred at 4 years requiring revision surgery to achieve stabilization.

In 2012, Van Tongel et al.[205] conducted a survey regarding treatment options in acute and chronic symptomatic anterior SC dislocation among three groups of orthopedic surgeons (from a general orthopedic society and from two societies with a special interest in shoulder and elbow surgery). There were a total of 212 respondents (212 of 753, or a 28% response rate). The majority of these surgeons would not perform an open reduction in an acute situation if a closed reduction failed or redislocation occurred. Concerning the treatment for chronic symptomatic anterior SC dislocation, 60% of the respondents chose conservative treatment. However, the majority of the surgeons (34 of 48, or 71%) from the American Shoulder and Elbow Surgeons indicated they would perform open treatment (i.e., ligamentous reconstruction or medial clavicle excision) for a chronic symptomatic anterior SC dislocation.

More recently in 2014, two large series have been published reporting the surgical outcomes following stabilization of the SC joint for chronic anterior instability in both adult and skeletally immature patients. Bak and Fogh[6] evaluated the results of a minimally invasive surgical technique (combined anterior capsular reinforcement and interposition arthroplasty) using autograft tendon on 32 consecutive patients with recurrent subluxation and dislocation. Twenty-seven patients (84.4%) were available for at least 2 years' follow-up (range, 24–120 months). The total median postoperative Western Ontario Shoulder Instability Index scores significantly improved compared to the preoperative scores; two surgical failures occurred requiring revision, and 40% of the patients complained of donor site morbidity at their latest follow-up. Uri et al.[203] reported the surgical results of 32 patients who underwent surgical reconstruction of the SC joint for chronic symptomatic anterior instability using the tendon of the sternal head of the ipsilateral sternocleidomastoid muscle. The patients were followed for a mean of 40 months. The etiology of the instability was posttraumatic in 14 patients, generalized hyperlaxity in 7 patients, and degenerative instability in 11. Postoperatively, clinical scores (Oxford Instability Shoulder score and Subjective Shoulder Value) and pain rating improved significantly in all three patient groups to the same extent; however, three patients from the posttraumatic group (21.4%), one patient from the generalized hyperlaxity group (14.3%), and three patients from the degenerative group (27.3%) reported the joint as being "unstable" or had persistent functional limitations. No complications were reported.

Injuries in the Skeletally Immature

Anterior Physeal Injuries of the Medial Clavicle

Many so-called dislocations of the SC joint in adolescents and young adults (≤25 years) are not dislocations but physeal injuries. Anterior physeal injuries can be managed expectantly when the displacement is mild, as most of these injuries will heal uneventfully. In time, the remodeling process usually minimizes bone deformity or displacement. If an anterior physeal injury is more displaced, closed reduction is performed. The shoulders should be held back in a clavicular strap or figure-of-eight dressing for 3 to 4 weeks, even if the reduction is stable. Healing is prompt, and remodeling will occur at the site of the deformity.

Anterior Dislocation

Few reports exist in the literature of true anterior SC joint dislocation in the adolescent and young adult population. Friedrich et al.[65] reported a case of painful recurrent anterior-superior SC joint instability in an 18-year-old male. After failing nonoperative treatment, the patient underwent surgical reconstruction of the SC joint using gracilis tendon autograft and repair of the intra-articular disk ligament with a successful outcome. In 2013, Gil-Albarova et al.[74] reported two cases of surgically confirmed anterior dislocation of the SC joint without associated physeal injury. Both adolescent patients underwent open reduction and stabilization of the SC joint using nonabsorbable sutures in a figure-of-eight fashion, followed by anterior capsulorrhaphy. Short-term follow-up (range, 27–32 months) revealed acceptable results, but one patient could not return to competitive sport.

Traumatic Injuries: Posterior

Nonoperative Treatment

Sprain/Subluxation

The treatment of a mild sprain (type I) or subluxation (type II) injury will be discussed in the "Authors' Preferred Treatment" section.

Acute Dislocation

Posterior SC dislocations can be life-threatening injuries, and thus are considered a true orthopedic emergency.[59] As a general rule, when a posterior dislocation of the SC joint is suspected, the physician must examine the patient very carefully to rule out damage to the structures posterior to the joint, such as the trachea, esophagus, brachial plexus, great vessels, and lungs. A CT scan of both medial clavicles allows the physician to compare the injured side with the normal side. Occasionally, when vascular injuries are suspected, the CT scan needs to be combined with an arteriogram of the great vessels (Fig. 10-31).

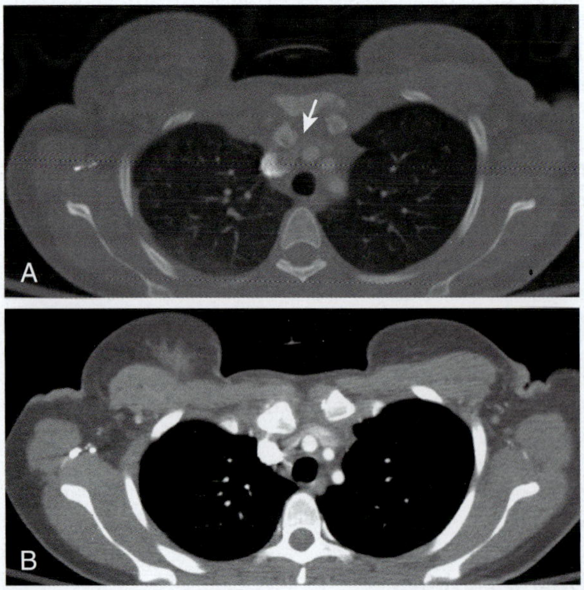

FIGURE 10-31: **A** and **B,** Computed tomographic scan with vascular contrast revealing a posterior dislocation of the right sternoclavicular joint with compression on the brachiocephalic vein.

Some posterior SC dislocations are successfully reduced closed if attempted within 24 to 48 hours of injury. Successful closed reduction after 48 hours is rare but has been noted even at 10 days postinjury.[78] Closed reduction should be performed in an operating room under general anesthesia with a cardiothoracic team immediately available.

Methods of Closed Reduction

Abduction Traction Technique

For the abduction traction technique (Fig. 10-32), the patient is placed on his or her back, with the affected shoulder near the edge of the table. A 3- to 4-inch-thick roll is placed between the shoulders. First, gentle traction is applied on the abducted arm in line with the clavicle while countertraction is applied by an assistant who steadies the patient on the table. The traction on the abducted arm is gradually increased while the arm is brought into extension. This may be all that is necessary to accomplish the reduction. The clavicle usually reduces with an audible snap or pop, and it is almost always

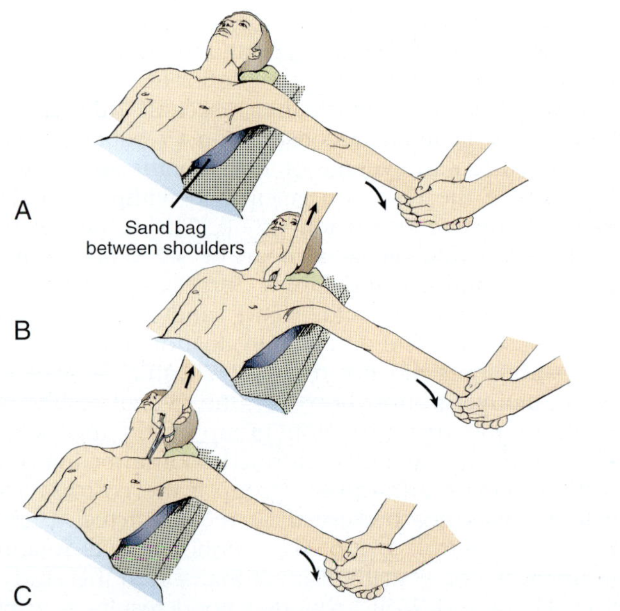

FIGURE 10-32: Technique of closed reduction of the sternoclavicular joint. **A,** The patient is positioned supine with a sandbag placed between the shoulders. Traction is then applied to the arm against countertraction in an abducted and slightly extended position. With anterior dislocations, direct pressure over the medial end of the clavicle can reduce the joint. **B,** With posterior dislocations, in addition to traction, it might be necessary to manipulate the medial end of the clavicle with the fingers to dislodge the clavicle from behind the manubrium. **C,** In stubborn cases of posterior dislocation, it may be necessary to sterilely prepare the medial end of the clavicle and use a towel clip to grasp around the medial clavicle to lift it back into position. (From Bucholz RW, Heckman JD, eds. *Rockwood and Green's Fractures in Adults.* 5th ed. Philadelphia: Lippincott Williams & Wilkins; 2001: 1264.)

stable. When traction alone is unsuccessful, closed reduction can be facilitated using a sterile towel clip or pointed reduction forceps (Fig. 10-33).

Adduction Traction Technique (Buckerfield and Castle Technique)

In this technique, the patient is supine on the table with a 3- to 4-inch bolster between the shoulders. Traction is then applied to the arm in adduction, while a posterior pressure is exerted on the shoulder. The clavicle is levered over the first rib into its normal position. Buckerfield and Castle[22] reported that this technique was successful in seven patients when the abduction traction technique had failed.

Operative Treatment

General Considerations

Once faced with the need for surgical stabilization of the joint, the surgeon must decide on one of the multiple techniques described to maintain the medial end of the clavicle in its normal articulation with the sternum. In general, most of these techniques can be used in the setting of either anterior or posterior instability, as the fundamental objective of each method is to stabilize the medial end of the clavicle. Surgical considerations not only include the tissue type (i.e., local tendon transfers vs. autograft or allograft tissue), but also the anatomic location of joint stabilization (i.e., stabilize to the first rib,

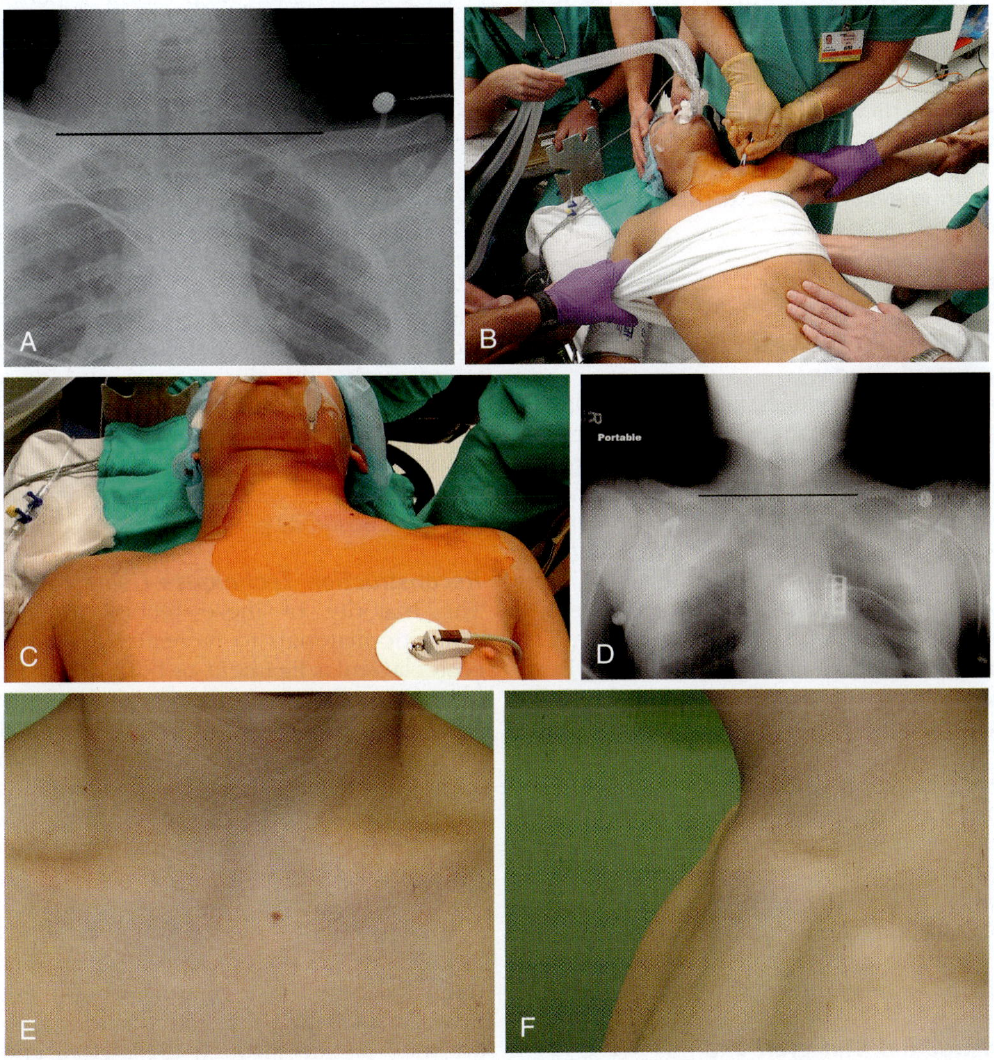

FIGURE 10-33: Posterior dislocation of the left sternoclavicular joint. **A,** The 40-degree cephalic tilt radiograph confirmed the presence of posterior displacement of the left medial clavicle in comparison with the right clavicle. **B,** We were unable to reduce the dislocation with simple traction on the arm. The left shoulder was surgically cleansed so that a sterile towel clip could be used. With the towel clip securely around the clavicle and with continued lateral traction, a visible and audible reduction occurred. **C,** Clinical appearance of the reduced left sternoclavicular joint. **D,** Postreduction radiograph showed that the medial part of the clavicle had been restored to its normal position. The reduction was quite stable, and the patient's shoulders were held back with a figure-of-eight strap. **E** and **F,** Clinical follow-up revealed that the left sternoclavicular joint remained reduced.

BOX 10-2. Surgical Techniques Used for Sternoclavicular Joint Stabilization

- Local tendon transfers using the subclavius tendon or sternocleidomastoid tendon
- Ligament reconstruction using autograft and allograft tissue
- Reconstruction techniques using synthetic materials
- Open reduction and internal fixation methods
- Interpositional arthroplasty
- Resection of the medial clavicle with or without costoclavicular ligament reconstruction

manubrium, or both). Among the plethora of surgical options available to stabilize the SC joint, more recent descriptions include "all-suture" techniques[195] and the use of specialized plate constructs.[62] Much like the AC joint, multiple surgical procedures have been described (Box 10-2); recent literature has focused on case series and case reports (level IV and V evidence) of technique descriptions and modifications of existing procedures, which are summarized below.

Reconstruction Techniques of the Sternoclavicular Joint

Local Tendon Transfers (Subclavius Tendon or Sternocleidomastoid Tendon)

In 1951, Burrows[23] recommended that the subclavius tendon be used to reconstruct a new costoclavicular ligament. In 1990, Tricoire et al.[197] reported six retrosternal dislocations of the medial end of the clavicle. Sternoclavicular joint capsulorrhaphy was performed in two patients and a subclavius tenodesis was used in the remaining four patients. All joints were temporarily stabilized with SC pins for 6 weeks. The results were satisfactory in all cases at a mean follow-up of 27 months.

Transfer of the sternocleidomastoid tendon has been revisited in different forms. Brown[21] used the clavicular head of the sternocleidomastoid as an anterior sling across the SC joint augmented with pins. Booth and Roper[17] described transferring the sternal head of the tendon around the first rib and through the clavicle and back upon itself. More recently, Armstrong and Dias[3] modified the sternocleidomastoid tendon transfer technique by using only a slip of the sternal head and passing it through a medial clavicle bone tunnel and back to the manubrium. The graft is sutured to itself to recreate the anterior SC ligament without exposure of the first rib.

Ligament Reconstruction (Autograft and Allograft Tissue)

Some of the earliest descriptions of soft tissue reconstruction of the SC joint involved the use of fascia lata. In 1928, Lowman[116] described using a loop of fascia in and through the SC joint, similar to the ligamentum teres in the hip (i.e., combination of ligament reconstruction and interposition arthroplasty). Bankart[7] used fascia lata between the clavicle and the sternum. Key and Conwell[105] reported on the use of a fascial loop between the clavicle and the first rib. In 1989, Eskola et al.[58] reported on 12 patients treated for painful chronic SC joint dislocation. The average time from injury was 1.5 years, and the average follow-up after surgery was 4.7 years. In five patients, the SC joint was stabilized with a palmaris longus or plantaris tendon graft placed from the medial clavicle to the first rib and the manubrium; in four patients, the medial 2.5 cm of the clavicle was resected without any type of stabilization; in three patients, the clavicle was fixed to the first rib with a fascia lata graft. They reported good results in four patients, three treated with tendon graft and one with a fascia lata graft. Another four patients had fair results, but all four patients treated with resection of the medial clavicle alone had poor results.

In 2004, Spencer and Kuhn[184] performed a biomechanical analysis of three different SC reconstruction techniques: a subclavius tendon reconstruction, an intramedullary ligament reconstruction, and a reconstruction with the use of a semitendinosus graft (placed in a figure-of-eight fashion through drill holes in the clavicle and manubrium). Each of the three reconstruction methods was subjected to anterior and posterior translation forces until failure, and the changes in stiffness compared statistically with the intact state. The figure-of-eight semitendinosus reconstruction demonstrated superior initial mechanical properties to the other two techniques. Spencer and Kuhn stated that this method reconstructs both the anterior and posterior joint capsules, providing an initial stiffness that is closer to that of the intact SC joint. This technique has now been reported with some success in young adults and in skeletally immature patients with refractory anterior and posterior instability.[4,28,147,178]

Reconstruction Techniques Using Synthetic Materials

The majority of these techniques use a variety of synthetic materials to recreate the capsular ligaments or costoclavicular ligament or both, in a figure-of-eight configuration or modification thereof. Thomas et al.[195] reported a safe surgical technique for stabilization of the SC joint using suture material. Their technique involved tying the suture material on the superficial aspects of the medial clavicle and manubrium. This avoids the exposure of the first rib and avoids drilling through the inner cortex of the clavicle and manubrium. Abiddin et al.[1] described a similar technique using suture anchors in the manubrium and drill holes in the clavicle. In 2010, Rotini et al.[161] described using a hybrid fixation technique for a traumatic anterior SC joint dislocation. Suture anchors are first placed within the manubrium; transosseous sutures are then passed through the medial end of the clavicle and secured through holes of a "rotator cuff miniplate" that is stabilized on the medial clavicle. More recent surgical techniques have been described with varying results using a polydioxanone ligament,[68] sternal tension cable system,[94] nonabsorbable synthetic ligament ("artificial ligament weave"),[146] and combined suture-ligament constructs.[66]

Open Reduction and Internal Fixation

Plate constructs are being used increasingly to manage unstable SC joint injuries. Franck et al.[62] reported using a plate (i.e., Balser plate) for traumatic SC joint instability. The plate was contoured to match the shape of the medial clavicle, and the hook of the plate was used for sternal fixation. A retrosternal hook position was used for seven anterior dislocations, and an intrasternal position was used for three posterior dislocations. For each patient, the plate was attached to the clavicle with screws and the torn ligaments were repaired. All plates were removed by 3 months. At the 1-year follow-up, 9 of 10 patients had excellent results with no cases of redislocation. One patient developed a postoperative seroma that required surgical drainage, and one patient developed arthrosis (Fig. 10-34). Using a similar technique, Hecox and Wood[84] described the use of a "ledge plate" for an unstable posterior SC joint dislocation. A standard 3.5-mm LC/DCP plate is contoured and fixed to the medial clavicle in a position that allows two holes of the plate to serve as a "ledge" over the manubrium. Two other plate techniques have recently been described. Shuler and Pappas[176] used two 3.5-mm locking reconstruction plates placed at 90 degrees across the SC joint for an unstable posterior dislocation. Pensy and Eglseder[141] described the use of combined suture anchor fixation and a long pelvic reconstruction plate that was contoured to the ipsilateral clavicle, manubrium, and contralateral clavicle for a posterior SC joint fracture-dislocation. No screws were placed in the manubrium, and fixation was achieved with three screws placed in each clavicle; after 5 months, the hardware was removed.

Interpositional Arthroplasty

Interpositional arthroplasty techniques have also emerged in recent years. Battaglia et al.[10] presented three cases of an Achilles tendon allograft and bone plug used to treat anterior instability in two patients and a medial clavicle fracture nonunion in one. The graft was placed within a bony trough created after medial clavicle excision and fixed with screws. The graft was then passed through bone tunnels in the manubrium and sutured upon itself. Meis et al.[124] reported using an intramedullary transfer of the sternocleidomastoid tendon as an interposition material after medial clavicle excision in patients with degenerative disease of the SC joint.

Combined Osteotomy of the Medial Clavicle and Ligament Repair

As described by Omer in 1967,[134] the SC ligaments are repaired and a step-cut osteotomy is made lateral to the SC joint to minimize stress on the reconstruction. The author also recommends releasing the clavicular head of the sternocleidomastoid muscle from the proximal fragment.

Resection of the Medial Clavicle (With and Without Costoclavicular Ligament Reconstruction)

Several authors have recommended excision of the medial clavicle when secondary degenerative changes are noted in the joint.[9,19,125] If the medial end of the clavicle is to be removed because of degenerative changes secondary to chronic instability, the surgeon must be careful not to damage the costoclavicular ligament, and when necessary should reconstruct this ligament.[156] Bisson et al.[15] performed an anatomic study using 86 cadavers, and recommended a resection length of the medial clavicle of no more than 1 cm in men and 0.9 cm in women to minimize disruption of the costoclavicular ligament. These findings have since been confirmed in an anatomic study performed by Lee et al.[110]

Arthrodesis

Arthrodesis was once reported[152] in the treatment of habitual dislocation of the SC joint. However, this procedure should *not* be performed because it prevents the previously described normal elevation, depression, and rotation of the clavicle. The end result would be severe restriction of shoulder movement.

Injuries in the Skeletally Immature

Acute Posterior Physeal Injuries of the Medial Clavicle

Physeal injuries can be more difficult to reduce than true dislocations of the SC joint.[111,212] Laffosse et al.[108] suggested that the closed reduction is hampered by the metaphyseal spike of the type II Salter-Harris fracture line. Furthermore, cases of redislocation may occur unexpectedly, even when the surgeon is confident of the intraoperative stability; late recurrences even after 1 week have been reported.[108] Fortunately, the vast majority of these injuries will remodel and rarely require surgery. However, if the posterior displacement is symptomatic and cannot be reduced by closed means, the displacement must be reduced surgically with repair or

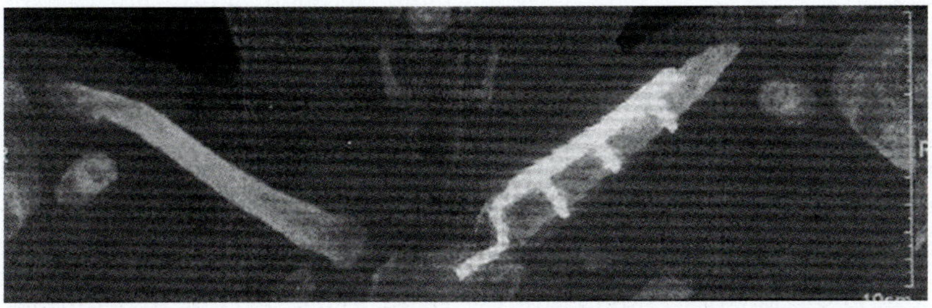

FIGURE 10-34: Computed tomography of the chest showing intrasternal placement of a Balser plate. (From Franck WM, Jannasch O, Siassi M, et al. Balser plate stabilization: an alternate therapy for traumatic sternoclavicular instability. *J Shoulder Elbow Surg.* 2003;12:276-281.)

reconstruction of the SC joint. Waters et al.[212] reported successful operative treatment of 13 traumatic posterior SC fracture-dislocations in children and adolescents, and other authors have also reported successful open treatment of similar injuries in adolescents.[111]

Chronic Posterior Physeal Injuries of the Medial Clavicle

Controversy persists in young adults and adolescents who have mild symptoms and present with chronic posterior physeal dislocations. In this situation, the physician can wait to see if the physeal plate remodeling process removes the posteriorly displaced bone; however, the potential for late complications must be emphasized, and patients should be followed clinically at regular intervals for several years. Zaslav et al.[221] reported on a 13-year-old male with a late presentation of a posterior physeal injury. At 6 months postinjury, the patient was asymptomatic and had complete remodeling on CT. In contrast, Emms et al.[54] reported on a subclavian thrombosis that occurred 2 years after the initial injury that was treated nonoperatively for what was originally diagnosed as a posterior subluxation. The patient had a new injury at 2 years, which precipitated vascular symptoms 3 weeks later, and CT revealed evidence of a remodeled medial physeal injury. The patient required a first rib resection to decompress the subclavian vein. Carbone et al.[26] reported a similar case of superior vena cava obstruction after abnormal remodeling (i.e., "asymmetric enlargement of the medial clavicle") following a medial physeal fracture, and a second injury precipitated the occlusion.

Posterior Dislocation (Acute and Chronic)

As previously discussed, posterior SC dislocations can occur in isolation without associated physeal fracture of the medial clavicle.[108,111,193,212] True posterior dislocations in the skeletally immature population are managed similarly to their adult counterparts. The only difference exists with respect to methods of surgical stabilization of the SC joint in skeletally immature patients; care should be taken to preserve the medial physis when at all possible.

Atraumatic Disorders

Spontaneous Subluxation or Dislocation (Anterior and Posterior)

As with glenohumeral joint instability, the importance of distinguishing between traumatic and atraumatic instability of the SC joint must be recognized if complications are to be avoided. Rowe[162] described several patients who had undergone one or more unsuccessful attempts to stabilize the SC joint. In all cases, the patient could voluntarily dislocate the clavicle after surgery.

Crosby and Rubino[42] reported a case of spontaneous atraumatic anterior dislocation secondary to pseudarthrosis of the first and second ribs. Despite a 6-month course of conservative treatment, this 14-year-old girl was still experiencing pain. A 3D CT scan of the chest revealed a pseudarthrosis anteriorly between the first and second ribs lying adjacent to the posterior aspect of the medial clavicle. Resection of the anterior portion of the first and second rib pseudarthrosis relieved her symptoms, and allowed her to return to her normal activities.

Spontaneous posterior subluxation or dislocation have only been noted in a few isolated case reports. Martin et al.[120] described a case of spontaneous atraumatic posterior dislocation of the SC joint. This occurred in a 50-year-old previously healthy woman who awoke one morning with a painful SC joint. A CT scan confirmed the posterior dislocation. She later developed dysphagia, and a closed reduction was unsuccessful. After 1 year without any other treatment, she was back to playing golf and was asymptomatic. More recently, Martinez et al.[121] described a 19-year-old woman with a symptomatic spontaneous posterior SC subluxation who was managed surgically. The posteriorly displaced medial clavicle was stabilized with a figure-of-eight soft tissue reconstruction using a gracilis autograft. At the 12-month follow-up, the patient was pain free; however, a repeat CT scan demonstrated posterior subluxation of the medial clavicle, with erosion of the clavicle and manubrium.

In our experience, spontaneous subluxations and dislocations of the SC joint are usually associated with laxity in other joints of the extremities. Rockwood and Odor[157] previously reviewed 37 cases, and reported a high incidence of operative complications, including recurrent instability and persistent or worsening pain.

Arthritis

Management of patients with OA, RA, condensing osteitis, and other inflammatory arthropathies can usually be accomplished with nonoperative treatment, including rest and activity modification, heat, and antiinflammatory agents (oral NSAIDs and corticosteroid injections). However, the patient must be thoroughly evaluated to rule out other conditions that mimic degenerative changes in the SC joint (i.e., tumor, metabolic, infectious, or collagen disorders). Patients with posttraumatic arthritic changes in the SC joint after fracture and previous attempts at reconstruction may require formal excision arthroplasty of the joint and careful stabilization of the remaining clavicle to the first rib. When performing an SC joint resection, 1 to 1.5 cm of the clavicle is resected, being careful to stay medial.

Pingsmann et al.[142] reported on the midterm results in eight women who did not respond to conservative therapy and underwent surgical treatment for primary arthritis of the SC joint. After limited resection of the medial clavicle and preservation of the costoclavicular and IC ligaments, they reported an improvement in symptoms and a low risk of complications.

Infection

Infections of the SC joint are managed as they are in other joints, except that during aspiration and surgical drainage, great care and respect must be directed to the vital structures that lie posterior to the joint. If aspiration demonstrates purulent material in the joint or the orthopedist has a high index of suspicion, formal arthrotomy is carried out. Arthrotomy is especially important with SC septic arthritis because of the significant risk of abscess formation in up to 20% of cases and the concern for subsequent spread of the infection to the mediastinal structures.[219] Care should be taken to preserve all supporting ligamentous structures when possible; only necrotic tissue is debrided. Occasionally, the infection arises in the medial end of the clavicle or the manubrium, or there is spread of the infection from the joint space into the adjacent bone, which necessitates resection of any necrotic bone.[38,133] Depending on the status of the wound after debridement, one can either close the wound loosely over a drain, pack the wound open followed by daily wound care (i.e., secondary intention) with or without negative-pressure wound therapy,[145] or close the wound at a later time (i.e., tertiary intention).

In 2002, Song et al.[181] presented seven patients who had SC joint infections. Predisposing factors included diabetes mellitus, HIV infection, immunosuppression, and pustular skin disease. All patients had local symptoms, including a medial clavicular mass and swelling. Antibiotic therapy and simple drainage and debridement were generally ineffective, with recurrence of infection in five patients. The patients were subsequently treated by resection of the SC joint and the involved portions of adjacent ribs with an advancement flap from the pectoralis major muscle. The response to therapy was excellent in all patients, and there were no wound complications. More recently, Joethy et al.[97] described a classification of postresection SC joint defects, and proposed a reconstructive algorithm based on the residual defect and vascularity of the wound bed.

Disorders Specific to the Sternoclavicular Joint

Most of these disorders are self-limiting, and treatment is directed at controlling local symptoms. For condensing osteitis, most patients do well with conservative treatment; however, Kruger et al.[107] recommend incisional or excisional biopsy in refractory cases. Patients diagnosed with SAPHO syndrome should be managed in conjunction with a rheumatologist. First-line treatments include NSAIDs, analgesics, and intra-articular corticosteroids. Other medications used include antibiotics, bisphosphonates, and immunosuppressant drugs (methotrexate, cyclosporine, and biologics). Wide excision of the ossified mass has been described for refractory cases, with limited success.[27]

AUTHORS' PREFERRED METHOD OF TREATMENT

Anterior Sternoclavicular Joint Injuries

Sprain/Subluxation

The initial treatment of a mild sprain (type I) or subluxation (type II) injury is nonoperative, and includes NSAIDs and ice. If an attempt is made to reduce the joint by drawing the shoulders backward, the deformity may be accentuated; for this reason, we rarely attempt closed reduction. A sling or shoulder immobilizer is used for support and comfort and to prevent further injury for 4 to 6 weeks.

Anterior Dislocation

In general, we manage acute anterior dislocations of the SC joint in adults by "skillful neglect" as most are unstable after closed reduction; therefore we accept the deformity since we believe it is less of a problem than the potential problems of operative repair and internal fixation. In contrast, we attempt a closed reduction in the skeletally immature population. In cases where symptoms persist and no other recourse exists outside of surgical management, the preferred technique is figure-of-eight ligament reconstruction as described in the section below.

Posterior Sternoclavicular Joint Injuries

Sprain/Subluxation

In mild sprains (type I) and subluxations (type II), the joint will be swollen and tender to palpation. Care must be taken to rule out the more significant posterior dislocation, which might have initially occurred and spontaneously reduced. When in doubt, it is best to protect the SC joint with a figure-of-eight bandage for 4 to 6 weeks and to repeat the CT imaging if symptoms persist.

Posterior Dislocation

It is important to obtain a thorough history, perform a careful physical examination, and obtain advanced imaging studies in all patients with a suspected posterior SC dislocation (Fig. 10-35). Without question, the CT scan is the best means to study injuries of the SC joint. While plain films may be suggestive of the nature of the injury, it is critical that a CT scan is obtained for the superior specificity and sensitivity of this study in the diagnosis of SC joint pathology. It is important to image both SC joints and the medial half of both clavicles so that the injured side can be compared with the normal side. The ability to reformat CT data to reconstruct various imaging planes (i.e., 3D reformatting) has been very helpful, particularly in preoperative planning (Fig. 10-36). If the patient has distention of the neck vessels, swelling of the arm, a bluish discoloration of the arm, or difficulty swallowing or breathing, the patient should be imaged with a contrast-enhanced CT scan and the appropriate cardiovascular or thoracic consult obtained (see Fig. 10-35).

Although we once thought that the diagnosis of an anterior or posterior injury of the SC joint could always be made on physical examination, one cannot rely on the anterior swelling and firmness as being diagnostic of an anterior injury. This reinforces our recommendation that the clinical impression always be supported with appropriate imaging studies, preferably a CT scan, to facilitate the treatment decision-making process.

We do not believe that open techniques are usually required to reduce *acute* posterior SC joint dislocations;

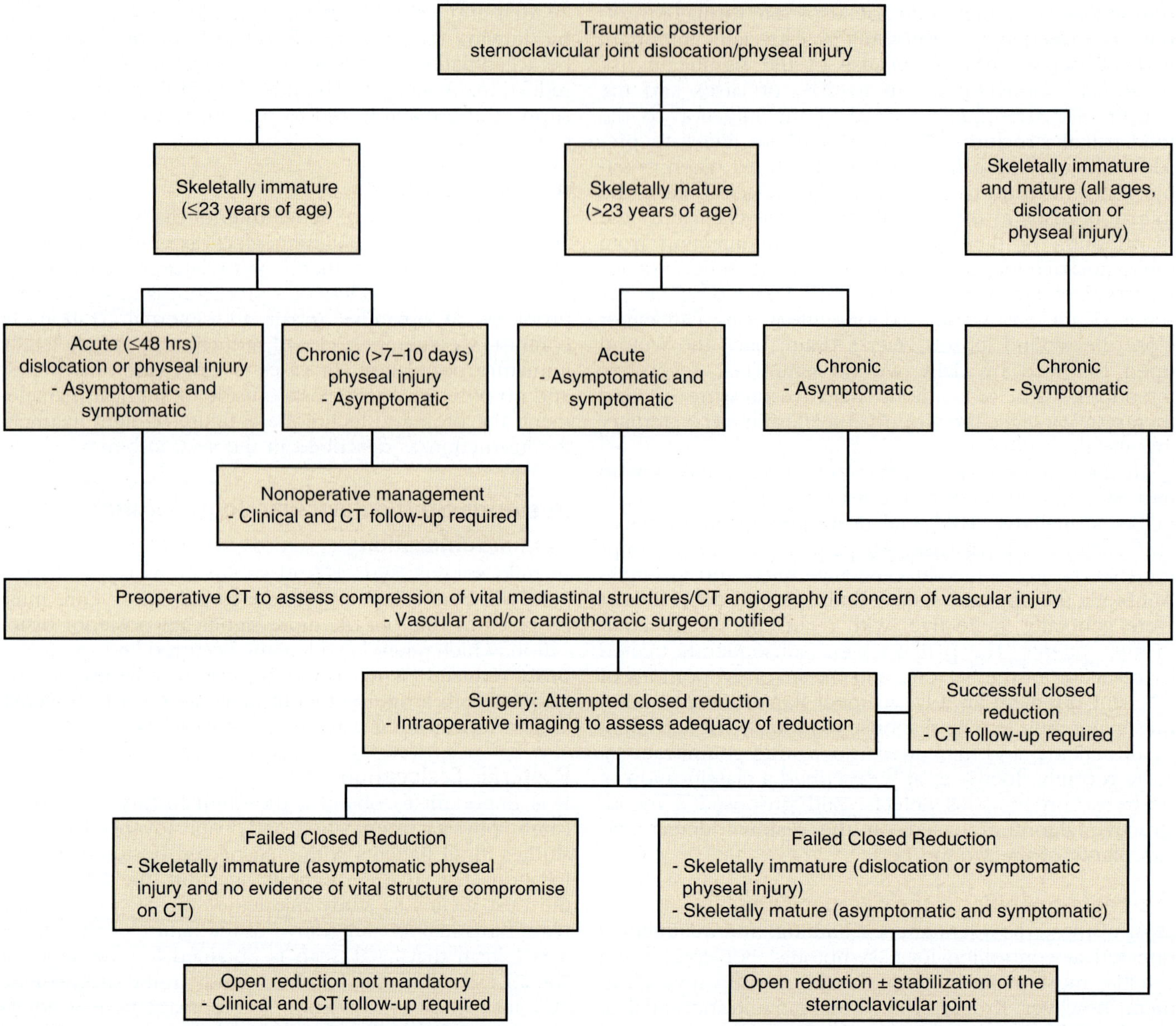

FIGURE 10-35: Treatment algorithm for traumatic posterior sternoclavicular joint dislocations or physeal injuries. *CT*, computed tomography. (Modified from Court-Brown CM, Heckman JD, McQueen MM, et al. *Rockwood and Green's Fractures in Adults*. 8th ed. Philadelphia: Lippincott Williams & Wilkins; 2015: 1631.)

however, the patient should always be consented for possible open reduction prior to the procedure in case closed reduction fails.

Method of Closed Reduction and Postreduction Care

Closed reduction of a posteriorly dislocated SC joint is performed in the operating room using the methods of closed reduction outlined previously (see Fig. 10-32). After the joint is reduced, we recommend supporting the shoulders in a gently retracted position using a well-padded figure-of-eight clavicle strap for 4 to 6 weeks to allow for soft tissue and ligamentous healing, even when the reduction is quite stable in the operating room.

Open Surgical Techniques

When considering operative intervention, the surgeon must decide whether to maintain the medial end of the clavicle and repair or reconstruct the surrounding ligaments or resect the medial 1 cm of the clavicle and anatomically stabilize the remaining clavicle to the first rib.[156] Resection alone cannot be performed in the setting of disrupted ligaments, as doing so may worsen the instability of the residual medial clavicle.[14,58]

It is also important to consider the timing of the surgery as the surrounding tissues scar to the posterior clavicle within 1 to 2 weeks of injury, which increases the risk of vascular injury during the reduction maneuver.[50,119,123] In these cases, it is especially critical to obtain

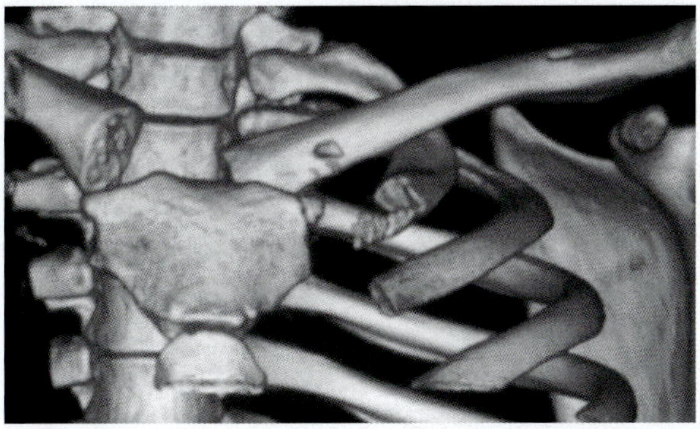

FIGURE 10-36: Three-dimensional CT scan revealing a posterior left sternoclavicular joint dislocation. Note the medial aspect of the clavicle posterior to the manubrium.

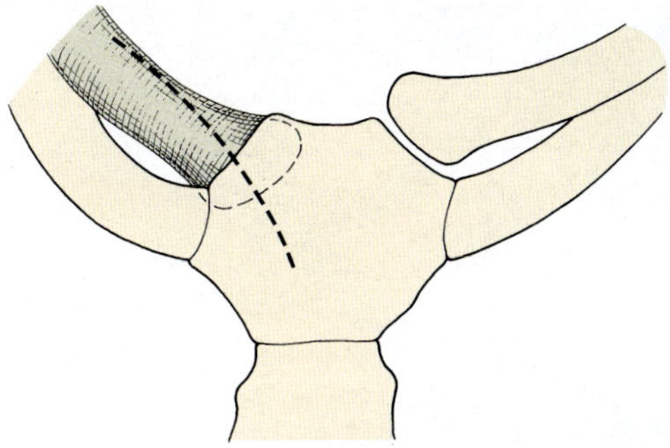

FIGURE 10-37: Proposed skin incision for open reduction of a posterior sternoclavicular dislocation.

a CT angiogram preoperatively to assess the vascular status and be prepared for vascular and/or cardiothoracic surgical assistance in the operating room.

The complications of an unreduced posterior dislocation are numerous: thoracic outlet syndrome, vascular compromise, and erosion of the medial clavicle into any of the vital mediastinal structures that lie posterior to the SC joint. Therefore in adults and in skeletally immature patients with posterior dislocations or symptomatic posterior physeal injuries, if closed reduction fails, an open reduction should be performed. It is critical that a vascular and/or cardiothoracic surgeon be immediately available when the patient is taken to the operating room to intervene if needed (see Fig. 10-35).

Acute Ligamentous Repair

The patient is positioned supine on a radiolucent operating table, and three or four towels or sandbags are placed between the scapulae. The upper extremity is draped out free so that lateral traction can be applied during the open reduction. An anterior incision is used that parallels the superior border of the medial 5 to 7 cm of the clavicle and then extends downward over the sternum just medial to the involved SC joint (Fig. 10-37). Skin flaps are elevated and the periosteum is incised in a horizontal fashion. Care is taken to preserve the anterior capsular ligament for later repair and closure (Fig. 10-38). The reduction can usually be accomplished with traction and countertraction while lifting up anteriorly with a sterile towel clamp or pointed reduction forceps around the medial clavicle. Occasionally, it may be necessary to use a blunt elevator to gently lever the clavicle back to its articulation with the manubrium (Fig. 10-39). Along with the intra-articular disk ligament, the posterior capsule is then incorporated into a running locking suture using No. 2 Ethibond (Johnson & Johnson) (Fig. 10-40). Drill holes are then passed through the clavicle from anterior to posterior, taking care to protect the neurovascular structures by passing a curved Crego or ribbon retractor around the posterior aspect of the medial clavicle. A Hewson suture passer is used to shuttle sutures from posterior to anterior through the clavicle (Fig. 10-41). Any

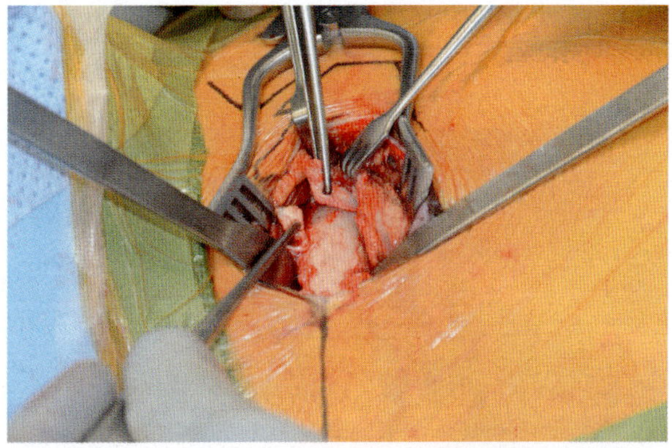

FIGURE 10-38: Initial elevation of the periosteum and capsule (held in forceps) and exposure of the medial clavicle (clinical example of right posterior sternoclavicular joint dislocation; patient's head at left of image). (From Court-Brown CM, Heckman JD, McQueen MM, et al, eds. *Rockwood and Green's Fractures in Adults*. 8th ed. Philadelphia, Lippincott Williams & Wilkins; 2015: 1632.)

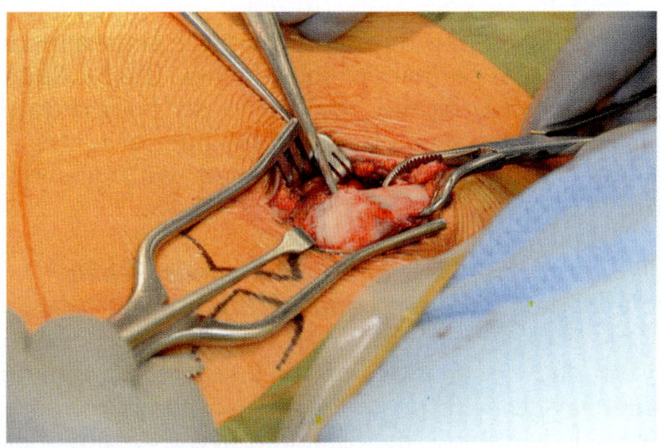

FIGURE 10-39: Elevation and open reduction of the medial clavicle with a reduction clamp (right sternoclavicular joint, viewed superiorly; patient's head at bottom right of image). (From Court-Brown CM, Heckman JD, McQueen MM, et al, eds. *Rockwood and Green's Fractures in Adults*. 8th ed. Philadelphia, Lippincott Williams & Wilkins; 2015: 1633.)

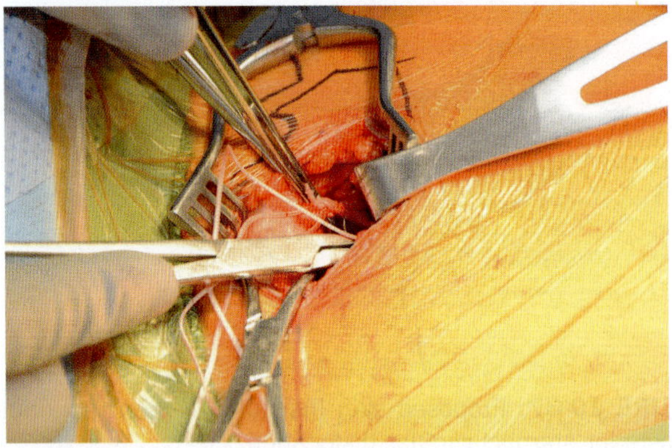

FIGURE 10-40: Grasping suture in the posterior capsule and intra-articular disk ligament (patient's head at left of image). (From Court-Brown CM, Heckman JD, McQueen MM, et al, eds. *Rockwood and Green's Fractures in Adults*. 8th ed. Philadelphia, Lippincott Williams & Wilkins; 2015:1633.)

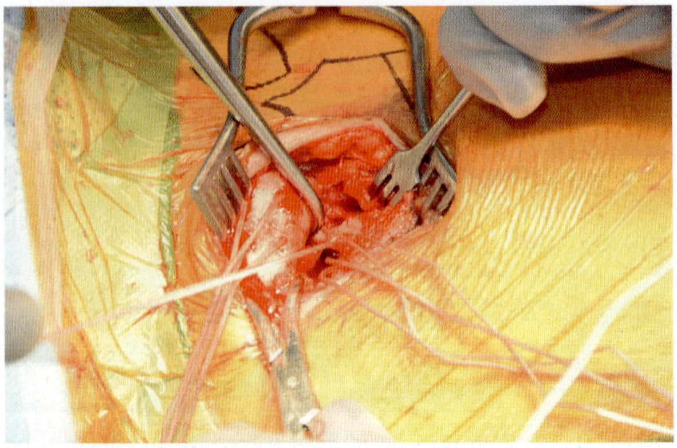

FIGURE 10-42: Repair of a posterior capsule defect with interrupted sutures (patient's head at left of image). (From Court-Brown CM, Heckman JD, McQueen MM, et al, eds. *Rockwood and Green's Fractures in Adults*. 8th ed. Philadelphia, Lippincott Williams & Wilkins; 2015: 1633.)

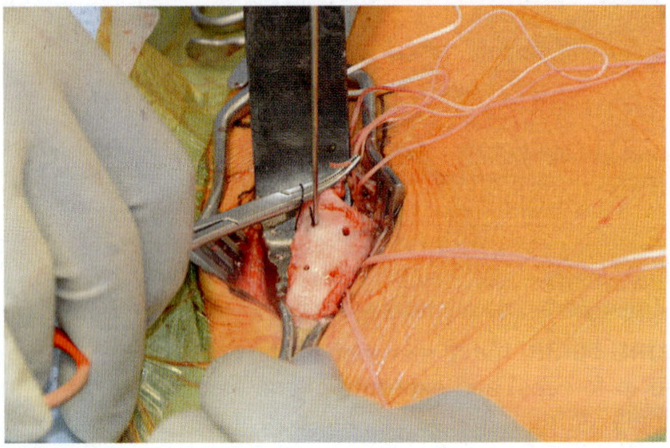

FIGURE 10-41: Drill holes through clavicle for the purpose of transosseous repair (patient's head at left of image). (From Court-Brown CM, Heckman JD, McQueen MM, et al. eds. *Rockwood and Green's Fractures in Adults*. 8th ed. Philadelphia, Lippincott Williams & Wilkins; 2015: 1633.)

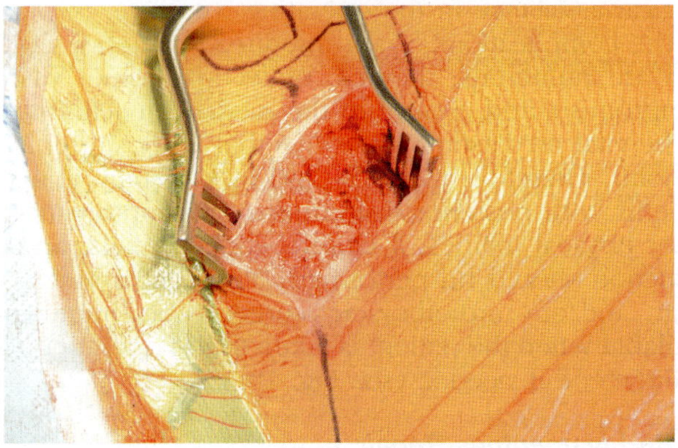

FIGURE 10-43: Completed repair after transosseous secured suture (patient's head at left of image). (From Court-Brown CM, Heckman JD, McQueen MM, et al, eds. *Rockwood and Green's Fractures in Adults*. 8th ed. Philadelphia, Lippincott Williams & Wilkins; 2015: 1634.)

remaining defect in the posterior capsule is then repaired with interrupted permanent sutures (Fig. 10-42). After the capsular defect is closed, the previously passed transosseous sutures are secured along the anterior cortex. The remaining capsular sleeve is closed with absorbable sutures to complete the repair (Fig. 10-43).

Resection Arthroplasty and Ligamentous Repair (Technique of Rockwood and Wirth)

In some situations, the medical clavicle may need to be excised. These scenarios include a severely comminuted medial clavicle with posterior displacement, pressure on the vessels within the mediastinum in the setting of acute trauma or in the chronic setting of posttraumatic degenerative arthritis of the SC joint. When the medial clavicle is excised, the SC joint is less stable, and the reconstruction can be reinforced by securing the residual clavicle to the first rib with 1-mm Dacron tape. The medial clavicle is exposed by careful subperiosteal dissection (Fig. 10-44). When possible, any remnants of the capsular or intra-articular disk ligaments are identified and preserved because these structures can be used to help stabilize the medial clavicle. The capsular ligaments are primarily attached to the epiphysis of the medial clavicle, and are usually avulsed from this structure with posterior SC dislocations. Similarly, the intra-articular disk ligament is usually avulsed from its attachment site on the medial clavicle. If the sternal attachment site of these ligaments are intact, nonabsorbable 1-mm cottony Dacron sutures are woven back and forth through the disk ligament so that the end of the sutures exits through the avulsed free end of the tissue. The medial 1 cm of the clavicle is resected while protecting the posterior structures with a ribbon retractor and preserving any remnants of the costoclavicular (rhomboid) ligament, which can be used to reinforce the repair.

Excision of the medial clavicle is facilitated by creating drill holes through both cortices of the clavicle at the intended site of clavicular osteotomy. Following this step, an air drill with a side-cutting bur is used to complete the osteotomy (Fig. 10-45). The anterior and superior corners of the clavicle are beveled smooth with an air bur for cosmetic purposes. The medullary canal of the medial clavicle is drilled and curetted to receive the transferred intra-articular disk ligament (Fig. 10-46). Two small drill holes are then placed in the superior cortex of the medial clavicle, approximately 1 cm lateral to the site of resection (Fig. 10-47). These holes communicate with the medullary canal, and will be used to secure the suture in the transferred ligament. The free ends of the suture are passed into the medullary canal of the medial clavicle and out the two small drill holes in the superior cortex of the clavicle (Fig. 10-48). While the clavicle is held in a reduced AP position in relation to the first rib and sternum, the sutures are used to pull the ligament tightly into the medullary canal of the clavicle. The suture is then tied over a bone bridge, thus securing the transferred ligament into the clavicle.

The stabilization procedure is completed by passing five or six 1-mm cotton Dacron sutures around the reflected periosteal tube, the clavicle, and any of the residual underlying costoclavicular ligament and periosteum on the dorsal surface of the first rib (Fig. 10-49); the intent of these sutures is to anatomically restore the normal space between the clavicle and the rib.

In 1997, Rockwood et al.[156] reported on a series of 15 patients who had undergone a resection of the medial end of the clavicle. The patients were divided into two groups:

Group 1: Those who underwent resection of the medial end of the clavicle with maintenance or reconstruction of the costoclavicular ligament (seven patients)

Group 2: Those who had a resection without maintaining or reconstructing the costoclavicular ligament (eight patients)

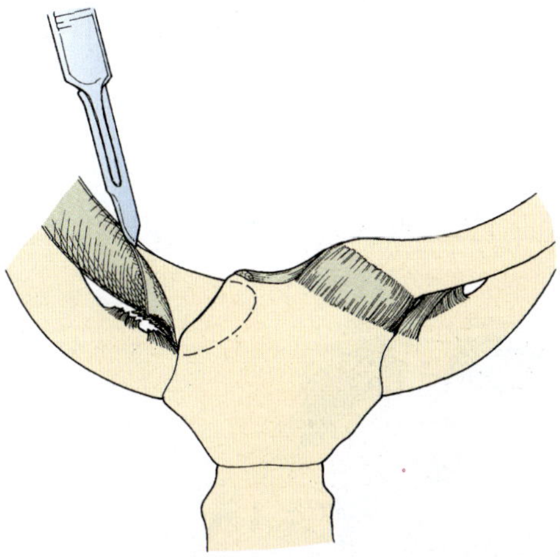

FIGURE 10-44: Subperiosteal exposure of the medial end of the clavicle. Note the posteriorly displaced medial clavicle. (From Bucholz RW, Heckman JD, eds. *Rockwood and Green's Fractures in Adults*. 5th ed. Philadelphia: Lippincott Williams & Wilkins; 2001: 1276.)

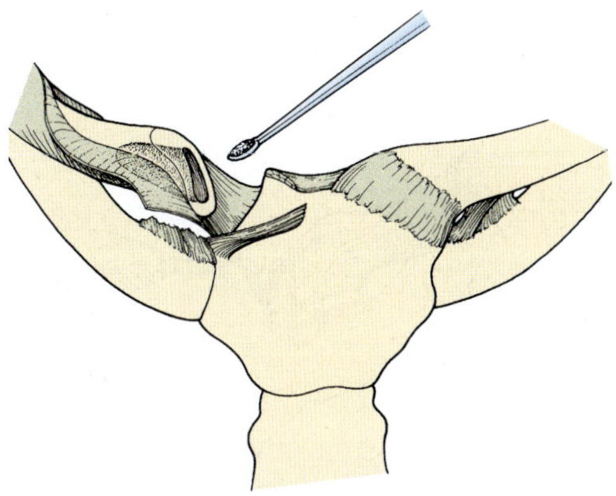

FIGURE 10-46: The medullary canal of the medial clavicle is prepared with a curette to receive the transferred sternoclavicular capsular ligament. (From Bucholz RW, Heckman JD, eds. *Rockwood and Green's Fractures in Adults*. 5th ed. Philadelphia: Lippincott Williams & Wilkins; 2001: 1276.)

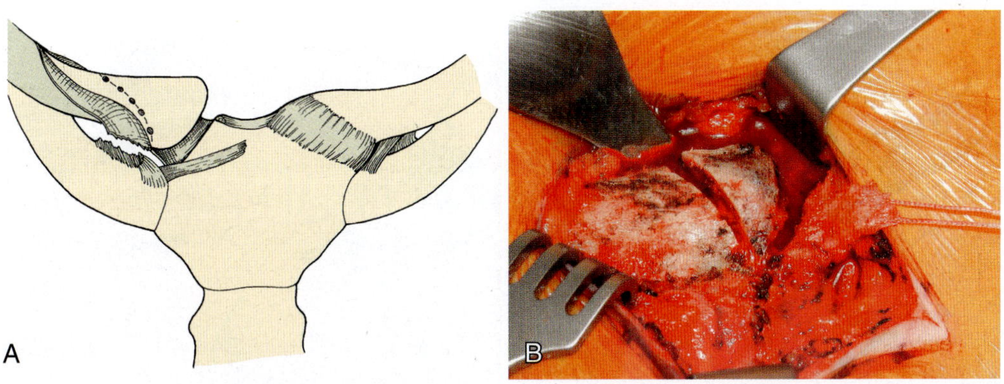

FIGURE 10-45: **A,** Excision of the medial clavicle is facilitated by drilling holes at the intended site of osteotomy. **B,** Intraoperative image following osteotomy of the right medial clavicle (patient's head at top of image) and identification of the intra-articular disk ligament avulsed from its attachment on the medial clavicle that is tagged with sutures. (**B,** Courtesy Charles E. Rosipal, MD, and R. Michael Gross, MD.)

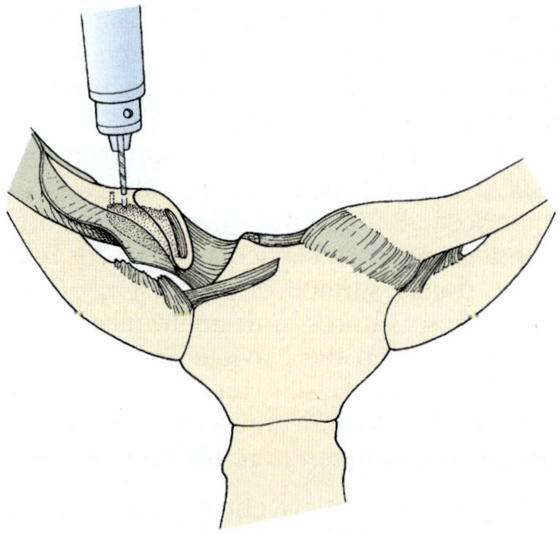

FIGURE 10-47: Drill holes are placed in the superior cortex of the clavicle approximately 1 cm lateral to the osteotomy site. (From Bucholz RW, Heckman JD, eds. *Rockwood and Green's Fractures in Adults*. 5th ed. Philadelphia: Lippincott Williams & Wilkins; 2001: 1277.)

The outcome in all but one of the seven patients in group 2 was poor, with persistence or worsening of preoperative symptoms (Fig. 10-50). The only patient of this group with a successful result suffered a posterior epiphyseal separation in which the costoclavicular ligament remained attached to the periosteum, thus preventing instability. All of the eight patients in group 1 who had a primary surgical resection of the medial end of the clavicle with maintenance of the costoclavicular ligaments had excellent results. When the operation was performed as a revision of a previous procedure with reconstruction of the costoclavicular ligaments, the results were less successful, but only one patient of seven was not satisfied with the outcome of the treatment.

Surgical Reconstruction With Graft (Figure-of-Eight Technique)

When the medial clavicle is intact we prefer the reconstruction method described by Spencer et al. for its superior biomechanical characteristics (Fig. 10-51).[185]

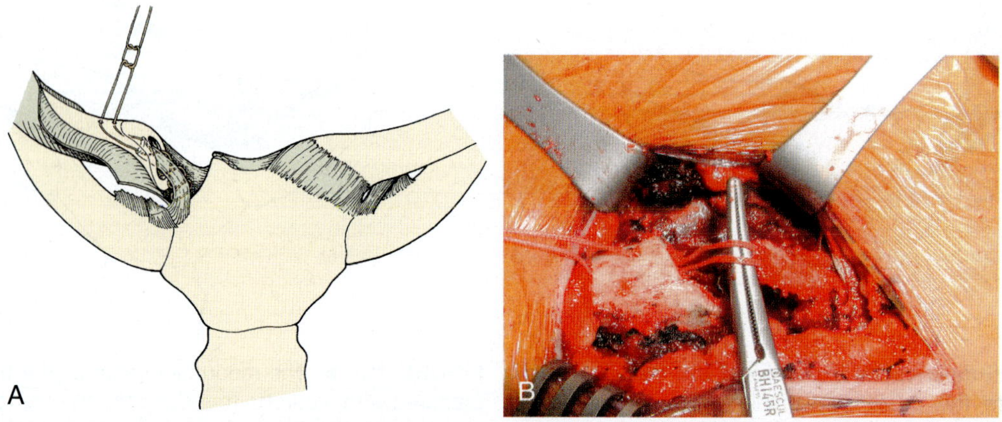

FIGURE 10-48: **A** and **B,** The free ends of the suture are passed into the medullary canal and out the two holes in the superior cortex. (**A,** From Bucholz RW, Heckman JD, eds. *Rockwood and Green's Fractures in Adults*. 5th ed. Philadelphia: Lippincott Williams & Wilkins; 2001: 1277. **B,** Courtesy Charles E. Rosipal, MD, and R. Michael Gross, MD.)

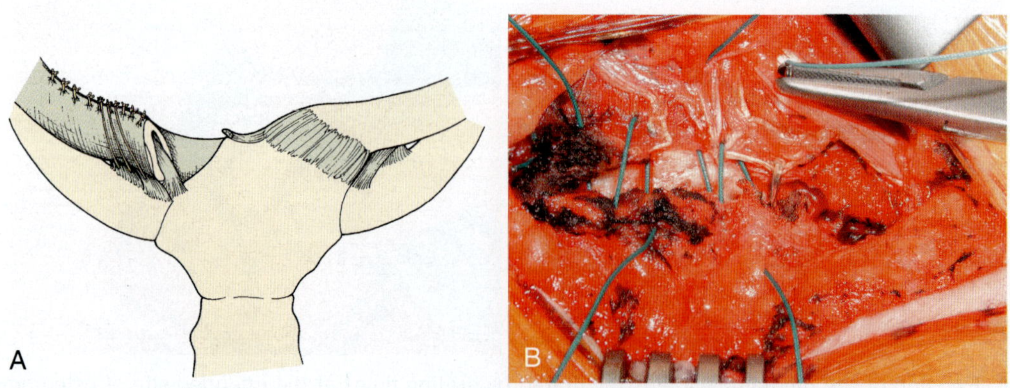

FIGURE 10-49: **A** and **B,** Closure of the periosteal sleeve around the medial clavicle and secure fixation of these structures to the costoclavicular ligament. (**A,** From Bucholz RW, Heckman JD, eds. *Rockwood and Green's Fractures in Adults*. 5th ed. Philadelphia: Lippincott Williams & Wilkins; 2001: 1277. **B,** Courtesy Charles E. Rosipal, MD, and R. Michael Gross, MD.)

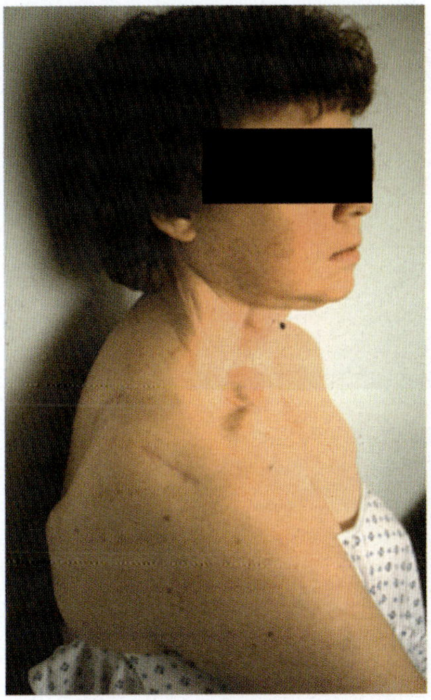

FIGURE 10-50: A 46-year-old patient with increased pain and an unsightly scar following medial clavicle resection that compromised the costoclavicular ligament. Note the postoperative scapular winging, which was associated with fatigue and spasm of the scapular-stabilizing musculature.

There are several key technical points to emphasize: (1) use of allograft over autograft tendon tissue to avoid the risk of donor site morbidity[6]; (2) proper sizing of the allograft tissue to ensure that the drill hole diameter matches the graft size; (3) use of a smaller tendon graft such as the gracilis tendon for smaller patients with smaller clavicular diameters; (4) avoid placement of drill holes too close to the end of the medial clavicle (i.e., careful drill hole position); and (5) avoid creating a large tendon knot anteriorly, which can be unsightly and symptomatic. Ensuring proper drill hole size and position is critical as the drill holes required for this technique weaken the bone and can lead to a stress fracture (Fig. 10-52).

Postoperative Care of Posterior Dislocations

A shoulder sling is used for 6 weeks. During this time, patients are instructed to work on active range of motion of the hand, wrist, and elbow and passive shoulder exercises below the horizontal plane (e.g., pendulum). They are permitted to use the hand for simple activities of daily living, but are to avoid using the arm for any activities of pushing, pulling, or lifting. They are also to avoid shoulder protraction and retraction at this time. At the 6-week point, they can begin active-assisted shoulder range of motion exercises in all planes and advance to active motion as tolerated. A progressive strengthening program begins at 3 months, and a full return to activities can be expected at 6 months if the SC joint is clinically stable and the patient is asymptomatic.

Injuries in the Skeletally Immature (Physeal Injuries and Dislocations)

Before the epiphysis ossifies at the age of 18 years, one cannot be sure whether a displacement about the SC joint is a dislocation or a fracture through the physeal plate. For this reason, we recommend performing a CT scan at the time of the initial clinical presentation. We still perform the closed reduction maneuvers as described earlier for anterior or posterior physeal injuries when they present acutely. The techniques for closed reduction of a posterior physeal injury are identical to those described for SC dislocations. After a stable reduction is achieved, the SC joint is protected with the shoulders held back in a figure-of-eight dressing for 3 to 4 weeks. Similar to dislocations in the adult population, steps must be taken to confirm the success of the closed reduction.

The single difference in treatment between posterior physeal separations and posterior SC dislocations occurs when a posterior physeal dislocation cannot be reduced by closed means and the patient is having *no significant symptoms*. Generally, this situation occurs when an attempted closed reduction is performed and postreduction CT reveals residual posterior displacement or when a patient presents after 48 hours with no significant symptoms but with a confirmed posterior fracture separation on imaging. Although there is significant displacement of the shaft with either a type I or type II physeal fracture, the periosteal tube remains in its anatomic position and the attaching ligaments are intact (i.e., the costoclavicular ligaments inferiorly and the capsular and intra-articular disk ligaments medially). As with other physeal injuries, the potential for remodeling is significant, and may extend until the 23rd to 25th years (Fig. 10-53).

Open reduction of a physeal injury is seldom indicated, except for an irreducible posterior displacement in a patient with significant symptoms or compression of the vital structures in the mediastinum. Open reduction is also indicated for irreducible posterior SC joint dislocations (see Fig. 10-35).

COMPLICATIONS OF INJURIES TO THE STERNOCLAVICULAR JOINT

A physician treating SC instability faces many challenges. Complications of the injury itself, improper selection of treatment, potential intraoperative misadventures, and postoperative problems such as migration of hardware and iatrogenic instability can all threaten the surgical outcome and, at times, even the patient's life. Thorough knowledge of the potential pitfalls is necessary if they

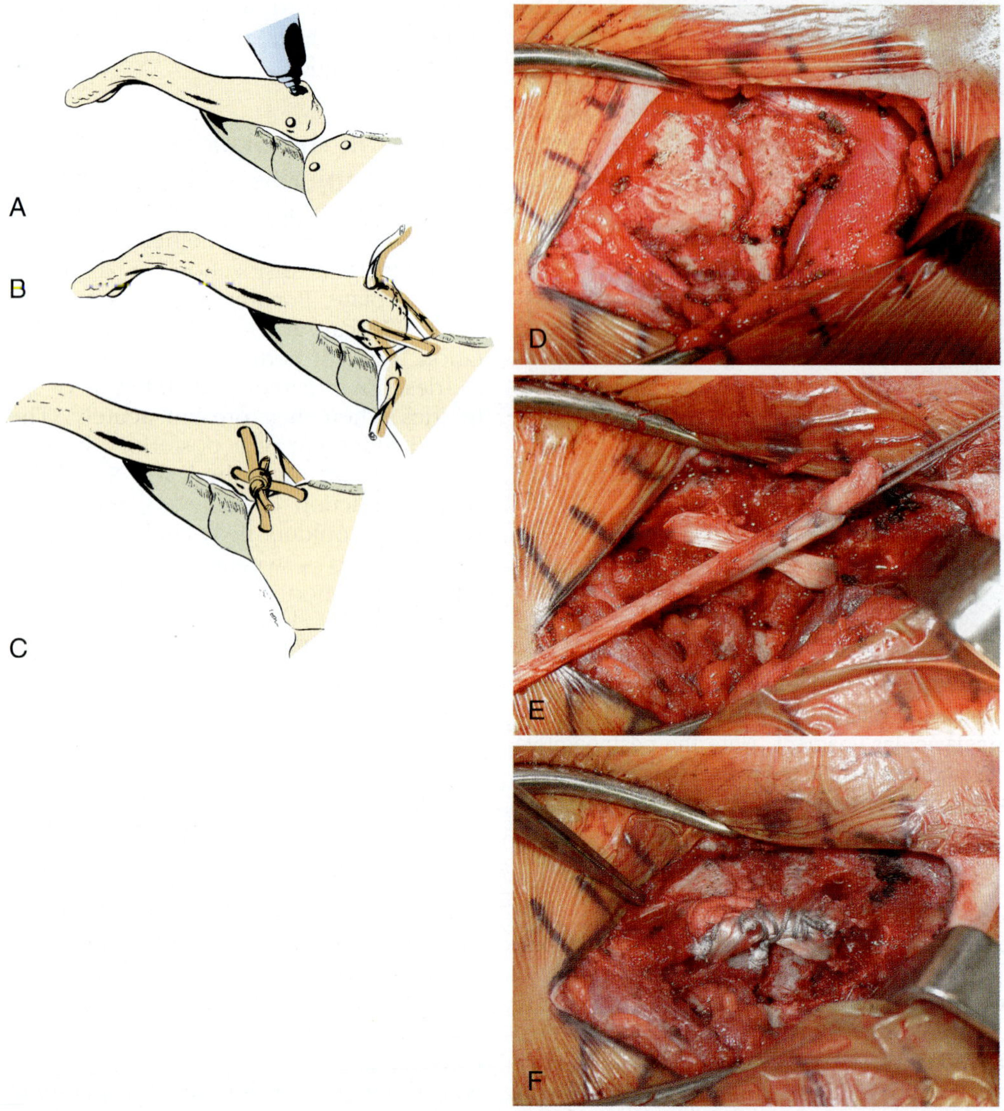

FIGURE 10-51: The figure-of-eight technique. **A,** Drill holes in the clavicle and manubrium. **B,** Placement of a semitendinosus graft. **C,** Final reconstruction. **D–F,** Intraoperative example of the figure-of-eight technique. (Courtesy Edwin E. Spencer Jr, MD.)

are to be avoided.[215-218] The serious complications that occur at the time of dislocation of the SC joint are primarily limited to posterior injuries (Box 10-3).

Worman and Leagus,[220] in an excellent review of the complications associated with posterior dislocations of the SC joint, reported that 16 of 60 patients (26.7%) reviewed from the literature had suffered complications of the trachea, esophagus, or great vessels. More recently in 2014, Tepolt et al.[193] performed a meta-analysis of posterior SC joint injuries in the adolescent population, and reported dysphagia or dyspnea in 30.4% of the patients. More serious complications including mediastinal hematoma, vessel laceration, stroke, pneumomediastinum, pneumothorax, and venous thromboembolism were all reported. Vessel compression was the most frequently reported serious complication (13.8%). Death secondary to the initial injury was reported in one case (0.72%).

BOX 10-3. Associated Injuries and Complications Following Posterior Sternoclavicular Joint Dislocation

- Airway compromise and breathing difficulties secondary to tracheal laceration, compression, or pneumothorax[128,139]
- Injury to the larynx causing stridor, hoarseness, snoring, and voice changes[104,126,167,201]
- Vascular injury (laceration, compression, occlusion, and thrombosis)[69,92,122,186]
- Esophageal injury (compression, perforation, and rupture) leading to dysphagia, abscess and osteomyelitis of the clavicle,[18] and fatal tracheoesophageal fistula[211]
- Brachial plexus injury/compression,[104,149] and thoracic outlet syndrome with swelling and cyanosis of the upper extremity[67]

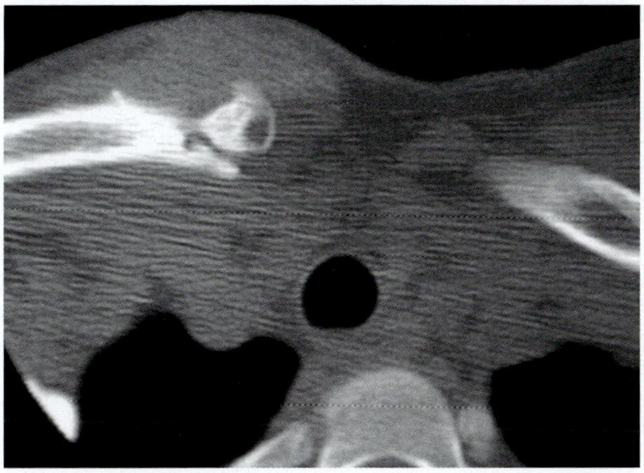

FIGURE 10-52: Computed tomographic scan of a 16-year-old patient whose sternoclavicular reconstruction was complicated by fracture of the medial clavicle in the early postoperative period.

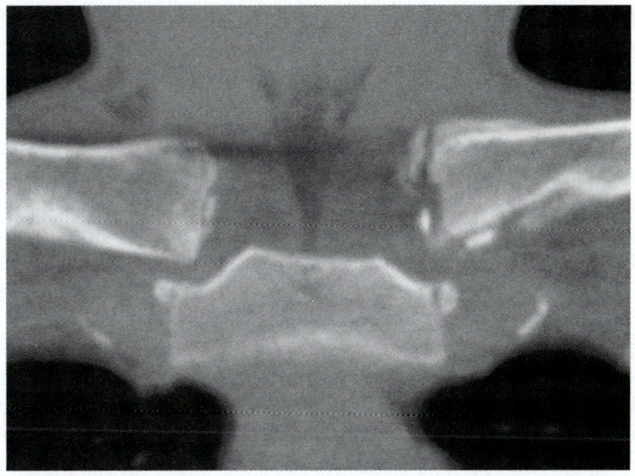

FIGURE 10-53: Computed tomographic scan (coronal image) 3 months following closed reduction of a left posterior sternoclavicular dislocation in an 18-year-old patient. New bone formation is readily apparent within the periosteal sleeve of the medial clavicle.

COMPLICATIONS OF OPERATIVE PROCEDURES

We are aware of eight deaths[39,70,112,129,153,167,179] and four near-deaths,[21,138,181,220] from complications of transfixing the SC joint with Kirschner wires or Steinmann pins. Numerous reports document migration of pins, either intact or broken, into the heart, pulmonary artery, subclavian artery, innominate artery, or the aorta.[21,95,112,115,132,138,163,171,173] *We do not recommend any type of transfixing pins—large or small—across the SC joint.*

EDITOR COMMENTARY

Michael A. Wirth

The authors of this chapter remind us that traumatic SC joint injuries are uncommon, accounting for less than 3% of all dislocations, and some orthopedic surgeons will never see or manage one of these potentially life-threatening injuries. Posterior SC dislocations are less common than their anterior counterpart, and often require surgical stabilization because of complications related to compression or injury to the critical mediastinal structures that lie within a few millimeters of the posterior aspect of the manubrium and medial clavicle. Although most anterior SC injuries are successfully treated without surgery, some patients will present with persistent or progressive symptomatic instability necessitating operative intervention.

Unfortunately, there are no clear evidence-based clinical or surgical practice guidelines to assist surgeons in the management of these injuries. The uncommon occurrence of SC joint injuries has made it nearly impossible to collect large-scale quality clinical outcome data and equally difficult to identify a gold standard reconstructive method when surgery is indicated. Regardless of the surgical technique employed, the poorest outcomes are associated with atraumatic injuries and patients with generalized ligamentous laxity.

The most significant impact in the last decade with respect to our understanding of SC instability was the result of a biomechanical study demonstrating the superiority of figure-of-eight tendon graft reconstruction.[184] This technique has emerged as the most widely accepted means to stabilize both anterior and posterior SC joint injuries, with favorable early follow-up and acceptable complication and reoperation rates. Several key points of this procedure were emphasized in this chapter. (1) Drill holes can be varied between 3 and 4.5 mm in diameter and should be based upon the SC anatomy as opposed to the graft size to minimize fracture. (2) An adequate cortical bridge of approximately 15 mm should be maintained between drill holes and the joint surfaces. (3) Superior-to-inferior drill holes may be preferred in both the clavicle and manubrium, as opposed to AP holes, to minimize injury to the critical mediastinal structures. (4) Secure the ends of the graft at the inferior aspect of the joint to avoid an anterior prominence, which is unsightly and often symptomatic. (5) Utilization of allograft to eliminate donor site morbidity, which has been noted in up to 40% of patients.

The current literature pertaining to SC joint surgery reveals promising results, even with reconstruction of anterior SC joint problems, but these reports are rarely prospective or randomized and the concern for overly aggressive surgical treatment must be mentioned. This is especially relevant to the management of physeal injuries in adolescents when they present with a fracture or dislocation of the medial clavicle that is not associated with injury to the mediastinal structures.

SENIOR EDITOR COMMENTARY

Frederick A. Matsen III

Combined, the three authors of this chapter have unmatched experience with this articulation—perhaps the most challenging of all. Many surgeons would prefer to look the other way when a patient presents with an SC joint problem because of its cosmetic prominence, its tenuous stability, its susceptibility to a wide range of symptomatic problems, and its close proximity to such structures as the innominate artery, brachiocephalic vein, vagus nerve, phrenic nerve, internal jugular vein, trachea, and esophagus. My own humbling experience has included substantial venous bleeding as I reduced a posteriorly dislocated medial clavicle in a 14-year-old Jehovah's witness and a pneumothorax as I attempted to place a screw across a very unstable SC joint.

I am fortunate in having a partner, Winston Warme, who has become a regional expert in the management of SC joint injuries. He observes that surgical reconstruction of unstable SC joints is associated with a risk of injury to the vital retrosternal structures. In an effort to increase the safety of reconstruction, he uses a posterior cruciate ligament drill guide in his reconstruction for anterior or posterior SC instability.[209] In his hands, this technique provides controlled drilling of the sternum and medial clavicle, and thus reduces the risk of iatrogenic injury to the structures found in the upper mediastinum. Despite the safety of this method, he recommends having thoracic surgery backup, especially when reconstructing posterior SC joint dislocations (Figs. 10-54 to 10-56).

Dr. Warme also points to the problem of "pseudoinstability" of the SC joint from a disrupted intra-articular disk. While the joint itself is not unstable, the patient may have a sense of recurrent subluxation after a major traumatic episode. This entity is best evaluated with MRI of both the affected joint and the opposite uninjured side for comparison. It can be readily treated with a partial diskectomy and capsulorrhaphy.

I appreciate all of the great guidance in the management of these complex conditions.

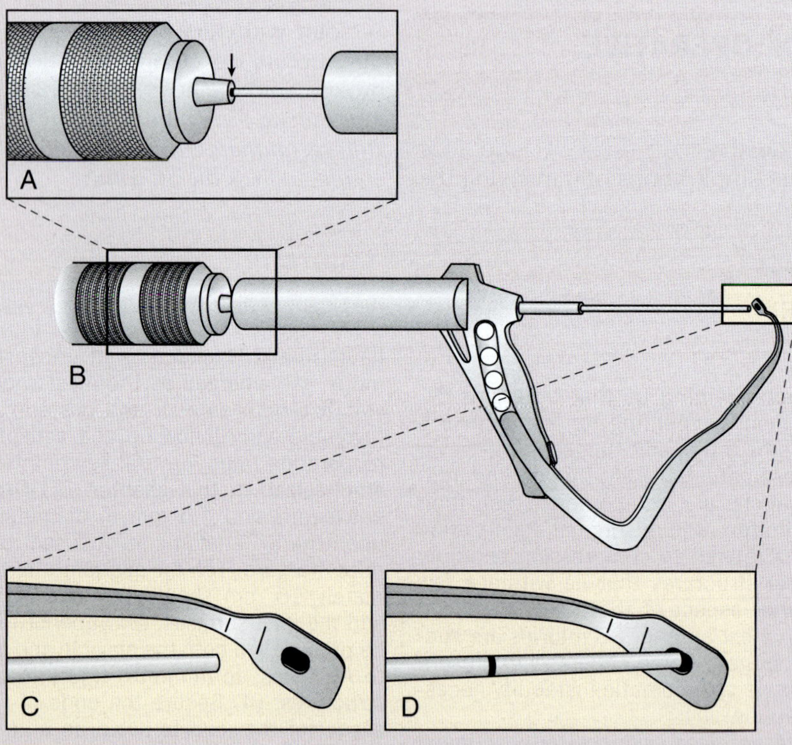

FIGURE 10-54: Chuck the posterior cruciate ligament (PCL) guide wire **(A)** to a safe length, and mark this on the guide wire **(A)**. Importantly, all measurements should be made off of this point. Care with this step precludes plunging beyond the posterior cortex of the bone **(B)**. Reverse the pin after penetrating the posterior cortex, such that the blunt end is advanced and captured in the wire catcher **(C)** and **(D)**. Once secured, the guide wire catcher can control the depth of the reaming to the correct diameter. (Modified from Warme WJ, Papadonikolakis A. The use of a PCL drill to increase safety in the reconstruction of unstable sternoclavicular joints. *Tech Shoulder Elbow Surg.* 2012;13[3]:142-144.)

SENIOR EDITOR COMMENTARY—cont'd

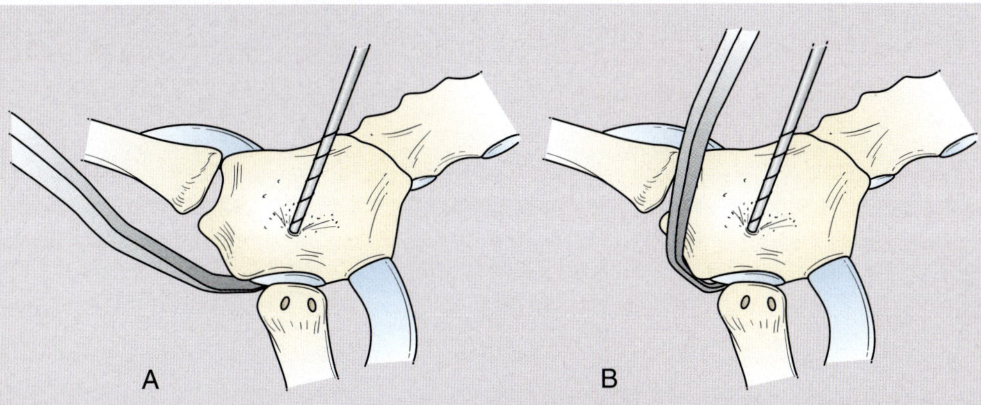

FIGURE 10-55: The manubrium is soft and spongy in comparison to the more dense clavicular cortical bone. With the posterior cruciate ligament (PCL) guide tip device resting on the posterior cortex of the manubrium (**A**), carefully advance the guide wire. Once through the posterior cortex, reverse the wire such that the blunt end inserted in the recess within the PCL guide wire catcher (**B**), then ream over the guide wire to the size of the graft, usually 5 mm. (Modified from Warme WJ, Papadonikolakis A. The use of a PCL drill to increase safety in the reconstruction of unstable sternoclavicular joints. *Tech Shoulder Elbow Surg.* 2012;13[3]:142-144.)

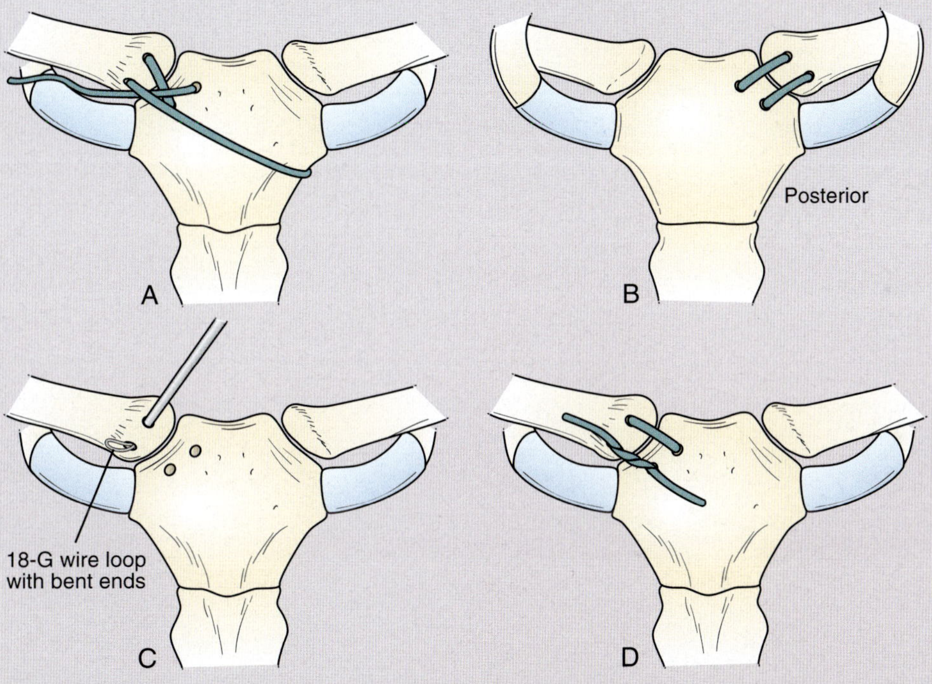

FIGURE 10-56: Suture the graft to itself with the sternoclavicular (SC) joint reduced **(A, B, D)**. Shuttle the graft through with 18-gauge wire loops that are first placed through the tunnels **(C)** and up out through the sternal notch. In posterior SC dislocations, ensure that two parallel strands are located on the posterior aspect of the SC joint **(B)**. Only the anterior cortex of the clavicle is drilled with anterior instability cases such that the parallel strands are anteriorly positioned **(D)**. (Modified from Warme WJ, Papadonikolakis A. The use of a PCL drill to increase safety in the reconstruction of unstable sternoclavicular joints. *Tech Shoulder Elbow Surg.* 2012;13[3]:142-144.)

CHAPTER 11

Sepsis of the Shoulder: Molecular Mechanisms and Pathogenesis

Robin R. Richards, Daniel S. Robertson

Shoulder sepsis can have a devastating impact on shoulder function, particularly if diagnosis and treatment are delayed or inadequate. The general principles in the pathogenesis of shoulder sepsis are similar to those pertaining to all intra-articular infections. There are three fundamental pathways for pathogens to enter a joint:

1. Spontaneous hematogenous seeding via the synovial blood supply
2. Contiguous spread from adjacent metaphyseal osteomyelitis via the intra-articular portion of the metaphysis
3. Penetration of the joint by trauma, therapy, or surgery (Fig. 11-1)

Susceptibility to infection is determined by the adequacy of the host defenses. Spontaneous bacteremia, trauma, and surgery present opportunities for inoculation of the joint, particularly if local or systemic conditions are favorable for infection to develop. However, shoulder sepsis is relatively uncommon due to the normal defense mechanisms, a good local blood supply, and the use of antibiotic prophylaxis.

Certain patient groups with immune system depression or aberrations are at increased risk for infection. Patients with rheumatoid disease can manifest a spontaneous and somewhat cryptic sepsis in joints.[71,93] Diabetics, infants, children, older people, patients with vascular disease, drug abusers, and patients with human immunodeficiency virus infection have an increased susceptibility to specific organisms, as have patients with hematologic dyscrasias or neoplastic disease.

Joint infection requires a threshold inoculum of bacteria and can be facilitated by damaged tissue, foreign body substrata, and the acellularity of cartilage surfaces. Total joint arthroplasties are at potential risk of infection because of the presence of metal and polymer biomaterials and the decreased phagocytic ability of macrophages in the presence of methylmethacrylate. Biomaterials and adjacent damaged tissues and substrates are readily colonized by bacteria in a polysaccharide biofilm that is resistant to macrophage attack and antibiotic penetration.[65,68] With antibiotic prophylaxis, infection rates of total joint arthroplasty have been reported to be low: 1% to 5%, depending on the device and the location.[69,119] However, once infected, biomaterials and damaged tissues are exceedingly resistant to treatment.

Clinical infection in immunosuppressed patients involves the maturation of an inoculum of known pathogens (e.g., *Staphylococcus aureus* or *Pseudomonas aeruginosa*) or the transformation of nonpathogens (e.g., *Staphylococcus epidermidis*) to a septic focus of adhesive virulent organisms. This transformation can occur in the presence of, and be potentiated by, the surface of biomaterials,[66,67] damaged tissue, and defenseless cartilage matrix surfaces.[170]

HISTORY

Experiences in shoulder infection have paralleled those of other large joints, although with less frequency. The work of outstanding scientists, such as Louis Pasteur (1822-1895), Joseph Lister (1827-1912), and Robert Koch (1843-1910), in the last quarter of the nineteenth century ushered in the modern age of bacteriology and an early understanding of intra-articular sepsis. Koch's experiments with culture media at the Berlin Institute for Infectious Disease verified the role of the tubercle bacillus in musculoskeletal infection.

The latter part of the nineteenth century also saw the development of the concept of antisepsis. Lister maintained that sepsis was the main obstacle to significant advances in surgery. He documented a dramatic reduction in cases of empyema, erysipelas, hospital gangrene, and surgical infection through the use of antiseptic techniques. Although the popularization of antiseptic techniques in the surgical theater greatly reduced the rate of complications resulting from infection, it was not until the 1930s that specific antimicrobial therapy was discovered. In 1935 a German bacteriologist, Gerhard Domagk, discovered that sulfonamides

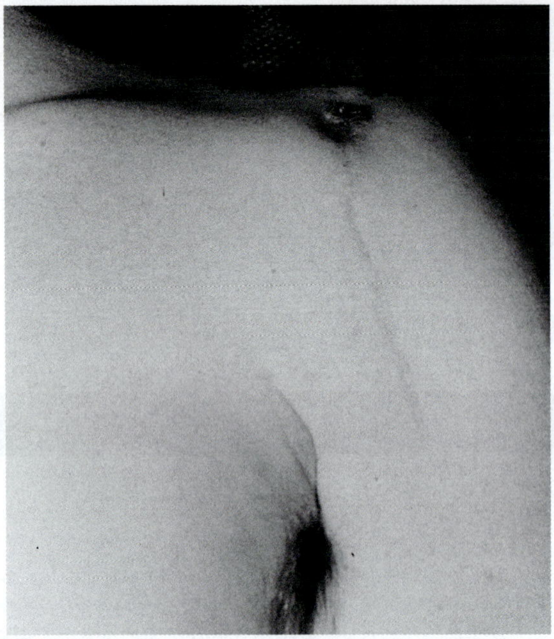

FIGURE 11-1: Sinus communicating with a prosthetic shoulder joint. This patient developed a chronic low-grade infection after undergoing a total shoulder arthroplasty.

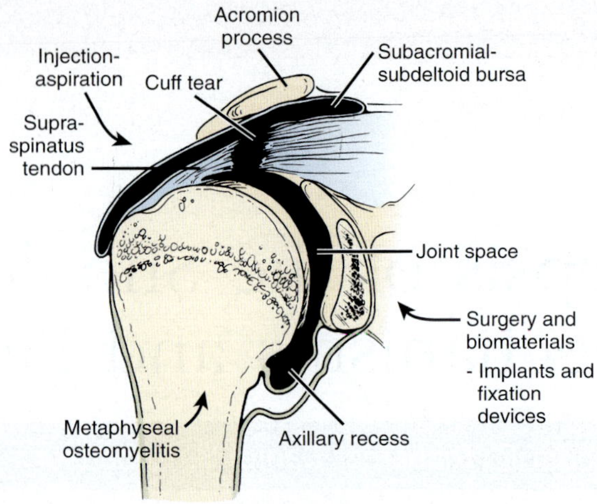

FIGURE 11-2: Routes of infection for intra-articular sepsis.

protected mice against fatal doses of hemolytic staphylococci. Sulfonamides were soon employed for infections in patients, with excellent results.

Although the history of bacteriology, antiseptic techniques in surgery, and the development of antibiotics are well documented, very little of the early literature relates specifically to infections about the shoulder. In Codman's book, *The Shoulder*, first published in 1934, infections of the shoulder and, in particular, osteomyelitis of the proximal humerus were considered to be very rare lesions.[28] Codman cited a report by King and Holmes in 1927 in which a review of 450 consecutive symptomatic shoulders evaluated at the Massachusetts General Hospital revealed five cases of tuberculosis of the shoulder, one luetic infection of the shoulder, three unspecified shoulder infections, and two cases of osteomyelitis of the proximal humerus. The rarity of tubercular lesions of the shoulder was documented through the results of four large series of tuberculosis involving the musculoskeletal system (Townsend, 21 of 3244 cases; Whitman, 38 of 1833 cases; Young, 7 of 5680 cases; and Billroth, 14 of 1900 cases). As microbial culturing and identification techniques developed in the early twentieth century, streptococcal and staphylococcal species were more often identified as the causative agents in shoulder infection.

SEPTIC ANATOMY OF THE SHOULDER

A review of shoulder anatomy reveals specific structural relationships that are intimately linked to the pathogenesis of joint sepsis and osteomyelitis. The circulation of the proximal humerus and periarticular structures (particularly the synovium) and the intricate system of bursae about the shoulder are critical factors.

Classically, the age-dependent presentations of hematogenous osteomyelitis and septic arthritis of the shoulder (and of other large joints, such as the hip and knee) have been attributed to vascular development about the growth plate and epiphysis. The most detailed studies of the vascular development in this area have involved the proximal femur; however, this is analogous to the same development about the proximal humerus. Experimental work by Trueta[167] demonstrated that before 8 months of age, there are direct vascular communications across the growth plate between the nutrient artery system and the epiphyseal ossicle. This observation was believed to account for the frequency of infection involving the epiphyseal ossicle and subsequent joint sepsis in infants. At some point between 8 and 18 months of age (an average of 1 year), the growth plate forms a complete barrier to direct vascular communication between the metaphysis and epiphysis. The last vestiges of the nutrient artery turn down acutely at the growth plate and reach sinusoidal veins. At this point the blood flow slows down, creating an ideal medium for the proliferation of pathogenic bacteria.[168]

In the adult shoulder, the intra-articular extent of the metaphysis is located in the inferior sulcus and is intracapsular for approximately 10 to 12 mm.[27] An infection of the proximal metaphysis, once established, can gain access to the shoulder joint via the haversian and Volkmann canals at the nonperiosteal zone (Fig. 11-2). With the obliteration of the growth plate at skeletal maturity, anastomoses of the metaphyseal and epiphyseal circulation are again established.

In his study of the vascular development of the proximal femur in fetuses and children up to 14 years and 8 months, Chung found no evidence of direct communications between the metaphyseal and epiphyseal circulation across the growth plate in any age group.[26] Chung's work demonstrated a persistent extraosseous anastomosis between the metaphyseal and epiphyseal circulation on the surface of the perichondrial ring. He found no evidence of vessels penetrating the growth plate in the infant population and attributed apparent changes in the arterial supply with age to enlargement of the neck and ossification center.

Branches of the suprascapular artery and the circumflex scapular branch of the subscapular artery from the scapular side of the shoulder anastomose with the anterior and posterior humeral circumflex arteries from the humeral side of the shoulder. This anastomotic system supplies the proximal humerus by forming an extra-articular and extracapsular arterial ring. Vessels from this ring traverse the capsule and form an intra-articular synovial ring. This fine anastomosis of vessels in the synovial membrane is located at the junction of the synovium and the articular cartilage. This subsynovial ring of vessels was first described by William Hunter in 1743 and named the *circulus articuli vasculosus*.[81] At the transitional zone, synovial cells become flattened over this periarticular vascular fringe. Fine arterioles at this boundary acutely loop back toward the periphery. Again, blood flow at this level can decrease, which provides a site for establishing an inoculum of pathogenic organisms. Rather than hemodynamic changes, however, it is more probable that receptor-specific, microbe-to-cell surface interactions potentiate the infectious process.

Another anatomic consideration in sepsis of the shoulder is the communication between the joint space and capsule and the system of bursae about the shoulder. Anteriorly, there is direct communication between the capsule and the subscapular bursa located just below the coracoid process. Posteriorly, the capsule communicates with the infraspinatus bursa. There is a third opening in the capsule at the point at which the tendon of the long head of the biceps enters the shoulder. From the transverse humeral ligament to its entry into the shoulder capsule, the tendon of the long head of the biceps is enveloped in folds of synovium. Intentional or inadvertent injection of the subscapular bursa, the infraspinatus bursa, or the tendon of the long head of the biceps provides the potential for intra-articular bacterial inoculation. Injection of the subacromial or subdeltoid bursa in the presence of a rotator cuff tear (degenerative or traumatic) provides further potential for bacterial contamination of the joint.

Ward and Eckardt[173] reported on four patients with subacromial or subdeltoid bursa abscesses. Three of these four patients were chronically ill and debilitated, the bursal abscesses coexisting with clinically diagnosed mild to resolving glenohumeral pyarthrosis. The symptoms and signs of the abscesses were minimal in all four patients. The authors found that computed tomography (CT) or magnetic resonance imaging (MRI) can help to detect abscesses and plan treatment.

MICROANATOMY AND CELL BIOLOGY

The hyaline cartilage of the articular surface is essentially acellular and consists of horizontally arranged collagen fibers in proteoglycan macromolecules. The boundaries of the joint cavity are composed of a richly vascularized cellular synovial tissue. It has been suggested that collagen fibers and the glycoprotein matrix, rather than the synovium, are the target substrata for microbial adhesion and colonization.[156,170]

Some synovial cells are phagocytic and appear to combat infection as part of the inflammatory response. Microscopic examination of infected joints in a lupine animal model indicated predominant colonization of cartilaginous, rather than synovial, surfaces.[170] Receptors for collagen have been identified on the cell surfaces of certain strains of *S. aureus*.[156] The infrequent occurrence of bacteria on synovial tissue might reflect the innate resistance of synovial cells to colonization, the lack of appropriate synovial ligands, or functional host defense mechanisms at a synovial level.[14] The subintimal vascularized layer contains fibroadipose tissue, lymphatic vessels, and nerves. Ultrastructural studies of the synovial subintimal vessels have revealed that gaps between endothelial cells are bridged by a fine membrane. There is no epithelial tissue in the synovial lining and, therefore, no structural barrier (basement membrane) to prevent the spread of infection from synovial blood vessels to the joint. The synovial lining in the transition zone is rarely more than three or four cell layers thick, placing the synovial blood vessels in a superficial position. Intra-articular hemorrhage caused by trauma, combined with transient bacteremia, may be implicated as a factor in the pathogenesis of joint sepsis. Hematogenous seeding can allow bacterial penetration of synovial vessels, producing an effusion consisting primarily of neutrophils that release cartilage-destroying lysosomal enzymes.

Articular (hyaline) cartilage varies from 2 to 4 mm in thickness in the large joints of adults. This avascular, aneural tissue consists of a relatively small number of cells and chondrocytes and an abundant extracellular matrix. The extracellular matrix contains collagen and a ground substance composed of carbohydrate and noncollagenous protein and has high water content. The chondrocytes are responsible for the synthesis and degradation of matrix components and are, therefore, ultimately responsible for the biomechanical and biologic properties of articular cartilage. Collagen (type II) produced by the chondrocytes accounts for more than half of the dry weight of adult articular cartilage. Individual collagen fibers, with a characteristic periodicity of 640 Å, vary from 300 to 800 Å in diameter, depending on their distance from the articular surface.

The principal component of the ground substance produced by chondrocytes is a protein polysaccharide complex termed *proteoglycan*. The central organizing molecule of proteoglycan is hyaluronic acid, with numerous glycosaminoglycans (mainly chondroitin sulfate and keratan sulfate) covalently bound from this central strand. Glycosaminoglycans carry considerable negative charge. The highly ordered array of electronegativity on the proteoglycan molecules interacts with large numbers of water molecules (small electric dipole). As a result, approximately 75% of the wet weight of articular cartilage

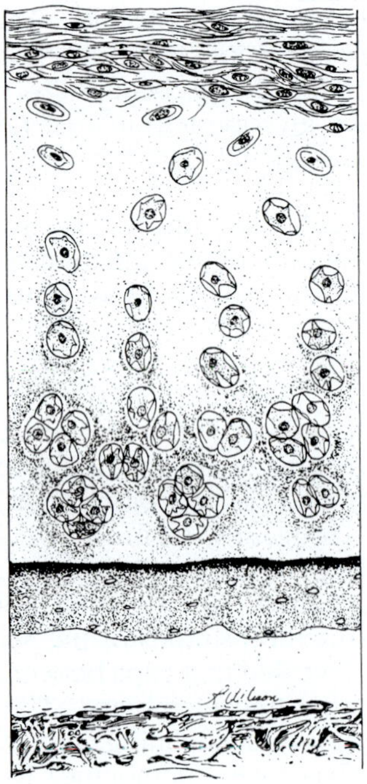

FIGURE 11-3: The zones of adult articular cartilage. (Modified from Turek SL. *Orthopaedics: Principles and Their Application.* Philadelphia: JB Lippincott; 1977.)

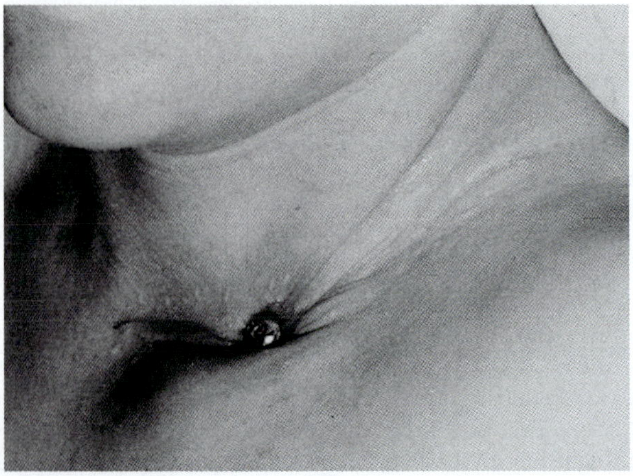

FIGURE 11-4: Internal fixation visible over the clavicle. The patient had a clavicular nonunion that was treated with internal fixation and bone grafting. Infection occurred, resulting in wound breakdown and exposure of the internal fixation. The patient was treated by removal of the internal fixation and by dressing changes. The wound healed with this treatment, with no recurrence of drainage over 6 years. Infection is not uncommon in the area of the clavicle and the acromioclavicular joint due to the thin soft tissue envelope that overlies these structures.

is water, the majority of which is structured by the electrostatic forces of the proteoglycan molecule.

The structure of articular cartilage varies relative to its distance from the free surface. For the purposes of description, the tissue can be subdivided into three zones that run parallel to the articular surface (Fig. 11-3). Electron microscopy of the free surface reveals a dense network of collagen fibers (40 to 120 Å in diameter) that is arranged tangentially to the load-bearing surface and at approximately right angles to each other. This dense, mat-like arrangement, the *lamina obscurans*, is acellular.

Zone 1, the superficial layer, contains large bundles of collagen fibers that are approximately 340 Å thick and lie parallel to the joint surface and at right angles to each other. This zone, the *lamina splendens,* has little or no intervening ground substance and contains the highest density of collagen. Chondrocytes in zone 1 are ellipsoid and are oriented parallel to the articular surface. Electron microscopy reveals little evidence of metabolic activity.

In zone 2 the collagen consists of individual, randomly oriented fibers of varying diameters. The chondrocytes in zone 2 tend to be more spherical and larger than those in zone 1, with abundant mitochondria and extensive endoplasmic reticulum, suggesting greater metabolic activity. The proteoglycan/collagen ratio in zone 2 is much higher than that near the surface.

In zone 3 the collagen fibers are thicker, often around 1400 Å in diameter, and tend to form a more orderly meshwork that lies radial to the articular surface. The chondrocytes in zone 3 are larger and tend to be arranged in columns, often appearing in groups of two to eight cells. The cells have been noted to have enlarged Golgi complexes, many mitochondria, and an extensively developed endoplasmic reticulum, indicating a high degree of metabolic activity.

Bone is a composite structure incorporating calcium hydroxyapatite crystals in a collagen matrix grossly similar to synthetic composites or to partially crystalline polymers. Devitalized bone provides a passive substratum for bacterial colonization as well as the ultimate incorporation of its proteinaceous and mineral constituents as bacterial metabolites.[68] *S. aureus* binds to bone sialoprotein, a glycoprotein found in joints, and it produces chondrocyte proteases that hydrolyze synovial tissue.[149]

CLASSIFICATION

Intra-articular sepsis may be classified in order of pathogenesis and frequency as direct hematogenous; secondary to contiguous spread from osteomyelitis; or secondary to trauma, surgery, or intra-articular injection (Fig. 11-4 and Box 11-1). Most joint infections are caused by hematogenous spread, although direct contamination is not uncommon with trauma. Inoculation of the joint with bacteria can occur in association with the intra-articular injection of steroid, local anesthetic, or synthetic joint fluid. Infection rates following arthroscopy are low, ranging from 0.4% to 3.4%.[15,130] Armstrong and Bolding reported that sepsis following arthroscopy could be associated with inadequate arthroscope disinfection and the use of intraoperative intra-articular corticosteroids.[4] Tosh

BOX 11-1. Classification of Osteomyelitis and Intra-articular Sepsis

Hematogenous
Contiguous spread
- Osteomyelitis
- Soft tissue sepsis
- Vascular insufficiency

Direct inoculation
- Surgery with or without a foreign body or biomaterials
- Trauma with or without a foreign body or biomaterials

reported that inadequate sterilization caused an outbreak of *Propionibacterium acnes* from retained tissue within the arthroscope.[165]

Osteomyelitis of the humerus can spread intra-articularly, depending on the age of the patient, the type of infecting organism, and the severity of infection. Osteomyelitis of the clavicle or scapula is uncommon, although it can occur after surgery and internal fixation, from retained shrapnel fragments, or in heroin addicts.[19,110,157,181] Brancos and colleagues reported that *S. aureus* and *P. aeruginosa* were the etiologic agents in 75% and 11% of episodes, respectively, of septic arthritis in heroin addicts.[18] The sternoclavicular joint was involved more commonly than the shoulder joint. Chaudhuri and colleagues have reported septic arthritis of the shoulder following mastectomy and radiotherapy for breast carcinoma.[25] Lymphedema was present in all cases. The onset of infection was subacute in all cases, and delays in diagnosis led to destruction of the joint in all but one patient.

Hematogenous osteomyelitis, although common in children,[118] is uncommon in adults until the sixth decade or later and is usually associated with a compromised immune system. Intravenous (IV) drug use is associated with the development of osteomyelitis in adults. Direct spread from wounds or foreign bodies, including total joint and internal fixation devices, is the most common etiology of shoulder sepsis in adults. Sepsis has been reported following shoulder arthrography, treatment for retroperitoneal abscess, and various gynecological surgeries.[21,37,136] In 1959 Gowans and Granieri reported the relationship between intra-articular injections of hydrocortisone acetate and the subsequent development of septic arthritis.[64] Kelly and colleagues reported that two of their six patients had a history of multiple intra-articular injections of corticosteroid.[95] Ward and Goldner reported that chronic disease was present in more than half of their 30 cases of glenohumeral pyarthrosis and that four cases were associated with ipsilateral forearm arteriovenous dialysis fistulas.[174] Soft tissue infection about the shoulder can also manifest in the form of pyomyositis, sometimes occurring as a result of hematogenous spread.[44] Aglas and colleagues reported sternoclavicular joint arthritis as a complication of subclavian venous catheterization.[2] Their two cases responded to antibiotic treatment. Glenohumeral pyarthrosis has been observed following acupuncture.[97] Lossos and colleagues reported that associated medical conditions were present in the majority of their patients with septic arthritis of the shoulder.[107]

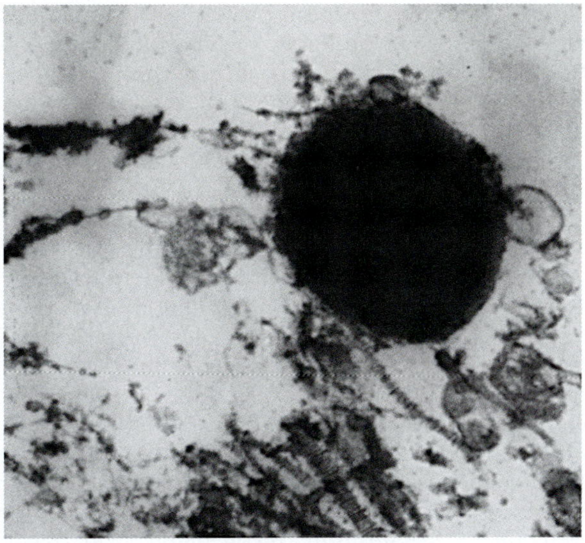

FIGURE 11-5: A photoelectron micrograph of rabbit articular cartilage illustrating direct bacteria-to-collagen fiber contact. (From Voytek A, Gristina AG, Barth E, et al. Staphylococcal adhesion to collagen in intra-articular sepsis. *Biomaterials.* 1988;9:107-110.)

PATHOGENIC MECHANISMS OF SEPTIC ARTHRITIS AND OSTEOMYELITIS

Surfaces as Substrata for Bacterial Colonization

The pathogenesis of bone and joint infections is related, in part, to the preferential adhesive colonization of inert substrata, such as the articular surface of joints or damaged bone, whose surfaces are not integrated with healthy tissue composed of living cells and intact extracellular polymers (Fig. 11-5).[16,68,77,88,147,176] Almost all natural biological surfaces are lined by a cellular epithelium or endothelium, with the exceptions being intra-articular cartilage and the surface of teeth. Mature enamel is the only human tissue that is totally acellular; it is primarily composed of inorganic hydroxyapatite crystals (96% by weight), with a small amount of water (3%) and an organic matrix (<1%).[5] Cartilage and enamel are readily colonized by bacteria because they lack the protection by natural desquamation or by intact extracapsular polysaccharides that is provided by an active cellular layer. Their acellular surfaces are similar to many of those in nature for which bacteria have developed colonizing mechanisms. Certain strains of *S. aureus* adhere to specific sites on collagen fibrils, a process that is mediated by specific surface receptor proteins. Dissimilarities in surface structure are probably responsible for the specificity of bacteria species in colonizing these surfaces.

Enamel is mostly crystalline and inorganic, whereas cartilage is noncrystalline and organic. Enamel contains no collagen, whereas collagen is ubiquitous in cartilage and bone. *S. aureus* is the natural colonizer of cartilage, but not of enamel, because it contains collagen receptors.[75,79,162] The specificity of colonization is also modulated in part by lectins and the host-derived synovial fluid, blood, and serum; by conditioning films of protein; and by polysaccharide macromolecules. The colonization of teeth by *Streptococcus mutans* and other organisms is a natural polymicrobial process and may be symbiotic or slowly destructive; however, bacterial colonization of articular cartilage is unnatural and rapidly destructive.

The acellular cartilage matrix and inanimate biomaterial surfaces offer no resistance to colonization by *S. aureus* and *S. epidermidis*, respectively. The observed invasion and gradual destruction of the cartilage over time supports clinical observations of the course of untreated septic arthritis (Fig. 11-6).[150,151] The acellular cartilaginous surfaces of joints are particularly vulnerable to sepsis because they allow direct exposure to bacteria from open trauma, surgical procedures, or hematogenous spread. This mechanism parallels previous observations on the mechanism of osteomyelitis, which suggest that the adhesion of bacteria to surfaces not protected by living cells, such as dead bone or cartilage, via receptors and extracellular polysaccharides is a factor in pathogenesis.[68,153]

Intra-articular Sepsis

The articular cavity is a potential dead space that can provide a favorable environment for bacterial growth. In this avascular and relatively acellular space, host defense mechanisms are at a disadvantage. Synovial cells are not actively antibacterial, although they are somewhat phagocytic. White blood cells (WBCs) must be delivered to the area and lack a surface for active locomotion. Under such conditions phagocytic action is expected to be impaired, especially against encapsulated organisms.

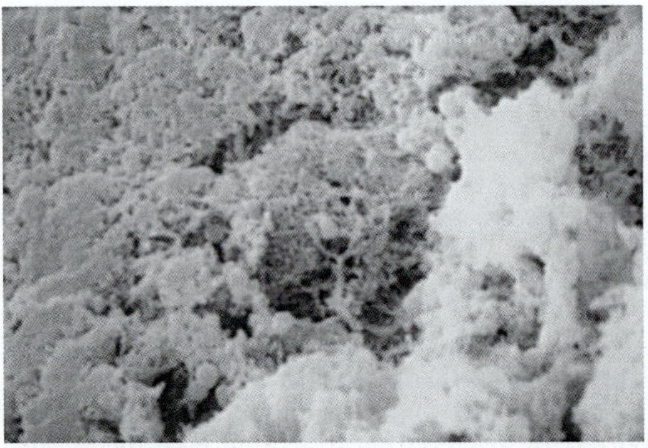

FIGURE 11-6: A photoelectron micrograph of articular cartilage 7 days after diagnosis of septic arthritis demonstrates destructive changes occurring beneath matrix-enclosed cocci. (From Voytek A, Gristina AG, Barth E, et al. Staphylococcal adhesion to collagen in intra-articular sepsis. *Biomaterials.* 1988;9:107-110.)

Spontaneous intra-articular sepsis of the shoulder results from random hematogenous bacterial seeding. The synovial vasculature is abundant, and the vessels lack a limiting basement membrane. Bacteremia, especially caused by *Neisseria gonorrhoeae*, increases the risk of intra-articular spread. Nosocomial infections in neonatal intensive care units are usually related to the presence of intravascular devices.[43] Contiguous spread from adjacent and intracapsular metaphyseal osteomyelitis also occurs. Surgery, arthroscopy, total joint replacement, aspirations, and steroid injections can also result in the direct inoculation of bacteria into the intra-articular space. The presence of foreign bodies from trauma or after surgery (stainless steel, chrome-cobalt alloys, ultra-high molecular weight polyethylene, and methylmethacrylate) increases the possibility of infection by providing a foreign body nidus for colonization, allowing antibiotic-resistant colonization to occur.[66,68] The presence of a foreign body also decreases the size of the inoculant required for sepsis and perturbs the host's defense mechanisms.

Septic arthritis of the shoulder most often involves the glenohumeral joint. The acromioclavicular and sternoclavicular joints are occasionally infected in specific patient groups or after steroid injections in arthritis. Direct contamination from open wounds is also possible. Sternoclavicular sepsis is more common in drug abusers and usually involves gram-negative organisms, specifically *P. aeruginosa*. The involvement of *S. aureus*, *Escherichia coli*, *Brucella* species, and *N. gonorrhoeae* has also been reported.

Septic arthritis of the shoulder has been reported to represent up to 14% of all septic arthritis cases.[112] In earlier studies the incidence was 3.4%.[94] Caksen and colleagues reported shoulder involvement in two of 49 joints involved in their series of pediatric patients with septic arthritis.[23] A more elderly population, increased trauma, and the common use of articular and periarticular steroids may be the factors in this epidemiology. The primary causal organism of shoulder sepsis is *S. aureus*. Sepsis in immunocompromised patients may be polyarticular as well as polymicrobial. Ten percent of septic arthritis cases involve more than one joint, and it is likely to occur in children.

Osteomyelitis

Hematogenous osteomyelitis accounts for most cases of osteomyelitis in children. Contiguous osteomyelitis is more common in adults, secondary to surgery and direct inoculation. In patients older than 50 years, contiguous osteomyelitis and diseases related to vascular insufficiency are predominant. Of the bones of the shoulder, the humerus is most commonly involved in osteomyelitis. In drug abusers the clavicle is occasionally involved due to hematogenous spread. The scapula is rarely involved; usually infection occurs by direct inoculation or contiguous spread (Fig. 11-7 and Table 11-1).

Epps and colleagues reviewed 15 patients with sickle cell disease and osteomyelitis affecting 30 bones.[45] On culture of specimens of bone, *S. aureus* was isolated from eight of these patients, *Salmonella* species from six, and *Proteus mirabilis* from one. This suggests that *Salmonella* species are not always the principle causative organisms of osteomyelitis in patients with sickle cell disease.

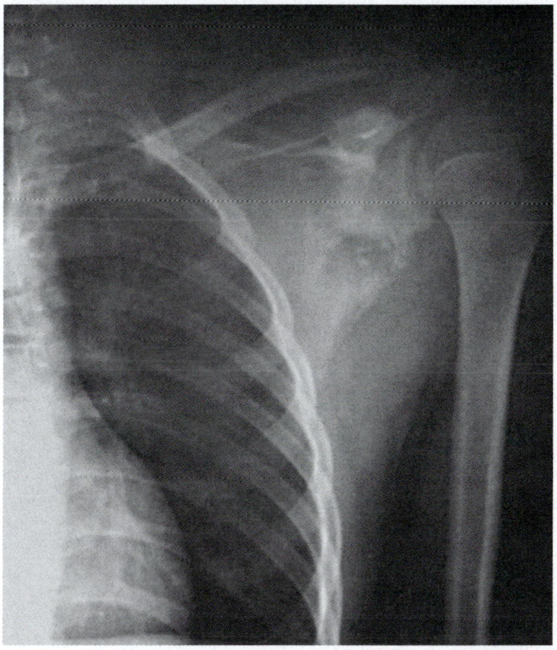

FIGURE 11-7: Staphylococcal osteomyelitis of the scapula secondary to closed trauma and hematogenous seeding with abscess formation. The shoulder joint is not involved. (Courtesy Department of Radiology, Wake Forest University Medical Center, Winston-Salem, NC.)

MICROBIAL ADHESION AND INTRA-ARTICULAR SEPSIS

An understanding of microbial adhesion is required for complete clinical and therapeutic insight into joint sepsis. Studies of bacteria in marine ecosystems indicate that they tend to adhere in colonies to surfaces or substrata. The number of bacteria that can exist in a given environment is related directly to stress and nutrient supply.[180] Surface attachment, rather than a floating or suspension population, is a favored survival strategy for bacteria; the major proportion of bacterial biomasses in most natural environments are therefore in an attached state, which is a common mode of microbial life in humans.

Bacterial attachment to surfaces is influenced by proteinaceous bacterial receptors and by an extracapsular exopolysaccharide substance—a biofilm—within which bacteria aggregate and multiply.[31] Once bacteria develop a biofilm-enclosed adhesive mode of growth, they become more resistant to antiseptics,[111] antibiotics,[63] and host defense systems.[7,63,176] Free-floating, nonadhesive bacteria or other microbes that lack a well-developed outer layer or exopolysaccharide are more susceptible to host-clearing mechanisms[145] and to lower concentrations of antibacterial agents.[63] Gibbons and van Houte first

TABLE 11-1 Frequency of Joint Involvement in Infectious Arthritis (%)

Joint	Bacterial (Suppurative) Children*	Bacterial (Suppurative) Adults†	Mycobacterial	Viral
Knee	41	48	24	60
Hip	23	24	20	4
Ankle	14	7	12	30
Elbow	12	11	8	20
Wrist	4	7	20	55
Shoulder	4	15	4	5
Interphalangeal and metacarpal	1.4	1	12	75
Sternoclavicular	0.4	8	0	0
Sacroiliac	0.4	2	0	0

From Mandell L, Douglas KG Jr, Bennett JE, eds. Principles and Practice of Infectious Diseases. 2nd ed. New York: John Wiley;1985:698.
More than one joint may be involved; therefore the total percentages can exceed 100%.
**Data from Nelson JD, Koontz WC. Septic arthritis in infants and children: a review of 117 cases. Pediatrics. 1966;38:966-971; and Jackson MA, Nelson JD. Etiology and medical management of acute suppurative bone and joint infections in pediatric patients. J Pediatr Orthop. 1982;2:313-323.*
†Data from Kelly PJ, Martin WJ, Coventry MD. Bacterial (suppurative) arthritis in the adult. J Bone Joint Surg Am. 1970;52:1595-1602; Argen RJ, Wilson DH Jr, Wood P. Suppurative arthritis. Arch Intern Med. 1966;117:661-666; Gifford DB, Patzakis M, Ivler D, Swezey RL. Septic arthritis due to Pseudomonas in heroin addicts. J Bone Joint Surg Am. 1975;57:631-635.
‡Data from Smith JW, Sanford JP. Viral arthritis. Ann Intern Med. 1967;67:651-659; Medical Staff Conference. Arthritis caused by viruses. Calif Med. 1973;99:38-44.

described the significance of this adhesive phenomenon in the formation of dental plaque.[58] In diseases, such as gonococcal urethritis,[175] cystic fibrosis,[179] and endocarditis, bacterial colonization and propagation occur along endothelial and epithelial surfaces. The association between bacterial growth on biomaterial surfaces and infection was first described in 1963.[70]

Microbial adhesion and associated phenomena also explain the foreign body effect, an increased susceptibility to infection experienced in the presence of a foreign body. Infections centered on foreign bodies are resistant to host defenses and treatment and tend to persist until the infecting locus is removed. Foreign bodies include implanted biomaterials, fixation materials, prosthetic monitoring and delivery devices, traumatically acquired penetrating debris and bone fragments, and compromised tissues.

Initial bacterial attachment or adhesion depends on the long-range physical force characteristics of the bacterium, the fluid interface, and the substratum. Specific irreversible adhesion, which occurs after initial attachment, is based on time-dependent adhesin-receptor interactions and on extracapsular polysaccharide synthesis.[87] Biomaterial surfaces present sites for environmental interactions that result from their atomic structures (Fig. 11-8).[166] Metal alloys have a thin (100 to 200 Å) oxide layer that is the true biological interface.[3,91] The surfaces of polymers and metals are modified by texture, manufacturing processes, trace chemicals, and wear debris and also by host-derived ionic, polysaccharide, and glycoproteinaceous constituents (conditioning films). The finite surface structure of conditioning films in humans is specific to each individual biomaterial, type of tissue cell, and local host environment.[6] Tissue cells and matrix macromolecules also provide substrata for bacterial colonization. Bacteria have developed adhesins or receptors that interact with tissue cell surface structures (Fig. 11-9).

Subsequent to or concomitant with the initial attachment, fimbrial adhesins (such as in *E. coli*) and substratum receptors can interact, as in bacteria-to-tissue cell pathogenesis or for the glycoproteinaceous conditioning films that immediately coat implants.[6] The production and composition of the extracellular polysaccharide polymer, which tends to act like a glue, is a pivotal factor.[180] After colony maturation, cells on the periphery of the expanding biomass can separate or disaggregate

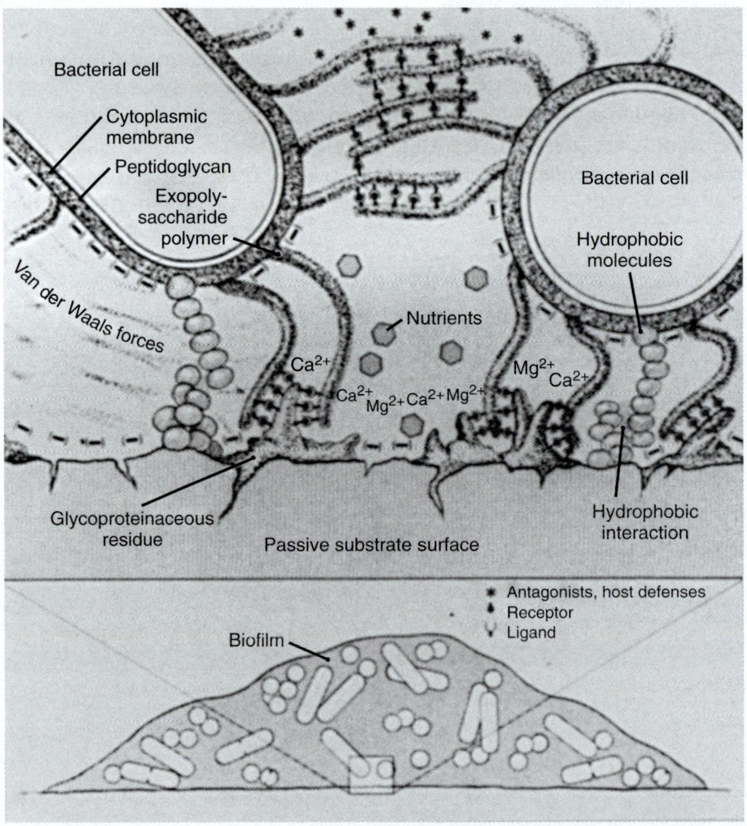

FIGURE 11-8: Mechanism of bacterial adherence to a biomaterial substrate. At specific distances, the initial repelling forces between like charges on the surfaces of bacteria and substrate are overcome by attracting van der Waals forces, and there are hydrophobic interactions between molecules. Under appropriate conditions, extensive development of exopolysaccharide polymers occurs, allowing ligand-receptor interaction and proteinaceous binding of the bacteria to the substrate. (From Gristina AG, Oga M, Webb LX, Hobgood CD. Adherent bacterial colonization in the pathogenesis of osteomyelitis. *Science.* 1985;228:990-993. Copyright 1985 American Association for the Advancement of Science.)

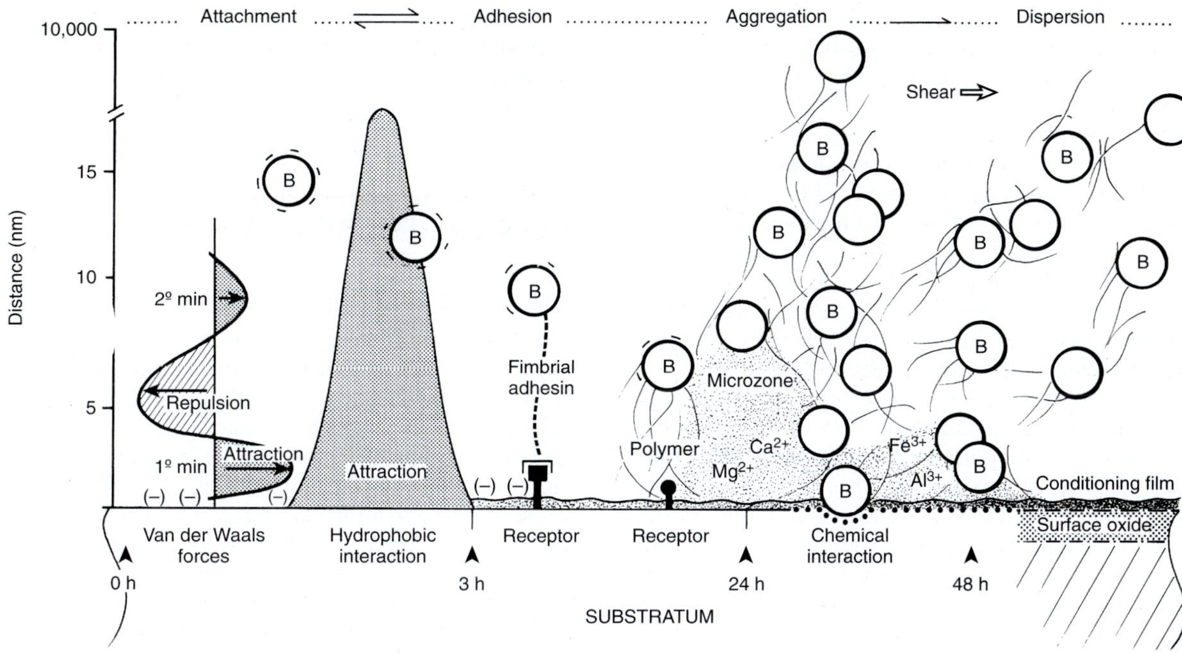

FIGURE 11-9: Molecular sequence for bacterial (*B*) attachment, adhesion, aggregation, and dispersion at the substratum surface. A number of possible interactions can occur, depending on the specific characteristics of the bacteria or substratum system (graphics, nutrients, contaminants, macromolecules, species, and materials). (From Gristina AG. Biomaterial-centered infection: Microbial adhesion versus tissue integration. *Science.* 1987;237:1588-1595. Copyright 1987 American Association for the Advancement of Science.)

and disperse, a process moderated by colony size, nutrient conditions, and hemodynamic or mechanical shear forces. In natural environments disaggregation is a survival strategy for the bacteria; in humans, however, it is involved in the pathogenesis of septic emboli. Disaggregation (dispersion) and its parameters might explain the phenomenon of intermittent or short-term bacterial showers or disseminated bacterial emboli.

BACTERIAL PATHOGENS

Organisms involved in septic arthritis and osteomyelitis of the shoulder include, in order of frequency,[95] *S. aureus, S. epidermidis, Streptococcus* group B, *E. coli, P. aeruginosa, Haemophilus influenzae* type B, *N. gonorrhoeae, Mycobacterium tuberculosis, Salmonella* and *Pneumococcus* species, and *Yersinia enterocolitica*.[164] Reported associations[42,47,52,54,89,139,169] and other etiologic pathogens are listed in Box 11-2.

S. aureus is now the most common cause of septic arthritis in children, followed by group A *Streptococcus*, and *Enterobacter* species. *H. influenzae*, previously a concern in those younger than 2 years, has significantly decreased with vaccination. The identification of *Kingella kingae* isolates in septic joints has increased with improved testing.[89] Lavy and colleagues reported on 19 children under the age of 2 years with *Salmonella* septic arthritis of the shoulder.[102] They concluded that low nutritional status was a factor in the development of bacteremia in their patients. Hematogenous septic arthritis

BOX 11-2. Organisms Involved in Septic Arthritis and Osteomyelitis of the Shoulder

Bacteria
Staphylococcus aureus
Staphylococcus epidermidis, Streptococcus group B
Escherichia coli, Pseudomonas aeruginosa, Haemophilus influenzae type B, *Neisseria gonorrhoeae, Mycobacterium tuberculosis,* and *Salmonella* and *Pneumococcus* species
Yersinia enterocolitica[66]

Fungi
Actinomyces species
Blastomyces species
Coccidioides species
Candida albicans
Sporothrix schenckii

Reported Associations
Rheumatoid arthritis: *Listeria monocytogenes*[67]
Renal transplant: *Aspergillus fumigatus*[68]
Newborns and pregnant women: group B β-hemolytic *Streptococcus agalactiae*[69]
Lymphedema: *Pasteurella multocida*[70]
Septic arthritis in systemic lupus erythematosus: *Mycobacterium xenopi*[71]
Chronic vesicoureteral reflux: *Escherichia coli*[72]
Sickle cell disease: *Salmonella* group G

in infants is primarily streptococcal, whereas hospital-acquired infections are primarily staphylococcal but can also feature *Candida* and gram-negative organisms, especially in infants.[144]

S. aureus is most common cause of septic arthritis in adults; *N. gonorrhoeae* is common in adults younger than 30 years.[56] Hemolytic streptococci are the most common streptococci in adults and children. Group B β-hemolytic streptococcal infection may rarely be associated with necrotizing fasciitis and death.[9] Necrotizing fasciitis has also been reported to be caused by *S. aureus*.[104] *Clostridium* septic arthritis has been reported to develop spontaneously and following intra-articular steroid injection.[62]

Gram-negative bacilli, such as *E. coli* and *P. aeruginosa*, are found in approximately 15% of joints and are especially prevalent in patients with urinary tract infections, diabetes,[8] or a debilitating disease. *Pseudomonas* sternoclavicular pyarthrosis is associated with IV drug abuse.[92] *M. tuberculosis* involves the knee, hip, ankle, and wrist more commonly compared with the shoulder. *Mycobacterium marinum* is found in marine environments. *Blastomyces* usually spreads from osteomyelitis to the intra-articular space. *Candida albicans* can spread via the hematogenous route in debilitated patients or directly from steroid injections. Shoulder girdle abscess formation due to *Streptococcus agalactiae* has been described as a complication of esophageal dilation.[129] *Aspergillus* arthritis of the glenohumeral joint has been reported in a renal transplant patient with associated neurologic involvement. Neutropenia and corticosteroid therapy have been associated with immunodeficiency-inducing risk factors. *Pneumococcal* septic arthritis seems to be predominantly a disease that affects the elderly.[12]

S. aureus is often the major pathogen in biometal, bone, joint, and soft tissue infections and is the most common pathogen isolated in osteomyelitis when damaged bone or cartilage acts as a substratum.[68] The predominance of *S. aureus* in adult intra-articular sepsis may be explained by its ubiquity as a tissue pathogen seeded from remote sites, its natural invasiveness and toxicity, and its receptors for collagen, fibronectin, fibrinogen, and laminin. *S. epidermidis* is most often involved when the biomaterial surface is a polymer or when a polymer is a component of a complex device (extended-wear contact lenses,[147] vascular prostheses,[176] and total joint prostheses). *S. epidermidis, S. aureus,* and *Propionibacterium* species are the most common organisms associated with deep infection following rotator cuff repair.[117]

Studies of chronic adult osteomyelitis have revealed polymicrobial infections in more than two thirds of cases.[68] The most common pathogens isolated include *S. aureus* and *S. epidermidis,* and *Pseudomonas, Enterococcus, Streptococcus, Bacillus,* and *Proteus* species. Polymicrobial infections, therefore, appear to be an important feature of substratum-induced infections; they are probably present more often than is realized, and can be a feature of chronic intra-articular sepsis and sinus formation.

In summary *S. aureus* is the most common organism in septic infections and is usually spread via hematogenous seeding. *S. epidermidis* is the principal organism in biomaterial-related infections, especially those centered on polymers. Mixed (polymicrobial), gram-negative, and anaerobic infections are often associated with open wounds and sinus tracts.

CLINICAL PRESENTATION

Symptoms and Signs

Pain, loss of motion, and effusion are early signs of infection. However, shoulder effusion is difficult to detect and is often missed. Motion is painful, and the arm is adducted and internally rotated. Radiographs might show a widened glenohumeral joint space and later signs of osteomyelitis (Fig. 11-10). Systemic signs include fever, leukocytosis, and sedimentation rate changes. The symptoms of immunosuppressed and rheumatoid patients may be muted. Delay in presentation is common, averaging greater than 7 days.[122] In a 50-patient case series by Sperling and colleagues, eight showed bilateral infection.[1]

The sternoclavicular joint may be involved and should be suspected in unilateral enlargement without trauma in patients younger than 50 years. Gonococcal and staphylococcal infections have been reported. IV drug abusers are susceptible to infection by gram-negative organisms, especially *P. aeruginosa* and *Serratia marcescens.* The acromioclavicular joint is rarely involved in sepsis but may be contaminated by steroid injections. Wound infection is not uncommon after surgical resection of the distal clavicle for osteoarthritis, probably due to the proximity of the joint to the overlying skin and the lack of an intervening muscle layer. Chanet and colleagues reported that a past history of radiation for breast cancer was a risk factor for the development of septic arthritis of the glenohumeral and sternoclavicular joints.[24] The mean

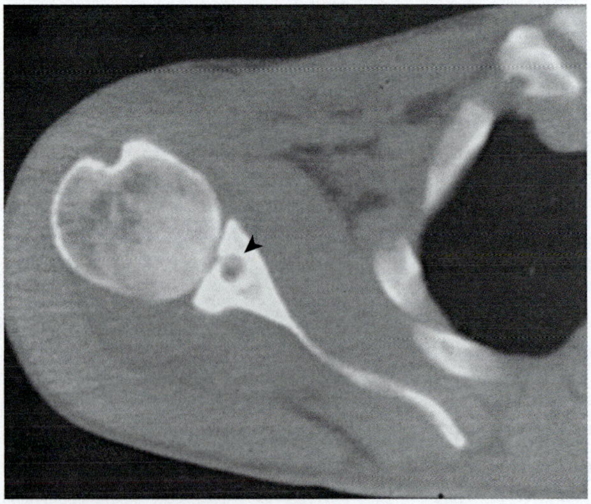

FIGURE 11-10: Staphylococcal osteomyelitis of the scapula. The *arrowhead* indicates an abscess secondary to infection caused by intra-articular steroid injection. (Courtesy Mark Warburton, MD, High Point, NC.)

time elapsed since radiation was 16 years (range, 3 to 34 years).

Gabriel and colleagues reported on a 5-week-old boy who had a brachial plexus neuropathy and paralysis of the upper extremity secondary to septic arthritis of the glenohumeral joint and osteomyelitis of the proximal part of the humerus.[53] They pointed out that pseudoparalysis of a limb associated with sepsis was a well-documented phenomenon. Similarly, muscular spasm associated with pain caused by infection can lead to apparent weakness. True nerve paralysis associated with osteomyelitis is uncommon, and its documentation by electrodiagnostic studies is rare. Permanent weakness persisted in the patient even though the glenohumeral joint and proximal humerus were surgically drained. The possible causes of the plexus neuropathy associated with infection included ischemic neuropathy from thrombophlebitis of the vasa nervorum, arterial embolism, hyperergic or hypersensitivity reactions, and local compression due to abscess formation. Rankin and Rycken reported bilateral dislocations of the proximal humerus as a result of septic arthritis.[131] Miron and colleagues have also reported transient brachial plexus palsy associated with suppurative arthritis of the shoulder.[116]

Total Shoulder Replacement

Sepsis after total joint replacement of the shoulder is relatively rare because of prophylactic antibiotic use and the excellent blood supply of the surrounding soft tissues. Symptoms of infection include pain, loss of motion, and subluxation. Pain relief is so universal after total shoulder replacement that infection should be suspected if there is pain or lucency around the cement mantle.

Rheumatoid Arthritis

Patients with chronic rheumatoid arthritis are susceptible to spontaneous septic arthritis.[71,93] Because the active destructive process of the rheumatoid arthritis masks the septic condition, detection of the infection is often delayed. The onset of septic arthritis should be suspected when the clinical course of the rheumatoid patient worsens acutely, especially if the disease is long term. When infection is present, the patient experiences a sudden aggravation of pain as well as swelling and increased temperature in the joint; sudden chills can also occur. The physician should emphasize to patients with chronic rheumatoid arthritis (and to caregivers) that a sudden exacerbation of symptoms warrants investigation.

Differential Diagnosis

Radiographs are not especially useful in the early diagnosis because septic arthritis does not significantly alter the bone destruction resulting from rheumatoid arthritis and because bone and joint radiographic changes are delayed. Other acute arthritic disorders can imitate or mask sepsis, including gout, pseudogout, rheumatic fever, juvenile rheumatoid arthritis, neuropathic arthropathy,[108] and the oligoarthritic syndromes. Trauma and tumors can cause adjacent joint effusions and must be considered.

LABORATORY EVALUATION

The culture and analysis of synovial fluid is critical for diagnosis. The joint should always be aspirated when sepsis is suspected. Radiographic control is indicated if the approach is difficult about total joints. The injection of saline or simultaneous arthrography of the glenohumeral joint may be helpful in certain cases. When the results of cultures are negative and the diagnosis is difficult to make, an arthroscopic biopsy can be useful. A synovial biopsy and culture for acid-fast organisms and fungi should be performed in patients with chronic monoarticular arthritis, especially those with tenosynovitis.

Viral infection must be considered when bacteria cannot be identified. Smith and Piercy report that viral arthritis is associated with rubella, parvovirus, mumps, hepatitis B, and lymphocytic choriomeningitis.[149] For a patient who presents with multiple joint involvement and systemic manifestations consistent with a viral infection, serologic confirmation of the infection should be obtained because it is not usually possible to isolate the virus from joint fluid.

Synovial Fluid Analysis

If septic arthritis is suspected, the synovial fluid should be examined. Septic arthritis is probable if the leukocyte count is greater than 50,000 cells/mm^3, the glucose level is low, and more than 75% of the cells are polymorphonuclear. These findings are beyond the range compatible with uncomplicated rheumatoid arthritis. In bacterial infections aspiration can yield 10 mL or more of fluid. Synovial joint fluid is usually opaque or brownish, turbid, and thick, but it may be serosanguineous in 15% of cases with poor mucin clot formation. Proteins are elevated primarily because of an elevated WBC count (usually >50,000/mm^3 and often as great as 100,000/mm^3, primarily of neutrophils). Half of adults and a less than half of children have a glucose level in the joint fluid that is 40 mg/L less than that in the serum glucose drawn at the same time.[83,146,172] These findings are more common later in infection. Polymorphonuclear leukocytes are dominant (90%); counts greater than 100,000/mm^3 are typical of staphylococcal and acute bacterial infection. Mehta and colleagues reported positive cultures in 96% of aspirates from patients with suspected septic arthritis when the polymorphonuclear differential count was greater than 85% of the total aspirate WBC count.[113] Monocytes are more predominant in mycobacterial infections. Crystal examination is needed to rule out gout or pseudogout. Rheumatoid, rheumatic, and crystalline joint diseases also elevate leukocytes, but the presence of these diseases does not exclude concomitant sepsis.[183]

The results of Gram staining are positive approximately 50% of the time, but false-positive results do occur. Positive joint cultures occur in 90% of patients with

TABLE 11-2 Synovial Fluid Findings in Acute Pyogenic Arthritis

Joint Fluid Examination	Noninflammatory Fluids	Inflammatory Fluids	
		Noninfectious	**Infectious**
Color	Colorless, pale yellow	Yellow to white	Yellow
Turbidity	Clear, slightly turbid	Turbid	Turbid, purulent
Viscosity	Not reduced	Reduced	Reduced
Mucin clot	Tight clot	Friable	Friable
Cell count (per mm^3)	200-1000	3000-10,000	10,000-100,000
Predominant cell type	Mononuclear	PMN	PMN
Synovial fluid to blood glucose ratio	0.8-1.0	0.5-0.8	<0.5
Lactic acid	Same as plasma	Higher than plasma	Often very high
Gram stain for organism	None	None	Positive*
Culture	Negative	Negative	Positive*

From Schmid FR. Principles of diagnosis and treatment of bone and joint infections. In: McCarty DJ, ed. Arthritis and Allied Conditions: A Textbook of Rheumatology. *Philadelphia: Lea & Febiger; 1985:1638.*

**In some cases, especially in gonococcal infection, no organisms may be demonstrated.*

PMN, polymorphonuclear neutrophil.

established bacterial septic arthritis and in 75% of patients with tubercular arthritis.[171] Blood cultures should also be obtained; the results are positive in approximately 50% of patients with acute infection. Some prosthesis-centered infections are difficult to detect unless tissue is biopsied and prepared for culture (Table 11-2). Protocols may need adjustment to allow adequate growth time to identify slower growing organisms, such as *P. acnes.* The current recommendations for isolating *P. acnes* state that it requires at least 13 days after collection.[22] Culture specimens should be taken for gram-positive, gram-negative, aerobic, and anaerobic bacteria, and for mycobacteria and fungi. Laboratory technique and media selection should be based on the type of antibiotic given to the patient and on the specific nutrient requirements of suspected bacteria. The magnitude of anaerobic septic arthritis has been underestimated in the past.[48]

Newer testing for infection, including serum markers for IL-6, alpha defensing, and leukocyte esterase, show promise, but clinical testing has shown mixed results.[35,36,73]

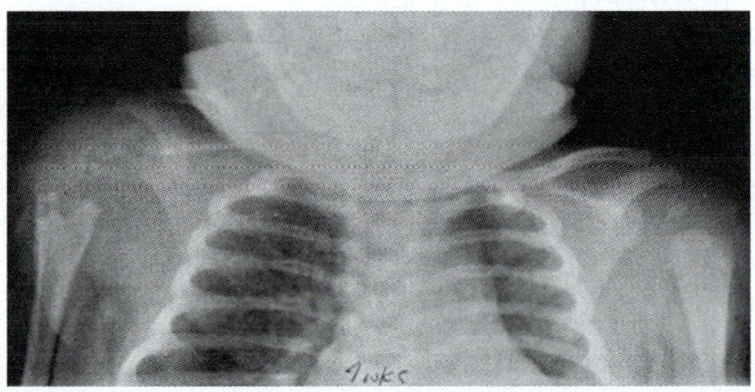

FIGURE 11-11: Septic arthritis of the right shoulder with destruction and widening of the proximal humerus. Note also the healing of a right clavicle fracture. The organism was β-hemolytic *Streptococcus.* (Courtesy Department of Radiology, Wake Forest University Medical Center, Winston-Salem, NC.)

Imaging Studies

Radiographs and CT scans of the septic shoulder can indicate changes ranging from widening to subluxation and from bone destruction to new bone formation (Figs. 11-11 to 11-13). Ultrasound is useful in assisting aspiration and in assessing the infected shoulder joints.[60] Technetium bone scanning has been reported to be positive in 75% to 100% of septic arthritis cases, but technetium, gallium, and indium scans are not always consistent.[57,114,182] Schmidt and colleagues found that the results of technetium bone scans performed on children with septic arthritis were often negative.[144] Indium scans may be more accurate indicators of sepsis, but conclusive data are lacking. Indium scintigraphy for osteomyelitis should be preceded by a positive result on a technetium scan. If the result of an indium scan is negative, infection is unlikely; a positive result on an indium scan increases the specificity of the diagnosis. Indium uptake should be evaluated against the normal reticuloendothelial background.[182] False-negative results can occur in neonates and during the acute phase of osteomyelitis.[55]

Gupta and Prezio[74] found that the specificity of nuclear scintigraphy using ^{99m}Tc phosphonates, ^{67}Ga citrate, or ^{111}In-labeled leukocytes for diagnosing musculoskeletal infection could be improved if two nucleotide studies

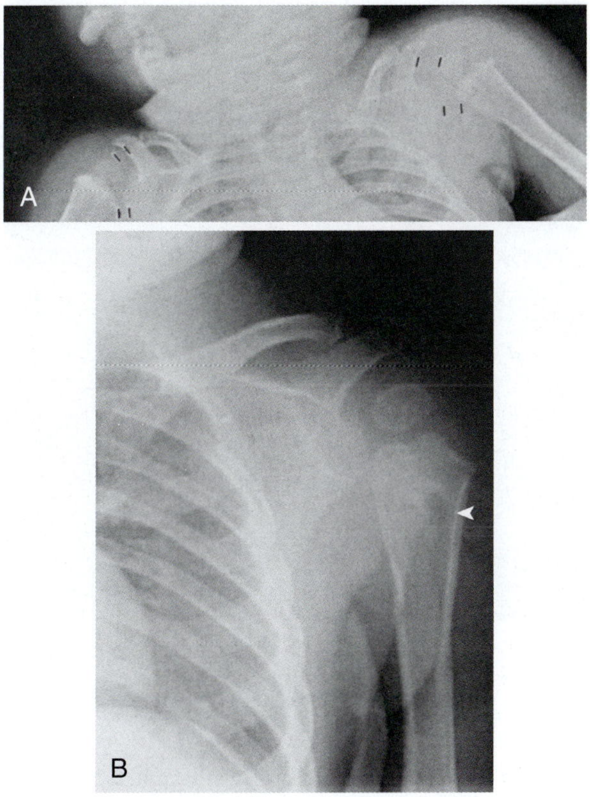

FIGURE 11-12: **A,** Early intra-articular sepsis of the left shoulder. Note the widening of the joint space (*markers*) compared with the opposite side. **B,** Late intra-articular sepsis. Note the lucent lesion and osteomyelitis of the proximal humerus (*arrowhead*). The organisms were *Staphylococcus epidermidis,* β-hemolytic *Streptococcus*, and *Bacillus subtilis.*

were used in conjunction. The main limitation of scintigraphic investigations is their limited spatial resolution, making the results inexact. Furthermore, such studies can take hours to days for completion.

CT is useful in identifying small early lytic lesions caused by osteomyelitis that might be obscured in ordinary radiographs. The diagnosis of sternoclavicular joint sepsis and clavicular osteomyelitis infections may be improved using CT because it overcomes the tissue-overlap problem that occurs with ordinary radiographs; however, CT does not offer much advantage in imaging the sepsis of humerus.

MRI can facilitate the differentiation of acute from chronic osteomyelitis and can help to detect evidence of active infection in the presence of chronic inflammation, rheumatologic disorder, or posttraumatic lesions.[11,163] Early changes of osteomyelitis cause accumulation of fluid, inflammatory cells, and exudate in the marrow, producing a focus of low signal intensity within bright, fatty marrow. In chronic osteomyelitis large areas of abnormal or low signals on MRI can indicate an area of possible sequestration and hyperemia, especially along sinus tracts.[33] The capsular distention of articular cartilage and fluid-filled spaces are clearly visible on MRI, as are damaged surfaces, loose bodies, and avascular regions. MRI can be sensitive in early detection and specific for localizing and identifying sequestra[49,78,143] (Figs. 11-14 and 11-15).

De Boeck and colleagues reported on the usefulness of MRI in detecting pyomyositis[34] and found it to be useful in excluding other pathologic processes, such as infectious arthritis, osteomyelitis, hematoma, thrombophlebitis, and malignant tumor. MRI is helpful for pregnant patients because it provides a highly sensitive

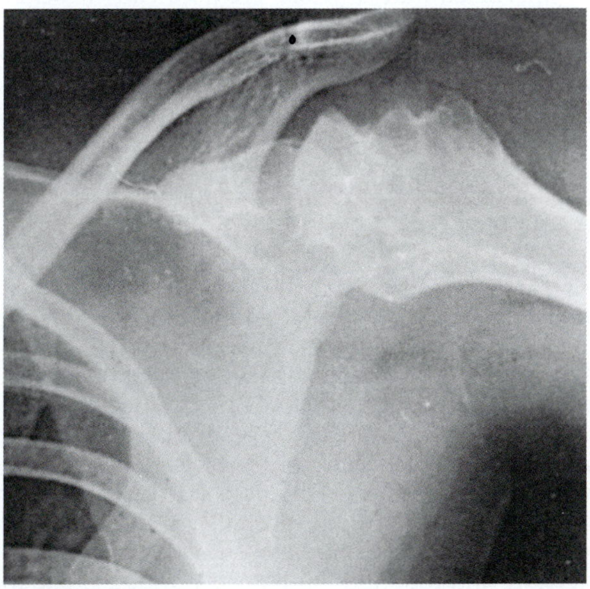

FIGURE 11-13: Cystic lesions in the humeral head consistent with tuberculosis sicca in a 19-year-old woman. (From DePalma AF, ed. *Surgery of the Shoulder.* 3rd ed. Philadelphia: JB Lippincott; 1983.)

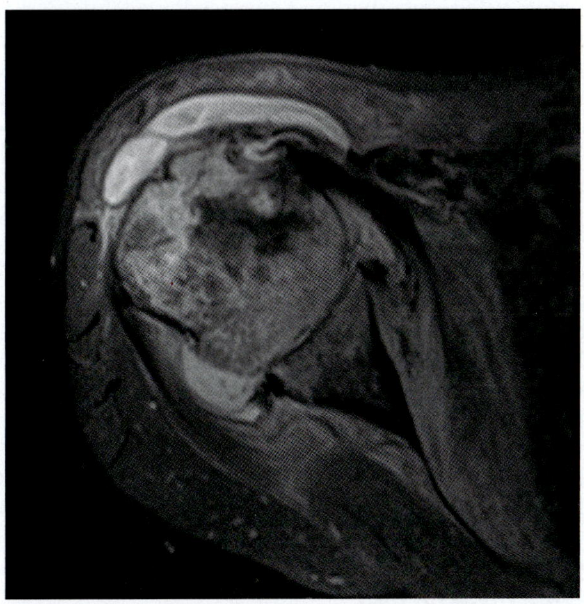

FIGURE 11-14: Axial T2-weighted image of diffuse shoulder infection in an adult. Abscess formation can be noted in the subdeltoid space and proximal humerus.

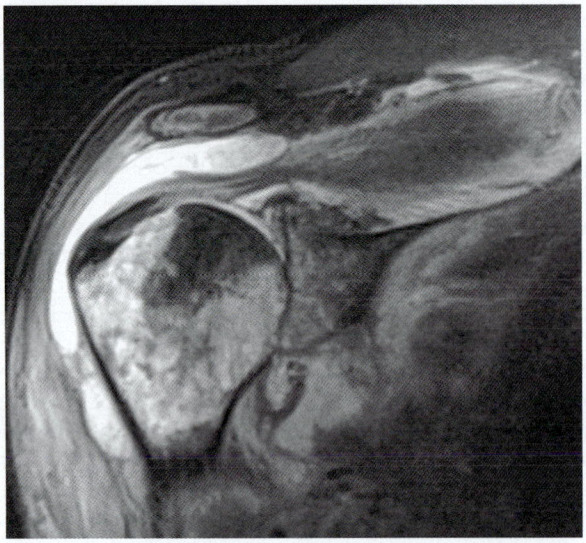

FIGURE 11-15: Coronal T2-weighted image of diffuse shoulder infection in an adult. Abscess tracks can be seen medially on the anterior and posterior surfaces of the body of the scapula.

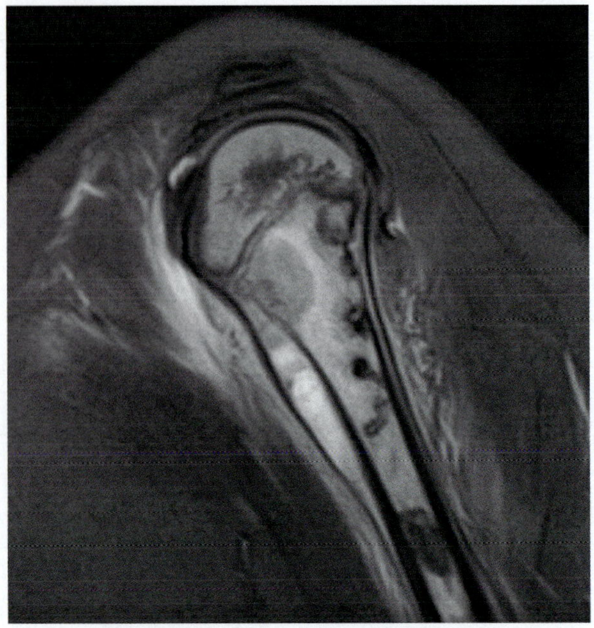

FIGURE 11-16: Sagittal magnetic resonance image of proximal humerus abscess formation in an adolescent.

method of detecting skeletal infection without exposing the fetus to ionizing radiation.

Ultrasound can also be used to advantage in defining abscess formation.[158] Widman and colleagues reported that ultrasound can be used to differentiate septic arthritis of the acromioclavicular joint from septic arthritis of the shoulder joint.[178]

Hopkins and colleagues assessed the role of gadolinium-enhanced MRI in providing diagnostic information beyond that given by nonenhanced MRI in the evaluation of musculoskeletal infectious processes.[80] They found that gadolinium-enhanced MRI was a highly sensitive technique that was especially useful in distinguishing abscesses from surrounding cellulitis or myositis. Lack of contrast enhancement ruled out infection with a high degree of certainty. However, these authors pointed out that contrast enhancement cannot be used to reliably distinguish infectious from noninfectious inflammatory conditions. In their study, gadolinium-enhanced MRI was found to have a very high sensitivity (89% to 100%) and high accuracy (79% to 88%) in the diagnosis of various infectious lesions in the musculoskeletal system. However, the specificities (46% to 88%) were not as high (Fig. 11-16).

Tehranzadeh and colleagues have reported on the use of MRI in diagnosing osteomyelitis.[163] In several comparative studies MRI has been reported to be more advantageous in detecting the presence and determining the extent of osteomyelitis compared with scintigraphy, CT, and conventional radiography.

COMPLICATIONS

Inadequately treated intra-articular sepsis or osteomyelitis can result in recurrent infection, contiguous spread, bacteremia, distant septic emboli, anemia, septic shock, and death. Delayed diagnosis and adequate treatment can result in joint surface destruction, contractures, subluxation, arthritis, and growth aberrations.[125] Inflammation, bacterial products, and lysosomal enzymes break down cartilage.[99] Within weeks, bacterial antigens stimulate destructive inflammation that can persist after the infection is treated. Bacterial endotoxins are chemotactic, and bacterial proteolytic enzymes further destroy surfaces. Increased intra-articular pressure causes ischemia. Thrombotic events are also stimulated by burgeoning infection, further destroying the joint and adjacent bone. Long-term complications of chronic osteomyelitis can include amyloidosis, the nephrotic syndrome, and epidermal carcinoma.

TREATMENT

Most clinicians agree that systemic antibiotic therapy should begin immediately after the diagnosis of septic arthritis, but there is less agreement on subsequent therapy. Repeated needle aspiration has been recommended as a primary treatment.[96,172] In our opinion, drainage by urgent arthroscopy or arthrotomy is the treatment of choice, especially for the shoulder.[90,133] Forward and Hunter have reported the use of a small arthroscope in the treatment of septic arthritis of the shoulder in infants.[51] They recommended insertion of the arthroscope posteriorly and reported full recovery with a single intervention in three patients. In a study of 78 joints (including 10 shoulders) Stutz and colleagues reported that septic arthritis could be treated with arthroscopic irrigation and systemic antibiotic therapy in 91% of the affected joints.[161]

Jerosch and colleagues reported the successful treatment of septic arthritis by arthroscopy in 12 patients between 4 and 57 years of age.[85] Jeon and colleagues reported on 19 patients who underwent arthroscopic irrigation and debridement for septic arthritis of the glenohumeral joint.[84] Fifteen patients had received an injection into the joint preceding the development of infection. The infection was eradicated completely with a single procedure in 14 patients. Sperling and colleagues found that 32% (16 of 50) patients required reoperation within 1 month due to recurrent infection.[1]

In general, the literature suggests that treatment of septic arthritis with repeated needle aspiration and appropriate IV antibiotics may be adequate, except for the hip. However, conclusive studies of initial surgical drainage versus needle aspiration are lacking. In a retrospective study comparing 55 infected joints treated by needle aspiration with 18 joints treated surgically, it was concluded that 60% of surgically treated patients experienced sequelae, whereas 80% of medically treated patients recovered completely.[59] However, it must be noted that there was no difference in outcome in the only randomized prospective study that compared aspiration to arthrotomy.[152] In this study of 61 children in Malawi who had septic arthritis of the shoulder, both groups received antibiotics for 6 weeks, and most of the infections were due to *Salmonella*.

Most orthopedic surgeons believe that the anatomy of the shoulder and the nature of shoulder sepsis demand surgical treatment. Septic arthritis that does not rapidly and progressively respond to medical management should be surgically drained. Sternoclavicular joint infections in drug abusers usually involve both bone and joint. For these patients, needle aspiration has not been useful in establishing the diagnosis. However, surgical drainage has been useful in identifying the pathogen. It also allows debridement of necrotic bone and permits drainage of abscesses, which are often present.[10,135] Intra-articular sepsis should be treated in a timely manner.[79] Variables that influence the selection of treatment methods include the duration of infection, host immune status, types of infecting organisms, and presence of foreign bodies, or adjacent osteomyelitis; of these, the most critical factors are the infecting organism and the presence of a foreign body.

Osteomyelitis of the proximal metaphysis can precede or be secondary to septic arthritis of the glenohumeral joint. Therefore, drilling of the metaphysis has been recommended for pediatric septic glenohumeral arthritis to rule out osteomyelitis and to allow adequate decompression of the bone.

Immobilization is usually recommended for septic arthritis. However, a study by Salter and colleagues of septic arthritis in a rabbit model indicated that the use of continuous passive motion was superior to immobilization or to intermittent active motion.[141] Possible explanations for this include prevention of bacterial adhesion, enhanced diffusion of nutrients, improved clearance of lysosomal enzymes and debris from the infected joints, and stimulation of chondrocytes to synthesize the various components of the matrix.

Gonococcal septic arthritis may be polyarticular. Fever is low grade, usually below 102° F; articular and periarticular structures become swollen, stiff, and painful, followed by desquamation of skin over the joints. During septicemia, a macular rash or occasionally a vesicular rash occurs in one third of patients, but such a rash can also be caused by *Neisseria meningitidis*, *Haemophilus* species, and *Streptobacillus* species. Organisms are not common in joint fluid and, therefore, are not isolated in most cases. The general picture of gonococcal septic arthritis is less acute than that of staphylococcal infection. Gonococcal arthritis responds well to systemic antibiotic therapy and needle aspiration; however, in refractory cases arthrocentesis may be required.

Antimicrobial agents used to treat joint infections generally achieve intra-articular levels that are equal to or greater than serum levels, except for erythromycin and gentamicin (Table 11-3). Thus, intra-articular antibiotics are generally not advocated. In osteomyelitis antibiotic penetration into bone is unreliable,[124] with clindamycin achieving higher bone levels than cephalothin or methicillin. When treating healthy (nonsequestrated) bone in children, delivery of antibiotics to the infected site is likely. However, the opposite situation exists in adults, older people, vascularly compromised patients, and patients with chronic osteomyelitis, sequestration, and sinus formation. Animal studies have suggested that antibiotic combinations (e.g., oxacillin and aminoglycosides) may be more effective than single antibiotics in osteomyelitis.[124] The quinolone group of antibiotics may be useful because of its broad spectrum of activity against staphylococci, *Pseudomonas* species, and gram-negative bacteria.[38] These agents achieve excellent local levels in living and dead bone. Mutant strains of organisms can emerge, but they can be reduced by the intelligent use of quinolones in combination with other antibiotics.

Mader and colleagues reported that antibiotic selection should be based on in vitro sensitivity testing, with the drug exhibiting the highest bactericidal activity with the least toxicity and lowest cost being chosen.[109] Surgical treatment must convert an infection with dead bone into a situation with well-vascularized tissues that are readily penetrated by blood-borne antibiotics. The duration of antibiotic therapy is empirical and depends on the clinical response of the patient. Several (4 to 6) weeks of treatment has become a standard length for empiric reasons. Dirschl and Almekinders reported that combined IV and oral antibiotic therapy has become accepted as a standard treatment for osteomyelitis in children.[39] The duration of IV antibiotic therapy ranges from 3 to 14 days in various series. Close outpatient follow-up is imperative, and treatment should be continued for 4 to 6 weeks; it should be prolonged if the erythrocyte sedimentation rate does not fall below 20 mm/hr after 6 weeks. Oral antibiotic therapy has obvious economic advantages over IV therapy. However, the route of antibiotic delivery is probably not important as long as the infecting organism is susceptible to the antibiotic and the antibiotic is delivered to the tissues in adequate concentration to eradicate the infection. The decision of whether to use oral or parenteral

TABLE 11-3 Empiric Antibiotic Therapy for Septic Arthritis

	Antibiotic	
Pathology	**Preferred**	**Alternative**
<2 Months		
No organism	Oxacillin and aminoglycoside	Cefazolin and aminoglycoside
Gram-positive cocci	Oxacillin *or* nafcillin	Cephalothin *or* cephapirin
Gram-negative bacilli	Aminoglycoside	Cefotaxime
2 Months to 5 Years		
No organism	Nafcillin and chloramphenicol	Cefuroxime
Gram-positive cocci	Nafcillin or oxacillin	Cefazolin, cephalothin, vancomycin, clindamycin
Gram-negative bacilli	Aminoglycoside	Cefotaxime
Gram-negative coccobacilli	Cefotaxime *or* ampicillin and chloramphenicol	Chloramphenicol alone; trimethoprim-sulfamethoxazole
5-15 Years		
No organism	Nafcillin *or* oxacillin	Cefazolin *or* vancomycin
Gram-positive cocci	Nafcillin *or* oxacillin	Cefazolin, cephalothin, vancomycin, clindamycin
Gram-negative bacilli*	Aminoglycoside	Cefotaxime
Gram-negative cocci	Treat for *Neisseria gonorrhoeae*	
>40 Years		
No organism	Nafcillin ± aminoglycoside	Cefazolin ± aminoglycoside
Gram-positive cocci	Nafcillin or oxacillin	Cefazolin, cephalothin, vancomycin, clindamycin
Gram-negative bacilli	Ticarcillin + aminoglycoside	Cefotaxime ± aminoglycoside

Modified from American Medical Association, Division of Drugs and Toxicology: Anti-microbial therapy for common infectious diseases. In American Medical Association: Drug Evaluations Annual 1995. *Chicago: American Medical Association, 1995, pp 1277-1282.*
**To 40 years.*

antibiotics should be based on microorganism sensitivity, patient compliance, infectious disease consultation, and the surgeon's experience.[103]

Antibiotic therapy is generally continued for more than 3 weeks in septic arthritis and for more than 4 to 6 weeks in osteomyelitis and is monitored by systemic signs, WBC count, and sedimentation rate.[123] Surgical debridement is the mainstay of treatment for septic arthritis and osteomyelitis of the shoulder as toxic products, damaged tissue, and foreign bodies must be removed to prevent damage and to treat infection effectively; laboratory studies have shown that the minimum inhibitory concentration and minimum bactericidal concentration levels needed to treat surface-adherent bacterial populations are 10 to 100 times higher than those needed to treat suspension populations.[67,101,125] These findings suggest that it is possible to clear a bacteremia or bacteria suspended in synovial fluid, but very difficult to sterilize an infected cartilaginous joint surface or sequestrum covered with debris without administering toxic levels of antibiotics (Fig. 11-17).

Antibiotic-impregnated beads (gentamicin or tobramycin) may be indicated in certain cases of osteomyelitis and articular sepsis[50,61]; removal at 6 to 12 weeks is suggested. Closed suction and irrigation may be used for short periods (<3 days) if necessary in special cases in septic joints, provided the system does not allow retrograde contamination. However, the literature does not indicate a definite advantage with this treatment, and it is seldom required in de novo joint sepsis because adequate antibiotic levels can be achieved systemically. IV amphotericin B remains the preferred drug in patients with deep systemic fungal infections.[39] Chronic osteomyelitis requires debridement to healthy viable tissue. Debridement should be performed until punctate bleeding is noted. Local muscle flaps or vacuum-assisted closure systems may be helpful if there is associated soft tissue deficiency.

OUTCOME

The prognosis for adults with septic arthritis of the shoulder is poor, but shoulders treated soon after the onset of symptoms may do well. Poor results are associated with delayed diagnosis, virulent (gram-negative) infecting

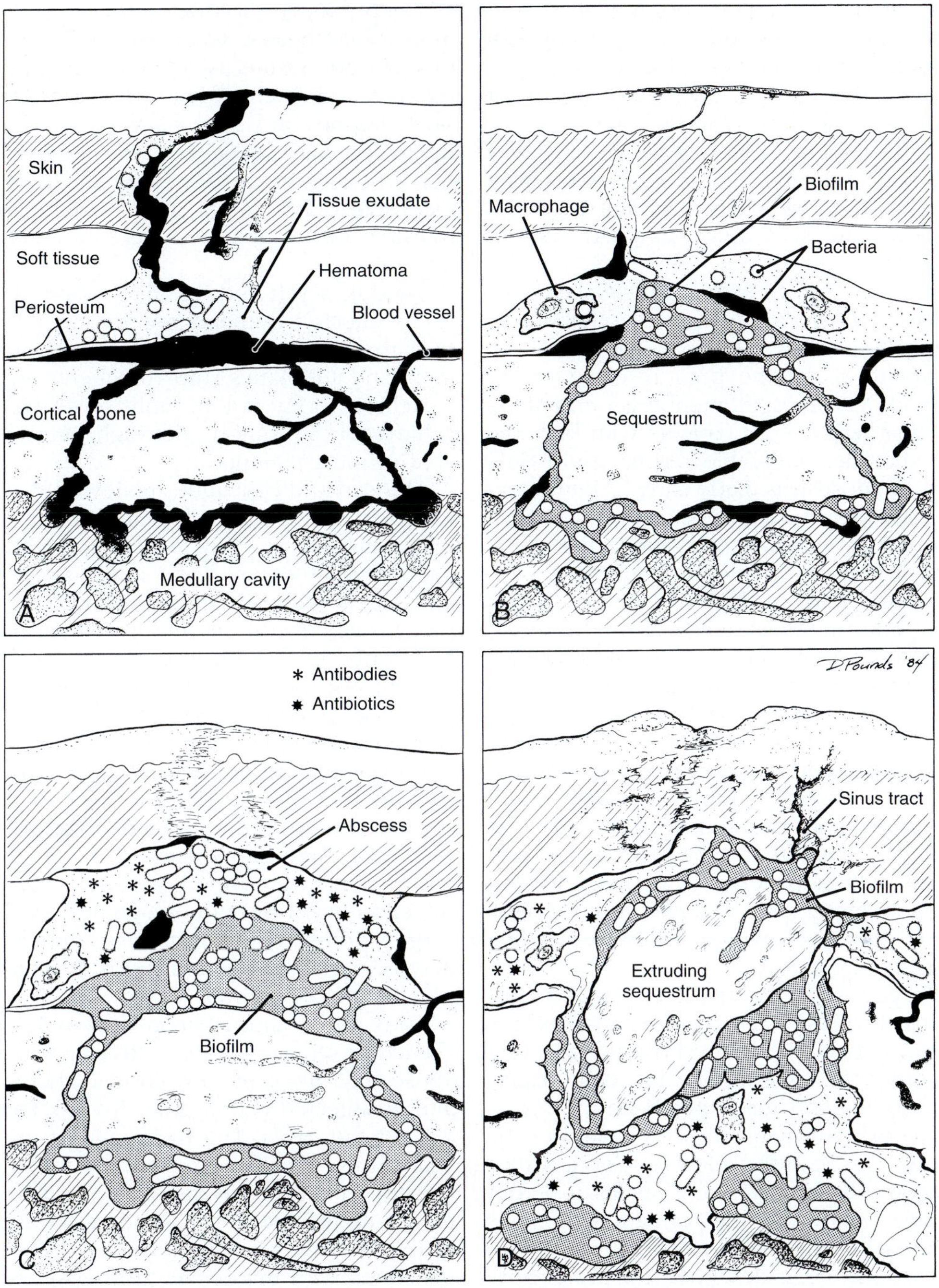

FIGURE 11-17: The sequence of pathogenesis in osteomyelitis. **A,** Initial trauma produces soft tissue destruction and bone fragmentation as well as wound contamination by bacteria. In closed wounds, contamination can occur by hematogenous seeding. **B,** As the infection progresses, bacterial colonization occurs within a protective exopolysaccharide biofilm. The biofilm is particularly abundant on the devitalized bone fragment, which acts as a passive substratum for colonization. **C,** Host defenses are mobilized against the infection but are unable to penetrate or act effectively in the presence of the biofilm. **D,** Progressive inflammation and abscess formation eventually result in the development of a sinus tract and, in some cases, ultimate extrusion of the sequestrum that is the focus of the resistant infection. (From Gristina AG, Barth E, Webb LX. Microbial adhesion and the pathogenesis of biomaterial-centered infections. In: Gustilo RB, Gruninger RP, Tsukayama DT, eds. *Orthopaedic Infection: Diagnosis and Treatment.* Philadelphia: WB Saunders; 1989:3-25.)

organisms, persistent pain, drainage, osteomyelitis, and destruction of the joint. In their series of eight children with neonatal septic arthritis of the shoulder, Bos and colleagues concluded that early diagnosis and treatment was associated with a more favorable outcome.[17]

In a series of 16 shoulders, Gelberman and colleagues reported a satisfactory outcome in 8 of 10 patients with septic arthritis of the shoulder when treatment was initiated 4 weeks or less after symptoms appeared.[56] Six of the eight satisfactory results from Gelberman's series were in patients infected with either *Streptococcus* or coagulase-negative *Staphylococcus* species. Gelberman attributed poor results in eight other patients to a delay in diagnosis, although six of the poor results were in patients infected with *S. aureus*. Pfeiffenberger and Meiss reported that in their series of 28 patients with bacterial infections of the shoulder, favorable results could only be obtained if the diagnosis was made early.[128] Bettin and colleagues also found early diagnosis to be the most important determining factor concerning the final outcome of septic arthritis in 35 elderly patients.[13]

Leslie and colleagues reviewed 18 cases of septic arthritis of the shoulder in adults aged 42 to 89 years.[106] All except one had at least one serious associated disease, and eight patients had received an injection or aspiration of the shoulder before the infection developed. Diagnosis was delayed in 17 of the 18 patients. On admission to hospital the erythrocyte sedimentation rate was elevated in all cases, but the body temperature and WBC count were not. After treatment, the functional result was usually poor. Only five patients regained forward flexion to 90 degrees or more; eight patients did not regain active motion of the glenohumeral joint, and two patients died. Arthrotomy appeared to have achieved better results than did repeated aspiration.

Leslie and colleagues reported that five of six patients with septic arthritis who had rotator cuff tears showed a marked discrepancy between active and passive shoulder motion.[106] They noted that the poor functional results recorded in these six patients may have been more of a reflection of the rotator cuff tear than of damage to the articular cartilage as a result of the infection. Septic arthritis following rotator cuff surgery rarely results in exposure of the humeral head and the formation of sinus tracts. In such cases the interposition of a muscle flap may be required, as has been described for the closure of infected sternotomy wounds.[46]

Smith and Piercy reported that the characteristics of patients with bacterial arthritis for whom a poor outcome is expected include age greater than 60 years, preexisting rheumatoid arthritis, infection in the shoulder, symptoms lasting for more than 1 week before treatment, involvement of more than four joints, and persistently positive cultures after a 7-day course with appropriate antibiotic therapy.[149] Smith and colleagues reported mortality in 3 of 15 rheumatoid patients with sepsis of the shoulder.[148] Nine of these patients had multiple joint infections. Unsatisfactory shoulder function was common, and the mean forward elevation was 100 degrees.

Deep infection following rotator cuff repair is uncommon. Nevertheless, when such infection occurs, numerous procedures are usually required in order to eradicate the infection. Such patients are often afebrile with normal WBC counts, but they have elevated erythrocyte sedimentation rates. Patients rarely recover overhead shoulder function. In the series of Mirzayan and colleagues, extensive debridement, often combined with a muscle transfer and antibiotics, were required to control the infection.[117]

Haidukewych and Sperling reported on the treatment of 15 infected humeral nonunions, of which four were proximal.[76] All the patients were treated with debridement and antibiotics, and 10 patients underwent attempts to achieve bony union. Only seven of these 10 patients achieved bony union, although pain relief was predictable in most patients.

Duncan and colleagues reviewed six patients who had infection following a clavicle fracture.[41] Five of the six infections occurred in association with open reduction and internal fixation. Three infections were polymicrobial and three were single-organism infections. Only two patients achieved bony union of their fractures. Infection following clavicle fracture is extremely difficult to treat and has a poor prognosis. Sperling and colleagues reviewed six patients who developed infection following shoulder instability surgery.[154] Three patients had late infections manifesting more than 8 months after surgery; each of these had a sinus leading to a retained nonabsorbable suture. Three patients had polymicrobial infections and three had single-organism infections. None of the patients developed recurrent shoulder instability. Infection may be acute or significantly delayed following surgery for shoulder instability, and if it occurs late, it may be associated with a nidus of infection surrounding nonabsorbable sutures.

Ross and Shamsuddin reviewed 180 cases of sternoclavicular septic arthritis.[138] Risk factors included IV drug abuse, a distant site of infection, diabetes mellitus, trauma, and an infected central line. No risk factor was found in 23% of the cases. The mean age of the patients was 45 years, and 73% of the patients were male. *S. aureus* was isolated in 49% of the cases. Sternoclavicular septic arthritis accounted for 1% of septic arthritis overall and 17% in the IV drug abusers, possibly due to attempted local injections with inadequate antisepsis. CT or MRI should be performed to rule out associated abscess formation or mediastinitis. Surgical drainage, antibiotics and, in some cases, pectoralis major muscle flap procedures were required to control the infection.

The majority of children do well after treatment of septic shoulder arthritis. In a study of nine children with glenohumeral arthritis, Schmidt and colleagues suggested surgical treatment with exploration of the biceps tendon sheath.[144] However, growth center damage is possible. Lejman and colleagues reported that almost all of their series of 42 pediatric patients experienced reduced motion as a sequela of septic arthritis that had occurred during the first 18 months of life.[105] Although only 7% of the humeral heads were normal in their patients, the range of motion could not be predicted from the shape of the humeral head. Saisu and colleagues reported humeral shortening and inferior subluxation as sequelae of septic arthritis of the shoulder in neonates and infants when arthrotomy was performed more than 10 days after the onset of the infection.[140]

Mileti and colleagues reported on 13 patients who underwent shoulder arthroplasty for the treatment of postinfectious glenohumeral arthritis.[115] None of the patients had a recurrence of infection; mean follow-up was 9.7 years, and pain decreased and motion improved in their patients. Shoulder abduction improved from 75 degrees to 117 degrees, and mean external rotation improved from 13 degrees to 36 degrees. The authors concluded that shoulder arthroplasty for the treatment of the sequelae of an infected shoulder can be performed with a low risk of reinfection.

Refractory clavicular infection may require clavicular resection. Krishnan and colleagues reported a high complication rate following claviculectomy, although functional outcome was good in their study group of six patients.[100]

Wick and colleagues treated 15 patients with septic arthritis by shoulder arthrodesis.[177] Antibiotics were administered for 6 weeks. A positive outcome was more common in patients younger than 50 years and in those who had undergone fewer than four previous procedures. We have rarely performed shoulder arthrodesis to treat infection.

Itamura and colleagues demonstrated that placement of an articulating antibiotic spacer is not only successful in eliminating infection but also potentially a final treatment in lower demand patients. Half of those treated elected to retain their implant rather than to undergo a revision surgery for reimplantation with a metal prosthesis (Fig. 11-18).[159]

Resection arthroplasty is a rare option for failed shoulder replacement and/or chronic infection of the shoulder joint. Rispoli and colleagues reported on 18 patients who underwent resection arthroplasty with a mean follow-up of 8.3 years.[134] Although pain was reduced by the procedure, 15 patients continued to experience moderate to severe pain. The mean active elevation was 70 degrees. Most shoulders were comfortable at rest, but with profound functional limitations.

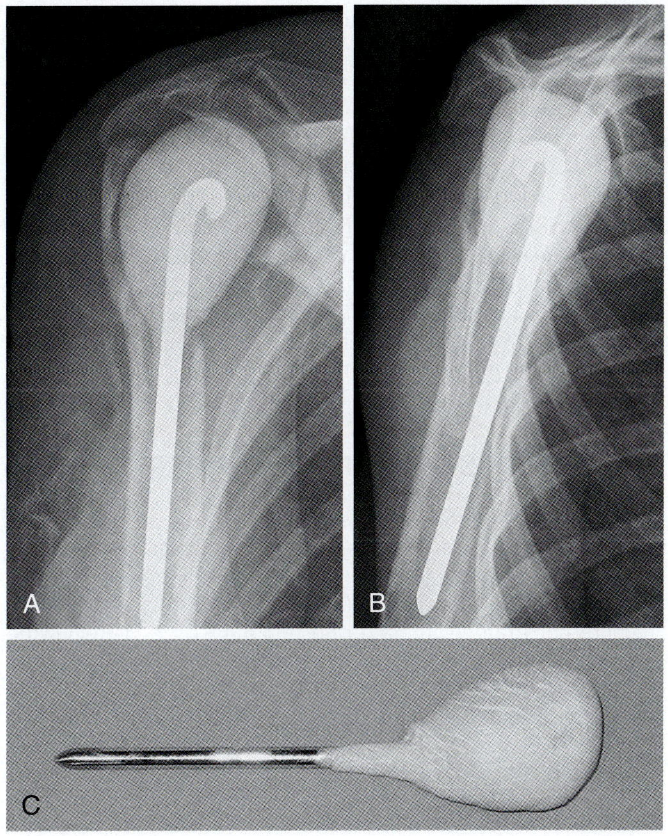

FIGURE 11-18: Gross and radiographic images of an antibiotic spacer used as part of staged treatment with future revision or in the final treatment of chronic infection in a low-demand patient.

PREVENTION

Antibiotic prophylaxis is effective because bacteria are cleared before they establish surface-adherent, rapidly growing populations at sites deep within bone or on biomaterials. We suggest using antibiotic prophylaxis, such as cefazolin 2 g IV, at anesthesia.[121] The use of prophylactic antibiotics is suggested for all implant surgeries, including prosthetic surgery and internal fixation of fractures. Not administering preoperative antibiotics has been shown to correlate with a six-fold increase in the risk of infection in shoulder arthroscopy.[159] The antibiotic used varies depending upon the specific conditions of each case and patient.[152] Treatment for 24 hours in clean cases is believed to be sufficient.

Open wounds that involve joints are, by definition, contaminated, even though bacteria are not always detected. Type 3 open fractures, especially those involving joints, have a very high rate of infection. Open fractures should be treated either with cefazolin or with a combination of cefazolin and gentamicin.[127]

AUTHORS' PREFERRED METHOD OF TREATMENT

Either an arthroscopic or an open approach can be used to drain the shoulder joint. If arthroscopy is used, the surgeon should use multiple portals to facilitate drainage and insert instruments for debridement.

When performing open drainage, we use an anterior deltopectoral approach. The deltoid and coracoid are not detached. Infected surfaces are debrided of adherent clot and other debris. Lavage of the joint with saline or saline mixed with bacitracin is an appropriate technique. In most cases, the wound may be loosely closed, and a large Hemovac is inserted for 24 hours to remove postsurgical accumulations. In cases of chronic sepsis or infection by gram-negative organisms, the wound is packed open and allowed to close spontaneously, with daily packing changes. Adequate intra-articular concentrations of antibiotics can be achieved by IV administration.[120] The duration of antibiotic treatment varies, depending on the host and organism; 3 weeks of IV therapy followed by 3 weeks of oral treatment is a reasonable base. The patient's response is the key to duration of treatment.

SUMMARY

Intra-articular shoulder sepsis presents many challenges in diagnosis and treatment. Sepsis following shoulder arthroplasty is seen more often now due to the number of arthroplasties inserted. The shoulder anatomy is unique in that bursae communicating with the joint can provide a pathway for bacteria for which cartilage is the target substratum. Successful treatment depends on the immune system response, the type of infecting organism, early surgical debridement, and effective antibiotic treatment.

INTERNATIONAL EXPERT COMMENTARY

Pierre Mansat

Introduction

The incidence of infection after shoulder surgery has been reported to be between 0% and 2.9%, with an increase in more constrained implants up to 15.4%.[29,30,155] Reviewing 3096 shoulder prostheses, Richards et al.[132] found that the risk of infection was lower with age and greater in males. Patients undergoing primary reverse shoulder arthroplasty were found to have six times greater risk of infection than patients undergoing primary unconstrained total shoulder arthroplasty. Arthroplasties for trauma were more at risk of infection than other etiologies.

The most common agents causing an infection are the same as those encountered in any other joint infection, such as coagulase-negative staphylococci (30% to 40%), *S. aureus* (12% to 23%), any of the streptococci family (9% to 10%), gram-negative bacilli and enterococci each 3% and 7%, respectively, and mixed flora approximately 10% to 12%.[86] However, *P. acnes* has been identified as a main pathogen involved in shoulder joint infections and has been shown to be sometimes difficult to detect.[20,142] The incidence of shoulder infection from this bacterium has been cited as being 16 times of that in other joints.[5] In Richard's study *P. acnes* was found in 31% of the cases.[132]

Infections are classified into early and late to guide the choice of therapeutic approaches for the patient. Early is classified as an event that occurs within the first 4 weeks after an intervention, and late as anything after this period. An infection that occurs within the first year might still be associated with the index surgery or intervention; infection developing after 1 year is considered to have followed the hematogenous pathway.[86]

Evaluation of the Patient

The clinical findings, symptoms, and signs of any infection are well known: erythema, pain, swelling, and warmth. The patient can present with signs of infection, such as fever and skin fluctuance.

After the clinical examination laboratory evaluation is performed, including the erythrocyte sedimentation rate, C-reactive protein value, and differential blood count. Synovial fluid analysis can be performed, and in a septic arthritis this will most likely show a high leukocyte count, a low glucose level, and more than 75% polymorphonuclear cells.

An intraoperative frozen section has been used for the presence of an infection. Sensitivity in diagnosing *P. acnes* is improved by utilizing a new histologic threshold value of 10 polymorphonuclear neutrophils (PMNs) per 5 hpf, while maintaining 100% specificity.[72]

Joint aspiration and culture is still the gold standard for identifying the causing agent. Any antibiotic therapy that the patient might have been started on erroneously will have to be stopped for at least 2 weeks in order to not compromise the results negatively. The culture must be followed for 15 to 21 days because of the slow-growing nature of some bacteria, such as *P. acnes*.[40]

Standard radiographs are taken to demonstrate any local erosions or secondary changes in an advanced infection. CT will help in demonstrating the amount of bone loss or loosening of the prosthesis. MRI will show the soft tissue involvement at the same time. Specific scans, such as an indium-labeled leukocyte scan, will also help in revealing activity at the local area.

Treatment Options

Therapy will depend on the extent and timing of detection of an infection. Arthroscopic lavage and open debridement might be chosen in acute early infection. An adequate history must prove that infection was present within only the previous 10 to 14 days to allow this therapy to be successful. If there is any doubt regarding its likely success, especially with a shoulder arthroplasty, open debridement should be performed, allowing mechanical cleansing of all joint surfaces and at the same time the replacement of any polyethylene components, if they are of a modular type. The exchange of all polyethylene inlays, if they are modular, should be performed to avoid increased adherence of bacteria to the surfaces.

One-Stage Exchange

Essential to the decision to perform a one-stage exchange is the identification of the underlying causative agent. The advantages of a one-stage surgery are as follows: less destruction of soft tissue and bone, immediate reconstruction, the avoidance of secondary adhesions that occur in the two-stage procedure, less anxiety for the patient, and lower hospitalization costs.

Two-Stage Revision

Two-stage revision is performed for patients in whom the underlying causative agent could not be identified. One needs to identify all the causative agents to effectively direct antibiotic therapy. After a first stage of aggressive debridement the patient's laboratory values as well as the clinical

INTERNATIONAL EXPERT COMMENTARY—cont'd

signs are monitored for minimum of 6 weeks before secondary replantation is considered. An antibiotic-free interval of approximately 2 weeks will demonstrate whether any increase in the infection-related parameters takes place. After surgery the same type of antibiotic is administered as before, but once the organisms have been reevaluated, an adjustment according to the pattern of resistance might be needed.

Resection Arthroplasty

Resection arthroplasty should be considered if a chronic fistula or a chronic infection has developed, or if the patient's health status is too fragile to sustain several surgical procedures. Resection arthroplasty gives relatively good pain relief, but function is usually poor.

Shoulder Arthrodesis

Arthrodesis is technically demanding. The limited function that has to be expected will induce many surgeons to attempt an arthroplasty revision before fusion or to prefer a resection arthroplasty.

Antibiotics

The choice of antibiotics will, in most cases, be second-generation cephalosporin for preoperative prevention. In patients with an allergy to beta-lactam agents, clindamycin may be chosen. Glycopeptide prophylaxis has also been considered, as a result of the rise of methicillin-resistant infection by *S. aureus* or *S. epidermidis*. Ideally, the antimicrobial agent should be bactericidal against biofilm-producing microorganisms. Rifampicin can do this in combination with ofloxacin or ciprofloxacin.[184]

Surgical Technique

One-Stage Exchange

The main problem with one-stage exchange is that the soft tissues and specifically the remaining rotator cuff will be affected. Furthermore, all suture material must be removed because this will act as a foreign body. Removal of the components can be challenging, especially if they are not loose.[82]

On the humeral side, one has to determine whether the components can be removed without further bone loss or destruction. This can be very challenging in the case of a well-fixed, uncemented arthroplasty stem. In such cases it is preferable to extend the deltopectoral approach in order to visualize the humeral shaft. A longitudinal split is performed in the humeral shaft, allowing the surfaces to be separated from the implants by long-bladed chisels. Other authors have proposed an anterior window. Gentle tapping from below will loosen the stem. A prophylactic cerclage may be used to prevent uncontrolled splitting distally, and a drill hole at the end of the split may prevent the stress riser extending any farther down the shaft. If the implant has been cemented, attempts should be made to remove all of the cement, which again can be challenging, especially below the tip of the stem of the prosthesis.

Removal of a well-fixed glenoid component can also be challenging, particularly if the glenoid bone stock is compromised. For an all polyethylene component, sectioning in different pieces can be useful for its removal while preserving the peripheral bone. It can be more difficult to remove a metal-backed component with ingrowth coating, and usually removal of such a component is associated with significant bone deficiency.

Once the implants have been removed, proper mechanical washing with a lavage system should be carried out. All mucosal layers must be removed from the joint surfaces, and the anterior and posterior walls along the glenoid neck should also be probed. In cases when a glenoid has been fixed with screws, the screw holes have to be drilled out to remove all debris within the old threads.

In a one-stage exchange the instruments are changed before the insertion of the new implant to avoid secondary contamination as far as possible.

In a two-stage procedure a temporary spacer is fashioned and an appropriate mix of antibiotics can be employed locally. Using a spherical molded spacer is more congruent with the joint surface and prevents the glenoid from further erosion.

Before the implantation of new implants, the bone and tissues should be rinsed to remove any remnants of the disinfectant from the joint surfaces. It is then decided whether a secondary implant is feasible and what type of implants may be used. Hemiarthroplasty has to be considered if the glenoid will not allow the safe seating of an implant. An autologous bone graft impacted safely in the glenoid cavity may be of help later to restore some bone stock. Reverse shoulder arthroplasty is another option with or without a bone graft to stabilize the glenoid component.

Evaluation and Complications

Debridement

The results of debridement with arthroscopic irrigation are rather disappointing as most authors agree that limited interventions are successful only if the infection was found early. Different series have shown persistent infection varying from 20% to 70%.[30,137] The functional result is often poor.

One-Stage Revision Arthroplasty

It seems that one-stage revision arthroplasty is the best option to eradicate infection and to preserve the shoulder function.[30,82,98] Using a reverse shoulder arthroplasty can give the best results for infection eradication and the preservation of function because debridement can be more extensive, with the deltoid muscle the only structure that needs to be protected.[32,82,98]

Two-stage Revision Arthroplasty

The two-stage revision procedure can be disappointing. According to different studies, persistent infection rates can vary from 25% to 40%.[30, 126, 160] The results seem superior to resection arthroplasty, but inferior to those of the one-stage procedure.

Resection Arthroplasty

Removing the implants and resecting the humeral head has been found to have a high success rate in treating infection. However, Rispoli et al.[134] found a high rate of patient dissatisfaction (89%), with persistent pain and poor functional recovery.

Conclusion

When confronted with the suspicion of an infected shoulder arthroplasty, the duration of infection from the initial

Continued

INTERNATIONAL EXPERT COMMENTARY—cont'd

arthroplasty procedure, the status of the patient, underlying pathologies, and the type of prosthesis must be considered. An early infection of less than 3 weeks might be treated with arthroscopic or open debridement with polyethylene exchange. Systemic antibiotics directed toward the pathogenic agent must be followed for at least 6 weeks. For painful shoulder arthroplasty, aspiration of the joint is the gold standard to isolate the pathogen. If the pathogen can be identified without major resistance to antibiotics, a one-stage exchange is preferred. Intraoperative frozen sections are also used to determine the presence of an infection. Reverse shoulder arthroplasty in this setting, if the local situation is favorable, seems to give better results as far as functional recovery is concerned. Systemic antibiotics are started for a duration of at least 6 weeks once tissue samples have been acquired during surgery. Adequate serum concentrations of the antibiotic have to be followed. In the event that negative cultures are present, and even a repeat aspiration cannot provide identification of the bacteria present, a two-stage revision is preferred. The decision to reimplant a new prosthesis will depend on clinical evaluation, biological evaluation, and aspiration of the joint after at least 2 weeks without antibiotics. Depending of the status of the patient and/or the local status of the joint, a decision will then be made regarding the placement of a new prosthesis or resection-arthroplasty.

EDITOR COMMENTARY

John W. Sperling

The authors should be acknowledged for their important contribution to this textbook. This chapter presents a comprehensive approach to the management of infection in the shoulder from the native joint to the post-operative setting. The diagnosis, classification, and treatment of shoulder infection remains highly controversial. The authors have done an outstanding job of outlining an all-inclusive approach to this very challenging problem.

There has been increasing awareness that *P. acnes* is a common cause of shoulder infection with rotator cuff repair, instability surgery, open reduction internal fixation, and shoulder arthroplasty. Infection in the shoulder is clearly different from the hip and knee periprosthetic infection. Whereas preoperative blood work and aspiration is thought to be of significant value in determining whether a hip or knee prosthesis is infected, these tests have been shown to be less reliable in the shoulder. It is also important for the reader to understand that, unlike other organisms, *P. acnes* can be slow growing and the average time to a positive culture can be greater than 5 days. Therefore it is imperative that a laboratory keep cultures for a minimum of 10 to 14 days to detect this organism. There are emerging technologies to detect low grade infection in the shoulder, and this clearly represents an opportunity to improve patient care.

The treatment of an infected shoulder arthroplasty also remains controversial. Two-stage reimplantation remains the gold standard for chronic infections. However, there has been some interest in one-stage exchange in these patients due to the significant scarring that can be present at the time of a delayed reimplantation. Additional data will be necessary to determine the outcome of one-stage procedures.

Overall, this chapter highlights how current thought can change rapidly over time. The diagnosis and treatment of infection has evolved into a major area of controversy in shoulder surgery. Additional research will be necessary to help guide our understanding of *P. acnes* and the role that it plays in shoulder infection.

CHAPTER 12

Fractures, Dislocations, and Acquired Problems of the Shoulder in Children

Peter D. Fabricant, John M. Flynn

FRACTURES OF THE PROXIMAL HUMERUS

Anatomy

Embryology and Development

The formation of the humerus begins with the appearance of the cartilage anlage, which is present by the fifth week of gestation. The primary ossification center for the humerus appears at about the sixth week.[87] By the time of birth, the entire humeral diaphysis is completely ossified.[88]

The proximal humerus is primarily cartilaginous at birth; however, the ossification centers can be detected with ultrasonography as early as the 38th week of gestation and are generally present between the 38th and 42nd week of gestation.[57,178]

The proximal humerus has three ossification centers: for the greater and lesser tuberosities and for the humeral head. The ossification center for the humeral head is usually present at birth; the greater tuberosity ossification center appears by 1 to 3 years of age, and the lesser tuberosity ossification center appears by 5 years of age.[88,188,222] These ossification centers fuse by 5 to 7 years of age to form the humeral head. The proximal humeral ossification center remains separated from the humeral shaft by the proximal humeral physis, which closes by 14 to 17 years of age in girls and by 16 to 18 years in boys.[22,88,200,201]

Humeral retroversion likewise gradually develops over time. While it has been shown to be highly variable in adults,[19,35,62,98,99,136,208] mean values are around 26 degrees in healthy adults.[165] In infants and young children humeral retroversion averages 65 degrees and gradually decreases, approaching adult values by 11 years of age.[61]

At birth, the body or shaft of the humerus is completely ossified.[88] Eighty percent of subsequent growth comes from the proximal humeral physis, accounting for approximately 40% of the growth of the entire upper extremity.[201,221] Growth derived from the proximal humerus varies with age: less than 75% of growth occurs before 2 years of age and more than 85% occurs by 8 years of age.[22,200,201]

Relevant Anatomy

The capsule of the glenohumeral joint extends from the glenoid rim, progressing laterally toward the surgical neck of the humerus and blending with the tendons of the rotator cuff musculature, where it surrounds the articular surface of the proximal humerus. Due to the limited amount of constraint conferred by the bony anatomy of the glenoid, static stability is maintained by the capsulolabral attachments and the intracapsular ligamentous thickenings (of the superior, middle, and inferior glenohumeral ligaments) while the rotator cuff and periscapular musculature afford dynamic stability to the glenohumeral joint. The posteromedial metaphysis, a portion of the physis, and the epiphysis are intracapsular. A large part of the physis is extracapsular, making it susceptible to traumatic injury. The proximal humeral physis is irregularly shaped, with its apex located on the posteromedial portion of the proximal humerus. The periosteum is also thicker and stronger in the posteromedial portion of the proximal humerus as opposed to the anterolateral portion, which is often quite thin.[47] This fundamental anatomy explains the tendency of proximal humeral metaphyseal fracture fragments to penetrate the anterolateral periosteum.

The proximal humerus is also the insertion site for the shoulder girdle musculature, which greatly influences fracture displacement, angulation, and rotation due to the forces exerted on the humeral head and neck.[31,107-109] The subscapularis originates from the anterior scapula and inserts anteriorly onto the lesser tuberosity. The greater tuberosity provides attachment superiorly and posteriorly for the supraspinatus, infraspinatus, and teres minor, all of which originate from the posterior scapula. The deltoid forward flexes and abducts the shoulder and courses from the clavicle and acromion superiorly, coalescing into a common tendinous insertion onto the lateral upper third of the humeral shaft. The pectoralis major powers adduction and internal rotation due to its tendinous insertion anteriorly onto the lateral wall of the bicipital groove and forms the roof of the distal continuation of the bicipital tunnel, which is a closed space that extends proximally to the glenohumeral joint.[240]

The anterior and posterior humeral circumflex arteries provide a rich blood supply to the proximal humerus. While it was thought in the past that the arcuate artery, which ascends from the anterior humeral circumflex artery, was the major vascular supply to the humeral head,[27,59,79,168] more recent quantitative assessment has shown that 64% of the humeral head blood supply arises from the posterior humeral circumflex artery.[101] This explains the exceedingly low rate of osteonecrosis associated with anterior shoulder dislocations. Due to its close proximity to the proximal humerus, the brachial plexus is prone to injury when the proximal humerus is injured in fractures or dislocations, or during traction. The axillary nerve, in particular, circles the humeral neck just inferior to the glenohumeral joint as it courses posteriorly.[21,78,122,270]

Fracture Incidence

Numerous studies have reported on the incidence of fractures in children. However, these studies have been affected by multiple factors, including cultural differences, climate, and environmental factors. Patient factors, such as age and gender, likewise influence various fracture patterns.

Fractures of the proximal humerus have been reported to comprise approximately 5% of all pediatric fractures.[103,104,114,142,214] The incidence of these fractures increases linearly with age, with Salter-Harris type I fractures predominating in younger children, metaphyseal fractures in children 5 to 11 years old, and Salter-Harris type II fractures in children older than 11 years. Fractures of the proximal humeral epiphysis represent 2% to 7% of all growth plate injuries in children.[162,171,199]

Mechanism of Injury

Shoulder dystocia is an infrequent cause of birth injuries and is associated with maternal diabetes, macrosomia, postterm pregnancy, and a previous history of shoulder dystocia. Gherman and colleagues reported the incidence of birth injuries associated with shoulder dystocia to be 24.9%, with a 4.2% incidence of proximal humeral fractures.[80] The mechanism of injury is related to arm position during delivery. Hyperextension and external rotation of the shoulder have been implicated in birth fractures, including separation of the proximal humeral physis.[44,96,160,224]

Fractures of the proximal humerus in older children and adolescents are more frequently caused by direct and indirect trauma to the shoulder and proximal humerus. Sports injuries, vehicular trauma, and falls are the most common cause of proximal humerus fractures in children.[134]

Repetitive injury can also cause damage to the proximal humeral physis (Fig. 12-1). Shoulder pain and proximal humeral epiphysiolysis has been frequently reported in gymnasts, baseball pitchers, and overhead athletes due to excessive repeated traction and torsional loads at the proximal humeral physis.[32,42,46,50,74,161,198,207,220,237]

Pathologic fractures occurring through benign lesions have been reported infrequently (Fig. 12-2) but are most commonly caused by aneurysmal and unicameral bone cysts.[55,92,128,191] Malignant lesions have been reported to cause pathologic fractures through the proximal humerus and, although infrequently seen, should be considered in the appropriate clinical setting.[51,60,95,191]

Metabolic conditions, such as pituitary gigantism, can cause weakening of the growth plate, leading to the development of deformity.[209] Underlying neuromuscular conditions, such as Arnold-Chiari malformation, syringomyelia, myelomeningocele, and cerebral palsy, have been identified as risk factors or etiologic agents in the

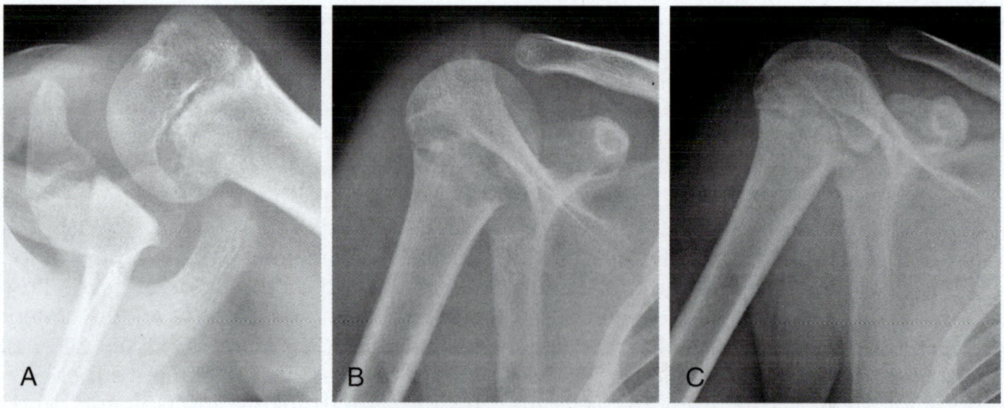

FIGURE 12-1: Epiphysiolysis in a 12-year-old right-hand-dominant male baseball pitcher evaluated for right shoulder pain. **A** and **B,** On initial evaluation, radiographs showed widening of the proximal humeral growth plate. **C,** The patient was managed conservatively with activity modification for 3 months; he went on to heal uneventfully.

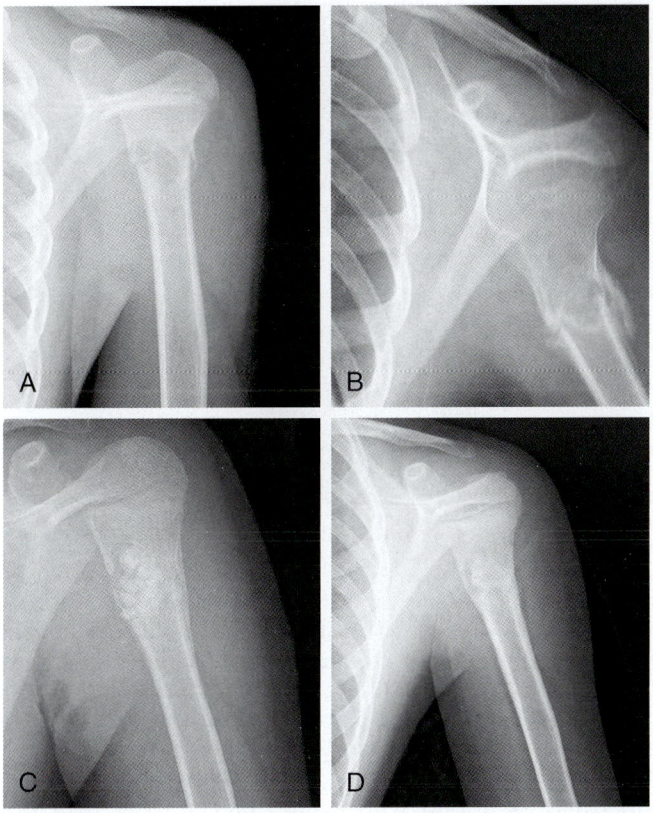

FIGURE 12-2: **A,** A 7-year-old boy who sustained a pathologic fracture through a simple bone cyst. This fracture was treated conservatively with a shoulder immobilizer. **B,** Follow-up radiographs show healing of the pathologic fracture, with the presence of a residual cystic lesion. **C,** The residual cystic lesion was treated with percutaneous biopsy, curettage, and bone grafting with calcium sulfate pellets. **D,** The latest follow-up films show progressive healing and remodeling through the lesion.

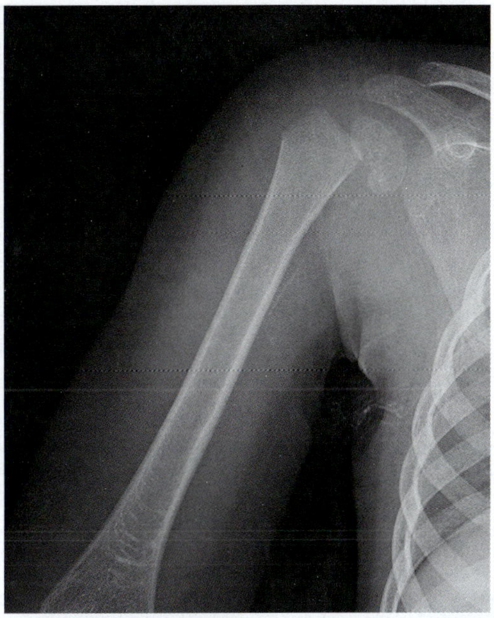

FIGURE 12-3: Anteroposterior radiograph of a 2-year-old who sustained a displaced Salter-Harris type I fracture through the proximal humeral growth plate.

development of growth plate injuries and fractures about the proximal humerus.[6,86,158,242]

Nonaccidental injury should also be considered when children present with a proximal humerus fracture, particularly if the underlying cause is unclear and multiple injuries are noted.[36,41,131,153,232]

Classification

Fractures of the proximal humerus in children can be classified according to the location of the injury. Growth plate injuries in children are classified according to the Salter-Harris classification.[221] In children under 5 years of age, Salter-Harris type I injuries predominate (Fig. 12-3), whereas in children older than 11 years, type II fracture patterns predominate (Fig. 12-4).[199] Salter-Harris types III, IV, and V are very rare, particularly in the proximal humerus, although cases of Salter-Harris type III injuries have been reported.[255]

The anatomic location of the fracture may also be used for classification. Dividing the fractures according to the area of involvement, such as the proximal humeral metaphysis (Fig. 12-5), physis, and lesser and greater tuberosities, eases communication regarding morphology and treatment of the fracture. Neer and Horwitz classified proximal humeral physeal fractures into four types according to the degree of displacement[180]:

Grade I fractures: less than 5 mm of displacement
Grade II fractures: displaced by more than 5 mm but less than one third of the width of the humeral shaft
Grade III fractures: displaced by up to two thirds of the width of the shaft
Grade IV fractures: displaced by more than two thirds of the width of the shaft

Open fractures of the proximal humerus, although uncommon, can occur and are frequently classified using the Gustilo-Anderson classification for open fractures.[89,90]

History and Physical Examination

In neonates and infants evaluation of the shoulder for injuries may be very difficult. An infant who presents with an inability to move the shoulder or an asymmetric Moro reflex should raise suspicion of brachial plexus birth palsy or pathology about the shoulder girdle or proximal humerus, such as fracture, dislocation, or infection. A detailed history should be obtained, including any abnormalities throughout the prenatal period, such as maternal diabetes or other maternal conditions that can predispose to macrosomia. Physical examination should include gentle palpation of the upper extremity, testing the passive range of motion (ROM), and evaluation for deformity or warmth.

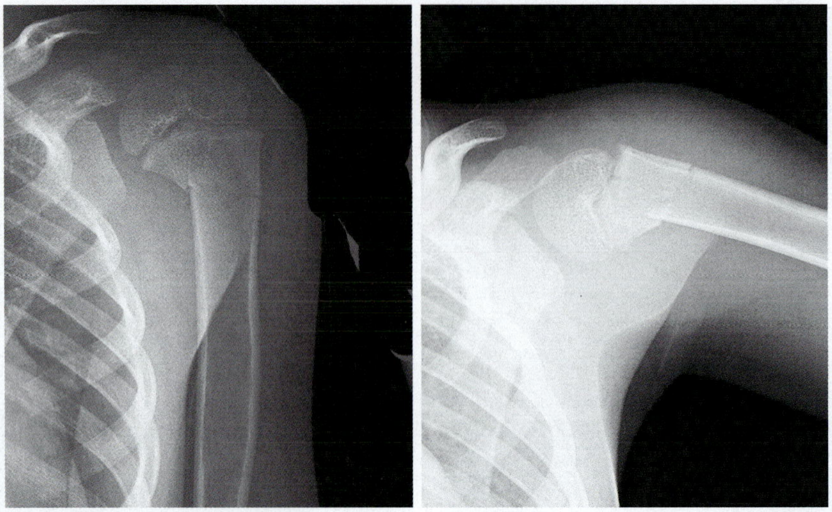

FIGURE 12-4: Radiographs of an 8-year-old who sustained a Salter-Harris type II growth plate injury secondary to a fall.

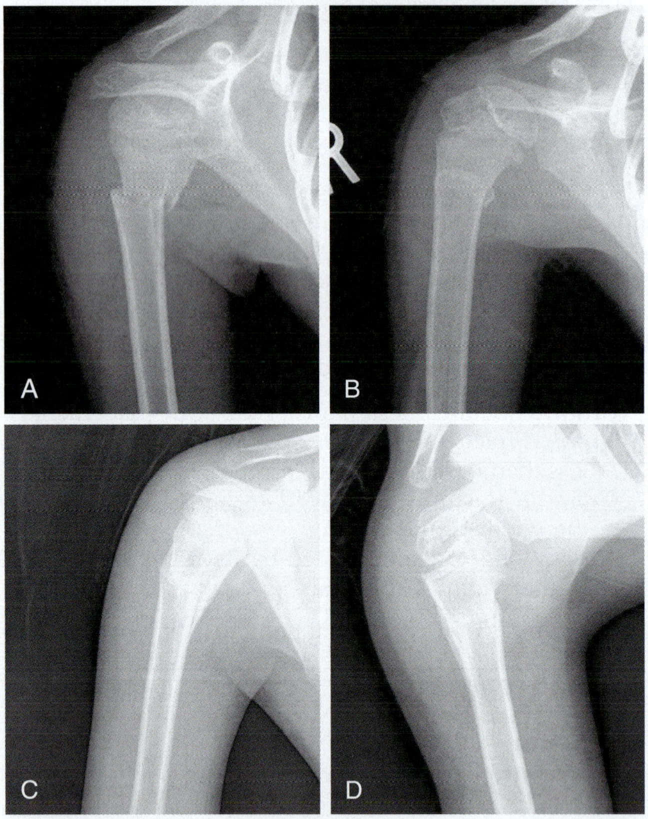

FIGURE 12-5: **A** and **B,** Radiographs of an 8-year-old boy who sustained a metaphyseal fracture through the proximal humerus. This fracture was treated conservatively. **C** and **D,** Radiographs taken at 7 weeks after injury show complete healing of the fracture.

In the older child, a history consistent with a traumatic event can usually be elicited. The most common presentation is limited ROM of the shoulder, with abnormal fullness or deformity of the affected shoulder compared with the contralateral shoulder. Depending on the degree of trauma, soft tissue injuries, ecchymosis, and swelling may also be present. The affected extremity is usually held in an internal rotation. In posterior fracture-dislocations there is painful, limited external rotation of the shoulder. In lesser tuberosity fractures there is limited active internal rotation and excessive passive external rotation of the shoulder.[149,154,215] Greater tuberosity fractures may be found with luxatio erecta,[73,135,267] whereby the shoulder is in fixed abduction with the elbow held flexed and the hand above the head.

Radiographic Evaluation

Imaging of the proximal humerus can be challenging in neonates and infants because it is primarily cartilaginous. Generally, in neonates and infants with a suspected fracture of the proximal humerus or proximal humeral physis, a single anteroposterior (AP) view of the chest and upper extremities may be used to screen for injuries. On these plain radiographs the relationship of the proximal humeral metaphysis, scapula, and acromion are evaluated, and these structures are compared with those on the contralateral side (Fig. 12-6). An abnormal relationship of the scapula and humerus has been reported as indicating a proximal humeral physeal injury with a posteriorly displaced proximal humeral fragment, termed the *vanishing epiphysis sign*.[133,224] Ultrasound examination may also be a valuable imaging tool.[26,68,119,226,269] Ultrasonography is quick and noninvasive, allowing the injury to be directly visualized, with the contralateral side serving as a comparison, although this technique is largely operator dependent. Arthrography can also be valuable but requires sedation.[54,261] Cross-sectional imaging, such as computed tomography (CT) or magnetic resonance imaging, may also be useful in evaluating shoulder injuries missed at birth, particularly those with posterior dislocation.[244]

Plain radiographs are still the mainstay of the initial evaluation of shoulder injuries in the older children. Well-taken radiographs obtained in orthogonal views should provide adequate clinical information. A true AP image

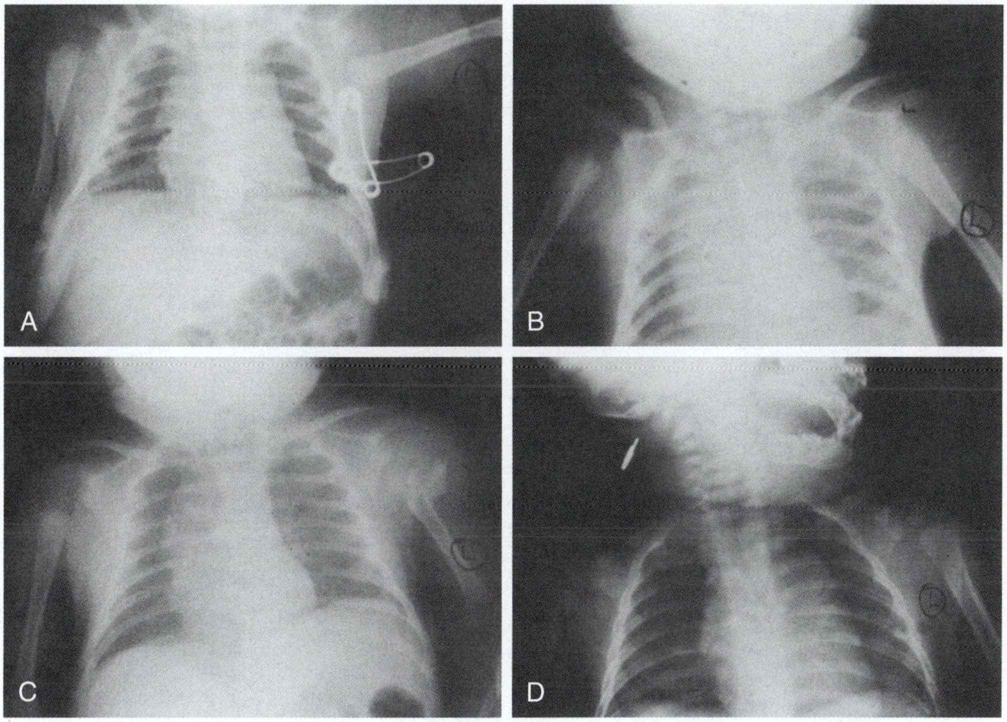

FIGURE 12-6: In a newborn injury to the proximal part of the humerus is usually a completely displaced physeal injury, which appears as a pseudodislocation. **A,** A radiograph of a newborn can sometimes be misleading because of the lack of ossification in the proximal epiphysis. **B,** Closed manipulation can be performed by applying longitudinal traction and gentle posterior pressure over the proximal end of the humerus. **C,** At 2.5 weeks, abundant callus is present and the patient is clinically asymptomatic. **D,** A 6-month follow-up radiograph shows symmetry when compared to the uninjured side.

of the shoulder is taken in the scapular plane with the beam parallel to the glenohumeral joint. The axillary lateral view is preferred, although it may be difficult to obtain in a setting where a child is acutely injured. In lieu of the axillary lateral view, alternative views, such as the Velpeau axillary, West Point axillary, transthoracic axillary, or scapular Y view may be obtained. The apical oblique, internal rotation, and external rotation views are also valuable in some cases.

Treatment

The treatment of fractures of the proximal humerus generally depends on the age of the patient and on the fracture type and location. In general, the prognosis for most proximal humerus fractures in children is good, with the vast majority amenable to nonoperative management. Because the proximal humeral physis contributes the most to the growth of the upper extremity and closes later in adolescence, there is tremendous remodeling potential for the proximal humerus (Fig. 12-7). One should be cautious, however, with fractures that may result in varus malunion, such as those which heal with the greater tuberosity above the level of the cartilage surface with physeal damage or with limited growth remaining. These may exhibit significant limitation of passive and active motion in abduction due to subacromial impingement and reduced power from limited rotator cuff excursion, necessitating corrective osteotomy.[245]

The prognosis is generally good in neonates with osseous birth injuries. Only the most severely displaced fractures require any attempt at reduction. If reduction is performed, gentle maneuvers without formal anesthesia generally work well. Reduction may be monitored using ultrasonography. In the vast majority of cases the shoulder can be immobilized efficiently by pinning the shirt sleeve or soft dressing to the shirt. These fractures heal rapidly, usually within 2 to 3 weeks.[47,160]

Most children with a slipped proximal humeral epiphysis do not need any form of reduction. These injuries generally respond well to nonoperative management.

In general, fracture treatment is determined by the degree of displacement and the amount of remodeling potential. Although there are no universally accepted criteria for acceptable limits of reduction for proximal humerus fractures in children, Beaty has classically recommended treatment guidelines based on the child's age (Table 12-1).[13] Trends in the contemporary peer-reviewed literature suggest that up to 60 to 70 degrees of angulation is acceptable in children under 10 to 11 years,[8,13,56] while children above 11 to 12 years should have less than 20 to 40 degrees of angulation and 50% displacement.[16,30,47,56,110] In young children excellent outcomes have been reported

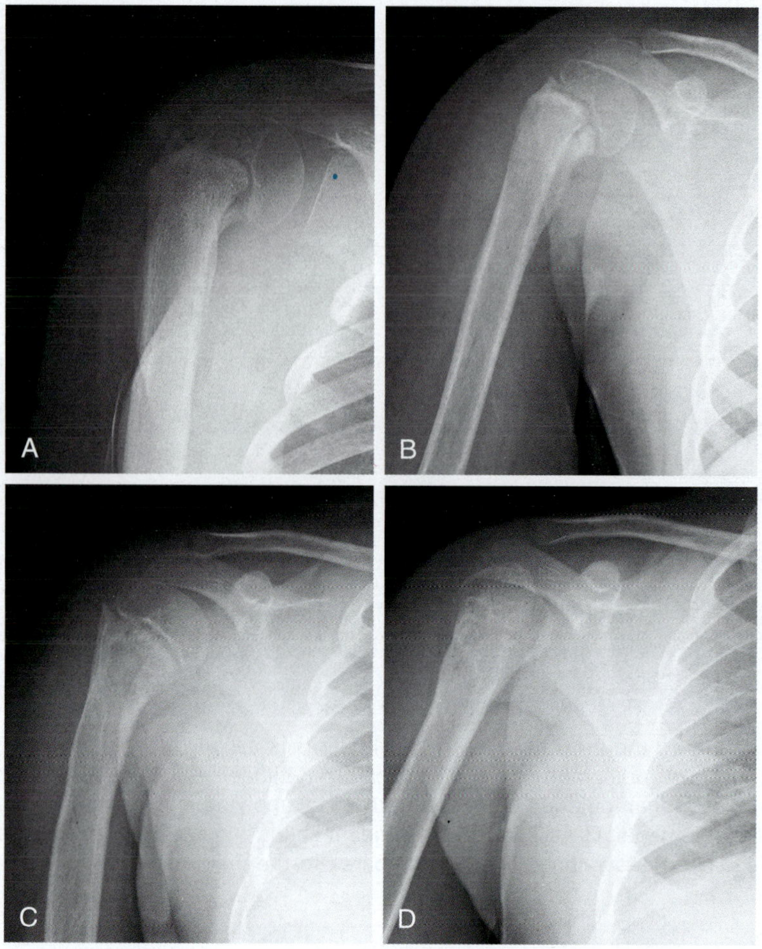

FIGURE 12-7: **A,** Radiograph of a 9-year-old boy who had sustained a Salter-Harris type II fracture of the proximal humerus, showing angulation of the proximal fragment in the anteroposterior plane. **B,** The patient was treated conservatively, and a follow-up radiograph taken 6 weeks after injury shows excellent callus formation and healing of the fracture. **C** and **D,** Radiographs taken 9 months after injury show full healing of the fracture with remodeling of the proximal humerus; continued remodeling would be expected as the patient progressed toward skeletal maturity.

TABLE 12-1 Guidelines for Reduction Acceptability

Age	Acceptable Angulation	Acceptable Displacement
<5 years	70 degrees	100%
5-12 years	40-70 degrees	—
>12 years	40 degrees	50%

Data from Beaty JH: Fractures of the proximal humerus and shaft in children. Instr Course Lect. 1992;41:369-372.

with nonoperative management.[47,143,180] Children approaching skeletal maturity who have Neer and Horwitz grade III and IV fractures may be considered for reduction and fixation, depending on angulation and expected residual deformity at skeletal maturity.[47,143,180,233] Older children with Neer and Horwitz grade I and II fractures are frequently treated successfully without surgery.

Reduction

In general, reduction is reserved for severely displaced or angulated fractures in older children. Potential blocks to reduction include the periosteum, capsule, and long head of biceps tendon.[13,45,150,252] Numerous reduction maneuvers have been recommended. Most fractures can be treated with gentle traction coupled with abduction, external rotation, and flexion of the shoulder. Neer and Horwitz recommended reduction with 90 degrees of forward flexion, abduction, and external rotation.[180] Others have recommended reduction with 135 degrees of abduction and 30 degrees of flexion and external rotation, with the fracture manipulated directly to obtain reduction.[23,117]

Once acceptable or adequate reduction is obtained, any of several immobilization techniques may be used. Immobilization methods described in the literature include the sling and swathe (Fig. 12-8), two-prong splint, thoracobrachial bandage, shoulder spica cast, Statue of Liberty cast, and hanging arm cast.[47,93,124,143,180] It is

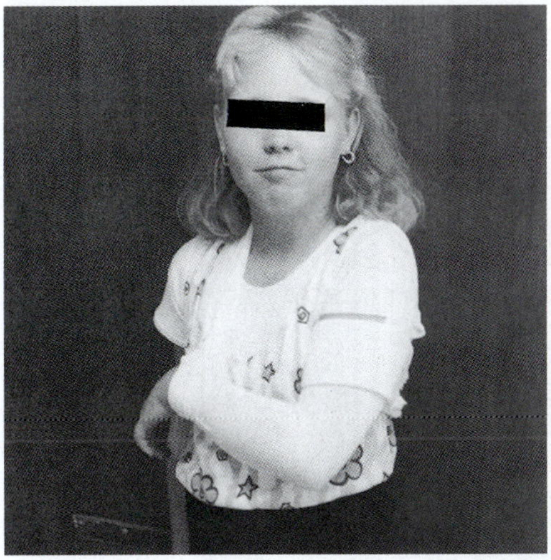

FIGURE 12-8: Clinical photograph of a 9-year-old girl wearing a sling and swathe used in the treatment of proximal humerus fractures. A stockinette is padded at pressure points with cast padding and held in position with safety pins.

important for the surgeon and family to understand that very displaced proximal humerus fractures in older children are generally quite unstable. Some loss of reduction is common if internal fixation is not used.

Operative Treatment

Operative management is infrequently indicated for children with fractures of the proximal humerus. However, occasionally, some fractures are not amenable to reduction due to soft tissue interposition. Specifically, the tendon of the long head of the biceps becomes interposed between fracture fragments in up to 10% of cases and precludes closed reduction.[195] These fractures often require an open reduction and internal fixation. Other indications for operative management include segmental fractures, floating shoulder injuries, displaced intra-articular fractures, open fractures requiring debridement, fracture-dislocations, and concomitant neurovascular injury, in addition to failure to obtain a closed reduction within acceptable limits of angulation and translation, as outlined previously. Open reduction of proximal humeral fractures is generally performed through a deltopectoral approach. A limited skin incision may be used to gain direct access into the joint space. One significant advantage of performing a reduction is that it lessens the amount of time needed for osseous remodeling.

There are numerous options for the internal fixation of proximal humerus fractures. Displaced fractures may be treated with closed reduction and percutaneous techniques or with open reduction and internal fixation.[30,56,229]

Percutaneous pin fixation may be performed once adequate reduction has been obtained (Fig. 12-9).[37,218] This can be carried out under image intensification. The patient is placed supine or in the beach chair position on a radiolucent operating table. A closed reduction is performed under image intensification, and once adequate reduction has been obtained, the pins are inserted laterally through the metaphysis in an inferior-to-superior direction. The surgeon should be careful to avoid the axillary nerve laterally and anteriorly, as well as other neurovascular structures more medially. The pinning technique can be challenging because the optimal trajectory is steep and the pin starting point may migrate while drilling. Smooth pins can be used, but they have a high risk of loosening. Alternatively, small external fixator pins with threaded tips can be used, with or without a fixator assembly.

Depending on the stability of the fracture after reduction, two or more pins may be used. In younger children

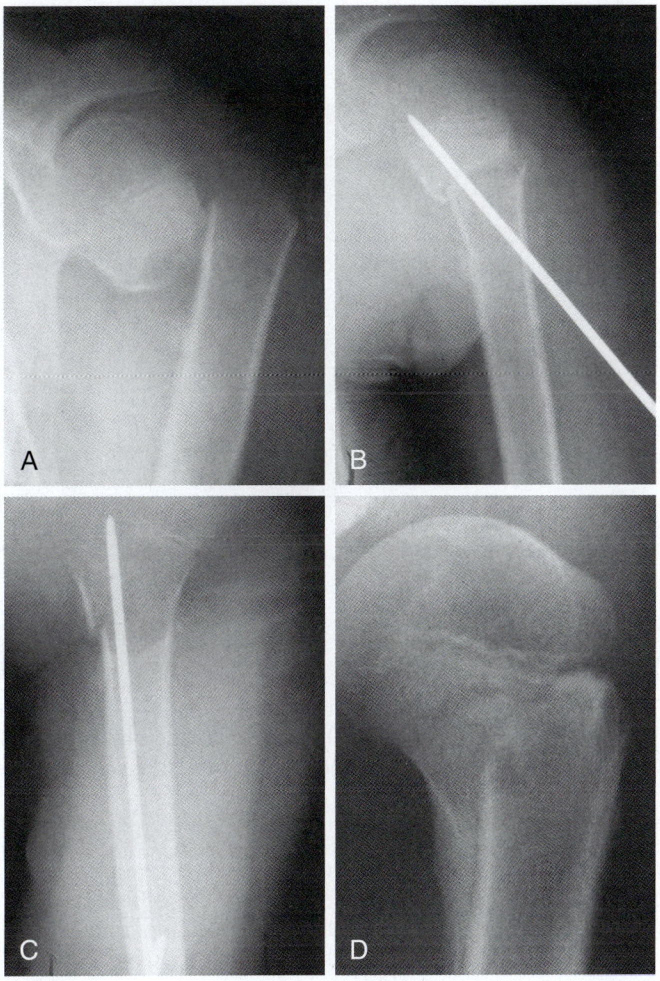

FIGURE 12-9: Technique of percutaneous pinning of a proximal humeral metaphyseal fracture from a distal approach to avoid the axillary nerve. **A,** Anteroposterior (AP) radiograph demonstrating a displaced proximal humerus metaphyseal fracture. **B** and **C,** Once satisfactory reduction is obtained, pins are inserted distally through the deltoid and advanced in an inferior-to-superior direction. **D,** AP radiograph after pin removal showing a healed fracture, which has started to remodel. (From Rockwood CA, Wilkins KE, Beaty J, eds. *Fractures in Children*. Philadelphia: JB Lippincott; 1996.)

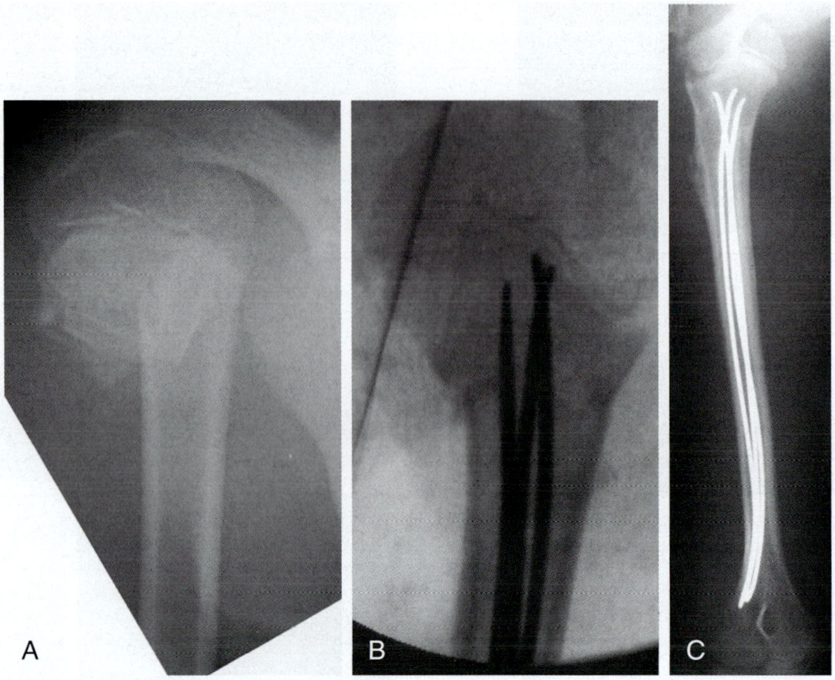

FIGURE 12-10: **A,** Radiograph of an 11-year-old boy with multiple trauma, including bilateral femoral fractures and a right proximal humerus fracture. **B,** The proximal end of the right humerus was treated by closed reduction with titanium elastic nail fixation to facilitate early mobility. **C,** The fracture was stabilized well with this internal splint. (Courtesy Richard L. Munk, MD.)

treated with smooth pins, the pins can be left in the percutaneous position and removed in the office. In older children treated with threaded pins and no fixator, the pins should be buried in the subcutaneous tissue and removed in the operating room once the fracture has healed.

Retrograde flexible intramedullary nails have also been used to stabilize proximal humerus fractures in children (Fig. 12-10).[254]

Tuberosity Fracture Treatment

The lesser tuberosity is the site of the insertion of the subscapularis, and good results have been reported with the nonoperative management of lesser tuberosity fractures with minimal displacement.[149,215,234] However, several authors have advocated open reduction and internal fixation in the acute setting.[132,154,260] Ogawa and Takahashi reported better results with operative management of lesser tuberosity fractures.[186] Options for fracture fixation depend on the size of the avulsed fragment. In most cases suture fixation is adequate; screw fixation may be performed in fractures with larger fragments. Good results have been reported after arthroscopic treatment of lesser tuberosity fractures and subscapularis tears.[141,225,258]

Greater tuberosity fractures in young children, particularly those that are nondisplaced, can often be treated nonoperatively with good outcomes. In adolescents a displaced greater tuberosity fracture often requires open reduction and internal fixation, with repair of any tears of the rotator cuff to prevent subsequent subacromial impingement.

Fracture-dislocations of the proximal humerus are rare injuries in children. However, they should be managed following the principles of adult urgent-emergent open reduction and fracture stabilization to minimize the risk of osteonecrosis.[116,185]

Glenohumeral Instability Treatment

The treatment of glenohumeral instability is covered at length elsewhere in this textbook, but clinical features unique to children and adolescents warrant special mention here. Primary shoulder dislocation and subluxation in children and adolescents is frequently treated nonoperatively with closed reduction, a short period of immobilization, and supervised physical therapy, resulting in an ultimate return to full activity.[43] Surgical intervention is reserved for adolescents with significant bony Bankart lesions, those who experience recurrent dislocations, those who fail conservative management, and those who participate in competitive overhead sports.[65,170,174] Although many surgeons continue to utilize open surgical techniques for instability repair (particularly in the presence of large bony lesions, poor-quality tissue, or revision settings), advances in arthroscopic fixation and instrumentation have made arthroscopy more desirable for many patients and surgeons.[196,235,268] Athletic adolescents and teenagers have good outcomes following arthroscopic stabilization,[137] with 87% reported as returning to competitive sports. However, it is important to note that the rate of recurrent instability is higher in younger patients than in adults, particularly in those with ligamentous laxity, multiple instability episodes, and Hill-Sachs lesions.[193,235]

Authors' Preferred Treatment

Nonoperative

Most proximal humerus fractures, including physeal fractures, can be managed nonoperatively. Our preferred method for treatment depends on the age of the patient. In neonates and infants we manage most fractures with simple immobilization, often by pinning the shirtsleeve to the front of the shirt or through use of a soft elastic bandage to secure the humerus to the infant's torso. In older children with a proximal humerus fracture, we follow the displacement guidelines of Beaty (see Table 12-1). Most fractures can be treated with immobilization alone. Initial management consists of a coaptation splint and an elastic bandage, and then at 10 to 14 days after injury, once the child is more comfortable, a change to a shoulder immobilizer or hanging cast (see Fig. 12-8).

Operative

We treat fractures that exceed the Beaty guidelines with closed reduction and internal fixation. The patient is placed supine or in a beach chair position on a radiolucent table. A bump may be placed under the scapula to allow greater ROM of the shoulder. The arm is sterilely prepped and draped free, and the fracture is reduced under fluoroscopic guidance, using the maneuvers described above. If closed reduction is unsuccessful, the deltopectoral interval can be opened to facilitate reduction.

Once adequate reduction is achieved, percutaneous pins are inserted through the lateral cortex. We prefer the small external fixator pins with a threaded tip to minimize the risk of migration. These pins are directed across the fracture site and into the head of the humerus, stopping short of the subchondral bone. Two or three pins are inserted until the fracture has been satisfactorily stabilized (Fig. 12-11). In older children (i.e., 13 years and older) we prefer either to affix the external fixation bar or to cut the pins and bury them beneath the skin because fracture healing can take 4 to 6 weeks. The extremity is placed in a shoulder immobilizer for 2 to 3 weeks.

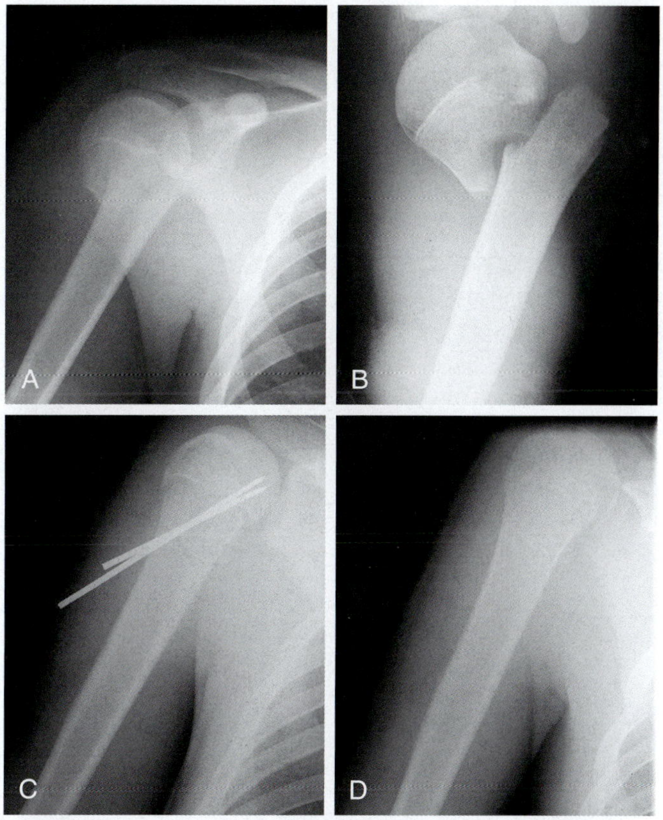

FIGURE 12-11: A 14-year-old male quarterback sustained an injury to his right shoulder when tackled. Anteroposterior (**A**) and lateral (**B**) radiographs show a displaced and angulated fracture of the proximal humerus. An attempt at treatment in a hanging cast failed, and a closed reduction was performed under anesthesia. **C,** The fracture was deemed unstable even after reduction, so percutaneous pinning was performed. The postoperative course was uneventful. **D,** A radiograph taken 6 weeks into the patient's postoperative course after pin removal shows excellent fracture healing.

Postfracture Care and Rehabilitation

Birth injuries and fractures in very young children tend to heal rapidly, frequently within 2 to 3 weeks. No formal rehabilitation is required in this age group.

In older children, injuries take longer to heal. In physeal injuries, the fracture stabilizes after 2 to 3 weeks, at which time gentle ROM and pendulum exercises can be instituted. After 6 weeks, active ROM exercises, which include flexion and extension, abduction, and internal and external rotation, can be started. This is followed by strengthening of the deltoid, periscapular, and rotator cuff muscles.

Metaphyseal fractures may take 4 to 6 weeks to heal. Rehabilitation should start with gentle ROM exercises, followed by strengthening exercises once motion is restored.

Complications

Both early and late complications from proximal humerus fractures have been reported. Early complications result directly from the fracture. These can be serious and can develop into potentially limb-threatening injuries, including neurovascular compromise.[7,58,249,251] Typically, these are injuries to the brachial plexus from fracture dislocation, which can often be diagnosed early after injury, with loss of strength and sensation in a specific nerve distribution. Most of these injuries are neurapraxias that recover within 4 to 6 months. If no sign of recovery is noted, an electromyography study is warranted to document whether there is tangible improvement in the status of the nerve palsy. If no improvement is noted, surgical exploration and possible repair or nerve grafting of the involved structure may be indicated.[7]

Vascular injuries are uncommon but have been reported.[11,157,259] Implant-related complications, such as hardware migration, have also been reported after the internal fixation of proximal humerus fractures.[156,159,243,254]

Loss of motion is another complication, seen particularly in patients who were treated surgically.

Late complications are often sequelae of the original injury. Humerus varus usually occurs in children and neonates after a history of trauma, infection, or metabolic or hematologic conditions (Fig. 12-12).[20,38,64,143,144,189,219,245]

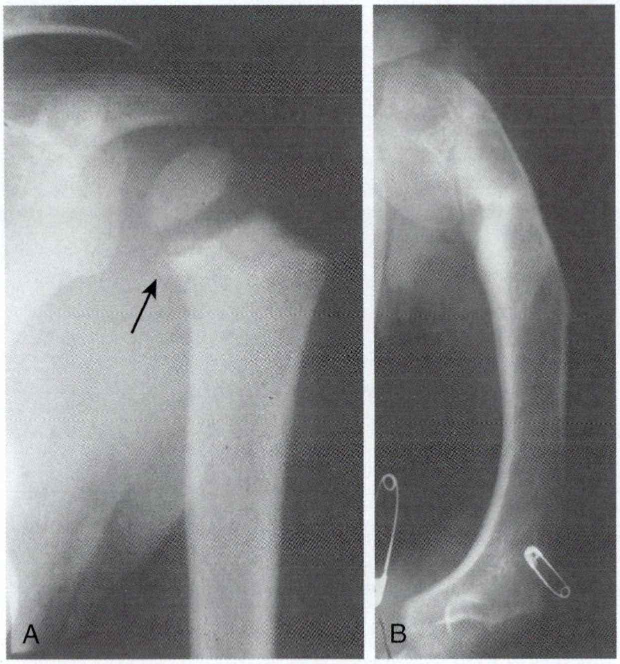

FIGURE 12-12: Proximal humeral varus resulting from an infection at 11.5 years of age. **A,** Early signs of infection and periosteal reaction (*arrow*). **B,** Varus and marked shortening. (From Rockwood CA, Wilkins KE, Beaty J, eds. *Fractures in Children*. Philadelphia: JB Lippincott; 1996.)

As previously mentioned these patients may occasionally exhibit significant limitation of passive and active motion in abduction due to subacromial impingement and reduced power from limited rotator cuff excursion, necessitating corrective osteotomy (Fig. 12-13).[14,64,82,219,245,259]

Growth arrest has been reported in children who sustain physeal fractures and in some pathologic conditions that cross the physis, such as chondroblastomas and bone cysts.[134,138,197,204,227,238,250,253] Complete physeal arrest has been reported but is relatively rare. More often, these cases do not result in any functional deficit, and most children do not need any form of surgical intervention.

Hypertrophic scar formation is a complication seen after surgical management.[47,72,81] To avoid this, some authors have proposed a more cosmetic axillary approach for the treatment of these injuries; however, full anatomic visualization may be impaired.[151] Osteonecrosis of the humeral head is a rare complication; however, even with osteonecrosis, good outcomes have been reported in the shoulder as it is a non–weight-bearing joint.[10] Glenohumeral subluxation has also been reported in children with proximal humerus fractures[185,255]; this often responds well to a period of nonoperative management, sling immobilization, and early rehabilitation.

FRACTURES OF THE CLAVICLE

Anatomy

Embryology and Development

The clavicle is one of the first bones to ossify, beginning from two primary ossification centers (medial and lateral) by 5 to 6 weeks of gestation, and by 7 to 8 weeks the

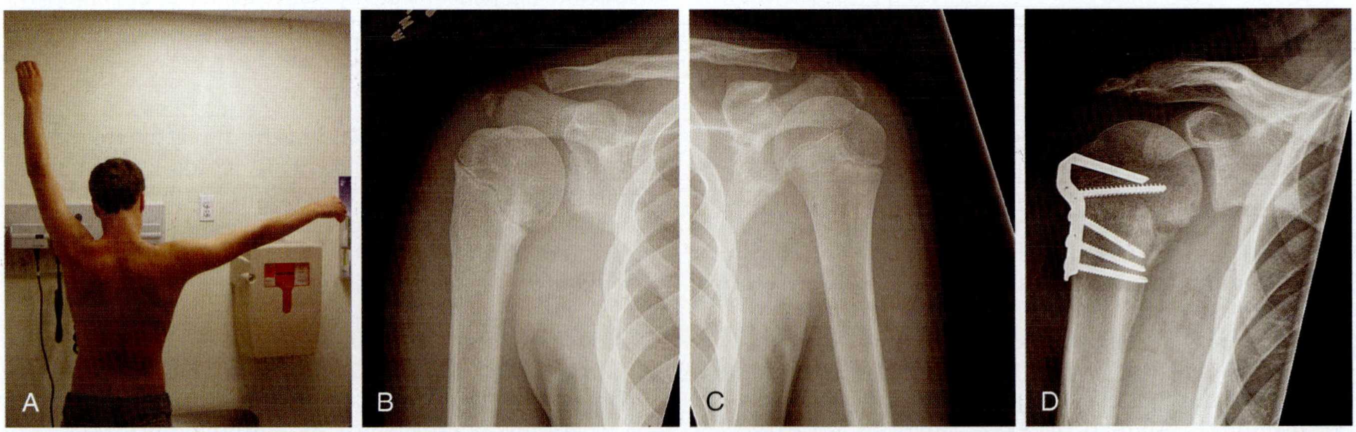

FIGURE 12-13: A 15-year-old male with posttraumatic proximal humerus varus malunion; this resulted in difficulty in performing activities of daily living and the inability to participate in sports. **A,** Clinical photograph showing a mechanical block to active and passive right shoulder abduction at 110 degrees. **B** and **C,** Anteroposterior (AP) radiographs of the right shoulder and uninvolved left shoulder, showing equal heights of the greater tuberosity and an articular surface resulting from 32 degrees of varus malunion. **D,** A 6-month postoperative AP radiograph showing the healed closing wedge osteotomy transfixed with a low-profile 3.5-mm blade plate and the restored neck-shaft angle, as well as the anatomic relationship between the greater tuberosity and articular surface. The patient regained full active abduction and returned to full activities. (Courtesy Daniel W. Green, MD, and Russell F. Warren, MD.)

clavicle has already assumed its overall contour and "S" shape. Most growth (80%) occurs from the medial physis.

Despite its early appearance, the clavicle is one of the last bones to complete ossification. The lateral epiphysis forms and fuses in a remarkably short time at around 18 to 19 years of age. The medial epiphysis is the last in the body to ossify, at the age of 18 to 20 years, and the last to complete ossification, at the age of 23 to 25 years.[76,173]

Relevant Anatomy

The clavicle is an S-shaped bone that articulates medially with the sternum and laterally with the scapula at the acromion. Through the sternoclavicular and acromioclavicular joints, the clavicle functionally links the axial skeleton and upper extremity, acts as a strut of the glenohumeral joint, and adds to the fluidity of shoulder motion through rotational motion, and proper positioning of the glenoid. The medial two thirds of the bone is round and tubular; the lateral third is flat. The anterosuperior aspect of the clavicle is subcutaneous. The subclavian vessels and brachial plexus lie posterior to the clavicle near the junction of the middle and lateral thirds (Fig. 12-14).

Numerous muscles and ligaments attach to the clavicle. Anteriorly, the pectoralis major originates on the medial two thirds of the clavicle and the deltoid on the lateral third. Posteriorly, the trapezius muscle inserts onto the lateral third of the clavicle. The clavicular head of the sternocleidomastoid muscle originates on the superior surface. The subclavius muscle and enveloping clavipectoral fascia attach to the inferior surface.

By providing stability for the muscular and ligamentous origins of the principal mobilizers of the upper arm, particularly the pectoralis major and deltoid muscles, the clavicle plays a significant role in the overall motion and function of the upper extremity. In addition, through the sternoclavicular joint, the clavicle itself is responsible for some motion.[1,113,175] Upward elevation of the clavicle through approximately 30 to 35 degrees contributes to shoulder abduction. The clavicle can also protract and retract approximately 35 degrees in the anterior-to-posterior plane, and it can rotate 45 to 50 degrees about its long axis.

Laterally, the clavicle articulates with the acromion of the scapula through the acromioclavicular joint, which is a diarthrodial joint, surrounded by a relatively weak capsule and supported superiorly and inferiorly by the acromioclavicular ligaments. In a child the lateral third of the clavicle is surrounded circumferentially by thick periosteum that confers stability against fracture displacement. The capsule and acromioclavicular ligaments blend with this periosteum. The primary stabilizing ligaments, the conoid and trapezoid portions of the coracoclavicular ligaments, arise from the coracoid and attach to the lateral end of the clavicle and its periosteum.

Medially, the clavicle articulates with the manubrium of the sternum and the first rib through the sternoclavicular joint. This joint is also diarthrodial and, similar to the acromioclavicular joint, it lacks inherent structural stability. The joint is stabilized by a group of ligaments that include the intra-articular disk ligament, the anterior and posterior capsular ligaments, the interclavicular ligament, and the costoclavicular ligament (Fig. 12-15). The anterior capsular ligament is heavier and stronger than the posterior.[216] The capsular ligaments attach mainly to the epiphysis of the medial clavicle; therefore the physis is extra-articular and susceptible to injury during injuries to the medial clavicle.[145] The sternoclavicular joint overlies several important mediastinal structures, including the great vessels, the vagus and phrenic nerves, and the trachea and esophagus.

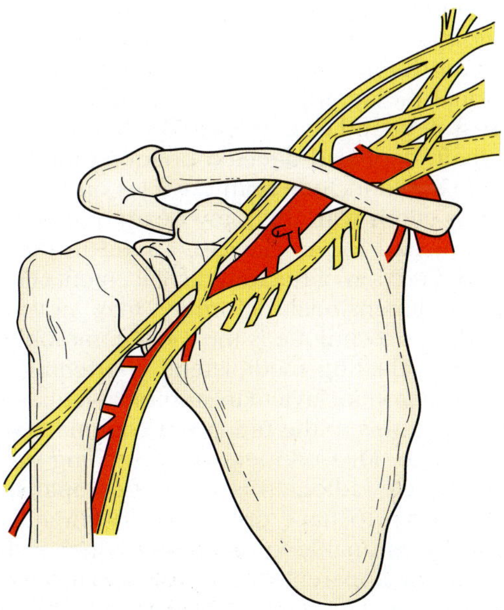

FIGURE 12-14: Relationship of the clavicle and scapula to the brachial plexus and subclavian artery. (From Sarwark JF, King EC, Luhmann SJ. Proximal humerus, scapula, and clavicle. In: Rockwood CA, et al, eds. *Fractures in Children.* 6th ed. Philadelphia: Lippincott Williams & Wilkins; 2006:703-771.)

Fracture Incidence

Fractures of the clavicle occur in 1% to 13% of all births.[40] The clavicle is also commonly injured during childhood,

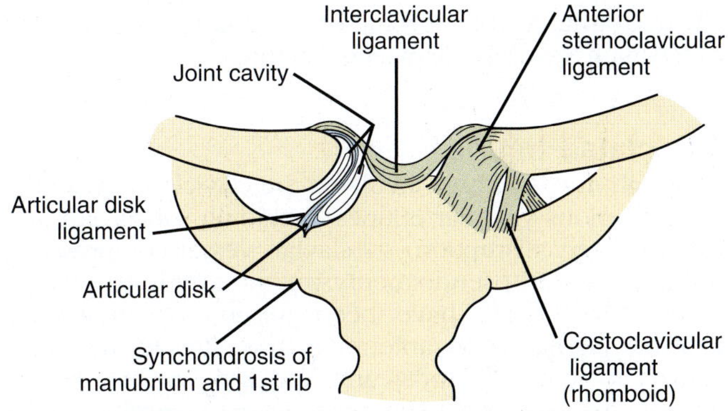

FIGURE 12-15: Anatomy of the sternoclavicular joint.

with the peak incidence of fractures observed between 10 and 19 years of age,[248] representing between 8% and 15.5% of all pediatric fractures.[184] Most fractures of the clavicle in children involve the middle third (76% to 85%), followed by the lateral third (10% to 21%); the incidence of lateral fractures increases with age. Fractures in the medial third are less common and account for only 1% to 5% of clavicle injuries in children.

Mechanism of Injury

The clavicle is the most commonly fractured bone during childbirth. The risk of birth-related clavicle fractures is increased for infants with larger birth weight (>4500 g), increased length (>52 cm), and shoulder dystocia.[12] However, the majority of birth-related clavicle fractures occur in uneventful deliveries of infants with average birth weights.

In children and adolescents, falls, especially onto the shoulder, are the most common cause of fractures of the clavicle.[184] Fractures of the clavicle can also occur in motor vehicle accidents and secondary to direct trauma sustained during sports activity. Nonaccidental trauma can also be a cause. Stress fractures are rare, but they do occur.

Signs and Symptoms

Fractures of the clavicle in newborns may be difficult to diagnose. One of the more reliable signs is difficulty with palpation of the margins of the injured clavicle due to generalized edema. Pain is usually present with movement about the shoulder or direct palpation of the clavicle. Newborns with clavicle fractures sometimes voluntarily splint or immobilize the ipsilateral arm, presumably to lessen pain. This pseudoparalysis can at times be misdiagnosed as a brachial plexus injury. To minimize pain related to the pull of the sternocleidomastoid muscle across the fracture site, affected infants might turn their head toward the side of the fracture. Infants with acute clavicle fractures typically have an asymmetric Moro reflex.

In older children the diagnosis of a clavicle injury is typically straightforward. Pain is present around the area of the fracture. Ecchymosis, swelling, and tenderness can also be present around the fracture site. Children with fractures of the clavicle resist and stop movement of the affected arm. A bony prominence or deformity may be noted with severely displaced fractures.

Associated Injuries

Although rare, fractures involving the clavicle increase the risk of serious vascular injuries, including subclavian and axillary artery disruption; subclavian vessel compression, thrombosis, and pseudoaneurysm; and arteriovenous fistulas.[106,230,239] There have been reports of anomalous external jugular veins anterior to the clavicle that were subject to injury.[206] Both early and late brachial plexus neuropathy has also been reported in association with injuries to the clavicle.[9,53,256] Thorough neurovascular examination of the upper extremity is warranted to rule out these injuries.

Fractures of the clavicle secondary to high-energy injuries can be associated with injuries to the ipsilateral lung and chest wall, such as pneumothorax, hemothorax, pulmonary contusion, and rib fractures. Additional injuries to the ipsilateral upper extremity and shoulder girdle are also possible in high-energy injury mechanisms.

Posterior displaced fractures of the medial clavicle and posterior dislocations of the sternoclavicular joint are at particular risk for concomitant injury to the retrosternal structures in the mediastinum, including the great vessels, the esophagus, and the trachea.[29,77,148,155,181,210,266] A child presenting with difficulty in speaking, breathing, or swallowing should raise suspicion of these. Signs of venous congestion and diminished distal pulse can also suggest associated injuries, some of which can be life threatening.

Fractures of the clavicle are rarely associated with atlantoaxial (C1-C2) rotatory subluxation (Fig. 12-16).[24,177] Clinically, the head is tilted laterally toward and rotated away from the fractured clavicle. The diagnosis of C1-C2 rotatory subluxation is difficult because of the masking of the torticollis by the acute symptoms of the fractured clavicle, but it should be suspected when there is asymmetrical cervical ROM. The diagnosis is best confirmed by dynamic CT.

Radiographic Evaluation

First-line radiographic imaging includes an AP radiograph of the clavicle (Fig. 12-17). In newborns, ultrasound examination is a reasonable alternative to conventional radiography in the diagnosis of fractures involving the clavicle.[17,126,127] Ultrasonographic imaging is particularly sensitive in detecting occult clavicle fractures and sternoclavicular injuries in this young demographic and can prove useful during follow-up to assess fracture healing.

Additional radiographic views are necessary for complete assessment and characterization. For fractures of the clavicle shaft, cephalad-directed oblique radiographs are useful and should include both clavicles on a single plate. This view is taken with the x-ray beam directed 20 to 45 degrees cephalad to the clavicle, an aid in defining the degree and direction of fracture displacement (Fig. 12-18). While three-dimensional deformity may not be easily recognized, this technique is the most commonly utilized method for evaluating mediolateral shortening by measuring the acromioclavicular–sternoclavicular distance and comparing this to the uninjured contralateral side on the same image. Measurement of shortening on isolated unilateral clavicle radiographs without comparison views has been shown to have only poor to fair reliability,[236] with the surgeon unable to determine whether the shortening is true or apparent due to a coronal-oblique fracture pattern (see Fig. 12-17). The apical oblique view, taken with the x-ray beam directed 45 degrees lateral to the axial axis of the body and 20 degrees cephalad to the clavicle, offers an additional oblique view of the clavicle shaft and is particularly effective for fractures involving the middle third of the clavicle.

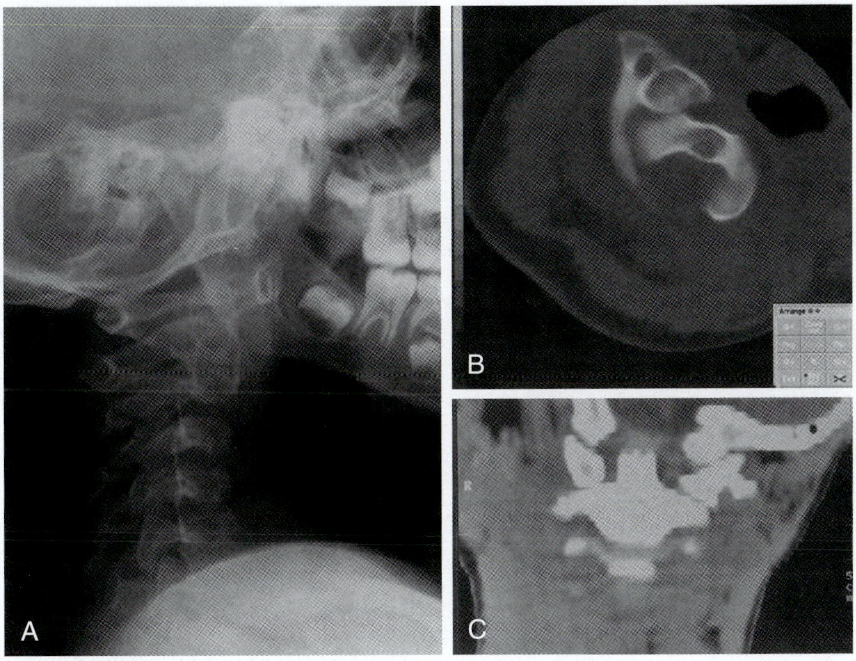

FIGURE 12-16: **A,** Lateral radiograph of the cervical spine with increased atlantodental interval and anterolisthesis of the atlas. **B,** Axial computed tomography (CT) showing significant atlantoaxial rotatory subluxation. **C,** Coronal CT reconstruction showing the eccentric axis of the dens in relation to the lateral masses of the atlas. (From Nannapaneni R, Nath FP, Papastefanou SL. Fracture of the clavicle associated with a rotatory atlantoaxial subluxation. *Injury.* 2001;32:71-73.)

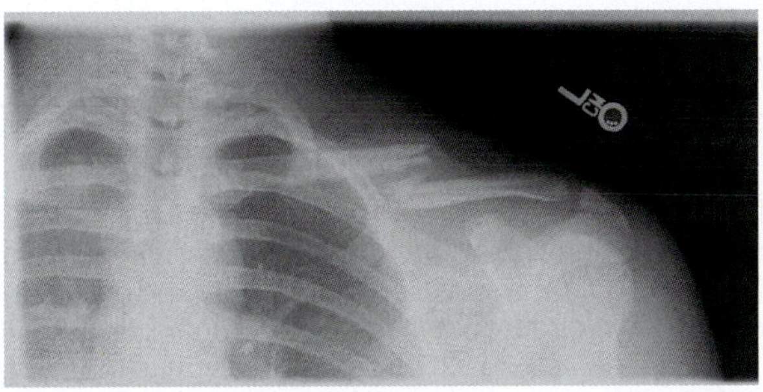

FIGURE 12-17: Anteroposterior radiograph of the left clavicle showing a midshaft fracture. Although this projection functions well for screening, it is difficult to determine whether there is true shortening or apparent shortening due to a coronal-oblique fracture pattern. Further radiographs are warranted to measure the sternoclavicular-acromioclavicular joint distances bilaterally.

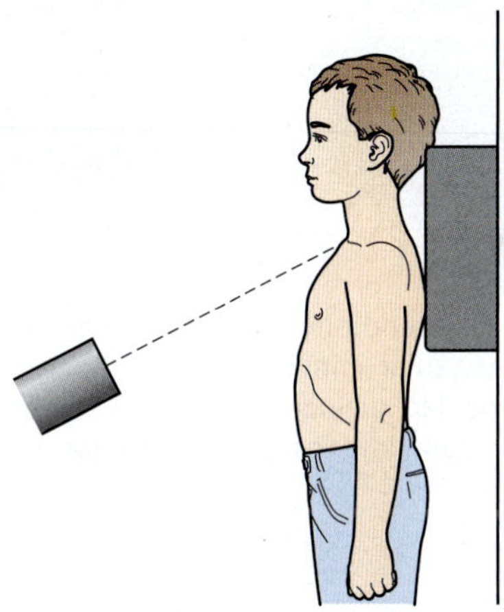

FIGURE 12-18: Technique for the cephalad-directed view of the clavicle. (From Sarwark JF, King EC, Luhmann SJ. Proximal humerus, scapula, and clavicle. In: Rockwood CA, et al, eds. *Fractures in Children.* 6th ed. Philadelphia: Lippincott Williams & Wilkins; 2006:703-771.)

For injuries to the lateral aspect of the clavicle and acromioclavicular joint, an AP radiograph centered on the acromioclavicular joint is recommended. In addition, cephalad-directed (15 to 20 degrees) and axillary lateral views are helpful for further delineation of the fracture. The Stryker notch view (a 10-degree cephalad radiograph of the shoulder with the patient's hand resting on top of the head) is helpful in detecting concomitant fractures of the coracoid (Fig. 12-19). Stress views (taken with the patient holding weights with the arms adducted) can reveal subtle injuries to the lateral clavicle or acromioclavicular joint but are not routinely indicated. A CT scan or MRI is indicated if additional detailed evaluation of the physis and acromioclavicular or sternoclavicular joints is needed.

Radiographic evaluation of injuries involving the medial third of the clavicle and sternoclavicular joint is difficult. A serendipity view, taken with the x-ray beam directed 40 degrees cephalad to the sternoclavicular joints, can be helpful (Fig. 12-20). CT, however, has

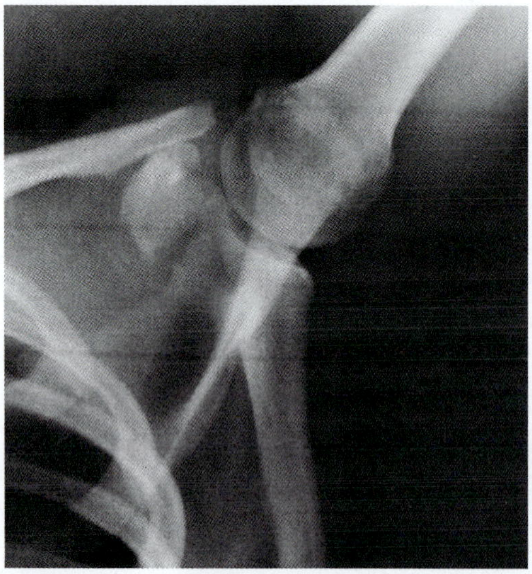

FIGURE 12-19: Stryker notch view showing a fracture of the base of the coracoid.

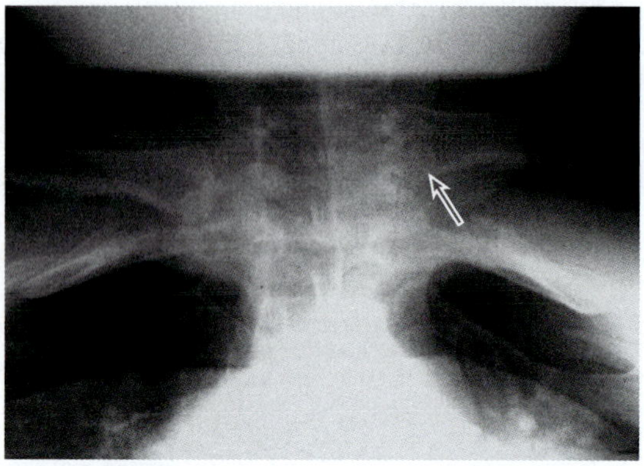

FIGURE 12-20: Serendipity view (40-degree cephalic tilt view of the sternoclavicular joints) showing an anteriorly displaced left sternoclavicular dislocation (*arrow*). (From Linnau KF, Blackmore CC: Bony injuries of the shoulder. *Curr Probl Diagn Radiol.* 2002;31:29-47.)

become the imaging modality of choice for quantifying posterior displacement and mediastinal encroachment (Fig. 12-21).

Differential Diagnosis

The differential diagnosis for fractures of the clavicle should include congenital pseudarthrosis of the clavicle.[15] This is rare and usually asymptomatic. Involvement is generally right sided, and left-sided involvement should raise suspicion of dextrocardia or situs inversus. Bilateral involvement is very rare. Clavicular abnormalities can also arise secondary to benign or malignant tumors; metabolic disorders, such as hyperparathyroidism; and renal osteodystrophy. Idiopathic hyperostosis may be difficult to differentiate from a fracture of the clavicle.

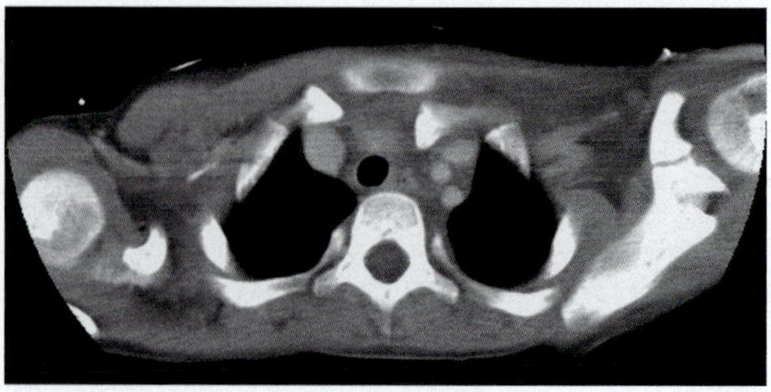

FIGURE 12-21: Axial computed tomography of a posteriorly displaced fracture of the medial end of the left clavicle. The close proximity of the trachea and great vessels can easily be appreciated.

Osteomyelitis of the clavicle is uncommon but can produce a periosteal reaction mimicking fracture healing.

Classification

The most common classification scheme for fractures of the clavicle is based on the anatomic location of the fracture (Fig. 12-22).[3] Type I fractures involve the middle third of the clavicle, lateral to the sternocleidomastoid muscle and medial to the coracoclavicular ligaments. Type II fractures involve the lateral third, including and lateral to the coracoclavicular ligaments. Type III fractures involve the medial third, medial to the sternocleidomastoid muscle. Separate classification schemata have been developed to categorize injuries involving the lateral and medial ends of the clavicle.

Lateral Clavicle Injuries

The most widely used classification scheme for injuries involving the lateral end of the clavicle and acromioclavicular joint in children is based on a similar classification for adults (Fig. 12-23).[211] In children displacement of the lateral clavicle occurs through the periosteal sleeve rather than through the coracoclavicular ligaments. True acromioclavicular dislocations are uncommon in children, although they do occur in older adolescents as they near skeletal maturity. Instead, most injuries to the lateral end of the clavicle in the immature skeleton are fractures involving the metaphyseal or physeal regions (Salter-Harris type I or II fractures) (Fig. 12-24). The lateral epiphysis of the clavicle does not ossify until the age of 18 or 19 years; therefore these metaphyseal and physeal injuries can manifest radiographically as an acromioclavicular dislocation (e.g., *pseudodislocation*).[66,187] The injuries are classified into following six types.

Type I injuries are caused by low-energy trauma, with mild strain of the acromioclavicular ligaments and no disruption of the periosteal tube. Radiographs appear normal except for occasional overlying soft tissue swelling.

In type II injuries the acromioclavicular ligaments are completely disrupted, with partial damage to the superolateral aspect of the periosteal sleeve. These injuries result in mild instability of the lateral end of the clavicle.

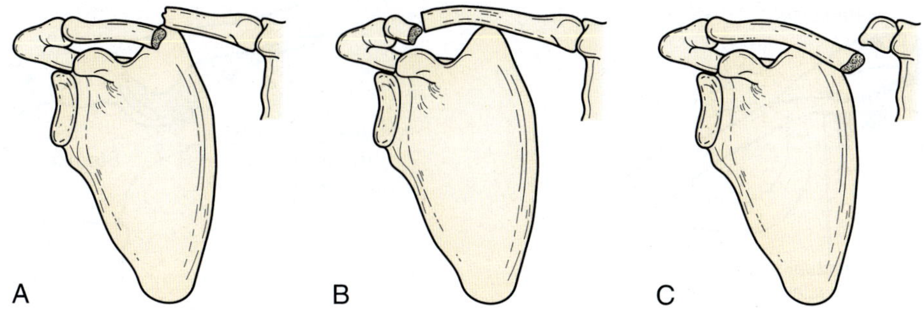

FIGURE 12-22: Anatomic classification scheme for fractures of the clavicle. **A,** Type I, fracture of the middle third of the clavicle. **B,** Type II, fracture of the lateral third of the clavicle. **C,** Type III, fracture of the medial third of the clavicle. (From Sarwark JF, King EC, Luhmann SJ: Proximal humerus, scapula, and clavicle. In: Rockwood CA, et al, eds. *Fractures in Children.* 6th ed. Philadelphia: Lippincott Williams & Wilkins; 2006:703-771.)

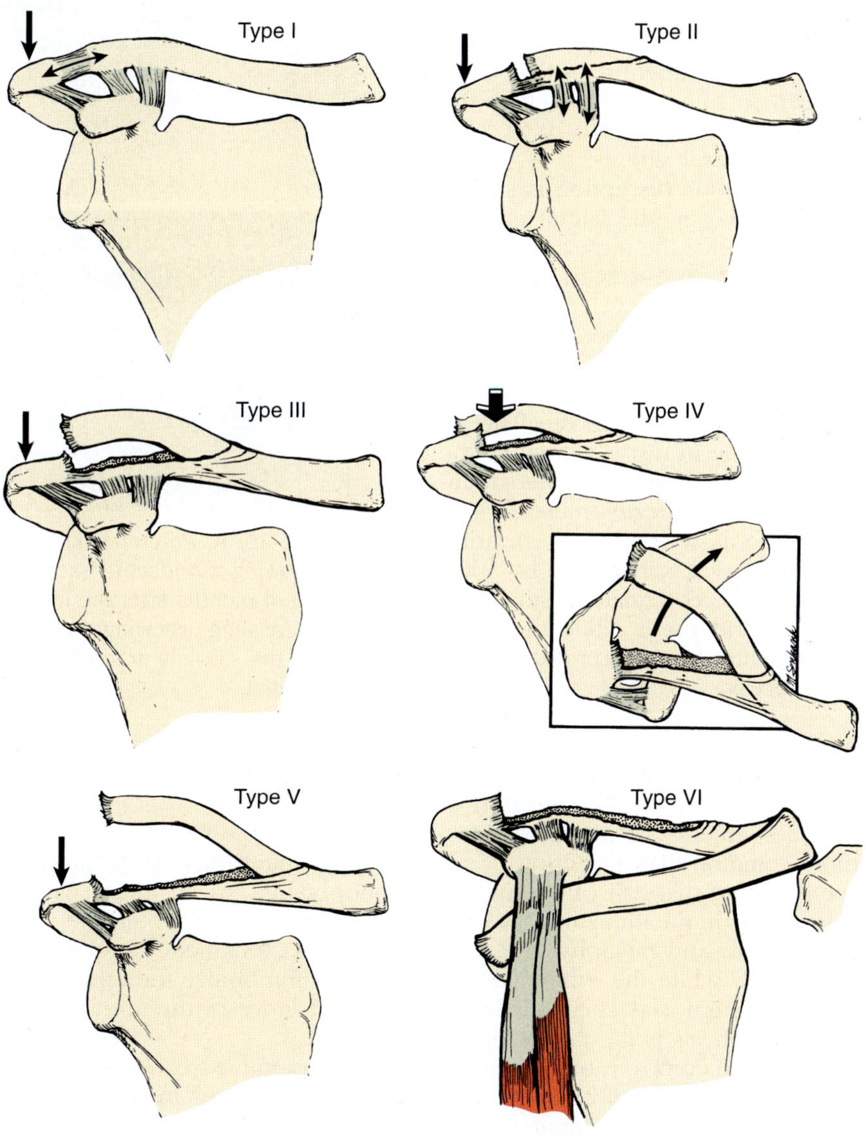

FIGURE 12-23: Dameron and Rockwood classification of fractures involving the lateral end of the clavicle and acromioclavicular joint in children (see text for description).

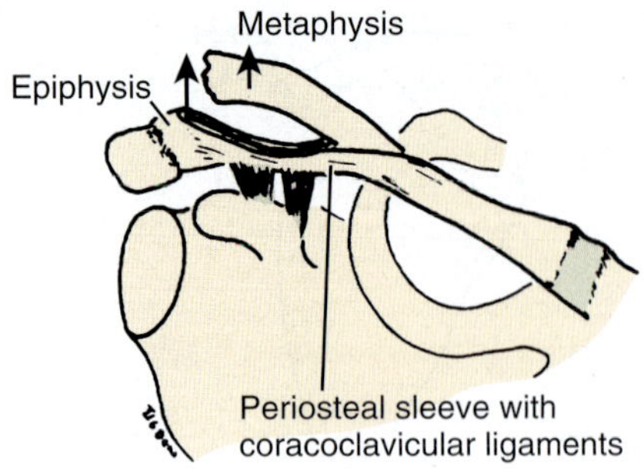

FIGURE 12-24: Most injuries to the lateral end of the clavicle in children are Salter-Harris type I or II fractures.

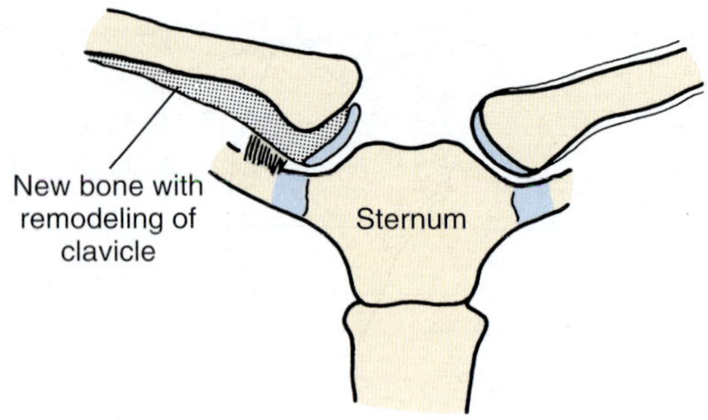

FIGURE 12-25: Half of medial clavicular injuries are Salter-Harris type I or II fractures as seen here, with the other half being true dislocations of the sternoclavicular joint.

Minimal widening of the acromioclavicular joint may be seen on radiographs.

In type III injuries complete disruption of the acromioclavicular ligaments occurs in addition to greater disruption of the periosteal sleeve, resulting in gross instability of the distal end of the clavicle. Superior displacement of the lateral clavicle is seen on AP radiographs, with the coracoid–clavicle interval increased by 25% to 100% compared to the uninjured contralateral side.

In type IV injuries the soft tissue disruption is similar to that in type III injuries; however, the lateral clavicle displaces posteriorly and can pierce the trapezius muscle and/or fascia. Little displacement may be seen on the AP radiograph, and the axillary lateral view is helpful for visualizing the posterior displacement of the clavicle relative to the acromion.

Type V injuries are similar to type III injuries but are more severe. The superior aspect of the periosteal sleeve is completely disrupted, resulting in displacement of the distal clavicle through the trapezial fascia into the subcutaneous tissues. The deltoid and trapezius muscles may be detached from the clavicle as well. On an AP radiograph the coracoid-clavicle interval is increased by 100% or more compared to that of the contralateral side.

Type VI injuries are rare and occur when the distal clavicle displaces inferiorly, with the distal end displaced inferior to the coracoid process.

Medial Clavicle Injuries

Injuries to the medial end of the clavicle and sternoclavicular joint are classified according to the direction of displacement of the clavicle—anterior or posterior. Anterior displacement is more common than posterior.[167,257,265] Recent case series have indicated that half of the injuries to the medial end of the clavicle in the immature skeleton are fractures through the physis and metaphysis (Salter-Harris type I and II fractures), while the other half are true dislocations through the sternoclavicular joint (Fig. 12-25).[145] The medial clavicle physis is the last physis in the body to close, and the medial epiphysis of the clavicle does not fuse completely to the shaft until 23 to 25 years of age. Because the sternoclavicular ligaments attach primarily to the epiphysis, the medial physis is extracapsular and left relatively unprotected.

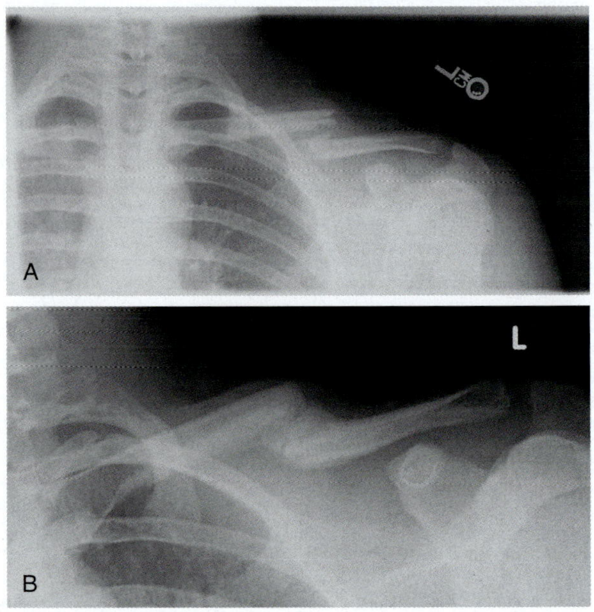

FIGURE 12-26: **A,** Anteroposterior (AP) radiograph of the left clavicle showing a midshaft fracture. **B,** AP radiograph of the left clavicle 4 months after the initiation of nonoperative treatment with a sling, showing significant callus formation and healing of the clavicle fracture. Remodeling continued over several months.

Treatment

Fractures of the Clavicle Shaft

The treatment for birth-related fractures of the clavicle is nonoperative. In an infant who appears uncomfortable, the affected arm should be immobilized for 10 to 14 days.[120] A stockinette or elastic stretch bandage may be used to immobilize the affected arm to the chest wall, or the shirtsleeve of the affected arm can be pinned to the shirt.

Nonoperative treatment is also effective for many clavicle shaft fractures in preadolescent and adolescent children (Fig. 12-26).[205,228] Treatment of nondisplaced and minimally displaced clavicle shaft fractures with a figure-of-eight splint or sling is effective; both methods result in equally excellent outcomes.[4,118] Caution is required with the use of a figure-of-eight splint, as too much tightening can lead to excessive swelling, compression of the axillary vessels, pain, and brachial plexus neuropathy.[71,118,147] Close weekly follow-up is required to monitor the skin and neurovascular status. If a sling is used, inadvertent migration around the neck can lead to choking and must be prevented.

Absolute indications for operative treatment include open fractures; severely displaced and irreducible clavicle fractures at risk for skin perforation; associated vascular injury requiring repair; and irreducible displaced fractures causing compression of mediastinal structures, such as the trachea and esophagus; and possibly compromise of the brachial plexus.[106,139] In addition, concomitant displaced fractures of the scapula (acromion, coracoid, or scapular neck)—a floating shoulder injury pattern—frequently require operative treatment.[52,115,192] More recently, indications for operative treatment of adolescent clavicle fractures have been broadened to include fractures with greater than 1.5 to 2.0 cm of shortening, complete displacement, and comminution,[33,102,118,246,262] although large survey studies have indicated that operative fixation in this demographic remains controversial.[34] Open fixation is typically performed with plate-and-screw constructs with either universal small fragment plates and screws or anatomic clavicle plating systems (Fig. 12-27). Fixation with percutaneous smooth Kirschner wires should be avoided because this technique has been associated with migration into vital structures and a high overall complication rate.[70,121,159]

Lateral Clavicle Injuries

Given the exceptional healing and remodeling potential in children for fractures involving the lateral end of the clavicle, most of these can be treated nonoperatively. Injuries to the lateral clavicle in the immature skeleton are typically physeal injuries. Moreover, the enhanced capacity to heal and remodel is related to the retained periosteal sleeve and to the usually undamaged and intact acromioclavicular joint and coracoclavicular ligaments.

Most surgeons agree that nondisplaced or minimally displaced injuries of the lateral clavicle (types I, II, and III) can be treated effectively without surgery by using a sling or a figure-of-eight splint (Fig. 12-28). Nonoperative treatment results in predictably excellent outcomes

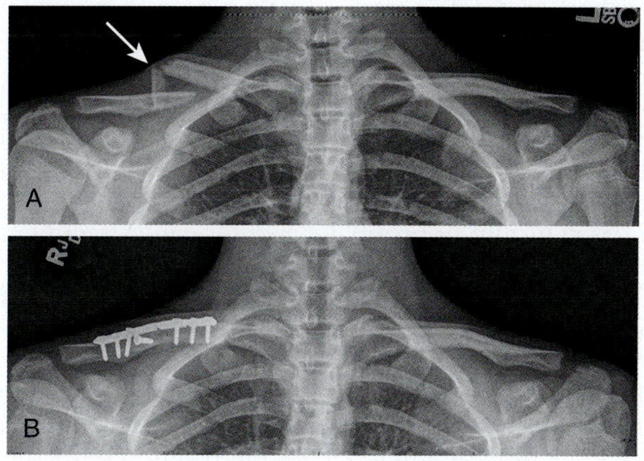

FIGURE 12-27: A, A 30-degree cephalic tilt anteroposterior view of bilateral clavicles revealing a comminuted, displaced, angulated, and significantly shortened right clavicle fracture with a "Z fragment" and tenting of the skin (*arrow*). The child was near skeletal maturity. **B,** Interval healing 6 weeks after open reduction and internal fixation with interfragmentary compression and anatomic clavicle plate fixation. (Courtesy Theodore J. Ganley, MD.)

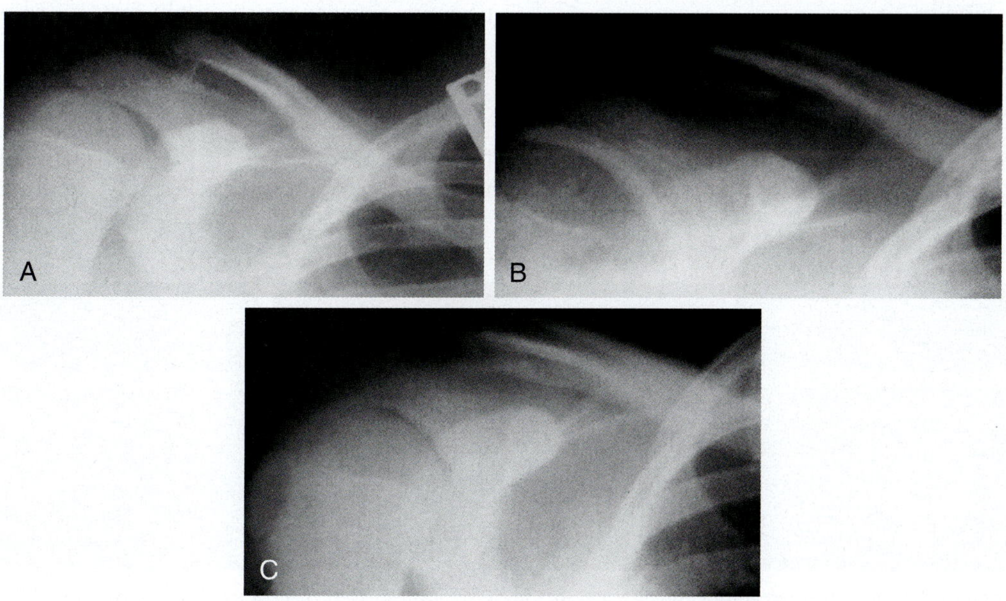

FIGURE 12-28: Plain radiographs showing the healing and remodeling of a fracture involving the lateral end of the clavicle. The periosteal sleeve remains in continuity but is invisible on radiographs. **A,** Two weeks after injury. **B,** One month after injury. **C,** Six months after injury.

without long-term functional disability.[18,63,97,187,211] The treatment of displaced type IV, V, and VI lateral clavicle fractures is controversial. In the past, recommendations have varied widely from nonoperative treatment to treatment with open reduction and internal fixation.[18,49,97,187,213] Currently, most recommendations advocate open reduction and stable fixation.[49,97,203,213] In younger children the lateral end of the clavicle can be reduced into its periosteal sleeve, and stable fixation can be achieved after repair of the periosteum.

Although rare, true acromioclavicular dislocations can occur in children. However, the vast majority of these are found in adolescents, and treatment recommendations overlap with those for the adult population.

Medial Clavicle Injuries

There is also significant potential for satisfactory healing and subsequent remodeling with fractures involving the medial end of the clavicle; therefore nonoperative treatment is typically appropriate. Symptomatic treatment is usually adequate for nondisplaced or minimally displaced fractures.[45,230] A sling can be worn for comfort, and early motion of the upper extremity is recommended.

Anteriorly displaced medial clavicle injuries can be expected to remodel; therefore reduction is not routinely performed. However, reduction may be attempted in the emergency department or operating room under local or general anesthesia. The reduction maneuver consists of longitudinal traction of the ipsilateral upper extremity while the shoulder is abducted to 90 degrees. Gentle posterior pressure is applied over the fracture. Limited immobilization with a figure-of-eight splint is recommended for 3 to 4 weeks. The reduction can be unstable, and redisplacement is not uncommon. Open reduction with internal fixation, however, is usually unnecessary, and reconstruction is reserved for patients with chronic symptomatic instability.

With posteriorly displaced medial clavicle injuries, evaluation for concomitant injuries of the airway, mediastinum, and great vessels should immediately be initiated. Acute posterior sternoclavicular dislocations are frequently treated with reduction and fixation; however, in the absence of any significant associated injuries, chronic and subacute minimally displaced sternoclavicular dislocations may be treated without reduction. Fractures and dislocations with significant displacement should be reduced. If the airway or great vessels are compromised, urgent reduction in the presence of vascular or thoracic surgery colleagues is warranted.

Reduction should be attempted under general anesthesia in an operating room setting, with a thoracic or general surgeon readily available in case of mediastinal, airway, or great vessel compromise. The patient is positioned supine with a bolster placed in the midline between the scapulae. Gentle longitudinal traction of the ipsilateral arm is applied while drawing the ipsilateral shoulder posteriorly and into abduction.

If attempts at closed reduction are unsuccessful, a sterile towel clip can aid reduction. After sterile preparation of the skin, the medial end of the clavicle is grasped and manipulated with a towel clip while longitudinal traction is applied to the ipsilateral upper arm (Fig. 12-29). If attempts at percutaneous reduction fail, open reduction is performed. Open reduction is also indicated for open fractures. At the surgeon's discretion, stable fixation can be achieved using heavy, nonabsorbable transosseous sutures, with concomitant repair of the overlying periosteum and ligaments. Internal fixation with metal implants is inadvisable because of the potential for migration into the mediastinum.

Complications

Malunions

Early malunion may be seen after a fracture with initial displacement, but significant deformity and long-term disability are unlikely given the remodeling potential of children. Clavicular reduplication and cleidoscapular synostosis can occur, but these are rare.[187,203] If the malunion is symptomatic, corrective osteotomy may be considered.

Nonunions

Nonunion following a traumatic fracture of the clavicle is uncommon; rates of nonunion have been reported to be 0.1% to 5.9%.[118,163,179,182,202,205,246,271] In most cases nonunions are asymptomatic. Rarely, operative intervention

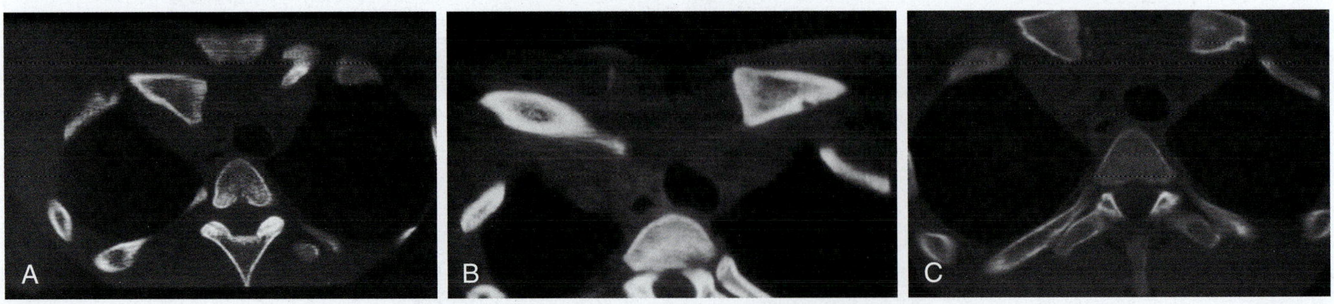

FIGURE 12-29: Axial computed tomography scans of a right posterior epiphyseal fracture of the medial clavicle in a 16-year-old male. **A,** On the first cut of the scan, the injury appears to be a posterior dislocation. **B,** Another cut faintly shows the epiphyseal fragment. **C,** After closed reduction with a towel clip, the epiphysis is realigned with the metaphysis. (From Bishop JY, Flatow AL: Pediatric shoulder trauma. *Clin Orthop Relat Res.* 2005;432:41-48.)

with bone grafting and stable fixation is required for unacceptable cosmetic deformity or pain.

Neurovascular Injuries

Numerous neurovascular complications have been reported in association with injuries to the clavicle: injury to the subclavian, axillary, and great vessels and brachial plexus palsy.[9,53,106,230,239,256] The majority of these neurovascular injuries occur concomitantly at or near the time of injury. Neurovascular complications, however, can also occur later, following nonoperative or operative treatment. Vascular complications include subclavian artery and vein compression, thrombosis, pseudoaneurysm, transection or laceration, arteriovenous fistulas, and thoracic outlet syndrome. Anomalous external jugular veins anterior to the clavicle have been reported; these can be subject to laceration at the time of injury or operative fixation.[206] Neurologic deficits related to brachial plexus neuropathy can also occur. Brachial plexus palsy has been reported in association with the inappropriate use of a figure-of-eight splint. Most brachial plexus neuropathies are self-limited and resolve spontaneously, but permanent deficits have also been reported.

FRACTURES OF THE SCAPULA

Anatomy

Embryology and Development

The scapula begins to form in the fifth week of gestation.[105,222] It first develops at the C4-C5 level, and then descends to its final position overlying the first through fifth ribs. Failure of the scapula to descend results in Sprengel's deformity.[105,129] Most of the scapula forms by intramembranous ossification and develops from multiple centers of ossification: three for the body, two to five for the acromion, two for the coracoid process, and one for the glenoid (Fig. 12-30).

Relevant Anatomy

The scapula is a triangular, flat bone that links the upper extremity to the axial skeleton. Seventeen distinct muscles attach to the scapula, and this overlying musculature leaves it relatively well protected. The scapular spine separates the inferior and superior fossae; the acromion is the lateral projection of the spine. The coracoid process is on the anterolateral portion of the scapular neck, and the glenoid is the lateral extension of the scapular neck. The scapula articulates with the clavicle at the acromioclavicular joint, with the humerus at the glenohumeral joint, and functionally with the chest wall at the scapulothoracic articulation (which is not a true joint). The scapula is highly mobile and provides approximately 60 degrees of shoulder elevation.

The brachial plexus and axillary artery course across the anterosuperior aspect of the scapula, passing posterior to the clavicle. These neurovascular structures continue past the tip of the coracoid process, first medially and then inferiorly. The suprascapular nerve and artery pass under and over the transverse scapular ligament, respectively; this ligament overlies the suprascapular notch medial to the base of the coracoid process. The axillary nerve travels immediately inferior to the glenoid.

The superior shoulder suspensory complex (SSSC) is a bone and soft tissue ring comprising the glenoid, coracoid process, coracoclavicular ligament, lateral part of the clavicle, acromioclavicular joint, acromion process, and coracoacromial ligament (Fig. 12-31).[52,84,192,264] The

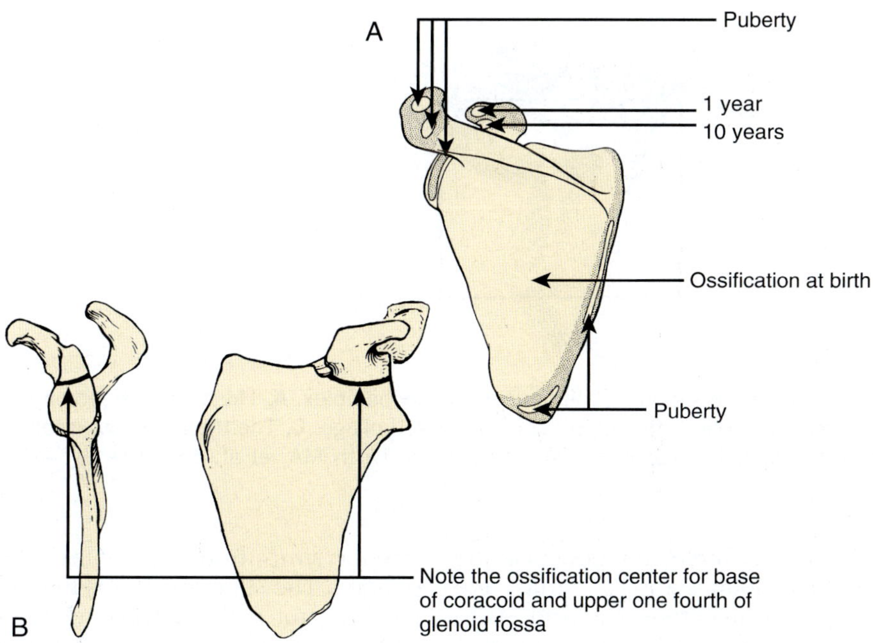

FIGURE 12-30: Multiple ossification centers of the scapula. **A**, Posterior view. **B**, Lateral and anterior views.

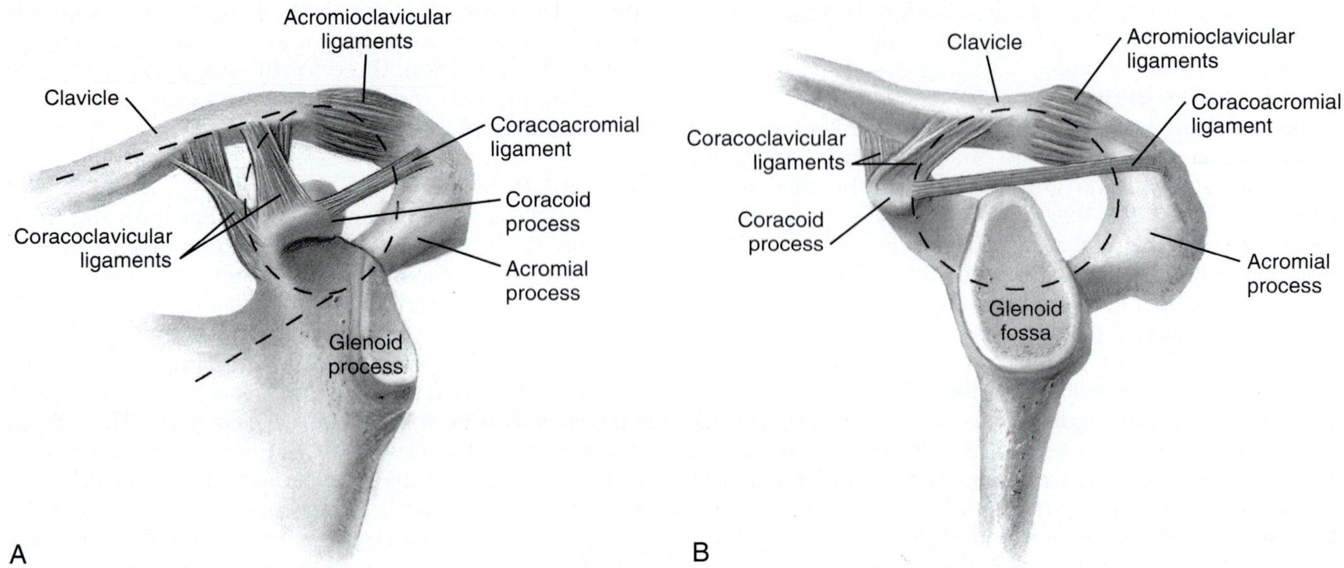

FIGURE 12-31: The superior shoulder suspensory complex. Anteroposterior (**A**) and lateral (**B**) views of the bone–soft tissue ring and the superior and inferior bone struts.

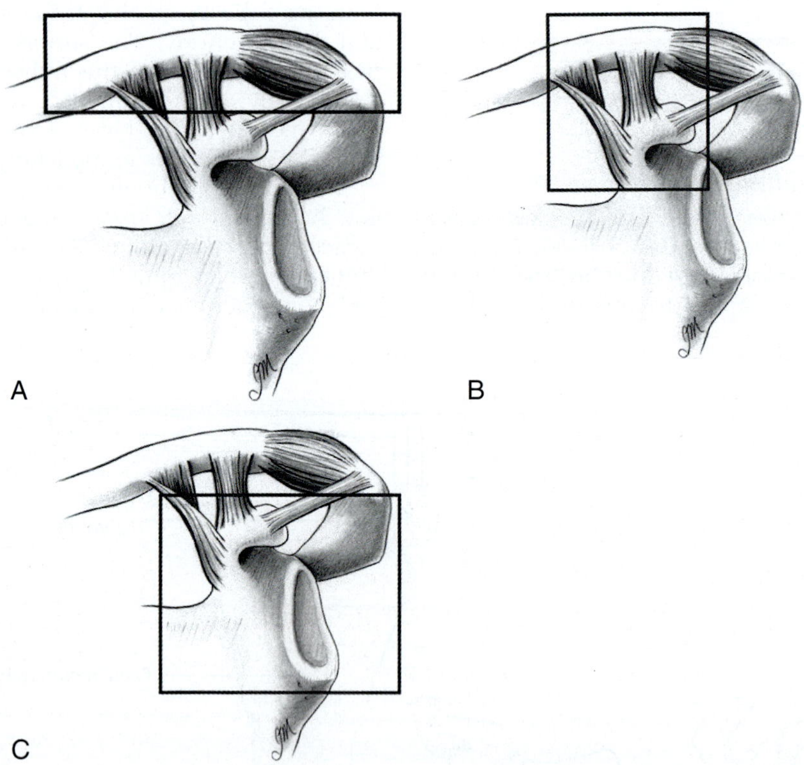

FIGURE 12-32: The three units of the superior shoulder suspensory complex. **A,** The clavicular–acromioclavicular joint–acromial strut. **B,** The clavicular–coracoclavicular ligamentous–coracoid (C4) linkage. **C,** The three-process–scapular body junction. (From Goss TP: Fractures of the scapula. In: Rockwood CA, Matsen FA, Wirth MA, et al, eds. *The Shoulder.* 3rd ed. Philadelphia: Saunders; 2004:413.)

complex can be divided into three components: the clavicular–acromioclavicular joint–acromial strut, the clavicular–coracoclavicular ligamentous–coracoid (C4) linkage, and the three-process–scapular body junction (Fig. 12-32). SSSC is secured to the trunk by superior and inferior struts from which the upper extremity is suspended. The superior strut is the middle clavicle, and the inferior strut is the junction of the lateral scapular body and medial scapular neck. Functionally, SSSC links the upper extremity and axial skeleton.

Fracture Incidence

Fractures of the scapula are rare and constitute only 1% of all fractures and 5% of shoulder fractures in the general population.[2,84] Fractures of the body and spine of the scapula are most common, and those of the coracoid are least common. According to one series in adults, the distribution of scapula fracture locations is 35% body, 27% neck, 12% acromion, 11% spine, 10% glenoid, and 7% coracoid.[2]

Mechanism of Injury

Injury to the scapula usually is a result of severe, high-energy trauma; therefore scapular injuries are rarely isolated. Scapular body fractures usually occur as a result of direct impact. In the absence of a clear traumatic cause, nonaccidental trauma must be excluded. Injury to the scapula, especially to the coracoid process, can also occur as a result of an avulsion mechanism. Stress fractures are rare. Fractures of the glenoid typically occur secondary to a fall onto the upper extremity. Scapulothoracic dissociations usually result from high-energy trauma with massive, direct force to the chest and shoulder regions accompanied by traction forces applied to the shoulder girdle.

Signs and Symptoms

Fractures of the scapula are characterized clinically by significant pain, swelling, ecchymosis, and tenderness around the shoulder girdle. The overall surface anatomy of the shoulder may be hidden by the localized swelling. Children with fractures of the scapula typically resist movement of the injured arm. Massive swelling is seen about the shoulder girdle following scapulothoracic dissociation, especially in the setting of an abnormal vascular examination and neurologic deficit. The presence of associated, sometimes life-threatening, injuries often leads to late diagnosis and delayed treatment of the injured scapula.

Associated Injuries

About 80% to 95% of fractures involving the scapula are associated with additional injuries, which may be life-threatening.[2,84,183,241] The most common injuries are to the head; chest; kidneys; and especially to the ipsilateral lung, chest wall, and shoulder girdle. In one series mortality associated with scapula fractures exceeded 14%.[241] Given the close anatomic relationship between the scapula and numerous neurovascular structures, associated neurovascular injury, particularly to the brachial plexus and axillary artery, can also occur. Scapulothoracic dissociations, in particular, are nearly universally associated with ipsilateral neurovascular injury.[125,164]

Radiographic Evaluation

Fractures involving the scapula are often first seen on the AP chest radiograph during the routine trauma series. If a scapula fracture is visible or suspected, AP and lateral radiographs of the scapula are necessary to define it (Fig. 12-33). Additional radiographic views can further characterize the scapula injury. Most trauma series to evaluate the shoulder region should include the axillary lateral view for confirmation of concentric reduction of the humeral head within the glenoid as well as for the assessment of fractures involving the glenoid face or neck. A 20-degree caudal tilt lateral view with the shoulder adducted may be helpful for injuries involving the acromion. The Stryker notch view (an AP radiograph of the shoulder with the patient's hand resting on top of the head) may be helpful for coracoid injuries (see Fig.

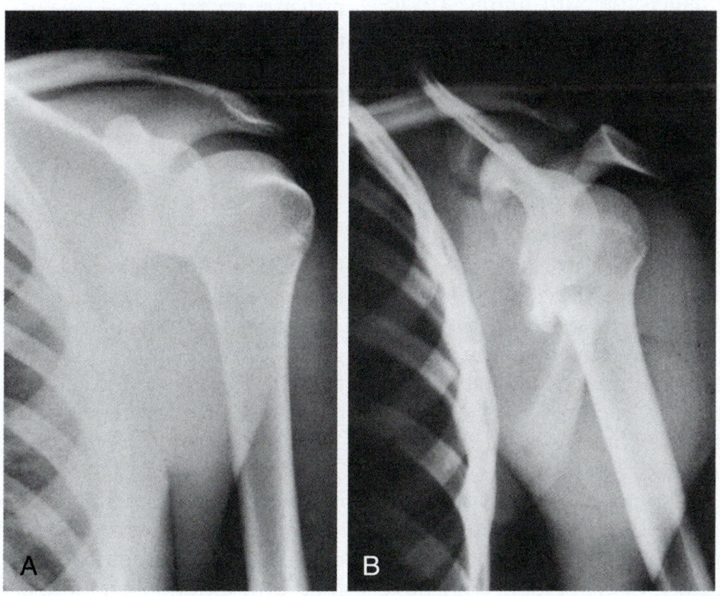

FIGURE 12-33: Anteroposterior (**A**) and lateral (scapular Y) (**B**) views of the scapula are able to define most scapular fractures.

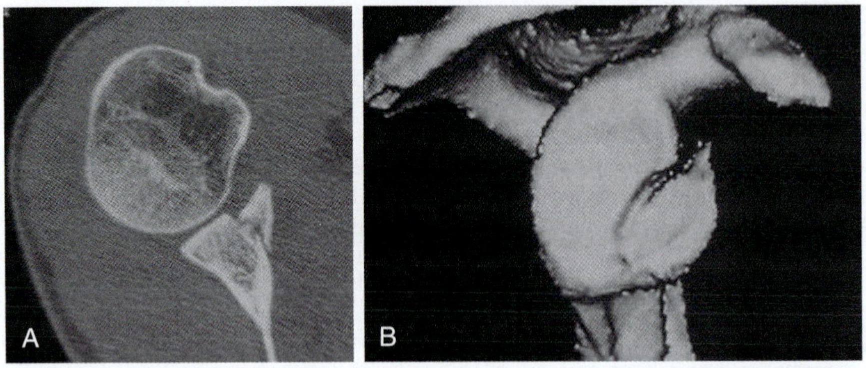

FIGURE 12-34: Computed tomography of an intra-articular glenoid fracture (bony Bankart lesion). **A,** Axial view, **B,** Three-dimensional reconstruction. (From Bauer T, Abadie O, Hardy P. Arthroscopic treatment of glenoid fractures. *Arthroscopy.* 2006;22:569.e1-e6.)

12-19). Given the complex anatomy of the scapula, CT scans with three-dimensional reconstructions are often necessary and are particularly useful for intra-articular glenoid fractures (Fig. 12-34).

Scapulothoracic dissociations are also identified initially on the AP chest radiograph. The index of suspicion for these injuries should be high, especially with high-energy injuries. Lateral displacement of the scapula (compared to the uninjured side) is pathognomonic (Fig. 12-35).[28,84] In addition to the lateral scapular displacement, severely displaced clavicle fractures, acromioclavicular joint injuries, and sternoclavicular injuries may be present.

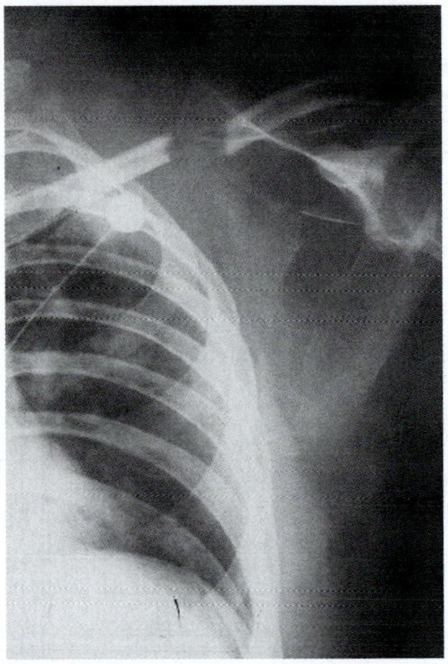

FIGURE 12-35: Anteroposterior radiograph showing scapulothoracic dissociation with concomitant fractures of the clavicle and scapula. (From Masmejean EH, Asfazadourian H, Alnot JY. Brachial plexus injuries in scapulothoracic dissociation. *J Hand Surg Br.* 2000;25:336-340.)

Differential Diagnosis

Developmental variations in scapular anatomy must be distinguished from a fracture or injury to the scapula. Os acromiale, a failure of the ossification centers in the acromion to unite, can be confused with a fracture (Fig. 12-36).[5] Other scapular anomalies that can mimic a fracture include Sprengel's deformity, an absent acromion, a bipartite or tripartite acromion, a bipartite coracoid, and coracoid duplication.[129,166,222,223]

Classification

Numerous classification schemata have been described for fractures of the scapula, although none are specific for the pediatric population. The majority are based on the anatomic location of the fracture. According to Ada and Miller, scapula fractures can be classified into fractures involving the scapular body, neck, acromion, spine, glenoid, and coracoid.[2] Thompson and colleagues relied on broader anatomic categories: fractures of the body, fractures of the acromion and the coracoid, and fractures of the glenoid and scapular neck.[241]

Fractures of the body and spine of the scapula are broadly divided into those with and without displacement. Fractures of the scapular neck are similarly classified into those with and without displacement and have also been classified by their anatomic location: anatomic neck (lateral to the base of the coracoid) and surgical neck (medial to the base of the coracoid) (Fig. 12-37).[94]

Isolated scapular neck fractures should be distinguished from those associated with an ipsilateral clavicle fracture. Ipsilateral fractures of the scapular neck and clavicle were first described by Ganz and Noesberger in 1975 and termed as *floating shoulder* (Fig. 12-38).[52,75,192] The definition of a floating shoulder has subsequently evolved, expanding to include injuries that result in a scapular neck fracture and additional disruption to SSSC: coracoid base fracture, acromion fracture, coracoacromial and coracoclavicular ligament disruption, and coracoclavicular and acromioclavicular ligament disruption

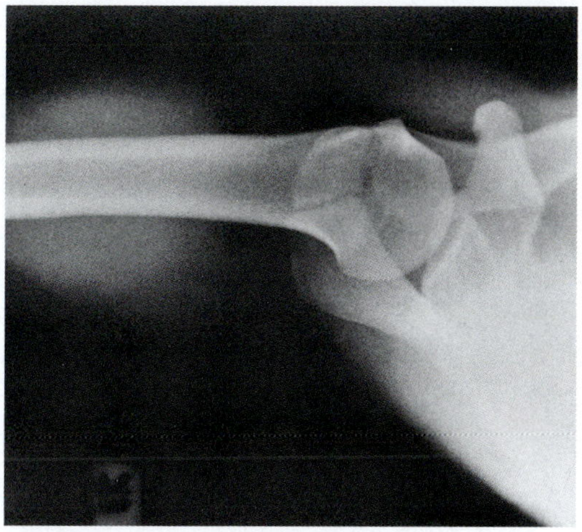

FIGURE 12-36: Axillary lateral radiograph showing a mesoacromion, one of several possible patterns of os acromiale.

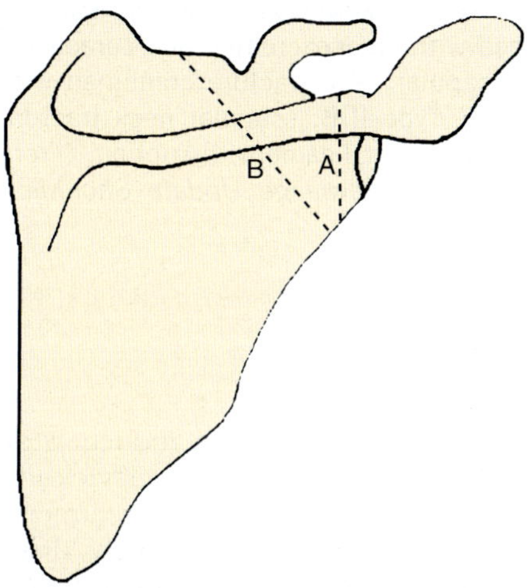

FIGURE 12-37: Classification of fractures of the scapular neck: Fracture through the anatomic neck (*A*) and fracture through the surgical neck (*B*). (From van Noort A, van der Werken C. The floating shoulder. *Injury.* 2006;37:218-227.)

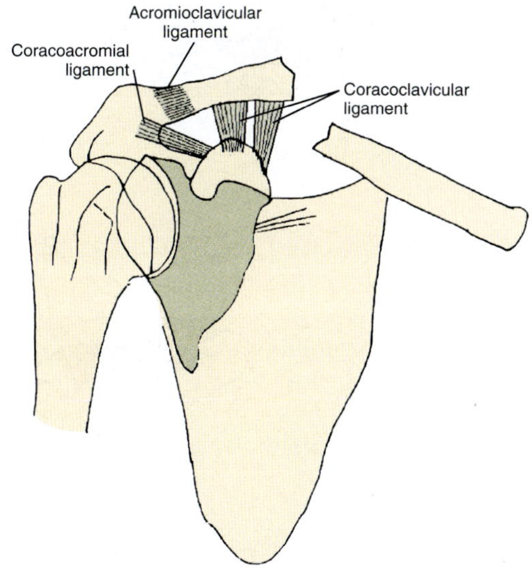

FIGURE 12-38: A floating shoulder with ipsilateral fractures of the clavicle and scapular neck. The glenoid has lost its attachment to the axial skeleton. (From van Noort A, van der Werken C: The floating shoulder. *Injury* 37:218-227, 2006.)

(Fig. 12-39).[75] These double-disruption injuries are significant for SSSC due to the risk of increased displacement and instability.

Fractures of the coracoid process are divided into those with and without associated injury to the lateral end of the clavicle or acromioclavicular joint.[85,172] A coracoid process fracture with such associated injury is considered to be a double-disruption injury to SSSC. Fractures of the acromion are classified into those with and without displacement.[85,140] If displacement is present, an additional disruption of SSSC is usually present—commonly an associated fracture of the coracoid process. Displaced fractures of the acromion are further categorized based on the presence or absence of subacromial narrowing.

Fractures of the glenoid are divided into six groups based on their location and the course of the fracture through the rest of the scapula (Fig. 12-40).[83,84,111] Type I fractures are isolated glenoid rim fractures, with type Ia involving the anterior rim and type Ib the posterior rim. Type II fractures are glenoid fractures with the fracture line through the glenoid fossa, exiting at the lateral border of the scapula. Type III fractures are glenoid fractures with the fracture line exiting at the superior aspect of the scapula. Type IV fractures are glenoid fractures with the fracture line exiting at the medial border of the scapula. Type V fractures are various combinations of type II, III, and IV fractures: type Va is a combination of types II and IV; type Vb is a combination of types III and IV; and type Vc is a combination of types II, III, and IV. Type VI fractures are glenoid fractures with severe comminution of the glenoid fossa.

Scapulothoracic dissociations are characterized by complete disruption of the scapulothoracic articulation with severe damage to the soft tissue supporting structures, including the deltoid, pectoralis minor, rhomboids, levator scapulae, trapezius, and latissimus dorsi. In the presence of a severe ipsilateral neurovascular injury, scapulothoracic dissociations are effectively termed *closed forequarter amputations.*

Treatment

Most scapular body fractures can be successfully treated nonoperatively—usually with sling immobilization.[112,183,217,263] Isolated fractures of the scapular body are inherently stable due to the overlying musculature, and so most fractures tend to be nondisplaced or minimally displaced. In adults scapular body fractures with significant displacement greater than 10 mm bring the risk of pain and disability when treated nonoperatively.[183] Thus although the rarity of these fractures precludes comparative study, operative treatment

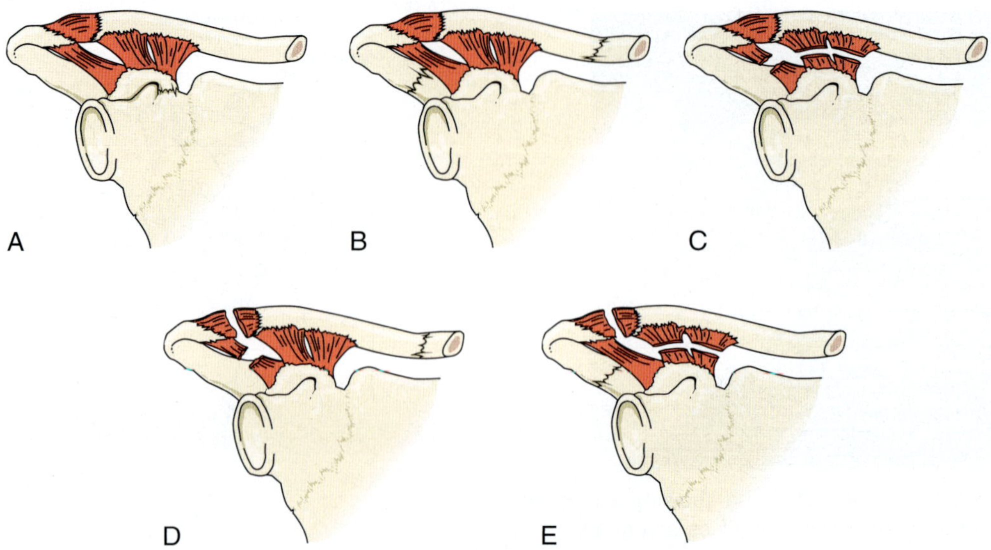

FIGURE 12-39: Floating shoulder injury patterns. Purely osseous injuries: **A,** Type IA, scapular neck fracture combined with a coracoid base fracture; **B,** Type IB, scapular neck fracture combined with a clavicle fracture and scapular spine or acromion fracture. Purely ligamentous injury: **C,** Type II, scapular neck fracture combined with coracoacromial and coracoclavicular ligament disruption. Combined osseous and ligamentous injuries: **D,** Type IIIA, scapular neck fracture combined with a clavicle shaft fracture plus coracoacromial and acromioclavicular ligament disruption; **E,** Type IIIB, scapular neck fracture combined with an acromion or scapular spine fracture plus coracoclavicular and acromioclavicular ligament disruption. (From Wong KL, Ramsey ML, Williams GR Jr. Scapular fractures. In: Norris TR, ed. *Orthopaedic Knowledge Update Shoulder and Elbow 2*. Rosemont, IL: American Academy of Orthopaedic Surgeons; 2002:227-236.)

may be indicated for widely displaced fractures of the scapular body in children.

Isolated nondisplaced or minimally displaced fractures of the scapular neck can be treated nonoperatively with satisfactory long-term outcomes.[130,183,247] Significantly displaced fractures of the scapular neck, however, appear to be associated with the risk of limited glenohumeral motion and glenohumeral instability.[84,130,183,194,212] In adults significant displacement has traditionally been defined as displacement greater than 10 mm or angulation greater than 40 degrees in either the axial or the coronal plane. More recently, angular displacement has been determined more accurately as a glenopolar angle of less than 20 degrees.[25,212,247] The glenopolar angle, measured on an AP radiograph, is the angle between the line connecting the most cranial with the most caudal point of the glenoid cavity and the line connecting the most cranial point of the glenoid cavity with the most caudal point of the scapular body (normal range, 30 to 45 degrees) (Fig. 12-41). Operative treatment should be considered for significantly displaced scapular neck fractures in children; a posterior approach to the scapular neck is recommended. After reduction, fixation can usually be achieved with a 2.7-mm or 3.5-mm contoured reconstruction plate or with interfragmentary compression screws.

The treatment of scapular neck fractures in the presence of associated injury to the clavicle is controversial. In the past, this combination of injuries necessitated operative intervention with open reduction and internal fixation of the scapular neck or clavicle fracture (or both).[2,84,152] Currently, nonoperative treatment is recommended for nondisplaced or minimally displaced fractures involving the scapular neck and clavicle. Significant fracture displacement and ligament disruption, however, lead to less predictable outcomes; therefore operative intervention should strongly be considered.[100] Operative intervention should also be considered for all floating shoulder injury patterns.

Isolated fractures of the coracoid process typically are nondisplaced or minimally displaced. In most cases nonoperative treatment with sling immobilization followed by early functional shoulder exercises is effective. Displaced coracoid fractures are commonly associated with injury to the acromioclavicular joint or lateral clavicle, and thus double disruption of SSSC. Displaced coracoid fractures near the suprascapular notch can also be associated with injury to the suprascapular nerve. Therefore for most displaced fractures of the coracoid, open reduction and internal fixation is recommended.[172,217,263]

Isolated fractures of the acromion in children are usually nondisplaced or minimally displaced; therefore they can be treated nonoperatively.[140] Indications for open reduction and internal fixation include displaced acromial fractures with narrowing of the subacromial space or with concomitant injury to SSSC.[84,140] In adults displaced acromial fractures with narrowing of the

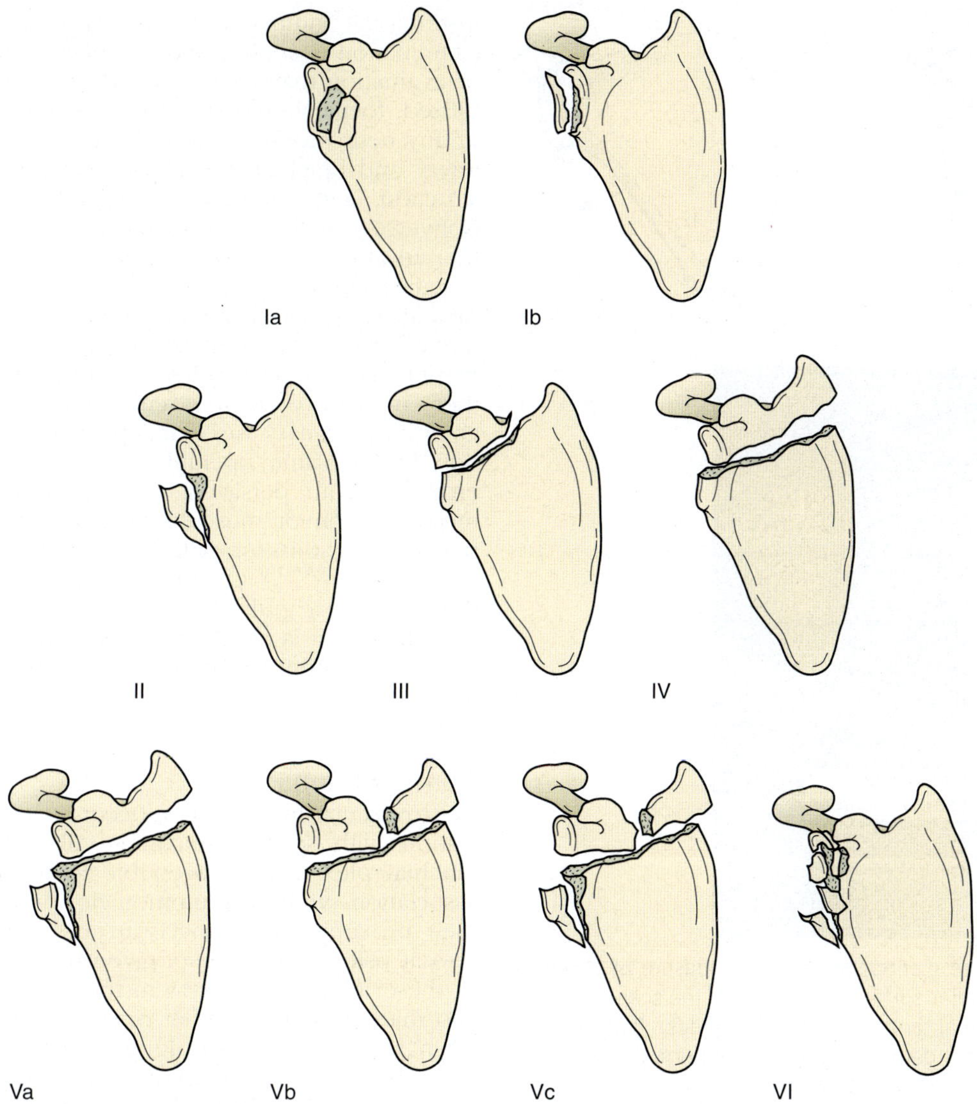

FIGURE 12-40: Classification of fractures of the glenoid (see text for description). (From Sarwark JF, King EC, Luhmann SJ. Proximal humerus, scapula, and clavicle. In: Charles CA, et al, eds. *Fractures in Children.* 6th ed. Philadelphia: Lippincott Williams & Wilkins; 2006:703-771.)

subacromial space have resulted in problems involving subacromial impingement.

Nondisplaced or minimally displaced glenoid rim fractures (types I and II) that are not associated with glenohumeral instability can be treated nonoperatively, typically with sling immobilization. Open reduction and internal fixation should be considered for glenoid rim fractures associated with glenohumeral instability. The surgical approach is anterior for fractures of the anterior rim and posterior for fractures of the posterior rim. Fixation options include interfragmentary compression screws or small plate fixation. Based on studies in adults, the risk of glenohumeral instability is increased with fracture displacement greater than 10 mm or with the involvement of at least one fourth of the anterior portion or one third of the posterior portion of the glenoid.[83,91,94]

Nondisplaced or minimally displaced glenoid fossa fractures (types III to VI) can also be treated nonoperatively. Open reduction and internal fixation should be considered for glenoid fossa fractures with intra-articular displacement greater than 5 to 10 mm, for significant separation between fracture fragments that makes nonunion likely, and for significant displacement of glenoid fragments that results in an incongruent relationship between the humeral head and glenoid cavity.[84,146] Fractures of the glenoid fossa are typically best approached posteriorly. The goals of operative intervention are anatomic restoration of the articular surface and stable fixation, usually by interfragmentary compression screw or contoured reconstruction plate, to allow early functional shoulder exercises. For severely displaced fractures of the glenoid fossa with significant comminution (type VI),

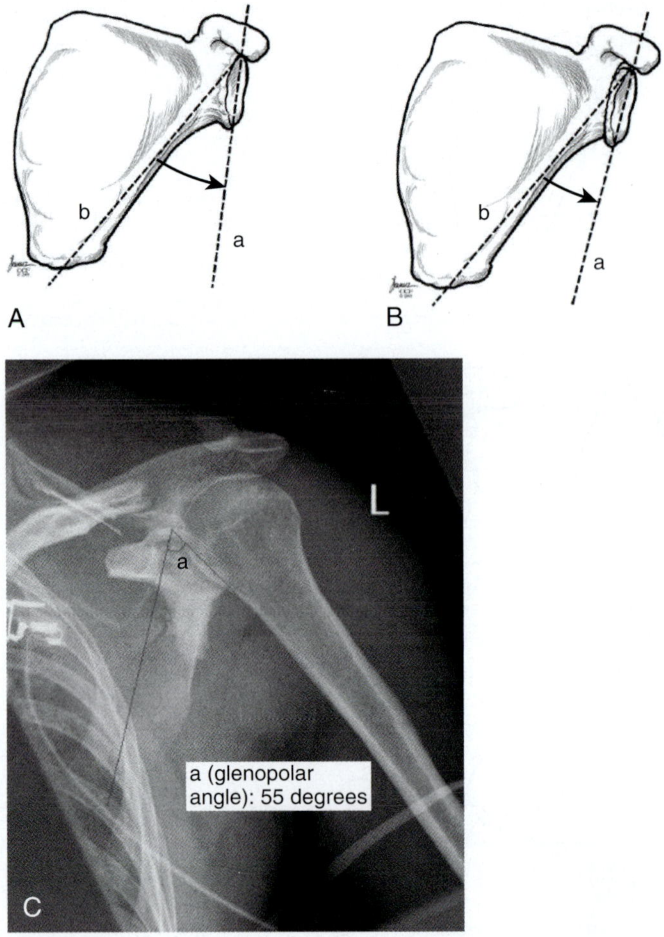

FIGURE 12-41: The glenopolar angle, a measure of obliquity of the glenoid articular surface in relation to the scapular body. **A,** Normal (the normal range is 30 to 45 degrees). **B,** Abnormal. **C,** Plain radiograph demonstrating an abnormal glenopolar angle of 55 degrees. (**A** and **B,** From DeFranco MJ, Patterson BM. The floating shoulder. *J Am Acad Orthop Surg.* 2006; 14:499-509. **C** from van Noort A, van der Werken C. The floating shoulder. *Injury.* 2006;37:218-227.)

nonoperative treatment should be considered because acceptable operative reduction and fixation are often difficult to achieve.

Because of the high-energy nature of these injuries, massive trauma to the entire extremity occurs with scapulothoracic dissociations. Initial management should focus on airway, breathing, and circulation, following standardized institutional trauma protocols. Thorough neurovascular examination is critical, and vascular surgery consultation or evaluation may be necessary. Once the patient is stabilized, focus should shift to the stabilization and repair of any neurovascular injury. If the injuries to the axillary artery and brachial plexus are beyond repair or reconstruction, early amputation should be considered.[28,190] Conversely, if the neurovascular injuries appear reparable, an attempt at limb salvage is recommended. When vascular injuries are identified, vascular repair should be prioritized to avoid life-threatening hemorrhage or prolonged upper extremity ischemia. Immediate exploration of brachial plexus injuries is not required. However, if there is a concomitant vascular injury that needs repair, combined primary vascular repair and nerve reconstruction in the same operative setting should be considered.[28,231] With persistent brachial plexus palsy, nerve reconstruction or musculotendinous transfer should be performed within 6 months to minimize muscle atrophy and fibrosis.[69,176,190] Operative stabilization of injuries to the clavicle, scapula, acromioclavicular joint, or sternoclavicular joint is necessary if the bony instability endangers the integrity of the neurovascular structures and/or reconstructions.[28,39,48]

Complications

Neurovascular injuries often occur concomitantly in association with scapula fractures. All or portions of the brachial plexus are susceptible to injury, especially in association with scapulothoracic dissociations. Given their proximity, the subclavian and axillary vessels are also at risk of injury. Also, given the high-energy nature of these injuries, multisystem trauma is not uncommon, and injuries occur to other organ systems, including the brain and especially the lungs, such as pneumothorax, hemothorax, and pulmonary contusion.

Fractures of the scapula can lead to disability of the shoulder complex and a poor functional outcome for the upper extremity.[2,84,183] Fractures with initial significant displacement and subsequent residual scapular deformity bring increased risk of long-term upper extremity weakness and pain. Displaced acromion fractures in particular increase the risk of pain and stiffness secondary to narrowing and impingement of the subacromial space.[85,140] Displaced intra-articular glenoid fractures are also associated with the risk of glenohumeral instability and early-onset degenerative arthritis.[84,91] Symptomatic nonunion of fractures involving the scapular body and acromion can also occur.[67,123,169]

EDITOR COMMENTARY

Jason Hsu

While few orthopedic surgeons specialize in the treatment of pediatric orthopedic disorders, the majority will have one or two distinct memories from their training years that exemplify the tremendous potential for bone remodeling in the pediatric population. It is not uncommon for a junior orthopedic resident to view films of a displaced proximal humerus fracture and look on in disbelief at the follow-up radiographs showing a proximal humerus that appears unharmed.

The majority of shoulder fractures in the pediatric population can be treated nonoperatively, but the physician must always be cautious and aware of the particular attributes that warrant the infrequent need for fixation—the authors of this chapter have done an excellent job of reviewing the appropriate nonoperative management as well as the fracture characteristics that require surgical management. Proximal humerus fractures can often be treated with immobilization in a simple sling. Fixation is generally reserved for severely displaced and angulated fractures in older children. Similarly, the majority of clavicle fractures can often be treated nonoperatively with excellent results. Although there has been a push by some surgeons toward more aggressive treatment of clavicle fractures, with operative fixation in adolescents, there is still insufficient evidence in the literature to support this approach.

Compared with the management of fractures, the management of soft tissue abnormalities in the shoulder can be more challenging. Patients with multidirectional instability can be difficult to manage, and recurrent instability can persist despite strengthening of dynamic stabilizers. We believe that in patients with a traumatic episode leading to instability, a trial of nonoperative treatment including cuff and deltoid strengthening is warranted. Some reports have suggested that operative fixation after the first dislocation may potentially fare better than that after recurrent instability. However, surgical management must be judicious—even when performed well, stabilization surgery in adolescents is often complicated by recurrent instability. An in-depth discussion with the patient and parents must therefore take into account the patient's activity level and expectations in order to preserve motion and function and prevent complications in the long term.

Such discussions can be a major challenge in managing a child with any orthopedic condition. On the one hand, the full support and engagement of the parents is crucial to the comfort and happiness of a child undergoing the daunting prospect of surgical intervention. On the other hand, the physician must be wary of red flags that may indicate parental involvement in physical or emotional child abuse. In both cases the physician must evaluate the interaction between parent and child and ensure this relationship is optimized for the successful treatment of the patient and his or her shoulder.

SENIOR EDITOR COMMENTARY

Frederick A. Matsen III

Shoulder problems in children present some distinct challenges, starting with the fact that the word "children" spans the spectrum from human beings as yet unborn to late teenagers that look more like adults than kids. The shoulder surgeon treating children may encounter conditions ranging from congenital absence of the clavicle or a rare genetic syndrome with shoulder manifestations on one hand to shoulder injuries that are a part of a polytraumatic motor vehicle accident on the other. In many cases the child is unable to provide a history of the problem and may not be able to cooperate fully for a physical examination. The parent has a unique and complex role, being a surrogate historian, a highly concerned family member, and occasionally a suspect in cases of possible child abuse. The bones of a child are relatively flexible and, with the exception of the growth plate, are resistant to fracture. However, these bones may be weakened by aneurysmal and unicameral bone cysts, which are rarely issues for adults. Fractures of the normal humeral shaft are rare and should arouse concern about possible adult-administered violence. Injuries that might cause joint dislocation in adults may result in growth plate fractures in children, such as those of the proximal humerus or medial clavicle. The delayed appearance of the epiphyses and the delayed closure of the growth plates may complicate the radiographic evaluation of possible fractures. Many pediatric fractures undergo remarkable remodeling with time, so that the view of "an acceptable deformity" in children is quite different from that in adults. The role of surgery is complicated by the potential risk of growth arrest. Children have greater flexibility of their shoulder and may become fascinated with their ability to "pop their shoulders out of joint." This type of instability requires management quite distinct from its adult counterpart. Finally, the context for treating a child is different than that for an adult. Usually, there is a concerned parent or guardian who wants to have a major role in the evaluation and management of the shoulder condition. "You need to understand, doctor, that my child has tremendous potential as a college athlete." In other cases Child Protective Services may be needed to ensure the safety of the child. For all these reasons and many more, the care of a child's shoulder is part science, part art, and especially deserving of those surgeons with skill, patience, and understanding.

CHAPTER 13

Glenohumeral Instability

Leslie Fink Barnes, Bradford O. Parsons, Steven B. Lippitt, Evan L. Flatow, Frederick A. Matsen III

A complementary discussion of the evaluation and management of glenohumeral instability with a particular emphasis on arthroscopic methods is found in Chapter 15.

> *It deserves to be known how a shoulder which is subject to frequent dislocations should be treated. For many persons owing to this accident have been obliged to abandon gymnastic exercises, though otherwise well qualified for them; and from the same misfortune have become inept in warlike practices, and have thus perished. And this subject deserves to be noticed, because I have never known any physician [to] treat the case properly; some abandon the attempt altogether, and others hold opinions and practice the very reverse of what is proper.*
>
> *Hippocrates, fifth century* BCE

> *In every case the anterior margin of the glenoid cavity will be found to be smooth, rounded, and free of any attachments, and a blunt instrument can be passed freely inwards over the bare bone on the front of the neck of the scapula.*
>
> *Perthes,[541] 1906*

> *The only rational treatment is to reattach the glenoid ligament (or the capsule) to the bone from which it has been torn.*
>
> *Bankart,[34] 1939*

HISTORICAL REVIEW

Early Descriptions

The first report of a shoulder dislocation is found in humankind's oldest book, the Edwin Smith Papyrus (3000-2500 BCE).[728] Hussein[294] reported that in 1200 BCE in the tomb of Upuy, an artist and sculptor to Ramses II, was found a drawing of a scene strikingly similar to Kocher's method of reduction (Fig. 13-1).

The most detailed early description of anterior dislocations came from the Father of Medicine, Hippocrates, who was born in 460 BCE on the island of Cos.[1] Hippocrates described the anatomy of the shoulder, the types of dislocations, and the first surgical procedure. In one of his classic procedures for reduction, he stressed the need for suitably sized, leather-covered balls to be placed into the axilla, for without them the heel could not reach the head of the humerus in his reduction maneuver. Other Hippocratic techniques are described by Brockbank and Griffiths (Fig. 13-2).[82]

Hippocrates criticized his contemporaries for improper burning of the shoulder, a treatment popular at the time. In this first description of a surgical procedure for recurrent dislocation of the shoulder, he described the manner in which physicians had burned the top, anterior, and posterior aspects of the shoulder, which only caused scarring in those areas and promoted downward dislocation. He advocated the use of cautery in which an oblong, red-hot iron was inserted through the axilla to make eschars, but only in the lower part of the joint. Hippocrates displayed considerable knowledge of the anatomy of the shoulder, and he warned the surgeon to not let the iron come in contact with the major vessels and nerves because it would cause great harm. Following the burnings, he bound the arm to the side, day and night, for a long time: "for thus more especially will cicatrization take place, and the wide space into which the humerus used to escape will become contracted."[273]

Interested readers are referred to the text by Moseley,[458] which has a particularly good section on the historical aspects of the management of shoulder instability.

Humeral Head Defect

In 1861, Flower[194] described the anatomic and pathologic changes found in 41 traumatically dislocated

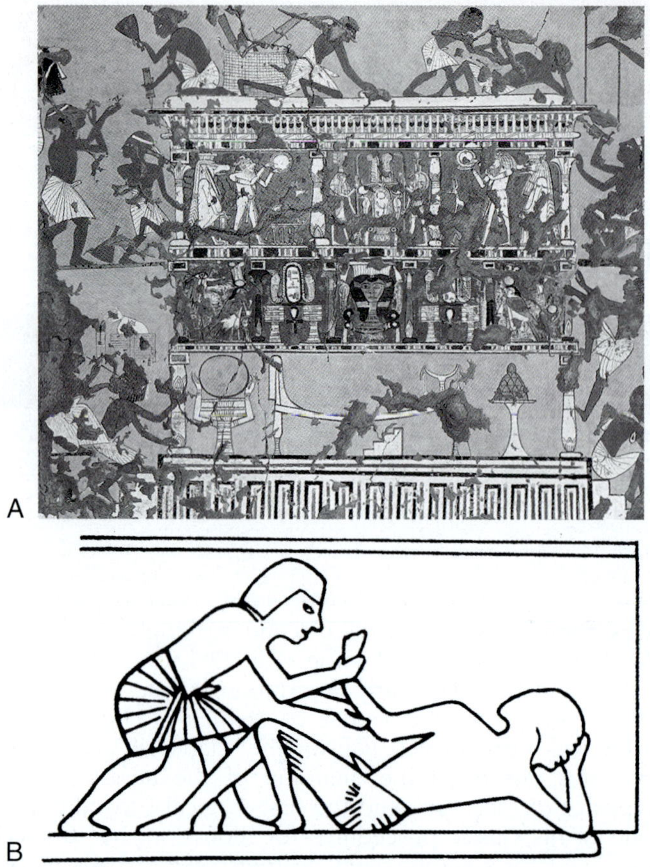

FIGURE 13-1: The Kocher technique is 3000 years old. **A,** Drawing from the tomb of Upuy in 1200 BCE. **B,** Schematic drawing of the picture in the upper right corner of the tomb painting depicting a patient on the ground while a man—possibly a physician—is manipulating a dislocated shoulder in the technique of Kocher. (**A,** From The Metropolitan Museum of Art. Egyptian Expedition of the Metropolitan Museum of Art, Rogers Fund, 1930. Photograph copyright 1978 The Metropolitan Museum of Art. **B,** From Hussein MK. Kocher's method is 3000 years old. *J Bone Joint Surg Br.* 1968;50:669-671.)

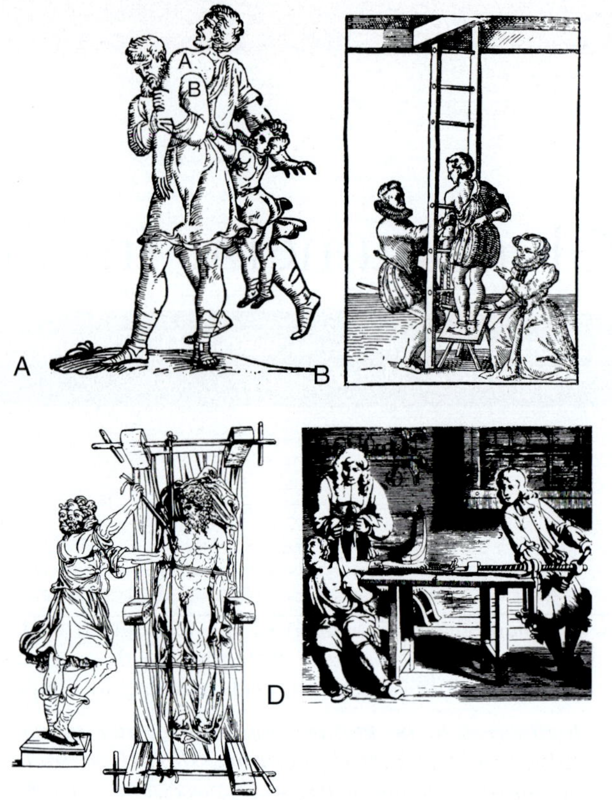

FIGURE 13-2: Modified techniques of Hippocrates to reduce dislocations of the shoulder. **A,** Reduction over the operator's shoulder (from the Venice edition of Galen in 1625). **B,** Reduction over the rung of a ladder. When the stepstool on which the patient is standing is withdrawn, the weight of the patient's body reduces the dislocation (from deCruce in 1607). **C,** Use of the rack to reduce a shoulder dislocation (Vidius). **D,** Reduction of a dislocation by a medieval type of screw traction (from Scultetus in 1693). (From Brockbank W, Griffiths DL. Orthopaedic surgery in the 16th and 17th centuries. *J Bone Joint Surg Br.* 1948;30:365-375.)

shoulders from specimens in London museums. He wrote that "where the head of the humerus rests upon the edge of the glenoid fossa absorption occurs, and a groove is evacuated, usually between the articular head and the greater tuberosity."[194] In 1880, Eve[172] reported an autopsy of a patient who died 12 hours after an acute anterior dislocation in which he found a deep groove in the posterolateral aspect of the head. Joessel[318] also observed the defect. According to Hill and Sachs,[271] beginning in 1882, publications by Kuster,[355] Cramer,[126] Löbker,[391] Schüller,[608] Staffel,[632] and Francke[195] described the finding of a posterolateral defect in humeral heads resected for relief of chronic or recurrent dislocation (Fig. 13-3).

In 1887, Caird[92] of Edinburgh concluded that a true subcoracoid dislocation must have an indentation fracture of the humeral head that is produced by the dense, hard anterior lip of the glenoid fossa. In cadaver experiments, he was able to produce the head defect. He said that the hard, dense glenoid lip would cut into the soft cancellous bone like a knife (Fig. 13-4).

Roentgen's discovery of x-rays in 1895 ushered in new evaluations and studies of the anatomy of the anterior glenoid and humeral head defects. The first description of the radiographic changes in the humeral head associated with recurrent instability is attributed to Francke[195] in 1898, only 3 years after Roentgen's discovery.[265] Hermodsson demonstrated that the posterolateral humeral head defect is the result of a compression fracture caused by the anterior glenoid rim following the exit of the humeral head from the glenoid fossa.[265] He also observed that the defect is seen in the majority of

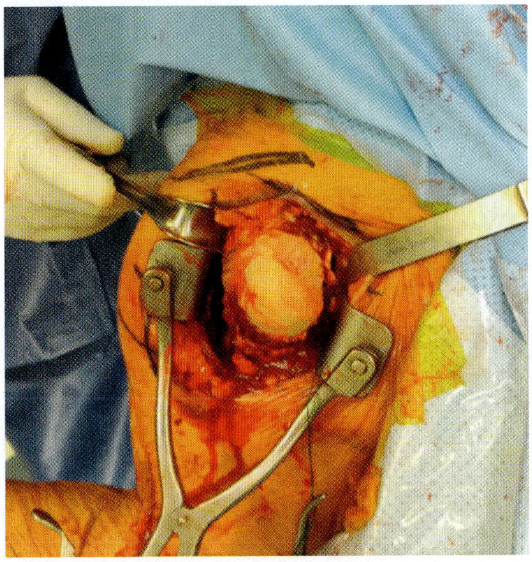

FIGURE 13-3: Hill-Sachs lesion in a patient with a chronic anterior dislocation.

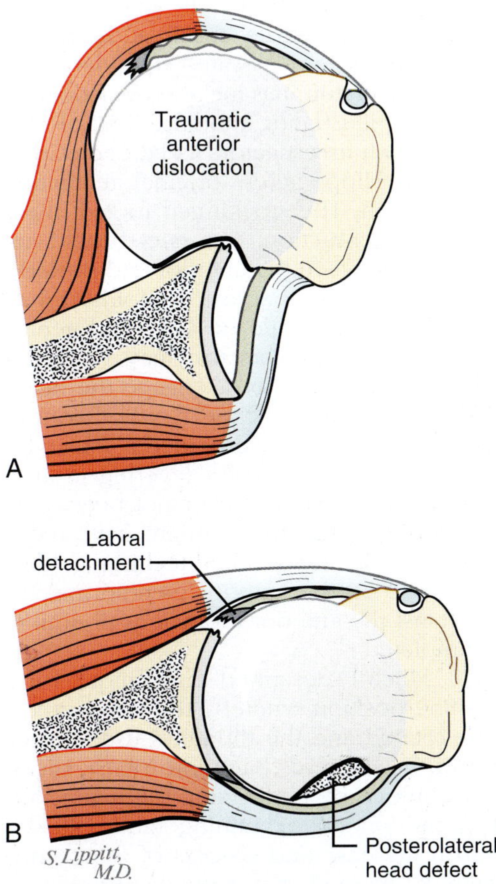

FIGURE 13-4: **A,** Anterior dislocation shown in an axillary projection with a posterolateral humeral head defect (Hill-Sachs defect) and a tear of the anterior capsule and labrum from the glenoid lip (Bankart lesion). **B,** The dislocation is reduced, but the humeral head and capsular lesions remain.

cases; the longer the head is dislocated, the larger the defect will be; the defects are generally larger in anteroinferior dislocations than in anterior dislocations; and the defect is usually larger in recurrent anterior dislocations of the shoulder.

In 1925, Pilz[543] reported the first detailed radiographic examination of recurrent dislocation of the shoulder and stated that routine radiographs were of little help. He stressed the need for an angled-beam projection to observe the defect. In 1940, Hill and Sachs[271] published a very clear and concise review of the available information on the humeral head compression fracture defect that now carries their names.

Anterior Capsule and Muscle Defects

According to the Hunterian Lecture given by Reeves in 1967, Roger of Palermo in the thirteenth century taught that the lesion in an acute dislocation was a capsular rupture. Bankart,[32] following the concepts of Broca and Hartmann,[81] Perthes,[541] Flower,[194] and Caird,[92] claimed that the essential lesion was detachment of the labrum and capsule from the anterior glenoid as a result of forward translation of the humeral head (referred to by subsequent authors as the *Bankart lesion*) (see Fig. 13-4). Later experimental and clinical studies by Reeves[559] and Townley[657] suggested that other lesions might be responsible for recurrent dislocation, such as failure of the initial injury to incite a healing response, detachment of the subscapularis tendon, and variance in attachment of the inferior glenohumeral ligament.

Moseley and Overgaard[461] found laxity in 25 consecutive cases, and DePalma et al.[148] reported subscapularis laxity, rupture, and decreased muscle tone in 38 consecutive cases. Several of their cases and some from Hauser[249] revealed a definite defect along the anterior or inferior aspect of the subscapularis tendon, as though it had been partially torn from its bone attachment, along with separation of the muscle fibers that insert into the humerus directly below the lesser tuberosity. McLaughlin,[427] DePalma et al.,[148] Jens,[312] and Reeves[560] noted at the time of surgery before arthrotomy that with abduction and external rotation, the humeral head would dislocate under the lower edge of the subscapularis tendon. Symeonides[642] took biopsy samples of the subscapularis muscle-tendon unit at the time of surgery and found microscopic evidence of "healed posttraumatic lesions." He stated that instability results because traumatic lengthening of the subscapularis muscle leads to loss of the power necessary to stabilize the shoulder.

Rotator Cuff Injuries

In 1880, Joessel[318] reported on his careful postmortem studies of four cases of known recurrent dislocation of the shoulder. In all cases, he found a rupture of the posterolateral portion of the rotator cuff from the greater tuberosity and a greatly increased shoulder joint capsule volume (Fig. 13-5). Moreover, he noted fractures of the humeral head and the anterior glenoid rim (Figs. 13-6 and 13-7). Joessel concluded that cuff

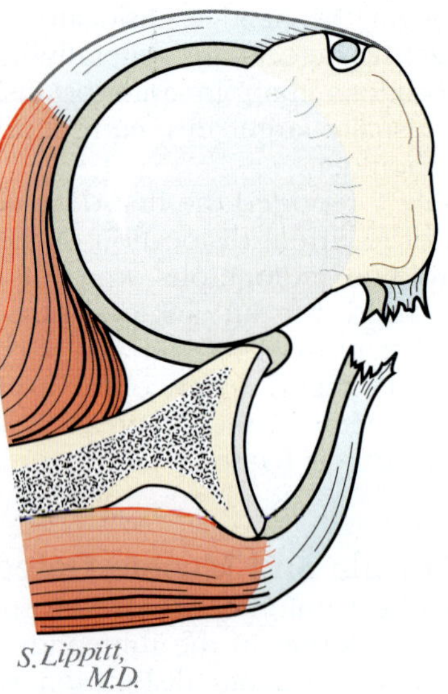

FIGURE 13-5: An anterior dislocation shown in an axillary view with a tear in the posterior rotator cuff.

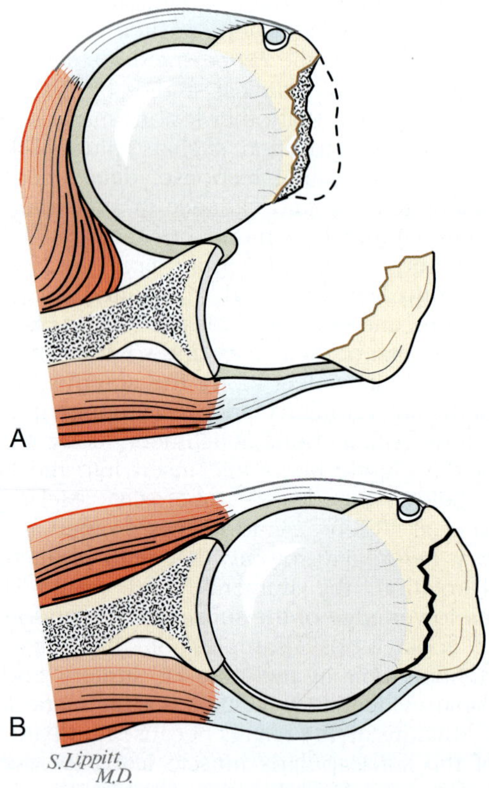

FIGURE 13-6: An anterior dislocation is shown in the axillary view with a displaced fracture of the greater tuberosity. **A,** Anterior dislocation with displaced tuberosity fracture. **B,** Tuberosity fracture is reduced when the dislocation is reduced.

disruptions that did not heal were predisposed to recurrence of the problem, that recurrences were facilitated by the enlarged capsule, and that fractures of the glenoid or the head of the humerus resulted in a smaller articular surface, which can tend to produce

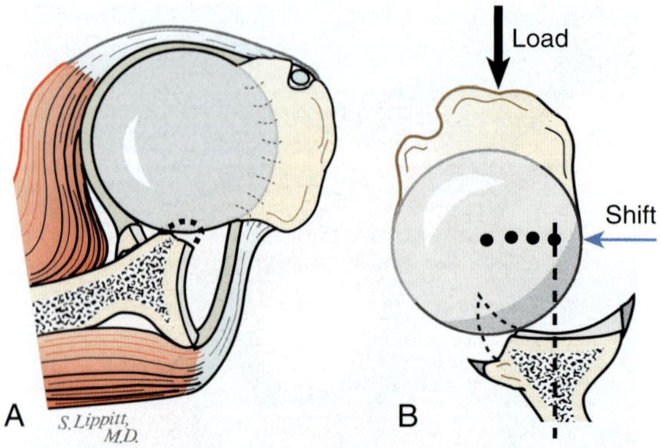

FIGURE 13-7: **A,** This anterior dislocation is shown in the axillary view with a displaced fracture of the anterior glenoid rim. **B,** This fracture reduces the intrinsic stability provided by the glenoid concavity.

recurrent dislocation. However, his four patients were elderly and might have had the degenerative cuff changes common in older people.

Treatment of Acute Traumatic Dislocations

Hippocrates[273] discussed in detail at least six different techniques to reduce a dislocated shoulder. From century to century, the literature has included woodcuts, drawings, and redrawings illustrating modifications of Hippocrates' teachings by such investigators as Paré, de Cruce, Vidius, and Scultetus. Hippocrates' original technique[1] is still used on occasion. The stockinged foot of the physician is used as countertraction. The heel should not go into the axilla (i.e., between the anterior and posterior axillary folds) but should extend across the folds and against the chest wall. Traction should be slow and gentle; as with all traction techniques, the arm may be gently rotated internally and externally to disengage the head.

In 1870, Theodore Kocher,[342] who won the Nobel Prize for medicine in 1909, provided a somewhat confusing report of his technique for levering in an anteriorly dislocated shoulder. Had Kocher not been as famous as a thyroid surgeon, his article might have received only scant attention. In the Kocher technique, the humeral head is levered on the anterior glenoid and the shaft is levered against the anterior thoracic wall until the reduction is completed.

In 1938, Milch[440] described a technique for reduction in the supine position whereby the arm is abducted and externally rotated and the thumb is used to gently push the head of the humerus back into place. Lacey[356] modified the technique by performing the maneuver with the patient prone on an examining table. Russell et al.[595] reported on the ease and success of this technique.

DePalma[145] warned that with the Kocher technique, undue forces used in rotation leverage can damage the soft tissues of the shoulder joint, the vessels, and the brachial plexus. Beattie et al.[44] reported a fracture of the humeral neck during a Kocher procedure. Other authors have described spiral fractures of the upper shaft of the humerus and further damage to the anterior capsular mechanism when the Kocher leverage technique of reduction was used. McMurray[433] reported that of 64 dislocations reduced by the Kocher method, 40% became recurrent, whereas of 112 dislocations reduced by gently lifting the head into place, only 12% became recurrent.

Since 1975, numerous articles have described simple techniques to reduce a dislocated shoulder: the forward elevation maneuver,[310,677] the external rotation method,[385,446] scapular manipulation,[11] the modified gravity method,[388] the crutch and chair technique,[525] the chair and pillow technique,[694] and others.[115,406]

Operative Reconstructions for Anterior Instability

Most of the published literature on shoulder dislocations is concerned with the problem of recurrent anterior dislocations. As mentioned previously, Hippocrates[273] described the use of a white-hot poker to scar the anteroinferior part of the capsule. Since then, hundreds of operative procedures have been described for the management of recurrent anterior dislocations. Readers who have a yearning for the detailed history should read the classic texts by Moseley[458] and Hermodsson.[265]

Various operative techniques have been based on the posterolateral defect and soft tissue disruptions on the front of the shoulder. Bardenheuer[37] in 1886 and Thomas[645,646] in 1909 and 1921 discussed capsular plication or shrinking. In 1898, Albert[6] performed arthrodesis, and in 1902, Hildebrand[268] deepened the glenoid socket.

In 1906, Perthes[541] wrote a classic paper on the operative treatment of recurrent dislocations. He stated that the operation should be directed at repairing the underlying lesion (i.e., repair of the capsule, the glenoid labrum detachment from the anterior bony rim, and the rotator cuff tear). He repaired the capsule with suture to the anterior glenoid rim through drill holes, and in several cases he used staples to repair the anterior capsular structures. This report gave the first description of repair of the anterior labrum and capsule to the anterior glenoid rim. Two patients were monitored for 17 years, one for 12 years, two for 3 years, and one for 1 year and 9 months. All had excellent function with no recurrence.

The muscle sling myoplasty operation was used in 1909 by Clairmont and Ehrlich.[111] The posterior third of the deltoid, with its innervation left intact, was removed from its insertion on the humerus, passed through the quadrilateral space, and sutured to the coracoid process. When the arm was abducted, the deltoid contracted, which held up the humeral head. Finsterer,[186] in a similar but reversed procedure, used the coracobrachialis and the short head of the biceps from the coracoid and transferred them posteriorly. Both operations failed, with high recurrence rates.

Beginning in 1929, Nicola[482-486] published a series of articles on management of recurrent dislocation of the shoulder. He used the long head of the biceps tendon and the coracohumeral ligament as a suspension checkrein to the front of the shoulder. Henderson[261,262] described another checkrein operation that looped half the peroneus longus tendon through drill holes in the acromion and the greater tuberosity. In 1927, Gallie and LeMesurier[199] described the use of autogenous fascia lata suture in treating recurrent dislocation of the shoulder. This procedure has been modified by Bateman.[42]

In 1923, Bankart[32] first published his operative technique and noted that only two classes of operations were used at that time for recurrent dislocation of the shoulder: those designed to decrease the size of the capsule by plication or pleating[645,646] and those designed to provide inferior support to the capsule.[111,112] Bankart condemned both in preference to his procedure. He stated that the essential lesion was detachment or rupture of the capsule from the glenoid ligament. He recommended repair with interrupted sutures of silkworm gut passed between the free edge of the capsule and the glenoid ligament. At that time, he did not repair the lateral capsule to the bone of the anterior glenoid rim.

In his 1939 article, Bankart[34] described the essential lesion as "detachment of the glenoid ligament from the anterior margin of the glenoid cavity" and stated, "the only rational treatment is to reattach the glenoid ligament (or the capsule) to the bone from which it has been torn." He further wrote that "the glenoid ligament may be found lying loose either on the head of the humerus or the margin of the glenoid cavity." He recommended repair of the lateral capsule down to the raw bone of the anterior glenoid and that it be held in place with suture through drill holes made in the anterior glenoid rim with sharp, pointed forceps. Although no references were listed in either article, Bankart must have been greatly influenced by the previously published work of Broca and Hartmann[81] and particularly that of Perthes,[541] which described virtually identical pathology and repair.

In 1980, Neer and Foster clarified the role of capsular pathology, delineated the clinical syndromes of anterior, posterior, and multidirectional instability (MDI), and described the inferior capsular shift procedure.[474] Later authors adopted the arthroscopic approaches to procedures described by Bankart and Neer. More recently, coracoid transfer, which was originally described by Latarjet and others, has had renewed popularity.[365,364]

Boileau and Walch have suggested the value of this procedure not only for glenoid bone loss but also for very loose capsules, failed instability repairs, and other high-risk cases.[50,326]

Posterior Glenohumeral Instability

In an 1839 Guy's Hospital report,[121] Sir Astley Cooper described in detail a dislocation of the os humeri on the dorsum scapulae. This report is a classic, for Cooper presented most of the characteristics associated with posterior dislocations: the dislocation occurred during an epileptic seizure; the pain was greater than with the usual anterior dislocation; external rotation of the arm was entirely impeded, and the patient could not elevate his arm from his side; the shoulder had an anterior void or flatness and a posterior fullness; and the patient was "unable to use or move his arm to any extent." In this report of a case in which Cooper had acted as a consultant, reduction could not be accomplished and the patient never recovered the use of his shoulder. Postmortem examination of the shoulder, performed 7 years later, revealed that the subscapularis tendon was detached and the infraspinatus muscles were stretched posteriorly about the head of the humerus. The report suggested that the detached subscapularis was "the cause of the symptoms." Cooper further described resorption of the anterior aspect of the humeral head where it was in contact with the posterior glenoid, probably the first description of the reverse Hill-Sachs lesion.

Another classic article on the subject was published in 1855 by Malgaigne,[405] who reported on 37 cases of posterior dislocation of the shoulder; three cases were his own and 34 were reviewed from the literature. This series of cases was collected 40 years before the discovery of x-rays, and it points out that with adequate physical examination of the patient, the correct diagnosis can be made.

RELEVANT ANATOMY

Skin

Shoulder stabilization surgery can usually be accomplished through cosmetically acceptable incisions in the lines of the skin (see Chapter 2). Anteriorly, the surgeon can identify and mark the prominent anterior axillary crease by adducting the shoulder. An incision placed in the lower part of this crease provides excellent access to the shoulder for anterior repair and yet heals nicely with subcuticular closure (Figs. 13-8 and 13-9). When cosmesis is a concern, the incision can be made more into the axilla, as described by Leslie and Ryan.[378]

Posteriorly, an analogous vertical incision in line with the extended posterior axillary crease (best visualized by extending the shoulder backward) also heals well (Fig. 13-10). Fortuitously, these creases lie directly over the joint to which the surgeon needs access.

First Muscle Layer

The shoulder is covered by the deltoid muscle arising from the clavicle, acromion, and scapular spine. The anterior deltoid extends to a line running approximately from the midclavicle to the midlateral portion of the humerus. This line passes over the cephalic vein, the anterior venous drainage of the deltoid, and the coracoid process. The deltoid is innervated by the axillary nerve, whose branches swoop upward as they extend anteriorly (Fig. 13-11). The commonly described safe zone 5 cm distal to the acromion does not take into account these anterior branches, which can come as close as 2 cm to the acromion.

At the deltopectoral groove, the deltoid meets the clavicular head of the pectoralis major, which assists the anterior deltoid in forward flexion. The medial and lateral pectoral nerves are not in the surgical field of shoulder stabilization. Splitting the deltopectoral interval just medial to the cephalic vein preserves the deltoid's venous drainage and takes the surgeon to the next layer. Extension of the shoulder tightens the pectoralis major and the anterior deltoid, as well as the coracoid muscles, and thus compromises the exposure. Accordingly, surgical assistants must be reminded to hold the shoulder in slight flexion to relax these muscles and facilitate access to the joint.

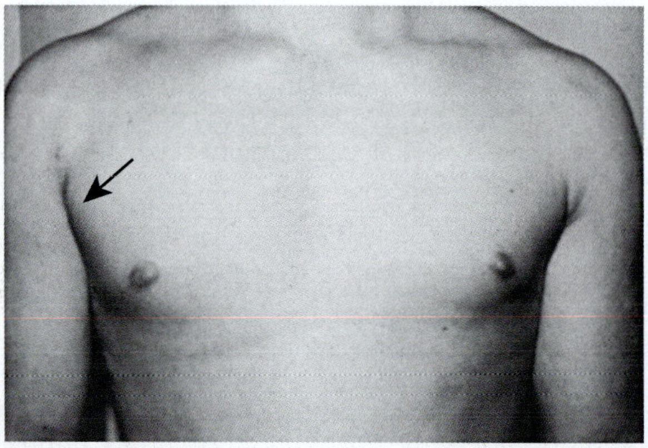

FIGURE 13-8: A cosmetic anterior approach on the patient's right shoulder. The incision is made in the axillary skin crease.

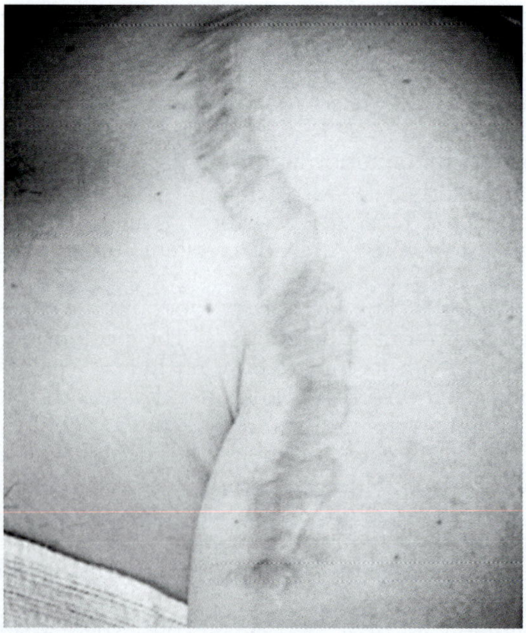

FIGURE 13-9: A noncosmetic approach across the front of the shoulder.

Posteriorly, the medial edge of the deltoid is too medial to provide useful access to the glenohumeral joint. Access must be achieved by splitting the deltoid, which is most conveniently done at the junction of its middle and posterior thirds. This junction is marked by the posterior corner of the acromion. The site is favorable for a split because it overlies the joint and also because the axillary nerve exiting the quadrangular space divides into two trunks (its anterior and posterior branches) near the inferior aspect of the split.

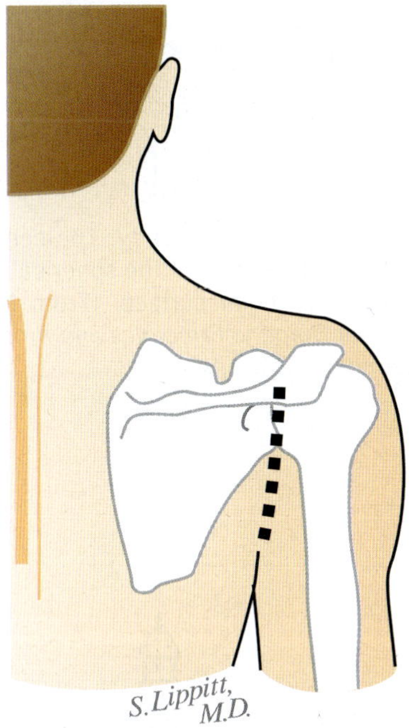

FIGURE 13-10: A posterior approach for treatment of posterior glenohumeral instability. The incision (*dashed line*) is centered over the posterior glenoid rim.

Coracoacromial Arch and Clavipectoral Fascia

The coracoacromial (CA) arch provides a concavity that articulates with the proximal humeral convexity (Figs. 13-12 to 13-14). The center of this articulation is identical to the center of the glenohumeral articulation in the normal shoulder. The radii of these two articulations differ by the thickness of the rotator cuff and tuberosity. The concentricity of the CA and glenohumeral spheres provides stable centering of the normal shoulder through an extremely wide range of positions.

The coracoid process has been described by Matsen as the lighthouse of the anterior aspect of the shoulder in that it provides a palpable guide to the deltopectoral groove, a locator for the CA arch, and an anchor for the coracoid muscles (the coracobrachialis and short head of the biceps) that separate, as Matsen has described, the lateral "safe side" from the medial "suicide" where the brachial plexus and major vessels lie (Fig. 13-15). The clavipectoral fascia covers the floor of the deltopectoral groove. Rotating the humerus enables the surgeon to identify the subscapularis moving beneath this fascial layer. Incising the fascia up to but not through the CA ligament preserves the stabilizing function of the CA arch.

The axillary nerve runs in the humeroscapular motion interface, superficial to the humerus and cuff and deep to the deltoid and coracoid muscles (Fig. 13-16; see also Fig. 13-11). Sweeping a finger in a superior-to-inferior direction along the anterior aspect of the subscapularis muscle catches the axillary nerve, which hangs like a watch chain across the muscle belly. Tracing this nerve proximally and medially leads the finger to the bulk of

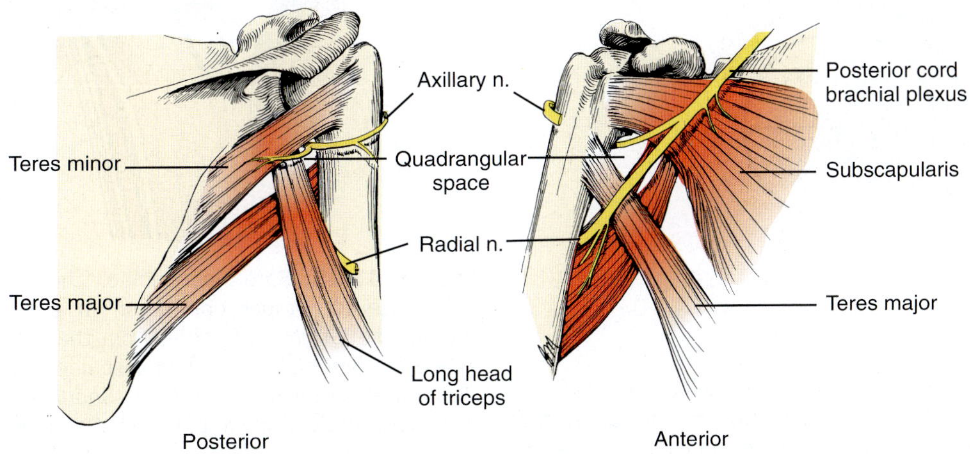

FIGURE 13-11: Relationships of the axillary nerve to the subscapularis muscle, the quadrangular space, and the neck of the humerus. With anterior dislocations, the subscapularis is displaced forward, which creates a traction injury in the axillary nerve. The nerve cannot move out of the way because it is held above by the brachial plexus and below where it wraps around behind the neck of the humerus. (From Rockwood CA, Green DP, eds. *Fractures*. 2nd ed. Philadelphia: JB Lippincott; 1984.)

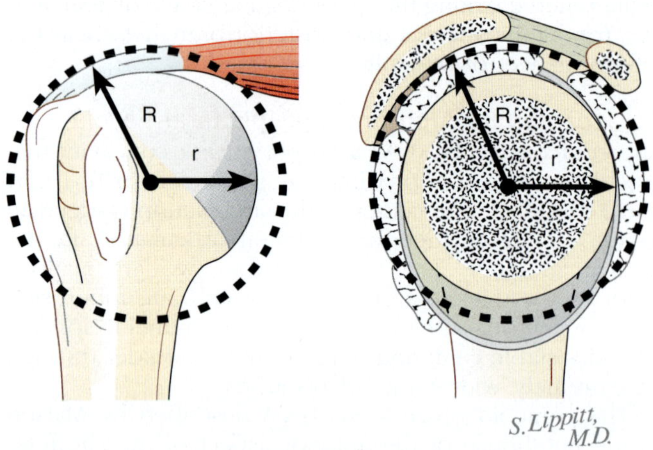

FIGURE 13-12: The proximal humeral convexity. *Left,* The rotational center of the proximal humeral convexity is the center of the sphere that best fits the tuberosities and the cuff tendons near their insertion. *Right,* The radius of the proximal humeral convexity (*R*) should be equal to the radius of the humeral articular surface sphere (*r*) plus the thickness of the rotator cuff tendons. (From Matsen FA III, Lippitt SB. *Shoulder Surgery: Principles and Procedures.* Philadelphia: WB Saunders; 2004:81.)

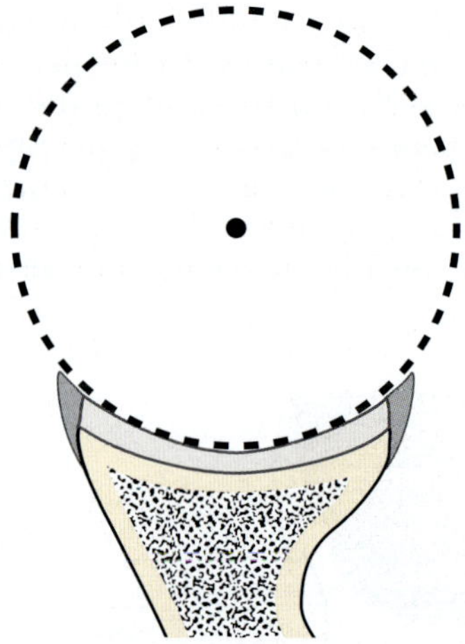

FIGURE 13-13: The glenoid concavity. The center of rotation of the glenoid (*dot*) is the center of the spherical concavity that best fits the glenoid articular surface. (From Matsen FA III, Lippitt SB. *Shoulder Surgery: Principles and Procedures.* Philadelphia: WB Saunders; 2004:82.)

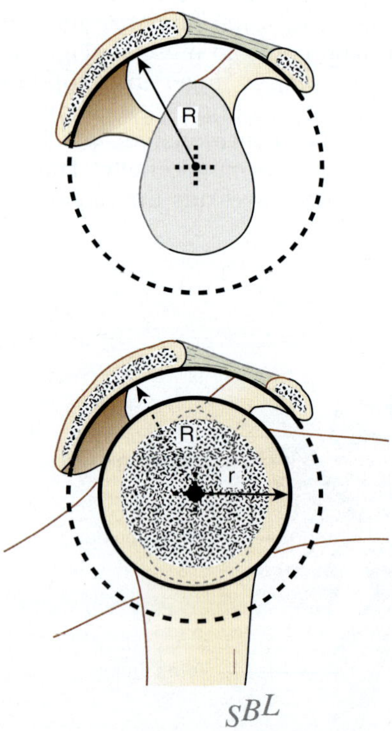

FIGURE 13-14: The coracoacromial concavity. The center of the coroacoacromial concavity is the center of the sphere that best fits the concave undersurface of the coracoacromial arch. *R,* radius of the proximal humeral convexity; *r,* radius of the humeral articular surface sphere. (From Rockwood CA, Matsen FA, eds. *The Shoulder.* 2nd ed. Philadelphia: WB Saunders; 1998:764.)

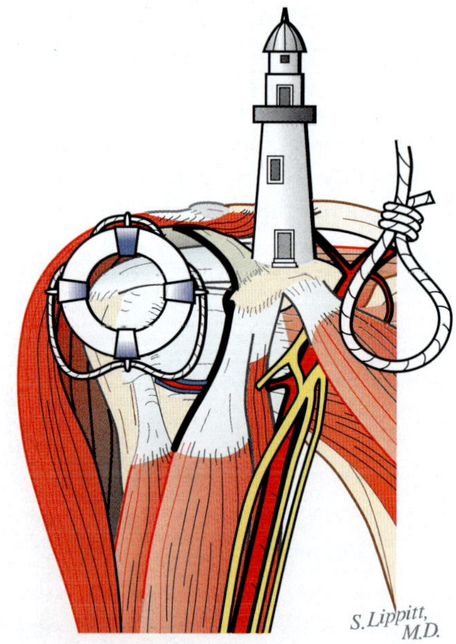

FIGURE 13-15: Safe side/suicide. The coracoid serves as a lighthouse for proper orientation in a scarred shoulder. It divides the lateral (safe side) from the medial side (suicide), where the brachial plexus and vascular structures are located. (From Matsen FA III, Lippitt SB. *Shoulder Surgery: Principles and Procedures.* Philadelphia: WB Saunders; 2004:663.)

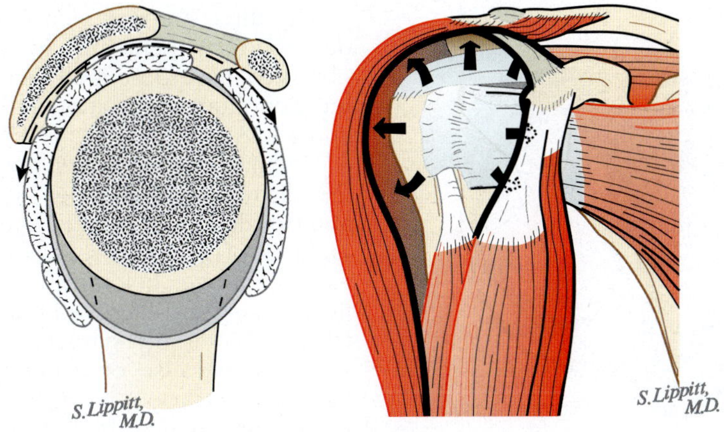

FIGURE 13-16: The axillary nerve in the humeroscapular motion interface between the cuff and the humerus on the inside and the coracoid muscles and the deltoid on the outside. (From Matsen FA III, Lippitt SB, Sidles JA, Harryman DT II. *Practical Evaluation and Management of the Shoulder*. Philadelphia: WB Saunders; 1994.)

the brachial plexus. Tracing it laterally and posteriorly leads the finger beneath the shoulder capsule toward the quadrangular space. From a posterior vantage, the axillary nerve is seen to exit the quadrangular space beneath the teres minor and extend laterally, where it is applied to the deep surface of the deltoid muscle. By virtue of its prominent location in close proximity to the shoulder joint anteriorly, inferiorly, and posteriorly, the axillary nerve is the most commonly injured structure in shoulder surgery.

The musculocutaneous nerve lies on the deep surface of the coracoid muscles and penetrates the coracobrachialis with one or more branches lying a variable distance distal to the coracoid.[190] The often-described 5-cm safe zone for the nerve beneath the process refers only to the average position of the main trunk and not to an area that can be entered recklessly. The musculocutaneous nerve is vulnerable to injury from retractors placed under the coracoid muscles and to traction injury during coracoid transfer. Knowledge of the position of these nerves can make the shoulder surgeon both more comfortable and more effective.

Rotator Cuff

The next layer of the shoulder is the rotator cuff. The tendons of these muscles blend in with the capsule as they insert into the humeral tuberosities.[113] Thus in reconstructions that require splitting of these muscles from the capsule, such splitting is more easily accomplished medially, before the blending becomes complete. The nerve to the supraspinatus and infraspinatus runs on their deep surfaces. The upper and lower subscapular nerve to the subscapularis runs on its anterior surface. Medial dissection can jeopardize their nerve supply. The superior portion of the subscapularis tendon has been found to have significantly higher stiffness and ultimate load than its inferior portion has.[239]

The capsule is relatively thin between the supraspinatus and the subscapularis (the rotator interval). This thinness allows the cuff to slide back and forth around the coracoid process as the arm is elevated and lowered. Splitting this interval toward the base of the coracoid may be helpful when mobilization of the subscapularis is needed.

The tendon of the long head of the biceps originates from the supraglenoid tubercle (Figs. 13-17 and 13-18). It runs beneath the cuff in the area of the rotator interval and exits the shoulder beneath the transverse humeral ligament and between the greater and lesser tuberosities. It is subject to injury when incising the upper subscapularis from the lesser tuberosity. In the bicipital groove of the humerus, this tendon is endangered by procedures that involve lateral transfer of the subscapularis tendon across the groove.

Scapulohumeral Ligaments

The primary passive stabilizers of the glenohumeral joint are the capsule and the scapulohumeral ligaments, which play a primary role in positions near the extremes of the allowed range of motion (Fig. 13-19). The thickness of the capsule decreases as it nears the humerus. The capsule is thickest in the inferior pouch at 2.8 mm, 2.4 mm in its anterior portion, and 2.2 mm in the posterior portion. The thickness ranges from 1.3 to 4.5 mm in cadaveric specimens.[110] The glenohumeral joint capsule is normally large, loose, and redundant, which allows full and free range of motion of the shoulder. By virtue of their mandatory redundancy, the capsule and its ligaments are lax throughout much of the range of joint motion, acting as checkreins when they come under tension as the joint approaches the limits of its range of motion. In the midrange of shoulder motion, the center of the humeral head remains within 2.2 mm of the center of the glenoid on magnetic resonance imaging (MRI).[605]

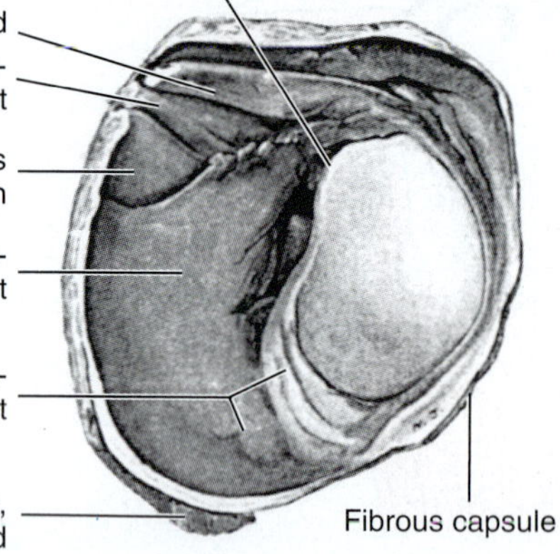

FIGURE 13-17: Anterior glenohumeral ligaments. The anterosuperior, anterior middle, and anteroinferior glenohumeral ligaments are shownj. The middle and inferior anterior glenohumeral ligaments are often avulsed from the glenoid or the glenoid labrum in traumatic anterior instability. (From Grant JCB. *Grant's Atlas of Anatomy.* 4th ed. Baltimore: Williams & Wilkins; 1956.)

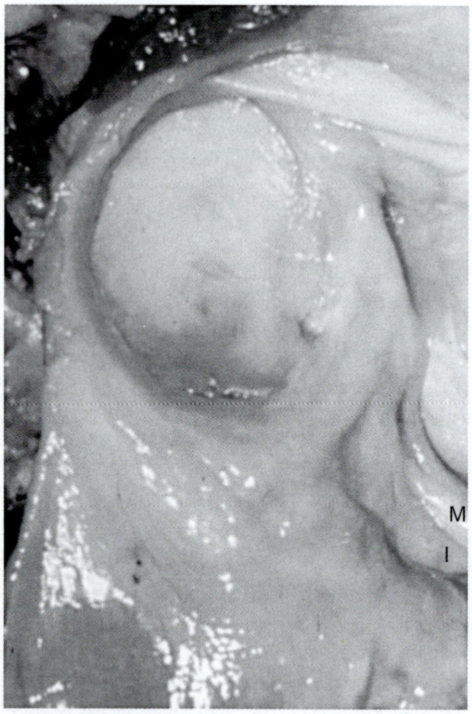

FIGURE 13-18: Cadaver dissection of the glenoid, biceps tendon insertion, and associated glenohumeral ligaments. This dissection demonstrates the anterior glenohumeral ligaments. Note the relationship of the anterior inferior (I) and the anterior middle (M) glenohumeral ligaments to the anterior rim of the glenoid.

This limited stabilizing effect shows the importance of mechanisms of glenohumeral stability other than the capsule and its ligaments. The capsular structures are also believed to contribute to stability through their proprioceptive functions.[466]

The three anterior glenohumeral ligaments were first described by Schlemm in 1853.[606] Since then, many observers have described their anatomy and role in limiting glenohumeral rotation and translation (see Figs. 13-17 and 13-18).[141,144,184,185,427,461,499,559]

Codman[116] and others pointed out the variability of the ligaments (see Fig. 13-18).[141,144,145,461,498,699] These authors also demonstrated great variation in the size and number of synovial recesses that form in the anterior capsule above, below, and between the glenohumeral ligaments. They observed that if the capsule arises at the labrum, few if any synovial recesses are present (in this situation, because of generalized blending of all three ligaments, no room is left for synovial recesses or weaknesses, and hence the anterior glenohumeral capsule is stronger). However, the more medially the capsule arises from the glenoid (i.e., from the anterior scapular neck), the larger and more numerous the synovial recesses are. The end result is a thin, weak anterior capsule. In an embryologic study involving 52 specimens, Uhthoff and Piscopo[663] demonstrated that the anterior capsule inserted into the glenoid labrum in 77% and into the medial neck of the scapula in 23%. This variation in anatomy was later classified into two different types, I and II. A type I attachment occurs when the fibers primarily originate from the labrum, with some fibers attaching to the glenoid, and it is seen 80% of the time. A type II origin of the capsuloligamentous structures occurs solely from the glenoid neck and is seen in 20% of cadaveric specimens.[163]

The superior glenohumeral ligament (SGHL) is identified as the most consistent capsular ligament.[147] It crosses the rotator interval capsule and lies between the supraspinatus and subscapularis tendons. Another interval capsular structure, the coracohumeral ligament, originates at the base of the coracoid, blends into the cuff tendons, and inserts into the greater and lesser tuberosities.[114,245,316,351,514,635]

Harryman et al. pointed out that these two ligaments and the rotator interval capsule come under tension with glenohumeral flexion, extension, external rotation, and adduction.[245] When they are under tension, these structures resist posterior and inferior displacement of the humeral head. Clinical and experimental data have shown that releasing or surgically tightening the rotator interval capsule increases or decreases the allowed posterior and inferior translational laxity, respectively.[38,245,476,491,679]

It is these ligaments and capsule, as well as the inferior glenoid lip, that provide static restraint against inferior translation.[38] It is of anatomic interest and clinical significance that when the lateral aspect of the scapula is allowed to droop inferiorly, the resulting passive abduction of the humerus relaxes the rotator interval capsule and the superior ligaments; as a result, the humeral head can be dumped out of the glenoid fossa (Fig. 13-20).[414] Drooping of the lateral part of the scapula is normally prevented by the postural action of the scapular stabilizers, particularly the trapezius and serratus. Elevation of the lateral aspect of the scapula with the arm at the side enhances inferior stability in two ways: the resulting glenohumeral adduction tightens the superior capsule

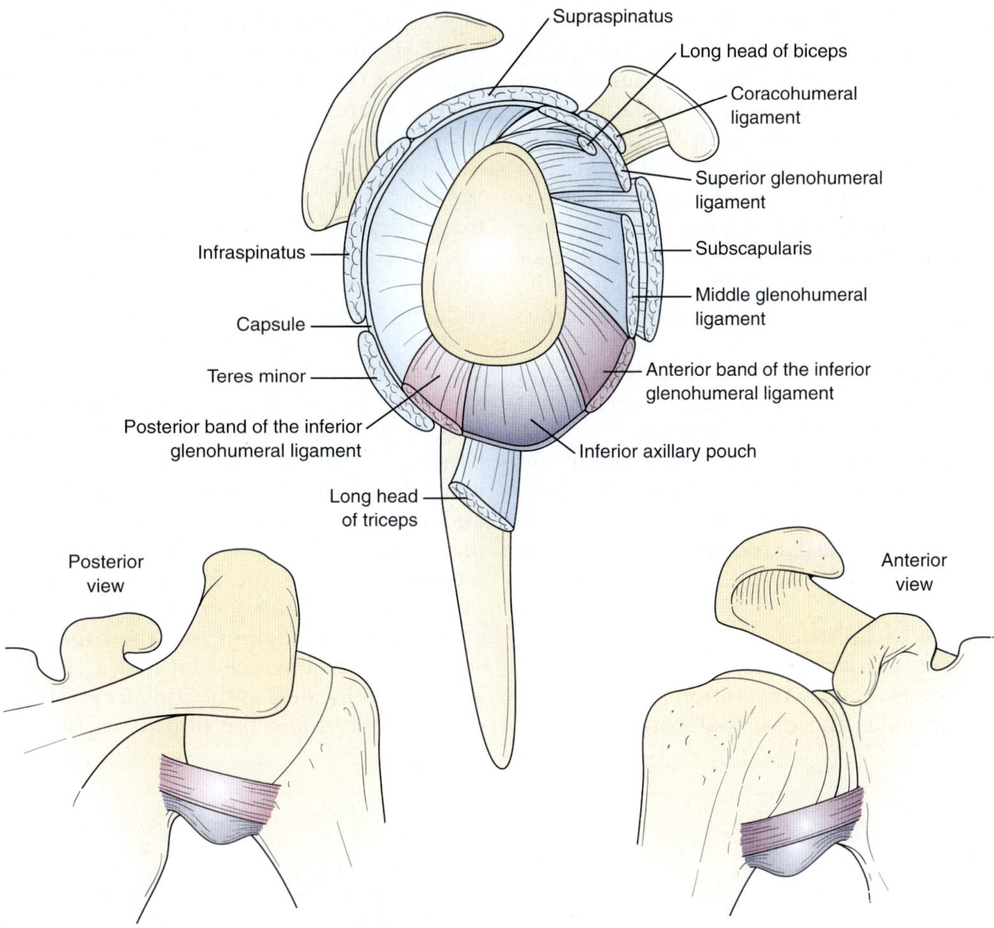

FIGURE 13-19: Static stabilizers for glenohumeral stability. (Modified from Bigliani LU, Pollock RG, McIlveen SJ, et al. Shift of the posteroinferior aspect of the capsule for recurrent posterior glenohumeral instability. *J Bone Joint Surg Am.* 1995;77[7]:1011-1020.)

and ligaments, and the scapular rotation places more of the inferior glenoid lip beneath the humeral head.[305,679]

SGHL and coracohumeral ligament come under tension with external rotation in adduction, whereas the middle glenohumeral ligament (MGHL) is tensioned by external rotation when the humerus is abducted to 45 degrees.[642,644] MGHL originates anterosuperiorly on the glenoid and inserts midway along the anterior humeral articular surface adjacent to the lesser tuberosity. In more than a third of shoulders, MGHL is absent or poorly defined, a situation that can place the shoulder at greater risk for anterior glenohumeral instability.[455]

With greater degrees of shoulder abduction, for example, in the apprehension position, the inferior glenohumeral ligament (IGHL) and the inferior capsular sling come into play (Fig. 13-21).[644,661] IGHL originates below the sigmoid notch and courses obliquely between the anteroinferior glenoid and its humeral capsular insertion.[498] O'Brien et al. have described an anterior thickening of IGHL, the anterior superior band.[498] The anterior

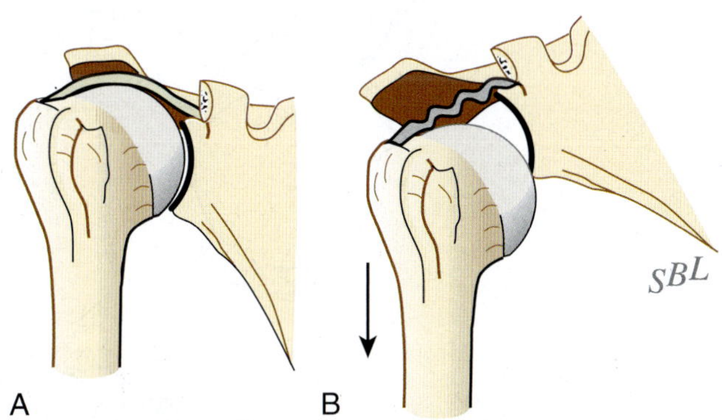

FIGURE 13-20: Scapular dumping. With the scapula in a normal position (**A**), the superior capsular mechanism is tight and supports the head in the glenoid concavity. Drooping of the lateral aspect of the scapula (**B**) relaxes the superior capsular structures and rotates the glenoid concavity so that it does not support the head of the humerus. (From Matsen FA III, Lippitt SB, Sidles JA, Harryman DT II. *Practical Evaluation and Management of the Shoulder*. Philadelphia: WB Saunders; 1994.)

and posterior aspects of IGHL are said to function as a cruciate construct in which they alternately tighten in external and internal rotation.[498,679,682] These ligaments can be stretched out with repeated use. The dominant shoulders of handball athletes were placed in 90 degrees of abduction and external rotation and then brought into extension while being observed using computed tomography (CT). The dominant shoulders were seen to have more external rotation of the humeral head and more of a shift from the posterior aspect of the glenoid to its center than noted in normal shoulders when brought into the late cocking position.[26]

When the humerus is elevated anteriorly in the sagittal plane (flexion), the posterior-inferior capsular pouch and the rotator interval capsule come into tension.[244,245,498,679] If the humerus is internally rotated while elevated in the sagittal plane, the interval capsule slackens but the posterior inferior pouch tightens. Posteroinferior capsular tension also limits flexion, internal rotation, and horizontal adduction.[244,245]

Glenoid Concavity and Labrum

The predominant method for centering the humeral head in the glenoid fossa is concavity compression.[411] The glenoid concavity provides the essential concavity (see Figs. 13-17 and 13-18). The deeper the concavity, the more stability results from compression of the humeral head in it (Fig. 13-22). The glenoid concavity is provided by the shape of the bony socket, which is functionally deepened as a result of the articular cartilage being thicker at the periphery than at the center (Fig. 13-23). Weldon et al.[691] showed that removal of the glenoid cartilage dramatically compromised the intrinsic stability offered by the glenoid fossa, especially in the posterior-inferior direction, where the balance stability angle was reduced almost 50% by cartilage removal.

The socket is further deepened by the presence of the labrum around the rim of the socket (Fig. 13-24). On average, the normal glenoid is 25 mm in width at its widest, with an average radius of 12.5 mm.[36] The glenoid labrum doubles the depth of the socket.[36] This structure is a fibrous rim that serves to deepen the glenoid fossa and allow attachment of the glenohumeral ligaments and the biceps tendon to the glenoid. Anatomically, the glenoid labrum is the interconnection of the periosteum of the glenoid, the glenoid bone, the glenoid articular cartilage, the synovium, and the capsule. Although microscopic studies have shown that a small amount of fibrocartilage is located at the junction of the hyaline cartilage of the glenoid and the fibrous capsule, the vast majority

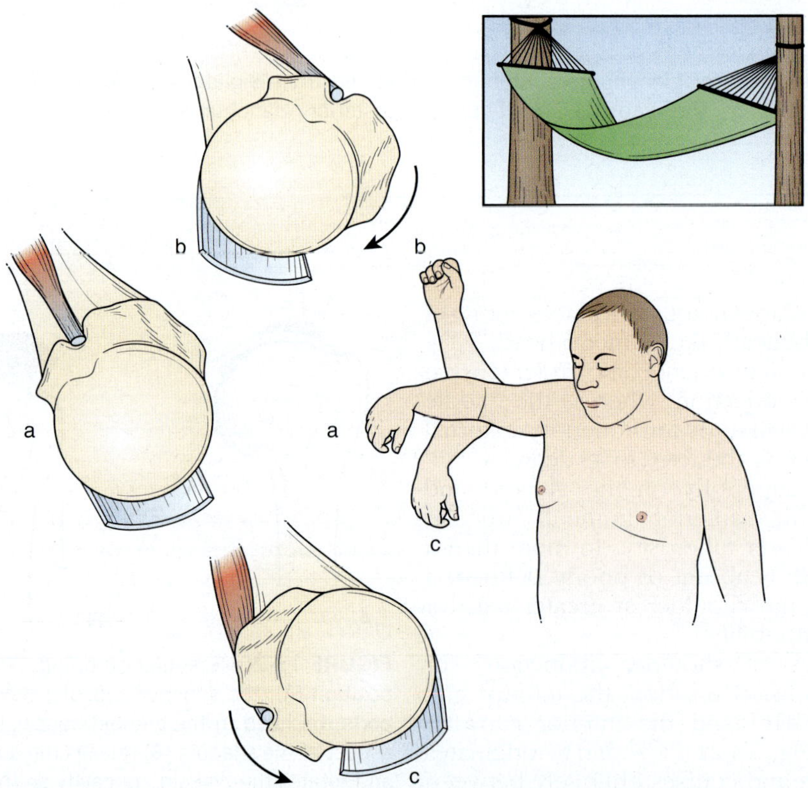

FIGURE 13-21: The interior glenohumeral ligament complex supports the humeral head like a hammock *(a)*. Reciprocal tightening *(b)* and external rotation and internal rotation *(c)* provide a barrier to anterior and posterior instability, respectively. (Modified from Warner JP, Caborn DNM. Overview of shoulder instability. *Crit Rev Phys Rehabil Med.* 1992;4:145-198.)

of the labrum consists of dense fibrous tissue with a few elastic fibers (Fig. 13-25).[203,461,657] The posterosuperior portion of the labrum is continuous with the tendon of the long head of the biceps. Anteriorly, it is continuous with IGHL (see Fig. 13-18).[222,457,460,659] Hertz et al.[266] detailed the microanatomy of the labrum, and Prodromos et al.,[549] DePalma,[145] and Olsson[506] have described changes in the glenoid labrum with age.

In cadavers, isolated labral lesions are not usually sufficient to allow complete glenohumeral dislocation.[521,558,560,657] However, cadaveric studies have shown diminished stability with labral lesions. Fehringer et al. have demonstrated that a simple incision in its attachment to the glenoid uncenters the humeral head.[181] Resection of the labrum was found to decrease the stability ratio of cadaveric shoulders by 9.6%.[238] Lazarus et al.[369] demonstrated that resection of the cartilage and labrum from the anteroinferior glenoid reduced the height of the glenoid by approximately 80% and the stability ratio by approximately 65% for translation in the direction of the defect. Halder et al.[238] again demonstrated the stabilizing effect of the labrum in a cadaver model. Clinical studies reveal a high incidence of labral

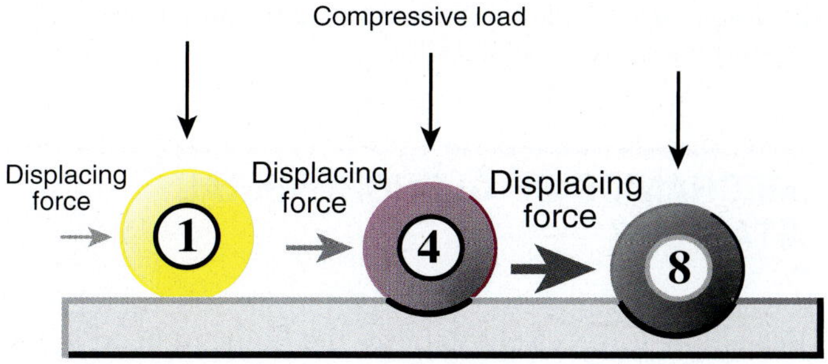

FIGURE 13-22: Concavity and compression. In the absence of a concavity, only a minimal translational force is required to displace the sphere. As the concavity becomes deeper, a greater displacing force is required for a given compressive load. (From Matsen FA III, Lippitt SB. *Shoulder Surgery: Principles and Procedures*. Philadelphia: WB Saunders; 2004:83.)

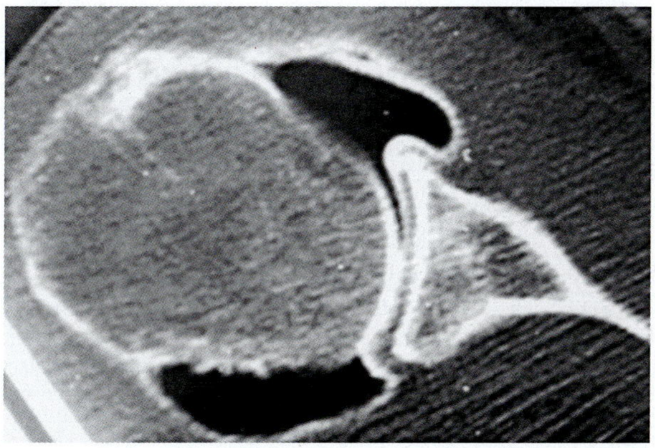

FIGURE 13-23: Computed tomographic arthrogram of the glenohumeral joint. The depth of the bony glenoid is enhanced by contributions of the articular cartilage and the glenoid labrum, which further increases the stability of the glenohumeral joint. Note that in this position, the anterior and posterior capsuloligamentous structures are relaxed and cannot contribute to stability.

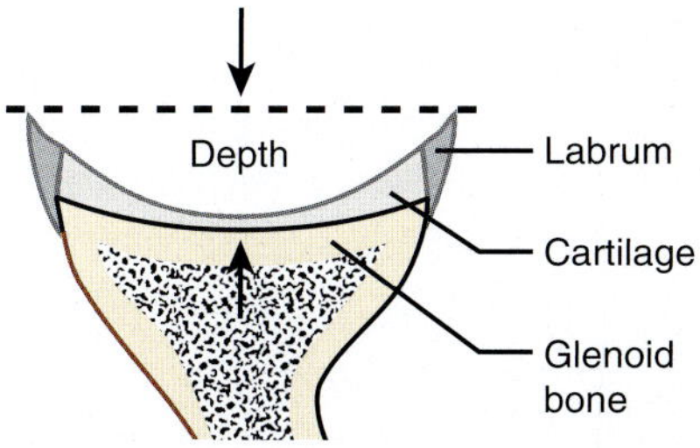

FIGURE 13-24: Components of the glenoid fossa. The glenoid fossa results from the relatively small concavity of the glenoid bone, deepened by the glenoid cartilage and by the labrum at its periphery. (From Matsen FA III, Lippitt SB. *Shoulder Surgery: Principles and Procedures*. Philadelphia: WB Saunders; 2004:88.)

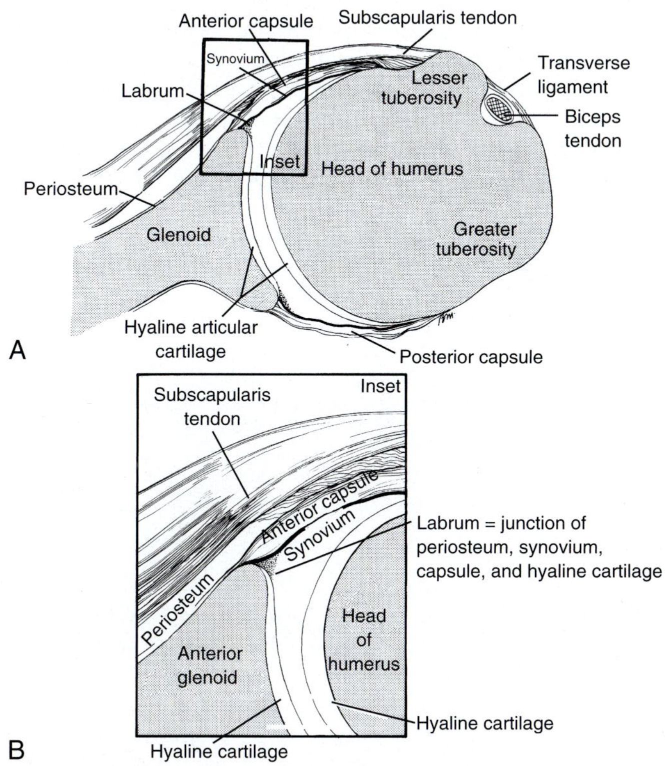

FIGURE 13-25: Normal shoulder anatomy. **A,** Horizontal section through the middle of the glenohumeral joint demonstrating normal anatomic relationships. Note the close relationship of the subscapularis tendon to the anterior capsule. **B,** Close-up view in the area of the labrum. The labrum consists of tissues from the nearby hyaline cartilage, capsule, synovium, and periosteum. (From Rockwood CA, Green DP, eds. *Fractures*. 2nd ed. Philadelphia: JB Lippincott; 1984.)

deficiency or detachment in patients with recurrent traumatic instability.[34,132,143,415,585,664]

Biomechanical studies have determined that 20% loss of the anteroinferior glenoid rim is the lowest significant threshold for changes in the force required to dislocate the shoulder.[721] Therefore estimating 20% of anterior bone loss from the center of the glenoid, roughly 10 mm in radius remains when 2.5 mm of the anterior glenoid is missing. In other words, the total diameter of the remaining glenoid will be 22.5 mm in the presence of 20% bone loss (Figs. 13-26 and 13-27).

In the glenoid track model, glenoid contact has been shown to shift with the humeral head from the inferomedial to the postero-superolateral portion of the humeral head, creating a roughly 2-cm arc zone of contact along the edge of the articular cartilage.[507] This observation provides the basis for understanding which Hill-Sachs lesion are "engaging"—in other words, significant during functional range of motion—and which areas of glenoid bone loss lead to glenohumeral instability.

Capsular Deformation

Capsular deformation after the first dislocation is also a key factor in perpetuating shoulder instability. Studies of capsular biology have shown that increased, deregulated, and abnormal expression of collagen genes occurred in the anteroinferior, anterosuperior, and posterior regionals of the joint capsule after a shoulder dislocation.[45] These changes at the molecular level impact collagen regeneration and likely play a role in the capsular deformation observed. Therefore many surgeons support capsular plication in addition to labral repair, while others bypass the issue of capsular deformation and favor bone block techniques to restore stability.

MECHANICS OF GLENOHUMERAL STABILITY

The most remarkable feature of the glenohumeral joint is its ability to precisely stabilize the humeral head in the center of the glenoid on the one hand and to allow a vast range of motion on the other. This balance of stability and mobility is achieved by a combination of mechanisms particular to this articulation.[412]

In contrast to the hip joint, the glenohumeral joint does not offer a deep stabilizing socket. An acetabulum-like socket would limit motion by contact of the anatomic neck of the humerus with its rim. Instead, the small arc of the glenoid captures relatively little of the humeral articular surface; thus neck-to-rim contact is avoided for a wide range of positions (Fig. 13-28).[135,404,414,597,661]

In contrast to hinge-like joints with shallow sockets, such as the knee, interphalangeal joints, elbow, and ankle, the glenohumeral joint does not offer isometric articular ligaments that provide stability as the joint is flexed around a defined anatomic axis. Instead, the glenohumeral ligaments play important stabilizing roles only at the extremes of motion; they are lax and relatively ineffectual in most functional positions of the joint (Fig. 13-29).[414,679]

In spite of its lack of a deep socket or isometric ligaments, the normal shoulder precisely constrains the humeral head to the center of the glenoid cavity

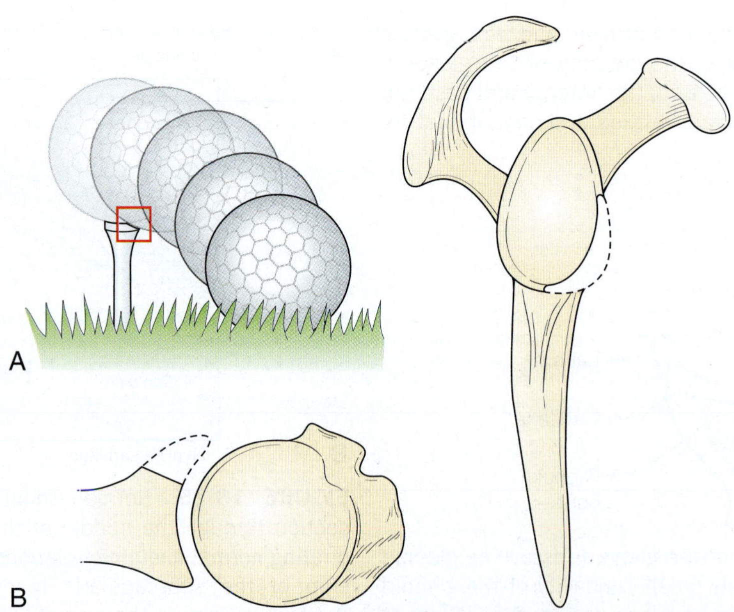

FIGURE 13-26: A and **B,** Glenoid concavity changes with loss of the anteroinferior glenoid rim. (Modified from Clavert PH, Millett P, Warner JP. Traumatic anterior instability: open solutions. In: Warner JP, Iannotti J, Flatow EL, eds. *Complex and Revision Problems in Shoulder Surgery.* 2nd ed. Philadelphia: Lippincott, Williams and Wilkins; 2005:26.)

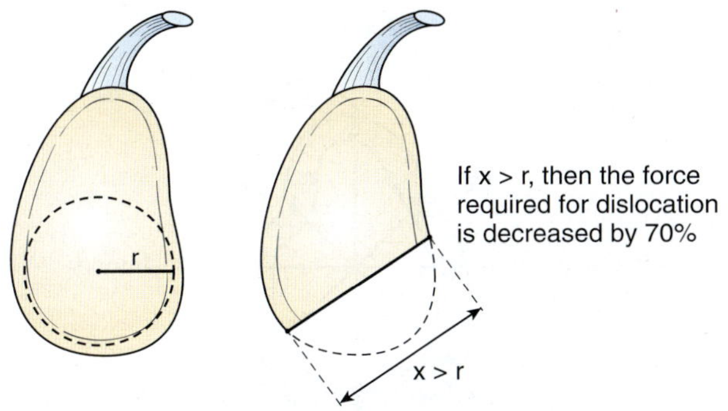

FIGURE 13-27: Biomechanical consequences of anteroinferior glenoid bone loss. If the diameter of the eroded region (x) is greater than the native glenoid radius (r), the force necessary for an anterior dislocation is decreased by at least 70% over the normal joint. (Modified from Gerber C, Nyffeler RW: Classification of glenohumeral joint instability. *Clin Orthop.* 2002;400:65.)

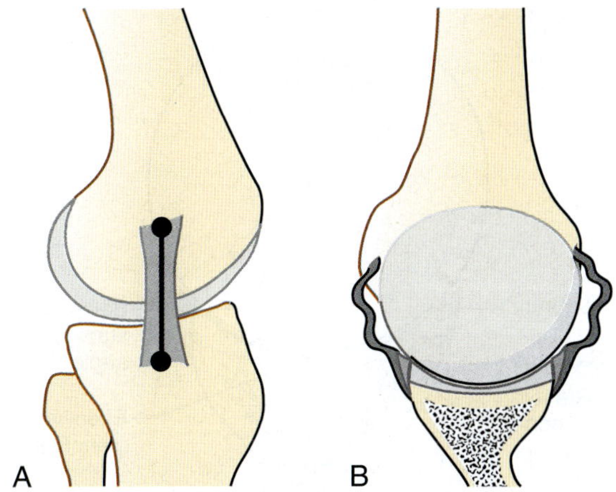

FIGURE 13-29: In contrast to the knee, where the ligaments remain isometric during joint motion (**A**), the glenohumeral ligaments must be slack in most of the joint's positions (**B**). (Modified from Matsen FA III, Lippitt SB, Sidles JA, Harryman DT II. *Practical Evaluation and Management of the Shoulder.* Philadelphia: WB Saunders; 1994.)

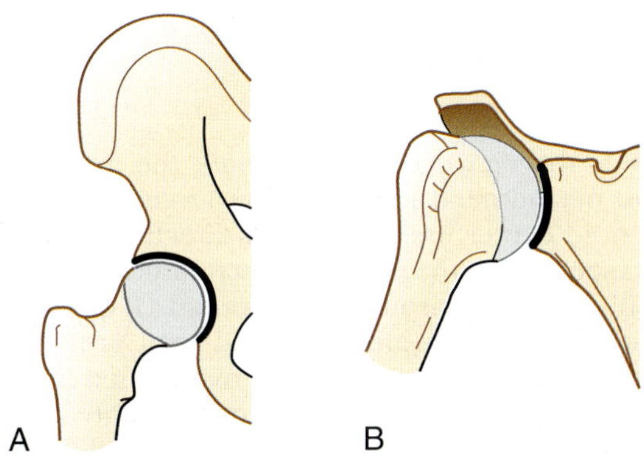

FIGURE 13-28: In contrast to the hip (**A**), the shallow glenoid captures relatively little of the articulating ball (**B**). (From Matsen FA III, Lippitt SB, Sidles JA, Harryman DT II. *Practical Evaluation and Management of the Shoulder.* Philadelphia: WB Saunders; 1994.)

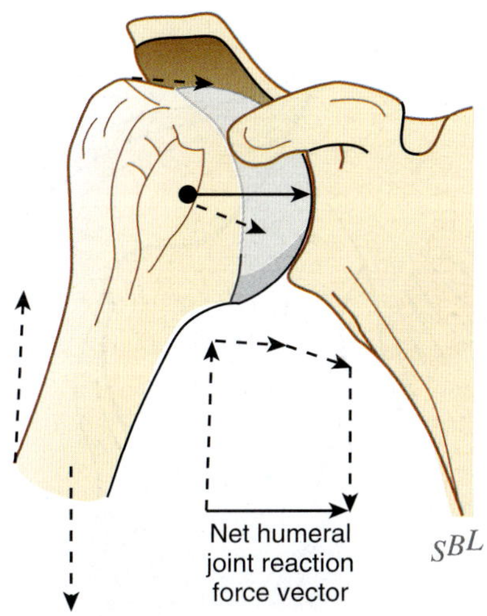

FIGURE 13-30: The net humeral joint reaction force is the vector sum of all forces acting on the head of the humerus relative to the glenoid fossa. (From Matsen FA III, Lippitt SB, Sidles JA, Harryman DT II. *Practical Evaluation and Management of the Shoulder.* Philadelphia: WB Saunders; 1994.)

throughout most of the arc of movement.[289,290,546,547,597,605] It is remarkable that this seemingly unconstrained joint can provide such precise centering, resist the gravitational pull on the arm hanging at the side for long periods, remain located during sleep, allow the lifting of large loads, permit throwing a baseball at speeds exceeding 100 miles per hour, and maintain stability during the application of an almost infinite variety of forces of differing magnitude, direction, duration, and abruptness.

The mechanics of glenohumeral stability can be most easily understood in terms of the relationship between the net force acting on the humeral head and the shape of the glenoid fossa. A working familiarity with the mechanics of glenohumeral stability will greatly enhance the clinician's understanding of the workings of the normal joint, laboratory models of instability, clinical problems of instability, and clinical strategies for managing glenohumeral instability.

The basic law of glenohumeral stability is that the glenohumeral joint will not dislocate as long as the net humeral joint reaction force* (Fig. 13-30) is directed

**The net humeral joint reaction force is the result of all muscular, ligamentous, inertial, gravitational, and other external forces applied to the head of the humerus (other than the force applied by the glenoid).*

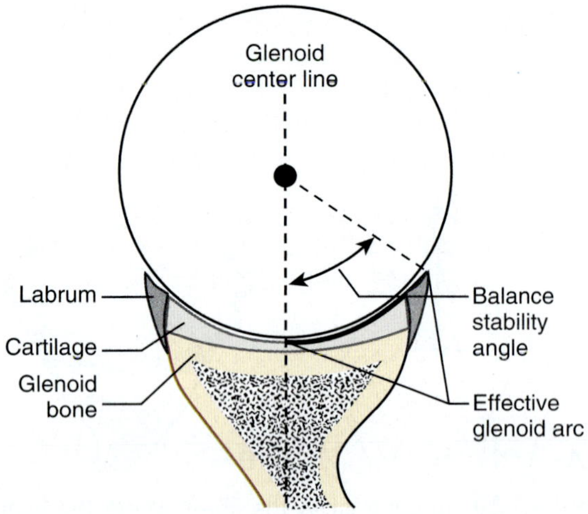

FIGURE 13-31: The effective glenoid arc is the arc of the glenoid able to support the net humeral joint reaction force. The balance stability angle is the maximal angle that the net humeral joint reaction force can make with the glenoid center line before dislocation occurs. The shape of the bone, cartilage, and labrum all contribute to the effective glenoid arc and the balance stability angle.

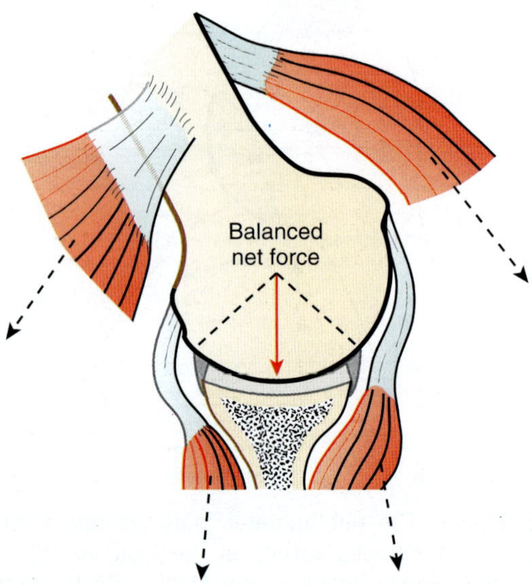

FIGURE 13-32: The deltoid and cuff muscle forces (*dotted arrows*) maintain the net humeral joint reaction force (*solid arrow*) within the balance stability angle (*dotted lines*). (Modified from Matsen FA III, Lippitt SB, Sidles JA, Harryman DT II. *Practical Evaluation and Management of the Shoulder.* Philadelphia: WB Saunders; 1994.)

within the effective glenoid arc* (Figs. 13-31 and 13-32).[289,629] If the net humeral joint reaction force passes outside the effective glenoid arc, the joint becomes unstable. The effective glenoid arc in a given direction is also

Because the rim of the glenoid is deformable under load, the effective glenoid arc is the arc of the glenoid available to support the humeral head under the specified loading conditions.

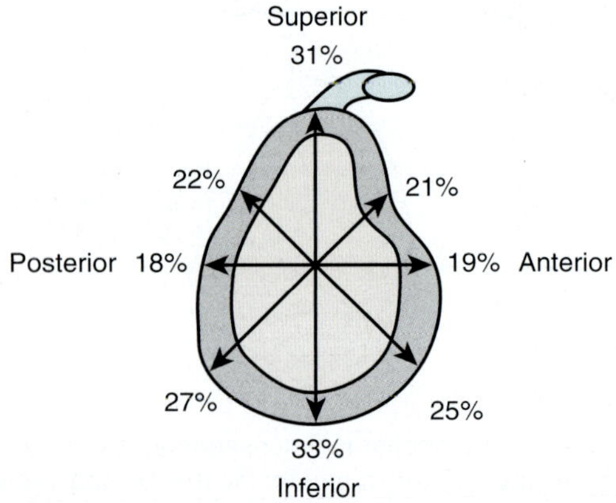

FIGURE 13-33: The balance stability angle varies around the face of the glenoid. For a normal glenoid, the superior and inferior balance stability angles are greater than the anterior and posterior balance stability angles. This figure shows the balance stability angles (*solid arrows*) measured in eight directions around the face of the glenoid. Values are means for 10 cadaver shoulders with a compressive load of 50 N. (Modified from Matsen FA III, Lippitt SB, Sidles JA, Harryman DT II. *Practical Evaluation and Management of the Shoulder.* Philadelphia: WB Saunders; 1994.)

known as the *balance stability angle,* the maximal angle that the net humeral joint reaction force can make with the glenoid center line in a given direction before dislocation (see Fig. 13-31). Balance stability angles vary for different directions around the glenoid (Fig. 13-33). The requisite for a stable glenohumeral joint is that the net humeral joint reaction force be maintained within the balance stability angles. The balance stability angle may be compromised by congenital deficiency (glenoid hypoplasia), excessive compliance, traumatic lesions (rim fractures or Bankart defects), or wear (Fig. 13-34).* The balance stability angle may be restored or augmented by anatomic repair of fractures or Bankart lesions (Fig. 13-35), by rim augmentation,[413] by congruent glenoid bone grafting,[454] and by glenoid osteotomy.[369]

Stability at Rest

It is apparent that a relaxed glenohumeral joint is held together without either active muscle contraction or ligament tension. The intact shoulder of a fresh anatomic specimen,[353] the anesthetized and paralyzed shoulder of a patient in the operating room, and the arm relaxed at the side[38] all maintain the normal relationships of the glenoid and humeral joint surfaces. This resting stability is conferred by a group of mechanisms, including adhesion and cohesion, the glenoid suction cup, and limited joint volume. These mechanisms save energy, as pointed out by Humphry in 1858[292]: "We have only to remember that this power is in continual operation to appreciate the amount of animal force that is economized."

References 6, 29, 33, 122, 131, 238, 289, 318, 390, 414-416, 474, 524, 585, 648.

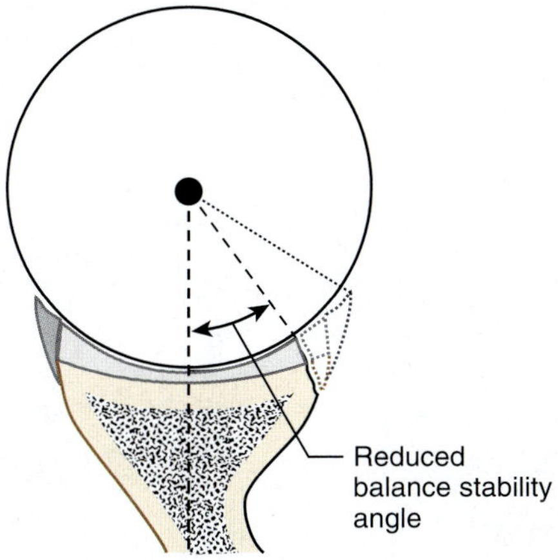

FIGURE 13-34: The balance stability angle and the effective glenoid arc are reduced by a fracture of the glenoid rim. (Modified from Matsen FA III, Lippitt SB, Sidles JA, Harryman DT II. *Practical Evaluation and Management of the* Shoulder. Philadelphia: WB Saunders; 1994.)

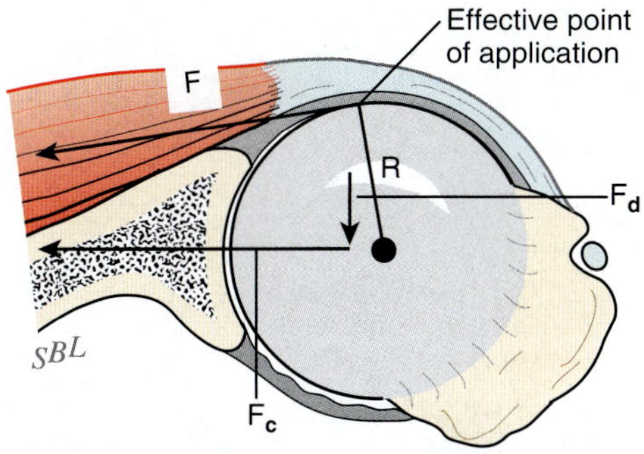

FIGURE 13-36: Each active muscle generates a force (*F*) whose direction is determined by the effective origin and insertion of that muscle. Note that the rotator cuff tendons wrap around the head of the humerus, so their effective point of attachment is on the humeral articular surface. Note also that each muscle force has a compressive (F_c) and a displacing (F_d) component. The product of the force multiplied by the radius (*R*) is the torque (F • R). (Modified from Matsen FA III, Lippitt SB, Sidles JA, Harryman DT II. *Practical Evaluation and Management of the Shoulder*. Philadelphia: WB Saunders; 1994.)

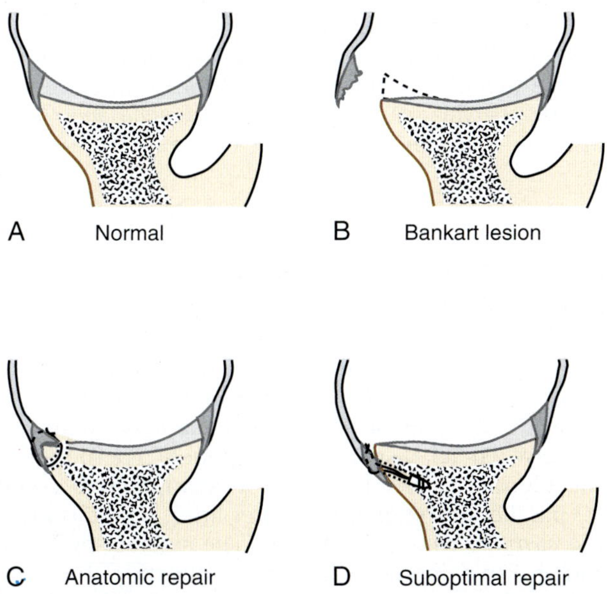

FIGURE 13-35: A, Normally, the capsule and labrum deepen the effective glenoid fossa. **B,** This effect is lost in the presence of a Bankart lesion, particularly if the articular cartilage is worn away. **C,** Anatomic repair of the detached glenoid labrum and glenohumeral ligaments to the glenoid rim helps restore the effective glenoid arc. **D,** By contrast, when the labrum and capsule heal to the neck, the effective glenoid arc is not restored. (Modified from Matsen FA III, Lippitt SB, Sidles JA, Harryman DT II. *Practical Evaluation and Management of the Shoulder*. Philadelphia: WB Saunders; 1994.)

Net Humeral Joint Reaction Force

The direction of the net humeral joint reaction force is controlled actively by elements of the rotator cuff and other shoulder muscles along with the weight of the arm and externally applied forces. Each active muscle generates a force whose direction is determined by the effective origin and insertion of that muscle (Fig. 13-36). Neural control of the magnitude of these muscle forces provides the mechanism by which the direction of the net humeral joint reaction force is controlled. For example, by increasing the force of contraction of muscles whose force directions are close to the glenoid center line, the direction of the net humeral joint reaction force can be aligned more closely with the glenoid fossa (Fig. 13-37). The elements of the rotator cuff are well positioned to contribute to this muscle balance.*

In addition to the compression provided by the rotator cuff musculature, the deltoid assists in this capacity as well. The middle and posterior portions of the deltoid have been shown to be more important than the anterior portion in producing concavity compression.[371,237] The long head of the biceps muscle might also contribute to shoulder stability, although electromyogram studies have shown little active biceps firing during shoulder use.[717,335]

In the healthy shoulder, strengthening and neuromuscular training help optimize neuromuscular control of the net humeral joint reaction force. Conversely, the net humeral joint reaction force is difficult to optimize when muscle control is impaired by injury, disuse, contracture, paralysis, loss of coordination, or tendon defects or when the glenoid concavity is compromised (Fig. 13-38). Neuromuscular training may be guided by proprioceptors in the labrum and ligaments.[229,247,313,670] Blasier et al.[59] and Kronberg et al.[347] showed that persons with generalized joint laxity have less-acute proprioception and altered

**References 39, 40, 60, 91, 243, 302, 306, 329, 521, 540, 574, 601, 667, 668, 671, 714.*

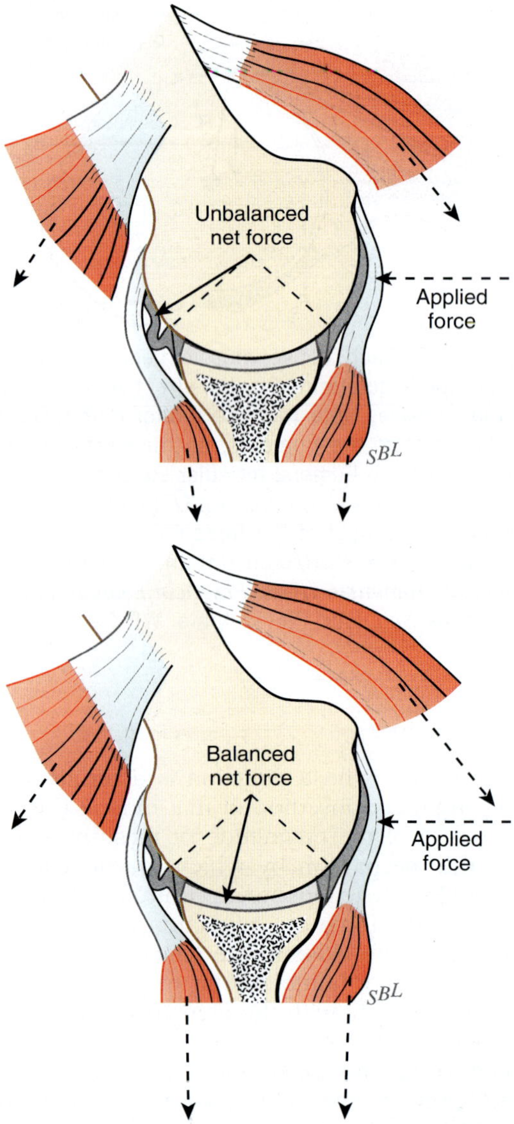

FIGURE 13-37: Stabilizing the glenohumeral joint against an applied translational force. *Top,* Weak contraction of cuff muscles results in an unbalanced net force and risk instability. *Bottom,* Strong contraction of the cuff muscles provides an increased compression force into the glenoid concavity. As a result, the net humeral force is balanced within the glenoid concavity.

muscle activation. Zuckerman et al. demonstrated that motion and position sense are compromised in the presence of traumatic anterior instability and are restored 1 year after surgical reconstruction.[731]

The reader is referred to reviews of neuromuscular stabilization of the shoulder by Lieber and Friden[412] and by Speer and Garrett.[412] In the same reference are found reviews of the role of capsular feedback and pattern generators in shoulder kinematics by Grigg[412] and the role of muscle optimization by Flanders.[412]

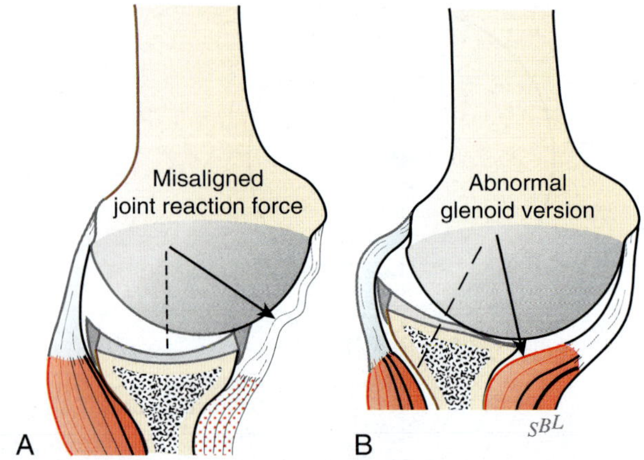

FIGURE 13-38: A, Stability is compromised by muscle imbalance. In this example, the humerus is aligned with the glenoid center line (*dotted line*), but the net humeral joint reaction force (*arrow*) is misaligned because of weakness of the posterior cuff musculature. **B,** Balance stability is compromised with abnormal glenoid version. In this example, the humerus is aligned with the plane of the scapula, but severe glenoid retroversion results in a posteriorly directed glenoid center line (*dotted line*) that is divergent from the net humeral joint reaction force (*arrow*). (Modified from Matsen FA III, Lippitt SB, Sidles JA, Harryman DT II. *Practical Evaluation and Management of the Shoulder.* Philadelphia: WB Saunders; 1994.)

Balance Stability Angle and the Stability Ratio

The balance stability angle is the maximal angle that the net humeral joint reaction force can make with the glenoid center line before glenohumeral dislocation occurs. The tangent of this balance stability angle is the ratio between its displacing component (perpendicular to the glenoid center line) and its compressive component (parallel to the glenoid center line), which is known as the *stability ratio* (Fig. 13-39). The stability ratio is the maximal displacing force in a given direction that can be stabilized by a specified compressive load, assuming frictional effects to be minimal.* The effective glenoid arc, the balance stability angle, and stability ratios vary around the perimeter of the glenoid (see Fig. 13-33). It is handy to note that for small angles, the stability ratio can be estimated by dividing the balance stability angle by 57 degrees (Fig. 13-40).

The stability ratio is often used in the laboratory because it is relatively easy to measure: A compressive load is applied, and the displacing force is progressively increased until dislocation occurs. For example, Lippitt et al.[390] found that a compressive load of 50 N resisted displacing loads of up to 30 N and that the effectiveness

**At small angles, the tangent of an angle is approximately equal to the angle expressed in radians. Thus the stability ratio (tangent of the balance stability angle) is approximately the balance stability angle divided by 57 degrees per radian.*

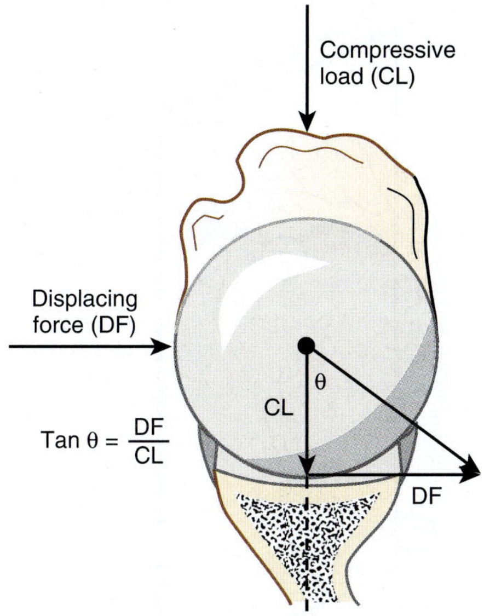

FIGURE 13-39: The relationship of the maximum local stability ratio to the balance stability angle. The tangent (Tan) of the balance stability angle is equal to the ratio of the displacing force and the compressive load. (From Matsen FA III, Lippitt SB. *Shoulder Surgery: Principles and Procedures*. Philadelphia: WB Saunders; 2004:108.)

of this stabilization mechanism varied with the depth of the glenoid (Fig. 13-41). Investigation of these parameters provides important information on stability mechanics. For example, resection of the labrum has been shown to reduce the stability ratio by 20%.[390] Furthermore, a 3-mm anterior glenoid defect has been shown to reduce the balance stability angle more than 25% from 18 to 13 degrees.[414] Bony defects of 21% of the anterior glenoid rim were noted to reduce the balance stability angle by 50%.[303,454]

Clinically, the stability ratio can be sensed using the load and shift test, wherein the examiner applies a compressive load pressing the humeral head into the glenoid while noting the amount of translating force necessary to move the humeral head from its centered position.[619] This test gives the examiner an indication of the adequacy of the glenoid concavity and is one of the most practical ways to detect deficiencies of the glenoid rim.

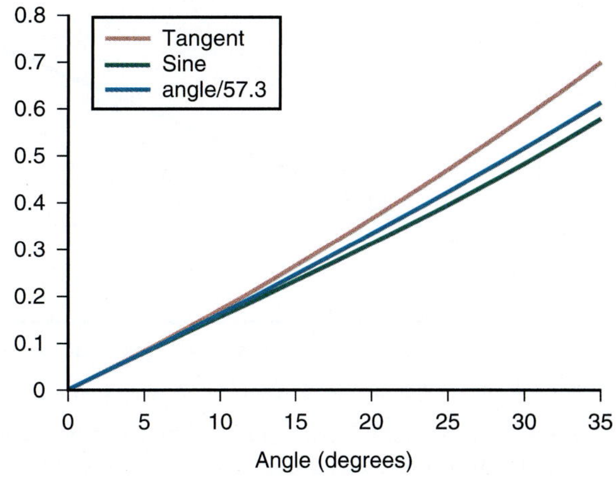

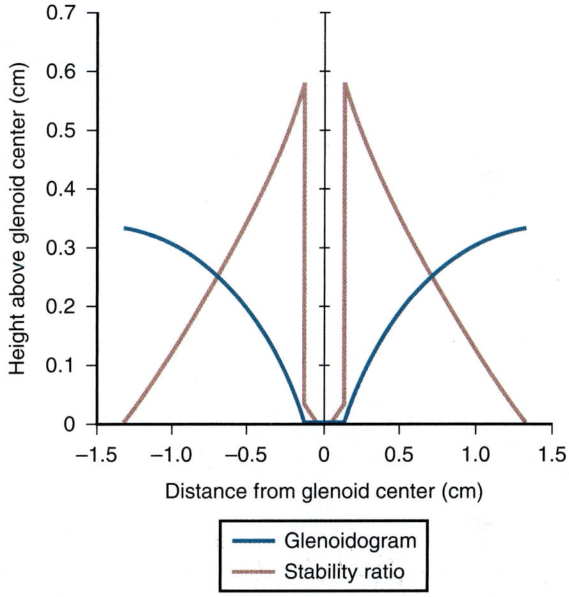

FIGURE 13-40: Small angle approximation. For small angles, the sine, the tangent, and the angle expressed in radians (57.3°) are all approximately the same, making it easy to predict the balance stability angle (BSA) without trigonometry calculations (BSA ≈ 57.3 × W/R, where *W* is width and *R* is radius of the glenoid). (From Matsen FA III, Lippitt SB. *Shoulder Surgery: Principles and Procedures*. Philadelphia: WB Saunders; 2004:97.)

Glenoidogram

The effective shape of the glenoid is revealed by the *glenoidogram*, which, rather than showing how the glenoid *looks*, shows how it *works*.[369,415] The glenoidogram is the path taken by the center of the humeral head as it is translated away from the center of the glenoid fossa in a specified direction. The shape of the glenoidogram indicates the extent of the effective glenoid arc in that direction. The glenoidogram is oriented with respect to the *glenoid center line*, a reference line perpendicular to the center of the glenoid fossa (Figs. 13-42 and 13-43). As the humeral head is translated from the center of the glenoid to the rim in a given direction, the center of the humeral head traces the glenoidogram, which has a characteristic "gull-wing" shape (Figs. 13-44 and 13-45). The glenoidogram is different for different directions of translation (Fig. 13-46) and presents data recorded for the superior, inferior, anterior, and posterior directions in a typical shoulder.

Glenoid Version

Glenoid version is the angle that the glenoid center line makes with the plane of the scapula. The glenoid center

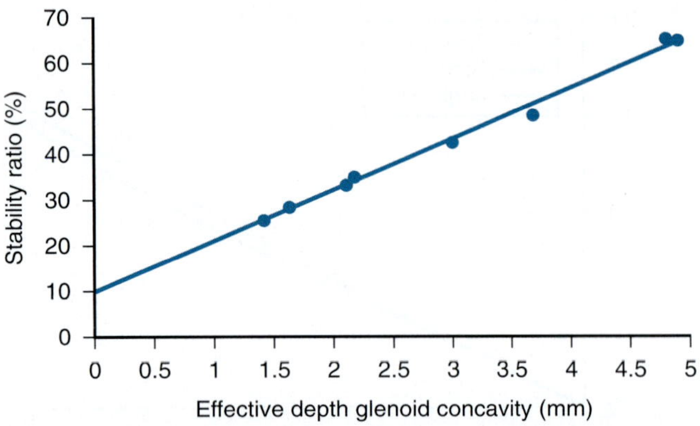

FIGURE 13-41: A nearly linear relationship exists between the effective depth of the glenoid concavity and the stability ratio with a 50-N compressive load. These data include points representing superior, inferior, anterior, and posterior translation before and after excision of the glenoid labrum. (From Matsen FA III, Lippitt SB, Sidles JA, Harryman DT II. *Practical Evaluation and Management of the Shoulder.* Philadelphia: WB Saunders; 1994.)

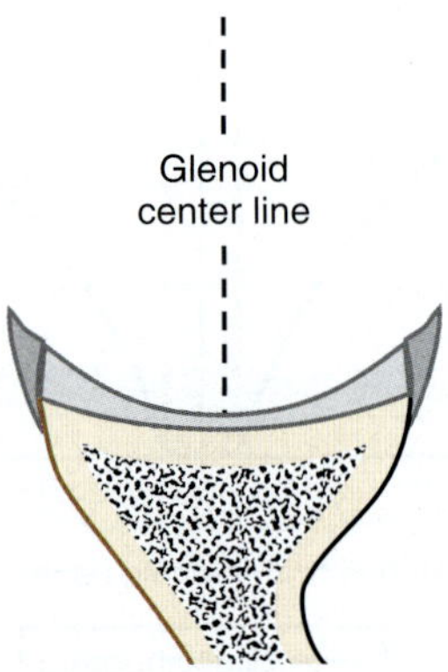

FIGURE 13-42: The glenoid center line is a line perpendicular to the surface of the glenoid fossa at its midpoint. (Modified from Matsen FA III, Lippitt SB, Sidles JA, Harryman DT II. *Practical Evaluation and Management of the Shoulder.* Philadelphia: WB Saunders; 1994.)

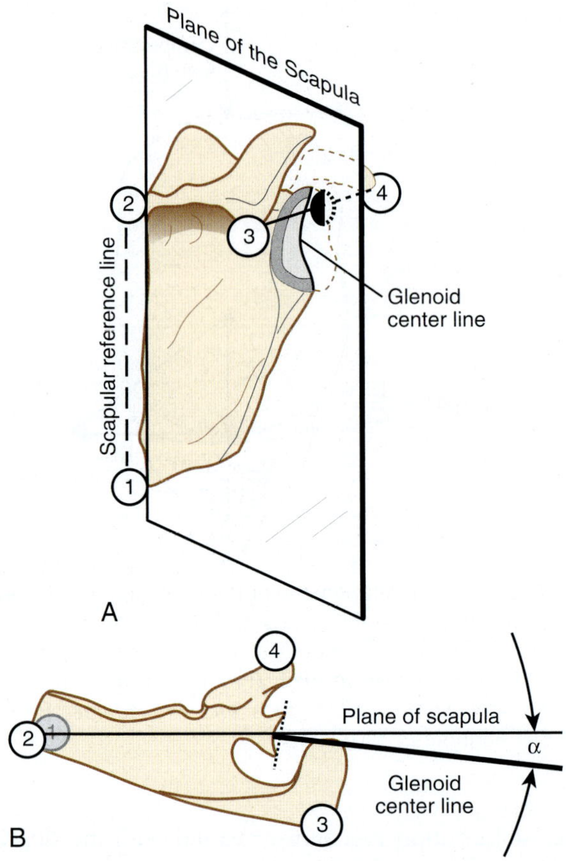

FIGURE 13-43: The glenoid center line can be related to scapular coordinates and the plane of the scapula. **A,** The plane of the scapula is the plane passing through the inferior pole of the scapula (*1*), through the medial extent of the spine of the scapula (*2*), and halfway between the coracoid tip (*4*) and the posterior angle of the acromion (*3*). **B,** The glenoid center line lies laterally approximately 10 degrees (α) posterior to this plane and perpendicular to the line connecting the inferior pole and the medial spine (the scapular reference line). (From Matsen FA III, Lippitt SB. *Shoulder Surgery: Principles and Procedures.* Philadelphia: WB Saunders; 2004:89.)

line usually points a few degrees posterior to the plane of the scapula (see Fig. 13-43). Changing the version of the glenoid articular surface imposes a corresponding change in the humeroscapular positions in which the net humeral joint reaction force will be contained by the effective glenoid arc. Glenoid version may be altered by glenoid dysplasia (Fig. 13-47),[707] glenoid osteotomy,[438,707] or glenoid arthroplasty.[691] Abnormal glenoid version positions the glenoid fossa in an abnormal relationship to the forces generated by the scapulohumeral muscles and changes the intrinsic stability provided by the glenoid concavity (Fig. 13-48). Normalization of abnormal glenoid version is often a critical step in glenohumeral reconstruction.

Apparent changes in glenoid version can arise from loss of part of the glenoid rim (see Figs. 13-34 and 13-38).[79,293,556] Dias et al. found no difference in apparent glenoid version between normal subjects and recurrent anterior dislocators.[151] Dowdy and O'Driscoll[160] found only minor variance in radiographic glenoid version among patients with and without recurrence after stabilization surgery. However, Hirschfelder and Kirsten[275] detected increased glenoid retroversion in both the symptomatic and asymptomatic shoulders of patients with posterior instability, and Grasshoff et al.[224] found increased anteversion in shoulders with recurrent anterior instability. The dominant shoulder of throwing athletes has been shown to have an average of 17 degrees of retroversion of the humeral head and 3 degrees of retroversion of the glenoid.[129] A cadaveric study by Churchill et al. demonstrated that black men and women have less glenoid retroversion than do white men and women: 0.2 and 2.65 degrees, respectively.[109] No significant difference was found between men and women. Patients with posterior instability were found to be more likely to have

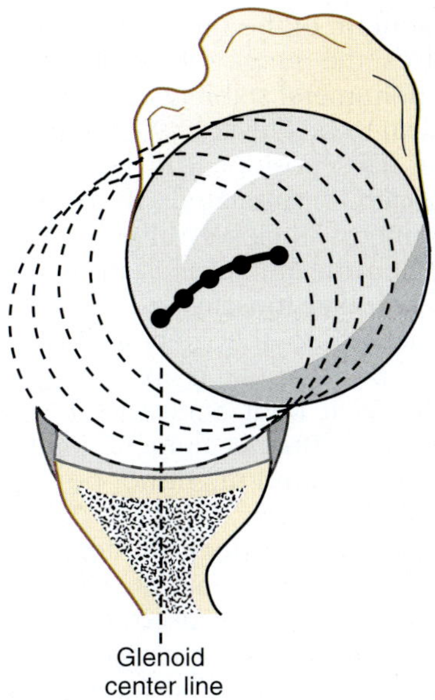

FIGURE 13-44: Glenoidogram. The glenoidogram is the path taken by the center of the humeral head as it translates across the face of the glenoid in a specified direction away from the glenoid center line. The height of the glenoidogram reflects the amount of work needed to dislocate the humeral head for a given compressive load. (From Matsen FA III, Lippitt SB. *Shoulder Surgery: Principles and Procedures*. Philadelphia: WB Saunders; 2004:100.)

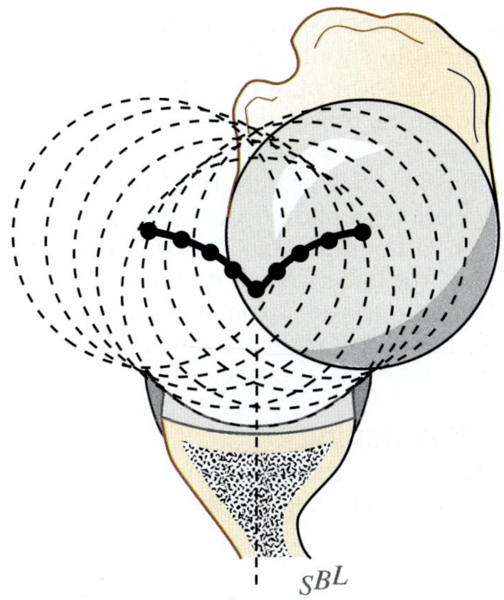

FIGURE 13-45: Paired glenoidograms. When the glenoidograms in two opposite directions are similar, they form a gull-wing shape together. The most stable position for the humeral head is that in which the two halves of the gull wing come together: at the center of the glenoid. (From Matsen FA III, Lippitt SB. *Shoulder Surgery: Principles and Procedures*. Philadelphia: WB Saunders; 2004:101.)

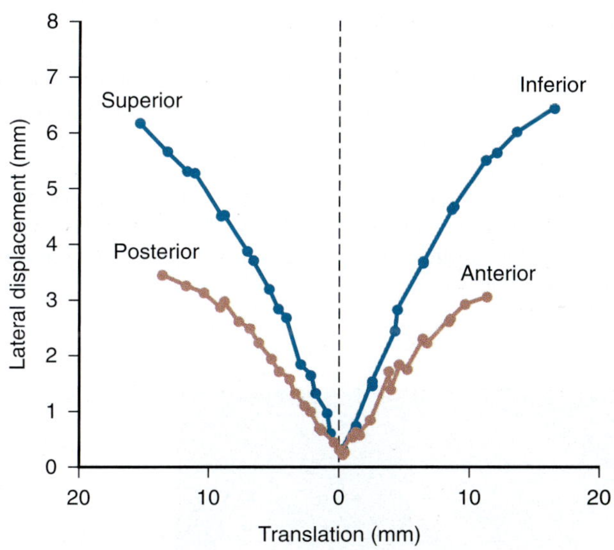

FIGURE 13-46: Measured glenoidograms for four different directions of translation in a young cadaver shoulder. The *dotted vertical line* represents the glenoid center line. The effective glenoid depth in this shoulder was 3.4 mm for translation in the posterior direction, 3.2 mm in the anterior direction, 6.2 mm in the superior direction, and 6.4 mm in the inferior direction. Note the high degree of symmetry about the glenoid center line and the deep valley when the head is exactly centered in the glenoid socket. (From Matsen FA III, Lippitt SB, Sidles JA, Harryman DT II. *Practical Evaluation and Management of the Shoulder*. Philadelphia: WB Saunders; 1994.)

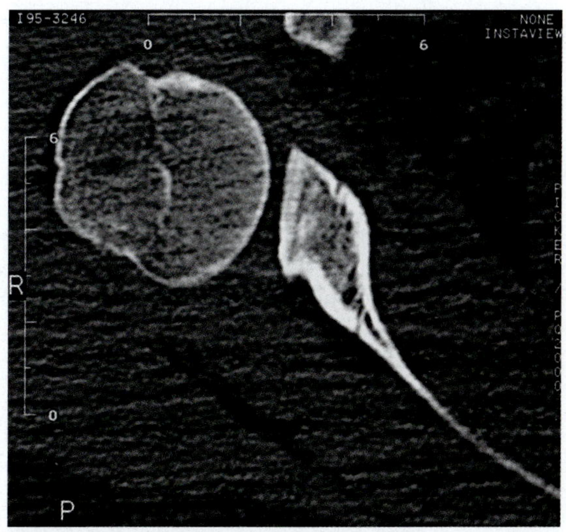

FIGURE 13-47: Computed tomographic scan of a shoulder with glenoid dysplasia manifested as absence of the posterior glenoid lip and glenoid retroversion. When the glenoid rim is hypoplastic, it cannot contribute normally to the glenoidogram.

glenoid rim deficiency than were those with normal or anteriorly unstable shoulders.[690]

Changes in version may be difficult to quantitate on axillary radiographs unless the view is carefully standardized (Fig. 13-49). Even with optimal radiographic technique, the important contributions of cartilage and labrum to the depth and orientation of the fossa[289,629] cannot be seen on plain radiographs or CT scans. When it is important to know the orientation of the cartilaginous joint surface in relation to the scapular body, a CT arthrogram or MRI may be necessary.

Scapular Positioning

A special feature of the glenohumeral joint is that the glenoid can be positioned on the thorax (in contrast to the fixed acetabulum of the hip). This scapular alignment greatly increases the range of positions in which the criteria for glenohumeral stability can be met (Fig. 13-50). Consider the arm to be elevated 90 degrees in the sagittal thoracic plane. This position can be achieved with the scapula protracted or retracted. If the scapula is protracted, the humerus is closely aligned with the glenoid center line. When the humerus is in this position, most of the humeroscapular muscles are oriented to compress the humeral head into the glenoid fossa (Fig. 13-51). Alternatively, if the scapula is maximally retracted, the humerus is almost at right angles to the glenoid center line. In this position, the net humeral joint reaction force is directed posteriorly and might not be contained within the balance stability angle.[75,216,299,517,629,680]

Scapular position also affects the tension in the glenohumeral capsule and ligaments (see Fig. 13-20). Which humeroscapular position is used to achieve a given humerothoracic position is a question of habit and training. Coordination of scapular position and glenohumeral muscle balance is an important element of the neuromuscular control of glenohumeral stability.

Atwater[24] has documented that in most throwing and striking skills, the shoulder abduction angle is usually 100 degrees. Higher and lower release points are achieved by tilting the trunk rather than by increasing or decreasing the shoulder abduction angle relative to the trunk.

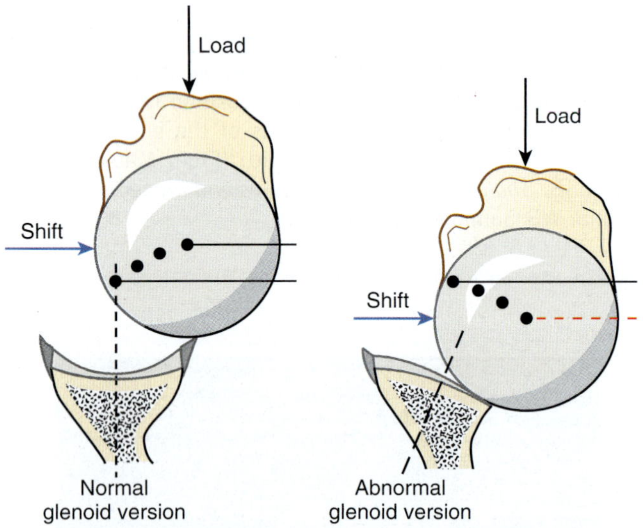

FIGURE 13-48: Glenoid hypoplasia. When the glenoid rim is hypoplastic, it cannot contribute normally to the glenoidogram. (From Matsen FA III, Lippitt SB. *Shoulder Surgery: Principles and Procedures*. Philadelphia: WB Saunders; 2004:111.)

Ligaments

Normally stable shoulders can demonstrate substantial laxity; consider the very lax but very stable glenohumeral joints of gymnasts. In a most important study, Emery and Mullaji[169] found that of 150 asymptomatic shoulders in schoolchildren, 50% demonstrated positive signs of increased laxity.

Some investigators have found increased laxity in patients with glenohumeral instability.[117,314,315,325,407] However, other studies suggest that these differences are not always significant.[246,389,414,631]

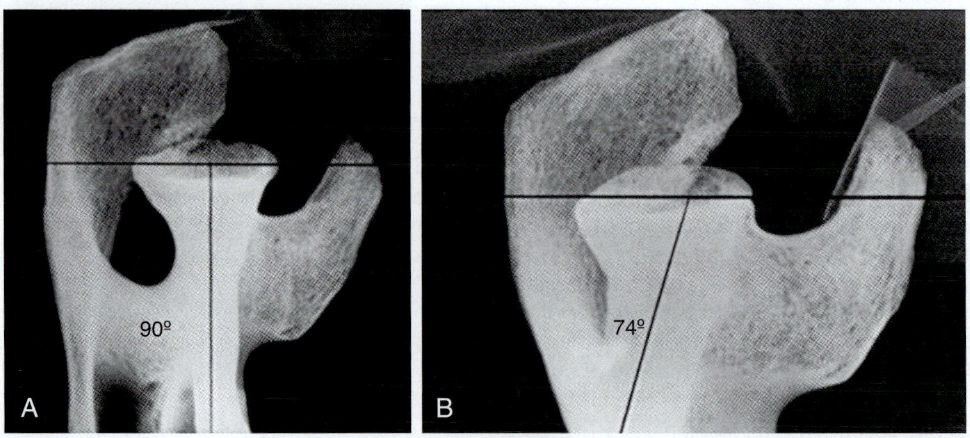

FIGURE 13-49: Two radiographs of the same cadaver scapula showing the variation in apparent glenoid retroversion, depending on the radiographic projection. **A,** Proper orientation. **B,** Oblique orientation.

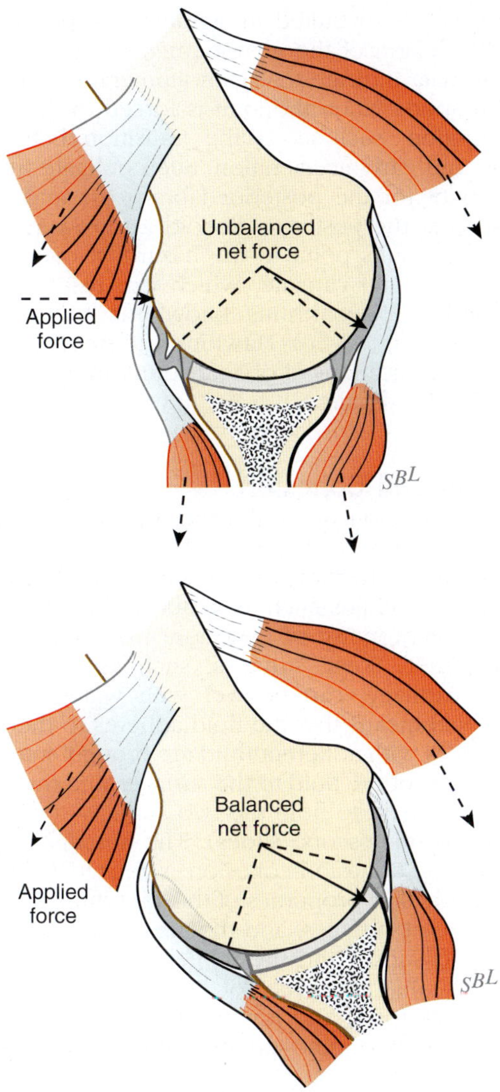

FIGURE 13-50: *Top,* Applied force results in an unbalanced net force. *Bottom,* Stabilization against an applied translational force by repositioning the glenoid concavity to support the net humeral force.

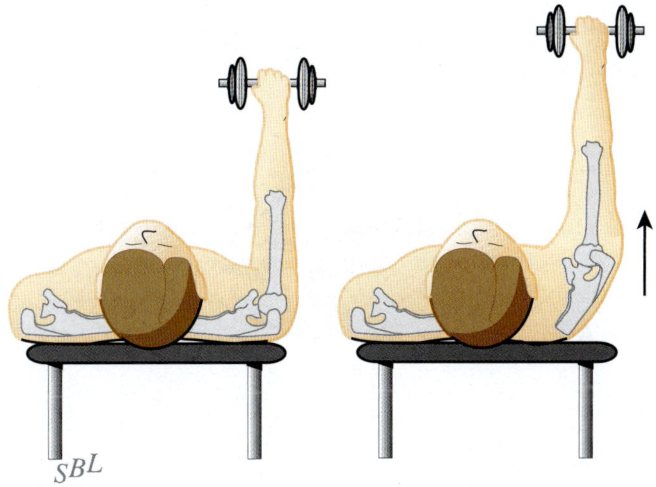

FIGURE 13-51: The glenoid can be moved to support the net humeral joint reaction force. Protraction of the scapula, as in the bench press, places the glenoid fossa squarely beneath the force exerted on it by the loaded humerus. (From Matsen FA III, Lippitt SB. *Shoulder Surgery: Principles and Procedures*. Philadelphia: WB Saunders; 2004:91.)

Biochemical composition (as in Ehlers-Danlos syndrome), anatomic variation (anomalies of attachment), use (or disuse), age, disease (e.g., diabetes, frozen shoulder), injury, and surgery (e.g., capsulorrhaphy) can affect the strength, laxity, and stretchiness of glenohumeral ligaments. See reviews of the material properties of IGHL by Mow et al.[412] (Chapter 2) and the role of ligaments in glenohumeral stability by Lew et al (Chapter 3).[412]

The glenohumeral ligaments serve as *checkreins* in which the range of joint positions is restricted to those that can be stabilized by muscle balance. This function is important because at extreme glenohumeral positions, the net humeral joint reaction force becomes increasingly difficult to balance within the glenoid (Fig. 13-52). For example, excessive abduction, extension, and external rotation of the shoulder may allow the net humeral joint reaction force vector to point beyond the anterior-inferior balance stability angle. Similarly, excessive posterior capsular laxity allows the net humeral joint reaction force to achieve large angles with the glenoid center line; these angles can exceed the posterior balance stability angle. At the extremes of motion, the muscles tend to be near their maximal extension, a position in which their force-generating capacity is diminished.[384] In these positions where muscles are disadvantaged, ligamentous forces can provide the necessary compression (Fig. 13-53).

Bigliani et al.[57] noted in 16 cadaver shoulders that IGHL could be divided into three anatomic regions: a superior band, an anterior axillary pouch, and a posterior axillary pouch, the thickest of which was the superior band (2.8 mm). With relatively low strain rates, the stress at failure was found to be nearly identical for the three regions of the ligament, an average of 5.5 mPa, which is 5.5 N/mm^2. The glenoid insertion was the most common site of failure, suggesting an analogy to the Bankart lesion, and significant capsular stretching occurred before failure, offering an analogy to capsular laxity seen clinically. This group has also shown that subfailure cyclic loading (simulating repetitive overhead sports) leads to irreversible glenohumeral ligament elongation.[545]

Excessive ligament tension can produce obligate translation of the humeral head. Harryman et al.[244] demonstrated that certain passive motions of the glenohumeral joint forced translation of the humeral head away from the center of the joint. This obligate translation occurs when the displacing force generated by ligament tension (quantity P in Fig. 13-54) overwhelms the concavity compression stability mechanism (Fig. 13-55). In Harryman's study, anterior humeral translation occurred at the extremes of flexion and cross-body adduction, whereas posterior humeral translation occurred at the extremes of

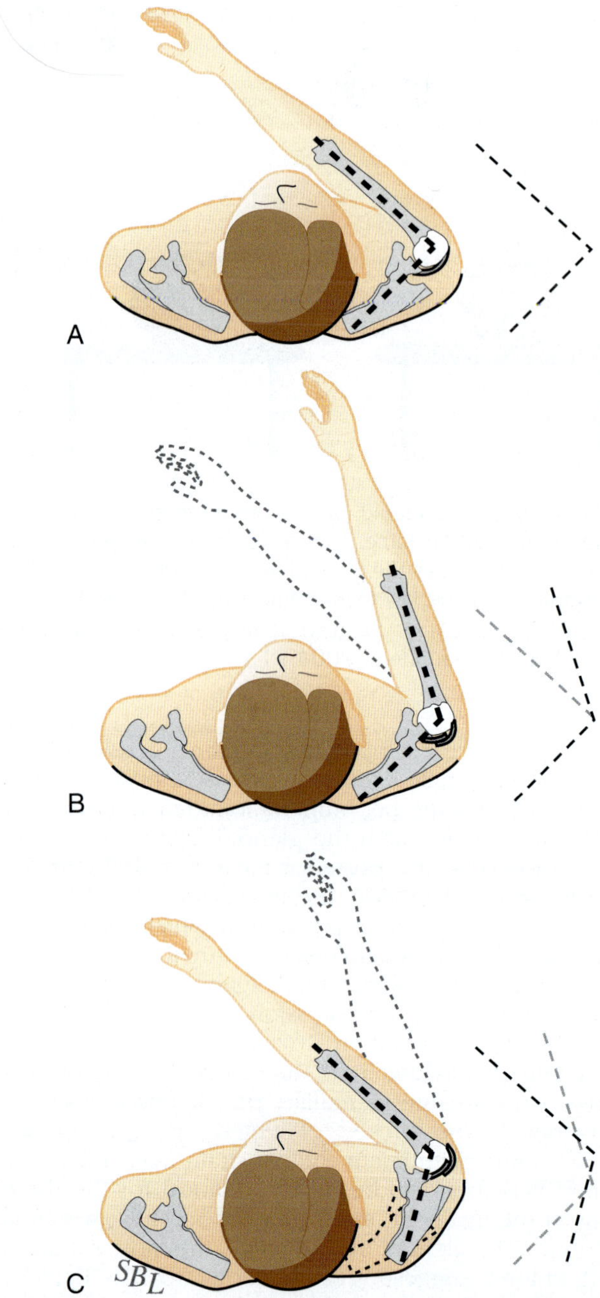

FIGURE 13-52: **A,** Excessive posterior capsular laxity allows an excessively small angle between the humerus and the plane of the scapula; as a result, posterior stability is challenged. **B,** Normal tightness appropriately limits the allowed angular position to the range that can be stabilized. **C,** Cross-body adduction is achieved by scapular protraction as well as by humeroscapular angulation.

extension and external rotation. Operative tightening of the posterior portion of the capsule increased anterior translation on flexion and cross-body adduction and caused it to occur earlier in the arc of motion than in an intact joint. Operative tightening of the posterior part of the capsule also resulted in significant superior translation with flexion of the glenohumeral joint.

These data indicate that glenohumeral translation can occur in sports when the joint is forced to the extremes of its motion, such as at the transition between late cocking and early acceleration. Such obligate translation can account for the posterior labral tears and calcifications seen at the posterior glenoid in throwers. In addition, these results point to the hazard of overtightening the glenohumeral capsule, which can result in a form of secondary osteoarthritis known as *capsulorrhaphy arthropathy* (Fig. 13-56). Hawkins and Angelo[250] pointed to these complications of obligate translation in overtightened capsular repairs.

Adhesion and Cohesion

Adhesion-cohesion is a stabilizing mechanism by which joint surfaces wet with joint fluid are held together by the molecular attraction of the fluid to itself and to the joint surfaces. Fluids such as water and joint fluid demonstrate the property of cohesion; that is, they tend to stick together. Some surfaces, such as clean glass or articular cartilage, can be wet with water or synovial fluid, which means that the fluid adheres to them. When two surfaces with adherent fluid are brought into contact, the adhesion of the fluid to the surfaces and the cohesion of the fluids tend to hold the two surfaces together (like two wetted microscope slides). The amount of stability generated by adhesion-cohesion is related to the adhesive and cohesive properties of the joint fluid, the wetability of the joint surfaces, and the area of contact between the glenoid socket and the humerus. Joint fluid has the highly desirable properties of high tensile strength (difficult to pull apart) and low shear strength (allows easy sliding of the two joint surfaces on each other with low resistance).[620]

The adhesion-cohesion effect is reduced by any factor that lowers the cohesion of joint fluid (such as in inflammatory joint disease), reduces wetability of the joint surfaces (as can occur in degenerative joint disease), or diminishes the glenohumeral contact area (such as in a displaced articular surface fracture or a congenitally small glenoid). It is also noteworthy that adhesion-cohesion forces do not stabilize a prosthetic shoulder replacement because metal and polyethylene are insufficiently compliant to provide the necessary nearly perfect congruence and because water does not adhere to their surfaces.

Glenohumeral Suction Cup

The glenohumeral suction cup provides stability by virtue of the seal of the labrum and capsule to the humeral head (Fig. 13-57). A suction cup adheres to a smooth surface by expressing the interposed air or fluid and then forming a seal with the surface. A rubber suction cup is noncompliant in the center but becomes more flexible toward its periphery. In a similar manner, the center of the glenoid is covered with a relatively thin layer of articular cartilage. At greater distances from the center,

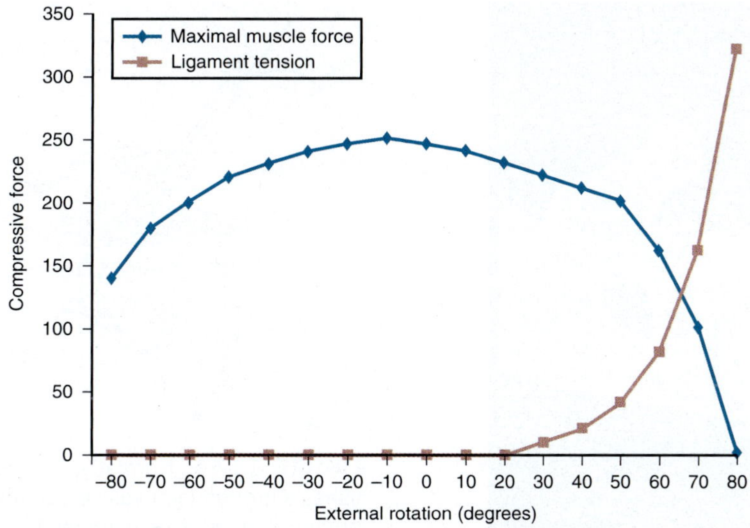

FIGURE 13-53: Hypothetical graph showing the interplay between muscular and capsular tension. As the humerus is passively externally rotated, the force that the subscapularis can generate drops off and the force generated by the anterior capsular ligaments increases in a complementary manner. (From Matsen FA III, Chebli C, Lippitt S. Principles for the evaluation and management of shoulder instability. *J Bone Joint Surg Am.* 2006;88:648-659.)

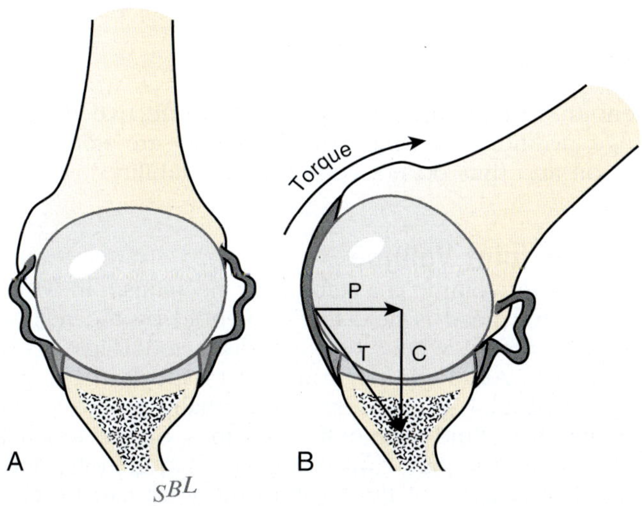

FIGURE 13-54: **A,** When the glenohumeral ligaments are slack, they exert no force. **B,** When torque is applied, the ligaments come under tension (*T*). This ligament tension exerts a compressive force (*C*) directed into the glenoid and a displacing force (*P*) pushing the humeral head away from the tight ligament.

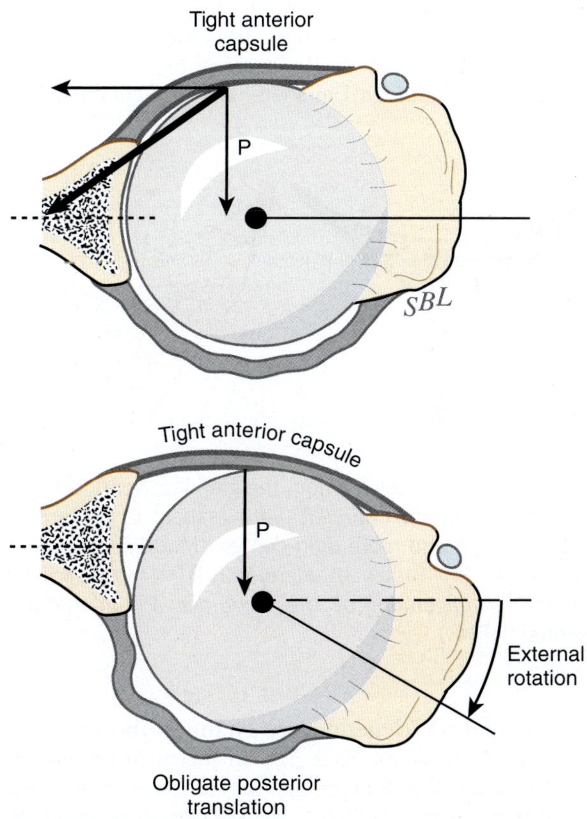

FIGURE 13-55: If the humerus is rotated beyond the point at which the ligaments become tight, the displacing force (*P*) can push the humeral head out of the glenoid center, a phenomenon known as *obligate translation.* (Modified from Matsen FA III, Lippitt SB, Sidles JA, Harryman DT II. *Practical Evaluation and Management of the Shoulder.* Philadelphia: WB Saunders; 1994.)

the articular cartilage becomes thicker and thus provides greater flexibility. More peripherally, the glenoid labrum and, finally, the capsule provide even more flexibility. This graduated flexibility permits the socket to conform and seal to the smooth humeral articular surface. Compression of the head into the glenoid fossa expels any intervening fluid so that a suction is produced that resists distraction.

The glenoid suction cup stabilization mechanism was demonstrated by Harryman et al.[390] In elderly cadaver

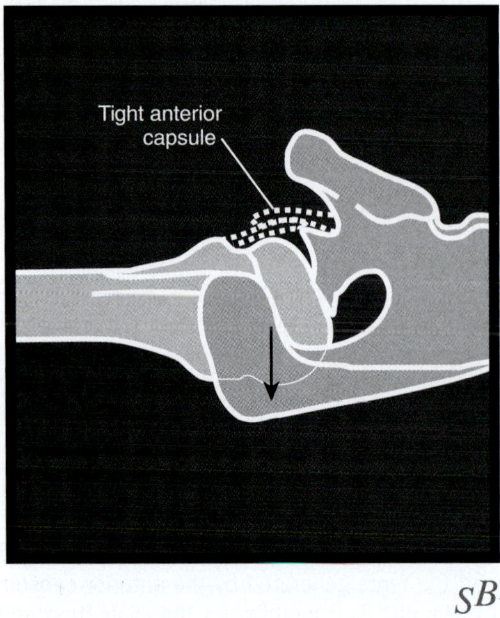

FIGURE 13-56: Axillary view of capsulorrhaphy arthropathy in which an excessively tight anterior capsular repair is forcing the head of the humerus posteriorly (*arrow*). This effect is accentuated by forced external rotation. Note also the typical posterior glenoid erosion. (Modified from Matsen FA III, Lippitt SB, Sidles JA, Harryman DT II. *Practical Evaluation and Management of the Shoulder*. Philadelphia: WB Saunders; 1994.)

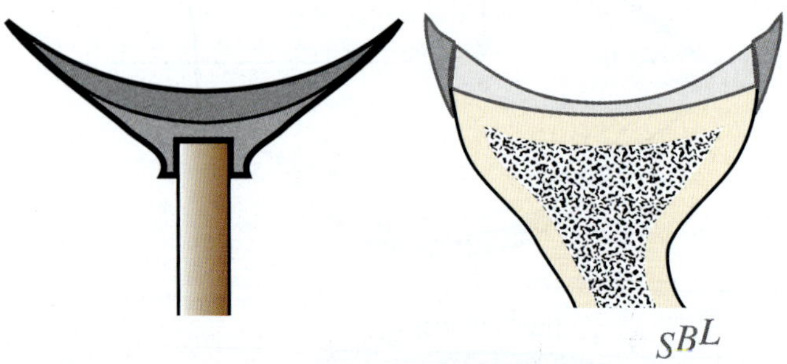

FIGURE 13-57: In cross section, the glenoid (*right*) looks much like a rubber suction cup (*left*) with respect to its feathered, compliant edges and more rigid center. (Modified from Matsen FA III, Lippitt SB, Sidles JA, Harryman DT II. *Practical Evaluation and Management of the Shoulder*. Philadelphia: WB Saunders; 1994.)

shoulders without degenerative changes, the suction cup resisted an average of 20 ± 3 N of lateral traction (about 4 lb). Creating a defect in the labrum completely eliminated the suction cup effect. No suction cup effect could be demonstrated in the two shoulders with mild degenerative change of the joint surface. This effect would likely be even stronger in younger living shoulders in which the articular cartilage, glenoid labrum, and joint capsule are larger, more hydrated, and more compliant. Like stabilization from adhesion-cohesion, the glenoid suction cup centers the head of the humerus in the

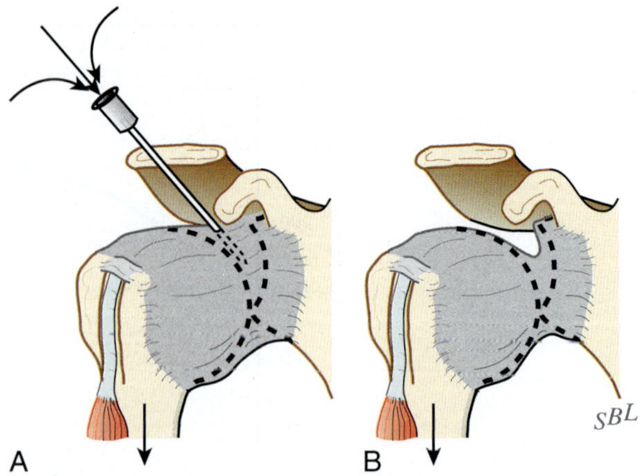

FIGURE 13-58: Normally, the glenohumeral capsule establishes a limited joint volume, so distraction of the humeral head produces a relative vacuum within the capsule that resists further displacement. **A,** Venting of the capsule eliminates the limited joint volume effect. **B,** The limited joint volume effect is reduced if the capsule is excessively compliant and can be displaced into the joint. (From Matsen FA III, Lippitt SB, Sidles JA, Harryman DT II. *Practical Evaluation and Management of the Shoulder*. Philadelphia: WB Saunders; 1994.)

glenoid without muscle action and is effective in midrange positions in which the ligaments are not under tension and thus do not contribute to stability.

Limited Joint Volume

Limited joint volume is a stabilizing mechanism in which the humeral head is held to the glenoid by the relative vacuum created when they are distracted (Figs. 13-58 and 13-59). Although it is common to speak of the glenohumeral joint space, there is essentially no space and minimal free fluid within the confines of the articular surfaces and the joint capsule of a normal glenohumeral joint. The scarcity of fluid within the joint can be confirmed on MRI of normal joints, on inspection of normal joints, and on attempts to aspirate fluid from normal joints. The appearance of the *potential* joint volume can only be demonstrated after instilling fluids such as air, saline, or contrast material into the joint. Osmotic action by the synovium removes free fluid, thus keeping slightly negative pressure within a normal joint.[620,380,463] This negative intra-articular pressure holds the joint together with a force proportional to the joint surface area and the magnitude of the negative intra-articular pressure. For example, if the colloid osmotic pressure of normal synovial fluid is 10 mm Hg and the colloid osmotic pressure of the synovial interstitium is 14 mm Hg, the equilibrium pressure in the joint fluid will be −4 mm Hg.[620] This negative intra-articular pressure adds a small amount of resistance to distraction (about 1 oz/in^2) to the limited joint volume effect. Because a normal joint is sealed, attempted distraction of the joint surfaces

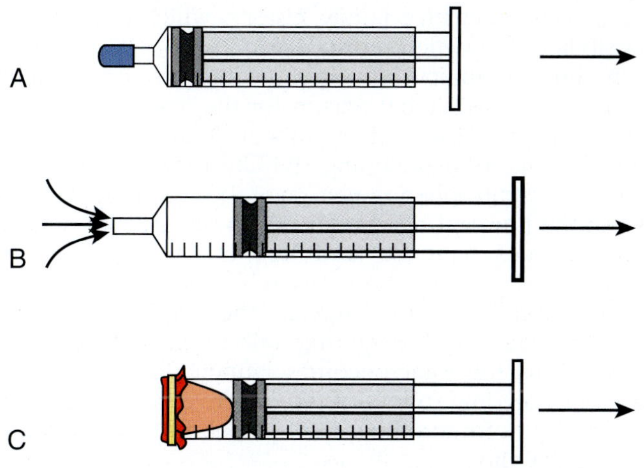

FIGURE 13-59: Limited joint volume effect demonstrated with a syringe model. Substantial force is required to pull the plunger from a plugged syringe (**A**). This stabilizing effect is lost if the syringe is uncapped (**B**) or if the end of the syringe is covered with compliant material (**C**). (From Matsen FA III, Lippitt SB, Sidles JA, Harryman DT II. *Practical Evaluation and Management of the Shoulder.* Philadelphia: WB Saunders; 1994.)

lowers the intra-articular pressure even more, thereby progressively adding substantial resistance to greater displacement.[243,304]

The limited joint volume effect is reduced if the joint is vented (opened to the atmosphere) or the capsular boundaries of the joint are very compliant. In the latter circumstance, attempted distraction draws the flexible capsule into the joint and produces a sulcus (see Figs. 13-58 and 13-59). The decreased stability from venting the joint was initially described by Humphry in 1858[292] and subsequently by others.[125,178,353,471,514,515,649,650,714] Gibb et al.[414,210] found that simply venting the capsule with an 18-gauge needle reduced the force necessary to translate the head of the humerus halfway to the edge of the glenoid by an average of 50%. Wulker et al.[715] found that venting the joint increased displacement of the joint with an applied load of 50 N by 50% in all directions.

From these results, it is expected that glenohumeral stability from limited joint volume is compromised by arthrography, arthroscopy, articular effusions, hemarthrosis, and other situations in which free fluid is allowed to enter the glenohumeral joint. In a very interesting study, Habermeyer et al.[234,235] found that the mean stabilizing force obtained by atmospheric pressure was 146 N (32 lb). In 15 stable, living shoulders, traction on the arm caused negative intra-articular pressure proportionate to the amount of force exerted. In contrast, unstable shoulder joints with a Bankart lesion did not exhibit this phenomenon.

These stabilizing mechanisms may be overwhelmed by the application of traction, as in cracking of the metacarpophalangeal joint. A crack is produced as the joint cavitates: subatmospheric pressure within the joint releases gas (>80% CO_2) from solution in the joint fluid. This release of gas is accompanied by a sudden increase in separation of the joint surfaces. Once a joint has cracked, it cannot be cracked again until about 20 minutes later when all the gas has been reabsorbed.[579,665]

TYPES OF GLENOHUMERAL INSTABILITY

Glenohumeral instability is an inability of the humeral head to remain centered in the glenoid fossa.[414,412] It is not the same as laxity, which is a physical finding often unassociated with clinical instability. As demonstrated by Largacha et al.,[362] glenohumeral instability is most commonly a functional disability and rarely a cause of pain in the absence of obvious functional difficulties. Clinical cases of instability can be characterized according to the circumstances under which they occur, the degree of instability, and the direction of instability.

Circumstances of Instability

Congenital instability may result from local anomalies such as glenoid dysplasia[704] or from systemic conditions such as Ehlers-Danlos syndrome. Instability is acute if seen within the first days after its onset; otherwise it is *chronic*. A dislocation is *locked* (or fixed) if the humeral head has been impaled on the edge of the glenoid, thus making reduction of the dislocation difficult. If a glenohumeral joint has been unstable on many occasions, the instability is *recurrent*. Recurrent instability can consist of repeated glenohumeral dislocations, subluxations, or both.

Instability can arise from a *traumatic* episode in which an injury occurs to the bone, rotator cuff, labrum, capsule, or a combination of ligaments. Recurrent traumatic instability typically produces symptoms when the arm is placed in a position near that of the original injury. Conversely, instability can arise from *atraumatic* decompensation of the stabilizing mechanisms.

Matsen has proposed that most patients with recurrent instability fall into one of two groups. On one hand, patients with a ***traumatic*** etiology usually have ***unidirectional*** instability, often have obvious pathology such as a ***Bankart*** lesion, and often require ***surgery*** when the instability is recurrent, thus the acronym TUBS. On the other hand, patients with ***atraumatic*** instability often have ***multidirectional*** laxity that is commonly ***bilateral*** and usually responds to a ***rehabilitation*** program. However, should surgery be performed, the surgeon must pay particular attention to performing an ***inferior*** capsular shift and closing the rotator ***interval***, thus the acronym AMBRII. Rowe[582] carefully analyzed 500 dislocations of the glenohumeral joint and determined that 96% were traumatic (caused by a major injury) and the remaining 4% were atraumatic. DePalma,[146] Rockwood,[571] and Collins and Wilde[119] also recognized the importance of distinguishing between traumatic and atraumatic instability of the shoulder.

In addition to major trauma and congenital laxity, Neer emphasized a third category of "acquired laxity," in which repetitive microtrauma from overhead use in gymnastics and sports results in gradual stretching of the capsule.[472,474] Trauma, congenital laxity, and acquired laxity are better thought of as etiologies of instability than as discrete patient groups. For example, a congenitally loose gymnast may further stretch his or her joint and also be injured by trauma. To use terminology pioneered by Matsen, the degree to which the shoulder was "torn loose" (traumatic) as opposed to "born loose" (atraumatic) or just "worn loose" (repetitive microtraumatic) is critical in determining the best management strategy.

Patients with atraumatic instability might have generalized joint laxity. Imazato[297] and Hirakawa[274] demonstrated that in patients with loose shoulders, the collagen fibers in the capsule, muscles, and skin are relatively immature, more soluble, and less cross-linked than those in controls; presumably, tissues such as the glenoid labrum contain immature collagen as well, thus making them more deformable under load but less likely to tear. Further evidence of constitutional factors is gained from numerous reports of positive family histories and bilateral involvement in patients with shoulder dislocations (Fig. 13-60). O'Driscoll and Evans[503] and Dowdy and O'Driscoll[159] found a family history of shoulder instability in 24% of patients who required surgery for anterior glenohumeral instability. Morrey and Janes[456] reported a positive family history in approximately 15% of patients who were operated on for recurrent anterior shoulder instability. A positive family history was also noted twice as often in patients whose postoperative course was complicated by recurrent instability as in those with successful surgery. Rowe et al.[585] reported a positive family history in 27% of 55 patients with anterior shoulder instability who were treated with a Bankart procedure. Bilateral instability was noted in 50% of patients with a positive family history versus 26% of those with a negative family history, which suggests the possibility of genetic predisposition.

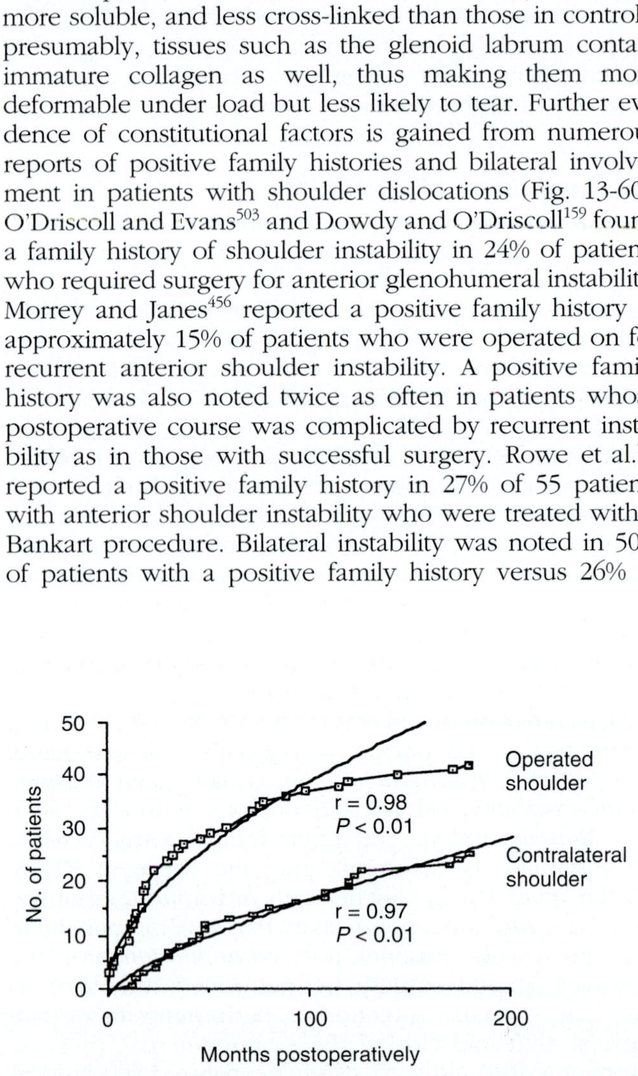

FIGURE 13-60: Incidence of contralateral shoulder instability from the data of O'Driscoll and Evans. In 13% of the patients with normal contralateral shoulders at the time of surgery, contralateral instability developed within the next 15 years. (From O'Driscoll SW, Evans DC. The DuToit staple capsulorrhaphy for recurrent anterior dislocation of the shoulder: Twenty years of experience in six Toronto hospitals. Presented at American Shoulder and Elbow Surgeons 4th Open Meeting; March 1988; Atlanta, GA.)

When instability develops with no or minimal injury,[205,550,589] the initial reason for the loss of stability is often unclear. However, it appears that once they are lost, the factors maintaining stability may be difficult to regain. Certain phenomena may be self-perpetuating: When the humeral head rides up on the glenoid rim, the rim becomes flattened and less effective and allows easier translation. Furthermore, when normal neuromuscular control is compromised, the feedback systems that maintain head centering fail to provide effective input. Thus the joint becomes launched on a cycle of instability leading to loss of the effective glenoid concavity and loss of neuromuscular control, further leading to more instability.

If a patient intentionally subluxates or dislocates the shoulder, the instability is described as *voluntary*. If the instability occurs unintentionally, it is *involuntary*. Voluntary anterior dislocation can occur with the arm at the side or in abduction and external rotation. Voluntary posterior dislocation can occur with the arm in flexion, adduction and internal rotation or with the arm at the side. The association of voluntary dislocation of the shoulder with psychiatric disorders has been noted by several authors (Figs. 13-61 and 13-62).[96,586] The desire to voluntarily dislocate the shoulder cannot be treated surgically. However, the fact that patients can voluntarily demonstrate their instability by putting their arum in an at-risk position (positional voluntary) does not necessarily mean that they are psychologically impaired. However, if the instability is produced at will by asymmetric muscle contraction (muscular voluntary), caution should be exercised.

Neuromuscular causes of shoulder instability have been reported as well. Percy[538] described a patient in whom posterior dislocation developed after an episode of encephalitis. Kretzler and Blue[345] discussed the management of posterior dislocation of the shoulder in children with cerebral palsy. Sever,[615] Fairbank,[177] L'Episcopo,[375] Zachary,[727] and Wickstrom[695] reported techniques for the management of neurologic dislocation of the shoulder as a result of upper brachial plexus birth injuries. Stroke is another important neurologic cause of instability.[730] Seizures, including those from alcoholism, glucose imbalance, head injury, and intracranial neoplasms can cause glenohumeral instability, both from the uncontrolled muscle activity at the time of the seizure and afterwards from bone and soft tissue injuries caused by the seizure.

Degree of Instability

Recurrent instability may be characterized as dislocation, subluxation, or apprehension. *Dislocation* of the glenohumeral joint is complete separation of the articular surfaces; immediate, spontaneous relocation might not occur. Glenohumeral *subluxation* is defined as symptomatic translation of the humeral head on the glenoid without complete separation of the articular surfaces.

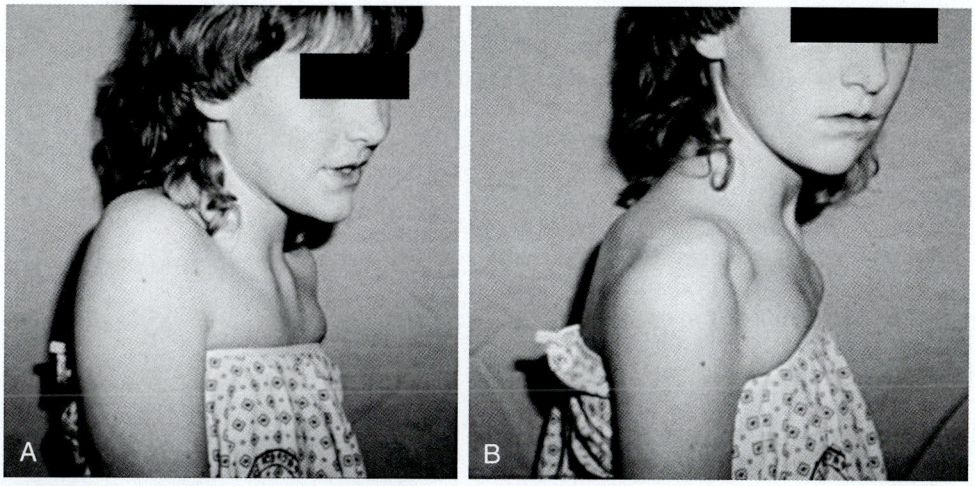

FIGURE 13-61: Voluntary instability. This patient had no significant history of injury but could voluntarily dislocate her shoulder with minimal discomfort. She is shown with the right shoulder reduced (**A**) and posteriorly dislocated (**B**).

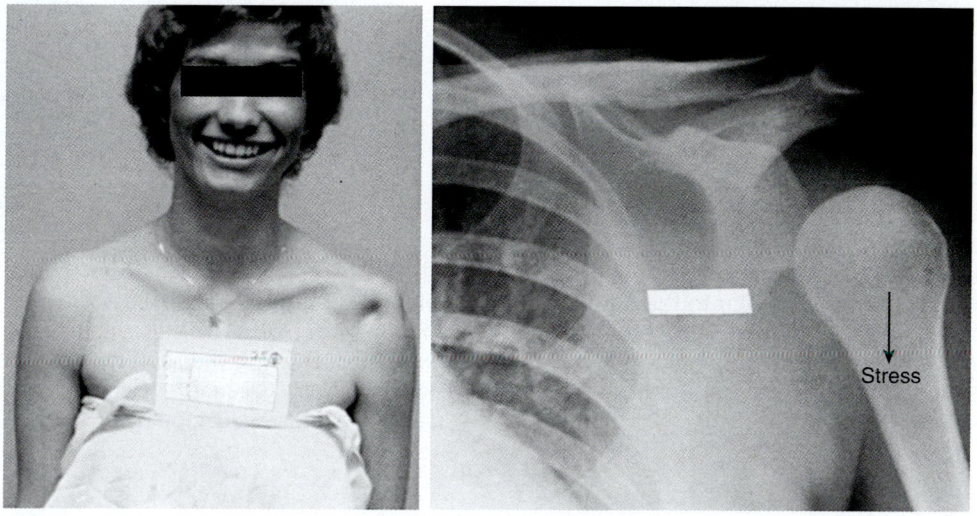

FIGURE 13-62: A patient with voluntary inferior instability. She performed this maneuver without discomfort. (From Rockwood CA, Green DP, eds. *Fractures*. 2nd ed. Philadelphia: JB Lippincott; 1984.)

Apprehension refers to the fear that the shoulder will subluxate or dislocate. This fear may prevent the person from participating fully in work or sports.

Subluxation of the glenohumeral joint is usually transient: the humeral head returns spontaneously to its normal position in the glenoid fossa. In a series of patients with anterior shoulder subluxation reported by Rowe and Zarins,[589] 87% of cases were traumatic, and more than 50% of patients were not aware that their shoulders were unstable. Like dislocations, subluxations may be traumatic or atraumatic; anterior, posterior, or inferior; or acute or recurrent; or they can occur after previous surgical repairs that did not achieve complete shoulder stability. Recurrent subluxations can coexist with or be initiated by glenohumeral dislocation. Rowe and Zarins[582,590] reported seeing a Hill-Sachs compression fracture in 40% of patients in their series on subluxation of the shoulder, an observation indicating that at some time these shoulders had been completely dislocated.

Traumatic Instability

Traumatic instability may have consequences beyond recurrent dislocation of the shoulder, including inability to return to work, inability to return to sport, or subsequent degenerative conditions. Nine percent of rugby players who stopped playing did so because of dislocation of the shoulder.[372] This figure was higher than the rate in players who abandoned rugby because of concussion (4%). The likelihood of glenohumeral arthrosis developing has been shown to be 10 to 20 times higher in patients who have had a shoulder dislocation.[410]

Direction of Instability

Dislocations of the shoulder account for approximately 45% of all dislocations.[331] Of these, almost 85% are anterior glenohumeral dislocations.[101]

Anterior Dislocations

Subcoracoid dislocation is the most common type of anterior dislocation. The usual mechanism of injury that causes a subcoracoid dislocation is a combination of shoulder abduction, extension, and external rotation producing forces that can challenge the anterior capsule and ligaments, the glenoid rim, and the rotator cuff mechanism. The head of the humerus is displaced anteriorly with respect to the glenoid and is inferior to the coracoid process (Fig. 13-63).

Other types of anterior dislocation include subglenoid (the head of the humerus lies anterior to and below the glenoid fossa), subclavicular (the head of the humerus lies medial to the coracoid process, just inferior to the lower border of the clavicle), intrathoracic (the head of the humerus lies between the ribs and the thoracic cavity) (Fig. 13-64),[214,459,534,628,692] and retroperitoneal (Figs. 13-65 and 13-66).[703] These rarer types of dislocation are usually associated with severe trauma and have a high incidence of fracture of the greater tuberosity of the humerus and rotator cuff avulsion. Neurologic, pulmonary, and vascular complications can occur, as can subcutaneous emphysema.

West[692] reported a case of intrathoracic dislocation in which on reduction, the humerus was felt to slip out of the chest cavity with a sensation similar to that of slipping a large cork from a bottle. His patient, who had an avulsion fracture of the greater tuberosity and no neurologic deficit, regained functional range of motion and returned to his job as a carpenter.

Posterior Dislocations

Posterior dislocations can leave the humeral head in a subacromial (head behind the glenoid and beneath the acromion), subglenoid (head behind and beneath the glenoid), or subspinous (head medial to the acromion and beneath the spine of the scapula) location. Subacromial dislocation is the most common by far (Fig. 13-67). Posterior dislocations are often locked. Hawkins et al.[255] reviewed 41 such cases related to motor vehicle accidents, surgery, and electroshock therapy.

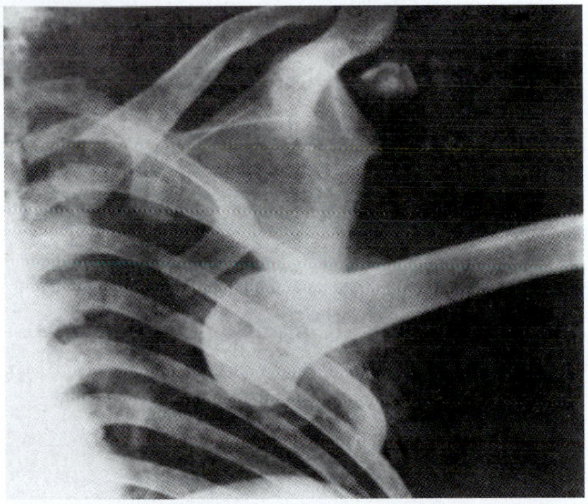

FIGURE 13-64: Intrathoracic anterior dislocation of the left shoulder. Note the wide interspace laterally between the third and fourth ribs and the avulsion fracture of the greater tuberosity, which remained in the vicinity of the glenoid fossa. (From Rockwood CA Jr, Green DP, Bucholz RW, eds. *Fractures in Adults*. Philadelphia: JB Lippincott; 1991.)

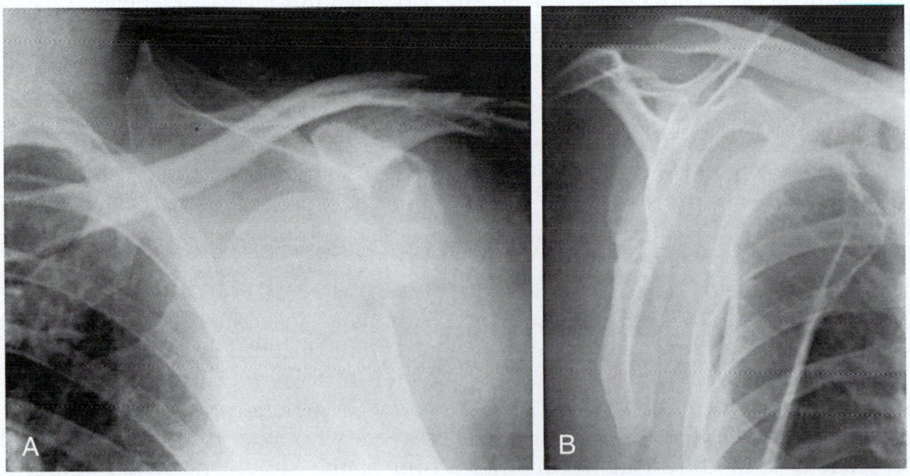

FIGURE 13-63: Subcoracoid dislocation. **A,** This anteroposterior view reveals that the head is medially displaced away from the glenoid fossa. With this view it is difficult to be sure whether the head is dislocated anteriorly or posteriorly. **B,** On a true scapular lateral view, the humeral head is completely anterior to the glenoid fossa. (From Rockwood CA, Green DP, eds. *Fractures*. 2nd ed. Philadelphia: JB Lippincott; 1984.)

Posterior instability is less common than anterior instability, with 1.1 occurring for every 100,000 people each year.[569] The overall incidence of posterior dislocations is estimated at 2% but is difficult to ascertain because of the frequency with which this diagnosis is missed. Thomas[647] reported seeing only four cases of posterior shoulder dislocation in 6000 radiographic examinations. The literature reflects that the diagnosis of posterior dislocation of the shoulder is missed in more than 60% of cases.[170,257,437,536,673] A 1982 article by Rowe and Zarins[590] indicated that the diagnosis was missed in 79% of cases. McLaughlin[425] stated that posterior shoulder dislocations are sufficiently uncommon that their occurrence creates a "diagnostic trap."

One of the largest series of posterior dislocations of the shoulder (37 cases) was recorded by Malgaigne[405] in 1855, 40 years before the discovery of x-rays. He and his colleagues made the diagnosis by performing a proper physical examination. Cooper[121] stated that the physical findings are so classic that he called it "an accident which cannot be mistaken."

Posterior dislocation can result from axial loading of an adducted, internally rotated arm,[449] from violent muscle contraction, or from electrical shock or convulsive seizures.[5,96,187,251,387,420,443,508,550,612] In the case of involuntary muscle contraction, the combined strength of the internal rotators (latissimus dorsi, pectoralis major, and subscapularis muscles) simply overwhelms the external rotators (infraspinatus and teres minor muscles) (Fig. 13-68). Heller et al. proposed a classification of posterior shoulder dislocations.[259]

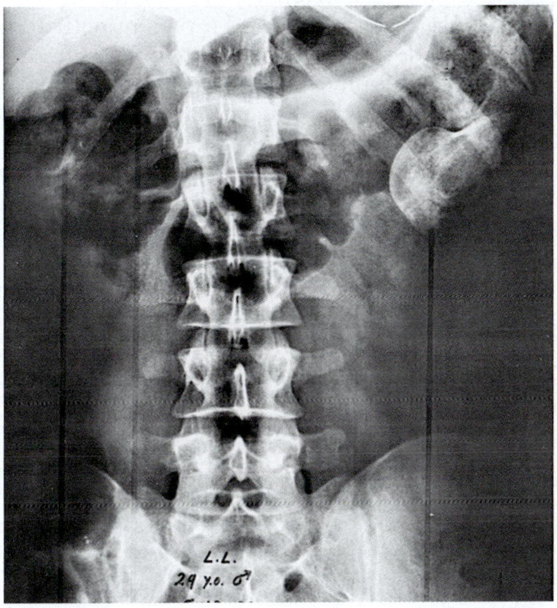

FIGURE 13-65: Abdominal radiograph revealing the proximal end of the humerus in the left upper quadrant.

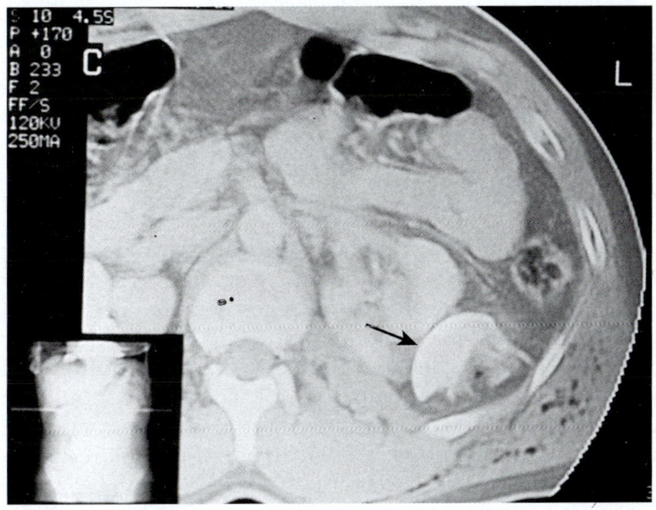

FIGURE 13-66: Enhanced computed tomographic scan of the abdomen. Note the retroperitoneal location of the humeral head posterior to the left kidney (*arrow*).

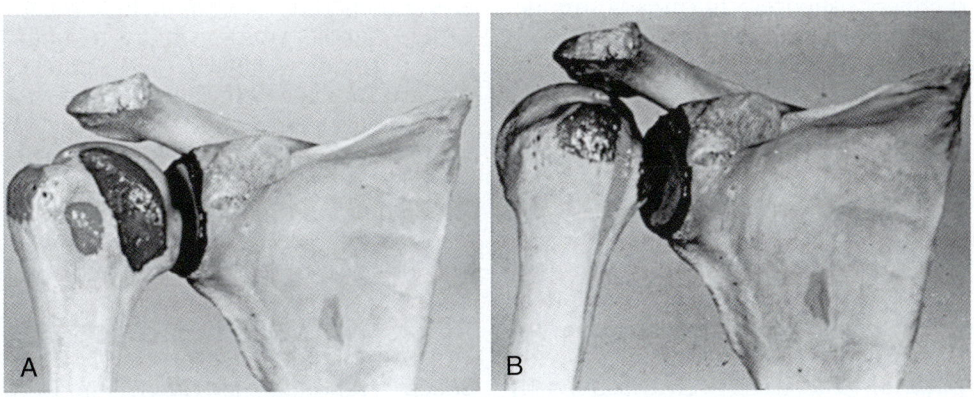

FIGURE 13-67: A subacromial posterior dislocation can appear deceptively normal on radiographs. **A,** Normal position of the humeral head in the glenoid fossa. **B,** In the subacromial type of posterior shoulder dislocation, the arm is in full internal rotation and the articular surface of the head is completely posterior, with only the lesser tuberosity left in the glenoid fossa. This positioning explains why abduction—and particularly external rotation—is blocked in posterior dislocations of the shoulder. (From Rockwood CA, Green DP, eds. *Fractures*. 2nd ed. Philadelphia: JB Lippincott; 1984.)

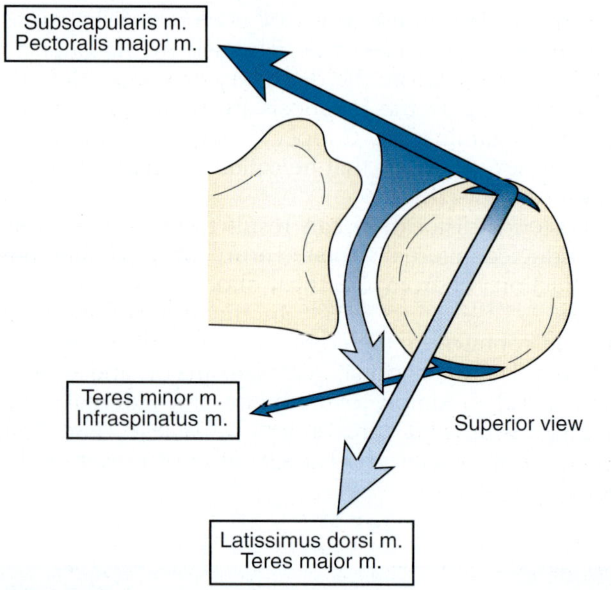

FIGURE 13-68: Mechanism of posterior dislocation of the shoulder caused by an accidental electrical shock or a convulsive seizure. The strong internal rotators simply overpower the weak external rotators.

Most traumatic "posterior dislocations" are actually impaction fractures of the anterior humeral articular surface from a fall, electroshock, or seizure. Because of the anterior impaction nature of the fracture, the posterior articular surface is left out the back of the glenohumeral joint. The nature of this injury indicates that it should be treated more like a fracture than a dislocation, with reduction and fixation or replacement of the injured fragments (Fig. 13-69).

After an overt, traumatic posterior shoulder dislocation, associated injuries occur in the majority of cases.[580] In addition to fracture, posterior labral tears, such as reverse Bankart lesions, posterosuperior tears, and posterior labrocapsular periosteal sleeve avulsions (POLPSA), are found in up to 58% of patients.[602] In cases of irreducible dislocation, MRI can identify interposed tissue, such as torn rotator cuff, avulsed capsule, or subluxed biceps tendon.[602]

Inferior Dislocations

The incidence of inferior shoulder dislocations is very low. Inferior dislocation of the glenohumeral joint was first described by Middeldorpf and Scharm[439] in 1859. Lynn[396] in 1921 carefully reviewed 34 cases, and Roca and Ramos-Vertiz[570] in 1962 reviewed 50 cases from the world literature. Laskin and Sedlin[363] reported a case in an infant. Three bilateral cases have been described by Murrard,[465] Langfritz,[361] and Peiro et al.[537] Nobel[490] reported a case of subglenoid dislocation in which the acromion-olecranon distance was shortened by 1.5 inches.

Inferior dislocation can be produced by a hyperabduction force that causes abutment of the neck of the humerus against the acromion process and subsequent leverage of the head out of the glenoid inferiorly (Figs. 13-70 to 13-73). The humerus is then locked with the head below the glenoid fossa and the humeral shaft pointing overhead, a condition called *luxatio erecta* (Fig. 13-74; see Figs. 13-70 to 13-73). The clinical picture of a patient with luxatio erecta is so clear that it can hardly be mistaken for any other condition. The humerus is locked in a position somewhere between 110 and 160 degrees of adduction (see Figs. 13-71 and 13-72). Severe soft tissue injury or fractures about the proximal end of the humerus occur with this dislocation (see Figs. 13-71 to 13-74). At the time of surgery or autopsy, various authors have found avulsion of the supraspinatus, pectoralis major, or teres minor muscles and fractures of the greater tuberosity.[350,363,396,439,465,570]

Neurovascular involvement is common.[202,379,396,434] Lev-El and Rubinstein[379] reported a patient with an injury to the axillary artery in whom a thrombus subsequently developed that required resection and a vein graft. Gardham and Scott[202] reported a case in 1980 in which the axillary artery was damaged in its third part and was managed with a bypass graft using the saphenous vein. Rockwood and Wirth found that in 19 patients with this condition, all 19 had a brachial plexus injury and some vascular compromise before reduction.

The force may be so great that it forces the head out through the soft tissues and skin. Lucas and Peterson[394] reported the case of a 16-year-old boy who caught his arm in the power takeoff of a tractor and suffered an open luxatio erecta injury.

Reduction of an inferior dislocation can often be accomplished by traction and countertraction maneuvers (Fig. 13-75). Acute reduction in the emergency department is accomplished with superior traction and a gradual decrease in abduction, or via conversion to an anterior dislocation with superior traction and forward manipulation. When closed reduction cannot be achieved, the buttonhole rent in the inferior capsule must be surgically enlarged before reduction can occur.

Common MRI findings in patients with a prior luxatio erecta humeri dislocation include rotator cuff tears, injury to the glenoid labrum, injury to both the anterior and posterior bands of IGHL, and humeral head contusions or focal cartilage defects in the antero-inferior glenoid.[349]

In a retrospective review spanning 42 years, 18 patients were identified with luxation erecta; half required only closed reduction as definitive treatment, while the other half required surgical treatment, usually for associated displaced humeral head fractures or for patients with a previous history of dislocation and recurrent instability.[227]

Superior Dislocations

Speed[630] reported that Langier, in 1834, was the first to record a case of superior dislocation of the glenohumeral joint; Stimson[638] reviewed 14 cases that had been reported in the literature before 1912. In the current literature, little is mentioned about this type of dislocation, but undoubtedly occasional cases do occur. The

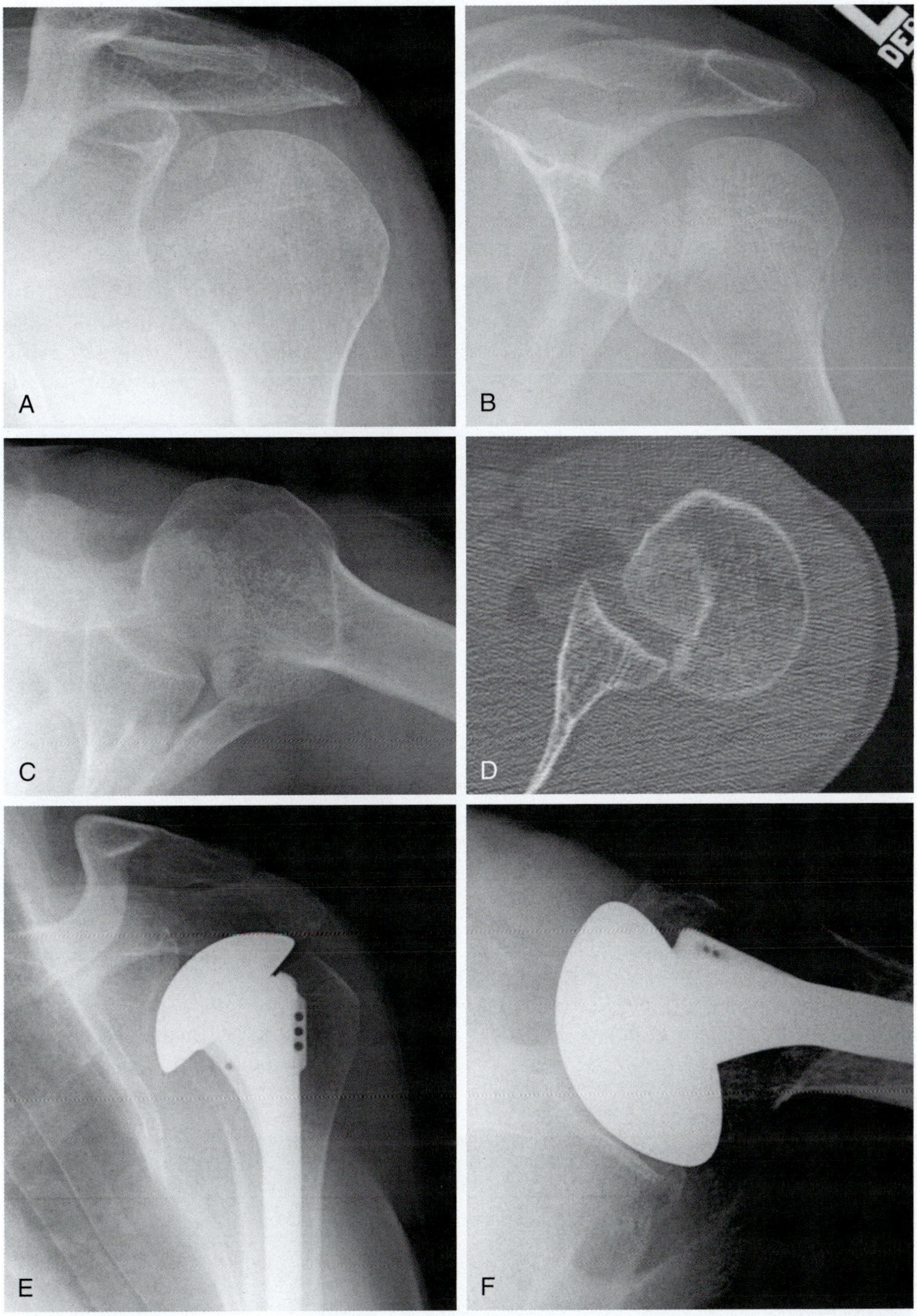

FIGURE 13-69: Images from a 40-year old cyclist who fell on the shoulder. Physical examination revealed an increased prominence of the coracoid anteriorly and inability to externally rotate the arm. **A,** Anteroposterior (AP) view showing reduced radiographic joint space and impaction fracture. **B,** AP view showing discontinuity of articular surface. **C,** Axillary view showing impaction fracture with intact articular surface posterior to the glenoid. **D,** Computed tomographic scan showing impaction of anterior articular surface with intact articular surface posterior to the glenoid. **E,** Postoperative AP view showing humeral head centered in the glenoid. **F,** Postoperative axillary view showing humeral prosthesis.

usual cause is an extreme forward and upward force on an adducted arm. With displacement of the humerus upward, fractures can occur in the acromion, acromioclavicular joint, clavicle, coracoid process, or humeral tuberosities (Fig. 13-76). Extreme soft tissue damage occurs to the capsule, rotator cuff, biceps tendon, and surrounding muscles. Clinically, the head rides above the level of the acromion. The arm is short and adducted to the side. Shoulder movement is restricted and quite painful, and neurovascular complications are usually present. Most cases of superior humeral translation are secondary to massive rotator cuff tears, which are not discussed in this chapter.

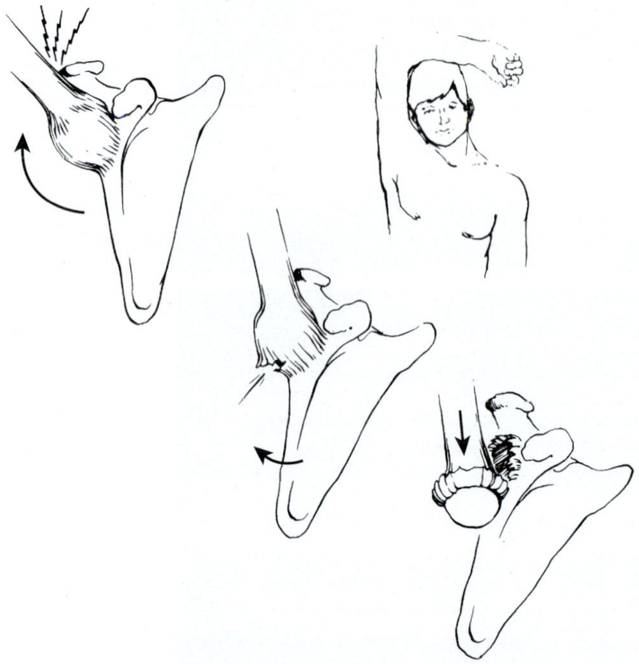

FIGURE 13-70: Mechanism of luxatio erecta. *Upper left,* With hyperabduction of the humerus, the shaft abuts the acromion process, which stresses and then tears the capsule inferiorly and levers the head out inferiorly. *Middle,* The head and neck may be buttonholed through a rent in the inferior capsule, or the entire capsule may be separated. *Lower right,* The rotator cuff muscles are always detached, and an associated fracture of the greater tuberosity may be present. (From Rockwood CA Jr, Green DP, Bucholz RW, eds. *Fractures in Adults.* Philadelphia: JB Lippincott; 1991.)

Bilateral Dislocations

Mynter[467] first described bilateral dislocation in 1902; according to Honner,[276] only 20 cases were reported

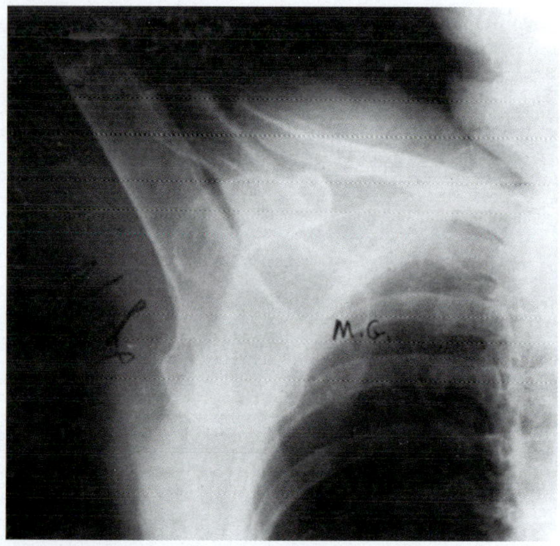

FIGURE 13-71: Anteroposterior radiograph of an inferior dislocation reveals that the entire humeral head and surgical neck of the humerus are inferior to the glenoid fossa. (From Rockwood CA Jr, Green DP, Bucholz RW, eds. *Fractures in Adults.* Philadelphia: JB Lippincott; 1991.)

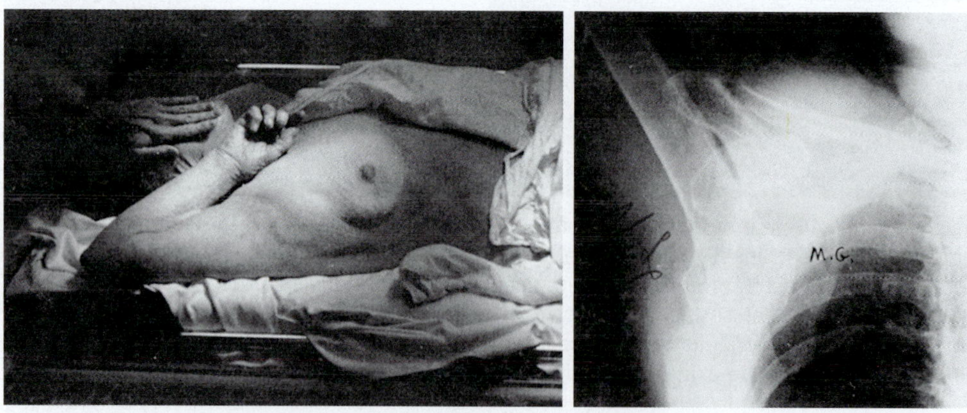

FIGURE 13-72: Inferior dislocation (*luxatio erecta*) of the right shoulder of a 75-year-old woman. Note that the arm is directed upward in relation to the trunk (*left*). The hand of the flexed elbow is lying on the anterior of the chest. An anteroposterior radiograph of the inferior dislocation reveals that the entire humeral head and surgical neck of the humerus are inferior to the glenoid fossa (*right*). (From Rockwood CA Jr, Green DP, Bucholz RW, eds. *Fractures in Adults.* Philadelphia: JB Lippincott; 1991.)

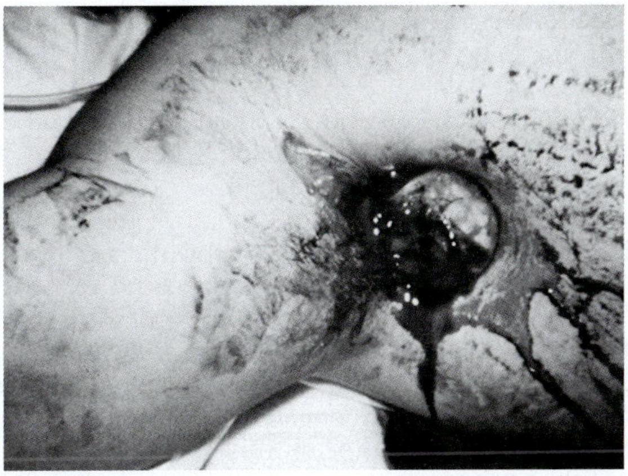

FIGURE 13-73: Photograph of the right shoulder and axilla of a patient who had an open inferior dislocation of the humeral head out through the axilla. (Courtesy George Armstrong.)

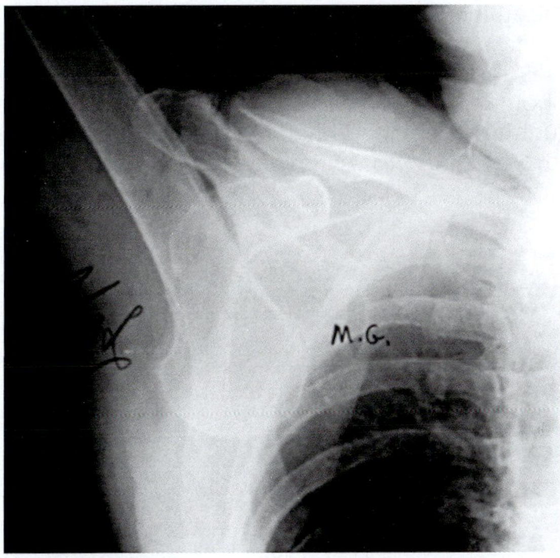

FIGURE 13-74: Anteroposterior radiograph of an inferior dislocation reveals that the entire humeral head and surgical neck of the humerus are inferior to the glenoid fossa.

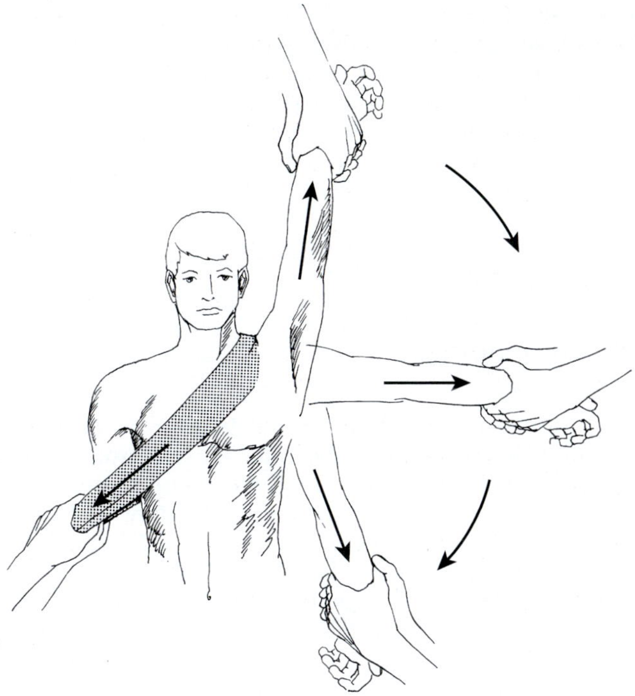

FIGURE 13-75: Technique of reduction of an inferior dislocation (*luxatio erecta*) of the glenohumeral joint. Countertraction is applied by an assistant using a folded sheet across the superior aspect of the shoulder and neck. Traction on the arm is first applied upward, and then gradually the arm is brought into less abduction and finally placed at the patient's side. (From Rockwood CA Jr, Green DP, Bucholz RW, eds. *Fractures in Adults*. Philadelphia: JB Lippincott; 1991.)

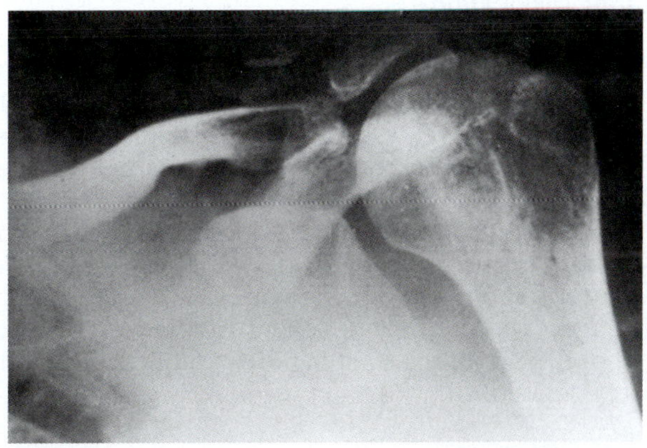

FIGURE 13-76: Superior dislocation of the left shoulder. Note that the head of the humerus is displaced superiorly from the glenoid fossa and that the fracture of the acromion process has also been displaced upward. (From Rockwood CA Jr, Green DP, Bucholz RW, eds. *Fractures in Adults*. Philadelphia: JB Lippincott; 1991.)

before 1969. Bilateral dislocations have been reported by McFie,[420] Yadav,[716] Onabowale and Jaja,[508] Segal et al.,[612] and Carew-McColl.[96] Most of these cases were the result of convulsions or violent trauma. Peiro et al.[537] reported bilateral erect dislocation of the shoulders in a man caught in a cement mixer. Bilateral dislocation of the shoulder secondary to accidental electrical shock has been described by Carew-McColl[96] and by Fipp.[187] Nicola et al.[487] reported cases of bilateral posterior fracture-dislocation after a convulsive seizure. Ahlgren et al.[5] reported three cases of bilateral posterior fracture-dislocation associated with a convulsion. Lindholm and Elmstedt[387] presented a case of bilateral posterior fracture-dislocation after an epileptic seizure, which was treated by open reduction and internal fixation with screws. Parrish and Skiendzielewski[528] reported a patient with bilateral posterior fracture-dislocation after status epilepticus. The diagnosis was missed for more than 12 hours. Pagden et al.[520] reported two cases of posterior shoulder dislocation after seizures related to regional anesthesia. Costigan et al.[124] reported a case of undiagnosed bilateral anterior dislocation of the shoulder in a 74-year-old patient admitted to the hospital for an unrelated problem. The patient had no complaints related to the shoulders and was able to place both hands on her head and behind her back.

DISLOCATION

Clinical Findings

History

The history should define the mechanism of the injury, including the position of the arm, the amount of force applied, and the point of force application.[550,589,590] Injury with the arm in extension, abduction, and external rotation favors anterior dislocation. Electroshock, seizures, or a fall on the flexed and adducted arm are commonly associated with posterior dislocation. If the instability is recurrent, the history defines the initial injury, the position or action that results in instability, how long the shoulder stays out, whether radiographs are available with the shoulder out of joint, and what means have been necessary to reduce the shoulder. The history also solicits evidence of neurologic or rotator cuff problems after previous episodes of shoulder instability. Previous treatment of the recurrent instability, as well as the effectiveness of this treatment, should be documented.

Physical Examination

Anterior Dislocation

An acutely dislocated shoulder is usually very painful, and muscles are in spasm in an attempt to stabilize the joint. The humeral head may be palpable anteriorly. The posterior and lateral aspect of the shoulder shows a hollow beneath the acromion. The arm is held in slight abduction. Passive and active motions are limited by pain. Because of the possible association of nerve injuries[138] and, to a lesser extent, vascular injuries,[62] an essential part of the physical examination of an anteriorly dislocated shoulder is assessment of the neurovascular status of the upper extremity and charting of the findings before reduction.

Posterior Dislocation

Because it is often more an impaction fracture than a dislocation, recognition of a posterior dislocation may be impaired by the lack of a striking deformity of the shoulder and by the fact that the shoulder is held in the traditional sling position of adduction and internal rotation. However, a directed physical examination will reveal the diagnosis. The classic features of a posterior dislocation include:

- Limited external rotation of the shoulder (often to <0 degrees)
- Limited elevation of the arm (often to <90 degrees)
- Posterior prominence and rounding of the shoulder in comparison to the normal side
- Flattening of the anterior aspect of the shoulder
- Prominence of the coracoid process on the dislocated side

Asymmetry of the shoulder contours can often best be visualized by viewing the shoulders from above while standing behind the patient (Fig. 13-77).

Motion is limited because the head of the humerus is fixed on the posterior glenoid rim by muscle forces, or the head might actually be impaled on the glenoid rim. With the passage of time, the posterior rim of the glenoid can further impact the fracture of the humeral head and produce a deep hatchet-like defect or a V-shaped compression fracture, which engages the head even more securely. Patients with old, unreduced posterior dislocations of the shoulder can have 30 to 40 degrees of glenohumeral abduction and some humeral rotation as a result of enlargement of the groove. With long-standing disuse of the muscles about the shoulder, atrophy will be present; such atrophy accentuates the flattening of the anterior portion of the shoulder, the prominence of the coracoid, and the fullness of the posterior portion of the shoulder.

Proper physical examination is essential. Rowe and Zarins[590] reported 23 cases of unreduced dislocation of the shoulder, 14 of which were posterior. Hill and McLaughlin[270] reported that in their series the average time from injury to diagnosis was 8 months. In the

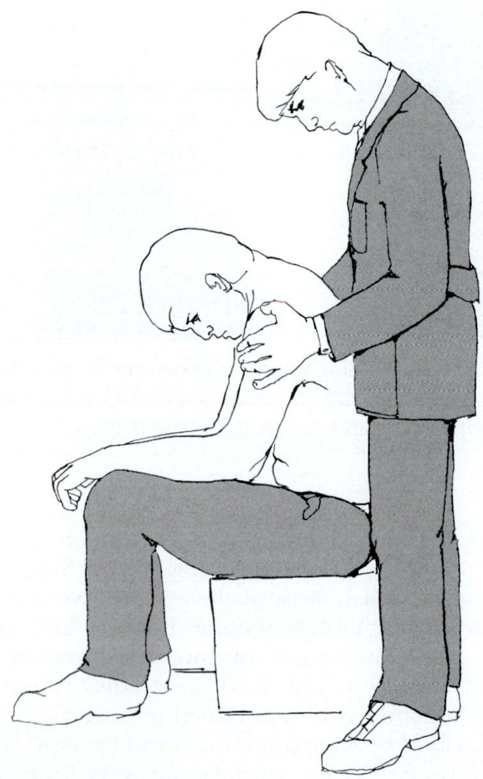

FIGURE 13-77: Inspection of the anterior and posterior aspects of the shoulders can best be accomplished by having the patient sit on a low stool with the examiner standing behind the patient. The injured shoulder can then be easily compared with the uninjured one. (From Rockwood CA, Green DP, eds. *Fractures*. 2nd ed. Philadelphia: JB Lippincott; 1984.)

interval before the diagnosis of posterior dislocation of the shoulder is made, the injury may be misdiagnosed as a frozen shoulder[270,428] for which vigorous therapy may be mistakenly instituted in an attempt to restore range of motion.

Radiographic Evaluation

When a shoulder is dislocated, radiographs need to demonstrate the direction of the dislocation, the existence of associated fractures (displaced or not), and possible barriers to relocation. Dorgan[158] and McLaughlin[425] have pointed out that reliance on anteroposterior (AP) and transthoracic radiographs will lead an unwary orthopaedist into a "diagnostic trap." The glenohumeral joint is most reliably imaged with three standardized views referred to the plane of the scapula. The complete series of three views oriented to the scapula provides much more information than does the commonly obtained view in the plane of the body (Fig. 13-78).

The first is an AP view in the plane of the scapula (Fig. 13-79). In 1923, Grashey[223] recognized that to take a true AP radiograph of the shoulder joint, the direction of the x-ray beam must be perpendicular to the plane of the scapula. This view is most easily accomplished by placing the scapula flat on the cassette (a position that the patient can help achieve) and passing the x-ray beam at right angles to this plane and centering it on the coracoid process (Fig. 13-80). This view can be taken with the arm in a sling and the body rotated to the desired position (Fig. 13-81). In a normal shoulder, this view reveals clear separation of the humeral subchondral bone from that of the glenoid. In an injured shoulder, it often reveals the pathology (Fig. 13-82).

The second is a scapular lateral view (Fig. 13-83). This view is taken at right angles to the AP view in the plane of the scapula (Figs. 13-84 and 13-85).[425,428,470] Like the AP

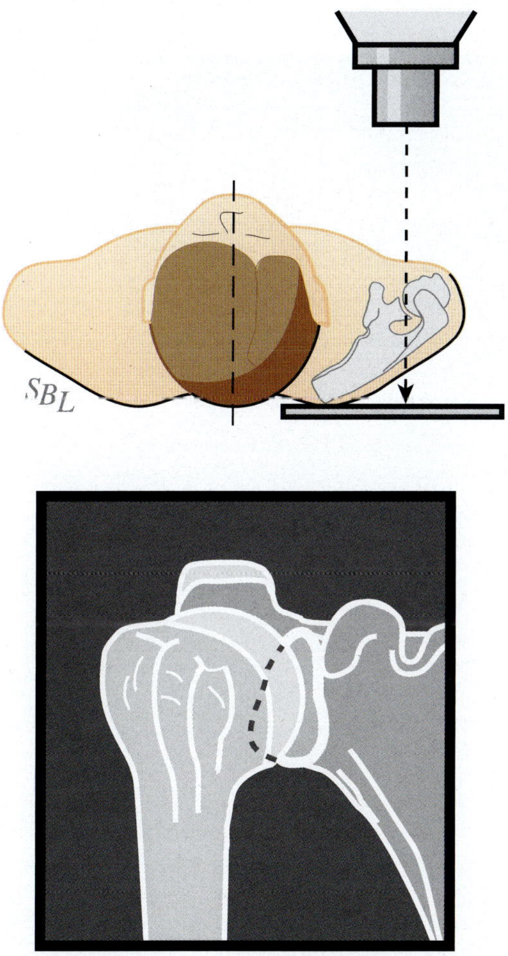

FIGURE 13-78: Anteroposterior (AP) radiograph in the plane of the body. An AP view in the coronal plane of the body is of limited use in the evaluation of the glenohumeral joint, the joint space, or the relationship of the humeral head to the glenoid fossa. (From Matsen FA III, Lippitt SB. *Shoulder Surgery: Principles and Procedures*. Philadelphia: WB Saunders; 2004:7.)

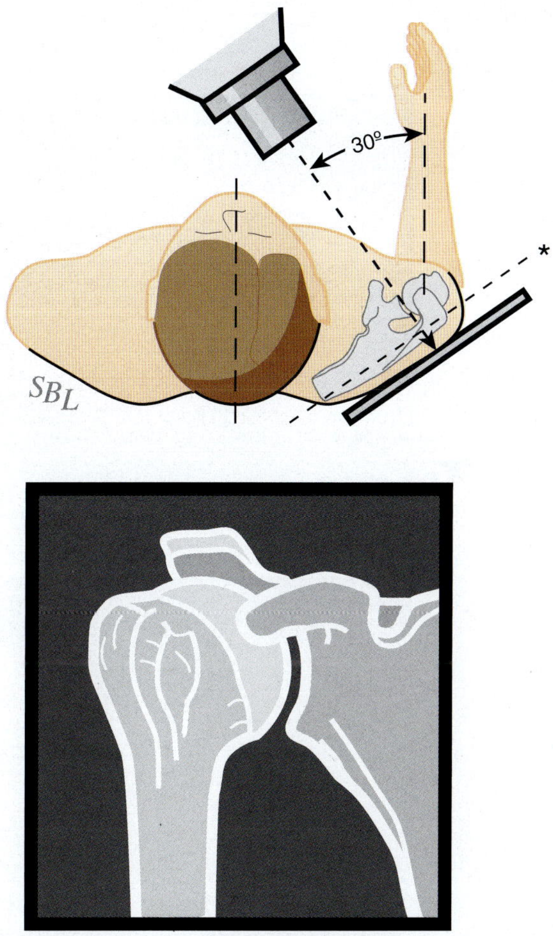

FIGURE 13-79: Anteroposterior (AP) radiograph in the plane of the scapula. An AP view in the plane of the scapula reveals the glenohumeral joint space and demonstrates whether the humeral head has a normal relationship to the glenoid fossa. It is most easily taken by positioning the patient's scapula flat on the cassette and then passing the x-ray beam at right angles to the film, aiming at the coracoid process. (From Matsen FA III, Lippitt SB. *Shoulder Surgery: Principles and Procedures*. Philadelphia: WB Saunders; 2004:7.)

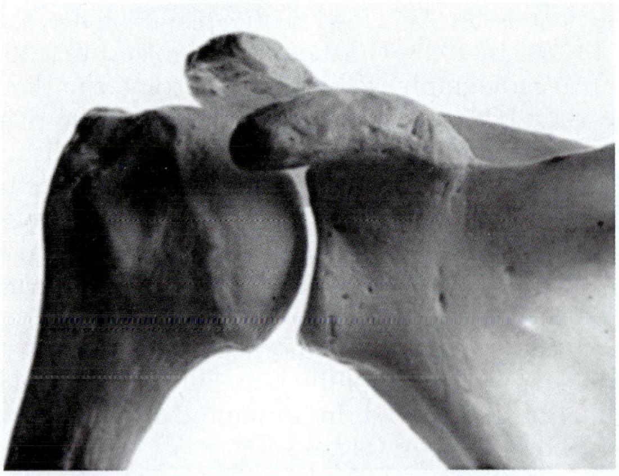

FIGURE 13-80: A simulated radiographic view of a scapular anteroposterior view using a backlighted skeletal model. This view reveals the radiographic glenohumeral joint space and provides a good opportunity to detect fractures of the humerus or glenoid lip.

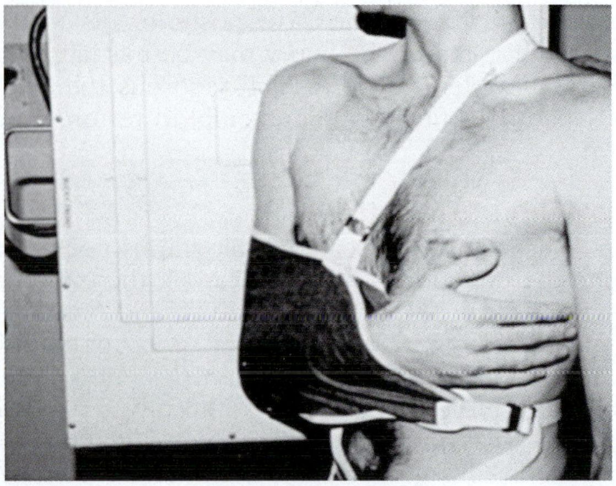

FIGURE 13-81: Positioning of the patient in a sling for an anteroposterior radiograph in the plane of the scapula. The scapula is placed flat on the cassette. The x-ray beam is positioned at right angles to the cassette and centered on the coracoid process.

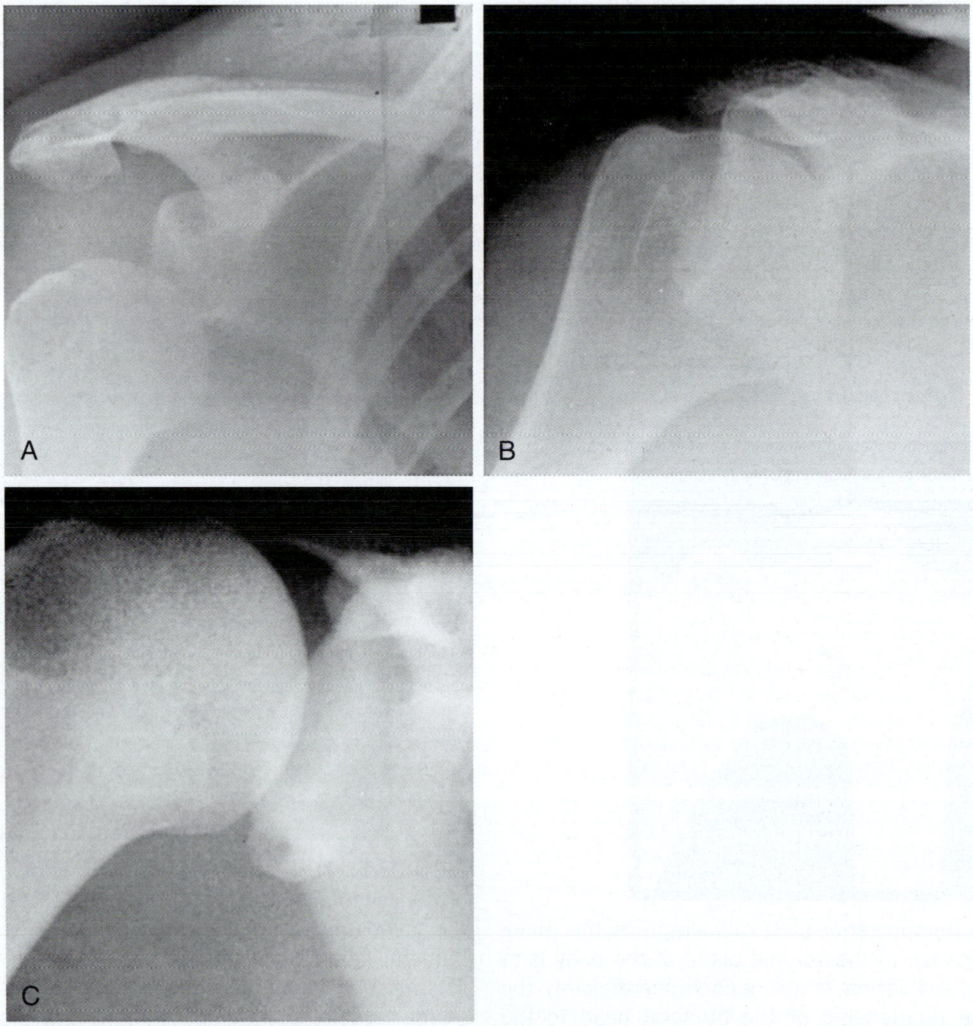

FIGURE 13-82: Anteroposterior radiographs in the plane of the scapula. **A,** Anteroinferior glenohumeral dislocation. **B,** Anterior glenohumeral dislocation. **C,** A radiograph showing inferior glenoid calcification as a result of previous anterior glenohumeral instability.

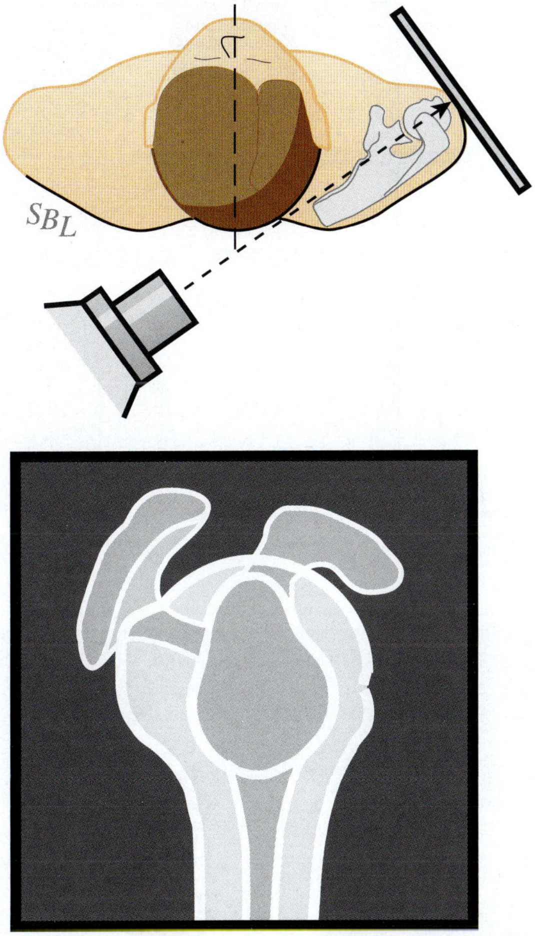

FIGURE 13-83: Scapular lateral position. The shoulder is placed against the radiographic cassette so that the scapular spine is perpendicular to it. The x-ray beam is passed parallel to the scapular spine and centered on the intersection of the coracoid process, the acromion process, and the plane of the scapular body. This intersection lies in the glenoid fossa. The humeral head should also lie centered at this intersection. (From Matsen FA III, Lippitt SB. *Shoulder Surgery: Principles and Procedures.* Philadelphia: WB Saunders; 2004:11.)

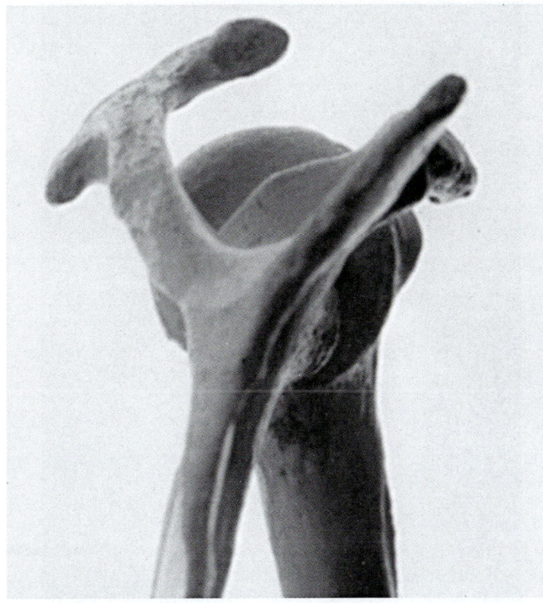

FIGURE 13-84: Simulated scapular lateral radiographic view with a backlighted skeletal model. The x-ray beam is passed parallel to the plane of the scapula and is centered on the scapular spine. The view reveals the anteroposterior relationship of the head of the humerus in the glenoid fossa. The glenoid fossa is identified as the intersection of the spine of the scapula, the coracoid process, and the body of the scapula.

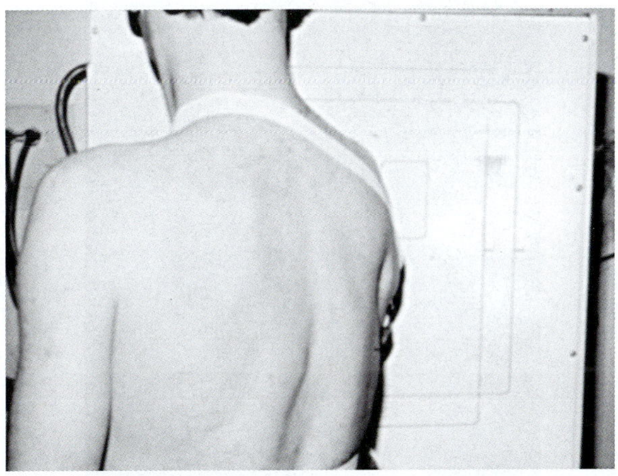

FIGURE 13-85: Position of the patient in a sling for a scapular lateral radiograph. The scapula is positioned perpendicular to the cassette. The beam should be placed parallel to the spine of the scapula and perpendicular to the cassette.

view, it can be obtained by positioning the body without moving the dislocated shoulder, which can remain in a sling. The radiographic beam is passed in a medial-to-lateral direction parallel to the body of the scapula while the cassette is held perpendicular to the beam at the anterolateral aspect of the shoulder. In this view, the contour of the scapula projects as the letter Y.[593] The downward stem of the Y is projected by the body of the scapula; the upper forks are projected by the coracoid process anteriorly and by the spine and acromion posteriorly (Figs. 13-86 and 13-87). The glenoid is located at the junction of the stem and the two arms of the Y. In a normal shoulder, the humeral head is at the center of the arms of the Y, that is, in the glenoid fossa. In posterior dislocations, the head is seen posterior to the glenoid (see Fig. 13-87); in anterior dislocations, the head is anterior to it (see Fig. 13-86).

The third is an axillary view (Fig. 13-88). In this view, first described by Lawrence in 1915,[367,436] the cassette is placed on the superior aspect of the shoulder. This view requires that the humerus be abducted sufficiently to allow the radiographic beam to pass between it and the thorax. Fortunately, sufficient abduction can be achieved by gentle positioning of the dislocated shoulder or by

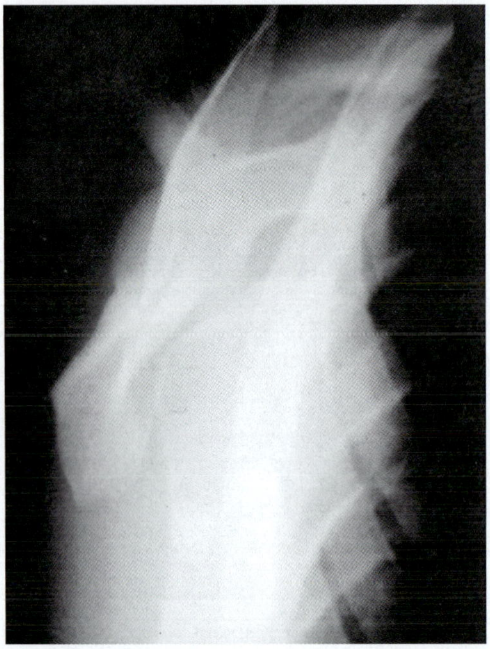

FIGURE 13-86: Scapular lateral view showing an anterior glenohumeral dislocation. Note that the humerus is no longer centered at the base of the Y.

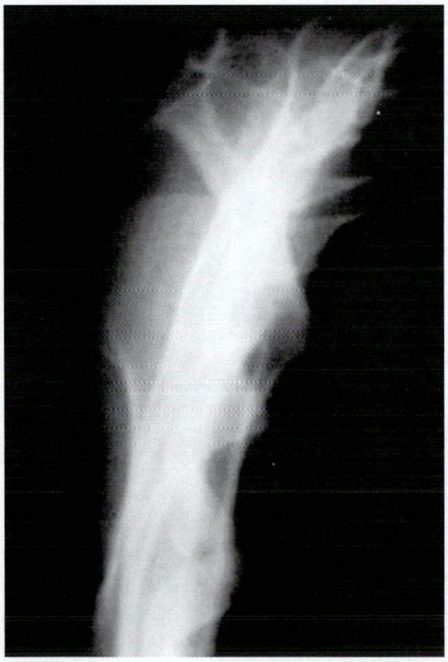

FIGURE 13-87: A scapular lateral view showing a posterior glenohumeral dislocation. The head of the humerus is dislocated posterior to the glenoid fossa and in this view appears to be sitting directly below the spine of the scapula.

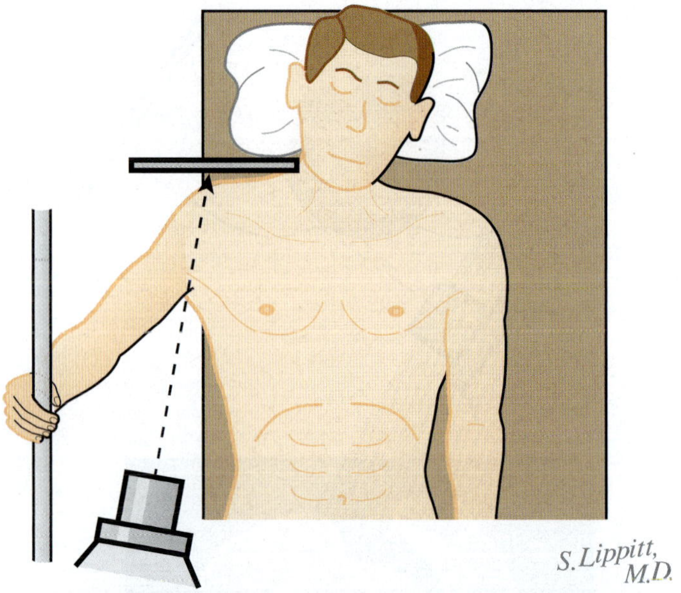

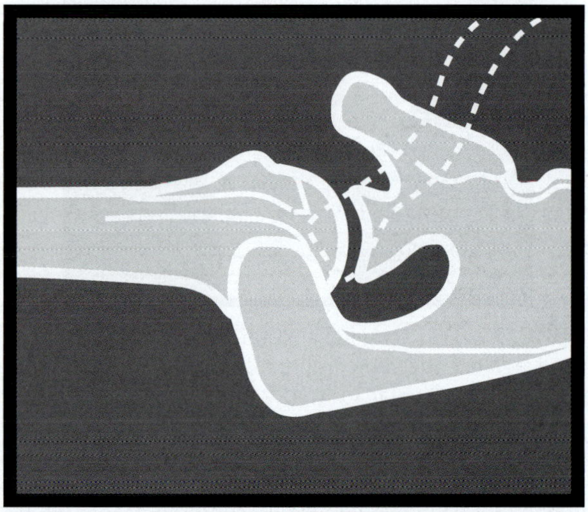

FIGURE 13-88: An axillary radiograph reveals the glenohumeral joint space and the anteroposterior position of the humeral head and glenoid fossa. It is obtained by having the patient's arm in abduction (e.g., holding onto an IV pole), the cassette on the superior aspect of the shoulder, and the x-ray beam passing up the axilla, aiming at the coracoid. (From Matsen FA III, Lippitt SB. *Shoulder Surgery: Principles and Procedures*. Philadelphia: WB Saunders; 2004:9.)

modifications of the technique (Figs. 13-89 to 13-92). The axillary radiograph is critical in evaluation of a dislocated shoulder: It unambiguously reveals not only the direction and magnitude of head displacement relative to the glenoid but also the presence and size of head compression fractures, fractures of the glenoid, and fractures of the humeral tuberosities (Figs. 13-93 to 13-97). The axillary view might also be helpful in judging the bony competence and version of the glenoid fossa, but the projection must be standardized to avoid misinterpretation (see Fig. 13-49).

In his text on radiographic positioning, Jordan demonstrated the various techniques for obtaining axillary lateral views.[324] Variations on this view have been described (see Fig. 13-90). Rockwood has pointed out that in a situation in which the patient cannot abduct the

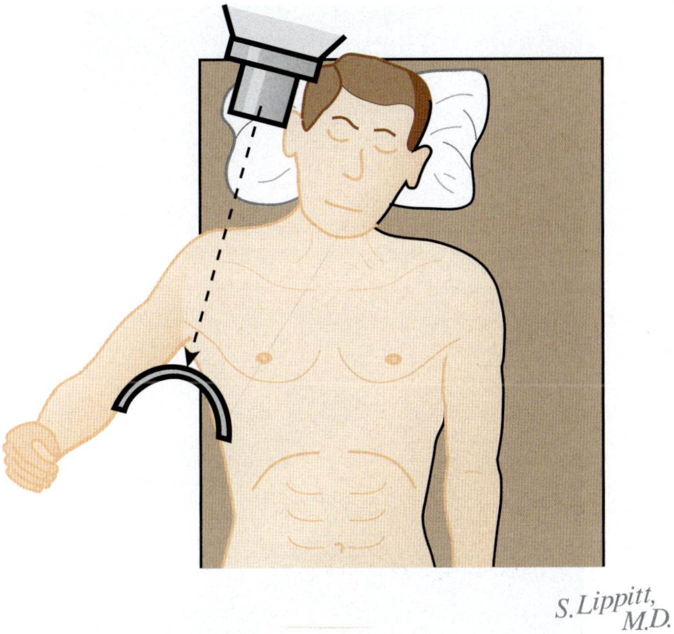

FIGURE 13-89: The axillary view with a curved cassette, a method that is useful if the arm cannot be adequately abducted for a routine axillary view.

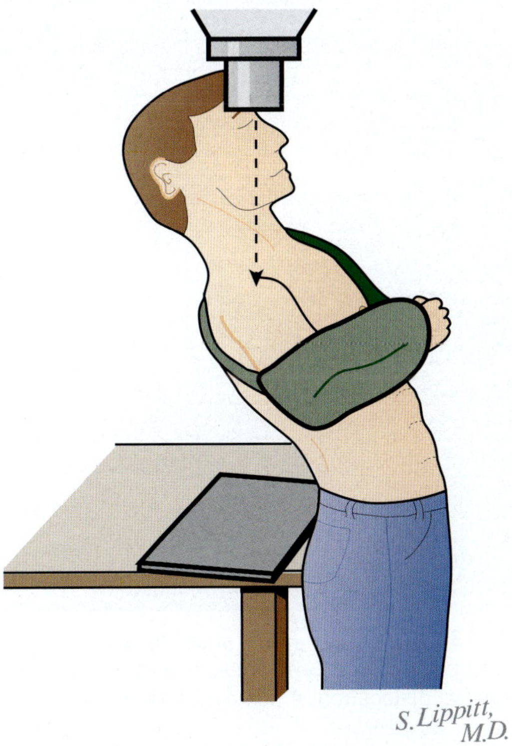

FIGURE 13-90: The Velpeau axillary lateral radiograph technique. With the arm in a sling, the patient leans backward until the shoulder is over the cassette. (Modified from Bloom MH, Obata WG. Diagnosis of posterior dislocation of the shoulder with use of the Velpeau axillary and angle-up roentgenographic views. *J Bone Joint Surg Am*. 1967;49:943-949.)

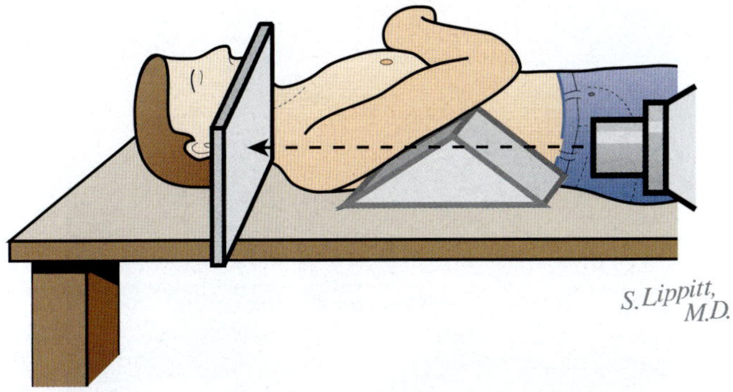

FIGURE 13-91: A trauma axillary lateral radiograph. This arm is flexed on a foam wedge.

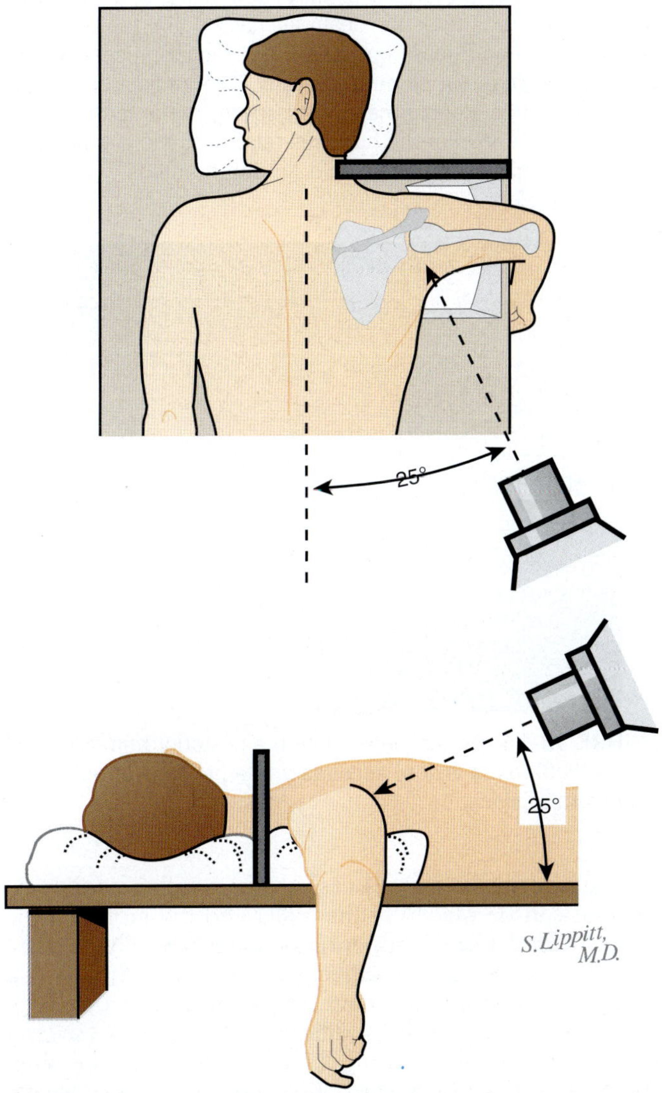

FIGURE 13-92: The West Point axillary lateral view. The patient is prone with the beam inclined 25 degrees down and 25 degrees medially. (Modified from Rokous JR, Feagin JA, Abbott HG. Modified axillary roentgenogram. *Clin Orthop Relat Res*. 1972;82:84-86.)

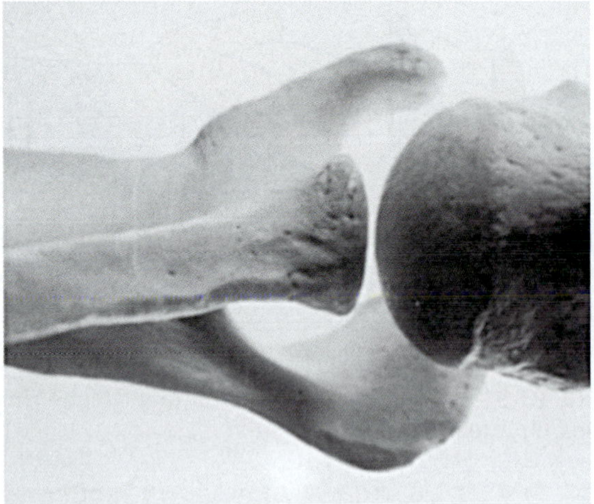

FIGURE 13-93: Simulated axillary view using a backlighted skeletal model. The x-ray beam is passed up the axilla to project the glenoid fossa between the coracoid process anteriorly and the scapular spine posteriorly. This projection reveals the radiographic glenohumeral joint space, the anteroposterior position of the head of the humerus relative to the glenoid, and a view of fractures of the glenoid lip and humerus.

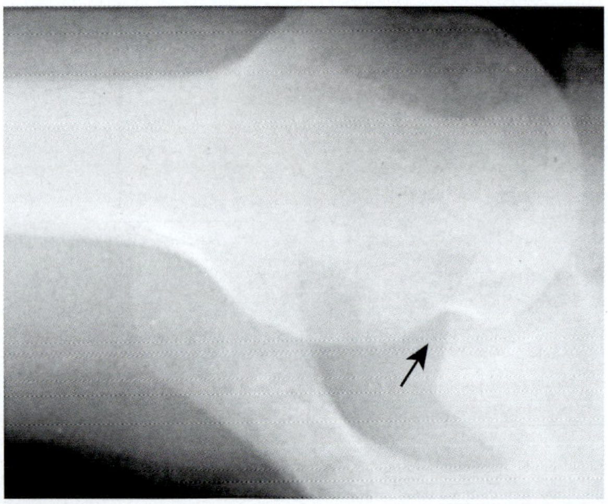

FIGURE 13-94: Axillary view. Note the posterior humeral head defect (Hill-Sachs lesion) secondary to a previous anterior glenohumeral dislocation.

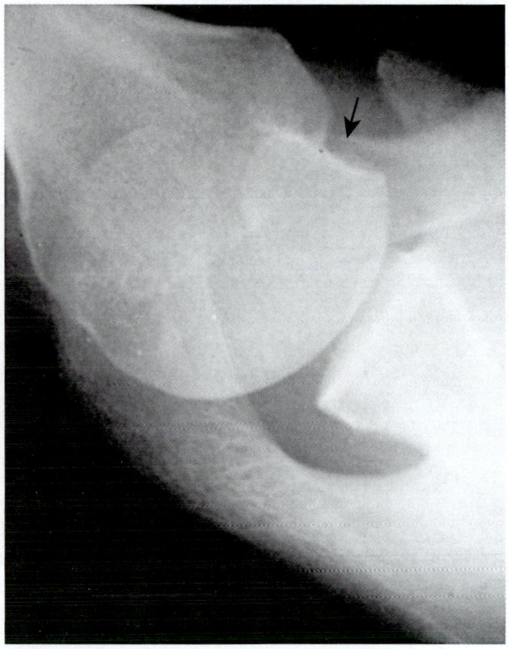

FIGURE 13-95: Axillary view. This patient has an anterior humeral head defect (*arrow*) that occurred as a result of a posterior glenohumeral dislocation.

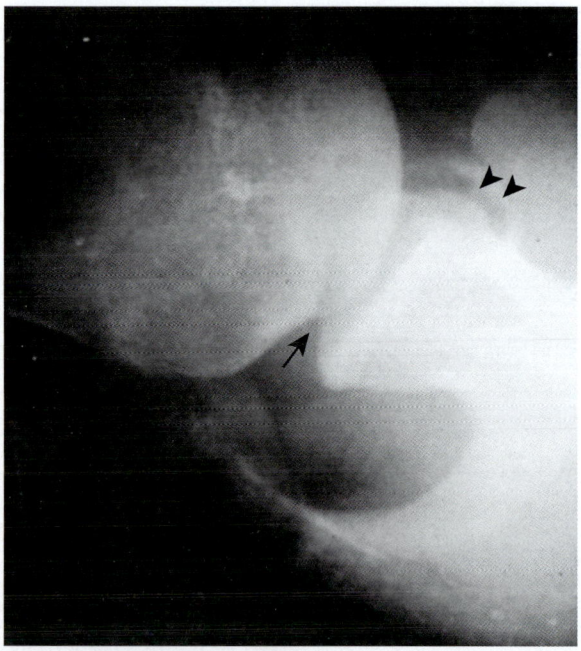

FIGURE 13-96: Axillary view showing an anterior glenoid defect and calcification (*arrowheads*) as a result of an anterior glenohumeral dislocation. A posterolateral humeral head defect is also seen (*arrow*).

arm sufficiently, a curved cassette or a rolled cardboard cassette can be placed in the axilla and the radiographic beam passed from a superior position (see Fig. 13-89). Bloom and Obata[63] modified the axillary technique so that the arm does not have to be abducted (see Fig. 13-90). They called this modification the *Velpeau axillary lateral view*. While wearing a sling or Velpeau dressing, the patient leans backward 30 degrees over the cassette on the table. The x-ray tube is placed above the shoulder and the beam is projected vertically down through the shoulder onto the cassette.

In summary, in the evaluation of a possibly dislocated shoulder or a fractured-dislocated shoulder, we recommend the three projections of the shoulder that provide a sensitive assessment of shoulder anatomy. The use of fewer views or other less-interpretable projections can obscure significant pathologic processes. If these views cannot be taken, if a question has arisen regarding the diagnosis,

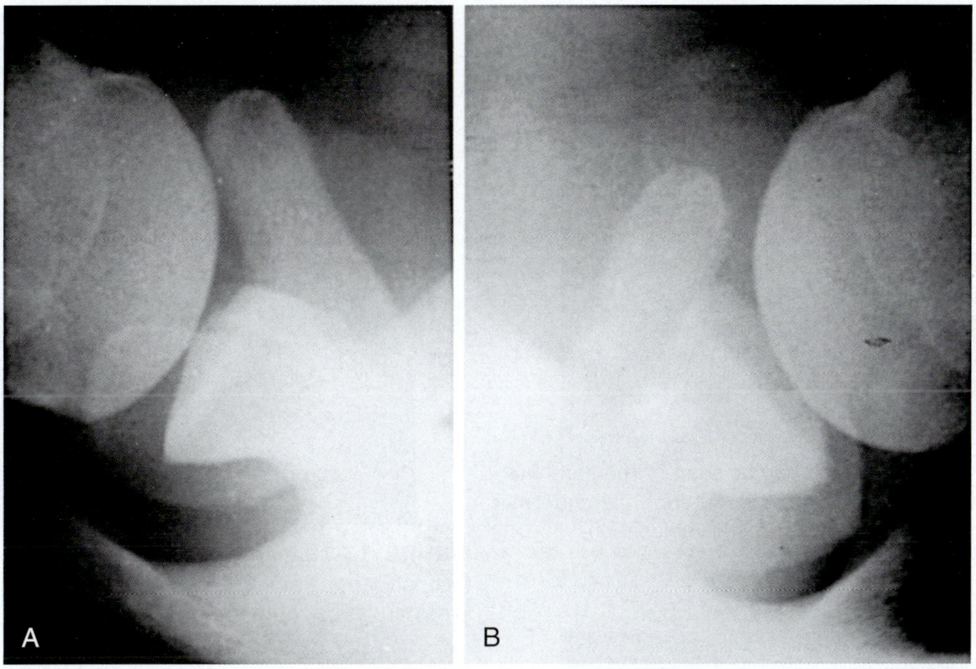

FIGURE 13-97: Bilateral axillary views. **A,** Rounding of the anterior glenoid rim as a result of recurrent anterior glenohumeral dislocation is evident on this axillary view. **B,** The normal side is shown for comparison.

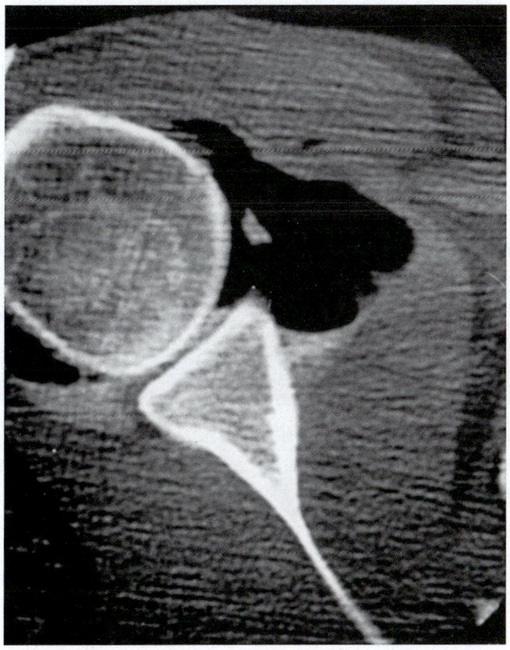

FIGURE 13-98: Computed tomographic scan of the glenohumeral joint with air contrast. This study demonstrates a bony avulsion from the anterior glenoid rim.

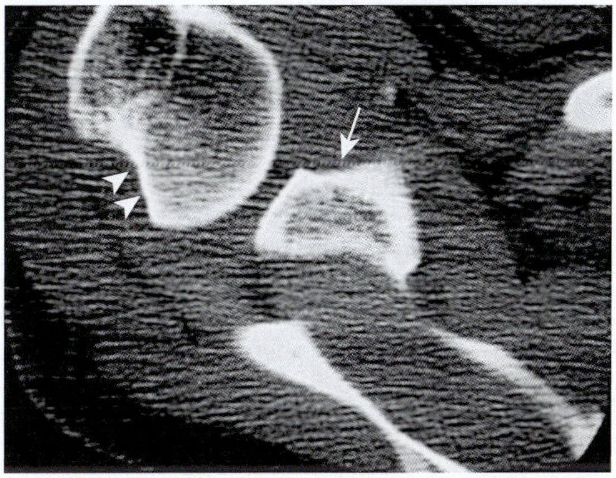

FIGURE 13-99: CT scan of the glenohumeral joint. The posterior humeral head defect (*arrowheads*) and the anterior glenoid defect (*arrow*) are well demonstrated.

or if the anatomy needs to be defined in greater detail, a CT scan may be of great assistance (Figs. 13-98 to 13-101; see Fig. 13-23).[337,561,618] Using modern methods of three-dimensional (3D) reconstruction, anterior-inferior glenoid lesions and posterior-lateral humeral head lesions can be shown in striking detail (Figs. 13-102 to 13-104). The patient whose shoulder is shown in these figures obtained an excellent result after nonoperative treatment in spite of the damage shown on the radiographic reconstructions.

INJURIES ASSOCIATED WITH ANTERIOR DISLOCATIONS

Ligaments and Capsule

A common feature of traumatic anterior dislocations is avulsion of the anteroinferior glenohumeral ligaments

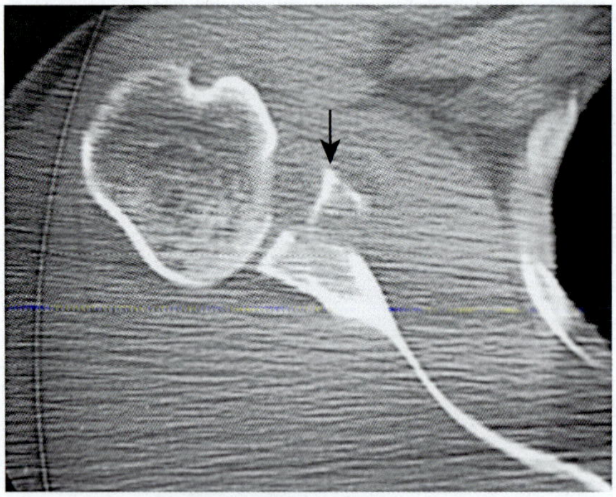

FIGURE 13-100: Computed tomographic scan of the glenohumeral joint showing a fracture of the anterior glenoid rim (*arrow*) secondary to anterior glenohumeral dislocation.

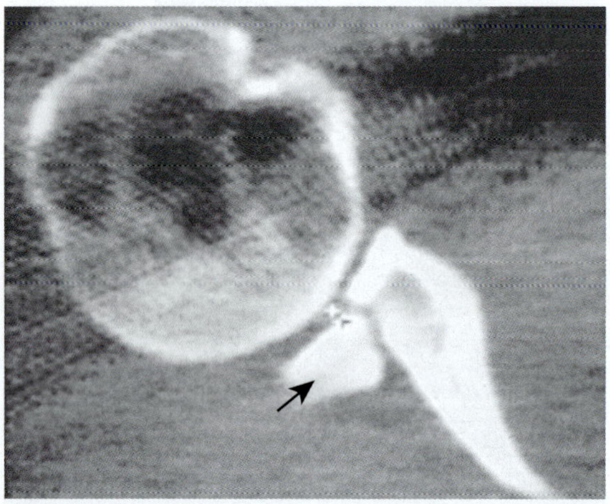

FIGURE 13-101: Computed tomographic scan of the glenohumeral joint demonstrating a fracture of the posterior glenoid rim (*arrow*) as a result of posterior dislocation of the glenohumeral joint.

and capsule from the glenoid lip, especially in younger persons (Fig. 13-105). Nonhealing of this avulsion is a major factor in recurrent traumatic instability. The capsule might also be avulsed from the anteroinferior portion of the glenoid, sometimes with a fleck of bone (see Fig. 13-103).

Fractures

Fractures of the glenoid (Fig. 13-106; see also Figs. 13-7 and 13-101), humeral head (see Figs. 13-94 and 13-95), and tuberosities (Figs. 13-107 to 13-109; see also Fig. 13-6) can accompany traumatic dislocations. A CT scan may be helpful in determining the degree of displacement of fractures (Figs. 13-110 and 13-111; see also Figs. 13-99 to 13-101).

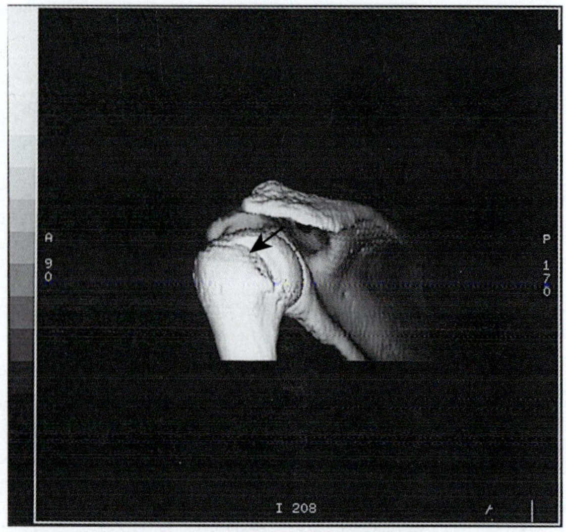

FIGURE 13-102: Three-dimensional computed tomographic reconstruction after reduction of a first-time dislocation showing a posterolateral humeral head defect (*arrow*).

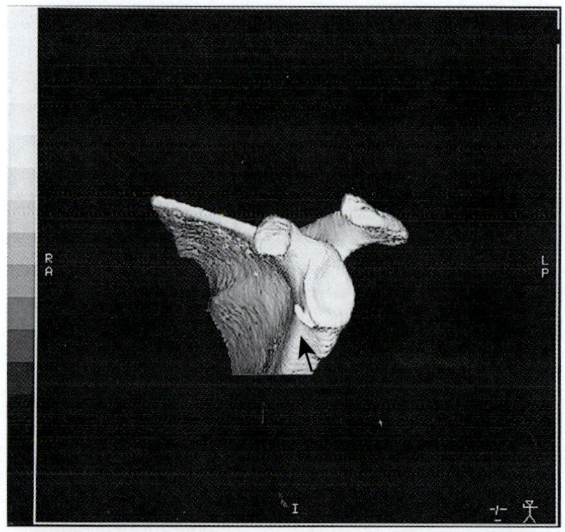

FIGURE 13-103: Three-dimensional computed tomographic reconstruction after reduction of a first-time dislocation showing anterior glenoid avulsion (*arrow*).

It is important to seek evidence of a nondisplaced humeral neck fracture on the prereduction radiographs lest this fracture be displaced during attempted closed reduction (see Fig. 13-109).[182]

Other fractures, such as those of the coracoid process, may be associated with glenohumeral dislocations.[47,711]

Cuff Tears

Rotator cuff tears can accompany anterior and inferior glenohumeral dislocations (see Fig. 13-5). The frequency of this complication increases with age: In patients older than 40 years, the incidence exceeds 30%; in those older than 60 years, it exceeds 80%.[308,532,542,560,642,653,695]

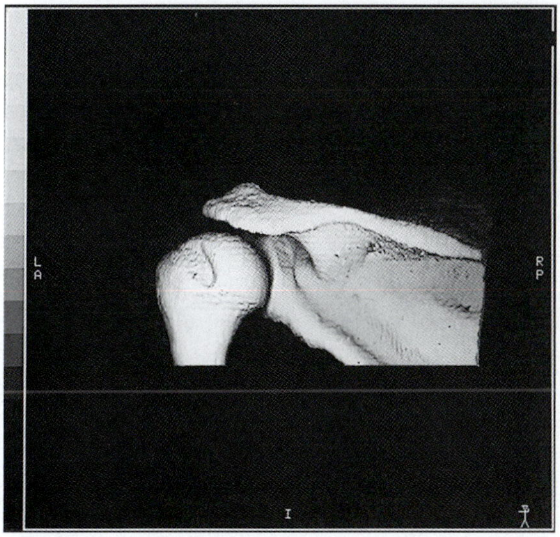

FIGURE 13-104: Three-dimensional computed tomographic reconstruction of the left shoulder of a 37-year-old man 3 days after his first traumatic glenohumeral dislocation. The patient recovered normal shoulder function with nonoperative management.

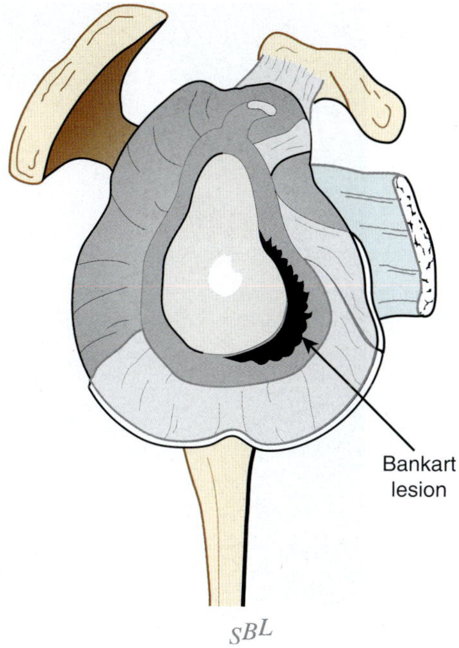

FIGURE 13-105: The capsulolabral detachment typical of traumatic instability. (Modified from Matsen FA III, Lippitt SB, Sidles JA, Harryman DT II. *Practical Evaluation and Management of the Shoulder*. Philadelphia: WB Saunders; 1994.)

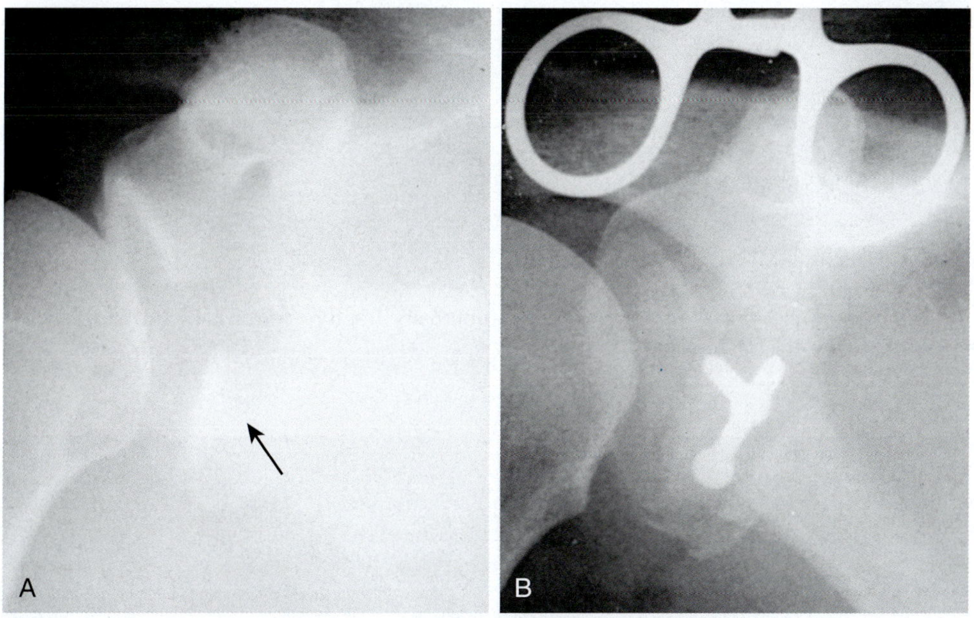

FIGURE 13-106: Anterior glenoid rim fracture. **A,** An anteroposterior (AP) radiograph demonstrates an anterior glenoid rim fracture secondary to traumatic anterior dislocation (*arrow*). **B,** An intraoperative AP radiograph shows reduction and screw fixation of an anterior glenoid rim fracture.

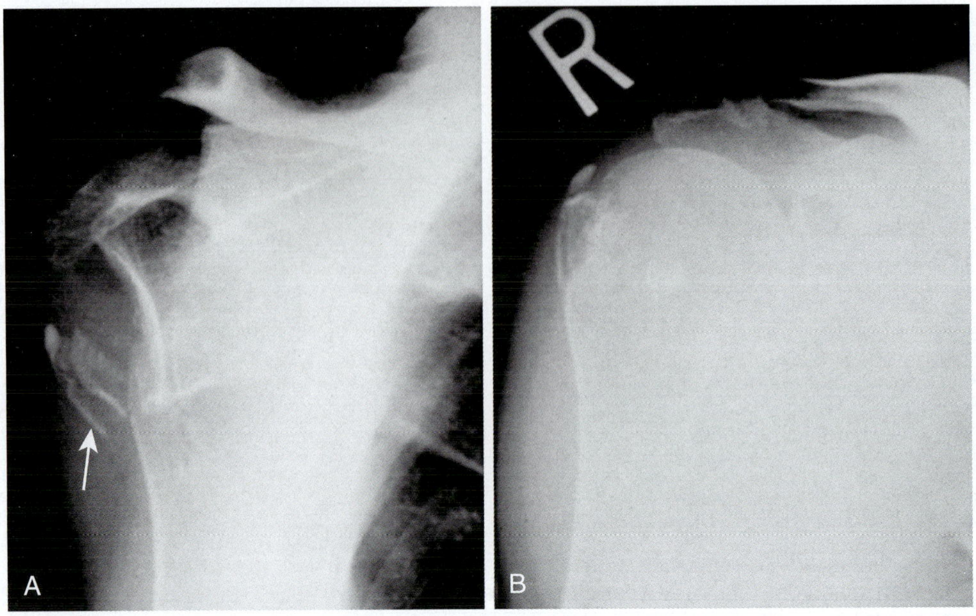

FIGURE 13-107: Greater tuberosity fracture. **A,** An anteroposterior (AP) radiograph before reduction shows a fracture of the greater tuberosity (*arrow*). **B,** Postreduction AP radiograph of a greater tuberosity fracture.

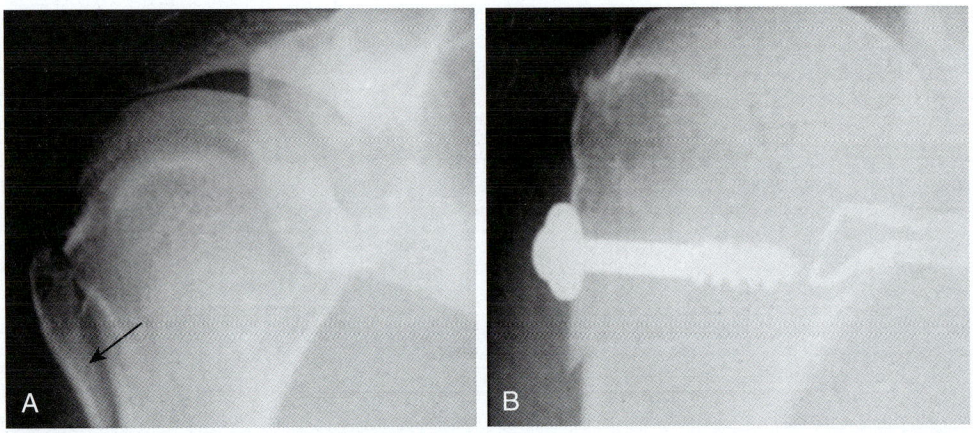

FIGURE 13-108: **A,** Radiograph showing a displaced greater tuberosity fracture (*arrow*). **B,** Intraoperative radiograph showing screw fixation of a greater tuberosity fracture.

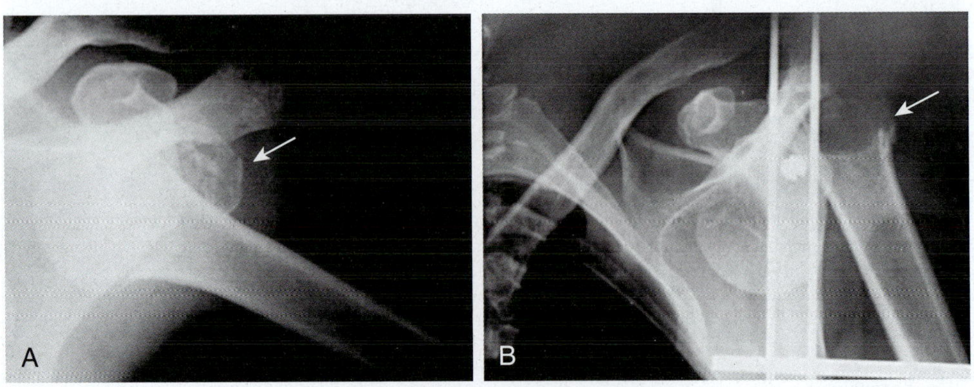

FIGURE 13-109: **A,** Anteroposterior (AP) view showing an anteroinferior dislocation with an associated greater tuberosity fracture (*arrow*). **B,** AP view after a reduction attempt showing displacement of a humeral neck fracture (*arrow*).

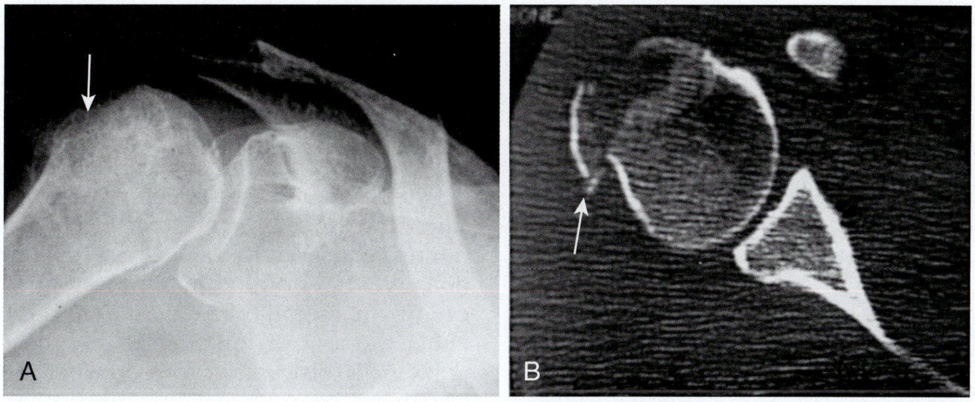

FIGURE 13-110: Minimally displaced greater tuberosity fracture. **A,** Anteroposterior radiograph shows a minimally displaced greater tuberosity fracture (*arrow*). **B,** Computed tomographic scan shows the position of the greater tuberosity (*arrow*).

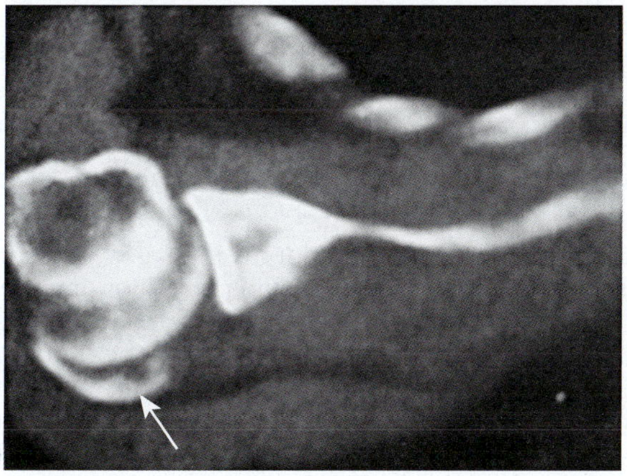

FIGURE 13-111: Computed tomographic scan of a significantly displaced greater tuberosity fracture (*arrow*).

Rotator cuff tears may be manifested as pain or weakness on external rotation and abduction.[252,479,542,558,694] Sonnabend reported a series of primary shoulder dislocations in patients older than 40 years.[628] Of the 13 patients who had complaints of weakness or pain after 3 weeks, 11 had rotator cuff tears. However, the presence of a rotator cuff tear may be masked by a coexisting axillary nerve palsy.[219,321]

Shoulder ultrasonography,[398] arthrography, or MRI is considered for evaluation of the possibility of an associated cuff tear when shoulder dislocations occur in patients older than 40 years, when initial displacement of the humeral head has been substantial (such as in a subglenoid dislocation), and when pain or loss of rotator cuff strength has persisted for 3 weeks after a glenohumeral dislocation. Toolanen found sonographic evidence of rotator cuff lesions in 24 of 63 patients older than 40 years at the time of anterior glenohumeral dislocation.[655]

Prompt operative repair of these acute cuff tears is usually indicated. Itoi and Tabata[308] reported 16 rotator cuff tears in 109 shoulders with a traumatic anterior dislocation. The cuff was surgically repaired in 11 shoulders, and the results were graded satisfactory in 73% of cases.

Neviaser et al.[480] reported on 37 patients older than 40 years in whom the diagnosis of cuff rupture was initially missed after an anterior dislocation of the shoulder. The weakness from the cuff rupture was often erroneously attributed to axillary neuropathy. Recurrent anterior instability caused by rupture of the subscapularis and anterior capsule from the lesser tuberosity developed in 11 of these patients. None of these shoulders had a Bankart lesion. Repair of the capsule and subscapularis restored stability in all of the patients. This study nicely points out that although younger patients with traumatic anterior instability often have anterior lesions (Bankart lesions or anterior rim fractures), older patients with traumatic anterior instability often have posterior lesions (cuff tears or tuberosity fractures). McLaughlin noted that there was usually either failure of the anterior or posterior supports, as "disruption of one tends to spare the other."[374]

Vascular Injuries

Several reports of arterial and neurologic injury with shoulder dislocation reinforce the importance of a thorough neurovascular evaluation.[260,409,509] Vascular damage most often occurs in elderly patients with stiffer, more fragile vessels. The injury may be to the axillary artery or vein or to branches of the axillary artery: the thoracoacromial, subscapular, circumflex, and, rarely, the long thoracic. Sometimes these injuries can be combined, as pointed out by Kirker, who described a case of rupture of the axillary artery and axillary vein along with a brachial plexus palsy.[338] Injury can occur at the time of either dislocation or reduction.[14,130,230,311]

Anatomy

The axillary artery is divided into three parts that lie medial to, behind, and lateral to the pectoralis minor muscle (Fig. 13-112). Injuries most commonly involve the second part, where the thoracoacromial trunk may be

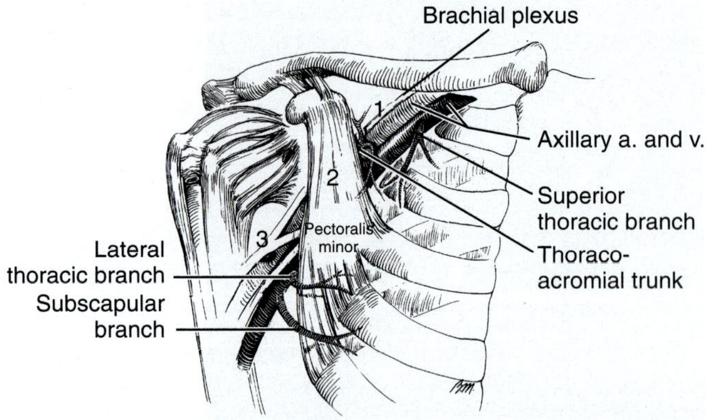

FIGURE 13-112: The axillary artery is divided into three parts by the pectoralis minor muscle. The first part (*1*) is medial to the pectoralis minor, the second part (*2*) is behind it, and the third part (*3*) is lateral to it. (From Rockwood CA, Green DP, eds. *Fractures*. 2nd ed. Philadelphia: JB Lippincott; 1984.)

avulsed, and the third part, where the subscapular and circumflex branches may be avulsed or the axillary artery may be totally ruptured.

Mechanism of Injury

Damage to the axillary artery can take the form of a complete transection, a linear tear of the artery caused by avulsion of one of its branches, or an intravascular thrombus, perhaps related to an initial tear. The artery is relatively fixed at the lateral margin of the pectoralis minor muscle. With abduction and external rotation, the artery is taut; when the head dislocates, it forces the axillary artery forward, and the pectoralis minor acts as a fulcrum over which the artery is deformed and ruptured.[85,311,445]

Watson-Jones[685] reported the case of a man who had multiple anterior dislocations that he reduced himself. Finally, when the man was older, the axillary artery ruptured during one of the dislocations and he died. Vascular injuries can occur either at the time of dislocation or during attempted reduction. Sometimes, it is unclear which is the case.[338,481,636]

Injury at the Time of Dislocation

Vascular injuries are commonly associated with inferior dislocation.[396,202,379,434] Gardham and Scott[202] reported occlusion of the axillary artery with an erect dislocation of the shoulder in a 40-year-old patient who had fallen headfirst down an escalator. Although vascular injuries are most common in older persons, they can occur at any age.[49,161,188,377,600,634] Baratta et al.[35] reported the case of a 13-year-old boy who ruptured his axillary artery after a subcoracoid dislocation sustained while wrestling.

Injury at the Time of Reduction

Vascular damage at the time of reduction occurs primarily in the elderly, particularly when a chronic old anterior dislocation is mistaken for an acute injury and closed reduction is attempted. The largest series of vascular complications associated with closed reduction of the shoulder has been reported by Calvet et al.,[94] who in 1941 collected 90 cases. This paper, which revealed the tragic end results, must have accomplished its purpose because very few reports have appeared in the literature since then dealing with the complications that occur during reduction. In their series, in which 64 of 91 reductions were performed many weeks after the initial dislocation, the mortality rate was 50%. The other patients lost either the arm or function of the arm. Besides the long delay from dislocation to reduction, these injuries might also have been caused by the use of excessive force. Delpeche observed a case in which the force of 10 men was used to accomplish the shoulder reduction; such force damaged the axillary vessel.[231]

Signs and Symptoms

Vascular damage may be obvious or subtle. Findings can include pain, expanding hematoma, pulse deficit, peripheral cyanosis, peripheral coolness and pallor, neurologic dysfunction, and shock. Doppler or an arteriogram should confirm the diagnosis and locate the site of injury.

Treatment and Prognosis

A suspected major arterial injury is managed as a surgical emergency, including establishing a major intravenous (IV) line and obtaining blood for transfusion. Jardon et al.[311] pointed out that bleeding can be temporarily controlled by digital pressure on the axillary artery over the first rib. These authors also recommend that the axillary artery be explored through the subclavicular operative approach, as described by Steenburg and Ravitch.[633]

The treatment of choice for a damaged axillary artery is either direct repair or a bypass graft after resection of the injury. Excellent results have been reported with prompt management of these vascular injuries.[85,128,157,202,211,264,311,379,422,564] The results of simple ligation of the vessels in elderly patients have been disappointing, probably because of poor collateral circulation and the presence of arteriosclerotic vascular disease in these typically older persons.[322,338,669] Even when ligation has been performed in younger patients with good collateral circulation, approximately two-thirds of these patients have lost function of the upper extremity because of complications such as upper extremity claudication.

Nerve Injuries

The brachial plexus and the axillary artery lie immediately anterior, inferior, and medial to the glenohumeral joint.[222] Therefore it is not surprising that neurovascular injuries often accompany traumatic anterior glenohumeral dislocations (Fig. 13-113).

Anatomy

The axillary nerve originates off the posterior cord of the brachial plexus. It crosses the anterior surface of

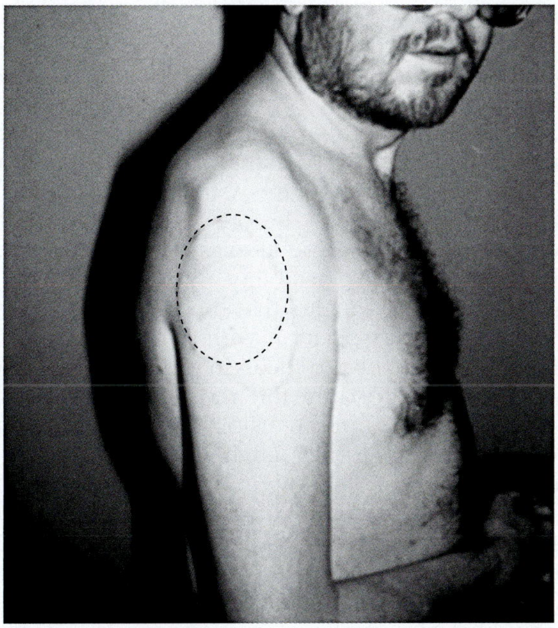

FIGURE 13-113: This patient sustained an axillary nerve palsy secondary to glenohumeral dislocation. The area of decreased sensation is marked on the lateral aspect of the proximal end of the humerus; note the significant wasting.

the subscapularis muscle and angulates sharply posteriorly to travel along the inferior shoulder joint capsule. It then leaves the axilla to exit through the quadrangular space below the lower border of the teres minor muscle, where it hooks around the posterior and lateral aspect of the humerus on the deep surface of the deltoid muscle.

Mechanism of Injury

The dislocated humeral head displaces the subscapularis and the overlying axillary nerve anteroinferiorly and creates traction and direct pressure on the nerve.[444,445] The injury to the nerve may be a neurapraxia (no structural damage, recovery in approximately 6 weeks), an axonotmesis (disruption of the axons, preservation of the nerve sheath, axonal regrowth at 1 inch per month), or a neurotmesis (complete nerve disruption, guarded prognosis for recovery).

Incidence

The reported incidence of nerve injuries in series of acute dislocations is substantial, often as high as 33%.[84,145,204,431,464,530,533,582,662,674,683] If careful electrodiagnostic studies are carried out prospectively, the incidence of nerve injury may be as high as 45%.[138]

The axillary nerve is most commonly involved; up to a third of first-time anterior dislocations are associated with axillary nerve involvement.[62,230,373,533,583] The likelihood of an axillary nerve injury increases with the age of the patient, the duration of the dislocation, and the amount of trauma that initiated the dislocation.[62,532] Other nerves injured are the radial, musculocutaneous, median, ulnar, and the entire brachial plexus.

Diagnosis

The diagnosis of nerve injury is considered in any patient with neurologic symptoms or signs such as weakness or numbness after a dislocation. A nerve injury can also be manifested as delayed recovery of active shoulder motion after glenohumeral dislocation. Blom and Dahlback[62] demonstrated that axillary neuropathy can exist without numbness in the usual sensory distribution of the axillary nerve. Electromyography provides objective evaluation of neurologic function, provided that 3 or 4 weeks has intervened between the injury and the evaluation.[62]

Treatment and Prognosis

Most axillary nerve injuries resulting from anterior dislocation are traction neurapraxias and will recover completely. However, if recovery has not occurred in 3 months, the prognosis is not as good.[22,62,84,138]

Recurrence of Instability After Anterior Dislocations

Effect of Age

The age of the patient at the time of the initial dislocation has a major influence on the incidence of redislocation.[582,621] Several authors have reported that patients younger than 20 years at the time of the initial dislocation have up to a 90% chance of recurrent instability.[18,263,278,282,340,430,431,458,582,587,621,693] In patients older than 40 years, the incidence drops sharply to 10% to 15%.[431,587] Hovelius et al.[280] reported a careful prospective study with a somewhat lower incidence of recurrence in each age group: 33% in those younger than 20 years, 25% between 20 and 30 years of age, and 10% between 30 and 40 years of age. The majority of all recurrences occur within the first 2 years of the first traumatic dislocation.[2,34,145,173,430,457,459,582,583,657]

A recent long-term, prospective study in Sweden investigated the natural history of nonoperatively treated primary anterior shoulder dislocation in patients younger than 40 years old. In this study, Hovelius et al. observed that more than half of those patients had a repeat episode of shoulder instability; although only 27% of the group received surgery, an additional 8% were experiencing multiple recurrent dislocations.[283] Furthermore, in the same cohort evaluated at 25 years after injury, more than half of the patients had developed glenohumeral arthritis from recurrent instability.[284] In a Danish study of patients under age 40 with 10 years of follow-up after a first-time traumatic anterior shoulder dislocation, more than half experienced a second dislocation and 75% of those treated nonoperatively reported unsatisfactory results because of recurrence, instability, and pain or stiffness; by contrast, 72% of the surgical group reported good or excellent results.[309]

Adolescent patients with a primary anterior dislocation of the glenohumeral joint have a high rate of recurrent dislocation, which usually occurs within two to five years of their initial injury.[565] During follow-up of 95.2 months on average, 102 (absolute incidence of 76.7%) patients had a recurrent dislocation. The median interval between primary and recurrent dislocation was ten months [95% confidence interval (CI), 7.4 to 12.6]. Applying survival analysis, the likelihood of having a stable shoulder one year after the initial injury was 59% (95% CI, 51.2 to 66.8), 38% (95% CI, 30.2 to 45.8) after 2 years, 21% (95% CI, 13.2 to 28.8) after 5 years, and 7% (95% CI, 1.1 to 12.9) after 10 years.[565] Longer-term follow-up reveals that the majority of all recurrences of shoulder dislocations will occur within 2 years, but 95% will occur within 5 years.[376]

Similar findings among freshmen in the U.S. Military Academy showed that cadets with a history of nonoperatively treated previous shoulder dislocation were over 5 times more likely to sustain an acute dislocation within the next 4 years of training.[95] This adolescent age group is particularly challenging, since the highest incidence of shoulder dislocations presenting to the emergency department is seen in patients aged 15 to 29 years; this group accounts for nearly half of all shoulder dislocations.[726]

Effect of Trauma, Sports, Sex, and Dominance

Rowe[582,587] has pointed out that the recurrence rate varies inversely with the severity of the original trauma; in other words, the more easily the dislocation occurred initially, the more easily it recurs. The recurrence rate in athletes may be higher than in nonathletes[621] and higher in men than women.[458] Dominance of the affected shoulder does not seem to have a major effect on the recurrence rate.[587] In a study of intercollegiate contact athletes, only 27% of the athletes with an instability episode successfully returned to play and completed the season without recurrence. By contrast, 64% of those who returned to in-season play had subsequent recurrent instability.[153]

Effect of Postdislocation Treatment

In many reports, the incidence of recurrence appears to be relatively insensitive to the type (sling vs. plaster Velpeau) and duration of immobilization (0 vs. 4 weeks) of the shoulder after the initial dislocation.[430,166,276,587] Most recent evidence indicates that immobilization other than that for comfort after dislocation does not have an impact on recurrence.[283,535]

By contrast, others have reported that longer periods of immobilization (over 3 weeks) are associated with a reduced incidence of recurrence.[20,331,639] Itoi et al.[307] have advocated immobilization in external rotation to hold the labrum in a reduced position to the anteroinferior glenoid rim during healing following reduction of a first time traumatic anterior dislocation. Subsequent studies have not demonstrated similar findings, and the value of external rotation immobilization remains controversial.

Effect of Fractures

The incidence of recurrence is lower when a first-time shoulder dislocation is associated with a greater tuberosity fracture.[142,278,280,431,579,582,586] Hovelius[278] reported that these fractures were three times as common in patients older than 30 years: 23% versus 8% in patients younger than 30 years. Other fractures, such as substantial posterolateral humeral head lesions and fractures of the glenoid lip, are likely to be associated with an increased incidence of recurrent instability.

In conclusion, it appears that the injuries sustained by young patients in association with traumatic dislocations are relatively unlikely to heal in a manner yielding a stable shoulder. Probably the most important of these nonhealing injuries are avulsion of the glenohumeral capsular ligaments from the anterior glenoid lip and defects of the posterolateral humeral head. Older patients tend to injure the posterior capsule or fracture the greater tuberosity, either of which is likely to heal and result in a stable shoulder unless the rotator cuff is substantially torn. In atraumatic instability, there is no traumatic lesion and thus a high chance of recurrence. The degree of trauma and the age of the patient seem to be the most important factors in determining the recurrence rate.

INJURIES ASSOCIATED WITH POSTERIOR DISLOCATIONS

Fractures

Fractures of the posterior glenoid rim and proximal part of the humerus (upper shaft, tuberosities, and head) are quite common in traumatic posterior dislocations of the shoulder.[500,501,647,700] The commonly associated compression fracture of the anteromedial portion of the humeral head is produced by the posterior cortical rim of the glenoid. It is best seen on an axillary view or a CT scan (Fig. 13-114; see also Fig. 13-95).

This lesion, sometimes called a *reverse Hill-Sachs lesion,* often occurs at the time of the original posterior dislocation. It becomes larger with multiple posterior dislocations of the shoulder. Large humeral head defects are also seen in old unreduced posterior dislocations.

The posterior rim of the glenoid may be fractured and displaced in posterior dislocations (see Fig. 13-101). Such injury occurs not only with direct forces from an anterior direction that pushes the humeral head out posteriorly but also with indirect types of dislocations such as those that occur during seizures or accidental electrical shock.

Fracture of the lesser tuberosity of the humerus can accompany posterior dislocations. The subscapularis muscle comes under considerable tension in this dislocation and can avulse the lesser tuberosity onto which it inserts. Although the fracture may be seen on AP and lateral radiographs of the glenohumeral joint, it is best seen on the axillary view and on CT scan.

Posterior dislocations of the humerus may be overlooked in the presence of a comminuted fracture of the

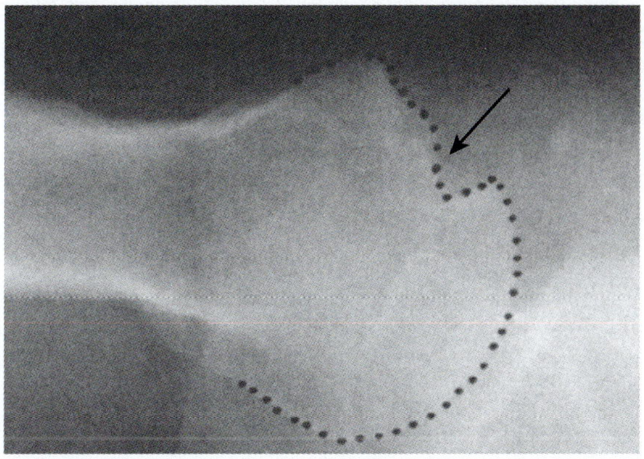

FIGURE 13-114: Axillary lateral radiograph demonstrating an anteromedial compression fracture (*arrow*) of the humeral head (*dotted outline*) (reverse Hill-Sachs lesion) after a traumatic posterior shoulder dislocation. (From Rockwood CA Jr, Green DP, Bucholz RW, eds. *Fractures in Adults*. Philadelphia: JB Lippincott; 1991.)

proximal end of the humerus or humeral shaft fractures. In the series of 16 cases of posterior dislocation of the shoulder reported by O'Conner and Jacknow,[501] 12 had comminuted fractures of the proximal part of the humerus. In eight of the 12 cases of fracture, the diagnosis of posterior dislocation was initially missed.

Other Associated Injuries

Injuries to the rotator cuff and neurovascular structures are less common with posterior than with anterior dislocations. However, they do occur. Moeller[449] reported a patient who had an open acute posterior dislocation of the left shoulder. The shoulder was totally unstable after reduction because of tears of the rotator cuff, biceps tendon, and subscapularis tendons. The patient had associated injury to the axillary and suprascapular nerves.

Recurrence of Instability After Posterior Dislocations

Recurrence of instability after posterior dislocation is less common. Recurrent posterior instability occurs at a rate of 17.7% of shoulders within the first year after initial dislocation. The risk is highest in patients who are younger than 40 years old, sustain the dislocation during a seizure, and have a large humeral head defect.[569]

TREATMENT

Anterior Dislocations

Acute Traumatic Anterior Dislocations

Timing of Reduction and Analgesia

Acute dislocations of the glenohumeral joint should be reduced as gently and expeditiously as possible, ideally after a complete set of radiographs is obtained to rule out associated bone injuries. Early relocation promptly eliminates the stretch and compression of neurovascular structures, minimizes the amount of muscle spasm that must be overcome to effect reduction, and prevents progressive enlargement of the humeral head defect in locked dislocations.

The extent of anesthesia required to accomplish a gentle reduction depends on many factors, including the amount of trauma that produced the dislocation, the duration of the dislocation, the number of previous dislocations, whether the dislocation is locked, and to what extent the patient can voluntarily relax the shoulder musculature. When seen acutely, some dislocations can be reduced without the use of medication. At the other extreme, reduction of a long-standing, locked dislocation can require a brachial plexus block or general anesthesia with muscle relaxation. Many practitioners use narcotics and muscle relaxants to aid in the reduction of shoulder dislocations. A potential trap exists: the doses required to produce muscle relaxation while the shoulder is dislocated may be sufficient to produce respiratory depression once the shoulder is reduced. Our recommendation is that if these medications are to be used, they should be administered through an established IV line. Such practice produces a more rapid onset, a short duration of action, and the opportunity to adjust the required dose more appropriately. Furthermore, resuscitation (if necessary) is facilitated by the prospective presence of such a route of access. Airway management tools should be readily available.

Milller et al.[441] compared two methods of analgesia for the reduction of anterior dislocations: IV analgesia plus muscle relaxation and intra-articular lidocaine. They found that the use of intra-articular lidocaine resulted in less use of manpower, money, and time in the emergency department.

Intra-articular lidocaine has been shown to be effective in reducing dislocations in other studies as well.[150,511] This technique may be particularly useful in patients with complicating factors such as medical problems or facial trauma and in whom respiratory depression with IV analgesia is not desired.

There is no need to put the patient through discomfort or potential risk by forcing a reduction in the emergency department. If a gentle, comfortable reduction cannot be obtained, we recommend reduction under formal anesthesia with muscle relaxation as needed. Once muscle relaxation is complete, reduction can usually be accomplished gently.

Methods of Reduction

Once the shoulder is relaxed, various gentle methods can be used to achieve reduction. Gentle traction on the arm is common to most (Figs. 13-115 and 13-116). One such method is known as the *Stimson technique*. Although the technique is named for Lewis A. Stimson,[638,637] Stimson credited Dr. Cole, a house staff physician of the Chambers Street Hospital. In the Stimson method, the patient is placed prone on the edge of the examining table while downward traction is gently applied.[637]

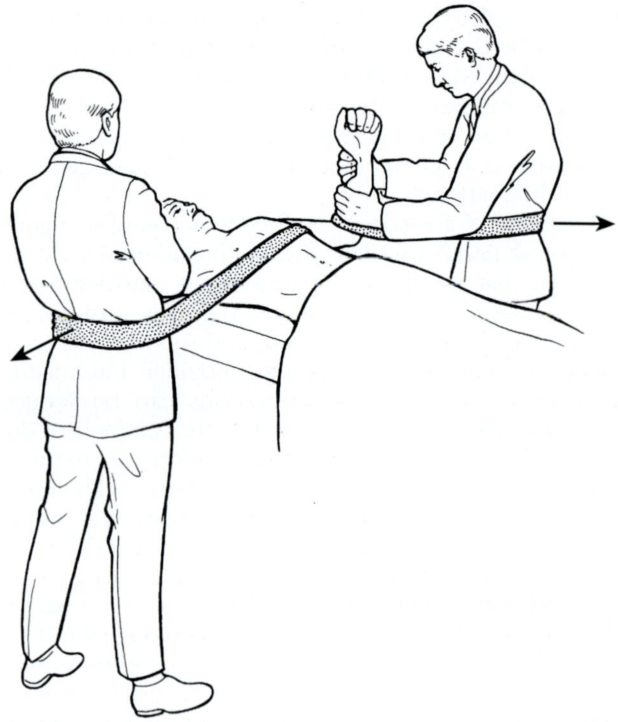

FIGURE 13-115: Reduction technique for an anterior glenohumeral dislocation. The patient lies supine with a sheet placed around the thorax and then around the assistant's waist to provide countertraction (*left arrow*). The surgeon stands on the side of the dislocated shoulder near the patient's waist with the elbow of the dislocated shoulder flexed to 90 degrees. A second sheet is tied loosely around the waist of the surgeon and looped over the patient's forearm, thus providing traction while the surgeon leans back against the sheet (*right arrow*) and grasps the forearm. Steady traction along the axis of the arm usually achieves reduction. The surgeon's hands are free to gently rock the humerus from internal to external rotation or provide gentle outward pressure on the proximal part of the humerus from the axilla.

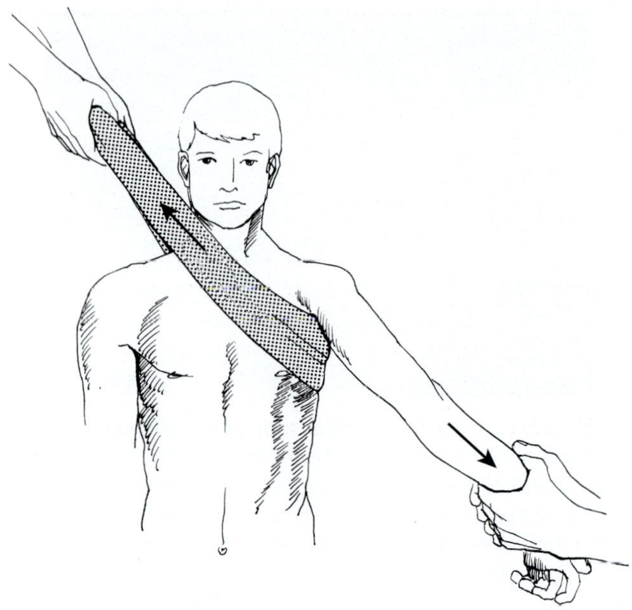

FIGURE 13-116: Closed reduction of the left shoulder with traction (*right arrow*) against countertraction (*left arrow*). (From Rockwood CA, Green DP, eds. *Fractures*. 2nd ed. Philadelphia: JB Lippincott; 1984.)

The traction-countertraction method is reliable: The patient is placed supine with a sheet around the thorax and the loose ends on the side opposite the shoulder dislocation, where they are held by an assistant. The surgeon stands on the side of the dislocated shoulder near the patient's waist. The elbow of the dislocated shoulder is flexed to 90 degrees (to relax the neurovascular structures), and traction is applied through a sheet looped over the patient's forearm, or traction can be applied directly. Steady traction along the axis of the arm usually effects reduction.

A new method of reducing shoulder dislocations has been described as the *Spaso technique*. This method places the patient in the supine position with the arm at the side. Longitudinal traction is applied as the arm is brought into forward flexion to produce an external rotational moment (Fig. 13-117).[724]

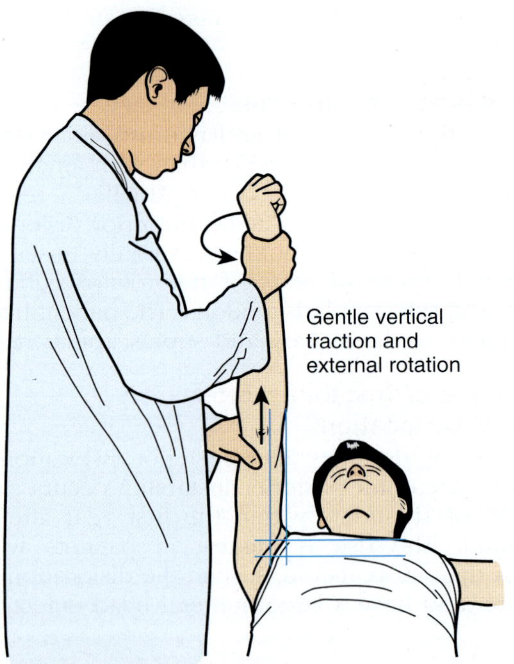

FIGURE 13-117: The Spaso technique for reducing anterior glenohumeral dislocations.

Authors' Preferred Method of Anterior Reduction

Although analgesia might not be necessary to achieve reduction, we are impressed with the safety and effectiveness of intra-articular lidocaine as described by Miller et al.[441] (Fig. 13-118). In this method, 20 mL of 1% plain

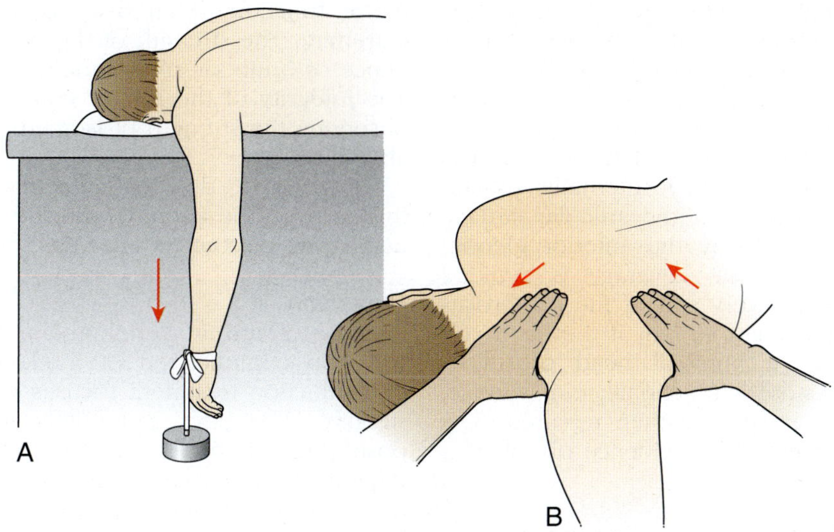

FIGURE 13-118: **A,** Stimson technique of prone gravity-assisted reduction of an anterior dislocation. **B,** Scapular manipulation during the Stimson reduction maneuver. (**A,** Modified from Rockwood CA. Fractures and dislocations of the shoulder. In: Rockwood CA, Green DP, eds. *Fractures in Adults.* 2nd ed. Philadelphia, JB Lippincott; 1984:722-805. **B,** Modified from Miller SL, Cleeman E, Auerbach J, et al. Comparison of intra-articular lidocaine and intravenous sedation for reduction of shoulder dislocations: a randomized, prospective study. *J Bone Joint Surg Am.* 2002;84-A[12]:2135-2139.)

lidocaine is injected with an 18-gauge needle placed 2 cm below the lateral edge of the acromion just posterior to the dislocated humeral head and directed toward the glenoid fossa. Placement of the needle in the joint is confirmed by a combination of feeling the needle penetrate the glenohumeral capsule, aspirating joint fluid or hemarthrosis and ensuring that the injection is not intravascular, gently palpating the glenoid fossa with the needle, and verifying easy flow on injection and return of the injected lidocaine solution. Fifteen minutes is allowed to maximize the analgesic effect of the lidocaine before manipulation.

The senior author (E.L.F.) prefers the Stimson method. In the Stimson method of reduction, the traction force may be applied by the weight of the arm, by weights taped to the wrist, or by the surgeon. It can take several minutes for the traction to produce muscle relaxation. It is important that patients not be left unattended in this position, particularly if narcotics and muscle relaxants have been administered (see Fig. 13-118).

To this basic maneuver, one may add gentle rocking of the humerus from internal to external rotation or outward pressure on the proximal end of the humerus from the axilla. These additions are particularly useful if prereduction axillary radiographs show the humeral head to be impaled on the glenoid rim. Postreduction radiographs are used to confirm reduction and detect fractures. A postreduction neurovascular examination and set of radiographs is routine.

Chronic Anterior Traumatic Dislocations

Reduction and Analgesia

A glenohumeral joint that has been dislocated for several days is a chronic dislocation. The principles and methods for reducing a chronic dislocation are similar to those relating to an acute dislocation, except that the patient and the shoulder are usually more fragile and the relocation is more difficult. As the chronicity of the dislocation increases, so do the difficulties and complications of reduction. When one encounters an elderly patient with pain in the shoulder whose radiographs reveal an anterior dislocation, a very careful history is needed to determine whether the initial injury occurred recently or quite a while earlier.

Chronic dislocations are seen most commonly in elderly people and in those whose general health or mental status might prevent them from seeking help for the injury. The event causing the injury may be relatively trivial.[48,446] Old age, chronicity of dislocation, and soft bone make closed reduction difficult and dangerous.[423] If closed reduction is to be performed, it should be done with minimal traction, without leverage, and with total muscle relaxation under controlled general anesthesia. If the dislocation is more than a week old, the humeral head is likely to be firmly impaled on the anterior glenoid with such soft tissue contraction that gentle closed reduction is impossible. When the risks of attempting reduction appear to outweigh the advantages, the dislocated position may be accepted.

Open Reduction

If a gentle attempt at closed reduction fails, open reduction may be considered. Open reduction can be a complex procedure because of the altered position of the axillary artery and branches of the brachial plexus and because the structures are tight and scarred. Sometimes the symptoms of chronic dislocation are surprisingly minimal.[201]

To perform an open reduction, the subscapularis and anterior portion of the capsule are incised near their insertion onto the lesser tuberosity to allow substantial external rotation of the dislocated shoulder. External rotation and lateral traction usually disimpact the humerus from the glenoid. While lateral traction is maintained, the humerus is gently internally rotated under direct vision to ensure that the articular surface of the humerus passes safely by the anterior glenoid lip and into the glenoid fossa. Leverage is avoided because the head is usually very soft. If the posterolateral head defect is greater than 40% or if the head collapses during reduction, a humeral head prosthesis may be necessary to restore a functional joint surface. The subscapularis and capsule are then repaired. The shoulder is carefully inspected for evidence of cuff tear or vascular damage.

Results of Treatment of Chronic Dislocations

Schulz et al.[609] reported a series of 17 posterior and 44 anterior chronic dislocations. These dislocations occurred primarily in elderly people, and more than half the dislocations were associated with fracture of the tuberosities, humeral head, humeral neck, glenoid, or coracoid process. More than a third involved neurologic deficits. Closed reduction was attempted in 40 shoulders and was successful in 20. Of the 20 shoulders successfully reduced (3 posterior and 17 anterior), the duration of dislocation exceeded 4 weeks in only 1 instance. Open reduction was performed in 20, humeral head excision was performed in 6, 8 patients were not treated, and 5 shoulders were not reducible.

Perniceni and Augereau[539] described reinforcement of the anterior shoulder complex in three patients after reduction of neglected anterior dislocations of the shoulder. They used the Gosset[220] technique, which places a rib graft between the coracoid and the glenoid rim. Rowe and Zarins[590] reported on 24 patients with unreduced dislocations of the shoulder and operated on 14 of them.

Flatow et al. reported on the treatment of 17 chronic, unreduced dislocations, of which 10 underwent surgery including one open reduction and nine arthroplasties.[192] They noted that if the dislocation is of fewer than 6 months' duration and if the head defect involves less than 40% of the articular surface, the articular surfaces may be preserved. When there is severe bone loss, reverse arthroplasty with bone grafting may need to be considered.

Management After Reduction of an Anterior Dislocation

Evaluation

After reducing the dislocation, AP and lateral radiographic views are obtained in the plane of the scapula to verify the adequacy of the reduction and provide an additional opportunity to detect fractures of the glenoid and proximal end of the humerus. The patient's neurologic status is again checked, including the sensory and motor function of all five major nerves in the upper extremity. The strength of the pulse is verified, and evidence of bruits or an expanding hematoma is sought.[230] The integrity of the rotator cuff is initially evaluated by observing the strength of isometric external rotation and abduction.

Trimmings[660] demonstrated that aspiration of hemarthrosis from the shoulder can be an effective means of decreasing discomfort after the shoulder is reduced.

Protection

Because recurrent glenohumeral instability is the most common complication of a glenohumeral dislocation, postreduction treatment focuses on optimizing shoulder stability. Thus two potentially important elements in postreduction treatment are protection and muscle rehabilitation. Reeves demonstrated that after repair of the subscapularis in primates, 3 months were necessary before normal capsular patterns of collagen bundles were observed, 5 months before the tendon was histologically normal, and 4 to 5 months before tensile strength was regained.[559] It is unknown whether labral tears or ligamentous avulsions from the glenoid heal or how long this might take. In any event, it is apparent that the shoulder cannot be immobilized for the full length of time required for complete healing. Immobilization in external rotation rather than the standard internally rotated position is suggested by Itoi et al., who used MRI to examine shoulders after dislocation and found the anterior labrum to have 1.9 mm of separation from the glenoid while the shoulder is in internal rotation but only 0.1 mm when the arm is externally rotated.[307]

We treat first-time dislocations in a manner similar to the postoperative management of dislocation repairs. Thus younger patients have flexion limited to 100 degrees and external rotation limited to 20 degrees for the first 3 weeks while strength is maintained with cuff and deltoid isometrics. The elbow is fully extended at least several times a day to prevent sling soreness. Because stiffness of the shoulder, elbow, and hand is more likely to develop in persons older than 30 years, the duration of immobilization is progressively reduced for persons of increasing age.[582,431,430,340,400] Patients are checked 3 weeks after relocation and examined for stiffness; if external rotation to 0 degrees is difficult, formal stretching exercises are started. Otherwise, the patient is allowed to increase use of the shoulder as comfort permits.

Strengthening

At 3 weeks, the patient institutes more vigorous rotator cuff–strengthening exercises using rubber tubing or weights. The patient is informed that strong subscapularis and infraspinatus muscles are ideally situated to increase glenohumeral stability.[597]

Burkhead and Rockwood,[90] Glousman et al.,[216] and Tibone and Bradley[651] emphasized the importance of strengthening not only the rotator cuff but also the scapular stabilizing muscles because of their vital importance in providing a stable platform for shoulder function. Even in the case of recurrent instability, Burkhead and Rockwood[90] found that a complete exercise program was effective in the management of 12% of patients with traumatic subluxation, 80% with anterior atraumatic subluxation, and 90% with posterior instability.

Swimming is recommended at 6 weeks to enhance endurance and coordination. By 3 months after the dislocation, most patients should have almost full flexion and rotation of the shoulder. Patients are not allowed to use the injured arm in sports or for overhead labor until they have achieved normal rotator strength, comfortable and nearly full forward elevation, and confidence in the shoulder with it in the positions necessary for the activity. Any deviation from the expected course of recovery requires careful reevaluation for occult fractures, loose bodies, rotator cuff tears, peripheral nerve injuries, and glenohumeral arthritis.

Early Surgery in Anterior Dislocations

According to conventional wisdom, nonoperative treatment is the conservative choice after an initial shoulder dislocation and, in general, surgery is reserved for recurrent instability. However, in a study of functional outcome and risk of recurrent instability after primary anterior shoulder dislocation in young patients (15 to 35 years old), Robinson et al.[567] found that within 2 years instability was present in more than half. Arciero et al.[18] showed in a randomized prospective study that early surgical repair significantly reduced the recurrence rate in young athletes after an acute, initial traumatic anterior dislocation. Their initial data indicated a decrease in recurrent instability from 80% with nonoperative management to 14% with early repair.[16-18]

Soft Tissue Interposition

Tietjen[652] reported a case in which surgery was required to retrieve the avulsed supraspinatus, infraspinatus, and teres minor from their interposition between the humeral head and the glenoid.

Bridle and Ferris[80] reported a case of apparent successful closed reduction of an anterior shoulder dislocation that appeared to be confirmed on an AP radiograph. However, the patient continued to experience severe pain, and a subsequent axillary lateral view demonstrated persistent anterior subluxation of the glenohumeral joint. At the time of open reduction, the ruptured muscle belly of the subscapularis was found interposed between the humeral head and glenoid. Inao et al.[298] reported a case of an acute anterior shoulder dislocation that was irreducible by closed treatment because of interposition of the posteriorly displaced tendon of the long head of the biceps.

Displaced Fracture of the Greater Tuberosity

Although fractures of the greater tuberosity are not uncommonly associated with anterior shoulder dislocation, the tuberosity usually reduces into an acceptable position when the shoulder is reduced (see Figs. 13-6 and 13-107). Occasionally, the greater tuberosity fragment displaces up under the acromion process or is pulled posteriorly by the cuff muscles. If the greater tuberosity remains displaced after reduction of the shoulder joint (see Fig. 13-111), consideration should be given to anatomic reduction and internal fixation of the fragment and repair of the attendant split in the tendons of the rotator cuff (see Fig. 13-108).[191]

Determining the amount of superior displacement of the tuberosity fragment is relatively easy on an AP radiograph in the plane of the scapula. Posterior displacement can be more difficult to discern.[529] It is important to look for the vacant tuberosity sign, wherein the normal contour of the greater tuberosity is lacking. If one is concerned about the AP position of the tuberosity on plain films, a CT scan should be considered. If the tuberosity is allowed to heal with posterior displacement, the functional equivalent of both a rotator cuff tear and a bony block to external rotation can result.

Glenoid Rim Fracture

Aston and Gregory[23] reported three cases in which a large anterior fracture of the glenoid occurred as a result of a fall on the lateral aspect of the abducted shoulder. A fracture of the glenoid lip can require open or arthroscopic reduction and internal fixation if an intra-articular incongruity or an inadequate effective glenoid arc is present (see Fig. 13-101).

Posterior Dislocations

Reduction

Reduction of acute traumatic posterior dislocations may be much more difficult than reduction of acute traumatic anterior dislocations. Hawkins et al.[255] reviewed 41 cases of locked posterior shoulder dislocations. The average interval between injury and diagnosis was 1 year! In seven of these cases, the shoulder deformity was acceptable to the patient. Closed reduction was successful in only six of the 12 cases in which it was attempted.

IV narcotics combined with muscle relaxants or tranquilizers can provide insufficient analgesia and muscle relaxation; general anesthesia with muscle paralysis may be required. Atraumatic closed reduction can usually be accomplished once the muscle spasm has been eliminated. With the patient in the supine position, longitudinal and lateral traction is applied to the arm while it is gently rocked in internal and external rotation. Once the head is disimpacted, it is lifted anteriorly back into the glenoid fossa. In locked posterior dislocations, it may be necessary to gently stretch out the posterior cuff and capsule by maximally internally rotating the humerus before reduction is attempted. Care should be taken not to force the arm into external rotation before reduction is achieved; if the head is locked posteriorly on the glenoid rim, forced external rotation could produce a fracture of the head or shaft of the humerus.

If gentle closed reduction of a locked posterior glenohumeral dislocation is not possible, open reduction may be accomplished through an anterior deltopectoral appr oach.[156,255,319,352,357,429,576,603] Because local anatomy is significantly distorted, the tendon of the long head of the biceps is used as a guide to the lesser tuberosity. The subscapularis is released either by osteotomy of the lesser tuberosity or by direct incision. With the glenoid thus exposed, open reduction is carried out by gently pulling the humeral head laterally and then lifting its articular surface up on the face of the glenoid.

If after closed reduction the shoulder is stable in the sling position, this type of postreduction management is most convenient for the patient. However, if recurrent instability is a concern, the shoulder is immobilized in a shoulder spica or brace with the amount of external rotation necessary to provide stability.[99,100] Scougall[611] has shown experimentally in monkeys that a surgically detached posterior glenoid labrum and capsule heal soundly without repair. He concluded that the best position of immobilization, to allow healing of all the posterior structures, was in abduction, external rotation, and extension and that the position should be maintained for 4 weeks.

Although some have recommended pin fixation for 3 weeks after reduction,[700] this method carries a risk of pin breakage and infection.

Surgery

Indications for surgery include a displaced lesser tuberosity fracture, a significant posterior glenoid fracture, an irreducible dislocation, an open dislocation, or an unstable reduction. If the shoulder cannot be maintained in a reduced position, reconstructive surgery to reduce the impaction fracture, a tendon or bone transfer, an allograft, or replacement of the humeral head can be considered.

A major cause of recurrent instability after reduction of a posterior dislocation is the presence of a large anteromedial humeral head defect. If at the time of reduction stability cannot be obtained because of such a defect, it may be rendered extra-articular by filling it with the subscapularis tendon as described by McLaughlin[379,424-426,429] or the lesser tuberosity as described by Neer.[486] If the humeral head defect involves more than 30% of the articular surface, replacement with a prosthesis may be indicated; otherwise, instability can recur with internal rotation. Hawkins et al. demonstrated the use of each of these techniques in a series of locked posterior dislocations.[255]

After surgery, the arm may be immobilized in a sling and swathe for 2 weeks as recommended by McLaughlin, the arm may be positioned at the side posterior to the coronal plane with a strip of tape or canvas restraint as recommended by Rowe and Zarins,[590] or a modified spica in neutral rotation may be used for 6 weeks, followed by an additional 3 to 6 months of rehabilitative exercises as recommended by Rockwood.

Keppler et al. suggested using rotational osteotomy of the humerus for the postreduction management of locked posterior dislocations.[334]

Authors' Preferred Method of Treatment

Our management of acute traumatic posterior dislocations begins with a thorough exploration of the cause of the dislocation, looking for evidence of seizures, substance abuse, or recurrent trauma. We then seek to define the extent and chronicity of the injury. A complete radiographic evaluation that includes AP and lateral views in the plane of the scapula and an axillary view is necessary. Careful note is made of associated fractures, including the extent of the impression fracture of the anteromedial humeral head. Under anesthesia and muscle relaxation, gentle closed reduction is attempted with the application of axial traction on the arm. If the head is locked on the glenoid rim, gentle internal rotation can stretch out the posterior capsule to facilitate reduction. Lateral traction on the proximal part of the humerus can unlock the humeral head. Once it is unlocked, the humerus is gently externally rotated. After reduction is achieved and confirmed by postreduction radiographs, a determination is made of the stability of the reduced shoulder and its bony anatomy.

If the shoulder appears to have a good chance of stability, the reduction is maintained for 3 weeks in a cummerbund handshake cast (Fig. 13-119) or orthotic (Fig. 13-120) in neutral rotation and slight extension. External rotation and deltoid isometrics are carried out during this period of immobilization. After removal of the cast, a vigorous *strengthening* program for the internal and external rotators is initiated. Range of motion is allowed to return with active use, beginning with elevation in the plane of the scapula. Vigorous physical activities are not resumed until the shoulder is strong and 3 months has elapsed since reduction. Swimming is

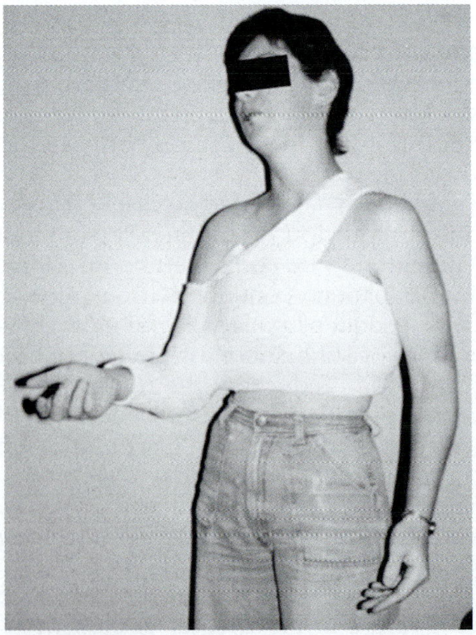

FIGURE 13-119: A handshake cast. After closed reduction of an acute traumatic posterior dislocation is confirmed by radiographs, a cast is applied in neutral rotation and slight extension for 3 weeks.

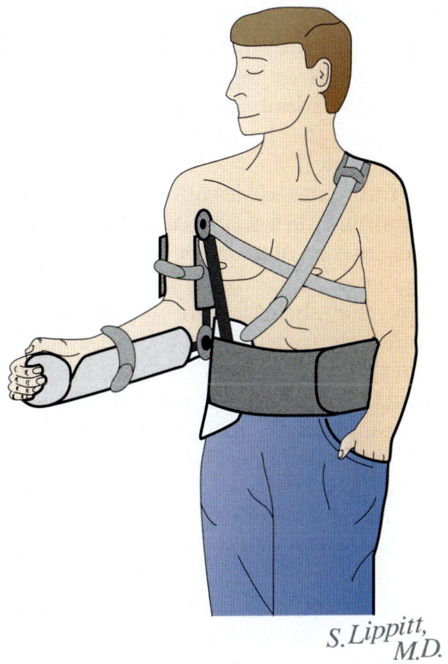

FIGURE 13-120: An orthosis is used to immobilize the arm after reduction of a posterior dislocation or a global capsular repair. (Modified from Matsen FA III, Lippitt SB, Sidles JA, Harryman DT II. *Practical Evaluation and Management of the Shoulder*. Philadelphia: WB Saunders; 1994.)

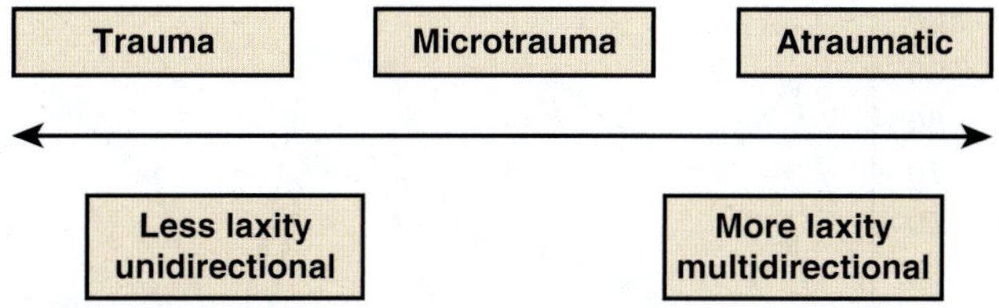

FIGURE 13-121: The spectrum of instability. (From Bigliani LU, Kurzweil PR, Schwartzbach CC, et al. Inferior capsular shift procedure for anterior-inferior shoulder instability in athletes. *Am J Sports Med*. 1994;22[5]:578-584.)

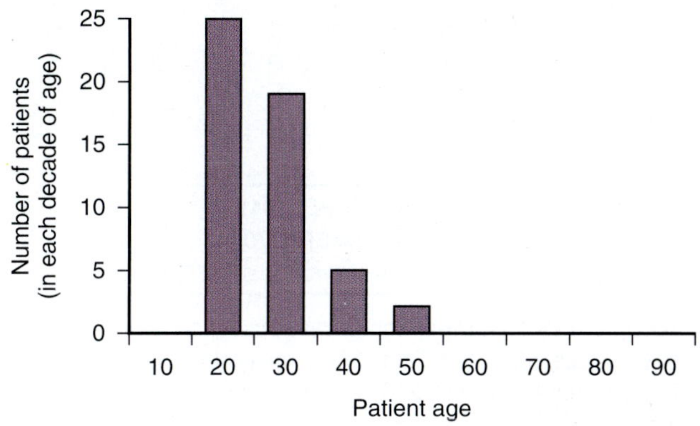

FIGURE 13-122: Age distribution of 51 patients with atraumatic instability. (From Matsen FA III, Lippitt SB, Sidles JA, Harryman DT II. *Practical Evaluation and Management of the Shoulder*. Philadelphia: WB Saunders; 1994.)

encouraged because it helps to develop endurance and muscle coordination.

When a humeral head defect involves 20% to 40% of the humeral head, a transfer of the lesser tuberosity with attached subscapularis into the defect can provide increased stability. When the humeral head defect is greater than 40% or the dislocation is of more than 6 months' duration, a proximal humeral prosthesis to replace the lost articular surface is often necessary to prevent the glenoid from falling into the humeral defect (see Fig. 13-69). In younger patients, an allograft segment or mini-resurfacing may be considered. In older patients or those with cuff loss, a reverse total shoulder replacement may be used. When the dislocation is obviously chronic, consideration may be given to accepting the dislocation and focusing on enhancing the patient's ability to carry out activities of daily living.

RECURRENT DISLOCATION

Evaluation

After an initial dislocation, the shoulder might return to functional stability, or it might fall victim to recurrent glenohumeral instability. Although intermediate forms of recurrent instability do occur, the great majority of recurrently unstable shoulders may be thought of as being either atraumatic or traumatic in origin.

Although Matsen has divided recurrent instability into atraumatic and traumatic categories, Bigliani et al.[55] described the "spectrum" of instability, from traumatic to microtraumatic to atraumatic, and from unidirectional to bidirectional to multidirectional (Fig. 13-121). Thus each patient is evaluated as to etiology (e.g., microtraumatic) and as to direction (e.g., anteroinferior). When primary repairs were performed open, this approach led to a laterally based capsular shift technique, with the dissection continued inferiorly and posteriorly as much as required for the degree of laxity found in each case.[544] In the arthroscopic era, the variable has been the degree to which posterior-inferior capsular "tucks" or plication stitches are added to the standard anteroinferior labral repair.

History

Most patients with atraumatic instability are younger than 30 years (Fig. 13-122). Because the instability occurs in the midrange positions of the shoulder, atraumatic instability typically causes discomfort and dysfunction in ordinary activities of daily living. Commonly, such patients have the greatest difficulty sleeping, lifting overhead, and throwing (Fig. 13-123).

The onset is usually insidious, but it can occur after a minor injury or period of disuse. The unwanted translations can range from a sensation of a minor slip in the

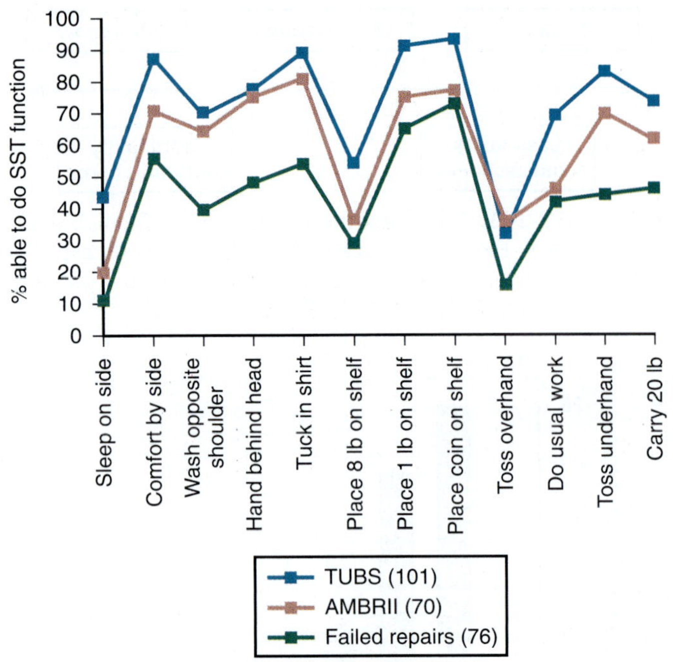

FIGURE 13-123: Comparison of responses to the 12 questions of the Simple Shoulder Test (SST) for groups of patients with traumatic instability (TUBS), atraumatic instability (AMBRII), and failed instability repairs.

joint to complete dislocation of the humeral head from the glenoid. The displacement characteristically reduces spontaneously, after which the patient is usually able to return to previous activities without much pain or problem. As the condition progresses, the patient notices that the shoulder has become looser and might feel it slip out and clunk back in with increasing ease and in an increasing number of activities. The shoulder can become uncomfortable, even with the arm at rest. Patients might volunteer that they can make the shoulder pop out and that at times the shoulder feels as though it needs to be popped out on purpose.

It is important to document the history and the circumstances surrounding the onset of the problem, as well as each and every position of the shoulder in which the patient experiences instability. Whether the opposite shoulder is symptomatic as well is also important to note. A family history might reveal other family members similarly affected, in addition to conditions known to predispose to atraumatic instability, such as Ehlers-Danlos syndrome.

Many patients admit that they had a habit of dislocating the joint but that they can now no longer control the stability of the joint. The surgeon must determine whether habitual dislocation remains a feature of the patient's problem. For surgery to cure habitual instability is clearly difficult.

In characteristic anterior traumatic instability, the usual mechanism of injury involves the application of a large extension-external rotation force to the arm elevated near the coronal plane. Such a mechanism can occur in a fall while snow skiing, while executing a high-speed cut in water skiing, in an arm tackle during football, with a block of a volleyball or basketball shot, or in relatively violent industrial accidents in which a posteriorly directed force is applied to the hand while the arm is abducted and externally rotated.

An initial traumatic dislocation often requires assistance in reduction rather than reducing spontaneously as is usually the case in atraumatic instability. Radiographs from previous emergency department visits may be available to show the shoulder in its dislocated position. Axillary or other neuropathy may have accompanied the glenohumeral dislocation. Any of these findings individually or in combination support the diagnosis of traumatic as opposed to atraumatic instability.

Traumatic instability can occur without a complete dislocation. In this situation, the injury produces a traumatic lesion, but the lesion is insufficient to allow the humeral head to completely escape from the glenoid. The shoulder may be unstable because as a result of the injury, it manifests apprehension or subluxation when the arm is placed near the position of injury. Such patients have no history of the need for reduction and have no radiographs with the shoulder in the dislocated position. Thus the diagnosis rests to an even greater extent on a careful history that focuses on the position and forces involved in the initial episode.

Characteristically, a shoulder with traumatic instability is comfortable when troublesome positions are avoided. However, the apprehension or fear of instability can prevent the patient from returning to work or sports. Recurrent subluxation or dislocation can occur when the shoulder is unexpectedly forced into the abducted, externally rotated position or during sleep when the patient's active guard is less effective. The patient might have a history of increasing ease of dislocation as the remaining stabilizing factors are progressively compromised.

Physical Examination

Demonstration of Instability

Because glenohumeral instability is defined as a condition wherein the patient cannot maintain the humeral head in a centered position in the glenoid, it is critical to allow the patient to demonstrate his or her functional problem to the examiner.

Laxity Tests

Laxity tests seek to define the amount of translation or rotation that an examiner can elicit in the relaxed shoulder. This translation is determined both by the position of the shoulder and by the properties of the ligaments and capsule. Translational and rotational laxity are closely related (Figs. 13-124 to 13-127). When interpreting the significance of the degree of translation on laxity tests, it is important to use the contralateral shoulder as an example of what is "normal" for the patient.

In the past, laxity was confused with instability; treatments were directed at managing laxity rather than at enabling the head to stay centered in the glenoid. Shoulders without clear evidence of instability were tightened

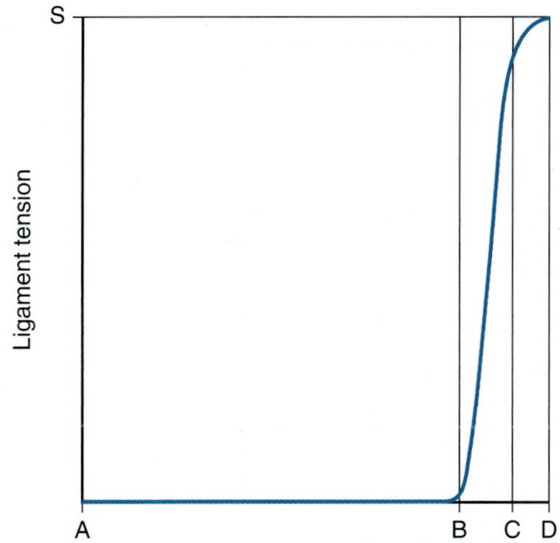

FIGURE 13-124: The properties of the glenohumeral ligament include its resting length, its elastic deformability, and its plastic deformability. These properties can be demonstrated as a plot of the ligament's tension versus the distance between the ligament's origin and insertion. At point *A*, the origin and insertion of the ligament are closely approximated. At point *B*, the origin and insertion have been separated enough to initiate tension in the ligament. Thus the resting length of the ligament is shown as *A* to *B*. Additional separation of the origin and insertion causes increasing ligament tension. Up to point *C*, this separation is elastic. Further separation of the origin and insertion plastically deforms the ligament up to point *D*, where the ligament fails at a tension of *S*.

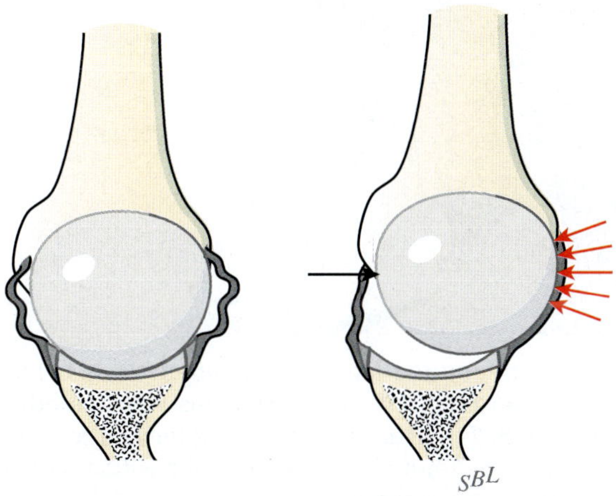

FIGURE 13-125: Glenohumeral translation is movement of the center of the humeral head with respect to the face of the glenoid. *Left*, The humeral head in mid glenoid with lax ligaments. *Right*, The amount of translation allowed (*black arrow*) is determined by the initial position of the joint and the length of the ligament that becomes tight (*red arrows*).

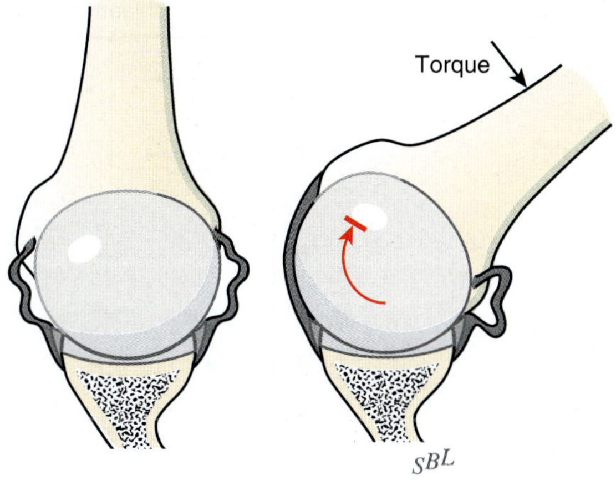

FIGURE 13-126: Glenohumeral rotation is movement of the humerus around the center of the humeral head, which remains centered in the glenoid fossa. *Left*, The humeral head in mid glenoid with lax ligaments. *Right*, The amount of rotation allowed (*red arrow*) in response to an applied torque (*black arrow*) is determined by the initial position of the joint and the length of the ligament that becomes tight.

because they were lax and painful; the results were not good. For this reason, it is important to recognize that normal shoulders are lax and that laxity is often not increased in unstable shoulders.[244] Many normally stable shoulders, such as those of gymnasts, demonstrate substantial translation on laxity tests even though they are asymptomatic.

In performing the tests described next, it is important for the examiner to note not only the amount of laxity but also any findings associated with the translation or rotation as well as the patient's subjective response to the test.

In the *drawer test* (Fig. 13-128), the patient is seated with the forearm resting on the lap and the shoulder relaxed. The examiner stands behind the patient. One of the examiner's hands stabilizes the shoulder girdle (scapula and clavicle) while the other grasps the proximal end of the humerus. These tests are performed with a minimal compressive load (just enough to center the head in the glenoid) and a substantial compressive load (to gain a feeling for the effectiveness of the glenoid concavity). Starting from the centered position with a minimal compressive load, the humerus is first pushed forward to determine the amount of anterior displacement relative to the scapula. The anterior translation of a normal shoulder reaches a firm end point with no clunking, no pain, and no apprehension. A clunk or snap on anterior subluxation or reduction can suggest a labral tear or Bankart lesion.[619]

In the *sulcus test* (Figs. 13-129 and 13-130), the patient sits with the arm relaxed at the side. The examiner centers the head with a mild compressive load and then pulls the arm downward. Inferior laxity is demonstrated if a sulcus or hollow appears inferior to the acromion.

In the *push-pull test* (Fig. 13-131), the patient lies supine with the shoulder off the edge of the table. The arm is in 90 degrees of abduction and 30 degrees of flexion. Standing next to the patient's hip, the examiner pulls up on the wrist with one hand while pushing down on the proximal part of the humerus with the other.

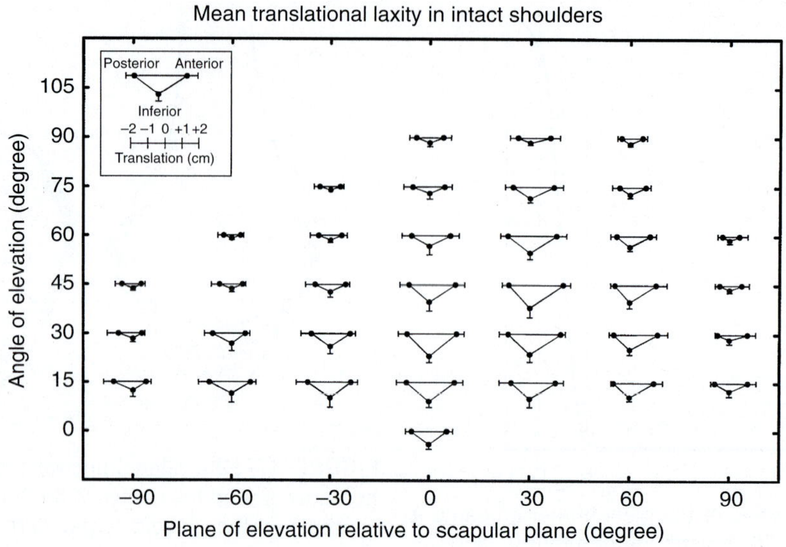

FIGURE 13-127: Mean translational laxity as measured in eight cadaveric shoulders. The applied translational force was 30 N (~6 lb), and it was applied along the anterior, posterior, and inferior axes. The planes of elevation are measured relative to the plane of the scapula (see Fig. 13-43), not the thoracic plane. The angles of elevation are measured relative to the scapular reference line (see Fig. 13-43). Standard deviations are shown at the vertex of each triangle. (From Matsen FA III, Lippitt SB, Sidles JA, Harryman DT II. *Practical Evaluation and Management of the Shoulder.* Philadelphia: WB Saunders; 1994.)

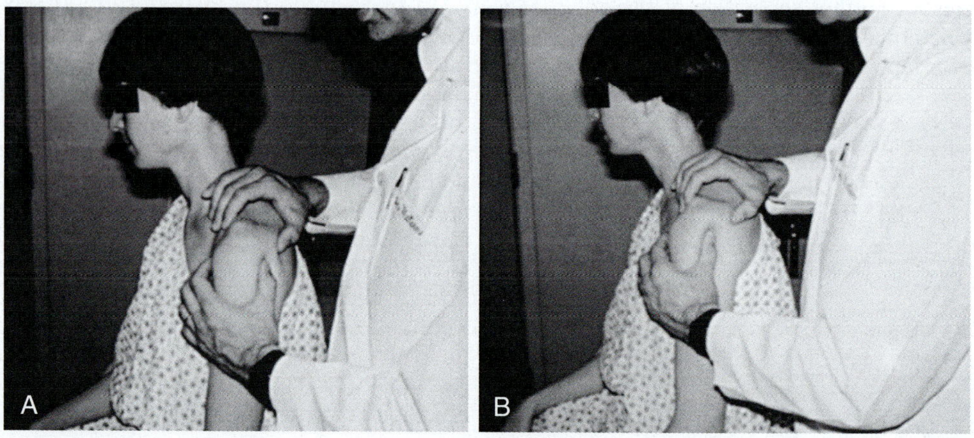

FIGURE 13-128: Drawer test. **A,** The patient is seated and the forearm is resting in the lap. The examiner stands behind the patient and stabilizes the shoulder girdle with one hand while grasping the proximal end of the humerus with the other and pressing the humeral head gently toward the scapula to center it in the glenoid. **B,** The head is then pushed forward to determine the amount of anterior displacement relative to the scapula. The head can then be returned to the neutral position, and a posterior force is applied to determine the amount of posterior translation relative to the scapula.

Normal shoulders of relaxed patients often allow 50% posterior translation on this test.

Provocative Stability Tests

Stability tests examine the ability of the shoulder to resist challenges to stability in positions in which the ligaments are normally under tension. A key element of these tests is noting if the maneuver reproduces the symptoms of concern to the patient.

In the *fulcrum test* (Fig. 13-132), the patient lies supine at the edge of the examination table with the arm abducted to 90 degrees. The examiner places one hand on the table under the glenohumeral joint to act as a fulcrum. The patient's arm is gently and progressively extended and externally rotated over this fulcrum. Maintaining gentle passive external rotation for a minute fatigues the subscapularis and thereby challenges the capsular contribution to anterior stability of the shoulder.

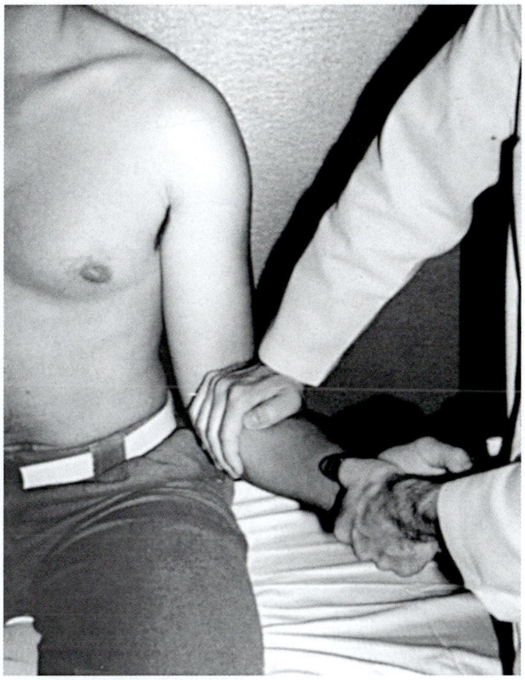

FIGURE 13-129: Sulcus test. The patient is seated with the arm relaxed and at the side. The examiner pulls downward on the arm. Inferior instability is demonstrated if a sulcus (or hollow) appears inferior to the acromion. The result of the sulcus test in this patient is negative.

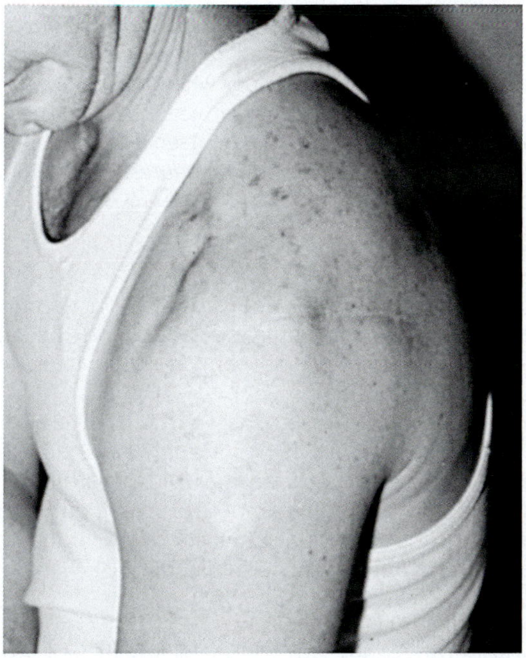

FIGURE 13-130: Sulcus sign. This patient had a posterior repair for glenohumeral instability. However, he continues to have inferior instability and demonstrates the sulcus (or hollow) just inferior to the anterior acromion during this sulcus test.

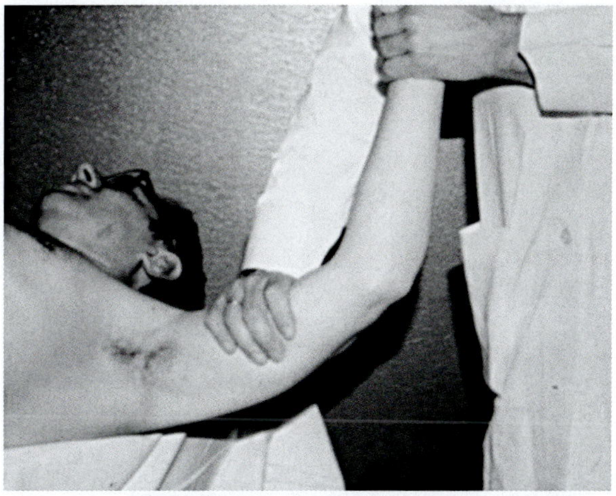

FIGURE 13-131: Push-pull test. The patient lies supine and relaxed with the shoulder at the edge of the examination table. The examiner pulls up on the wrist with one hand while pushing down on the proximal part of the humerus with the other. Approximately 50% posterior translation of the humerus on the glenoid is normal in relaxed patients.

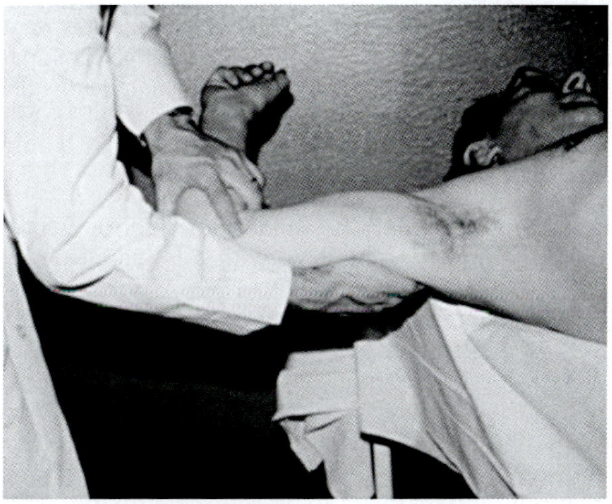

FIGURE 13-132: Fulcrum test. With the patient supine and the shoulder at the edge of the examination table, the arm is abducted to 90 degrees. The examiner's right hand is used as a fulcrum while the arm is gently and progressively extended and externally rotated. In the presence of anterior instability, the patient becomes apprehensive or the shoulder translates with this maneuver.

Normally, no apprehension or translation occurs because the anterior ligaments are intact. A patient with anterior instability usually becomes apprehensive as this maneuver is carried out; this finding suggests deficiency in the anterior stabilizing structures.

In the *crank* or *apprehension test* (Fig. 13-133), the patient sits with his or her back toward the examiner. The patient's arm is held in 90 degrees of abduction and external rotation. The examiner pulls back on the patient's wrist with one hand while stabilizing the back of the

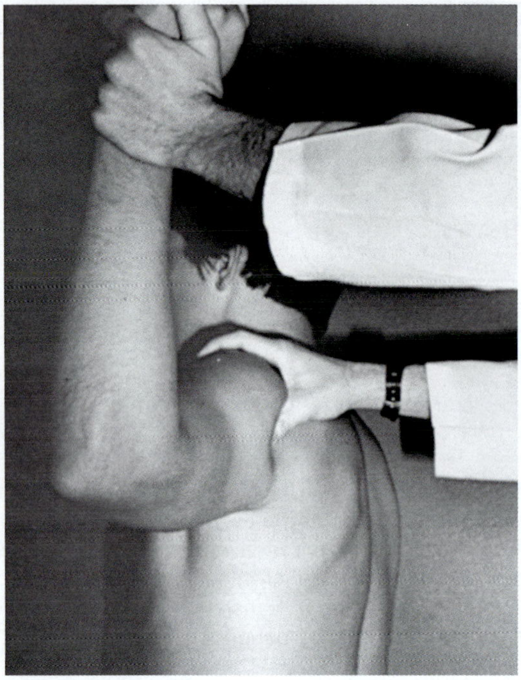

FIGURE 13-133: Crank test. The arm is held in 90 degrees of abduction and external rotation. The examiner's left hand is pulling back on the patient's wrist while the right hand stabilizes the back of the shoulder. A patient with anterior instability becomes apprehensive with this maneuver.

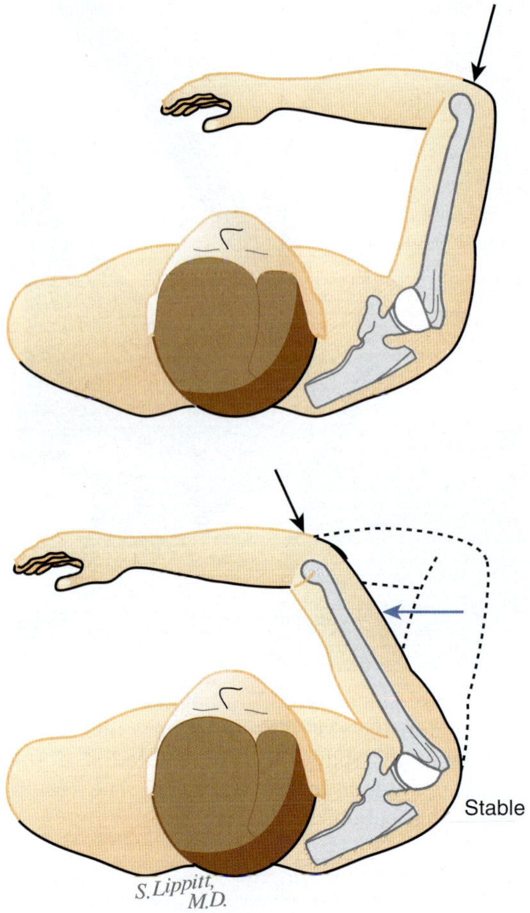

FIGURE 13-134: *Top,* Negative jerk test. The humeral head of the axially loaded arm remains centered in the glenoid fossa even with axial loading of humerus (*black arrow*). *Bottom,* Positive jerk test. The humeral head of the axillary loaded arm slides out the back of the shoulder when the arm is adducted across the body and clunks back in when the arm position is aligned with the scapula. (From Matsen FA III, Lippitt SB. *Shoulder Surgery: Principles and Procedures.* Philadelphia: WB Saunders; 2004:115.)

shoulder with the other. A patient with anterior instability usually becomes apprehensive with this maneuver.

In the *jerk test* (Figs. 13-134 to 13-137), the patient sits with the arm internally rotated and flexed forward to 90 degrees. The examiner grasps the elbow and axially loads the humerus in a proximal direction. While axial loading of the humerus is maintained, the arm is moved horizontally across the body. A positive test is indicated by a sudden jerk as the humeral head slides off the back of the glenoid. When the arm is returned to the original position of 90-degree abduction, a second jerk may be observed, that of the humeral head returning to the glenoid.

The magnitude of translation on standard tests of glenohumeral laxity (see Figs. 13-128 to 13-131) does not necessarily distinguish stable from unstable shoulders. However, an experienced examiner can detect diminished resistance to anterior translation on the drawer test when the humeral head is compressed into the glenoid fossa; the diminished resistance in this case indicates loss of the anterior glenoid lip. This maneuver can also elicit grinding as the humeral head slides over the bony edge of the glenoid from which the labrum has been avulsed or elicit catching as the head passes over a torn glenoid labrum.

Pain on abduction, external rotation, and extension is not specific for instability. Such pain can relate to shoulder stiffness or alternatively to abutment of the glenoid against the cuff insertion to the head posteriorly.[414,578] Relief of this pain by anterior pressure on the humeral head can result from diminished stretch on the anterior capsule or from relief of the abutment posteriorly (Fig. 13-138).

In all patients with instability, particularly those older than 35 years, the strength of internal and external rotation must be examined to explore the possibility of cuff weakness or tear. Finally, a neurologic examination is performed to determine the integrity of the axillary nerve and other branches of the brachial plexus.

Radiographs and Other Tests

Full radiograph series are obtained, including true AP, axillary, and the Stryker notch view. For gross instability despite reduction, and/or obvious glenoid fracture, CT scan is obtained to assess for fracture. For patients over 40 years of age with a shoulder dislocation, noncontrast

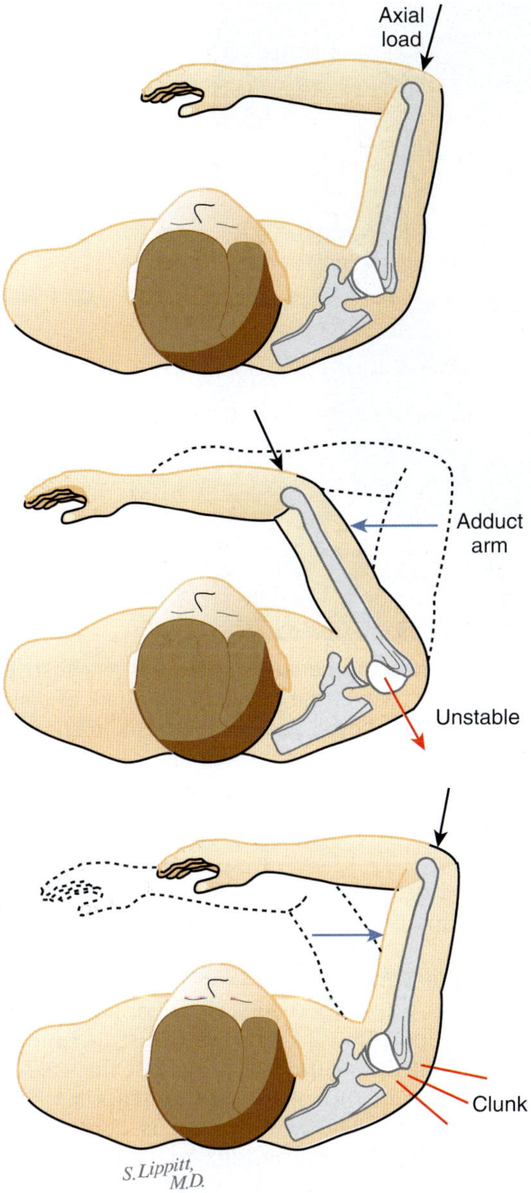

FIGURE 13-135: Positive jerk test. The humeral head of the axially loaded arm slides out the back of the shoulder when the arm is adducted across the body and clunks back in when the arm position is aligned with the scapula. (From Matsen FA III, Lippitt SB. *Shoulder Surgery: Principles and Procedures*. Philadelphia: WB Saunders; 2004:115.)

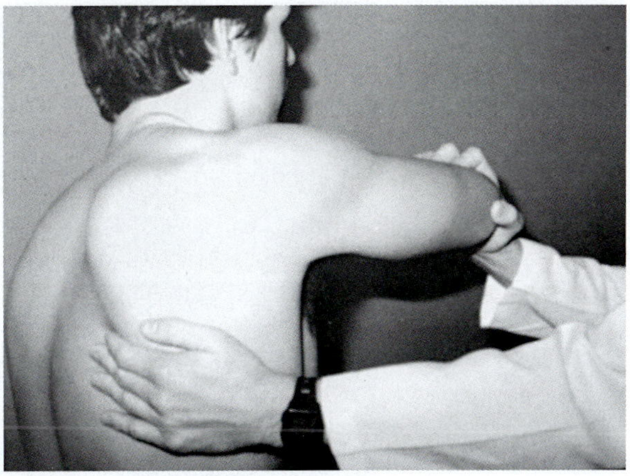

FIGURE 13-136: Jerk test. The patient's arm is abducted to 90 degrees and internally rotated. The examiner axially loads the humerus while the arm is moved horizontally across the body. The left hand stabilizes the scapula. A patient with a recurrent posterior instability might demonstrate a sudden jerk as the humeral head slides off the back of the glenoid or when it is reduced by moving the arm back to the starting position.

MRI is indicated routinely to evaluate the integrity of the rotator cuff. For recurrent instability, MR arthrogram is essential to fully assess the labrum and injury to capsular structures, and CT scan should be considered to assess for glenoid bone loss. Especially helpful is the view of the glenoid en face in the 3D reconstruction series with the humerus removed.[108] However, it is equally important to recognize normal anatomic variants of the anterior glenoid labrum. A normal labrum may not be fully inserted into the anterior glenoid in the normal variants such as a sublabral foramen or a Buford complex.

In atraumatic instability, shoulder radiographs characteristically show no bony pathology—specifically, no posterolateral humeral head defect, no glenoid rim fracture or new bone formation, and no evidence of tuberosity fracture. Because these patients typically demonstrate midrange instability, radiographs can show translation of the humeral head with respect to the glenoid; for example, the axillary view can show posterior subluxation. Occasionally, radiographs can suggest factors underlying the atraumatic instability, such as a relatively small or hypoplastic glenoid or a posteriorly inclined or otherwise dysplastic glenoid. The bony glenoid fossa can appear quite flat; however, it is difficult to relate the apparent depth of the bony socket to the effective depth of the fossa formed by cartilage and labrum covering the bone.

Recurrent traumatic dislocations more commonly have radiographic findings.

Humeral Head Changes

One of the most common findings is indentation or impaction in the posterior aspect of the humeral head from contact with the anteroinferior corner of the glenoid when the joint was dislocated (Fig. 13-139; see Figs. 13-4 and 13-95). In their classic article,[271] Hill and Sachs evaluated the relationship of humeral head defects to shoulder instability. They concluded that more than two-thirds of anterior shoulder dislocations are complicated by a bony injury of the humerus or scapula.

Compression fractures as a result of impingement of the weakest portion of the humeral head, that is, the posterior lateral aspect of the articular surface against the anterior rim of the glenoid fossa, are found so frequently

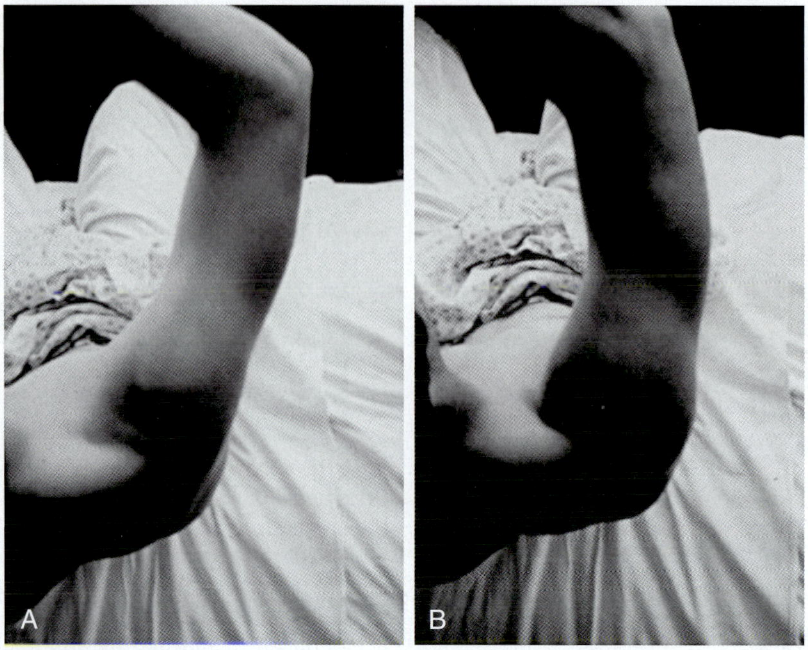

FIGURE 13-137: Voluntary jerk test. **A,** Normal appearance of the shoulder before the patient performs a jerk test. **B,** With movement of the arm horizontally across the body, the humeral head slides off the back of the glenoid with a jerk of dislocation and a prominence in the posterior aspect of the patient's shoulder. When the arm is moved back to the position shown in **A,** a jerk of reduction occurs.

in cases of habitual dislocation that they have been described as a typical defect. These defects are sustained at the time of the original dislocation. A special sign is the sharp, vertical, dense medial border of the groove known as the line of condensation, the length of which is correlated with the size of the defect.[271]

They reported the defect in only 27% of 119 acute anterior dislocations but in 74% of 15 recurrent anterior dislocations. However, they stated that the incidence of the groove defect was low, undoubtedly because it was only in the last 6 months of their 10-year study (1930 to 1940) that they used special radiographic views. The size of the defect varied in length (cephalocaudal) from 5 mm to 3 cm, in width from 3 mm to 2 cm, and in depth from 10 mm to 22 mm.[269]

A number of special projections have been used to enhance visualization of the Hill-Sachs defect.[3,154,240,265,458,510,536,642] Two of these views bear special mention.

Stryker Notch View

The patient is supine on the table with the cassette placed under the shoulder.[240] The palm of the hand of the affected shoulder is placed on top of the head, with the fingers directed toward the back of the head. The elbow of the affected shoulder should point straight upward. The x-ray beam tilts 10 degrees toward the head and is centered over the coracoid process (Fig. 13-140). This technique was developed by William S. Stryker and reported by Hall et al.[240] They stated that they could demonstrate the humeral head defect in 90% of 20 patients with a history of recurring anterior dislocation of the shoulder.

Apical Oblique View

Garth et al.[205,206] described the apical oblique projection of the shoulder (Fig. 13-141). In this technique, the patient sits with the scapula flat against the cassette (as for the AP view in the plane of the scapula). The arm may be in a sling. The x-ray beam is centered on the coracoid and directed perpendicular to the cassette (45 degrees to the coronal plane), except that it is angled 45 degrees caudally. The beam passes tangential to the articular surface of the glenohumeral joint and the posterolateral aspect of the humeral head. This view is likely to reveal both anterior glenoid lip defects and posterolateral impression fractures of the humeral head.

The incidence of the Hill-Sachs defect reported depends on both the radiographic technique and the patient population. Symeonides[642] reported the humeral head defect in 23 of 45 patients who had recurrent anterior dislocations of the shoulder. However, at the time of surgery, he could confirm only 18 of 45.

Eyre-Brook[175] reported a 64% incidence of the Hill-Sachs defect in 17 recurrent anterior dislocations, and Brav[78] recorded a rate of 67% in 69 recurrent dislocations. Rowe et al.[584] noted the defect in 38% of 125 acute dislocations and in 57% of 63 recurrent dislocations. Adams[2] reported that the defect was found at the time of surgery in 82% of 68 patients. Palmer and Widen[523] found the defect at surgery in all 60 patients.

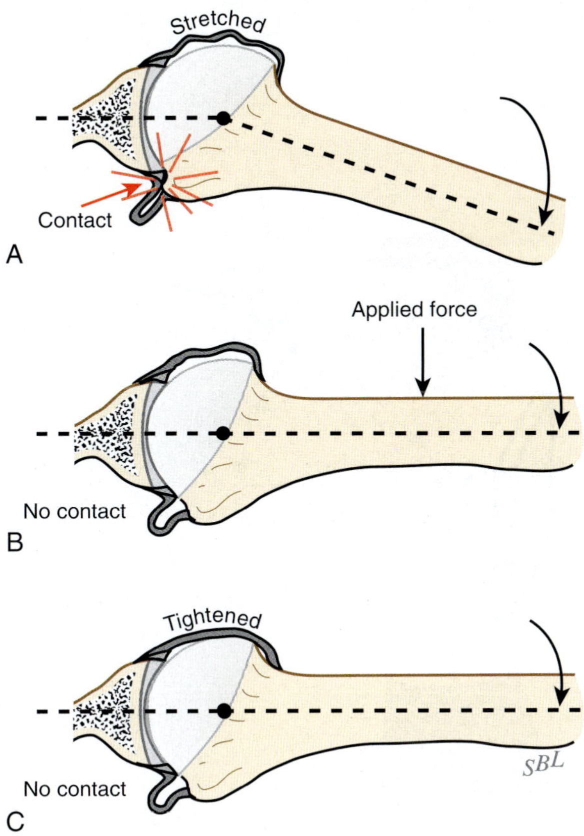

FIGURE 13-138: Posterior contact between the glenoid lip and the insertion of the cuff onto the tuberosity occurs in the apprehension, or fulcrum, position, especially if the anteroinferior aspect of the capsule has been stretched and is allowing the humerus to extend to an unusually posterior scapular plane. This contact can challenge the integrity of the posterior cuff insertion and the tuberosity (**A**). Application of a posteriorly directed force on the front of the shoulder can change the humeroscapular position enough to relieve this posterior abutment. This maneuver is similar to that described as the relocation test; however, this diagram suggests that the mechanism for relief of discomfort is avoidance of posterior abutment rather than elimination of subluxation (**B**). A similar protection from posterior abutment may be achieved by tightening the anterior part of the capsule, thus preventing extension of the humerus to a substantially posterior scapular plane (**C**). (From Matsen FA III, Lippitt SB, Sidles JA, Harryman DT II. *Practical Evaluation and Management of the Shoulder*. Philadelphia: WB Saunders; 1994.)

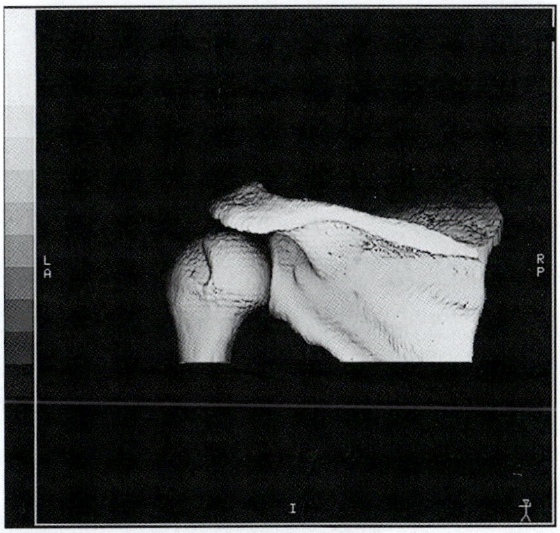

FIGURE 13-139: Three-dimensional computed tomographic reconstruction of the left shoulder of a 37-year-old man 3 days after his first traumatic glenohumeral dislocation. The bony defect in the posterolateral aspect of the humeral head is clearly shown. The patient recovered normal shoulder function with nonoperative management.

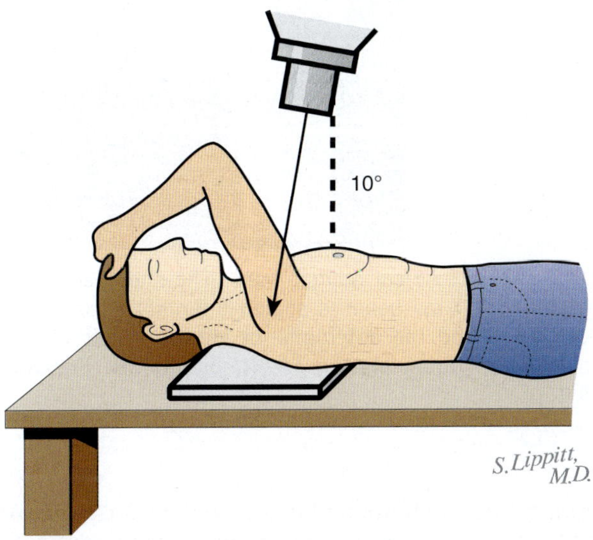

FIGURE 13-140: Stryker notch view. (Modified from Hall RH, Isaac F, Booth CR. Dislocations of the shoulder with special reference to accompanying small fractures. *J Bone Joint Surg Am*. 1959;41:489-494.)

Calandra et al.[93] used diagnostic arthroscopy to prospectively study the incidence of Hill-Sach lesions. In a young population of 32 patients with a mean age of 28 years, the frequency of this lesion was 47% for initial anterior shoulder dislocations.

Danzig et al.[133] reported that in cadaveric and clinical studies, no single view always reveals the humeral head compression fracture. Pavlov et al.[536] and Rozing et al.[592] found that the Stryker notch view taken in internal rotation best revealed the posterolateral humeral head defect (see Fig. 13-140).

The demonstration of a posterolateral humeral head defect strongly indicates that the shoulder has been subjected to a traumatic anterior dislocation. When these factors are already known—for example, in a 17-year-old whose recurrent anterior dislocations began with a well-documented abduction–external rotation injury in football—it is not necessary to spend a great deal of effort

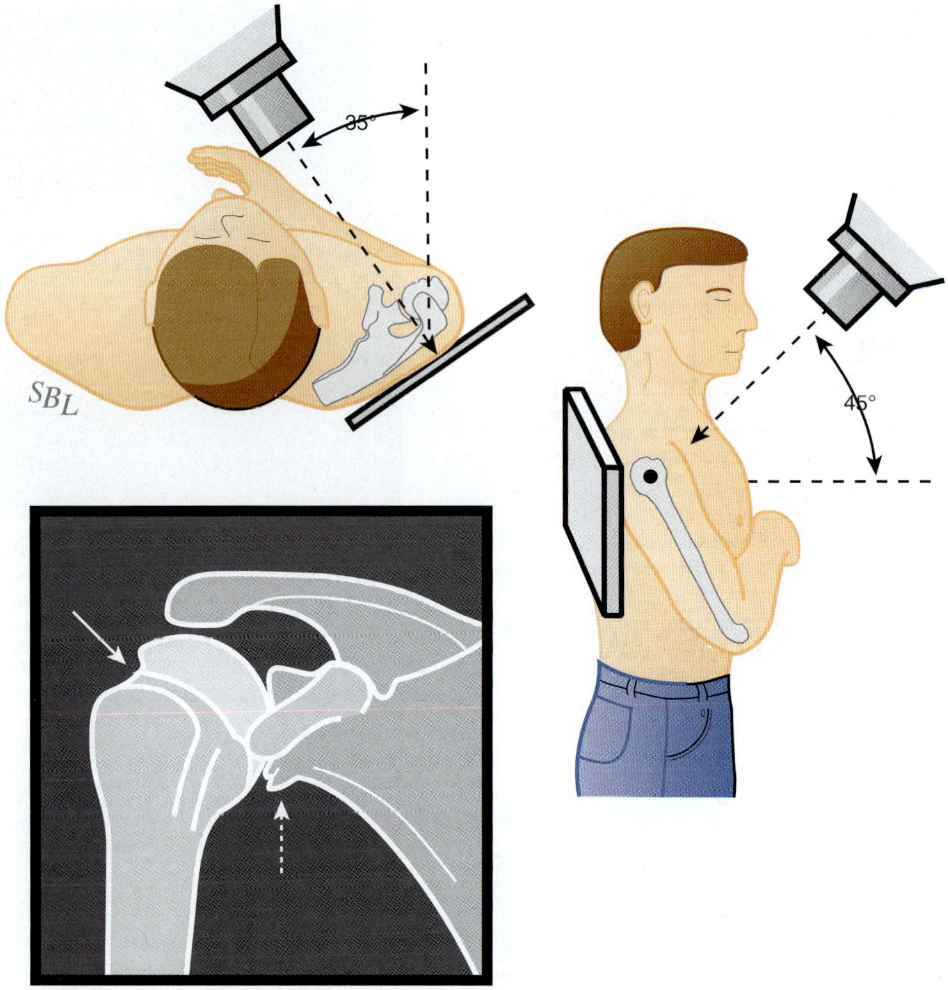

FIGURE 13-141: Apical oblique view. The shoulder is positioned as for an anteroposterior view in the plane of the scapula except that the x-ray beam is angled inferiorly at an angle of 45 degrees. This view reveals the contour of the posterolateral humeral head and the anteroinferior glenoid. *Solid arrow* indicates Hill-Sachs defect. *Dashed arrow* indicates anteroinferior glenoid defect. (From Matsen FA III, Lippitt SB. *Shoulder Surgery: Principles and Procedures*. Philadelphia: WB Saunders; 2004:12.)

demonstrating the humeral head defect because it is very likely to be present even if not seen on radiographs and the existence of such a lesion does not in itself alter management of the patient.

Glenoid Changes

Standard radiographs can reveal a periosteal reaction to the ligamentous avulsion at the glenoid lip or a fracture (see Figs. 13-7 and 13-100), erosion (see Fig. 13-97), or new bone formation (see Figs. 13-82 and 13-96) at the glenoid rim. Modifications of the axillary view can help in identifying glenoid rim changes. Rokous et al.[575] described the West Point axillary view. In this technique, the patient is placed prone on the x-ray table with the involved shoulder on a pad raised 7.5 cm from the top of the table. The head and neck are turned away from the involved side. With the cassette held against the superior aspect of the shoulder, the x-ray beam is centered on the axilla, 25 degrees downward from the horizontal and 25 degrees medial. The resulting radiograph is a tangential view of the anteroinferior rim of the glenoid (see Fig. 13-92). Using this view, Rokous et al. demonstrated bony abnormalities of the anterior glenoid rim in 53 of 63 patients whose histories indicated traumatic instability of the shoulder. Cyprien et al.[131] demonstrated lessening of the glenoid diameter and shortening of the anterior glenoid rim in shoulders with recurrent anterior dislocation. Blazina and Satzman[61] also reported anteroinferior glenoid rim fractures seen on the axillary view in nine of their cases. We have found that high-quality AP and axillary radiographs can give substantial information about the condition of the anterior glenoid lip (Figs. 13-142 and 13-143).

Special Radiographic Techniques

Most often the diagnosis of recurrent traumatic instability is clear from a careful history, physical examination, and

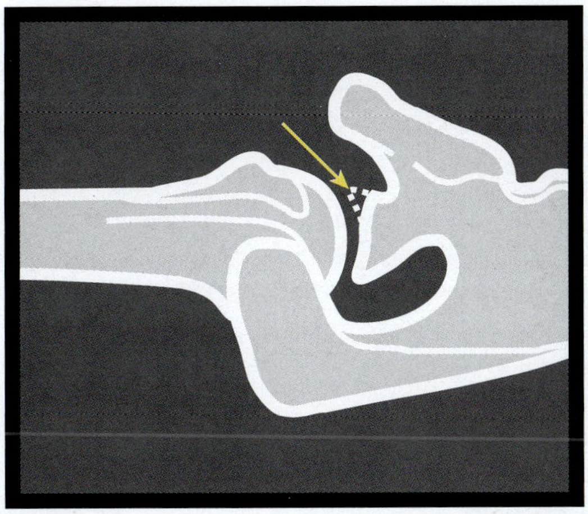

FIGURE 13-142: Axillary view showing anterior glenoid deficiency. This axillary view shows a bony defect (*arrow*) of the anterior glenoid lip. (From Matsen FA III, Lippitt SB. *Shoulder Surgery: Principles and Procedures*. Philadelphia: WB Saunders; 2004:117.)

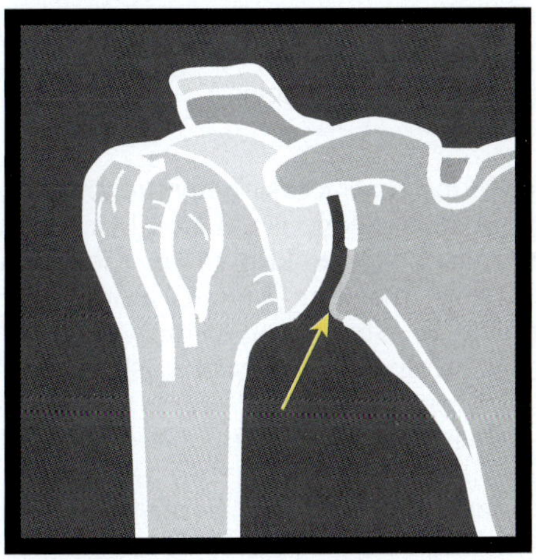

FIGURE 13-143: Anteroposterior view showing loss of the anterior inferior cortical line. The normally sclerotic border of the anterior inferior glenoid lip has been worn away (*arrow*). (From Matsen FA III, Lippitt SB. *Shoulder Surgery: Principles and Procedures*. Philadelphia: WB Saunders; 2004:117.)

plain radiographs. Nevertheless, related pathology can be best seen with additional radiographic views,[225,447,525,558] CT arthrography,[77,127,167,332,341,421,432,555,554,617] fluoroscopy,[494] or MRI. CT scans with 3D reconstructions can be useful in defining the magnitude of bone loss when sizable humeral head or glenoid defects are suggested on plain radiographs (see Figs. 13-99 and 13-100).[221,613] When previous glenoid bone blocks have been carried out or hardware inserted, CT scans are useful for examining the possibility of their encroachment on the humeral head.[126,127,134]

MRI is the gold standard for imaging the labrum and capsule of an unstable shoulder[104,228,296,523] (Fig. 13-144). Iannotti et al.[296] reported that the sensitivity and specificity of MRI in the diagnosis of labral tears associated with

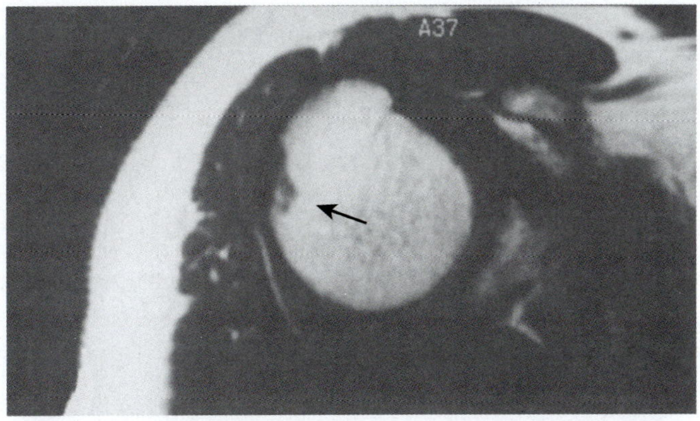

FIGURE 13-144: Magnetic resonance image demonstrating a focal abnormality in the posterolateral aspect of the humeral head (*arrow*) that is consistent with a recent episode of anterior glenohumeral instability. The plain radiographs were interpreted as normal. (From Rockwood CA Jr, Green DP, Bucholz RW, eds. *Fractures in Adults*. Philadelphia: JB Lippincott; 1991.)

glenohumeral instability were 88% and 93%, respectively (Fig. 13-145).

MRI after postoperative recurrence of instability is less accurate than on unoperated shoulders. For imaging of recurrent labral lesions, MR arthrography has a higher sensitivity for detecting recurrent labral lesions than does MRI, 100% versus 71%, respectively.[676] The specificity of MR arthrography in this study was 60% versus 80% for standard MRI. Indirect MR arthrography in this study had 100% sensitivity and specificity in six shoulders, two of which had recurrent labral tears.

Rotator Cuff Imaging

Patients whose onset of traumatic instability occurred after the age of 35 years might have evidence of rotator cuff pathology on the history and physical examination. Particular concern arises if weakness of external rotation or elevation persists longer than a week or so. In these situations, preoperative imaging of cuff integrity can play an important role in surgical planning; for example, the approach for rotator cuff repair is quite different from the approach for repair of an anteroinferior capsular lesion. Ultrasound or MRI can be useful in this situation.

Electromyography

Electromyography may be helpful in evaluating a patient with recurrent traumatic instability if the history and physical examination suggest residual brachial plexus lesions such as an axillary or suprascapular nerve palsy.

Arthroscopy

Because of the information gained from the history, physical examination, and plain films, diagnostic arthroscopy is not a necessary prelude to surgical repair of documented recurrent traumatic instability if an open approach is selected. If an arthroscopic repair is planned, the procedure begins with a diagnostic arthroscopy. Shoulder arthroscopy has helped define some of the pathology associated with recurrent

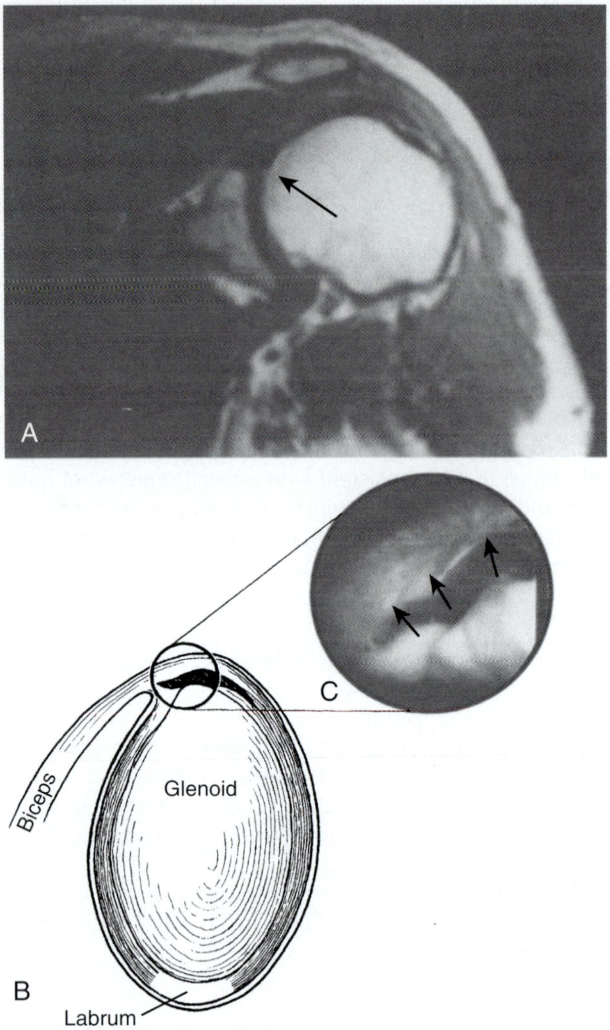

FIGURE 13-145: Lesion of the long head of the biceps tendon origin and superior glenoid labrum. **A,** Lesion (*arrow*) as seen on magnetic resonance image. **B,** Anatomic diagram. **C,** Lesion (*arrows*) as seen on arthroscopic examination. (From Rockwood CA Jr, Green DP, Bucholz RW, eds. *Fractures in Adults*. Philadelphia: JB Lippincott; 1991.)

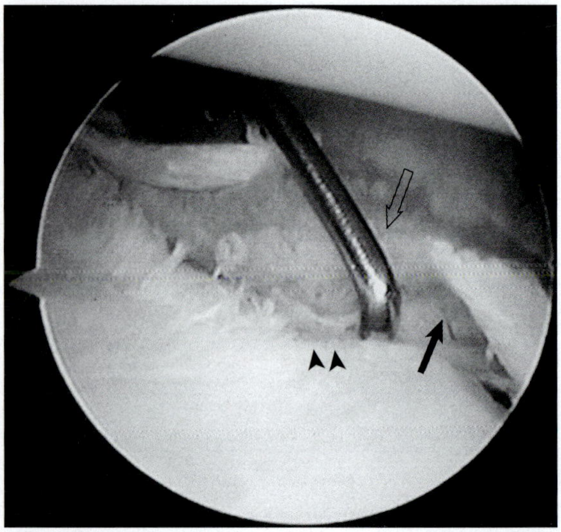

FIGURE 13-146: A Bankart lesion in a patient with recurrent anteroinferior instability. Note the traumatic disruption of the glenoid labrum (*solid arrow*), fraying of articular cartilage at the glenoid rim (*arrowheads*), and anterior capsular scarring with synovitis along the inferior glenohumeral ligament (*open arrow*). (Courtesy Douglas T. Harryman II, MD, Department of Orthopaedics, University of Washington.)

instability. Such lesions include labral tears, capsular rents, humeral head defects, and rotator cuff defects (see Fig. 13-145).[12,96,198,205,236,272,320,386,432,448,505,526,696,697,729]

An arthroscopic classification of anterior labral Bankart lesions was proposed by Green and Christensen.[226] In 37 cases, they described the arthroscopic appearance common to five separate groups:

Type I is the normal intact labrum.
Type II is a simple detachment of the labrum from the glenoid.
Type III is an intrasubstance tear of the glenoid labrum.
Type IV is a detachment of the labrum with significant fraying or degeneration.
Type V is complete degeneration or absence of the glenoid labrum.

Neviaser found that occasionally the anterior labroligamentous periosteal sleeve is avulsed from the glenoid.[478] This injury has become known as the anterior labral periosteal sleeve avulsion (ALPSA) lesion. The posterior labral periosteal sleeve avulsion (POLPSA lesion) described by Simons et al. has been shown to be associated with posterior instability,[622] tends to occur in younger patients, and is similar to the anterior version, the ALPSA lesion. The labrum is intact but separated from the glenoid by an avulsion of its periosteum. The POLPSA lesion has been seen on MRI evaluation.[723]

Gleyze and Habermeyer noted that shoulders with more than five recurrent dislocations had erosion of the anterior articular cartilage.[215] Harryman detected labral damage in all patients treated for recurrent anterior traumatic instability (Fig. 13-146) and in 20% of patients treated for significant articular erosion to subchondral bone (Fig. 13-147).[242]

Other lesions may be associated with Bankart lesions. Snyder et al.[625] and Warner et al.[681] found an association of superior labral detachment and Bankart lesions.

Wolf et al. reported that six of 64 patients with anterior instability had avulsion of the glenohumeral ligaments from the humerus, whereas 47 had true Bankart lesions (73.5%).[710]

Arthroscopy has revealed defects in the articular cartilage of the posterolateral humeral head that would not be detected on radiographs (Figs. 13-148 to 13-150).

Glenoid bone loss can also be assessed at the time of arthroscopy. Using arthroscopy, Burkhart et al. have shown the bare spot of the glenoid to be a consistent reference point for the center of the glenoid.[89] Adequacy of the glenoid may be assessed by determining the

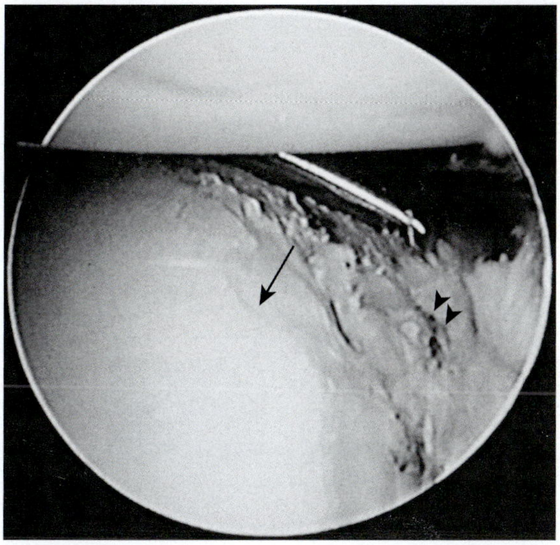

FIGURE 13-147: Chronic anteroinferior instability with evidence of erosion of articular cartilage to subchondral bone (*arrow*) and degenerative erosion of the labrum (*arrowheads*). (Courtesy Douglas T. Harryman II, MD, Department of Orthopaedics, University of Washington.)

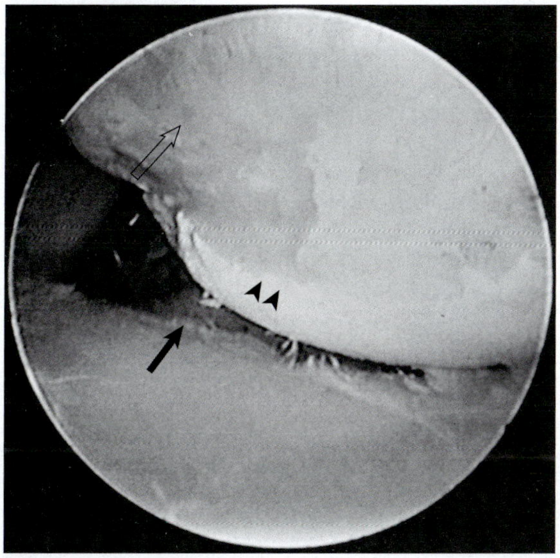

FIGURE 13-148: Visualizing the anterior rim of the glenoid (*solid arrow*) and the posterior edge of the humeral articular surface (*arrowheads*) adjacent to a large Hill-Sachs defect (*open arrow*) with the humerus in abduction and external rotation. (Courtesy Douglas T. Harryman II, MD, Department of Orthopaedics, University of Washington.)

amount of glenoid surrounding the bare area. The drive-through sign has been used as an indicator of laxity. In a study of 339 patients undergoing shoulder arthroscopy for any reason, the drive-through sign was found to have a sensitivity of 92% but only 37.6% specificity for the diagnosis of instability. The positive and negative predictive values were 29.9% and 94.2%, respectively.[419]

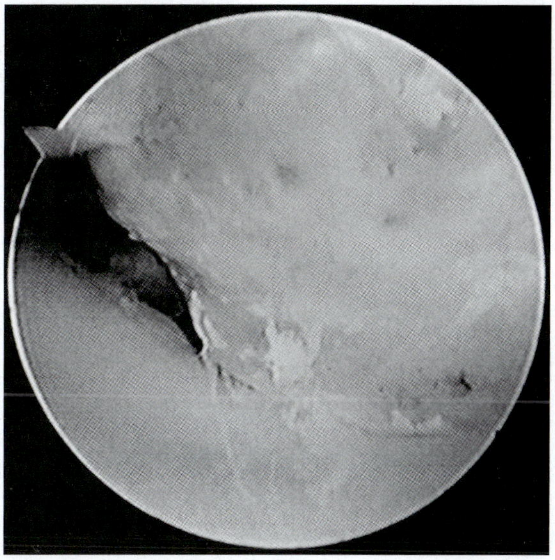

FIGURE 13-149: External rotation is increased until the humeral head suddenly dislocates over the edge of the anterior glenoid rim. After repair, external rotation of the glenohumeral joint must be checked adequately to maintain articular contact. (Courtesy Douglas T. Harryman II, MD, Department of Orthopaedics, University of Washington.)

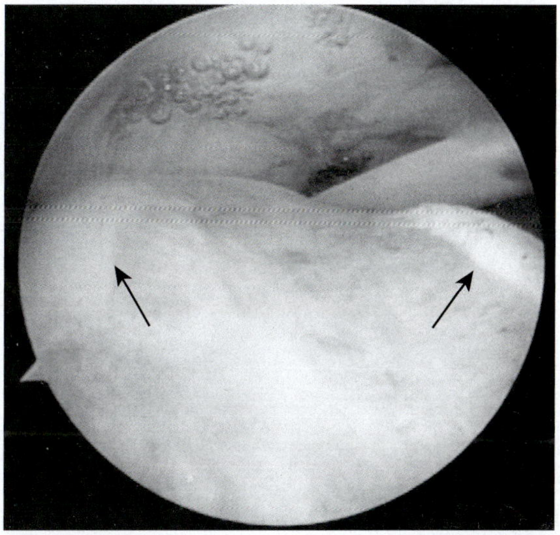

FIGURE 13-150: An extensive Hill-Sachs defect that crosses the superior humeral articular surface (*arrows*). Even with this degree of articular surface loss, an arthroscopic Bankart repair was performed with use of the Seattle Bankart guide and has been entirely successful. (Courtesy Douglas T. Harryman II, MD, Department of Orthopaedics, University of Washington.)

TREATMENT

Nonoperative Management

Strengthening of the rotator cuff, deltoid, and scapular motors can be accomplished with a simple series of exercises (Figs. 13-151 to 13-153; see also Fig. 13-51).

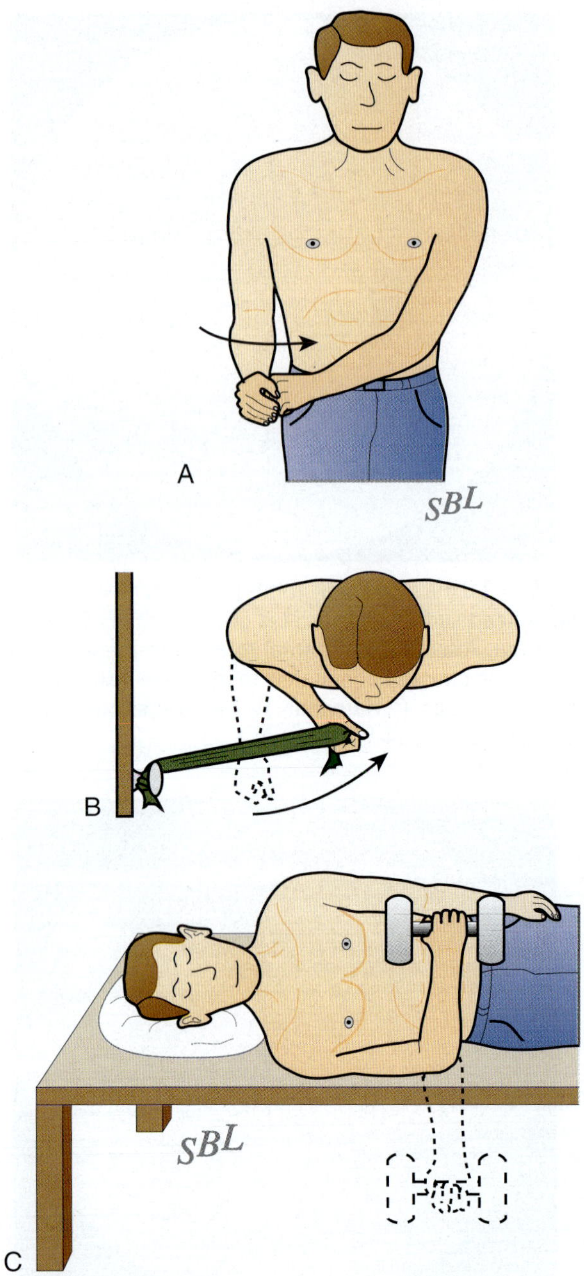

FIGURE 13-151: Internal rotation can be strengthened with isometrics (**A**), rubber tubing (**B**), or free weights (**C**). (From Matsen FA III, Lippitt SB, Sidles JA, Harryman DT II. *Practical Evaluation and Management of the Shoulder*. Philadelphia: WB Saunders; 1994.)

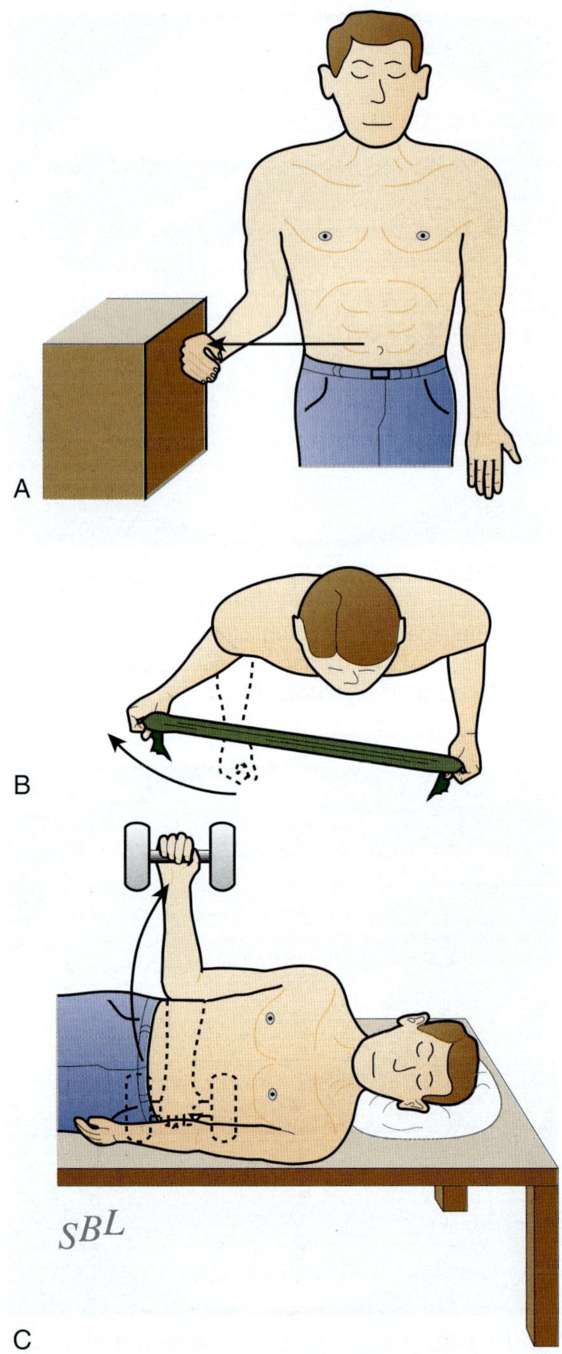

FIGURE 13-152: External rotation strengthening with isometrics (**A**), rubber tubing (**B**), or free weights (**C**). (From Matsen FA III, Lippitt SB, Sidles JA, Harryman DT II: Practical Evaluation and Management of the Shoulder. Philadelphia: WB Saunders; 1994.)

During the early phases of the program, the patient is taught to use the shoulder only in the most stable positions, that is, those in which the humerus is elevated in the plane of the scapula (avoiding, for example, elevation in the sagittal plane with the arm in internal rotation if the patient has a tendency to posterior instability). As coordination and confidence improve, progressively less intrinsically stable positions are attempted. Taping can provide a useful reminder to avoid unstable positions (Fig. 13-154). The shoulder is then progressed to smooth repetitive activities such as swimming or rowing, which can play an essential role in retraining the neuromuscular patterns required for stability.

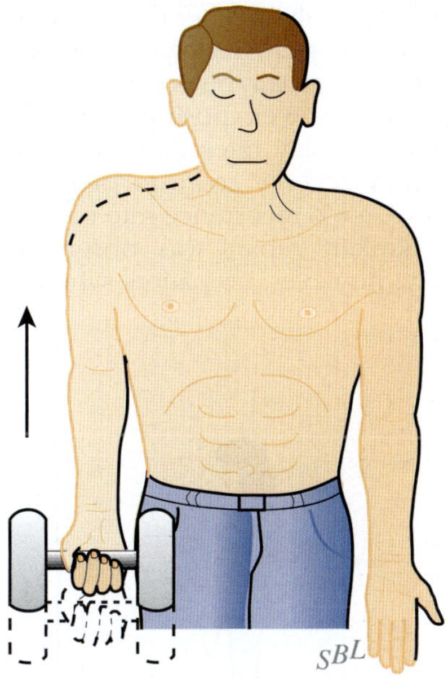

FIGURE 13-153: Trapezius shrug. The trapezius is strengthened by shrugging the shoulder upward while a weight is held in the hand. (From Matsen FA III, Lippitt SB. *Shoulder Surgery: Principles and Procedures*. Philadelphia: WB Saunders; 2004:345.)

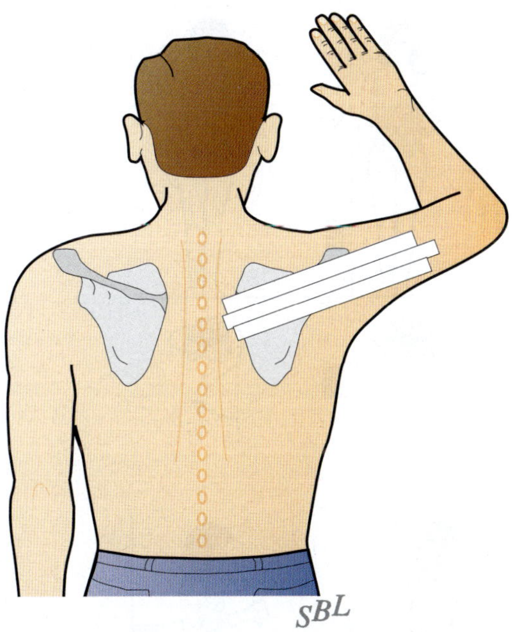

FIGURE 13-154: Training tape is applied across the back of the shoulder as a reminder to avoid unbalanced positions. (Modified from Matsen FA III, Lippitt SB, Sidles JA, Harryman DT II. *Practical Evaluation and Management of the Shoulder*. Philadelphia: WB Saunders; 1994.)

Finally, it is important to avoid all activities and habits that promote glenohumeral subluxation or dislocation; patients are taught that each time their shoulder goes out, it gets easier for it to go out the next time.

Rockwood et al.[572] and Burkhead and Rockwood[90] found that 16% of patients with traumatic subluxation, 80% of those with anterior atraumatic subluxation, and 90% of those with posterior instability responded to a rehabilitation program (Fig. 13-155). Brostrom et al.[83] found that exercises improved all but 5 of 33 unstable shoulders, including traumatic and atraumatic types. Anderson et al. demonstrated the effectiveness of an exercise program that used rubber bands to improve internal rotator strength.[10]

Wirth et al. demonstrated that nonoperative management can be successful even in patients with a congenital factor in their instability. They reported 16 patients with hypoplasia of the glenoid.[704] A subset of this group consisted of five patients with bilateral glenoid hypoplasia and MDI as indicated by symptomatic increased translation of the humeral head during anterior, inferior, and posterior drawer testing. Generalized ligamentous laxity of the metacarpophalangeal joints, elbows, or knees was noted in all five patients in the subset. Four of the patients had been involved in occupational or recreational activities, or both, that had placed heavy demands on the shoulders. All four had considerable improvement in ratings for pain and the ability to carry out work and sports activities at an average of 3 months after they had begun a strengthening program designed by Rockwood. None of the patients needed vocational rehabilitation despite the heavy demands on their shoulders associated with their occupational or recreational activities.

These results again support the concept of concavity compression and point out that when the concavity is compromised, stability can often be restored by optimizing balance of the compression mechanism.

Surgical Management of Traumatic Anterior Instability

Chalmer et al. conducted a systematic review of overlapping metanalyses and concluded that the best available evidence shows no difference in failure rates between open and arthroscopic repair.[103] Of course, appropriate patient selection may play a role in eliminating the differences seen in meta-analyses. However, arthroscopic approaches resulted in better early function as reflected by the Rowe scores in the randomized clinical trials for dislocators without glenoid bone loss. This finding is especially important for young athletes. In a study by Ozturk et al., 87% of their athletes under age 25 had returned to sport at 2 years' average follow-up.[518] They further noted that multiple instability episodes were associated with failure of arthroscopic surgery, suggesting that arthroscopic treatment is more successful in first-time dislocators.

The shoulder Instability Severity Score (ISS) was developed following examination of patient characteristics with recurrent instability that failed arthroscopic Bankart repair: at 31.2 months (24 to 52) postoperatively, 19 (14.5%) had recurrent instability.[30] The following risk factors were identified: patient age under 20 years at the time of surgery; involvement in competitive or contact sports or those involving forced overhead activity; shoulder hyperlaxity; a Hill-Sachs lesion present on an AP radiograph of the shoulder in external rotation and/or loss of the sclerotic inferior glenoid contour. Patients received 2 points for each, and those patients with a score over 6 points had an unacceptable recurrence risk of 70% ($P < .001$) after arthroscopic stabilization. Therefore for patients with ISS score more than 6 points, open stabilization with Latarjet is suggested.[30] ISS has been independently validated but not always correlated with the Western Ontario Shoulder Instability index (WOSI).[581] Unfortunately, neither the preoperative ISS nor WOSI predicted recurrent dislocation within 2 years of arthroscopic Bankart repair, but lower preoperative WOSI scores did predict lower postoperative function and decreased return to play rates. In a study attempting to use the instability severity score to predict arthroscopic treatment failure, a 6% recurrence rate of dislocation after arthroscopic Bankart repair was observed at 2 years postoperatively; however, no patient who dislocated had

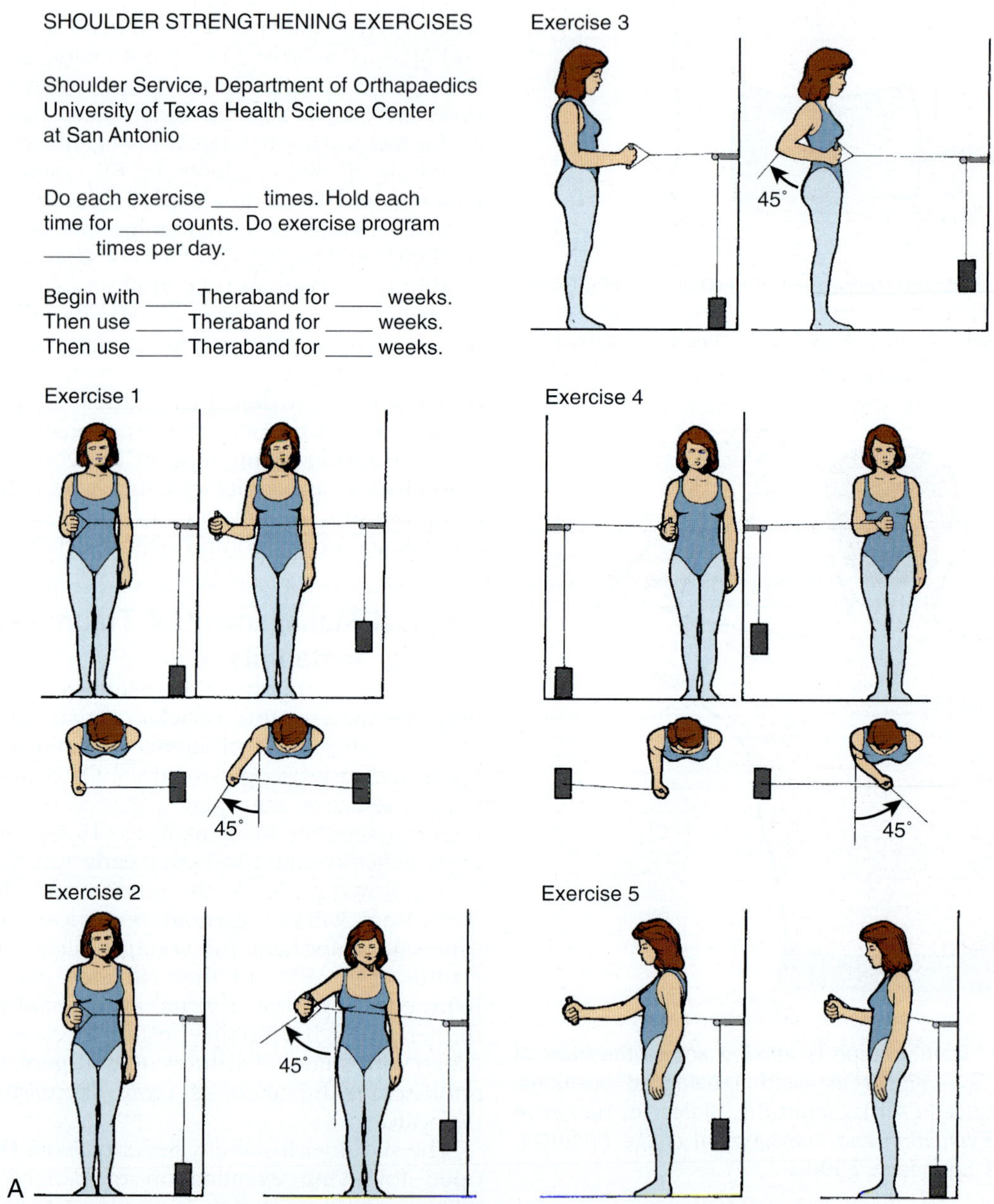

FIGURE 13-155: Shoulder-strengthening exercises. **A,** Initially, the patient is given rubber exercise bands to strengthen the rotator cuff muscles and the three parts of the deltoid. After achieving proficiency in rubber resistance with exercises 1 to 5, the patient is given an exercise kit that consists of a pulley, hook, rope, and handle. The pulley is attached to the hook, which is fixed to the wall, and the five exercises are performed. Initially, the patient is instructed to use 5 or 10 lb of weight; the weight is gradually increased over a period of several months to as much as 25 lb. The purpose of the five exercises is to strengthen the three parts of the deltoid muscles, the internal rotators, and the external rotators.

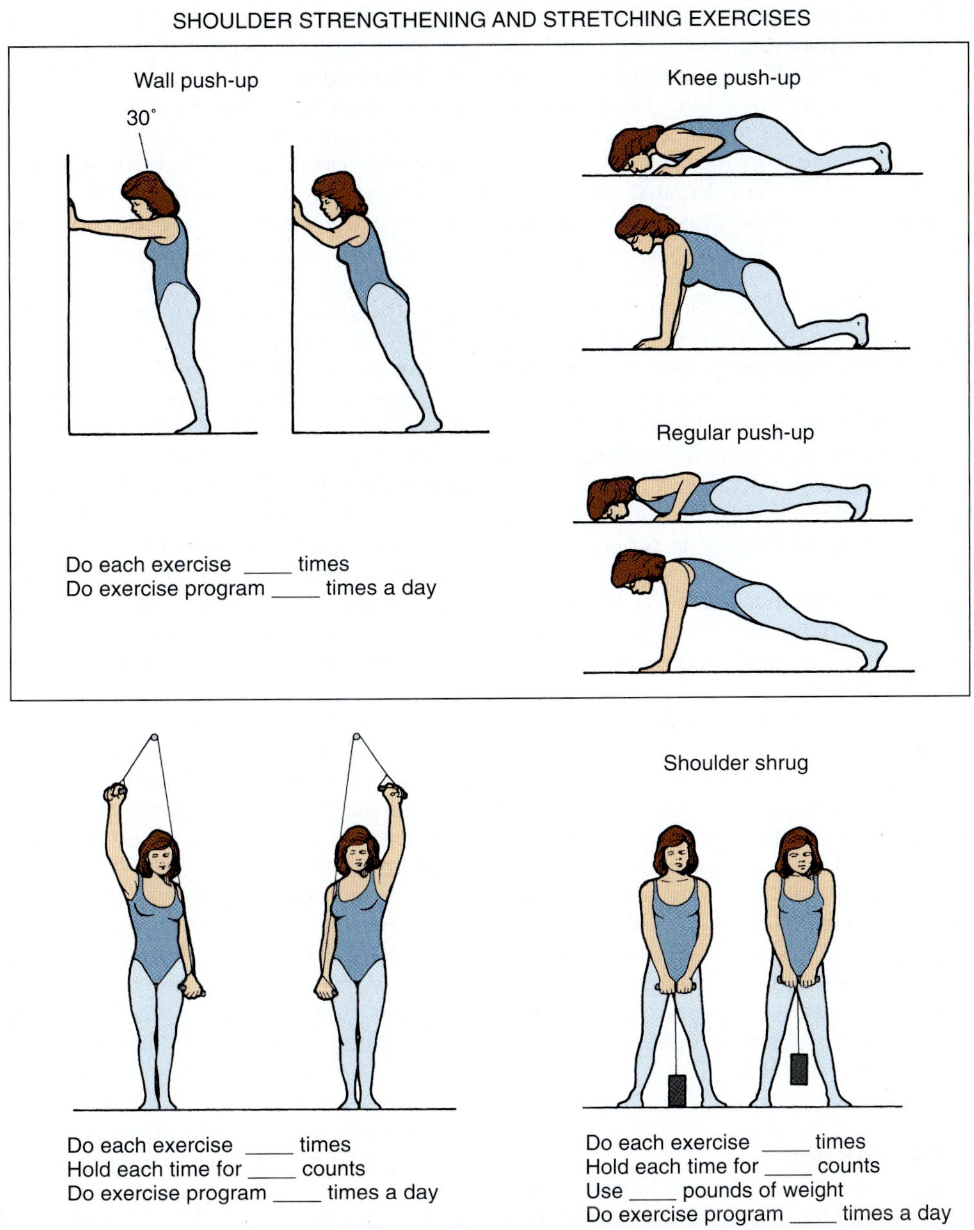
SHOULDER STRENGTHENING AND STRETCHING EXERCISES
Wall push-up
30°
Knee push-up
Regular push-up
Do each exercise ____ times
Do exercise program ____ times a day
Shoulder shrug
Do each exercise ____ times
Hold each time for ____ counts
Do exercise program ____ times a day
Do each exercise ____ times
Hold each time for ____ counts
Use ____ pounds of weight
Do exercise program ____ times a day

B

FIGURE 13-155, cont'd B, In addition, the patient is instructed in exercises to strengthen the scapular stabilizer muscles. To strengthen the serratus anterior and the rhomboids, the patient is instructed to first do wall pushups, then gradually do knee pushups, and later do regular pushups. The shoulder-shrug exercise is used to strengthen the trapezius and levator scapulae muscles.

a preoperative ISS greater than 6 points, although the authors conceded that only few patients had ISS greater than 6 points preoperatively in their study and follow-up was limited to 2 years.[70]

Examination Under Anesthesia

Examination with the patient under anesthesia is the first step of any procedure to address instability. Such examination is an important adjunct to the physical examination in the office, as it allows for full assessment of shoulder instability without guarding or apprehension. Comparison with the contralateral side is performed but is not always helpful in cases of bilateral instability.

Operative Management

In the past, many surgical procedures have been described for treating recurrent anterior glenohumeral instability. Tightening and, to some degree, realigning the subscapularis tendon and partially eliminating external rotation were the goals of the Magnuson-Stack and the Putti-Platt procedures. The Putti-Platt operation also tightened and reinforced the anterior capsule. Reattachment of the capsule and glenoid labrum to the glenoid lip was the goal of the DuToit staple capsulorrhaphy and the Eyre-Brook capsulorrhaphy.[173,174] The Bristow procedure transferred the tip of the coracoid process with its muscle attachments to create a musculotendinous sling across the anteroinferior glenohumeral joint. An anterior glenoid bone buttress was the objective of the Oudard and Trillat procedures. Augmentation of the bony anterior glenoid lip was the goal of anterior bone block procedures such as the Eden-Hybbinette procedure. Haaker et al.[233] added an autogenous bone graft to the glenoid rim for recurrent instability. In their series of recurrent instabilities in 24 young soldiers, they used screws to fix an anterior iliac crest graft to the anterior glenoid rim. At the conclusion of graft placement, the glenoid labrum is replaced over the graft.

Large posterolateral humeral head defects have been approached by limiting external rotation, filling the defect with the infraspinatus tendon, and performing a rotational osteotomy of the humerus.[99,100,640,687]

Most of the reported series on the various types of reconstruction have yielded "excellent" results. However, it is very difficult to determine how each author graded the results. For example, if the patient has no recurrence after repair but has loss of 45 degrees of external rotation and cannot throw, is that a fair, good, or excellent result? The simple fact that the shoulder no longer dislocates cannot be equated with an excellent result. Although the older literature suggested that the goal of surgery for anterior dislocation of the shoulder was to limit external rotation, more modern literature suggests that a reconstruction can both prevent recurrent dislocation and allow nearly normal range of motion and comfortable function.

Capsulolabral Reconstruction

Reconstruction of the avulsed capsule and labrum at the glenoid lip is often referred to as a *Bankart repair*. This was apparently first performed in 1906 by Perthes,[541] who recommended repair of the anterior capsule to the anterior glenoid rim. He was not in doubt about the pathology of traumatic instability: "In every case the anterior margin of the glenoid cavity will be found to be smooth, rounded, and free of any attachments, and a blunt instrument can be passed freely inwards over the bare bone on the front of the neck of the scapula." He reattached the capsule to the glenoid rim by placing drill holes through the bone.

Credit for this type of repair should go to Perthes, but the popularity of the technique is based on the work of Bankart,[32,34] who first performed the operation in 1923 on one of his former house surgeons. The procedure commonly used today is based on Bankart's 1939 article in which he discusses repair of the capsule to the bone of the anterior glenoid through the use of drill holes and suture. The subscapularis muscle, which is carefully divided to expose the capsule, is reapproximated without any overlap or shortening. Bankart reported 27 consecutive cases with "full movements of the joint and in no case has there been any recurrence of the dislocation."[61,575,583,589]

There are several significant differences between Bankart's original method and the capsulolabral reconstruction currently recommended. Today we do not osteotomize the coracoid, we do not shave off bone from the anterior glenoid, and we strive to reattach the capsule and any residual labrum up on the surface of the glenoid lip rather than on the anterior aspect of the glenoid, as shown by Bankart.[648]

Hovelius et al.[287] found a 2% redislocation rate after the Bankart procedure versus a 19% rate after the Putti-Platt procedure. More than one-third of the patients younger than 25 years were dissatisfied with the results of the Putti-Platt procedure. Rowe and Zarins[589] reported a series of 50 subluxating shoulders in which good or excellent results were achieved in 94% after a Bankart repair. A Bankart lesion was found in 64% of these shoulders. Rowe et al.[584] reported on 51 shoulders with a fracture of the anterior rim of the glenoid; 18 shoulders had a fracture involving one-sixth or less of the glenoid, 26 involved one-fourth of the glenoid, and seven had one-third of the anterior glenoid fractured off. In this group of patients, who were treated with a Bankart repair without particular attention paid to the fracture, the overall incidence of failure was 2%. Prozorovskii et al.[552] reported no recurrences in the long-term follow-up of 41 Bankart repairs. Martin et al.[408] reported excellent results and minimal degenerative change in a 10-year follow-up of 53 patients managed with a Bankart repair.

Bigliani et al. adapted the inferior capsular shift developed by Neer to the entire spectrum of instability, titrating the capsulorraphy to the degree of capsular redundancy present and adding repair of the Bankart lesion. They credited this approach to their success in athletes.[55] Additional evidence indicates that open approaches are superior at preventing recurrent instability and enabling patients to return to work or sports.[450,522,688]

Open Bankart Repair With Open Capsular Shift

Many authors have advocated the addition of a capsular shift or capsulorrhaphy to the Bankart repair.[9] Stretching of the capsular ligaments occurs at the time of injury; therefore these ligaments should be plicated along with repair of the labrum. In a series of cadaveric simian shoulder dislocations, capsular microtears were seen in addition to a Bankart lesion in all shoulders.[123]

When pathologically increased anterior laxity is combined with a Bankart lesion, the addition of capsular plication to reattachment of the capsulolabral avulsion has been recommended. Jobe et al.[317] and Montgomery and Jobe[453] achieved good or excellent results in athletes with shoulder pain secondary to anterior glenohumeral subluxation or dislocation. Two years after surgery, more than 80% had returned to their preinjury sport and level of competition.

Wirth et al. reported their results in 108 patients (142 shoulders) with recurrent anterior shoulder instability.[701] All patients were managed by repair of the capsulolabral injury, when present, and reinforcement of the anteroinferior capsular ligaments by an imbrication technique that decreases the overall capsular volume. According to the grading system of Rowe et al., 93% of the results were rated good or excellent at an average follow-up of 5 years (range, 2 to 12 years). The incidence of recurrent instability was approximately 1%.

Open capsular shift is especially favored in contact athletes. Athletes in collision sports who were treated with open Bankart repair and capsulorrhaphy had a 3% redislocation rate.[688] In a report by Pagnani and Dome, American football players were able to return to their sport 89% of the time after open anterior capsulorrhaphy along with repair of a Bankart lesion, if present.[522] When the labrum is flattened or excessively compliant, a method of labrum augmentation using autologous blood has been described (Figs. 13-156 to 13-163).[413]

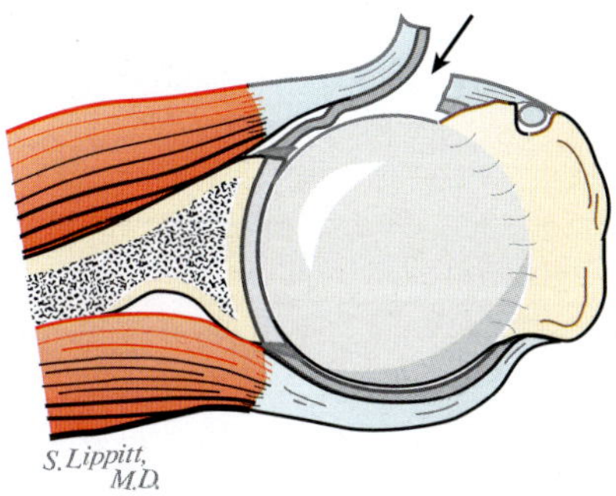

FIGURE 13-156: Subscapularis and capsular incision. The subscapularis and subjacent capsule are incised *(arrow)* so that strong tendinous tissue remains on either side of the incision. Sufficient tissue is left attached to the lesser tuberosity so that repair at the end of the case is facilitated. The subscapularis and capsule are not separated. (From Matsen FA III, Lippitt SB. *Shoulder Surgery: Principles and Procedures*. Philadelphia: WB Saunders; 2004:199.)

Excessive tightening of the anterior capsule and subscapularis can lead to limited comfort and function, as well as a form of secondary degenerative joint disease known as *capsulorrhaphy arthropathy*.[58,250,346,395] Rosenberg et al.[577] found that 18 of 52 patients had at least minimal degenerative changes at an average follow-up of 15 years. As a cautionary note against unnecessary capsular tightening, these authors found a correlation between loss of external rotation and the incidence of degenerative changes. To help guard against postoperative loss of motion, Rowe et al.[585] limit immobilization to just 2 to 3 days, after which the patient is instructed to gradually increase the motion and function of the extremity.

In open Bankart repair with capsular shift, the loss of external rotation was observed to be 13 degrees compared with the contralateral side and glenohumeral osteoarthritis incidence increased from 4% preoperatively to 17% postoperatively.[65] Another long-term study by Fabre et al. reported on the results of open Bankart repair after a mean of 28 years in a group in which two thirds were contact athletes.[176] In the study, 82% had returned to their preoperative level of sports activity, and 96% were satisfied with the surgery despite a 10 degree loss of external rotation and 6 degree loss of forward elevation.[176] The only recurrences in that group occurred as a result of new traumatic episode, but approximately 20% experienced radiographic arthritis of stage 2, 3, or 4. Another study with an average of 22 years of follow-up on primary and revision patients treated with open Bankart repair with capsular shift showed similar results of durable stability with no recurrent dislocations and no revision surgery.[106] Six percent underwent subsequent total shoulder replacement, and active forward elevation averaged 169 degrees, external rotation, 65 degrees, and internal rotation to T12.[106]

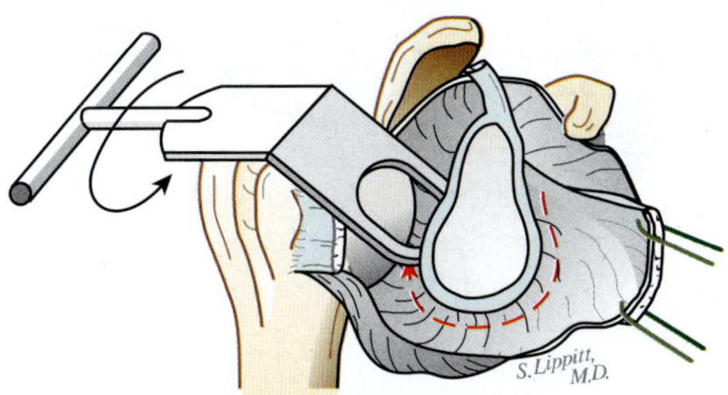

FIGURE 13-157: Capsular exposure. Twisting the inferior part of the humeral head retractor away from the glenoid exposes the inferior capsule. (From Matsen FA III, Lippitt SB. *Shoulder Surgery: Principles and Procedures*. Philadelphia: WB Saunders; 2004:201.)

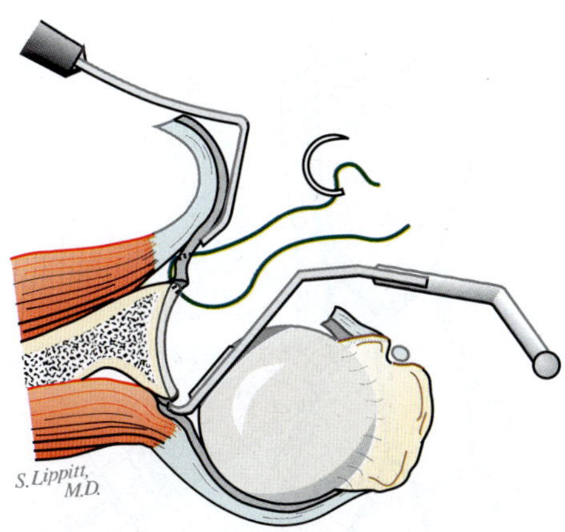

FIGURE 13-158: Suture passage. The suture is passed through the margin of the articular cartilage, around the labrum, and around 1 cm of capsule. (From Matsen FA III, Lippitt SB. *Shoulder Surgery: Principles and Procedures*. Philadelphia: WB Saunders; 2004:201.)

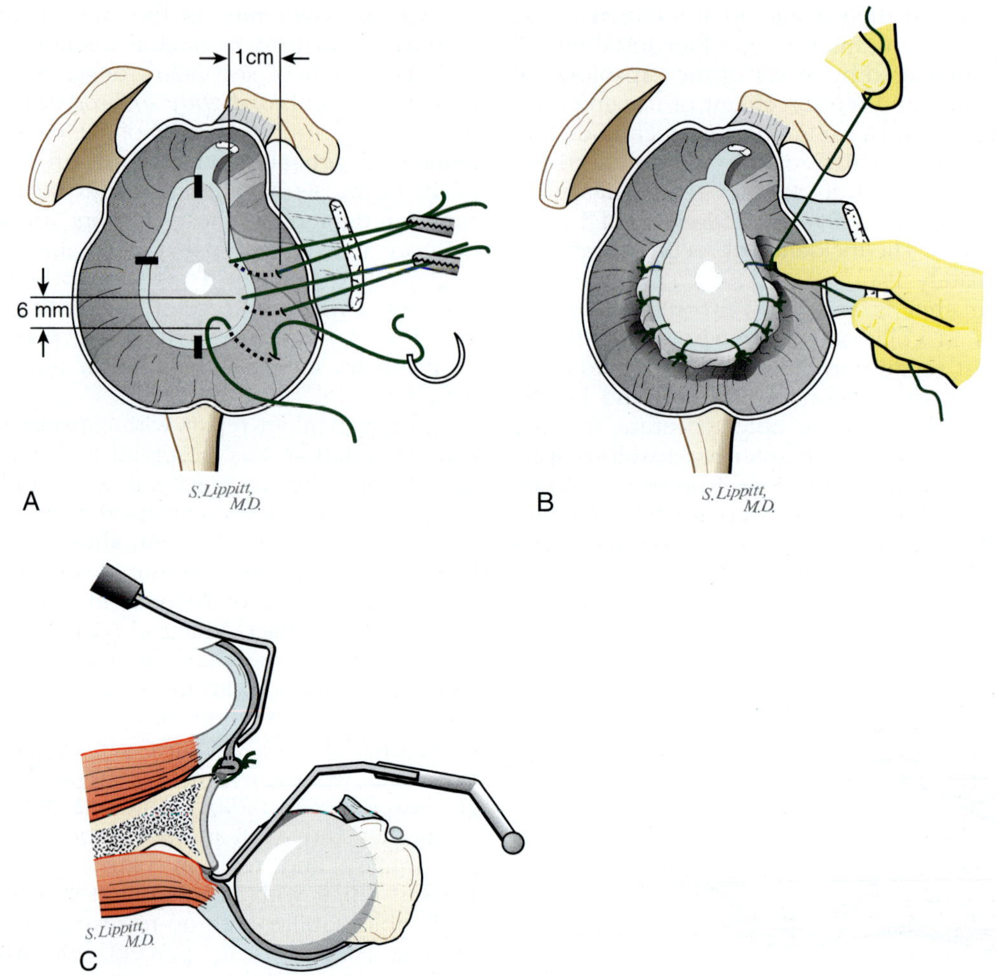

FIGURE 13-159: Suture placement and tying. **A,** Sutures are placed around the perimeter of the glenoid from the 3 o'clock position to the 9 o'clock position. **B,** These sutures are tied so that the knots overlie the capsule. **C,** Tying these sutures creates a substantial bumper, augmenting the glenoid concavity. (From Matsen FA III, Lippitt SB. *Shoulder Surgery: Principles and Procedures*. Philadelphia: WB Saunders; 2004:202-204.)

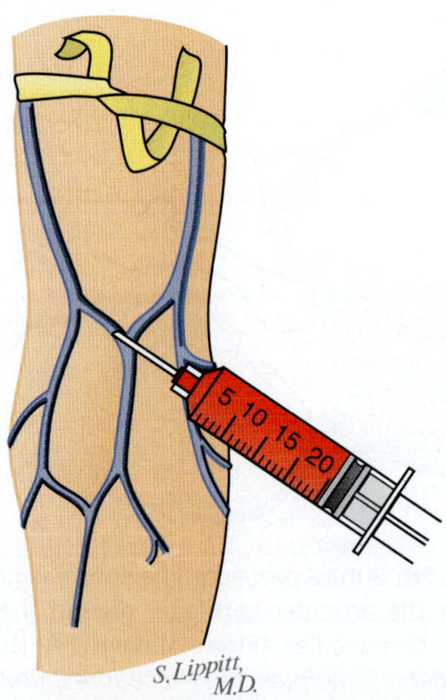

FIGURE 13-160: Blood harvest. From the ipsilateral antecubital fossa, 20 mL of blood is withdrawn. (From Matsen FA III, Lippitt SB. *Shoulder Surgery: Principles and Procedures*. Philadelphia: WB Saunders. 2004:205.)

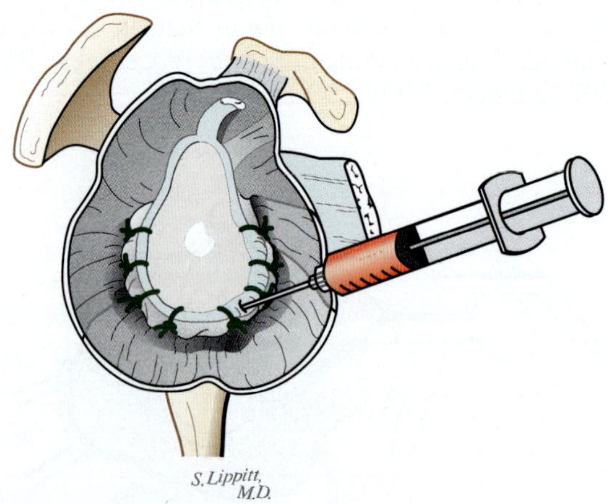

FIGURE 13-161: Labral inflation. The harvested blood is immediately injected into the rolled up capsule and labrum before it clots. A flat, beveled needle is helpful here. (From Matsen FA III, Lippitt SB. *Shoulder Surgery: Principles and Procedures*. Philadelphia: WB Saunders; 2004:206.)

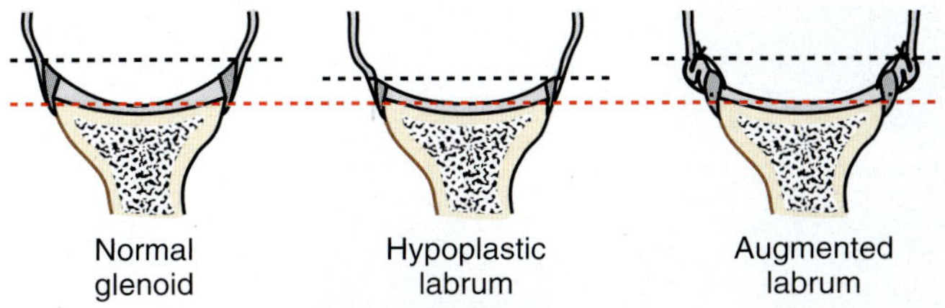

FIGURE 13-162: Augmented glenoid depth. The functional depth of the glenoid is increased by this labral augmentation. (From Matsen FA III, Lippitt SB. *Shoulder Surgery: Principles and Procedures*. Philadelphia: WB Saunders; 2004:207.)

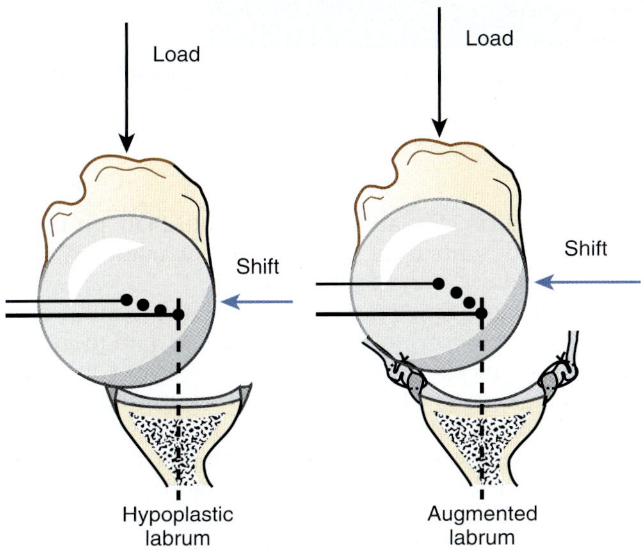

FIGURE 13-163: Restoration of centering. The augmented labrum restores the centering effect of the concavity, as demonstrated on the load and shift test. (From Matsen FA III, Lippitt SB. *Shoulder Surgery: Principles and Procedures*. Philadelphia: WB Saunders; 2004:207.)

Other Anterior Repairs

Many other anterior repairs have been described, but most are of historical interest only. The reader is also referred to a review of glenohumeral capsulorrhaphy by Friedman.[197]

Staple Capsulorrhaphy

In the DuToit staple capsulorrhaphy, the detached capsule is secured back to the glenoid with staples.[162,624] Actually, the staple repair had been described 50 years earlier by Perthes. Rao et al.[557] reported the follow-up of 65 patients who underwent DuToit staple repair for avulsion of the capsule from the glenoid rim; two patients showed radiographic evidence of loose staples. Ward et al.[678] reviewed 33 staple capsulorrhaphies at an average of 50 months postoperatively; 50% continued to have apprehension, and 12 had staple malposition.

O'Driscoll and Evans[503,502] reviewed 269 consecutive DuToit capsulorrhaphies in 257 patients at a median follow-up of 8.8 years; 53% had postoperative pain, and internal and external rotation was limited. Recurrence was reported in 28% if stapling alone was performed and in 8% if a Putti-Platt procedure was added; staple loosening, migration, or penetration of cartilage occurred in 11%. Staple complications contributed to pain, physical restriction, and osteoarthritis. Zuckerman and Matsen pointed out that the use of staples for surgical repair may be associated with major complications (Figs. 13-164 and 13-165).[732]

Capsular Reconstruction

In scenarios of capsular insufficiency, such as in revisions of failed previous stabilization or especially following previous thermal capsulorrhaphy, hamstring autograft and tibialis tendon allograft have been used to reinforce the anterior capsule, but available evidence is limited. Alcid et al. found in their series of 15 patients that there were no postoperative dislocations at 2 years after

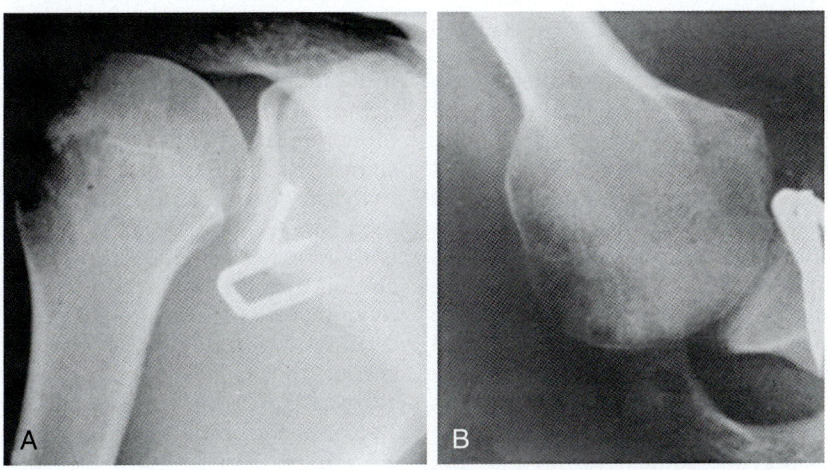

FIGURE 13-164: Complications of staple capsulorrhaphy. **A,** Anteroposterior radiograph showing a prominent staple on the inferior glenoid rim. **B,** Axillary view showing impingement of a staple on the head of the humerus.

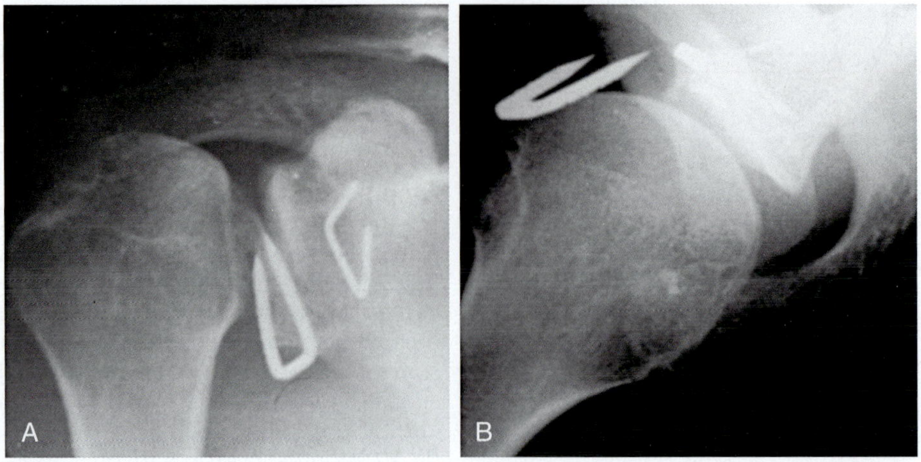

FIGURE 13-165: A loose staple after staple capsulorrhaphy. **A,** AP radiograph showing a loose staple in the glenohumeral joint. **B,** Axillary view.

employing this technique, but there was significant loss of motion, leading to early glenohumeral arthritis.[7] The patients lacked 10 degrees of forward flexion, 21 degrees of external rotation at the side, 24 degrees of external rotation with the arm in abduction, and four spinal levels of internal rotation. Two patients required total shoulder arthroplasty for painful glenohumeral arthritis. Clinical failure was related to glenohumeral arthritis or residual anterior shoulder apprehension.

Subscapularis Muscle Procedures

Putti-Platt Procedure

In 1948, Osmond-Clarke[512] described this procedure, which was used by Sir Harry Platt of England and Vittorio Putti of Italy. Platt first used this technique in November 1925. Some years later, Osmond-Clarke saw Putti perform essentially the same operation, which had been his standard practice since 1923. Scaglietta, one of Putti's pupils, revealed that the operation may well have been performed first by Codivilla, Putti's teacher and predecessor. Neither Putti nor Platt ever described the technique in the literature.

In the Putti-Platt procedure, the subscapularis tendon is divided 2.5 cm from its insertion. The lateral stump of the tendon is attached to the "most convenient soft tissue structure along the anterior rim of the glenoid cavity." If the capsule and labrum have been stripped from the anterior glenoid and neck of the scapula, the tendon is sutured to the deep surface of the capsule, and "it is advisable to raw the anterior surface of the neck of the scapula, so that the sutured tendo-capsule will adhere to it." After the lateral tendon stump is secured, the medial muscle stump is lapped over the lateral stump to produce substantial shortening of the capsule and subscapularis muscle. The exact placement of the lateral stump into the anterior soft tissues and the medial stump into the greater tuberosity is determined so that after conclusion of the procedure, the arm should externally rotate to the neutral position. Variations on the Putti-Platt procedure have been described by Blazina and Satzman,[61] Watson-Jones,[684] Müller,[463] and Symeonides.[642]

Quigley and Freedman[553] reported the results of 92 Putti-Platt operations; of these patients, 11 had more than 30% loss of motion and seven had recurrent instability after their surgery. In 1982, Leach et al.[370] reported a series of 78 patients who had been treated with a modified Putti-Platt procedure. Loss of external rotation averaged between 12 and 19 degrees. Collins et al.[118] reviewed a series of 58 Putti-Platt procedures and 48 Putti-Platt-Bankart procedures. The redislocation rate was 11% (some because of significant trauma), 20% had residual pain, and the average restriction of external rotation was 20 degrees. Hovelius et al.,[287] in a follow-up of 114 patients who underwent either a Bankart or Putti-Platt reconstruction, found a recurrence rate of 2% in 46 patients treated with the Bankart procedure and 19% in 68 patients treated with a Putti-Platt procedure. Follow-up was between 1.5 and 10 years.

Fredriksson and Tegner[196] reviewed 101 patients who had had a Putti-Platt procedure with a mean follow-up of approximately 8 years (range, 5 to 14 years). Recurrent instability occurred in 20% of cases, and all patients demonstrated a decrease in the range of all measured movements, especially external rotation. Additionally, a significant decrease in strength and power was noted by Cybex dynamometer assessment. The authors stated that the restricted motion after this procedure did not improve with time as previous reports had suggested and concluded that this method of reconstruction should not be recommended for young, active patients.

It is important to recognize that if this operation is carried out as described, a 2.5-cm lateral stump of subscapularis tendon is attached to the anterior glenoid. Because the radius of the humerus is approximately 2.5 cm, a 2.5-cm stump of subscapularis fused to the anterior glenoid would limit total humeral rotation to 1 radian, or 57 degrees. Angelo and Hawkins[13,250] presented a series of patients in whom osteoarthritis developed an average of 15 years after a Putti-Platt repair. Limitation of external rotation after repair for anterior instability is now recognized as a factor predisposing to capsulorrhaphy arthropathy.[346,395]

Magnuson-Stack Procedure

Transfer of the subscapularis tendon from the lesser tuberosity across the bicipital groove to the greater tuberosity was originally described by Paul Magnuson and James Stack in 1940.[328,401-403,442,557] In 1955, Magnuson recommended that in some cases the tendon should be transferred not only across the bicipital groove but also distally into an area between the greater tuberosity and the upper shaft. DePalma[145] recommended that the tendon be transferred to the upper shaft below the greater tuberosity. Karadimas et al.,[328] in the largest single series of Magnuson-Stack procedures (154 patients), reported a 2% recurrence rate. Badgley and O'Connor[25] and Bailey[27] reported on a combination of the Putti-Platt and the Magnuson-Stack operations; they used the upper half of the subscapularis muscle to perform the Putti-Platt procedure and the lower half of the muscle to perform the Magnuson-Stack procedure.

Complications of the Magnuson-Stack procedure include excessive anterior tightening with posterior subluxation or dislocation (Fig. 13-166), damage to the biceps (Fig. 13-167), and recurrent instability.

Bone Block Procedures

Historically, bone block procedures were unpopular because of concerns of humeral articular contact with nonarticular bone on the glenoid side and early posttraumatic arthrosis. However, recent appreciation of the impact of glenoid and humeral bone loss on the failure of other stabilization procedures[87] has led to resurgence in the value and utilization of bone block procedures, particularly the Latarjet procedure. Many options for bone block procedures have been described, including autologous coracoid transfer, tricortical iliac crest, frozen glenoid allograft, or fresh osteochondral distal tibial allograft. Biomechanical studies analyzing the best fit for recreation of glenoid curvature have shown that the inferior coracoid and an osteochondral allograft of the lateral distal tibia are the best matches,[137] whereas tibial plafond and iliac crest allografts more adequately restore depth compared with standard Latarjet reconstruction.[493] The

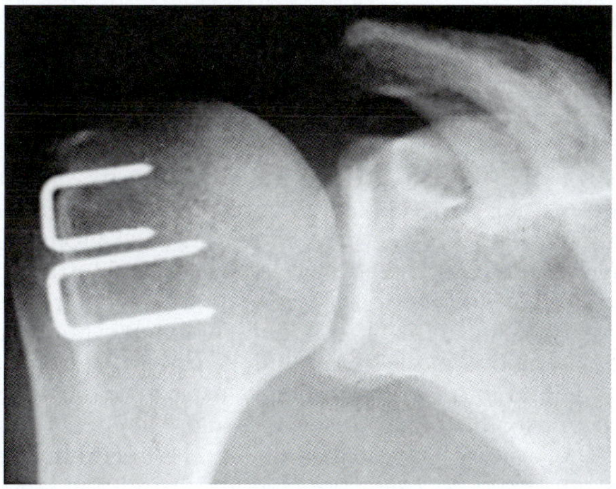

FIGURE 13-167: Impingement of a staple on the long head of the biceps tendon. This anteroposterior radiograph shows the position of the staple resulting in tendon impingement. The patient's anterior shoulder pain resolved when the staple was removed.

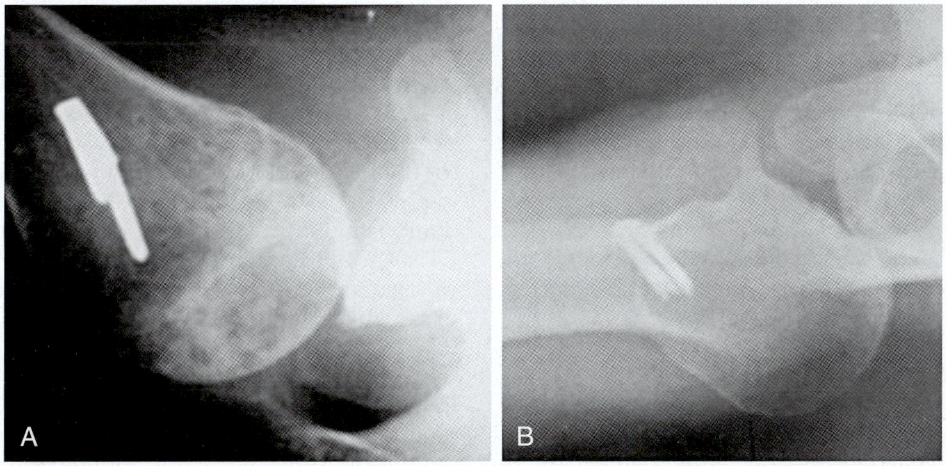

FIGURE 13-166: The Magnuson-Stack procedure. **A,** This axillary view shows posterior subluxation of the humeral head on the glenoid as a result of excessive anterior tightening with the Magnuson-Stack procedure. **B,** Another patient's axillary view shows excessive anterior tightening from the Magnuson-Stack procedure that resulted in posterior glenohumeral displacement of the humeral head.

following sections delineate the options for bony procedures to treat recurrent anterior instability.

Eden-Hybbinette Procedure

The Eden-Hybbinette procedure was performed independently by Eden[164] in 1918 and by Hybbinette[295] in 1932. Eden first used tibial grafts, but both authors finally recommended the use of iliac grafts. This procedure, which is supposed to extend the anterior glenoid, has been used by Palmer and Widen,[523] Lavik,[366] and Hovelius et al.[279] to treat shoulder subluxation and dislocation. Lavik modified the procedure by inserting the graft into the substance of the anterior glenoid rim. Lange[359] inserted the bone graft into an osteotomy on the anterior glenoid. Hehne and Hubner[257] reported a comparison of the Eden-Hybbinette-Lange and the Putti-Platt procedures in 170 patients; their results seemed to favor the latter. Paavolainen et al.[519] reported on 41 patients treated with the Eden-Hybbinette procedure; three had recurrent instability, and external rotation was diminished an average of 10%. They found the results to be similar to those in their series of Putti-Platt operations. Degenerative joint disease developed in 10% in each group!

Niskanen et al.[489] reported a series of 52 shoulders with a mean follow-up of 6 years that had been treated using a modification of the Eden-Hybbinette procedure. The operation involved creating a trough through the capsule and into the anteroinferior aspects of the scapula neck. A tricortical iliac crest bone graft was then wedged into the trough without fixation. A 21% recurrence rate was attributed to one spontaneous dislocation and 10 traumatic redislocations. Postoperative arthrosis was noted in nine shoulders and early degenerative changes in an additional 18 shoulders.

Oudard Procedure

In 1924, Oudard[513] described the original method in which the coracoid process was prolonged with a bone graft from the tibia. The graft (4 × 3 × 1 cm) was inserted between the sawed-off tip and the remainder of the coracoid and was directed laterally and inferiorly. The graft acted as an anterior buttress that served to prevent recurrent dislocations. Oudard also shortened the subscapular tendon. Later, he published another method of achieving elongation of the coracoid: oblique osteotomy of the coracoid with displacement of the posterolateral portion to serve as a bone block. Matsen and Thomas[415] described a technique for using a contoured bone graft covered with joint capsule or other soft tissue to replace the missing glenoid bone in order to offer a smooth surface to articulate with the humeral head.

Fresh Osteochondral Allograft From the Distal Tibia

Provencher[551] has investigated the use of osteochondral allograft distal tibia to reconstruct large defects in the anterioinferior glenoid, that is, lesions greater than 30% of the articular surface, in cases of recurrent anterior shoulder instability (Fig. 13-168). The distal tibial plafond has been found to have an arc of curvature that nearly matches that of the glenoid face. Use of a fresh allograft offers the potential of viable articular cartilage to restore the glenoid arc of curvature, which is not possible with autologous tricortial iliac crest graft or fresh frozen allografts. Biomechanical analysis[53,208,698] demonstrates that distal tibia allograft can improve stability similar to tricortical iliac crest.

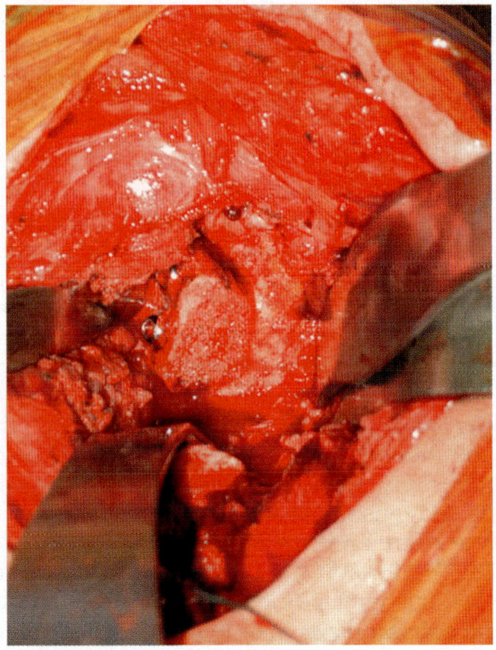

FIGURE 13-168: Tricortical iliac crest graft is used to fill large glenoid defects.

The risks of coracoid transfer are avoided, although the benefits of the "sling effect" mentioned below are also absent. In biomechanical studies, iliac crest and distal tibial allograft have been shown to improve stability even in patients without significant glenoid bone loss.[698,208,53] Additionally, the risk of infection or disease transmission is increased with the use of fresh allograft rather than autologous grafts or coracoid transfer.

In their initial series of three patients, Provencher et al.[551] reported on three patients treated with the lateral portion of the distal tibia as a fresh osteochondral allograft for the treatment of substantial glenoid bone loss measuring 30% of the radius on average. All three patients demonstrated incorporation of the graft on postoperative CT scan, but no clinical results were reported. More clinical data are required to validate the utilization of the fresh distal tibial allograft.

Coracoid Transfer

In transfer of the coracoid process to the anterior glenoid, an attempt is made to create an anteroinferior musculotendinous sling with an added bone block effect to restore glenoid bone loss and prevent dislocation. However, the procedure is technically demanding, revision options are limited, and subsequent surgery is challenging: The subscapularis, musculocutaneous, and axillary nerves are scarred in abnormal positions; the subscapularis muscle is scarred and tethered; and the axillary artery may be displaced in scar tissue.

Trillat Procedure

Trillat and Leclerc-Chalvet[64,492,658,659] performed an osteotomy at the base of the coracoid process and then displaced the coracoid downward and laterally. The displaced coracoid is held in position by a special nail-pin or screw. The pin is passed into the scapula above the inferiorly displaced subscapularis muscle, effectively shortening the muscle.

Bristow-Helfet Procedure

In 1958, Helfet published his results on a modified bone block technique using a procedure he named after his mentor, Rowley Bristow of South Africa.[258] Helfet originally described detaching the tip of the coracoid process from the scapula just distal to the insertion of the pectoralis minor muscle and leaving the conjoined tendons (the short head of the biceps and the coracobrachialis) attached. Through a vertical slit in the subscapularis tendon, the joint is exposed and the anterior surface of the neck of the scapula is "rawed up." The coracoid process with its attached tendons is then passed through the slit in the subscapularis and kept in contact with the raw area on the scapula by suturing the conjoined tendon to the cut edges of the subscapularis tendon. In effect, a subscapularis tenodesis is performed. A later modification secured the coracoid process to the anterior glenoid rim with a screw.

May[417] modified the Bristow procedure further by vertically dividing the entire subscapularis tendon from the lesser tuberosity; after exploring the joint, he attached the tip of the coracoid process with the conjoined tendon to the anterior glenoid with a screw. The subscapularis tendon was then split horizontally and reattached—half the tendon above and half below the transferred conjoined tendon—to the site of its original insertion. Again, the net effect is a tenodesis of the subscapularis due to the small size of the coracoid transferred.

Bonnin[68,67] modified the Bristow procedure in the following way: He did not shorten or split the subscapularis muscle tendon unit, but for exposure, he divided the subscapularis muscle at its muscle-tendon junction; after attachment of the coracoid process to the glenoid with a screw, he reattached the subscapularis on top of the conjoined tendon. The results of this modification in 81 patients have been reported by Hummel et al.[291]

Torg et al.[656] reported their experience with 212 Bristow procedures. In their modification, the coracoid was passed over the superior border rather than through the subscapularis. Their postoperative instability rate was 8.5% (3.8% redislocation and 4.7% subluxation). Ten patients required reoperation for screw-related problems; 34% had residual shoulder pain, and 8% were unable to do overhead work. Only 16% of athletes were able to return to their preinjury level of throwing.

Carol et al.[97] reported on the results of the Bristow procedure performed for 32 recurrently dislocating shoulders and 15 "spontaneous" shoulder instabilities. At an average follow-up of 3.7 years, only one patient had recurrent instability, and the average limitation of external rotation was 12 degrees.

Banas et al.[31] reported a 4% recurrence rate with an 8.6-year follow-up; however, additional surgery was required in 14%. Wredmark et al.[713] found only two of 44 recurrent dislocations at an average follow-up of 6 years, but 28% of patients complained of pain.

Hovelius et al.[279] reported follow-up on 111 shoulders treated with the Bristow procedure. At 2.5 years, the postoperative instability rate was 13% (6% dislocation and 7% subluxation). External rotation was limited an average of 20 degrees, and 6% required a reoperation because of screw-related complications. Muscle strength was 10% less in the operated shoulder.

Chen et al.[105] found that after the Bristow procedure, the reduced strength of the short head of the biceps was compensated for by increased activity in the long head. Other series of Bristow procedures have been reported, each of which emphasizes the potential risks.[686]

Lamm et al.[358] and Lemmens and de Waal Malefijt[374] described four special x-ray projections to evaluate the position of the transplanted coracoid process: AP, lateral, oblique lateral, and modified axial. Lower et al.[393] used CT scans to demonstrate impingement of a Bristow screw on the head of the humerus. Collins and Wilde[119] and Nielsen and Nielsen[488] reported that although they had minimal problems with recurrence of dislocation, they did encounter problems with screw breakage, migration, and nonunion of the coracoid to the scapula. Hovelius et al.[277,281] reported only a 50% union rate of the coracoid to the scapula.

Norris et al.[495] evaluated 24 patients with failed Bristow repairs; only two had union of the transferred coracoid. Causes of failure included residual subluxation and osteoarthritis from screw or bone impingement or an overtight repair. They pointed to the difficulty of reconstructing a shoulder after a failed Bristow procedure. Singer et al.[623] conducted a 20-year follow-up study of the Bristow-Latarjet procedure; in spite of an average Constant-Murley score of 80 points, radiographic evidence of degenerative joint disease was detected in 71%.

Ferlic and DiGiovine[183] reported on 51 patients treated with the Bristow procedure. They had a 10% incidence of redislocation or subluxation and a 14% incidence of complications related to the screw. An additional surgical procedure was required in 14% of the patients. In a long-term follow-up study of 79 shoulders, Banas et al.[31] also reported complications necessitating reoperation in 14% of patients; 73% of reoperations were for hardware removal secondary to persistent shoulder pain.

Recurrent subluxation after the Bristow procedure also appears to be a significant problem.[420,281,495,183,400] Hill et al.[269] and MacKenzie[399] noted failure to manage subluxation with this procedure. Schauder and Tullos[604] reported 85% good or excellent results with a modified Bristow procedure in 20 shoulders at a minimum of 3 years of follow-up. Interestingly, the authors attributed the success to healing of the Bankart lesion because in many instances, the position of the transferred coracoid precluded it from containing the humeral head. The authors suggested that the 15% fair or poor results were secondary to persistent or recurrent subluxation.

In 1989, Rockwood and Young[573,722] reported on 40 patients previously treated with the Bristow procedure. They commented on the danger and the technical difficulty of these repairs. Of the 40, 31 underwent subsequent reconstructive procedures: 10 had a capsular shift reconstruction, four required capsular release, four had total shoulder arthroplasty, one had an arthrodesis, and the rest had various combined procedures. The authors concluded that coracoid transfers are technically demanding and can be associated with serious complications, and thus recommended that it not be performed for routine anterior reconstruction of the shoulder.

Latarjet Procedure

The Latarjet procedure,[365,364,531] described in 1954, involves the transfer of a larger portion of the coracoid process than used with the Bristow procedure, with the biceps and coracobrachialis tendons transferred along with it to the anteroinferior aspect of the neck of the scapula. Instead of the raw cut surface of the tip of the coracoid process being attached to the scapula, as is done in the Bristow-Helfet procedure, the coracoid is laid flat on the neck of the scapula and held in place with two screws.

Biomechanical differences in joint stability have been found to favor the Latarjet, in that it confers more stability than the Bristow procedure, likely secondary to the larger volume of bone for glenoid reconstruction.[213] A critical stabilizing mechanism of the Latarjet procedure is the sling effect at both the end-range and the mid-range arm positions.[720,212] If the coracoid is fractured intraoperatively, it may still be worthwhile to transfer the strap muscles to the anteroinferior glenoid rim for this dynamic sling effect.[333]

Orientation of the coracoid graft has been studied when performing the Latarjet procedure. In the original description, the inferior surface of the coracoid is decorticated and placed along the glenoid neck. Another option described by Burkhart and De Beer[88] places the medial decorticated surface of the coracoid against the glenid neck, thereby rotating the graft 90 degrees on its long axis and placing the inferior coracoid surface flush with the glenoid articular surface superiorly. This modification has been termed the "congruent arc" technique, which may better restore the native glenoid coronal radius of curvature because the coracoid graft is 30% wider in this orientation due to the increased width of the coracoid relative to its thickness.[19,208] However, the fixation surface is reduced by 30% as well, and this may carry a higher risk of coracoid fracture or graft failure.[69]

However, postoperative arthritis is a concern with misplaced bone grafts. Therefore many surgeons opt to place the bone block extra-articular, where the humeral head is not expected to glide across the graft surface in continuity with the native glenoid. Extra-articular coracoid graft placement is achieved by repairing the capsulobral complex to the native glenoid anteroinferior rim or to the stump of the CA ligament retained during coracoid harvest. Regardless, the best position for the graft is within 1 cm medial to the glenoid rim.[285]

Tagliabue and Esposito[643] reported on the Latarjet procedure in 94 athletes. Wredmark et al.[713] analyzed 44 patients at an average follow-up of 6 years after a Bristow-Latarjet procedure for recurrent shoulder dislocation; 72% had no discomfort, but the remaining 28% complained of moderate exertional pain. Vittori has modified the procedure by turning the subscapularis tendon downward and holding it displaced downward with the transferred coracoid. Pascoet et al.[531] reported on use of the Vittori modification in 36 patients and noted one recurrence.

More recent studies have demonstrated improved results with the Latarjet procedure and have helped highlight some critical technical aspects of the procedure.[87,285,286] These include placement of the coracoid graft flush with glenoid articular surface such that there is no lateral overhang or excessive medialization, repair of the capsulobral complex, either to the native glenoid or to the CA ligament stump, and meticulous subscapularis management.

Following these principles, a study by Schmid et al. on outcomes 3 years after Latarjet showed that no patients had recurrent dislocation or required revision surgery and 88% were graded as excellent, demonstrating the importance of proper graft placement.[607] Another recent study retrospectively compared the results of arthroscopic Bankart repair to Latarjet, demonstrating lower recurrence rates following Latarjet. At 4-year follow-up, 10% (nine of 93) in the Latarjet group and 22% (20 of 93) in the Bankart group demonstrated recurrent instability. Reoperation rate was 6% and 7% in the Bankart and Latarjet groups, respectively. In both groups, patients younger than 20 years had higher recurrence risk. In the Bankart group, independent factors predictive for recurrence were practice of competitive sports and shoulder hyperlaxity, but these were not significant factors affecting outcome after Latarjet.[50]

Other Open Repairs

Gallie Procedure

Gallie and LeMesurier[199,200] originally described the use of autogenous fascia lata to create new ligaments between the anteroinferior aspect of the capsule and the anterior neck of the humerus in 1927. Bateman[41] of Toronto has also used this procedure. Although fascia lata might not be the ideal graft material, exogenous autograft or allograft may be necessary for reconstructing deficient capsulolabral structures in the management of failed previous surgical repairs.

Nicola Procedure

Toufick Nicola's name is usually associated with this operation, but the procedure was first described by Rupp[594] in 1926 and Heymanowitsch[267] in 1927. In 1929, Nicola[482] published the first article in which he described the use of the long head of the biceps tendon as a checkrein ligament. The procedure has been modified several times.[483-485,487] Recurrence rates are reported to be between 30% and 50%.[98,323,687]

Saha Procedure

Saha[596-599] has described transfer of the latissimus dorsi posteriorly into the site of the infraspinatus insertion on the greater tuberosity. He reported that during abduction, the transferred latissimus reinforces the subscapularis muscle and the short posterior steering and depressor muscles by pulling the humeral head backward. He has used the procedure for traumatic and atraumatic dislocations, and in 1969 he reported 45 cases with no recurrence.

Boytchev Procedure

Boytchev first described this procedure in 1951 in the Italian literature,[72,73] and later modifications were developed by Conforty.[120] The muscles that attach to the coracoid process along with the tip of the coracoid are rerouted deep to the subscapularis muscle between it and the capsule. The tip of the coracoid with its muscles is then reattached to its base in the anatomic position. Conforty[120] reported on 17 patients, none of whom had a recurrence of dislocation. Ha'eri and Maitland[236] reported 26 cases with a minimum of 2 years' follow-up.

Osteotomy of the Proximal Humerus

Debevoise et al.[136,346] stated that humeral torsion is abnormal in a repeatedly dislocating shoulder. B.G. Weber[330,442,557,687,689] of Switzerland reported a rotational osteotomy whereby he increased the retroversion of the humeral head and simultaneously performed an anterior capsulorrhaphy. The indications were a moderate to severe posterolateral humeral head defect, which he found in 65% of his patients with recurrent anterior instability. By increasing the retroversion, the posterolateral defect is delivered more posteriorly and the anterior undisturbed portion of the articular surface of the humeral head then articulates against the glenoid. It is recognized that the effective articular surface of the humerus is reduced by the posterolateral head defect and that the osteotomy realigns the remaining articular surface in a position more compatible with activities of daily living. Weber et al.[689] reported a redislocation rate of 5.7%, with good to excellent results in 90%. Most patients required a reoperation for plate removal.

Osteotomy of the Neck of the Glenoid

In 1933, Meyer-Burgdorff reported on decreasing the anterior tilt of the glenoid with a posterior closing wedge osteotomy.[596] Saha has written[596] about an anterior opening wedge osteotomy with a bone graft placed into the neck of the glenoid to decrease the tilt.

Complications of Anterior Repairs

Complications of surgical repairs for anterior glenohumeral instability may be grouped into several categories.[368]

The first includes complications that can follow any surgical procedure. Of primary importance in this category is postoperative infection. Thorough skin preparation, adhesive plastic drapes, and prophylactic antibiotics are useful in reducing contamination by axillary bacterial flora. It is also important to prevent the accumulation of significant hematoma by achieving good hemostasis, obliterating any dead space, and using a suction drain if significant bleeding persists. It is important to keep the axilla clean and dry postoperatively by using a gauze sponge as long as the arm is held at the side.

The second category of complications consists of postoperative recurrent instability. The published incidence of recurrent dislocation after anterior repairs ranges from 0% to 30%. It is noteworthy that many of the reports in their tally included only recurrent dislocation rather than recurrent subluxation or recurrent apprehension. A 1975 review of 1634 reconstructions compiled from the literature revealed that the incidence of redislocation averaged 3%. In a 1983 review of 3076 procedures, the incidence was unchanged.[570] This review included 432 Putti-Platt operations, 571 Magnuson-Stack operations or modifications, 513 Bankart operations or modifications, 45 Saha operations, 203 Bankart-Putti-Platt combinations, 639 Bristow operations, 115 Badgley combined procedures, 254 Eden-Hybbinette operations, 277 Gallie operations or modifications, and 27 Weber operations.

The incidence of recurrence is underestimated by studies with only 2 years of follow-up. Morrey and Janes,[456] in a long-term follow-up study of 176 patients that averaged 10.2 years, found a redislocation rate of 11%. The operative reconstructions were of the Bankart and Putti-Platt types. In seven of the 20 patients, redislocation occurred 2 or more years after surgery. The need for long-term follow-up was further emphasized in a study by O'Driscoll and Evans,[502] who monitored 269 consecutive patients undergoing staple capsulorrhaphy for a minimum of 8.8 years. Twenty-one percent of 204 shoulders demonstrated redislocation; this incidence increased progressively with the length of follow-up.

Factors that have been shown to be significantly associated with a poor outcome after open surgical anterior stabilization are workers' compensation, voluntary instability, previous instability surgery, age of the patient, and shorter periods of postoperative immobilization.[248] Immobilization for less than 6 weeks and age 32 years or older were associated with significantly lower Rowe scores. The sex of the patient, Hill-Sachs lesions, type of instability, labral tears, and the surgeon's experience were not statistically significant. The majority of these patients had Bankart repairs or capsular shifts.

Rowe et al.[591] reported on the management of 39 patients with recurrence of instability after various surgical repairs. Of 32 who underwent reoperation, 84% did not have an effective repair of the Bankart lesion at the initial surgery. When the previously unrepaired Bankart lesion was repaired at revision surgery, almost all (22 of 24) the shoulders became stable and remained so for at least 2 years. Excessive laxity was thought to be the primary cause of instability in only four shoulders. Ungersbock et al.[664] also found that rounded or deficient glenoid rims and large unhealed Bankart lesions were associated with failure of surgical repair for anterior instability. Zabinski et al. reported similar findings: over half of their failed instability repairs were associated with unhealed Bankart lesions; most regained stability after revision repair.[725] By contrast, only nine of the 21 shoulders with recurrent MDI obtained a good or excellent result from revision surgeries. All 17 patients who had a significant traumatic event subsequent to instability surgery had excellent results after revision open stabilization. Of 33 patients with recurrent instability and no significant trauma after initial surgery, only 67% had good or excellent results.[381]

Refractory instability can be a major problem, whether caused by bone deficiency, poor-quality soft tissue, musculotendinous failure, or decompensation of neuromuscular control (Fig. 13-169). Richards et al.[562] described the challenges associated with trying to manage such cases of refractory or terminal instability by glenohumeral arthrodesis.

The third major category of complications arises from failure of diagnosis. Differentiating traumatic unidirectional instability (TUBS syndrome) from atraumatic MDI (AMBRII syndrome) is essential before carrying out any surgical repair. The consequences of mistaking MDI for pure anterior instability are substantial. In this situation, if only the anterior structures are tightened, limited external rotation along with the resulting obligate posterior subluxation can lead to rapid loss of glenohumeral articular cartilage and capsulorrhaphy arthropathy.[250,346,395] This complication can be prevented only by accurate preoperative diagnosis and appropriate surgery that avoids unnecessary capsular tightening.

The importance of an accurate diagnosis and subsequent treatment cannot be overemphasized: 20 shoulders (53%) in the study of Cooper and Brems[122] and 22 shoulders (15%) in the report of Wirth and Rockwood[706] had previously been operated on for a mistaken diagnosis. In the latter report, diagnostic errors included (in order of decreasing frequency) rotator cuff disease, biceps tendinitis, thoracic outlet syndrome, and cervical disk herniation.

The fourth category of operative complications consists of neurovascular injuries. The musculocutaneous nerve runs as a single or multipartite structure obliquely through the coracobrachialis at a variable distance distal to the coracoid process. In this location, it can be injured by dissection to free up the coracoid process, by retraction, or by inclusion in sutures.[617] Helfet[258] described one case in which the nerve had high penetration into the coracobrachialis and became injured where the conjoined tendon entered the slit made in the subscapularis tendon for a Bristow procedure. The axillary nerve can be injured during dissection and suture of the inferior capsule and subscapularis.[392]

Richards et al.[563] presented nine patients who sustained nerve injuries during anterior shoulder repair (three Bristow and six Putti-Platt procedures). Seven involved the musculocutaneous nerve, and two involved the axillary nerve. Two of the nerves were lacerated, five were injured by suture, and two were injured by traction. These nerve injuries are relatively more common during reoperation after a previous repair; in this situation, the nerves are tethered by scar tissue and are thus more difficult to mobilize out of harm's way. Neurovascular complications can best be avoided by good knowledge of local anatomy (including the possible normal variations), good surgical technique, and a healthy respect for the change in position and mobility of the neurovascular structures after a previous surgical procedure in the area. We recommend that the axillary nerve be routinely palpated and protected during all anterior reconstructions.[476]

The fifth category of complications includes those related to hardware inserted about the glenohumeral joint.[102,256] The screw used to fix the coracoid fragment in Bristow procedures has a particular potential for being

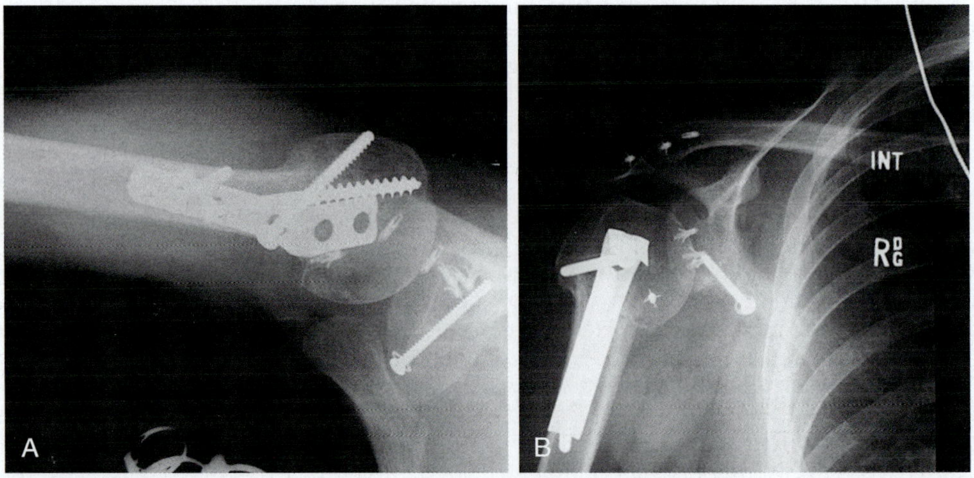

FIGURE 13-169: Axillary (**A**) and anteroposterior (**B**) radiographs of the shoulder of a young woman. The shoulder remained unstable after six surgeries for glenohumeral instability, including Bankart repairs, capsular shifts, and a Bristow and derotational osteotomy.

problematic.[488,553] Loosening of the screw can result from rotation of the coracoid fragment as the arm is raised and lowered (Fig. 13-170). Artz and Huffer[21] and Fee et al.[180] reported a devastating complication in which the screw became loose and caused a false aneurysm of the axillary artery with subsequent compression of the brachial plexus and paralysis of the upper extremity. Similar complications have been reported as late as 3 years after surgery.[165] In other instances, the Bristow screw has damaged the articular surface of the glenoid and humeral head when placed too close to the glenoid lip, irritated the infraspinatus or its nerve when too long, or affected the brachial plexus when it became loose (Figs. 13-171 to 13-176).

Staples used to attach the capsule to the glenoid can miss their target and damage the humeral or glenoid articular cartilage (Fig. 13-177; see also Figs. 13-164 to 13-166). Staples also can become loose from repeated pull of the muscles and capsule during shoulder use, particularly if they were not well seated in the first place. O'Driscoll and Evans[502] reported an 11% incidence of staple complications after the DuToit procedure. If screws and staples migrate into the intra-articular region, significant damage to the joint surfaces can result (Fig. 13-178). Metal fixation can injure the biceps tendon in a Magnuson-Stack procedure (see Fig. 13-167).

Zuckerman and Matsen[732] reported a series of patients with problems related to the use of screws and staples about the glenohumeral joint; 21 had problems related to the Bristow procedure and 14 to the use of staples (either for capsulorrhaphy or subscapularis advancement). The time between placement and symptom onset ranged from 4 weeks to 10 years. Screws and staples had been incorrectly placed in 10 patients, had migrated or loosened in 24, and had fractured in three. Almost all patients required reoperation, at which time 41% had a significant injury to one or both of the joint surfaces.

Recent attempts to lessen the potential complications of hardware by using bioabsorbable implants have been described. However, Edwards et al.[165] reported the adverse effects of a polyglyconate polymer in six shoulders after repair of the glenoid labrum. All patients had increasing pain and loss of motion requiring arthroscopic debridement. Dual-contrast arthrotomography revealed bony cystic changes around the implant, and histologic evaluation was consistent with a granulomatous reaction.

The depth and variable orientation of the glenoid at surgery provide substantial opportunity for hardware misplacement (into the joint, under the articular cartilage, subperiosteally, out the back, too high, too low, too medial, too prominent anteriorly, and too insecurely). The large range of motion of the shoulder with frequent vigorous challenge to its stability creates an opportunity for loosening of hardware and for surface and neurovascular damage.

The sixth category of complications is limited motion. Limited range of motion, especially external rotation, has been reported after the Magnuson-Stack and the Putti-Platt procedures. It has also been noted after the Bristow procedure, which was supposed to be free of this problem.[37,76,397] Hovelius et al.[287] reported an average loss of external rotation of 21 degrees with the arm in abduction. In their series of 46 patients with continuing problems after shoulder reconstruction, Hawkins and Hawkins[251] found that 10 had stiffness related to limited external rotation.

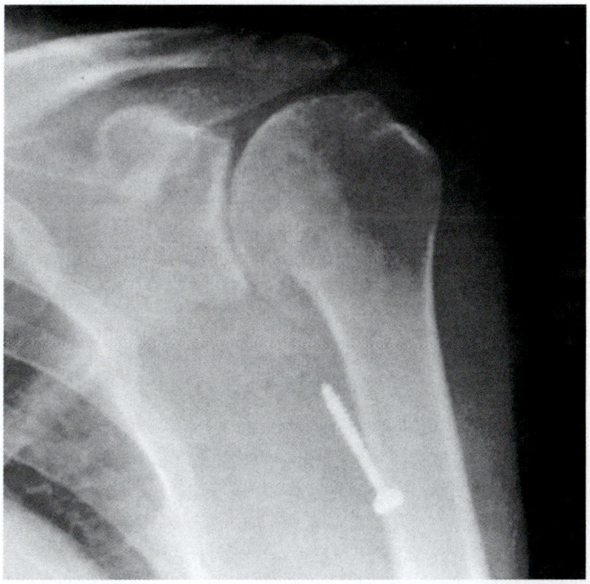

FIGURE 13-170: This patient experienced a pop while externally rotating the shoulder 5 months after a Bristow procedure. Shortly after this episode, he palpated a bump in his axilla while applying deodorant. (From Rockwood CA Jr, Green DP, Bucholz RW, eds. *Fractures in Adults*. Philadelphia: JB Lippincott; 1991.)

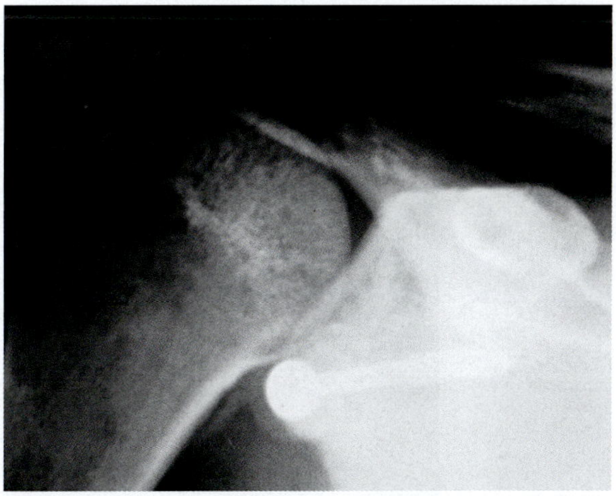

FIGURE 13-171: Anteroposterior radiograph showing impingement of a screw on the humeral head after the Bristow procedure.

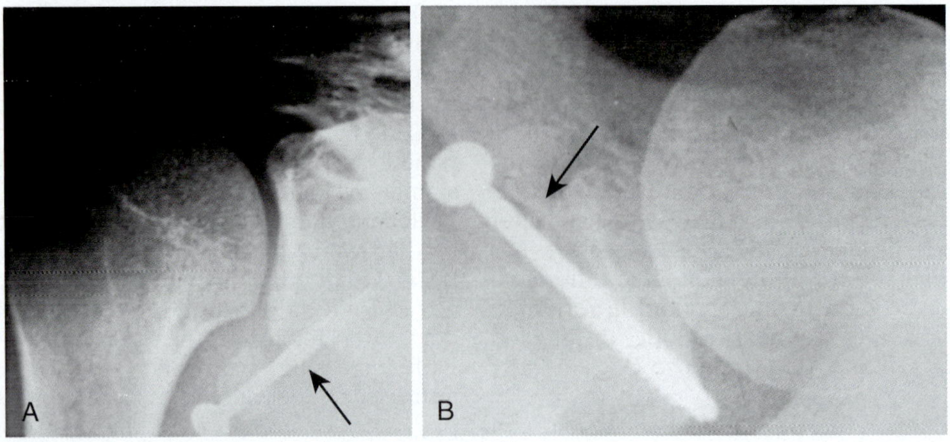

FIGURE 13-172: Nonunion of the coracoid process after the Bristow procedure. **A,** Anteroposterior radiograph shows nonunion of the coracoid process (*arrow*). **B,** An axillary view in a different patient shows nonunion of the coracoid process after the Bristow procedure (*arrow*).

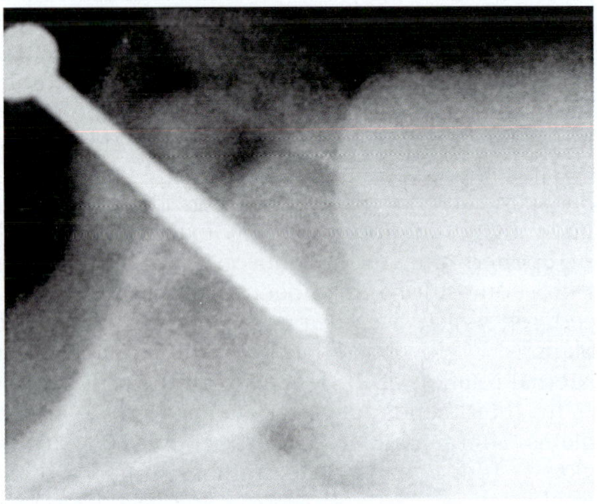

FIGURE 13-173: This axillary view shows the screw backing out of the glenoid after the Bristow procedure.

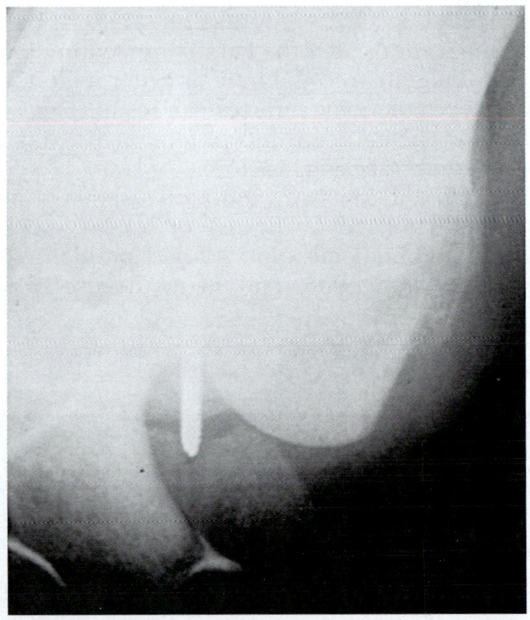

FIGURE 13-174: Axillary view showing an excessively long screw used during the Bristow procedure. The patient had an infraspinatus palsy as a result of injury to the nerve to this muscle.

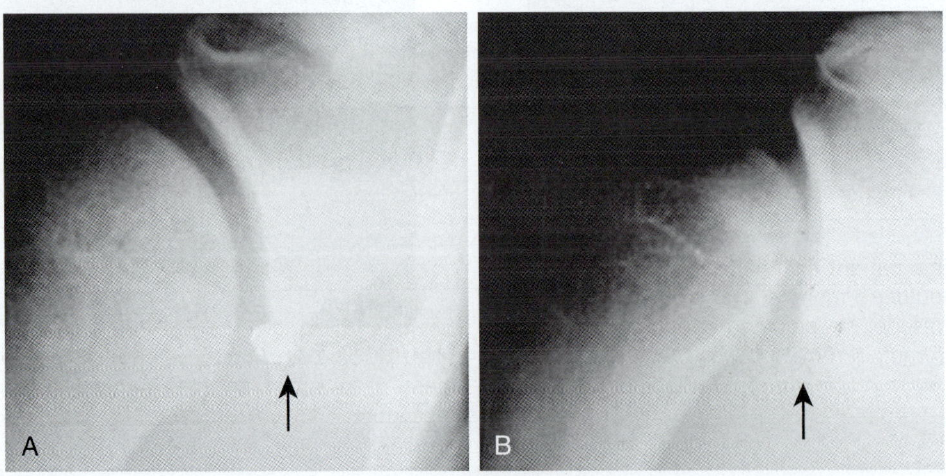

FIGURE 13-175: Anteroposterior radiographs showing broken screws with the humerus in external rotation (**A**) and internal rotation (**B**).

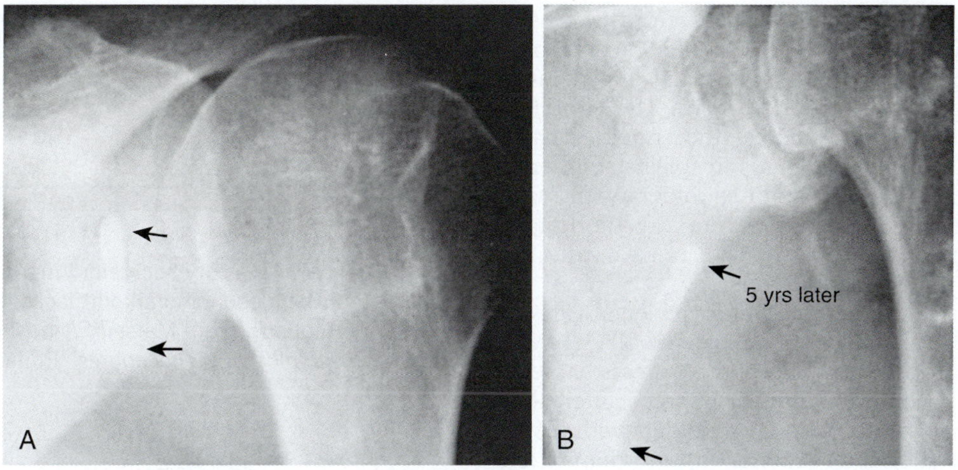

FIGURE 13-176: Late screw loosening after the Bristow procedure. **A,** Anteroposterior (AP) radiograph shows the position of the screw (*arrows*) in the transferred coracoid process. **B,** AP radiograph taken 5 years later shows the screw had backed out (*arrow*) as well as significant glenohumeral arthropathy.

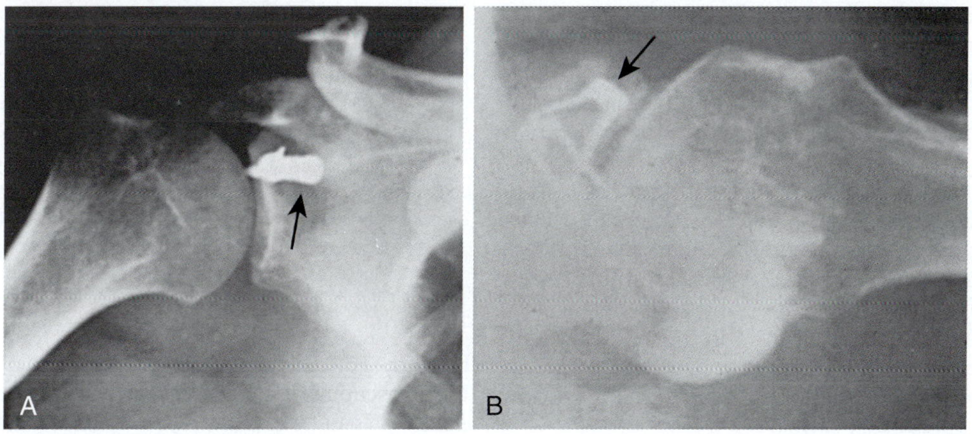

FIGURE 13-177: **A,** Anteroposterior radiograph shows the position of an arthroscopically placed staple (*arrow*). Contact of the staple with the humeral head is suggested by this view. **B,** An axillary view with contrast material demonstrates impingement of the staple on the humeral head (*arrow*).

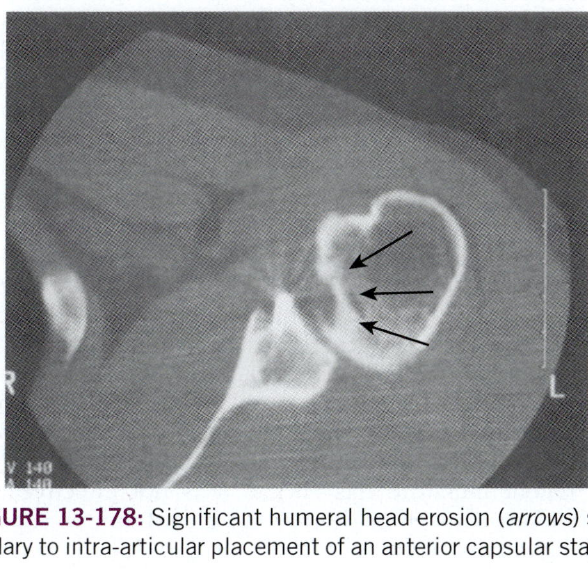

FIGURE 13-178: Significant humeral head erosion (*arrows*) secondary to intra-articular placement of an anterior capsular staple.

MacDonald et al.[397] described release of the subscapularis muscle in 10 patients who had an internal rotation contracture after shoulder reconstruction for recurrent instability. At an average follow-up of 3 years, all patients reported less pain and demonstrated an average increase of 27 degrees of external rotation.

Lazarus and Harryman[368] pointed out that each centimeter of surgical lengthening of an excessively tightened capsule regains approximately 20 degrees of rotation.

Lusardi et al. reported on 19 patients (20 shoulders) who had been treated for severe loss of external rotation of the glenohumeral joint after a previous anterior capsulorrhaphy for recurrent instability.[395] All 20 shoulders were managed by release of the anterior soft tissue. The average increase in external rotation was 45 degrees (range, 25 to 65 degrees).

The seventh complication is that of capsulorrhaphy arthropathy, or secondary degenerative joint disease resulting from surgery for recurrent instability.[13,346,368,395,414]

This condition most commonly arises from excessive surgical tightening of the anterior capsule, causing obligate posterior translation with secondary degenerative joint disease (see Figs. 13-55 and 13-56). The condition can be prevented by ensuring that the shoulder has a functional range of motion after repair for instability and by performing a surgical release of shoulders with major limitations in external rotation. Severe capsulorrhaphy can require shoulder arthroplasty with normalization of the posteriorly inclined glenoid version.[346,368,395,396]

Angelo and Hawkins[13] reported eight patients with disabling degenerative arthritis seen an average of 15.1 years after a Putti-Platt procedure. None of the patients had ever gained external rotation beyond 0 degrees after their repair. Lusardi et al.[395] described 20 shoulders with severe loss of external rotation after anterior capsulorrhaphy and spoke about the risk of posterior subluxation and secondary degenerative joint disease in these circumstances.

Lusardi et al.[395] also reported on seven shoulders in which the humeral head had been subluxated or dislocated posteriorly and 16 shoulders that had been affected by mild to severe degenerative joint disease after surgical repair for recurrent anterior dislocation. Nine required shoulder arthroplasty because of severe joint surface destruction. At a mean follow-up of 48 months, all shoulders had an improvement in ratings for pain and range of motion.

The eighth complication after surgical repair is failure of the subscapularis. As pointed out by Lazarus and Harryman,[368] the clinical manifestations of subscapularis failure can include pain, weakness of abdominal press and lumbar pushoff, apprehension, and frank instability. A failed subscapularis can sometimes be repaired directly and on other occasions might require a hamstring autograft, allograft, or transfer of the pectoralis major tendon (Figs. 13-179 to 13-186).

Wirth et al.[708] reported a series of failed repairs in which the subscapularis was completely disrupted and contracted medially into a dense connective tissue scar that precluded mobilization. Most of the shoulders had undergone multiple previous procedures. The subscapularis deficiency was reconstructed by transfer of either the upper portion of the pectoralis major or the pectoralis minor in five shoulders.

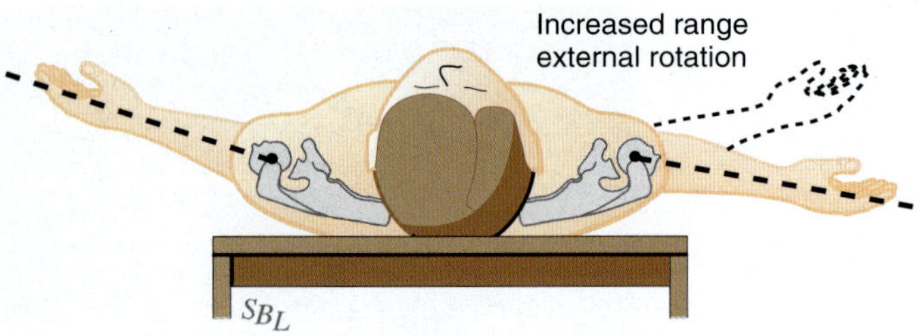

FIGURE 13-179: Loss of checkrein. When the anterior capsule is disrupted, the glenohumeral joint lacks its normal limitation of external rotation. (From Matsen FA III, Lippitt SB. *Shoulder Surgery: Principles and Procedures*. Philadelphia: WB Saunders; 2004:225.)

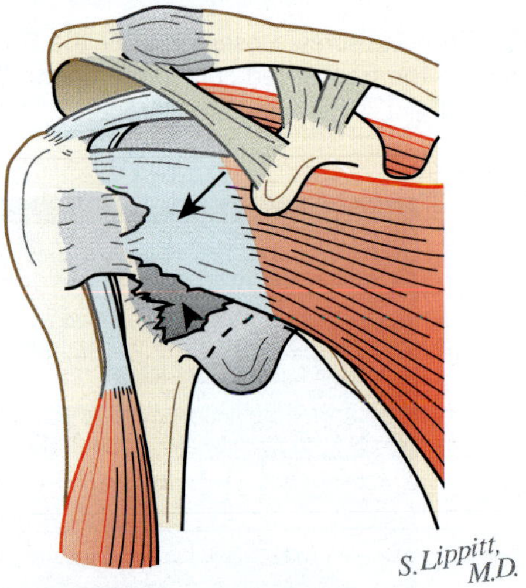

FIGURE 13-180: Compromised tissue quality. The quality of the subscapularis tendon (*arrow*) and anterior capsule (*arrowhead*) is insufficient for repair. (From Matsen FA III, Lippitt SB. *Shoulder Surgery: Principles and Procedures*. Philadelphia: WB Saunders; 2004:227.)

Arthroscopic Bankart Repair

Although initially felt to yield inferior results to open anatomic Bankart or capsulolabral repair, modern arthroscopic stabilization procedures, with improved techniques, implants, and appreciation of the pathoanatomy of recurrent instability, have been effective for the treatment of anterior instability.[103,241,343,418,516,654] Among first-time traumatic anterior dislocators, the recurrence rate after arthroscopic Bankart repair was 14.3% at a mean follow-up of over 11 years.[516] Favorable results have also been reported among pediatric and adolescents with shoulder instability who underwent arthroscopic stabilization.[343]

Among patients with a bony Bankart treated with arthroscopic repair, a lower recurrence has been observed if the bony Bankart heals after surgery; larger fragments more likely to heal. The recurrence rate for postoperative instability was only 6.1% for shoulders with complete union by 1 year, while it was 50% for shoulders with partial union, nonunion, no fragment, and no fragment on CT.[468] The recurrence rate was significantly higher (36.4%) in shoulders with small fragments.[468] A systematic review did not find a difference in the rate of recurrent instability, clinical outcome scores, return to sport, or incidence of postoperative arthritis.[241]

However, a randomized clinical trial evaluated open stabilization with arthroscopic stabilization and found that there was a significantly lower risk of recurrence at two years with open repair: 11% in the open group versus 23% in the arthroscopic group.[450] Arthroscopic electrothermal capsulorrhaphy was advocated by some as an option for management of recurrent dislocation, but recent literature has shown it is not effective and further can damage or destroy the glenohumeral capsule and ligaments, making success of subsequent revision

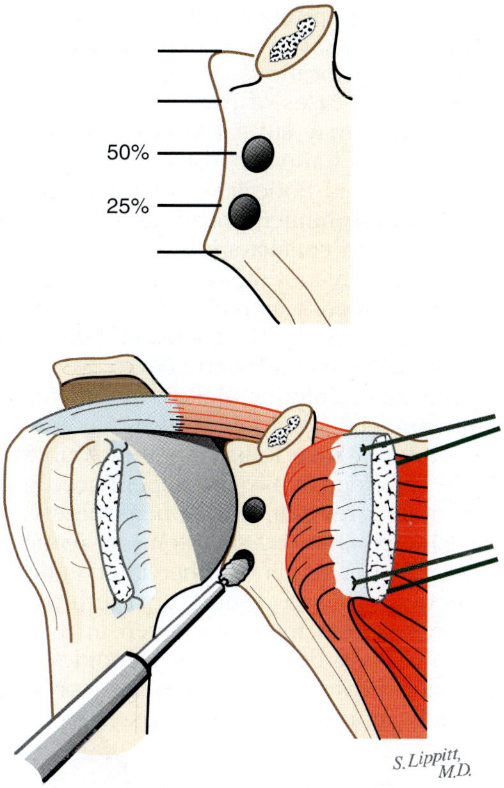

FIGURE 13-181: Glenoid drill holes. Using a pinecone bur, drill holes are placed in the middle and inferior aspects of the anterior glenoid, near the lip. (From Matsen FA III, Lippitt SB. *Shoulder Surgery: Principles and Procedures*. Philadelphia: WB Saunders; 2004:229.)

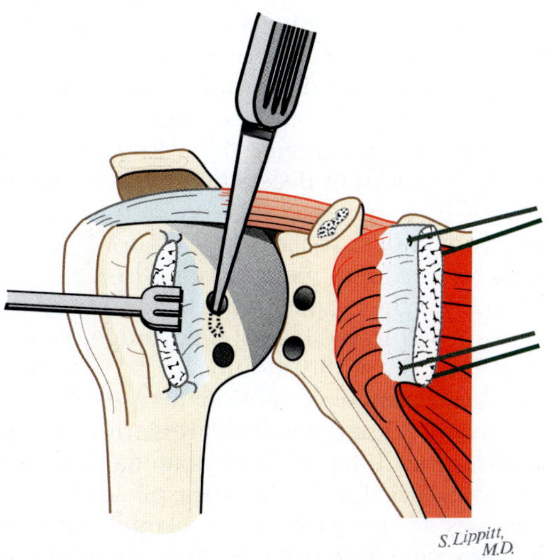

FIGURE 13-182: Humeral drill holes. Similarly, holes are made in the middle and inferior aspects of the proximal humerus, near the articular surface. (From Matsen FA III, Lippitt SB. *Shoulder Surgery: Principles and Procedures*. Philadelphia: WB Saunders; 2004:229.)

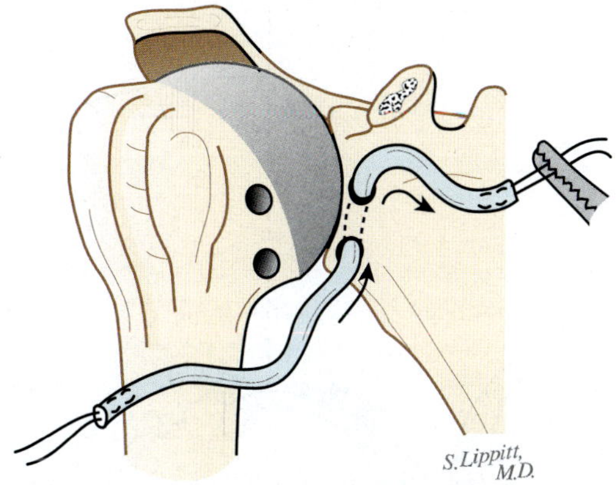

FIGURE 13-183: Passing the graft through the glenoid holes. The hamstring tendon graft is passed through the glenoid holes. (From Matsen FA III, Lippitt SB. *Shoulder Surgery: Principles and Procedures*. Philadelphia: WB Saunders; 2004: 230.)

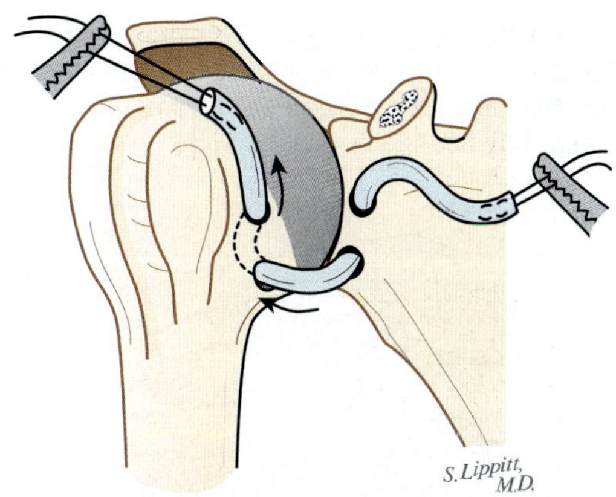

FIGURE 13-184: Passing the graft through the humeral holes. The hamstring tendon graft is then passed through the humeral holes. (From Matsen FA III, Lippitt SB. *Shoulder Surgery: Principles and Procedures*. Philadelphia: WB Saunders; 2004:231.)

stabilization procedures, either open or arthroscopic, guarded.[253]

Arthroscopy enables repair of extensive 270 degree labral tears, which historically may have been underappreciated with open techniques. Recent studies have demonstrated favorable results in the arthroscopic management of these injuries.[418] Three of the 20 shoulders (in 19 patients) had subsequent episodes of instability for a failure rate of 15%. One required a second procedure for continued instability for a revision rate of 5%. Two patients developed adhesive capsulitis postoperatively, one of who required an arthroscopic arthrolysis.[418] In a similar study of 41 circumferential labral tears repaired arthroscopically with a mean of 7.1 suture anchors, there were two revisions for instability, two for biceps tendonitis, and two for tightness.[654]

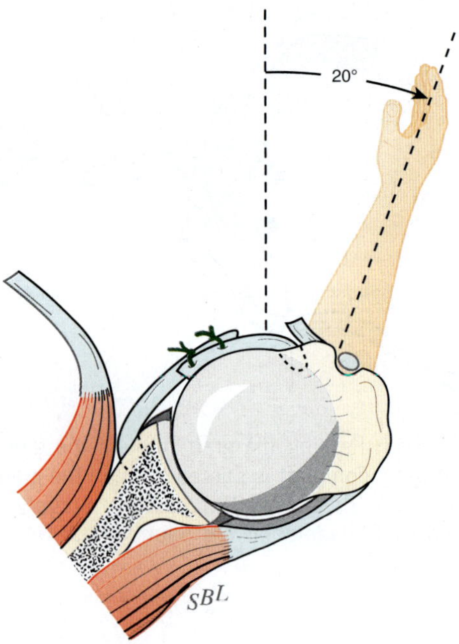

FIGURE 13-185: Tying the graft. The graft is tied so that external rotation is checked at 20 degrees. (From Matsen FA III, Lippitt SB. *Shoulder Surgery: Principles and Procedures.* Philadelphia: WB Saunders; 2004:231.)

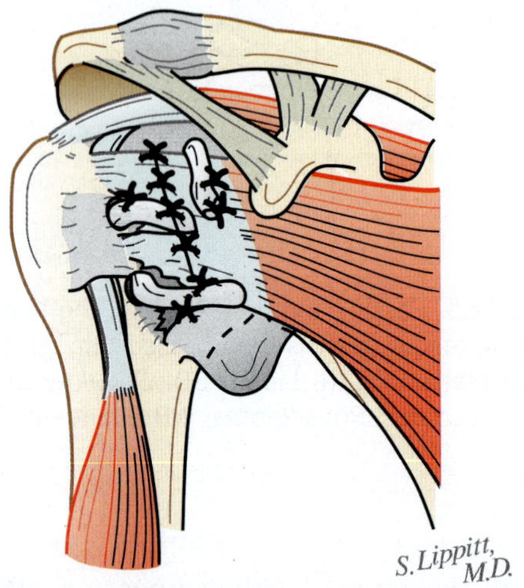

FIGURE 13-186: Reinforcing the graft. Any available capsular or tendon tissue is anchored to the graft. (From Matsen FA III, Lippitt SB. *Shoulder Surgery: Principles and Procedures.* Philadelphia: WB Saunders; 2004:231.)

Recurrence of instability after arthroscopic treatment can be affected by younger age at the time of the first dislocation, male gender, and the longer duration of time from the first dislocation until surgery (>6 months), all of which have been identified as significant risk factors for recurrence.[518,548] Postoperative increase in anterior capsular volume has been observed in these cases as well.[527] For this reason, some surgeons advocate capsular plication in addition to labral repair in cases of anterior instability, especially in those with a component of capsular laxity as evidenced by a pathologic sulcus sign from either repeated dislocations or contralateral/systemic signs of laxity.[382] In cases of revision instability surgery, arthroscopic repair may still yield good results if unidirectional, in cases of traumatic instability, in patients with less than 25% glenoid bone loss, for a Hill-Sachs lesion less than 30% of the humeral head, and in patients who are willing to forego contact sports.[15]

In patients with recurrent instability, attritional bone loss of the anteroinferior glenoid becomes a concern. In a study by Mologne et al., 21 patients in the military with a mean age of 25 years and with 20% to 30% bony deficiency of the anteroinferior glenoid were treated with arthroscopic anterior stabilization using an average of 3 anchors.[451] At 2- to 4-year follow-up, they found that 85% had a stable shoulder, while 5% experienced a dislocation that required revision with open surgery, and an additional 10% experienced symptoms of recurrent subluxation but did not require further intervention during the study period. They concluded that arthroscopic stabilization for recurrent instability, even in the presence of a significant bony defect of the glenoid, can yield a stable shoulder; however, outcomes are not as predictable, especially in attritional bone loss cases.[87]

Arthroscopic Remplissage With Arthroscopic Bankart Repair

Although most attention is placed on the impact of glenoid bone loss on success of open or arthroscopic capsulolabral repair, humeral head defects (Hill-Sachs lesions), especially those that can engage the anterior glenoid rim in relatively minimal external rotation or abduction (the glenoid track), can result in failure as well. In an effort to prevent Hill-Sachs engagement, some authors have advocated performing a Remplissage procedure. Remplissage, French meaning "to fill" involves imbrication of the infraspinatus tendon into the Hill-Sachs defect.

Research has indicated that the value of Remplissage may be indicated only in scenarios with substantial humeral head defects greater than 30% of the articular surface.[66,168,496] Recurrent dislocation after combined remplissage with Bankart repair are reported to be as low as 4% at an average of 6 years of follow-up.[709] Remplissage is not indicated to treat glenoid bone loss.

Additionally, other series have demonstrated that remplissage can result in the loss of an average of 10 degrees of external rotation of the shoulder.[66,168,496,709] This restriction in external range of motion may explain the low recurrence rate. Other concerns regarding remplissage include posterior cuff pain and potential rupture at the muscle-tendon junction of the infraspinatus.

Alternatives to remplissage for large humeral sided bone deficiency include osteoarticular allograft transplantation or partial humeral head resurfacing.[348] This procedure can be performed in a single operative setting or as a staged procedure via posterior approach to avoid takedown of the repaired anterior structures. Osteoarticular allografts carry additional risk of infection owing to the requirements that they be fresh in order to avoid chondral damage after flash-freezing or irradiation.

Authors' Preferred Method of Management of Anterior Shoulder Instability

A patient with traumatic anterior glenohumeral instability usually has symptoms primarily when the arm is elevated near the coronal plane, extended, and externally rotated. Characteristically, the shoulder is relatively asymptomatic in other extreme positions or in midrange positions. Thus appropriate management for some patients consists solely of education about the nature of the lesion and identification of the positions and activities that need to be avoided.

Strengthening the shoulder musculature can help prevent the shoulder from being forced into positions of instability. The exercise program previously described for atraumatic instability may be considered as an option for traumatic instability as well.

The option of surgical repair is discussed when careful clinical evaluation has documented the diagnosis of refractory anterior instability after an initial episode that was sufficiently traumatic to tear the anterioroinferior glenohumeral ligament and produce significant functional deficits (recurrent apprehension, subluxation, or dislocation) when the arm is in abduction, external rotation, and extension.

A patient desiring surgical stabilization is presented with a frank discussion of the alternatives and the risks of infection, neurovascular injury, stiffness, recurrent instability, pain, and the need for revision surgery.

Preoperative radiographs are obtained, including an AP view in the plane of the scapula (see Fig. 13-79), an apical oblique (Garth) view (see Fig. 13-141), and an axillary view (see Fig. 13-88). A preoperative rotator cuff MRI is obtained if cuff disease is suspected, for example, in a patient older than 40 years with pain between episodes of dislocation or with weakness of internal rotation, external rotation, or elevation. An electromyogram is performed if clinical evaluation suggests the possibility of nerve injury.

In recent years, we have treated most primary cases with arthroscopic repair, discussed in Chapter 15. Revisions, cases with glenoid bone loss, and those returning to contact sports are considered for Latarjet reconstruction. Nevertheless, the senior author has had good experience with open reconstruction; for completeness, this technique is described below.

Flatow's Preferred Method for Open Management of Traumatic Shoulder Instability

Before surgery, all of our patients are instructed in a series of exercises designed to strengthen the rotator cuff, deltoid, and scapular stabilizers (see Fig. 13-155). Our preferred method of surgical repair has been a modification of Neer's inferior capsular shift with an added capsulorraphy tailored to each individual.[55,360] This procedure reduces capsular volume by retensioning capsular tissue on the side of greatest instability and reducing overall tissue redundancy. For anterior inferior instability, we use a modified inferior capsular shift procedure, in essence a laterally based T-shaped capsulorraphy.

The rationale behind this approach to instability is based on several factors. First, the capsule is shaped like a funnel with a broader insertion on the humeral side. Implementing a laterally based capsolotomy allows the tissue to be shifted a greater distance for reattachment to the broader lateral insertion. Second, following intraoperative assessment of the inferior pouch and capsular redundancy, the inferior shift procedure permits variable directions of capsular mobilization around the humeral neck to treat different aspects of capsular laxity. Third, use of a T-shaped capsulotomy permits independent tensioning of the capsule in the medial-lateral and superior-inferior directions. Medial-lateral tensioning is usually a secondary concern, and, if overdone, may result in loss of external rotation. Fourth, a lateral capsular incision affords some protection to the axillary nerve, particularly during an inferior dissection as the nerve traverses under the inferior capsule. Finally, capsular tears/avulsions from the humeral insertion, although rare, are more readily identified and repaired with a laterally based incision. The procedure is performed in the semiupright beach chair position.

Surgical Incision

The standard anterior axillary incision begins in the anterior axillary crease and extends up toward and usually stops at the coracoid process (Fig. 13-187A). We use the modified axillary incision described by Leslie and Ryan.[378]

The skin is undermined subcutaneously in the proximal medial and distal lateral corners to expose the deltopectoral interval (Fig. 13-187B). Usually, this interval is identified by the presence of the cephalic vein (Fig. 13-187C), which may be absent or lying deep in the interval out of sight. When the vein is not present, we can define the deltopectoral interval proximally because in this area, it is easier to see the difference in angles of the muscle fibers between the pectoralis major and the deltoid.

The interval should be very carefully opened, with the vein taken laterally with the deltoid muscle. Routine ligation of the vein produces venous congestion in the area and in the upper extremity and increases postoperative discomfort. Preservation of the vein contributes to an easier postoperative course (less pain and swelling). We use 8-0 nylon suture to repair any inadvertent nicks in the vein. The deltopectoral interval is developed all the way up to the clavicle with no need to detach any of the deltoid from the clavicle. If needed, the upper 1 to 2 cm of the pectoralis major tendon is detached to allow better visualization of the inferior capsule and make it easier to locate and protect the axillary nerve, which passes just inferior to the capsule. We do not find it necessary to detach the coracoid process or the conjoined tendon (Fig. 13-187D). With the deltopectoral muscles retracted out of the way, the clavipectoral fascia is seen covering the conjoined tendon. This fascia is divided vertically along the lateral border of the conjoined tendon. Proximally, the clavipectoral fascia blends into the CA ligament.

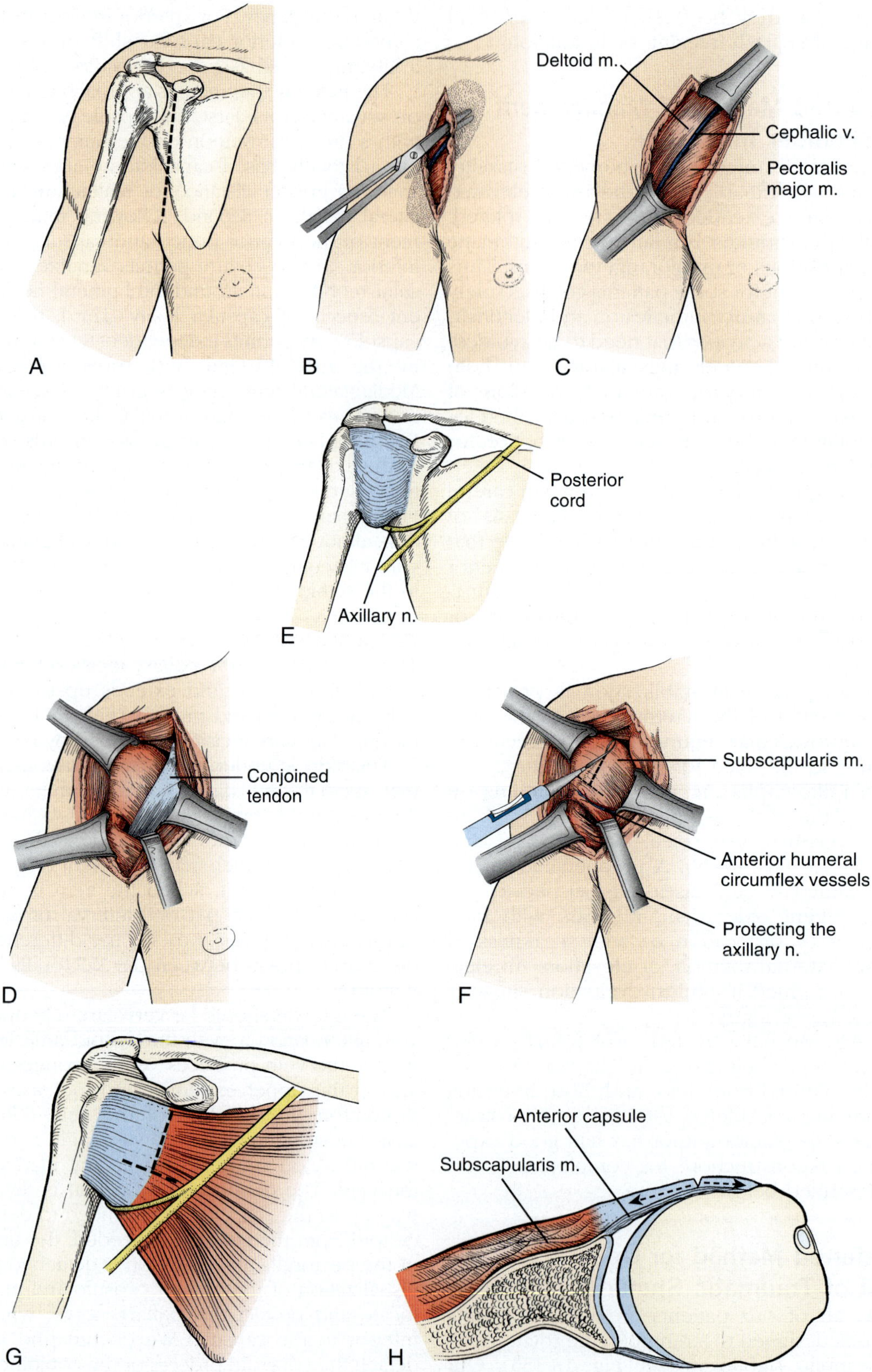

FIGURE 13-187: A–H. The authors' technique of open management of traumatic shoulder instability. The details of the procedure are described in the text. (From Wirth MA, Blatter G, Rockwood CA Jr. The capsular imbrication procedure for recurrent anterior instability of the shoulder. *J Bone Joint Surg Am.* 1996;78:246-259.)

Identification and Protection of the Axillary Nerve

Next, we locate the axillary nerve—an especially important step when performing the capsular shift procedure—by passing the finger down and along the lower and intact subscapularis muscle–tendon unit (Fig. 13-187E). The right index finger should be used to locate the nerve in the left shoulder, and the left index finger should be used to locate the nerve in the right shoulder. When the finger is as deep as it will go, the volar surface of the finger should be on the anterior surface of the muscle. Then the distal phalanx is flexed and rotated anteriorly, which hooks under the axillary nerve before it dives back posteriorly under the inferior capsule. With the arm in external rotation, the nerve is displaced medially and is difficult to locate. This large nerve can easily be located with the arm in adduction and neutral rotation. A second finger may be placed under the deltoid laterally, and the circumflex branch of the axillary nerve palpated. A gentle tug may be transmitted between the fingers, confirming that the palpated structures are indeed the axillary nerve. This has been coined the "tug test."[189]

Division of the Subscapular Tendon

The arm is positioned in external rotation so that the upper and lower borders of the subscapularis tendon can be visualized and palpated. The soft spot at the superior border of subscapularis tendon is the interval between the subscapularis and supraspinatus tendons. The lower border of the tendon is identified by the presence of the anterior humeral circumflex artery and veins, which are ligated and divided (see Fig. 13-187F). The subscapularis tendon will be vertically transected, usually 0.75 to 1 inch medial to its insertion into the lesser tuberosity. We prefer to incise the subscapularis tendon with a sharp scalpel (see Fig. 13-187F and G). We are very careful to divide only the tendon and usually try to leave a little of the subscapularis tendon on the capsule to add to its strength (see Fig. 13-187H).

Once the vertical cut in the tendon has been completed, we very carefully reflect the medial part of the tendon off the capsule with curved Mayo scissors until there are no further connections between the tendon and the capsule. The tendon should have a rubbery bounce to it when lateral traction is applied to it. Three or four stay sutures are placed in the medial edge of the tendon; these sutures are used initially for retraction and later at the time of tendon repair.

The lateral stump of the subscapularis tendon is reflected off the capsule with a small sharp knife. This step is easy with the capsule intact when the arm is in external rotation and difficult when the capsule has been divided. Failure to perform this step will make the two-layer closure of the capsule and the subscapularis tendon more difficult.

Division of the Capsule

A laterally based T capsular incision is made with the extent of capsular dissection and mobilization dictated by the extent of redundant capsular found at surgery (Figs. 13-188 and 13-189).

Capsular Shift and Bankart Repair

If the capsule has secure fixation on the glenoid rim, capsular reconstruction can then be performed. However,

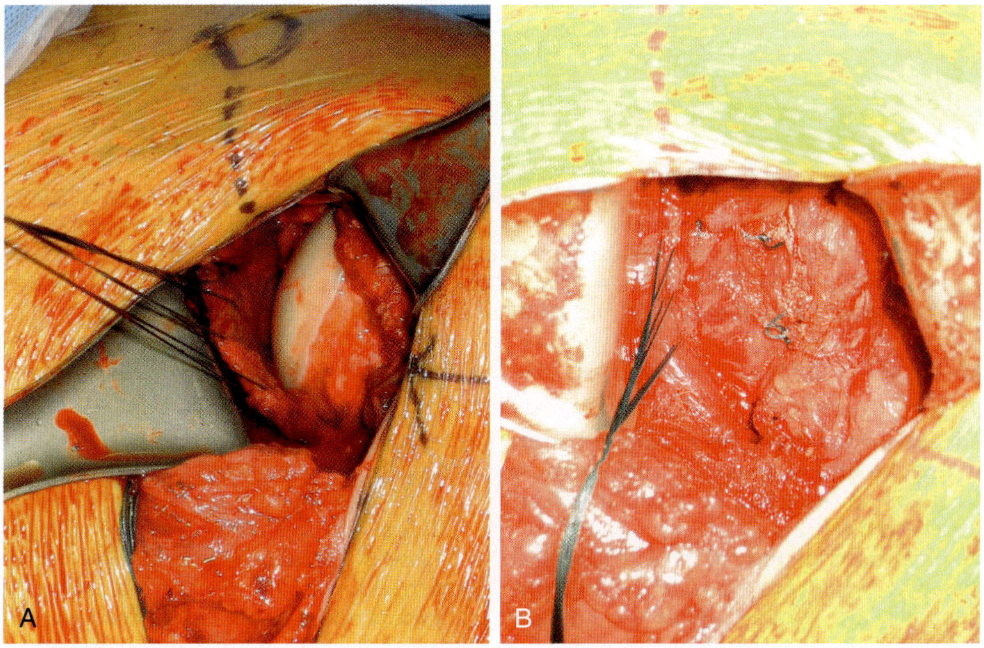

FIGURE 13-188: **A** and **B,** Bone tunnels through the glenoid rim secure the labrum, followed by capsular repair in pants over vest fashion. The inferior leaf of the capsule is pulled up and secured first, followed the superior leaf, and lastly the medial leaf.

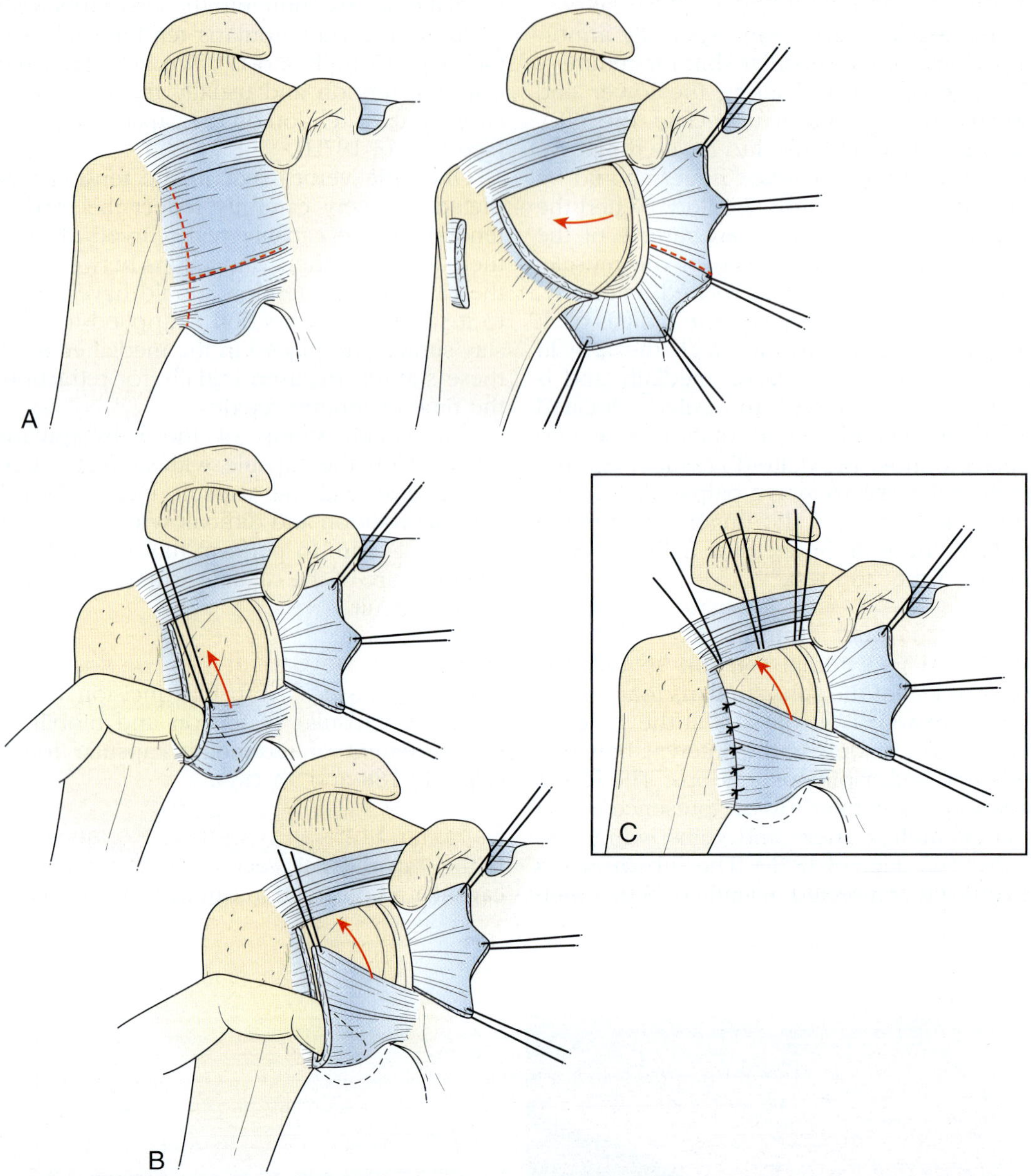

FIGURE 13-189: **A** and **B,** Open capsular shift with laterally based T-shaped capsulotomy. The surgeon's finger is placed in the inferior pouch to assess capsular laxity, and to determine the degree of tightening desired. **C,** Inferior capsular shift. (**A,** Modified from Bigliani LU. Recurrent anterior instability: open surgical repair. In: Bigliani LU, ed. *AAOS Monograph Series: The Unstable Shoulder,* Rosemont, IL: AAOS; 1996. **B–C,** Modified from Pollock RG, Owens JM, Flatow EL, et al. Operative results of the inferior capsular shift procedure for multidirectional instability of the shoulder. *J Bone Joint Surg.* 2000;82-A[7]:919-928.)

if the capsule and periosteum have been stripped from the glenoid rim and neck of the scapula, the capsule must first be reattached before proceeding to capsular reconstruction (Figs. 13-190 to 13-192).

A forked retractor is used to retract the capsule and muscles out of the way while the anterior glenoid rim and neck of the scapula are abraded. With the Fukuda retractor holding the humeral head out of the way and the forked retractor holding the medial capsule and subscapularis, an osteotome or bur is used to abrade the anterior surface of the neck of the scapula. Traditionally, bone tunnels were used to repair the labrum, but suture anchors may also be used.

Before closure of the capsule, the joint is thoroughly irrigated with saline. Next, the rotator interval closure is performed with the arm in an adducted and externally rotated position. This is followed by shifting the inferior capsular flap up with the arm initially positioned in 45 degrees of abduction and usually about 45 degrees of external rotation. With the arm at the side and the same

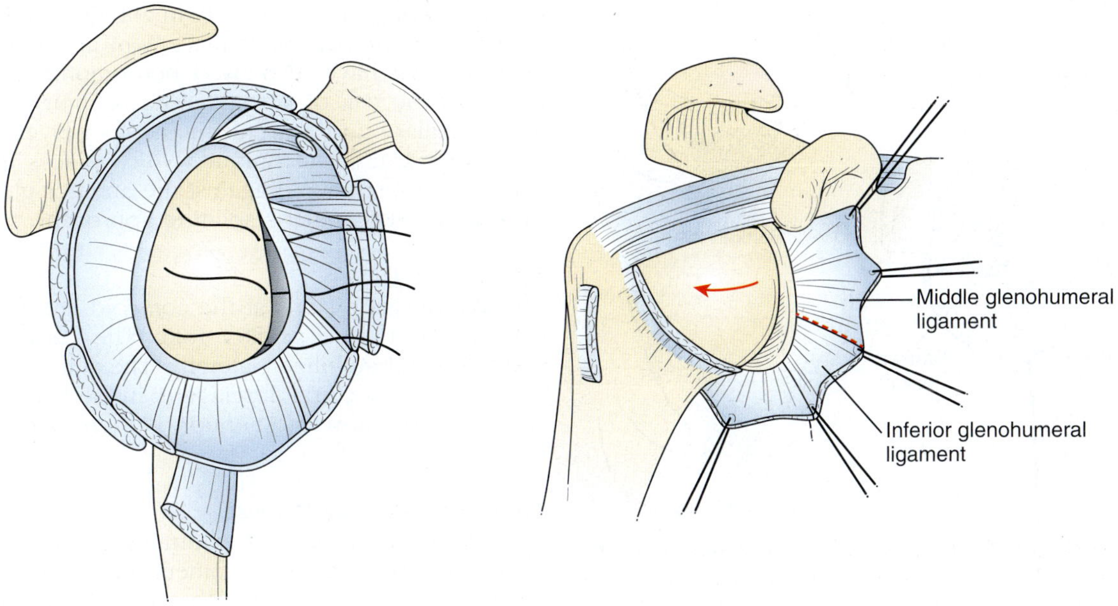

FIGURE 13-190: Open capsular shift with T-shaped capsulotomy between the middle and inferior glenohumeral ligaments. (Modified from Bigliani LU. Recurrent anterior instability: open surgical repair. In: Bigliani LU, ed). *AAOS Monograph Series: The Unstable Shoulder*. Rosemont, IL: AAOS; 1996.)

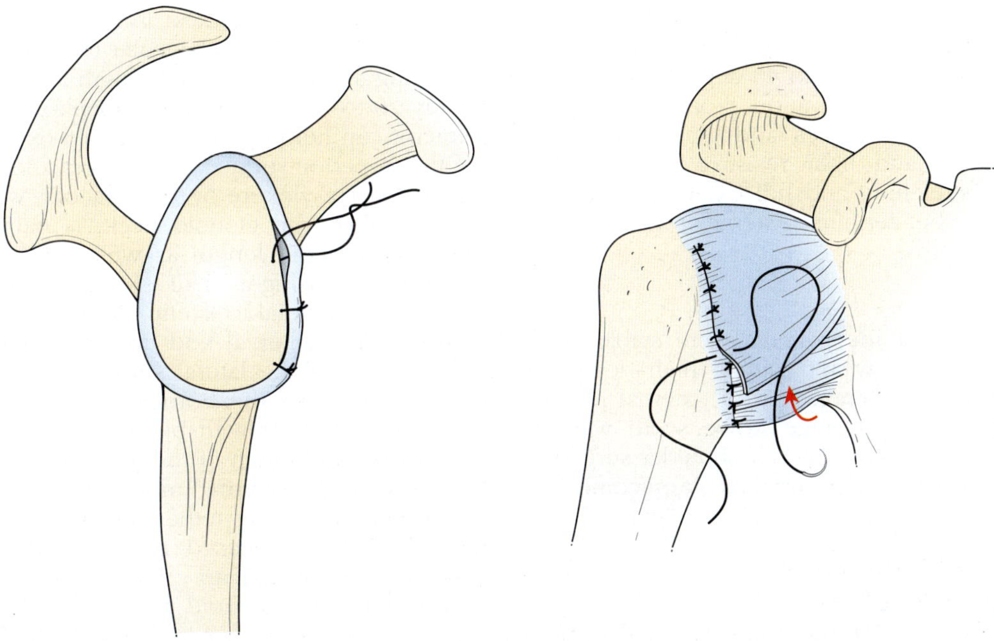

FIGURE 13-191: Open Bankart repair with capsular shift. (Modified from Langford J, Bishop J, Lee E, et al. Outcomes following open repair of Bankart lesions for recurrent, traumatic anterior glenohumeral dislocations. *Orthopedics* 2006;29[11]:1008-1013.)

external rotation, the superior flap is repaired. The supscapularis is then repaired anatomically (see Fig. 13-189B,C).

Wound Closure

A layered wound closure is then performed. The skin is approximated with a 4.0 resorbable monofilament subcuticular suture.

Postoperative Management

The postoperative regimen is individualized for each patient—faster for traumatic cases without generalized ligamentous laxity, slower in overlap cases with underlying laxity. In general, patients are protected in a sling for 6 weeks with immediate hand, wrist, and elbow motion. At 10 days, gentle assisted motion is begun with external rotation with a stick to 20 degrees and elevation in the

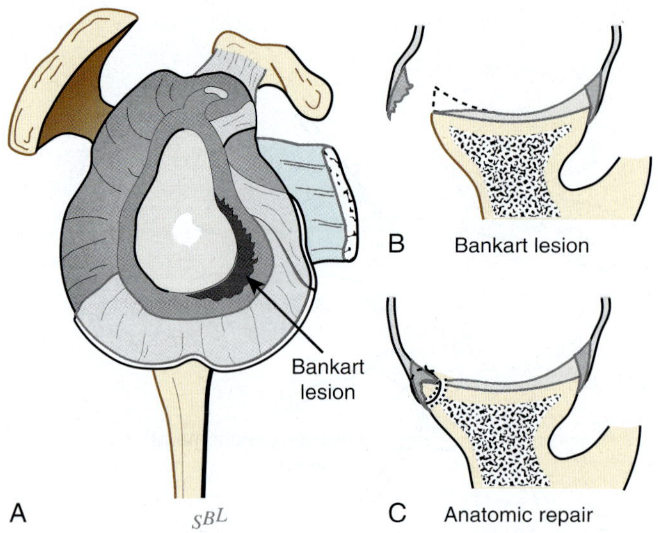

FIGURE 13-192: Anatomic repair of labral avulsion. If the labrum is avulsed from the glenoid (**A** and **B**), anatomic repair of the attachment of the labrum to the glenoid lip restores normal rotational laxity (**C**). Videos 13-1 through 13-10 demonstrate this technique. (From Matsen FA III, Lippitt SB. *Shoulder Surgery: Principles and Procedures.* Philadelphia: WB Saunders; 2004:125.)

forward plane of the scapula to 100 degrees. From 2 to 4 weeks, motion is progressed to 40 degrees of external rotation and 140 degrees of elevation. From 4 to 6 weeks, external rotation to 60 degrees and elevation to 160 degrees is allowed, and light resistive exercises are begun. Terminal stretching and full external rotation is begun at 6 weeks, but terminal external rotation is not allowed until 3 months.

Results

In our series,[360] 98% of the patients were stable at an average follow-up of 6.5 years, with a high degree of patient satisfaction. The average loss of external rotation was 4 degrees, and the average Rowe score was 96. Despite this success, revision anterior shoulder surgery is a formidable challenge with a less-predictable outcome.[193,381]

Parsons' Preferred Technique for the Latarjet Procedure

Our primary indication for the Latarjet is failed prior arthroscopic or open soft tissue anterior glenohumeral stabilization, especially in patients with associated anterior glenoid bone loss and engaging Hill-Sachs lesions, or in patients without a history of prior surgery but with substantial glenoid bone loss of greater than 20% of the diameter (Fig. 13-193).

Procedure

Patients are positioned semirecumbent in a beach chair with a small pad placed under the ipsilateral scapula to help protract the scapula, and the forequarter is draped free. We routinely use a pneumatic arm holder to control the arm during the procedure, in addition to fluoroscopy to evaluate coracoid graft placement and hardware orientation. We have also used neuromonitoring to help minimize the risk of iatrogenic nerve injury, particularly to the axillary and musculocutaneous nerves.[139] We use the classic Latarjet technique, which places the inferior surface of the coracoid against the anterior glenoid neck through a subscapularis splitting approach.

Surgical Incision

The skin incision starts at the coracoid and travels vertically down to the axillary fold. The cephalic vein is identified and mobilized laterally. The deltopectoral interval and clavipectoral fascia are incised, exposing the subscapularis muscle. Attention is then placed on coracoid harvest.

Coracoid Autograft Harvest

The arm is abducted and externally rotated to relax the deltoid and place the CA ligament under tension. The CA ligament is incised lateral to the coracoid, leaving a 1-cm stump of tissue attached to the coracoid for later repair to the capsule. Medially, the pectoralis minor is reflected off the medial surface of the coracoid base using electrocautery because of the numerous perforating vessels. Care must be taken to protect the underlying brachial plexus. The coracoid base is exposed posterior to the insertion of the coracoclavicular (CC) ligaments, thereby providing as much coracoid length as possible (approximately 20 to 25 mm in most patients). A forked Darrach retractor can help optimize coracoid exposure, placing it on the superior surface of the coracoid against the CC ligaments. The flexure of the coracoid, where the undersurface meets the glenoid neck, is palpated to ensure maximal coracoid length as well. The coracoid is then osteotomized using a small 90-degree angled microsagittal saw from medial to lateral. Residual deep attachments of the rotator interval and coracohumeral ligament are reflected off of the lateral surface of the coracoid with cautery. Medially, the border of the conjoint tendon is carefully mobilized with blunt dissection distally to the most proximal branch of the musculocutaneous nerve to further provide optimal mobilization. Often there are fascial slips that may tether the medial coracoid proximally and, if not released, compress the underlying brachial plexus or axillary nerve once the coracoid is transferred to the glenoid neck.

Preparation of the Coracoid Autograft

Following osteotomy and mobilization, the inferior coracoid surface is decorticated with a burr to provide an optimal healing surface. Proximally and distally, the coracoid is flattened with the burr to further match the orientation of the glenoid neck. Care must be taken to protect the distal origin of the conjoint tendon. Two 3.0-mm drill holes are then made in the center of the coracoid, one 5 mm proximal to the distal tip and another 1 cm proximal to that (assuming a 20-mm coracoid length). A suture is placed in the proximal screw hole to allow for control of the coracoid later.

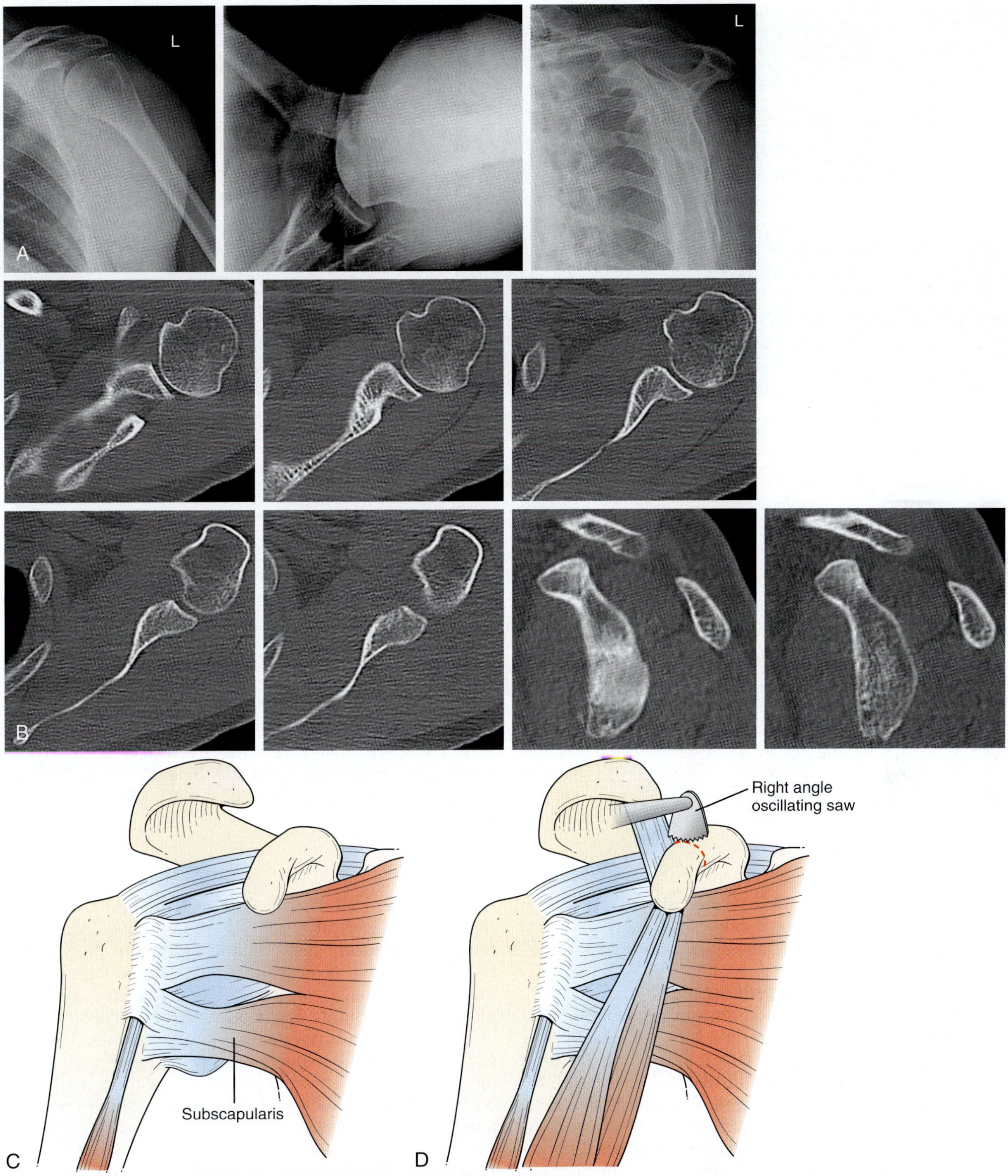

FIGURE 13-193: A 34-year-old male with recurrent glenohumeral instability. **A–B,** Preoperative radiographic and computed tomographic images demonstrate significant glenoid bone loss. **C,** The subscapularis is split longitudinally at the junction of the upper two-thirds and inferior one-third. The split is extended laterally to the level of the lesser tuberosity. **D,** The coracoid is osteotomized at the "knee" with a right angle oscillating saw.

Continued

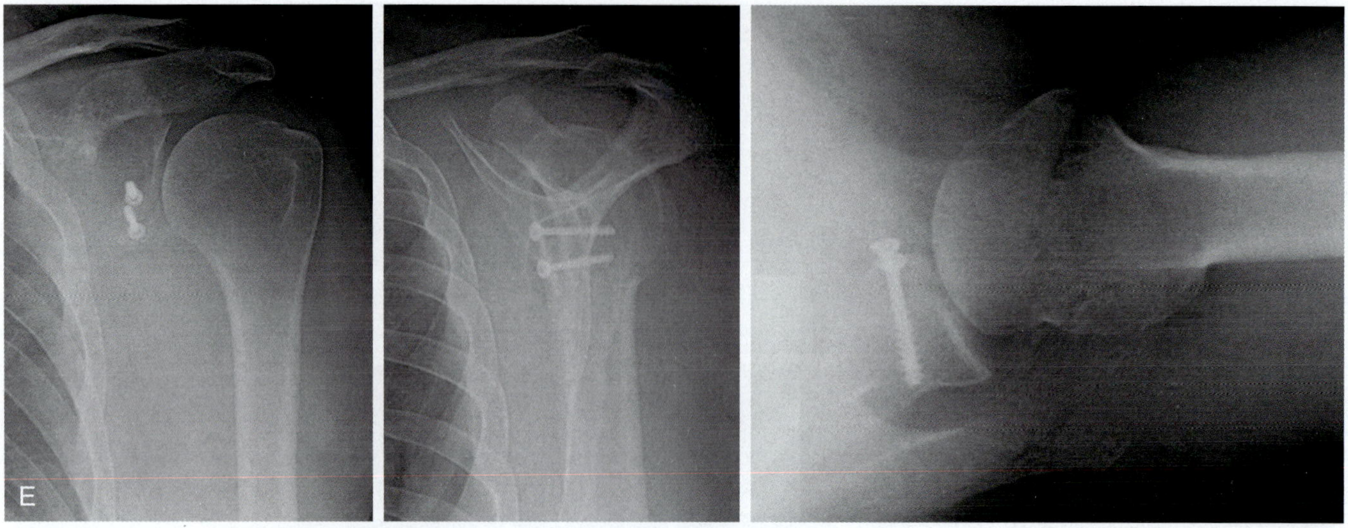

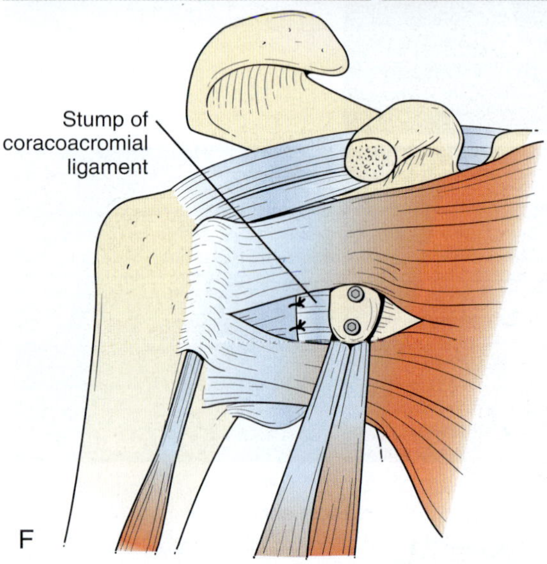

FIGURE 13-193, cont'd **E,** Postoperative radiographs after Latarjet procedure show the coracoid autograft secured in place with 4.0 mm partially threaded cancellous screws. **F,** The stump of the coracoacromial ligament is sutured to the capsule. The split in the subscapularis is not repaired. (**C, D, F** Modified from Obermeyer T, Parsons B: Bone block/latarjet procedure. In: Dodson CC, Dines DM, Dines JS, et al. *Controversies in Shoulder Instability,* Philadelphia: Lippincott, Williams & Wilkins; 2014:89-98.)

The coracoid is then placed medially, deep to the pectoralis muscle to keep it out of the way of deep exposure of the glenohumeral joint.

Subscapularis Split and Capsulotomy

The arm is placed in adduction and 30 degrees of external rotation to place the subscapularis under tension. The subscapularis is then split horizontally along its long axis between the upper two thirds and inferior third, often demarcated by a small raphe. The split is dissected deeply to the underlying anterior capsule and extended laterally to the tendinous insertion on the lesser tuberosity. Occasionally, if additional exposure of the glenoid is needed, a vertical tenotomy just medial to the insertion from the muscular split superiorly to the rotator interval can be made, reflecting the upper subscapularis tendon medially off of the lesser tuberosity. Medially, a small sponge is placed deep to the subscapularis muscle along the glenoid neck to provide hemostasis from perforating vessels.

The subscapularis split is then held open with three retractors: superiorly with a right-angled Army-Navy retractor, inferiorly with a blunt Hohmann placed deep to the muscle to protect the axillary nerve superficial to this, and medially with a Bankart retractor along the glenoid neck. Blunt dissection with a sponge or lap pad helps expose the underlying anterior capsule. The anterior glenoid rim is palpated deep to the capsule, and a medially based vertical capsulotomy is then made flush with the glenoid face and anterior rim along the entire length of the glenoid.

Fixation of the Coracoid Autograft

Following capsulotomy, the medial capsule, glenoid periosteum and any residual labrum is resected off of the anteroinferior glenoid neck. The glenoid neck is then roughened to punctate bleeding bone with a motorized burr. A Fukuda retractor is then placed within the glenohumeral joint to help retract the humeral head laterally, thereby exposing the glenoid articular surface.

Careful measurement of the exact orientation of the previously made coracoid drill holes are then checked, including the distance from the lateral surface and inferior tip to the inferior drill hole to help insure appropriate placement of the lateral aspect of the coracoid flush or just medial to the articular surface of the glenoid. Proud or lateral overhang of the coracoid is to be avoided.

Once proper orientation is confirmed, the inferior docking drill hole is made in the native glenoid neck at the appropriate distance medial to the glenoid face and superior to the inferior glenoid rim. Drill-hole orientation should be parallel to the glenoid face, exiting the posterior glenoid neck, and care must be taken not to penetrate the articular surface of the glenoid. The depth of the glenoid tunnel added together with the depth of inferior tunnel in the coracoid graft will determine the appropriate screw length, most commonly 30 to 36 mm depending on the severity of glenoid bone loss. We commonly incorporate a washer under the screw heads to minimize graft fracture risk. While the inferior screw is tightened to bicortical purchase, the long axis of the coracoid is positioned flush with the anterior glenoid rim and held with a clamp to prevent rotation of the graft during screw tightening, and the tagging suture is removed. The superior glenoid tunnel is then drilled through the previously made superior coracoid tunnel into the glenoid, again bicortically. The appropriate length screw with washer is then seated with good purchase.

Appropriate coracoid placement is then confirmed with digital palpation and fluoroscopy. The lateral stump of CA ligament is then repaired with nonabsorbable sutures to the laterally reflected glenohumeral capsule with the arm still held in 30 degrees of external rotation. The deep sponge placed for hemostasis is removed and the subscapularis split closed with absorbable sutures laterally. If a vertical tenotomy was performed, this is repaired as well. The shoulder is then brought through a range of motion, checking abduction, external rotation, and stability. The axillary nerve is carefully palpated to ensure no undue tension or pressure from the transferred coracoid or conjoint tendon is present.

Wound Closure

A layered closure of the subcutaneous tissues and skin is then completed with absorbable monofilament suture.

Postoperative Management

Postoperatively, the patient's arm is placed in a sling. Passive exercises are initiated 1 to 2 weeks postoperatively, including pendulums, passive external rotation to 30 degrees, and passive forward elevation in the plane of the scapula to 120 degrees. Patients can discontinue the sling at 4 to 6 weeks and begin active range-of-motion exercises. Strengthening exercises begin at 3 months postoperatively.

Operative Management of Posterior Instability

Considerations in the Decision for Surgery

In a current concepts review, Robinson et al.[566] concluded that recurrent posterior instability is a relatively uncommon debilitating condition that requires careful evaluation, vigorous nonoperative management, and carefully selected surgical approaches. In an important study, Kim et al.[336] performed MR arthrography on posteriorly unstable shoulders. They found that posterior glenoid depth was significantly reduced in the inferior and middle aspects of posteriorly unstable shoulders. The loss of depth was caused by diminished osseous and chondrolabral height. Their findings might help explain recurrent instability after repairs that do not address the lack of what they refer to as chondrolabral containment.

Recent findings indicate that posterior instability does occur with high frequency in association with combined traumatic anterior instability at a higher rate than previously thought.[627] In a study by Song et al., 40% of operative instability cases contained posterior instability combined with anterior instability identified at the time of surgery; this rate is double the incidence in previous reports, and MRI was furthermore inadequate for detecting this pathology.[627] Failure to recognize the posterior instability element will lead to potential failure of repair, recurrent instability, and patient dissatisfaction after surgery.

Many shoulders with posterior instability can be well managed by education, muscle strengthening, and neuromuscular retraining. Surgical stabilization of posterior glenohumeral instability may be considered when recurrent involuntary posterior subluxation or dislocation occurs in spite of a concerted effort at a well-structured rehabilitation program.[547] Before surgery, it is essential to identify all directions of instability and any anatomic factors that can predispose the joint to recurrent instability, such as humeral head or glenoid defect, abnormal glenoid version, rotator cuff tears, neurologic injuries, or generalized ligamentous laxity.[705,706]

Arthroscopic techniques have shown promising results, and results are generally more favorable than those after anterior instability repair.

Arthroscopic Posterior Instability Repair

Posterior instability is amenable to arthroscopic treatment.[140] In a prospective cohort study of 200 shoulders in 183 athletes who underwent arthroscopic posterior capsulolabral repair, results were durable at 3 years with 90% of athletes returning to sport and a majority at the same level of play.[74] In the adolescent population, 92% of patients who underwent posterior capsulolabral repair were stable at 5 years follow-up.[712] Arthroscopic techniques for posterior instability repair will be described in Chapter 15. Below we describe our preferred technique for open repair of posterior instability.

Open Posterior Surgical Approaches

Several surgical approaches have been described for treating recurrent posterior glenohumeral instability, including the posterior deltoid-splitting approach (Fig. 13-194).[702] Shaffer et al.[616] described a surgical approach to the posterior glenohumeral joint through an infraspinatus-splitting incision that they found to offer safe and excellent exposure of the posterior capsule, labrum, and glenoid without requiring tendon detachment or causing neurologic

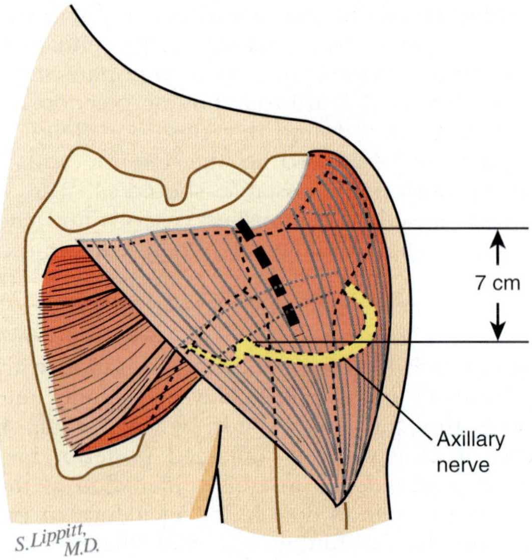

FIGURE 13-194: Posterior deltoid split. The deltoid is split (*heavy dashed line*) between the anterior two-thirds and the posterior third of the muscle, being mindful of the axillary nerve inferiorly. (From Matsen FA III, Lippitt SB. *Shoulder Surgery: Principles and Procedures*. Philadelphia: WB Saunders; 2004:211.)

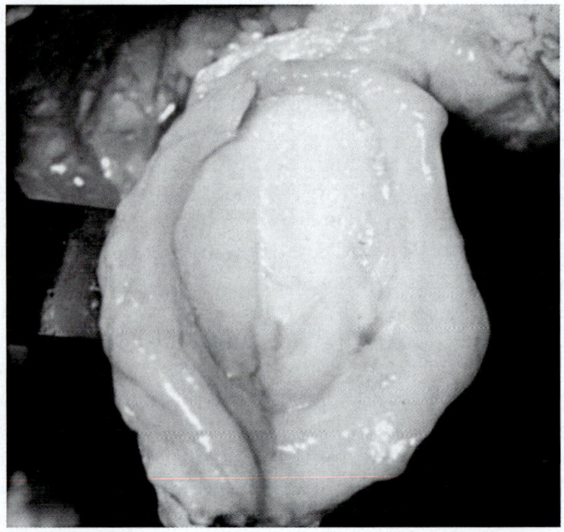

FIGURE 13-195: The articular surface of the glenoid after a posterior opening wedge osteotomy in a cadaver specimen.

compromise. Most surgeons prefer to split the deltoid at the posterior corner of the acromion and incise the infraspinatus tendon near its attachment to the greater tuberosity.

Open Posterior Soft Tissue Repairs

The goal of these procedures is to tighten the posterior capsule (the infraspinatus and posterior capsule) to restrict the range of positions attainable by the humerus in relation to the scapula.[218,288,383,475,591,666] In some cases, the infraspinatus and teres minor tendons may be used together in the plication. Boyd and Sisk[71] described transplanting the long head of the biceps tendon posteriorly around the humerus to the posterior glenoid rim.

One of the difficulties with these procedures is that the repair tends to stretch out as the shoulder resumes normal use. Hurley et al.[293] retrospectively reviewed 50 patients with recurrent posterior shoulder instability. Of the 25 patients treated surgically, 72% experienced recurrent instability. Tibone and Bradley[651] reported a failure rate of 30% after posterior staple capsulorrhaphy. Bayley and Kessel[43] stated that failure to distinguish between traumatic and habitual (atraumatic) types of instability led to inappropriate surgery and was a major cause of recurrence after operative repair.

Tibone and Bradley[651] reviewed their experience with the management of posterior subluxation in athletes. They pointed out the difficulty in diagnosis, the unclear pathology, the importance of nonoperative management with exercises, and a 40% failure rate of surgical management with a posterior capsular shift. Of the failures, 11 were secondary to instability; eight were a recurrence of posterior instability and three demonstrated anterior subluxation. These cases of conversion of posterior instability to anterior instability emphasize the importance of recognition and the challenge of management of MDI.

Bigliani et al.[56] reported reliable results for management of recurrent posteroinferior instability with a posterior capsular shift; most of the failures were in patients who had undergone previous attempts at surgical stabilization.

Rotation Osteotomy of the Humerus[642,550]

Surin et al.[641] evaluated 12 shoulders that had recurrent posterior shoulder instability treated by external rotation osteotomy of the humerus. Recurrent instability developed in one shoulder with MDI.

Glenoid Osteotomy

Kretzler and Blue,[345,344] Scott,[610] English and Macnab,[171] Bestard,[51] Vegter and Marti,[672] Ahlgren et al.,[4] and others[177,209,232,368,469] have reported using a posterior opening wedge glenoid osteotomy for recurrent posterior dislocations of the shoulder. In 1966, Kretzler and Blue[345] reported the use of this procedure in six patients with cerebral palsy. They used the acromion as the source of the graft to hold the wedge open. Kretzler[344] reported on 31 cases of posterior glenoid osteotomy in patients with voluntary (15 cases) and involuntary (16 cases) posterior dislocations, with recurrence in four patients, two from each category.

Extreme care must be taken during this procedure to prevent the osteotome from entering the glenoid, although cracks in subchondral bone are often experienced as the osteotomy is opened (Fig. 13-195). The suprascapular nerve above and the axillary nerve below are also at risk. English and Macnab[171] pointed out that the humeral head might have a tendency to subluxate anteriorly after osteotomy of the glenoid. Gerber et al.[207] demonstrated that with major angular changes, posterior glenoid osteotomy can thrust the humeral head forward and potentially cause abutment of the humeral head against the coracoid and produce pain and dysfunction. Their cadaver studies demonstrated that glenoplasty consistently resulted in squeezing of the subscapularis between the coracoid tip and the humeral head. In cadaveric shoulders, posteroinferior glenoplasty increased the posteroinferior glenoid depth from 3.8 to 7.0 mm and shifted the center of the humeral head anteriorly and superiorly by an average of 2.2 and 1.8 mm, respectively. This, along with an increase in the posterior slope, resulted in an increase in the stability ratio in the posteroinferior direction from 0.47 to 0.81.[438]

Posterior Glenoid Bone Blocks

Open posterior stabilization of the shoulder is possible with the use of a posterior bone block, although it is a relatively uncommon procedure. Servien et al. reported on a series of 21 patients with a mean follow-up of 6 years and found a low risk of recurrent dislocation with 71% return to sports at their preinjury level.[614] Three patients were considered clinical failures; one with a recurrent posterior dislocation and two with substantial posterior apprehension on follow-up examination. Two shoulders had glenohumeral arthritis on radiographs at the latest follow-up.

The posterior bone block, or glenoid osteotomy, has been combined with various soft tissue reconstructions.[152] Mowery et al.[462] reported a series of five patients treated with a bone block for recurrent posterior dislocation. One patient had a subsequent anterior dislocation. Wirth et al.[707] reported the use of glenoid osteotomy to manage recurrent posterior glenohumeral instability (Fig. 13-196).

Complications of Posterior Repairs

The principal cause of failure after a posterior soft tissue repair is recurrent instability.[254,477] Unless excellent dynamic stabilization is regained so that concavity compression rather than capsular restraint is the dominant mechanism of stability, the tightened posterior soft tissues are likely to stretch out as motion is regained. Even in its normal state, the posterior capsule is thin and often translucent. Its stretching out after surgical tightening is hastened if the posterior soft tissues are of poor quality, if the patient voluntarily or habitually tries to translate the shoulder posteriorly, or if large bony defects cause unphysiologic dependency on soft tissues for stability.

Occasionally, the opposite outcome can occur: posterior repair can produce a shoulder that is too tight, which can push the shoulder out anteriorly. Insufficient posterior laxity can limit flexion, cross-body adduction, and internal rotation.

Complications can also result from bony procedures for posterior instability. Attempted posterior opening wedge osteotomy of the glenoid can result in an intra-articular fracture, in avascular necrosis of the osteotomized fragment, or in excessive anterior inclination and anterior instability. Posterior bone blocks placed in an excessively prominent position can cause severe degenerative joint disease.

Neurovascular injuries can also complicate posterior instability surgery. The axillary nerve may be injured as it exits the quadrangular space, or the nerve to the infraspinatus may be injured in the spinoglenoid notch.[299,475]

Authors' Preferred Method for Open Repair of Recurrent Posterior Glenohumeral Instability

Preoperative Considerations

Care is taken to identify the circumstances and directions of instability, the presence of generalized ligamentous laxity, and any anatomic factors that might potentially compromise the surgical result. We evaluate the possibilities of multidirectional and voluntary instability in each patient with posterior instability. All patients with posterior instability are started on the rehabilitation program described previously for atraumatic instability. A substantial number of patients with recurrent posterior instability respond to this program, particularly those with relatively atraumatic initiation of their condition. Straightforward patients who continue to have major symptomatic posterior instability after a reasonable rehabilitation effort may be considered for surgery. The type of posterior repair is influenced by the degree of trauma that initiated the repair and the quality of the posterior glenoid lip on the load and shift test and on imaging.

Shoulders with traumatic posterior instability might have pathology very similar to that of traumatic anterior instability (avulsion of the capsule and labrum from the glenoid rim or a capsular tear), which is amenable to primary repair. This condition must be diagnosed primarily from a history of an initial forcible posterior displacement of the humeral head on the glenoid, but it may be corroborated by a painful snap on the posterior drawer test.

Shoulders with lax posterior capsules may be managed with posterior capsulorrhaphy, but this capsular tightening is subject to stretching out again postoperatively, with resultant recurrent instability. This condition is suggested if the shoulder has an excessive range of cross-body adduction or internal rotation in abduction.

Procedure

Bigliani et al. describe a technique for posterior capsular shift, adapted from Neer and Foster.[54,56,474] As in the anterior capsular shift described above, the degree of modification is determined at the time of surgery depending on the extent of capsular laxity. The procedure is performed in the lateral decubitus position or in the semiupright beach-chair position with care taken to drape the operative site far medially to the midline posteriorly.

Surgical Incision

The surgical incision is centered on the posterolateral corner of the acromion and extended obliquely from the scapular spine toward the deltoid insertion. The deltoid is split in line with the incision between the posterior third and middle third. The deltoid is detached from the scapular spine sharply and tagged with sutures for later repair (Fig. 13-197).

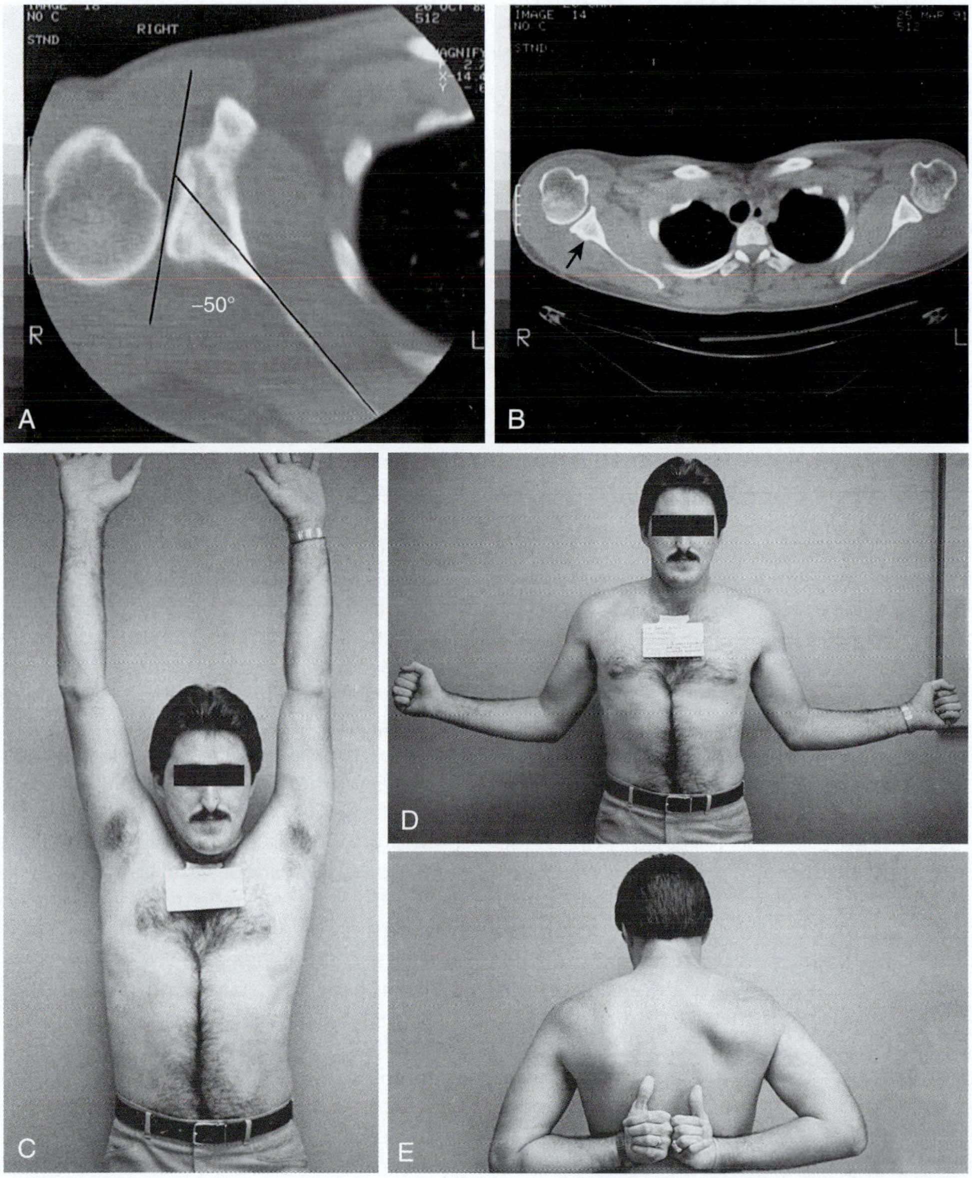

FIGURE 13-196: **A,** Preoperative computed tomographic (CT) scan demonstrating moderate glenoid retrotilt. **B,** Postoperative CT scan revealing a significant degree of correction of the glenoid version and incorporation of the tricortical bone graft after a posterior opening wedge osteotomy of the glenoid. **C–E,** Clinic photographs demonstrating full and symmetric motion. (From Wirth MA, Seltzer DG, and Rockwood CA Jr. Recurrent posterior glenohumeral dislocation associated with increased retroversion of the glenoid. *Clin Orthop Relat Res*. 1994;308:98-101.)

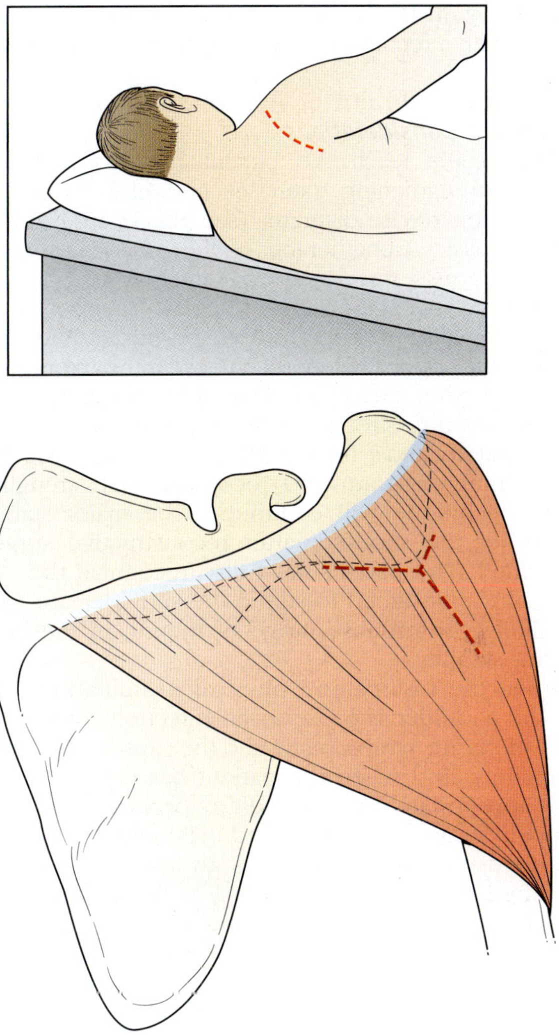

FIGURE 13-197: Posterior capsular shift. The patient is placed in a lateral position, and an oblique incision is made starting at the posterolateral corner of the acromion and extending distally. The deltoid is split along the raphe between the posterior and middle third at the posterolateral border of the acromion and extended for 4 cm. (Modified from Bigliani LU, Kelkar R, Flatow EL, et al. Glenohumeral stability: biomechanical properties of passive and active stabilizers. *Clin Orthop Relat Res.* 1996;330:13-20.)

Identification and Elevation of the Infraspinatus Tendon

Next, the infraspinatus tendon is identified and differentiated from the supraspinatus and teres minor tendons. The infraspinatus lies in the infraspinatus fossa, below the scapular spine; while the supraspinatus is above the scapular spine in the supraspinatus fossa. The infraspinatus is a bipennate muscle with a large insertional footprint on the posterior greater tuberosity, while the teres minor is unipennate with a small footprint just inferior to the infraspinatus on the posterior aspect of the greater tuberosity. The axillary nerve is located in the quadrangular space below the teres minor.

Once identified, the infraspinatus tendon is sharply elevated off of the underlying capsule and tagged with sutures for later repair.

Division of the Capsule

The capsule is then incised with a laterally based T-shaped incision starting just medial to its insertion on the humerus. Care should be taken to protect the axillary nerve inferiorly. The arm is internally rotated and extended to maximize dissection into the inferior capsular pouch, thereby enhancing the degree of capsular shift available. The capsular flaps are tagged with sutures for control and later repair.

Capsular Shift

If the capsule has been adequately mobilized, the surgeon should be able to palpate the effect of the capsular shift with his or her index finger in the inferior axillary pouch by pulling superiorly on the capsular sutures. The posterior labrum is repaired at this point if detached, using transosseous bone tunnels[588] or suture anchors.

The arm is placed in 5 degrees of external rotation and 15 degrees of abduction. The superior capsular flap is shifted inferiorly first and reattached to the lateral cuff remaining with nonabsorbable heavy suture. The inferior flap is then shifted superiorly to obliterate the inferior pouch, thereby creating a reinforced pants-over-vest capsular repair.

The infraspinatus is repaired back to the greater tuberosity via transosseous tunnels, and the deltoid muscle is reattached to the scapular spine.

Wound Closure

A layered wound closure is then performed, starting with the split in the deltoid muscle. The skin is approximated with a 4.0 resorbable monofilament subcuticular suture.

Postoperative Management

The postoperative consists of a 6-week period of immobilization with the arm in a brace held in slight external rotation, slight abduction, and slight extension. The brace is removed after 6 weeks, and gradual range of motion as well as isometric exercises are then initiated but not to exceed 150 degrees of forward elevation in the plane of the scapula or internal rotation to the side. Internal rotation and forward elevation greater than 150 degrees are avoided until 3 months postoperatively. Strengthening begins at 3 months and return to sporting activity at 6 months.

Results

At an average of 5 years follow-up, 35 shoulders in 34 patients were evaluated following superior capsular shift for posterior glenohumeral instability.[55] Ninety percent of shoulders were stable at follow-up; among those not satisfactory at follow-up, 86% had been revisions. The remaining unsatisfactory results were attributed to preexisting glenohumeral arthrosis that was treated with prosthetic replacement and improvement in symptoms in one case and with observation in the other case, which was undergoing workers' compensation litigation. Labral detachment was found in only 11% of cases, and none of these patients had increased glenoid retroversion.

Multidirectional Instability

Multidirectional instability is instability in all three directions: anterior, posterior, and inferior.[544] In some cases, it has been defined as dislocation in two directions, with subluxation in the remaining direction; for example, anterior combined with inferior instability or posterior combined with inferior instability. True MDI, in that the translations are symptomatic in all directions, is uncommon. Multidirectional instability can have a traumatic or atraumatic etiology, or a combination. Patients with instability in multiple directions can have voluntary or involuntary dislocations, and a traumatic component can exist from recurrent instability episodes and accrued microtrauma or also from a traumatic injury in a patient with ligamentous laxity and preexisting evidence of MDI.

Patients with MDI may exhibit symptomatic instability of the glenohumeral joint in the presence of physical exam findings such as positive anterior and posterior apprehension, a pathologic sulcus sign with no history of trauma, and no history of dislocation requiring reduction. Multidirectional instability is characterized by generalized ligamentous laxity, as well as abnormal shoulder and scapular kinematics. The contralateral shoulder may exhibit many of the same characteristics, but may or may not be symptomatic for the patient.

Capsular laxity is the essential lesion in MDI. Increased capsular volume and cross-sectional area are nonspecific findings common to many patients with capsular laxity and recurrent instability.[149] Injury to the rotator interval is an important component of anterior capsular injury in general. Shallow glenoid morphology has also been identified as a contributing factor in some cases.[675] Voluntary dislocators with a component of natural laxity and untreated skeletal dyskinesis, can become involuntary dislocators with labral tears or capsular pathology. In other words, patients who are "born loose" may become patients who are "worn loose" or "torn loose."

Nonoperative Treatment of Multidirectional Instability

The goal of nonoperative treatment for patients with MDI is restoration of shoulder function by increasing the effectiveness of coordinated humeroscapular positioning. Altered scapular motion has been found in patients with MDI; specifically, Ogsten et al. found that people with MDI demonstrated a significant decrease in scapular upward rotation and increased internal rotation when performing scapular plane.[504] Interestingly, glenohumeral translation was not altered. Therefore scapular rehabilitation exercises and proprioception are the mainstay of initial treatment for atraumatic MDI patients. However, up to 40% may experience treatment failure with physical therapy alone, with an improvement in kinematics subsequently seen after open capsular shift and additional physical therapy to a level comparable to normal controls.[339] Thus the mainstay of nonoperative treatment is physical therapy with a reconditioning program as described earlier.

Operative Treatment of Atraumatic Instability

Presurgical Considerations

We personally teach the patient how to perform the shoulder-strengthening exercises and give the patient a copy of the exercise diagrams (see Fig. 13-155). When we start the basic strengthening of the rotator cuff and the deltoid, we also instruct the patient how to perform the exercises to strengthen the scapular stabilizer muscles. Pushups (wall pushups, knee pushups, and regular pushups) are used to strengthen the serratus anterior, rhomboids, and other muscles, and shoulder-shrugging exercises are performed to strengthen the trapezius muscles.

The patient must have participated in a strengthening and training program and recognize that strength and proper technique will continue to be major stabilizing factors for the shoulder after reconstructive surgery is performed. The patient must also recognize that capsulorrhaphy is designed to stiffen the shoulder: the surgery will likely compromise range of motion in the hope of gaining stability.

When the history and physical examination indicate that the shoulder is loose in all directions, and that the translations are symptomatic and the cause of the patient's complaints, and when the patient has failed to respond to an appropriate physical therapy program, arthroscopic or open surgery is considered. The original procedure described for this problem was an inferior capsular shift described by Neer and Foster.[474,544] The principle of the procedure is to symmetrically tighten the anterior, inferior, and posterior aspects of the capsule by advancing its humeral attachment (see Fig. 13-189).

Surgical repair of atraumatic MDI is often erroneously assumed to be an operation principally of the inferior capsule. In fact, this procedure tightens the capsule on three sides: anterior, inferior, and posterior. The inferior capsular shift was named for its novel feature of shifting the inferior capsule as a way of tightening the capsule on the opposite side of the approach, which is performed on the side of greatest instability, since the capsular overlap and scarring will be on the side of the approach.

Open Capsular Shift for Multidirectional Instability

A capsular shift procedure has produced good results in appropriate patients with MDI.[122,474,9] Cooper and Brems[122] reported a 2-year follow-up of inferior capsular shift procedures and found that 91% were stable at follow-up. Altchek et al.[9] used a T-plasty modification of the Bankart procedure for MDI on 42 shoulders injured during athletics. Four patients experienced episodes of instability after the procedure, and throwing velocity decreased in the throwing athletes. Despite these shortcomings, patient satisfaction was noted to be excellent in 95% of shoulders.

Bigliani et al.[55] used an inferior capsular shift procedure to manage 68 shoulders in 63 athletes with anterior and inferior instability. Fifty-eight patients returned to their major sports, 75% at the same competitive level, but only 50% of elite throwing athletes returned to their previous level of competition. In contact athletes, 92% had no further dislocations after an anterior-based capsular shift, and 88% of patients who underwent a posterior-based capsular shift had no further dislocations.

In the series of Choi and Olgivie-Harris, 82% of athletes returned to their sport after an anterior procedure; 75% of athletes were able to return to their sport after a posterior procedure. However, only 17% of patients with combined inferior, anterior, and posterior procedures were able to return to their sport.[107]

At an average 61-month follow-up by Pollack et al., 94% of patients with primarily anterior MDI remained stable after the anterior capsular shift procedure, and all 15 patients with primarily posterior instability remained stable after posterior capsular shift.[544]

Obremskey et al.[497] reviewed 26 patients with no history or radiographic or surgical evidence of a traumatic etiology. The patients in this series had failed an average of 17 months of vigorous physical rehabilitation before proceeding with surgery. Fifty-seven percent of the patients had bilateral symptoms. The average age was 22 ± 6 years (range, 13 to 34 years). Twenty-nine percent had generalized ligamentous laxity, and 15% had an industrial claim. At an average of 27 months after inferior capsular shift was performed, 74% of the patients were satisfied with the condition of their shoulder; 46% were able to return to recreation, and 69% returned to their previous job. Thirty-nine percent had persistent pain, and 57% had night pain that interfered with sleeping. Sixty-eight percent had at least occasional symptoms of instability, and 10% required further surgery. By regression analysis, the most important correlate of patient dissatisfaction was not recurrent instability but rather persistent pain and stiffness.

Arthroscopic Stabilization for Multidirectional Instability

Given the number of dislocation events, the labral tears seen in involuntary MDI patients can be nearly circumferential around the glenoid. Arthroscopic stabilization with or without capsular plication is then recommended. These procedures are designed to improve glenoid concavity while removing pathologic capsular redundancy. After arthroscopic stabilization, recurrence rates of involuntary dislocations are generally low in the short term, with good pain relief and improvement in shoulder strength.[8] Loss of motion is not as commonly seen, and return to sports in the athletic population is possible in up to 86%.[28]

No clear clinical data support the amount of arthroscopic capsular plication necessary in addition to arthroscopic labral repair. In the presence of excessive capsular volume even after labral repair with capsulorrhaphy, some surgeons advocate additional capsular plication via rotator interval closure based on biomechanical studies.[179,452] However, concerns over limitations in external rotation limit its use.

The arthroscopic techniques for this procedure are described in Chapter 13. Below is the description for the open approach to a patient with MDI.

Authors' Preferred Technique for Open Treatment of Multidirectional Glenohumeral Instability

Procedure

The principle underlying MDI repair is balanced capsular plication. Overtightening of one side of a shoulder with MDI will exacerbate any instability in the direction left undertreated. Examination under anesthesia is performed before incision to confirm the diagnosis and office-based physical examination.

The approach is determined based on the primary direction of instability. An anterior approach is used for shoulders in which the anteroinferior direction was the predominant component of instability or if the shoulder dislocates frankly in all three directions. A posterior approach is used in shoulders where the posteroinferior direction is the predominant component of instability.

Details regarding the incision, surgical approach, and protection of the axillary nerve are essentially the same as described above for the management of posterior and anterior instability, with the addition of formally detaching the inferior capsular around the humeral neck until reaching the opposite side, then shifting the inferior capsule to tighten the opposite side. For example, in an anterior approach, the capsule is detached along the neck of the humerus and then the inferior capsule is drawn forward, tightening the posterior capsule.

Postoperative Management

After MDI repair, muscle strengthening and kinematic training is crucial to protect the surgically tightened glenohumeral capsule from excessive loading that could lead to failure of the surgical reconstruction. The patient is initially immobilized in a sling with a pillow to place the arm in slight abduction and neutral rotation for six weeks. Passive range of motion exercises begin at 6 weeks postoperatively. Strengthening begins at 3 months, and return to sporting activity at 6 months.

Results

Pollock and colleagues[544] reported the results of inferior capsular shift with anterior and posterior capsular shift for 49 shoulders with MDI at an average of 5 years follow-up. 96% of the shoulders remained stable, and 92% achieved full overhead function. 86% of the athletes were able to return to sports, but 31% returned at a lower level of participation.

INTERNATIONAL EXPERT COMMENTARY

Eiji Itoi

I would like to comment on the most common type of shoulder instability: an anterior shoulder dislocation. There are two pathologic entities: first-time dislocation and recurrent dislocation. While they look similar, they are quite different from the therapeutic point of view. The first-time dislocation is an acute injury caused by a significant trauma, whereas recurrent dislocation, a consequence of a first-time dislocation, is of a pathologic status known as chronic instability. Once the initial dislocation has been reduced, we never know whether the patient will have chronic instability (recurrent dislocation) in the future. We know that the recurrence rate is very high among the young males involved in vigorous activities.[587]

Surgical stabilization provides the best stability to the shoulder among all the treatment options.[217] For this reason, some surgeons recommend surgical stabilization after an initial dislocation.[18] The number of patients needing surgical stabilization after an initial dislocation is calculated to be 7.0 for the general population and 2.6 for high-risk patients.[568] This means that if you perform surgical stabilization in all patients after an initial dislocation, you will end up doing unnecessary surgery in 60% to 85% of them. The surgery used for recurrent dislocation is a therapeutic surgery for chronic instability. However, the surgery for an initial dislocation is a preventive surgery for chronic instability, which may or may not occur. Thus discretion is required when selecting a surgical procedure for a patient with an initial dislocation. I prefer to wait until the second dislocation occurs. Then, it is a recurrent dislocation, for which surgical stabilization is a therapeutic surgery and is 100% warranted. Surgical stabilization is the treatment of choice only when a high-risk patient strongly requires a stable shoulder in the shortest amount of time. Patients who are in-season athletes usually prefer to go back to sports with a protective brace. After the season, If the shoulder remains stable through the season, this treatment is sufficient. If the shoulder becomes unstable, then surgical stabilization should be considered. For off-season athletes and nonathletes, I prefer immobilization in external rotation. The outcome of this conservative treatment is still controversial. Recently, we reported that adding abduction to external rotation improves reduction of the Bankart lesion to the glenoid.[301] We need to have complete protocols for both conservative and surgical treatment options. The best conservative treatment needs to be determined in terms of position and length of immobilization.

Bipolar lesions of the shoulder (glenoid bony defect and Hill-Sachs lesion) are very common and are observed in 81% of patients with recurrent anterior dislocation of the shoulder.[354] The question remains as to what size of defect requires treatment. The critical size of a glenoid defect is reported to be 25% to 26% of the glenoid width.[89,303,718,721] These studies determined that the acceptable defect size is less than 17% and the unacceptable defect size more than 25%.[718,721] As a result, the size between 17% and 25% remains a gray zone. The decision whether to perform a bone graft for a gray-zone bony defect depends on the patient's background, including age, gender, joint laxity, sports involved, daily activity level, and occupation. The critical size of a Hill-Sachs lesion, on the other hand, is controversial. Several studies report a critical size for Hill-Sachs lesions.[86,327,585,626] However, these investigators overlooked the interaction between the Hill-Sachs lesion and the glenoid. A Hill-Sachs lesion that never engages with an intact glenoid could engage if the glenoid has a large bony defect. In other words, the risk of engagement depends on the relative location of the medial margin of the Hill-Sachs lesion to the anterior rim of the glenoid. For the purpose of assessing the risk of engagement, we introduced a new concept called the "glenoid track."[719] The glenoid track is the zone of contact between the glenoid and the humeral head during arm movement along the posterior end-range of motion. If the Hill-Sachs lesion stays within the glenoid track, there is no chance that it will engage with the anterior rim of the glenoid, whereas if the medial margin of the Hill-Sachs lesion travels outside the glenoid track, there is a risk of engagement.[300] The latter has been called an engaging Hill-Sachs lesion. Theoretically, all Hill-Sachs lesions engage with the anterior rim of the glenoid before Bankart repair. Only those that engage after Bankart repair should be called "engaging" Hill-Sachs lesions, which need treatment. However, many surgeons call those that engage before Bankart repair "engaging." This inconsistency has caused a great deal of confusion. To avoid such confusion, we propose the use of new terms: "on-track" and "off-track" Hill-Sachs lesions.[155] A Hill-Sachs lesion that stays on the glenoid track is an "on-track" lesion, while one that goes outside the glenoid track is an "off-track" lesion. Treatment selection depends on whether the Hill-Sachs lesion is on or off the glenoid track. For an on-track Hill-Sachs lesion, soft tissue repair alone, such as arthroscopic Bankart repair, is sufficient. For an off-track lesion, we have to look at the glenoid bony defect. If the glenoid defect is smaller than the critical size, remplissage may be indicated; however, the Latarjet procedure may be preferable in the case of a throwing athlete or with high risks of recurrence as in a collision athlete. If a glenoid defect is larger than the critical size, it must be fixed by iliac bone graft or coracoid transfer. In our series of 100 patients with recurrent anterior dislocation, 93% had an on-track Hill-Sachs lesion and were treated by arthroscopic Bankart repair. The remaining 7% had an off-track Hill-Sachs lesion: 5% with a small glenoid defect and 2% with a large defect. All of these cases were treated by the Latarjet procedure.[354]

EDITOR COMMENTARY

Michael A. Wirth

The Rubicon River of northern Italy formed a boundary between Cisalpine Gaul and Italy, the crossing of which by Julius Caesar in 49 BC was regarded by the Roman Senate as an act of war. For many orthopaedic surgeons, the management of shoulder instability complicated by glenoid and humeral bone loss, capsular deficiency, subscapularis tears, and failed surgery is one of the most challenging problems in orthopedics, and treating some of these conditions is comparable to crossing the Rubicon. The journey irrevocably leads down a path ending with great satisfaction, conquest or disappointment, and obvious casualties!

We have provided an extensive array of topics including historical perspectives, mechanics of stability, types of instability and associated injuries, evaluation and clinical decision making in failed or complex instability, and methods of surgical repair.

This chapter highlights the importance of glenoid and/or humeral bone loss as a significant risk factor for postoperative recurrence. The effect of glenoid bone loss has been shown biomechanically to affect the balance stability angle by decreasing the effective glenoid arc. The consensus of most authors suggests that clinically significant glenoid bone loss involves 25% or more of the width of the glenoid at the level of the bare spot or greater that 20% of the surface area of the inferior glenoid face. Additionally, an anterior glenoid defect as small as 3 mm can reduce the balance stability angle by more than 25%. In light of the importance of reestablishing an effective glenoid arc, there has been a resurgence of bulk bone graft procedures, particularly the Latarjet technique. A 2014 systematic review of open Latarjet procedures revealed a risk of recurrent instability ranging from 0% to 8% with good to excellent patient satisfaction in more than 90% of patients.[52] Risk factors for glenohumeral arthritis following this procedure included age over 40 years and placement of the graft lateral to the glenoid rim.

Over the past decade, modern arthroscopic stabilization procedures have emerged as a viable and often preferred surgical option for glenohumeral instability. The increased use of this procedure is attributed to new technology, additional insight into shoulder pathology, and the increasing number of fellowship-trained shoulder surgeons technically able and confident to perform complex procedures.[46] Historically, open shoulder stabilization procedures have shown superior results to arthroscopic methods, but with the evolution of arthroscopic implants, instrumentation, and techniques, the outcomes have become comparable. At the present time, a review of the most recent literature provides insufficient data to conclude that one of these methods results in better outcomes. This might at first glance seem perplexing in light of the orthopedic literature that is replete with publications pertaining to the surgical management of shoulder instability. However, there is a paucity of meaningful data to guide open vs arthroscopic treatment of these injuries because of differing classification schemes, the variability of inclusion/exclusion criteria of associated pathology such as ALPSA and humeral avulsion of the glenohumeral ligament, lack of consensus for a definition of what constitutes failure of a repair, the use of multiple outcome measures, and crossover rates between arthroscopic and open treatment arms.

In summary, the road to conquest of the unstable shoulder was paved by the wisdom of Charles Neer, who urged surgeons not to be wedded to one standard operative procedure but to be prepared to correct the pathology present when performing surgical repairs, striving to return the joint to as near the normal anatomic condition as possible.[473] To this end, the authors offer this chapter in hopes of improving patient outcomes and increasing surgeon satisfaction with these common and yet sometimes perplexing injuries.

CHAPTER 14

The Rotator Cuff

Jason E. Hsu, Albert O. Gee, Steven B. Lippitt, Frederick A. Matsen III

HISTORICAL REVIEW

It is often difficult to ascertain where concepts begin. It is not obvious who first used the term *rotator cuff* or *musculotendinous cuff*. Credit for first describing ruptures of this structure is often given to J.G. Smith, who described the occurrence of tendon ruptures after shoulder injury in the *London Medical Gazette* in 1834.[303] In 1924, Meyer published his attrition theory of cuff rupture.[217] In his 1934 classic monograph, Codman summarized his 25 years of observations on the musculotendinous cuff and its components, and discussed rupture of the supraspinatus tendon.[51] Beginning 10 years after the publication of Codman's book and for the next 20 years, McLaughlin wrote on the etiology of cuff tears and their management.[212,213] Arthrography, with air used as the contrast medium, was first carried out by Oberholtzer in 1933.[252] Lindblom and Palmer[190] used radiopaque contrast and described partial-thickness, full-thickness, and massive tears of the cuff.

Codman recommended early operative repair for complete cuff tear and carried out what may have been the first cuff repair in 1909.[50] Current views of cuff tear pathogenesis, diagnosis, and treatment are quite similar to those that he proposed. Codman[52] and numerous well-known surgeons, including Armstrong,[6] Hammond,[115,116] McLaughlin,[212] Moseley,[234] Smith-Petersen et al.,[304] and Watson-Jones[341] suggested that subacromial abrasion may be an element in rotator cuff disease. Some of these surgeons proposed complete acromionectomy for relief of these symptoms,[6,63,115,116,341] whereas others advocated lateral acromionectomy.[212,304]

The term *impingement syndrome* was popularized by Charles Neer in 1972.[242] Neer emphasized that the supraspinatus insertion to the greater tuberosity and the bicipital groove lie anterior to the coracoacromial arch with the shoulder in the neutral position, and also noted that with forward flexion of the shoulder, these structures must pass beneath the arch, thereby providing the opportunity for abrasion. He suggested a continuum from chronic bursitis and partial tears to complete tears of the supraspinatus tendon that can extend to involve rupture of other parts of the cuff. He pointed out that physical examination and plain radiographic findings were not reliable in differentiating chronic bursitis and partial tears from complete tears. Importantly, he emphasized that patients with partial tears seemed more prone to increased shoulder stiffness and that surgery in this situation was inadvisable until the stiffness had resolved.

In 1972, Neer[242] described the indications for acromioplasty as complete tears of the supraspinatus or long-term disability from chronic bursitis and partial tears of the supraspinatus tendon. He described operating on only 50 shoulders over a 5-year period, demonstrating his great discretion regarding the removal of "impinging" bone. If surgery was performed, Neer pointed out the importance of preserving a secure acromial origin of the deltoid, performing a smooth resection of the undersurface of the anteroinferior acromion, carefully inspecting for other sources of abrasion (e.g., the undersurface of the acromioclavicular joint), and ensuring careful postoperative rehabilitation.[242-244] He also reported that patients with an irreparable rotator cuff tear could be made more comfortable and could gain surprising function after acromioplasty, as long as the deltoid origin was preserved.[243]

He described the lateral acromion as "an innocent part," and recommended removing only the anterior edge. But what if all of the acromion is innocent? In his commentary on Neer's article, Zarins stated:

> *Neer believed that impingement causes rotator cuff tears. This hypothesis does not appear to have withstood the test of time. It is more likely that rotator cuff dysfunction results in upward displacement of the humeral head and causes impingement of the humeral head against the acromion with shoulder use rather than the reverse.*

Over time, strict adherence to Neer's original indications for acromioplasty has relaxed. With the advent of arthroscopic acromioplasty initially popularized by Ellman,[76] the frequency with which this procedure was performed had increased dramatically,[360] and became one of the most common of all orthopedic procedures to treat "impingement syndrome." Additional approaches to subacromial abrasion had been proposed, including section of the coracoacromial ligament,[121,135,150,265] resection arthroplasty of the acromioclavicular joint,[137] extensive acromionectomy,[6,63,115,116,212,218,234,304,341] and combined procedures such as acromioplasty, incision of the coracoacromial ligament, acromioclavicular resection arthroplasty, and excision of the intra-articular portion of the biceps tendon with tenodesis of the distal portion to the bicipital groove.[111,247,274]

Subsequently, a vast body of evidence over the next couple of decades did not support extrinsic compression of the rotator cuff as the cause for cuff pathology but rather age-related intrinsic degeneration of the tendon. Numerous studies on the outcomes of isolated acromioplasty and rotator cuff repair with and without acromioplasty have demonstrated no difference in outcomes.[1,123,200,221,300] With the most recent evidence demonstrating its limited role, the enthusiasm for and prevalence of acromioplasty for impingement syndrome has since diminished.[142,260]

Recently, Papnikodolakis et al.[261] summarized:

> *The concept of impingement syndrome was originally introduced to cover the full range of rotator cuff disorders, as it was recognized that rotator cuff tendinosis, partial tears, and complete tears could not be reliably differentiated by clinical signs alone. The current availability of sonography, magnetic resonance imaging (MRI), and arthroscopy now enable these conditions to be accurately differentiated. Nonoperative and operative treatments are currently being used for the different rotator cuff abnormalities. Future clinical investigations can now focus on the indications for and the outcome of treatments for the specific rotator cuff diagnoses. It may be time to replace the nonspecific diagnosis of so-called impingement syndrome by using modern methods to differentiate tendinosis, partial tears, and complete tears of the rotator cuff.*

RELEVANT SHOULDER ANATOMY

Deltoid Muscle

The deltoid arises from the lateral half of the clavicle, the acromion, and posteriorly from the scapular spine. The deltoid has an important and constant tendon of origin separating its anterior and lateral thirds. This tendon attaches to the anterolateral corner of the acromion, in which location it provides the key to the anterior deltoid-splitting approach to the cuff (Fig. 14-1).

Open rotator cuff surgery can usually be accomplished with this deltoid split approach through cosmetically acceptable incisions in the lines of the skin without taking down the deltoid origin. By splitting the deltoid down the center of the tendon, the surgeon can be assured of having strong tendinous handles on the muscle to use in closing the deltoid. Although it is often said that the location of the axillary nerve is on average 5 cm distal to the acromion,[44,312] its anterior branches turn upward, so it is desirable to limit the inferior extent of the deltoid split to minimize the risk of injury to the axillary nerve branches.

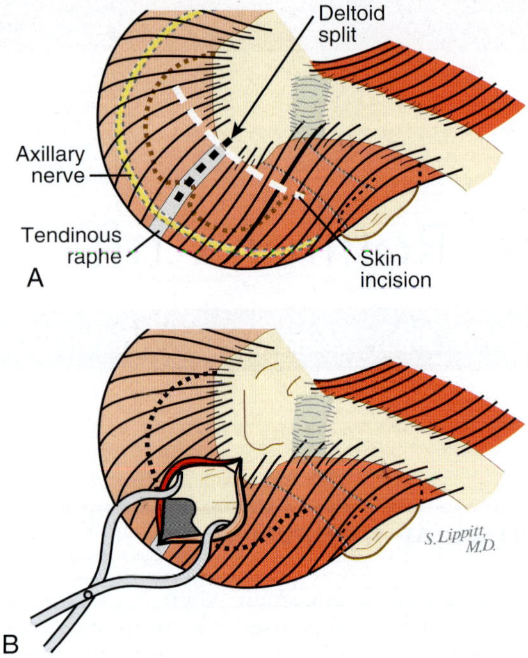

FIGURE 14-1: Deltoid split. **A** and **B,** The deltoid-on approach to the rotator cuff includes a cosmetic skin incision in Langer's lines and a deltoid split in the tendinous raphe between the anterior and lateral thirds of the deltoid. This approach preserves all of the deltoid origin, avoiding the risk of failure of a repair. (From Matsen FA III, Lippitt SB. *Shoulder Surgery: Principles and Procedures.* Philadelphia: Saunders; 2004.)

Rotator Cuff

The rotator cuff is a complex of four muscles that arise from the scapula and whose tendons blend in with the subjacent capsule as they attach to the tuberosities of the humerus.[47] The *subscapularis* arises from the anterior aspect of the scapula and attaches over much of the lesser tuberosity. It is innervated by the upper and lower subscapular nerves.[361] The *supraspinatus* muscle arises from the fossa that lies superior to the scapular spine on the posterior portion of the scapula, passes beneath the acromion and the acromioclavicular joint, and attaches to the superior aspect of the greater tuberosity. The suprascapular nerve innervates the supraspinatus after the nerve passes through the suprascapular notch. The *infraspinatus* muscle arises from the fossa below the scapular spine on the posterior portion of the scapula and attaches to the posterolateral aspect of the greater tuberosity. The suprascapular nerve innervates the infraspinatus after the nerve passes through the spinoglenoid notch. The suprascapular nerve is at risk of compression from paraglenoid cysts at both the suprascapular and spinoglenoid notches. The *teres minor* arises from the lower lateral aspect of the scapula and attaches to the

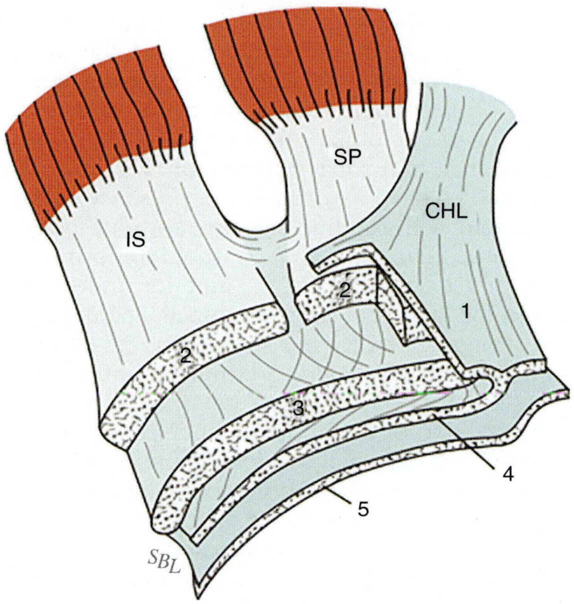

FIGURE 14-2: Schematic diagram of a cross-section of the supraspinatus (SP) and infraspinatus (IS) tendons and capsule demonstrating five distinct layers. *1,* superficial extension of CHL; *2,* fibers of the SP/IS tendons parallel to the tendon; *3,* fibers of the SP/IS tendons obliquely oriented to layer 2; *4,* deep extension of CHL; *5,* true joint capsule. CHL, Coracohumeral ligament. (From Clark JM, Harryman DT, 2nd. Tendons, ligaments, and capsule of the rotator cuff. Gross and microscopic anatomy. *J Bone Joint Surg Am.* 1992;74[5]:713-725.)

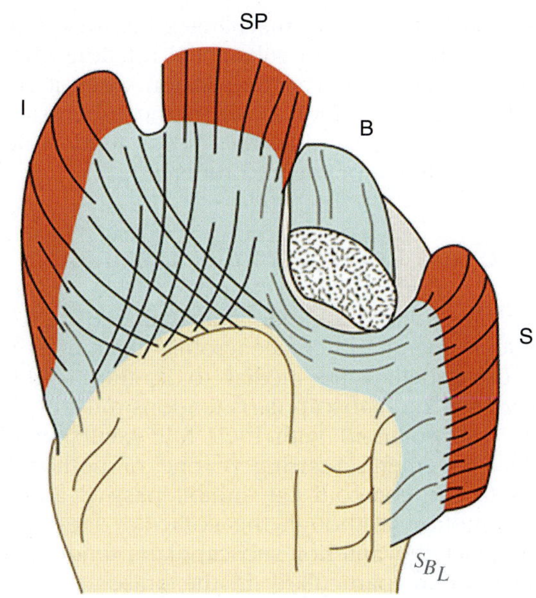

FIGURE 14-3: The normal interweaving of the fibers from the subscapularis (S), supraspinatus (SP), and infraspinatus (I) tendons near the humeral insertion. B, Long head of biceps tendon. (From Clark JM, Harryman DT, 2nd. Tendons, ligaments, and capsule of the rotator cuff. Gross and microscopic anatomy. *J Bone Joint Surg Am.* 1992;74[5]:713-725.)

lower portion of the greater tuberosity. It is innervated by a branch of the axillary nerve. The tendons of the rotator cuff blend together to form a continuous cuff around the humeral head.

Histologic studies by Clark and Harryman described the rotator cuff tendons as having five distinct layers (Fig. 14-2).[47] The most superficial layer is the coracohumeral ligament fibers, which are obliquely oriented to the axis of the muscle and span the interval between the subscapularis and supraspinatus tendons. The second layer is composed of tendon fibers grouped into large bundles that extend from the supraspinatus tendon and form a layer over the biceps tendon in its groove. The third layer contains tendon fascicles that are smaller in size and less tightly packed than the bundles in the second layer and also have less uniform orientation. The fourth layer is composed of loose connective tissue with thick bands of collagen fibers. This tissue merges with the coracohumeral ligament at the anterior edge of the supraspinatus. The fifth and last layer is the continued sheet of collagen fibrils that composes the superior joint capsule.

The footprint of the rotator cuff has been a subject of numerous cadaveric studies. While the rotator cuff muscles were often thought to run in parallel and insert onto discrete portions of the greater and lesser tuberosity, we now know that there is significant overlap of the tendinous portions of each rotator cuff onto the tuberosities. Clark and Harryman have demonstrated significant interdigitation of the supraspinatus and infraspinatus tendons occurring near the footprint (Fig. 14-3).[46,47,48] Minagawa et al. also demonstrated a significant overlap of the posterior supraspinatus with the infraspinatus cuff tendon.[225] Mochizuki et al. studied 113 cadaveric specimens, and found that the portion of the greater tuberosity occupied by the supraspinatus insertion was much smaller than previously believed, and that the infraspinatus insertion occupied the preponderance of the footprint on the greater tuberosity.[227]

The long head of the biceps tendon may be considered a functional part of the rotator cuff. It attaches to the supraglenoid tubercle of the scapula, runs between the subscapularis and the supraspinatus, exits the shoulder through the bicipital groove under the transverse humeral ligament, and attaches to its muscle in the proximal part of the arm. The coracohumeral ligament and the transverse humeral ligament keep the biceps tendon aligned in the groove.[302] Although electromyographic studies on the long head of the biceps have demonstrated that it may be inactive during shoulder movements,[352] it may serve as a passive restraint during most shoulder motions and contribute to anterior stability in abduction and external rotation. Changes in elbow position and loading of the biceps can lead to altered shoulder motion and muscle recruitment.[358,359] This tendon also has the potential for guiding the head of the humerus as it is elevated, with the bicipital groove traveling on the biceps tendon like a monorail on its track. This mechanism helps explain why the humerus is capable of substantial rotation when it is adducted and allows very little rotation when it is maximally abducted (in which position the tuberosities are constrained as they straddle the biceps tendon near its attachment to the supraglenoid tubercle).

Coracoid and Coracoacromial Ligament

The *coracoid* arises from two or three ossification centers.[289] It provides the medial attachment site for both the coracohumeral and coracoacromial ligaments. In that their muscle bellies lie medial to it, the neighboring supraspinatus and subscapularis tendons must be able to glide by the coracoid with their full excursion during shoulder movement. Scarring of one or both of these tendons to the coracoid can inhibit passive and active shoulder motion. Although the coracoid does not normally contact the anterior subscapularis tendon, forced internal rotation, particularly in the presence of a tight posterior capsule, can produce such contact as a result of the obligate translation.[99,119]

The *coracoacromial ligament* spans from the undersurface of the acromion to the lateral aspect of the coracoid and is continuous with the less dense clavipectoral fascia. It forms a substantial part of the superficial aspect of the humeroscapular motion interface (Figs. 14-4 and 14-5). This ligament may be thought of as the spring ligament of the shoulder in that it maintains the normal relationships between the coracoid and the acromion. Separation of these two scapular processes has been observed on sectioning this ligament in cadavers.[81] Calcification in the acromial end of this ligament can give the appearance of a subacromial spur (Fig. 14-6). Radiographic studies have associated the presence of such an acromial spur with full-thickness rotator cuff tears.[85,114,254]

The *coracoacromial arch* is the inferiorly concave smooth surface consisting of the anterior undersurface of the acromion and the coracoacromial ligament. It provides a strong ceiling for the shoulder joint, along which the cuff tendons must glide during all shoulder movements (see Fig. 14-5). Passage of the cuff tendons and the proximal end of the humerus under this arch is facilitated by the subacromial-subdeltoid bursa, which is not normally a space, as often shown on diagrams, but rather two serosal surfaces in contact with each other, one on the undersurface of the coracoacromial arch and deltoid and the other on the cuff. These sliding surfaces are lubricated by the bursal surfaces and synovial fluid.

Scapular and Acromial Anatomy

The acromion is a scapular process arising from four separate centers of ossification: a basi-acromion, a meta-acromion, a meso-acromion, and a pre-acromion (Fig. 14-7). The basi-acromion typically fuses to the scapular

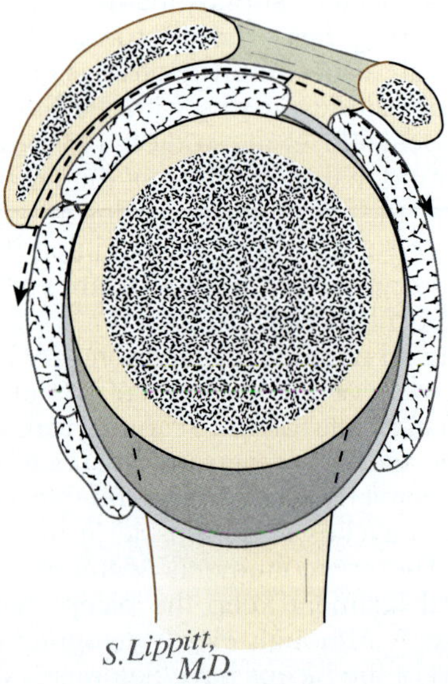

FIGURE 14-4: The humeroscapular motion interface beneath the coracoacromial arch. The external surface of the rotator cuff articulates with the undersurface of the coracoacromial arch. This articulation is part of the humeroscapular motion interface. Smooth, unrestrained movement at this interface is required for normal shoulder function. (From Matsen FA III, Lippitt SB. *Shoulder Surgery: Principles and Procedures.* Philadelphia: Saunders; 2004:42.)

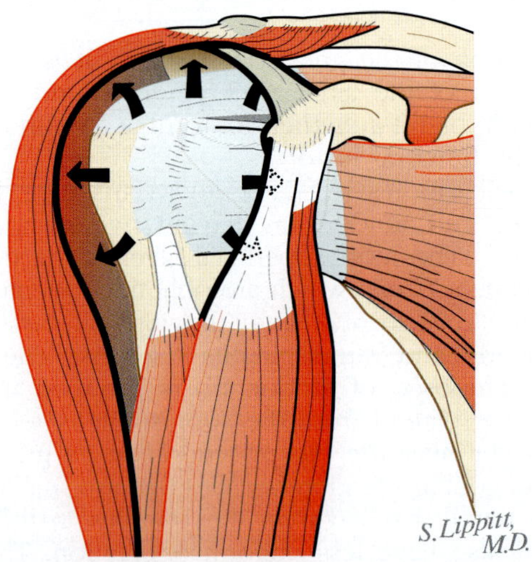

FIGURE 14-5: The humeroscapular motion interface. The humeroscapular motion interface is the set of gliding surfaces between the proximal humerus covered by the rotator cuff tendons and the overlying structures attached to the scapula, including the deltoid, the acromion, the coracoacromial ligament, the coracoid, and the tendons of the coracoid muscles. Approximately 4 cm of motion takes place at this interface in normal shoulder movement. (From Matsen FA III, Lippitt SB. *Shoulder Surgery: Principles and Procedures.* Philadelphia: Saunders; 2004:42.)

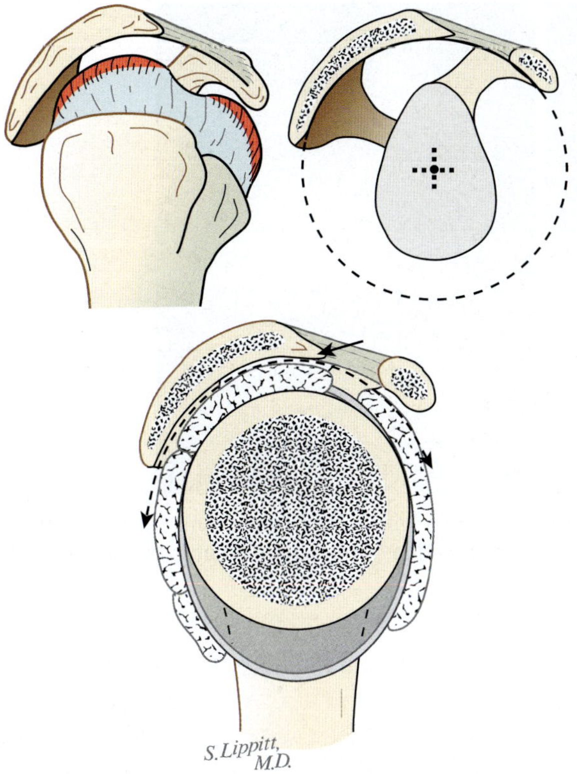

FIGURE 14-6: Calcification in the coracoacromial ligament. *Top left,* Calcification of the coracoacromial ligament does not encroach on the rotator cuff. *Top right,* The center of the coracoacromial arch lies in the center of the glenoid. *Bottom,* The proximal humeral convexity articulates smoothly with the coracoacromial arch, even if there is calcification in the ligament (*solid arrow*). (From Matsen FA III, Lippitt SB. *Shoulder Surgery: Principles and Procedures*. Philadelphia: Saunders; 2004:417.)

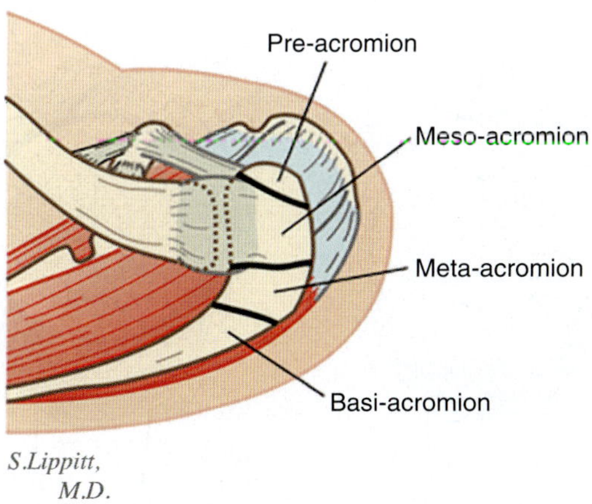

FIGURE 14-7: Superior view of the scapula and clavicle demonstrating the four ossification centers of the acromion.

spine by 12 years of age, and the other centers of ossification are usually united by 22 years of age but may occur as late as 25 years.[210]

When these centers fail to unite, the ununited portion is referred to as an *os acromiale*. The unfused segment directly anterior to the nonunion site defines the type of os acromiale. An unfused segment between the meso- and pre-acromion ossification centers is termed a pre-acromiale. The most common lesion is a failure of fusion of the meso-acromion to the meta-acromion.[73,210,248,291] Most studies have reported the incidence of os acromiale to be approximately 2% to 8%,[73,185,236,291] and they often occur bilaterally.[185] It can be difficult to differentiate a fused os acromiale from a free ossicle in the clinical setting.[291] Clinicians must be cautious about diagnosing and surgically treating an os acromiale before the age of 25 years given the potential for the ossification centers to unit. Resection of a large fragment creates a challenge for deltoid reattachment.

The notion that an os acromiale is a pathologic condition and the association of os acromiale with rotator cuff tears is controversial. Norris et al.[251] and Bigliani et al.[29] pointed to an association of cuff degeneration and an unfused acromial epiphysis. Boehm et al. assessed 62 patients with an os acromiale in the axillary radiographs of 1000 patients undergoing rotator cuff repair.[24] The average number of tendons and average age was similar between those with and without the os acromiale. They concluded that the prevalence of os acromiale in patients with tears is comparable to that in a standard population with an unknown rotator cuff status. A subsequent MRI study found similar results.[258]

Our understanding of the individual anatomy of the scapula and acromion and its association with rotator cuff pathology is continuing to evolve. Bigliani et al.[28] described three acromial shapes: type I (flat) in 17%, type II (curved) in 43%, and type III (hooked) in 40%. In this study, 58% of the cadavers had the same type of acromion on each side. Thirty-three percent of the shoulders had full-thickness tears, 73% of which were seen in association with type III acromia, 24% with type II, and 3% with type I. The anterior slope of the acromion in shoulders with cuff tears averaged 29 degrees, slightly more than the slope of those without cuff tears, which averaged 23 degrees. The clinical significance of this relatively small difference is unknown. Numerous other authors have reported that patients with cuff defects are more likely to have hooked or angled acromia.[327,329]

Subsequent studies of acromial morphology have not found the same relationships, and have suggested that the initial correlations between acromial morphology and cuff disease may be confounded by age. Nicholson et al.[248] demonstrated in a review of 420 scapulae that spur formation on the anterior acromion was an age-related process such that persons younger than 50 years had less than one-fourth the prevalence of those older than 50 years. The status of the cuffs of these shoulders is unknown. A study by Gill et al.[101] showed that in patients older than 50 years, no significant association between acromial morphology and rotator cuff pathology could be found. However, there was a significant correlation with age and rotator cuff tears. Older patients were more likely to have type II and III acromia, although this study did not comment on whether this trend was significant. These findings imply that apparent correlations between

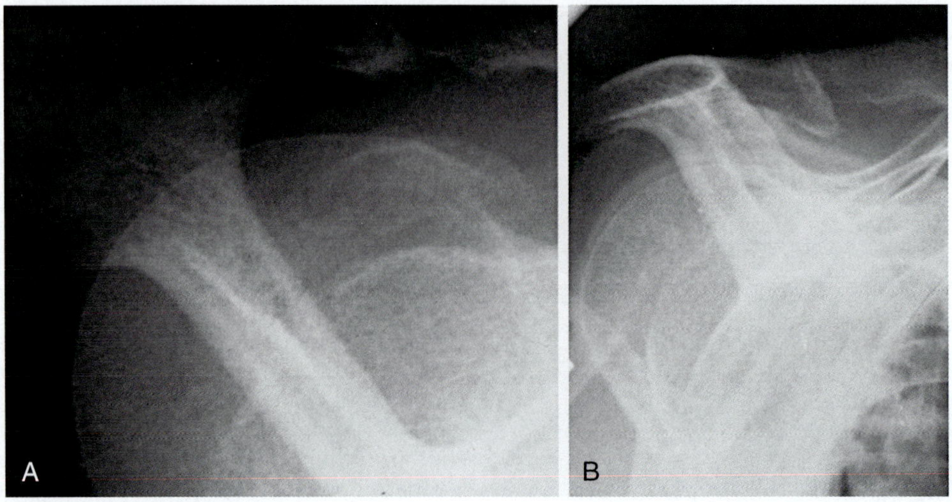

FIGURE 14-8: A, Variations in acromial shape are commonly observed in patients with cuff disease. The supraspinatus outlet view is helpful in defining this anatomy. **B,** In this arthrogram (*lateral view*), indentation of the supraspinatus by the anteroinferior acromion can be seen.

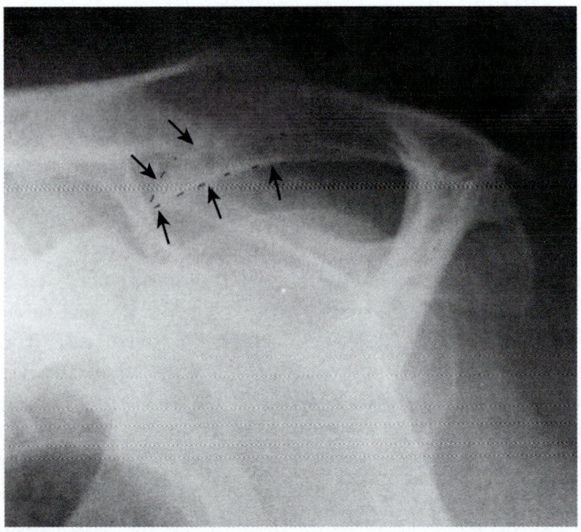

FIGURE 14-9: Supraspinatus outlet radiograph demonstrating a large anteroinferior osteophyte (*arrows*). (From Iannotti JP. *Rotator Cuff Disorders: Evaluation and Treatment.* Rosemont, IL: American Academy of Orthopaedic Surgeons; 1991.)

acromial morphology and rotator cuff tears may be exaggerated because of the confounding variable of age.[129]

Other studies have suggested that type II and III acromia are acquired rather than developmental.[357] Because most acromial hooks lie within the coracoacromial ligament (Figs. 14-8 and 14-9), it seems likely that they are actually traction spurs in this ligament (Fig. 14-10). The traction loads producing this hook can result from loading of the arch by the cuff, and may be increased with increasing dependency on the coracoacromial arch for superior stability in the presence of cuff

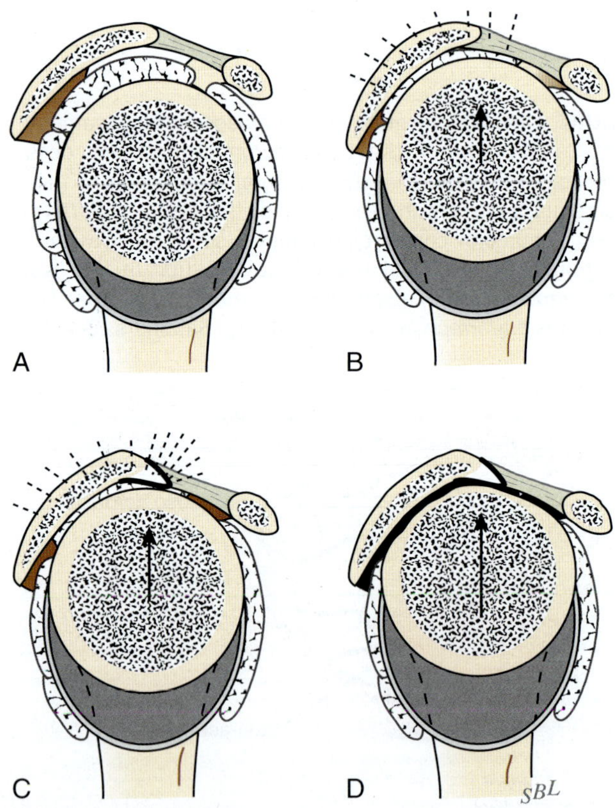

FIGURE 14-10: Acromial traction spur. **A,** Normal relationships. **B,** As the humeral head moves upward, the coracoacromial arch becomes progressively loaded. **C,** The result is a traction spur in the coracoacromial ligament. Because it lies within the substance of the ligament, this spur does not encroach on the rotator cuff, even though it can look impressive on radiography. **D,** Cuff tear arthropathy. (From Matsen FA III, Lippitt SB. *Shoulder Surgery: Principles and Procedures.* Philadelphia: Saunders; 2004:280.)

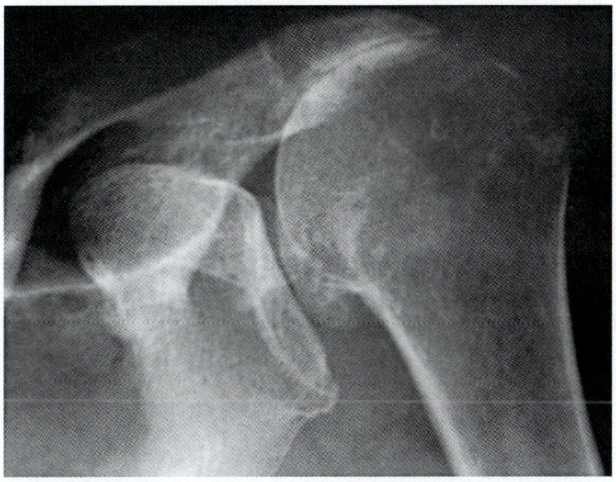

FIGURE 14-11: Chronic massive tears result in upward displacement of the humeral head until it articulates with the acromion. Humeral osteophytes result from abnormal glenohumeral articulation. Note the smooth undersurface of the coracoacromial arch.

degeneration.[81,82,365] The concept of the hook as a traction phenomenon was first put forward by Neer more than 30 years ago.[242] Because this hook lies within the ligament and points toward the coracoid (see Fig. 14-9), it seems unlikely that it would jeopardize passage of the cuff beneath the coracoacromial arch. Even in cases of cuff tear arthropathy, the undersurface of the coracoacromial arch commonly presents a smooth articulating concavity (see Fig. 14-10 and Fig. 14-11).

More recent radiographic and biomechanical studies have suggested that scapular morphology may predispose certain individuals to rotator cuff tears. Moor et al. performed a radiographic study that suggested that the individual anatomy of the scapula seen on plain radiographs is associated with degenerative rotator cuff tears.[229] They found that the acromion index, the lateral acromion angle, and the "critical shoulder angle" (an angle that accounts for both glenoid inclination and lateral acromial extension) could accurately predict the presence of a degenerative cuff tear, but that acromial slope as described by Bigliani et al.[28] was not predictive.[230] A biomechanical study suggested that overloading of the supraspinatus tendon can occur with a higher critical shoulder angle.[98] Considering all the available evidence, it seems most likely that loading of the coracoacromial arch over the years by the rotator cuff and proximal humerus can cause age-related calcification *within* the coracoacromial ligament. This intraligamentous calcification can present the radiographic appearance of an acromial "spur," but because the calcification does not extend beyond the ligament, it does not "impinge" on the rotator cuff.

Our practice is to downplay the importance of the appearance of the acromion on radiographs and to perform acromial surgery only if there is a substantial prominence on the inferior aspect of the coracoacromial arch.

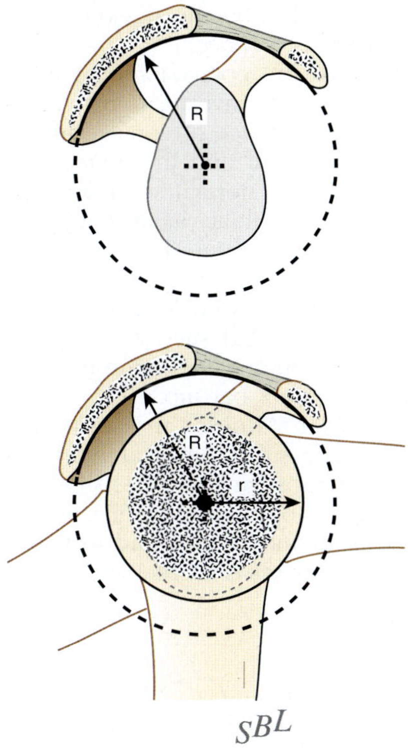

FIGURE 14-12: Concentric spheres. The spherical proximal humeral convexity is formed by the tuberosities and the superficial surface of the rotator cuff tendons. It has a radius of *R* and articulates with the undersurface of the coracoacromial arch. The spherical humeral articular surface has a radius of *r* and articulates with the glenoid. The difference between these two radii is made up by the height of the tuberosities and the thickness of the cuff tendons. The centers of these two spheres and the concavities with which they articulate must be superimposed in normal shoulder function. These two mating spheres enable the shoulder to have both great mobility and stability. (From Matsen FA III, Lippitt SB. *Shoulder Surgery: Principles and Procedures.* Philadelphia: Saunders; 2004:43.)

Humeroscapular Motion Interface

Matsen et al. described the humeroscapular motion interface as an articulation (see Figs. 14-4 and 14-5) between the cuff, the humeral head, and the biceps on the inside and the coracoacromial arch, the deltoid, and the coracoid muscles on the outside.[207] Up to 4 cm of gliding can occur at this articulation in normal shoulders in vivo. It is instructive to consider the humeroscapular articulation as consisting of two concentric spheres, the glenohumeral sphere and the sphere represented by the articulation between the inferior surface of the coracoacromial arch and the proximal humeral convexity. Together, these two spheres enhance both shoulder stability and the surface available for scapulohumeral load transfer (Fig. 14-12).[51] Normally, the spheres of the humeral head and the coracoacromial arch share the same center. The difference in radius of the two spheres (*R* and *r* in

Fig. 14-12) is provided by the thickness of the rotator cuff, which serves as a spacer.

Contact beneath the coracoacromial arch is present in normal shoulders.[354] Investigations[42,81,82,280,348,365] have pointed out the importance of contact and load transfer between the rotator cuff and the intact coracoacromial arch in the function of normal shoulders, including the provision of superior stability against superiorly directed loads applied to the humerus. This backstop preventing superior translation of the proximal humerus is particularly important when upward loads are applied parallel to the face of the glenoid such as when the arms are used to press up from a seated lying position or in performing exercises like a bar dip.

Posterior capsular stiffness can lead to higher contact pressures under the subacromial arch.[237,238] In the presence of posterior capsular tightness, shoulder flexion or internal rotation (or both) cause obligate anterosuperior translation of the humeral head and loss of the concentricity of the two spheres (Fig. 14-13).[54,119] As a result, the proximal humeral convexity is forced against the anterior undersurface of the concave coracoacromial arch rather than rotating concentrically beneath it (see Figs. 14-12 and 14-13). In the presence of degeneration of the cuff tendon, the shoulder can lose the concentricity of the humeral head and coracoacromial arch spheres (Figs. 14-14 and 14-15). Taken together, these observations reinforce the shoulder's need for normal posterior capsular laxity; a smooth, concentric, and congruent coracoacromial undersurface; and a normally thick and uniform cuff interposed between the humeral head and the coracoacromial arch.

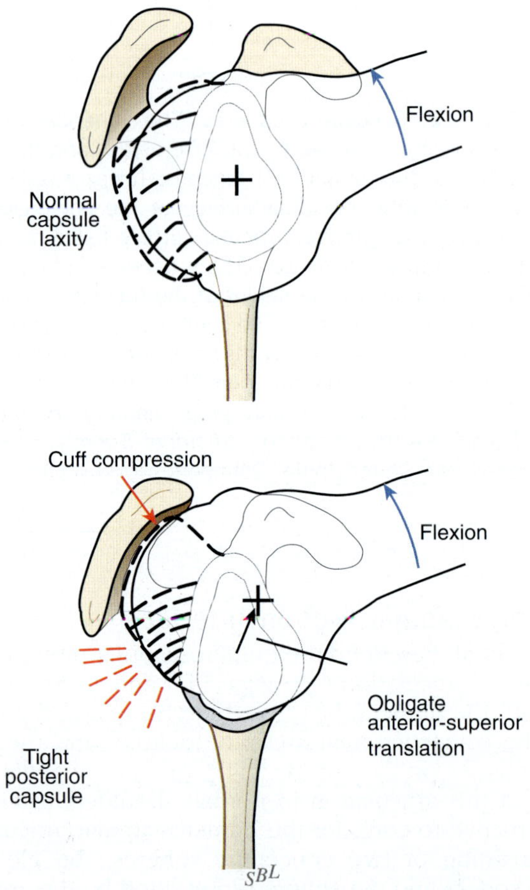

FIGURE 14-13: Posterior capsule tightness. Tightness of the posterior inferior capsule causes obligate anterosuperior translation on flexion. As a result, the centers of the humeral articular surface and proximal humeral convexity are no longer the same as the centers of the coracoacromial arch and the glenoid concavity. (From Matsen FA III, Lippitt SB. *Shoulder Surgery: Principles and Procedures*. Philadelphia: Saunders; 2004:418.)

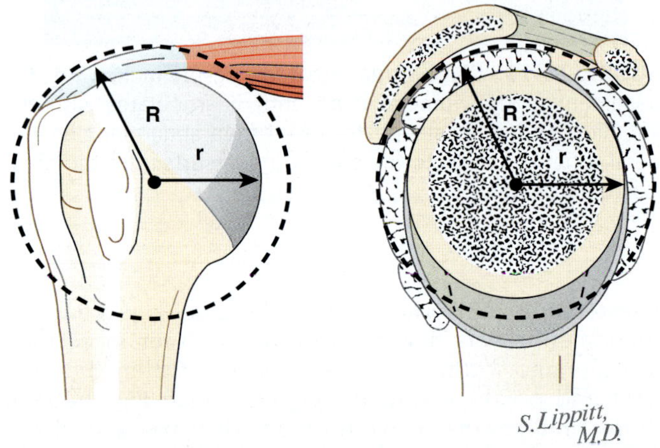

FIGURE 14-14: The proximal humeral convexity. The rotational center of the proximal humeral convexity is the center of the sphere that best fits the tuberosities and the cuff tendons near their insertion. The radius of the proximal humeral convexity (R) should be equal to the radius of the humeral articular surface sphere (r) plus the thickness of the rotator cuff tendons. (From Matsen FA III, Lippitt SB. *Shoulder Surgery: Principles and Procedures*. Philadelphia: Saunders; 2004:81.)

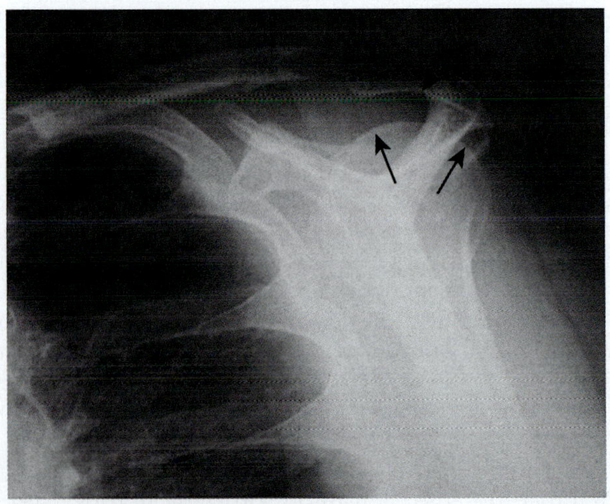

FIGURE 14-15: Congruence of the humeral head (*arrows*) and coracoacromial arch (*arrowhead*) spheres in a scapular lateral radiograph of the normal left shoulder of a 58-year-old man.

Acromioclavicular Joint

Theoretically, osteophytes from the acromioclavicular joint may encroach on the space normally occupied by the cuff tendons (Figs. 14-16 and 14-17). However, these spurs are usually too medial to contact the tendons. In a series of 47 patients with arthrographically confirmed supraspinatus tendon rupture, Peterson and Gentz[266] found that 51% had distally pointing acromioclavicular joint osteophytes. A similar incidence was found in their series of 170 autopsy specimens with cuff defects. The incidence of distally pointing acromioclavicular osteophytes in normal shoulders was 14% in the clinical studies and 10% in the cadaver studies. It is recognized, however, that degenerative changes in the cuff and degenerative changes in the acromioclavicular joint can coexist in the aging population without the former being causally related to the latter. Steinbeck et al. pointed out in their retrospective study of 102 patients in whom cuff repair was performed with resection of the lateral end of the clavicle in 20, that the results were not significantly influenced by the clavicle resection.[313] Again, it is recognized that acromioclavicular osteophytes are usually sufficiently medial that they do not jeopardize the cuff.

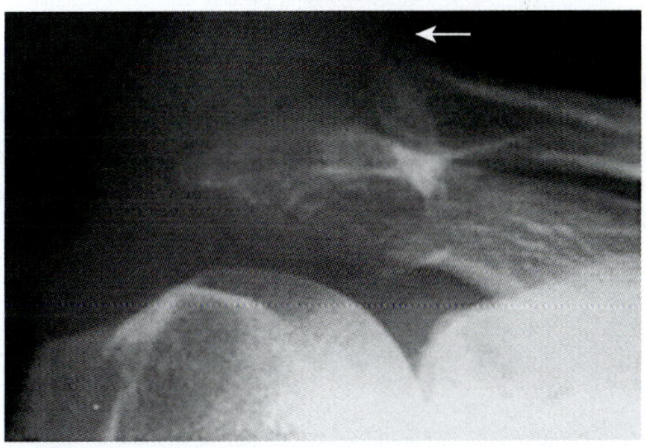

FIGURE 14-16: An anteroposterior radiograph showing acromioclavicular joint arthritis (*arrow*).

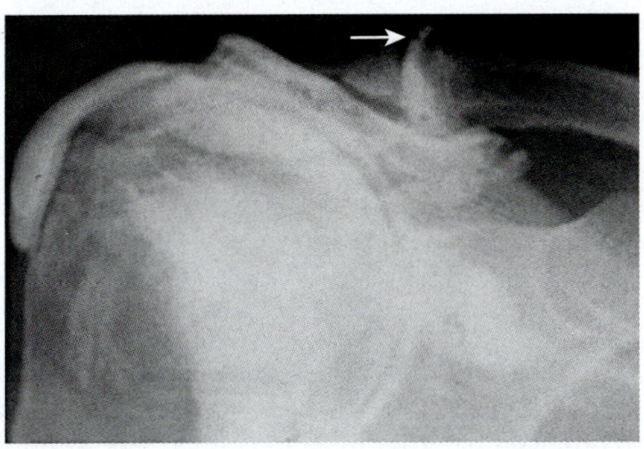

FIGURE 14-17: An arthrogram in the same patient shown in Fig. 14-16 reveals leakage of dye into the acromioclavicular joint (geyser sign; *arrow*), thereby confirming the clinical suspicion of a rotator cuff tear. Note the indentation of the cuff caused by the acromioclavicular joint osteophytes.

Vascular Anatomy

The vascular anatomy of the cuff tendons has been described by numerous investigators.[32,198,235,279,283] Lindblom[188,189] described an area of relative avascularity in the supraspinatus tendon near its insertion. Rothman and Parke[283] found contributions to the cuff vessels from the suprascapular, anterior circumflex, and posterior circumflex arteries in all cases. The thoracoacromial artery contributed to the cuff's blood supply in 76%, the suprahumeral in 59%, and the subscapular in 38%. These authors found the area of the supraspinatus just proximal to its insertion to be markedly under vascularized in comparison to the remainder of the cuff. Recent studies have suggested an age-related decrease in vascularity that is consistent with the increasing prevalence of cuff pathology with aging.[87,285] Uhthoff et al.[331] observed relative hypovascularity of the deep surface of the supraspinatus insertion as compared with its superficial aspect. Nixon and DiStefano[250] suggested that the critical zone of Codman corresponds to the area of anastomoses between the osseous vessels (the anterolateral branch of the anterior humeral circumflex and the posterior humeral circumflex) and the muscular vessels (the suprascapular and subscapular vessels).

An additional anatomic feature of importance is the acromial branch of the thoracoacromial artery. This artery is closely related with the coracoacromial ligament, and is often transected in the course of acromioplasty and section of the coracoacromial ligament. This artery is invariably encountered during arthroscopy if sectioning of the coracoacromial ligament is performed.

BIOMECHANICS OF THE ROTATOR CUFF

The rotator cuff musculature may be thought of as having three functions: rotation of the humerus with respect to the scapula, muscular balance, and compression of the head into the concavity of the glenoid fossa. This concavity compression concavity mechanism is important in providing glenohumeral stability through range of motion of the shoulder in the many functional positions where the capsular ligaments are lax.[191,192]

The concept of the rotator cuff "force couple" has been described in the coronal and transverse planes.[35,40,41] In the coronal plane, the pull of the deltoid must be balanced with the inferior portion of the rotator cuff including the infraspinatus, teres minor, and subscapularis. This couple will be balanced only if the line of action of the inferior cuff is below the center of rotation of the humeral head to oppose the deltoid moment. The transverse force couple is composed anteriorly of the subscapularis and posteriorly of the infraspinatus and teres minor (Fig. 14-18). Clinically, these force couples are important in the treatment of massive rotator cuff tears in which the goal is not necessarily to repair all torn tendons to the cuff insertion but rather to balance the coronal and transverse force couples so that the humeral head is stable within the glenoid concavity and a stable fulcrum is maintained throughout range of motion.[41] Without adequate stability imparted by the force couples, the power

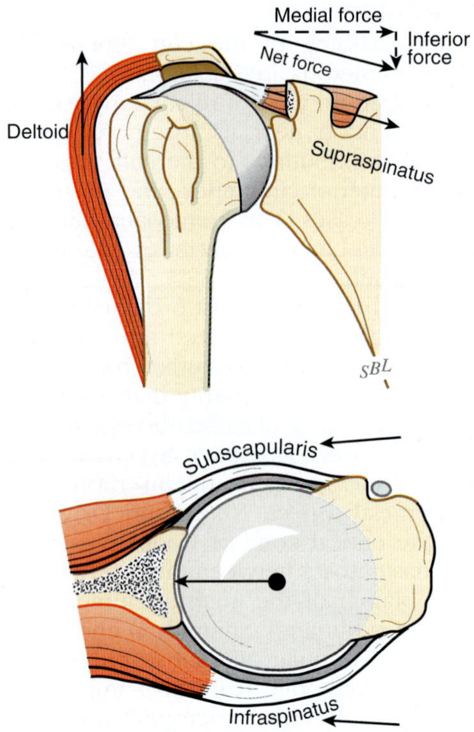

FIGURE 14-18: Balanced anteroposterior cuff forces compress the humeral articular convexity into the glenoid concavity. (From Matsen FA III, Lippitt SB. *Shoulder Surgery: Principles and Procedures*. Philadelphia: Saunders; 2004:85.)

of the deltoid muscle cannot be used efficiently for elevation of the shoulder.

This concept of force couples around the shoulder is important but may oversimplify the complex interactions between the cuff and the different heads of the deltoid, trapezius, latissimus dorsi, and pectoralis muscles. The timing and magnitude of these balancing muscle effects must be precisely coordinated to avoid unwanted directions of humeral motion. In a specified position, activation of a muscle creates a unique set of rotational moments. For example, the anterior deltoid can exert moments in forward elevation, internal rotation, and cross-body movement (Fig. 14-19). If forward elevation is to occur without rotation, the cross-body and internal rotation moments of this muscle must be neutralized by other muscles, such as the posterior deltoid and infraspinatus (Fig. 14-20).[299] As another example, use of the latissimus dorsi in a movement of pure internal rotation requires that its adduction moment be neutralized by the superior cuff and deltoid. Conversely, use of the latissimus dorsi in a movement of pure adduction requires that the posterior cuff and posterior deltoid muscles neutralize their internal rotation moment. Thus the simplified view of muscles as isolated motors, or as members of force couples, must give way to an understanding that all shoulder muscles function together in a precisely coordinated way, with opposing muscles canceling out undesired elements and leaving only the net torque that

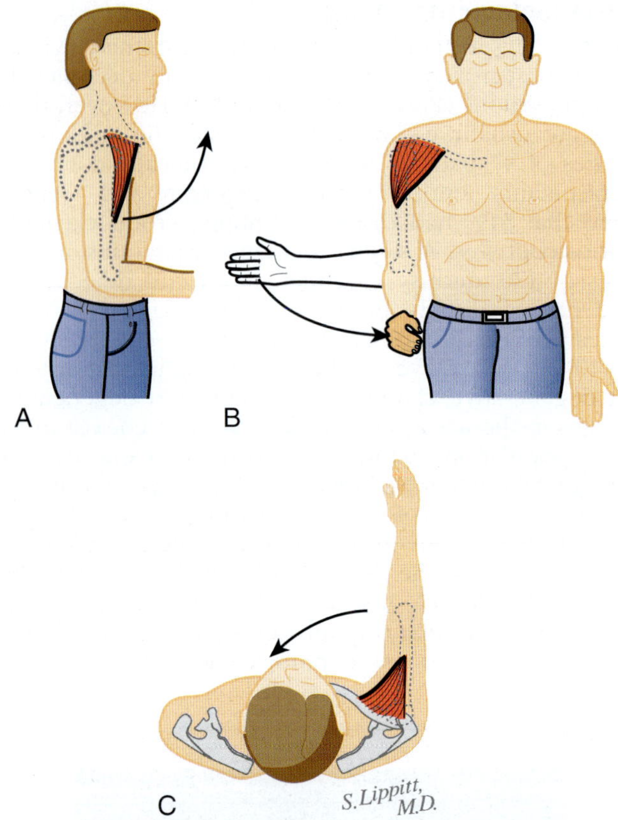

FIGURE 14-19: Deltoid moment. The anterior deltoid generates moments in forward elevation (**A**), internal rotation (**B**), and cross-body movement (**C**). (From Matsen FA III, Lippitt SB. *Shoulder Surgery: Principles and Procedures*. Philadelphia: Saunders; 2004:261.)

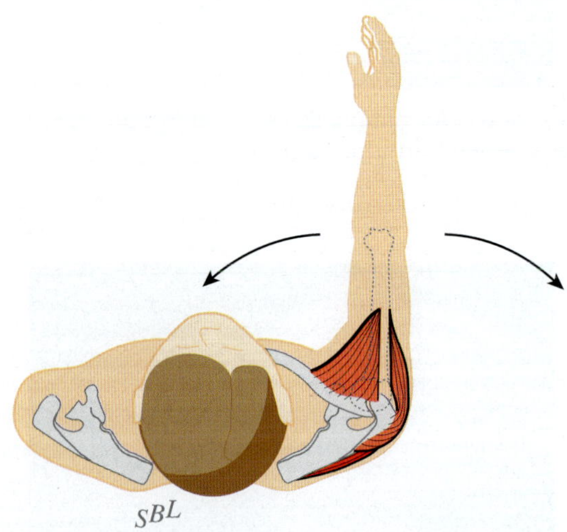

FIGURE 14-20: Deltoid balance. Pure elevation requires that the internal rotation and cross-body moments of the anterior deltoid be opposed by other muscle actions. For example, even though it is an antagonist to the anterior deltoid, the posterior deltoid must contract during elevation to resist the cross-body moment of the anterior deltoid. (From Matsen FA III, Lippitt SB. *Shoulder Surgery: Principles and Procedures*. Philadelphia: Saunders; 2004:261.)

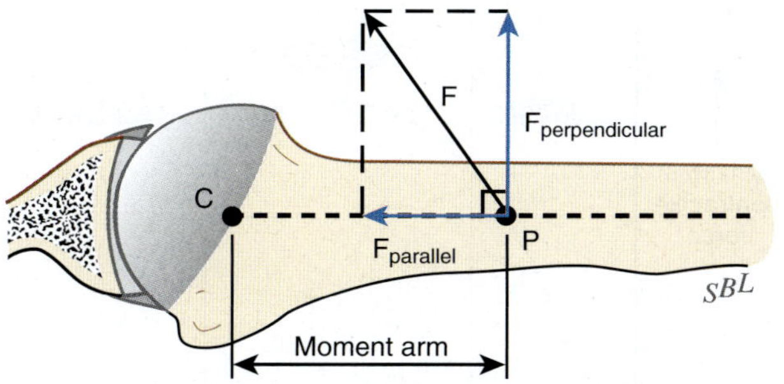

FIGURE 14-21: Torque. The magnitude of the torque resulting from a muscle force is the product of the moment or lever arm (the length of the line connecting the center of rotation to the effective attachment of the muscle, *C* to *P*) and the magnitude of the force perpendicular to this line *(F perpendicular).* (From Matsen FA III, Lippitt SB. *Shoulder Surgery: Principles and Procedures.* Philadelphia: Saunders; 2004:252.)

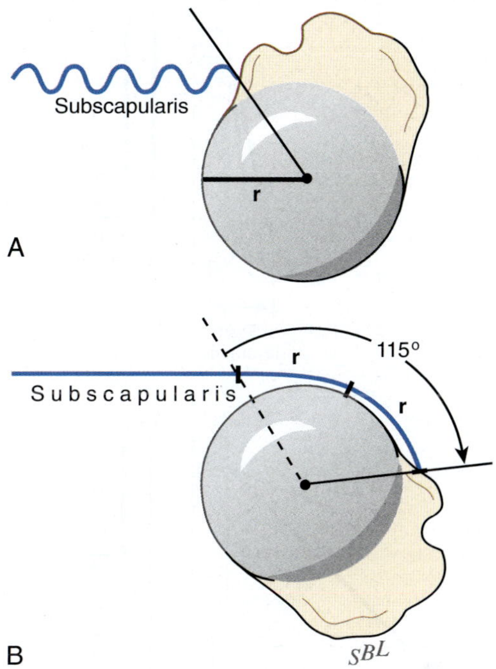

FIGURE 14-22: Subscapularis excursion. **A,** To power the shoulder through a range of motion, the excursion of a muscle must equal the product of the effective lever arm (in the case of the subscapularis, the radius of the humeral head, *r*) multiplied by the rotational range of motion in the direction of action of the muscle divided by the number of degrees in a radian (57.3). **B,** Thus if the subscapularis is to power the shoulder through a 115-degree arc of rotation acting through a lever arm equal to the radius of the humeral head (e.g., 25 mm), its excursion would need to be 115 degrees × 25 mm/57.3 degrees, or 50 mm. (From Matsen FA III, Lippitt SB. *Shoulder Surgery: Principles and Procedures.* Philadelphia: Saunders; 2004:256.)

is needed to produce the desired action.[284] This degree of coordination requires a preprogrammed strategy of muscle activation that must be established before the motion is carried out. The rotator cuff muscles are critical, but not the only, elements of this shoulder muscle balance equation.[15,62,80,106,133,137,141,187,288,310,315,339]

The humeral torque resulting from contraction of a cuff muscle is determined by the moment arm (the distance between the effective point of application of this force and the center of the humeral head) and the component of the muscle force that is perpendicular to it (Fig. 14-21).[349] The magnitude of force that can be delivered by a cuff muscle is determined by its size, health, and condition, as well as the position of the joint. The cuff muscles' contribution to shoulder strength has been evaluated by Colachis et al.,[55,56] who used selective nerve blocks and found that the supraspinatus and infraspinatus provide 45% of the abduction and 90% of the external rotation strength. Howell et al.[125] found that the supraspinatus and deltoid muscles are equally responsible for producing torque about the shoulder joint in the functional planes of motion. Generation of force in abduction of the arm decreased only 5% after a simulated tear of one-third and two-thirds of the supraspinatus. Detachment of the entire tendon resulted in a 17% loss of strength. Simulation of retraction of tears of one-third, two-thirds, and the entire supraspinatus resulted in losses of 19%, 36%, and 58%, respectively. These losses were almost completely regained with side-to-side repair.[113] Other estimates of the relative contributions of the rotator cuff to shoulder strength have been published.[28,53,336]

Bey et al.[23] found that the strain within the rotator cuff increased in positions of greater abduction, even when the same force was applied through the rotator cuff. No significant difference in strain on the superficial and deep portions of the cuff was detected. The compressive stiffness of the articular side of the supraspinatus tendon was found to be significantly less than that of its bursal side.[173] This difference in stiffness might be one reason that most tears begin on the articular surface.

At least three factors complicate analysis of the contribution of a given muscle to shoulder strength. The moment arms of each rotator cuff muscle vary with the increasing angles of elevation and abduction,[164,194,257] and therefore the torque that a muscle can generate varies with joint position. Muscles are usually stronger near the middle of their excursion and weaker at the extremes (Figs. 14-22 to 14-24).[186] The direction of a given muscle force is determined by the position of the joint. For example, the supraspinatus can contribute to abduction or external rotation, or both, depending on the initial position of the arm.[257] The effective humeral point of application for a cuff tendon wrapping around the humeral head is not its anatomic insertion but rather at the point where the tendon first contacts the head, a point that usually lies on the articular surface (Fig. 14-25).

Early studies reported that the rotator cuff, specifically the supraspinatus, contributed most to abduction of the arm at low abduction angles, and that cuff contribution was insignificant at higher abduction angles.[299] However, subsequent data have demonstrated that the supraspinatus and infraspinatus have smaller torque in the scapular

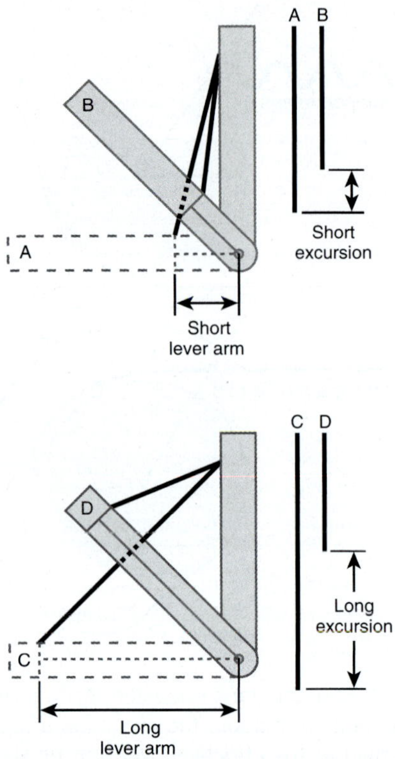

FIGURE 14-23: Lever arm and excursion. Muscles acting through longer lever arms (*bottom*) generate more torque per unit force (torque = force × lever arm), but they require greater excursion for a given arc of motion (see the difference between the dark lines to the right representing muscle length in extension and flexion) than muscles acting through shorter lever arms, which require less excursion but result in less torque (*top*). (From Matsen FA III, Lippitt SB. *Shoulder Surgery: Principles and Procedures*. Philadelphia: Saunders; 2004:257.)

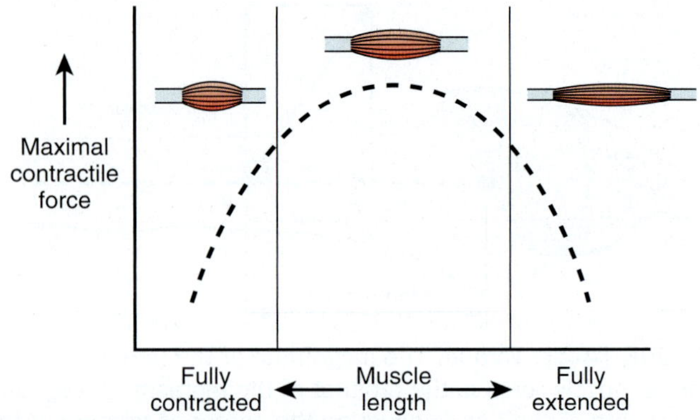

FIGURE 14-24: Muscle length and force. A typical relationship between a muscle's length and the maximal force that it can produce. Note that the maximal force is less at the extremes of the range of motion. (From Matsen FA III, Lippitt SB. *Shoulder Surgery: Principles and Procedures*. Philadelphia: Saunders; 2004:257.)

plane than previously reported.[164] A significant increase in the middle deltoid torque is required to initiate abduction in the presence of supraspinatus paralysis, but glenohumeral kinematics and motion are not affected when the transverse force couple is intact.[214,325] The subscapularis and infraspinatus are not only internal and external rotators of the glenohumeral joint but also play a role in elevation in the plane of the scapula.[257] The subscapularis enhances abduction in external rotation while the infraspinatus enhances abduction in internal rotation.

The concept of the "rotator cable" and "suspension bridge" should be considered when evaluating the biomechanics of a shoulder with a rotator cuff tear. A thickening of tissue seen on the articular side of the rotator cuff that runs in a crescent shape was originally described as a "transverse band" by Clark and Harryman[47] and termed the "rotator cable" by Burkhart et al. (Fig. 14-26).[40] This thickening of tissue runs from within the anterior supraspinatus at the biceps groove towards the posterior infraspinatus near the middle facet of the greater tuberosity. The "suspension bridge" concept proposes a protective role of the rotator cable in which the free margins

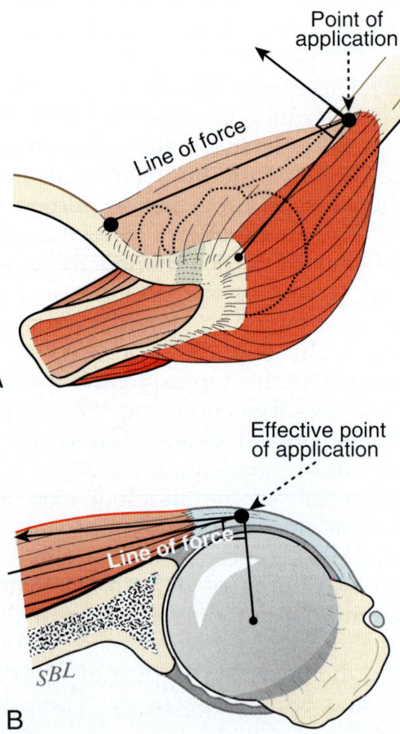

FIGURE 14-25: Effective point of application of muscle force. The torque the muscle exerts is the product of the length of the line from the center of rotation to the effective point of application of the force times the component of the muscle force vector perpendicular to this line. As shown for the deltoid muscle **(A)**, the part of the muscle force vector contributing to adduction torque is only the component of the vector perpendicular to the moment arm. The effective point of application of a muscle force is not necessarily its anatomic insertion **(B)**. (From Matsen FA III, Lippitt SB. *Shoulder Surgery: Principles and Procedures*. Philadelphia: Saunders; 2004:253.)

of the tear correspond to the supports of the cable (Fig. 14-27).[34,40] A tear that occurs within the crescent tissue more lateral to the cable should be shielded from stress as long as the thicker cable tissue is intact. In these tears, the function of the superior cuff would still be intact due to distribution along the length of the cable of the suspension bridge.[216]

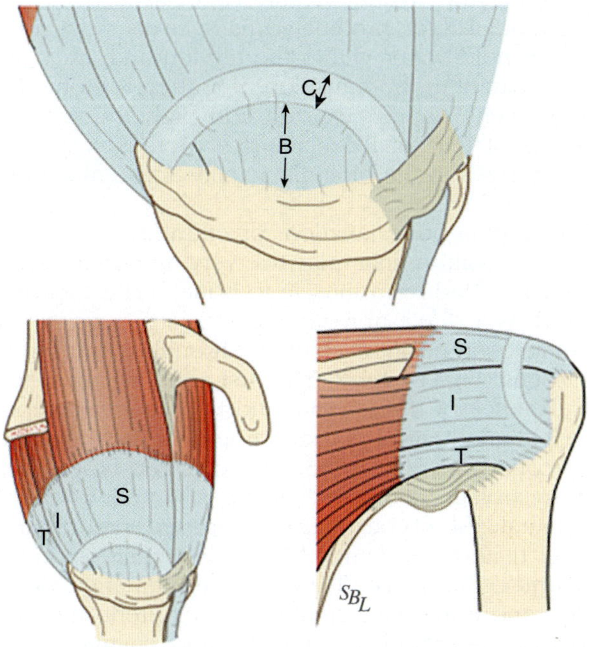

FIGURE 14-26: Superior and posterior views of the rotator cable and crescent. B, Mediolateral diameter of rotator crescent tissue; C, width of rotator cable; I, infraspinatus; S, supraspinatus; T, teres minor. (Modified from Burkhart SS, Esch JC, Jolson RS. The rotator crescent and rotator cable: an anatomic description of the shoulder's "suspension bridge." *Arthroscopy.* 1993;9[6]:611-616.)

Consideration of the biomechanics of the rotator cuff is not limited to the glenohumeral joint but must also include the complex interaction between several other articulations, including the scapulothoracic, acromioclavicular, and sternoclavicular joints. The humeroscapular interface is of particular importance. Smooth, unrestricted motion must occur at this articulation, which consists of the proximal humeral convexity formed by the tuberosity and rotator cuff on one side and the inferior surface of the coracoacromial arch. Because the scapula is the origin of the rotator cuff muscles and the deltoid, it serves as the base for glenohumeral motion.

Nerve lesions, muscle damage, fatigue, or weakness can lead to dyskinetic movement of the scapula on the chest wall. This can lead to a mechanical disadvantage for the cuff muscles, and treatment that involves strengthening the scapular stabilizers can improve rotator cuff function. The scapula is the origin of the cuff musculature, and is supported and stabilized only by muscular and ligamentous (acromioclavicular and coracoclavicular) attachments. The position of the scapula is controlled by scapulothoracic muscles, including the trapezius, levator scapulae, serratus anterior, pectoralis minor, and rhomboids. Fatigue of these stabilizers can lead to inability of the scapula to rotate, subsequently preventing the acromion from clearing when the arm is elevated. Patients treated for scapular dyskinesia with strengthening of the scapular stabilizers can show improvement in rotator cuff mechanics.

BASIC SCIENCE OF CUFF TENDON AND HEALING

Only recently has the basic science behind rotator cuff pathogenesis and healing been investigated. Much of the focus has been on the tendon-to-bone insertion of the cuff, and recent advances and innovation in molecular biology have allowed us to investigate biologic changes that occur

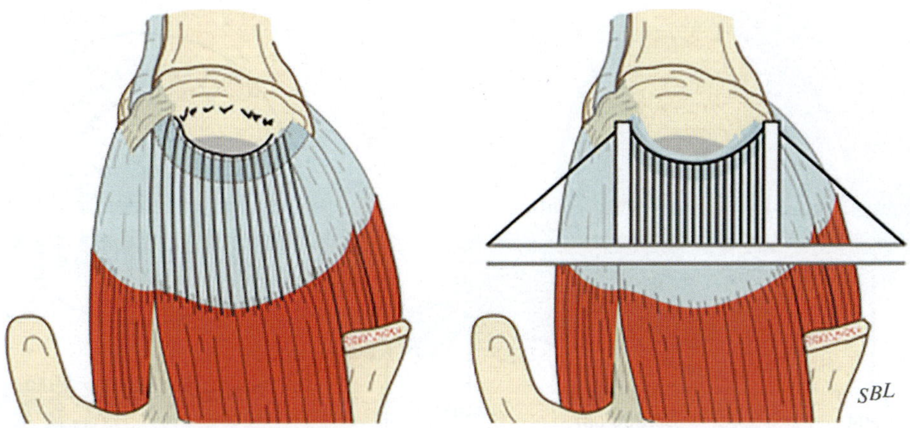

FIGURE 14-27: The rotator cable produces a similar configuration to a suspension bridge. The free margin of the tear corresponds to the cable, and the anterior and posterior attachments of the tear correspond to the supports at the end of each cable. (Modified from Burkhart SS, Esch JC, Jolson RS. The rotator crescent and rotator cable: an anatomic description of the shoulder's "suspension bridge." *Arthroscopy.* 1993;9[6]:611-616.)

during the progression of disease as well as during the healing process. Numerous animal models have been utilized to study healing of this particular enthesis.

Tendon Composition and Structure

The rotator cuff tendons are dense fibrous connective tissue structures with approximately 85% of its dry weight composed of collagen.[193] Of the various collagen types, the majority (95%) is type I with lower levels of type III collagen. Collagen molecules in tendon typically consist of a triple-chain helix composed of a characteristic tripeptide sequence of glycine, proline, and hydroxylproline. Covalent intramolecular and intermolecular crosslinks are produced by the action of various enzymes—this process is the key characteristic that is responsible for the high tensile strength of tendons.[103,144] Collagen molecules are aligned with the longitudinal axis of the tendon to form a collagen fibril, which is the basic structure of tendons. The multiunit hierarchical structure of the tendon proceeds from a collagen fibril to a collagen fiber to a tendon bundle and a tendon fascicle that is bound by endotenon.[150] Tendon fascicles are then grouped to form the tendon unit (Fig. 14-28).[340]

The predominant cell types in tendon are tendon fibroblasts, or tenocytes, which are elongated spindle-shaped cells that are located between the collagen bundles. These fibroblasts have prominent cytoplasmic processes that allow for a complex three-dimensional structural network and cell-to-cell communication.[215,344] This may be important in the tendon's ability to change structure, composition, and mechanical properties in response to mechanical loading. When mechanically loaded, the tendon cells can alter their gene expression and protein synthesis, which subsequently leads to changes in the composition of the extracellular matrix proteins. These cellular mechanisms for mechanotransduction are still being elucidated.

Between these collagen fibers and tendon fibroblasts are numerous noncollagenous matrix components.[326] This extracellular matrix plays a crucial role in the ability of the tendon to transfer large loads from muscle to bone. The matrix/cell ratio in tendon is very high when compared with that in other musculoskeletal tissues. An integral part of the extracellular matrix of tendon is proteoglycans, which are glycoproteins composed of glycosaminoglycan chains. These chains are important for maintaining the hydration and viscoelastic behavior of the tendon. Larger proteoglycans such as versican and aggrecan hold water within the tendon and are particularly important at the transition of tendon to bone. Small proteoglycans such as decorin and biglycan, which are members of the small leucine-rich proteoglycan family, play key roles in the biologic activity and remodeling of tendons.[68,249,290,295]

The tendon-bone junction, or enthesis, is a complex area of transition that plays a very important role in transferring load from muscle to bone.[20] The rotator cuff insertion is a direct fibrocartilaginous structure in which the tissue composition changes through a transition of four zones (Fig. 14-29).[363] The first zone is similar to the midsubstance of the tendon, and is primarily composed of well-aligned type I collagen fibers. In the transition to the second and third zones, the collagen type changes to fibrocartilage composed of types II and III collagen to mineralized fibrocartilage composed predominantly of type II and X collagen.[167] The last zone is primarily bone and contains type I collagen and minerals. Because tendon and bone have significantly different mechanical properties, this gradual transition and change in collagen composition is crucial in dissipating mechanical load as stress is applied to the insertion site.[322] These specialized transition zones are typically not recreated after a rotator cuff repair, and therefore the strength and durability of the repair does not emulate the native enthesis.

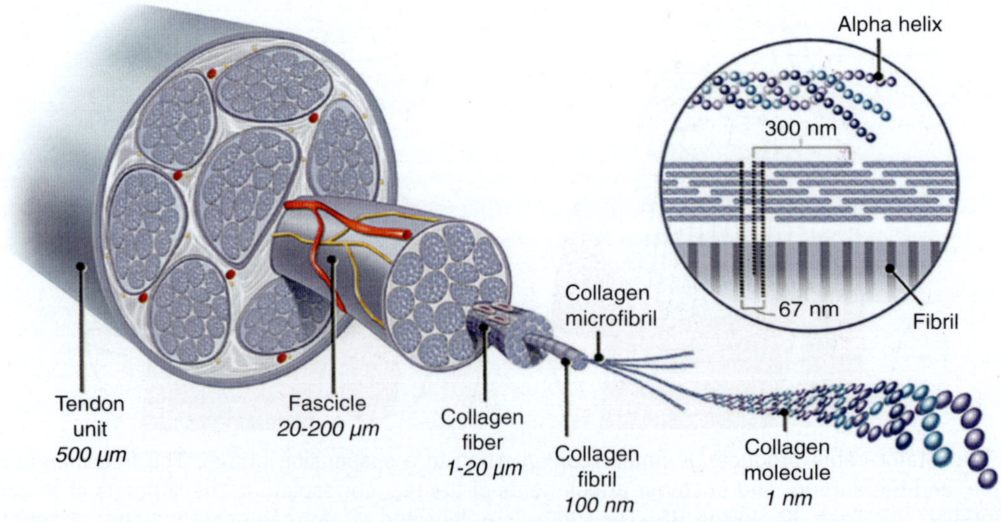

FIGURE 14-28: Schematic of the multiunit hierarchical structure of tendon. (Courtesy University of Washington.)

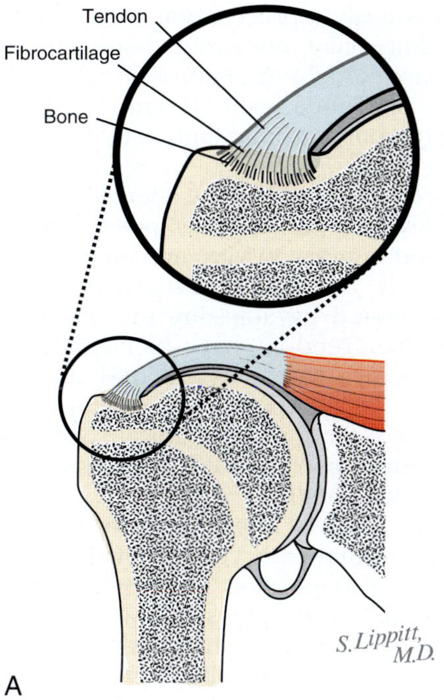

A

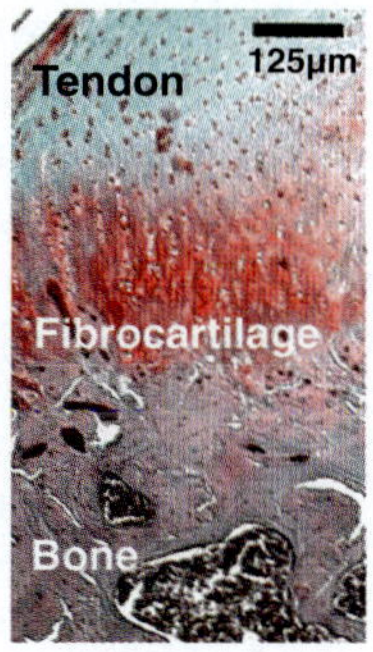

Tissue Region	Cell Type	Major Matrix Componemt
Tendon	Fibroblasts	Collagen types I, III (diameter: 40-400 nm)
Nonmineralized fibrocartilage	Fibrochondrocytes	Collagen types I, II, III
Mineralized fibrocartilage	Hypertrophic Fibrochondrocytes	Collagen types I, II, X
Bone	Osteoblasts Osteocytes Osteoclasts	Collagen types I (diameter: 34.5-39.5 nm)

B

FIGURE 14-29: A, Transition from cuff to bone. The normal tendon insertion to bone is a smooth transition from tendon fibers to fibrocartilage and then to bone. **B,** Structure and composition of tendon-to-bone insertion site with Masson's trichrome staining in a rat. (**A,** From Matsen FA III, Lippitt SB. *Shoulder Surgery: Principles and Procedures*. Philadelphia: Saunders; 2004:250. **B,** From Zhang X, Bogdanowicz D, Erisken C, et al. Biomimetic scaffold design for functional and integrative tendon repair. *J Shoulder Elbow Surg*. 2012;21[2]:266-277.)

Biomechanical Properties

The rotator cuff must be able to transmit large forces with minimal deformation. The biomechanical characteristics of a tendon can be described by its structural and material properties. Structural properties refer to the tensile capacity of the overall structure, and are dependent on the size and shape of the tendon. Material properties refer to the intrinsic quality of the tendon itself, and therefore characterize the tendon independent of size and shape. The structural properties of a tendon are represented by a load displacement curve (Fig. 14-30), while the material properties are best described by their stress-strain relationship (Fig. 14-31). The slope between two defined points of elongation on a load displacement curve represents the stiffness. The slope between two limits of strain represents the elastic modulus of the tendon.

An important characteristic of tendon is its viscoelastic nature. Viscoelastic properties allow for smooth movement during normal joint motion. This characteristic is dependent on the extracellular composition of the tendon. Hysteresis is a viscoelastic characteristic that represents energy that is dissipated during cyclic loading of tendon.

A fundamental biologic response of living musculoskeletal tissue is the ability of the cells to respond to mechanical loading. As load is transferred from the muscle unit through the tendon to bone, the tendon senses external force and will adjust its biomechanical properties in a coordinated response.[14,171,296] Physiologic loads are typically healthy and are required to maintain tendon homeostasis.[92,117] Excessive, repetitive loading or excessive immobility can both have detrimental effects on the structural and material properties of tendon; repetitive loading can result in a catabolic response leading

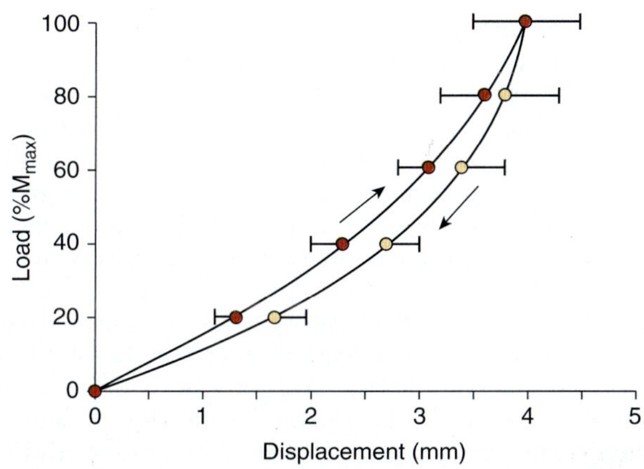

FIGURE 14-30: Load displacement plots of tendon with arrows indicating the loading and unloading directions. The area between the loading and unloading curves is the energy dissipated by viscous damping. (From Maganaris CN, Paul JP. Hysteresis measurements in intact human tendon. *J Biomech*. 2000;33[12]:1723-1727.)

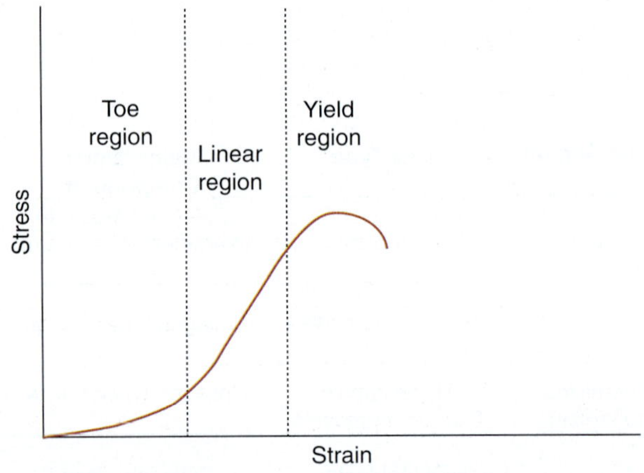

FIGURE 14-31: Stress-strain behavior of ligament showing the toe, linear, and yield regions. (From Freeman JW, Woods MD, Laurencin CT. Tissue engineering of the anterior cruciate ligament using a braid-twist scaffold design. *J Biomech.* 2007;40 [9]:2029-2036.)

to tendinopathy.[5,7,202] This also becomes particularly important when we consider the benefits of controlled loading in prescribing rehabilitation after rotator cuff repair. Determining the optimal magnitude, frequency, and duration of controlled loading has been the focus of numerous animal studies on the pathogenesis of tendinopathy and the healing response after tendon repair.

Tendon Healing

The local environment of the tendon dictates its healing potential. Because rotator cuff tendons are intrasynovial, they do not undergo the spontaneous healing that can be seen in extrasynovial tendons such as the Achilles tendon.

Healing of tendon or ligament typically progresses through three phases: an inflammatory phase that lasts a few days, a proliferative phase that lasts a few weeks, and then a longer remodeling phase that lasts months.[337] In the first phase, inflammatory cells release cytokines and growth factors that lead to recruitment of tendon fibroblasts that proliferate and produce, deposit, and crosslink collagen fibrils. Despite some remodeling, the resultant collagen scar is relatively disorganized and fails to replicate the normal zonal transition at the tendon-bone insertion site.

Modulation of the healing environment has the potential to improve healing rates. The primary targets are the biologic environment and the mechanical environment. Biologic factors can be used to stimulate healing at the time and after surgical repair. Basic fibroblast growth factor can improve angiogenesis and matrix synthesis. Transforming growth factor-β (TGF-β), various bone morphogenetic proteins, vascular endothelial growth factor, and platelet-derived growth factor are all involved in the healing response. Much effort has gone into investigating methods of modulating these growth factors in order to convert a typically reparative scar-forming process to the regenerative scarless healing process that is seen in fetal tendon healing. Additionally, numerous tissue engineering approaches have sought to improve cuff healing using various types of aligned scaffolds aimed at delivering biofactors or promoting cellular ingress to the tendon healing site.[18,245,161]

The mechanical environment can be affected by modifying the activity level of the shoulder postoperatively, and has been studied in many in vitro and animal model studies. Because cuff healing is a mechanosensitive process, it can be altered by adjusting the mechanical load to the repair site. Tendons have biochemical and biomechanical properties that respond and adjust to mechanical loading.[13,154,321,340] Appropriate exercise-related loading can enhance tendon mechanical properties, while repetitive overuse or complete load removal from tendon can lead to deterioration.[90,324,330,345]

When mechanical load is imparted onto a tendon, biochemical changes within tenocytes are evident, along with increased collagen deposition and upregulation of growth factors important in collagen synthesis. Expression of TGF-β and scleraxis, both of which are involved in differentiation and proliferation, is altered with mechanical load.[239,273,294] On the other hand, chronic, repetitive loads on tendons (overuse/overload) can lead to microtrauma and the production of inflammatory mediators such as PGE_2 and LTB_4,[184,346,347] which causes further tendon degeneration and soft tissue edema. The magnitude of load is also important; repetitive mechanical load can have two opposite effects that are dependent on load magnitude.[356] A smaller magnitude decreases MMP-1, COX-2, and IL-1β and has an anti-inflammatory effect, while the opposite is seen with larger magnitudes.

Disuse and immobilization can decrease the stiffness and tensile strength of tendons. Stress deprivation at the repair site induces a catabolic state. mRNA expression of collagenase (MMP-1) is markedly increased in load-deprived tendon cells but significantly inhibited with increasing load to the tendon cells.[9] This suggests that upregulation of MMP-1 expression can be inhibited through a cytoskeletal-based mechanotransduction pathway. A subsequent study by the same group has suggested that load deprivation decreases the mechanoresponsiveness of tendon cells.[8]

CLASSIFICATION OF ROTATOR CUFF PATHOLOGY

The requisites for normal cuff function are stringent, and include healthy, strong cuff muscles, normal capsular laxity, intact cuff tendons, a smooth contour of the undersurface of the coracoacromial arch, a thin, lubricating bursa, a smooth upper surface of the cuff and tuberosities, and concentricity of the glenohumeral and cuff-coracoacromial spheres of rotation. Disorders of this complex mechanism are the most common source of shoulder problems.[45,131]

Rotator cuff pathology spans a spectrum of severity that includes rotator cuff tendinopathy, partial-thickness tears, full-thickness tears, and rotator cuff arthropathy. Physical examination can assist in making the diagnosis, but oftentimes, advanced imaging is required to distinguish tendinosis, partial-thickness tears, and small full-thickness tears—all of which can cause anterolateral shoulder pain.

The terms rotator cuff "tendinitis" and "tendinopathy" are often used interchangeably to describe a broad range of painful conditions of the shoulder. The term "tendinitis" implies inflammation and may be misleading however, because numerous studies have shown that little inflammation is actually present in these syndromes.[151,308] Symptoms related to acute bursitis or tendinitis may respond well in the short term to oral or local antiinflammatories.[208,268,269] However, there is no clear evidence that antiinflammatory medications can reliably improve symptoms related to more chronic "tendinitis," indicating that the terms "tendinosis" or "tendinopathy" may be more appropriate in this setting. Treatment should be focused on therapeutic exercises that can relieve pain and improve function.[206]

Numerous different classification systems have been devised to try to better describe rotator cuff pathology. Neer initially described three different stages of cuff lesions[243]:

- *Stage 1:* Reversible edema and hemorrhage are present in a patient younger than 25 years.
- *Stage 2:* Fibrosis and tendinitis affect the rotator cuff of a patient typically in the 25- to 40-year-old age group. Pain often recurs with activity.
- *Stage 3:* Bone spurs and tendon ruptures are present in a patient older than 40 years.

Neer's original classification of rotator cuff pathology has been subsequently modified by many other classification systems to include the structural integrity of the tendon and also to differentiate between articular-sided partial-thickness tears, bursal-sided partial-thickness tears, and intrasubstance delamination. As imaging techniques and technology advanced with time, classification systems began incorporating more tear characteristics, including tear size, tear shape, and muscular atrophy.

Partial-Thickness Tears

A commonly referenced classification system for partial-thickness tears was described by Ellman, and is based on tear location, depth, and area (Table 14-1)[77]; this is considered a subclassification of the stage 3 cuff lesion described by Neer. Grade 1 involves less than 3 mm of tendon or a quarter of the footprint thickness, grade 2 involves 3 to 6 mm or less than half of the footprint thickness, and grade 3 involves greater than 6 mm of the footprint. Tears are also divided into articular sided, bursal sided, or interstitial.

Snyder et al. devised a more detailed classification system based on arthroscopic findings.[306] In this system, A, B, and C represent articular-sided, bursal-sided, and complete tears. Grade 0 represents a normal rotator cuff, grade 1 is superficial fraying less than 1 cm in size, grade 2 involves fraying 1 to 2 cm in size, grade 3 is tissue disruption in 2 to 3 cm of tendon, and grade 4 is a substantial cuff tear that involves a sizable flap and more than one tendon.

TABLE 14-1 Ellman Classification for Partial-Thickness Rotator Cuff Tears

	Location	Grade	Size
A	Articular	1	<3 mm
B	Bursal	2	3-6 mm
C	Interstitial	3	>6 mm

Modified from Ellman H. Diagnosis and treatment of incomplete rotator cuff tears. Clin Orthop Relat Res. *1990;254:64-74.*

Habermayer et al. also developed a classification for articular-sided tears based on arthroscopic findings that not only accounts for size in the coronal plane but also accounts for sagittal tear extension.[112] In this classification, type A tears involve the coracohumeral ligament up to the medial border of the supraspinatus, type B tears are isolated within the crescent tissue, and type C tears extend from the lateral border of the pulley system over the medial border of the supraspinatus to the crescent tissue.

Despite the numerous types of classifications for partial-thickness tears, studies have demonstrated poor interobserver reliability in distinguishing tears that are greater than and less than 50% using both MRI and arthroscopic examinations.[165,311] Interobserver reliability for distinguishing full-thickness from partial-thickness tears in these studies was much higher.

Full-Thickness Tears

There are numerous classification schemes of full-thickness tears, all of which are extremely diverse in their attempts to describe the tear size, number of tendons involved, tear shape, chronicity, tendon quality, and muscle atrophy.

Tear Size/Number of Tendons Torn

One of the most commonly used classifications for the size of full-thickness rotator cuff tears was described by DeOrio and Cofield.[61] Groups are stratified by tear size from anterior to posterior: less than 1 cm is small, 1 to 3 cm is medium, 3 to 5 cm is large, and more than 5 cm is massive.

A classification system described by Harryman et al. is based on the size and number of tendons involved.[118] Stage 0 is an intact rotator cuff, stage IA is a partial-thickness tear of the supraspinatus, and stage IB is a full-thickness tear involving only the supraspinatus. Stage II includes the supraspinatus and a portion of the infraspinatus. Stage III includes the supraspinatus, infraspinatus, and subscapularis tendons. Stage IV is used to describe rotator cuff arthropathy.

Tear Shape

A classification developed by Ellman and Gartsman attempted to characterize tears by their three-dimensional shapes.[78] This classification includes crescent, reverse L, L-shaped, trapezoidal, and massive tears (Fig. 14-32).

Burkhart also described a classification system based on tear pattern. Type 1 tears are crescent tears that are short on the coronal image but wide on the sagittal image. Type 2 tears are U- or L-shaped tears that are wide on the coronal image and short on the sagittal image. Type 3 tears are massive tears that are wide on both coronal and sagittal imaging. Type 4 tears are massive tears with concomitant glenohumeral arthrosis. The advantage of this classification is the potential for guiding repair technique: type 1 tears may benefit most from tendon-to-bone repair, while type 2 tears may benefit from margin convergence.

Patte Classification

Patte developed a complex and comprehensive classification system that incorporates both tear size coronal and sagittal imaging, tendon retraction, muscle atrophy, and integrity of the long head of the biceps tendon (Box 14-1).[264] Topography in the frontal plane is grouped into three stages (Fig. 14-33A): stage 1 is minimal retraction, stage 2 is tendon retraction to the level of the humeral head, and stage 3 is tendon retraction at the level of the glenoid. In the sagittal plane, tears were grouped into six segments (see Fig. 14-33B and 14-33C).

Muscle Atrophy and Fatty Infiltration

The most common reference for classification of fatty infiltration of the rotator cuff musculature is that described by Goutallier et al.[104] Advanced muscle atrophy typically indicates chronic retraction of a tear, which has been shown to be of prognostic importance and should be considered in all rotator cuff tears. Table 14-2 shows the successive stages of fatty infiltration that were originally described by Goutallier on a sagittal CT cut that incorporates the tip of the coracoid and the inferior glenoid. This classification has since been adapted for use on T1 sagittal oblique imaging on MRI, and Fuchs has simplified the original Goutallier classification to three categories by combining grades 0 and 1 as normal and grades 3 and 4 as advanced degeneration.[84]

Two other methods have been described to characterize the amount of muscle atrophy. Zanetti's "tangent sign" is a simple binary method of defining atrophy. A line is

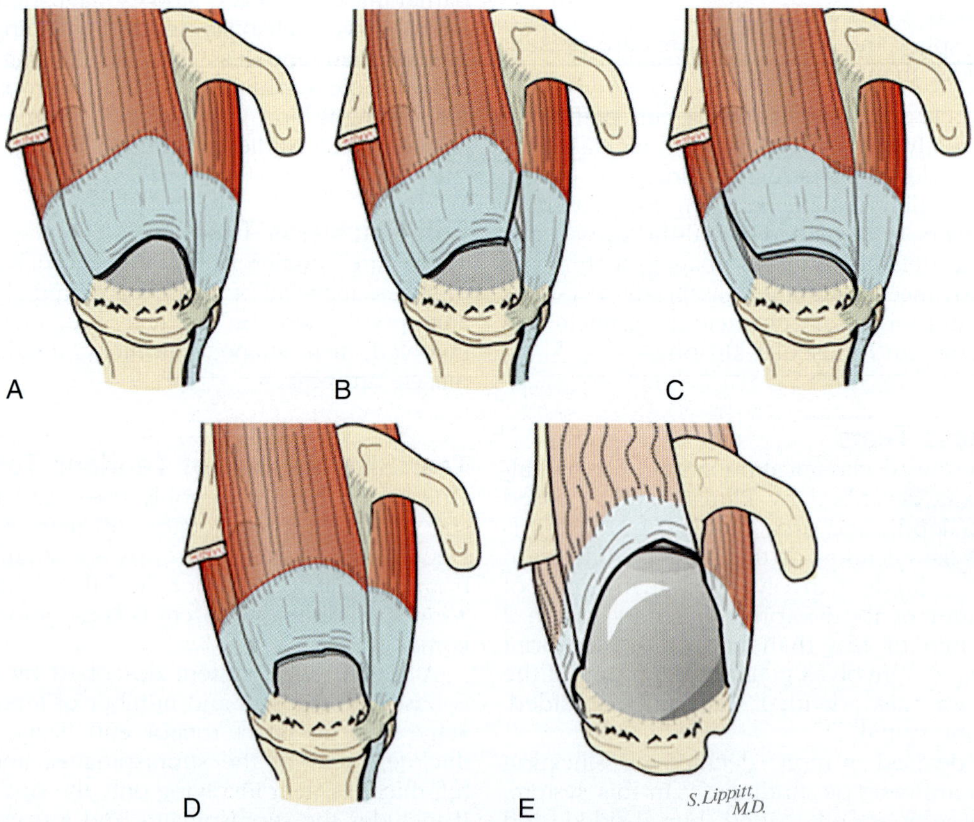

FIGURE 14-32: The Ellman and Gartsman classification of full-thickness rotator cuff tears. A, Crescent; B, reverse L; C, L-shaped; D, trapezoidal; E, massive full-thickness rotator cuff tear. (Modified from Ellman H. Rotator cuff disorders. In: Ellman H, Gartsman GM, eds. *Arthroscopic Shoulder Surgery and Related Disorders*. Philadelphia: Lea & Febiger; 1993.)

BOX 14-1. Patte Classification for Full-Thickness Rotator Cuff Tears

1. Extent of Tear
Group I: Partial tears and full-thickness tears <1 cm in sagittal diameter
A: Deep, partial tears
B. Superficial tears
C. Small, full substance tears
Group II: Full substance tears of the entire supraspinatus
Group III: Full substance tears involving more than one tendon
Group IV: Massive tears with secondary osteoarthritis

2. Topography of Tear in Sagittal Plane
Segment 1: Subscapularis tear
Segment 2: Coracohumeral ligament tear
Segment 3: Isolated supraspinatus tear
Segment 4: Entire supraspinatus and half of infraspinatus tear
Segment 5: Entire supraspinatus and infraspinatus tear
Segment 6: Subscapularis, supraspinatus, and infraspinatus tear

3. Topography of Tears in Frontal Plane
Stage 1: Proximal stump close to bony insertion
Stage 2: Proximal stump at level of humeral head
Stage 3: Proximal stump at level of glenoid

4. Trophic Quality of Muscle of Torn Tendon

5. State of Long Head of Biceps

Modified from Patte D. Classification of rotator cuff lesions. Clin Orthop Relat Res. *1990;254:81-86.*

TABLE 14-2 Goutallier Classification of Fatty Infiltration

Grade 0	Normal muscle without fatty streaks
Grade 1	Muscle has some fatty streaking
Grade 2	Fatty infiltration present, but less than muscle
Grade 3	Equal amount of fat and muscle tissue
Grade 4	More fat than muscle

Modified from Goutallier D, Postel JM, Bernageau J, et al. Fatty muscle degeneration in cuff ruptures. Pre- and postoperative evaluation by CT scan. Clin Orthop Relat Res. *1994;304:78-83.*

drawn from the superior border of the coracoid to the superior border of the scapular spine (Fig. 14-34).[362] If the muscle belly of the supraspinatus fails to intersect this line; the "tangent sign" is positive and indicates significant muscular atrophy. Thomazeau et al. described an "occupation ratio" that takes into account the cross-sectional area of the muscle belly in relation to the size of the fossa.[320] This measurement is performed on a sagittal oblique cut at the level of the medial border of the coracoid process. An occupation ratio between 0.6 and 1.0 is considered normal or indicates slight atrophy; 0.4 to 0.6 indicates moderate atrophy; and less than 0.4 indicates severe atrophy.

Subscapularis Tears

A grading system specific for subscapularis tears was described by LaFosse et al.[168] Type I involves a partial-thickness tear of the superior third of the subscapularis, type II involves a complete tear of the superior one-third, type III involves a complete tear of the superior two-thirds, type IV is a complete tear of the entire tendon with a well-centered head and less than 50% fatty infiltration, and type V is a complete tear with significant fatty infiltration.

CLINICAL EVALUATION AND PHYSICAL EXAMINATION

A comprehensive history is the first and arguably the most important aspect of a complex decision-making process in evaluating a patient with a suspected rotator cuff tear. It will form the foundation of any ongoing diagnostic and therapeutic decisions.

It is now recognized that rotator cuff tears—even ones of substantial size—can be asymptomatic.[232] Furthermore, it is known that the amount of shoulder discomfort experienced by the patient is not related to the size of the tear.[228,69] Pain may not be the primary symptom of rotator cuff failure, which may also produce weakness, stiffness, crepitus, or instability.

The patient's physiologic and chronologic age should be considered throughout history and examination. Degenerative tearing typically occurs in older patients, while a greater injury is required to tear the cuff of persons at the younger end of the age distribution. Traumatic glenohumeral dislocations in persons older than 40 years have a strong association with rotator cuff tears. Age is thought to be a strong predictor of rotator cuff healing if operative intervention is a consideration—older patients are less likely to achieve a durable repair.

Chronicity is one of many important tear characteristics that have an impact on healing potential. Acute rotator cuff tears from a distinct injury causing weakness often do well, and have good healing potential with early surgery. In these patients, the acute component of their shoulder pain must be differentiated by history and imaging from more chronic symptoms that may have preceded the injury. More often, patients who present with a painful shoulder problem have endured their symptoms for months or years as a result of cuff degeneration rather than injury.

Activity level and expectations of treatment are an essential part of the overall decision-making process and discussion with the patient. An inactive patient without

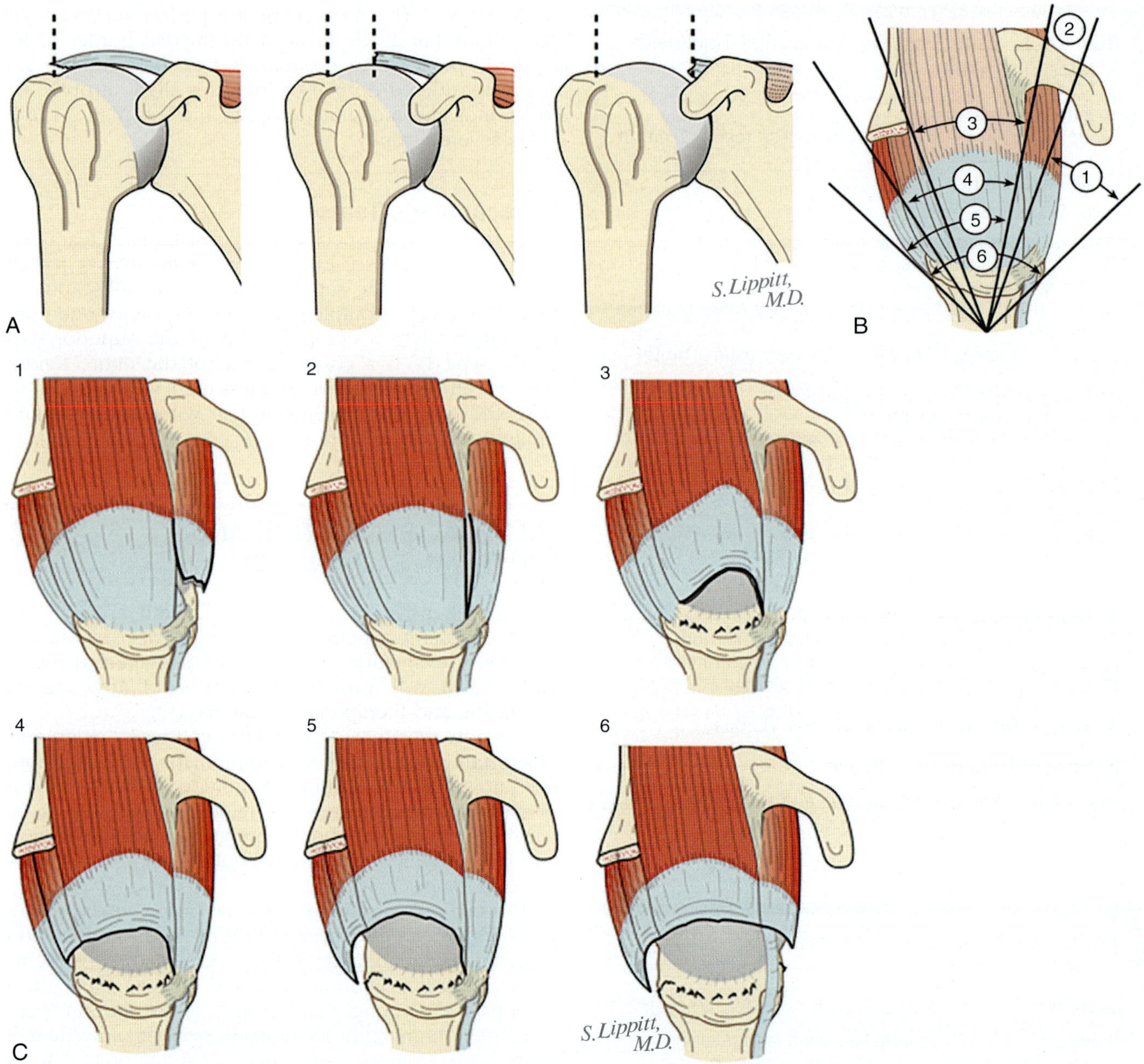

FIGURE 14-33: Patte classification of full-thickness rotator cuff tears in the (**A**) frontal and (**B** and **C**) sagittal planes. 1, Subscapularis tear; 2, coracohumeral ligament tear; 3, isolated supraspinatus tear; 4, tear of entire supraspinatus, half of infraspinatus; 5, tear of supraspinatus and infraspinatus; 6, tear of subscapularis, supraspinatus, and infraspinatus. (Modified from Patte D. Classification of rotator cuff lesions. *Clin Orthop Relat Res.* 1990;254:81-86.)

high functional demands will likely be able to perform activities of daily living without difficulty even with a full-thickness rotator cuff tear treated nonoperatively. On the other hand, even a small full-thickness tear could present difficulties to a young laborer with high functional demands who requires overhead strength. Hand dominance, smoking, genetic predisposition, medical comorbidities, and social factors affecting rehabilitation after potential surgery are variables that should be taken into account when deciding between nonoperative and operative care.

In all patients, prior treatment including physical therapy, injections, and previous surgery should be noted. Also, any neck pain, numbness and tingling in the arm, symptoms radiating below the elbow, or medial scapular pain may be a sign of cervical radiculopathy. In these patients, a comprehensive cervical spine examination should follow.

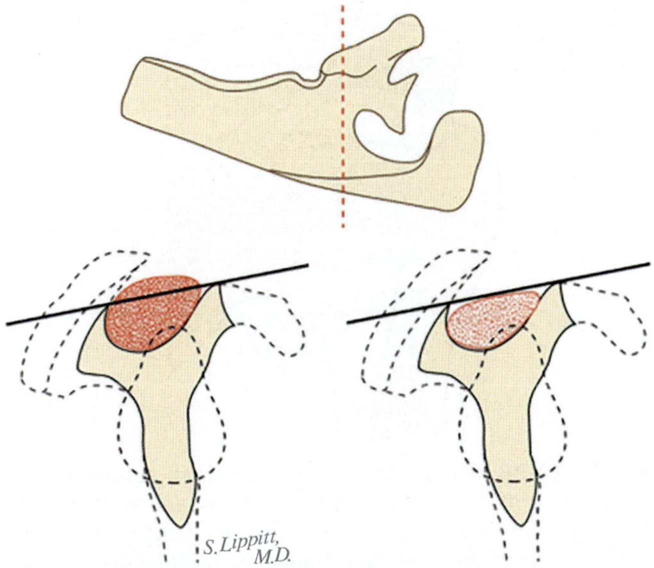

FIGURE 14-34: Zanetti's "tangent sign" for defining muscular atrophy. (Modified from Zanetti M, Gerber C, Hodler J. Quantitative assessment of the muscles of the rotator cuff with magnetic resonance imaging. *Invest Radiol*. 1998;33[3]:163-170.)

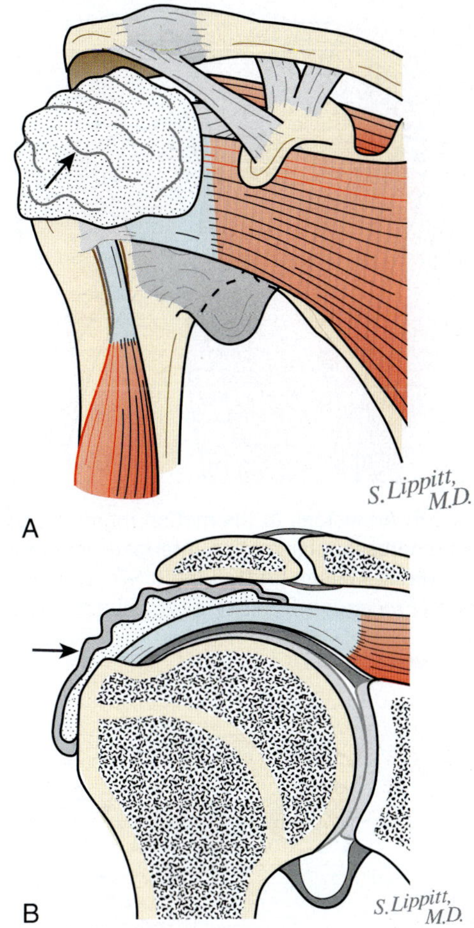

FIGURE 14-35: Thick bursa. Thickened bursa (*arrow*) interferes with the smooth articulation of the proximal humeral convexity with the coracoacromial concavity. **A,** Frontal view. **B,** Cross-sectional view. (From Matsen FA III, Lippitt SB. *Shoulder Surgery: Principles and Procedures*. Philadelphia: Saunders; 2004:419.)

Physical Examination

A standardized physical examination should include inspection, range of motion, and strength testing in order to assess the various clinical manifestations of cuff disease including stiffness, weakness, instability, and roughness. An especially relevant point in the physical examination is an accurate assessment of the strength of the rotator cuff musculature, deltoid muscle, and scapular stabilizers. This physical assessment often forms the basis of any ongoing management program.

The patient's shoulder should be exposed for inspection and palpation. If cuff dysfunction has been present for more than a few months, it may be accompanied by supraspinatus and infraspinatus muscle atrophy. Subtle atrophy can be seen most easily by casting a shadow from a light over the patient's head. Clear visualization of the supraspinatus and infraspinatus fossae can be a distinct sign of chronic atrophy. Additionally, the location of any surgical incisions can help the examiner determine the nature of any previous surgeries, particularly if the patient's history of previous shoulder surgery was remote.

Crepitus should be noted with palpation of the shoulder during range of motion. *Roughness* associated with cuff disease is manifested as symptomatic crepitus on passive glenohumeral motion. Bursal hypertrophy (Fig. 14-35), adhesions (Fig. 14-36), secondary changes in the undersurface of the coracoacromial arch, loss of integrity and smoothness of the upper aspect of the cuff tendons (Figs. 14-37 and 14-38), and uncovering of the tuberosities (Fig. 14-39) can all contribute to *subacromial abrasion*. Crepitus from subacromial abrasion is easily detected by placing the examiner's thumb and fingers on the anterior and posterior aspects of the acromion while the humerus is moved relative to the scapula (Figs. 14-40 and 14-41). Because many shoulders demonstrate asymptomatic subacromial crepitus, it is important during the examination to ask whether the crepitus noted by the examiner reproduces the patient's complaints.

Tendon defects can also be assessed by palpation of the shoulder. As pointed out by Codman,[51] defects in the cuff can often be palpated by rotating the proximal end of the humerus under the examiner's finger placed at the anterior corner of the acromion. The perimeters of the divot left by a defect in the supraspinatus are particularly easy to palpate. The defect is usually just posterior to the bicipital groove and medial to the greater tuberosity (Figs. 14-42 to 14-44).

Limitations in passive and active range of motion should be documented. Restriction in motion due to arthritis or adhesive capsulitis needs to be ruled out. Stiffness often presents as a result of partial-thickness cuff lesions, but it can also be associated with full-thickness

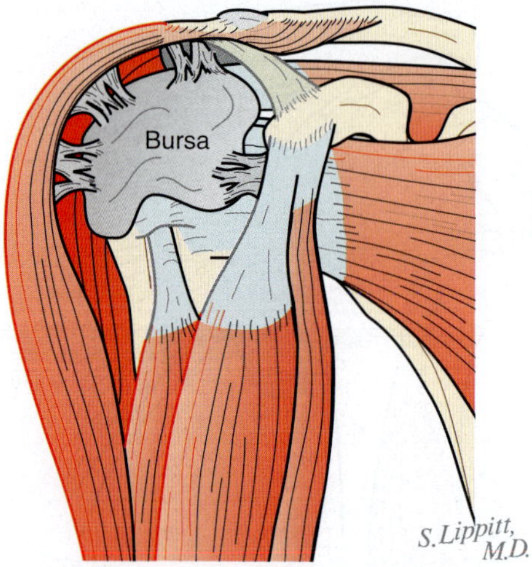

FIGURE 14-36: Adhesions in the motion interface. Scar tissue across the humeroscapular motion interface limits motion and smoothness. (From Matsen FA III, Lippitt SB. *Shoulder Surgery: Principles and Procedures*. Philadelphia: Saunders; 2004:333.)

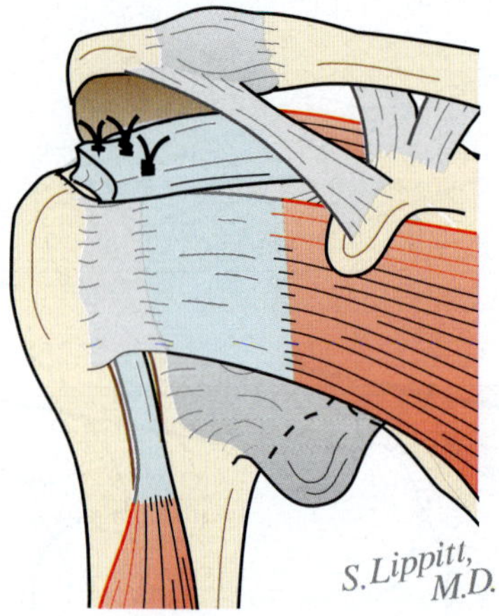

FIGURE 14-38: Suture knots. The knots from sutures tied on top of the cuff can contribute to humeroscapular roughness. (From Matsen FA III, Lippitt SB. *Shoulder Surgery: Principles and Procedures*. Philadelphia: Saunders; 2004:420.)

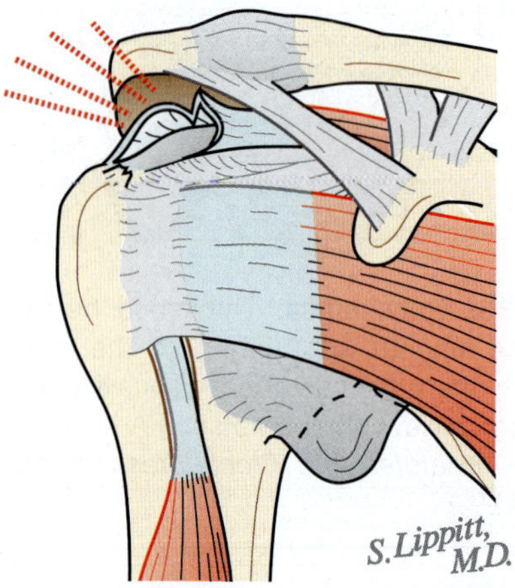

FIGURE 14-37: Cuff tear edge. The edges of a torn cuff are a common cause of subacromial roughness (*red dotted lines*). (From Matsen FA III, Lippitt SB. *Shoulder Surgery: Principles and Procedures*. Philadelphia: Saunders; 2004:420.)

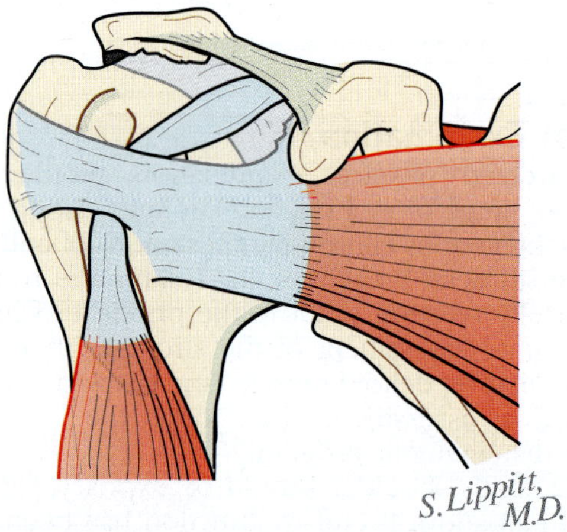

FIGURE 14-39: Prominent tuberosity. When the cuff is absent from its insertion, the tuberosity is proud relative to the humeral convexity and disrupts smooth motion. (From Matsen FA III, Lippitt SB: *Shoulder Surgery: Principles and Procedures*. Philadelphia: Saunders; 2004:421.)

cuff defects.[135] Stiffness may be demonstrable as limitations in the following:

- Flexion—degrees from the neutral position (Fig. 14-45)
- External rotation—degrees from the neutral position (Fig. 14-46)
- Internal rotation reaching up the back—posterior segment reached with thumb (Fig. 14-47)
- External rotation in abduction—degrees from neutral position (Fig. 14-48)
- Internal rotation in abduction—degrees from neutral position (Fig. 14-49)
- Cross-body adduction—centimeters from the ipsilateral antecubital fossa to the contralateral acromion or coracoid (Fig. 14-50).

Although patients with full-thickness cuff defects might still retain the ability to actively abduct the arm,[246] significant tendon fiber failure is usually manifested by weakness on manual muscle testing.[122,30,175,176] *Isometric* testing of muscle strength prevents confusion with symptoms that can arise from shoulder movement (such as those associated with subacromial abrasion). Although individual cuff muscles are difficult to specifically isolate

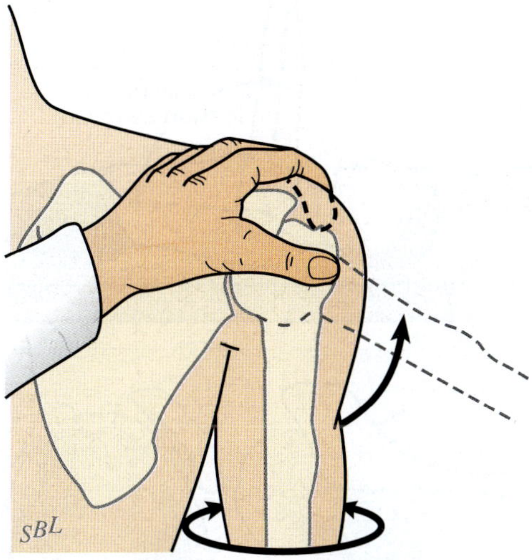

FIGURE 14-40: Palpation for crepitus. The examiner can palpate the rotator cuff for crepitus by placing one hand on the scapula with the index finder just anterior to the acromion while the arm is moved through its full range of motion. (From Matsen FA III, Lippitt SB. *Shoulder Surgery: Principles and Procedures*. Philadelphia: Saunders; 2004:282.)

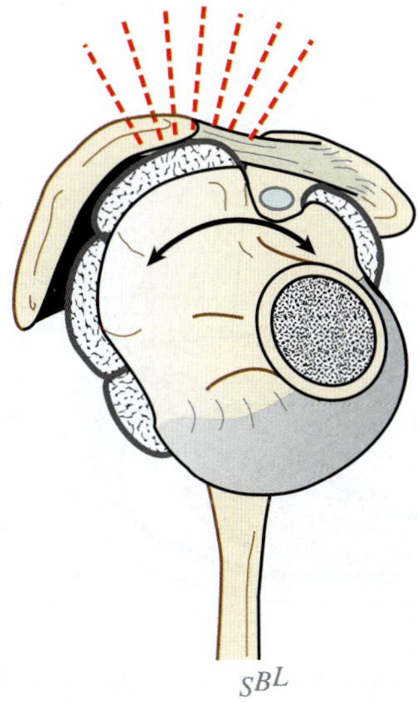

FIGURE 14-41: Abrasion test. The existence and location of the cause of subacromial abrasion (*red dashed lines*) can be detected at surgery by passively rotating the proximal humerus beneath the coracoacromial arch in different positions of flexion and abduction *(arrow)*. The cause of the roughness is almost universally on the proximal humeral convexity rather than on the coracoacromial concavity. (From Matsen FA III, Lippitt SB. *Shoulder Surgery: Principles and Procedures*. Philadelphia: Saunders; 2004:298.)

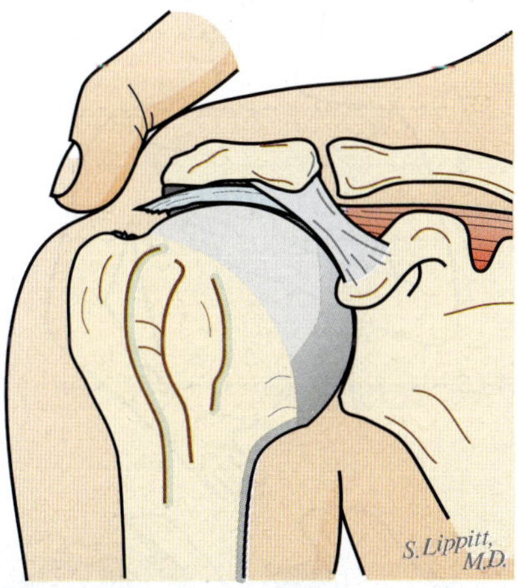

FIGURE 14-42: Palpation of cuff defect. Defects in the tendinous cuff can often be palpated through the overlying skin and deltoid. (From Matsen FA III, Lippitt SB. *Shoulder Surgery: Principles and Procedures*. Philadelphia: Saunders; 2004:283.)

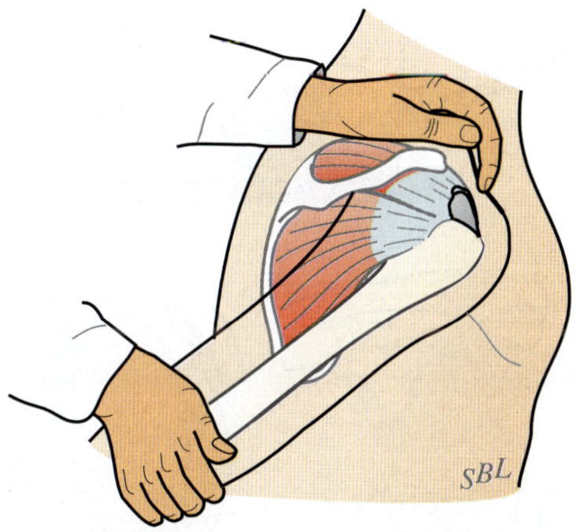

FIGURE 14-43: Palpation of supraspinatus defect. The accessibility of the supraspinatus tendon for palpation can be enhanced by extending the arm. (From Matsen FA III, Lippitt SB. *Shoulder Surgery: Principles and Procedures*. Philadelphia: Saunders; 2004:283.)

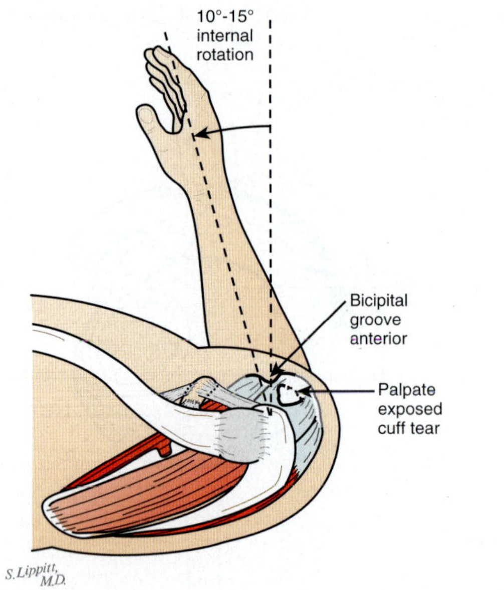

FIGURE 14-44: Reference to bicipital groove. The bicipital groove is normally straight anterior when the arm (with a flexed elbow) is in 10 to 15 degrees of internal rotation. Reference to these anatomic landmarks can help locate the tear. (From Matsen FA III, Lippitt SB. *Shoulder Surgery: Principles and Procedures*. Philadelphia: Saunders; 2004:283.)

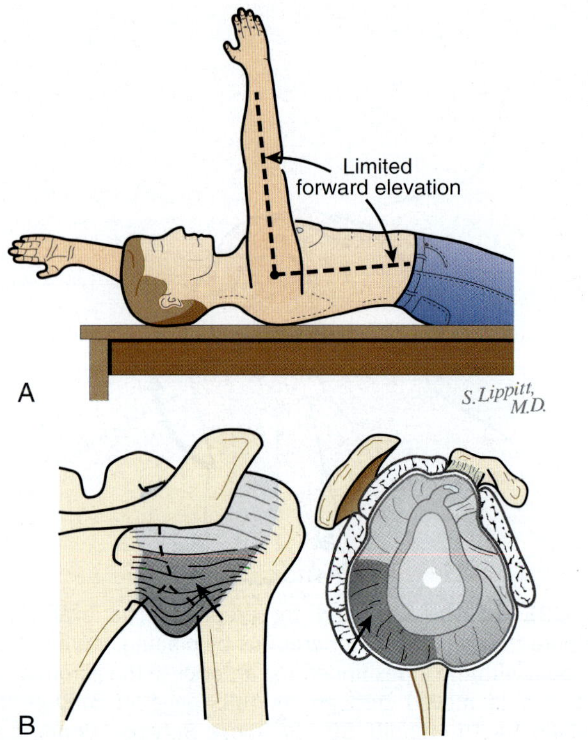

FIGURE 14-45: Limited forward elevation. **A,** Tightness of the posteroinferior capsule can limit glenohumeral forward elevation, also known as flexion. **B,** Tight portion of the capsule. (From Matsen FA III, Lippitt SB. *Shoulder Surgery: Principles and Procedures*. Philadelphia: Saunders, 2004;50.)

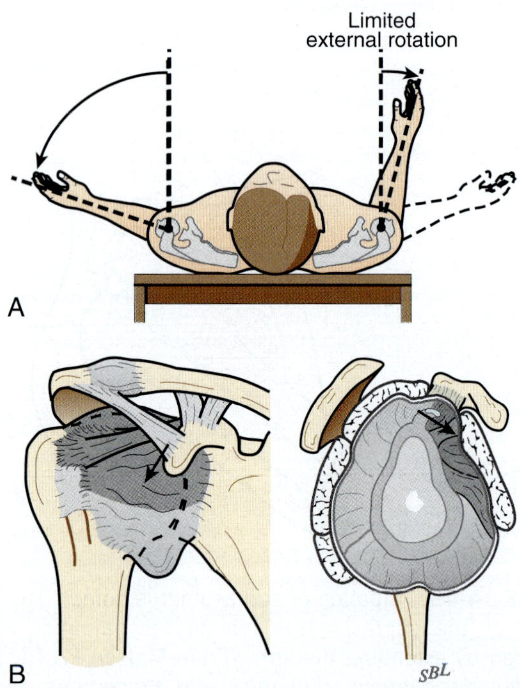

FIGURE 14-46: Limited external rotation in adduction. **A,** Tightness of the anterior-superior capsule and coracohumeral ligament can limit external rotation of the arm at the side. **B,** Tight portion of the capsule. (From Matsen FA III, Lippitt SB. *Shoulder Surgery: Principles and Procedures*. Philadelphia: Saunders, 2004:52.)

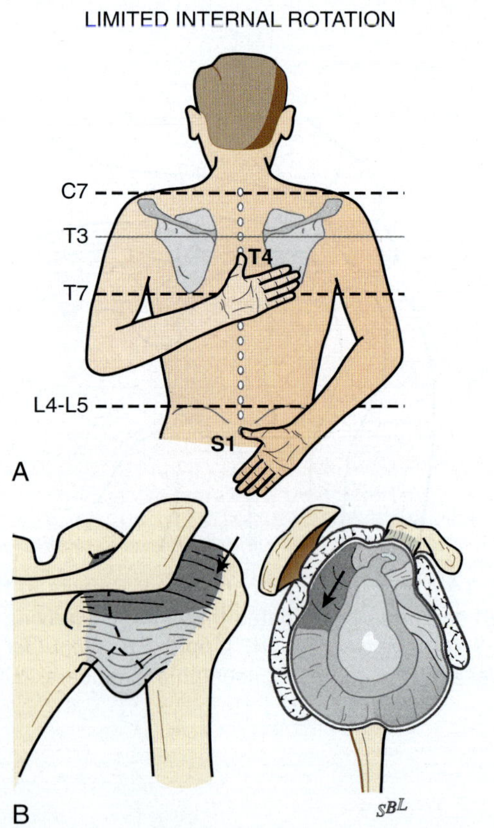

FIGURE 14-47: Limited internal rotation. **A,** Tightness of the posterior-superior capsule can limit glenohumeral internal rotation. **B,** Tight portion of the capsule. (From Matsen FA III, Lippitt SB. *Shoulder Surgery: Principles and Procedures*. Philadelphia: Saunders; 2004:51.)

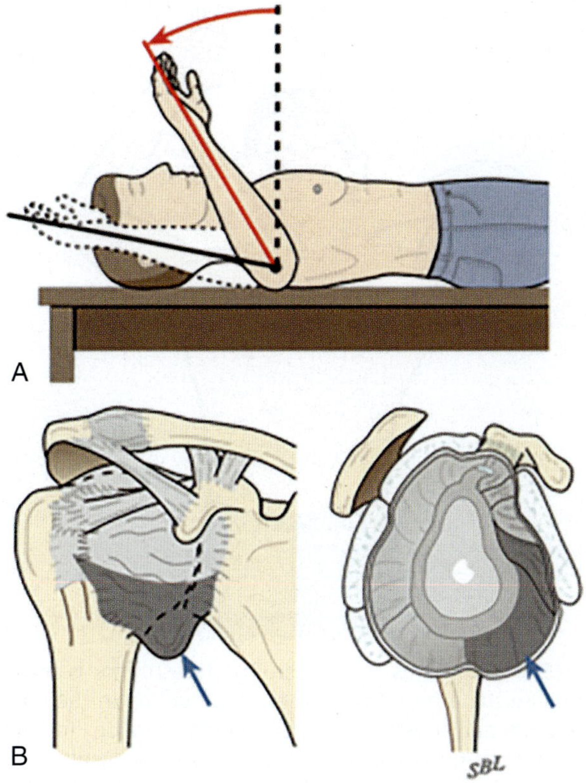

FIGURE 14-48: Limited external rotation in abduction. **A,** Tightness of the anterior-inferior capsule can limit external rotation of the arm in abduction. **B,** Tight portion of the capsule.

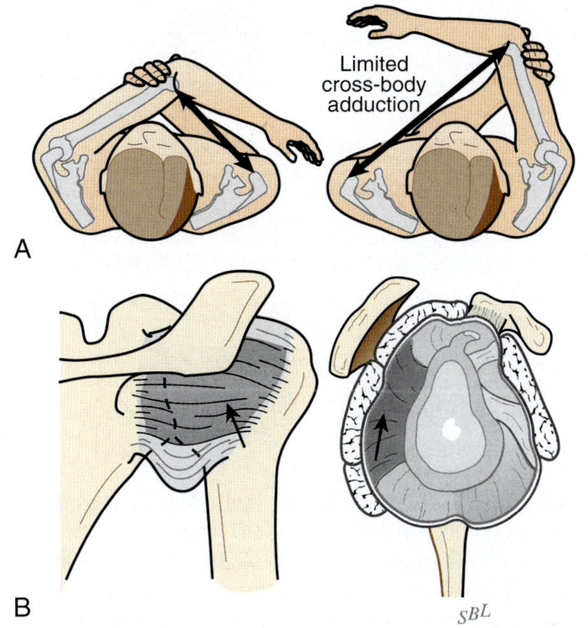

FIGURE 14-50: Limited cross-body adduction. **A,** Tightness of the posterior capsule can limit adduction of the arm across the body. **B,** Tight portion of the capsule. (From Matsen FA III, Lippitt SB. *Shoulder Surgery: Principles and Procedures*. Philadelphia: Saunders; 2004:53.)

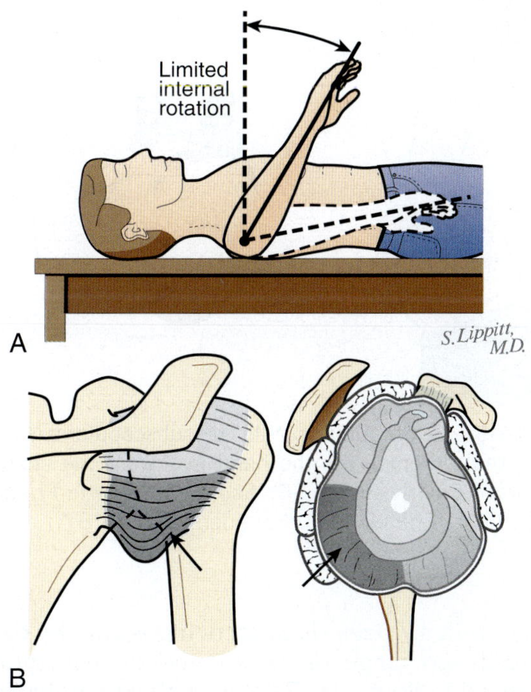

FIGURE 14-49: Limited internal rotation in abduction. **A,** Tightness of the posterior-inferior capsule can limit internal rotation of the abducted arm. **B,** Tight portion of the capsule. (From Matsen FA III, Lippitt SB. *Shoulder Surgery: Principles and Procedures*. Philadelphia: Saunders; 2004:55.)

given the interdigitation of their tendon insertions, the following isometric tests are reasonably selective:

- *Supraspinatus:* Isometric elevation of the arm held in 90 degrees of elevation in the plane of the scapula and in mild internal rotation (Fig. 14-51)
- *Infraspinatus:* Isometric external rotation of the arm held at the side in neutral rotation with the elbow flexed to 90 degrees (Fig. 14-52)
- *Teres minor:* Isometric external rotation of the arm in 90 degrees of abduction with the elbow flexed to 90 degrees (Fig. 14-53)
- *Subscapularis:* Isometric internal rotation of the arm with the elbow flexed to 90 degrees and the hand pressing in toward the stomach (Fig. 14-54); alternatively, isometric internal rotation of the arm with the back of the hand on the lumbar area (Fig. 14-55)

These simple manual tests are helpful for characterizing the size of the tendon defect, from single tendon tears involving only the supraspinatus to two-tendon tears involving the supraspinatus and infraspinatus, as well as three-tendon tears involving the subscapularis. Some have suggested that weakness from pain inhibition can be distinguished from weakness from a tendon defect by subacromial injection of a local anesthetic.[190,19] It is important to keep in mind, notes Kibler et al., that apparent supraspinatus weakness on clinical examination can depend on scapular position. The weakness can result from other factors besides supraspinatus muscle

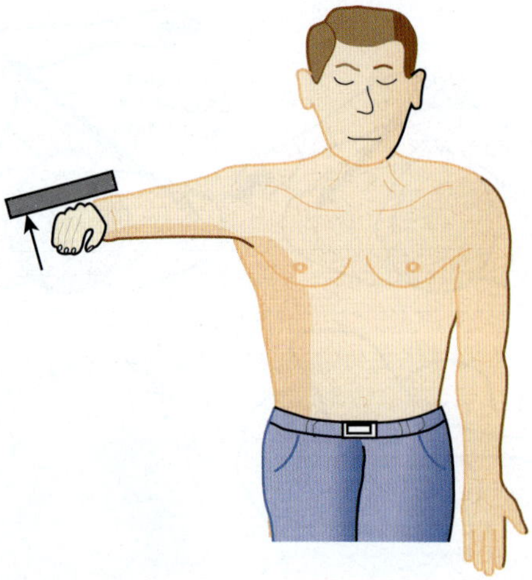

FIGURE 14-51: Supraspinatus test. The supraspinatus is tested by positioning the arm in 90 degrees of abduction in the plane of the scapula and in slight internal rotation; this puts the supraspinatus tendon on top of the humeral head. The patient holds this position while the examiner attempts to adduct the arm. (From Matsen FA III, Lippitt SB. *Shoulder Surgery: Principles and Procedures*. Philadelphia: Saunders; 2004:286.)

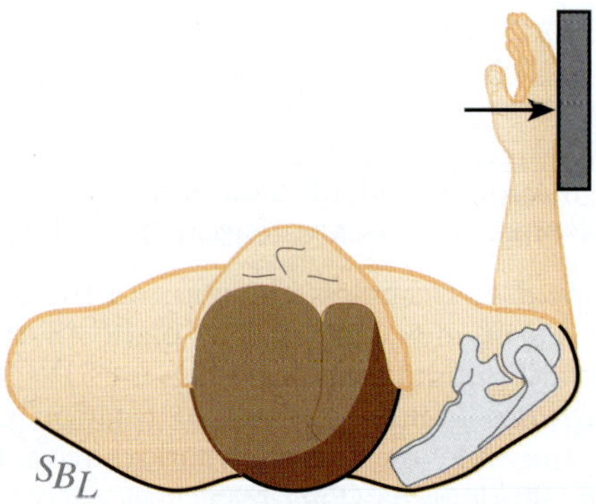

FIGURE 14-52: Infraspinatus test. The infraspinatus is tested by positioning the humerus with the elbow at the side and the forearm pointing straight ahead. The patient holds this position while the examiner attempts to push the arm into internal rotation. (From Matsen FA III, Lippitt SB. *Shoulder Surgery: Principles and Procedures*. Philadelphia: Saunders; 2004:287.)

weakness, such as a lack of a stable base in the kinetic chain or scapula.[153]

Differential Diagnosis

Traditionally, it has been stated that rotator cuff tears must be differentiated from cuff *tendinitis* and *bursitis*, and that tests such as arthrography and ultrasonography are necessary to make this distinction. Perhaps a more realistic view is that many of the symptoms often attributed to tendinitis and bursitis are, in actuality, episodes of acute fiber failure that are not clinically detected.

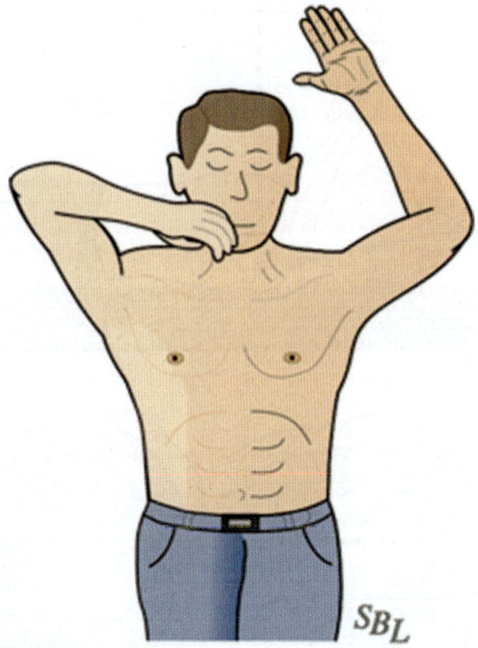

FIGURE 14-53: Teres minor test. The teres minor is tested by positioning the arm in 90 degrees of abduction in the plane of the scapula and in 90 degrees of external rotation. Inability to hold this position is considered a positive test result.

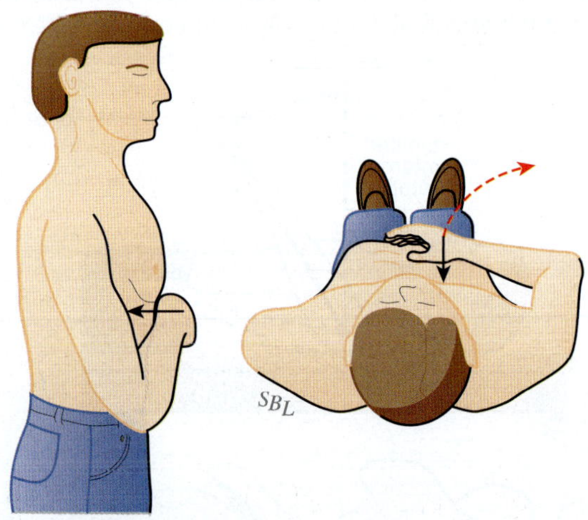

FIGURE 14-54: Subscapularis test. The subscapularis is tested by having the patient press the hand in toward the stomach. (From Matsen FA III, Lippitt SB. *Shoulder Surgery: Principles and Procedures*. Philadelphia: Saunders; 2004:287.)

Patients with a *frozen shoulder* demonstrate, by definition, a restricted range of passive motion with normal glenohumeral radiographs. Patients with partial-thickness cuff defects might similarly demonstrate motion restriction, whereas patients with major full-thickness defects usually have a good range of passive shoulder motion but may be limited in strength or range of active motion. An arthrogram in the case of frozen shoulder shows a

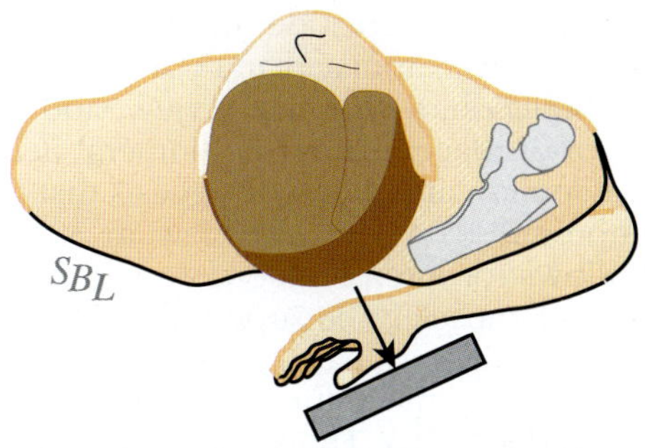

FIGURE 14-55: Lift-off test. The subscapularis can also be tested by having the patient push the hand away from the lumbar area posteriorly against resistance. (From Matsen FA III, Lippitt SB. *Shoulder Surgery: Principles and Procedures.* Philadelphia: Saunders; 2004:287.)

diminished volume and obliteration of the normal recesses of the joint.

A *snapping scapula* can produce shoulder pain on elevation and a catching sensation somewhat reminiscent of the subacromial snap of a cuff tear. However, the latter can usually be elicited with the scapula stabilized while the arm is rotated in the flexed and somewhat abducted position. Scapular snapping generally arises from the superomedial corner of the scapula and produces local discomfort; scapular movement without glenohumeral motion elicits it.

Glenohumeral arthritis can also produce shoulder pain, weakness, and catching. This diagnosis can be reliably differentiated from rotator cuff disease by a careful history, physical examination, and roentgenographic analysis.

Acromioclavicular arthritis can imitate cuff disease. Characteristically, however, the shoulder is most painful with cross-body movements and with activities requiring strong contraction of the pectoralis major. Tenderness is commonly limited to the acromioclavicular joint. Relief of pain on selective lidocaine injection and coned-down radiographs can help establish the diagnosis of acromioclavicular arthritis.

Suprascapular neuropathy and cervical radiculopathy are common imitators of cuff disease. The suprascapular nerve and the fifth and sixth cervical nerve roots supply two of the most important cuff muscles: the supraspinatus and infraspinatus. Thus patients with involvement of these structures can have lateral shoulder pain, and can lack strength of elevation and external rotation.

In the presence of weakness, the neurologic examination should test the cutaneous distribution of the nerve roots from C5 to T1. The biceps reflex and the triceps reflex help screen C5-C6 and C7-C8, respectively. The next component of the neurologic examination requires verifying the integrity of the segmental innervation of joint motion: Abduction, C5; adduction, C6, C7, and C8; external rotation, C5; internal rotation, C6, C7, and C8; elbow flexion, C5 and C6; elbow extension, C7 and C8; wrist extension and flexion, C6 and C7; finger flexion and extension, C7 and C8; and finger adduction and abduction, T1.

A set of screening tests checks the motor and sensory components of the major peripheral nerves; the axillary nerve: the anterior, middle, and posterior parts of the deltoid and the skin just above the deltoid insertion; the radial nerve: the extensor pollicis longus and the skin over the first dorsal web space; the median nerve: the opponens pollicis and the skin over the pulp of the index finger; the ulnar nerve: the first dorsal interosseous and the skin over the pulp of the little finger; and the musculocutaneous nerve: the biceps muscle and the skin over the lateral aspect of the forearm. The long thoracic nerve is checked by having the patient elevate the arm 60 degrees in the anterior sagittal plane while the examiner pushes down on the arm and looks for winging of the scapula posteriorly. Observing the strength of the shoulder shrug checks the nerve of the trapezius. Lesions of the suprascapular nerve produce weakness of elevation and external rotation without sensory loss.

Clinical conditions affecting these structures include cervical spondylosis involving C5 and C6, brachial plexopathy involving the suprascapular nerve, traction injuries (as in the mechanism of Erb's palsy), suprascapular nerve entrapment at the suprascapular notch, pressure on the inferior branch of the suprascapular nerve from a ganglion cyst at the spinoglenoid notch, traumatic severance in fractures, or iatrogenic injury.*

Cervical spondylosis involving the fifth and sixth cervical nerve roots can imitate or mask rotator cuff involvement by producing pain in the lateral aspect of the shoulder as well as weakness of shoulder flexion, abduction, and external rotation. Cervical radiculopathy is suggested if the patient has pain on neck extension or on turning the chin to the affected side. Pain of cervical origin more commonly includes the area of the trapezius muscle along with the area of the deltoid, and can radiate down the arm to the hand. Sensory, motor, or reflex abnormalities in the distribution of the fifth or sixth cervical nerve root provide additional support for the diagnosis of cervical radiculopathy. Inasmuch as many asymptomatic patients have degenerative changes at the C5-C6 area, cervical spine radiographs are not a specific diagnostic tool. When mild cervical spondylosis is suspected, it is practical to implement a rehabilitation program without an extensive diagnostic workup. This program includes gentle neck mobility exercises, isometric neck-strengthening exercises, home traction, and protection of the neck from positions that aggravate the condition during sleep. If the condition is unresponsive or severe, additional evaluation by electromyography or MRI, or both, may be indicated.

Suprascapular neuropathy is characterized by dull pain over the shoulder that is exacerbated by movement of the shoulder, weakness in overhead activities, wasting of the supraspinatus and infraspinatus muscles, weakness of external rotation, and normal radiographic

---

References 12, 17, 31, 49, 65, 66, 72, 79, 94, 136, 162, 163, 201, 240, 271, 278, 281, 292, 293, 307, 314, 332, 342.

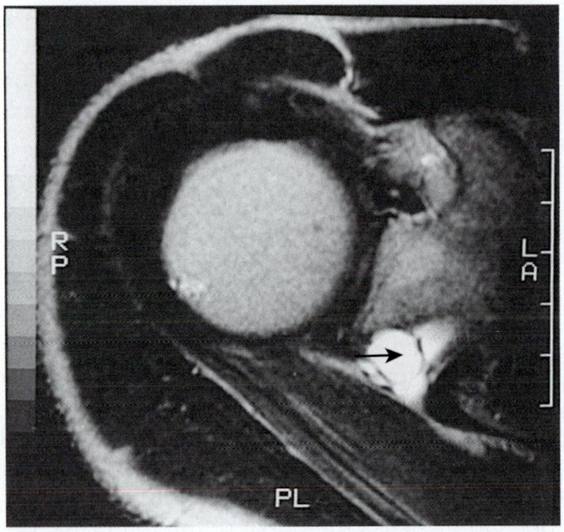

FIGURE 14-56: Magnetic resonance image showing a ganglion cyst in the spinoglenoid notch (*arrow*). Cysts in this location can press on the nerve to the infraspinatus, which runs through this notch. Symptoms can include pain and weakness of external rotation, somewhat similar to the symptoms of cuff disease.

evaluation. This condition can arise from suprascapular nerve traction injuries, suprascapular nerve entrapment, brachial neuritis affecting the suprascapular nerve, or a ganglion cyst in the spinoglenoid notch. The first three should involve the nerve supply to both the supraspinatus and infraspinatus, and are most easily differentiated by the history. Traction injuries to the suprascapular nerve are usually associated with a history of a violent downward pull on the shoulder, and may be a part of a larger Erb's palsy–type injury to the brachial plexus. Suprascapular nerve entrapment can produce chronic recurrent pain and weakness aggravated by shoulder use. Brachial neuritis often produces a rather intense pain lasting for several weeks, with the onset of weakness being noted as the pain subsides.

A ganglion cyst in the spinoglenoid notch usually arises from a defect in the posterior shoulder joint capsule, and can press on the nerve to the infraspinatus as it passes through the notch. These cysts are well seen on MRI (Fig. 14-56). Depending on the site of the suprascapular nerve lesion, electromyography can indicate involvement of the infraspinatus alone or involvement of this muscle along with the supraspinatus.

None of these conditions should produce cuff defects on shoulder MRI, ultrasonography, or arthrography. However, as shown by Albritton et al., the degree of rotator cuff muscle atrophy commonly observed after a massive tear may be explained by increased tension on the suprascapular nerve due to muscle retraction.[2]

IMAGING OF THE ROTATOR CUFF

Plain radiographs of the shoulder can be obtained as a standard evaluation of any patient with suspected rotator cuff abnormality. These include an anteroposterior (AP) view, true AP in the scapular plane (Grashey view) in 30 degrees of abduction, a scapular Y view, and an axillary view. Superior displacement of the humeral head in relation to the acromion and glenoid suggests that the rotator cuff is compromised. A Grashey view in 30 degrees of abduction allows for interpretation of plain films with an activated deltoid muscle. The superiorly directed force of the activated deltoid can make proximal humeral migration more evident in the setting of a large, chronic tear (Fig. 14-57A and 14-57B). The scapular Y view can characterize acromial morphology. An axillary view should be obtained with the arm in the scapular plane in neutral rotation. Adequate visualization of "the eye" or the spinoglenoid notch is important in ensuring correct rotation. This axillary view is important in assessing joint space narrowing associated with arthritis and anterior or posterior joint subluxation.

MRI

MRI is now the most often used imaging modality for comprehensive assessment of the shoulder. It can be used to assess the rotator cuff, labrum, capsule, and cartilage. A standard protocol for the rotator cuff should include T1-weighted, fat-saturated proton-density (PD)-weighted, and fat-saturated T2-weighted imaging in the oblique coronal, oblique sagittal, and axial planes. PD- and T2-weighted imaging are useful in assessing the integrity of the rotator cuff tendons. Fat saturation is useful to highlight fluid edema only. T1-weighted images highlight fat, and are useful for assessing fatty infiltration associated with chronic rotator cuff tears.

The rotator cuff tendons should demonstrate low signal intensity on all pulse sequences. Cuff tendinopathy shows intermediate signal intensity on T2-weighted images, and partial- and full-thickness tears demonstrates high signal intensity. It should be noted that in many asymptomatic patients over the age of 60 years, intermediate signal will be seen in the tendon and does not necessarily imply a pathologic state. Rotator cuff tears typically initiate in the superior cuff and can be initially assessed on PD-weighted and T2-weighted coronal imaging (Fig. 14-58, *A*). Additional evaluation of sagittal and axial imaging can allow for three-dimensional characterization of the tear. If a tear is identified, fatty infiltration and atrophy of the muscle belly should be evaluated on the T1-weighted sagittal oblique images as a method to grade chronicity and the likely reparability of the tear (see Fig. 14-58, *B*).

The accuracy of MRI as a diagnostic tool for full-thickness rotator cuff tears is excellent, and it has high sensitivity and specificity. The utility of MRI for partial-thickness tears is more limited, but because of the limitations of physical examination for diagnosing partial-thickness tears, it does provide useful information for the clinician. MR arthrography may improve the diagnosis of subtler cuff pathology such as partial-thickness rotator cuff tears, but the necessity of injecting gadolinium through normal cuff structures may occasionally lead to interpretative errors.

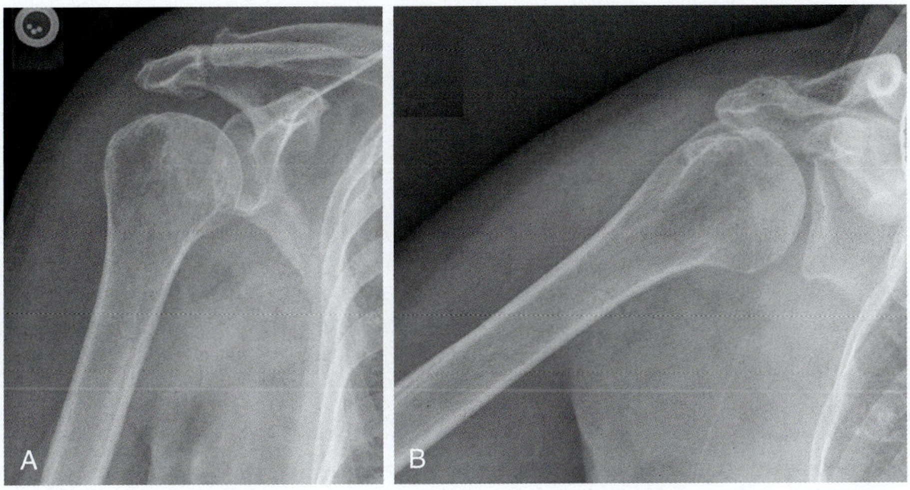

FIGURE 14-57: **A,** Anteroposterior (AP) view of the shoulder may not reveal proximal humeral migration. **B,** True AP (Grashey) view with 30 degrees of abduction activates the deltoid and provides a superiorly directed vector that may make proximal humeral migration more evident.

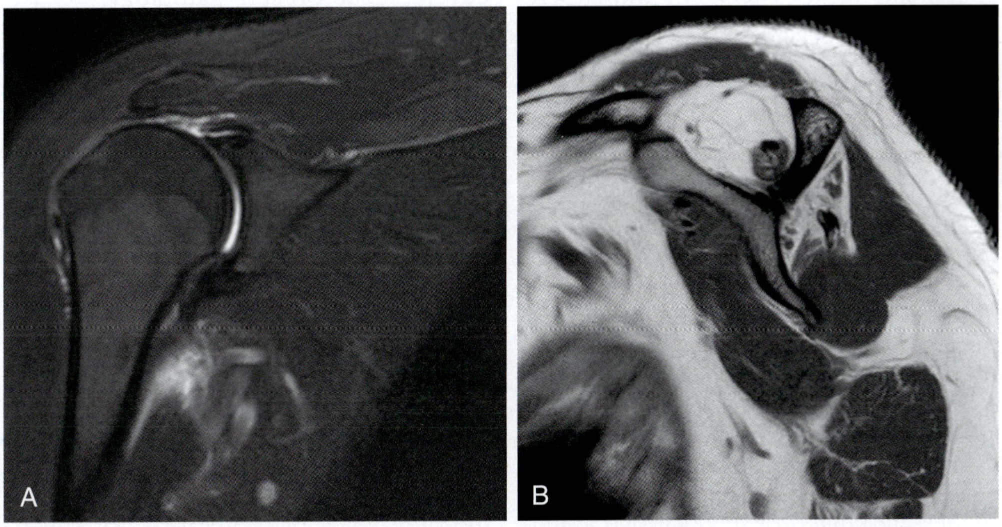

FIGURE 14-58: **A,** Coronal T2-weighted image demonstrating a massive retracted full-thickness rotator cuff tear. **B,** Sagittal oblique T1-weighted image demonstrating severe atrophy of the supraspinatus and infraspinatus muscle bellies.

Ultrasonography

Ultrasound is an imaging modality that can be utilized to perform dynamic evaluation of the cuff and long head of the biceps tendon. It is less expensive than MRI but is more highly dependent on the operator and the interpretation of the ultrasound images. High frequency (10 to 18 MHz) transducers are used for the shoulder. Because ultrasound is more subject to interpretation errors, the physician evaluating the images should be aware of artifacts that can cause false-negative or false-positive interpretations.

Normal tendon should appear as uniform echogenicity with a fibrillar pattern when the transducer is perpendicular to the tendon axis. Because normal tendon is anisotropic, when the beam is not perpendicular to the tendon, a hypoechoic signal will appear. This should be differentiated from tendinosis, which also produces a heterogeneous echotexture. The tendon should be interpreted as abnormal only if the area maintains a hypoechoic signal as the transducer is moved perpendicular to the tendon axis. A focal area of hypoechogenicity can diagnose partial- and full-thickness tearing with discontinuity of the normal fibrillation pattern of tendons (Fig. 14-59). Compression of the transducer into the area in question can increase the gap size between the tendon fibers and bone and assist in evaluation.

Ultrasonography has also been reported to have similar accuracy to MRI in the detection of full-thickness rotator

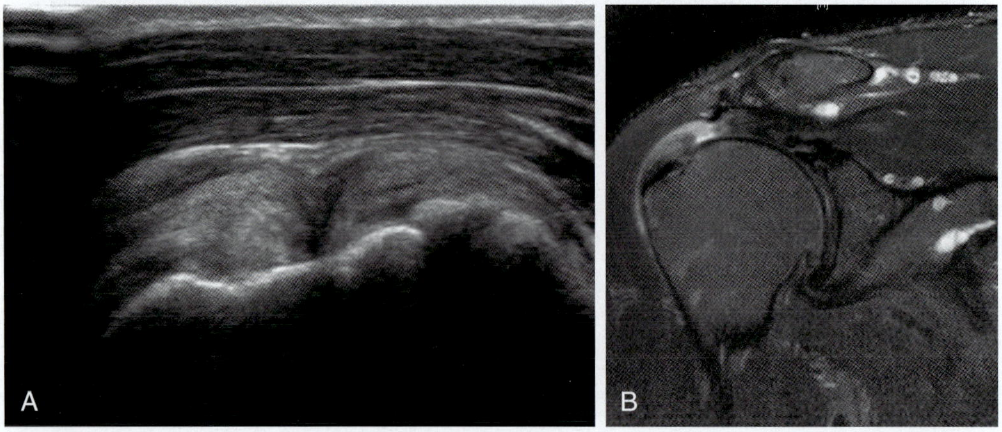

FIGURE 14-59: Ultrasound image demonstrating a focal area of hypoechogenicity and discontinuity of tendon fibers indicative of a full-thickness rotator cuff tear (**A**) and correlation with magnetic resonance imaging (**B**).

cuff tears. As mentioned previously, this modality has more significant variability in interpretation, and experience may play a larger role in decreasing the number of false-positive and false-negative interpretations.

NATURAL HISTORY OF ROTATOR CUFF PATHOLOGY AND IMPLICATIONS ON SURGICAL INDICATIONS

Considerable controversy exists on the optimal management of rotator cuff pathology. Orthopedic surgeons have significant variation in their decision-making process for the management of rotator cuff tears.[70] This is evidenced by the lack of high-quality evidence available to surgeons to help guide management. The majority of the clinical practice guidelines set out by the American Academy of Orthopaedic Surgeons are limited or inconclusive.[3] Similarly, the Cochrane reviews fail to provide an evidence basis for the treatment of cuff disease.[152]

There is a need to understand the epidemiology and natural history of rotator cuff disease. Numerous studies have demonstrated a high prevalence of rotator cuff pathology in the aging population.[138,259,319,351,355] While the exact prevalence varies among studies, a consistent finding is that increased age is associated with a higher prevalence of rotator cuff pathology. In a study using bilateral shoulder ultrasound in patients with unilateral shoulder pain, the average age of patients with bilaterally intact cuffs, unilateral cuff tears, and bilateral cuff tears formed an almost perfect 10-year distribution of 48.7, 58.7, and 67.8 years, respectively.[260] Population-based studies have shown that one-quarter of patients above 60 years of age and half of patients above 80 years will have a rotator cuff tear.[355] These and many other studies have suggested that tendon degeneration and tearing occur with aging.[222,231,319]

A strong genetic influence may also contribute to the development of cuff pathology.[110,120,316] An investigation utilizing the Utah Population Database has demonstrated a significant heritable predisposition to rotator cuff disease in first- and second-degree relatives of patients with cuff pathology.[316] Other studies have demonstrated increased risk in siblings as well as a genetic predisposition to tear progression.[110,120]

Natural History of Asymptomatic Rotator Cuff Tears

Studying the natural history of rotator cuff disease is difficult, as patients may or may not have related symptoms. Those with symptoms may request treatment that interrupts disease progression. Ideally, asymptomatic patients that do not require physiotherapy, injections, or surgery can be followed to better understand the natural history of rotator cuff disease. As mentioned previously, the prevalence of bilateral rotator cuff pathology is substantial, and often, patients presenting with pain in one shoulder will have a rotator cuff tear on the contralateral shoulder that is asymptomatic. By performing bilateral ultrasounds, a large number of asymptomatic rotator cuff tears "at risk" for pain development and tear progression can be identified. This model has been used to prospectively follow a large cohort of asymptomatic tears, and has given us a wealth of information regarding tear initiation, location, enlargement, and symptomatic development.[204,232,351]

Essential to characterizing rotator cuff pathology is to understand the location and initiation of degenerative rotator cuff tears. The common understanding of rotator cuff tears was that they initiated at the anterior edge of the supraspinatus adjacent to the biceps tendon and propagated posteriorly (Fig. 14-60). This conventional theory has been challenged by ultrasound data from Kim et al. measuring the distance from the posterior edge of the biceps to the anterior edge of a rotator cuff tear as

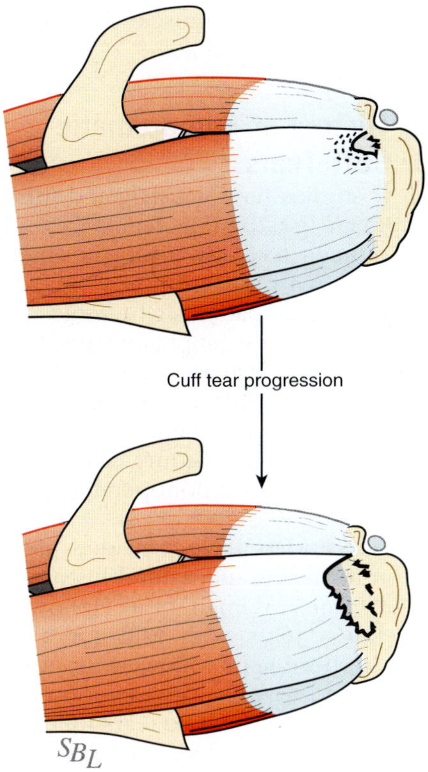

FIGURE 14-60: Degenerative rotator cuff tears were thought to initiate at the anterior edge of the supraspinatus and propagate posteriorly. (From Matsen FA III, Lippitt SB. *Shoulder Surgery: Principles and Procedures*. Philadelphia: Saunders; 2004:271.)

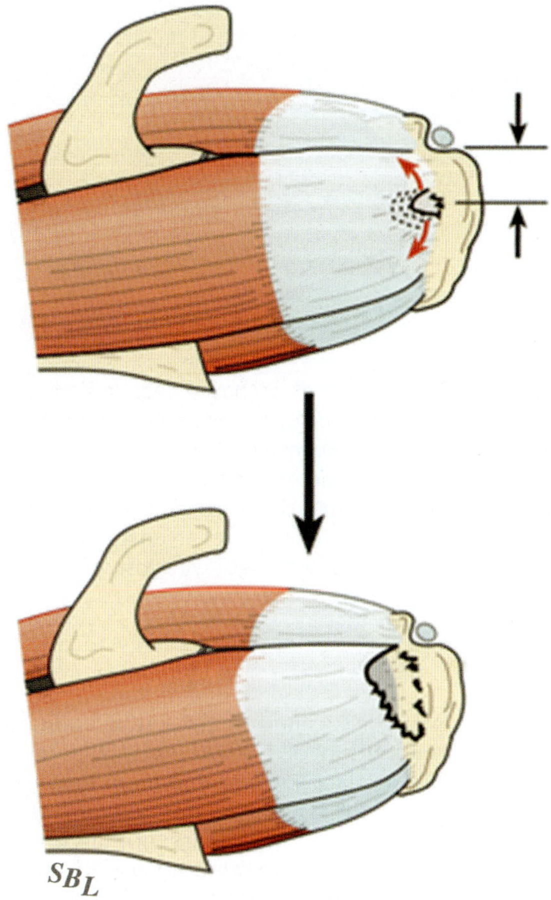

FIGURE 14-61: Ultrasound studies have suggested the initiation of degenerative rotator cuff tears to be approximately 13 to 17 mm posterior to the long head of the biceps tendon followed by propagation anteriorly and posteriorly.

well as the sagittal plane width of a rotator cuff tear.[158] By analyzing the frequency of tear involvement at each millimeter posterior to the biceps tendon, the area around 15 mm posterior to the biceps tendon was found to be most frequently involved, suggesting that degenerative rotator cuff tears initiate at this location (Fig. 14-61).

Anatomically, this location of initiation is interesting from two aspects. First, depending on the anatomic definition of the insertion of the supraspinatus and infraspinatus that is used,[60,225,227] 15 mm posterior to the biceps tendon may correlate to the posterior supraspinatus and even anterior infraspinatus. Clark and Harryman demonstrated that significant interdigitation of the supraspinatus and infraspinatus fibers exists in this region of the rotator cuff.[47] Mochizuki et al. have shown that the area of the anterior cuff footprint that involves only the supraspinatus tendon is relatively small, and that the infraspinatus tendon footprint is larger than previously thought.[227] The average AP width of the medial and lateral margins of the supraspinatus were 12.6 ± 2.0 mm and 1.3 ± 1.4 mm, respectively. Using measurements from this study, 15 mm posterior to the biceps tendon involves the anterior infraspinatus. This could potentially explain why isolated infraspinatus muscle atrophy can sometimes be encountered in tears that appear to involve the supraspinatus.

Second, this area of the rotator cuff is within the "rotator crescent" tissue described by Burkhart et al. (Fig. 14-62).[40] He described the "rotator cable" as a thicker band of rotator cuff tissue spanning from the anterior supraspinatus to the posterior supraspinatus and the "rotator crescent" as a thinner tissue lateral to the cable. This crescent tissue is not only thinner but more avascular. The "suspension bridge" configuration of this cable theoretically shields the crescent tissue from stress. The ultrasound data suggest that these rotator cuff tears initiate towards the middle of the crescent tissue and propagate in both directions from the initiation site.

Propagation or involvement of the anterior cable of the rotator cuff have been shown to have significant impact on the rate of irreversible muscle degeneration associated with rotator cuff tears.[157] Based on the suspension bridge concept of the rotator cable, the anterior supraspinatus tissue is important for distributing the forces along the cable. Loss of integrity of this tissue may lead to accelerated retraction and degeneration of muscle tissue that is associated with lower rates of tendon healing. In ultrasound studies, tears involving the anterior

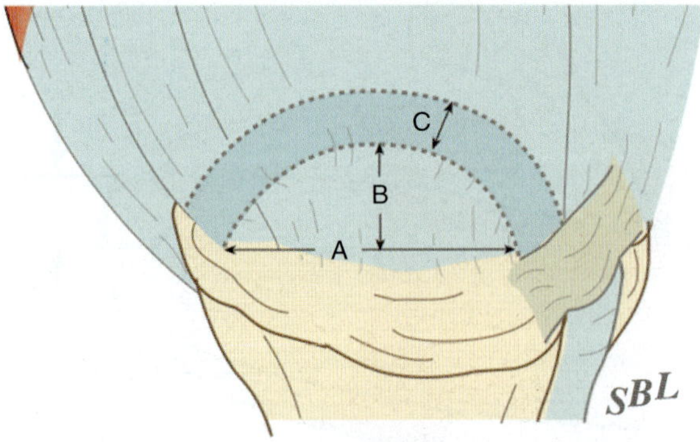

FIGURE 14-62: The area of proposed tear initiation (13 to 17 mm posterior to the biceps tendon is within the rotator crescent tissue). A, Anteroposterior diameter of rotator crescent; B, mediolateral diameter of rotator crescent; C, width of rotator cable. (Modified from Burkhart SS, Esch JC, Jolson RS. The rotator crescent and rotator cable: an anatomic description of the shoulder's "suspension bridge." *Arthroscopy.* 1993;9[6]: 611-616.)

cable tissue were associated with significantly greater rates of fatty infiltration of both the supraspinatus and infraspinatus. These data suggest that tears involving the anterior portion of the supraspinatus may need earlier surgical intervention, and that tears not involving but close to the cable may need to be more closely monitored if being treated nonoperatively.

Normal glenohumeral kinematics may be disrupted by larger rotator cuff tears. The infraspinatus may help maintain coronal plane kinematics, and increasing rotator cuff tear size may lead to the development of proximal humeral migration.[148] Using a combination of ultrasound data for tear size and plain radiographs to measure relationships of the humeral head center to the glenoid, Keener et al. found that larger, symptomatic tears involving the infraspinatus had increased superior migration compared with asymptomatic, smaller tears.[148] A critical tear area of 175 mm^2, which correlates to tear dimensions of approximately 15 mm ×12 mm, was found to be associated with proximal humeral migration.

Longitudinal studies of tear degeneration and pain development in asymptomatic tears are helpful in defining the risks of nonoperative management of degenerative tears. Moosmayer et al. and Mall et al. have reported on longitudinal studies of tear degeneration in asymptomatic shoulders. Moosmayer et al. found that 18 of 50 tears (36%) developed symptoms and that an increase in tear size was associated with symptoms.[232] These results are similar to the findings of Mall et al., who also found that tears that became symptomatic over time also significantly increased in size, while tears that did not become symptomatic did not increase in size.[204] A subsequent study by Keener et al.[147] demonstrated that approximately 50% of asymptomatic tears have a significant increase in size at a median time of 2.8 years. Full-thickness tears are more likely to enlarge, become painful, and progress to muscle degeneration compared with partial-thickness tears.

Natural History of Symptomatic Rotator Cuff Tears

Only a few studies have investigated the natural history of symptomatic rotator cuff tears.[83,205,287] These patients are more difficult to study given the interruption of the natural history with any proposed treatment. Fucentese et al. reported on 24 patients who refused operative treatment for full-thickness supraspinatus tears, and found that there was no increase in the average size of the rotator cuff tears on MRI at 3.5 years after the initial MR arthrogram.[83] Of the 24 patients, 8 (33%) had an increase in tear size, and 4 (17%) had no change in tear size. This group of patients treated nonoperatively had a high level of satisfaction.

Two other studies have provided us with additional information regarding the natural history of symptomatic rotator cuff tears. Maman et al. followed 59 full and partial-thickness tears with MRI for a minimum of 6 months.[205] In those tears followed for at least 18 months, 48% were found to have progression of tear size, compared with only 19% in those tears followed for less than 18 months. Similar to findings in asymptomatic tears, full-thickness tears were more likely to progress than partial-thickness tears. Also, age was an important factor, with progression in 54% of tears in patients over the age of 60 years versus 17% in patients under 60 years. Safran et al. studied a cohort of patients under the age of 60 years that were treated nonoperatively for full-thickness rotator cuff tears, and found that 49% of the tears increased in size.[287]

Valuable information has been derived from a longitudinal cohort of more than 400 patients with atraumatic, full-thickness rotator cuff tears followed by the Multicenter Orthopaedic Outcomes Network Shoulder Group.[33,166,228,333] Data from this multicenter group have suggested that pain and duration of symptoms are not associated with the severity of rotator cuff tears.[69,228] These data are in contrast to those from other studies that have shown stronger correlations between tear size and pain development.[204,232] The differences are likely due to variations in study design. The Multicenter Orthopaedic Outcomes Network group has found that nonoperative treatment of these full-thickness tears is effective in 75% of patients after 2 years.[166] A patient's perception of whether physical therapy would be beneficial was a strong predictor of whether conservative treatment would be successful.

Indications for Rotator Cuff Repair

As noted previously, neither the clinical practice guidelines set out by the American Academy of Orthopaedic Surgeons nor the Cochrane systematic reviews provide guidance on the management of rotator cuff tears.[3,152] Clinical decision-making for the management of rotator cuff tears can be complex and lacks consensus among orthopedic surgeons.[70] As we continue to improve our understanding of the natural history of rotator cuff disease, this complex decision-making process will continue to be refined over time. Based on our current understanding of the natural history of rotator cuff disease and the results of operative repair in a multitude of age groups and tear characteristics, we can generate general guidelines regarding operative indications and the importance of surgical timing.

Patients can generally be divided into three main categories that are based on the potential risk of nonoperative treatments and the proposed benefits of surgical intervention. These categories include those patients needing urgent or early operative repair, those patients that can benefit from a trial of conservative treatment, and those patients that may be best suited for nonoperative treatment.

Group I: Early Operative Repair—Acute Tear

Perhaps the clearest indication for repair of the rotator cuff is the young patient that presents with shoulder pain and weakness after a distinct, acute injury and imaging consistent with an acute full-thickness rotator cuff tear. A thorough history should be performed and should evaluate for preexisting shoulder pain or dysfunction that could be a sign of an acute-on-chronic tear. Additionally, review of imaging should confirm the absence of fatty infiltration on ultrasound or T1 oblique sagittal MRI. Imaging with severe muscle atrophy would suggest more chronic rotator cuff disease that would not be as amenable to surgical repair. Although the supporting literature is limited to case series, urgent repair in the setting of an acute rotator cuff tear typically has positive results.[16,169,267]

Operative repair should also be considered in acute subscapularis tears as well as more chronic subscapularis tears with biceps tendon instability.[74,203] More urgent surgical repair should be considered for acute, retracted subscapularis tears due to the potential for muscle degeneration and fixed degeneration that can occur as a result of these injuries. Repair of more chronic subscapularis tears can be complicated by scar formation and the risk of neurovascular injury due to the proximity to the brachial plexus and associated vasculature. Concomitant biceps tenotomy or tenodesis at the time of subscapularis repair is associated with improved subjective and objective results.[74]

Early surgical repair should be considered in select, higher functioning patients under the age of 60 to 65 years with a full-thickness tear. The impetus for repair comes from the established risk for tear enlargement, muscle degeneration, and change in glenohumeral kinematics over time. Around half of degenerative full-thickness tears will continue to enlarge more than 5 mm at a median of 2.8 years.[147] Additionally, multiple studies have shown that the rates of rotator cuff healing decrease with aging. Therefore early repair may give the patient the best chance at healing. These data should be considered along with short-term follow-up data regarding symptomatic full-thickness tears.[83,166] However, it is important to note that there have not been any studies that have demonstrated that operative repair for degenerative tears provides any long-term structural or functional advantage over nonoperative management of these degenerative tears. Thus while we can identify shoulders at risk for tear propagation, we cannot be confident that performing surgery on these shoulders will prevent progression of the cuff defect.

Therefore an individualized approach to patients with small full-thickness tears is required, and a thorough discussion with the patient regarding the risks of nonoperative and operative treatment is necessary for this subset.

Group II: Trial of Nonoperative Treatment—Nonacute Tear

A trial of nonoperative treatment aimed at retaining comfort, motion, and strength should be considered in any patient with chronic rotator cuff tendinitis, partial-thickness tear, or full-thickness tear. While such shoulders carry a risk for tear enlargement for full-thickness tears (61%), partial-thickness tears (44%), and intact cuffs (14%),[147] there is time and opportunity to explore the effectiveness of a gentle progressive rehabilitation program.

Articular- and bursal-sided partial-thickness tears can be more painful than full-thickness tears, because in contrast to full-thickness tears, partial-thickness defects of the cuff give rise to stiffness and nonphysiologic tension on the remaining fibers. Because they are unlikely to progress acutely, these tears should be initially treated with nonoperative management. Articular- and bursal-sided partial-thickness should be differentiated, however, because the rates of improvement with nonoperative options in these two groups are different. Articular-sided tears often respond well to physical therapy. On the other hand, bursal-sided tears have a higher failure rate with nonoperative treatment. These lesions can be associated with *subacromial abrasions*, producing subacromial crepitus on passive joint motion. Because of the limited success with nonrepair strategies for bursal-sided tears, prolonged conservative treatment may be more appropriate for articular-sided tears than for bursal-sided tears.

There is an abundance of literature regarding operative treatment for full-thickness rotator cuff tears, but literature regarding nonoperative treatment of full-thickness tears was lacking until recently; it is now recognized that a nonoperative approach to full-thickness rotator cuff tears can lead to clinical improvement.[83,166,205] This subset of patients requires an individualized approach in which the surgeon discusses the risks of tear progression and irreversible muscle changes with nonoperative treatment on one hand versus the risks and chances of a better outcome with surgery on the other.

Group III: Maximize Conservative Care—Irreparable Tear

It is of interest that elderly patients with massive defects in the rotator cuff can realize a comfortable and functional range of motion without surgery. Patients over the age of 60 years with large degenerative tears are unlikely to heal from an attempted cuff repair.[26] In an elderly patient (60 years and older) with a complete or partial rotator cuff defect, administration of a physician-directed, home-based rehabilitation program has proved to be an effective, reproducible, and reliable method of attaining significant clinical and functional improvement.

NONOPERATIVE MANAGEMENT OF ROTATOR CUFF TEARS

The nonoperative program consists of four distinct, progressive phases: pain control, gentle progressive stretching, strengthening, and maintenance.

Phase I: Pain Control

This phase uses modalities such as small doses of pain medications, including antiinflammatories, rest, activity modification, and the use of either ice packs or moist heat to address the acute pain in the affected shoulder joint.

Phase II: Stretching

The second phase consists of a gentle, progressive stretching program with the patient being his or her own therapist. The treating physician or trusted therapist educates the patient on gentle progressive assisted forward flexion, extension, internal and external rotation, posterior capsular stretching, and pendulum exercises (Figs. 14-63 to 14-70). Each stretch is performed only to the point of a comfortable stretch that the patient holds for 20 seconds before relaxing and performing the next repetition.

Phase III: Strengthening Program

The strengthening phase of the program is commenced when the patient has achieved a comfortable passive range of motion in the affected shoulder. It focuses on strengthening exercises for the deltoid, scapular stabilizers (pectoralis, teres major and minor, trapezius, serratus anterior, and latissimus dorsi) and the parts of the rotator cuff that remain intact.

A simple exercise that needs no equipment and that develops integrated strength for the deltoid, residual cuff, and periscapular muscles is the progressive press (see Fig. 16-151 from Chapter 16). The patient starts supine and presses the arm up toward the ceiling as far up as it can go. When this can be accomplished for 20 repetitions, the torso is inclined slightly upwards on pillows, giving the shoulder added resistance. When 20 repetitions can be accomplished at this new level, the angle of inclination is increased until the arm can be actively elevated towards the ceiling in the sitting and then the standing position. Light weights can be held in the hand for added resistance.

Strengthening exercises can also be carried out with resistance bands. The resistance of these bands can be increased incrementally as progression is made through the various colors (Figs. 14-71 to 14-75). The directed movements are forward flexion, extension, internal and external rotation, and abduction. We advise patients to avoid pushing the strength of flexion and external

Text continued on p. 690

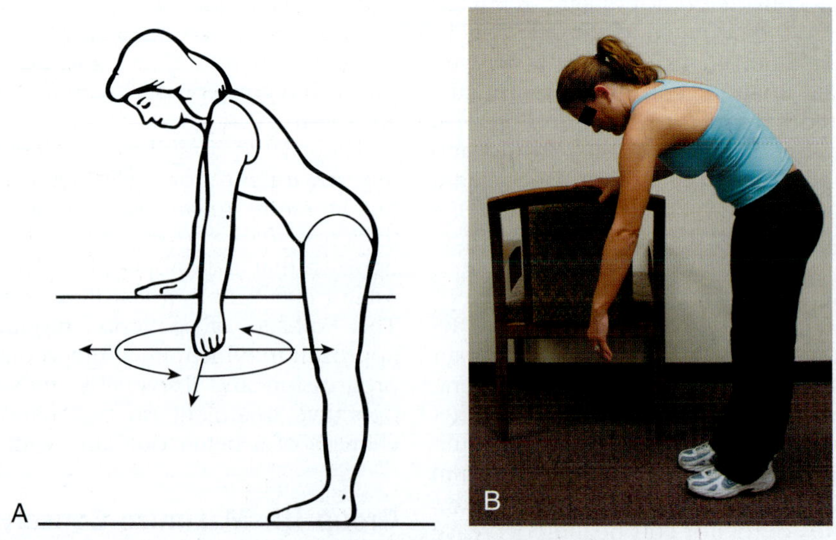

FIGURE 14-63: The pendulum exercise. **A,** The technique of supporting the upper body on a firm table, countertop, or stable chair back. **B,** A patient demonstrates the exercise using a stable chair back; the involved arm is moved in a side-to-side, a backward-and-forward, and a circular motion, but always in a loose swinging arc.

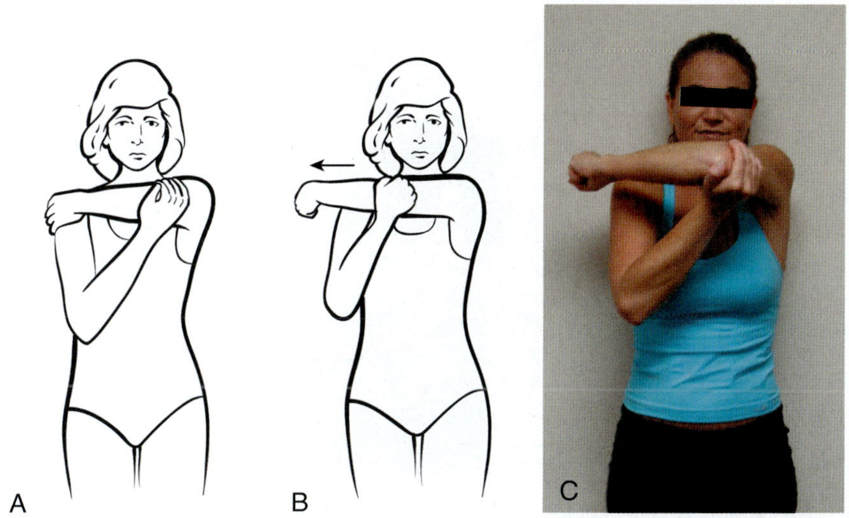

FIGURE 14-64: The posterior shoulder–stretching exercise. **A,** The affected shoulder should be just in front of the chin. **B,** The good arm grasps the affected elbow and gently pulls the elbow across the chest toward the good shoulder (*arrow*). The affected elbow is pulled as far as possible to the point of stretching, but not to the point of pain. **C,** A patient demonstrates the posterior shoulder–stretching exercise.

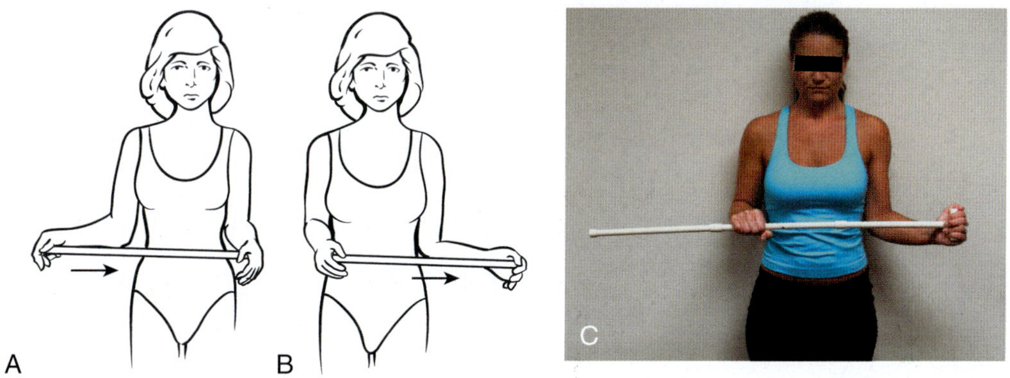

FIGURE 14-65: The external rotation stick exercise. **A** and **B,** The good arm (the right arm in these drawings) uses its power to move the affected shoulder into external rotation using a stick. **C,** A patient demonstrates the pain-free endpoint of external rotation using the stick.

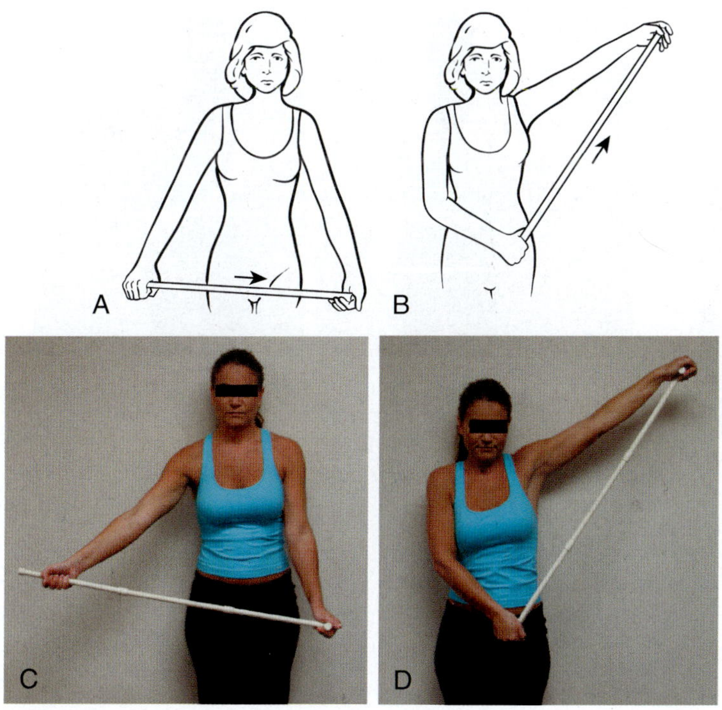

FIGURE 14-66: The abduction stick exercise. The stick is used to passively abduct the affected arm (the left arm in these drawings) using the strength of the good arm. **A,** Starting position. **B,** Ending position. **C,** A patient demonstrates the starting point of this exercise. **D,** A patient demonstrates the ending point of this exercise.

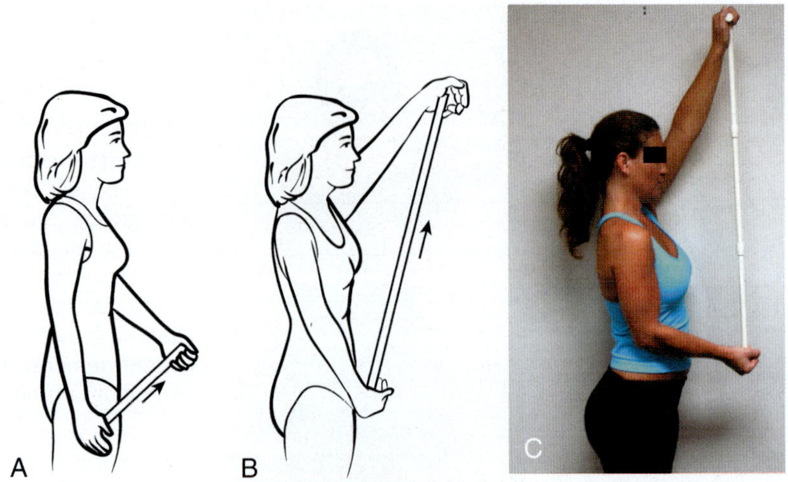

FIGURE 14-67: The forward elevation stick exercise. **A** and **B,** The stick is used to passively elevate the affected arm. **C,** A patient demonstrates the exercise.

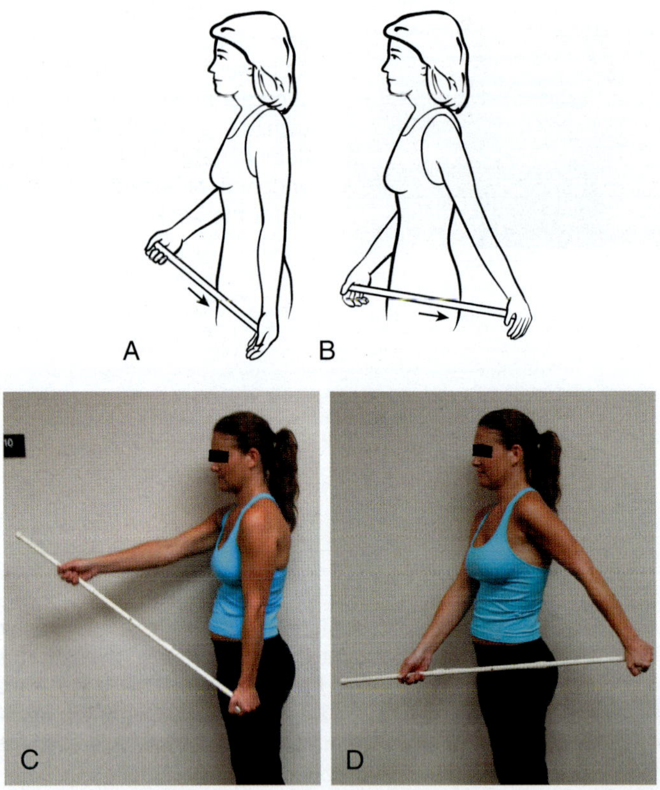

FIGURE 14-68: The extension stick exercise. **A** and **B,** The stick is used to passively extend the affected shoulder. **C** and **D,** A patient demonstrates this shoulder extension exercise.

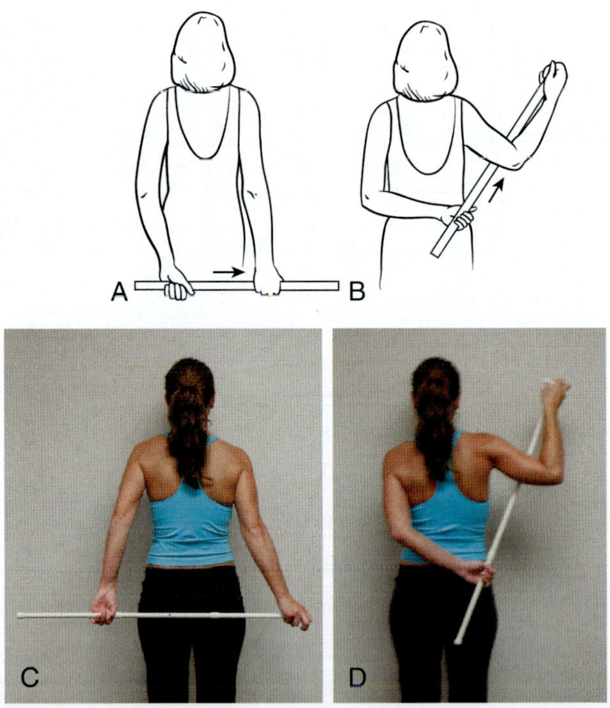

FIGURE 14-69: The internal rotation stick exercise. **A** and **B,** The stick is used to passively stretch the affected shoulder in internal rotation. **C** and **D,** A patient demonstrates how the stick is used to passively stretch the affected shoulder in internal rotation.

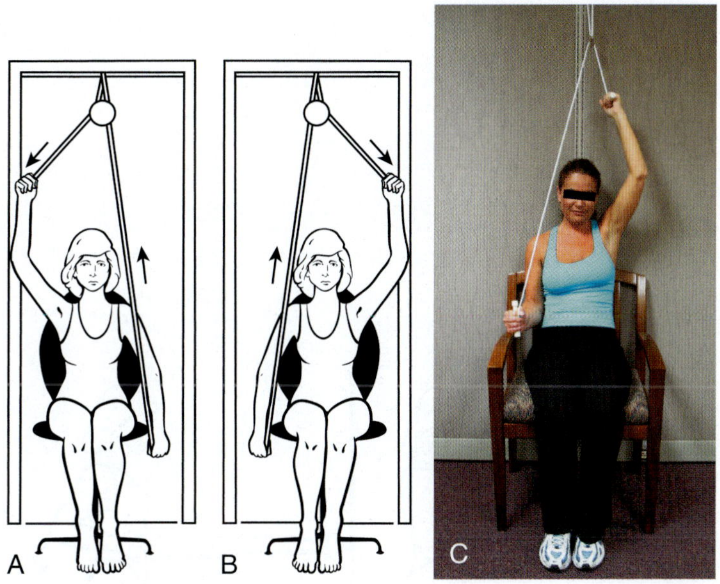

FIGURE 14-70: The pulley system. **A** and **B,** The good arm provides the motor power to pull the involved arm into the overhead position. **C,** A patient demonstrates that when she pulls down with the good arm, the affected arm is passively lifted into the overhead position to the point of stretching but not pain.

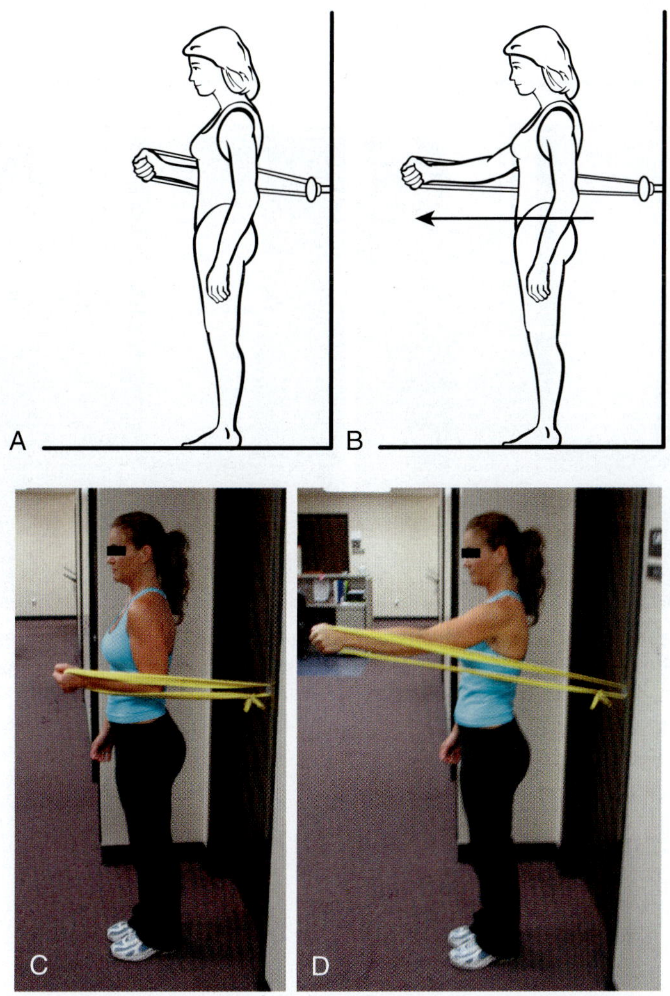

FIGURE 14-71: Exercise band anterior deltoid–strengthening exercise. **A** and **B,** A loop of the exercise band is placed around a doorknob or a similar fixed object. The exercise band provides resistance as the affected shoulder is flexed forward. **C** and **D,** A patient demonstrates how the exercise band is used while forward flexing the affected shoulder.

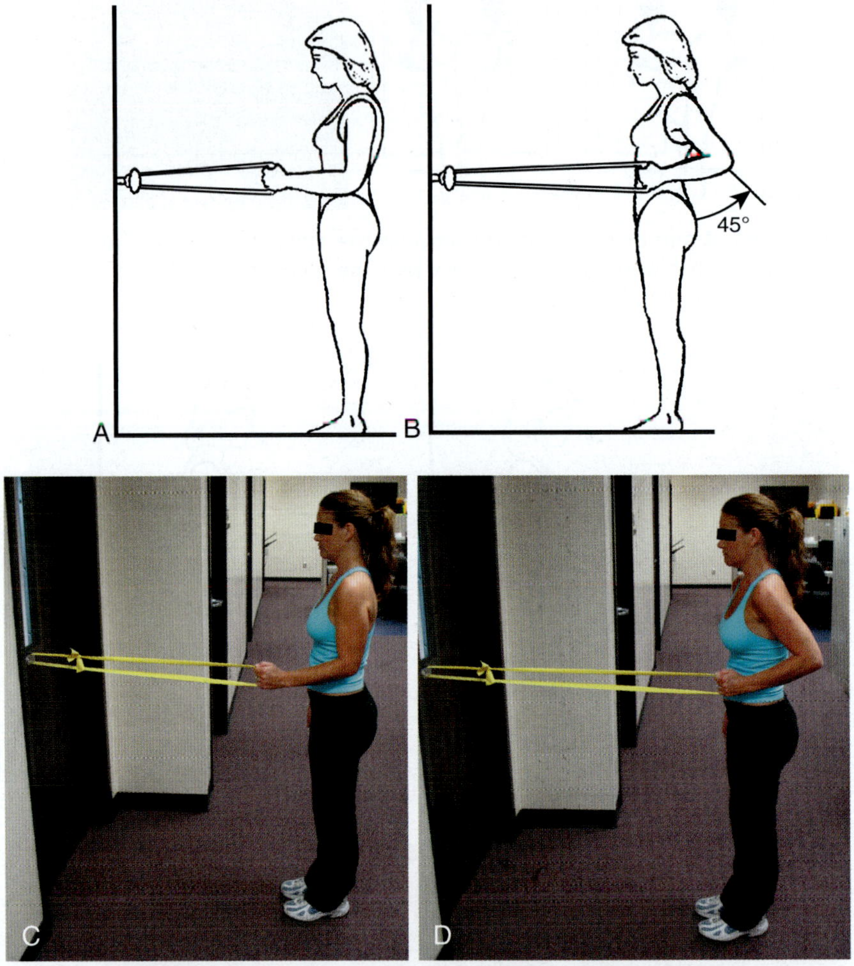

FIGURE 14-72: The exercise band posterior deltoid–strengthening exercise. **A** and **B,** The exercise band is used to provide resistance as the shoulder is extended. **C** and **D,** A patient demonstrates how the exercise band is used while extending the affected shoulder.

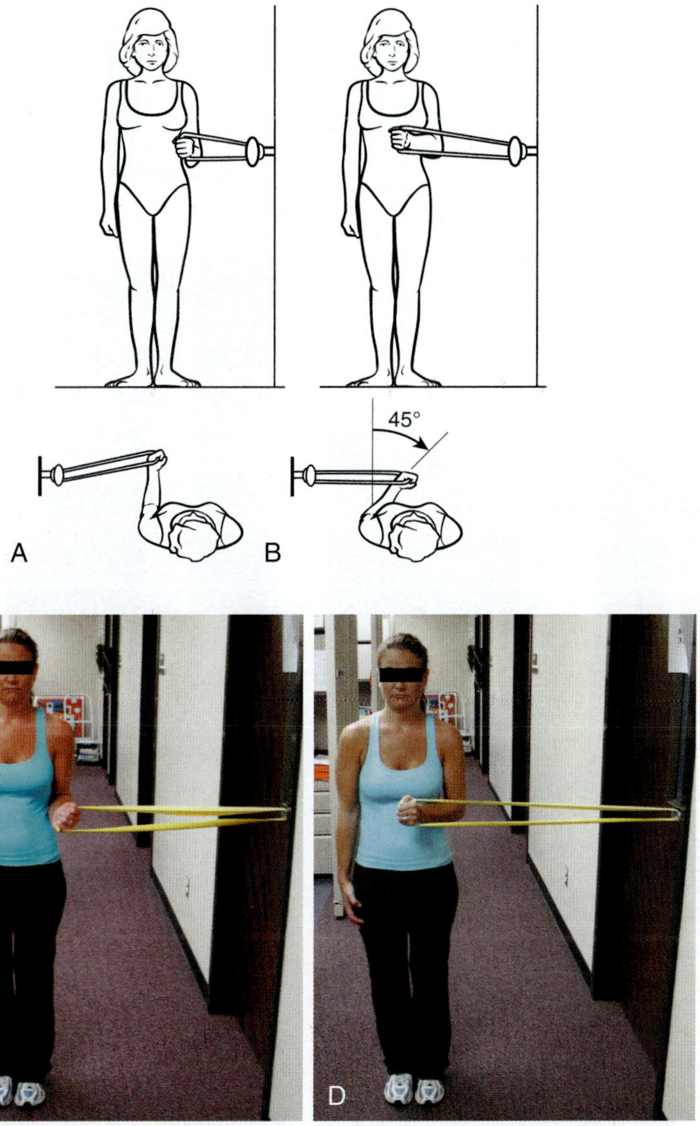

FIGURE 14-73: The exercise band deltoid- and subscapularis-strengthening exercise. **A** and **B,** A loop of the exercise band is placed around a doorknob or a similar fixed object. The exercise band provides resistance as the affected shoulder is internally rotated. **C** and **D,** A patient demonstrates how the exercise band is used while internally rotating the affected shoulder against resistance.

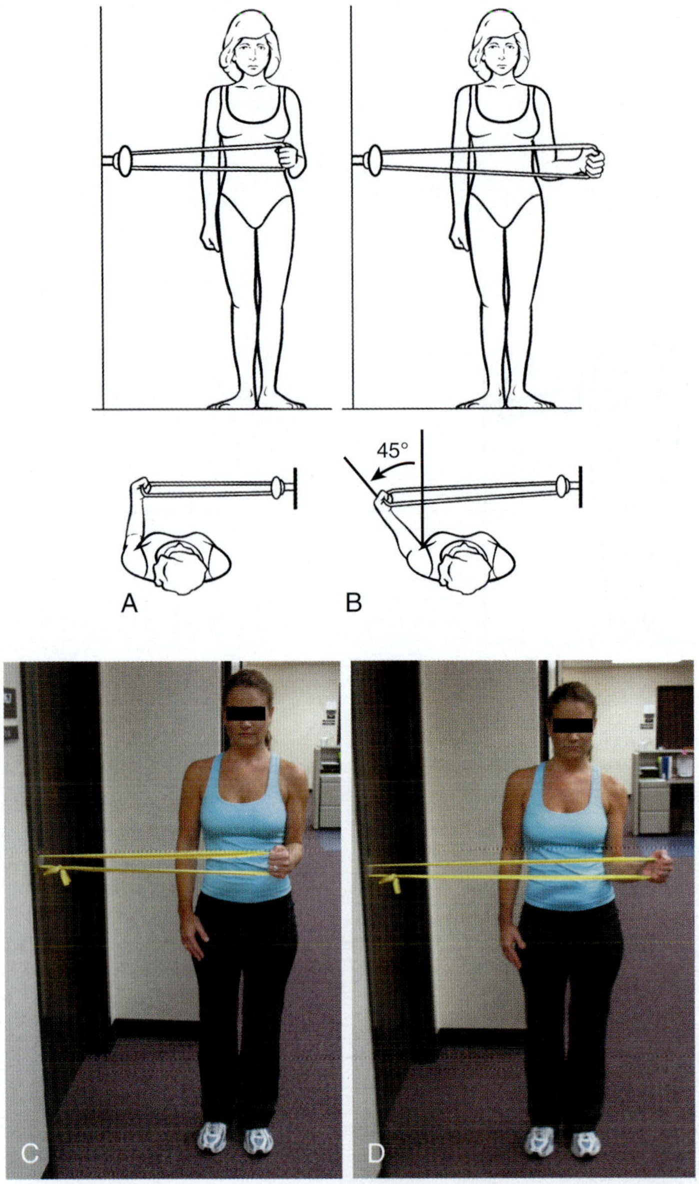

FIGURE 14-74: The exercise band deltoid- and teres minor–strengthening exercise. **A** and **B,** The exercise band provides resistance as the affected shoulder is externally rotated. **C** and **D,** A patient demonstrates how the exercise band is used while externally rotating the affected shoulder against resistance.

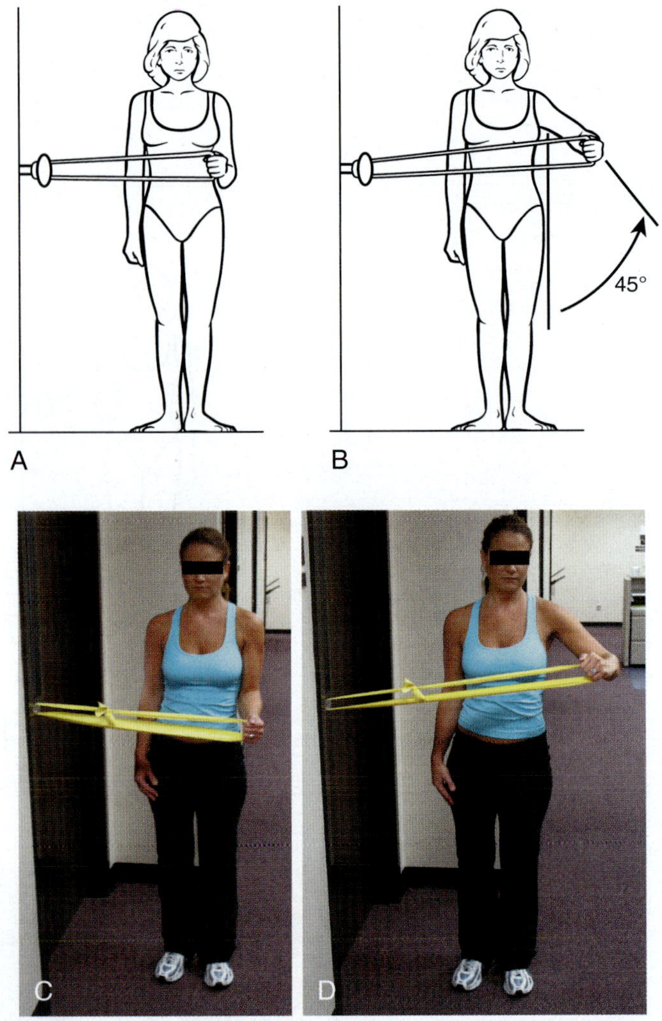

FIGURE 14-75: The exercise band lateral deltoid–strengthening exercise. **A** and **B,** The exercise band provides resistance as the affected shoulder is abducted while the elbow is kept bent at 90 degrees. **C** and **D,** A patient demonstrates how the exercise band is used while abducting the affected shoulder against resistance.

rotation out of concern for aggravating a rotator cuff tear. The patient does not progress to the next colored band until exercises on the current band are easy and painless.

Strengthening of the shoulder stabilizer muscles is also important. This includes a series of shoulder shrug movements and exercises for the trapezius (Fig. 14-76). These exercises are augmented by a program including wall pushups, and occasionally, knee pushups, to strengthen the serratus anterior and rhomboid muscles (Figs. 14-77 and 14-78). Seated chair press-ups are also used to enhance this strengthening of the very important latissimus dorsi muscles (Fig. 14-79). These additional techniques have been used to enhance the overall clinical improvements in shoulder strength and range of motion.

If acute shoulder pain is exacerbated at any stage during the strengthening phase, the patient is directed to either slow or cease progression through the strengthening exercises. The patient may also be advised to return to the stretching phase (phase II) of the rehabilitation program.

Phase IV: Maintenance and Prevention

The final phase of the program consists of resumption of activities and maintenance of the improvements in pain control, flexibility, and strength. To achieve this, the

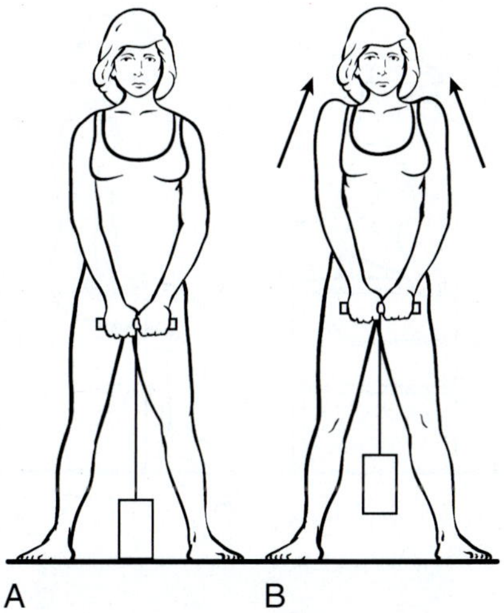

FIGURE 14-76: The shoulder shrug: Trapezius- and levator scapulae muscle–strengthening exercise. **A,** The elbows are kept straight and the shoulders are relaxed. **B,** Weight is lifted by shrugging the shoulders up, not by bending the elbows.

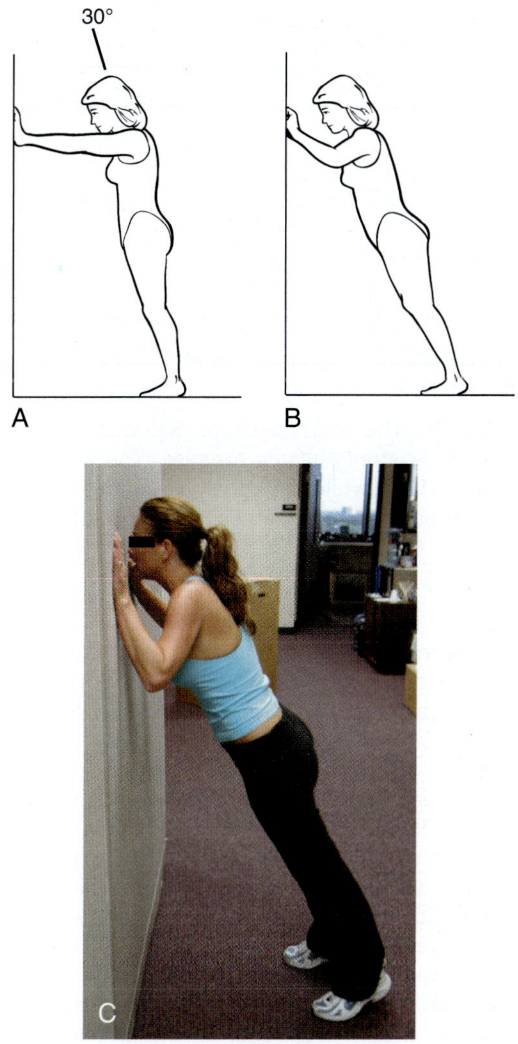

FIGURE 14-77: The wall pushup: Serratus anterior– and rhomboid muscle–strengthening exercise. The patient's feet are kept about 2 ft away from the wall. Both hands are placed in front on the wall. The elbows are bent to allow the body to lean forward until the nose almost touches the wall. **A,** Starting position. **B,** Ending position. **C,** A patient demonstrates the endpoint of the wall pushup.

patient is instructed to continue with the stretching and strengthening exercises at a frequency of two to three times per week and to maintain this pattern of exercise indefinitely. If the symptoms recur, they can often be managed by resumption of the stretching and then strengthening exercises.

An important aspect of the long-term management of patients with cuff disorders is education in the protection of the cuff. Patients are taught that sudden, heavy jerky movements of the shoulder, lifting with the arm away from the side, and falls can injure their rotator cuff. Lifting with two hands, lifting with the elbow close to the body, and avoiding sudden movements can protect the cuff from additional injury.

ARTHROSCOPIC ROTATOR CUFF REPAIR

Advances in arthroscopic equipment and increased surgeon familiarity with shoulder arthroscopy have made arthroscopic surgery the preferred method of rotator cuff repair for many shoulder surgeons. It offers numerous advantages over traditional open repair techniques. More thorough visualization, diagnosis, and treatment of lesions within the joint are facilitated, which is critical because a high prevalence of concomitant intra-articular pathology has been reported in patients undergoing rotator cuff repair.[223] Arthroscopy allows a more comprehensive assessment of intra-articular pathology and rotator cuff tear configuration by viewing from multiple angles. Tendon mobilization is also facilitated by precise releases of adhesions that limit tendon excursion, leading to an improved ability to anatomically reduce the edge and create a tension-free repair. Injury to the deltoid muscle is minimized. The acromial deltoid origin is preserved, eliminating the risk of deltoid dehiscence, a potentially devastating complication. Another key theoretical benefit of arthroscopic repair is decreased postoperative pain secondary to less soft tissue trauma. This aids in postoperative rehabilitation, leading to earlier resumption of range of motion and possibly less pain-induced muscle inhibition.

A potential disadvantage of arthroscopic repair had historically been the inability to completely mirror the open procedure with regard to fixation options. Concerns due to the necessity of using suture anchors as fixation and the inability to use tissue-grasping stitches have eased with the advent of improved implants, suture materials, suture-passing devices, and techniques. Anatomic

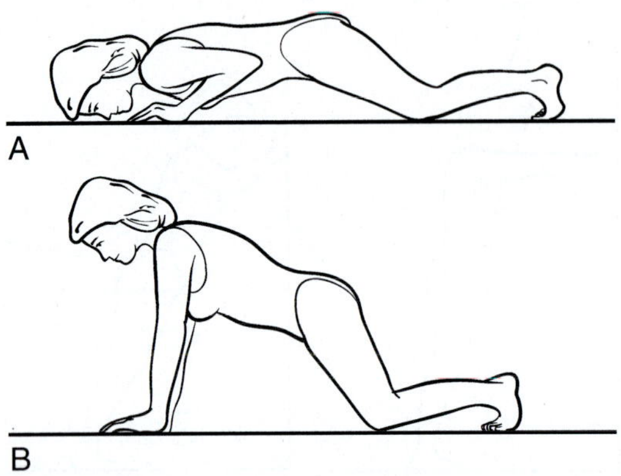

FIGURE 14-78: The knee pushup: Serratus anterior– and rhomboid muscle–strengthening exercise. The knees and feet are kept on the floor, while the upper extremities lift the upper body from the floor. **A,** Starting position. **B,** Ending position.

footprint restoration is now possible, with fixation at both the suture-tendon interface and the anchor-bone interface that approximates traditional open transosseous repairs.

Historically, arthroscopic repair was performed using a single row of bone anchors placed within the tuberosity (Fig. 14-80A). The double-row technique involved the use of two rows of suture anchors, one medially and one laterally, with the sutures tied separately (Fig. 14-80B). This allows for additional points of fixation of the tendon down to the bone and better coverage of the footprint area. Newer techniques have involved using a medial row of suture anchors, with suture strands passed medially to a lateral row of anchors in order to compress the tendon down to the bone (Fig. 14-80C). The double-row technique has been advocated as a better biomechanical construct and a more anatomic repair strategy.[199,275,334] While in biomechanical studies, the double-row repair outperforms single-row repair in failure strength, superior clinical results with double-row fixation over single-row fixation is still controversial.[170,224,350,364]

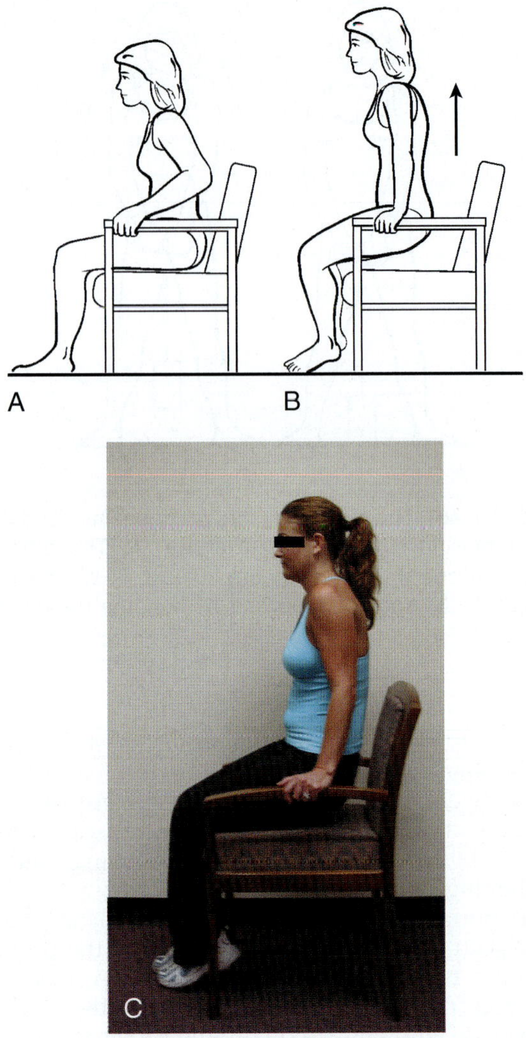

FIGURE 14-79: The seated press-up: Latissimus dorsi–strengthening exercise. The easiest way to perform this exercise is to sit in a chair and put the hands on the arms of the chair. Keeping the feet on the floor, the patient pushes their body up and out of the chair. The elbows are kept slightly bent. **A,** Starting position. **B,** Ending position. **C,** A patient demonstrates a seated press-up exercise.

SURGICAL TECHNIQUE

The goal of surgical repair is to restore the attachment of the torn cuff tendon(s) back to its (their) insertion on the tuberosity in a near anatomic fashion with minimal tension in order to best restore the proper muscular balance of the rotator cuff and allow for a durable repair. The outcomes in terms of pain, function, and range of motion after arthroscopic repair have been shown to be similar to those of open repair.[140]

The basics of shoulder arthroscopy are further discussed in Chapter 15. Arthroscopic rotator cuff repair can be performed with the patient in either the beach chair or lateral decubitus position. The beach chair position allows for easier movement of the surgical extremity and the ability to convert to an open procedure if needed. General or regional anesthesia can be used depending on the surgeon's and anesthesiologist's preferences. Bursal bleeding may limit visualization in the subacromial space, and this may be minimized by hypotensive general anesthesia. The use of a regional nerve block (interscalene block) in conjunction with general anesthesia is useful in postoperative pain control and may also help intraoperatively with blood pressure management.

After a sterile prep and drape and administration of appropriate perioperative intravenous antibiotics, a standard posterior portal is created to initiate arthroscopy. While most surgeons have advocated a posterior portal

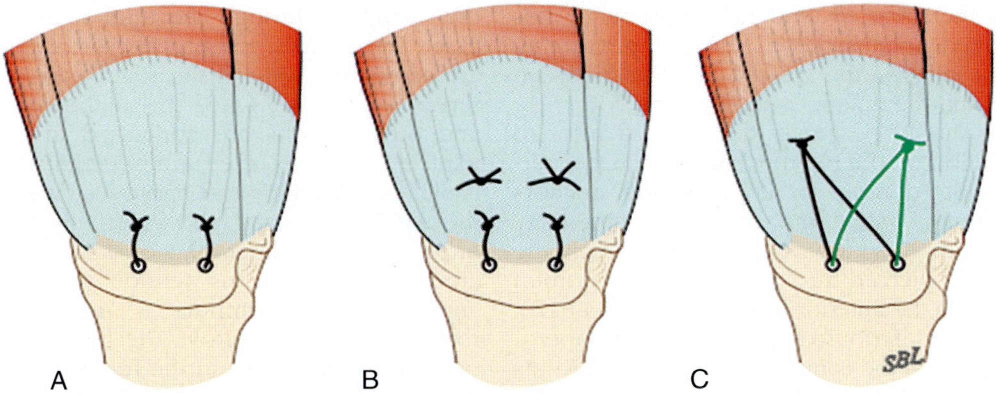

FIGURE 14-80: Arthroscopic repair can be performed using a single-row repair (**A**), a double-row repair using separate anchors (**B**), or using sutures spanning the medial and lateral row (**C**).

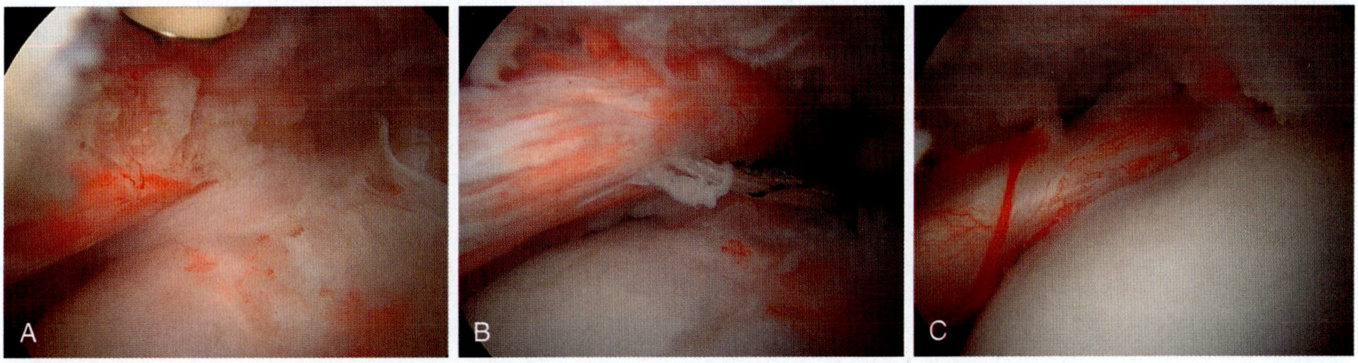

FIGURE 14-81: A, A tear of the upper border of the subscapularis can be visualized with a 70-degree arthroscope from the intra-articular space. **B,** A combination of an anterior and anterosuperolateral portal can be used to pass sutures from inferior to anterior through the tendon. **C,** The knots are tied sequentially from inferior to superior to complete a single-row repair.

that is 2 cm distal and 2 cm medial to the posterolateral border of the acromion, we prefer to place our portal more distal than this. As soft tissue swelling increases during the procedure, the angle of approach to the subacromial space may be affected, and having a portal too superior may lead to contact between the arthroscope and the posterior border of the acromion. We also prefer our posterior portal to be placed slightly more laterally for rotator cuff repairs to improve visualization.

The glenohumeral joint is first entered with the arthroscope, and localizing both the placement and trajectory using a spinal needle creates an anterior portal. The anterior portal is placed just lateral to the tip of the coracoid. This allows for evaluation and management of any concomitant intra-articular pathology such as articular cartilage lesions, labral tears, rotator cuff tears (particularly the subscapularis), and long head biceps tearing or subluxation.

Subscapularis Repair

A 70-degree arthroscope should be used interchangeably with a 30-degree arthroscope to assess the subscapularis and its footprint. Any tearing of the upper subscapularis may be accompanied by instability of the long head of the biceps tendon, both of which should be addressed while in the intra-articular space (Fig. 14-81A). Due to the limited working space in the anterior shoulder, subscapularis tears should be addressed before any posterosuperior cuff tears. The biceps tendon can be treated with either tenotomy or tenodesis after the rotator cuff tear has been repaired (see Chapter 17).

Repair of a subscapularis tear can be performed intra-articularly using a 70-degree arthroscope to better visualize the tendon and its footprint. A spinal needle near the anterolateral border of the acromion should be used to begin establishing an anterosuperolateral portal (through the superior and lateral rotator interval); this will be used primarily as a working portal. In retracted subscapularis tears, identification of the "comma sign," which represents the superior glenohumeral/coracohumeral ligament complex and medial sling of the biceps, will mark the superolateral border of the subscapularis tendon. Release of adhesions around the anterior, superior, and posterior tendon should be performed to obtain enough lateral excursion to perform a tension-free repair. A grasper can be used to pull the retracted tendon laterally while this release is performed. Some surgeons advocate performing a coracoplasty to increase the amount of space between the coracoid tip and the anterior subscapularis.[39]

The footprint should be gently decorticated prior to repair. Either single- or double-row repairs can be performed by placing double- or triple-loaded anchors through the anterior portal into the lesser tuberosity about 10 mm apart. A suture is retrieved through the anterolateral portal, pierced through the inferior portion of the tear, and exits the anterior portal (see Fig. 14-81B). This is repeated from inferior to superior until the superolateral border medial to the comma sign is reached. Knots are then tied sequentially from inferior to superior through either of the anterior portals to complete the repair (see Fig. 14-81C).

Focus is turned to the superior and posterior rotator cuff. The tear can be visualized first from the articular side, which will confirm whether the tear is partial or full thickness. Estimation of the extent of partial-thickness tearing can be performed during arthroscopy by visualizing the amount of exposed tuberosity lateral to the articular margin. The average medial-lateral width of the superior rotator cuff insertion on the tuberosity varies along the length of the tuberosity. It has been traditionally thought to be about 15 mm or more,[140,39] but a subsequent study of a large number of cadaver specimens has suggested this to be smaller.[60,67,227] A tagging suture can be placed while in the intra-articular space for bursal-sided evaluation. For full-thickness rotator cuff tears, the next step usually involves placement of the arthroscope into the subacromial space. A thorough bursectomy should be performed in order to fully visualize the rotator cuff tear and to facilitate repair. We typically do not perform an acromioplasty unless there is a large spur present anteriorly (which can usually be identified on preoperative scapular Y views) and there is clear fraying or damage to the coracoacromial ligament. Most high-level studies regarding rotator cuff repair with and without acromioplasty have not shown a benefit of acromioplasty.[1,200,300]

Partial-Thickness Repair

Articular-sided partial-thickness tears involving only a small portion of the cuff footprint can be treated with debridement with or without acromioplasty.[57,197] More extensive partial-thickness articular-sided tears can typically be repaired without removal of the intact bursal-sided tendon, although good results have been reported with detachment of the remaining tendon before repair.[143] After debridement of the footprint, the quality of the intact bursal-sided tendon tissue should be evaluated. If the tissue tears easily with probing, it may be best to detach the degenerative tendon. If the tissue quality is good, the repair technique should keep the tendon intact.

For tears under 15 mm from anterior to posterior, a single double-loaded suture anchor can be introduced through the rotator cuff just off the articular margin after localizing with a spinal needle. This can be done while viewing from the intra-articular space. Suture strands are then shuttled through the tendon in order to create a tissue bridge. Alternatively, for partial-thickness tears that are commonly seen in the rotator crescent, an all-inside repair is possible. Once this pathoanatomy is observed and other lesions are addressed in the glenohumeral joint, the arm is placed in abduction (Fig. 14-82A). This facilitates the repair and improves visualization similar to the ABER (abducted and externally rotated) MRI view improving the radiographic conspicuity of PASTA (partial articular supraspinatus tendon avulsion) lesions. The anterior-superior cannula is introduced through the rotator interval just above the biceps tendon. The footprint is decorticated and the frayed edges of the tear are debrided with a shaver. A 60- or 90-degree suture-passing device is then passed through the detached flap of the tendon and out the articular side. A shuttling suture is grasped through the anteroinferior cannula. A high-strength polyethylene suture is then shuttled through the tendon and back out the anterior-superior cannula. The maneuver is repeated, and the other end of the suture is brought out in a similar fashion 5 mm away from the first pass to affect a horizontal mattress configuration (see Fig. 14-82B). A knotless suture anchor is threaded with the sutures and inserted through the anterior-superior cannula with the shoulder in internal rotation (see Fig. 14-82C). This allows the appropriate trajectory to deploy the anchor into the footprint, achieve secure fixation, and restore the anatomy without disrupting intact cuff fibers (see Fig. 14-82D).

For large articular-sided tears (>15 mm), two suture anchors can be placed through the intact tendon to span the tear. One suture limb from each anchor can be tied together to create a bridge of suture over the rotator cuff, and subsequent tying of the other suture will compress the rotator cuff down onto the medial insertional footprint.

Full-Thickness Repair

Mobilization and release of tendon must first be performed, particularly in retracted tears, to assess whether repair is possible and to ensure a repair with minimal tension. One or two lateral portals (depending on tear size) should be established based on the location of the tear. These portals are usually two or three fingerbreadths lateral to the lateral edge of the acromion. Adhesions often develop between the articular side of the rotator cuff and the superior aspect of the glenoid and labrum. This can be released with a radiofrequency device. Bursal-sided adhesions can also be released using the undersurface of the acromion and the scapular spine as bony guides.

Assessment of rotator cuff tear configuration can be performed from the posterior portal. Larger tears can be more accurately assessed from an additional lateral portal. Determining the rotator cuff tear pattern is important in order for the surgeon to plan the appropriate method of repair. Most tears can be classified as (1) crescent shaped, (2) U-shaped, 93) L-shaped, or (4) massive, contracted tears. Our preference is to perform double-row repairs

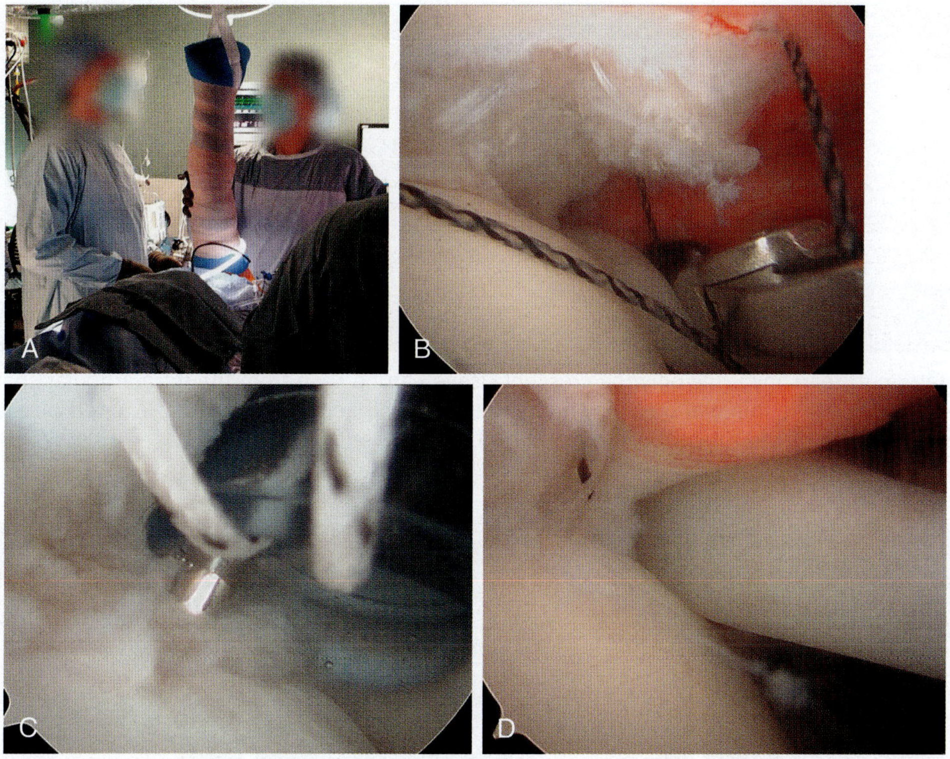

FIGURE 14-82: **A,** All-inside partial-thickness rotator cuff repair can be performed with the arm in abduction. **B,** A curved suture-passing device is used to pass sutures through the detached tendon flap. **C,** This is repeated, and the tendon is brought down to the insertion with a knotless suture anchor. **D,** This can restore the tendon anatomy without disrupting intact cuff fibers.

when possible and to use an inverted mattress technique for small crescent-shaped tears.

Before anchor placement and tendon fixation, the tuberosity footprint should be prepared. This involves removing residual soft tissue and exposing the underlying cortical bone surface. The bone surface can be gently burred to promote punctate bleeding in order to maximize the local biology for healing without violating the structural integrity of the bone, which could compromise anchor purchase. Others have described a microfracture technique at or near the footprint of the repair to allow for egress of bone marrow elements to augment the local healing response.[305]

Crescent-shaped tears are considered simple tears that have minimal medial retraction (Fig. 14-83A and 14-83B). Often, these tears have good lateral mobility and can be fixed back to the tuberosity with minimal tension. For these types of tears, we consider using an inverted mattress configuration of sutures. Through the lateral portal, an arthroscopic suture-passing device can be used to pass the suture from inferior to superior through the anterior portion of the torn tendon. This is repeated with the other suture limb a few millimeters posterior to the initial pass. This can be repeated with more sutures. After the sutures have been passed through the tendon, the suture limbs are brought out through the lateral cannula, tensioned appropriately, and inserted into an anchor on the lateral aspect of the greater tuberosity. When the anchor is seated, the sutures should provide compression of the rotator cuff tendon down onto the bone (see Fig. 14-83C).

L-shaped and U-shaped tears are more complex, and are more medially retracted tears than the simple crescent configuration. In U-shaped tear patterns, often the apex of the tear cannot simply be brought straight laterally to the tuberosity without a large amount of tension. Side-to-side suturing from medial to lateral will allow the free margin of the tear to converge toward the insertion, thus the name "margin convergence." This technique can decrease strain on the repair site. In L-shaped and reverse L-shaped tears, one portion of the tear will be more readily mobile. Gentle traction of the tendon edge with a grasper should be used to determine which direction the tendon mobilizes. A common L-shaped tear will have a more mobile leaf posteromedially, and the reduction maneuver will require bringing that apex to the anterolateral corner. Side-to-side sutures can be used in a margin convergence technique between the longer medial-lateral components of the tear before repairing the converged margin to the bone (Fig. 14-84).[37,38]

Arthroscopic double-row repairs of large rotator cuff tears (Fig. 14-85A) can be performed by placing anchors at the medial margin of the cuff footprint. The appropriate angle for anchor insertion is first confirmed using a spinal needle along the lateral edge of the acromion (see Fig. 14-85B). Once the appropriate angle is confirmed, a small skin incision is made with an 11-blade scalpel, and

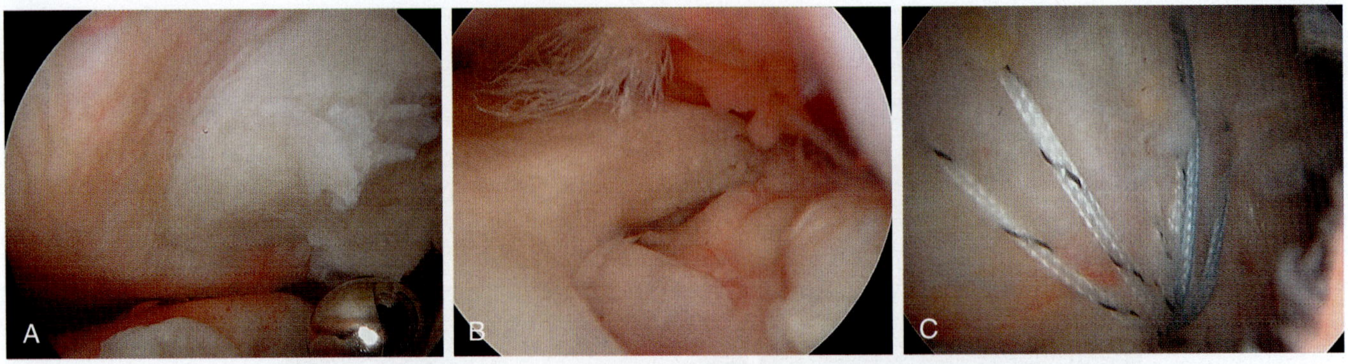

FIGURE 14-83: Rotator cuff tears involving only the crescent tissue can be seen from the intra-articular space (**A**) and subacromial space (**B**). They typically have minimal medial retraction and can be addressed with an inverted mattress configuration of sutures to provide compression of the rotator cuff tendon down onto bone (**C**).

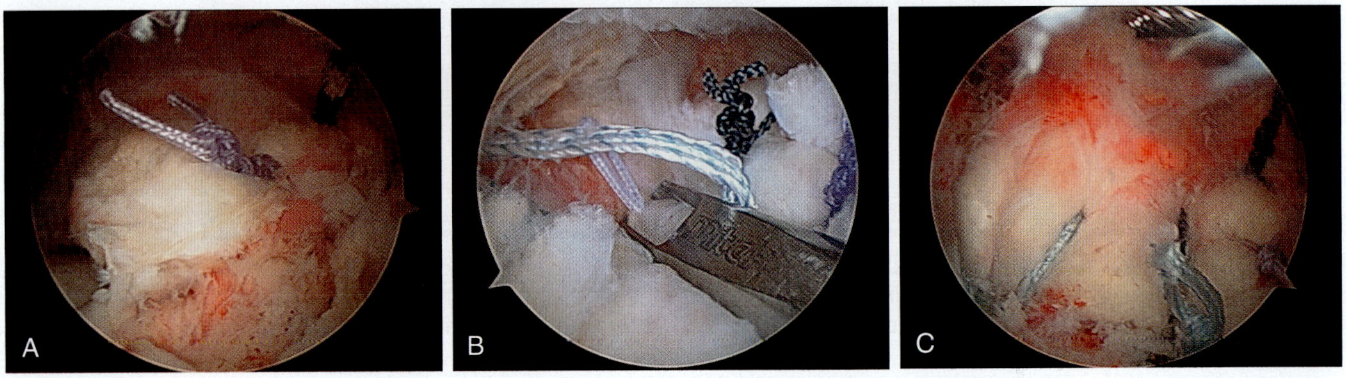

FIGURE 14-84: For a reverse L-shaped tear, side-to-side sutures can be placed through the posterior leaflet (**A**), then the suture can be passed through the free margin (**B**) and tied down to the bone in order to repair the converged margin down to the bone (**C**).

a small hemostat is used to open up the tissue to accept the anchor (see Fig. 14-85C). Anchor insertion is repeated with one or two more anchors depending on the size of the tear. Each limb of the suture is passed through the tendon about 2 to 3 mm lateral to the musculotendinous junction using a suture-passing device and retrieved from an anterior portal. A traction stitch is often helpful to gain access to retracted tears. This is repeated with each suture strand from anterior to posterior (see Fig. 14-85D). Care should be taken to ensure that the sutures are not passed too medially in the tendon, as this can put the patient at risk for overtensioning, postoperative stiffness, and repair failure. Matching suture limbs are tied arthroscopically from posterior to anterior (see Fig. 14-85E). Any dog ears can be addressed with inverted mattress sutures prior to insertion of the lateral row of anchors. Suture limbs from each anchor are crossed and inserted into a lateral row of suture anchors to compress the tendon down to the bone (see Fig. 14-85F and G).

Anterior and posterior interval slides have been described to free up the contracted muscle-tendon units of both the supraspinatus and infraspinatus.[195,317] The anterior interval slide involves releasing the interval between the supraspinatus tendon anteriorly and the rotator interval, effectively cutting through a contracted coracohumeral ligament. Posterior interval release involves dividing the interval between the supraspinatus and the infraspinatus, and can also be utilized to improve excursion of the tendon(s) back to the tuberosity. Care must be taken not to damage the suprascapular nerve as it curves around the base of the scapular spine.

The repair of the tendon back to the bone surface of the tuberosity is most commonly performed using suture anchors in an arthroscopic approach. These anchors come in various materials from nonabsorbable metals and inert plastics to fully absorbable polymers to all-suture anchors. They also come in various sizes depending on the type of anchor and the manufacturer. There is debate about the different materials from which anchors are made and how they perform clinically. Studies have shown that some anchors such as poly-L-lactic acid anchors may be associated with pain, synovitis, and early failure.[209,262]

MINI-OPEN ROTATOR CUFF REPAIR

Mini-open rotator cuff repair has the advantages of allowing direct assessment of the nature of the cuff tear, the quality of the remaining tissue, and the ease with which the tendon edge can be restored to the normal insertion

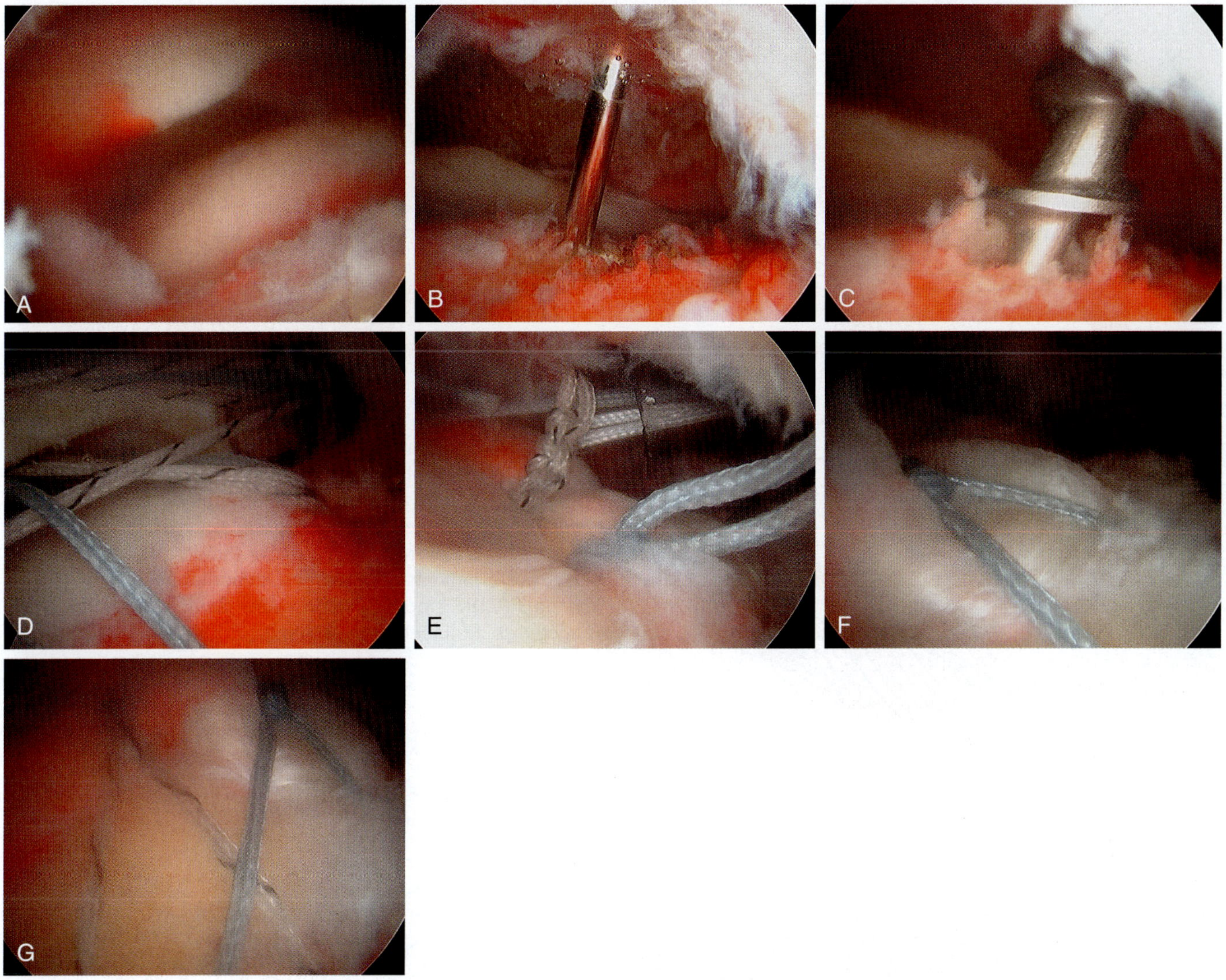

FIGURE 14-85: Arthroscopic double-row repair of a large rotator cuff tear (**A**) can be performed by first localizing the proper anchor insertion point with a spinal needle just off the lateral border of the acromion (**B**). Medial row anchors are then inserted (**C**), and the suture limbs are passed sequentially through the tendon from anterior to posterior (**D**). Matching suture limbs are tied from posterior to anterior (**E**). Strands from each anchor are then crossed to two different lateral row anchors to complete the repair (**F** and **G**).

site with the arm in an adducted position. The transosseous technique for attachment of the tendon to the tuberosity is simple, expeditious, avoids issues related to suture anchors, and enables the surgeon to find sufficiently strong bone to hold the sutures. The creation of a trough into which the tendon is inserted increases the surface area of the repair, stimulates local stem cells and growth factors, excludes joint fluid from the repair site, and places sutures laterally so that they do not rub beneath the coracoacromial arch.

The patient is positioned in a semisitting (beach chair) position. Both the anterior and posterior aspects of the chest and the arm are prepared to allow access to the posterior shoulder and full arm motion. Surgery begins with an inspection of the cuff through a deltoid-on approach (Fig. 14-86). Great care is taken to avoid deltoid detachment and preserve the tendon fibers of the deltoid origin so that a strong repair can be achieved at the conclusion of the procedure. The deltoid has an important tendon of origin between its anterior and middle thirds. Arising from the anterior lateral corner of the acromion, this tendon is a guide to exposure of the cuff shoulder be repaired at the conclusion of cuff repair. This tendon is split longitudinally for 3 to 4 cm distal to the acromion in line with its fibers, with care taken to leave some of the tendon on each side of the split (Fig. 14-87). The humeroscapular motion interface is mobilized (Figs. 14-88 and 14-89).

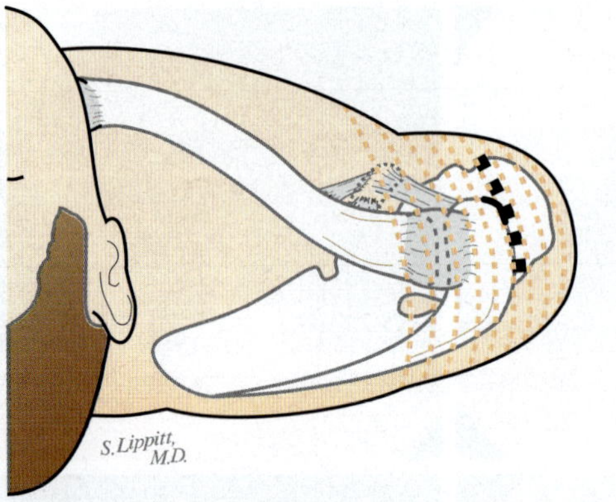

FIGURE 14-86: The deltoid-on approach, showing the skin incision in Langer's lines. (From Matsen FA III, Lippitt SB. *Shoulder Surgery: Principles and Procedures.* Philadelphia: Saunders; 2004:330, 312, 349.)

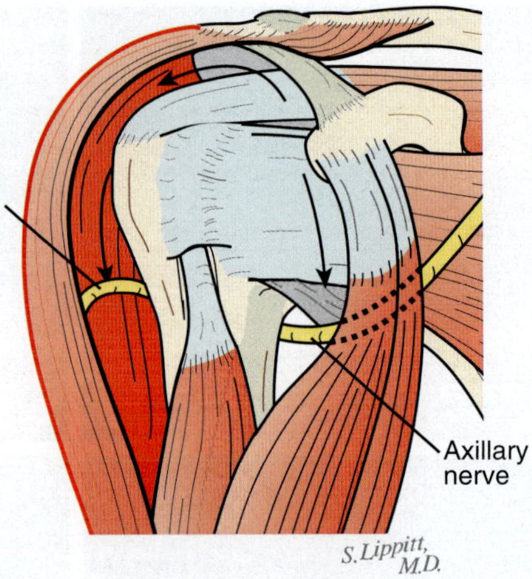

FIGURE 14-88: Nerve-to-nerve release. All scar tissue in the humeroscapular motion interface is released from the axillary nerve medially as it crosses the subscapularis, then under the coracoid, then under the coracoacromial ligament, then under the acromion, and then finally, under the deltoid to the axillary nerve posteriorly as it exits the quadrilateral space. (From Matsen FA III, Lippitt SB. *Shoulder Surgery: Principles and Procedures.* Philadelphia: Saunders; 2004:334.)

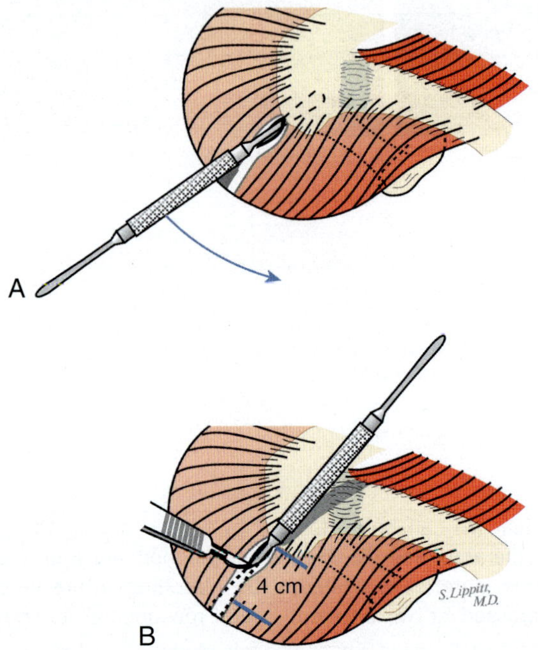

FIGURE 14-87: Inserting an elevator in the deltoid split. **A,** Once the subdeltoid bursa is entered, a small blunt elevator is inserted through the split and then underneath the deltoid. **B,** This elevator is then rotated 180 degrees while still in the bursa. The incision in the deltoid and bursa is then extended 4 cm distal from the acromion. (From Matsen FA III, Lippitt SB. *Shoulder Surgery: Principles and Procedures.* Philadelphia: Saunders; 2004:332.)

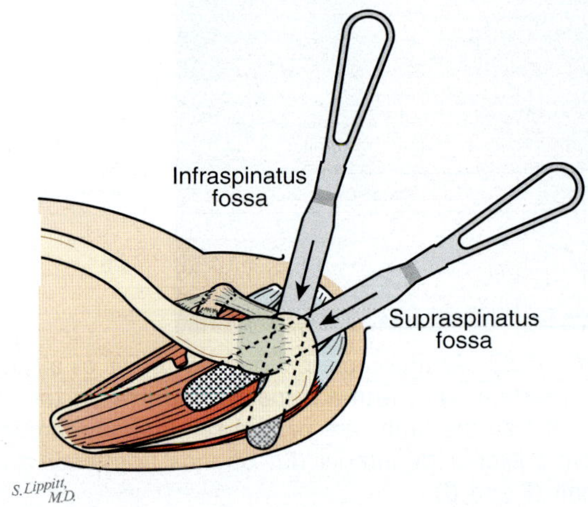

FIGURE 14-89: Verifying complete release. A smooth elevator is passed superficially to the supraspinatus and infraspinatus to ensure their freedom from the overlying coracoacromial arch. (From Matsen FA III, Lippitt SB. *Shoulder Surgery: Principles and Procedures.* Philadelphia: Saunders; 2004:299.)

Hypertrophic bursa and scar tissue are resected to allow a good view of cuff tendon involvement, tendon quality, and tendon tissue loss (Fig. 14-90). The undersurface of the coracoacromial arch is palpated to detect any points of roughness. Any rough spots are smoothed with a pinecone bur (Fig. 14-91). It is essential to preserve the integrity of the coracoacromial arch.

The goal of repair is strong fixation of the tendon to the humerus under normal tension with the arm at the side while leaving a smooth surface on the proximal humeral concavity to articulate with the undersurface of the coracoacromial arch. The desired attachment site is at the sulcus near the base of the tuberosity. This goal is facilitated using three stages of sequential release. These releases are required because the cuff is usually retracted and tissue is lost in chronic cuff disease. Unless these releases are carried out, increased tension in the repaired

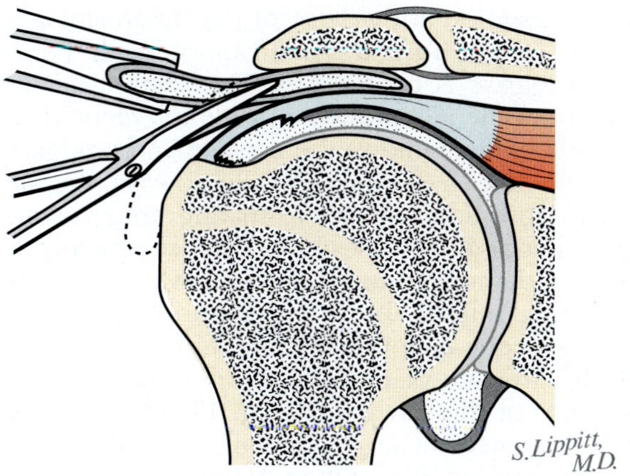

FIGURE 14-90: Removal of bursa. The hypertrophic bursa is removed by sharp dissection. (From Matsen FA III, Lippitt SB. *Shoulder Surgery: Principles and Procedures.* Philadelphia: Saunders; 2004:333.)

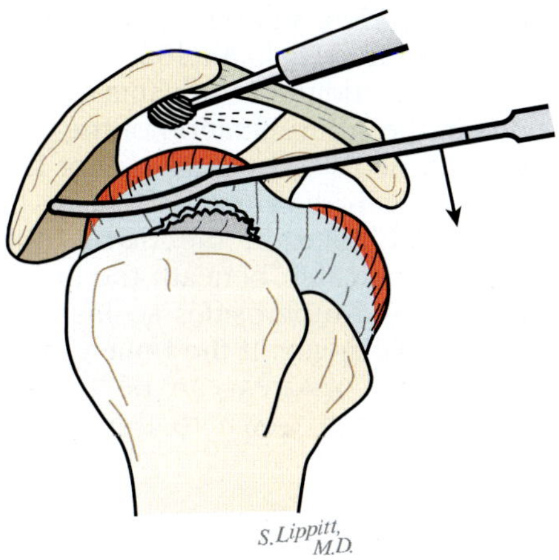

FIGURE 14-91: Smoothing of the coracoacromial arch. If there is roughness on the underside of the coracoacromial arch (although this is rarely the case), it can be smoothed with a pinecone bur, leaving the arch intact. (From Matsen FA III, Lippitt SB. *Shoulder Surgery: Principles and Procedures.* Philadelphia: Saunders; 2004:355.)

tendon will predispose to tightness of the glenohumeral joint and will additionally challenge the repair site.[366] The humeral head is rotated to successively present the margins of the cuff defect through the incision (Fig. 14-92) rather than enlarging the exposure to show the entire lesion at one time.

The deep surface of the cuff is searched for retracted laminations. All layers of the cuff are assembled and tagged with sutures (Fig. 14-93). Traction is applied to these sutures, by which the cuff is mobilized sequentially as necessary to allow the torn tendon edge to reach the desired insertion at the base of the tuberosity. First, the humeroscapular motion interface (see Figs. 14-88 and 14-89) is freed between the cuff and the deltoid, acromion, coracoacromial ligaments, coracoid, and coracoid

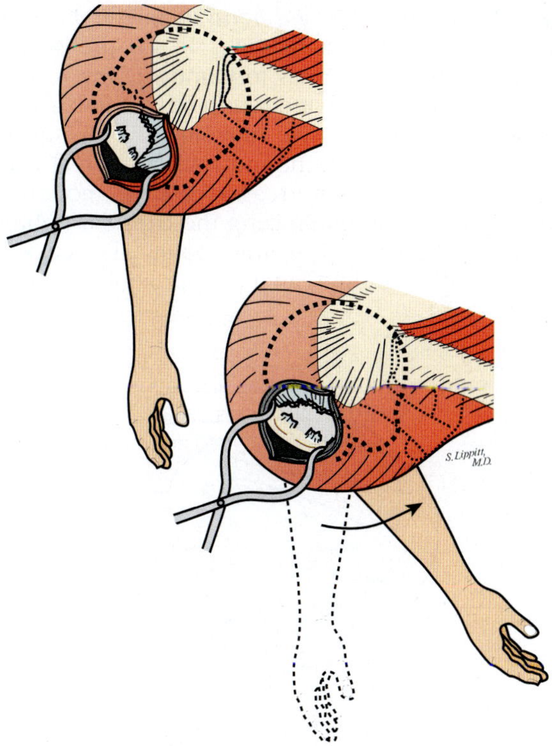

FIGURE 14-92: Viewing the cuff tear. By rotating the arm, the different elements of the cuff can be brought to this split, rather than making a bigger exposure by detaching the deltoid origin. (From Matsen FA III, Lippitt SB. *Shoulder Surgery: Principles and Procedures.* Philadelphia: Saunders; 2004:356.)

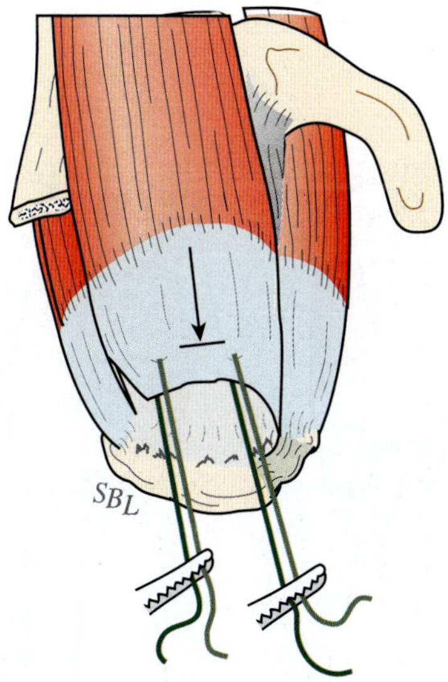

FIGURE 14-93: Traction sutures are placed in the cuff tendon. These sutures should be able to withstand a strong pull (*arrow*) without pulling through the tendon. (From Matsen FA III, Lippitt SB. *Shoulder Surgery: Principles and Procedures.* Philadelphia: Saunders; 2004:357.)

muscles. Next, the *coracohumeral* ligament (Fig. 14-94) and rotator interval capsule (Fig. 14-95) are sectioned around the coracoid process to eliminate any restriction to excursion of the cuff tendons and minimize tension on the repair during passive movement. This release of the *coracohumeral* ligament and rotator interval capsule also contributes to comfort and ease of motion after the surgical repair by minimizing the capsular-tightening effect of cuff repair.[366] At this point, the ease with which the cuff margins can be approximated to their anatomic insertion at the base of the tuberosity is evaluated (Fig. 14-96). If good tissue cannot reach the sulcus, the third release is carried out. This release divides the capsule from the glenoid just outside the glenoid labrum (Fig. 14-97), which allows the capsule and tendon of the cuff to be drawn farther laterally toward the desired tuberosity insertion without restricting range of motion. After the necessary releases have been completed, a judgment is made concerning the site at which the cuff can be implanted into the bone without undue tension while the arm is at the side (Figs. 14-98 and 14-99).

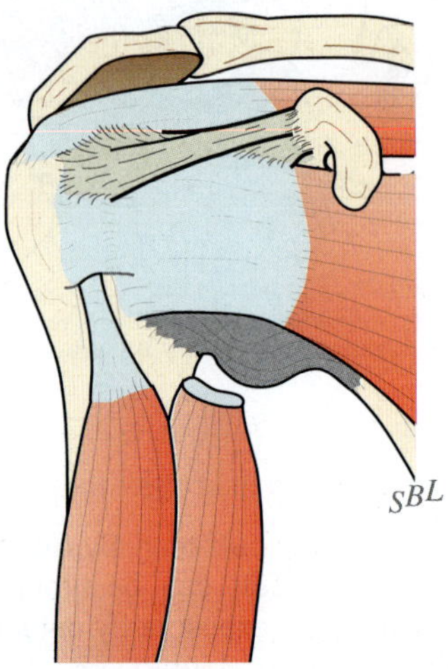

FIGURE 14-94: Coracohumeral ligament. The coracohumeral ligament runs from the base of the coracoid to the transverse humeral ligament. It can restrict external rotation and internal rotation when the arm is in adduction. It is most easily released at the base of the coracoid process. (From Matsen FA III, Lippitt SB. *Shoulder Surgery: Principles and Procedures*. Philadelphia: Saunders; 2004:335.)

Ideally, the site of implantation will be in the sulcus at the base of the tuberosity (Fig. 14-100). In large cuff defects, a somewhat more medial insertion site may be necessary (Fig. 14-101). Often, when a medial insertion site is required for a large cuff defect, the new insertion lies in an area where the articular cartilage has been damaged by abrasion against the undersurface of the acromion.

The repair is accomplished as a tongue-in-groove type of repair, with the cuff tendon drawn into a trough near the tuberosity to provide a smooth upper surface to glide beneath the acromion (Figs. 14-102 to 14-111). This groove provides the additional advantage that if some slippage occurs in the suture fixation of the cuff to bone, contact between these two structures is not lost. Nonabsorbable sutures woven through the tendon margin are passed through drill holes in the distal tuberosity so that the knots will not catch beneath the acromion. The knots are tied over the tuberosities so that they will lie out of the subacromial space. If the bone of the tuberosities is osteopenic, the sutures can be passed through bone more distally, even down to the junction of the

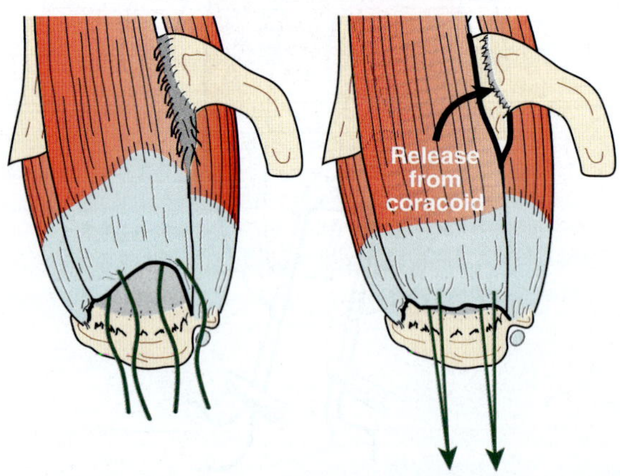

FIGURE 14-95: Release of the cuff tendon from the coracoid allows lateral advancement of the tendon edge toward the desired insertion site. (From Matsen FA III, Lippitt SB. *Shoulder Surgery: Principles and Procedures*. Philadelphia: Saunders; 2004:300.)

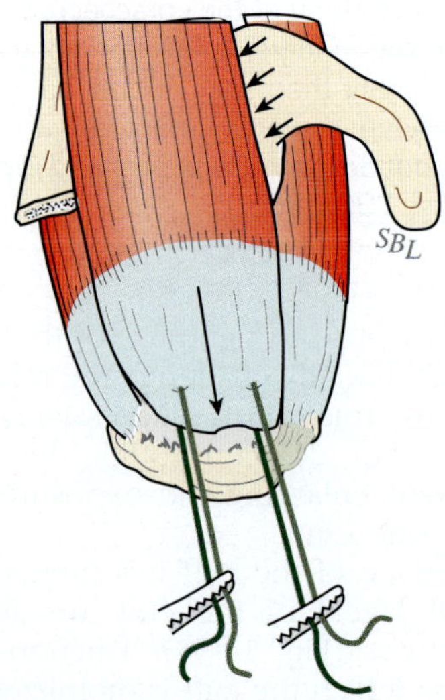

FIGURE 14-96: After the release (*small horizontal arrows*). The lateral edge of the supraspinatus can now reach the base of the greater tuberosity (*large vertical arrow*). (From Matsen FA III, Lippitt SB. *Shoulder Surgery: Principles and Procedures*. Philadelphia: Saunders; 2004:360.)

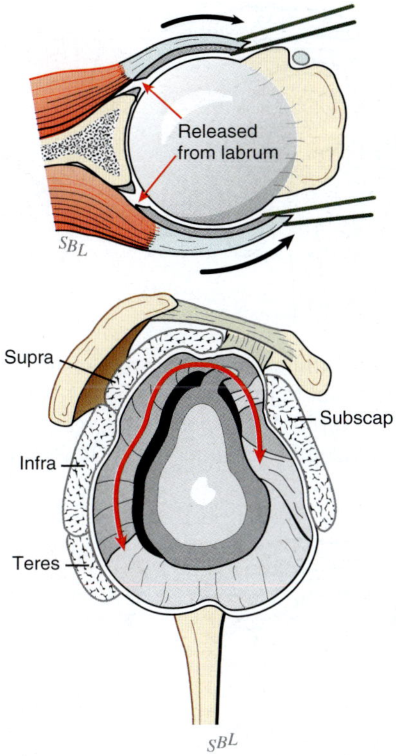

FIGURE 14-97: Release of the capsule from the labrum allows further lateral advancement of the tendon edge. *Infra,* infraspinatus; *Subscap,* subscapularis; *Supra,* supraspinatus; *Teres,* teres major. (From Matsen FA III, Lippitt SB. *Shoulder Surgery: Principles and Procedures*. Philadelphia: Saunders; 2004:301.)

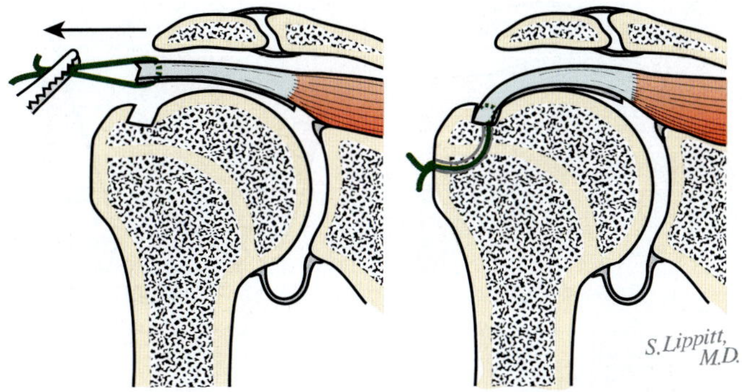

FIGURE 14-98: Adequate excursion. If a durable repair is to be carried out, the tendon margin should reach the insertion site with the arm in adduction without the application of excess tension. (From Matsen FA III, Lippitt SB. *Shoulder Surgery: Principles and Procedures*. Philadelphia: Saunders; 2004:360.)

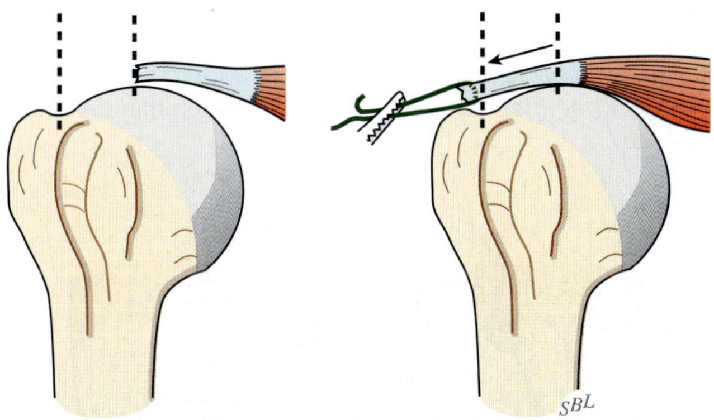

FIGURE 14-99: Cuff bounce. Once the tendon is freed of adhesions, the muscle should have a springy feel when traction is applied and released. (From Matsen FA III, Lippitt SB. *Shoulder Surgery: Principles and Procedures*. Philadelphia: Saunders; 2004:361.)

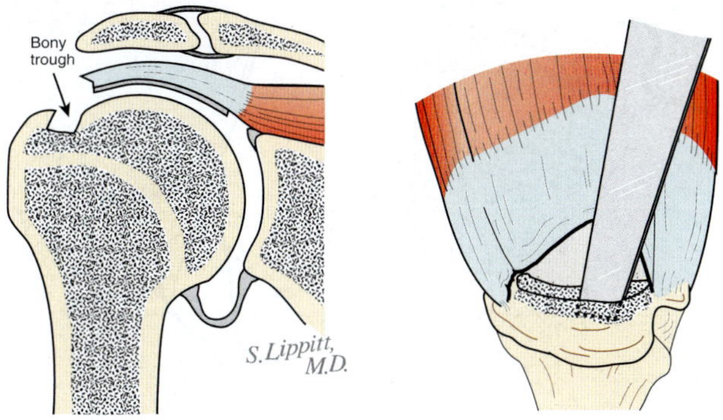

FIGURE 14-100: A bony trough is made at the base of the greater tuberosity, just lateral to the articular surface. The trough extends the full length of the tendon detachment. (From Matsen FA III, Lippitt SB. *Shoulder Surgery: Principles and Procedures*. Philadelphia: Saunders; 2004:302.)

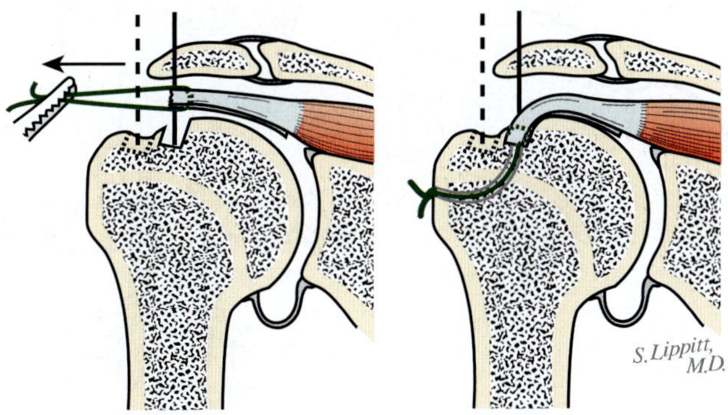

FIGURE 14-101: Medializing the trough. If the tendon will not reach the normal insertion site with the arm in adduction, the trough can be moved medially on the head if this will allow a robust attachment. (From Matsen FA III, Lippitt SB. *Shoulder Surgery: Principles and Procedures*. Philadelphia: Saunders; 2004:365.)

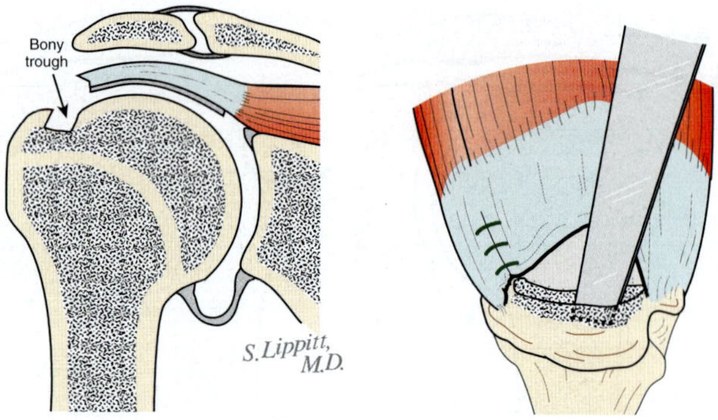

FIGURE 14-102: Creating a trough. Using a flat osteotome, a 7-mm wide trough is created at the base of the tuberosity at the margin of the articular cartilage for the length of the cuff tear. (From Matsen FA III, Lippitt SB. *Shoulder Surgery: Principles and Procedures*. Philadelphia: Saunders; 2004:364.)

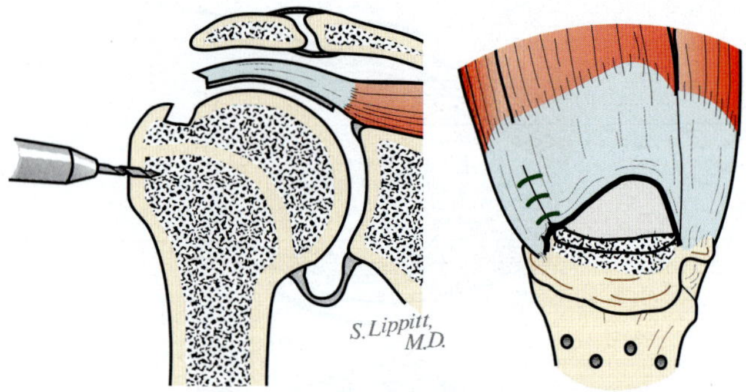

FIGURE 14-103: Drilling the greater tuberosity. Staggered drill holes are made distal to the trough using a 1.8-mm drill. (From Matsen FA III, Lippitt SB. *Shoulder Surgery: Principles and Procedures*. Philadelphia: Saunders; 2004:365.)

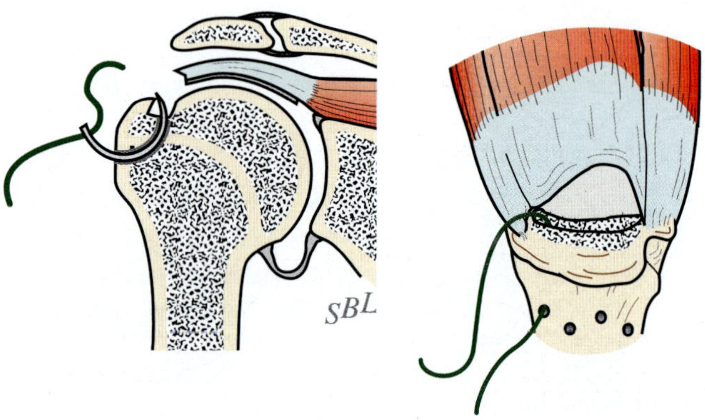

FIGURE 14-104: Placement of the first suture. The first suture of No. 2 braided nonabsorbable suture is passed from the tuberosity into the groove using a No. 3 trocar needle. (From Matsen FA III, Lippitt SB. *Shoulder Surgery: Principles and Procedures*. Philadelphia: Saunders; 2004:366.)

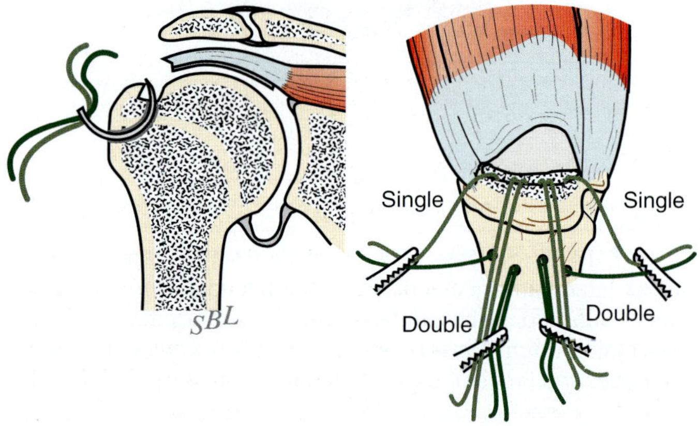

FIGURE 14-105: Placement of the double sutures. Double sutures are passed through the remainder of the holes except for the last one. (From Matsen FA III, Lippitt SB. *Shoulder Surgery: Principles and Procedures*. Philadelphia: Saunders; 2004:367.)

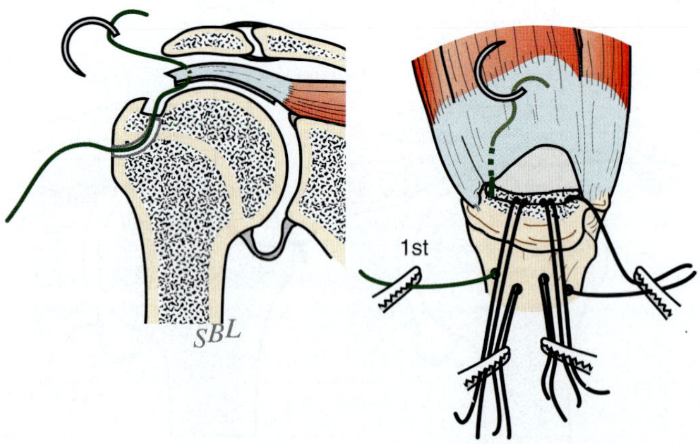

FIGURE 14-106: Passing the first suture through tendon. The first suture is passed through the tendon edge, making sure that the full-thickness of the cuff and capsule are included and that the bite is sufficiently medial so that the tissue is robust. (From Matsen FA III, Lippitt SB. *Shoulder Surgery: Principles and Procedures*. Philadelphia: Saunders; 2004:367.)

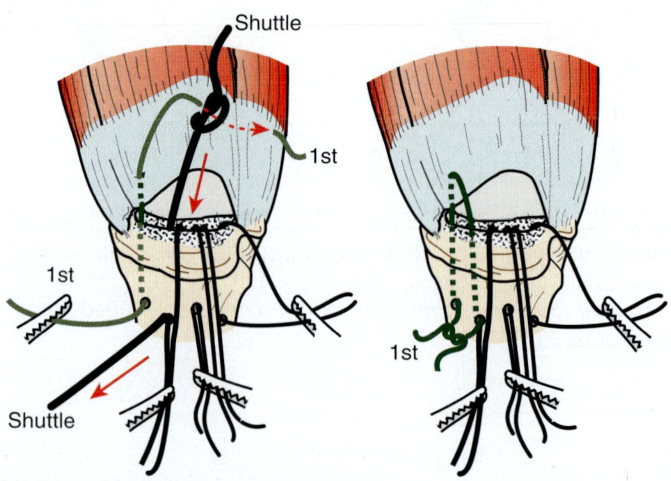

FIGURE 14-107: Shuttling the first suture. One of the two sutures in the second hole is used to shuttle the free end of the first suture through it. The *solid arrows* indicate the direction of shuttling; the *dotted arrow* indicates the direction of the suture through the shuttle. (From Matsen FA III, Lippitt SB. *Shoulder Surgery: Principles and Procedures*. Philadelphia: Saunders; 2004:368.)

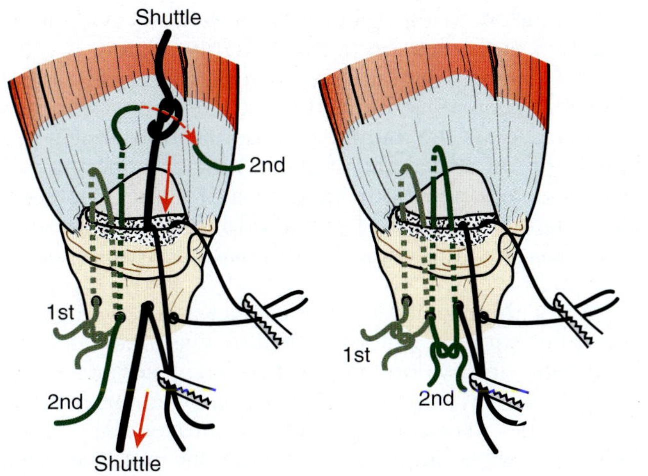

FIGURE 14-108: Shuttling the second suture. The second suture is passed through the tendon and out the adjacent hole. The *solid arrows* indicate the direction of shuttling; the *dotted arrow* indicates the direction of the suture through the shuttle. (From Matsen FA III, Lippitt SB. *Shoulder Surgery: Principles and Procedures*. Philadelphia: Saunders; 2004:369.)

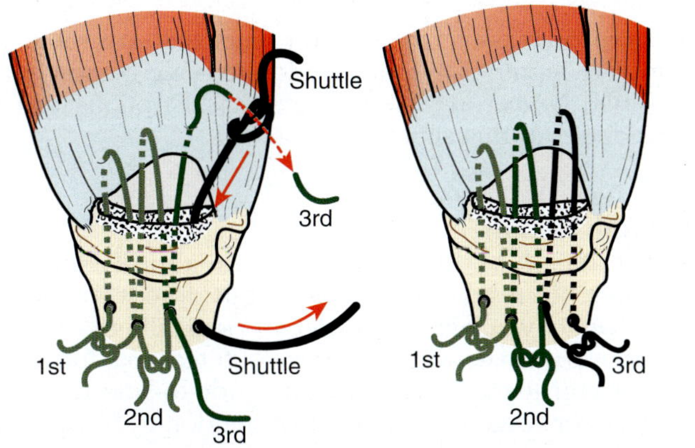

FIGURE 14-109: Shuttling the third suture. The process is continued until the final single suture is used to shuttle the end of the last suture through the last hole. The *solid arrows* indicate the direction of shuttling; the *dotted arrow* indicates the direction of the suture through the shuttle. (From Matsen FA III, Lippitt SB. *Shoulder Surgery: Principles and Procedures*. Philadelphia: Saunders; 2004:370.)

metaphysis and diaphysis (Fig. 14-112). If the tear has a longitudinal component, it is repaired in a side-to-side fashion with the knots buried out of the humeroscapular motion interface. The repair is checked throughout a range of motion to 140 degrees of elevation and 40 degrees of external rotation to ensure that it is strong, that it is not under excessive tension, and that it will permit smooth subacromial motion. If additional debridement is required to allow smooth passage of the repaired tendon, it is performed at this time (Fig. 14-113).

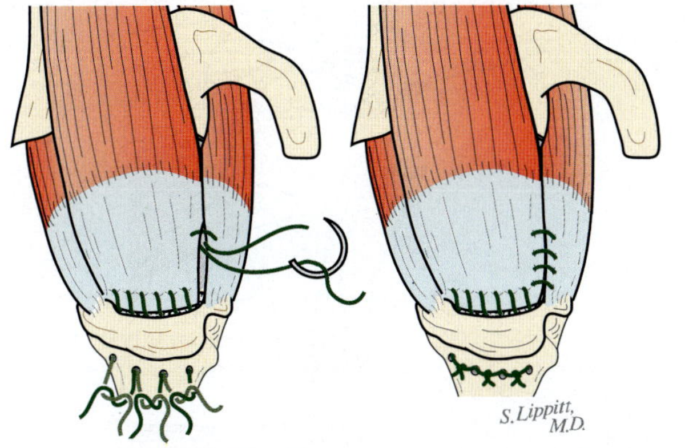

FIGURE 14-110: The side-to-side repair of the split between the supraspinatus and subscapularis is carried out using a buried knot technique so that when the knots are tied there will be no roughness on the outer aspect of the proximal humeral convexity. (From Matsen FA III, Lippitt SB. *Shoulder Surgery: Principles and Procedures*. Philadelphia: Saunders; 2004:371.)

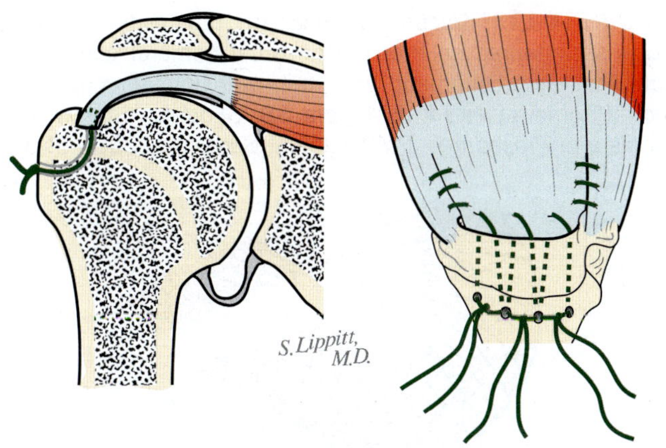

FIGURE 14-111: Tying these sutures brings the tendon into the trough and places the knots out of the way of the coracoacromial arch. (From Matsen FA III, Lippitt SB. *Shoulder Surgery: Principles and Procedures*. Philadelphia: Saunders; 2004:372.)

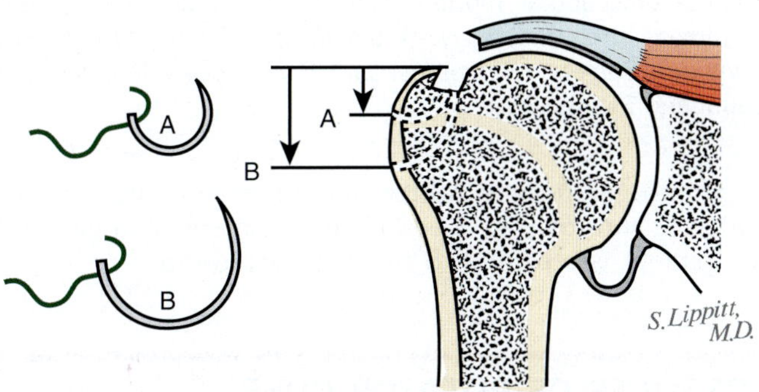

FIGURE 14-112: Finding adequate bone. If the bone of the proximal tuberosity is weak, the holes are made more distally in solid bone. (From Matsen FA III, Lippitt SB. *Shoulder Surgery: Principles and Procedures*. Philadelphia: Saunders; 2004:366.)

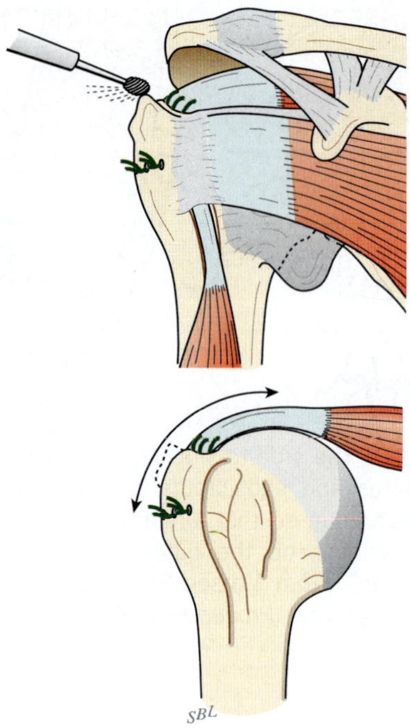

FIGURE 14-113: Smoothing the greater tuberosity. The tuberosity is contoured so that the proximal humeral concavity is spherical and congruent with the overlying coracoacromial arch. (From Matsen FA III, Lippitt SB. *Shoulder Surgery: Principles and Procedures*. Philadelphia: Saunders; 2004:373.)

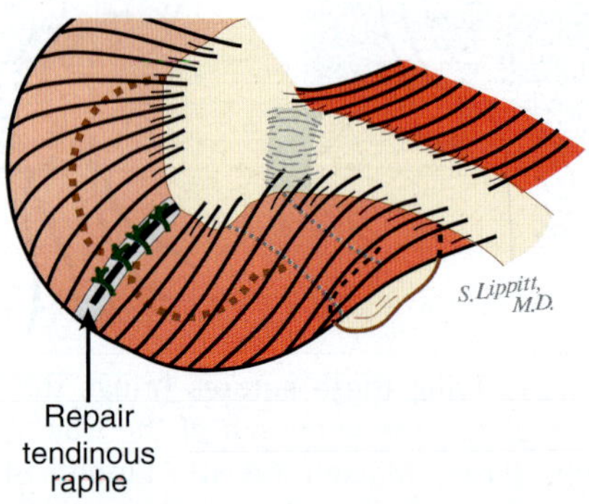

FIGURE 14-114: Deltoid split repair. The tendinous raphe of the deltoid split is repaired, ensuring that the knots are out of the humeroscapular motion interface and that they are not prominent subcutaneously. (From Matsen FA III, Lippitt SB. *Shoulder Surgery: Principles and Procedures*. Philadelphia: Saunders; 2004:338.)

After a careful and robust deltoid repair using nonabsorbable sutures (Fig. 14-114) and cosmetic skin closure, the patient is returned to the recovery room.

RESULTS OF ROTATOR CUFF REPAIR SURGERY

There are two aspects of the results of cuff repair surgery: functional improvement and success of the reattachment of the tendon to the tuberosity. It is now evident that these two outcomes are not necessarily related. A recent review[211] found 2383 articles on rotator cuff repair published between 1980 and 2012, with an almost exponential increase in the number of publications each year. One hundred and eight of these articles covering 8011 shoulders reported both imaging and clinical outcomes after rotator cuff repair. Despite efforts to advance surgical techniques, the clinical and anatomic results did not show improvement over the period of study. Over one-quarter of the repairs were not intact at an average of 2 years after surgery. Failure of healing was associated with more fatty infiltration, larger tear size, advanced age, and double-row repairs. Clinical improvement averaged 72% of the maximum possible improvement. Clinical outcomes were improved whether or not the repair attempt was successful in restoring the integrity of the rotator cuff. These findings led us to consider options other than repair for cuff tears that are unlikely to heal after attempted repair.

SURGICAL OPTIONS FOR IRREPARABLE CUFF TEARS

In large or massive rotator cuff tears that are retracted, complete repair of the torn tendon to bone is usually not possible. Numerous alternative surgical options can be considered in this situation.

Partial Repair

Partial repair of the rotator cuff is a procedure that attempts to restore the rotator cuff force couples to improve active elevation. Burkhart originally described a partial repair to convert a massive cuff tear to a functional rotator cuff tear.[36] This involved a side-to-side repair for margin convergence followed by tendon-to-bone repair to decrease strain at the free margin of the tear.

In a rat rotator cuff model of a two-tendon rotator cuff tear, repair of the infraspinatus only was superior to no repair and equivalent to repair of both the infraspinatus and supraspinatus.[127] A comparative clinical study of partial and complete repairs for massive cuff tears by Iagulli et al. demonstrated similar improvements in University of California at Los Angeles scores between both groups.[130]

Numerous case series have reported on the clinical results after partial repair of the rotator cuff for massive cuff tears. Duralde and Bair noted high patient satisfaction and excellent or good results in two-thirds of patients undergoing partial repair.[71] Kim et al. investigated partial repair in tears over 3 cm, and found that all patients improved in terms of Simple Shoulder Test (SST), University of California at Los Angeles, and Constant scores, but muscle strength was not restored to the level of the contralateral side.[159] Porcellini[367] reported a minimum 5-year follow-up after partial repairs and found good results in terms of patient satisfaction, and also suggested that acromiohumeral distance can be increased with a partial repair. Wellmann et al.[368] found that pain and function improved significantly with partial repair, but that acromiohumeral distance decreased and active external rotation motion decreased.

Despite the positive results of these case series, others have reported high rates of structural failure after partial repair.[22,233] Mori et al. reported a 41.7% re-tear rate with partial repair, which was significantly higher than that of a cohort of patients treated with a patch graft.[233] Berth et al. noted that over half (52%) of their partial repairs were re-torn at the latest follow-up.[22] Shon et al. reported that despite initial improvement in most patients, about half of the patients in their study had deterioration over time and were unsatisfied with the results.[301]

The disadvantages of attempting a partial repair are that (1) the tissue quality is often poor, so re-tears are likely, and (2) protection of the repair is necessary for months after surgery, delaying the resumption of rehabilitation and daily activities.

Nonrepair Strategies

Bigliani et al.[27] and Galatz et al.[91] have reported improved shoulder function after attempting surgery for massive rotator cuff defects. Their studies, however, failed to demonstrate convincing evidence that the cuff tissue healed. Other authors have also reported good clinical outcomes following attempted repair of massive cuff defects, but follow-up studies have demonstrated failure of the cuff to heal in 60% to 90% of cases.[43,93,118,353] These studies pose the inevitable question that if the cuff tissue did not heal, what factors contributed to the reported improvement in clinical status of these patient populations? Possible contributing factors include removal of inflamed bursal tissue and smoothing of the articulation between the proximal humerus and the acromion.

In patients with refractory pain, stiffness, and crepitus with large rotator cuff tears, we have found that addressing subacromial pathology without repair of the cuff tear can decrease pain and allow for smooth, unrestricted motion at the humeroscapular interface; we refer to this as the "smooth and move procedure."

Smooth and Move Procedure

Surface irregularities producing subacromial roughness are almost always on the humeral side of the humeroscapular motion interface rather than on the side of the coracoacromial arch. The goal of the smooth and move procedure is to smooth the surface of the proximal humeral convexity while preserving the integrity of the coracoacromial arch and deltoid.

Our experience suggests that the optimal candidate for a smooth and move procedure is a well-motivated patient with symptoms of pain, crepitus, and stiffness associated with an irreparable tear or a failed prior repair who wishes to avoid the risks of failure and the extended rehabilitation associated with an attempted surgical reconstruction. The procedure is not appropriate for shoulders with pseudoparalysis or anterior-superior escape, glenohumeral arthritis, or instability. Patients who are depressed or have problems attributed to their employment tend to do less well.

A mini-open approach to subacromial smoothing is utilized so that the passage of the proximal humeral convexity beneath the coracoacromial arch can be evaluated directly. The patient is positioned with the head up at 30 degrees and the arm draped free so that full motion is possible. Before incision, the surgeon notes the positions and motions in which subacromial crepitus can be palpated through the acromion. The shoulder is approached through an incision in the skin lines over the anterolateral corner of the acromion (see Fig. 14-86). The strong deltoid raphe is split between the anterior and middle thirds of this muscle (see Fig. 14-87). This technique allows two strong handles on the deltoid for repair. In most cases, no detachment of the deltoid origin is needed. This split is deepened under direct vision until the bursa is entered. Rotating the humerus provides easy differentiation between the deltoid surface of the bursa (which does not move with humeral rotation) and the superficial surface of the cuff (which does).

On entering the subacromial aspect of the humeroscapular motion interface, the surgeon can observe the subacromial space while the preoperatively identified crepitus-producing movements are carried out. This step reveals the cause of the crepitus, which is usually some combination of hypertrophic bursa, adhesions between the cuff and acromion, roughness of the superior surface of the rotator cuff, frayed edges of torn tendons, residual suture anchors, and sutures and prominence of the greater tuberosity. By gently rotating the arm, the surgeon can bring most of the cuff to the incision, as pointed out by Codman[52] (Fig. 14-115). The rotator cuff is thoroughly explored and palpated for evidence of superior surface blisters, partial tears, thinning, or full-thickness defects. Although deep surface cuff fiber failure cannot be seen through this approach, it is also true that such fiber disruption cannot be causing the subacromial crepitus. The methylene blue dye test of Hiro Fukuda[86] or, more recently, the Fukuda-lite test with saline is used to evaluate shoulders with suspicious cuff integrity (there are some reports that intra-articular dye injections have been associated with chondrolysis). In this test, fluid is injected to distend the glenohumeral joint to further explore suspected thinning or small cuff defects.

Hypertrophic bursa is resected (see Fig. 14-90) so that there is complete freedom of the humeroscapular motion interface. If it is contracted, the coracohumeral ligament is released (see Fig. 14-94). Superior surface cuff defects are smoothed either by resecting their protruding aspects or, occasionally, by reattaching a superior surface cuff flap. Prominences of the tuberosity are smoothed so that the tuberosity passes easily beneath the coracoacromial arch (Fig. 14-116). The undersurface of the coracoacromial arch is palpated to identify areas of roughness or prominence. Roughness of the undersurface of the coracoacromial arch is actually rare despite radiographic suggestions of spurs. If irregularities are identified by

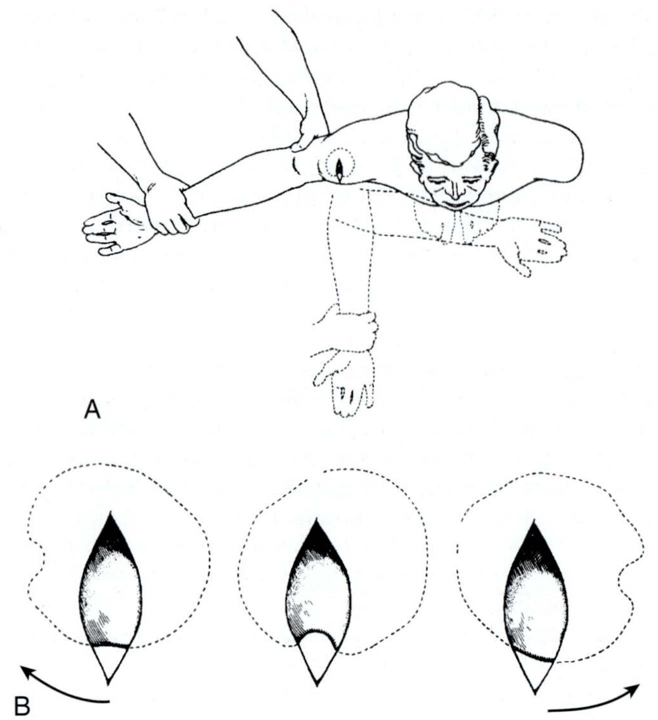

FIGURE 14-115: **A,** Operative position, superior view. **B,** The underlying cuff is systematically explored and palpated by rotating the arm to bring the different parts of the cuff into view (rather than by extending the incision). (From Codman EA. *Rupture of the Supraspinatus Tendon and Other Lesions in or About the Subacromial Bursa.* Malabar, FL: Robert E. Krieger; 1984.)

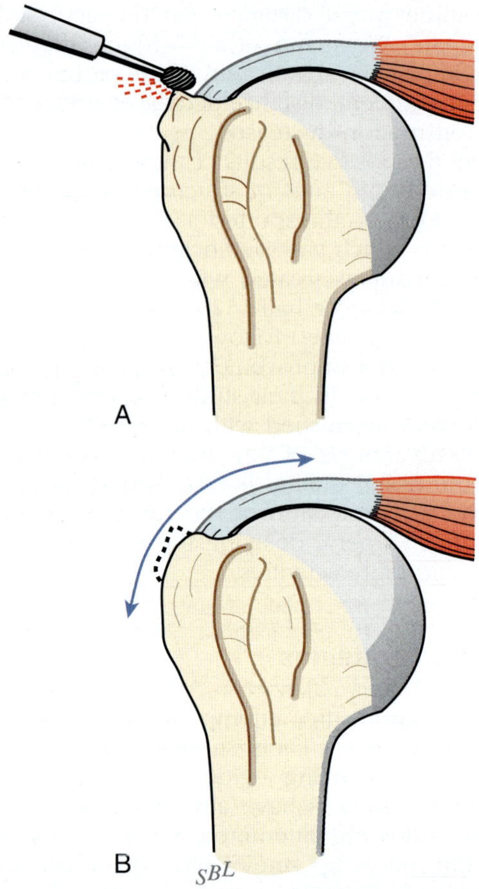

FIGURE 14-116: Smoothing of the greater tuberosity. Any prominence of the greater tuberosity is smoothed with a bur or rongeur (**A**), leaving a smooth surface on the proximal humeral convexity (**B**). (From Matsen FA III, Lippitt SB. *Shoulder Surgery: Principles and Procedures.* Philadelphia: Saunders; 2004:336.)

palpation, they can be smoothed with a pinecone bur (Fig. 14-117). Inferiorly directed acromioclavicular osteophytes are resected if they scrape on the cuff but they rarely contact the cuff tendon. The long head of the biceps is left undisturbed unless it appears to be seriously inflamed, obviously unstable, or partially torn, in which case we perform a tenotomy or tenodesis to the proximal part of the humerus. The entire humeroscapular motion interface (see Fig. 14-89) is carefully inspected to assure that all adhesions are lysed between the humerus on one hand and the coracoid muscles, the acromion and the deltoid on the other.

The shoulder is gently manipulated through a complete range of motion to ensure the absence of stiffness or additional adhesions. Before the procedure is concluded, the upper surface of the cuff and tuberosities and the undersurface of the coracoacromial arch are carefully palpated to ensure the absence of residual roughness. The entire range of passive shoulder motion must be free of stiffness or crepitus.

On closure, a secure deltoid reconstitution is of top priority so that early postoperative passive and active motion may be instituted. The deltoid is repaired by side-to-side closure of the medial and lateral aspects of the tendon split with No. 2 nonabsorbable sutures. If the deltoid origin has been partially detached, the area of

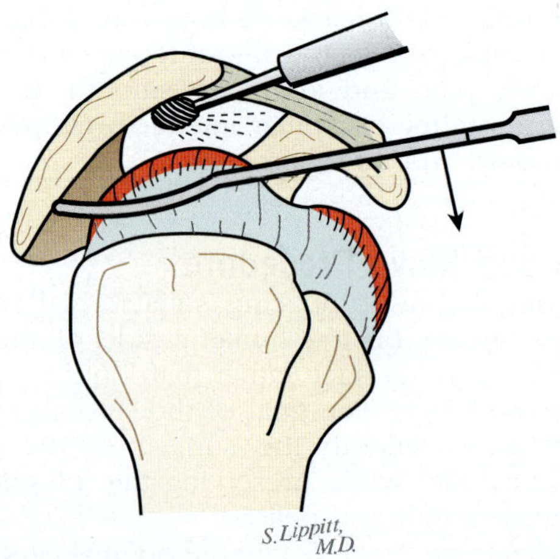

FIGURE 14-117: Smoothing of the coracoacromial arch. If, as is rarely the case, there is roughness on the underside of the coracoacromial arch, it can be smoothed with a pinecone bur, leaving the arch intact. (From Matsen FA III, Lippitt SB. *Shoulder Surgery: Principles and Procedures.* Philadelphia: Saunders; 2004:337.)

detachment is secured to the acromion by suturing it to bone as necessary. Sutures from the medial hole are passed through the lateral part of the deltoid tendon, and sutures from the lateral hole are passed through the medial part of the deltoid. This technique avoids the telltale "V" defect that indicates poor deltoid closure. All knots are placed on the superficial aspect to avoid recreating the subacromial roughness.

Postoperative Program

After any type of subacromial surgery, there is potential for adhesions between the cuff and the arch. To avoid these problems, we begin motion as soon as possible, possibly using continuous passive motion in the recovery room. Continuous passive motion can set to move the arm slowly through an arc of 0 to 90 degrees of elevation and from 50 to 0 degrees of internal rotation. On the day of surgery, assisted motion is instituted: the patient is instructed in the 140/40 passive program, in which the opposite hand is used to assist the operated shoulder in achieving 140 degrees of elevation (Figs. 14-118 to 14-120) and 40 degrees of external rotation (Fig. 14-121). Emphasis is also placed on posterior capsular stretching, including cross-body adduction (Fig. 14-122), reaching up the back (Fig. 14-123), and internal rotation of the abducted arm (Fig. 14-124).

The patient is allowed active use of the shoulder within the realm of comfort, unless the strength of the deltoid reattachment is a concern. Exercises for strengthening internal (Fig. 14-125) and external rotation (Fig. 14-126) are also begun immediately. Strengthening

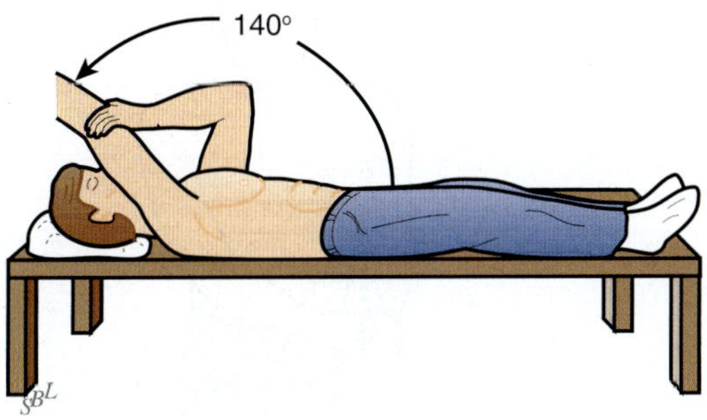

FIGURE 14-118: Assisted forward elevation. With the patient comfortable in the supine position, the sound arm helps stretch the affected arm to 140 degrees of forward elevation. (From Matsen FA III, Lippitt SB. *Shoulder Surgery: Principles and Procedures*. Philadelphia: Saunders; 2004:20.)

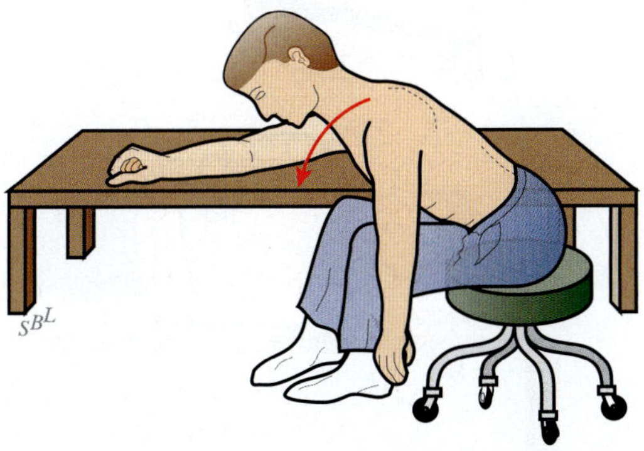

FIGURE 14-119: The forward lean. We use this exercise to gain the final 30 degrees of forward elevation. The patient places the arm on a table and slides it forward while sliding the stool backward and leaning forward. The stretch is sustained for 1 minute. (From Matsen FA III, Lippitt SB. *Shoulder Surgery: Principles and Procedures*. Philadelphia: Saunders; 2004:22.)

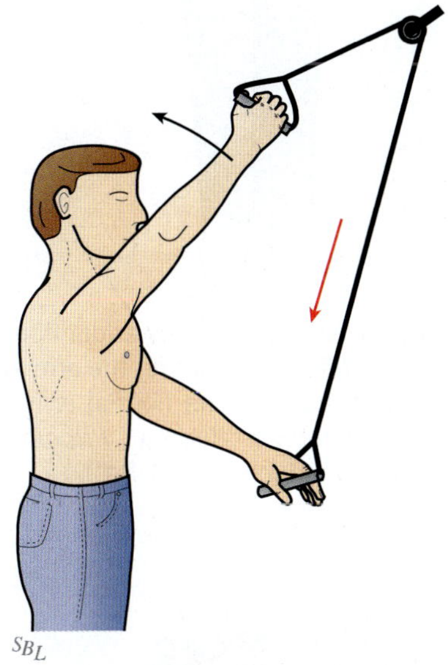

FIGURE 14-120: Door pulley. A pulley mounted on the door can be helpful in achieving elevation, especially when both shoulders are involved. (From Matsen FA III, Lippitt SB. *Shoulder Surgery: Principles and Procedures*. Philadelphia: Saunders; 2004:343.)

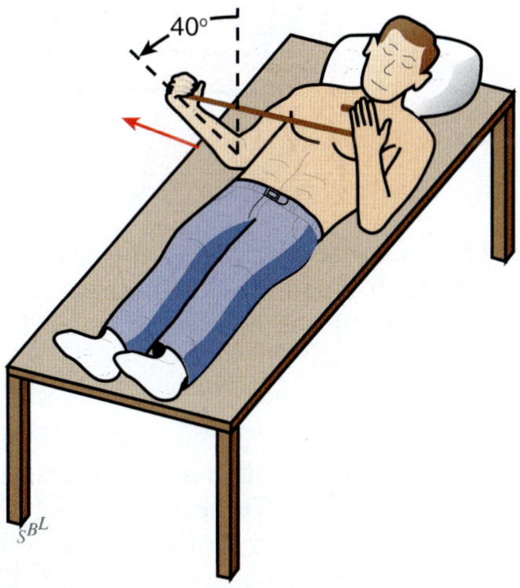

FIGURE 14-121: Assisted external elevation. The sound arm helps the operated arm to 40 degrees of external rotation using a cane or yardstick. Each elbow should be held in a position of 90 degrees of flexion. (From Matsen FA III, Lippitt SB. *Shoulder Surgery: Principles and Procedures*. Philadelphia: Saunders; 2004:21.)

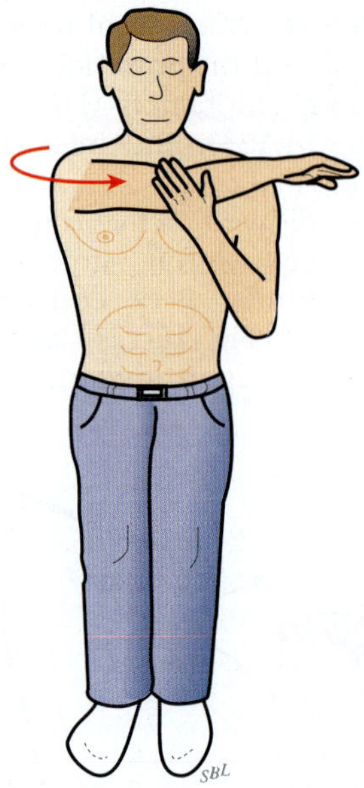

FIGURE 14-122: Assisted cross-body adduction. The posterior capsule can be stretched by adducting the arm across the body to the point where it matches the normal arm. (From Matsen FA III, Lippitt SB. *Shoulder Surgery: Principles and Procedures*. Philadelphia: Saunders; 2004:24.)

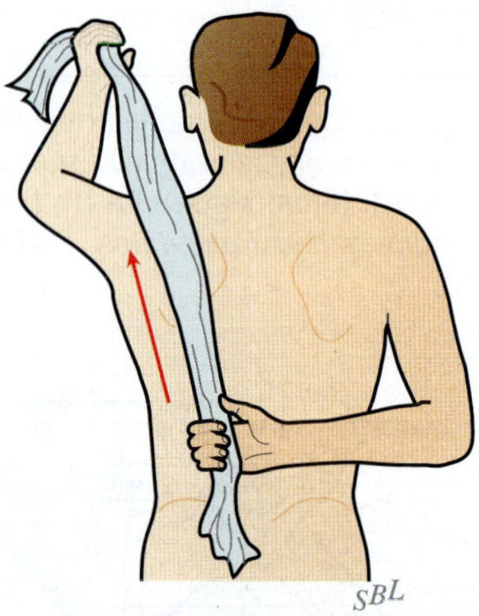

FIGURE 14-123: Internal rotation up the back. We use this exercise to gain reach up the back. The patient's sound arm pulls the affected arm up the back using a towel.

in elevation may also be initiated immediately because no cuff repair has been performed (Fig. 14-127). As soon as they can be performed comfortably, exercises to strengthen the scapular stabilizers are added (Figs. 14-128 and 14-129). Athletic activity is not allowed for 3 months after surgery and until normal motion and near-normal strength are regained.

In summary, the smooth and move procedure is used for cuff problems where repair surgery is either not indicated or not desired by the patient. It has the advantage

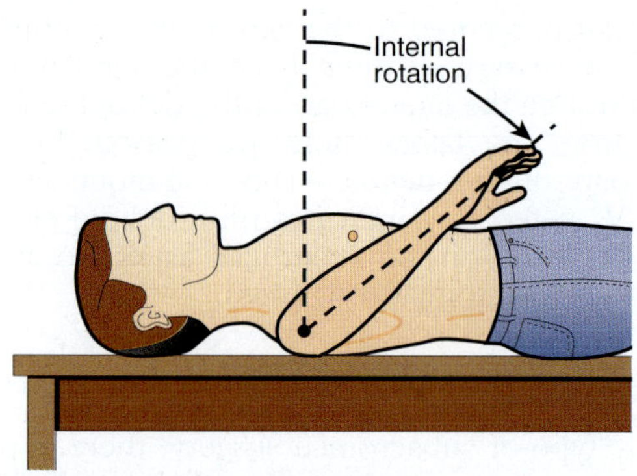

FIGURE 14-124: Internal rotation in abduction. The abducted arm is passively internally rotated to stretch the posterior capsule. (From Matsen FA III, Lippitt SB. *Shoulder Surgery: Principles and Procedures*. Philadelphia: Saunders; 2004:78.)

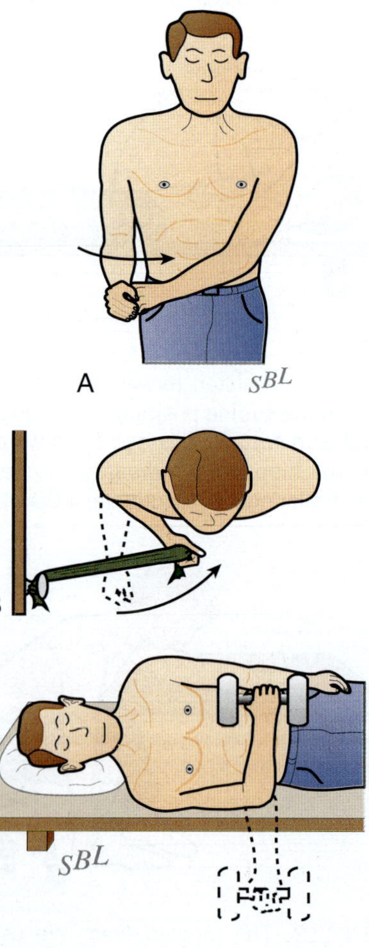

FIGURE 14-125: Internal rotator strengthening. The muscles of internal rotation are strengthened by exercising them against isometric resistance (**A**), against elastic tubing (**B**), and against weights (**C**). (From Matsen FA III, Lippitt SB. *Shoulder Surgery: Principles and Procedures*. Philadelphia: Saunders; 2004:25.)

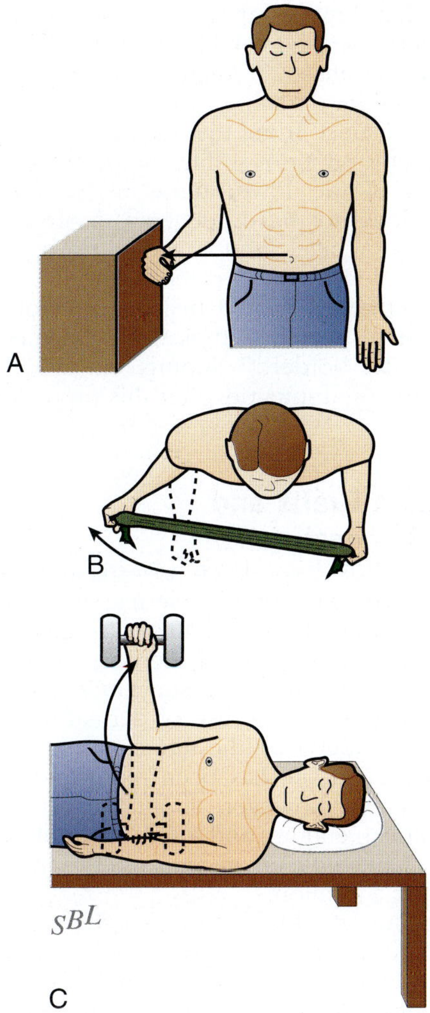

FIGURE 14-126: External rotator strengthening. The muscles of external rotation are strengthened by exercising them against isometric resistance (**A**), against elastic tubing (**B**), and against weights (**C**). (From Matsen FA III, Lippitt SB. *Shoulder Surgery: Principles and Procedures.* Philadelphia: Saunders; 2004:26.)

of allowing resumption of passive exercises and active use of the shoulder starting immediately after surgery.

Tendon Transfers

Gerber described latissimus dorsi tendon transfers for the treatment of irreparable rotator cuff tears.[95,100] It has been suggested that this procedure has the potential to improve active external rotation and depress the humeral head, although the mechanism for the latter is unclear. The surgical technique involves detaching of the latissimus dorsi tendon from its insertion on the humeral shaft and bringing the tendon through the plane between the deltoid and external rotators.[100] The edge of the tendon is then anchored into the greater tuberosity. Postoperative rehabilitation requires immobilization in an abduction splint for 6 weeks followed by active abduction and

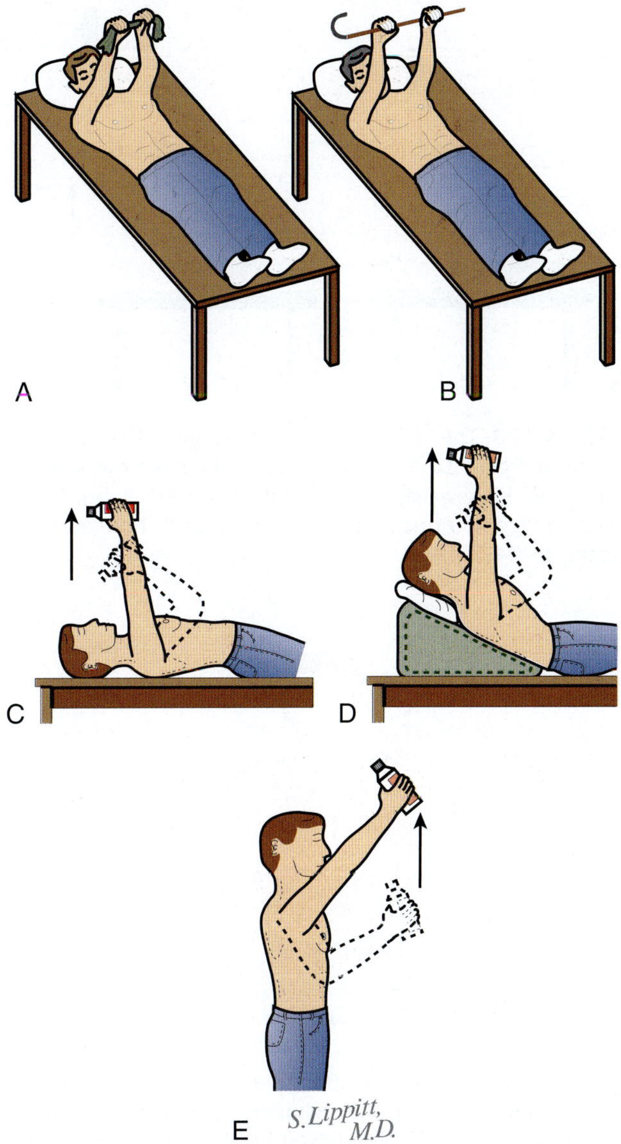

FIGURE 14-127: The progressive tilting supine press. Integrated forward elevation is developed by a series of exercises that can be progressed in small increments. **A,** Two hands are placed close to each other on a light stick and both hands are pressed upward toward the ceiling while the patient is in the supine position. **B,** Next, the same exercise is repeated with the arms progressively farther apart. **C,** The arm does the supine press unassisted. Small amounts of weight are added to the hand until 2 lb can be pressed upward 20 times. **D,** The patient's back is elevated slightly while the weight is pressed vertically upward. **E,** The amount of elevation is increased when 2 lb can be pressed upward 20 times. The progression is continued until the exercise can be performed with the back in a vertical position. (From Matsen FA III, Lippitt SB. *Shoulder Surgery: Principles and Procedures.* Philadelphia: Saunders; 2004:28.)

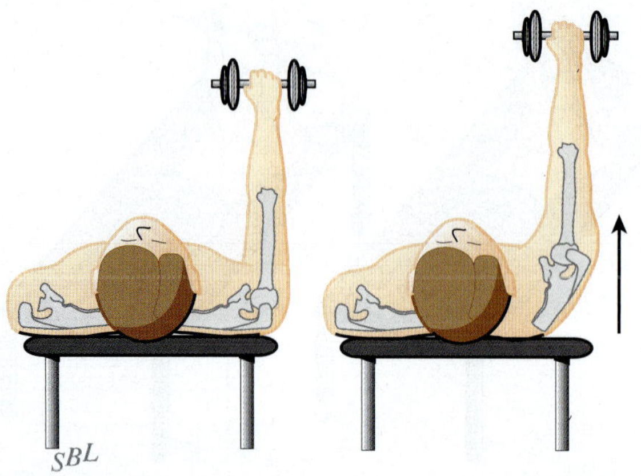

FIGURE 14-128: The press plus. At each stage of the exercises described in Figure 14-127, each press is finished by protracting the scapula upwards. (From Matsen FA III, Lippitt SB. *Shoulder Surgery: Principles and Procedures.* Philadelphia: Saunders; 2004:29.)

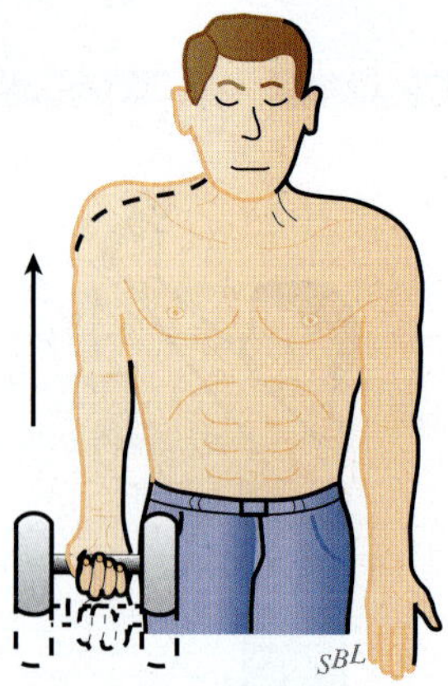

FIGURE 14-129: Trapezius strengthening. The trapezius is strengthened by shrugging the shoulders upward while weights are held in the hands. (From Matsen FA III, Lippitt SB. *Shoulder Surgery: Principles and Procedures.* Philadelphia: Saunders; 2004:27.)

external rotation exercises. Strengthening exercises are started at 3 months and continued for 6 to 9 months.[96]

Most studies have reported approximately 75% to 85% patient satisfaction with this procedure.[4,95,96,226,335] Recent reports have suggested that this tendon transfer is an effective and durable treatment for posterosuperior rotator cuff tears, with a 10% failure rate.[97] The integrity of the subscapularis and teres minor appear to be important predictors of good function after the latissimus transfer.[58,96,97]

Lower trapezius transfer is another potential option for massive rotator cuff tears. This transfer was originally described as a technique to address pediatric brachial plexus palsy,[21] but has been used to address massive rotator cuff tears and external rotation weakness.[75] A cadaveric biomechanical study performed by Omid et al. suggested that lower trapezius transfer is superior at restoring intact glenohumeral kinematics when compared with latissimus transfer.[256] Anatomically, the lower trapezius inserts on the dorsum of the scapular spine, and its insertion is distinct from the middle trapezius, which inserts along the superior surface of the scapular spine.[255] The tendon of the lower trapezius is released, and because it does not have adequate excursion to reach the tuberosity, Achilles tendon allograft is used to bridge the lower tendon to the greater tuberosity. During this procedure, surgeons should be cognizant of the spinal accessory nerve, which is typically 2 cm medial to the medial scapular border.[105] Reports of clinical improvement and structural integrity after this procedure are still pending.

Interposition Grafts and Capsular Reconstruction

Biologic scaffolds have been investigated as possible interposition grafts for irreparable massive tears. Porcine xenograft had previously been tested to augment rotator cuff repair, but had issues with sterile inflammatory reactions.[132] Since then, newer tissue engineered strategies have been proposed. The use of dermal tissue allograft to span the gap between the retracted tendon edge and the bony insertion site has been reported recently.[107,108] Concern remains, however, about the ability of these scaffolds to heal, endure, and improve shoulder functionality in the challenging environment between the humeral head and the acromion.

The superior shoulder capsule has been suggested as being an important passive stabilizer of the glenohumeral joint.[134,219] A cadaveric biomechanical study has demonstrated an increase in glenohumeral translation in all directions with a defect in the superior capsule.[134] The use of a graft to reconstruct the superior capsule from the superior glenoid medially to the greater tuberosity laterally may allow adequate restoration of the superior stability of the glenohumeral joint, more so than a patch graft that is attached medially to the supraspinatus tendon.[219] Mihata et al. described a technique of reconstructing the superior shoulder capsule with fascia lata.[220] Clinical results after arthroscopic superior capsule reconstruction are limited.[220] Acellular dermal extracellular matrix has been used by some surgeons as an alternative to fascia lata. Again there is concern about the ability of a graft to endure as an interposition in this challenging environment. Furthermore, it is recognized that a graft attaching the superior glenoid to the tuberosity will only be under tension when the arm is adducted, but will not be functional as a restraint when the arm is abducted.

APPROACH TO FAILED CUFF SURGERY

Surgical management of rotator cuff tears (both repair and nonrepair surgery) leads to successful outcomes in the majority of patients. For arthroscopic repair, greater than 90% of patients report satisfactory outcomes in terms of improvements in pain and shoulder function. However, approximately 25% of rotator cuff repairs will re-tear at a mean of about 2 years after surgery.[211] Of these patients that have re-tears, approximately half will still have a "successful" outcome.[241] Patients with labor-intensive occupations will most often be symptomatic.[241] In addition, those with a lower education level and a Workers' Compensation claim are more likely to do poorly.[155]

Patients with continued pain and dysfunction after rotator cuff repair present a significant diagnostic and therapeutic challenge as the etiology of their persistent symptoms can often be difficult to identify and treatment outcomes of revision surgery can be unpredictable.[145] The possible etiologies for pain and shoulder dysfunction after prior rotator cuff surgery can be categorized into those that are extrinsic and intrinsic to the shoulder itself (Box 14-2). The differential diagnosis can be narrowed down by detailed history and thorough physical examination aided by appropriate radiographic assessment.

The evaluation begins with a good history. The patient will often present with ongoing shoulder pain and weakness. Details should be sought regarding the location of the pain, duration before and after the index surgery, and the current intensity and quality. Radiation of pain past the elbow into the distal extremity, numbness, tingling, and burning symptoms may indicate an extrinsic etiology, such as cervical radiculopathy.

Whether there was a period of time after the initial surgery and rehabilitation when the patient was pain-free and regained shoulder function should be determined.

BOX 14-2. Common Causes of Persistent Pain After Rotator Cuff Surgery

Extrinsic Causes of Pain
Brachial plexopathy
Cervical radiculopathy
Long thoracic neuropathy
Neoplasm
Reflex sympathetic dystrophy
Spinal accessory neuropathy
Suprascapular neuropathy
Thoracic outlet syndrome

Intrinsic Causes of Pain
Acromial stress fracture
Acromioclavicular arthropathy
Adhesive capsulitis
Articular cartilage defect
Biceps or labral pathology
Deltoid insufficiency
Infection
Osteoarthritis
Persistent subacromial impingement
Rotator cuff defect

Modified from Williams GR. Painful shoulder after rotator cuff surgery. J Am Acad Orthop Surg. *1997;5(2):97-108.*

History of a new traumatic event versus insidious onset of shoulder pain and dysfunction is also important in determining possible failure mechanisms. The length of physical therapy and rehabilitation after the initial cuff surgery as well as compliance with sling immobilization, the duration of immobilization, and compliance with physical therapy should be assessed.

Additionally, the specifics of the index surgery should be sought from the patient as well as reviewing the reports of the previous surgeries. Original imaging prior to surgery may also help in determining the size of the original tear, the degree of muscle atrophy, and fatty infiltration.

The social history and review of systems are important factors to assess as well. The use of tobacco products, history of diabetes, and obesity may have bearing on the likelihood of cuff healing. The patient should be asked about fevers, chills, or malaise, and whether there were any problems with wound healing after the initial surgery as possible indications of postoperative infection. In addition, the patient's work and recreational activity status are important considerations when discussing therapeutic options.

Following history, a thorough physical examination of the shoulder should be performed as detailed in the physical examination section. The neck should also be examined as cervical spine radiculopathy is a common extrinsic etiology for shoulder pain. Proper evaluation of the cervical spine should include range-of-motion and specific tests for nerve root compression such as Spurling's test and upper motor neuron signs such as Hoffman's sign and clonus. A thorough neurovascular examination of both upper extremities will help identify possible brachial plexus lesions, and rare conditions such as thoracic outlet syndrome may be detected.

The shoulder exam should progress in the usual systematic fashion, starting with observation of both shoulders and noting asymmetry. Atrophy of the supraspinatus and infraspinatus musculature should be closely evaluated on visualization of both fossae on the posterior shoulder. Palpation of the acromioclavicular joints and the biceps within the intertubercular groove may elucidate possible intrinsic etiologies of pain. Bilateral shoulder motion is checked actively and passively. Particular attention is directed at the examination for stiffness in flexion, internal rotation, and external rotation. Bilateral rotator cuff strength is tested and compared for deficits. Biceps tension tests such as Speed's, Yergason's, and O'Brien's active compression test can be helpful to assess the long head of the biceps. Cross-body adduction may confirm the acromioclavicular joint as an origin of pain. Evaluation of scapulothoracic motion to assess for scapular winging and/or scapular dyskinesis is important, as these conditions may cause chronic shoulder pain.

Imaging studies should begin with standard radiographs of the shoulder, including AP, Grashey, scapular Y, and axillary lateral views. Radiographs will help to diagnose other sources of pain such as AC joint arthropathy, glenohumeral joint arthritis, superior humeral head migration, and acromial stress fracture. Often, MRI is helpful in the setting of prior cuff repair surgery as it can detect failed cuff repair while also providing information about the size of the re-tear, degree of tendon retraction, muscle atrophy, and fatty infiltration. Other possible etiologies such as the long head of the biceps tendon and labral pathologies, AC joint degeneration, articular cartilage injuries, and rare conditions such as neoplasm can be identified by MRI. Ultrasound has been proven useful in diagnosing rotator cuff tears in both the primary and postoperative setting,[318,272] and may be particularly useful in the setting of prior tuberosity anchor placement, which can cause signal degradation and image artifact with MRI.

Once the etiology for failed cuff surgery has been determined, treatment should be individualized based on the diagnosis and patient characteristics and expectations. If an extrinsic cause for pain from failed cuff surgery is identified, the appropriate treatment should be instituted or appropriate referral made to a subspecialist for further management. The remainder of this chapter will focus on the intrinsic causes of failed cuff surgery and emphasize the more common etiologies among this group.

MANAGEMENT

Patients over the age of 65 years who continue to be symptomatic following previous surgery for a massive cuff defect should not be considered candidates for revision repair surgery. Surgical repair of the tendons in this age group is typically unsatisfactory given the intraoperative observation of the tissue paper-like strength and consistency of the involved tendon tissue. Multiple reports of revision cuff repair have noted that increasing age, poor tissue quality, and increased tear size are predictors of failure.[64,149] In patients in this age range, a structured home-based rehabilitation program should be considered before any potential surgical intervention.

If one believes that the reason for shoulder pain after prior cuff repair is due to recurrent tear, it is important to rule out other potential etiologies for the painful shoulder (especially stiffness/adhesive capsulitis, biceps pathology, and infection). If after appropriate evaluation, the surgeon remains convinced that the source of pain and dysfunction is caused by failed cuff repair, then treatment must take into account patient-related factors. This includes age, activity level required for work and recreation, medical comorbidities (diabetes, smoking), and the degree of shoulder weakness and function loss. Additional considerations include the tear size, degree of retraction, and muscle quality determined on MRI. The presence or absence of glenohumeral joint arthritis and proximal migration of the humerus are also crucial considerations in treatment planning.

Initial management of the vast majority of recurrent cuff tears should be a trial of nonoperative treatment. This includes physical therapy and rehabilitation, activity modifications, and possibly cortisone injection if pain is limiting the patient's ability to undergo therapy. If at the end of this period, the patient continues to have pain and dysfunction, they may be a candidate for revision surgery. However, the same conditions and factors that have been shown to negatively impact rotator cuff healing apply in the recurrent tear setting as well, and should be considered to be magnified in the revision situation. Previous studies of revision arthroscopic repair have demonstrated that patients with retained elevation above 90 degrees will have good outcomes.[64,145,149,270] Patients with pseudoparalysis and glenohumeral arthritis do poorly after revision repair surgery and may be better served by arthroplasty.

Arthroscopic revision repair surgery is our method of choice when attempting to re-repair the cuff. The benefit of arthroscopy is improved visualization of the tear and help in determining the tear pattern. It also allows for the identification and treatment of other lesions within the shoulder joint (long head of biceps tendon, labral degeneration, capsular adhesions/contractures). In the vast majority of cases we will release the biceps tendon at the time of revision surgery as this is a known source of pain in the setting of cuff repair.[25,338] A 70-degree scope can be used to fully assess the subscapularis tendon, and repair should be performed if a tear of the tendon is identified.

Once these concomitant pathologies have been addressed, the scope is placed into the subacromial space, and the cuff tear and tendon must be visualized and assessed for retraction, excursion, and tissue quality. The principles for repair remain the same as those detailed above in the section on primary arthroscopic cuff repair. The goal is to achieve robust fixation of quality tendon tissue to bone without undue tension. This requires a thorough release of bursal adhesions within the subacromial, subdeltoid, and subcoracoid spaces. This must be done carefully, as there is often thickened bursal-sided scar tissue that can obscure the identification of the tendon edge.

The posterosuperior cuff tendon, which often requires continued dissection from within the subacromial space, is dissected free from bursal adhesions and scar tissue. This area may be best viewed from the lateral portal while maneuvering a shaver from the posterior portal in a plane of section just inferior to the acromion and working medial to lateral to free up the tendon edge. The scapular spine can also be used to define the supraspinatus from the infraspinatus. At this point, analogous to primary repair techniques, the tear pattern and degree of tendon excursion are determined, and anterior and posterior interval slides are performed in order to free up the tendon further to achieve tendon-to-bone repair. If this is not possible, many authors recommend repairing as much tendon to tuberosity as possible even in a partial repair.[36,41] This emphasizes repairing the posterior cuff in order to reestablish the force couple.

As to be expected, the outcomes after revision rotator cuff repair are less predictable than those after primary repair.[298] Early results of revision rotator cuff repair described by DeOrio and Cofield demonstrated pain relief in the majority of patients, but the overall outcomes were unsatisfactory.[61] Djurasovic et al. reported improved results after open revision rotator cuff repair, with about 50% of the patients achieving excellent or good results.[64] They also described predictors of poor results, including detachment of the deltoid, poor tendon quality, multiple prior procedures, and preoperative elevation below horizontal. Similarly, Keener et al. reported on the results after revision cuff repair, and found that about half remained intact at a minimum of 1 year of follow-up.[149] Advanced age and the number of tendons involved were associated with re-tear, and those with re-tears often had decreased abduction strength and Constant scores.

Arthroscopic revision rotator cuff repair can be technically demanding, and the complication rates, including failure, are high.[263,298] Numerous reports have noted that pain relief and improvement in function can be attained in appropriately selected patients.[149,196] Shamsudin et al. noted that the short-term clinical outcomes are equivalent to those of primary repair but that these outcomes were not durable.[298] Parnes et al. reported that the complication rate after revision cuff repair is significantly higher than that after primary surgery.[263] Keener et al. noted that about 50% of revision repairs are intact at 1 year, and the patient age and number of torn tendons were related to the failure rate.[149] Others have attempted to use augmentation grafts to improve outcomes, but success in terms of structural integrity has been limited.[174,297]

Because of the high failure rate following re-repairs of failed cuff repair attempts, we often present the option of a smooth and move procedure to patients with painful stiffness and crepitus after prior cuff surgery. The surgical findings often include thick bursa, prominent suture and suture anchors, adhesions between the coracoid muscles and the subscapularis, and scarring in the humeroscapular motion interface. Once these are resolved and after gentle manipulation, full smooth motion is often restored. After surgery, the patient is ready to start immediate postoperative passive and active motion exercises.

Rehabilitation After Rotator Cuff Repair

Two important and surgeon-controlled factors that can affect the outcomes of rotator cuff repair are surgical technique and the postoperative rehabilitation protocol. There is an abundance of literature regarding various techniques for rotator cuff repair, and despite advances in technology and techniques, the rate of recurrent rotator cuff tears has not changed significantly over time. With re-tear rates reported to be about 20%[211,224,286] and even greater for larger tears,[89] it is important for surgeons to consider the postoperative rehabilitation protocol as another important modifiable factor in the patient's care.

Significant variation of these protocols exists—some surgeons prefer to immobilize the shoulder for a period of time after surgery to protect the repair site from excessive force that may damage the repair construct. This risks shoulder stiffness and decreased shoulder function. Other surgeons prefer early mobilization to improve early shoulder function, but this approach may put the repair construct at risk.

Basic Science Evidence

Optimization of the mechanical environment for tendon-to-bone healing has been the focus in numerous in vitro and animal studies. These studies, in combination with recent high-quality clinical studies, have helped guide our understanding of the role of mechanobiology, early mobilization, and immobilization after repair. During the remodeling phase of tendon-to-bone healing, mechanical traction plays a role in the generation of organized tissue at the cuff footprint.[13,321,340] Like many other musculoskeletal tissues, tendon-bone healing is affected by the transmission of force across the healing interface. This force may promote the formation of collagen in an organized manner that more closely models the anisotropic material properties of native tendon, and may increase the strength of the repair site over time.

Numerous in vitro studies have supported the theory that appropriate exercise-related loading can enhance the mechanical properties of tendon and that removal of a load from tendon can lead to deterioration.[8,9,90,324,330,345] Studies using the rat rotator cuff model have investigated the role of immobilization on cuff healing. Initial rat studies by Thomopoulos et al. had quantified tendon-to-bone healing under numerous different loading conditions and found superior material properties and better tendon organization in immobilized rats.[323] A follow-up study also demonstrated superior mechanical properties with decreased activity level.[102] However, subsequent studies from other groups have shown that complete load removal is detrimental to the healing site.[90,124] Galatz et al. used the same rat model with a combination of immobilization and Botox to inhibit muscle contraction.[90] They found inferior structural properties in rats treated with immobilization combined with botulinum toxin (Botox), suggesting that complete load removal was detrimental to tendon healing.

To summarize, the basic science evidence suggests that both complete removal of load and chronic overload are detrimental to tendon healing. Removal will understimulate the repair site, while chronic overload may activate a catabolic environment that is detrimental to healing. Controlled loading and a balance between understimulation and overload of the repair site will lead to the best mechanical environment for tendon-to-bone healing.

Clinical Evidence

Until recently, literature regarding postoperative mobilization and immobilization after rotator cuff repair was almost nonexistent. Clinicians were dependent on personal experience and intuition when formulating protocols for postoperative motion. Recently, however, there have been numerous prospective, randomized trials comparing commonly used protocols. It should be noted that the individual protocols in each of the studies are distinct, and readers must familiarize themselves with the details of each protocol in order to understand the differences.

Lee et al.[172] treated 64 patients with arthroscopic single-row repair for medium- to large-sized full-thickness cuff tears and randomized them to two different rehabilitation protocols: early passive motion including manual therapy by a therapist without limitation versus the use of a continuous passive motion machine for 3 weeks followed by passive forward flexion as tolerated. No differences were seen at 1 year, but the aggressive, early motion group had better gains in motion at 3 months. Notably, the integrity of the repair site as documented by MRI demonstrated a re-tear rate of 23.3% in the aggressive motion group versus 8.8% in the limited exercise group.

Cuff and Pupello[59] randomized 68 patients' status after arthroscopic suture-bridge repair of full-thickness supraspinatus tears into a group that had early passive forward elevation and external rotation and a group that performed pendulums and delayed therapy until 6 weeks. The two groups had similar satisfaction, range of motion, American Shoulder and Elbow Surgeons (ASES) scores, and SST scores as well as no differences in cuff healing as documented by ultrasound.

Kim et al.[156] randomized 105 patients with small-to-medium-sized full-thickness rotator cuff tears to early and delayed passive motion. Early passive motion was started the day after surgery in one group. The other group started passive motion at 4 weeks for a small tear and 5 weeks for a medium tear. Range of motion and pain and Constant, SST, and ASES scores were similar between the two groups, and re-tear rates were 12% in the early group and 18% in the delayed group.

Similarly, Keener et al.[146] randomized 124 patients who were treated with double-row repairs for small- or medium-sized full-thickness tears. One group started pendulums immediately and passive range-of-motion exercises 1 week after surgery, while the other group delayed motion for 6 weeks. Motion was significantly worse in the immobilized group at 3 months, but this resolved at later time points. Pain and SST, ASES, and Constant scores were similar between groups at all time points. Healing rates were similar between the two groups, with an overall healing rate of 92%.

Koh et al.[160] investigated the effect of increased immobilization time on healing rates after rotator cuff repair in 100 patients that were randomized to either 4 or 8 weeks of immobilization with no passive or active range-of-motion exercises. A higher proportion of patients immobilized for 8 weeks (38%) were stiff compared with the patients immobilized for 4 weeks (18%). No difference was seen in the re-tear rates between the groups.

The information provided by these randomized, prospective controlled trials helps surgeons formulate a postoperative rehabilitation plan. Early mobilization may result in better function at early time points without risking re-tear. However, these studies do not suggest any difference in healing rates or motion when comparing early and delayed motion at later time points. Of these studies, one study reported a relatively high re-tear rate (23.3%)[172] in a group that received aggressive therapist-guided manual therapy without limitation. This high re-tear rate may be a result of mechanical overload to the repair site. Patient-controlled, self-directed range-of-motion exercises may be preferable to prevent overloading of the repair site.

The results of these randomized trials can be interpreted and utilized differently. In young patients with small- or medium-sized tears with good potential for healing, early mobilization may result in better function at earlier time points without risking re-tear. In contrast, patients with risk factors for re-tearing (older age, larger tears, revision repair) may benefit from a delayed rehabilitation protocol in which the repair site is protected from mechanical overload for a longer period of time.

Our practice is to optimize the circumstances for tendon healing after cuff repair surgery because stiffness after a repair can usually be managed by stretching exercises or, if necessary, by a smooth and move procedure. On the other hand, if early implementation of rehabilitation exercises causes failure of the repair, the salvage is more complicated.

INTERNATIONAL EXPERT COMMENTARY

Ofer Levy

The authors have written an excellent chapter educating and updating us on rotator cuff pathology, assessment, diagnosis, and management. They present a comprehensive description of the anatomy, physiology, and biomechanics of the rotator cuff and the shoulder.

The rotator cuff conflict against the acromion and the coracoacromial arch may be the "common final pathway" causing impingement due to either intrinsic or extrinsic causes of cuff degeneration. The degenerate cuff fails to appropriately compress the humeral head during movements of elevation and abduction, leading to the rubbing of the rotator cuff against the acromion and the coracoacromial arch. When examined arthroscopically, the different degrees of acromial lesions on the acromion and the bursal side of the rotator cuff can be observed, as classified by Copeland and Levy.[88,182]

The rate of rotator cuff tears associated with os acromiale is unknown. However, different studies have shown that a 6.2% to 9.8% incidence of os acromiale was evident in patients with symptomatic cuff tears.[24,139,236] In the Reading Shoulder Unit database,[177] we have found a 12% incidence of os acromiale in patients with massive rotator cuff tears (16/135) and a 31.5% incidence in those with cuff tear arthropathy. Therefore the question remains: Does the presence of an os acromiale (with a step-off) predispose patients to a massive rotator cuff tear? In addition, do anatomic alignment and fusion at an earlier stage prevent the progression to a cuff tear? Furthermore, is the presence of an os acromiale in cuff arthropathy due to preexisting nonunion or superior migration of the humeral head causing erosion and eventual disruption to the acromion: a "chicken and egg" scenario? Despite these unanswered questions, the simple finding of a higher occurrence of os acromiale in the

INTERNATIONAL EXPERT COMMENTARY—cont'd

presence of rotator cuff disease should guide the management of these patients with concomitant rotator cuff tear repair and fusion of the os acromiale.[11,179] The authors alluded to the combination of posterior capsule tightness and impingement that should be diagnosed and treated.

AC joint excision arthroplasty should be considered in cases of AC joint pain or tenderness or when there are arthritic changes in the AC joint. Although the AC joint may not cause symptoms while patients avoid movements above shoulder height due to cuff disease, after surgery, when they regain a high arc of movement, they may become symptomatic from the AC joint.

Laser Doppler flowmetry analyses[181] of the rotator cuff blood supply indicate a significant difference between the vascularity of the normal and pathologic rotator cuff.[181] We were unable to demonstrate a functional hypoperfusion area, or so-called "critical zone," in the normal cuff. The mean laser Doppler flowmetry flux was significantly higher at the edges of the tear in torn cuffs (43.1; 95% confidence interval [CI], 37.8 to 48.4) compared with normal cuffs (32.8; 95% CI, 27.4 to 38.1; $P = .0089$). It was significantly lower across all anatomic locations in cuffs with impingement (25.4; 95% CI, 22.4 to 28.5) compared with normal cuffs ($P = .0196$), and significantly lower in cuffs with impingement compared with torn cuffs ($P < .0001$). The measured flux decreases with advancing impingement, but there is a substantial increase at the edges of rotator cuff tears. This may reflect an attempt at repair.[181]

The importance of the "force couple" of the rotator cuff was well described by the authors.

The section on clinical evaluation and physical examination is comprehensive and very well written, as was the differential diagnosis. They emphasized the importance of good history and the patient's main complaint: pain, weakness, loss of motion, or stiffness. The importance of the patient's physiologic age versus chronologic age, the activity level, and expectations are all important. Hand dominance, occupation, smoking, comorbidities, and social problems should all be considered. I would evaluate and examine the patient in a similar way. I perform ultrasound of the shoulder as part of my clinical examination ("one-stop clinic"),[109] and I rarely use MRI.

Fatty degeneration of the rotator cuff muscles has a prognostic importance in the recovery of rotator cuff strength following repair. However, in my view, the presence of high-grade fatty degeneration is not a contraindication for rotator cuff repair. Even in the presence of high-grade fatty degeneration, patients will improve substantially following surgery, although they may not recover good strength.

The authors give special attention to acute traumatic tears with the need for urgent repair. Although the majority of rotator cuff tears occur in degenerate cuffs, any acute deterioration in shoulder function following an episode of trauma (even minor trauma) should be considered as an acute traumatic tear and should receive early operative repair for better outcomes.

For chronic atraumatic tears, the treatment is tailored to the patient according to the parameters mentioned earlier. In elderly patients or patients with a partial-thickness tear, a course of conservative treatment is tried first. If this fails, then surgery is considered. In young and active patients with a full-thickness tear and weakness, surgical repair is offered earlier. In patients with a massive irreparable tear, nonoperative treatment is initiated first. This includes pain management with subacromial injections of local anesthetic and steroids, stretching exercises, and the deltoid rehabilitation regimen (The Reading Deltoid regimen) (Fig. 14-130).[180]

My preferred surgical technique is arthroscopic rotator cuff repair. I perform the procedure with the patient in the lateral decubitus position. I initially use the posterior portal for viewing with the lateral and anterior working portals and additional portals as needed. I tend to change the viewing and working portals as needed. It is often better to understand the shape and size of the tear when viewing from the lateral portal.

After assessment of the rotator cuff from the joint side and the bursal side, and understanding the size and shape of the tear (L, C, or U shape) and its mobility and reparability, I have a clear idea of how I will repair it at that stage. The approach to repair the different tear shapes is different. U-shaped tears are sometimes longstanding L-shaped tears. This is well described by the authors in this chapter.

I assess the impingement lesions[88,182] and, if the cuff is reparable, I usually perform arthroscopic subacromial decompression. AC joint excision arthroplasty will be performed as well in cases with symptomatic or arthritic AC joints to open the space for the rotator cuff muscle and for the reasons mentioned earlier. A thorough and good release of the rotator cuff from both the joint and bursal sides should be performed. I perform release of the contracted coracohumeral ligament as well as interval slides if necessary.

When repairing the cuff, care must be taken to ensure that all layers of the cuff are repaired. Repairing only one layer will fail to achieve good outcomes. It is important, as the authors describe, to refresh the footprint on the tuberosity to encourage better healing of the tendon to bone.

My preferred technique for rotator cuff repair for small- to medium-sized tears is the "parachute" technique.[183] It is a single-row technique with one or two suture anchors and consists of a suture and knot configuration that resembles a parachute (Fig. 14-131), which increases the contact area and pressure between the tendon and its footprint. After debridement of the tear, mobilization of the cuff, and preparation of the footprint, one or two suture-loaded anchors are inserted into the area of the footprint. Using penetrating graspers, the two limbs of each suture are passed through the healthy edge of the tear anteriorly, creating a configuration of a horizontal mattress suture. The same technique is applied to the remaining suture in the anchor, but the sutures are pulled out posteriorly, creating another horizontal mattress suture. By doing this alone, the cuff is approximated to the footprint. In order to increase the contact area between tendon and bone, the trailing ends of each mattress suture are tied to each other and then cut.

For larger tears, or after a repair with the parachute technique, where there was a flap of cuff tissue laterally, we used a double-row technique in a ratchet-loop configuration (Fig. 14-132).[183] In this technique, a second double suture-loaded anchor is placed laterally. One pair of sutures is used for the anterior leaf of the tear and the other pair for the posterior leaf. Using a penetrating grasper, the suture is

Continued

INTERNATIONAL EXPERT COMMENTARY—cont'd

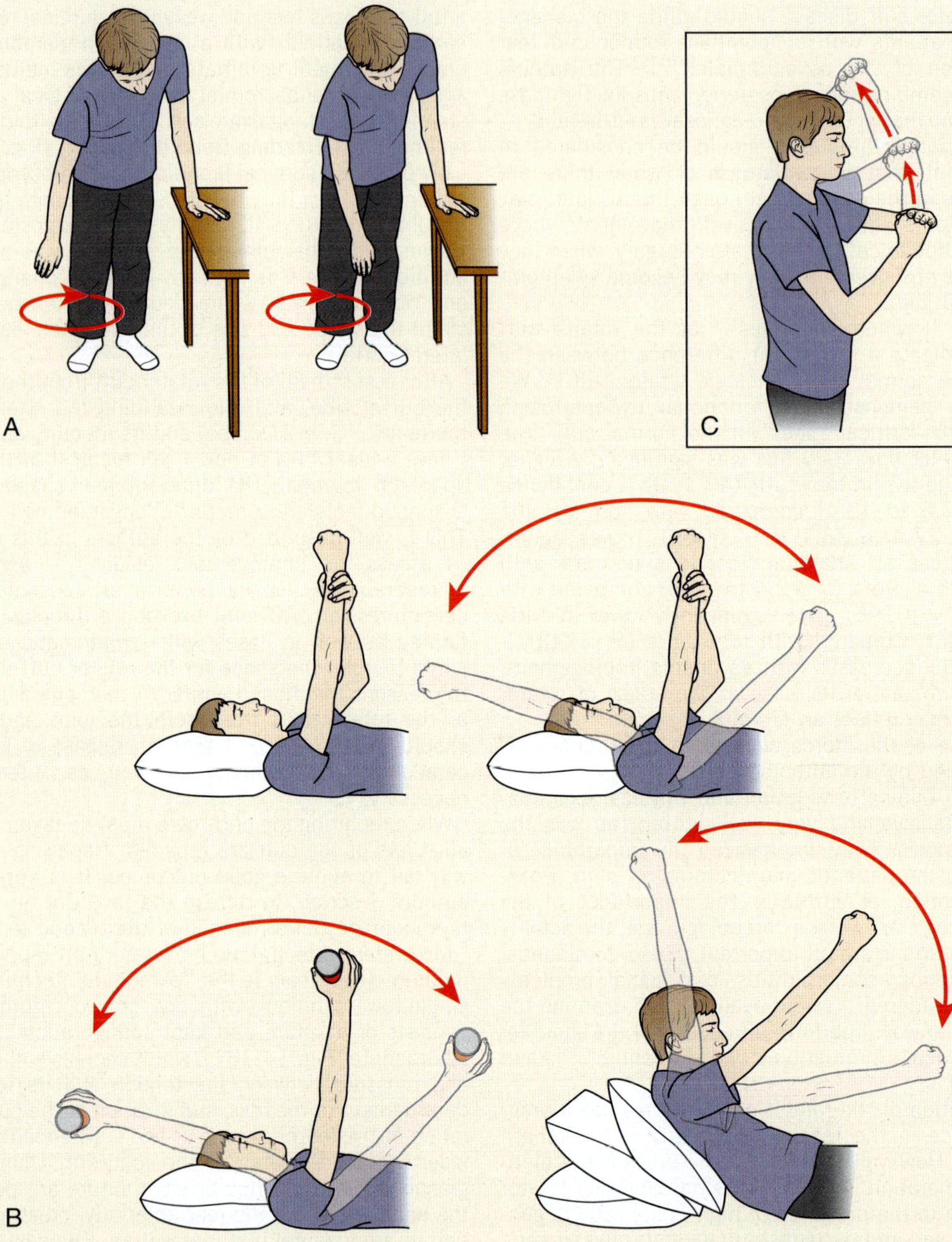

FIGURE 14-130: A-C, The deltoid rehabilitation regimen (the Reading deltoid regimen). (From the Reading Shoulder Unit, Reading, United Kingdom. www.readingshoulderunit.com.)

taken through the cuff, creating a loop of suture that is left out through the cuff. The free end of the same suture limb that has been passed through the cuff is then passed through the loop. It is then tied to the limb of the suture that has not been passed through the cuff using a nonsliding knot, creating a ratchet-loop (pulley) configuration. The procedure is repeated for the posterior leaf of the cuff. This suture configuration multiplies the lateral pull on the cuff by four times. The ratchet-loop technique doubles the load on the cuff tendon for each suture by creating a pulley system; there are two sutures per anchor, and hence the load is multiplied by four. This follows the basic principles of force equilibrium and mechanical statics in the use of pulley systems.[309] Another option for the lateral row is to use the trailing ends of the sutures from the medial row parachute technique and fix them to a knotless suture-locking anchor placed laterally. In order to reduce tension on the sutures and the rotator cuff when tying the knots, I

INTERNATIONAL EXPERT COMMENTARY—cont'd

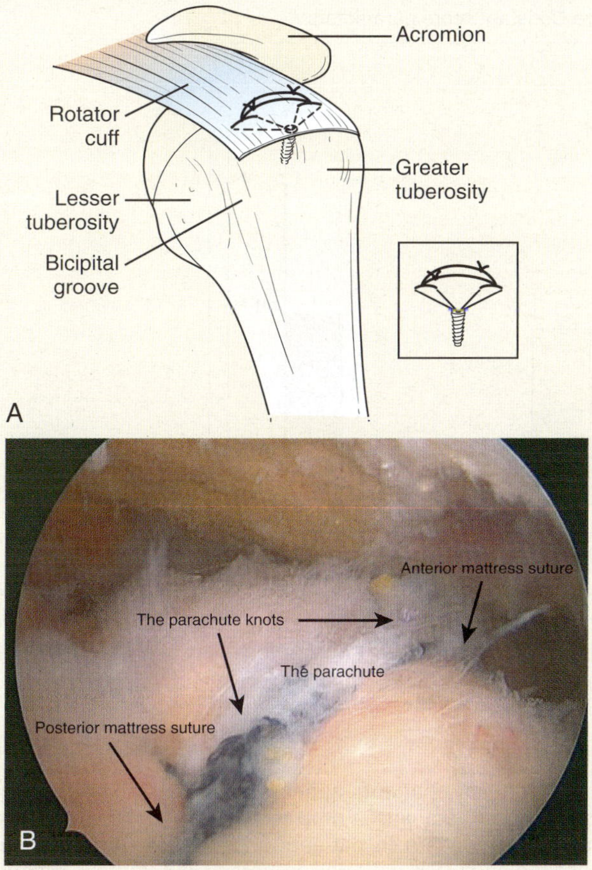

FIGURE 14-131: A, The "parachute" technique for arthroscopic rotator cuff repair. The configuration of the sutures after they are tied resembles a parachute. **B,** Arthroscopic view of the parachute technique. (**A,** From Levy O, Venkateswaran B, Even T, et al. Mid-term clinical and sonographic outcome of arthroscopic repair of the rotator cuff. *J Bone Joint Surg Br.* 2008;90-B[10]:1341-1347. Copyright the British Editorial Society of Bone and Joint Surgery.)

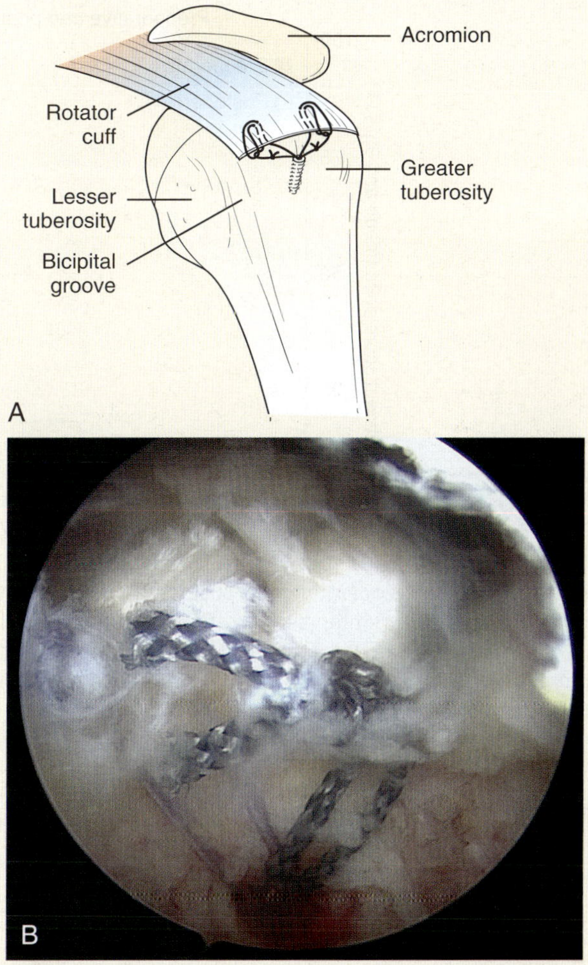

FIGURE 14-132: A, The "ratchet-loop technique" for lateral-row arthroscopic rotator cuff repair. **B,** Lateral arthroscopic view of double-row repair with the "parachute" technique medially and the ratchet-loop technique laterally. (**A,** From Levy O, Venkateswaran B, Even T, et al. Mid-term clinical and sonographic outcome of arthroscopic repair of the rotator cuff. *J Bone Joint Surg Br.* 2008;90-B[10]:1341-1347. Copyright the British Editorial Society of Bone and Joint Surgery.)

ask the operating room staff to release the weights from the arm traction and ask my assistant to abduct the arm.

For massive U-shaped tears, a marginal convergence repair with side-to-side sutures can be used, with preferably complete or partial repair. This can be augmented by a lateral suture anchor repair if needed. For partial-thickness tears, I prefer to use an all-inside transtendon repair, leaving the outer intact layer of the cuff as a "scaffold" for cuff healing. The cuff is repaired using penetrating graspers ("sixters") from the bursa by triangulation. The advantage of this all-inside repair is better visualization of all the cuff layers. I do not use cannulas.

Recently, several arthroscopic transosseous techniques and devices to perform it were introduced.

The rotator cuff repair results in one of our studies[183] show significant improvement of the Constant score to 84.5 (Fig. 14-133), with a significant inverse association between the size of the tear and the postoperative Constant score and patients with smaller tears attaining higher Constant scores after repair. Postoperatively, 80 patients (78.4%) were able to resume their occupations, and 84 (82.4%) returned to their preinjury leisure activities. Ninety-four cases (92%) were highly satisfied with their results, and only eight (7.8%) of 102 patients were not satisfied with the outcome.[183]

Re-tears (or nonhealing) were detected by ultrasound in 19 (18.6%) patients, and were generally smaller than the original ones. All the patients including the ones with re-tears improved substantially after repair; however, the patients with intact repairs were significantly better (Fig. 14-134).[183]

Continued

INTERNATIONAL EXPERT COMMENTARY—cont'd

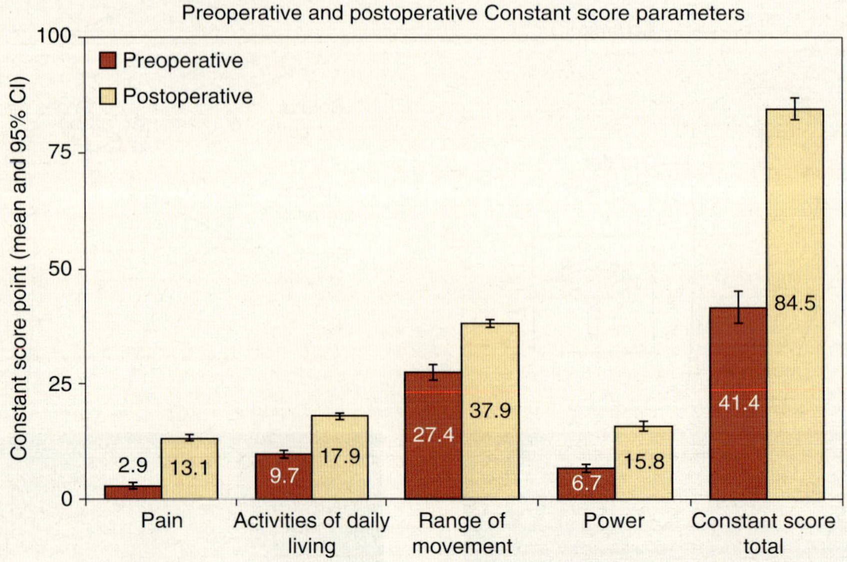

FIGURE 14-133: Preoperative and postoperative Constant scores. The box height represents the mean value; the whiskers show 95% confidence intervals ($P < .0001$, paired *t* test for each parameter). CI, confidence interval. (Modified from Levy O, Venkateswaran B, Even T, et al. Mid-term clinical and sonographic outcome of arthroscopic repair of the rotator cuff. *J Bone Joint Surg Br.* 2008;90-B[10]:1341-1347. Copyright the British Editorial Society of Bone and Joint Surgery.)

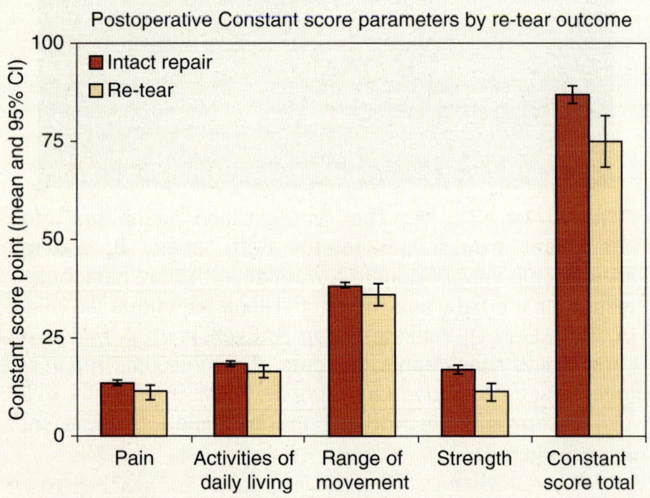

FIGURE 14-134: Comparison of the Constant score and its parameters between patients with intact rotator cuff repair and patients with re-tear. CI, confidence interval. (Data from Levy O, Venkateswaran B, Even T, et al. Mid-term clinical and sonographic outcome of arthroscopic repair of the rotator cuff. *J Bone Joint Surg Br.* 2008;90-B[10]:1341-1347.)

It is important to remember and advise the patients that the length of time needed to recover after rotator cuff repair is long and takes 6 to 12 months. We have found that although there is highly significant improvement in the overall function (Constant score) and strength 6 months postoperatively, patients appear to take a step back before improving, in fact with a drop in strength at 3 months. This may cause concern in patients and may require assurance that time and effort with physiotherapy will improve function and symptoms.[128]

In recent years, the use of platelet-rich plasma (PRP) has been advocated by several authors.[126,276,277,328] PRP can potentially regenerate tissue via multiple mechanisms as it is rich in many growth factors that have important implications in healing. However, there is limited reliable clinical evidence to guide the use of PRP, and studies have obtained conflicting results with different preparations of PRP.[126,276,277,282,343] We have been using a specific leukocyte-poor PRP with mononuclear cells to supplement our rotator cuff repair in the last few years. When compared with a matched historic cohort without PRP, we found that the patients who received the PRP injection at the time of rotator cuff repair reported significantly less pain at 3 weeks postsurgery (pain score 12.67 vs. 12.29; $P = .02$). The majority (93.6%) of the PRP group patients stopped taking painkillers or only occasionally took painkillers (paracetamol) at 3 weeks postoperatively, whereas 57% of the non-PRP patients were still on a painkiller regimen at 3 weeks post-operatively. At 3 and 6 months postsurgery, pain and the Constant score were slightly better in the PRP group than in the non-PRP group but with no statistical significance,[328] which is similar to the results of Randelli et al.[277] Future larger randomized trials will hopefully provide better answers.

The surgical options for irreparable cuff tears are well described in this chapter. Another option to add for treatment is biceps tenotomy, following the French school.

Personally, I have found the results of tendon transfers (latissimus dorsi transfer) to be disappointing. There may

INTERNATIONAL EXPERT COMMENTARY—cont'd

be improvement in external rotation but no improvement in elevation.

I use a synthetic mesh as a scaffold for tissue ingrowth combined with PRP containing high concentrations of growth factors as an interposition graft or for augmentation in all arthroscopic techniques in young and active patients with massive irreparable cuff tears.[253] This technique seems to be a useful and successful method. However, it is a demanding and highly skilled procedure with a failure rate of 40%.[253]

My approach to failed cuff surgery is similar to how the authors have very nicely described. It is important to define the failure: is it pain, limitation of movement, weakness, stiffness, pseudoparalysis, and/or other? One must perform a thorough examination and assess other causes for pain such as neck problems, AC joint, biceps, stiffness, and so forth. As many details as possible must be gathered about previous operations, the state and quality of the rotator cuff at the time of the previous surgery, the tension of the repair, and so forth. The use of imaging with plain radiographs, ultrasound, and MRI scans is necessary to assess the integrity of the cuff and to explore other pathologies. Once the etiology for the failed surgery has been determined, the treatment should be individualized. As the authors described, the first line of treatment is conservative, with stretching exercises and the deltoid rehabilitation regimen.[180]

If the patient develops postoperative stiffness, with stiffness remaining after 6 months, I consider arthroscopic release (not earlier). It is important to explain to the patients that we know to deal with stiffness better than we know how to deal with nonhealing. I consider revision rotator cuff repair in younger, active patients (physiologic age) who had reasonable cuff tissue in the previous operation. I consider the use of a synthetic patch with PRP.[253] Contraindications for revision rotator cuff repair are anterosuperior escape and/or pseudoparalysis. In these cases, I consider reverse total shoulder replacement.[178,10] For elderly patients, I consider reverse total shoulder replacement rather than revision rotator cuff repair, as it will allow them early recovery with good predictable outcomes.[178,10]

During postoperative rehabilitation, the patient has the operated arm in a sling with a small pillow for 6 weeks to hold the arm in neutral rotation with minimal abduction. In this position, the tension on the repaired cuff is reduced. Patients should avoid active exercises for 6 weeks. According to the size of the tear and the quality and tension of the repair achieved, pendulum and passive exercises will commence immediately for small tears, at 3 weeks for medium tears, and at 6 weeks for large and massive tears. I start strengthening exercises at 6 weeks. All the patients are recommended to perform the deltoid-strengthening regimen[180] and undergo hydrotherapy if possible.

EDITOR COMMENTARY

Edward V. Fehringer

The authors have done a fantastic job of educating and updating readers on the rotator cuff as well as management of its pathology. Since I originally read the rotator cuff chapter as a fourth-year resident in 1998 (in the second edition of this text), the study and understanding of rotator cuff pathology and its treatment options have evolved significantly. The current chapter is a succinct yet comprehensive discussion of a structure that has been studied and presented extensively.

The understanding of intrinsic versus extrinsic sources of cuff degeneration is paramount to better treatment of patients, most of whom never seek care for their rotator cuff problems. Theories of extrinsic tear causes have slowly given way to theories of intrinsic tear causes, as clinical and basic science research have supported. With the advent of shoulder arthroscopy, the rates of arthroscopic acromioplasty soared. With more clinical research calling into question the role of acromioplasty with concomitant cuff repair, its role as an isolated procedure for rotator cuff pathology has been questioned. More work is clearly necessary to better understand the sources of shoulder pain and rotator cuff disease. Along with that, a clearer understanding of the necessity for concomitant procedures at the time of rotator cuff repair would be beneficial.

Arthroscopic rotator cuff repair has evolved from arthroscopic-assisted mini-open approaches to all-arthroscopic approaches. Yet the goal of repair remains what it has always been: secure fixation to the humerus, with a relatively tension-free repair that respects several disciplines, including biology and biomechanics. Improved instrumentation has probably been the greatest advancement that has facilitated approaches to repairing cuff tendons through cannulas. While the national and international trend has been toward all-arthroscopic approaches, I prefer the mini-open approach without the routine acromioplasty or suture anchors that Matsen has advocated. It is safe, reliable, reproducible, effective, inexpensive, and efficient; utilizes simple tools; and has been proven successful in many studies and clinical practices. It allows the surgeon to address concomitant long head of the biceps pathology and contractures. Moreover, without compelling evidence that concomitant acromioclavicular joint or perilabral surgery are advantageous, I continue to find it well tolerated and beneficial to patients in whom rotator cuff repair is a viable option.

Professor Levy has graciously shared his work and thoughts on the diagnosis and treatment of rotator cuff disease. He has shown an association between os acromiale and rotator cuff tears. As an intrinsic cause advocate, I have tended to ignore the acromial side both with repair and arthroplasty with success. His thoughts on the utilization of ultrasound for assessing rotator cuff and the minimal use of MRI should encourage continued study. Ultrasound is less expensive, may be used by the examiner, and may be used to evaluate bilateral shoulders. Concomitant procedures along with rotator cuff repair also require continued study. While it may seem plausible that patients do well following concomitant procedures, it could be asked whether they need to be performed to achieve good outcomes and/or whether doing them may compromise reconstruction efforts in the future if the repairs fail to heal. All in all, his international perspective confirms the great work on rotator cuff disease being done in many areas of the globe and our need for continued study and collaboration.

CHAPTER 15

Shoulder Arthroscopy

Edited by Frank A. Cordasco

Contributors

General Principles

Xavier A. Duralde, Scott D. Pennington

Shoulder arthroscopy has been revolutionary in advancing the understanding of shoulder anatomy and pathology. It has given orthopedic surgeons the ability to evaluate and address shoulder pathology utilizing minimally invasive techniques and to develop a new array of techniques in managing complex shoulder problems. Clear visualization of anatomy and pathoanatomy has allowed an improved understanding of the pathophysiology of multiple processes about the shoulder in a way previously not possible. It is also associated with less pain postoperatively leading to easier postoperative rehabilitation, and it decreases the risk of deltoid muscle damage seen with open surgery.[767]

However, arthroscopic surgery takes away from the surgeon the tactile feedback of open surgery. In many ways, it is similar to building a ship inside a bottle, and increases the difficulty of certain procedures. It forces the surgeon to carefully visualize pathology and maintain appropriate orientation of the camera throughout the procedure. These challenges are increased in obese patients. Hemostasis is a greater challenge in shoulder arthroscopy compared with that associated with arthroscopic interventions for other joints and requires special maneuvers to maintain visual access to the operative field.

Although rare, complications associated with shoulder arthroscopy can be averted by meticulous surgical preparation.[434] As with open surgery, the key to success is careful planning for the entire procedure beginning with the positioning, portal placement, and equipment.

This chapter discusses our preferences and makes brief references to alternative methods of conducting shoulder arthroscopy. There are many ways to achieve any given goal. Surgeons must understand what works best in their hands and also understand their own level of ability in shoulder arthroscopy. They must be ready to open the shoulder if necessary to complete the surgery. Timely completion of surgery is critical to minimize complications associated with fluid extravasation and edema; nothing good happens in shoulder arthroscopy after 2 hours.

ANESTHESIA AND MONITORING

Shoulder arthroscopy is commonly performed using a combination of interscalene regional block and general anesthesia. When compared with general anesthesia alone, interscalene blocks have been demonstrated to decrease postoperative pain and opioid requirements and shorten anesthesia recovery times.[766] Postoperative pain scores are typically 2 or less in 99% of patients[175] with this technique.

Interscalene blocks are safe and effective, with an associated complication rate of approximately 1% for experienced anesthesiologists who have performed more than 100 blocks.[398] Reported complications have included pneumothorax, nerve injury, and respiratory compromise from phrenic nerve paralysis.[87] Interscalene blocks are relatively contraindicated in patients with bleeding disorders or lung disease because of the associated risk of hemi-diaphragmatic paralysis. Inadvertent intravascular injection of the block agent induces seizures, cardiac arrest, and death.

Awake anesthesia under interscalene block alone can be performed; however, we do not routinely utilize this method due to concerns regarding the patient's discomfort and motion during surgery, especially in longer procedures. The beach chair position does allow us to use interscalene anesthesia alone in cases where general anesthesia increases patients' risks, such as with airway problems or severe asthma, or in cases of patient preference. Isolated interscalene block anesthesia may require intravenous sedation, and there is a risk that sedation with a hemi-diaphragmatic paralysis without airway support may cause respiratory compromise. In addition, any axillary incision such as that required for open subpectoral biceps tenodesis lies outside the cutaneous coverage area of an interscalene block and requires supplementation with infiltration of local anesthesia.

Patients undergoing shoulder arthroscopy in the beach chair position with hypotensive anesthesia may be at risk for cerebral desaturation, which can result in stroke and even death.[495] A cerebral desaturation event is defined as an intraoperative decrease in regional cerebral tissue oxygenation saturation of 20% or more. Although this rare catastrophic complication can occur in young healthy patients, obesity is a major risk factor.[625] The risk of cerebral desaturation appears to correlate with the degree of elevation in the beach chair position.[543] Unfortunately, the typically utilized brachial noninvasive blood pressure measurements and estimated temporal mean arterial pressure measurements are unreliable for detection of cerebral desaturation events.[714] Near-infrared spectroscopy measures regional cerebral tissue oxygenation and is a promising potential warning device for cerebral desaturation. It is still unknown what degree and duration of cerebral desaturation is necessary to produce a measurable neurocognitive decline[543] and the exact incidence of this complication is unknown. We have not instituted the routine use of infrared spectroscopy for shoulder arthroscopy but are extremely cautious with the use of hypotensive anesthesia, especially in obese patients.

EQUIPMENT

"Good workmen never quarrel with their tools."
—*Lord Byron, 1818*

Having the correct arthroscopic equipment and tools in good working order is critical to the success of arthroscopy. Detailed surgical planning identifies all necessary tools including those that might not be used routinely. Good communication with staff is critical to identify any equipment technical difficulties. Much like a pilot's preflight checklist, it is wise to review the equipment and tools before surgery. Affirmation that the correct equipment is in the room is part of our surgical time out prior to making an incision. This routine can also result in cost savings to assure that unneeded disposable equipment is not inadvertently opened. The necessary equipment can be divided into arthroscopic equipment and surgical tools (Box 15-1).

BOX 15-1. Arthroscopic Equipment

- Arthroscopes:
  - 30 degree
  - 70 degree (rarely utilized)
- Light cord
- Monitor
- Printer
- Irrigation and suction tubing
- Irrigation tower or pump
- Power equipment:
  - Shavers (5.5 and 4.5 mm)
  - Burrs (5.5 mm)
  - Power drill (labral surgery)
- Cautery/ablation device
- Cannulae (8 mm and 5 mm)
- Switching stick
- Surgical tools:
  - Probe
  - Graspers
  - Ringed retrievers
  - Tissue penetrators
  - Arthroscopic scissors
  - Soft tissue elevator
  - Rasp
- Suture passers

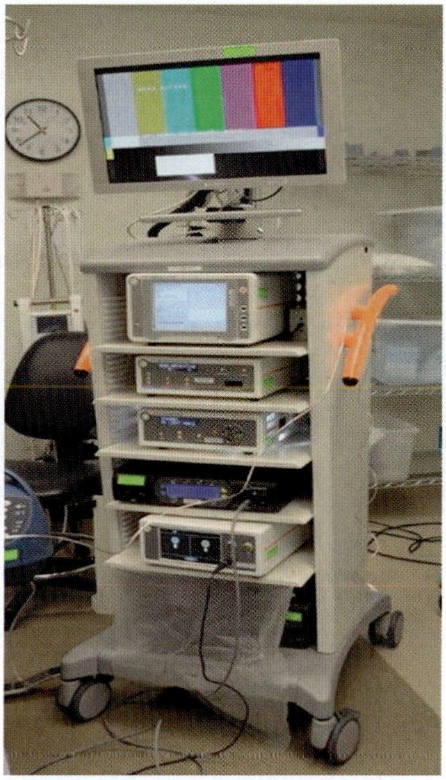

FIGURE 15-1: Arthroscopic tower with monitor, light source, electrocautery, shaver/burr motor, and printer.

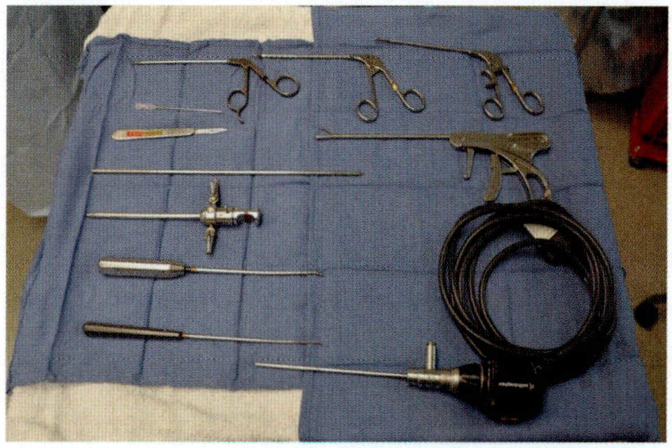

FIGURE 15-2: Standard arthroscopic instruments: camera, blunt trochar, switching stick, probe, elevator, grasper, ringed retriever, biter, penetrators, and needle-projecting suture passer.

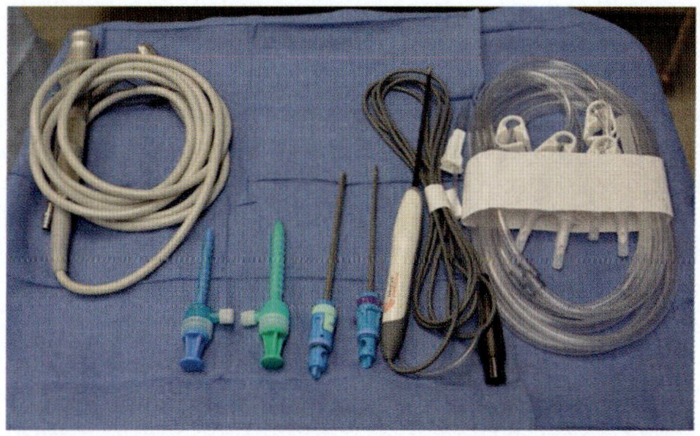

FIGURE 15-3: Disposable arthroscopic equipment: electrocautery device/ablator, 4.5-mm shaver, 5.5-mm burr, and cannulae.

Arthroscopic equipment includes the camera, light cord, light source, monitor, printer, arthroscopy irrigation tubing, suction tubing, and a pump or tower for gravity flow (Fig. 15-1). Prior to surgical incision, the scrub technologist attaches the light cord to the 4-mm 30-degree camera and performs white balancing and focusing of the camera after confirming that the light source and monitor are functioning correctly. The camera should be exchanged if the lens is cracked or the image is not otherwise clear. A 70-degree scope may be utilized for distal clavicle resection, subscapularis repair, acromioclavicular (AC) reconstruction, bony Bankart repair, and other procedures where a more perpendicular view is helpful. The printer should be functioning with sufficient ink and paper. Irrigation tubing should be as short as possible to limit the resistance of fluid flow but long enough to prevent contamination of the surgical field. The pump setting should be confirmed or the bags of irrigation elevated to the correct height. A well-functioning suction is mandatory for both the surgeon and the anesthetist. The correct electrocautery ablation and cauterization levels should be confirmed and functioning of the pedals or buttons of the shaver checked.

Routine shoulder arthroscopy tools include a blunt trocar, 18-gauge spinal needle, hooked probe, arthroscopic grasper, arthroscopic ringed retriever, arthroscopic biter or scissors, Bankart elevator, and a switching stick (Fig. 15-2). Most arthroscopic procedures also utilize 5.5-mm and 8.25-mm cannulas though the sizes may vary. For debridement or decompression procedures, a bipolar electrocautery device, motorized shaver, and burr are necessary (Fig. 15-3). The size, shape, and teeth of the shaver and burr depend on surgeon preference. We typically use 5.5-mm shavers and burrs for subacromial decompression (SAD) but often use smaller shavers to prepare the glenoid neck during labral repair. Suture passing tools are necessary for procedures such as rotator cuff repair, Bankart repair, and capsular plication. These tools include a needle projecting device to drive suture through soft tissue, cannulated penetrators that project a suture passage wire or monofilament, and hooked penetrators for grabbing suture after traversing soft tissue. If anchors are utilized, the correct power drill or awl is essential and the surgeon should confirm the availability of the anchors before surgery. More specialized tools include arthroscopic rasps, arthroscopic dilators, and bone punches. Arthroscopic Latarjet and AC reconstructions often require specialized instrument sets.

Preoperative planning and attention to detail may prevent equipment issues that could delay or compromise an arthroscopic procedure and will allow the surgeon to focus on the dexterous technical demands of the surgery rather than being distracted by equipment problems.

POSITIONING

Both the beach chair[660] and the lateral decubitus positions[12] are used commonly in the United States. There are advantages and disadvantages to both. We prefer the beach chair position for multiple reasons. The orientation of the shoulder is in a more understandable position for the surgeon allowing a more clear evaluation of arthroscopic intra-articular anatomy. In the beach chair position, surgery can be performed with the patient under regional block alone and does not necessarily require general anesthesia. The position facilitates intraoperative examination of the shoulder under anesthesia due to the favorable arm position and the stabilization of the scapula by the operating table. Moreover, it is easier to convert to open surgery if necessary following arthroscopy.[563] Fluid extravasation during arthroscopy occurs in the arm and upper chest and does not generally extravasate to the neck or airway as can occur in the lateral decubitus position.[70] The arm does not block the surgeon's access to the anterior portal and there has been a lower incidence of nerve injuries associated with this technique compared with the lateral decubitus position.[610] We have found this position to be compatible with most arthroscopic interventions but admit that access to the most inferior portion of the glenoid, as may be needed during some instability operations, is relatively more difficult in the beach chair position than in the lateral decubitus position. However, the beach chair position has been associated with a rare complication of cerebral ischemia[544] and the surgeon must be conscious of this with cautious use of hypotensive anesthesia especially in obese patients.

The patient is initially placed supine on a conventional operating table. A padded articulated headrest such as the Mayfield headrest, which has a long cross bar, is used (Fig. 15-4). This operation can be performed on a standard operating table without the use of an expensive shoulder positioner. Following intubation, the patient is moved laterally so that the operative shoulder and about half the scapula hangs off the lateral aspect of the table for access. The hips are brought to the edge of the table. A padded articulated head rest with a long bar to allow translation of the headrest to the lateral border of the operating table is ideal to allow access to the superior aspect of the shoulder, to account for any kyphotic deformity of the chest, and to maintain the neck in neutral rotation. The headrest can be brought to the far lateral position on the table to allow excellent support of the head with the body shifted over the edge of the table. A bolster usually consisting of two folded towels is placed at the medial border of the scapula to prevent medial migration of the scapula during surgery. A pillow is placed underneath the knees and gel pads placed underneath the heels. The table is first flexed at the level of hips to approximately 30 degrees. The knees are then flexed approximately 30 to 40 degrees so that the foot of the table is just past parallel to the ground. The head of the bed is then brought into as far an upright position

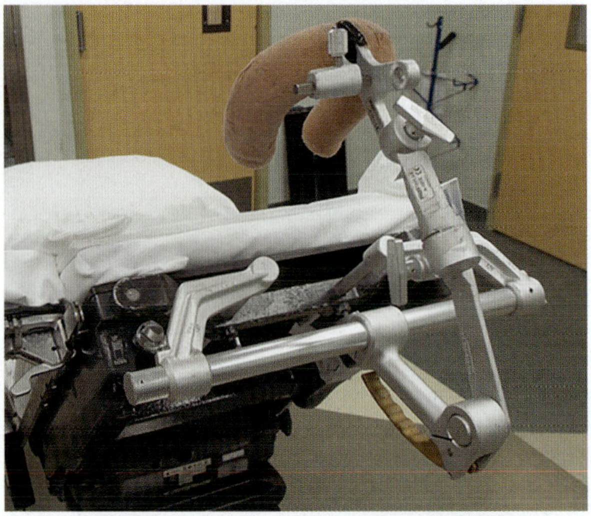

FIGURE 15-4: A padded articulated headrest allows the head to be positioned comfortably, reduces stress on the patient's neck, and allows excellent access to the shoulder. Note the long cross bar on the headrest that extends to the edge of the table.

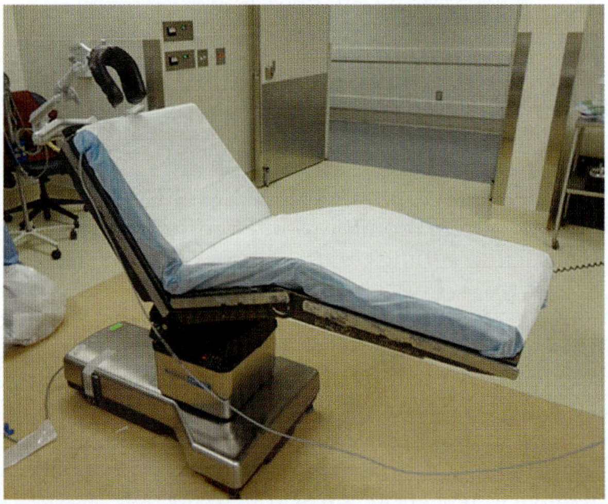

FIGURE 15-5: A standard operating table with an articulated headrest can be used to place the patient in the beach chair position.

as possible usually approximately 60 to 80 degrees (Fig. 15-5). If the patient appears to be unsteady falling towards the operative shoulder, the table can be slightly "airplaned" in the opposite direction. The headrest is adjusted to allow neutral positioning of the neck without stress. The anesthesiologist is responsible for maintaining the head in neutral position throughout the positioning of the table. The head is then fixed to the head rest with either tape or self-adhesive wrap. Care is taken to avoid any pressure to the orbits and eye protection such as goggles may be of some benefit. The strap across the patient's thighs must be checked as this may tighten during positioning and may lead to pressure to the lateral femoral cutaneous nerve and resultant meralgia paresthetica if not adjusted properly. The contralateral arm is supported on pillows to avoid pressure along the cubital tunnel and to assure adequate flow of the intravenous fluids. This arm is carefully secured resting along the patient's lap. The operative arm is hung from an IV pole to allow prep and drape. It is important to avoid pressure to the carpal tunnel during this step (Fig. 15-6). Following the prep, the forearm is wrapped sterile and the arm is placed in an arm holder. Use of a mechanical arm holder obviates the need for an assistant to hold the arm during the procedure. It is important to avoid prolonged traction on the arm to avoid neurological injury that can occur with use of this type of mechanical device (Fig. 15-7). The arm holder should be well padded to avoid skin injury. Neurological injury in the beach chair position is avoided with careful hanging of the arm for prep and drape, careful positioning of the neck in neutral position with a padded articulated head rest, avoiding trunk migration away from or towards the operative side during surgery that can strain the neck, avoiding prolonged traction on the arm with the arm holder, and by careful portal placement. Segmental compression devices are placed on the legs not only to decrease the possibility of deep venous thrombosis (DVT) but also to help maintain cerebral blood flow during hypotensive anesthesia.[383]

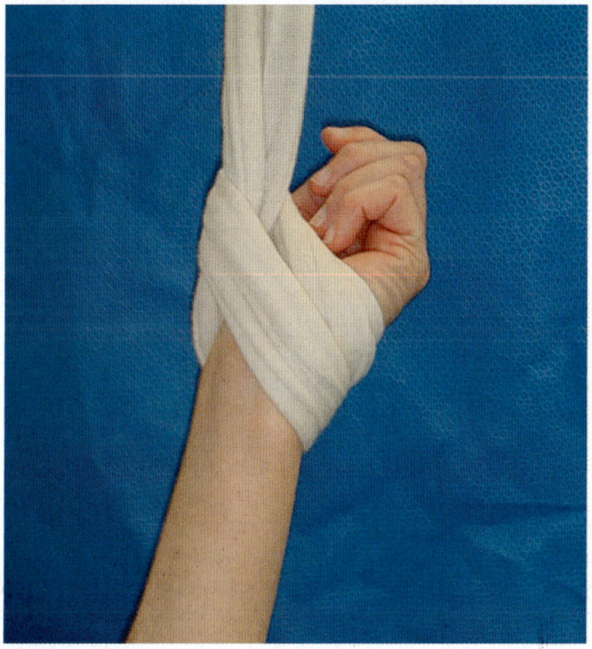

FIGURE 15-6: When the arm is hung for prepping, the loop of the stockinet is placed over the volar aspect of the wrist to avoid pressure on the carpal canal.

EXAMINATION UNDER ANESTHESIA

Examination under anesthesia is an invaluable diagnostic maneuver as the patient is now completely relaxed. Examination in the office is often limited by guarding and pain. Once the joint has been vented with a needle, the surgeon loses the opportunity to perform a meaningful examination under anesthesia. This procedure therefore is performed after positioning of the patient but prior to prep and drape. Initially, range of motion (ROM) in elevation, external rotation at the side, and external and internal rotation in abduction are evaluated. The sulcus sign is elicited by placing axial traction on the arm in line with the trunk of the body. The sulcus sign is evaluated with the arm in neutral and then external rotation looking for inferior laxity in the shoulder. A

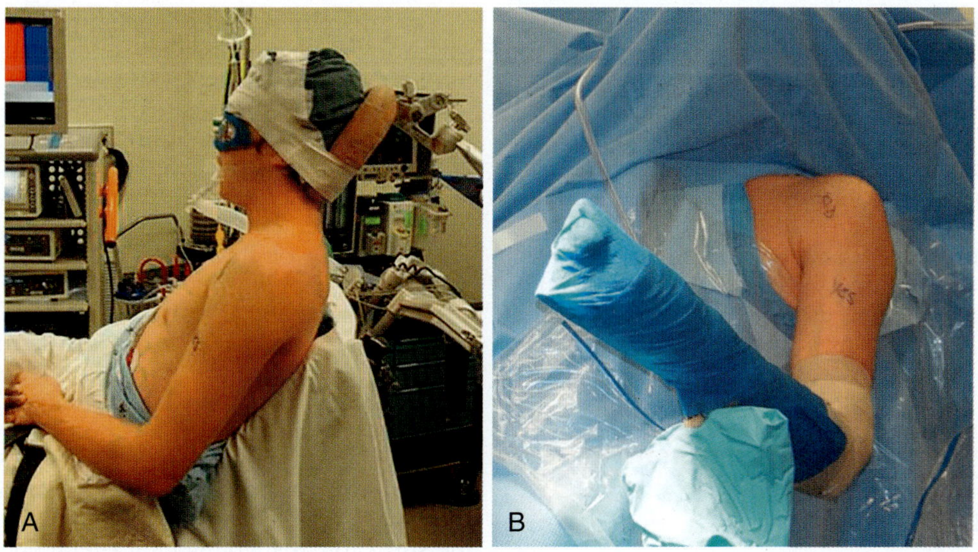

FIGURE 15-7: **A** and **B,** A patient in the beach chair position following prep and drape with the arm in an articulated arm holder. Note the unobstructed access to the shoulder that this position allows.

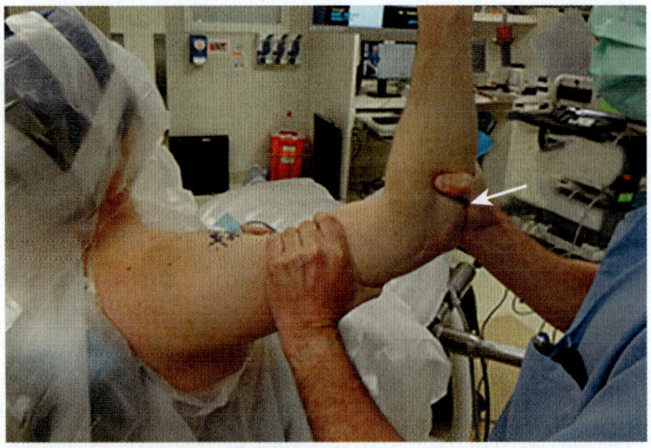

FIGURE 15-8: Axial loading of the humeral shaft through the elbow with use of the examiner's outside hand while the inner hand stresses the glenohumeral joint anteriorly and posteriorly.

sulcus sign that does not improve with the arm in external rotation indicates a deficiency in the rotator interval. Tensioning of the superior glenohumeral ligament (SGHL) that occurs in external rotation should typically decrease the sulcus sign unless there is some incompetency of this ligament.

If the patient is large, the arm can be supported by an assistant who holds the wrist while the surgeon holds the humerus and elbow. However, typically, this maneuver can be performed without assistance. The first critical step is to assure that the examination begins with the humeral head in a located position. The joint is loaded by placing axial pressure through the elbow and down the humeral shaft. The elbow is grasped by the surgeon's outer hand and the humeral shaft by the inner hand. The upper arm is grasped at the site of deltoid insertion, and pressure is applied anteriorly, inferiorly, and posteriorly to determine laxity in those directions (Fig. 15-8). Laxity is generally graded on a 3 point scale as described by Hawkins. Grade 1 laxity implies that the humeral head cannot be translated onto the rim of the glenoid. Grade 2 laxity implies that the humeral head can be translated onto the rim of the glenoid. Grade 3 laxity implies that the humeral head can be dislocated over the rim of the glenoid. Crepitus elicited during these maneuvers usually indicates a labral tear. Other important findings on examination under anesthesia include whether the shoulder locks out of the joint and does not reduce on its own on release of pressure. Both direction and degree is critical in planning instability surgery. Examination under anesthesia also allows determination of true stiffness as opposed to guarding that may occur due to pain in the office setting.

PORTALS AND DIAGNOSTIC ARTHROSCOPY

The bony landmarks of the acromion, clavicle, and coracoid are marked on the skin for points of reference for portal placement. Primary portals are used in most shoulder arthroscopy and consist of the posterior, anterior, midlateral, and anterolateral portals. Accessory portals are utilized depending on the pathology being treated.

Portal placement is planned to allow direct access to the structure being treated while minimizing the risk of injury to adjacent structures, especially nerves. The relative location of the surrounding neurovascular structures has been well outlined. The axillary nerve passes along the undersurface of the deltoid muscle approximately 5 cm distal to the lateral border of the acromion especially with any lateral portals. The safe zone for anterior portals is superior and lateral to the coracoid to avoid the brachial plexus, axillary nerve, and musculocutaneous nerve. The posterior portal is 2 cm away from both the suprascapular nerve and the axillary nerve. Nerve location can be altered by arm abduction and edema, which requires adjustments on the part of the surgeon.

STANDARD PORTALS

The posterior portal is approximately 2 to 3 cm inferior and 1 to 2 cm medial to the posterolateral corner of the acromion in the "soft spot." Translating the humeral head anteriorly and posteriorly can also provide an estimation of the location of glenohumeral articulation as well as the angle of the glenoid relative to the portal. An 18-gauge spinal needle is passed from the posterior portal directed towards the coracoid. The glenohumeral joint is normally under negative pressure and the creation of pressure equilibrium can often be heard. The joint is insufflated with 40 mL of irrigation fluid. The skin is incised with a No. 11 blade and a blunt trocar is directed toward the coracoid until it penetrates the posterior capsule and enters the joint. We feel that insufflation of the joint decreases the chances of cartilage damage during insertion of the trocar.

The anterior portal is generally located immediately superior and lateral to the coracoid entering the joint through the rotator interval; however, its location can vary (Fig. 15-9). An 18-gauge spinal needle is used in an outside-in fashion to confirm the location and trajectory of the portal while viewing from the posterior portal. A No. 11 blade is used to create the anterior portal with care taken not to damage the biceps tendon or the upper border of the subscapularis. If an arthroscopic subscapular repair is planned, the anterior portal is made a few millimeters lateral to allow more direct access to the lesser tuberosity. If a Bankart repair is planned, two anterior portals are typically needed. One portal is made slightly more medial and superior than normal, which leaves room for a second portal that is placed at the lateral apex of the rotator interval. This second anterior portal is made more lateral and inferior such that the spinal needle enters the rotator interval just above the subscapularis while being lateral enough to allow the spinal needle to reach the anteroinferior glenoid with the trajectory needed for glenoid anchors.

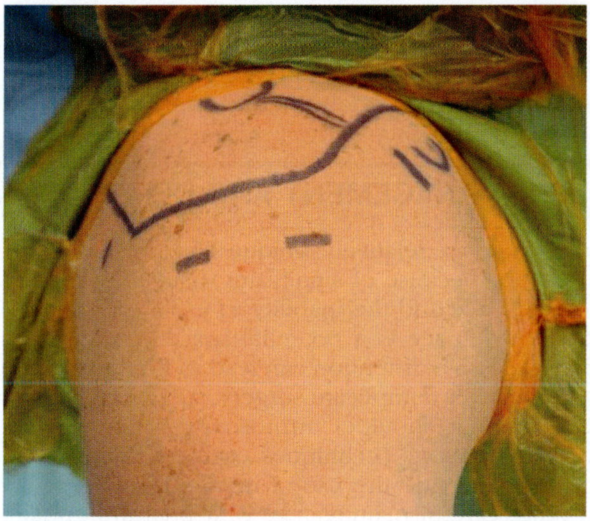

FIGURE 15-9: Standard arthroscopy portals with the acromion, clavicle, and coracoid references drawn out.

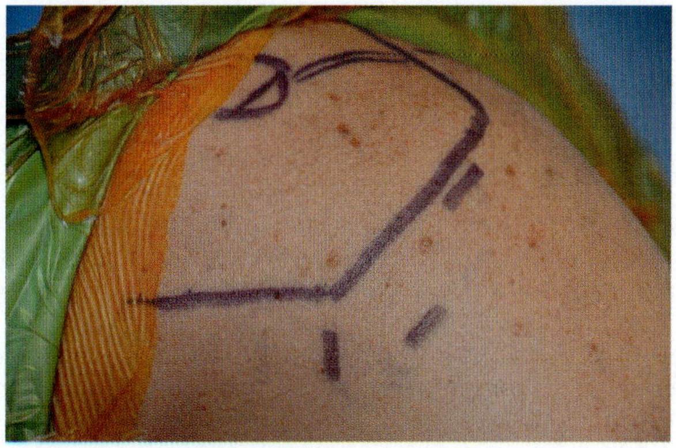

FIGURE 15-10: Approximate locations of accessory portals. These portals are made using an outside-in technique with an 18-gauge spinal needle to establish the portal location on the skin and its trajectory.

The midlateral portal is made 2 to 3 cm below the lateral acromion midway between the anterior and posterior corners of the acromion. This portal is created with a spinal needle observed from the subacromial space. The midlateral portal is useful for SAD as well as a lateral viewing portal for rotator cuff repair. If this portal is made too proximally, the surgeon cannot adequately lower his or her hand to present the burr to the bone. In obese patients, this portal must be made slightly lower to accommodate for the increased thickness of the subcutaneous tissues.

The anterolateral portal is made 2 to 3 cm below the anterolateral corner of the acromion. A spinal needle is used to plan the trajectory for mobilizing the rotator cuff, passing sutures through the cuff, and placement of suture anchors.

ACCESSORY PORTALS

Accessory portals include the posterolateral portal, axillary pouch portal, lateral transtendinous rotator cuff portal, anteromedial portal, and the Neviaser portal (Fig. 15-10).

The posterolateral portal is made approximately 2 cm posterior and lateral to the posterolateral corner of the acromion. This portal is useful for a different approach trajectory for massive cuff tear repairs and is also a good transtendinous rotator cuff portal for posterior labral repairs. This portal also allows the appropriate trajectory for the posterior glenoid anchors. This portal is typically made while viewing from either the subacromial space or glenohumeral joint and allows for appropriate modification to optimize the trajectory.

The site of axillary pouch portal is 2 to 3 cm inferior to the posterolateral corner of the acromion and 2 cm lateral to the posterior portal. This portal is useful for removal of loose bodies and for anchor placement on the posteroinferior glenoid. This portal is made using the outside-in technique with a spinal needle, and is thought to be safer with respect to the axillary nerve than other posteroinferior portals.[559]

The lateral transtendinous rotator cuff portal is made just inferior to the lateral border of the acromion, with the spinal needle directed inferomedially to penetrate the rotator cuff for an optimal trajectory to the superior and posterosuperior glenoid for superior labrum anterior to posterior (SLAP) lesion repairs. This portal is typically 1 cm superior to the midlateral portal and allows adequate inclination necessary for placement of suture anchors at the superior rim of the glenoid. Attempts to place a suture anchor via the midlateral portal would result in a trajectory that is parallel to the superior glenoid neck, which does not allow safe insertion of the anchor.

The Neviaser portal is made at the soft spot superiorly where the spine of the scapula meets the posterior edge of the clavicle just medial to the body of the acromion. The spinal needle is directed in an inferolateral and anterior direction and is useful for passing suture around the biceps anchor, although the suprascapular nerve can be in jeopardy with this portal. It is also useful for excision of osteophytes from the posterosuperior aspect of the AC joint in large patients if this area cannot be adequately accessed via the anterior portal. This technique does require incision of the posterior AC joint capsule, may destabilize the joint further, and is not recommended in routine cases.

The anterosuperior portal is made just anterior to the biceps tendon and used in concert with a low lateral anterior portal for Bankart repairs as a suture management portal.

DIAGNOSTIC ARTHROSCOPY

An organized diagnostic arthroscopy examination is essential to prevent missing any unrecognized shoulder pathology that could compromise surgical outcomes. Magnetic resonance imaging (MRI) is not entirely reliable in identifying all the pathology present in the shoulder and physical exam itself is not definitive in many cases. All potential sources of pain in the shoulder must be ruled out by a systematic examination and ideally documented photographically. This is critical in cases in which patients have ongoing problems after surgery and the surgeon wants to review any possible source of ongoing pain. Once the anterior and posterior portals are established, the chondral surfaces of the glenoid and humeral head are assessed. The superior and anterior labrums are probed to rule out any detachment, with care taken not to confuse anatomic variants like a sublabral foramen or a Buford complex with labral pathology. The biceps is probed and then depressed into the joint to visualize the portion of the tendon that lies in the superior aspect of the bicipital groove (Fig. 15-11). The upper border of the subscapularis and the articular surfaces of the supraspinatus and infraspinatus are probed. The arm is placed in forward flexion and abduction to allow a thorough assessment of the cuff attachments (Fig. 15-12). The camera is then placed in the axillary pouch to look for loose bodies. Finally, the camera is placed through the anterior portal and probe through the posterior portal to evaluate the posterior labrum and capsule.

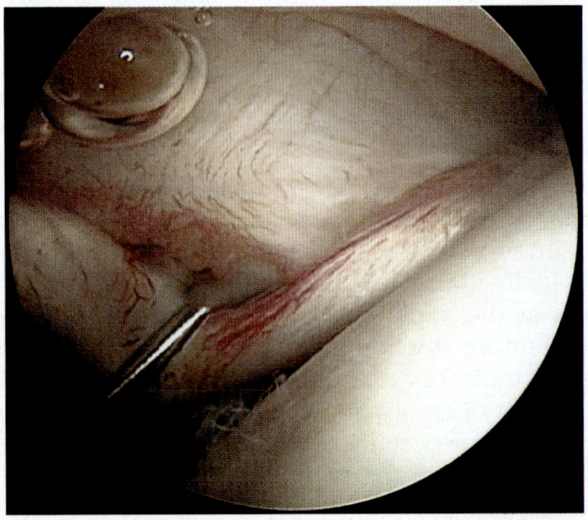

FIGURE 15-11: Arthroscopic view of the glenohumeral joint with the biceps being depressed with a probe to evaluate the portion of the tendon that lies in the bicipital groove.

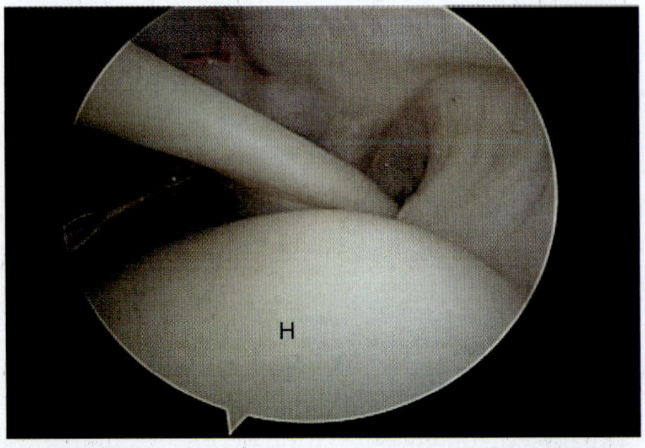

FIGURE 15-12: Arthroscopic view of the articular attachment of the supraspinatus tendon with the arm forward flexed and abducted. H, Humeral head.

FLUID MANAGEMENT AND HEMOSTASIS

Hemostasis is a relatively unique challenge in shoulder arthroscopy because of significant vascularity in the subacromial space and the inability to use a tourniquet. The subacromial space is a potential space without synovial lining; excessive distention can lead to fluid extravasation that can further complicate surgery. Adequate hemostasis is essential for shoulder arthroscopy because it allows clear visualization. Techniques used for maintenance of hemostasis include the use of epinephrine in the irrigation fluid, careful maintenance of a pressure gradient in the subacromial space, avoiding injury to blood vessels in the subacromial space, and by appropriate preoperative medication.

Little direction exists in the orthopedic literature regarding the use of epinephrine in the irrigation fluid for shoulder arthroscopy.[344] Epinephrine must be used cautiously. Excessive absorption of epinephrine can lead to paradoxical increase in blood pressure and increased bleeding during surgery. Potentially lethal arrhythmia has been reported from excessive absorption of epinephrine.[356] We prefer to use a 1/300,000 mixture of epinephrine in the first two irrigation bags. This is achieved by placing 1 mL of 1:1000 mixture of epinephrine in the first two 3-L bags of saline used for irrigation. No other epinephrine is utilized and adequate hemostasis is achieved with this minimal amount of epinephrine in the irrigation.

An adequate gradient between the patient's blood pressure and hydrostatic pressure is necessary to limit bleeding, especially from smaller vessels during the course of surgery.[490] Hypotensive anesthesia may be beneficial in this situation but must be used cautiously to avoid the rare cases of cerebral hypoperfusion, which could lead to stroke or death.[270] This is especially true in the beach chair position. Patient's with morbid obesity and those with a body mass index (BMI) greater than 35 are at a higher risk for this potential complication; however, at this point, it is difficult to completely understand all the risk factors that could potentially lead to this devastating complication.[625] Interscalene block anesthesia results in venous dilatation and increased venous capacitance in the extremity that can also limit bleeding. This form of anesthesia also decreases afferent pain sensations and helps keep the systolic blood pressure low thereby also limiting bleeding.[84]

Irrigation fluid in arthroscopy allows clear visualization by expanding the cavity that is being observed and increasing hydrostatic pressure, which limits bleeding. However, fluid extravasation can lead to edema, which can limit the surgeon's ability to perform surgery and lead to a multitude of complications. Fluid extravasation is more difficult to control in situations in which the glenohumeral joint is not sealed such as in patients with rotator cuff tears, than it is in situations in which capsular and labral surgery are being performed and the fluid is well contained within the glenohumeral joint capsule. In particular, this is true in cases of massive rotator cuff tears in which extravasation of the fluid begins immediately upon insertion of the arthroscope into the glenohumeral joint. Risk factors for the development of edema during shoulder arthroscopy include extended duration of procedure over 2 hours, high pump pressures, loss of fluid containment as is seen in the subacromial space or after capsular release, obesity, and increased fluid volumes. Edema has been linked with almost all complications following shoulder arthroscopy. Surgeons should be ready to abort to an open procedure at the point where it appears that the operation will take more than 2 hours.

Inflow pressure can be maintained either through use of a commercially available pump or through gravity by elevation of the saline bags (Fig. 15-13). Either technique is acceptable. We typically use gravity alone as this appears to be adequate in maintaining visualization without excessive extravasation. We utilize four 3-L bags of saline solution generally elevated two at 8 feet and two at 7 feet. This ensures that two bags will empty first, allowing the circulating nurse time to exchange these with full bags prior to the complete loss of all irrigation fluid. If a pump is utilized, pressures of 50 to 60 mm Hg are generally recommended. Adequate fluid inflow is critical to maintain joint and bursal distention and maintain hydrostatic pressure. This inflow must match fluid outflow through suction shavers and burs, while maintaining adequate pressure at the same time. Gravity flow through the arthroscopic camera cannula is often not sufficient to allow use of shavers with suction. If gravity flow is utilized, a separate 5-mm inflow cannula allows adequate flow and maintains subacromial pressure during shaving and burring. There is no particular advantage of use of gravity inflow over that of pump except for the financial savings if a pump is not utilized. Increased hydrostatic pressure results in decreased bleeding but is also associated with fluid extravasation. A fine balance is necessary to maintain visualization but avoid excessive edema.

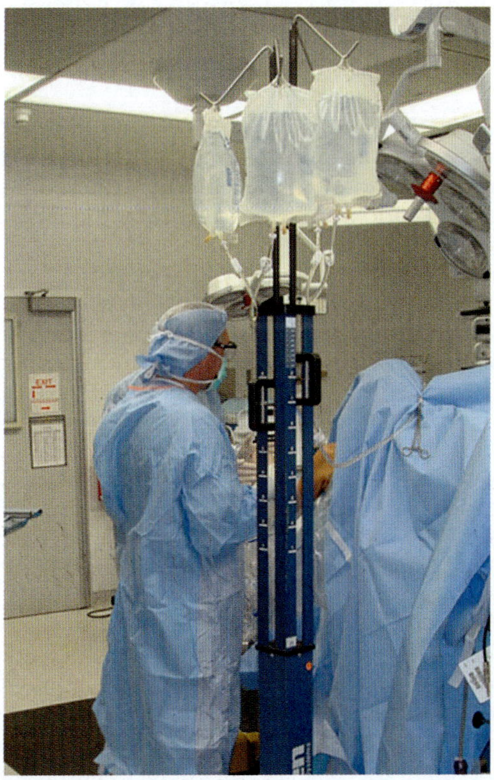

FIGURE 15-13: Three-liter bags of saline placed at a height of 7 and 8 feet to generate enough hydrostatic pressure to facilitate shoulder arthroscopy.

One advantage of the beach chair position is that fluid extravasation occurs into the chest wall and through it into the upper arm. It does not typically extravasate into the neck as seen in the lateral decubitus position. There are less airway problems associated with the beach chair position due to fluid extravasation than in the lateral decubitus position.

Hemostasis is achieved not only with hydrostatic pressure but with judicious and careful use of a thermal ablation probe. Many of these devices are available in the market and are useful both in ablating tissues and attaining hemostasis. Bleeding issues are more common in the subacromial space than in the glenohumeral joint itself. There are three main sources of bleeding in the subacromial space. These include blood vessels in the deltoid muscle, the acromial branch of the thoracoacromial artery, which lies in the coracoacromial ligament, and blood vessels in the fatty tissue adjacent to the AC joint. Bleeding is avoided by staying out of the deltoid as much as possible, cautious takedown of the coracoacromial ligament and slow ablation of fatty tissues in the area of the AC joint.

Shaving and ablation in the subacromial space should always be performed under direct vision. In the event of bleeding, the surgeon has a good idea of its source based on his or her most recent surgical step, and can direct actions to control hemostasis. Several maneuvers are available to the surgeon if bleeding does occur. If a separate inflow is being utilized, outflow through the scope allows removal of some of the bloody irrigation fluid and will improve visualization so that the ablation probe can be maneuvered into position. Placement of an outflow cannula adjacent to the bleeding vessel allows the blood to pass directly out of the subacromial space and allows the surgeon more clear visualization of the bleeding vessel. Increasing the pressure of the irrigation is also an option but must be used diligently to avoid excessive extravasation. Hypotensive anesthesia can also be utilized with caution.

Patients should be cautioned to stop taking any medications that affect coagulation including warfarin, aspirin, and other antiinflammatory medications as these will lead to an increase in bleeding during arthroscopic surgery.

The steps outlined above can help set up any shoulder arthroscopic procedure for success. As case complexity increases, the tools required and sequence of steps will change but if the surgeon is prepared through careful planning, patient positioning, and portal placement, delays and surgical complications can be minimized and the chances of successful outcome improved. There are a variety of options available when performing shoulder arthroscopy and each surgeon must develop a routine that allows for a thorough evaluation and expert treatment of all pathology encountered. The steps outlined in this chapter have been developed over many years and helped achieve those goals in our hands.

Arthroscopic Treatment of Shoulder Instability

Peter D. Fabricant, Frank A. Cordasco

Arthroscopic treatment of shoulder instability has continued to gain wide acceptance as refined techniques have improved clinical outcomes. Arthroscopy confers distinct advantages in the treatment of glenohumeral instability; these include improved visualization and examination of pathoanatomy,[129,457] confirmation of preoperative imaging findings,[395] and the facility for minimally invasive treatment. While open stabilization continues to have a role in the surgical management of glenohumeral instability (particularly in the presence of a large osseous lesion, poor quality tissue, hypermobility, or in the revision setting), advanced arthroscopic techniques continue to offer expanded indications for arthroscopic stabilization.

In addition to maximal surgical visualization achieved with minimal surgical dissection, arthroscopic interventions are associated with significant reduction in operative and hospitalization time and perioperative complications.[282] In recent years, shoulder surgeons have reported results that are comparable with those of traditional open techniques in patients with traumatic anterior instability.

This chapter reviews the indications and contraindications to arthroscopic management of unidirectional anterior and posterior shoulder instability and multidirectional instability (MDI). Recent evidence pertaining to arthroscopic treatment of first-time anterior shoulder dislocation in typical high-risk athletes is presented, and outcomes of open and arthroscopic stabilization are compared. Finally, we discuss our preferred techniques for arthroscopic stabilization of anterior instability, posterior instability, and MDI.

PATHOANATOMY

Historically, surgical treatment of shoulder instability focused on preventing recurrent dislocations rather than restoring joint anatomy, which was frequently achieved by limiting external rotation (Putti-Platt, Magnusson-Stack) or by providing a bony block to anterior instability (Bristow, Latarjet). Although often effective in preventing further dislocations, these procedures decrease shoulder mobility, especially in external rotation, and may cause early osteoarthritis. Arthroscopy has provided improved visualization and understanding of the pathoanatomy of shoulder instability and has enabled surgeons to focus on arthroscopic or open restoration of anatomy, reserving nonanatomic stabilization only for complex or revision situations.

History, mechanism of injury, physical examination findings, and imaging studies all play a role in determining the direction, severity, and chronicity of instability. Contact sports (e.g., football, lacrosse, wrestling, and ice hockey), especially those that involve forcible overhead activity, place the athlete at a greater risk of dislocation compared with that associated with noncontact sports. Males are at a greater risk than females, in part due to their higher rate of participation in contact sports. Ligamentous laxity further increases the risk of dislocation and subluxation of the glenohumeral joint.[538,730] Finally, younger patients are at higher risk than those who are older than 30 years.[17,268,318,376,538,609,616,743]

Biomechanical and clinical studies have shown that traumatic dislocation or subluxation of the shoulder leads to an anteroinferior capsulolabral detachment from the glenoid—the so-called Bankart lesion. It has also been shown that the glenohumeral ligaments fail in continuity (stretching and attenuation of the capsulolabral complex, whose osseous attachments remain intact) as well as from bone.[55,677]

Although the Bankart lesion is the most common pathoanatomic pattern in traumatic anterior instability, it is important to recognize less-common causes of anterior instability. In addition to labral detachment, capsular injury is often an inherent component in anterior instability, especially in cases of chronic or recurrent instability. Rotator interval capsular injury or deficiency can also contribute to anterior instability. Addressing both labral detachment and capsular laxity is critical to successful surgical treatment of anterior shoulder instability. Occasionally, in patients with traumatic anterior instability, the capsule can avulse from the humeral side, producing a humeral avulsion of the glenohumeral ligament (HAGL) or the capsule can rupture in the midsubstance.[25,67,602,762]

Bone injury or defect also contributes to anterior instability. Acute fracture of the anterior-inferior glenoid (bony Bankart lesion) or bony erosion of the glenoid due to recurrent instability affects surgical decision making and can require grafting. The size of Hill-Sachs defects (posterior superior compression fractures of the humeral head) must be noted during surgical planning for instability repairs. The location of the Hill-Sachs lesion may be more important than the size of the defect. For lesions that extend more medial (away from the articular cartilage–rotator cuff insertion), an engaging, or so-called "off-track," defect may exist.[197,769] Engaging lesions will increase the likelihood of failure with a standard arthroscopic Bankart repair in the high-risk athlete. Furthermore, the relationship between glenoid bone loss and humeral head bone loss is complex. Smaller amounts of bone loss in combination with the so-called bipolar lesions have a compounding effect.[16] DiGiacomo has developed a guideline for a more objective assessment of the Hill-Sachs lesion and has suggested that if the Hill-Sachs interval is greater than the glenoid track in high-risk athletes, a remplissage[583] is indicated.[197] Failure to recognize and properly address the bone loss and the bipolar lesions can lead to failure of arthroscopic Bankart repair and likely requires more advanced arthroscopic or open techniques.

MDI is recognized as a separate entity and is not generally associated with a classic Bankart lesion or with bony injury. This syndrome is not limited to the anterior inferior instability in abduction and external rotation. Congenital or pathologic attenuation of the capsule and ligaments can result in repetitive and painful subluxation. Repetitive microtrauma in a susceptible shoulder is also considered to play a role in the pathophysiology of this condition.

Frank posterior dislocation is uncommon in the absence of high-energy trauma or seizure or in the setting of electrical shock. Isolated or repetitive posterior subluxation is more common in athletes, particularly among football linemen who sustain repeated posteriorly directed force to their shoulders. Posterior instability pathoanatomy manifests as labral detachment and capsular injury, which allows increased posterior translation of the humeral head. Pain is often the predominant complaint in many patients with posterior instability.

DIAGNOSIS AND DIAGNOSTIC ARTHROSCOPY IN SHOULDER INSTABILITY

Although history and physical examination is covered elsewhere in this book, it is important to revisit this topic here as it pertains to shoulder instability and arthroscopic stabilization. A failed arthroscopic stabilization procedure often starts not in the operating room but with the failure to identify red flags in the patient's history and physical examination that might preclude a successful arthroscopic repair. The risk factors associated with treatment failure (recurrent instability or functional deficits) include age, gender, presence of osseous Bankart, and/or large Hill-Sachs (cortical depression in the posterolateral humeral head)[309] lesions, participation in competitive collision or forced overhead sports, hypermobility, time lapse between dislocation and reduction, and the number of instability episodes prior to operation.[130,185,538,576,730] A brief summary of our approach in diagnosing shoulder instability is presented in Box 15-2.

A thorough history and physical examination should allow the examiner to understand the etiology, direction, degree, and frequency of a patient's shoulder instability. Radiographs and MRI are used as adjuncts to diagnosis, to determine whether a patient is a candidate for arthroscopic stabilization, and for preoperative planning. MRI has proven to be useful in identifying capsulolabral avulsions (HAGL and reverse HAGL lesions) and rotator cuff pathology, which is common in patients over 40 years old with glenohumeral dislocation[509,652] and at times coexist with a Bankart lesion. Unless such lesions are actively sought, correctly identified, and appropriately addressed, the treatment is likely to fail. While plain radiography is able to capture any substantial bone loss on the glenoid and humerus, computed tomography (CT) allows for a more precise quantification of bone loss. Using CT, the best views to evaluate the glenoid are sagittal cuts and three-dimensional (3D) reconstructed en face glenoid views with humerus subtracted.[328,517,692] The inferior two thirds of the glenoid forms a circle; any bone loss is liable to result in circumferential asymmetry. A 1.5-mm osseous lesion corresponds to 5% glenoid bone loss.[191] Glenoid bone loss greater than 18% to 25% of the glenoid surface area increases risk of failure of

BOX 15-2. History and Physical Examination for Shoulder Instability

History Taking
- Age
- Handedness
- Sport or recreational activity
- Unilateral or bilateral complaint
- Family history of shoulder dislocation
- Initial traumatic event
- Position of arm during subluxation or dislocation
- Number of previous episodes of dislocations or subluxations
- Was the dislocation reduced in the emergency department?
- Interval of time between dislocation and reduction
- Degree of trauma required for recurrence
- Voluntary dislocation
- Dislocation during sleep
- Presence of and location of pain
- Presence or absence of mechanical symptoms
- Sensory disturbance or motor weakness
- Previous shoulder surgery

Physical Examination
- Inspection
- Constitutional ligamentous laxity (e.g., Marshall test, Beighton score)
- Neck range of motion and Spurling's maneuver
- Shoulder range of motion and scapular symmetry
- Strength testing of shoulder girdle muscles
- Lift-off and belly press tests
- Sulcus sign
- Anterior apprehension test and position of arm (include evaluation for mid-range instability)
- Relocation test
- Load and shift (anterior and posterior)
- Jerk test
- O'Brien's active compression test
- Hawkin's and Neer's impingement tests
- Cross-body adduction

nonoperative and operative management that does not address the bone loss.[105,339,770] Recent analysis of the combined effects of glenoid and humeral head bone loss in the so-called bipolar lesions suggests 18% bone loss as the threshold for concern in these cases.[16] This threshold may be even lower as reported in a series of high demand military personnel following arthroscopic Bankart repair who had unacceptably low Western Ontario Shoulder Instability (WOSI) scores, when the anteroinferior glenoid bone loss was greater than 13.5%.[649] However, the critical limits are yet to be defined.

An examination under anesthesia is also critical to the success of arthroscopic stabilization, and is more sensitive for determining both the degree and direction of instability. The pattern of instability can be determined without getting affected by patient apprehension or guarding. The axial load test or load-and-shift test is conducted and the translation noted in the anterior, inferior, and posterior directions. Grading reflects the degree of humeral head translation anterior and posterior to the glenoid rim. Grade 1+ corresponds to the translation of the humeral head to the edge of the glenoid, 2+ if the humeral head can be subluxated over the glenoid rim but reduces spontaneously, and 3+ if a frank dislocation of the humeral head over the glenoid rim does not reduce spontaneously.[8]

After examination under anesthesia, diagnostic arthroscopy is critical for finalizing the surgical plan and includes evaluation of the glenoid labrum, the capsular redundancy and tissue quality, size of the humeral Hill-Sachs defect, anterior-inferior bony defects of the glenoid, osteochondral loose bodies, and glenohumeral ligament detachment (either glenoid or humeral). Detachment or tearing of the glenoid labrum, depending on the site, can confirm the presence and indicate the direction of the dominant instability vector.

Arthroscopic inspection of the intra-articular and bursal surfaces of the rotator cuff should also be performed, particularly in older patients who tend to have a high prevalence of concomitant rotator cuff pathology. Snyder and Strafford noted that approximately 20% to 25% of patients with instability undergoing arthroscopy have associated loose bodies, rotator cuff tears, biceps tendon pathology, or SLAP lesions.[670] These lesions, if unrecognized or untreated, may compromise the surgical outcome. Thus arthroscopic examination can both clarify the diagnosis in ambiguous cases and identify associated pathology that may require surgical management in complex settings. In a study by Mok et al., arthroscopic examination altered the diagnosis in 40% of patients with atraumatic instability and in 8% of those with traumatic anterior instability.[482] Adolfsson and Lysholm found concurrent pathology at the time of diagnostic arthroscopy that could have influenced the outcome of surgery in 44% of 39 dislocating shoulders.[2]

As understanding of the complex and highly interdependent interactions of the glenoid, humerus, labrum, glenohumeral ligaments, and rotator cuff has become more refined, arthroscopy has become a valuable diagnostic and therapeutic tool. At our institution, we routinely use diagnostic arthroscopy as part of the management of glenohumeral instability, even when open stabilization is planned.

ARTHROSCOPIC MANAGEMENT OF POSTTRAUMATIC ANTERIOR INSTABILITY

Overview

Most shoulder specialists consider arthroscopic anterior stabilization as the first-line treatment for recurrent glenohumeral instability. This has not always been the case as the outcomes of earlier arthroscopic techniques were inferior to those of open repair.[399] This in large part was attributable to incomplete treatment of the entire spectrum of pathology associated with anterior instability. Successful arthroscopic management of posttraumatic unidirectional instability must be able to independently address several coexisting pathologic entities: the Bankart lesion (labral detachment), anterior labroligamentous periosteal sleeve avulsion (ALPSA lesion),[510] HAGL lesion,[25,762] and capsular attenuation. Despite historical data indicating the superiority of primary open stabilization, it has, however, fallen out of favor as it is more invasive and risks subscapularis insufficiency, along with recent data showing equivalence or superiority of modern arthroscopic techniques.[72,296,565,743]

An anteroinferior Bankart labral detachment is present in the majority of recurrently unstable shoulders after an initial traumatic dislocation. However, most of these shoulders have a certain degree of coexisting capsular redundancy at the time of surgery. As the acute dislocation evolves into chronic, recurrent instability, further capsular attenuation is likely to occur. In this setting, isolated labral reattachment is usually inadequate and results in failure. Thus patients with more than two or three instability episodes and/or significant capsular attenuation require capsular shifting in conjunction with Bankart repair to regain and maintain stability.

Results of Arthroscopic Treatment of Anterior Shoulder Instability

Historically, early arthroscopic repairs reported higher failure rates than open techniques. Staples or transglenoid sutures were used,[280,487,539] with a high incidence of recurrence and hardware migration.[166,190,385,442] Transglenoid suturing of the Bankart lesion showed some success but fell out of favor due to variable recurrence rates, technical difficulty, and the risk of injuring the suprascapular nerve by tying sutures over the posterior fascia.[150] Bioabsorbable tacks were unable to adequately treat capsular redundancy[227,679] and resulted in synovitis as the device loosened with time.[679,739]

With advances in suture anchor technology, clinical outcomes have improved significantly. Arthroscopic techniques have the advantage of approximating the methods routinely used during open shoulder stabilization. Anchors can be placed more precisely at the margin of the articular surface and the glenoid neck to anatomically recreate the labrocapsuloligamentous origin. McEleney et al. demonstrated that suture anchor techniques are biomechanically the strongest of eight repair techniques (including single and multiply placed tacks, sutures, and transglenoid sutures) in a canine Bankart model.[454]

Early clinical outcomes of suture anchor repair were promising and realized similar results to open stabilization,[310] even in high demand athletes, with redislocation rates of 6% and an 85% return to previous level of sporting activity.[26]

Prospective evaluation of midterm outcomes have shown durability of these clinical results; Carreira et al. evaluated a consecutive series of 85 patients with Bankart lesions treated arthroscopically with suture anchors loaded with nonabsorbable sutures.[127] Over a mean follow-up period of 46 months, the overall recurrence rate was 10%, while in 90% of cases the subjective outcome measures were graded as good to excellent. Recurrent dislocation occurred in two of 18 athletes involved in collision sports at 22 and 60 months postoperatively after return to sport. The variables associated with successful outcomes were use of a low anterior portal (5 o'clock position), repair of tear extension into the superior labrum, and placement of the suture anchors 2 mm in on the glenoid face articular cartilage.

Advanced arthroscopic techniques include double-row labral repair, posteroinferior capsulolabral repair, and remplissage. While arthroscopic single row techniques are commonly employed for primary surgical management in patients with capsulolabral avulsions, recent cadaveric studies have shown that double-row fixation may better restore normal anatomy.[3,365,368,486] These techniques may be indicated in the setting of small (<20%) bony Bankart lesions as well.[470] Arthroscopic approaches to shoulder stabilization may benefit from use of these advanced techniques in the clinical setting of the high-risk male athlete[221]; however, their superiority over traditional techniques has not been evaluated in comparative clinical studies.

Arthroscopic Versus Open Anterior Stabilization

Although open anterior stabilization has a successful track record, the trend in recent years among many shoulder specialists has been to repair uncomplicated Bankart lesions arthroscopically. As mentioned above, the two principle advantages of arthroscopy are decreased surgical morbidity, including avoiding subscapularis takedown, and improved ROM, especially terminal external rotation. Studies that have evaluated the early outcomes of arthroscopic stabilization have largely involved use of first-generation techniques and implants, which do not perform as well as the current instrumentation.[286] These studies are further perpetuated in the orthopedic literature through meta-analyses that combine results from heterogeneous cohorts,[243] thus leading to open repair being described as the gold standard for shoulder stabilization. This should be interpreted with caution as there is significant noncomparability between first generation arthroscopic techniques and those performed today.

More recent studies have shown that outcomes of arthroscopic stabilization using modern techniques and fixation methods for recurrent traumatic anterior shoulder instability are comparable to those of open stabilization and involve minimal bone loss.[72,296,565] This has resulted in a relative increase in the use of arthroscopic stabilization techniques and a decline in open stabilization techniques on the whole.[171,779] While there is a paucity of adequately powered randomized controlled trials comparing current arthroscopic stabilization techniques versus open stabilization, a recent large study of a cohort of 3854 active duty military personnel who underwent Bankart repair revealed a 4.5% rate of recurrence after arthroscopic stabilization as against a 7.7% recurrence rate associated with open stabilization.[743] There remains some controversy in the literature with a recent randomized controlled trial demonstrating a higher failure rate in the arthroscopic stabilization group (23% vs. 11% in the open stabilization group).[481]

Contraindications

In current practice, patients with recurrent anterior instability tend to be well informed and expect successful outcomes of arthroscopic stabilization. More important, therefore, is deciding which patients are *not* candidates for arthroscopic stabilization. Risk factors for failure of operative stabilization include: age younger than 20 years, competitive overhead or contact athlete, shoulder capsular attenuation (due to a genetic collagen disorder and/or poor quality capsulolabral tissue), a Hill-Sachs lesion present on the anteroposterior (AP) radiograph in external rotation, and loss of the anteroinferior glenoid contour on the AP radiograph.[29,130,481,576,730,743] These factors have been used to develop the instability severity index score (ISIS), which identifies patients for whom open stabilization may be more effective.[29] When the interval of time between the dislocation and reduction approaches 5 hours or more, stabilization techniques that address bone loss such as the Latarjet reconstruction should be considered.[185] The number of formal reductions required for anterior dislocation has been shown to directly correlate with failure following arthroscopic repair as well.[538,741]

Patients with demonstrable bone loss from the glenoid or humeral head that warrants bone augmentation or transfer (e.g., Latarjet procedure,[387] Bristow procedure,[304] free allograft or autograft[582]), patients with capsular injury, and those who require a revision stabilization through an open approach may still benefit from a diagnostic arthroscopy prior to open surgery to document all pathology.[138,658] Although capsular avulsions of the glenohumeral ligaments have been successfully repaired arthroscopically, many arthroscopic shoulder surgeons still consider HAGL lesions as a relative contraindication to an all-arthroscopic stabilization (Fig. 15-14).

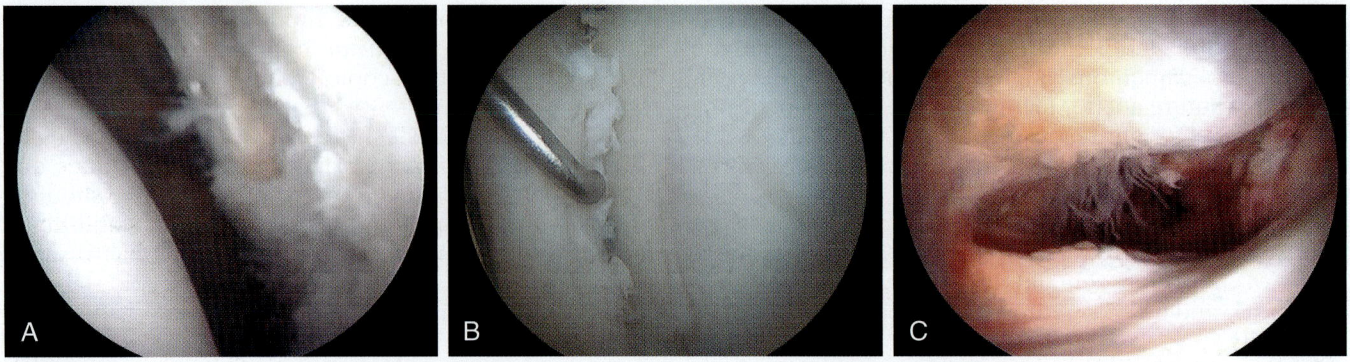

FIGURE 15-14: Example of a patient indicated for a combined open and arthroscopic repair. This patient was a 25-year-old National Football League cornerback who sustained a traumatic anterior glenohumeral dislocation. **A,** Evaluation with a 30-degree arthroscope from the posterior portal in the beach chair position revealed an anterior capsulolabral tear. **B,** The tear was repaired using a mattress technique with knotless suture anchors. **C,** Arthroscopy confirmed the preoperative imaging finding of a humeral avulsion of the glenohumeral ligament lesion that was repaired through an open anterior deltopectoral approach with a subscapularis split.

Traumatic Humeral Avulsion of the Glenohumeral Ligaments

At times, traumatic subluxation or dislocation can result in avulsion of the glenohumeral ligament complex at the humeral insertion. This pathology was first described by Nicola[516] but was first reported arthroscopically by Bach et al. in 1988.[25] Like Bankart lesions at the glenoid, the HAGL lesion may involve soft tissue or bony avulsion.[523] In a published series, the incidence of HAGL lesions was between 7.5%[67] and 9.3%[762]; the lesion occurs in the setting of high-velocity sports injury or violent traumatic injury and generally in an older patient population.[67] It is important for the surgeon to identify this lesion on MRI[313] or during diagnostic arthroscopy for shoulder instability, as these lesions may occur in conjunction with Bankart lesions,[736] a condition termed a *bipolar* or *floating* anterior-inferior glenohumeral ligament (IGHL). If a floating capsule is addressed only on the glenoid side, the Bankart repair will fail because the procedure will advance but not repair the capsule.

The HAGL lesion has received more attention in recent years because the advent of arthroscopy has allowed direct visualization of lesions that may otherwise have been neglected during open stabilization. In their retrospective review of 547 shoulders treated for instability, Bokor et al. reported a 39% incidence of HAGL as the cause of anterior instability in the subset of patients who had a posttraumatic primary dislocation without a discrete Bankart lesion and a purely unidirectional instability.[67] In addition, HAGL has been reported as a cause of recurrent instability after arthroscopic Bankart repair.[639] Although repair of HAGL lesions arthroscopically has been reported by several authors,[137,375,602,675] there are no large case series to suggest that the arthroscopic repair of HAGL is routinely reliable. Therefore many surgeons continue to treat HAGL lesions via an open approach.

Treatment of the First-Time Dislocator

Although the historical treatment for first-time glenohumeral dislocation has been immobilization, this has been debated in the recent literature. Due to the high recurrence of anterior instability in the younger population (<25 years old), some authorities have recommended operative stabilization for first-time dislocators who intend to return to high-risk activities. Evidence from several recent studies support operative intervention for the first-time dislocators in populations who are at high risk for recurrent dislocation (e.g., active duty military, overhead and contact athletes). Clinical outcomes have generally been good, with redislocation rates in these high risk groups dropping from as high as 75% to 11% to 12%.[177]

In our practice, a young patient with a first-time anterior dislocation and a documented Bankart lesion on MRI is counseled that the recurrence rate with nonoperative treatment will likely be higher than 75%, in the event of the patient returning to high-risk activities. A detailed discussion is conducted with the athlete (and parents of young athletes) to delineate the sport, position and level of competition as well as the optimal time for operative intervention based on the athlete's season and goals. The in-season athlete with an anterior shoulder dislocation can occasionally be managed with bracing depending upon the sport and position; however, subsequent subluxation or dislocation is common. Buss et al. reported their results of physical therapy and bracing for 30 in-season athletes who had acute or recurrent anterior dislocation.[115] They reported an average of 1.4 instability episodes per athlete per season. About half of these patients underwent anterior stabilization after the season was over. The importance of competing must be weighed against the risk of further damage to the shoulder in these cases. Surgery is recommended if there is evidence of recurrent instability. There is compelling evidence to demonstrate that the failure rate with arthroscopic stabilization increases substantially with each subsequent instability episode.[538,741]

Summary of Indications

We routinely perform primary arthroscopic anterior stabilization for recurrent anterior instability and uncomplicated revision surgery without significant bone loss. We do not consider participation in contact or overhead athletics as a contraindication to arthroscopic stabilization. We do counsel athletes involved in collision sports that recurrence after stabilization depends on the repair type and on the activity level chosen after surgery. In general, we have been satisfied with our arthroscopic results (even in contact athletes) when the following conditions are met:

- The patient has unidirectional instability of traumatic origin that consists of anterior or isolated anteroinferior instability without more than 1+ sulcus sign on examination under anesthesia.
- Arthroscopic examination shows a discrete Bankart lesion. The lesion in some cases has migrated and healed medially and inferiorly (ALPSA lesion).[510] When the capsule and labrum have healed in the medialized position, it must be elevated off the glenoid and brought to a functionally appropriate position on the anterior-inferior glenoidal rim.
- The capsule is robust, and the IGHL complex does not exhibit signs of attrition.
- No humeral avulsion of the glenohumeral ligament is present.
- No off-track or engaging bony Bankart, Hill-Sachs, or combined lesion is contributing to instability within the functional ROM.

It is important to be prepared to convert to open surgery if examination under anesthesia and diagnostic arthroscopy reveal any of the aforementioned diagnoses that are not amenable to successful arthroscopic reconstruction (see Fig. 15-14).

Authors' Preferred Technique

Based on results from our institution and results published using suture anchors for arthroscopic anterior stabilizations, we routinely use an arthroscopic approach for Bankart repair. The goal of arthroscopic anterior stabilization or Bankart repair is to restore the glenoid labrum and the attached capsule and ligaments back to the anatomic position on the face of the anterior-inferior glenoid and reduce capsular redundancy associated with recurrent dislocation. A preoperative MRI is routinely obtained to confirm the pathology and to avoid any unforeseen pathology on arthroscopy (Fig. 15-15). In male athletes younger than 25 years engaged in contact or forced overhead sports who have more than one instability episode or when more than 2 hours have elapsed since the occurrence of dislocation, CT is performed with 3D reconstruction en face view with the humerus subtracted.

Regional anesthesia with an interscalene block combined with general anesthesia is administered. The patient is placed in the beach chair (modified Fowler) position. Arthroscopic landmarks are palpated and marked on the skin of the shoulder: acromion, AC joint, clavicle, and coracoid. Supplementary local anesthesia in the area of the posterior portal is injected.

An examination with the patient under anesthesia is performed to determine the pattern of instability. In our experience, examination in the operating room is more sensitive in determining both the degree and direction of instability. The axial load test or load-and-shift test is conducted and translation is noted in the anterior, inferior, and posterior directions. Grading reflects the degree of humeral head translation anterior and posterior to the glenoid rim. The grade is 1+ if the translation of the humeral head is to the edge of the glenoid, 2+ if the humeral head can be subluxated over the glenoid rim but reduces spontaneously, and 3+ if a frank dislocation of the humeral head over the glenoid rim does not reduce spontaneously.[8]

The arm is positioned using a mechanical arm positioner. The arthroscope is introduced through the posterior portal, 2 cm below and 1 cm medial to the posterolateral corner of the acromion. The anterior working portal 1 cm lateral to the coracoid is localized using a spinal needle and established with a 5.5-mm cannula. Diagnostic arthroscopy is performed to confirm the presence of a Bankart lesion. It is important to rule out any associated pathology, such as rotator cuff tears, anterosuperior labral tears, and posterior labral tears. We also ascertain any bone loss before committing to an arthroscopic repair. The bare area of the glenoid has

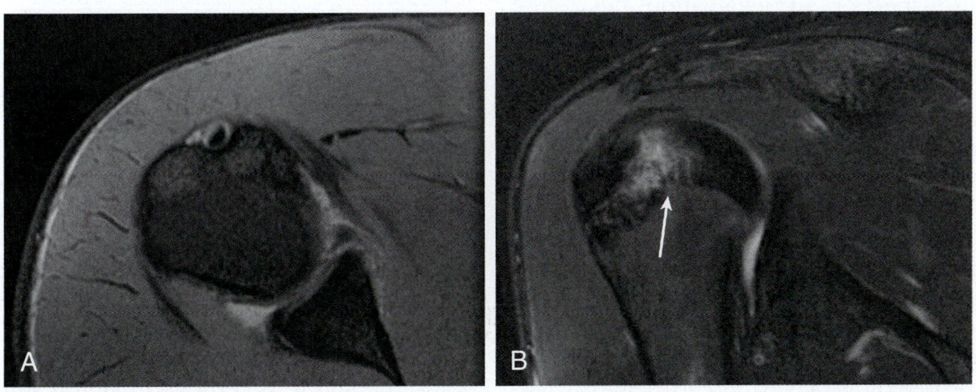

FIGURE 15-15: Preoperative magnetic resonance image of a 21-year-old contact athlete with an acute shoulder dislocation showing detachment of the anterior labrum (Bankart lesion) (**A**) and Hill-Sachs defect (*arrow*) (**B**).

been advocated as a useful landmark to assess for bone loss[106] and while we use this technique we incorporate it in the overall assessment along with the preoperative imaging and examination under anesthesia as recent publications have demonstrated variability of this arthroscopic assessment tool.[28,36,517] If there is an off-track/engaging lesion with less than a 20% anterior glenoid bone defect, an arthroscopic stabilization is performed with a remplissage. If there is an off-track/engaging lesion with a greater than 20% anterior glenoid defect an open Latarjet Reconstruction is performed.

After ruling out any significant bone loss involving the glenoid or an engaging Hill-Sachs lesion that may prevent successful arthroscopic repair, a second anteroinferior portal is placed under direct vision using a spinal needle. The angle of approach of this portal is critical. Before inserting an 8.25-mm clear, twist-in cannula, we use the spinal needle to be certain that the direction afforded by the portal is both inferior enough to reach the 5:30 o'clock position on the glenoid with an anchor, and lateral enough to place anchors on the face of the glenoid rather than on the glenoid neck. In addition, ensuring an appropriate distance between the two anterior portal skin incisions (2 to 3 cm) facilitates instrument and suture management. We have found that a "bump" in the axilla in conjunction with the arm holding device can provide improved access to and visualization of the inferior portion of the glenohumeral joint (Fig. 15-16).

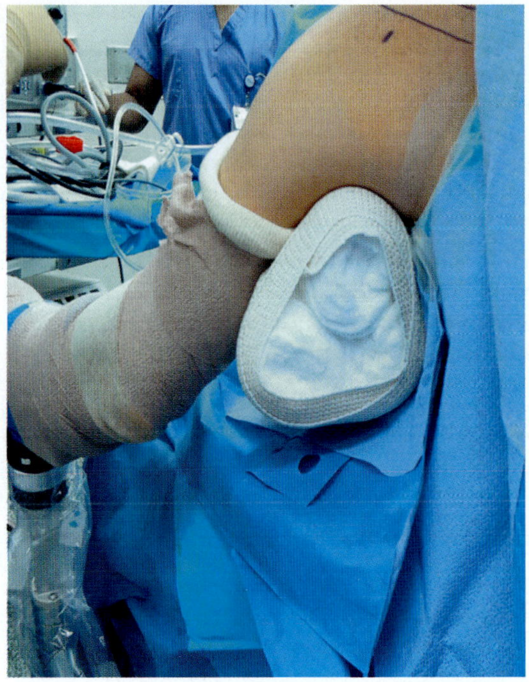

FIGURE 15-16: By utilizing an axillary "bump" in conjunction with a pneumatic arm holding device, glenohumeral distraction may be provided, affording improved access and visualization of the inferior portion of the joint. (From Moran CJ, Fabricant PD, Kang R, et al. Arthroscopic double-row anterior stabilization and Bankart repair for the "high-risk" athlete. *Arthrosc Tech*. 2014;3[1]:e65-e71.)

Once the second anterior portal is established, the labrum and capsule are mobilized from the glenoid using a sharp elevator (Samurai) in chronic cases and a rasp in acute cases. In an acute dislocation, the tissue is easily reducible, but in a chronic dislocator the capsulolabral complex may be scarred down medially and inferiorly on the glenoid neck (Fig. 15-17A, B). We routinely utilize a 70-degree lens while visualizing the anteroinferior and posteroinferior capsulolabral structures. The 70-degree lens is used for viewing via the posterior portal while the labrum is elevated from the anterosuperior portal, especially if the labrum has healed in a medialized (ALPSA) position. In this setting, we have found a sharp elevator (Samurai) to be useful in dealing with the scar. We will often place the arthroscope in the anterosuperior portal also for additional inspection and evaluation.

Proper mobilization of the tissue is critical for arthroscopic stabilization; the glenoid labrum and capsule complex should be elevated to the 6 o'clock position to ensure restoration of the tension of these structures, and closure of the axillary pouch. A probe is used to assess the mobility of tissue before the placement of anchors. Another indicator of sufficient mobilization of the capsule and labrum is the visualization of the subscapularis muscle under the mobilized capsule and labrum. After satisfactory mobilization, the labrum should float up to its near anatomic position (see Fig. 15-17B, C). Next, a motorized shaver is used to gently decorticate the glenoid neck to prepare a bleeding bed to aid in healing. This maneuver should be performed with the shaver suction off to prevent damage to the soft tissues.

It is quite common for the capsulolabral damage to extend into the posteroinferior zone.[672] When this is noted, we believe it is imperative to include this area in the repair and reconstruction by switching portals, and viewing via the anterosuperior portal and reattaching the posteroinferior capsulolabral tissue. This in effect restores the posterior attachment of the "hammock." When we perform this associated repair, the anteroinferior sutures are not secured to the glenoid with the knotless anchor until the posteroinferior sutures have been placed.

Single-Row Repair

We use a knotless anchor mattress technique (see Fig. 15-17). The 70-degree lens while viewing posteriorly is particularly helpful at this stage. Suture shuttling devices in the anteroinferior portal are used to pass stiff suture material through the capsule and into the defect between the labrum and the glenoid. The first suture is placed inferiorly. The limb is grasped and brought out through the anterosuperior portal. Without removing the shuttling device from the cannula, it is advanced through the capsule more superiorly and once again advanced into the defect between the labrum and the glenoid. At this point, the suture is retrieved using a suture retriever and brought out through the anterosuperior portal. Before securing the suture to a knotless anchor, the next stitch

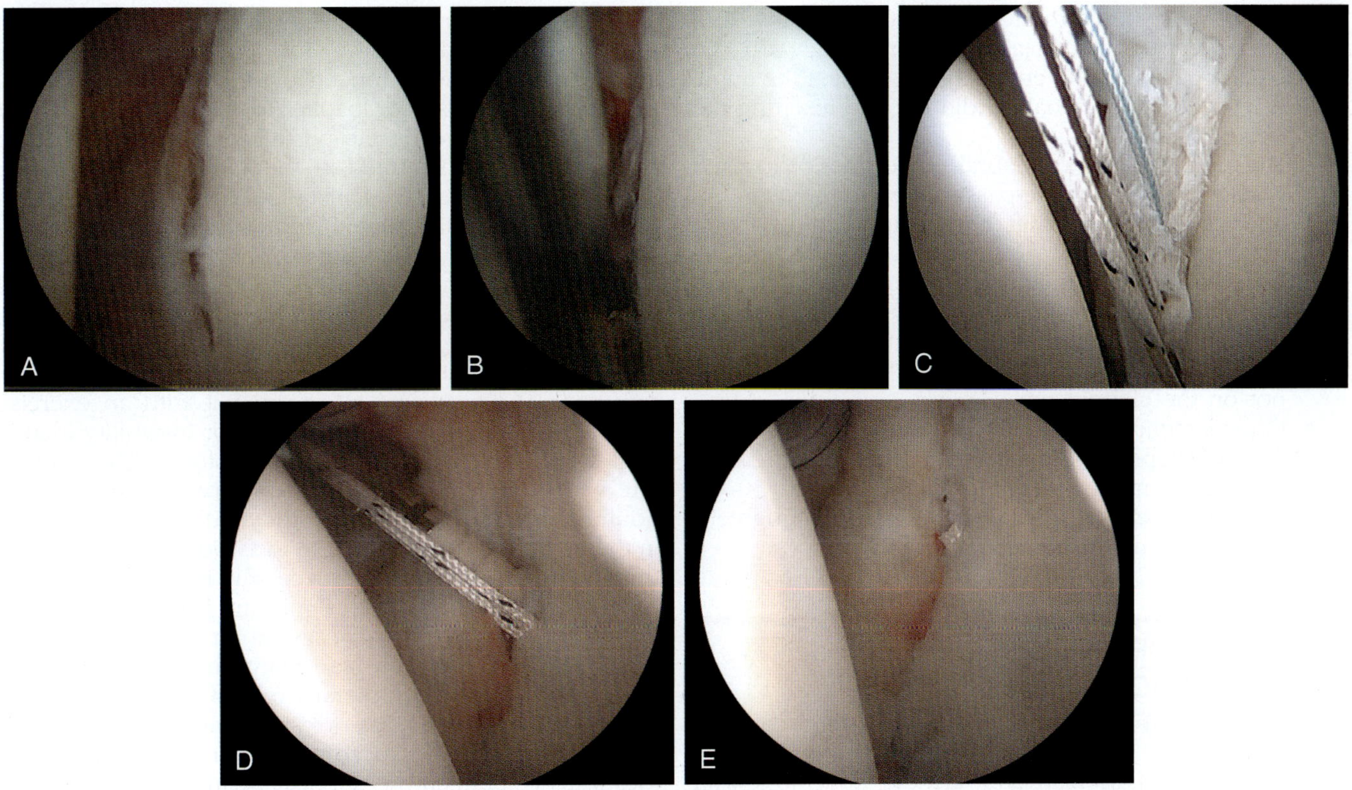

FIGURE 15-17: This patient was a 24-year-old National Football League player with acute traumatic anterior glenohumeral instability. **A,** Evaluation with a 30-degree arthroscope from the posterior portal revealed an anterior capsulolabral avulsion. **B,** An arthroscopic blade (Samurai) is used to sharply elevate and mobilize the retracted capsulolabral tissue off the anterior glenoid, followed by preparation of the glenoid neck with a shaver to stimulate bony bleeding. **C,** Nonabsorbable mattress sutures are placed at the anteroinferior glenoid as viewed from the posterior portal with a 70-degree arthroscope. **D,** A knotless anchor is deployed with attached mattress suture construct. **E,** Completed mattress repair with three knotless suture anchors.

is passed. Depending upon the location of the capsulolabral injury, the repair can move from the most inferior 6 o'clock position to as far superiorly as is necessary. Care is taken to ensure that the suture anchors are placed on the glenoid face, centered about 2 mm from the edge of the glenoid cartilage. Anchors placed more medial than this risk restoration of the glenoid labrum in a nonanatomic medialized position that will not restore the normal bumper effect of the anterior labrum. Conversely, if placed too far out on the face of the glenoid, significant articular cartilage injury can occur.

Double-Row Repair

This technique, shown in Video 15-1, is indicated for high-risk athlete (<25 years old, male, contact or forced overhead sports, higher levels of competition, more than two or three dislocations) and acute bony Bankart lesions that are amenable to arthroscopic repair.[486] We use a percutaneous long needle while staying lateral to the conjoint tendon. A guide wire and cannulated drill are introduced. The correct location for medial row anchors 10 to 15 mm medial to articular surface of glenoid is identified. Each of two to four anchors (depending on size of the lesion) are placed without removing the drill guide, progressing from inferior to superior. The anchor suture limbs are passed from the medial row using outside-in or inside-out technique. Sutures are prepared on knotless anchors for lateral-row fixation at the articular margin.

After completion of the arthroscopic Bankart repair, anterior stability is reassessed. The subacromial space is always inspected to evaluate the bursal surface of the rotator cuff and coracoacromial arch.

Remplissage is a technique we often employ for management of Hill-Sachs defects in off-track/engaging lesions (defined by a Hill-Sachs interval greater than the glenoid track).[197] This technique is presented in Chapter 13.

Key components of a successful arthroscopic repair include the following:

- Thorough diagnostic arthroscopy to identify any associated pathology that requires concomitant treatment.
- Mobilization of the capsulolabral tissue using a combination of arthroscopic blade and rasp and performing a trial reduction of the tissue to the glenoid to ensure that the mobilization is adequate.

- A well-placed anteroinferior portal that is low and lateral enough to obtain a proper angle on the glenoid. This can be ensured by assessing the angle of entry using a spinal needle prior to inserting the large cannula.
- Grasping capsule and labral tissue inferior to each anchor with the suture-passing device to ensure an adequate capsular shift and restoration of labral anatomy.
- Knotless fixation methods to prevent mechanical abrasion of the knots on the glenohumeral cartilage and restore the bumper effect of the labrum.
- Anchors placed on the edge of the glenoid face, not on the glenoid rim or neck.
- Capsular plication to address capsular stretch performed (depending upon the athlete being treated) with the arm in 30-degree abduction and 30- to 40-degree external rotation to prevent overtightening of the anterior structures.

ARTHROSCOPIC ANTERIOR STABILIZATION GUIDELINES FOR HIGH-RISK ATHLETES

1. Scenario 1: Less than 20% glenoid bone loss with on track/nonengaging lesion: advanced arthroscopic techniques (single- vs. double-row labral repair and/or posteroinferior capsulolabral repair and plication)
2. Less than 20% glenoid bone loss with off track/engaging lesion: advanced arthroscopic techniques (single- vs. double-row labral repair and/or posteroinferior capsulolabral repair and plication) with remplissage
3. Greater than 20% glenoid bone loss or larger bipolar lesions: Latarjet
4. HAGL, larger capsular injury, documented connective tissue disorder, or poor-quality capsulolabral tissue: open stabilization

ARTHROSCOPIC MANAGEMENT OF POSTERIOR INSTABILITY

Posterior instability is relatively rare (2% to 4% of all dislocations) compared with anterior instability and is therefore less well studied.[608] Acute posterior shoulder dislocations are usually caused by higher-energy injuries and can be associated with electrical shock and seizure.[301] These are liable to be missed on plain AP radiographs if not actively sought out; routine lateral and axillary views should be obtained to document the diagnosis or for confirmation of reduction. Acute reduction is accomplished by traction, external rotation, and gentle abduction.

A more common presentation of posterior instability is in athletes who undergo repeated load to a flexed, adducted, and internally rotated arm (e.g., rugby, hockey, weightlifting, American football).[246,704] Athletes often present with recurrent subluxation and pain rather than acute posterior dislocation.[246,496,641] Posterior labral detachment can occur with repetitive trauma among football linemen due to posterior loading of the shoulder joint that creates a shear force at the posterior labrum.[430] This type of injury has been termed as the *reverse Bankart lesion* and is often encountered in unidirectional posterior glenohumeral instability. Operative treatment in this population is indicated if conservative management fails.[430,458,757]

Initial treatment of posterior instability is physical therapy.[113] As with anterior instability, physical therapy is more likely to be successful in the absence of a large reverse Bankart lesion or bony deficits. Fronek et al. reported a 63% success rate achieved with an exercise program in patients who had posterior instability associated with moderately disabling symptoms. The success rate was higher in those with posterior instability and a nontraumatic etiology. In that study, 10 out of 16 patients in the exercise group were able to avoid surgery. Physical therapy is unlikely to be successful in patients with a traumatic etiology and with significant labral injury. Physical therapy was more successful in patients with an MDI-type picture of capsular laxity. In patients who did not respond to physical therapy or had severe symptoms, success rate of open posterior stabilization was 91%.[246] If physical therapy fails to control recurrent posterior dislocation or subluxation, surgical treatment is successful in controlling symptoms and preventing recurrence in the majority of patients.

At our institution, arthroscopic stabilization is preferred for uncomplicated posterior Bankart lesions due to reproducible clinical success and because the open posterior approach to the shoulder is associated with higher morbidity.[19,182,757] Open treatment is considered in revision settings and for patients with a voluntary component to their instability.[761] Other relative contraindications to arthroscopic management of posterior instability include shoulders with significant capsular attenuation not amenable to arthroscopic plication (e.g., 3+ posterior and inferior instability assessed on examination under anesthesia or MDI picture) or with capsular or bony deficiency.

Arthroscopic posterior stabilization has been successful for returning athletes to sport in a vast majority of cases. Bradley et al. reported a prospective evaluation of 91 athletes with unidirectional posterior instability who were treated with arthroscopic capsulolabral reconstruction; 89% athletes returned to sport.[74] The same authors more recently reported similar results in professional football players (93% return to sport; 79% at same level)[19] as well as excellent results in meta-analysis of studies that used suture anchor fixation.[182]

A diverse constellation of pathologic characteristics may be encountered in posterior instability. Bradley et al.[74] noted that at arthroscopy, 43% of patients had only a patulous posterior capsule without labral tear, which often manifests itself as increased visualization of the posterior glenoid neck upon initial diagnostic arthroscopy via the posterior portal. The other 57% of patients had partial or complete posterior labral tears. Furthermore, 23% of patients had both labral tear and capsular laxity.

Arthroscopic findings in posterior instability are therefore less consistent than anterior Bankart lesions. These authors pointed out that the arthroscopic stabilization of posterior shoulder instability can consist of labral repair with suture anchors, capsular plication, or both, depending on the pathologic characteristics observed at arthroscopy.

In summary, unidirectional posterior instability with a posterior Bankart lesion and a mild to moderate capsular attenuation can be successfully treated arthroscopically without the morbidity associated with a formal posterior approach. Athletes whose sport requires loading of the shoulder in flexion, adduction, and internal rotation (e.g., football linemen) are at high risk for unidirectional, recurrent, painful shoulder subluxation. According to the current literature, these patients can successfully return to active sports after an arthroscopic posterior stabilization in up to 80% to 90% of the time. For an arthroscopic approach to be successful, both labral detachment and capsular laxity must be addressed at the time of surgery. In our experience, it is difficult to obtain enough capsular shift arthroscopically to treat a patient with both 3+ inferior and 3+ posterior instability detected on examination under anesthesia; an open approach may be required in this rare clinical setting.

Authors' Preferred Technique

We conduct repair of a posterior Bankart lesion in a manner similar to that used for anterior stabilization. Preoperative MRI confirms the diagnosis of a posterior Bankart and reverse Hill-Sachs lesion (Fig. 15-18). A standard posterior portal is established and diagnostic arthroscopy is carried out. Posterior capsular laxity can manifest itself as increased visualization of the posterior capsule, labrum, and the glenoid neck. To improve visualization of the posterior glenoid, it is helpful to establish the anterosuperior portal and utilize a 70-degree lens. Upon completion of a satisfactory diagnostic arthroscopy viewed posteriorly, including inspection for a reverse Hill-Sachs lesion noted at the anterior humeral head, the arthroscope is moved to the anterosuperior portal to evaluate the posterior labrum and capsule (Fig. 15-19). The posterior capsulolabral complex is usually detached from the glenoid rim at the 6 to 10 o'clock position in the affected right shoulders and at the 2 to 6 o'clock position in the affected left shoulders.[757]

Upon confirmation that a posterior Bankart repair is necessary, we have found that three portals are required: an anterosuperior viewing portal, a standard posterior portal with an 8.25-mm cannula to allow passage of a suture shuttling device through tissue, and an accessory portal (4.5-mm cannula) that is more lateral and superior to obtain a proper angle for posterior glenoid drilling and placement of suture anchors (see Fig. 15-19B). This portal is often more lateral than is intuitive (often lateral to the posterolateral acromion), and the angle should be confirmed with a spinal needle before the cannula is inserted in the proper orientation for placement of suture anchors. This portal should not pass through the rotator cuff tendon tissue close to its insertion, but rather medially, closer to the muscle-tendon junction and in line with the fibers to avoid significant transtendon injury.

The preparation of the labrum and capsule as well as suture passage is similar to anterior stabilization. After debridement to a bleeding bed of bone on the posterior glenoid rim, we reattach the capsule and labrum to the glenoid margin using a knotless suture anchor and mattress technique.

Anchor placement and suture management is as follows. A suture with a stiff end is shuttled through the capsule and labrum with use of a curved suture hook via the posterior portal. This suture limb is grasped via the posterolateral portal and the shuttling device is passed through the capsule and labrum a second time and

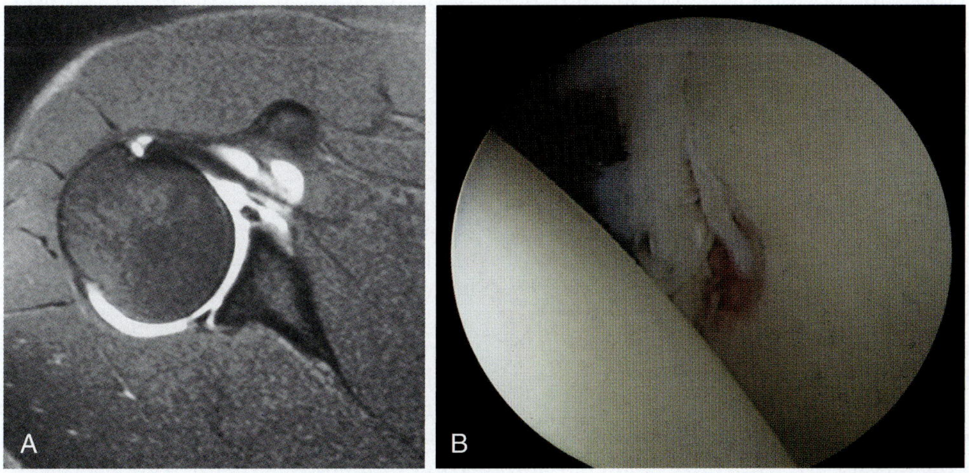

FIGURE 15-18: A, Magnetic resonance arthrogram demonstrating a preoperative posterior Bankart lesion in a 24-year-old National Football League defensive lineman with recurrent shoulder subluxation and pain in adduction and internal rotation. **B,** Corresponding arthroscopic image demonstrating a posterior Bankart lesion and posterior articular cartilage injury to the glenoid.

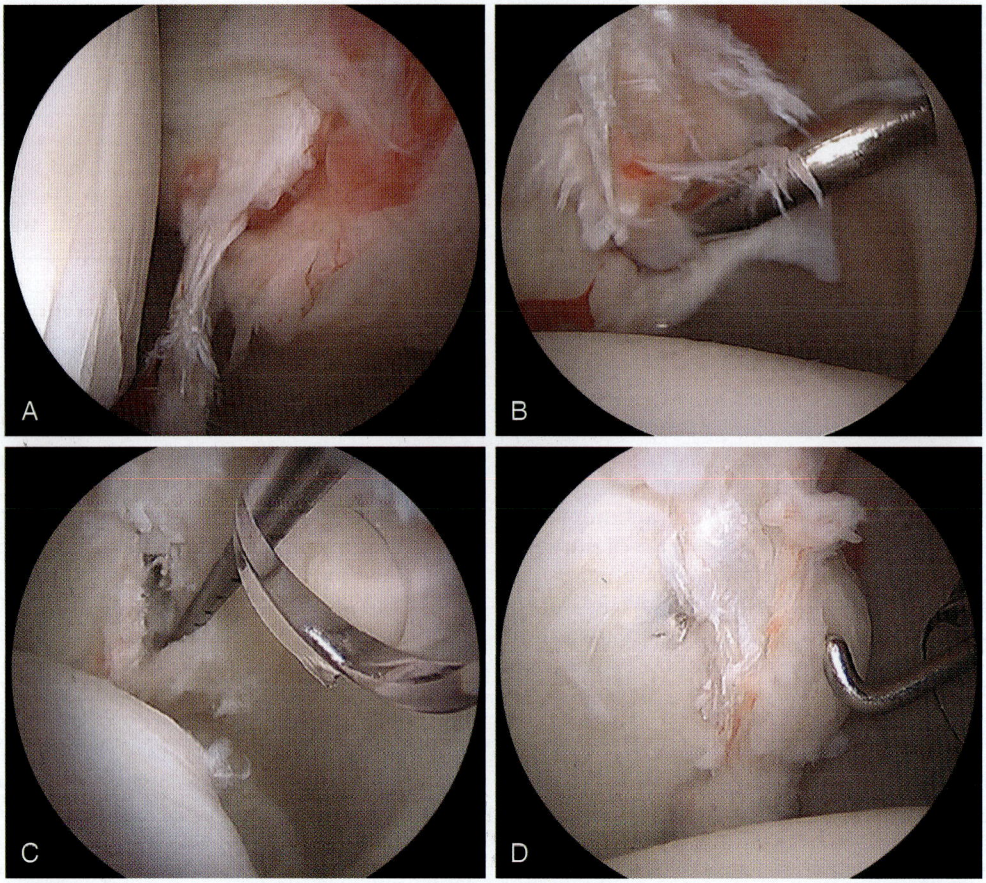

FIGURE 15-19: Posterior glenohumeral instability in a 26-year-old National Football League guard who had sustained two posterior dislocations that required formal reduction. A posterior capsulolabral avulsion is viewed with a 70-degree arthroscope via both the posterior **(A)** and anterosuperior **(B)** portals. **C,** The inferior portion of the defect has been repaired. **D,** A completed posterior repair using a mattress suture construct with knotless anchors is seen with a 70-degree arthroscope from an anterosuperior viewing portal.

retrieved through the same posterolateral portal. Depending upon the size of the capsulolabral defect, multiple sutures are passed through the capsulolabral tissue. A knotless suture anchor is then placed via the posterolateral portal after attaching the suture limbs and is secured via the most inferior anchor first. Three suture anchors are usually adequate for repair (see Fig. 15-19D). The subacromial space is inspected to assess the integrity of the rotator cuff and the coracoacromial arch.

ARTHROSCOPIC MANAGEMENT OF MULTIDIRECTIONAL INSTABILITY

When discussing a management approach to gross shoulder instability, it is useful to categorize patients into subsets that Matsen has termed as the TUBS and AMBRI populations.[439] Patients with TUBS have a ***t***raumatic etiology for their ***u***nidirectional (anterior) instability, a ***B***ankart lesion is central to their pathoanatomy, and they respond well to ***s***urgical repair of this lesion when indicated. Conversely, patients with AMBRI have an ***a***traumatic ***m***ultidirectional instability, which is often present ***b***ilaterally and often responds best to ***r***ehabilitation; if surgery proves necessary, ***i***nferior capsular shift is preferred.[439] Since the pathophysiology and anatomy of glenohumeral instability represents a broad continuum rather than two discrete entities, the TUBS/AMBRI classification in effect represents two opposite poles on a spectrum of patients with shoulder instability. McIntyre et al.[458] further subdivided MDI types. One group is composed of contact athletes, predominantly male, with anterior and posterior Bankart lesions. A second includes athletic patients, often male, with traumatic anterior Bankart lesions but also an increased inferior or posterior laxity (or both).[8] A third group is composed of athletic or nonathletic patients (predominantly female) with excessive capsular attenuation in all planes; this is the true AMBRI type.

Clearly, patients with traumatically induced focal pathology can be expected to respond to surgical repair differently than patients with systemic tissue disorders, global capsular redundancy, or a volitional component resulting in atraumatic attenuation without discrete pathology. In this section, we discuss the arthroscopic treatment of MDI in patients who have congenital ligamentous redundancy or repetitive microtrauma in a susceptible shoulder (e.g., swimmers).[561] In this population, the condition is usually atraumatic and bilateral, but symptoms may be dissimilar for each shoulder.[703] Diagnosis is made by history and physical examination; the common findings include 2+ instability in more than one direction and a sulcus sign. Treatment initially relies on physical therapy, which is successful in the majority of cases but needs to be continued for 6 to 12 months. Burkhead and Rockwood reported successful nonoperative management with an exercise program in 80% of 66 patients with atraumatic shoulder subluxation, thereby making physical therapy a mainstay of treatment.[113]

Results of Open Inferior Capsular Shift

When rehabilitation fails, arthroscopic[308] or open[148] capsular plication can result in improved stability of the shoulder and decreased pain. Acceptance of arthroscopic management of MDI has been tentative because MDI has classically been considered a relative contraindication to arthroscopic management. However, studies have shown that arthroscopic treatment success is approaching that of open surgery, and most studies demonstrate a low recurrence rate and few complications.[124,308,458]

The results of all-arthroscopic treatment must be interpreted in the context of the results reported for comparable open procedures. Neer and Foster were the first to report the success of open inferior capsular shifting for MDI.[502] Of their 40 patients, 17 had a follow-up of at least 2 years; one of these patients had recurrent instability, one had disabling pain, and three had sustained axillary nerve neurapraxia. Cooper and Brems subsequently applied Neer's technique to 43 shoulders. At a minimum of 2 years of follow-up, 13 patients (30%) had recurrent instability or episodic apprehension of instability; 40% of this cohort had to change or cease sports, but 86% were thought to have been improved by the surgery.[162] Subsequent studies of open capsular shift in patients with MDI have reported recurrence rates of 10% and high levels of patient satisfaction and return to sport.[8] In short, instability can be eliminated in 70% to 96% of patients undergoing open capsular shift with various techniques, and these results appear to be durable over the mid to long term.

Arthroscopic Capsular Plication

Arthroscopic management of MDI was first described in the early 1990s. Duncan and Savoie initially reported on 10 patients with MDI treated with the Caspari technique in an arthroscopic modification of the medially based inferior capsular T-plasty.[8] At a minimum of 1 year of follow-up, none had recurrent instability. All had satisfactory results according to Neer's criteria,[502] and the average Bankart score was 90. Subsequent studies have reported 5% to 12% recurrent instability[458,712] without significant loss of external rotation.[255,256]

Cadaveric studies have validated that arthroscopic capsular plication can result in a significant capsular volume reduction. Flanigan et al. confirmed that the size of the capsular pleat affected the amount of volume reduction: four 5-mm capsular pleats resulted in a decrease in capsular volume of 16% compared with 33% for four 10-mm capsular pleats.[235] Other studies have documented a 19% to 58% reduction in capsular volume with various plication techniques and pleat sizes[124, 355]; this reduction in volume is comparable to that of an open shift control model reported in two studies that decreased volume by 45% or 50%.[124,148] Currently, we use a pneumatic shoulder holder to position the shoulder in a 30-degree abducted and 30- to 45-degree externally rotated position during plication to avoid overtightening. We use multiple factors to gauge our degree of capsular plication during arthroscopic treatment of MDI; these include the size of the inferior pouch, tension on capsular tissue, centering of the humeral head, and elimination of the "drive-through" sign. Despite these arthroscopic indicators of a successful plication, the amount of capsular tightening is still subjective and based on the surgeon's preference and experience.

Arthroscopic Thermal Capsulorrhaphy

The modern use of nonablative thermal energy to shrink collagenous soft tissue dates from the early 1980s[459] and is largely of historical significance. Radiofrequency probes impart heat to soft tissues, which causes unwinding of the normal triple-helix architecture of the collagen molecules, with a resultant net decrease in length. This tissue would then act as a scaffold onto which fibroblasts migrate and initiate repair. Catastrophic complications including adhesive capsulitis, capsular necrosis, chondrolysis, and axillary neuritis have caused thermal capsulorraphy to fall out of favor in recent years.[157,267,275,402,418,680,710,764]

Rotator Interval Closure

Rotator interval closure can be a useful procedure both as an adjunct to arthroscopic stabilization and as a standalone procedure for a mild form of MDI (microinstability).[134,232,379] Many technical papers detailing techniques for rotator interval closure have been published,[119,257,354,379,405,696,711] with the commonality of suture fixation of the medial glenohumeral ligament (MGHL) to the SGHL. Numerous biomechanical studies performed at the Hospital for Special Surgery,[641,678] the Mayo Clinic,[338] and elsewhere[298,671] have identified the contribution of the rotator interval to shoulder stability and have more clearly defined the mechanics of a rotator interval capsular shift. The rotator interval capsule provides significant restraint to inferior (and to a lesser degree, superior) translation of the humerus on the glenoid.[338,671] Plausinis et al. evaluated three different rotator interval closure techniques in a cadaveric model and found that interval closure decreased flexion

(6 degrees), external rotation (10 degrees), and anterior translation (3 mm) of the adducted shoulder.[570]

Although there is no level I evidence that suggests that rotator interval closure can improve the results of routine anterior stabilization, we close the rotator interval in cases of MDI if the shoulder is still objectively loose (especially inferiorly) after the capsulolabral reconstruction is complete.

Authors' Preferred Technique

Despite good results of open capsular shift for MDI, our institutional preference favors less-invasive arthroscopic capsular plication to stabilize shoulders with MDI. The operation begins with an examination under anesthesia, which can guide the amount and direction of capsular plication necessary. A typical examination in a patient requiring stabilization is 2+ or 3+ anteriorly, 2+ posteriorly, and a 2+ or 3+ sulcus sign. Diagnostic arthroscopy shows a drive-through sign and patulous capsule, usually with an intact labrum (Fig. 15-20).

We use a mattress technique with knotless anchors. Capsular plication begins anteroinferiorly, incorporating an appropriate amount of capsule laterally with a curved suture-passing hook. A second pass through the capsule near the capsule-labrum transition with the suture-passing hook creates a pleat in the tissue. The size of the pleat and degree of volume reduction in the capsule increases with increased distance between bites. A stiff-ended suture is then passed into the joint and grasped via the anterosuperior portal. The suture shuttling device is then passed a second time and retrieved via the anterosuperior portal. Multiple sutures are passed and prepared for knotless fixation. Portals are switched and while viewing anterosuperiorly with a 70-degree lens, the posteroinferior and posterior capsule are prepared in a similar manner. To avoid overtightening of the soft tissue and losing external rotation, it is important that capsulolabral reconstructions and plications be tensioned in 30 to 45 degrees of external rotation and 30 degrees of abduction.

We strongly consider open stabilization when instability is 3+ to the front or back and 3+ inferiorly because the degree of capsular shift obtainable arthroscopically might not be great enough to stabilize a shoulder with this degree of capsular redundancy and attenuation. We believe it is more effective to shift the capsule from the lateral (humeral side) approach in cases of global and extensive capsular redundancy.

Summary of Indications

Critical review of the previously mentioned literature regarding arthroscopic glenohumeral stabilization underscores several key points. First, the results of arthroscopic stabilization of MDI have begun to approach those of comparable open procedures. However, longer term follow-up intervals are required because most results of arthroscopic stabilization of MDI are 2-year result studies only. Second, although significant volume reduction of the shoulder capsule can be accomplished arthroscopically, the number of sutures and the way they are placed varies significantly between techniques; therefore the degree of capsular plication required for a successful result remains based on surgical opinion rather than on well-done biomechanical or clinical studies. Lastly, the most critical element in successful arthroscopic stabilization of MDI is appropriate patient selection. The outcome is vitally dependent on the surgeon's understanding of the character and quality of the pathoanatomy, the patient's activity level and expectations, and the patient's psychology and compliance with rehabilitation protocols.

It is important for the surgeon to remain familiar with open capsular shift techniques and capsular augmentation techniques because arthroscopic techniques might not be sufficient to address MDI in the revision setting, severe capsular attenuation, or capsular deficiency. We routinely use open capsular shift techniques at our institution in these difficult clinical situations.

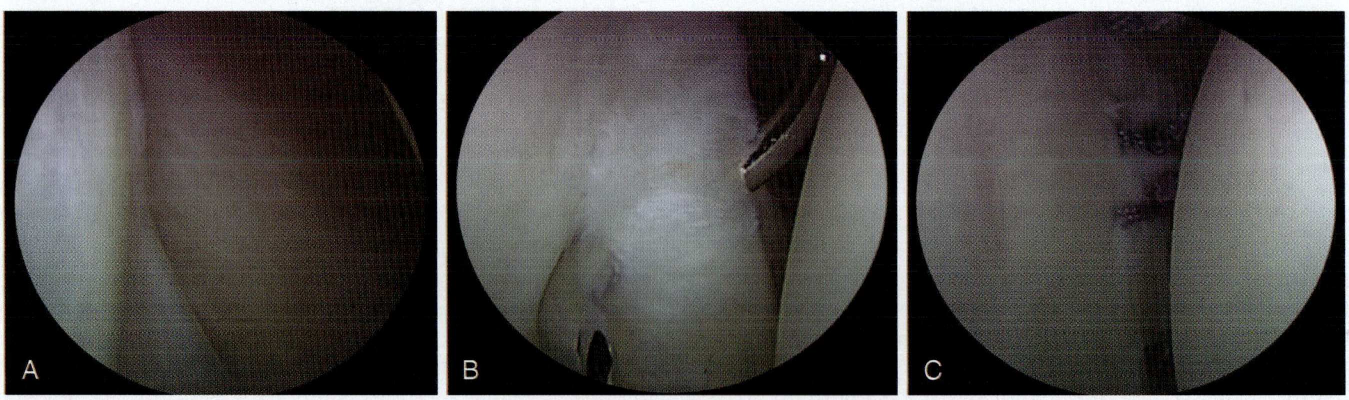

FIGURE 15-20: Arthroscopic stabilization of multidirectional instability. **A,** Drive-through sign and redundant anterior inferior capsule. **B,** Suture hook at 5:30 o'clock position drawing the inferior pouch of the capsule superiorly and medially. **C,** Elimination of the drive-through sign and centering of the humeral head after placement of four anterior sutures through the capsule and intact anterior labrum to plicate the capsule. A single capsular plication suture was placed posteriorly.

POSTOPERATIVE MANAGEMENT AND RETURN TO PLAY

Postoperative management after arthroscopic or open stabilization surgery is critical and must be individualized based on the type of surgery performed and quality of the repaired tissue. We immobilize the shoulder in a sling for 3 to 4 weeks after a labral repair and up to 5 to 6 weeks for a capsular plication. If a subscapularis takedown was performed for an open repair, this is generally protected as well for 4 weeks.

Pendulum exercises in a sling and passive forward elevation in the plane of the scapula to 45 degrees are allowed immediately. Passive external rotation is permitted to 0 degrees. Distal ROM is also started immediately. Active ROM is allowed after the sling immobilization is discontinued. Terminal passive stretching exercises are delayed until 8 to 10 weeks after surgery. After ROM is near full, strengthening is started. Return to sport is generally delayed until 4 to 6 months after surgery, depending upon the sport, position, and level of competition.[450]

McCarty et al. reviewed rehabilitation and return-to-play guidelines after shoulder surgery.[450] These authors divided the rehabilitation after shoulder surgery into four phases:

- *Phase one* is primary healing of capsulolabral tissue, consisting of sling immobilization, active-assisted range-of-motion exercise, distal ROM, and isometrics.
- *Phase two* spans weeks 6 to 12 and involves gaining full ROM.
- *Phase three* involves strengthening of the shoulder, including dynamic strengthening.
- *Phase four* takes place 4 to 8 months after surgery, when the patient has sport-specific rehabilitation and then returns to sport when appropriate.

COMPLICATIONS OF STABILIZATION SURGERY

Complications of open shoulder instability surgery include recurrence of instability, stiffness, subscapularis rupture, arthrosis, neurovascular injury, hardware failure, and capsular necrosis.[389,468] The risk factors for recurrence after stabilization include MDI, large Hill-Sachs or glenoid rim fractures, and voluntary instability.[66,191,719]

The key to avoiding recurrence is proper diagnosis and proper surgical technique in addressing the constellation of pathology observed on imaging and arthroscopy.

Arthrosis of the glenohumeral joint is a known sequela of recurrent shoulder dislocation in some shoulder joints with or without surgery. There is evidence that dislocation of the shoulder alone is associated with development of osteoarthritis,[319,627] with 10 to 20 times greater odds of developing severe arthrosis in for persons who have had a dislocation of the shoulder versus patients with no dislocation.[437] Despite this, there is limited long-term evidence that shoulder surgery for instability prevents osteoarthritis. While arthritis after shoulder stabilization was common after nonanatomic repairs,[242,319,449] the incidence after modern open Bankart repair is thought to be lower.[613]

Stiffness can complicate shoulder stabilization surgery, especially with overtensioning of the soft tissues and prolonged immobilization. To avoid overtightening of the soft tissues and losing external rotation, it is important that capsulolabral reconstructions be tensioned in 30 to 45 degrees of external rotation and 30 degrees of abduction.[468]

The incidence of neurovascular complications in open stabilization surgery has been reported as 1% to 8%.[62] Neurovascular complications and subscapularis rupture are rare but devastating complications of open stabilization surgery and are best prevented by meticulous surgical technique and deliberate exposure of surgical planes during revision surgery. Subscapularis rupture and neurologic injury are exceedingly rare in arthroscopic stabilization.

When failure of an arthroscopic stabilization is excluded (apprehension or redislocation), the surgical complication rate for this procedure is low and complications are generally thought to be less common than in open stabilization and self-limited or resolved with nonoperative measures.[149,367] Most cases of early osteoarthritis after arthroscopic stabilization have been associated with anchor complications or chondrolysis from thermal capsulorrhaphy.[402] Rhee et al. treated five cases of early glenohumeral osteoarthritis an average of 12 months after arthroscopic stabilization and found intra-articular metal anchors in all cases.[600] Absorbable suture anchors can also displace, break, and cause chondral injury or synovitis.[545,631] Infection rarely complicates arthroscopic stabilization procedures.[545]

CONCLUSIONS

Improved instrumentation and understanding of the anatomy, pathoanatomy, and biomechanics of the shoulder have allowed surgeons to advance arthroscopic stabilization techniques for the unstable shoulder. A thorough history and physical examination most often diagnose the degree, direction, frequency, and etiology of shoulder instability. The cornerstone of treatment for instability remains immobilization followed by rehabilitation, but the optimal nonoperative treatment of a shoulder dislocation is still unknown and deserves further study.

Early arthroscopic stabilization can decrease recurrence rates and improve functional outcomes in young (>25 years old), high-risk patients with first-time anterior dislocations and an associated Bankart lesion. In the absence of severe capsular laxity or bony deficiency, we also consider arthroscopic stabilization a first-line therapy in recurrent anterior and posterior instability of traumatic origin. Recent evidence also suggests that participation in a contact sport is not a contraindication to arthroscopic stabilization. Athletes may return to play after a shoulder dislocation or after stabilization surgery when strength and mobility have normalized.

Proper mobilization of capsulolabral tissue, placement of an accessory portal low and lateral to aid in placement of suture anchors, and addressing the associated capsular injury are critical to the success of arthroscopic stabilization surgery. Results of arthroscopic surgery using modern suture-anchor techniques and shoulder-specific instrumentation have yielded results comparable to those of open surgery; however, many believe that open surgery has a slightly lower recurrence rate at the cost of some loss of external rotation. Open surgery should also be strongly considered in cases of severe capsular laxity or deficiency, glenoid or humeral bone loss, avulsion of the capsule from the humeral side, documented connective tissue disorders, and for revision stabilizations.

MDI often manifests as bilateral shoulder subluxations in a susceptible patient and should be treated with an extended course of physical therapy. Arthroscopic and open capsular shifts have been successful in restoring stability and decreasing pain, but thermal capsulorrhaphy has recently shown a high complication rate. Generally, the results of arthroscopic treatment are less predictable in patients with greater than 2+ instability in two or more directions, patients with 3+ (locking) unidirectional patterns without evidence of capsular injury, and those with atraumatic posterior instability. In these patients, an open capsular shift may provide a more predictable outcome.

Arthroscopic treatment of instability continues to evolve. With increased surgical skills and improved implants and instrumentation, a greater proportion of instability cases can be successfully treated via arthroscopy than that in the past. However, improved clinical research, more randomized trials, and longer-term follow-up are needed for understanding the true impact of arthroscopic treatment on the natural history of shoulder instability.

Arthroscopic Management of Rotator Cuff Disease

Brian T. Feeley, Richard J. Han, C. Benjamin Ma

EVOLUTION OF ARTHROSCOPIC ROTATOR CUFF REPAIR

Over the past 3 decades, arthroscopic surgery for rotator cuff repair has evolved to become the modality of choice for rotator cuff repairs. In 1918, Takagi used a cystoscope to examine knees affected by tuberculosis.[693] Watanabe, a student of Takagi, improved the design of the arthroscope and allowed this technique to become popular.[183] Shoulder arthroscopy was first reported by Ellman, who performed SAD in 50 patients,[213] and Andrews, who reported his results on rotator cuff debridement in the 1980s.[9] The transition from open rotator cuff repair to arthroscopic rotator cuff repair occurred in 1990s when Levy reported the possibility of combining shoulder arthroscopy and mini-arthrotomy to better diagnose and repair rotator cuff pathology.[404] Snyder, one of the pioneers of arthroscopic shoulder surgery, was the first to report arthroscopic repair of rotator cuff tears.[667] Since the 1990s, the technique has evolved to repair small to massive rotator cuff tears. With advanced arthroscopic tools, repair rotator cuff tears can be repaired with much more efficiency. In the 1990s, there were numerous reports on the initial success of arthroscopic rotator cuff repairs. In the 2000s, the focus was largely on the different repair techniques and configurations along with reports of early failures of arthroscopic rotator cuff repairs of larger tears. More recently in the 2010s, the discipline has focused more on clinical outcomes and on other alternatives to primary repairs such as augmentation and biologic modulation. This chapter focuses on arthroscopic management of rotator cuff tears. Tear recognition, repair techniques, advanced approaches to tears, and outcomes of rotator cuff repairs are addressed.

TEAR RECOGNITION

Approach

Arthroscopic rotator cuff surgeries can be performed in both the beach chair and lateral positions. Both are popular techniques and have their pros and cons. Beach chair position allows for easier conversion to an open or mini-open rotator cuff repair. It is also more convenient in cases where manipulation of the shoulder is needed such as that required for subscapularis tendon repair.[563] However, although it is rare, there has been concern with cerebral blood flow in a sitting position under anesthesia.[572] In the lateral position, the arm needs to be in traction during surgery. The position allows easier access to the inferior part of the shoulder while doing shoulder stabilization or removing loose bodies. While it is extremely rare, there have been reports of brachial plexus injuries.[587] In our opinion, both approaches are appropriate and the use between the two depends much on the skill set and experience of the surgeon.

Diagnostic Arthroscopy and Tear Recognition

Rotator cuff repairs start with a thorough and comprehensive diagnostic arthroscopy and tear recognition. The operation starts with an appropriate position for diagnostic arthroscopy. After establishing appropriate portals and performing a diagnostic arthroscopy, a thorough evaluation and characterization of the tear is necessary to determine the repair strategy. Partial articular sided rotator cuff tears and isolated subscapularis tendon tears are best visualized within the joint. Adequate bursectomy is needed in the subacromial space to identify the tear. In particular, the shape of the tear, its configuration, size, and the extent of retraction and quality of tissue should be assessed. A thorough characterization of the tear helps in determining the best repair strategy and predicting the healing rates.

Tear shape has been best classified by Burkhart.[96,99,104,173,410] This classification system divides rotator cuff tears into crescent-shaped, U-shaped, L-shaped, reverse L-shaped, and massive, contracted, immobile tears and is most useful in guiding the choice of technique for repair of the rotator cuff. Preoperative MRI or other advanced imaging modalities should be utilized to characterize the tear, but ultimate confirmation will come intraoperatively to delineate the pattern and subsequent repair.

When addressing an intra-articular problem such as partial-thickness articular-sided rotator cuff tear, isolated subscapularis tendon tear, labral tear or loose bodies, a standard portal through the soft spot of the shoulder is often appropriate. When addressing a tear that involves the superior or posterosuperior cuff, such as partial-thickness bursal-sided tear, isolated supraspinatus or combined supraspinatus and infraspinatus tendon tear, it is advisable to place the diagnostic arthroscopic portal in a high lateral position. This is a portal that is based off the posterolateral edge of the acromion. The portal is higher and more lateral than the traditional soft spot portal. This allows the arthroscope to be above the greater tuberosity where the tendon needs to be repaired. This ensures adequate visual access after the tendon is mobilized and pulled back to the insertion site.

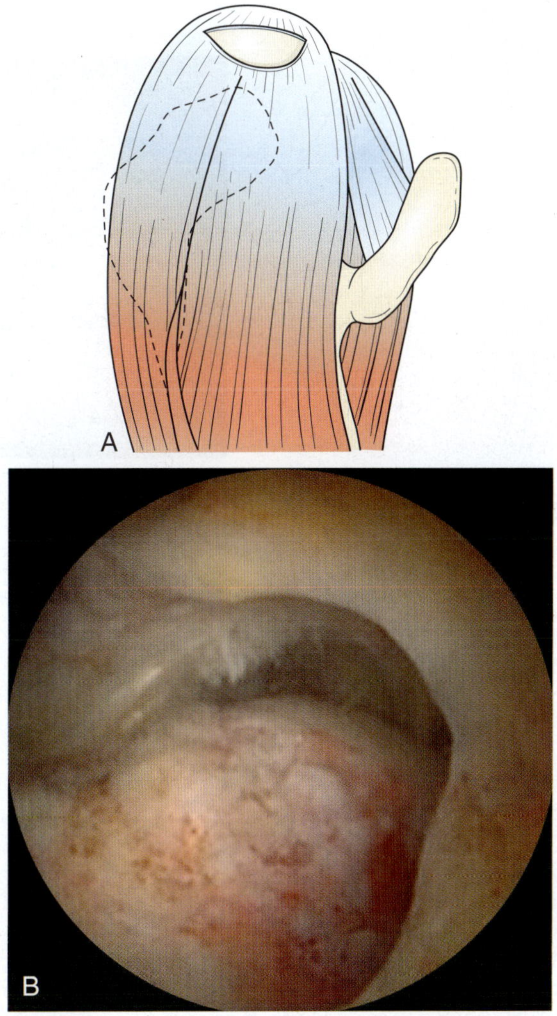

FIGURE 15-21: Illustration **(A)** and intraoperative image **(B)** of crescent-shaped tear.

Rotator Cuff Tear Classification

Tear Shape

Crescent Tears

Crescent tears (Fig. 15-21) are the most common form of small and medium-sized rotator cuff tears. These tears tend to be mobile and the medial-to-lateral width is less than the anterior-to-posterior width. In other words, this type of tear is relatively small with minimal retraction. Direct repair from the end of the tendon to bone can be performed with good functional restoration.[104]

U-Shaped Tears

U-shaped tears (Fig. 15-22) are wider in the mediolateral aspect compared with their AP axis. It is important to recognize the difference between this and a crescent tear as an attempt to fix the medial margin of this tear directly to the bone increases the strain at the site of the repair[103] as well as creates a “dog ear” effect in which the tear edge does not completely reduce to bone. Instead, a side-to-side repair/margin convergence technique must be used to convert the U-shaped tear to a crescent-shaped tear followed by direct repair of the tear edge to the bone.

L-Shaped Tears

L-shaped tears (Fig. 15-23) are similar to the U-shaped tear in that they are longer than they are wide from anterior-to-posterior, except that the elongated portion of the tear occurs at the most anterior or posterior portion of the tear (L or reverse-L tear). This usually occurs when the anterior supraspinatus tendon tear is pulled posteriorly by the infraspinatus tendon or when a supraspinatus tendon tear leads to a split between supraspinatus and infraspinatus junction. Recognizing and fixing the side-to-side portion of the L and reverse-L tears allow the surgeon to take the tension off while fixing the lateral edge to the bone. This also allows more anatomic repair of the tendon to the bone. The same repair techniques of margin convergence apply to this type of tear, followed by a standard direct repair of the remaining edge to the greater tuberosity. When treated in this manner, U-shaped and L-shaped tears demonstrate good to

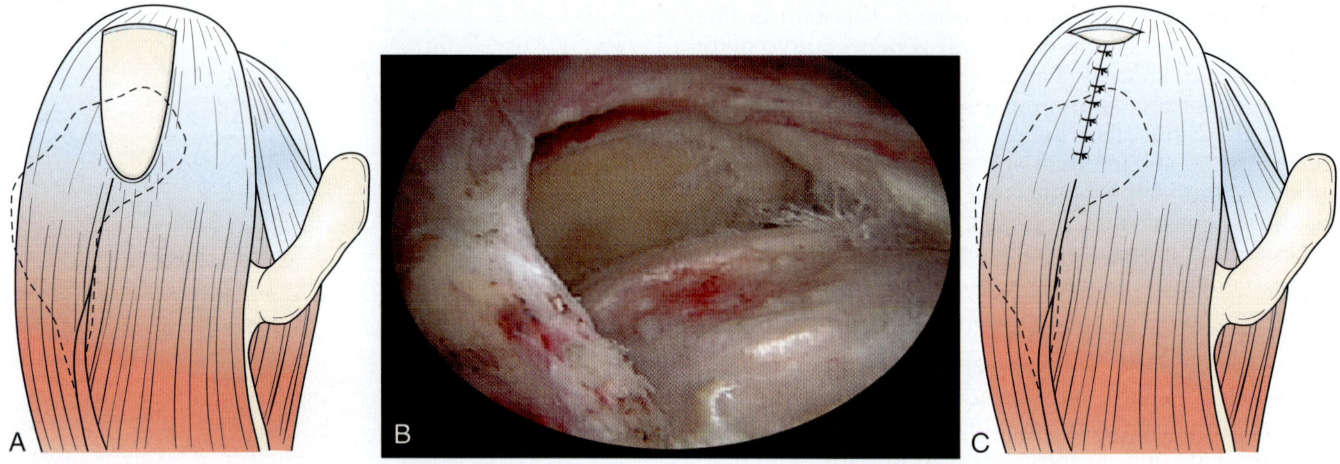

FIGURE 15-22: Illustration **(A)** and intraoperative image **(B)** of U-shaped tear. **C,** Margin convergence utilized to fix the tear; a standard rotator cuff tear can now be repaired.

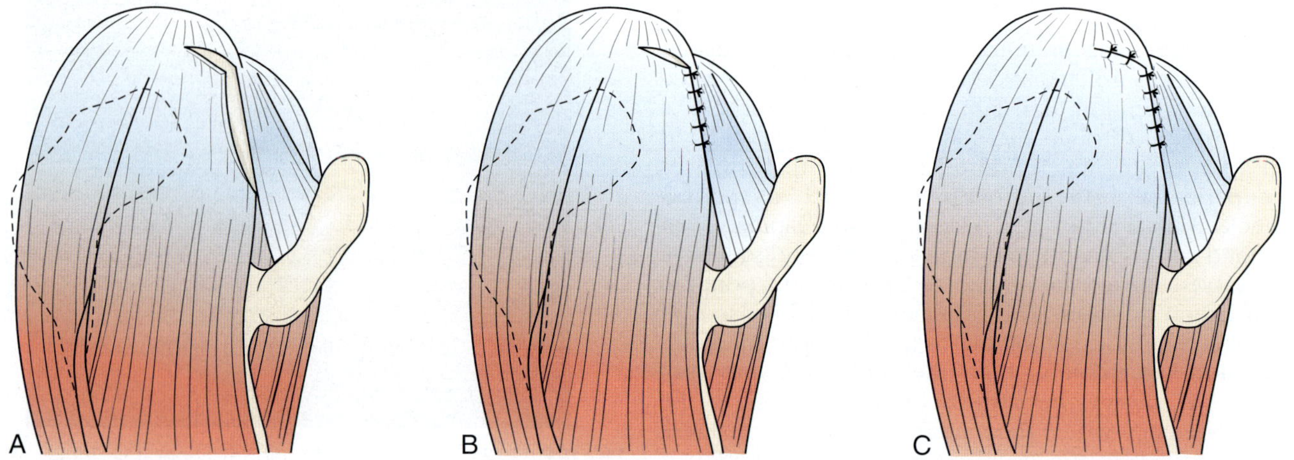

FIGURE 15-23: **A,** An L-shaped tear. **B,** Margin convergence of tear. **C,** Remaining tear can be fixed with standard technique with suture anchors.

excellent functional results that are comparable to crescent tears.[104]

Massive, Contracted, Immobile Tears

Repair of this type of tear (Fig. 15-24) is typically challenging and often requires advanced arthroscopic techniques to mobilize the tendon; complete repair may still be impossible to achieve. Massive tears are usually not amenable to direct repair without compromising the integrity of the fixation; additional techniques such as margin convergence, interval slides and partial repair are often required. Functional outcomes after repair are typically poor.[104] It should be noted that a subset of these rotator cuff tears may be irreparable and may require tendon transfer or reverse total shoulder arthroplasty (TSA) for functional restoration.

Tear Size

Another commonly used classification system developed by DeOrio and Cofield uses size of the tear along the AP direction.[188] The original description relied on intraoperative findings to classify the tear, but we have found that this can be assessed preoperatively with MRI on sagittal images. The sizes are small (<1 cm), medium (1 to 3 cm), large (3 to 5 cm), and massive (>5 cm) (Table 15-1). The limitation of this scheme is that it characterizes a 3D tear in a single plane. Nonetheless, this is a common classification system used for rotator cuff tears.

Tear Retraction

Patte further categorized tears in a second dimension by measuring the amount of retraction of the tear in the coronal plane (Fig. 15-25).[552] This was broken down into three categories of retraction: stage 1 (little retraction, stump close to insertion), stage 2 (retraction to the level of the humeral head), and stage 3 (retraction to the glenoid). This classification system has been reported by the Multi-Centre Orthopaedic Outcome Network (MOON) shoulder group of having the best agreement in tear classification.[380]

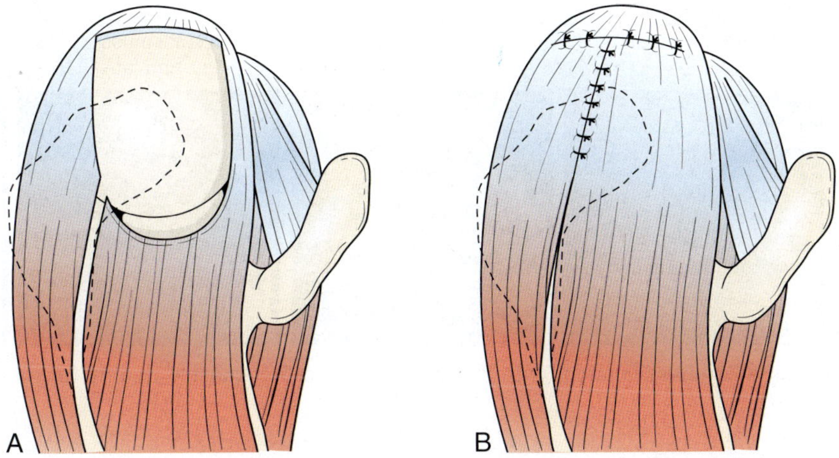

FIGURE 15-24: **A,** Illustration of massive, contracted, immobile tear. **B,** Multiple advanced techniques may be necessary for this repair.

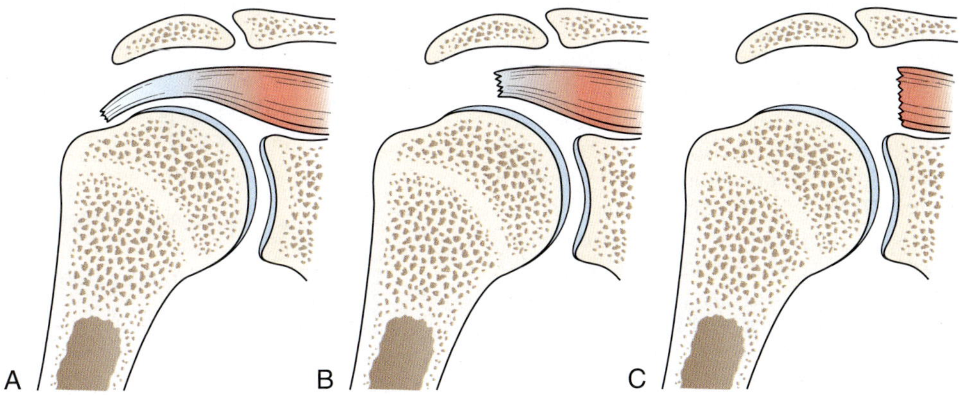

FIGURE 15-25: **A** to **C,** Rotator cuff tear classification based on retraction of the tendon in the coronal plane.

TABLE 15-1 Rotator Cuff Classified by Size*

Size	Length (cm)
Small	<1
Medium	1-3
Large	3-5
Massive	>5

Measured in the sagittal plane from anterior to posterior.

Rotator Cuff Muscle Quality

A final classification method that is often utilized is based upon the quality of the tissue itself. Goutallier introduced a system based on the degree of fatty infiltration in the supraspinatus muscle belly.[278] Although originally based on CT findings, Fuchs et al. introduced the use of MRI[248] for this evaluation (Fig. 15-26). Five stages of muscle fatty infiltration have been defined in this classification system: stage 0 (normal muscle), stage I (muscle with fatty streaks), stage II (more muscle than fat), stage III (equal muscle and fat), and stage IV (more fat than muscle). Several other classification schemes have been developed over time, but the above grading scheme is the one that most surgeons are able to recognize. This is a subjective classification system and is limited by a low intraobserver and interobserver reliability.

REPAIR TECHNIQUES

The development of suture anchors has significantly improved the ability to perform arthroscopic rotator cuff repair. While most open rotator cuff repairs were performed with transosseous sutures with and without suture anchors, the initial reports of arthroscopic rotator cuff repairs have all relied on suture anchors repairs. With fixation of the rotator cuff tear, there are three potential points of failure in the repair: (1) anchor-bone interface, (2) suture-anchor interface at the eyelet, and (3) the suture-tendon interface.

Suture anchors are the point of fixation of the tendon to the bone. Several types of anchors have been developed, with metal and bioabsorbable anchors being the

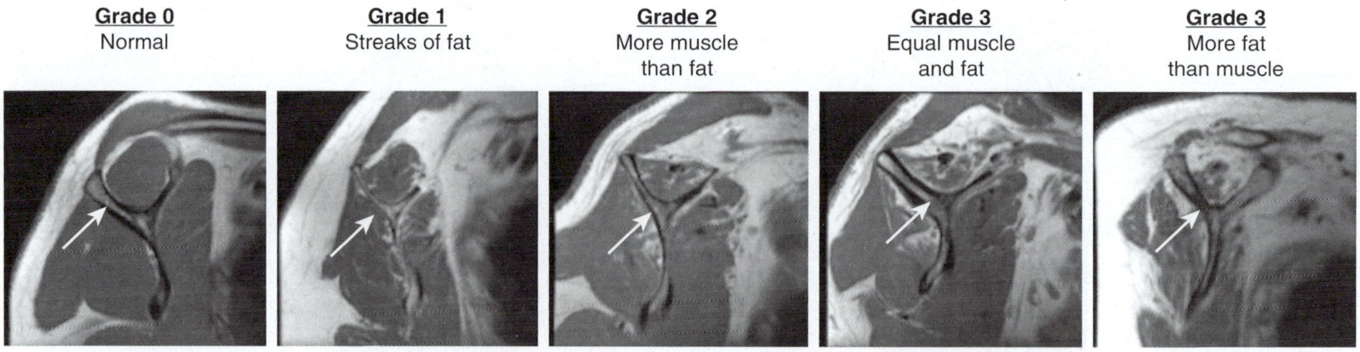

FIGURE 15-26: Goutallier classification (with Fuchs modification) of muscle quality for rotator cuff tears.

most common. Metal anchors minimize the steps involved in placement by obviating the need for predrilling whereas bioabsorbable anchors require predrilling or use of an awl to create a path for anchor placement. Early metal anchors were associated with suture failure because of cutout through the eyelet[513]; however, more recent designs have used improved suture material and eyelet designs to reduce this risk. Metal anchors also carry the risk of loosening, migration, cartilage injury, and interference with subsequent MRI.[249,511,656] In contrast, bioabsorbable anchors have been reported to cause osteolysis, stiffness and arthropathy.[21,245,451] More recently, composite anchors have been developed and have the advantage of minimal tissue reaction and the possibility for replacement with bone ingrowth. These have been shown to have good mechanical strength but the long term clinical data in shoulder surgery are still lacking at this point.[382,513]

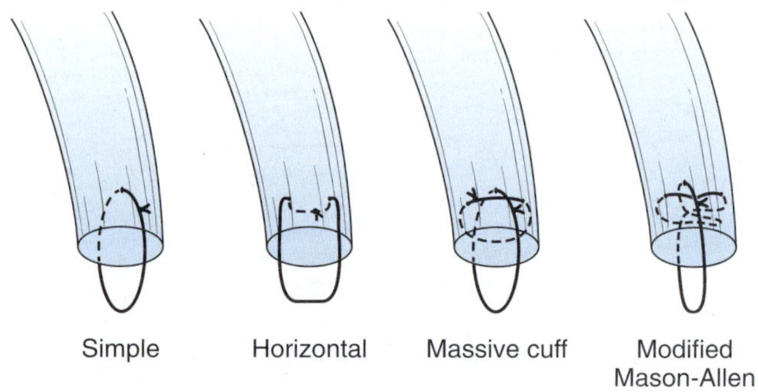

FIGURE 15-27: Various suture configurations.

Proper anchor placement is essential to the fixation of the repair and to prevent pullout of the anchor regardless of the material type used. In 1995, Burkhart popularized the idea of the "dead man's angle" in suture anchor placement. He demonstrated that the ideal angle for anchor fixation is 45 degrees or less with respect to the pull of the tendon and the humeral surface.[100] Although a number of subsequent studies have shown that an anchor placed at 90 degrees or greater may have superior biomechanical pullout properties,[144,283,689] we continue to utilize the dead man's angle in the placement of our suture anchors.

Sutures can be placed through tissue via different methods. Antegrade suture passage utilizes any of the commercially available devices to pass the suture from the articular side of the cuff to the bursal side. This method requires the fewest steps in suture passage as the surgeon is able to grasp the tissue and pass the suture through it in a single step; however, this requires the use of a cannula as the device tends to be bigger. Furthermore, the trajectory of suture passage and the depth of tissue grasped can be limited by the device. In contrast, retrograde passage requires penetration of the tissue with an instrument followed by grasping the suture in a second step. The advantage of retrograde passage is that allows for precise placement of the suture without a limitation in depth of tissue taken. This method is helpful in subscapularis repair, particularly if there is a component of retraction. Both types of suture passing instruments are helpful and can be used for different areas of the shoulder and in different steps of the repair.

With the strong fixation provided by properly placed anchors, the weakest point in the fixation is the suture-tendon interface.[168,265,266] The earlier reports of arthroscopic rotator cuff repairs have all utilized simple suture or horizontal mattress configurations, but these have lower pullout strengths. In order to address this, various suture configurations have been developed to provide better pullout strength within the tissue (Fig. 15-27). Historically, with open rotator cuff repair, the Mason-Allen stitch was considered to have superior tensile strength and ultimate tensile load compared with simple and mattress configurations.[184,265,266,422] However, owing to the technical challenge of placing the Mason-Allen stitch in arthroscopic repair, several modified techniques based on the principles of the Mason-Allen stitch have been developed. Both the arthroscopic Mason-Allen stitch for suture anchors[637] and the massive cuff (Mac) stitch[426] have been described as alternatives to the Mason-Allen stitch. Ma et al. demonstrated that the strength of the Mac stitch was comparable to that of the Mason-Allen stitch for open rotator cuff repairs and that both were significantly stronger than the simple or horizontal mattress configuration.[422]

However, a recent meta-analysis found no difference in rerupture rates associated with use of simple, mattress, and modified Mason-Allen sutures, regardless of the tear size.[86] Furthermore, with the emergence of double-row and transosseous-equivalent (TOE) techniques, suture configuration has become a less critical determinant of the biomechanical properties of the repair.

The final step in fixation of the tendon to bone is the arthroscopic knot. It is essential that the surgeon ties a secure knot to avoid gapping between the tendon and bone during the healing phase. This is a variable of the repair that the surgeon can completely control, and in our opinion should never be a point of failure. A multitude of knot-tying techniques have been described in the literature and can broadly be divided into three categories: nonsliding, sliding, and sliding-locking. Nonsliding knots are utilized when the suture does not slide through the anchor and the tissue thereby retaining the same length of the suture throughout the knot tying. These are typically half hitches or combinations of half hitches, as in the Revo knot. Sliding and sliding-locking knots require a post limb, which is the limb that has been passed through the rotator cuff, to slide down upon and reduce the tissue to bone. Sliding knots use the friction of the knot to prevent slippage whereas locking knots require countertension on the non–post limb to flip the knot and lock it in place. Examples of common sliding knots are the Duncan loop, Tennessee slider, and Roeder knot. Commonly used sliding-locking knots are the Samsung medical center (SMC) knot, Nicky's knot, and the Weston knot. Typically these knots are then backed up with several alternating half hitches to secure it in place. Ultimately, surgeons must be comfortable tying one type of sliding knot and one nonsliding knot in order to be able to address any situation faced in the operating room. Additionally, utilization of a knot pushing device and a cannula allow for ease of knot passage through the overlying subcutaneous fat and muscle without entrapment of tissue within the knot during tensioning.

The concept of loop security and knot security has been popularized by Burkhart. Loop security is the ability of a knot to maintain a tight suture loop while the knot is tied whereas knot security is the ability to resist knot slippage as a load is applied; the ideal knot configuration would have both.[111,413] In his study, he found that a sliding knot alone had poor knot security and the addition of reverse half hitches with alternating posts significantly improved both knot and loop security. However, a static surgeon's knot provides the best security of all knots tested.

AUTHORS' PREFERRED METHOD

In our practice, we utilize a knot similar to that described by Burkhart. We utilize a double half hitch tied in the same direction as a sliding knot. This is followed by another half hitch also in the same direction. The repair can still be tightened during the tying of the third knot. This is then followed by three alternating half hitches that are made to lie square on the knot by equalizing tension on the post and non–post limb as each successive knot is secured in place.

Standard arthroscopic repair of the rotator cuff utilizes a single row of sutures to reduce the tear edge to the greater tuberosity. Typically, one to three anchors are placed from anterior to posterior just lateral to the articular margin in the greater tuberosity, spaced about 1 cm apart. These anchors can be double loaded with sutures to minimize the number of anchors in bone while maximizing fixation points within the tendon. Having multiple fixation points by using a double loaded suture anchor can increase fixation within the tissue, thereby increasing the strength of the repair. Sutures are passed through the tendon edge in an anterograde or retrograde fashion from anterior to posterior and then tied down from posterior to anterior. The limitation of single-row fixation is that it essentially acts a spot weld of fixation to bone at each knot but does not restore an anatomic footprint of the rotator cuff repair. Concerns about recurrent defects in larger tears arose in this setting[250] and thus additional means of fixation were sought out. This led to the advent of double-row and TOE rotator cuff repair that provides a broader base of fixation for the tendon.

Much attention has been paid to the anatomic footprint of the individual tendons of the rotator cuff as anatomic restoration was thought to improve healing rates and outcomes. As will be discussed later, this is particularly helpful in determining the amount of tendon involved in partial-thickness tears, but can also guide the surgeon in restoring an anatomic attachment in posterior-superior cuff repairs. There has been much variability in the reported dimensions of the anatomic footprints of the rotator cuff. In particular, Mochizuki et al. determined that the supraspinatus insertion is much smaller, and the infraspinatus insertion much larger than previously reported (Table 15-2). Despite these findings, the key takeaway point is that there is a broad insertion of the rotator cuff and SR cuff repair may not be able to restore this.

Double-row repair of the rotator cuff sought to establish a more anatomic repair of the footprint with the hope that the increase in contact surface area and the initial fixation strength would lead to higher rates of healing.[411] In double-row repair, two rows of anchors, medial adjacent to the articular margin, and lateral, at the end of the greater tuberosity, are used. Prior to utilizing this technique, the surgeon must confirm that the tendon can reach the lateral edge of the greater tuberosity. Next, one to two double-loaded suture anchors are placed from anterior to posterior just adjacent to the articular margin. At the time of anchor placement, we plan our stab incision and the anchor trajectory using an 18-gauge spinal needle under direct visualization to ensure precise anchor placement. The sutures from the medial row can then be passed through the rotator cuff at least 10 to 12 mm medial to the tendon edge in a horizontal mattress fashion. The lateral row of anchors is then placed along the lateral edge of the greater tuberosity, just medial to the "drop off" of the bone. Care must be taken at this

TABLE 15-2 Anatomic Footprint Dimensions of the Posterior-Superior Rotator Cuff

	Supraspinatus		Infraspinatus	
Study	Mediolateral length (mm)	Anteroposterior length (mm)	Mediolateral length (mm)	Anteroposterior length (mm)
Curtis et al.[169]	23	16	29	19
Dugas et al.[204]	12.7	16.3	13.4	16.4
Mochizuki et al.[479]	6.9	12.6	10.2	32.7

step to allow for a sufficient bone bridge between the rows of anchors to prevent overcrowding of anchors and the risk of failure. The sutures from the lateral row anchors are passed in a simple suture configuration over the lateral edge of the tendon. The lateral row of sutures is then tied down first followed by the medial row to allow for proper tensioning. Although this technique does provide a larger area of fixation and initial strength of repair, it does require longer operative times and an associated increase in cost for additional anchors.

Double-row rotator cuff repair has been shown to restore the footprint of the rotator thereby increasing the potential surface area for healing.[411,447] Brady et al. compared single- and double-row repair and found that single-row cuff repair left a 52.7% uncovered footprint, but that the entire footprint was covered after securing the medial row, essentially doubling the coverage with a second row.[75] Similarly, Meier utilized 3D mapping to show that the double-row repair restored 100% of the footprint, and which was significantly greater than single-row or transosseous fixation.[460] Despite this anatomic restoration of the rotator cuff attachment, the theorized biomechanical and clinical results remain mixed.

Biomechanically, double-row repair does appear to show improved results compared with single-row repair. Ma et al. showed that double-row had a significantly higher ultimate tensile load compared with several SR repair configurations.[421] Several other studies have supported these findings with improved initial strength and stiffness, resistance to gap formation, higher yield load, higher ultimate load, and higher energy absorbed at yield load with double-row compared with single-row repair.[364,585,663] Although there are some contradicting data that suggest that there may not be a difference in some of these biomechanical properties,[447] the bulk of the literature does support that double-row repair is a stronger construct in rotator cuff repair; however, the clinical data are not quite as clear.

Double-row repair has taken a step forward with the development of TOE rotator cuff repairs. Transosseous fixation is the gold standard in open rotator cuff repair, in which the sutures are passed through a bony tunnel in the greater tuberosity. As arthroscopic rotator cuff repair was emerging, this was the standard to which it was compared. This led to the development of a TOE repair in which the sutures of the medial row are linked to the lateral row, acting as a "suture bridge" (Fig. 15-28). This is performed using a medial row of suture anchors with the sutures placed 10 to 12 cm medially through the tear edge in mattress fashion. The sutures are then left intact and tied to an interference screw placed about a centimeter lateral to the footprint.[546] The benefit of this method is that sutures from the lateral row do not need to be passed through the tissue allowing for fewer steps in suture passage and less suture material to be interposed between the tendon and the bone. Additionally, rather than having two rows of spot welds, the bridging sutures act to compress the intervening rotator cuff tissue. In theory, this helps to enhance the healing process of the rotator cuff TOE repair and aids in compression of the tendon to the footprint.[102,473,475,547,550]

A more recent potential advancement in TOE repair of rotator cuff repair has been the introduction of knotless TOE constructs where only the lateral row of fixation is tied down. This method was developed to address concerns with the need to tie knots in the medial row and the subsequent tendon strangulation, the increased surgical time, and the associated increased costs.[475] The early results of this are varied. Knotless TOE may have worse biomechanical properties compared with a tied medial row,[432] and complications have been reported due to suture slippage and loosening.[140,753] However, MRI-diagnosed re-tear rates were found to be higher in knotted TOE compared with knotless TOE.[73,599] In a series of 22 patients, Hug et al. reported good to excellent clinical results using knotless TOE,[325] but sufficient clinical data are lacking at this point and this will need to be further evaluated in years to come.

For small rotator cuff tears less than 1 cm, we prefer to use a single-row repair using simple suture configurations. For medium, large, or massive rotator cuff tears, we prefer to use TOE-type repair with or without side-to-side repair stitches for margin convergence if the tear pattern dictates the need. We recommend a complete bursectomy prior to the repair to identify the tear pattern accurately and to determine the best repair method. When placing anchors and sutures for repair, we tend to place the sutures from an anterior-to-posterior fashion while tying them from posterior-to-anterior fashion. This will allow better visualization while the arthroscope is used to view the rotator cuff tendon through the posterior portal.

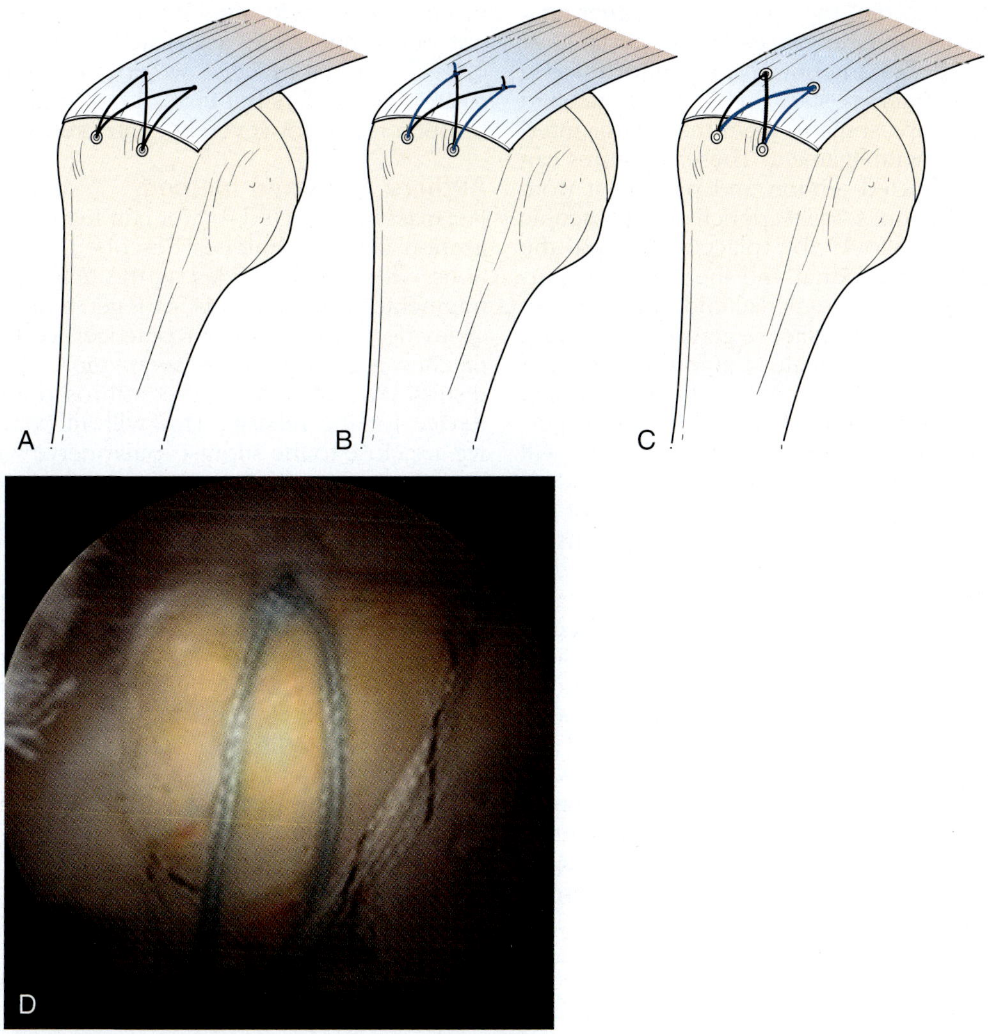

FIGURE 15-28: **A,** Transosseus-equivalent (TOE) repair. **B,** Knotted TOE repair. **C,** Knotless TOE repair. **D,** Arthroscopic image of knotted TOE repair.

ADVANCED ARTHROSCOPIC REPAIRS

Massive Rotator Cuff Tears

Large and massive contracted rotator cuff tears remain a daunting challenge for the orthopedic surgeon. Although tendon transfers and reverse TSA have provided a solution for truly irreparable rotator cuff tears, the term *irreparable* remains a moving target. The following section describes some techniques to mobilize a retracted rotator cuff and convert what may seem to be an irreparable cuff tear to a well-functioning repair.

Mobilization

For the posterosuperior rotator cuff, large and massive tears may retract beyond the glenoid. Adequate mobilization of the tear is key to a tensionless repair without damaging the overlying suprascapular nerve. After a thorough SAD is performed, the edge of the retracted tear should be visualized. The undersurface of the tendon is relatively safe, so an arthroscopic elevator can be placed in the interval between the tendon and glenoid neck/scapula to break up any adhesions that have formed. For the superior aspect of the cuff, we prefer to use the arthroscopic cautery device to free adhesions, as any ablation in proximity of the nerve will cause the muscle to contract. For the subscapularis, a thorough release of tissue using arthroscopic cautery from the inferolateral coracoid is essential. We also perform a release of the rotator interval from the tendon to aid in mobilization. A coracoidplasty can also be performed to prevent further impingement on the subscapularis tendon and provide easier access to the retracted tendon. A combination of cautery and use of the arthroscopic elevator can help free up the tendon. However, for severely retracted subscapularis tears beyond the glenoid margin, open repair should be considered.

Interval Slides

When mobilizing the tendon by performing a lysis of the adhesions does not provide enough mobility, interval slides can be utilized to free the tendon from other anatomic attachments to provide excursion. Two types of slides can be utilized: the anterior and posterior interval slides. The anterior interval slide frees the contracted leading edge of the supraspinatus from the rotator interval and the coracohumeral ligament. These structures can be scarred to the retracted tendon and prevent it from further lateral mobilization. A basket punch or arthroscopic electrocautery device should be placed through the lateral subacromial (LSAC) portal and the release is performed from lateral towards the medial end. An accessory lateral portal can be made to place a grasper to provide countertension on the supraspinatus tendon by pulling it laterally. The rotator interval and coracohumeral ligament should be released until tension free repair can be performed. The posterior edge of the tear typically will require a margin convergence followed by a standard repair of the tendon to bone. If complete release of the anterior interval is performed and there is residual tension on the supraspinatus, a posterior interval slide can also be used. Also through the lateral portal, the interval between the supraspinatus and infraspinatus is incised to free up the tendon. The scapular spine should be visualized during this procedure to prevent migration anteriorly that could lead to inadvertent injury to the suprascapular nerve. This technique should be used sparingly as the intact cuff is being incised to release the tendon. After the release, a margin convergence between the infraspinatus and advanced supraspinatus should be performed, followed by a standard tendon to bone repair. Despite initial reports of good outcomes, we are still guarded regarding the outcomes in patients that have tears that require interval slides.

Patches/Tissue Augmentation

Despite thorough mobilization and use of anterior and posterior interval slides, there can be residual tension on the rotator cuff that makes it impossible to reduce it to the greater tuberosity. In these cases, a patch can be used to bridge the remaining gap or augment a repair with tenuous tissue. Various grafts have been utilized including fascia lata autograft, xenograft, and synthetic grafts including Gore-Tex and poly-L-lactide patches. The area of the remaining defect or area to be augmented is measured and the patch is cut to match this size. If the patch has some elasticity, the patch can be cut slightly smaller than the area to account for this. Free sutures are placed in the medial margin of the native tendon and these are passed through the medial margin of the patch. The lateral edge of the patch can then be fixed to the greater tuberosity in single- or double-row fashion to complete the repair. There are limited data on this repair method, and the current data are mixed in outcomes. Malcarney et al. reported on 4 cases of an early inflammatory reaction with a porcine graft which they felt had the potential to break down the repair.[431] Other studies have demonstrated significant improvement in functional scores with use of this graft,[464] but an MRI follow-up study by Sclamberg et al. demonstrated re-tears in 10 of 11 patients at 6 months.[642] Poly-L-lactide synthetic grafts have shown some promise in early studies with significant improvement in functional outcomes but were associated with a re-tear rate of 62%.[397,581] In our practice, we do not use these patches for rotator cuff repairs but instead opt to utilize partial repair or open repair for severely contracted tears.

Authors' Preferred Method

For massive retracted rotator cuff tears, we perform mobilization using techniques described above. We are cautious with interval slides as the tear can become more fragmented and patients can get worse if the interval slides do not heal. In our practice, we have not utilized patches regularly as we await more definitive positive results. We do utilize the arthroscopic electrocautery device for the release. This will allow us to know that we are close to the suprascapular nerve when performing the release.

Partial Rotator Cuff Tears

Partial rotator cuff tears account for a significant percentage of patient visits, and often represent a diagnostic and treatment dilemma for the surgeon. In many cases, the partial tear can be only mildly symptomatic and treated with nonoperative modalities including rest, physical therapy, and modification of activities. For those that do not respond to nonoperative treatment, current management can consist of either transtendonous repair or takedown of the remaining fibers and standard arthroscopic rotator cuff tear as described previously.

Classification

The most common classification of partial rotator cuff tear was proposed by Ellman.[214] In this system, the tear is classified by location (articular, bursal, interstitial), and grade (grade 1, <3 mm deep; grade 2, 3-6 mm deep; grade 3, >6 mm deep). This has important treatment implications as grade 3 tears represent more than half of the width of the supraspinatus footprint. Snyder popularized the term partial articular supraspinatus tendon avulsion (PASTA) lesion for the articular sided tear with delamination of the articular portion of the supraspinatus, particularly in the throwing population.[476,669] Conway popularized the partial articular tear with intratendinous extension (PAINT) lesion to incorporate this subset of partial-thickness tears with intratendinous involvement.[156] Others have confirmed that this is an important component of partial cuff tears as the repairs should include the intratendinous portion of the tear.

Treatment Options

Currently, there is no well-established clinical practice guideline that dictates treatment of partial-thickness rotator cuff tears. Furthermore, it is still unclear if these tears represent a unique entity or a part of a broader spectrum of disease in the shoulder that encompasses impingement and full-thickness cuff tears. The first line of treatment in a majority of patients should consist of activity modification with avoidance of overhead sports or other pain-provoking activities, a short course of nonsteroidal antiinflammatory drugs (NSAIDs), and either home exercises or physical therapy programs directed by a physical therapist. In many cases of throwers with a PASTA lesion, a tight anterior capsule will be found, and focused stretching that addresses this functional limitation can lead to significant improvement in both the short and long term. On failure of these initial modalities, subacromial injections of corticosteroid can be considered. Currently, there is a lack of high-quality literature evaluating the efficacy of subacromial corticosteroid injections (SAIs) for the treatment of partial-thickness rotator cuff tears. However, some patients certainly receive some benefit, particularly those with bursal-sided tears.

Operative Management

The indications for surgery for patients with partial-thickness rotator cuff tears include patients with symptoms consistent with a rotator cuff tear, a documented partial-thickness cuff tear on imaging, and an attempted and failed period of nonoperative management. Biomechanical data provide a strong rationale for treatment as partial tears result in differential shear stresses and likelihood of tear propagation of larger tears. Surgical treatment has evolved to an all-arthroscopic approach, with debridement of Ellman grade I and II tears. The results of debridement in low-grade partial tears have been good[93,163,690] and should remain the treatment of choice for small partial tears.

The optimal treatment strategy for PASTA lesions remains a controversial topic. Some surgeons prefer in situ transtendon repair of the rotator cuff, while others prefer removal of the remaining rotator cuff tissue and treatment of the tear in a manner similar to that used for a full-thickness tear. Recent biomechanical studies have evaluated both techniques. Gonzalez-Lomas et al. found that the in situ transtendon repair had less gapping and a higher failure strength, which suggests its biomechanical superiority.[274] Mihata et al. evaluated transtendon repair in a cadaveric throwing shoulder model, and found that there was decreased anterior translation and external rotation, which may place the cuff at risk for further injury over time.[466]

Clinically, there are data to support either technique, and the chosen method is often a judgment call based on surgeon preference and experience. Porat et al. described their results in 51 patients with an arthroscopic takedown and repair of the partial supraspinatus tear. They found that this technique resulted in a good/excellent result in 83% of patients.[575]

Authors' Preferred Method

When a partial rotator cuff tear is encountered, the decision of debridement versus repair depends on the depth and quality of the remaining rotator cuff tendon. In general, any tear that has less than 25% of the depth of the insertion will be treated with debridement alone. For tears that are more than 25% but less than 75% of the depth of the insertion, these tears are usually repaired in situ if the remaining tendon is not degenerative (Fig. 15-29). In the event of suboptimal tendon quality, the tear is completed and a standard full-thickness repair performed. For tears that are more than 75% of the depth of the insertion, the tear is usually completed and a standard repair performed. In general, bursal-sided rotator cuff tears tend to be more symptomatic and cause more subacromial bursitis; these tears are usually treated aggressively with surgical repair. Cordasco et al. reported that even grade 1 and grade 2 bursal-sided tears have a higher rate of failure with SAD alone.[163]

Subscapularis Tears

The subscapularis is the largest and strongest of the rotator cuff tendons. It is responsible for active internal rotation of the humerus and contributes to the stability of the shoulder. As a component of the dynamic stabilization mechanism of the glenohumeral joint, it forms the anterior portion of the transverse plane "force couple" of the rotator cuff, and serves to balance the forces generated across the joint to maintain glenohumeral congruency throughout movement.[41,264,291]

Tears of the subscapularis can occur by a degenerative process or less commonly, from acute traumatic injury. These can often lead to significant pain and functional disability. Subscapularis tears are relatively rare, with a reported incidence of 2.1% to 10.5% in patients with rotator cuff tears.[15,192,237] However, with the development of a better diagnostic capability, the actual prevalence of subscapularis tears may be higher than previously reported.[41] Untreated subscapularis tears go on to develop persistent pain and disability, and in addition to this, can lead to dynamic anterior instability and glenohumeral arthrosis. Early operative treatment is therefore recommended for most tears.[237]

Diagnosis

The clinical diagnosis of subscapularis tendon tears can be difficult as the presenting complaint is often nonspecific anterior shoulder pain. Provocative physical exam maneuvers specific for subscapularis tears are designed to isolate various aspects of the subscapularis that contribute to the strength of internal rotation of the shoulder. These maneuvers include the lift-off test,[264] the belly press test,[263] and the bear hug test.[40] While these examination maneuvers have a high specificity for detecting a tear when used individually, they tend to have a low sensitivity. The bear hug test has been shown to be the most sensitive (60% sensitivity). Despite these specific maneuvers to isolate the subscapularis, up to 40% of tears are not detected on physical exam; therefore advanced imaging should be obtained in case a tear is suspected.[40]

MRI is the imaging modality of choice for diagnosing subscapularis tears and should be performed early if there is any concern of an injury. Axial sequences are best to demonstrate subscapularis tendon disruption, muscle edema, and biceps tendon subluxation or dislocation. Full-thickness tears can be seen on MRI axial images as complete defects in the tendon attachment, with or without medial retraction of the entire musculotendinous

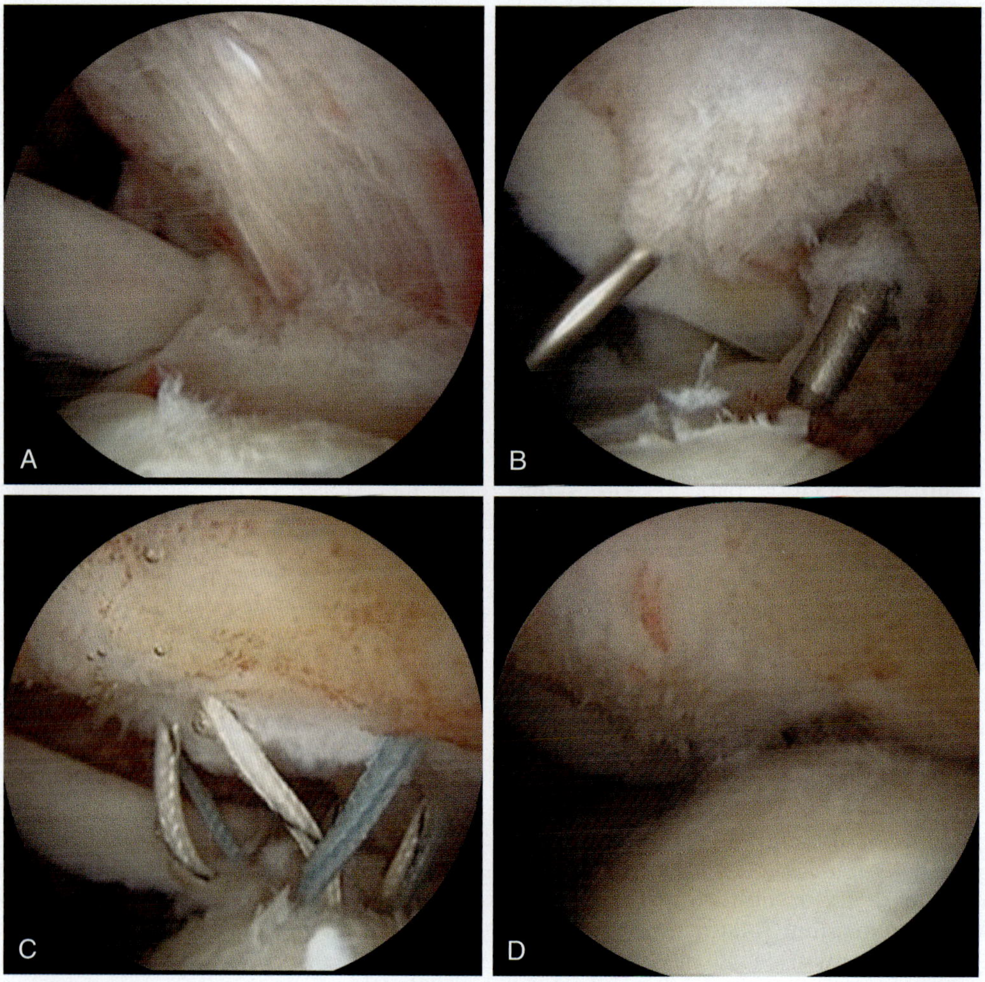

FIGURE 15-29: **A,** Partial articular-sided supraspinatus tear. **B,** Metal anchor placed through tear with spinal needle for suture shuttling. **C,** Passed sutures prior to being tied down. **D,** In situ transtendon repair.

unit. Complete or partial disruption of the insertion can be better visualized by positioning the arm in external rotation during the MRI. Partial-thickness tears manifest as increased signal in the rotator cuff, especially in T2-weighted images, that incompletely traverse the tendon substance.[223] The coronal sequences should be reviewed to assess for biceps and labral lesions, particularly in the younger patient, which often coexist with subscapularis injuries. The diagnosis of subscapularis tendon tears on the basis of MRI remains challenging. The tendon attaches to the lesser tuberosity which is medial to the bicipital groove. A dislocation or subluxed biceps tendon is usually indicative of a tear of the subscapularis tendon.

MRI can provide valuable information about the size of the tear, amount of medial retraction of the leading edge of the tendon, and the presence of muscular fatty infiltration. The presence of fatty infiltration in the muscle belly may be used as a surrogate marker of the chronicity of the tear and the quality of the torn musculotendinous tissue.[248,278] The presence of fatty infiltration may lead to higher rates of rerupture and poorer surgical outcomes.[41]

Ultrasound has been successfully used for diagnosing subscapularis tears but is operator dependent and offers limited visualization of other glenohumeral joint structures.

Operative Indications

As the natural progression of subscapularis injuries is persistent pain, weakness, and subsequent development of anterior dynamic instability that can lead to glenohumeral arthrosis, it is generally accepted that most symptomatic subscapularis tears will require operative management.[192,237,264] Early operative intervention is recommended, as several authors have found that time to surgical treatment can influence success rates.[41,237,263,378] Small partial-thickness tears may be treated nonoperatively, especially those that are chronic, mildly symptomatic, or in poor surgical candidates such as patients with other medical comorbidities or patients unwilling or unable to undergo the rehabilitation protocol.

Arthroscopic Repair Outcomes

While there are numerous studies on the treatment outcomes of rotator cuff pathology, the literature on arthroscopic management of subscapularis tears is relatively sparse. Burkhart et al. reported the early results of 25 arthroscopic subscapularis repairs (average follow-up duration of 10.7 months) using the University of California–Los Angeles (UCLA) shoulder outcome score. In their series, the average UCLA score improved from 10.7 preoperatively to 30.5 postoperatively, with 92% of patients achieving "good-excellent" results.[110] Bennett reported on a prospective cohort of patients with isolated subscapularis tears 2 and 4 years postoperatively and found that the outcomes were maintained over time.[48,49] Regardless of the treatment method employed, several studies have shown that early management of subscapularis tears is preferable to conservative management—the latter being associated with tendon degeneration and fatty infiltration of the muscle belly.[737] For this reason, we favor treatment of subscapularis tendon injuries in the acute phase once the diagnosis is confirmed. There is also an association between concomitant rotator cuff pathology involving the posterosuperior cuff and poorer outcomes when compared with isolated subscapularis repair that warrants consideration.[110]

Biceps Tendon

The biceps tendon remains a source of controversy in the shoulder, especially in the setting of a subscapularis tear. Edwards et al. suggested that a biceps tenodesis or tenotomy should be performed at the time of repair of a subscapularis tendon tear, regardless of any identified biceps tendon or pulley pathology.[209] In certain subsets of patients such as younger patients with simple rupture of the pulley sling or those with acute injuries, comparable results have been reported with isolated repair of the biceps pulley.[41,429] There is a general consensus that if there is evidence of biceps pathology or if the tendon is subluxated or dislocated, a tenodesis or tenotomy is the preferred treatment.

There is no clear consensus regarding the decision between tenodesis and tenotomy. Evidence of superiority of one procedure over the other with respect to pain relief, functional outcomes, or strength is largely inconsistent.[64,209,239,269,361,534]

Biceps tenotomy has the advantage of being a fast and relatively simple procedure, with fewer restrictions on postoperative rehabilitation and the avoidance of potential complications associated with further surgical dissection and hardware placement involved in the tenodesis.[65,247,269] However, in patients undergoing a concomitant subscapularis repair, the rehabilitation protocol will be dictated by the cuff repair.

The benefits of biceps tenodesis over tenotomy are the avoidance of a "Popeye deformity," which can occur in up to 70% of patients after a tenotomy, and the avoidance of persistent biceps spasm and fatigue that can be seen in up to 40% of patients. However, recent literature suggests no difference in the outcome from these procedures.[361,534,603] Some authors recommend tenodesis in young or athletic patients in order to restore the length-tension relationship and maximize the function of the elbow; however, there is limited evidence to support this in the literature.[247,361,446]

Authors' Preferred Method

When subscapularis tendon tears are encountered, we usually perform an intra-articular approach for repair. The rotator interval is exposed and the coracoid is identified. A beach chair positioned patient can help tremendously as forward flexing the arm can expose the entire lesser tuberosity and does not require moving the arthroscope to the anterior shoulder. A coracoidplasty is performed if there is evidence of impingement with shoulder internal rotation. The biceps tendon is closely evaluated for any instability. The presence of an intact SGHL usually represents a stable biceps tendon. If the biceps tendon is subluxated or dislocated, the biceps tendon will be tagged and released. This will later be tenodesed or tenotomized based on the condition of the biceps tendon and on the patient's preference.

The tear is then identified. If this is a significantly retracted tear, a traction suture can be placed to apply lateral tension. We then place metal anchors from the inferior part of the lesser tuberosity first and move superiorly. We pass sutures individually as we place the anchors. For the inferior part of the tendon, we place horizontal mattress sutures to advance the tendon laterally. We then tie the sutures as we pass them from an inferior to superior fashion. This will allow us to adequately reduce the tear to its anatomic position. For the most superior stitch, we usually place a simple suture to tie the superior edge of the subscapularis down to the lesser tuberosity. This also serves to re-create the SGHL. For most full width subscapularis tendon tears, two double-loaded metal anchors will be used. This allows us to place three horizontal mattress sutures and one simple suture configuration for repair. Most superior-half subscapularis tendon tears can be repaired with just one double-loaded metal anchor utilizing one horizontal and one simple suture configuration (Fig. 15-30). For tears that are retracted to the glenoid rim or those that have a significant amount of scarring, an open deltopectoral approach is used for repair.

If the patient desires to have a biceps tenodesis and the tendon allows a repair, a small incision is made by extending the anterior portal and utilizing a mini-deltopectoral split in line with the bicipital groove. We usually place an anchor or a bioabsorbable interference screw on the inferior most aspect of the bicipital groove for biceps tenodesis. We prefer to perform the tenodesis outside the bicipital groove to avoid any residual pain along the groove. Biceps tenotomy can be performed, but older patients should be warned about the cosmetic deformity ahead of time.

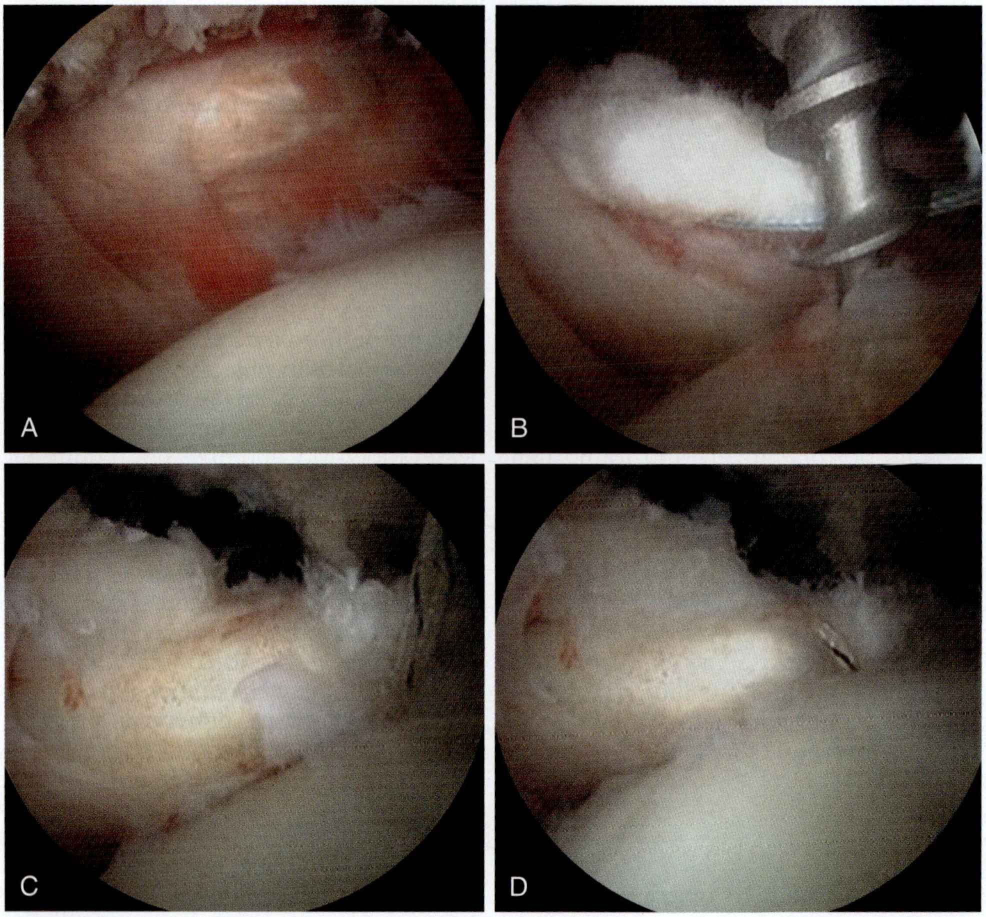

FIGURE 15-30: **A,** Upper border of the subscapularis tendon tear. **B,** Placement of suture anchor in lesser tuberosity (blue traction suture in place). **C,** Tear is reduced to footprint with single horizontal mattress suture. **D,** Simple suture configuration used to fold down uppermost edge of tendon.

OUTCOMES OF ARTHROSCOPIC ROTATOR CUFF REPAIRS

Over the past decade, the outcomes of arthroscopic cuff repairs have improved with advances in our knowledge of rotator cuff biomechanics and increased comfort level with arthroscopic techniques. Several recent systematic reviews have suggested that results are comparable to those of mini-open repairs. For example, Ji et al. evaluated five randomized controlled trials (n = 166 for arthroscopic repair; n = 163 for mini-open repair group), and found significant differences in operation time, weighted 100-point shoulder score, and visual analog score (VAS) for pain and ROM.[348] This study did not evaluate healing rates.

In one recent randomized controlled trial, van der Zwaal et al. found that shoulder functional outcomes, pain, ROM, and complications did not significantly differ between patients treated with all-arthroscopic repair and those treated with mini-open repair in the first year after surgery.[722] Other studies have found similar findings, but a lack of robust data on postoperative healing is a significant limitation.

Biomechanical Repair Strategies

The choice of treatment strategy for rotator cuff repair is a contentious subject. Many surgeons prefer single-row repair for smaller tears and double-row or TOE for larger tears. Biomechanical studies support the use of double-row or TOE repair strategies to improve the footprint contact area, which may improve outcomes in larger rotator cuff tears.[394] Furthermore, TOE techniques have been shown to better restore the footprint and contact pressure, especially with respect to rotational movements.[548,549]

There remains a relative paucity of clinical data to support use of multiple-row repair techniques. Shen et al. recently performed a literature review to determine whether a double-row repair results in a lower incidence of recurrent cuff tears. Aggregate analysis of data from six studies (n = 428) revealed no difference in outcomes with respect to American Shoulder and Elbow Surgeons

(ASES), Constant, or UCLA scores between different repair techniques; however, DR cuff repairs were associated with a lower incidence of re-tears.[651] DeHaan et al. performed a systematic review of functional outcomes after single and double row repairs. In the seven studies that met the inclusion criteria, functional ASES, Constant, and UCLA outcome scores revealed no difference between single- and double-row rotator cuff repairs. The total re-tear rate, which included both complete and partial re-tears was 43% for the single-row repair and 27% for the double-row repair (P = .057).[180] Saridakis and Jones also found superior healing with double-row repair compared with that with single-row repair, but with no difference in functional outcomes. In larger tears, double-row repair tend to improve healing rates.[630] Ma et al. followed 53 patients who had undergone a cuff repair (27 single row and 26 double row) and found that arthroscopic rotator cuff repair with double-row fixation showed better shoulder strength in patients with larger tear size (>3 cm) compared with those who had undergone single-row fixation. However, no significance difference in terms of healing rates was observed.[424]

TOE techniques were originally described for open cuff repair and were then adapted for arthroscopic use. Recently, outcomes from TOE repairs have begun to be reported. McCormick et al. found that all repair strategies (single row, double row, TOE) yielded statistically significant improvement 2 years after cuff repair, with no differences in functional outcomes.[452] The study also found decrease in re-tear rates from single row (22%) to double row (18%) to TOE (11%); however, this difference was not statistically significant. Gartsman et al. performed a prospective randomized study that assessed healing after single-row and TOE treatment techniques using ultrasound.[254] Eighty-three patients were available for ultrasound examination (40 single row and 43 suture bridge). Thirty of 40 patients (75%) who had undergone single-row repair showed a healed rotator cuff compared with 40 of 43 (93%) patients who had undergone suture bridge repair (P = .024). Thus there appears to be structural advantages to TOE repair.

SUMMARY

In summary, arthroscopic rotator cuff repairs have made significant advances over the past 3 decades. We believe that we can achieve very strong initial repairs with good restoration of the tendon bone interface. The repair outcomes for small and medium size tears are good; however, the outcomes for degenerated muscles or for large rotator cuff tears remain poor. Future research imperatives include development of means to improve soft tissue-to-bone healing and biologic modulation to minimize degeneration of the muscle and tendon before and after repairs.

Arthroscopic Treatment of Acromioclavicular Joint Osteolysis, Arthritis, and Instability

Justin S. Yang, Andreas Voss, John Apostolakos, Augustus D. Mazzocca

ANATOMY

The AC joint, located in the anterior, medial-most aspect of the subacromial space, is evident by its glistening white joint capsule. The capsule is reinforced by superior, inferior, anterior, and posterior AC ligaments; the superior ligaments are significantly thicker than the inferior ligaments.[596] The superior and posterior AC ligaments are the most significant restraints to posterior motion of the distal clavicle,[373] with both collectively accounting for 81% of the resistance against posterior displacement (superior ligament 56%, posterior ligament 25%).[373] The inferior ligament appears to be the major restraint against anterior displacement.[392]

The AC joint is a diarthrodial joint with a freedom of motion in three different axes with a limitation due to the passive stabilizers. Therefore the joint offers a wide capacity of rotation up to a total of 50 degrees.[624] Furthermore, the AC joint with its ligamentous reinforcements of the capsule shows a capacity of superior translation of approximately 5.4 mm, that of anterior translation of 6.6 mm, and of posterior translation of 7.8 mm.[44]

To prevent superior displacement, the AC joint is reinforced by the coracoclavicular (CC) ligaments, which comprise the conoid and trapezoid ligaments. The mean distance of the conoid ligament center from the lateral edge of the clavicle is 46.3 mm and 24.9 mm for the trapezoid ligament.[604] The mean widths of these ligaments are 15.6 mm and 16.0 mm, respectively. Furthermore, the conoid ligament has a more posterior insertion on the inferior aspect of the clavicle and the trapezoid ligament a more anterior insertion.[687] The distance between the clavicular insertions is an average of 20 mm compared with a mean distance of 10.1 mm on the coracoid base; the ligaments form a rectangular V-shape to reinforce stability (Fig. 15-31).[297,604]

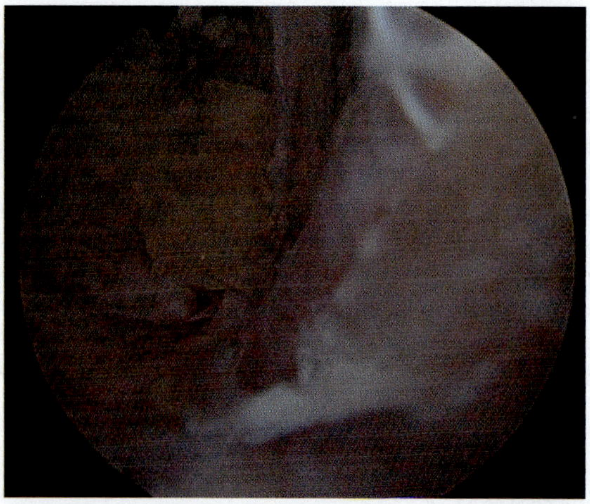

FIGURE 15-31: The conoid ligament, as seen arthroscopically during a suprascapular nerve decompression.

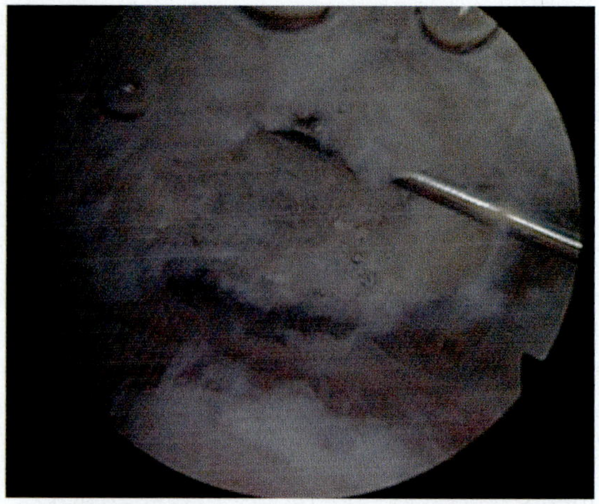

FIGURE 15-32: When viewing from the lateral subacromial portal, a needle can be used to localize the anterior subacromial portal.

Depending on the presence or absence of an articular disk, the AC joint can be classified into three types. The first type shows a complete disk, which divides the articulating surfaces completely with a more prominent thicker superior portion compared with the lower portion. In the second type, the disk is incomplete and a subclassification characterizes the shape of the articulating surfaces. Furthermore, the disk compensates for the incongruity of the articular facets. The third type is characterized by the absence of articular disk and is also subclassified depending on their articulating facets.[218]

The disk, which is attached to the superior ligament, is usually reduced to a fibrocartilage remnant by early adulthood.[647] The subacromial bursa and rotator cuff are in direct contact with the inferior surface of the joint.[765]

Distal Clavicle Osteolysis

Indications

Distal clavicular osteolysis is a well-known cause of shoulder pain in adults. Patients present with isolated pain at the distal clavicle and AC joint that tends to worsen with activity. There are two forms: posttraumatic distal clavicular osteolysis, caused by a direct traumatic injury,[205] and atraumatic distal clavicular osteolysis, which is attributable to repetitive stress.[210] In adults, the most common risk factor for stress-induced distal clavicular osteolysis has been shown to be weightlifting.[118]

After a careful history taking and physical examination, imaging should be performed to confirm the diagnosis. Radiographic findings may range from mild osteopenia to overt osteolysis. The bilateral Zanca view is especially helpful in this setting, as it profiles the AC joint and also allows for comparison with the contralateral side. The MRI characteristics include distal clavicular bone marrow edema that is out of proportion to the edema at the acromion, as well as a subchondral cystic change; in advanced cases, periostitis may be observed at the distal clavicle.[358] Activity modification, NSAIDs, and physical therapy should be the first line treatment for this condition. In our practice, we perform an intra-articular injection of lidocaine and corticosteroids into the AC joint, which is both diagnostic and therapeutic. Nonoperative treatment with injections, medication, and physical therapy is a good option for in-season athletes. Failing this, the definitive operative treatment is a distal clavicle resection.

Technique: Distal Clavicular Resection

As distal clavicle osteolysis occurs primarily in younger patients, there is typically minimal arthrosis on the acromial cartilage surface. Thus we believe that resection should be limited to the distal clavicle for this condition. The subacromial approach is preferred as it allows for diagnosis of any missed bursal issues.

Diagnostic arthroscopy is performed starting in the glenohumeral joint using a standard posterior portal. This portal should be put in line with the lateral border of the acromion to facilitate future work in the subacromial space. Concomitant rotator cuff, bicep, or labral pathology is addressed first. The scope is then introduced into the subacromial space from the posterior portal. We recommend using the blunt scope trocar to sweep directly under the acromion in a medial to lateral direction. This breaks up any subacromial adhesions and clears away the bursa. Under direct visualization, an LSAC portal is established. This should be made at the "50 yard line" or at the AP midpoint of the acromion. It should be approximately 3 to 4 cm distal to the acromial border. A needle can be used to confirm the trajectory, which should be directly parallel to the rotator cuff below. The scope is placed with a switch stick into the LSAC portal.

Next, a needle is used to localize the AC joint from the anterior part of the shoulder joint (Fig. 15-32). The anterior subacromial (ASAC) portal is made slightly medial to this needle, and a cautery device is introduced into the joint. The trajectory should allow complete access to the posterior distal clavicle. A switching stick may be introduced from the posterior portal to allow for retraction of the medial bursa with a help of an assistant. The inferior AC capsule on the distal clavicle is removed from anterior to posterior. Care is taken to protect the coracoacromial ligament and the cartilage surface on the acromion. A 4.5-mm burr or bone cutting shaver is then introduced through the ASAC portal. A trough from the anterior to posterior on the inferior distal clavicle is resected until the posterior AC capsule is visualized. The hood of the burr protects the acromial cartilage. This is then carried inferior to superior until we can see the superior AC capsule. Then the resection is carried progressively more medial in a similar fashion until 5 to 8 mm of resection is achieved. From the LSAC portal, a 70-degree scope is very helpful to visualize the superior and posterior resection to ensure enough bone has been removed, without violating the superior and posterior capsule. A curved curette can be used in the superior and posterior portion of the distal clavicle to ensure the superior and posterior capsule is protected. At the end, the scope can be switched to the ASAC portal to check that the cut is even. Before completing the procedure, good hemostasis should be obtained using electrocautery.

Some surgeons prefer the superior or direct approach to distal clavicle excision. This allows for minimal disruption of the subacromial space and tends to aid visual access in the setting of AC joint arthrosis. The technique involves placing the scope in the ASAC portal to start the case. A smaller 2.7-mm scope may be needed to get into the joint. The working portal is either directly superior, or posterosuperior to the AC capsule.

After the resection is completed, an intraoperative fluoroscope view is recommended to confirm that enough bone has been removed, and there are no residual spurs. This is especially helpful in visualizing any remaining bone in the superior capsule. Two needles can be placed on the medial and lateral AC joint to measure the gap.

Outcome

Several biomechanical studies have examined the optimal extent of distal clavicle resection to prevent abutment of the AC joint. Edwards et al. recommend a 5-mm arthroscopic resection to prevent contact between the acromion and clavicle.[208] Beitzel and Mazzocca subsequently showed that 10 mm of resection increased the extent of anterior translation of the distal clavicle, rendering both the superior and posterior AC capsules as well as the CC ligaments as intact.[45]

Several studies have looked at the results of arthroscopic resection of the distal clavicle for osteolysis. Flatow et al. compared the results of distal clavicle resection for osteolysis in six patients who underwent an open Mumford resection from those of six patients who underwent an arthroscopic procedure.[236] There was no difference in terms of the amount of resection (18 mm in the open group vs. 17 mm in the arthroscopic group), pain relief, and function. Patients who underwent arthroscopic resection were discharged the same day and were symptom free 3 months earlier than those treated by open resection.

Zawadsky et al. reported 92% good and excellent results at an average 6.2-year follow-up after arthroscopic resection of 4 to 7 mm of distal clavicle.[778] All 41 shoulders had a diagnosis of distal clavicular osteolysis, although onset of symptoms occurred after trauma in 18 of the shoulders. All three failures occurred among the shoulders that became symptomatic following trauma.

Auge reported their results in a cohort of 10 weight lifters and body builders with osteolysis treated with distal clavicle resection via the direct arthroscopic approach.[23] Resection of an average of 4.5 mm of bone allowed all of the patients to resume training within the first week (mean, 3.2 days). Patients had regained their preoperative level of training by the second week (mean, 9.1 days) and all were able to return to active sport over a mean follow-up period of 18.7 months.

Acromiclavicular Arthritis

Indication

Posttraumatic arthritis is the most common form of AC arthritis, although primary osteoarthritis has also been described.[647] Pain induced by palpation over the AC joint as well as on cross-body adduction is the characteristic physical finding. Radiographs typically show joint space narrowing, spur formation, and subchondral cysts. It is important to realize that radiographs often do not correlate with symptoms, as many asymptomatic individuals have AC joint degenerative changes on radiographs and increased signals on MRI. Thus physical exam and a diagnostic injection are most helpful to establish a diagnosis. Randomized controlled studies have shown that asymptomatic AC joint arthrosis in the setting of a rotator cuff tear does not need to be addressed.[531]

Similar to distal clavicle osteolysis, activity modification, NSAIDs, and physical therapy should be the first line treatment. In our practice, intra-articular injection of lidocaine and corticosteroids is the standard diagnostic and therapeutic intervention. Failing this, AC resection is the only definitive operative treatment.

Technique: Acromioclavicular Joint Resection

We first start with a diagnostic examination of the glenohumeral joint to identify additional lesions. AC joint arthritis has been found to be associated with rotator cuff tears (81%), labral fraying or tears (33%), and biceps tendon pathology (23%).[85]

Diagnostic arthroscopy is performed starting in the glenohumeral joint from a standard posterior portal. This portal should be put in line with the lateral border of the acromion to facilitate further work in the subacromial space. Concomitant rotator cuff, bicep or labral pathology is addressed first. The scope is then introduced into the

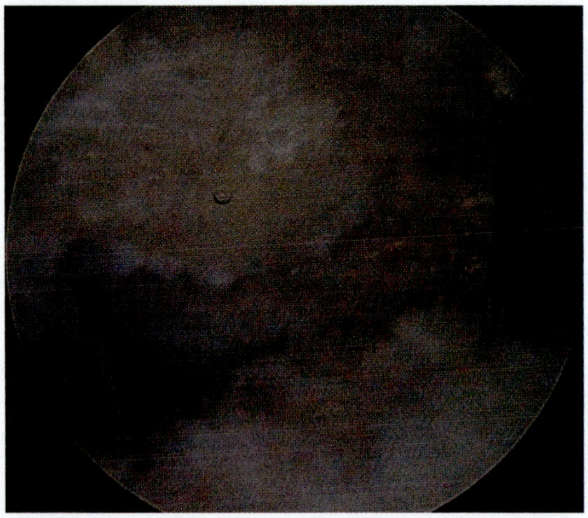

FIGURE 15-33: When viewing from lateral subacromial portal, two needles can be used to localize the anterior and posterior distal clavicle.

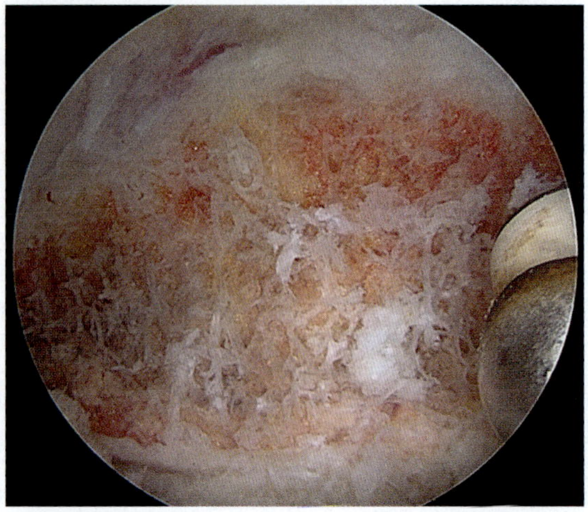

FIGURE 15-34: View from the lateral subacromial portal of the resection of 8 mm of distal clavicle with preservation of the superior and posterior capsule.

subacromial space from the posterior portal. We recommend using the blunt scope trocar to sweep directly under the acromion in a medial to lateral direction. This breaks up any subacromial adhesions and clears away the bursa. Under direct visual access, an LSAC portal is established. This should be made at the "50 yard line" or at the midpoint of the acromion anterior-posteriorly. It should be approximately 3 to 4 cm distal to the acromial border. A needle can be used to confirm the trajectory, which should be directly parallel to the rotator cuff below.

Next, using the LSAC portal as the working portal, a subacromial bursectomy is performed to visualize the AC joint. A 5-mm burr is used to remove any spurs on the inferior AC joint to aid examination. The anterior and posterior portions of the distal clavicle should be clearly visualized for proper resection, and two needles placed adjacent to the anterior/posterior distal clavicles can be helpful landmarks (Fig. 15-33). A needle is used to localize the AC joint from the anterior shoulder. The trajectory should allow complete access to the posterior distal clavicle. The ASAC portal is made directly in line with this needle, and a cautery device is introduced into the joint. The inferior AC capsule on the acromion and the distal clavicle is removed. A 5-mm burr or bone cutting shaver is then introduced through the ASAC portal. The burr is used to remove bone from both the acromion and distal clavicle until 8 to 10 mm of joint space is created. We believe the resection should be symmetrical and should remove 4 to 5 mm of bone on both the acromion and distal clavicle. The posterior and superior capsule should be preserved (Fig. 15-34). From the LSAC portal, a 70-degree scope is very helpful to visualize the superior and posterior resection to ensure enough bone has been removed, without violating the superior and posterior capsule. Alternatively, the scope can be switched to the ASAC portal to check that the cut is even. Before completing the procedure, good hemostasis should be obtained using electrocautery.

Outcome

There is biomechanical evidence to support excision of the acromion and distal clavicle, instead of the distal clavicle alone, for AC joint arthritis. In a study of 20 cadaveric shoulders, specimens were randomly assigned to one of two groups: 1-cm distal clavicle excision or symmetric (5-mm excision of acromion and distal clavicle) AC joint resection.[542] The specimens were then loaded in the anterior-posterior plane. The peak load to failure was significantly higher in the AC joint resection group, though there was no increase in anterior-posterior translation in either of the group.

Originally described by Mumford,[494] open resection of the distal end of the clavicle is a long-established treatment for symptomatic AC joint arthrosis and is associated with a successful outcome in 85% to 95% of patients.[564,623] Arthroscopic resection has led to similar results based on short- to intermediate-term follow-up in several series of patients treated in this fashion.[54,164,253,607] Arthroscopic resection lessens the degree of surgical trauma, which facilitates a swifter postoperative functional recovery.[607] Martin reported 100% patient satisfaction over an average follow-up duration of 4 years and 10 months after arthroscopic distal clavicle resection as an adjunct to SAD in patients with subacromial impingement and concomitant AC pathology.[436] Of the competitive athletes in the cohort, 22 of 25 (88%) were able to return to competition at the same level. Robertson reported a retrospective comparison of open versus arthroscopic distal clavicle excisions in 48 patients over a 5-year follow-up period. Arthroscopic patients had significantly less pain by VAS compared with open resection patients at final follow-up. There was no significant difference between the groups with regard to ASES, percentage of shoulder with normal function, average operative time, or extent of radiographic resection. The authors concluded that although both are effective treatments, less residual pain was found using the arthroscopic technique.[607]

Although the results are generally excellent when the procedure is properly indicated and complete resection is performed, incomplete resection has been reported to lead to disappointing results.[233] The traditional teaching has been that resection of 8 to 10 mm of distal clavicle is necessary for an adequate resection, but Branch et al. demonstrated that as little as 5 mm of resection may be enough to ensure that there is no contact between the clavicle and acromion on elevation of the arm.[77] The amount of resection may vary with the obliquity of the AC joint. With a more vertical AC joint, less resection might suffice, while AC joints with superolateral overhang of the distal clavicle typically require greater resection.

Acromioclavicular and Coracoclavicular Instability

Indication

The AC joint is the second most commonly dislocated joint around the shoulder. These injuries are typically characterized using the Rockwood classification. Less-severe type I and II injuries are typically treated conservatively; higher-grade type IV to VI injuries are surgically treated. The role of surgical treatment for type III injuries is much contested. One study revealed comparable clinical outcomes with surgical and conservative treatment but rates of subsequent osteoarthritis were higher in patients treated operatively.[120] Other studies have suggested that patients may not do as well as previously thought with nonoperative treatment.[35,640,760]

The general consensus regarding these grade III injuries is to utilize nonoperative treatment for 8 to 12 weeks followed by reexamination to evaluate residual pain and/or dysfunction.[604] In our practice, the primary indicator for operative treatment is pain. Secondary factors that may be indicative of operative treatment include weakness and loss of motion in the extremity. The rationale behind this management strategy is that after an initial period of nonoperative treatment many patients report improvements in pain and arm movements. It is important to note the primary importance of residual pain in the evaluation of AC joint treatment. Patients who continue to experience significant residual pain after the initial period of nonoperative management are then considered for operative intervention.

The differentiation between grade III and grade V separations can be difficult to make. Based on simple definitions, grade III separations are described as those with 100% displacement of the clavicle on radiographs compared with the contralateral side. Grade V separations, however, are described as the exaggerated superior dislocation of the AC joint between 100% and 300% as seen radiographically (Fig. 15-35).[59,445] A differential diagnosis of grade III versus V may also be made during the physical examination by use of the shrug test. The AC joint of type III injuries may reduce during the shrug test, but tearing of the deltotrapezial fascia makes it impossible for type V injuries to reduce during this test (Fig. 15-36).[59] We also like to use the cross-body adduction test as a decision tool. If the distal clavicle

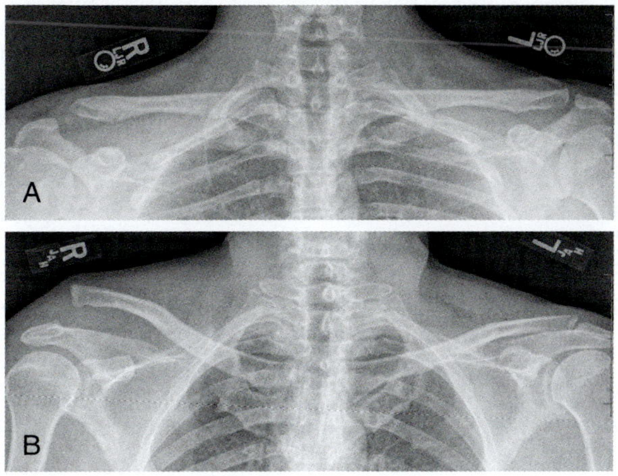

FIGURE 15-35: **A,** Right acromioclavicular (AC) Rockwood grade III joint dislocation. **B,** Right AC joint Rockwood grade V dislocation.

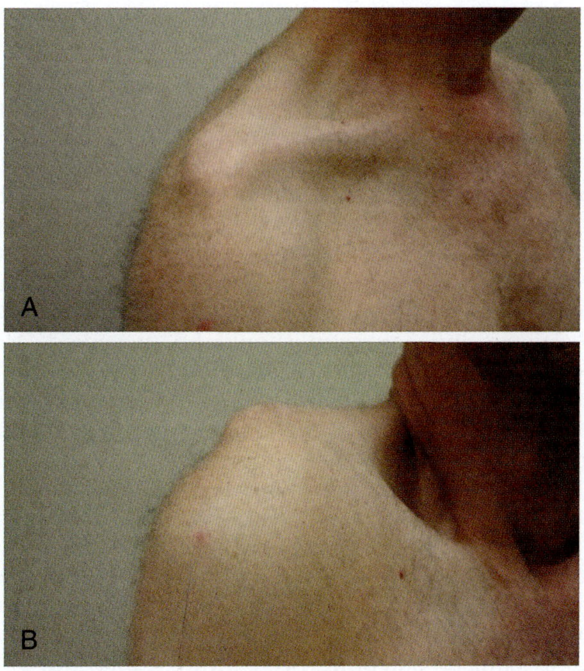

FIGURE 15-36: Right acromioclavicular Rockwood grade V joint dislocation shown at rest **(A)** and shrugging **(B)**.

displaces superiorly with pain on adduction of the arm across the body, the patient may do better with operative management.[139]

Benefits and Disadvantages of Arthroscopic Versus Open Surgical Approaches

Due to the lack of a gold standard operative technique for AC joint repairs, various procedures exist for both arthroscopic and open techniques. The basis of the conflicting opinions regarding surgical approach is largely related to visualization. Advocates of the arthroscopic approach note that ideal visualization remains elusive even during open procedures, leaving the patient susceptible to neurovascular injury during passage of suture or graft regardless of surgical approach.[782,783] An additional argument for these advocates is the minimization of soft tissue damage compared with dissection techniques required during open approaches. This advantage is particularly apparent in regard to the minimal takedown of the deltotrapezial fascia, which acts as a secondary stabilizer to the joint.

Proponents of the open procedure argue that increased visualization of both the clavicle and coracoid are essential. To begin, optimal exposure of the clavicle allows more precise dissection of the trapezius and deltoid insertions while also providing more exact placement of tunnels, which has been shown to affect repair integrity.[259] We are proponents of open procedures for these reasons, in addition to the benefit of a more robust pants-over-vest advancement of the deltotrapezial fascia during closure, which may contribute to increased AC stability. While the lack of deltotrapezial disruption may be of benefit in the acute setting, it is important to point out that in many high-grade (or chronic) AC lesions the damage to the deltotrapezial fascia has already occurred and therefore needs a robust repair to maintain the stability of the joint.[783]

Based on the current literature, and given the heterogeneity among study populations and surgical techniques, it is difficult to draw valid inferences on to the superiority of a particular approach. Irrespective of the surgical approach used, the experience of the senior author (A.D.M.), when considered in the context of multiple clinical and biomechanical investigations, has led to the development of the following principles when operatively managing the AC joint. (1) The bony anatomy of the clavicle and acromion should be preserved. More specifically, the distal clavicle should be preserved when possible because any disruption may result in further instability to the joint. (2) Anatomic reconstruction of the conoid and trapezoid ligaments should most reliably replicate the native CC ligamentous structures, which act as stabilizers to the joint. (3) The goal of management is to effectively reproduce the native three-dimensional motion pattern while simultaneously reestablishing substantial stability to the joint.[782,784] A subanalysis of a recent paper on clavicular bone tunnel position revealed comparable clinical outcomes with arthroscopic and open techniques.[158]

Technique: Arthroscopic Coracoclavicular Reconstruction

Arthroscopic CC reconstruction can be approached from either within the glenohumeral joint or from the subacromial space. Both approaches allow access to the inferior coracoid.

Glenohumeral Approach for Arthroscopic Coracoclavicular Reconstruction

This approach can be performed both in beach chair and lateral decubitus position but only the former is described. A standard posterior portal is used and a 30-degree arthroscope is inserted in the glenohumeral joint. This allows for additional examination to exclude any injuries to the glenohumeral joint and presents an advantage over the other approaches. A working portal in a low anterolateral position is carried out in an outside-in technique with a flexible cannula to allow instrumentation to the anterior-inferior surface of the base of the coracoid process. To have access to the coracoid base, dissection through the glenohumeral joint capsule is performed with a shaver or electrocautery device. The subscapularis tendon serves as the direct visual guide passing the rotator cuff interval between the superior and middle glenohumeral ligaments (Fig. 15-37). The debridement should be focused on the lateral part of the coracoid process to avoid neurovascular injury (Fig. 15-38). Once the coracoid process is reached, the arthroscope can be switched to an anterior-superior portal to afford superior visualization. Alternatively, a 70-degree arthroscope can be used from the posterior portal. To perform a safe

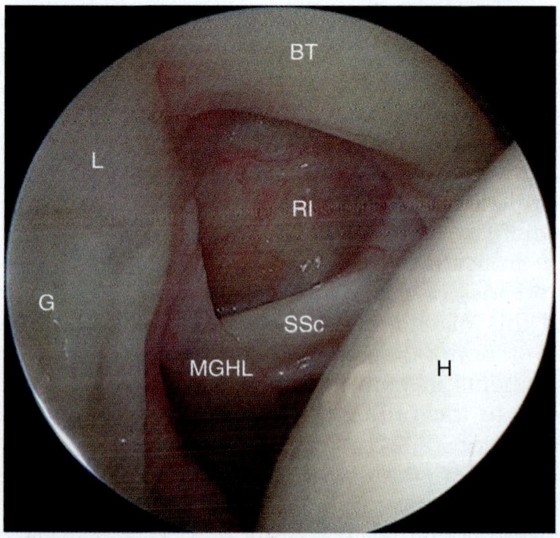

FIGURE 15-37: Intra-articular anatomy with special attention to the medial glenohumeral ligament (MGHL) and subscapularis (SSc), which will guide the surgeon to the coracoid base. BT, Biceps tendon; G, glenoid; H, humeral head; L, superior labrum; RI, rotator interval.

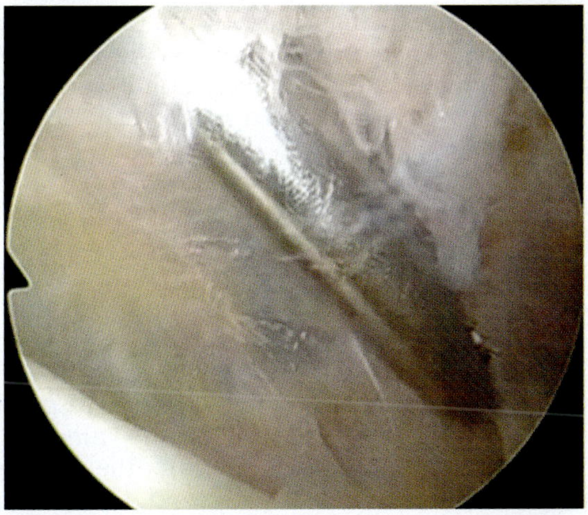

FIGURE 15-38: While viewing within the glenohumeral joint from the posterior portal, the base of the coracoid is debrided through an anterolateral working portal.

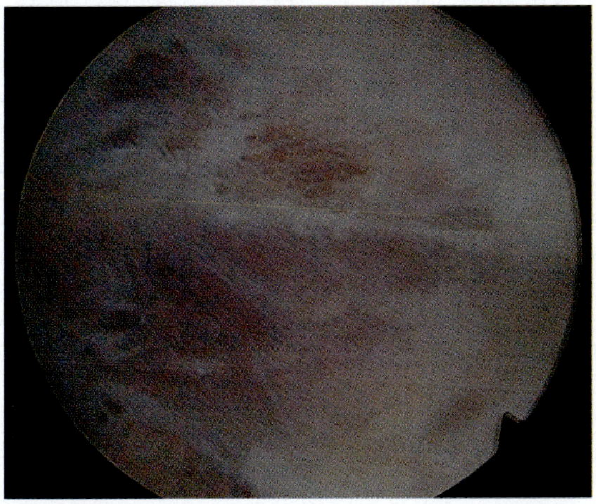

FIGURE 15-39: The inferior portion of the coracoid as seen from the lateral subacromial portal.

reconstruction, the inferior coracoid base has to be clearly visualized.[178]

Lateral Subacromial Approach for Acromioclavicular Joint Reconstruction

The patient is placed in the beach chair position using a special arm holder to secure the desired position. A straight lateral portal is established and a 30-degree arthroscope is placed in the subacromial space, if this is an isolated case of AC joint dislocation. To allow instrumentation during surgery, a second anterolateral portal is placed to visualize the coracoacromial (CA) ligament. The electrocautery device is used to debride down to the base of the coracoid process following along the CA ligament to the tip (Fig. 15-39). To perform a safe reconstruction, the inferior coracoid base has to be clearly visualized.[178]

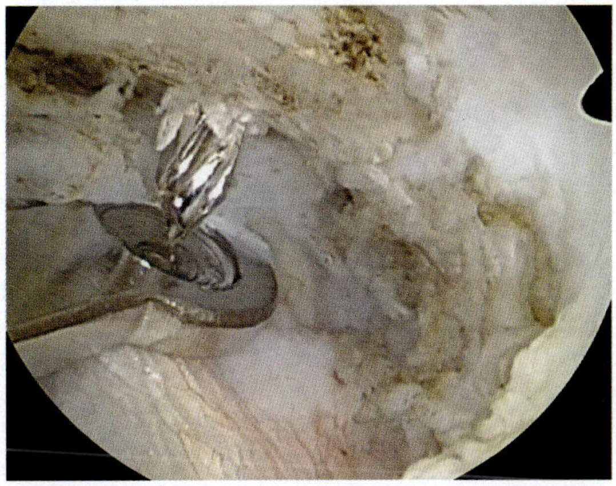

FIGURE 15-40: The pin should be clearly visualized and protected by the guide.

Coracoid Drilling

With undersurface of the base of the coracoids clearly visualized, the drill guide is placed via the anterolateral portal under the base of the coracoids. Care is directed at making sure the guide is centered under the coracoid to avoid eccentric drilling or notching of the coracoids. The drill sleeve of the guide is directed over the lateral clavicle approximately 4 cm medial to the AC joint. A small 2-cm saber incision is centered over the posterior aspect of the clavicle.

Minimal sharp and blunt dissection between the deltoid and trapezius muscles provides direct access to the superior cortex of the clavicle. Using a 2.4-mm canulated drill, all four cortices of the clavicle and coracoid are passed. Once the tip of the drill is visualized the core pin is removed and a flexible looped passing wire is delivered down the reamer (Fig. 15-40).

Coracoid and Clavicle Button

The coracoid button is loaded with two limbs of ultrahigh tensile suture. The sutures are then passed into the looped wire in the anterolateral portal. The sutures are delivered through the coracoid and out the top of the clavicle. A second clavicle button is then loaded onto the sutures and the AC joint is reduced. The sutures are then tensioned while the reduction is held manually, and the sutures tied over to secure the reduction.

Graft Passage

Some surgeons prefer to use a graft at this point to reinforce the fixation. The saber incision may have to be extended for dissection to the coracoid. The medial and lateral coracoid is dissected free of soft tissue. A coracoid passer, right angle clamp, or free needle can be used to pass a suture from medial to lateral, taking care to protect the nerves and vessels medial to the coracoid. The passing suture can then be used to pass a 5- to 6-mm graft around the coracoid. The limbs of the graft can then be docked into a small socket on the clavicle, or tied over the clavicle based on surgeon preference.

Surgical Technique for Anatomic Coracoclavicular Reconstruction

Patient Positioning and Preparation

The patient is placed in a beach-chair position with a bump placed underneath the medial border of the ipsilateral scapula for stabilization and to elevate the coracoid anteriorly. In the senior author's practice, 3-inch cloth tape and a safety belt are used to further stabilize the patient during the procedure. For optimal intraoperative repositioning, the head is left mobile. The patient is then draped in a standard fashion with wide exposure for adequate visualization of the sternoclavicular joint to allow the surgeon to work medially when placing the conoid tunnel. The patient is then prepped with a solution containing 2% chlorhexidine gluconate and 70% isopropyl alcohol.[783,785,788]

Exposure of the AC Joint

The skin incision for the ACCR is purposefully more medial than the Weaver-Dunn procedure to allow for adequate exposure of the medial clavicle. A 6.5-cm longitudinal incision is initiated approximately 3.5 cm medial to the AC joint starting at the posterior clavicle and progressing directly over or slightly medial to the underlying coracoid (Fig. 15-41). A needle-tipped bovie is then used to elevate skin flaps medially and laterally for adequate visualization while also maintaining adequate hemostasis. The deltotrapezial fascia is then dissected out in line with the demarcation between the posteriorly inserted trapezius and anteriorly inserted deltoid further exposing the underlying clavicle. The dissection should extend medially to expose the conoid ligament. This dissection is continued by splitting the intramuscular plane of the trapezius and deltoid insertions onto the clavicle using the needle-tipped bovie device. The posteriorly inserted trapezius and the anteriorly inserted deltoid muscles are peeled off as atraumatically as possible using an elevator, and full-thickness flaps are tagged with suture for later repair. Gelpi retractors are then used to retract the flaps and ensure proper visualization. Once the clavicle and acromion have been fully exposed, adequate anatomical reduction is confirmed by manual intraoperative reduction of the clavicle without restriction.[783,785-789]

Clavicular Tunnel Placement

Determination of proper placement of the conoid and trapezoid ligaments begins with measurement and marking of the clavicle with a surgical pen. The conoid and trapezoid tunnels will be roughly 45 and 25 mm medial to the lateral end of the clavicle, respectively, thereby leaving 20 mm separating the tunnels (Fig. 15-42). The basis for these distances is the progressive increase in bone mineral density and load to failure measurements of the clavicle from lateral to medial in addition to the approximate correlation to the anatomic locations of the CC ligaments.[783]

Next, a 2.4-mm guide pin is placed along the posterior-superior cortex at the marked site of the conoid tunnel. The pin should be directed roughly 30 degrees anterior in the direction of the coracoid process. Similarly, another 2.4-mm guide pin is placed on the anterosuperior aspect of the clavicle at the marked site of the trapezoid tunnel. Again the pin is directed roughly 30 degrees anterior in the direction of the coracoid process. Next, a 5.0-mm cannulated reamer is used in a "ream-in, pull out" manner for both tunnels—meaning the reamer is advanced under power and removed by hand to prevent eccentric reaming on removal. A 5.5-mm tap is then used to create thread holes for the screw. If needed based on size of the graft, the tunnel can be increased by 0.5-mm increments. However, small tunnel size is optimal to ensure a tight fit between tunnel and graft. A potential pitfall to consider during reaming is to carefully ensure the reamer does not "blow out" the posterior or anterior cortex of the clavicle when preparing the conoid and trapezoid tunnels, respectively. For preventative measures, irrigation is used while reaming to avoid thermal necrosis of the clavicular bone, and a Cobb

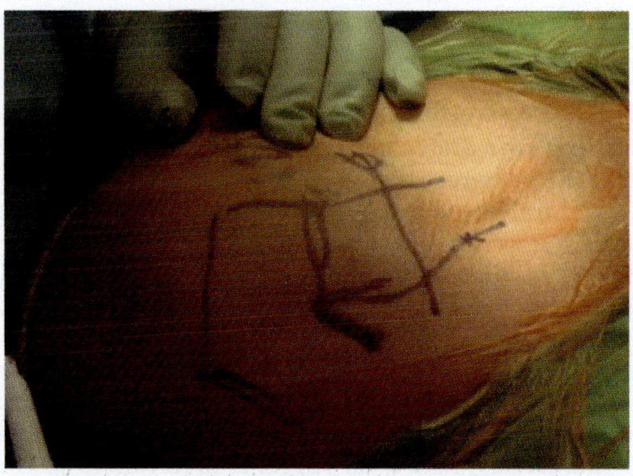

FIGURE 15-41: Planned incision and anatomic landmarks.

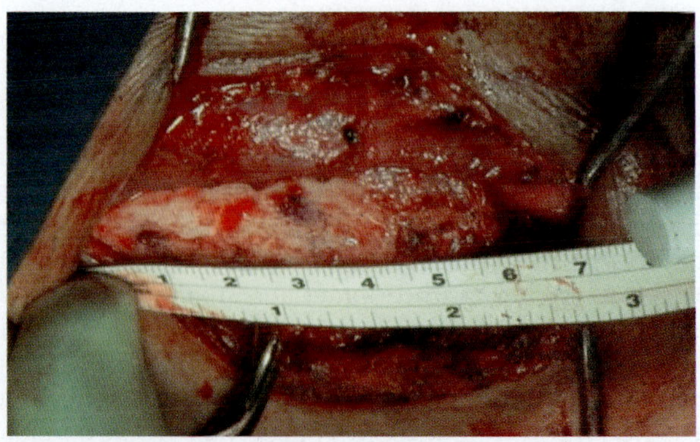

FIGURE 15-42: Measuring and marking for coracoclavicular tunnel placement.

retractor is placed underneath the clavicle to protect the underlying soft tissue.[783,785-789]

Preparation, Passage, and Fixation of the Graft

We prefer to use peroneus longus allograft for reconstruction, as it is typically easier to obtain compared with other grafts. Other possibilities for the graft include semitendinosus (allograft or autograft) or anterior tibialis (allograft). The graft is prepared with a whipstitch or grasping suture placed in both free ends using collagen-coated nonabsorbable suture (Arthrex, Inc.). The ends of the graft are then "bullet tipped" by making the diameter of the distal ends of the graft as small as possible, thereby easing passage of the graft through tunnels while also preventing fraying. The tendon is sized (typically 5 to 6 mm) and is ready for passage and fixation.

The first step in the passage of the graft is preparation of the coracoid graft fixation. A looped suture is passed underneath the coracoid base using a curved cannulated passing device (Arthrex, Inc.), which is loaded with a nonabsorbable high-strength suture. This suture is typically passed medial to lateral underneath the coracoid with the intention of minimizing risk to neurovascular structures. The looped end of the suture is then used for passage of the graft and collagen-coated nonabsorbable suture. The graft serves as the biologic portion of the repair while the suture acts as an internal brace during healing and is considered the nonbiologic portion of the repair. When passing the graft it is important to consider the diameter of both ends; the surgeon should attempt to have the thicker end passed into the trapezoid tunnel because the lateral clavicle is more prone to failure.

After passing underneath the coracoid the thinner graft is pulled in an inferior to superior direction through the conoid tunnel until roughly 2 cm of excess graft extends superiorly above the clavicle. The thicker end of the graft is passed in a similar inferior-to-superior fashion through the trapezoid tunnel. At this time, adequate reduction of the AC joint is achieved by provisional fixation via pointed reduction forceps and verified with an intraoperative mini C-arm. It is recommended to over reduce the AC joint by 2 to 3 mm to compensate for anticipated loss of reduction postoperatively. After confirmed reduction, both ends of the graft are cyclically tightened to remove slack from the system. The conoid ligament is then secured using a 5.5 × 8 mm cannulated polyetheretherketone (PEEK) tenodesis screw. The trapezoid ligament in then secured in a similar fashion. Finally, the nonabsorbable suture previously shuttled underneath the coracoid is passed through the cannulated PEEK screws in an inferior-to-superior manner. The suture is then tied together over the superior aspect of the clavicle.[783,785-789]

Acromioclavicular Joint Capsule Repair and Wound Closure

The excess graft of the trapezoid ligament is then sewn to the posterior acromion, replicating the posterior AC ligament. The remaining graft is then wrapped around the anterior clavicle, bringing the graft up posteriorly to create a sling effect that replicates the superior AC ligament. Any remaining graft is then sewn onto itself. Finally, the conoid limb of the graft is sewn to the trapezoid limb for further strengthening of the repair (Fig. 15-43).

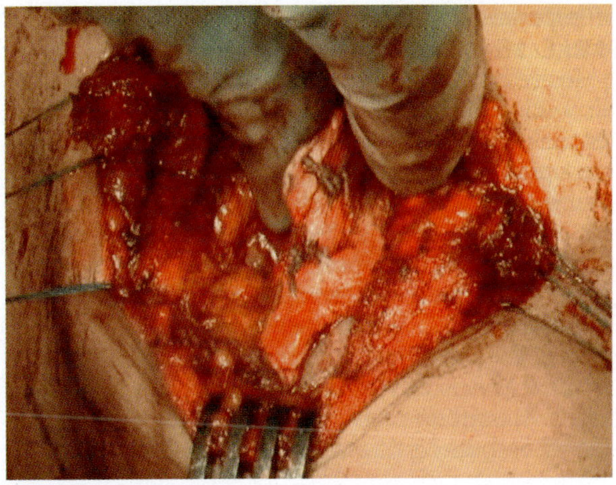

FIGURE 15-43: Stabilized acromioclavicular joint capsule after repair. Deltotrapezial flaps are tagged and will be closed with interrupted nonabsorbable polyester suture.

The deltotrapezial flaps are then closed with interrupted nonabsorbable polyester suture. Braided absorbable suture is then used for deep dermal closure followed by absorbable monofilament for a running subcuticular wound closure.[783,785-789]

Rehabilitation Protocol

See Table 15-3.

Outcome

Historically, many articles have been published on the modified Weaver-Dunn and other nonanatomic techniques. However, clinical outcomes of dual tunnel anatomic CC reconstruction are not well documented in literature. In a retrospective cohort analysis of 28 military personnel who underwent both arthroscopic and open CC reconstructions, the overall failure rate was 28.6% (8/28) at an average of 7.4 weeks postoperatively.[158] Comparison of bone tunnel position showed that a medialized bone tunnel was a significant predictor of early loss of reduction for the conoid and trapezoid bone tunnels. Failed reconstructions had tunnels which were on average 7 to 9 mm more medial. Conoid tunnel placement was also a statistically significant predictor of return to duty of the military population. There were no differences between the arthroscopic and open techniques on subgroup analysis. As this technique becomes more popular in the future, data on clinical outcome studies should become more plentiful and shed light on proper treatment.

TABLE 15-3 Rehabilitation Protocol After Anatomic Coracoclavicular Reconstruction

	0-8 Weeks	8-12 Weeks	12-20 Weeks	24 Weeks
ROM	Shoulder completely immobilized. Home exercise program may involve movements of the distal arm (hand, wrist, forearm, elbow).	Active assisted ROM	Full ROM	Full ROM
Strengthening	No strengthening exercises during this period.	Closed-chain scapular exercises and kinetic chain activities.	Resistance training can begin with rowing exercises initiated and progressing to isotonic scapular strength exercises (Blackburn exercises).	Full activity as tolerated.
Important considerations	This is a time for biological healing of the operative repair. Patients remain immobilized in a platform brace for support.	This period is focused on restoring ROM and scapular control. Painful activity resulting from increased load to the AC joint should be approached cautiously as tolerated.	Strengthening is focused on scapular strengthening, thereby reducing stress on the AC joint. When the patient can demonstrate active forward elevation while maintaining control of the scapula, isometric scapular holds are prescribed.	Higher load activities may be initiated, such as bench press, shoulder press, overhead lifts, and pectoral fly exercises. Patients may begin full contact athletics and heavy labor; however, full strength may not return until 9-12 months postoperatively.

AC, Acromioclavicular; ROM, range of motion.

Arthroscopic Treatment of Shoulder Stiffness and Rotator Cuff Calcific Tendinitis

Amit Nathani, Ryan A. Mlynarek, Asheesh Bedi

The stiff shoulder is a common and challenging problem for treating surgeons. The terms *adhesive capsulitis* and *frozen shoulder* are often used interchangeably in the literature, although these refer to distinct pathologies that cause shoulder stiffness. Numerous surgical and nonsurgical treatment options have been proposed, which reflect the lack of complete understanding of the disease process. The development of a responsible treatment plan requires accurate diagnosis of the various etiologies of shoulder stiffness due to dissimilar treatment approaches. The etiologies include primary adhesive capsulitis, secondary adhesive capsulitis, and iatrogenic (i.e., shoulder stiffness secondary to surgical intervention). Natural history and clinical outcome studies comparing surgical and nonsurgical management are rather limited, and there is a consensus need for robust studies to refine indications and improve clinical decision-making. This section describes the continued evolution of treatment as it relates to shoulder stiffness, focusing primarily on the technical aspects and outcomes of arthroscopic management.

PRIMARY ADHESIVE CAPSULITIS

Overview

The term *frozen shoulder* was initially coined by Codman in 1934 to describe a condition that is characterized by pain and reduced ROM at the shoulder.[146] Neviaser described the term as a "waste-can diagnosis" and stressed the importance of differentiating between a painful and stiff shoulder and a distinct pathologic entity termed *adhesive capsulitis*; his assertion was based on intraoperative findings of capsular fibrosis and inflammation.[505-508] Nevertheless, the terms *frozen shoulder* and *adhesive capsulitis* continue to be used interchangeably. A recent survey of the American Shoulder and Elbow Society resulted in a consensus definition of frozen shoulder: "a condition characterized by functional restriction of both active and passive shoulder motion for which radiographs of the glenohumeral joint are essentially unremarkable except for the possible presence of osteopenia or calcific tendinitis."[781] Adhesive capsulitis is classified as primary or idiopathic, wherein an underlying etiology cannot be identified, or secondary, which has a similar histopathologic appearance but results from a known intrinsic or extrinsic cause.

The estimated incidence of adhesive capsulitis is between 2% and 5%, and the condition primarily affects women between the ages of 40 and 60 years.[80,285,292,323,763] Other risk factors for adhesive capsulitis include diabetes,[80,438,467,529] thyroid disease,[759] and autoimmune disorders.[94,606] The disease is poorly understood but thought to be a combination of synovial inflammation and capsular fibrosis that results from an imbalance in the local cytokine milieu. Increased expression of transforming growth factor β, platelet-derived growth factor, interleukin 1β, tumor necrosis factor α, and vascular endothelial growth factor are found in the synovium.[611,620] The result is a hyperplastic and neovascular tissue response leading to a capsule with highly fibroblastic properties, similar to that seen in Dupuytren disease.[95] The microscopic changes in tissue architecture parallel the four stages of adhesive capsulitis proposed by Neviaser and Neviaser, which are based on arthroscopic evaluation.[293] Stage 1 and 2 are characterized by hypervascular synovitis, most prominently in the rotator interval, whereas stage 3 and 4 lack the acute inflammatory signs but show dense synovial thickening that typically involves the rotator interval, coracohumeral ligament, and anterior capsule extending into the inferior capsular recess.[508,754] Clinical staging is more commonly used. Reeves described the stages of progression from painful freezing, through frozen, to thawing over a duration of 2 to 3 years.[592] The stages represent a continuum of disease, rather than discrete, well-defined phases.

The diagnosis of adhesive capsulitis is primarily one of exclusion, made from the history and physical exam. Though formal diagnostic criteria have not been developed, commonly referenced clinical findings include (1) a painful stiff shoulder for at least 4 weeks, (2) severe shoulder pain that interferes with activities of daily living or work, (3) nocturnal pain, (4) painful restriction of both active and passive shoulder ROM (forward elevation in scapular plane <100 degrees, >50% restriction of external rotation compared with contralateral side), and (5) normal radiographic appearance.[88] Plain radiographs should be obtained for all patients to rule out alternative sources of pain and stiffness, that may include osteoarthritis, calcific tendinitis, or rotator cuff disease. Though not routinely recommended, relevant MRI findings may include thickening of the coracohumeral ligament and rotator interval; the "subcoracoid triangle sign" or obliteration of the fat triangle, or subcoracoid fat between the coracohumeral ligament and the coracoid process, and a loss of the axillary recess indicative of contracture of the joint capsule and reduced joint volume (Fig. 15-44).[128,217,462,694] The extent of shoulder range restriction tends to correlate with joint volume reduction.[419]

Management

Adhesive capsulitis is a painful and debilitating disease, typically with a protracted course. In 1934, Codman stated that "recovery is always sure and may be confidently expected" in patients with frozen shoulder, while advocating for nonoperative management. While many authors have characterized the natural history since then, management approach is still evolving and remains controversial. Some studies suggest initial management with benign neglect, supervised neglect, home stretching programs, or formal physical therapy generally results in good outcomes,[195,284] while others report long-term pain and a residual loss of motion.[57,285,292,532] Miller et al. reported the disease process as completely self-limiting with all 50 patients followed for 10 years obtaining resolution of the disease, as measured by pain and ROM testing, with a home rehabilitation program and antiinflammatory medication.[467] Shaffer et al., on the other hand, reported residual pain and/or loss of motion in up to 50% of patients over a mean of 7 years of follow-up.[646] The majority of the cited studies are case series that describe a single therapeutic approach, thus direct comparison is difficult. Studies commonly describe outcomes at time points greater than 1 year, which can be too long of a time period for patients to wait for relief of symptoms; thus clinical decision-making becomes further complex.

Nonoperative Management

Given the self-limiting natural history, the mainstay of initial treatment for adhesive capsulitis is nonsurgical. A number of nonoperative options exist and all have been shown to have positive short-term results. These include physiotherapy/home therapy,[401,467,514] supervised neglect,[195] steroid injection,[90,341] hydrodilatation,[569,586,715] oral steroids,[91] and nerve blockade.[170,353] In our practice, we prefer formal physical therapy in combination with a home program. Intra-articular steroid injections are offered in cases where pain is a limiting factor. This corresponds to stages 1 and 2, where an inflammatory component is present. In a randomized study that looked at 93 patients, the combination of steroid injection and physical therapy was more effective treatment than injection alone, physical therapy alone, or placebo.[125] We do not routinely use the other aforementioned techniques. In refractory cases in which patients continue to have a passive mechanical block to motion after 6 months of therapy, we consider manipulation under anesthesia (MUA) and arthroscopic release.

Closed Manipulation

We do not routinely perform closed manipulation in isolation; however, in cases of refractory pain and stiffness in patients with primary adhesive capsulitis, it can be considered. Our preferred technique is manipulation followed by arthroscopy. Under general anesthesia or interscalene block, the patient is placed in the beach chair position. First, a gentle examination of passive shoulder motion is compared with that of the contralateral side. With the scapula stabilized with one hand, the other is used to grasp the distal humerus and manipulate

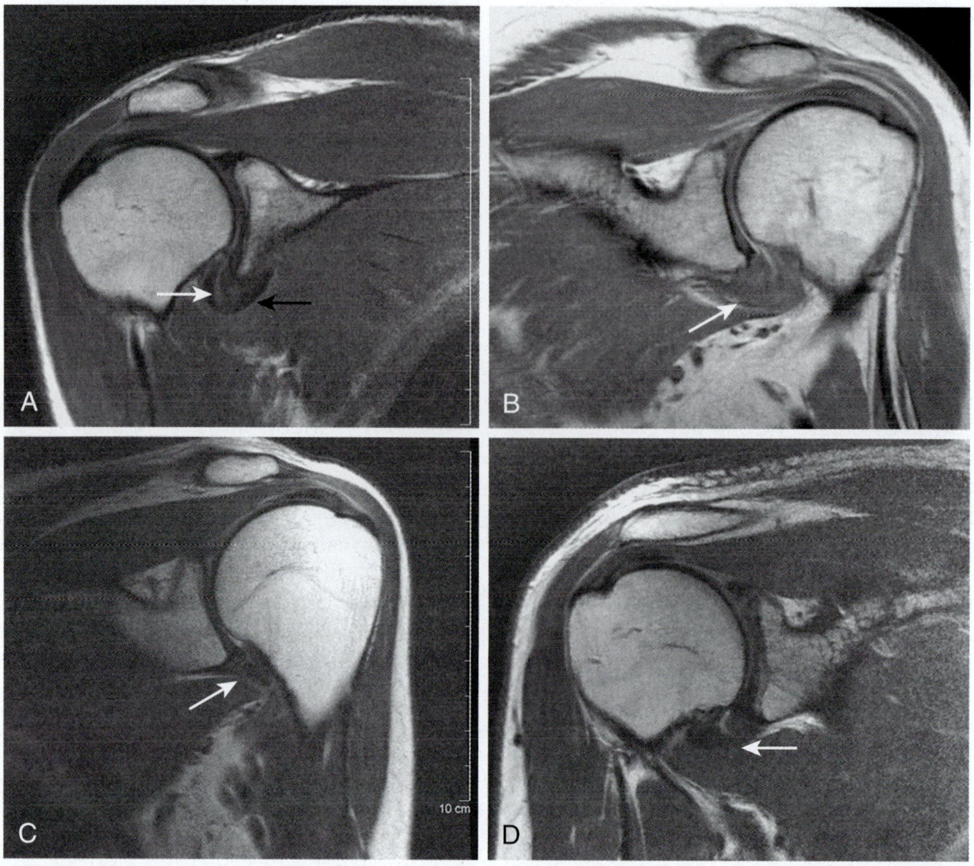

FIGURE 15-44: Magnetic resonance images demonstrating adhesive capsulitis. **A,** Stage 1 adhesive capsulitis. The inferior capsule (*black arrow*) is thickened. The synovium (*white arrow*) can be distinguished from the capsule and the inferior recess is maintained. **B,** Stage 2 adhesive capsulitis. The inferior capsule (*arrow*) is hyperintense and now markedly thickened. **C,** Stage 3 adhesive capsulitis. The inferior capsule (*arrow*) is hypointense, representing mature capsular scar. There is complete loss of the axillary pouch. **D,** Stage 4 adhesive capsulitis, with partial reconstitution of the axillary pouch and reappearance of synovium. The inferior capsule (*arrow*) is less thickened compared with stage 3. (Courtesy Hospital for Special Surgery, New York, NY.)

the extremity with a short moment arm to decrease chance of a torsional humeral fracture. First, forward flexion in the scapular plane is performed followed by external rotation with arm at the side. Often, audible and palpable yielding of tissue with minimal force confirms an effective manipulation. Passive terminal ROM is repeated and recorded. Outcomes of closed manipulation have largely been reported to be excellent[201,225]; however, comparative studies have shown equivocal benefit when compared with home exercise therapy.[371] Farrell et al. showed patients who underwent closed manipulation for frozen shoulder achieved sustained improvements in ROM over a mean follow-up of 15 years.[225] However, a more recent randomized controlled trial that compared patients undergoing MUA with a control group failed to show a benefit to manipulation; both groups showed similar improvement at all-time points up to 1 year.[371] A recent systematic review found an overall complication rate of 0.4% with MUA, with proximal humerus fracture being the most common.[279] Others have reported complications such as glenohumeral dislocation, rotator cuff and labral tears, and brachial plexus injuries. Typical findings during postmanipulation arthroscopy are hemarthrosis and capsular tearing.[415] If ligament or tendon tearing is noted, this may suggest a need for improvement in the manipulation technique.

Arthroscopic Treatment

As stated earlier, our preferred technique for refractory stiffness is closed manipulation followed by arthroscopy. Arthroscopy has several advantages, including the opportunity to address any concomitant pathology such as debridement of synovitis, biceps-related pathology, and allows for a more controlled and complete capsular release not achieved with manipulation. The order of arthroscopy before or after manipulation is controversial. Performing the manipulation first may facilitate placement of the arthroscope into the joint and decrease the risk for chondral damage. Others advocate performing arthroscopy before manipulation, as any capsular tearing during manipulation will cause a hemarthrosis and make visualization more difficult. The plane of the traumatic capsular tearing created during manipulation may be unfavorable as well.

Arthroscopy is initiated using a standard posterior portal. A spinal needle-guided anterior portal is established under direct vision above the leading edge of the subscapularis and just lateral to the middle glenohumeral ligament. Depending on the stage of disease, there may be extensive synovitis in addition to capsular thickening (Fig. 15-45). A synovectomy can be atraumatically performed with a 4.5-mm motorized shaver. Next, the capsular release is performed with the aid of an arthroscopic radiofrequency device. The rotator interval is first released under direct visualization starting the capsular division anterior and inferior to the biceps tendon and continuing inferior to the upper edge of the subscapularis tendon (Fig. 15-46).[298] In the prearthroscopic era, experience from open capsular release of the rotator interval has been reported to restore external rotation in patients with refractory adhesive capsulitis.[536] With adequate release, the humeral head begins to become more mobile, moving inferiorly and laterally, thus allowing improved access to the anterior and inferior capsule. The release is now carefully continued anteriorly and inferiorly to include the middle glenohumeral ligament and anterior band of the IGHL all the way to the 6 o'clock position, and releasing the capsule in layers to protect the underlying subscapularis muscle belly and the adjacent labrum (Fig. 15-47). As one moves inferiorly, care is taken to perform this release in layers under direct visualization, to work from an "outside-in" technique, and to place the arm in adduction and external rotation to protect and minimize risk of injury to the axillary nerve. The arthroscope is removed and motion again tested. The arthroscope can then be switched to the anterior portal to examine the posterior capsule and to debride synovitis or release any capsular contracture to perform a complete 360-degree release if necessary, though our experience suggests that this is usually not required (Fig. 15-48). A recent systematic review found an overall complication rate of 0.6% during or following an arthroscopic capsular release, with superficial wound infection and brachial plexopathy cited as most common.[279] We have had no cases of axillary nerve injury using the above technique.

Postoperatively, the goal is to maintain the intraoperative ROM that was achieved, provide adequate pain control, and begin immediate supervised therapy. An interscalene nerve block or indwelling catheter in the recovery room has been shown to be beneficial in allowing the patient to tolerate early motion following shoulder arthroscopy.[84,370] Physical therapy with aggressive ROM and hydrotherapy is recommended 5 days per week for the first 2 weeks and three times per week until

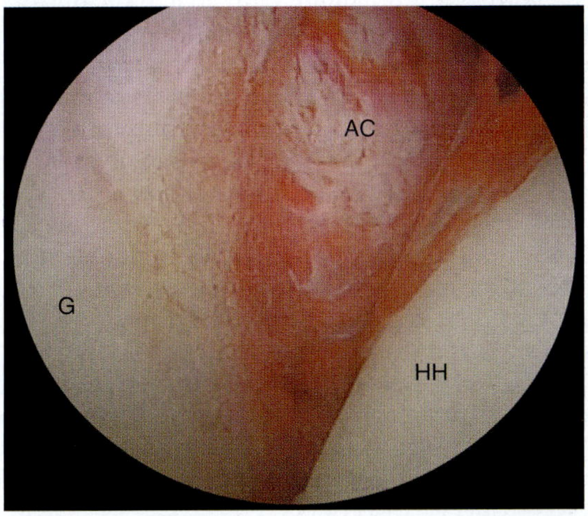

FIGURE 15-45: Arthroscopic view of a glenohumeral joint with stage 2 adhesive capsulitis prior to synovectomy or capsular release. The anterior capsule (AC) shows hypervascular synovitis and capsular proliferation. *HH,* humeral head; *G,* glenoid.

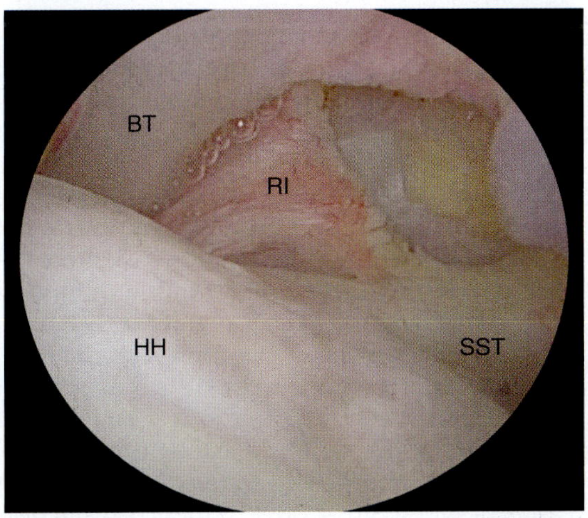

FIGURE 15-46: Arthroscopic view following rotator interval (RI) release between the long head of the biceps tendon (BT) and subscapularis tendon (SST). *HH,* humeral head.

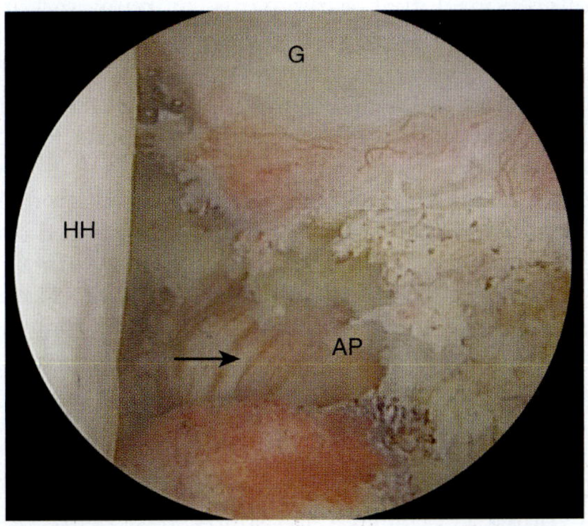

FIGURE 15-47: Arthroscopic view following release of the inferior capsule in the axillary pouch (AP) using an outside-in technique. Underlying muscle fibers (*arrow*) can be visualized following adequate release. *HH,* humeral head; *G,* glenoid.

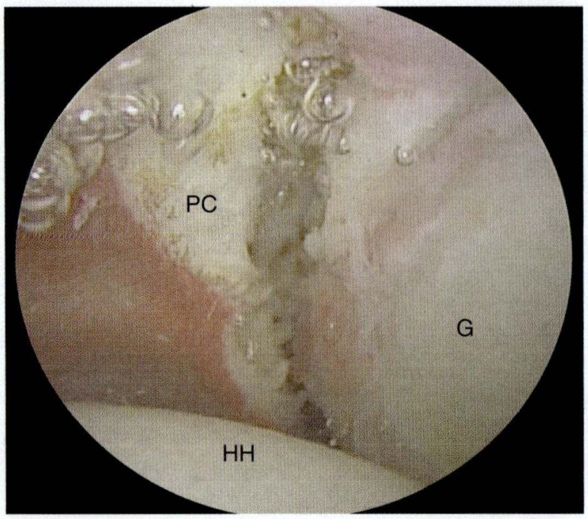

FIGURE 15-48: Arthroscopic view from the anterior portal shows posterior capsule (PC) release. *HH,* humeral head; *G,* glenoid.

treatment is completed. A home program of stretching is also a critical component to optimize outcomes.

Outcomes

Arthroscopic capsular release has become more commonplace. The techniques have been well described and limit the scope for any intra-articular damage.[573,734] A multitude of studies in the past few years have supported the role of arthroscopic release as safe and effective, particularly for the treatment of recalcitrant cases of frozen shoulder.[43,52,142,212,665] In a level III comparison of MUA and arthroscopic division of the joint capsule, patients treated with arthroscopy were twice as likely to be pain free at 2 years' follow-up. Additionally, nine of the 20 patients treated with MUA alone had residual functional deficit compared with three of 20 patients treated with arthroscopy.[528] Most recently, Le Lievre and Murrell reported that early gains in pain and motion after arthroscopic capsular release were maintained or enhanced over a mean follow-up duration of 7 years.[396] There is some debate about how much of the capsule should be released. Jerosch described a 360-degree capsular release,[345,535] as the posterior release is thought necessary to alleviate significant internal rotation deficit. However, a recent level III study that compared anterior release with anterior plus posterior release did not show any benefit to the more extensive technique.[665] Another study showed early gains with combined anterior and posterior release, but longer-term outcomes were similar to those of isolated anterior release.[135]

Secondary Adhesive Capsulitis

While primary adhesive capsulitis has been used to describe the idiopathic global capsular inflammation and fibrosis that occurs in the absence of other lesions, secondary adhesive capsulitis by definition is associated with intrinsic or extrinsic conditions that limit shoulder mobility. Intrinsic conditions that have been implicated include rotator cuff tears, bursitis, and tendinitis, while extrinsic factors may include trauma, repetitive overuse injuries, and surgical procedures, including arthroscopic thermal capsulorrhaphy, resection of calcific tendinitis, and capsular shift procedures.[261,483] These conditions demonstrate isolated areas of capsular contracture that are histopathologically indistinguishable from idiopathic adhesive capsulitis, but occur concurrently with other known injuries or diseases.[504] Distinguishing between idiopathic and secondary disease can be difficult and there is frequent overlap. Yoo et al. reported partial-thickness supraspinatus tears in 62% of patients with stage 2 idiopathic adhesive capsulitis diagnosed on MR arthrography.[775] Clues from the history and physical examination can allow discrimination between primary and secondary disease. Patients with secondary adhesive capsulitis typically have a more acute onset of symptoms, present with day and night pain that typically occurs a few weeks after the insult. Physical therapy at this stage to prevent stiffness is often unsuccessful as any manipulation tends to exacerbate the symptoms. Treatment options include pain control and gentle stretching until the initial painful stage subsides. There is a paucity of literature regarding secondary adhesive capsulitis, but typically aggressive manipulation or surgery has not been recommended.[508,733] Indeed, following the initial painful stage and after appropriate treatment of the patient's underlying etiology, the prognosis tends to be good. In some cases of recalcitrant frozen shoulder secondary to a posttraumatic or a postsurgical etiology, circumferential arthroscopic capsular release has shown good results, though the data are limited.[515] More research is needed to define surgical indications, if any, for this very heterogeneous group of disorders.

SECONDARY SHOULDER STIFFNESS

Overview

Shoulder stiffness following surgical intervention has numerous etiologies and should be distinguished from primary or secondary adhesive capsulitis. Shoulder stiffness is common following instability procedures, fracture surgery, and in the context of rotator cuff tears. Stiffness is typically preceded by a course of prolonged immobilization. While guided physical therapy is often the first-line treatment to regain motion, some authors advocate for a more aggressive approach given more unfavorable outcomes in the literature.[733] Holloway et al. compared the results of arthroscopic capsular release in patients with primary frozen shoulder to those with postoperative and postfracture stiffness. Over a mean follow-up duration of 20 months, the postoperative stiffness group had significantly lower pain scores, patient satisfaction, and functional restoration compared with those in the other two groups.[312] Gerber et al. reported similar findings on comparing the same three groups following arthroscopic capsular release. At 26 months' follow-up, the Constant score, pain, ROM, and quality of sleep were least favorable in the posttraumatic group.[262]

Stiffness After Instability Procedures

Stiffness is one of the most common problems following shoulder arthroscopy, with overall rates estimated to be between 2.7% and 15%.[745] Beyond postoperative morbidity, some patients are left with significant residual functional deficits.[648] Stiffness following instability procedures can result from an excessively tightened anterior capsule, errant closure of an anatomic variant or sublabral foramen, and can lead to an internal rotation contracture. The humeral head is forced posterior, and this change in position can lead to failure of the posterior capsule and degeneration of the articular cartilage, a devastating result in the young patient (Fig. 15-49).[420] Historical procedures that shortened the subscapularis tendon also led to this complication ("postcapsulorrapy" arthritis). Following a failed course of nonoperative treatment, arthroscopy has a role when stiffness is secondary to a capsular contracture. When external rotation is limited to less than 60% of the contralateral shoulder following these procedures, arthroscopic capsular release has shown good results.[262,733,735]

Stiffness After Fracture

Fractures of the proximal humerus commonly lead to stiffness. Physical therapy is usually successful following fractures treated nonoperatively in the absence of malunion and secondary osseous impingement. Stiffness following open reduction and internal fixation can be due to a number of causes, which may include poor reduction and capsular, subdeltoid, and subscapularis tendon scarring. Though arthroscopy has a limited role, it can be considered prior to considering corrective osteotomy or arthroplasty. Burkhart described an arthroscopic subscapularis tenolysis for refractory stiffness following open fixation of a proximal humerus fracture. ROM was reestablished following arthroscopic capsular release of the middle glenohumeral ligament and of adhesions surrounding the subscapularis.[97] With proper patient selection, we have had good results in our practice with anterior-inferior arthroscopic capsular release and synovectomy in patients who have postfracture stiffness due to capsular contracture. More customary treatment is open surgical hardware removal with lysis of adhesions.

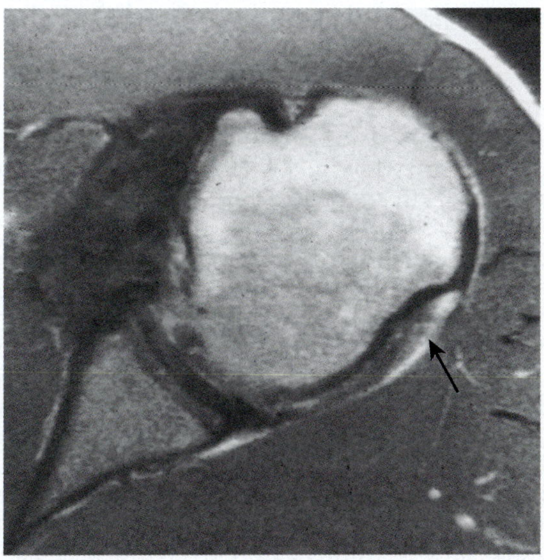

FIGURE 15-49: Axial magnetic resonance image demonstrating posterior capsular failure (*arrow*) following open capsular shift. (Courtesy Hospital for Special Surgery, New York, NY.)

Stiffness and Rotator Cuff Disease

With respect to stiffness, rotator cuff surgery represents several challenges for the treating surgeon. An aggressive rehabilitation program in the early postoperative period places the repair at risk for failure, whereas prolonged immobilization may increase the likelihood of arthrofibrosis. Correctly identifying patients who are stiff preoperatively is equally as important as recognizing the postoperative patient who is developing stiffness. Stiffness and the presence of rotator cuff pathology is common.[775] Regardless of etiology, the decision of whether or not to restore ROM before rotator-cuff repair is controversial. Tauro reported on 66 patients who underwent arthroscopic rotator cuff repair with a preoperative total ROM deficit less than 70% of the uninvolved extremity. All patients had improved ROM postoperatively, and none required manipulation or further surgery. Of the six patients who underwent rotator cuff repair with a preoperative deficit greater than 70%, three required arthroscopic capsular release at an average of 5.5 months to regain ROM. He thus recommended repair after resolution of stiffness in such patients.[695] Trenerry et al. reviewed 209 patients who had preoperative stiffness and who underwent rotator cuff repair and found that the only preoperative predictor of postoperative stiffness was hand behind the back motion.[713]

Despite the best efforts of patients and surgeons, a small percentage of patients undergoing rotator cuff surgery become stiff and fail conservative management. In this group, closed manipulation or arthroscopic capsular release is supported to effectively restore motion and relieve pain.[735] Care should be taken to ensure that the rotator cuff was not malreduced, and which may serve to limit postoperative passive and active ROM.

CALCIFIC TENDINITIS

Overview

Calcific tendinitis is a relatively common disorder of unknown etiology characterized by a cyclical progression of reactive calcium hydroxyapatite crystal intratendinous deposition, which is followed by spontaneous resorption and healing of the tendon. First described in the early 1900s, the condition may affect any tendon in the body; however, rotator cuff is most commonly involved.[145,540,629] Reported prevalence of the disease varies between 2% and 20%, often identified as an incidental finding on chest radiographs.[71,676] Welfling et al. examined 925 patients presenting with a painful shoulder, and found an overall prevalence of 6.8%; the highest prevalence was amongst patients aged 31 to 60 years.[676,748] Calcific tendinitis most commonly affects the "critical zone" of relative hypovascularity of the supraspinatus tendon (70% to 83%) as described by Moseley and Goldie[322,416,491,571] (Fig. 15-50). Recent studies have indicated it is the result of a metaplastic cell-mediated transformation of tenocytes into chondrocytes, which then induce calcification.[717] These foci of metaplasia are then phagocytized by giant cells and ultimately, the tendon remodels to reform normal tendon.[179] There are several classification and staging schemes to characterize the disease process, the details of which are beyond the scope of this chapter.[189,224,252,276,417,483,553]

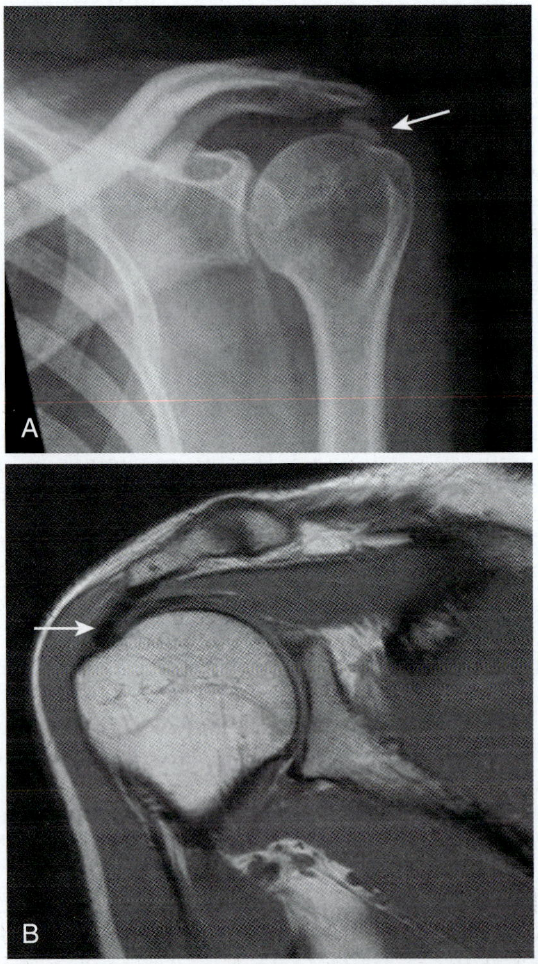

FIGURE 15-50: A, Anteroposterior radiograph of the left shoulder demonstrating a calcific deposit (*arrow*) located superior to the greater tuberosity. **B,** Magnetic resonance image of the right shoulder demonstrates an intratendinous calcific deposit (*arrow*) within the supraspinatus tendon. (Courtesy Hospital for Special Surgery, New York, NY.)

Nonoperative Treatment

Typically, calcific tendinitis is a self-limiting disease that causes low-grade pain and may be associated with concomitant shoulder stiffness. The condition tends to respond well to oral analgesics such as NSAIDs, physical therapy, and activity modifications. However, symptoms can be severe and long lasting and confer substantial disability.[258] In patients who do not respond to conservative management, more invasive treatment options may be considered. There is no consensus on the preferred treatment, and therefore several options are available. The most common include SAI, ultrasound-guided needling and lavage (barbotage), and extracorporeal shock wave therapy. SAI is inexpensive, relatively low risk, and easy to perform. Many studies have shown an improvement in pain, ROM, and function after SAI when compared with placebo.[1,4,61,566] In a randomized controlled trial by de Witte et al., patients in both SAI and ultrasound-guided barbotage treatment groups experienced improved pain and functional scores at 1-year follow-up. However, clinical outcome scores and radiographic calcification size was significantly better after barbotage.[193] Kim et al. recently published a randomized controlled trial that compared barbotage with extracorporeal shock wave therapy, finding improved clinical outcomes and decreased calcium deposit size in both groups, but the barbotage group experienced greater pain relief in the initial 6-month follow-up period.[369] Although all above treatments are relatively safe with low complication rates, there is no evidence to assess their effectiveness when compared with a placebo control group given that this is a self-limiting disease.[258]

Arthroscopic Treatment

In our practice, patients presenting with signs and symptoms consistent with calcifying tendinitis of the rotator cuff are initially treated with NSAIDs and physical therapy. They are offered a SAI to improve pain, decrease inflammation, and facilitate better participation in physical therapy focusing on ROM exercises. They are counseled regarding the natural history of the disease process and the expected peak of inflammation and pain often experienced during the acute resorptive phase of the disease.[717] For those patients with severe, recalcitrant pain affecting ROM at the 6-month period, surgical treatment can be considered.

Surgical decompression was historically performed in an open fashion, but with advances in surgical technique and instrumentation over the past 20 years, arthroscopic decompression has become the gold standard treatment. Rubenthalar et al. performed a prospective randomized controlled trial of open versus arthroscopic decompression in 38 patients and found equivalent clinical outcomes at 17-month follow-up.[618]

We perform arthroscopic decompression in the beach chair position under general anesthesia combined with preoperative regional anesthesia for postoperative pain control. We obtain adequate orthogonal radiographs and MRI prior to surgical incision to ensure adequate localization of the calcified deposits intraoperatively. Fluoroscopy is used if deposits are difficult to localize. The glenohumeral joint is first accessed using the posterolateral portal. A thorough diagnostic arthroscopic examination of the shoulder is performed and any concurrent pathology is addressed. Special attention is paid to the integrity of the rotator cuff insertion, and any partial- or full-thickness tears are noted for consideration of subsequent repair. If the calcium deposits can be visualized from the articular side, a passing suture is used to tag the location for evaluation from the bursal side. The subacromial space is then accessed via the same posterolateral portal. An anterolateral working portal is then established and an adequate bursal debridement is performed with a motorized shaver to maximize visualization and mobility within the subacromial space. The bursal surface of the rotator cuff is then evaluated for intratendinous calcium deposits. A probe is used from the anterolateral portal to evaluate the integrity of the rotator cuff and to palpate for intratendinous deposits. The location of the calcium deposits is compared with the preoperative radiographs, to ensure that all areas have been located intraoperatively. A needle can assist in localization of deposits, which often have the appearance of powdered sugar within the tendon. If necessary, fluoroscopy or ultrasound may be used.

Sabeti et al. reported that the use of intraoperative ultrasound facilitates the detection of calcium deposits and significantly reduces the number of needle punctures to detect the deposits, thus decreasing operative time and increasing shoulder function outcome scores and pain relief at 2 weeks and 9 months of follow-up.[621] However, we appreciate the learning curve associated with using intraoperative ultrasound and therefore use fluoroscopy when localization is challenging. Once all deposits are localized, a percutaneous spinal needle is then used from the lateral approach in line with the rotator cuff fibers to approximate portal placement. A linear incision is made in the tendon, with careful attention paid not to violate the articular side of the tendon. A probe, switching stick, or arthroscopic grasper is then used to mobilize the calcium deposits, while exercising due diligence to minimize iatrogenic damage to the tendon. Once the deposit is removed, a motorized shaver is used in oscillation mode with suction to remove any small fragments and floating debris. Confirmatory fluoroscopy may be performed to ensure adequate excision.

Whether all calcium deposits must be excised is controversial in the literature. Porcellini et al. performed arthroscopic excision of calcium deposits in 63 patients and found that patients with residual calcifications detected on postoperative ultrasound at 2 years' follow-up achieved satisfactory functional outcomes, but a significant decrease in pain relief when compared with those patients without residual calcifications.[578] Other studies have failed to reproduce a significant difference in clinical functional outcomes or pain relief when residual calcifications are appreciated on postoperative imaging.[18,428,644] It is our opinion that a balance must be achieved to excise as much of the calcium deposit as possible without compromising the integrity of the rotator cuff tendon that would then necessitate a large rotator cuff repair and rehabilitation course for the patient.

Once the calcium deposits have been removed, the integrity of the rotator cuff tendon is evaluated. Typically, the calcium deposits are localized from the bursal side alone and do not violate the articular side of the tendon. If there is only a small, partial-thickness defect of the bursal-sided tendon, we do not typically perform a repair. However, if the defect is full thickness or if the rotator cable is violated, then the rotator cuff is repaired. Often the defect is intratendinous and can be fixed with simple sutures across the linear tear. However, if the defect is U-shaped and has compromised a portion of the footprint, anchors are utilized and generally single-row fixation is sufficient.

After addressing the rotator cuff, attention is turned to the CA ligament and the acromion process. These are evaluated for fraying and signs of mechanical outlet impingement to assess the potential need for concomitant SAD. The need to perform a SAD is controversial in the literature.[18,578,618,644,706] Authors generally agree that when subjective signs of mechanical impingement (fraying of the underside of acromion or CA ligament, presence of acromial osteophyte) are present, a SAD is warranted. However, Jacobs et al. performed arthroscopic excision of calcium deposits in 61 shoulders and concomitant SAD in those patients with fraying or degeneration of the CA ligament (14 of 61 shoulders) and found no significant difference in functional outcome scores between patients in whom a SAD was performed.[342] Balke et al. have recently published an attempt to objectively define radiographic parameters of the acromiohumeral relationship to better define the indication for SAD.[30] They found that the acromion index (AI) (described by Nyffeler et al.) in patients with calcifying tendinitis is similar to those patients presenting with subacromial impingement, but no difference in Bigliani classification, acromial tilt (AT), or lateral acromial angle (LAA) when patients with calcifying tendinitis were compared with a control group.[56,522] Therefore we combine preoperative radiographic evaluation of the coracoacromial arch (AI, AT, LAA calculations) with the patient's history, physical examination for signs of impingement, and intraoperative findings to determine whether SAD is warranted on an individualized basis. If a SAD is planned, calcific deposit excision and possible rotator cuff repair is performed first to prioritize procedures prior to joint swelling and bleeding from acromioplasty.

Several studies have reported on the outcomes of arthroscopic calcium excision.[18,31,216,347,483,578,591,644] Balke et al. published mid-term results of arthroscopic treatment of calcifying tendinitis in 70 shoulders with 6-year follow-up. They report a significant improvement in functional outcome scores and improvement in pain.[31] Although most commonly identified in the supraspinatus and infraspinatus tendons, calcific tendinitis has been successfully treated arthroscopically in various other locations.[20,238,335] Vinanti et al. recently published excellent short-term results after arthroscopic calcium deposit excision from atypical locations about the shoulder (medial supraspinatus muscle belly, subscapularis tendon, and the long head of biceps tendon).[728] Complications following arthroscopic treatment of calcifying tendinitis are infrequently encountered, but may include infection, stiffness, neurovascular injury and rarely, ossifying tendinitis.[463,520] Merolla et al. reported two cases of ossifying tendinitis following arthroscopic treatment of calcifying tendinitis, both of which were treated successfully with arthroscopic excision of the hydroxyapatite crystals in a histologic pattern of lamellar bone.[463]

Arthroscopic Management of Prearthritic and Arthritic Conditions of the Shoulder and the Postarthroplasty Shoulder

Adam J. Seidl, Alexa Narzikul, Joseph A. Abboud

INDICATIONS FOR ARTHROSCOPIC TREATMENT

The utility of arthroscopy for treating glenohumeral arthritis has been recently questioned. The current American Academy of Orthopaedic Surgeons clinical practice guidelines classifies the use of arthroscopy for the treatment of glenohumeral arthritis as grade I, implying that they are unable to recommend for or against this option.[340] Furthermore, a systematic review of the literature by Namdari et al. showed that arthroscopic debridement for glenohumeral arthritis lacks high-quality evidence to support its routine use.[501] Despite this, we have found that the utility and benefits of arthroscopic treatment of glenohumeral arthritis in certain clinical scenarios.

Any surgical treatment should be preceded by an adequate trial of conservative management that includes activity modification, physical therapy, antiinflammatory medication, and corticosteroid injections. Injectable viscosupplemention is an additional nonoperative treatment option, although there is a paucity of evidence that supports its use in the shoulder, and it is not currently approved by the U.S. Food and Drug Administration for injection in joints other than the knee.[153] When these nonoperative measures fail, TSA is considered the gold standard for treating severe glenohumeral arthritis. However, in some patients, a joint reconstruction is not desirable, possible, or practical, and arthroscopic treatment may be the best alternative. Elderly patients with significant medical comorbidities might be unable to tolerate the stresses involved with a major surgery; in these patients an arthroscopic intervention might be more suitable. Conversely, a young patient who has developed early onset arthritis might not be the best candidate for TSA due to concerns related to prosthesis longevity and/or the high functional demands of the patient.[281] Sperling et al. studied the long-term outcomes of TSA and hemiarthroplasty in patients aged under 50 years and noted a 59% rate of glenoid lucency after TSA and a 68% rate of radiographic glenoid erosions after hemiarthroplasty. At a minimum follow-up of 5 years, more than 50% of patients in both the groups had radiographic findings that were of some concern.[681,682] Finally, some patients (of any age) have significant pain, but diagnostic studies reveal only mild arthritic changes in the glenohumeral joint, making it difficult to justify the utility of arthroplasty in these patients.

Studies have shown that coexistent soft tissue pathology is common in patients with osteoarthritis.[747] Arthroscopy provides an opportunity to diagnose and treat these secondary conditions, perhaps eliminating the need for arthroplasty. The benefits of a lower complication rate and quicker return to normal activities after arthroscopy compared with TSA make this scenario quite appealing.[58,747]

Patients with shoulder pain do not frequently undergo arthroscopic surgery, and intraoperatively, significant arthritis is noted that was not observed on preoperative workup.[288] Cameron et al. and Guyette et al. also found that preoperative radiographs and clinical examination were unreliable in predicting osteoarthritis that was intraoperatively documented.[121,288] In these patients, it is crucial to know what can be arthroscopically performed to address unexpected osteoarthritis.

TECHNIQUE AND OUTCOMES

Standard Setup and Overview

At our institution, we typically perform shoulder arthroscopy in the beach chair position. A standard posterior arthroscopic portal is first established, approximately 1 cm medial and 2 cm distal to the posterolateral border of the acromion. With the arthroscope in the posterior portal, a standard anterior interval portal is established under direct visualization using a spinal needle. Coexisting pathology observed on preoperative workup should be considered before placing this portal because minor changes in position can significantly aid certain procedures such as distal clavicle excision.

We utilize an arthroscopic pump for these cases as this facilitates lavage of the joint throughout the procedure. The pump is also helpful for parts of the procedure that cause bleeding such as synovectomy. Accessory portals may be required depending on the pathology.

We perform a systematic diagnostic arthroscopic evaluation followed by treatment that involves the following procedures: debridement and loose body removal, capsular release, microfracture for focal full-thickness chondral defects, biceps treatment (tenotomy or tenodesis) if warranted, and finally SAD and acromioplasty. We do not routinely take up patients with large osteophytes for arthroscopic treatment, and thus do not perform aggressive procedures such as osteophytecomy or axillary neurolysis. In addition, we do not currently perform glenoidplasty or glenoid recontouring because we consider a significant asymmetric wear as a contraindication to arthroscopic treatment. Lastly, we rarely perform biologic resurfacing in our practice because the inherent risk of complications and the lack of documented favorable mid- and long-term results. The following sections detail a comprehensive list of possible arthroscopic procedures for the treatment of glenohumeral arthritis and the outcomes associated with these procedures. Although we do not use all of these procedures, we believe that a competent shoulder surgeon should be aware of all possible options and the documented success or failure of these options.

Debridement

The components of arthroscopic debridement include lavage, synovectomy, removal of small to moderate osteophytes, debridement of chondral flaps, debridement of degenerative labrum or partial rotator cuff tears, and removal of loose bodies. The extent and aggressiveness of the debridement depends on the location and nature of the pathology found on systematic diagnostic evaluation.

Debridement of osteophytes is performed using an arthroscopic shaver and/or burr. The goal of debridement is to remove potential points of impingement of the glenohumeral joint and synovium. Authors have argued that osteophytes are a result of degeneration and not a significant cause of pain and that osteophytectomy is ill conceived.[732] While there are no objective data clarifying periarticular osteophytes as being a source of pain, their removal does has mechanical benefits. Osteophytes tend to restrict excursion of the capsule, and their removal can confer an immediate increase in ROM. Osteophytes of the inferior humeral head are most common and can be particularly problematic clinically. Use of an accessory low anterior or posterior portal can be helpful in removing these bone spurs. These portals are safe when spinal needle localization is employed and appropriate anatomic landmarks are recognized. The accessory posterior portal is established approximately 2 cm inferior to the site of the standard posterior portal, and the view is obtained by moving the camera anteriorly. The shaver or bur tip must be maintained intra-articular at all times to avoid injury to the axillary nerve.

Flaps of cartilage should also be debrided to alleviate mechanical causes of symptoms and potentially slow the progression of the injury (Fig. 15-51). In the case where there is an area of full-thickness focal cartilage loss, beveling the edges of the lesion has been shown to be detrimental. Instead, a perpendicular cartilage margin should be created.[619] This debridement may be combined with microfracture, as discussed later in this section.

Removal of loose bodies can be performed using an arthroscopic grasper or a pituitary rongeur. Removal of loose bodies can be one of the greatest sources of relief for the patient having mechanical (locking or blocking) symptoms, so it is important that they not be overlooked.

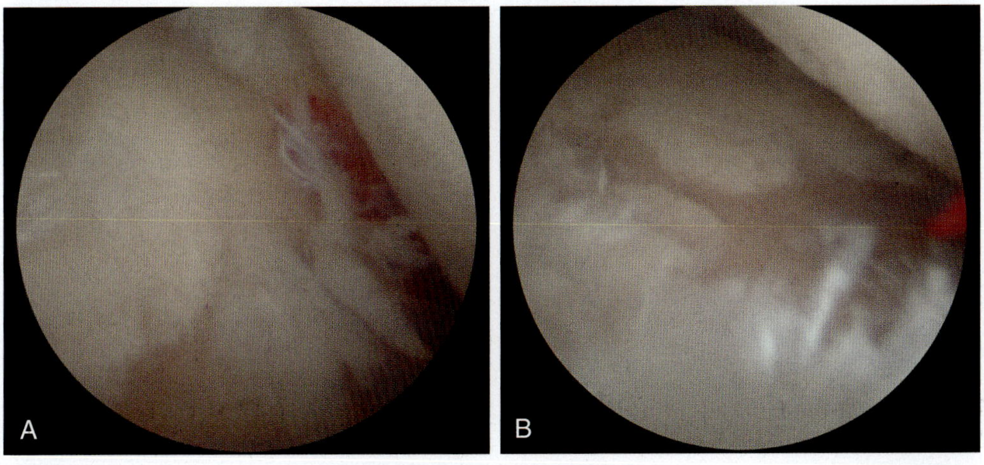

FIGURE 15-51: A, Full-thickness cartilage wear with chondral flap. **B,** Debridement of chondral flap.

Loose bodies often lodge in the subscapularis recess or axillary pouch and can be removed with a grasper (Fig. 15-52). An appropriate-size skin incision should be made before retrieving the loose body to avoid difficulties delivering it through the soft tissue.

Debridement of degenerative partial tears of the rotator cuff, labrum, and biceps are likely to alleviate mechanical symptoms and can contribute to pain-relief by elimination of a source of inflammation.[690] Degenerative labral tears are extremely common in the arthritic shoulder and should be debrided back to a stable rim (Fig. 15-53). Caution should be exercised when considering a superior labral repair in a patient with glenohumeral arthritis, because postoperative stiffness is common in this group. Any partial tear of rotator cuff encountered in the arthritic shoulder should be debrided. Tears involving less than 50% thickness of the biceps should be debrided as needed to improve tracking in the groove. Treatment of more significant biceps pathology, such as extensive tearing, subluxation, scarring, or immobility, ideally mandates either tenotomy or tenodesis and is discussed later in this chapter (see "Arthroscopic Management of Biceps/Labral Complex Injuries of the Shoulder") as well as in Chapter 17. In our hands, the biceps is critically evaluated and treated on a case-by-case basis according to the specific pathology.

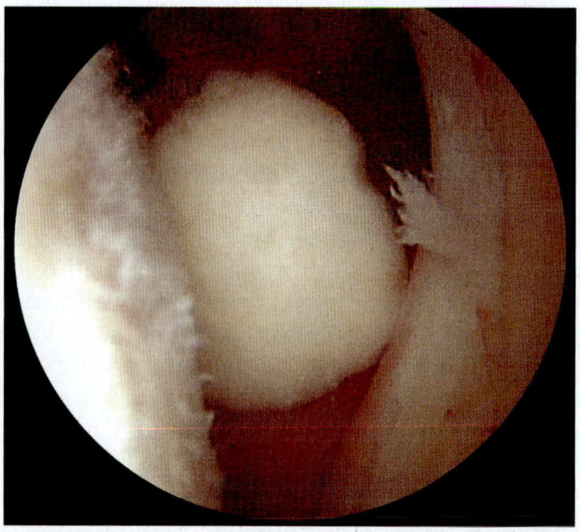

FIGURE 15-52: Loose body delivered by palpation from the subscapularis recess.

Given the high incidence of coexistent soft tissue pathology, outcome studies looking at isolated arthroscopic debridement in glenohumeral osteoarthritis are limited. In the knee literature, there is evidence that lavage alone can benefit patients with osteoarthritis.[220,320,336] In evaluating the role of arthroscopic debridement in the shoulder, Weinstein et al.[747] reported on 25 patients with Outerbridge grades II to IV osteoarthritis of the glenohumeral joint who underwent arthroscopic treatment including lavage, removal of loose bodies, partial synovectomy, and subacromial bursectomy, as well as debridement of cartilage lesions, degenerative labrum, and osteophytes. None of these patients had undergone a capsular release. Over an average follow-up of 34 months, 80% of the cases had excellent or good results with respect to pain relief. Patients who had return of pain at the final follow-up had a temporary pain relief lasting a minimum of 7 months. Of the 25, 92% stated they would undergo the procedure again. Out of the 13 recreational athletes, seven were able to return to preinjury level of play. Of note, a statistically significant correlation was observed between radiographic and arthroscopic grade of injury and patient satisfaction.[747]

Cameron et al. reported on the outcomes of 61 patients, 88% of whom had a mean duration of pain relief for 28 months. In addition to lavage and debridement, capsular release was performed in 22 of 61 patients. This study also found that patients with cartilage lesions larger than 2 cm^2 had increased incidence of pain recurrence after debridement.[121]

Safran and Baillargeon reported 80% good or excellent results in their series of 19 patients with grade IV changes, in whom simple arthroscopic lavage, chondral flap

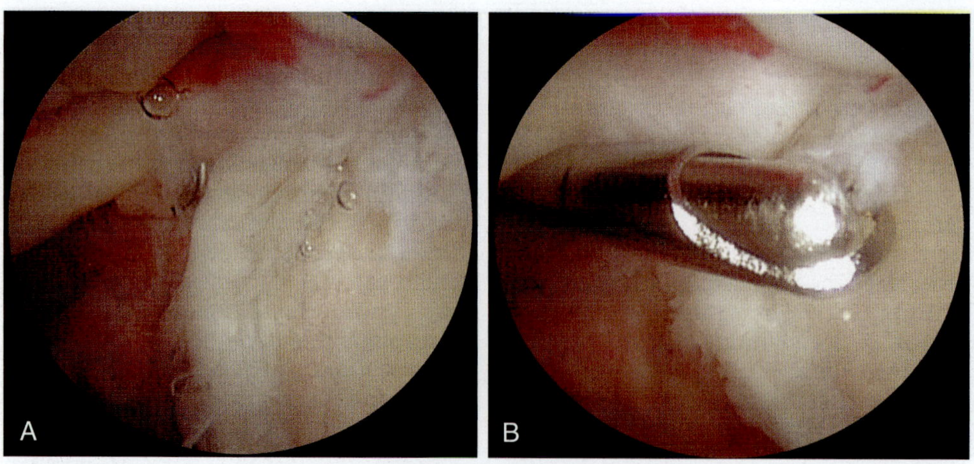

FIGURE 15-53: **A,** Degenerative superior labral tear. **B,** Debridement of superior labrum.

debridement, and bursectomy were performed. They downplayed the role of capsular release and bony procedures such as osteophyte removal, glenoidplasty, and SAD.[622]

Kerr and McCarty evaluated 19 patients (20 shoulders) all under the age of 55 that underwent arthroscopic treatment for glenohumeral arthritis, which included debridement and loose body removal without capsular release. They found that poor outcome was not related to the grade of the lesion, but was related to lesions being bipolar. Patients with unipolar lesions had higher outcome scores than those associated with bipolar lesions.[362]

Van Thiel et al.[725] published the largest series to date was composed of 71 patients treated with arthroscopic debridement for glenohumeral arthritis. In this series, all patients underwent glenohumeral debridement of whom a number of patients required concomitant procedures (44 capsular release, 15 biceps tenotomy/tenodesis, 11 microfractures, 28 SADs). Sixteen (22%) of their patients went on to arthroplasty after a mean interval of 10 months after arthroscopy. In the patients that did not require arthroplasty, they found significant improvement in ASES, simple shoulder test (SST), and VAS scores as well as improved ROM. On comparing patients who required arthroplasty with those treated successfully with arthroscopy, the presence of grade 4 bipolar arthritis, a joint space of less than 2 mm, and presence of large osteophytes appeared to be risk factors for failure of arthroscopic treatment.[725]

Millet has published on his technique and outcomes for what he terms the comprehensive arthroscopic management (CAM) procedure for glenohumeral arthritis.[469,471] This technique involves a combination of debridement, chondroplasty, removal of loose bodies, humeral osteoplasty and osteophyte resection, capsular release, SAD, axillary nerve neurolysis, and biceps tenodesis.[469] Axillary neurolysis is justified in that author's opinion as the axillary nerve is often in close proximity to the inferior humeral osteophytes and that compression of this nerve could contribute to posterior shoulder pain in a manner similar to that in quadrilateral space syndrome.[469] Results of the CAM procedure have been promising; Millet et al. reported on a group of 30 patients, of which 24 did not require arthroplasty over an average follow-up period of 2.6 years. ASES score and pain levels improved significantly for those patients not going on to arthroplasty. Survivorship analysis for the CAM procedure showed 1-year survival rate of 92% and 2-year survival rate of 85%.[471] Similar to the conclusions of Van Thiel et al., they found that patients with less than 2 mm of joint space had a significantly higher rate of failure.[471,725]

Capsular Release

Routine capsular release during arthroscopy for glenohumeral arthritis has been advocated. Capsular tightness, as evidenced by decreased ROM, increases joint contact pressures, and thus can be a source of pain. Release of the capsule alleviates the joint contact pressure. At our institution, we routinely perform a capsular release as part of the arthroscopic treatment of glenohumeral arthritis.

Capsular release is performed through well-placed standard portals. Once the diagnostic arthroscopy and intra-articular debridement (described above) are complete, the capsular release is performed. Arthroscopic cautery is used to release the rotator interval first. This includes transection of the coracohumeral ligament and the SGHL. To perform the anterior release, the capsule is released with an arthroscopic biter approximately 1 cm lateral to the glenoid starting at the level of the interval (Fig. 15-54). This release is carried down through the middle glenohumeral ligament and capsule covering the subscapularis, the anterior band of the IGHL and into the axillary pouch. Great care is taken to identify the axillary nerve and stay posterior and medial to it as the release extends into the pouch. Some authors have suggested use of arthroscopic scissors that offers the advantage of tactile feedback that is quite handy while working in this area.[39] Freeing up any adhesions between the subscapularis and capsule can help optimize motion. The posterior and superior capsule can be released in a

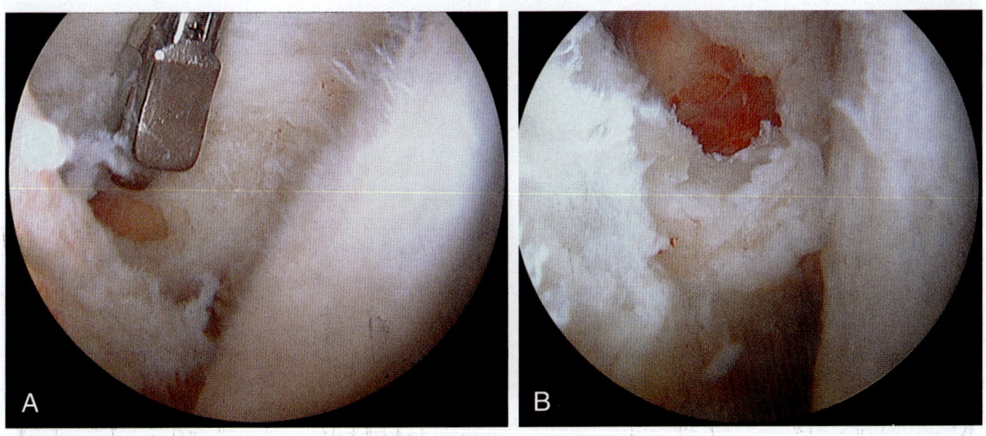

FIGURE 15-54: A, Arthroscopic biter used for capsular release. **B,** Extension of release to axillary pouch.

similar fashion by viewing through the anterior portal. Of note, posterior release is contraindicated in the setting of posterior extrusion of the humeral head.[521]

Ogilvie-Harris and Wiley, in an early retrospective review of their 10-year experience with shoulder arthroscopy, supported capsular release when stiffness coexists with osteoarthritis; 14 of their 54 patients with osteoarthritis had stiffness that required manipulation and/or capsular release. Without providing specifics, the authors stated that these patients benefited more than those in whom only debridement was performed.[530]

As previously mentioned, Cameron et al. performed capsular release in 22 of 61 patients undergoing arthroscopic debridement for grade IV osteochondral lesions. Their indication for capsular release was a 15-degree loss of passive motion. Pain relief was achieved in 88% of their patients overall. In the 22 patients who had capsular release, the mean forward flexion increased from 119 degrees to 157 degrees, external rotation from 23 degrees to 46 degrees, and internal rotation from L2 to T11.[121]

Nowinski and Burkhead reported 77% good or excellent results in a series of 13 patients with grade IV arthritis who were treated with debridement, capsular release, and manipulation under anesthesia. The release was not dependent on preoperative ROM; 12 out of 13 patients underwent SAD and distal clavicle excision as well.[521]

Skelley et al. demonstrated potential short-lasting benefit of debridement and capsular release. They reviewed outcomes in 33 patients who underwent isolated arthroscopic debridement and capsular release by a single surgeon and found initial improvement in ROM and pain that lasted only 3.8 months, before a relapse to preoperative values. A significant number of patients (42%) went on to TSA at an average of 8.8 months after arthroscopy.[659]

MICROFRACTURE

Microfracture involves penetration of the subchondral bone to promote bleeding from cancellous bone. This blood, that contains pluripotent marrow-derived mesenchymal cells, forms a clot in the cartilage defect, which ultimately leads to fibrocartilage formation at the site.[92,374,377,478,684] Steadman first described the technique of microfracture of the knee in 1997.[685] In his experience with 1200 cases, Steadman achieved a 75% success rate, with pain being the factor most affected by the surgery.[684] On review of the literature, success rates have tended to range between 60% and 95%.[92]

We perform microfracture for the treatment of focal full-thickness cartilage defects of either the glenoid or humerus (Outerbridge grade IV or ICRS grade 3/4). In our experience, accessory portals are often unnecessary but should be considered if a lesion cannot be easily approached through standard portals. Anterosuperior glenoid lesions are most easily addressed through a laterally placed anterior portal, while inferior lesions may require a lower portal just proximal to the subscapularis. Posterior accessory portals are often useful for posterior glenoid lesions. Humeral lesions can be treated through standard portals by rotating the arm.

Following debridement and capsular release, a shaver is used to remove any additional cartilage flaps and to confirm containment of the lesion. As discussed previously, beveling of the cartilage should be avoided and curettes can be used to create a perpendicular margin. Arthroscopic awls (with varying angulation) are then used to penetrate the subchondral plate perpendicular to its surface. Awls can be impacted in a controlled fashion with a mallet or gently levered on the humerus in case of an osteoporotic bone (Fig. 15-55). Attention should first be paid to the periphery of the lesion and proceeding towards the center of the lesion with holes (2 to 3 mm deep) placed approximately 3 to 4 mm apart (Fig. 15-56). Appropriate spacing between holes is crucial to avoid fracture between the penetrations. Decreasing pump pressure or temporarily shutting off the inflow allows for confirmation of the release of marrow elements.

In the knee, factors that have been associated with decreased success of microfracture include BMI greater than 30 kg/m^2, age older than 35 to 45 years, and preoperative symptoms lasting more than 12 months.[27,377,478] Additionally, the size of the lesion has also been shown

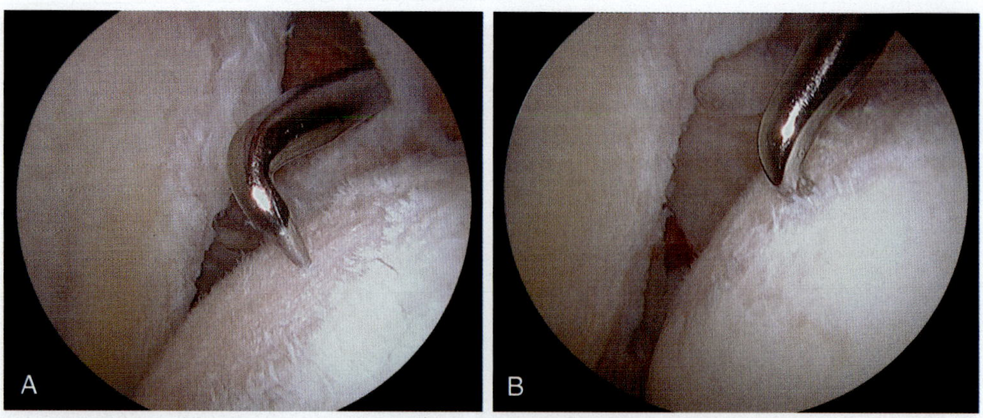

FIGURE 15-55: A, Arthroscopic awl used for microfracture of humeral head. **B,** Levering of awl in osteoporotic bone to penetrate subchondral plate.

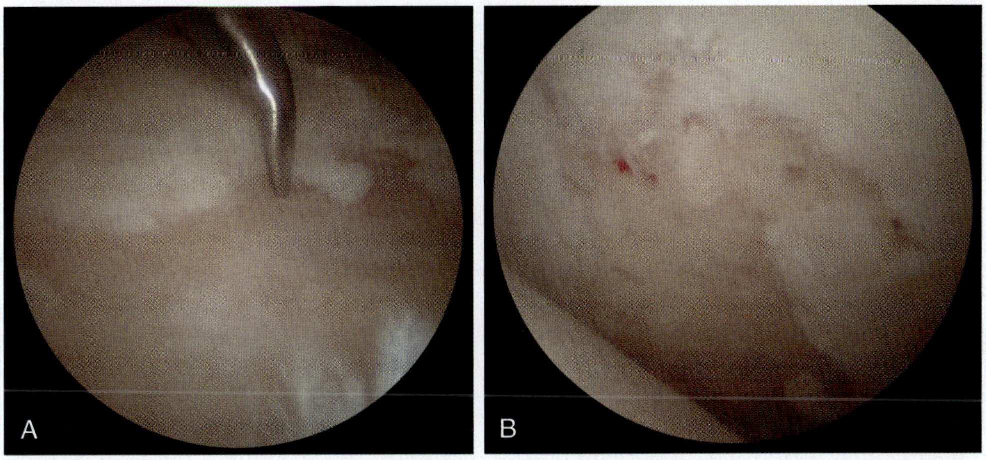

FIGURE 15-56: **A,** Arthroscopic awl used for microfracture of glenoid. **B,** Glenoid after microfracture, showing spacing of holes.

to affect results in the knee. Bae et al. found healing rates of 99% when the lesion of the femoral condyle was less than 3.0 cm^2, and 86% when these were greater than 3.0 cm^2. Notably, they also found variable amounts of type II collagen in all of the 18 patients who had second-look biopsies, with 22% of these demonstrating staining greater than 75% that of normal cartilage.[27]

Evidence supporting microfracture in the shoulder is still somewhat limited, but reports of a favorable experience exist with both open and arthroscopic techniques.[121,122,241,655] Frank et al. reported on the outcomes of 14 patients (15 shoulders) who underwent arthroscopic microfracture of the humeral head and or glenoid. In this series, the mean age was 37 years; the average size of humeral cartilage defect was 5.07 cm^2, and the glenoid cartilage defect was 1.66 cm^2. Microfracture produced significant improvement in pain, SST and ASES scores, over an average follow-up duration of more than 2 years. Three patients required subsequent surgery, which included osteochondral allograft placement and hemiarthroplasty. Overall, 92% of patients expressed their willingness to undergo repeat microfracture surgery.[241]

Millet et al. reviewed 30 patients (31 shoulders) who underwent arthroscopic microfracture procedure. In their series, 13 patients had an isolated glenoid lesion (mean size, 1.37 cm^2), 12 had an isolated humeral lesion (mean size, 4.22 cm^2), and 6 had a combination of humeral and glenoid lesions (mean size, 4.42 cm^2 and 2.73 cm^2, respectively). They reported significant improvement in VAS, ASES, and ROM overt a mean follow-up duration of 47 months. Lower outcome scores were associated with a history of prior shoulder surgery and that of two or more concomitant procedures performed at the time of microfracture. Location of lesion was found to be an important predictor of outcome scores. Patients who were treated for an isolated humeral head lesion experienced the greatest improvement, while those treated for bipolar lesions or isolated glenoid lesions showed less improvement. Six patients required subsequent shoulder surgery, three of whom went on to undergo TSA.[472]

Glenoidplasty

Patients with osteoarthritis often have asymmetric wear of the glenoid with more wear occurring posteriorly.[492] Nowinski and Burkhead listed a biconcave glenoid as a contraindication to arthroscopic treatment of glenohumeral arthritis.[521] However, other authors suggest that arthroscopic recontouring of the glenoid can be beneficial in selected cases.[58,683] O'Driscoll reported good to excellent results in 80% of the 14 patients who underwent arthroscopic glenoidplasty at 36 months.[526]

Although there are no peer-reviewed publications on arthroscopic glenoid recountouring, there is some published work concerning open glenoidplasty. Levine et al. emphasized the importance of addressing glenoid wear in patients with posterior glenoid wear. They documented inferior results in patients with type II glenoids who underwent hemiarthroplasty.

When the arm is raised in the scapular plane, the humeral head shifts to the posterior glenoid. In a healthy shoulder, the dynamic muscle stabilizers and static constraints of the glenoid contour prevent posterior subluxation.[673] When the posterior glenoid is eroded, posterior subluxation occurs, which can cause pain on arm elevation. A patient who has more advanced osteoarthritis and opts for arthroscopic treatment as a palliative measure can benefit from recontouring the glenoid using an arthroscopic bur or bone-cutting shaver. Some authors recommend planing down the inferior 20% of the glenoid as well to relieve pressure on the inferior humeral head.[673] However, if TSA is conceivable in the future, the surgeon should preserve as much bone on the glenoid as possible. In addition, severe retroversion generally requires open glenoid osteotomy rather than arthroscopic treatment.

Resurfacing

Several authors have described arthroscopic resurfacing of the glenoid. Brislin et al. described a technique that involved implantation of a porcine graft material prepared on the back table to fit the glenoid, which was attached using suture anchors. In their preliminary series of 10 patients, decreased pain, increased forward flexion and abduction, and reconstitution of joint space on plane radiograph was noted.[81]

Arthroscopic resurfacing with lateral meniscal allograft has also been described. This arthroscopic technique evolved in response to promising results with open meniscal interposition.[32,562] The arthroscopic technique involves shaping the meniscal allograft into an appropriate-size ring with sutures. This is then manipulated into position arthroscopically and fixed with anchors to the glenoid. Preliminary results in 10 patients showed an enhanced quality of life due to alleviation of pain and improved function. However, it should be noted that in addition to the resurfacing, extensive debridement of osteophytes, cartilage, and soft tissue as well as capsular release were performed. These procedures alone have been associated with benefit.

More recently, De Beer et al., Savoie et al., and Porcellini et al. have published on their technique and results of biologic resurfacing.[176,632] De Beer et al. reported on a series of 32 patients who underwent arthroscopic debridement and biologic glenoid resurfacing with acellular, allograft human dermal matrix-based scaffold. They documented a significant improvement in Constant and Murley score with a "successful outcome" in 72% of patients and "failure" in the remaining 28% of patients over a minimum follow-up of 2 years. Twenty-two of the 23 patients with a successful outcome had a postoperative MRI, which identified glenoid cartilage in 12 of these 22 patients.

Savoie et al. reported on 20 patients with grade IV glenohumeral arthritis who underwent arthroscopic resurfacing with a biologic patch. Over a minimum follow-up of 3 years, they reported an overall success rate of 75%; five patients went on to humeral head surface replacement at 1 to 5 years after the index operation. Despite the need for conversion to a humeral head resurfacing, four of the five "failures" expressed willingness to undergo the arthroscopic procedure again. This study demonstrated that most patients did not show improvement until 3 to 4 months postoperatively but after this time period significant improvement was seen in ROM as well as with respect to several validated outcome scores (VAS, ASES, UCLA, Constant, Rowe, and SF-12).

Porcellini et al. recently reported on a series of 47 patients with early glenohumeral arthritis (Samilson-Prieto stage I or II), of which 11 patients had engineered hyaluronic acid membrane placed over a microfractured glenoid defect without use of any fixation. They found significant improvement in subjective outcome scores (Constant and SST) in the majority (93.6%) of their patients; however, the use of hyaluronic acid membrane had no effect on the final outcome when compared with the effect of debridement, capsular release, and microfracture alone.[577]

Techniques described and used for arthroscopic glenoid resurfacing involve a high level of complexity and require advanced arthroscopic skills. Surgeons attempting to perform these techniques should feel comfortable with this procedure and understand the inherent associated risks.

Subacromial Decompression and Distal Clavicle Excision

Just as soft tissue pathology can coexist with glenohumeral arthritis, so can extra-articular pathology such as impingement and AC arthrosis. It is important to not focus in on glenohumeral arthritis as the sole source of pain until the other potential etiologies have been ruled out. Failure to recognize these issues can result in failure to treat a significant portion of the patient's symptom-complex. We routinely perform SAD when arthroscopically treating glenohumeral arthritis. The technique we use for SAD and distal clavicle excision is similar to that described earlier in this chapter.

Arthroscopic decompression has been shown to be an effective treatment for subacromial impingement.[215,558,686] Guyette et al.[288] retrospectively reviewed 36 patients who underwent arthroscopic SAD and had coexisting glenohumeral arthritis. In these patients, removal of loose bodies, debridement of unstable articular margins, and partial synovectomy to address the glenohumeral arthritis were also performed. The authors reported an average postoperative L'Insalata score of 78 at 5-year follow-up, which indicates that satisfactory results with decompression can be achieved even in the presence of glenohumeral arthritis. However, there was a negative correlation between L'Insalata scores and the grade of chondromalacia.[288] Distal clavicle excision has been shown to be effective in the treatment of symptomatic AC arthrosis. In our hands, the decision to perform a distal clavicle excision is made prior to the surgery and is based primarily on clinical evidence of pain at the AC joint. The incidence of radiographic AC arthritis is very high (>50%) but the majority of these patients are asymptomatic.[317] Furthermore, a recent study appeared to refute the case for prophylactic distal clavicle excision in asymptomatic patients who have radiographic evidence of AC arthritis.[531]

INFLAMMATORY SYNOVITIS AND ARTHRITIS

Most of the inflammatory conditions respond well to medical therapy and can be treated conservatively. In cases that are refractory to conservative management, arthroscopic synovectomy should be considered.

Pigmented villonodular synovitis is an inflammatory condition that is most commonly treated by arthroscopic or open synovectomy. It is a benign proliferation of synovial fibroblasts and histiocytes that should be treated much like a benign tumor. All affected tissue must be removed analogous to a marginal excision of any other benign soft tissue tumor. Recurrence can occur in up to one third of patients with a diffuse form of pigmented villonodular synovitis.[234]

Synovial chondromatosis is also commonly treated with arthroscopic excision. The cartilage bodies associated with this condition are thought to represent abnormal metaplasia of the synovium. Loose body removal is helpful in alleviating mechanical symptoms, but when done without synovectomy the recurrence rate is 25%.[159]

An inflammatory disorder of the shoulder should be considered when the joint aspirate contains high protein level, a white blood cell count in the 2000 to 40,000 range, with 50% to 90% neutrophils.[441] Rheumatoid arthritis, like the primary synovial disorders, will benefit from synovectomy when surgery is performed before significant joint destruction has occurred and before destruction involves the rotator cuff and other soft tissues.

Bleeding is always a concern when performing arthroscopic synovectomy. Measures such as hypotensive anesthesia, large-bore cannulas for increased flow, electrocautery, and epinephrine in irrigation fluid are often employed. Special attention should be paid to the subacromial bursa and AC joint when performing synovectomy. Both are lined with synovium and are often involved in synovial disorders.[116,744]

RENAL ARTHROPATHY

Arthropathy can occur in up to 50% to 69% of patients on chronic dialysis therapy, with one third involving the shoulder.[37,593] Conservative management of this condition is often not successful, because these patients do not respond to physical therapy and cannot tolerate antiinflammatory medication. Shiota et al. reported success with open synovectomy in patients with amyloid deposition resulting from dialysis.[653] Coleman et al. performed arthroscopic synovectomies in six patients with noninfectious renal arthropathy. Over an average follow-up duration of 5.5 years, five of the six were satisfied with the results of the surgery having maintained the improved function noted immediately after arthroscopy.[152]

OSTEONECROSIS

Osteonecrosis of the shoulder is staged radiographically according to the Cruess modification of the classification developed by Ficat and Arlet for the hip.[167,231] Although prosthetic replacement is the gold standard for treating stage III, IV, and V osteonecrosis, there are case reports of these patients who benefitted from simple arthroscopic debridement of loose bodies and synovium. This technique might delay the need for arthroplasty in a younger patient.[294,302] There is potential to halt the progression of avascular necrosis if it is diagnosed earlier in its course.

Although conservative treatment is a viable option for early stages of osteonecrosis, L'Insalata et al. reported poor outcomes in nearly three quarters of these patients treated conservatively. Furthermore, once the disease progresses to stage III, the prognosis tends to worsen.[408]

Core decompression has been successfully used in the hip to treat stage I and II disease.[315] La Porte et al. subsequently reported on open core decompression in 63 patients with avascular necrosis of the humeral head over a mean follow-up duration of 10 years. In patients with stage I and II disease, 91% had good or excellent results, but only 70% of the patients with stage III and 14% with stage IV disease did as well.[386,484] These findings, combined with those from current arthroscopically assisted techniques for core decompression, make early surgical treatment an attractive option for stages I and II and possibly stage III disease.

In the arthroscopically assisted technique, an anterior cruciate ligament tibial guide is placed through the anterior portal. Localization of the affected area is achieved by palpation of the cartilage with a probe to identify soft areas and by using fluoroscopic imaging. Once the guide is appropriately positioned, a guide wire is inserted into the lesion with the tip at the level of subchondral bone. A 7-mm cannulated drill is then used to create a tunnel into the area of avascular necrosis. Multiple smaller tunnels can also be made. The arthroscopically assisted technique simplifies the procedure, minimizes radiation exposure, malpositioned tunnels, and incisions as well as allowing diagnostic arthroscopy for ruling out any other pathology.[133,200]

Arthroscopy After Shoulder Arthroplasty

Arthroscopy can serve as both a diagnostic and therapeutic tool for patients who have pain after shoulder arthroplasty. Failure of standard investigations to identify the cause of pain after shoulder arthroplasty is an indication for diagnostic arthroscopy. Arthroscopy allows the surgeon to directly visualize and evaluate the intra-articular and extra-articular parts of the shoulder. Indications for the use of arthroscopy as a therapeutic tool are extensive and have been well documented in the literature. These range from removal of a loose glenoid component to treatment of shoulder instability.[260,307,500,527]

Use of the arthroscope in the postarthroplasty shoulder utilizes the same general concepts and techniques as in a native joint with a few notable exceptions. When performing arthroscopy after arthroplasty, care should be taken to avoid damage to the metal or polyethylene surfaces. O'Driscoll noted visual damage to the humeral head after arthroscopic excision of loose glenoids.[527] A 30-degree arthroscope should be used and turned away from the humeral head or glenosphere (for reverse shoulder arthroplasty [RSA]) as a method to avoid the "mirror effect" that can distort anatomy and confuse the surgeon (Fig. 15-57).

Bonutti et al. in 1993 published the first report of arthroscopy after shoulder arthroplasty.[69] They reviewed nine cases of arthroscopy for painful arthroplasty, all of whom had subsequent open evaluation to correlate arthroscopic findings. In this series, serial radiographs correctly predicted glenoid loosening in only two of six patients, while arthrography did so only in one out the three cases. Arthroscopic examination for more than

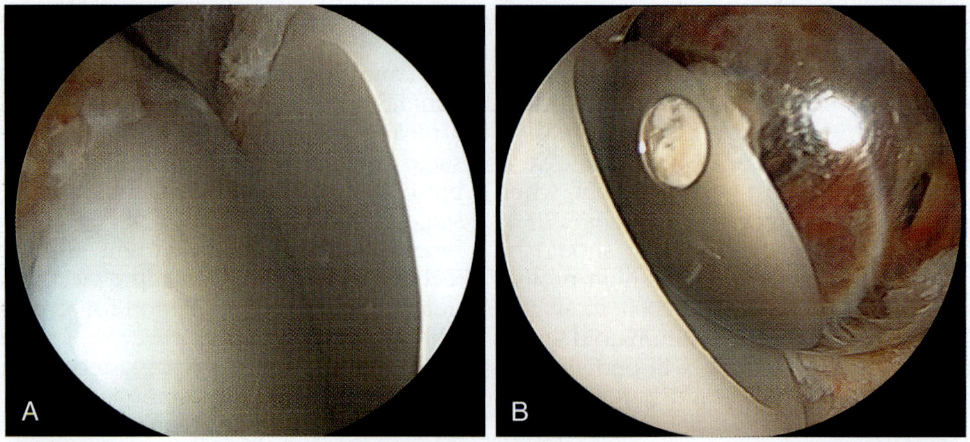

FIGURE 15-57: A, Arthroscopic appearance of total shoulder arthroplasty. **B,** Arthroscopic appearance of reverse shoulder arthroplasty.

2 mm of motion at the interface correctly diagnosed all five of the loose glenoid components. Additionally, the authors correctly identified one patient with a rotator cuff tear and another with extensive adhesions that required surgical treatment.[69]

In 2005, O'Driscoll et al. reported a novel technique for conversion of a failed TSA with a loose glenoid component to a hemiarthroplasty via arthroscopic removal of an all-polyethylene glenoid component.[527] The scenario for this technique is uncommon and should only be considered when glenoid loosening occurs in a patient with a large rotator cuff defect or those with associated medical comorbidity that precludes a revision arthroplasty. Standard posterior and anterior portals are established and a 7-mm plastic cannula is placed anteriorly. A 4- to 6-mm osteotome is inserted through the anterior cannula and is used to make three or four consecutive diagonal cuts from the anterosuperior to posteroinferior glenoid. After each cut, a segment of the glenoid is freed from the remaining cement mantle with the osteotome and removed through the anterior portal with a large grasper. The cement mantle is removed using a curved osteotome and curette. This technique provided some pain relief and increased function in all five patients, three of whom had complete relief of symptoms.[527] Namdari and Glaser reported the use of a similar technique for removing a glenoid component and an additional arthroscopic bone grafting of the defect. This technique involves removal of the glenoid component, and debridement of the contained defect followed by drainage of the intra-articular fluid and use of a trephine to deliver cancellous bone graft, which is packed into the defect with the aid of a bone tamp or reverse curette.[500]

Impingement syndrome after TSA is relatively rare and can sometimes be prevented with prophylactic acromioplasty at the time of shoulder arthroplasty. In a series of 203 cases of TSA, of which 5% had prophylactic acromioplasty, Freedman et al. found that 3% had impingement refractory to conservative management. Diagnosis was based on anterior shoulder pain with positive Neer and Hawkins signs as well as on positive impingement tests. Arthroscopic SAD yielded excellent or good results in five of six patients.[244]

Herschet al. reported their experience with arthroscopy in 12 painful shoulder arthroplasties. Procedures performed included, SAD (8), distal clavicle excision (4), capsular release (3), mini-open rotator cuff repairs (4), biceps tenodesis or debridement (6), and loose body or suture granuloma removal (3).[307] All patients had significant improvement in Hospital for Special Surgery shoulder scores. Particular attention was given to the biceps tendon pathology, which was described for the first time. The tendon was described as bowstringing over the humeral head component in several cases, leading to pain and degeneration. Tytherleigh-Strong et al. reported a similar array of procedures in 29 patients with comparable results.[716]

There has been one report to date on the use of arthroscopy after RSA. Garberina and Williams described a case in which the cause of failure after RSA was identified by diagnostic arthroscopy. In this report, the patient was having continued pain after RSA without significant radiographic, laboratory, or aspirations findings. Arthroscopy revealed obvious motion of the polyethylene component which confirmed its dissociation from the metaphyseal component. This patient was then converted to a revision arthroplasty to address the problem.[251]

Summary

It is unlikely than any combination of the described procedures will help in all cases of glenohumeral arthritis. Instead, there is likely to be a unique combination of procedures for each patient depending on the symptom complex and pathology. Our preference is to address each aspect of the patient's pathology individually, rather than use a standard technique to treat all patients with arthritis of the shoulder.

Arthroscopic Surgery for Biceps-Labral Complex Disease

Samuel A. Taylor, Stephen J. O'Brien

INTRODUCTION

Previous editions of this text included separate chapters for biceps and superior labrum surgery, which represents an antiquated notion of the long head of the biceps tendon (LHBT) and the glenoid labrum as being clinically independent. Emerging clinical and basic science studies, however, suggest a clinically significant interdependence. We now appreciate these to encompass the biceps-labral complex (BLC). Successful surgical intervention for BLC disease is predicated upon a comprehensive understanding of the relevant anatomy and the available diagnostic approaches to ensure accurate surgical indications and selection of patient specific techniques.

Traditionally held beliefs that the LHBT and labrum be considered independently have been challenged by emanating evidence both in the clinical[230,485,584,628,699] and basic science domains.[697,723] The new approach is based on enhanced understanding of the clinically relevant anatomy, pathoanatomy, and biomechanical considerations. For example, Provencher et al.[584] and others[277,453,752] described successful salvage in cases of failed SLAP repairs performed via open subpectoral biceps tenodesis. The etiology of failed SLAP repair is likely multifactorial (Fig. 15-58), and results from technical errors,

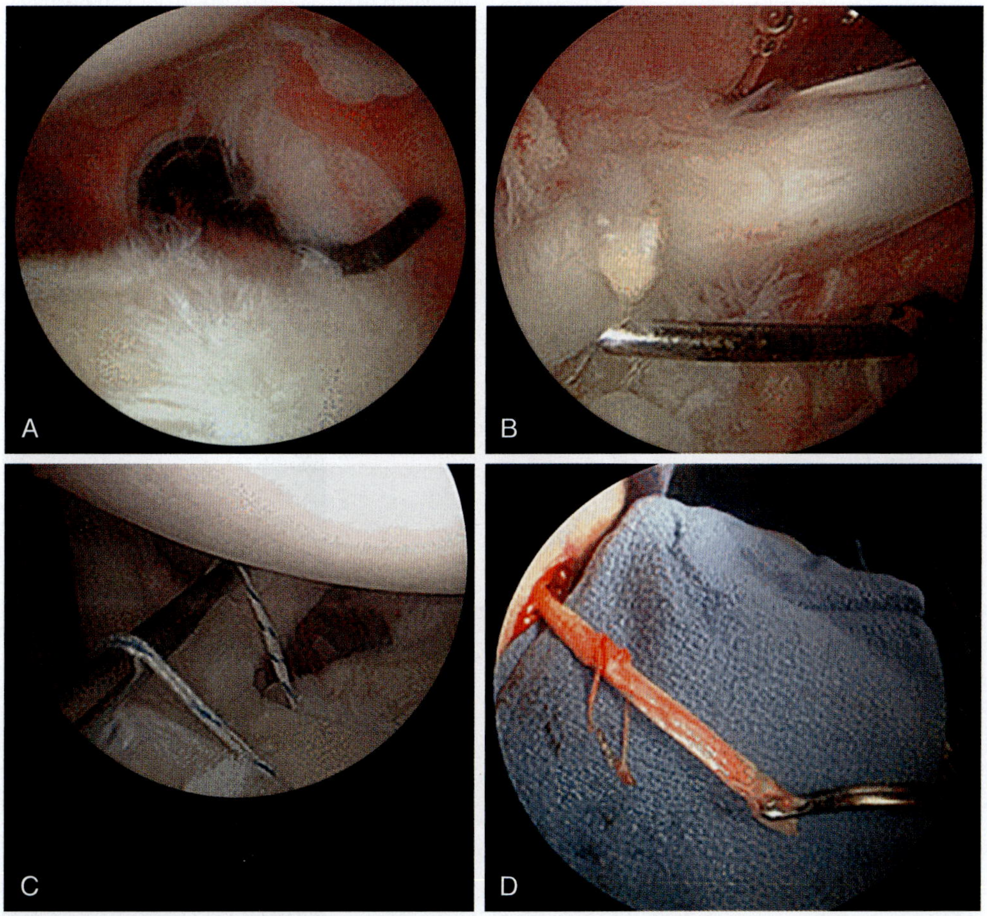

FIGURE 15-58: Arthroscopic images of four patients with failed type II superior labrum anterior to posterior (SLAP) lesion surgery who underwent biceps tenodesis. **A,** Arthroscopic view from the posterior portal of a 32-year-old man who underwent type II SLAP repair 9 months earlier, showing evidence of synovitis of the rotator interval, scarring of the long head of the biceps tendon (LHBT) to the capsule, and superior and posterosuperior capsulitis. **B,** Arthroscopic view from the posterior portal of a 34-year-old man who underwent failed type II SLAP repair 13 months earlier. There is evidence of a loose anchor (under probe), scarring of the long head of the biceps to the superior and anterosuperior capsule, synovitis in the rotator interval, and loosened sutures. **C,** Arthroscopic view from the posterior portal of a 35-year-old man who underwent type II SLAP repair 7 months earlier, showing evidence of loose sutures and an unstable LHBT attachment. **D,** Failed SLAP undergoing mini-open subpectoral tenodesis. Note significant tendon degeneration and fraying.

nonadherence to postoperative rehabilitation guidelines, kinematic deficiencies, biological factors that impair healing, or perhaps due to concomitant unrecognized extra-articular bicipital tunnel syndrome.[697,699]

Dozens of surgical techniques have been described to address symptomatic BLC disease. These have included labral repairs, biceps debridement, tenotomy, and a variety of tenodeses. The latter techniques tend to vary with respect to location (proximal vs. distal), type (bony vs. soft tissue), bicipital tunnel (decompressing vs. non-decompressing), and the hardware used (suture only, anchors, buttons, and/or interference screws). The sheer magnitude of surgical techniques described in the literature reflects an ongoing and evolving quest for an optimal surgical solution to BLC disease.

We have reorganized the chapter to provide the most current and comprehensive view of the BLC, its clinically relevant anatomic considerations, the offending lesions, commonly employed surgical techniques, and our evidence-based algorithm for selection of patient-specific interventions.

REDEFINING THE ANATOMY OF THE BICEPS-LABRAL COMPLEX

The BLC has three clinically relevant zones: inside, junction, and bicipital tunnel (Fig. 15-59).[699] *Inside* includes the superior labrum and the biceps anchor. *Junction* includes the intra-articular portion of the LHBT, which is visualized during standard glenohumeral arthroscopy and its stabilizing pulley. *Bicipital tunnel* represents the extra-articular segment of LHBT from the articular margin through the subpectoral region and its fibro-osseous confinement referred to as the bicipital tunnel.[697,699] Understanding the normal anatomy, pathoanatomy, and the limitations of diagnostic arthroscopy of these three zones is imperative.

INSIDE

The inside (see Fig. 15-59B) represents the labrum and the proximal biceps anchor. Careful consideration must

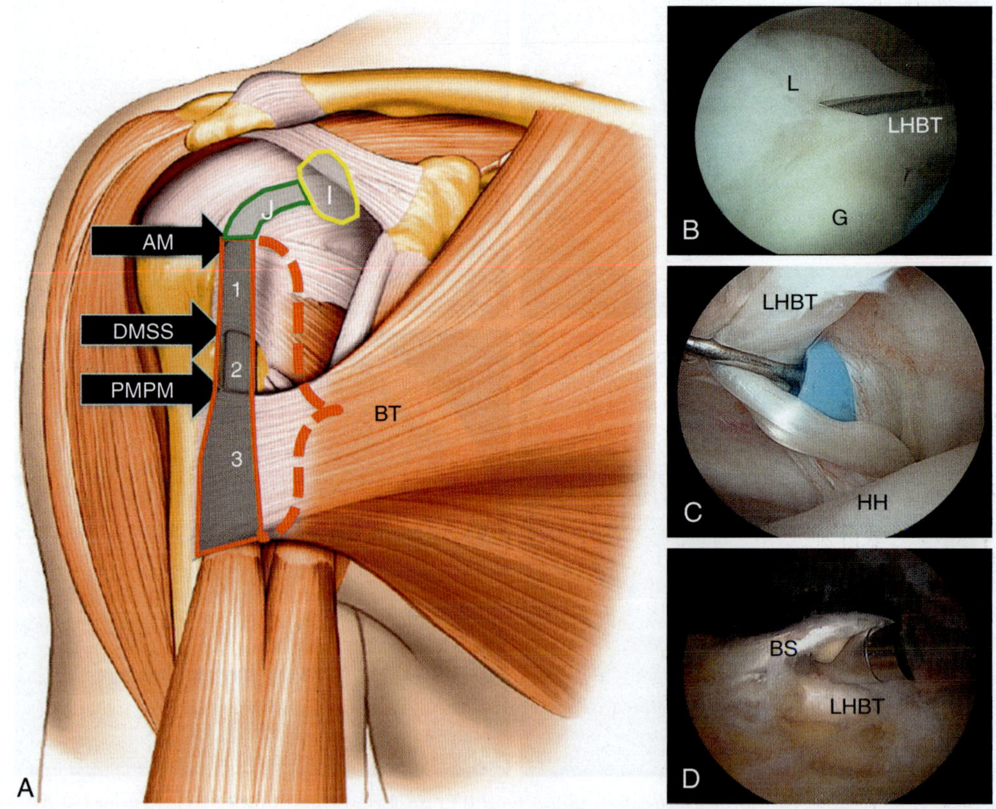

FIGURE 15-59: The biceps-labrum complex consists of three zones. **(A)** Inside (*yellow,* I) encompasses the superior labrum and the biceps anchor **(B)**, junctional (*green, J*) represents the intra-articular segment of the long head of the biceps tendon (LHBT) **(C)**. Bicipital tunnel (*red,* BT) includes the extra-articular biceps tendon and its fibro-osseous enclosure **(D)**. The bicipital tunnel is further divided into three zones. Zone 1 extends from the articular margin (AM) to the distal margin of the subscapularis (DMSS) and represents the traditional bony groove; zone 2 extends from the DMSS to the proximal margin of the pectoralis major tendon (PMPM) and is referred to as "no man's land" because it is completely hidden from diagnostic arthroscopy; zone 3 is the subpectoral region. L, labrum; G, glenoid; HH, humeral head; BS, biceps sheath.

be given to differentiate between normal anatomic variations and pathoanatomy during glenohumeral arthroscopy. Thorough diagnostic arthroscopy includes probe retraction of the labrum and the arthroscopic active compression test.[727] The inside pathology tends to be readily identifiable during diagnostic arthroscopy.

Normal Anatomy

The triangular-shaped collagenous glenoid labrum connects circumferentially to the glenoid to deepen the shallow fossa without altering its radius of curvature.[160] It is approximately 4 to 6 mm wide and 4 mm thick[579] and is intimately associated with capsular ligaments[524] and the LHBT anchor. Labral vascularity emanates from an anastomotic network receiving contributions from the suprascapular, anterior humeral circumflex, and the posterior humeral circumflex arteries[160] without any direct vascularity emanating from the glenoid bone. Of particular interest is the superior labrum, which has limited inherent healing potential due to its relative vascular deprivation.

The superior labrum shows great variability in its attachment morphology. It has a more meniscal-type, loose attachment, which consists of thin elastic connective tissue as opposed to a more firm inelastic tissue in the case of inferior labrum.[160] Normally, there is a synovial reflection at the superior aspect of the glenoid deep to the superior labrum, which is of variable depth and has been confused with a type II SLAP tear. Stoller[688] also reported variations in superior labral attachment. Type 1 represents a solid attachment to the glenoid rim. Type 2 and 3 attachments are separated by a small synovium-lined recess. The depth of the recess serves to differentiate between the two. Meniscoid superior labrum is represented by redundant labrum with a deep synovial reflection without tearing of its attachment. Rispoli et al.[605] identified 2.6 mm to 7.3 mm overlap of the labrum onto the bony surface of the glenoid. This is a variation of normal anatomy and should not be mistaken for a SLAP tear. A mobile and loosely attached superior labrum should not be considered abnormal unless there is a definitive detachment and the tear is visible.[155]

The LHBT anchor attaches to both the superior glenoid labrum[160] and the supraglenoid tubercle at the 12 o'clock position approximately 5 mm medial to the superior edge of the glenoid rim. There is a particularly intimate association between the LHBT and the glenoid labrum with blending of fibers.[324] Vangsness et al.[723] evaluated the biceps anchor in 105 cadaveric specimens and demonstrated that the LHBT attached to the supraglenoid tubercle in 50% of the specimens and only to the superior labrum in the remaining 50% specimens. They described four types of biceps attachments to the glenoid labrum: attached entirely to the posterior labrum (type I), predominately posterior with some anterior labral attachment (type II), attached equally to the anterior and posterior labrum (type III), and a mostly anterior labral contribution (type IV). Grossly, the majority of biceps tendons that originate from the superior labrum do so posterior to the supraglenoid tubercle (type I or II).[541,723] The fibers of the LHBT and glenoid labrum blend in this region[160] regardless of their gross appearance. Another cadaveric study determined that 83% of the LHBT origins were either entirely posterior (28%) or posterior dominant (55%).[314]

Several variations of normal anatomy such as sublabral foramen and Buford complex have been described and must be differentiated from pathologic lesions at arthroscopy.[160,333,337,568,756] The Buford complex is a variation marked by a lack of anterosuperior labrum; a cord-like middle glenohumeral ligament arises from the base of the biceps tendon and attaches to the capsule. The reported incidence of the Buford complex was 1.5% in a series comprising 200 patients.[756] A more common variant is the sublabral foramen in which a well-defined hole is visible beneath the anterosuperior labrum in 12% of patients, and the authors found an associated cord-like middle glenohumeral ligament in most of these holes.[756] Fixation of either of these variants is not advisable as it produces significant loss of external rotation. Variations of the biceps anchor have been described ranging from mesotendon that is freely movable and unattached to the rotator cuff, to an adherent type LHBT where the LHBT is attached to the supraspinatus and/or labrum,[196] congenital absence,[240] extra-articular origin,[330] and others.[731]

Pathological Lesions

In 1985, Andrews first described injury to the anterior-superior labrum near the origin of the LHBT in overhead throwing athletes in 1985.[11] Later, Snyder et al.[668] coined the term SLAP lesion (superior labrum anterior and posterior) in 1990 to describe the tearing of the intra-articular origin of the biceps tendon. Since then, this term has universally been accepted and used to describe a spectrum of injuries affecting the biceps tendon anchor and the surrounding glenoid labrum. Hwang et al.[329] showed that humeral head translation had a greater effect on superior glenoid labrum strain than did biceps tension, which supports the notion that SLAP tears result primarily from superior migration of the humeral head rather than biceps tension. Patzer et al.[555] suggested that SLAP repair improves glenohumeral stability as long as the LHBT remains in continuity, based on their cadaveric study. If the biceps was tenotomized, then subsequent SLAP repair had no impact on the glenohumeral translation. Strauss et al.[691] used a cadaveric model to demonstrate that type II SLAP tears increased glenohumeral translation in all directions, and that biceps tenodesis in the setting of type II SLAP did not magnify glenohumeral instability induced by the type II SLAP tear. While their results suggested that biceps tenodesis as a treatment for type II SLAP would not adversely impact stability, one may consider concomitant superior labral repair in throwing athletes in an effort to restore stability.

Snyder's classification for SLAP tears, types I to IV, remains the most widely recognized (Fig. 15-60)[668]:

- Type I lesions are characterized by marked fraying and a degenerative appearance of the superior labrum. The labrum remains firmly attached to the glenoid with an intact biceps anchor attachment. These lesions are commonly seen in middle-aged population and may be asymptomatic. Surgical treatment is debridement and not surgical repair.

- Type II lesions are defined by the visible detachment of the biceps anchor from the supraglenoid tubercle. These must be carefully distinguished from biceps anchors with normal meniscal variant attachments. Although mobile on probing, the meniscal variant will reveal normal articular cartilage beneath the anchor that is contiguous with the smooth synovial lining of the biceps anchor. Pathological findings include inflammatory tissue under the anchor and an anchor that can be lifted off the glenoid. These lesions require surgical repair versus biceps tenodesis depending on clinical findings and patient age.
- Type III lesions consist of a bucket handle tear of the biceps anchor and a normal biceps tendon and anchor attachment. Mechanical locking can occur from mobile fragments of the flap and is treated with debridement of the loose fragment.
- Type IV lesions include a bucket handle tear of the superior labrum that extends into the biceps tendon and/or the anchor. These lesions can cause mechanical symptoms and may be treated with debridement and/or repair, or biceps tenodesis, again depending on clinical examination findings and patient's age.

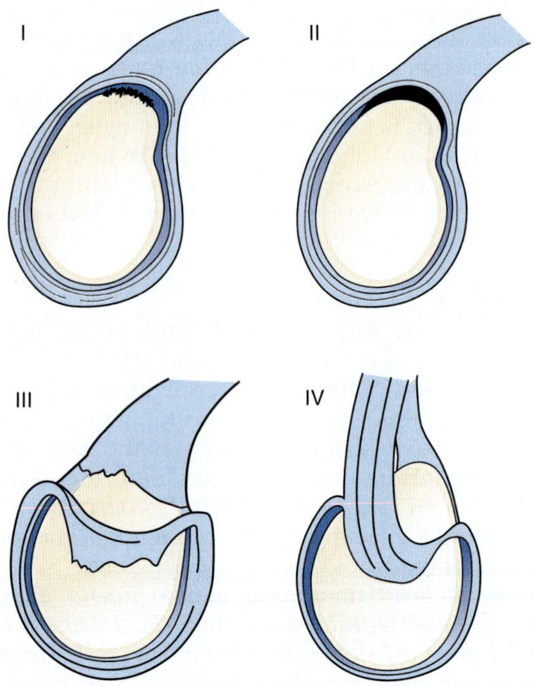

FIGURE 15-60: Types I to IV superior labrum anterior to posterior lesion tears as classified by Snyder.

Several others have modified Snyder's original classification. Morgan subclassified type II lesions based on the predominant area of instability under the biceps anchor.[488] Type IIA lesions have an anterosuperior lesion, IIB lesions have a posterosuperior lesion, and IIC lesions have combined anterior and posterior lesions (Fig. 15-61). Maffet et al. expanded the classification to include types V to VII.[427] Type V includes a Bankart lesion with a separation of the biceps anchor, type VI adds an unstable flap tear of the labrum to a biceps anchor separation, and type VII has a biceps anchor separation that continued beneath the middle glenohumeral ligament. Nord and Ryu added types VIII to X.[518] Type VIII was a SLAP tear with posterior extension to the inferior glenoid, type IX was a circumferential labral detachment, and type X was a SLAP tear with a bridge of normal labrum immediately posterior followed by a posteroinferior labral tear. Pfahler et al.[568] suggested that SLAP tears may normally occur during the aging process, with fissuring reported in the fourth decade and spontaneous detachments occurring in the seventh decade and beyond. The biceps anchor and anterosuperior labrum were the most common sites for detachment.

In addition to the superior labral tears, inside lesions include dynamic incarceration and medial biceps chondromalacia (Fig. 15-62). Incarceration of the LHBT

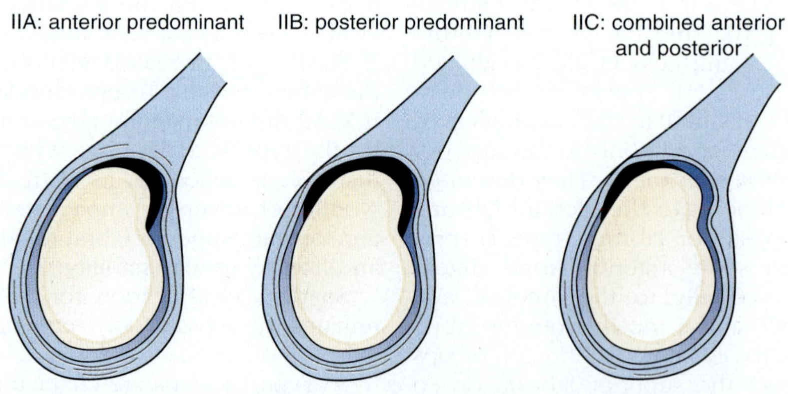

FIGURE 15-61: Subclassification of type II superior labral anterior to posterior tears as classified by Morgan.

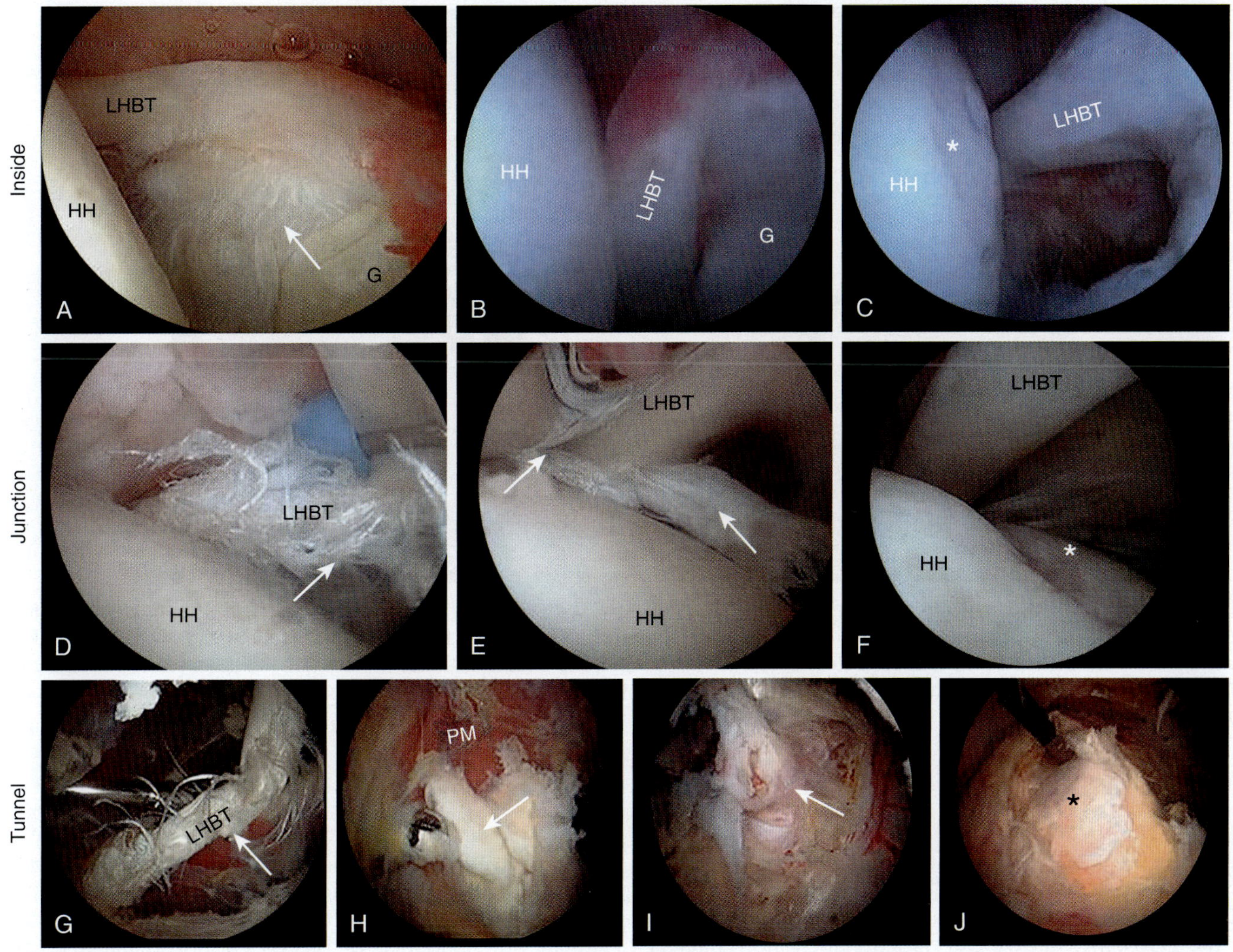

FIGURE 15-62: The three zones of the biceps-labral complex harbor unique pathologic lesions. Inside lesions (**A-C**) include superior labral anterior to posterior tears (**A,** *arrow*), incarceration of the long head of the biceps tendon (LHBT) within the glenohumeral joint (**B**), and medial biceps chondromalacia, which is attritional wear of the medial humeral head from a windshield wiper effect of the LHBT (**C,** *asterisk*). Junctional lesions include partial tears of the LHBT (**D,** *arrow*), pulley lesion (**E,** *arrows*), and junctional biceps chondromalacia which occurs below the LHBT near the articular margin (**F,** *asterisk*), among other lesions. Bicipital tunnel lesions are a diverse group which includes partial tears (**G,** *arrow*), loose bodies (**H,** *arrow*), dense synovitis (**I,** *arrow*), and extra-articular osteophytes (**J,** *asterisk*), among others. HH, humeral head; G, glenoid; PM, pectoralis major.

between the humeral head and the glenoid fossa may occur in a subset of patients. Verma and O'Brien[727] described a subset of symptomatic patients who had arthroscopically normal LHBT, but who demonstrated incarceration of the tendon between the glenoid and humeral head when the arm is positioned in forward flexion and internal rotation (i.e., mimicks the Active Compression Test or O'Brien sign) as viewed from the standard posterior portal (see Fig. 15-62B). We believe that the arthroscopic active compression test should be a part of routine diagnostic arthroscopy in any patient with preoperative BLC symptoms. For certain, incarceration is not in and of itself pathologic, but may become symptomatic. In our clinical experience, patients who incarcerate the LHBT often do so bilaterally. As such, we suggest performing the active compression test (O'Brien sign) bilaterally during the preoperative evaluation. Discomfort deep within the shoulder produced by this test on the unaffected contralateral shoulder may indicate that the patient is an incarcerator. In a patient with a SLAP tear who is also an incarcerator, even a perfectly performed SLAP repair may inadequately address the pathology and leave the patient with persistent symptoms. In such a situation, we recommend that biceps tenodesis should be preferred over a SLAP repair.

We define medial biceps chondromalacia as attritional chondral wear along the anteromedial aspect of the humeral head articular surface due to chronic incarceration of the LHBT between the humeral head and glenoid (see Fig. 15-62C). It corresponds to the area of contact

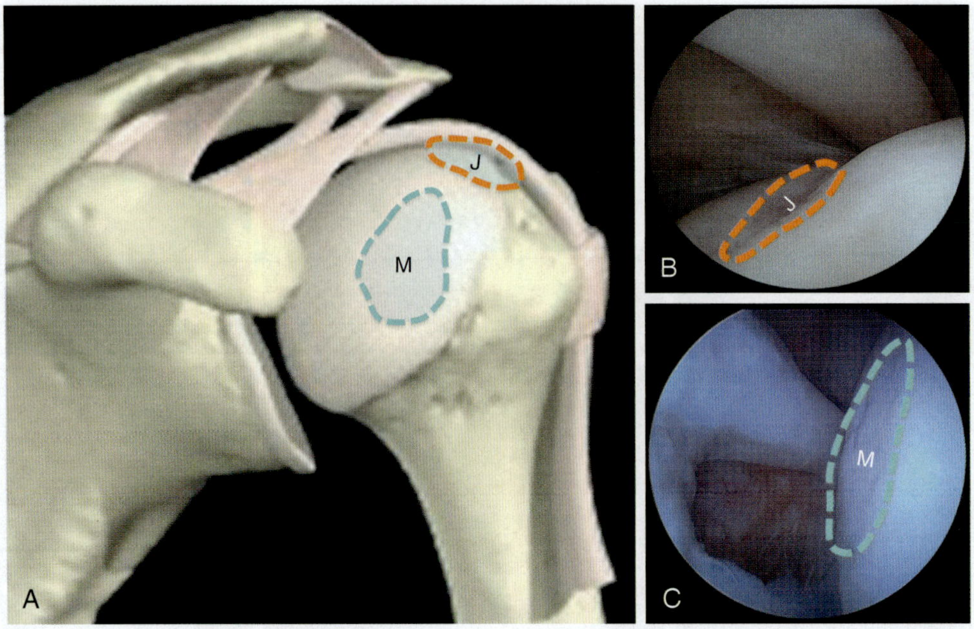

FIGURE 15-63: A, Biceps chondromalacia presents in two locations, either medial (M) or junctional (J). Both represent attritional wear of the articular cartilage but have different etiologies such that junctional **(B)** occurs from repeated sawing action of the long head of the biceps tendon (LHBT) near the articular margin and medial **(C)** stems from the "windshield wiper" effect of the LHBT on the anteromedial humeral head due to biceps instability caused by a pulley lesion or biceps anchor disruption or dynamic incarceration.

between the LHBT and humeral head during a positive arthroscopic active compression test. Other authors have observed this phenomenon at the articular margin deep to the LHBT in what we call "junctional chondromalacia" (described later in this chapter). Sistermann[657] reported "biceps tendon footprint" in 16% of 118 shoulder arthroscopies, which had a strong correlation with biceps synovitis, MDI and rotator cuff tears. As discussed later, biceps chondromalacia presents in two distinct locations: medial and junctional (Fig. 15-63).

A recent study by our group retrospectively compared preoperative MRI evaluation for three groups of patients who underwent shoulder arthroscopy to assess the diagnostic accuracy of MRI for biceps chondromalacia (Figs. 15-64 and 15-65).[654] Group 1 had symptomatic BLC disease *with* grossly visible biceps chondromalacia at arthroscopy. Group 2 had symptomatic BLC disease *without* grossly visualized biceps chondromalacia at arthroscopy. Group 3 served as a control population and consisted of patients with an asymptomatic BLC who underwent an anterior arthroscopic stabilization procedure. Preoperative MRI radiographs of each patient were reviewed by a musculoskeletal trained radiologist, blinded to all clinical and intraoperative data, for evidence of biceps chondromalacia. MRI evidence of cartilage loss, subchondral signal changes, and proximal biceps signal abnormalities were significantly different among the three groups. The results demonstrated very good sensitivity (61% to 82%) and moderate positive (51% to 53%) and negative (58% to 67%) predictive value for arthroscopically confirmed biceps chondromalacia. Interestingly, the two symptomatic groups (groups 1 and 2) demonstrated similar MRI evidence of biceps chondromalacia regardless of whether a lesion was evident at arthroscopy. These two groups differed significantly from the control population. As such, the aforementioned MRI features proved an excellent diagnostic tool for identification of symptomatic BLC disease (groups 1 or 2) with sensitivity 60% to 84%, specificity 48% to 66%, positive predictive value (PPV) 76% to 78%, and negative predictive value (NPV) 46% to 64%.

JUNCTION

The "junction" represents the intra-articular segment of LHBT and its constraining biceps pulley. Junctional pathology can be identified during standard diagnostic glenohumeral arthroscopy (see Fig. 15-62D-F).

Normal Anatomy

The LHBT has an average length of 99 to 138 mm from its origin at the supraglenoid tubercle to the musculotendinous junction[186,327,699] and an average intra-articular and extra-articular diameter of 6.6 mm and 5.1 to 6 mm, respectively.[186,384] Braun et al.[78] reported an average 6 mm diameter of LHBT at arthroscopy in their series

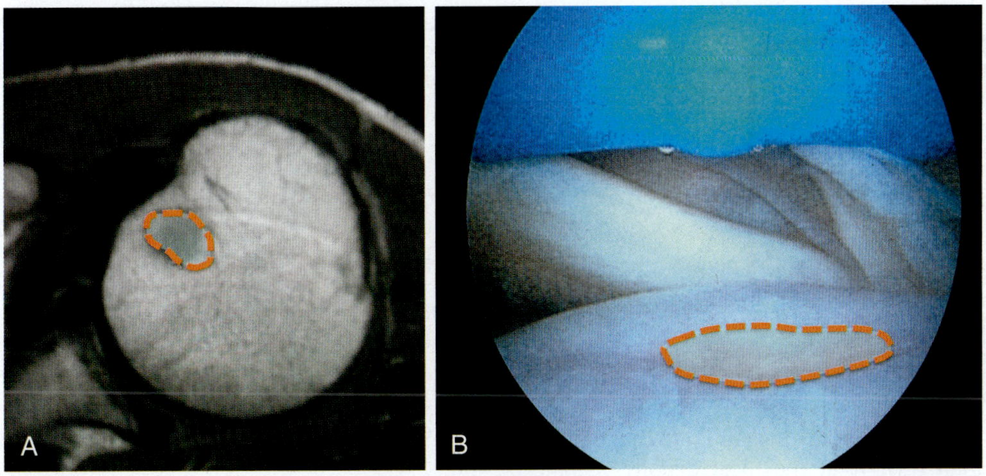

FIGURE 15-64: **A** and **B,** Junctional biceps chondromalacia can be identified on preoperative magnetic resonance imaging scans.

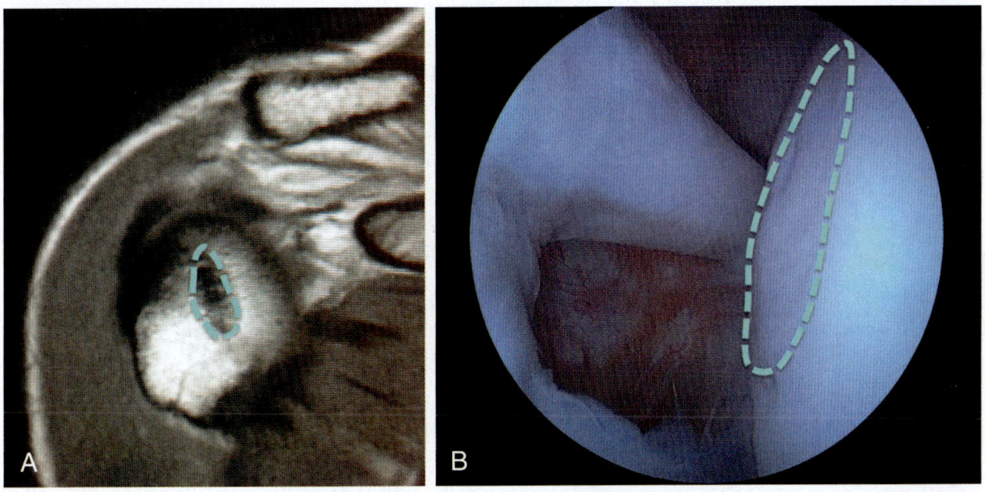

FIGURE 15-65: **A** and **B,** Medial biceps chondromalacia can be identified on preoperative magnetic resonance imaging scans.

comprising more than 200 patients. Excursion of 19 mm occurs during normal glenohumeral motion.[456] Its blood supply emanates from superior labrum tributaries proximally[160] and ascending branches of the anterior humeral circumflex artery distally as well as from the vincular attachments. As such, there is a hypovascular zone or watershed region present 12 to 30 mm from the LHBT origin, which corresponds with the segment of tendon that crosses the articular margin marked by a particular susceptibility to rupture.[136]

Alpantaki et al.[6] demonstrated an extensive sensory and sympathetic network within the LHBT, which was densest within the proximal segment of the tendon, thus supportive of the widely accepted notion that LHBT can be a source of pain in a variety of shoulder pathologies. A follow-up study also identified neural cell adhesion molecules that play an important role in nociception within several samples of LHBT harvested from six patients who underwent shoulder surgery.[7] Tosounidis et al.[709] used immunohistochemical analysis and identified increased sympathetic innervation of the LHBT and alpha-1 adrenergic receptors among patients with acute (proximal humerus fracture) and chronic pathology (rotator cuff disease), compared with cadaveric controls.

Intra-articular delivery of the LHBT during glenohumeral arthroscopy with a probe is considered the gold standard diagnostic modality for the discovery of pathologic lesions[50] with ideal arm positioning in 30 degrees forward flexion, 40 degrees abduction, and 90 degrees of elbow flexion.[299] Several studies have recently reported the limitation of diagnostic arthroscopic pull-test for visualization of the LHBT (Fig. 15-66). The average LHBT excursion afforded by arthroscopic pull-test was only 15 to 19 mm in a cadaveric studies[230, 699] and 14 mm in vivo.[271]

The biceps pulley is a capsulo-ligamentous stabilizing complex formed by coalescing fibers from the SGHL, the coracohumeral ligament, and contributions from the subscapularis and supraspinatus tendons (Fig. 15-67).

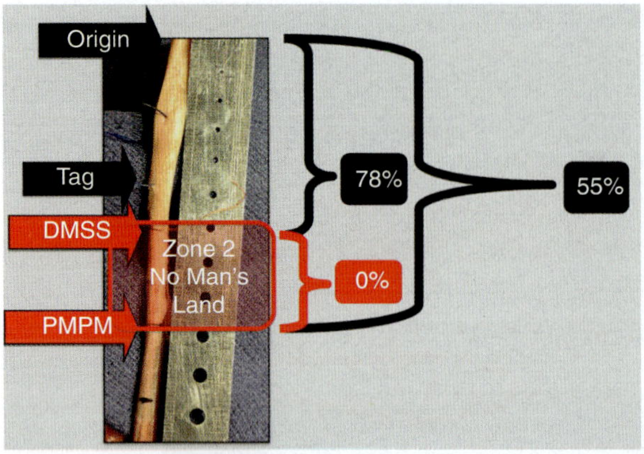

FIGURE 15-66: An anatomic study tagged (Tag) the long head of the biceps tendon (LHBT) at the most distally visualized segment of the tendon during standard glenohumeral diagnostic arthroscopy. The specimens were dissected and marked at the distal aspect of the traditional bicipital groove, indicated by the distal margin of subscapularis (DMSS) and the proximal margin of the pectoralis major tendon (PMPM). The researchers demonstrated that under the best-case scenario, 78% of the LHBT could be visualized relative to the DMSS, and only 55% could be visualized relative to the PMPM. In other words, none of the tendon could be visualized within zone 2 of the bicipital tunnel; hence the term "no man's land."

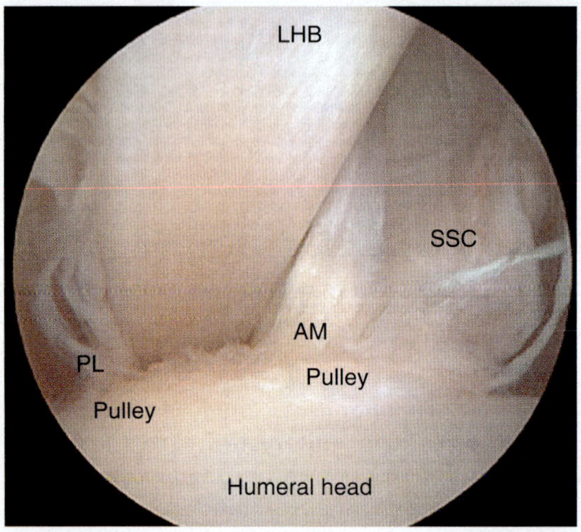

FIGURE 15-67: Standard arthroscopic view of the left shoulder from the standard posterior portal using a 30-degree lens with the arm positioned in 30 degrees forward flexion and neutral rotation. There is good visualization of the long head of the biceps tendon (LHB), the subscapularis tendon (SSC), and the anteromedial biceps reflection pulley (AM pulley). PL, posterolateral.

Together these structures stabilize the LHBT as it turns 35 to 40 degrees along the articular margin en route to its extra-articular course.[289] The coracohumeral ligament stretches from the coracoid process to the greater tuberosity and partially to the lesser tuberosity, and is an inferior stabilizer of the glenohumeral joint. The SGHL originates with or just anterior to the origin of the long head of the biceps and consists of oblique and direct fibers, which arise from the supraglenoid tubercle and labrum, respectively, that course in parallel with the biceps tendon and insert onto the fovea capitis just superior to the lesser tuberosity. Some fibers continue to insert into the base of the bicipital groove, while the remainder contribute to the transverse humeral ligament.[14,357,772]

Braun et al.[78] defined the arthroscopic anatomy of the biceps pulley as having an anteromedial biceps reflection pulley and a posterolateral biceps reflection pulley, either of which may be compromised. In their series of 207 patients who underwent shoulder arthroscopy for a wide variety of indications 32% of patients had a pulley tear, which was highly associated with proximal LHBT instability/subluxation. Interestingly, there was only a slightly higher predominance of anteromedial pulley lesions than that of posteromedial ones. The average age of patients with pulley tears was 13 years higher than those without and there was a significant association of pulley lesions with rotator cuff tears and SLAP tears. Biceps excursion at the level of the biceps pulley is 10 to 13 mm; the highest shear forces occur with the arm in internal rotation, with the arm at the side, and forward flexion with the humerus in either internal or neutral rotation.[79] These cadaveric findings suggest a vulnerability of the biceps pulley to injury due to increased shear stress sustained in the aforementioned positions as well as attritional abrasion secondary to repeated excursion of the LHBT against the pulley.

Pathological Lesions

Partial and complete tears of the LHBT are common, particularly those along the articular margin, which is approximately 2.5 cm from the origin[186] and is a vascular watershed region.[136] Boileau et al.[63] described an "hourglass biceps" lesion in which the tendon hypertrophy occurs proximal to the bicipital groove, and cause symptoms related to entrapment of the tendon within the glenohumeral joint. Moon et al.[485] reported that 79% of proximal, arthroscopically visualized LHBT tears propagated distally into the bicipital tunnel and were often accompanied by extensive tenosynovitis.

In their cadaveric study (see Fig. 15-67), Taylor et al.[699] demonstrated that on standard diagnostic arthroscopy, the pull-test was only able to visualize 78% and 55% of the LHBT relative to the inferior margin of the subscapularis tendon (bicipital tunnel zone 1) and the proximal margin of the pectoralis major tendon (PMPM) (bicipital tunnel zone 2), respectively. In a study by Gilmer et al.,[271] diagnostic arthroscopy with inclusion of the pull test was able to visualize 30 mm (range, 15 to 45 mm) of LHBT compared with 95 mm (75 to 130 mm) during open subpectoral biceps tenodesis among a series of patients who underwent open subpectoral biceps tenodesis for BLC disease. Others drew similar conclusions regarding diagnostic limitations of arthroscopy for visualizing the full extent of clinical pathology. Gilmer et al.[271] showed that diagnostic arthroscopy only identified 67% of

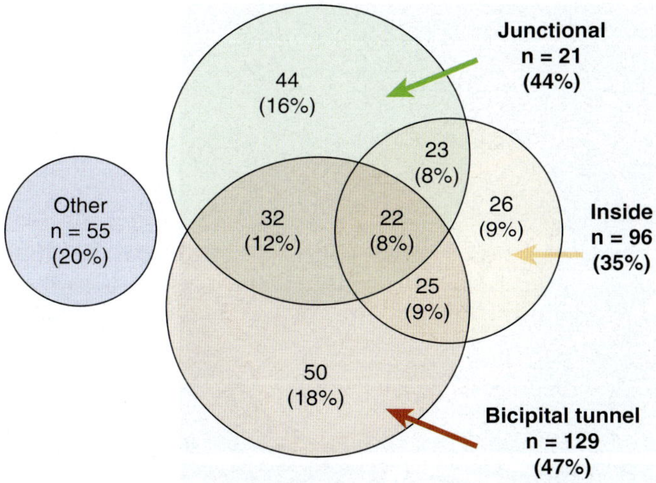

FIGURE 15-68: The distribution of biceps-labral complex lesions in a series of 277 symptomatic shoulders that underwent subdeltoid transfer of the long head of the biceps tendon to the conjoint tendon showed that lesions often occurred in multiple anatomic zones (inside, junction, and bicipital tunnel) concomitantly. Biceps chondromalacia and the arthroscopic active compression test, which were not included in our analysis, are represented as "other."

pathology and tended to underestimate the extent of the injury in up to 56% of patients.

It is important to note that junctional lesions not only occur in isolation, but may also occur concomitantly with lesions in other zones. For example, nearly half of patients with a junctional lesion *also* had a hidden bicipital tunnel lesion (Fig. 15-68).[699] As will be evident later, concomitantly occurring disease and hidden bicipital tunnel disease plays an important role in surgical decision making.

Lesions of the biceps pulley described by Bennett[50] produce proximal LHBT instability. The investigators identified resulting instability among 165 patients who underwent shoulder arthroscopy for subscapularis tears (28%) and rotator interval lesions (19%). Several signs of interval/pulley insufficiency have been described in the imaging literature such as displacement of the LHBT relative to the subscapularis tendon on oblique sagittal images, medial subluxation of the LHBT on axial images, discontinuity of the SGHL, and the presence of biceps tendinopathy. Overall, MR arthrography has demonstrated a high sensitivity (82% to 89%) and specificity (87% to 98%) for detection of pulley lesions.[635]

Junctional biceps chondromalacia is a term coined by the senior author (SJO) to describe attritional wear of the humeral head below the LHBT along the articular margin. Other authors have recognized this phenomenon as well though by different names. Sistermann[657] reported on "biceps tendon footprint" which was observed in 16% of 118 shoulder arthroscopies and identified a high correlation with biceps synovitis, MDI and rotator cuff tears. Byram et al.[117] identified a group of patients with humeral head abrasion below the intra-articular portion of the LHBT, and 33 of the 127 patients in their retrospective series had humeral head abrasions. While this lesion was most common among patients with failed SLAP repairs, it was also seen in the presence of other biceps pathologies. Chondral lesions on the humeral head below the LHBT called "bicipital chondral print" were observed in 78% of 182 patients with SLAP tears (type I excluded)[556] and the association was independent of age of the patient or type of trauma. Furthermore, in a follow-up study, the authors found that SLAP lesion tends to increase the anterior and anteroinferior translation and is associated with greater LHBT tension.[554]

BICIPITAL TUNNEL

Taylor et al.[697] recently defined the "bicipital tunnel" as the extra-articular segment of LHBT and its fibro-osseous enclosure extending from the articular margin through the subpectoral region.[699] The bicipital tunnel has been subdivided into three distinct zones (Fig. 15-69). It is a *closed space* that commonly harbors lesions that are hidden during standard diagnostic glenohumeral arthroscopy (Fig. 15-70). Patients with bicipital tunnel disease producing bicipital tunnel syndrome, who undergo proximal BLC surgical techniques, may remain symptomatic due to residual distal lesions.

Normal Anatomy

Zone 1 is the osseous bicipital groove defined proximally by the aperture created by the biceps pulley at the articular margin and distally by the distal margin of the subscapularis (DMSS). While the osseous morphology of zone 1 has been described as widely variable,[567] Cone et al.[154] reported the average medial wall angle to be 56 degrees, depth to be 4.3 mm, proximal width to be 8.8 mm, and middle width to be 5.4 mm. Nearly a third of specimens had gross osteophytic changes.

The constraining roof of zone 1 can be described as the "transverse humeral ligament," though this term has been debunked after recent cadaveric studies suggested that this ligament is actually the coalescence of fibers from the subscapularis and coracohumeral ligament medially, the supraspinatus laterally, and the falciform ligament inferiorly. Gleason et al.[273] used cadavers to show that the transverse humeral ligament consisted of a continuation of the superficial fibers of the subscapularis tendon that stretches over the intertubercular groove and meshed with longitudinal fibers from the supraspinatus and the coracohumeral ligament. MacDonald et al.[425] reported similar findings among 85 cadaveric specimens. They demonstrated subscapularis fibers extending deep to the LHBT along the floor of the groove in approximately one-third of the specimens. Taylor et al.[697] identified a deep osseous morphology of zone 1 that is covered by periosteum and extending fibers of the subscapularis tendon. In keeping with previous reports, the authors identified synovium in all specimens. They

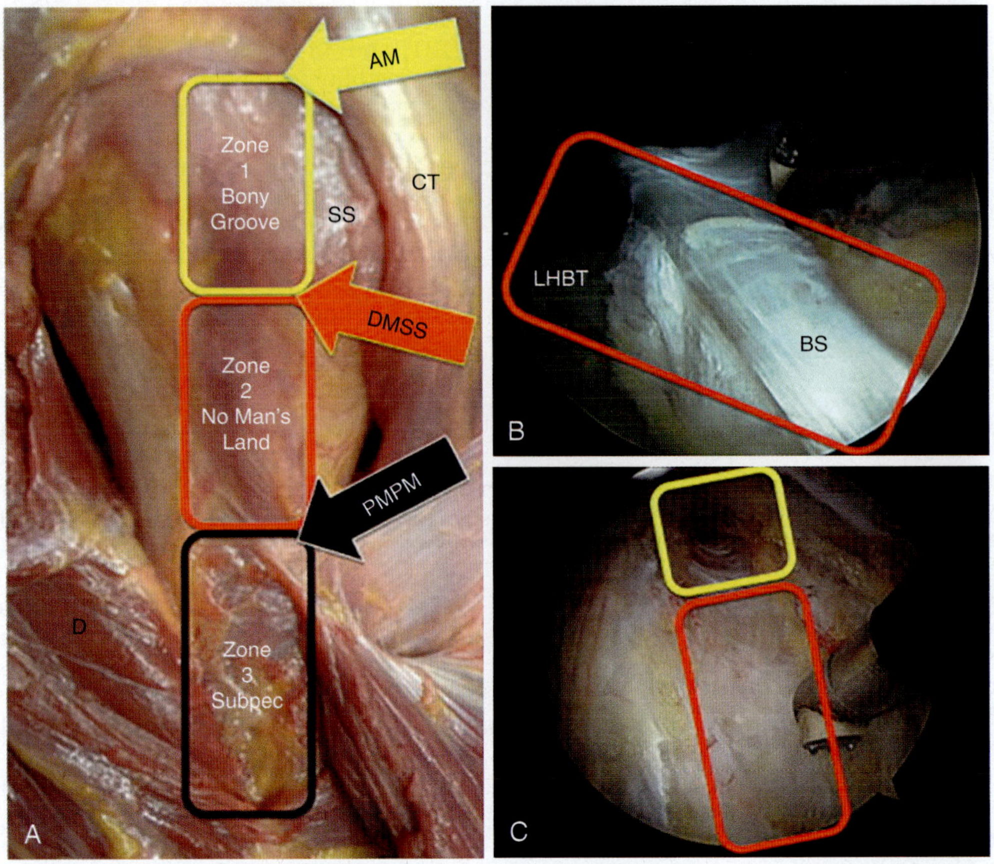

FIGURE 15-69: A soft tissue sheath **(A** and **B)** consistently covers the long head of the biceps tendon (LHBT) to the level of the proximal margin of the pectoralis major tendon (PMPM) and contributes to the roof of the bicipital tunnel. The sheath is clearly visible during open procedures **(A)** and extra-articular arthroscopic procedures within the subdeltoid space **(B** and **C)**. The fibro-osseous bicipital tunnel consists of three distinct anatomic zones **(A)**. Zone 1 represents the traditional bony bicipital groove (yellow) that begins at the articular margin (AM) and ends at the distal margin of the subscapularis tendon (DMSS). Zone 2 (red) extends from the DMSS to the PMPM and represents "no man's land" because it is not viewable on arthroscopy above or from subpectoral exposure below. Zone 3 is distal to the PMPM and represents the subpectoral region. The sheath overlying zone 2 can be robust **(B)**. D, deltoid; SS, subscapularis; CT, conjoint tendon; BS, bicipital sheath.

also found that the roof (transverse humeral ligament) was formed by a meshwork of subscapualris, supraspinatus, and falciform fibers. Interestingly, when proximal extension of the falciform ligament was present (33% of specimens), the fibers were oriented perpendicularly (parallel to the LHBT).

Zone 2, referred to as "no man's land," is defined proximally by the DMSS and distally by the PMPM (Fig. 15-71). Identification of offending lesions in zone 2 is particularly challenging due to its relative invisibility from arthroscopic visualization above and from open subpectoral exposure below. The osseous morphology of the floor is that of a shallow trough with overlying periosteum and proximal expansion of latissimus dorsi fibers and distal expansion of subscapularis fibers. In zone 2, the roof is made up of fibers from the bicipital sheath and the falciform ligament. Previous reports have suggested that the falciform ligament was the bicipital sheath;[112, 612, 768] however, recent histological evaluation[697] clearly demonstrates that the bicipital sheath and falciform ligament are independent structures with perpendicularly oriented fibers. The falciform ligament is an expansion of the sternocostal head of the pectoralis major, but has substantial variability with regard to the location of fibers, its proximal extension, and thickness. The authors also demonstrated that 67% of specimens had synovium in zone 2, which stands in contrast to the traditional notion[112] of a synovial reflection in the groove (zone 1).

Zone 3 is the subpectoral region, which begins at the PMPM.[697] The osseous floor here is predominately flat and is covered by periosteum and fibers of the latissimus dorsi. The roof of zone 3 is formed by the PMPM, which inserts on the humerus lateral to the LHBT. Importantly, the medial enclosure of the LHBT here consists of loose areolar connective tissue and was shown to have significantly increased percent empty tunnel (% ET) as determined by cross-sectional quantitative analysis in contrast

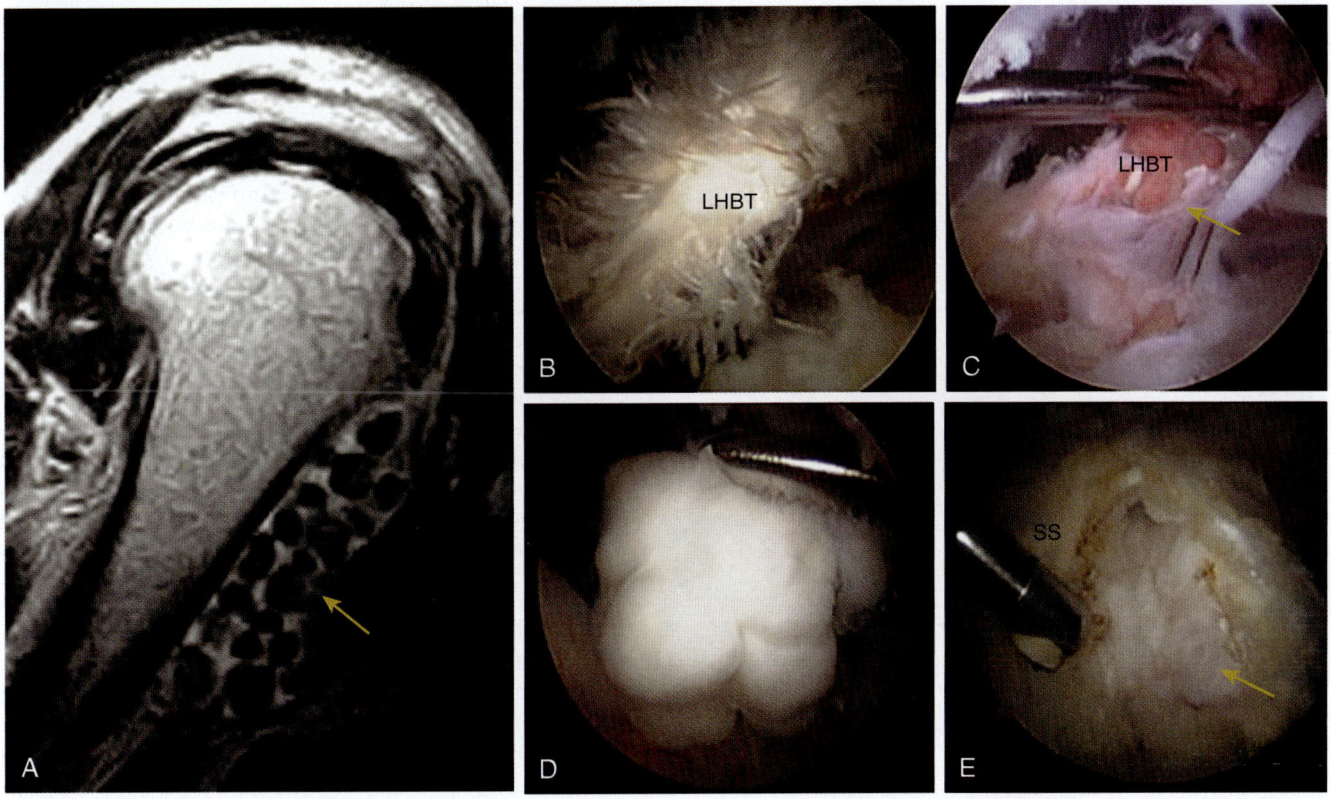

FIGURE 15-70: The extra-articular bicipital tunnel is a closed space in which lesions such as loose bodies can aggregate (**A,** *arrow*), as seen on this sagittal view magnetic resonance image. Several different space-occupying extra-articular lesions have been identified within the bicipital tunnel at the time of transfer of the long head of the biceps tendon (LHBT) to the conjoint tendon in symptomatic patients that would not have been visualized arthroscopically; these have included partial tears **(B)**, adhesion and scar formation (**C,** *arrow*), loose bodies **(D)**, and osteophyte formation (**E,** *arrow*). *SS*, subscapularis.

to that in zone 1 and zone 2, which had similarly constrained % ET. As a consequence, space occupying lesions such as scar, osteophytes, and loose bodies likely have less of a clinical impact in zone 3 than they do in zones 1 and 2.

Pathological Lesions (Bicipital Tunnel Syndrome)

The bicipital tunnel commonly harbors lesions in chronically symptomatic patients and conceals them from standard glenohumeral arthroscopic evaluation.[699] Such lesions confer a diagnosis of bicipital tunnel syndrome as described by Taylor and O'Brien,[699] with a reported prevalence of up to 47% (Fig. 15-72). Gilmer et al.[271] reported that the bicipital tunnel concealed 33% BLC lesions and that glenohumeral arthroscopy frequently underestimated the magnitude of pathology. Recently, Moon et al.[485] found that 79% of proximally identified LHBT tears propagated distally into the bicipital tunnel and were accompanied by dense synovitis.

According to Taylor et al.,[699] the bicipital tunnel disease includes a wide variety of lesions such as loose bodies, scar, partial LHBT tears, osseous stenosis, osteophytes, instability, synovitis, and inflamed vincula (see Fig. 15-72). In their retrospective evaluation of 277 patients, 47% patients had bicipital tunnel syndrome. The most common lesion was adhesion/scar (22%), followed by instability (11%), bony stenosis (8%), LHBT partial tearing (6%), loose bodies (4%), and inflamed vincula (3%). Scar and adhesion formation in zones 1 and 2 of the bicipital tunnel are most prevalent.[699] McGahan et al.[456] demonstrated that such simulated adhesions produce a 47.3-degree loss of glenohumeral internal rotation.

We believe that several anatomic features, namely the dense connective tissue sheath, presence of synovium, and functional bottleneck imposed by the PMPM, contribute to the pathogenesis of bicipital tunnel syndrome. First, the dense connective tissue sheath encloses the tunnel in zones 1 and 2, thus rendering it particularly vulnerable to synovial hypertrophy, scar formation, osteophytes and loose bodies. Secondly, the synovial extension exists further than what was previously thought. We identified it in zone 2 in the majority of specimens and even in zone 3 in one specimen. As such, synovitis may occur more distally than previously thought in areas hidden from traditional arthroscopic view. Finally, PMPM defines the transition from zone 2 to zone 3 of the

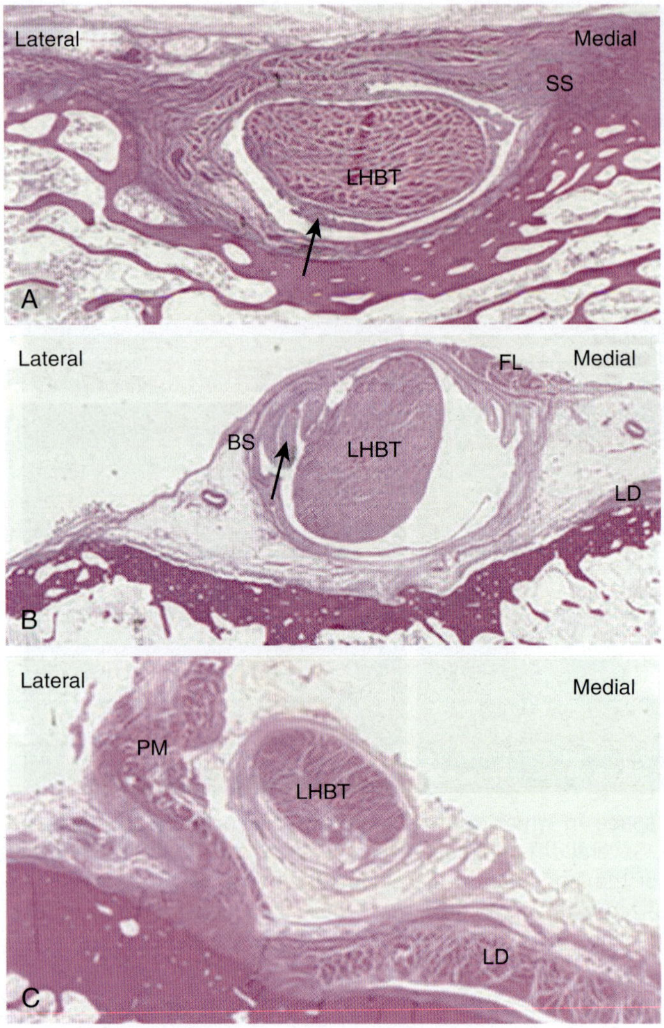

FIGURE 15-71: Hematoxylin and eosin stained sections from each of the three anatomic zones of the bicipital tunnel. Zone 1 **(A)** shows continuation of the subscapularis (SS) fibers superficial and deep to the long head of the biceps tendon (LHBT), which blend with fibers of the supraspinatus laterally. Synovium *(arrow)* completely envelops the LHBT. Zone 2 **(B)** demonstrates the axially oriented circumferential fiber of the bicipital sheath (BS), which extended laterally to bone. The falciform ligament (FL) can be seen as a discrete superficial bundle of longitudinally oriented fibers along the medial aspect of the bicipital tunnel. Partial synovial extension is seen *(arrow).* Proximal extension of latissimus dorsi (LD) fibers is also seen in a subset of specimens. Zone 3 **(C)** shows thick fibers of the LD along the floor with a roof of pectoralis major tendon (PM). Medially, loose areolar connective tissue predominated.

bicipital tunnel and is particularly important as it forms a bottleneck for many lesions such as loose bodies and synovitis which migrate distally but cannot decompress into the subpectoralis region (zone 3), and tend to aggregate in zone 2.[697,699]

SURGICAL OPTIONS

Surgeons are increasingly aware of BLC disease and its clinical implications as evidenced by an increased rate of both isolated and concomitant biceps tenodeses, tenotomies, and SLAP repairs.[588] For example, Werner et al.[749] queried a large surgical database to assess modern trends in BLC surgery in the United States. They identified 44,932 biceps tenodeses. During the study period, there was a 1.7-fold increase in concomitantly performed biceps tenodesis and a 1.8-fold increase in isolated biceps tenodesis from 2008 to 2011. The most common diagnoses associated with biceps tenodesis were rotator cuff tear, biceps tenosynovitis, biceps tendon rupture, superior labral lesion, and osteoarthritis. Vogel et al.[729] showed that there was a large increase in SLAP repairs during the period from 2002 to 2010 based upon the New York Statewide Planning and Research Cooperative System for Ambulatory Surgery and the California Office of Statewide Health Planning and Development Ambulatory Surgery Database, but relative stability among American Board of Orthopaedic Surgery (ABOS) candidates. The phenomenon was attributed to the greater awareness of new surgeons and their preference for narrow and defensible indications. We believe this paradigm change to be the cornerstone of the successful management of BLC disease. Nevertheless, BLC surgery has been broadly categorized as (1) SLAP repair, (2) biceps tenotomy, or (3) biceps tenodesis.

Labral Procedures

Today, much controversy surrounds the appropriate indications for SLAP repair, and for good reason. Sayde et al.[634] reported low return to play results following surgical repair of type II SLAP tears. While 83% of the 506 patients included in their review reported good to excellent results, return to play rates were only 73% overall and only 63% among throwing athletes. More recently, Fedoriw et al.[228] retrospectively evaluated a series of professional baseball players who had painful shoulders and MRI evidence of SLAP tear that were either treated with rehabilitation or surgical intervention. Outcomes included return to same level of play and return to prior level of performance. Pitchers in both groups demonstrated frighteningly low rates of return to play (40% rehabilitation vs. 48% surgery) and return to prior performance (22% rehabilitation vs. 7% surgery). Denard et al.[187] looked at the 2-year clinical outcomes for patients over age 35 years who underwent type II SLAP repair or biceps tenodesis and concluded that satisfaction rates and time to return to activity were higher among those undergoing biceps tenodesis. Conversely, Ek et al.[211] demonstrated similar ASES scores and return to play rates for patients with type II SLAP tears who underwent either SLAP repair or biceps tenodesis.

Biceps tenodesis has been shown to be an effective salvage option for failed SLAP repairs. McCormick et al.[453] suggested that open subpectoral biceps tenodesis was a

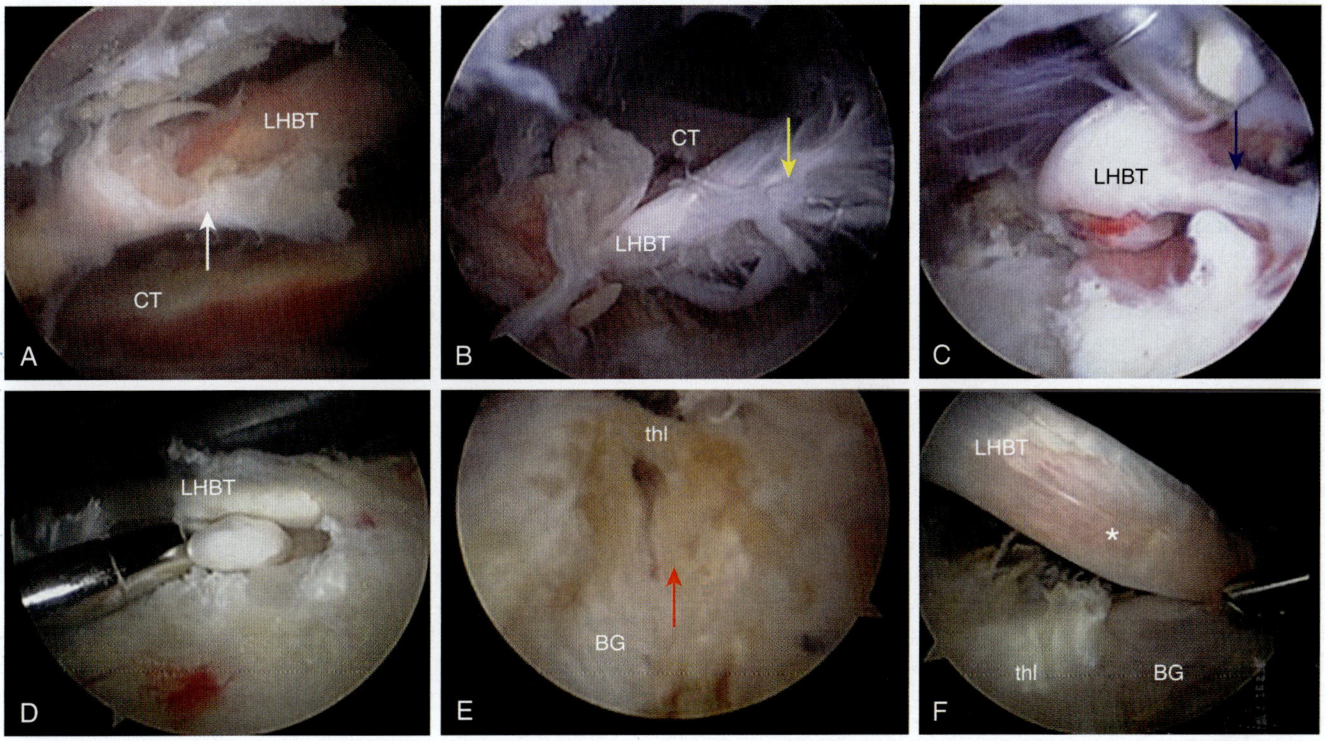

FIGURE 15-72: Several abnormal lesions were identified in the fibro-osseous extra-articular segment of the long head of the biceps tendon (LHBT) from within the subdeltoid space during arthroscopic transfer of the LHBT to the conjoint tendon (CT), despite a normal intra-articular arthroscopic examination. Representative examples included scarring (**A,** *white arrow*), partial tear (**B,** *yellow arrow*), symptomatic vincula (**C,** *blue arrow*), loose bodies **(D)**, bony stenosis of the bicipital groove (BG) (**E,** *red arrow*), and instability characterized by a shallow broad osseous floor, gossamer transverse humeral ligament (thl), and the resultant irritation of the LHBT (**F,** *asterisk*).

viable option for failed SLAP repairs in the military population. Their retrospective review of 42 patients (predominantly male; average age 39 years) revealed an 81% rate of return to active duty and clinically and statistically significant improvements in all measured outcome scores (ASES, SANE, and WOSI) at a minimum of 2-year follow-up. Similarly, Werner et al.[752] concluded that biceps tenodesis was an effective salvage operation for failed SLAP repairs.

The effectiveness of biceps tenodesis in the setting of failed SLAP repairs has led some other authors to advocate primary use of biceps tenodesis to treat SLAP tears. In their retrospective case series of 29 shoulders (average age, 47 years) with SLAP II of SLAP IV diagnoses treated with open subpectoral biceps tenodesis, Gottschalk et al.[277] reported final ASES score of 88 and 90% return to play at 40 months postoperatively. Similarly, Gupta et al.[287] evaluated 28 patients who underwent primary open subpectoral biceps tenodesis for patients with SLAP tears and clinical signs for biceps tendonitis at 2 years postoperatively. The cohort averaged 44 years old at time of surgery and demonstrated significant improvements for all validated outcome measures.

While Ek et al.[211] reported equally good to excellent results for SLAP repairs and biceps tenodesis in their retrospective review of 25 patients; the tenodesis group was significantly older (average age, 47 years) than the SLAP repair group (average age, 31 years), and had a higher rate of degenerative SLAP tears than traumatic types, which echoes the importance of appropriate patient selection. To this end, Provencher et al.[584] determined in a landmark paper that there was a 37% failure rate for SLAP repairs performed on patients older than 36 years (relative risk, 3.45).

We believe that age is an important determinant in the choice of surgical selection, largely because older patients have a higher prevalence of hidden extra-articular bicipital tunnel disease. In our recent study of 277 chronically symptomatic patients, we found bicipital tunnel disease to be significantly more common among older patients than younger patients (average age of 44 years for tunnel disease vs. 38 years for those negative for tunnel disease; $P < .003$).[699]

As the current trend in the field shifts towards tenodesis, its impact on the biomechanics is an obvious question. Chan et al.[132] found that biceps tenotomy at the superior labrum decreased the threshold force required to superiorly subluxate the humeral head by 8.6%, and resection of the superior labrum resulted in 15.2% decrease in threshold force required. Strauss et al.[691]

found that SLAP tears generated an increase in glenohumeral translation that was unchanged by biceps tenodesis and partially restored with SLAP repair. Specifically, SLAP repair restored posterior, abduction, and maximal external rotation translations, but did not restore anterior translation. The authors urged caution in resorting to biceps tenodesis as a primary treatment for SLAP tears in the throwing athletes as abnormal translation persisted in their cadaveric model. Similarly, Patzer et al.[555] reported that SLAP repair in conjunction with tenotomy of the LHBT did not normalize glenohumeral translation.

In vivo, Chalmers et al.[131] used motion analysis and surface EMG to evaluate the impact of SLAP repair and open subpectoral biceps tenodesis on the throwing mechanics. They determined that both surgical techniques restored neuromuscular control with the exception of thoracic rotation and normal lead-knee flexion patterns, which remained significantly altered in the SLAP repair group compared with healthy controls. Furthermore, Laughlin et al.[388] also used motion analysis tools to compare 13 elite baseball pitchers who had a history of SLAP repair with a matched healthy control group of pitchers. The authors found significantly less horizontal abduction, less external rotation, and decreased forward trunk tilt at the time of ball release among those who underwent SLAP repair. We hypothesize that the compensatory throwing mechanics subsequent to SLAP repair adversely affect velocity and accuracy and induce adjacent structure stress, which contributed to the relatively low return to play rates.

The literature clearly demonstrates a decreased enthusiasm for SLAP repair, particularly in higher age groups (>36 years)[584] and those with suspected bicipital tunnel syndrome.[697,699] SLAP repair likely has the advantage of restoring more normal shoulder kinematics based on cadaveric models, but motion analysis studies appear to suggest otherwise.[131, 388] The controversy surrounding the ideal treatment for SLAP tears bespeaks the evolving understanding of the BLC.

Biceps Procedures

Tenodesis and tenotomy of the LHBT have been shown similarly effective as treatment modalities in three separate systematic reviews.[247,321,661] It should be noted, however, that among both groups only 74% to 77% of patients achieved good to excellent results and 19% to 24% of patients had persistent biceps symptoms. Many factors ultimately contribute to outcomes, including tenodesis location, type of fixation, and surgical exposure among others. We believe that, for many patients, persistent symptoms following a biceps procedure results from unrecognized and thus unaddressed bicipital tunnel disease.

Therefore, while considering the selection of surgical technique, we prefer to group these as either bicipital tunnel decompressing or bicipital tunnel nondecompressing. This triage strategy is clinically supported by a retrospective cohort study by Sanders et al.[628] who reported a threefold higher failure rate for surgical techniques that did not include release of the extra-articular bicipital sheath when compared with those where the sheath was released.

To further elucidate the role of the bicipital tunnel, we recently completed a meta-analysis that compared biceps procedures that compared bicipital tunnel decompression (group 1, n = 1017) and nondecompression (group 2, n = 864).[701] We identified a total of 30 studies (n = 1881 subjects) who met inclusion and exclusion criteria. Between-group differences with respect to standardized, validated clinical outcome measures (Constant, UCLA, SST, VAS pain, and ASES) as well as revision rates were compared. Constant scores were the most widely reported outcome measures. Group 1 (tunnel decompression) was associate with significantly better Constant scores compared with group 2 (88.3 vs. 81.7; $P = .001$). No significant differences were identified with respect to revision rates, SST, VAS pain, or ASES ($P > .05$ for all). While the findings were not conclusive, it is important to recognize that the majority of included studies were level IV, which underscores the need for more robust studies.

The mere fact that dozens of biceps techniques have been reported in the literature speaks of the lack of consensus as to the optimal tenodesis location and technique. In general, we consider mode of fixation (soft tissue to soft tissue vs. soft tissue to bone), surgical exposure (open vs. arthroscopic), and bicipital tunnel status (decompressed vs. nondecompressed).

Bicipital Tunnel Decompressing Techniques

Bicipital tunnel decompressing techniques include arthroscopic subdeltoid transfer to the conjoint tendon, open subpectoral biceps tenodesis, arthroscopic suprapectoral biceps tenodesis, and proximal techniques that include release of the bicipital sheath in zones 1 and 2.

Our preferred biceps procedure is arthroscopic subdeltoid transfer of the LHBT to the conjoint tendon, which was developed by the senior author (S.J.O.) (Fig. 15-73). Its advantages include soft tissue–to–soft tissue tenodesis fixation and ability to visualize and thoroughly decompress the bicipital tunnel, while preserving the anatomic contour of the biceps and avoiding hardware-related complications (which obviates the need for bone tunnels), and tends to limit postoperative inflammation. Drakos et al.[202] reported an average UCLA score of 28 and an average ASES score of 80. In a large cohort of 56 patients at 77 months follow-up, Taylor et al.[698] reported an average UCLA score of 31.1, ASES score of 86, and VAS pain of 1.5.

A recent study by our group that evaluated the histological healing and inflammatory response in a rat model of LHBT tenodesis to metaphysis, to diaphysis, and to soft tissue (conjoint tendon) demonstrated a significantly lower inflammatory response in the soft tissue tenodesis group compared with that in either of the tendon to bone groups. Furthermore, in both tendon-to-bone groups, healing seemed to occur at the bony aperture with degeneration of the intramedullary portion of the tendon.

Open subpectoral biceps tenodesis has recently been popularized as it allows for removal of the LHBT from

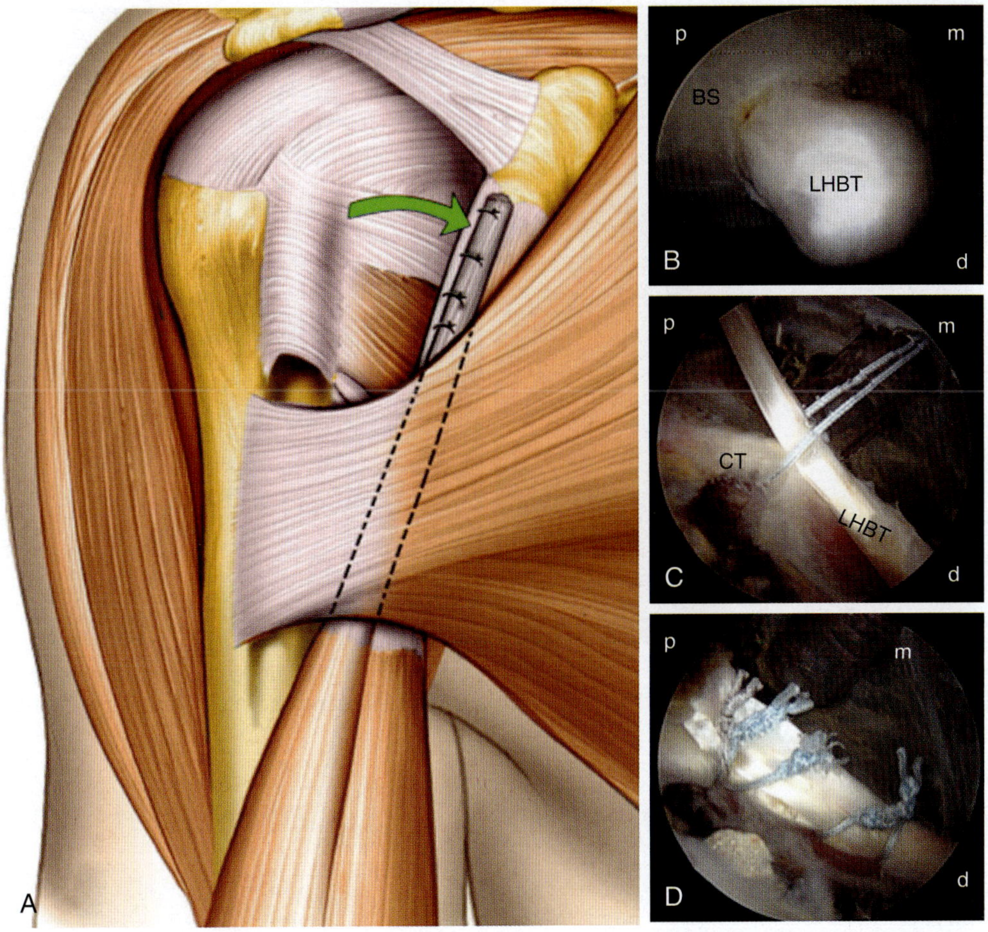

FIGURE 15-73: **A,** Subdeltoid transfer *(arrow)* of the long head of the biceps tendon (LHBT) to the conjoint tendon (CT). **B,** An aperture is created in the overlying bicipital sheath (BS) to allow delivery of the LHBT into the subdeltoid space. **C,** The LHBT is then tensioned in parallel with the conjoint tendon and **(D)** secured with sutures. d, distal; m, medial; p, proximal.

zones 1 and 2 of the bicipital tunnel, its relatively fascicle open exposure, and secure fixation of tendon to bone. Mazzocca[448] reported their case series of 41 shoulders, which had an average ASES score of 81, SST of 9.2, and low revision rate (2.4%). Nho et al.[512] reported a revision rate less than 1% in 353 cases of open subpectoral biceps tenodesis. Ek et al.[211] reported an average ASES score of 88 among 36 patients at 40 months of follow-up. With regard to fixation, Millett et al.[474] found no difference in failure (pain at tenodesis site or Popeye sign) rates or validated clinical outcome measures (VAS, ASES, or Constant) among 88 consecutive patients who underwent open subpectoral biceps tenodesis with use of either interference screw fixation or suture anchors.

Giphart et al.[272] evaluated the kinematic impact of open subpectoral biceps tenodesis on glenohumeral translation by performance of a series of dynamic maneuvers under the scrutiny of biplane fluoroscopy. Each maneuver was performed using the postoperative extremity and compared with the contralateral side as an internal control. The average difference between postoperative and control side with regard to translation was less than 1.0 mm, which included 0.7 mm anterior during abduction and 0.9 mm anterior during late cocking motion. The authors concluded that subpectoral biceps tenodesis had little effect on glenohumeral kinematics.

While open subpectoral biceps tenodesis has been shown by Nho et al.[512] to have a very low complication rate, it is important to consider the nearby neurovascular structures at risk, of ways to minimize infection rates with a peri-axillary incision, and the stress riser implications of a diaphyseal cortical breach caused by drilling a socket. During open subpectoral biceps tenodesis, external rotation of the arm increased the distance of the musculocutaneous nerve from 8.1 mm to 19.4 mm from the tenodesis site. Radial nerve and deep brachial artery were within 7.5 mm of the medial retractor. The median nerve, brachial artery and brachial vein were all greater than 25 mm from the tenodesis location.[194] Sethi et al.[645] suggested that bicortical guide wire placement was safe during a subpectoral approach and was on average 37 mm, 48 mm, and 37 mm from the axillary, radial, and

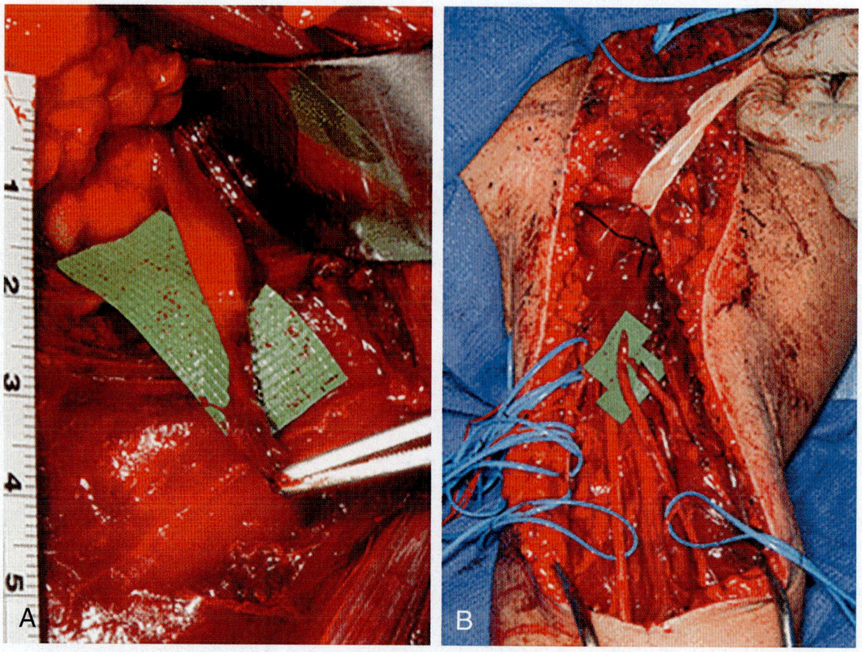

FIGURE 15-74: Intraoperative images illustrating the inadvertent tenodesis of the musculocutaneous nerve (sutures within the proximal stump) **(A)** and resultant transection of the musculocutaneous nerve and the motor branch to the biceps muscle **(B)**.

musculocutaneous nerves, respectively. Alternatively, they advised against bicortical penetration of a guide wire during a suprapectoral approach as it reportedly came into contact with the axillary nerve in 20% of the cadaveric specimens. Though uncommon, significant neurovascular injury has been reported by Rhee et al.,[598] Carofino et al.,[126] and Ma et al.[423] (Fig. 15-74).

While rarely reported in the literature, fracture is a potential risk of open subpectoral biceps tenodesis due to the stress riser created by the diaphyseal drill hole. Sears et al.[643] reported humeral fracture occurring within 6 months of open subpectoral biceps tenodesis. Dein et al.[181] described humerus fracture occurring in a 46-year-old recreational baseball pitcher 10 months following open subpectoral biceps tenodesis with an 8-mm diaphyseal aperture (Fig. 15-75). Reiff et al.[594] similarly reported a fracture in a 50-year-old woman. Recently Euler et al.[219] assessed the implications of eccentric 8-mm unicortical screw malposition on humeral strength during subpectoral tenodesis in a cadaveric model. They found that laterally eccentric malposition decreased the humeral strength during axial loading by 25% compared with that in the contralateral intact internal control ($P = .017$) while concentrically placed aperture did not significantly reduce strength ($P = .059$). As such, the authors recommended careful attention to concentric placement of the drill hole to mitigate the stress riser effect.

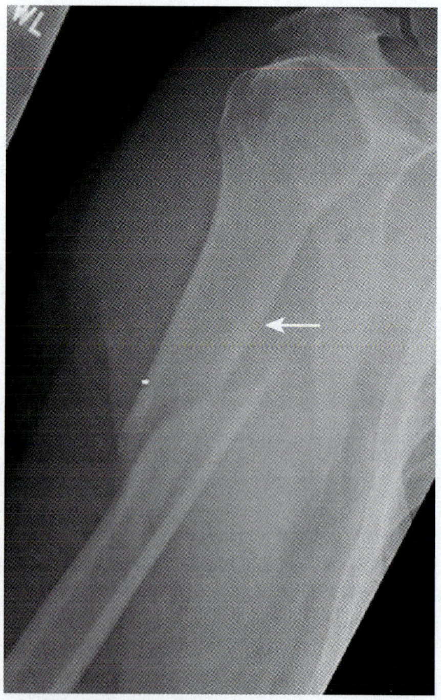

FIGURE 15-75: A preoperative view of the humerus showing a spiral fracture that enters the drill hole of the biceps tenodesis site (*arrow*). There were no signs of a pathological lesion or stress fracture.

Some advocate arthroscopic suprapectoral biceps tenodesis into metaphyseal bone with a tenodesis location approximately 2.2 cm more proximal to that used for open subpectoral biceps tenodesis.[351] Similar to that for subdeltoid transfer of the LHBT to the conjoint tendon, this technique can be performed arthroscopically and allows for decompression of zones 1 and 2 of the bicipital tunnel. Werner et al.[750] evaluated clinical outcomes for patients who underwent either open subpectoral biceps tenodesis (n = 27) or arthroscopic suprapectoral biceps tenodesis (n = 35) and found no significant differences in any of the assessed clinical outcome measures at 2 years postoperatively. A follow-up study by the same authors[751] revealed an increased rate of postoperative stiffness among patients who underwent arthroscopic suprapectoral biceps tenodesis compared with those who underwent open subpectoral tenodesis. Female sex, smoking status, and more proximal tenodesis location positively correlated with risk of stiffness.

Bicipital Tunnel Nondecompressing Techniques

Bicipital tunnel nondecompressing techniques include simple biceps tenotomy and proximal tenodeses to bone or soft tissue with the sheath left intact.

Biceps tenotomy has the advantage of not being technically demanding, being efficient, producing similar outcomes to biceps tenodesis procedures, and is associated with a low morbidity.[661] However, the associated high rates of Popeye deformity, the occasional subjective fatigue/discomfort complaints, and slight decrease in overall supination strength are some of the disadvantages. Tenotomy has been shown to be an effective treatment modality for chronic symptomatic BLC disease. Kelly et al.[361] retrospectively reviewed 40 patients who underwent LHBT tenotomy, either concomitantly or in isolation, and found 68% good to excellent results, 70% Popeye sign, and 38% with fatigue/discomfort symptoms at greater than 2 years of follow-up. Gill et al.[269] reported 90% rate of return to sport, 97% for to work, and an average ASES score of 82% among 30 shoulders evaluated at 2 years. Duff and Campbell[203] evaluated 117 patients 1 year after LHBT tenotomy and found no significant difference between the younger active patients and the older more sedentary ones, with regard to overall satisfaction, cosmetic deformity, strength, or cramps. The mechanical implications of simple tenotomy are relatively minimal. While peak supination torque was lower among patients who underwent tenotomy compared with those that underwent tenodesis, the same was not true for peak flexion torque or flexion/supination endurance.[758] In another study, Shank et al.[650] found no significant difference in supination or flexion strength among 19 patients who either underwent tenotomy or tenodesis.

Brady et al.[76] recently reported the largest retrospective cohort in the literature, the results of 1,083 proximal arthroscopic soft tissue-to-bone biceps tenodesis procedures along the articular margin. Final follow-up averaged 2.6 years. While the overall revision rate was 4.1%, only 0.4% of patient underwent revision surgery for persistent biceps symptoms. Final VAS pain scores were 1.1, UCLA score was 30.1, and SST was 10.2. While these results are indeed quite compelling and suggest that we do not need to decompress the bicipital tunnel to obtain excellent outcomes, not all proximal techniques have found similar success.[628,636]

In our clinical practice, bicipital tunnel nondecompressing techniques are used when bicipital tunnel disease is of low suspicion. Furthermore, simple tenotomy is typically reserved for older (>65 years), low demand patients, or those unwilling or unable to comply with postoperative rehabilitation and restrictions following tenodesis.

Reproducing Length-Tension Relationship

Regardless of the selected tenodesis location or technique, one should consider restoration of the normal length-tension relationship. Avoidance of undertensioning of the LHBT during tenodesis seems important to prevent subjective sense of fatigue, discomfort, and cramping as well as an aesthetically displeasing subsidence or frank Popeye sign. While our experience suggests that overtensioning of the LHBT is less of a problem due to the muscle's dynamic ability to accommodate over time, pullout forces at the tenodesis site are increased and thus overtensioning may in theory increase the failure rate.

The LHBT distance from its origin at the supraglenoid tubercle to the articular margin is 25 to 36 mm (Fig. 15-76), that from the origin to the DMSS tendon (zone 1 of the bicipital tunnel) is 52 to 63 mm, from the origin to the PMPM (zone 2 of the bicipital tunnel) is 74 to 90 mm, and from the origin to the musculotendinous junction is 99 to 138 mm (Fig. 15-77).[186,327,699] It should be noted that the musculotendinous junction is quite variable and often begins further proximal than may be appreciated at the time of open subpectoral biceps tenodesis.[384] That being said, Jarrett et al.[343] found that the musculotendinous junction of the LHBT began 2.2 cm distal to the PMPM. In their cadaveric study, LaFrance et al.[384] reported that the musculotendinous junction began 3.2 cm distal to the PMPM and that this junction extends for an average of 7.8 cm before complete conversion to muscle such that the junction may be extended for an average of 3.3 cm distal to the inferior margin of the PMPM.

Given the variability in the musculotendinous junction and the landmark measurements noted above, one of the authors of this section (S.A.T.) developed a way to reliably reproduce a patient's anatomic length-tension relationship during open subpectoral biceps tenodesis, as follows:

- The arm is positioned in neutral forward flexion and abduction such that it is at the patient's side.

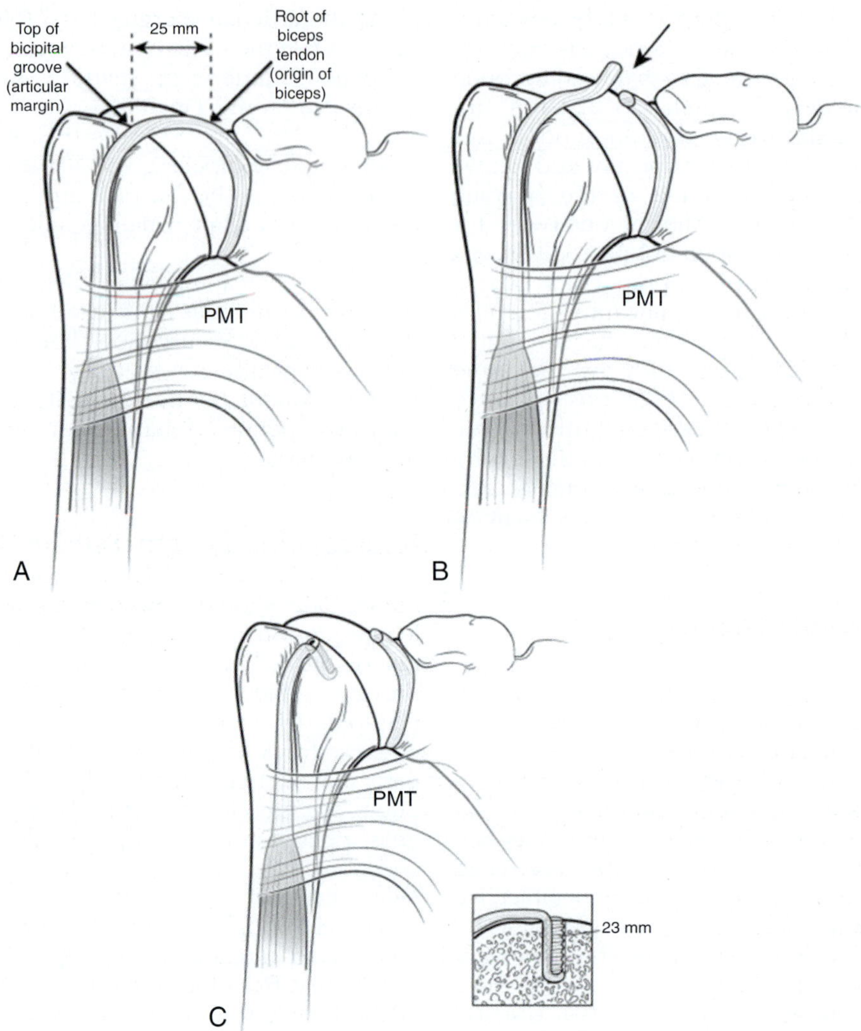

FIGURE 15-76: A biceps tenodesis at the top of the bicipital groove, adjacent to the articular margin of the humeral head. **A,** The normal biceps tendon averages 25 mm in length from its origin to the articular margin of the humeral head. **B,** The biceps undergoes tenotomy *(arrow)* at the level of the glenoid. **C,** A bone socket is created adjacent to the articular margin of the humeral head, and the tendon is secured in this socket with a tenodesis screw. As shown in the inset, allowing for 2 mm of tendon to be at the tip of the screw, a 23-mm tenodesis screw at this location will maintain the length-tension relation of the biceps because the native tendon is 25 mm long from its origin to this location of tenodesis. PMT, pectoralis major tendon.

- Prior to tenotomy, two 18-gauge spinal needles are placed percutaneously through the rotator interval tissue and LHBT near the articular margin while ensuring that the arm is in a neutral position.
- A PDS suture is placed through each of these two needles and retrieved through the anterior portal.
- A No. 2 nonabsorbable suture is then shuttled back through the LHBT and the rotator interval such that the loop remains on the undersurface of the LHBT and two free ends of suture have passed percutaneously through the site of spinal needle entry.
- This loop suture though biceps and interval tissue allows the surgeon to reapproximate the anatomic position of the LHBT after tenotomy by pulling tension on the sutures.
- LHBT is tenotomized arthroscopically.
- Open subpectoral exposure is then performed.
- Tension is pulled on the proximal suture, which reduces the LHBT to the rotator interval tissue in a patient-specific and anatomic length-tension relationship.
- A spade tip guide wire is then passed into the humeral diaphysis at the tenodesis location and the adjacent LHBT is marked.
- The LHBT is then pulled distally to decompress the bicipital tunnel.
- A whip-stitch is then placed such that the sutures end at the previously placed mark on the tendon, which are then secured to the bone via a unicortical tenodesis button.

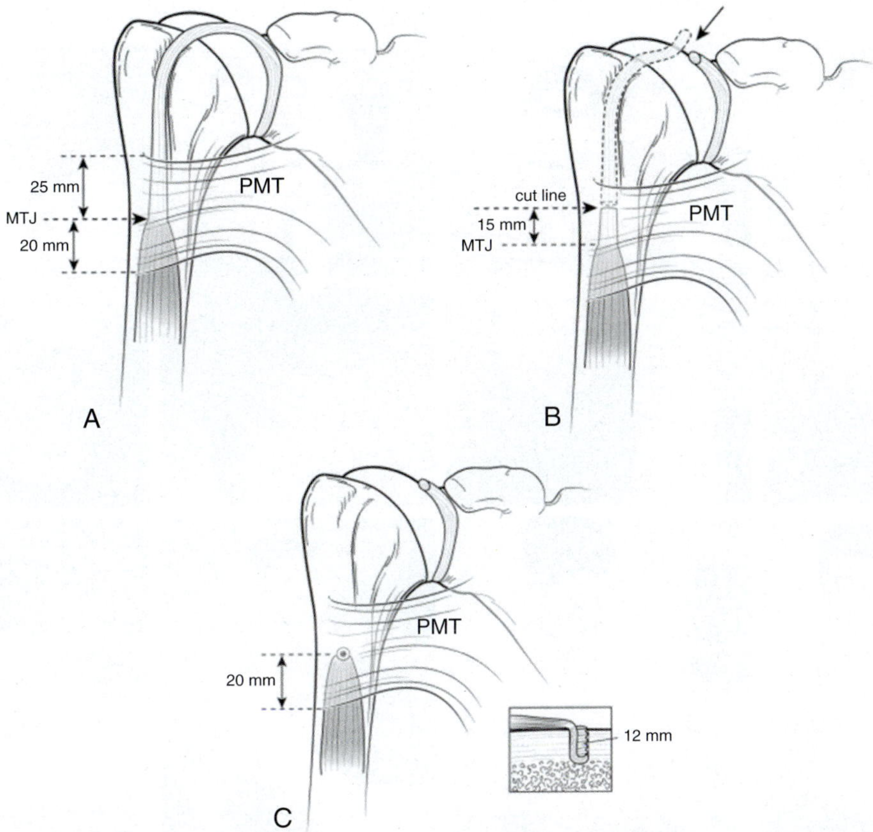

FIGURE 15-77: The proper location for a subpectoral biceps tenodesis. **A,** The musculotendinous junction (MTJ) of the long head of the biceps tendon is located beneath the pectoralis major tendon (PMT). The MTJ is approximately 25 mm below the upper border of the PMT and 20 mm above the lower border of the PMT. **B,** The biceps undergoes tenotomy *(arrow)* at the level of the glenoid, and a proximal portion of the tendon is resected until there is only 15 mm of tendon remaining above the MTJ. **C,** A bone socket is created 20 mm above the lower border of the PMT, and tenodesis performed at this location to maintain the normal position of the biceps tendon. As shown in the inset, a 12-mm-long tenodesis screw at this location will allow for a small part of tendon at the base of the screw and maintain the length-tension relation of the biceps.

SELECTING THE OPTIMAL SURGICAL TECHNIQUE

Preoperative Evaluation

The presence of bicipital tunnel disease must be considered during the selection of a surgical technique as bicipital tunnel nondecompressing procedures such as SLAP repairs, simple tenotomy, and proximal tenodeses that do not release the sheath in zones 1 and 2 may not fully address the clinically relevant pathology. As bicipital tunnel decompressing procedures potentially add surgical time and morbidity, the onus is on the surgeon to select the most appropriate procedure for a given patient.

MRI has been shown to be unreliable in determining the presence or absence of bicipital tunnel disease. Taylor et al.,[700] retrospectively reviewed 277 shoulders with chronic refractory BLC symptoms that underwent arthroscopic subdeltoid transfer of the LHBT to the conjoint tendon. Attending radiologist-generated MRI reports were graded dichotomously as positive or negative for biceps and labrum damage and then compared with intraoperative findings. Sensitivity, specificity, PPV, and NPV of MRI were calculated in the light of intraoperative findings. The overall sensitivity, specificity, PPV, and NPV of MRI for inside lesions were 77.3%, 68.2%, 57.3%, and 84.5%, respectively. The corresponding figures for junctional lesions were 43.3%, 55.6%, 73.1%, and 26.0%, respectively. For the bicipital tunnel, MRI had sensitivity, specificity, PPV, and NPV of 50.4%, 61.4%, 48.7%, and 63.0% respectively. MRI offered a limited assessment of the BLC and should not be relied upon as a screening diagnostic tool; rather it should serve as an adjunct to a detailed history and physical examination. MRI performed reasonably well for labral lesions, but not for biceps lesions.

Physical examination remains the mainstay diagnostic modality (Fig. 15-78). In a prospective study by our group (n = 145),[525] we sought to evaluate the sensitivity, specificity, PPV, and NPV for the "three-pack" examination

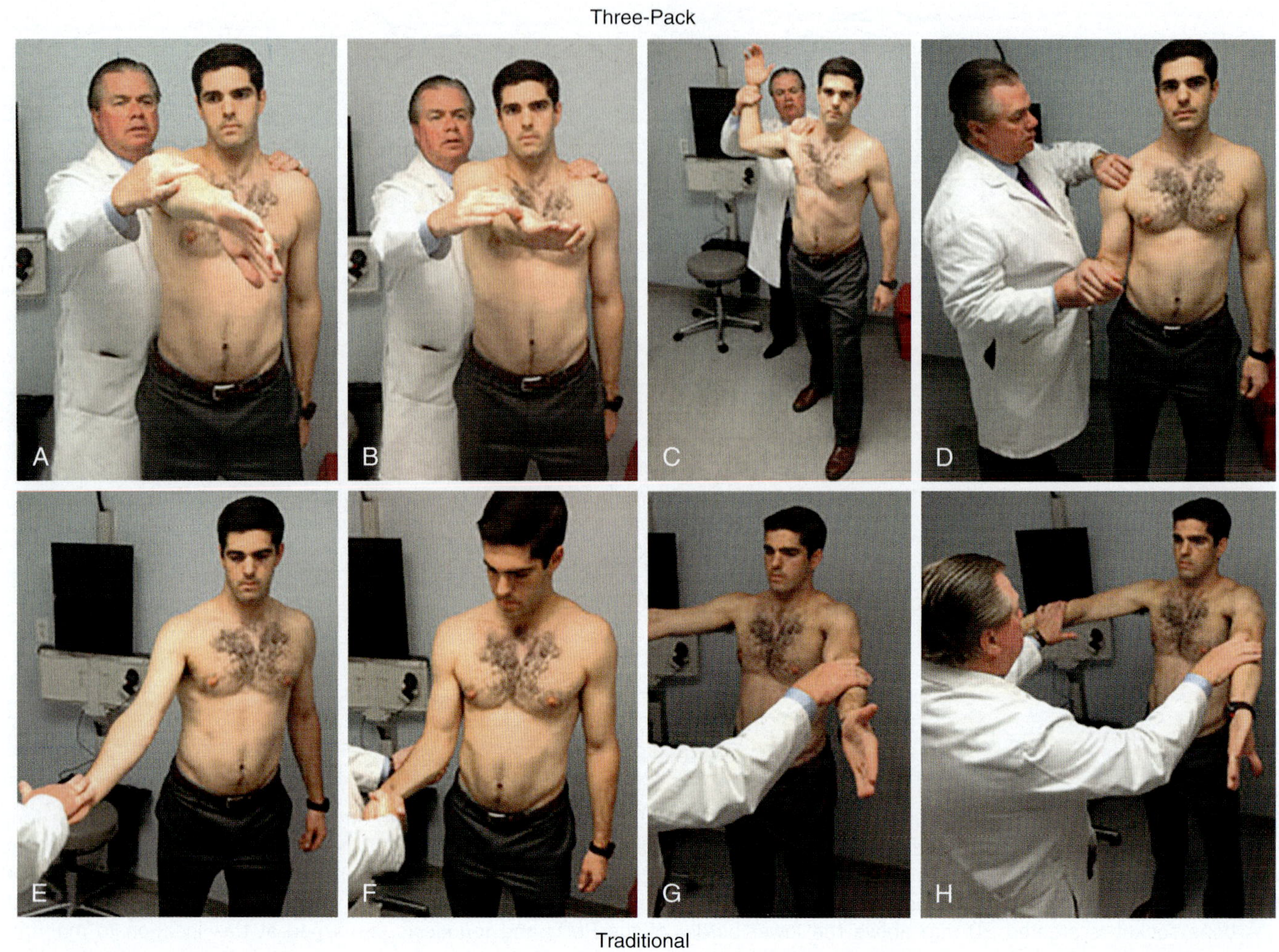

FIGURE 15-78: A-D, The three-pack examination includes the active compression test **(A-B)**, the throwing test **(C)**, and palpation of the bicipital tunnel **(D)**. **E-H,** Traditional physical examination maneuvers include Speed's **(E)**, Yergason's **(F)**, full-can **(G)**, and empty-can **(H)** tests.

(bicipital tunnel palpation, throwing test, and O'Brien sign) as well as the more traditional tests (Speed's, Yergason's, and Jobe's). The three-pack tests were highly sensitive (73% to 98%), but were less specific (46% to 79%) for BLC disease in all three locations (inside, junction, and tunnel) than the traditional tests, which were less sensitive (20% to 67%), but more specific (83% to 100%) for BLC disease in all three locations (Fig. 15-79). Of particular importance for the choice of surgical technique, palpation and O'Brien sign were highly sensitive (97.8% and 95.7%, respectively) for hidden bicipital tunnel disease and had a high NPV (96.4% and 92.6% respectively), which essentially allows the surgeon to rule out bicipital tunnel disease if negative. Speed's and Yergason's tests, conversely, were poorly sensitive but had high specificity (86.7% and 97.9%, respectively) and PPV (76% and 92.3%, respectively), which suggests that a positive examination should prompt the selection of a bicipital tunnel decompressing tenodesis technique.

We have also found corticosteroid injections combined with a local anesthetic delivered to the extra-articular bicipital tunnel to be a powerful therapeutic and diagnostic tool. While such injections can be given via landmark localization, we advocate their administration under ultrasound guidance to ensure their delivery to the bicipital tunnel. Hashicuchi et al.[300] clearly demonstrated improved accuracy with use of the ultrasound. Among 30 shoulders in their study, only 27% of unguided injections were accurately delivered as against 87% in the ultrasound group ($P > .05$).

Authors' Preferred Algorithm

BLC disease remains a preoperative diagnosis as does the selection of the most appropriate surgical technique. The accompanying algorithm relies heavily upon preoperative physical examination and guides the surgeon to select either a bicipital tunnel decompressing or a

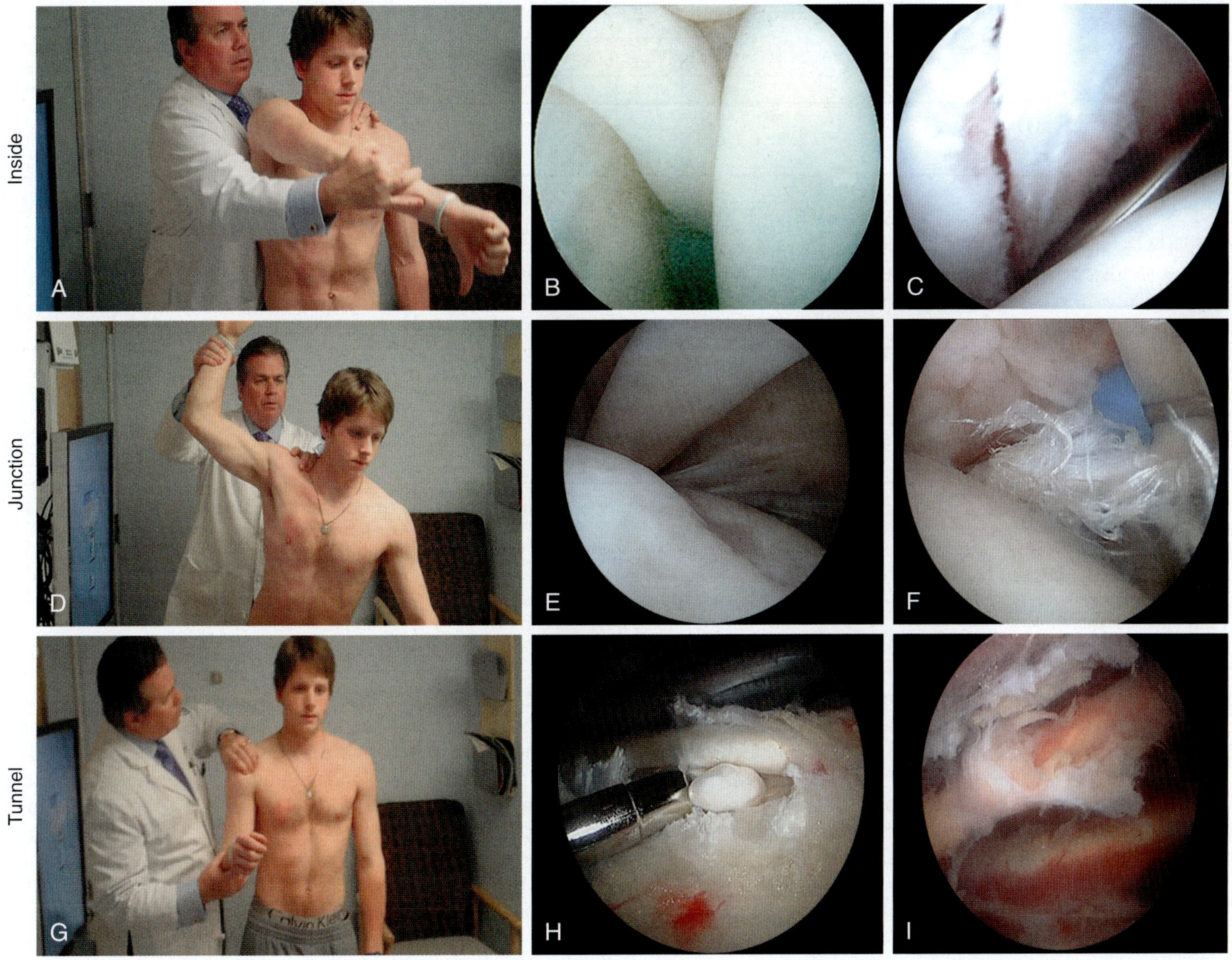

FIGURE 15-79: The active compression test (O'Brien sign; **A**) is particularly useful for picking up inside lesions such as incarceration of the biceps **(B)** and labral tears **(C)**. The throwing test **(D)** is helpful for junctional lesions such as junctional biceps chondromalacia **(E)** and partial tears of the biceps tendon **(F)**. Palpation **(G)** is very sensitive for bicipital tunnel disease, which may include a heterogeneous set of lesions such as loose bodies **(H)** and adhesion/scar **(I)**.

nondecompressing technique (Fig. 15-80). Based on the aforementioned study,[525] a patient with no tenderness on palpation of the bicipital tunnel and/or a negative O'Brien sign can safely undergo a nondecompressing surgical technique, given their NPV of 96% and 93%, respectively. If both of these examination maneuvers are positive, bicipital tunnel disease cannot be excluded and should prompt selection of a decompressing technique to ensure adequate treatment of the offending pathology.

SUMMARY

The BLC represents the shared anatomic and clinical features of the biceps *and* labrum. The BLC has three clinically relevant zones: inside, junction, and bicipital tunnel. Any one or a combination of these zones may harbor clinically significant lesions. Of emerging relevance are lesions within the bicipital tunnel because they are hidden from standard glenohumeral arthroscopy. Therefore surgical techniques can be categorized as either bicipital tunnel decompressing or bicipital tunnel nondecompressing, the latter of which should only be selected when there is low preoperative index of suspicion for bicipital tunnel disease. Bicipital tunnel palpation and the O'Brien sign are highly sensitive for bicipital tunnel disease and more importantly have a very high NPV. As such, surgeons may safely select a nondecompressing technique if preoperative palpation and/or the O'Brien sign are negative.

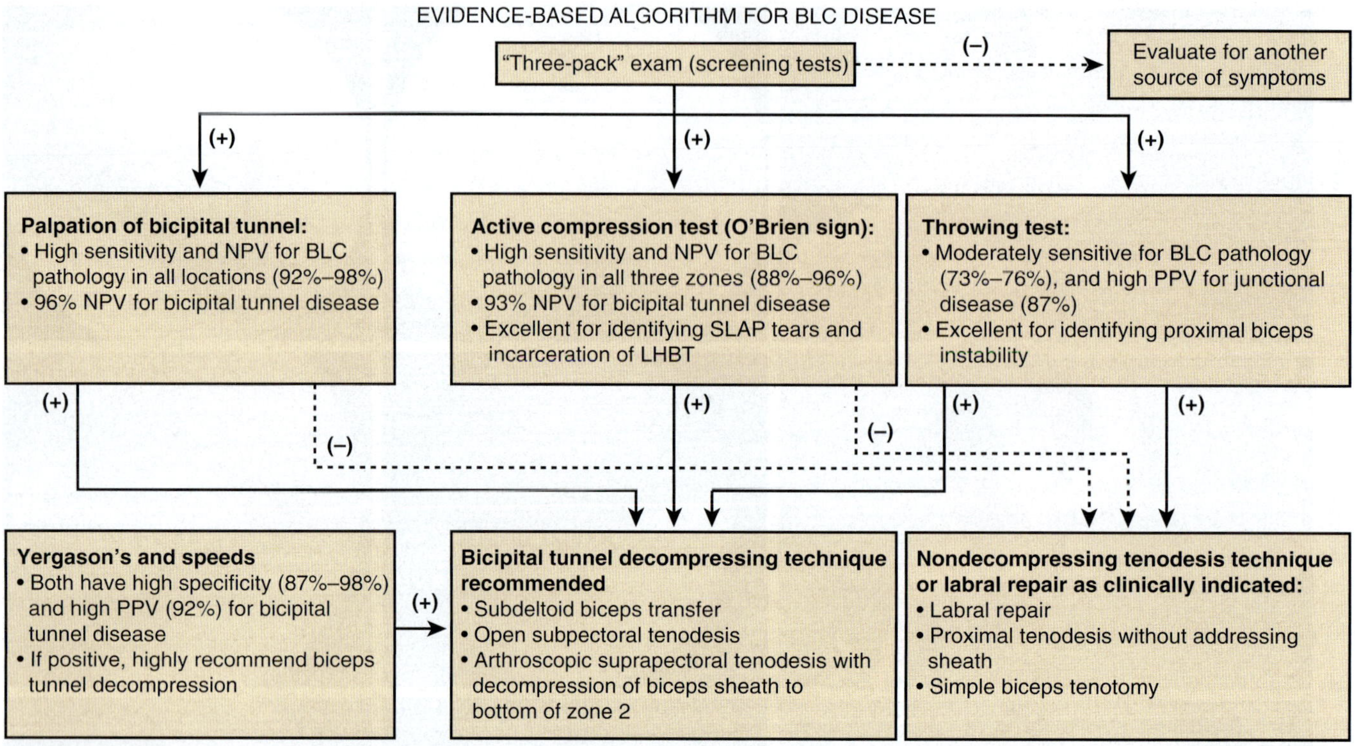

FIGURE 15-80: This treatment algorithm helps the clinician determine the most appropriate surgical technique in a particular patient based on their physical examination. Techniques can be divided into those that decompress and those that do not decompress the bicipital tunnel. Bicipital tunnel decompressing techniques include open subpectoral tenodesis, transfer to conjoint and proximal tenodesis with sheath release to the pectoralis major tendon. Nondecompressing techniques include tenotomy, proximal tenodesis without sheath release, and superior labral anterior to posterior (SLAP) lesion repair. The most important factor is identifying the bicipital tunnel disease when present. Both the active compression test (O'Brien sign) and tenderness to palpation are particularly sensitive and have high negative predictive values which allows a surgeon to identify such disease when present and to rule it out when one or both of these tests are negative. BLC, biceps-labral complex; LHBT, long head of the biceps tendon; NPV, negative predictive value; PPV, positive predictive value.

Arthroscopic Management of the Thrower's Shoulder

Curtis Bush, John Conway, George LeBus

INTRODUCTION

Diagnosis and treatment of problems in the thrower's shoulder remains a significant clinical challenge. The repetitive stress of pitching can lead to a range of adaptive pathologic changes and chronic overuse degeneration as well as acute injury. Adaptive pathology of osseous and soft tissue structures allows the shoulder to accommodate the extremes of horizontal extension and external rotation required for high-velocity throwing and can result in a shoulder that is relatively "loose in the front" and "tight in the back." The corresponding pathology often includes anterior inferior capsular laxity, posterior inferior capsular contracture, humeral retroversion, altered range of glenohumeral rotation, scapular drooping and protraction, PASTA tears, PAINT tears, and SLAP tears. In some cases, these adaptive changes may ultimately lead to structural failure, such as that seen in case of PASTA tears and chronic SLAP tears. Identification and treatment of symptomatic pathology in the context of asymptomatic adaptive or chronic change makes effective intervention difficult for the treating physician. Despite abnormal imaging findings, the primary cause of a thrower's shoulder pain are typically from being "too loose in the front," "too tight in the back," to poor muscle balance and impaired mechanics. Anatomic abnormality identified on imaging may be the result of the problem rather than being the problem itself; in such cases, treatment of the structural defect as the primary problem without redress of the underlying pathology is liable to fail.

Effective treatment requires recognition of symptomatic pathology in the context of biomechanics as well as that of adaptive changes. In symptomatic patients who do not respond to extensive, appropriate nonoperative treatment, surgical repair may be warranted given that a certain pathology, such as a rotator cuff tear or SLAP tear, will not heal spontaneously and may progress to worsen the pain and disability. On the other hand, the rotator cuff tear or SLAP tear may reach equilibrium whereupon progression or disability does not occur. As many as 50% of asymptomatic, professional-level pitchers were recently shown to have a partial-thickness rotator cuff tear and/or a SLAP lesion on MRI in one study.[400] As many as 80% of asymptomatic, mature pitchers had MRI changes and 45% had a labral tear in another study.[477] In asymptomatic individuals with pathologic findings on imaging, restoration of normal anatomy may even be detrimental and may potentially lead recurrent tear, loss of motion, and worsening of performance. This fact may explain why results of SLAP repair, rotator cuff repair, or combined SLAP and rotator cuff repair are less favorable in throwers compared with those in the general population.

Restoration of anatomy is important in the correct context. While surgical treatment of adaptive, asymptomatic pathology may create additional problems in this patient population, acute injury and symptomatic chronic pathology may warrant surgical intervention. Nonoperative treatment is the first-line therapy for the injured thrower's shoulder regardless of the source of pain. This consists of rest, activity modification, and a well-conceived rehabilitation program. The evaluation should focus on commonly acquired, overuse kinetic chain deficits, which may include the throwing mechanics; hamstring tightness; landing leg quad weakness/lunge strength; landing leg hip flexion; loss of internal rotation; stance leg hip extension; loss of external rotation; pelvic obliquity and rotation limitations; poor posture; poor core/trunk/spine flexibility, strength, and endurance; scapular malposition and dyskinesis (SICK scapula); shoulder motion loss (GIRD, total arc of motion loss, cross-body adduction); shoulder weakness, dynamic instability; pectoralis major/latissimus mismatch; pectoralis major/minor tightness; and muscle inactivation (C5 nerve dysfunction, thoracic outlet syndrome, suprascapular nerve palsy, long thoracic nerve palsy). A good throwing rehabilitation program should focus on the deficits above, with particular emphasis on restoration of the kinetic chain, internal and external rotation recovery, scapular repositioning (i.e., pectoralis minor stretching) and strengthening, lower extremity flexibility and strengthening, core strengthening, and a controlled return to throwing exercises. If initial rehabilitation yields little improvement then targeted injections, such as subacromial, intra-articular, AC joint, and biceps tunnel, are invaluable diagnostic cum therapeutic tools to distinguish and treat potential pain generators. If these conservative measures fail, operative treatment may be necessary. Surgical strategies are diverse and continue to evolve. This chapter describes the range of surgical techniques used for the treatment of symptomatic shoulder pathology in the throwing athlete, which includes rotator cuff tear, SLAP tear, glenohumeral motion loss, instability, biceps tunnel disease, subacromial impingement, and posterior shoulder ossification.

Rotator Cuff Tears

The rotator cuff sustains significant stress with repetitive acceleration, deceleration, and a wide range of overhead motion that is required of the throwing athlete. Most rotator cuff tears in the throwing athlete are partial-thickness, articular-sided injuries caused by supraphysiologic eccentric, torsional, and shear forces due to repetitive throwing motion as well as to the repeated undersurface compression from posterosuperior glenohumeral internal impingement. One of the most challenging aspects in treating rotator cuff pathology in overhead throwers is to determine whether the rotator cuff tear is indeed the primary source of pain. Rotator cuff tears may be asymptomatic or only a minor contributor to the overall symptomatology, and the pain may in fact result from other concomitant pathologies. Without question, the presence of a rotator cuff tear seems to make treatment of other coexisting pathology more difficult. Rotator cuff tears may also contribute to kinematic dysfunction in general and lead to other painful conditions such as bursitis. In order to establish a cuff tear as being truly symptomatic and to verify that surgical intervention is justified, the evaluation of the thrower with a rotator cuff tear must be comprehensive. The treating physician should rule out all other potential sources of symptoms, such as glenohumeral motion loss, SLAP tear, biceps pain, thoracic outlet syndrome, lower extremity weakness or poor flexibility, core weakness, scapular dyskinesis, and other shortcomings in the throwing mechanics. If these conditions are present, they may be addressed with a rehabilitation program prior to specific intervention for the rotator cuff tear. In our experience, the rotator cuff pathology is not commonly the source of pain; however, when it is, a subacromial injection may provide relief. A good response may also indicate the presence of commonly associated painful subacromial bursitis.

When the rotator cuff tear is ultimately determined to be the main pain generator and when conservative measures have failed, surgical intervention is warranted. Prognosis with surgery may be strongly influenced by patient factors such as age, position, level of the athlete, future potential, and history of surgery on the shoulder in question as well as other surgical factors such as the quality of the tissue, depth of the tear, and the extent of tear delamination. The surgeon should establish realistic expectations both for himself or herself and for the patient. Both parties must communicate effectively so that realistic goals of surgery and recovery are clearly understood.

Surgical Findings

Arthroscopic findings in a thrower with a rotator cuff tear typically include a posterior, L-shaped, undersurface articular sided tear/avulsion of variable depth at the junction of the posterior and anterior infraspinatus tendons. The greater tuberosity footprint is usually partially exposed, and delamination may occur within the tendon between the torn articular-sided flap and the residual attached cuff. Conway et al. described this injury pattern as PAINT lesion, which is essentially a posterior variant of the Snyder type A4 PASTA lesion.[156,666] Detachment can be variable ,with its greatest extent typically at the posterior supraspinatus tendon. Delamination can be seen between the retracted articular margin flap and the remainder of the attached cuff. The posterior margin of the tear is mobile and appears as a flap of tendon, with the tear often extending medially, well into the middle layers of the infraspinatus tendon (Figs. 15-81 to 15-84; Video 15-2). One factor that may contribute to the intratendinous location of this tear type is the shear stress created between the tangential and perpendicularly directed forces which act within the five-layered architecture of the rotator cuff tendon. The degree of delamination is difficult to assess accurately arthroscopically, but a thin-section, high-resolution MRI with intra-articular contrast in abduction–external rotation views may help predict the extent of delamination.[393] The surgeon must also be suspicious for the presence of a concealed tear, which is an anterior variant of a Snyder type A4 PASTA lesion that is primarily intratendinous and often unseen on arthroscopic exam. Preoperative MRI is essential to the detection of this lesion (Fig. 15-85).

The pathophysiological basis of the PAINT lesion is not entirely clear. Some of the factors thought to contribute

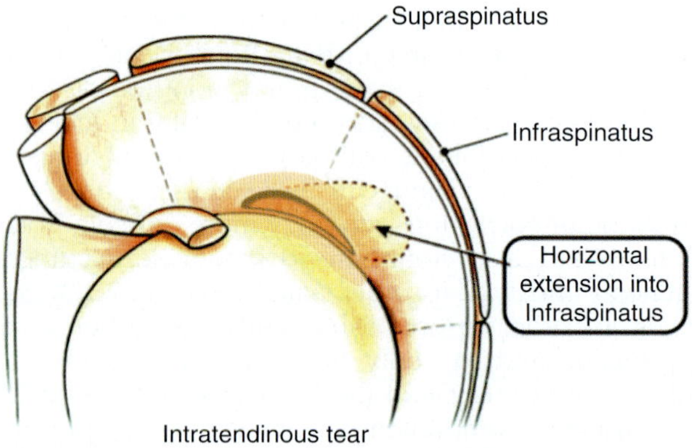

FIGURE 15-81: Diagram depicting a posterior articular intratendinous rotator cuff tear at its typical location at the posterior aspect of the supraspinatus tendon and anterior aspect of the infraspinatus tendon.

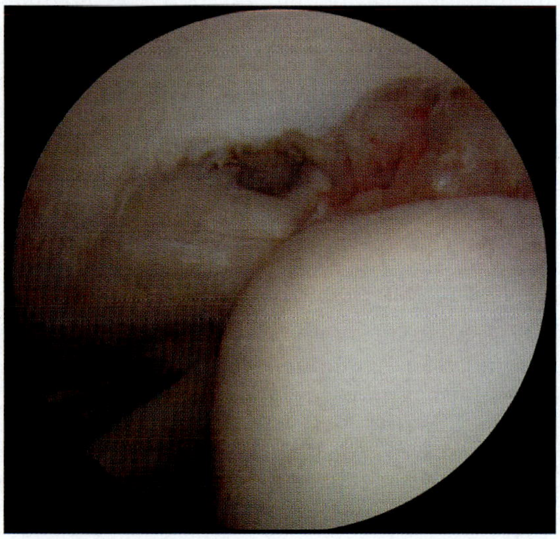

FIGURE 15-83: Arthroscopic view of a partial articular tear with intratendinous extension lesion.

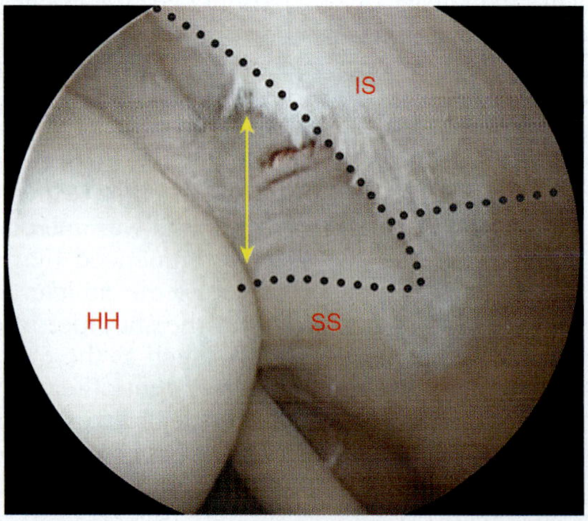

FIGURE 15-82: Arthroscopic view of a partial articular tear with intratendinous extension. The arrow indicates retraction of the partial-thickness rotator cuff tear. HH, humeral head; IS, infraspinatus; SS, supraspinatus.

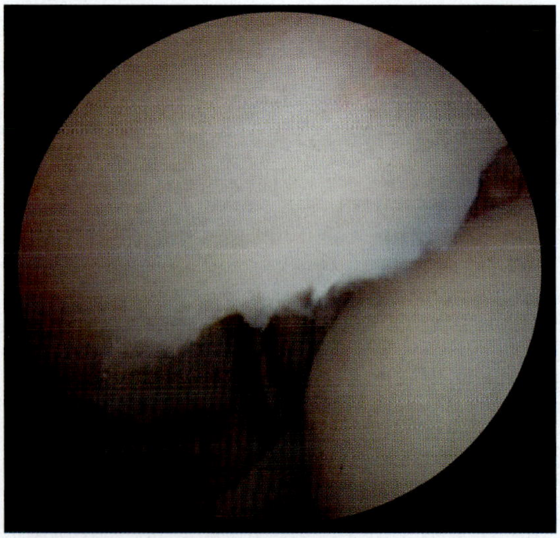

FIGURE 15-84: An additional arthroscopic view demonstrating the mobile flap of the posterior margin of the tear and evidence of the substantial delamination that can occur in these lesions.

to these tears include internal impingement (excessive glenohumeral laxity, glenohumeral external rotation, and horizontal extension); intrinsic tendon degeneration; local tissue hypovascularity; anterior-inferior glenohumeral instability; rotator interval and coracohumeral ligament laxity; subacromial outlet impingement; SLAP lesions, shoulder motion loss, humeral retroversion, trunk and shoulder girdle muscle dysfunction; neurologic conditions; impaired mechanics, and excessive throwing volume. Additionally, the articular side of the cuff is less vascular and has a higher modulus of elasticity, greater stiffness, and a less favorable stress-strain curve compared with the bursal surface. Furthermore, eccentric forces tend to be concentrated more along the articular surface fibers.[143,491,590,615,718]

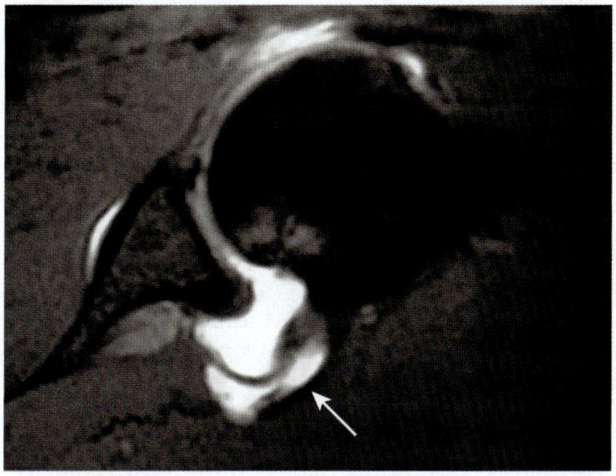

FIGURE 15-85: Axial image from abduction–external rotation magnetic resonance image demonstrating an intratendinous tear, which may be difficult to visualize arthroscopically (*arrow*).

Other associated findings on arthroscopic examination of the thrower's shoulder may include type II SLAP tears; posterior-superior labral tears; posterior-inferior labral tears, avulsions or Kim lesions, anterior-inferior labral tears, anterior-inferior glenohumeral laxity, contracted and thickened posterior-inferior capsule, inflammatory and hypertrophic subacromial bursa, excessive glenohumeral external rotation with concomitant deficient glenohumeral IR/ER loss, and scapular dyskinesis or malposition.

Surgical Technique

Three surgical options that are typically discussed for the treatment of rotator cuff tears in the throwing athlete include debridement, in situ tendon-to-tendon repair of delamination, and repair of partial tear to bone. Specific controversies include whether the decision to repair should be based on the depth of tear, on the extent of delamination, the location of the tear with respect to the rotator cable insertion, or on some other factor. Debridement has produced return to throw rates of 16% to 85% (Table 15-4). In these cases, healing may be limited by continued separation of torn tendon edges, poor vascularity, presence of degenerative tissue, and repetitive contact between the rotator cuff tear and glenoid rim while throwing.

If repair is warranted, the choice of the method and the healing potential are key considerations. A number of methods have been described. The broad goals of repair should be to restore the integrity of the rotator cable, to repair the delamination component of the tear, and to avoid overconstraining the shoulder.[82] In general, a side-to-side tendon-to-tendon or tendon-to-bone repair technique is rarely indicated. When repair is necessary, we most commonly employ a lateral tendon-to-tendon vertical mattress to stabilize the free margins of the tear (Videos 15-3 and 15-4) or rotator cable articular repair (Videos 15-5 and 15-6).

TABLE 15-4 Outcomes of Rotator Cuff Debridement Surgery

Citation	LOE	No. of Patients	Technique	Associated Pathology	Follow-up (Months)	Return to Play (Same or Higher Level)
Andrews et al., 1985[9]	IV	34 athletes (23 pitchers), mean age 22 y	Debride PTRCT	All had labral tears, 6 with partial biceps tear, 3 with tendonitis	13.1	76%
Payne et al., 1997[560]	IV	29 overhead athletes, aged <40 y	Debride PTRCT	17 had labral tears; 11 posterior, 3 anterior, 3 SLAP lesions	24	45%
Reynolds et al., 2008[597]	IV	67 professional pitchers, mean age 25.6 y	Debride PTRCT	Only 4% isolated cuff; labral debridement in 26%, labral repair in 60%, thermal shrinkage in 33%, capsule release in 6%	39.2	55%
Riand et al., 2002[601]	IV	67 throwing athletes	Debride PTRCT	90% had labral lesions, most posterior	22.3	16%

LOE, level of evidence; PTRCT, partial thickness rotator cuff tear; SLAP, superior labral anterior to posterior.
Modified from Kibler WB, Juhn JE, Wilk K. The disabled throwing shoulder: spectrum of pathology-10 year update. Arthroscopy. *2013;29(1):141-161.*

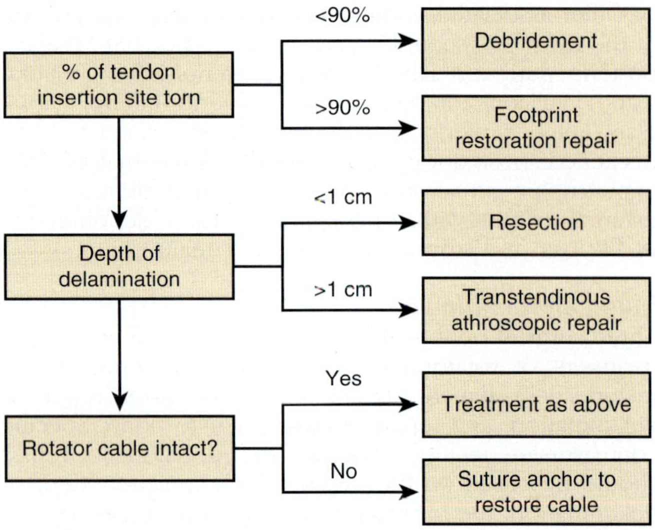

FIGURE 15-86: The authors' algorithm for surgical treatment of rotator cuff injuries in throwers.

Our algorithm is based primarily on the depth of the tear and extent of delamination as well as on the integrity of the rotator cable as described by Burkhart et al.[107] (Fig. 15-86). Debridement is performed if the tear involves less than 90% of the tendon insertion site. Arthroscopic partial footprint restoration repair is considered for tears that have more than 90% of the footprint. When the depth of delamination is less than 1 cm and involves poorly vascularized, degenerative tissue, resection of the articular-sided segment is performed. When delamination is greater than 1 cm and involves tissue that is amenable to repair, transtendinous arthroscopic repair of the lateral margin of the tear is the procedure of choice.

With regard to the rotator cable, if the anterior or posterior cable anchor is disrupted, a suture anchor is placed to restore the cable anatomy at the anchor site (see Videos 15-5 and 15-6). Any detachment or partial detachment of the cuff between the anterior and posterior cable anchor sites is usually left unrepaired. The goal is to establish a tear that is contained between the anterior and posterior cable anchors and that does not overconstrain the cuff. The thrower's PASTA/PAINT is probably well tolerated as long as it is less than full thickness, is contained within the rotator crescent, and when both rotator cable anchors are intact.

We recommend performing a bursectomy prior to suture passage, which aids in passing and tying of suture knots in the subacromial space. Care should be taken to avoid injury to the coracoacromial ligament during bursectomy. Although some recent studies[83,151] have shown favorable results of acromioplasty, we strongly discourage this technique as outlet impingement is rarely the primary cause of pain in the overhead throwing athlete. Furthermore, published reports that have included acromioplasty with treatment of rotator cuff tears have failed to yield excellent results.[222,560,617,705] We recommend preservation of the subacromial arch in the throwers unless there is obvious enthesopathy that contributes to the pathology. The addition of biologics to the repair is somewhat controversial at present and we do not favor it; however, further research may establish it as an accepted part of the armamentarium.[13]

Outcomes

Neither the outcomes of rotator cuff debridement nor those of repair have yielded particularly favorable results in the throwing athlete. Published results of rotator cuff debridement are listed in Table 15-4 and those of repair in Table 15-5. In an early report of debridement of partial-thickness rotator cuff tears, Andrews et al. documented an 85% return to play rate after surgical intervention.[9] More recent studies of debridement have not been as favorable with Tomlinson and Payne both reporting 45% return to play rates at the same level.[560,708] For repair, published outcomes are limited to small series that have involved various surgical techniques and limited follow-up. Ide reported on 17 patients with mean age of 42 (range, 17-51 years) with partial articular-sided rotator cuff repair. In the study, the authors describe a transtendinous repair technique using one or two doubly loaded suture anchors placed at the medial footprint. Sutures are passed through cuff tissue in mattress fashion and tied in the subacromial space in order to reduce the torn tendon to the footprint. Only six of the 17 patients in this study group were overhead athletes. Of these, three were baseball players and the remaining three played tennis, volleyball, and badminton, respectively. Five of the six athletes participated in competitive sports and one in organized recreational sports. Two athletes, the badminton player and tennis player, returned to their previous level of sports competition, three returned at a lower level, and one baseball player was unable to return to active sports. The mean time to return was 8.4 months. Overall, 14 of 17 patients (82%) had excellent results, and two of 17 (12%) had good results; however, the results were less favorable among the baseball players.[332] Based on this study, tendon-to-bone transtendinous repairs in throwers may not be reliable.

Brockmeier et al. described a transtendinous repair technique with encouraging early results.[82] Their report included eight patients, five baseball players (three Major League pitchers and two collegiate-level pitchers) and three tennis players (one high-level prospect and two competitive amateur players) with a mean follow-up of 5 months. Their technique calls for the reduction of the partial-thickness flap using a grasper placed through the anterior rotator interval portal. With the reduction held in place, two percutaneous spinal needles are placed through the full thickness of the cuff, one anterior and one posterior to create a horizontal mattress configuration. Passing sutures or wire snares are passed through the needles and retrieved from an anterior intra-articular portal. The passing suture and/or snare are used to pass one limb of a nonabsorbable suture through each site in which the needles were initially passed. The suture limbs are then retrieved in the subacromial space, where they are tied.

TABLE 15-5 Outcomes of Rotator Cuff Repair in Throwing Athletes

Citation	LOE	No. of Patients	Technique	Associated Pathology	Follow-up (Months)	RTP (Same or Better Level)
Conway et al., 2001[156]	IV	14 professional baseball players (13 pitchers)	Repair delaminated tendon, not to bone	100% with SLAP tears; 50% with anterior instability; 57% had subacromial bursitis	16	8/9 players; RTP <12-month follow-up; 89% RTP
Ide et al., 2005[332]	IV	17 athletes, 6 throwing athletes; mean age 42 y	Repair PTRCT to bone	None	39	2/6 RTP same level; 3/6 RTP lower level; 1/6 did not return
Liem et al., 2008[406]	III	21 amateur throwing athletes; mean age 58.9 y; isolated supraspinatus tear	FTRCT repair to bone	Distal clavicle excision in 4/21; biceps tenotomy in 4/21	25.7	No difference between preinjury and postoperative participation levels; re-tear rate 29% but no influence on RTP
Mazoue and Andrews, 2006[444]	IV	16 professional baseball players (12 pitchers)	Mini-open repair of FTRCT to bone	2 SLAP repair plus thermal capsulorrhaphy; 2 labral debridement plus thermal capsulorrhaphy; 2 thermal capsulorrhaphy; 4 labral debridement	66.6	1/12 (8%) RTP; 1/2 (50%) position players with dominant arm involved RTP
Van Kleunen et al., 2012[724]	IV	17 collegiate and high school baseball players	3 suture anchor repairs to bone; 14 intratendinous repairs	Posterior inferior capsular release in 11; SLAP repair in all 17	37	6/17 (35%) RTP similar or better level; 5/17 (29%) RTP at lower level; 6/17 (35%) no RTP

LOE, level of evidence; PTRCT, partial thickness rotator cuff tear; FTRCT; full thickness rotator cuff tear; RTP, return to play; SLAP, superior labral anterior to posterior tear.

Modified from Kibler WB, Juhn JE, Wilk K. The disabled throwing shoulder: spectrum of pathology-10 year update. Arthroscopy *2013;29(1):141-161.*

Conway et al. reported on their technique in nine baseball players. The average age was 26 (range, 19 to 36 years); seven were professional players, and two played at the college level. At 1-year follow-up, 8/9 (89%) had returned to throwing. At the 2-year follow-up, excellent outcomes were recorded in seven of the nine (78%) who had returned to play by 1 year.[156] Finally, Van Kleunen et al. reported on a case series that consisted of 17 baseball players treated for concomitant rotator cuff and SLAP tears with repairs of both. The SLAP tear was treated with glenoid based repair with use of suture anchors, and the rotator cuff tear was treated with PDS suture (14/17 patients) or suture anchor (3/17). Only 35% of the players were able to return to the same or higher level of play, while 29% returned to a lower level or other position with persistent arm problems; 35% were unable to return to baseball due to arm problems. Both the Kerlan-Jobe Orthopaedic Clinic overhead athlete scores (KJOC) and return to play status were significantly worse in patients in whom a suture anchor was used compared with those in whom a PDS suture for used for rotator cuff repair.[724] The small sample size in this series prevents any definitive conclusions; however, these results underscore the notion that a minimalistic approach may limit deleterious, iatrogenic injury of the rotator cuff or overconstrained throwing shoulder. Rotator cuff tears have also been shown to be predictive of poor outcomes in the context of SLAP tears in throwing athletes. Neri et al. recently demonstrated that although 80% of patients with an isolated SLAP tear returned to play at the same level, only 12.5% of throwers with a combined SLAP and rotator cuff tear were able to reach their former level of competition.[503]

Full-thickness rotator cuff tears are less common in throwing athletes and are associated with significantly worse outcomes than the previously described partial-thickness tears. Only two clinical studies have discussed full-thickness rotator cuff tears in throwers. Mazoué and Andrews reported on 16 professional baseball players who were treated with mini-open rotator cuff repair for full-thickness tear, 12 of whom were pitchers who had sustained injury to their dominant shoulder. Only one pitcher (8%) was able to return to a highly competitive level of baseball without significant shoulder dysfunction.[444] Tibone et al. reported on 45 athletes, 15 of whom had full-thickness tears. Of their patients, only 7 of 22 (32%) returned to compete at the same level.[705]

Many questions remain regarding the ideal treatment for rotator cuff tears in the thrower's shoulder. For example, little is known in terms of what player-specific factors place athletes at higher risk for symptomatic rotator cuff injury. Some athletes may be "high contact throwers" who place excessive force and torque on their rotator cuff or who have increased humeral head translation. These patients may perhaps have better outcomes if rotator cuff repair is performed in conjunction with capsular procedures to favorably alter the glenohumeral kinematics. Overall, due to the limited follow-up of the current studies, long-term results of rotator cuff debridement or repair and the state of the thrower's shoulder 5 or 10 years after treatment are as yet unknown. Furthermore, the surgical philosophy for symptomatic rotator cuff tears in throwers is controversial. One argument claims that repair of a rotator cuff tear is justified based on the fact that rotator cuff tears do not heal on their own, may progress, and aggravate pain and functional decline. The counterpoint to this view proposes that the rotator cuff tear, as an element of adaptive pathology, may allow for greater horizontal extension and external rotation which may lead to better performance. The tear may reach an equilibrium at which progression no longer occurs and restoration of the normal footprint anatomy may actually be detrimental, and lead to recurrent tear, motion loss, and poorer performance. In general, most throwing athletes who require surgical intervention for rotator cuff tear will have an optimal outcome if the proceduralist considers the adaptive, chronic changes in the throwing shoulder and the notion proposed by Jobe that often "less is more." Surgery that minimizes soft tissue trauma, avoids overconstraint of the shoulder, and aims to establish a stable partial-thickness tear that is contained between the intact anterior and posterior cable anchors may have the best result.

SLAP Tears

SLAP tears are among the most common anatomic derangements associated with pain and dysfunction in the thrower's shoulder. The pathogenesis of SLAP tears in throwers remains unknown although several theories have been expounded in the literature. Nonoperative treatment of SLAP tears is the mainstay of treatment, particularly in throwers, and has achieved good success.[207] Even with initial failure of nonoperative treatment, Fedoriw et al. demonstrated reasonable success with a second course of physical therapy specifically designed to improve glenohumeral internal rotation deficit (GIRD), scapular dyskinesia, posterior capsular contracture, and any concomitant injuries.[228] Surgical treatment of SLAP tears, whether by repair or biceps tenotomy/tenodesis, has overall been successful in the general population, but surgical results are far less favorable in overhead athletes. Emphasis should certainly be placed on conservative treatment, namely rest and physical therapy for this condition. Intra-articular injection of anesthetic agents/steroids serves both therapeutic and diagnostic roles and may help determine if the SLAP tear is indeed the pain generator. Failed nonoperative treatment may warrant surgical intervention; however, success may be largely influenced by factors independent of the quality of surgical repair, such as age, associated pathology, position in sport, and the competitive level. For instance, Fedoriw et al. showed that higher level pitchers return to play and at a higher level than lower level pitchers regardless of whether they undergo nonoperative or operative treatment.[228]

Surgical Findings

Examination under anesthesia is an important diagnostic tool and should be incorporated into the operative plan for SLAP lesions. Common findings may include increased anterior-inferior laxity, increased or decreased external rotation at 90 degrees abduction, increased or decreased internal rotation at 90 degrees abduction, total arc of motion difference relative to contralateral side, and diminished horizontal (cross-body) adduction at 90 degrees of forward flexion (indicative of posterior capsular contracture). In the evaluation of ROM the surgeon must also take into account humeral version, as external/internal rotation and total arc of motion differences may, in part, be attributable to humeral version, which may be different between the thrower's dominant and nondominant upper extremity.

The arthroscopic evaluation may be performed in either the beach chair or lateral decubitus position using traditional posterior and anterior portals. The surgeon may encounter several different tear types, which were initially described using a classification by Snyder et al.[668] The Snyder classification has since been modified by others with the incorporation of several tear patterns.[427,488] The BLC may be evaluated for the "peel back" phenomenon, which is indicative of glenoid detachment and loss of washer and bumper effect (Video 15-7).[34,109,668,726] One should be familiar with the anatomic variants such as sublabral foramina, Buford complex, or meniscoid-like labral attachment that lacks evidence of peel back.[101] Other associated findings may include articular cartilage damage, which is indicated by increased translation of the humeral head[633]; anterior inferior capsular laxity, loss of tension in posterior IGHL; increased posterior labral thickness and fraying indicated by increased translation and consequent shear and compression on the labrum (Figs. 15-87 and 15-88); posterior capsular thickness, representative of the capsular changes that contribute to motion loss; and biceps tenosynovitis (Fig. 15-89). SLAP tears and rotator cuff tears are linked by their pathologic mechanisms in overhead throwing athletes, and as a result, rotator cuff pathology is commonly present as well (Video 15-8). Morgan et al. found 31% incidence of partial-thickness rotator cuff tears in association with SLAP tears,[488] and Fedoriw et al. found that 12 of 45 (27%) professional pitchers with a SLAP tear had a coexisting rotator cuff tear of at least 30% thickness.[228] In these circumstances, the challenge for the treating physician is

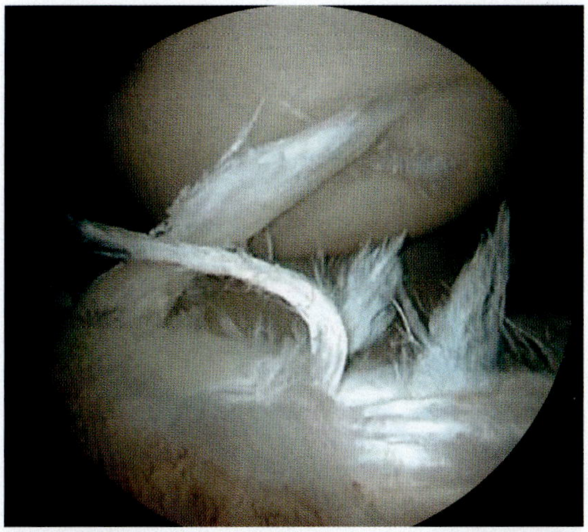

FIGURE 15-87: Posterior labral thickening and fraying in the setting of a superior labral anterior to posterior tear caused by increased translation of the humeral head and the consequent shear on and compression of the labrum.

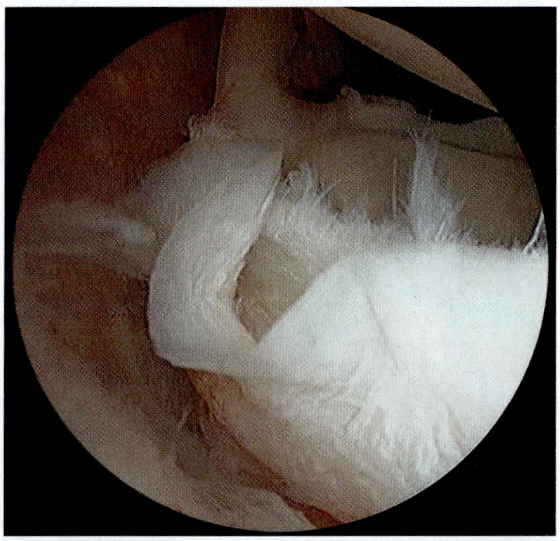

FIGURE 15-88: Posterior labral fold tear in the setting of a superior labral anterior to posterior tear.

to ascertain the true etiology of pain in the elite overhead throwing athlete.

Surgical Technique

The labral repair begins with appropriate portal placement. A traditional posterior portal is used in conjunction with an anterior interval portal. Some surgeons utilize a second anterior portal through either the superior anterior interval or a transtendinous (through supraspinatus) portal. We prefer to use a single anterior interval portal and place anchors percutaneously through a transtendinous portal through the muscular portion of the rotator cuff. We believe that a transtendinous portal is essential to proper anchor placement; however, we discourage the use of a transtendinous cannula.

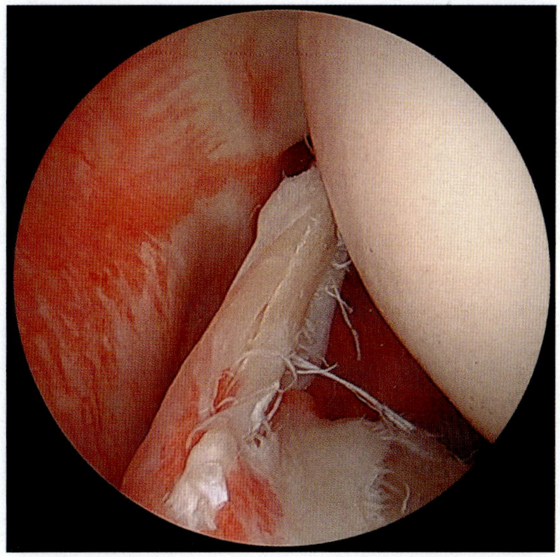

FIGURE 15-89: Fraying of the long head of the biceps tendon representative of biceps tenosynovitis.

The sequence of repair is as follows. First, the surgeon should look out for the peel back phenomenon. The meniscoid rim, which is often frayed, is debrided. The superior-posterior glenoid is then primed for repair by creation of a bleeding bony bed for reattachment of the labrum. Anchor drill sites are placed on the rim of the glenoid but not onto the face. At this point, anchor is placed followed by reaffixation of the labrum with a goal of at least two separate points of fixation. A typical repair will incorporate two to three anchors, spaced approximately 5 mm apart; however, the number of anchors may vary. Suture placement should be posterior to the biceps insertion site and care should be taken to avoid overconstraining the biceps. Sutures at the 12 and 11 o'clock positions are passed through the superior surface of the labrum, within the substance of the labrum, and great care is taken to prevent capture or strangulation of the biceps tendon. It is also important to avoid capture or cause trauma to the superior capsule to avoid postoperative fibrosis of the superior glenoid recess. We no longer tie knots due to the risk of chondral and/or rotator cuff abrasion; we routinely use knotless anchors because of their ease and to avoid the problems associated with bulky, abrasive knots (Figs. 15-90 to 15-95; Video 15-9). Though we recommend against use of knots for SLAP repairs, if knots are used they should be placed medially away from the glenoid and humeral articular surfaces. Following repair, the biceps is reevaluated for mobility to make sure it is not overconstrained in abduction and external rotation. An anterior-superior anchor (at the 12:30 to 2 o'clock position in the right shoulder) is rarely used to avoid biceps tethering, but this anchor may be necessary in the setting of instability with middle glenohumeral ligament avulsion of the glenoid. Special attention is needed to prevent against any loss of external rotation compared with the preoperative assessment.[363] With respect to the thrower's shoulder, "too loose" is better than "too tight."

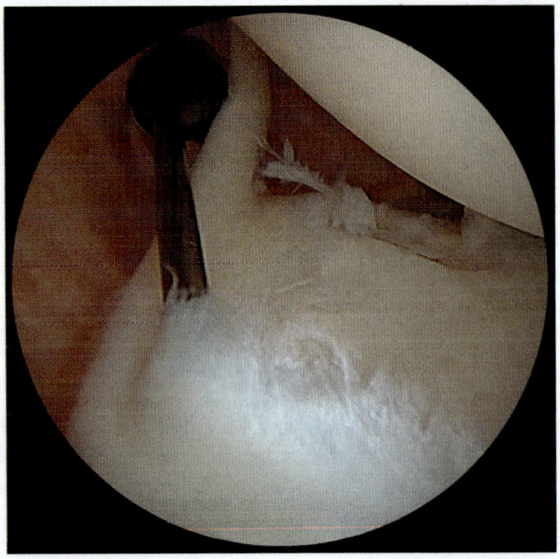

FIGURE 15-90: Probe placed through the anterior interval portal demonstrating superior labral anterior to posterior tear.

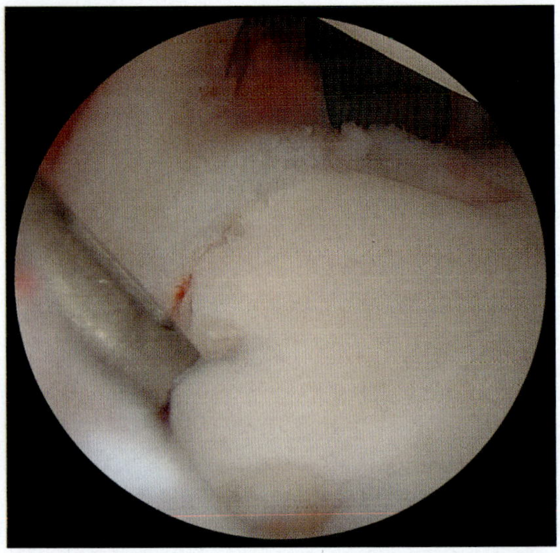

FIGURE 15-92: Drill for anchor placement for superior labral anterior to posterior lesion repair.

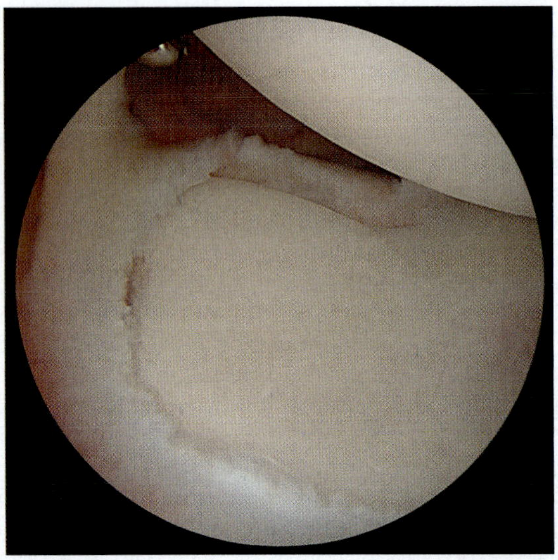

FIGURE 15-91: Superior labral anterior to posterior tear before repair.

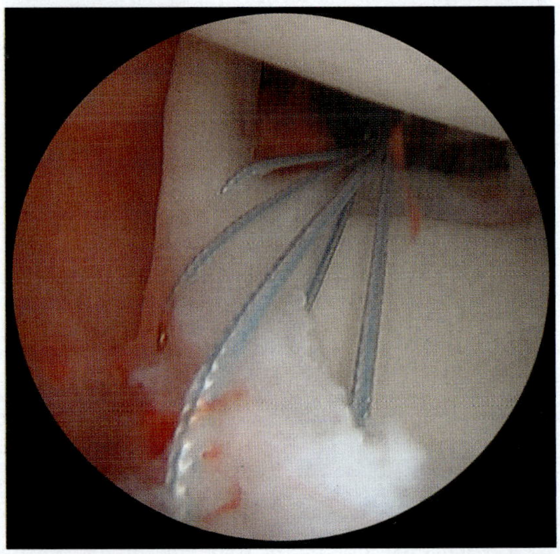

FIGURE 15-93: Suture passage for superior labral anterior to posterior lesion repair.

Outcomes

The published results of surgical treatment of SLAP tears in throwers are summarized in Table 15-6. If return to play at the same or higher level is used as the criteria for success, only 5 of 22 series have reported success rates above 85%. Successful outcomes have ranged from 22% to 94%.[147,228,334,366] Most published series represent a low level of evidence, which likely contributes to the wide variability in the results.

Determining the isolated outcomes of SLAP lesions is also made difficult by the fact that most studies assess SLAP treatment in conjunction with treatment of other lesions. SLAP tears may be associated with or predispose to other pathology in the shoulder as well, such as partial-thickness rotator cuff tears,[488] chondral injury,[554] or posterosuperior glenoid bone fragment (superior Bennett lesion).[498] Van Kleunen et al. showed that in a series of 17 patients with SLAP tears treated in conjunction with GIRD and infraspinatus tears, only 6 (35%) returned to their previous level of performance.[724] In areport by Neri et al., only 13 out of 23 (57%) throwers were able to achieve preinjury performance levels 1 year after arthroscopic repair of type II SLAP lesions. Moreover, a concomitant partial-thickness rotator cuff tear was a negative predictor of the ability to return to play[503]; however, the authors did not report routine inspection of the

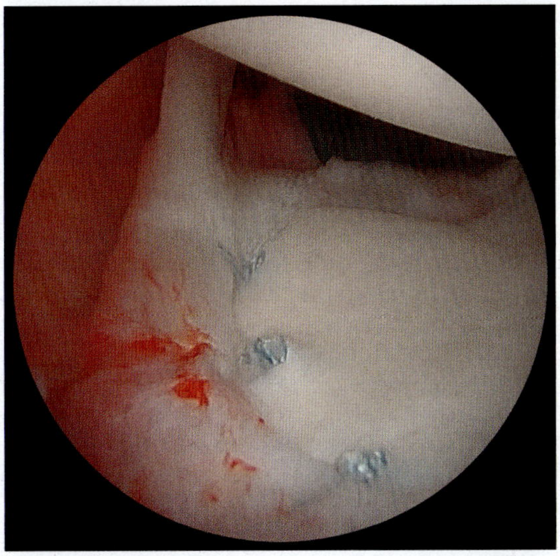

FIGURE 15-94: Superior labral anterior to posterior repair viewed from the posterior portal after anchor placement and cutting of suture.

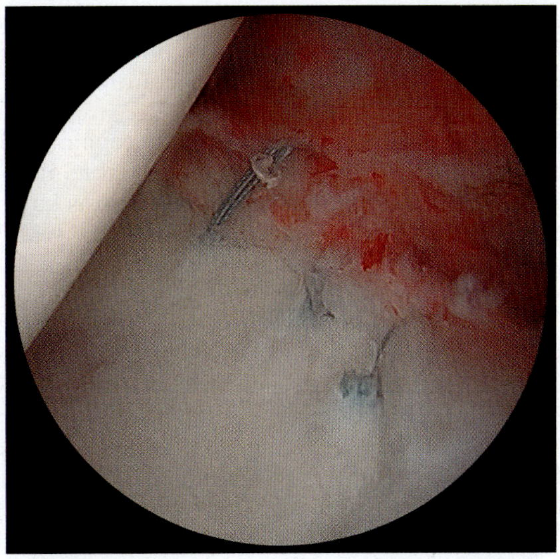

FIGURE 15-95: Superior labral anterior to posterior lesion repair viewed from the anterior interval portal.

TABLE 15-6 Outcomes of SLAP Repairs in Throwing Athletes

Citation	LOE	No. of Patients	Technique	Associated Pathology	Follow-up	RTP (Same or Better Level)
Brockmeier et al., 2009[83]	IV	47 total, 34 athletes (28 overhead throwing athletes)	Suture anchor	24/47 PTRCT debridement; 33/47 subacromial bursectomy; 4/47 DCE	2.7 yr	71% of athletes; 11/12 with acute injury; 14/22 with chronic injury
Cohen et al., 2011[147]	IV	23 baseball players	Suture anchor	None	>24 mo	32% RTP overall; 17% RTP for AA or higher level
Ide et al., 2005[334]	IV	40 overhead throwing athletes	Suture anchor	30/40 with PTRCT debridement	41 mo	60% RTP for baseball players with overuse SLAPs
Fedoriw et al., 2014[228]	IV	40 baseball players (27 pitchers)	Suture anchor or debridement	None	>1 season	40% RTP for pitchers; 85% for nonpitchers
Kim et al., 2002[366]	IV	34 patients (18 throwing athletes)	Suture anchor	None	33 mo	4/18 (22%) RTP for throwers

DCE: distal clavicle excision; LOE, level of evidence; PTRCT, partial thickness rotator cuff tear; RTP, return to play; SLAP, superior labral anterior to posterior tear.
Modified from: Kibler WB, Juhn JE, Wilk K. The disabled throwing shoulder: spectrum of pathology-10 year update. Arthroscopy 2013;29(1):141-161.

subacromial bursa or bursectomy in these patients. We recommend subacromial inspection if symptoms are suggestive of bursitis, and bursectomy in the event that a thick, inflamed bursa is encountered.

Whereas acromioplasty has had poor results documented in the literature in conjunction with rotator cuff treatment, two reports have demonstrated more favorable results with acromioplasty performed in conjunction with treatment of type II SLAP lesions. Brockmeier et al. reported higher level of satisfaction among throwers who underwent SAD in addition to SLAP repair, when compared with those who underwent SLAP repair alone.[83] Similarly, Coleman et al. also compared outcomes of isolated SLAP repair with those of SLAP repair plus acromioplasty. Over a mean follow-up of 3 years, although functional outcomes scores were identical in the two groups, SLAP repair plus acromioplasty was associated with better subjective satisfaction (81% patients claimed "good" or "excellent" outcome in the latter group).[151]

Given the unfavorable results of SLAP repairs in throwers, biceps tenodesis has emerged as a viable alternative to SLAP repair. Biceps tenotomy and tenodesis have been described for the treatment of nonthrowers with SLAP tears. In these patients, tenotomy or tenodesis may be performed either in addition to or in lieu of SLAP repair with the goal of treatment to remove the traction force acting on an unstable, torn superior labrum. Indeed, outcomes for primary treatment of SLAP tears or revision surgery for failed SLAP repairs with biceps tenodesis or tenotomy have been generally favorable.[277,752] There is insufficient data on either technique in throwers, particularly for tenotomy. The impact of biceps tenodesis or tenotomy on the stability and kinematics of the throwing shoulder is still unclear,[5,555] and its precise role in the treatment of these patients is controversial.

In general, we attempt to treat superior labral disease with superior labral surgery (debridement or repair) and to treat biceps or biceps tunnel disease with biceps tunnel surgery. Accordingly, our approach is to perform a biceps tenodesis if there is obvious pathology in the biceps tendon, such as frank tear or marked tenosynovitis (see Fig. 15-89). In such a case we would typically perform an arthroscopic suprapectoral tenodesis, although the tenodesis site may be altered in the presence of zone 3 biceps tunnel disease. Biceps tunnel disease is discussed in further detail elsewhere. Biceps tenodesis may also be considered for revision SLAP surgery in case of considerable fibrosis of the superior glenoid recess or where debridement is likely to compromise the superior labrum and the base of the biceps tendon. Owing to the stress riser, proximal humerus fracture is a potential risk to the throwing athlete after biceps tenodesis.[181] Further research on the benefits and risks associated with biceps tenodesis in throwers is certainly warranted.

GIRD/MOTION LOSS

Glenohumeral rotation deficit is a consistent finding in the disabled throwing shoulder. Typically glenohumeral internal rotation (GIR) is asymmetrically diminished on the dominant side in throwers while glenohumeral external rotation (GER) is asymmetrically increased. The total ROM (TROM = GIR + GER) should be symmetric between dominant throwing arm and nondominant arm. Alterations in GIR or TROM of certain magnitudes have been implicated in causing shoulder and elbow injury.[199,497,755] No clear consensus exists on the threshold for abnormal GIR deficit (GIRD) and TROM loss. Though the traditional definition of GIRD is a side-to-side internal rotation deficit of 20 degrees, studies have shown that GIRD of 11 degrees and 18 degrees is associated with increased risk of injury.[497,755] Side-to-side alterations in TROM seem to be less tolerated as a 5-degree asymmetry was shown to increase the risk of injury.[755] Alterations in GIRD and TROM may not directly cause shoulder injury, but they may alter the normal GH kinematics by increasing the load and stress on the adjacent glenohumeral structures. Therefore GIRD and TROM should be considered important targets of treatment in the at-risk throwing shoulder.

In our opinion, evaluation of side-to-side ROM differences at the shoulder is not complete without accounting for the difference in side-to-side humeral torsion. Not accounting for torsion precludes detection of an actual motion deficit, because for some pitchers, the side-to-side humeral torsion difference will completely account for even a very large side-to-side internal rotation difference. For these throwers, values that would have suggested GIRD now may suggest external rotation loss when taking into account torsion. Therefore estimation of arm injury risk based on an absolute value or standard side-to-side internal rotation difference is an inherently flawed method. The internal rotation difference, the external rotation difference, the total ROM difference, and the humeral torsion should all be considered.

Treatment

Treatment of GIRD is essentially nonoperative and consists of rest and physical therapy aimed at posterior capsular stretching. Burkhart et al. reported their favorable experience wherein most throwers with GIRD responded well to diligent posterior capsule stretching program such as the sleeper stretch; however, they noted the rare instances where an athlete may not improve. These cases typically involved throwers at the extreme of the GIRD spectrum who also tend to have associated intra-articular pathology such as type II SLAP tears. In these cases, intraoperative findings have typically included a thickened posterior inferior capsule up to 6 mm or greater. We proposed selective posterior inferior capsular release in these patients (Fig. 15-96).[108] Yoneda et al. reported results of posterior capsular release in 16 overhead throwing athletes who had throwing pain. Pain disappeared in 14 and decreased notably in two; 11 throwers returned to preinjury activity level.[774] Morgan et al. reported a 100% successful return to the same or higher level of play after posterior inferior capsular release in 11 pitchers (eight professional, three college level) who did not respond to stretching. The mean preoperative and postoperative GIRD were 56 degrees (range, 35 to 67 degrees) and 16 degrees (2 to 20 degrees), respectively. All pitchers returned to the same or higher level of play.[489]

Instability

Instability typically manifests in the throwing shoulder as anterior microinstability due to attenuation of the IGHL from repetitive throwing cycles.[350] Increased laxity of these structures reduces anterior restraint and alters the normal glenohumeral kinematics, which may contribute to intra-articular injury such as rotator cuff and labral pathology in the form of internal impingement. Similar to the other pathologic conditions of the throwing

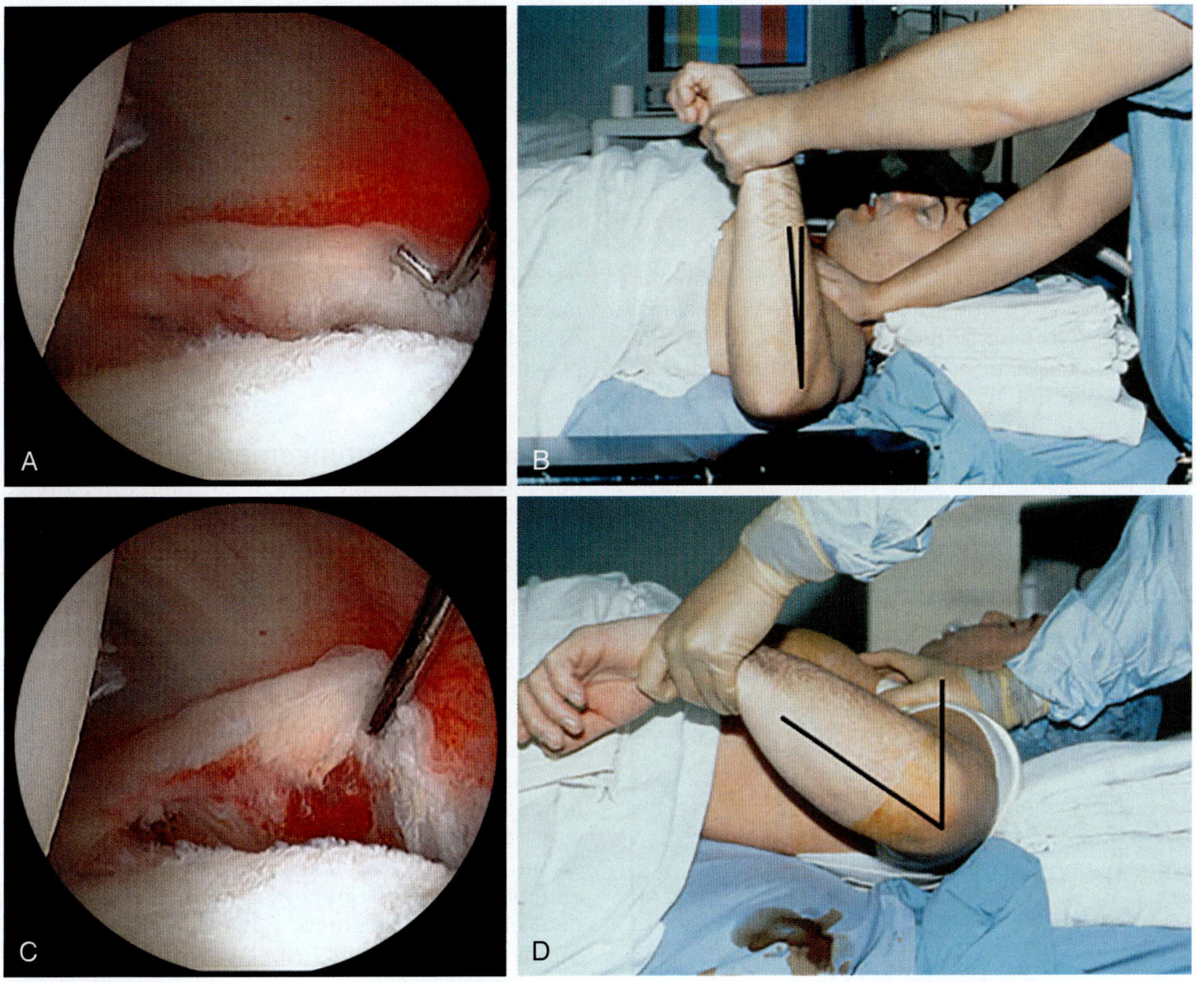

FIGURE 15-96: **A,** Posterior inferior capsule prior to release. **B,** Preoperative internal rotation deficiency. **C,** Posterior-inferior capsule after arthroscopic release. **D,** Improvement in internal rotation clinically immediately after posterior inferior capsular release.

shoulder, initial treatment for anterior instability consists of nonoperative measures which include physical therapy for posterior capsular stretching, scapular stabilization, and general strengthening and ROM of the shoulder girdle. A vast majority of patients improve on this regimen. Surgical treatment may be necessary for the minority of patients who do not respond to conservative treatment. Originally described by Jobe et al., surgical intervention has included open capsulolabral reconstruction,[349] modified Bankart procedure and anteroinferior capsular shift,[8,53,738] and arthroscopic thermal capsulorrhapy.[403] Overall, results have been inconsistent with a significant proportion of athletes unable to return to preinjury performance levels postoperatively.

Currently, the most accepted method for treatment of anterior instability in the overhead athlete is arthroscopic plication of the anteroinferior capsule to the intact labrum. Surgical treatment should always include an examination under anesthesia to document degree of instability. Following plication, humeral head translation must once again be assessed. Caution should be exercised to prevent overconstraining the anterior capsule as some degree of laxity in the throwing shoulder may represent an important form of adaptive pathology. We consider the instability in the throwing shoulder as a microinstability; therefore our approach when performing surgery is to perform "microcapsulorrhaphy" (Figs. 15-97 and 15-98; Videos 15-10 and 15-11). Our mantra, in keeping with the teachings of Frank Jobe, is that less is more and that it is better to be "too loose" than to be "too tight."

Biceps Tunnel Disease

Biceps tunnel disease is discussed elsewhere but deserves mention in the context of the throwing athlete, as the long head of the biceps can be a significant pain generator. These patients typically present with pain in the proximity of zones 1 or 2 of the biceps tunnel that is predictably relieved by ultrasound-directed tunnel injection. Collectively known as biceps tunnel disease, the spectrum of pathology that may affect the biceps tendon in this region includes space occupying lesions (such as hypertrophic tenosynovium, loose bodies, scarring, osteophytes), biceps tear, tenosynovitis, or stenosing tenosynovitis, which results from a tight pectoralis major or loss of normal restraint that maintains the biceps tendon deep to the pectoralis major. Nonoperative treatment regime includes rest, NSAIDs, pectoralis major stretching, and biceps tunnel steroid/anesthetic injections. Cases refractory to nonoperative measures deserve consideration of biceps tunnel surgery.

Intraoperative evaluation of the biceps tendon may be limited. A useful technique to analyze the tendon from inside the joint is to take a smooth grasper (e.g., Arthrex KingFisher) with space wide enough to capture the whole biceps without traumatizing it and then roll the tendon to draw it further into the joint for analysis. It may then be pushed further with a grasper or a probe. This technique provides a better look at the portion of tendon that courses through the groove. If the biceps tendon is clearly fissured, torn, or significantly frayed, then it should be treated with a biceps tenodesis. If it is merely inflamed, then nonoperative treatment is usually suitable. In our opinion, a lower zone 2 biceps tunnel suprapectoral tenodesis is likely the most appropriate option in the thrower, although others have argued in favor of a subpectoralis approach. As mentioned earlier, holes drilled into the humeral shaft for the purpose of biceps tenodesis have been complicated by humeral shaft fracture.[181] If pathology is isolated to the superior labrum instead of the biceps tunnel, we prefer superior labral debridement or repair over biceps tenodesis whenever possible.

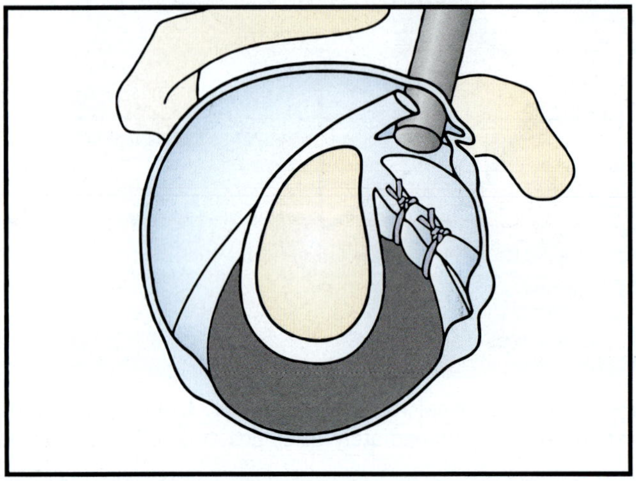

FIGURE 15-97: A diagram illustrating "microcapsulorrhaphy" technique via limited superior shift of the anterior band of the inferior glenohumeral ligament.

Subacromial Impingement

Subacromial impingement is a common pain generator in the throwing shoulder. Patients often have equivocal physical examination and positive impingement tests. A diagnostic, subacromial injection with anesthetic is perhaps the most valuable diagnostic and therapeutic modality in our experience. Throwers typically respond to conservative treatment including rest, dedicated physical therapy programs, antiinflammatory drugs, and subacromial steroid injection. Rarely, these conservative treatments are unsuccessful, and patients may undergo shoulder arthroscopy with SAD. SAD is typically performed via standard portals. An anterior interval portal can be used to access both the intra-articular and subacromial space. Typical operative findings may include extensive, perhaps hypertrophic subacromial bursal formation and CA ligament fraying (Video 15-12). We recommend a thorough inspection of hypertrophic bursa, including the lateral, posterior, posterolateral, and anterior subdeltoid space. If pain is anterior, we recommend clearing the entire subcoracoid region of bursa, the full surface of the biceps retinaculum down to the falciform ligament, the deep surface of the CA ligament, and medially so that the conjoint tendon can be visualized. If pain is more posterior, we recommend placing the scope

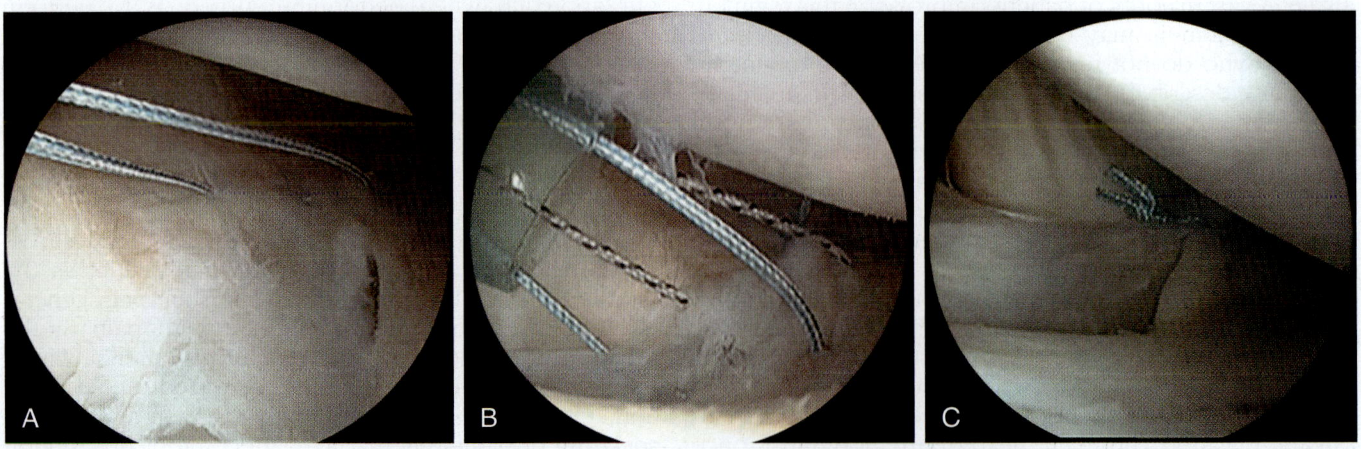

FIGURE 15-98: Arthroscopic views of "microcapsulorrhaphy" technique for suture passage (**A** and **B**) and tied knot (**C**).

anterior to look posteriorly to treat any posterolateral acromial bursal fibrosis. Care must be taken to protect the coracoacromial ligament at the time of bursectomy. If we find the coracoacromial ligament to be hypertrophic or abraded, then we may perform a coracoacromial ligament sculpting/thinning procedure, but we do not recommend CA ligament resection. In order to preserve the subacromial arch, we do not recommend acromioplasty even in the face of variant acromion morphology (e.g., downward sloping posterior to anterior or medial to lateral morphologies or even true type 3 acromion morphology). The exception to this rule is the case of obvious enthesopathy that likely contributes to the pathology.

Posterior Ossification of the Shoulder

Throwers with symptomatic posterior glenoid exostoses tend to have posteriorly located shoulder pain during throwing, usually at the late cocking or early acceleration phase. First documented in 1941, posterior ossification of the shoulder, also known as the Bennett lesion or thrower's exostosis (Figs. 15-99 and 15-100), was classically thought to be induced by traction of the triceps muscle. Surgical outcomes tend to be poor and nonoperative treatment is recommended.[46,47] More recent reports have documented better results with surgical intervention.[229,537] There are sparse reports of this clinical entity in the literature overall. In 1999 Meister et al. documented a case series of 18 patients treated with details arthroscopic excision and debridement of coexisting partial-thickness rotator cuff and labral tears. Over an average follow-up duration of 6.3 years, 10 patients (58%) returned to their same level of play for greater than 1 year, and one patient had a recurrent exostosis 8 years after surgery. The authors of this report found partial-thickness rotator cuff tears in all patients except one at the time of arthroscopic intervention and concluded that posterior glenoid exostosis was a cause of internal impingement. They noted that osteophytes larger than 100 mm^2 at the time of surgery were predictive of inability to return to former level of play.[461] More recently Yoneda et al. prospectively evaluated 16 baseball players who underwent arthroscopic removal of posterior Bennett lesions. Eleven returned to preinjury playing status at 1-year follow-up.[773] In another study involving 51 consecutive baseball players treated arthroscopically, Yoneda et al. sought to identify characteristics that distinguish symptomatic Bennett lesions from asymptomatic ones. Thirteen athletes had a painful lesion while 11 had an asymptomatic lesion. Characteristic features of painful lesions were posterior laxity, no deficit of internal rotation, and avulsed fragment on CT.[499] We recommend arthroscopic resection of exostosis and labral repair in such patients (Figs. 15-101 and 15-102).

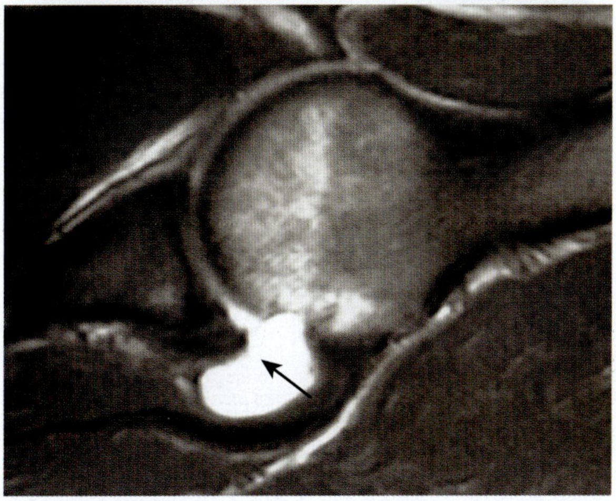

FIGURE 15-100: Axial magnetic resonance image demonstrating posterior glenoid exostosis, a known cause of posterior shoulder pain in the thrower.

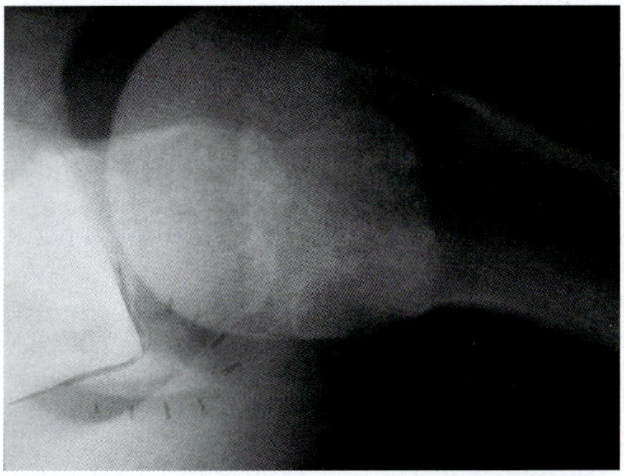

FIGURE 15-99: Axillary radiograph demonstrating posterior glenoid exostosis or Bennett lesion (*dashed lines*).

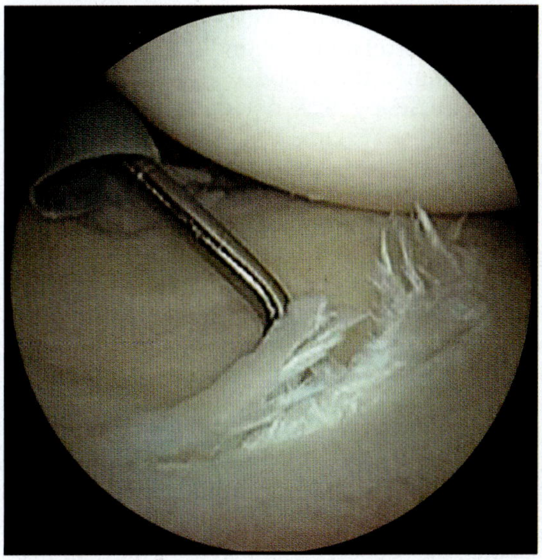

FIGURE 15-101: Posterior glenoid labrum damage due to Bennett lesion.

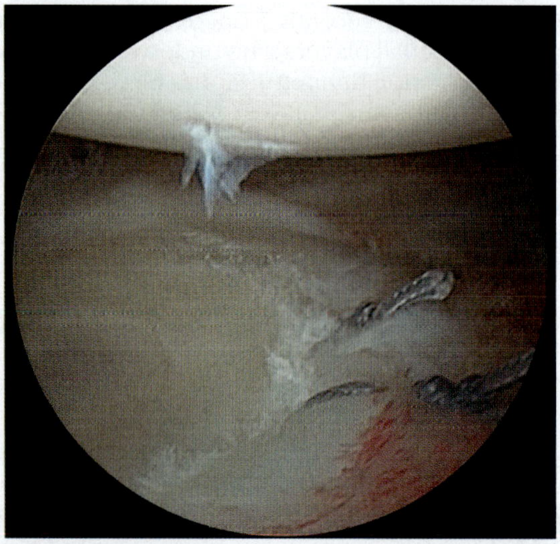

FIGURE 15-102: Repair of posterior glenoid labrum after resection of Bennett lesion.

CONCLUSION

The throwing shoulder is subject to a wide range of pathology, all of which may coexist on a spectrum of adaptive chronic change to acute injury. Given the prevalence of asymptomatic pathology that can be identified on imaging,[400] great diagnostic diligence is required to accurately identify the pain generator and to avoid overtreatment. Generally, nonoperative measures remain the mainstay of management of the painful throwing shoulder; however, surgical intervention may become necessary in some patients. Those who do undergo surgery will likely have the best outcome if the surgeon adheres to the notion that "less is more" rather than heroic attempts at restoration of normal anatomy. Overtreatment and overconstraint should be avoided as "too loose" is often better than "too tight." Despite our best efforts at this point, a significant percentage throwers requiring surgery do not return to their former level of play. Strategies for the surgical treatment of this difficult entity continue to evolve.

Complications of Shoulder Arthroscopy

Robert W. Westermann, Brian R. Wolf

INTRODUCTION

Shoulder arthroscopy has been gaining popularity over the past 30 years. Bircher, who evaluated the shoulders of 25 cadavers at the New York University in the 1920s, first described the arthroscopic examination of the shoulder joint. He correlated his findings that he observed through a 3-mm arthroscope with an open dissection. Shoulder arthroscopy was not described clinically until the late 1970s by Watanabe.[742] Shoulder arthroscopy is currently one of the most common orthopedic procedures. Many conventional shoulder procedures previously performed with open techniques are now accomplished arthroscopically. Early proponents of the trend towards arthroscopic shoulder management suggested that the technique is associated with fewer complications compared with open surgery. Overall, complications of shoulder arthroscopy are low. Most of the literature describing complications is limited to single-institution case series with conflicting data in several areas. Surgeons must have a thorough understanding of the potential arthroscopic complications in shoulder surgery to prevent, recognize, and manage them when they occur. This section describes the potential preoperative, intraoperative, and postoperative complications of shoulder arthroscopy.

PREOPERATIVE COMPLICATIONS

Anesthesia

Regional Anesthesia

Several anesthetic options exist for pain control during and following shoulder arthroscopy. Regional anesthesia is associated with improved recovery times[290] and decreased pain[771] on the day of surgery, as well as reduced costs[326] compared with general anesthesia. Regional nerve blocks have generally been well accepted[60,89,326,625] but are not without risk. Adverse events associated with regional shoulder anesthesia include total spinal anesthesia, hemidiaphragmatic paralysis and respiratory distress, hematoma, local anesthetic systemic toxicity (LAST) that may induce seizures and cardiac arrest, peripheral nerve injury, recurrent laryngeal nerve blockade, and Horner syndrome.[84,359,360,381,720]

Interscalene brachial plexus block is the most common form of regional anesthesia used for shoulder procedures. Bishop evaluated the efficacy of interscalene regional anesthesia for shoulder surgery.[60] They evaluated 478 patients undergoing interscalene regional anesthesia. They concluded that 3% of procedures were converted to a general anesthetic because the block was unable to provide adequate anesthesia to begin or complete the operation. Moreover, they noted 2.3% of patients had peripheral nerve injuries or complex regional pain syndrome postoperatively because of the brachial plexus block. They concluded that interscalene blocks are safe and effective for shoulder surgery.

Hemidiaphragmatic paralysis on the side of the interscalene/brachial plexus block is commonly encountered after shoulder arthroscopy.[206,398,533,702] The reported incidence of transient paralysis has been reported to range from 33% to 100%.[391,721] Healthy patients are able to compensate for this transient stress to the pulmonary system, and the diaphragm tends to recover functionality without any adverse outcomes. Permanent phrenic nerve injury following shoulder arthroscopy with regional anesthesia can be devastating, affect the patient's quality of life, significantly limit activity, and predispose patients to respiratory infections and pulmonary fibrosis.[359] Patients with preexisting pulmonary conditions should be counseled regarding the inherent risks of regional anesthesia prior to shoulder arthroscopy.

Severe cardiac and neurologic events from LAST are rare but well-described complications of shoulder surgery.[595] Di Gregorio et al. evaluated the 77 documented cases of LAST reported between 1979 and 2009.[198] Local anesthetic systemic toxicity most commonly occurs within 1 minute of block placement but can occur up to 15 minutes or even longer after block placement.[198] Toxicity mainly affects the cardiovascular and neurologic systems. The central nervous system was affected in 89% of cases, with seizure being the most common manifestation. Cardiovascular events occurred in 55% of cases; bradycardia and asystole were the most common adverse events.[198] LAST is effectively treated with 20% lipid emulsion infusion for resuscitation along with symptomatic care.[409,614] The incidence of LAST is low at about 0.1%.[38] Early recognition and supportive care by the operative team are essential in treating those affected by local anesthetic toxicity.

Peripheral Nerve Injury

Peripheral nerve injuries may occur from the use of regional anesthesia. These are usually transient, but permanent cases are on record.[51,746] The incidence of permanent neurological injury from regional anesthesia is rather low. Data from an Australian regional anesthesia database, when queried between 2006 and 2008, revealed 30 cases of peripheral nerve injuries from regional anesthesia in a total of 6069 patients for whom follow-up data were available (0.49% of patients).[38] Regional anesthesia has several benefits, as previously discussed. These benefits must be weighed against the risks of the procedure for each patient.

Positioning

Regardless of the preference (beach chair or lateral), proper patient positioning prior to surgery is important to avert complications (Fig. 15-103). Some have suggested positioning to be the topmost contributor to complications of shoulder arthroscopy.[161,480] All four extremities are vulnerable to peripheral nerve injuries, paresthesias, and palsies depending on the patient positioning or malposition. When placing a patient in the lateral position, attention should be paid to the padding beneath the head to keep the hips in neutral position. An axillary roll should be used to prevent injury of the contralateral (down side) brachial plexus. Careful inspection of the lower extremities and nonoperative upper extremity to ensure adequate padding is crucial. Careful attention to the peroneal nerve is needed while preparing a patient for a laterally positioned shoulder arthroscopy. In the beach chair position, gentle hip flexion would prevent excessive stretch of the sciatic nerve and also prevent the patient from migrating caudally.[480]

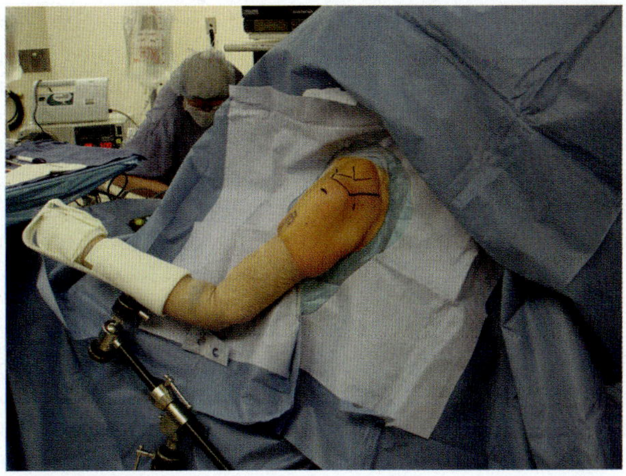

FIGURE 15-103: Proper beach chair position with the anterior and posterior aspects of the shoulder exposed for access. The arm is supported by an arm holder. The exposure and arm support decrease the risk of neurologic injury secondary to traction.

TRACTION

Traction injuries to the brachial plexus can occur during shoulder arthroscopy.[161] The brachial plexus is tethered proximally at the spinal column and prevertebral fascia, and distally in the arm's axillary fascia. With the administration of anesthesia, protective muscular tone is lost between these two points. Therefore persistent nonphysiological position may subject nerves to traction injury or ischemia.

Operative side upper extremity peripheral nerve paresthesias and palsies have been reported with both beach chair and lateral decubitus positions. The operative arm is commonly held in a mechanical arm holder in the beach chair position, and in a traction device for lateral position. Distraction and longitudinal traction may increase risk of traction-related paresthesias in the lateral position. Early reports of neuropraxia following shoulder arthroscopy have ranged from 3% to 20% where the traction used in the lateral setup was attributed to several injuries.[10,557] Traction padding around the forearm and wrist when applied too tight in the lateral position may cause digital neuropraxia and radial sensory nerve paresthesias.[213] Paresthesias are far less common in the beach chair position, perhaps because little or no traction is applied across the joint.[563] Cutaneous cervical plexus nerve and hypoglossal nerve palsies have been reported following beach chair surgery.[493,551] These have been attributed to poor head and neck positioning, excessive rotation, or compression.[480] Therefore, in the beach chair position, careful attention should be paid to safely secure the head and maintain the cervical spine in a neutral position.

Finally, arm perfusion has been studied in the setting of traction in the lateral decubitus position.[305] The combined use of longitudinal traction and joint distraction lateral decubitus position may decrease arm perfusion.[305] Decreased blood flow to peripheral nerves may be a contributing factor in the development of nerve paresthesias in this position. Strain across the brachial plexus appears to be associated with the arm position.[372] In a cadaveric study, Klein et al. evaluated the effect of arm position on brachial plexus strain; the strain was lowest at 90 degrees of forward flexion and 0 degrees of abduction.[136] The authors also noted that this arm position did not lend easy access to the glenohumeral joint for arthroscopy and concluded that the two arm positions that lends access to the shoulder while having relatively low stresses on the brachial plexus are (1) 45 degrees of flexion and 90 degrees of abduction and (2) 45 degrees of flexion and 0 degrees of abduction.[372] Paresthesias from traction typically resolve within 6 weeks postoperatively. Careful attention to patient positioning, padding, and judicious use of traction may help avoid certain traction related injuries following arthroscopic surgery.

INTRAOPERATIVE COMPLICATIONS

Neurovascular Injury and Portal Placement

Neurovascular injuries must be avoided across all surgical procedures; fortunately these are rare events in shoulder arthroscopy.[662] Iatrogenic injuries to nerves can result in significant morbidity and disability.[126] The etiology of nerve injury following shoulder arthroscopy can be difficult to understand, as injuries can result from traction, regional anesthesia, as previously discussed, or from direct injury. Direct injury to certain nerves during portal placement or surgery are uncommon.[662] However, cases of nerve transection and nerve suturing are on record.[126] Carofino et al. reported data from Mayo Clinic's brachial plexus referral practice of patients with iatrogenic injuries from shoulder surgery. There were nine cases of nerve injuries from shoulder arthroscopy.[126] Of these, three cases involved injuries to the proximal brachial plexus, one case was that of a radial nerve palsy that completely recovered, and one case was a permanent median nerve injury that required tendon transfer surgery. They reported four axillary nerve injuries, which included transections, and one case where the nerve was sutured to the anterior capsule during an arthroscopic Bankart repair.[126] Injuries to the suprascapular and musculocutaneous nerves have been described in the setting of shoulder arthroscopy. Good understanding of the relevant anatomy at the time of portal placement is the key to avoid iatrogenic neurovascular injuries during shoulder arthroscopy.

The axillary nerve's anatomic course and variants have been well described.[33,580] The portal that is nearest to the proximal portion of the axillary nerve is the standard "soft spot" posterior portal, located 2 cm medial and 2 cm inferior to the posterior corner of the acromion. This standard portal is usually safe, and is typically about 3 to 5 cm from the axillary nerve and circumflex artery.[414,465] The suprascapular artery and nerve are located 2.5 to 3 cm from the standard posterior portal.[465] The accessory posterolateral portal is, on average, about the same distance to the axillary nerve, and is generally safe.[174] Lateral portal placement depends on the goals of the operation. Lateral portals are considered safest with respect to the risk of from neurovascular injury as long as they are created within 3 cm of the lateral boarder of the acromion in Burkhead's "safe zone."[114] Depending on the AP position, lateral portals are typically placed between 5.5 and 7 cm of the axillary nerve.[465]

Anterior portal placement poses the greatest risk to neurovascular structures. Anatomic studies suggest that outside-in anterior portal placement lateral to the coracoid and through the rotator interval is safe (Fig. 15-104).[443] The axillary nerve courses close to the inferior glenoid and is often adjacent to the inferior glenohumeral capsule. The axillary nerve is between 1.4 and 2.5 cm from the anterior joint capsule and depends on the arm position.[346] In a cadaveric study by Meyer, 25% of standardized anterior portals were placed within 1 cm of the cephalic vein.[465] Injury to the cephalic vein has been described in clinical settings and can result in a hematoma; however, no long term consequences have been reported. Surgeons must consider the anatomic course of neurovascular structures around the shoulder at the time of

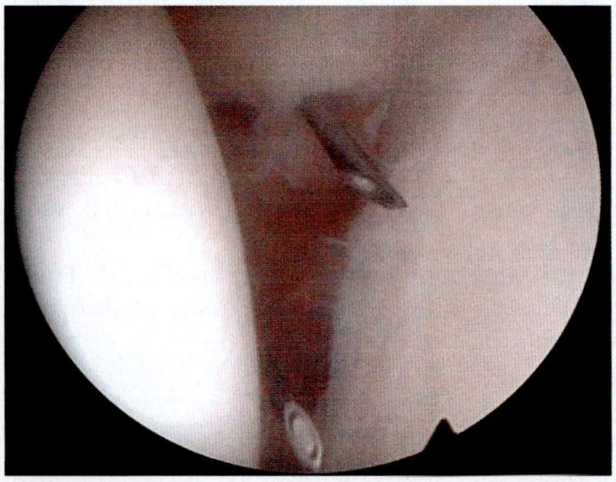

FIGURE 15-104: The rotator interval is bordered by the biceps tendon superiorly and the subscapularis tendon inferiorly. Needles can be placed as markers to ensure proper incision and portal placement.

portal placement to safeguard against iatrogenic neurovascular injury.

Suprascapular (SS) nerve is at risk during shoulder arthroscopy, which is not necessarily linked to portal placement. The nerve is particularly at risk from blind glenoid drilling for instability operations, a practice almost completely eliminated with use of anchors. Currently, mobilization of large rotator cuff tears poses some risk to the SS nerve. The SS nerve runs an oblique course across the floor of suprascapular fossa and commonly passes under the transverse scapular ligament. The rotator cuff can tolerate about 3 cm of lateralization before compromising the SS nerve.[740] Zanotti et al. describe outcomes of 10 patients in whom mobilization was required to repair massive rotator cuff tears. They report only one of the 10 patients had a suprascapular nerve palsy confirmed by electromyography at mean 2.5-year follow-up.[777] Caution should be exercised during mobilization of retracted rotator cuffs near the SS in preparation for the repair.

Air Embolism

Fatal venous air embolism is an extremely rare complication of shoulder arthroscopy, with only a few cases having been reported.[226,303,780] The first two reports of this phenomenon involved arthroscopic procedures where air was used to pressurize the joint.[226,303] A recent report described a similar case; however, in this patient only arthroscopic fluid was used for joint dilation and pressurization.[780] Air embolism can occur when venous systems are exposed to ambient air above the level of the heart. These can also occur at any point where air is forced into a closed body cavity under pressure, as described above. The source of air in the third case (arthroscopic fluid only) is unknown, although preexisting air in saline bags was thought to have been the source of air introduced into the closed arthroscopic system.[24]

The diagnosis of venous air embolism is usually not straightforward and is usually a diagnosis of exclusion. Presenting symptoms include a decrease in end-tidal CO_2 followed by hypotension and cardiopulmonary collapse. When venous air returns to the heart and goes on to cause pulmonary obstruction, pulmonary gas exchange diminishes (decreasing end-tidal CO_2), which induces right heart strain and eventual cardiopulmonary failure. When air embolism is suspected, patients are best managed in the Trendelenburg position. An intraoperative transesophageal echocardiogram will demonstrate right heart strain, and in some cases air in the right side of the heart.[780] The operative field should be irrigated and filled with fluid, and hemostasis ensured by the operating surgeon. Supportive care is essential to maintain blood pressure during the event. Although a rare event, limiting the air infiltration during shoulder arthroscopy may help prevent this terrible complication. Evacuation of air from arthroscopy fluid bags prior to their connection to the closed system will prevent introduction of air into the closed arthroscopic system.[24]

Fluid Extravasation and Airway Compromise

Arthroscopic fluid is used to expand and pressurize the working area of the shoulder (glenohumeral or subacromial space) during surgery. Extravasation of this fluid into surrounding soft tissues is common. Typically, patients gain 2 to 4 pounds of weight during arthroscopic surgery due to fluid extravasation.[412,664] Factors associated with increased weight gain include length of surgery, quantity of arthroscopic fluid used, and size/complexity of rotator cuff tears. While commonly benign, extravasation may compromise airway during shoulder arthroscopy.[70,331,776] When this occurs, the procedure must be aborted and the airway expeditiously managed. Additional factors that are thought to contribute to this phenomenon include procedures that are extracapsular or involve capsular resection, high pump pressures, lateral positioning and prolonged procedures.[70,331] Subcutaneous emphysema may also occur during shoulder arthroplasty. Relative changes in subacromial pressure are thought to introduce air into the subcutaneous space. While this can be benign, cases of pneumomediastinum and tension pneumothorax have been reported.[390] Limiting the pump pressures and being efficient with operative time may help decrease fluid extravasation and its related complications.

Hemodynamics

Maintenance of appropriate blood pressure and hemodynamic control can be a challenging task in the beach chair position. Due to the upright position, patients may experience sudden bradycardia and hypotensive events.[407] These episodes reportedly occur in more than one in five beach chair positioned cases.[407] Other more profound consequences of hypotension during beach chair surgery, although rare, have been reported. These include stroke, spinal cord ischemia, ophthalmoplegia, and temporary visual loss.[544,572] Close hemodynamic monitoring during patient positioning and surgery, and open communication with the anesthesia teams is essential in preventing hemodynamic-related complications during shoulder arthroscopy.

Tendon and Osseous Injuries

Structures within the shoulder and subacromial space are theoretically at risk for injury during portal placement and surgery. Iatrogenic muscle and tendon injuries during shoulder arthroscopy are well described. Norwood and Fowler reported four instances of iatrogenic injury to the rotator cuff during the creation of the posterior portal.[519] These injuries occurred in young athletes undergoing shoulder arthroscopy for indications that were not related to the rotator cuff; all were eventually treated with open repair. The less commonly used supraclavicular fossa portal, also known as the Neviaser's or the superomedial portal, may place the supraspinatus tendon at risk of injury during its placement. Souryal et al. determined that portal placement subjected the rotator cuff to iatrogenic risk when the arm was abducted 45 degrees or more.[674] Osseous injuries have also been described. Acromial fractures may occur during or shortly after aggressive acromioplasty.[440,648,745] This is typically due to technical error but may result from inability to recognize a patient with a thin acromion prior to surgery. Technical error is the reason for most iatrogenic tendon and osseous injuries in the shoulder; appropriate planning and careful attention to portal placement may help avoid these complications.

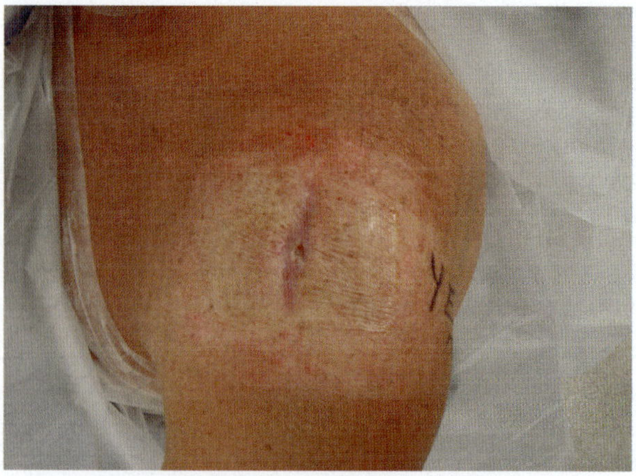

FIGURE 15-105: A draining wound as a result of an infection after combined arthroscopic and mini-open rotator cuff repair.

POSTOPERATIVE

Infection

The incidence of postoperative infection following shoulder arthroscopy is low. Infection rates have ranged from 0 to 3.4%.[435,455,745] Martin et al. reported 30-day complications following elective shoulder arthroscopy from the American College of Surgeon's NSQIP database. They determined the superficial infection rate to be 0.16% and the deep infection rate to be 0.01% after reviewing 9410 cases.[435] Certain superficial infections may be treated with oral or parenteral antibiotics, while others are better treated additionally with incision and drainage. Deep-seated infections should be managed with arthroscopic or open irrigation and debridement along with antibiotic therapy. Preoperatvie antibiotic administration has been associated with lower infection rates, and should be used routinely.[172,589] Proper arthroscopic instrument sterilization prior to surgery is important in preventing infection.[352]

Intra-articular *Propionibacterium acnes* infection has become increasingly recognized in the setting of primary and revision shoulder arthroscopy.[316] It has been identified, recently, as the most commonly isolated infecting organism following rotator cuff repair.[22] *P. acnes* is a gram-positive, microaerophilic non–spore-forming bacillus. It often takes longer than 10 to 14 days for cultures to turn positive. The bacterium is of inherently low virulence; infection with *P. acnes* can present with a relatively benign clinical picture such as persistent pain and stiffness following shoulder arthroscopy.[316] It may colonize the skin of up to 72.5% of patients undergoing shoulder arthroscopy prior to preparation.[141] Chlorhexidine plus alcohol (ChloraPrep) skin preparation has proven most effective in eradicating skin flora prior to shoulder surgery in a prospective series by Saltzman.[626] When *P. acnes* was evaluated separately, the rates of colonization after skin prep were 7% for ChloraPrep, 12% for DuraPrep, and 15% for povidone-iodine, but the difference was not statistically significant likely due to the small sample size. We recommend skin preparation with ChloraPrep prior to shoulder arthroscopy.

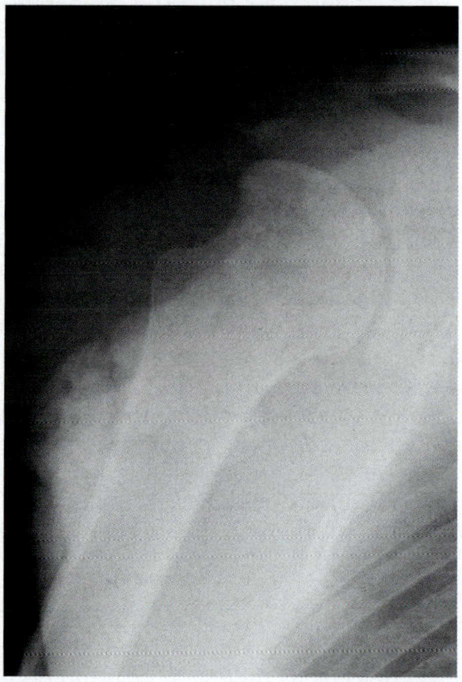

FIGURE 15-106: In case of infection, all foreign material must be removed. The greater tuberosity in this patient was deformed after substantial bone loss secondary to the infection and difficulty in removing the anchors.

Conversion from an arthroscopic procedure to an open procedure has been associated with postoperative infection (Figs. 15-105 and 15-106).[306] Herrera et al. reported a 1.9% incidence of infection among 360 patients in whom arthroscopically assisted rotator cuff repair required conversion to mini-open procedures. All cases were treated with irrigation and debridement, long-term antibiotic therapy, and revision rotator cuff repair where required. After this finding, these authors changed their practice. Patients who were converted to mini-open repairs had a second skin prep performed, a new drape, and a change of surgical gloves prior to making a new incision. Following these changes, the authors reported a 0% infection rate in 200 cases.[306]

Thromboembolism

Venous thromboembolism (VTE) is a rare complication following shoulder arthroscopy with an estimated incidence of 0.15%.[638] To date, fewer than 100 cases have been reported in the literature.[638] Although robust data has been largely lacking, factors associated with the development of VTE following shoulder arthroscopy in the current literature include cancer history, thrombophilia, smoking history, prolonged operative time, and lateral positioning.[68,98,295,574] In a multicenter study, Schick et al.[638] evaluated 22 cases of VTE following shoulder arthroscopy, all in the beach chair position. After multivariate analysis, they found no correlation between age, sex, operative time, use of compression devices, or use of postoperative chemoprophylaxis with development of VTE.[638] DVT may occur in the upper or lower extremities following shoulder arthroscopy. The lower extremities DVTs are more common than upper extremity DVTs. While DVT rates may be higher in the lower extremities, more complications may occur with upper extremity DVT. Up to 36% The pulmonary embolism rate with upper extremity DVT has been reported to be as high as 36%.[165] Although uncommon, VTE events occur after shoulder arthroscopy. They must be recognized early and treated aggressively.

EDITOR COMMENTARY

Frank A. Cordasco

Chapter 15 has been organized into nine subchapters, beginning with "General Principles" and finishing with "Complications of Shoulder Arthroscopy." These subchapters have been authored by an internationally recognized group of academic orthopedic shoulder surgeons. My comments are intended to augment and add an international perspective to the great contributions these authors have provided.

"General Principles" provides a thorough and concise overview of the anesthesia and monitoring, equipment, positioning, examination under anesthesia, portals, diagnostic arthroscopy, fluid management, and hemostasis. These general principles provide a great foundation for the remaining components of Chapter 15.

With respect to anesthesia, my approach at the Hospital for Special Surgery is to use a regional block alone for nonrepair arthroscopies, rotator cuff repairs, and biceps tenodeses. For arthroscopic stabilizations and AC reconstructions, I prefer a combined anesthesia approach using both regional and general anesthesia.

Like the authors, I prefer the beach chair position for most arthroscopic approaches. The primary advantage of the lateral decubitus approach described by advocates relates to inferior access during instability repairs. I have found the use of an axillary bump and a traction arm holder to facilitate and enhance the exposure for these instability operations. Although an appropriate surgical plan is developed preoperatively based upon history, physical exam, and imaging, occasionally a decision is made to proceed to an open stabilization, which is an easy transition from the beach chair position. In general I prefer the beanbag for instability repairs and a device attached to the table that lifts the patient from the waist up for all of the other arthroscopic procedures.

"Arthroscopic Management of Rotator Cuff Disease" provides a comprehensive review of the tear recognition and classification, repair techniques, treatment of partial rotator cuff tears, subscapularis tears, and biceps tendon injuries. I agree with the authors' description of tear recognition and use of the Burkhart classification technique to determine the best approach and strategies for repair.

The authors' technique for small to large rotator cuff tears is one that I use as well. For all but the smallest tears (high-grade bursal-sided partial-thickness tears), I prefer the TOE technique using a knotless construct.

I no longer perform SAD routinely in all rotator cuff repairs. I prefer to repair the rotator cuff tear first before considering a decompression. In my experience, this has helped to maintain distension and diminish swelling. Bursae that compromise visualization and/or mobilization are debrided before the repair. After the repair has been completed, if a large impingement lesion is present on the undersurface of the CA ligament, I will perform a CA ligament release and consider an acromial smoothing. Particularly when performing massive repairs or repairs in which the tissue is of poor quality, I prefer to leave the CA arch undisturbed.

I agree with the authors' discussion regarding patches; I do not use them in my practice either and prefer to perform partial repairs when a complete repair is not possible despite appropriate mobilization techniques and extra-articular releases.

Regarding subscapularis tears and dislocated LHBT pathology, in patients who are not candidates for tenotomy (either by age and level of activity or choice) I prefer to perform the tenodesis first and keep it attached at the origin to maintain the length-tension relationship. After the tenodesis, I will release it at the origin and excise the intra-articular portion. The subscapularis repair is then performed. My repair technique uses a knotless construct that begins by passing tapes via an anterolateral portal using a suture shuttling device. The mattress tapes are then secured to the lesser tuberosity from inferior to superior using an anterior portal. A 70-degree lens is very helpful to facilitate visualization.

"Arthroscopic Treatment of Acromioclavicular Joint Osteolysis, Arthritis, and Instability" provides a thorough review of the anatomy of the AC joint, distal clavicle osteolysis, AC joint arthritis, the technique of AC joint resection, and AC joint instability and techniques for repair and reconstruction.

Distal clavicle resection is often performed in conjunction with associated subacromial pathology. When distal clavicle resection is indicated, an indirect or subacromial approach is preferred. In the case of isolated distal clavicular osteolysis in the young athlete, a direct or superior approach may be optimal. If the surgeon chooses this approach, care must be taken in establishing the posterior portal to avoid injury to the posterior superior AC joint capsule that has been shown to be the important and strong stabilizer of the joint.

Continued

EDITOR COMMENTARY—cont'd

When I select the direct or superior approach, I develop the posterior portal inferiorly to protect the posterosuperior AC joint capsule.

The authors discuss and review arthroscopic, open, and arthroscopic-assisted approaches to the AC joint reconstruction in cases of complete separation. I prefer the arthroscopic-assisted approach as it allows arthroscopic assessment of the glenohumeral and subacromial aspects of the shoulder and facilitates the passage of sutures and/or grafts whether the surgeon's preference is to pass around the coracoid or to use a transcoracoid fixation technique.

"Arthroscopic Treatment of Shoulder Stiffness and Rotator Cuff Calcific Tendinitis" provides a broad overview of primary and secondary adhesive capsulitis as well as posttraumatic and postsurgical stiffness, calcific tendinitis, and the respective nonoperative and operative treatments.

Arthroscopic controlled capsular release and lysis of adhesions followed by MUA is my preferred approach to idiopathic adhesive capsulitis because it has been most successful in my experience with refractory cases.

Calcific tendinitis can be effectively managed nonoperatively, in my experience, with an ultrasound-guided aspiration and injection in the majority of cases. This has been more effective than corticosteroid injection alone and often obviates the need for arthroscopic management when provided upon presentation.

"Arthroscopic Management of Prearthritic and Arthritic Conditions of the Shoulder and the Postarthroplasty Shoulder" describes the indications and outcomes of debridement, capsular release, microfracture, glenoidplasty, resurfacing, decompression, and distal clavicle resection for patients in whom arthroplasty is not indicated. The authors also review systemic problems associated with these conditions, including PVNS, renal arthropathy, and avascular necrosis as well as the diagnostic and therapeutic uses for arthroscopy in patients who have had arthroplasty of the shoulder.

The authors have identified many associated pathologic entities that may coexist in the setting of arthritic conditions of the shoulder and may in fact be contributing to the patient's symptoms. I do not use arthroscopic glenoidplasty and biologic resurfacing in this setting and agree with the authors' comments and conclusions in this regard.

"Arthroscopic Surgery for Biceps-Labral Complex Disease" provides a comprehensive review of evolving concepts involving these associated structures that, as pointed out by the authors in their introduction, were covered in separate chapters in previous editions of this text. The authors have described a novel and thoughtful classification system of anatomic zones as well as pathology based upon their line of research. With respect to treatment of biceps tendon pathology, the role of biceps tendon transfer remains to be determined as the options of tenotomy and tenodesis at the top of the groove, in the groove, below the grove, but above the pectoralis and subpectoral have all demonstrated indications and advocates. My preferences are to perform tenotomy in low-demand elderly and sedentary patients, usually in the setting of rotator cuff repair. I prefer tenodesis at the top of the groove in active patients undergoing rotator cuff repair. In younger patients with isolated biceps tendinosis or partial-thickness tears I will generally perform either an arthroscopic infragroove suprapectoral tenodesis or an open subpectoral biceps tenodesis depending upon the intraoperative findings.

"Arthroscopic Management of the Thrower's Shoulder" reviews in a concise and thorough approach, the complex treatment algorithm for rotator cuff tears, SLAP tears, GIRD, instability, biceps tunnel disease, subacromial impingement, and posterior ossification of the shoulder in this high-demand subpopulation of athletes.

"Complications of Shoulder Arthroscopy" completes Chapter 15 in this broad and thorough overview of the preoperative, intraoperative, and postoperative complications. Fortunately, these complications are rare but it is critical that every surgeon performing shoulder arthroscopy be thoroughly familiar with the preventative, diagnostic, and management options available in the event that they do occur.

SENIOR EDITOR COMMENTARY

Frederick A. Matsen III

The authors of Chapter 15 have provided a wonderful, almost encyclopedic, presentation of the opportunities, challenges, and risks of arthroscopic surgery. In this commentary my purpose is not to critique contributions of the large number of surgeons striving to improve the care of patients using arthroscopic methods, but rather to provide a provide a perspective from a surgeon who does not do shoulder arthroscopy, but has for the last 30 years been referred patients with the various problems that can arise from these procedures.

General

There are many attractive features of the arthroscopic approach to shoulder pathology, including the potential for less-invasive interventions, outpatient surgery in a surgeon-owned surgery center, and an ability to see pathology that may not be evident with open approaches. Each of these potential advantages may encourage surgeons to lower the threshold for offering a procedure to patients with shoulder problems, even if the pathology is not clearly defined preoperatively. Like a preoperative MRI done for nondescript shoulder symptoms, the arthroscope will almost always reveal "findings." The challenge for the arthroscopist is to first determine if these findings are likely to be responsible for the patient's symptoms, and second whether the surgeon can safely and effectively manage the findings in a way that will benefit the patient. As the saying goes, "seeing more doesn't of itself give us license to do more." For example, the statement that "a sulcus sign that does not improve with the arm in external rotation indicates that there is deficiency in the rotator interval" needs to be interpreted in light of the fact that many asymptomatic shoulders have positive sulcus signs[297C]; this finding should not tempt a surgeon to perform a rotator interval closure unless it is clearly related to the patient's symptoms. Laxity is *not* the same as

SENIOR EDITOR COMMENTARY—cont'd

instability; every female gymnast has incredible joint laxity and, simultaneously, incredible joint stability through the mechanism of concavity compression.[408A,408B] We have seen a number of minimally symptomatic shoulders that were converted to stiff, very painful shoulders by arthroscopic tightening.

There is a current tendency to rely on MRI to establish the nature of the shoulder problem. Because an MRI will almost always reveal findings that may tempt treatment, there is a risk that treatment be directed at these findings rather than on the results of the history and the physical examination with the patient awake (so that the dynamic stability can be assessed rather than an examination under anesthesia, when the dynamic stabilizers are defunctionalized). If the diagnosis is so occult that it is not evident on this standard examination and plain radiographs, it is less likely that it will respond well to operative treatment. Better to focus on having the patient describe and demonstrate the activities or positions that produce symptoms rather than on what the MRI, the examination under anesthesia, or a diagnostic arthroscopy "shows."

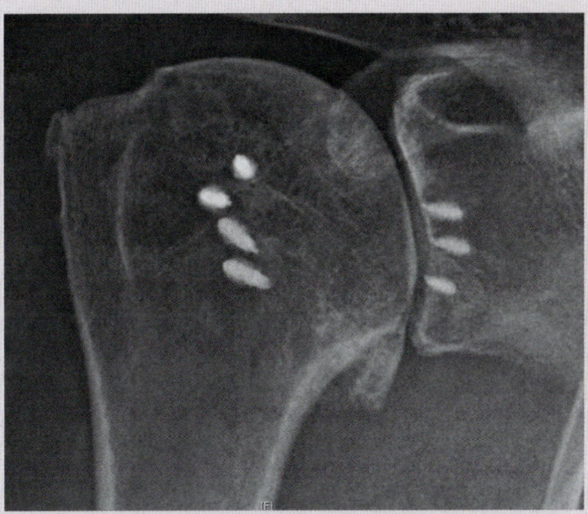

FIGURE 15-107: Anchor arthropathy. Anteroposterior radiograph showing prominent suture anchors.

Instability

Arthroscopic surgery is frequently used for shoulders with apparent instability. It is important to note, however, that recent randomized trials and systematic reviews have not shown the superiority of modern arthroscopic techniques compared with open repairs. Mohtadi et al. noted, "There was no difference between open and arthroscopic repair in terms of patient quality of life. Open repair resulted in a significantly lower risk of recurrence. Secondary outcome data from this trial suggest that open surgical repair may be recommended to reduce the risk of recurrent instability in younger male patients with a Hill-Sachs lesion."[481] Cole et al. stated, "Arthroscopic and open repair techniques for the treatment of recurrent traumatic shoulder instability yield comparable results if the procedure is selected on the basis of the pathologic findings at the time of surgery."[149] Lenters et al. noted, "The available evidence indicates that arthroscopic approaches are not as effective as open approaches in preventing recurrent instability or enabling patients to return to work."[399] Furthermore, while the argument is often made that arthroscopy is minimally invasive and provides "improved visualization" and improved patient safety, it is not uncommon for us to see shoulders in which suture anchors were misplaced and have given rise to secondary degenerative joint disease or "anchor arthropathy" (Figs 15-107 to 15-109). In addition, use of intra-articular infusion of local antibiotics via a pain pump after arthroscopic instability repairs results in a risk of a most severe complication: glenohumeral chondrolysis[438B] (Figs. 15-110 and 15-111). Finally, although arthroscopic stabilization spares the incision of the subscapularis, the healing time for a labral reattachment is likely to be essentially the same as the time to heal a subscapularis tenotomy; healing of both proceeds concurrently so the time to return to activity should not be different with the two approaches.

Confusion exists regarding the terms *instability* and *laxity*. Traumatic anterior instability usually affects shoulders that are not lax, enabling the applied force to avulse the labrum from the anteroinferior glenoid. The capsule of these shoulders is not excessively stretchy, and an anatomic repair[703,389A]

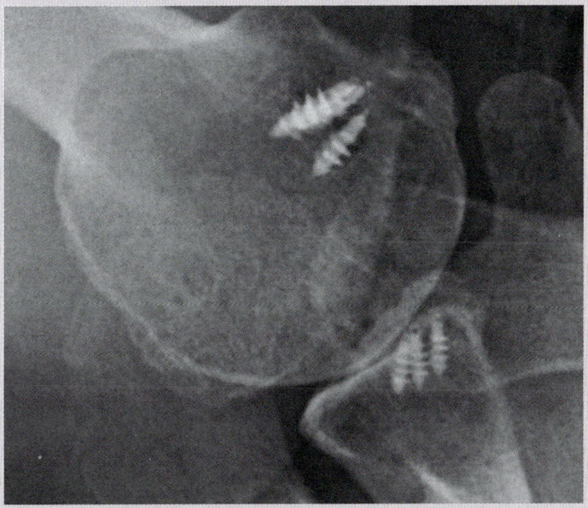

FIGURE 15-108: Anchor arthropathy. Axillary radiograph showing prominent suture anchors and joint space narrowing not visible on the anteroposterior radiograph.

usually suffices to manage the instability; additional capsular tightening or shifting can result in a stiff shoulder. By contrast, lax shoulders may be dislocatable but typically do not have labral avulsions; thus the management of relatively less-traumatic instability in more stretchy shoulders may require some combination of labral augmentation and capsular tightening with great care to avoid excessive or asymmetrical tightening. The goal is always a flexible and stable shoulder.

For reasons that are unclear, we are in an era where it is popular to use a Latarjet or other bone transfer procedure to treat shoulders with glenohumeral instability in the absence of major glenoid bone loss. While bone transfers surely have a role in cases where a third of the glenoid is missing and in patients whose anatomic repairs have failed,

Continued

SENIOR EDITOR COMMENTARY—cont'd

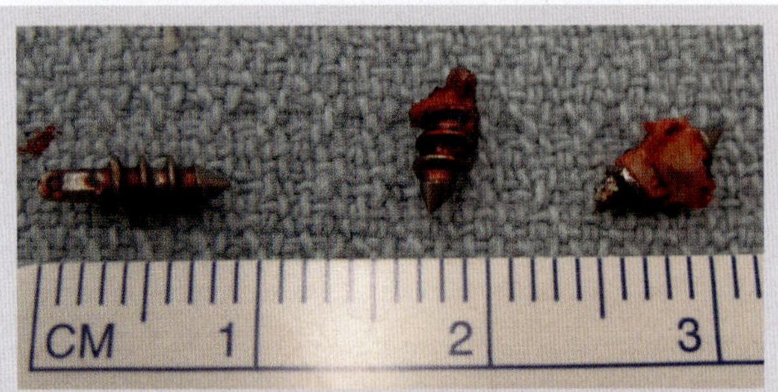

FIGURE 15-109: Anchor arthropathy. Three suture anchors that were prominent on the glenoid surface, where they were excoriating the humeral articular cartilage.

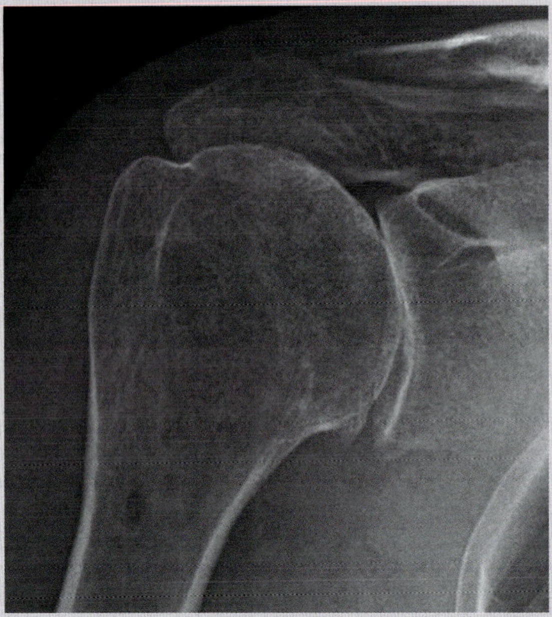

FIGURE 15-110: Anteroposterior radiograph of chondrolysis after arthroscopic stabilization surgery and postoperative infusion of local anesthetic with a pain pump.

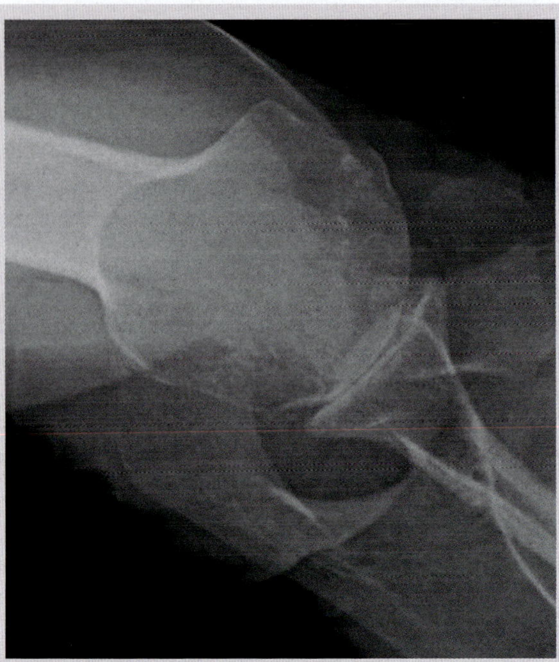

FIGURE 15-111: Axillary radiograph of chondrolysis after arthroscopic stabilization surgery and postoperative infusion of local anesthetic with a pain pump.

the routine use of bone transfers does not seem advisable because of the increased risk of arthritis, screw-related problems, damage to the subscapularis, and difficulty in revision. One of the first shoulder papers I wrote was in 1984 for Joe Zuckerman in which we cautioned about the potential hazards of screws about the shoulder.[780A] We are now seeing these same complications with the Latarjet procedure, whether done open or arthroscopically.

While this chapter advocates "regional anesthesia with an interscalene block combined with general anesthesia," it seems that this exposes the patient to the risks of both types of anesthetic and might be overkill, especially in view of the minimally invasive nature of arthroscopic surgery and the potentially serious complications of interscalene blocks.[398] Nerve injuries can be forever.

The management of shoulders with the AMBRI type of instability continues to be an interesting challenge. By definition, compared with the TUBS type of instability, it is more a constitutional than a traumatic entity. Fortunately, most many cases can be managed nonoperatively by patient education and rehabilitation. When surgery is considered, the surgeon needs to recognize that the capsule is likely to be more stretchy than usual and the labrum is likely to be more compressible than usual; this combination allows the humeral head to translate due to failure of the concavity compression mechanism.[408A] So, rather than risking over-tightening of the shoulder with capsular plication that may result in a stiff, painful shoulder, the surgeon has the opportunity to use the redundant capsule to augment the labrum, creating a deeper stabilizing concavity.[439A] In managing shoulders with the AMBRI type of instability, rotator interval closure may be another useful adjunct.[298]

Rotator Cuff

Rotator cuff tears are common, and their characteristics vary widely among different practices.[438A,664A] While it used to be thought that cuff tears resulted from "impingement" by the acromion, this etiology has been largely put to rest in favor of the recognition that most tears result from tendon degeneration and that acromioplasty is not a necessary part of surgical management.[543A,449A] Many rotator cuff tears can be successfully managed without surgery.[273A] Currently, there is great interest in arthroscopic management of cuff tears and the rate of publication of new methods and case series is rising exponentially; however, the rates of clinical improvement and the rates of anatomically durable repairs have not noticeably improved (Fig. 15-112).[454A] Furthermore, it has been repeatedly documented that the comfort and function of shoulders with failure of the anatomic repair have results that are not significantly different from those in which the repair attempt was successful.[454A,297A] Thus the AAOS

SENIOR EDITOR COMMENTARY—cont'd

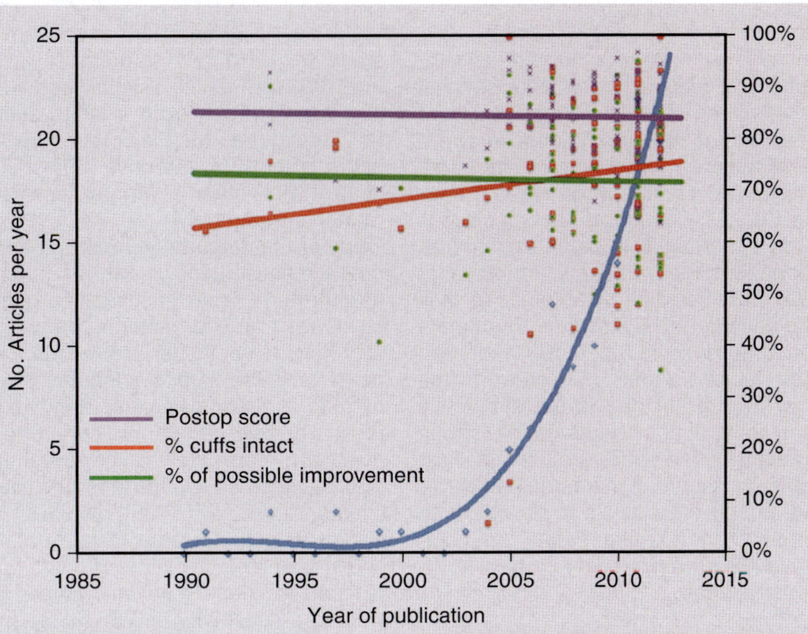

FIGURE 15-112: Lack of improvement in clinical outcomes or cuff integrity after rotator cuff repair over time in spite of exponential increase in the number of articles published on this topic. (From McElvany MD, McGoldrick E, Gee AO, et al: Rotator cuff repair: published evidence on factors associated with repair integrity and clinical outcome. *Am J Sports Med.* 2015;43[2]:491-500.)

current evidence-based guidelines for rotator cuff surgery are in a state of uncertainty: there is only *limited* evidence that "rotator cuff repair is an option for patients with chronic, symptomatic full-thickness tears" and only *limited* evidence that "early surgical repair after acute injury is an option for patients with an acute rotator cuff tear" and *inconclusive* evidence "for or against a specific technique (arthroscopic, mini-open, or open repair) when surgery is indicated for full-thickness rotator cuff tears. Interestingly, the only recommendation with *moderate* support was that "routine acromioplasty is not required at the time of rotator cuff repair."[8A]

While there are many approaches to classifying cuff tears—size, shape, degree of fatty infiltration—perhaps the most important is to determine the amount of trauma that it took to produce the tear. I try to determine to what degree was the cuff "torn" and to what degree was it "worn." It is intuitive that a cuff tendon that failed with little or no force being applied to it is made of weak stuff, the quality of which will not be enhanced by putting thread in it. Alternatively, a tendon that required substantial force to tear it has a much better chance of holding suture and facilitating a strong repair. While it is said that "there are three potential points of failure within the repair: (1) anchor-bone interface, (2) suture-anchor interface at the eyelet, and (3) the suture-tendon interface," my experience indicates that the preponderance of re-tears are from suture pullout through worn tendon.[319A] Because of the potential frailty of the repairs of chronic degenerative tears, there is uncertainty about the optimal postoperative program: should the arm be abducted in a splint to off-load the repair? When should passive ROM be started? How long before the shoulder can be used actively? One gets the sense that the outcome of cuff surgery is much more dependent on the quality of the cuff tissue and the characteristics of the patient than whether the method used to in the repair attempt is a single row, double row, TOE, or marginal convergence.

It will take high-quality evidence to guide the management of patients with rotator cuff tears. A recent randomized trial concluded that in patients older than 50 years with a degenerative rotator cuff tear there is no difference in clinical effectiveness or cost-effectiveness between open repair and arthroscopic repair at 2 years for the primary outcome (OSS) and all other prespecified secondary outcomes." The rate of re-tear was not significantly different across the randomized groups (46.4%!) and 38.6% (!) for arthroscopic and open surgery, respectively.[126A] A recent level I randomized controlled trial of the management of degenerative supraspinatus rotator cuff tears in patients older than 55 years with 2 years of clinical and imaging follow-up compared treatment with (1) physiotherapy only, (2) acromioplasty plus physiotherapy group, and (3) arthroscopic rotator cuff repair, acromioplasty, and physiotherapy.[380A] Although at 2 years the mean sagittal size of the tendon tear was slightly (7 mm) smaller in the repair group compared with the two no-repair groups, there were no significantly or clinically important differences in the Constant score, the VAS for pain, or patient satisfaction among the three groups. Because arthroscopic repair and physiotherapy were significantly more expensive, the value (clinical benefit/cost) of arthroscopic repair was less than physical therapy alone. Obviously we need to continue to learn.

Continued

SENIOR EDITOR COMMENTARY—cont'd

Acromioclavicular Joint

Only a few comments to make here. The diagnosis of AC joint arthritis needs to be made by a good history and physical exam. MRIs and bone scans often show "findings" at the AC joint in shoulders where this joint presents no clinical symptoms, potentially tempting surgery on an asymptomatic joint. In the resection of the distal clavicle it is important to check to ensure there is no residual AC contact as the shoulder is ranged and that the wound is thoroughly irrigated to minimize the risk of heterotopic bone formation. Patients with AC joint resection not infrequently have residual symptoms, so it is important that the job be done right the first time. In managing AC instability, recall that (1) holes in the clavicle can weaken it, increasing the risk of fracture, (2) screws in the coracoid have a tendency to pull out due to the distractive force applied, (3) the reconstruction needs to be strong enough to support the weight of the entire arm, (4) in most cases, it seems desirable to secure a hamstring allograft around the coracoid and around the clavicle to provide both immediate support and new tissue to enhance the torn coracoacromial ligaments, and (5) smokers seem to have difficulty healing these reconstructions.

The Stiff Shoulder

Evaluation of the stiff shoulder requires careful assessment of the motion of the humerus in relation to the scapula.[297C] Limitation of glenohumeral motion can result from a wide range of conditions, including idiopathic frozen shoulder, adhesions in the humeroscapular motion interface,[611A] glenohumeral arthritis, diabetes, and iatrogenic stiffness from surgical capsulorrhaphy. I find that physicians often overlook limitation of internal rotation with the arm in abduction—a sign of tightness of the posterior-inferior glenohumeral capsule—referred to by some as glenohumeral internal rotation deficit (GIRD).

Many cases of shoulder stiffness may be responsive to a gentle home stretching program.[532] If the articular surfaces are intact, arthroscopic release of the contracted capsule may be considered as described by our late partner Doug Harryman[297B] and others. I continue to use MUA and succinylcholine muscle relaxation in the management of refractory idiopathic frozen shoulders when the bone is of good quality and the shoulder radiographs are normal.

In the management of calcific tendinitis, the surgeon needs to be careful to decompress the deposit while carefully preserving the integrity of the rotator cuff. It is possible to weaken the cuff in the process of excision of the cuff, giving rise to a subsequent rotator cuff failure.

Arthritis

Arthroscopic procedures have been used in the management of glenohumeral arthritis. While there are many level IV reports of patient improvement after these procedures, we must recall one of the few randomized controlled trials of arthroscopic surgery for arthritis. In that level I study a total of 180 patients with osteoarthritis of the knee were randomly assigned to receive arthroscopic debridement, arthroscopic lavage, or placebo surgery. Patients in the placebo group received skin incisions and underwent a simulated debridement without insertion of the arthroscope. The results were that the patients in each of the three groups were improved, but at no point did either of the intervention groups report less pain or better function than the placebo group that had sham surgery.[491A] From this study we learn two cautions in interpreting the results of level IV case series: (1) patients are likely to improve after *any* intervention—even a sham surgery—and (2) it cannot be concluded that a procedure, such as arthroscopic debridement, is effective unless it is compared with a control (for other examples see the commentary on the rotator cuff section).

One of the potentially important applications of arthroscopy in the management of arthritis is its use for taking biopsies for culture in cases of suspected periprosthetic infection. We recognize that the bacteria commonly recovered from failed shoulder arthroplasties are *Propionibacterium* and coagulase-negative *Staphylococcus*, neither of which is easily recovered by fluid aspiration because they are often embedded in biofilms. Thus tissue cultures and cultures of explanted components are more likely to be revealing. In a level I study on arthroscopic tissue culture for the evaluation of periprosthetic shoulder infection,[198A] all 19 biopsy culture results were consistent with the culture results obtained during the revision surgery, yielding 100% sensitivity, specificity, PPV, and NPV. In contrast, fluoroscopically guided glenohumeral aspiration yielded a sensitivity of 16.7%, specificity of 100%, PPV of 100%, and NPV of 58.3%.

Biceps-Labral Complex

This topic requires a great deal of careful thought. As with the rotator cuff, biceps and labral pathology can be traumatic or degenerative. Labral "pathology" can also represent developmental differences that may be normal for the individual person and not productive of symptoms. While there are many classification systems, it seems important to recognize the importance of the history and the physical examination. Patients that seem to do the best are those with identifiable mechanisms of injury that can "push off" or "pull off" the labrum, followed by an identifiable "clunk" as the humeral head translates over the destabilized labrum. Patients who seem to do poorly are those without a history of injury, nonspecific pain, no definite mechanical signs, and questionable pathology on MRI. Attempting repair of degenerative lesions of the labrum can lead to unwanted shoulder tightness. Placement of suture anchors for labral repairs is critical to avoid problems with "anchor arthropathy."

While it is common to refer to the biceps as a "pain generator," and some surgeons pride themselves in being "biceps killers," it is also an important part of the functional anatomy of the normal shoulder. There are many tests for biceps pathology, but in evaluating these tests it is important to recall that the biceps only slides in the grove with shoulder motion—thus the "saw test," in which the biceps is contracted and the shoulder is flexed and extended can reveal symptoms from fraying or instability. Biceps instability (including the pulley lesion of the upper subscapularis), tendon fraying, and labral avulsion are potential indications for surgical intervention. Thanks to the powerful magnification of the arthroscope, biceps changes that might appear minor at open surgery may appear substantial at arthroscopy, so good judgment is necessary to decide when to pull the trigger on biceps tenodesis or tenotomy. As the authors of this subchapter point out, biceps surgery—whether bursectomy, tenotomy, soft tissue tenodesis, or tenodesis to bone—may not satisfy the patient because of cosmetic

SENIOR EDITOR COMMENTARY—cont'd

concerns, muscle cramping, pain at the tenodesis site, bone reaction at the anchor site, fracture, and more.

Thrower's Shoulder

It is always refreshing to read statements such as these authors make, that "Nonoperative treatment of SLAP tears is the mainstay of treatment, particularly in throwers, and has achieved good success. Even with initial failure of nonoperative treatment...demonstrated reasonable success with a second course of physical therapy specifically designed to improve glenohumeral internal rotation deficit (GIRD), scapular dyskinesia, posterior capsular contracture, and any concomitant injuries. ... Failed nonoperative treatment may warrant surgical intervention; however, success may be largely influenced by factors independent from the quality of surgical repair, such as age, associated pathology, position in sport, and competitive level."

The authors of this section obviously have the greatest respect for the throwing shoulder. Adaptive changes necessary for a high-level throwing shoulder may resemble pathologic changes in other shoulders. They state that "as many as 50% of asymptomatic, professional-level pitchers have recently been shown to have a partial-thickness rotator cuff tear and/or a SLAP lesion on MRI in one study, and as many as 80% of asymptomatic, mature pitchers had MRI changes and 45% had a labral tear." "In asymptomatic individuals with pathology on imaging, restoration of normal anatomy may even be detrimental, potentially leading to the recurrent tear, loss of motion, and worsening of performance." They caution against anything that may interfere with this fine motion, such as prominent knots, constraint of the biceps, or tightening the capsule any more than absolutely necessary. This makes one wonder if this same conservatism might be applicable to nonthrowing shoulders.

Complications

Patients and surgeons considering shoulder arthroscopy need to consider the possible complications that can follow the minimally invasive arthroscopic approach to shoulder surgery. In my referral practice, the most common complications I see after arthroscopic surgery are related to improper placement of suture anchors (usually on the articular face of glenoid leading to anchor arthropathy), excessive tightening in surgery for SLAP lesions or perceived instability, weakening of the cuff in excision of calcium deposits (leading to cuff rupture), failed repair of degenerative cuff tears, or anterosuperior escape from acromioplasty to decompress irreparable cuff tears.

CHAPTER 16

Glenohumeral Arthritis and Its Management

Frederick A. Matsen III, Steven B. Lippitt, Charles A. Rockwood Jr, Michael A. Wirth

OVERVIEW

Glenohumeral arthritis may be defined as a condition in which the normal articular surfaces of the humeral head and glenoid are compromised by degeneration, inflammation, or injury. The healthy glenohumeral joint has excellent smoothness, strength, and stability, features that humble the surgeon's attempt to restore them once they are altered by arthritis. Many different philosophies, surgical approaches, and implants are used to manage glenohumeral arthritis. Rather than providing a superficial overview of the many alternatives, this chapter presents in detail the techniques we have evolved over 4 decades of evaluating and managing shoulder arthritis. The lead author (F.A.M.) has no financial relationship with or allegiance to any implant company; the principles and procedures presented in this chapter are generic and applicable to many different arthroplasty systems. There are many ways to spend money in the evaluation and management of glenohumeral arthritis. This chapter emphasizes value (i.e., benefit to the patient divided by the cost) over more expensive diagnostic and therapeutic approaches unless they have proven value for the patient.

The normal articular surfaces are concentric, smooth, and securely bonded to the underlying bone.[88] The two essential functions of these articular surfaces are (1) to distribute the glenohumeral joint reaction force across the broadest possible articular contact area throughout the range of shoulder motion and (2) to optimize stability without compromising motion. Even with the translation of the humeral head that occurs at the extremes of motion, the glenoid fossa, with its thick peripheral articular cartilage and labrum, still maintains full surface contact with it for optimal load transfer (Fig. 16-1).* The unique design of the glenohumeral joint allows a great range of motion with a large humeral head (Fig. 16-2) and a small glenoid socket (Fig. 16-3). This potentially unstable anatomy is stabilized by the action of the rotator cuff, which compresses the humeral articular surface into the glenoid concavity—a mechanism referred to as "concavity compression" (Fig. 16-4).[303,307] This is similar to the stabilization of a golf ball on a small golf tee by the compressive force of gravity. When there is a sufficient concavity in the glenoid fossa, the concavity compression mechanism can provide glenohumeral stability even if the supraspinatus is deficient (Fig. 16-5). However, if the glenoid concavity is compromised, the humeral head is no longer stabilized (Fig. 16-6).

In the arthritic glenohumeral joint, the smooth, concentric joint surfaces are lost because of damage to the articular cartilage and the underlying bone (Figs. 16-7 and 16-8). This chapter will discuss important differences among the different types of arthritis, but a brief overview is provided here. *Degenerative joint disease* (also known as osteoarthritis or osteoarthrosis) is a common type of glenohumeral arthritis in which the articular cartilage fails from heavy use, cumulative minor traumatic episodes, underlying structural defects in the joint, anomalies in cartilage composition, or a combination of these factors. *Capsulorrhaphy arthropathy* is one of the most common forms of glenohumeral arthritis in younger patients; it is a complication of a prior repair for glenohumeral instability with some combination of (1) overtightening of the anterior capsule that causes posterior humeral subluxation and/or (2) prominent suture anchors, staples, screws, or transferred coracoid bone that cause excoriation of the humeral articular cartilage.[364,600] In *rheumatoid and other types of inflammatory arthritis* the cartilage of the humeral head and glenoid is uniformly destroyed by an autoimmune reaction, with characteristic periarticular osteopenia, marginal erosions, and minimal osteophyte formation. *Chondrolysis* is an iatrogenic condition in which the glenohumeral articular cartilage is destroyed, most commonly due to the toxic effects of local anesthetics infused by a pain pump after arthroscopic surgery, particularly after procedures involving the use of glenoid suture anchors in young individuals.[339,489,581] In *avascular necrosis* the bone supporting the humeral articular

References 19, 105, 140, 155, 201, 202, 287, 303, 305, 307, 308, 338, 426, 490.

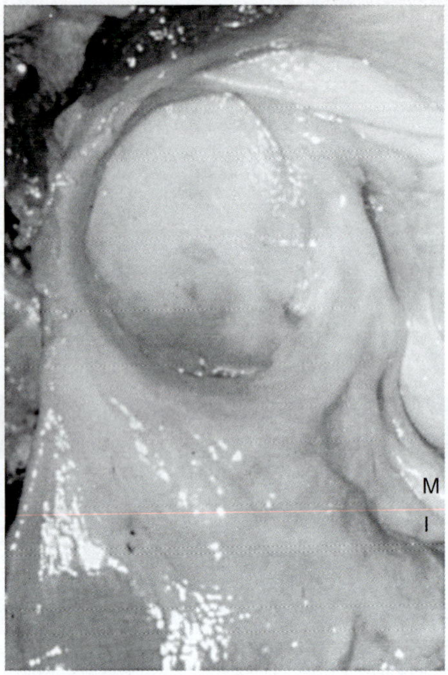

FIGURE 16-1: Cadaver dissection of the glenoid, biceps tendon insertion and associated glenohumeral ligaments. This dissection demonstrates the anterior glenohumeral ligaments. Note the relationship of the anterior inferior (I) and the anterior middle (M) glenohumeral ligaments to the anterior rim of the glenoid.

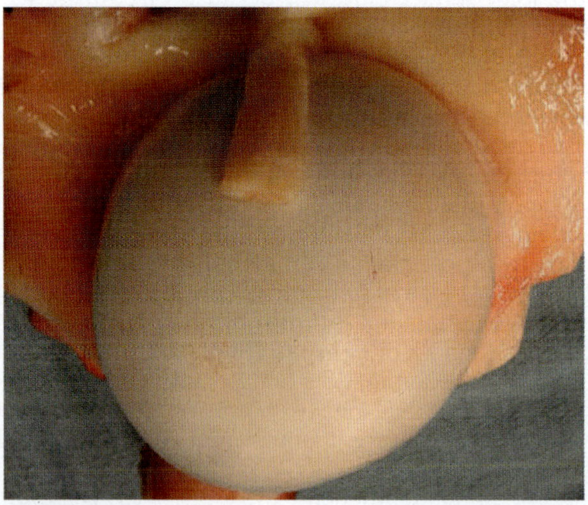

FIGURE 16-2: The smooth articular surface of the humeral head surrounded by the insertion of the tendons of the rotator cuff, with the long head of the biceps entering the bicipital groove at top center.

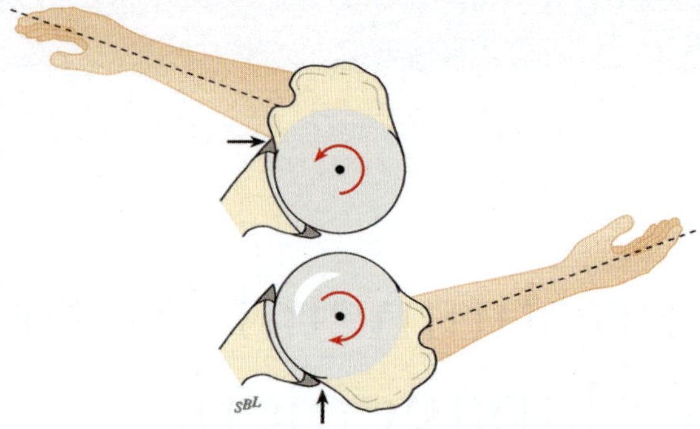

FIGURE 16-3: The relatively smaller surface area of the glenoid socket allows a large range of humeral motion before contact occurs between the humeral tuberosities and the glenoid rim (arrows).

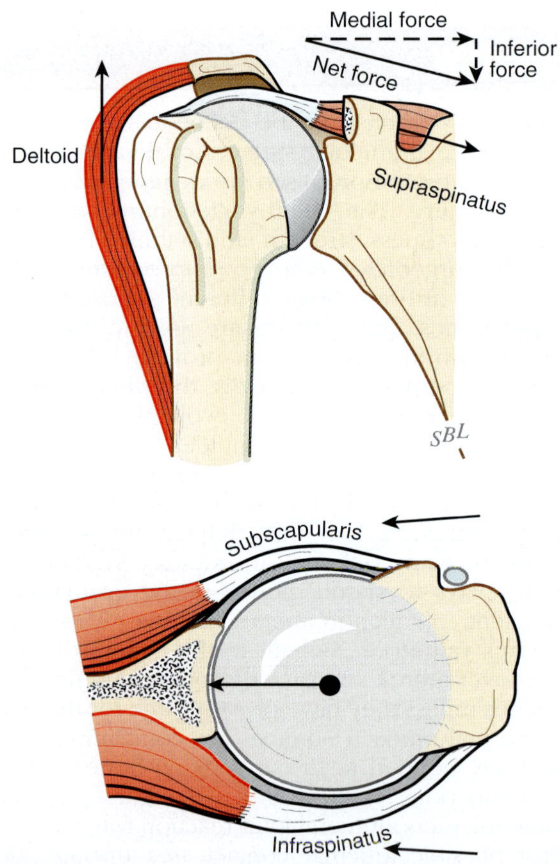

FIGURE 16-4: Compression into the glenoid concavity. The rotator cuff compresses the humeral articular convexity into the glenoid concavity, as shown by the arrows. (From Matsen FA III, Lippitt SB. *Shoulder Surgery: Principles and Procedures.* Philadelphia: Saunders; 2004:85.)

cartilage collapses, often because of corticosteroid use, alcoholism, or prior trauma. In *posttraumatic arthritis* the anatomy of the glenohumeral joint is distorted due to a prior fracture with malunion or nonunion. *Rotator cuff tear arthropathy* is the combination of an irreparable rotator cuff defect and glenohumeral arthritis, which may lead to anterosuperior escape and pseudoparalysis.[331] *Neurotropic arthropathy* arises in association with syringomyelia, diabetes, or other causes of joint denervation; the joint and subchondral bone are destroyed due to the

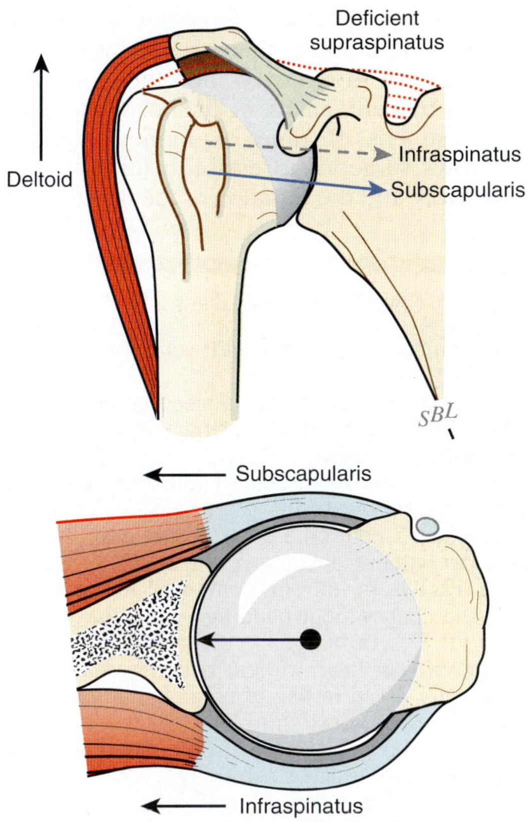

FIGURE 16-5: Intact glenoid concavity. If the glenoid concavity is intact, the compressive action of the subscapularis and infraspinatus can stabilize the humeral head in the center of the glenoid socket against the upward pull of the deltoid, even in the absence of the supraspinatus (red dotted lines). (From Matsen FA III, Lippitt SB. *Shoulder Surgery: Principles and Procedures.* Philadelphia: Saunders; 2004:263.)

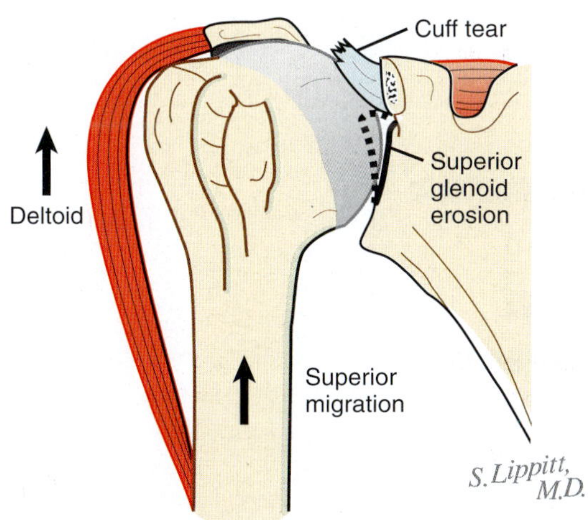

FIGURE 16-6: Loss of centering. A loss of both the rotator cuff and the superior glenoid concavity (dotted line) allows the destabilized humeral head to move upward rather than abduct on deltoid contraction. (From Matsen FA III, Lippitt SB. *Shoulder Surgery: Principles and Procedures.* Philadelphia: Saunders; 2004:263.)

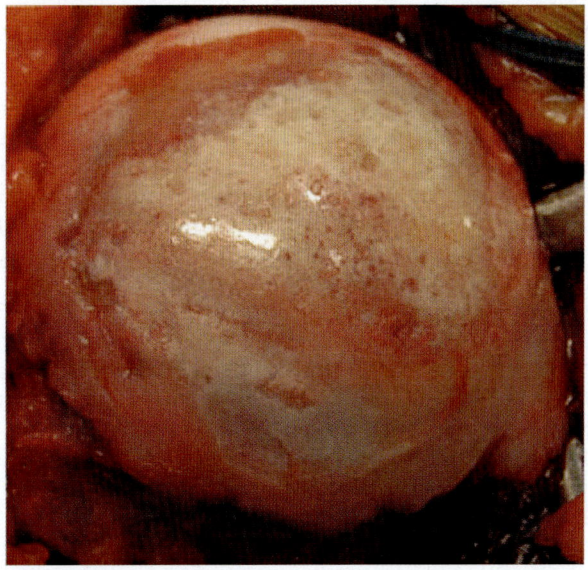

FIGURE 16-7: The arthritic head devoid of articular cartilage and surrounded by osteophytes.

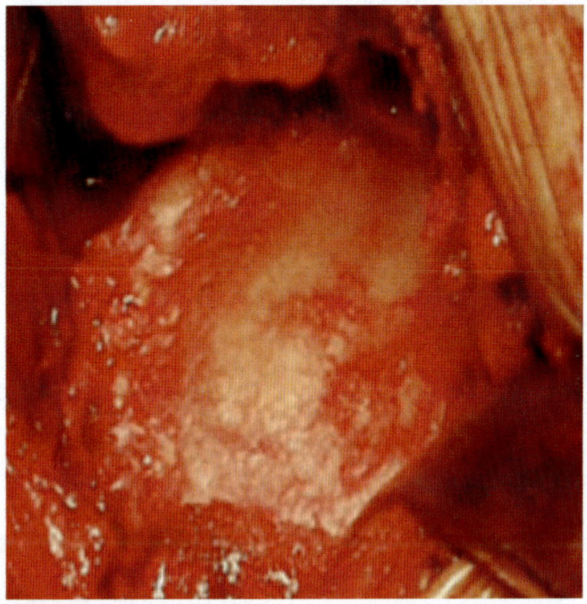

FIGURE 16-8: An arthritic glenoid with loss of cartilage on the posterior 75% of the surface (to the right of the image).

loss of the trophic and protective effects of their nerve supply.

CLINICAL EVALUATION

Patients suspected of having glenohumeral arthritis should be evaluated with a history, a physical examination, and standardized plain radiographs. In the great majority of cases this basic evaluation is sufficient to establish the diagnosis and enable surgical planning without the additional expense of computed tomography (CT) or magnetic resonance imaging (MRI).[335,344]

History

Chief Complaint

A useful way to open the clinical evaluation is to ask a question, such as "What can I help you with today?" This allows the patient to describe the problem in their own words without interruption. Patients with symptomatic glenohumeral arthritis will often complain of pain, stiffness, crepitation on movement, loss of function, difficulty sleeping, and discomfort with changes in barometric pressure. Glenohumeral arthritic pain is commonly felt over the posterior aspect of the glenohumeral joint in contrast to pain from cervical radiculopathy that is commonly felt in the area of the trapezius. It is important to document the circumstances surrounding the onset of the problem, its pattern of progression over time, and its response to prior medical and surgical treatment.

Because it is important to get a "snapshot" of the condition of the shoulder at the time of initial presentation, we ask all our new patients to characterize their shoulder comfort and function using the Simple Shoulder Test (SST) (Box 16-1),[284,338,342,345,421,470] a practical, efficient, sensitive, and extensively validated tool that we developed based on the chief complaints of patients presenting to us with shoulder arthritis. The major functional deficits for the common types of glenohumeral arthritis include difficulty with sleeping comfortably on the affected side, washing the back of the opposite shoulder, placing eight pounds on a shelf, and throwing overhand (Fig. 16-9; Table 16-1).

As a patient-reported assessment, SST serves as the baseline for documenting the presenting status of the shoulder and tracking its response to treatment over time, and it removes concern over variability related to different observers. Importantly, this assessment tool does not require the patient to return to the office, but rather can be submitted by mail, email, or online. Without any substantial investment of time or money, this practical method allows surgeons to establish for themselves the time to recovery and the duration of the functional benefit

BOX 16-1. Simple Shoulder Test

Is your shoulder comfortable with your arm at rest by your side?
Does your shoulder allow you to sleep comfortably?
Can you reach the small of your back to tuck in your shirt with your hand?
Can you place your hand behind your head with the elbow straight out to the side?
Can you place a coin on a shelf at the level of your shoulder without bending your elbow?
Can you lift 1 lb (a full pint container) to the level of your shoulder without bending your elbow?
Can you lift 8 lb (a full gallon container) to the level of the top of your head without bending your elbow?
Can you carry 20 lb (a bag of potatoes) at your side with the affected extremity?
Do you think you can toss a softball underhand 10 yards with the affected extremity?
Do you think you can throw a softball overhand 20 yards with the affected extremity?
Can you wash the back of your opposite shoulder with the affected extremity?
Does your shoulder allow you to work full time at your regular job?

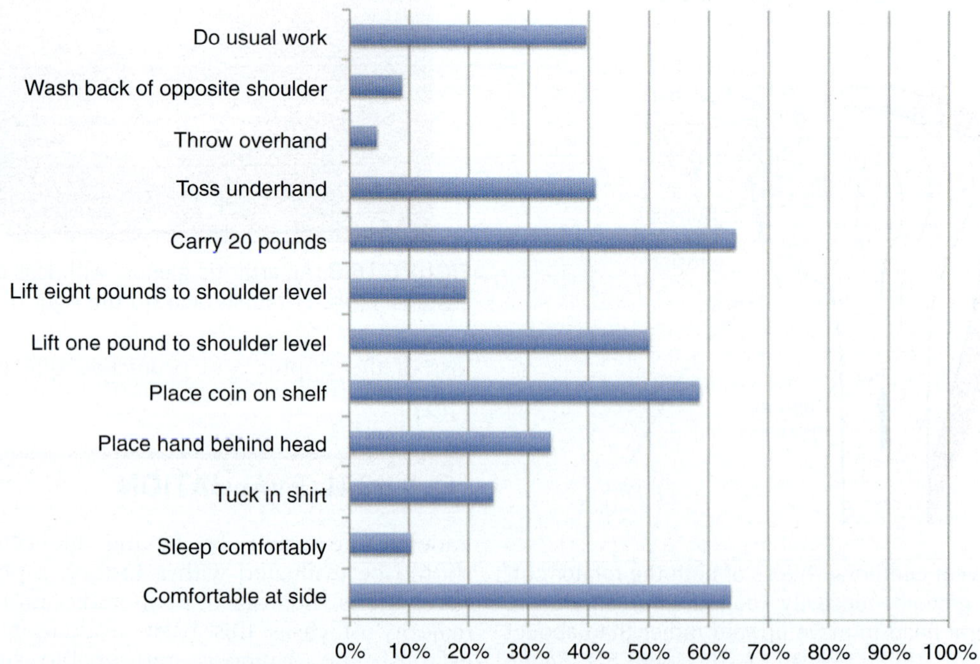

FIGURE 16-9: Percentage of 3128 patients with primary degenerative joint disease of the shoulder able to perform each of the 12 functions of the Simple Shoulder Test.

TABLE 16-1 Percentage of Patients Able to Perform Functions of the Simple Shoulder Test at the Time of Initial Evaluation, According to Type of Glenohumeral Arthritis

Function	DJD	SDJD	RA	CTA	CA	AVN
Sleep comfortably	12	13	18	8	0	29
Arm comfortable at side	67	36	61	33	65	79
Wash back of shoulder	13	20	13	0	18	7
Hand behind head	35	38	26	21	35	50
Tuck in shirt	32	33	39	38	29	50
8 lb on shelf	19	16	3	0	18	7
1 lb on shelf	54	36	26	21	53	50
Coin on shelf	59	44	29	29	53	64
Throw overhand	7	9	3	4	0	0
Do usual work	39	44	21	17	41	21
Throw underhand	53	44	13	42	29	21
Carry 20 lb	62	62	21	33	41	29

AVN, avascular necrosis; CA, capsulorrhaphy arthropathy; CTA, cuff tear arthropathy, DJD, degenerative joint disease; RA, rheumatoid arthritis; SDJD, secondary degenerative joint disease.

of different procedures and share these results with prospective patients. Perhaps even more importantly, monitoring changes in SST after surgery enables the surgeon to identify individual arthroplasty procedures that were not successful in restoring comfort and function for the patient, and to learn from these "with a view to preventing similar failures in the future," as recommended by Codman.[93,94]

The second important self-assessment tool is the Short Form-36 Health Survey (SF-36), which enables patients to document their overall health status.[284,329,342,345,470] The SF-36 scales of emotional role function, mental health, and social function are more closely correlated with pain and functional impairment than the "objective" measures of the severity of the disease.[162,338,345,533] For patients with osteoarthritis presenting for shoulder arthroplasty, the SF-36 scores are inversely correlated with the number of comorbidities.[470] The greatest compromise in the self-assessed overall health status of patients with glenohumeral arthritis is found in the SF-36 domains of physical role function and overall comfort (Table 16-2). For patients with primary or secondary degenerative joint disease or cuff tear arthropathy (CTA), scores for the other SF-36 parameters (such as vitality and overall health) are relatively close to those of population-based age- and sex-matched controls. In contrast, the health status of patients with rheumatoid arthritis, capsulorrhaphy arthropathy, or avascular necrosis is poorer than that of controls of the same age and sex.[284,342] The overall well-being of the patient, including preoperative physical function, general health, social function, and mental health, has been shown to be strongly correlated with the quality of the outcome after shoulder arthroplasty.[329,421] The recognition of the importance of the overall condition of the patient in influencing the outcome of treatment recalls the quote often attributed to Sir William Osler: "It is much more important to know what sort of a patient has the disease than what sort of a disease the patient has." SF-36 provides a convenient and standardized way of knowing "what sort of a patient has the disease."

Medical History

When taking the patient's history, the surgeon attempts to elicit all factors that may influence the patient's situation and recovery from surgery, such as use of nicotine, alcohol, and narcotics; complications of prior surgeries and anesthetics; medical comorbidities; depression; the patient's living situation; social and family support; the relationship of the shoulder condition to work; and insurance coverage for surgical and postoperative care.[80,118,397,482,488,497] Shoulder arthroplasty is an elective procedure, which allows time to optimize pain medication control, respiratory health (including obstructive sleep apnea), diabetic control, blood pressure, cardiac health, and urinary function. We encourage our patients to partner with us in optimizing their surgical and postoperative care, starting by asking them to complete a presurgery checklist (Box 16-2).

Physical Examination

Perhaps the most important part of the physical examination looks at the overall person: is the individual happy or depressed, healthy or chronically ill, fit or frail, well nourished or malnourished, actively engaged or passive? Who accompanied the patient to the visit: spouse, friend, caregiver, caseworker, or lawyer? Does the patient smell

TABLE 16-2 Self-Assessed Health Status of Patients, Revealed by SF-36, According to the Type of Glenohumeral Arthritis*

SF-36 Parameter	DJD	SDJD	RA	CTA	CA	AVN
Physical role function	44	33	23	30	39	28
Comfort	54	47	34	39	40	47
Physical function	78	73	38	81	62	50
Emotional role function	83	76	58	100	64	40
Social function	84	73	63	81	71	62
Vitality	86	83	44	81	65	60
Mental health	92	90	87	97	76	84
General health	100	93	65	100	71	63

**Data presented as the mean percentage of the value for an age- and sex-matched control population.[28]*

AVN, avascular necrosis; CA, capsulorrhaphy arthropathy; CTA, cuff tear arthropathy; DJD, degenerative joint disease; RA, rheumatoid arthritis; SDJD, secondary degenerative joint disease; SF-36, Short Form-36 Health Survey.

BOX 16-2. Checklist for Patients Considering Shoulder Joint Replacement

Habits

____ Engage in 3 hours of aerobic exercise per week unless your primary care physician deems it unsafe.

____ Avoid smoking or use of any nicotine-containing products for 3 months prior to surgery.

____ Avoid any narcotic medications stronger than hydrocodone for 3 months prior to surgery. If heavier narcotics have been used, detoxification under physician supervision is recommended 3 months before the surgery.

____ For 3 months before surgery, restrict alcohol consumption to one drink per day.

Planning

____ Formulate a plan for postoperative care well in advance of surgery, recognizing that the shoulder may be less useful than it was before for a period of weeks or longer after surgery. Understand the limitations on activities after surgery, such as restrictions on driving (usually for 6 weeks after surgery), as well as the need for someone to be with you for days or weeks after the procedure. Identify the possible need for a temporary stay at a skilled nursing facility and secure the funding for this stay well in advance of the procedure.

____ Identify a primary care physician who will manage your nonsurgical concerns and medications after surgery. If you live at a distance from your surgeon, identify a physician locally who will be available to check the wound and obtain follow-up radiographs as necessary.

____ Understand and plan for the rehabilitation program after surgery as well as the plan for follow-up with the surgeon. Ask your surgeon if a local therapist will be needed after this procedure; if so, identify one before surgery.

Physical and Emotional Health

____ Obtain a current dental evaluation. Optimize dental hygiene, including gum care. The mouth can be a source of bacteria leading to infection. Dental concerns need to be tended to at least 4 weeks before surgery.

____ Identify any skin lesions anywhere on the body, especially on the arm that will undergo surgery. These need to be completely healed at least 2 weeks before surgery. Be particularly careful to check the skin in the arm pit and under the breasts.

____ Ensure that any infections are completely resolved and antibiotics discontinued at least 6 weeks prior to surgery.

____ Optimize control of health conditions, such as sleep apnea, anxiety, depression, diabetes, hypertension, heart conditions, and urinary tract function.

Communication With the Surgical Team

____ Discuss the surgeon's personal experience with the problem and the procedure, along with possible risks, alternatives, and anticipated outcomes.

____ Notify the team if prior experience suggests that it will be difficult to establish an intravenous (IV) line for surgery, that it has been difficult for an anesthesiologist to establish an airway, or if you have had any problems with prior anesthetics, the control of pain, excessive bleeding, or blood clots.

____ Let the surgical team know if any family member or blood relative ever had a serious problem with anesthesia; if they did, what was the problem?

____ Discuss with the surgeon any heart conditions, strokes, kidney disease, liver disease, lung disease, bleeding tendencies, prior surgical complications, reactions to anesthetics, or seizures. Do you have a pacemaker?

BOX 16-2. Checklist for Patients Considering Shoulder Joint Replacement—cont'd

____ Document and communicate all medical allergies, especially allergies to antibiotics and latex.

____ Could you be pregnant? If so, we would recommend that you have a pregnancy test performed before coming for surgery, and, if you are pregnant, that you not undergo elective surgery until after delivery.

____ Compile and share with your surgeon a complete list of all prescription and over-the-counter medications you are taking.

____ Recognize that antiinflammatory medications, blood thinners (e.g., aspirin, ibuprofen, Advil, warfarin, Coumadin, or Plavix), fish oil, omega-3 fatty acids, and some herbal supplements can increase the risk of bleeding and their use may need to be modified well in advance of surgery. If you are taking drugs to prevent blood clotting, you should consult with your cardiologist and the preanesthesia clinic or your surgeon at least 10 days in advance to obtain instructions regarding when these medications need to be stopped or modified.

____ Identify and discuss with your surgeon any legal issues regarding the shoulder problem well in advance of surgery.

____ Verify insurance coverage well in advance of surgery. This is especially important for patients from a different state than the one where the surgery will be performed, for those for whom an extended care facility may be needed after surgery, and for patients making Workers' Compensation insurance claims.

of cigarettes or alcohol, or have pinpoint pupils suggestive of narcotic use? Does the patient use a cane or crutch, and if so, in which hand? Is the patient steady or unsteady on his or her feet? Can the patient get up on the examination table unassisted? Does he or she use the involved arm to slip off a coat or to talk or to shake hands?

Inspection of the shoulder requires it to be exposed by appropriate disrobing so that the examiner can evaluate the health of the skin over the shoulder, in the axilla, and down the arm, as well as the presence and location of previous skin incisions and the manner in which they healed. Is the arterial, venous, and lymphatic circulation of the limb intact, or has the patient had prior lymph node dissections and lymphedema? Are the deltoid, cuff, and periscapular muscles of normal or diminished size compared with the opposite side? Are there signs of inflammation (warmth, tenderness, and erythema)? Is there swelling suggestive of infection, CTA, or Charcot arthropathy?

After the inspection, it is useful to start the physical examination with a "no-touch" opening: "Can you show me the movements that are the biggest problem for you?" These patient-identified limitations allow initial consideration about which treatment may be of benefit. Next, we ask the patient to demonstrate the ability to actively abduct, flex, and rotate the shoulder as well as reach across the body and up the back, first with the normal shoulder and then with the symptomatic one. In a patient-friendly way this provides an initial broad assessment of the function of the shoulder and the degree of discomfort associated with motion. After asking permission to physically examine the shoulder, we palpate it, seeking evidence of effusion, tenderness, or glenohumeral instability, as well as subacromial, glenohumeral, scapulothoracic crepitance, or rotator cuff and subscapularis defects (Figs. 16-10 to 16-12).

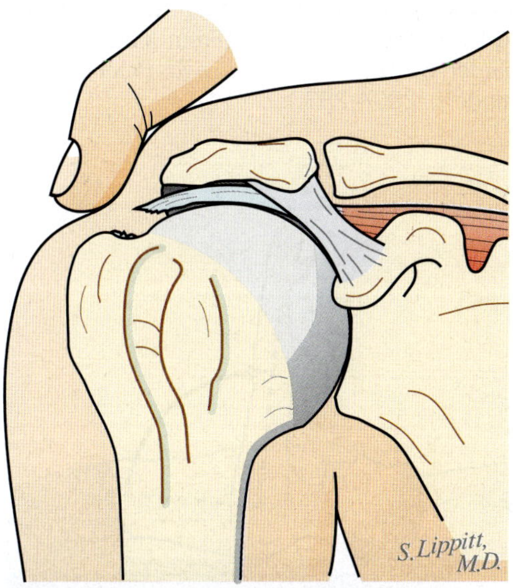

FIGURE 16-10: Palpation of cuff defects. Defects in the tendinous cuff can often be palpated through the overlying skin and deltoid. (From Matsen FA III, Lippitt SB. *Shoulder Surgery: Principles and Procedures.* Philadelphia: Saunders; 2004:283.)

We then proceed with the formal evaluation of shoulder mobility, including the assessment of forward elevation (Fig. 16-13), abduction (Fig. 16-14), external rotation at the side (Fig. 16-15), external rotation in abduction (Fig. 16-16), internal rotation up the back (Fig. 16-17), internal rotation in abduction (Fig. 16-18), and cross-body adduction (Fig. 16-19). These tests evaluate the range of motion of the humerus relative to the thorax. A more specific assessment of the range of glenohumeral motion can be obtained if the examiner uses one hand to stabilize the scapula while establishing flexion and extension and internal and external rotation of the humerus, relative to the scapula, with the other hand. It is useful to show the patient and family members the contrast between the motion of the affected shoulder and that of the contralateral normal or less affected shoulder. Whereas most arthritic shoulders show reduced range of motion, those

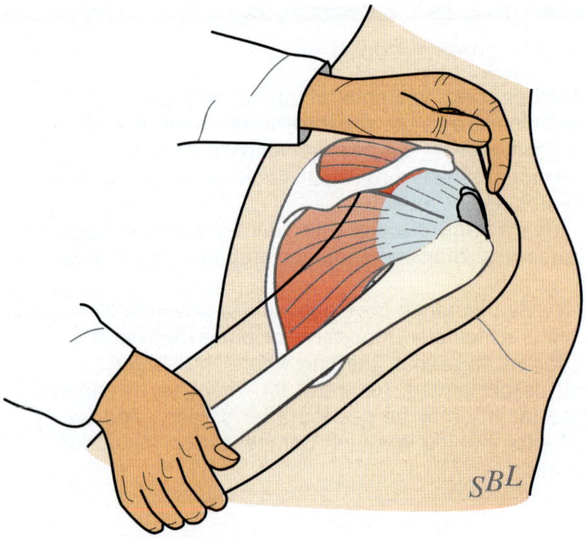

FIGURE 16-11: Palpation of supraspinatus defects. The accessibility of the supraspinatus tendon for palpation can be enhanced by extending the arm. (From Matsen FA III, Lippitt SB. *Shoulder Surgery: Principles and Procedures.* Philadelphia: Saunders; 2004:283.)

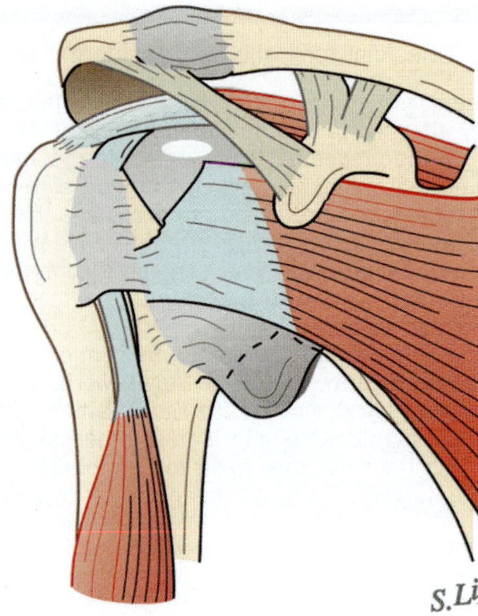

FIGURE 16-12: A defect in the superior subscapularis tendon insertion may be palpable at the anterior shoulder.

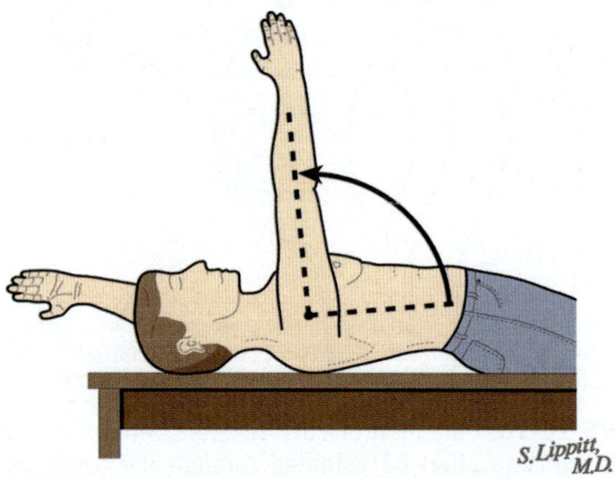

FIGURE 16-13: Limited humeral forward elevation relative to the thorax.

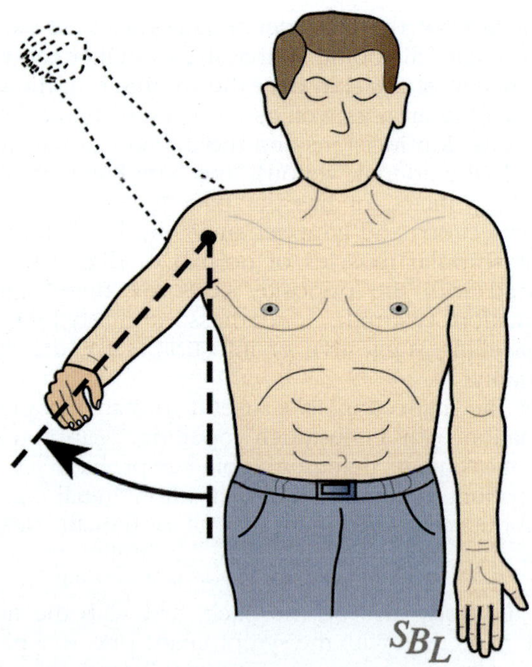

FIGURE 16-14: Limited humeral abduction.

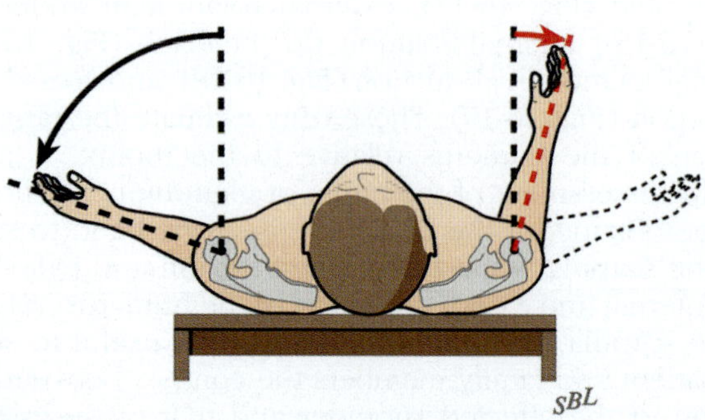

FIGURE 16-15: Limited humeral external rotation with the arm adducted at the side.

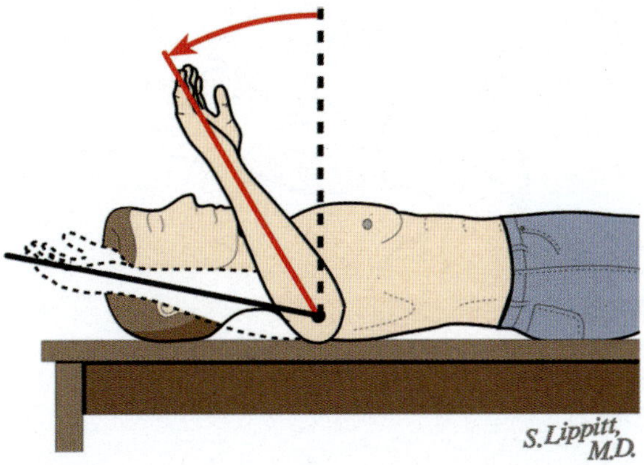

FIGURE 16-16: Limited humeral external rotation with the arm in the 90-degree abducted position.

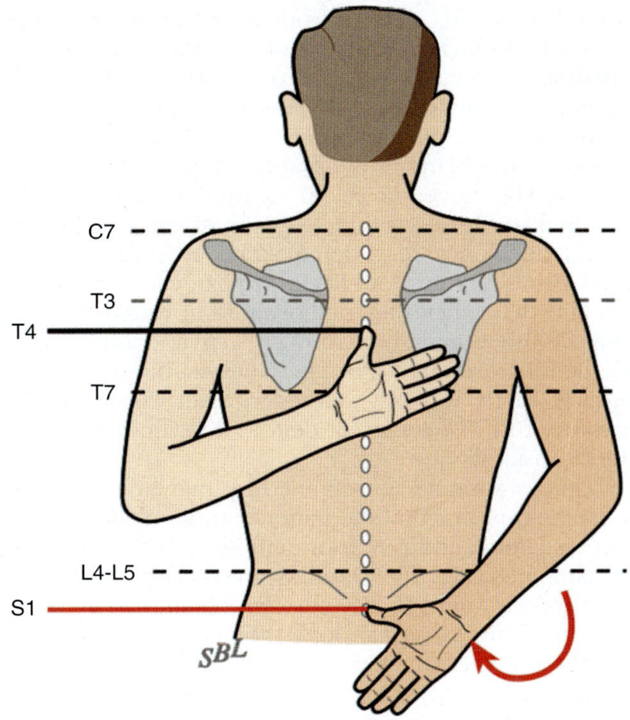

FIGURE 16-17: Limited humeral internal rotation behind the back as measured by the level of the thumb position relative to the level of spine.

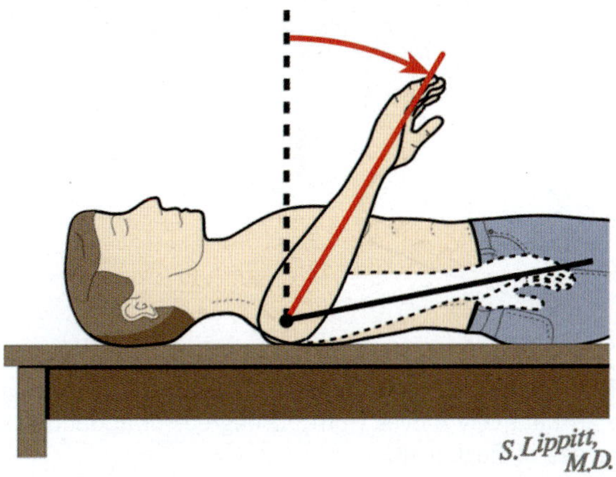

FIGURE 16-18: Limited humeral internal rotation with the arm in the 90-degree abducted position.

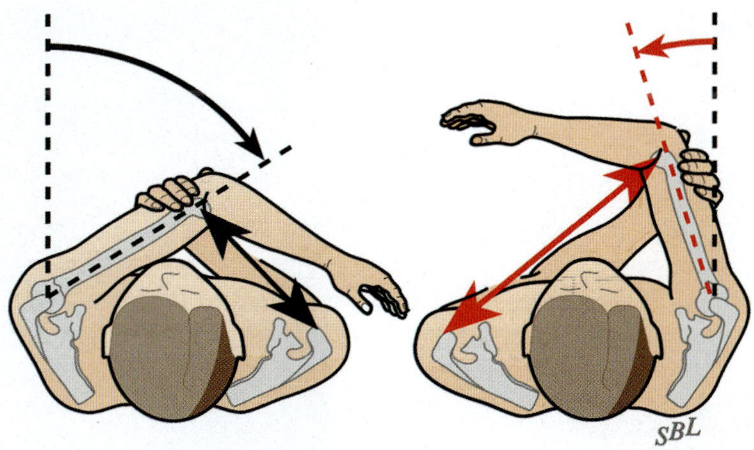

FIGURE 16-19: Limited cross-body adduction as measured by the distance between the elbow antecubital crease and the opposite shoulder.

with subscapularis defects from injury or prior surgery may show an increased range of external rotation.

Arthritic shoulders may be unstable. Shoulders with degenerative joint disease or capsulorrhaphy arthropathy may demonstrate posterior humeral translation as the arm is raised in the plane of the scapula (Fig. 16-20) or when it is actively moved from 90 degrees of abduction to 90 degrees of flexion (Fig. 16-21). Shoulders with anterior glenoid deficiency may demonstrate anterior instability as the arm is moved from flexion to extension. Shoulders with cuff deficiency may demonstrate upwards displacement of the humeral head with active contraction of the deltoid, referred to as "anterosuperior escape" (Figs. 16-22 to 16-25).[331] Shoulders with distorted bony anatomy, cuff deficiency, or deltoid deficiency may have inferior instability.

Shoulder strength is examined by manually assessing the isometric force that the patient can generate with the anterior, lateral, and posterior deltoid, as well as with the supraspinatus (Fig. 16-26), infraspinatus (Fig. 16-27), and subscapularis (Fig. 16-28) muscles. Examination of the function of suprascapular, long thoracic, axillary, musculocutaneous, median, radial, and ulnar nerves is important both for identifying possible neurologic contributions to the patient's symptoms as well as establishing the integrity of these nerves before surgical intervention.

Finally, examination of the neck may reveal evidence of cervical spondylopathy that may be contributing to the patient's symptoms, or restriction of the range of neck

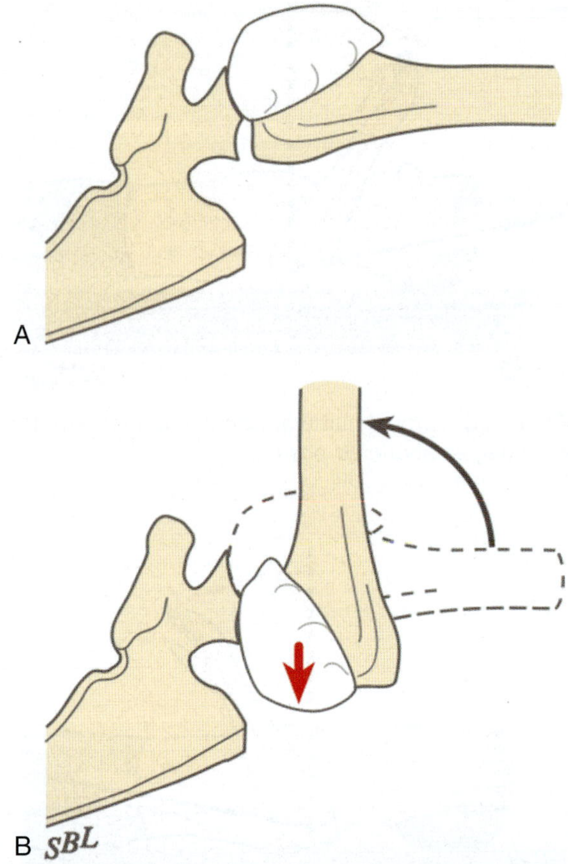

FIGURE 16-21: Posterior humeral head subluxation (*red arrow*) as the arm actively moves from 90 degrees of abduction (**A**) to 90 degrees of flexion (**B**).

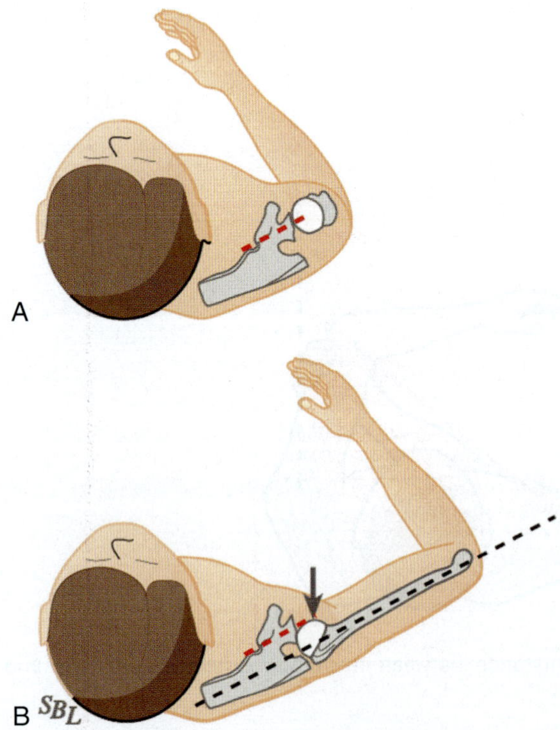

FIGURE 16-20: Posterior humeral head subluxation as the arm moves from adduction at the side (**A**) to abduction in the scapular plane (**B**), referred to as "scaption."

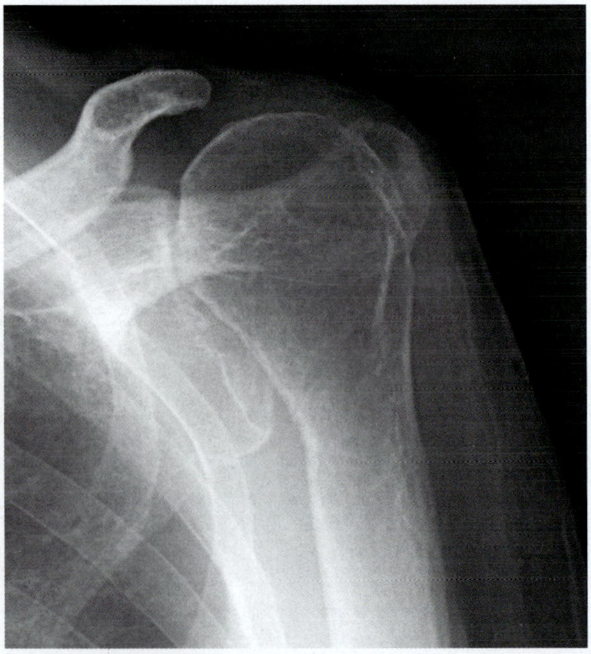

FIGURE 16-22: Anterosuperior escape.

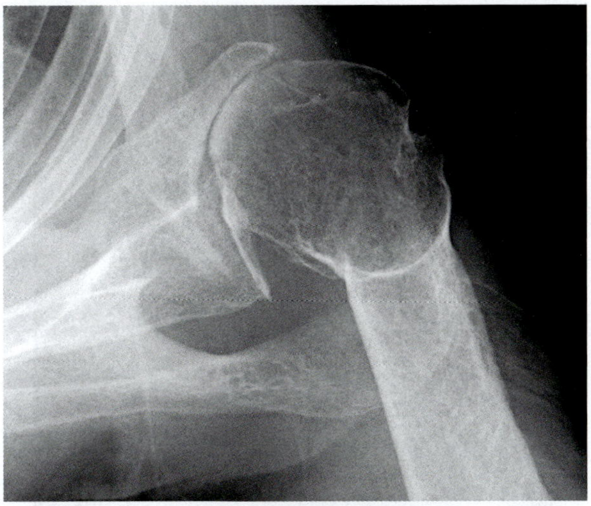

FIGURE 16-23: Rotator cuff tear arthropathy with anterior instability.

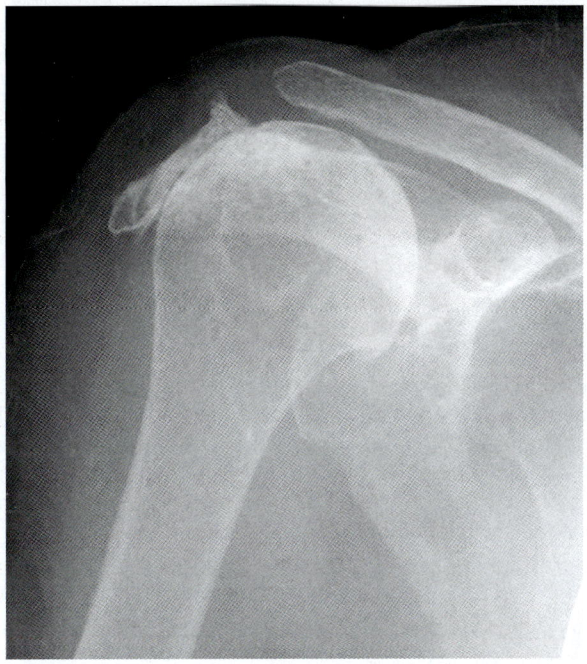

FIGURE 16-24: Rotator cuff tear arthropathy with severe acromial erosion that predisposes to acromial fracture.

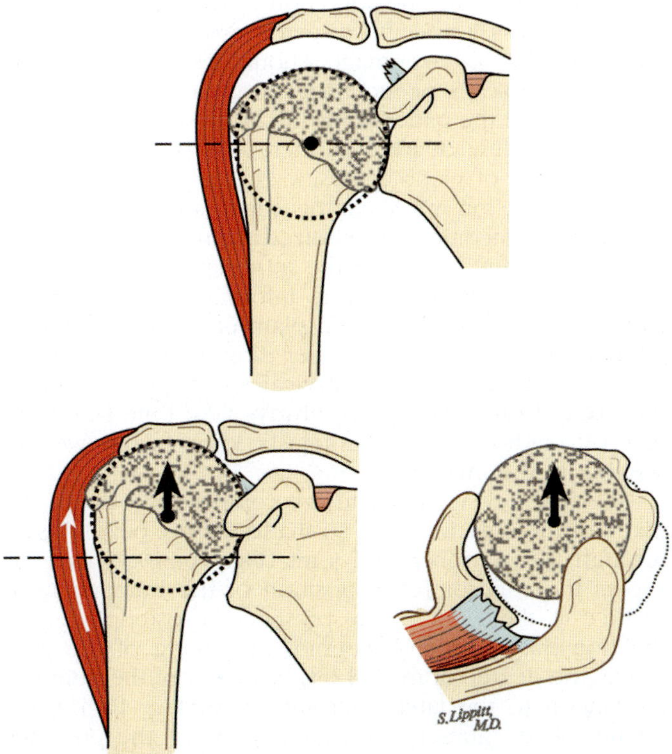

FIGURE 16-25: In shoulders with rotator cuff deficiency the humeral head demonstrates superior displacement with active contraction of the deltoid (*bottom left*). If the coracoacromial arch is also impaired, anterior displacement from beneath the acromion may occur, referred to as "anterosuperior escape" (*bottom right*).

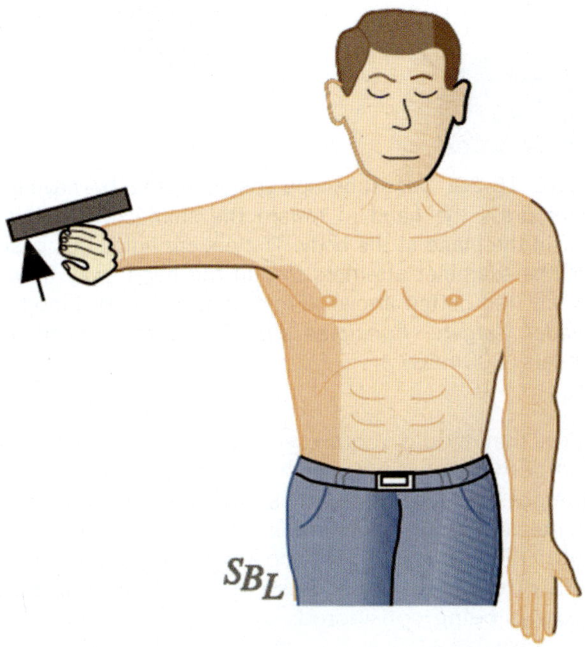

FIGURE 16-26: The supraspinatus is tested by positioning the arm in 90 degrees of abduction in the plane of the scapula and in internal rotation; this puts the supraspinatus tendon on top of the humeral head. The patient holds this position while the examiner attempts to adduct the arm.

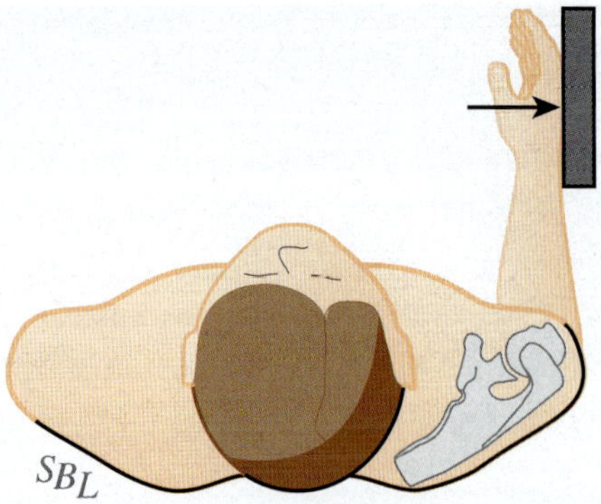

FIGURE 16-27: The infraspinatus is tested by positioning the humerus with the elbow at the side and the forearm pointing straight ahead. The patient holds this position while the examiner attempts to push the arm into internal rotation. (From Matsen FA III, Lippitt SB. *Shoulder Surgery: Principles and Procedures.* Philadelphia: Saunders; 2004:287.)

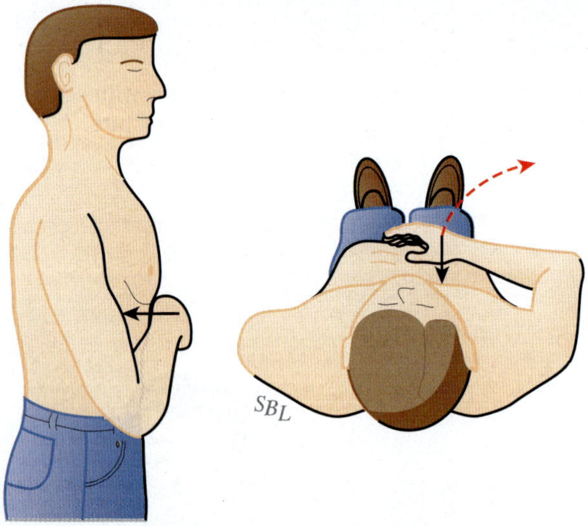

FIGURE 16-28: The subscapularis is tested by having the patient press the hand in toward the stomach, keeping the elbow in the plane of the body. The patient holds this position while the examiner attempts to pull the hand away from the stomach (red dotted arrow). (From Matsen FA III, Lippitt SB. *Shoulder Surgery: Principles and Procedures.* Philadelphia: Saunders; 2004:287.)

motion that would require special attention at the time of surgery. In patients with rheumatoid arthritis it is important to determine neck stability as well as the patient's ability to open their mouth to a degree that would allow anesthetic intubation. In all patients the health of the teeth and gums is particularly important if surgery is being considered.

Radiographic Evaluation

The purpose of imaging of the shoulder is to help establish the diagnosis, determine the severity of the pathoanatomy, assist in surgical planning, and enable the

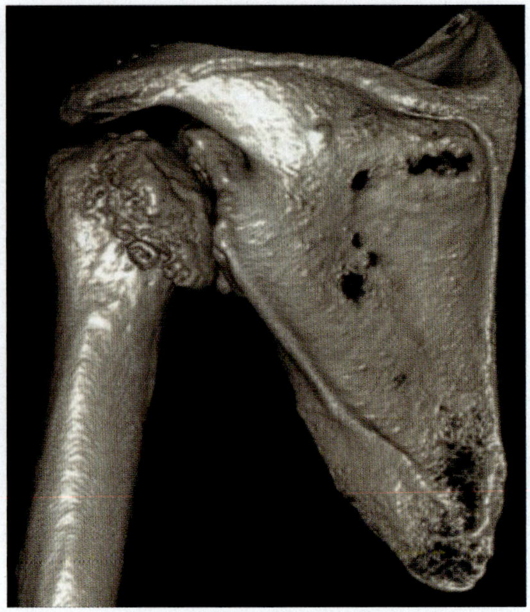

FIGURE 16-29: Three-dimensional reconstructions can reveal fine details of the shoulder anatomy, but this additional information rarely changes the planning or conduct of the arthroplasty.

surgeon to illustrate the condition of the shoulder to the patient. Unless a specific research protocol is in place, the temptation to "overimage" should be resisted, obtaining only the scans or reconstructions that are necessary for the care of the patient (Fig. 16-29). Although CT scans may offer a few degrees of increased precision in the measurement of glenoid version, we are not convinced that this precision improves the quality of the surgery or the clinical outcome. Standardized plain films are almost always sufficient to garner the information needed and, as described below, there is information that can be gathered from properly taken plain films that cannot be obtained from CT scans. Proper radiographic technique is as important as proper surgical technique to achieve the desired outcome, so we always take time to ensure that our radiograph technologists know what we are seeking in the images.

The first key view is the anteroposterior (AP) in the plane of the scapula taken so that the x-ray beam passes through the glenohumeral joint (Fig. 16-30). This view shows the superoinferior position of the humeral head relative to the glenoid, the presence of osteophytes on the humeral head and glenoid, narrowing of the joint space, the degree of medial displacement of the humerus in relation to the lateral acromial line (Fig. 16-31), the quality of the humeral and glenoid bone, the presence of loose bodies, and whether there is humeral head collapse or deformity.

The second key view is the axillary view taken with the arm in the functional position of elevation in the plane of the scapula (Fig. 16-32) and oriented so that both the spinoglenoid notch and the scapular neck are visible. This view shows a different perspective of the

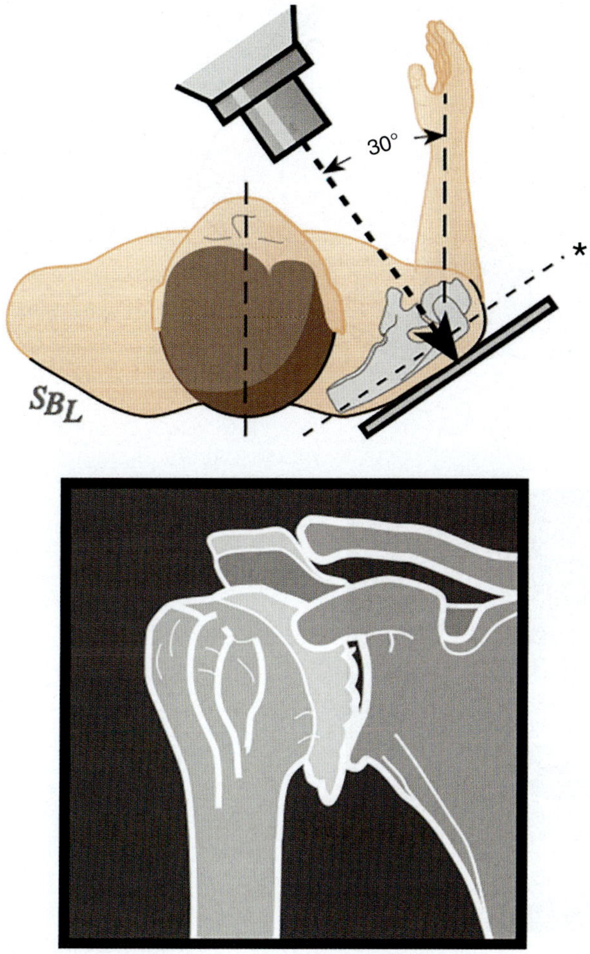

FIGURE 16-30: Anteroposterior radiograph in the plane of the scapula taken 30 degrees medial to the lateral of body's sagittal plane such that the x-ray beam passes through the glenohumeral joint. It is most easily taken by positioning the patient's scapula flat against the cassette (asterisk) and then passing the beam at right angles to the film, aiming at the coracoid process.

humeral anatomy, the amount of glenoid bone, the shape of the glenoid, its version in relation to the plane of the scapula, and the relationship of the humeral head to the glenoid fossa. We refer to this view as the "truth view"[335] because it demonstrates the glenohumeral relationships in the functional position of elevation. This is in contrast to CT scans,[564,568] which have the disadvantage of being taken with the arm in the adducted position (Fig. 16-33). Unfortunately, many of the "axillary views" sent to us for consultation are taken without standardization, making it impossible to determine the important features of the glenohumeral joint (Fig. 16-34).

When taken properly, the standardized anteroposterior and axillary views indicate the thickness of the cartilage space between the humerus and the glenoid, relative positions of the humeral head and the glenoid, presence of osteophytes (Fig. 16-35), degree of osteopenia, and extent of bony deformity and erosion.

Since arthritis usually involves the central aspect of the humeral head (Figs. 16-36 and 16-37; see Fig. 16-7), joint space narrowing is most evident on the truth view[335] as opposed to images made with the arm at the side. Of even greater importance is the ability of the axillary truth view to show posterior subluxation or "functional decentering" that is not evident in images taken with the arm at the side (Figs. 16-38 to 16-44).[335,344,560] The degree of posterior subluxation can be measured as (1) the position of the center of the humeral head in relation to the plane of the scapula (Fig. 16-45), (2) the position of the center of the humeral head in relation to the glenoid face (Fig. 16-46), or (3) the point of contact of the humeral articular surface on the glenoid articular surface (Figs. 16-47 and 16-48). We prefer the last of these because this point of contact reflects the degree of centering of the net humeral joint reaction force on the glenoid (see Fig. 16-47).[335,344] It is the malcentering of this joint reaction force that leads to posterior instability, posterior glenoid wear, and "rocking horse" loosening of prosthetic glenoid components. The standardized axillary view also enables

Text continued on p. 849

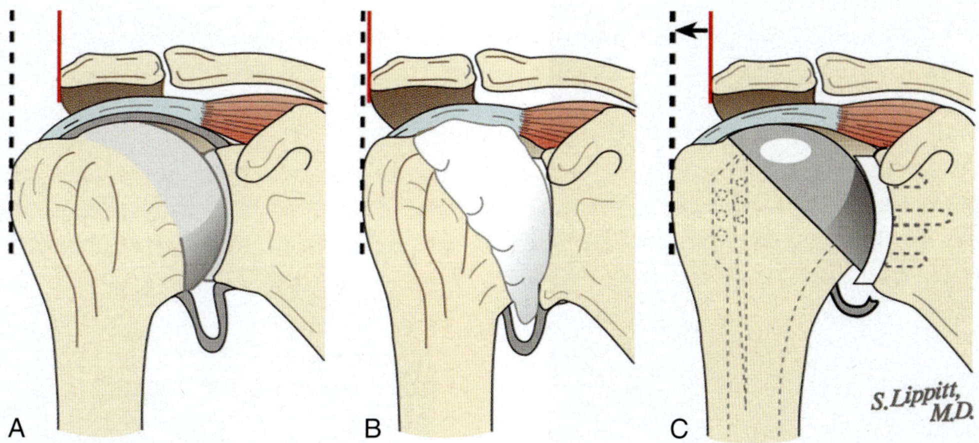

FIGURE 16-31: **A,** Normal humeral lateral offset with the greater tuberosity lateral to the lateral acromial line (red line). **B,** Loss of humeral lateral offset due to medial joint erosion in glenohumeral arthritis. **C,** Improved humeral lateral offset following an anatomic total shoulder arthroplasty.

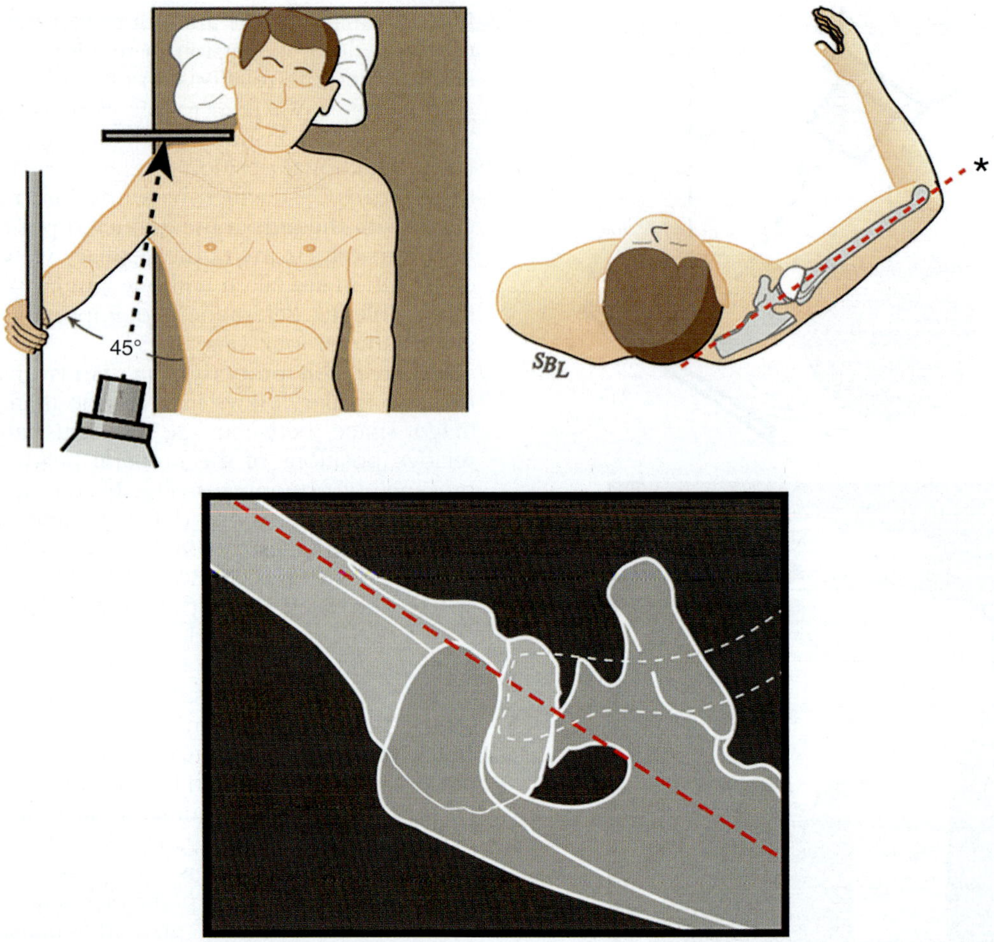

FIGURE 16-32: Axillary view taken with the arm in the functional position of elevation in the plane of the scapula. This is referred to as the axillary "truth view."

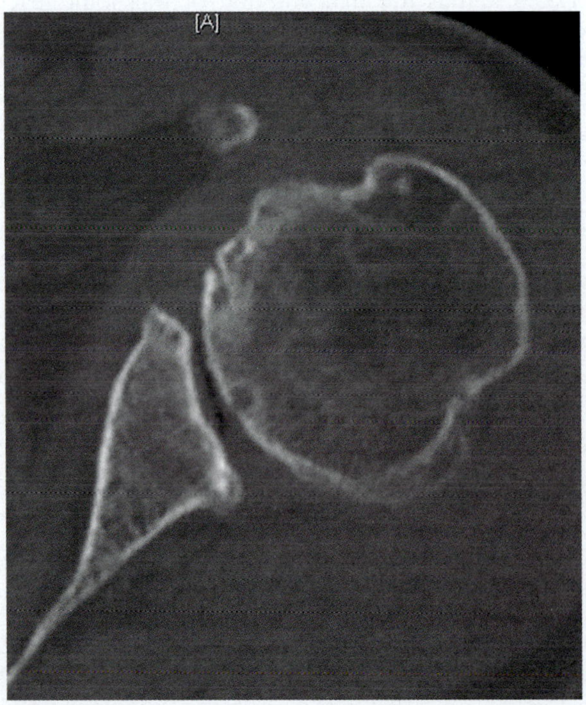

FIGURE 16-33: Computed tomographic scan taken with the arm at the side.

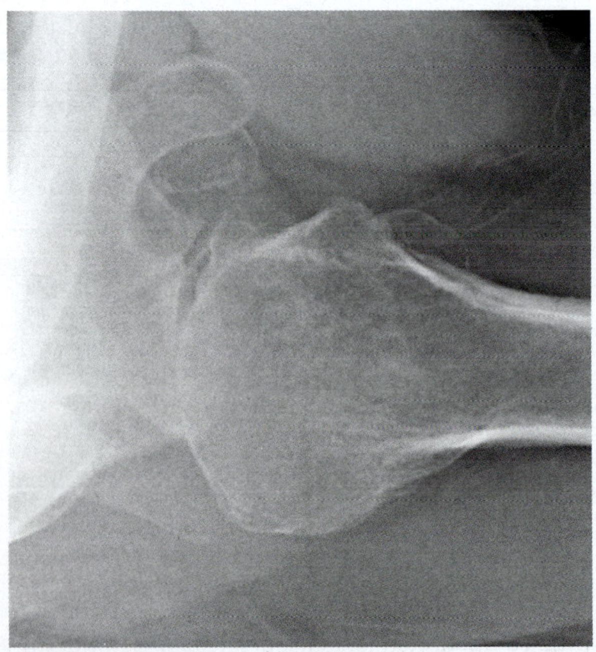

FIGURE 16-34: A nonstandardized axillary view from which it is difficult to determine the glenohumeral pathoanatomy.

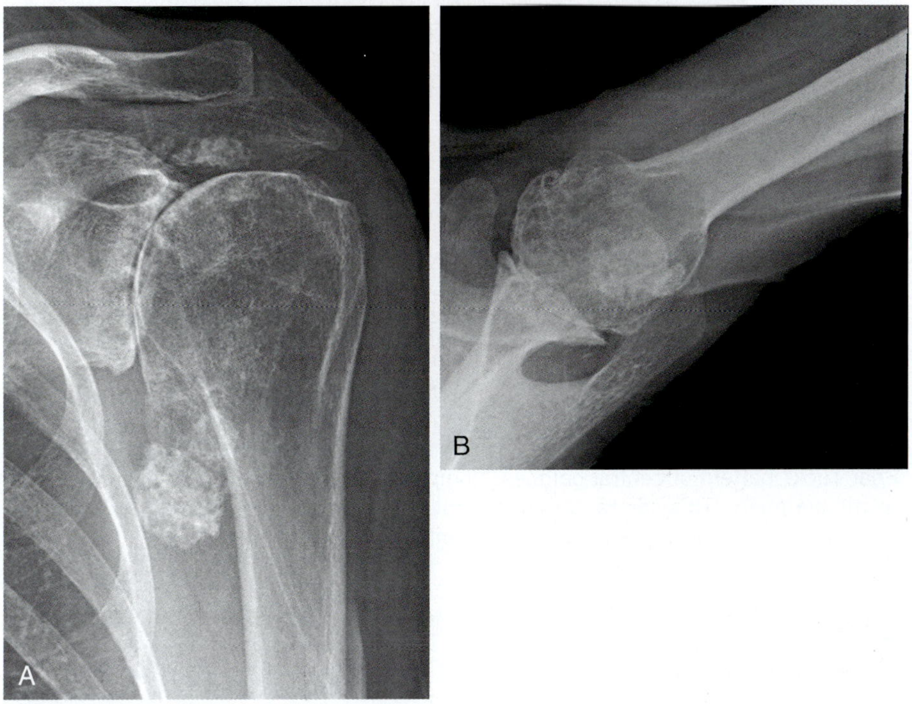

FIGURE 16-35: **A,** A large "goat's beard" osteophyte shown on the anteroposterior view. **B,** A medially eroded glenoid seen on the axillary view.

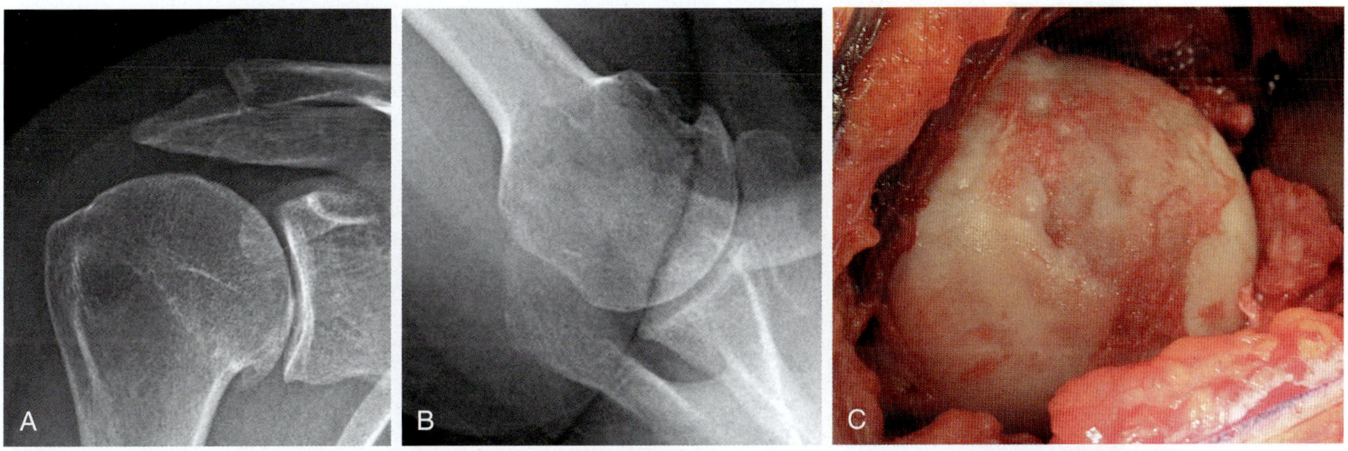

FIGURE 16-36: Secondary degenerative joint disease with a central humeral defect from contact with suture anchors. **A,** Anteroposterior radiograph showing minimal joint space narrowing. **B,** Axillary view showing minimal joint space narrowing. **C,** Intraoperative image showing substantial central defect.

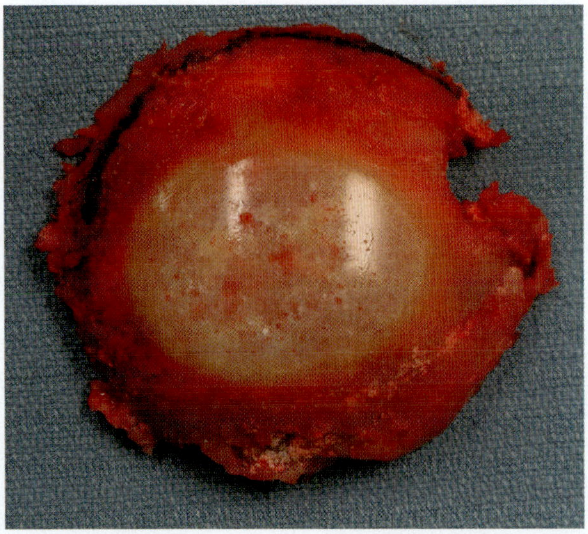

FIGURE 16-37: The "Friar Tuck" pattern of central baldness commonly seen in primary degenerative joint disease, with remaining articular cartilage at the periphery. This central loss of articular cartilage is only evident on radiographic images taken with the arm in abduction, a position that places the bald spot in contact with the glenoid.

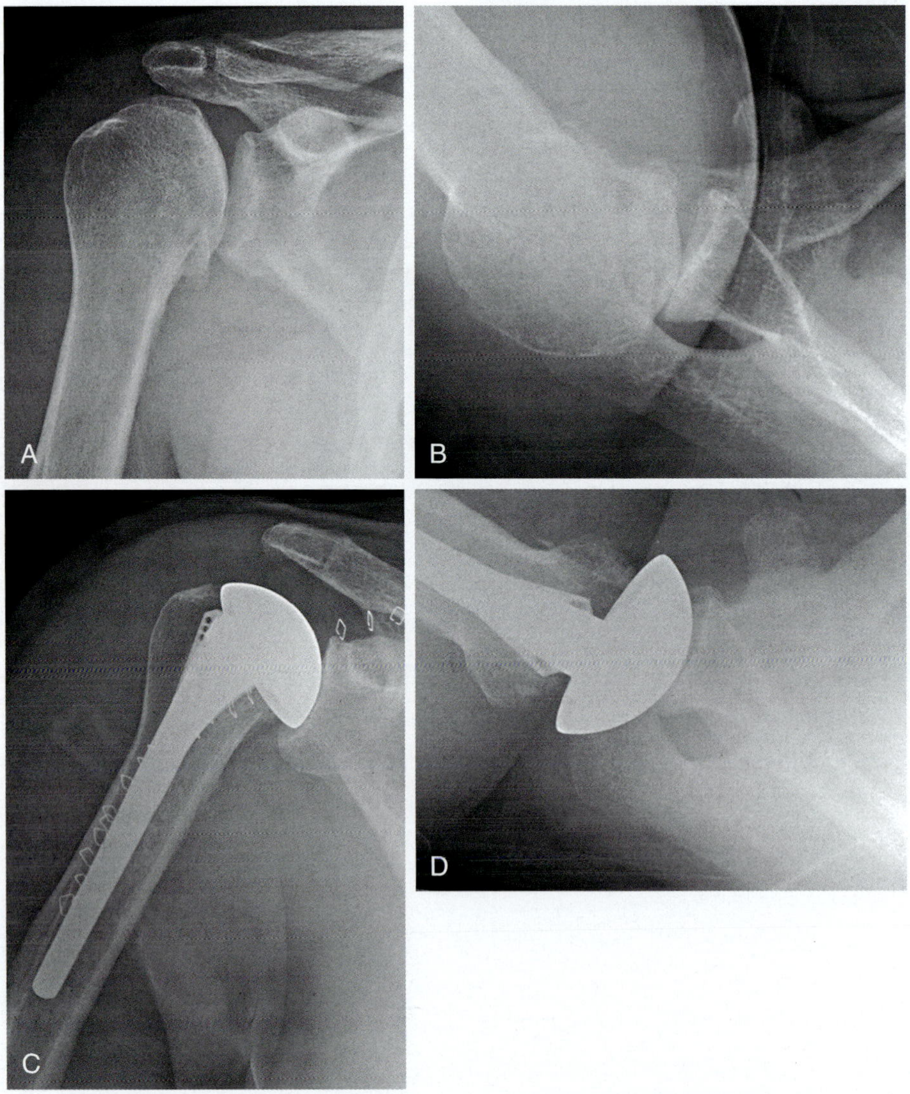

FIGURE 16-38: Functional decentering revealed by the "truth view" that was managed with a ream and run arthroplasty using an anteriorly offset humeral component. **A,** Anteroposterior radiograph showing degenerative changes. **B,** Axillary view showing functional decentering of the humeral head on the glenoid. **C,** Anteroposterior view showing reconstruction with the ream and run procedure. **D,** Axillary view showing improved centering achieved with an anteriorly eccentric humeral head component.

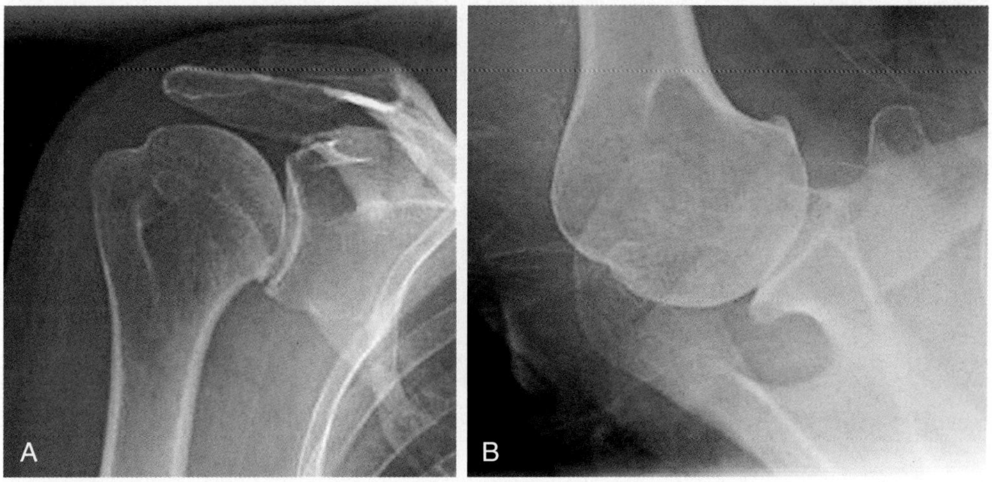

FIGURE 16-39: Functional decentering in the absence of substantial glenoid retroversion. **A,** The anteroposterior view suggests minimal pathology. **B,** The truth view shows decentering of the humeral head, as indicated by a posterior contact point of the humeral head on the glenoid face.

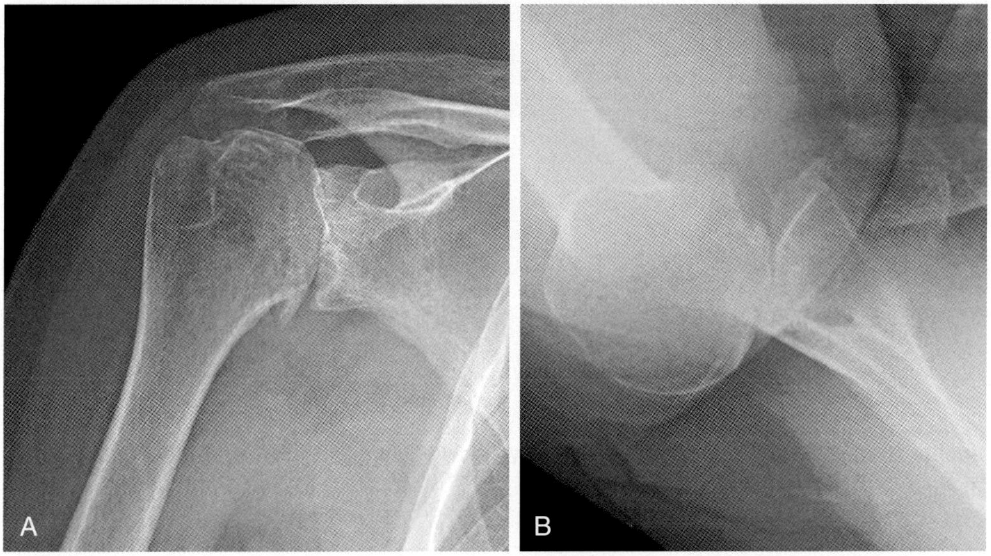

FIGURE 16-40: The axillary truth view reveals pathology without computed tomography. **A,** Anteroposterior view showing loss of glenohumeral joint space. **B,** Axillary view showing severe posterior subluxation in a biconcave glenoid.

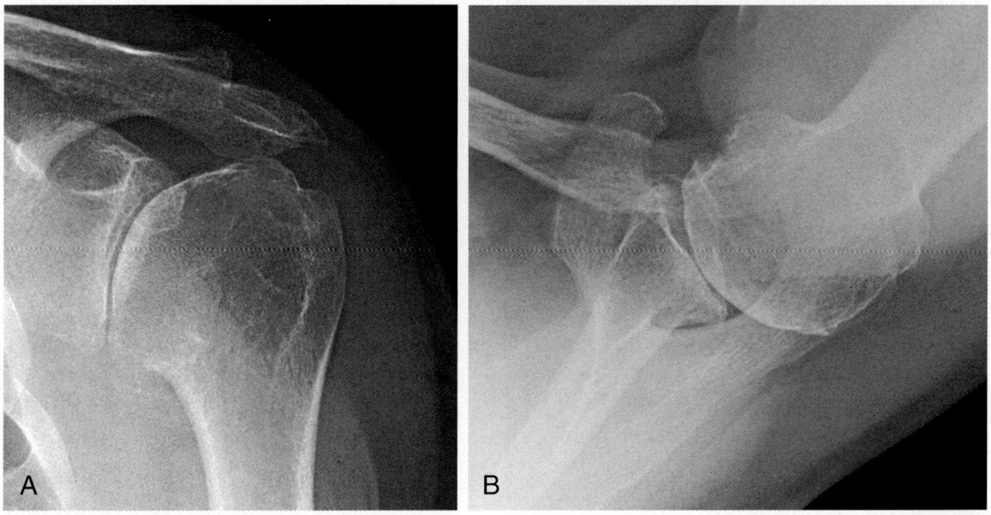

FIGURE 16-41: Functional decentering. **A,** Anteroposterior view showing an arthritic glenohumeral joint. **B,** Axillary view showing posterior humeral head subluxation into a biconcave glenoid.

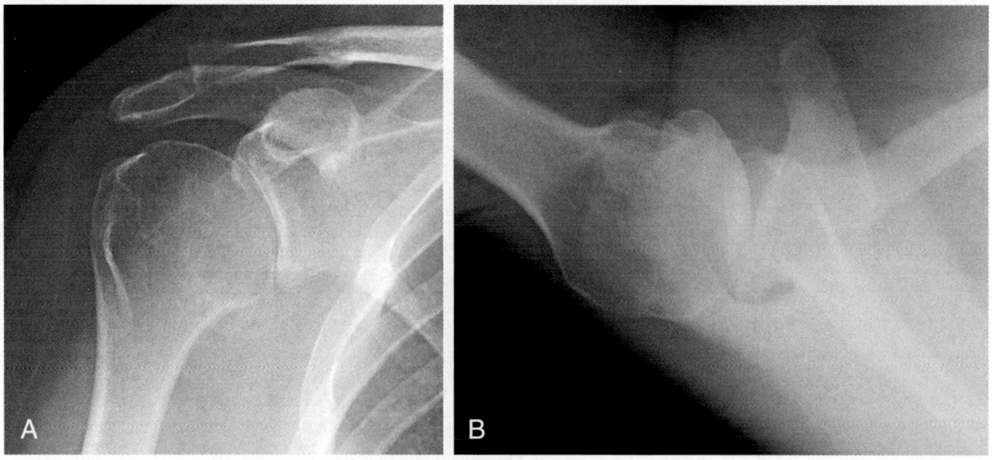

FIGURE 16-42: Functional decentering. **A,** Anteroposterior view showing an arthritic glenohumeral joint. **B,** Axillary view showing posterior humeral head subluxation into a biconcave glenoid.

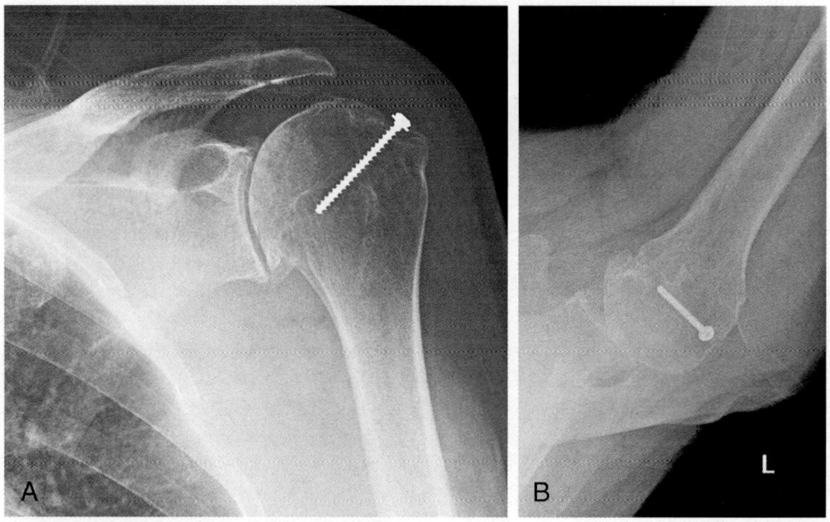

FIGURE 16-43: Functional decentering. **A,** Anteroposterior view showing an arthritic glenohumeral joint. **B,** Axillary view showing posterior humeral head subluxation into a biconcave glenoid.

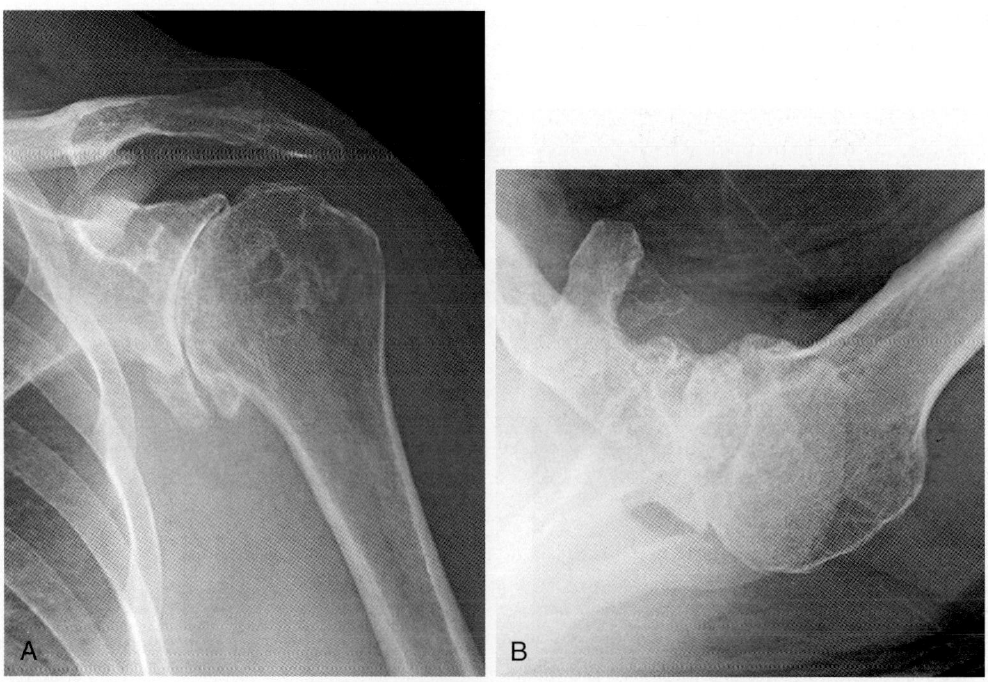

FIGURE 16-44: Functional decentering. **A,** Anteroposterior view showing an arthritic glenohumeral joint. **B,** Axillary view showing posterior humeral head subluxation into a biconcave glenoid.

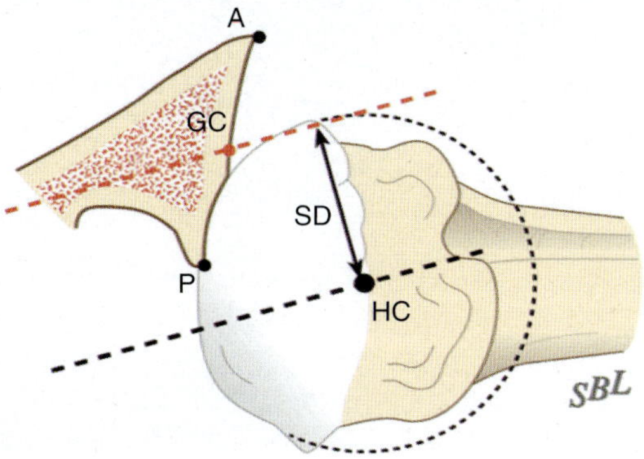

FIGURE 16-45: Measure of humeral posterior subluxation as the distance (SD) from the humeral head center (HC) relative to the scapular plane (red dotted line) through the mid glenoid, that is, glenoid center (GC), which is point midway between the anterior (A) and posterior (P) glenoid rim. The humeral head center is determined from the best circle for the humeral head curvature (circular black dotted line).

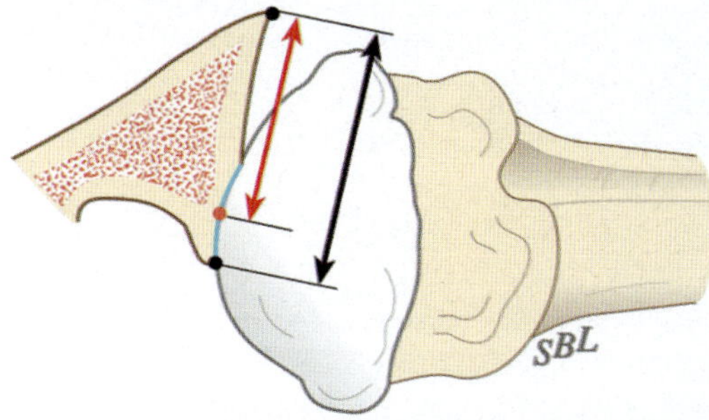

FIGURE 16-47: Measure of humeral posterior subluxation as determined by the point of contact of the humeral articular surface on the glenoid articular surface. The point of contact is characterized as the ratio of the distance from the anterior lip of the glenoid to the center of glenohumeral contact (red arrow) divided by the distance between the anterior and posterior lips of the glenoid (black arrow).

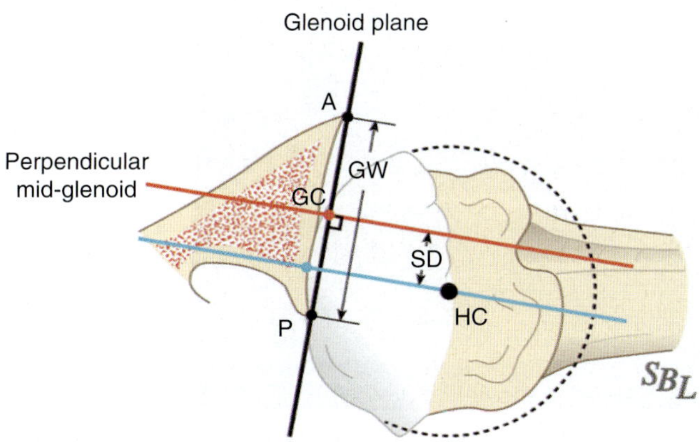

FIGURE 16-46: Measure of humeral posterior subluxation as the distance (SD) from the humeral head center (HC) relative to the mid-glenoid axis (red line). The glenoid plane (black line) is the line between the anterior (A) and posterior (P) glenoid rim. The glenoid center (GC) is the midpoint of the glenoid plane. The mid-glenoid axis (red line) is a line perpendicular to the glenoid plane through the GC. Posterior humeral subluxation is calculated as SD divided by the glenoid width (GW).

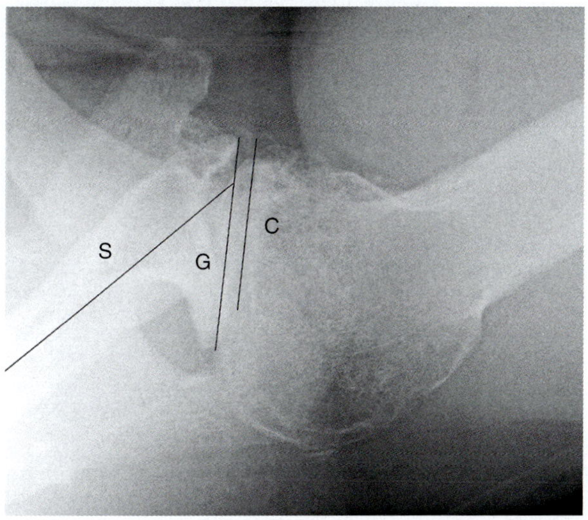

FIGURE 16-48: Measurements of the pathoanatomy of the arthritic glenohumeral joint. S is the axis of the scapular body. G is the line connecting the anterior and posterior lips of the glenoid. C is the distance between the anterior lip of the glenoid and the center of the contact area between the humeral head and the glenoid. The angle between G and S reflects the glenoid version. The ratio of C to G reflects the position of the center of contact point on the face of the glenoid; a centered contact point has a ratio of 0.5.

the surgeon to see the shape of the glenoid surface. Three main surface types have been described[564]: concentric wear (type A) (see Fig. 16-35; Fig. 16-49), eccentric posterior wear (type B) (Fig. 16-50), and dysplastic (type C) (Fig. 16-51). In practice there are so many intermediate types of glenoid pathoanatomy that rigorous categorization into a few distinct classes is difficult (see Fig. 16-50; Figs. 16-52 to 16-58).[405] An important aspect of glenoid pathology is the amount of the glenoid that is involved in the pathologic concavity, known as the "neoglenoid" (Fig. 16-59). Finally, the standardized axillary view enables measurement of the degree of glenoid retroversion in relation to the body of the scapula (Figs. 16-60 and 16-61). Thus, on the standardized axillary view, the surgeon can usually determine the major important characteristics of glenohumeral arthritic pathoanatomy: the amount of joint space narrowing, degree of retroversion, degree of posterior subluxation with the arm in a functional position, shape of the glenoid, percentage of the glenoid involved in the pathologic concavity, and angle of retroversion (see Figs. 16-45 to 16-47,

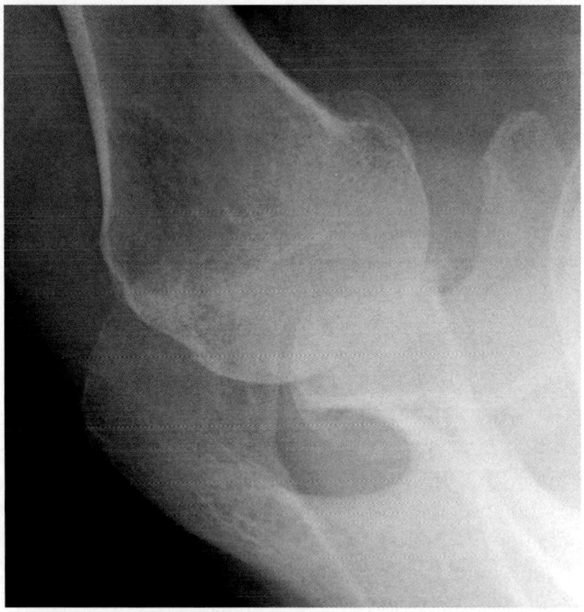

FIGURE 16-49: Axillary view showing an A2 glenoid.

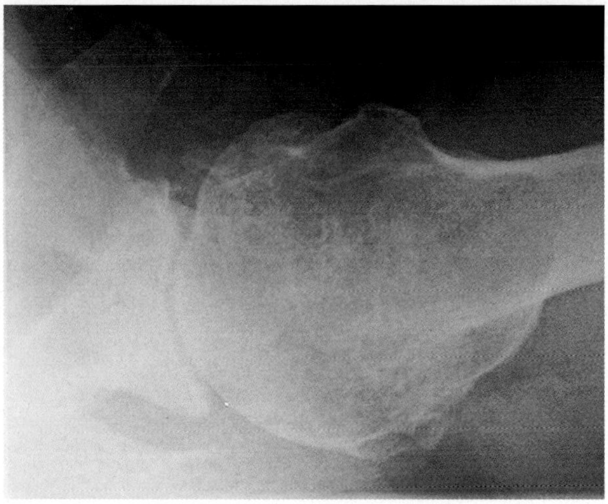

FIGURE 16-50: Axillary view showing a major biconcavity with a relatively small amount of posterior subluxation.

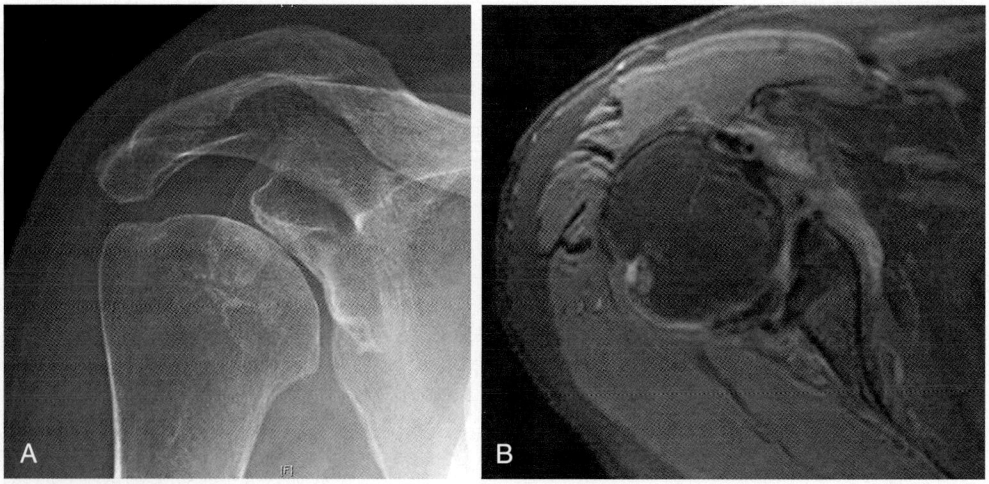

FIGURE 16-51: Glenoid dysplasia. A, Anteroposterior radiograph showing glenoid deformity. B, Magnetic resonance image showing failure of formation of the posterior glenoid bone.

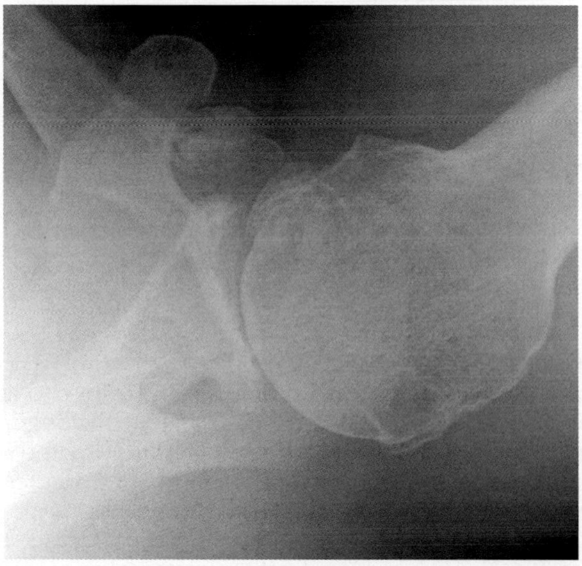

FIGURE 16-52: Axillary view showing a small biconcavity illustrating the high degree of variability in glenoid pathoanatomy.

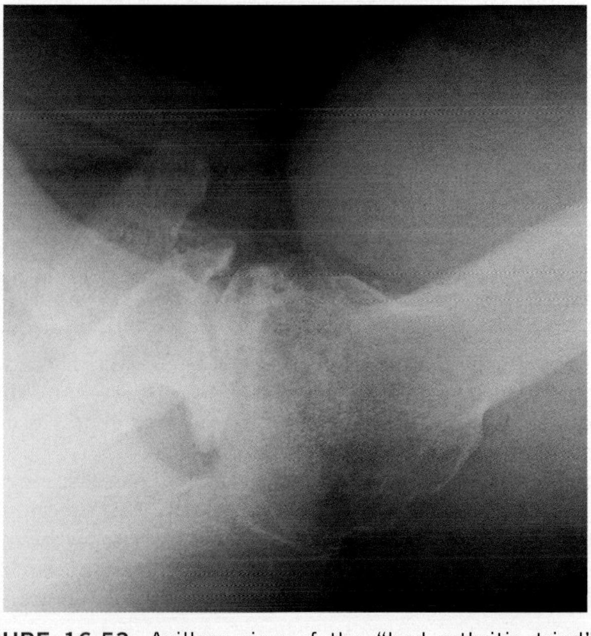

FIGURE 16-53: Axillary view of the "bad arthritic triad": a biconcave glenoid, glenoid retroversion, and posterior subluxation of the humeral head on the glenoid.

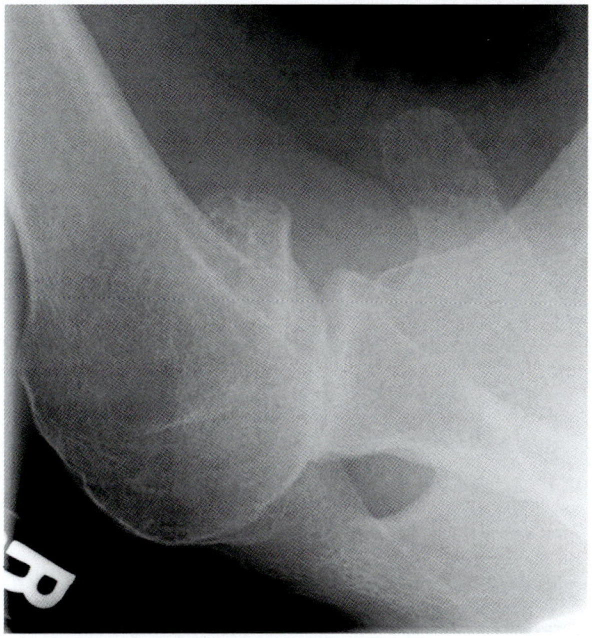

FIGURE 16-54: Axillary view of a mildly biconcave glenoid, with minimal glenoid retroversion but substantial posterior subluxation of the humeral head on the glenoid.

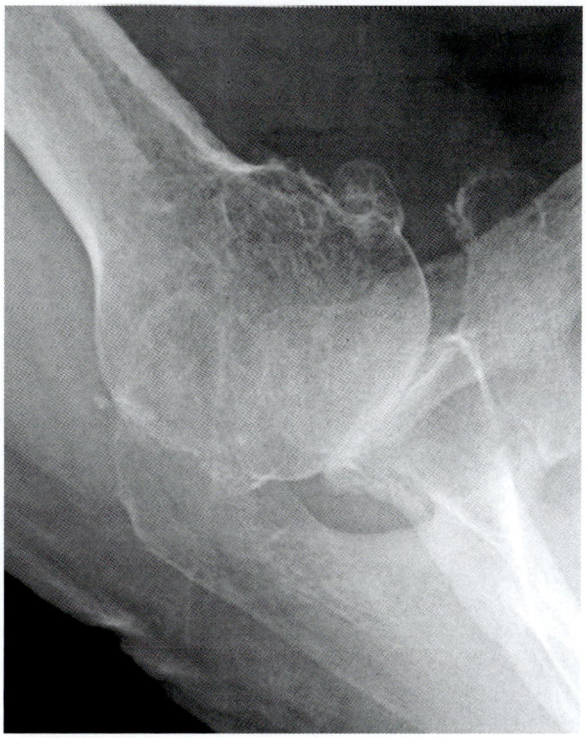

FIGURE 16-55: Axillary view showing a small biconcavity illustrating the high degree of variability in glenoid pathoanatomy.

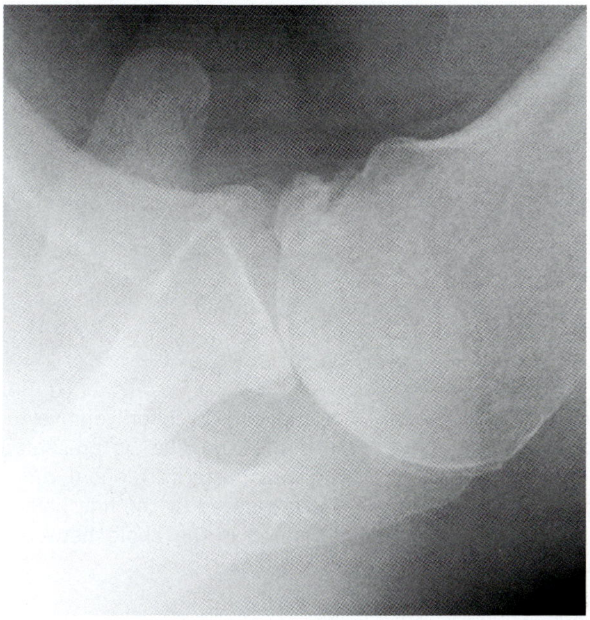

FIGURE 16-56: Posterior subluxation with minimal glenoid biconcavity and mild retroversion.

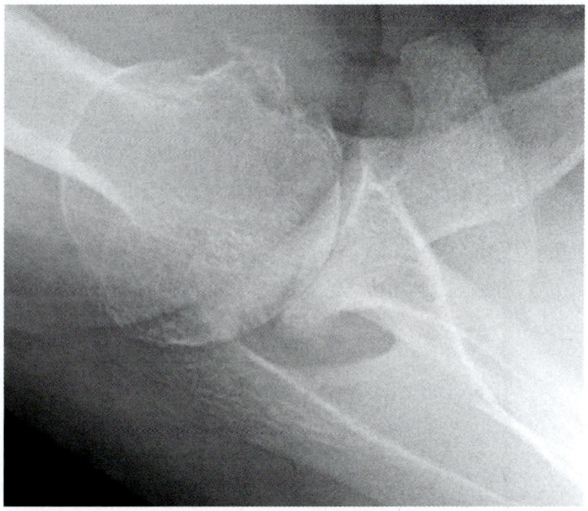

FIGURE 16-57: Axillary view showing a small biconcavity illustrating the high degree of variability in glenoid pathoanatomy.

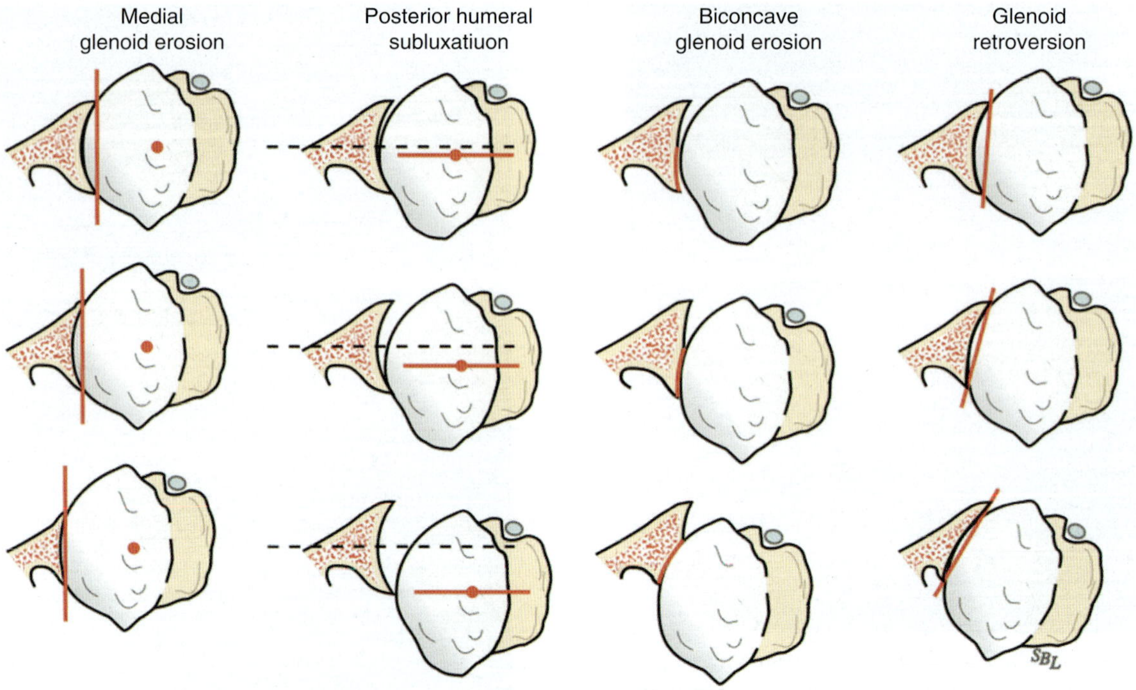

FIGURE 16-58: Various intermediate types of glenoid pathology depend on the extent of medial glenoid erosion, posterior humeral subluxation, biconcave glenoid morphology, and glenoid retroversion.

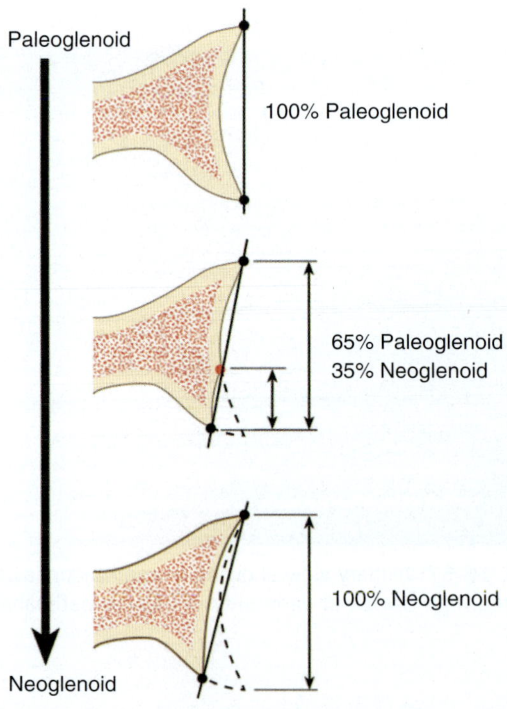

FIGURE 16-59: An important aspect of glenoid pathology is the amount of glenoid fossa that is involved in the pathologic concavity, known as the "neoglenoid."

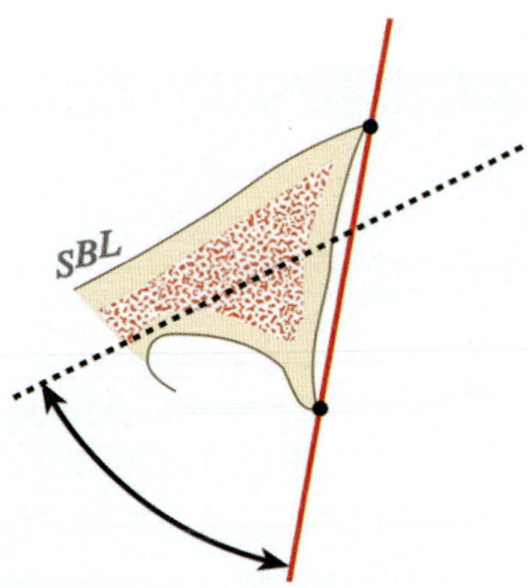

FIGURE 16-60: Degree of glenoid retroversion relative to the scapular plane. The glenoid plane (red line) is presented by the line through the anterior and posterior glenoid rim. The scapular plane (dotted line) is presented by the line parallel to the scapular body. Glenoid version is the angle between the scapular plane and the glenoid plane.

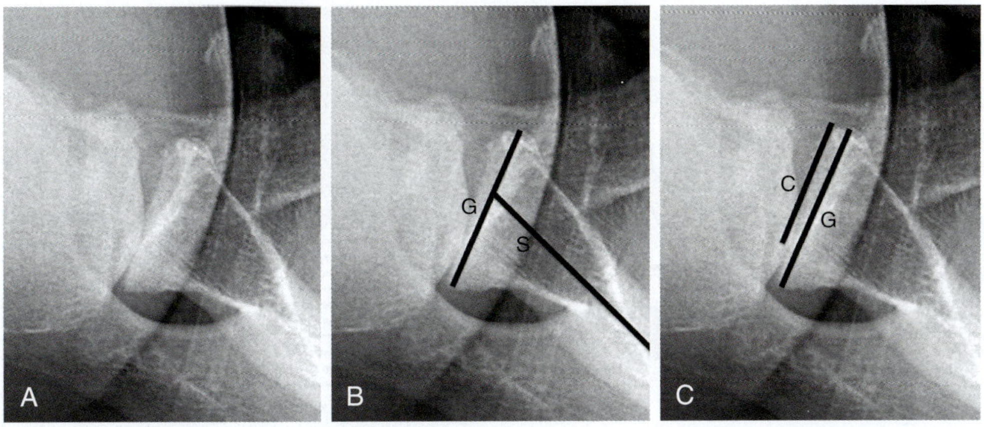

FIGURE 16-61: A, The important characteristics of glenohumeral pathoanatomy can be quantified on the standardized axillary view. **B,** Glenoid version is the angle between the axis of the scapular body (S) and the line connecting the anterior and posterior lips of the glenoid (G). **C,** The degree of centering is indicated by the ratio between the distance between the anterior lip and the point of glenohumeral contact (C) and the distance between anterior and posterior lips of the glenoid (G). A well-centered articulation has a ratio of 0.5.

and 16-61). Because of their low cost and freedom from metal artifacts, standardized axillary views provide a practical and reliable way to document the postoperative anatomy sequentially over time and to compare it to the anatomy before surgery.[222,335,344]

A third view, the templating view, is obtained when humeral arthroplasty is being considered. This view is an anteroposterior (AP) view of the humerus taken with the arm in 30 degrees of external rotation relative to the x-ray beam, with a magnification marker added (Fig. 16-62). This view places the humeral neck in maximal profile and allows the comparison of potential humeral prostheses with the proximal humeral anatomy (Fig. 16-63). In templating, it is important to recognize that the humeral canal is not cylindrical; the mediolateral dimension is usually wider than the anteroposterior dimension and so the AP view may overestimate the size of the stem that will fit the diaphysis (Fig. 16-64).[288] The templating view is also useful for determining whether sufficient osteoporosis is present to merit special consideration at the time of arthroplasty (Fig. 16-65).

Advanced imaging may be useful for unusual cases where the anatomy is distorted by prior injury or surgery, when there is concern about the amount of bone available for reconstruction, or when the standardized plain radiographs cannot be obtained. In the great majority of cases, however, the extra cost and radiation dose of the CT scan can be avoided through the use of standardized plain films. We can learn what we need to know about the status of the rotator cuff from physical examination and plain radiographs, so shoulder MRIs are rarely needed unless indicated to exclude avascular necrosis or tumor. However, MRI of the neck may be useful in evaluating patients suspected of having cervical radiculopathy, myelopathy, stenosis, or a syrinx.

Laboratory Evaluation

We do not usually obtain blood or joint fluid laboratory tests in the assessment of the arthritic shoulder. There are two exceptions: cases of suspected inflammatory or septic arthritis (where tests, such as the rheumatoid factor, sedimentation rate, C-reactive protein, and antinuclear antigen may be useful) and suspected malnutrition (where tests, such as a complete blood count, hemoglobin A1C, metabolic chemistry panel, iron binding capacity, transferrin, albumin, and prealbumin may be useful in addition to assessment of the body mass index).[49]

DISEASE CHARACTERISTICS

A number of diseases can destroy the glenohumeral joint surface. This section describes the characteristics of the most significant of these.

Degenerative Joint Disease

Degenerative joint disease is also known as osteoarthritis, osteoarthrosis, or wear and tear arthritis. The pathogenesis of this condition results from the age-related loss of the ability of articular cartilage to sustain itself against seemingly minor mechanical imbalances and years of use. Degenerative joint disease typically affects healthy and active individuals. In our practice most patients with degenerative glenohumeral joint disease are of Northern European rather than Asian, Southern European, Hispanic, or African ancestry. The disease results in progressive loss of the glenoid cartilage and subchondral bone, typically in one of two patterns: concentric medial loss, which is more characteristic of female shoulders and

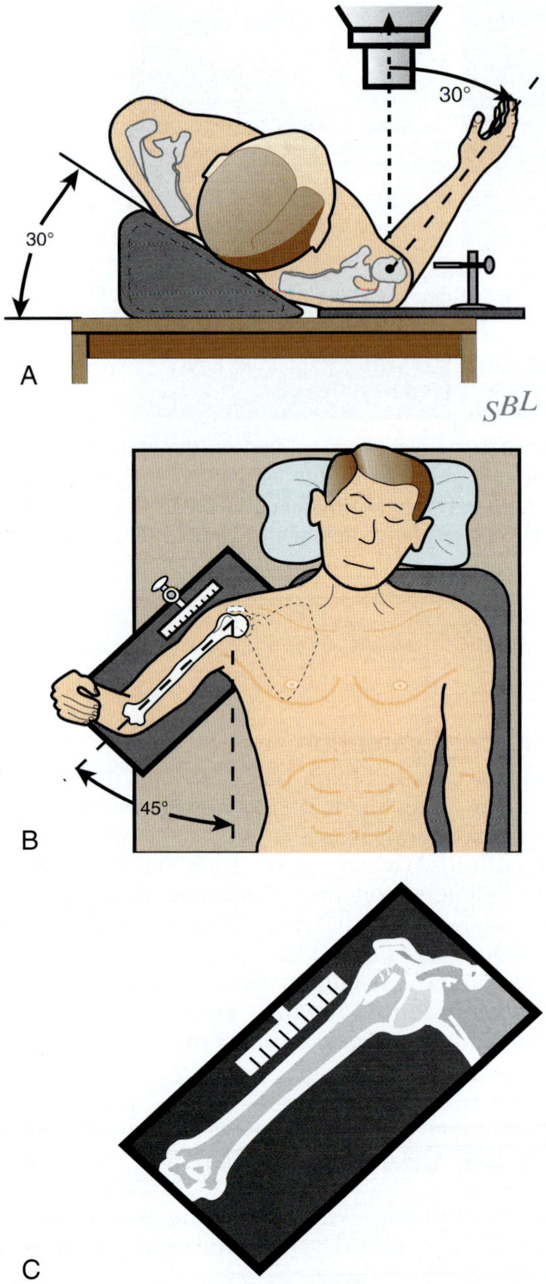

FIGURE 16-62: **A** and **B,** The humeral templating view is obtained by having the flexed forearm externally rotated 30 degrees with respect to the x-ray beam. **C,** The humeral templating view shows the humeral shaft with the humeral head and neck in maximal profile. A calibrated marker helps correct for magnification in templating. (From Matsen FA III, Lippitt SB. *Shoulder Surgery: Principles and Procedures.* Philadelphia: Saunders; 2004:11.)

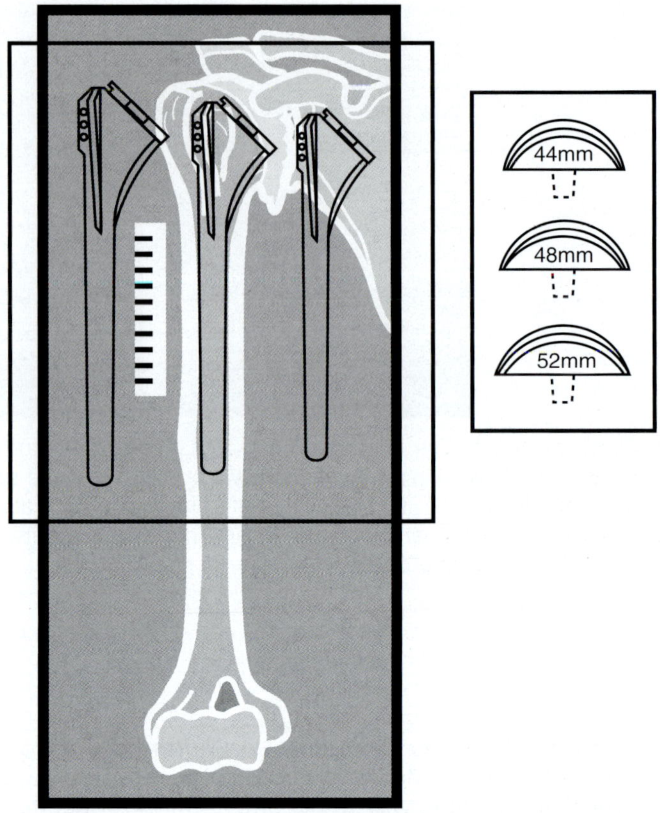

FIGURE 16-63: Templating view. The templating view enables the surgeon to preview the procedure and estimate the required component size and fit. (From Matsen FA III, Lippitt SB. *Shoulder Surgery: Principles and Procedures.* Philadelphia: Saunders; 2004:513.)

shoulders with inflammatory arthritis; or eccentric posterior loss (with the articular cartilage often left intact anteriorly), which is more characteristic of male shoulders and shoulders with degenerative joint disease or capsulorrhaphy arthropathy (Fig. 16-66). The concern with the eccentric wear pattern is that the diminished articular contact area results in increased force per unit area leading to increased posterior wear, which in turn results in even less contact area (Fig. 16-67). The cartilage of the humeral head is eroded in a so-called "Friar Tuck" pattern: central baldness often surrounded by a rim of remaining cartilage and osteophytes (see Figs. 16-7 and 16-37). The bone underlying the joint surfaces is usually sclerotic, but degenerative cysts can occur in the humeral head or glenoid. When severe, glenoid cysts may jeopardize the fixation of prosthetic glenoid components (Fig. 16-68).

In its early stages degenerative glenohumeral joint disease may be visible only on the truth view radiograph (see Fig. 16-38). Later, it is typical for osteophytes to surround the anterior, inferior, and posterior aspects of the humeral head and the inferior and posterior glenoid; as a result, the humeral and glenoid articular surfaces may take on a flattened configuration that blocks rotation (Fig. 16-69). We refer to the commonly seen inferior humeral osteophyte as the "goat's beard" (see Fig. 16-35; Fig. 16-70). Loose bodies are often found in the axillary or subscapularis recesses. The pathoanatomy of the arthritic glenoid may include medial erosion, posterior

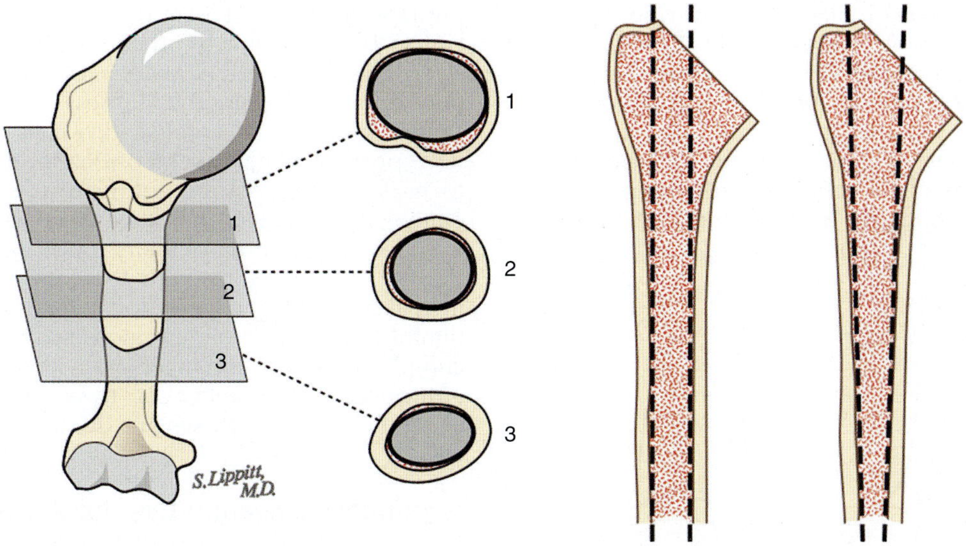

FIGURE 16-64: The varying shape and orientation of the humeral canal cross sections from proximal to distal make it impossible to fit the endosteal surface with a defined shape of prosthetic body (left). There is also wide variety between humeral medullary canals that are more cylindrical or more funnel-shaped (right). A tapered stem would not fit well in a cylindrical canal, and a cylindrical stem would not fit well in a funnel-shaped canal.

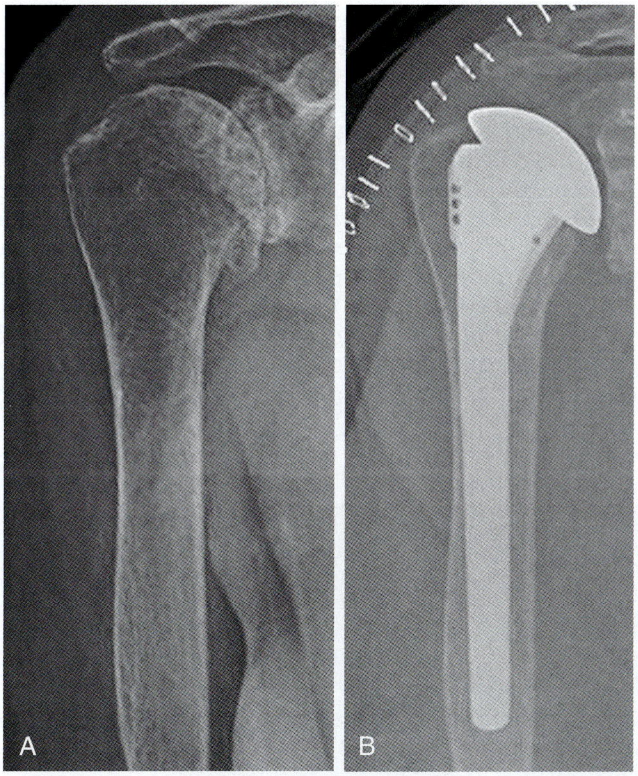

FIGURE 16-65: Impaction bone grafting for an osteopenic humerus. **A,** Anteroposterior radiograph showing very thin bone. **B,** Humeral prosthesis secured with impaction grafting without reaming to a press-fit, bone ingrowth, or cement.

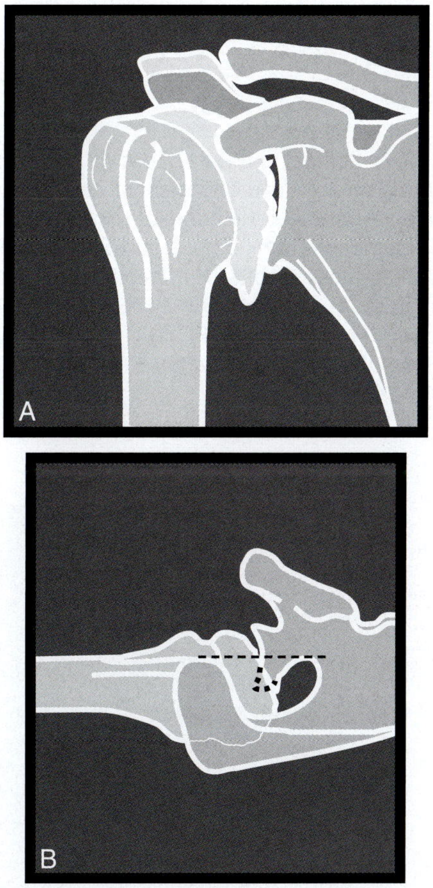

FIGURE 16-66: Degenerative arthritis. **A,** Anteroposterior view in the plane of the scapula. **B,** Axillary view showing posterior erosion typical of degenerative arthritis and capsulorrhaphy arthropathy. The humeral head is displaced posterior to the glenoid centerline (dotted line). (From Matsen FA III, Lippitt SB. *Shoulder Surgery: Principles and Procedures.* Philadelphia: Saunders; 2004:425.)

erosion, and retroversion along with varying degrees of posterior humeral subluxation (see Fig. 16-58). The triad of glenoid biconcavity, glenoid retroversion, and posterior humeral subluxation—the "bad arthritic triad"—is commonly found together in primary degenerative joint disease.[335,344] Progressive contracture of the anterior capsule limits external rotation and compounds the tendency of the humeral head to translate posteriorly (Fig. 16-71). Major biceps pathology and substantial rotator cuff defects are uncommon in patients with primary degenerative joint disease. The common clinical course is one of slowly progressive loss of the ability to sleep and to use the shoulder for work and recreation due to shoulder pain and stiffness.

It is of note that young individuals are less likely to have primary glenohumeral osteoarthritis and more likely to have capsulorrhaphy arthropathy, secondary degenerative joint disease, or other more complex forms of arthritis, often a result of injury, prior surgery, or systemic disease.[482] This, along with their greater longevity and increased activity expectations, may help explain the diminished satisfaction and increased rate of arthroplasty complications for younger individuals after shoulder arthroplasty. A number of these important but less straightforward diagnoses are discussed later.

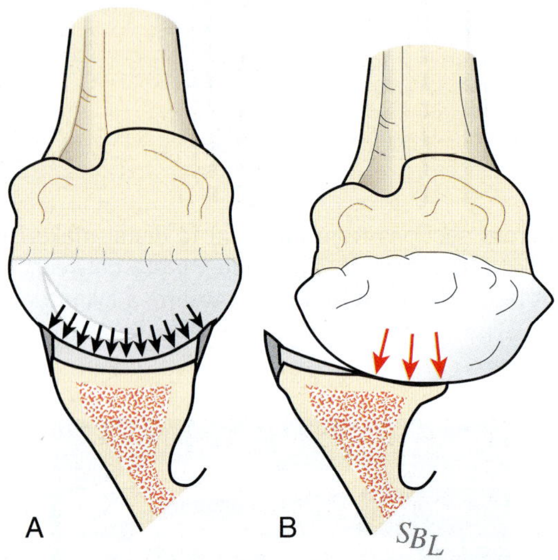

FIGURE 16-67: Contact pressure. Loss of the articular cartilage from the humeral head and glenoid results in the loss of the uniform distribution of the humeral joint reaction force over the face of the glenoid. **A,** Normal load transfer. **B,** Load transfer after cartilage loss results in a locally large joint pressure and a steep pressure gradient between the loaded and unloaded glenoid bone. (From Matsen FA III, Lippitt SB. *Shoulder Surgery: Principles and Procedures.* Philadelphia: WB Saunders; 2004:424.)

Secondary Degenerative Joint Disease

In contrast to primary degenerative joint disease—that arises spontaneously without a specific cause—secondary degenerative joint disease develops when a prior injury or surgery affects the joint surface, precipitating its degeneration. The presentation and clinical course of each case of secondary arthritis depend on the underlying etiology.

Anchor arthropathy is a type of secondary degenerative joint disease in which the glenohumeral joint surfaces are destroyed by prominent suture anchors used for the repair of superior labral anterior to posterior (SLAP) lesions (Fig. 16-72; see Fig. 16-36) or for Bankart repairs (Figs. 16-73 to 16-75). In this condition the suture anchors excoriate the humeral joint surface, which then erodes the glenoid surface.[600] In cases of anchor arthropathy—or with any prior glenohumeral surgery—it is important to be alert to the possibility of infection with *Propionibacterium* species (Fig. 16-76).

Posttraumatic arthropathy is a condition in which prior injury has damaged the joint surfaces or given rise to malunion with joint incongruity (Fig. 16-77), instability,

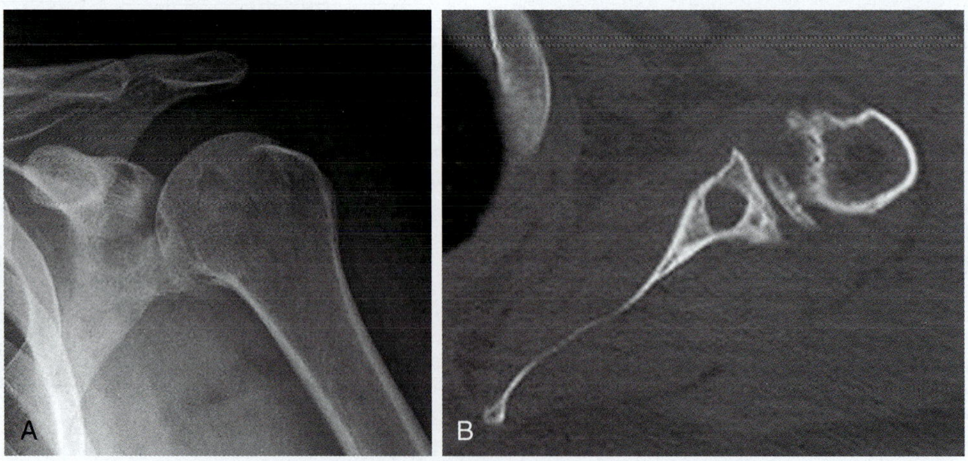

FIGURE 16-68: Cyst formation within the glenoid may compromise glenoid component fixation, requiring the use of bone graft or cement. **A,** Anteroposterior radiograph. **B,** Computed tomographic scan.

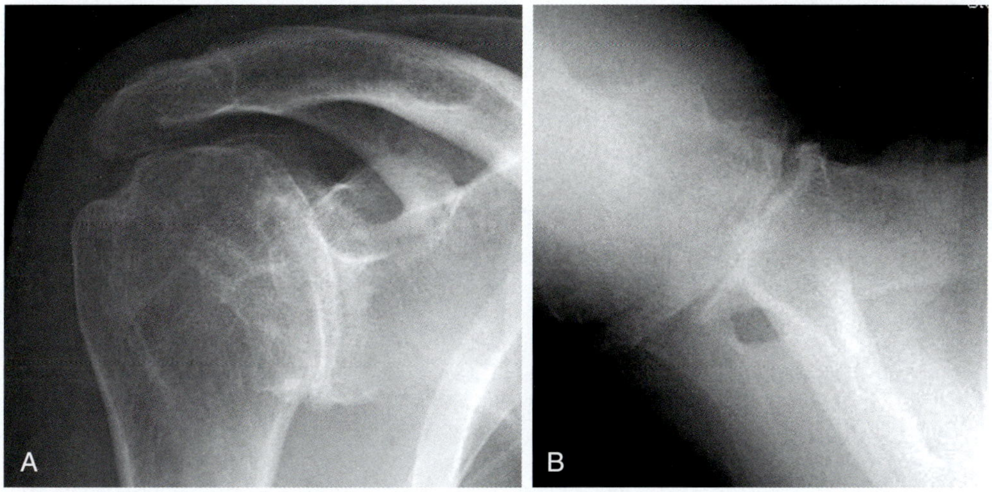

FIGURE 16-69: Flattening of the humeral and glenoid articular surfaces. **A,** Anteroposterior view. **B,** Axillary view.

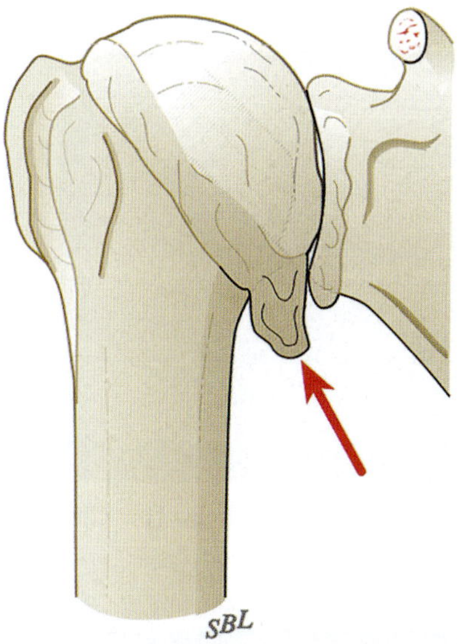

FIGURE 16-70: The commonly seen inferior humeral osteophyte is referred to as the "goat's beard" osteophyte (red arrow).

nonunions, and/or posttraumatic avascular necrosis (Fig. 16-78), without or with problems related to fixation hardware (Figs. 16-79 to 16-81).[97,125,154,192,368,401,538]

Anterior or posterior dislocations may be followed by *dislocation arthropathy* (Fig. 16-82).[215,291,323,407,440,483,537] In unreduced dislocations the humeral head may be indented and worn (Figs. 16-83 and 16-84).The cartilage of the joint surfaces may be replaced by scar tissue, or the subchondral bone may be so weakened by bone atrophy that it collapses after reduction, resulting in an incongruous joint surface (Fig. 16-85).

Shoulders with secondary degenerative joint disease often have complex pathology that can challenge surgical management. Each case presents its own particular combination of capsular contracture, scarring, malunion, nonunion, bone loss, bone fragility, nonanatomic location of neurovascular structures, and the presence of hardware from prior procedures.

Capsulorrhaphy Arthropathy

Capsulorrhaphy arthropathy is a specific type of secondary degenerative joint disease in which deterioration of the joint surface is related to a prior repair for recurrent dislocations[338] and is one of the most common causes of severe arthritis in individuals younger than 55 years.[482] It may be caused by overtightening the anterior capsule; when external rotation is limited by a Putti-Platt repair (Fig. 16-86),[211,267,312,316,555] a Bankart repair,[224] or a Bristow-Latarjet procedure,[177,224,364] obligate posterior translation can force the humeral head out of its normal concentric relationship with the glenoid fossa (Figs. 16-87 and 16-88).[201] This chronic posterior humeral subluxation typically erodes the posterior glenoid, and major posterior bone deficiencies can result (Figs. 16-89 and 16-90). Shoulder arthroplasty for capsulorrhaphy arthropathy is associated with high rates of revision surgery and unsatisfactory outcomes because of instability, subscapularis failure, glenoid component failure after total shoulder arthroplasty, and pain from glenoid arthrosis after hemiarthroplasty.[36,139,176,181,211,312,346,420,503,514] The importance of these poor results is heightened as commonly the individuals affected are young.

Rheumatoid and Other Types of Inflammatory Arthritis

Rheumatoid arthritis is a systemic disease with highly variable clinical manifestations. It can appear to be isolated to the glenohumeral joints or it can affect most of the tissues in the body. In rheumatoid arthritis and many other types of inflammatory arthritis, the cartilage is characteristically destroyed evenly across all joint surfaces of both glenohumeral joints. The glenoid is eroded medially

Text continued on p. 865

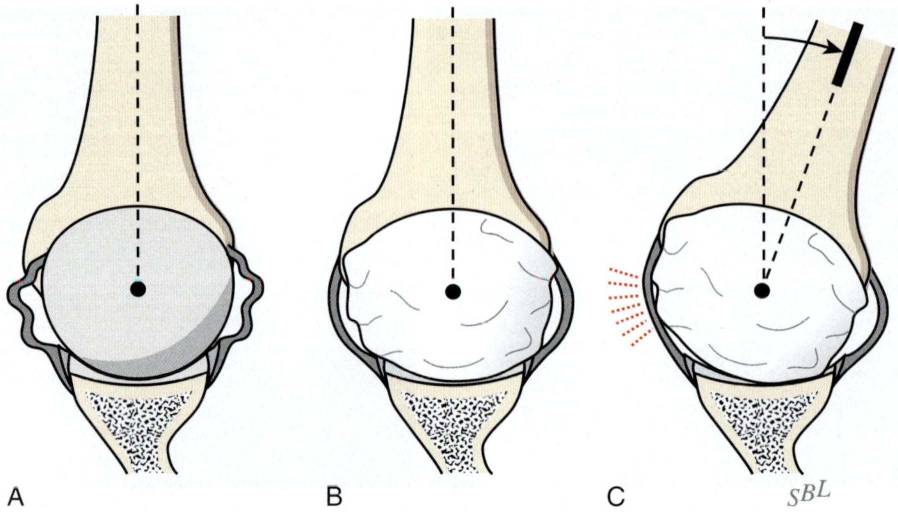

FIGURE 16-71: **A,** Normal capsular laxity allows unrestricted range of motion. **B,** The capsule may be contracted in degenerative joint disease and must course over osteophytes. **C,** As the joint approaches the limit of its range, the tension in the capsule and ligaments increases sharply, thereby limiting the range of rotation.

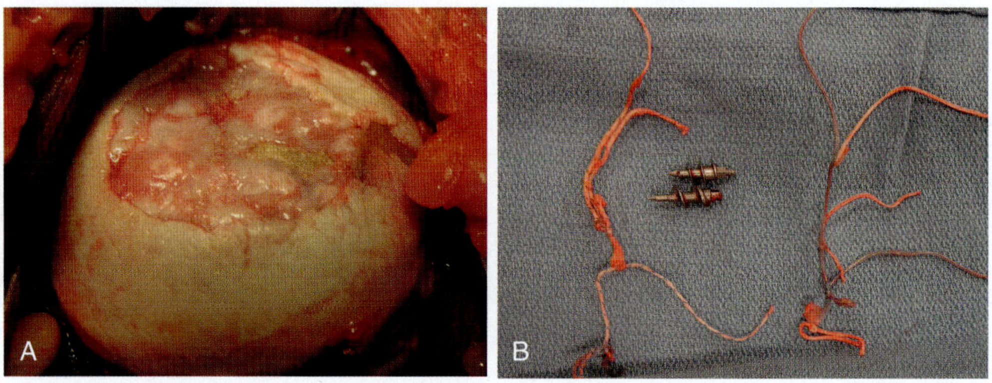

FIGURE 16-72: Anchor arthropathy. **A,** Destruction of the central aspect of the humeral head. **B,** The cause was prominent suture anchors.

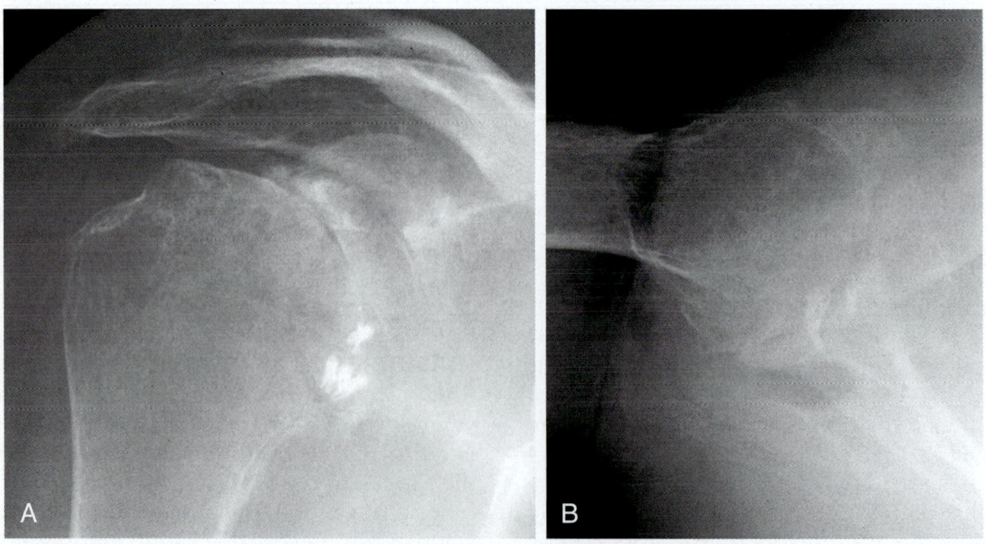

FIGURE 16-73: Anchor arthropathy. Metallic suture anchors can be seen in the joint on the anteroposterior (**A**) and axillary (**B**) view.

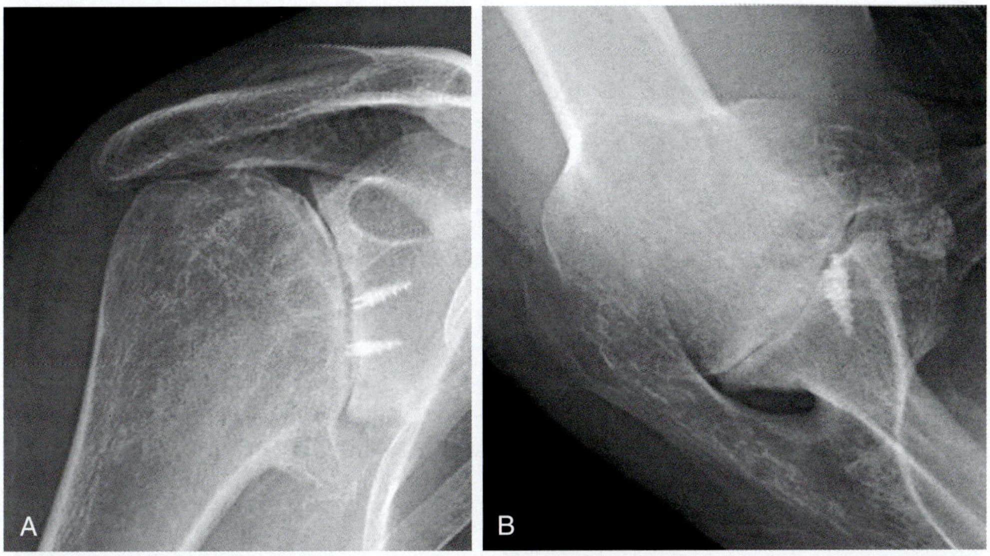

FIGURE 16-74: Anchor arthropathy with excoriation of the articular surface of the humeral head by prominent suture anchors, with secondary loss of the glenoid and humeral articular cartilage. **A,** Anteroposterior view. **B,** Axillary view.

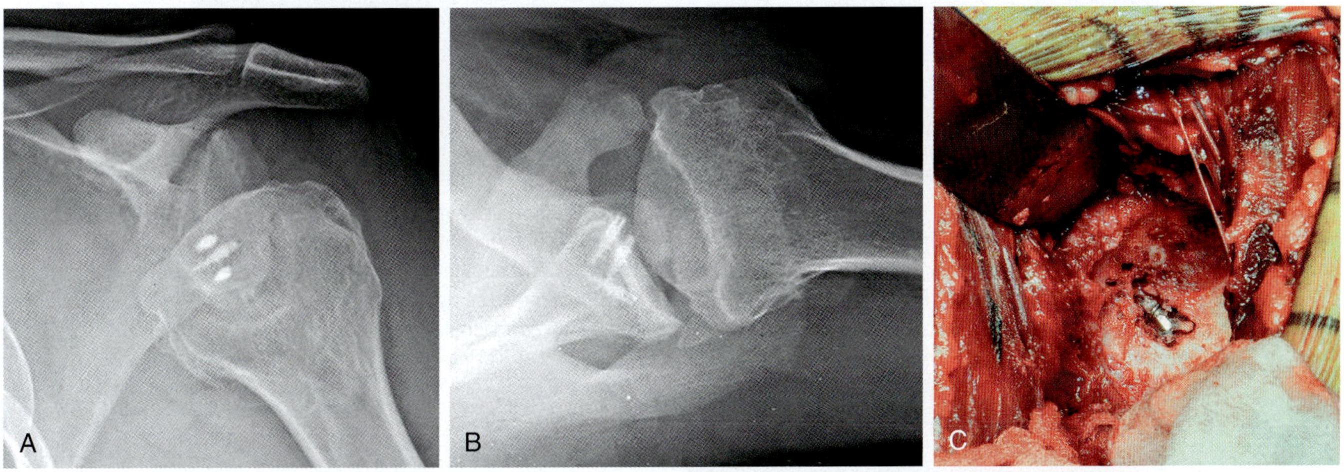

FIGURE 16-75: Anchor arthropathy caused by placement of suture anchors on the glenoid surfaces. **A,** Anteroposterior view. **B,** Axillary view. **C,** Intraoperative image.

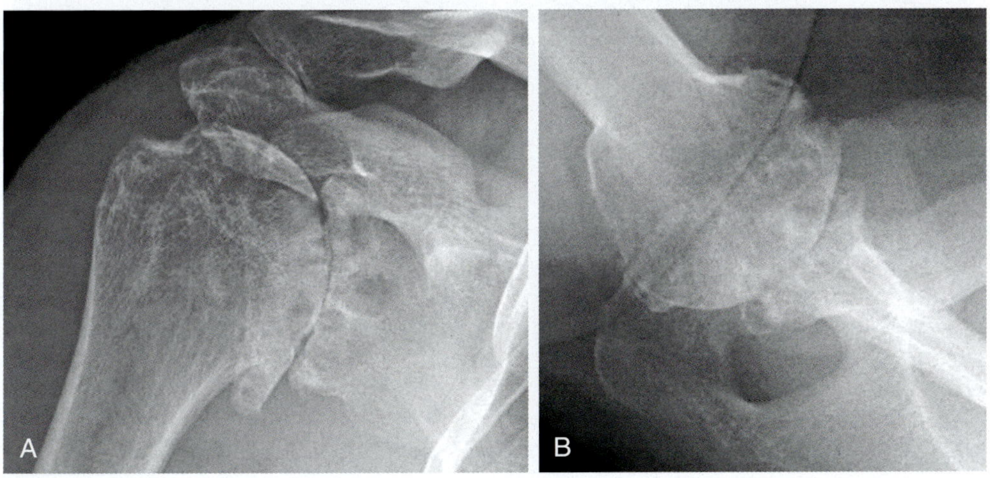

FIGURE 16-76: Septic arthritis from *Propionibacterium* species after a labral repair, with loss of joint space. **A,** Anteroposterior view. **B,** Axillary view.

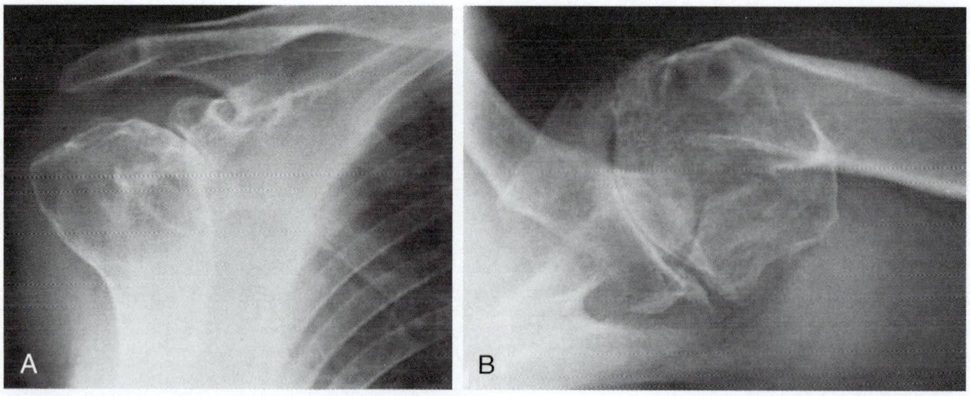

FIGURE 16-77: Traumatic arthritis with a loss of glenohumeral cartilage developed after malunion of a comminuted proximal humeral fracture. **A,** Anteroposterior view in the plane of the scapula. **B,** Axillary view.

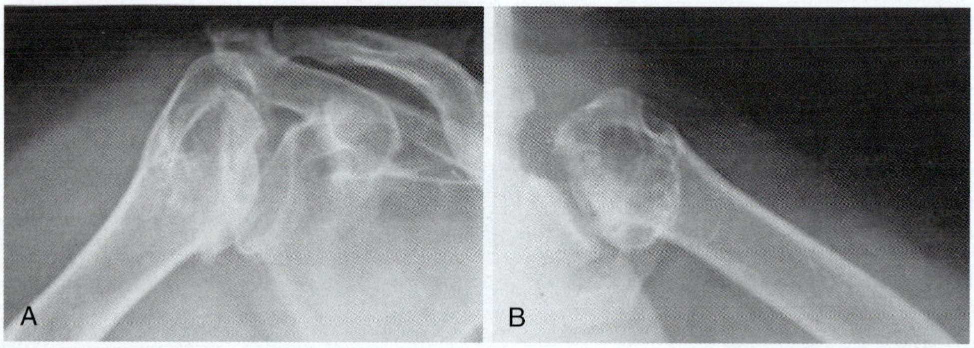

FIGURE 16-78: Traumatic arthritis with malunion and osteonecrosis of the head segment. **A,** Radiograph showing collapse of the head segment and a slight malunion of the greater tuberosity relative to the shaft. **B,** Radiograph showing the collapse of the humeral head segment, but with the tuberosities in reasonable positions on this view. Damage to the glenoid articular surface is underestimated on these projections. Proximal humeral prosthetic replacement or total shoulder arthroplasty might be needed as reconstructive surgery for such situations, depending on the extent of glenoid surface involvement.

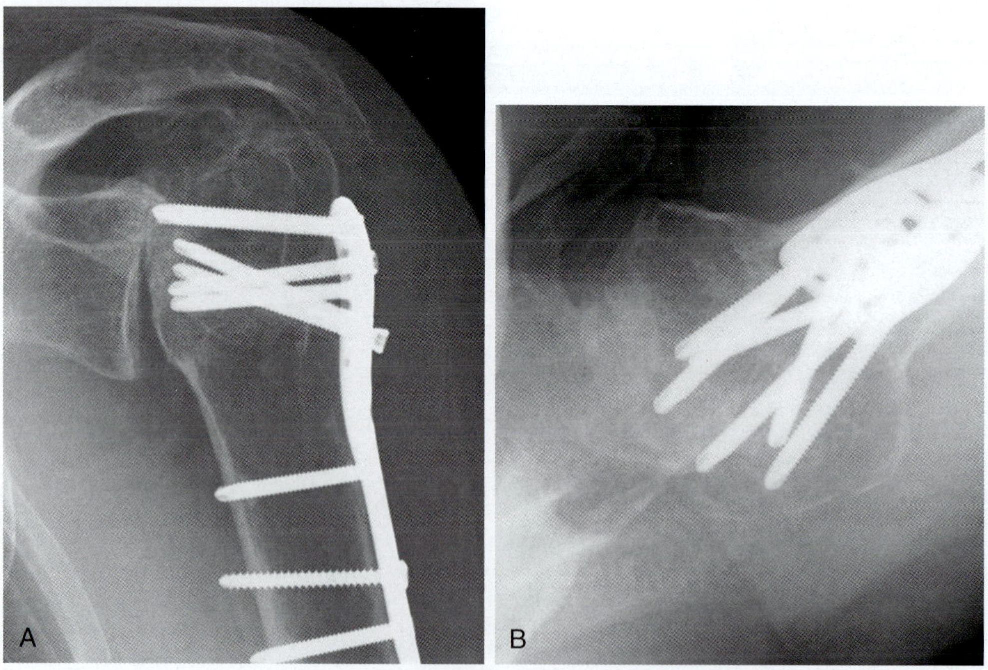

FIGURE 16-79: Posttraumatic arthritis with humeral head deformity and prominent intra-articular screws. **A,** Anteroposterior view showing head deformity. **B,** Axillary view showing head deformity with screw penetration.

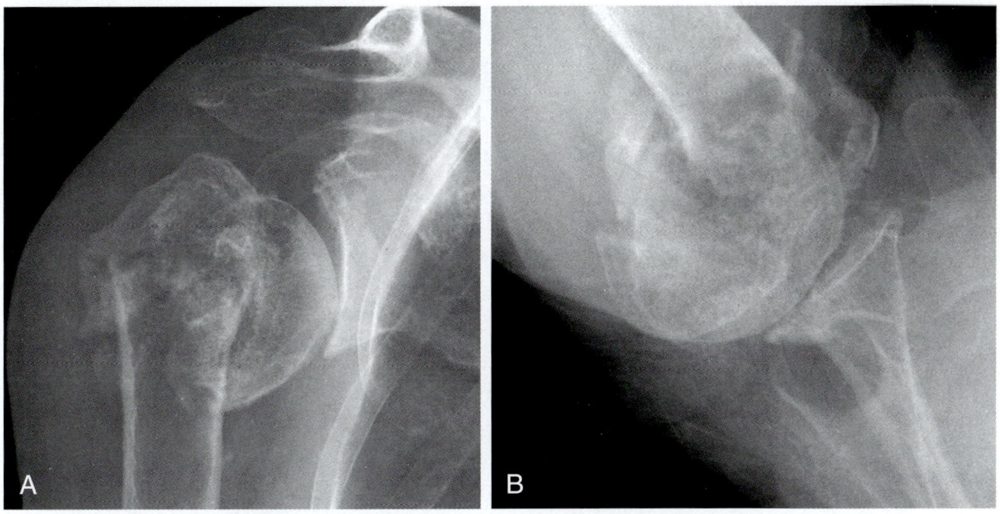

FIGURE 16-80: Subtuberous nonunion. **A,** Anteroposterior view. **B,** Axillary view.

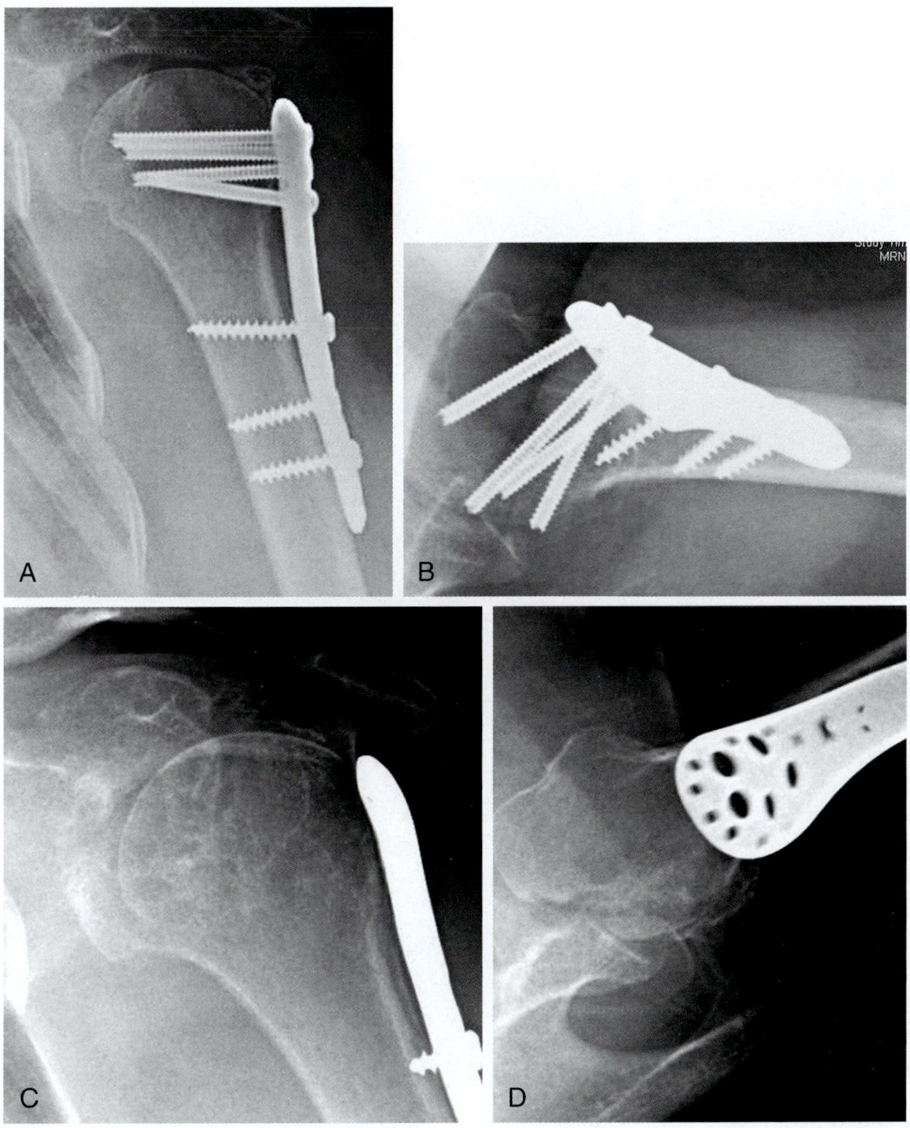

FIGURE 16-81: Posttraumatic arthropathy with screws eroding the joint surfaces and the anterior glenoid bone. **A** and **B,** Anteroposterior and axillary views with the hardware in place. **C** and **D,** anteroposterior and axillary views with the hardware removed.

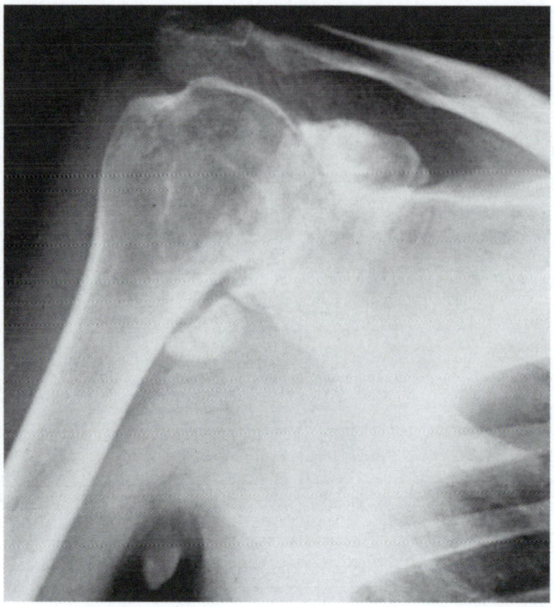

FIGURE 16-82: An elderly man had a 5- to 10-year history of progressively severe shoulder pain and limitation of motion. As an adolescent, he experienced recurrent dislocations of this shoulder; his current arthritis presumably developed subsequent to his recurrent instability.

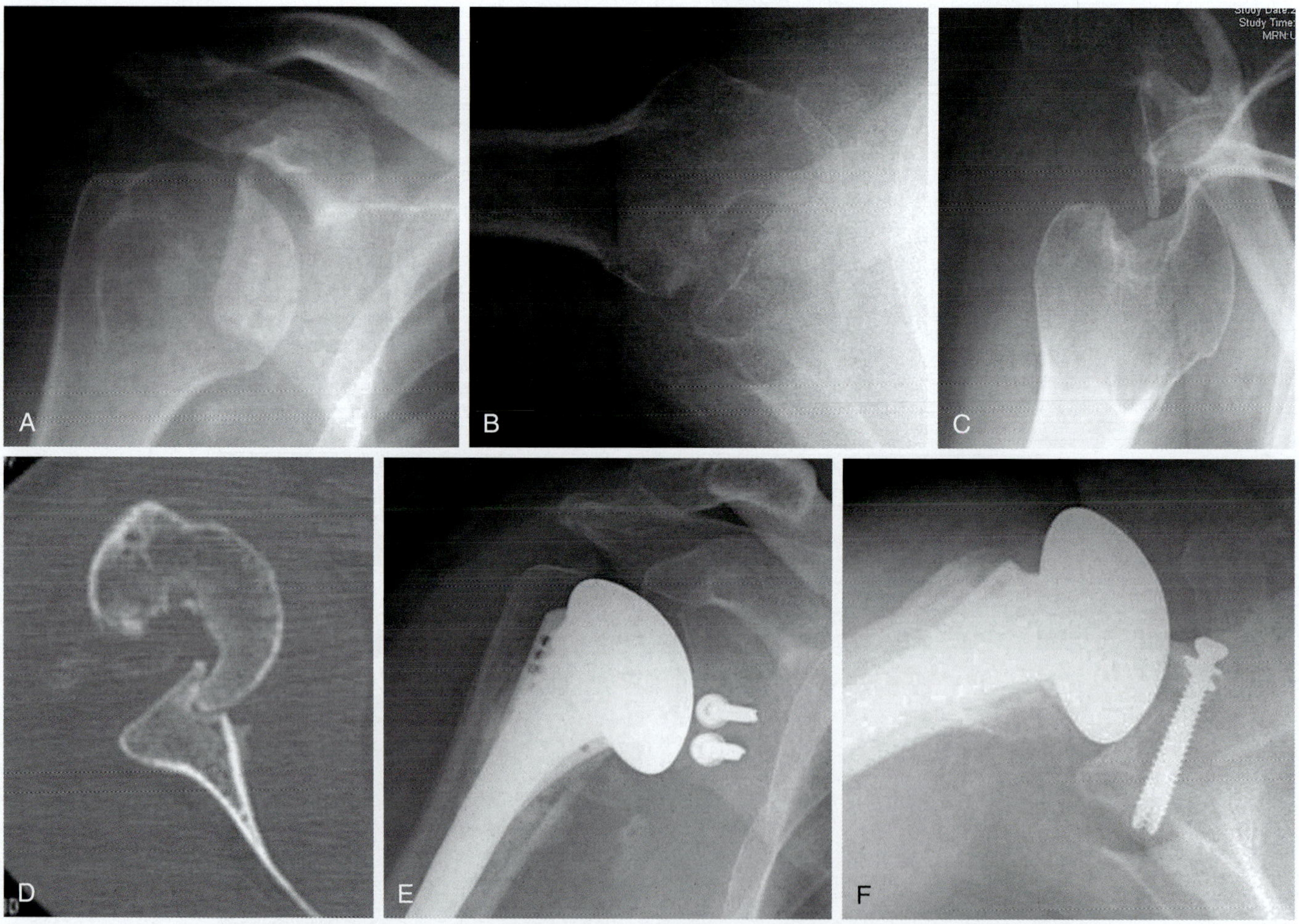

FIGURE 16-83: Arthroplasty for chronic shoulder dislocation. **A,** Anteroposterior view showing anterior dislocation. **B,** Axillary view showing posterior humeral and anterior glenoid bone loss. **C,** Apical oblique view showing posterior humeral and anterior glenoid bone loss. **D,** CT scan showing posterior humeral and anterior glenoid bone loss. **E,** Anteroposterior view showing hemiarthroplasty after an iliac crest graft to the anterior glenoid. **F,** Axillary view showing hemiarthroplasty after an iliac crest graft to the anterior glenoid.

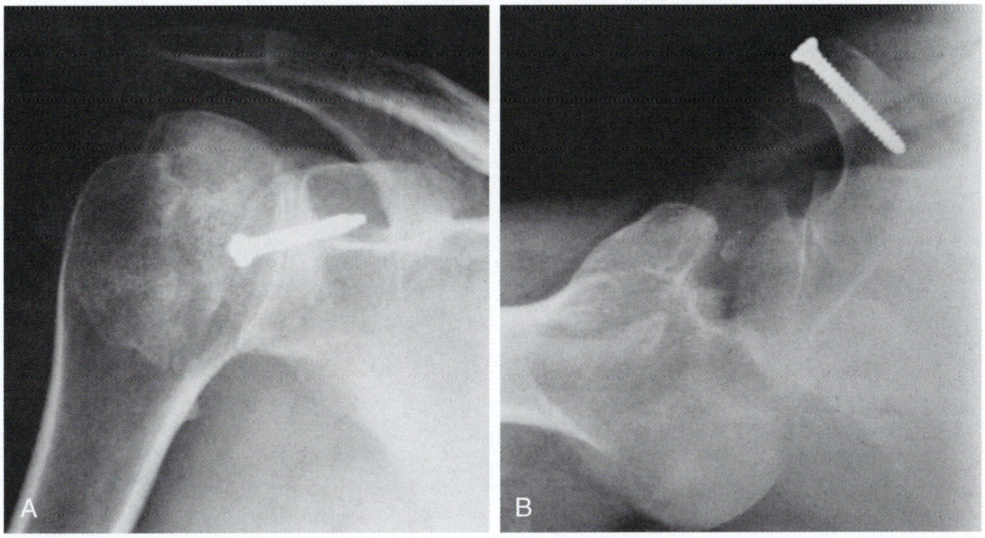

FIGURE 16-84: Chronic posterior shoulder dislocation in a 26-year-old man. The injury occurred approximately 1 year prior to obtaining the radiographs. A recent previous anterior approach to the shoulder was ineffective in reducing the dislocation. The shoulder was reduced during a second surgical procedure, but the cartilage of the humeral head was replaced with fibrous tissue. A proximal humeral prosthesis was placed as a part of the reconstructive procedure. **A,** A 40-degree posterior oblique view illustrating the overlap between the humeral head and the glenoid. **B,** Clearly illustrated are the posterior dislocation, the slight malunion between the head and shaft fragments, and evidence of fracturing of the lesser tuberosity and healing of this tuberosity to the shaft, although somewhat displaced from the humeral head segment.

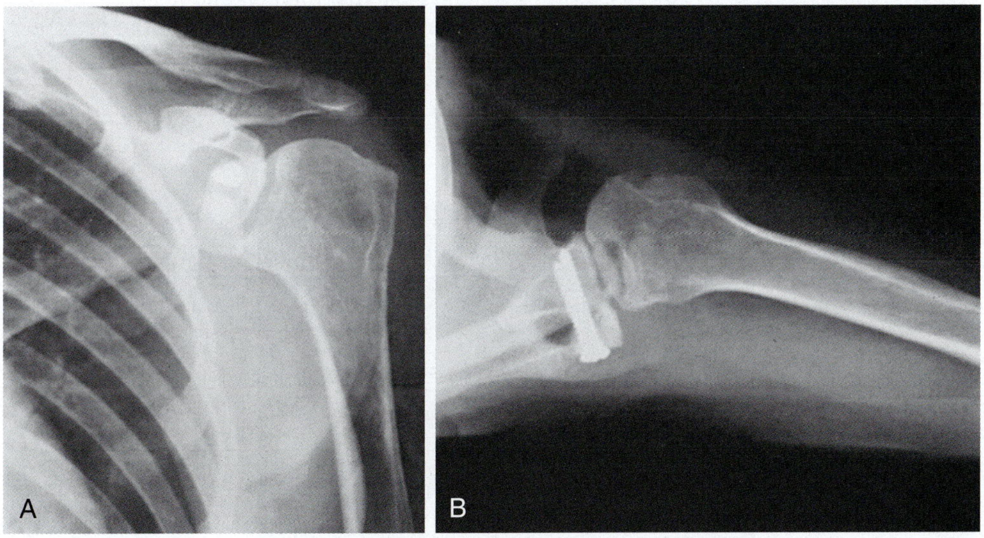

FIGURE 16-85: This young woman underwent open reduction of a posterior shoulder dislocation that had been unreduced for approximately 2 months. At the time of reduction, the cartilage surfaces were intact, but the humeral head was noted to be somewhat softened. A bone graft was added to the posterior aspect of the shoulder to substitute for an area of glenoid wear. Within the first month after open reduction, it was apparent on the anteroposterior and axillary view that because of its softness, the humeral head had collapsed and traumatic arthritis was developing. A proximal humeral prosthesis was subsequently placed. **A,** Anteroposterior view. **B,** Axillary view.

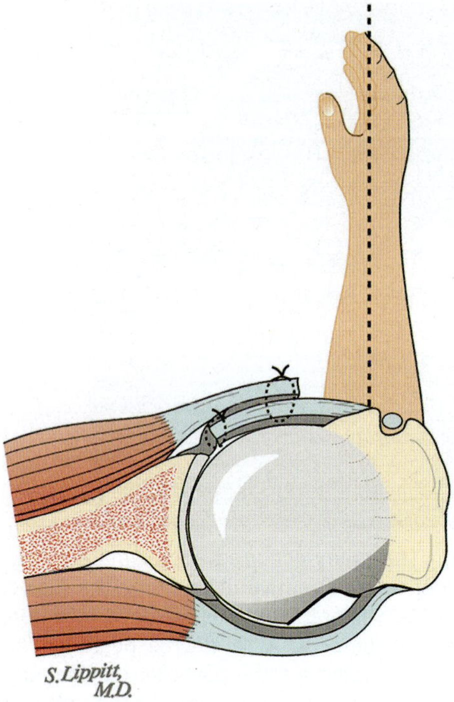

FIGURE 16-86: Putti-Platt repair consisting of shortening of the anterior capsule and subscapularis tendon, limiting humeral external rotation.

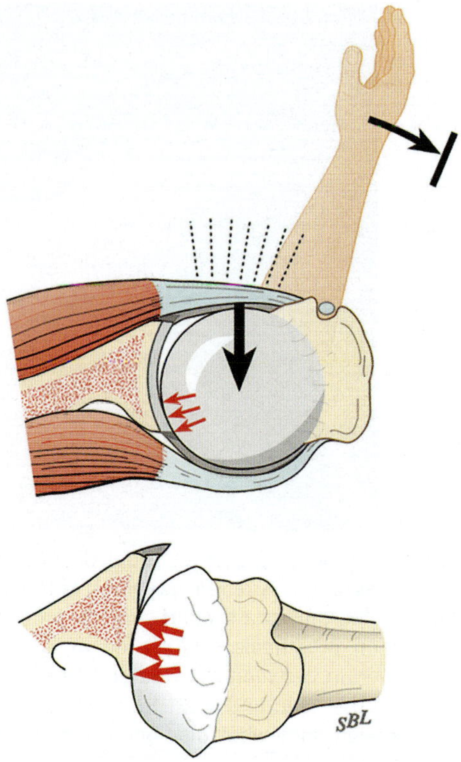

FIGURE 16-87: Progressive contracture of the anterior capsule limits external rotation and leads to obligate posterior humeral translation, increased force on the posterior glenoid, and eventual posterior glenoid erosion.

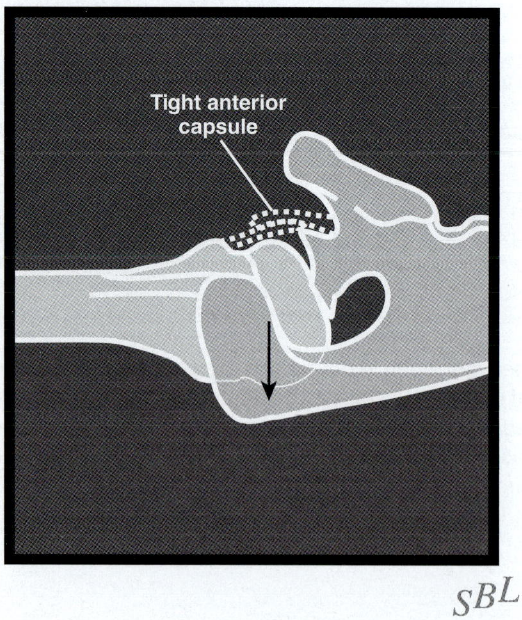

FIGURE 16-88: Axillary view of capsulorrhaphy arthropathy in which an excessively tight anterior capsular repair is forcing the head of the humerus posteriorly (arrow). This effect is accentuated by forced external rotation. Note also the typical posterior glenoid erosion. (From Matsen FA III, Lippitt SB, Sidles JA, Harryman DT II. *Practical Evaluation and Management of the Shoulder.* Philadelphia: Saunders; 1994.)

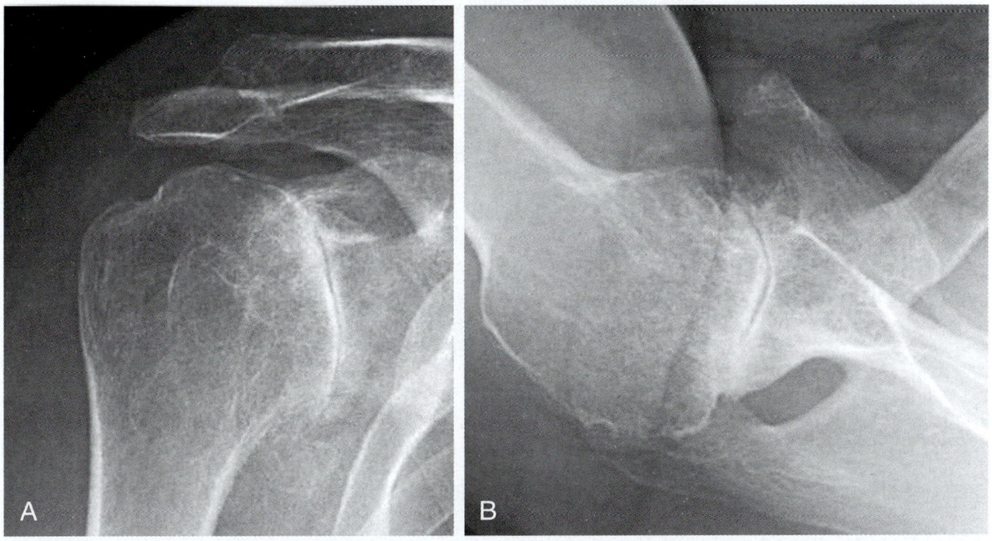

FIGURE 16-89: Capsulorrhaphy arthropathy, that is, arthritis after a prior repair for anterior glenohumeral instability. **A,** Anteroposterior view. **B,** Axillary view.

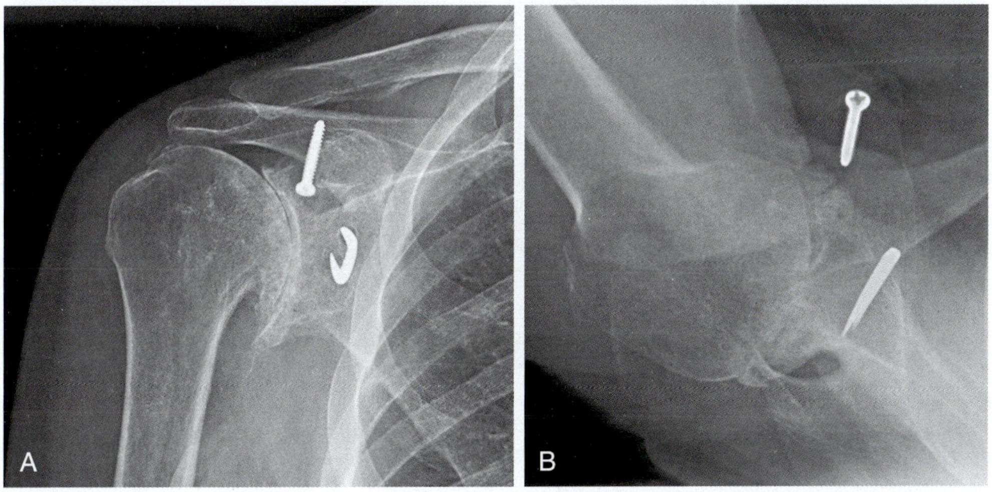

FIGURE 16-90: Capsulorrhaphy arthropathy. **A,** Anteroposterior view showing loss of joint space and hardware from a prior repair for anterior instability. **B,** Axillary view showing glenoid retroversion, a biconcave glenoid, and posterior humeral subluxation.

(Fig. 16-91) rather than posteriorly, as in degenerative joint disease (see Fig. 16-66). The arthritic process erodes not only cartilage but also subchondral bone, rendering it osteopenic and at risk of fracture (Fig. 16-92). Rheumatoid arthritis can be associated with major bone loss and rotator cuff deficiency, even in young individuals (Fig. 16-93).[379] When the onset of the disease occurs during youth, the joint volume may be small (Fig. 16-94) and the humerus curved, with a thin medullary canal (Fig. 16-95).[292] The restoration of comfort and function to the rheumatoid glenohumeral joint is often complicated by concurrent involvement of the rotator cuff* as well as the acromioclavicular, sternoclavicular, elbow, wrist, and hand articulations and the joints of the opposite upper extremity.[429,587] Arthritis in the lower extremities may demand the use of ambulatory aids and that in the upper extremities may demand wheelchair transfers. Even the skin of an individual with rheumatoid arthritis may be fragile and subject to compromised wound healing. The fragility of a patient with rheumatoid arthritis is often compounded by long-term use of steroids and other antimetabolic medications. The physician should remain aware of the possible coexistence of joint infection as rheumatoid arthritis involves the immune system due to the patient often receiving immunosuppressive medication, and the clinical manifestations of this condition are similar to those of infectious arthritis. Methotrexate may also increase the risk of nerve dysfunction after shoulder arthroplasty.[315]

**References 1, 2, 10, 33, 47, 50, 107, 133, 158, 161, 189, 261, 264, 301, 342, 394, 429, 430, 455, 471, 475, 510, 511, 513, 526, 542, 551, 562, 597.*

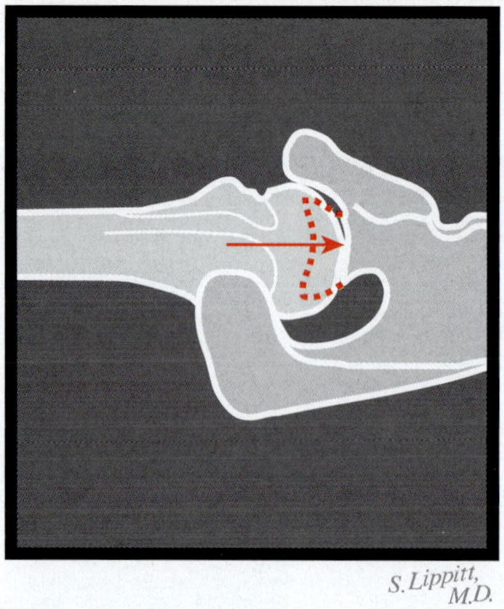

FIGURE 16-91: Inflammatory arthritis. Medial erosion (arrow) typical of inflammatory arthritis. The original contour of the glenoid is shown (dotted line). (From Matsen FA III, Lippitt SB. *Shoulder Surgery: Principles and Procedures.* Philadelphia: Saunders; 2004:425.)

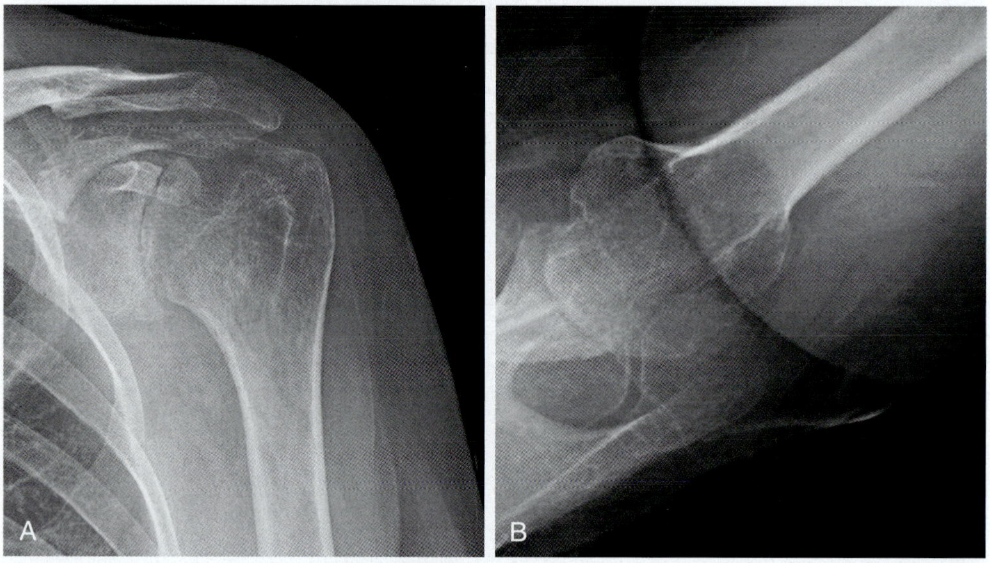

FIGURE 16-92: A shoulder with rheumatoid arthritis. Sclerosis and osteophytes typical of osteoarthritis are absent. The bone is osteopenic with erosions at the margins of the articular surface. The humeral head is displaced upwards, suggesting cuff deficiency, and the glenoid is eroded medially. **A,** Anteroposterior view. **B,** Axillary view.

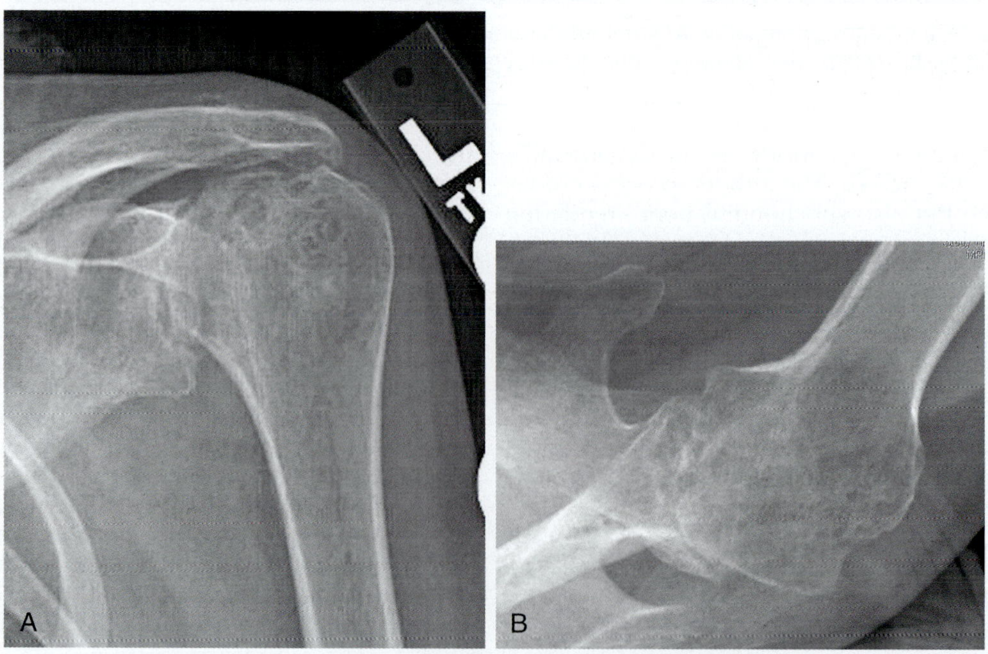

FIGURE 16-93: A shoulder with findings of rheumatoid arthritis more advanced than those shown in Figure 16-92. **A,** Anteroposterior view. **B,** Axillary view.

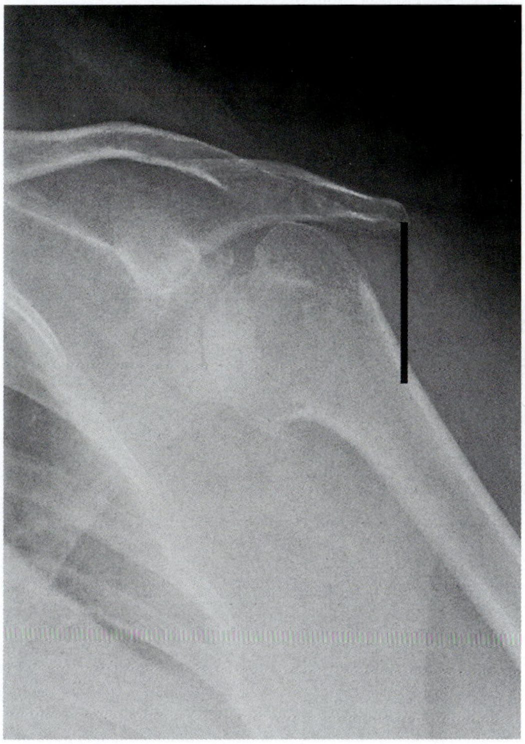

FIGURE 16-94: Severe medial erosion in rheumatoid arthritis. Note that the entire proximal humerus is medial to the lateral acromial line. Normally, the lateral acromial line passes through the lateral humeral articular surface.

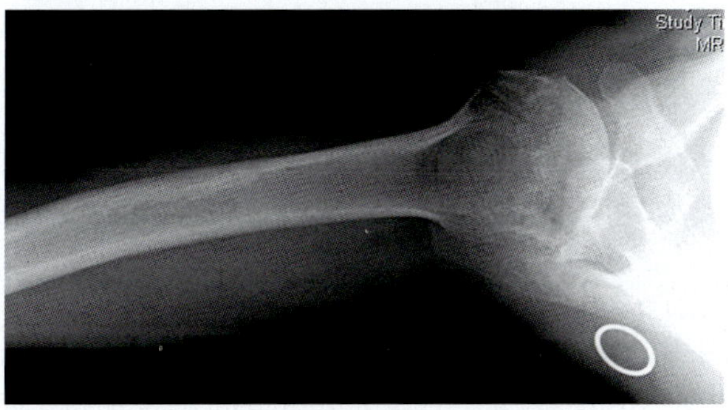

FIGURE 16-95: Lateral view of the humerus of a patient who experienced the onset of rheumatoid arthritis as a child. The radiograph shows a bend; this was included in the preoperative planning.

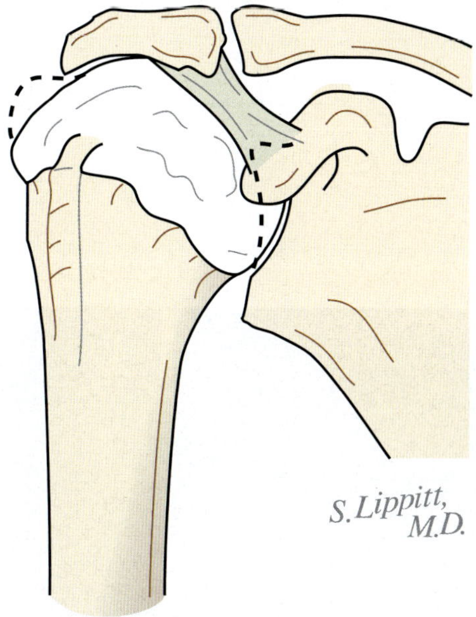

FIGURE 16-96: Cuff tear arthropathy. In cuff tear arthropathy the shoulder takes on a form similar to that of the hip: the greater tuberosity becomes eroded such that the proximal humerus is "femoralized" (dotted lines on the humerus), and the coracoacromial arch and upper glenoid erosion results in their "acetabularization" (dotted lines on the upper glenoid).

Because of the fragility of the skin and other soft tissues, osteopenia, and the severe bone erosion common with this condition, a patient with substantial involvement of rheumatoid arthritis or similar types of arthritis must be treated with extreme gentleness and thoughtfulness. Shoulder arthroplasty for rheumatoid arthritis has a high rate of glenoid component loosening and rotator cuff failure.[50,107,511,513] Patients with rheumatoid arthritis characteristically have substantially lower self-assessed vitality and overall physical function than do those with other causes of glenohumeral arthritis. The compromised general health and strength of patients with rheumatoid arthritis must be considered in planning their surgical and postoperative management.[342] Special preoperative evaluation and intraoperative care should be directed at the potentially tenuous stability of the cervical spine.

Cuff Tear Arthropathy

CTA is a compound degenerative condition of the shoulder that involves tendon, cartilage, and bone.[75,138,247,391,394,406,559] In this condition, chronic, massive rotator cuff defects are associated with loss of the humeral articular cartilage and superior displacement of the humeral head so that it articulates with the undersurface of the coracoacromial arch. The humeral head becomes "femoralized" by rounding off of the tuberosities, whereas the coracoacromial arch and upper glenoid fossa become "acetabularized" when the humerus sculpts a concentric concavity from these structures (Figs. 16-96 to 16-106).

In CTA the glenohumeral joint is deprived of several of its major stabilizing factors: the normal cuff muscle force vector compressing the humeral head into the glenoid (see Fig. 16-5); the superior lip of the glenoid concavity, which is typically worn away by chronic superior subluxation (see Fig. 16-6); and the cuff tendon that is normally interposed between the humeral head and the coracoacromial arch (Fig. 16-107). The superior displacement of the humeral head slackens the deltoid,

Text continued on p. 872

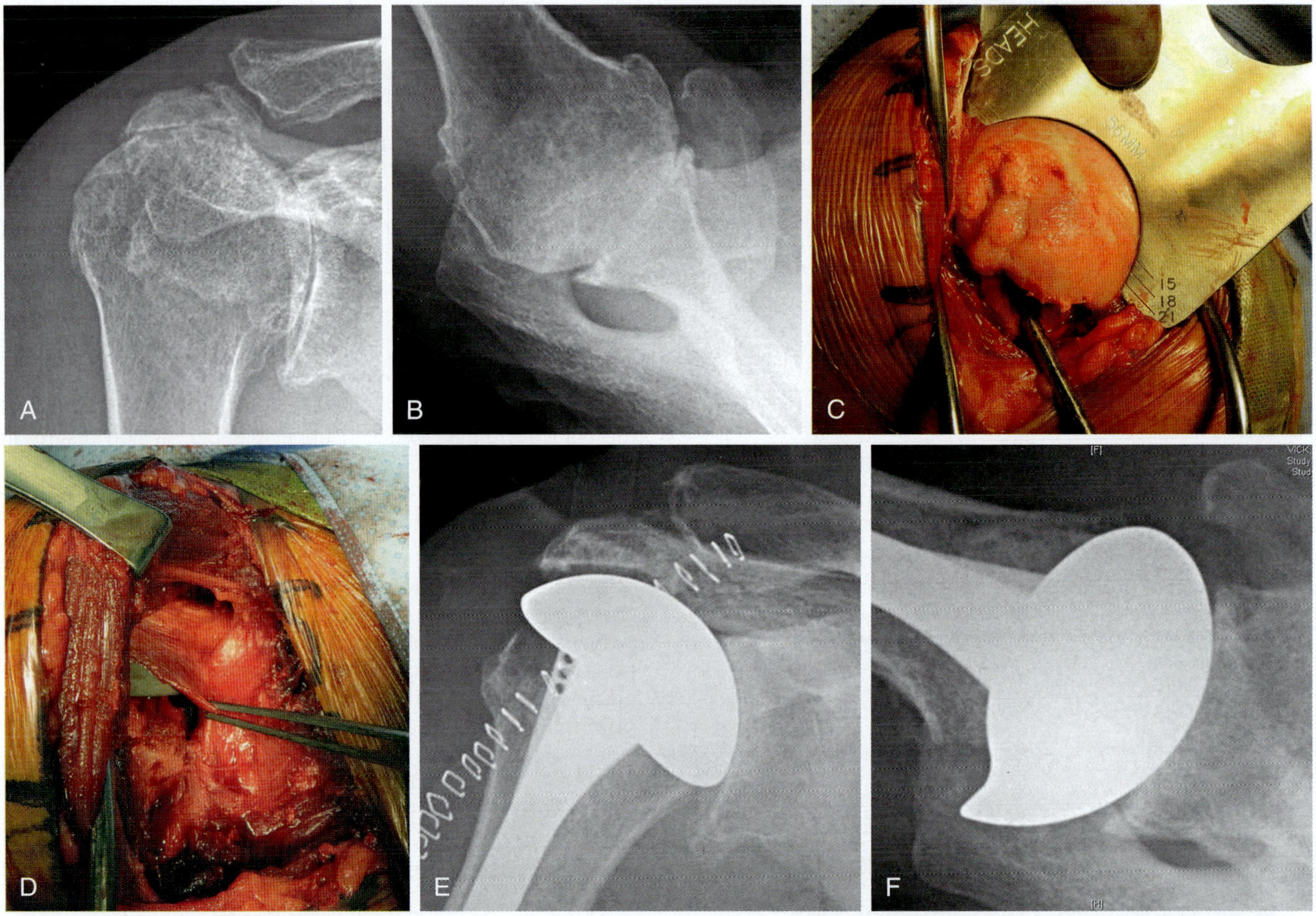

FIGURE 16-97: Rotator cuff tear arthropathy (CTA) treated with a CTA prosthesis. **A,** Preoperative anteroposterior radiograph showing superior displacement of the humeral head that has resulted in contact with the acromion as well as the loss of humeral and glenoid articular cartilage and a secondary superior glenoid concavity. The proximal humerus has been "femoralized" and the coracoacromial arch and upper glenoid have been "acetabularized." **B,** Preoperative axillary radiograph showing medial but not posterior erosion of the glenoid. **C,** Intraoperative photo showing measurement of the humeral diameter of curvature. **D,** Intraoperative photo showing preservation of the clavipectoral fascia coming off the coracoacromial ligament (the "CA+") to enhance anterosuperior stability. **E,** Postoperative anteroposterior view after implantation of the CTA prosthesis. Note the congruent fit of the prosthesis in the socket. **F,** Postoperative axillary view after implantation of the CTA prosthesis.

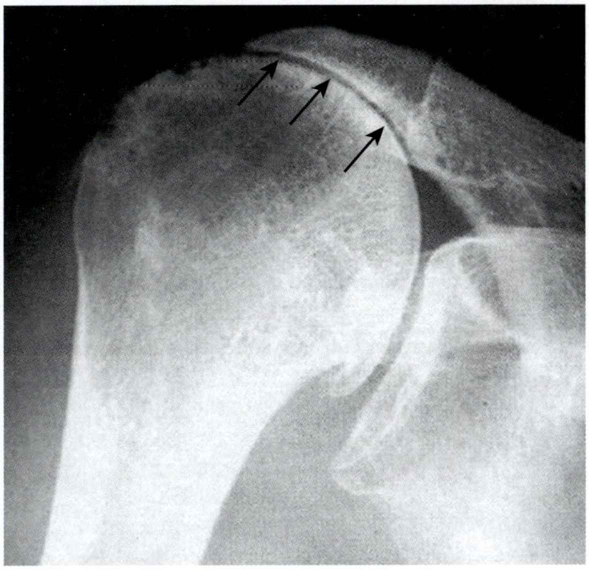

FIGURE 16-98: Rotator cuff tear arthropathy with acetabularization of the coracoacromial arch and upper glenoid.

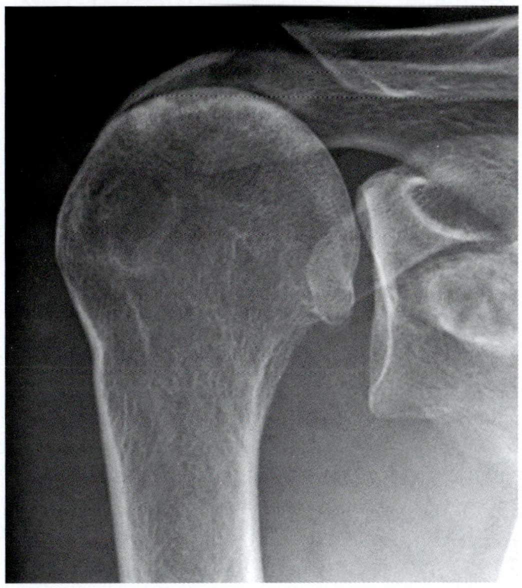

FIGURE 16-99: Rotator cuff tear arthropathy with femoralization of the proximal humerus and actetabularization of the coracoacromial arch and upper glenoid.

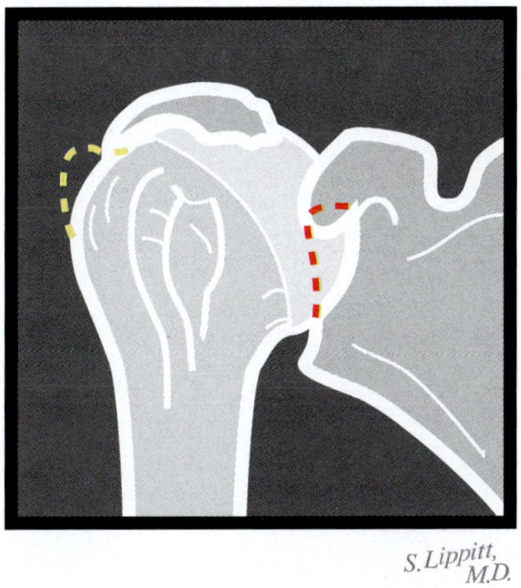

FIGURE 16-100: Cuff tear arthropathy. Superior medial erosion (dotted red line) typical of cuff tear arthropathy. (From Matsen FA III, Lippitt SB. *Shoulder Surgery: Principles and Procedures*. Philadelphia: Saunders; 2004:426.)

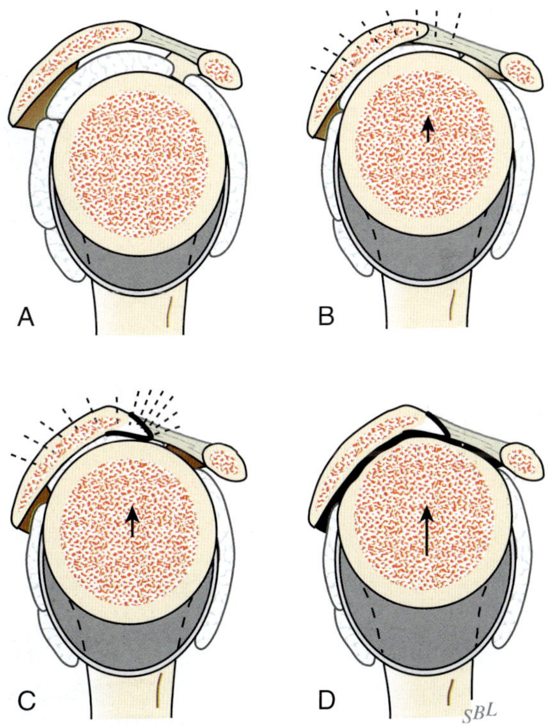

FIGURE 16-101: Acromial traction spur. **A,** Normal position. **B,** As the humeral head moves upwards, the coracoacromial arch becomes progressively loaded. **C,** The result is a traction spur in the coracoacromial ligament. Because it lies within the substance of the ligament, this spur does not encroach on the rotator cuff, even though it might look impressive on the radiograph. **D,** Rotator cuff tear arthroplasty. (From Matsen FA III, Lippitt SB. *Shoulder Surgery: Principles and Procedures*. Philadelphia: Saunders; 2004:280.)

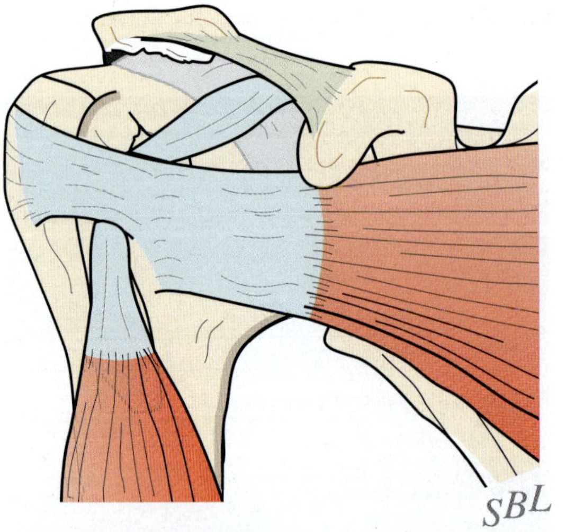

FIGURE 16-102: The boutonnière deformity, in which the subscapularis and infraspinatus tendons slide below the center of the humeral head. (Modified from Matsen FA III, Lippitt SB, Sidles JA, Harryman DT II. *Practical Evaluation and Management of the Shoulder.* Philadelphia: Saunders; 1994.)

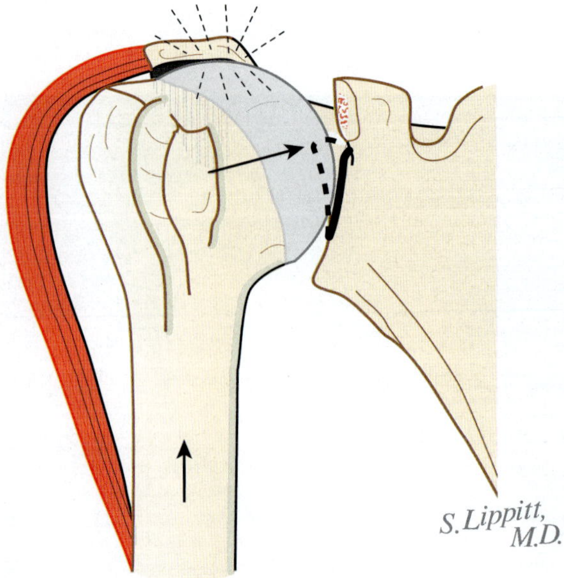

FIGURE 16-103: Erosion of the superior glenoid concavity (dotted line and horizontal arrow) compromises the concavity compression stability mechanism and allows upward translation of the humeral head (vertical arrow) when the deltoid contracts. (Modified from Matsen FA III, Lippitt SB, Sidles JA, Harryman DT II. *Practical Evaluation and Management of the Shoulder.* Philadelphia: Saunders; 1994.)

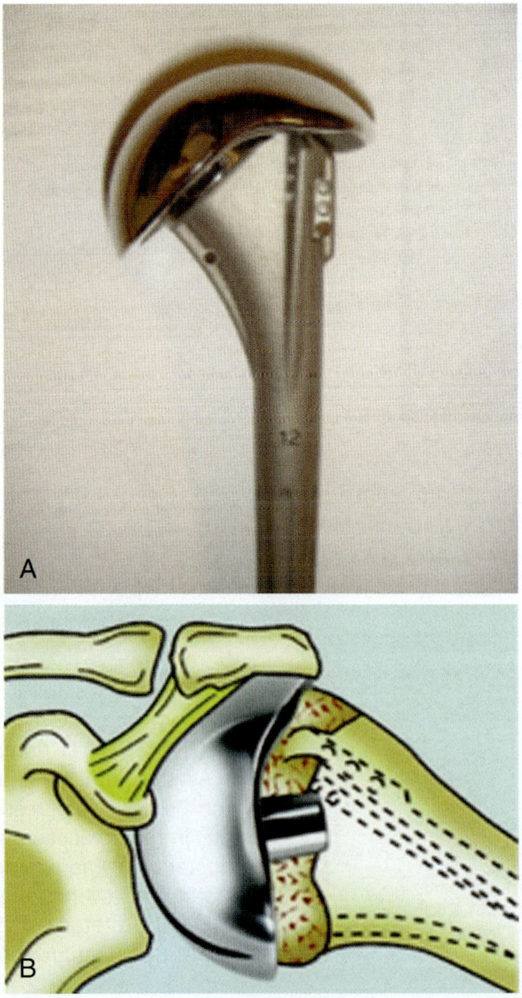

FIGURE 16-104: Hemiarthroplasty with a laterally extended cuff tear arthropathy (CTA) head. **A,** CTA prosthesis. **B,** The installed prosthesis.

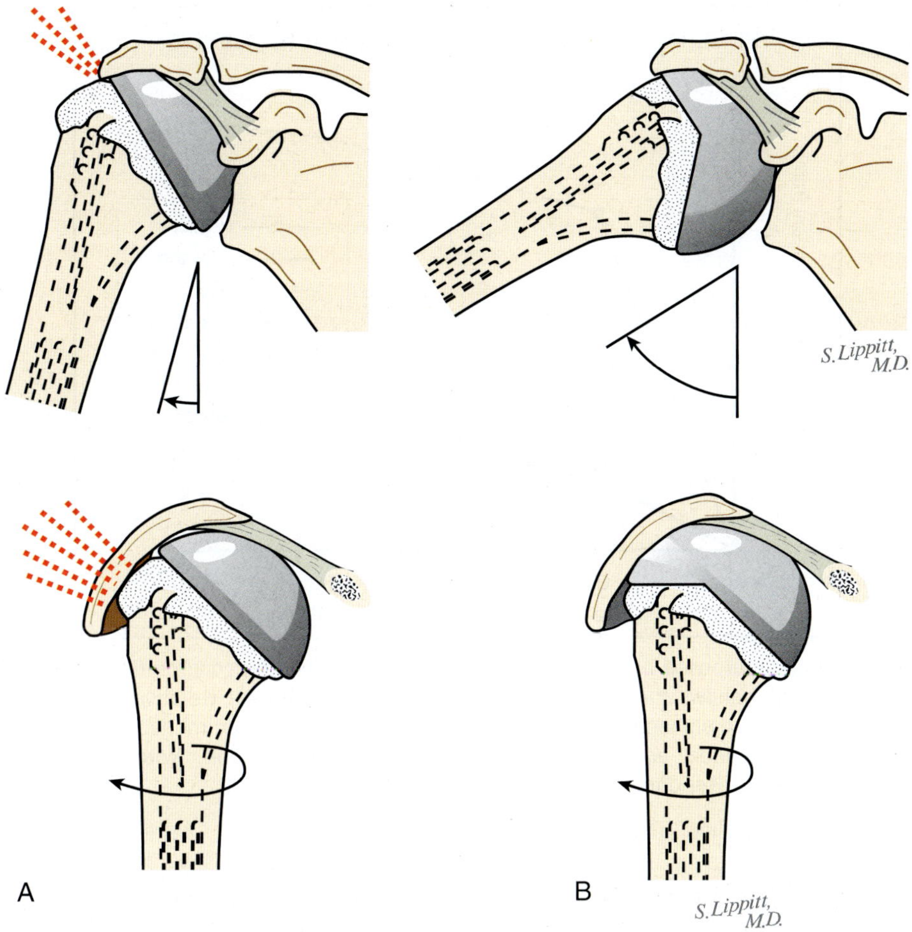

FIGURE 16-105: Rationale for a laterally extended cuff tear arthropathy (CTA) head. **A,** Abduction and external rotation are limited due to painful impingement against the uncovered greater tuberosity. Impingement is indicated by the dashed red lines radiating up and to the left. **B,** The laterally extended CTA head allows a greater arc of motion in abduction and greater external rotation by coverage of the greater tuberosity.

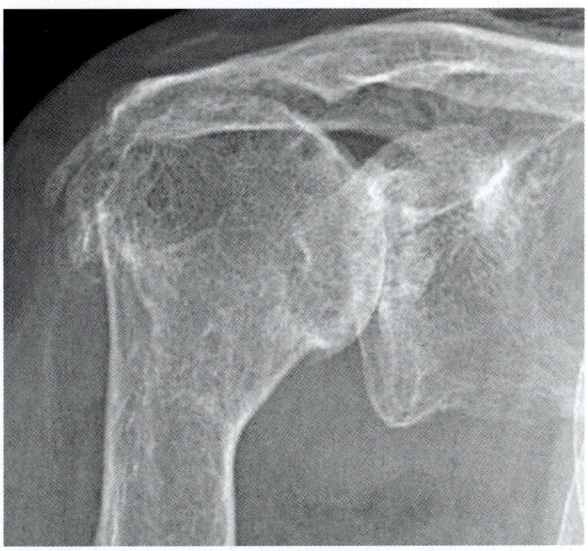

FIGURE 16-106: Rotator cuff tear arthropathy. The humeral head is displaced superiorly and medially, eroding into the acromion and upper glenoid. The thinning of the acromion will predispose it to fracture at the time of or after arthroplasty.

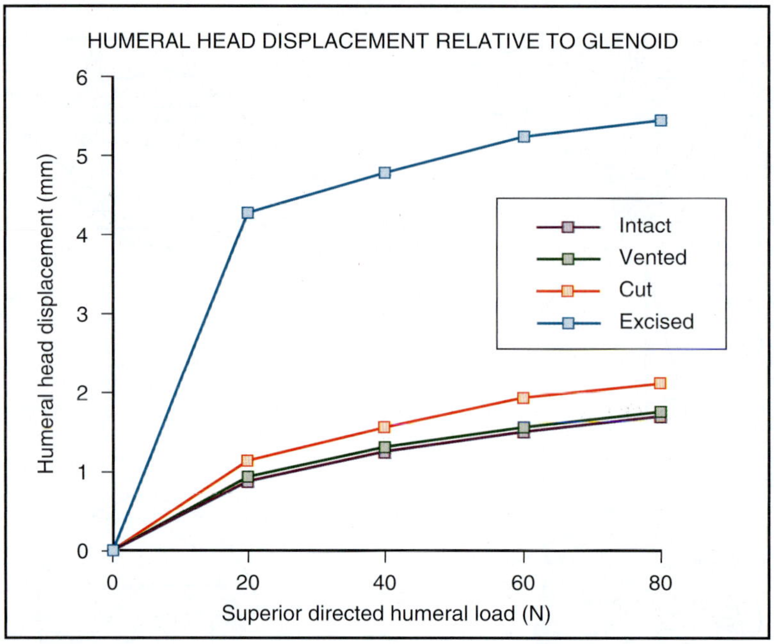

FIGURE 16-107: The cuff tendon interposed between the humeral head and the coracoacromial arch stabilizes the head against superiorly directed loads. The graph shows the mean superior humeral displacement (relative to the scapula) as a function of the superior humeral load, comparing displacements under four conditions: intact specimens, after venting the joint to air, after cutting (but not excising) the cuff tendon, and after excising the superior cuff tendon. Note the markedly increased superior displacement after excision of the cuff tendon.

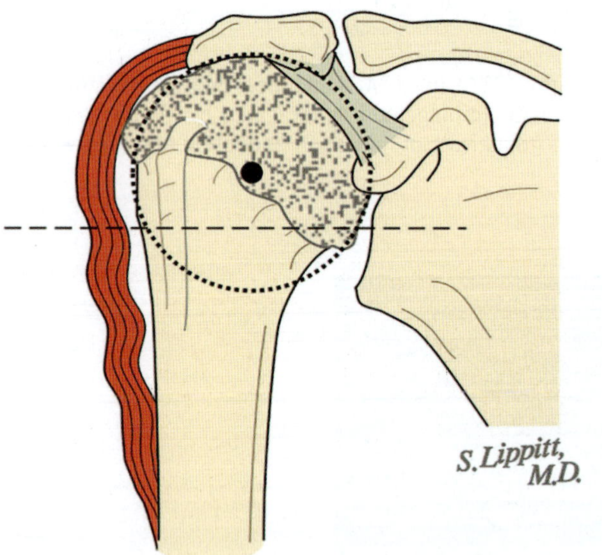

FIGURE 16-108: Superior displacement of the humeral head slackens the deltoid so that its ability to flex or abduct the shoulder is weakened.

weakening its ability to flex or abduct the shoulder (Fig. 16-108). As the condition progresses, the coracoacromial arch may become compromised, allowing anterosuperior escape (Fig. 16-109). Prior acromioplasty and section of the coracoacromial ligament further compromise glenohumeral stability and contribute to anterosuperior escape (Figs. 16-110 and 16-111). These consequences of loss of integrity of the coracoacromial arch are reminders of the need to preserve the integrity of the acromion and coracoacromial ligament in all shoulder procedures.

CTA provides several challenges for the surgeon. In the absence of an intact rotator cuff, total shoulder arthroplasty has been shown to have an early failure rate from glenoid loosening through the so called "rocking horse" phenomenon (Fig. 16-112).[152,309,432,436] Standard hemiarthroplasty may provide only partial pain relief and partial improvement in function.[11,391,432,484,585,601] Currently, the surgical management of CTA commonly involves either a CTA prosthesis (see Fig. 16-105) or a reverse total shoulder arthroplasty (Fig. 16-113).[43,506,579]

Several systems for the classification of the pathoanatomy of CTA have been proposed as guides to treatment.[138,258,506,559] However, we have found the following factors to be even more critical than radiographic classification in determining the treatment: (1) the stability of the humeral head beneath the coracoacromial arch (i.e., the presence or absence of anterosuperior escape) (Figs. 16-114 and 16-115; see also Figs. 16-109 and 16-111); (2) the amount of active elevation provided by the deltoid (i.e., the presence or absence of pseudoparalysis, defined as the inability to actively raise the arm to 90 degrees despite a good passive range of motion); (3) the strength of the residual internal and external rotator musculature; (4) the amount and quality of glenoid, humeral, and

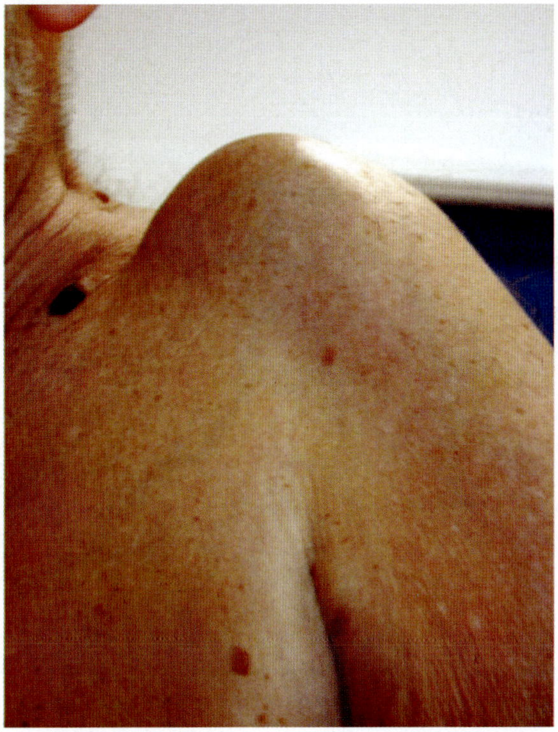

FIGURE 16-109: Patient with long-standing cuff tear arthropathy with anterosuperior escape of the humeral head when active elevation is attempted.

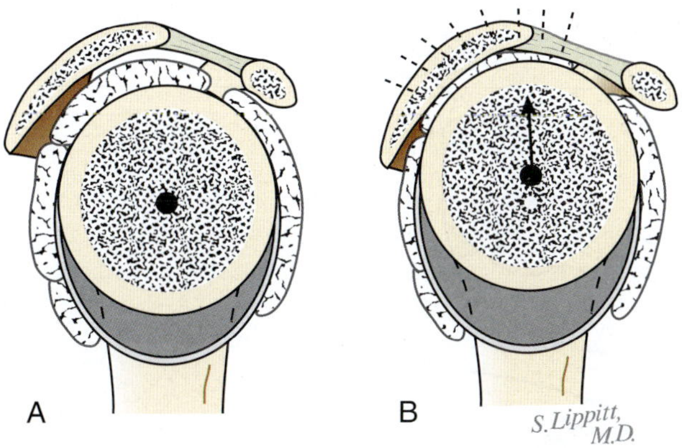

FIGURE 16-110: **A,** Normal shoulder. **B,** Cuff-deficient shoulder with an intact coracoacromial arch. If the coracoacromial arch remains intact (i.e., not damaged by acromioplasty or coracoacromial arch section), the arch may provide secondary stabilization for the humeral head against the upward pull of the deltoid. (From Matsen FA III, Lippitt SB. *Shoulder Surgery: Principles and Procedures.* Philadelphia: Saunders; 2004:264.)

acromial bone stock available for surgical reconstruction (Fig. 16-116); (5) the patient's fall risk, which is a particular concern in individuals with Parkinson disease or other problems of balance; (6) the patient's dependency on the upper extremities for mobility; and (7) the patient's activity expectations.

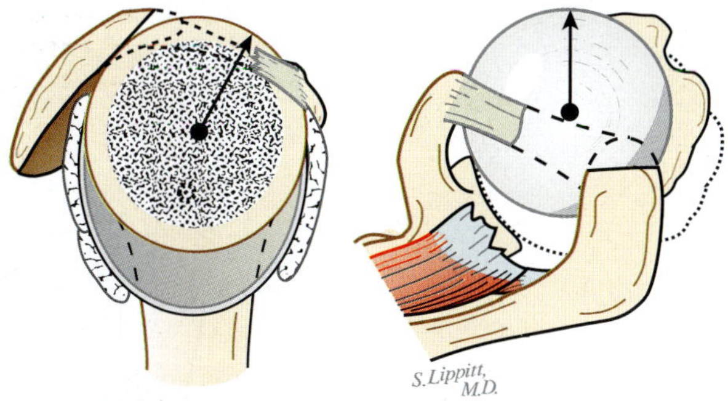

FIGURE 16-111: Anterosuperior escape of the humeral head. Resection of the coracoacromial ligament and anterior acromioplasty can allow the humeral head of the cuff-deficient shoulder to escape anterosuperiorly. (From Matsen FA III, Lippitt SB. *Shoulder Surgery: Principles and Procedures.* Philadelphia: Saunders; 2004:265.)

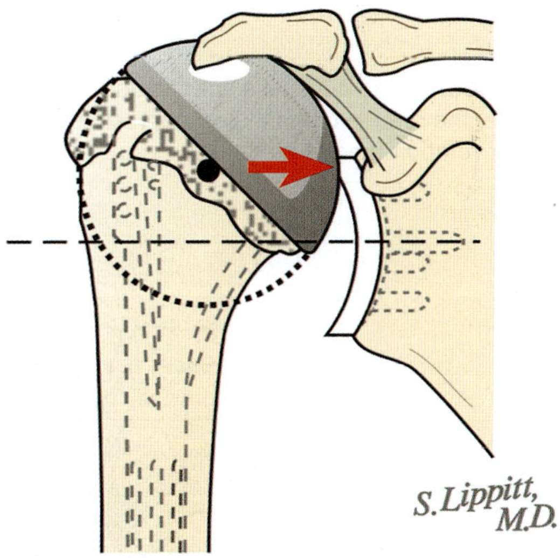

FIGURE 16-112: Total shoulder arthroplasty in the absence of an intact rotator cuff has been shown to result in early glenoid loosening by the "rocking horse" mechanism of the superior migrated humeral component on the superior glenoid component.

Avascular Necrosis

Nontraumatic or primary avascular necrosis of the humeral head may be idiopathic or may be associated with systemic steroids, trauma, dysbaric conditions, renal or other organ transplantation, or systemic illnesses with vasculitis. Other implicated conditions include alcoholism, sickle cell disease, hyperuricemia, Gaucher disease, pancreatitis, familial hyperlipidemia, and lymphoma.[19,52,113,114,208,320,369,370,411,466] Avascular necrosis has also been reported as a result of section of the anterior humeral circumflex artery in open instability surgery.[423]

Avascular necrosis of the humeral head may be seen on plain radiographs or MRI before collapse of the joint surface occurs (Figs. 16-117 to 16-120). Often, a fracture superocentrally through the abnormal subchondral bone

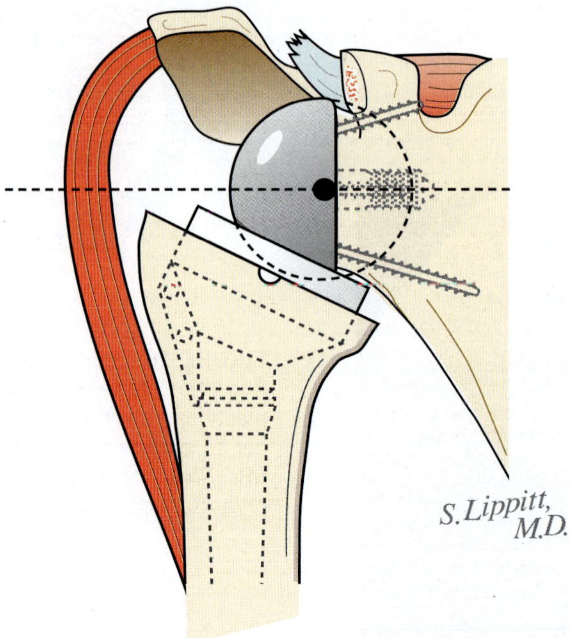

FIGURE 16-113: In the cuff-deficient shoulder with a compromised coracoacromial arch and subsequent functional anterosuperior escape, the reverse ball-and-socket prosthesis helps provide glenohumeral stability by retensioning the deltoid and moving the center of rotation medially.

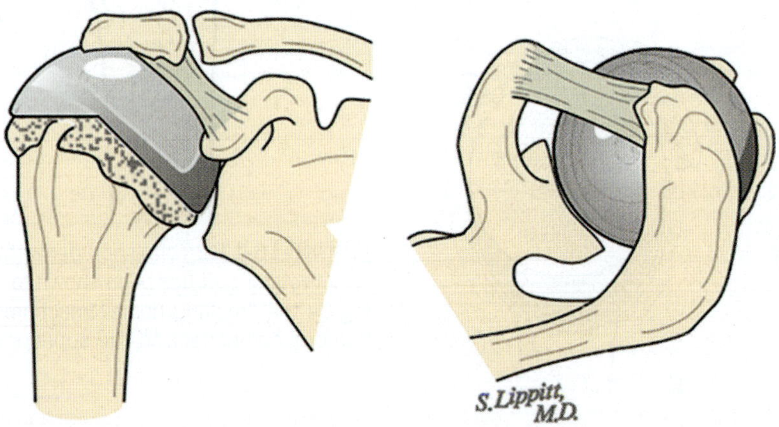

FIGURE 16-114: Hemiarthroplasty with cuff tear arthropathy. The head component is stable beneath the intact coracoacromial arch.

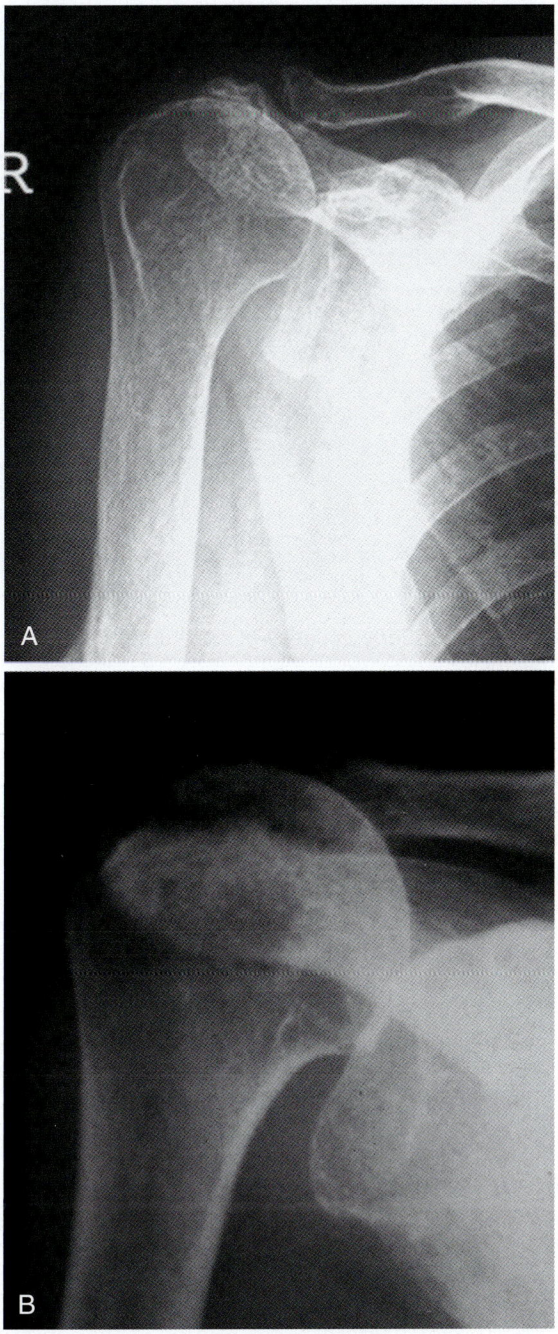

FIGURE 16-115: Anteroposterior radiographs, static and dynamic with fluoroscopy. **A,** Superior displacement with the arm resting at the side. **B,** Superior dislocation with the arm under resisted abduction.

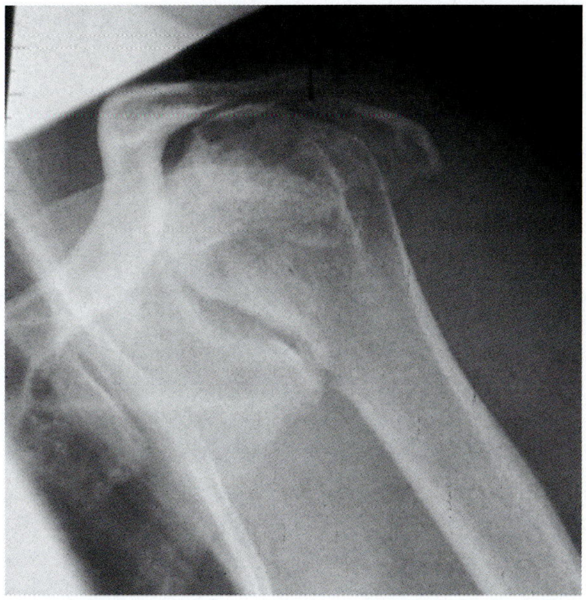

FIGURE 16-116: Typical radiograph of a progressive cuff tear arthropathy. It shows superior migration of the head with secondary superior glenoid erosion.

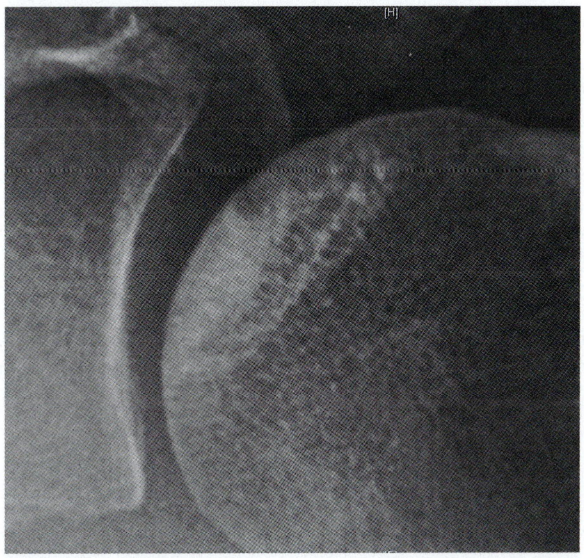

FIGURE 16-117: Early avascular necrosis revealed as sclerosis of the superior medial aspect of the humeral head. The humeral head has not collapsed.

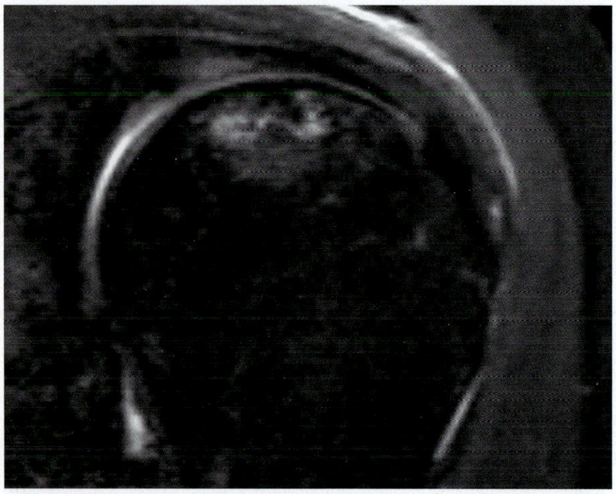

FIGURE 16-118: Magnetic resonance imaging findings of early avascular necrosis, shown on a sagittal T2-weighted image.

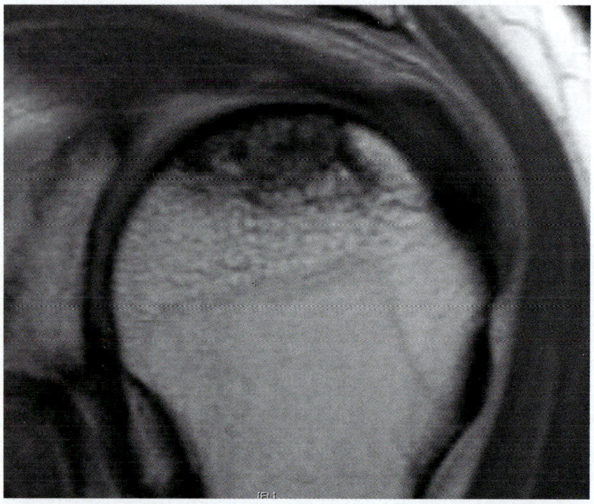

FIGURE 16-119: Magnetic resonance imaging findings of early avascular necrosis, shown on a coronal T1-weighted image.

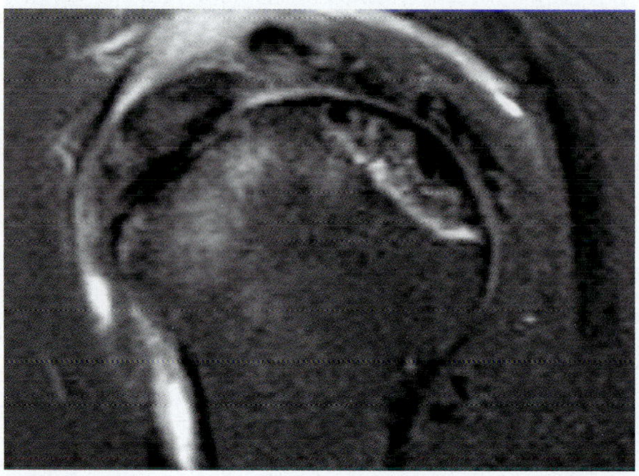

FIGURE 16-120: Magnetic resonance imaging findings of early avascular necrosis, shown on a coronal T2-weighted image.

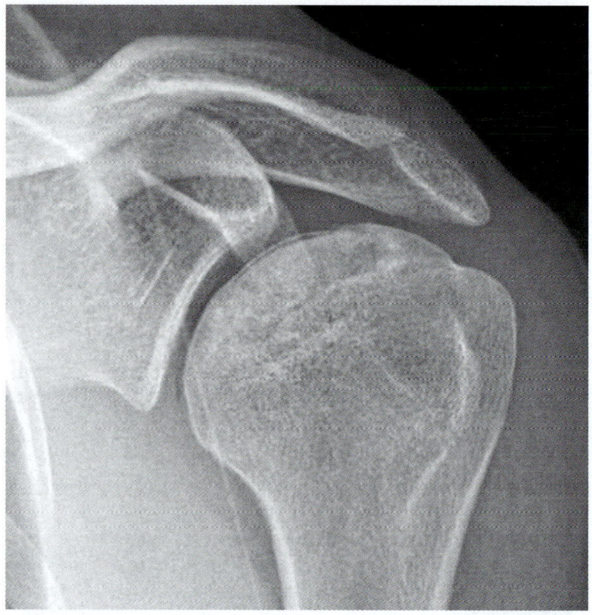

FIGURE 16-121: Early collapse of the humeral head in avascular necrosis.

is noted (Fig. 16-121). Subsequently, collapse of the subchondral bone can occur, putting the glenoid articular surface at risk for secondary erosion (Fig. 16-122). In end-stage avascular necrosis the irregular humeral head destroys glenoid articular cartilage, resulting in glenohumeral joint disease (Fig. 16-123).[114]

Core decompression may be of benefit early in the course of the disease.[369] When the process involves only the humeral head, a humeral hemiarthroplasty is considered, but when the glenoid is involved, a glenohumeral arthroplasty may be needed (Fig. 16-124).[320,411]

Glenohumeral Chondrolysis

Glenohumeral *chondrolysis* is a condition the etiology of which unfortunately was formerly referred to as being "speculative,"[441,596] but is now clearly recognized as being most commonly caused by the intra-articular infusion of local anesthetics using a "pain pump." This condition is particularly a risk after arthroscopic procedures in which suture anchors are placed in the glenoid.[339,489,581] Chondrolysis has also been associated with radiofrequency or laser procedures within the joint.[441,596] The diagnosis is made from a history of pain pump use, the postoperative onset of pain and stiffness, and radiographs showing loss of the joint space without osteophytes (Figs. 16-125 and 16-126). This iatrogenic condition primarily affects young individuals, often leaving them without options other than arthroplasty; even with arthroplasty the prognosis for the recovery of comfort and function is poor. The condition can largely be prevented by avoiding the use of pain pumps and heat energy, which are not necessary for the treatment of shoulder disorders.

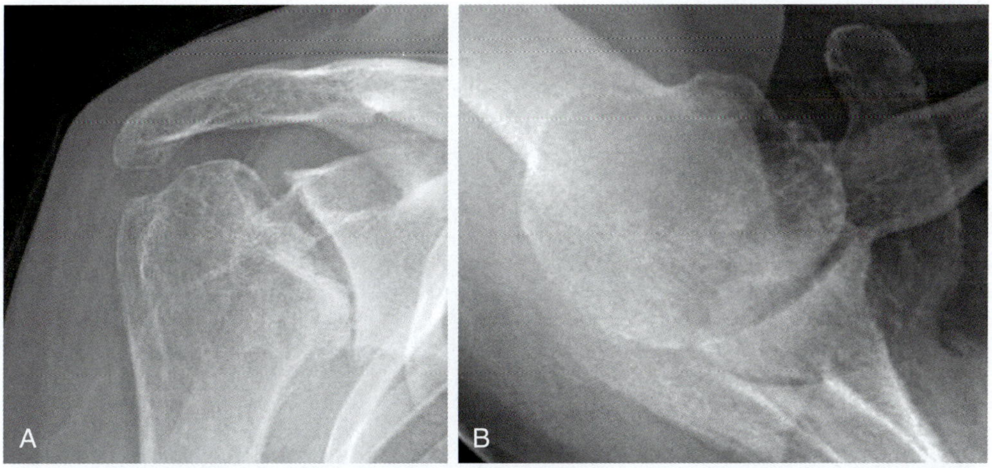

FIGURE 16-122: Avascular necrosis with humeral head collapse and secondary destruction of the glenoid articular surface. **A,** Anteroposterior view. **B,** Axillary view.

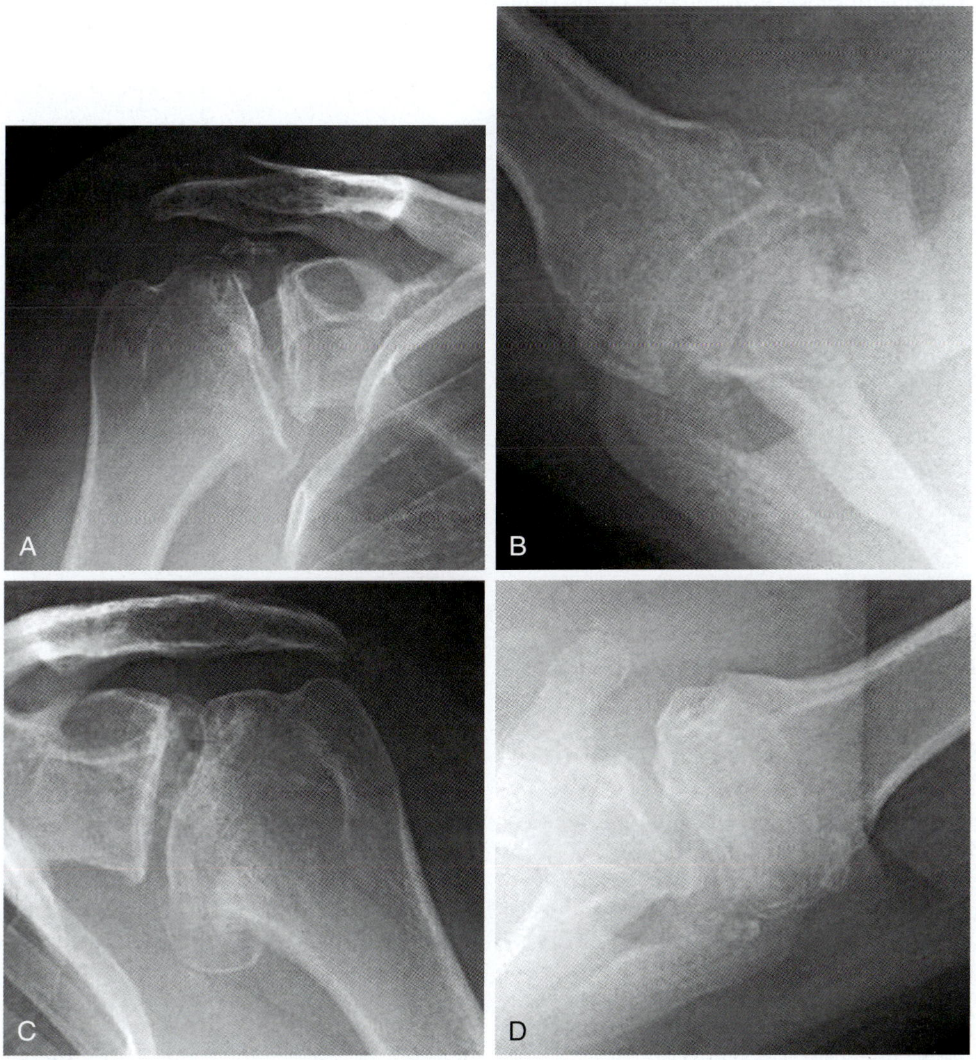

FIGURE 16-123: Bilateral avascular necrosis with collapse of the humeral articular surface. **A** and **C,** Anteroposterior views. **B** and **D**, Axillary views.

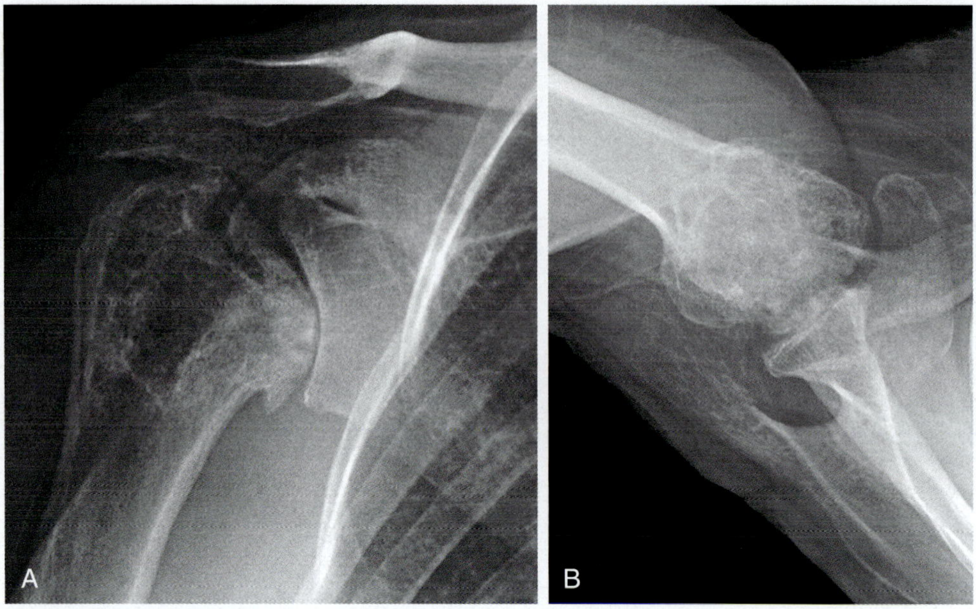

FIGURE 16-124: Avascular necrosis with collapse of the humeral head and secondary glenohumeral arthritis. **A,** Anteroposterior view. **B,** Axillary view.

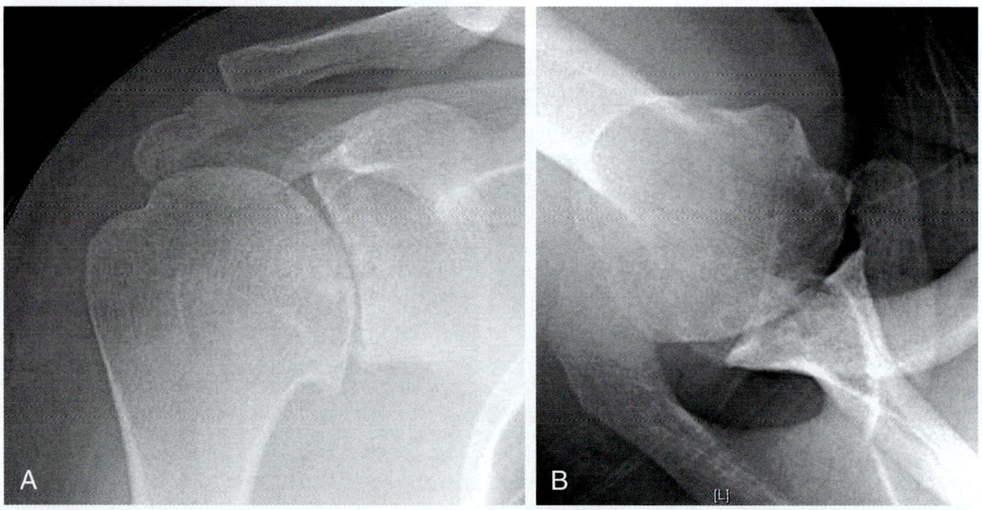

FIGURE 16-125: Chondrolysis in the right shoulder of a 22-year-old man resulting from the intra-articular infusion of local anesthetics with a pain pump. There was a complete loss of articular cartilage but without the osteophytes or sclerosis typical of osteoarthritis. **A,** Anteroposterior view. **B,** Axillary view.

Other Types of Arthritis

Neurotropic (Charcot) Arthropathy

Neurotropic (Charcot) arthropathy arises in association with syringomyelia, diabetes, or other causes of joint denervation. The joint and subchondral bone are destroyed because of the loss of the trophic and protective effects of its nerve supply. The individual may have experienced cervical spine trauma in the past,[448] or there may be unrecognized syringomyelia.[348,553] Other causes include diabetes, leprosy, syphilis, and chronic alcoholism, and it has been suggested that injection of corticosteroids might accelerate the development of this condition.[417] The Charcot joint is characterized by functional limitation and pain, despite the denervation. There is usually significant bone destruction and osseous debris about the joint area (Figs. 16-127 and 16-128). A useful mnemonic for the characteristic features of Charcot arthropathy is given by the three Ds: ***d***enervation, ***d***estruction, and ***d***ebris. This condition can resemble infectious arthritis.[311] The longevity of an arthroplasty performed for Charcot arthropathy may be jeopardized by the lack of a protective nerve supply.

Radiation Arthropathy

Radiation, especially for the treatment of breast cancer, can cause a number of shoulder problems: brachial plexopathy, osteonecrosis, secondary malignant bone

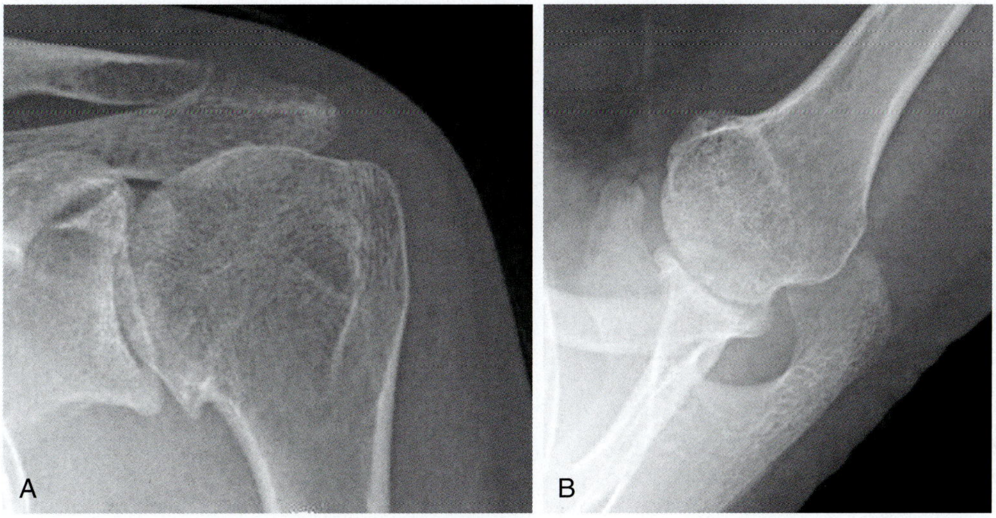

FIGURE 16-126: Chondrolysis in the left shoulder of a 24-year-old woman resulting from the intra-articular infusion of local anesthetics with a pain pump. There was a complete loss of articular cartilage but without the osteophytes or sclerosis typical of osteoarthritis. A, Anteroposterior view. **B,** Axillary view.

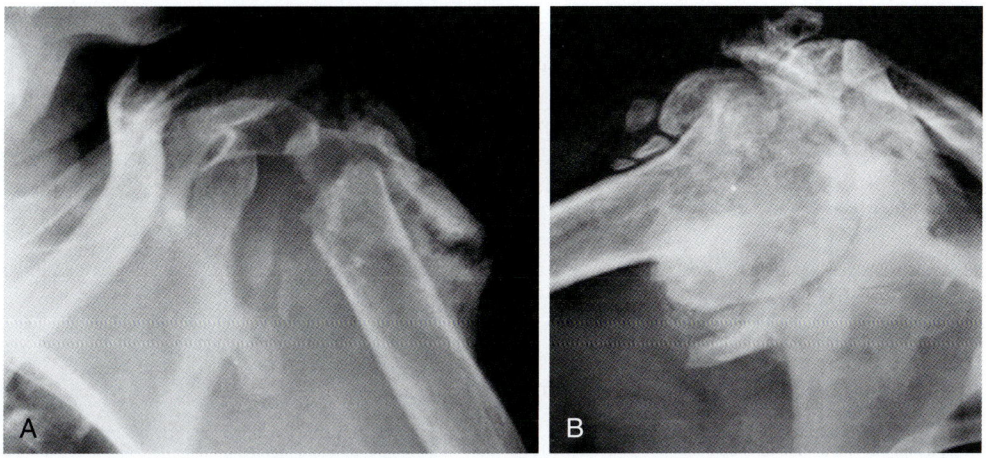

FIGURE 16-127: Occasionally, neuropathic arthritis can be confused with more common forms of glenohumeral arthritis. **A,** Fragmentation of the proximal end of the humerus with bone debris scattered throughout the joint region. **B,** Bone fragmentation is shown, but in addition, there is a predominantly sclerotic response associated with neuropathic arthritis. The underlying condition in both this patient and the one shown in Fig. 16-126 was syringomyelia of the cervical portion of the spinal cord.

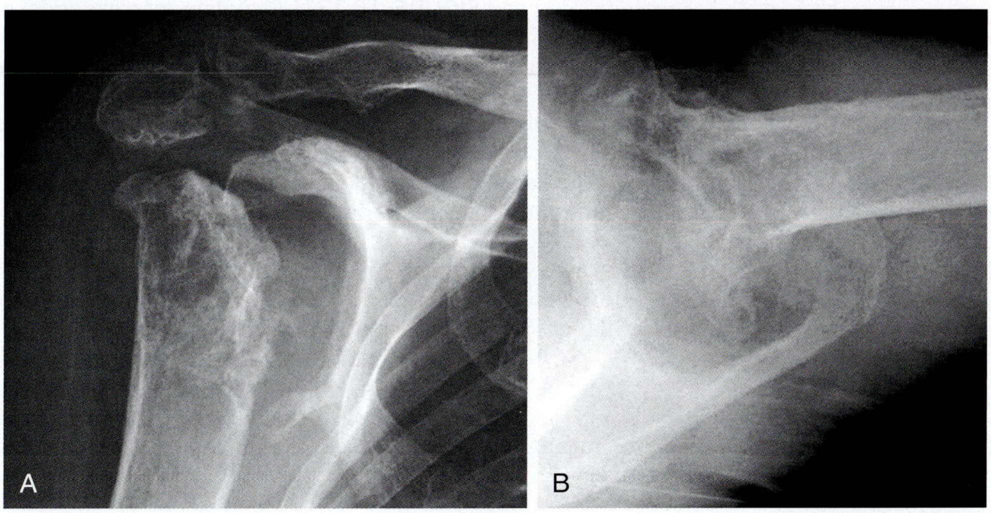

FIGURE 16-128: A shoulder with Charcot arthropathy characterized by massive bone destruction. **A,** Anteroposterior view. **B,** Axillary view.

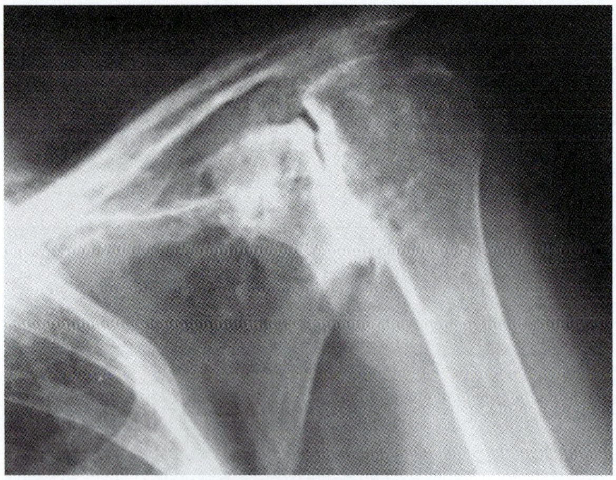

FIGURE 16-129: Cartilage loss, alteration in the shape of subchondral bone with segmental collapse, and a change in bone texture secondary to irradiation performed as part of treatment for breast cancer. Symptoms were quite significant in this elderly woman and were relieved effectively by total shoulder arthroplasty.

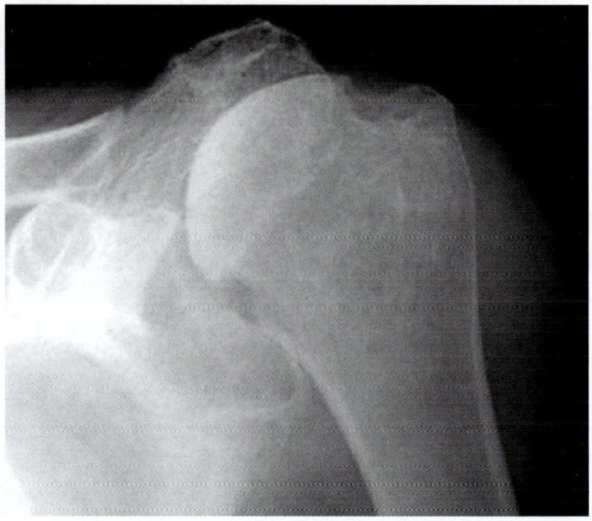

FIGURE 16-130: Septic arthropathy characterized by loss of the joint surface, marginal erosions around the humeral articular surface, rotator cuff destruction, and superior migration of the humerus.

tumors, and fibrous scarring. Glenohumeral cartilage and subchondral bone are occasionally affected by these changes and can require treatment by prosthetic arthroplasty (Fig. 16-129). A lack of normal soft tissue suppleness, scars from prior surgery, or lymphedema may complicate surgical management.

Septic Arthritis

Septic arthritis of the shoulder may arise from bacteria in the patient's dermis, from hematogenous spread from a remote infection, from injections into the joint, or from surgery on the joint itself. Patients with reduced immunologic defenses—from chronic systemic disease[17,67] or from immunosuppressive medications—are particularly at risk.[9,90,275,294] Radiographs may show bone destruction and instability (Figs. 16-130 to 16-132). Treatment must be directed at resolving the infection before considering arthroplasty for the management of the resulting arthritis.

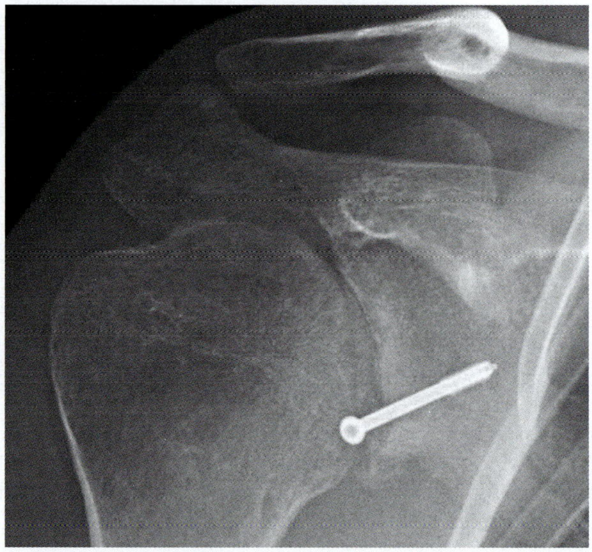

FIGURE 16-131: Complete loss of articular cartilage after a coracoid transfer for instability. The shoulder showed multiple positive cultures for *Propionibacterium* species at revision surgery.

Neoplastic Joint Destruction

Neoplastic joint destruction may present insidiously and is often characterized by nonmechanical pain, that is, pain at rest.[31,356] Alternatively, tumors may present acutely as a pathologic fracture. The diagnosis will depend on knowledge of the patient's general health; high-quality plain radiographs; and possibly additional imaging modes, such as tomography, CT, bone scanning, or MRI. Identification of the primary lesion in metastatic disease is desirable, but sometimes biopsy of the shoulder lesion is the most direct route when making a diagnosis (Fig. 16-133).

Miscellaneous Arthropathies

Miscellaneous arthropathies include crystalline arthritis (such as calcium pyrophosphate deposition disease or hydroxyapatite deposition disease),[194,196,197,270] dialysis arthropathy,[493] hemophilic arthropathy, hemochromatosis,[134,445] synovial chondrometaplasia,[220] alkaptonuria, gouty arthropathy,[132] acromegalic arthropathy,[431] spondyloarthropathy,[89] Milwaukee shoulder,[160,195,352,353] rapidly destructive articular disease (Fig. 16-134),[74,398] amyloid arthropathy,[117] pseudogout,[230] primary hyperparathyroid arthropathy,[83] psoriatic arthropathy,[90] ulcerative colitis, Crohn disease, Reiter syndrome, pigmented villonodular synovitis,[126] and Lyme arthritis.[117]

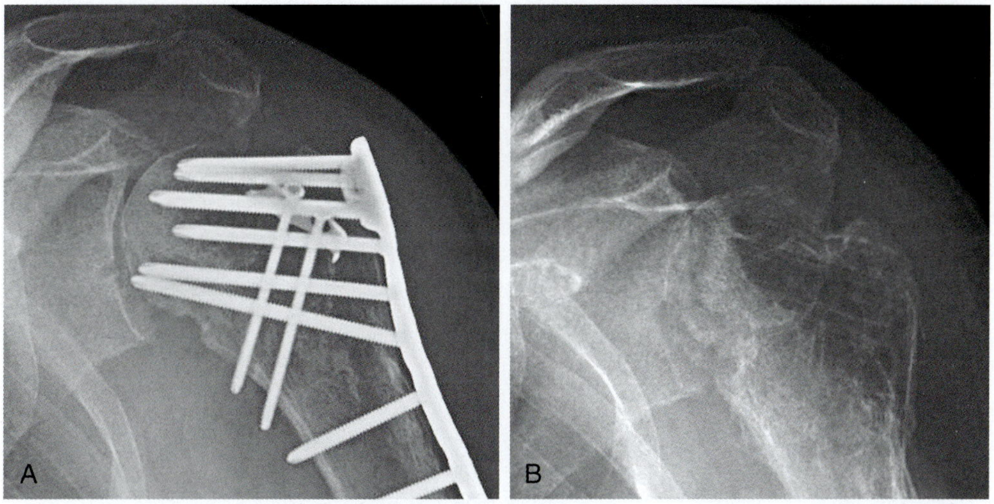

FIGURE 16-132: Septic arthritis due to *Propionibacterium* species after internal fixation of a proximal humeral fracture. **A,** An internal fixation removed because of the concern for screw penetration into the joint. **B,** Progressive destruction of the articular surface leading to shoulder hemiarthroplasty, at which time cultures were positive for *Propionibacterium* species.

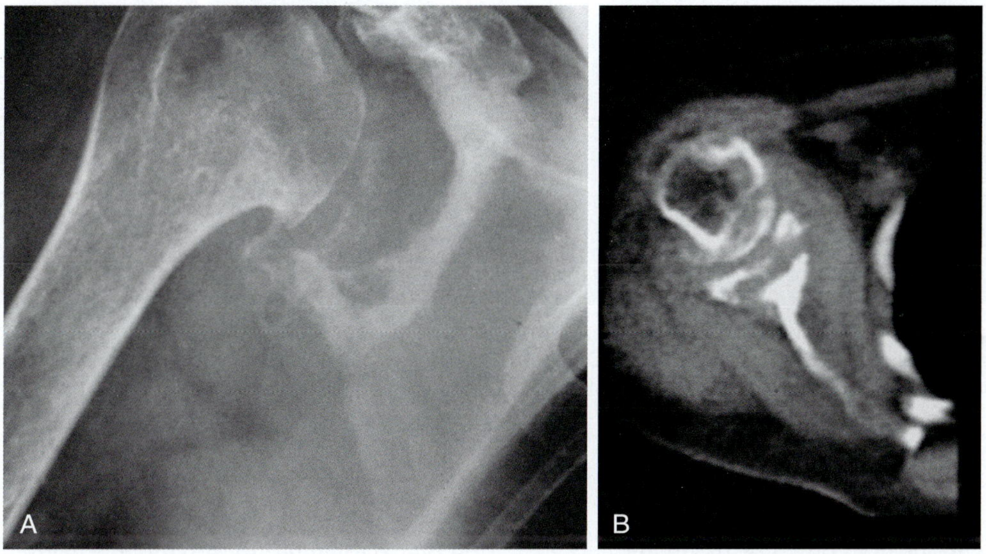

FIGURE 16-133: An upper-middle-aged woman with gradual onset of shoulder pain and reduction in movement. The shoulder was more painful with use but was also painful at rest. She had no known systemic illness. **A,** Involvement of the glenohumeral joint is shown, with some collapse of the humeral head articular surface. More importantly, this radiograph shows destruction of the bone of the glenoid. **B,** Computed tomographic image showing the bone destruction quite well. A biopsy revealed metastatic thyroid carcinoma.

TREATMENT

Communication

Treatment should begin with a dialogue between the surgeon and the patient regarding the diagnosis; the probable natural history of the condition, if untreated; and the potential risks and benefits of the different treatment options. The likely outcomes are discussed in light of the patient's expectations and the surgeon's personal experience in treating the patient's condition.[179] A partnership is formed. Because glenohumeral arthritis is usually insidious in onset and chronic in duration, there is ample opportunity to try nonoperative management. A period of nonoperative treatment offers the patient and surgeon the opportunity to get to know each other better and gives the patient time to learn some of the exercises that will be a part of the postoperative rehabilitation should surgery be elected. Patients may have difficulty recalling the nature of these discussions; thus our practice is to provide illustrated handouts (Fig. 16-135) and our

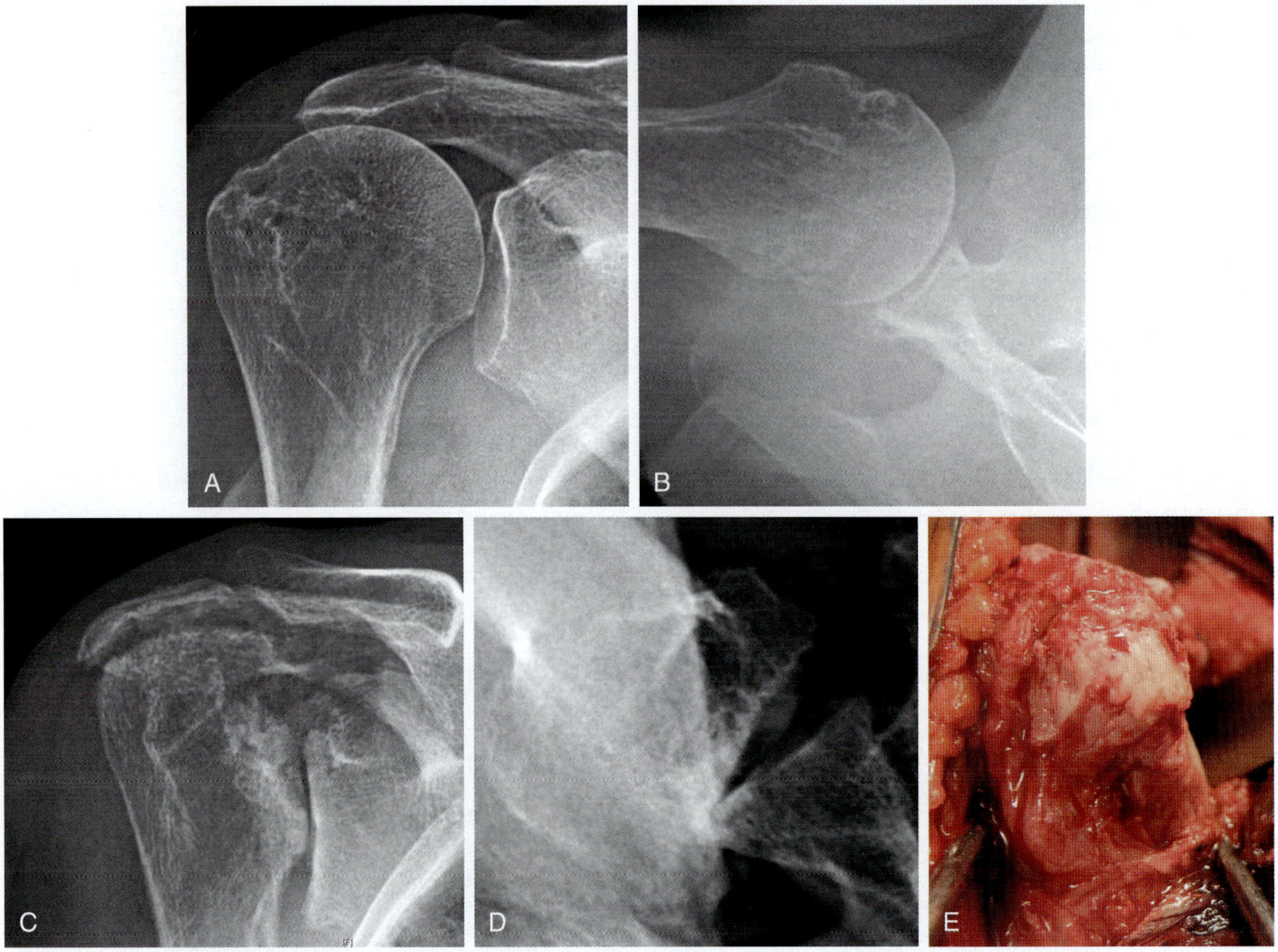

FIGURE 16-134: Rapid-onset glenohumeral arthritis. **A,** Anteroposterior view showing findings typical of a chronic cuff tear. **B,** Axillary view showing slight joint space narrowing. **C,** Anteroposterior view taken 10 months later with no intercurrent injury or evidence of infection. **D,** Axillary view. **E,** Intraoperative image showing destruction of the humeral head.

personal email contact information in case questions arise before and throughout the course of treatment.

Nonoperative Treatment

Activity Modification and Fitness

Most patients with glenohumeral arthritis wish to continue their activities of daily living, work, and recreation, but continued full participation in these activities may lead to aggravation of the arthritis symptoms. As a general principle, work that involves pushing heavy loads or impact loading as well as recreational activities, such as wood chopping or bench pressing, may hasten the progression of the disease process and symptoms. Eliminating these activities through vocational and recreational modification may lessen the symptoms and extend the survival of the natural joint. Occupational therapy may help effect changes in the workplace, as well as suggesting adaptive changes in the home. Modification of sports activity may also be helpful; for example, rowing, swimming, paddling, and two-handed tennis strokes may be better tolerated than handball, martial arts, and vigorous bench pressing. Activities that are disallowed after a surgical reconstruction should be disallowed before surgery to observe the effect on the patient's symptoms. Another important aspect of nonoperative management is optimizing the overall fitness of the patient through regular aerobic exercise; withdrawing from nicotine, alcohol, and narcotics; a healthy diet; and achieving a body mass index less than 25. Improved fitness can improve the feeling of well-being and optimism as well as the safety of surgical intervention, should that become necessary.

Exercises

Glenohumeral joint arthritis is commonly accompanied by stiffness related to contracture and adhesions involving the glenohumeral capsule, the cuff muscles, and the nonarticular humeroscapular motion interface. Disuse or tendon failure can result in weakness of the deltoid and

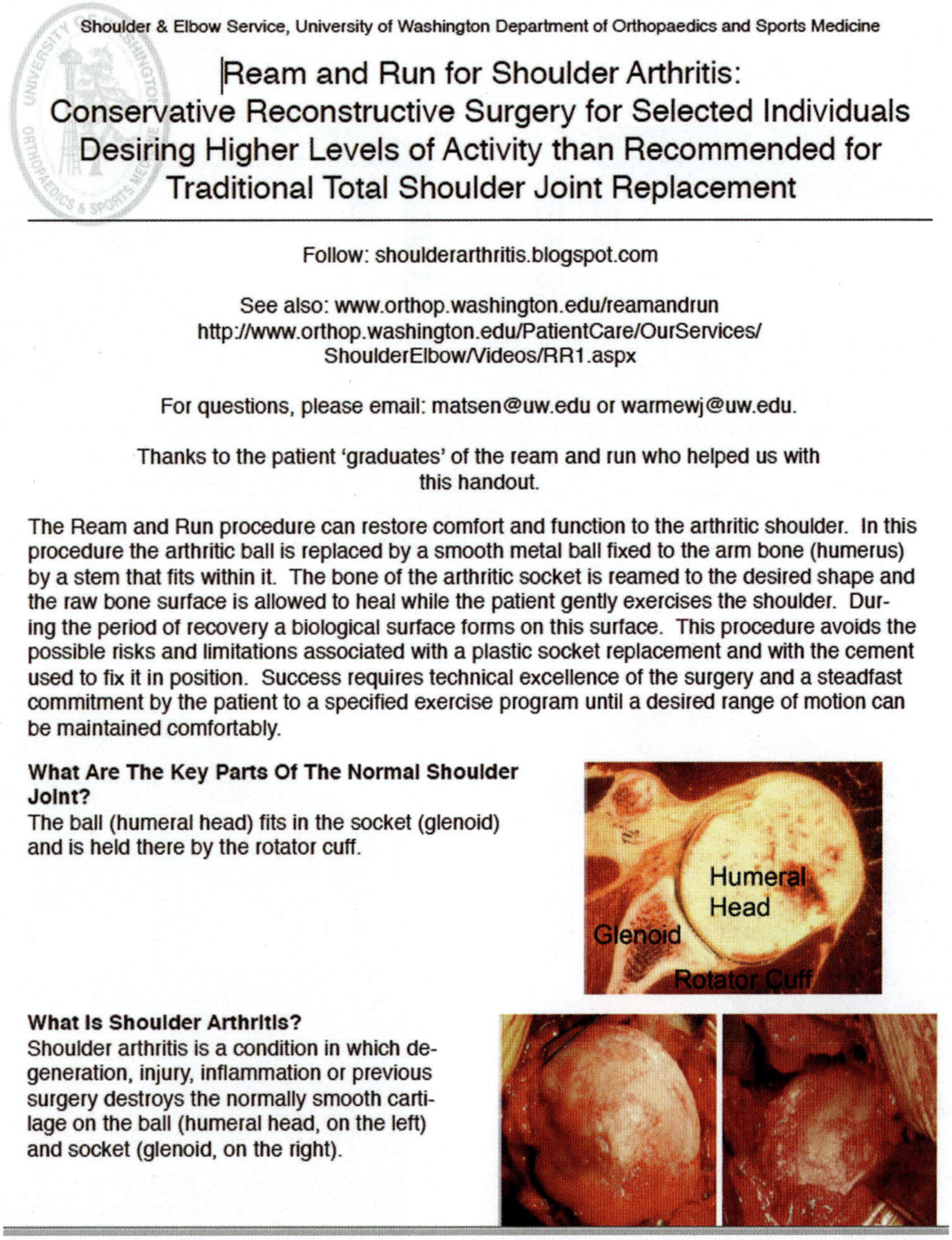
Shoulder & Elbow Service, University of Washington Department of Orthopaedics and Sports Medicine

Ream and Run for Shoulder Arthritis: Conservative Reconstructive Surgery for Selected Individuals Desiring Higher Levels of Activity than Recommended for Traditional Total Shoulder Joint Replacement

Follow: shoulderarthritis.blogspot.com

See also: www.orthop.washington.edu/reamandrun
http://www.orthop.washington.edu/PatientCare/OurServices/ShoulderElbow/Videos/RR1.aspx

For questions, please email: matsen@uw.edu or warmewj@uw.edu.

Thanks to the patient 'graduates' of the ream and run who helped us with this handout.

The Ream and Run procedure can restore comfort and function to the arthritic shoulder. In this procedure the arthritic ball is replaced by a smooth metal ball fixed to the arm bone (humerus) by a stem that fits within it. The bone of the arthritic socket is reamed to the desired shape and the raw bone surface is allowed to heal while the patient gently exercises the shoulder. During the period of recovery a biological surface forms on this surface. This procedure avoids the possible risks and limitations associated with a plastic socket replacement and with the cement used to fix it in position. Success requires technical excellence of the surgery and a steadfast commitment by the patient to a specified exercise program until a desired range of motion can be maintained comfortably.

What Are The Key Parts Of The Normal Shoulder Joint?
The ball (humeral head) fits in the socket (glenoid) and is held there by the rotator cuff.

What Is Shoulder Arthritis?
Shoulder arthritis is a condition in which degeneration, injury, inflammation or previous surgery destroys the normally smooth cartilage on the ball (humeral head, on the left) and socket (glenoid, on the right).

FIGURE 16-135: Educational handouts are useful for informing patients about their disease, the treatment alternatives, and the risks of the different options.

cuff muscles. Instability patterns can also complicate glenohumeral roughness, such as the posterior subluxation characteristic of degenerative joint disease and capsulorrhaphy arthropathy, or the superior subluxation characteristic of CTA.

The mechanics of the shoulder may often be improved by a physician-directed program of gentle range-of-motion and strengthening exercises (Figs. 16-136 to 16-146).[498] Stretching exercises are performed slowly with a full 2-minute hold, allowing time for the muscles to relax and for the tight capsule to be plastically deformed. One of our patients used his electric toothbrush to time his stretches. It is important that vigorous torque and force not be applied in an attempt to regain mobility because of the possibility of causing obligate translation and accelerated wear (see Fig. 16-71; Fig. 16-147). Strengthening exercises must also be gentle, with the resistance limited to a level that allows at least 20 comfortable repetitions. Activities that apply gentle repetitive traction to the joint, such as the pulley (Fig. 16-148), swimming, latissimus pulls (Fig. 16-149), and rowing (Fig. 16-150), seem to be particularly well tolerated. When forward elevation is weak, gentle progression of the

Text continued on p. 888

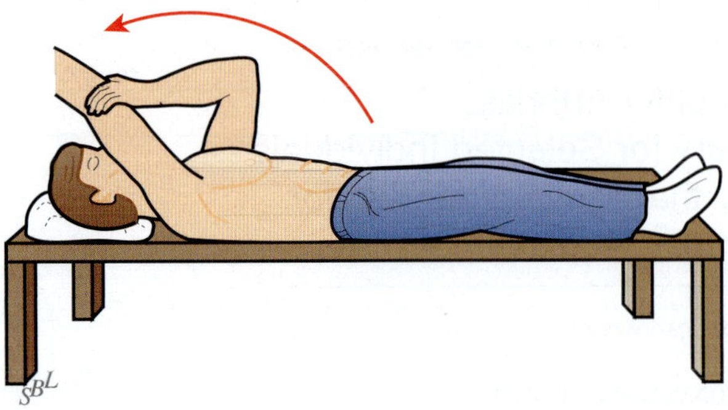

FIGURE 16-136: Stretching in overhead reach, with the opposite arm assisting the movement in place of the therapist. (From Matsen FA III, Lippitt SB, Sidles JA, Harryman DT II. *Practical Evaluation and Management of the Shoulder.* Philadelphia: Saunders; 1994.)

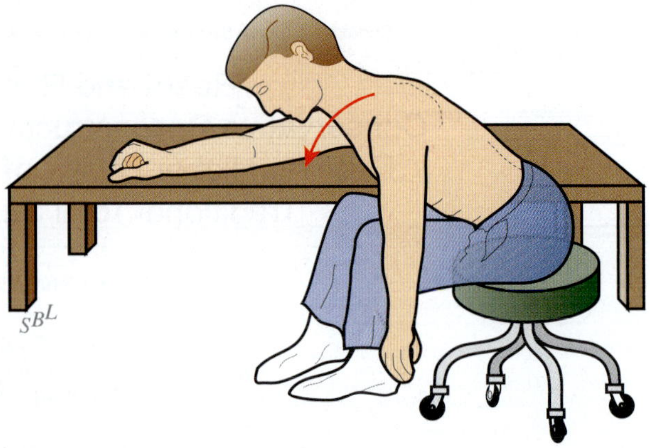

FIGURE 16-137: Stretching in overhead reach with progressive forward leaning used to apply gentle force to the arm. (From Matsen FA III, Lippitt SB, Sidles JA, Harryman DT II. *Practical Evaluation and Management of the Shoulder.* Philadelphia: Saunders; 1994.)

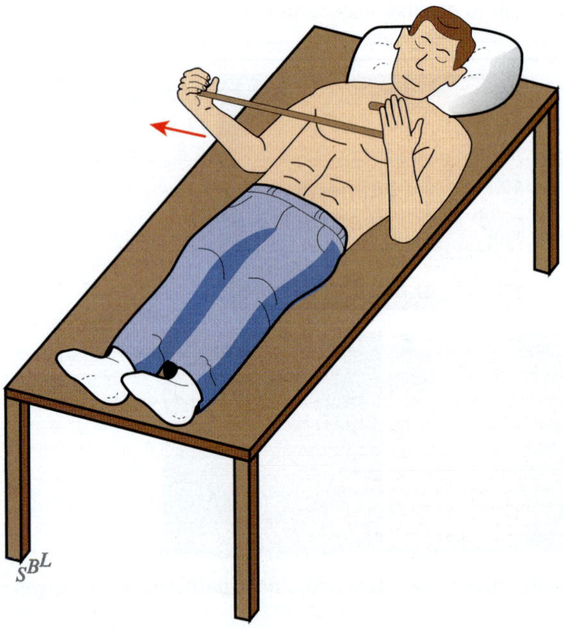

FIGURE 16-138: Stretching in external rotation with the opposite hand used in place of the therapist. (From Matsen FA III, Lippitt SB, Sidles JA, Harryman DT II. *Practical Evaluation and Management of the Shoulder.* Philadelphia: Saunders; 1994.)

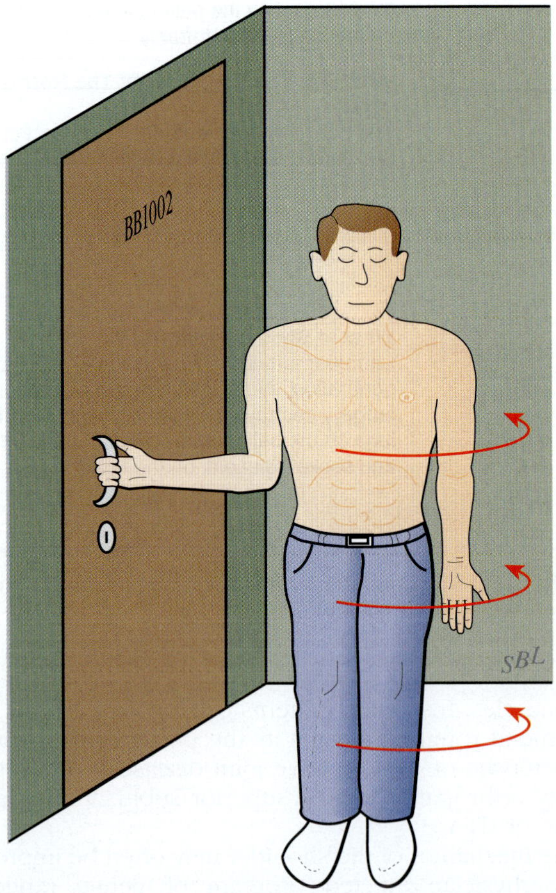

FIGURE 16-139: Stretching in external rotation by turning the body away from a fixed object to apply a gentle stretching force. (From Matsen FA III, Lippitt SB, Sidles JA, Harryman DT II. *Practical Evaluation and Management of the Shoulder.* Philadelphia: Saunders; 1994.)

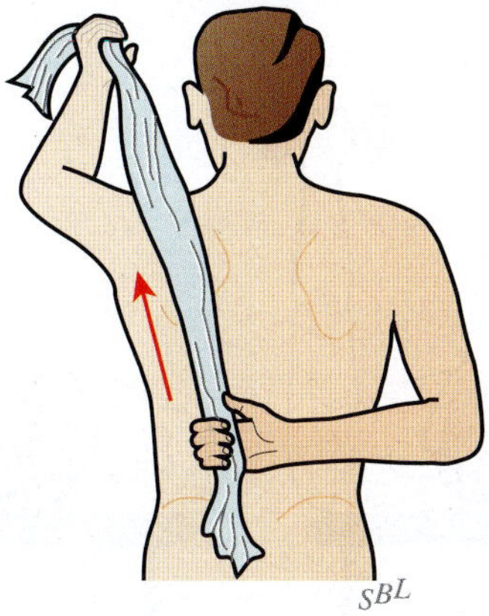

FIGURE 16-140: Stretching in internal rotation with a towel used to apply a gentle stretching force. (From Matsen FA III, Lippitt SB, Sidles JA, Harryman DT II. *Practical Evaluation and Management of the Shoulder.* Philadelphia: Saunders; 1994.)

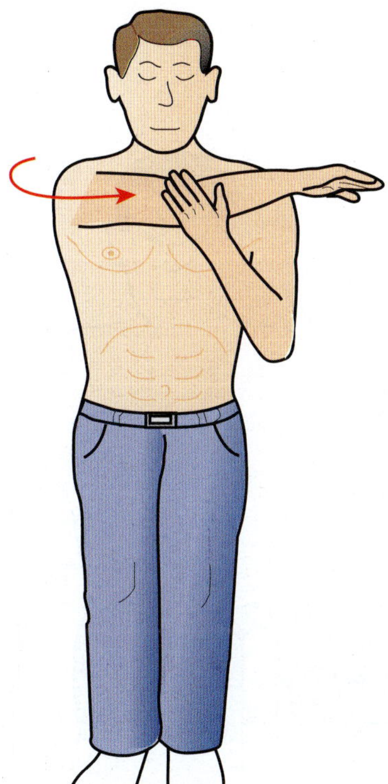

FIGURE 16-141: Stretching in cross body reach with the opposite arm serving in place of the therapist. (From Matsen FA III, Lippitt SB, Sidles JA, Harryman DT II. *Practical Evaluation and Management of the Shoulder.* Philadelphia: Saunders; 1994.)

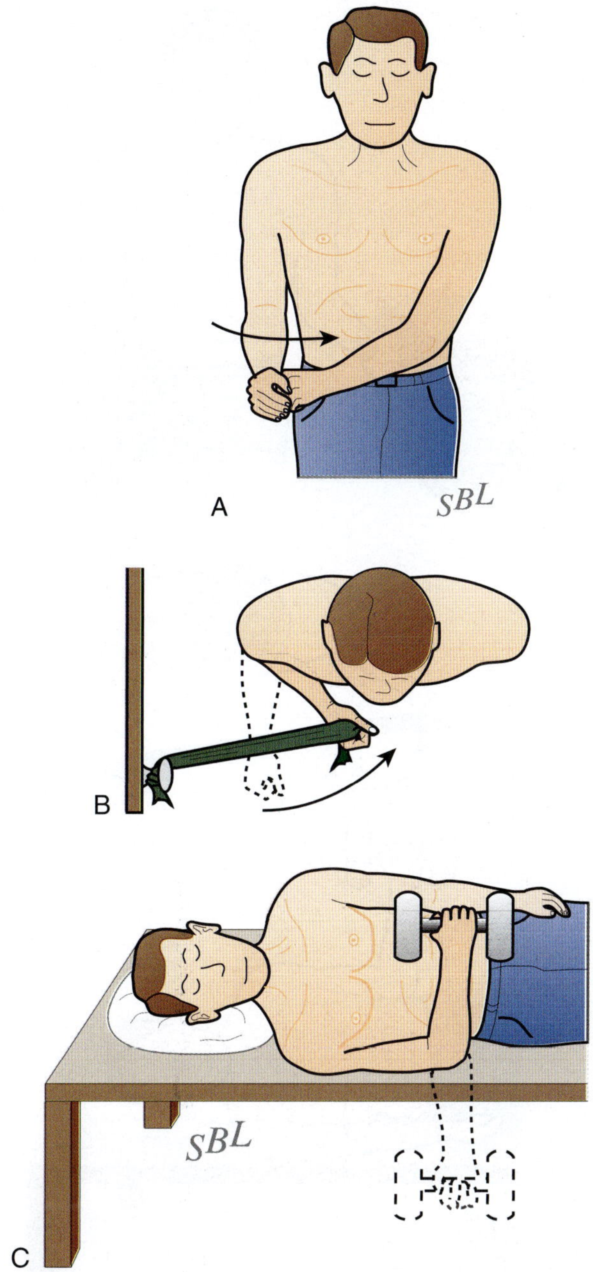

FIGURE 16-142: Internal rotation can be strengthened with **A,** isometrics, **B,** rubber tubing, or **C,** free weights. (From Matsen FA III, Lippitt SB, Sidles JA, Harryman DT II. *Practical Evaluation and Management of the Shoulder.* Philadelphia: Saunders; 1994.)

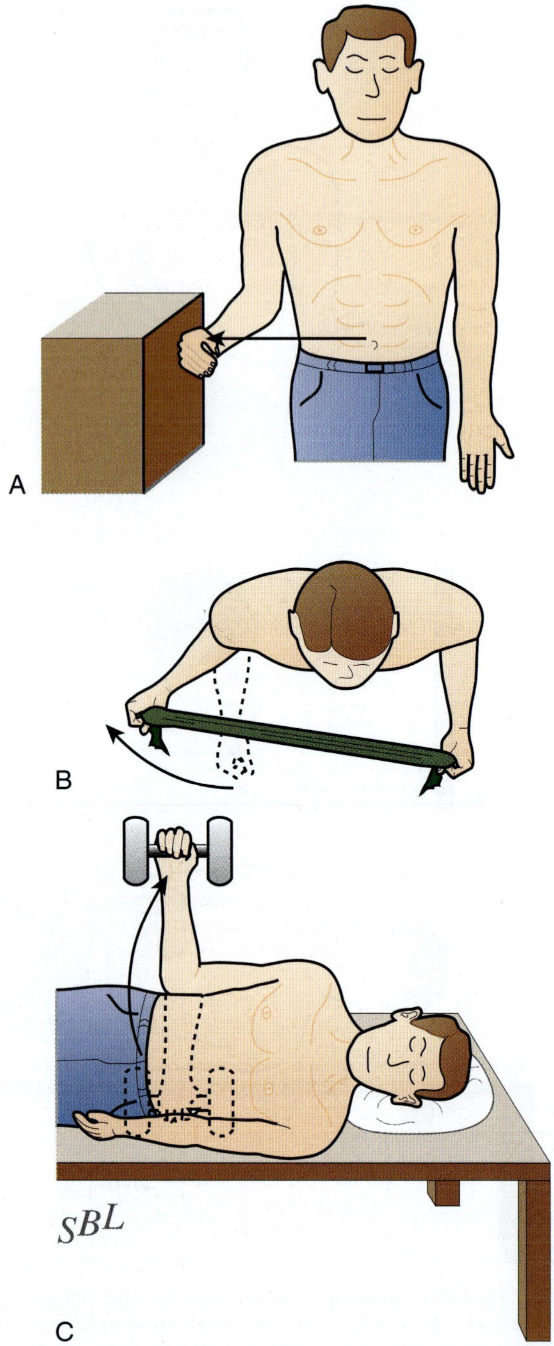

FIGURE 16-143: External rotation strengthening with **A,** isometrics, **B,** rubber tubing, or **C,** free weights. (From Matsen FA III, Lippitt SB, Sidles JA, Harryman DT II. *Practical Evaluation and Management of the Shoulder.* Philadelphia: Saunders; 1994.)

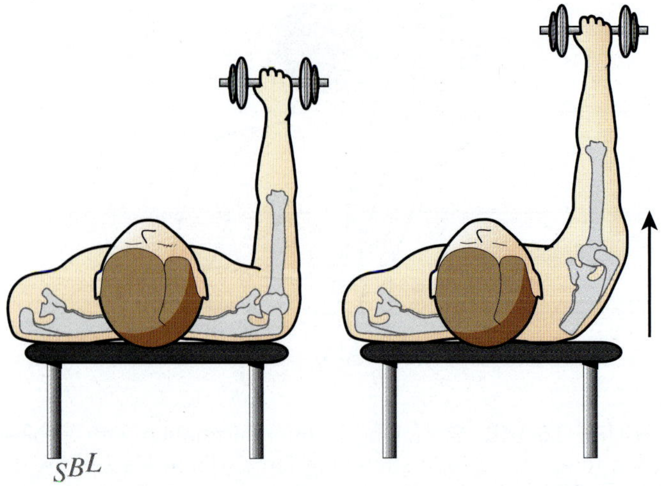

FIGURE 16-144: In the press plus the arm is pushed upward until the shoulder blade is lifted off the table or bed. (From Matsen FA III, Lippitt SB, Sidles JA, Harryman DT II. *Practical Evaluation and Management of the Shoulder.* Philadelphia: Saunders; 1994.)

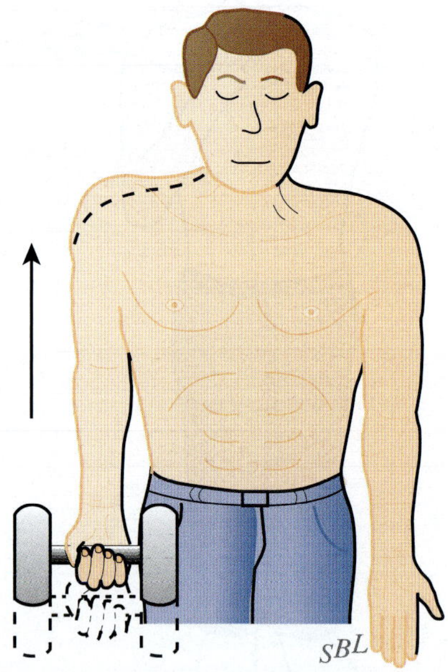

FIGURE 16-145: In the shoulder shrug exercise the tip of the shoulder is lifted toward the ear while the elbow is held straight. (From Matsen FA III, Lippitt SB, Sidles JA, Harryman DT II. *Practical Evaluation and Management of the Shoulder.* Philadelphia: Saunders; 1994.)

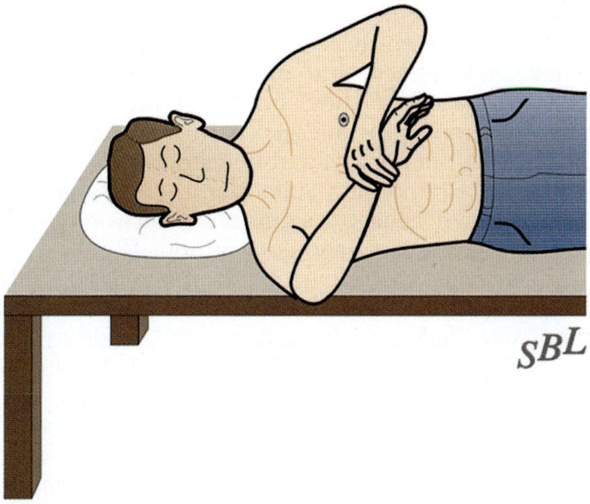

FIGURE 16-146: Sleeper stretch. A gentle internal rotation force is applied to the arm abducted to 90 degrees.

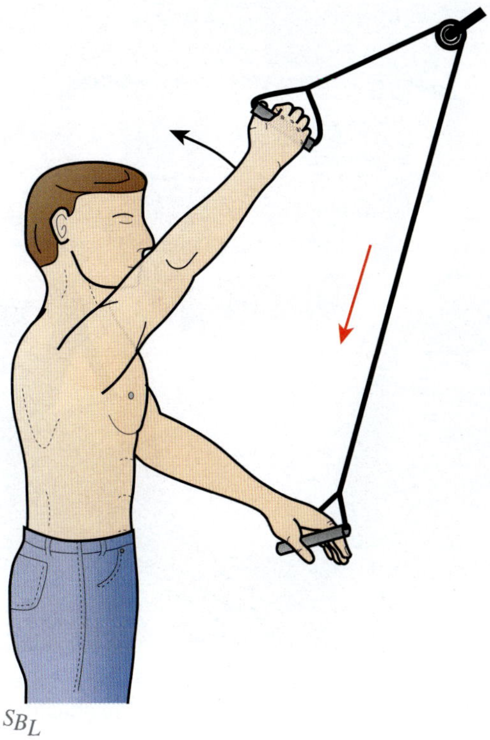

FIGURE 16-148: Door pulley. If the opposite arm is weak or painful, a pulley is useful in helping the arm in elevation. (From Matsen FA III, Lippitt SB. *Shoulder Surgery: Principles and Procedures.* Philadelphia: Saunders; 2004:549.)

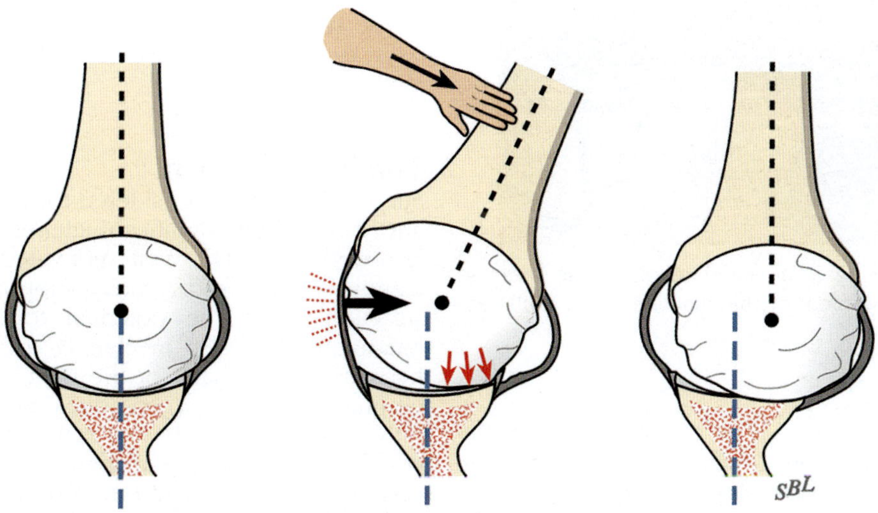

FIGURE 16-147: Forceful torque causes obligate translation leading to accelerated glenoid wear.

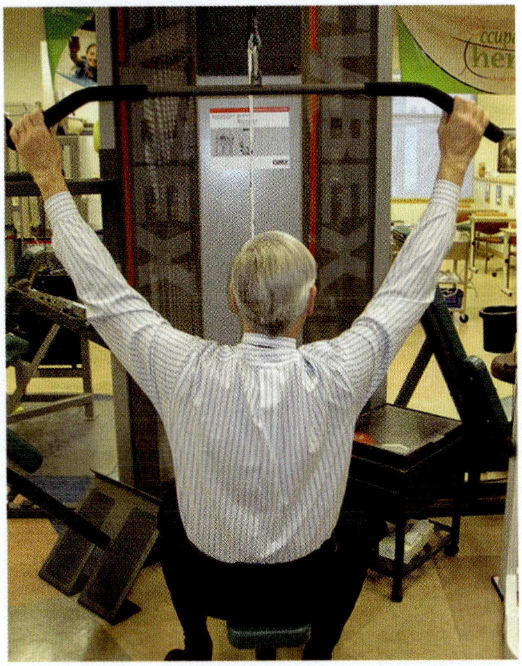

FIGURE 16-149: The lateral pulldown is a useful rehabilitative exercise because it enables movement of the shoulder while a distraction force is applied.

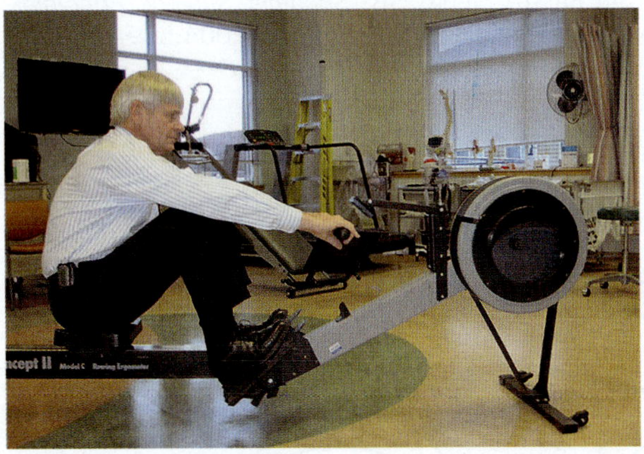

FIGURE 16-150: Rowing is a useful rehabilitative exercise because it enables movement of the shoulder while a distraction force is applied.

supine press (Fig. 16-151) can be helpful in improving active shoulder motion, even with what seems to be pseudoparalysis. When posterior stability is compromised, gentle external rotator strengthening may help restore the centering of the humeral head (Fig. 16-152).

Medication

In the management of most forms of arthritis, nonsteroidal antiinflammatory medication and mild analgesics may be useful adjuncts to the exercise program. In our practice we often recommend that the patient discuss with their primary care physician the use of naproxen 275 mg to 550 mg orally twice a day or another similar medication. However, even these relatively benign medications can have side effects and unwanted interactions with other medications; if they are taken for an extended period, monitoring for allergic, gastrointestinal, hepatic, renal, cardiac, pulmonary, and hematopoietic side effects is important. Chondroitin sulfate and glucosamine have not been shown to have a significant effect on the symptoms or progression of shoulder arthritis.[148]

The medical management of rheumatoid arthritis includes traditional disease-modifying drugs, including methotrexate, leflunomide, sulfasalazine, hydroxychloroquine, cyclosporine, azathioprine, D-penicillamine, and gold (oral or intramuscular). For patients who do not respond to this class of medications, rheumatologists may turn to biologic response modifying agents. These drugs are engineered proteins designed to inhibit specific components of the immune system that fuel the inflammation in rheumatoid arthritis. They include tocilizumab (Actemra), certolizumab pegol (Cimzia), etanercept (Enbrel), adalimumab (Humira), anakinra (Kineret), abatacept (Orencia), infliximab (Remicade), rituximab (Rituxan), and golimumab (Simponi). Both classes of drugs may affect the safety of surgical interventions, reducing healing time and increasing the risk of neurologic complications and infection; consultation is therefore recommended to determine the recommended time for preoperative dosage modification or discontinuance.[225]

Injections

Although injections of steroids[528] or viscosupplementation[55,400,499,529] have been used in pursuit of the temporary relief of symptoms, the evidence in support of their use is weak at best.[239,278] We generally avoid them because of the risk of cartilage damage and allergic reactions as well as the possibility of introducing bacteria into the joint.[135,294,447]

Surgical Treatment

Surgery should be considered for patients with refractory and functionally significant glenohumeral arthritis who are well informed, well motivated, cooperative, sufficiently healthy, and socially supported. Surgical reconstruction offers the potential to optimize soft tissue balance and muscle mechanics as well as the smoothness, size, and shape of the joint surfaces. It should be emphasized that surgery does not "fix" the problem; rather, it provides a basis for the patient to improve the comfort and function of their shoulder through a concerted rehabilitation effort. Although prosthetic arthroplasty is the primary surgical option to be considered when major pain and functional loss result from glenohumeral arthritis, other surgical alternatives may be useful in selected cases.

Arthroscopic

Considerations

Patients sometimes ask, "Why can't you just use an arthroscope to clean the arthritis out of my shoulder?" We know,

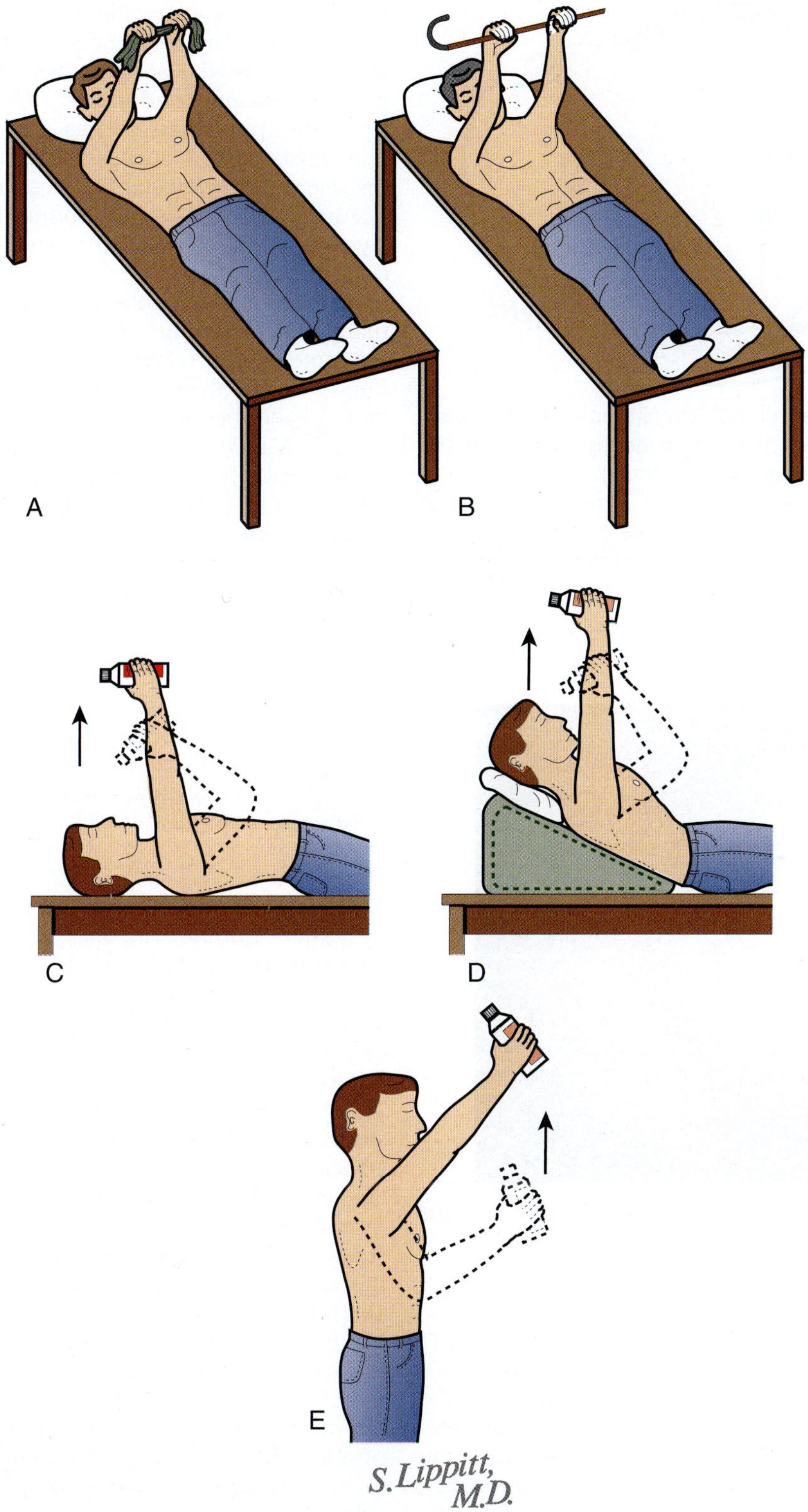

FIGURE 16-151: Incremental press. Integrated forward elevation is developed through a series of exercises that can be progressed in small increments. **A,** With the patient in the supine position, the two hands are placed close to each other on a light stick and both are pressed upward toward the ceiling. **B,** The same exercise is repeated with the arms progressively farther apart. **C,** The arm performs the supine press unassisted. Small amounts of weight are added to the hand until 2 lb can be pressed upward 20 times. **D,** The patient's back is elevated slightly while the weight is pressed vertically upward. The amount of elevation is increased when 2 lb can be pressed upward 20 times. **E,** The progression is continued until the exercise can be performed with the back in a vertical position. (From Matsen FA III, Lippitt SB. *Shoulder Surgery: Principles and Procedures.* Philadelphia: WB Saunders; 2004:344.)

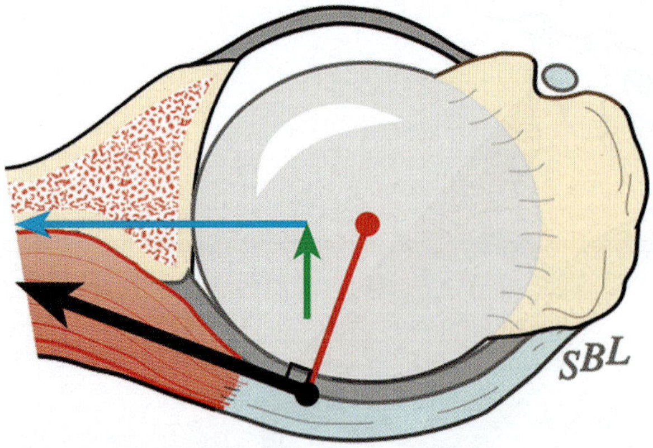

FIGURE 16-152: External rotation strengthening helps center the posterioriorly subluxed humeral head by increasing the anterior displacement force (green arrow). Contraction of the infraspinatus causes a force (black arrow) tangential to the point of contact with the humeral head. The force vector can be resolved into an anterior displacement force on the humeral head (green arrow) and a compression force into the glenoid (blue arrow).

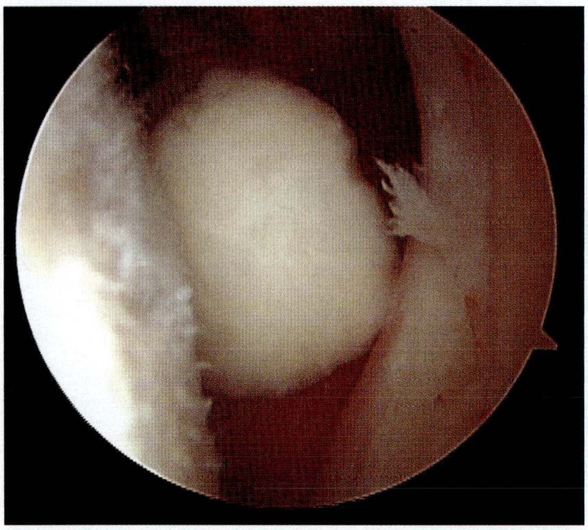

FIGURE 16-153: Loose body delivered by palpation from the subscapularis recess.

however, that because glenohumeral arthritis is a condition in which articular cartilage is lost, the arthritis cannot be "cleaned out." In most cases simply removing the osteophytes will not improve shoulder comfort and function unless the osteophytes are clearly restricting the range of motion and the joint surfaces are functional. Aspects of glenohumeral arthritis that could potentially be addressed arthroscopically include loose body removal (Fig. 16-153), the release of capsular contracture, and resection of synovitis in cases of inflammatory arthropathy refractory to medical management.[509] Beneficial results have been reported from arthroscopic debridement for glenohumeral arthritis without or with microfracture and without or with glenoid recontouring.[4,22,32,249,297,310,507,584] However, rigorous evaluation of the outcome is complicated by the inconsistent inclusion of procedures, such as surgery on the subacromial space, acromioclavicular joint, or biceps tendon.[351,361,371,512] It can be concluded from the published results for arthroscopic treatment that this can be successful in early instances of the disease before substantial destruction of the joint has occurred or for osteochondral lesions that are localized.[38,120,187,249,371,435] Because such mildly involved shoulders may also improve with nonoperative management, it is important to determine the value of arthroscopic management using carefully controlled studies. The outcome of arthroscopic debridement is worse for shoulders with involvement of the joint surfaces of both the glenoid and the humerus, that is, true glenohumeral arthritis.[265,557] A recent systematic review found that there was insufficient evidence to support the routine use of arthroscopic debridement for glenohumeral arthritis.[385] Another concluded that isolated arthroscopic debridement and capsular release did not provide sufficient benefit to justify its use in most patients.[507] Microfracture appears to be of little benefit except for small localized defects in either the humeral or the glenoid joint surface.[149,362] It is important to note that arthroscopic surgery is still surgery, carrying costs and risks. A carefully controlled trial found that arthroscopic surgery for arthritis of the knee was no more effective than sham surgery (which, by the way, resulted in significant clinical improvement, illustrating the need for surgical controls).[374]

Open

Debridement and Capsular Release

In a small number of cases of early arthritis—especially where there is substantial limitation of motion with relatively preserved joint surfaces—a debridement and capsular release may be considered for patients who wish to avoid a prosthetic arthroplasty, although it should be recognized that subsequent surgery may well be needed. This procedure is performed through the same skin incision as would be used for a joint replacement (Fig. 16-154). The shoulder is approached through a subscapularis tenotomy (Fig. 16-155), and adhesions in the humeroscapular motion interface are released (Fig. 16-156). The subscapularis is released from the glenoid along with the attached subjacent anterior capsule (Figs. 16-157 to 16-160) to allow a good range of passive motion (Fig. 16-161). If there is a tendency for posterior instability, the capsular release is limited to the anterior aspect of the glenoid (Fig. 16-162). Loose bodies, osteophytes, and interfering soft tissue are removed. The joint is thoroughly irrigated and gently manipulated to achieve the maximum possible range of passive motion, and the subscapularis is securely repaired (Fig. 16-163). After surgery, a range of assisted motion exercises are immediately implemented. As with arthroscopic debridement, data on the effectiveness of this procedure are limited. We use it sparingly in cases of relatively early arthritis, especially in capsulorrhaphy arthropathy, where the anterior soft tissues have previously been tightened in the treatment of anterior instability (see Fig. 16-87).[211,316]

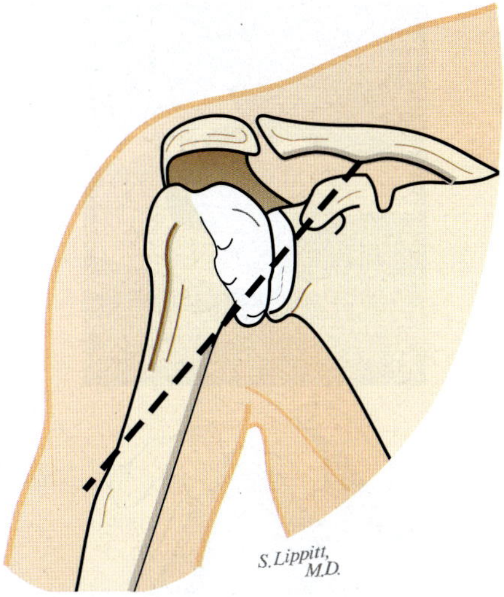

FIGURE 16-154: Incision. The skin incision for the extended deltopectoral approach (dashed line) uses the mid-clavicle, the tip of the coracoid process, and the deltoid tuberosity of the midhumerus as landmarks. It is important that the incision avoid the axillary crease; otherwise, painful scarring might result. (From Matsen FA III, Lippitt SB. *Shoulder Surgery: Principles and Procedures.* Philadelphia: Saunders; 2004:515.)

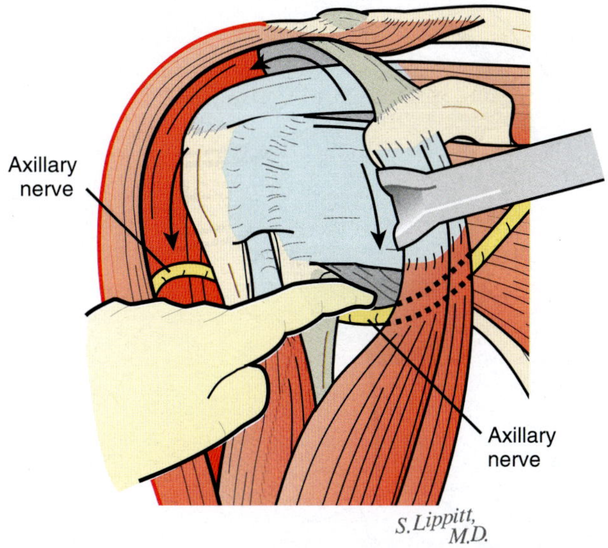

FIGURE 16-156: Nerve-to-nerve release. All scar tissue in the humeroscapular motion interface (arrows) is released medially from the axillary nerve as it crosses the subscapularis, then under the coracoid, under the coracoacromial ligament, under the acromion, and finally under the deltoid to the axillary nerve posteriorly as it exits the quadrilateral space. (From Matsen FA III, Lippitt SB. *Shoulder Surgery: Principles and Procedures.* Philadelphia: Saunders; 2004:517.)

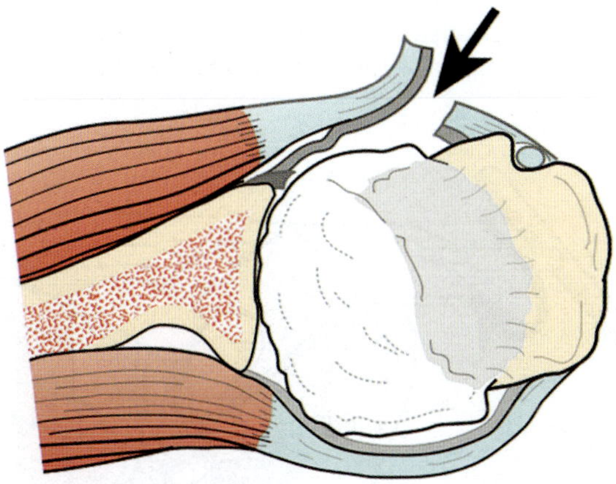

FIGURE 16-155: Subscapularis tenotomy approach. The subscapularis tendon is divided medial to its insertion on the lesser tuberosity.

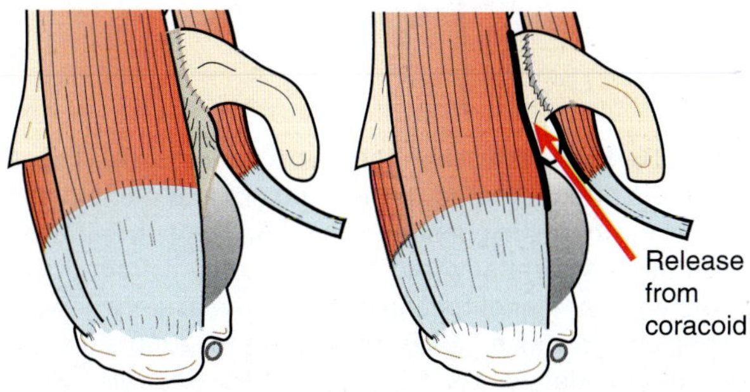

FIGURE 16-157: Releasing the coracohumeral ligament. The coracohumeral ligament is released from the base of the coracoid process, allowing unrestricted gliding of the supraspinatus as well as the subscapularis. (From Matsen FA III, Lippitt SB. *Shoulder Surgery: Principles and Procedures.* Philadelphia: Saunders; 2004:519.)

Synovectomy

The management of rheumatoid arthritis has been substantially improved through the use of disease-modifying agents (e.g., Plaquenil, cyclosporine, methotrexate, Cytoxan, Imuran, and Azulfidine) and biologics (e.g., Enbrel, Humira, Orencia, Remicade, and Rituxan). Before the availability of these medications, synovectomy and other nonprosthetic options were commonly used to remove inflammatory tissue from the glenohumeral joint.[33,263,264,510,542,562] Currently, synovectomy is used primarily to manage refractory synovitis and bursitis in the absence of major joint surface damage (Fig. 16-164).[413,509]

Resection

Before prostheses were available, resection of the humeral head was used to manage arthritis and severe fractures.[161,324,358,523,561] In general, comfort and function after resection arthroplasty are poor and so its current use is

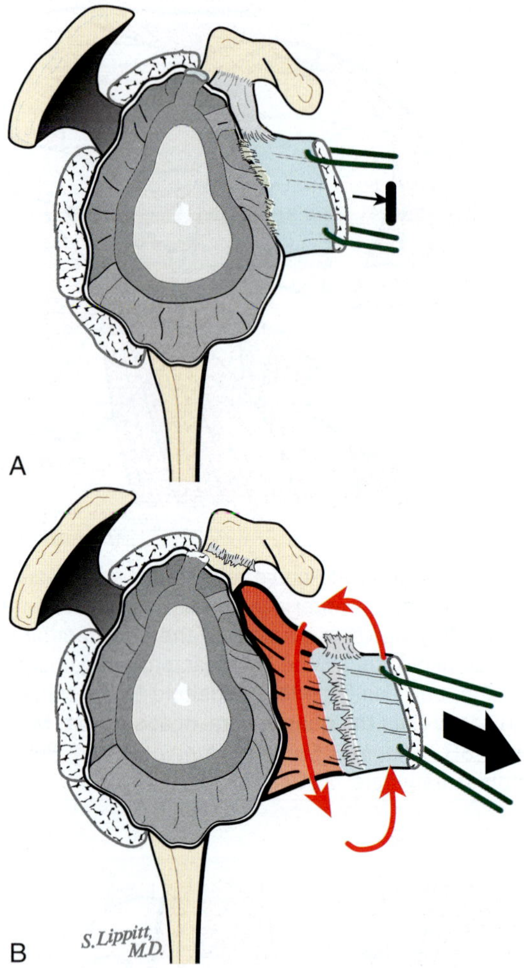

FIGURE 16-158: Releasing the subscapularis. **A,** The subscapularis is often tethered to the coracoid and glenoid via the capsule, limiting its excursion (arrow). **B,** The subscapularis is released circumferentially (red arrow), freeing it from the coracoid, the anterior glenohumeral capsule, the axillary nerve, and the coracoid muscles, allowing increased excursion (black arrow). (From Matsen FA III, Lippitt SB. *Shoulder Surgery: Principles and Procedures.* Philadelphia: Saunders; 2004:519.)

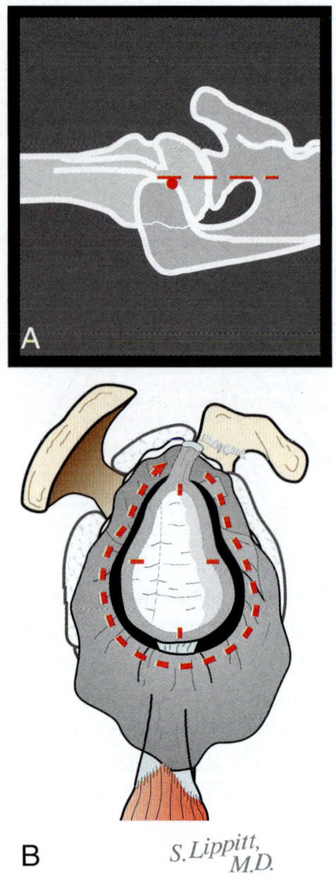

FIGURE 16-159: A 360-degree capsular release. **A,** The glenoid here is concentrically worn and the shoulder is tight. **B,** An extralabral release is therefore performed 360 degrees around the perimeter of the glenoid (red dashed line).

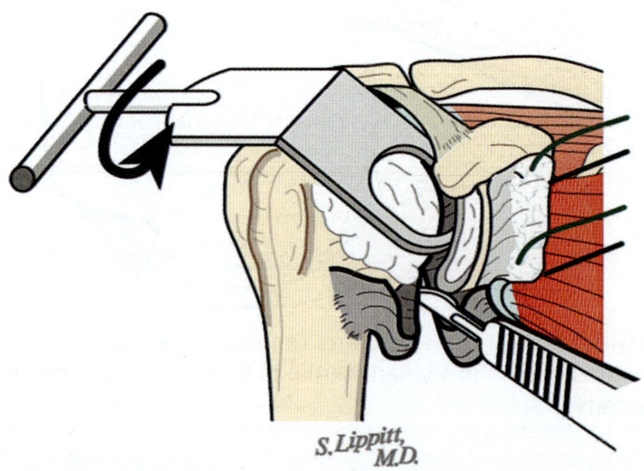

FIGURE 16-160: Posterior capsular release. If the posterior capsule is tight, it can be released under direct vision by rotating the inferior aspect of the retractor away from the glenoid and gently internally rotating the humerus.

primarily for refractory infection or for failed arthroplasty without other means of reconstruction (Figs. 16-165 to 16-167).[376]

Arthrodesis

Considerations

Glenohumeral arthrodesis is usually reserved for attempts at salvaging septic arthritis or complex deficiencies of the joint surface associated with permanent loss of the cuff and deltoid.[37,102,475] The best candidates for this procedure are shoulders that meet the following criteria: (1) permanent and severe weakness because of loss of cuff and deltoid function; (2) good scapular motors (e.g., trapezius, levator scapulae, pectoralis, serratus anterior, and rhomboids); and (3) sufficient residual glenoid and humeral bone stock to enable the fusion. Patients considering this procedure should have a strong motivation to succeed, minimal complaints of pain, and a good understanding of the following: (1) the potential complications of a shoulder fusion (including fracture of the

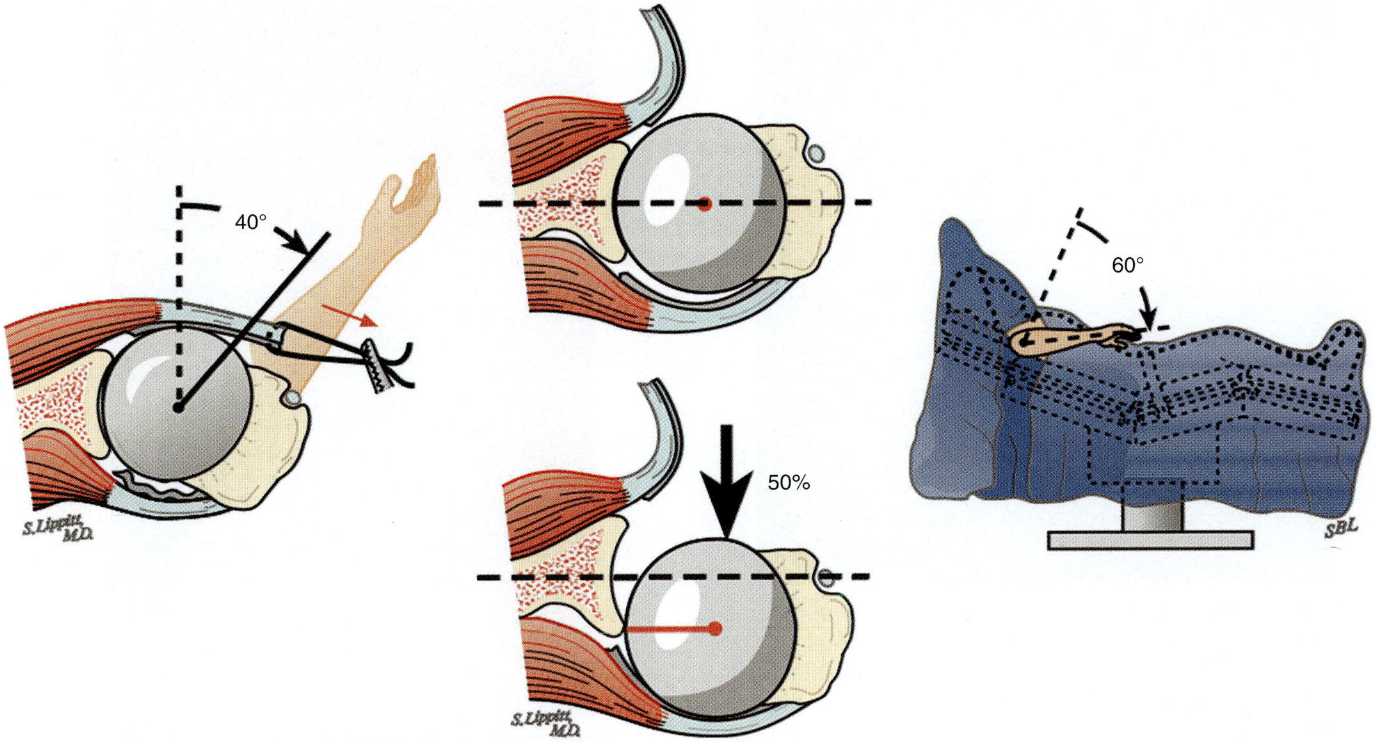

FIGURE 16-161: The 40-50-60 rule for appropriate soft tissue tensioning is as follows: at least 40 degrees external rotation with a reapproximated subscapularis tendon (left), 50% posterior subluxation on the posterior drawer test (middle), and 60 degrees of internal rotation of the 90-degree abducted arm (right).

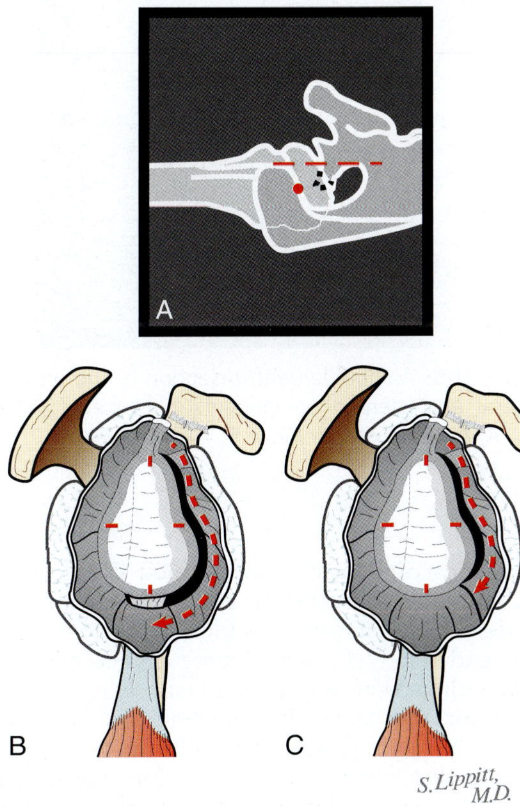

FIGURE 16-162: A, The preoperative axillary view shows posterior subluxation of the humeral head and posterior glenoid wear. **B,** The extralabral release (red dashed line) then includes only the anterior capsule. **C,** If the posterior instability is substantial, the release (red dashed line) stops at the inferior glenohumeral ligament.

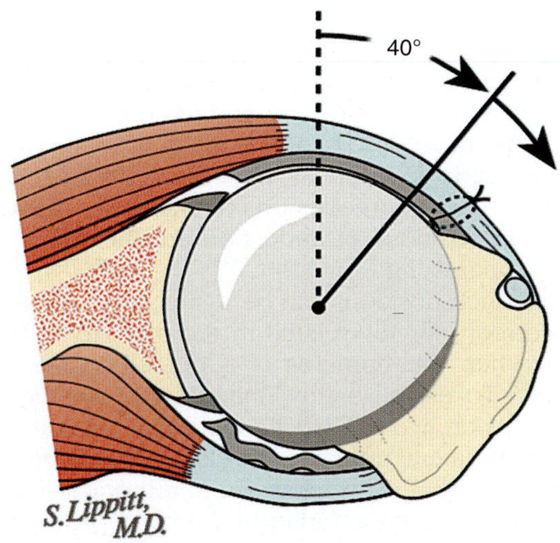

FIGURE 16-163: Anatomic repair of the subscapularis tendon should allow at least 40 degrees of external rotation.

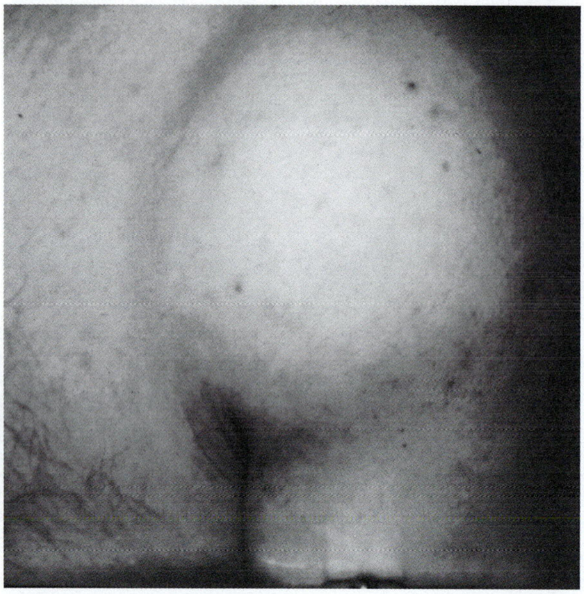

FIGURE 16-164: The shoulder of a young man with rheumatoid arthritis and primary rheumatoid involvement of the subacromial-subdeltoid bursa. The rotator cuff was intact, and the glenohumeral joint had minimal involvement with rheumatoid synovitis. The patient had a full, minimally painful range of motion in the shoulder, with excellent shoulder strength. The hypertrophic bursitis did not respond to medical management, and the bursa was surgically excised.

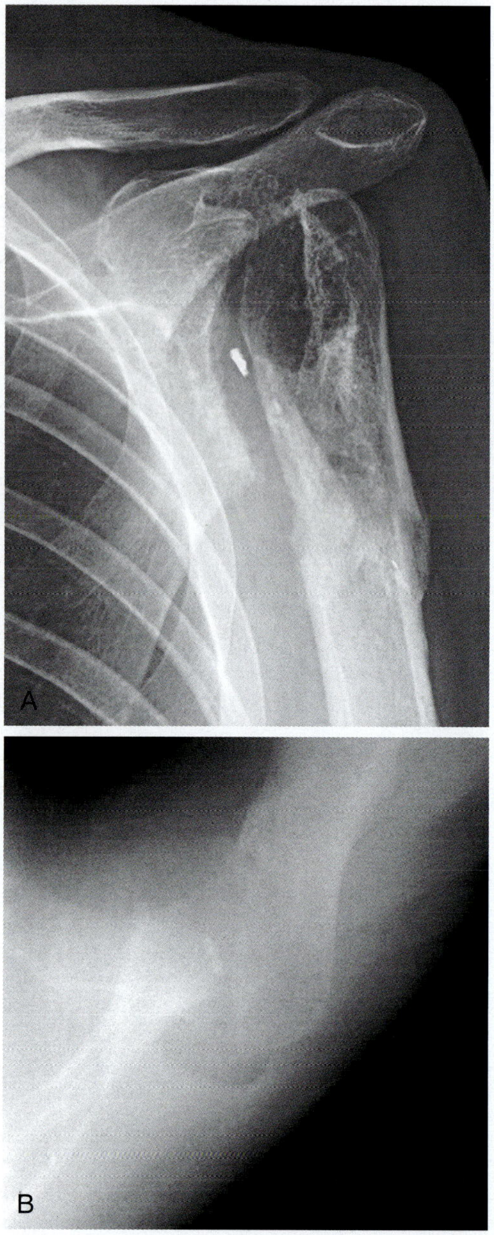

FIGURE 16-165: A shoulder with resection of the total shoulder humeral and glenoid components because of refractory infection. **A,** Anteroposterior view. **B,** Axillary view.

humerus below the fusion); (2) the resultant limitation of internal and external rotation; and (3) the possible need for a second procedure to add bone graft to augment the fixation if the fusion does not "take" on the first attempt.

In the past, surgeons recommended fusing the shoulder in positions of abduction and flexion with the aim of optimizing function.[28,214,349,453,467,468,472,475,554,575,583] However, such positions can be associated with substantial discomfort, largely related to the need to "wing" the scapula when the humerus is adducted to the resting position.[87] To establish the limitations of function after shoulder fusion, we studied 12 shoulders that had undergone glenohumeral arthrodesis at least 2 years before the time of study.[205,338] The mean humerothoracic elevation in the plus 90-degree (anterior sagittal) plane was 47 degrees, the mean elevation in the minus 90-degree (posterior sagittal) plane was 22 degrees, the mean humerothoracic external rotation was 9 degrees, and the mean internal rotation was 46 degrees. These ranges of motion were similar to the scapulothoracic motion measured in normal subjects.[205] Only one patient could reach his hair without bending his neck forward, five could reach their perineum, six could reach their back pocket, seven could reach the opposite axilla, and ten could reach their side pocket. We conducted a second study of normal in vivo shoulder kinematics to predict the functions that would be allowed by various positions of glenohumeral arthrodesis.[338] This indicated that activities of daily living could best be performed if the joint was fused in 15 degrees of flexion, 15 degrees of abduction, and 45 degrees of internal rotation. This low angle of elevation and relatively high degree of internal rotation facilitated sitting comfortably on a chair; lying flat in bed; and reaching the face, the opposite axilla, and the perineum. Thus our preferred position is the "15,15,45" combination described above, a position that minimizes protrusion of the shoulder blade posteriorly into the chair or bed when the arm is at the side.[205] This position has the additional advantages of being easy to determine at surgery and needing only a sling for postoperative immobilization rather than a cast or brace. It is most important to avoid fusing the shoulder in neutral or external rotation because this position precludes reaching the mouth or perineum.

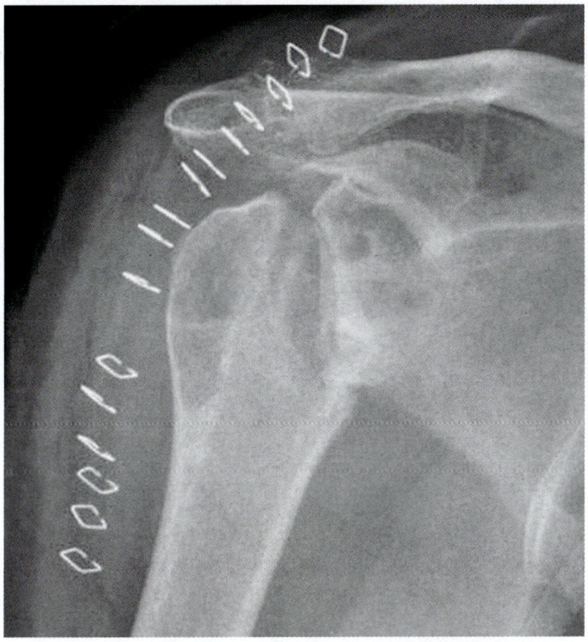

FIGURE 16-166: Resection for a failed arthroplasty.

Many techniques have been described for shoulder arthrodesis.* When possible, our preferred method is an intra-articular fusion that preserves the deltoid, most of the rotator cuff, and most of the bone of the glenohumeral joint, allowing the potential for later conversion to a reverse shoulder arthroplasty. If necessary for stability, however, a neutralization plate can be contoured over the scapular spine and down the humerus, but this risks denervating the anterior and part of the lateral deltoid. A vascularized fibular graft has been recommended when there is bone deficiency.[37]

Technique

The patient is placed in the beach chair position with the scapula in the prepared field and the arm draped free. The operative approach is through an anterior deltopectoral incision, with superior extension of the incision if plate fixation is used. We have used a low anterior axillary incision when cosmesis is a concern and intra-articular fusion is planned.

Any residual articular cartilage on the humerus or glenoid is curetted down to raw subchondral bone, as removing the subchondral bone weakens the construct and makes solid glenohumeral compression more difficult to achieve (Figs. 16-168 and 16-169). The supraspinatus tendon is resected from between the humeral head and the acromion, and the undersurface of the acromion

References 28, 30, 39, 61, 77, 83, 87, 98, 102, 122, 210, 229, 251, 256, 301, 347, 349, 380, 450-453, 467, 472, 473, 475, 554, 575, 583.

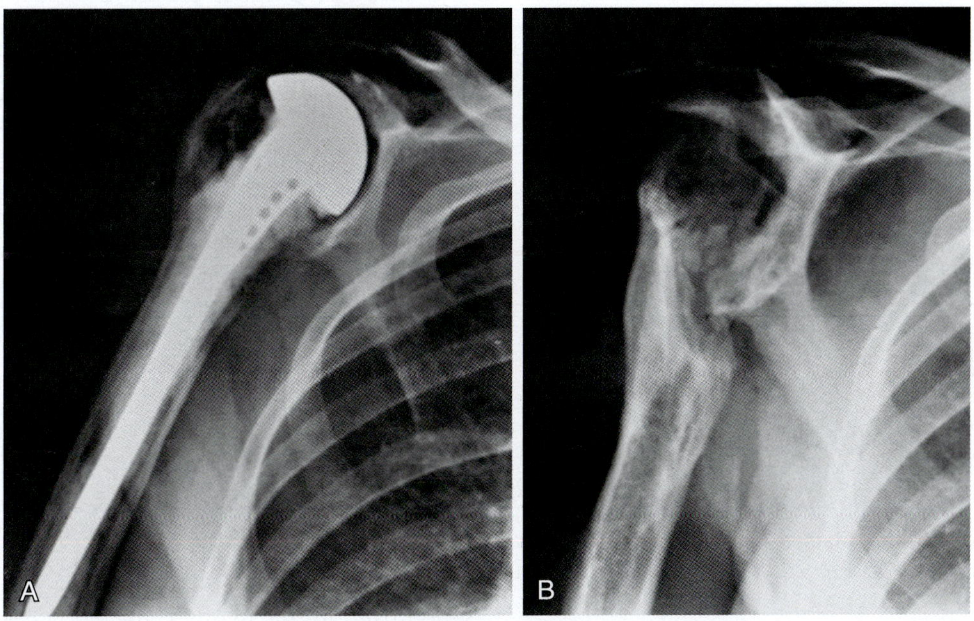

FIGURE 16-167: A proximal humeral prosthetic replacement had previously been placed in an elderly woman with multiple-joint osteoarthritis. **A,** Her total knee arthroplasty became infected, and the infection spread to the proximal humeral prosthetic replacement. The shoulder region was brawny and erythematous, with a draining sinus on the anterolateral aspect of the arm. The region was debrided and the prosthesis and cement removed. **B,** Radiographic appearance of the joint after delayed primary closure. At follow-up, the patient had only mild pain, and the shoulder was stable because of fibrosis. She had active abduction of 65 degrees and external rotation of 10 degrees.

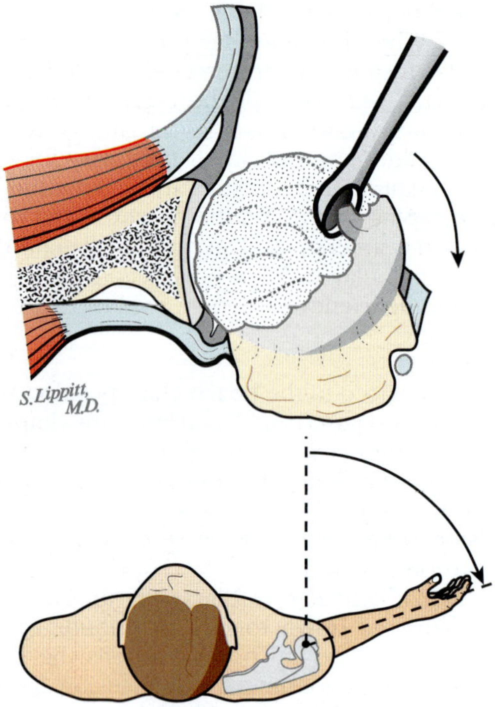

FIGURE 16-168: Humeral head curettage. The articular cartilage is removed from the head of the humerus without sacrificing subchondral bone. Access to the joint surface is achieved by external rotation. (From Matsen FA III, Lippitt SB. *Shoulder Surgery: Principles and Procedures.* Philadelphia: Saunders; 2004:236.)

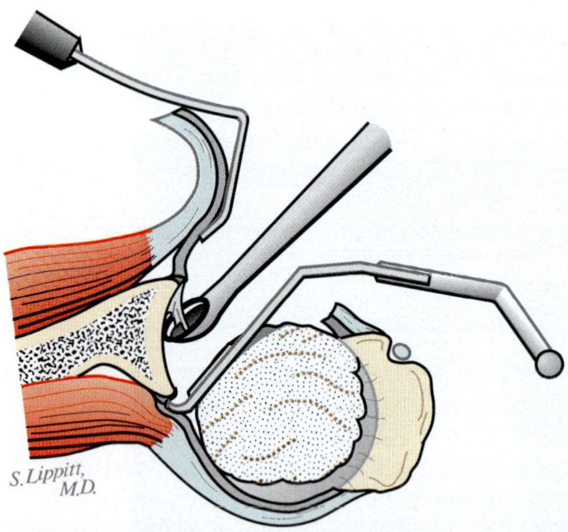

FIGURE 16-169: Glenoid curettage. The articular cartilage of the glenoid is removed with a curette without compromising the subchondral bone. (From Matsen FA III, Lippitt SB. *Shoulder Surgery: Principles and Procedures.* Philadelphia: Saunders; 2004:237.)

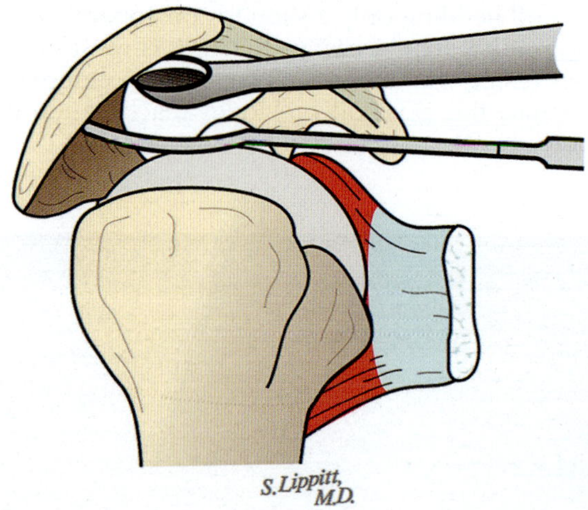

FIGURE 16-170: Acromion curettage. The periosteum of the acromial undersurface is curetted without compromising the cortical bone.

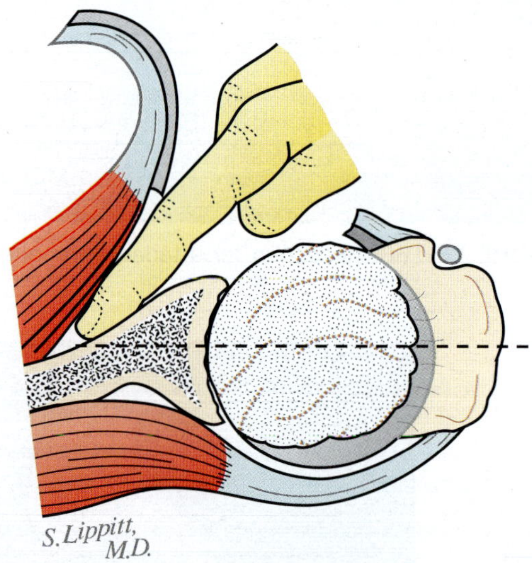

FIGURE 16-171: Identifying the subscapularis fossa. The anterior aspect of the glenoid neck is palpated. This area will be the target for the compression screws. (From Matsen FA III, Lippitt SB. *Shoulder Surgery: Principles and Procedures.* Philadelphia: Saunders; 2004:239.)

is stripped down to raw bone (Fig. 16-170). The soft tissues are lifted from the anterior glenoid neck so that the subscapularis fossa can be palpated (Fig. 16-171).

The humeral head is centered in the glenoid with the arm in 15 degrees of abduction, 15 degrees of flexion, and 45 degrees of internal rotation (Fig. 16-172). It is temporarily fixed with three long 3.2-mm drill bits; these should exit the neck of the scapula anteriorly approximately 2 cm medial to the glenoid lip, where their tips can be palpated and controlled (Figs. 16-173 and 16-174). When used in this manner, the known length of the drill bits can serve as depth gauges to determine the length of screws needed. The position of the arm is checked by making sure that the hand can reach the mouth, the anterior perineum, and the contralateral axilla. The 3.2-mm drill bits are sequentially replaced by fully threaded 6.5-mm cancellous screws with washers

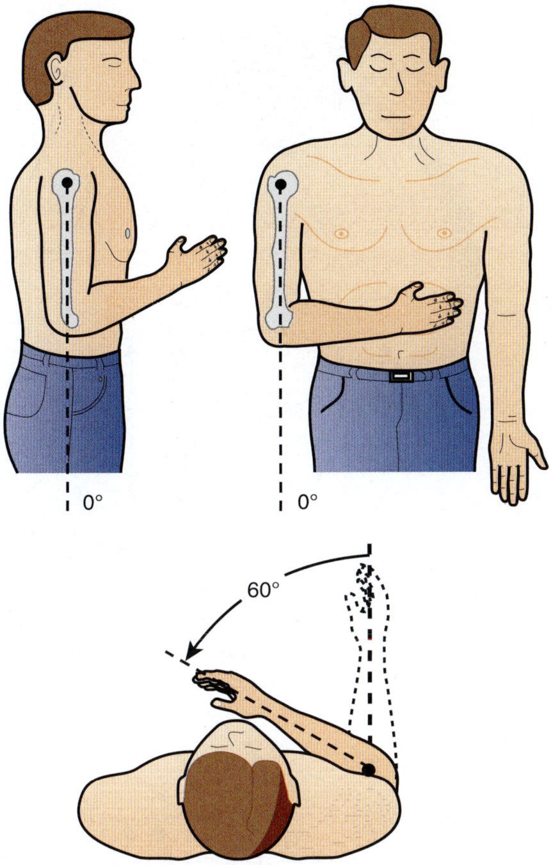

FIGURE 16-172: For many patients, the most comfortable position of fusion is that of 0 degrees of flexion, 0 degrees of abduction, and 60 degrees of internal rotation. This position allows the scapula to sit in its normal position on the chest wall while the arm is at the side. (From Matsen FA III, Lippitt SB. *Shoulder Surgery: Principles and Procedures.* Philadelphia: Saunders; 2004:239.)

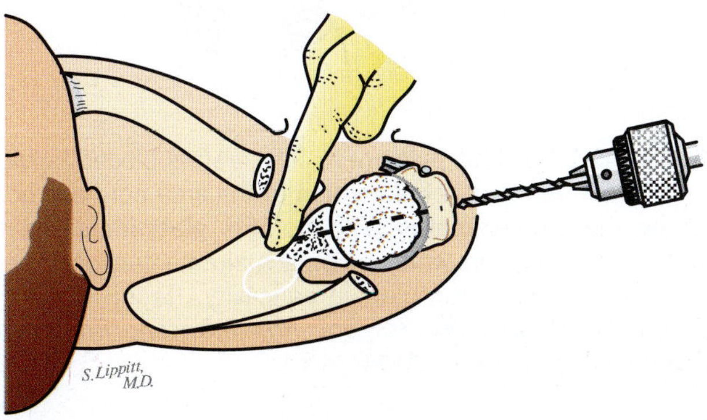

FIGURE 16-173: While the humeral head is held reduced in the glenoid fossa in its proper position, a drill bit is passed through a stab incision then through the deltoid, the proximal humerus, and the glenoid, before exiting anteriorly from the neck. (From Matsen FA III, Lippitt SB. *Shoulder Surgery: Principles and Procedures.* Philadelphia: Saunders; 2004:240.)

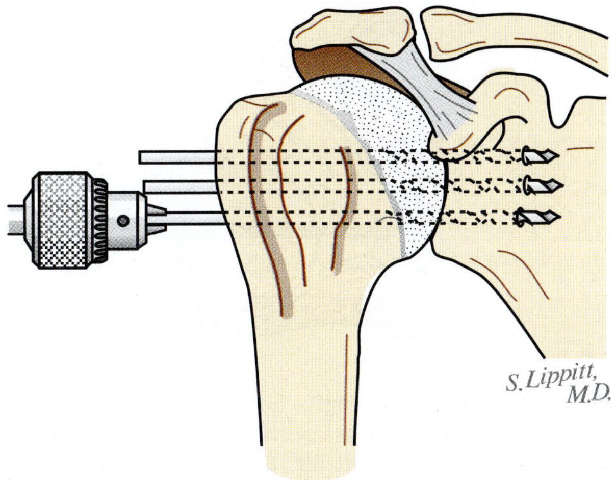

FIGURE 16-174: Subsequent drill placement. Two additional drill bits are placed parallel to the first, equally spaced across the glenohumeral joint. The position and orientation of the humerus in relation to the glenoid is checked again. (From Matsen FA III, Lippitt SB. *Shoulder Surgery: Principles and Procedures.* Philadelphia: Saunders; 2004:241.)

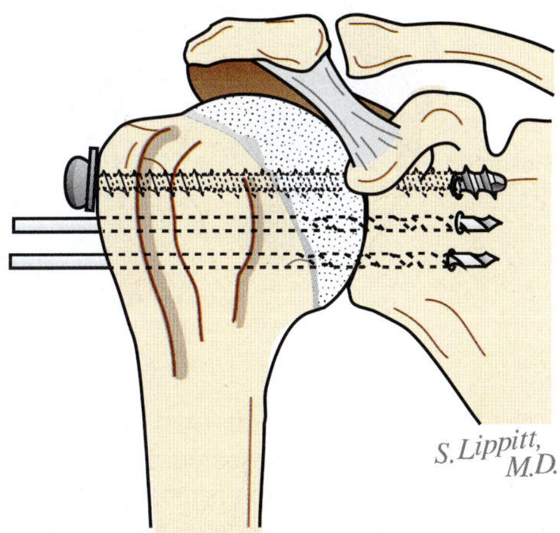

FIGURE 16-175: Screw placement. The drill bits are sequentially replaced with 6.0-mm fully threaded cancellous screws with washers. (From Matsen FA III, Lippitt SB. *Shoulder Surgery: Principles and Procedures.* Philadelphia: Saunders; 2004:242.)

(Figs. 16-175 and 16-176). Because the humeral head is softer than the glenoid, compression can usually be achieved without formally lagging the screw or needing to use a smooth shank.

An iliac crest bone autograft is fashioned to fit between the humeral head and the acromion; it rests in the position normally occupied by the supraspinatus tendon (Figs. 16-177 to 16-179). Interposition of the iliac crest graft maximizes humeroscapular contact by preserving the normal concave-convex glenohumeral relationships while allowing stabilizing contact between the head, the graft, and the acromion. If the humeral head is moved

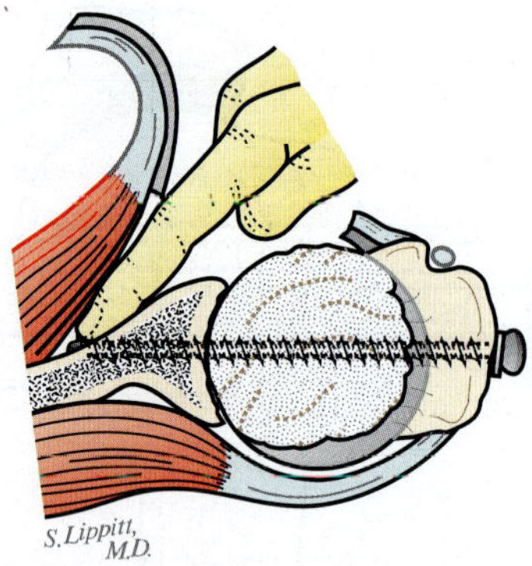

FIGURE 16-176: Screw length. Each screw should just penetrate the subscapularis fossa at the base of the glenoid neck. (From Matsen FA III, Lippitt SB. *Shoulder Surgery: Principles and Procedures.* Philadelphia: Saunders; 2004:243.)

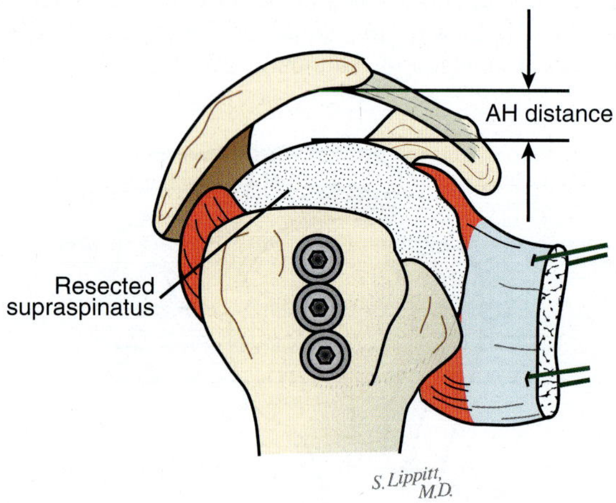

FIGURE 16-177: Acromiohumeral (AH) distance. After the supraspinatus tendon has been resected, the distance between the humeral head and the acromion is measured. (From Matsen FA III, Lippitt SB. *Shoulder Surgery: Principles and Procedures.* Philadelphia: Saunders; 2004:243.)

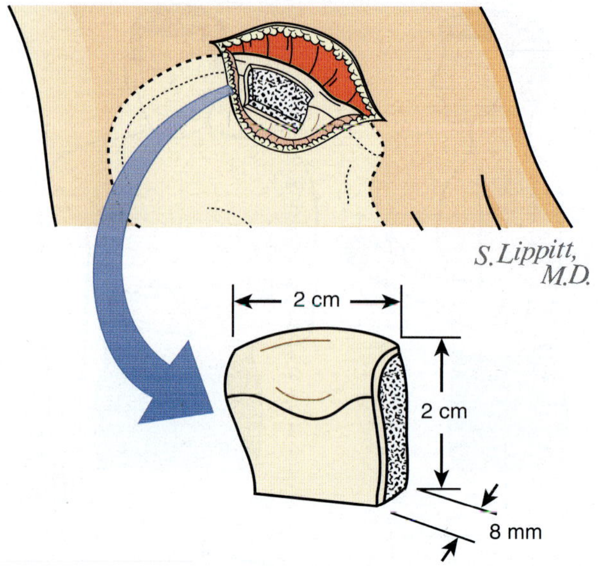

FIGURE 16-178: Graft harvest. A segment of graft measuring 20 × 20 × 8 mm is harvested from the iliac crest. (From Matsen FA III, Lippitt SB. *Shoulder Surgery: Principles and Procedures.* Philadelphia: Saunders; 2004:244.)

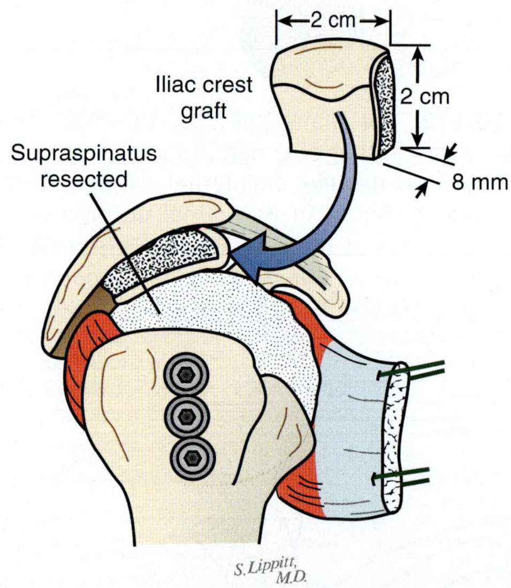

FIGURE 16-179: Graft placement. The graft is placed between the humeral head and the acromion in the area normally occupied by the supraspinatus tendon. This graft increases the quality of the fixation while helping maintain the position of the humeral head in the glenoid concavity. (From Matsen FA III, Lippitt SB. *Shoulder Surgery: Principles and Procedures.* Philadelphia: Saunders; 2004:245.)

upward to make contact with the acromion without a graft, the glenohumeral contact area for fusion gets reduced. The graft is held in position by another screw placed from the acromion through the graft and out through the anteromedial aspect of the humeral neck (Figs. 16-180 and 16-181). Additional bone graft is added around the fusion area to optimize healing.

Depending on the circumstances, a neutralization plate (usually an 8- to 12-hole dynamic compression plate or pelvic reconstruction plate) may be used (Fig. 16-182). If so, several points need to be emphasized. The plate needs a bend of about 90 degrees at the acromion and often an internal rotation twist of about 45 degrees to fit on the anterior of the humerus. The strongest fixation for the plate on the scapula is obtained by a screw down the base of the spine of the scapula just medial to the spinoglenoid notch. The arm is protected in a sling until the fusion is clinically and radiographically healed. When the fusion is solid, function and comfort can be enhanced by strengthening the periscapular musculature.

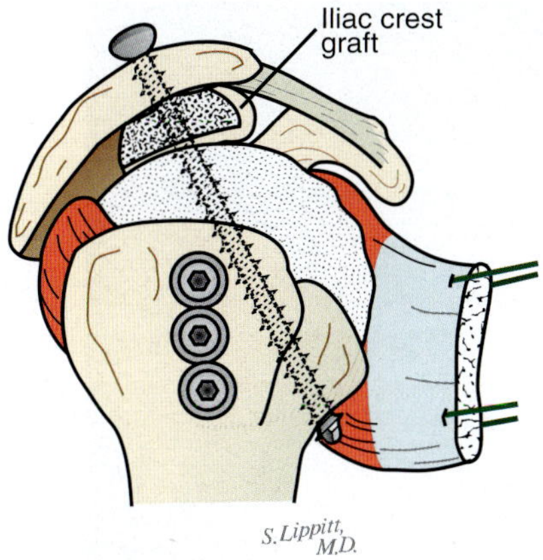

FIGURE 16-180: Graft fixation. A fourth screw is passed through the acromion, the graft, and out the firm bone at the humeral neck. (From Matsen FA III, Lippitt SB. *Shoulder Surgery: Principles and Procedures.* Philadelphia: Saunders; 2004:247.)

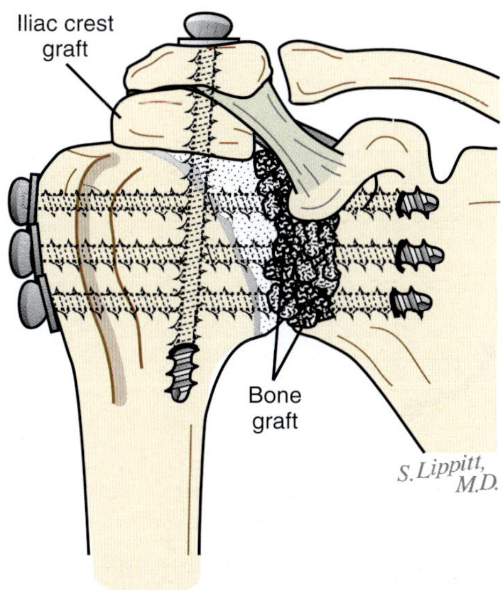

FIGURE 16-181: Cancellous grafting. Cancellous bone graft is added across the area of glenohumeral arthrodesis. (From Matsen FA III, Lippitt SB. *Shoulder Surgery: Principles and Procedures.* Philadelphia: Saunders; 2004:247.)

Complications of shoulder arthrodesis include nonunion, infection, malposition, prominence of the internal fixation plates, and fracture. Nonunion can be treated by freshening the arthrodesis site, repeat fixation, and bone grafting. It can sometimes be difficult to be sure from radiographs whether or not the fusion is solid; in such cases a reexploration may be helpful in evaluating the completeness of the fusion and the security of the internal fixation. Infection is treated by incision, drainage, and antibiotics, attempting to maintain the hardware stabilizing the fusion. Malposition is most commonly in excessive flexion, abduction, or external rotation. It is often preferable to manage malposition by humeral osteotomy

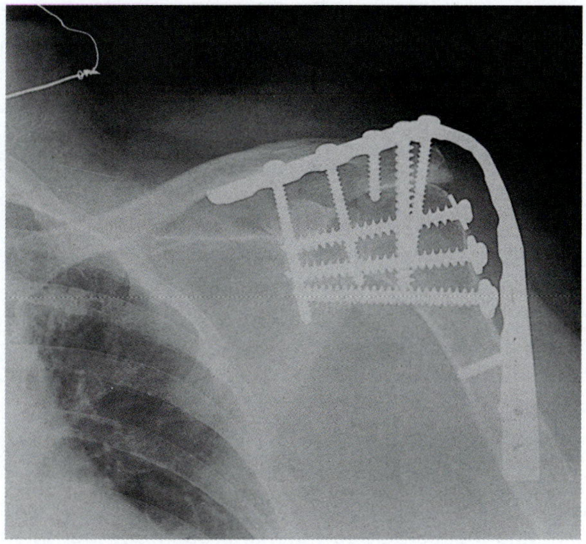

FIGURE 16-182: Glenohumeral and acromiohumeral arthrodesis performed using a contoured iliac crest bone graft inserted between the acromion and the humeral head. The arthrodesis is stabilized securely with the following components: three washered, fully threaded cancellous humeroglenoid screws; one fully threaded cancellous screw through the acromion, graft, and humeral head; and a contoured reconstruction plate.

(Fig. 16-183), rather than by taking down a solid fusion and attempting to reposition it. Care must be taken in removing prominent hardware unless the fusion is absolutely solid. Humeral shaft fracture is a particular risk because the fused shoulder lacks the normal shoulder's ability to absorb load without damage.

Arthroplasty

Considerations

Under optimal circumstances, glenohumeral arthroplasty can be a powerful approach for reconstructing an arthritic shoulder. In considering the advisability of a shoulder arthroplasty and the selection of a specific procedure, it is important to consider the four Ps.

1. Is the *problem* (diagnosis and associated aspects of the shoulder) one that can be well managed with arthroplasty? Are the essential bone, deltoid, cuff, nerve, and skin tissues in sufficiently good condition for a safe and effective arthroplasty? Is the severity of the problem typical of patients presenting for shoulder arthroplasty (Fig. 16-184)?
2. Is the *patient* informed and in sufficiently good physical, social, and emotional health to succeed with the procedure and its postsurgical rehabilitation? Comorbidities, level of education, type of insurance, age, sex, and the patient's overall well-being have all been shown to influence the outcome of the arthroplasty.[80,118,329,482,488,497]
3. Is the *physician* sufficiently experienced in shoulder reconstruction to optimize the chance of a good outcome? Many shoulder arthroplasties are performed

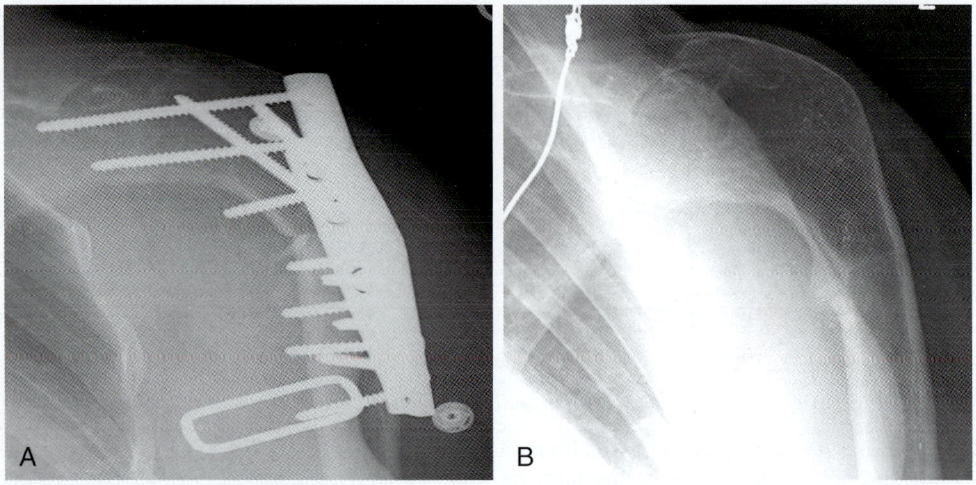

FIGURE 16-183: Subtuberous humeral osteotomy performed for a shoulder that was fused in excessive abduction, excessive flexion, and malrotation. **A,** Internal fixation. **B,** After internal fixation has been removed.

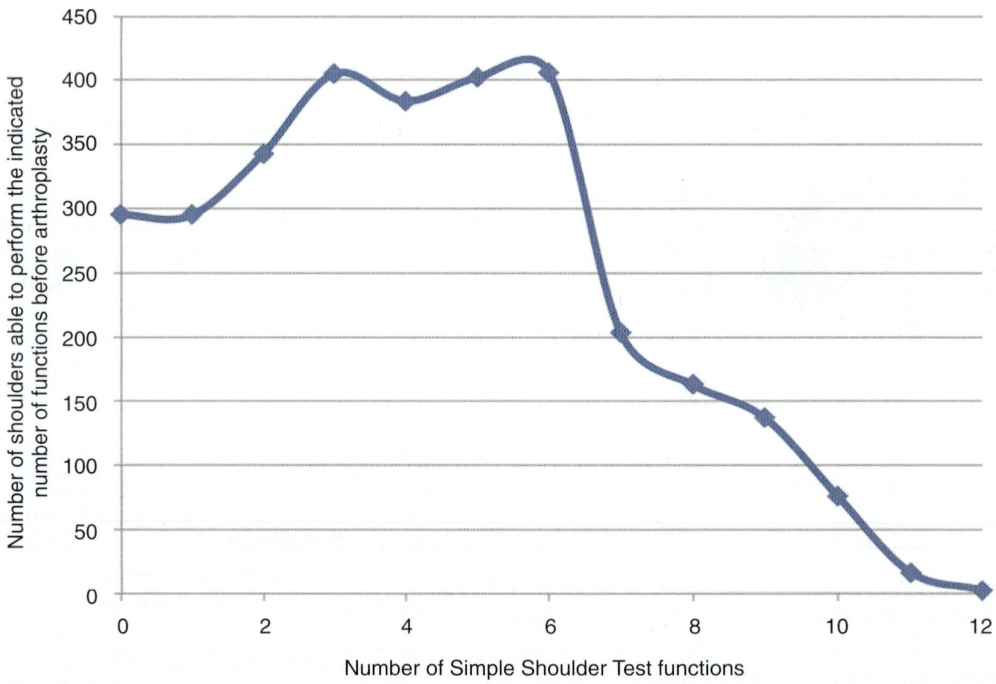

FIGURE 16-184: Frequency distribution of the number of Simple Shoulder Test functions that a sample of patients was able to perform immediately prior to shoulder arthroplasty. We use this chart to help the patient consider the question, "When is my arthritic shoulder bad enough to justify a joint replacement?" As shown by this graph, the great majority of these patients were able to perform less than half of the 12 functions.

by surgeons who perform only a small number of these cases each year,[207] yet case volume has a strong influence on the outcome of the surgery.[199,243,502] As we say, "The surgeon is the method," and "Experience is the great teacher."[328]

4. Is the *procedure* appropriate for the problem, patient, and physician? Among the variations of shoulder arthroplasty available, which is the best fit for the shoulder, the patient, and the surgeon?

Types of Arthroplasty

There are four basic types of shoulder arthroplasty: the humeral hemiarthroplasty, the ream and run arthroplasty (humeral hemiarthroplasty with a nonprosthetic glenoid arthroplasty), the anatomic total shoulder arthroplasty (humeral hemiarthroplasty with a prosthetic glenoid arthroplasty), and the reverse total shoulder arthroplasty.

Prosthetic humeral hemiarthroplasty is considered under the following circumstances: (1) when the glenoid articular surface is intact (as in avascular necrosis before collapse of the humeral head and before secondary destruction of the glenoid surface); (2) when there is insufficient joint volume or glenoid bone stock to allow for secure placement of a glenoid component; (3) in cases of rotator CTA when the humeral head is stabilized by an intact coracoacromial arch (see Fig. 16-110) and active elevation exceeds 90 degrees[11,92,100,143,261,432,514,585]; and (4) in cases where concern about infection discourages the use of a glenoid component. In glenohumeral arthritis—that is, when both the humeral and glenoid articular surfaces are involved—a hemiarthroplasty alone may be insufficient treatment.[186] There are two types of humeral hemiarthroplasty implants: a humeral head prosthesis fixed with a stem inserted down the medullary canal of the humerus (Fig. 16-185) and a partial or complete resurfacing prosthesis mounted on the retained biologic humeral head (Fig. 16-186).

Ream and run arthroplasty (humeral hemiarthroplasty with a nonprosthetic glenoid arthroplasty) is considered for the treatment of glenohumeral arthritis when the patient, after being informed, wishes to avoid the potential risks[334] and activity restrictions[317] associated with a prosthetic glenoid component. Initially there was interest in biologic resurfacing of the glenoid with capsule or cadaveric meniscus (Fig. 16-187) as a way to avoid the risks of prosthetic glenoid component failure; however, recent experience with this approach has not been encouraging.[18,60,70,375,531] The ream and run procedure is a glenohumeral arthroplasty in which a humeral hemiarthroplasty is combined with conservative reaming of the glenoid to a single concentric concavity without substantially modifying glenoid version and without the use of biologic interposition.[173,314,327,333,335,337,344] Because the ream and run procedure modifies both the humeral and glenoid articular surfaces, it is a glenohumeral arthroplasty; this should not be confused with a hemiarthroplasty in which only the humeral side of the joint is addressed. We refer to it as a radically conservative procedure because it involves the removal of less glenoid bone than would be required for the insertion of a glenoid component.[327]

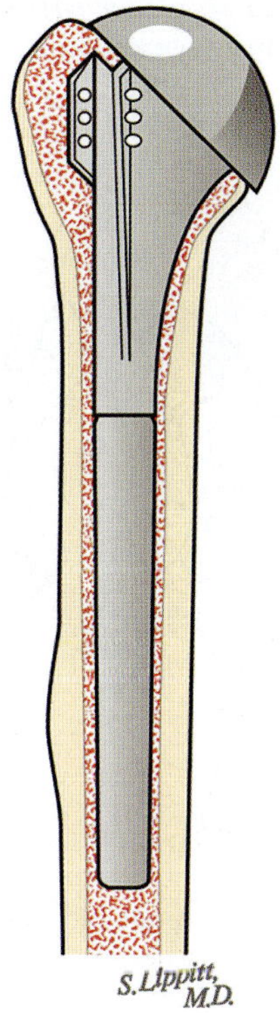

FIGURE 16-185: Humeral head prosthesis fixed with a stem inserted down into the humeral medullary canal.

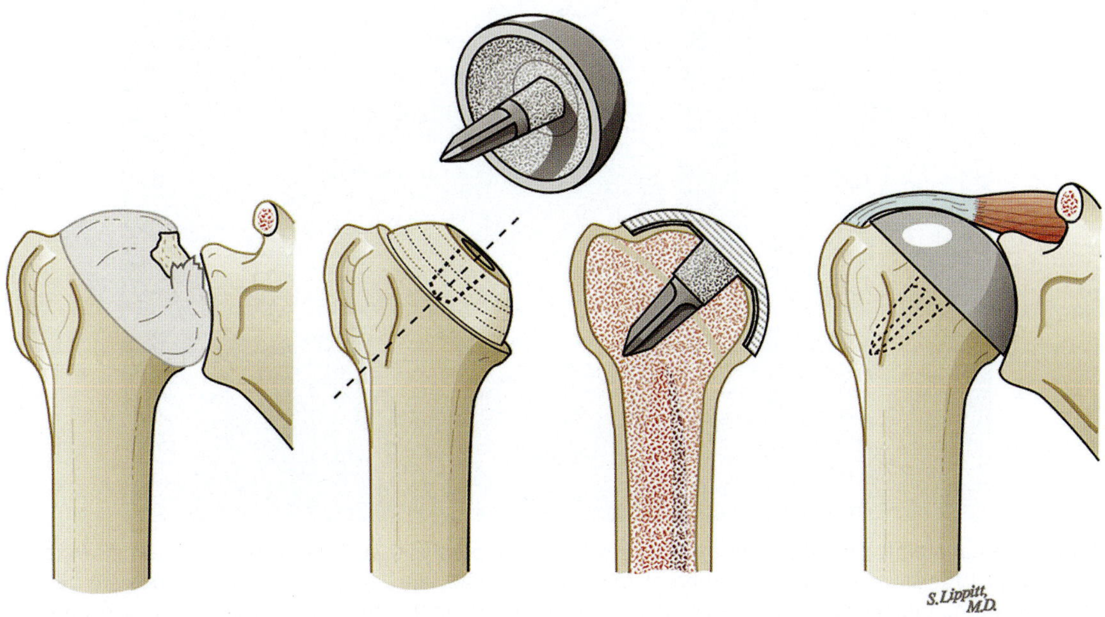

FIGURE 16-186: Complete resurfacing head prosthesis mounted on the retained biologic humeral head.

In the *anatomic total shoulder arthroplasty*, a humeral hemiarthroplasty is combined with a prosthetic glenoid component. The total shoulder arthroplasty is the most commonly used approach to glenohumeral arthritis when the rotator cuff is intact and when sufficient glenoid bone is available for fixation of the glenoid prosthesis.[29,51,64,89,104,164,388,389,394,403,433]

In the *reverse total shoulder arthroplasty*,[331] the positions of the ball and socket are reversed from the anatomic arrangement. This type of prosthesis is used when the arthritic shoulder demonstrates instability that cannot be managed with an anatomic prosthesis or when the shoulder is "pseudoparalytic," meaning that the shoulder cannot be actively elevated to 90 degrees despite a good range of passive motion and intact deltoid function. Reverse total shoulder arthroplasty is used to manage rotator CTA and anterosuperior escape after a failed attempt at rotator cuff repair (see Figs. 16-109 to 16-111 and 16-115). Reverse arthroplasty is also used to manage comminuted proximal humeral fractures in the osteopenic bone of older individuals, massive cuff tears without arthritis, and failed anatomic arthroplasty with instability or pseudoparalysis (Fig. 16-188).[43,115,150,298,571,579]

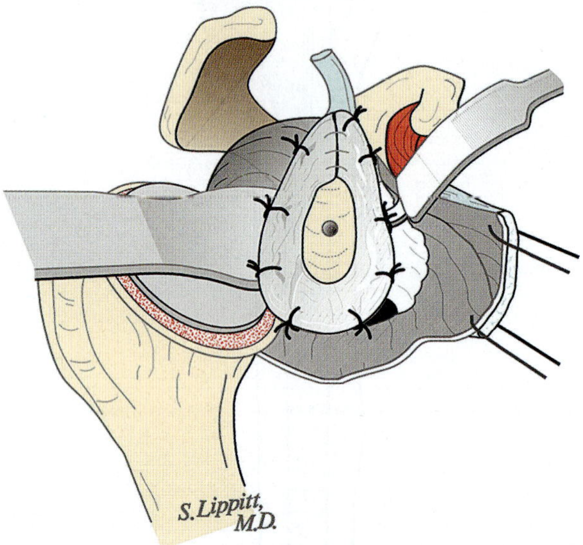

FIGURE 16-187: Biologic glenoid resurfacing with a knee meniscal allograft.

Mechanics of Anatomic Arthroplasty

Four basic mechanical characteristics are essential to shoulder function: mobility, stability, strength, and smoothness. Commonly, each of these characteristics is compromised in an arthritic shoulder, and each can potentially be improved by shoulder arthroplasty. The approach to glenohumeral arthritis is guided by an understanding of these elements necessary for optimal shoulder mechanics. Restoration of glenohumeral mobility and stability is the priority rather than trying to recreate "normal anatomy." In performing glenohumeral reconstruction it is often necessary to modify the humeral head size, thickness, and eccentricity to achieve the desired joint mechanics while preserving glenoid and humeral bone stock.[40] Thus templating systems or patient-specific instrumentation systems based on a preconceived "normal" shoulder are less helpful than learning to use

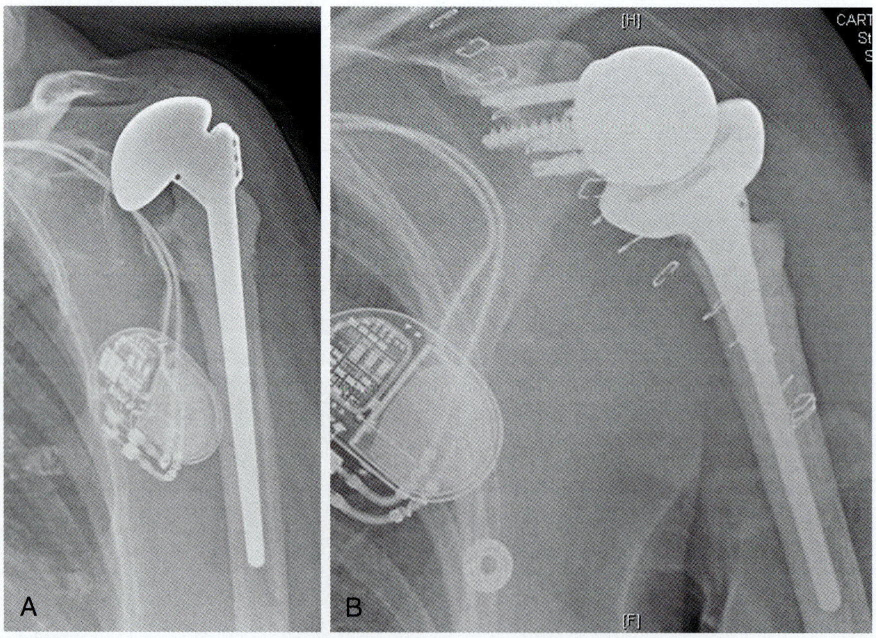

FIGURE 16-188: Failed anatomic prosthesis for a fracture with pseudoparalysis. **A,** Anteroposterior view showing superior placement of the humeral prosthesis, superior subluxation of the humeral head, and an absent greater tuberosity. **B,** Because of the high position of the stem, the humeral prosthesis had to be removed at the time of conversion to a reverse total shoulder arthroplasty.

techniques, such as those involving eccentric humeral heads, humeral heads of different thickness, and rotator interval plication to manage the wide range of arthritic pathologies.[127,335,337,344]

Mobility

The requisites for a normal range of glenohumeral motion include normal capsular laxity, appropriately sized and shaped concentric articular surfaces, and the absence of osteophytes or other unwanted sources of contact between the proximal humerus and the lateral scapula.

Capsular Laxity. In normal shoulders ample capsular laxity allows the full range of rotation at the glenohumeral joint. The glenohumeral capsule normally remains lax through most of the functional range of motion.[202,305] As the joint approaches the limit of its range, the tension in the capsule and its ligaments increases sharply, checking the range of motion (Fig. 16-189). However, in most conditions that require shoulder arthroplasty, the capsule and ligaments are contracted; this prematurely limits the range of motion and increases the joint pressure at the limits of motion (Fig. 16-190). In 1994 we introduced

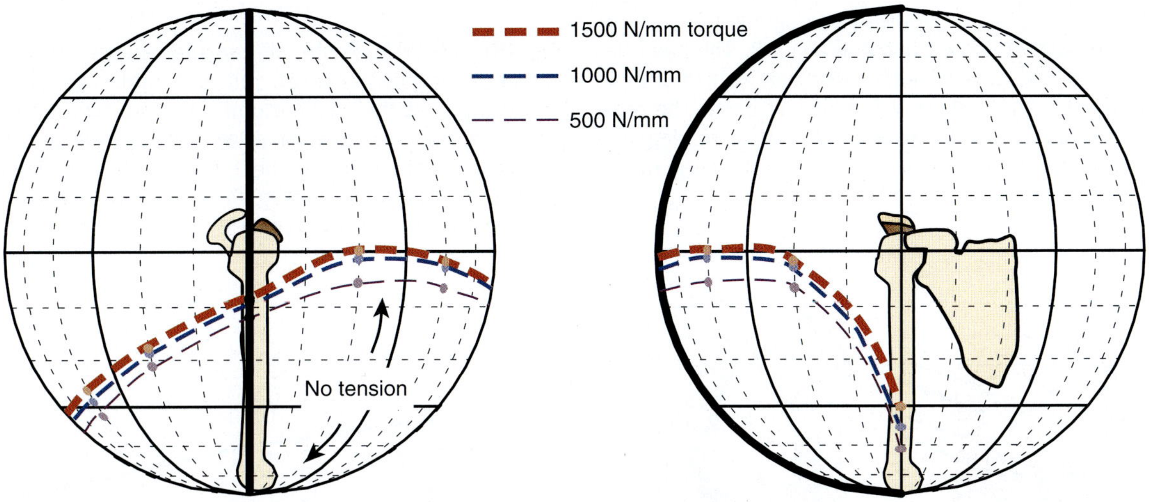

FIGURE 16-189: Range of humeroscapular elevation with no capsular tension. This global diagram represents data from a cadaver experiment in which the humerus was elevated in a variety of scapular planes and free axial rotation was allowed. Elevation was performed until the torque reached 500, 1000, and 1500 N/mm. The positions associated with these torques are indicated by the isobars (gray, red, and blue dashed lines). The area within the 500 N/mm isobar indicates the range of positions in which there was effectively no tension in the capsuloligamentous structures. For further details, see reference 338.

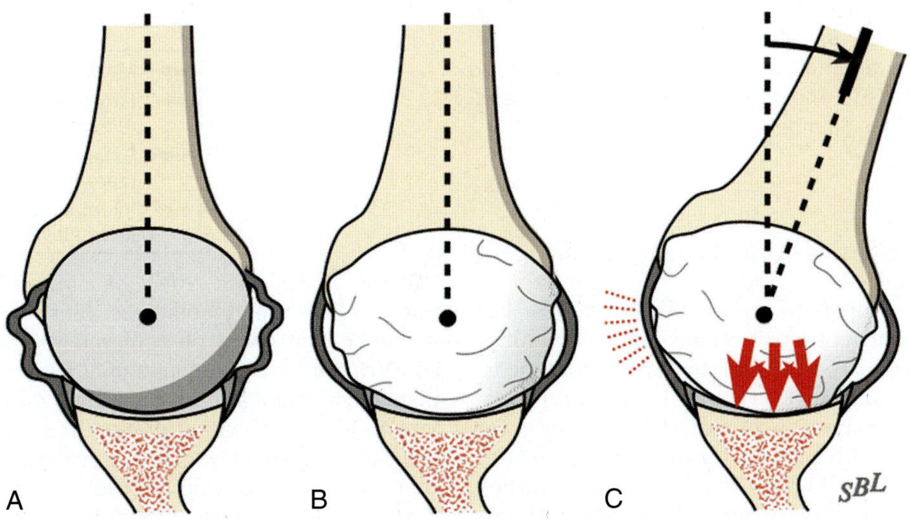

FIGURE 16-190: **A,** Normal capsular laxity allows an unrestricted range of motion. **B,** In degenerative joint disease the capsule may be contracted and has to course over osteophytes. **C,** As the joint approaches the premature limit of its range, the tension in the capsule and ligaments increases sharply, increasing the joint pressure (red arrows).

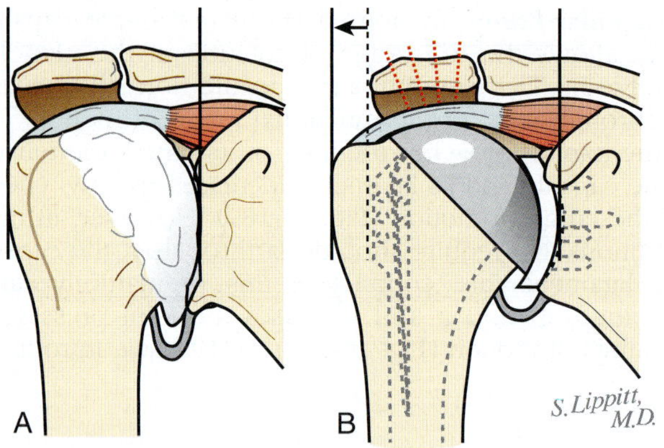

FIGURE 16-191: Shoulder arthroplasty can tighten the capsule. **A,** A degenerated and collapsed humeral head. **B,** The head has been replaced by a relatively larger prosthesis with a glenoid component added to the surface of the glenoid bone. The prosthetic components take up a greater volume than the degenerated surfaces they replace and consequently stuff the joint.

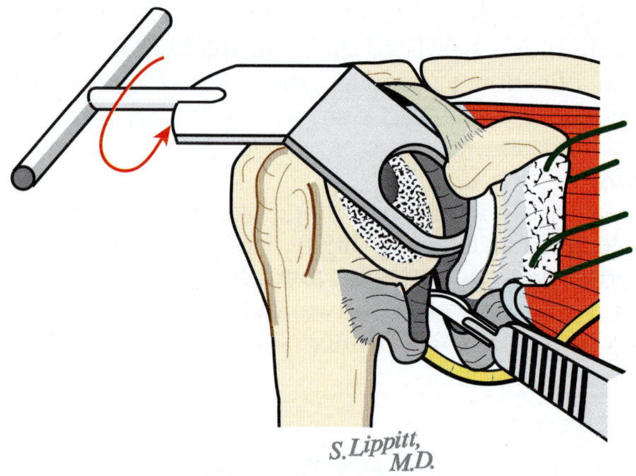

FIGURE 16-193: Posterior capsule release. If the posterior capsule is tight, it can be released under direct vision. The surgeon places the capsule under tension by rotating the inferior aspect of the retractor away from the glenoid (arrow) and gently internally rotating the humerus. (From Matsen FA III, Lippitt SB. *Shoulder Surgery: Principles and Procedures.* Philadelphia: WB Saunders; 2004:555.)

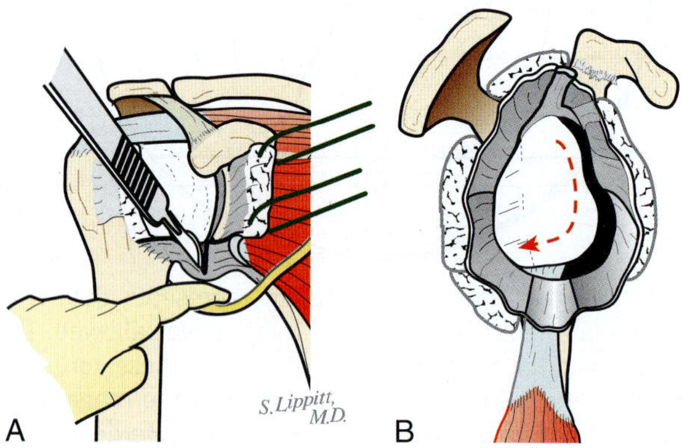

FIGURE 16-192: Release of the anterior capsule from the glenoid while the axillary nerve is protected. **A,** Anteroposterior view showing incision of the inferior capsule while the axillary nerve (yellow) is retracted. **B,** Lateral view showing release of the capsule from the anterior and inferior glenoid. (From Matsen FA III, Lippitt SB. *Shoulder Surgery: Principles and Procedures.* Philadelphia: Saunders; 2004:520.)

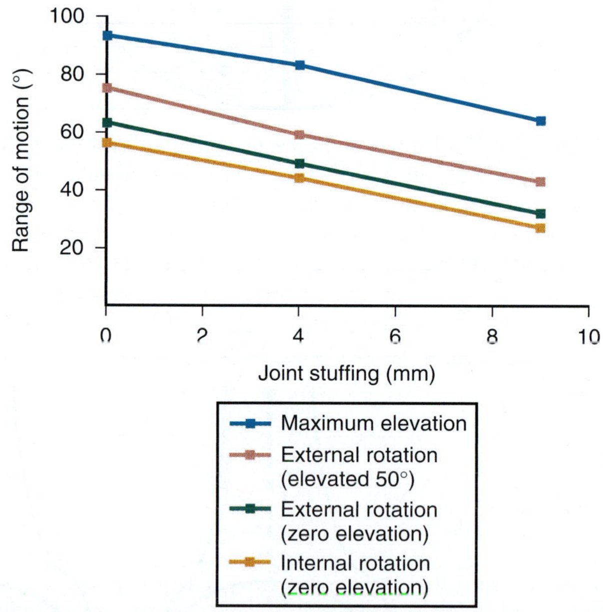

FIGURE 16-194: The effect of joint stuffing on the range of motion. This graph compares four humeroscapular ranges of motion that could be achieved with an applied torque of 1500 N/mm for an anatomic joint (0 mm of joint stuffing), an anatomic humeral arthroplasty with a 4-mm-thick glenoid component (4 mm of overstuffing), and an arthroplasty with a 4-mm-thick glenoid and a 5-mm oversized humeral neck (a total of 9 mm of overstuffing). Note the sequential loss of range of motion as the degree of stuffing increases. (From Matsen FA III, Lippitt SB, Sidles JA, Harryman DT II. *Practical Evaluation and Management of the Shoulder.* Philadelphia: WB Saunders; 1994.)

the term "stuffing" referring to additional tightening of the capsule that results from the insertion of prosthetic components that take up more space than that afforded by the available joint volume[338] (Fig. 16-191). Unless capsular releases (Figs. 16-192 and 16-193) sufficient to accommodate this additional volume have been performed, the joint becomes "overstuffed," limiting joint motion (Fig. 16-194), with greater torque (muscle force) required to move the arm (Fig. 16-195).[203] Cadaver studies have indicated that less than 10 mm of overstuffing can reduce normal capsular laxity by as much as 50% (Fig. 16-196).[203] Overstuffing also causes obligate translation of the humeral head on the glenoid, resulting in eccentric

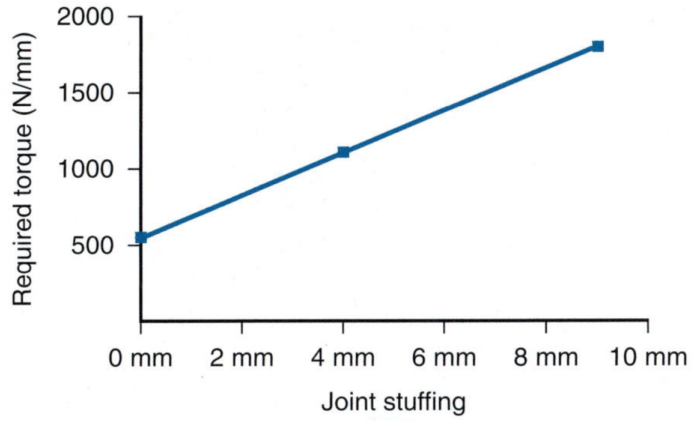

FIGURE 16-195: The average torque necessary to achieve 60 degrees of elevation in the +90-degree scapular plane for an anatomic shoulder (0 mm of stuffing), an anatomic shoulder arthroplasty with 4 mm of glenoid stuffing, and an arthroplasty with 4 mm of glenoid and 5 mm of humeral overstuffing (a total of 9 mm of overstuffing). The required torque is almost three times higher for the joint overstuffed with 9 mm of component than for the anatomic joint. (From Matsen FA III, Lippitt SB, Sidles JA, Harryman DT II. *Practical Evaluation and Management of the Shoulder.* Philadelphia: WB Saunders; 1994.)

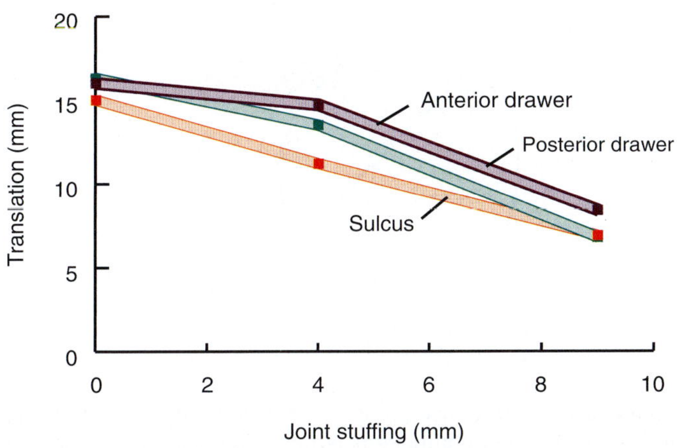

FIGURE 16-196: The effect of overstuffing on capsular laxity in eight cadaver shoulders (mean age, 73 ± 8.5 years). The intact shoulders (0 mm of stuffing) demonstrated 15 mm of translational laxity on the anterior drawer, posterior drawer, and sulcus tests. Overstuffing by 9 mm reduced this normal joint laxity by approximately 50% in all directions. (From Matsen FA III, Lippitt SB, Sidles JA, Harryman DT II. *Practical Evaluation and Management of the Shoulder.* Philadelphia: WB Saunders; 1994.)

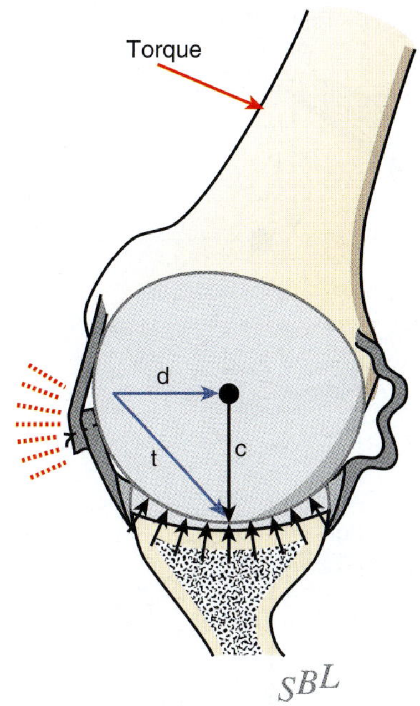

FIGURE 16-197: Ligament shortening (red dotted lines) can cause increased joint pressure (short arrows). If the capsule and ligaments on one side of the joint are shortened, applying torque against them (red arrow) can increase the compressive force (c) applied to the joint surface. This increased joint pressure can damage the joint surface. *d*, Displacing force; *t*, total force. (From Matsen FA III, Lippitt SB. *Shoulder Surgery: Principles and Procedures.* Philadelphia: Saunders; 2004:40.)

TABLE 16-3 Range of Angular Motion Before Onset of Obligate Translation*

Angular Motion	Anatomic Shoulder	Joint Overstuffed 9 mm
Elevation in the +90-degree scapular plane	60 degrees	30 degrees
External rotation of the arm elevated 50 degrees	60 degrees	32 degrees

**Values represent the maximal elevation achieved with no more than 2 mm of obligate translation.*

glenoid loading (Table 16-3); for example, the compressive load increases and forced posterior translation occurs when external rotation is attempted against a tight anterior capsule, accounting for the pathology common seen in capsulorrhaphy arthropathy (see Fig. 16-88; Figs. 16-197 and 16-198).

In total shoulder arthroplasty, the contribution of the components to joint stuffing can be estimated by adding the thickness of the glenoid component to the net added thickness of the humeral component (i.e., the difference between the amount of intra-articular humerus resected and the amount of humerus added) (see Fig. 16-191; Figs. 16-199 to 16-201). The amount of stuffing from the humeral component is also influenced by the position in which it is placed: a humeral stem inserted in varus will increase the stuffing of the joint when the arm is at the

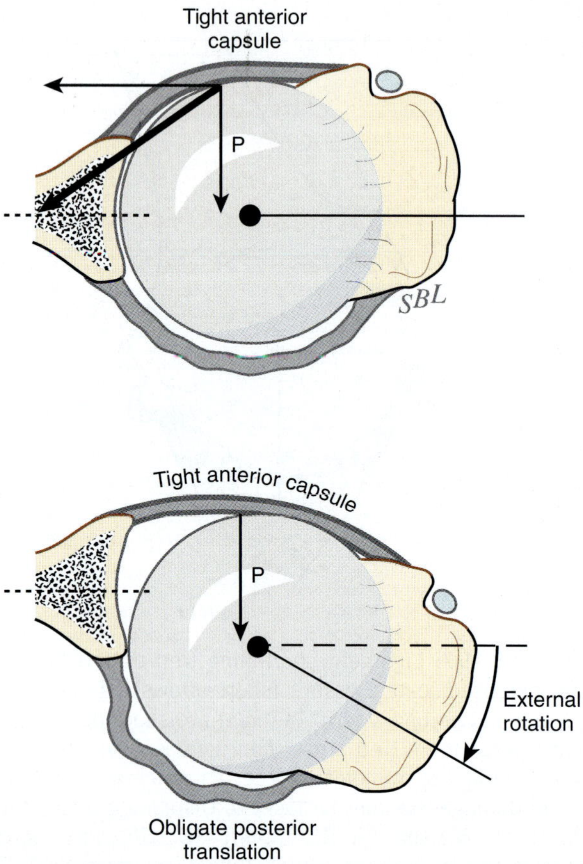

FIGURE 16-198: If the humerus is rotated beyond the point at which the ligaments become tight, the displacing force (P) can push the humeral head out of the glenoid center, a phenomenon known as "obligate translation." (Modified from Matsen FA III, Lippitt SB, Sidles JA, Harryman DT II. *Practical Evaluation and Management of the Shoulder.* Philadelphia: Saunders; 1994.)

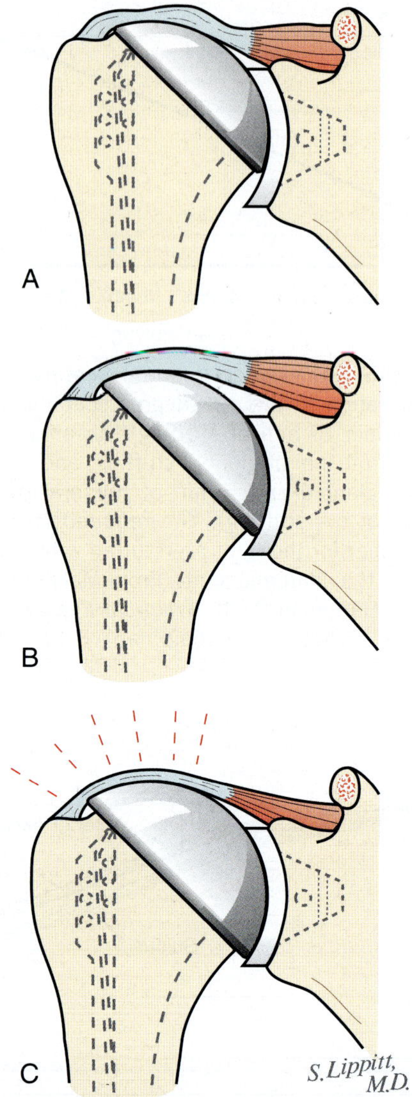

FIGURE 16-199: Consequences of the amount of joint stuffing. **A,** When the head component is too small, the cuff is slack at rest. **B,** With a properly sized head component, there is appropriate tensioning of the rotator cuff. **C,** Overstuffing the joint with a head component that is too large places excessive tension on the rotator cuff.

side (Fig. 16-202). A component inserted in an excessively high position tightens the capsule in adduction (Fig. 16-203) and in abduction (Fig. 16-204). The incremental thickness of the glenoid is determined by the thickness of the component, as well as by the amount of reaming, the presence or absence of cement between the component and the bone, and the effect of bone grafts (Fig. 16-205). The thickness of currently available glenoid components varies from 3 mm to more than 15 mm.

Overstuffing can be avoided by ensuring adequate capsular laxity at the time of surgery using the "40, 50, 60" rule of thumb to guide the selection of the prosthetic sizes: the arm should allow 40 degrees of external rotation at the side after the anterior structures have been approximated (Fig. 16-206), the humeral head should translate approximately 50% of the width of the glenoid in the posterior drawer test (Fig. 16-207), and the abducted arm should allow 60 degrees of internal rotation (Fig. 16-208).

If the humeral head translates posteriorly by more than 50%, three strategies may be considered individually or in combination: (1) selecting a humeral head component of greater width (Fig. 16-209); (2) using an anteriorly eccentric head component (Fig. 16-210); or (3) performing a rotator interval plication (Fig. 16-211).

Humeral Articular Surface. A substantial, properly located humeral articular surface area allows a large unimpeded range of motion (Fig. 16-212). Humeral articular surfaces that are nonspherical (Figs. 16-213 and 16-214) or that comprise a reduced portion of the sphere (Figs. 16-215 to 16-218) reduce the amount of range of motion that can take place with full surface contact at the glenohumeral joint (Fig. 16-219).[19,20,338,586]

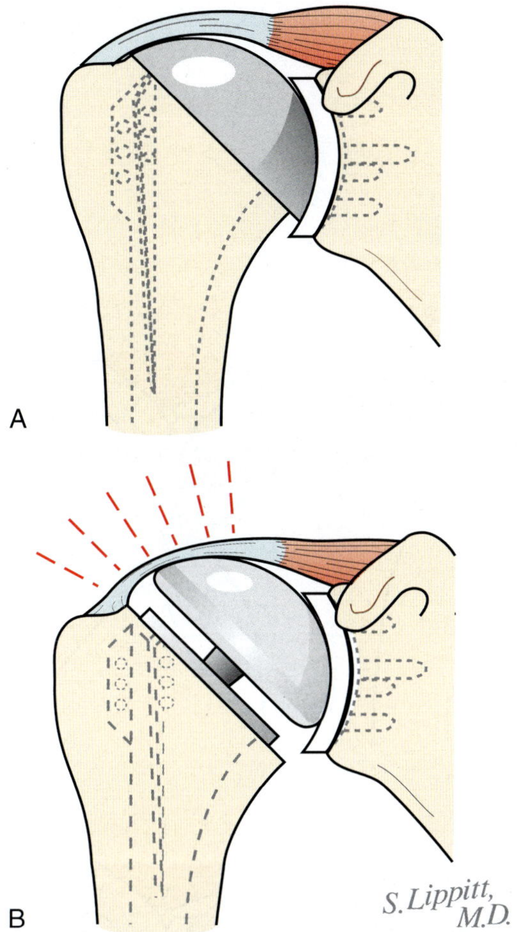

FIGURE 16-200: Neck length. **A,** Normal relationships. **B,** A prosthesis with a collar and gap increases the total neck length. (From Matsen FA III, Lippitt SB. *Shoulder Surgery: Principles and Procedures.* Philadelphia: Saunders; 2004:458.)

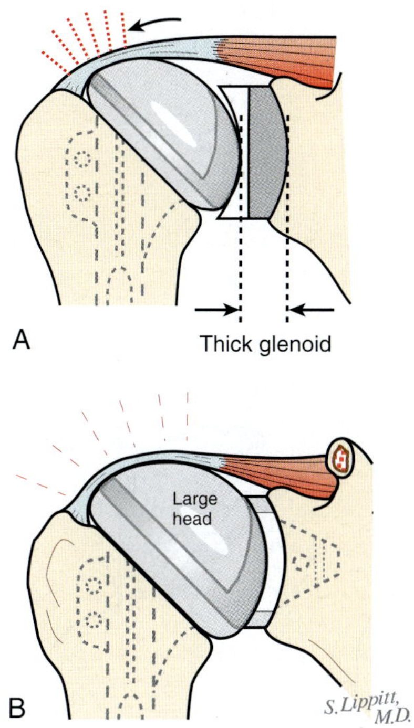

FIGURE 16-201: Overstuffing. Excessive height of the humeral articular surface, from either a thick glenoid (**A**) or a large head (**B**), overstuffs the joint and places the rotator cuff under greater tension when the arm is in adduction. (From Matsen FA III, Lippitt SB. *Shoulder Surgery: Principles and Procedures.* Philadelphia: Saunders; 2004:702.)

Glenoid Articular Surface. The glenoid surface encompasses a relatively small portion of the articulating sphere when compared with the articular surface of the humerus. If the prosthetic joint surface area of the glenoid is large compared with that of the humerus, abutment of the prosthesis against the humeral neck or tuberosities can restrict joint motion (Fig. 16-220).

Concentricity of the Coracoacromial and Glenohumeral Spheres. Two spheres are involved in glenohumeral motion: one represented by the articular surfaces of the humeral head and the glenoid, and the other by the proximal humeral convexity and the coracoacromial arch (Figs. 16-221 and 16-222). The difference in the radius of these two spheres is made up by the height of the tuberosities and the thickness of the rotator cuff. For optimal shoulder kinematics, the centers of these spheres need to match.

Absence of Unwanted Bone Contact. Osteophytes predispose to unwanted contact between the humerus and the glenoid and can impair motion (Figs. 16-223 to 16-225). Any blocking osteophytes must be completely resected at the time of joint reconstruction (Figs. 16-226 and 16-227). A malunited greater tuberosity can also limit rotation (Fig. 16-228).

Unrestricted Humeroscapular Motion Interface. Normally, 4 to 5 cm of excursion takes place at the upper aspect of the interface between the coracoid muscles and the subscapularis (Fig. 16-229 and 16-230).[464] Bursal hypertrophy, adhesions, or spot welds between the proximal aspect of the humerus and the cuff on the one hand and the deltoid and coracoacromial arch on the other can limit motion, even when the intra-articular aspect of the arthroplasty is perfectly balanced (Fig. 16-231). Lysis of humeroscapular spot welds is an important early step in arthroplasty of the shoulder.

Stability

The primary mechanism for glenohumeral stability is "concavity compression," described earlier (see Fig. 16-4).[307,338] Concavity compression is optimized by an ample humeral articular surface area, a stabilizing glenoid concavity, and muscular control of the net humeral joint reaction force such that it compresses the humeral articular surface into the glenoid concavity (Fig. 16-232). This mechanism is commonly altered in osteoarthritis, with some degree of posterior humeral head subluxation present in most cases.[16,167,221,560]

Text continued on p. 917

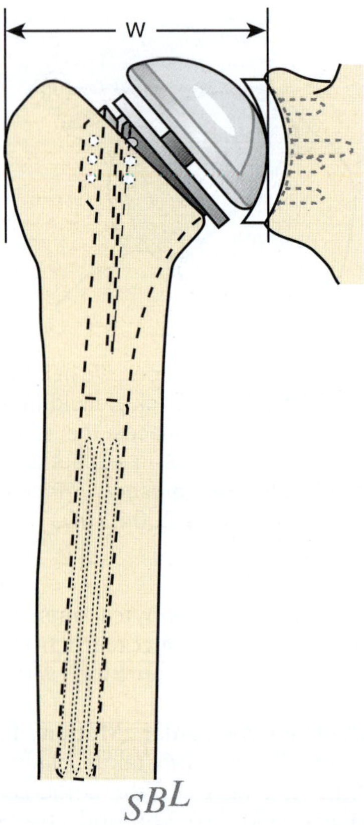

FIGURE 16-202: Varus position of the humeral component can increase the distance between the greater tuberosity and the glenoid (W), effectively overstuffing the joint. (From Matsen FA III, Lippitt SB. *Shoulder Surgery: Principles and Procedures.* Philadelphia: Saunders; 2004:703.)

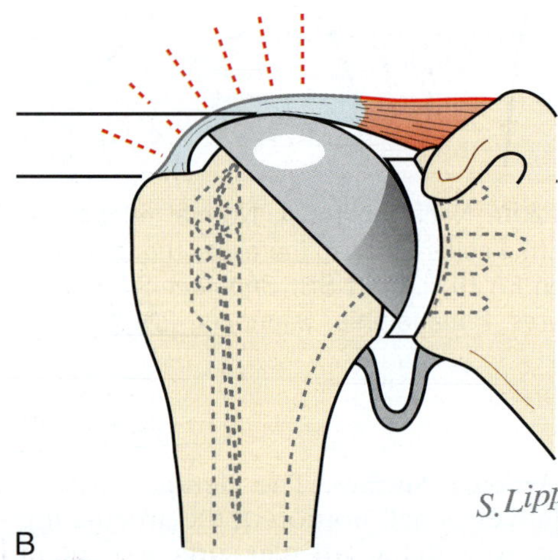

FIGURE 16-203: Head height and adduction. **A,** The ideal position. **B,** Positioning the humeral prosthesis in an excessively superior position causes excessive tension in the superior cuff when the arm is in adduction (dotted lines). (From Matsen FA III, Lippitt SB. *Shoulder Surgery: Principles and Procedures.* Philadelphia: Saunders; 2004:454.)

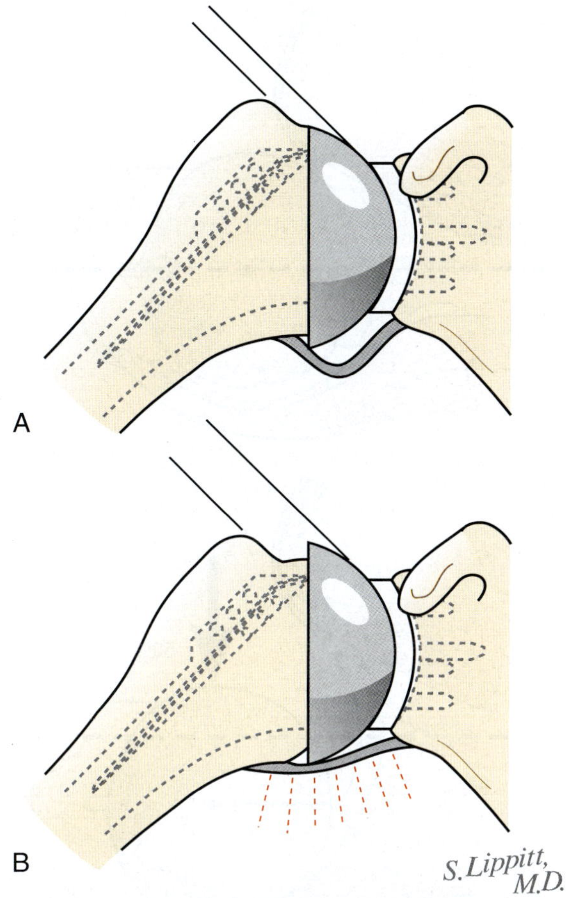

FIGURE 16-204: Head height and abduction. **A,** The ideal position. **B,** Positioning the humeral prosthesis in an excessively superior position causes excessive tension in the inferior capsule when the arm is in abduction. (From Matsen FA III, Lippitt SB. *Shoulder Surgery: Principles and Procedures.* Philadelphia: Saunders; 2004:455.)

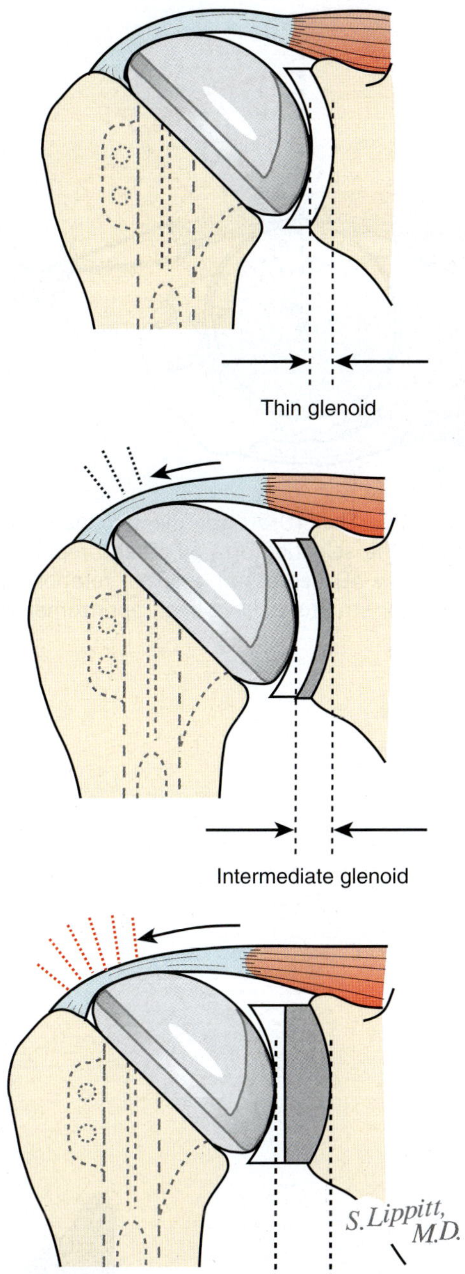

FIGURE 16-205: The glenoid thickness contributes to the relative stuffing of the joint. This is particularly an issue with some metal-backed components, where a minimum thickness of 3 to 4 mm of polyethylene is superimposed on a metal base. As a result, some components are up to 1.25 cm thick. Insertion of such a component can be predicted to reduce the range of rotation in each direction by about 28 degrees (12.5 mm of increased thickness is half a radian for an average humeral head of radius 25 mm; in degrees, half a radian is $0.5 \times 360/2\pi$, or 28 degrees). Thus the restoration of motion to an arthritic shoulder can require a combination of soft tissue releases and avoiding the insertion of a thick glenoid component. (From Matsen FA III, Lippitt SB. *Shoulder Surgery: Principles and Procedures.* Philadelphia: Saunders; 2004:504.)

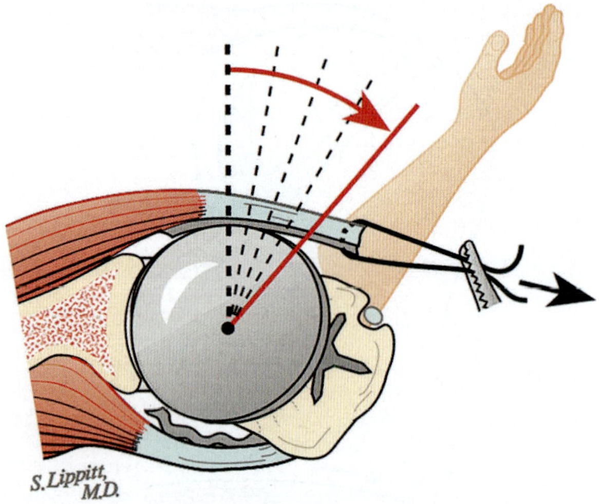

FIGURE 16-206: The 40-50-60 rule for adequate capsular laxity to guide the selection of a prosthetic replacement. The arm should allow 40 degrees of external rotation at the side after the anterior structures have been approximated.

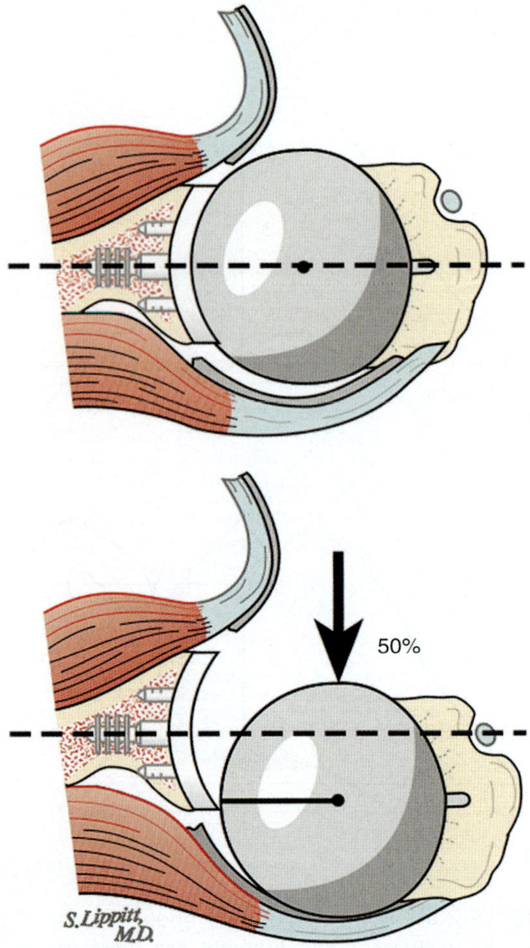

FIGURE 16-207: The 40-50-60 rule for adequate capsular laxity to guide the selection of a prosthetic replacement. The humeral head component should translate approximately 50% of the glenoid width on the posterior drawer test.

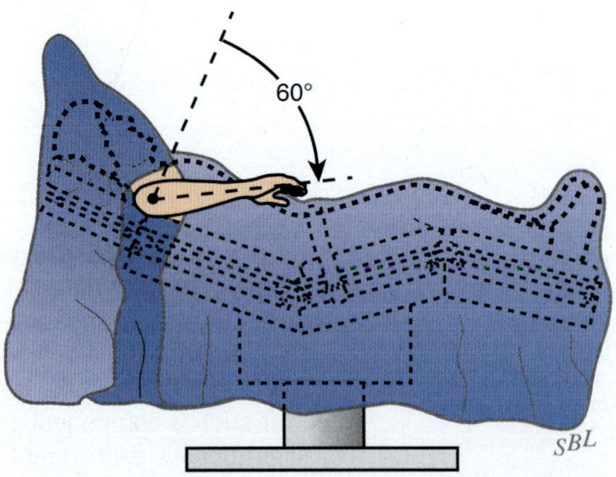

FIGURE 16-208: The 40-50-60 rule: internal rotation. There should be 60 degrees of internal rotation of the arm abducted to 90 degrees. (From Matsen FA III, Lippitt SB. *Shoulder Surgery: Principles and Procedures.* Philadelphia: Saunders; 2004:480.)

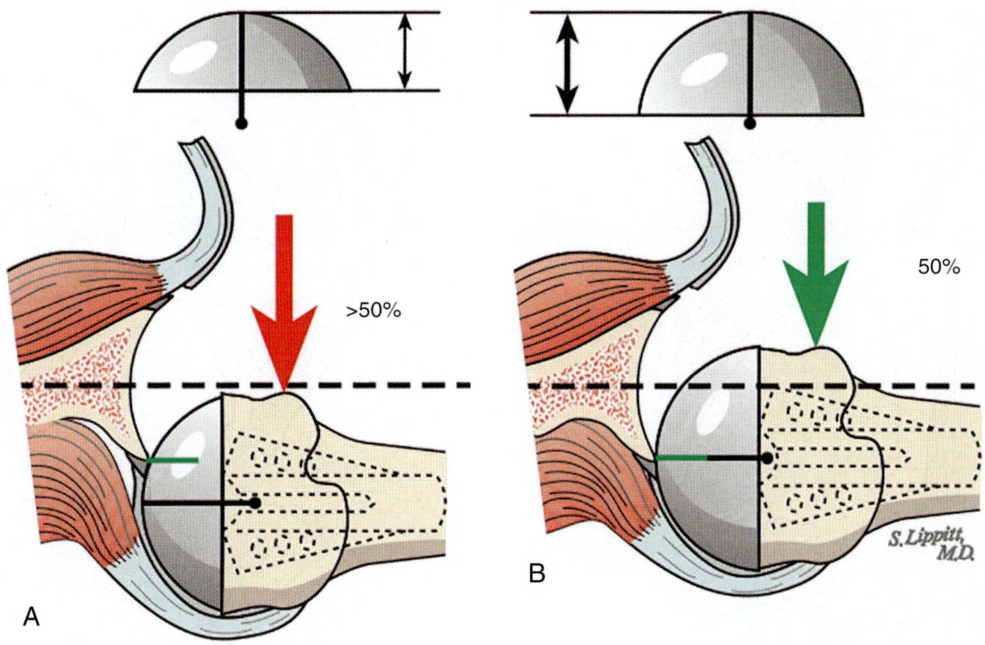

FIGURE 16-209: **A,** The humeral head translates further than 50% posteriorly. **B,** A larger width head component may improve the balance of the reconstruction.

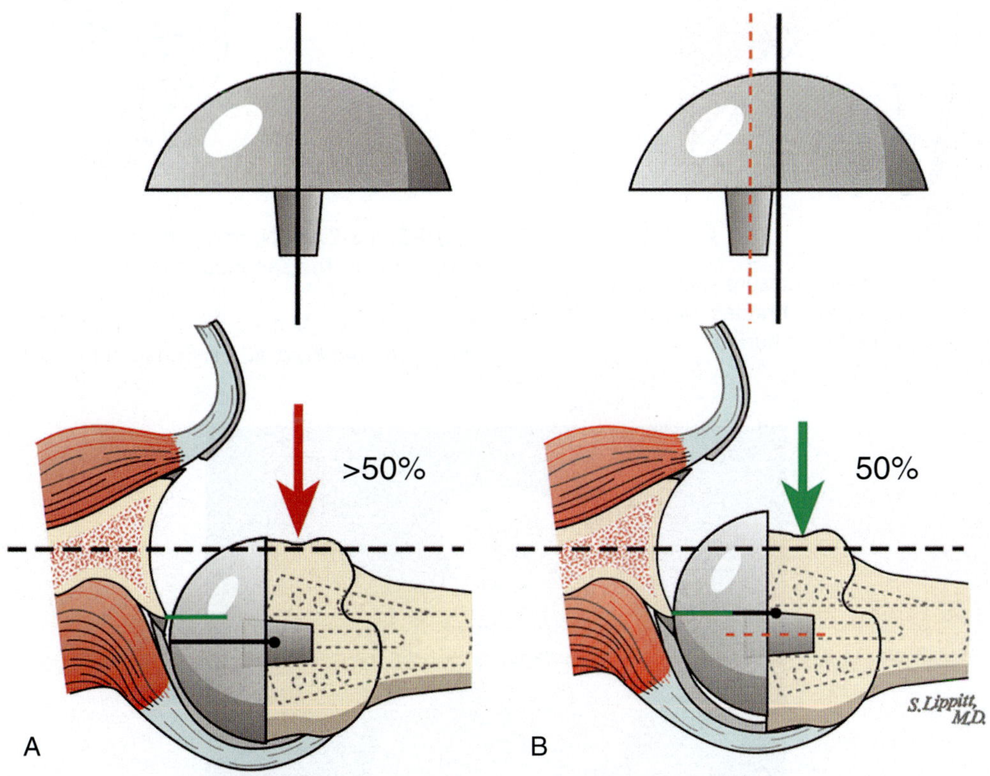

FIGURE 16-210: **A,** The humeral head translates further than 50% posteriorly. **B,** An eccentric head component oriented anteriorly may improve the balance of the reconstruction.

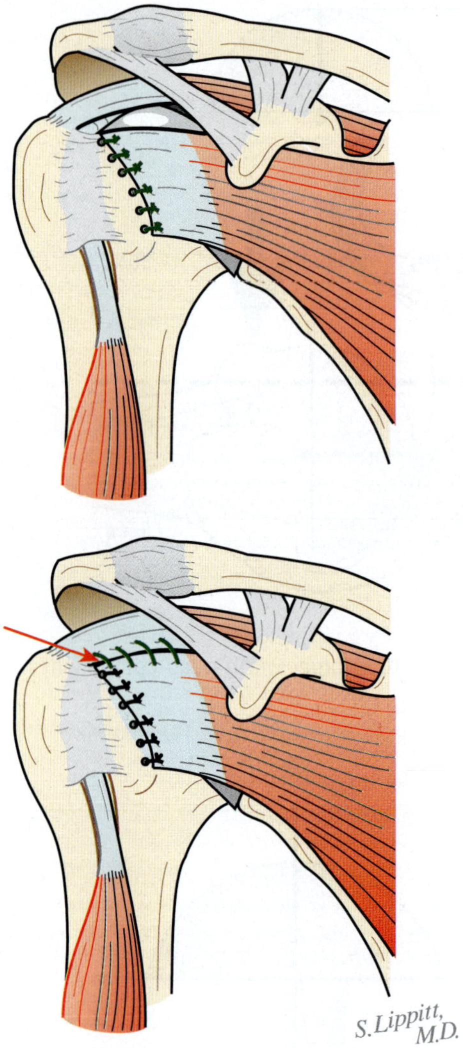

FIGURE 16-211: Rotator interval closure, anterior view. The rotator interval is closed using four braided No. 2 nonabsorbable sutures inserted with the knots buried.

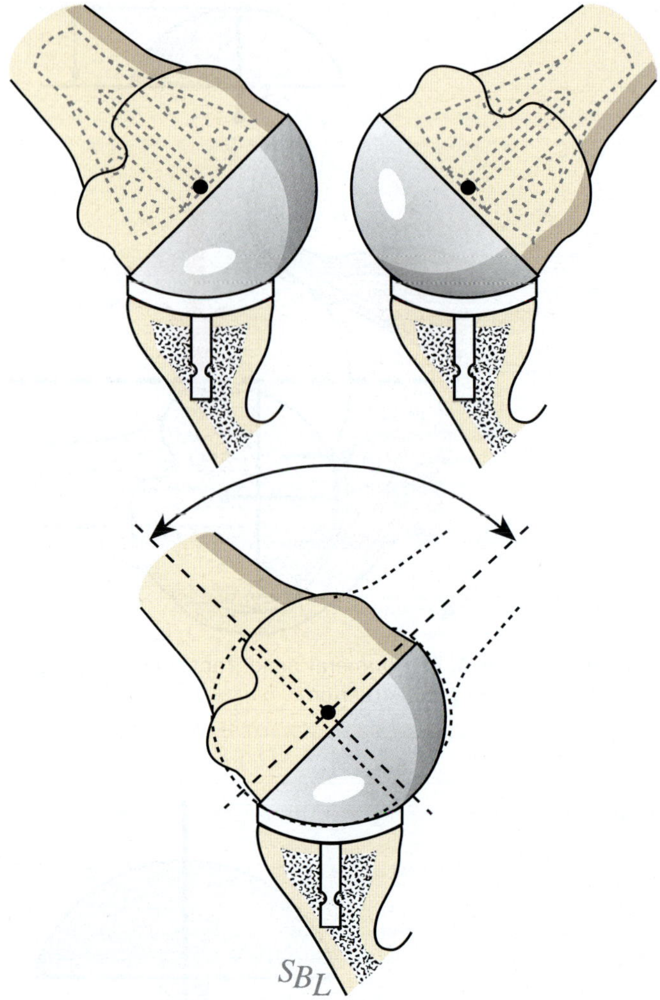

FIGURE 16-212: Normal spherical cap. Restoration of the entire area of the spherical cap maximizes the range of motion with full surface contact between the humeral head and glenoid. (From Matsen FA III, Lippitt SB. *Shoulder Surgery: Principles and Procedures.* Philadelphia: Saunders; 2004:430.)

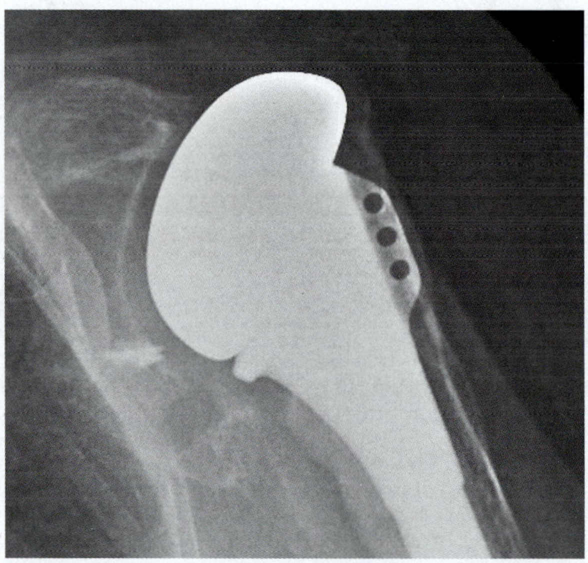

FIGURE 16-213: Nonspherical humeral head prosthesis.

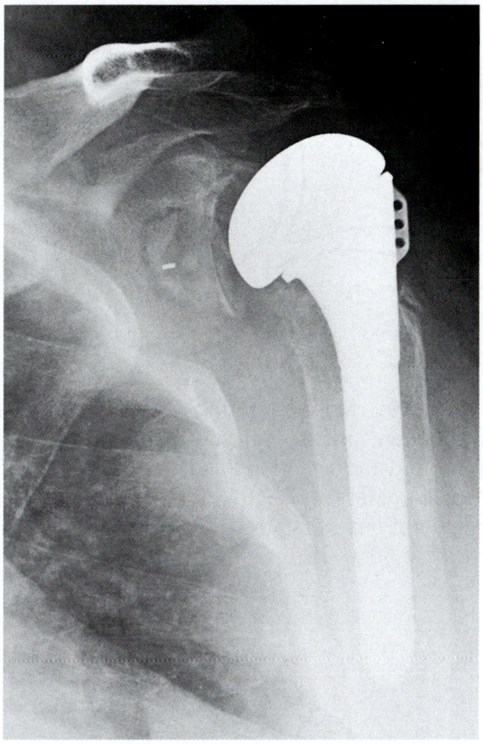

FIGURE 16-214: "Rocking horse" glenoid loosening with a nonspherical humeral head.

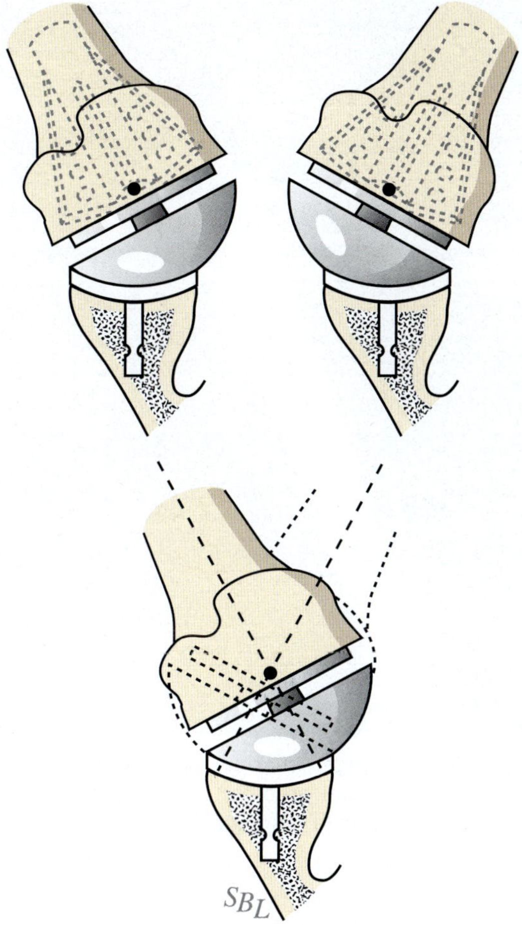

FIGURE 16-215: Spherical cap reduced by collar and gap between the head and collar of the prosthesis. A prosthesis with a collar and a gap sacrifices the height of the spherical cap and the range of motion with full surface contact. (From Matsen FA III, Lippitt SB. *Shoulder Surgery: Principles and Procedures.* Philadelphia: Saunders; 2004:432.)

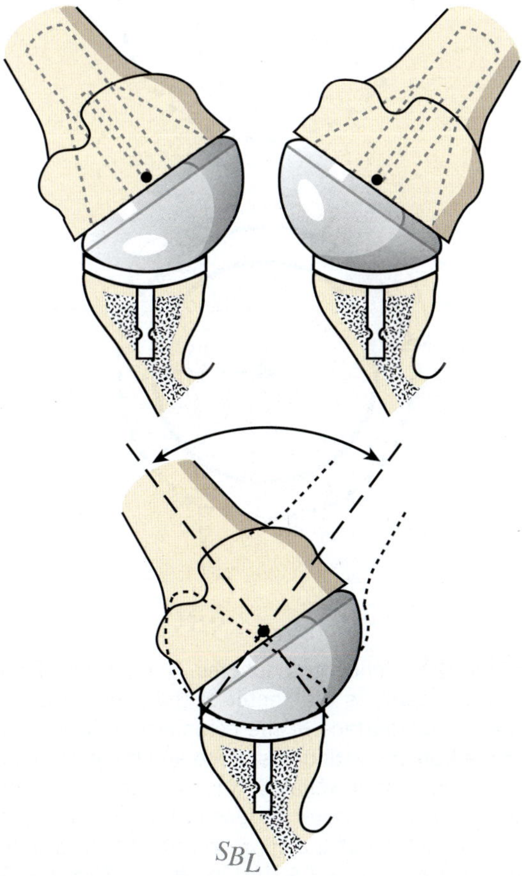

FIGURE 16-216: Spherical cap reduced by chamfering. A chamfered humeral head prosthesis has a reduced height of the spherical cap and reduced range of motion with full surface contact. (From Matsen FA III, Lippitt SB. *Shoulder Surgery: Principles and Procedures.* Philadelphia: Saunders; 2004:431.)

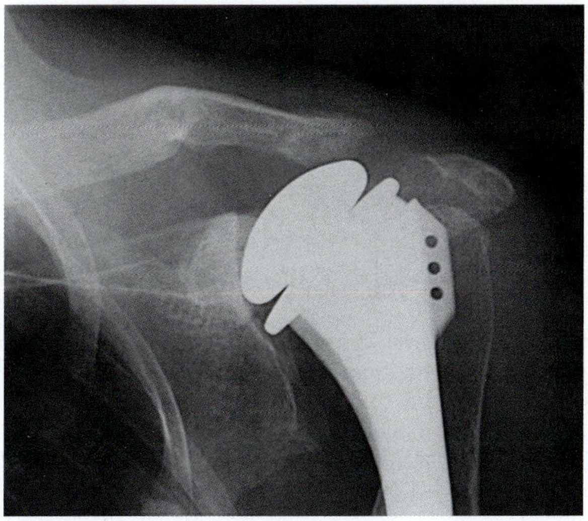

FIGURE 16-217: A humeral component with an articular surface that encompasses only a small portion of the potential spherical articular surface can predispose the prosthesis to unwanted translation as well as unwanted contact between the prosthetic collar and the glenoid.

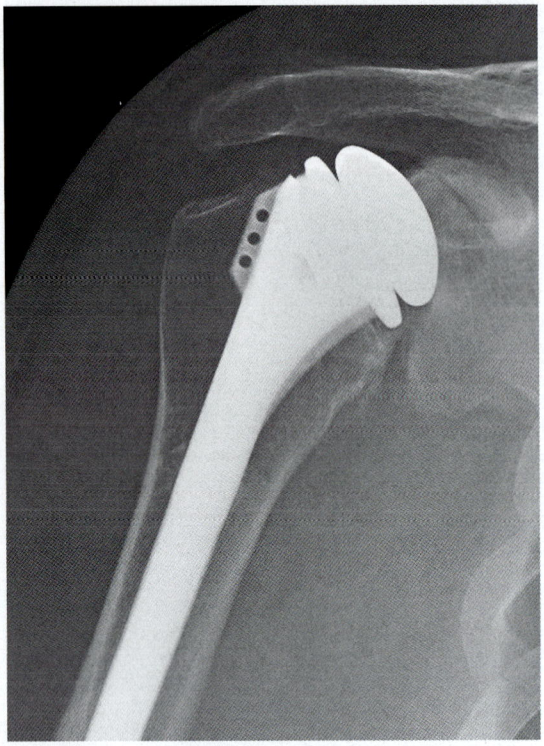

FIGURE 16-218: A large collar and a small articular surface provide minimal humeral articular surface area. In addition, this prosthesis was placed too high.

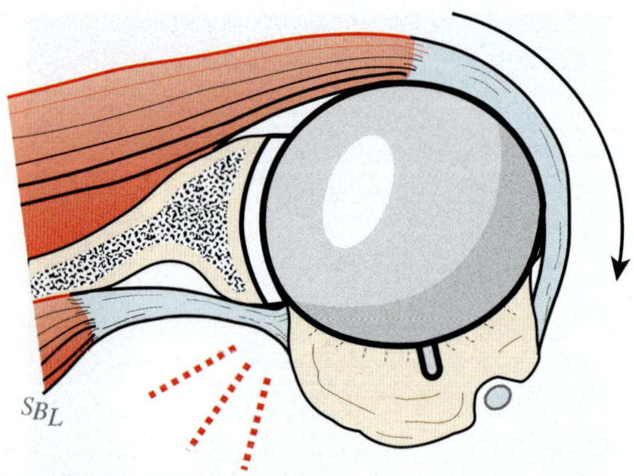

FIGURE 16-219: Motion-limiting abutment between the glenoid component and soft tissue or bone when the arm is externally rotated (arrow). (Modified from Ballmer FT, Lippitt SB, Romeo AA, Matsen FA III. Total shoulder arthroplasty: Some considerations related to glenoid surface contact. *J Shoulder Elbow Surg.* 1994;3:299-306.)

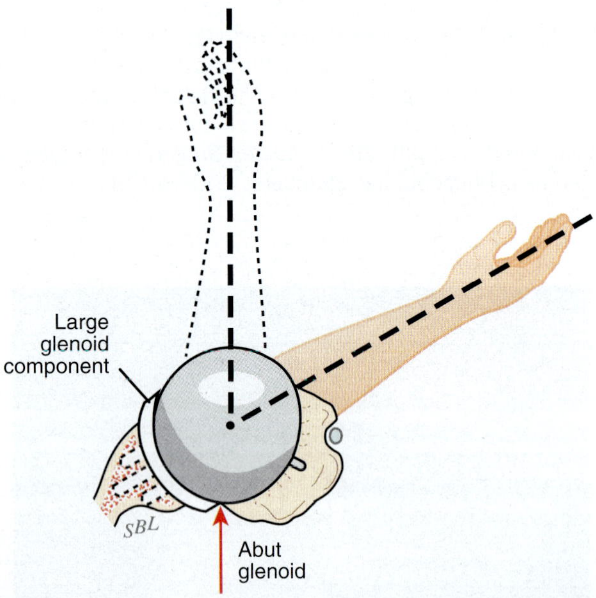

FIGURE 16-220: If the prosthetic glenoid joint surface area is large compared with that of the humerus, abutment of the prosthesis against the humeral neck or tuberosities can restrict joint motion.

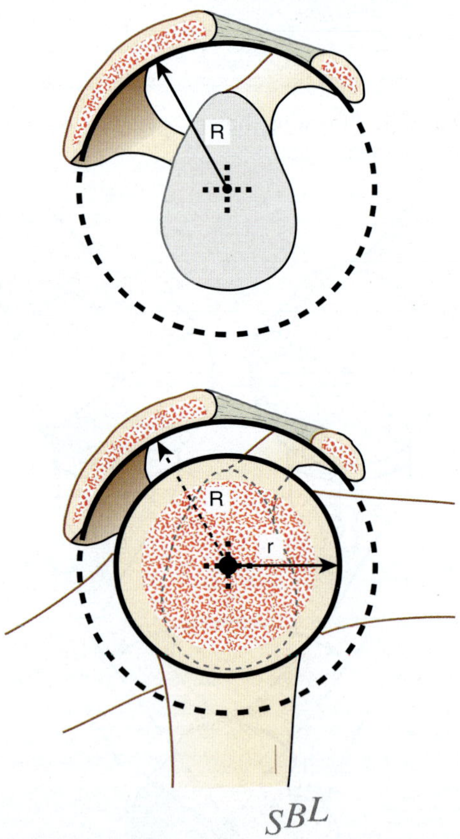

FIGURE 16-221: Concentric spheres. The center of the coracoacromial concavity is the center of the sphere that best fits the concave undersurface of the coracoacromial arch. *r* is the radius of the humeral articular surface and the glenoid articular surface with which it articulates; *R* is the radius of the proximal humeral convexity (the outer surface of the cuff and tuberosity) and the undersurface of the coracoacromial arch with which it articulates. (From Matsen FA III, Lippitt SB. *Shoulder Surgery: Principles and Procedures.* Philadelphia: Saunders; 2004:413.)

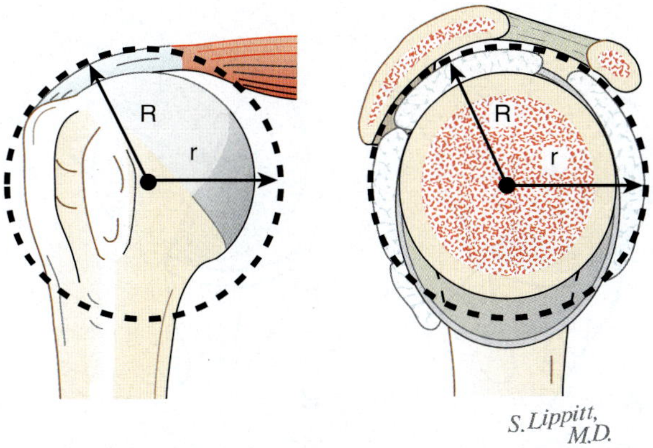

FIGURE 16-222: Proximal humeral convexity. The center of the proximal humeral convexity is the center of the sphere that circumscribes the cuff tendons and the tuberosity. The radius of the proximal humeral convexity (R) differs from the radius of the humeral head (r) by the thickness of the rotator cuff. (From Matsen FA III, Lippitt SB. *Shoulder Surgery: Principles and Procedures.* Philadelphia: Saunders; 2004:415.)

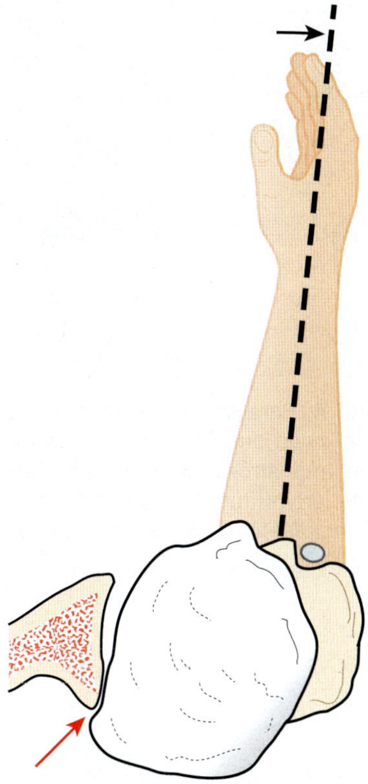

FIGURE 16-224: Blocking osteophytes. Humeral osteophytes can abut against the glenoid lip (red arrow), limiting the range of rotation. (From Matsen FA III, Lippitt SB. *Shoulder Surgery: Principles and Procedures.* Philadelphia: Saunders; 2004:47.)

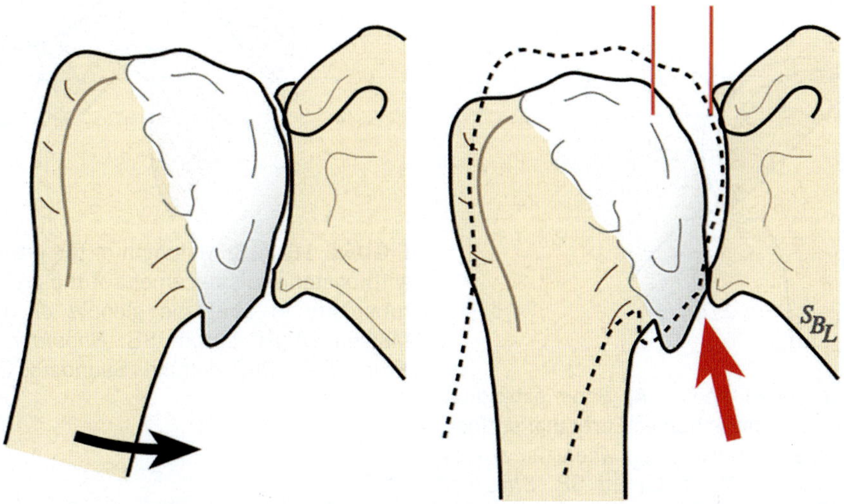

FIGURE 16-223: When the arm is adducted (black arrow), humeral inferior osteophytes can abut the inferior glenoid (red arrow), causing the glenohumeral joint to "open book" superiorly (red lines).

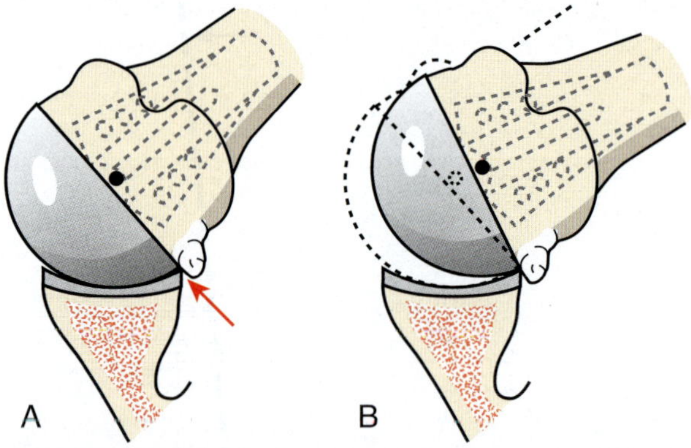

FIGURE 16-225: **A,** Care should be taken to ensure that the posterior humeral head does not abut the posterior glenoid in external rotation (red arrow). **B,** This can cause the joint to "open book" anteriorly. (From Matsen FA III, Lippitt SB. *Shoulder Surgery: Principles and Procedures.* Philadelphia: Saunders; 2004:585.)

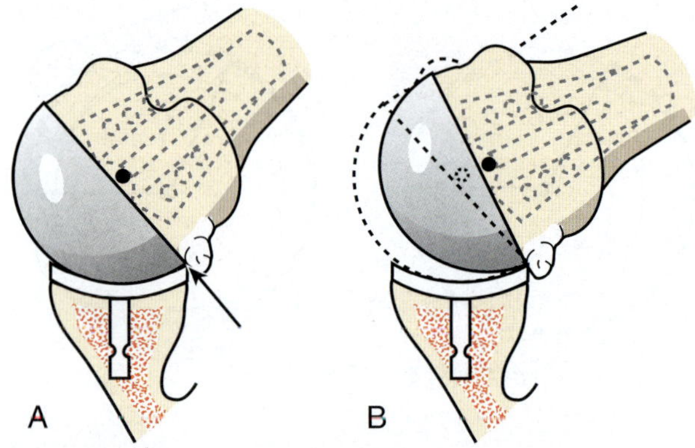

FIGURE 16-226: Posterior "open book." **A,** If the posterior nonarticular humerus abuts against the posterior corner of the glenoid, the joint will "open book" on external rotation (**B**). (From Matsen FA III, Lippitt SB. *Shoulder Surgery: Principles and Procedures.* Philadelphia: Saunders; 2004:579.)

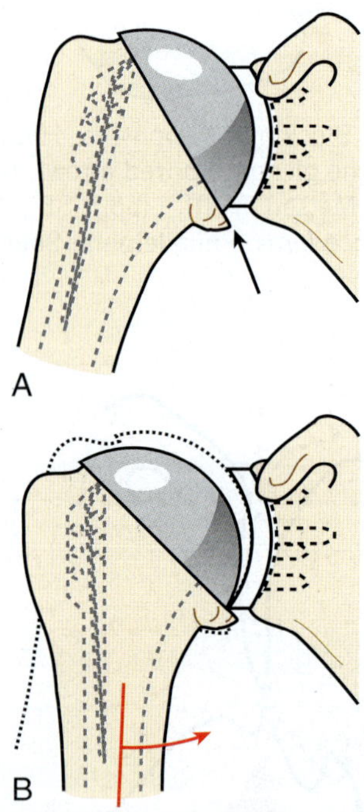

FIGURE 16-227: Inferior "open book." **A,** Bone extending beyond the curvature of the prosthetic humeral articular surface (arrow). **B,** This can abut the inferior glenoid when the arm is adducted (arrow). (From Matsen FA III, Lippitt SB. *Shoulder Surgery: Principles and Procedures.* Philadelphia: Saunders; 2004:701.)

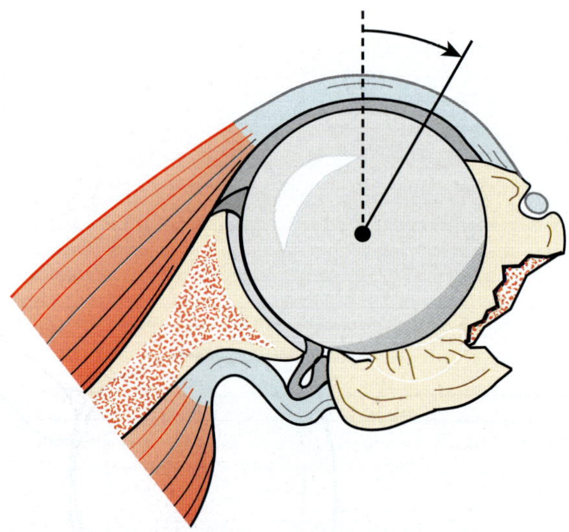

FIGURE 16-228: Malunion of the greater tuberosity. Malunion with posterior displacement of the greater tuberosity allows the tuberosity to abut the glenoid on external rotation. (From Matsen FA III, Lippitt SB. *Shoulder Surgery: Principles and Procedures.* Philadelphia: Saunders; 2004:701.)

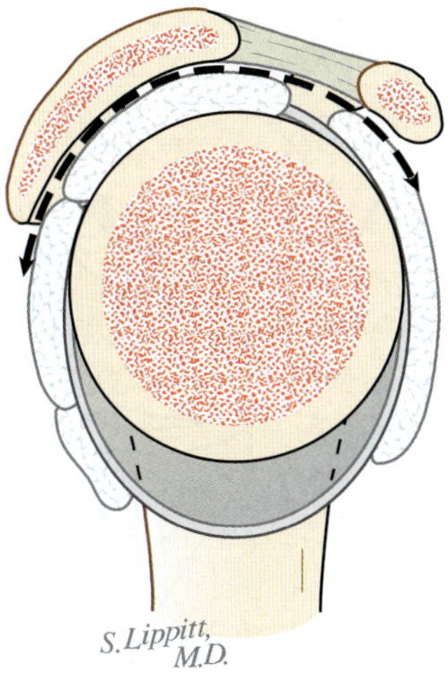

FIGURE 16-229: Humeroscapular motion interface (dotted line). The external surface of the rotator cuff articulates with the undersurface of the coracoacromial arch. This articulation is part of the humeroscapular motion interface. Smooth, unrestrained movement at this interface is required for normal shoulder function. (From Matsen FA III, Lippitt SB. *Shoulder Surgery: Principles and Procedures.* Philadelphia: Saunders; 2004:412.)

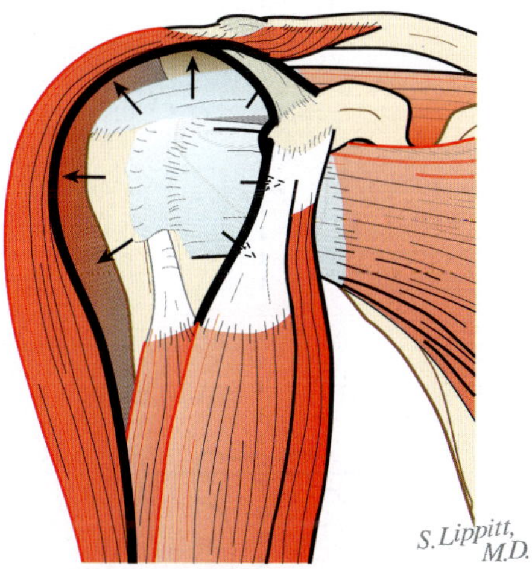

FIGURE 16-230: Humeroscapular motion interface. The humeroscapular motion interface is the set of gliding surfaces (arrows) between the proximal humerus covered by the rotator cuff tendons and the overlying structures attached to the scapula, including the deltoid, acromion, coracoacromial ligament, coracoid, and the tendons of the coracoid muscles. Approximately 4 cm of motion takes place at this interface in normal shoulder movement. (From Matsen FA III, Lippitt SB. *Shoulder Surgery: Principles and Procedures.* Philadelphia: Saunders; 2004:413.)

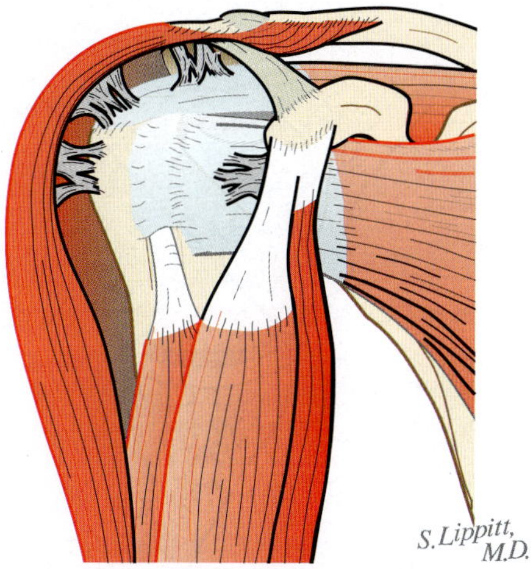

FIGURE 16-231: Spot welds. Adhesions from the external to the internal surface of the humeroscapular motion interface can restrict the range and smoothness of motion. (From Matsen FA III, Lippitt SB. *Shoulder Surgery: Principles and Procedures.* Philadelphia: Saunders; 2004:45.)

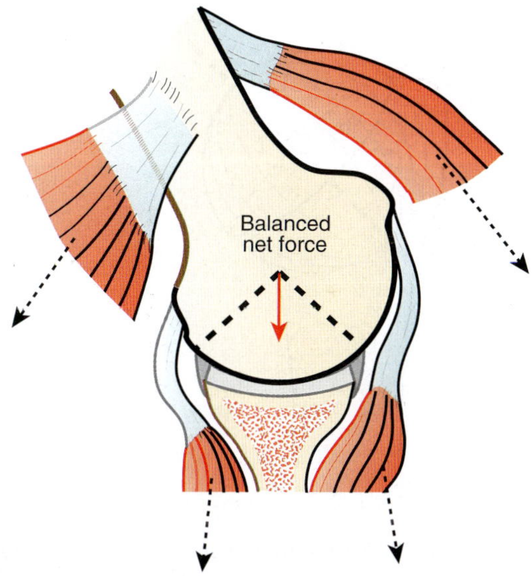

FIGURE 16-232: Balanced net forces. The direction of the forces exerted by the scapulohumeral muscles (dashed arrows) is determined by their effective attachments to the scapula and humerus. (From Matsen FA III, Lippitt SB. *Shoulder Surgery: Principles and Procedures.* Philadelphia: Saunders; 2004:488.)

Humeral Articular Surface Area. The function of the humeral articular surface is to apply the net humeral joint reaction force evenly across the glenoid throughout the normal range of glenohumeral motion. A prosthetic surface area that represents only a small part of the total sphere can predispose to instability in the same way that a Hill-Sachs defect does in traumatic instability by offering less contact area for joint surface contact (see Figs. 16-213 to 16-218; Fig. 16-233).

The orientation of the humeral articular surface can be described in terms of the humeral head centerline, a line that passes through the center of the humeral joint surface and the center of the anatomic neck (Fig. 16-234). This line usually makes a valgus angle of about 130

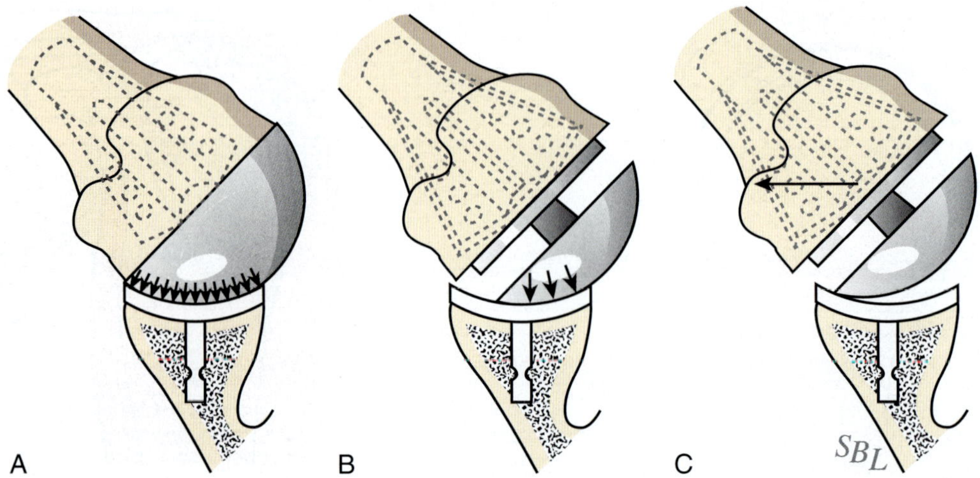

FIGURE 16-233: Surface contact. **A,** Full surface contact provides broadly distributed load transfer and maximal joint stability. **B** and **C,** Without full surface contact, the humeral component can be translated in the direction of the empty part of the glenoid. (From Matsen FA III, Lippitt SB. *Shoulder Surgery: Principles and Procedures.* Philadelphia: Saunders; 2004:433.)

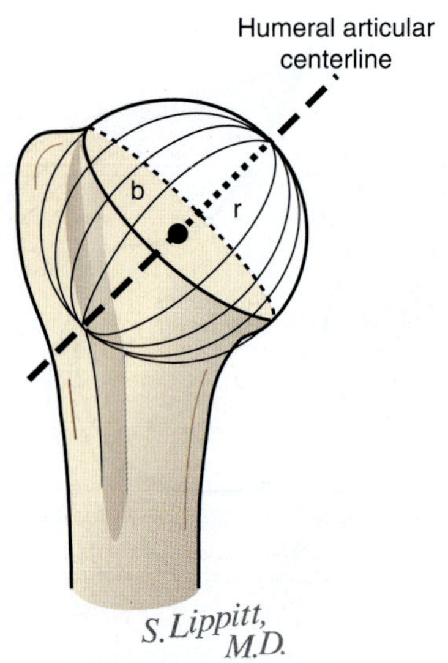

FIGURE 16-234: Humeral articular surface. The humeral articular surface can be considered as a spherical cap described by its radius of curvature (r), base (b), height along the humeral articular centerline, and surface area. (From Matsen FA III, Lippitt SB: *Shoulder Surgery: Principles and Procedures.* Philadelphia: WB Saunders; 2004:429.)

degrees with the humeral shaft, and it generally makes a retroversion angle of about 30 degrees with the plane of the humerus (Figs. 16-235 and 16-236).[106,276,427,456] In contrast to the situation with the femoral component in hip arthroplasty where rotational alignment is critical (Fig. 16-237), changing the version of the humeral component has relatively little effect on the effective position of the articulating surface of the humerus. This is because in most situations the center of rotation of the spherical humeral articular surface is close to the center of rotation

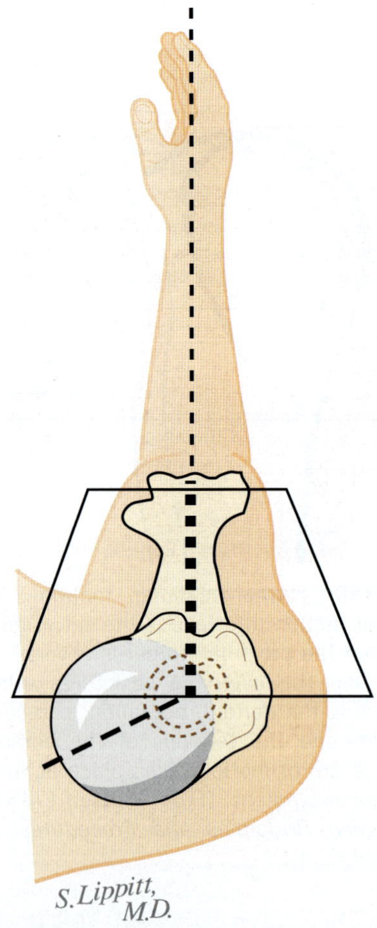

FIGURE 16-235: Plane of the humerus and humeral centerline. The humeral articular centerline (running to the lower left) usually points posteriorly and medially to the humeral plane. (From Matsen FA III, Lippitt SB. *Shoulder Surgery: Principles and Procedures.* Philadelphia: Saunders; 2004:438.)

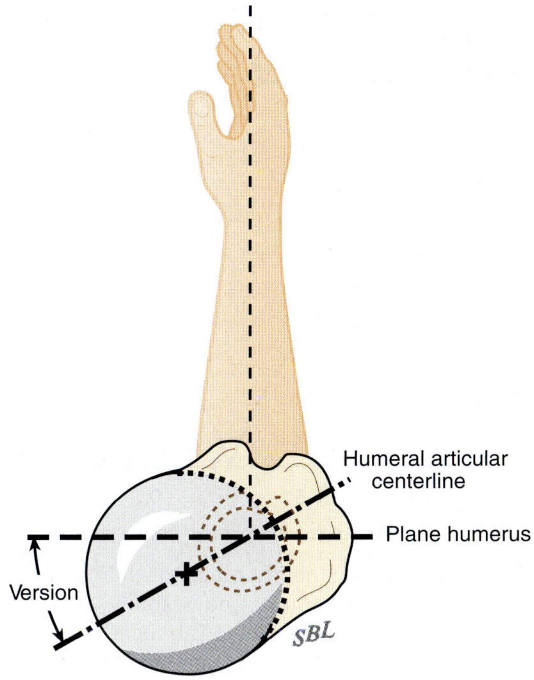

FIGURE 16-236: Retroversion. This retroversion is usually about 30 degrees. (From Matsen FA III, Lippitt SB. *Shoulder Surgery: Principles and Procedures.* Philadelphia: Saunders; 2004:439.)

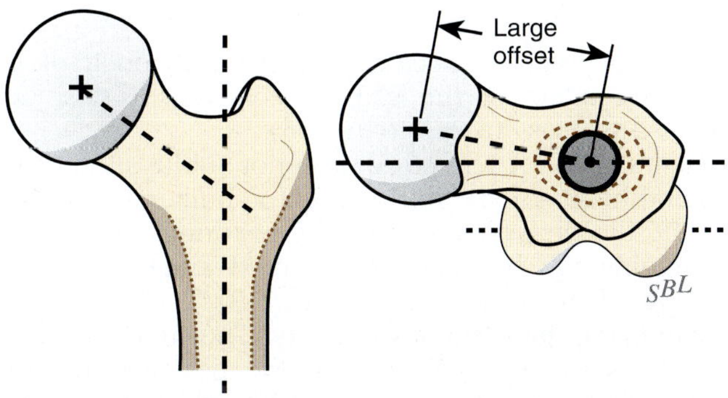

FIGURE 16-237: The center of the femoral head is substantially offset. In the femur the large offset and the lack of restricting soft tissue attachments allow a substantial effect on the articular surface position from changes in version. (From Matsen FA III, Lippitt SB. *Shoulder Surgery: Principles and Procedures.* Philadelphia: Saunders; 2004:441.)

of the stem of the prosthesis in the diaphysis (Fig. 16-238). Thus alteration of humeral version is relatively ineffective in managing glenohumeral instability.

Effective use of the available glenoid concavity requires the humeral articular surface to be aligned with the socket, which we refer to as proper "register" (Fig. 16-239). If the ball is centered in the glenoid concavity, the socket provides the maximal stabilizing effect as shown by the glenoidogram (Figs. 16-240 to 16-242). If the humeral component is placed too high

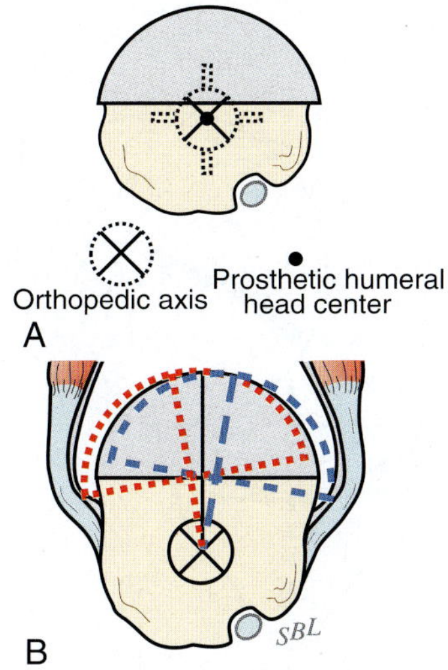

FIGURE 16-238: Modifying humeral version. The ability of the surgeon to change the position of the articular surface by changing the humeral component version is restricted by two factors. **A,** Because the offset between the center of rotation of the humeral head and the orthopedic axis is small, the effect of changing version on the position of the articular surface is small. **B,** With a press-fit humeral stem, the amount by which the version of the prosthesis can be changed without compromising the cuff insertion is small. (The red and blue dotted lines show the maximum excursion possible without compromising cuff insertion.) (From Matsen FA III, Lippitt SB. *Shoulder Surgery: Principles and Procedures.* Philadelphia: Saunders; 2004:440.)

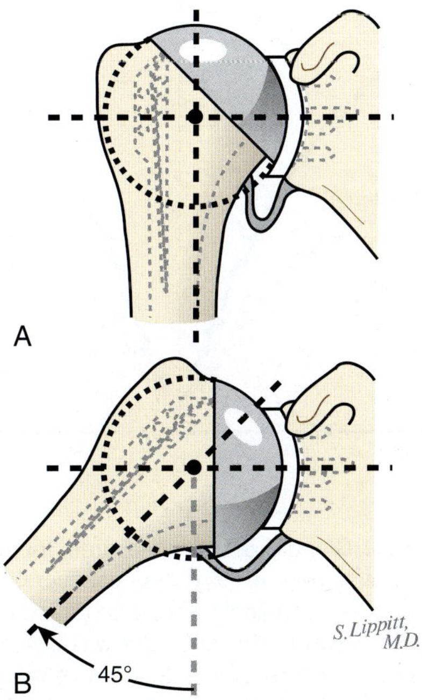

FIGURE 16-239: If the components are in proper register, the humeral articular surface should seat fully in the glenoid in adduction (**A**) andin 45 degrees of abduction (**B**). (From Matsen FA III, Lippitt SB. *Shoulder Surgery: Principles and Procedures.* Philadelphia: Saunders; 2004:461.)

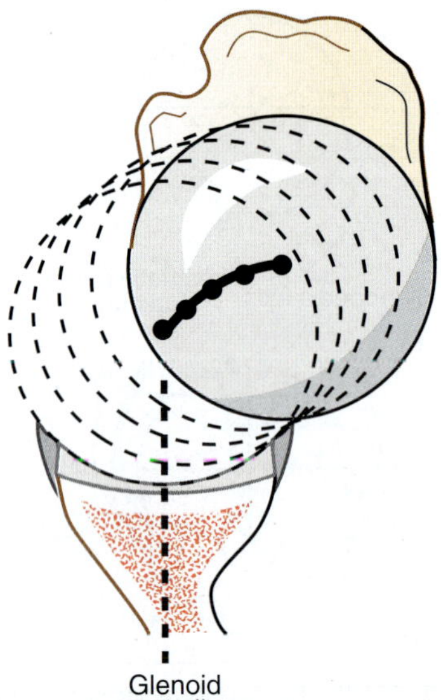

FIGURE 16-240: The functional shape of the glenoid surface in a given direction is best characterized by the glenoidogram, that is, the path taken by the head of the humerus as it passes from the center of the glenoid over its rim in that direction. (The black dot indicates the center of the head of the humerus.) (From Matsen FA III, Lippitt SB. *Shoulder Surgery: Principles and Procedures.* Philadelphia: Saunders; 2004:483.)

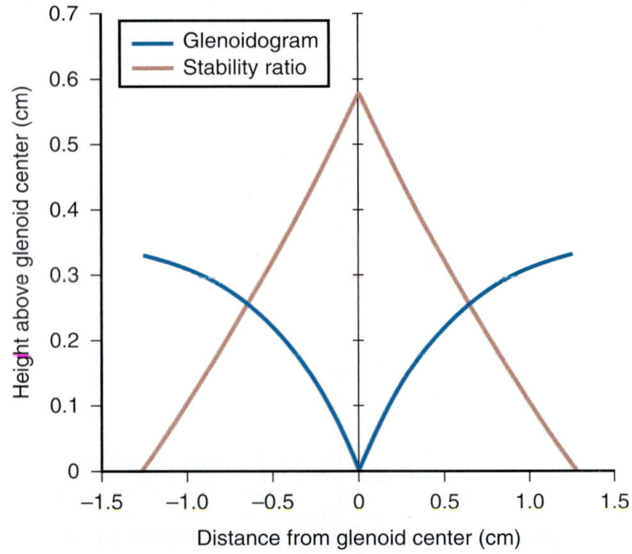

FIGURE 16-242: Local stability ratio: the humeral head and glenoid have the same radius. The stability ratio does not remain constant across the glenoid. The local stability ratio is at its maximum where the glenoidogram has the greatest slope. When the glenoid and humerus have the same radius, there is a peak in the local stability ratio at the center of the glenoid. Thus the humerus is most stable in the center of the glenoid. (From Matsen FA III, Lippitt SB. *Shoulder Surgery: Principles and Procedures.* Philadelphia: Saunders; 2004:106.)

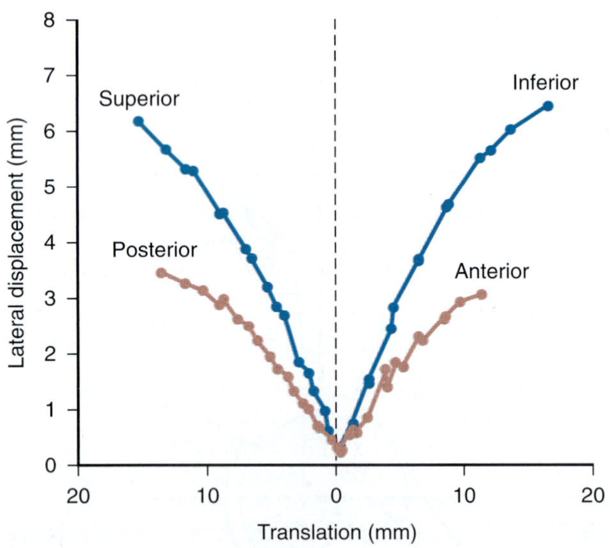

FIGURE 16-241: Glenoidograms measured for four different directions of translation in a young cadaver shoulder. The dotted vertical line represents the glenoid center line. The effective glenoid depth in this shoulder was 3.4 mm for translation in the posterior direction, 3.2 mm in the anterior direction, 6.2 mm in the superior direction, and 6.4 mm in the inferior direction. Note the high degree of symmetry about the glenoid center line and the deep valley when the head is exactly centered in the glenoid socket. (From Matsen FA III, Lippitt SB, Sidles JA, Harryman DT II. *Practical Evaluation and Management of the Shoulder.* Philadelphia: WB Saunders; 1994.)

or too low with respect to the glenoid, much of the stabilizing effect of the glenoid concavity is lost (see Fig. 16-218; Figs. 16-243 to 16-255).

In situations of refractory posterior subluxation of the humeral head, an anteriorly eccentric humeral head may provide the necessary stability by restoring register, that is, aligning the humeral and glenoid articular surfaces (see Fig. 16-38; Figs. 16-256 to 16-259).[344]

Stabilizing the Glenoid Concavity. The function of the glenoid concavity is to contain the net humeral joint reaction force, enabling stability from concavity compression, and to distribute this load uniformly to the subjacent bone.[330] In normal shoulders the glenoid centerline (the line perpendicular to the center of the glenoid fossa) is usually within 15 degrees of the plane of the scapula (Figs. 16-260 and 16-261). The arc of the glenoid determines the maximum angles for which the net humeral joint reaction force is supported by the glenoid articular surface (Fig. 16-262).

In an arthritic glenohumeral joint the effective glenoid arc and stability are often compromised by abnormal glenoid shape and orientation.[16,156,379,563] Central erosion of the glenoid is typical of rheumatoid arthritis (see Figs. 16-91 to 16-94); superior erosion is typical of CTA (see Figs. 16-24, 16-98 to 16-100, and 16-106); and posterior erosion is typical of glenohumeral osteoarthritis and capsulorrhaphy arthropathy (see Figs. 16-42, 16-66, 16-89, and 16-90; Fig. 16-263). The effect of posterior glenoid

Text continued on p. 929

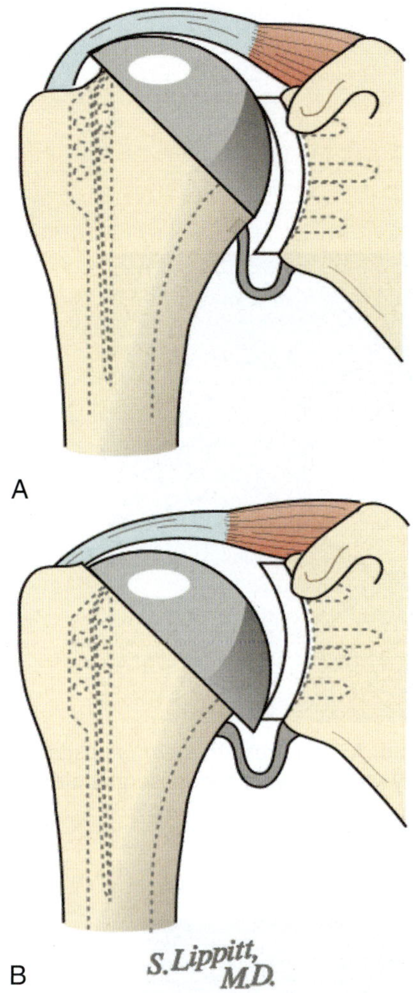

FIGURE 16-243: When the humeral and glenoid components articulate, it is important that they are in proper register. If the humeral head component sits too superiorly or too inferiorly with respect to the glenoid component, eccentric loading can jeopardize the durability and stability of the arthroplasty. **A,** Head too superior. **B,** Head too inferior.

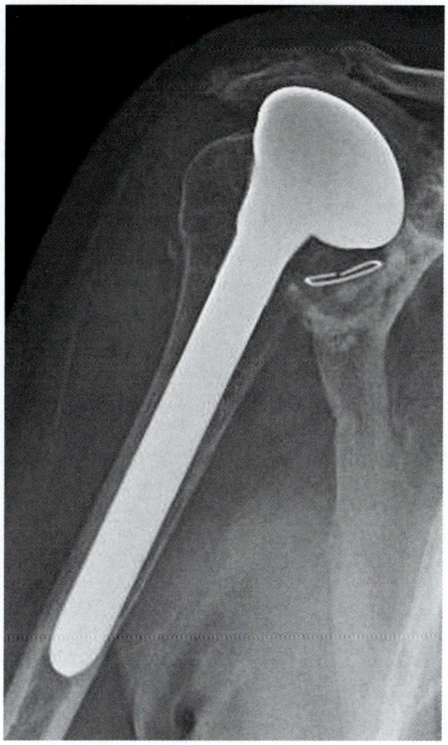

FIGURE 16-245: Implantation of a humeral stem with an excessively large diameter resulted in diaphyseal incarceration, a humeral component that was too high, and "rocking horse" loosening of the glenoid.

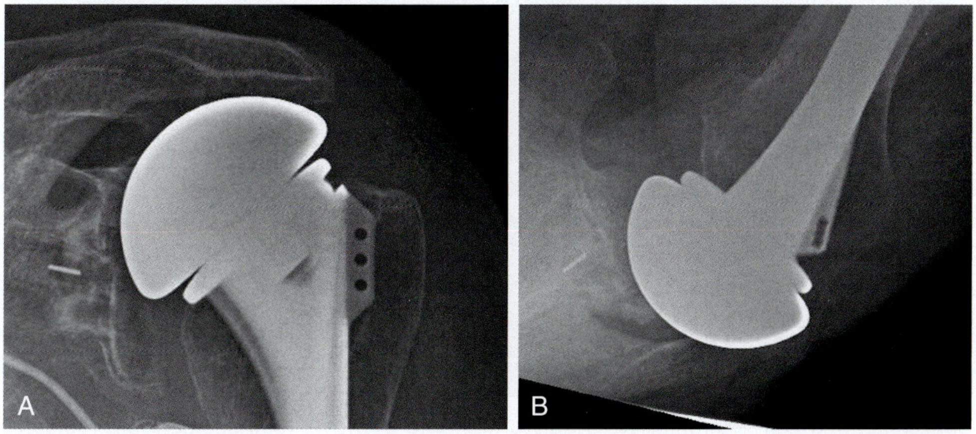

FIGURE 16-244: Problems resulting from too high positioning of a humeral prosthesis. **A,** Glenoid component loosening due to the "rocking horse" mechanism. **B,** Posterior instability.

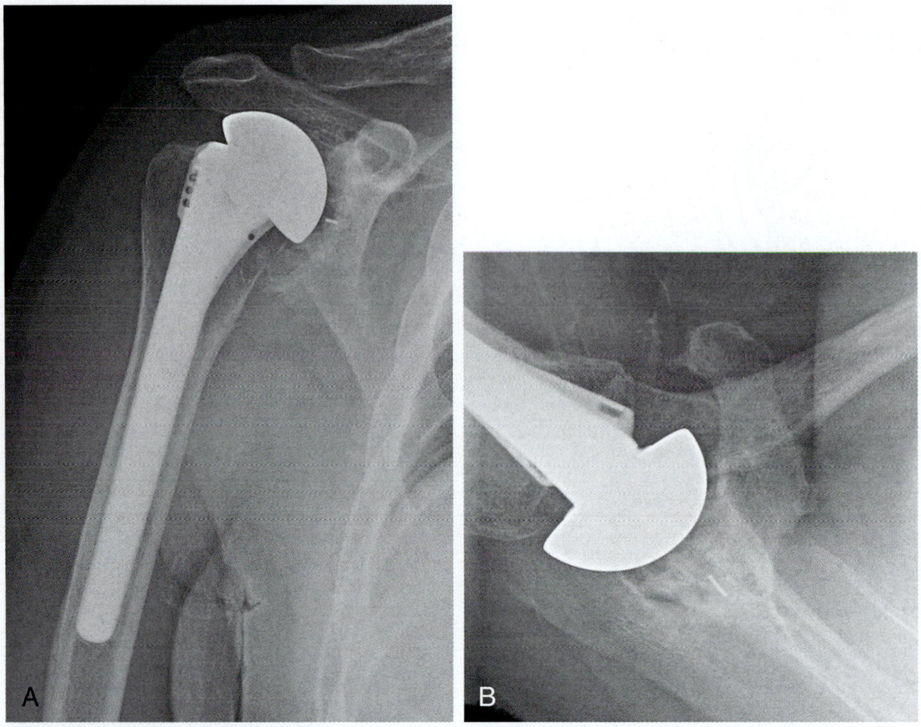

FIGURE 16-246: High humeral head positioning associated with a loose glenoid. **A,** The press-fit stem is positioned high in the humerus because of a tight diaphyseal fit that prevents full seating. **B,** Axillary view showing the loose glenoid component.

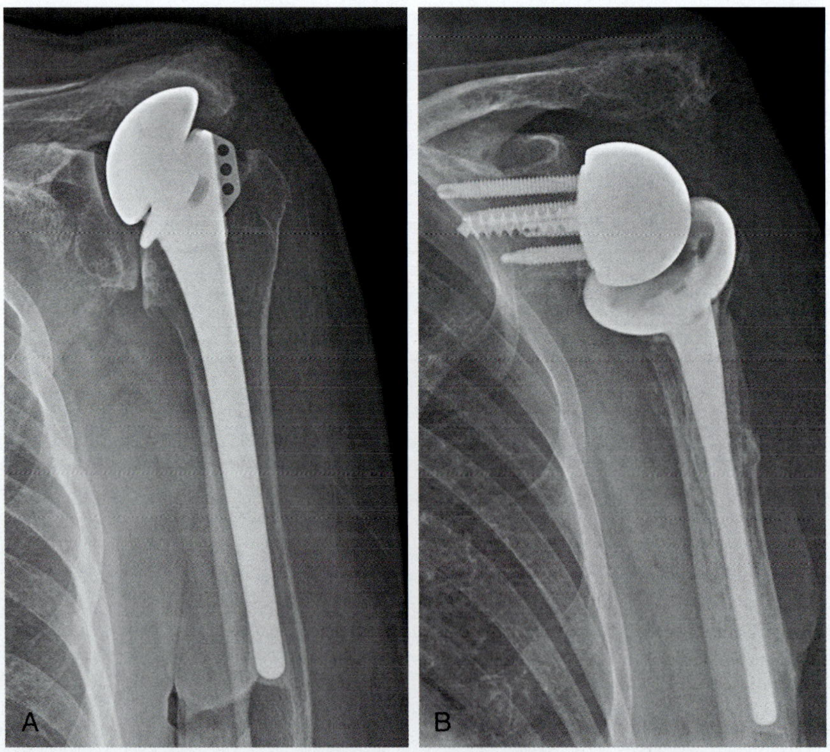

FIGURE 16-247: Conversion of a hemiarthroplasty that is too high into a reverse total shoulder arthroplasty. **A,** Anteroposterior radiograph showing a humeral component that is too high with upper glenoid and acromial erosion. **B,** Monoblock reverse total shoulder arthroplasty inserted with impaction grafting.

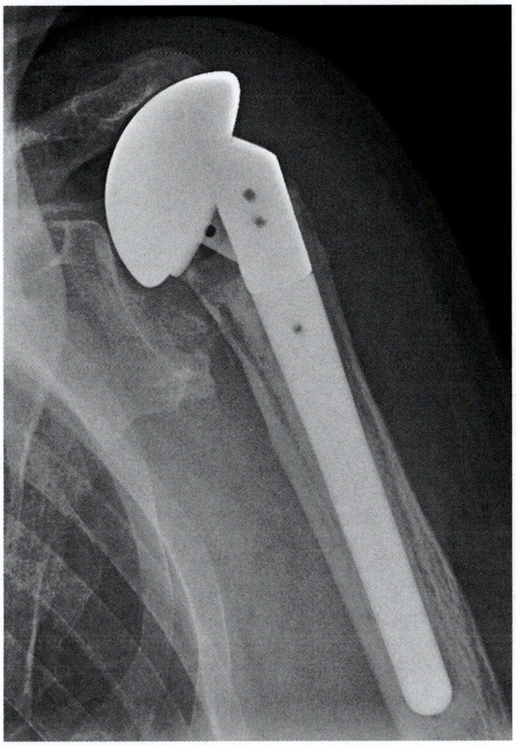

FIGURE 16-248: Platform prosthesis cemented in a high position that complicates revision to a reverse arthroplasty without the complex removal of the cemented stem.

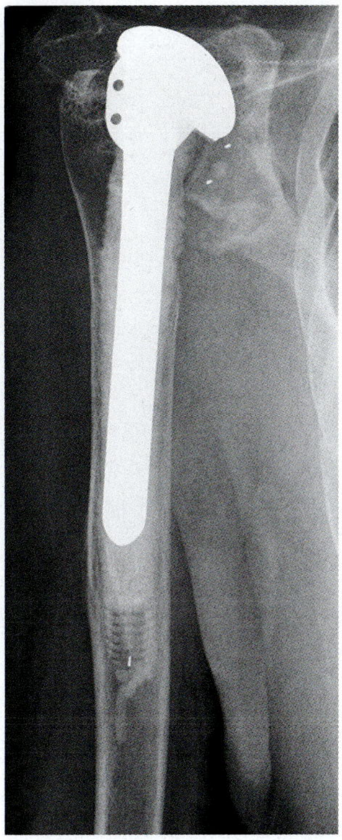

FIGURE 16-249: Humeral prosthesis cemented in a position that is too high, with "rocking horse" loosening of the glenoid component.

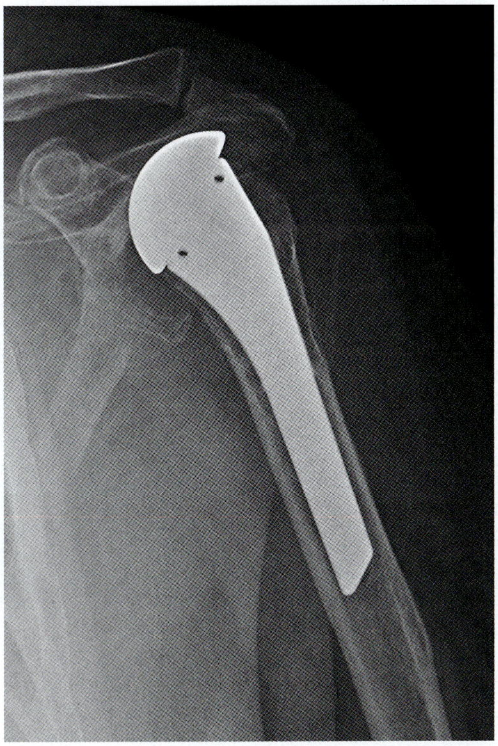

FIGURE 16-250: A too-high humeral stem with superior instability.

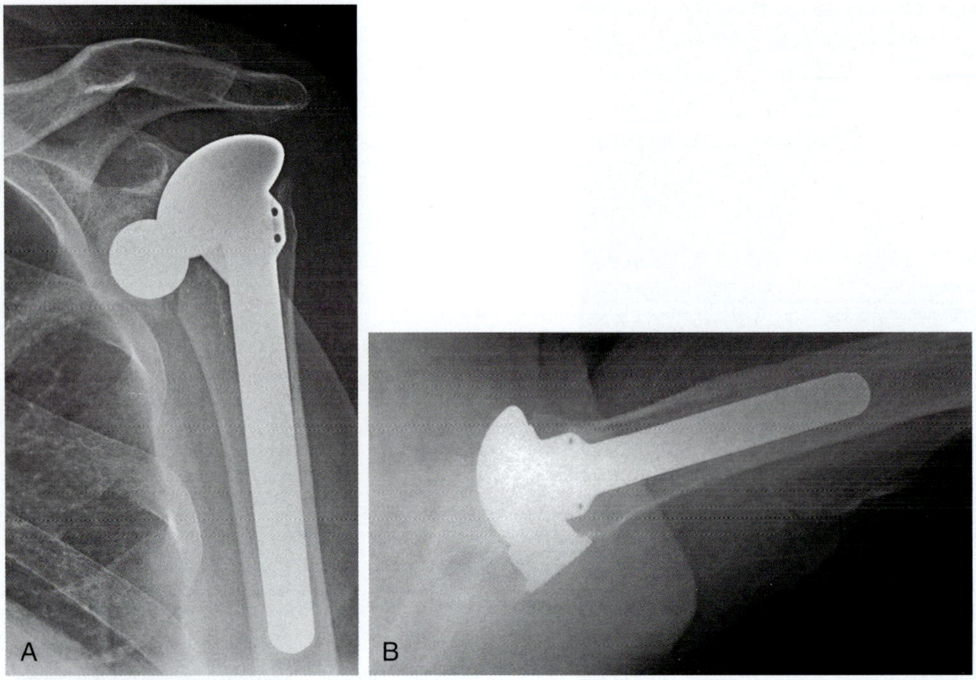

FIGURE 16-251: A too-high humeral stem with the tip wedged in the diaphysis and a dislocated metal-backed glenoid component. **A,** Anteroposterior view. **B,** Axillary view.

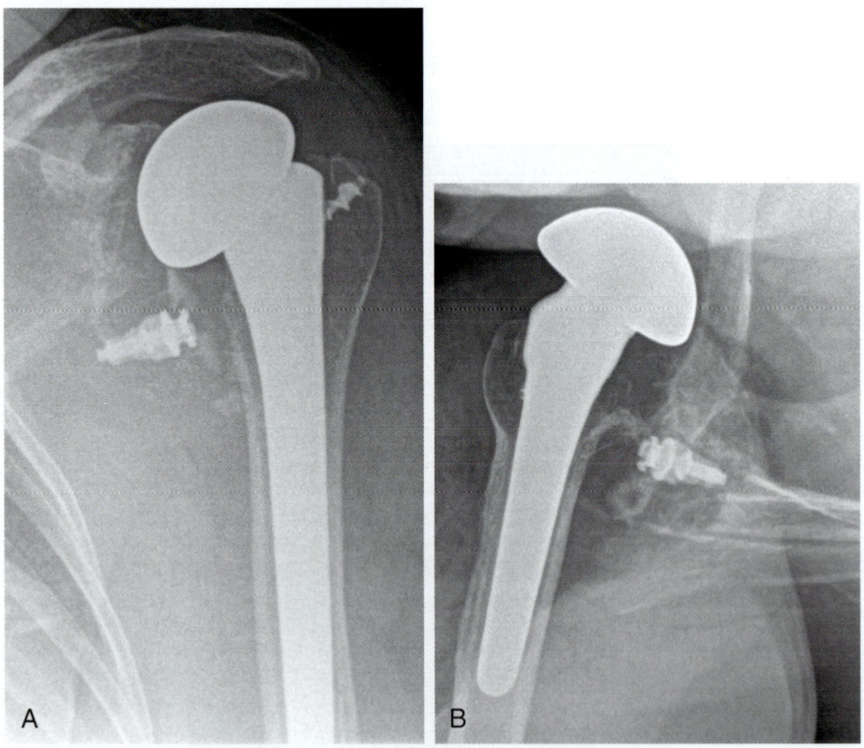

FIGURE 16-252: A too-high humeral head (**A**) and a loose glenoid (**B**) with anterior dislocation of the total shoulder.

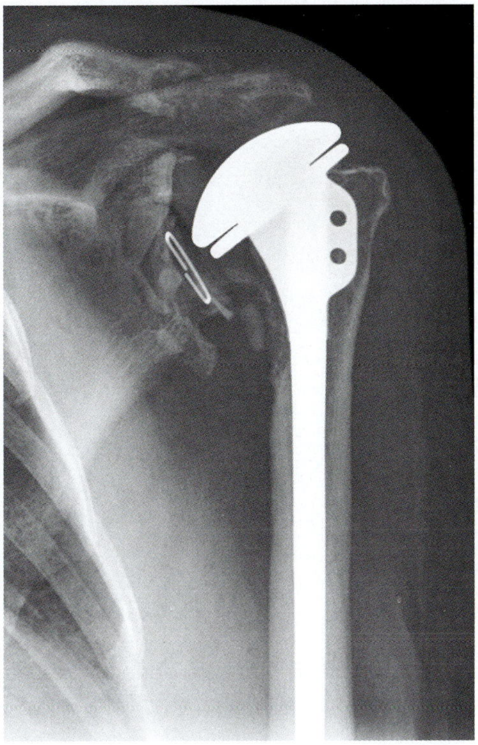

FIGURE 16-253: A too-high humeral head with "rocking horse" loosening of the glenoid component.

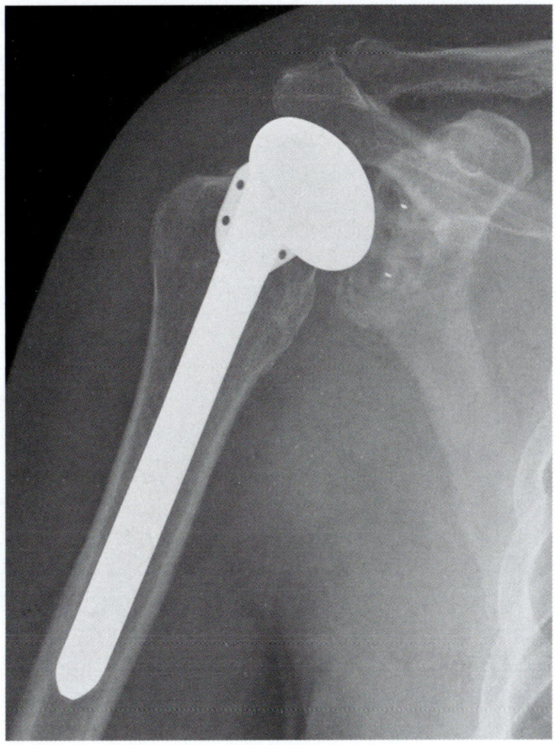

FIGURE 16-255: A too-high humeral component and loose glenoid.

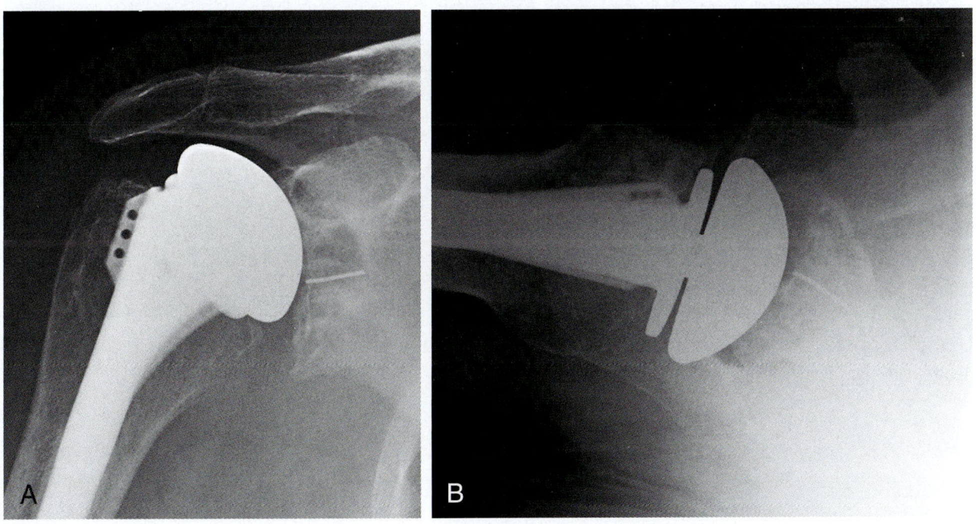

FIGURE 16-254: A too-high humeral head with superior glenoid wear. **A,** Anteroposterior view. **B,** Axillary view.

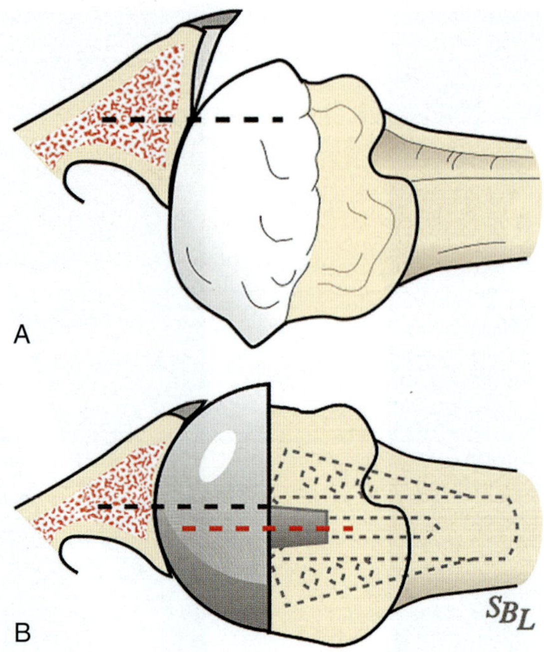

FIGURE 16-256: **A,** Preoperative posterior humeral subluxation on a biconcave glenoid. **B,** Anteriorly oriented eccentric head component with proper alignment on a concentric reamed glenoid.

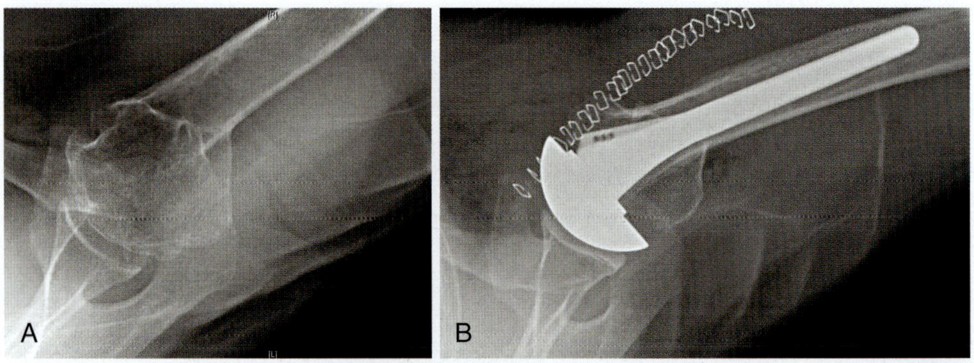

FIGURE 16-257: Use of a posteriorly eccentric humeral head to manage a postfracture offset of the humeral head on the shaft. **A,** Preoperative radiograph. **B,** Postoperative radiograph.

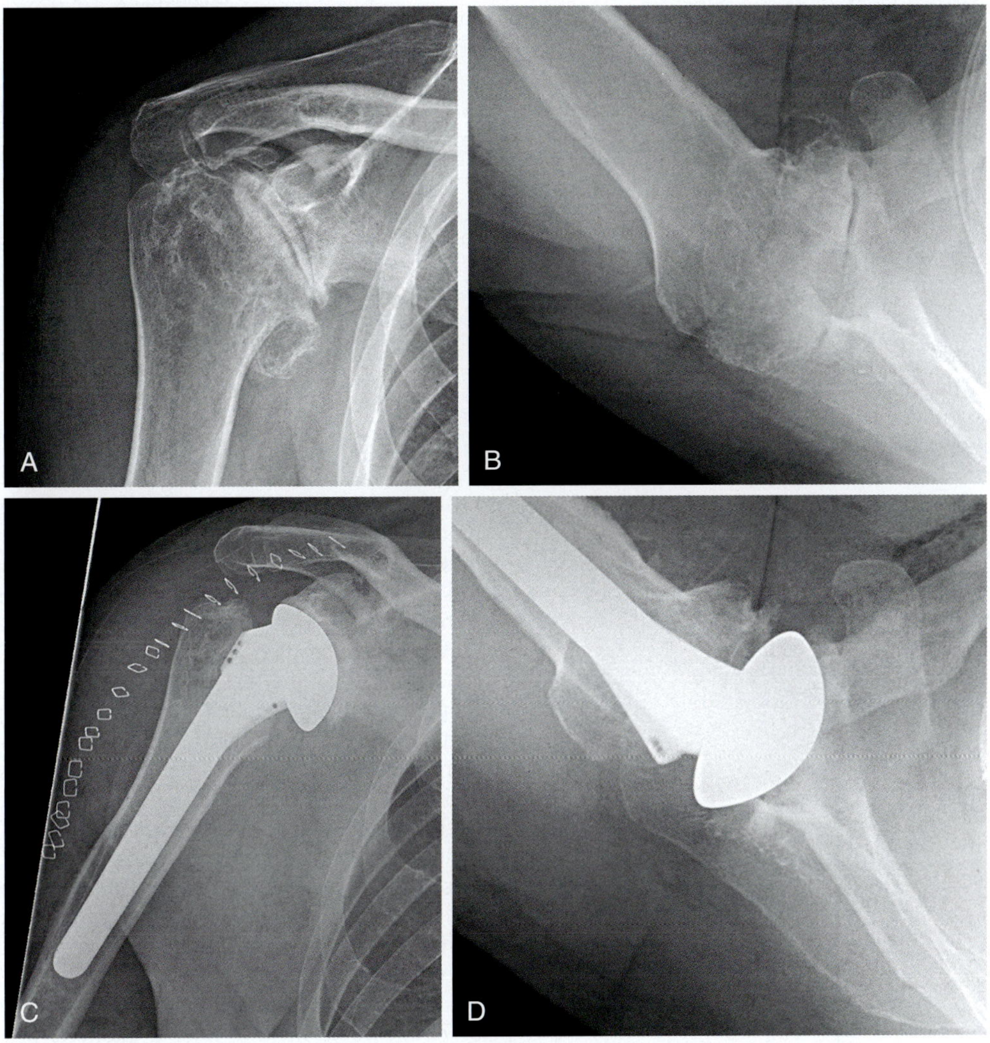

FIGURE 16-258: Management of severe retroversion with a ream and run procedure. **A,** Preoperative anteroposterior view. **B,** Preoperative axillary view. **C,** Postoperative anteroposterior view. **D,** Postoperative axillary view showing centering of the anteriorly eccentric humeral head in the retroverted glenoid.

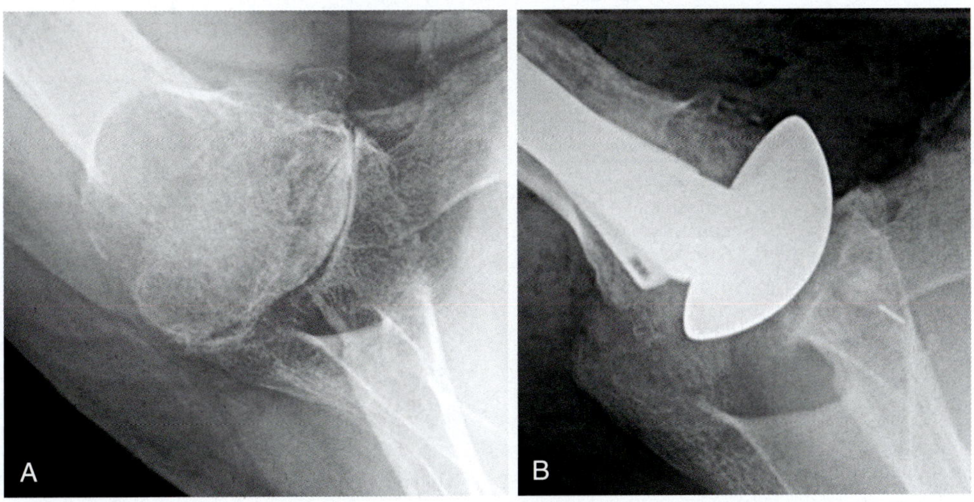

FIGURE 16-259: **A,** Preoperative axillary view showing glenoid retroversion. **B,** Axillary view after a total shoulder arthroplasty showing an anteriorly eccentric humeral head centered on the retroverted glenoid component.

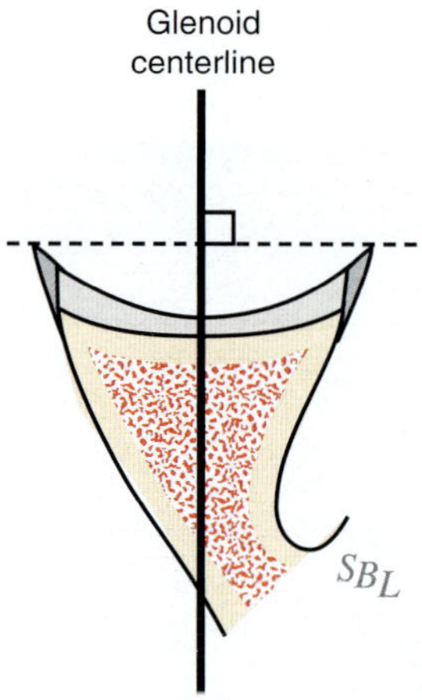

FIGURE 16-260: The glenoid centerline is perpendicular to the center of the glenoid fossa. (From Matsen FA III, Lippitt SB. *Shoulder Surgery: Principles and Procedures.* Philadelphia: Saunders; 2004:481.)

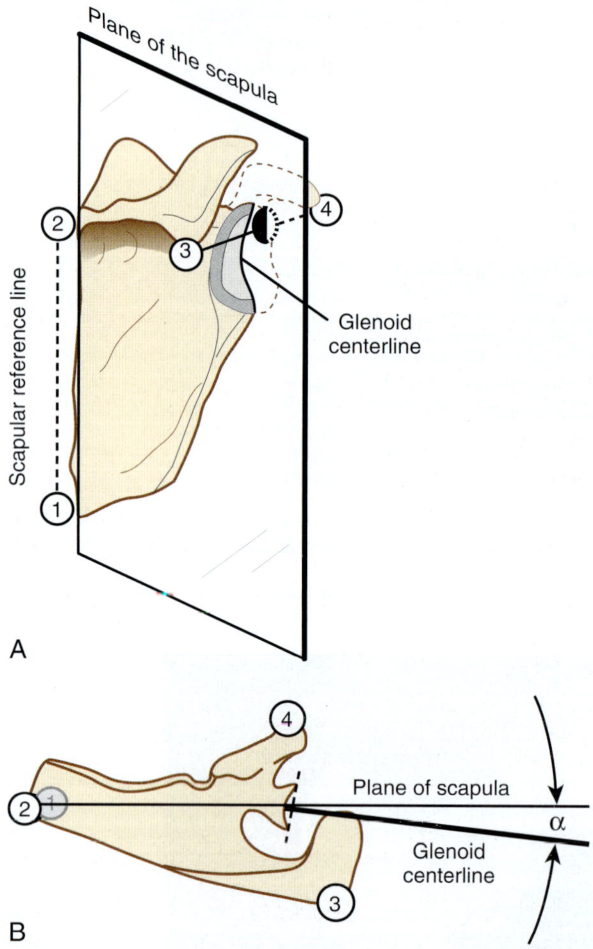

FIGURE 16-261: Orientation of the glenoid centerline with respect to the scapula. **A,** The plane of the scapula is the plane that passes through the inferior pole of the glenoid (1), the medial extent of the spine of the scapula (2), and halfway between the coracoid tip (3) and the posterior angle of the acromion (4). **B,** Laterally, the glenoid centerline passes approximately 10 degrees posterior to this plane and perpendicular to the line that connects the inferior pole and the medial spine (the scapular reference line). (From Matsen FA III, Lippitt SB. *Shoulder Surgery: Principles and Procedures.* Philadelphia: Saunders; 2004:89.)

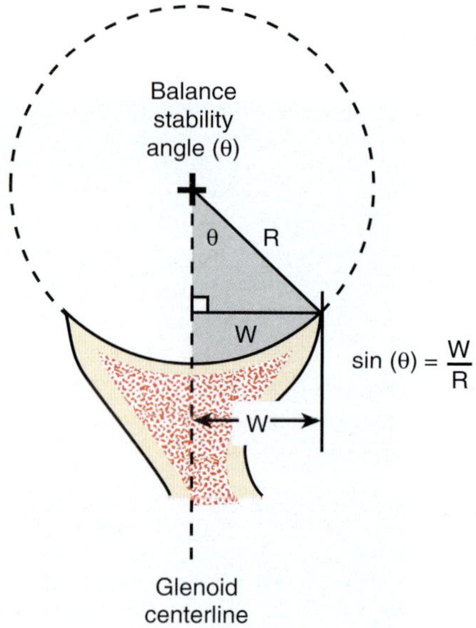

FIGURE 16-262: Calculating the balance stability angle. The predicted balance stability angle (BSA) for a spherical glenoid in a specified direction is given by the arcsine of the ratio of the glenoid width (W) in the direction of interest (the distance from the glenoid center to the reamed edge) and the radius of curvature of the glenoid. BSA = arcsine W/R, where R is the radius of the spherical glenoid. Because the sine and the tangent are about equal for small angles (e.g., <30 degrees), and the tangent is approximately equal to the angle expressed in radians (~57.3 degrees), a convenient general rule is BSA > 57.3 × W/R. For a normally directed glenoid concavity, the desired stability angle is at least 20 degrees. So if the glenoid width from the center to the edge is W, the radius should be less than three times the width (20 = 57.3 × W/R or R = 3 × W), or the diameter should be less than six times the width from the center to the edge. Thus a glenoid with a width of 10 mm would have the desired intrinsic stability if it had a diameter of less than 60 mm, whereas a glenoid with a width of 7 mm would need to have a diameter of less than 42 mm. (From Matsen FA III, Lippitt SB. *Shoulder Surgery: Principles and Procedures.* Philadelphia: Saunders; 2004:499.)

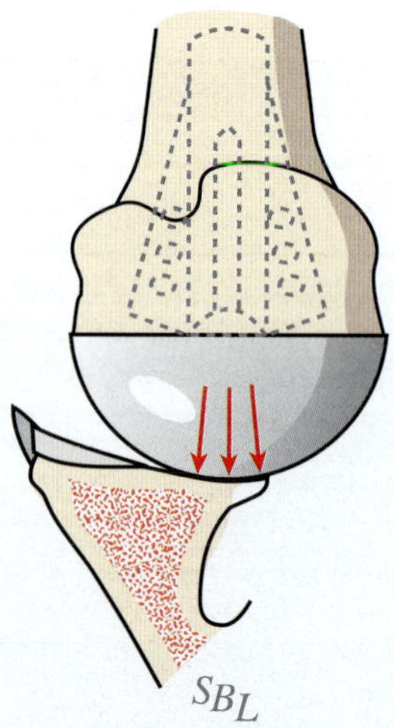

FIGURE 16-263: Biconcave glenoid. Unless a biconcave glenoid is addressed at the time of shoulder arthroplasty, the prosthetic humeral head will sit in the abnormal part of the glenoid (arrows). (From Matsen FA III, Lippitt SB. *Shoulder Surgery: Principles and Procedures.* Philadelphia: Saunders; 2004:483.)

erosion can be seen from the normal and pathologic glenoidograms (see Fig. 16-240; Fig. 16-264). It is important to note that the direction and severity of arthritic glenoid erosion are highly variable (see Figs. 16-50 and 16-52 to 16-58).[274,566]

While glenoid retroversion can be associated with posterior instability (see Figs. 16-42 and 16-53),[167,564,567] shoulders with normal version can also be posteriorly unstable (see Figs. 16-38 and 16-39) and shoulders with substantial retroversion can have the humeral head relatively centered in the glenoid fossa (Fig. 16-265).[221] Although shoulders with increased retroversion have an increased rate of glenoid component failure,[42,334,415] it has not been shown that "correction" of glenoid retroversion reestablishes stability or improves longevity of the prosthetic glenoid arthroplasty. Shoulders with greater glenoid deformity have a more severe form of arthritis, so the results of reconstruction may not measure up to what is achieved for shoulders with milder forms of the disease.[227,548]

The goal of surgical reconstruction is to center the humeral head in the glenoid fossa, rather than to align the humeral head with the body of the scapula (Fig. 16-266). Experience has taught us that centering of the posteriorly subluxated humeral head can be achieved without attempting to change glenoid version, as is described in some detail later in this chapter. Although we do not prioritize changing glenoid version during a glenohumeral arthroplasty, we will briefly review some of the approaches that other surgeons have advocated for altering glenoid retroversion (Figs. 16-267 to 16-269).

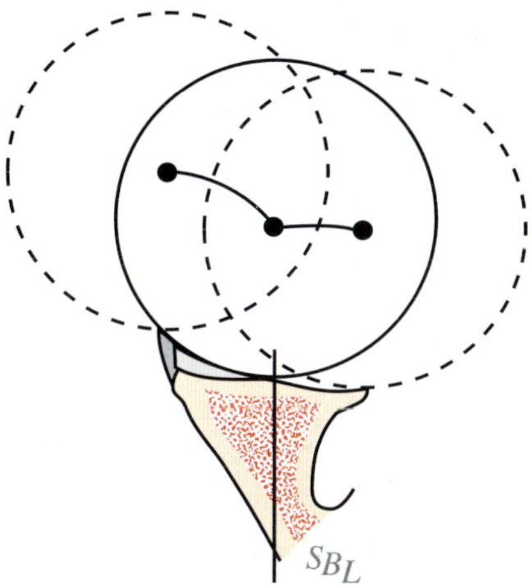

FIGURE 16-264: Glenoidogram with posterior erosion. The normal glenoid concavity creates a glenoidogram that rises dramatically as the humeral head (black dot indicates center) is translated from the center (the left half of the curve). When the glenoid is flattened, this rise is lost, indicating a loss of intrinsic stability of the glenoid (the right half of the curve). (From Matsen FA III, Lippitt SB. *Shoulder Surgery: Principles and Procedures.* Philadelphia: Saunders; 2004:483.)

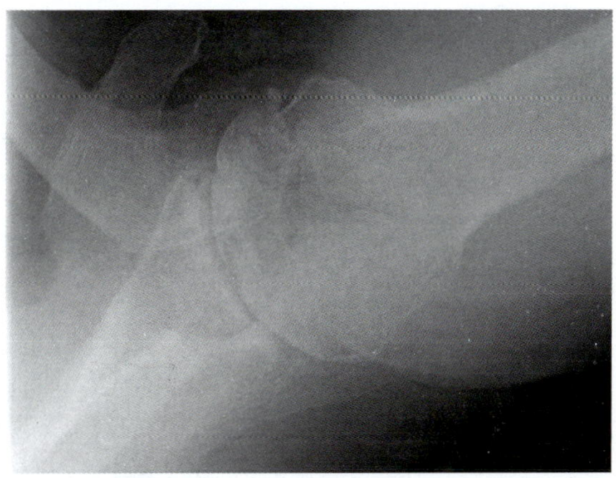

FIGURE 16-265: Humeral head centered in a retroverted glenoid.

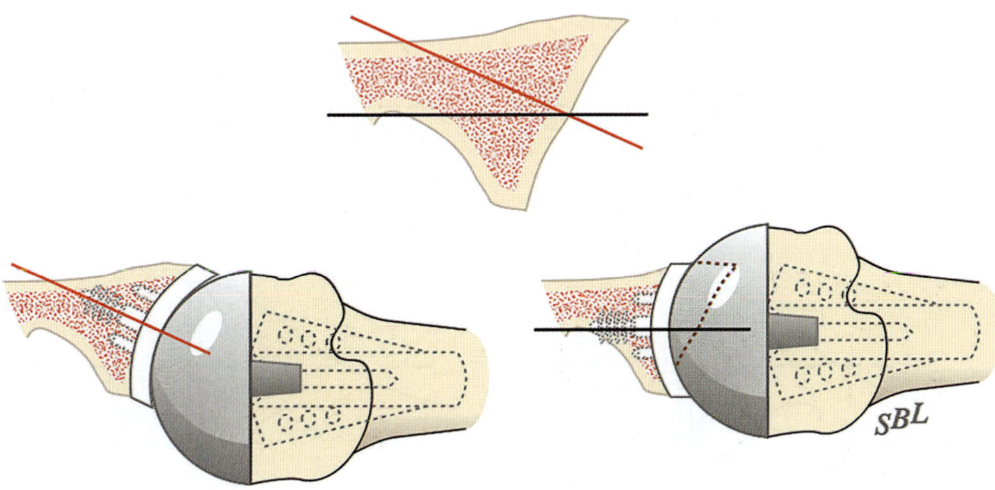

FIGURE 16-266: The goal of surgical reconstruction is to center the humeral head in the glenoid fossa along the glenoid axis (red line), rather than to align the humeral head with the scapular plane (black line).

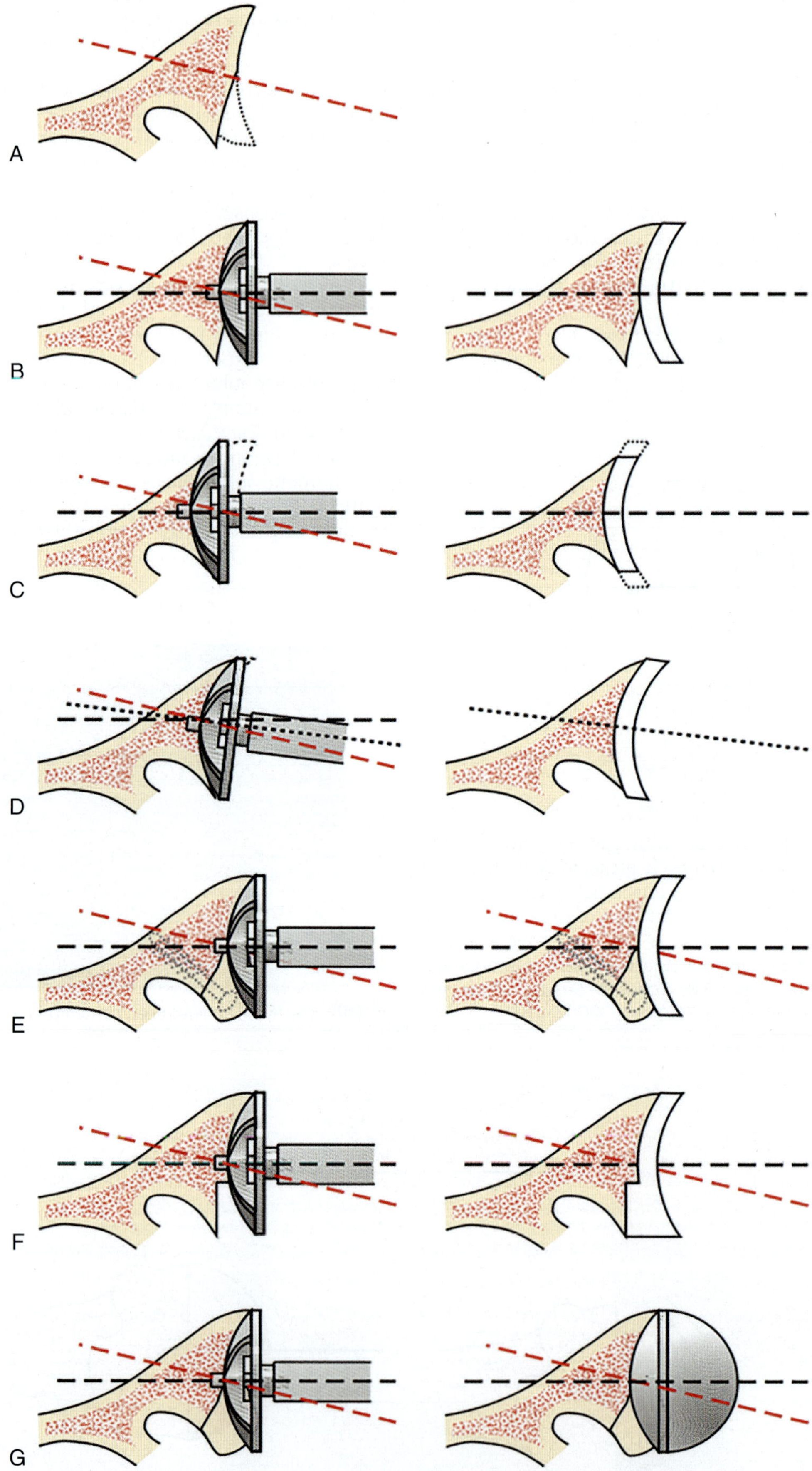

FIGURE 16-267: Different approaches advocated for a biconcave glenoid. **A,** Biconcave glenoid. **B,** Partial glenoid reaming in neutral version leaves a posterior glenoid deficiency with no support for the posterior glenoid component. **C,** Further glenoid reaming in neutral version removes excess bone, medializing the joint center and reducing the glenoid width. **D,** Partial correction glenoid retroversion preserves the glenoid bone stock. **E,** Posterior glenoid bone graft. **F,** Posterior build-up glenoid component. **G,** Glenosphere for reverse shoulder arthroplasty.

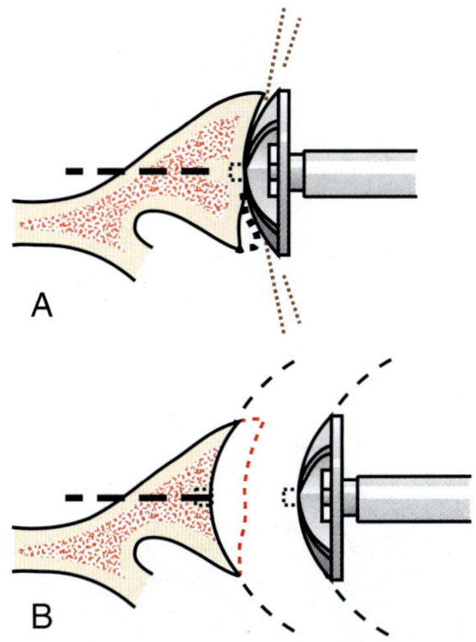

FIGURE 16-268: Glenoid reaming for nonprosthetic glenoid arthroplasty. If posterior erosion of the glenoid is minimal, the glenoid is reamed along the glenoid centerline until the full anterior and posterior extent of the surface has the desired spherical contour. (From Matsen FA III, Lippitt SB. *Shoulder Surgery: Principles and Procedures.* Philadelphia: Saunders; 2004:561.)

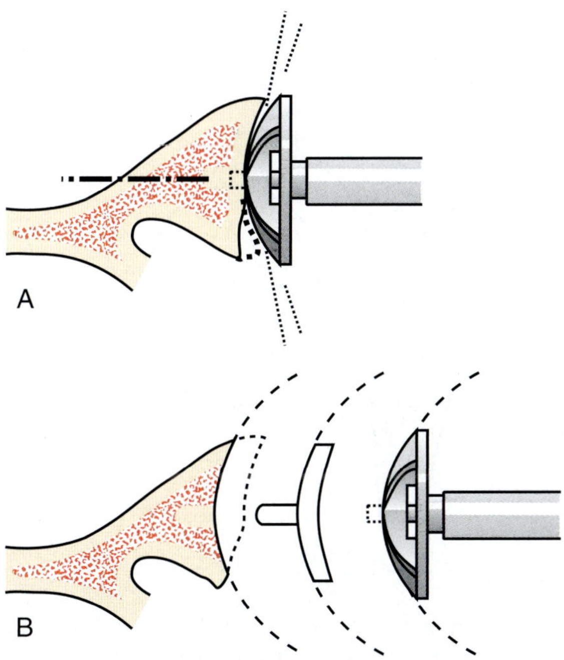

FIGURE 16-269: Glenoid reaming. A biconcave glenoid bone is spherically reamed to a diameter of curvature that matches the back of the prosthetic glenoid. (From Matsen FA III, Lippitt SB. *Shoulder Surgery: Principles and Procedures.* Philadelphia: Saunders; 2004:571.)

One method is to remove bone from the relatively high anterior side of the glenoid until the effective glenoid version is "normal." However, this method results in loss of glenoid bone stock (Fig. 16-270).[566,570] Posterior bone grafts[218,477] have been used to reduce retroversion, but the clinical effectiveness and durability of this approach is uncertain (Fig. 16-271).[218,228,268,477,525] Some surgeons have used extra cement to build up the posterior glenoid component; however, cement between the back of the component and the bone is at risk of cracking and loosening, leading to the failure of component fixation (Figs. 16-272 to 16-274). Posteriorly augmented glenoid components have also been used to "normalize" glenoid version (Fig. 16-275).[86,216,228,231,425,449,478,525] These posteriorly augmented components appear to have diminished lift-off resistance with posterosuperior loading and to be more susceptible to cold flow of the polyethylene compared with nonaugmented glenoid components.[235,425] Furthermore, changing glenoid version with posteriorly augmented glenoid components may involve the removal of glenoid bone to accommodate the particular shape of the back of the glenoid component.[273] This sacrifice of posterior bone stock can worsen the problem of posterior instability should the implant fail (Fig. 16-276).

In shoulders with glenoid retroversion we prefer to preserve glenoid bone stock by conservatively reaming the glenoid to a single concavity, whether for a ream and run procedure or to support a glenoid component in total shoulder arthroplasty; we do not strive to "correct" the retroversion (Fig. 16-277). Stability is achieved through a combination of soft tissue balancing, humeral component sizing, the use of eccentric humeral components, and rotator interval plication[334,335,337] (see Figs. 16-38, 16-211, and 16-257 to 16-259; Figs. 16-278 to 16-281).

Control of the Net Humeral Joint Reaction Force. The net humeral joint reaction force is the vector sum of all the forces acting on the humeral articular surface in relation to the glenoid. It includes the force vectors of the weight of the arm, the cuff, deltoid, and other scapulohumeral and thoracohumeral muscles as well as the effect of capsular tension. In the normal shoulder this net force is balanced within the glenoid concavity (see Fig. 16-232). The direction of the net humeral joint reaction force is modulated by neural control of the magnitudes of the different muscle forces. For example, by increasing the force of contraction of muscles, such as the infraspinatus and the subscapularis, whose direction of force is parallel to the glenoid centerline, the direction of the net humeral joint reaction force can be changed to an orientation that is in closer alignment with the glenoid fossa.[8]

In glenohumeral arthritis the desired alignment of the net humeral joint reaction force may be compromised by tendon rupture, tuberosity detachment, capsular contracture, or muscle imbalance. A most striking example is CTA, where the normally stabilizing cuff muscle forces are compromised, allowing the deltoid muscle to pull the humerus superiorly (see Fig. 16-102). In this situation the superior glenoid may be flattened, compromising the concavity and further increasing the resulting instability (see Figs. 16-6 and 16-103).

If the net humeral joint reaction force is not centered in the glenoid fossa after a total shoulder arthroplasty, rim loading can produce a "rocking horse" loosening of

Text continued on p. 936

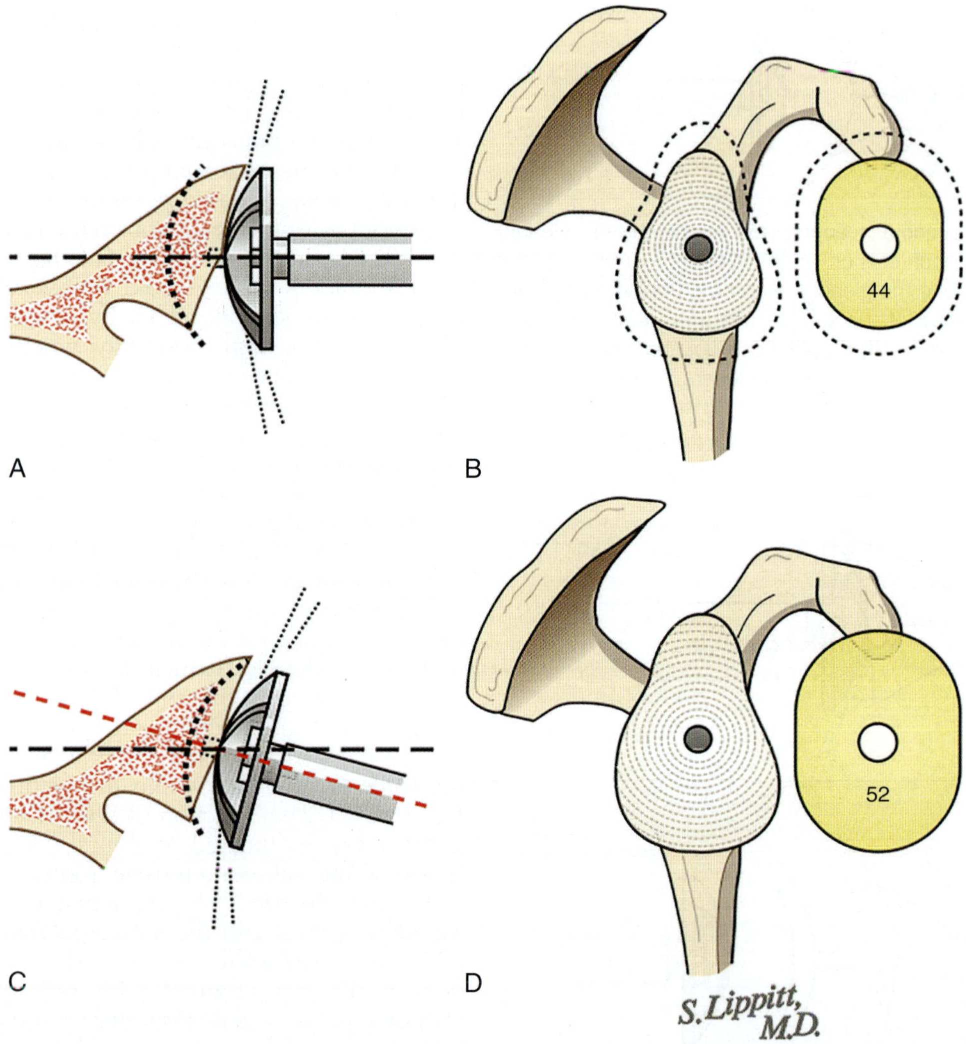

FIGURE 16-270: **A,** Reaming the anterior high side of a posterior eroded glenoid in neutral version results in the loss of glenoid bone stock and subsequently a relatively small glenoid component size. **B,** Reaming without changing glenoid version preserves more glenoid bone and allows for a larger glenoid component (**D**).

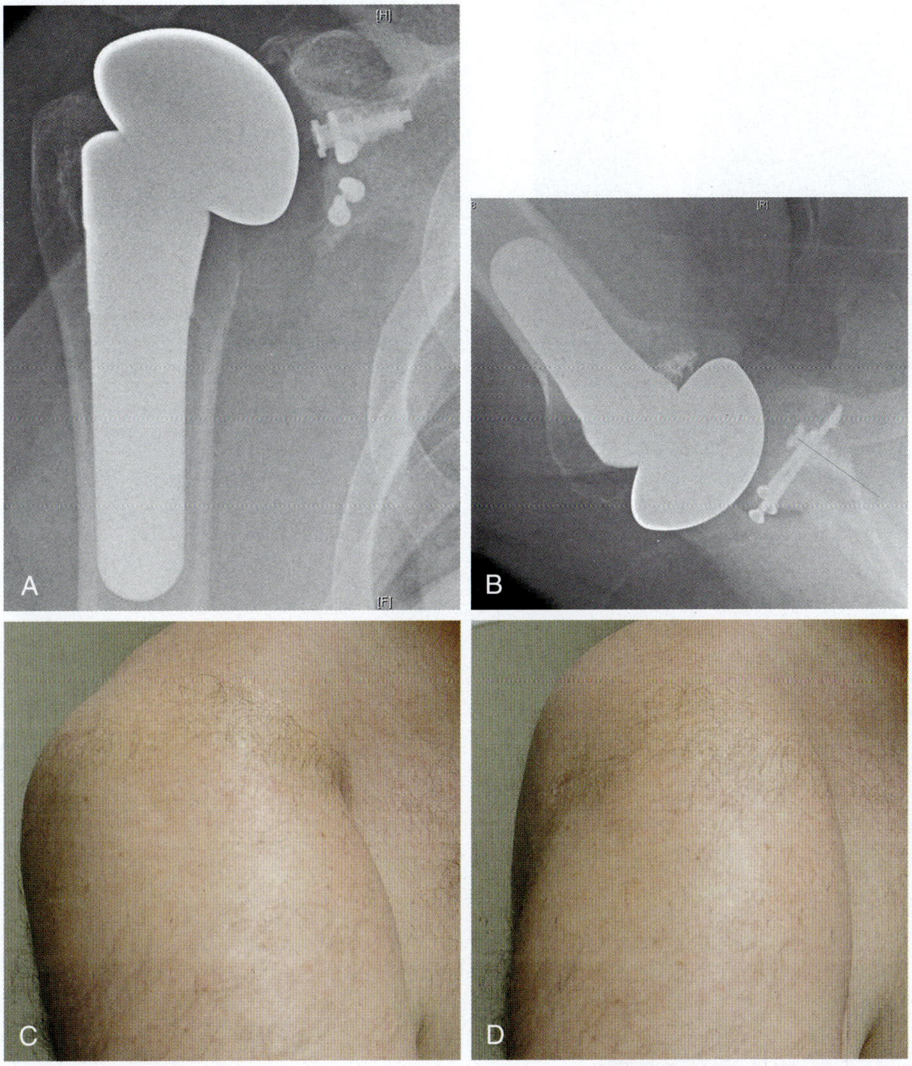

FIGURE 16-271: Posterior instability in a 40-year-old patient less than 1 year after total shoulder arthroplasty for a failed resurfacing and posterior bone block. **A,** Anteroposterior view showing a high humeral component with a bone-ingrowth stem incarcerated in the diaphysis. **B,** Axillary view showing chronic posterior subluxation of the humeral prosthesis on the glenoid, suggesting either cold-flow or fracture of the posterior aspect of the polyethylene. **C,** Clinical image showing posterior subluxation with attempted active elevation of the arm. **D,** Clinical image showing reduction of the humeral head when the arm is relaxed at the side.

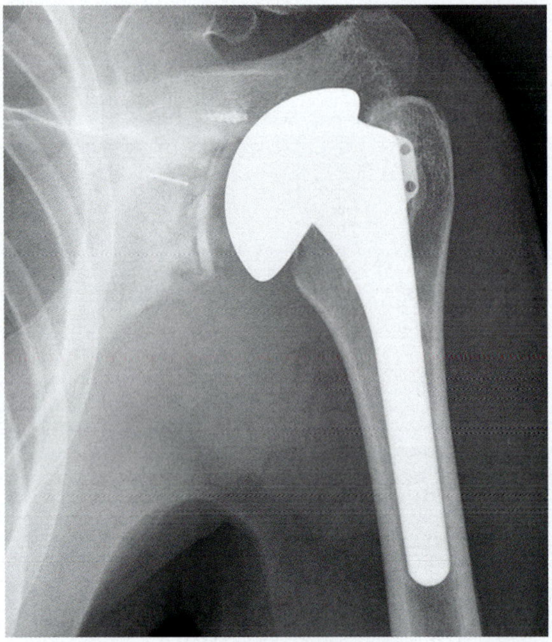

FIGURE 16-272: Poor cement technique and "rocking horse" loosening. Anteroposterior view showing a wedge of cement that was applied to the face of the glenoid beneath the glenoid component. Both it and the glenoid component have become loose.

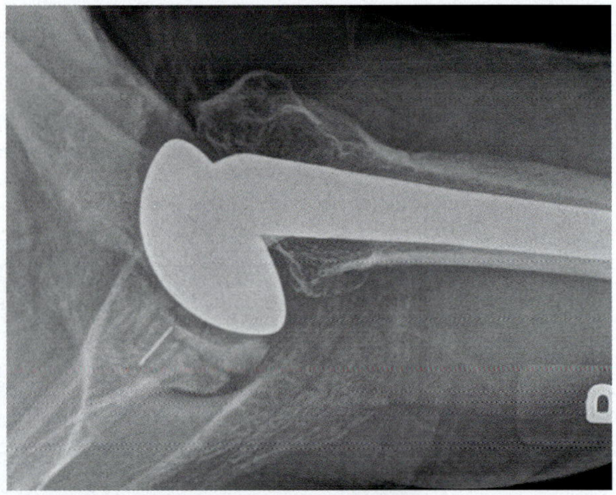

FIGURE 16-273: Faulty fixation of the glenoid component with a wedge of cement between the back of the component and the glenoid bone. Note that this wedge of bone and the entire glenoid have loosened.

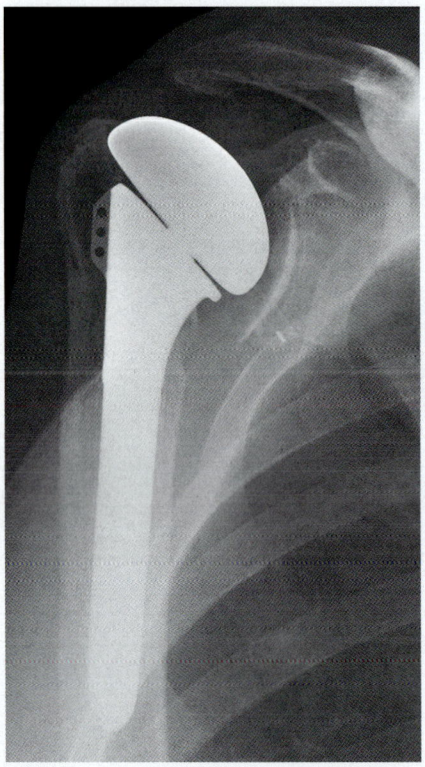

FIGURE 16-274: "Rocking horse" loosening of the glenoid component with failed cement that had been inserted beneath the glenoid face.

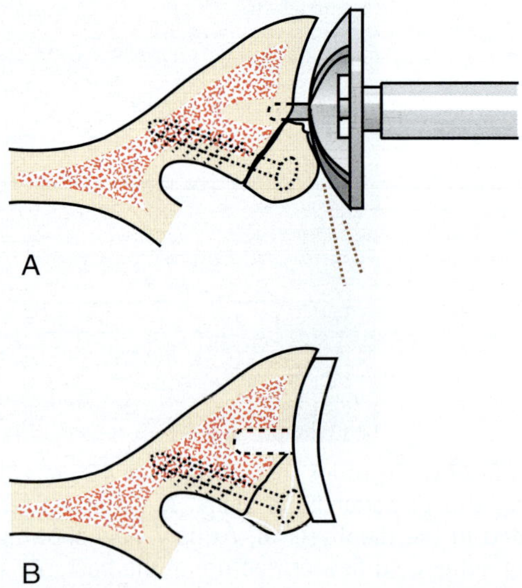

FIGURE 16-275: Posterior glenoid bone grafting. **A,** When a major defect of the posterior glenoid is present, a humeral head or iliac bone graft can be used to replace a deficient glenoid lip. **B,** If the fixation screw is recessed, the bone graft can be contoured and reamed for balanced support of the glenoid component. (Modified from Matsen FA III, Lippitt SB, Sidles JA, Harryman DT II. *Practical Evaluation and Management of the Shoulder.* Philadelphia: WB Saunders; 1994.)

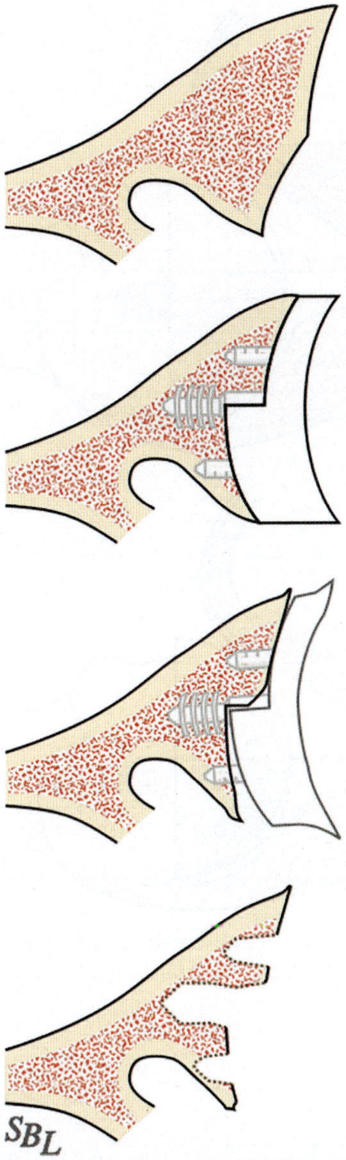

FIGURE 16-276: The sacrifice of posterior glenoid bone stock for an augmented glenoid component can exacerbate the problem of posterior instability if the implant fails.

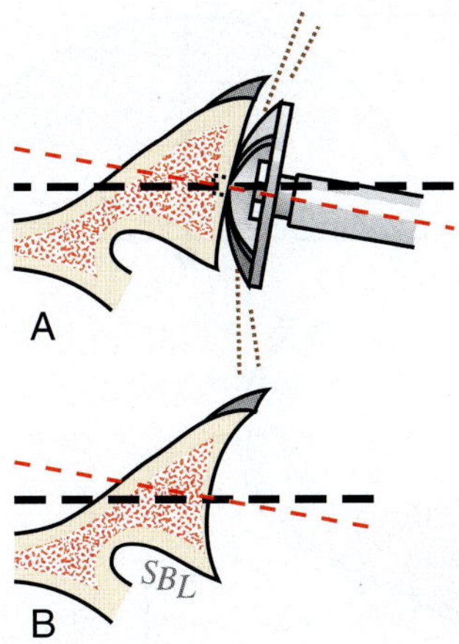

FIGURE 16-277: A, If posterior erosion of the glenoid is more significant, the angle of glenoid reaming is not completely corrected to the glenoid centerline in order to preserve glenoid subchondral bone. **B,** The process of glenoid reaming converts the surface to a single concavity, which improves glenohumeral joint congruity and balance.

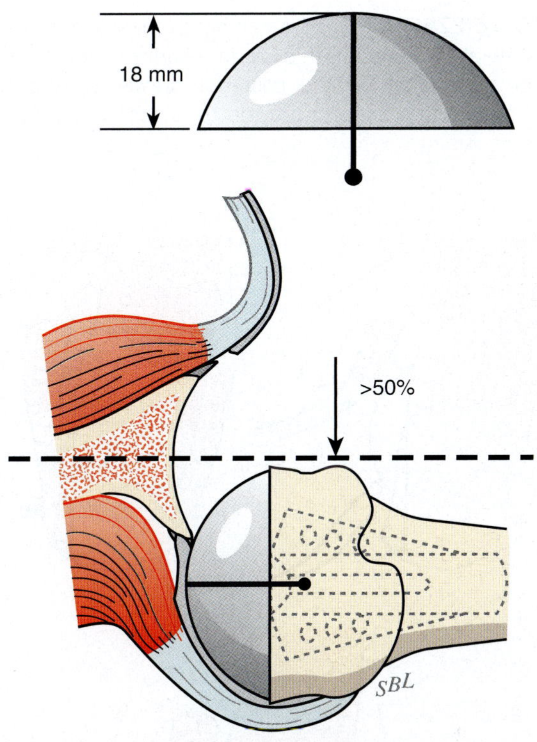

FIGURE 16-278: In this example, a humeral head component with a height of 18 mm allowed more than 50% posterior translation of the humeral head on the posterior drawer test.

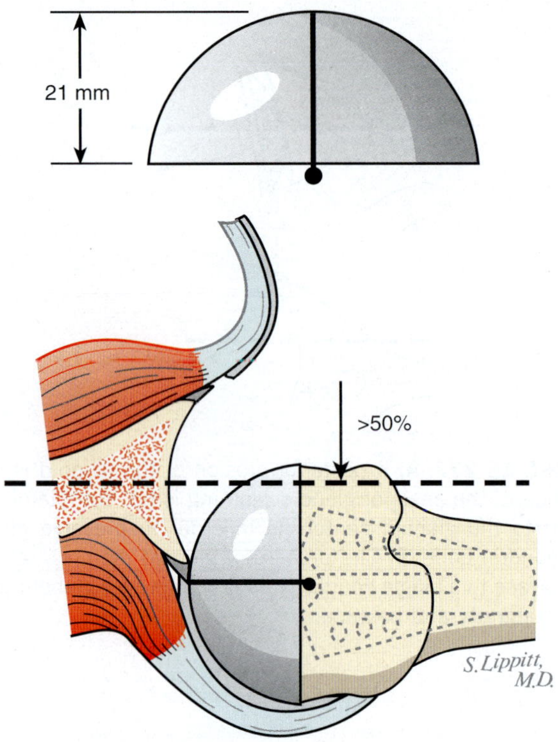

FIGURE 16-279: If the humeral head component with the greatest height (21 mm in this example) allows more than 50% posterior translation on the posterior drawer test, a rotator interval plication is used to provide the needed stability.

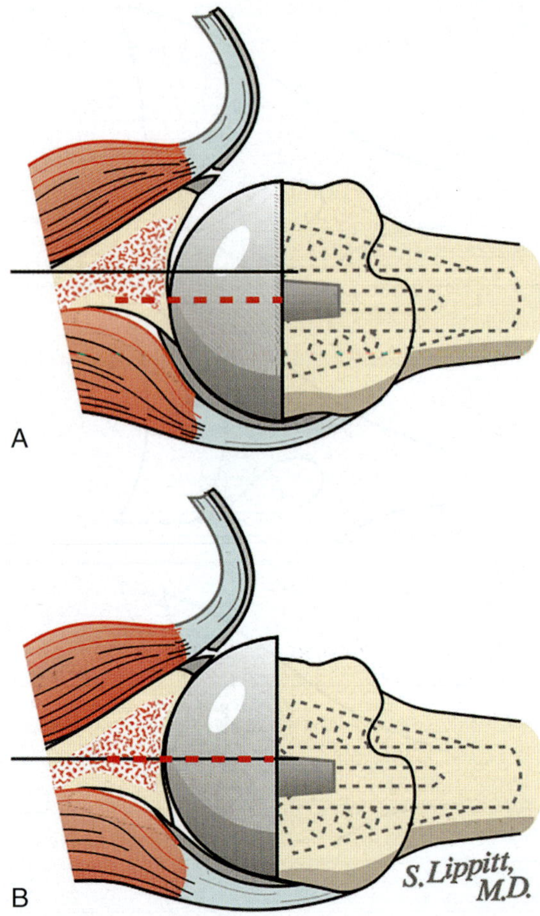

FIGURE 16-281: **A,** Eccentric head component with an anterior offset. **B,** This corrects standard head component posterior subluxation.

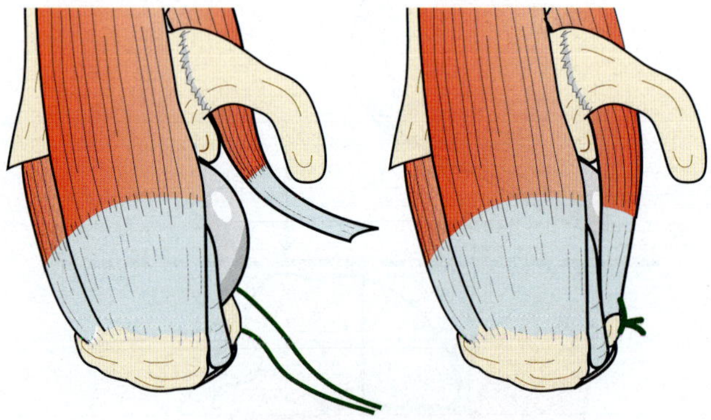

FIGURE 16-280: Rotator interval closure, superior view.

the glenoid component (see Figs. 16-214, 16-244, 16-245, 16-249, 16-253, 16-272, and 16-274; Figs. 16-282 to 16-285).[5,152,260,309,338,494] The effect of an off-center humeral joint reaction force depends on the degree of mismatch between the diameter of curvature of the humeral head and that of the glenoid. A slight degree of mismatch between these diameters of curvature allows minor amounts of humeral translation before rim contact occurs (Figs. 16-286 and 16-287).[565] However, a severe degree of mismatch can dramatically reduce the glenohumeral contact area (Fig. 16-288) and increase the peak stresses in the polyethylene component and its fixation to bone (Figs. 16-289 and 16-290).[110,539] Conversely, no mismatch results in rim loading even with small amounts of translation (Fig. 16-291).[260] Thus component selection represents a compromise between the factors favoring greater mismatch between the diameters of curvature of the glenoid and that of the humerus (lower translational loads on the glenoid component and less risk of rim loading with translation) and those favoring greater conformity (more stability and less contact stress). In

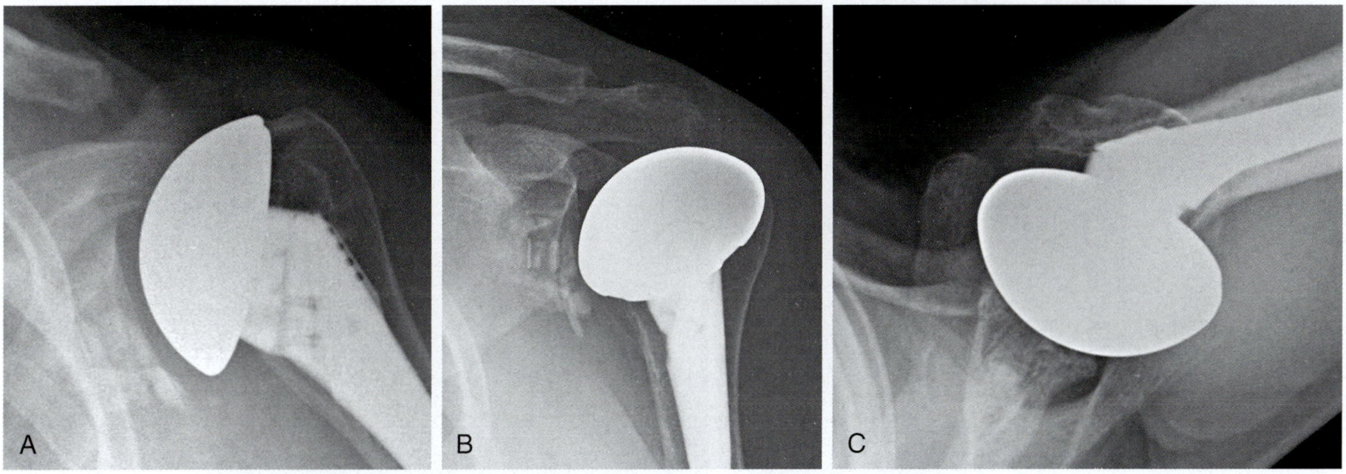

FIGURE 16-282: Total shoulder arthroplasty complicated by a loose glenoid and *Propionibacterium* species infection. **A,** "Rocking horse" loosening of the glenoid component. **B,** A loose fragment of cement. **C,** Radiolucent lines around the glenoid component.

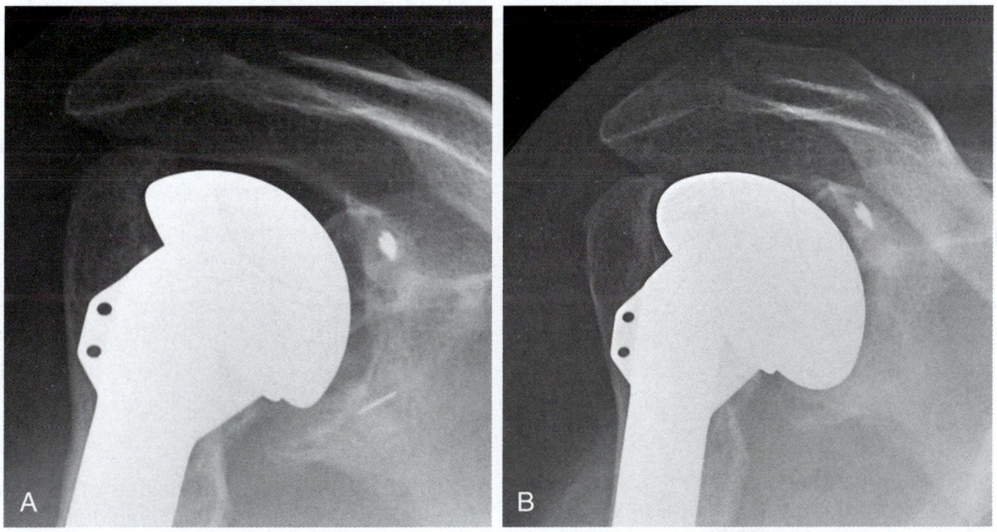

FIGURE 16-283: **A,** Inferior placement of the glenoid component facilitates "rocking horse" loosening. **B,** This shoulder was treated by the removal of the glenoid component.

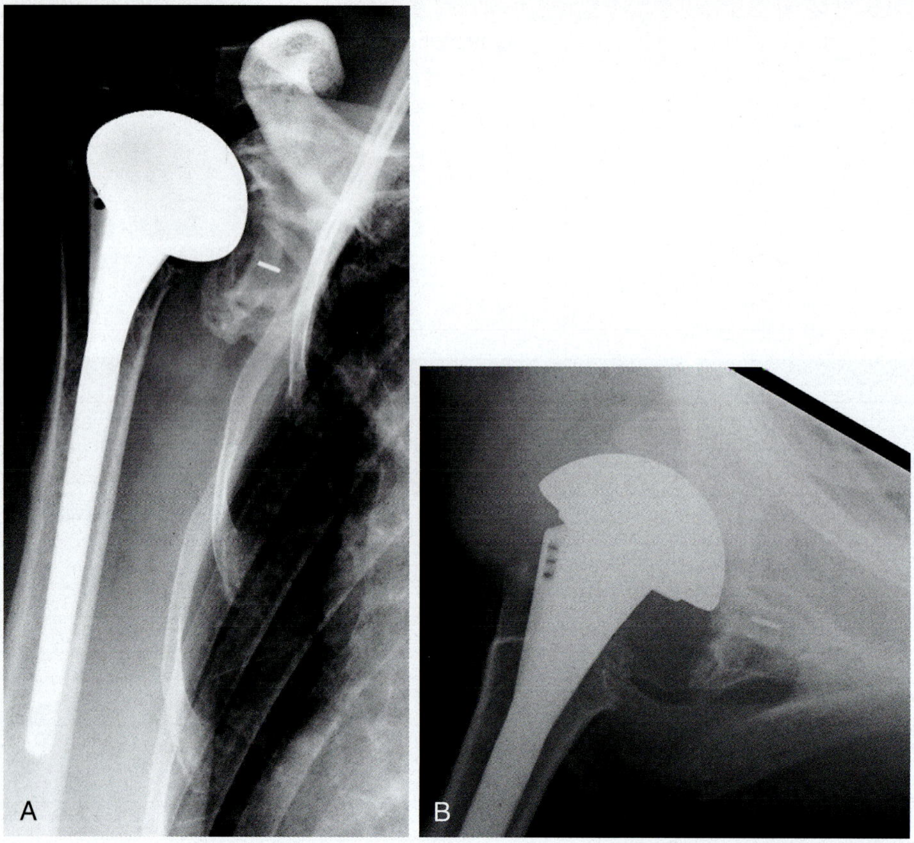

FIGURE 16-284: "Rocking horse" loosening of a glenoid component. **A,** Anteroposterior view. **B,** Axillary view.

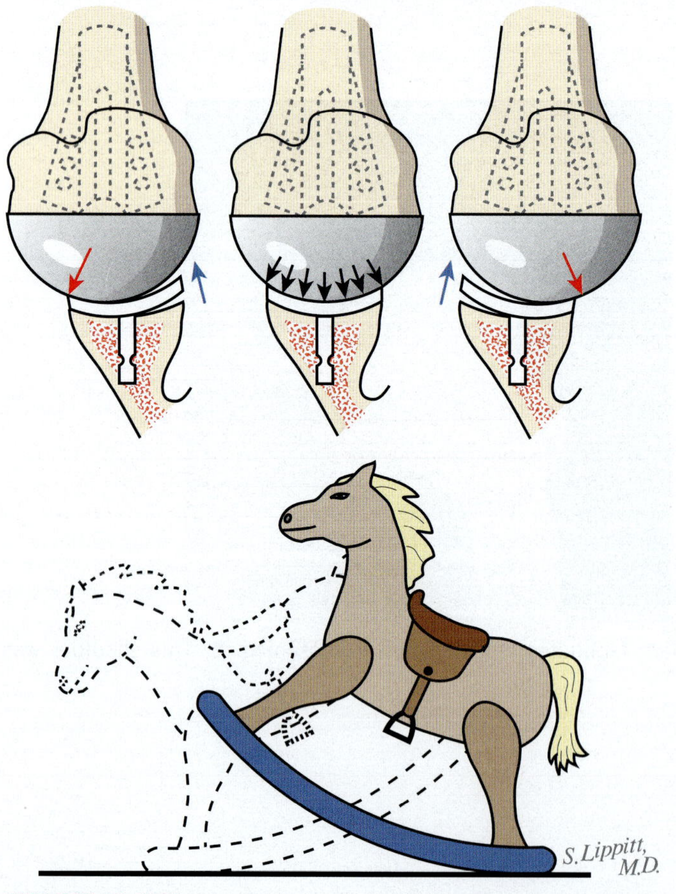

FIGURE 16-285: Eccentric loading of the glenoid (red arrows and blue arrows) exposes it to risk via the "rocking horse" mechanism. The middle diagram shows normal loading (black arrows). (From Matsen FA III, Lippitt SB. *Shoulder Surgery: Principles and Procedures.* Philadelphia: Saunders; 2004:508.)

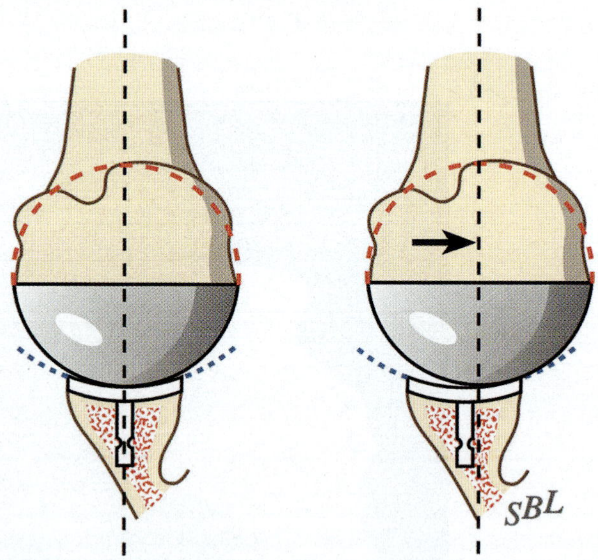

FIGURE 16-286: A slight degree of mismatch between the diameters of curvature of the glenoid and humeral components allows a minor amount of humeral translation before rim contact occurs.

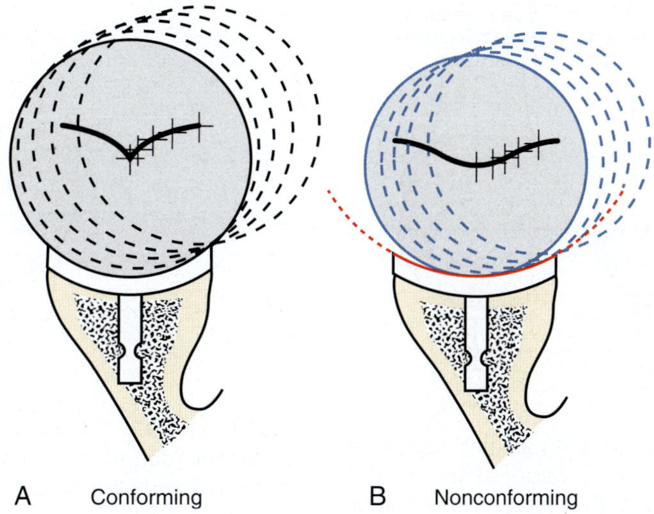

FIGURE 16-287: Conforming and nonconforming glenoidograms. Glenoid arthroplasty offers the opportunity to restore the concavity, orientation, and stability of the glenoid surface. **A,** In a glenoidogram for a conforming set of glenohumeral joint surfaces, each of the two convex halves of the glenoidogram has a radius equal to that of the humeral head, and each half is centered on the respective glenoid edge. In this situation the steepest part of each half of the glenoidogram is where the humeral head just begins to leave the center of the glenoid. **B,** In a glenoidogram for a glenoid surface with a radius of curvature slightly greater than that of the humeral head, each of the convex parts of the glenoidogram describes a curve centered on the glenoid edge, with a radius equal to that of the humeral head. These two convex parts are connected by a concave segment with a radius equal to the difference between the glenoid and the humeral radii of curvature. The stability against translation in each direction is at its maximum where the glenoidogram is steepest, which is a short distance from the glenoid center. This configuration allows some translation of the humeral head in the well of the glenoid. (From Matsen FA III, Lippitt SB. *Shoulder Surgery: Principles and Procedures.* Philadelphia: Saunders; 2004:485.)

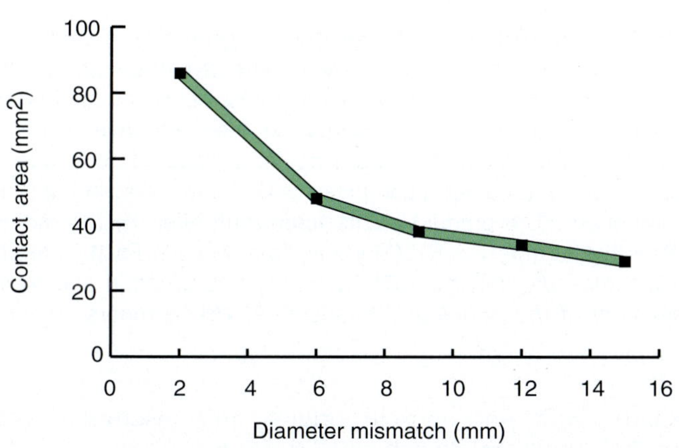

FIGURE 16-288: Results of a finite element model analysis of a polyethylene glenoid showing the effect of diameter mismatch on the contact area. Even a slight increase in the diameter of the glenoid relative to that of the humerus dramatically reduces the contact area. Any further increase in the mismatch further reduces the contact area. (From Matsen FA III, Lippitt SB, Sidles JA, Harryman DT II. *Practical Evaluation and Management of the Shoulder.* Philadelphia: WB Saunders; 1994.)

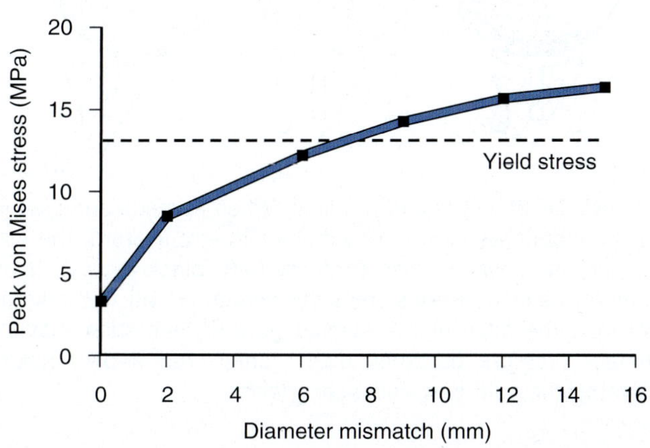

FIGURE 16-289: Results of a finite element model analysis of the effect of diameter mismatch on peak contact stresses (pressure-modified von Mises stress) in a polyethylene glenoid component. The applied compressive load is 625 N (equivalent to approximately one body weight). The predicted yield stress for the component is shown. A load of one body weight with diameter mismatch in excess of 6 mm is predicted to exceed the yield stress of ordinary polyethylene. (From Matsen FA III, Lippitt SB, Sidles JA, Harryman DT II. *Practical Evaluation and Management of the Shoulder.* Philadelphia: WB Saunders; 1994.)

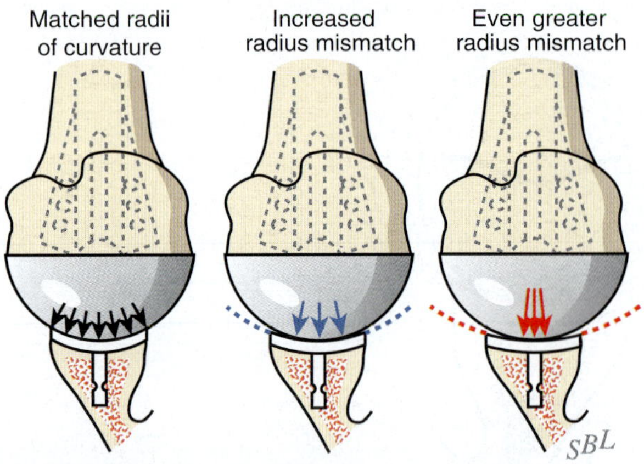

FIGURE 16-290: Diameter mismatch. With greater degrees of mismatch between the diameters of curvature of the glenoid and the humeral head, there is a decreased contact area, increased contact pressure, and increased pressure gradient between the loaded and unloaded polyethylene. (From Matsen FA III, Lippitt SB. *Shoulder Surgery: Principles and Procedures.* Philadelphia: Saunders; 2004:493.)

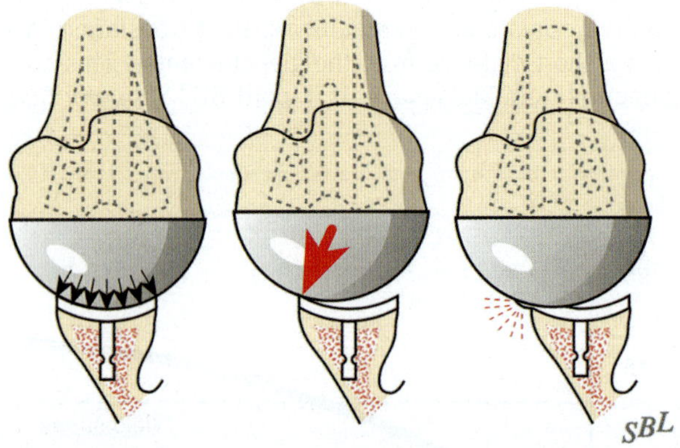

FIGURE 16-291: Glenoid rim load. When humeral and glenoid components have conforming diameters of curvature, the load is distributed evenly when centered (left, black arrows). If the humeral head translates from the center, it will immediately rim load the edge of the glenoid polyethylene such that the contact pressure becomes high (center, red arrow), risking polyethylene cold flow and wear (right).

performing a total shoulder arthroplasty we select components so that the diameter of curvature of the humeral component is 6 mm smaller than that of the glenoid component (Fig. 16-292).

When the net humeral joint reaction force cannot be contained by the shallow socket of an anatomic arthroplasty, the more constrained geometry of a reverse total shoulder arthroplasty can be considered.[331,365]

Strength

Shoulder strength after an anatomic shoulder arthroplasty depends on having a functional deltoid, a functional rotator cuff, and muscle origins and insertions with normal length relationships (Fig. 16-293).

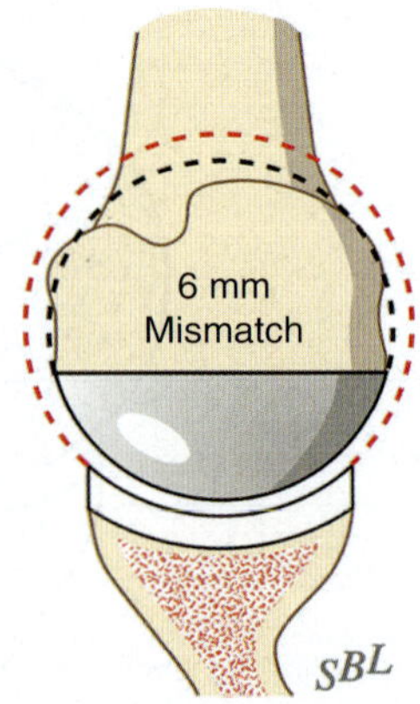

FIGURE 16-292: The diameter of curvature of the humeral component (dotted black line) is 6 mm smaller than that of the glenoid component (dotted red line).

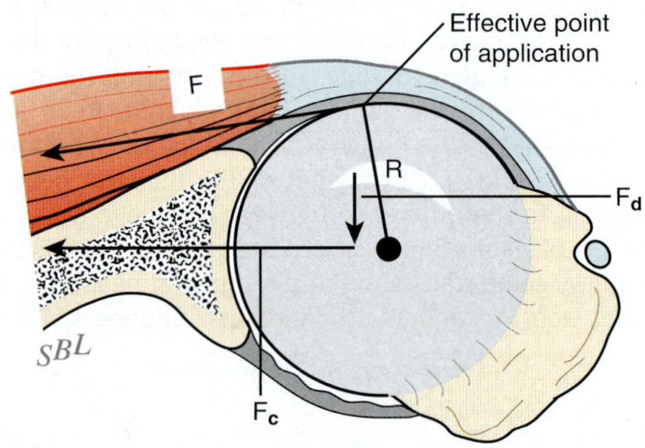

FIGURE 16-293: Each active muscle generates a force (F) whose direction is determined by the effective origin and insertion of that muscle. Note that the rotator cuff tendons wrap around the head of the humerus, so their effective point of attachment is on the humeral articular surface. Note also that each muscle force has a compressive (Fc) and a displacing (Fd) component. The product of the force multiplied by the radius (R) is the torque (F × R). (Modified from Matsen FA III, Lippitt SB, Sidles JA, Harryman DT II. *Practical Evaluation and Management of the Shoulder.* Philadelphia: WB Saunders; 1994.)

In an arthritic shoulder, strength is often compromised by a combination of cuff deterioration, disuse, injury, prior surgery, nerve damage, cervical radiculopathy, and comorbidities. The surgeon may be able to provide a basis for improved strength of the shoulder through appropriate muscle tensioning. The selection of component thickness for the humeral head establishes the resting length and lever arms of the cuff muscles and the deltoid.[226,240] If the component is too small, the cuff will be slack at rest and the length-tension relationship of the muscles will be at the low end of the ideal curve. If the joint is overstuffed, the cuff muscles may be at the high end of their length-tension curve. Overtensioning of the cuff may increase the risk of rotator cuff failure (see Fig. 16-199). After surgical optimization of the shoulder kinematics, the principal method for improving strength is effective postoperative rehabilitation.[58,498]

Smoothness

The anatomic requisites for smooth motion include distributed load transfer, smooth joint surfaces, and smooth and unimpaired humeroscapular motion.

Distributed Load Transfer. In a normal shoulder the humeral load is distributed evenly across the glenoid articular surface. When there is erosion of the glenoid surface, the contact area is reduced and the local joint pressure is increased (see Fig. 16-67). In performing a hemiarthroplasty it is important to optimize the load transfer by selecting a prosthetic humeral head with a diameter of curvature that is equal to or slightly greater than that of the glenoid (Fig. 16-294). In a total shoulder arthroplasty the load transfer is related to the diameter mismatch between the humeral head and the glenoid (see Fig. 16-290; Fig. 16-295). In a total shoulder arthroplasty our preference is for a mismatch in which the diameter of curvature of the glenoid component is 6 mm greater than that of the articular surface of the humeral head prosthesis; this geometry provides stability while allowing some translation of the head on the glenoid. In a ream and run procedure we ream the glenoid to a diameter 2 mm greater than that of the articular surface of the humeral head prosthesis so that load transfer and stability for the metal-on-bone articulation are optimized (Fig. 16-296).

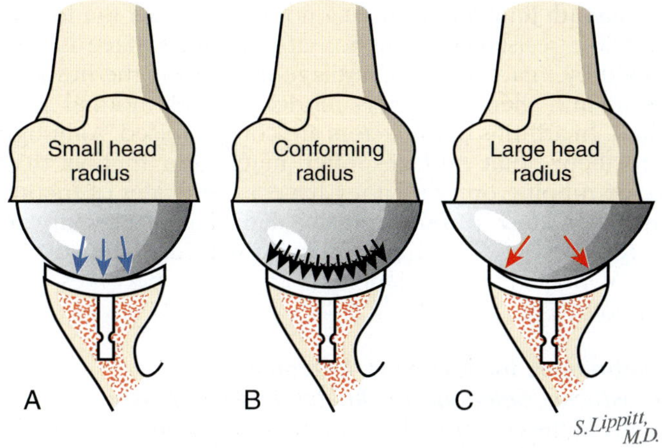

FIGURE 16-295: Support of glenoid and load transfer. **A,** The relative curvatures of the head and glenoid affect the load transfer and stability at the glenohumeral articulation. If the diameter of curvature of the head is smaller than that of the glenoid, there is focal loading in the center of the glenoid and the opportunity for small amounts of translation before rim loading. **B,** If the head conforms to the glenoid, the load is evenly distributed and no translation can occur without rim loading. **C,** If the head is larger than the glenoid, the load is concentrated on the glenoid rim, subjecting it to cold-flow and wear. The humeral head does not seat completely in the glenoid, which reduces glenohumeral stability. Laboratory and clinical experience suggest that for a polyethylene glenoid component, the relationships are optimized when the diameter of curvature of the glenoid is 6 mm greater than that of the humeral head that articulates with it. (From Matsen FA III, Lippitt SB. *Shoulder Surgery: Principles and Procedures.* Philadelphia: Saunders; 2004:503.)

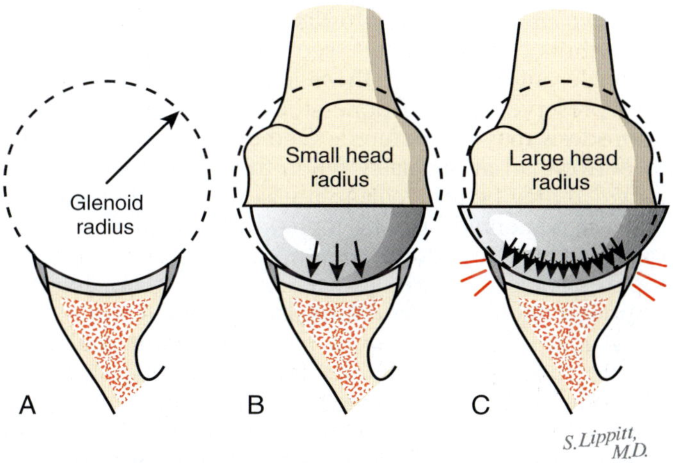

FIGURE 16-294: Optimizing head curvature. **A,** In hemiarthroplasty it is desirable to match the humeral head size to the size of the cartilage-covered biologic head that is removed so that the prosthesis fits well in the glenoid. **B,** If the prosthesis head is too small, the hard center of the glenoid cannot distribute the load, which then becomes concentrated on a small part of the glenoid surface area. **C,** If matching of the head size cannot be achieved, it is preferable to slightly oversize the head because the compliance of the glenoid periphery can accommodate the mismatch. (From Matsen FA III, Lippitt SB. *Shoulder Surgery: Principles and Procedures.* Philadelphia: Saunders; 2004:435.)

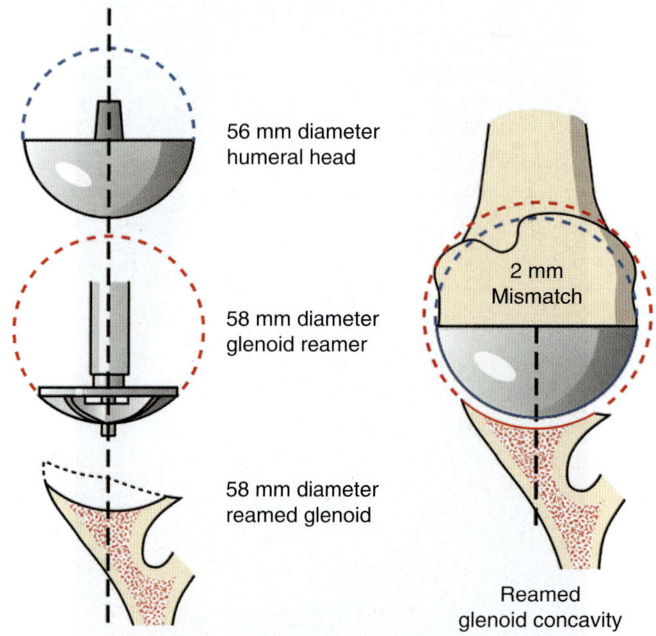

FIGURE 16-296: In a ream and run procedure the glenoid is reamed to a diameter 2 mm greater than that of the humeral head component.

Smooth Joint Surfaces. In a normal shoulder the lowest possible resistance to motion at the joint surface is provided by intact articular cartilage that covers the humeral head and glenoid and is lubricated with normal joint fluid. In arthritis these factors are compromised. Although prosthetic joint surfaces offer much less friction than bone rubbing on bone, they have a coefficient of friction approximately 10 times greater than that of normal cartilage moving on normal cartilage. With use, the surface of a polyethylene glenoid component becomes less smooth (Fig. 16-297).[53,399,487,578]

Techniques for Anatomic Arthroplasty

Prosthesis Selection for Anatomic Arthroplasty

Many different shoulder arthroplasty systems are on the market, with more being introduced each year. New "advances" in prosthetics and techniques have been promoted, advances that are often more expensive, have more parts, and are more complicated than the systems they are intended to replace. What is lacking, in many instances, is evidence that these newer, more costly, and more complicated approaches yield better outcomes for the patient. In our practice we have chosen relatively simple implants that in most cases have been available for a decade or so. We try to use the same basic approach for all arthroplasties; this allows our discussions with patients, preoperative work up, surgical procedures, and rehabilitation to be efficiently standardized. The principles for prosthesis selection discussed below are based on this philosophy and are not specific to any particular manufacturer or component design.

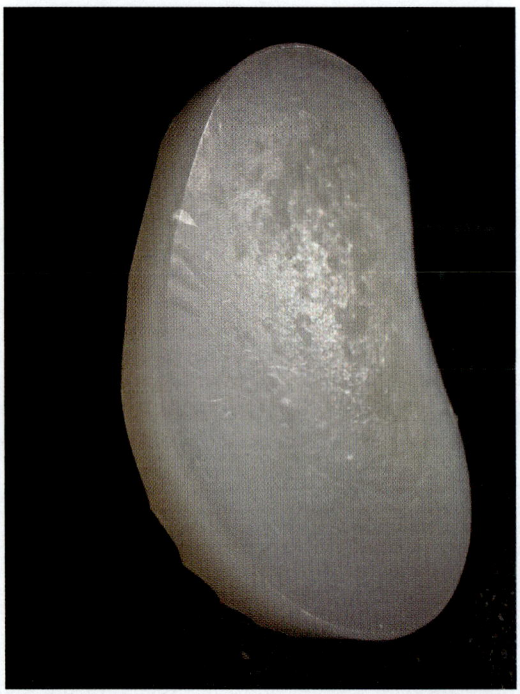

FIGURE 16-297: Pitting on the surface of a glenoid retrieved from a failed total shoulder arthroplasty.

Humeral Component. The ideal humeral component is one that allows secure and durable placement of an ample articular surface in the position that optimizes glenohumeral motion and stability. It should also allow for complete removal of the component—should revision become necessary—without the risk of damage to the bone of the humerus by attempting to remove a cemented or bony ingrowth implant. The humeral implant is modular, allowing the head and body components to be selected independently. In selecting the humeral component we prioritize optimization of glenohumeral mechanics over attempting to "restore normal anatomy."[426,427] By adjusting the humeral diameter of curvature, head thickness, and head offset with respect to the stem, the surgeon has the opportunity to modify both the capsular tension and the fit of the component to the glenoid articular surface. There are two aspects of the humeral component that deserve consideration: the articular surface and the way the articular surface is connected to the humerus.

Humeral Articular Surface. There are three types of prosthetic humeral articular surfaces: partial resurfacing (Fig. 16-298), complete resurfacing (see Fig. 16-186), and head replacement (see Fig. 16-185).

Partial resurfacing prostheses may seem an attractive choice for covering partial articular surface defects. However, the modulus of elasticity varies by a factor of 200,000 between the metal prosthesis (about 200,000 MPa) and the surrounding intact articular cartilage (0.5 to 0.9 MPa); this creates a major discontinuity in the deformation of the joint surface under load at the margin of the prosthesis (Fig. 16-299).

Complete resurfacing prostheses are intended to cover the arthritic humeral head (see Fig. 16-186).[300,301,543] The rationale put forward for these implants is as follows: (1) they preserve humeral bone stock in case a subsequent arthrodesis may be required; (2) they enable the surgeon to perform an arthroplasty when there is humeral deformity; (3) they better facilitate revision than do prostheses that use cemented or bone ingrowth humeral stems; and (4) they facilitate restoration of normal anatomy, although the restoration is not always anatomic (Fig. 16-300). Although attempting to reestablish normal anatomy may be a goal of arthroplasty, a more important goal is to restore functional mechanics for the arthritic shoulder. This often requires adjustments in the diameter of curvature, thickness, and orientation of the head and also requires glenoid arthroplasty—adjustments where there is no attempt to exactly duplicate the normal glenohumeral anatomy. As a result, we do not use resurfacing prostheses in our practice for the following reasons: (1) the need for arthrodesis after prior arthroplasty is extremely rare; (2) almost all cases of arthritic and posttraumatic deformity can be managed with a conventional stemmed prosthesis (see Fig. 16-257); (3) the difficulties associated with the removal of cemented or ingrowth components can be avoided by humeral stem fixation with impaction grafting; (4) by retaining the humeral head, resurfacing implants limit the surgeon's ability to modify the orientation and thickness of the component;

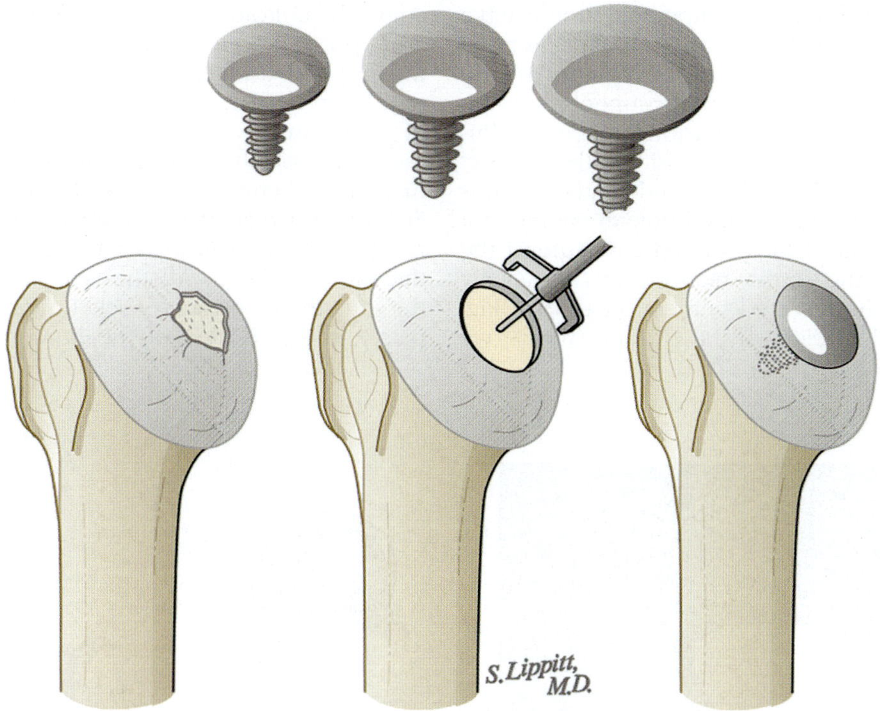

FIGURE 16-298: Example of partial resurfacing of a central humeral head cartilage defect.

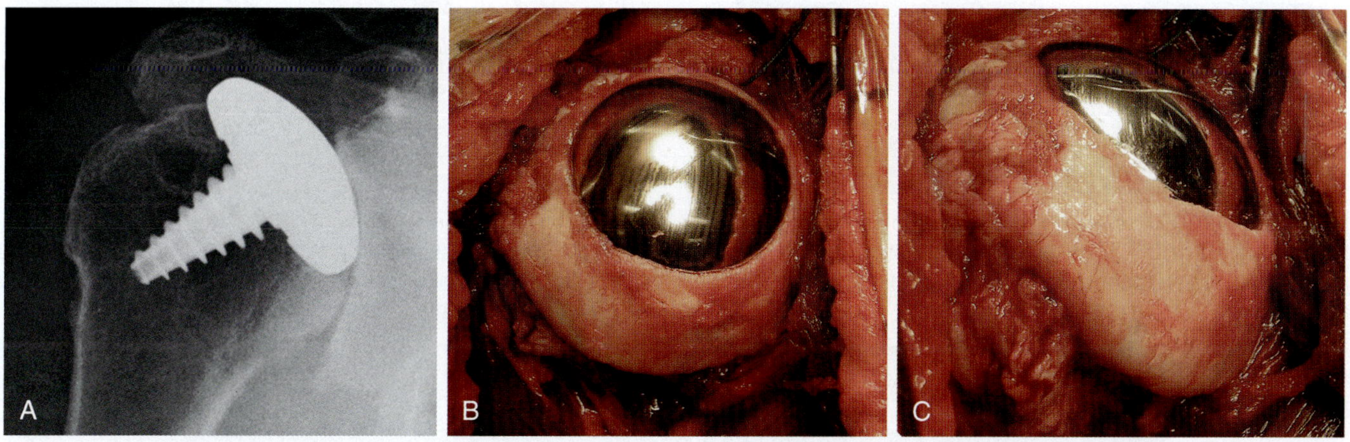

FIGURE 16-299: Failed partial joint resurfacing. **A,** Anteroposterior radiograph. **B** and **C,** Intraoperative images showing articular surface discontinuity at the margins of the prosthesis.

and (5) retention of the anatomic humeral head compromises access to the glenoid, making it difficult to address the glenoid pathology encountered in glenohumeral osteoarthritis (Figs. 16-301 and 16-302).[302] Finally, it is worth noting that registry data indicate a 2.5-year revision rate for resurfacing prostheses; this is more than three times the revision rate for stemmed hemiarthroplasty.[7]

Head replacement prostheses allow extensive versatility in the selection of the humeral head component. The humeral head cut for these prostheses allows excellent access to the glenoid bone so that an appropriate glenoid arthroplasty can be carried out. Some prostheses are nonspherical (see Figs. 16-213 and 16-214), but these do not appear to be superior to the spherical design found in nature. In our practice the selection of the diameter of curvature of the spherical humeral articular surface (Fig. 16-303) depends on the management of the socket side of the articulation (Fig. 16-304). With a *hemiarthroplasty* in the absence of any form of glenoid arthroplasty, the shape of the socket is not changed and so the articular surface of the humeral component should have the same diameter of curvature as the resected humeral head (Figs. 16-305 and 16-306). In a *CTA humeral arthroplasty* without pseudoparalysis or anterosuperior escape, a humeral head with a lateral extension can be used to resurface the articulation of the tuberosity with an intact coracoacromial arch (see Figs. 16-103 and 16-104). In this case the diameter of curvature of the humeral component is selected to match that of the sculpted curvature of the coracoacromial arch and upper glenoid; this is usually the same as that of the resected humeral head (see Fig. 16-97). In selecting the height of the CTA prosthesis, we adjust the deltoid tension such that the passively adducted arm springs about 20 degrees away from the side when the applied adduction force is removed (Figs. 16-307 and 16-308). In a *ream and run arthroplasty* the diameter of curvature of the humeral component is 2 mm less than that of the reamed glenoid; in most cases the diameter of curvature of the humeral head prosthesis is 56 mm and that of the reamed glenoid is 58 mm. In a *total shoulder arthroplasty* the diameter of curvature of the humeral head prosthesis is 6 mm less than that of the prosthetic glenoid socket. For all types of arthroplasty, the thickness of the humeral head prosthesis is

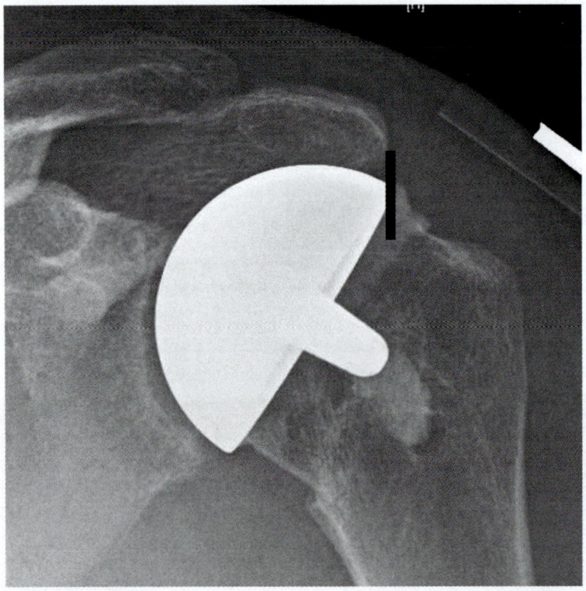

FIGURE 16-300: Resurfacing hemiarthroplasty that resulted in overstuffing of the joint due to poor seating of the component. Note the relationship of the tuberosity to the lateral acromial line.

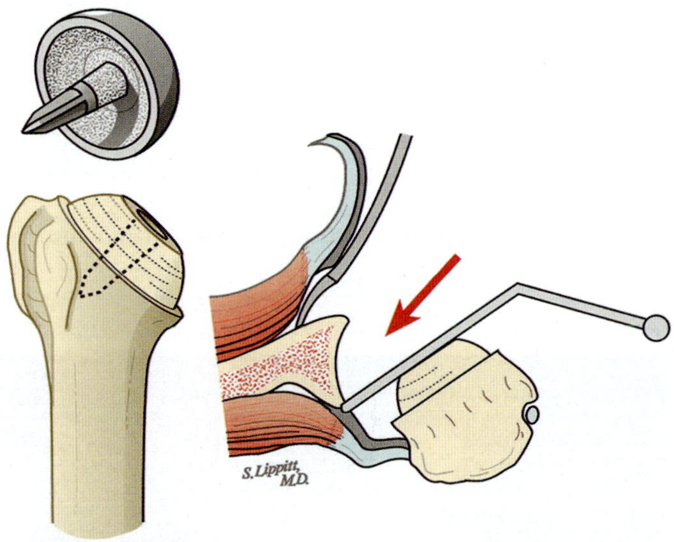

FIGURE 16-301: The retention of the anatomic head convexity within a humeral resurfacing arthroplasty compromises access to the glenoid, making it difficult to address the glenoid pathology encountered in glenohumeral arthritis.

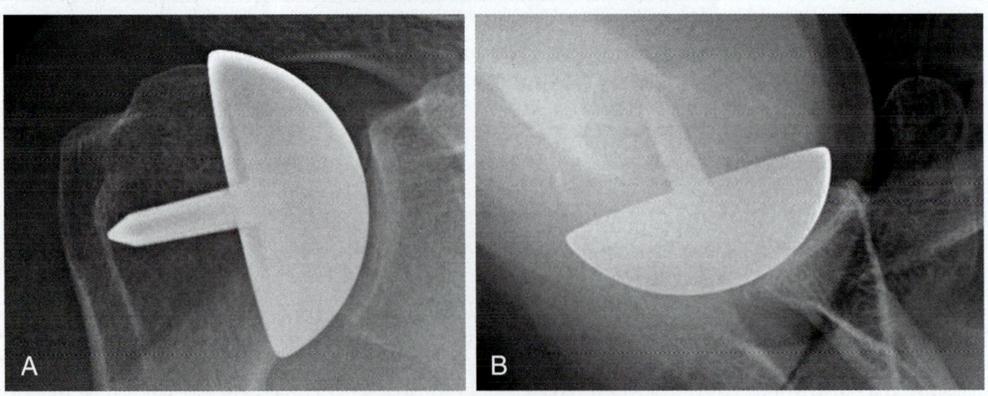

FIGURE 16-302: Resurfacing hemiarthroplasty. **A,** The anteroposterior view shows apparently intact glenoid articular cartilage. **B,** However, the axillary "truth view" reveals loss of articular cartilage and functional decentering. The patient had multiple positive cultures for *Propionibacterium* species at the time of surgical revision.

selected such that the glenohumeral joint meets the "40, 50, 60" guideline described earlier (Fig. 16-309), which avoids overstuffing on the one hand and excessive laxity on the other. To maximize the articular area, the articular surface of the prosthesis should not be sacrificed to a chamfer and should minimize the gap between the articular area and the humeral neck cut (see Fig. 16-218; Fig. 16-310). The humeral head prosthesis should have eccentric options to help control excessive translation posteriorly or anteriorly (Fig. 16-311; see Figs. 16-38, 16-258, and 16-259) and for the management of malunited fractures (see Fig. 16-257). The humeral head should attach to the body with a Morse taper that has the male part on the head rather than the body of the prosthesis so that the taper does not interfere with access to the glenoid (Fig. 16-312).

Fixation of the Head Component to the Humeral Bone. The humeral head component is fixed to the humeral bone by methods that range from stemless[34] and mini-stemmed (Fig. 16-313)[261] to long stemmed (Fig. 16-314) and include fixation with cement, press-fit, tissue ingrowth, and impaction grafting. There are at least three issues to consider. (1) The humeral canal is curved longitudinally and is elliptical in cross section, with some canals cylindrical and others funnel-shaped (see Fig. 16-64). (2) Fixation needs to be achieved without either the risk of loosening or the risk of fracture (Figs. 16-315 to 16-317). Intramedullary reaming to achieve a diaphyseal press-fit preferentially removes bone from the anterior and posterior endosteal cortex[288] (see Fig. 16-315; Fig. 16-318); this endosteal notching at the prosthesis tip creates a risk of periprosthetic fracture. (3) With any shoulder arthroplasty, there is a potential risk—as high as 10%—that revision surgery will be needed to manage infection, loosening, malposition, fracture, or instability,[137,142,223,386] and so it is important that the humeral component be completely removed without seriously damaging the humeral bone stock. We have found that these three issues are best addressed by using a 120- to 140-mm–long smooth (non-ingrowth) humeral stem (Fig. 16-319; see Fig. 16-185) that fits in the canal without diaphyseal reaming (Figs. 16-320 and 16-321) and that is fixed with impaction autografting using bone harvested from the resected humeral head rather than with cement (Figs. 16-322 to 16-325).[46,193,336,591] Cancellous allograft is used in revision cases or where the amount of bone

Text continued on p. 951

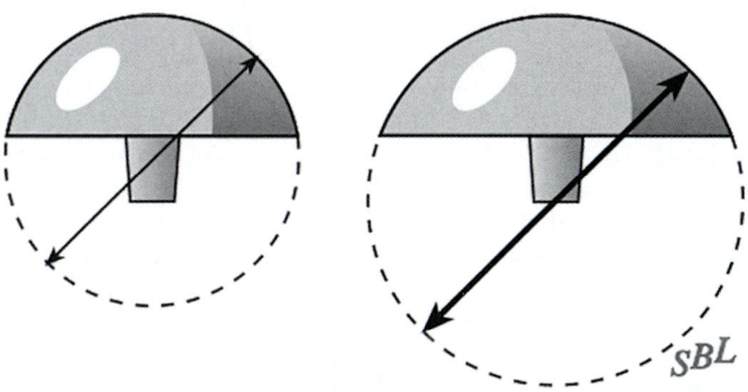

FIGURE 16-303: Conceptual diameter of curvature of the humeral head component.

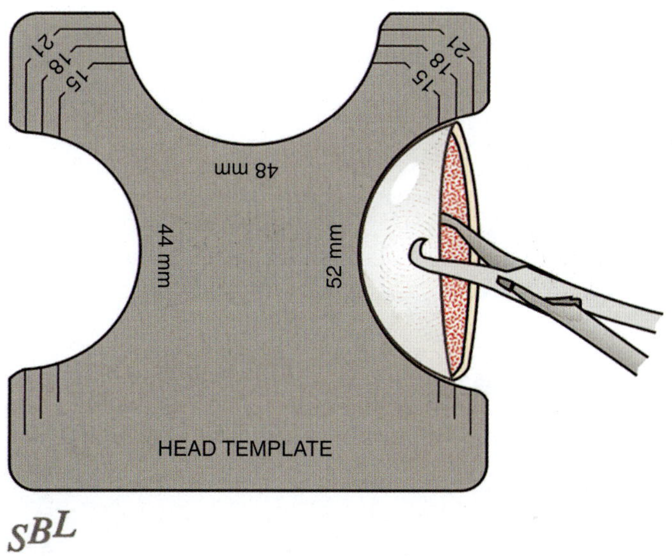

FIGURE 16-305: The humeral component articular surface should have the same diameter of curvature of that measured for the resected humeral head.

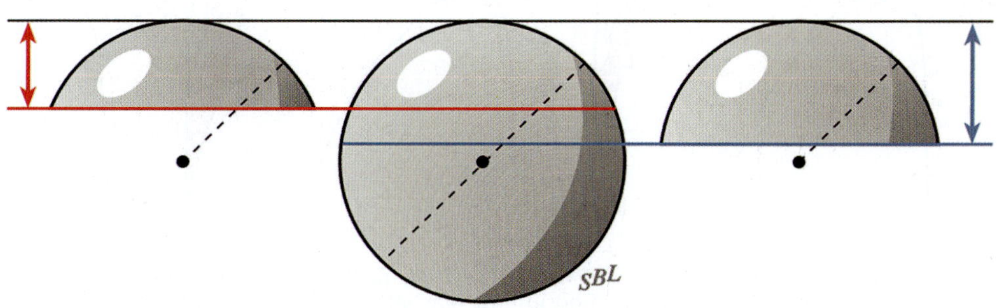

FIGURE 16-304: Conceptual width of the humeral head component.

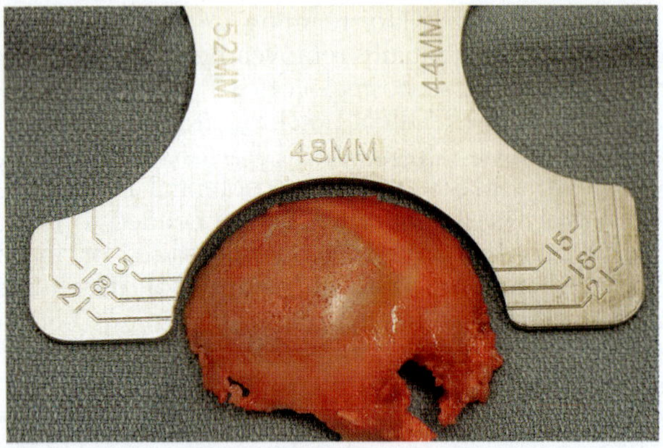

FIGURE 16-306: When performing a hemiarthroplasty, it is important to match the diameter of curvature of the resected humeral head. If the measurement lies between the available prosthetic sizes, we use a prosthesis with a diameter of curvature slightly larger than the measurement so that the prosthetic head can rest on the softer perimeter of the glenoid socket.

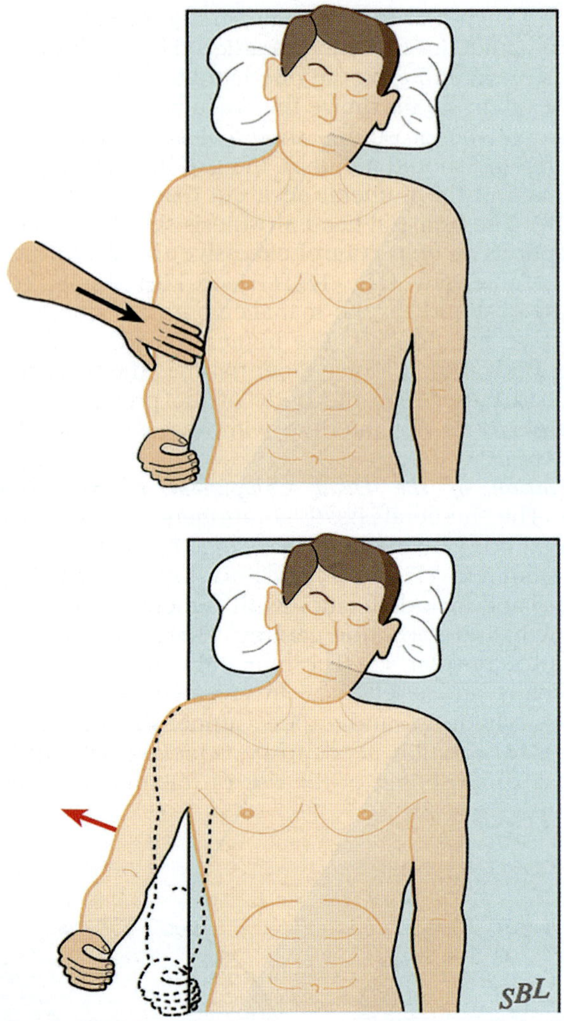

FIGURE 16-308: Deltoid spring test. In selecting the height of the cuff tear arthropathy prosthesis, the deltoid tension is adjusted such that the passively adducted arm springs about 20 degrees away from the side when the applied adduction force is removed.

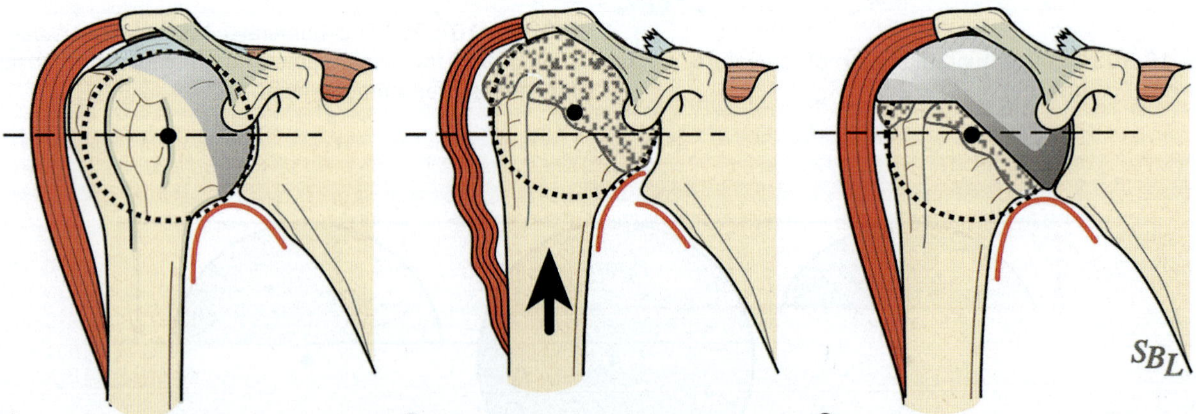

A B C

FIGURE 16-307: Hemiarthroplasty for cuff tear arthropathy. **A,** Normal glenohumeral mechanics with an intact cuff. **B,** Lax deltoid and superiorly displaced humeral center of rotation in cuff tear arthropathy. **C,** A cuff tear arthropathy head component of increased thickness can help restore the deltoid tension and the superiorly displaced humeral center of rotation.

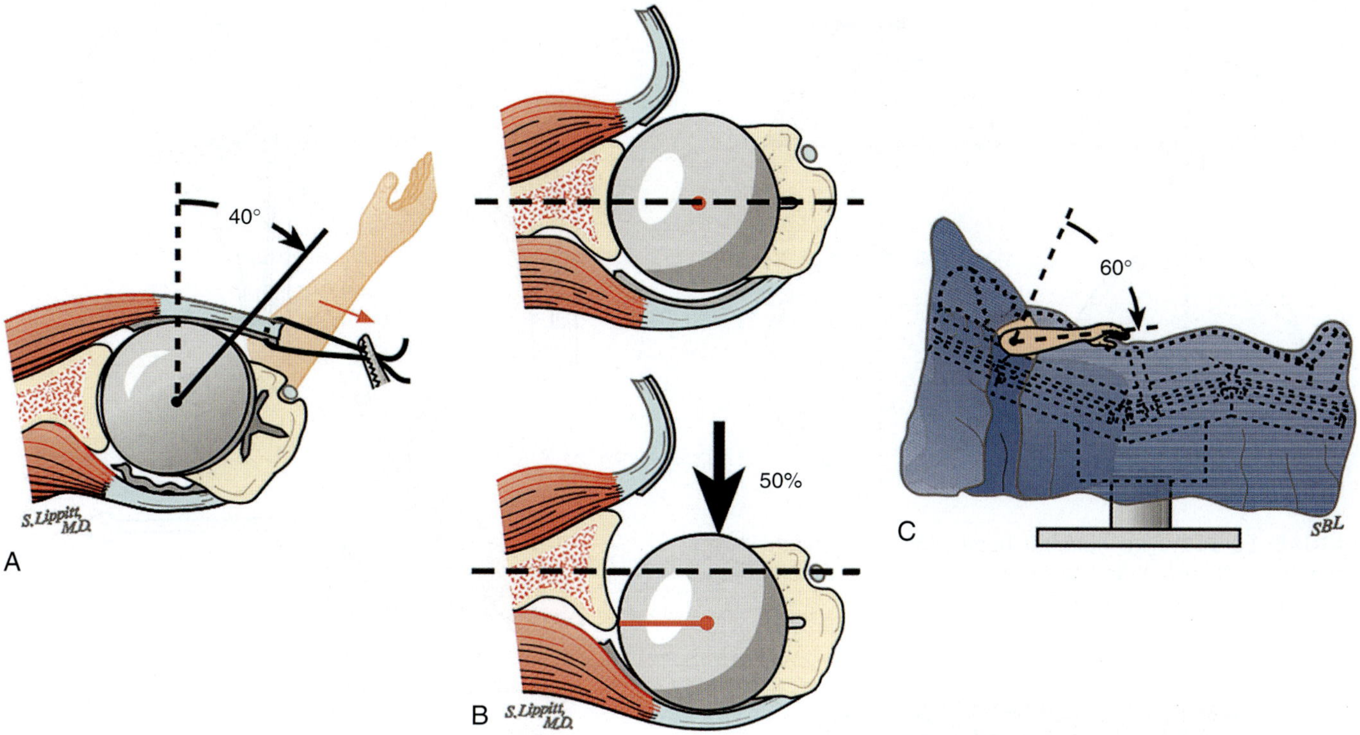

FIGURE 16-309: The 40-50-60 rule involves 40 degrees of external rotation with the subscapularis approximated (**A**), 50% posterior subluxation of the humerus relative to the glenoid on the posterior drawer test (**B**), and 60 degrees of internal rotation of the arm abducted to 90 degrees (**C**).

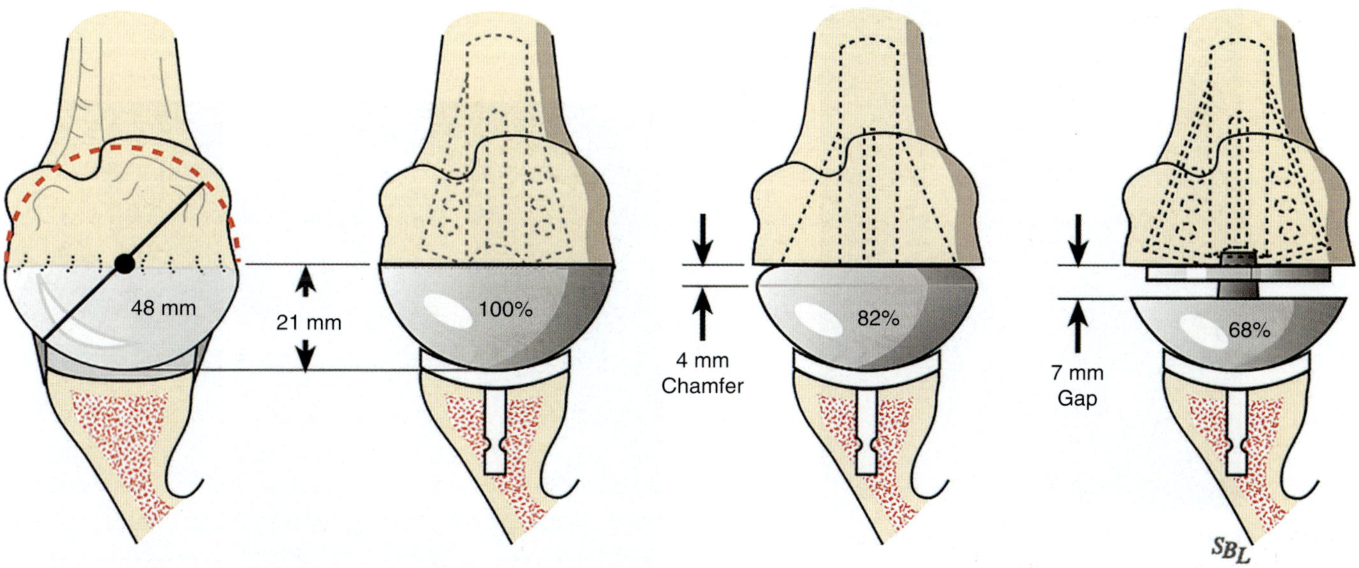

FIGURE 16-310: Peripheral chamfering or the presence of a collar and a gap can reduce the effective articular area of the humeral head spherical prosthesis compared with the normal biologic head. (Modified from Matsen FA III, Lippitt SB. *Shoulder Surgery: Principles and Procedures.* Philadelphia: WB Saunders; 2004.)

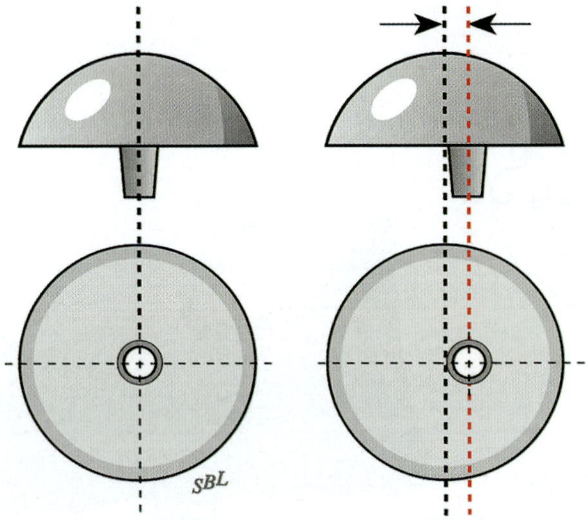

FIGURE 16-311: The humeral head prosthesis should have eccentric options to help control excessive translation anteriorly or posteriorly.

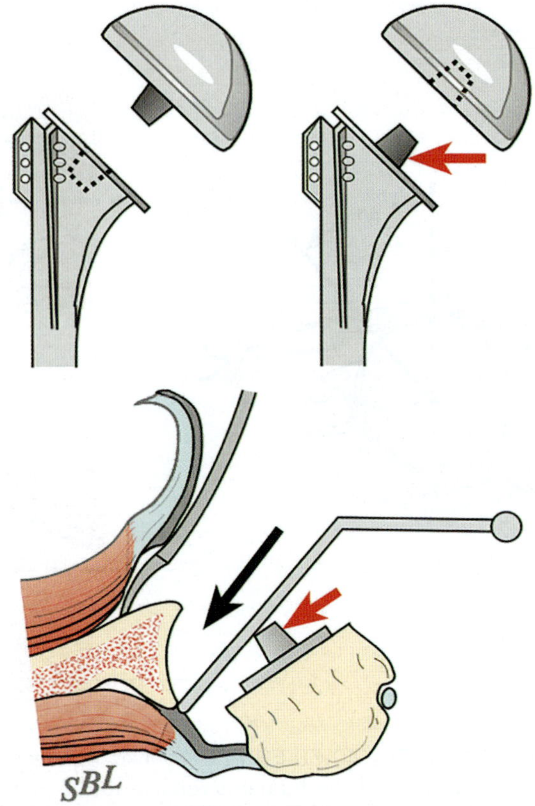

FIGURE 16-312: The Morse taper design should have the male part on the humeral head rather than on the body of the prosthesis (red arrow) so that this taper does not interfere with access to the glenoid when the stem is in situ.

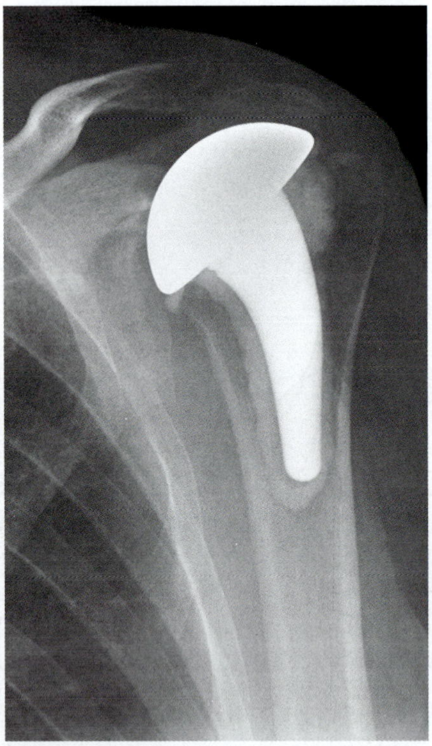

FIGURE 16-313: Superiorly unstable and loose cemented, short-stemmed humeral component.

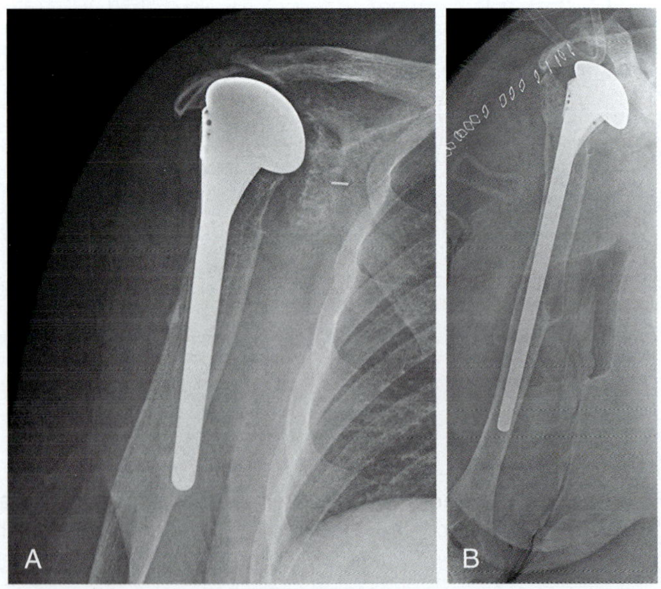

FIGURE 16-314: Prosthesis migration in osteopenic bone managed with a long stemmed prosthesis and impaction grafting. **A,** Anteroposterior view showing the migrating humeral stem. **B,** Long stem bypassing the weak spot in the humeral shaft after insertion with impaction grafting.

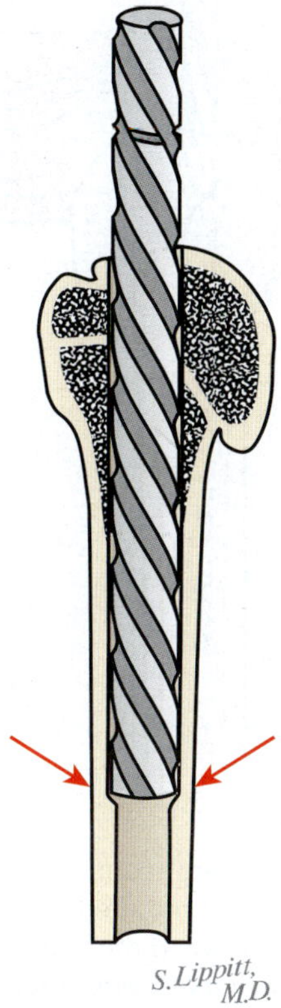

FIGURE 16-315: Stress riser from reaming. Cylindrical reaming of a funnel-shaped canal can create a stress riser (arrows) distally in the diaphysis. (From Matsen FA III, Lippitt SB. *Shoulder Surgery: Principles and Procedures.* Philadelphia: Saunders; 2004:463.)

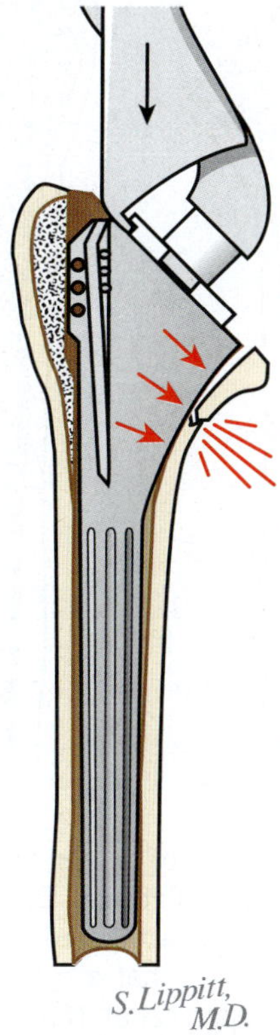

FIGURE 16-316: Press-fit fracture. Attempting to impact the prosthesis (arrow) to achieve a cortical press-fit in the metaphysis runs the risk of fracture (red arrows). (From Matsen FA III, Lippitt SB. *Shoulder Surgery: Principles and Procedures.* Philadelphia: Saunders; 2004:464.)

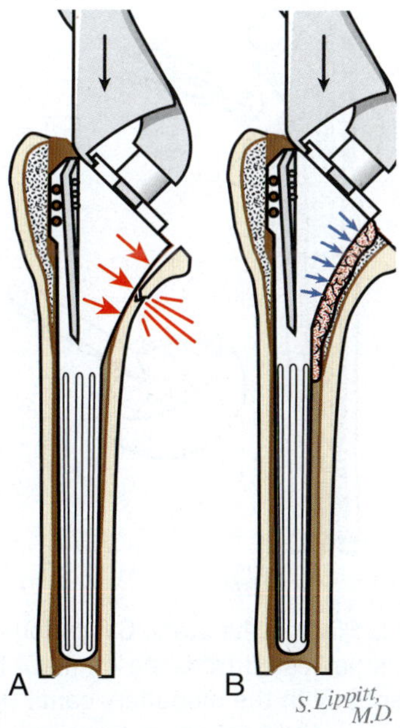

FIGURE 16-317: Safety with cancellous grafting. **A,** Press-fitting carries a risk of fracture. **B,** The voids have been filled with impacted cancellous bone (red stippled areas), enabling a more even distribution of loads during press-fitting and minimizing the risk of fracture. (From Matsen FA III, Lippitt SB. *Shoulder Surgery: Principles and Procedures.* Philadelphia: Saunders; 2004:465.)

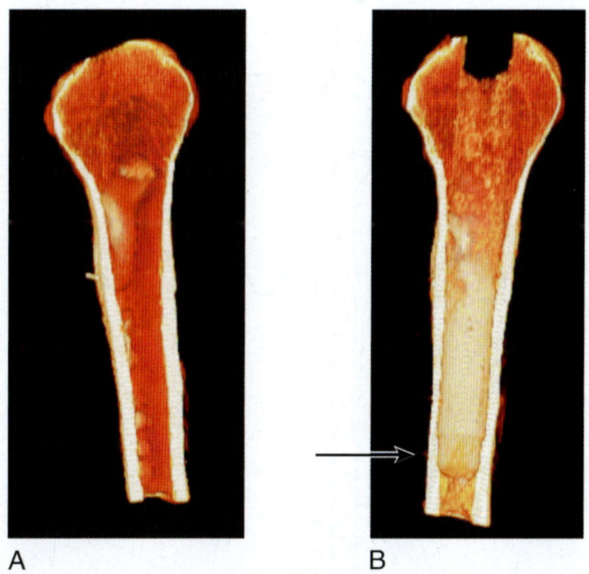

FIGURE 16-318: **A,** Cross section of the humerus before conservative intramedullary reaming. **B,** Note that even with conservative reaming, the endosteal cortex is thinned distally, creating a stress riser (arrow) in the humeral diaphysis.

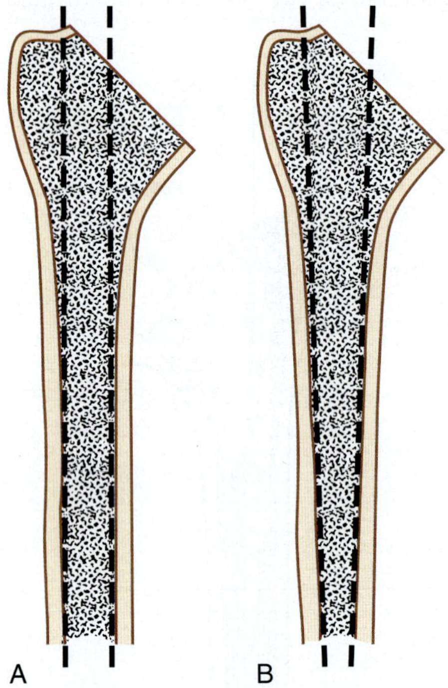

FIGURE 16-319: The shape of humeral medullary canals varies widely. **A,** Some are more cylindrical. **B,** Others are more funnel shaped. It is apparent that a tapered stem would not fit well in the cylindrical canal and that a cylindrical stem would not fit well in the funnel-shaped canal. (From Matsen FA III, Lippitt SB. *Shoulder Surgery: Principles and Procedures.* Philadelphia: Saunders; 2004:462.)

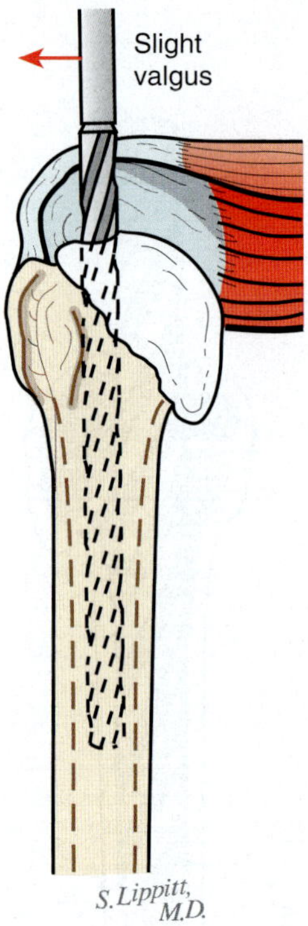

FIGURE 16-320: Medullary reaming. Cylindrical reamers are inserted down to the depth required by the prosthesis, exerting a slight valgus bias (arrow). (From Matsen FA III, Lippitt SB. *Shoulder Surgery: Principles and Procedures.* Philadelphia: Saunders; 2004:523.)

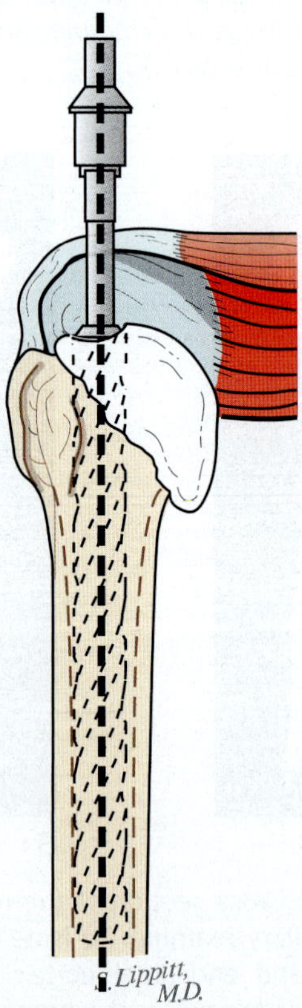

FIGURE 16-321: Medullary reaming. Progressively larger reamers are used until one just achieves a bite in the cortex distally. The orthopedic axis is the central axis of this reamer (dark dotted line). (From Matsen FA III, Lippitt SB. *Shoulder Surgery: Principles and Procedures.* Philadelphia: Saunders; 2004:524.)

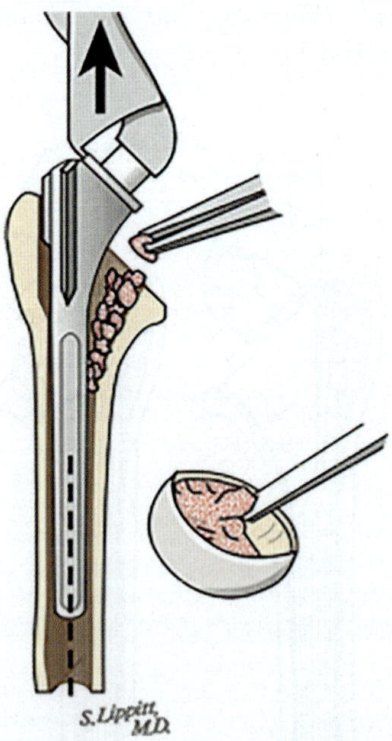

FIGURE 16-322: Placing the graft. Cancellous bone graft (red stippled areas) is harvested from the humeral head (right) and impacted sequentially in the medullary canal (left) to fill in the voids. This improves the fixation and corrects any malorientation of the prosthetic body. (From Matsen FA III, Lippitt SB. *Shoulder Surgery: Principles and Procedures.* Philadelphia: Saunders; 2004:537.)

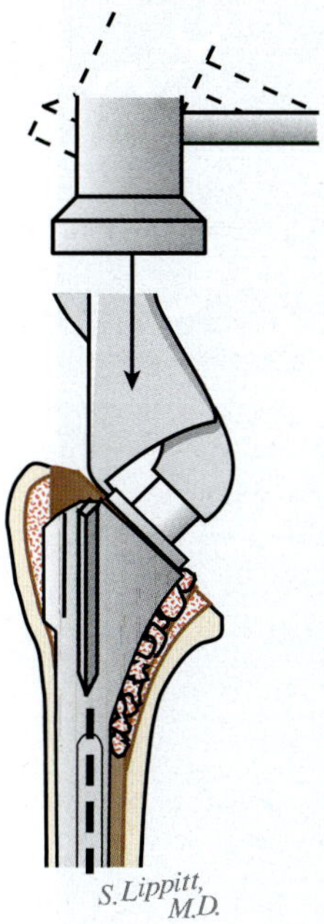

FIGURE 16-323: Smoothing the graft. Seating the impactor (arrow) compresses the cancellous graft (red stippled areas) against the walls of the medullary canal. (From Matsen FA III, Lippitt SB. *Shoulder Surgery: Principles and Procedures.* Philadelphia: Saunders; 2004:537.)

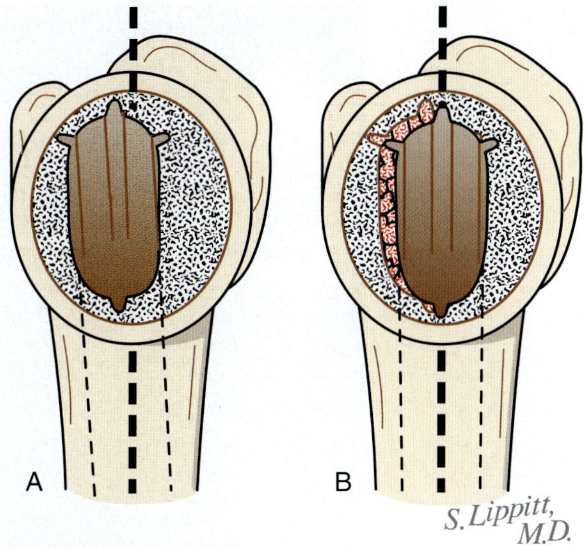

FIGURE 16-325: Anterior grafting. **A,** An apparent posterior offset of the neck related to anterior inclination of the prosthesis. **B,** This can be eliminated by selective anterior grafting. (From Matsen FA III, Lippitt SB. *Shoulder Surgery: Principles and Procedures.* Philadelphia: Saunders; 2004:538.)

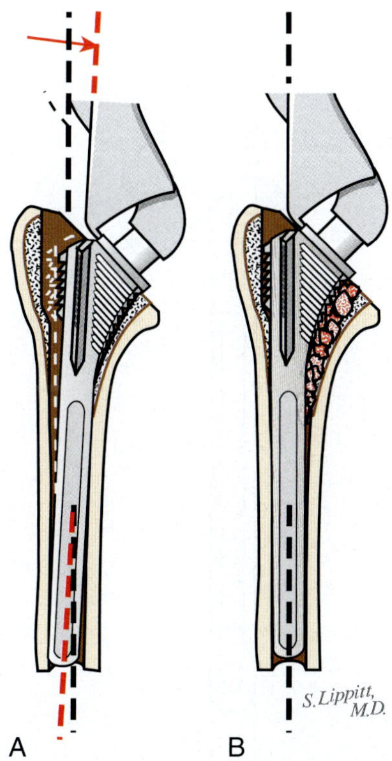

FIGURE 16-324: Medial grafting. **A,** Selective medial grafting can eliminate the tendency of the prosthesis to angulate into varus. **B,** Cancellous bone graft (red stippled areas) fills the medullary canal. (From Matsen FA III, Lippitt SB. *Shoulder Surgery: Principles and Procedures.* Philadelphia: Saunders; 2004:538.)

available for grafting is insufficient (Fig. 16-326). Because it is difficult to achieve secure impaction with a cylindrical humeral body (Fig. 16-327), we use a stem with a proximal flare. The metaphyseal portion of the prosthetic body is thicker in the anteroposterior and mediolateral dimensions than the diaphyseal portion, a configuration that enables secure fixation without driving the stem tightly into the humeral cortex distally (Figs. 16-328 to 16-334; see Fig. 16-185). The effectiveness of this technique has been documented by a laboratory study that showed an increase in quality of fit and fill[193] and by clinical follow-up studies.[336,591] This method of conservative reaming and broaching combined with impaction grafting avoids the most common problem with press-fit humeral components: if the prosthesis is positioned too high because of incarceration of the distal end of the stem in the humeral diaphysis, this leaves the prosthesis prominent with respect to the tuberosities and the glenoid (see Figs. 16-244, 16-245, 16-247, and 16-252). Tip incarceration and incomplete seating of the humeral component may result from choosing a stem-size based on the AP radiograph (see Fig. 16-63); because of its oval shape, the humeral canal usually appears to be wider on the AP view than on the axillary view (see Fig. 16-64). Obviously, the problem of a too high and tight stem fit cannot be solved by trying to hammer the prosthesis down further; instead, our solution is to change to a smaller implant stem diameter and fill the void by impaction grafting. We like to say that the impaction grafting approach allows the surgeon to "get it wrong, but still get it right." In a way this is similar to the method used

Text continued on p. 956

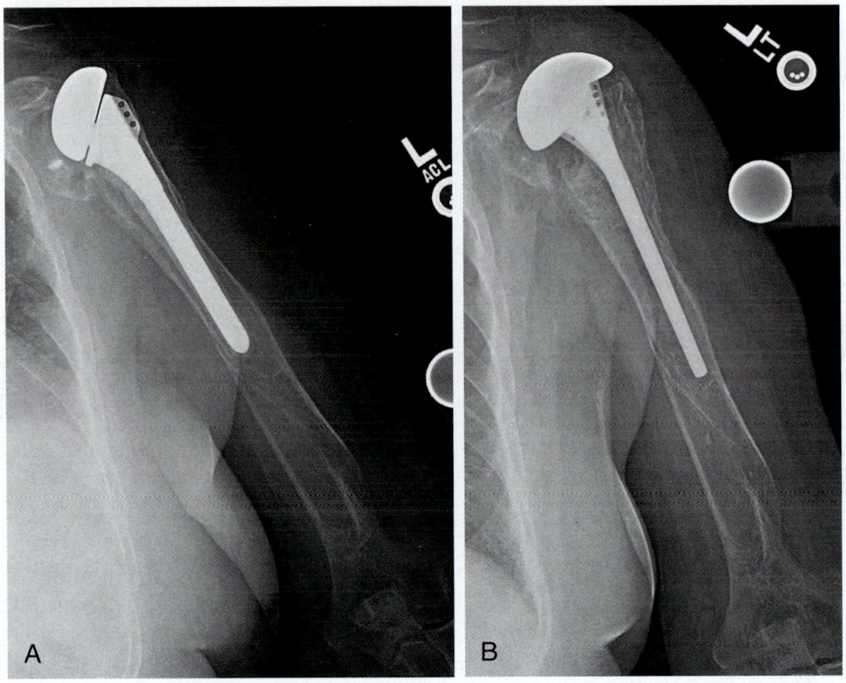

FIGURE 16-326: **A,** Loose humeral and glenoid components in very osteopenic bone. **B,** This was treated by the removal of both components followed by impaction allografting of a cuff tear arthropathy prosthesis.

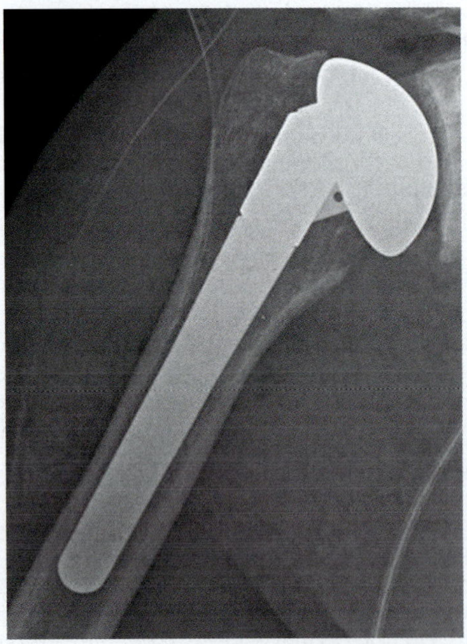

FIGURE 16-327: A cylindrical stem on the humeral implant does not allow for effective impaction grafting.

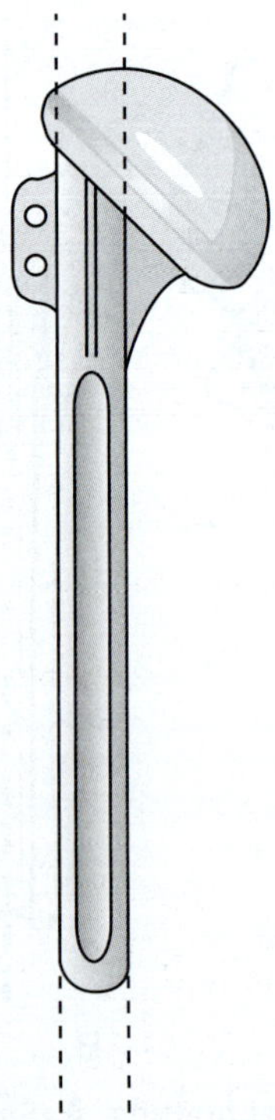

FIGURE 16-328: Cylindrical stem. A cylindrical body can slide within a cylindrical canal. This configuration can allow distal migration of the component. (From Matsen FA III, Lippitt SB. *Shoulder Surgery: Principles and Procedures.* Philadelphia: Saunders; 2004:463.)

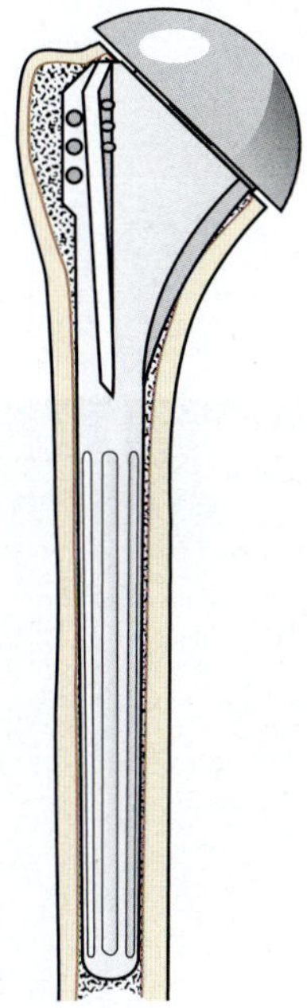

FIGURE 16-329: Humeral press-fit. A prosthetic body with a tapered metaphyseal section achieves a press-fit in the tapered humeral metaphysis. (From Matsen FA III, Lippitt SB. *Shoulder Surgery: Principles and Procedures.* Philadelphia: Saunders; 2004:463.)

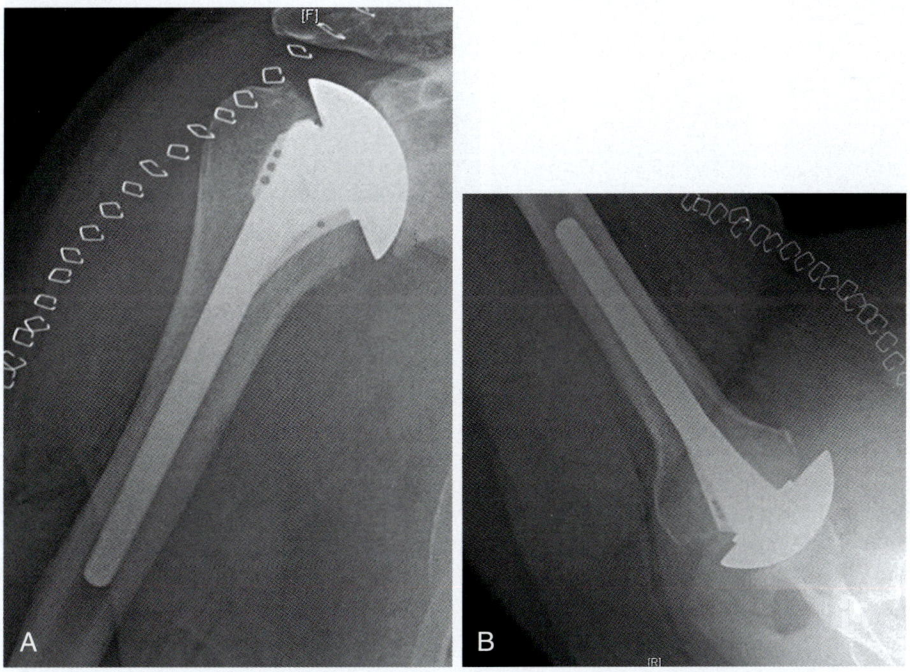

FIGURE 16-330: A prosthetic stem with a metaphyseal flare in the mediolateral (**A**) and the anteroposterior (**B**) dimensions facilitates impaction grafting. Note that the impacted graft has filled the funnel-shaped metaphysis.

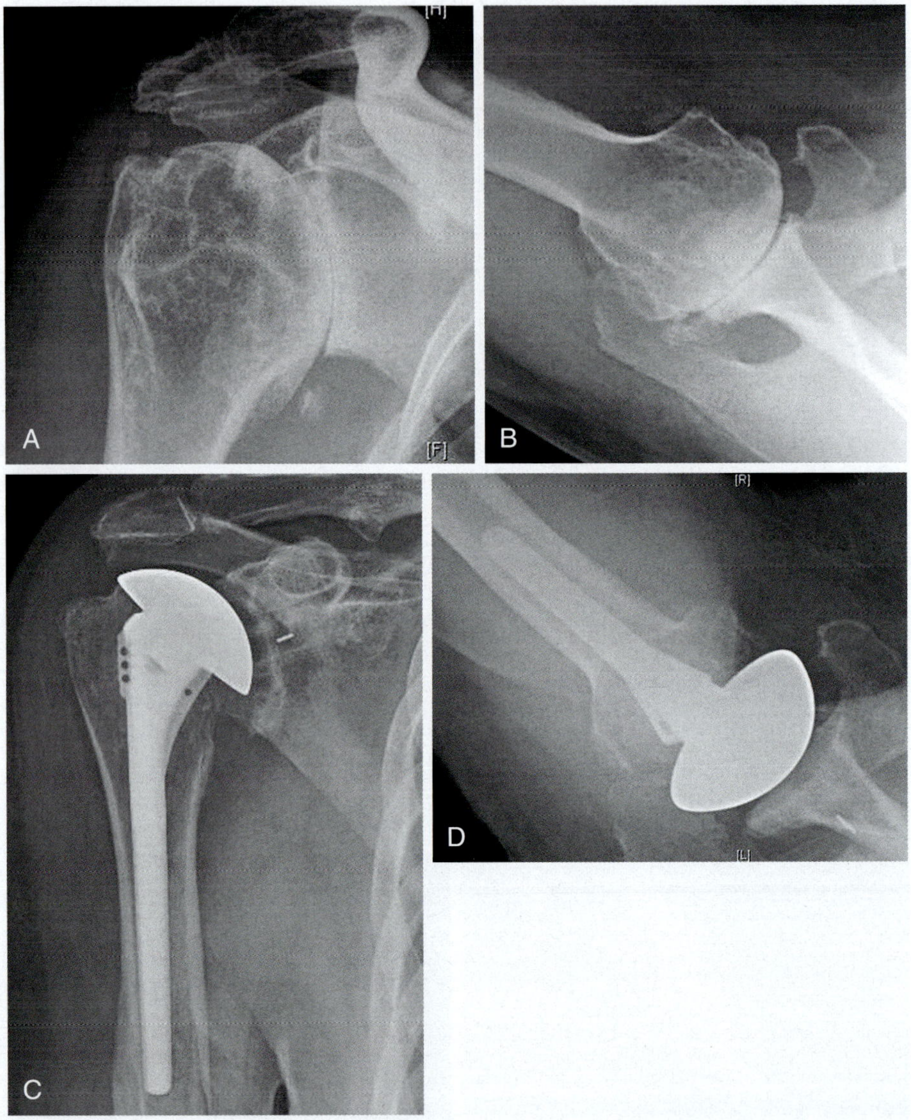

FIGURE 16-331: Glenohumeral arthritis with glenoid anteversion. **A,** Preoperative anteroposterior view. **B,** Preoperative axillary view showing anteversion. **C,** Postoperative anteroposterior view at 2 years after surgery showing a stable impaction-grafted humeral stem. **D,** Postoperative axillary view showing a humeral prosthesis centered in the glenoid component which was inserted without changing version.

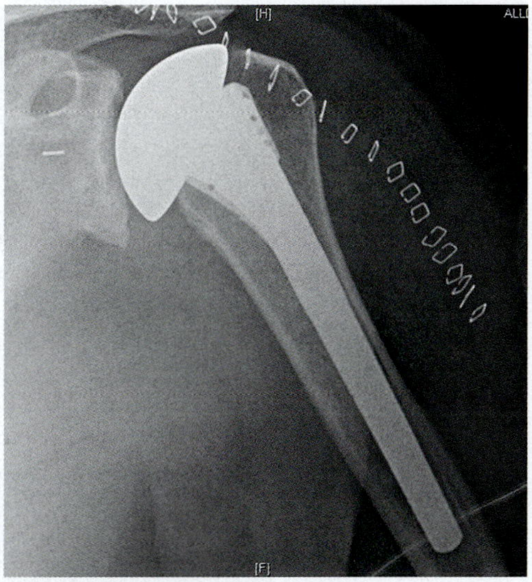

FIGURE 16-332: Total shoulder arthroplasty showing fixation of a glenoid component with no radiolucent lines and the fixation of humeral component with impaction grafting.

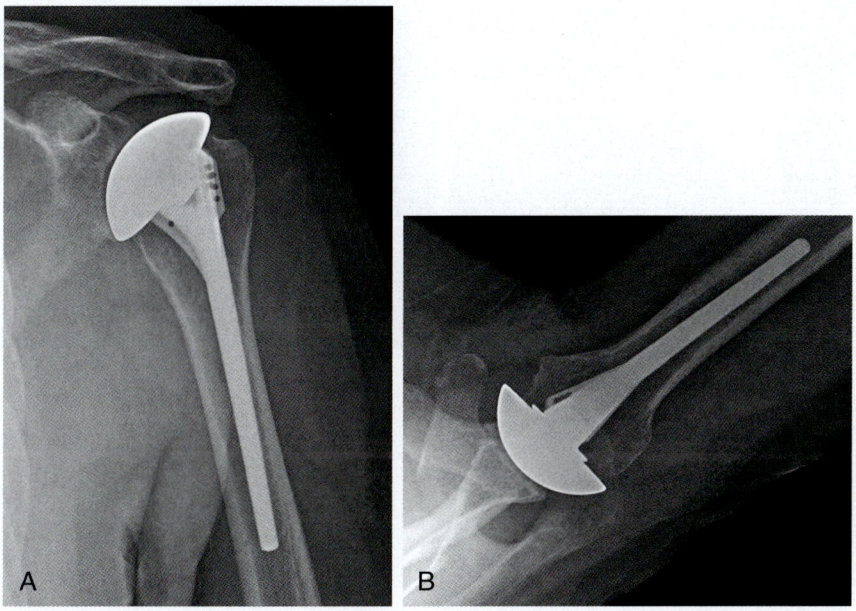

FIGURE 16-333: Stable ream and run procedure 2 years after surgery. **A,** Anteroposterior view showing secure fixation of a prosthesis inserted with impaction grafting. **B,** Axillary view indicating the presence of fibrocartilage between the humeral prosthesis and the reamed glenoid face.

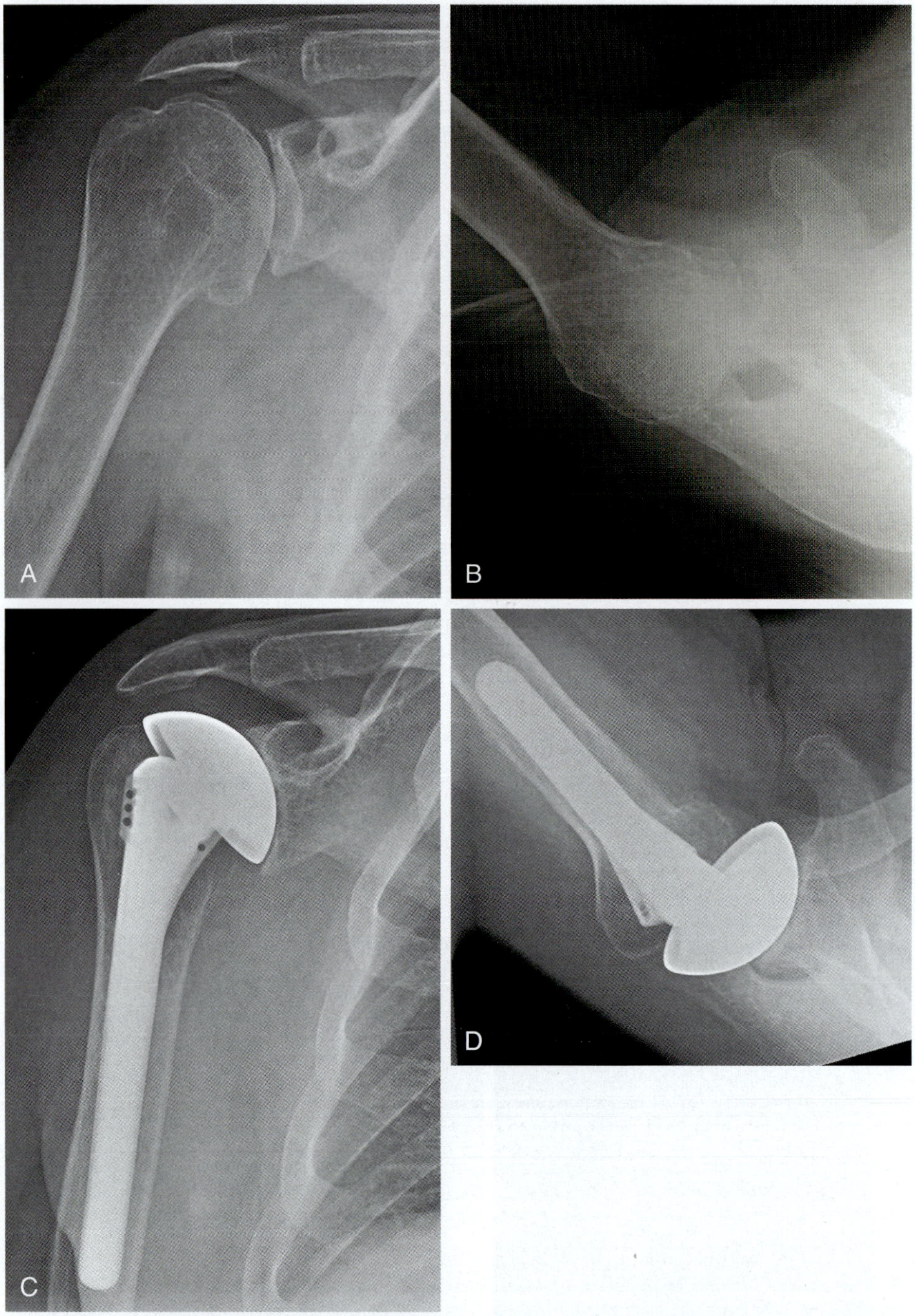

FIGURE 16-334: Functionally decentered humeral head managed with an anteriorly eccentric humeral prosthesis. **A,** Preoperative anteroposterior view. **B,** Preoperative axillary view. **C,** Postoperative anteroposterior view. **D,** Postoperative axillary view.

by Procrustes, the legendary Greek innkeeper, who "fitted" his "guest" to his bed, rather than fitting the bed to the guest. If the prosthesis sits too far distally, the problem is solved by adding more autograft. If it sits too far proximally, a smaller stem can be used. If the position of the prosthesis is not ideal, it can be fine-tuned by selective placement of the graft (see Figs. 16-324 and 16-325). If an impaction grafted, uncemented, nonporous coated stem needs to be revised, it can usually be disimpacted (Fig. 16-335) without concern about cement removal (see Fig. 16-247) and without the need to perform a humeral osteotomy (Fig. 16-336) as may be necessary when removing a prosthesis with ingrowth surfaces,[517,547] trabecular metal,[303] or platform (modular) stems.[582] In some specific situations it may be necessary to saw off the tip of the prosthesis to the necessary length

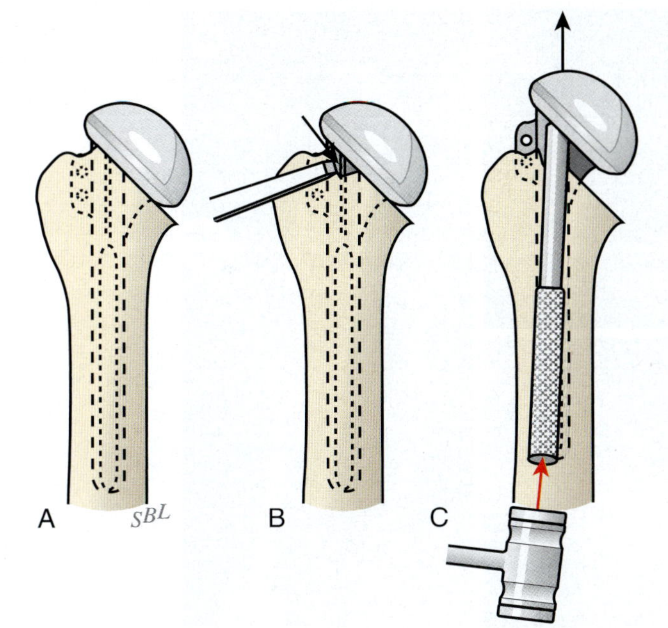

FIGURE 16-335: Removing a humeral component. **A** and **B,** A simple, effective method for removing a humeral component is to create a notch (arrow) in the shaft beneath the head of the humeral component. **C,** A bone tamp can then be placed in this notch and used to drive the humeral prosthesis out of the shaft with slaps of the hammer in line with the prosthetic stem. (From Matsen FA III, Lippitt SB. *Shoulder Surgery: Principles and Procedures.* Philadelphia: Saunders; 2004:719.)

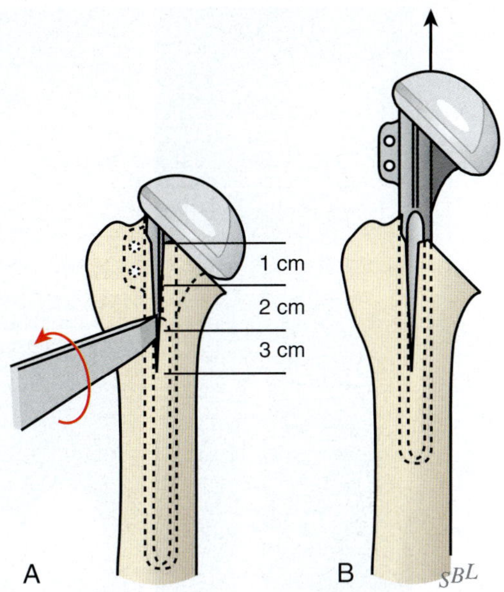

FIGURE 16-336: Osteotomy of the humeral shaft. **A,** When the humeral prosthesis cannot be freed from the humerus, an osteotomy is created, starting at the upper edge of the bicipital groove. The osteotomy is pried open by turning the osteotome in the bone cut (red arrow) to increase the cross section of the humerus. **B,** After each cut, the bone tamp is placed in the osteotomy and a hammer is used to try to drive the prosthesis out proximally (black arrow). If the component cannot be removed, the osteotomy is extended distally by another centimeter and these steps are repeated until the prosthesis becomes loose. (From Matsen FA III, Lippitt SB. *Shoulder Surgery: Principles and Procedures.* Philadelphia: Saunders; 2004:720.)

and fix it with cement (Fig. 16-337). We reserve the use of long stems for cases in which an area of cortical weakness needs to be bypassed (see Fig. 16-314).

We are not convinced of the value of systems with "platform" stems because many failures of anatomic arthroplasties are related to improper placement of the stem (see Fig. 16-248). It seems doubtful that a platform design would facilitate revision of such cases to a reverse arthroplasty (see Figs. 16-188 and 16-247; Figs. 16-338 to 16-340). As long as the stem is not cemented and does not have a bony ingrowth surface, conversion to a reverse total shoulder arthroplasty is usually straightforward (Fig. 16-341).

Although some systems offer adjustable neck shaft angles (Fig. 16-342), in our experience this added complexity is unnecessary as a standard 45-degree cut can accommodate normal (Fig. 16-343), varus (Fig. 16-344), and valgus (Fig. 16-345) anatomy.

Glenoid Component. Anatomic total shoulder arthroplasty involves the insertion of a prosthetic glenoid component. Without question, this component is the weakest link in total shoulder arthroplasty.[334,414,415] The reasons for its high rate of failure are apparent: (1) a prosthetic component cannot duplicate the basic structure of the normal glenoid (Fig. 16-346), with its firm center and compliant periphery that allows small amounts of translation without damage to the rim (Figs. 16-347 and 16-348)[578]; (2) a prosthetic component cannot duplicate the wear resistance of normal articular cartilage (Fig. 16-349)[53,487]; and (3) the prosthetic joint component cannot duplicate the natural secure fixation of hyaline cartilage to the underlying bone,[88] especially in its ability to withstand eccentric loading (see Fig. 16-285).

The goal of glenoid component insertion is to optimize the support of the component through excellent shaping, rather than by using cement "putty" (Fig. 16-350; see Figs. 16-272 to 16-274). The optimal glenoid insertion technique involves the following: (1) conservatively reaming the glenoid bone surface so that it has congruent contact with the back of the prosthesis without interposed cement that can crack and fail (Figs. 16-351 to 16-353); (2) selecting a prosthesis that covers the maximum amount of prepared glenoid bone surface (Fig. 16-354) and which is relatively thin (3 to 4 mm) so as to avoid contributing to overstuffing and to minimize the loosening moment (see Fig. 16-205); (3) precisely aligning the prosthesis with the prepared bone, minimizing the need for large amounts of cement that can kill bone (Fig. 16-355)[85]; (4) achieving firm fixation; and (5) preserving glenoid bone stock, the most precious commodity in total shoulder arthroplasty.[570]

Text continued on p. 965

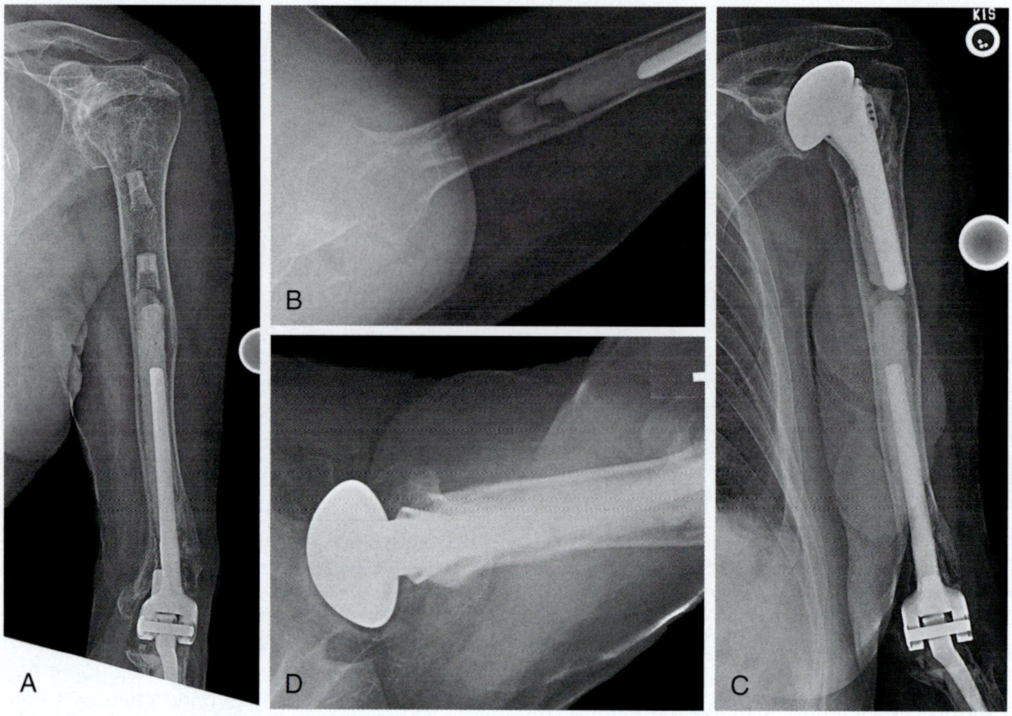

FIGURE 16-337: Shoulder arthroplasty after a prior elbow arthroplasty. **A** and **B,** Anteroposterior and axillary views of glenohumeral arthritis and a prior total elbow arthroplasty with a long humeral stem. **C** and **D,** Anteroposterior and axillary views of glenohumeral reconstruction using a hemiarthroplasty with a prosthesis that was shortened with a high-speed saw and then cemented such that the upper and lower cement mantles were in contact. This minimized the risk of fracture at the junction.

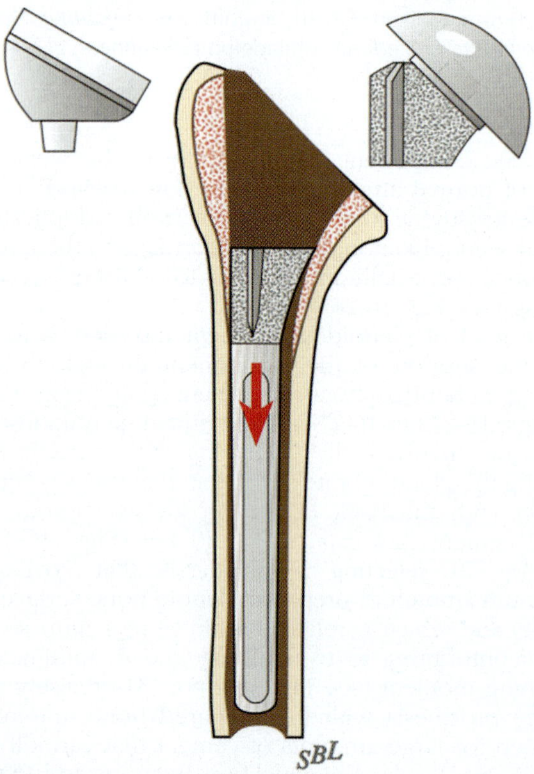

FIGURE 16-338: If a platform stem is fixed too far distally, conversion to a reverse arthroplasty may require removal of the platform stem.

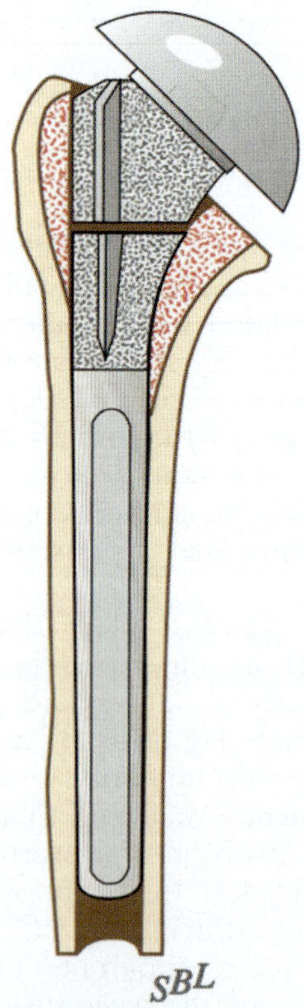

FIGURE 16-339: If a platform stem is fixed too proximally, conversion to a reverse arthroplasty may require removal of the platform stem.

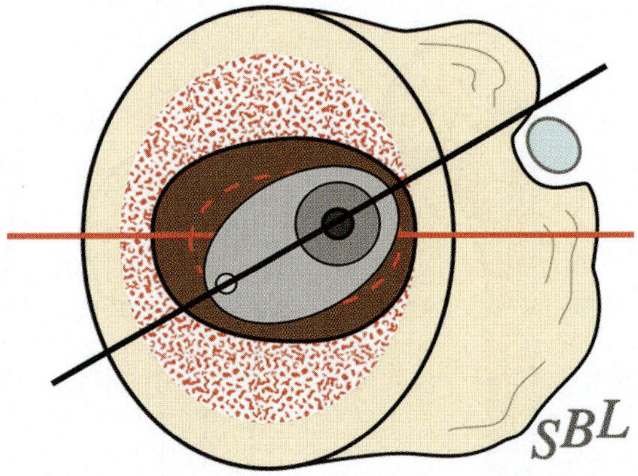

FIGURE 16-340: If a platform stem is fixed in malrotation, conversion to a reverse arthroplasty may require removal of the platform stem.

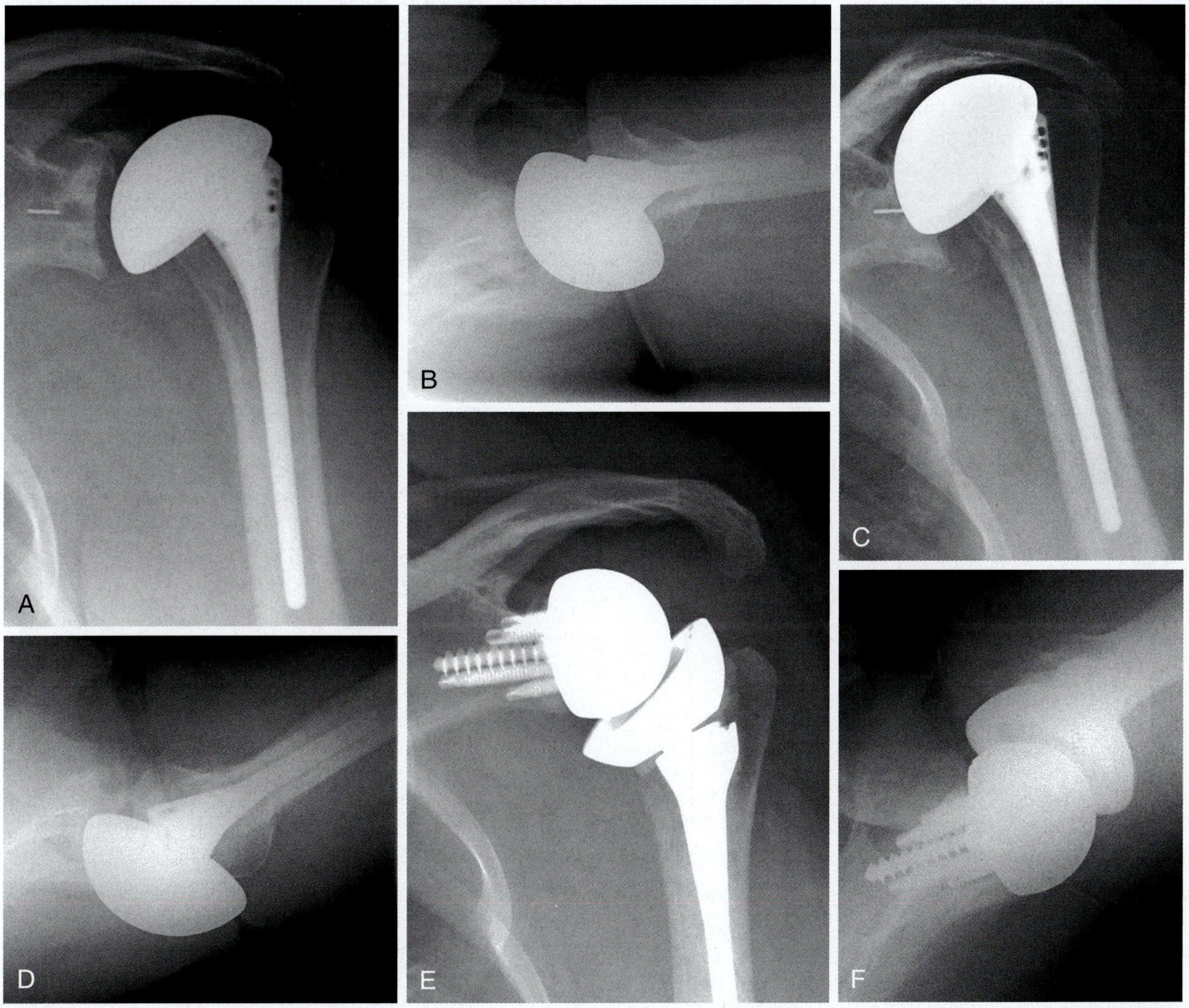

FIGURE 16-341: Dislocated total shoulder arthroplasty managed by conversion to a reverse total shoulder arthroplasty. **A** and **B,** Anteroposterior and axillary views of a total shoulder arthroplasty that functioned well until the patient awoke with sudden onset of pain 6 years after the index surgery. **C** and **D,** A posterior dislocation was noted on the anteroposterior and axillary views. **E** and **F,** The impaction grafted stem and glenoid were removed and the shoulder converted to a reverse total shoulder arthroplasty as shown on the anteroposterior and axillary views.

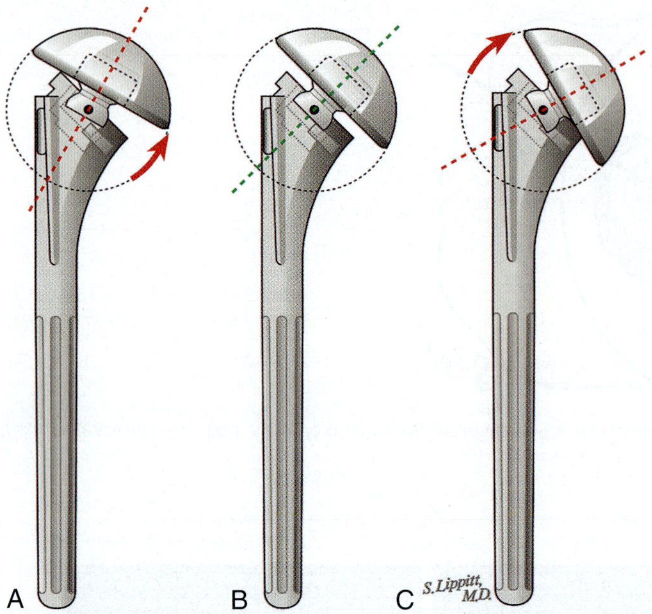

FIGURE 16-342: Example of a modular prosthetic design with an adjustable humeral head component. This can be placed into varus and valgus positions relative to the standard 135 degree head-shaft angle. **A,** Valgus position. **B,** Standard angle. **C,** Varus position.

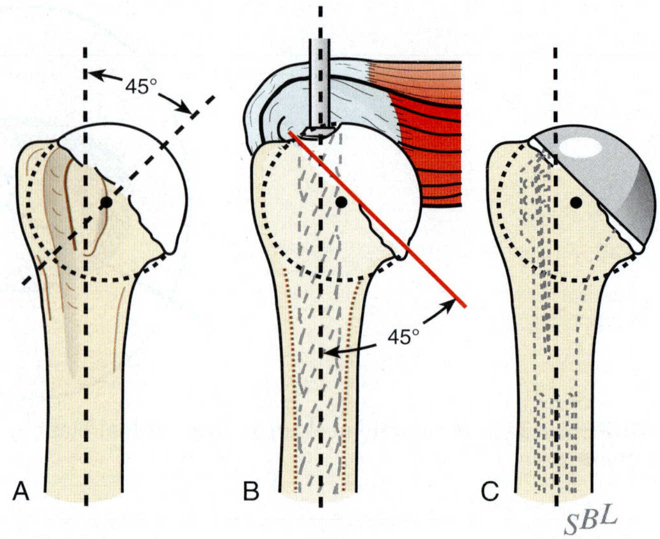

FIGURE 16-343: Neck-shaft angle and humeral prosthesis. **A,** In the great majority of cases, a surgeon can use a prosthesis with a fixed 45-degree neck-shaft angle, an appropriate head height and diameter of curvature, and a small offset to restore the articular surface anatomically. Prostheses with variable neck–shaft angles do not seem to be necessary. **B,** The humeral neck cut plane passes just inside the cuff insertion and makes a 45-degree angle with the orthopedic axis. **C,** Insertion of the prosthesis along the orthopedic axis restores the articular surface. (From Matsen FA III, Lippitt SB. *Shoulder Surgery: Principles and Procedures.* Philadelphia: Saunders; 2004:449.)

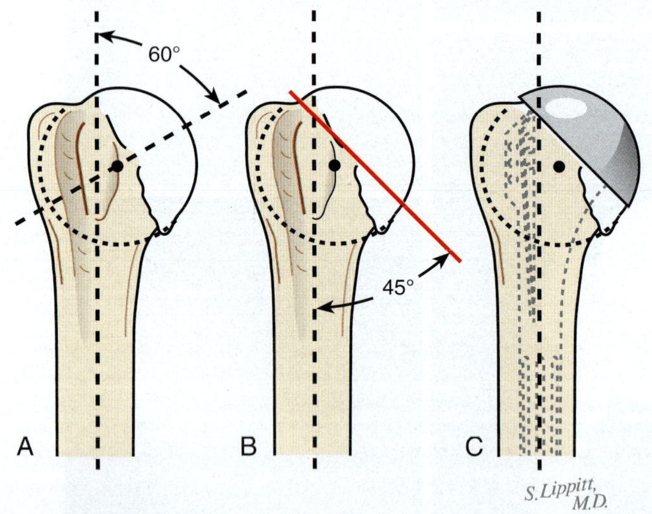

FIGURE 16-344: Varus humeral head. **A,** The biologic humeral head in a varus configuration. **B** and **C,** A prosthesis with a 45-degree angle cut can still result in an anatomic restoration of the joint surface by leaving a small amount of the medial head unresurfaced. (From Matsen FA III, Lippitt SB. *Shoulder Surgery: Principles and Procedures.* Philadelphia: Saunders; 2004:450.)

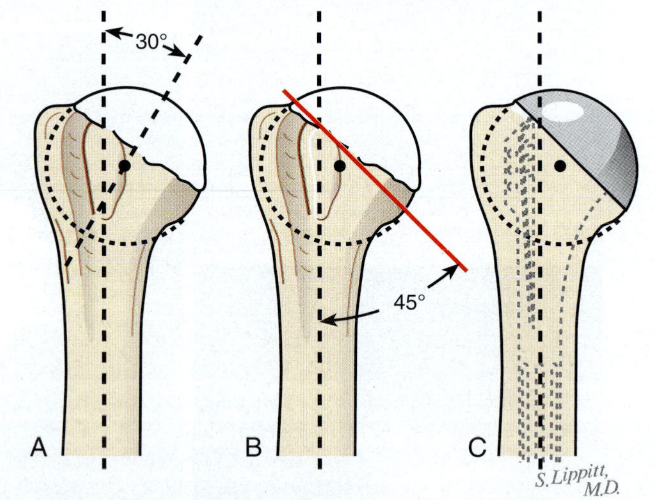

FIGURE 16-345: Valgus humeral head. **A,** The biologic humeral head in a valgus configuration. **B** and **C,** A prosthesis with a 45-degree angle cut can still result in an anatomic restoration of the joint surface by resecting and resurfacing a small amount of the medial metaphysis. (From Matsen FA III, Lippitt SB. *Shoulder Surgery: Principles and Procedures.* Philadelphia: Saunders; 2004:451.)

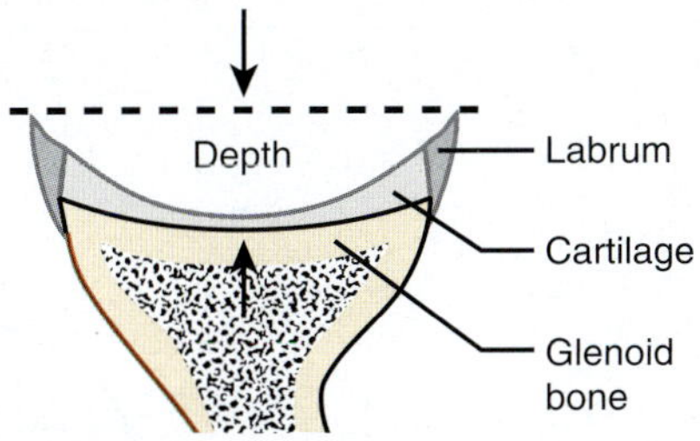

FIGURE 16-346: Components of the glenoid fossa. The glenoid fossa results from the relatively small concavity of the glenoid bone, deepened by the glenoid cartilage and by the labrum at its periphery. (From Matsen FA III, Lippitt SB. *Shoulder Surgery: Principles and Procedures.* Philadelphia: Saunders; 2004:88.)

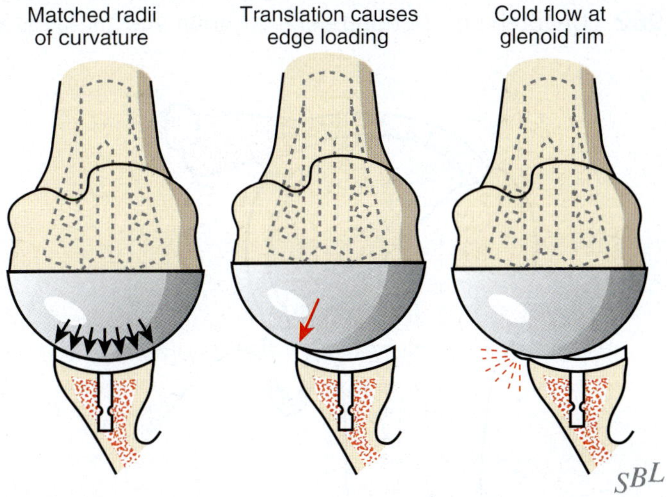

FIGURE 16-348: Glenoid rim load. If the humeral head translates from the center (black arrows) to a position where it is up on the glenoid rim (red arrow), the contact area becomes very small (involving only the sharp edge of the polyethylene) and the contact pressure therefore becomes very high, risking polyethylene cold flow and wear. (From Matsen FA III, Lippitt SB. *Shoulder Surgery: Principles and Procedures.* Philadelphia: Saunders; 2004:493.)

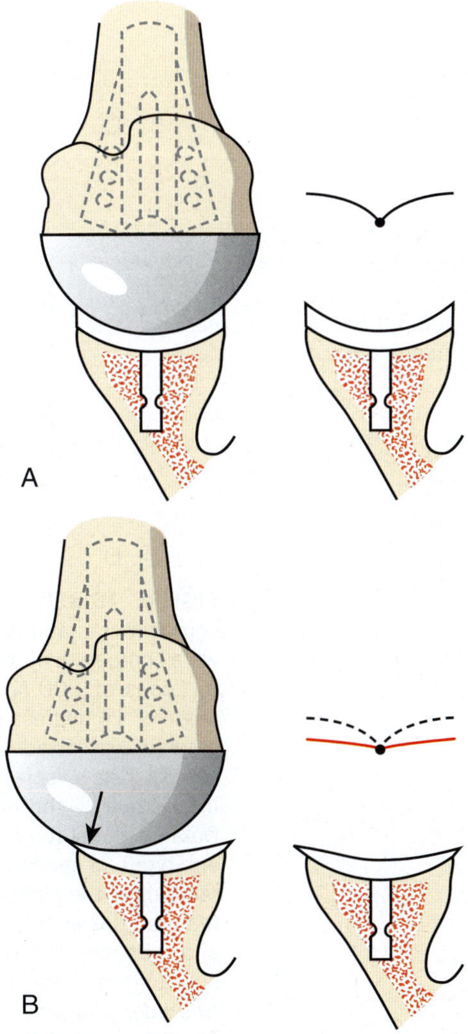

FIGURE 16-347: Worn glenoid lips. **A,** The intact glenoid. **B,** Cold flow or edge wear can result in loss of the glenoid depth, increased shallowness of the glenoidogram, and loss of intrinsic glenoid stability. (From Matsen FA III, Lippitt SB. *Shoulder Surgery: Principles and Procedures.* Philadelphia: Saunders; 2004:487.)

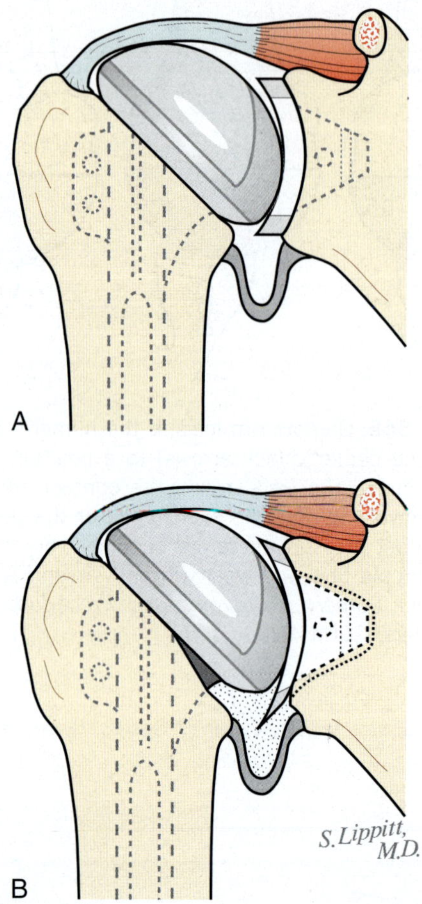

FIGURE 16-349: Polyethylene wear. Wear of the glenoid polyethylene results in loss of the normal glenoid shape, but the wear particles can cause osteolysis around the glenoid and humeral components. (From Matsen FA III, Lippitt SB. *Shoulder Surgery: Principles and Procedures.* Philadelphia: Saunders; 2004:697.)

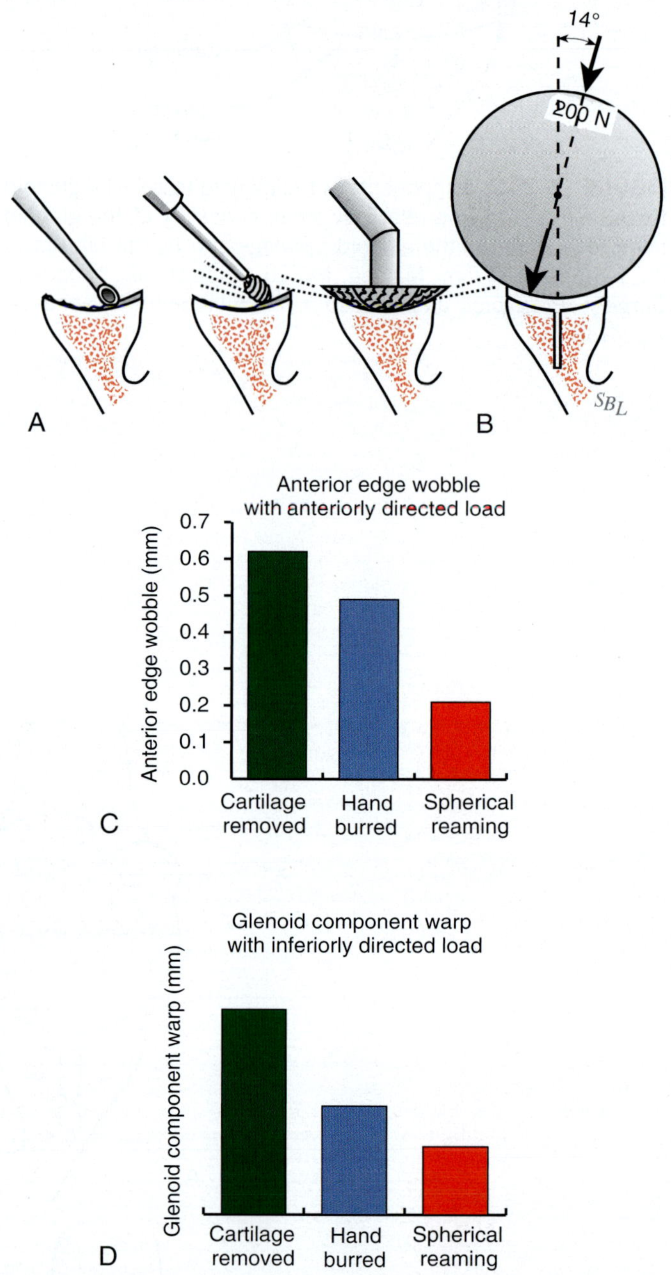

FIGURE 16-350: The effect of glenoid bone preparation on component stability. **A,** Three methods of bone preparation were compared: curettage, hand burring, and spherical reaming. **B,** Loads of 200 N were applied through a metal ball at an angle of 14 degrees with respect to the glenoid centerline. The glenoid was fixed only with a single, uncemented flexible central peg. Displacement transducers measured the change in position of the edges of the glenoid component. **C** and **D,** Data on the stability of a glenoid component with three different types of glenoid surface preparation show that spherical reaming of the glenoid along the glenoid centerline significantly reduced the wobble (**C**) and warp (**D**) of the glenoid component and thus provided greater glenoid component stability than did curettage or hand burring. (From Matsen FA III, Lippitt SB. *Shoulder Surgery: Principles and Procedures.* Philadelphia: Saunders; 2004:510.)

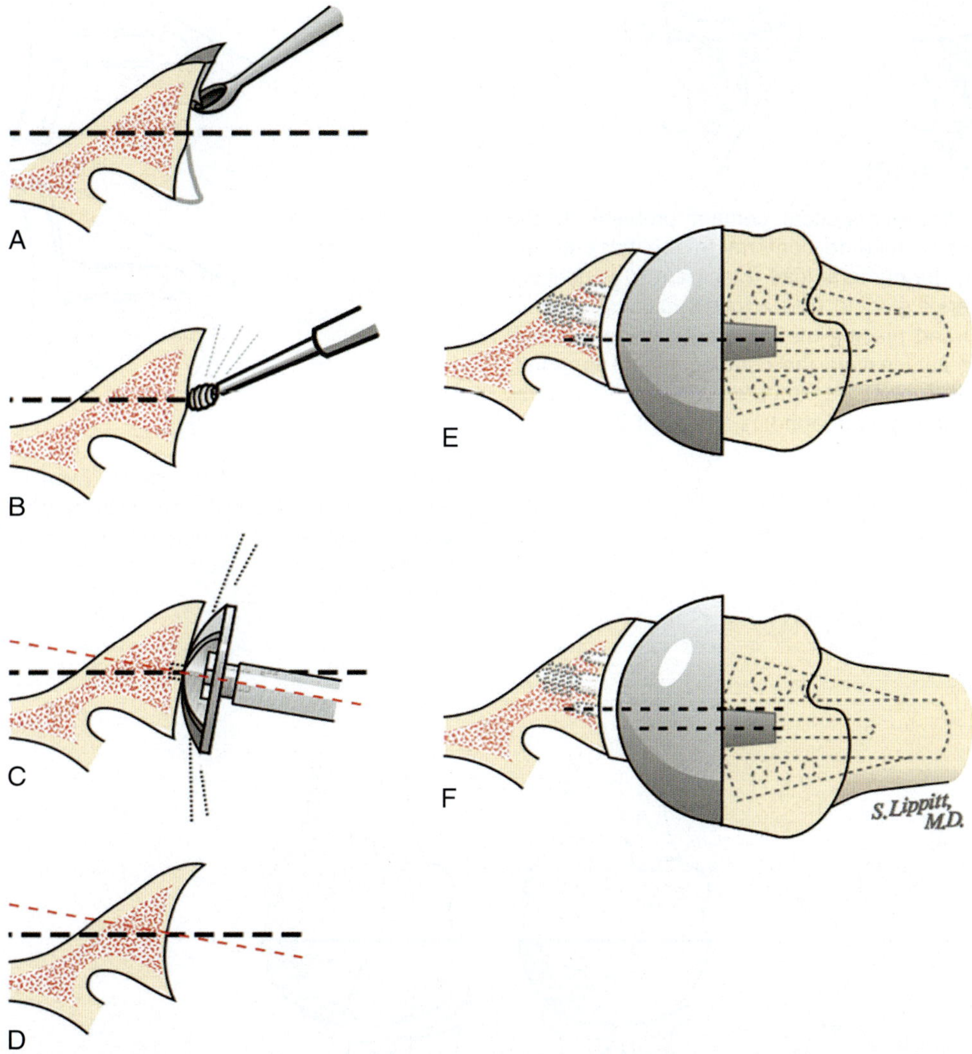

FIGURE 16-351: Optimal technique for glenoid reaming. **A,** Curette the remaining anterior glenoid cartilage. **B,** Burr the central ridge of the biconcave glenoid. **C,** Conservative reaming accepting glenoid retroversion. **D,** Concentric reamed glenoid with remaining retroversion. **E**, Total shoulder arthroplasty (TSR) stabilized with a concentric head component. **F,** TSR stabilized with an anterior eccentric head component.

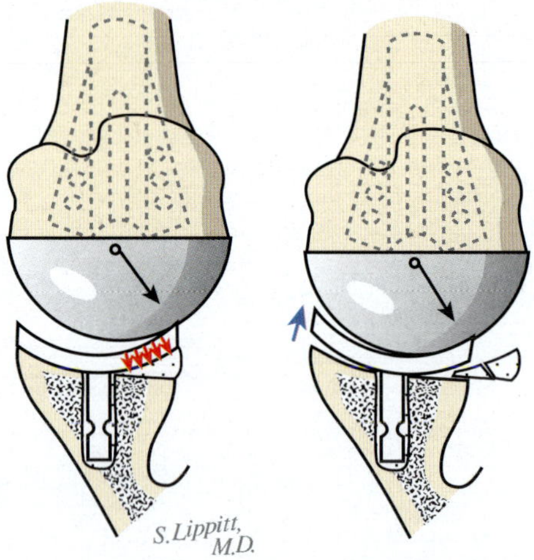

FIGURE 16-352: Posterior glenoid cement problem. If the glenoid bone is not reamed to conform to the back of the glenoid component, the humeral load (black arrow) is concentrated on the posterior glenoid (red arrows), causing anterior lift-off (blue arrow) and placing the interposed cement wedge at risk for cracking out, leaving the component unsupported. (From Matsen FA III, Lippitt SB. *Shoulder Surgery: Principles and Procedures.* Philadelphia: Saunders; 2004:507.)

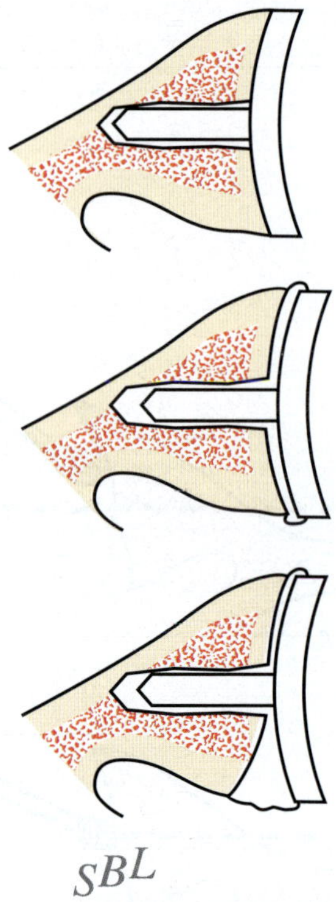

FIGURE 16-353: Glenoid seating. Even if the fixation of the glenoid keel appears solid, the seating of the component onto the bone may be suboptimal. (From Matsen FA III, Lippitt SB. *Shoulder Surgery: Principles and Procedures.* Philadelphia: Saunders; 2004:723.)

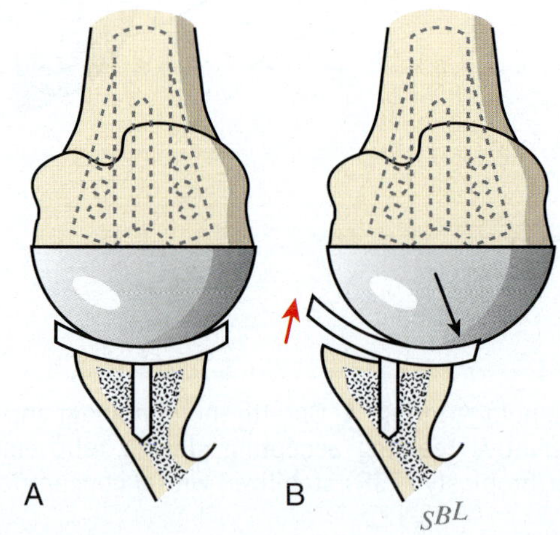

FIGURE 16-354: Glenoid overhang. **A,** The edges of the prosthetic glenoid are unsupported by bone. **B,** This brings an increased risk of loosening when rim loading occurs. (From Matsen FA III, Lippitt SB. *Shoulder Surgery: Principles and Procedures.* Philadelphia: Saunders; 2004:503.)

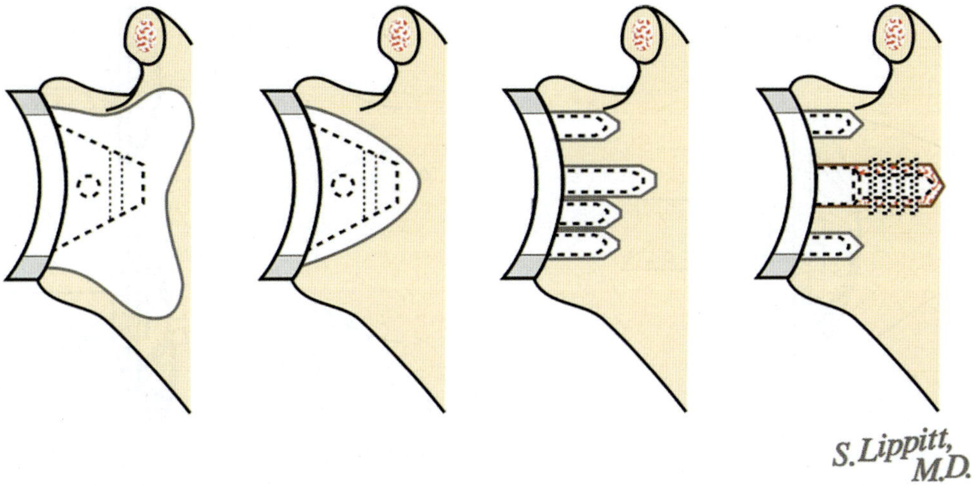

FIGURE 16-355: Glenoid peg fixation preserves bone stock and minimizes the need for large amounts of cement fixation. This lessens the risk of cement thermal bone necrosis.

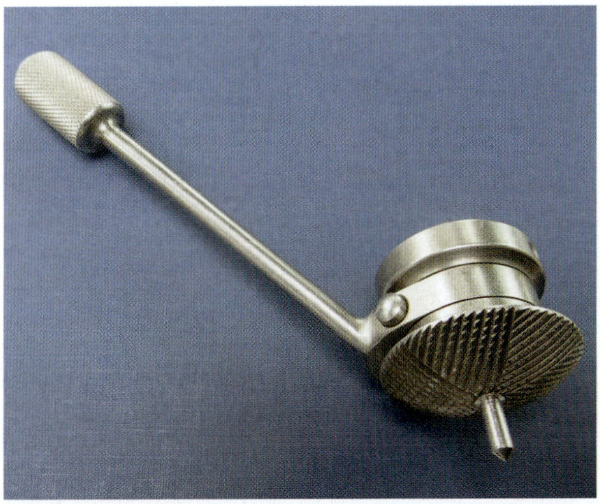

FIGURE 16-356: The first spherical reamer we developed in 1992. Note the nub to maintain the centered position of the reamer. This allows for inclination of the reamer to minimize the amount of bone removed in achieving a single glenoid concavity.

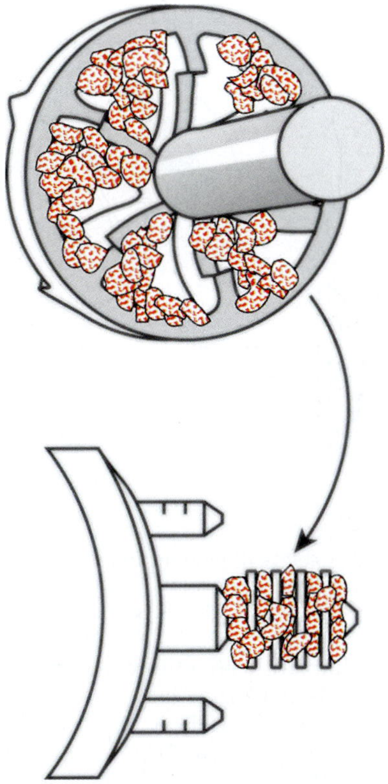

FIGURE 16-357: Finely morselized bone (red stippled areas) retrieved during the glenoid preparation (reaming and drilling) is interposed as a bone paste between the flanges of the central anchor peg to facilitate bone integration.

The purpose of glenoid reaming is to conservatively conform the bone to the back of the glenoid component for maximal component stability and load transfer. This should be done without needlessly sacrificing glenoid bone stock to accommodate complex back side geometry or in an attempt to "normalize" glenoid version by reaming down the high side. The use of sharp reamers is important to avoid thermal damage in preparing the glenoid bone.[409] In 1991 we started using a spherical reamer stabilized by a nub placed in a hole centered on the glenoid face (Fig. 16-356). The modern version of the reamer is bladed and collects bone that can be used as fine bone graft to enhance the fixation of the glenoid central peg (Fig. 16-357). The nubbed reamer (Fig. 16-358) allows the surgeon to make small changes in the superior/inferior and anterior/posterior inclination of the reamer to ensure the entire glenoid surface is reamed (see Figs. 16-234 and 16-269). Because conservative reaming requires this fine-tuning of the reamer's orientation so that a single

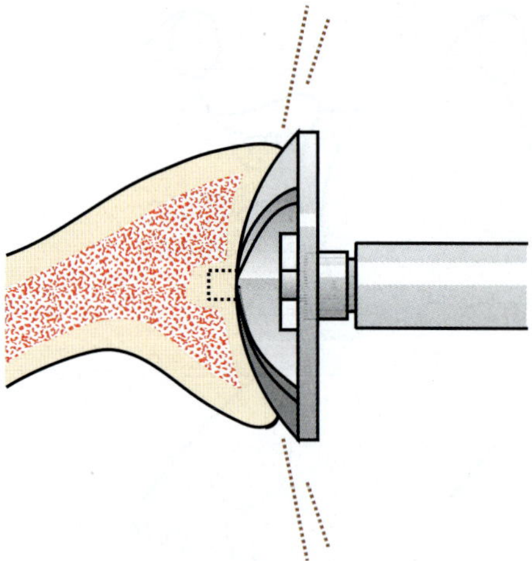

FIGURE 16-358: The orientation of the glenoid face is normalized using a spherical reamer that corresponds with the previously selected glenoid sizing disk. Overreaming is avoided to preserve sufficient glenoid subchondral bone for secure support of the glenoid implant.

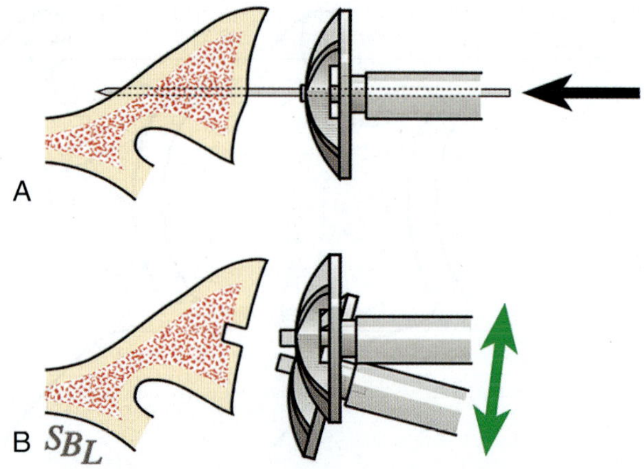

FIGURE 16-360: **A,** A guide pin rigidly defines the direction of reaming. **B,** In contrast, the nubbed reamer allows the surgeon to make changes in the superior/inferior and anterior/posterior inclination of the reamer, ensuring that the entire glenoid surface is reamed while minimizing the amount of glenoid bone that is removed.

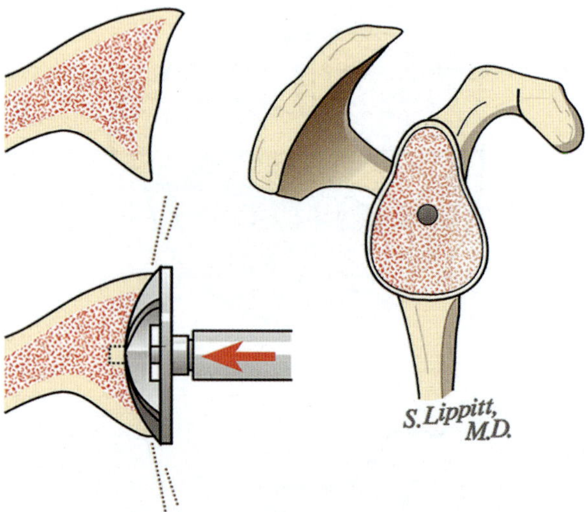

FIGURE 16-359: Excessive glenoid reaming results in the loss of subchondral bone support.

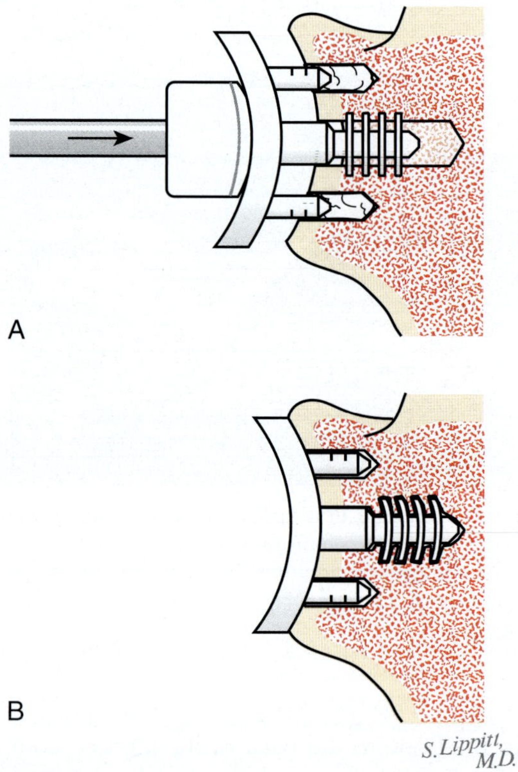

FIGURE 16-361: Insertion of the anchor peg glenoid prosthesis. **A,** The glenoid impactor is used to seat the component until there is complete contact with the perimeter of the glenoid. **B,** The inserted prosthesis. Pressure must be maintained directly on the glenoid component until the cement has hardened.

concavity is achieved with minimal bone removal (Fig. 16-359; see Fig. 16-270), we have not been attracted to approaches that rigidly define the orientation of the reamer with a guide pin based on a theoretical preoperative plan.[165,233,237,486,546,568] A guide pin not only prevents fine-tuning of the reamer's orientation, but is also at risk of bending, breakage, or inadvertent advancement into the chest (Fig. 16-360).

Because of their precise geometry and the spread of points of fixation across the glenoid face, fixation systems using pegs (Fig. 16-361) provide more secure fixation and require less cement compared with keeled components (Figs. 16-362 to 16-368; see Fig. 16-332).[105,273,286,558] Interference-fit pegs (Figs. 16-369 and Fig. 16-370) enhance initial fixation and allow for subsequent bone ingrowth (see Fig. 16-370).[185,590,592]

Although several metal-backed components have been designed, such components are reported to have a three times higher rate of revision than all-polyethylene components (see Fig. 16-251).[7,42,414] One of the intrinsic difficulties with metal-backed glenoid components relates

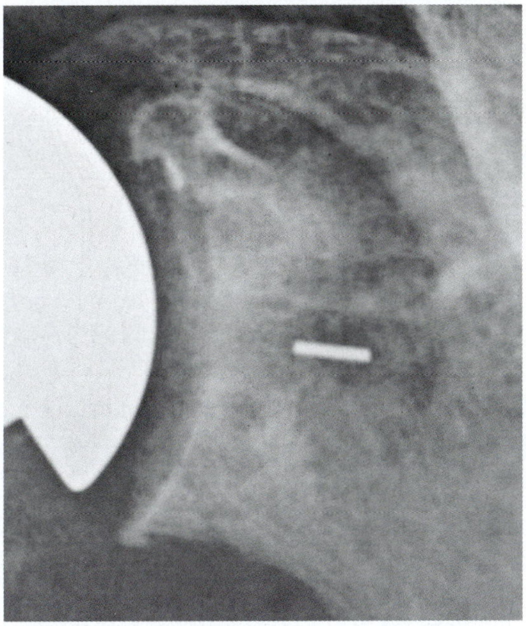

FIGURE 16-362: Radiograph taken 2 years after a total shoulder arthroplasty, showing no radiolucent lines.

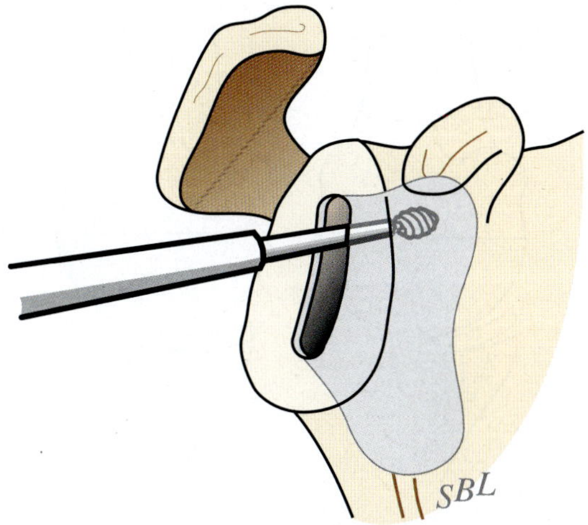

FIGURE 16-364: An air bur, rongeur, or curette is used to make a vertical slot in the glenoid concavity to accept the keel of the glenoid component. Bone is excavated from the base of the coracoid and down the lateral border of the scapula to help lock the keeled prosthesis with cement.

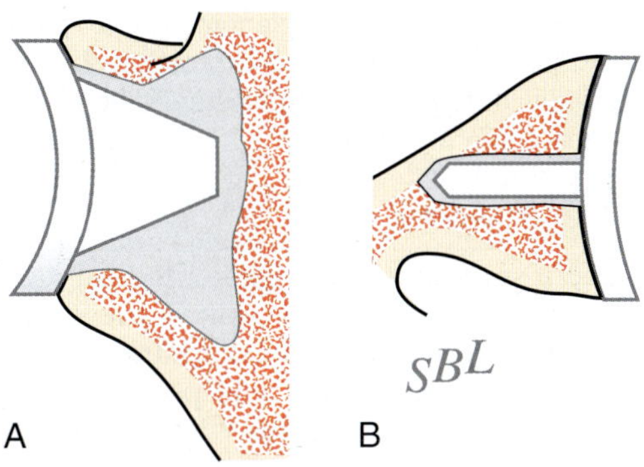

FIGURE 16-363: Example of the keeled glenoid component. **A,** Anteroposterior view. **B,** Axillary view.

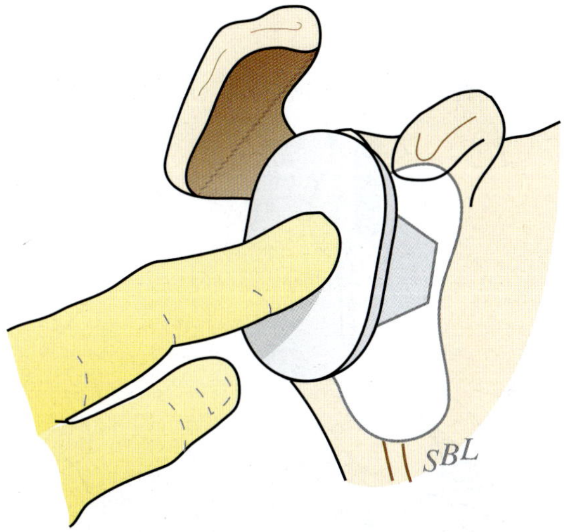

FIGURE 16-365: The glenoid slot is cleaned, dried, and packed with cement. The keeled prosthesis is held in place with finger pressure until the cement has set.

to the difference in the modulus of elasticity (Young's modulus) between metal and the other materials involved, as can be seen from the following examples:[414]

Cobalt chrome	200.0 GPa
Titanium	112.0 GPa
Cortical bone	8.0 GPa
PMMA cement	2.0 GPa
Polyethylene	0.5 GPa
Cancellous bone	0.4 GPa

The wide differences in these values indicate that different materials will deform differently under load. This results in shear stresses at the interfaces, especially that between metal and polyethylene.[157,530] This cannot be avoided when glenoids are made of substantially dissimilar materials. Notably, the closest match for modulus of elasticity is between polyethylene and bone; this may contribute to the lower revision rate of all-polyethylene components. Other issues with metal-backed glenoid components include their greater thickness (see Fig. 16-205), which may limit the range of motion and predispose the reconstruction to instability, increased contact stresses, and polyethylene cold flow.[414,537]

Surgical Technique for Anatomic Arthroplasty

Preparation of the Patient. It is helpful if surgical teams standardize the preoperative, operative, and postoperative protocols for shoulder arthroplasty; standardization improves both patient safety and efficiency. Because so much is common to the majority of shoulder joint

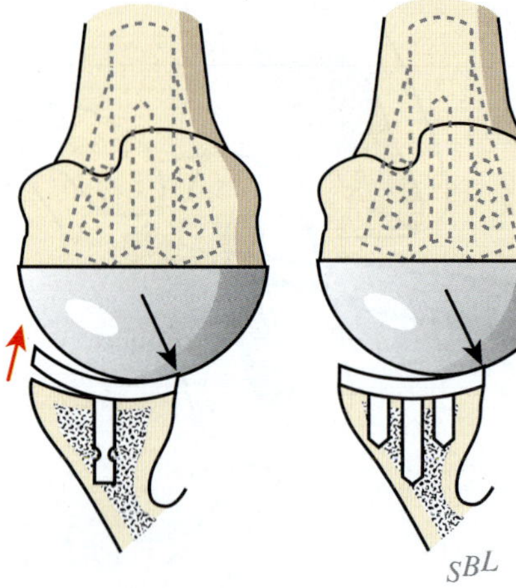

FIGURE 16-366: Peg fixation. A glenoid-fixation design that has pegs anterior and posterior to the glenoid midline helps to minimize the problem of lift-off (red arrow) with eccentric loading (black arrows). (From Matsen FA III, Lippitt SB. *Shoulder Surgery: Principles and Procedures.* Philadelphia: Saunders; 2004:509.)

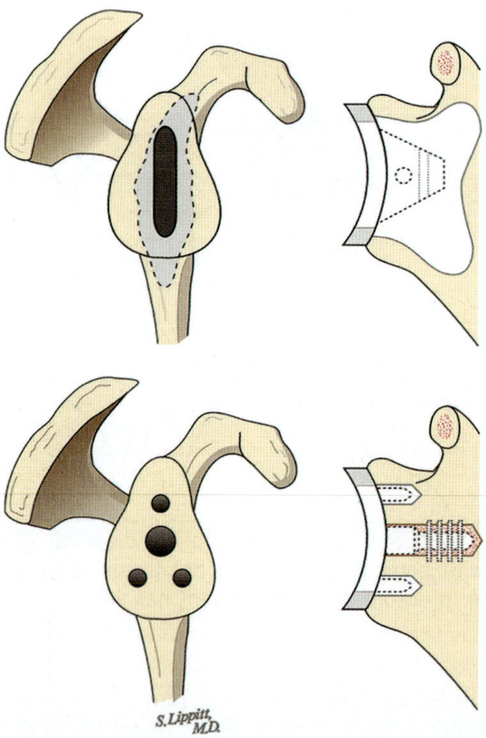

FIGURE 16-367: The precise geometry and multiplanar points of fixation in pegged glenoid components provide fixation that is more secure and require less cement compared with keeled components.

replacements, this presents an opportunity for the surgical team to establish "the way we always do it." Although the protocol is a matter of individual surgeon choice, the key is standardization to minimize any unnecessary uncertainty. The following is one possible approach.[337]

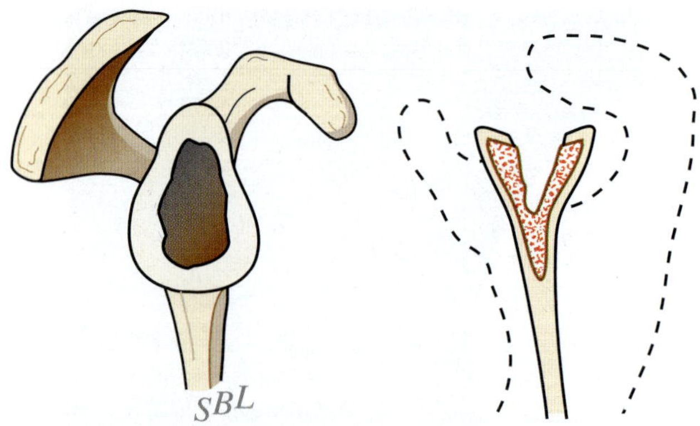

FIGURE 16-368: A cemented keeled glenoid may be indicated when a deficient central glenoid vault will not allow firm fixation of the central anchor peg.

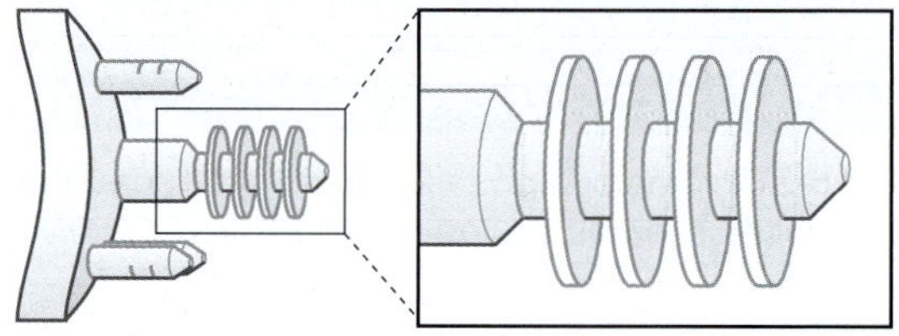

FIGURE 16-369: The anchor peg glenoid is an all-polyethylene, minimally cemented, pegged glenoid prosthesis. It features a circumferentially fluted central interference-fit peg for tissue integration and three small cemented peripheral pegs.

The patient's identity, allergies, medical conditions, side of surgery, condition of the skin of the shoulder and axilla, diagnosis, procedure, and discharge plan are confirmed with the patient awake. The presence or absence of a pacemaker is verified along with its recommended management.

The requisite plain radiographs (Figs. 16-371 and 16-372; see Fig. 16-62), including a template view (see Fig. 16-63), are displayed to confirm the side of surgery (Fig. 16-373) and reviewed to reveal the amount, quality, and orientation of the glenoid bone, as well as the size and configuration of the humerus down to where the tip of the humeral prosthesis will rest. The aim is to anticipate the final position of the humeral and glenoid components and any particular problems in their placement. Is there significant glenoid erosion or altered version? Are any potentially confusing glenoid osteophytes present? Is enough bone available to support a glenoid component or is there a large glenoid cyst (see Fig. 16-68)? What is the diameter of curvature of the humeral joint surface? Is the humeral canal straight? Is it cylindrical or funnel-shaped (see Fig. 16-319)? What size is it? Does the bone appear to be fragile? Is there anything that may block stem insertion (Fig. 16-374)? How are the tuberosities positioned in relation to the canal and the joint surface? How much humeral bone will need to be excised? Are there other major abnormalities of bone structure that could change the procedure

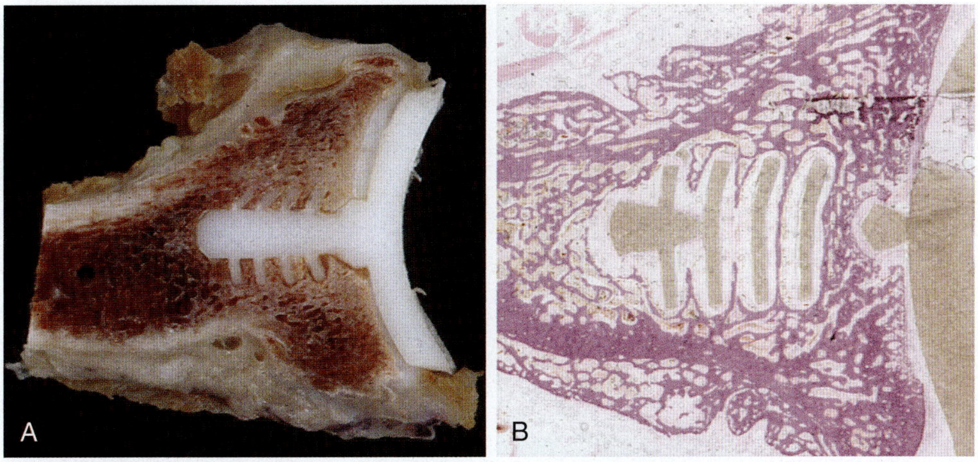

FIGURE 16-370: **A,** Cross section of one of the canine models that demonstrated bone ingrowth around the peg flanges of the central fluted peg of the glenoid anchor peg component. **B,** Histologic demonstration of the bone ingrowth around the peg flanges of the anchor peg glenoid.

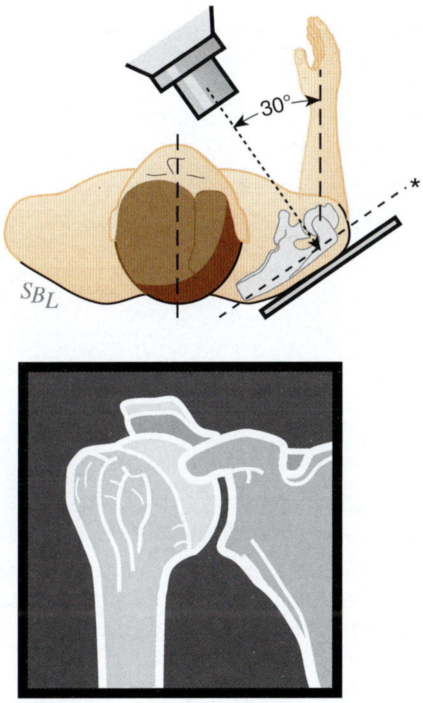

FIGURE 16-371: Anteroposterior (AP) radiograph in the plane of the scapula. The AP view in the plane of the scapula reveals the glenohumeral joint space and demonstrates whether the humeral head has a normal relationship to the glenoid fossa. The view is most easily taken by positioning the patient's scapula flat on the cassette and then passing the x-ray beam at right angles to the film, aimed at the coracoid process. (From Matsen FA III, Lippitt SB. *Shoulder Surgery: Principles and Procedures.* Philadelphia: Saunders; 2004:7.)

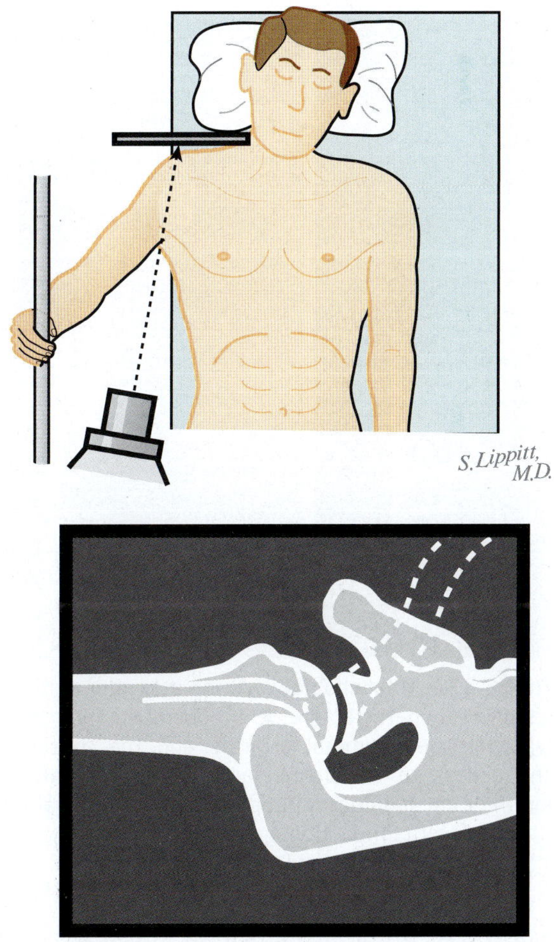

FIGURE 16-372: An axillary radiograph reveals the glenohumeral joint space and the anteroposterior position of the humeral head and glenoid fossa. This view is obtained with the patient's arm in abduction (for example, holding onto an IV pole), the cassette on the superior aspect of the shoulder, and the x-ray beam passing up the axilla, aimed at the coracoid. (From Matsen FA III, Lippitt SB. *Shoulder Surgery: Principles and Procedures.* Philadelphia: Saunders; 2004:9.)

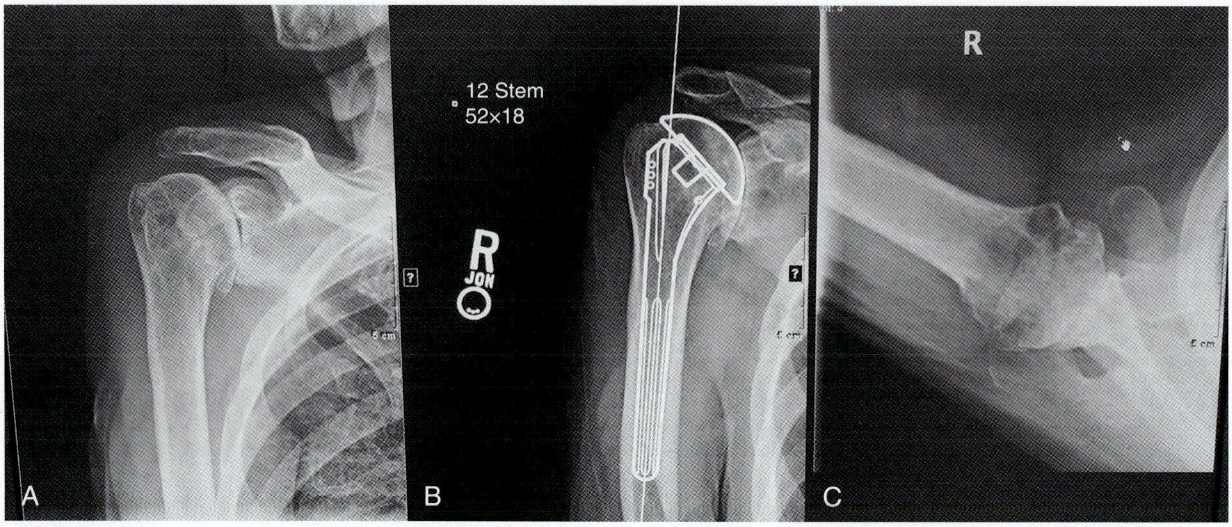

FIGURE 16-373: Anteroposterior (**A**), templating (**B**), and axillary (**C**) radiographs as displayed in the operating room.

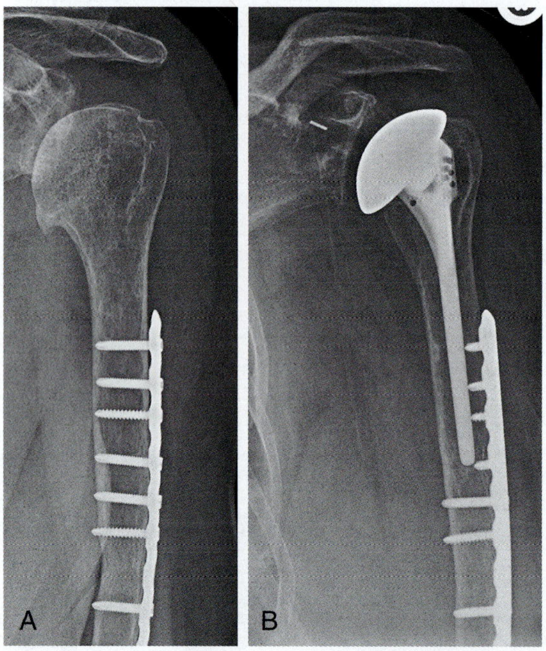

FIGURE 16-374: Total shoulder arthroplasty after a prior internal fixation of a shaft fracture. **A,** Preoperative anteroposterior view showing glenohumeral arthritis and the fixation plate blocking access to medullary canal. **B,** Postoperative view showing the total shoulder arthroplasty with a humeral component inserted with impaction grafting after proximal screws were converted from bicortical to unicortical.

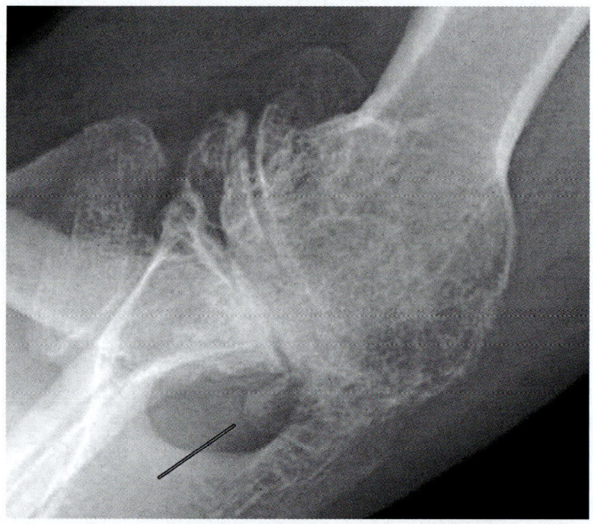

FIGURE 16-375: Large posterior humeral osteophyte that blocked external rotation and complicated dislocation of the humeral head at the time of arthroplasty.

(see Fig. 16-257)? Is it likely that an in situ humeral cut will be needed to prevent locking osteophytes from complicating the dislocation of the proximal humerus (Fig. 16-375)? Might a high-speed saw be needed to modify the humeral stem (see Fig. 16-337)? Would cancellous allograft be needed to augment the bone available for impaction grafting? Is there a reason to withhold antibiotics until cultures can be obtained?

Patients are not routinely cross-matched unless they are anemic or extraordinary blood loss is anticipated, but blood specimens are sent preoperatively for "type and hold."

An 18-gauge intravenous (IV) line is placed in the opposite upper extremity, avoiding the antecubital fossa (so as not to encumber postoperative use of the contralateral arm). If the IV line cannot be established, access is established through the external jugular vein. IVs in the foot are avoided so as not to impair ambulation after surgery. Ceftriaxone (2 g) and vancomycin (15 mg/kg every 12 hours × 2) are administered in normal saline (to prevent precipitation) as the routine preoperative antibiotic prophylaxis against the most common shoulder arthroplasty pathogens, *Propionibacterium* species, and coagulase-negative staphylococci.[73,289,332,341,355,438] These antibiotics are discontinued after 24 hours.

General anesthesia is used for three reasons: to avoid the cost and potential risks of nerve blocks,[293] to enable immediate postoperative neurologic examination, and to facilitate rapid transition to oral analgesics as the patient is weaned off IV narcotics on the evening of surgery.

The preoperative ranges of motion are measured and posted on a white board in full view of the surgical team. A Foley catheter is placed for most male patients and for female patients with voiding or ambulation difficulties; the Foley is discontinued the morning after surgery. Pneumatic compression stockings are used during surgery. Pharmacologic thromboembolic prophylaxis is used only in patients at substantial risk, following consultation with the medicine service.

The patient is placed in a comfortable, relaxed beach chair position with the thorax at an angle of 30 degrees (Fig. 16-376). The shoulder is placed just off the edge of the operating table so that the arm can be moved freely through a full range of motion. The anesthesiologist takes a position at the side of the neck that is opposite to the shoulder being operated on. The skin over the incision is cut with a clipper not a razor; the axillary hair is not cut.[321] A careful double skin preparation with chlorhexidine gluconate and isopropyl alcohol includes the entire arm and forequarter, anteriorly and posteriorly. Pooling of the preparation solution is avoided. After the skin incision is marked, the surgical site is covered with a sterile adherent plastic drape. The draping should allow access to the entire scapula, clavicle, and humerus as well as free movement of the arm. The draped arm is supported on a padded portable stand in a horizontal and slightly abducted position to relax the deltoid muscle.

The skin incision is made over the deltopectoral groove along a line connecting the midpoint of the clavicle to the midpoint of the lateral aspect of the humerus and crossing over the coracoid process (see Fig. 16-154). The skin knife is discarded after the skin incision because of possible contamination with *Propionibacterium* species from the dermal sebaceous glands. It is important that the incision passes lateral to the axillary crease so that it will not come under tension as the arm is moved immediately after surgery. The coracoid serves as a lighthouse to the deltopectoral interval (Fig. 16-377). The coracoid usually lies deep to the deltopectoral groove, and palpating it provides a landmark for the position of the cephalic vein and the brachial plexus; the

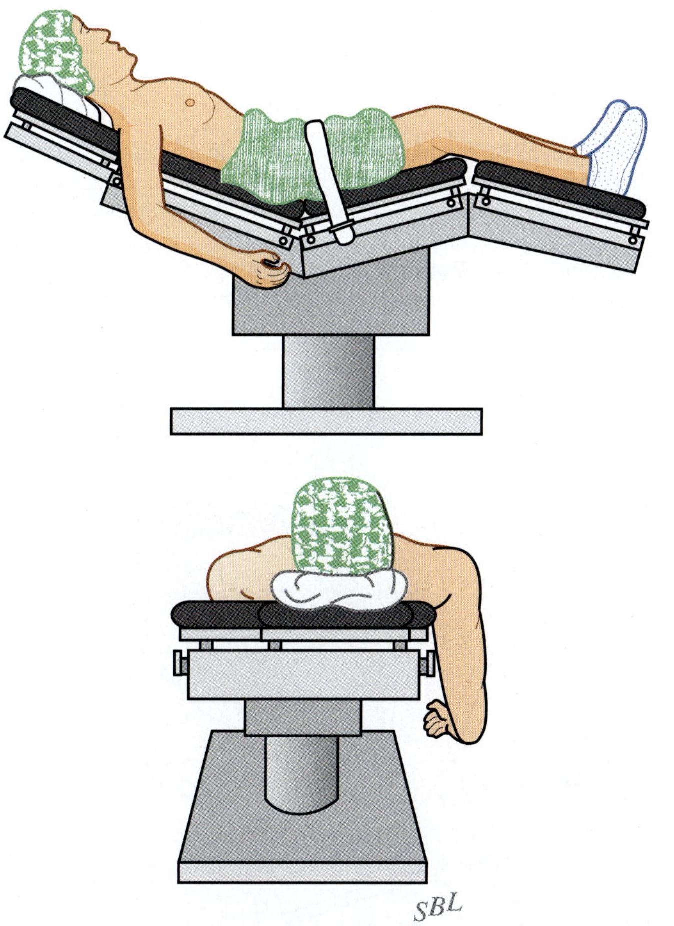

FIGURE 16-376: The patient is placed in the beach chair position, with the thorax angled 30 degrees above the horizontal. The neck is in a neutral position. The glenohumeral joint is at the edge of the table and the arm is completely free. Compressive stockings (not shown here) are applied to the legs. (From Matsen FA III, Lippitt SB. *Shoulder Surgery: Principles and Procedures.* Philadelphia: Saunders; 2004:514.)

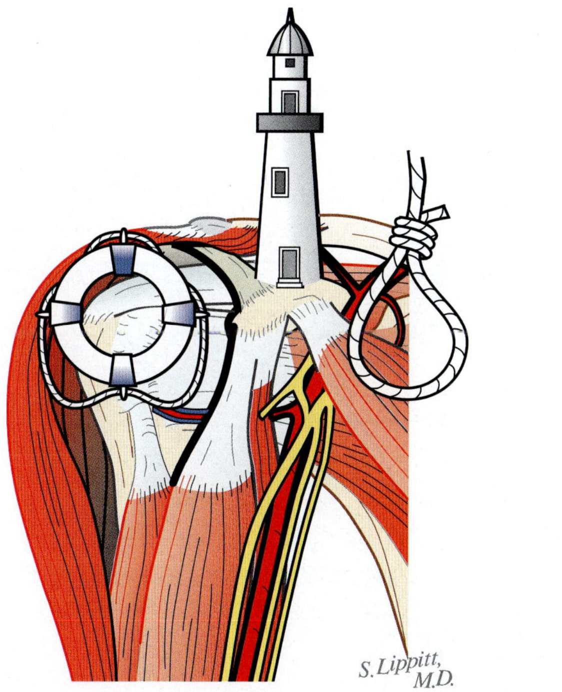

FIGURE 16-377: "Safe side/suicide." The coracoid serves as a "lighthouse" for proper orientation in a scarred shoulder. It divides the lateral side ("safe side") from the medial side ("suicide"), where the brachial plexus and vascular structures are located. (From Matsen FA III, Lippitt SB. *Shoulder Surgery: Principles and Procedures.* Philadelphia: Saunders; 2004:663.)

cephalic vein is intimately attached to the deltoid and directly overlies the coracoid, and the brachial plexus and its terminal divisions lie medial to the base of the coracoid. The deltopectoral interval is developed medial to the cephalic vein, with preservation of its major tributaries from the deltoid muscle (Fig. 16-378). The anterior portion of the deltoid must be preserved because no other muscle can effectively compensate for loss of this powerful shoulder flexor.[71,103,589] Incising the clavipectoral fascia at the lateral edge of the conjoined tendon up to, but not through, the coracoacromial ligament provides entry to the humeroscapular motion interface (Fig. 16-379). All adhesions in this interface are lysed from the axillary nerve medially to the point at which the axillary nerve exits the quadrilateral space posterolaterally (see Fig. 16-156; Fig. 16-380).[71] Care should be taken to avoid damage to the musculocutaneous nerve from sharp instruments, compression during retraction of the conjoined tendons, or traction.[63,146,304]

Several methods have been described for detaching the subscapularis to allow access to the glenohumeral joint (Fig. 16-381). Of these, our preference is to incise the tendon and the subjacent capsule directly off of the lesser tuberosity just medial to the bicipital groove. The capsule is retained on the deep surface of the tendon to reinforce the quality of the repair (Fig. 16-382); it should be noted that the inferior 40% of the belly of the subscapularis extends all the way to the bone rather than inserting as a tendon.[219] The anterior humeral circumflex vessels on the lower third of the subscapularis tendon are identified and cauterized. Great care is taken to protect the axillary nerve running at the lower extent of the subscapularis muscle and the biceps tendon at the superior edge of the subscapularis insertion (see Figs. 16-192 and 16-193).[63,69,71,304] Because of its role in

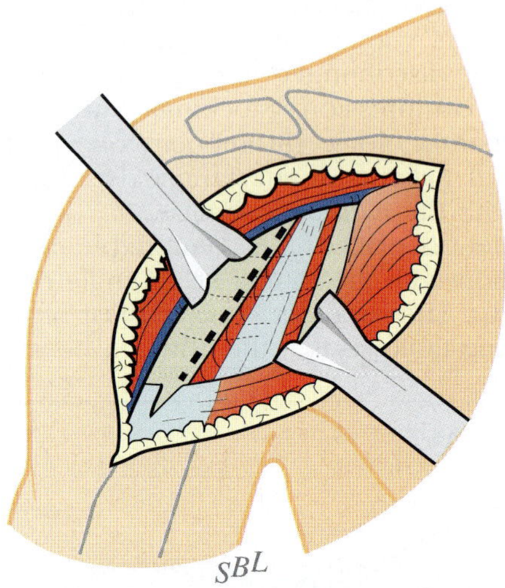

FIGURE 16-379: The clavipectoral fascia is incised just lateral to the conjoined tendons of the coracoid muscles. If necessary, a small amount of the upper edge of the pectoralis major tendon may be incised to assist in exposure and gaining external rotation. (From Matsen FA III, Lippitt SB. *Shoulder Surgery: Principles and Procedures.* Philadelphia: Saunders; 2004:516.)

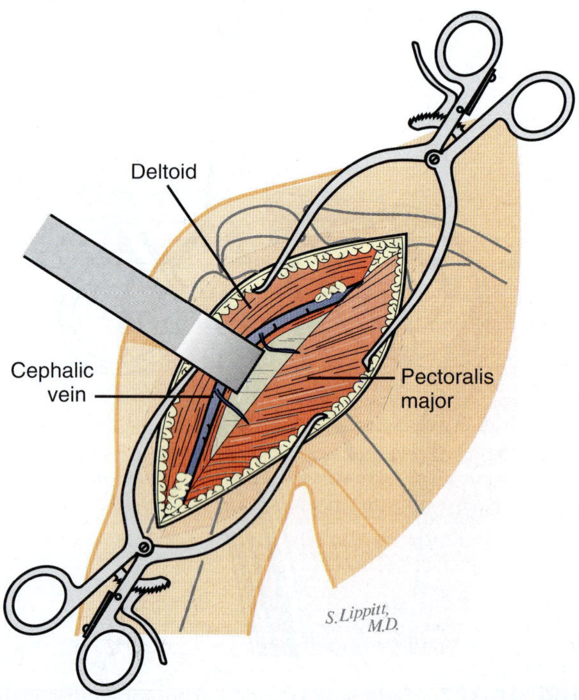

FIGURE 16-378: The cephalic vein is identified in the deltopectoral groove. It is retracted laterally along with the deltoid to expose the clavipectoral fascia. (From Matsen FA III, Lippitt SB. *Shoulder Surgery: Principles and Procedures.* Philadelphia: Saunders; 2004:516.)

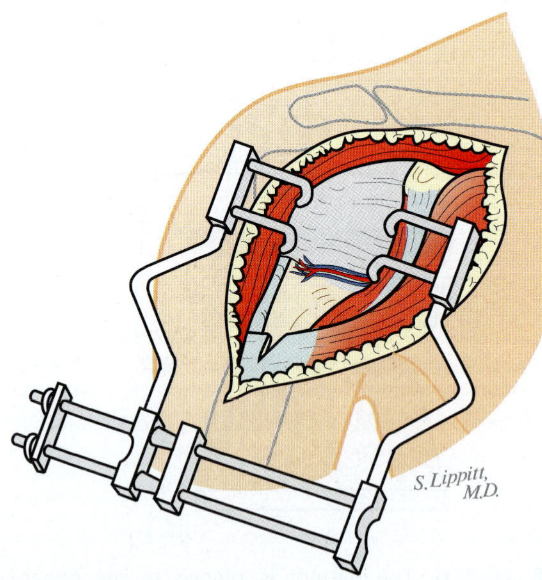

FIGURE 16-380: Self-retaining retractor. A self-retaining retractor placed below the conjoined tendons medially and the deltoid muscle laterally. The subscapularis can now be seen, with the anterior humeral circumflex vessels marking its inferior border. (From Matsen FA III, Lippitt SB. *Shoulder Surgery: Principles and Procedures.* Philadelphia: Saunders; 2004:517.)

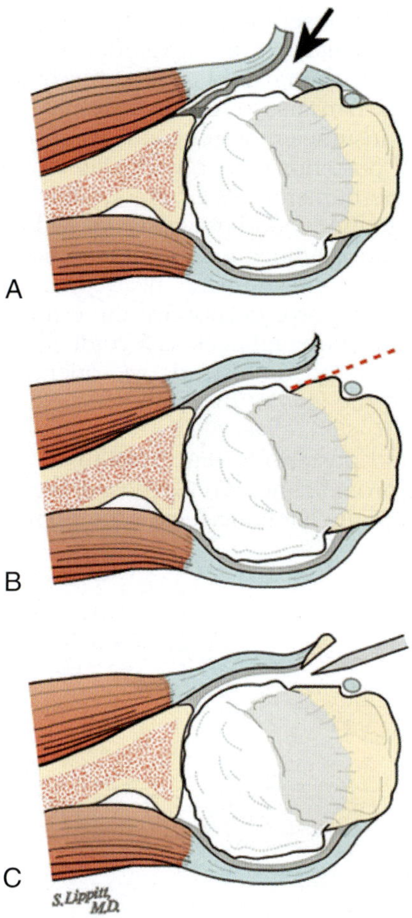

FIGURE 16-381: Methods for detaching subscapularis tendon. **A,** Tenotomy medial to the lesser tuberosity. **B,** Osseotendinous release from the lesser tuberosity. **C,** Lesser tuberosity osteotomy.

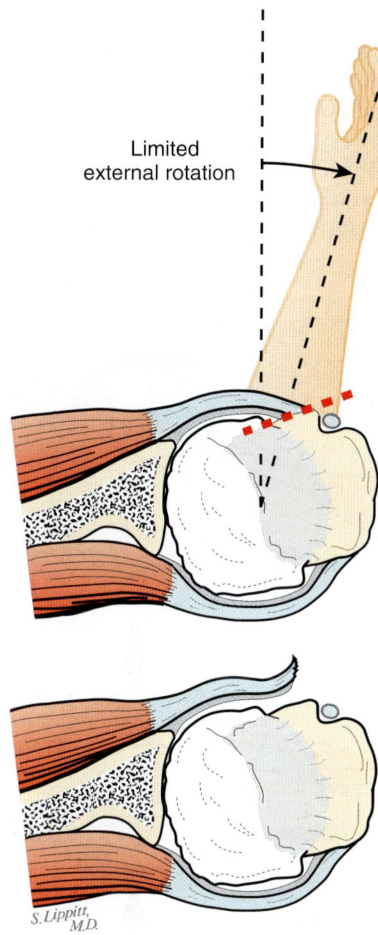

FIGURE 16-382: Incising the subscapularis. The subscapularis and the subjacent capsule are incised directly from the lesser tuberosity (red dashed line), striving for the maximal length of the tendon so that external rotation can be regained. (From Matsen FA III, Lippitt SB. *Shoulder Surgery: Principles and Procedures.* Philadelphia: Saunders; 2004:518.)

stabilizing the humeral head in abduction (Fig. 16-383), the long head of the biceps tendon should be preserved unless it is substantially degenerated or subluxated. If the biceps tendon is frayed or unstable, an in-and-out biceps tenodesis is performed at the time of prosthesis insertion (Fig. 16-384).

Although there has been some enthusiasm for using a lesser tuberosity osteotomy as an approach for accessing the joint[170,171,244] (Fig. 16-385) instead of the less invasive direct incision of the subscapularis tendon from bone, we have not adopted this approach for the following reasons: (1) lesser tuberosity osteotomy requires sacrifice of the long head of the biceps tendon, irrespective of its health; (2) it compromises the ability to achieve a press-fit of the metaphysis of the humeral component by breaking the circumferential continuity of the proximal humerus; (3) healing of the osteotomy may be problematic,[496] especially if the bone is osteopenic; (4) the direct incision of the tendon from the lesser tuberosity allows adjustment in its tension at the time of repair; (5) with a careful repair, failure of the repair of a direct tendon incision from bone is rare; and (6) comparison studies have not demonstrated any advantage of the lesser tuberosity osteotomy.[282,283]

A 360-degree release of the subscapularis tendon is then performed so that the tendon moves freely with respect to the glenoid, the coracoid, the coracoid muscles, the axillary nerve, and the inferior capsule (see Figs. 16-157 and 16-158). An anterior capsular release is performed, taking care to protect the axillary nerve (see Fig. 16-192). The release is not continued beyond the inferior glenohumeral ligament if posterior subluxation of the humeral head on the glenoid is observed on the preoperative axillary view radiograph (see Fig. 16-38).

Despite surgical skin preparation and IV antibiotic prophylaxis, bacteria from the skin—notably *Propionibacterium* species—can be introduced into the surgical field and have the potential for establishing a biofilm on the implanted prostheses.[289,332,341,438] Adhering to the dictum "dilution is the solution to pollution," we irrigate the wound throughout the procedure with at least

3 L of saline solution containing ceftriaxone and vancomycin. All prostheses are handled with clean gloves and inserted without allowing them to touch the skin edge. It may be helpful to keep the exposed skin edge covered with sponges kept moist with antibiotic-containing solution (Fig. 16-386).

Initial Preparation of the Humerus. The humeral head is exposed anteriorly by *gentle* external rotation and slight extension, inserting a large, flat retractor behind it (Fig. 16-387). Special care is exercised in older patients and those with rheumatoid arthritis or other causes of fragile bone. Barriers to gentle external rotation may include an insufficiently released anterior capsule or blocking by posterior osteophytes (Fig. 16-388; see Fig. 16-375). If the humeral head cannot safely be dislocated anteriorly into the wound, we consider making a preliminary conservative humeral neck cut with the head in situ. Because the arthritic humeral head often has severely distorted anatomy, we do not use the estimated location of the anatomic humeral neck as a guide for the resection of the humeral head. Instead, we orient the humeral osteotomy to the axis of the humeral canal as described below (Fig. 16-389). Osteophytes are removed anteriorly, inferiorly, and posteriorly (Fig. 16-390).

With the proximal humerus exposed, the starting point is identified at the lateral aspect of the humeral head just

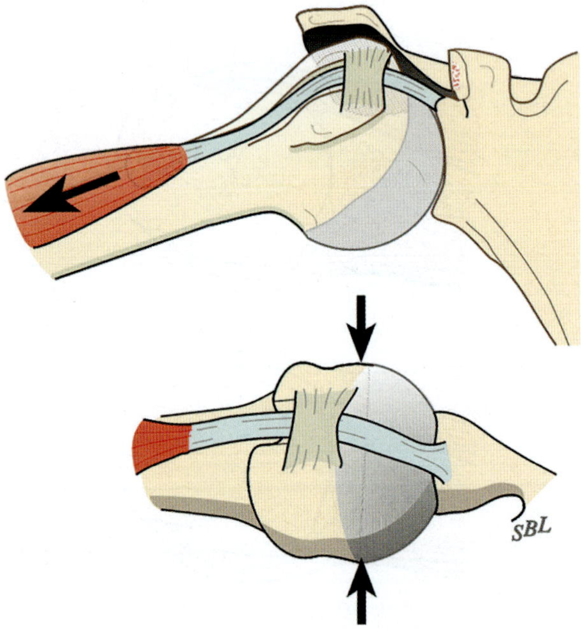

FIGURE 16-383: The long head of the biceps tendon plays a role in stabilizing the humeral head in abduction.

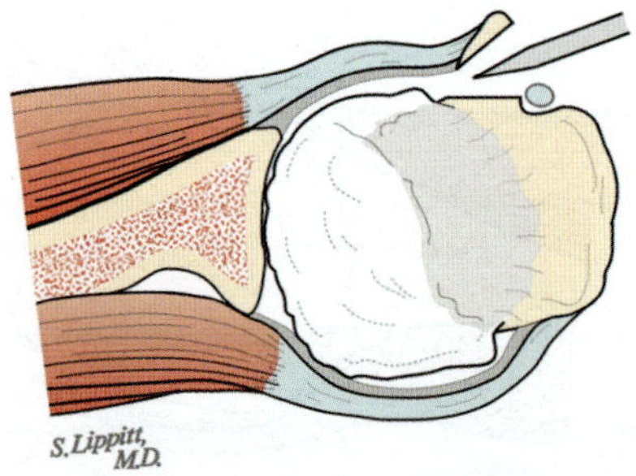

FIGURE 16-385: Lesser tuberosity osteotomy compromises the stability of the long head of the biceps tendon in the bicipital groove and weakens the anterior bone continuity, which may compromise humeral component metaphyseal press-fit.

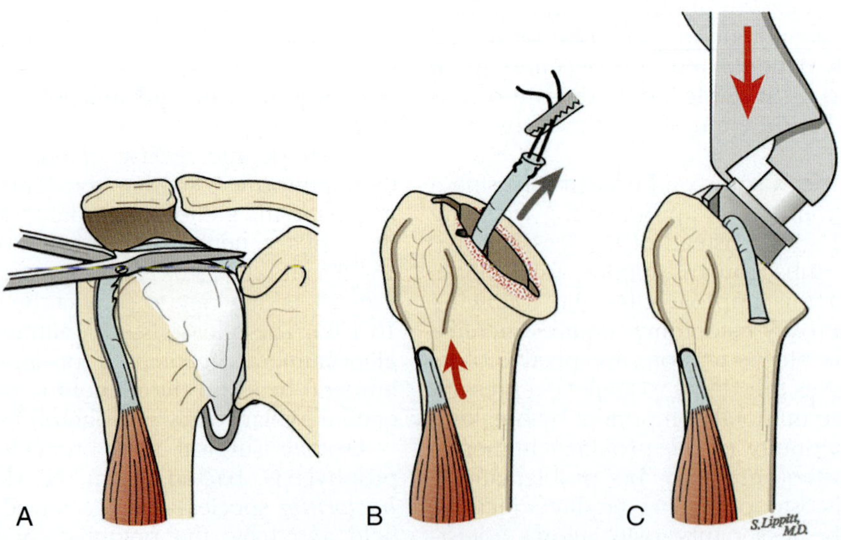

FIGURE 16-384: Technique for in-and-out long head of the biceps (LHB) tenodesis. **A,** The origin of the LHB tendon is released. **B,** The tendon is passed through an 8-mm hole in the distal bicipital groove 10 cm distal to the humeral osteotomy and passed out the canal. **C,** The tendon is then secured by the press-fit humeral stem.

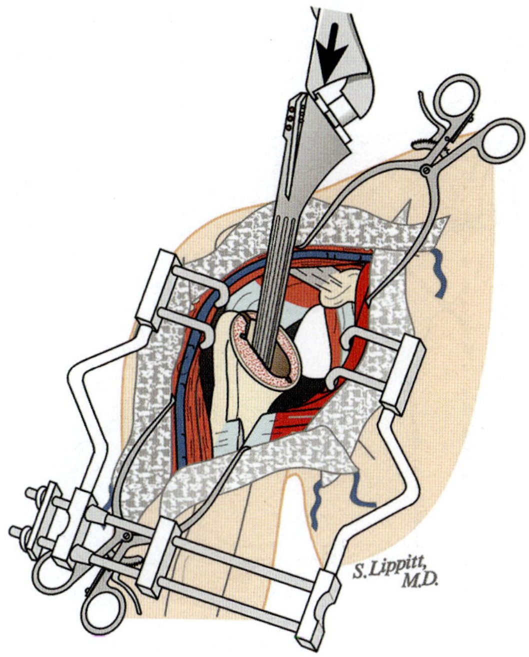

FIGURE 16-386: The wound edges are covered with sponges kept moist with antibiotic solution to prevent skin contact during insertion of the prosthesis.

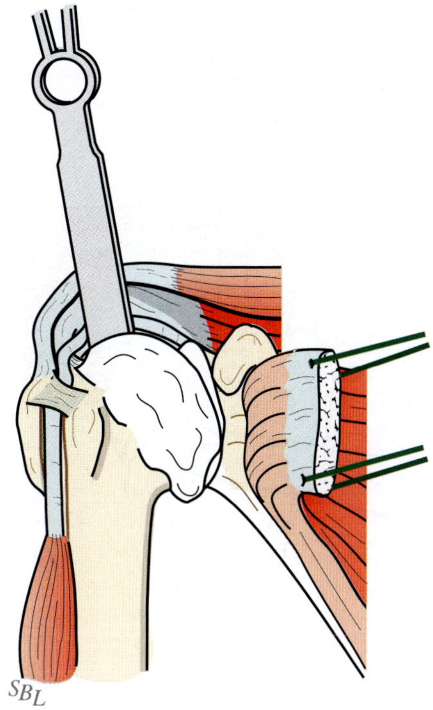

FIGURE 16-387: Exposing the humeral head. A broad, smooth retractor is inserted beneath the supraspinatus and levered gently against the deltoid and acromion to expose the proximal humerus. (From Matsen FA III, Lippitt SB. *Shoulder Surgery: Principles and Procedures.* Philadelphia: Saunders; 2004:521.)

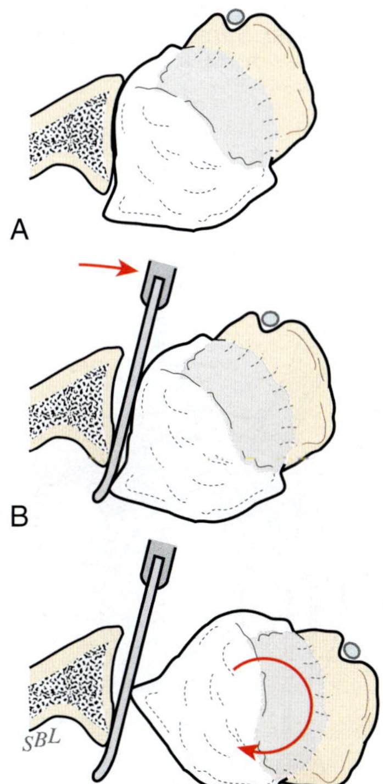

FIGURE 16-388: Osteophytes. **A,** Large posterior humeral osteophytes can form a barrier to external rotation and result in dislocation of the humeral head. **B,** Rotation of the osteophytes onto the joint face can usually be accomplished by placing a broad smooth retractor through the joint (arrow) while the humerus is in internal rotation. **C,** The humerus is then gently externally rotated (arrow). (From Matsen FA III, Lippitt SB. *Shoulder Surgery: Principles and Procedures.* Philadelphia: Saunders; 2004:521.)

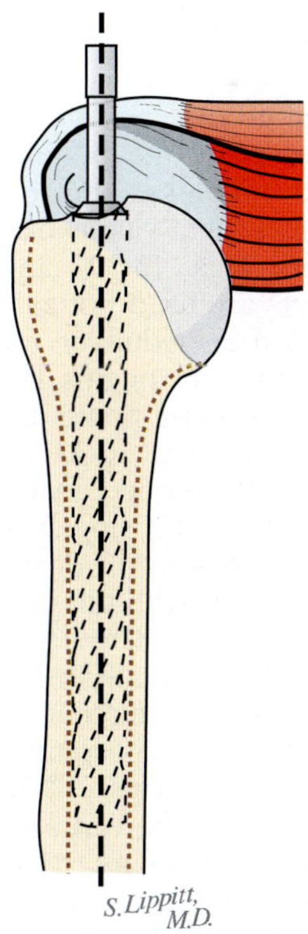

FIGURE 16-389: The orthopedic axis (dashed line) is the axis of a cylindrical reamer that just engages the endosteal surface of the humeral shaft. (From Matsen FA III, Lippitt SB. *Shoulder Surgery: Principles and Procedures.* Philadelphia: Saunders; 2004:437.)

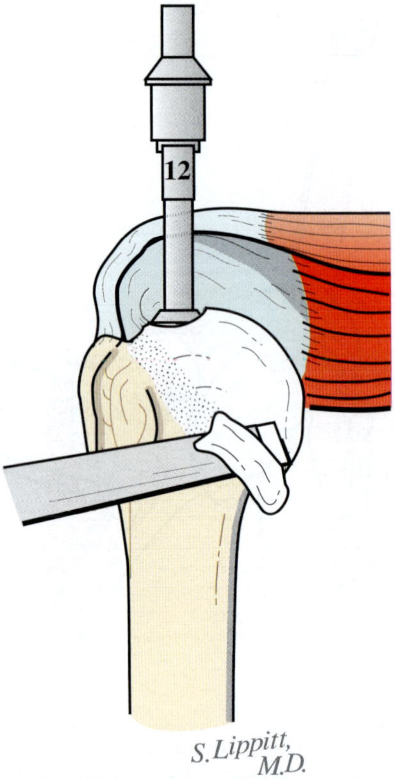

FIGURE 16-390: Removing osteophytes. The osteophytes around the neck of the humerus are removed using a rongeur and an osteotome. (From Matsen FA III, Lippitt SB. *Shoulder Surgery: Principles and Procedures.* Philadelphia: Saunders; 2004:525.)

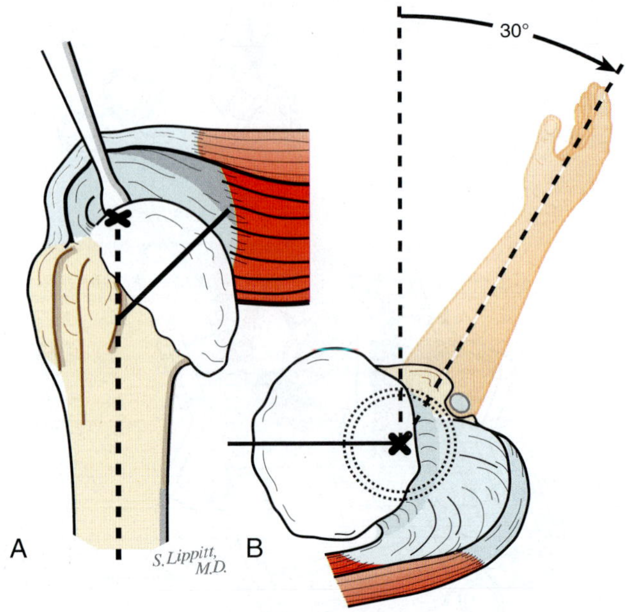

FIGURE 16-391: Intraoperative planning. Two orienting lines are drawn. **A,** One line is parallel to the humeral articular centerline. **B,** The other line splits the humeral articular surface into its anterior and posterior halves (humeral bisecting line). The starting point for entering the canal is along the second line near the cuff insertion to the tuberosity. (From Matsen FA III, Lippitt SB. *Shoulder Surgery: Principles and Procedures.* Philadelphia: Saunders; 2004:522.)

behind the bicipital groove, close to the cuff insertion. A hole is burred at this point, the medullary canal is opened with a curette, and a 6-mm medullary reamer is inserted into the canal using a slight valgus bias (see Figs. 16-320, 16-387, and 16-388; Figs. 16-391 and 16-392). Successively larger reamers are used not as reamers per se but rather as sizers of the medullary canal, passing them down the canal until one begins to engage the distal endosteal cortex at the appropriate depth for the implant ("love at first bite") (see Fig. 16-321). When in position, the largest reamer that fits the canal defines the "orthopedic axis" of the humerus. Using an oscillating saw, the humeral head is resected in 30 degrees of retroversion at an angle of 45 degrees with the orthopedic axis of the medullary canal (Figs. 16-393 to 16-395). The cut plane passes just inside the rotator cuff insertion to the tuberosity under direct vision, ensuring that the humeral articular surface is resected without damaging the cuff attachment superiorly or posteriorly (Figs. 16-396 to 16-398). No attempt is made to match the varus or valgus angulation of the native humerus (see Figs. 16-343 to 16-345).

The full circumference of the neck cut is inspected to ensure that the osteophytes have been completely resected. Because access to posterior osteophytes may require substantial external rotation of the humerus, placing tension on the median and musculocutaneous

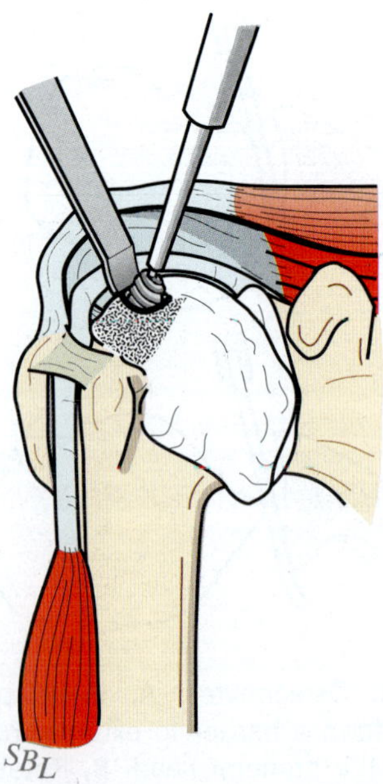

FIGURE 16-392: Burr start. The medullary space of the humeral head is entered at the starting point using a pinecone burr. (From Matsen FA III, Lippitt SB. *Shoulder Surgery: Principles and Procedures.* Philadelphia: Saunders; 2004:523.)

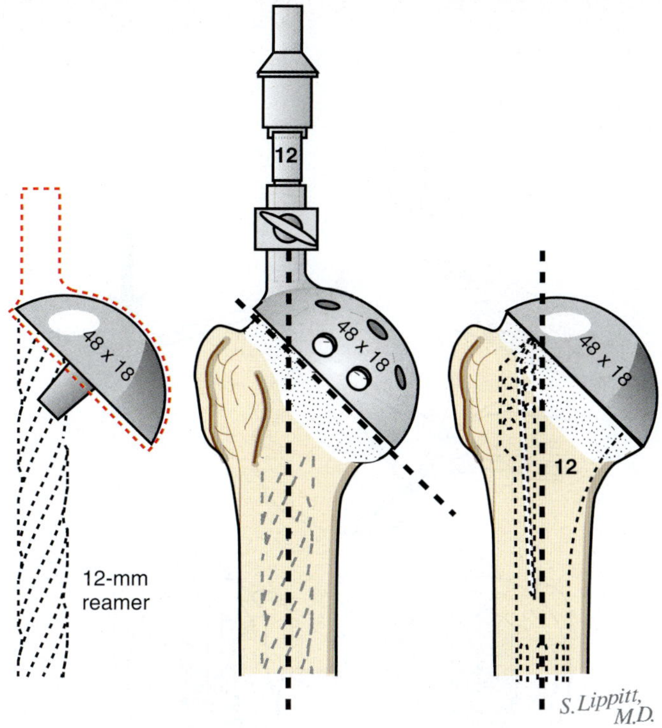

FIGURE 16-393: Selecting a mask. A mask that represents the three-dimensional geometrical relationships of the prosthetic articular surface to the prosthetic stem can be used. A mask placed on the reamer inserted into the canal enables the surgeon to see the resulting position of the articular surface and the location of the plane for humeral head resection before committing to a prosthesis size or neck cut. (From Matsen FA III, Lippitt SB. *Shoulder Surgery: Principles and Procedures.* Philadelphia: Saunders; 2004:526.)

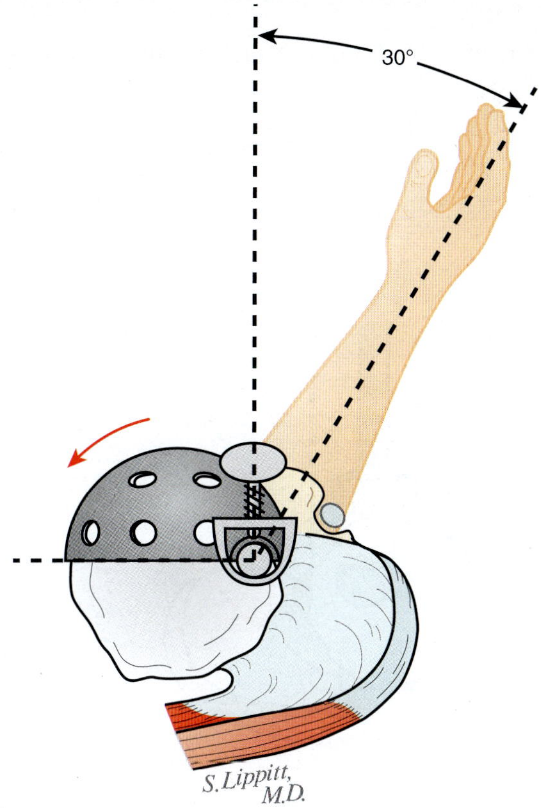

FIGURE 16-394: Position of the mask. When the mask is in position, its posterior edge should align along the humeral bisecting line drawn previously. (From Matsen FA III, Lippitt SB. *Shoulder Surgery: Principles and Procedures.* Philadelphia: Saunders; 2004:527.)

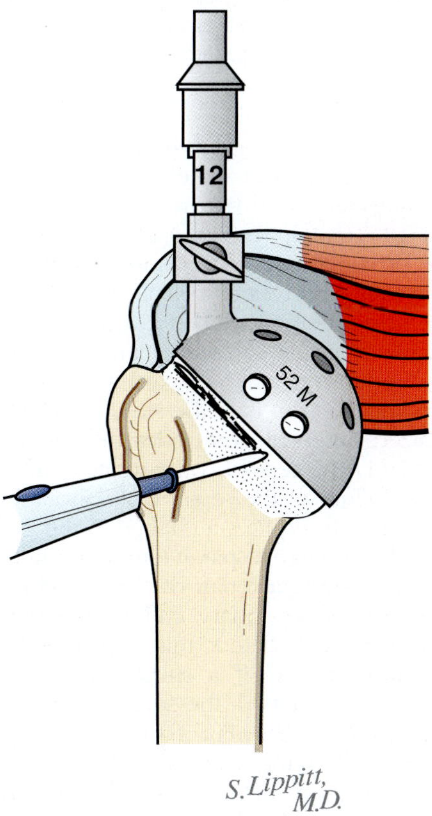

FIGURE 16-395: Marking the osteotomy. Once the position of the mask is determined to be acceptable, the cut plane is marked on the humeral neck with electrocautery. (From Matsen FA III, Lippitt SB. *Shoulder Surgery: Principles and Procedures.* Philadelphia: Saunders; 2004:528.)

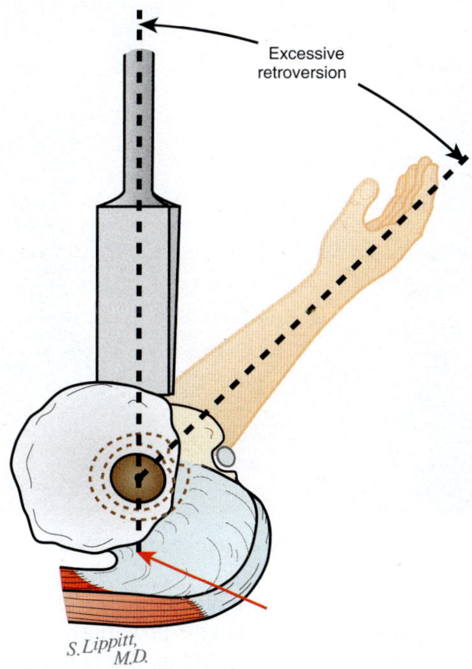

FIGURE 16-396: Retroversion of the cut. Excessive retroversion of the cut jeopardizes the integrity of the tuberosity and the cuff insertion. (From Matsen FA III, Lippitt SB. *Shoulder Surgery: Principles and Procedures.* Philadelphia: Saunders; 2004:529.)

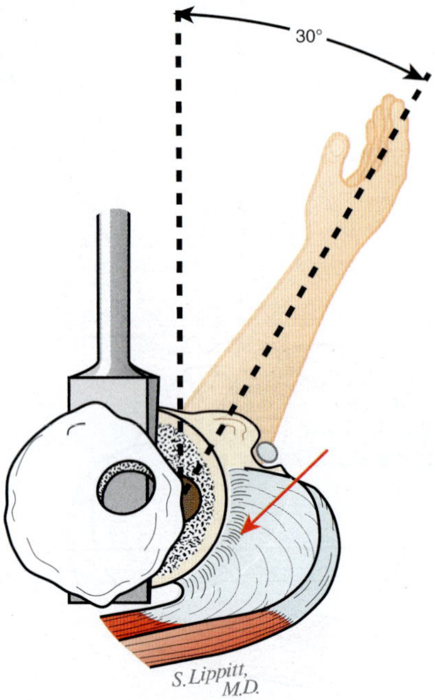

FIGURE 16-397: Extending the cut line. The osteotomy passes just inside the cuff insertion. (From Matsen FA III, Lippitt SB. *Shoulder Surgery: Principles and Procedures.* Philadelphia: Saunders; 2004:529.)

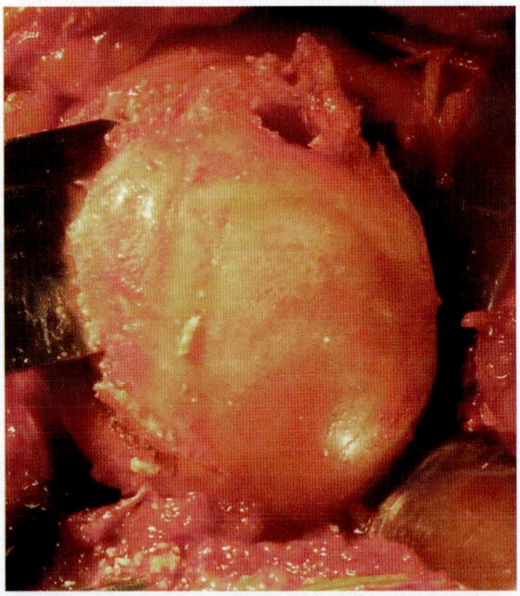

FIGURE 16-398: The humeral neck cut is made at an angle of 45 degrees to the orthopedic axis. Great care should be taken to preserve the long head of the biceps tendon and the rotator cuff insertions superiorly and posteriorly. These structures need to be seen and protected as the cut is made.

nerves, we try to ensure that the arm is not maintained in this "danger" position for longer than 20 seconds or so at a time, especially in shoulders that have had internal rotation contractures preoperatively. When a humeral hemiarthroplasty alone or a CTA prosthesis is planned, there is no change in the socket anatomy; thus it is important to measure and match the diameter of curvature of the resected head before it is converted to bone graft (see Figs. 16-305, 16-306, and 16-397).

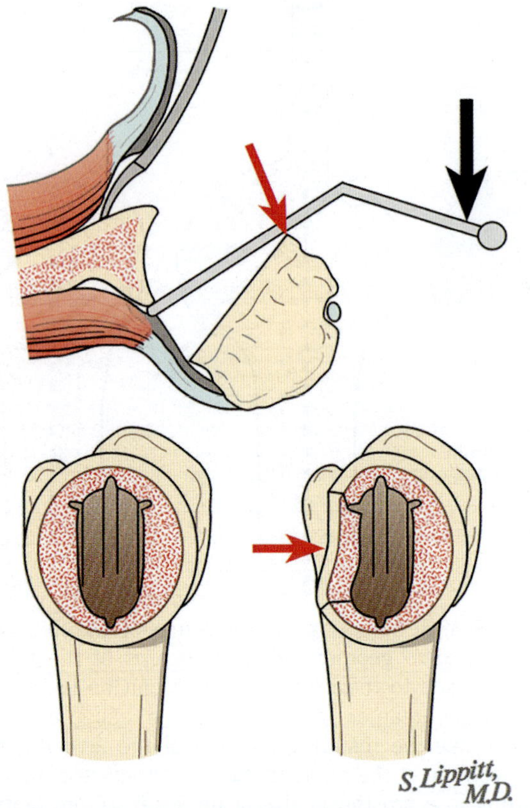

FIGURE 16-399: Do not prepare the humeral metaphysis before exposing and placing the glenoid component. Posterior humeral retraction after humeral bone preparation may fracture or crush the anterior humeral cortex (red arrow). This is especially at risk with osteoporosis and lesser tuberosity osteotomy.

With the proximal end of the humerus displaced medially into the joint, the rotator cuff is observed to establish its integrity. Consideration can be given to repairing a cuff defect if excellent quality cuff tissue can reach the tuberosity without undue tension when the arthroplasty components are in place and the arm is at the side. However, there are two recognized potential downsides of cuff repair in this circumstance: (1) the tension of a rotator cuff repair may predispose to failure of the repair or to shoulder tightness, and (2) a cuff repair requires a change in the postoperative rehabilitation from active to passive motion until the tendon has healed. Attempting a repair of tenuous cuff tissue may increase the risk of secondary cuff dysfunction.[598] If it is elected to repair a cuff defect, this step is performed after the glenoid arthroplasty. If a substantial and irreparable rotator cuff tear is identified, the surgeon may consider the use of CTA prosthesis (see Fig. 16-104).

To avoid challenging the integrity of the proximal humerus during exposure for the glenoid arthroplasty, no further preparation of the humerus is carried out until after the work on the glenoid is complete (Fig. 16-399).

Glenoid Arthroplasty. Accurate preparation of the glenoid surface for a ream and run arthroplasty or for the glenoid component of a total shoulder arthroplasty requires excellent exposure (Figs. 16-400 and 16-401). In either case the exposure needs to allow reaming of the face of the glenoid to a single concavity (Figs. 16-402 and 16-403). Rather than using a guide wire in an attempt to guide the angle of glenoid reaming to a specific theoretical orientation, we use a nubbed glenoid reamer placed in a central drill hole, a technique that enables the orientation of the reamer to be adjusted such that a concentric concavity is achieved with minimal bone removal (see Figs. 16-359 and 16-360). The insertion of the reamer is facilitated by using a humeral head retractor as a "shoehorn," which is removed once the reamer is in place (Fig. 16-404).

Ream and Run Arthroplasty. The goal of the glenoid aspect of the ream and run arthroplasty is to ream the glenoid face concentrically and conservatively until glenohumeral stability and the contact area for distribution of the humeral load to the glenoid are optimized (Figs. 16-405 and 16-406). The glenoid is exposed by an

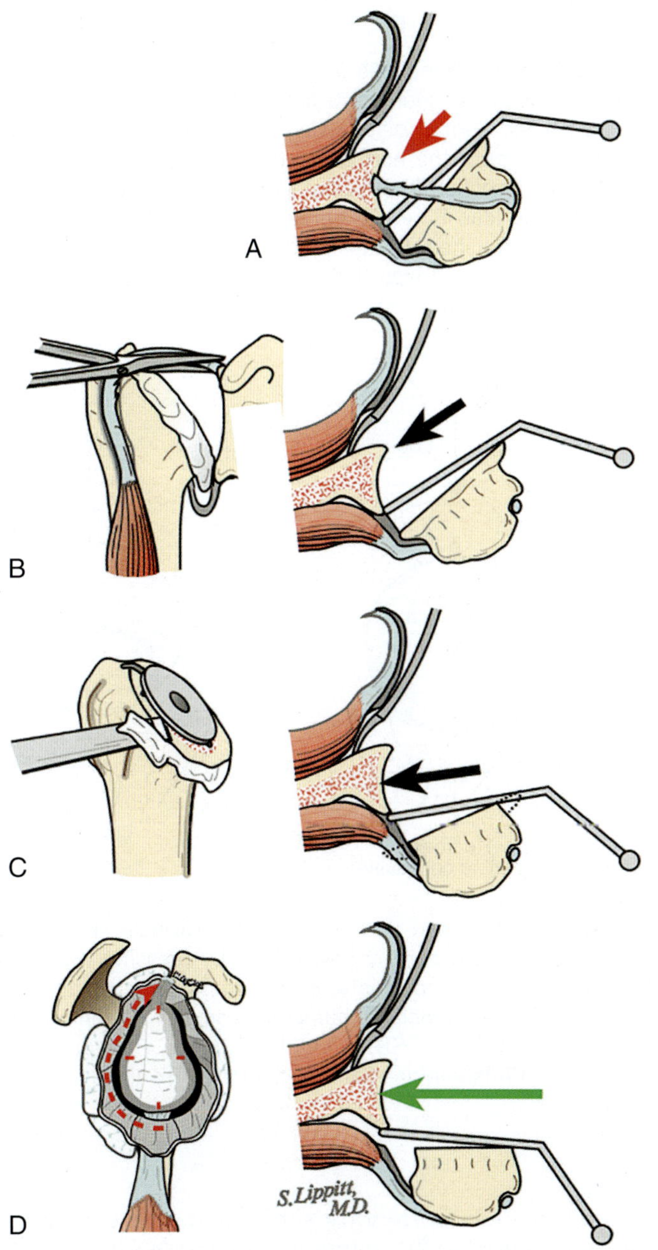

FIGURE 16-400: Improving glenoid exposure. **A,** Initial poor glenoid fossa exposure. **B,** Release the tethered long head biceps tendon. **C,** Remove the peripheral humeral osteophytes. **D,** Release the posterior capsule at the glenoid.

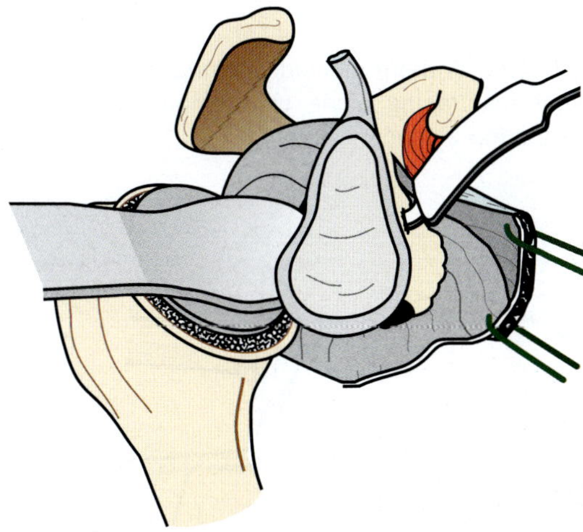

FIGURE 16-401: Glenoid exposure. By placing a broad, smooth retractor behind the glenoid and a spiked retractor anteriorly, an excellent exposure of the glenoid is achieved. (From Matsen FA III, Lippitt SB. *Shoulder Surgery: Principles and Procedures.* Philadelphia: Saunders; 2004:555.)

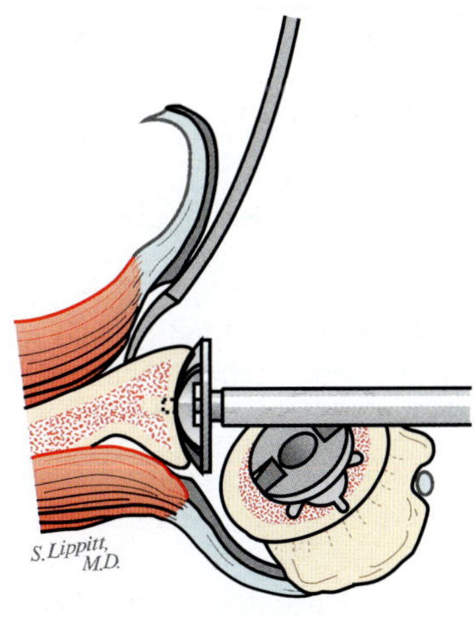

FIGURE 16-402: Exposure of the glenoid for reaming can be gained using a combination of retractors and a straight or angled reamer handle. (The straight handle is shown here.) (From Matsen FA III, Lippitt SB. *Shoulder Surgery: Principles and Procedures.* Philadelphia: Saunders; 2004:561.)

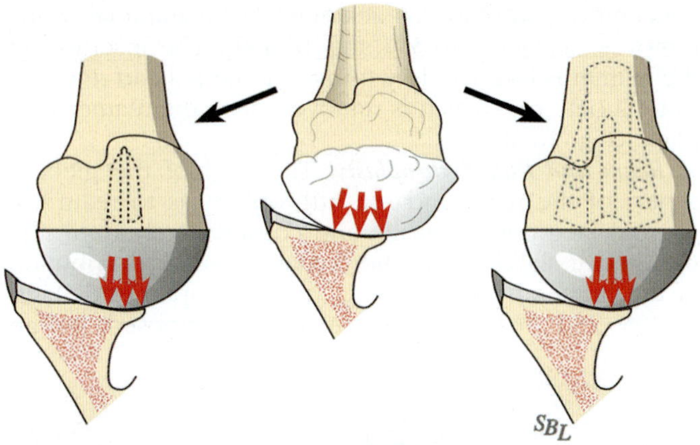

FIGURE 16-403: Without glenoid reaming to a single concavity, humeral resurfacing alone will remain subluxed in the posteriorly eroded biconcave glenoid.

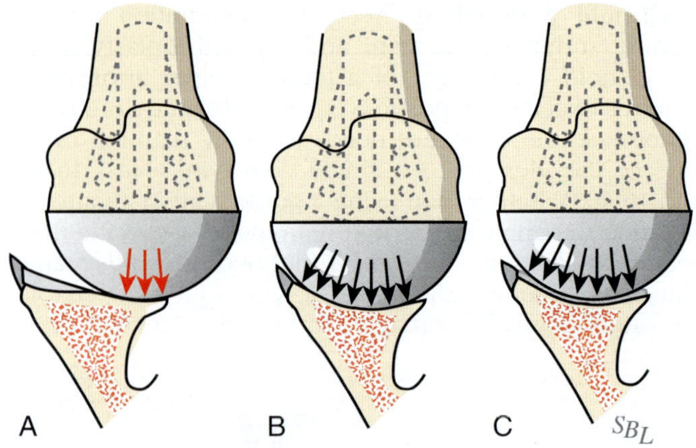

FIGURE 16-405: Principles of ream and run. **A,** In the presence of a biconcave glenoid, a hemiarthroplasty alone cannot reestablish the normal distribution of load across the glenoid surface (arrows) or the normal centering of the humeral head on the glenoid socket. **B,** By reaming the glenoid to a concentric concavity, the load is redistributed (arrows) and the centering effect is reestablished. **C,** Ideally, the reamed surface becomes covered with fibrocartilage that remodels under the loading by the humeral head (arrows).

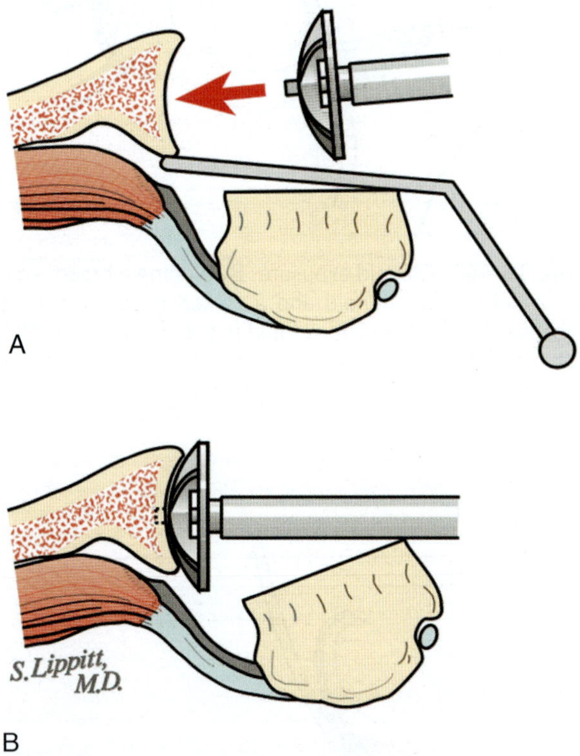

FIGURE 16-404: **A,** Insertion of the glenoid reamer is facilitated by using a humeral head retractor as a "shoehorn." **B,** The retractor is removed once the reamer is in place.

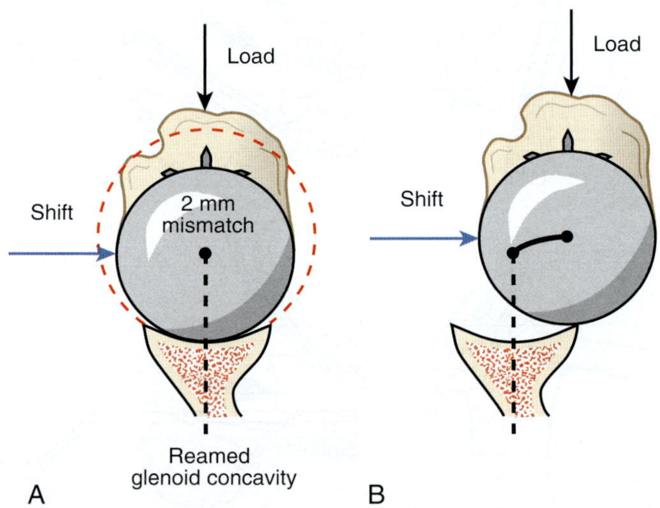

FIGURE 16-406: Load and shift. **A,** The intrinsic stability of the reamed glenoid can be determined by pressing the prosthetic head into the concavity. **B,** It is then verified that there is substantial resistance to humeral head translation. (From Matsen FA III, Lippitt SB. *Shoulder Surgery: Principles and Procedures.* Philadelphia: Saunders; 2004:563.)

extralabral capsular release, that is, by leaving the labrum attached to the glenoid to help preserve its contribution to the depth of the socket. When the shoulder is symmetrically tight and without posterior erosion, a 360-degree extralabral capsular release is performed (see Fig. 16-159). When the shoulder is tight anteriorly and the humeral head is posteriorly subluxated, the extralabral release is limited to the anterior capsule (see Fig. 16-162). Any remaining articular cartilage is curetted from the face of the glenoid (Fig. 16-407). Frequently, the removal of the remaining anterior cartilage reveals a biconcavity of the bony surface, in which case the ridge between these

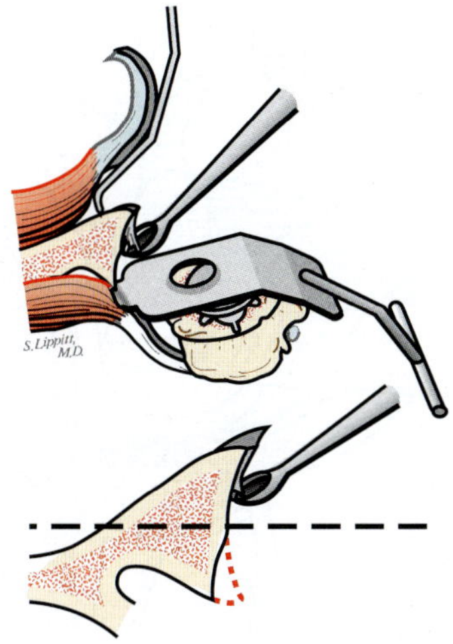

FIGURE 16-407: Curetting the residual articular cartilage reveals the biconcavity of the underlying glenoid bone.

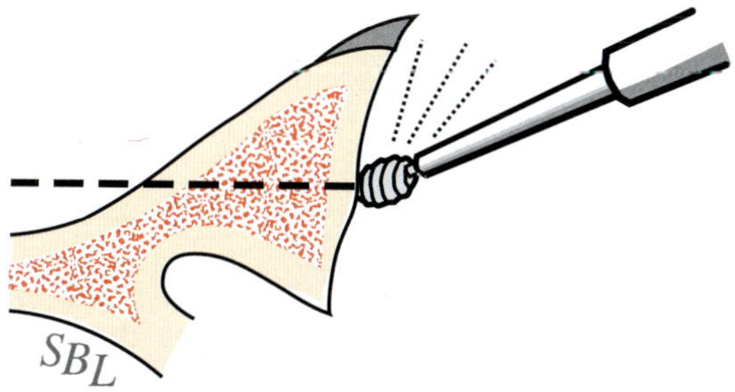

FIGURE 16-408: Concentric reaming of the glenoid is facilitated by first burring down the ridge between the two concavities.

concavities is burred to facilitate reaming (Fig. 16-408). The center of the glenoid is identified and burred (Figs. 16-409 and 16-410) to center the drill for the nub of the reamer.

It should be emphasized that the reaming of the glenoid face must be conservative—only enough bone is removed to establish a single glenoid concavity. As no holes are made in the glenoid surface for component fixation, less bone is removed with the ream and run than for a total shoulder arthroplasty. The angle of glenoid reaming is adjusted to preserve as much glenoid subchondral bone as possible (see Figs. 16-277 and 16-360). The adequacy of the glenoid bone preparation is checked by inserting a round-back glenoid trial component and ensuring that it does not rock even when eccentric loads are applied to the rim (Figs. 16-411 and 16-412). The diameter of curvature of the humeral head is chosen to be 2 mm less than that of the reamed glenoid surface. In most cases we pair a reamed glenoid of 58-mm diameter of curvature with humeral head prosthesis of 56-mm diameter of curvature, yielding a 2-mm mismatch in the diameters (see Fig. 16-296).

Total Shoulder Arthroplasty. As with the ream and run procedure, the goals for total shoulder arthroplasty

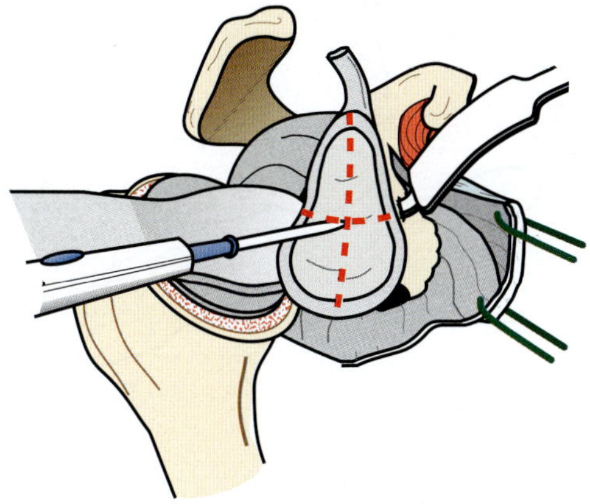

FIGURE 16-409: Cautery of the glenoid center. The center of the exposed glenoid (intersection of the dashed lines) is marked with electrocautery. It is important that the glenoid is fully exposed superiorly so that the mark is not placed too low. (From Matsen FA III, Lippitt SB. *Shoulder Surgery: Principles and Procedures.* Philadelphia: Saunders; 2004:557.)

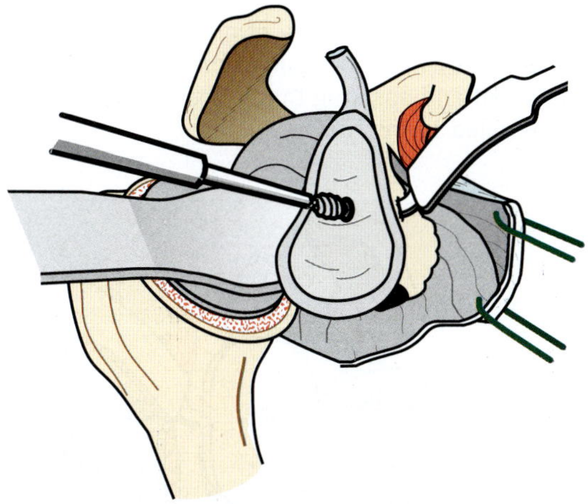

FIGURE 16-410: Burring the glenoid center. The starting point for drilling the glenoid centerline is established with a pinecone burr. (From Matsen FA III, Lippitt SB. *Shoulder Surgery: Principles and Procedures.* Philadelphia: Saunders; 2004:557.)

include establishing both maximum stability and maximum contact area for distribution of the humeral load to the glenoid. In addition, the procedure needs to achieve support of the prosthetic glenoid by precisely contouring the bone that supports it and by ensuring secure and durable fixation of the component to the underlying bone. Preservation of glenoid bone is a high priority as glenoid bone stock is a precious commodity when performing shoulder arthroplasty and because excessive reaming has been associated with increasing rates of glenoid component failure[570] (see Figs. 16-351 and 16-360). The precise drilling of the holes for peg fixation of a glenoid component is better than the less precise preparation for a keeled component for both bone

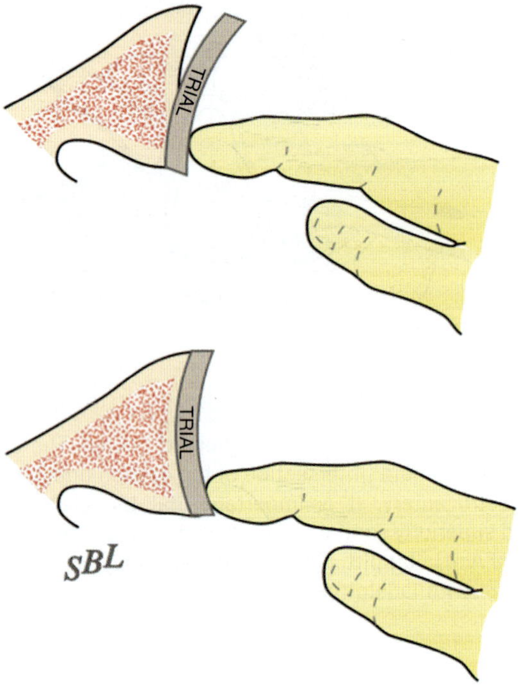

FIGURE 16-411: The adequacy of glenoid concavity preparation is checked by inserting a concentric, round-back glenoid trial component and ensuring that it does not rock with eccentric loads applied to the rim.

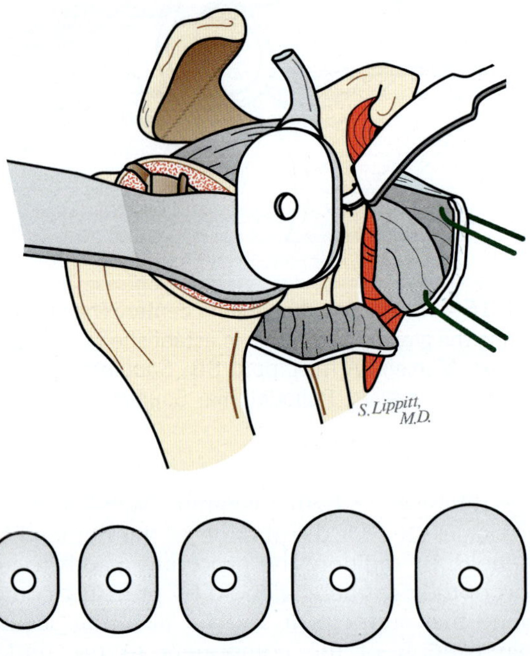

FIGURE 16-412: Round-back glenoid trials. Transparent glenoid-sizing disks with the same diameter of curvature as the back of the glenoid component are used to ensure complete reaming of the glenoid surface and complete seating of the disk on the reamed glenoid and to establish the size of the glenoid component that completely covers the reamed bone. (From Matsen FA III, Lippitt SB. *Shoulder Surgery: Principles and Procedures.* Philadelphia: Saunders; 2004:573.)

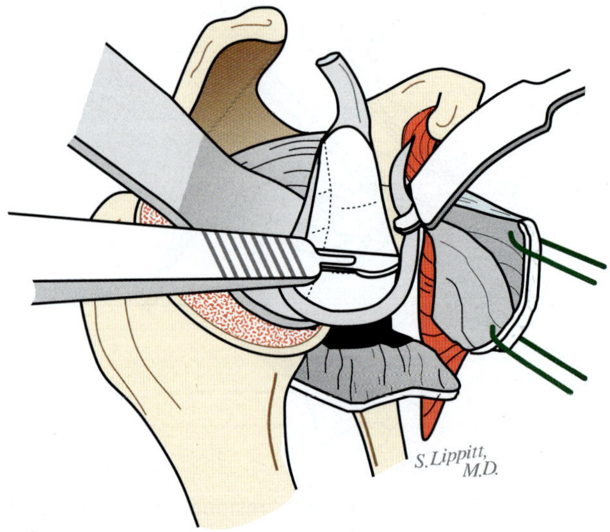

FIGURE 16-413: Excising the labrum. The labrum is progressively detached from the anterior glenoid by sharp dissection, moving the sharp-tipped retractor inferiorly in small successive steps. (From Matsen FA III, Lippitt SB. *Shoulder Surgery: Principles and Procedures.* Philadelphia: Saunders; 2004:567.)

preservation and the quality of fixation. This precision has the additional benefit of minimizing the amount of cement used, thus reducing the risk of thermal damage.[85]

In contrast to the ream and run technique, during total shoulder arthroplasty, the glenoid is exposed by excising the labrum from the bony glenoid, removing any tissue that may interfere with complete glenoid component seating (Fig. 16-413). As with the ream and run procedure, if the preoperative axillary view shows posterior humeral head subluxation, the inferior glenohumeral capsule is left intact (Fig. 16-414).

The size of the glenoid component is determined using round-back glenoid trials (Fig. 16-415). The center of the glenoid face is marked (Fig. 16-416) and a burr hole is made at this point (Fig. 16-417) to guide the drill for the reamer (see Fig. 16-358). The angle of glenoid reaming is adjusted to preserve as much glenoid subchondral bone as possible (see Figs. 16-277 and 16-360). Glenoid bone is preserved by orienting the reaming and the component along the glenoid axis rather than the scapular axis (Fig. 16-418). Reaming is always started by hand; power is used very sparingly except in hard bone. Appropriate positioning of retractors facilitates this reaming (Fig. 16-419; see Fig. 16-402). As the goal of reaming is to conservatively establish a single glenoid concavity (see Fig. 16-351), it is important to frequently check the progress of the reaming so that the reamer does not inadvertently remove more bone than necessary. The adequacy of the glenoid bone preparation is checked by inserting the round-back glenoid trial component and ensuring that it does not rock even when eccentric loads are applied to the rim (see Fig. 16-411).

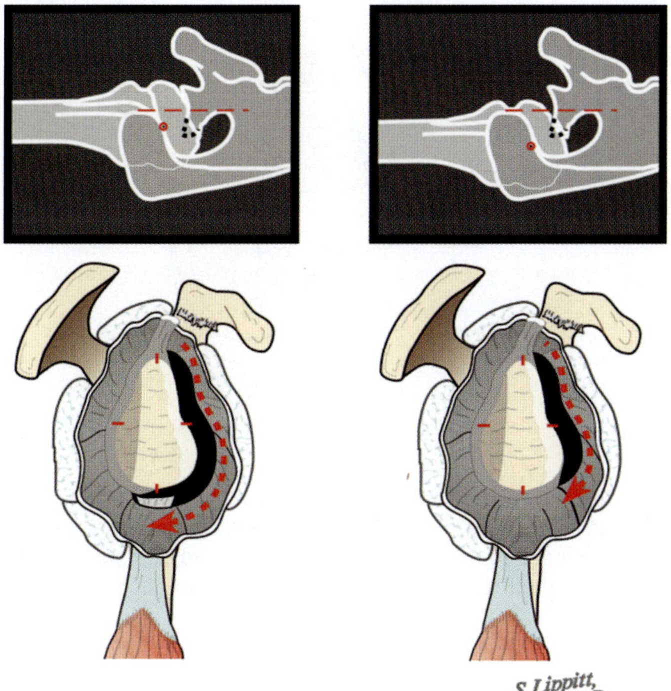

A B

FIGURE 16-414: **A,** If the preoperative axillary view reveals posterior subluxation of the humeral head and posterior glenoid wear, the release includes only the anteroinferior capsule. **B,** If the preoperative axillary view reveals substantial posterior humeral head subluxation greater than 50%, the anterior release stops at the inferior glenohumeral ligament.

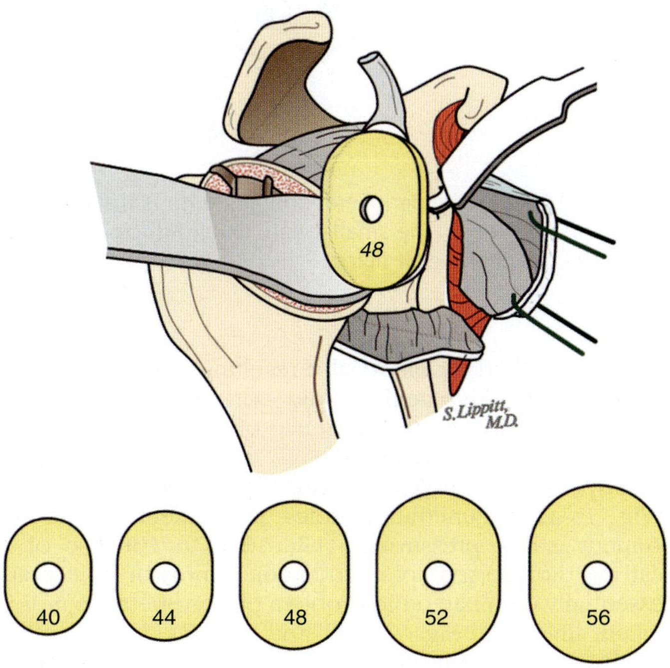

FIGURE 16-415: The planned size of the glenoid component is determined by best fit using round-back glenoid trials.

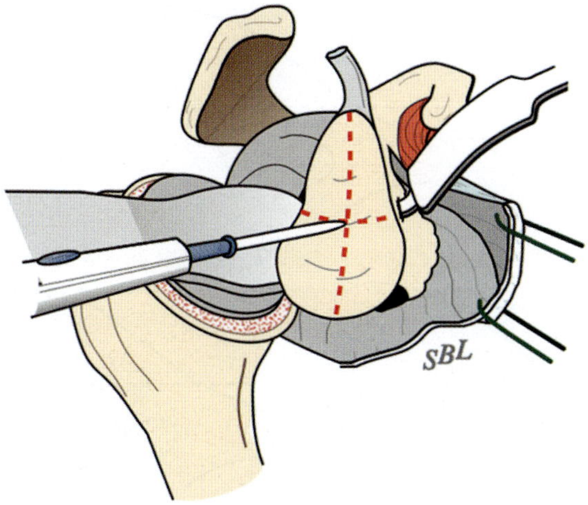

FIGURE 16-416: The glenoid center is determined by marking the superoinferior and anteroposterior glenoid axes with electrocautery. It is important that the glenoid fossa is fully exposed superiorly so that the mark is not placed too low.

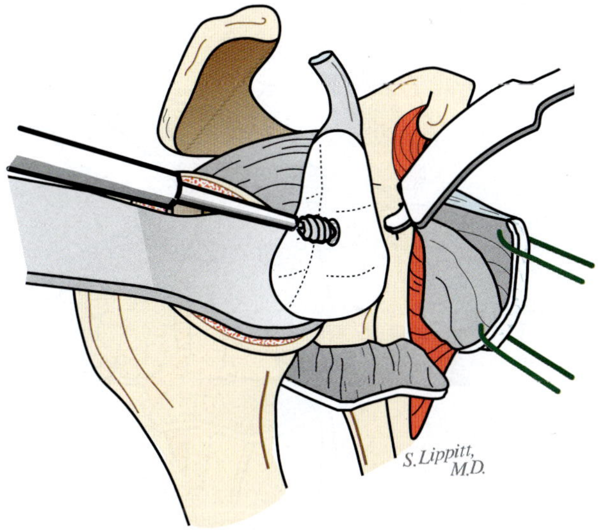

FIGURE 16-417: Burring the glenoid center. The starting point for drilling the glenoid centerline is established with a pinecone bur. (From Matsen FA III, Lippitt SB. *Shoulder Surgery: Principles and Procedures.* Philadelphia: Saunders; 2004:569.)

After the hole for the central peg is drilled (Fig. 16-420), the peripheral drill guide is inserted into the central peg hole and set firmly on the reamed glenoid surface to precisely guide the drilling of the additional holes for the peripheral pegs (Fig. 16-421). The drill guide should be oriented to take maximum advantage of the available glenoid bone (Fig. 16-422); care must be taken to ensure that the drill guide sits flush on the reamed glenoid surface so that the hole position will match the position of the component pegs. After each peripheral hole is drilled, a derotation peg is placed into it to maintain the

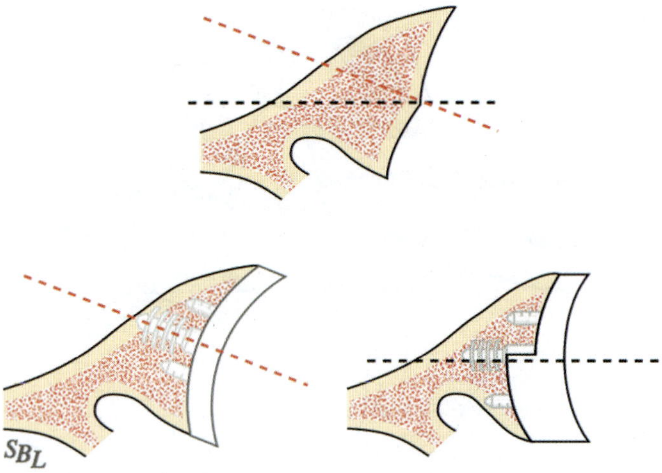

FIGURE 16-418: Rather than orienting the glenoid reaming and the glenoid component to the scapular axis (black line) by removing extra bone and using a posterior augmented glenoid component (right), we orient the reaming and component to the glenoid axis (red line) with minimal bone removal (left).

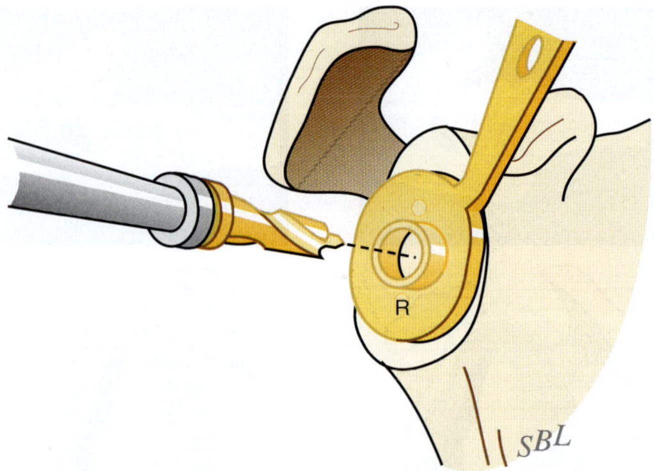

FIGURE 16-420: With the gold central guide, the drill guide hole is aligned with the previously created central drill hole that was used to ream the glenoid. The central anchor peg hole is then drilled with the appropriately sized anchor peg center drill bit.

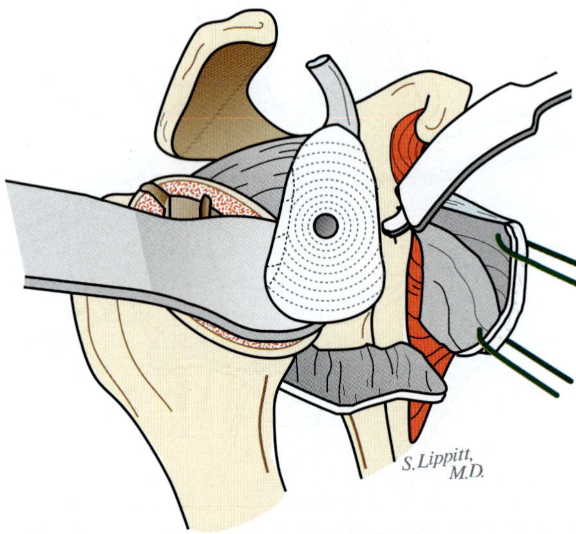

FIGURE 16-419: Reamed glenoid. Reaming is continued until the smooth reamed surface extends to the anterior and posterior margins of the glenoid. Often, concentric circular marks are left by the reamer, indicating the extent of the reamed surface. (From Matsen FA III, Lippitt SB. *Shoulder Surgery: Principles and Procedures.* Philadelphia: Saunders; 2004:572.)

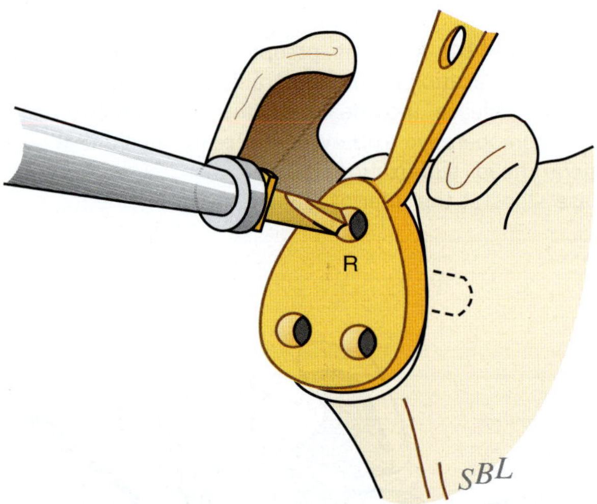

FIGURE 16-421: The peripheral drill guide tip is inserted into the anchor peg hole. The smaller peripheral drill bit is used to make the peripheral drill holes.

alignment of the guide while the subsequent holes are completed and to make sure that the hole is of the proper depth (Fig. 16-423). Each hole is checked to determine whether it penetrates the scapula.

After irrigation with antibiotic-containing saline solution, the holes are cleaned and dried with a spray of sterile carbon dioxide gas (Figs. 16-424 and 16-425), removing all tissue and fluid from the holes so that the injected cement will contact the bone directly without interposed fluid or blood clot resulting from the use of thrombin. Clearly, neither fluid nor clot will turn into bone or cement, so the presence of either will compromise the quality of fixation.

Unpenetrated holes are pressurized with a syringe (Fig. 16-426). Penetrating holes are cemented, but the cement is not pressurized (Fig. 16-427). The use of a carbon dioxide gas spray and cement pressurization has essentially eliminated the problem of postoperative radiolucent lines (see Figs. 16-331 and 16-362).

No cement is placed on the bony face of the glenoid; if the back of the glenoid component matches the prepared bony face, there is no advantage to an interposed

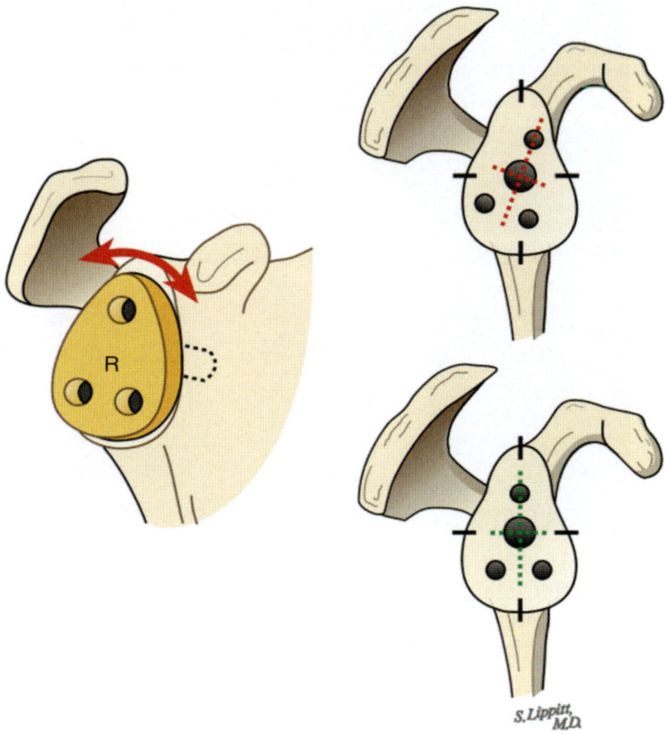

FIGURE 16-422: The peripheral hole drill guide needs to be oriented properly (as in the lower illustration) to take maximum advantage of available glenoid bone.

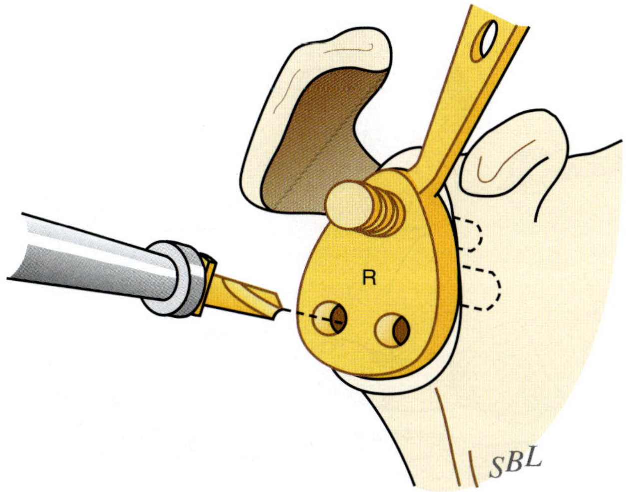

FIGURE 16-423: After the initial peripheral hole is drilled, a derotation peg is inserted to maintain alignment of the guide while subsequent holes are completed.

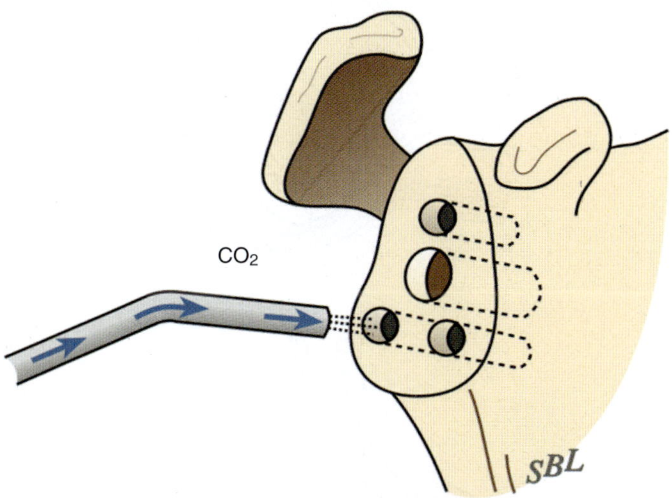

FIGURE 16-424: After irrigation with saline solution containing antibiotic, the glenoid holes are cleaned and dried with a spray of sterile carbon dioxide gas. This removes interposed fluid and blood clot from the holes so that the injected cement will directly contact bone.

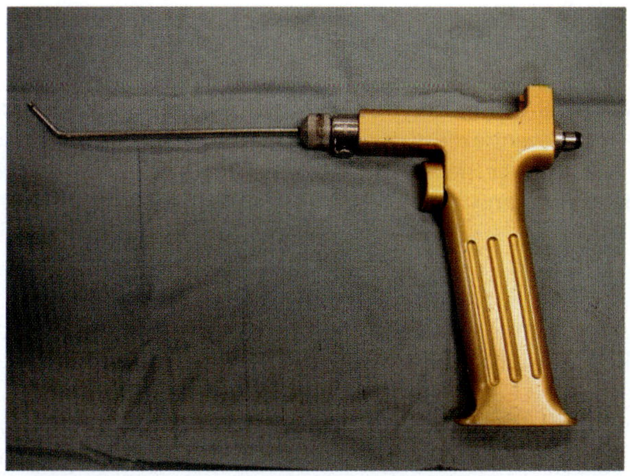

FIGURE 16-425: Instrument that uses a sterile carbon dioxide jet for cleaning and drying glenoid fixation holes before cementing.

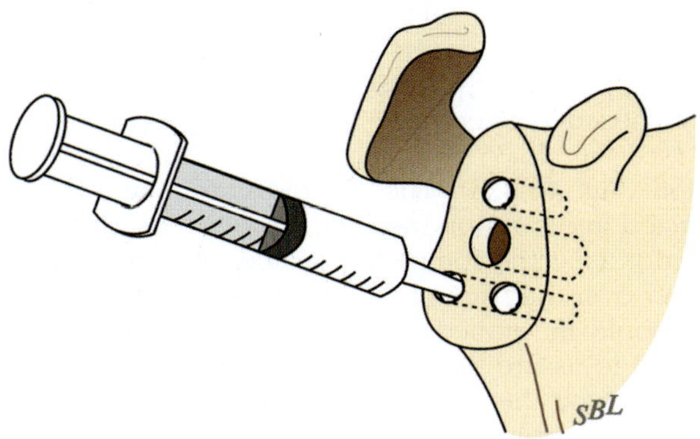

FIGURE 16-426: Cement is pressurized into an unpenetrated glenoid hole immediately after that hole is cleaned and dried with the carbon dioxide spray.

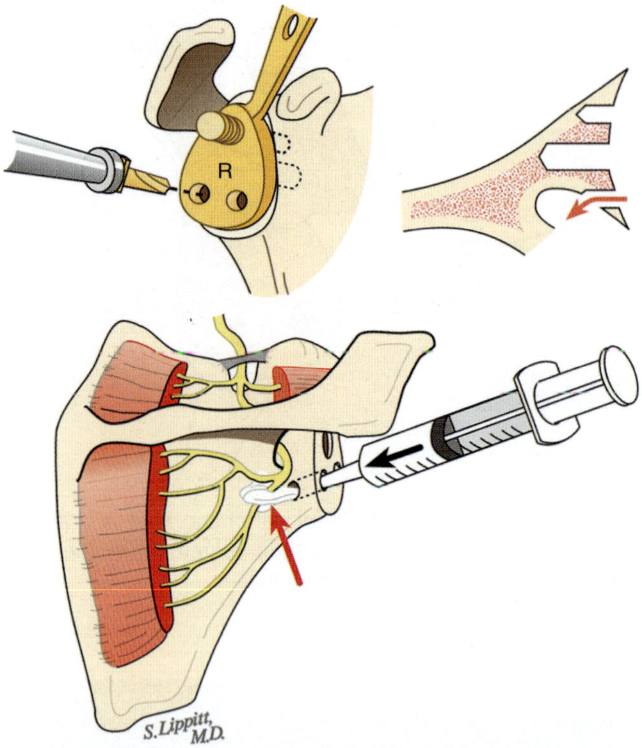

FIGURE 16-427: Cement is not pressurized into penetrating holes to prevent excess cement extrusion. Pressurizing cement into a posterior penetrating peg hole may result in excess cement extruding around the suprascapular nerve (red arrow).

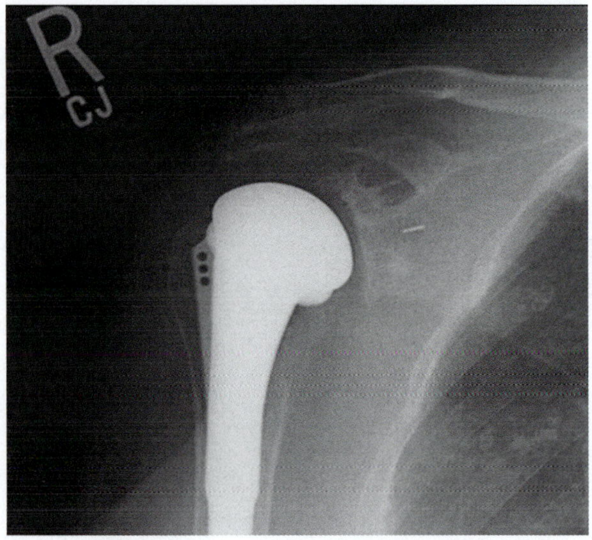

FIGURE 16-428: Anteroposterior radiograph of a patient 12 months after total shoulder arthroplasty using the anchor peg glenoid component. This demonstrates bone integration between the flanges of the central anchor peg.

layer of cement, which could fail and become displaced and consequently leave the glenoid component relatively unsupported (see Figs. 16-272 and 16-352). Some surgeons have been concerned about avoiding penetration of the holes for glenoid fixation,[227,548] but glenoid perforation does not appear to affect the clinical outcome of total shoulder arthroplasty.[439] It is evident however that penetration is more likely to occur in severely pathologic glenoids that have substantial medial or posterior bone erosion,[548] and for this reason, rather than the penetration itself, shoulder arthroplasty may be less successful in cases of particularly severe arthritic deformity.[227]

Reamed bone retrieved during the glenoid preparation (reaming and drilling) is used to create a bone paste that is interposed between the flutes of the central anchor peg (see Fig. 16-357) to help facilitate bone tissue integration (Fig. 16-428). The glenoid component is firmly impacted into position (see Fig. 16-361), ensuring that its posterior aspect is completely seated on bone by sliding a finger over the back of the component to feel the bone that should lie immediately beneath. The joint space is checked to assure that no fragments of cement or bone remain. Once the glenoid component is in place, it is important to prevent the humerus from dislodging it by the "bottle cap" mechanism; we use a broad flat retractor to safely deliver the proximal humerus into the wound after the glenoid has been implanted (Fig. 16-429).

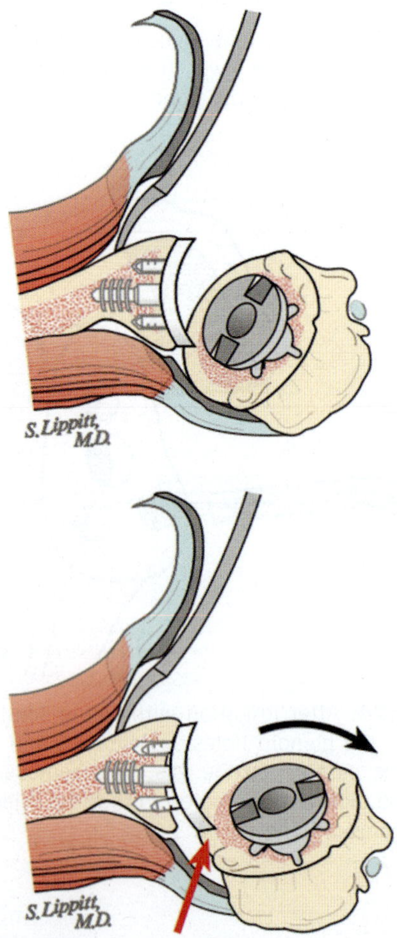

FIGURE 16-429: From the time the glenoid component is in place, care is taken not to pry apart the posterior edge of the glenoid component (red arrow) while repositioning the humerus.

Humeral Arthroplasty. The humeral preparation is completed after the glenoid arthroplasty. The goal is to achieve secure fixation without creating a stress riser at the tip of the component. Impaction grafting enables the use of a prosthetic humeral stem that is smaller in diameter than the humeral diaphysis so that diaphyseal loading is avoided. The canal is shaped to receive the humeral body (Figs. 16-430 to 16-433), ensuring that the component will be oriented in 30 degrees of retroversion (see Fig. 16-236). It is important to note that in an osteoporotic humerus the endosteal diaphyseal diameter may be disproportionately enlarged; a prosthesis with a stem sized to the diaphysis may therefore not fit into the metaphysis without fracture (see Fig. 16-316). If this is a concern, the prosthetic stem diameter can be downsized and the void filled with impaction grafting (see Fig. 16-322). Any remaining osteophytes are then resected (Fig. 16-434). If a plate is present on the humeral shaft, we prefer to leave it in place to minimize the risk of fracture, shortening the screws to allow passage of the stem (see Fig. 16-374).

The final selection of the humeral head prosthesis is made after the glenoid aspect of the surgery is complete. The trial body is inserted with humeral head prosthesis trials of the appropriate diameter of curvature and different thicknesses until the desired soft tissue balance is achieved: 150 degrees of elevation, 40 degrees of external

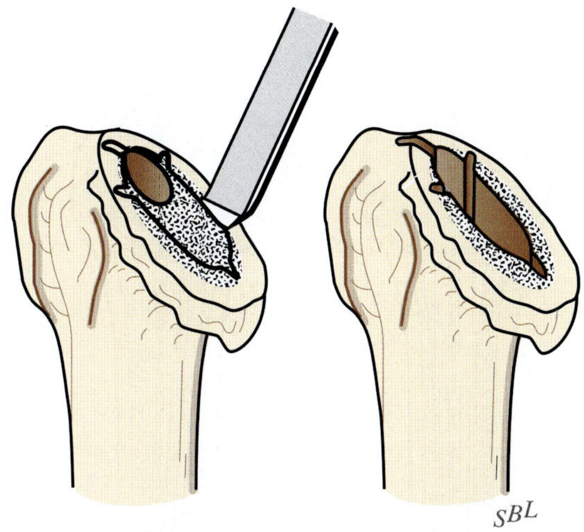

FIGURE 16-431: After body sizing, a 0.25-inch osteotome is used to remove the bone outlined by the "cookie cutter." (From Matsen FA III, Lippitt SB. *Shoulder Surgery: Principles and Procedures.* Philadelphia: Saunders; 2004:531.)

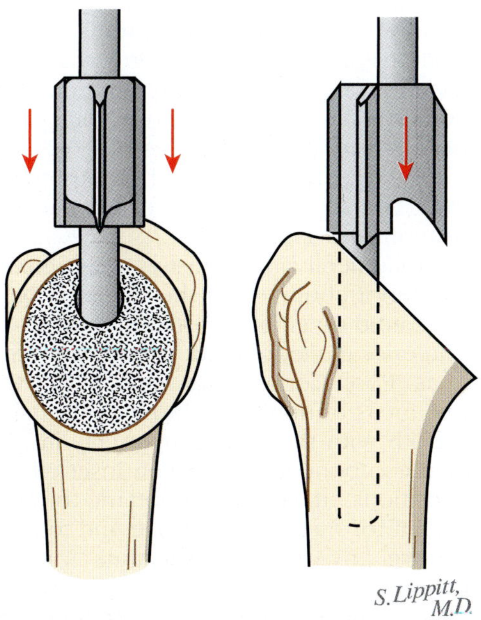

FIGURE 16-430: Orienting the humeral osteotome. A broach osteotome, or "cookie cutter," is placed down the medullary canal so that it is centered in the anteroposterior direction and held with a valgus bias so that the lateral bone will not force it into varus. Its rotation is oriented such that it is aligned with the neck and so that the anterior and lateral fins straddle the bicipital groove. This osteotome is then driven into the metaphysis (arrows) to mark the resection of the metaphyseal bone. (From Matsen FA III, Lippitt SB. *Shoulder Surgery: Principles and Procedures.* Philadelphia: Saunders; 2004:530.)

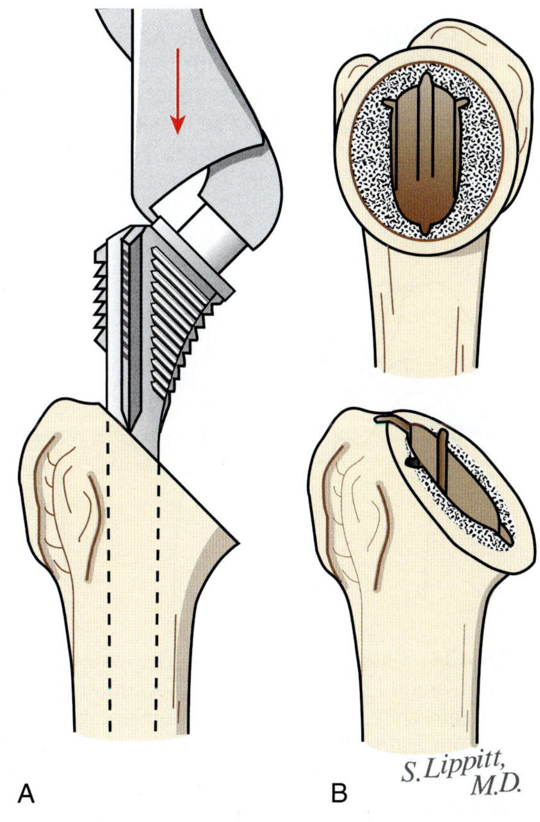

FIGURE 16-432: A, The medullary broach corresponding to the size of the medullary reamer is inserted in proper retroversion. **B,** Care should be taken that the center of the broach is positioned in the center of the neck cut. (From Matsen FA III, Lippitt SB. *Shoulder Surgery: Principles and Procedures.* Philadelphia: Saunders; 2004:532.)

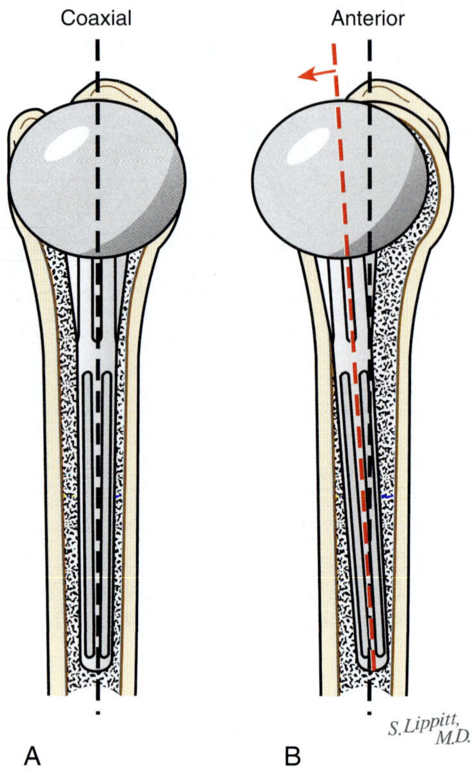

FIGURE 16-433: Positioning the broach. **A,** Particular care is needed to keep the broach coaxial with the medullary canal. **B,** It should not be inserted with its upper end too anterior. Such anterior angulation gives the false impression of posterior offset of the humeral neck. (From Matsen FA III, Lippitt SB. *Shoulder Surgery: Principles and Procedures.* Philadelphia: Saunders; 2004:533.)

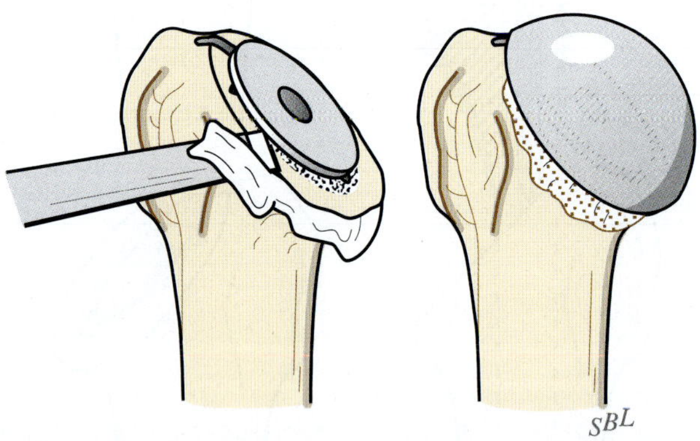

FIGURE 16-434: Osteophyte removal. The osteophytes are removed from around the neck using the centered humeral broach as a reference. Placing a trial humeral head on the broach can help guide this resection. (From Matsen FA III, Lippitt SB. *Shoulder Surgery: Principles and Procedures.* Philadelphia: Saunders; 2004:533.)

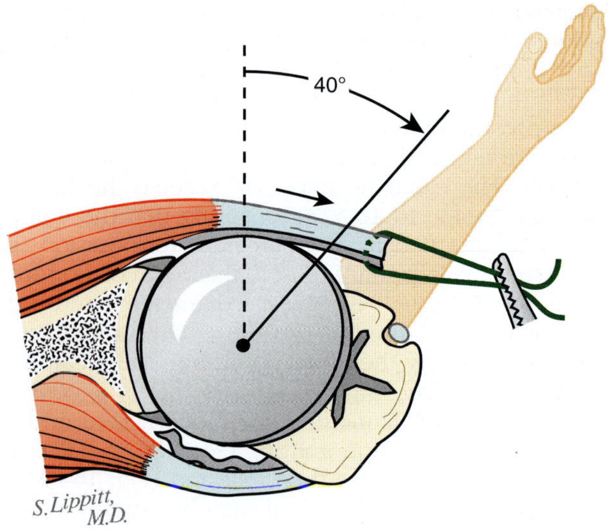

FIGURE 16-435: The 40-50-60 rule: external rotation. Forty degrees of external rotation with the subscapularis approximated. (From Matsen FA III, Lippitt SB. *Shoulder Surgery: Principles and Procedures.* Philadelphia: Saunders; 2004:478.)

rotation of the adducted arm with the subscapularis approximated (Fig. 16-435), 50% posterior subluxation of the humeral head on the posterior drawer test (Fig. 16-436), and 60 degrees of internal rotation of the arm elevated in the coronal plane ("scarecrow test") (see Figs. 16-208 and 16-309). Restricted range of motion might require a head prosthesis of lesser thickness or additional soft tissue releases.

If there is more than 50% posterior translation or if the shoulder demonstrates a positive "drop back" sign on passive elevation (Fig. 16-437), the surgeon can adopt one or more of three strategies: (1) using a thicker humeral head component (Fig. 16-438); (2) using an anteriorly eccentric humeral head component (Figs. 16-439 and 16-440; see Fig. 16-334); or (3) using a rotator interval plication (see Fig. 16-280).

In all glenohumeral arthroplasties it is important to check for posterior abutment of the humerus against the back of the glenoid on external rotation (Fig. 16-441) and against the inferior glenoid on adduction; we refer to this critical area as "Pooh Corner" (see Fig. 16-227). Checking for these two areas of unwanted bone contact should be carried out both with the trial components in place and after the final components have been inserted into their definitive positions. It is also important to thoroughly inspect the joint for fragments of bone and to irrigate the joint to remove any potential substrate for unwanted bone formation.

After the definitive humeral component has been selected, it is assembled securely on the back table. This assures a tighter fit of the Morse taper than can be achieved by impacting the head on the stem after the stem has been placed in the humerus. Assembling the head on an implanted stem runs the risk of incomplete seating or of changing the position of the stem. Impaction grafting is carried out using cancellous bone harvested from the resected humeral head and soaked in a vancomycin solution during the time between harvest and insertion (see Figs. 16-322 and 16-323).[46,193] Selective graft

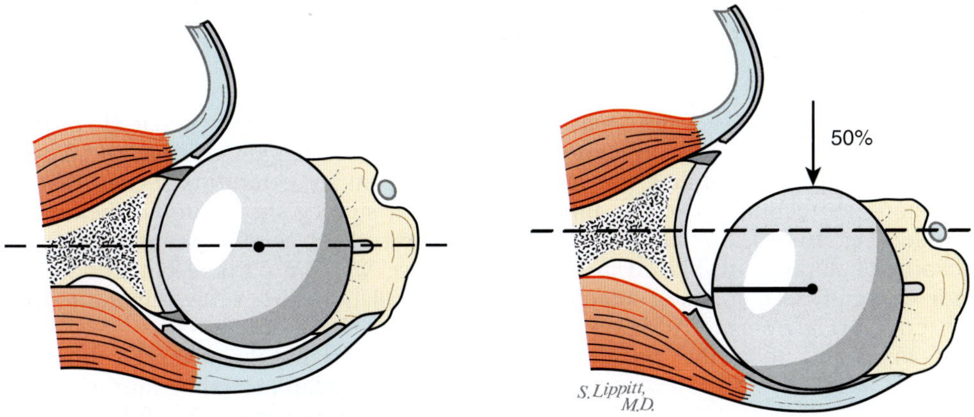

FIGURE 16-436: The 40-50-60 rule: posterior drawer. Fifty percent posterior subluxation on the posterior drawer test. (From Matsen FA III, Lippitt SB. *Shoulder Surgery: Principles and Procedures.* Philadelphia: Saunders; 2004:479.)

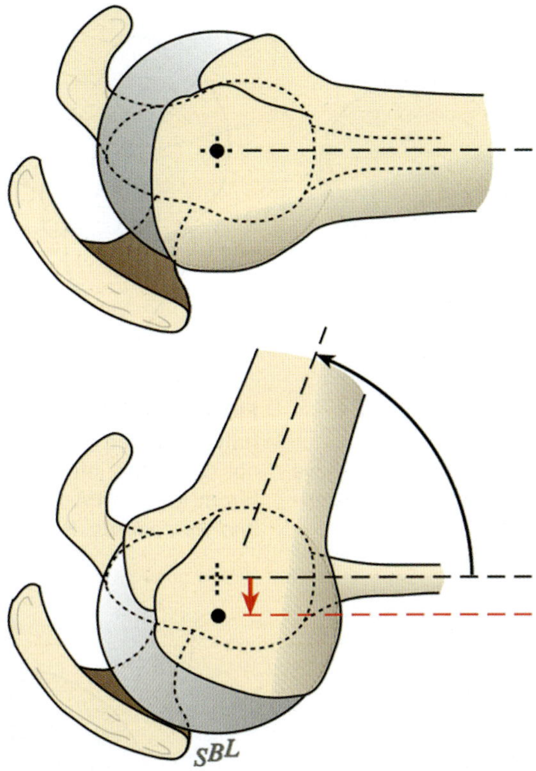

FIGURE 16-437: Drop back sign. Check for unstable posterior humeral translation on passive elevation of the arm.

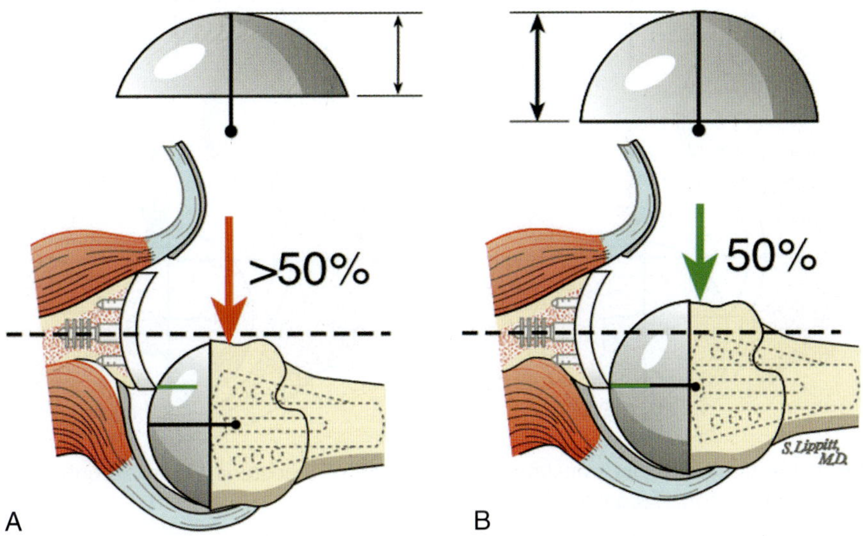

FIGURE 16-438: **A** and **B,** If the humeral head translates greater than 50% posteriorly, a wider head component may improve the balance of the reconstruction.

placement can fine-tune the position of the stem (see Figs. 16-324 and 16-325). If the biceps tendon is in need of tenodesis because of fraying or instability, this is performed using an in-and-out technique at the time of prosthesis insertion (see Fig. 16-384).

Six No. 2 nonabsorbable sutures are placed in secure bone at the anterior humeral neck for later attachment of the subscapularis tendon (Fig. 16-442). Additional graft is inserted (Fig. 16-443), and then the prosthesis is press-fitted into the prepared proximal end of the humerus. The height, version, and fixation of the humeral component are carefully checked. The lateral edge of the articular surface should lie just below the cut edge of the humeral neck, which we refer to as the "berm" (Fig. 16-444). We pay particular attention to the register, that is, the relationship of the humeral to the glenoid articular surface (see Fig. 16-239).

Before closure, the wound is thoroughly irrigated with antibiotic-containing saline and inspected for debris. The joint is again put through a full range of motion to verify

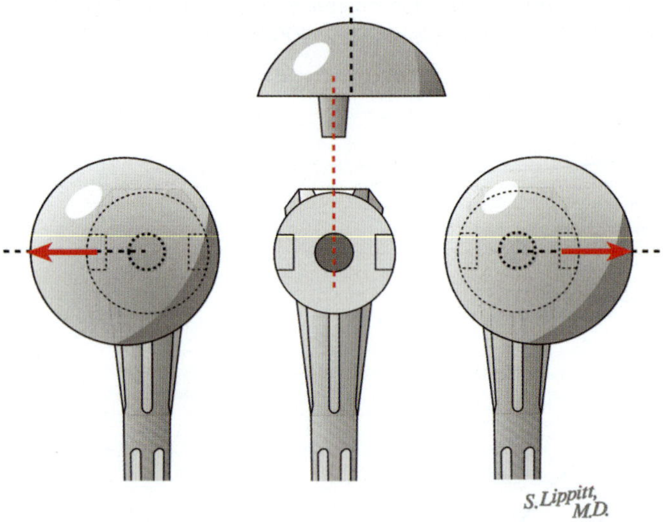

FIGURE 16-439: The humeral head prosthesis should have eccentric options to help control excessive translation posteriorly or anteriorly.

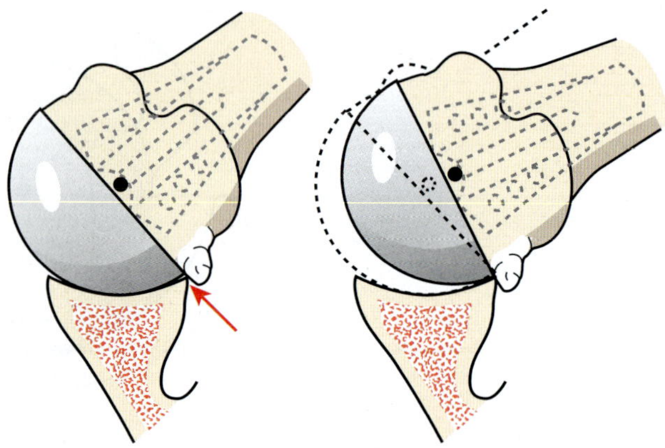

FIGURE 16-441: Posterior "open book." The shoulder is carefully examined to ensure that posterior abutment (arrow) does not cause the joint to "open book" (right) in external rotation. (From Matsen FA III, Lippitt SB. *Shoulder Surgery: Principles and Procedures.* Philadelphia: Saunders; 2004:563.)

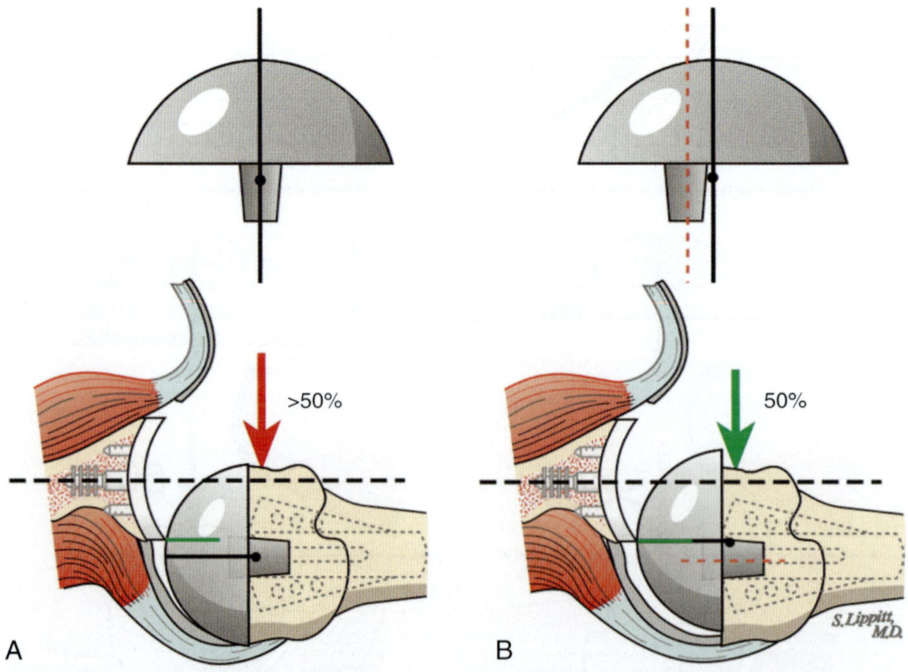

FIGURE 16-440: **A** and **B,** If the humeral head translates greater than 50% posteriorly, an eccentric head component oriented anteriorly may improve the balance of the reconstruction.

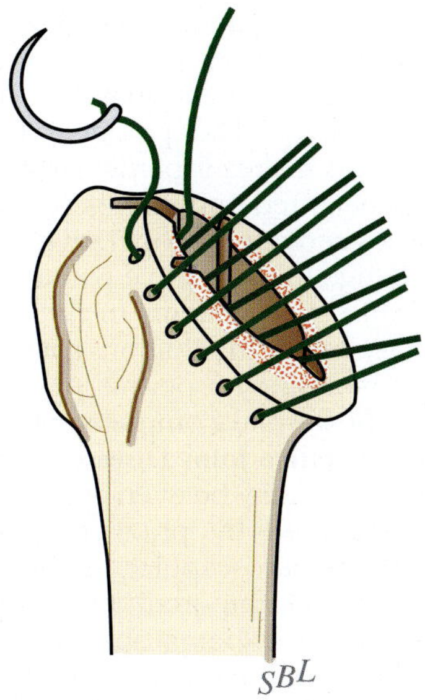

FIGURE 16-442: At least six No. 2 braided nonabsorbable sutures are placed through drill holes in the anterior neck for reattachment of the subscapularis. Moving the subscapularis insertion from the lesser tuberosity to the neck gains about 1 cm in subscapularis length, which is an increase in external rotation of about 20 degrees. (From Matsen FA III, Lippitt SB. *Shoulder Surgery: Principles and Procedures.* Philadelphia: Saunders; 2004:539.)

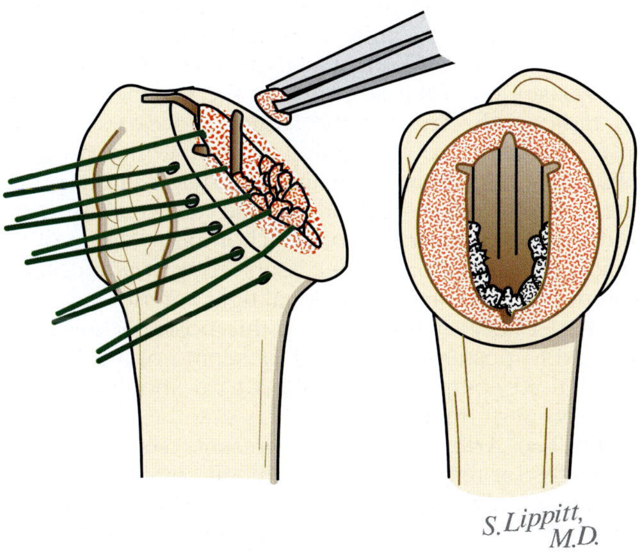

FIGURE 16-443: If the components are in proper register, the humeral articular surface should seat fully in the glenoid in adduction and in 45 degrees of abduction. (From Matsen FA III, Lippitt SB. *Shoulder Surgery: Principles and Procedures.* Philadelphia: Saunders; 2004:461.)

smoothness and lack of contact, such as between the medial aspect of the humerus and the inferior glenoid (see Fig. 16-227) or posteriorly (see Fig. 16-441). The wound is not drained. After a gram of vancomycin powder is placed deep in the wound, the subscapularis

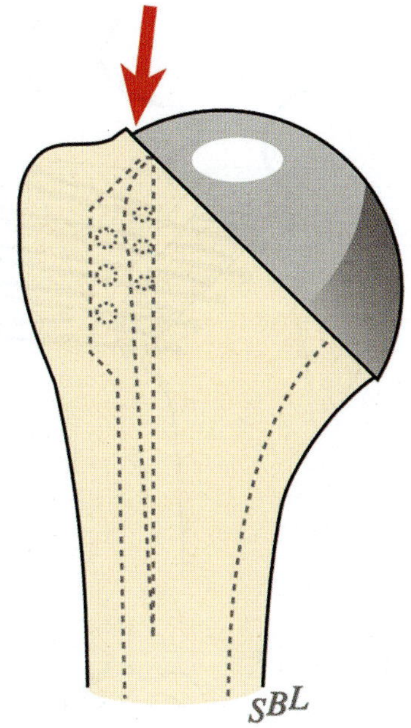

FIGURE 16-444: The lateral edge of the humeral head component articular surface should lie just below the cut edge of the humeral neck. We refer to this as the "berm."

is repaired securely to the humeral neck (Fig. 16-445). Another gram of vancomycin powder is placed on the repaired tendon. The wound is then closed in layers. We usually use skin staples to create a secure closure that will tolerate immediate postoperative motion.

AP and lateral radiographs are obtained in the recovery room to document the immediate postoperative status of the shoulder and to show the patient and family what procedure was done. The radiographs are repeated at 6 weeks and at 2 years (see Figs. 16-38, 16-331, and 16-333). Videos 16-1 to 16-6 demonstrate this procedure.

Special Considerations

Degenerative Joint Disease. In degenerative joint diseases, the glenoid face is typically flattened and often eroded posteriorly as a result of chronic posterior subluxation (see Fig. 16-66). The glenoid may be distorted by peripheral osteophytes that mask the location of the anatomic fossa. The humeral head may be flattened in a corresponding manner and effectively enlarged by the proliferation of goat's beard osteophytes from the anterior, inferior, and posterior articular rim (see Figs. 16-35 and 16-375). Intra-articular loose bodies may lie hidden in the subcoracoid or axillary recess. Anterior capsular and subscapularis contractures are common in degenerative joint disease and require release; however, posterior capsular release is not performed if posterior humeral subluxation was noted preoperatively.

Rheumatoid Arthritis. The basic principles of shoulder arthroplasty for rheumatoid arthritis are similar to those for degenerative arthritis, but some important differences exist. Rheumatoid tissue is much more fragile: the bone

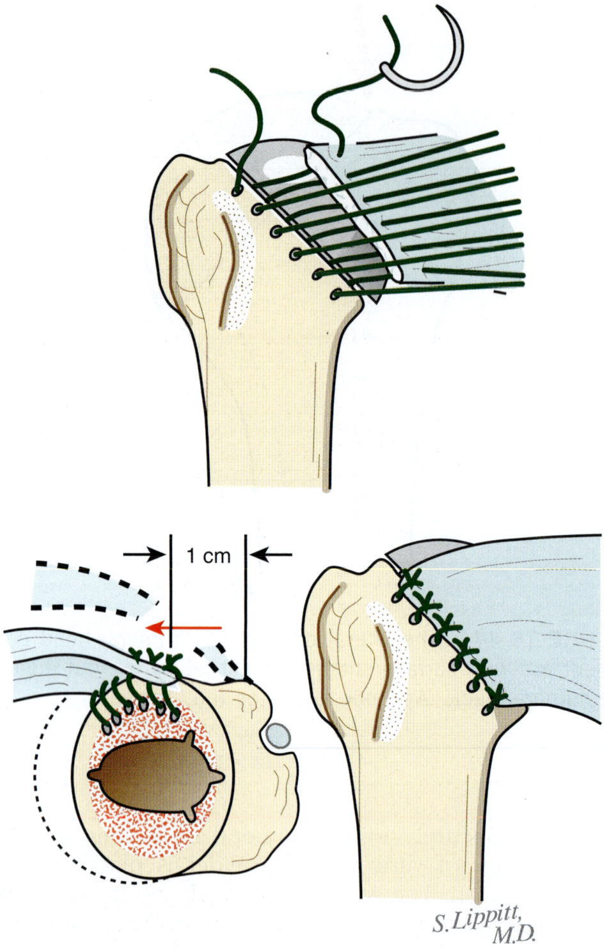

FIGURE 16-445: The subscapularis is repaired to the anterior humeral neck cut. (From Matsen FA III, Lippitt SB. *Shoulder Surgery: Principles and Procedures.* Philadelphia: Saunders; 2004:544.)

is more likely to fracture, and the muscle and tendons are more susceptible to tear. Thus, from the outset, extreme care must be taken to preserve bone and soft tissue integrity. We refer to these requirements for extraordinary gentleness as the "rheumatoid rules"; they guide each step of our management of the patient.

Because rheumatoid arthritis is an erosive and destructive disease, deficiencies of bone and the rotator cuff are more likely than in degenerative joint disease. The glenoid bone may be so eroded that insufficient stock is available to support a glenoid component. The rotator cuff may be partially or totally deficient. The shoulder may be so limited in volume that it will accept only a thin humeral component and no glenoid component. Thus all these factors need to be considered in the preoperative evaluation and in discussions with the patient concerning the possible outcomes of surgery.

The standard preoperative scapular AP and axillary radiographs are required to evaluate the humeral and glenoid bone stock (see Fig. 16-91). In rheumatoid arthritis the glenoid erosion is usually medial (rather than posterior, as in degenerative joint disease). For this reason, only minimal glenoid reaming by hand may be needed to achieve an excellent-quality fit to the back of the glenoid component. The potential fragility of the bone and soft tissues makes it particularly important that the joint is not overstuffed and that there is adequate soft tissue laxity for immediate postoperative motion. This is a particular challenge in diminutive patients with juvenile rheumatoid arthritis; such patients might also have a tiny humeral medullary canal. In addition, some patients have insufficient joint volume to permit the insertion of a glenoid component despite complete soft tissue release.

Secondary Degenerative Joint Disease. In posttraumatic arthritis, the challenges may be even greater. The anatomy is likely to be distorted by prior fracture or surgery. The nonarticular humeroscapular motion interface is likely to be scarred, with important neurologic structures, such as the axillary nerve, being obscured. The tuberosities, humeral shaft, and glenoid may be ununited or malunited. Each case requires consideration of the complexities of the shoulder and the needs of the patient (Fig. 16-446).

Capsulorrhaphy Arthropathy. Shoulders affected by capsulorrhaphy arthropathy present additional challenges, such as neurovascular scarring from prior surgery, soft tissue contractures, bone deficiencies, implants from prior surgery, changes in glenoid version, and an increased potential for glenohumeral instability after the arthroplasty. Patients with capsulorrhaphy arthropathy are typically younger than those with primary degenerative or inflammatory arthritis conditions; they also tend to desire a higher level of activity after their shoulder arthroplasty. Careful assessment of the preoperative axillary radiograph can alert the surgeon to excessive posterior capsular laxity resulting from chronic posterior humeral subluxation after anterior stabilization procedures. Such laxity can predispose the reconstructed shoulder to posterior instability. Thorough release of the subscapularis tendon is necessary to prevent obligate posterior translation from residual tight anterior structures (see Fig. 16-87). If unmanaged, this posterior instability can lead to posterior wear and loosening of a polyethylene glenoid component should a total shoulder arthroplasty be performed.

Cuff Tear Arthropathy. CTA presents several unique challenges for regaining glenohumeral comfort and function. The humeral head may be in a superior position such that it articulates with the coracoacromial arch (see Figs. 16-100, 16-101, 16-103, 16-110, and 16-224) or it may escape the arch altogether (see Figs. 16-109, 16-111, and 16-115). The rotator cuff is almost never amenable to a repair, and the glenoid is eroded superiorly so that an acetabular-like structure is formed in continuity with the coracoacromial arch. Under these circumstances, a standard anatomic arthroplasty is unlikely to be successful.

If the coracoacromial arch is intact and if the shoulder is capable of 90 degrees or more of active elevation, a shoulder with CTA can often be reconstructed with a hemiarthroplasty designed to provide a smooth articulation between the proximal humerus on one side and the

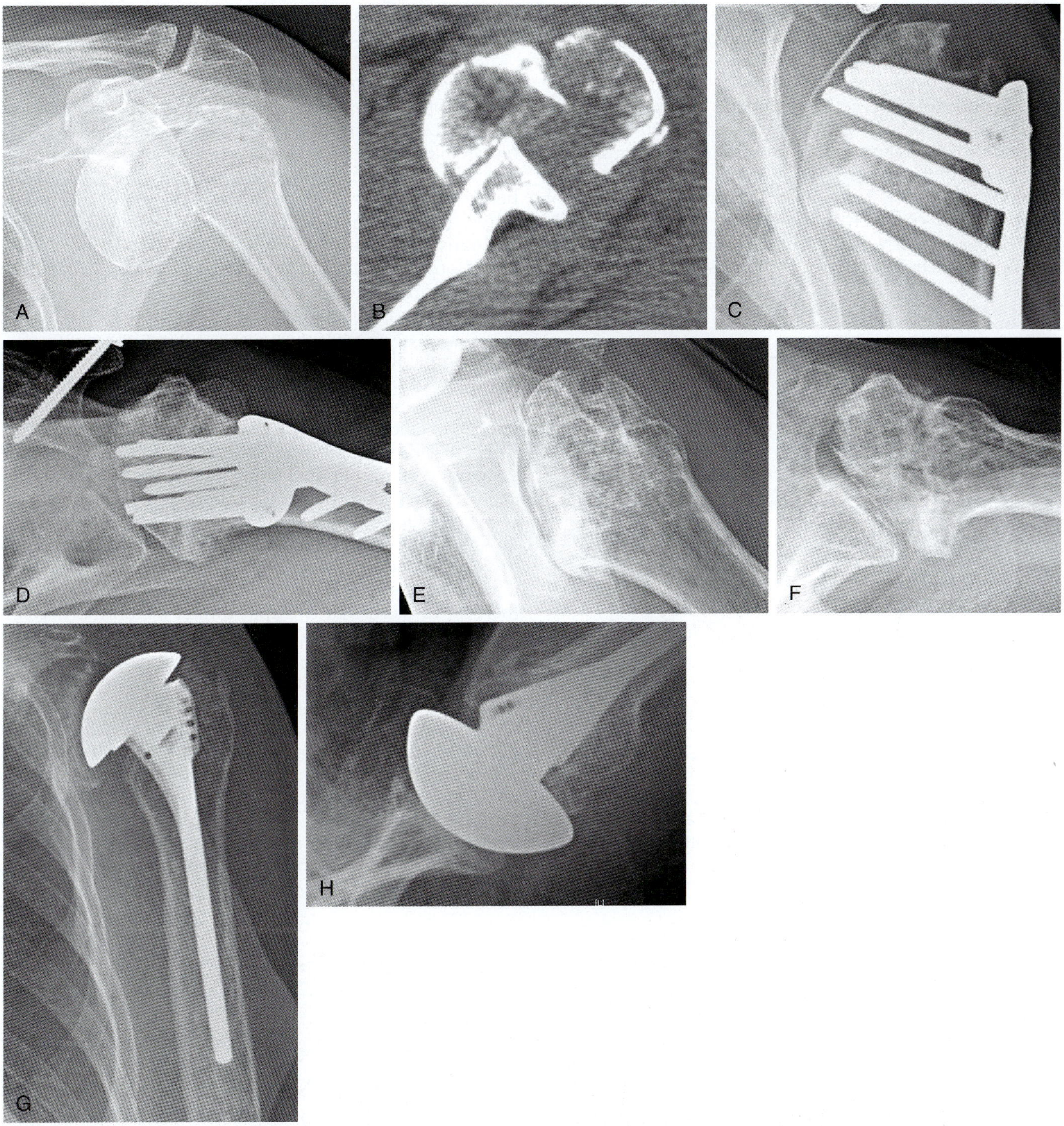

FIGURE 16-446: Posttraumatic arthritis. **A,** Displaced humeral neck fracture. **B,** Computed tomographic scan showing dislocation of the head fragment. **C,** Anteroposterior view after internal fixation. **D,** Axillary view after internal fixation showing screws engaging the glenoid. **E,** Anteroposterior view after hardware removal showing deformity of the head. **F,** Axillary view showing collapse of the head. **G,** Anteroposterior view after reconstruction with impaction grafted humeral component without a glenoid arthroplasty. **H,** Axillary view after reconstruction with an impaction grafted humeral component.

coracoacromial arch and glenoid on the other. In this situation we prefer using a special humeral prosthesis with an articular surface that extends over the area of the greater tuberosity (see Figs. 16-97 and 16-104; Figs. 16-447 and 16-448), with a diameter of curvature that matches that of the resected head (see Fig. 16-305). This type of prosthesis may also be useful in managing post-traumatic deformity (Fig. 16-449). When there is antero-superior instability from acromial erosion or a prior acromioplasty or when the patient is unable to actively raise the arm above 90 degrees despite good passive motion (i.e., there is pseudoparalysis) (Fig. 16-450), a reverse total shoulder arthroplasty may be considered (see Fig. 16-113).

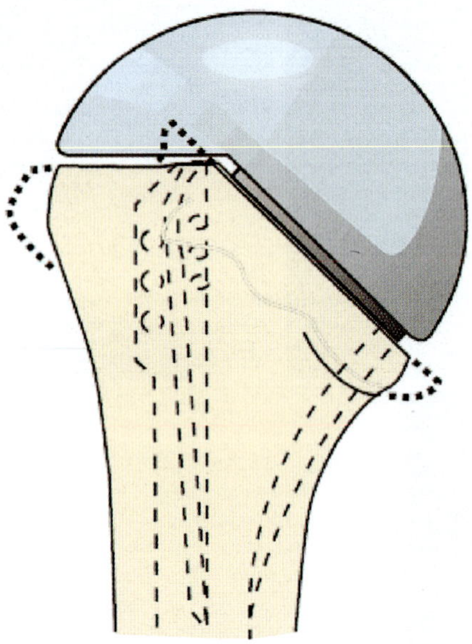

FIGURE 16-447: Attaching the trial head and adjusting the bony contours for perfect articulation beneath the coracoacromial arch.

Postoperative Rehabilitation

It is helpful for patients and for the entire care team to standardize the postoperative program as much as possible. While variations may be needed for special circumstances, we describe the program we usually use for hemiarthroplasties, CTA prostheses, ream and run procedures, and total shoulder arthroplasties. Our overall goals are early ambulation, early shoulder motion, and early transition to oral analgesics. The patient is encouraged to use the arm for gentle activities, such as eating, using a keyboard, and squeezing a foam ball (Fig. 16-451). A sling is used only for comfort or support when necessary.

The rehabilitation goal is a 150-degree range of assisted elevation prior to hospital discharge. We emphasize that the patient must accept responsibility for the success of the rehabilitation program. Patients are given access to a website with videos of the key exercises.[498] The exercise program is started immediately after surgery in the recovery room with the initiation of slow and gentle continuous passive motion for 30 minutes each hour (Figs. 16-452 and 16-453). Continuous passive motion is avoided in arms that are large and heavy, when there is concern about the strength of the subscapularis repair, or when there is concern that a carpal tunnel syndrome may be aggravated by pressure from the gauntlet. The patient-conducted rehabilitation program starts on the day of surgery under instructions given by the surgeon or therapist. Elevation stretching is performed in the supine position (lying flat on the back) by grasping the wrist or elbow of the relaxed operative shoulder with the hand of the unoperated arm, pulling it up toward the ceiling, and then reaching overhead as high as possible aiming to achieve the goal of 150 degrees (Fig. 16-454). This stretch is most effective if the patient relaxes the shoulder musculature while holding the position for 2 minutes.

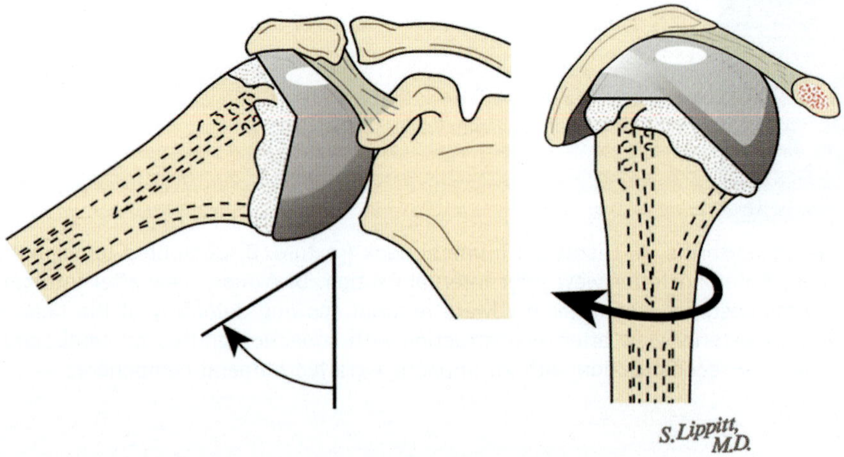

FIGURE 16-448: Hemiarthroplasty with a cuff tear arthropathy (CTA) head component that is stable beneath an intact coracoacromial arch. The laterally extended CTA head allows a greater arc of motion in abduction and greater external rotation by coverage of the greater tuberosity.

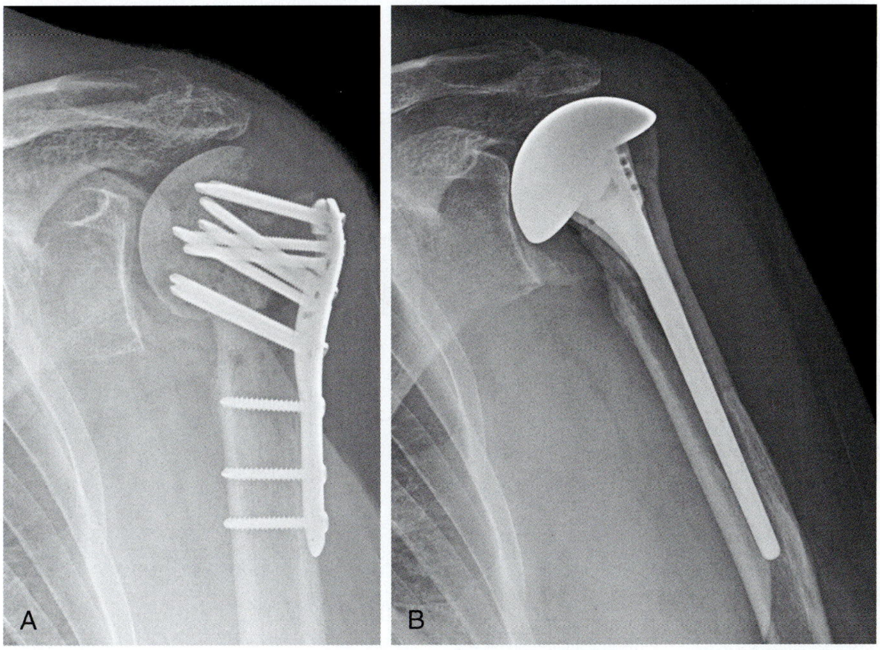

FIGURE 16-449: Posttraumatic arthritis with humeral nonunion, treated with a cuff tear arthropathy prosthesis.

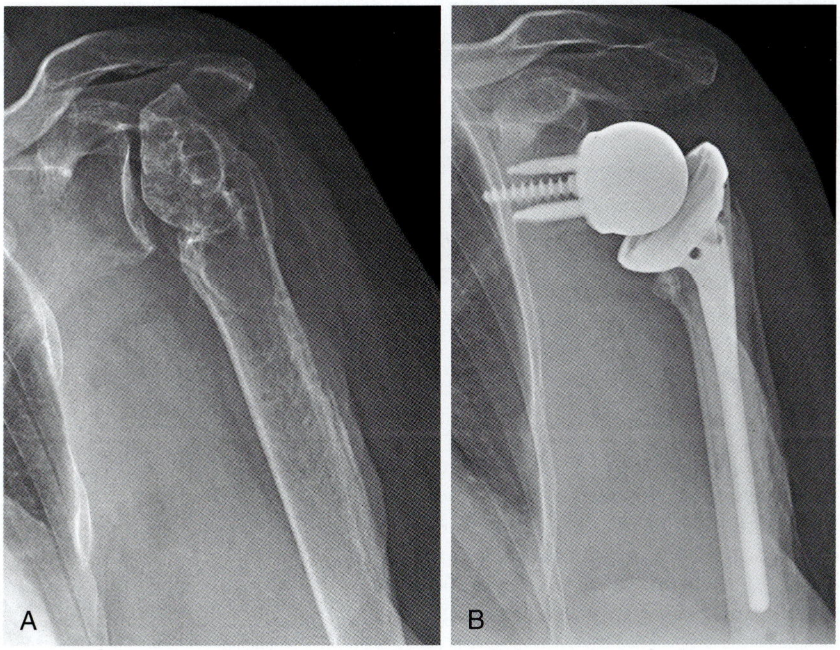

FIGURE 16-450: **A,** Posttraumatic arthritis. **B,** The condition was managed with reverse total shoulder arthroplasty. In this case cement was necessary for rotational control of the prosthesis in the distorted humeral anatomy.

The pulley (see Fig. 16-148) and the forward lean (see Fig. 16-137) are also very useful, particularly if the opposite upper extremity is not healthy. Passive external rotation stretching is restricted to zero degrees initially (Fig. 16-455). The daily range of elevation as measured by the surgeon or therapist is displayed on a wall chart in full view of the patient, staff, and visitors (Fig. 16-456) to provide the patient with feedback on their rehabilitation progress. Because the desired range was achieved while the patient was on the operating table, the patient's task is simplified: the achieved range has only to be maintained during the postoperative period. It is important to warn the patient that the arm may swell during the first week after surgery (Fig. 16-457), but this usually subsides

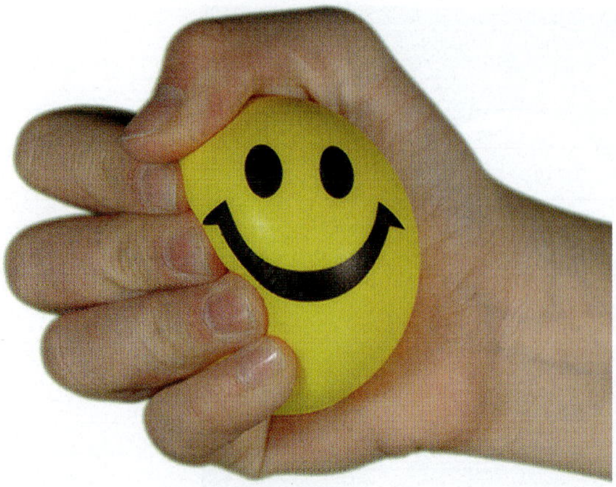

FIGURE 16-451: Squeeze ball used to reduce swelling after surgery.

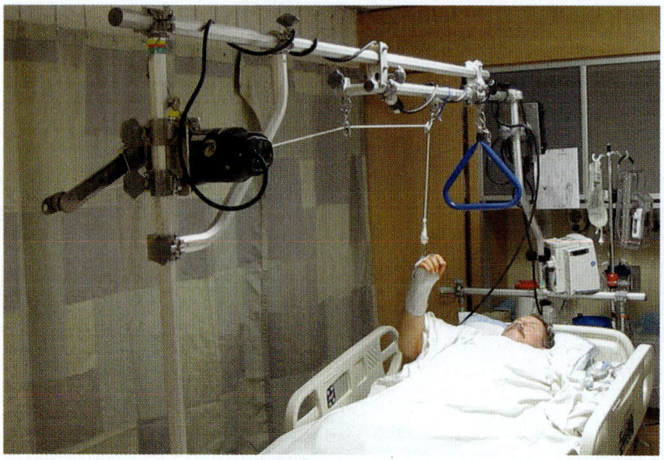

FIGURE 16-452: Continuous passive motion is implemented immediately after surgery for most anatomic arthroplasties.

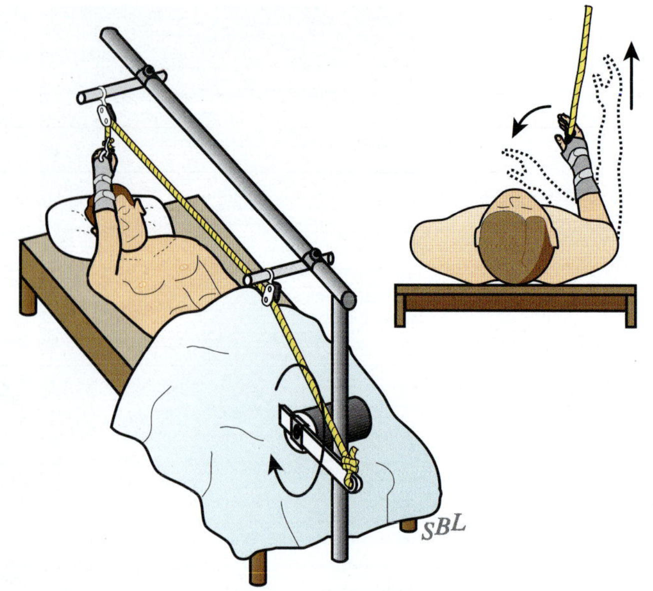

FIGURE 16-453: Continuous passive motion for the first 36 hours after surgery helps ensure that healing of the humeroscapular motion interface proceeds in a way that yields smooth articulating surfaces, preventing the adhesions that can develop rapidly if the shoulder is immobilized during the early healing response after surgery. Continuous passive motion provides mechanical signals to the healing cells, differentiating those that are to heal the subscapularis tendon to the bone from those that are to facilitate sliding of the proximal humeral convexity on the undersurface of the coracoacromial arch. (From Matsen FA III, Lippitt SB. *Shoulder Surgery: Principles and Procedures.* Philadelphia: Saunders; 2004:547.)

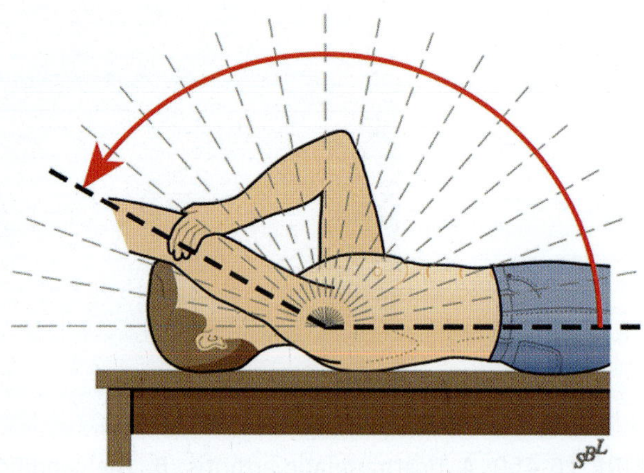

FIGURE 16-454: Postoperative forward elevation exercise. Using the opposite arm for assistance as necessary, the patient works to forward elevate the arm to the rehabilitation goal of 150 degrees.

by the second week and should not deter performance of the range of motion exercises. The exercises are to be performed five times a day (Fig. 16-458) both while the patient is in the hospital and at home after discharge.

At 6 weeks after surgery, the assisted elevation program still continues but we add stretching in abduction (Fig. 16-459), the sleeper stretch (see Fig. 16-146), cross-body adduction (see Figs. 16-19 and 16-141), internal rotation up the back (see Fig. 16-140), and gentle external rotation (see Fig. 16-138).

Strengthening exercises are also started at 6 weeks. The most important of these is the two-hand supine press series (see Fig. 16-151) which is progressed to the "press plus" with a 1-lb weight, starting in the supine position and progressing to increasingly vertical positions, adding the "press plus" at the top of each exercise (see Fig. 16-144). This exercise, along with the shoulder shrug, helps to develop the scapular musculature (see Fig. 16-145). We indicate to patients that they should be able to repeat these strengthening exercises comfortably 20 times before they advance to a greater weight or a more upright position. Slow, steady progression is the goal. In most cases strengthening exercises that isolate the cuff muscles are avoided so as to minimize the risk of delayed

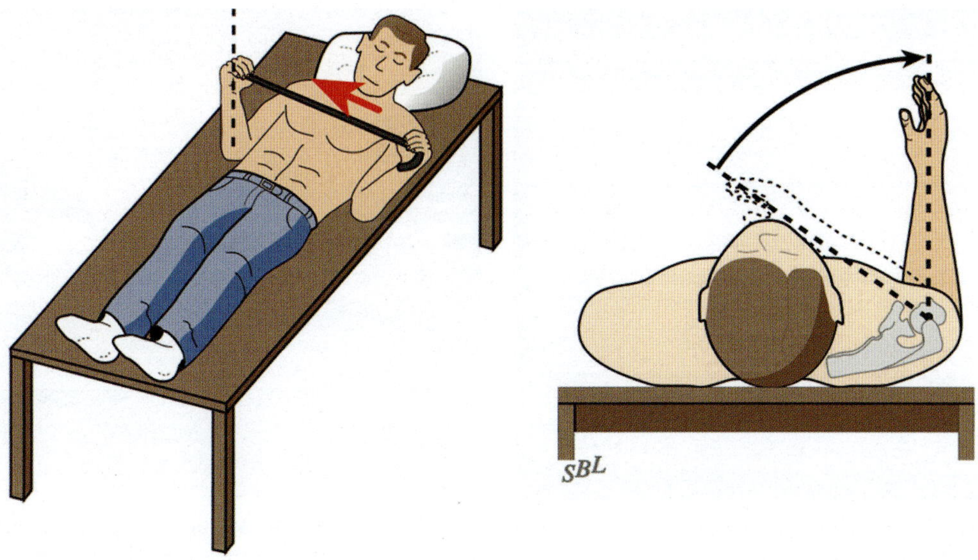

FIGURE 16-455: Postoperative external rotation exercise. Using the opposite arm for assistance, as necessary, the patient works to externally rotate the arm to a limit of zero degrees for the first 6 weeks.

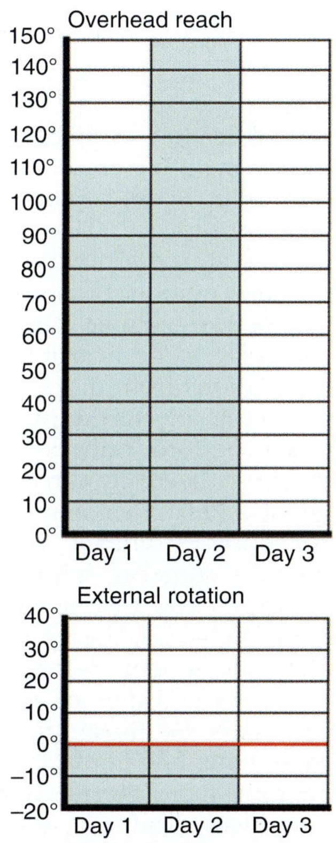

FIGURE 16-456: Daily range of motion as measured by the surgeon or therapist is recorded on a wall chart kept in full view of the patient, staff, and visitors.

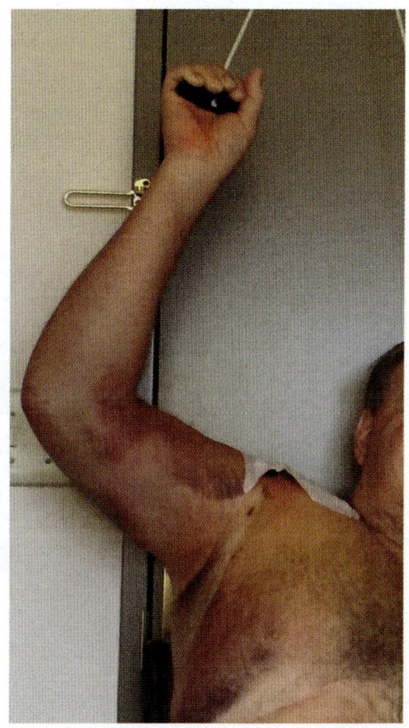

FIGURE 16-457: Ecchymosis may occur if there is early motion after arthroplasty.

cuff failure.[598] Activities are added progressively. We allow driving and gentle water exercises at 6 weeks. Golf and tennis may be started at 3 to 6 months if the shoulder is comfortable, flexible, and strong. Impact activities, such as chopping wood, are precluded for total shoulder arthroplasties but are permitted for the ream and run once the patient has achieved a good range of motion, comfort, and strength.

Because successful rehabilitation is critical to the outcome of shoulder arthroplasty, we encourage patients to give us regular progress reports and to feel welcome to contact us by email if they have questions or concerns. A most effective way to monitor progress in range of

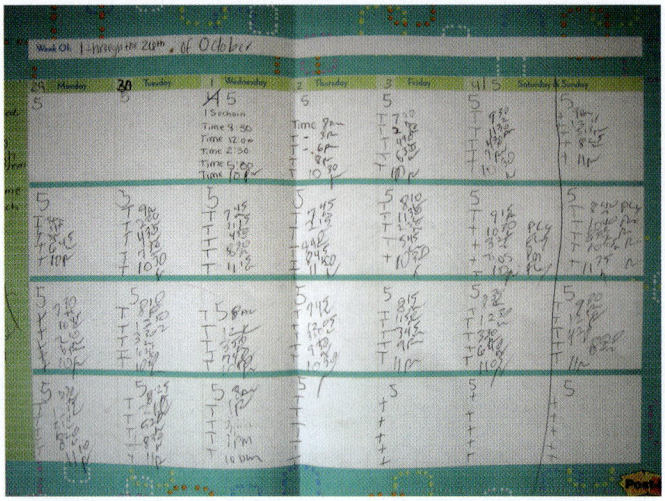

FIGURE 16-458: The most successful patients keep a careful calendar of their rehabilitation exercises.

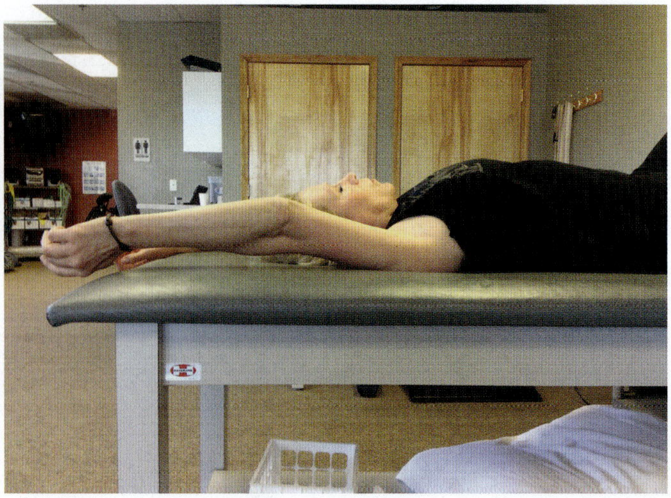

FIGURE 16-460: A lateral photograph of the supine patient elevating the arm overhead provides an easy way to track the progress of rehabilitation. This photo was emailed to us 2 weeks after the patient had undergone a ream and run procedure on the right shoulder.

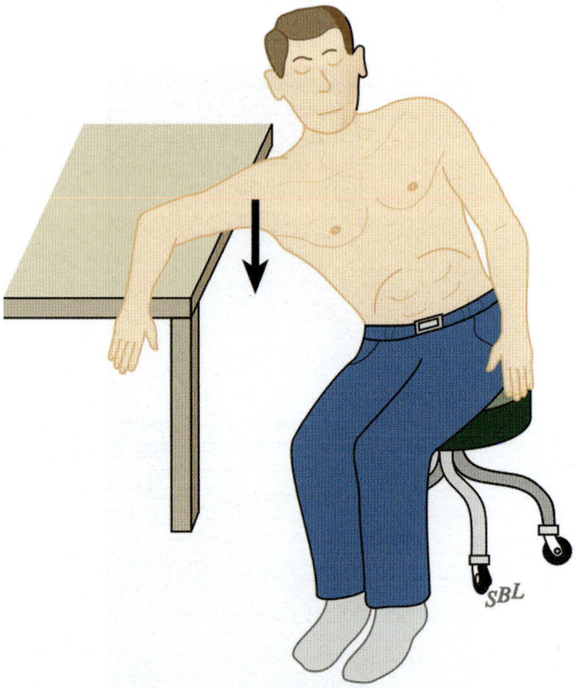

FIGURE 16-459: At 6 weeks after surgery, stretching in abduction is added to the assisted exercise program.

motion is to ask the patient to email a lateral photograph with the arm in maximal elevation (Fig. 16-460).

Results

A PubMed search for "shoulder + arthroplasty + outcome" in early 2015 returned more than 1500 articles, most of which were case series from surgeons with substantial experience. These demonstrated substantial improvement in comfort and function after shoulder arthroplasty for a variety of arthritic conditions and with a wide variety of implants. As expected, the results were worse for more complex pathologies[236,477] and for patients who were less healthy.[48,183] However, the additional knowledge to be gained from these publications is limited. In spite of the sheer volume of this literature, most of the published studies did not represent a valid sample of the overall results of shoulder arthroplasty. The great majority of shoulder arthroplasties are performed by surgeons who operate on only a small number of cases each year[199,207]; the results from these low volume surgeons are highly relevant but are unlikely to be available in the surgical literature. The observations from major shoulder centers are not necessarily applicable to the practice of the surgeons who may each perform only occasional shoulder arthroplasties but who collectively carry out the majority of joint replacements. Reliable comparisons of results with different procedures is difficult without a prospective study that involves surgeons who are adept at the techniques under study, who treat similar patients with similar problems, and who use the same metrics before and sequentially after treatment.[164] This is particularly a problem in evaluating the value of newer and more costly approaches, such as those that involve novel designs (e.g., stemless humeral implants or metal-backed glenoids), more complex prostheses (higher degrees of adjustability or modular, platform stems), or patient-specific guidance systems developed from three-dimensional scans with special software. Many articles present data from computer models, sawbones surgery, or cadaver models. Others present Level IV data, concluding that the procedure discussed is a "viable treatment," without putting it in context with other alternatives for similar patients. Thus much of the literature describing arthroplasty outcomes is not very helpful in guiding practice. A few inclusive arthroplasty registries are becoming available and hold promise of providing a more comprehensive view of the practice of shoulder arthroplasty in the future.[15,255,396,536]

Conversely, it is always possible to learn from studying failure. The study of airplanes that crash is more informative than the study of those that land on time. The study of football games lost teaches more than the recordings of games won. In the science of shoulder arthroplasty, recognition of the problem of delayed failure of the rotator cuff after shoulder joint replacement[443,598] led to reconsideration of the recommended rehabilitation and activity levels following shoulder arthroplasty. Similarly, studies showing the persistent problem of glenoid prosthesis failure after total shoulder arthroplasty[334,414,415,443,531] motivated the exploration of nonprosthetic options for managing the glenoid side of the arthritic glenohumeral joint.

Definitions of arthroplasty failure vary widely; they include radiographic loosening, lack of clinical improvement, and surgical revision. *Radiographic loosening* is evaluated by follow-up radiographs,[570,598] but because loosening is not often evident until many years after the arthroplasty,[414,415,443,531] it becomes difficult to know the rate of these changes in the absence of a strict annual and prolonged follow-up protocol. The most common types of failure of total shoulder arthroplasty are related to the glenoid component.[153,334,443] Increased rates of radiographic glenoid component failure have been associated with excessive glenoid reaming,[570] the use of keeled components,[572] the use of metal-backed components,[42,414] delayed rotator cuff disruption,[443,598] a biconcave glenoid,[119] and humeral component malposition (see Figs. 16-218 and 16-243 to 16-255).

Lack of clinical improvement can be defined in terms of failure to change an outcome score by the minimal clinically important difference (e.g., three points on the SST)[469] or by failure to improve by a certain percent of the maximum possible improvement.[173,354] *Surgical revision* rates can be obtained from national databases,[21,243] registries,[7,137,142,223,255,386,396,536] or systematic reviews of case series.[415] The proportion of arthroplasties that are revised increases with time after surgery, so protracted follow-up is needed to understand the durability of an arthroplasty. The mean time to revision for component loosening is approximately 8 years[59,78,121,218,302,443,519,550,570,598]; the commonly used 2-year minimum follow-up may therefore miss the majority of revisions. A particular issue in studying revision rates is that the threshold for performing a revision may vary widely, and it has been pointed out that the rate of revision underestimates the rate of clinical failure.[66,153,206] Some patients with loose glenoid components or rotator cuff failure may accept their symptoms rather than undergoing another procedure.[66] Poor patient health may preclude additional surgery, and some surgeons may be less eager than others to perform revisions after the failure of the initial procedure.[511] In addition, high revision rates with certain procedures may not be related to the procedure itself, but rather to its use by less skilled surgeons or its application to more complex problems. Finally, the definition of "revision" is not standardized: do revisions include manipulations and procedures in which the implants are not changed (such as washouts for infection, soft tissue releases, cuff repair, subscapularis repair, and neurolysis) or only those in which the implants were "revised"?

The challenge in evaluating arthroplasty failure relates to the need for good data on each of the four Ps: (1) the *problem* (i.e., the diagnosis and aspects of the shoulder itself)[217]; (2) the *patient*, including their physical, emotional, and social health, age, sex, occupation, comorbidities, level of education, and type of insurance[66,80,118,329,482,488,497,505]; (3) the *physician*, including their training, relevant case volume, and practice environment[199,207,242,243,313,502]; and (4) the *procedure*, including the surgical technique, perioperative care, and rehabilitation.[153,206,334,414,415] The analysis of failure seeks to determine whether the surgery failed because the *problem* was one that could not be well managed by the arthroplasty, because the *procedure* was not optimally selected or performed, because the *patient* was not a good candidate for the procedure, or because the *physician* (i.e., the surgeon) had received insufficient training, experience, or support. These factors can be interrelated; for example, inexperienced surgeons may be more likely to use hemiarthroplasty rather than total shoulder arthroplasty for treating more complex problems, creating three reasons why a systematic review comparing hemiarthroplasties to total shoulders might tend to favor the latter.[199,242,243,502] As it is the surgeon that selects the problem and patient to treat and the procedure to use in the treatment, the effect of the surgeon is the dominant factor—"the surgeon is the method."[328]

The most important studies of failure are those conducted by each individual surgeon seeking to determine the specific factors that may have contributed to the inability of a patient who is undergoing treatment involving a certain procedure for a specific problem to realize the expected benefit. Codman spoke of the "common sense notion that every hospital should follow every patient it treats, long enough to determine whether or not the treatment has been successful, and then to inquire 'If not, why not?' with a view for preventing similar failures in the future."[93,94] Note the emphasis that this quotation places on failures. As Codman pointed out, determining which patients fail requires the surgeon to use practical yet sensitive methods to follow the treated patients over time. For this purpose, our approach is to use the SST. This enables individuals to document the comfort and function before and sequentially after treatment using a validated and extensively used patient-reported metric that takes 1 minute to complete and that—in contrast to measurements of strength and range of motion—is relatively free of physician influence. It has also been shown to be stable across cultures.[357,395,556] By using this tool we have been able to learn what procedures in our hands are helpful in managing which diagnoses.[91,173,176,306,314,338,469,480] A convenient way to display these data is by using the Codman graph (Fig. 16-461), which shows the initial (preoperative) data and the outcome (postoperative) data for each patient. We can use these results to pick out the individual patients who did not benefit from our surgery and to see what could have been done better.[329] This is helpful in studying

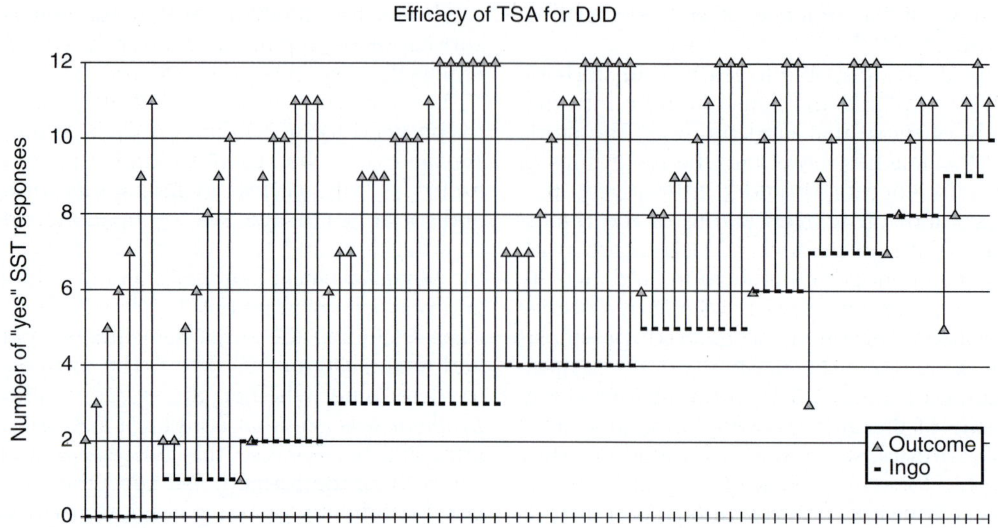

FIGURE 16-461: Codman graph showing the efficacy of total shoulder arthroplasty (TSA) for 82 patients with glenohumeral degenerative joint disease (DJD) monitored for at least 1 year. The ordinate indicates the number of the 12 Simple Shoulder Test questions answered "yes." Each patient is represented by a mark on the abscissa. The ingo for each patient is indicated by the short horizontal line. The outcome for each patient is indicated by the arrowhead. For each patient, efficacy is the height of the vertical line connecting the ingo to the outcome. The graph indicates that most but not all patients improved substantially after shoulder arthroplasty. *Ingo*, State of the shoulder before treatment.

established procedures, such as total shoulder arthroplasty,[139,176,420] as well as newer ones, such as the ream and run.[173]

Another critical tool for evaluating the quality and durability of an arthroplasty is serial standardized plain radiographs (see Figs. 16-371 and 16-372). It is obvious that CT scans are not useful for this purpose due to the cost, radiation exposure, and problems associated with artifact from the metal humeral head. A good example of the utility of plain films is in the evaluation of the quality of fixation and seating of the glenoid component after total shoulder arthroplasty (Fig. 16-462; see Fig. 16-353).[23,99,180,286,394,508] These studies showed that difficulties with glenoid component fixation and seating are common, especially with keeled components and for less experienced surgeons.

Modes of Failure

In the spirit of learning from failures of shoulder arthroplasty, it is informative to review the adverse outcomes that occur after these procedures and to consider how they could be avoided. The most commonly reported complications of shoulder arthroplasty include prosthetic loosening, glenohumeral instability, periprosthetic fractures, rotator cuff tears, infection, neural injury, and deltoid dysfunction. The reported complication rate associated with total shoulder arthroplasty is highly variable (0% to 62%),[340,594] with a mean value of around 10% to 16%.* With any type of presentation of failed arthroplasty,

References 41, 42, 47, 64, 72, 78, 121, 128, 130, 164, 173, 209, 218, 245, 257, 319, 320, 322, 338, 340, 346, 359, 403, 410, 418, 485, 513, 514, 518-520, 526, 550, 551, 572, 593, 594.

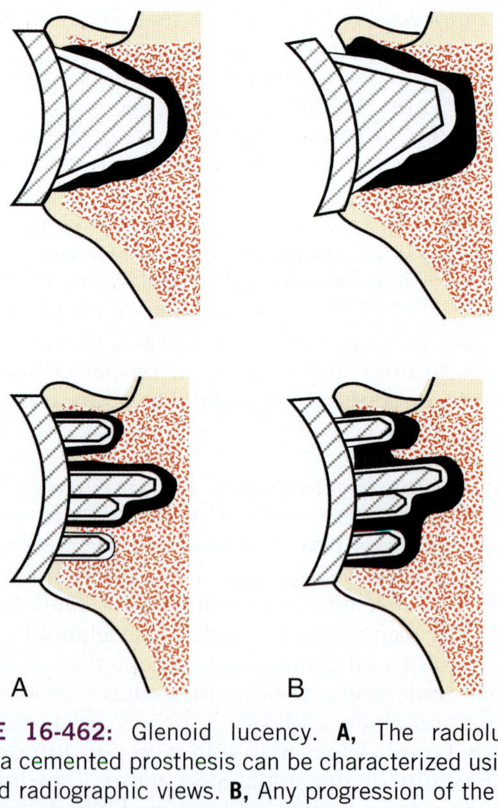

FIGURE 16-462: Glenoid lucency. **A,** The radiolucencies around a cemented prosthesis can be characterized using standardized radiographic views. **B,** Any progression of the lucency can be documented. (From Matsen FA III, Lippitt SB. *Shoulder Surgery: Principles and Procedures.* Philadelphia: Saunders; 2004:723.)

there is a substantial chance of a "stealth" infection; therefore, to exclude this possibility, we obtain cultures at any revision arthroplasty, as discussed in the section on infection below.

Stiffness. Although it is rarely listed as a complication of shoulder arthroplasties, stiffness is probably the most common adverse outcome of these procedures, reported by up to 75% of patients who were dissatisfied with their results.[153,206] Postarthroplasty stiffness has been an issue since the early days of the Neer arthroplasty, even to the extent that some cynics referred to it as a "Neer fusion." The evaluation of the stiff arthroplasty includes establishing a history of the initial diagnosis, the prearthroplasty range of motion, and the rehabilitation effort as well as review of the prior operative report. A physical examination documents the motion in flexion, abduction, external rotation, cross body adduction, and internal rotation in abduction. Radiographs are used to assess the size of the components compared with the preoperative glenohumeral anatomy, the component fixation, any evidence of infection, and the presence of unwanted bone contact between the humerus and the glenoid.

Gentle persistent stretching exercises are the first line of treatment for the stiff arthroplasty (see Figs. 16-136, 16-137, 16-140, and 16-141).[498] If the rehabilitation effort seems to be failing early (i.e., in the first month or so) after the arthroplasty, a gentle manipulation under anesthesia and complete muscle relaxation can be considered as long as the quality of the bone and soft tissues is excellent. Refractory shoulder stiffness uncomplicated by other factors can be managed by an open capsular release (Figs. 16-463 to 16-465; see Fig. 16-441); this may include resection of any blocking bone (see Figs. 16-226 to 16-228 and 16-434; Figs. 16-466 and 16-467). Stiffness may be caused by overstuffing of the joint by components that are relatively large (see Fig. 16-201) or malpositioned (see Fig. 16-202), in which case downsizing or repositioning the humeral head may help restore capsular laxity. Stiffness may also be a result of an indolent infection with *Propionibacterium* species, especially if it has an onset after an apparently normal postoperative course—a "honeymoon."

Infection. The reported incidence of infection in the literature for unconstrained primary shoulder arthroplasty ranges from 0% to 4%.[109,412,422,438,522] The actual rate may be much higher because many cases of "aseptic loosening" are now being found to be infected with

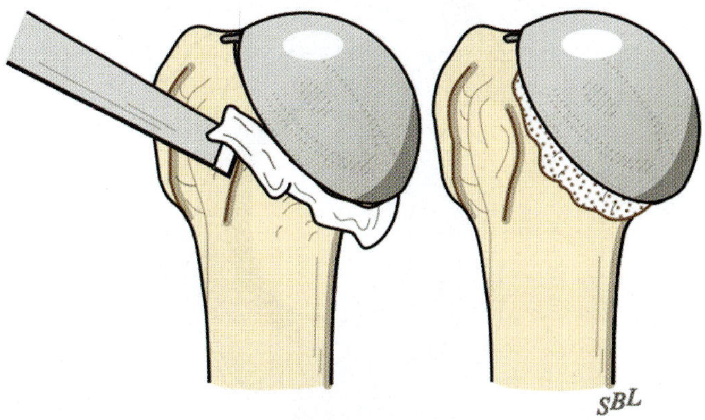

FIGURE 16-464: Any osteophytic bone that protrudes beyond the margin of the humeral head component and may block motion needs to be resected.

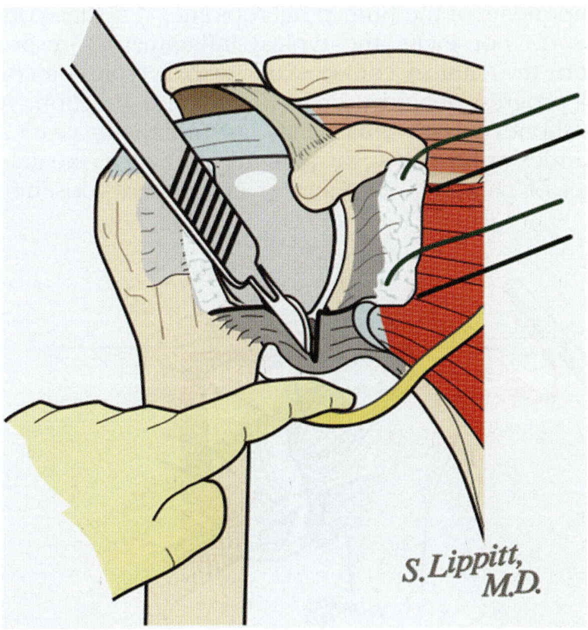

FIGURE 16-463: The axillary nerve should be protected during inferior capsular release, especially during altered anatomy in revision surgery.

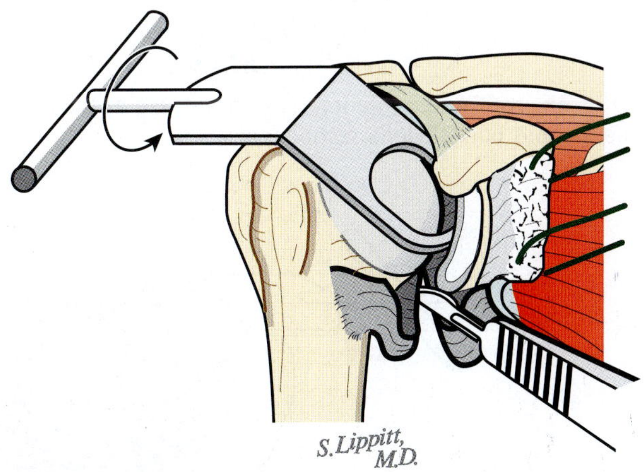

FIGURE 16-465: The posterior capsule is placed under tension by slightly internally rotating the humerus while a twist is applied to the retractor (arrow) so that the inferior humerus is pushed away from the glenoid. This tensioning facilitates the safe and selective release of the capsule. (From Matsen FA III, Lippitt SB. *Shoulder Surgery: Principles and Procedures.* Philadelphia: Saunders; 2004:674.)

slow-growing organisms that live on the patient's skin and hair follicles and sebaceous glands, such as *Propionibacterium* species and coagulase-negative staphylococci.[289,332,341,438]

Patients with infected arthroplasties may present with some combination of the classic symptoms and signs of infection: nonmechanical pain (i.e., pain when the arm is at rest), stiffness, fevers, chills, warmth, swelling, tenderness, redness, draining sinuses, an elevated white blood cell count, elevated serum C-reactive protein, and an elevated erythrocyte sedimentation rate. The laboratory values may be elevated early in a benign recovery, but persistently elevated values along with other clinical manifestations require further investigation.[281,549,580] Radiographs may reveal progressive bone loss and prosthetic loosening (Figs. 16-468 to 16-472; see Fig. 16-302). Fluoroscopically guided aspiration of the joint can provide fluid for culture, although the most common organism to be recovered from the shoulder, i.e., *Propionibacterium* species is characteristically ensconced in biofilms and thus fluid aspirates are often falsely negative. Arthroscopic tissue biopsy may have a higher yield of positive cultures than fluid aspiration.[124] It is important to appreciate that whereas *positive* cultures support the diagnosis of infection, *negative* cultures cannot exclude the possibility of infection. Surgical exploration may reveal cloudy joint fluid; acute or chronic inflammation; frozen sections with increased white blood cells per high-power field; and inflammatory markers in the joint fluid, such as leukocyte esterase, interleukin-6, and C-reactive protein, but again normal test results do not exclude the possibility of infection.[109,522,594]

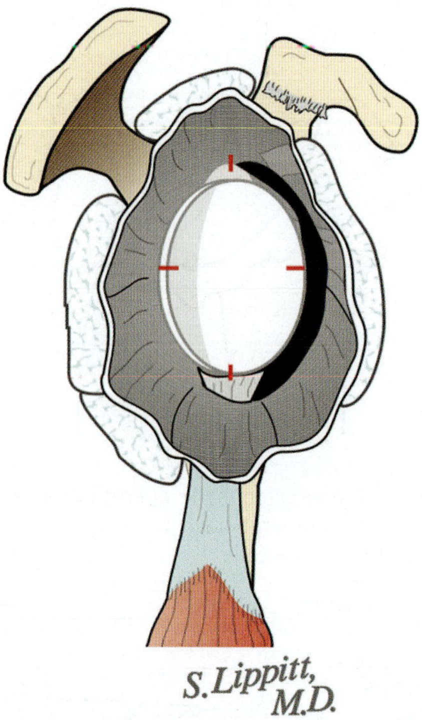

FIGURE 16-466: Anteroinferior capsular release at the margin of the glenoid polyethylene component.

Over the last several years it has become clear that there are two types of infection that can complicate shoulder arthroplasty. The "classic" type is similar to the infections that complicate hip and knee arthroplasty,[422,446,552] where organisms, such as *Staphylococcus aureus,* streptococci, or enterococci, infect total joints, especially in patients at increased risk because of diabetes, rheumatoid arthritis, systemic lupus erythematosus, chemotherapy, systemic corticosteroid administration, repeated intra-articular steroid injections, poor skin coverage, or distant sites of hematogenous spread.

Recently, the "stealth" type of infection has been identified; that is, an infection caused by commensal organisms from the patient's skin, such as *Propionibacterium* species and coagulase-negative staphylococci.[13,14,153,206,289,341,438,521,522,549] As they are normal components of the human microbiome,[182,408] these organisms do not incite the typical inflammatory response. Often, the clinical course starts with a typical recovery and progress in increasing comfort and function. After this "honeymoon," which may last months or years after the index arthroplasty, the patient experiences the gradual onset of pain, stiffness, and/or component loosening.[355]

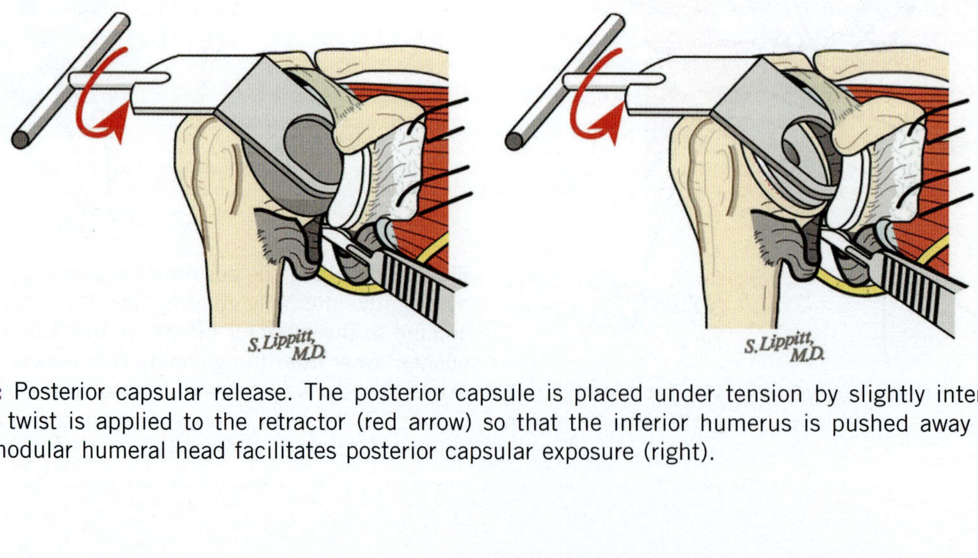

FIGURE 16-467: Posterior capsular release. The posterior capsule is placed under tension by slightly internally rotating the humerus while a twist is applied to the retractor (red arrow) so that the inferior humerus is pushed away from the glenoid. Removal of the modular humeral head facilitates posterior capsular exposure (right).

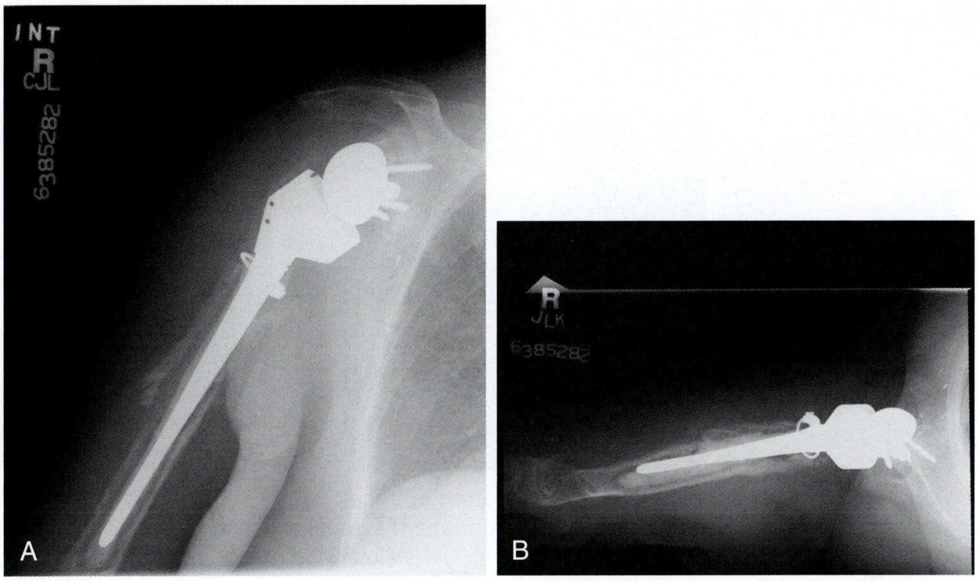

FIGURE 16-468: Radiographs of a 60-year-old patient with an infected long stem reverse prosthesis. There is significant periprosthetic lucency as well as periosteal new bone formation. **A,** Anteroposterior view. **B,** Axillary view.

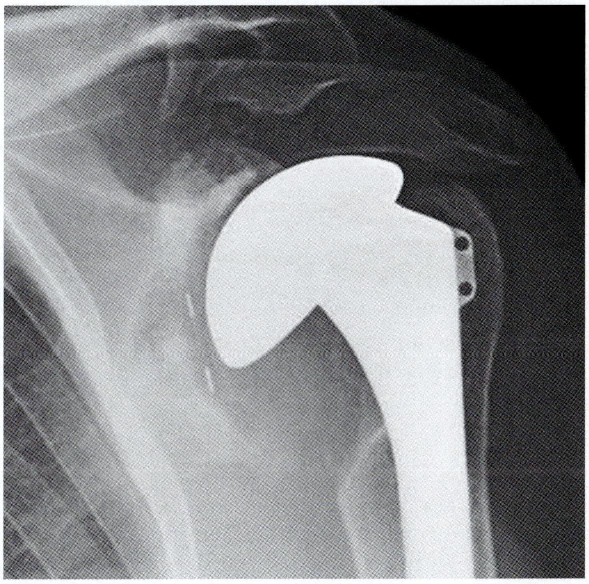

FIGURE 16-469: Shoulder arthroplasty complicated by an infection with *Propionibacterium* species. Note the loose glenoid and the medial humeral osteolysis.

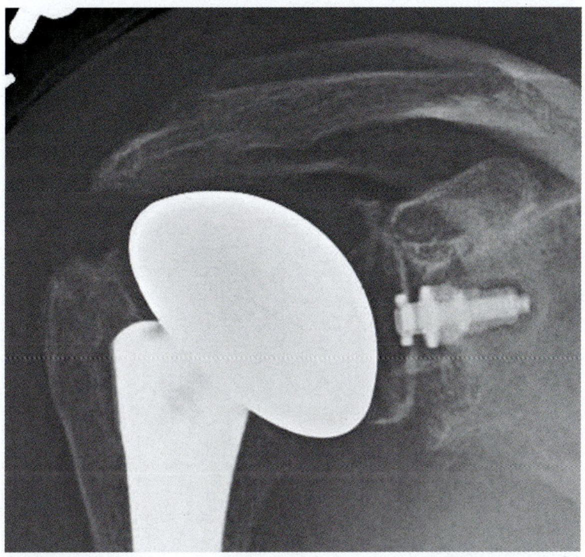

FIGURE 16-470: Loose glenoid with *Propionibacterium* species infection.

The indolent yet pernicious nature of these infections is related to the organisms' tendency to form a biofilm on the surface of the implants where they can exist chronically, protected from the body's immune systems and from antibiotic treatment (see Fig. 16-282). The characteristic signs of infection (warmth, redness, swelling, and abnormal serum laboratory tests) are typically absent, and so the finding of positive cultures may be unexpected.[147,188] These organisms require special methods for their identification, including the harvest of at least five specimens of tissue or explant, culturing on aerobic and anaerobic media, and observation for 17 days.[73,332]

Early in their course, acute periprosthetic shoulder infections may be treated with irrigation, debridement, and antibiotics; however, the results of this approach are often unsatisfactory.[109,522] Because periprosthetic shoulder infections are usually chronic at the time of diagnosis, treatment usually requires removal of the implants that have become coated with antibiotic-resistant biofilms. The ever-present risk of the need to remove an infected

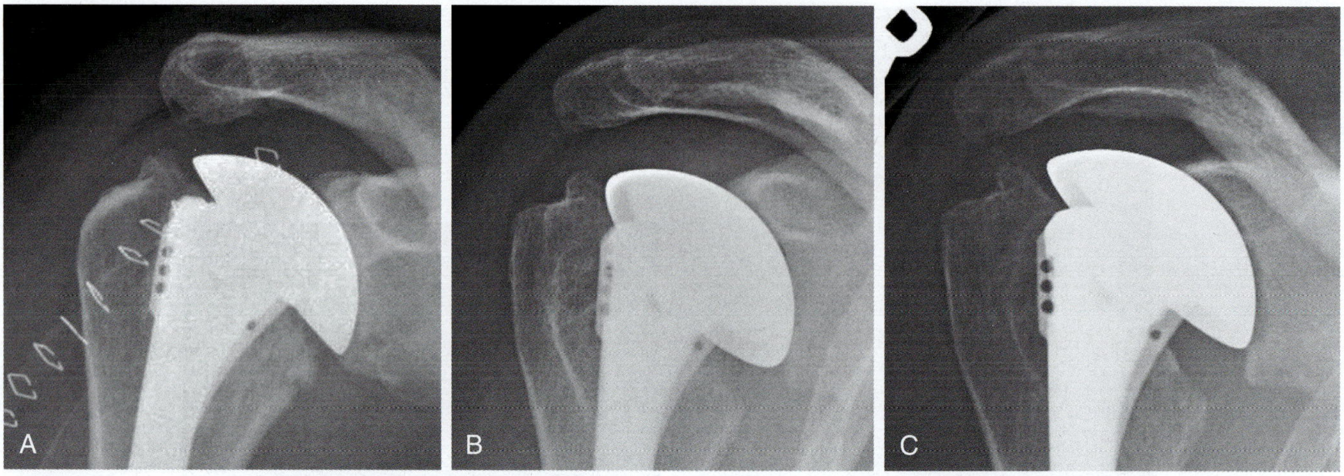

FIGURE 16-471: Delayed *Propionibacterium* species infection after an initially successful ream and run procedure. **A,** Immediate postoperative radiograph. **B,** Radiograph at 9 months, at which time the patient had returned to all physical activities without difficulty. **C,** Radiograph at 18 months, at which time the patient had shoulder pain and stiffness, glenoid resorption, and multiple positive cultures for *Propionibacterium* species at revision surgery.

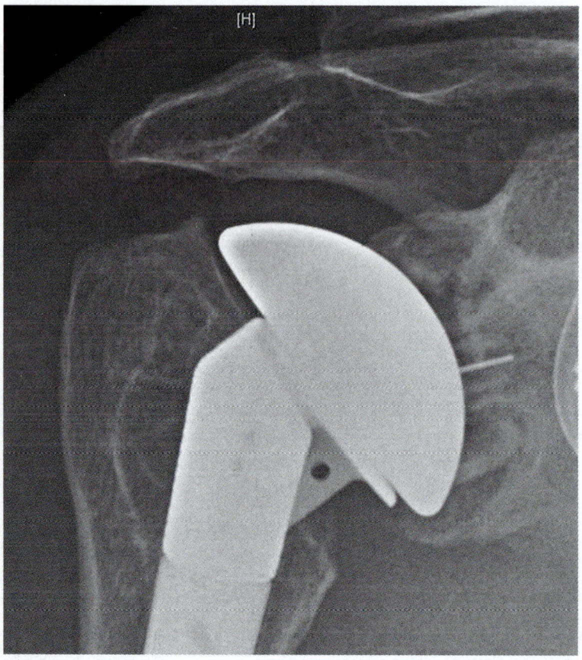

FIGURE 16-472: Loose glenoid component with osteolysis. The shoulder had multiple positive cultures for *Propionibacterium* species at revision surgery.

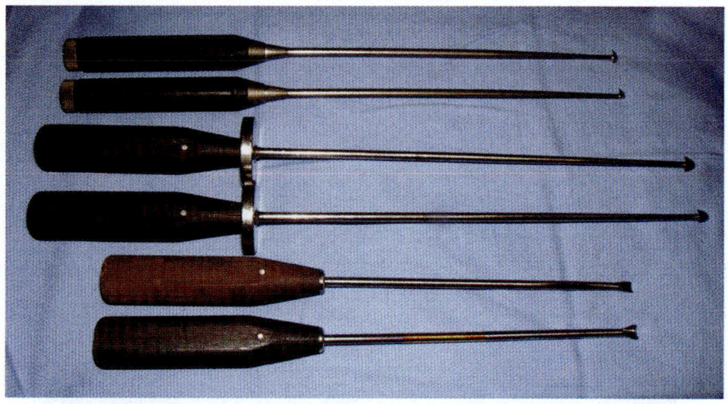

FIGURE 16-473: An assortment of instruments and cement-removal tools may be necessary to ensure complete removal of cement.

implant is one of the major reasons to avoid cemented humeral stems, bone ingrowth humeral stems, and platform prostheses, each of which can be very difficult to remove without humeral osteotomy (Figs. 16-473 and 16-474).[515] Cement removal is very hazardous even with the use of special osteotomes, sonic devices,[175] and fluoroscopic guidance.

In performing a revision of any failed arthroplasty, it should be recognized that the risk of positive cultures is high,[438] even though clinical evidence and observations at the time of surgery are usually insufficient to make or exclude a diagnosis of infection. Preoperative antibiotics are therefore withheld before revision surgery to allow for the harvest of at least five explant or tissue samples for culture. Ceftriaxone and vancomycin are then administered. Unhealthy tissue is thoroughly debrided. Every attempt is made to preserve the rotator cuff and to restore the suppleness of the subscapularis for repair at the conclusion of the case. Frozen sections of suspicious tissue are submitted to determine the number of white blood cells per high-power field.

Because the results of intraoperative cultures obtained at the time of revision arthroplasty cannot be known until well after the patient has left the operating room, the surgeon needs to make a judgment at the time of surgery between two protocols: (1) the "yellow" protocol, in which the prostheses are retained and the patient is placed on oral antibiotics (usually Augmentin) until the culture results are finalized and the therapeutic plan

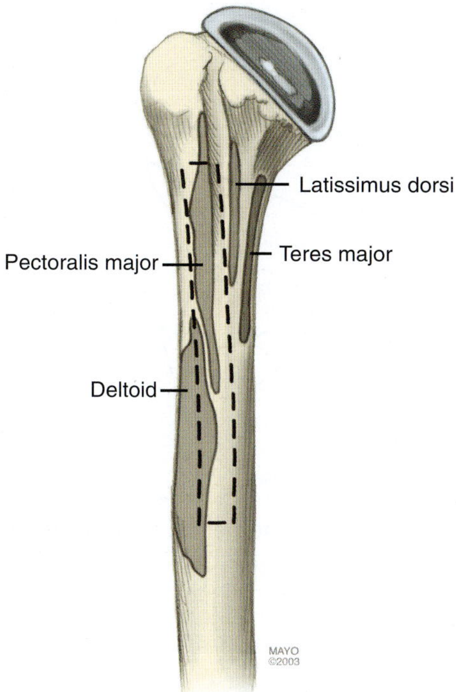

FIGURE 16-474: A humeral window may be necessary to remove a well-fixed component. (From Sperling JW, Cofield RH. Humeral windows in revision shoulder arthroplasty. *J Shoulder Elbow Surg.* 2005;14:258-263.)

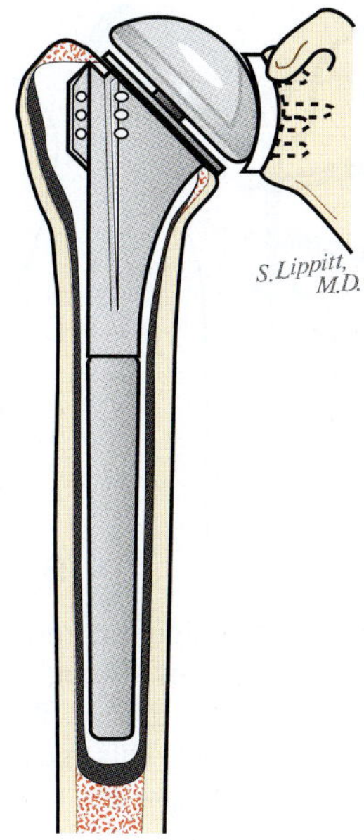

FIGURE 16-475: Loose cemented stem. When there is a lucent zone completely around the humeral component and any cement used for fixation, component removal is usually straightforward. (From Matsen FA III, Lippitt SB. *Shoulder Surgery: Principles and Procedures.* Philadelphia: Saunders; 2004:717.)

adjusted accordingly, or (2) the "red" protocol, in which the prostheses are removed, a thorough debridement carried out, a primary humeral exchange performed with vancomycin-soaked allograft, and 6 weeks of IV antibiotics administered (usually ceftriaxone, unless the cultures are positive for *mecA* staphylococcus, in which case vancomycin is maintained). At 3 weeks, the program is adjusted according to the culture findings. Active culture yogurt and probiotics are recommended for all patients on antibiotics.

In the red protocol, the humeral component is removed (Figs. 16-475 to 16-477; see Figs. 16-335 and 16-336) and the canal thoroughly curetted to remove the infected membrane that often forms between the bone and the prosthesis. The glenoid component is removed, usually leaving a substantial defect in the glenoid bone (Figs. 16-478 to 16-481). Rather than considering reimplantation, the residual glenoid surface is smoothed to provide a surface congruent with the humeral component (Fig. 16-482). Although some surgeons routinely use a two-stage humeral exchange—prosthesis is removed with the insertion of an antibiotic-impregnated spacer (Figs. 16-483 and 16-484), followed by a second procedure that reinserts a humeral component (Fig. 16-485)[248,372,444,479,527]—we reserve this two-surgery approach for cases with particularly virulent infections. For most cases we perform a primary humeral component exchange[238] after vigorous debridement of all explants, cement, and unhealthy tissue and after irrigation with 3 to 6 L of saline that contains ceftriaxone and vancomycin. A humeral prosthesis that articulates well with the residual glenoid and provides proper mobility and stability is then selected. To avoid the use of cement, this component is inserted with vancomycin-soaked allograft (see Fig. 16-323). This approach has several

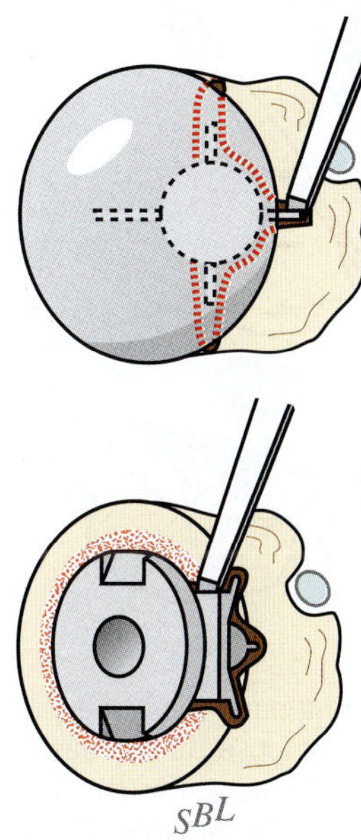

FIGURE 16-476: Freeing the fins. If the stem must be removed, the first step is to remove all bone and cement from the path for backing out the fins. Care should be taken to protect the rotator cuff during this dissection. (From Matsen FA III, Lippitt SB. *Shoulder Surgery: Principles and Procedures.* Philadelphia: Saunders; 2004:718.)

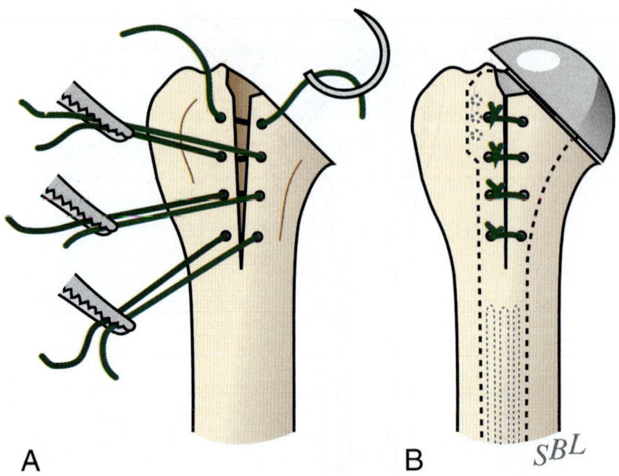

FIGURE 16-477: A, The osteotomy is repaired by passing No. 2 braided nonabsorbable sutures through drill holes on either side of the split in the bicipital groove. **B,** Tying these sutures reconstitutes the humeral shaft. This repair technique is safer than cerclage, which can endanger the radial nerve posteriorly. (From Matsen FA III, Lippitt SB. *Shoulder Surgery: Principles and Procedures.* Philadelphia: Saunders; 2004:722.)

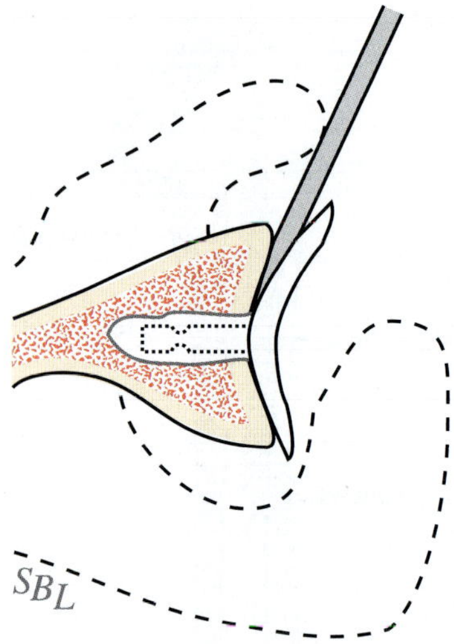

FIGURE 16-479: Cutting the glenoid component. When a polyethylene glenoid component is well fixed, the surface of the component can be cut with an osteotome, allowing access to the pegs or keel and the cement. (From Matsen FA III, Lippitt SB. *Shoulder Surgery: Principles and Procedures.* Philadelphia: Saunders; 2004:725.)

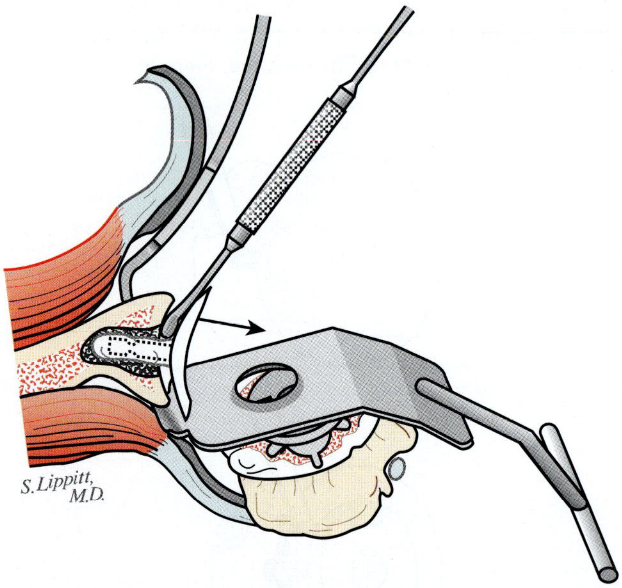

FIGURE 16-478: Prying out a loose glenoid component. When a glenoid component is loose, it can easily be lifted from the glenoid bone. (From Matsen FA III, Lippitt SB. *Shoulder Surgery: Principles and Procedures.* Philadelphia: Saunders; 2004:725.)

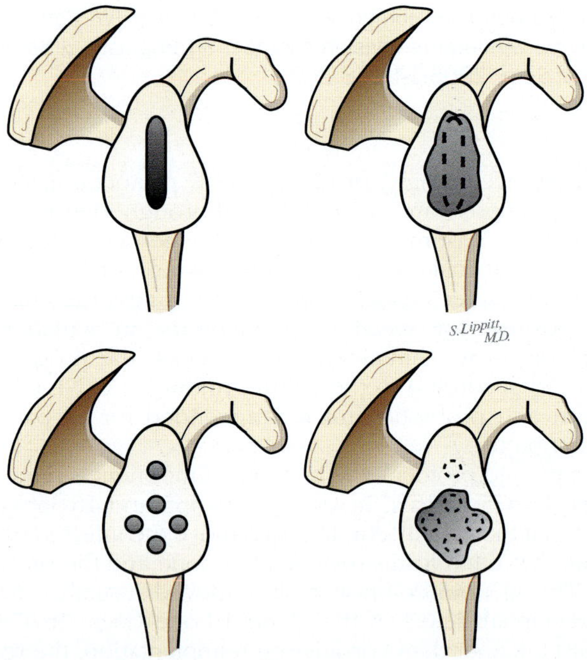

FIGURE 16-480: The potential for reinserting a glenoid prosthesis is determined in large part by the amount of subchondral bone that remains intact to support the component. (From Matsen FA III, Lippitt SB. *Shoulder Surgery: Principles and Procedures.* Philadelphia: Saunders; 2004:726.)

advantages: it potentially avoids another surgical procedure, it enables routine postoperative rehabilitation to restore motion, and it provides secure fixation with reinforcement of the residual humeral bone without compromising any further revision surgery that may become necessary. Unless cultures are negative at 3 weeks after surgery, IV antibiotics administered through a peripherally inserted central catheter are continued for 6 weeks, after which the patient is placed on 1 year of oral antibiotic suppression. Again, active culture yogurt and probiotics are recommended for all patients on antibiotics.

Other approaches to infection have included resection arthroplasty (see Figs. 16-71 and 16-165),[145,454] arthrodesis, and amputation. Long-term antibiotic suppression is

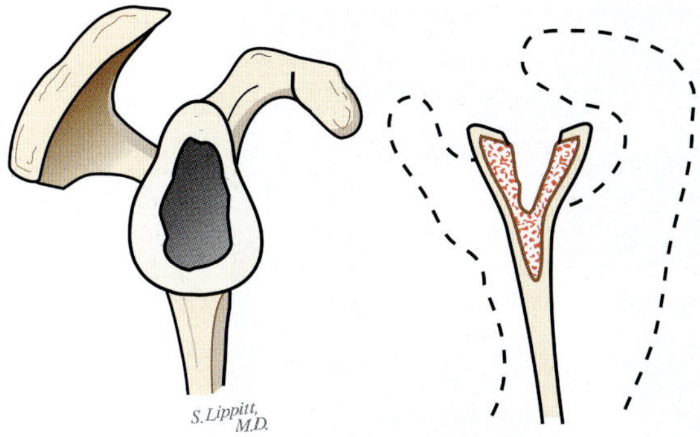

FIGURE 16-481: When the glenoid defect is large, refixation of a glenoid component may be difficult. (From Matsen FA III, Lippitt SB. *Shoulder Surgery: Principles and Procedures.* Philadelphia: Saunders; 2004:727.)

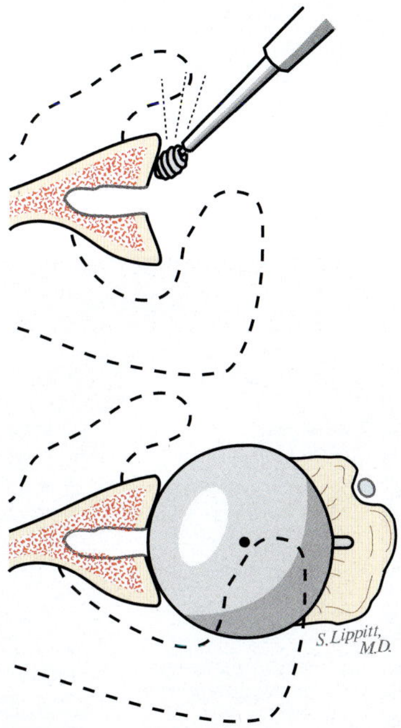

FIGURE 16-482: When the revision arthroplasty does not allow a secure glenoid component reimplantation, it is usually possible to smooth off the remaining bony glenoid surface with a bur (as shown here) or with a reamer and possibly fill the void with cancellous graft. (From Matsen FA III, Lippitt SB. *Shoulder Surgery: Principles and Procedures.* Philadelphia: Saunders; 2004:727.)

considered for patients too fragile for the challenges of revision surgery.

Although there has been much effort to define a "true" infection[372] as opposed to a "contaminant," it is simpler and clearer to present the results of cultures in a manner that records both the number of specimens that were culture-positive from each source and the total number of specimens taken from each source. As an example, "*Propionibacterium*: explant 2+/2, tissue 4+/5, fluid 0+/1" would indicate that two explant specimens, five tissue specimens, and one fluid specimen were submitted and

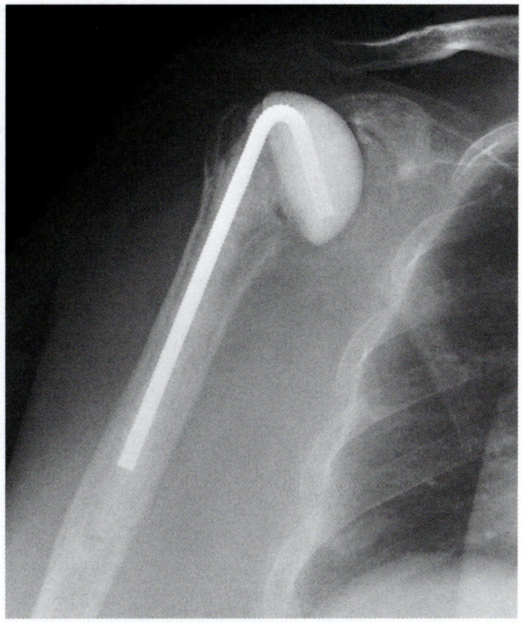

FIGURE 16-483: Tightly cemented cement spacers do not usually provide a durable humeral articular surface and may be difficult to remove at the time of revision arthroplasty.

that two, four, and zero of these, respectively, were positive for *Propionibacterium* species (see Fig. 16-282). Using this system permits clearer interpretation of the significance of culture results.

Glenoid Failure. The glenoid side of the joint remains the weakest link in shoulder arthroplasty (see Figs. 16-274 and 16-284). Glenoid arthrosis after a hemiarthroplasty may be managed by revision with a total shoulder arthroplasty.[78,186] After a total shoulder arthroplasty, glenoid component failure can take place in the form of polyethylene deformity or loosening. With polyethylene deformity, the original shape of the articular surface becomes progressively distorted over time from wear (see Fig. 16-254), fracture, or cold flow (see Figs. 16-271, 16-297, and 16-349; Fig. 16-486).[53,399,487,578] Polyethylene wear particles that are approximately three microns in size can elicit a phagocytic response that mimics low-grade infection (Fig. 16-487). Occasionally, this process can lead to detritic synovitis that can strongly resemble infection, even down to the presence of cloudy joint fluid (see Fig. 16-487).

Polyethylene failure appears to be more common with metal-backed glenoid components.[414] Polyethylene deformities can compromise the stabilizing effect of the prosthetic glenoid conformity.[53,399,487,578] The management of significant glenoid component wear requires removal of the glenoid component.

Loosening of the glenoid component is one of the most common complications of total shoulder arthroplasty (see Figs. 16-253 and 16-486).* Despite many different

**References 6, 42, 64, 72, 78, 121, 128-130, 152, 164, 174, 181, 209, 218, 245, 309, 319, 320, 322, 326, 334, 346, 359, 403, 410, 414, 415, 418, 485, 487, 513, 514, 518-520, 526, 550, 551, 565, 570, 572, 594, 598.*

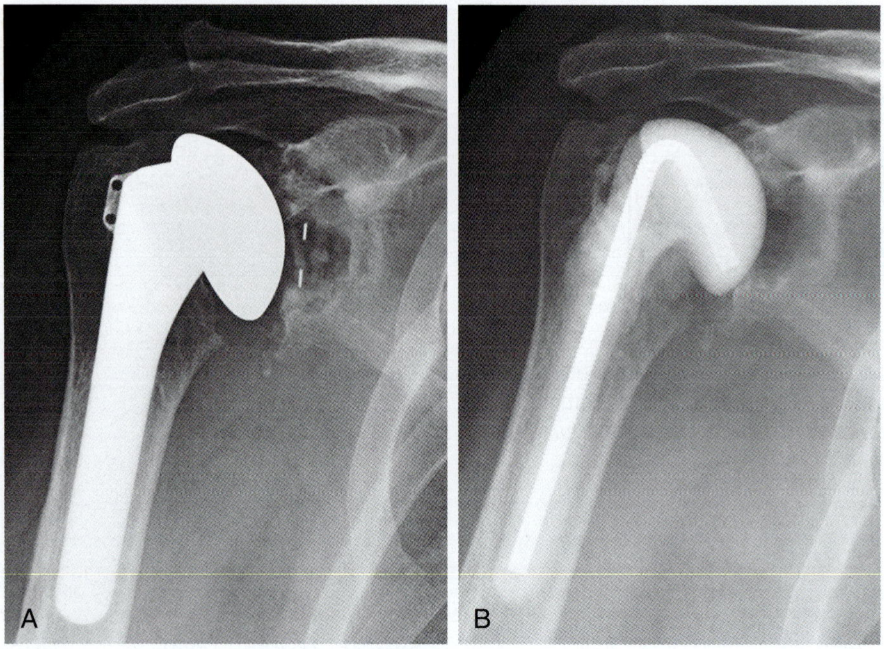

FIGURE 16-484: **A,** Infected loose glenoid component. **B,** This was treated with excision and a spacer.

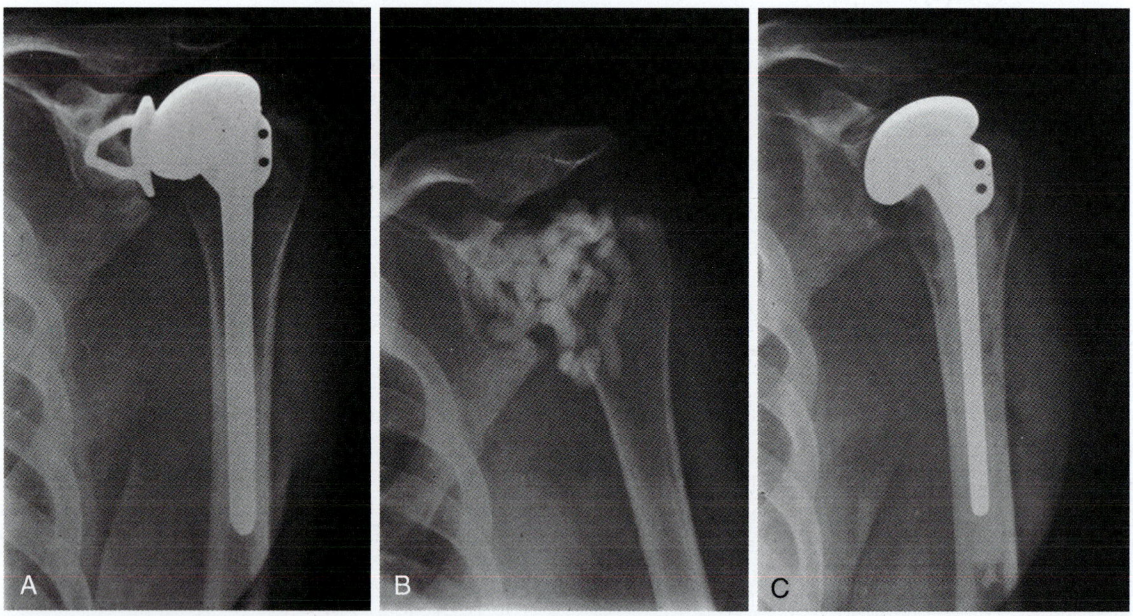

FIGURE 16-485: Radiographs of a patient who underwent a total shoulder arthroplasty for osteoarthritis. He presented with pain and a fever 6 years after surgery. **A,** The radiograph demonstrates glenoid component loosening and humeral osteolysis. **B,** The patient underwent component removal and placement of antibiotic-impregnated beads. **C,** He underwent delayed reimplantation 2 months following component removal. (From Sperling JW, Kozak TKW, Hanssen AD, Cofield RH. Infection after shoulder arthroplasty. *Clin Orthop Relat Res.* 2001;383:206-216.)

approaches attempting to improve long-term glenoid stability,[42,234,322,565,572,588,590,594] radiolucencies at the cement-bone interface of the glenoid remain common and progressive[23,29,51,56,99,163,269,286,590] (see Figs. 16-214 and 16-249). In studies with an average follow-up of 10 years or more, glenoid radiolucent lines are evident in nearly 80% of shoulders, and radiographic loosening (migration, tilt or shift of the component, or a complete radiolucent line greater than 1.5 mm[322]) is noted in more than one third.[526,550] Early enthusiasm for metal-backed glenoid implants has been tempered by longer follow-up studies revealing radiolucent line progression, severe osteolysis, polyethylene–metal

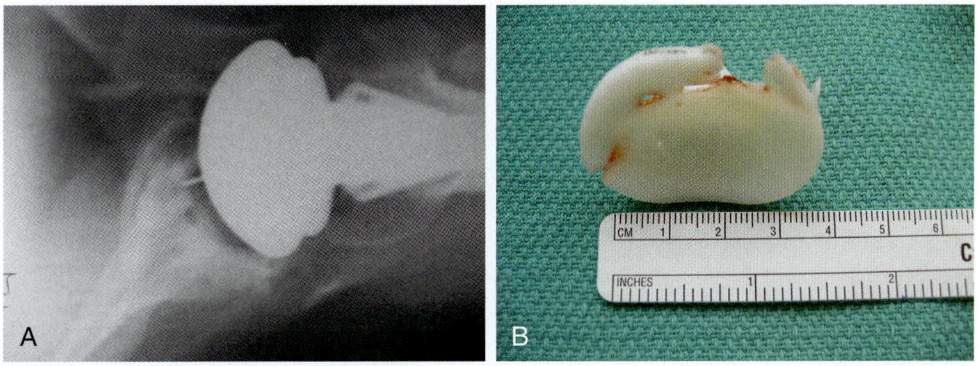

FIGURE 16-486: **A,** Axillary view of a circumferential glenoid radiolucent line in a 63-year-old patient with a 6-month history of persistent shoulder pain. **B,** Gross specimen of explanted keeled glenoid component with macroscopic structural damage and polyethylene wear. (From Bohsali KI, Wirth MA, Rockwood CA. Complications of total shoulder arthroplasty. *J Bone Joint Surg Am.* 2006;88:2279-2292.)

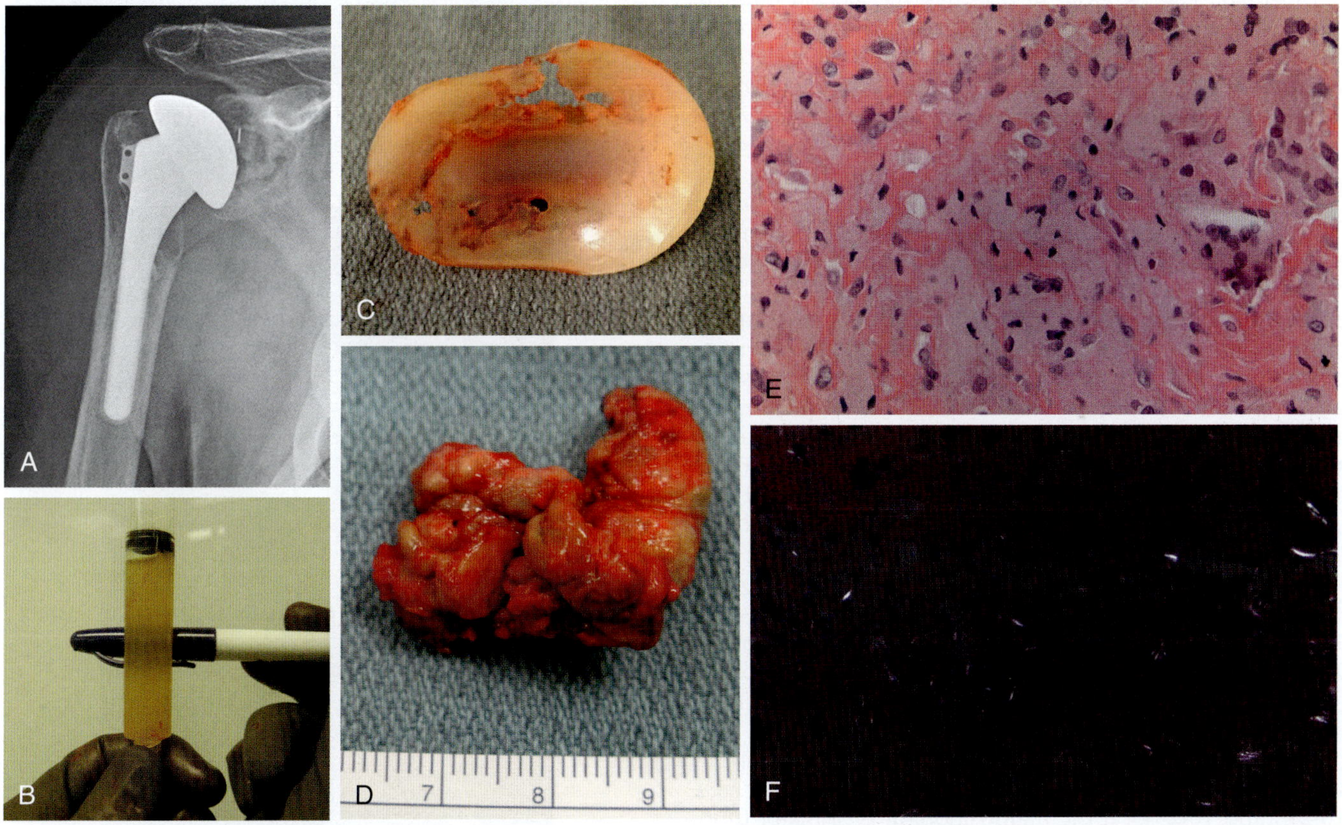

FIGURE 16-487: Detritic synovitis with negative bacterial cultures. **A,** Loose glenoid component and humeral osteolysis, suggesting infection. **B,** Cloudy joint fluid, suggesting infection. **C,** Fragmented glenoid component. **D,** Glenoid membrane. **E,** High-power microscopy showing multinucleated giant cells. **F,** Polarized microscopy showing fragments of polyethylene.

tray dissociation, glenoid tray fracture, screw breakage, and a reported revision rate three times that of all-polyethylene components.[42,86,322,414,461-463,572]

In considering a shoulder with a loose glenoid it is important to recall that a substantial number of these cases will have cultures positive for *Propionibacterium* species—a loose glenoid component in the absence of obvious evidence of infection cannot be assumed to represent "aseptic" loosening.[438] Our practice is to obtain tissue and explant cultures for *Propionibacterium* species in all cases of revision for glenoid loosening. The surgeon must then select between the yellow and red protocols as described previously.

Whether the glenoid component is removed due to wear, loosening, or infection, we usually do not reimplant a new one[6,131] because of the problem of bone

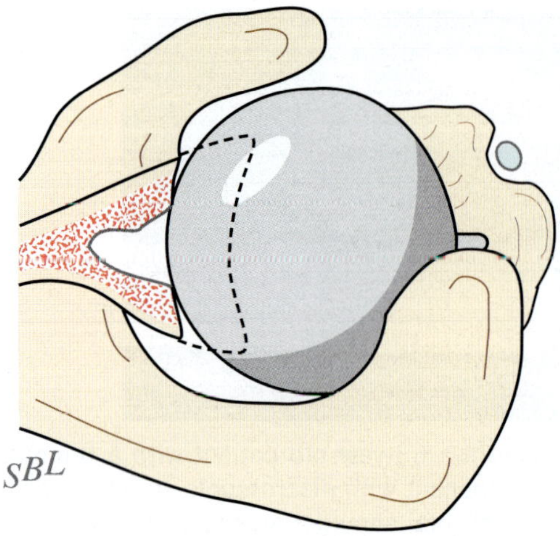

FIGURE 16-488: Excising the glenoid. When there is insufficient bone for reaming to an effective concavity or for grafting, consideration can be given to resecting the glenoid down to the base of the coracoid and scapular spine, leaving a deep dish for articulation with a humeral head of relatively large diameter. (From Matsen FA III, Lippitt SB. *Shoulder Surgery: Principles and Procedures.* Philadelphia: Saunders; 2004:711.)

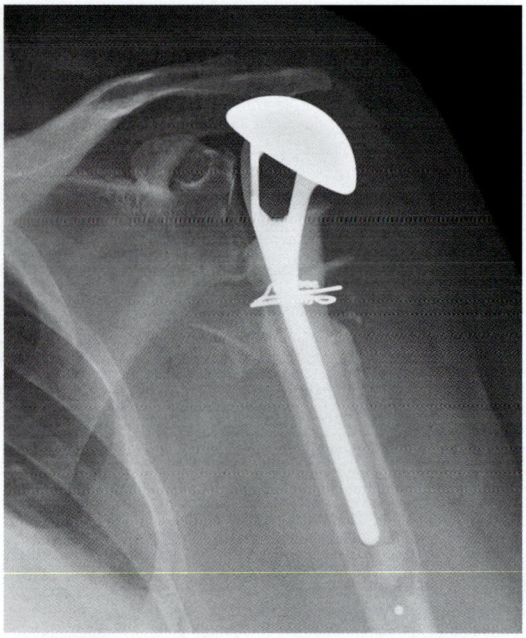

FIGURE 16-489: Loosening of a cemented fracture prosthesis in a proximally deficient humerus.

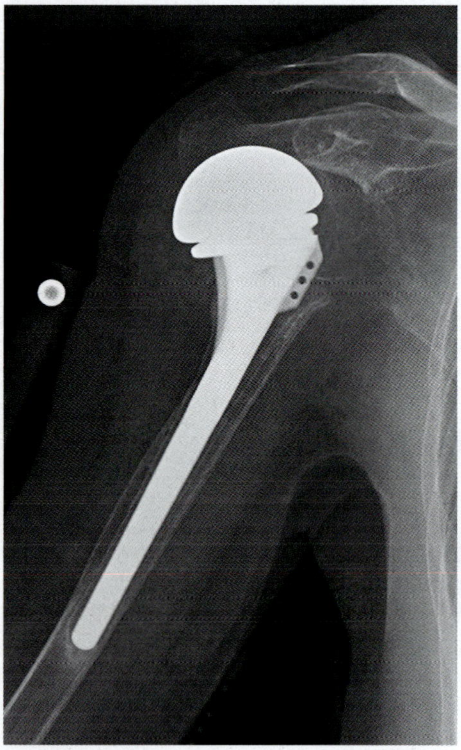

FIGURE 16-490: Loosening of an uncemented prosthesis in a proximally deficient humerus.

deficiency and the high risk of repeat glenoid component failure[44,84] (see Figs. 16-283 and 16-478 to 16-482). Instead, we prefer to smooth the residual glenoid bone and shape it to articulate with a humeral component of large diameter of curvature (see Fig. 16-283). We have not found it useful to add bone graft (see Fig. 16-482). If the insertion of the original glenoid component required posterior glenoid bone resection to accommodate a posteriorly augmented glenoid component, restoration of posterior stability may be very difficult (see Fig. 16-276). In extreme situations it may be necessary to excise the glenoid and position a large humeral head between the coracoid and the scapular spine (Fig. 16-488).

Humeral Component Failure. Humeral component failure can be related to malpositioning (see Fig. 16-255) or loosening (Figs. 16-489 and 16-490). Malpositioning includes incorrect version, varus, or valgus malpositioning (see Fig. 16-202). The most common form of malpositioning is when the humeral component is excessively high (see Figs. 16-244 and 16-335), often due to an attempt to insert a stem that is too large for the diaphysis (see Figs. 16-245 and 16-271). If the malpositioning is of major functional significance, the prosthesis may need to be removed (see Figs. 16-335 and 16-476), and a new prosthesis—usually one with a smaller stem diameter—repositioned using impaction allografting (see Fig. 16-323). If a humeral osteotomy is required (see Fig. 16-336), we prefer to close it using a bodice repair (see Fig. 16-477) rather than a cerclage wire that can endanger the radial nerve and crush the bone when it is tightened.

Humeral component loosening is much less common than glenoid component loosening, but it is not rare.* As described earlier for glenoid component loosening, each case of apparently "aseptic" humeral component loosening may actually be infected with *Propionibacterium* species,[438] and thus explant and tissue cultures should be taken at the time of revision surgery, even if clinical

References 108, 121, 128-130, 174, 181, 209, 218, 245, 271, 319, 320, 322, 336, 350, 359, 367, 410.

evidence of infection is lacking. The surgeon must then select between the yellow and red protocols as described in the section on infection.

Because humeral component loosening is a result of bone loss around the implant (see Fig. 16-475), our approach to reinsertion is to avoid additional reaming and cementing, as each of these methods carries the risk of additional bone loss. Instead, we carefully curette any residual soft tissue from the medullary cavity and insert the new component with a vancomycin-soaked allograft (see Fig. 16-323) for both fixation and bone augmentation (see Figs. 16-314 and 16-326).

Instability. Glenohumeral instability may involve the humeral head displacing anteriorly, posteriorly, superiorly, or inferiorly (Fig. 16-491). Instability may result from soft tissue or component positioning issues, or both. If the stability of an anatomic shoulder arthroplasty cannot be restored, a reverse total shoulder arthroplasty may be considered (see Fig. 16-113).

Anterior instability is usually associated with some combination of subscapularis deficiency, glenoid anteversion, humeral component anteversion, anterior deltoid dysfunction, anterior capsule failure, and loss of the stabilizing effect of the coracoacromial arch (see Fig. 16-252).[57,366,485,574,594] Subscapularis failure may result from a weak tendon, a weak repair, external rotator stretching during the early postoperative period, premature forceful contraction of the subscapularis, falls, or tendon compromise from lengthening techniques.[57,360] Individuals with heavy arms and those with prior subscapularis incisions seem to be at particular risk. Because the first subscapularis repair is always the best repair, we take great care in repairing good tendon to good bone with six nonabsorbable sutures at the time of the primary arthroplasty (see Fig. 16-445), and we avoid external rotator stretching past zero degrees for 6 weeks and internal rotator strengthening for 3 months.

Subscapularis failure is indicated by increased external rotation (Fig. 16-492), a lack of internal rotation strength (Fig. 16-493), and the palpable absence of the tendon when the shoulder is rotated (Fig. 16-494; see Fig. 16-12). An axillary radiograph may reveal anterior translation of the head on the glenoid (Fig. 16-495). If revision surgery is performed, our preference is to reinforce the repair of a previously failed subscapularis reattachment. As long as there is sufficient subscapularis muscle, the failed tendon can usually be reconstructed by a hamstring allograft passed through the residual subscapularis tendon and attached either to humeral soft tissue (Fig. 16-496) or to drill holes in the lesser tuberosity (see Fig. 16-495). If the subscapularis is not amenable to reconstruction, we use a tendon allograft to create an anterior checkrein to limit external rotation (Figs. 16-497 to Fig. 16-502). If excessive glenoid anteversion is indicated by the axillary view, consideration can be given to a revision glenoid arthroplasty, either by reaming the high posterior side (Fig. 16-503) or by bone grafting the anterior aspect of the socket (Fig. 16-504). Excessive humeral anteversion can be managed by humeral component repositioning.

Posterior instability (see Fig. 16-244) can arise from inadvertent transection of the rotator cuff or tuberosity when performing the humeral osteotomy, from overtightened anterior soft tissues (see Figs. 16-88 and 16-197), from excess humeral component retroversion, from glenoid retroversion (Fig. 16-505), or from posterior glenoid bone deficiency (Fig. 16-506).[57,218,366,383,574,594] Unless it is recognized and repaired at the time of the

Text continued on p. 1016

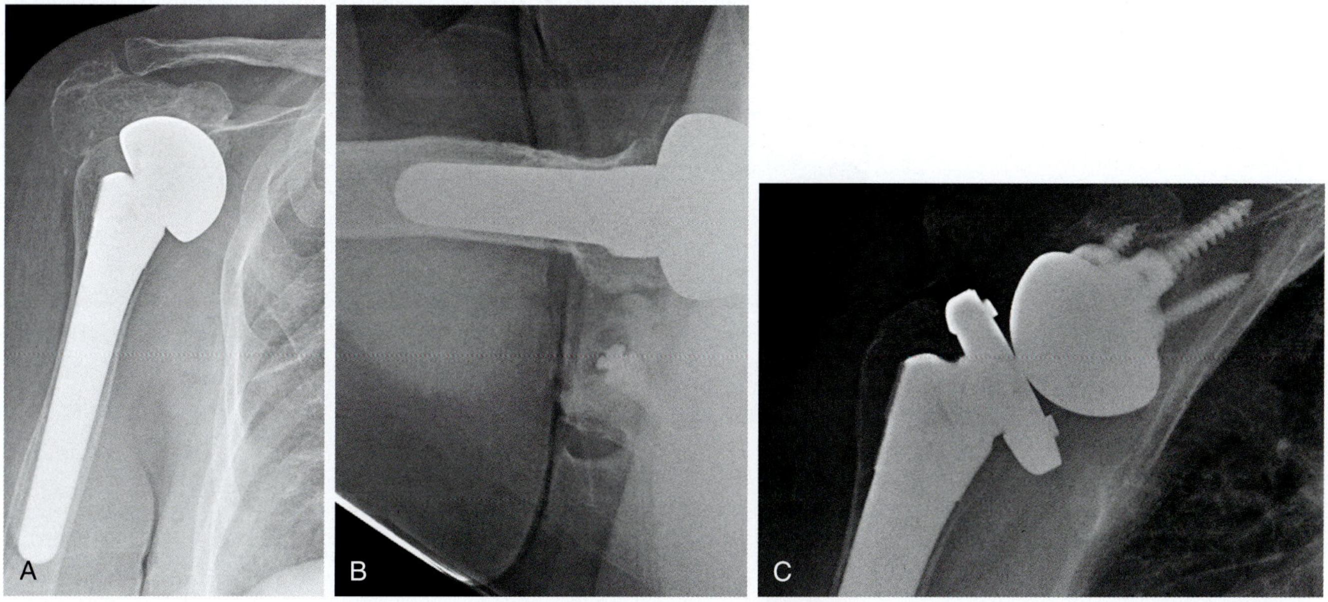

FIGURE 16-491: **A** and **B,** Anteroposterior and axillary views of an anteriorly dislocated total shoulder arthroplasty. **C,** This was managed with conversion to a reverse total shoulder arthroplasty, accomplished without needing to remove the humeral stem.

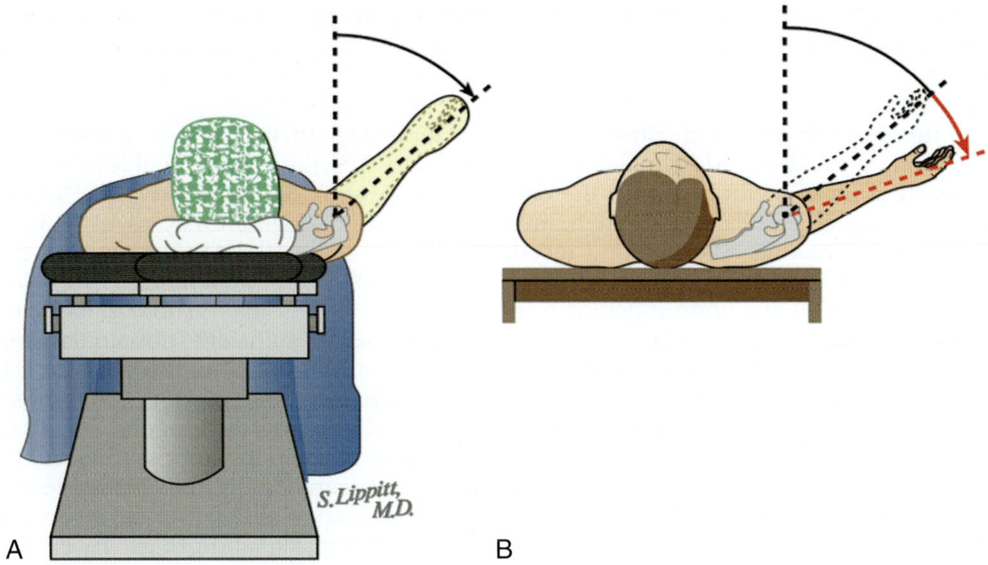

FIGURE 16-492: **A,** The limit to passive external rotation should be recorded after intraoperative subscapularis tendon repair. **B,** Excessive postoperative passive external rotation indicates loss of subscapularis attachment.

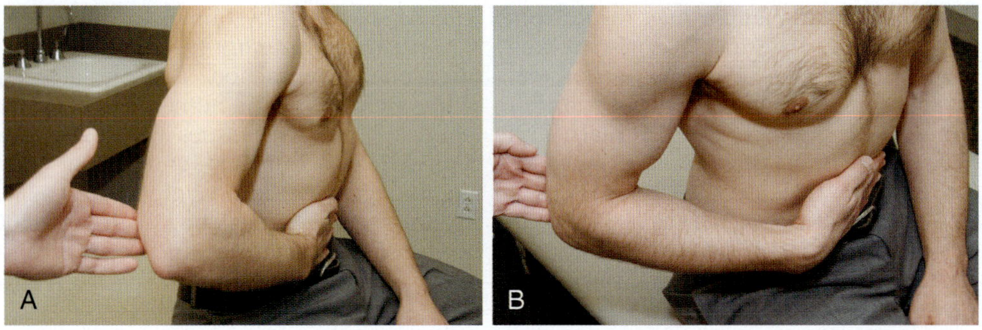

FIGURE 16-493: The belly-press test. **A,** The test is negative when the patient can press the hand against the abdomen while keeping the wrist straight and the elbow in front of the plane of the body. **B,** The test is positive when the patient must flex the wrist to press against the abdomen.

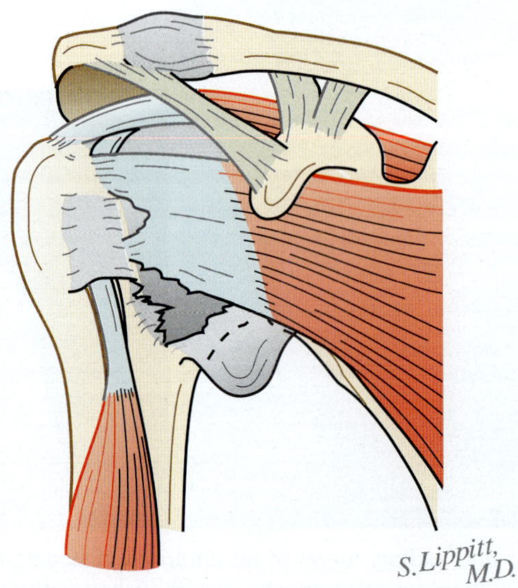

FIGURE 16-494: Defects in the anterior capsule and subscapularis may be substantial due to loss of tendon and capsular tissue. (From Matsen FA III, Lippitt SB. *Shoulder Surgery: Principles and Procedures.* Philadelphia: Saunders; 2004:685.)

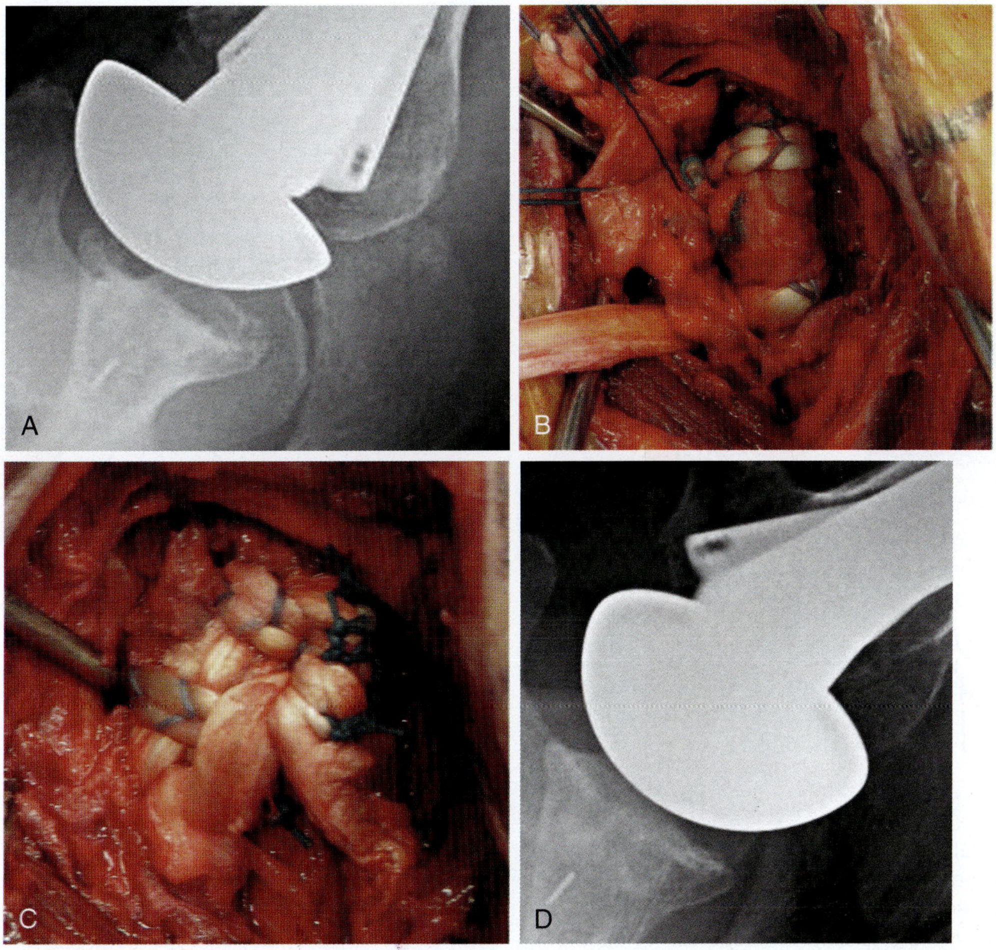

FIGURE 16-495: Subscapularis failure from a fall on the abducted arm shortly after a total shoulder arthroplasty. The patient had weak internal rotation, increased passive external rotation, and a palpable defect at the subscapularis insertion. **A,** Anterior subluxation of the humeral head on the glenoid. **B,** Semitendinosus graft passed through drill holes in the lesser tuberosity and then through the lateral margin of the torn subscapularis tendon. **C,** Secured graft. **D,** Restored centering of the humeral head after repair.

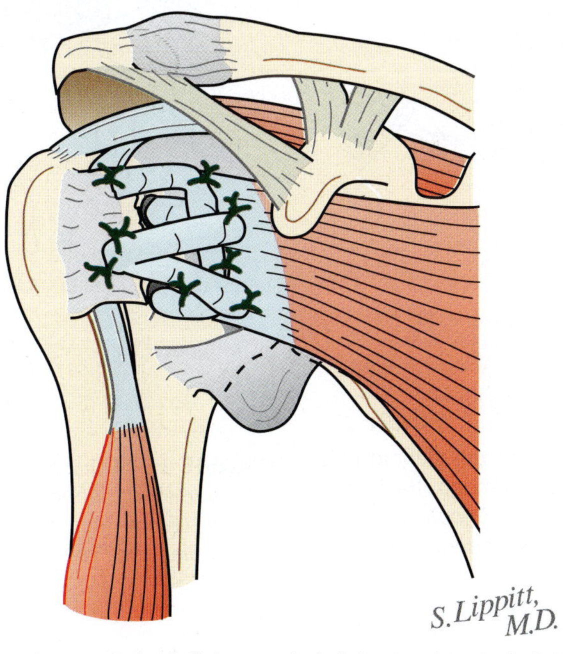

FIGURE 16-496: Hamstring graft for subscapularis deficiency. A deficient subscapularis tendon may be reconstructed using a hamstring autograft woven between the residual tendon and the soft tissue or bone at the lesser tuberosity. (From Matsen FA III, Lippitt SB. *Shoulder Surgery: Principles and Procedures.* Philadelphia: Saunders; 2004:669.)

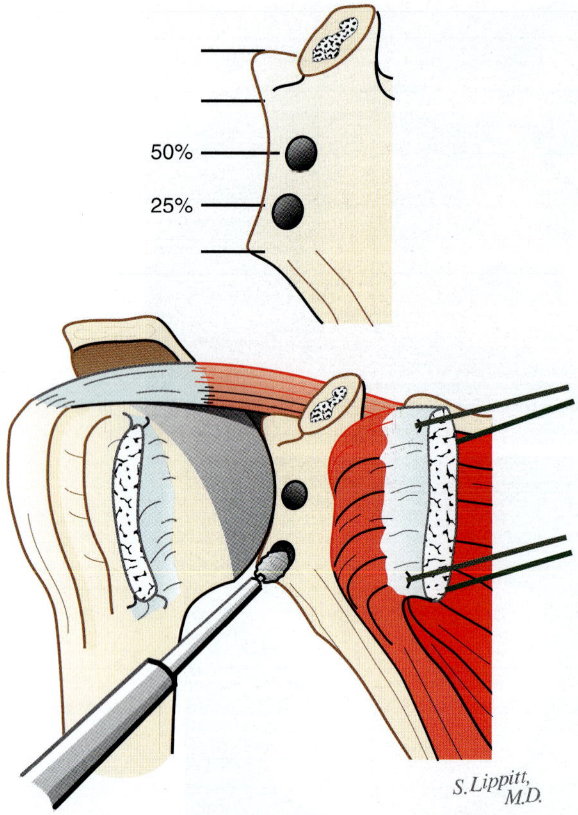

FIGURE 16-497: Glenoid drill holes. Using a pinecone bur, drill holes are placed in the middle and inferior aspects of the anterior glenoid, near the lip. (From Matsen FA III, Lippitt SB. *Shoulder Surgery: Principles and Procedures.* Philadelphia: Saunders; 2004:229.)

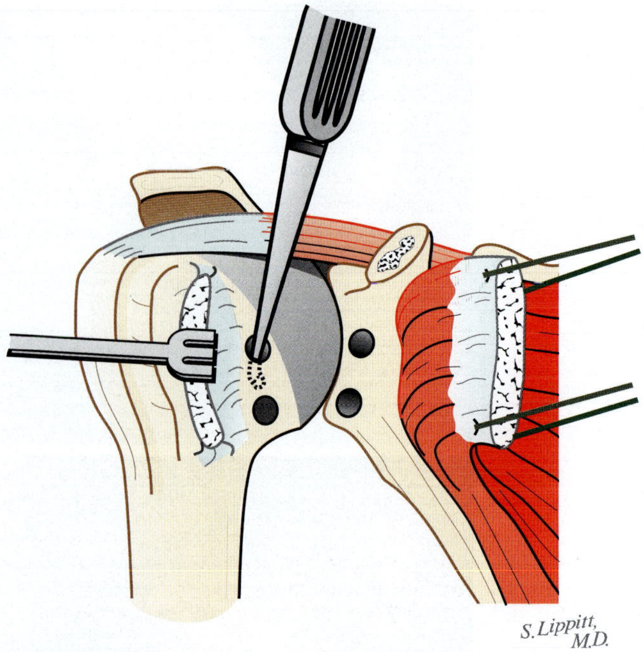

FIGURE 16-498: Humeral drill holes. Holes are made in the middle and inferior aspects of the proximal humerus, near the articular surface. (From Matsen FA III, Lippitt SB. *Shoulder Surgery: Principles and Procedures.* Philadelphia: Saunders; 2004:229.)

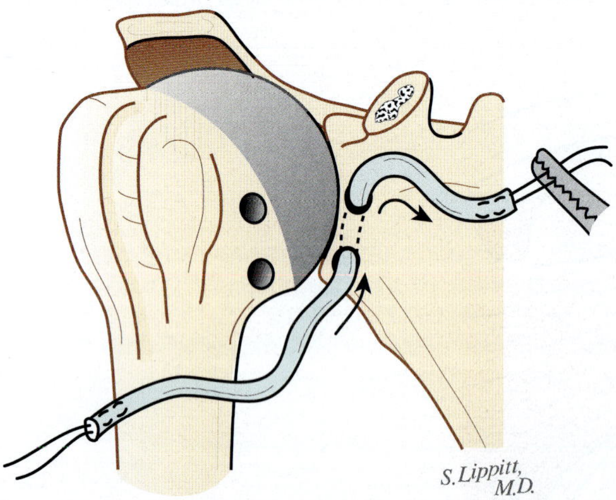

FIGURE 16-499: Passing the graft through the glenoid holes. The hamstring tendon graft is passed through the glenoid holes. (From Matsen FA III, Lippitt SB. *Shoulder Surgery: Principles and Procedures.* Philadelphia: Saunders; 2004:230.)

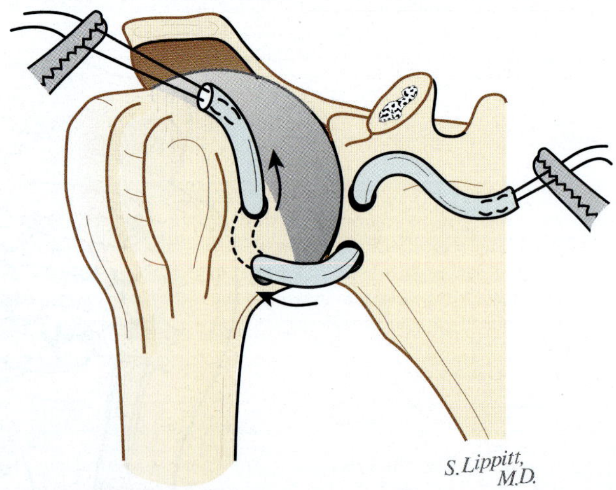

FIGURE 16-500: Passing the graft through the humeral holes. The hamstring tendon graft is then passed through the humeral holes. (From Matsen FA III, Lippitt SB. *Shoulder Surgery: Principles and Procedures.* Philadelphia: Saunders; 2004:231.)

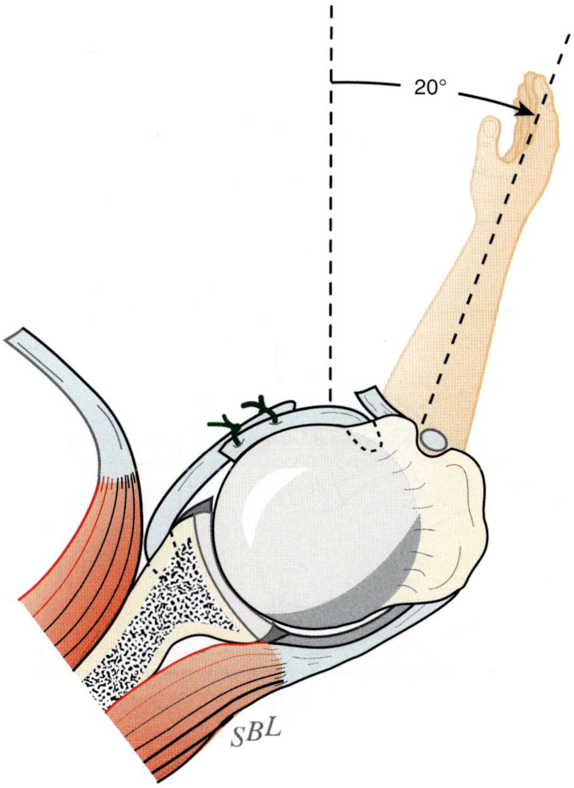

FIGURE 16-501: Tying the graft. The graft is tied such that external rotation is checked at 20 degrees. (From Matsen FA III, Lippitt SB. *Shoulder Surgery: Principles and Procedures.* Philadelphia: Saunders; 2004:231.)

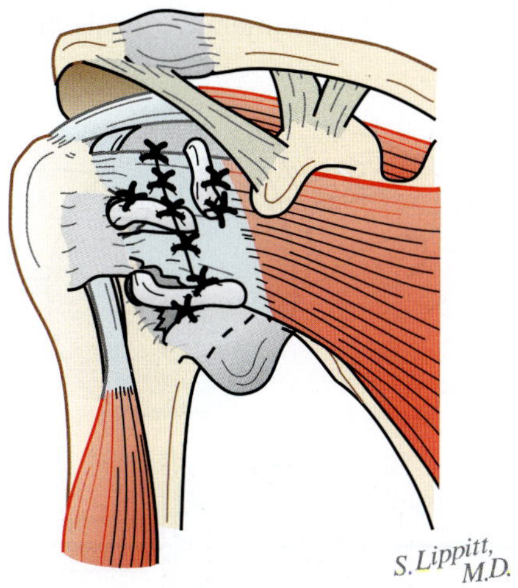

FIGURE 16-502: Reinforcing the graft. Any available capsular or tendon tissue is anchored to the graft. (From Matsen FA III, Lippitt SB. *Shoulder Surgery: Principles and Procedures.* Philadelphia: Saunders; 2004:231.)

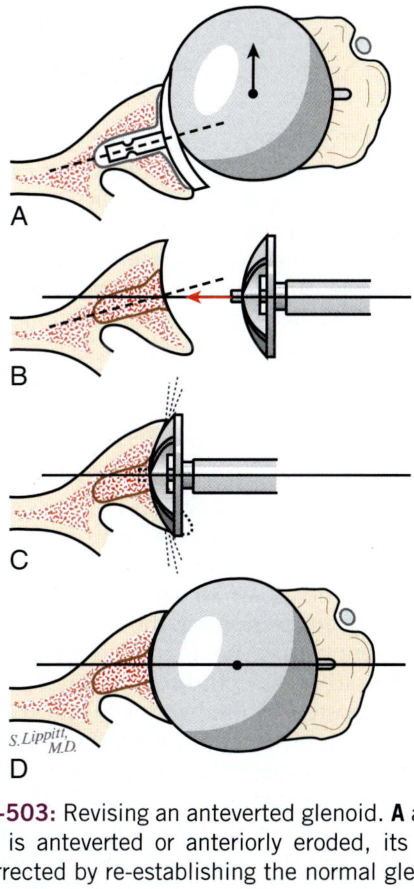

FIGURE 16-503: Revising an anteverted glenoid. **A** and **B,** When the glenoid is anteverted or anteriorly eroded, its version can often be corrected by re-establishing the normal glenoid centerline. **C,** It is then reamed along this new axis. **D,** Completed revision. (From Matsen FA III, Lippitt SB. *Shoulder Surgery: Principles and Procedures.* Philadelphia: Saunders; 2004:705.)

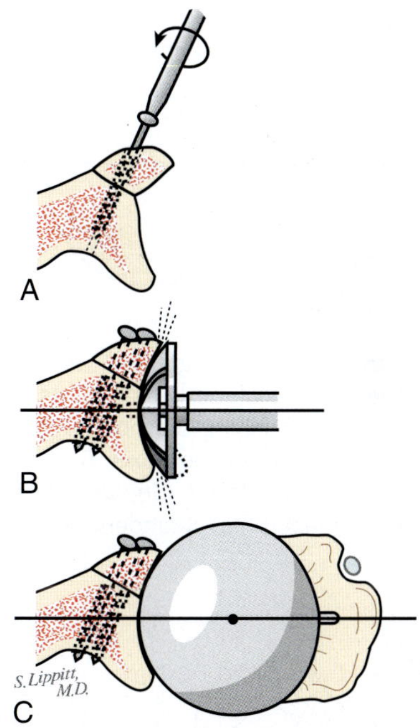

FIGURE 16-504: Anterior glenoid graft. **A,** When the anterior glenoid is deficient, an anterior iliac crest graft can be placed and fixed with screws. **B,** The grafted assembly is reamed for either a nonprosthetic or a prosthetic glenoid arthroplasty. **C,** Completed repair. (From Matsen FA III, Lippitt SB. *Shoulder Surgery: Principles and Procedures.* Philadelphia: Saunders; 2004:706.)

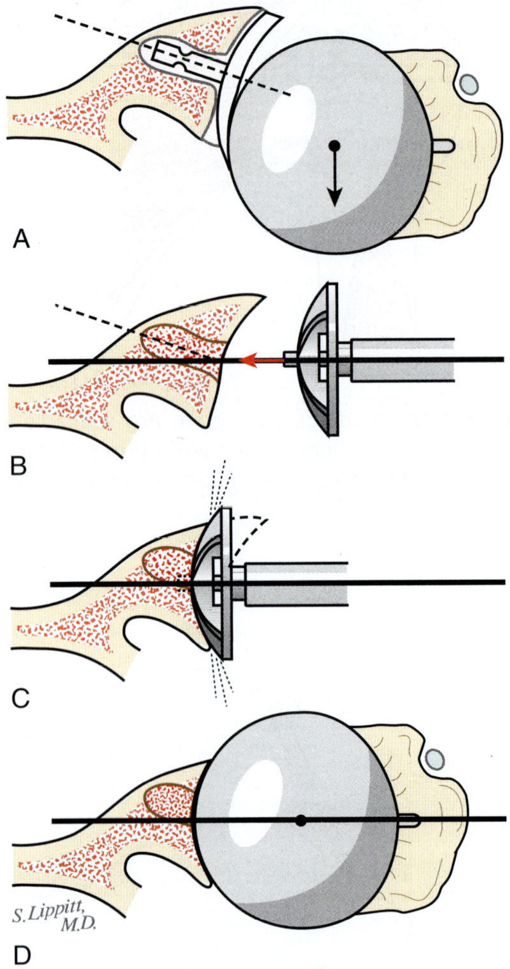

FIGURE 16-505: Retroverted glenoid. **A** and **B,** When the glenoid is retroverted or posteriorly eroded, its version can often be corrected by re-establishing the normal glenoid centerline. **C,** It is then reamed along this new axis. **D,** Completed revision. (From Matsen FA III, Lippitt SB. *Shoulder Surgery: Principles and Procedures.* Philadelphia: Saunders; 2004:708.)

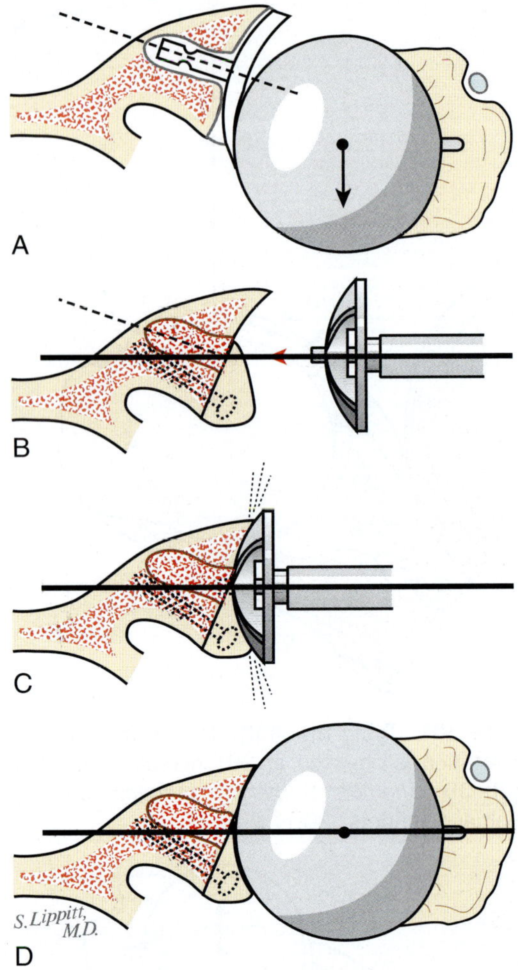

FIGURE 16-507: Posterior glenoid graft. **A,** When the posterior glenoid is deficient, a posterior iliac crest graft can be placed, but rigid fixation of the graft is technically challenging. **B** and **C,** If the graft can be secured, it can be reamed to the appropriate version and concavity for a nonprosthetic or prosthetic glenoid arthroplasty. **D,** Completed revision. (From Matsen FA III, Lippitt SB. *Shoulder Surgery: Principles and Procedures.* Philadelphia: Saunders; 2004:710.)

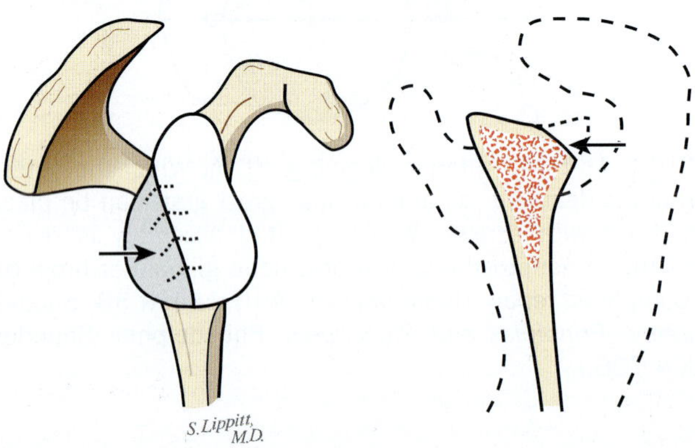

FIGURE 16-506: Posterior erosion and rim deficiency. Posterior glenoid deficiency (arrows) is a commonly encountered problem in revision arthroplasty. (From Matsen FA III, Lippitt SB. *Shoulder Surgery: Principles and Procedures.* Philadelphia: Saunders; 2004:707.)

initial arthroplasty, posterior instability from transection of the cuff is difficult to manage and may require conversion to a reverse total shoulder arthroplasty. Tight soft tissues can be released during revision surgery (see Figs. 16-463, 16-466, and 16-467). Humeral retroversion can be managed by repositioning the prosthesis. Posterior glenoid deficiency may be managed by attempting to normalize glenoid version through anterior reaming (see Fig. 16-505) or posterior bone grafting (Fig. 16-507); when possible, our preference is to ream the glenoid conservatively to a single concavity, to accept substantial glenoid retroversion, and to stabilize the head in the retroverted socket with an anteriorly eccentric humeral head component (see Fig. 16-281), a rotator interval plication (see Figs. 16-211 and 16-280), or both.[344] If this cannot be

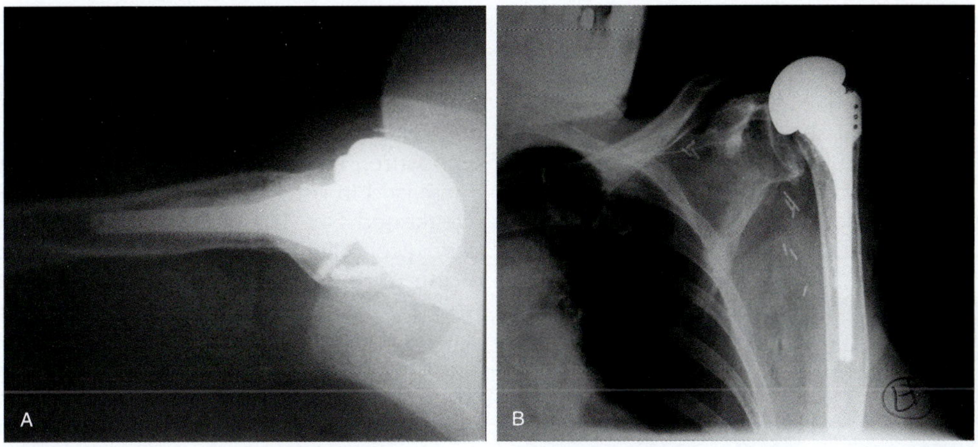

FIGURE 16-508: Combined anterior subluxation of the glenohumeral joint and superior escape of the humeral head due to rotator cuff dysfunction and compromise of the coracoacromial arch. **A,** Axillary lateral view. **B,** Anteroposterior view. (From Bohsali KI, Wirth MA, Rockwood CA. Complications of total shoulder arthroplasty. *J Bone Joint Surg Am.* 2006;88:2279-2292.)

accomplished, conversion to a reverse total shoulder may be required (see Figs. 16-247 and 16-341).

Superior instability most commonly arises with rotator cuff deficiency, fractures, or failed arthroplasty (see Figs. 16-101 to 16-103 and 16-188; Fig. 16-508).[50,51,103,241,598] The risk of superior instability is increased if the humeral component is placed too high above the tuberosities (see Figs. 16-218, 16-244, and 16-250).

The situation is further compounded if an acromioplasty has been performed, removing the secondary stabilizing effect of the coracoacromial arch (Fig. 16-509) and resulting in anterosuperior escape (see Figs. 16-109 and 16-115). For this reason, we preserve the acromion and the coracoacromial ligament in all shoulder surgeries. If the coracoacromial arch is intact, superior instability may be managed in some cases using CTA prosthesis (see Figs. 16-104 and 16-105). In the presence of anterosuperior escape we consider a reverse total shoulder arthroplasty (see Fig. 16-113).

Inferior instability can result from rotator cuff deficiency; deltoid injury; paresis or atony; or failure to restore the humeral length when replacement is performed for proximal humeral fractures, tumors, or arthritis.[485,594] Clinically, patients with inferior instability lack the ability to raise the arm above the horizontal plane due to poor deltoid tensioning.[594] If the deltoid and cuff are intact, stability may be restored by repositioning the humeral component.

Rotator Cuff Failure. Postoperative failure of the rotator cuff is a recognized complication of shoulder arthroplasty.* This problem is not unexpected for at least four reasons: (1) shoulder arthroplasty is commonly performed on individuals who are of an age where cuff failure is common; (2) shoulder arthroplasty restores motion to joints that may previously have been disused, abruptly placing new loads on cuff tissue that had been inactive for years; (3) some postarthroplasty rehabilitation programs focus on rotator cuff strengthening using exercises that put the cuff at a mechanical disadvantage; and (4) the cut to remove the humeral head may inadvertently weaken the cuff or the tuberosity to which it attaches. Recognition of the problem of delayed failure of the rotator cuff after shoulder joint replacement[129,443,598] has led to reconsideration of the recommendations for rehabilitation and activity levels following shoulder arthroplasty. Although it may be tempting to try to repair cuff tears that occur after shoulder arthroplasty, this is a most challenging undertaking due to poor tendon quality and limited tuberosity reattachment sites. In cases where there is secondary superior stability provided by an intact

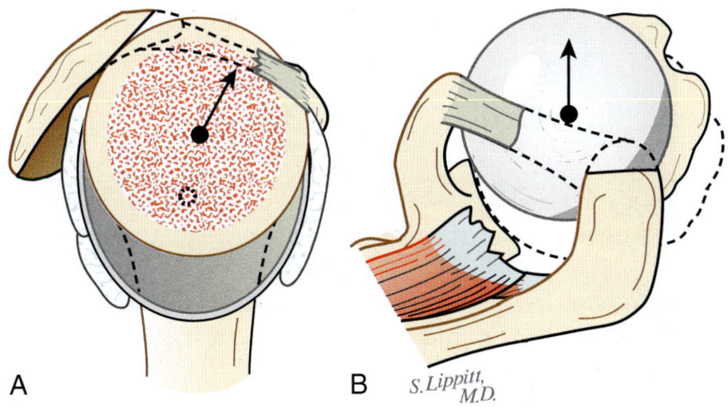

FIGURE 16-509: Anterosuperior escape. **A,** The integrity of the anterior coracoacromial arch compromised by prior surgery. **B,** This allows the humeral head to escape anterosuperiorly when the deltoid contracts. (From Matsen FA III, Lippitt SB. *Shoulder Surgery: Principles and Procedures.* Philadelphia: Saunders; 2004:713.)

**References 6, 42, 64, 121, 128-130, 164, 174, 181, 209, 218, 245, 319, 320, 322, 346, 359, 403, 410, 418, 506, 513, 514, 519, 520, 526, 550, 551, 572, 579, 598.*

coracoacromial arch, conversion to a CTA prosthesis may be considered (Fig. 16-510; see Figs. 16-104 and 16-105). If the shoulder demonstrates anterosuperior escape or the inability to perform active elevation (Fig. 16-511), conversion to a reverse total shoulder is considered (see Figs. 16-113 and 16-188).

Fractures. Periprosthetic fractures represent an important complication of shoulder arthroplasty, whether they occur intraoperatively or after surgery.[45,172,277,495,505,594]

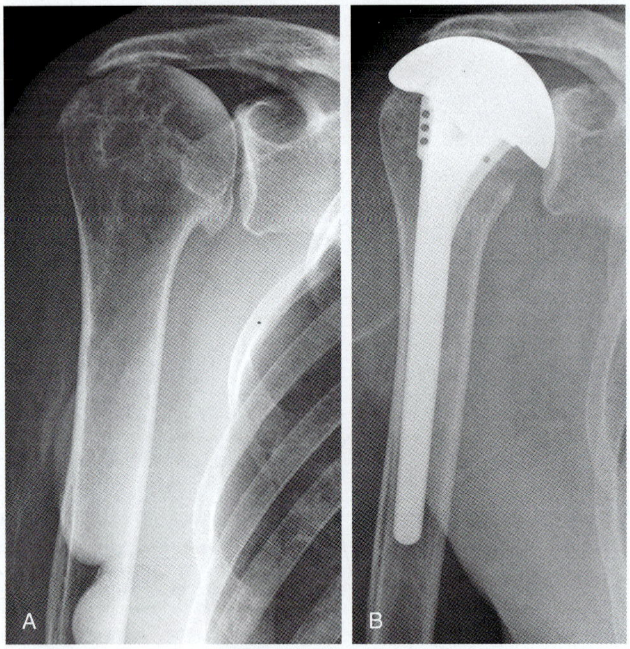

FIGURE 16-510: A, Cuff tear arthropathy. **B,** Treatment with a prosthesis.

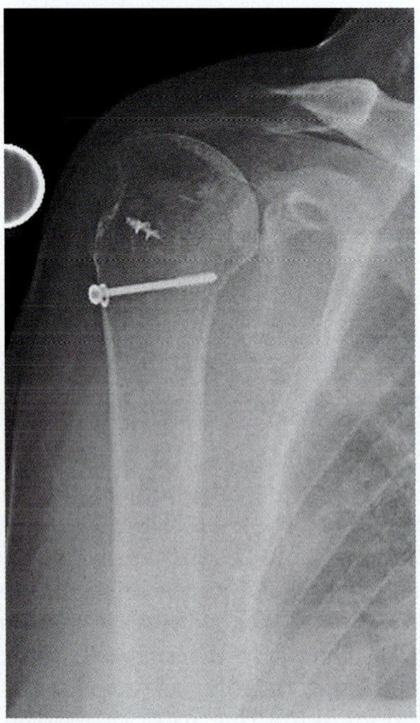

FIGURE 16-511: Superior glenohumeral instability after failed rotator cuff reconstruction.

Intraoperative fractures of the humerus generally arise from attempting to externally rotate the humerus without adequate soft tissue releases, overvigorous reaming, attempts to fully seat the component in a tight canal, or manipulation of the upper extremity during glenoid exposure. The risk of intraoperative humeral fracture is increased in osteopenic bone or when the shaft has been weakened (see Fig. 16-318) or perforated during medullary preparation or cement removal. When fractures occur during surgery, immediate stabilization is desirable so that rehabilitation of the shoulder arthroplasty can proceed. Fixation methods for shaft fractures may include cerclage (Fig. 16-512) or plating (Figs. 16-513 and 16-514). Cerclage must be performed with great care because the radial nerve is hidden in the musculospiral groove behind the humerus. Conversion to a long-stemmed humeral implant can be considered (Fig. 16-515), but this may not improve torsional stability. Intraoperative fractures of the tuberosity may be treated by suturing the tuberosity fragments to the prosthesis.

Intraoperative fractures of the glenoid may result from overzealous reaming, drilling, or retraction or from forcing the component into position. Glenoid fractures rarely require internal fixation, but they may preclude the insertion of a glenoid component.

Postoperative fractures can often be managed nonoperatively by splinting the arm against the body without or with a circumferential brace (Fig. 16-516). This method is particularly applicable for spiral fractures resulting from forced external rotation. If satisfactory reduction cannot

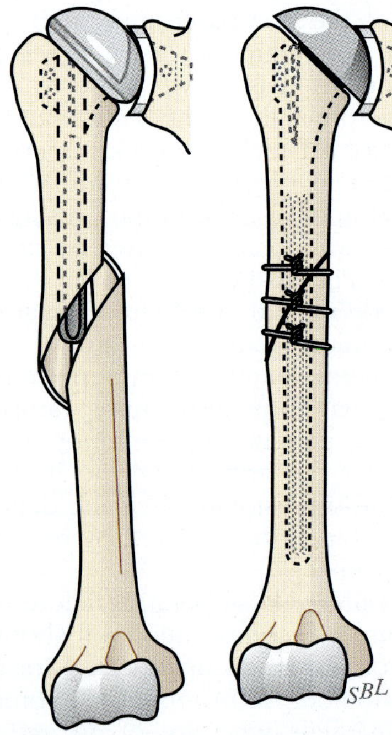

FIGURE 16-512: Spiral fracture. Spiral fractures at the level of the prosthesis tip can be stabilized by removing the original humeral prosthesis, inserting a long-stem prosthesis, and cerclage wiring. (From Matsen FA III, Lippitt SB. *Shoulder Surgery: Principles and Procedures.* Philadelphia: Saunders; 2004:698.)

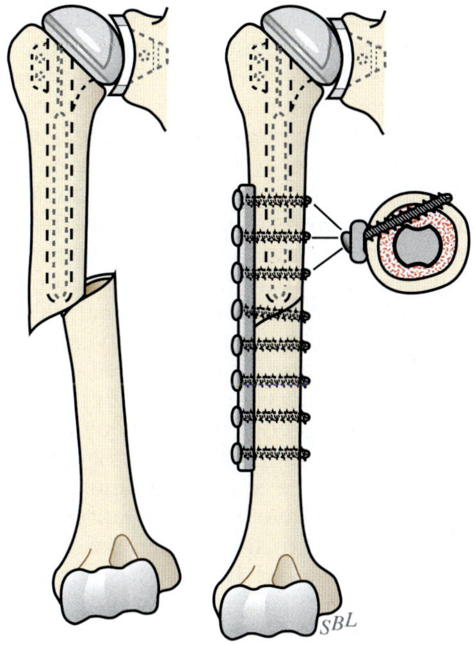

FIGURE 16-513: Oblique fracture. It is often possible to fix short oblique fractures at the tip of a well-fixed prosthesis by using a plate and angling the proximal screws around the prosthesis. (From Matsen FA III, Lippitt SB. *Shoulder Surgery: Principles and Procedures.* Philadelphia: Saunders; 2004:699.)

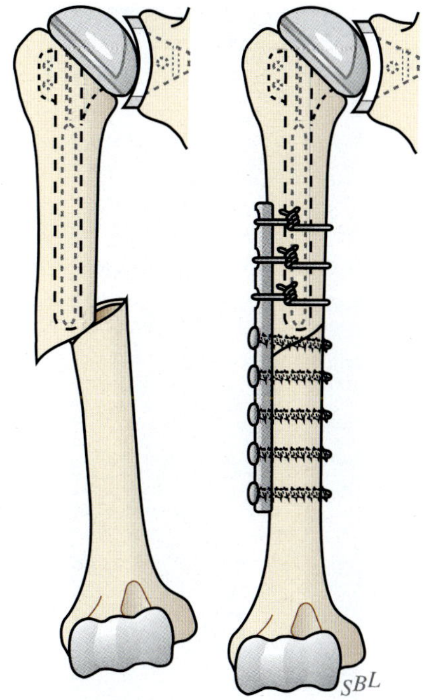

FIGURE 16-514: Oblique fracture. Alternatively, a plate can be screwed to the distal fragment and cerclaged around the proximal fragment. (From Matsen FA III, Lippitt SB. *Shoulder Surgery: Principles and Procedures.* Philadelphia: Saunders; 2004:700.)

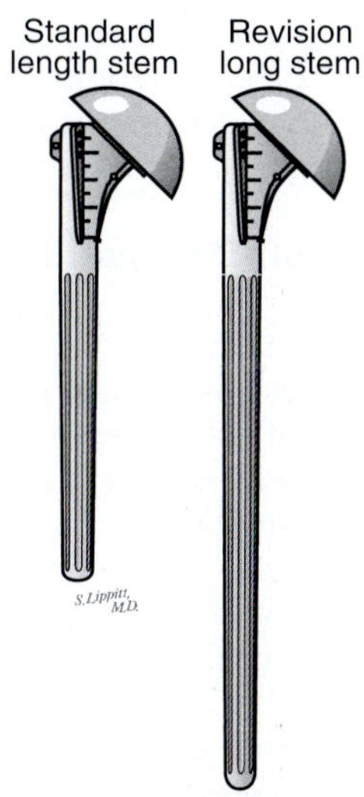

FIGURE 16-515: Standard versus long stem. In preparing for a revision arthroplasty, it is always prudent to have a long-stem prosthesis available. Because the exact prosthesis length may be difficult to judge and because optimizing the fit in the distal humerus may be critical (for example, when there is a fracture of the proximal humerus), we often start with a 300-mm long implant and cut it in the operating room to the desired length. (From Matsen FA III, Lippitt SB. *Shoulder Surgery: Principles and Procedures.* Philadelphia: Saunders; 2004:721.)

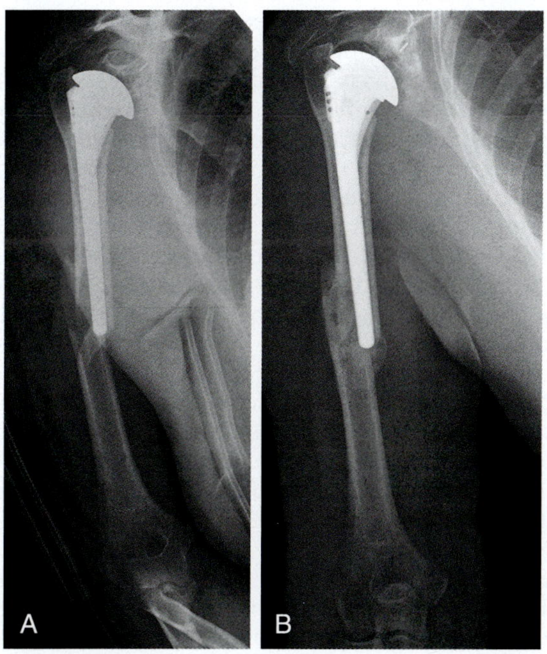

FIGURE 16-516: A, Fracture at the tip of the humeral prosthesis. **B,** Fracture healed with nonoperative management.

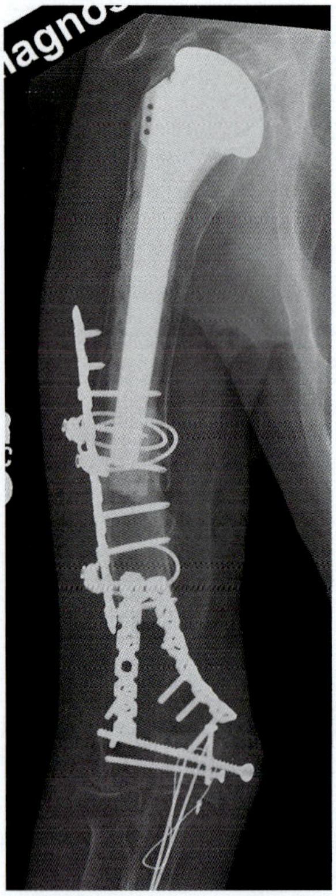

FIGURE 16-517: Failed fixation of a periprosthetic fracture distal to humeral prosthetic tip.

be maintained or if healing does not occur as expected, operative approaches can be considered,[45,277] although reconstruction can be complex (Fig. 16-517).

The risk of periprosthetic fractures is minimized through preoperatively identifying shoulders that have fragile bone, that are tight, or that have undergone prior surgery and then carefully planning for these conditions.[1] The forces applied to the humerus should be minimized and soft tissue releases should be complete to facilitate exposure. Humeral bone is preserved by minimizing reaming and broaching of the humeral canal (see Figs. 16-315 and 16-316). The risk of fracture is minimized by using stems that are smaller than the endosteal diameter of the diaphysis and by using impaction grafting—rather than cement or ingrowth—for fixation (see Figs. 16-317, 16-322, 16-323). Glenoid bone is preserved by limiting the reaming only to what is necessary to provide a smooth concave surface. In revision surgery the risk of fracture is minimized by performing careful repairable longitudinal osteotomies (see Figs. 16-336 and 16-477) rather than cortical windows.

Nerve Injuries. We suspect that nerve injuries during shoulder arthroplasty are more common than is generally realized.[41,76,280,491,532,535,593] Studies using intraoperative nerve monitoring during shoulder arthroplasty have helped elucidate the situations in which nerves are particularly at risk.[318,381] These are as follows: the axillary nerve is at risk when freeing up the capsule and subscapularis or during lateral dissection around the greater tuberosity; the musculocutaneous nerve is at risk when the coracoid muscles are retracted to expose the glenoid; the radial nerve is at risk during the cerclage fixation of fractures; the median nerve is at risk from traction when the arm is externally rotated and extended; the suprascapular nerve and nerves to the subscapularis are at risk when attempting to free up retracted tendons (see Fig. 16-158); the ulnar nerve is at risk from external pressure during the procedure; and the upper plexus is at risk when the head is inclined to the opposite side and traction applied to the arm and when brachial plexus block anesthesia is used. Failure to protect nerves in the surgical field is a leading cause of malpractice claims.[343]

Some patients incur nerve injuries prior to their arthroplasty, so a thorough preoperative evaluation is always required. Shoulders with postsurgical or posttraumatic arthritis may have nerves scarred at unusual positions. Shoulders with preoperative internal rotation contractures and prior open surgery are at particular risk as the motion of the shoulder is restored by soft tissue releases and bone resection. Patients who take methotrexate appear to be at increased risk of nerve injury.[315] Nerve transection is best avoided by ensuring that the nerves are kept out of the way of the knife and electrocautery (see Fig. 16-156). Nerve injury from traction or compression is best avoided by minimizing the number of seconds that the arm is held in any extreme position and by relaxing the retractors frequently to "give the nerves a drink."

It is important to document the integrity of the *motor* components of the axillary, musculocutaneous, median, radial, and ulnar nerves before and immediately after surgery; this is yet another reason we avoid nerve block anesthesia. Most traction and compression injuries will recover spontaneously. If recovery is not evident at 6 weeks after surgery, electromyography and nerve conduction studies can help document the site of the injury and suggest the prognosis.

Arthroplasty for the Cuff-Deficient Shoulder

Considerations

As with the normal shoulder, the anatomic shoulder arthroplasty is stabilized by concavity compression: the action of the rotator cuff compressing the humeral head into the glenoid concavity (see Fig. 16-232)[25,259,266,290,308,419,573] as well as by the articulation of the cuff-covered head against the coracoacromial arch (see Figs. 16-221, 16-222, and 16-229). In some cases this stabilizing mechanism remains functional even though the cuff is no longer completely intact (Fig. 16-518). However, in the absence of a sufficiently functional cuff, the humeral head is not stabilized in the socket (see Figs. 16-102 and 16-115), and thus contraction of the deltoid pulls the humerus superiorly (see Figs. 16-101, 16-103, and 16-109; Fig. 16-519).[123,266,545] This superior displacement can compromise the effectiveness of the superior lip of the glenoid concavity (Fig. 16-520; see Fig. 16-116). Over time, this process can lead to rounding of the humeral tuberosities—which we have termed "femoralization"—along with the creation of a socket that includes the acromion, coracoacromial arch, and upper glenoid—which we have

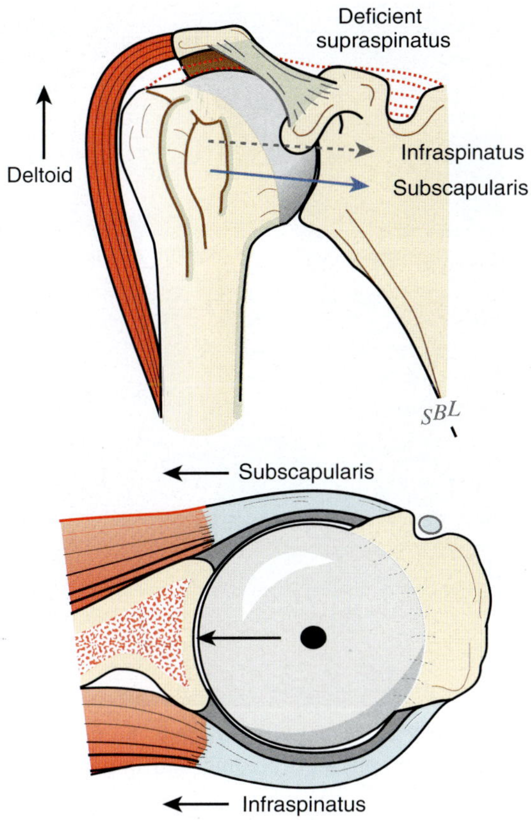

FIGURE 16-518: Intact glenoid concavity. If the glenoid concavity is intact, the compressive action of the subscapularis and infraspinatus can stabilize the humeral head in the center of the glenoid socket against the upward pull of the deltoid. (From Matsen FA III, Lippitt SB. *Shoulder Surgery: Principles and Procedures.* Philadelphia: Saunders; 2004:263.)

termed "actetabularization" (see Figs. 16-97 to 16-100). The combination of a deficient rotator cuff and shoulder arthritis is referred to as cuff tear arthropathy (CTA) (see Figs. 16-96 and 16-100).[3,143,247,258,309,391,559,599] Instability from cuff deficiency also arises when the cuff tendons fail after shoulder arthroplasty* and when tuberosity fractures have compromised the ability of the cuff to insert securely into the humerus. In the absence of the normal stabilizing

References 42, 64, 121, 128-130, 164, 174, 181, 209, 218, 245, 319, 320, 322, 346, 359, 403, 410, 418, 506, 513, 514, 519, 520, 526, 550, 551, 572, 579, 598.

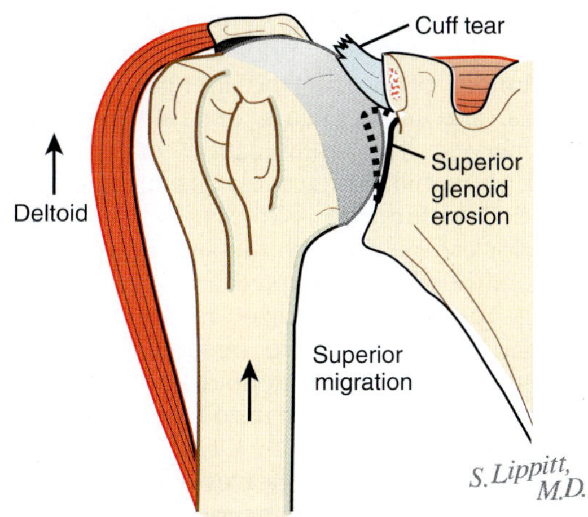

FIGURE 16-520: Loss of centering. The combination of loss of both the rotator cuff and the superior glenoid concavity allows the destabilized humeral head to move upward (arrows), rather than abduct, on deltoid contraction. (From Matsen FA III, Lippitt SB. *Shoulder Surgery: Principles and Procedures.* Philadelphia: Saunders; 2004:263.)

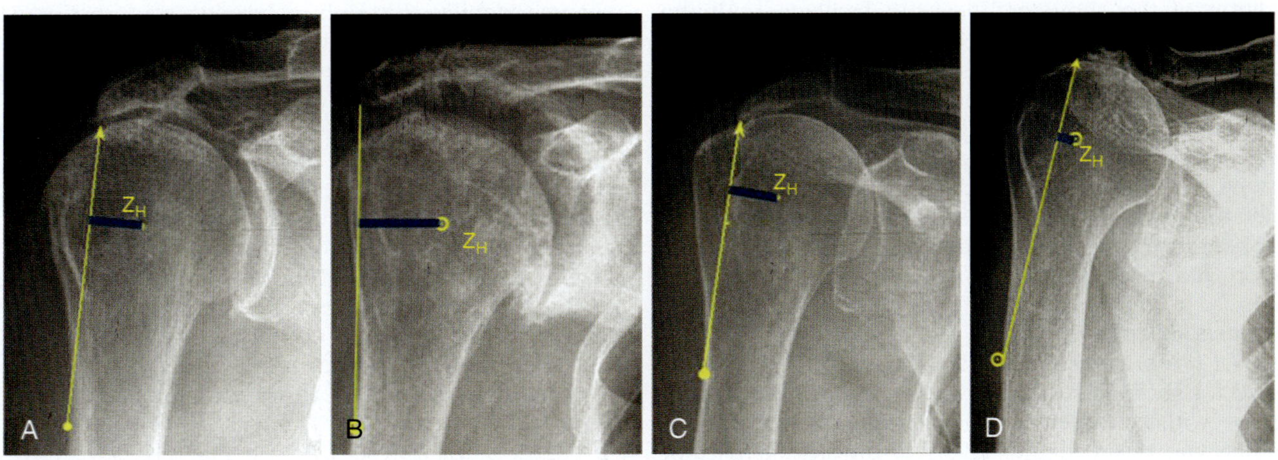

FIGURE 16-519: Typical radiographs of the four types of cuff tear arthropathy according to our classification. **A,** Type Ia. **B,** Type Ib. **C,** Type Iia. **D,** Type Iib. The blue bar indicates the lever arm of the deltoid muscle; the yellow lines indicate the orientation of the deltoid force sum vector in abduction. Z_H, Center of humeral head.

effect of the rotator cuff, the coracoacromial arch may provide secondary stabilization of the humeral head in the glenoid (see Figs. 16-101, 16-107, and 16-110) unless the arch has been compromised by acromioplasty or wear (see Figs. 16-111 and 16-509).

When the head is superiorly displaced relative to the glenoid, an anatomic total shoulder arthroplasty is often unsuccessful. Superior displacement of the humeral head places an anatomic prosthetic glenoid component at risk of "rocking horse" loosening from eccentric loading (see Figs. 16-214, 16-244, 16-245, 16-249, 16-253, 16-272, 16-274, and 16-282 to 16-285).[152,309]

In evaluating a shoulder with major cuff deficiency, it is important to document any history of prior injury, surgery, or infection. Physical examination should include evaluation of the skin and prior incisions; the passive and active ranges of motion; the strength of the deltoid, subscapularis, and infraspinatus; and the function of all peripheral nerves. The combination of good passive motion and an inability to actively elevate the arm even with intact deltoid function is known as pseudoparalysis. Anterosuperior escape refers to the superior displacement of the humeral head on attempted active elevation of the arm (see Fig. 16-109). Standardized radiographs (see Figs. 16-62, 16-371, and 16-372) are needed to evaluate the integrity of the humeral and glenoid bone. A number of different approaches have been used to classify the various degrees of pathology seen with CTA.[138,178,198,258,492,500,506,559] Our approach to rotator CTA however is based primarily on the history, physical examination, plain radiographs, and the characteristics and needs of the patient.

In considering treatment, one must not overlook the potential value of nonoperative management. Many patients have been referred to us for consideration of reverse total shoulder arthroplasty whose primary problem was shoulder stiffness or weakness from disuse. A gentle progressive range of motion and strengthening program (see Figs. 16-136 to 16-145)[498] can substantially increase the comfort and function of shoulders with large cuff tears, despite the presence of a degree of arthritis. Even if these exercises do not sufficiently improve the condition of the shoulder, they can facilitate both the surgery and the postsurgical recovery. Before proceeding to surgery, a detailed discussion with the patient is needed to understand his or her functional goals as well as the risks of falling, especially if Parkinson disease or other issues with balance are present. Because individuals with cuff-deficient shoulders are often older and debilitated, careful planning is needed to minimize the risk of surgery as well as to optimize their postdischarge support and recovery.

Prosthesis Selection

The *CTA prosthesis* (see Figs. 16-104 and 16-105) is considered for shoulders with active elevation of 90 or more degrees without anterosuperior escape, especially for patients who desire higher levels of physical activity or those who are at increased risk of falls. Importantly, this prosthesis has an extended lateral joint surface for articulation with the undersurface of the coracoacromial arch; thus it is distinct from the usual hemiarthroplasty prosthesis. The implant system should allow selection of the appropriate diameter of curvature (see Fig. 16-305) and should enable fixation by impaction grafting (see Fig. 16-323).

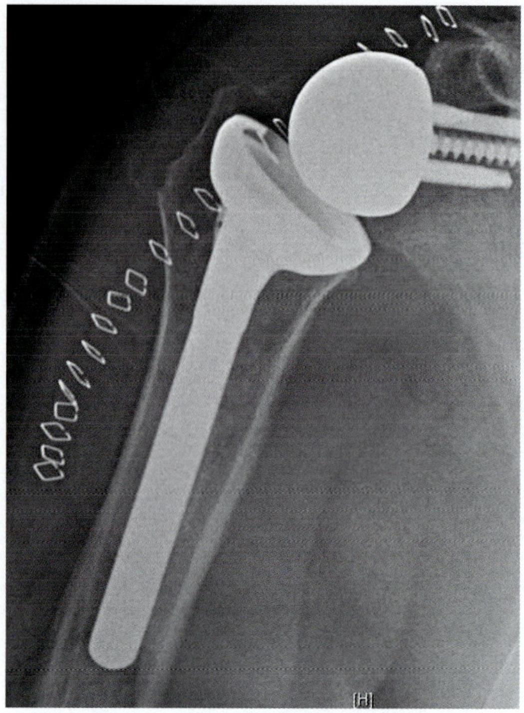

FIGURE 16-521: Monoblock reverse humeral component secured with metaphyseal reaming and impaction grafting of the canal.

The *reverse total shoulder arthroplasty* (Fig. 16-521)* is considered for individuals with pseudoparalysis and anterosuperior escape—findings that are evident on physical examination. The reverse total shoulder arthroplasty, like the anatomic total shoulder arthroplasty, achieves stability through concavity compression (Fig. 16-522). The glenoid component manages the compressive force applied to it by a combination of compressive and tensile loading of the glenoid bone (Fig. 16-523). As long as the net glenohumeral joint reaction force is contained within the humeral socket, the articulation is stable (Fig. 16-524). Conversely, if the net glenohumeral joint force is not contained within the humeral socket, the joint is unstable (Fig. 16-525).

Our preferred implant (Fig. 16-526) meets the following criteria. (1) It enables a relatively anatomic reconstruction (Fig. 16-527) in contrast to those that result in distal displacement of the humerus with the associated increased risk of fracture of the acromion (Figs. 16-528

References 3, 12, 43, 79, 81, 112, 115, 116, 136, 150, 151, 166, 169, 183, 190, 191, 200, 268, 279, 296, 298, 299, 331, 365, 373, 377, 378, 382, 384, 416, 434, 455, 457, 481, 492, 500, 501, 524, 540, 541, 569, 571, 579, 582, 597, 599.

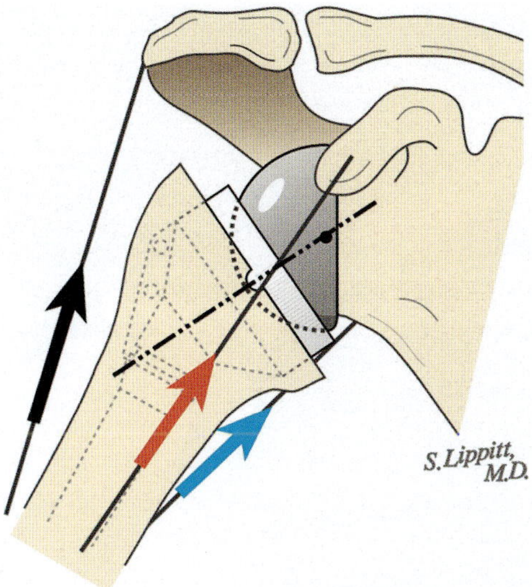

FIGURE 16-522: The reverse total shoulder arthroplasty uses the concavity compression mechanism by providing a relatively deep socket on the humeral side into which the glenosphere is compressed by the combined action of the deltoid (black arrow), conjoined tendon (red arrow), and the long head of the triceps (blue arrow).

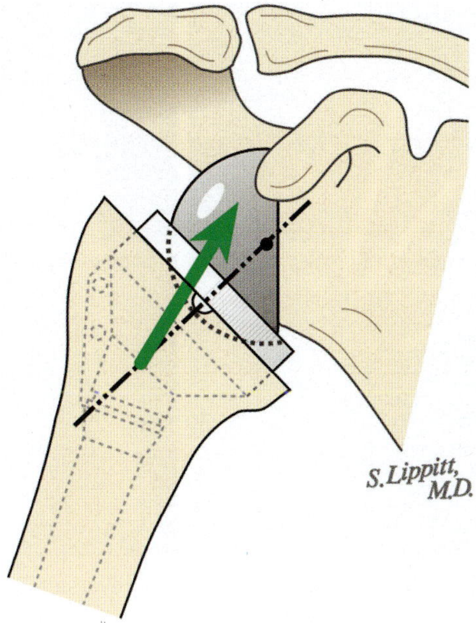

FIGURE 16-524: In order for a reverse arthroplasty to be stable, the net glenohumeral joint reaction force (green arrow) must be contained within the humeral concavity.

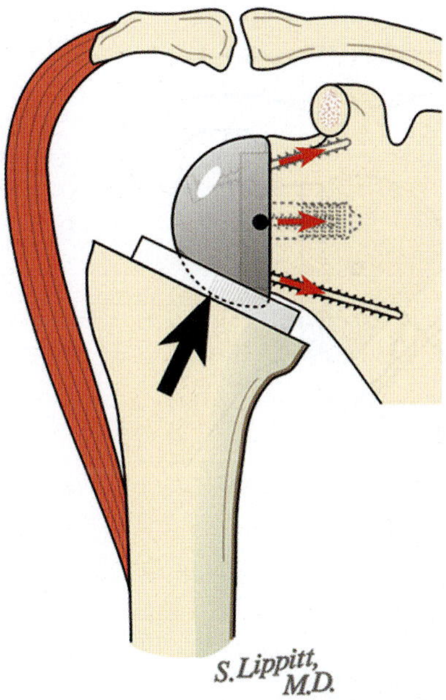

FIGURE 16-523: Secure, immediate fixation of the glenoid baseplate with compression screws helps resist the upward shear force (black arrow) applied by the humerus, without having to wait for bone ingrowth.

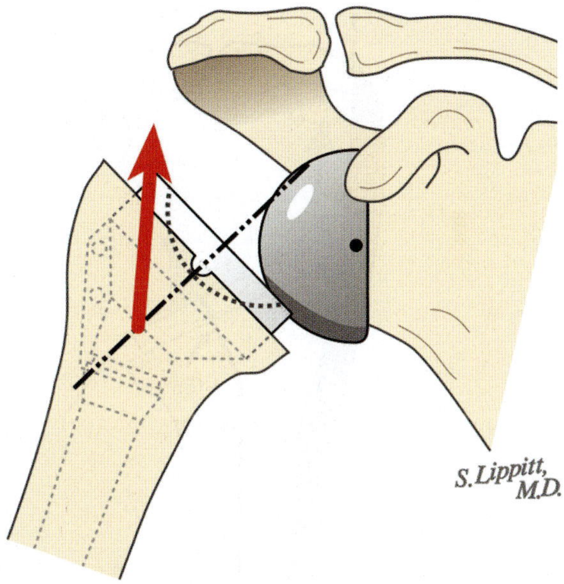

FIGURE 16-525: If the net glenohumeral joint reaction force is not contained within the humeral concavity (red arrow), the reverse arthroplasty dislocates.

and 16-529), instability (Fig. 16-530), or neurologic injury from lengthening the arm.[279] (2) It preserves glenoid bone stock. (3) It provides immediate glenoid fixation with a screw that engages the cortex of the subscapularis fossa, compressing the baseplate against the prepared glenoid bone without having to wait for tissue ingrowth. (4) It has sufficient lateral offset to prevent unwanted contact between the medial aspect of the humeral component and the glenoid without the need for bone graft interposed between the baseplate and the glenoid to achieve

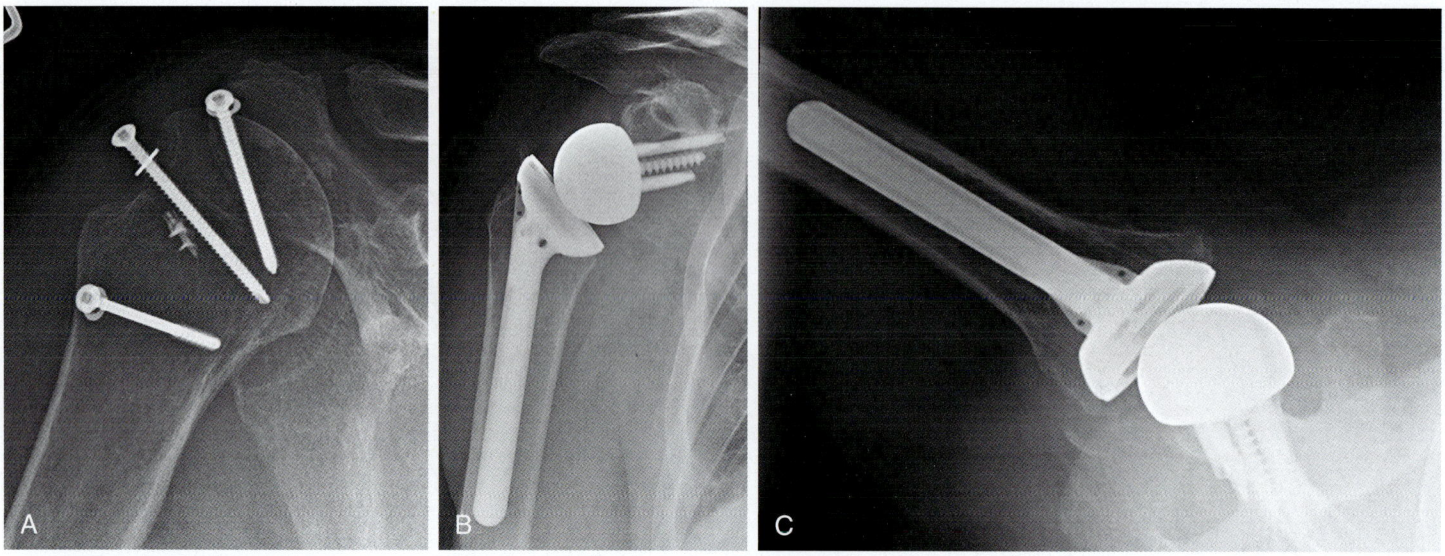

FIGURE 16-526: Cementless monoblock reverse total shoulder arthroplasty for posttraumatic cuff deficiency and superior instability. **A,** A humeral head that is superiorly unstable. **B,** Impaction grafted monoblock stem. **C,** Fixation of the glenosphere with secure fixation of glenoid screws.

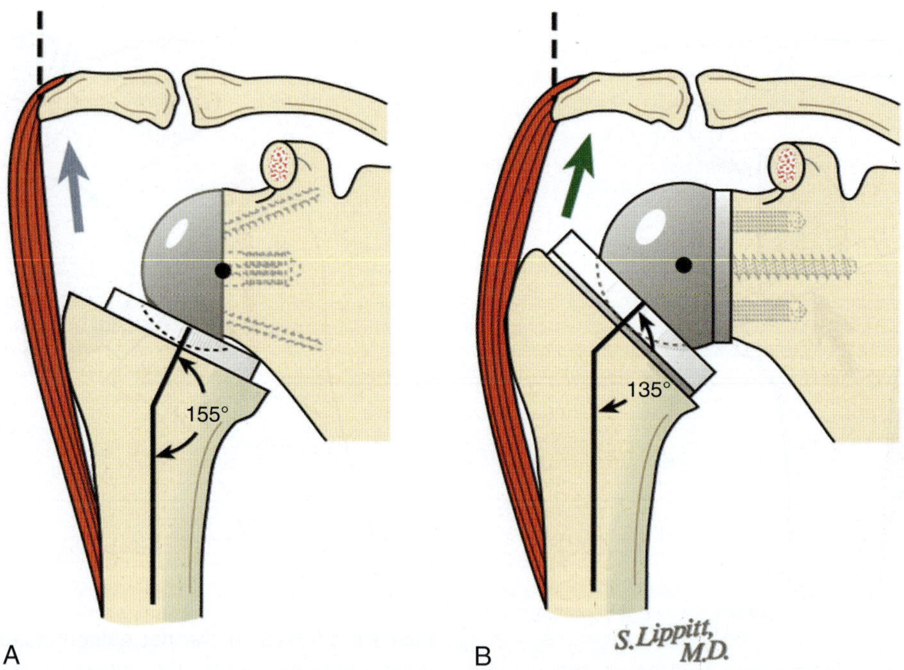

FIGURE 16-527: **A,** When the center of rotation is placed medially on the glenoid bone and a valgus humeral cup are used, the humerus is moved medially and the deltoid is tensioned by moving it distally or "south." **B,** With an extended glenoid neck and a less valgus humeral cup, a more anatomic reconstruction is achieved with "east-west" tensioning of the deltoid.

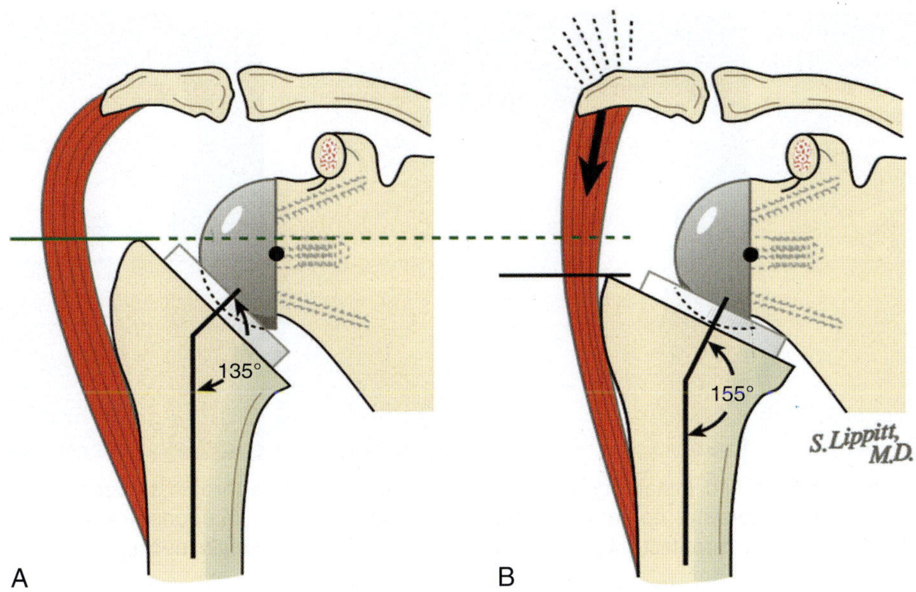

FIGURE 16-528: **A,** Reverse shoulder arthroplasty with relatively anatomic humeral inclination. **B,** This contrasts with a design that results in distal displacement of the humerus with increased risk of acromial stress fracture.

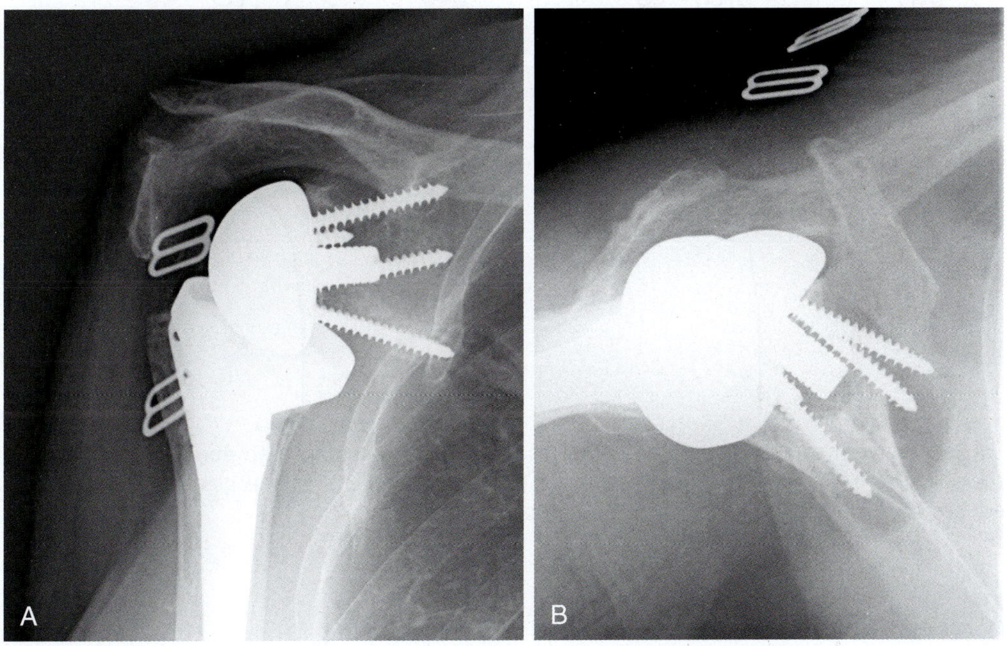

FIGURE 16-529: Acromial fracture and scapular notching after a reverse total shoulder arthroplasty performed with a non-offset glenosphere. **A,** Anteroposterior view. **B,** Axillary view.

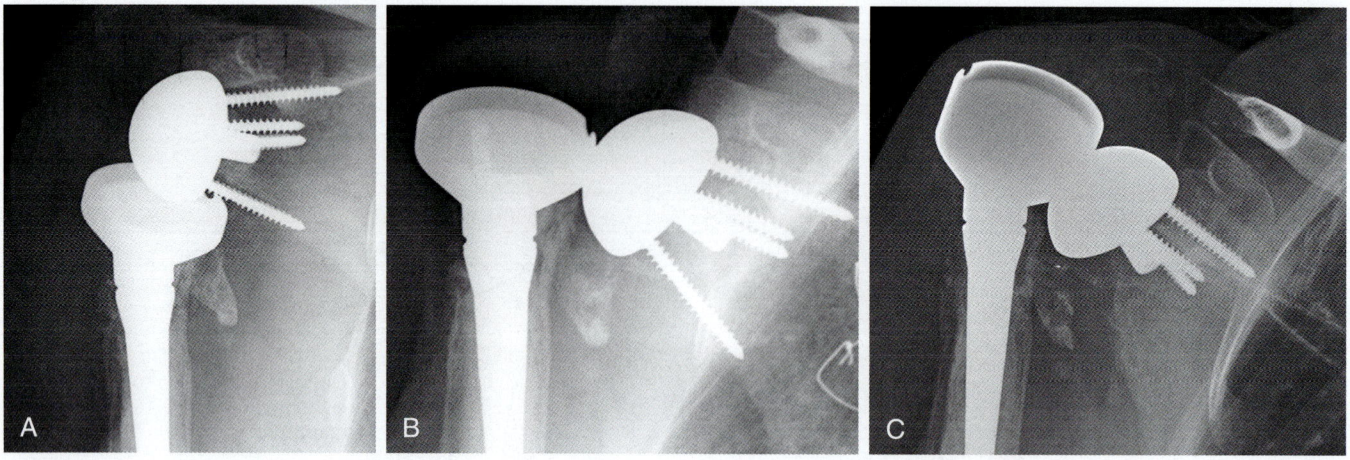

FIGURE 16-530: Scapular notching and instability after a reverse total shoulder arthroplasty performed with a non-offset glenosphere. **A,** Anteroposterior view showing contact between the medial humeral component and an inferior glenoid screw. **B,** Dislocated reverse total shoulder arthroplasty. **C,** Dislocation after revision to a longer necked humeral component.

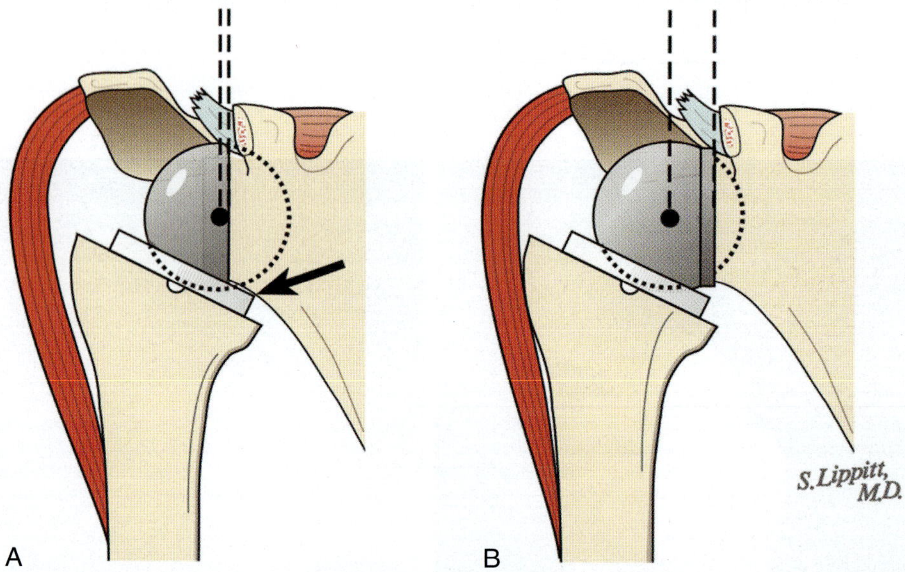

FIGURE 16-531: **A,** Excessive medialization of the center of rotation risks contact between the medial aspect of the humeral component and the scapula. **B,** Because of this, we prefer a design with a neck on the glenosphere that lateralizes the center of rotation and reduces the risk of unwanted humeral–scapular contact.

this (Fig. 16-531). (5) Finally, it allows fixation of a monoblock humeral stem with impaction grafting (see Fig. 16-521; Fig. 16-532), avoiding the stress riser that would otherwise exist between the end of the cement or press-fit stem tip and the often weak bone distal to that point (Figs. 16-533 and 16-534) and obviating the risk of failure at the juncture between the metaphyseal and diaphyseal parts of the prosthesis (Fig. 16-535).

Surgical Technique

Cuff Tear Arthropathy Prosthesis. The two key surgical elements to a successful CTA arthroplasty are as follows: (1) optimizing stability and (2) matching the diameter of curvature of the prosthesis to that of the resected humeral head (Fig. 16-536; see Fig. 16-97).

The patient position, anesthetic, prophylactic antibiotics, skin preparation, and skin incision are identical to those described earlier for an anatomic arthroplasty. In exposing the humeral head, we retain as much as possible of the clavipectoral fascia attached to the coracoacromial ligament (the "CA+") as an additional barrier to anterosuperior instability. The subscapularis is carefully incised from the lesser tuberosity, taking care to keep the subjacent capsule attached to its deep side. The humerus is exposed by gentle external rotation, allowing debridement of cuff tendon remnants and osteophytes as well as sectioning of the long head of the biceps tendon if it remains intact. The humeral head's height and diameter of curvature are measured, ideally before the head is resected (see Fig. 16-306). The medullary canal is entered and progressively larger reamers inserted as sizers until the diaphyseal endosteal cortex is encountered at a depth corresponding to the length of the prosthetic stem ("love at first bite") (see Figs. 16-320, 16-321, 16-387, 16-388, and 16-390 to 16-392); this reamer defines the orthopedic axis. The humeral head is resected at an angle of 45 degrees to the orthopedic axis and the proximal humerus prepared as for a standard humeral arthroplasty (see Figs. 16-393 to 16-397, and 16-430 to 16-434). The lateral tuberosity is resected (Fig. 16-537), the diameter of curvature of the humeral head chosen to match that of the resected head (see Fig. 16-305), and a trial reduction is performed (see Fig. 16-447). The height of the prosthesis is selected so that the deltoid is under mild-to-moderate tension when the arm is adducted (see Fig. 16-308). Impaction grafting is carried out using bone from the resected humeral head (see Fig. 16-323). If the biceps tendon is available, an in-and-out biceps tenodesis is performed (see Fig. 16-384). Drill holes are placed for reattachment of the subscapularis, the prosthesis is assembled and inserted, and the subscapularis is securely repaired.

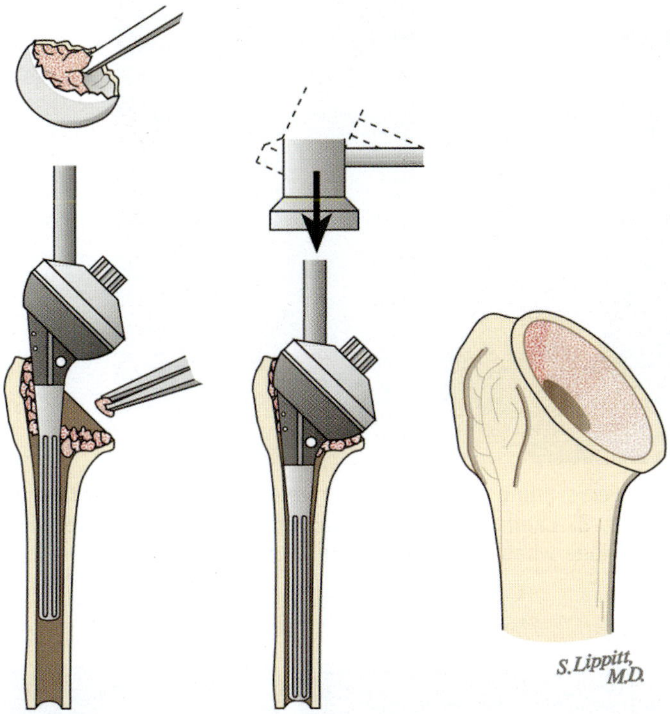

FIGURE 16-532: Reverse arthroplasty system with monoblock humeral stem allowing stable fixation with metaphyseal impaction bone grafting.

Rehabilitation is as for an anatomic arthroplasty, with special emphasis on subscapularis protection.

Reverse Total Shoulder Arthroplasty. The key surgical elements to a successful reverse total shoulder arthroplasty are as follows: (1) immediate, secure glenoid and humeral component fixation; (2) the absence of unwanted contact between the medial proximal humeral component and the scapula; (3) preservation of humeral and glenoid bone stock; (4) stability throughout the range of motion; and (5) a functional range of motion.

The patient position, anesthetic, prophylactic antibiotics, skin preparation, and skin and subscapularis incisions

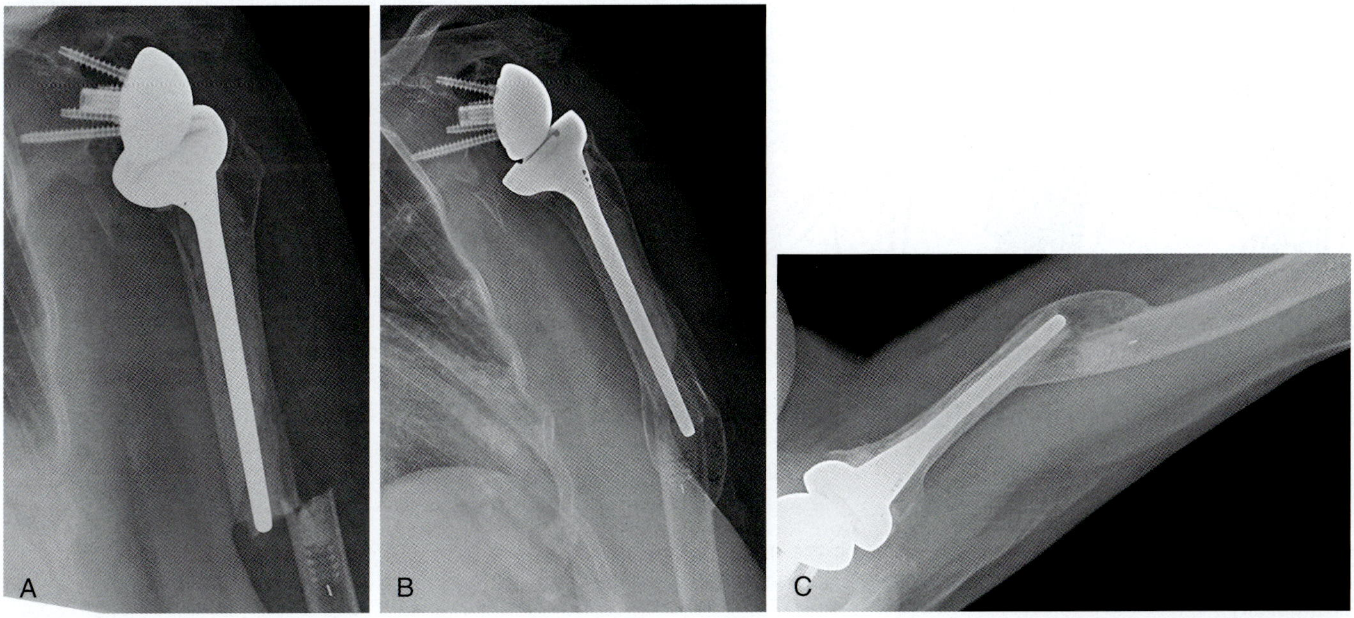

FIGURE 16-533: Periprosthetic fracture just distal to the tip of a reverse humeral component, managed with sling immobilization. **A,** Radiograph soon after fracture. **B,** Anteroposterior view of the healed fracture at 3 months. **C,** Lateral view of the healed fracture at 3 months.

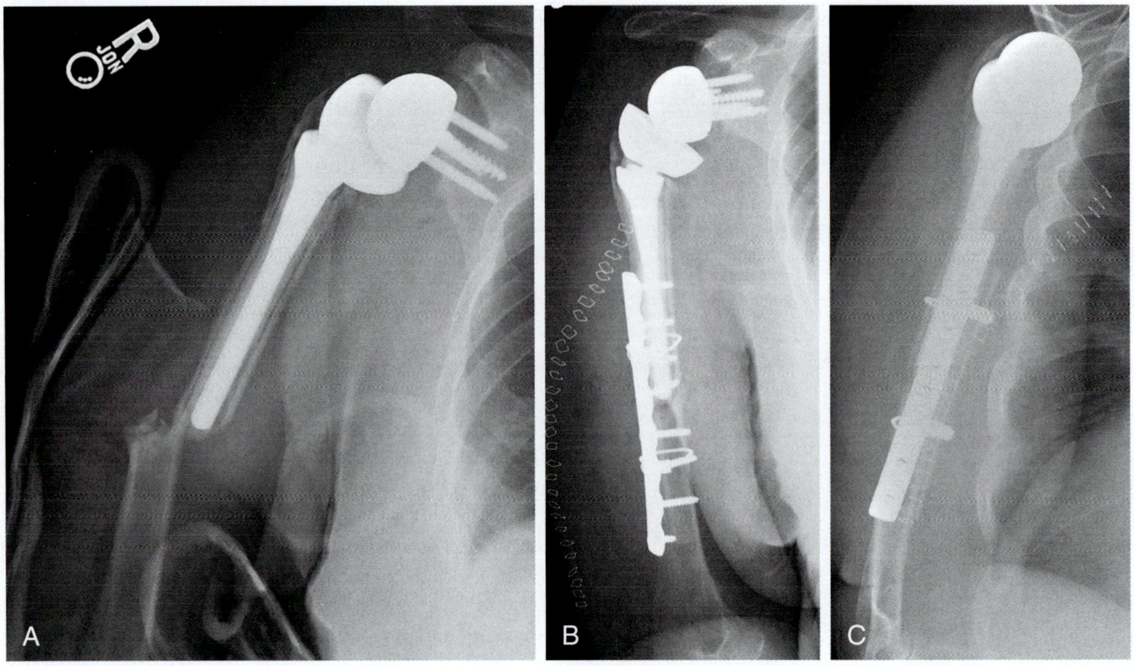

FIGURE 16-534: Periprosthetic fracture just distal to the tip of a reverse humeral component, managed with internal fixation because of fracture instability. **A,** Anteroposterior view of the fracture. **B,** Lateral view of the fracture. **C,** Anteroposterior view showing fixation with a plate, screws dodging the prosthesis, and cerclage wires around a structural allograft.

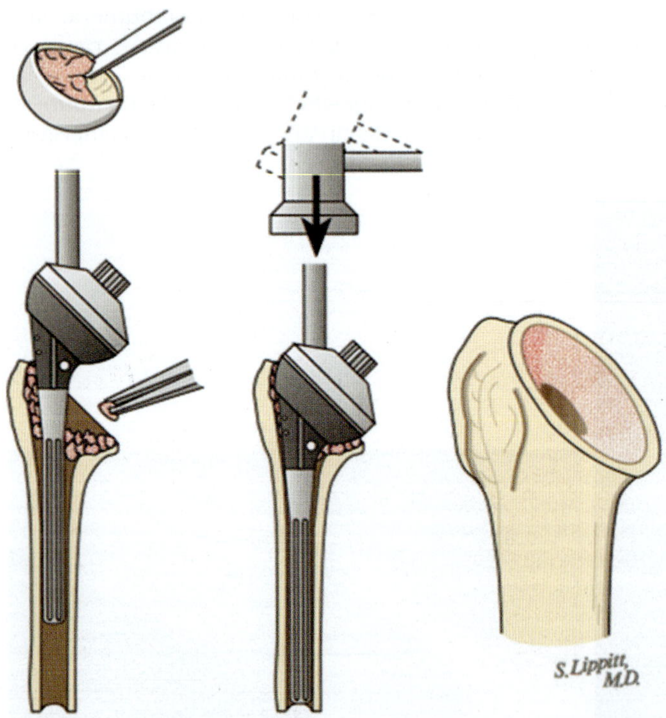

FIGURE 16-535: Failure of the junction between the humeral shaft and the humeral stem of a reverse total shoulder arthroplasty.

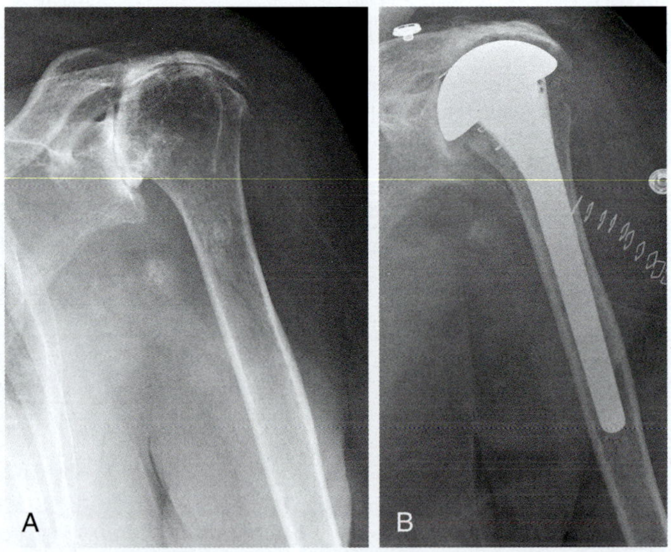

FIGURE 16-536: **A,** Cuff tear arthropathy. **B,** Treatment with a prosthesis.

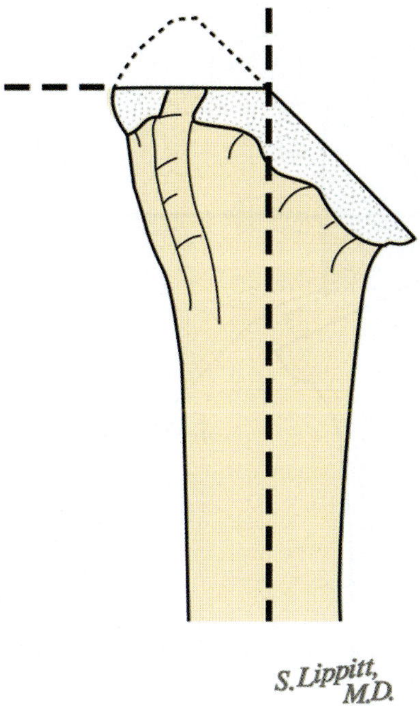

FIGURE 16-537: Resection of the superior aspect of the greater tuberosity in the preparation of a cuff tear arthropathy head component.

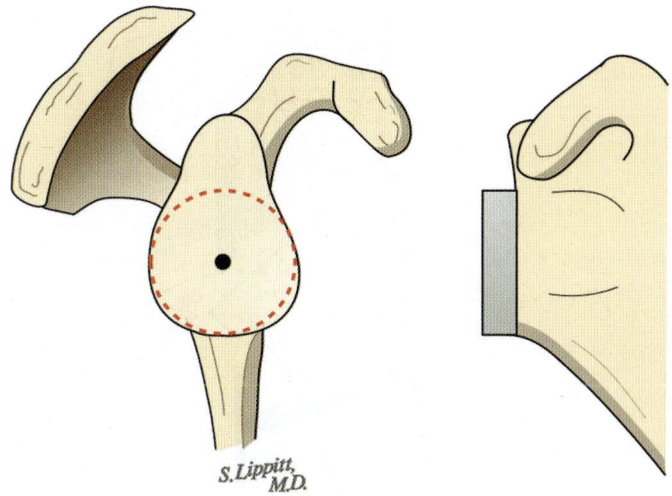

FIGURE 16-538: The starting point for the glenoid drill is selected such that the base plate will cover the maximum amount of good glenoid bone surface.

are identical to those for an anatomic arthroplasty. A deltopectoral approach is used, paying careful attention to protection of the deltoid and the axillary nerve. Care should also be taken to identify, preserve, and protect the subscapularis. The intrinsic stability of the reverse arthroplasty allows the adhesions and scar tissue to be completely removed. As anterior instability can be a complication, it is important to perform sufficient posterior soft tissue releases to accommodate the prosthesis and prevent unwanted anterior pressure on the back of the humeral component. This can be a particular challenge in the revision of anteriorly unstable anatomic prostheses and in diminutive individuals. It is also important to release the contracted inferior capsule, which is frequently present when the humerus has been chronically displaced upwards.

In performing the humeral resection, there are three priorities: (1) leaving as much of the tuberosities as possible for rotational control of the prosthesis; (2) resecting enough bone so that the glenoid arthroplasty can be performed effectively; and (3) enabling reconstruction at the proper length. Our practice is to begin with a very conservative cut to keep our options open. Osteophytes and other unwanted bony prominences are removed. Further humeral preparation is delayed until after the glenoid arthroplasty to avoid weakening the humerus and risking fracture during the glenoid part of the arthroplasty.

A complete circumferential release of the soft tissues from around the glenoid allows excellent visualization. The glenoid is curetted free of cartilage and the inferior lip of the glenoid fossa is smoothed so that it is flush with the glenoid face. The starting point for the glenoid drill is selected such that the base plate will cover the inferior glenoid where the best bone support exists (Figs. 16-538 and 16-539). Excessive inferior positioning of the glenosphere is avoided. Although some surgeons advocate an inferior inclination of the glenoid, we prefer to orient the baseplate squarely on the face of the glenoid to optimize the quality and quantity of the bone supporting the baseplate. Minimal glenoid reaming allows for the preservation of the denser bone at the glenoid surface (Fig. 16-540). The baseplate is fixed securely using the central screw that engages the strong bone of the subscapularis fossa followed by insertion of the peripheral screws (see Fig. 16-523). Care is taken to remove any bone or soft tissue from around the baseplate that may prevent complete seating of the glenosphere. In general, we use a 32-mm glenosphere for smaller individuals, a 36-mm glenosphere for larger individuals, and a 40-mm glenosphere for cases where there is concern about instability. The glenosphere is placed over the cleaned and dried baseplate and vigorously impacted into place, again ensuring complete seating without blockage from bone or soft tissue. The seating can be verified as complete by the inability to distract or turn the seated glenosphere using the insertion handle. The set screw is then placed.

Attention is then directed to the humerus. The goal is to achieve secure fixation without creating a stress riser at the tip of the component. Impaction grafting enables the use of a prosthetic humeral stem that is smaller in diameter than the humeral diaphysis in order to avoid diaphyseal loading. The medullary canal is conservatively reamed to remove cancellous bone but retain cortical bone. The humeral metaphysis is reamed to 42 mm to accommodate the metaphyseal aspect of the humeral component (Figs. 16-541 and 16-542). A trial component is inserted to ensure

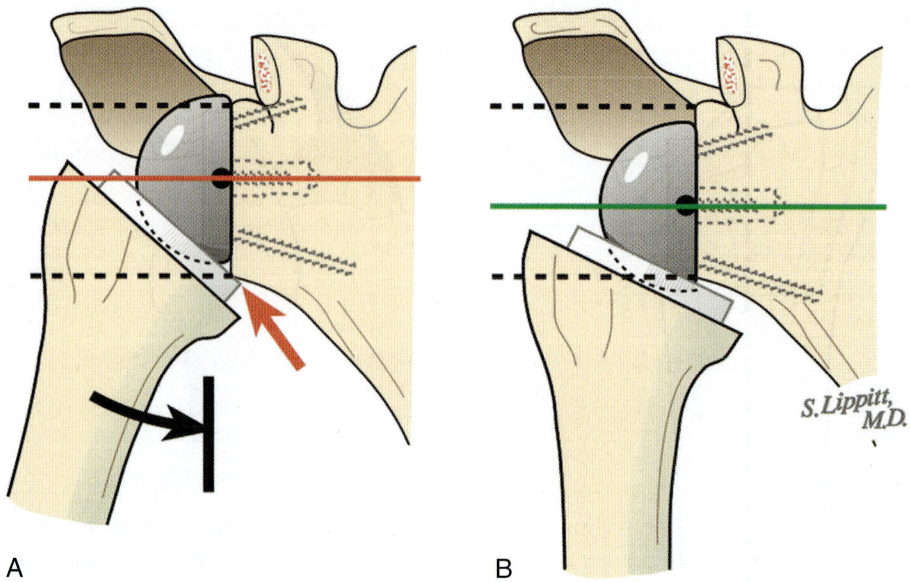

FIGURE 16-539: **A,** Superior placement of the glenoid base plate will tend to cause abutment of the humeral component with the glenoid neck (red arrow), blocking shoulder adduction. **B,** Inferior placement of the glenoid base plate helps prevent the risk of scapular notching.

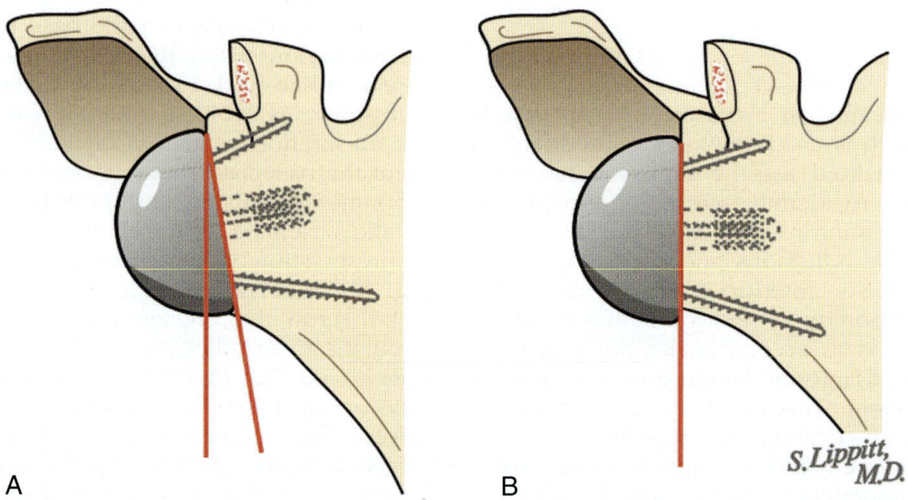

FIGURE 16-540: **A,** Some advocate an inferior inclination of the glenoid achieved by reaming the inferior bone. **B,** We prefer to orient the baseplate squarely on the face of the glenoid to optimize support of the glenoid component without having to sacrifice inferior glenoid cortical bone.

that reduction can be accomplished, that the joint is stable, and that there is no unwanted contact between the prosthesis and the scapula. Impaction grafting is carried out with an impactor of the same size and shape as the monoblock humeral component (see Fig. 16-533; Fig. 16-543). If sufficient tendon is available, drill holes are placed in the lesser tuberosity for reattachment of the subscapularis. The wound is thoroughly irrigated. The humeral prosthesis is then driven into the impaction grafted canal, ensuring a snug fit and rotational stability (Fig. 16-544; see Figs. 16-521 and 16-526). The joint is reduced, and range of motion and stability are again verified to assure the absence of factors that limit mobility.[191] The subscapularis is repaired to the previously placed sutures. A standard wound closure is followed by the application of dry sterile dressings. The goal is a reconstruction with stability, mobility, bone preservation, and optimization of the length-tension relationships of the deltoid and residual cuff muscles (Fig. 16-545).

Postoperative rehabilitation consists of the use of a sling for comfort and support for 6 weeks. Gentle activities of daily living are allowed during this period. After 6 weeks, a progressive increase in active use of the

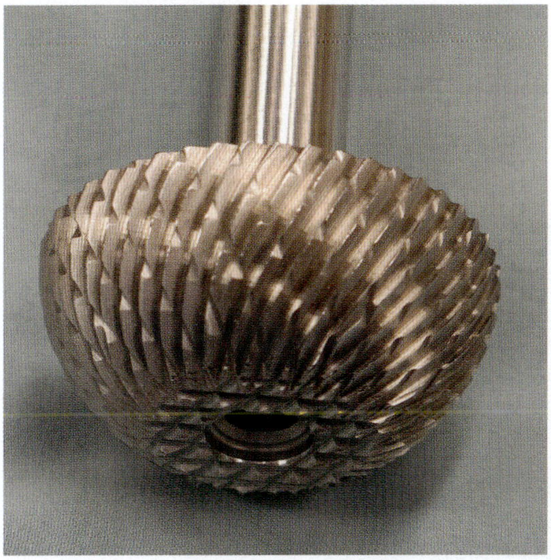

FIGURE 16-541: The "pineapple" reamer used to ream the humeral metaphysis for an impaction grafted monoblock reverse humeral component.

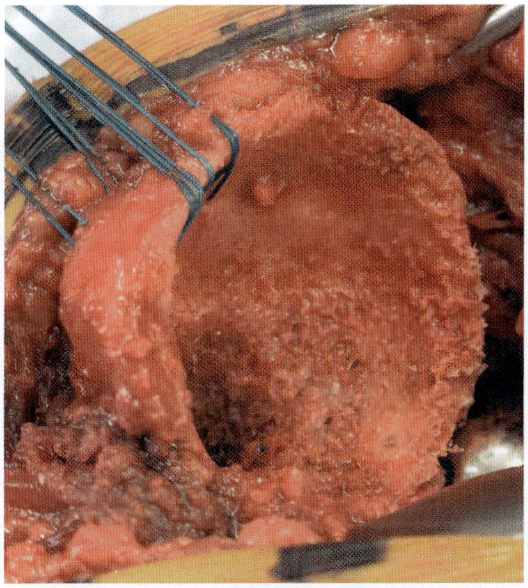

FIGURE 16-542: Humeral metaphysis reamed to fit the metaphyseal aspect of a monoblock reverse humeral component.

shoulder is encouraged; stretching exercises are usually unnecessary.

Results

Cuff Tear Arthropathy Prosthesis. There have been few reports published on the CTA prosthesis, and we suspect that it is underused because of the current enthusiasm for the reverse total shoulder arthroplasty. However, because of its robustness, the CTA prosthesis remains our favored option for active individuals without anterosuperior escape and with more than 90 degrees of active elevation before surgery (Fig. 16-546).

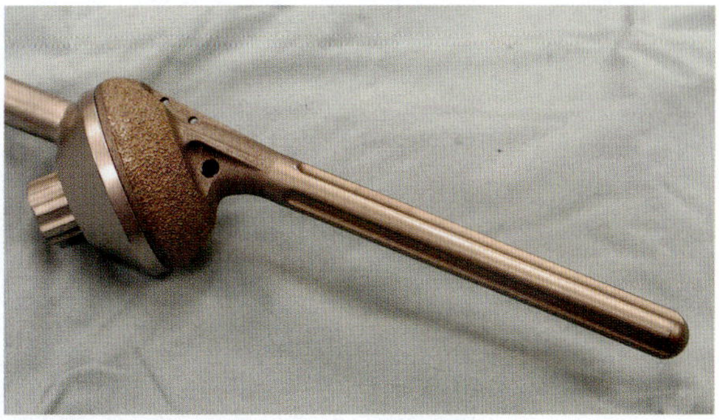

FIGURE 16-543: Trial component used to impaction graft a monoblock reverse humeral component.

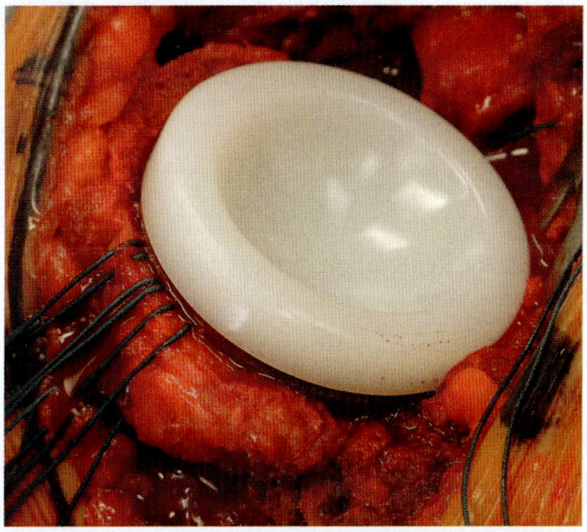

FIGURE 16-544: Impaction grafted reverse humeral component. The sutures at the left were placed prior to prosthesis insertion and would later be used to reattach the subscapularis tendon.

In such patients the resulting functional level can be excellent (Fig. 16-547). Maintaining the integrity of the subscapularis appears to be important to the outcome (Fig. 16-548). The primary causes of failure of the CTA prosthesis are weakness and instability.

Reverse Total Shoulder Arthroplasty. The reverse total shoulder arthroplasty offers a treatment option for a problem that previously had no solution: the unstable, cuff-deficient shoulder. There are now substantial reports of the use of this type of prosthesis to manage a wide range of pathologies, including rotator cuff deficiency without arthritis (see Fig. 16-526),[115,116,200,378,579] rotator CTA,[3,43,150,151,190,416,434,599,601] rheumatoid arthritis,[455,597] failed anatomic arthroplasties,[43,79,298] posttraumatic arthritis[43] (see Fig. 16-450), fractures,[382,384] and arthritis with glenoid bone deficiency.[365,567] Specific methods have been developed for the management of bone defects on the humeral and glenoid sides of the arthroplasty.[79,268]

Complication rates are higher and functional improvement more modest when reverse shoulder arthroplasty is performed as a revision of a prior arthroplasty.[43,79,166,184,524] There are several important modes of failure following reverse total shoulder arthroplasty.[136,166,280,457,569] Infection

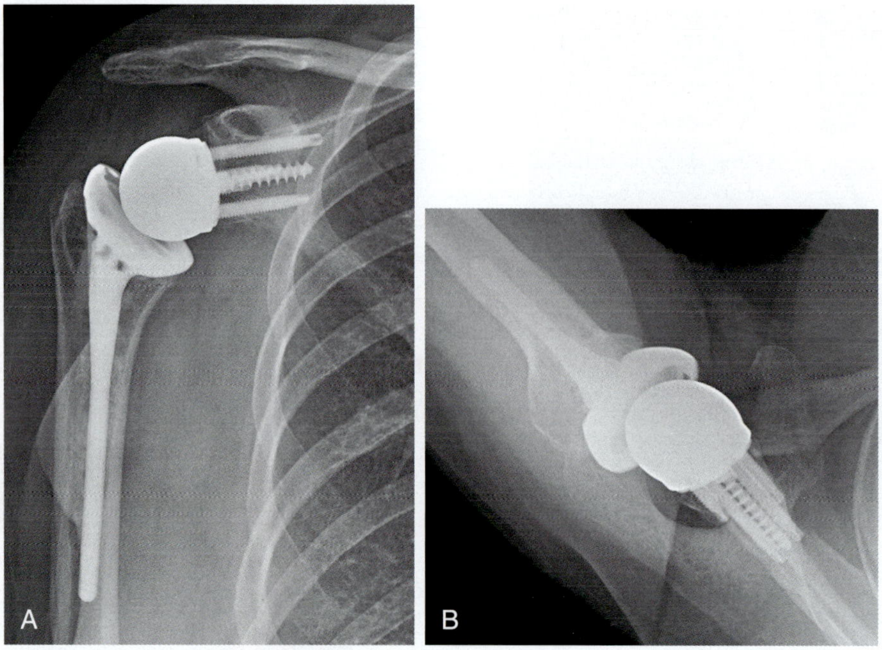

FIGURE 16-545: Restoration of near normal anatomy with impaction grafted monoblock reverse total shoulder. **A,** Anteroposterior view. **B,** Axillary view.

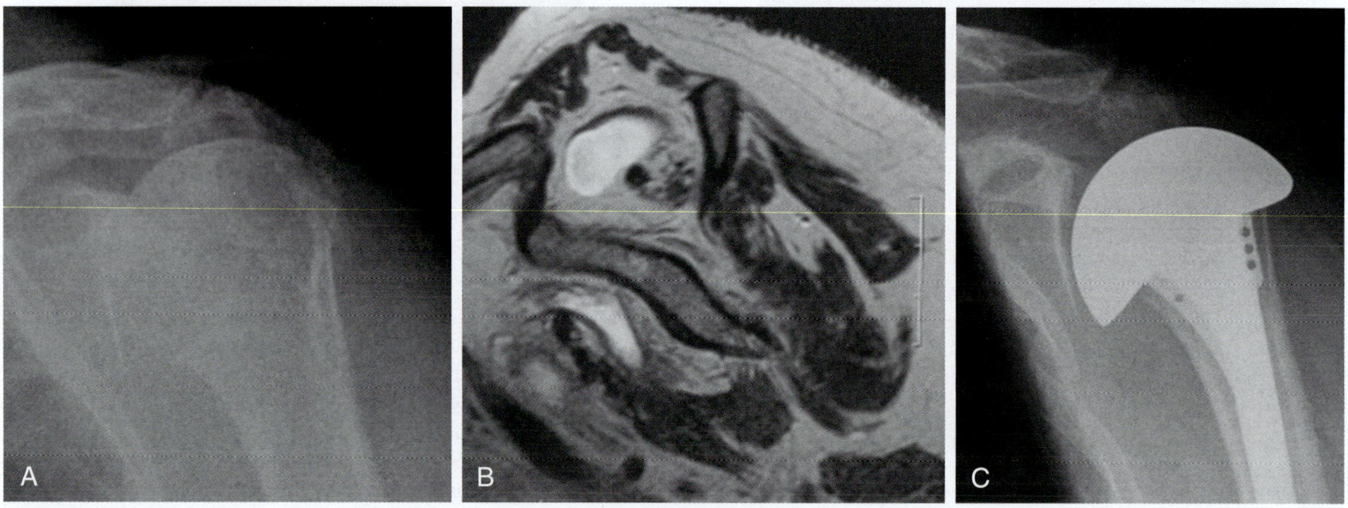

FIGURE 16-546: Typical indication for cuff tear arthropathy (CTA) in a 55-year-old man with balanced (compensated) rotator cuff defect. **A,** Type Ia CTA (minimal superior migration, no significant instability). **B,** Preoperative magnetic resonance image shows some atrophy and secondary fatty degeneration of the superior part of the subscapularis and infraspinatus and advanced atrophy of the supraspinatus. **C,** Radiograph taken 6 months after surgery shows a centered joint without any signs of superior migration.

is one of the most common[373,412] and is probably related to many reverse total shoulder arthroplasties being performed as revisions after multiple prior surgeries coupled with the dead space created when the humerus is displaced distally by the procedure. As with anatomic shoulders, *Propionibacterium* species is a frequently cultured organism from failed reverse total shoulders, which can present with loosening in the absence of the usual clinical signs of infection (Fig. 16-549). Instability[81,541] can result from falls, suboptimal component selection, component malposition (see Fig. 16-530), bulky tissues in the posterior shoulder, leverage of the humeral component

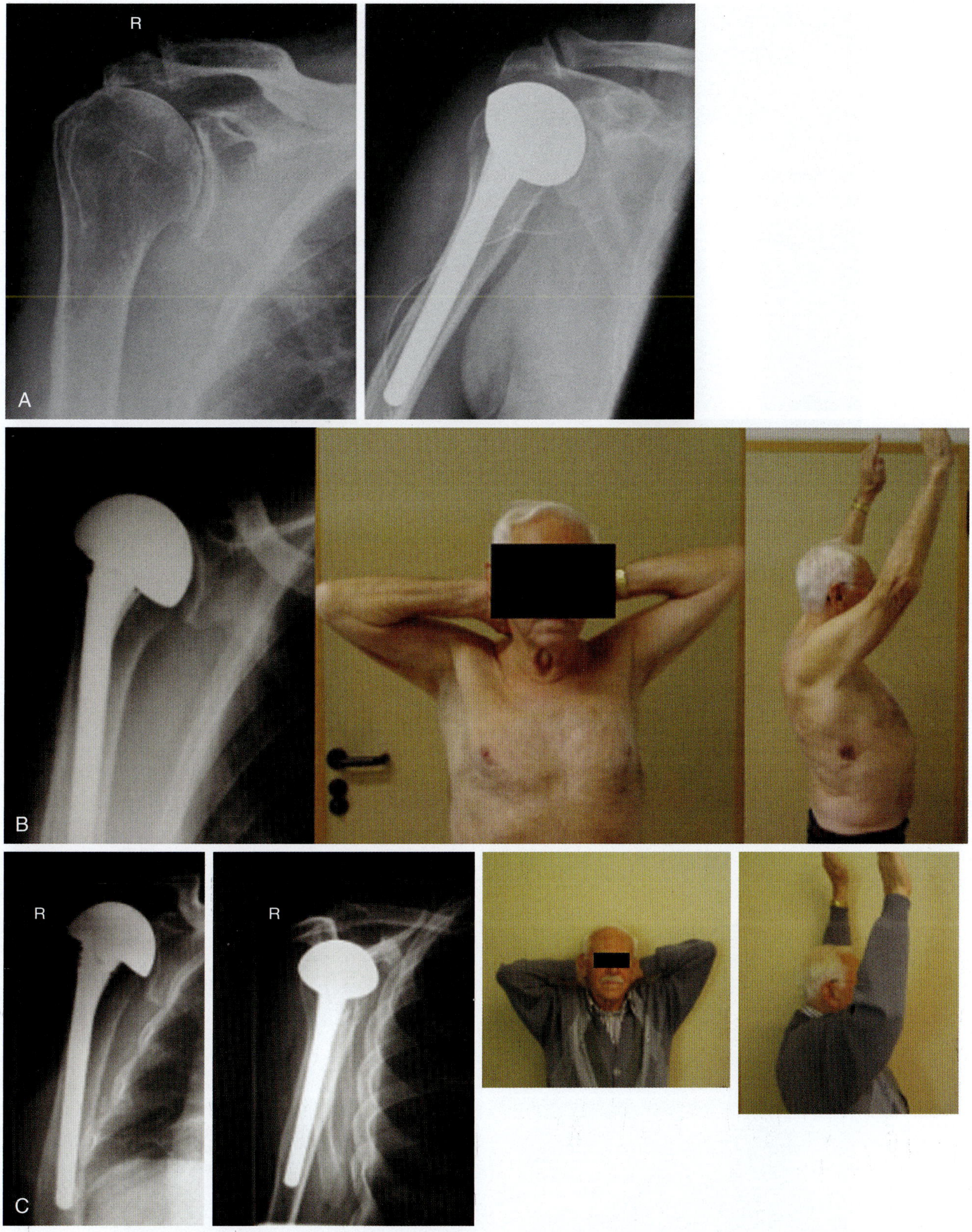

FIGURE 16-547: An 81-year-old man with type IIa cuff tear arthropathy. **A,** Radiographs taken preoperatively (left) and on the first day postoperatively (right). The postoperative radiograph shows good centering of the head. The patient experienced almost no superior migration due to weakness of the deltoid postoperatively because of a continuous postoperative indwelling interscalene catheter delivering pain therapy. **B,** The same patient 6 months after surgery. The radiograph shows some superior migration of the head (left). Photographs show a very good clinical result (center and right). **C,** The same patient 2 years after surgery. The radiographs show increasing superior migration, but the photographs still show a very good clinical result. There is no anterosuperior translation in the Y view (right radiograph), proof of a good functioning subscapularis-infraspinatus force couple.

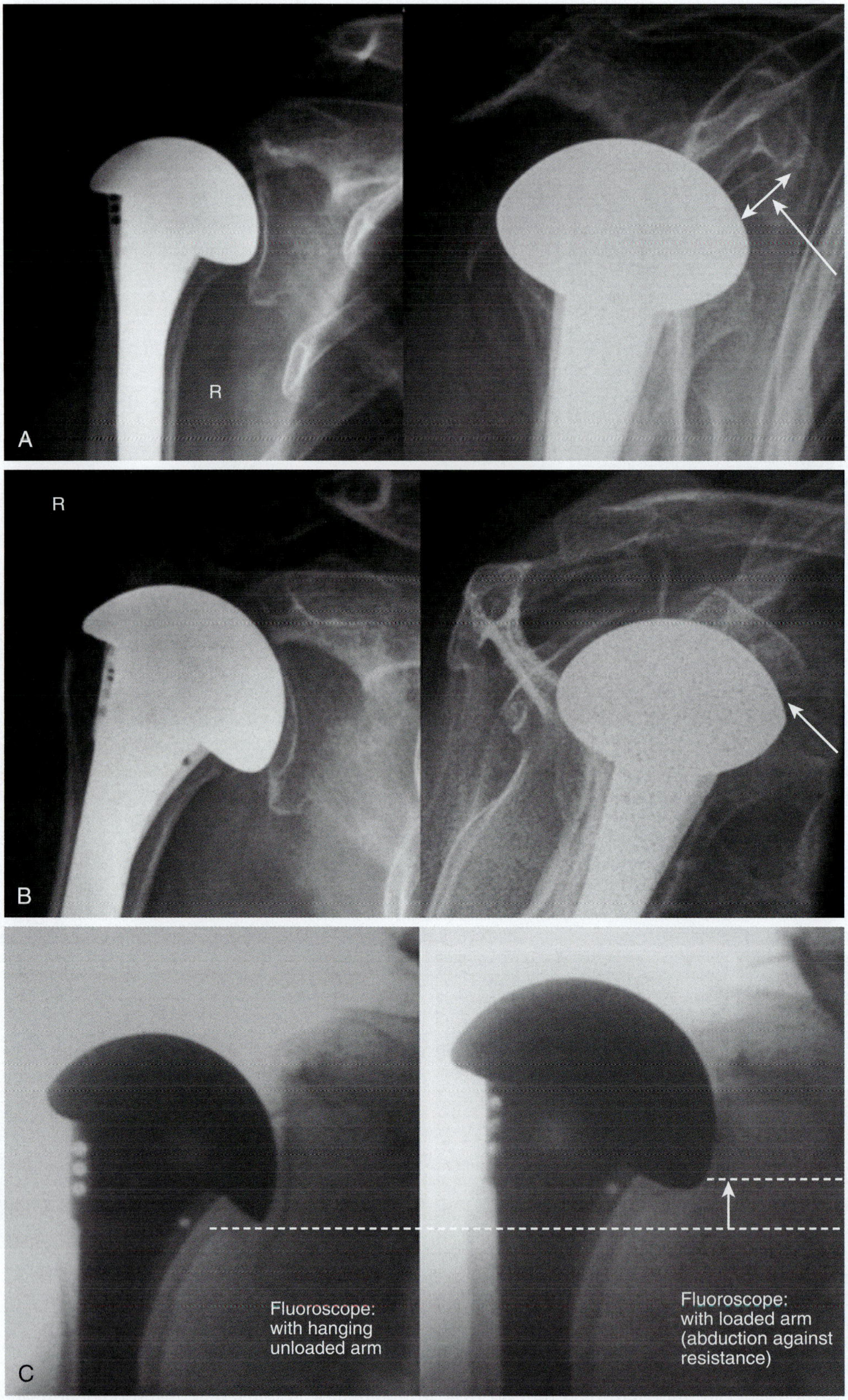

FIGURE 16-548: Failed cuff tear arthropathy head arthroplasty. **A,** Radiograph 6 months after surgery showing a stable joint; the patient had good clinical function. The double-headed arrow indicates the distance between the humeral head and coracoid process. **B,** Radiographs 12 months after treatment show slight superior migration and significant anterior displacement. The arrow indicates contact between the humeral head and coracoid process. **C,** Fluoroscopy 12 months after surgery demonstrates dynamic anterosuperior instability. Deterioration of function was indicated by a positive belly press sign. Revision surgery proved the failure of the subscapularis tendon. The arrow indicates the degree of superior migration.

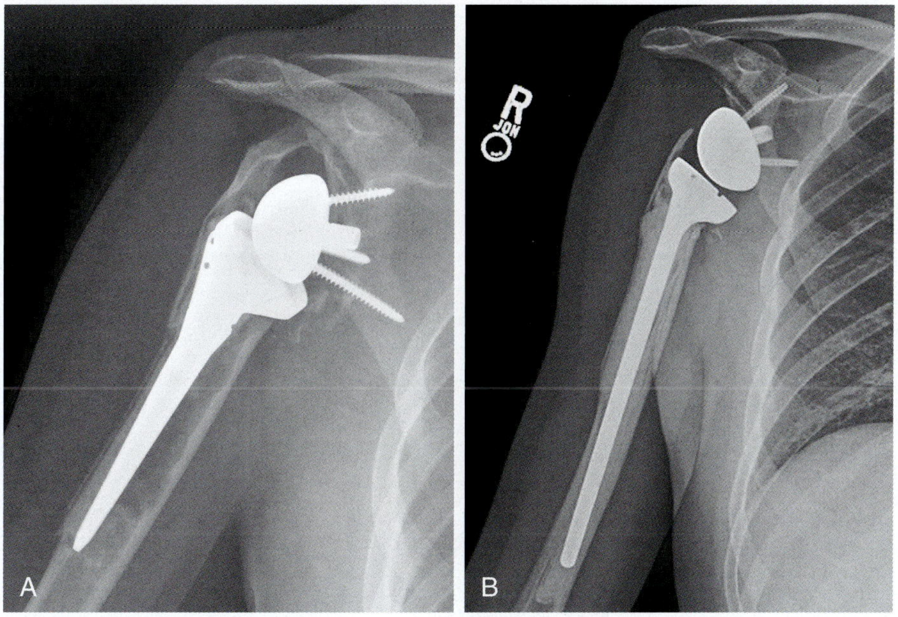

FIGURE 16-549: *Propionibacterium* species infection in a reverse total shoulder arthroplasty. **A,** Four years after a complex reverse arthroplasty for failed hemiarthroplasty, the patient presented with pain in the arm and radiographs showed humeral osteolysis with a cortical break, heterotopic bone formation, and glenoid notching after a reverse total shoulder arthroplasty. **B,** The shoulder was treated with a single-stage revision to a long-stem prosthesis along with 6 weeks of intravenous and 1 year of oral antibiotics. At 6 years there was no evidence of the recurrence of infection and shoulder function was excellent.

against the glenoid (Fig. 16-550), or lack of a sufficient compressive effect by the deltoid (Fig. 16-551). Early closed reduction can be successful.[541] Recurrent or chronic instability may require surgical revision (Fig. 16-552). Stability may be restored by changing to a larger diameter of curvature and increasing the thickness of the polyethylene humeral cup (Fig. 16-553).

The risk of humeral fracture is increased by revision surgery and by falls. It is also increased when the humeral component fixation results in an abrupt transition between a cemented or press-fitted diaphyseal stem tip and osteopenic bone distal to the prosthetic tip. These fractures deserve a trial at closed management (see Fig. 16-533), as surgical revision can be very complex (see Fig. 16-534). Scapular and acromial fractures can result from excessive deltoid tension producing a fatigue fracture or from bone weakened by screw placement.[112,299,540] These fractures are preferably treated nonoperatively.

Scapular notching is a prominent complication and is particularly common in prosthetic designs that medialize the humerus (Figs. 16-554 and 16-555; see Figs. 16-529 and 16-531) or when the glenoid component is positioned high on the glenoid bone (see Fig. 16-539).[3,12,296,501] The issue with notching is not so much the "notch" in the scapula but rather the radiographically unseen damage to the polyethylene of the humeral component (Fig. 16-556) and to glenoid component fixation (Fig. 16-557). Notching may also be associated with unwanted bone formation that limits the range of motion (Fig. 16-558).

Text continued on p. 1040

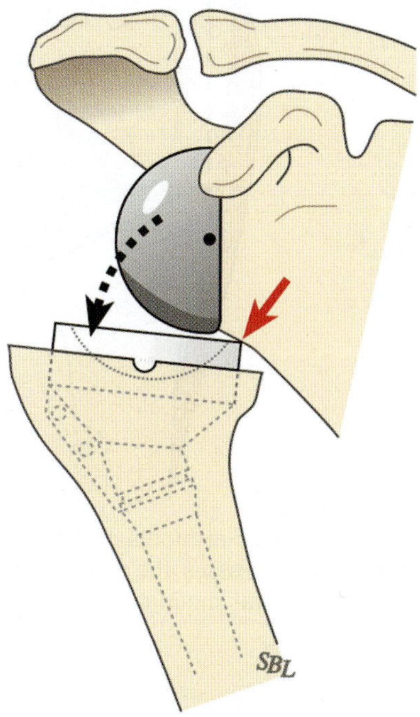

FIGURE 16-550: Leverage of the humeral component against the inferior scapular neck in shoulder adduction (red arrow), resulting in reverse arthroplasty instability.

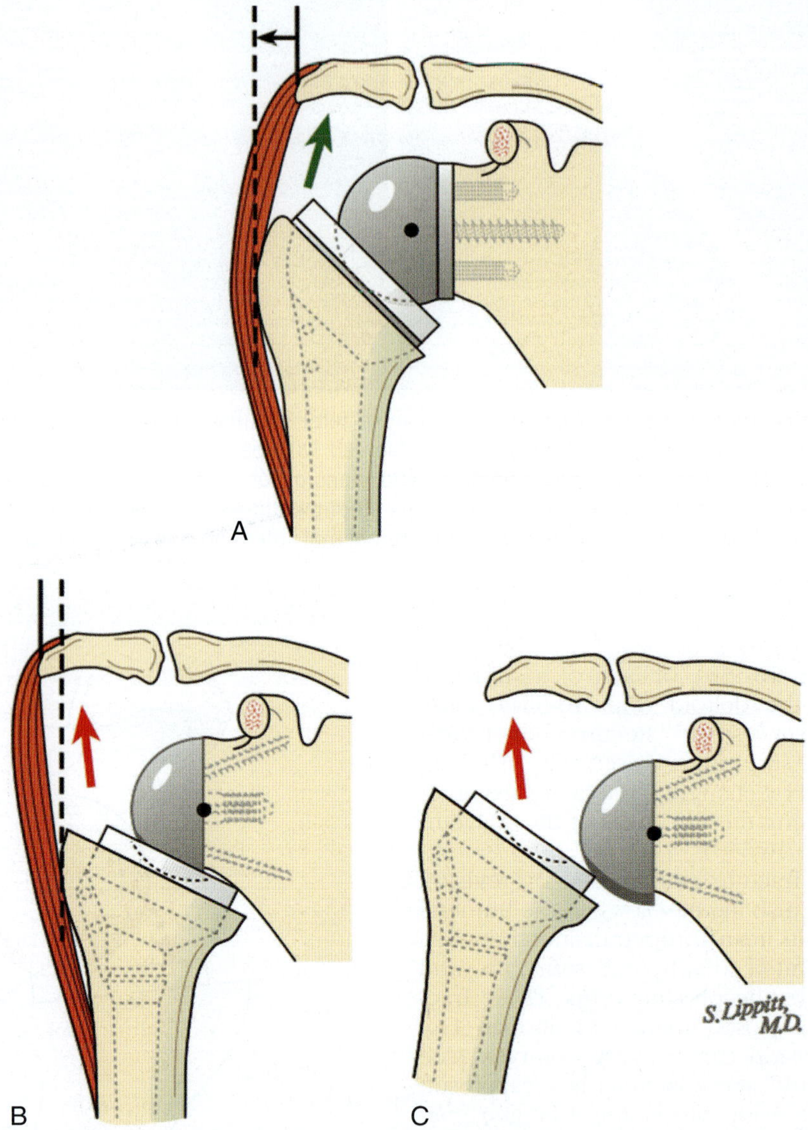

FIGURE 16-551: **A,** Reverse arthroplasty with a lateralized center of rotation and anatomic humeral neck inclination produces a compressive force that presses the humeral cup onto the glenosphere. **B,** Reverse arthroplasty with a medialized center of rotation and valgus humeral inclination produces a force more tangential to the glenosphere. **C,** This situation can lead to instability.

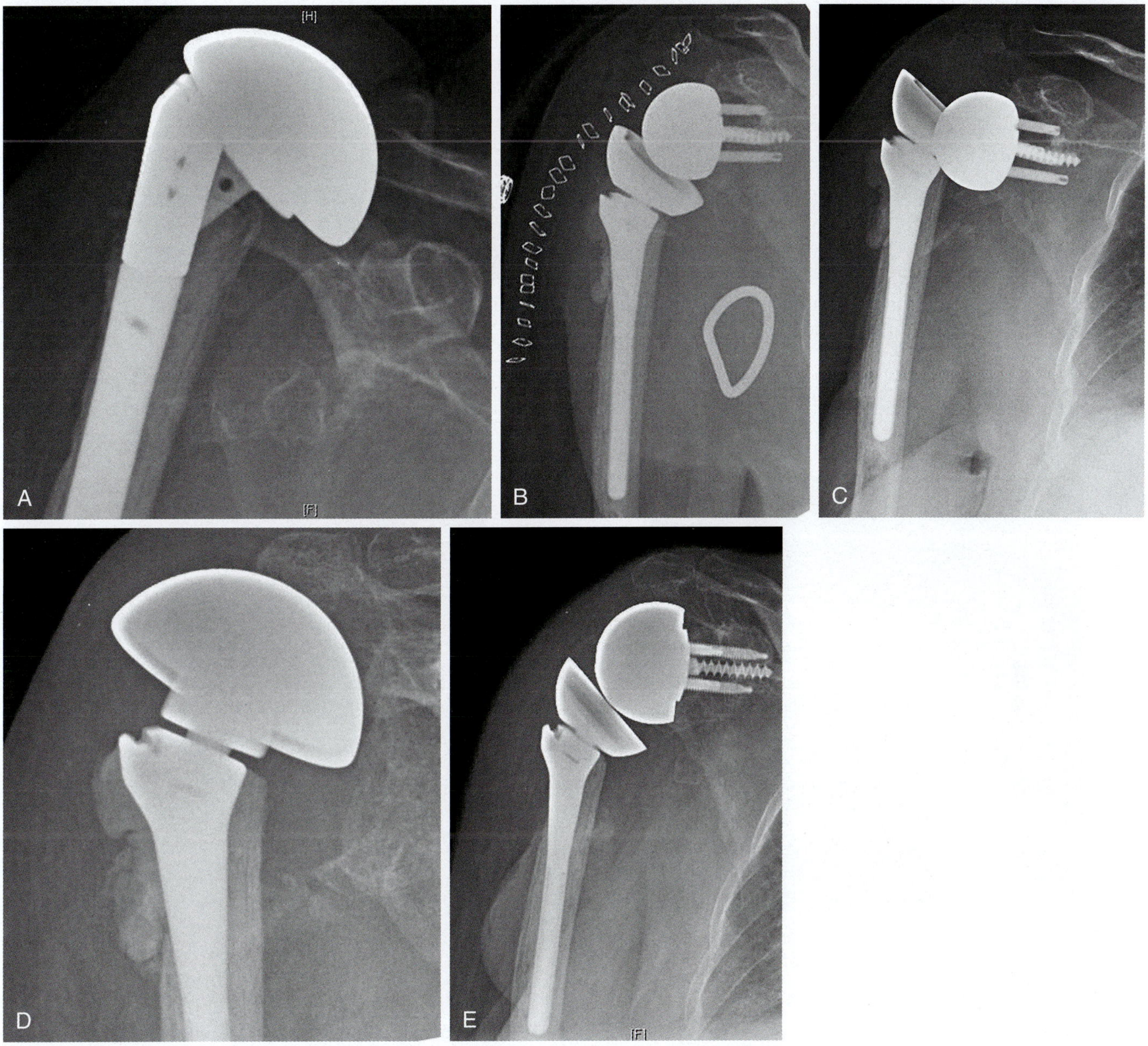

FIGURE 16-552: Problematic instability after reverse total shoulder arthroplasty performed for unstable hemiarthroplasty. **A,** Superiorly unstable hemiarthroplasty. **B,** Reverse total shoulder arthroplasty. **C,** Dislocation of reverse total shoulder arthroplasty. **D,** Recurrent instability after conversion back to hemiarthroplasty. **E,** Successful management after conversion to a large glenosphere.

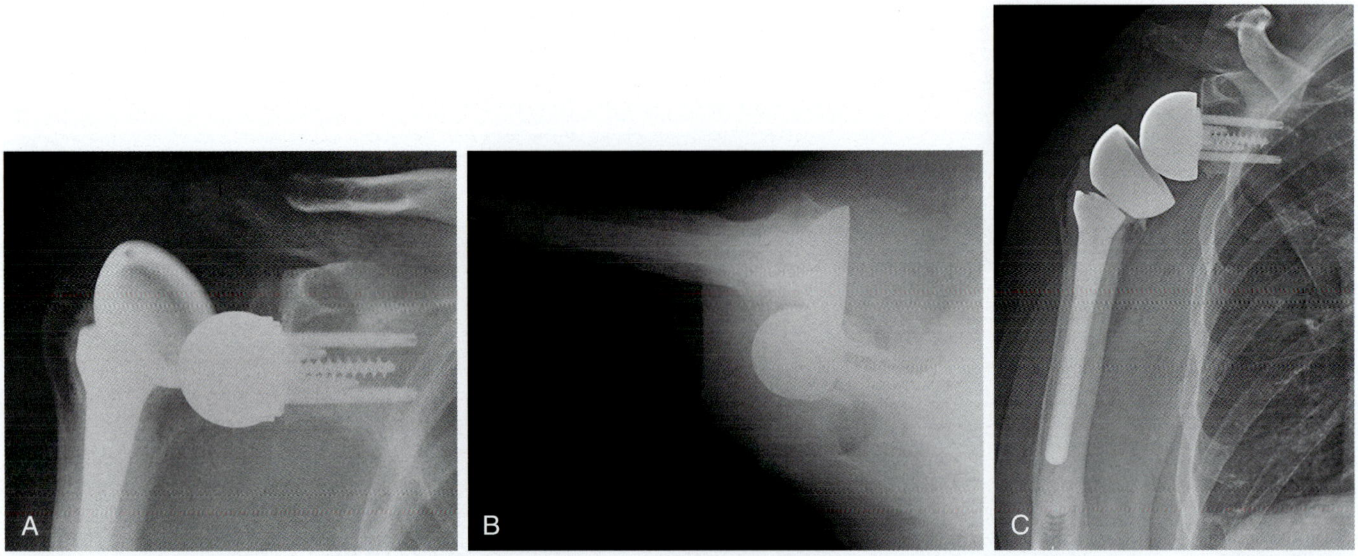

FIGURE 16-553: Dislocation of reverse total shoulder arthroplasty. **A,** Anteroposterior view. **B,** Axillary view. **C,** Stabilization by conversion to a larger sized glenosphere.

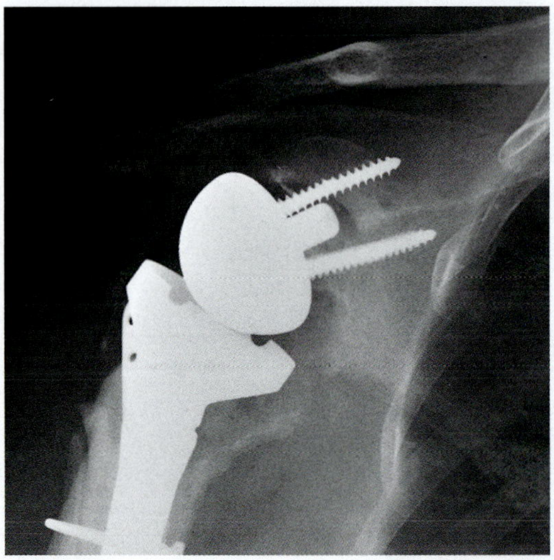

FIGURE 16-554: Scapular notching after a reverse total shoulder arthroplasty performed with a non-offset glenosphere.

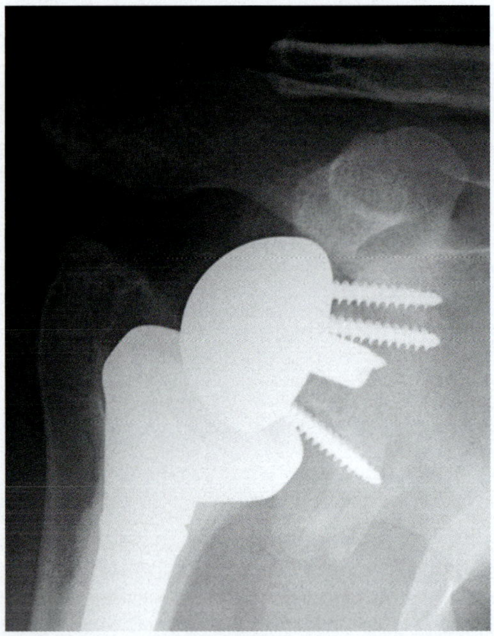

FIGURE 16-555: Scapular notching after a reverse total shoulder arthroplasty performed with a non-offset glenosphere.

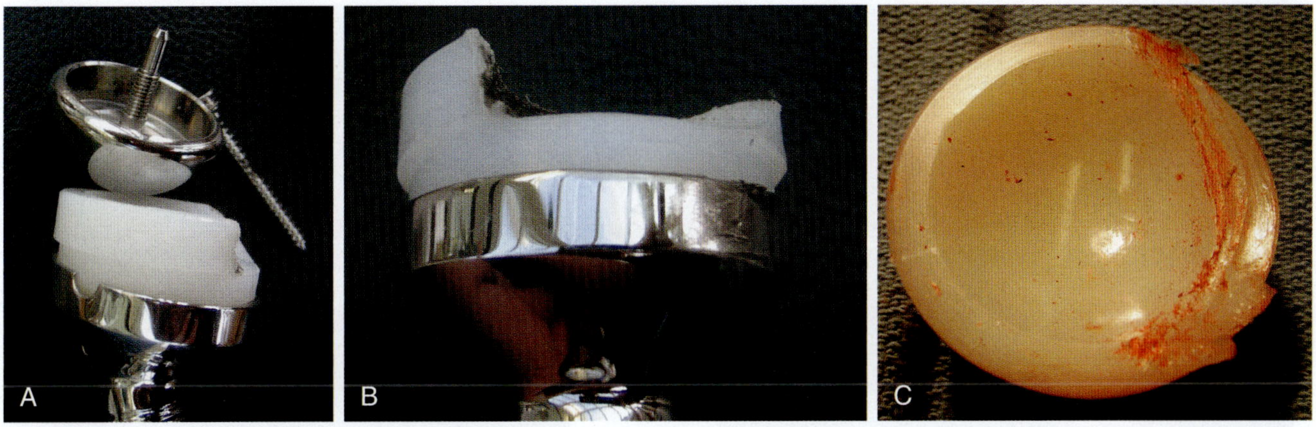

FIGURE 16-556: Polyethylene damage from "notching." The "notch" in the scapula is not the concern; rather, it is the damage to the polyethylene. **A** and **B,** Damage to the humeral cup and screw. **C,** Damage to the humeral cup.

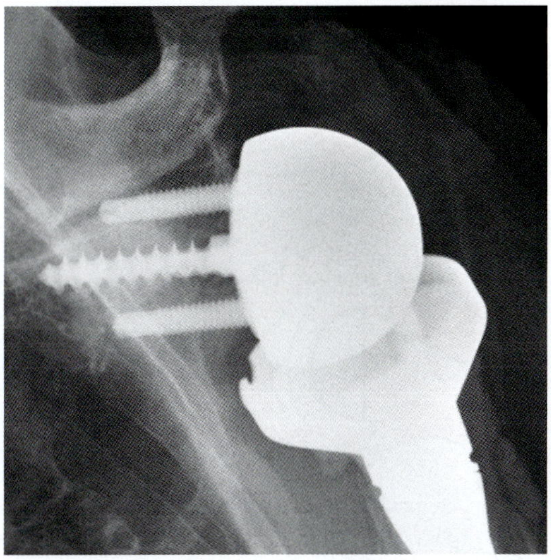

FIGURE 16-557: Scapular notching and glenoid bone loss after a reverse total shoulder arthroplasty performed with a non-offset glenosphere.

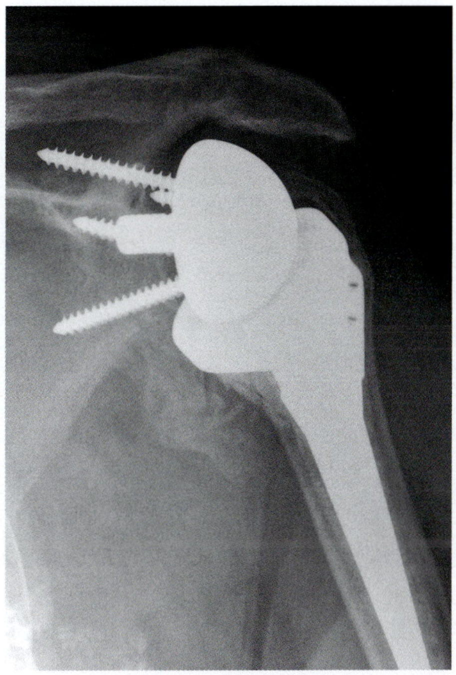

FIGURE 16-558: Scapular notching and heterotopic bone formation after a reverse total shoulder arthroplasty performed with a non-offset glenosphere.

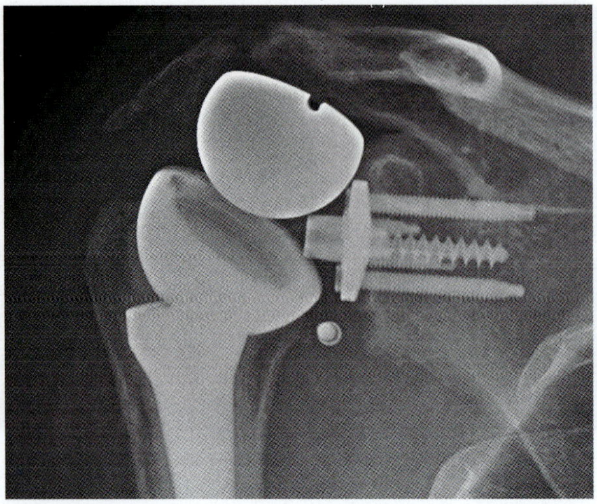

FIGURE 16-559: Dissociation of the glenosphere from the baseplate, the result of bone around the baseplate blocking the complete seating of the glenosphere.

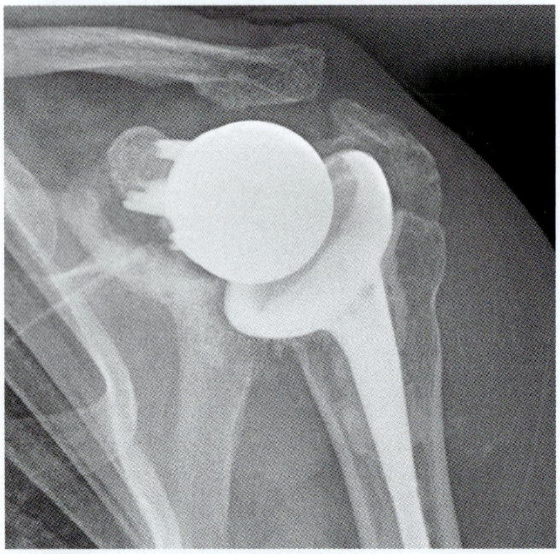

FIGURE 16-560: Fatigue fracture of the glenoid bone after a reverse total shoulder arthroplasty in a woman with severe osteopenia.

Humeral component failure may result from dissociation of the cup from the stem (see Fig. 16-538). Glenoid failure may result from glenosphere-baseplate dissociation (Fig. 16-559), glenoid fracture (Fig. 16-560), or a failure of fixation (Fig. 16-561). While some cases can be reconstructed, others require salvage conversion to a hemiarthroplasty after glenoid component removal. The clinical results of this conversion are generally poor.

Neurologic lesions can result from dissection, retraction, or overlengthening of the arm.[279,280]

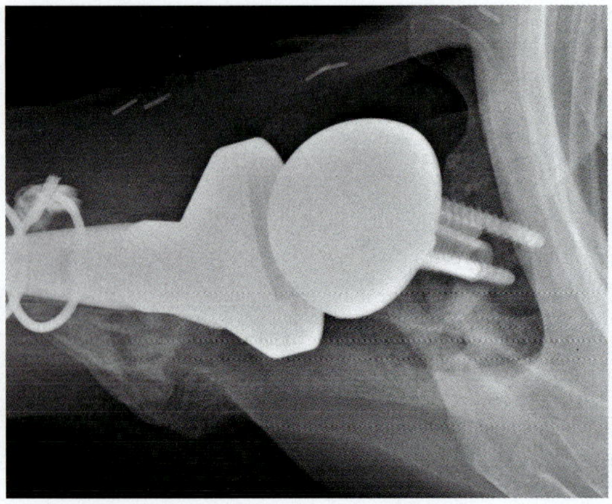

FIGURE 16-561: Failure of glenoid fixation in a reverse total shoulder.

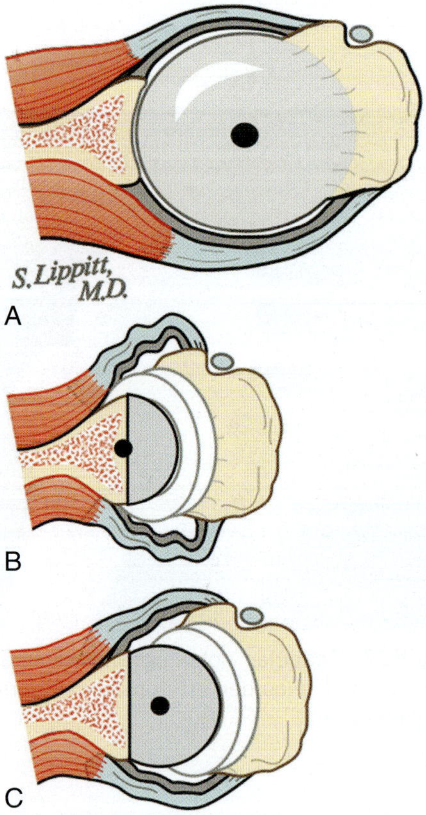

FIGURE 16-562: Tensioning of the rotator cuff. **A,** Normal cuff tensioning in anatomic glenohumeral joint. **B,** Loss tensioning of residual cuff with medialized reverse arthroplasty. **C,** Better tensioning of the residual cuff in lateralized reverse arthroplasty, which contributes to better active external rotation.

There has been some concern about the loss of active external rotation with reverse total designs that medialize the tuberosity, prompting the consideration of latissimus dorsi transfers.[169] This problem seems less of an issue with designs that maintain "east-west" tensioning of the residual cuff posteriorly (Fig. 16-562).

INTERNATIONAL EXPERT COMMENTARY

Gilles Walch

The authors should be congratulated for this extremely well-organized and thorough chapter. Throughout the text, the extraordinary experience of the senior authors, who have performed several thousand shoulder arthroplasties during their careers, provides a very valuable perspective. One can appreciate this invaluable teaching based mainly on experience: what the authors have written is based on first-hand experience, and this piece of work differs greatly from a standard book chapter.

The authors outline or describe their philosophy of shoulder arthroplasty using their experience as background. Although they express strong ideas and opinions throughout the manuscript, their knowledge of the international literature is exhaustive and allows them to comment on the other options available, even though the reader may disagree.

The first part of the chapter is about clinical and radiologic evaluation, and great emphasis is placed on the patient interview and observation. The protocol for radiographs is simple, with the authors' view being that there is no need for secondary imaging, such as MRI or CT. My experience has been different, and over time I have learned to focus more on (1) the state of the rotator cuff muscles, (2) the amount of glenoid wear and retroversion, and (3) the position of the humeral head with respect to the glenoid in the frontal and axial planes.

Although it is true that a perfectly taken axillary view may allow the surgeon to assess the pathology quite nicely in some instances, most of the time the plain radiographs are not usable either because the radiologist or the technician does not know how to take the radiographs correctly or because the patient is too stiff or in too much pain to abduct the arm. Moreover, these radiographs do not allow the surgeon to reliably assess the amount of symmetric or asymmetric glenoid wear, the glenoid retroversion, and the humeral head subluxation. All these parameters have been shown to significantly influence the long-term outcomes of shoulder arthroplasty. I believe that alongside correct standard plain radiographs, the systematic CT scans is very useful before the surgery, allowing assessment of the bony anatomy of the shoulder. Furthermore, a preoperative CT scan is also crucial because it allows an assessment of the state of the rotator cuff muscles.

It has been shown that a small supraspinatus tendon tear does not affect the outcome of total shoulder arthroplasty, and there is no need, indeed, to perform a costly imaging study to detect it. However, it has been shown that fatty infiltration of muscles does have a considerable influence, particularly fatty infiltration of the subscapular, infraspinatus, and teres minor muscles. It is not always possible to reliably assess by clinical examination the rotator cuff in cases of arthritis because of the stiffness and pain. Particularly, it is important to preoperatively detect the absence or atrophy or severe fatty infiltration of the teres minor, associated with fatty infiltration of the infraspinatus, to inform the patient about the postoperative consequences of palsy of the external rotator. This offers the opportunity to discuss with the patient the option of performing a latissimus dorsi transfer simultaneously with implanting the reverse prosthesis.

The second point concerns the definition of CTA. The authors did not describe the Hamada-Fukuda classification, which in my experience is useful for distinguishing between massive rotator cuff tears without glenohumeral arthritis (stages 1, 2, and 3), which are not a good indication for an arthroplasty, and massive rotator cuff tears with glenohumeral chondrolysis with or without osteolysis (stages 4 and 5), for which an arthroplasty must be discussed. Hamada stages 1, 2, and 3 are massive rotator cuff tears; normal active mobility is frequent, and rather than proposing an arthroplasty for pain relief, I prefer to propose a rotator cuff repair (complete or not) and biceps release.

Regarding the mechanics and the stability of the shoulder joint, the authors focus more on the stabilizing glenoid concavity and concavity compression. However, I believe that the state of the internal-external rotators is just as important for explaining the loss of the glenohumeral fulcrum. In cases of complete fatty infiltration of the infraspinatus, the humeral head will always migrate superiorly, whereas in cases of subscapularis insufficiency, the humeral head will be anteriorly unstable. The biomechanics of total and reverse shoulder arthroplasties are mixed: unfortunately the concepts of stability and range of motion are very different for both prosthesis and biomechanical concepts, and the efficiencies of both the systems differ greatly.

Treatment Options

I do not use CTA prosthesis in cases of CTA even if the shoulder can be raised to 90 degrees of elevation. If there is correct active elevation, I believe that it is not a good indication for an arthroplasty. Acromiohumeral contact is rarely a cause of pain. In cases of massive rotator cuff tear I propose either a partial rotator cuff repair with biceps release if there is normal active elevation or a reverse shoulder arthroplasty if there is loss of active elevation. I pay particular attention to the preoperative quality of the external rotator muscles to inform the patient about the risk of paralysis of external rotation or about the possibility of performing a latissimus dorsi transfer.

I prefer to use standard hemiarthroplasty with or without a stem. I also do not use a regular or long-stem prosthesis: metaphyseal stability with or without impaction grafting has been proven to be an excellent option. Therefore there is no need to use long stems, which introduce a risk either of fracture or of stress shielding.

Technique

I do not preserve the long head of the biceps in cases of shoulder prosthesis, regardless of the type of prosthesis implanted. To have an intact long head of the biceps is extremely rare in cases of primary or secondary osteoarthritis; the biceps is one of the main pain generators and does not influence shoulder function.

I do not consider the concept of "soft tissue balancing" easy to apply and relevant for shoulder function. It is very difficult for an inexperienced surgeon, and even for an experienced one, to intraoperatively assess good stability and range of motion. No clinical studies have proven that a thicker humeral head can achieve better stability or range of motion than an anatomic humeral head. Moreover, its influence on overstuffing and a secondary subscapularis tear has never really been explored. The concept of matching normal anatomy is much simpler: adapting the diameter and the thickness of the prosthetic head, its inclination, and retroversion to the normal anatomy does not require

Continued

INTERNATIONAL EXPERT COMMENTARY—cont'd

tremendous experience and does not introduce multiple potential reasons for failure.

Ream and Run

It has never been proven that conservative reaming and flattening of the glenoid without careful correction of version and inclination can prevent progressive erosion of the cancellous bone or even recurrence of posterior humeral head translation. I prefer to use either hemiarthroplasty with a pyrocarbon head or total shoulder arthroplasty.

Postoperative Rehabilitation

I ask my patients not to actively use the affected arm for activities of daily living for the first month postoperatively to allow correct healing of the subscapularis. Early active external-internal rotation at the side will likely create a subscapularis rupture, such as after rotator cuff repair if the patient is allowed to move right away. For the same reason, I focus the rehabilitation program on self-stretching in forward elevation. I never recommend strengthening exercises at any time; I have observed that if the patient is able to stretch several times a day and recover at least 150 degrees of forward elevation within 3 months postoperatively, he or she will recover active mobility easily and rapidly without a strengthening program.

Regarding prevention, evaluation, and the treatment of complications, I enjoyed reading the authors' excellent opinions.

EDITOR COMMENTARY

John W. Sperling

The authors should be congratulated on an extremely well-written and centrally important addition to this book. This comprehensive chapter covers arthritis of the shoulder in great detail and highlights key areas for the physician to be aware of in treating patients with specific causes of shoulder arthritis. The authors have described in significant detail the clinical and radiographic evaluation, with great attention towards directing the surgeon to potential pitfalls and areas to be particularly aware of in treating these patients. The authors have also included less common types of arthritis, which will allow this chapter to serve as an important reference for physicians who have a special interest in shoulder arthroplasty.

The authors have tremendous experience in the management of arthritis of the shoulder. Although I have a stronger preference for anatomic total shoulder arthroplasty and reverse arthroplasty in the treatment of shoulder arthritis, the authors have pioneered alternate options that may be valuable in the young active patient who wishes fewer restrictions following surgery. Overall, this chapter will serve as a central repository for an all-inclusive review of arthritis of the shoulder that will be extremely valuable for physicians who have a strong interest in caring for these patients.

CHAPTER 17

The Biceps Tendon

Todd C. Moen, Wayne Z. Burkhead Jr

In the early 1980s it was not uncommon to see patients who had undergone isolated biceps tenodesis when in reality their symptoms emanated from rotator cuff disease and impingement syndrome. It is quixotic to think, however, that the biceps escapes the degenerative process or is unable to produce symptoms either on its own or in conjunction with other pathologic entities of the shoulder.

The long head of the biceps brachii is the proverbial stepchild of the shoulder. Kessell and Watson[112] described the tendon as "somewhat of a maverick, easy to inculpate but difficult to condemn." Lippman[123] likened the long head of the biceps to the appendix: "An unimportant vestigial structure unless something goes wrong with it." At various times in history, surgeons have subjected this tendon to tenodesis, translocation, pulling it through drill holes in the humeral head, debridement with an arthroscope, and tenotomy. Still others have worshipped at the altar of the biceps, keeping it sacrosanct, contending that it must be there for a reason, even if it is unclear what exactly that reason is or ever was.

The advent of magnetic resonance imaging (MRI), ultrasound, and arthroscopy has allowed clinicians to visualize this tendon through noninvasive and minimally invasive modalities. These techniques have provided fundamental insights into various shoulder pathologies, which in turn have influenced thinking about how lesions of the long head of the biceps tendon (LHBT) are treated. Specifically, the LHBT is intimately related—both anatomically and pathologically—to the superior labrum proximally and to the bicipital groove and beyond distally. Understanding these relationships is crucial to making an accurate diagnosis and devising an appropriate treatment plan for patients with shoulder problems.

This chapter discusses how these lesions have been treated historically, reviews the pertinent anatomy, and attempts to understand the function of this unique tendon. The chapter also reviews current concepts on the etiology, diagnosis, and management of lesions involving the long head of the biceps.

HISTORICAL REVIEW

The history of our understanding of the long head of the biceps is long and full of controversy. The long head of the biceps has at times been indicted as the source of all shoulder pain; at other times it has been seen as an incidental structure of no real consequence. Hippocrates was the first to call attention to the pathologic displacement of muscles and tendons in dislocations. Accurate depictions of the anatomy of the biceps region and intertubercular groove appeared in the 1400s (Fig. 17-1A).

The first reported case of a long head of the biceps brachii tendon dislocation was in 1694 by William Cowper.[42] He presented a case of a woman who was wringing clothes when she suddenly felt something displace in her shoulder. When Cowper examined her 3 days after the injury, he noted a depression of the deltoid, rigidity in the lower biceps, and an inability to extend the forearm. According to Cowper's report, the tendon was reduced by manipulation, and with reduction, the patient immediately recovered use of the arm. Such sudden disabling episode followed by a miraculous recovery is seldom seen in our practice, but so are women who wring clothes, for that matter. Cowper had his supporters, and his theory was accepted by Boerhaave and Bromfield.[20] His observations came under suspicion, however, because of his plagiarism of the Dutch anatomist Godfried Bidloo.[14] Before Cowper's description, many biceps injuries were undoubtedly the result of a direct trauma (see Fig. 17-1B).

In 1803 Monteggia[160] reported a second case of dislocation, but one in which the mechanism was habitual. Subsequently, numerous additional clinical reports appeared in the literature.[87,92,184,196,197] Soden[218] reported one such case in 1841 and was able to confirm the diagnosis at autopsy. Hueter,[100] in 1864, very nicely documented the signs and symptoms of lesions of the LHBT.

However, even during this relatively early period of our knowledge, there was controversy. Jarjavey[104] believed that most of the symptoms were attributable to

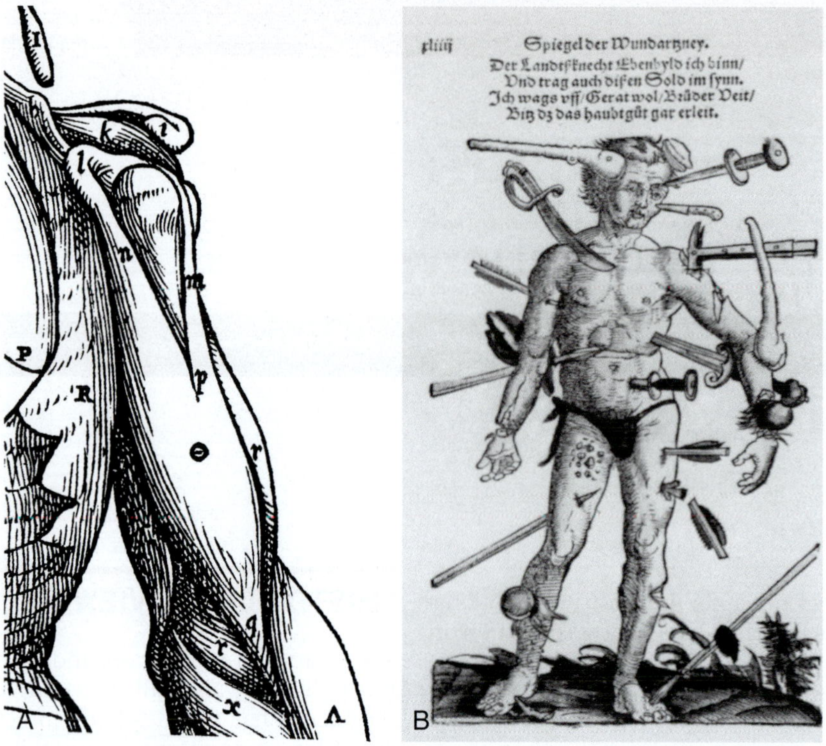

FIGURE 17-1: A, Three tendons of the biceps brachii: short head *(n)*, long head *(m)*, and distal tendon *(q)*. **B,** Anonymous wound manikin, 1517. Probable mechanism of injury to the biceps before Cowper's description. Note the saber-type incision in the opposite shoulder. (**A,** From the Sixth Plate of Muscles. Possibly by Jan Stevenz van Calcar [Flemish ca. 1499-1550]. **B,** From Karp D. *Ars Medica: Art, Medicine, and the Human Condition*. Philadelphia: University of Pennsylvania Press; 1985.)

subacromial bursitis and did not believe in the existence of simple luxation as a clinical phenomenon. Some authors[7,20] believed that the biceps lesion was in fact secondary to arthritis or other concomitant pathology. Callender[28] mentioned one case of recurring dislocation, which he attributed to fibrous tissue within the groove. Duplay[57-59] described *périarthrite scapulo-humérale*, a syndrome that included tendinitis of the biceps. McClellan[137] believed the LHBT to be an important depressor of the humeral head. He wrote:

> Furthermore, the long tendon of the biceps muscle which is lodged below the tuberosities pierces the capsular ligament and passes over the head of the humerus to the top of the glenoid cavity, strengthens the upper anterior part of the joint and prevents the head of the humerus from being brought against the acromion, processing the normal upward movements of the arm. In fact it is mainly by the normal position of this tendon, assisted somewhat by atmospheric pressure, that the head of the humerus is retained in its natural position.

Bera,[12] in 1910, believed that osteitis reduced the height of the lesser tuberosity and thus led to biceps instability. In the 1920s valuable contributions were made by Meyer,[145-152] who discussed observations based on 59 spontaneous dislocations and 20 complete ruptures of the LHBT. He was the first to describe the supratubercular ridge (Fig. 17-2), degenerative changes on the undersurface of the acromion, the acromioclavicular joint, and the coracoacromial ligament. Meyer thought that attrition, particularly after the use of the extremity in abduction and external rotation, led to a gradual destruction of the capsule proximal to the lesser tuberosity and in the region around it. Dislocation resulted as a consequence of capsular weakness in this region.

According to Schrager,[208] F. Pasteur[185] recognized all facets of biceps tendinitis and described it fully, elevating its status as a distinct clinical entity. In 1934 the diagnosis of biceps tendinitis was questioned by Codman,[34] who wrote, "Personally, I believe that the sheath of the biceps is less apt to be involved than are other structures. I have never proved its involvement in a single case. I think that the substance of the tendon of the supraspinatus is most often involved." In the 1940s Lippmann,[123,124] Tarsy,[221] and Hitchcock and Bechtol[96] all believed that biceps tendinitis was an important cause of shoulder pain, and each independently described tenodesis procedures. In 1950 DePalma[47] described degeneration of the biceps tendon with aging and reported on both

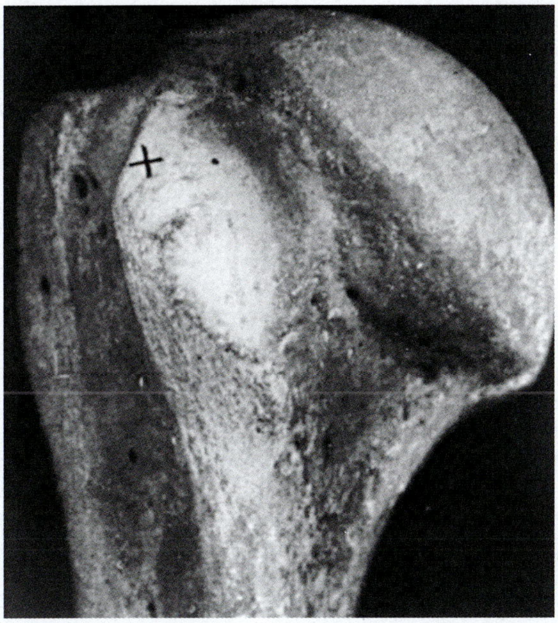

FIGURE 17-2: Original photograph of the supratubercular ridge taken by Meyer. (From Gilcreest EL. Dislocation and elongation of the long head of the biceps brachii. Analysis of six cases. *Ann Surg.* 1936;104:118-138.)

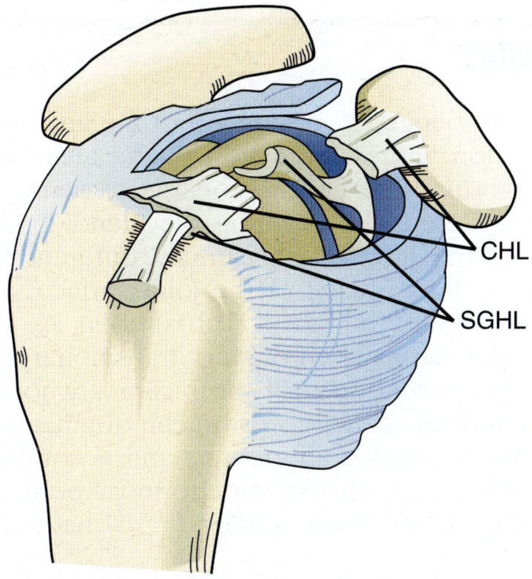

FIGURE 17-3: Diagram of the biceps pulley. The coracohumeral ligament (CHL) and superior glenohumeral ligament (SGHL) blend together to form the reflection pulley, which encloses the long head of the biceps at the entrance of the intertubercular groove.

operative and nonoperative care. Based on gross and microscopic examination of 78 cases, he believed bicipital groove tenosynovitis was the most common cause of a painful and stiff shoulder.

In 1972 Neer[163] described the anterior impingement syndrome, in which anterior acromial spurring with thickening and fibrosis of the coracoacromial ligament causes impingement wear on the rotator cuff and biceps tendon. He pointed out a close association between rupture of the biceps tendon and rotator cuff tears.

Although in the 1970s and 1980s the focus moved away from primary biceps tendinitis and isolated biceps tendon instability, these have definitely regained attention in the last 20 years. Even during the period of skepticism about isolated biceps tendinitis and dislocation, there still were advocates of the significance of these conditions, and several authors published the results of their diagnosis and treatment. Post[194] presented a series of patients with primary bicipital tenosynovitis, and O'Donoghue[174] reported on surgical techniques for treating the subluxating biceps tendon in athletes.

Since the late 1980s and early 1990s, the increased use of MRI and arthroscopy has provided valuable information about the LHBT and its lesions. In 1985 Andrews[5] described tears in the superior labrum of the glenohumeral joint at the attachment of the biceps tendon. In 1990 Snyder[217] first coined the term *SLAP lesion* (superior labrum anterior and posterior lesion) and described a classification system for it.

In the early 1990s Walch[240,242] classified various subluxations and dislocations of the biceps tendon. Since then, he has described the biceps pulley and pulley lesions (Fig. 17-3). Pulley lesions involve the rotator interval and cuff and therefore affect the stabilizers of the LHBT. These hidden lesions,[244] as described by Walch, are not always visible on arthroscopic examination, and open exploration of the rotator interval is sometimes required to identify them. Study of these lesions has directly implicated the superior glenohumeral and coracohumeral ligaments and the subscapularis and supraspinatus in allowing biceps subluxation and dislocation. Bennett[11] has shown that good visualization of the rotator interval, including the coracohumeral and superior glenohumeral ligaments, is possible with the arthroscope.

Further study has helped to delineate the relationship between the LHBT and its anatomic neighbors—the superior labral complex proximally and the bicipital tunnel and beyond distally. Romeo, Provencher, Mazzocca, and colleagues have extensively studied the use of biceps tenodesis as a treatment for superior labral injuries.[88,89,134-136,138,170,198,199,207,213,225] O'Brien and colleagues have defined the anatomy and histology of the bicipital tunnel,[222] studied the validity of arthroscopy as a tool to diagnose bicipital lesions,[224,225,236] and established arthroscopic biceps transfer as a useful treatment for bicipital lesions.[55,223,235] Increasingly, lesions of the biceps are seen more in a proximal and distal continuum of the biceps-labral complex rather than in isolation.[40,88,199,222,223]

It has been more than 300 years since Cowper described his first case. Despite an ever-increasing amount of research, the role of the LHBT and the clinical significance of the lesions associated with it remain controversial.

ANATOMY

It is fitting to begin any discussion of the anatomy of the biceps tendon with a discussion of the anatomy of the superior labrum. The labrum consists of dense fibrocartilage circumferentially covering the glenoid. The fibrocartilage of the labrum is distinctly different from the hyaline articular cartilage of the joint surface, and from tendinous tissue of the biceps. Labral fibers are confluent with articular cartilage through a transitional zone and with the biceps tendon near the biceps anchor.[40]

The long head of the biceps brachii originates, in most cases, at the supraglenoid tubercle and is confluent with the glenoid labrum in the superiormost portion of the glenoid (Fig. 17-4). Some authors[66,129,176] have described the absence of the intra-articular portion of the long head of the biceps or an extra-articular structure. The tendon itself is approximately 9 cm long. At its origin, it varies in insertion: it may be bifurcated or trifurcated, or it can have a single insertion point.[62]

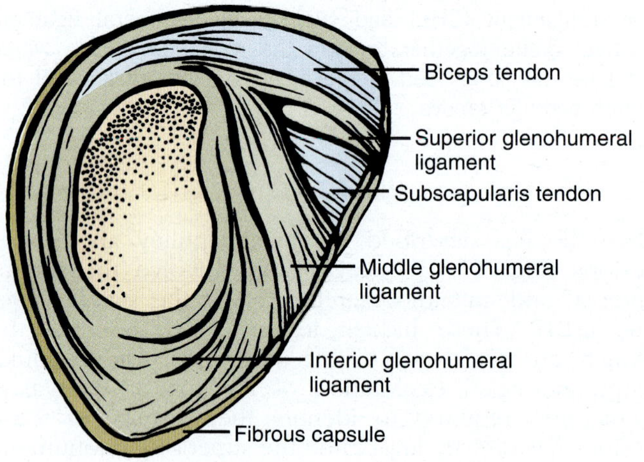

FIGURE 17-4: The biceps tendon is seen inserting on the superior-most portion of the glenoid labrum. Its origin may be simple, bifurcated, or trifurcated.

In a study by Habermeyer and colleagues[90] the biceps was found to originate off the supraglenoid tubercle in 20% of specimens studied. In 48% of the specimens the origin was off the superoposterior aspect of the labrum, and in 28% of the specimens the origin was from both the tubercle and the labrum.

Classically, the anterior-to-posterior distribution of the biceps attachment has been classified into four types as described by Vangsness (Fig. 17-5A to D). The attachment is primarily posterior most of the time, with fewer specimens showing contributions from the anterior labrum.[40,183,233] Tuoheti and colleagues questioned whether the anterior labrum contributes at all to the biceps origin.[229] They looked macroscopically as well as microscopically at the attachment site of the LHBT in a series of 101 cadaveric specimens. When the attachment of the biceps was assessed macroscopically, they found the distribution to be 27% all posterior, 55.4% posterior dominant, 16.8% equal anterior and posterior, and 0% all anterior. However, when these same specimens were assessed microscopically, the attachment site of the LHBT was seen to be predominantly posterior in all cases. This was the case even in specimens that had macroscopically appeared to have equal contributions from anterior and posterior. The authors noted that the macroscopic assessment was often influenced by the variable attachment of the inferior glenohumeral ligament to the labrum. When this attachment was close to that of the long head of the biceps, the macroscopic impression given was of a posterior-dominant or equal anteroposterior (AP) insertion. Microscopic examination however revealed that the attachment, even in these cases, was predominantly posterior.

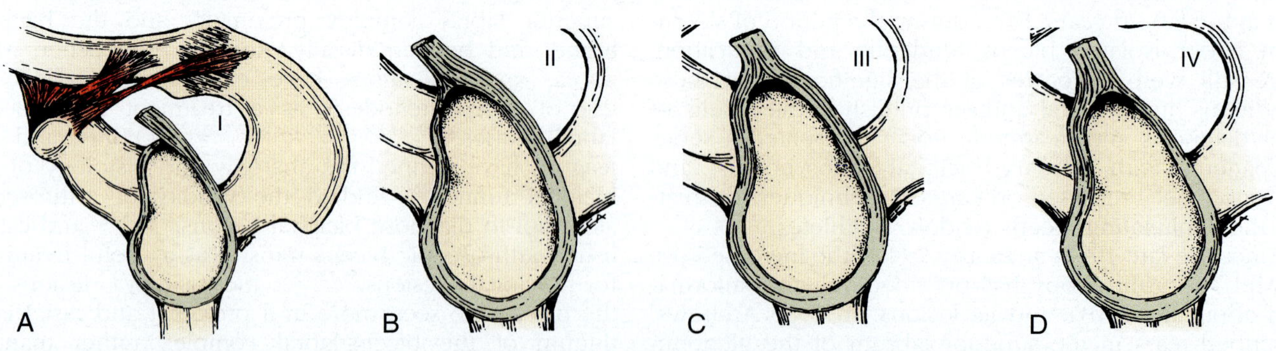

FIGURE 17-5: Distribution of the biceps attachment. **A,** Type I: the labral attachment is entirely posterior, with no contribution to the anterior labrum (22%). **B,** Type II: most of the labral contribution is posterior (33%). **C,** Type III: there are equal contributions to the anterior and posterior parts of the labrum (37%). **D,** Type IV: most of the labral contribution is anterior, with a small contribution to the posterior labrum (8%). (From Vangsness CT Jr, Jorgenson SS, Watson T, Johnson DL. The origin of the long head of the biceps from the scapula and glenoid labrum. An anatomical study of 100 shoulders. *J Bone Joint Surg Br.* 1994;76:951-954.)

The cross-sectional characteristics of the long head of the biceps change during its course from the supraglenoid tubercle down to the musculotendinous junction.[94] The shape of the proximal tendon differs from that of the middle and distal portions. The proximal part is flatter and becomes more circular as it enters the bicipital groove.

McGough and colleagues tested the tensile properties of the LHBT in normal specimens.[142,143] They measured the cross-sectional area of the biceps tendon at three regions: proximal (22.7 ± 9.3 mm^2), middle (22.7 ± 3.5 mm^2), and distal (10.8 ± 2.8 mm^2). There was no significant difference between these three regions. The mean ultimate tensile strength, ultimate strain, and strain energy density for the specimens were found to be 32.5 ± 5.3 MPa, 10.1% × 2.7%, and 1.9 ± 0.4 MPa, respectively. The modulus of elasticity was calculated to be 421 ± 212 MPa. The mode of failure of the tendons in all cases was complete rupture within the midpoint of the tendon substance.

The course of the LHBT is oblique over the top of the humeral head and down into the bicipital (intertubercular) groove. Once out of the groove, the tendon continues down the ventral portion of the humerus and becomes musculotendinous near the insertion of the deltoid and the pectoralis major.

The angle formed by a line from the bottom of the groove to a central point on the humeral head is constant and corresponds to the retrotorsion angle measured from the epicondyles (Fig. 17-6).[83] This angle can be referenced as a guide when placing a humeral head prosthesis. The bicipital tendon, although intra-articular, is extrasynovial. The synovial sheath reflects on itself to form a visceral sheath that encases the biceps tendon (Fig. 17-7). The sheath is open; it communicates directly with the glenohumeral joint and ends in a blind pouch at the level of the bicipital groove.

The long head of the biceps muscle receives its blood supply from the brachial artery. Three arteries supply blood to the bicipital tendon. The distal portion of the tendon receives branches from the deep brachial artery. The proximal part of the tendon also receives branches from the anterior humeral circumflex artery. In the intertubercular sulcus a branch of this artery gives rise to two small branches running in cranial and caudad directions.

The LHBT can be divided into two zones. The first is the traction zone, in which the tendon of the biceps closely resembles a normal tendon. The second is the sliding zone, the fibrocartilaginous portion of the tendon that is in contact with the bony groove. The density of intratendinous vessels in the traction zone is comparable to the vascularization of other tendons, but vascularization of the biceps tendon is markedly decreased in the sliding zone. There are no vessels in the part of the tendon on which the humerus slides. A difference in blood supply between the sliding and intra-articular portions has been reported.[116] This area has also been shown to be composed of fibrocartilage. The portion of the long head of the biceps inside the bicipital groove possesses a mesotendon that arises from the posterolateral portion of its groove.[90] Vascularization appears to play a minor role in the pathogenesis of biceps tendon rupture.

The biceps tendon has classically been described as having an intra-articular portion and a groove portion. Experimental studies have shown that this type of classification is not entirely accurate. Because of the humeral head sliding on the biceps tendon, the position of the arm dictates the amount of intra-articular tendon present. The maximal amount of intra-articular tendon occurs with the arm in adduction and extension, whereas very little of the tendon actually resides within the joint in extremes of abduction.

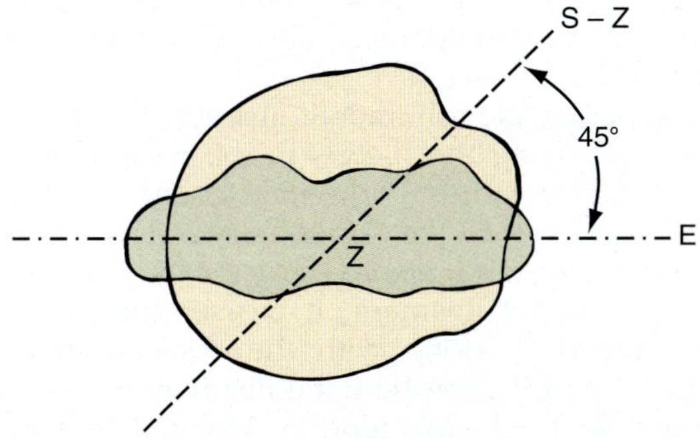

FIGURE 17-6: A line (*S–Z*) through the center of the bottom of the bicipital groove and intersecting with a line drawn across the humeral condyles (*E*) accurately depicts retroversion of the humeral head. (Modified from Habermeyer P, Kaiser E, Knappe M, et al. Functional anatomy and biomechanics of the long biceps tendon. *Unfallchirurg.* 1987;90:319-329.)

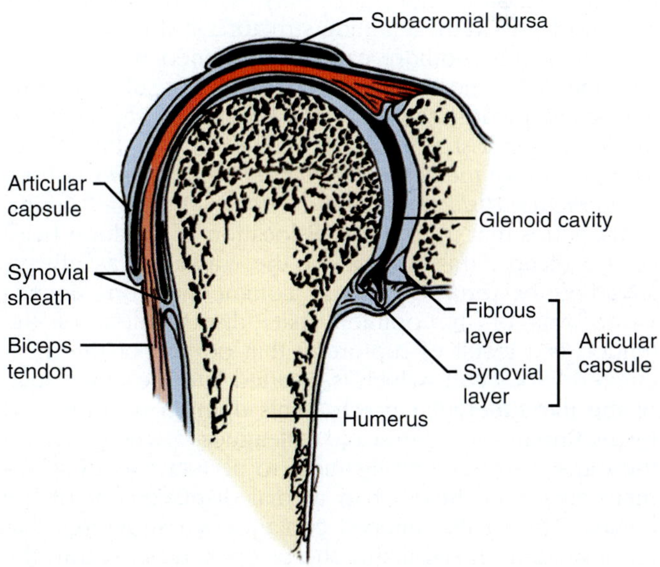

FIGURE 17-7: The insertion of the biceps onto the superior glenoid labrum and the supraglenoid tubercle and the reflection of the synovial sheath, which maintains the tendon as an extracapsular structure while on its intra-articular course.

Distally, the long and the short head of the biceps come together to form a common tendon before inserting onto the radial tubercle. A third muscle belly has been described in some specimens. Mercer[144] and Gilcreest[77] measured the tensile strength of the distal biceps tendon and found it to range from 150 to 200 lb. The blood supply of the muscle belly of the long head of the biceps is via the brachial artery.[90] The nerve supply to this muscle is via the musculocutaneous nerve arising from C5-C7.

Soft Tissue Restraint

As the LHBT courses from its origin on the superior aspect of the glenoid labrum and supraglenoid tubercle to its muscular insertion, it is kept in its anatomic position by several structures. Among the most important of these structures are the capsuloligamentous tissues, which play a major role in keeping the LHBT in the groove. The supraspinatus, subscapularis, coracohumeral ligament, and superior glenohumeral ligament all play a vital role in stabilizing the biceps.

Rotator Interval

The rotator interval is the area bounded by the anterior edge of the supraspinatus superiorly, the superior border of the subscapularis tendon inferiorly, and the coracoid process medially. This triangular area includes both the coracohumeral and the superior glenohumeral ligaments. In its anatomic position, the intra-articular portion of the biceps tendon runs underneath the coracohumeral ligament, which lies within the interval between the subscapularis and supraspinatus, increasing its strength.

The rotator interval is an integral part of the cuff and capsule and is distinguishable only by sharp dissection.[162] The most important retaining structure in this area is the portion of the shoulder capsule thickened by the coracohumeral ligament and the edges of the subscapularis and supraspinatus tendons; this bridges the tuberosities in the uppermost portion of the sulcus (see Fig. 17-3). *This portion of the capsule is the first and foremost obstacle to medial dislocation of the tendon.* Meyer[149,151] found in his series that in cases of dislocation of the long head of the biceps, this portion of the capsule was always stretched or torn. Codman,[34] commenting on Meyer's work, was of the opinion that "displacement of the tendon is a result of rupture at that portion of the musculotendinous cuff, which is inserted into the inner edge of the intratubercular notch." This opinion is supported by the findings of Sakurai and colleagues,[206] who observed the transverse humeral ligament to be intact in 25 specimens that nonetheless had medial displacement of the biceps. The rotator interval contains two structures that are important in stabilizing the biceps tendon within the groove: the coracohumeral ligament and the superior glenohumeral ligament.

The coracohumeral ligament has a broad, thin origin on the coracoid along its lateral border. As the ligament passes laterally, it divides into two main bands. One band

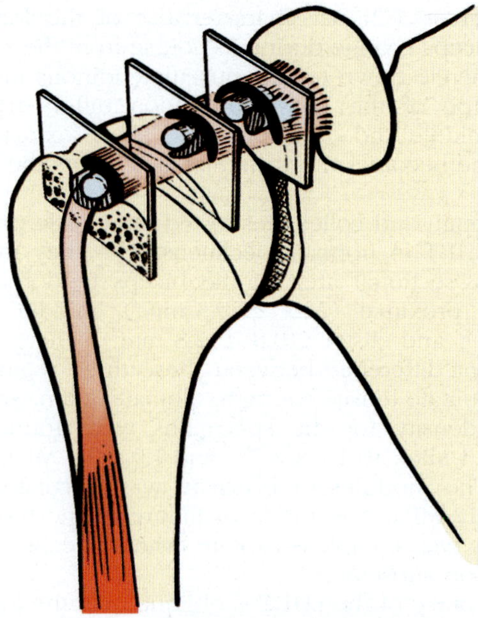

FIGURE 17-8: The interrelationship between the coracohumeral ligament, superior glenohumeral ligament, and long biceps tendon at several planes in the rotator interval. The long biceps tendon (*pale blue*) is positioned centrally. The coracohumeral ligament (*black*) forms a crescent-shaped roof above it, and the superior glenohumeral ligament (*hatched area*) forms a U-shaped trough. (From Habermeyer P, Walch G. The biceps tendon and rotator cuff disease. In: Burkhead WZ Jr, ed. *Rotator Cuff Disorders.* Baltimore: Williams & Wilkins; 1996:142-159.)

inserts onto the anterior edge of the supraspinatus tendon and the greater tuberosity. The other inserts onto the superior border of the subscapularis, the transverse humeral ligament, and the lesser tuberosity (Figs. 17-8 and 17-9). The coracohumeral ligament has extensions that envelop the cuff tendons and blend into the superficial and deep layers of the supraspinatus and subscapularis tendons and the articular capsule. These extensions reinforce the capsule in the rotator interval at the border of the tendinous cuff.[35] The coracohumeral ligament is superficial to the shoulder capsule and overlies the biceps tendon.

The superior glenohumeral ligament is the second structure stabilizing the biceps in the rotator interval. It arises from the labrum adjacent to the supraglenoid tubercle, inserts onto the superior lateral portion of the lesser tuberosity, and blends into the medial aspect of the coracohumeral ligament. It crosses the floor of the rotator interval.[172] Along with the coracohumeral ligament, the superior glenohumeral ligament forms a reflection pulley for the biceps tendon. This pulley is in direct contact with the insertion of the subscapularis tendon. All of these structures blend together to form a sleeve above the entrance to the bicipital groove that is analogous to the flexor tendon pulleys of the hand.[240] This sleeve prevents medial dislocation of the long biceps tendon. Although the superior glenohumeral ligament

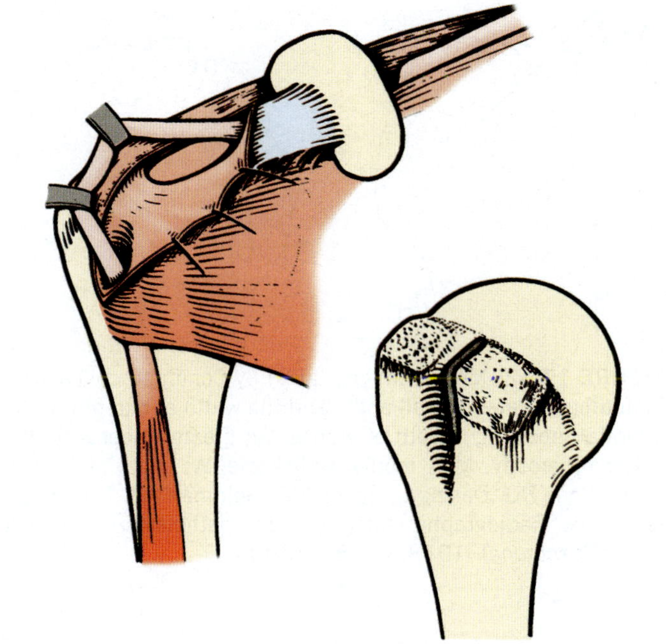

FIGURE 17-9: The rotator interval has been opened to demonstrate the common attachment of the coracohumeral ligament and superior glenohumeral ligament on the humeral head. (From Habermeyer P, Walch G. The biceps tendon and rotator cuff disease. In: Burkhead WZ Jr, ed. *Rotator Cuff Disorders.* Baltimore: Williams & Wilkins; 1996:142-159.)

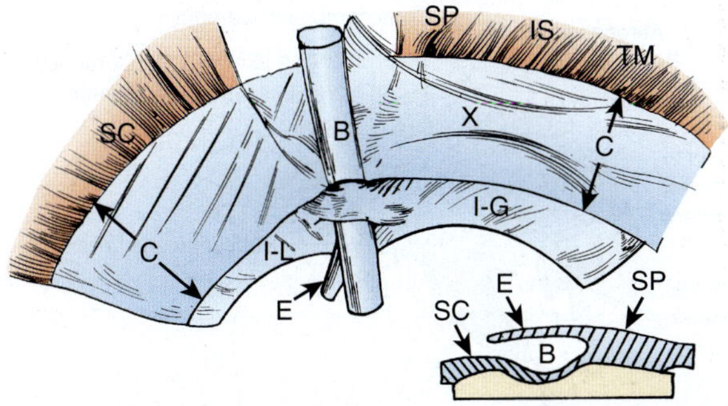

FIGURE 17-10: The deep surface of the rotator cuff–capsule complex after it has been detached from the humerus. The inset shows a cross section of the bicipital groove and related structures. Note the relationships of the capsule (*C*), subscapularis (*SC*), supraspinatus (*SP*), infraspinatus (*IS*), and teres minor (*TM*) tendons, as well as the confluence of the supraspinatus and subscapularis tendons proximal to their insertions on the lesser (*I-L*) and greater (*I-G*) tuberosities. *Inset,* The complex sheath surrounding the biceps tendon (*B*) is shown in cross section. The deep portion of this sheath is formed by the subscapularis tendon, and a slip (*E*) from the supraspinatus tendon forms a roof over the biceps tendon. (From Clark JM, Harryman DT II. Tendons, ligaments, and capsule of the rotator cuff. Gross and microscopic anatomy. *J Bone Joint Surg Am.* 1992;74:713-725.)

has previously been considered insignificant, it is now considered an important stabilizer for the biceps tendon.

Cole and colleagues[36] described the anatomy of the rotator interval in both adults and fetuses. They found two distinct types. Type I intervals have a contiguous layer of capsule in the region of the superior and middle glenohumeral ligaments. In contrast, type II intervals have a defect in the capsule between the superior and middle glenohumeral ligaments. The type II interval was more common (observed in 28 of 37 specimens). Their study results suggest that interval defects may be a congenital phenomenon. In Werner and colleagues' study[251] of the rotator interval, the superior glenohumeral ligament was found to make a U-shaped sling that stabilized the biceps tendon in the groove. The fasciculus obliquus also plays a significant role in investing the biceps tendon, as has been revealed on microscopic examination. The subscapularis was not found to be involved in this suspensory sling, a mechanism that protects the biceps against anterior shearing stresses. The authors concluded that the superior glenohumeral ligament is the most important stabilizing structure for the biceps tendon and that injury to this sling may lead to anterior bicipital instability.

The Groove

The supraspinatus and subscapularis tendons fuse to form a sheath that surrounds the biceps tendon at the proximal end of the groove. Fibers from the superior portion of the subscapularis tendon pass below the biceps tendon and join with fibers from the superior part of the supraspinatus to form the floor of the sheath (Fig. 17-10). A slip from the supraspinatus forms the roof of the sheath along with the superior glenohumeral and coracohumeral ligaments. The deep portion of the sheath runs adjacent to the bone and forms a fibrocartilaginous lining in the groove that extends approximately 7 mm distal to the entrance of the groove.[38]

The role of the transverse humeral ligament in stabilizing the biceps in its sulcus has been disputed by several authors.[149,179,206] Traditionally, the LHBT was thought to be maintained within the sulcus by the action of the transverse ligament (Fig. 17-11), but Meyer[149] found that this ligament was in fact either too weak or often entirely absent. Gleason and colleagues[81] even disputed the very existence of the transverse ligament as a separate discrete structure, showing continuation of fibers from the supraspinatus and subscapularis tendons even in the distal portion of the groove. Paavolainen and colleagues[179] were unable to dislocate the biceps even after sectioning the intertubercular transverse ligament, provided the rotator cuff was intact.[169]

Once the tendon has entered the groove, the principal structure maintaining the tendon within the groove is the falciform ligament, a tendinous expansion from the sternocostal portion of the pectoralis major. It forms a margin with the deep aspect of the main tendon that stabilizes

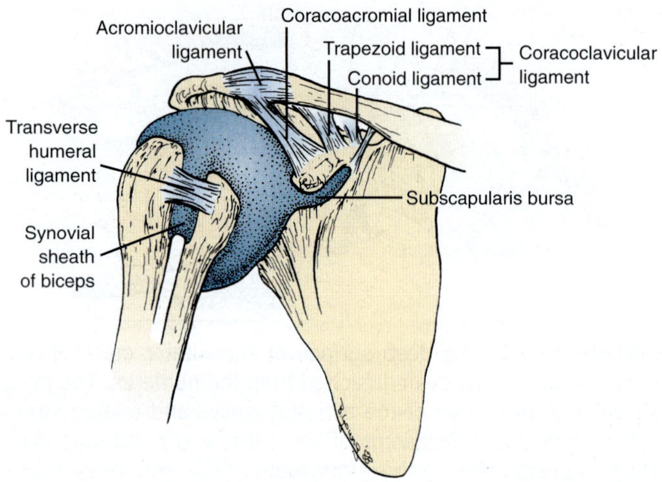

FIGURE 17-11: The ligaments around the shoulder. Meyer[23] found the transverse ligament to be too weak or entirely absent.

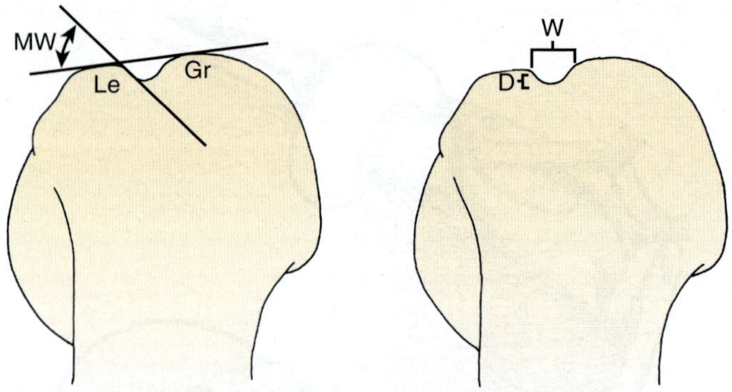

FIGURE 17-12: Measurements taken by Cone and colleagues, including the medial wall angle and the width and depth of the bicipital groove. D, depth of groove; Gr, greater tuberosity; Le, lesser tuberosity; MW, medial wall angle; W, width of groove. (From Cone RO, Danzig L, Resnick D, Goldman AB. The bicipital groove: Radiographic, anatomic, and pathologic study. *AJR Am J Roentgenol.* 1983;41:781-788.)

the biceps. The falciform ligament is attached to both lips of the groove and blends with the capsule at the shoulder joint.

O'Brien and colleagues have rigorously studied the anatomy of the biceps, both where it traverses through the bicipital groove and distally.[40,222,224,225] They defined the bicipital tunnel as a specific fibro-osseous structure that encloses the long head of the biceps.[222,225] The bicipital tunnel begins at the articular margin of the humeral head and ends in the subpectoral region; it has three zones. Zone 1 begins at the articular margin and ends at the distal end of the subscapularis tendon. Zone 2 begins at the distal margin of the subscapularis and ends at the proximal portion of the pectoralis major tendon. Zone 3 is defined as the subpectoral region. This zoning is clinically significant as zone 2 is a "no man's land" in which pathology cannot be visualized at arthroscopy or in open subpectoral surgery.[222-225,235]

Osseous Anatomy

The bicipital groove is formed between the lesser tuberosity medially and the greater tuberosity laterally. Cone and colleagues[37] have extensively studied the bicipital groove, measuring the width and depth of the intertubercular groove and the angle of the medial wall (Fig. 17-12). In assessing the width of the intertubercular sulcus, they obtained two separate measurements from the bicipital groove view. The first of these was the top width or the distance between the medial and lateral lips of the intertubercular sulcus. The second was the middle width or the distance between the walls of the sulcus but taken at a depth halfway into the sulcus. The difference between measurements varied, but the ratio of the top width to the middle width was constant at 1.6. The average depth of the groove was found to be 4.3 mm (range, 4 to 6 mm), and the mean medial wall angle was 56 degrees (range, 40 to 70 degrees).

In a separate study Ueberham and Le Floch-Prigent[230] measured the intertubercular sulcus in dry bones. They found the total length of the groove to be 27.5 mm. On average, the proximal part of the intertubercular sulcus was 12.4 mm, and the most distal part was 15.1 mm. They noted that the groove was deepest in the middle and shallower at its proximal and distal ends. They measured the angle between the proximal segment of the groove and the distal segment and found it to have a mean of 142 degrees but with a high degree of variability. A supratubercular ridge was present in 45% of specimens and was thought to force the biceps anteriorly, thereby increasing the risk of dislocation. This abnormality was found in isolation in 17% of specimens and in association with one other lesion in 18%.

Variability in the medial wall angle was confirmed in studies by Hitchcock and Bechtol,[96] Habermeyer,[90] and Cone.[37] Hitchcock and Bechtol found that the medial wall angle was 90 degrees in 10% of specimens, 75 degrees in 35%, 60 degrees in 34%, 45 degrees in 13%, 30 degrees in 6%, and 15 degrees in 2% (Fig. 17-13). They found (as did Habermeyer) that the medial wall angle correlated with the probability of subluxation of the LHBT. Cone, however, did not find a correlation between the incidence of subluxation and low medial wall angles.

Vettivel and colleagues[238] found that the shape of the intertubercular sulcus correlated with hand dominance: the intertubercular sulcus on the dominant extremity was wider and had a more acute medial wall angle. They attributed this difference to greater stress passing through the tendon in the dominant extremity, especially during manual activities.

Comparative Anatomy

Hitchcock and Bechtol,[96] using specimens from the Field Museum of Natural History in Chicago, outlined changes in the relationship between the scapula and

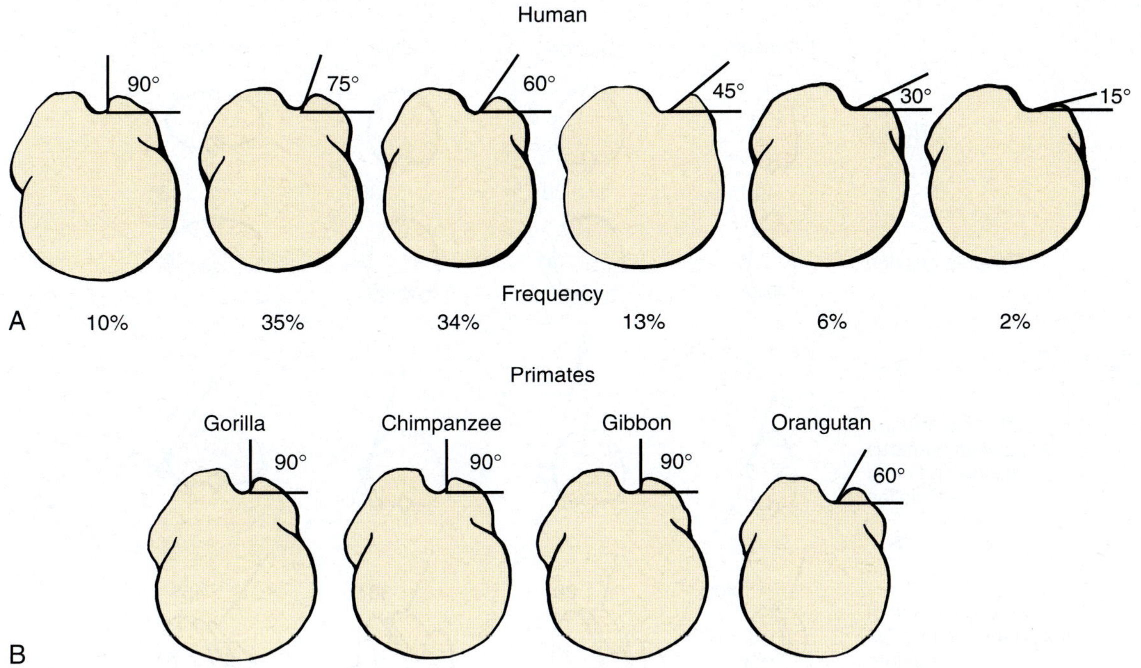

FIGURE 17-13: A, Humans are unique in having variations in the bicipital groove. **B,** The groove of the biceps in primates is constant within species. (Modified from Hitchcock HH, Bechtol CO. Painful shoulder. Observations on the role of the tendon of the long head of the biceps brachii in its causation. *J Bone Joint Surg Am.* 1948;30:263-273.)

bicipital groove from the quadruped to the erect biped (Fig. 17-14). They described a progressive AP flattening of the thorax that resulted in an increased angle between the scapula and the thorax and a relative lateral displacement of the scapula. Humans have a relatively short forearm and lateral part of the scapula. Such anatomy necessitates greater medial rotation of the humerus to enable the hand to reach the midline. The AP flattening of the thorax and the short forearm were compensated for, but only incompletely, by torsion of the humerus. In the quadruped opossum, the biceps tendon takes a straight course through the bicipital groove and is an effective abductor of the forelimb in the forward plane. In contrast, in humans the tendon is lodged against the lesser tuberosity, where a supratubercular ridge or shallow groove can traumatize the tendon. Humans are unique among the primates in having marked variation in the configuration of the bicipital groove.

The human arm is derived from the foreleg of the quadruped. Whereas in the quadruped the forelimb is designed to bear weight, the upper limb in humans is moved away from the body. For effective use of the limb, it must move not only against its own weight but also against the weight of other objects. This short power arm has to act against a long lever arm, a situation that produces unfavorable mechanical conditions that can lead to tendinitis of the rotator cuff and biceps.

Developmental Anatomy

During the ninth week of gestation, the limbs undergo rotation. The upper limb rotates dorsally at the elbow. This rotation is reflected in the shoulder as humeral retroversion, which averages 35 degrees. In essence, this rotation leaves the biceps tendon behind on the anterior aspect of the shoulder in the groove and requires the biceps to cross the joint obliquely at an angle of 30 to 45 degrees rather than proceeding in a lateral straight line, as in quadrupeds.

The development of the glenohumeral joint is similar to that of other synovial joints in the human body. According to Gardner and Gray,[72] it involves two basic processes. Initially, an inner zone forms between the two developing bones of the joint. This is followed by the creation of cavities by enzymatic action. The inner zone often comprises three layers: a chondrogenic layer on either side of a looser layer of cells. The joint capsule and many of the intra-articular structures, such as the synovial membrane, the ligaments, the labrum, and the biceps tendon, are formed from this inner zone of tissue. Giuliani and colleagues[80] confirmed that the tendon of the long head of the biceps brachii arises in continuity with the anlage of the glenoid labrum. At approximately 7 weeks of gestation, the joint is well formed; the humeral head is spherical; and the tendons of the infraspinatus, subscapularis, and biceps, as well as the glenoid labrum can be seen (Fig. 17-15).

Pathologic Anatomy

Some authors[47,49-51] consider tenosynovitis to be the chief cause of pain in biceps tendinitis and believe that it leads to an altered gliding mechanism of the tendon sheath. They describe gradual pathologic changes in the area of

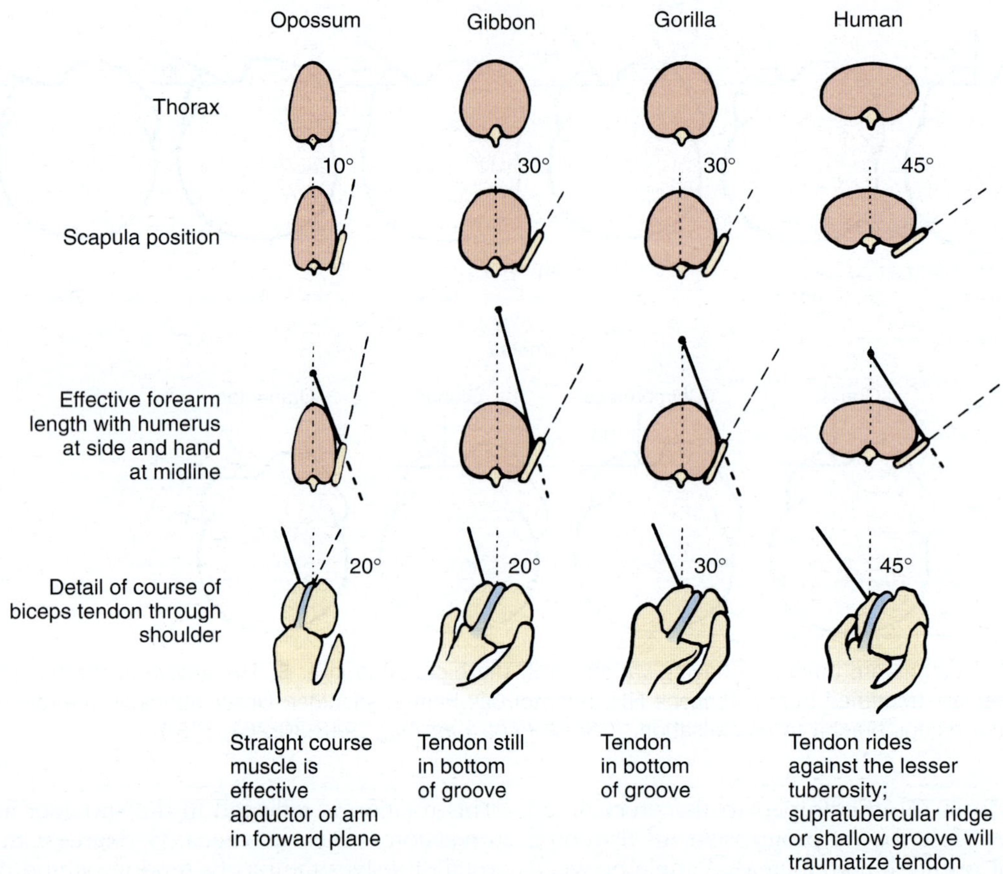

FIGURE 17-14: Progressive changes in anteroposterior flattening of the thorax, scapular position, and migration of the biceps tendon from the quadruped to the biped. (Modified from Hitchcock HH, Bechtol CO. Painful shoulder. Observations on the role of the tendon of the long head of the biceps brachii in its causation. *J Bone Joint Surg Am.* 1948;30:263-273.)

the biceps tendon. Initially, there can be capillary dilation, and edema of the tendon with progressive cellular infiltration of the sheath and synovium. Filmy adhesions can then form between the tendon and the tendon sheath. In the chronic stage fraying and narrowing of the biceps tendon occurs along with minimal to moderate synovial proliferation and fibrosis. Ultimately, the tendon is replaced by fibrous tissue, and dense fibrous adhesions become organized. The biceps tendon passes directly under the critical zone of the supraspinatus tendon.

Claessens and Snoek[33] described microscopic changes consistent with a relatively avascular state, including atrophic irregular collagen fiber, fissuring and shredding of tendon fibers, fibrinoid necrosis, and a productive inflammatory reaction with an increase in fibrocytes. Refior and Sowa[201] found that the origin of the tendon and the portion of the tendon that exits the sulcus were predisposed to microscopic degeneration and concluded that these areas were at the highest risk for tendon rupture. Cadaver studies by DePalma[47-51] and by Claessens and colleagues[32,33] noted a number of macroscopic changes, including the following: tendinitis with shredding of the tendon by osteophytes, adhesions of the synovial sheaths and of the tendon and its osteofibrous compartment, subluxation or dislocation of the tendon, and rupture of the tendon with retraction of the distal portion or adhesion of the distal portion to the sulcus.

Although it was commonly believed that the dislocated tendon always displaces medially and rides over the subscapularis tendon, Petersson[190] found only one such case in his series. In most cases he noted internal degeneration of the subscapularis in the region of the lesser tuberosity, which allowed the tendon to dislocate medially and under the subscapularis. Similar pathologic findings were described by DePalma.

Sakurai and colleagues[206] studied three groups of patients with chronic shoulder pathology. Patients with an intact rotator cuff (group 1) had no flattening of the tendon in the intertubercular region. Half of the patients with partial-thickness tearing or small rotator cuff tears (group 2) had flattening of the tendon in the intertubercular groove. For the patients with massive rotator cuff tears (group 3), tendon flattening was observed in 66% of the specimens. Bicipital fraying was seen in 16% of these cases. Medial displacement was noted in 12% of group 2 and 38% of group 3. Rupture of the biceps tendon was seen in 16% of group 3 specimens. These authors measured bicipital height, which included the

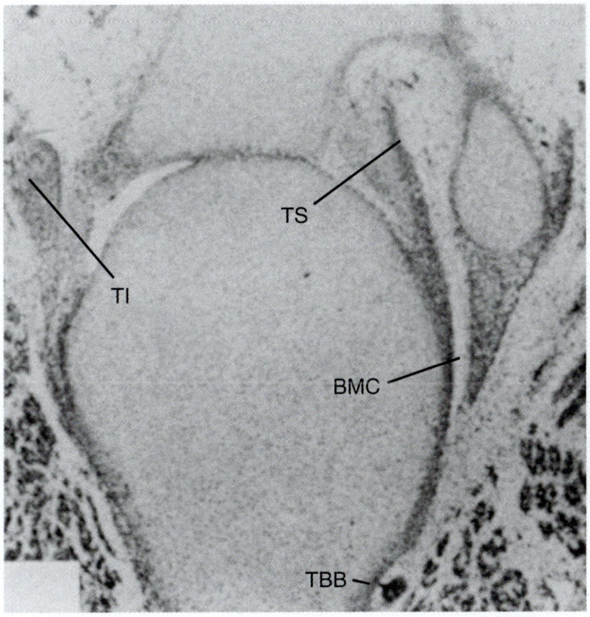

FIGURE 17-15: At approximately 7 weeks of gestation, the joint is well formed and the humeral head is spherical. The biceps tendon (TBB) is seen clearly in the groove. This image was obtained before rotation occurred; the biceps tendon will eventually assume a position less lateral than shown here. The other structures are the tendons of the infraspinatus (TI) and subscapularis (TS), and the bursa of the coracobrachialis (BMC). (From Gardner E, Gray DJ. Prenatal development of the human shoulder and acromioclavicular joint. *Am J Anat.* 1953;92:219.)

height of the soft tissues, demonstrating a significant difference in height of the medial wall between patients with medial displacement of the biceps and those without instability. The authors were unable to show differences in height of the medial wall between the three groups. They concluded that the LHBT could potentially compensate for deficient rotator cuff function, resulting in relative stenosis of the tendon in the groove. Other gliding disorders can also result from this mismatch between the enlarged tendon size and the noncompliant bony groove. The mismatch may be responsible for degeneration of the soft tissue along the medial wall of the sulcus, causing a pulley lesion and resulting instability.

The biceps tendon and its enveloping synovial sheath can be affected by inflammatory or infectious processes of the glenohumeral joint as a result of their anatomic location and course. Tumorous conditions affecting the synovium of the shoulder can also involve the sheath of the tendon.[41] Therefore tenosynovitis of the biceps accompanies septic arthritis of the shoulder. Similarly, rheumatic inflammation, osteoarthritis, hemodialysis arthropathy,[208] and crystalline arthritis of the glenohumeral joint affect the biceps tendon. The clinical syndrome in such cases is dominated by the articular pathology. Biceps rupture has been reported to occur in conjunction with tuberculosis and syphilis.

Osteochondromatosis has also been reported in the shoulder and bicipital sheath.[45] This disorder causes pain and the formation of loose bodies in the shoulder. Detection of loose bodies in the bicipital sheath on radiography or MRI should arouse suspicion of this pathologic process. Treatment by synovectomy has been successful.

Osseous Pathoanatomy

The shape of the groove has often been implicated in the pathogenesis of biceps tendon ruptures.[47,49-51,83,96,192] A shallow, flattened groove (Fig. 17-16) is commonly associated with subluxation or dislocation of the biceps tendon, and a narrow groove with a sharp medial wall. An osteophyte at the aperture is often associated with biceps tendinitis and rupture (Fig. 17-17). Spurs on the floor of the groove can erode the tendon. Although these groove abnormalities can contribute to bicipital tendon problems, it is likely that some are changes in response to pathology of the soft tissues around the shoulder rather than to the underlying cause. In all degenerative conditions about the shoulder, soft tissue changes precede bony changes. For instance, in rotator cuff disorders, the formation of spurring in the anterior acromion is preceded by fibrosis, bursitis, and tendinosis or enthesopathy. Synovitis and cartilage degeneration precede spur formation in the acromioclavicular joint. It seems logical that changes in the bicipital groove and the entrance to the groove would follow changes in the tendon, capsule, ligaments, and synovium around it.

Bony anomalies and variations have been proposed as a cause of subluxation and tendinitis of the biceps tendon. The supratubercular ridge has been described by Meyer[149] as a ridge that extends forward and downward from the region of the articular cartilage to the upper and dorsal portions of the lesser tuberosity (Fig. 17-18). According to Cilley,[31] the incidence of this structure in 200 humeri examined was 17.5%. The ridge decreases the depth of the sulcus and diminishes the effectiveness of the tuberosity as a trochlea. Meyer believed that the ridge pushes the biceps tendon against the transverse ligament, thereby favoring dislocation.

In Hitchcock and Bechtol's series[96] the supratubercular ridge was found to be markedly developed in 8% and moderately developed in 59%. They found a direct correlation between the presence of a supratubercular ridge and spurs on the lesser tuberosity (medial wall spurs). In their series medial wall spurs were found in approximately 45% of patients with a supratubercular ridge. When no supratubercular ridge was present, only 3% of the humeri had spurs on the lesser tuberosity (see Fig. 17-18C). The authors concluded that spurs on the lesser tuberosity developed in response to the biceps tendon being pressed against the tuberosity by the supratubercular ridge.

A supratubercular ridge was found in approximately 50% of patients in a study by Cone and colleagues.[37] They did not however find a correlation between its presence and the presence of bicipital groove spurs. It was their belief that the medial wall spur was related more to a

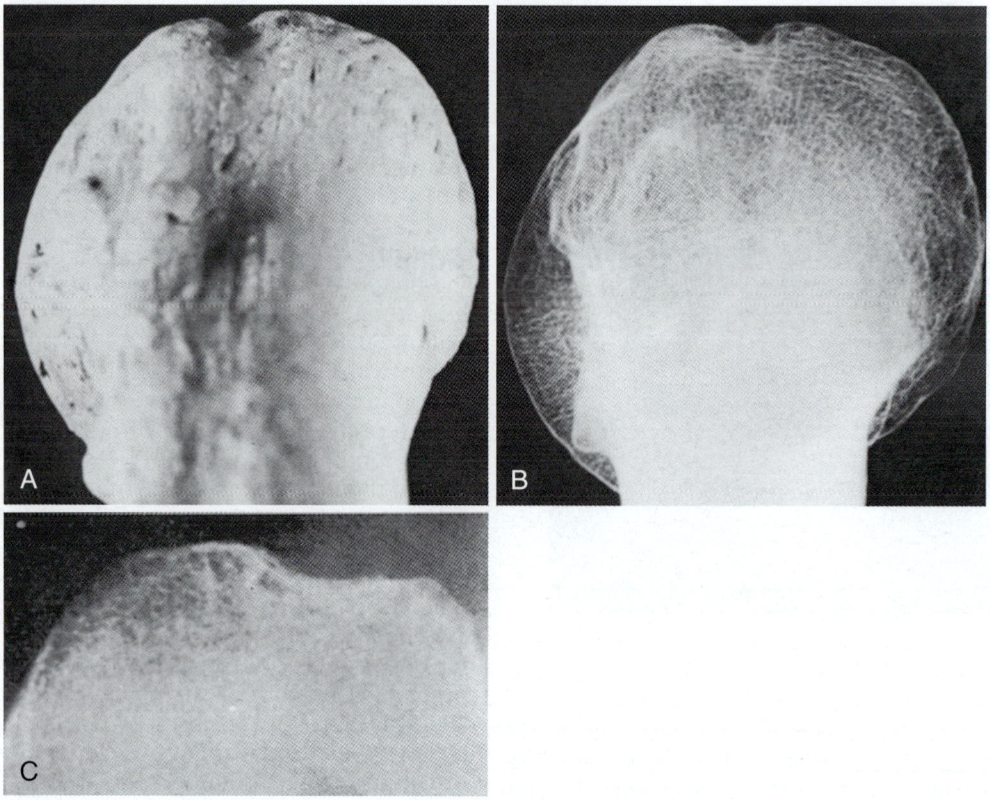

FIGURE 17-16: Image (**A**) and radiograph (**B**) of a cadaver specimen reveal a shallow sulcus. **C,** An even shallower bicipital groove. (**A** and **B,** From Cone RO, Danzig L, Resnick D, Goldman AB. The bicipital groove: Radiographic, anatomic, and pathologic study. *AJR Am J Roentgenol.* 1983;141:781-788. **C,** From Ahovuo J, Paavolainen P, Slatis P. Radiographic diagnosis of biceps tendinitis. *Acta Orthop Scand.* 1985;56:75-78.)

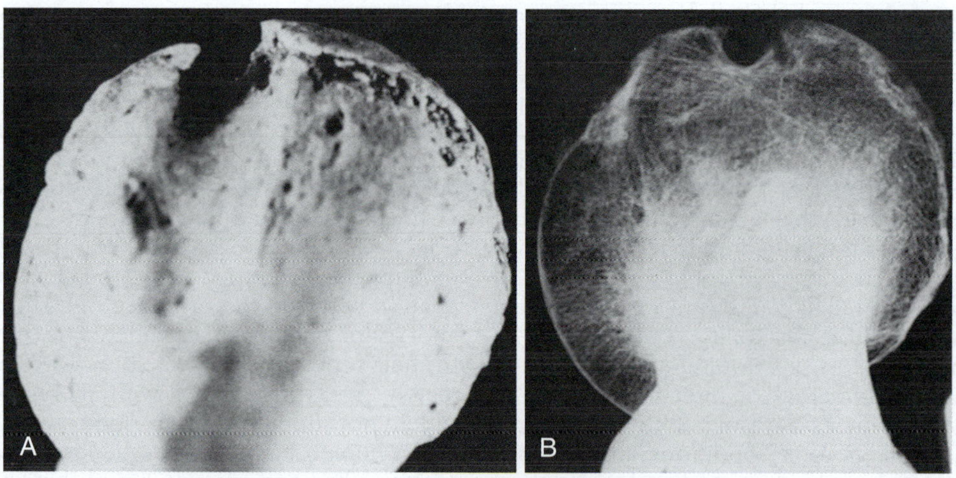

FIGURE 17-17: Pathologic specimen (**A**) and radiograph (**B**) of the bicipital groove with a 90-degree medial wall angle and a medial osteophyte at the aperture, seen commonly with biceps tendinitis and rupture. (From Cone RO, Danzig L, Resnick D, Goldman AB. The bicipital groove: Radiographic, anatomic, and pathologic study. *AJR Am J Roentgenol.* 1983;141:781-788.)

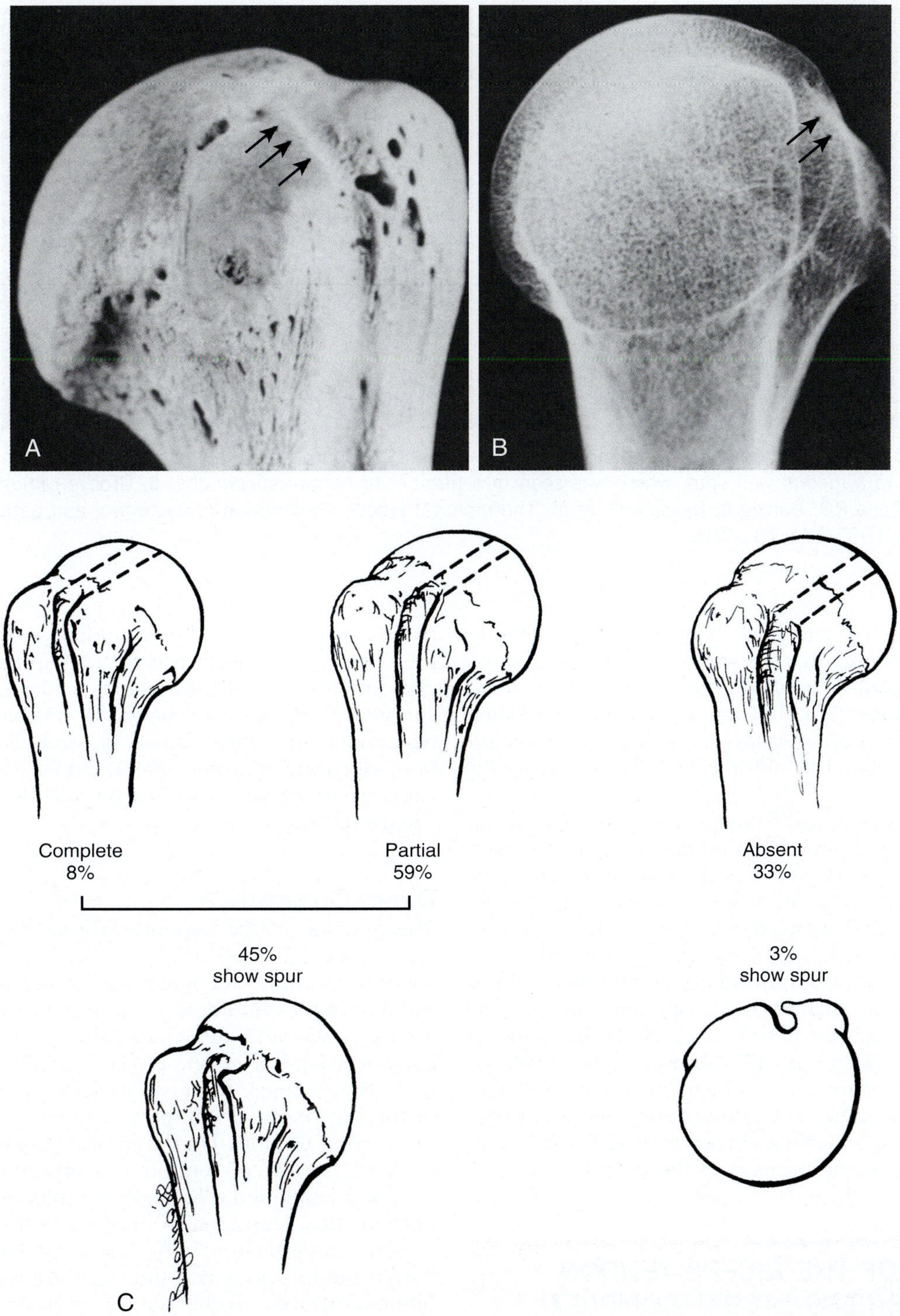

FIGURE 17-18: **A,** Externally rotated view of a cadaveric specimen showing the supratubercular ridge (arrows). **B,** Internally rotated radiograph showing a prominent supratubercular ridge (arrows). **C,** The presence of the supratubercular ridge (seen extending from the lesser tuberosity and altering the angle of the biceps tendon) and narrowing of the groove, both partial and complete, in the specimens of Hitchcock and Bechtol. Medial wall spurs are much more common in specimens with supratubercular ridges. (**A** and **B,** From Cone RO, Danzig L, Resnick D, et al. The bicipital groove: Radiographic, anatomic, and pathologic study. *AJR Am J Roentgenol.* 1983;141:781-788. **C,** Modified from Hitchcock HH, Bechtol CO. Painful shoulder. Observations on the role of the tendon of the long head of the biceps brachii in its causation. *J Bone Joint Surg Am.* 1948;30:263-273.)

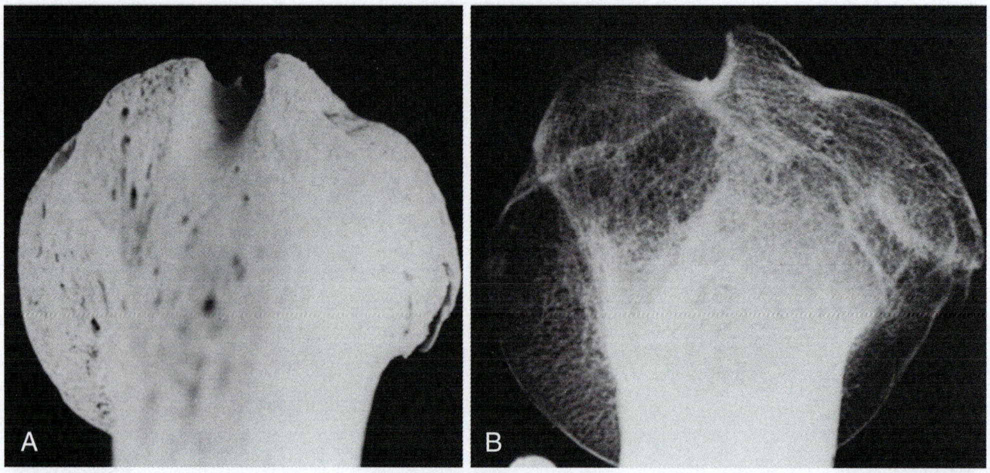

FIGURE 17-19: **A,** A spur in the floor of the bicipital groove, thought by Cone and colleagues to be significant in biceps tendinitis, as opposed to a medial wall spur, which was seen in a number of normal specimens. **B,** Groove radiograph of the same structure. (From Cone RO, Danzig L, Resnick D, et al. The bicipital groove: Radiographic, anatomic, and pathologic study. *AJR Am J Roentgenol.* 1983;141:781-788.)

traction enostosis or a reactive bone formation. In one specimen they found that the transverse humeral ligament had completely ossified, converting the bicipital groove into a bony tunnel. They agreed with DePalma that the presence of bony spurs on the floor of the bicipital groove was related to chronic bicipital tenosynovitis (Fig. 17-19).

Pfahler and colleagues[192] prospectively compared the ultrasound and radiographic findings of patients with chronic shoulder pain to those of normal control subjects. They found that 43% of those with radiographically evident degenerative changes of the bicipital groove also had sonographic evidence of biceps tendon inflammation. Conversely, ultrasound findings of biceps tendinitis correlated with a smaller total opening angle (<80 degrees) on radiographs in 65% of cases. Of the patients with a flatter medial angle, 47% showed signs of biceps tendinitis. Among patients with bicipital rupture 61% had a shallow medial angle. The authors concluded that 65% of patients in their series with anterior shoulder pain had "conspicuous anatomic findings of the bicipital groove."

FUNCTION OF THE BICEPS TENDON (AND THE BICEPS-LABRAL COMPLEX)

Basmajian and Latif[8] characterized the action of the biceps brachii muscle as flexion of the elbow joint when the forearm is in the neutral or supinated position but contributing little when the forearm is in a pronated position. They also considered the biceps to be important in decelerating the rapidly moving arm, such as occurs during forceful overhand throwing. There is now general agreement that the biceps brachii is in fact a strong supinator of the forearm and only a weak flexor of the elbow. Debate continues, however, on the exact function of the biceps proximally at the shoulder, and the function of the biceps in connection with the superior labrum. Most anatomy texts regard the biceps as a weak flexor of the shoulder.[97] Studies on function of the biceps tendon can be divided into three broad categories: direct observation, electromyographic (EMG) studies, and biomechanical cadaver studies. The first two of these categories are discussed below.

Direct Observation

The function of the superior labrum, in both intact and torn states, has been the focus of extensive study. The superior labrum is recognized as contributing to the static stability of the shoulder.[219] The role of the biceps tendon on the static and dynamic stability of the shoulder is controversial, but in one of the seminal papers on superior labral injuries, Andrews[5] noted a dynamic tensioning of the biceps-labral complex with electric stimulation of the biceps tendon. However, the dynamic relationship between the biceps tendon and superior labral complex and their combined role in glenohumeral stability remains unclear; this is an area in need of further study.

Many investigators[96,123-125] have pointed out that the biceps tendon does not slide in the groove. Rather, the humerus moves on the stationary biceps tendon during shoulder motion like a monorail car on a track. From full adduction to full elevation of the arm, the groove moves a distance of up to 2 to 5 cm along the tendon. Maximal excursion of the humeral head along the tendon results when the shoulder is in a position of maximal external rotation. Minimal excursion is seen when the shoulder is in a position of maximal internal rotation. To facilitate excursion along the tendon, the synovial pouch extends from the shoulder joint, lining the greater part of the intertubercular groove (see Fig. 17-7). Within this bursa, the tendon glides through its peritendineum.

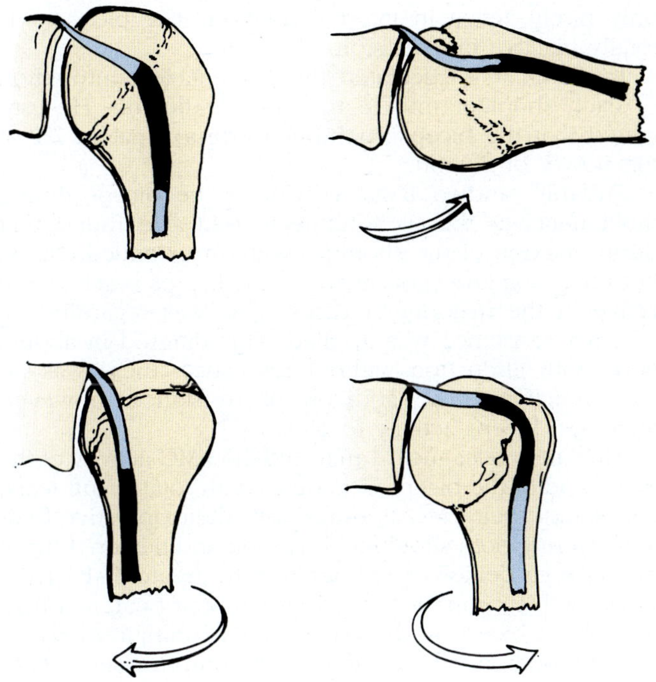

FIGURE 17-20: Lippmann found by direct observation under local anesthesia that the biceps tendon slid freely in its sheath during motion of the shoulder. Motion of the tendon in its groove appears only with motion of the shoulder joint. The amount of the biceps tendon that can be found within the joint changes according to the given position. (Modified from Lippmann RK. Bicipital tenosynovitis. *N Y State J Med.* 1944;90:2235-2241.)

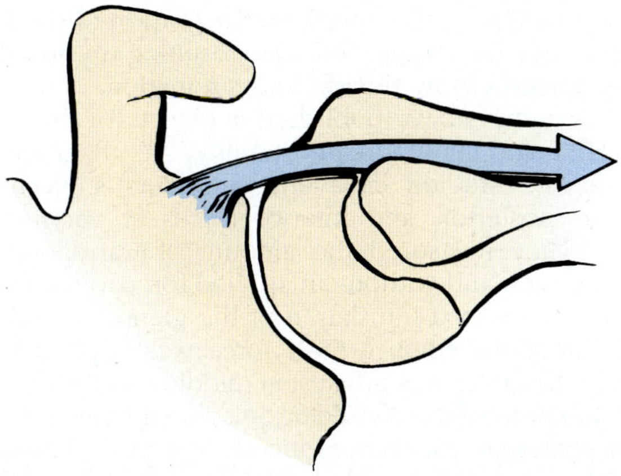

FIGURE 17-21: The biceps tendon is at least a static head depressor. Given the line of pull and the resultant vector (arrow), the tendon is an active head depressor, although undoubtedly a weak one as shown by the percentage of recruitment on electromyographic analysis. (Modified from Habermeyer P, Kaiser E, Knappe M, et al. Functional anatomy and biomechanics of the long biceps tendon. *Unfallchirurg.* 1987;90:319-329.)

The LHBT is sometimes divided into an intra-articular portion and an intratubercular portion. Lippman[123] noted that with the arm in a position of full abduction, 1.3 cm of the LHBT lies within the shoulder joint. This changes however when the arm is adducted and externally rotated such that the length of tendon within the joint increases to 5 cm. He therefore questioned the utility of such a distinction given that the portions of the tendon that are intracapsular or within the groove depend on the position of the arm (Fig. 17-20).

When the arm is in full external rotation, the tendon occupies the floor of the groove, and its more proximal portion presses on the humeral head. Because of this, it was originally believed that in external rotation the long head of the biceps acted as a head depressor at the shoulder to enhance abduction strength at the shoulder. Lucas[126] used a force vector diagram to demonstrate how the long head of the biceps could act as a dynamic humeral head depressor. In addition, the biceps can potentially act as a static humeral head depressor, preventing migration of the humeral head into the acromion with contraction of the deltoid (Fig. 17-21). Rowe[204] believed that the function of the biceps tendon as a humeral head depressor increased in the context of a chronic rotator cuff tear. He pointed to the hypertrophy often seen in the tendon in these situations as evidence. Bush[27] went as far as to transfer the LHBT laterally when repairing cuff defects and claimed that humeral head depression increased with this procedure.

Andrews and colleagues[5] arthroscopically observed the biceps tendon and the superior glenoid-labrum complex during electrical stimulation of the biceps. They noted superior lifting of the labrum and compression of the glenohumeral joint and concluded that in this respect the biceps is a “shunt muscle of the shoulder” and that it helps to stabilize the glenohumeral joint during throwing. They agreed that its primary role during throwing is still to decelerate the elbow. It is this sudden deceleration that leads to tearing of the superior glenoid-labrum complex by the biceps tendon.

In a study by Itoi and colleagues[103] both the long and short heads of the biceps were shown to function as anterior stabilizers of the glenohumeral joint with the arm in abduction and external rotation. They further demonstrated that with increasing instability from sectioning of the inferior glenohumeral ligament (as occurs with the development of a Bankart lesion), both heads of the biceps have an increased stabilizing function to resist anterior displacement of the humeral head. They concluded that during rehabilitation of patients with chronic anterior instability, biceps strengthening should be included in the nonoperative treatment of these lesions.

Kumar and colleagues[117] also studied the stabilizing role of the biceps tendon. They were able to show that severing the LHBT while both heads were tensed caused significant upward migration of the humeral head. The long head of the biceps is therefore important in stabilizing the humeral head in the glenoid during powerful elbow flexion and forearm supination. They warned against sacrifice of the intra-articular portion of the LHBT because of the danger of this resulting in instability during forced elbow flexion and supination.

Other authors have published evidence for the role of the LHBT in glenohumeral stability.[131,182] Pagnani and colleagues[182] studied cadaveric shoulders subjected to anterior, posterior, and inferior forces at varying arm angles. They measured the amount of translation that occurred with and without an applied force to the biceps, showing decreased translation of the glenohumeral joint in all directions when a 55-N force was applied to the biceps. The effect was greatest at middle and lower elevations. Rotation of the shoulder joint also influenced translation: external rotation reduced posterior translation, whereas internal rotation reduced anterior translation. This applied force to the biceps also reduced superior and inferior translation of the glenohumeral joint. The authors concluded that the biceps helped to center the humeral head on the glenoid, thus stabilizing the fulcrum at which motion can occur.

Malicky and colleagues[131] showed that the biceps provided a 30-N stabilizing force to the humeral head when the arm was in neutral rotation. This stabilizing force depended on the relative position of the groove, with the stabilizing effect at its minimum when the arm was in external rotation. In neutral rotation the biceps added concavity compression as well as a posteriorly directed force on the head against the glenoid. In external rotation the biceps applied an anteriorly directed force on the humeral head and could actually destabilize the joint.

Warner and McMahon[247] studied seven patients with isolated rupture of the LHBT, documented either surgically or with MRI. They demonstrated an increased superior translation of the humeral head at all angles of humeral abduction when compared with the contralateral (control) side. This increased superior translation was not present with the arm at 0 degrees of elevation. They concluded that isolated loss of the biceps could lead to impingement.

Electromyographic Evaluation

Basmajian and Latif[8] were pioneers in evaluating the musculoskeletal system, including the shoulder, with integrated-function and dynamic-spectrum EMG. They reported that both heads of the biceps are active during shoulder flexion, with the long head being the more active of the two. Habermeyer and colleagues[90] found clear EMG activity in the biceps during abduction, greatest at 132 degrees of abduction. Interestingly, he found the muscle to be active even with the arm in neutral rotation; that is, the biceps is active in abduction even when the arm is not externally rotated. The authors found the greatest activity in flexion during the first 90 degrees of flexion and showed that the biceps was active in external but not internal rotation. The effectiveness of the long head of the biceps is greatest in external rotation when its tension is maximal. With the arm adducted and internally rotated, the long head was always inactive; the short head was active in half the cases of adduction and only rarely active in internal rotation. The biceps was totally inactive in extension.

Laumann[120,121] calculated the percentage contribution of each shoulder muscle to shoulder flexion. He estimated that the biceps contributed approximately 7% of the power of flexion.

Furlani[70] studied EMG activity of the biceps during movements at the glenohumeral joint. He found that during flexion of the shoulder with an extended elbow, both the long and short heads of the biceps brachii were active in the majority of cases. This was regardless of whether resistance was applied. This differed in abduction. With abduction without resistance, there was no biceps activity. The addition of resistance, however, increased biceps activity to 10%.

Ting and colleagues[227] analyzed the EMG activity of the long head of the biceps in patients with rotator cuff tears, correlating their EMG findings with their operative findings. During both shoulder abduction and flexion, four of five subjects demonstrated significantly greater EMG activity of the biceps in the presence of a rotator cuff tear than that of the biceps in the contralateral (uninjured) shoulder. In addition, all shoulders with compromised rotator cuffs proved to have a significantly larger tendon at the time of surgery than those observed in controls. (This finding correlates with the observations of Rowe.[204]) Ting and colleagues suggested that the lateral head of the biceps may be more important to abduction and flexion in the compromised shoulder than in the normal shoulder and that the concomitant enlargement of the tendon may represent use-induced hypertrophy. They therefore recommended against sacrificing the intracapsular portion of the tendon (e.g., for graft material) or tenodesing the tendon indiscriminately in the groove as a routine part of rotator cuff repair and acromioplasty.

The contribution of the biceps to the shoulder during throwing has been evaluated by Jobe and colleagues[106] and by Perry.[189] In these studies biceps function correlated with motion that occurred at the elbow but not in the shoulder. A relatively stable elbow position during acceleration was accompanied by a marked reduction in the muscle's firing intensity. During follow-through, the need for deceleration of the rapidly extending elbow and pronating forearm was accompanied by peak biceps action. There was no activity in the biceps muscle during the act of throwing, except in conjunction with elbow activity. Peak activity was only 36% of maximum. With a 9-cm^2 cross section and only half of the muscle related to the long head, the humeral force is small. In Perry's words, "It seems doubtful that the long head (biceps tendon) is a significant stabilizing force at the glenohumeral joint." Conversely, Glousman and colleagues[82] reported increased activity in the biceps during throwing in patients with unstable shoulders, suggesting that the biceps may increase in importance if the primary stabilizers are injured.

EMG activity in patients with rotator cuff tears of less than 5 cm was found by Ozaki[178] to be higher than activity in healthy subjects. This increased activity could be an attempt to compensate for the decreased function of the torn rotator cuff. Ozaki, like Ting, postulated that this increased activity could be responsible for the hypertrophy of the tendon often seen accompanying small and medium rotator cuff tears. Patients with massive rotator cuff tears and dislocated biceps tendons did not show a similar increase in activity.

EMG activity of the biceps and rotator cuff was found to precede motion of the glenohumeral joint in a study by David and colleagues.[44] They found that the EMG activity in these muscles occurred before actual internal or external rotation movement (preceding the movement by 0.092 ± 0.038 to 0.215 ± 0.045 seconds). The deltoid and pectoralis major muscles were also active before glenohumeral motion, but significantly later (at 0.030 ± 0.047 to 0.12 ± 0.053 seconds before the movement). They postulated that the biceps and rotator cuff muscles were stiffening the joint, providing a stable platform before the initiation of movement. Once movement was initiated, the activity of the biceps depended on the direction of motion. Little activity was found in the biceps during internal rotation, whereas greater activity was seen during external rotation.

Sakurai and colleagues[205] studied EMG activity in the biceps while maintaining the elbow in neutral rotation in a brace. Surface electrodes were used to measure EMG activity of the deltoid and biceps muscles. Their results showed there to be EMG activity in both the long and short heads of the biceps with all types of motion of the shoulder, independent of elbow position. This indicated that the biceps acted as an active flexor and abductor of the shoulder. There was also activity with rotation, and external rotation induced more activity than internal rotation did. In addition, they demonstrated greater fatigability of the biceps compared with the deltoid. Accordingly, they considered the biceps at higher risk of injury than the deltoid.

In direct contradiction two other studies found no significant dynamic role for the biceps in glenohumeral stability. Yamaguchi and colleagues[257,258] fixed the elbow at 100 degrees of flexion and held the forearm in neutral rotation with a brace in an attempt to relax the elbow flexors. EMG activity of the brachioradialis was used as a control for biceps EMG activity. They found little to no activity in the biceps tendon with shoulder motion, even in patients in whom the head-depressor effect of the cuff musculature had been compromised. Furthermore, they observed no difference in EMG activity between the brachioradialis and the biceps. They concluded that the role of the biceps in shoulder stability was probably a passive one.

Using a similar experimental design, Levy and colleagues[122] studied the EMG activity of the biceps and rotator cuff muscles with intramuscular electrodes during motion of the shoulder. Again, a brace was used to control elbow motion. Three different elbow positions were tested. The shoulders were moved in flexion, external rotation, and internal rotation at two different speeds and with a 5-lb weight. They found no activity in the biceps when elbow motion was controlled. The authors pointed out that many activities performed by the arm require both elbow and shoulder motion. Their experimental design intentionally eliminated elbow motion, and the lack of biceps activity seems to have been a reflection of the elbow being controlled. The EMG activity of the biceps in other studies may therefore have been a consequence of active motion or stabilization of the elbow and not the shoulder. Based on this, they concluded that the biceps was not active in isolated motion of the shoulder.

Summary

It appears from a review of the literature that the biceps tendon might have a weak active head depressor or stabilizing effect that is clinically insignificant in the normal shoulder. Because of its anatomic position, the tendon serves as a superior checkrein to humeral head excursion and therefore acts as a weak static head depressor as long as it is anatomically positioned. Attempts to understand the dynamic role of the biceps at the shoulder have been confounded by its associated function at the elbow. Immobilization of the elbow with a brace has been used in various studies to circumvent this, but at the same time this creates an artificial scenario that only approximates how the arm is actually used in activities of daily living. Nonetheless, these studies offer compelling evidence that the role of the biceps is minimal during shoulder motion.

The tendon's importance seems to increase in pathologic states of the shoulder, such as rotator cuff tears and shoulder instability; this is evidenced by the increased EMG activity and by the observed hypertrophy and resistance to translation. The observation of increased superior translation of the humeral head in patients with confirmed bicipital rupture reinforces these findings. However, the clinical relevance of this is questionable given that measurable deterioration in shoulder function has not been demonstrated in patients who have undergone biceps tenotomy or tenodesis. Therefore if the LHBT is implicated as a possible source of a patient's symptoms (either through physical examination or at surgery), the risk of decreased shoulder function from tenotomy or tenodesis is negligible compared with the risk of continued pain from biceps pathology.

CLASSIFICATION OF BICIPITAL AND LABRAL LESIONS

Superior labral anterior posterior (SLAP) lesions were first described by Snyder and colleagues in 1990.[217] Their original classification divided SLAP lesions into four types. A type I lesion is characterized by superior labral degeneration. Type II lesions involve a detachment of the superior labrum and biceps anchor. A type III lesion is typified by a bucket handle tear of the superior labrum, with the biceps anchor still attached, and a type IV lesion is a type III lesion in which the tear extends into the biceps tendon root.

Maffet and colleagues[130] expanded Snyder's original classification to include three additional types (types V through VII): type V is an extension of a superior labral injury to include an anteroinferior labral tear, type VI is characterized by an unstable labral flap and biceps tendon separation, and type VII represents a detachment of the biceps-labral complex, with extension to the middle glenohumeral ligament. The most recent expansion of SLAP classification was devised by Knesek et al.[115] to include VIII to X: type VIII is a posterior extension of a type II lesion to the 6 o'clock position, type IX represents a circumferential labral tear, and type X is type II tear with a reverse Bankart lesion.

Morgan and colleagues subclassified type II lesions into anterior, posterior, and AP variants.[161]

Biceps lesions have historically been divided into biceps tendinitis and biceps instability. Often, however, much like with rotator cuff tears or lateral epicondylitis, a preponderance of inflammation is not present and the lesion would more accurately be termed *tendinosis* or *tendinopathy*. Biceps tendinitis has been subdivided into primary tendinitis (due to pathology of the biceps tendon sheath) and secondary biceps tendinitis (resulting from associated pathology, such as osteoarthritis or rheumatoid arthritis.) Many authors[41,50,163-166,194,195] believe that the pathology seen in the biceps is directly related to its intimate relationship with the rotator cuff. As they pass under the coracoacromial arch, both can be involved in the impingement syndrome. A classification by anatomic locale has been offered by Walch.[241]

Primary biceps tendinitis has been likened to de Quervain's tenosynovitis by Lapidus and Guidotti,[119] who demonstrated the presence of thickening and stenosis of the transverse ligament and sheath as well as narrowing of the tendon underneath the sheath. Post[194] found consistent inflammation within the intertubercular portion of the tendon, a proliferative tenosynovitis, and irregularity of the walls of the groove. This inflammation can be visualized arthroscopically if the extra-articular portion of the tendon is pulled into the joint; it has been referred to as the *lipstick sign*. There are no reports of inflammation involving the intra-articular portion of the biceps. Codman[34] believed that primary biceps tendinitis was a rare entity. In contrast, DePalma[47-51] considered it to be a common cause of stiff and painful shoulders. In DePalma's series 39% of cases had associated disorders. Crenshaw and Kilgore[43] were also proponents of the significance of primary biceps tendinitis, although 40% of their patients also had an associated lesion. They concluded that whether the biceps tendon or its sheath was involved primarily or secondarily was not important. The important point was that tenosynovitis was the chief cause of pain and limitation of motion.

Isolated rupture of the biceps tendon has been described by several authors.[39,97,151,181] Neer believed that most biceps tendon ruptures were associated with supraspinatus tendon tears.[163-165] Some studies have shown isolated rupture of the biceps tendon to occur in 25% of patients.[46] When computed tomography (CT) arthrograms are performed for patients who meet the clinical criteria for isolated long head of the biceps rupture, the incidence of isolated lesions decreases to 6%.[43] In an arthroscopically controlled study of isolated LHBT lesions, a 2.2% rate of isolated rupture was documented. These studies show that isolated rupture is rare. Many authors have described bicipital groove osteophytes that were thought to be the cause of rupture of the long head of the biceps.[39,102,151,180] Studies using CT scans have shown that the depth and width of the bicipital groove do not have pathognomonic significance.[46]

Although primary biceps tendinitis was commonly recognized as the cause of shoulder pain in the 1940s and 1950s, today it is a much less frequent diagnosis. We do not doubt its existence, but it is clinically very uncommon and should be considered a diagnosis of exclusion.

Slatis and Aalto Classification

Slatis and Aalto[214] have offered a useful clinical classification of biceps lesions (Box 17-1) based on pathoanatomy. According to their review, this appears to have prognostic significance.

Type A: Impingement Tendinitis

Type A is tendinitis secondary to impingement syndrome and rotator cuff disease. The torn cuff exposes the biceps to the rigid coracoacromial arch, and such exposure results in tendinitis (tendinosis) (Figs. 17-22 and 17-23).

BOX 17-1. Slatis and Aalto Classification

Type A: Impingement tendinitis
Type B: Subluxation of the biceps
Type C: Attrition is primary

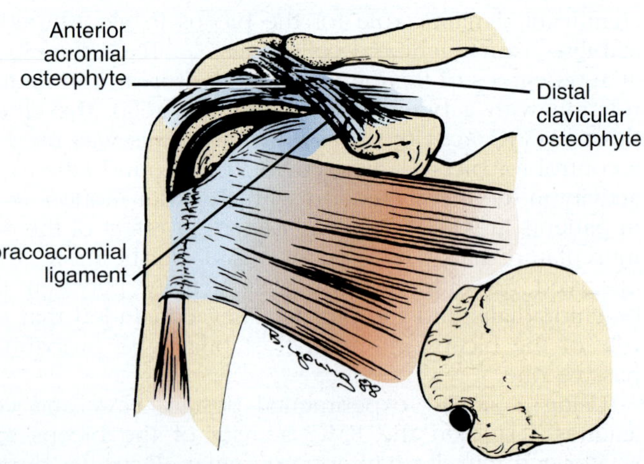

FIGURE 17-22: Type A: impingement tendinitis. Rupture of the rotator cuff exposes the tendon to compression between the acromion above and the humeral head below. The tendon normally lies in its groove. (Modified from Paavolainen P, Slatis P, Aalto K. Surgical pathology in chronic shoulder pain. In: Bateman JE, Welsh RP, eds. *Surgery of the Shoulder*. Philadelphia: BC Decker; 1984.)

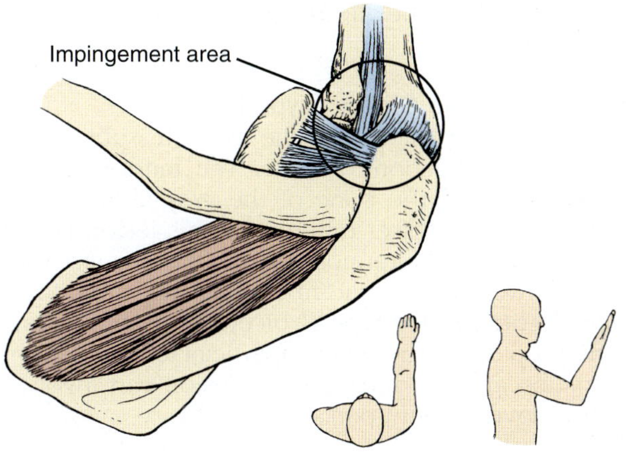

FIGURE 17-23: When the arm is flexed forward, the impingement area (i.e., the groove, biceps tendon, and anterior cuff) comes into contact with the coracoacromial arch. The longer the acromial process, the more likely it is that the biceps will be involved. (Courtesy Charles A. Rockwood Jr, MD.)

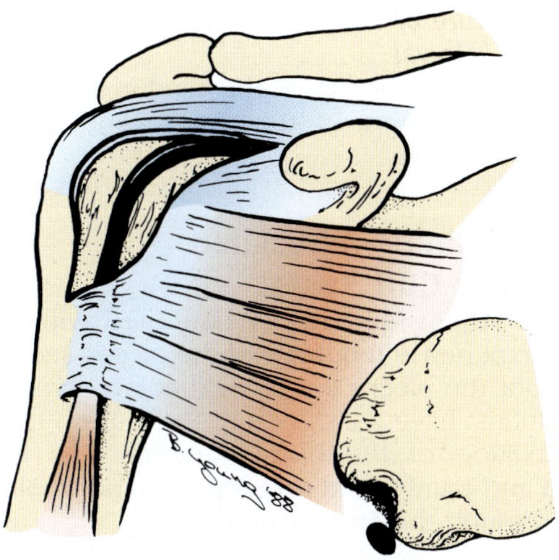

FIGURE 17-24: Type B: subluxation of the biceps. A tear in the medial portion of the coracohumeral ligament causes subluxation and medial displacement of the tendon from the bicipital groove. Note the filling of the groove with fibrous tissue. (Modified from Paavolainen P, Slatis P, Aalto K: Surgical pathology in chronic shoulder pain. In: Bateman JE, Welsh RP, eds. *Surgery of the Shoulder.* Philadelphia: BC Decker; 1984.)

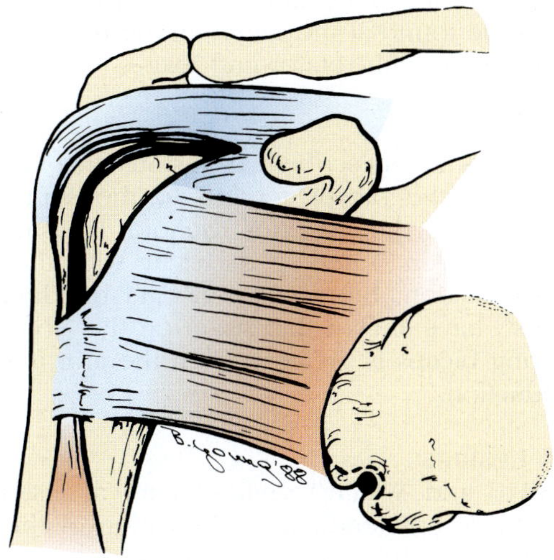

FIGURE 17-25: Type C: attrition tendinitis. The cuff is exposed to show the pathology of constriction of the biceps tendon within the groove. The local formation of new bone and connective tissue causes stenosis of the bicipital groove and subsequent attrition of the tendon of the long head of the biceps.

BOX 17-2. Habermeyer and Walch Classification of Biceps Lesions

I. Origin
II. Interval Lesions
  A. Biceps tendinitis
  B. Isolated ruptures
  C. Subluxation
    Type I: Superior
    Type II: At the groove
    Type III: Malunion or nonunion of the lesser tuberosity
III. Associated with RCT
  A. Tendinitis
  B. Dislocation
    Type IA: Extra-articular with a partial subscapularis tear
    Type IB: Extra-articular with an intact subscapularis
    Type II: Intra-articular
  C. Subluxation with RCT
  D. LHB rupture with RCT

LHB, long head of the biceps; RCT, rotator cuff tear.

Type B: Subluxation of the Biceps Tendon

The type B category includes all pathologies of the biceps that involve subluxation and dislocation of the tendon (Fig. 17-24). In this category, lesions of the coracohumeral ligament allow the biceps tendon to gradually become displaced medially.

Type C: Attrition Tendinitis

Type C represents lesions of the biceps tendon that occur within the groove. These are associated with inflammation, stenosis, spur formation, and shredding of the biceps tendon (Fig. 17-25). This condition is considered to be rare but extremely painful.

Habermeyer and Walch Classification

Habermeyer and Walch[91] classified lesions of the biceps tendon in a different way (Box 17-2). They noted that the biceps tendon could be involved in pathology in different anatomic locations. In their classification lesions of the biceps are found at the origin, in the rotator interval, or in association with rotator cuff tears.

Origin Lesions

Origin lesions are described as lesions that affect the attachment of the biceps tendon to the supraglenoid tubercle and to the superior glenoid labrum. These lesions have been observed to occur with the use of muscle stimulation. Biomechanical data by Grauer and colleagues[85] have shown that strain on the labrum from the working biceps is greatest when the arm is in overhead abduction.

Interval Lesions

Habermeyer and Walch[91] divided interval lesions into three types: biceps tendinitis, subluxation of the LHBT, and isolated rupture.

Biceps Tendinitis

Biceps tendinitis is clinically characterized by chronic shoulder pain with tenderness over the bicipital groove and a positive Speed test. When these criteria are used, 90% of all painful shoulders could be considered to have biceps tendinitis, but pathologic examination of biceps tendons in these shoulders rarely shows degenerative or microtraumatic lesions. Such changes of the biceps tendon have been reported in only 5% of cases.

According to Habermeyer and Walch,[91] primary biceps tendinitis can be diagnosed only by arthroscopy. Findings of erythema and a vascular reaction around the long head of the biceps and in the groove are usually observed. For this diagnosis to be made, the shoulder must have a complete passive range of motion. The tendon should not be subluxated or dislocated out of its groove. Mechanical fraying of the bicipital tendon caused by osteophytes or narrowing of the groove from fracture is considered secondary. Habermeyer and Walch reported that although they looked specifically for isolated biceps tendinitis during more than 3 years of arthroscopy of the shoulder, they were unsuccessful in finding a single case. Isolated biceps tendinitis remains a diagnosis of exception.[240]

Subluxation of the Long Head of the Biceps Tendon

The definition of instability of the LHBT is poorly standardized and controversial.[53,132,174,180,190] Walch[240] defined *subluxation of the LHBT* as partial or incomplete loss of contact between the tendon and its bony groove and defined *dislocation* as complete loss of contact between these two. He divided subluxation into three types.

Superior Subluxation (Type I)

Superior subluxation occurs when the superior glenohumeral and the coracohumeral ligaments are partially or completely torn. The result of this tearing is that the LHBT above the entrance of the groove is subluxated superiorly. The subscapularis tendon remains intact, and this prevents true dislocation of the tendon. A type I lesion is a discontinuity of the tendoligamentous rotator interval sling surrounding the LHBT that allows the tendon to migrate superiorly.

Subluxation in the Groove (Type II)

The lesion responsible for the type II subluxation is located inside the bony groove. The tendon slips over the medial rim of the bone of the groove and rides on the border of the lesser tuberosity. This lesion is caused by tearing of the outermost fibers of the subscapularis tendon as well as of some fibers that line the floor. The principal criterion for type II biceps tendon subluxation is partial rupture of the outer superficial tendinous portion of the subscapularis muscle. This lesion can involve the whole groove or only part of it.

Malunion and Nonunion of the Lesser Tuberosity (Type III)

Fracture-dislocation of the lesser tuberosity with malunion or nonunion can allow the biceps tendon to slip in and out of its groove. This lesion is seen after proximal humeral fractures. Affected patients complain of pain with internal rotation of the humerus.

Isolated Rupture of the Biceps Tendon Occurring in the Rotator Interval

Severe primary tendinitis of the tendon in the interval can cause weakening of the tendon and its eventual rupture in this area.

Biceps Tendinitis Associated With Rotator Cuff Tears

Patients in whom tendinitis is associated with a rotator cuff tear experience tendinitis of the biceps secondary to exposure of the biceps to the rigid coracoacromial arch. These patients have a rotator cuff tear but no dislocation or subluxation of the biceps tendon. The biceps is inflamed and painful and can appear hypertrophic when viewed through the arthroscope.

Dislocation Associated With Rotator Cuff Tears

Extra-Articular Dislocation Associated With Subscapularis Lesions (Type IA)

Extra-articular dislocation combined with a partial tear of the subscapularis tendon occurs when the biceps tendon is completely dislocated over the lesser tuberosity. Despite superficial tearing of the subscapularis tendon, the deep portion of the subscapularis is intact, allowing the biceps tendon to line up over the lesser tuberosity and preventing the biceps from entering the joint. In this type of dislocation the outer layer of the subscapularis tendon is always torn. This injury is an evolutional type II subluxation.

Extra-Articular Dislocation of the Long Head of the Biceps Tendon Associated With an Intact Subscapularis (Type IB)

The biceps tendon can dislocate over an intact subscapularis tendon. This condition is extremely rare. The LHBT is found lying superficial to the intact subscapularis tendon, and an associated tear of the supraspinatus tendon is always seen. Type IB was found in 3% of 70 patients with biceps dislocations.[171]

Intra-Articular Dislocation of the Long Head of the Biceps Tendon (Type II)

This type involves intra-articular dislocation of the long biceps tendon combined with a complete tear of the subscapularis tendon. Complete dislocation of the biceps is found in the intra-articular location. This usually occurs in conjunction with extensive tearing of the rotator cuff. The subscapularis tendon is torn completely from its attachment on the lesser tuberosity, and the biceps tendon can become interposed into the joint. The biceps tendon is then apposed to the glenoid labrum and can be entrapped in the anterior joint space during rotational movements of the humerus. Subluxation of the biceps can also be associated with rotator cuff tearing.

Ruptures of the Biceps Associated With Rotator Cuff Tears

The biceps can also rupture as a consequence of rotator cuff tears. Walch[242] has shown the frequency with which these lesions are associated. An isolated rupture of the biceps tendon is extremely rare; most biceps tendon ruptures are associated with rotator cuff tears, usually as a result of impingement of the biceps and supraspinatus tendons in the area of the biceps sulcus.

TLC Classification

In an attempt to simplify how best to think about these complex lesions, one of the authors of this chapter (W.Z.B.) uses the simple mnemonic "TLC." The TLC system (Box 17-3) takes into account three distinct factors: the status of the biceps tendon (T), the anatomic location (L) of the pathologic process, and associated pathologic conditions of the rotator cuff (C). With this classification, subtypes, such as I, IIA, IIB, IIC, III, or IV do not need to be memorized; there are merely three entities to remember when assessing the biceps.

BOX 17-3. TLC Classification

Tendon
Stable
Unstable
Tendinitis
Rupture

Location
Origin
Interval
Groove
Musculotendinous junction

Cuff
Intact
Partial tear
Complete tear
Tendinosis

INCIDENCE

In 1934 DePalma[47-51] stated that tenosynovitis of the long head of the biceps brachii tendon was the most common antecedent of painful and stiff shoulders. He believed that this was true in both younger and older patients. In his 1954 series[51] he observed the lesion in 77 men and 98 women ranging in age from 16 to 69 years. The highest incidence was between the ages of 45 and 55 years. Bilateral involvement was observed in 8% of cases. Lesions of greater severity were found in the later decades of life, when more severe degenerative changes prevail. In 61.2% of cases the bicipital tenosynovitis was a localized pathologic process; in the remaining 38.8% of cases, inflammation in the biceps tendon and sheath was part of a generalized and chronic inflammatory process. DePalma believed that bicipital tenosynovitis was the initiating agent in 80% of cases of frozen shoulder. Regardless of the cause, bicipital tenosynovitis was always seen in conjunction with a frozen shoulder.

Calcific tendinitis of the long head of the biceps brachii is uncommon.[202] This lesion has been described at two locations: the first is at the insertion of the biceps tendon into the supraglenoid tubercle and superior labrum, and the second is in the distal portion of the groove near the musculotendinous junction. Calcific tendinitis occurred more often in a series by Goldman.[83] He found 9 cases of insertion tendinitis in 119 cases of calcific tendinitis of the shoulder, as opposed to 11 of 19 for the more distal location.

Injuries to the superior labrum and biceps tendon complex are uncommon. In a series by Andrews and colleagues,[5] 7 of 73 throwing athletes had associated partial tears of the biceps tendon and labral pathology. Burkhart and Fox[22] described two cases of complete tears of the biceps associated with SLAP lesions.

According to McCue and colleagues[140] and O'Donoghue,[174] biceps tendinitis and subluxation are common causes of anterior shoulder pain in throwing athletes. They are common in football quarterbacks because of the weight of the ball and the need for additional pushing action and in softball pitchers because of the forceful supinator strain with arm and forearm flexion.

Lapidus and Guidotti[119] identified 89 patients with tendinitis of the long head of the biceps in a total of 493 patients treated for shoulder pain (an incidence of 18%). Paavolainen and colleagues[180] reported on patients who failed to respond to conservative care and were referred to a shoulder center. A preoperative diagnosis of biceps tendinitis was made before arthrotomy in 38 (30%) of 126 cases. Postoperatively, the incidence was much higher, with 54% of operative specimens showing some evidence of biceps tendinitis. In patients with cuff ruptures the incidence was as high as 60%. If the rotator cuff was intact (with no full-thickness tear), the incidence was approximately 50%. Although this study defined cuffs without a full-thickness rotator cuff tear at surgery as being intact, most of these cuffs showed some evidence of degeneration, edema, and signs of type I and II impingement. Medial dislocation of the biceps tendon occurred in 12 of 51 patients with a ruptured rotator cuff and in 9 of 75 patients when the cuff was intact, for an overall incidence of dislocation of 17%. Frank rupture of the biceps tendon was seen in 8 (6%) of the 126 patients.

Because bicipital tenosynovitis occasionally accompanies impingement syndrome, it remains a relatively common cause of anterior shoulder pain. However, as an isolated entity (i.e., as primary bicipital tenosynovitis), it is much less common.

ETIOLOGY

Although the majority of biceps tendon dislocations occur secondarily as a result of degeneration and attrition of the anterior cuff and coracohumeral ligament,[68-72,145-152,163,164,166,167] there have been reports of acute traumatic dislocation of the tendon. Abbott and Saunders[2] presented six such cases in 1939 along with their operative findings. Four were caused by a fall, resulting in either a direct blow to the shoulder or an indirect blow after falling on the outstretched hands. Two occurred during heavy lifting. All but one of these patients had a concomitant injury to the rotator cuff.

DePalma[47-51] and later Michele[153] divided the etiology of biceps tendinitis according to age group. In younger patients anomalies of the bicipital groove together with repeated trauma are the major inciting factors. In older patients degenerative changes in the tendon are the predominant etiologic factor.

As with most other musculoskeletal problems, the etiology of biceps pathology is most likely to be multifactorial. Chief among the causes is the anatomic location of the tendon. The blood supply of the tendon has been studied by Rathbun and Macnab,[200] who showed it to be diminished, with a critical zone similar to that seen in the supraspinatus. In abduction there is a zone of avascularity in the intracapsular portion of the tendon. This is thought to be caused by pressure from the head of the humerus, the "wringing out" phenomenon. Occupational causes also exist because patients who perform repetitive overhead lifting and throwing are more prone to rupture, elongation, and dislocation of the biceps. Meyer[145-152] reasoned that capsular defects leading to problems with the biceps resulted from repeated and continual use of the arm in a position of marked abduction and external rotation. Borchers[18] and later DePalma[47-51] explained spontaneous rupture within the groove in terms of osteophytic excrescences, which eventually wear through the tendon. Etiologic factors based on variations in the groove have been discussed earlier.

The etiology of calcific deposits in the biceps may be active or passive. Hydroxyapatite deposition disease has been described and can occur in various tendons throughout the body. In a study by Refior and Sowa,[201] histologic analysis of the biceps tendon showed degeneration at the biceps origin and in the region in which the biceps tendon exits the groove. They noted kinking and destruction of the collagen fibers in both these areas. Whether this degeneration is responsible for inducing calcification in some susceptible patients is debatable.

Intra-articular lesions of the biceps and superior labrum can be caused by several mechanisms. The first is a fall on the outstretched hand that drives the humeral head up into the labrum and the tendon.[217] Andrews and colleagues[5] noted that excessive and forceful contraction of the biceps in throwing athletes, especially baseball pitchers and quarterbacks, can induce traction and avulsion of the biceps and superior labral complex in the deceleration phase of throwing. SLAP lesions can also be created by traction on an adducted arm. Burkhart described a "peel-back" mechanism in the etiology of SLAP tears.[24] This phenomenon of superior labral injury is the end result of a pathologic chain of events that begins with functional deficiencies in the core and includes pathologic glenohumeral internal rotation deficit and the SICK scapula syndrome (***s***capular malposition on rib cage, ***i***nferior medial scapular winging, ***c***oracoid tenderness, and scapular dys***k***inesis).[23-26]

Gerber and Sebesta[75] described an anterior internal impingement syndrome similar to the posterior internal impingement syndrome described by Walch and colleagues.[243] In their study, contact between the superior glenohumeral ligament and the anterior rim of the glenoid occurred while performing the Hawkins modified impingement test at 120 degrees of anterior elevation. The undersurface of the subscapularis tendon came into contact with the anterior glenoid rim when the arm was placed between flexion of 80 and 100 degrees. Contact of the superior glenohumeral ligaments and subscapularis on the anterior glenoid rim could explain fraying of these deep structures that do not come into contact with the anterior acromion. These findings were most commonly found in the dominant arm of manual laborers.

Patients maintained on dialysis with long-standing kidney failure can have shoulder pain and symptoms similar to biceps tendinitis. Often, the etiology of this syndrome is a synovitis caused by the deposition of amyloid-like substances. This is a rare cause of shoulder pain.[220] Another rare cause of bicipital pain and degeneration is a tumoral condition, such as osteochondromatosis of the bicipital sheath.

PREVENTION

Prevention of biceps tendon injuries includes warmup, passive stretching, strengthening exercise, and avoidance of painful activities while symptomatic. Strengthening should include all the muscles of the rotator cuff to improve the force couple and reduce impingement. The parascapular muscles should also be rehabilitated. Better balance of the shoulder musculature will theoretically diminish the vicious circle of tendinitis, irritation, and muscle weakness, followed by altered biomechanics, cuff tears, subluxation, and further impingement. Manual laborers, such as carpenters, who do a lot of heavy lifting or repetitive overhead work should probably spend as much time stretching before undertaking their jobs as football and baseball players do before undertaking theirs. Stretching of the biceps tendon is maximal when the shoulder is fully extended and externally rotated and the elbow is fully extended as well.

Overhand athletes, especially pitchers and quarterbacks, should warm up and stretch their capsule to avoid glenohumeral internal rotation deficit and its attendant consequences for the superior labrum and biceps. They should be encouraged to strengthen the muscles of their upper extremity, especially the rotator cuff. Athletes should also be monitored closely to prevent overuse syndromes and capsular contracture.

CLINICAL FEATURES OF BICIPITAL LESIONS

As with all medical conditions, an accurate history and physical examination is vital. This is especially true for subtle lesions of the shoulder, such as biceps tendinitis and biceps instability.

Patients with biceps tendinitis typically complain of chronic pain in the proximal anterior shoulder. The pain can extend down the arm into the muscle belly of the biceps or radiate to the deltoid insertion. It is less likely to radiate into the neck or distally beyond the biceps. Typically, patients have no history of major trauma. They tend to be young or middle-aged and have a history of repetitive overhead activity. The pain is less intense at rest and worse with use. There is disagreement regarding night pain associated with biceps tendinitis: Neviaser[168] stated that there is significant night pain, whereas Simon[212] stated that nocturnal exacerbation is common. In our experience all painful conditions of the shoulder are worse at night, possibly because of compression loading and the supine position placing the shoulder at or below the level of the heart.

Bicipital symptoms are often seen in patients who participate in sports. Any activity at or above shoulder level brings the tuberosities, the bicipital groove, the biceps tendon, and the rotator cuff into close proximity and potentially in direct contact with the anterior acromion, the coracoacromial ligament, and the anterior edge of the glenoid. This can lead to trauma to the intervening biceps tendon.

Biceps instability is most commonly seen in throwing athletes. A palpable snap or pop is often felt at certain positions in the arc of rotation. The patient complains again of pain in the front of the shoulder. This pain is usually reproduced when the arm is raised to 90 degrees.

Patients with rupture of their biceps tendon sometimes also report an audible pop in the shoulder followed by acute onset of pain. The patient then often notes a change in contour of the arm and formation of ecchymosis over the next several days.

Calcific tendinitis in the distal part of the LHBT can also clinically manifest as anterior shoulder pain in young and middle-aged adults. The duration and severity of this pain varies.

Superior labral injuries and injuries to the biceps-labral complex can occur in isolation or in parallel with any of the above conditions. Overhead athletes may report pain during throwing, serving, or other overhead activity, but a paucity of pain at rest. In more severe injuries throwers may report a “dead arm” and the inability to throw.[25,26]

Physical Examination

Clinical evaluation of the superior labrum and biceps-labral complex can be challenging due to relatively poor specificity for a number of clinical tests.[9,141] Many of the tests described below for evaluating the biceps can also be utilized to test the superior labrum. However, multiple maneuvers can be performed in isolation and in combination with other tests to specifically evaluate the superior labrum. The original and modified O’Driscoll dynamic labral shear test[9,113] is performed by stabilizing the scapula, placing the humerus in the location that evokes symptoms, and then applying a compressive and shear load.[113]

The active compression test—commonly known as O’Brien’s test—evaluates the superior labrum and can help distinguish pain emanating from the superior labrum from pain from the acromioclavicular joint.[173] The test is performed by placing the shoulder in 90 degrees of forward flexion, 10 to 15 degrees of adduction and internal rotation, and applying a downward force. This maneuver is then repeated with the arm in external rotation. The test is considered positive for labral pathology if the first maneuver caused pain localized deep in the shoulder and the second maneuver (the arm in external rotation) resulted in less pain. O’Brien and colleagues have extended the original active compression test to include the “three-pack” physical examination of the biceps-labral complex.[224] This consists of (1) palpation of the bicipital tunnel, (2) an active compression test, and (3) a throwing test that consists of placing the arm in 90 degrees of abduction and the elbow in 90 degrees of flexion and then passively placing the arm in external rotation, thus simulating a throwing motion. The three-pack examination can be used in conjunction with diagnostic or therapeutic injections into the glenohumeral joint to diagnose or rule out symptomatic biceps-labral complex lesions.[173,219,222-225,235,236]

Physical examination can reveal point tenderness in the bicipital groove. With the arm in 10 degrees of internal rotation, the biceps tendon faces directly anterior and sits 7 cm distal to the acromion (Fig. 17-26).[133,164] This point tenderness would be expected to move as the arm is rotated and the position of the bicipital groove changes. Tenderness from subdeltoid bursitis can also localize to the anterior shoulder but is generally more diffuse and should not travel with arm rotation. In our opinion this tenderness in motion is the most specific test for bicipital lesions. It does not however differentiate biceps instability from tendinitis. Many authors have suggested that the biceps tendon can be manipulated and, in the presence of instability, can be felt subluxating out of the groove. In our opinion what is perceived by the examiner as the biceps tendon subluxating may in fact be muscle bundles of the deltoid rolling against the humerus. Palpable subluxation might therefore be an inaccurate test for biceps instability.

Slight restrictions of abduction and internal rotation may be noted. This loss of motion is usually a result of pain rather than a capsular constriction and should thus improve with a diagnostic injection of local anesthetic. Pain is felt with abduction and internal rotation, abduction and external rotation, and resisted forward flexion of the shoulder.

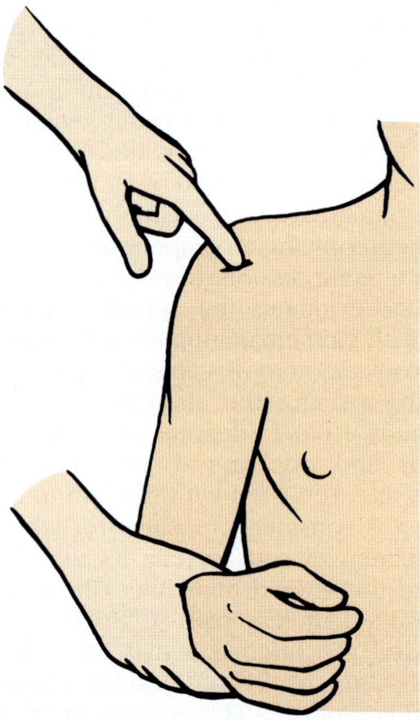

FIGURE 17-26: Matsen and Kirby[148] found that the biceps tendon can be palpated directly anteriorly with the arm in 10 degrees of internal rotation. This position is the same as that used before performing the deAnquin and Lippmann tests.

Several tests have been described in the literature for biceps pathology. However, scant literature is available regarding the sensitivity or specificity of these tests, with the available literature indicating poor specificity. As with all provocative maneuvers, the most important question is not "Does the maneuver produce pain?" but rather "Does the maneuver specifically reproduce the pain that the patient is complaining of?" Selective injections that result in obliteration of this pain are then an extremely important tool for localizing and confirming the patient's diagnosis. Several tests have been described in the past for isolating lesions in the biceps tendon. These include Speed's test, Yergason's sign, the biceps instability test, Ludington's test, deAnquin's test, Lippmann's test, and Hueter's sign.

In Speed's test (Fig. 17-27)[73] the patient flexes the shoulder against resistance with an extended elbow and supinated forearm. Pain should localize to the bicipital groove. Bennett[10] assessed the sensitivity and specificity of Speed's test by correlating preoperative results from the test with pathology seen intraoperatively during arthroscopy. He considered Speed's test to be correctly positive only when a macroscopic lesion was found on the biceps or superior labrum. On the basis of these criteria, he found that Speed's test was 90% sensitive for shoulder pain but only 13% specific for bicipital pathology; furthermore, whereas the negative predictive value was 83%, the positive predictive value of Speed's test was only 23%. Therefore only limited conclusions can be made on the basis of a positive Speed's test.

The test for Yergason's sign (Fig. 17-28)[2] is performed with the patient's elbow flexed. The patient forcibly supinates against resistance, and pain referred to the front and inner aspect of the shoulder in the bicipital groove constitutes a positive sign. Post[194] found the incidence of this positive sign to be 50% in patients with primary biceps tendinitis. The advantage of Yergason's test is that the shoulder is not moving, allowing the possibility of a more isolated examination of the biceps.

The biceps instability test (Fig. 17-29)[2] identifies dislocation of the tendon, complete or incomplete, which may be differentiated from peritendinitis by the test of Abbott and Saunders.[2] After full abduction of the shoulder, the arm, held in complete external rotation, is slowly brought down to the side in the plane of the scapula. A palpable

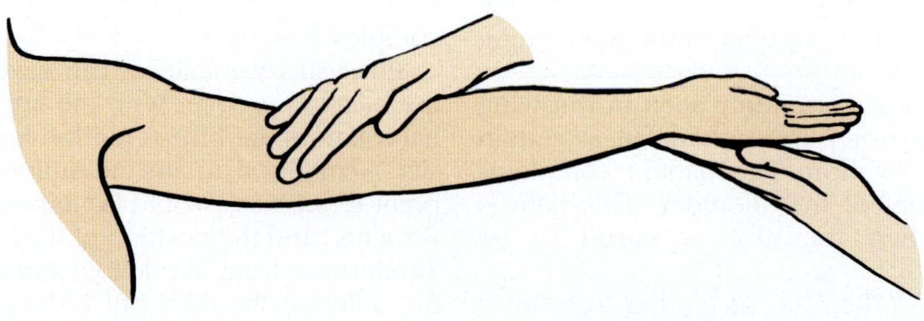

FIGURE 17-27: Speed's test. The biceps resistance test is performed with the patient flexing the shoulder against resistance with the elbow extended and the forearm supinated. Pain referred to the biceps tendon area constitutes a positive test.

or audible click, sometimes accompanied by pain, is noted as the biceps tendon, now forced against the lesser tuberosity, becomes subluxated or dislocated from the groove.

In Ludington's test (Fig. 17-30)[127] the patient puts his or her hands behind the head. In this position of abduction and external rotation the patient flexes the biceps isometrically, and pain is felt in the region of the bicipital groove in those with tendinitis. If the examiner's finger is in the groove at the time of the contraction, subluxation can sometimes be felt. Subtle differences in the contour of the biceps in cases of elongation are best noted in this fashion.

In deAnquin's test (Fig. 17-31)[203] the arm is rotated with the examiner's finger on the most tender spot. Pain is felt immediately as the tendon glides beneath the finger.

Lippmann's test[124] produces pain when the tendon is displaced from one side to the other by the probing finger and then released. The probing is performed about

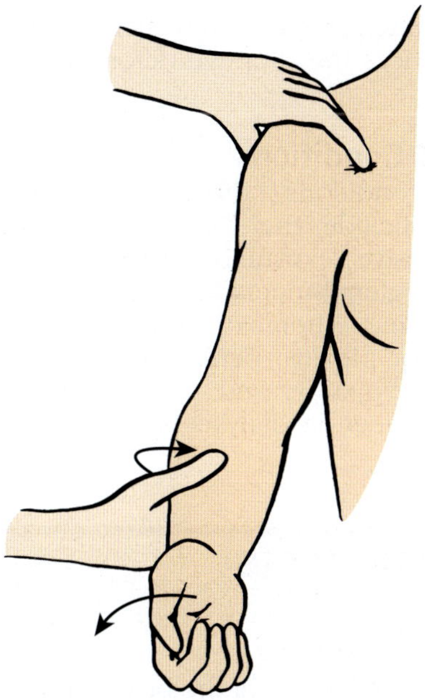

FIGURE 17-28: Yergason's sign. With the arm flexed, the patient attempts to forcefully supinate against resistance from the examiner's hand. Pain referred to the anterior aspect of the shoulder in the region of the bicipital groove constitutes a positive test.

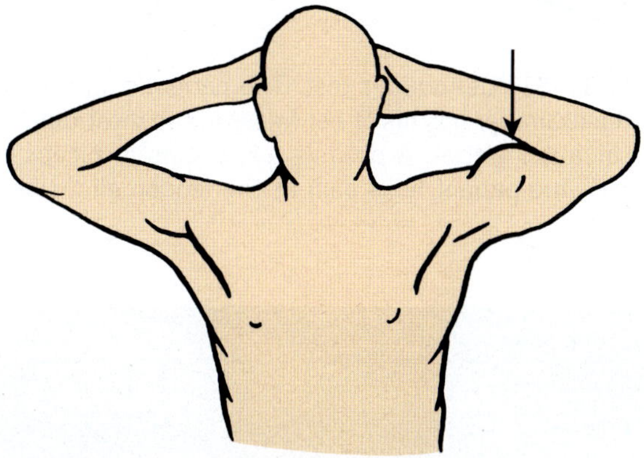

FIGURE 17-30: Ludington's test. The patient puts his or her hands behind the head and flexes the biceps. The examiner's finger can be in the bicipital groove at the time of the test. Subtle differences in the contour of the biceps are best noted with this maneuver. In this illustration the patient has a ruptured biceps at the left shoulder (arrow).

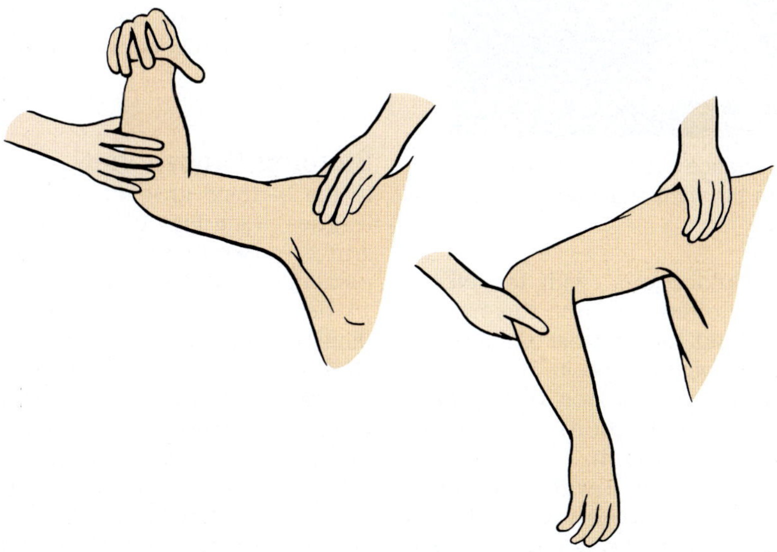

FIGURE 17-29: Biceps instability test (described by Abbott and Saunders). During palpation of the biceps in the groove while taking the arm from an abducted, externally rotated position to a position of internal rotation, a palpable or audible painful click is noted as the biceps tendon is forced against or over the lesser tuberosity.

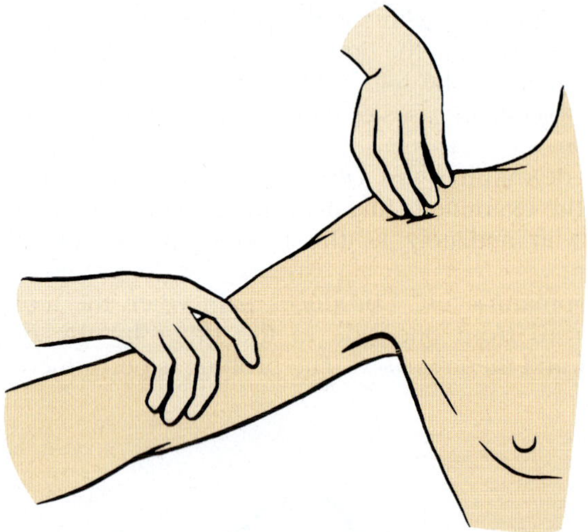

FIGURE 17-31: DeAnquin's test. The patient's arm is rotated while the examiner has his or her finger in the most tender spot in the bicipital groove. A positive test occurs in biceps tendinitis when the patient feels pain as the tendon glides beneath the finger.

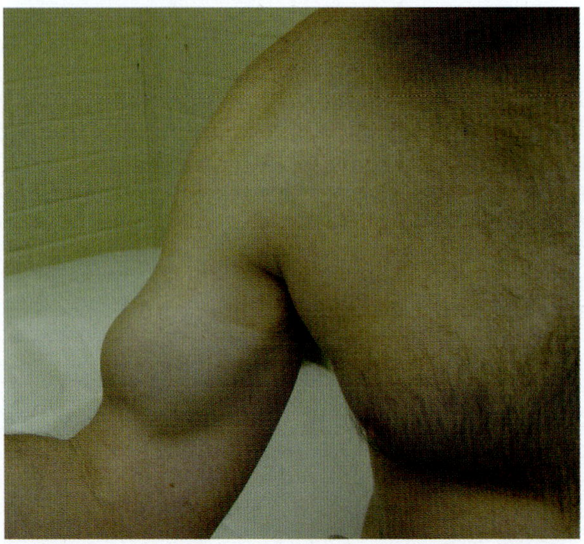

FIGURE 17-32: Clinical appearance of a biceps tendon rupture with a "Popeye deformity" in the right shoulder.

7.5 cm (3 in) from the shoulder joint, with the elbow flexed at a right angle. More often than not, this may in fact be a rolling of the deltoid muscle that is palpated and not a subluxation of the biceps tendon.

Hueter's sign[100] is positive when flexion of the supinated forearm (primarily a biceps function) is less forceful than flexion of the pronated forearm.

The examination findings associated with a complete rupture of the long head of the biceps are much less subtle. A hollowness is evident in the anterior portion of the shoulder, and a "Popeye deformity" develops from the balling up of the biceps below the midbrachium (Fig. 17-32). It is important in such ruptures to look carefully for any atrophy of the rotator cuff musculature, because there is often an associated attrition-type tear in the rotator cuff. Such tears often precede the biceps rupture and may or may not have been symptomatic before the rupture. On careful questioning however patients commonly recall a remote history of treatment for bursitis. With complete rupture of the LHBT, some patients actually experience relief of their prior shoulder pain symptoms. These patients often do not seek medical attention, and it is not until they are seen for unrelated complaints, often in the contralateral shoulder, that the examiner notices the "Popeye deformity."

Associated Conditions

Associated conditions, discussed under "Differential Diagnosis," include the following: impingement syndrome; adhesive capsulitis; rheumatoid arthritis and osteoarthritis; glenohumeral instability; coracoid impingement syndrome; thoracic outlet syndrome, brachial plexopathy, or plexitis; peripheral nerve entrapment or cervical radiculopathy; and rare tumors. Similar symptoms are also seen in dialysis patients.

DIAGNOSTIC TESTS

Plain Film Radiology

When evaluating lesions of the biceps, routine plain films of the shoulder are typically normal. Consequently, special views have been developed for more careful evaluation of the bicipital groove.

Fisk Method

In the Fisk method[65] (Fig. 17-33A) the patient holds the cassette and leans over the table. The biceps groove is marked, and the central beam is perpendicular to the groove.

Bicipital Groove View

In the bicipital groove view described by Cone and colleagues[37] (see Fig. 17-33B), the patient is supine and the arm is in external rotation. The central beam is directed parallel to the coronal axis of the humerus and angled 15 degrees medially. The film cassette is held perpendicular to the superior aspect of the shoulder. This view allows assessment of the medial wall angle, the width of the bicipital groove, and possible spurring in the bicipital groove. Degenerative changes in the greater or lesser tuberosity as well as the presence of a supratubercular ridge can also be determined (Fig. 17-34).

Ahovuo[3] correlated radiographic findings of the bicipital groove with surgical findings. He found that 50% of patients with surgically confirmed biceps tendinitis had radiographic findings of degenerative changes in the walls of the groove. Furthermore, patients with attrition

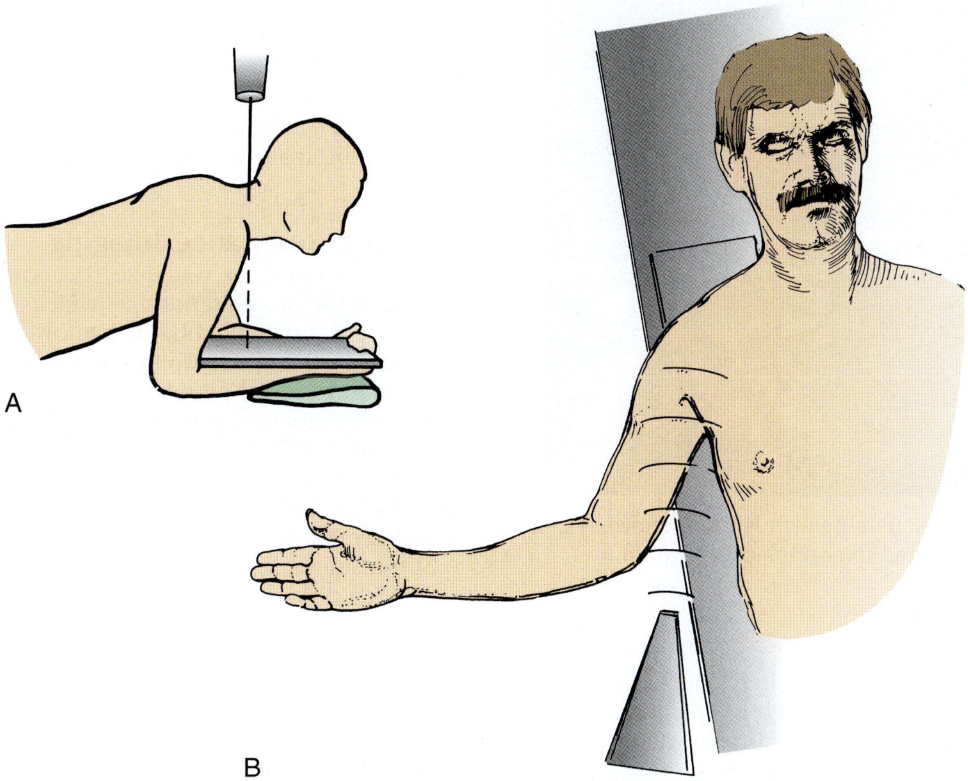

FIGURE 17-33: **A,** Fisk's method. The patient holds the cassette while leaning over the table to bring the bicipital groove perpendicular to the central beam of the x-ray. **B,** Bicipital groove view. The central beam is directed parallel to the coronal axis of the humerus and angled 15 degrees medially. The patient is supine with the arm in the externally rotated position.

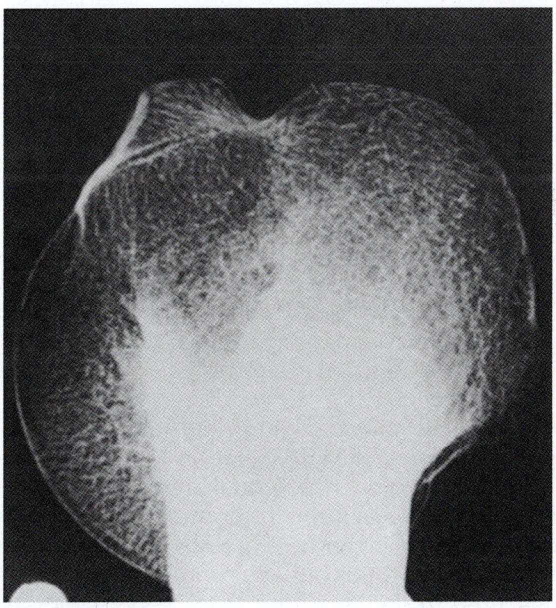

FIGURE 17-34: Normal bicipital groove projection. (From Cone RO, Danzig L, Resnick D, et al. The bicipital groove: Radiographic, anatomic, and pathologic study. *AJR Am J Roentgenol.* 1983;141:781-788.)

tendinitis tended to have deeper grooves (with a depth of 4.8 mm or more and inclination of 58 degrees or more). A shallow groove was seen more often with bicipital dislocation.

Two additional views that can be helpful are the caudal tilt view[191] and the outlet view of Neer and Poppen.[167] The caudal tilt view is a standing anteroposterior view of the shoulder with a 30-degree caudal tilt of the x-ray beam. With this technique, the degree of anterior acromial prominence or spurring can be appreciated. The outlet view is a transscapular radiograph performed with a 10-degree caudal tilt. The easiest way to take this radiograph is to have the patient stand with the spine of the scapula perpendicular to the cassette. The x-ray beam should be parallel to the spine, but with a 10-degree caudal tilt.

Arthrography

Shoulder arthrography has classically been used to evaluate the biceps tendon and bicipital groove. For example, contrast within the groove can outline the presence or absence of the biceps tendon. Today, shoulder arthrography is typically used in combination with MRI or CT (Fig. 17-35). MRI alone can provide excellent imaging of

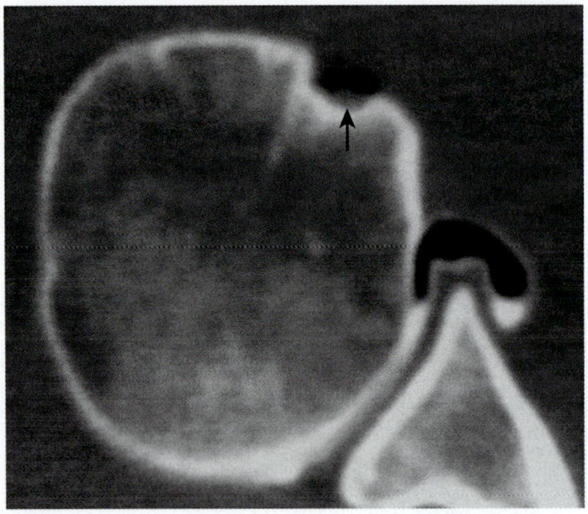

FIGURE 17-35: The bicipital tendon is seen (arrow) seated in the groove on a computed tomographic arthrogram.

the soft tissues. The addition of a gadolinium arthrogram can further define labral pathology, such as superior labral avulsions and tearing of the bicipital attachment.

Reflection pulley lesions can also be diagnosed with MRI arthrography. Weishaupt and colleagues[250] evaluated MRI criteria for diagnosing pulley lesions and found three MRI findings to be useful. A thickened superior border of the subscapularis tendon three to five sections below the humeral head on axial gradient echo images can indicate a pulley lesion. This was the most sensitive and specific sign. Likewise, a poorly defined superior border of the subscapularis tendon at its insertion site on the lesser tuberosity was suspicious for a pulley lesion. Finally, a collection of contrast material anterior to the superior border of the subscapularis above the level of the coracoid process on axial images in the expected area of the rotator interval also indicated a pulley lesion.

Ultrasonography

Ultrasonography is a noninvasive imaging modality for the shoulder. Although highly operator dependent, it has been shown to be useful in evaluating the rotator cuff. It can also be helpful in evaluating lesions of the biceps tendon. Middleton and colleagues[154] compared ultrasonography with arthrography and found them to be equally successful in evaluating the bony anatomy of the bicipital groove. Sonography however provided a superior image of the biceps tendon within the groove (Fig. 17-36A to D).

Armstrong and colleagues[261] looked at the efficacy of ultrasound in diagnosing pathology of the long head of the biceps. They prospectively evaluated 71 patients using standard ultrasonography and correlated findings with the results of subsequent arthroscopic examination. Not surprisingly, ultrasound showed high specificity and sensitivity (100% and 96%, respectively) for subluxation or dislocation. However, it failed to identify any of the 23 partial-thickness tears of the biceps tendon in this study. Overall, ultrasound had a sensitivity of 50% for biceps pathology and a specificity of 100%. It had a positive predictive value of 100% and a negative predictive value of 71%. Therefore a normal ultrasound does not preclude an anatomic biceps tendon lesion.

Magnetic Resonance Imaging

MRI can be used to visualize the normal intra-articular portion of the biceps tendon as well as the portion within groove. For optimal MRI evaluation, images should be obtained in the axial, oblique, and sagittal planes. The oblique and sagittal planes provide the best visualization of the intra-articular portion of the biceps tendon in the rotator interval.[228] The axial plane is best for showing the descending portion of the biceps in the groove. MRI is also useful for imaging the concomitant rotator cuff pathology that is often associated with biceps lesions.[111,151]

Subluxations or dislocations can be identified with MRI. With dislocations, the tendon is usually shown displaced out of its groove and is seen lying medial to the lesser tuberosity (Fig. 17-37). Subluxation can be identified when the tendon is observed to overlie the lesser tuberosity on some images. Care must be taken because osteophytes and scar tissue can be misinterpreted as tendon within the groove.[234]

MRI is also useful in diagnosing biceps ruptures (Fig. 17-38). Ruptures are easier to diagnose than partial tears, clinically as well as on MRI. They are diagnosed by the absence of the tendon at any point along its anatomic course. Klug and Moore[114] refer to this as the *empty groove sign*. Occasionally, an intra-articular stump can be seen. Clearly, care should be taken to ensure that the biceps tendon is not simply dislocated out of the groove rather than ruptured. With ruptures of the tendon, atrophy and retraction distally may be seen.

Partial tears, on the other hand, are more difficult to diagnose. On MRI, partial tearing can appear as an irregular or notched appearance of the tendon. A partial tear may be inferred from a sudden change in cross-sectional diameter of the tendon between adjacent cuts on a scan.[123] Longitudinal tears may be easier to identify than transverse tears because they can often be identified on several coronal and sagittal cuts, whereas focal transverse tears may be dismissed as artifact because they appear only on one cut, or may be missed altogether because the interval between cuts is too great. When transverse tears are visualized, partial tearing of the tendon can appear as signal changes within the tendon. Focal lines and globular zones of high signal on long transient echo sequences are two such potential signal changes.[114]

Biceps tendinitis is a much more difficult diagnosis to make on MRI, but it can be suggested by certain criteria. One criterion is fluid out of proportion to the intra-articular fluid in the shoulder. In shoulders with a large joint effusion, fluid surrounding the tendon can be a normal finding; but the presence of a large amount of fluid in the biceps sulcus with only a small quantity of intra-articular fluid can indicate tendinitis. Thickening

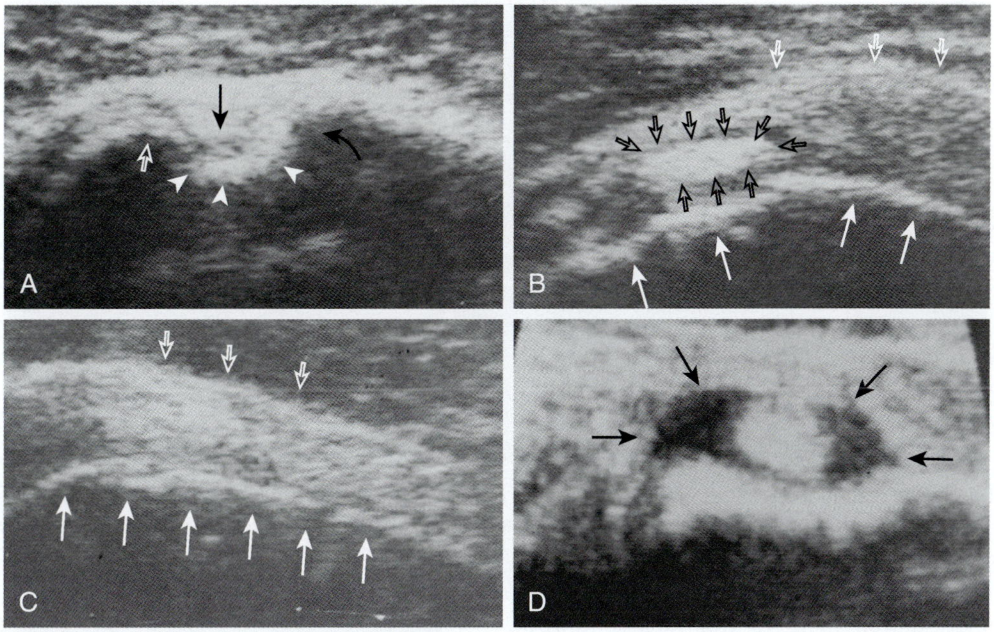

FIGURE 17-36: A, Transverse sonogram of the anterior aspect of the shoulder showing the bicipital groove (arrowheads) as a semicircular depression in the proximal part of the humerus, formed by the lesser tuberosity medially (open arrow) and the greater tuberosity laterally (curved arrow). The biceps tendon is seen as an echogenic ellipse within the groove (black arrow). **B,** Sonogram perpendicular to the long axis of the intra-articular portion of the biceps tendon (open black arrows), seen between the subscapularis anteriorly and the supraspinatus posteriorly. The deep surface of the deltoid muscle is indicated by open white arrows and the humeral head by solid white arrows. **C,** On longitudinal scans, the biceps tendon appears as an echogenic band sandwiched between the upper portion of the humeral head (solid arrows) and the lower portion of the deltoid (open arrows). **D,** Transverse sonogram of the distal part of the biceps tendon showing biceps sheath effusion (arrows) surrounding the biceps tendon. (From Middleton WD, Reinus WR, Tetty WG, et al. Ultrasonographic evaluation of the rotator cuff and biceps tendon. *J Bone Joint Surg Am.* 1986;68:440-450.)

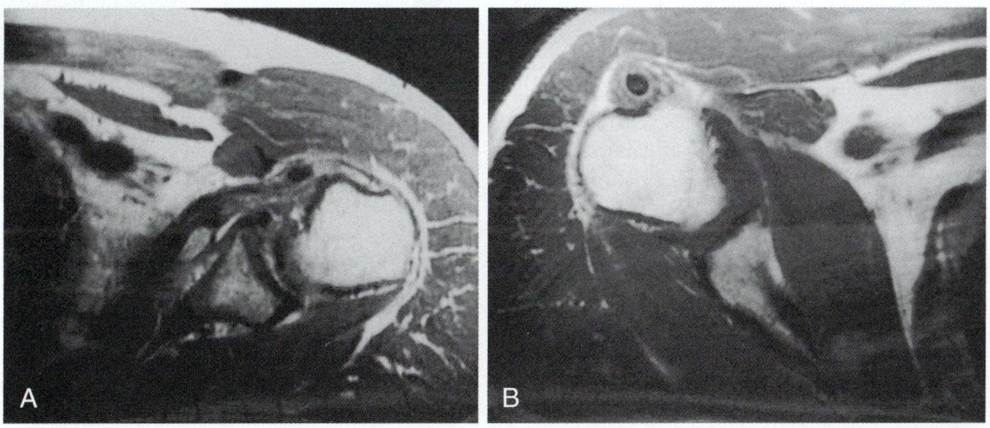

FIGURE 17-37: Axial magnetic resonance images demonstrating the biceps tendon medially displaced out of the bicipital groove (**A**) and the biceps tendon located within the bicipital groove (**B**).

of the tendon and increased intensity on T1- and T2-weighted images can suggest degenerative changes in the tendon. This degeneration may be diffuse or can occur in segmental areas.[228] Clearly, such assessments are often very difficult to make.

In a prospective double-blinded study Mohtadi and colleagues[159] looked at the clinical accuracy of MRI in evaluating patients with shoulder pain. They used MRI with intravenous contrast to evaluate 58 patients whose conservative management of their shoulder pain had failed. The findings on MRI were compared to subsequent findings at arthroscopy, with 53 of the patients reviewed with regard to pathology of the long head of the biceps. Tendons were assessed as normal, inflamed, partially torn, or ruptured. Of the 53 patients studied, 35 ultimately had tendon pathology noted at arthroscopy, a

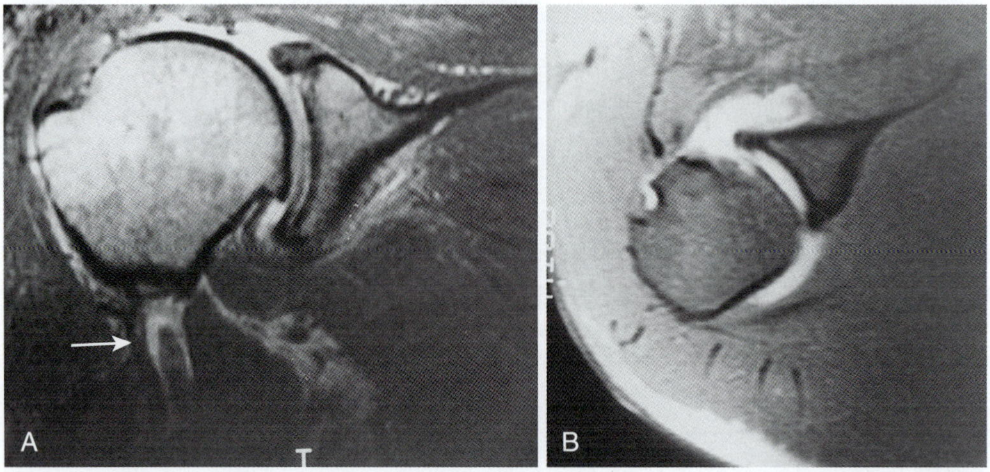

FIGURE 17-38: Magnetic resonance images (MRI) showing a biceps tendon rupture. **A,** Coronal MRI demonstrating the distal retraction of the biceps tendon stump. **B,** Axial MRI demonstrating the absence of the biceps tendon in the bicipital groove.

prevalence of 66%. Partial tears of the biceps tendon were difficult to diagnose. Half (five out of 10) of the partial tears identified at arthroscopy were misdiagnosed on MRI, and 12 of the patients thought to have partial tearing in fact merely had an inflamed or even normal tendon. MRI likewise missed three nonretracted complete ruptures. Overall there was 37% concordance between MRI and arthroscopy. They concluded that although MRI was highly accurate in detecting full-thickness tears of the cuff and acromioclavicular joint pathology, it was less reliable in diagnosing biceps tendon pathology.

MRI is often ordered before consultation with a specialist. The radiologists who read these MRIs may be inexperienced in assessing subtle lesions of the biceps tendon, and errors and omissions can sometimes occur. Because biceps pathology or a suspicion of biceps pathology can alter a surgeon's surgical plan (or can require the availability of special equipment or implants), we recommend that surgeons review all studies themselves. The surgeon will then be able to correlate findings on MRI with findings at arthroscopy and hone his or her interpretive skills.

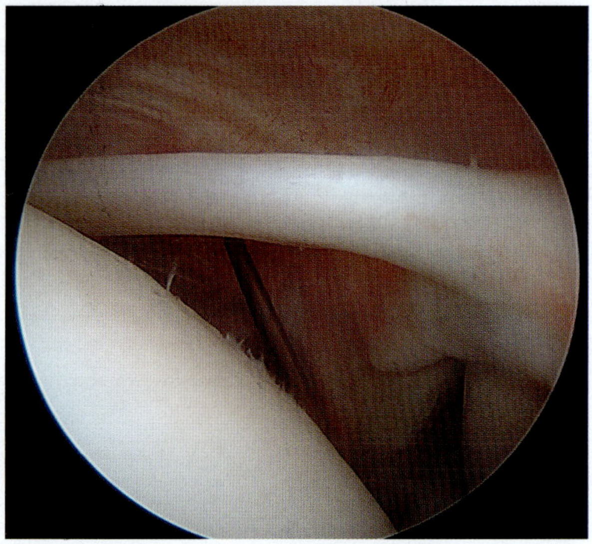

FIGURE 17-39: Arthroscopic view of the biceps tendon.

Arthroscopy

Arthroscopy remains the best method for visualizing the intra-articular biceps tendon (Fig. 17-39). It is also useful in identifying other causes of chronic anterior shoulder pain.[4,5,175,256] It provides the examiner with both static and dynamic examinations that can reveal lesions of the biceps, biceps anchor, and superior labrum, or subtle instability of the biceps.

A disadvantage of arthroscopy is that it is an invasive procedure that normally requires general anesthesia and thus, as with all surgical procedures, carries with it the usual risks (such as infection, or risks from anesthesia). Another disadvantage is that extra-articular lesions of the biceps might not be appreciated. Positioning the arm to relax the biceps tendon however allows more of the tendon to be visualized. This can be done by flexing the elbow and supinating the forearm while flexing and externally rotating the shoulder. A probe can then be used to pull more of the biceps tendon into the joint and into the arthroscopist's field of vision.[64] In this way an extra 3 to 5 cm of tendon can be visualized (Fig. 17-40). This can sometimes reveal fraying of the intertubercular portion of the tendon.

Boileau and colleagues[15] described the *hourglass biceps*, in which hypertrophy of the proximal, intra-articular portion of the long head of the biceps prevents this portion of the tendon from entering the bicipital groove. Clinically, patients complain of pain in the anterior shoulder and loss of 10 to 20 degrees of passive elevation. Intraoperatively, the mechanical block to elevation is confirmed arthroscopically. With the elbow fully

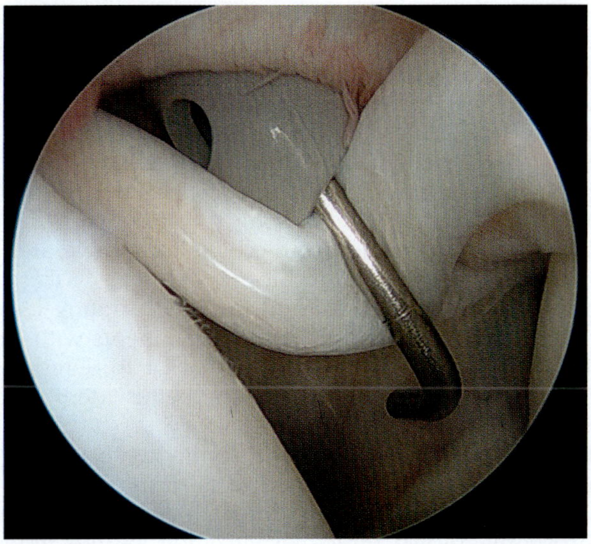

FIGURE 17-40: Arthroscopic view of the biceps tendon pulled into the joint.

extended and the arm passively elevated, the hypertrophic biceps tendon is seen with the arthroscope as buckling and unable to enter the bicipital groove. Treatment requires excision of the hypertrophic, intra-articular portion of the tendon, which is left as a tenotomy or subjected to tenodesis.

Evaluation of the rotator interval for potential pulley lesions is also important.[10] Flexing the shoulder 60 to 90 degrees with the arthroscope advanced anteriorly in the joint allows the surgeon to visualize the interval structures. Internal rotation of the arm relaxes the subscapularis and allows access to the interval ligaments, rotator cuff tendons, and biceps pulley. A 70-degree scope can aid this examination. A careful and systematic examination is the best way to ensure identification of these lesions.

Arthroscopy has limitations in diagnostic evaluation. O'Brien and colleagues have shown that there is a "no man's land" distally along the biceps tunnel that cannot be visualized either at arthroscopy or via an open subpectoral approach. This "no man's land" adds an element of uncertainty to diagnostic arthroscopy and the treatment of biceps lesions.[224,225,236]

COMPLICATIONS

The most common complication of treating biceps tendon lesions is, as has already been emphasized previously, the failure to recognize a concomitant disruption of the rotator cuff. The majority of rotator cuff tears are secondary to chronic impingement and tendinitis, with only a minority of patients sustaining an acute massive cuff avulsion as a result of trauma. Consequently, given the intimate relationship between the rotator cuff and the biceps tendon, it could be expected that impingement of one would result in impingement on the other. Although the results of cuff debridement and decompression are impressive in terms of pain relief and restoration of range of motion, early diagnosis and aggressive surgical intervention are preferable for patients younger than 60 years who wish to maintain strength above shoulder level.

Adhesive capsulitis can follow a number of painful conditions about the shoulder including lesions of the biceps. Because biceps tendinitis has been associated with adhesive capsulitis, early recognition and treatment is important. Antiinflammatory agents; moist heat; and early, gentle, and patient-directed range-of-motion exercises can prevent or at least shorten the potentially long and painful course of adhesive capsulitis.

DIFFERENTIAL DIAGNOSIS

Because it is typical for tendinitis of the long head of the biceps to be seen in association with other conditions, primary, isolated biceps tendinitis is a diagnosis of exclusion. Therefore the need to identify these other clinical entities that can mimic or are commonly seen with biceps tendinitis should be foremost in the examiner's mind. These include impingement syndrome, adhesive capsulitis, rheumatoid arthritis and osteoarthritis, glenohumeral instability, coracoid impingement syndrome, thoracic outlet syndrome or brachial plexopathy or plexitis, peripheral nerve entrapment, and cervical radiculopathy. Distinguishing these conditions from one another starts, of course, with a thorough history in which an accurate understanding of the mechanism of injury (if present) can be helpful. Examination, as described earlier in this chapter and in other chapters, can further clarify the pathology, and imaging can be ordered as necessary. We review here some techniques of differentiating these various clinical entities.

Impingement Syndrome

Patients with impingement syndrome without bicipital involvement complain of more proximal pain with tenderness primarily over the anterior acromion, coracoacromial ligament, and supraspinatus tendon insertion. The impingement and impingement reinforcement signs are positive. Selective injection with a local anesthetic is helpful in differentiating primary biceps tendinitis from impingement tendinitis. In patients with impingement syndrome, injection of lidocaine into the subacromial space typically relieves all of their pain, whereas patients with associated biceps tendinitis complain of more distal pain over the bicipital groove. Subacromial injection in these patients fails to alleviate all of their symptoms, and they continue to experience pain over the groove. Subsequent injection of lidocaine into the sheath itself that obliterates this residual pain confirms biceps tendinitis involvement in pain production.

It is important to remember that the subdeltoid bursa (which covers the groove) is continuous with the subacromial bursa. Therefore inadvertent injection of anesthetic into the subdeltoid bursa will also anesthetize the subacromial bursa and confuse the examination. We therefore recommend first injecting the subacromial bursa at the level of the midlateral acromion. A clinical diagnosis of primary biceps tendinitis can only be made if subacromial injection has absolutely no effect on the patient's pain and subsequent injection of the bicipital groove relieves all of the patient's pain and restores 100% of the motion. A positive response to injection has been found to be a predictor of good long-term results.[13]

A technique for injecting the bicipital groove has been described by Kerlan.[111] The patient is placed supine with the arm over the table. The elbow is bent and the shoulder extended with the arm in external rotation to reduce the distance from the groove to the surface. The biceps tendon is located anteriorly, and a mark is made on the skin. The area is prepared in a sterile fashion and injected. It is extremely important, especially if corticosteroids are used, that the injection be placed into the sheath and not into the tendon itself. Directing the needle superiorly at an angle tangential to the tendon should eliminate this potential complication. Fluid must flow easily from the syringe; if any resistance is encountered, the needle should be repositioned. Because of the anatomy of the sheath and its communication with the joint, a very low volume of local anesthetic (only 2 to 3 mL of 1% lidocaine) is used.

Claessens and Snoek[33] considered intra-articular injection of an anesthetic to be important in differentiating rotator cuff tendinitis from biceps tendinitis. Although this may be true of bursal-side lesions, undersurface tears of the rotator cuff or labral lesions are also anesthetized with this technique. Imaging studies should therefore be used to confirm the surgeon's clinical impression.

Shoulder Instability

Subluxation of the glenohumeral joint can cause anterior shoulder pain. This pain is episodic and generally lasts for several days after a major episode of subluxation. If the brachial plexus is stretched and inflamed, then pain and paresthesias can be experienced transiently or, depending on their severity, for several weeks or even months.

The mechanism of injury for lesions of the biceps and for anterior shoulder instability can be similar in that both can occur with forced external rotation. However, biceps lesions are more likely to occur with forced external rotation of the adducted arm. When differentiating shoulder instability from subluxation of the biceps tendon, provocative tests are helpful. In anterior shoulder instability the maximal point of apprehension and clicking should be in 90 degrees of abduction and maximal external rotation (a positive apprehension sign).

The humeral head translating across a torn glenoid labrum causes pain in the anterior part of the shoulder. This pain may be felt anteriorly due to internal impingement of the subscapularis and anteromedial humeral head in cases of posterior instability. Pain may also be felt posteriorly at this time, secondary to cuff stretching. In a patient with a subluxating biceps tendon, pain is not maximal until the arm is brought down from the position of maximal abduction and external rotation, and the click occurs as the examiner begins to internally rotate the arm (the biceps instability test). Yergason's and Speed's signs should be negative in patients with anterior shoulder instability, but positive if the biceps is inflamed.

Special radiographic views for shoulder instability should be obtained (see Chapter 4). MRI or CT arthrograms allow visualization of the bicipital groove and the presence or absence of the biceps tendon. A CT arthrogram can be extremely helpful in demonstrating lesions of the anterior cartilaginous labrum in patients with instability. Although MRI is not as good as CT in demonstrating Bankart-type lesions, it can better demonstrate inflammation of the tendon itself.

In cases where the diagnosis continues to be unclear even after the aforementioned tests, arthroscopy or an examination under anesthesia or both can be performed. Arthroscopy allows direct visualization of the anterior labrum, the intra-articular portion of the biceps tendon, and the aperture of the sulcus and the surrounding cuff; evaluation for possible glenohumeral instability can be performed at the same time. For example, a Bankart lesion and a positive drive-through sign can suggest glenohumeral instability as the cause of pain, especially in the absence of any biceps tendon findings.

Glenoid Labrum Tears Without Instability

Tears of the glenoid labrum without instability, such as those that occur in the superior third of the labrum in close proximity to the biceps, can show symptoms similar to those of biceps tendon subluxation. These superior labral tears can occur in baseball players and other overhead-throwing athletes and often cause symptoms very similar to those of a subluxating bicipital tendon or of a rotator cuff tear (see Chapter 20). An audible or palpable clunk occurs during rotation above the horizontal as the tear flips in and out of the joint and impinges on the humeral head.

There should be a high index of suspicion for this lesion when dealing with shoulder pain in a throwing athlete. These patients sometimes have more pain with release because of the deceleration effect of the biceps pulling on the torn labrum. CT arthrography occasionally misses this lesion. MRI with or without gadolinium can be helpful in making this diagnosis. However, the best way to differentiate it from a subluxating biceps tendon is by glenohumeral arthroscopy.

Adhesive Capsulitis

Patients with adhesive capsulitis often have tenderness in the anterior aspect of the shoulder in the region of the bicipital groove and anterior portion of the subdeltoid bursa. In evaluating patients with a painful, stiff shoulder and point tenderness over the bicipital groove, it is useful to administer a diagnostic lidocaine injection in this area, initially without cortisone, to observe its effect on motion. If injection of the tendon sheath with 2 to 3 mL of lidocaine results in the obliteration of the patient's pain but does not appreciably improve motion, then the underlying problem is an adhesive capsulitis or frozen shoulder. If this same injection eliminates the patient's pain and results in a return of full motion, then biceps tendinitis is more likely to be the underlying problem.

Glenohumeral Arthritis

Glenohumeral arthritis often manifests as anterior shoulder pain with decreased range of motion. Because the biceps tendon is an intra-articular structure, it is involved in any process involving the joint. Inflammatory changes occur in the visceral layers of the synovium of the biceps recess just as in the subscapular and axillary recesses. Plain radiographs can show spurring of the proximal end of the humerus with a ring osteophyte and flattening of the glenoid.

Coracoid Impingement Syndrome

Warren[248,249] and Gerber and colleagues[76] described the role of the coracoid process in coracoid impingement syndrome. Symptoms of coracoid impingement are similar to those of biceps tendinitis and instability. Using CT scan data, Gerber established the *normal coracoid-to-humeral distance* to be 8.6 mm and noted that this distance decreased in those with *coracoid impingement* (to an average of 6.7 mm). The syndrome has been described in patients with an excessively long or laterally placed coracoid process and in those who have undergone bone block and osteotomy procedures for instability.

The symptom of coracoid impingement is dull pain in the front of the shoulder referred to the anterior upper arm and occasionally extending into the forearm. The pain can be consistently elicited by bringing the arm into forward flexion and internal rotation or adduction and internal rotation. In contrast to subacromial impingement, forward flexion is most often painful between 120 and 130 degrees rather than 60 to 120 degrees. The diagnosis is established clinically by obliteration of the patient's pain by subcoracoid injection.

The importance of considering this entity before surgery on the biceps tendon has been pointed out by Dines and colleagues.[53] In their series one third of biceps tenodesis failures were related to undiagnosed coracoid impingement syndrome.

TREATMENT

Nonoperative Treatment

History

In 1773 Bromfield[20] discussed the technical aspects of reducing dislocations of the biceps tendon. Treatment of tendinitis was initially discussed by Schrager[208] in the 1920s. Recommendations during the 1920s and 1930s included morphine, sudden traction, diathermy, massage, faradization, and light and x-ray treatment. Milgram[155-158] and later Lapidus[118] were proponents of procaine hydrochloride (Novocain) infiltration and aspiration of the calcific deposits in cases of acute calcific tendinitis.

DePalma[50] initially treated bicipital tenosynovitis conservatively with hydrocortisone injections directly into the tendon under the transverse ligament, noting improvement in 10 of 18 cases. He recommended, as a rule, three or four 1-mL injections into the tendon under the transverse ligament at weekly intervals. It is now apparent from the data of Kennedy and Willis[110] that such frequent steroid injection is ill advised. Injections should be made only in the tendon sheath, and the tendon itself should be avoided. Of the patients treated in this way, 29% had excellent results, 45% good, 9% fair, and 16% poor.

Habermeyer and Walch[91] also recommend nonoperative therapy for isolated tendinitis of the LHBT. They recommend a single intra-articular injection of cortisone and oral antiinflammatory medication in the acute stages of the disease; this is carried out in conjunction with limited immobilization and local ice therapy along with a conservative regimen of physical therapy. Physical therapy, including isometric and isokinetic strengthening of the rotator cuff, is the key to rehabilitate these patients.

Biceps tendinitis secondary to impingement syndrome can respond to conservative treatment aimed at treating the primary rotator cuff pathology. Subacromial injections of corticosteroids may be of assistance in a patient with a large rotator cuff tear who is not interested in or not a candidate for surgery. Because the intra-articular and subacromial spaces communicate with the rotator cuff tear, there is less need to specifically inject the area of the biceps tendon in these cases.

SLAP tears can also be successfully treated nonoperatively. In a retrospective review Edwards and colleagues[60] showed significant improvements in pain and functional scores following nonoperative treatment of SLAP lesions. Nonoperative treatment was less successful in younger patients and in overhead athletes.

Results

Nontreatment of the LHBT ruptures (especially in the elderly) can still lead to outcomes acceptable to most patients. Predictably, patients with a bicipital rupture who have an intact brachialis muscle experience no decrease in flexion strength at the elbow. Loss of supination strength has been estimated by Warren and colleagues to be between 10% and 20% with Cybex testing.[248,249] Phillips and colleagues[193] did not find a significant difference between patients who had proximal biceps tendon ruptures treated operatively and those who underwent nonoperative treatment. All the patients in this study were middle aged and older. After a period of conservative care, including range-of-motion exercises, moist heat, and strengthening, most patients have relatively normal flexion strength and only minimal loss of supination power.[98-102] Carroll and Hamilton[29] studied 100 patients who sustained a rupture of the biceps brachii as a result of forced extension. Follow-up function was ascertained by assessing the patient's ability to lift weights. The authors concluded that a patient could return to work earlier and suffered no residual disability with conservative treatment. Patients in their series returned to work at an average of 4 weeks. Warren and colleagues,[249] using Cybex testing in 10 patients with chronic biceps rupture, failed to find any significant loss of elbow flexion strength and observed only a 10% loss of elbow supination strength. Phillips and colleagues[193] compared patients treated with long-term nonoperative therapy to those treated with operative therapy and found no significant difference in supination or elbow flexion strength in 19 patients.

Long head of the biceps tendon rupture may not be completely benign. Deutch and colleagues[52] assessed pain and disability in patients following nonoperative treatment of ruptures of the long head of the biceps. They followed 11 patients with a mean age of 59 years for a minimum of 6 months (range, 6 months to 3.5 years) and found objective decreases in supination, pronation, and flexion strength of 23%, 29%, and 29%, respectively. Subjectively, all patients complained of some degree of pain or disability or both from their rupture. Whether surgical treatment would have resulted in a superior outcome was beyond the scope of this study.

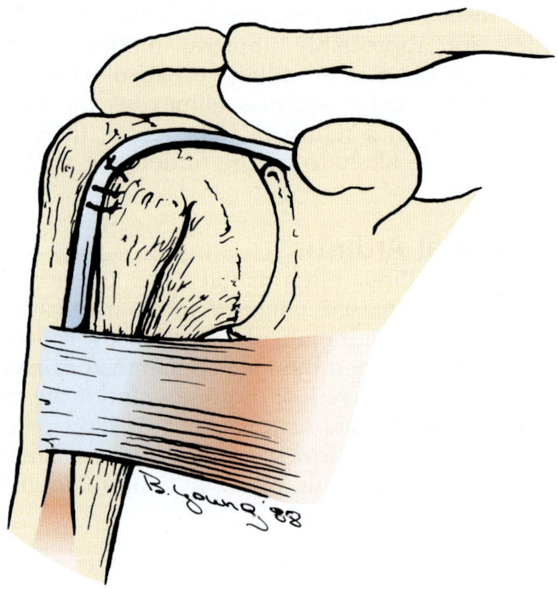

FIGURE 17-41: Lippmann's technique of suturing the biceps tendon to the lesser tuberosity for adhesive capsulitis.

Operative Treatment: Open

Review

Surgical treatment of the biceps tendon received little attention before Gilcreest[78] in 1926. He was the first to suggest suturing the stump of the tendon to the coracoid process. In 1939 Abbott and Saunders[2] reported on a series of six cases of biceps dislocation treated by surgically fixing half of the tendon through drill holes, leaving the intracapsular tendon intact. In their series four of the six patients required reoperation for pain, and all patients ultimately experienced some pain, weakness, and decreased range of motion. The poor results from their procedure stemmed from two problem areas: the procedure as described prevented the normal sliding of the humerus on the biceps tendon, and too much attention was paid to the biceps lesion, with insufficient attention paid to concomitant cuff tears and impingement.

Lippmann[123,124] recommended tenodesis of the long head of the biceps to the lesser tuberosity (Fig. 17-41) to shorten the course of frozen shoulder. He strongly believed (based on 12 operative cases) that frozen shoulder was the result of tenosynovitis of the long head of the biceps.

Hitchcock and Bechtol[96] in 1948 described tenodesis of the biceps tendon within the groove with an osteal-periosteal flap (Fig. 17-42). Hitchcock's name has become synonymous with tenodesis of the biceps tendon in the bicipital groove. According to the authors, solid fixation of the LHBT to the floor of the intertubercular groove decreased time to recovery and improved pain relief. However, no objective measures were provided to support this statement, and results were based on a subjective review of 26 such cases. The authors did note an association with other lesions, such as tears of the rotator cuff. However, in contrast to our earlier warnings, their primary admonition was that peritendinitis of the biceps tendon should not be overlooked in light of associated pathology.

In 1954 DePalma and Callery[51] reported on 86 cases of bicipital tenosynovitis managed operatively, the majority of which were treated by suturing the LHBT into the coracoid process (Fig. 17-43). Shortly before publication, several patients underwent tenodesis of the tendon in the groove using a staple for fixation. The rationale cited for this change was that the three-pronged staple provided sufficient fixation while eliminating the extensive dissection needed to expose the coracoid process. Of 86 cases, 59 were available for follow-up (on average for 27 months); 23 of the cases were complicated by a frozen shoulder. Excellent results were achieved in 64%, good in 16%, fair in 8%, and poor in 10%. Thus 80% of the patients experienced a good or excellent result. Examination of those with a poor result revealed errors in diagnosis and technique and cases of reflex sympathetic dystrophy.

Michele[153] described keystone tenodesis in 1960. In this technique a rectangular block of bone (which includes the bicipital groove) is removed. The bone is decorticated and a bony trough is prepared for the tendon. Two semilunar holes are placed on either side of the trough to allow the tendon to enter and exit. The biceps tendon is then placed into the trough, and the bone block is returned to its original position. The periosteum is sutured back to secure the bone block in place. Michele reported on 16 cases in which radiographs demonstrated persistence of the entrance and exit holes and "smooth gliding of the biceps through the holes." Range of motion was complete in all planes and was

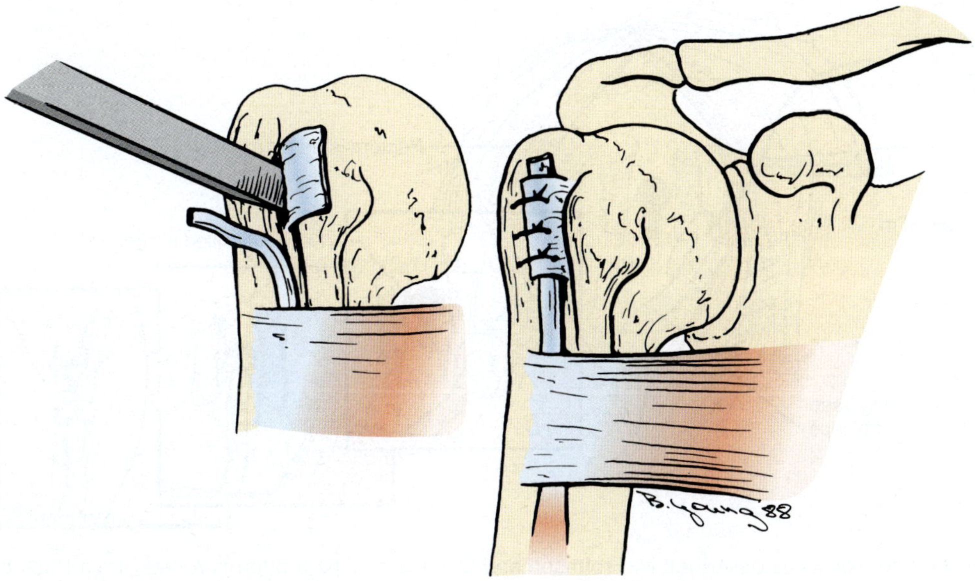

FIGURE 17-42: Hitchcock's procedure. With an osteotome, a bed is made in the intertubercular groove by elevating a portion of the floor from the outside inward (left). The tendon is roughened and then sutured beneath this osteal periosteal flap with heavy nonabsorbable sutures. The transverse humeral ligament is laid down over the tendon and the osteal periosteal flap (right).

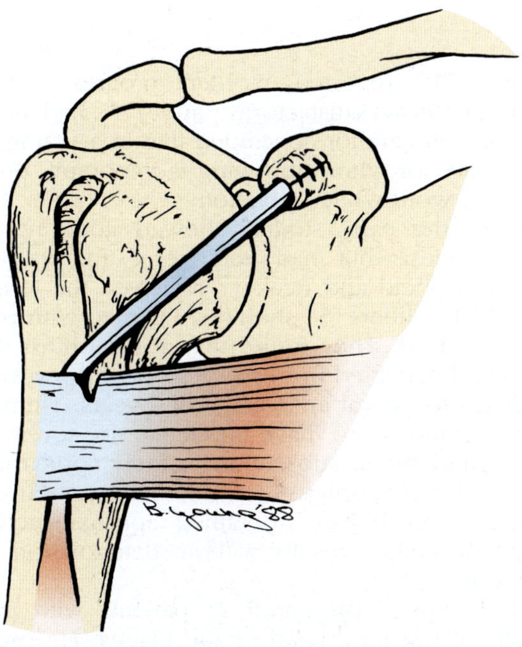

FIGURE 17-43: Tenodesis of the long head of the biceps to the coracoid process. This procedure was initially described by Gilcreest and popularized by DePalma. It involves medial dissection and potential denervation of the deltoid if performed through a deltoid-splitting approach. It also theoretically changes the long head from a static head depressor to an active head elevator. (Modified from Crenshaw AH, Kilgore WE. Surgical treatment of bicipital tenosynovitis. *J Bone Joint Surg.* 1966;45:1496-1502.)

asymptomatic, and the patients experienced no recurrence of their symptoms.

In 1966 Crenshaw and Kilgore[43] reported on their experience using the Hitchcock technique in 65 cases, the DePalma technique in five cases, and the Lippmann technique in three cases. Relief of moderate-to-severe pain was good in 90% of the patients, but 2% continued to complain of "mild, nagging pain." In their series restoration of motion was often disappointing, with patients having only 85% of their normal motion at follow-up. Interestingly, half of the patients who had good preoperative motion actually lost motion after the Hitchcock procedure. It has to be wondered what the addition of an acromioplasty would have done to these results.

Keyhole tenodesis (Fig. 17-44) of the biceps was originally described in 1974 by Froimson and Oh[69] for the treatment of rupture, instability, and tendinitis of the biceps. They reported on 12 shoulders in 11 patients with an average follow-up of 24 months. The results were satisfactory in all their patients, but those with tenosynovitis enjoyed less than excellent results because of associated pericapsulitis. The authors cited several advantages of keyhole tenodesis: the procedure avoids hardware and undue medial dissection; it removes the remnant of the biceps tendon, thereby allowing motion of the humeral head and avoiding intra-articular derangement; and the inherent stability of the method engenders confidence to begin the early, gentle range of motion of both the shoulder and elbow. Humeral fractures have been reported without keyhole tenodesis.[260]

Dines and colleagues[53] in 1982 reviewed 17 patients treated with keyhole tenodesis and 3 treated with tenodesis to the coracoid. (Excision of the coracoacromial ligament was also performed in 14 of their 20 patients.)

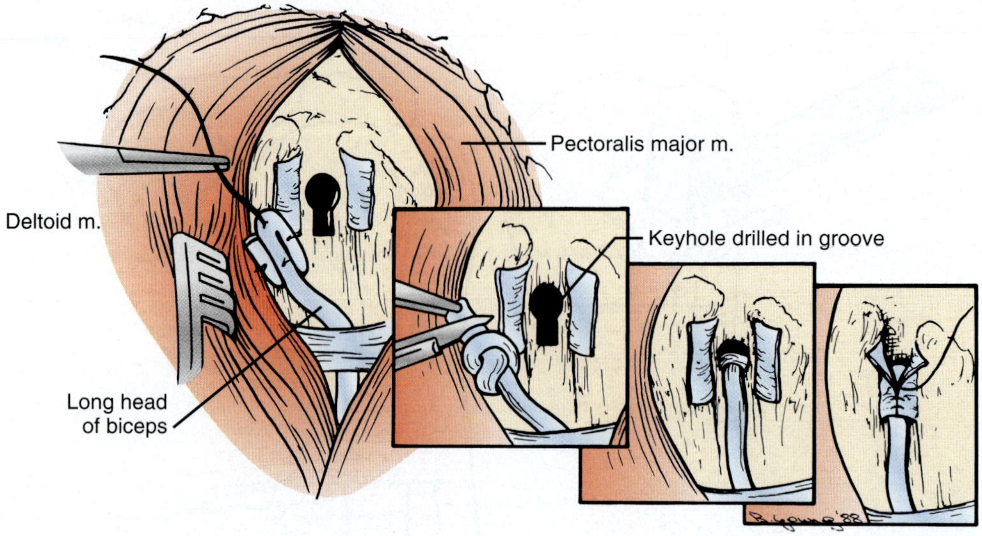

FIGURE 17-44: Keyhole tenodesis as described by Froimson and Oh. The biceps tendon is rolled into a thick ball in the proximal stump and then sutured together into a knot. A keyhole is made in the groove with a dental bur. The tendon is then inserted into the keyhole, and the transverse ligament is repaired over the tendon with nonabsorbable sutures. Post has recommended marking the groove and the tendon with methylene blue before incision of the tendon to determine the normal tension of the tendon postoperatively. (Modified from Froimson AI, Oh I. Keyhole tenodesis of biceps origin at the shoulder. *Clin Orthop.* 1974;112:245-249.)

In their series there was a 30% failure rate (six of 20 patients), and revision surgery was necessary in four of the six patients. Four of the failures occurred in patients with tendinitis, three of whom were found to have an impingement syndrome: one patient had typical anterior impingement, two had coracoid impingement, and the remaining patient was later noted to have glenohumeral instability. The patients who did well in their series were those who were older, averaging 41 years of age. In these patients excision of the coracoacromial ligament was performed as part of the procedure. However, it is their current recommendation that acromioplasty and coracoacromial ligament release be performed. The most salient recommendation and lesson from this review is that at the time of surgery, if biceps tenodesis is planned, the subacromial space and the interrelationship of the coracoacromial arch and the tendon must be assessed. In addition, careful preoperative evaluation and examination under anesthesia will reveal concomitant anterior instability. It was their impression that isolated inflammation of the long head of the biceps was an infrequent finding unless injury to the biceps tendon in the groove had occurred. They also believed that whether a subluxating biceps tendons actually occurred was still questionable. They concluded, "The role of the biceps tendon in the production of shoulder pain is difficult to assess and easily overestimated. Biceps tendon inflammation may be a secondary manifestation of an impingement syndrome. Unless treated, surgery for impingement syndrome will not be successful."

O'Donoghue[174] looked at athletes with biceps instability treated surgically with the Hitchcock procedure. At follow-up, 71% reported excellent progress, 77% said they could throw satisfactorily, and 77% had resumed their sport. The author concluded that in a young, motivated athlete for whom throwing is important, this procedure is a worthwhile operation.

Most of the early studies showed good results of biceps tenodesis but had very scant and very short follow-up. Cofield and Becker[35] reviewed the long-term results of 51 patients (54 shoulders) treated with isolated biceps tenodesis. They found that at 6 months, 94% of patients had benefited from the procedure; however, this number fell to 52% at an average of 7 years. Thirty-three percent continued to have moderate to severe pain, and 15% underwent subsequent surgery (primarily cuff repairs and acromioplasty). In another long-term study Berlemann and Bayley[13] obtained approximately 70% good and excellent results without deterioration in the longer term.

In 1987 Post[194] presented 21 patients with primary tendinitis of the long head of the biceps. He excluded patients with any associated impingement syndrome, rotator cuff pathology, recurrent anterior shoulder instability, or repeated biceps tendon subluxation. All patients in his series had marked tenderness over the long head of the biceps, a negative impingement sign, and little or no relief of pain with subacromial injection; 50% showed a positive Yergason sign. In this series, 17 patients underwent keyhole biceps tenodesis and four had transfer of the tendon to the coracoid process. In the Transfer group, two excellent and two good results were achieved. One patient required manipulation under anesthesia. Of 17 patients who underwent a keyhole tenodesis, 13 results were excellent, two were good, and one failed. Two patients in this group required manipulation. In the single patient whose surgery was considered a failure, symptoms and findings of impingement syndrome developed postoperatively and eventually required a partial anterior acromioplasty. In the tenodesis group 88.3% good and excellent results were achieved. On the basis of his experience, it is Post's conviction that primary biceps tendinitis does occur as an isolated entity. Moreover, when it does occur, it is observed in the intertubercular groove alone.

Habermeyer and Walch[91] stated that chronic biceps tendinitis combined with chronic subacromial impingement syndrome was best treated by subacromial decompression. They recommended biceps tenodesis only in patients who are younger than 40 years and who have isolated biceps tendinitis refractory to conservative treatment.

For the subluxating or dislocating bicipital lesions, Habermeyer and Walch recommended two approaches to treatment. The first of these is reconstruction of the rotator interval sling and repair of the subscapularis tendon. In this procedure the extensions of the supraspinatus and subscapularis tendons are formed into a lasso at the entrance of the groove to prevent resubluxation of the biceps tendon. The second approach is a biceps tenodesis (using any of the various previously described techniques) or the Walch tubularization technique (Fig. 17-45). In this technique the widened and damaged tendon is formed and fixed into a tube with a running suture. The groove is then deepened with an impactor, and the tendon is relocated into the groove. The damaged rotator interval, subscapularis tendon, and supraspinatus tendon are then repaired.

Subpectoral biceps tenodesis has emerged as a popular technique to treat biceps lesions, superior labral lesions, and lesions of the biceps-labral complex.[86,88,89,93,134,135,170,198,210] Originally described by Mazzocca,[134] subpectoral biceps tenodesis secures the biceps tendon distal to the bicipital groove through a mini-open incision. A variety of methods can be utilized for fixation of the biceps to the humerus.[134,198,207,210,213]

Biceps pathology is usually associated with other pathologic lesions of the shoulder; this point cannot be overemphasized. Berlemann and Bayley[13] reviewed a series of patients who underwent keyhole biceps tenodesis, and they noted that multiple pathologies were encountered in most shoulders. Walch and colleagues[245] reviewed 445 patients who underwent rotator cuff repair. They found that the incidence of concomitant bicipital instability in these patients was 16%. In 80% of these cases a fibrous fascia extending from the subscapularis to the bicipital groove was present, giving the superficial impression of normal anatomy. Once opened however the subscapular lesions and dislocation of the biceps were apparent. Bicipital subluxations were associated with limited lesions of the subscapularis and supraspinatus tendons. In contrast dislocations were found in conjunction with massive tears of the subscapularis, supraspinatus, and infraspinatus. Clinically, these patients had pseudoparalysis of their arm. According to Walch, dislocation of the biceps tendon over an intact subscapularis tendon was rare. He maintained that opening the rotator interval was an essential part of open rotator cuff repair to avoid missing bicipital subluxation.

Chen and colleagues[30] evaluated 122 complete tears of the rotator cuff treated arthroscopically. At the time of arthroscopy, the biceps tendon was also evaluated and lesions noted. In this retrospective review the authors found 76% of these patients had some lesion of the biceps: 41% had tendinitis, 8% subluxation, 10% dislocation, 12% a partial tear, and 5% a complete tear. Larger tears (>5 cm^2) were associated with advanced lesions.

Zimmerman and colleagues investigated the biomechanical strength of four different forms of biceps tenodesis[260] and found simple techniques, such as anchor fixation or suture to soft tissue alone to be stronger than the more complex keyhole or Hitchcock techniques. The authors found that the tendon was the weakest link in the chain. Doubling the biceps at the time of tenodesis improved the pullout strength of the surgical construct.

Operative Treatment: Arthroscopic

Review

The surgical treatment of superior labral lesions has evolved since the initial description by Andrews and colleagues in 1985.[5] As the recognition and understanding of SLAP lesions improved, surgeons refined their treatment from simple debridement towards anatomic reconstruction. This can be seen in Snyder's initial series on the treatment of SLAP tears. Early in the series, type II lesions were initially treated with debridement of the labral tear and abrasion of the superior glenoid; later, such lesions were treated by repair with absorbable tacks and eventually with a suture anchor reconstruction.[215-217] Many authors have subsequently reported results of the surgical repair of SLAP lesions. With the proliferation of superior labral surgery came a better understanding of the complications that follow this procedure, namely stiffness, persistent pain, incomplete restoration of function, and lower rates of return to previous levels of performance.[239] Recognizing these complications, many authors now advocate primary biceps tenodesis as a superior alternative to SLAP repair.[17,67,88,89,138,139,219,237] Currently, authors are synthesizing the above experience and refining the specific indications for labral repair versus tenodesis in patients with type II SLAP lesions.[199]

The current treatment of biceps tendinitis focuses on arthroscopic tenotomy and tenodesis. The use of arthroscopic biceps tenotomy for the treatment of biceps tendinitis originated with Walch and colleagues as an adjunct procedure during the repair of massive rotator cuff tears.[244] The technique is a simple release of the tendon at its origin on the superior glenoid labrum. The distal end of the tendon is allowed to retract into the bicipital groove. Walch and colleagues reviewed 307 patients with irreparable rotator cuff tears and shoulder pain. The source of their shoulder pain was thought to be the intact LHBT and therefore these patients were treated with an arthroscopic tenotomy of the biceps

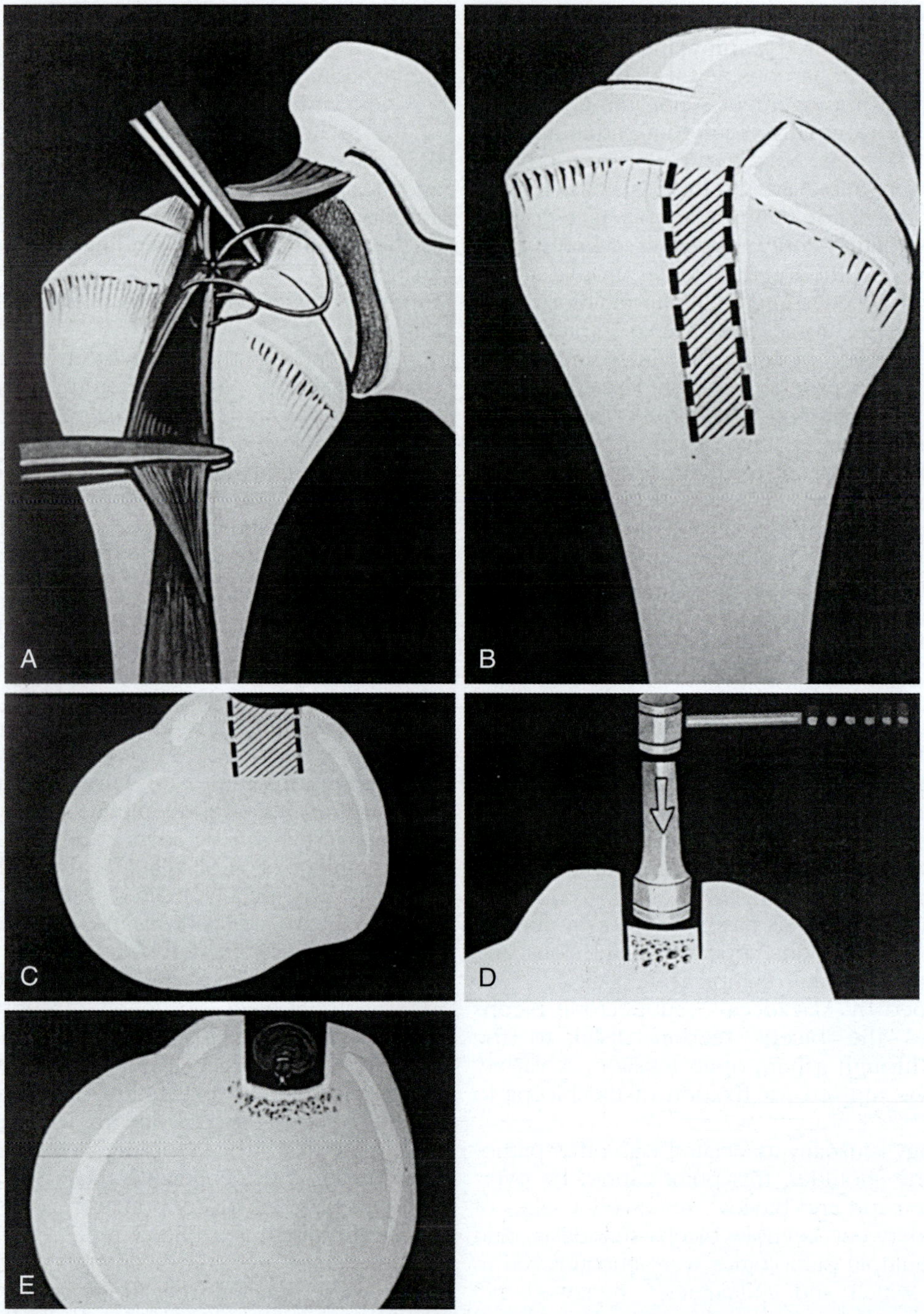

FIGURE 17-45: Walch's tubularization technique for a widened, thinned, long biceps tendon. **A,** Inverting sutures are used to fashion the widened biceps tendon into a tube. **B** to **E,** The bicipital groove is deepened by impaction, and the tubularized tendon is returned to the groove. (From Habermeyer P, Walch G. The biceps tendon and rotator cuff disease. In: Burkhead WZ Jr, ed. *Rotator Cuff Disorders.* Baltimore: Williams & Wilkins; 1996:142-159.)

tendon. At follow-up (at an average of 57 months), mean Constant scores showed improvement (48.4 points preoperatively compared with 67.6 points postoperatively), and 87% of the patients were satisfied or very satisfied. Acromiohumeral distance decreased (mean, 1.3 mm), as would be expected, and glenohumeral arthritis was noted in more patients at follow-up after the procedure (67%) than was noted before the procedure (38%).

Kempf and colleagues, in a multicenter study,[109] found that biceps tenotomy resulted in an improved level of physical activity, improved active mobility, and improved pain. Statistical analysis showed that the benefits of biceps tenotomy were especially evident in patients with a two-tendon rotator cuff tear.

Gill and colleagues[79] showed good results from biceps tenotomy based on American Shoulder and Elbow Surgeons scores. Significant improvements in pain and function were noted after the procedure, and the complication rate was low, at 13%. Two patients developed impingement after the procedure. One patient was not satisfied with the cosmetic result and ultimately received tenodesis. From these results, the authors concluded that tenotomy was a good treatment option. Thomazeau and colleagues[226] also showed good results in their study when bicipital pathology (encountered during the treatment of a rotator cuff tear) was treated with a tenotomy.

Osbahr and colleagues[177] looked retrospectively at the subjective patient self-assessment results after tenotomy versus tenodesis in 80 patients and found no difference in anterior shoulder pain, muscle spasm of the biceps, or cosmetic deformity. In this study the two patient populations were dissimilar: patients younger than 50 years were treated with tenodesis, whereas those older than 50 years were treated with tenotomy. Similarly, Walch and colleagues also used age as a criterion for selecting patients for tenotomy. They described three criteria[246]:

1. Patients were older than 50 years.
2. Patients' humeral head-to-acromion distance had to be less than 7 mm.
3. Tenotomy was not performed if anterosuperior subluxation was present.

Biceps tenotomy therefore is a good treatment option when applied to the appropriate patient.

Arthroscopic bicipital tenodesis has continued to evolve as arthroscopic instrumentation and techniques continue to improve. A multitude of tenodesis techniques, both open and arthroscopic, have been described, including fixation with sutures, screws, and anchors. Whatever the method of fixation, tenodesis of the tendon within the groove has been shown to give good results. Arthroscopic techniques have been advocated to reduce the morbidity associated with shoulder surgery and to speed recovery.

Techniques

The first arthroscopic technique for biceps tenodesis was described by Boileau and colleagues.[16] The arthroscope is positioned in the glenohumeral joint and the biceps tendon is marked with a suture or needle as it enters the groove. The biceps is released from its origin. The arthroscope is moved to the subacromial space, and the previously placed suture or needle is localized. The transverse ligament over the bicipital groove is opened, exposing the underlying tendon. The biceps tendon is delivered out of the groove and through a skin incision directly over the groove. At least 25 mm of tendon is retained to ensure good fixation. A guide pin from an anterior cruciate ligament set is then driven into the humeral head, keeping it parallel to the acromion and tangential to the chest wall, with the arm at approximately 10 degrees of external rotation so that the bicipital groove is facing anterior. The pin is tapped out through the deltoid and skin once it has pierced the posterior cortex of the humerus. An absorbable stitch is placed through the biceps tendon so that the tendon can be pulled into the hole. Using a cannulated drill, an appropriately sized opening is then made in the anterior cortex of the humerus to allow entry of the tendon. Only the anterior cortex is drilled, and the posterior cortex is left intact. The previously placed guide pin is then used to pull the tendon into the bone tunnel. An appropriately sized screw is then placed over a second guide pin placed in the tunnel. The screw is driven into place and the tendon held by an interference fit (Fig. 17-46).

A variation of this technique of biceps tenodesis uses a similar approach, but the use of instruments specifically designed for the procedure obviates the need for a pin passing out of the posterior humerus. This reduces the risk of injury to the axillary nerve, chest wall, and blood vessels (Fig. 17-47A to E).

A second technique uses two suture anchors placed in the groove approximately 1 cm apart to fix the tendon in the groove.[65] A mattress-type suture is used in conjunction with the anchors to secure the biceps in the groove. Advantages of the suture anchor technique are that it involves little risk to the nerves and blood vessels of the arm, and no special instruments are required other than those used to perform arthroscopic rotator cuff repairs. The open variation of this technique is performed by a large number of surgeons and seems to give good results (Fig. 17-48).

Biceps tenodesis can also be performed in situ simply by using sutures to fix the tendon to the capsule. The biceps is inspected with an arthroscope through the posterior portal. A needle is placed through the bicipital tendon distal to the pathology. A suture is passed through the needle and brought out through the anterior portal. A second suture is placed through the biceps in the same manner, and the biceps is cut with scissors. The proximal suture ends are retrieved with a clamp through a tunnel in the subcutaneous tissue. The sutures are tied and the tenodesis is complete. Any remaining biceps anchor is removed and smoothed to a stable base (Fig. 17-49). Lerner and colleagues reviewed the results of 28 patients treated with this tenodesis procedure at 6-year follow-up. They had four failures of tenodesis (14%) diagnosed by a positive Popeye deformity; of these, only one reported cramping with resisted supination. One patient whose tenodesis was successful complained of cramping with resisted elbow flexion.

A number of alternative techniques and variations of biceps tenodesis have been described in the literature. An open subpectoral biceps tenodesis with an interference screw has been described by Mazzocca and colleagues.[136] Paulos has described an arthroscopic wedge tenodesis technique in which the proximal tendon is sutured to itself to prevent it from entering the groove and retracting distally. O'Brien has championed the technique of arthroscopic transfer of the long head of the biceps to the conjoint tendon.[235] The rationale for the

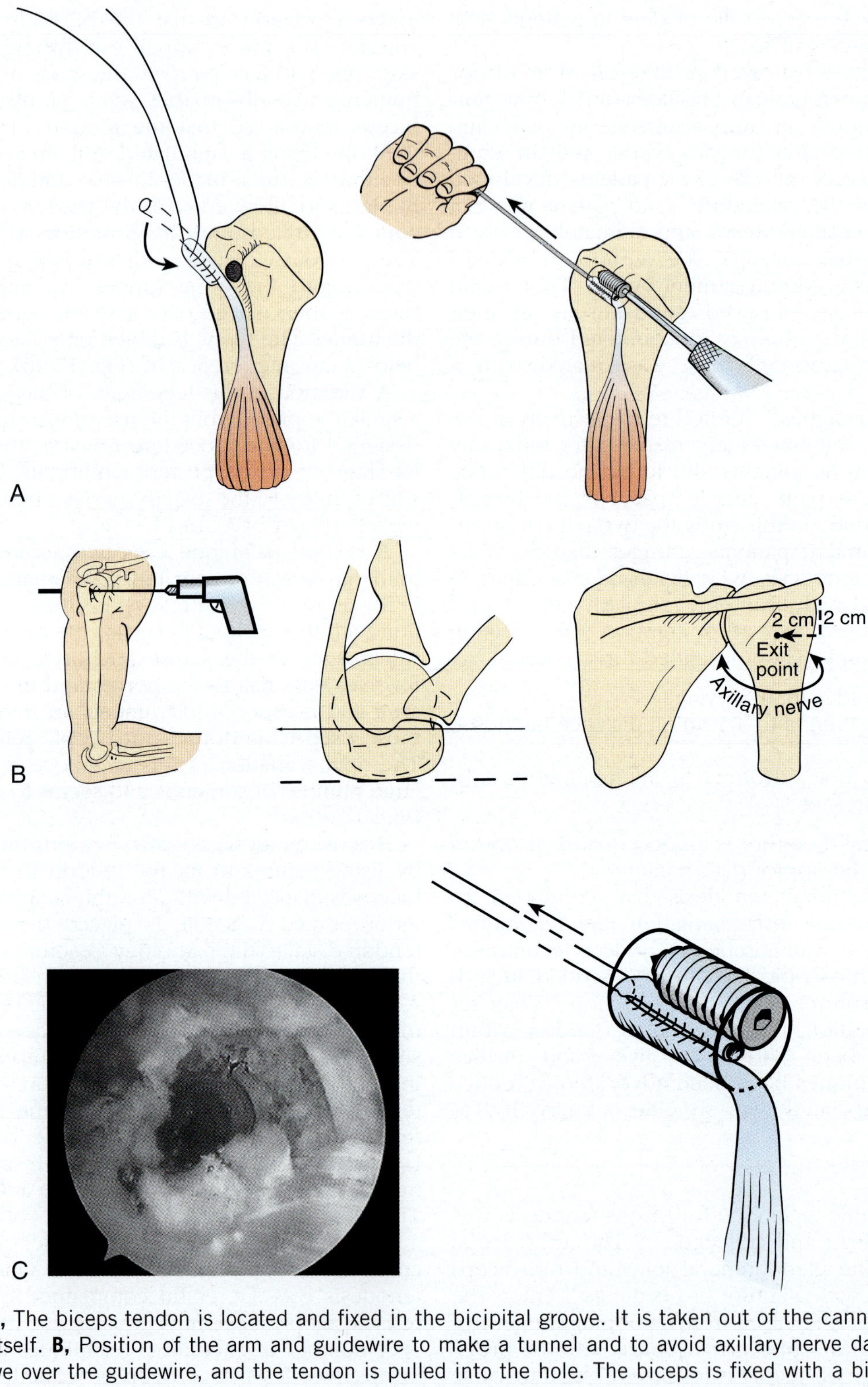

FIGURE 17-46: A, The biceps tendon is located and fixed in the bicipital groove. It is taken out of the cannula to prepare it by doubling it onto itself. **B,** Position of the arm and guidewire to make a tunnel and to avoid axillary nerve damage. **C,** A hole is made in the groove over the guidewire, and the tendon is pulled into the hole. The biceps is fixed with a bioabsorbable screw.

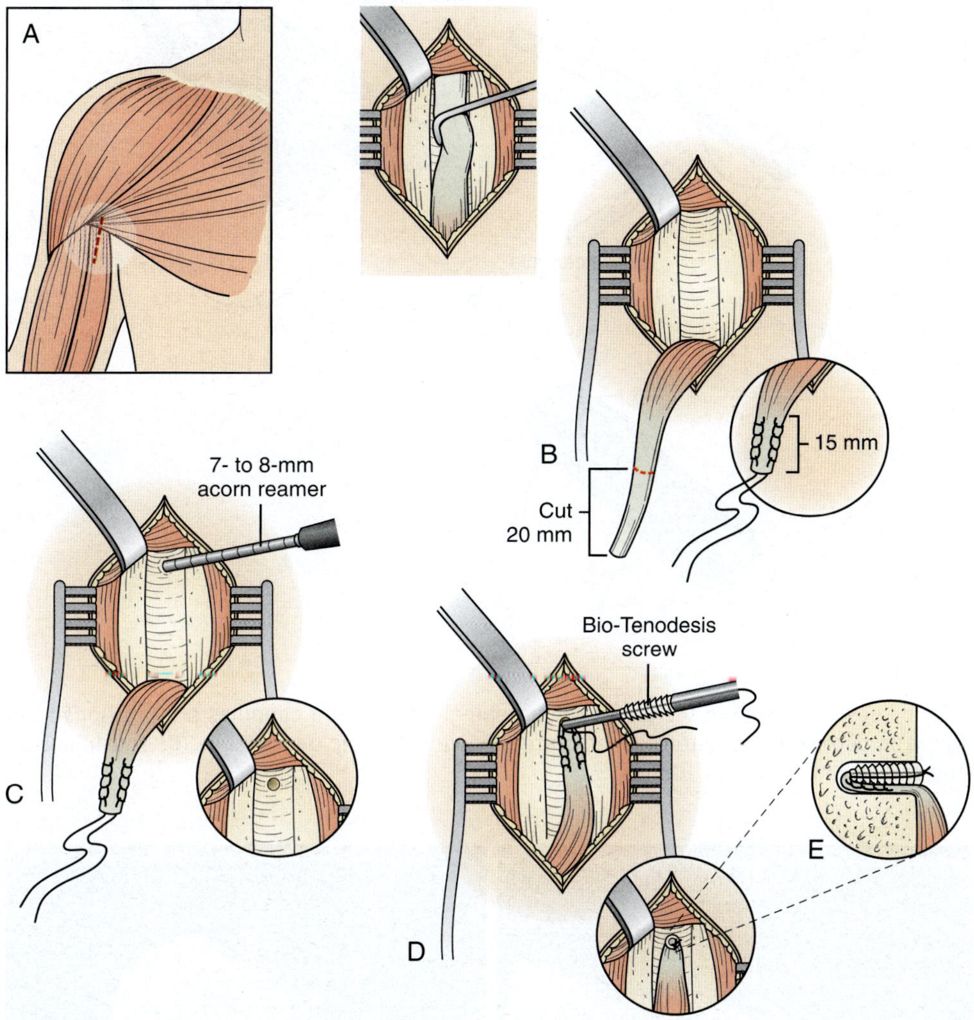

FIGURE 17-47: **A,** The skin incision for the subpectoral open biceps tenodesis is made in the medial third of the arm. It extends 1 cm superior to the inferior border of the pectoralis tendon to 3 cm below this border. This tendon can be palpated by resisted internal rotation with the arm abducted and internally rotated through 10 to 15 degrees. **B,** *Top,* A probe is used to withdraw the tendon from the joint and out of the incision. *Bottom,* To ensure appropriate tensioning, 20 mm of the diseased portion of the tendon is excised. The musculotendinous border of the biceps muscle is directly under the inferior edge of the pectoralis tendon. A Krackow or other type of interrupted tendon or whipstitch is placed in 10 to 15 mm of tendon proximal to the musculotendinous junction. This amount of tendon is placed into the bone tunnel, allowing the musculotendinous junction to rest in its exact anatomic location underneath the inferior border of the pectoralis major tendon. **C,** A guidewire is placed in the center of the bicipital groove. This is usually at the junction of the middle and distal thirds of the intertubercular groove between the lesser and greater tuberosities. A 7- or 8-mm acorn reamer is then placed over this and it is reamed to approximately 25 to 30 mm. **D,** Once the bone debris has been removed from this hole, one suture is placed through the Arthrex Bio-Tenodesis driver and one suture is left out. The driver is then placed with the tendon into the hole so there is a secure fit with the driver in the tendon placed within the bone tunnel. In general, the size of screw used is the size of the reamer (e.g., an 8-mm reamer warrants an 8 × 23 mm Bio-Tenodesis screw). **E,** After the tenodesis driver has inserted the Bio-Tenodesis screw into the bone tunnel, the suture that is left out of the driver is then tied to the suture that is within or passing through the cannulated portion of the tenodesis screw. This allows for both interference and suture anchor fixation. (Modified from Mazzocca AD, Rios CG, Romeo AA, et al. Subpectoral biceps tenodesis with interference screw fixation. *Arthroscopy.* 2005;21[7]:866.e1-896.e7.)

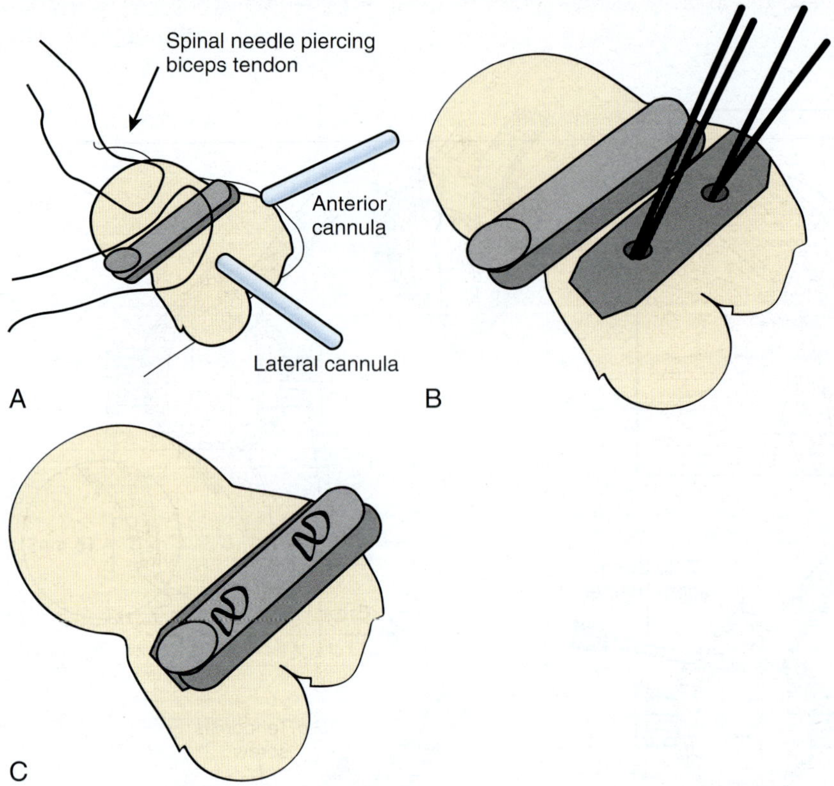

FIGURE 17-48: **A,** The biceps is secured in the groove with a spinal needle, and cannulas are positioned to perform the biceps tenodesis. **B,** The groove is debrided and suture anchors are placed in the bicipital groove. **C,** The final repair with the biceps sutured down into the groove with mattress sutures.

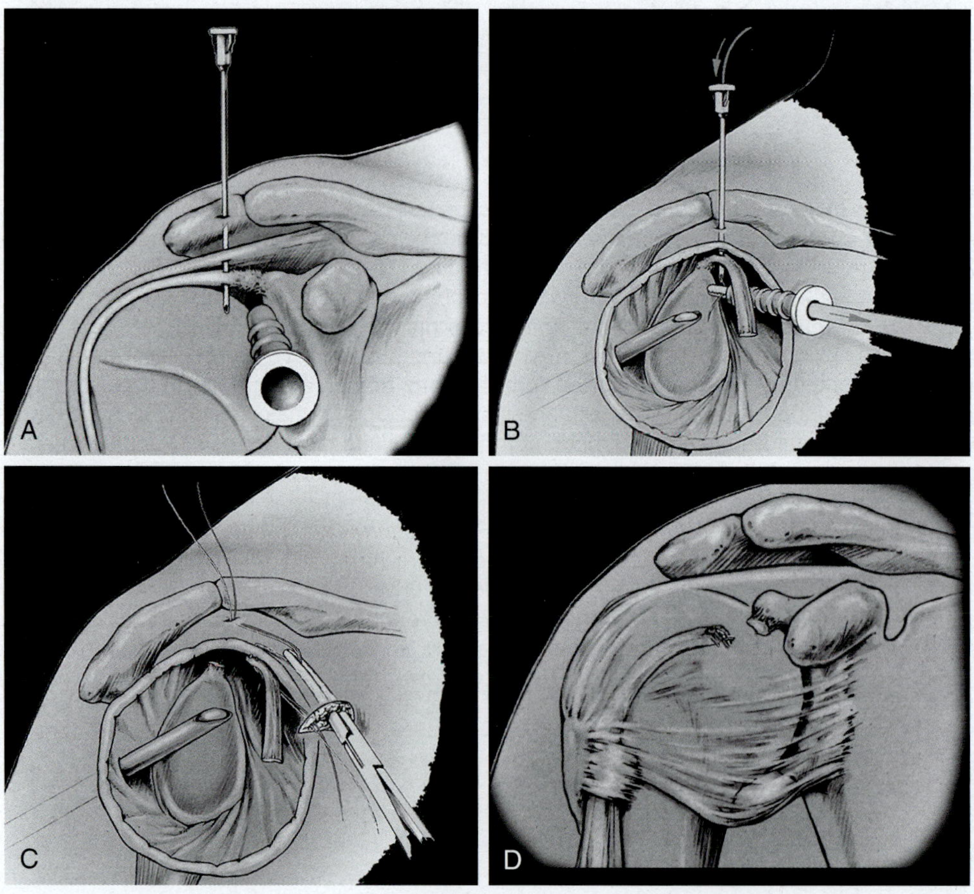

FIGURE 17-49: **A,** From a separate stab hole anterior to the acromion, a needle is placed into the biceps tendon distal to the pathology on the biceps. **B,** A suture is passed into the needle and retrieved from the lateral or anterior portal. A second suture is placed via the same method. **C,** The proximal part of the biceps is resected. The proximal suture limbs are retrieved subcutaneously and tied. **D,** The sutures are cut and the tenodesis is complete. (Courtesy Dr. Peter Habermeyer.)

arthroscopic transfer is that this technique can successfully address extra-articular scarring in the bicipital tunnel that would otherwise lead to the failure of other techniques.[222-225,235]

Operative Treatment: Current Controversies

The treatment of lesions of the biceps and biceps-labral complex has generated significant interest and controversy. A relevant recent debate centered on a suprapectoral versus subpectoral location for patients undergoing biceps tenodesis.[84,107,128,186-188,211,252,253,255] Both techniques have shown comparable clinical, biomechanical, and functional results. Proponents of the suprapectoral technique[19] argue that this technique is less invasive, more efficient, and can accurately restore the length-tension relationship of the biceps muscle. They also reason that the suprapectoral approach avoids the risk to neurovascular structures, namely the musculocutaneous nerve, inherent in the open subpectoral approach. Advocates of the subpectoral approach cite lower rates of postoperative pain as the main reason to perform a subpectoral tenodesis. Pain in the bicipital groove is a recognized complication of suprapectoral tenodesis. However, when the biceps tunnel is decompressed, rates of postoperative pain diminish. The suprapectoral versus subpectoral debate remains unresolved.

Another controversy in the treatment of biceps-labral complex lesions is whether to perform a labral repair or primary biceps tenodesis for type II SLAP tears. Boileau and colleagues[17] proposed biceps tenodesis as an alternative to SLAP repair, citing higher rates of return to play and superior clinical outcomes in patients who underwent biceps tenodesis. Other authors have shown biceps tenodesis to be a useful treatment for failed SLAP repairs.[6,17,88,89,138,139,199,237] Provencher[199] has argued that the answer to the question of whether to perform SLAP repair or tenodesis may be more nuanced, with patients under 35 years of age achieving more acceptable results with SLAP repair, and patients above 35 years of age having higher failure rates. Further research is required to refine the specific indications for repair versus tenodesis.

Authors' Preferred Methods

The treatment of lesions of the biceps tendon and associated pathology must be individualized to the patient. Factors, such as the age of the patient and his or her demands, the quality of the tendon to be tenodesed, and the position at which tenodesis is possible must all be taken into account. Surgeons need therefore to be acquainted with various techniques so that they can match the individual patient with the most appropriate surgery.

Except for young patients with an acute traumatic rupture of the tendon and active patients with an associated massive cuff tear, management should begin with prolonged conservative, nonoperative treatment, during which time the patient should constantly be reevaluated for progress. As long as the patient is improving (however gradually), surgical intervention is not recommended. Surgery is indicated only after a minimum of 6 months of conservative care.

As has been emphasized throughout this chapter, given the high incidence of associated pathology, other lesions should be identified and addressed appropriately and not overlooked. The biceps pathology is then addressed, and usually the decision must be made between tenotomy and tenodesis. In older patients, relatively low demand patients, and patients in whom a Popeye deformity is not a concern, tenotomy is a simple and effective treatment with few postoperative restrictions. In younger patients and high-demand patients, such as heavy laborers or those in whom a Popeye deformity would be unacceptable, tenodesis is considered.

The technique for tenodesis and the requisite strength of the tenodesis can likewise be individualized to the patient. For example, in older, less active patients in whom tenodesis is considered simply for cosmesis rather than for flexion and supination strength, a soft tissue tenodesis may suffice. Alternatively, in a young patient who performs heavy labor and who wishes to return to work as quickly as possible, the tenodesis can be expected to be subjected to high loads and therefore a more rigid fixation with a tenodesis screw may be more appropriate. We review here some common scenarios for biceps pathology along with our preferred treatment.

Superior Labral Tears

A symptomatic superior labral tear resulting from a traumatic injury in a patient younger than 30 years old is an indication for surgery. The labrum is repaired arthroscopically, utilizing knotless suture anchor fixation of the labrum to the glenoid. Horizontal mattress stitches are placed to minimize suture abrasion of the glenohumeral joint.

For symptomatic superior labral tears in patients over 40 years old, our preferred technique is a primary biceps tenodesis. If the patient has additional symptoms localized to the bicipital groove, we perform a subpectoral tenodesis to minimize the risk of postoperative groove pain.

For symptomatic superior labral tears in patients between 30 and 40 years old, we discuss the pros and cons of profile of both SLAP repair and primary tenodesis and allow the patient to decide which procedure they would prefer.

Impingement Tendinitis

When biceps tendinitis is associated with coracoacromial arch impingement (enthesopathy) we recommend that treatment of the impingement be performed as outlined by Neer in his original and follow-up articles. This can be performed arthroscopically or open and is discussed in depth in Chapter 14.

After the impingement is addressed, the long head of the biceps is tenodesed into the groove with screw-type anchors and permanent sutures. The proximal end is sutured into the rotator interval. Alternatively, if there is significant tendinosis and the tissue quality is poor, the tendon can be doubled back on itself to strengthen the construct.

Post and colleagues[195] recommended marking the exposed biceps tendon in its native position in the groove before releasing the biceps tendon. By doing so, the relative position and tension of the muscle can be reapproximated. We simply tension the repair such that the arm can be fully extended without placing undue pressure on the surgical construct.

In cases where the impingement has been treated arthroscopically, it is our preference also to perform the biceps tenodesis arthroscopically. This obviates the need for a takedown of the deltoid and avoids violating the rotator interval. In arthroscopic tenodesis the marking suture or a needle is passed through the tendon at the entrance of the groove, often at the level of the cuff insertion. Marking the tendon in this way provides us with a reference point for fixation, much like Post's methylene blue technique. After the biceps is released proximally, the tendon has a tendency to retract and become distally located in the groove. Driving a spinal needle into the bone can prevent retraction of the biceps after release. The tendon is then delivered into the cannula, and we the suture can be used to measure the distance between the tendon, the point where the tendon should be fixed, and the position of the bone tunnel. If the point of fixation is 1 cm distal to the suture, the tunnel must be 1 cm distal to the entry point of the bicipital groove. When the biceps tendon is held in position by a needle, the biceps can be fixed in situ because it did not retract when the release was performed.

Type III impingement by definition includes a full-thickness tear of the rotator cuff. Patients with type III impingement generally have severe spurring in the anterior acromion and distal clavicle. Often, if the anterior cuff is involved, subluxation, hypertrophy, degenerative changes, or frank rupture of the biceps tendon may be present. In these patients a formal open anterior acromioplasty and cuff repair are performed with reconstruction of the rotator cuff.

If the biceps is dislocated but otherwise completely normal, it is replaced in the groove, and after the supraspinatus is sutured the rotator interval is closed. In doing this the edges of the subscapularis and the coracohumeral ligament complex are sutured to the repaired supraspinatus to recreate the stabilizing effect at the aperture of the tuberosities (Fig. 17-50). Alternatively, if any attritional wear is noted we perform a tenodesis or tenotomy.

In cases of chronic ruptures (those lasting longer than 6 weeks) there is seldom an attempt to repair the tendon. Patients are warned preoperatively that they will continue to have a bulge in the lower portion of the brachium. The intra-articular stump is removed to prevent possible impingement in the joint.

When arthroscopic repair is used to treat full-thickness defects in the rotator cuff, the aforementioned techniques for bicipital tenodesis can be used. We are very careful to avoid destabilizing the coracoacromial arch when decompressing the subacromial space. Even when using arthroscopic techniques we must remain vigilant of the superior stabilization afforded by an intact LHBT. The larger the rotator cuff tear, the more likely we are to preserve the biceps.

Biceps Instability

In our experience, surgically proven biceps instability is always related to a degenerative cuff, restraining capsule, and coracohumeral ligament in the proximal portion of the groove. As with impingement tendinitis, primary attention should be given to repair of the rotator cuff and to careful decompression of the coracoacromial arch. It is well established that the main stabilizer of the biceps tendon is the musculotendinous cuff and the

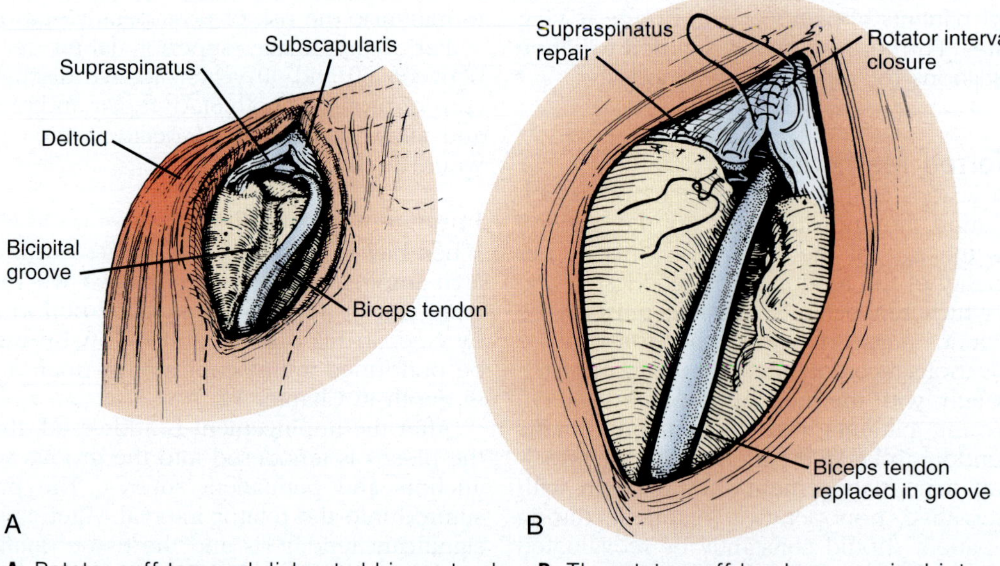

FIGURE 17-50: A, Rotator cuff tear and dislocated biceps tendon. **B,** The rotator cuff has been repaired into a bony trough and the rotator interval closed with the tendon replaced in the groove.

coracohumeral ligament. These structures can be injured acutely or by the mechanisms previously described, and fixed or recurrent subluxation of the biceps tendon can occur. If the injury is acute and the patient is younger than 65 years, an MRI is recommended to help with diagnosis and to evaluate the status of the rotator cuff. If the biceps is dislocated, we recommend early open reduction of the tendon with reconstruction of the fibrous roof, supraspinatus, and subscapularis, combined with an acromioplasty if indicated.

Once the diagnosis of a dislocated biceps tendon is made, a rotator cuff tear is also diagnosed. Whereas in patients older than 65 years this injury can be accepted and treated nonoperatively, patients younger than 50 years will fare better if the tendon is relocated and the fibrous roof reconstructed. Alternatively, if significant tenderness is present, biceps tenodesis can be performed. Because older patients tend to be more active now than in the past, chronologic age is not an absolute guide for treatment. Active older patients with a dislocated biceps tendon can also benefit from relocation and stabilization of the tendon and rotator cuff repair. We continue to treat biceps instability nonoperatively, if possible, in less active older patients.

Isolated Biceps Lesions

Patients with isolated biceps lesions generally respond to rest, nonsteroidal antiinflammatory medications, moist heat, and gentle, patient-directed exercises. The judicious use of corticosteroids by injection can also be helpful. The injection should be within the bicipital sheath; it should require only minimal pressure and a low volume (2 to 3 mL of lidocaine and 1 mL of water-soluble steroid). The injection technique is described under "Differential Diagnosis."

Numerous case reports have described tendon ruptures related to corticosteroid injections. Such ruptures have been described in the patellar tendon, the Achilles tendon, the flexor and extensor tendons of the hand, and the LHBT. Although some tendons (especially in older patients with systemic disease or attrition tendinitis) spontaneously rupture as a result of their disease process, there is a strong indication that injection within the tendon contributes to tendon degradation. Kennedy and Willis[110] showed collagen necrosis as well as disorganization and loss of the normal parallel collagen arrangement in Achilles tendons injected with corticosteroids. In addition, they noted a 35% loss of failure strength at approximately 48 hours after injection. The failure strength of the tendon returns at approximately 2 weeks; however, ultrastructural changes in the tendon persist for up to 6 weeks. Consequently, patients are asked to avoid any strenuous activity for at least 3 weeks. We typically perform steroid injections at intervals of at least 6 weeks and then only two or, rarely, three times. Injections have been shown to be more efficacious than placebo or naproxen (Naprosyn) in the treatment of chronic shoulder pain and shown to be equivalent to the use of indomethacin (Indocin).[231,232] Unfortunately, some patients cannot tolerate nonsteroidal antiinflammatory agents in the doses required, and steroid injections are a beneficial alternative.

If the patient fails to respond to nonoperative care over a 6- to 12-month period, surgery is recommended. Because the results of isolated biceps tenodesis have not been spectacular in the long term and impingement syndrome has developed after biceps tenodesis, subacromial decompression is routinely performed.

Isolated Biceps Rupture in Patients Younger Than 50 Years

In younger, active patients, particularly those involved in overhead sports, weightlifting, or jobs that require forceful supination, a sudden overload can result in an isolated biceps rupture. The rupture may be within the muscle-tendon junction rather than the long head tendon. Physical examination and ultrasonography of the biceps should enable isolation of the point of rupture. At the same time, sonography or MRI should be used to evaluate the rotator cuff. Early repair is recommended for these patients, who typically have high functional expectations. If the rupture is musculotendinous, early repair is performed using a Bunnell-type weave suture through a deltopectoral incision. This is the only group of patients in whom use of the deltopectoral approach is recommended.

Acute Biceps Rupture in Patients Older Than 50 Years

If the patient is relatively inactive, a graduated leave-alone method protocol of treatment is recommended. This involves rest, antiinflammatory medications, and moist heat. The patient is also instructed in how to maintain motion through passive-motion exercises. For patients who are physically active, an early aggressive diagnostic work-up should be performed. Such a work-up usually consists of an MRI, but arthrography or sonography can also be performed.

It is usual to find a so-called acute cuff tear in addition to the biceps tendon rupture. This acute cuff tear may in reality be an acute extension of a chronic tear or simply a chronic, asymptomatic tear that suddenly became symptomatic. The two-incision approach in these cases is used if the rupture is less than 6 weeks old (Fig. 17-51A). If there is a tear in the rotator cuff, anterior acromioplasty, rotator cuff repair, and biceps tenodesis are performed. The biceps tendon is exposed through a separate incision in the brachium (see Fig. 17-51B). The subcutaneous tissue is incised and edema and hemorrhage are evacuated. The tendon may be curled up in this area or adhered proximally to the pectoralis insertion. With a suture passer inserted from proximal through the bicipital groove and passed distally into the lower wound, the tendon is advanced into the superior wound (see Fig. 17-51C). A biceps tenodesis in the groove is then performed.

Postoperative Care

Unless there is some tension on the cuff repair with the arm at the side, a Velcro elastic immobilizer is used postoperatively for 3 weeks. On the night of the surgery, the

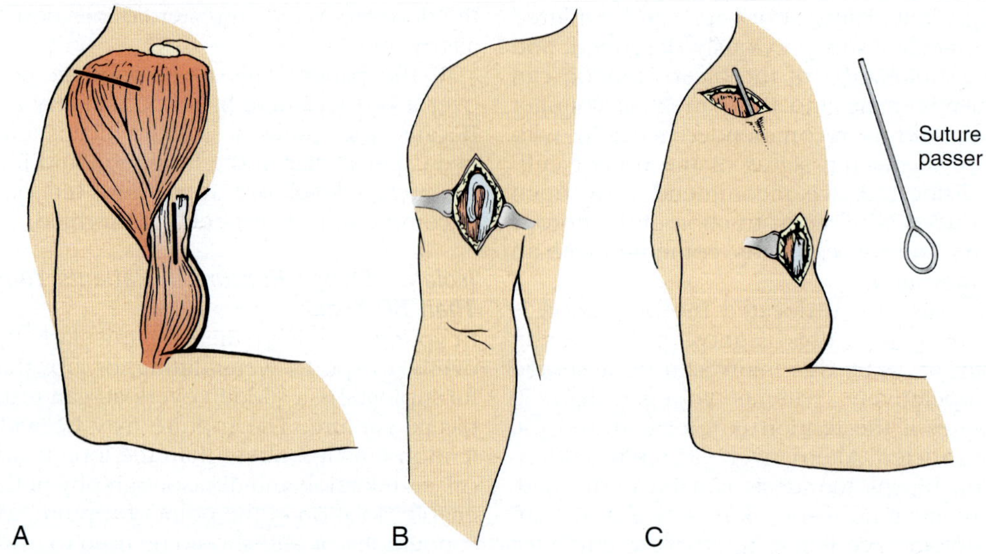

FIGURE 17-51: A, Two-incision approach to bicipital tendon rupture. The proximal incision is exactly the same as used for an anterior acromioplasty. The distal incision allows pick up of the tendon of the biceps in the sulcus created by the defect in the biceps. The incision does not have to be long, and only subcutaneous tissue and fascia need to be incised; a suture passer can then be used. **B,** Exposure of the ruptured biceps tendon through the counterincision in the sulcus, magnified in this view. A 3-cm incision is all that is required to pick up the end of the tendon in this region. **C,** A suture passer is used to bring the tendon into the proximal wound for tenodesis or repair.

patient is encouraged to take the elbow out and gently flex and extend it passively with the opposite hand. Gentle pendulum exercises are initiated on the first postoperative day. Passive flexion performed by the patient (with the other arm), nurse, or therapist is begun on the second postoperative day. Because holding onto a pulley handle requires some active contraction of the biceps, we generally instruct a family member in how to administer gentle, passive forward flexion and external rotation. At 1 month, the pulley can safely be used, and gentle, active elbow flexion may begin. Strengthening of the repaired cuff, deltoid, and biceps generally begins at 2 months and becomes more vigorous at 3 months. Patients with jobs that require moderate lifting usually return to work at approximately 6 months.

Failed Biceps Tenodesis or Tenotomy

Rarely, patients are dissatisfied with the cosmetic or functional results from tenotomy or with a tenodesis that has failed. These patients mostly present several months postoperatively, and so reconstruction at the level of the groove cannot be accomplished. In these patients the biceps can be restored to its resting length by imbrication of the tendon combined with tenodesis to the humeral shaft at whichever level is possible.

If the tendon itself is available and capable of holding suture, a Mitek Super Anchor, which works well in cortical bone with an attached 1-mm Cottony Dacron suture, can be used to fix the imbricated tendon to the roughened humeral cortex at the brachialis origin. If only the musculotendinous junction remains, the broad tissue in this area can be advanced on the humeral shaft and fixed to the roughened humeral shaft with a cortical screw and a soft tissue washer of the surgeon's preference.

The elbow must be kept flexed for 3 weeks, and full elbow extension is discouraged for 6 weeks. In a small group of patients treated by one of the authors (W.B.Z.), this method has been successful in eliminating cramping in the biceps and producing satisfactory cosmesis.

SUMMARY

Inflammation and degeneration of the LHBT often accompany rotator cuff pathology. The LHBT's close anatomic relationship to the coracoacromial arch makes it uniquely susceptible to secondary injury and inflammation.

Biomechanically, the LHBT in normal shoulders seems to contribute little to shoulder stability. However, in the presence of a rotator cuff tear, in vitro studies suggest an increased role of the biceps as a humeral head depressor. Accordingly, routine tenodesis of the biceps tendon or its use as a free graft in rotator cuff repair is not recommended.

The biceps tendon's primary restraints against dislocation are the coracohumeral ligament, the superior glenohumeral ligament, and the rotator cuff proximal to the groove. Because of its intimate relationship to the coracoacromial arch, whenever a diagnosis of biceps pathology is under consideration, rotator cuff pathology should also be considered. When possible, subluxation of the biceps can be treated by replacement of the tendon into the groove and reconstruction of the rotator cuff combined with subacromial decompression.

Isolated biceps tenodesis or tenotomy is not recommended except for treatment of a massive cuff tear. The addition of anterior acromioplasty with excision of the coracoacromial ligament adds little morbidity in patients with an intact cuff and improves clinical results. It cannot be overemphasized that isolated biceps tendon pathology is a diagnosis of exclusion. Recognizing associated pathology and addressing it appropriately are the keys to successful treatment.

Finally, a note of caution is in order. Although biceps tenotomy has gained popularity, patients must be prepared to live with the attendant deformity, and some experience significant pain for several months at the site of tendon relocation. Others complain of chronic pain, fatigue, and cramping if their activities of daily living require repetitive forceful supination. Careful informed consent and patient selection are necessary to avoid medicolegal entanglements.

Acknowledgements

Dr. Burkhead wishes to recognize past contributors to this chapter: Michele Arcand, Peter Habermeyer, Kenneth Lin, and Gilles Walch.

INTERNATIONAL EXPERT COMMENTARY

Thomas Lawrence

It is a great pleasure to provide commentary on this excellent and very thorough chapter on proximal biceps tendon problems.

The anatomy, function, and pathologic process of the LHBT are well detailed in the initial half of the chapter. As the authors have demonstrated, the exact function of the LHBT in glenohumeral biomechanics is not clearly understood despite extensive research. It is, however, well recognized that the LHBT is a pain generator that deserves the attention of any surgeon managing shoulder problems. Thus the LHBT should be considered as a potential source of pain in all patients ranging from the young elite throwing athlete through to the elderly person with a massive rotator cuff tear.

This commentary serves to compare and contrast my approach to problems related to the LHBT to those presented by the authors in the chapter.

Patient Evaluation

The authors highlight the importance of history and examination to help determine the contribution of the biceps to shoulder pain. Patient age, speed of onset, and duration of symptoms as well as the possibility of a precipitating injury should be ascertained. The young athlete with pain only on throwing or heavy use raises the suspicion of a SLAP tear. This contrasts with an elderly individual with a degenerate biceps tendon related to concomitant pathology, such as chronic impingement and rotator cuff tears.

Inspection may reveal the loss of biceps muscle contour following LHBT rupture. This is particularly important in the young, physically active patient, where acute tenodesis may be indicated to restore the normal biceps length-tension relationship. Palpation can help distinguish the location of pain, which is typically felt more anteriorly in the shoulder over the bicipital groove with the arm in internal 10-degree rotation. However, lesions more proximal to the groove may not reveal tenderness. There are numerous biceps-specific shoulder tests that have been well described in the chapter. Of those documented, I find O'Brien's active compression test and O'Driscoll's dynamic labral shear test the most useful for SLAP pathology. However, where there is coexisting pathology involving the subacromial space, acromioclavicular joint, and rotator cuff, other tests have poor specificity and are not conclusive for biceps pathology. It is crucial therefore to formally assess cuff integrity, including of the subscapularis that is intimately related to the LHBT. Occasionally in my practice, to help differentiate the source of pain, patients are referred for local anesthetic injections, with or without steroid, around the biceps in the groove, using ultrasound guidance.

Imaging modalities of the proximal biceps, including the pros and cons of MRI versus ultrasound, are well discussed in the chapter. I am in agreement that while ultrasound scan is useful to assess for tendinopathy, partial tears, and subluxation, this modality is user dependent and does not visualize the intra-articular portion or the superior labrum. For this reason, in the younger, more active patient where more subtle lesions may be present, MRI provides distinct advantages. Furthermore, if there is any clinical concern about SLAP pathology then MRI enhanced with a gadolinium arthrogram is my investigation of choice.

Treatment Options and Selection

I concur with the authors that initially conservative management is preferred for isolated biceps lesions. This includes activity modification, rest, nonsteroidal antiinflammatory drugs, physical therapy, and occasionally steroid injections. The most common indications for surgery are partial tearing, instability, tenosynovitis, and SLAP tears. Where a trial of nonoperative treatment has failed, there are several surgical treatment options, including SLAP repair, tenotomy, and tenodesis. The authors have discussed the current controversies surrounding these options and comment that treatment is individualized to each patient depending on age, activity levels, and operative findings.

Tenotomy

Arthroscopic biceps tenotomy is a quick and easy procedure that simplifies postoperative rehabilitation and allows patients to return to activity as soon as possible. Many authors have reported high satisfaction rates with little or no loss of strength.[56] However, patients should be made aware of the potential for persisting cosmetic deformity, fatigue, and cramping.[108] For these reasons, I agree with the authors that tenotomy should be reserved for the lower-demand/older age group in the setting of associated impingement and cuff tears.

Tenodesis

As a result of the disadvantages associated with tenotomy, some surgeons advocate biceps tenodesis that aims to restore

Continued

INTERNATIONAL EXPERT COMMENTARY—cont'd

the normal length-tension relationship of the biceps anatomy. In doing so tenodesis may result in a better ability to return to full activity and a decreased rate of cosmetic deformities and cramping pain.[74] As the authors have discussed, this is particularly important in the younger, more active patient with higher demands. Tenodesis is also typically the preferred surgical option in the management of failed SLAP repair.[254]

Repair of SLAP Tears

Although the pathology and surgical treatment of SLAP lesions are not the main remit of the chapter, they are worthy of brief discussion as such problems may only be identified at arthroscopy and a high index of suspicion is required. There is continued debate over how to manage SLAP tears, due to the reported failure rates of arthroscopic repairs.[61] This has led to some authors recommending tenodesis as a primary treatment in certain patient groups. It is my preference, similar to that of the authors, to perform a SLAP repair over tenodesis in the younger age group. This is particularly the case for those who have sustained a traumatic (rather than degenerative) lesion of the superior labrum or for high-level athletes involved in overhead sports. Although being above 35 to 40 years is frequently quoted as a cutoff for SLAP repair,[63] I personally make a case-by-case decision depending on intraoperative findings, including labral tissue quality, reparability, and associated damage to the biceps tendon itself. The presence of any adverse features would influence me away from SLAP repair and toward tenodesis. Careful informed discussion and consent preoperatively with patients is essential in the decision-making process.

Technique Used for Surgery

As discussed, the decision to proceed with SLAP repair, tenotomy, or tenodesis depends on patient factors and operative findings. The surgeon must careful inspect the intra-articular portion of the tendon, looking specifically for partial tearing, inflammatory changes, and hourglass deformity. The use of a probe through an anterior portal to deliver more of the tendon into the joint allows for a more complete assessment as well as for instability around the pulley. The attachment of the superior labrum on the glenoid is carefully inspected, and finally the rotator cuff is assessed for associated tears. Normal anatomic variants of the superior labral attachment must be differentiated from the pathologic process.

SLAP Repair

A detailed description of the technique is beyond the remit of this commentary. In brief, I prefer a knotted ("all suture") anchor fixation technique ahead of the knotless systems. A percutaneous portal of Wilmington is utilized to give the optimal trajectory for anchor drilling and placement. A shuttling technique is used to pass the suture through the labral tissue in a simple suture configuration. For a typical SLAP tear, two anchors placed behind the biceps tendon are used. I ensure that the knots are tied over the superior-medial side of the labrum to minimize knot related abrasion on the cuff.

Arthroscopic Tenotomy

The LHBT is divided from the superior labrum using a punch or radiofrequency device from the anterior interval portal. If the tendon fails to retract outside of the joint, a segment can be removed. Additional pathology, such as impingement or cuff tears, can then be addressed.

Tenodesis

As the authors have commented, the location and technique of tenodesis continues to be hotly debated. Broadly, this is categorized into proximal (in the groove) and subpectoral (below the groove) tenodesis. The authors have experience in and preference of arthroscopic tenodesis in the groove. However, in some series revision rates for chronic pain are high after arthroscopic proximal tenodesis,[128] and therefore I prefer the mini-open subpectoral tenodesis popularized by Mazzocca.

Arthroscopic tenotomy is performed initially as described above. Subpectoral tenodesis utilizes a small cosmetic axillary incision in line with the inferior aspect of the pectoralis major. The intermuscular plane between the short head of biceps and pectoralis major is developed to locate the LHBT, which is gently pulled out from the shoulder. Anatomic studies have demonstrated the musculotendinous junction to be around 3 cm above the inferior border of the pectoralis major[105] and have shown that tenodesis at this level offers a safe window to minimize nerve injury.[54,211] To optimize the length-tension relationship of the biceps, I start the whipstitch suture at the musculotendinous junction for a distance of 2.5 cm, remove the residual biceps, and drill the hole for the tendon 2 to 3 cm above the inferior border of the pectoralis major. The common fixation methods are the interference screw and cortical button that offer comparable strength.[21] I personally prefer the use of the button using a "tension slide technique," which allows for the use of a slightly smaller drill hole that may lessen the risk of fracture.[209] Furthermore, the intraosseous placement of the tendon optimizes the surface area for tendon to bone healing. Ultimately, surgeons should employ the technique they are most comfortable using.

Approach to Postsurgical Rehabilitation

Postoperative care and rehabilitation depends entirely upon the surgical procedure that has been performed as well as upon any additional procedures, such as rotator cuff repair. A detailed description of rehabilitation protocols is beyond the scope of this commentary.

In brief, for patients that have undergone simple tenotomy of the biceps, no specific restrictions are applied unless concomitant rotator cuff repair has been performed. Patients are advised to use the elbow to the extent pain allows but to avoid heavy lifting during the initial few months to minimize associated cramping.

For patients that have had subpectoral tenodesis, a sling is worn to protect the repair for 4 weeks. During this time, the shoulder and elbow can be mobilized gently as pain allows. A weight restriction of 5 lb is applied for the initial 6 weeks, after which gradual strengthening can be commenced. Heavy lifting should be avoided for at least 3 months after the surgery.

EDITOR COMMENTARY

John W. Sperling

The authors have succeeded in bringing together in one chapter a comprehensive review of the biceps tendon. There is perhaps no area in shoulder surgery that is more controversial than the evaluation and management of the biceps. Significant controversy still exists on whether the biceps should be addressed routinely in shoulder surgery and if it is addressed, which surgical technique should be used. The authors have provided great insight that helps the reader determine whether the biceps is the cause of pain in an individual patient or whether other structures are the source of the discomfort.

One of the unique aspects of this chapter is the historical overview. It provides a perspective and reference not equally available elsewhere. It becomes clear when reading the history of the biceps tendon that many surgeons in the past have sought an ideal solution for bicipital pain; however, there is still no consensus on the preferred treatment options.

It is my experience that determining whether the biceps is a source of pain is difficult. In addition, some procedures that have been designed to alleviate the biceps as a cause of pain can result in continued disability and pain. Although I have a less-aggressive view on the treatment of the biceps tendon compared with most shoulder surgeons, the authors have clearly outlined a very well thought out approach to treating this potential pain generator. The authors should be congratulated for a fantastic addition to this book.

CHAPTER 18

Nerve Problems Related to the Shoulder

Scott P. Steinmann, Bassem T. Elhassan

Patients with shoulder pain or injuries not infrequently have concomitant neurologic conditions, and orthopedic surgeons caring for such patients must be aware of them. In addition, the practice of reconstructive shoulder surgery carries an inherent risk of iatrogenic injury to neighboring neurologic structures. Knowledge of the common nerve lesions about the shoulder allows surgeons to recognize these entities when they see them, and familiarity with the relevant neural anatomy will help surgeons avoid potential neural injuries when they operate. Surgeons must adopt a systematic approach to the challenges of evaluating and treating patients with nerve-related disorders about the shoulder region.

CLINICAL EVALUATION

Patients with nerve injuries are often seen in situations involving significant trauma. Commonly, the patient is confused, incoherent, sedated, or even unconscious, and it can be difficult to perform a satisfactory neurologic examination before initiating surgical care. Nonetheless, a good neurologic examination should be attempted in the emergency department. If for any reason an adequate examination cannot be performed, this should be noted in the patient's medical record. Specifically, if the function of a particular nerve cannot be properly assessed preoperatively, the record should include such information. Too often in the emergency setting, the patient receives only a cursory evaluation, and perhaps the most junior person on the orthopedic surgical team writes in the clinical record that the extremity was "neurovascularly intact." These two words, if inaccurate, are sometimes the origin of unnecessary litigation. Such general terms should not be used when recording a patient's examination; instead, individual muscle strength, sensory examination, and deep tendon reflexes should be carefully documented in the patient's record.

A detailed neurologic evaluation of the upper extremity can be performed on a coherent patient in a relatively short time, even if the patient has a shoulder dislocation or proximal humeral fracture. It is often easiest to start at the hand and progress proximally during the examination. Radial, median, and ulnar nerve function can all be assessed by a thorough evaluation of the hand and wrist, which should take less than 1 minute. Elbow flexion and extension strength are relatively simple to determine. The examiner should be aware, however, that it is possible to flex the elbow strongly with the action of the brachioradialis without having any function of the biceps. Loss of motor or sensory function in the distal end of the extremity can help direct examination of the more proximal musculature. For example, loss of radial nerve function should make the examiner look closely at axillary nerve function because both nerves are derived from the posterior cord. Likewise, loss of median nerve function might also affect the musculocutaneous nerve if the lesion is in the lateral cord.

Progressing up the arm, the condition of the medial and lateral pectoral nerves can be assessed by individually testing the strength of each of the major portions of the pectoralis major. The deltoid and rotator cuff muscles are then examined. The deltoid can be assessed even in the case of a painful proximal humeral fracture or glenohumeral dislocation. With the arm at the side, the patient is instructed to push out or "elbow" the examiner's hand (which is placed at the lateral aspect of the elbow, with the other hand over the deltoid region to feel for contracture). If the patient is in a great deal of pain and the examiner cannot adequately determine the condition of the axillary nerve, this information should be recorded in the clinical record. Do not assume that it "might be okay."

Examining shoulder abduction is an important part of the examination both to record muscle strength and to visualize shoulder kinesis through the arc of motion. Two important points are relevant here. First, some patients are able to abduct the shoulder through a full arc of motion by using either just the supraspinatus or the deltoid in the face of complete paralysis of either of them. Ensuring muscle contraction is a critical element in this part of the examination. Second, visualizing and palpating the scapula are a necessary part of the examination, especially when there is possible dysfunction. For example, patients with winged scapulae due to weakness of the serratus anterior or trapezius may have difficulty abducting the arm fully without the scapula stabilized and may compensate with trick motions. The examiner should recognize the clinical appearances and know the techniques to examine winging of the scapula, particularly with respect to distinguishing serratus anterior, trapezius, and rhomboid muscle dysfunction. In addition, a useful test for serratus anterior function that can be applied even in a patient with a complete brachial plexus lesion is to stabilize the inferior pole of the scapula while the patient pushes the arm forward; patients unable to perform this test would not be able to perform the more standard push-off test with the arms extended against a wall.

The examiner needs to evaluate the patient for other conditions besides a neurologic etiology that can cause lack of movement. In particular, it should be considered whether the inability of a patient to externally rotate the arm or perform the lift-off test might represent a neurologic lesion affecting the infraspinatus or subscapularis, a rotator cuff tear, or both. A patient who is feigning paralysis in the upper limb for secondary gain issues cannot voluntarily stop the latissimus dorsi from contracting while coughing.

Examination of the shoulder should include examination well above the shoulder and even above the neck, as well as the distal portion of the limb. Proximal and distal lesions should always be considered when examining a patient with shoulder pain or weakness and establishing a differential diagnosis. Cervical radiculopathy is a common cause of pain in the shoulder accompanied by motor weakness and sensory loss in the upper extremity. In this situation flexion and extension of the cervical spine or Spurling's maneuver might reproduce or exacerbate the patient's symptoms. Upper motor neuron lesions can also result in shoulder weakness. In these cases the deep tendon reflexes may be hyperreflexic, pathologic reflexes may be present, and tone may be increased. The clinical examination should exclude referred pain as a possibility, because cardiac and other intrathoracic as well as intraabdominal complaints may manifest as shoulder pain.

Finally, examination of the shoulder should always be performed with both shoulders exposed. Visualization is the first component of a physical examination, but this step is often neglected because of time constraints or modesty issues. If the bare scapula is not examined, it is easy to miss atrophy of the spinatus muscles. Bilateral atrophy or weakness would certainly change the differential diagnosis and force the examiner to consider an underlying neurogenic or myopathic condition.

MUSCULOCUTANEOUS NERVE INJURY

Etiology

Musculocutaneous nerve injury is most commonly associated with severe brachial plexus trauma. Although the nerve can be injured in glenohumeral dislocation, it is unusual to diagnose such injury as an isolated neuropathy.[45] When seen as an isolated nerve injury, it is most often associated with a form of penetrating trauma, open surgical reconstruction, or a direct blow to the chest (near the coracoid). Occasionally, musculocutaneous neuropathy can occur after strenuous physical activity, such as rowing.[122]

The musculocutaneous nerve travels obliquely below the coracoid process and enters the coracobrachialis. The anatomy of this juncture has been investigated in several studies. Small branches of the nerve can be found inserting into the coracobrachialis as close as 1.7 cm below the coracoid.[3] The main trunk of the musculocutaneous nerve enters the coracobrachialis approximately 5 cm from the coracoid and exits at 7 cm.[73,60] The nerve then enters the biceps, typically more than 10 cm from the coracoid.[60] The nerve is at risk during anterior shoulder procedures that result in significant retraction medially, and during medial surgical dissection. The Bristow procedure has been thought to be associated with injury to this nerve,[11] although such injury is probably related less to the transfer and more to manipulation of the nerve.[34]

It is important for the operating surgeon to recognize the protective value of maintaining the origins of the coracobrachialis and biceps. When these muscles are allowed to remain on the coracoid during surgery, they act as a tether to overzealous medial retraction. In fact, exposure of the posterior cord or the axillary nerve can lead to musculocutaneous nerve palsy as a result of retraction. Care must be taken to avoid excessive traction on the musculocutaneous nerve during dissection. As an alternative, detachment of the conjoined tendon allows excellent exposure as well as potentially decreased pressure in the entire brachial plexus. Actual detachment of these muscles from the coracoid and reattachment to the anterior glenoid (the Bristow procedure) relaxes the musculocutaneous nerve. Nonetheless, the surgical manipulation required can result in damage to the nerve.

The nerve can also be damaged during arthroscopic surgery, although such injury is very uncommon. Anterior portals that stray medial to the coracoid put the musculocutaneous nerve and other branches of the brachial plexus at potential risk for injury. Low anterior portals, such as the 5-o'clock portal, can bring instruments to within 10 mm of the nerve.[145] Carofino and colleagues reported on iatrogenic nerve injuries during shoulder surgery.[32] In their report out of 26 patients with iatrogenic nerve injuries, 4 had undergone arthroscopic surgery and 10 had undergone combined arthroscopic and open shoulder surgery.

A patient with a musculocutaneous nerve lesion typically has a mixed sensory and motor lesion. Less commonly, a pure sensory lesion of the lateral antebrachial cutaneous nerve, the distal sensory termination of the musculocutaneous nerve, can occur. Lesions of the lateral antebrachial cutaneous nerve at the level of the elbow often have an atraumatic etiology and should be distinguished from more proximally occurring (incomplete) musculocutaneous lesions manifesting with sensory loss. These patients might have numbness or paresthesia along the lateral elbow crease that extends distally along the anterolateral aspect of the forearm. Treatment involves splinting or corticosteroid injection and, possibly, surgical exploration.[184] Occasionally, surgical exploration reveals a thickened aponeurosis that is compressing the lateral antebrachial cutaneous nerve as it transits between the biceps and brachioradialis muscles. Patients might respond to surgical decompression of the nerve in this area.[49]

Nonoperative Treatment

Patients seen after trauma or surgery with an injury to the musculocutaneous nerve should be observed for 3 to 4 weeks. If no improvement in function is noted in that period, electromyography (EMG) and nerve conduction study (NCS) may be performed to assess the extent of nerve damage. Most postoperative musculocutaneous neuropathies are traction injuries that resolve over a period of weeks to months, depending on the extent of the injury.

Operative Treatment

If no improvement in biceps and brachialis function is seen on clinical examination or electrophysiologic studies, surgical exploration should be undertaken, ideally within 6 months from the injury. Surgical treatment options vary for persistent musculocutaneous neuropathy. If at surgical exploration the nerve appears intact but is compressed by scar tissue and demonstrates electrical conduction across the lesion, neurolysis may be indicated. If surgical exploration reveals a neuroma in continuity that does not conduct a nerve action potential (NAP)[101] or reveals a rupture or transection of the nerve, additional treatment options should be considered.

In patients who have an isolated musculocutaneous nerve injury, a standard approach is to perform interpositional nerve grafting across the lesion. However, nerve transfers can also be used to shorten the distance (and time) for reinnervation or to bypass a scarred or avascular segment. A possible nerve transfer is the Oberlin transfer, a technique in which one or two fascicles of the ulnar nerve are transferred directly to the motor branch to the biceps.[107,139] The distance to achieve reinnervation is extremely short because the site of repair is in the proximal part of the arm (several centimeters from the biceps end-organ) rather than a more lengthy repair from the neck or shoulder region. This technique can be used in patients with upper plexus lesions. In two large series each with more than 30 patients, grade 3 or 4 Medical Research Council (MRC) function was achieved in more than 90% of the patients treated with this technique.[139,183] Reinnervation in the biceps was noted approximately 3 months after the procedure. Importantly, no patient suffered loss of distal ulnar nerve function or sensation. Recent modifications of this procedure have been reported with double reinnervation of elbow flexion: an ulnar nerve fascicle may be transferred to the biceps motor branch and a median nerve fascicle to the brachialis branch.[114,116]

If patients are seen for more than 1 year after musculocutaneous nerve injury, nerve repair or reconstruction is significantly less likely to be effective.[40,75,98,141,161,165,172] Nevertheless, nerve transfer techniques can be considered in select cases.

Some patients with little or no biceps or brachialis strength still function extremely well by using their brachioradialis alone for elbow flexion. The majority of patients however need augmentation. A number of tendon or muscle transfer procedures that achieve good results can be used. Popular options include Steindler flexorplasty (proximal advancement of the flexor-pronator muscle group) and triceps, pectoralis major, pectoralis minor, and latissimus dorsi transfer. Free muscle transfer is also a possibility in patients in whom these other potential donor muscles are not available.

AXILLARY NERVE

Anatomy

The axillary nerve is one of the more commonly injured nerves about the shoulder. It is a terminal branch of the posterior cord and is derived from the fifth and sixth cranial nerves. The axillary nerve lies lateral to the radial nerve, posterior to the axillary artery, and anterior to the subscapularis muscle. It enters the quadrilateral space accompanied by the posterior humeral circumflex artery and is in close contact with the inferior shoulder capsule.

The axillary nerve is easy to locate at surgery during an anterior exposure by sweeping an index finger inferiorly over the anterior subscapularis and gently hooking the nerve while simultaneously palpating it on the underside of the deltoid with the other index finger.[72] As it exits the space, the axillary nerve continues to the posterior aspect of the humeral neck and divides into anterior and posterior branches. The position of the anterior branch is commonly reported as lying 4 to 7 cm inferior to the anterolateral corner of the acromion.[28] The posterior branch innervates both the teres minor and the posterior portion of the deltoid. The branch to the teres minor usually arises within or just distal to the quadrilateral space and enters the posteroinferior aspect of the teres minor muscle.

The internal topography of the axillary nerve has been studied by Aszmann and Dellon.[8] As the nerve leaves the posterior cord, it is monofascicular, but as it enters the quadrilateral space, it has three distinct groups of fascicles: motor groups to the deltoid and teres minor and the sensory group of the superior lateral cutaneous nerve. The deltoid motor fascicles are found in a superolateral position; those of the teres minor and superior lateral cutaneous nerve are located inferomedially.

Etiology and Clinical Manifestation

Most axillary nerve injuries occur as part of a combined brachial plexus injury; isolated axillary nerve injury occurs in only 0.3% to 6% of brachial plexus injuries.[180] Injury to the axillary nerve most often follows closed trauma

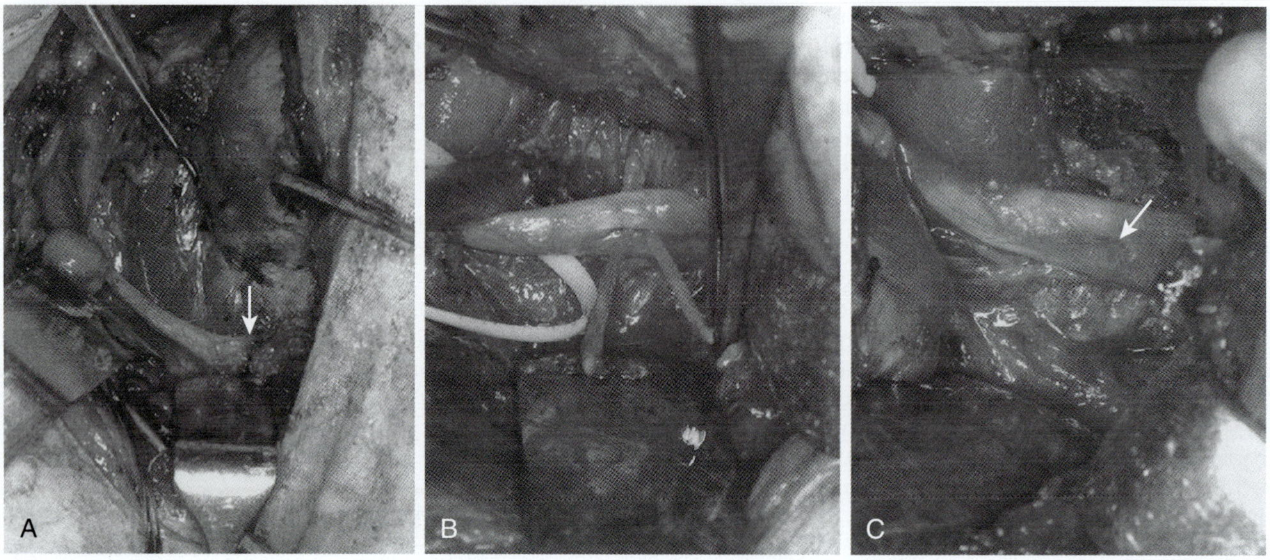

FIGURE 18-1: Axillary nerve palsy. This 21-year-old man underwent arthroscopic repair for recurrent left anterior shoulder dislocation. Postoperatively, new shoulder weakness and deltoid atrophy developed, and the patient was referred to examination 6 months after the operation. He had 120 degrees of abduction and 160 degrees of forward flexion. Electromyography demonstrated dense fibrillations in the deltoid without voluntary activation. A severe axillary nerve lesion was diagnosed. **A,** At surgery, the conjoined tendon was taken down. The axillary nerve was encased in scar tissue (*arrow*) and was decompressed. **B,** At the inferior portion of the glenoid, a suture anchor splitting the axillary nerve in half was noted. **C,** Stimulation across the lesion resulted in a deltoid response. The indentation within the nerve from which the suture anchor was removed can be seen (*arrow*).

involving traction on the shoulder. Axillary nerve paralysis is the most common neurologic complication of shoulder dislocations. Some patients with a proximal humeral fracture or shoulder dislocation have a subclinical axillary nerve lesion that is evident by EMG/NCS but which is not apparent clinically because of the associated discomfort.[86,134,144,189,198] The vast majority of these patients recover from the nerve injury as they rehabilitate from the dislocation or fracture. Blunt trauma to the anterolateral aspect of the shoulder has also been noted to cause injury to the axillary nerve as it travels on the deep surface of the deltoid muscle.[149]

Open reconstructive surgery (Fig. 18-1) and some newer arthroscopic techniques can put the axillary nerve at risk. For example, capsular shrinkage procedures can create a local increase in temperature in the inferior capsule that can lead to nerve injury.[82,83] Injury to the nerve has been reported in 1% to 2% of thermal capsular shrinkage procedures, but fortunately, the vast majority of these injuries seem to be only temporary.[203] The axillary nerve is also at risk during capsular resection for adhesive capsulitis.[94] Because the nerve is in close proximity to the anteroinferior capsule, great care should be taken when resecting in this area. A safer method of inferior capsular resection in this area is to visualize the axillary nerve with the arthroscope during the procedure.

Nonoperative Treatment

Young patients may be able to compensate for complete deltoid paralysis and can often perform activities of daily living with only partial disability. The shoulder can easily maintain a full range of motion with an intact rotator cuff. However, most patients experience early fatigue in the involved side if asked to perform repetitive activities. Although deltoid atrophy is quite evident in a fit person, it can sometimes be difficult for the examiner to detect deltoid atrophy in a less fit patient. Injury to the superior lateral cutaneous nerve of the arm can lead to sensory loss over the lateral aspect of the shoulder. It is possible for patients with a complete deltoid motor deficit to experience only a mild loss of sensation over the lateral part of the shoulder. The diagnosis of axillary neuropathy should not be determined by the presence or absence of lateral shoulder sensation. It is unclear whether the sensory branch is spared from injury or whether the sensory zone is supplied by overlapping innervation from other cutaneous branches.

Another potential cause of posterior shoulder pain that has been described is the quadrilateral space syndrome, which presumably results from compression of the axillary nerve within the quadrilateral space. This syndrome is a controversial clinical entity; it might simply be a manifestation of Parsonage-Turner syndrome (brachial neuritis). Tenderness may be noted posteriorly along the shoulder joint; otherwise, the clinical examination is often normal. Deltoid atrophy or lateral sensory changes are uncommon, and EMG examination is usually normal. Magnetic resonance imaging (MRI) may demonstrate signal change indicating denervation in the deltoid and teres minor muscles.[113] Observation is the usual treatment for quadrilateral space syndrome, and the vast majority of patients improve with time.[112] Surgical exploration of the quadrilateral space and release of scar or fibrous bands to achieve decompression of the axillary nerve are rarely needed.[30]

Patients with a history of blunt trauma to the axillary nerve should be observed over at least a 3-month period before operative treatment is considered. At 3 to 4 weeks, a baseline EMG/NCS examination should be obtained. Physical therapy, including active and passive exercises, should be initiated to preserve the maximal range of motion and prevent joint contracture while awaiting return of function. Electrical stimulation of the deltoid has been used in an attempt to preserve muscle viability, although it is unclear whether this approach has any genuine effect.

The results of nonoperative treatment of a blunt traumatic lesion have generally been good. Leffert reported that axillary nerve injury after fracture or dislocation is more common than is usually appreciated, yet the majority of patients progress to full recovery.[110] In a study of 73 patients with proximal humeral fracture or dislocation, 33% were noted on EMG to have an axillary nerve injury, with 9 complete and 15 partial lesions.[22] All of the patients, including those with complete nerve lesions, recovered with no objective loss of function. In a series of 108 elderly patients with anterior shoulder dislocation, 9.3% were found to have an axillary nerve injury, but all went on to full recovery by 12 months.[86] However, some patients do not make the expected recovery. In these patients surgical exploration with neurolysis or possibly nerve grafting can be undertaken if no clinical or EMG recovery is evident by 3 to 4 months.[5,42,137,156] If the patient has experienced a sharp penetrating wound or a surgical injury, surgical exploration should be performed at an earlier date.

Operative Treatment

The proximal monofascicular structure of the axillary nerve with primarily motor fibers and its relatively short length from the posterior cord to the deltoid motor end plate are characteristics that lend themselves to surgical intervention. Alnot and Valenti reported on 37 axillary nerve surgeries, including 33 cases of sural nerve grafting, 3 neurolysis procedures, and 1 direct repair.[5] In 23 of the 25 isolated axillary nerve lesions M4 or M5 strength was achieved. The fact that 33 of the 37 patients required sural nerve grafting illustrates the difficulty in adequately mobilizing the nerve for direct repair. The small number of patients undergoing neurolysis (3 of 37) is an indication that mild nerve compression by scar or fibrous bands is not common. Repair of the axillary nerve with a short interposed cabled sural nerve graft has been the most common method and has demonstrated the most consistent results.[4,26,42,147,150,157]

We have found the use of intraoperative NAPs and EMG techniques to be invaluable in evaluating neuromas and helping us decide whether to perform neurolysis alone or to resect the neuroma and perform a graft. In all cases we are also prepared to expose the axillary nerve posteriorly. In selected cases such exposure is necessary to identify normal nerve more distally for grafting.

Other techniques for repair of the axillary nerve include nerve transfer. Direct neurotization with a donor nerve, such as the medial pectoral, thoracodorsal, or radial, has yielded satisfactory results in cases in which direct repair or short cable grafting of the axillary nerve itself is not possible or not preferable.[47,78,164] Nerve transfers using the spinal accessory nerve or upper intercostal nerves have been described, but these require an interpositional sural nerve graft[38,164] and have demonstrated less optimal results.[164,176] A nerve transfer using a triceps branch to the anterior division of the axillary nerve has been described in cases of upper trunk brachial plexopathy[106]; because of promising results, it is now being used by some surgeons instead of nerve grafting techniques in cases of isolated axillary paralysis.

Patients seen longer than 15 to 18 months after trauma usually do not benefit from surgical repair of the nerve because of the poor condition of the deltoid muscle and its motor end plates. In patients with poor shoulder function that limits their activities of daily living but a normal rotator cuff, muscle transfer procedures can be considered. Potentially, if the posterior deltoid and middle deltoid are innervated and the anterior deltoid is not functioning, the posterior-middle deltoid can be rotated anteriorly on the clavicle. This procedure however has the potential to harm the remaining deltoid and is not strongly recommended.

Pedicled pectoralis major transfer can be performed to reconstruct the anterior deltoid (Fig. 18-2). The clavicular head of the pectoralis major alone or combined with the upper two thirds of the sternal head can be rotated on its pedicle to reconstruct mostly the anterior deltoid. Another option is the transfer of pedicled latissimus dorsi based on the thoracodorsal neurovascular bundle to reconstruct the anterior deltoid (Fig. 18-3). One of the authors of this chapter (B.T.E.) has performed the first of these procedures on 17 patients and the second on 23 patients, with very promising results. Alternatively, to reconstruct middle deltoid function, the upper/middle trapezius can be transferred to the proximal humerus.[62,63] Different techniques have been described for this transfer, including transfer of the muscle on top of the acromion, prolonged with Achilles tendon allograft, or transfer of the acromial bony insertion to the proximal humerus. The outcome of this transfer has been very marginal, especially in patients with no rotator cuff function. We favor pedicled muscle transfers, as described above, when these are available because of the more predictable improvement of shoulder function.

SPINAL ACCESSORY NERVE

Etiology

Injury to the spinal accessory nerve can occur after penetrating trauma to the shoulder. Blunt trauma can also cause loss of trapezius function. Most commonly, surgical dissection in the posterior triangle of the neck, such as

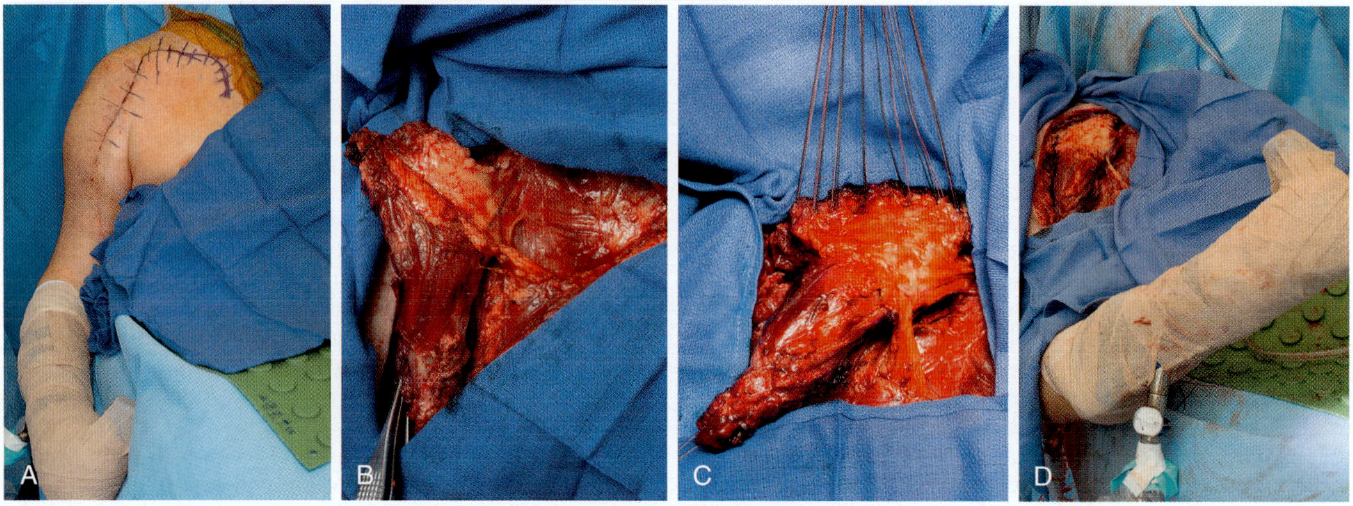

FIGURE 18-2: **A,** A patient positioned in the beach chair position for the pedicled pectoralis transfer. The incision starts at a scar from prior surgery and extends in a curved way distal to the clavicle at the level of the pectoralis major origin. **B,** The upper two thirds of the pectoralis major is elevated on its pedicle and turned (almost as if turning the page of a book) to insert it at the level of anterior deltoid. **C,** The muscular portion of the pectoralis is attached to the lateral clavicle and anterior acromion. **D,** How the muscle looks after its final transfer and attachment. The tendinous portion is attached distally at the level of the deltoid insertion.

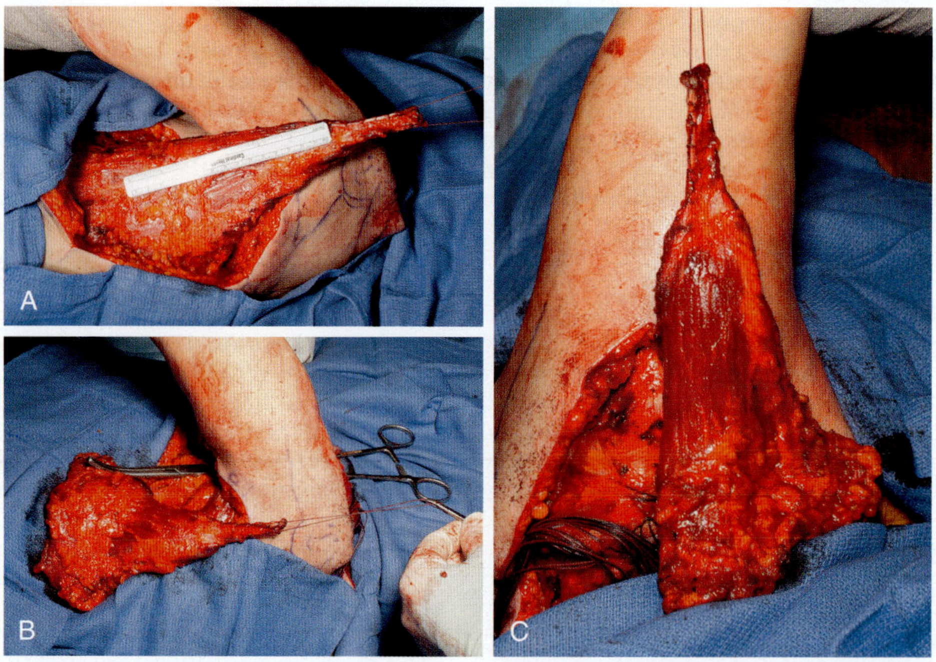

FIGURE 18-3: **A,** Harvesting the latissimus dorsi bipolar muscle for transfer. **B,** Passing the latissimus deep to the pectoralis from posterior to the anterior wound at the site of the planned transfer. **C,** The pedicled latissimus is transferred to the level of the anterior deltoid where the muscular portion will be attached to the lateral portion of the clavicle and acromion, and the tendinous portion is inserted distally at the site of deltoid insertion.

for lymph node biopsy, can expose the nerve to possible damage (Fig. 18-4).[102,123,131,193,202]

Anatomy

The spinal accessory nerve passes through the upper portion of the sternocleidomastoid muscle, which it innervates. It then crosses the posterior cervical triangle, which is bordered anteriorly by the sternocleidomastoid muscle, posteriorly by the trapezius, and inferiorly by the clavicle. The nerve lies on the floor of the posterior triangle with only the overlying fascia as protection against injury.[48] It abuts the posterior cervical lymph nodes. The nerve enters the anterior surface of the trapezius and

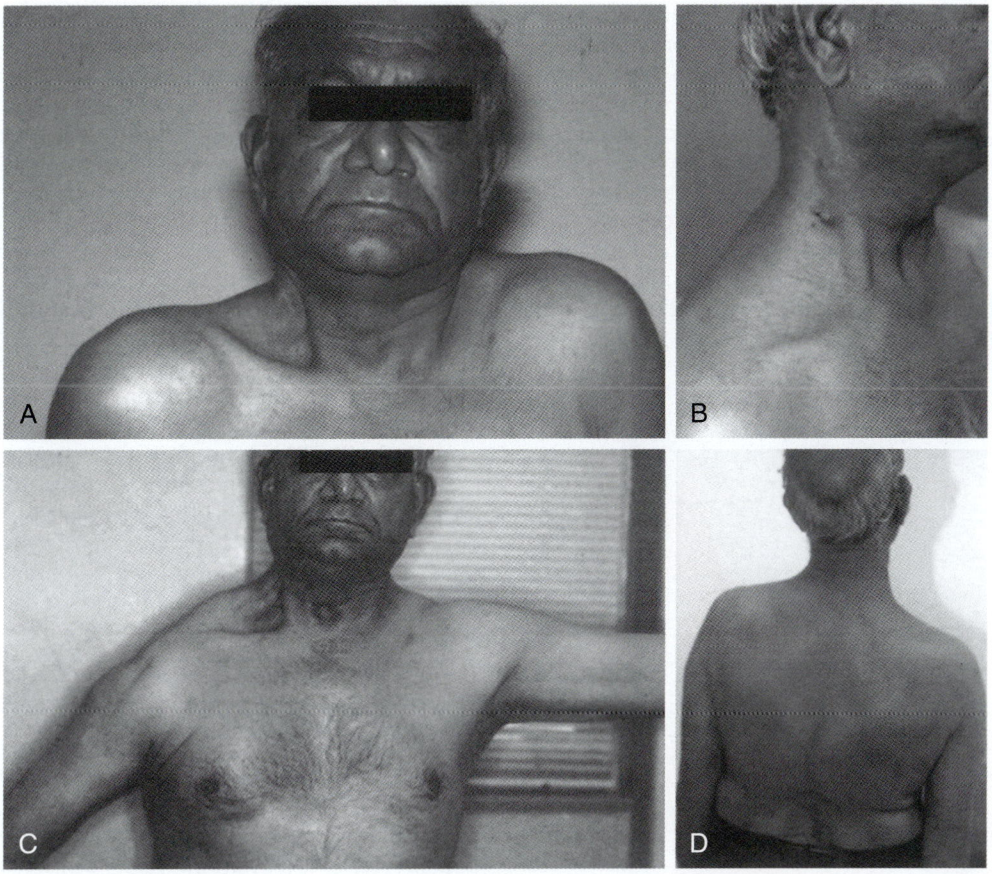

FIGURE 18-4: Spinal accessory nerve paralysis. This 53-year-old man underwent a cervical lymph node biopsy to exclude tuberculous lymphadenitis. The specimen was nondiagnostic. Severe pain and deformity developed in the affected shoulder after surgery and a postoperative pain syndrome was thought to have developed. The diagnosis of spinal accessory nerve paralysis was not made until several months later. **A,** An asymmetric shoulder shrug and trapezius atrophy are evident. **B,** A small transverse incision from the lymph node biopsy is seen directly posterior to the sternocleidomastoid muscle. This incision is directly over the oblique course of the accessory nerve. **C,** The patient had significant difficulty with shoulder abduction. **D,** Resultant shoulder droop can be seen from loss of the trapezius.

travels inferiorly, parallel to the medial border of the scapula.[95] The trapezius has a broad origin from the ligamentum nuchae to the 12th thoracic vertebra and inserts over the lateral part of the clavicle, acromion, and spine of the scapula. The upper trapezius is the prime elevator of the scapula, acting to upwardly rotate the lateral aspect of the bone (Fig. 18-5).

Diagnosis

A diagnosis of injury to the spinal accessory nerve is often missed, and appropriate treatment may be delayed.[102] Patients usually have vague shoulder pain as their primary complaint. Loss of motion may be a secondary concern. Unless trapezius function is specifically tested, the diagnosis may not be recognized. Because of the common occurrence of anterior shoulder pain in these patients, with occasionally only slight visible wasting of the trapezius muscle, the pain may be assumed to represent postoperative pain, or it may be misinterpreted as resulting from another condition associated with shoulder pain, such as rotator cuff pathology. The trapezius receives some innervation from the upper cervical nerve roots; thus complete atrophy of the muscle might not occur.

The spinal accessory nerve supplies the sole innervation to the lateral portion of the muscle, which is critical in supporting abduction of the shoulder. If the patient is carefully observed, the scapula appears to be rotated forward at the shoulder. The shoulder might hang lower or droop in comparison to the contralateral side; this difference can even cause symptoms of thoracic outlet syndrome. Winging of the scapula often occurs but is not as dramatic as that associated with injury to the long thoracic nerve. Usually, a shoulder shrug produces the deformity; however, a strong levator scapula can compensate well, and only minimal deformity may be noted. The patient might not be able to abduct the arm fully with the forearm either pronated or supinated.

Some of the pain that patients experience might come from strain of the other parascapular muscles as they attempt to compensate for the lack of trapezius function. Additionally, because the scapula cannot properly rotate the acromion away from the humerus as the arm is elevated, impingement of the rotator cuff can cause secondary rotator cuff tendinopathy. If attention is directed only at the rotator cuff, the underlying nerve pathology will be missed. In addition, the spinal accessory nerve, although mainly a motor nerve, still has sensory fibers. Injury to the nerve can also produce neuropathic pain. Finally, examination should also cover possible concomitant injury to other neighboring nerves, such as the cervical plexus or great auricular nerve.

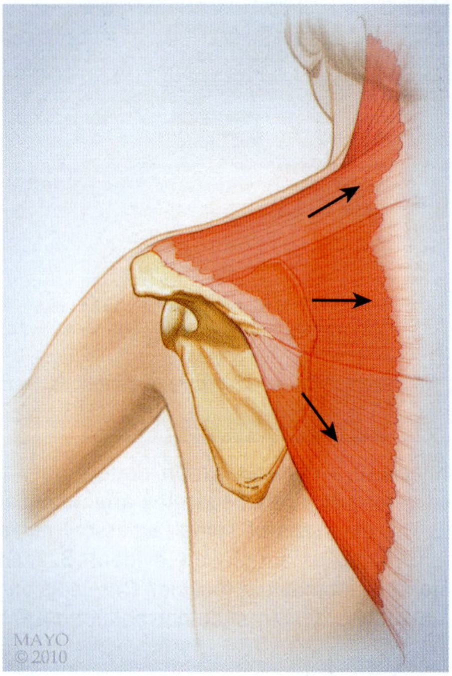

FIGURE 18-5: The trapezius, showing its broad origin on the 12th spinous process of the thoracic spine and insertion on the clavicle, acromion, and spine of the scapula. The three parts of the trapezius, including the upper, middle, and lower, work together in stabilizing the scapula on the chest wall. (Courtesy Mayo Foundation for Medical Education and Research.)

Operative Treatment

Whenever possible, surgical exploration of the nerve should be performed within 6 months. Although surgical reconstruction of the nerve may be considered up to 1 year after injury, better results occur with treatment as soon after injury as possible.[102,123,193] We favor early exploration of these nerve injuries when they occur immediately after surgery, especially when the nerve was not identified and protected as part of the operation.[123]

Surgical options include neurolysis, direct repair, or nerve grafting, depending on intraoperative observations and electrophysiologic testing.[140] During surgical reconstruction, it is important to consider the acromion-mastoid distance in the anesthetized patient. If direct repair of the nerve is performed with the head tilted toward the operated shoulder, significant traction can occur when the patient is awakened after surgery and transported to the recovery room, and this can disrupt the repair. If the nerve ends are found to have retracted at surgery, it is best to use an intervening graft, such as a sural nerve or the great auricular nerve, to reduce tension on the repair (Fig. 18-6).

Nerve Transfer

Nerve transfer using a pectoral branch can be performed in cases of proximal injury to the accessory nerve, inability to identify proximal stump, or late referral.[136] If more than 12 to 18 months have passed since injury to the spinal accessory nerve, nonoperative treatment may be considered if the patient has compensated reasonably well. The degree of disability varies from patient to patient, even despite aggressive physical therapy. Some patients experience only a persistent ache in the shoulder, whereas others feel and act completely disabled with respect to the upper extremity. Braces have been advocated as adjunctive treatment, but they are bulky and not used consistently by the patients.[197] A patient symptomatic enough to attempt to use a brace is potentially a candidate for surgical reconstruction.

Muscle Transfer

Modern surgical procedures currently involve dynamic muscle transfer techniques. Earlier historical procedures however initially involved mostly static repairs. Henry

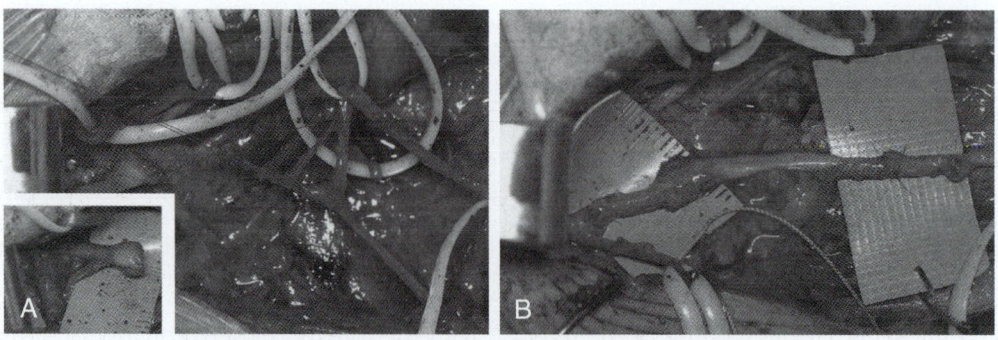

FIGURE 18-6: Spinal accessory nerve paralysis. **A,** The spinal accessory nerve was transected. A neuroma (*inset*) can be seen. A suture marks the distal stump. **B,** An interpositional graft repair (backgrounds) was performed using the sural nerve.

and others advocated static stabilization of the medial aspect of the scapula to the vertebral spine with strips of fascia lata.[51,90,201] Dewar and Harris described lateral transfer of the levator scapulae to the lateral part of the scapula, combined with a static fascial sling from the vertebral spine to the medial part of the scapula.[50] However, static repairs with fascia, tendon, or artificial materials tend to stretch out or rupture over time.[105]

Dynamic transfer of the levator scapulae along with the rhomboid major and rhomboid minor was described in Germany by Eden and Lange.[58,103,104] Bigliani reported good results with this technique.[18,20,202]

Elhassan and Wagner proposed a modification of the Eden-Lange (EL) procedure, called the "triple transfer," with good to excellent results in 22 patients.[65] The authors reported that the line of pull of the rhomboid major and minor when transferred to the body of the scapula worked in almost the opposite direction to the lower trapezius, and for this reason these muscles should independently be transferred more proximally for better replication of the line of pull of the middle/lower trapezius.

The surgical approaches for the EL procedure and the Elhassan-Wagner (EW) modified transfer are similar and involve an inverted L-incision with a vertical incision placed midway between the vertebral spine and the medial edge of the scapula and a horizontal incision extended laterally to the mid-aspect of the supraspinatus fossa. The atrophied trapezius is detached from the spine of the scapula and acromion and can be used to cover the muscles' transfer at the end of the case. The levator scapulae and rhomboidei are exposed and dissected. If the EL procedure is performed then the levator scapulae is detached with a small bony insertion, and the rhomboid minor and major are detached together with small bony insertions. This release can be accomplished with a small saw or an osteotome. At this time the spine of the scapula is debrided to prepare it for the bony insertion of the muscle transfer. With the EL procedure (Fig. 18-7), the levator scapulae is attached laterally on the spine of the scapula, posterior to the acromion. The levator should be placed as far laterally as possible on the spine of the scapula, usually 5 to 7 cm medial to the posterolateral edge of the acromion. The rhomboid major and minor can be elevated individually or together from the medial edge of the scapula. The dorsal scapular nerve is potentially at risk during this part of the procedure. The infraspinatus is partially elevated from the scapula in a medial-to-lateral direction. The rhomboids are then placed as far laterally as possible—at least 4 cm—on the posterior aspect of the scapula and secured in place via suture and drill holes through the scapula. Alternatively, the rhomboid minor can be transferred cephalad to the spine of the scapula into the supraspinatus fossa. The infraspinatus is then sutured back in position over the transferred rhomboids.

With the EW transfer, the levator scapula is placed as lateral as possible on the spine of the scapula (as described above), the rhomboid minor is attached on the spine of

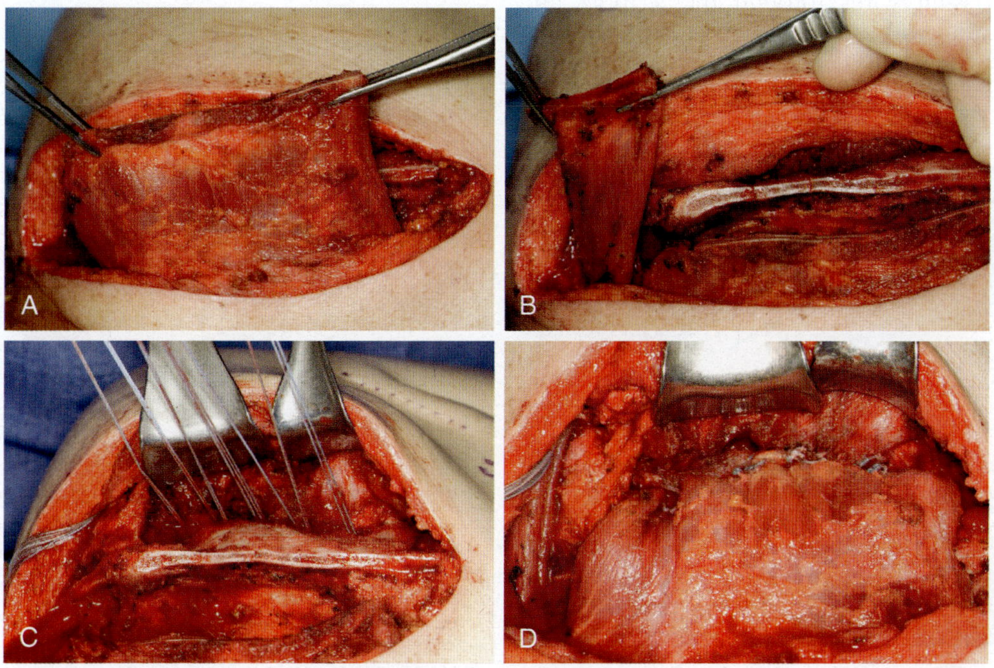

FIGURE 18-7: A 60-year-old woman with spinal accessory paralysis after lymph node biopsy undergoing an Eden-Lange procedure of the rhomboid and a levator scapulae transfer. **A,** Right shoulder rhomboid major and minor elevated. **B,** Levator scapulae elevated for transfer. **C,** Sutures passed through drill holes in the scapula for rhomboid fixation. **D,** Rhomboid muscle sutured to the scapula.

the scapula just medial to the levator scapulae, and the rhomboid major is attached on the spine of the scapula just medial to the rhomboid minor. Because of the wider insertion of the rhomboid major, its attachment on the medial spine of the scapula is better performed by breaking the bony attachment in its middle part and then closing the two edges of the bone (like closing a fish's mouth) around the medial spine of the scapula (Fig. 18-8).

Postoperatively, patients are placed in a shoulder abduction brace that holds the arm at approximately 70 degrees of abduction for 6 to 8 weeks, depending on the preference of the treating surgeon. Because of the smaller size of the levator scapulae and rhomboidei, we prefer 8 weeks of immobilization to allow full healing of the transfers and to reduce the risk of stretch injuries from early mobilization. At 8 weeks, patients are started on progressive range of motion for 6 weeks followed by gentle strengthening and aquatherapy for 8 weeks; they are allowed unrestricted activities at 6 months.

Good outcomes have been reported with both techniques, but the EW procedure has been reported to have a better outcome and less risk of failure.[65,104] If an EL procedure fails, the only possible remaining muscle transfer option available is to transfer the lower contralateral trapezius origin to the lateral spine of the scapula to restore scapula retraction.[66] One of the authors (B.T.E.) has performed this procedure on five patients with a failed prior EL procedure and the results were promising in all five cases. The main salvage procedure to stabilize the scapula in symptomatic patients with failed EL procedure is scapulothoracic fusion. Different techniques have been used to perform scapulothoracic fusion, but most involve passing wires through the scapula and around several ribs, with a broad iliac crest bone graft or metallic plate for support. The complication rate can be high, with the potential for pneumothorax or hardware failure.

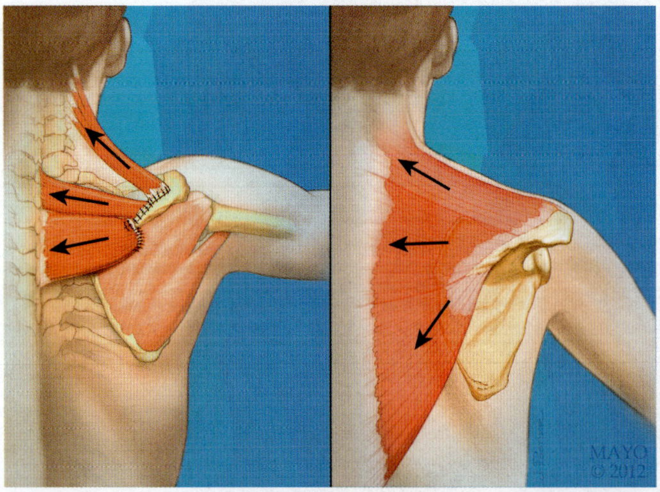

FIGURE 18-8: The Elhassan-Wagner transfer showing that the levator scapulae, rhomboid minor, and rhomboid major are transferred separately on the spine of the scapula in a pattern that is meant to replicate the line of pull of the trapezius. (Courtesy Mayo Foundation for Medical Education and Research.)

LONG THORACIC NERVE

Anatomy

The serratus anterior originates from the upper nine ribs and inserts on the anteromedial border of the scapula. This insertion is only a few millimeters wide at the midportion of the scapula, but it becomes more substantial at the inferior pole of the scapula (Fig. 18-9). It is the inferior portion of the muscle that is important in maintaining protraction and upward rotation of the scapula during forward elevation of the shoulder. The long thoracic nerve has a relatively long course after taking origin from the C5, C6, and C7 nerve roots. After crossing over the first rib, it travels 10 to 20 cm to its motor end plate in the serratus anterior. It is vulnerable to blunt trauma over the first rib along the lateral chest wall and can be crushed by forceful displacement of the scapula.

Etiology

The nerve is rarely injured as a result of penetrating trauma, but injury can occur during thoracic outlet surgery in the region of the first rib, breast surgery, or lateral chest wall procedures, such as axillary node dissection.[194,205] Spontaneous cases of entrapment at the scalenus medius have been described.[52] The most common cause of serratus anterior dysfunction is probably Parsonage-Turner syndrome; indeed, this condition is most likely the underlying cause of long thoracic

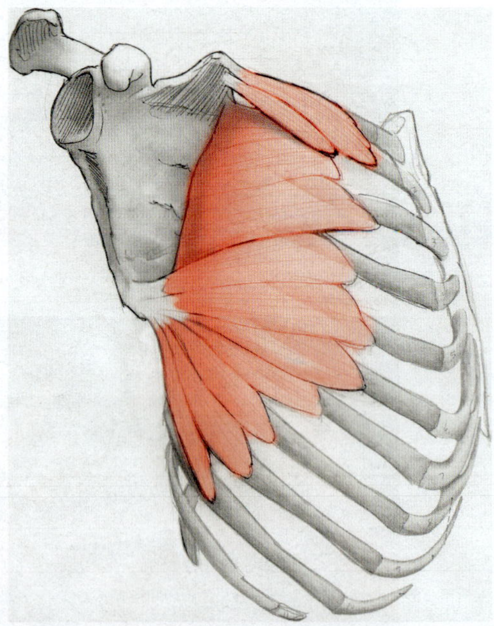

FIGURE 18-9: Anatomy of the serratus anterior showing its broad origin and insertion over the medial scapula body. The most important part is the lower part that inserts on the distal border of the scapula and has the largest cross-sectional area of the muscle.

nerve dysfunction attributed to overexertion, including athletic activities.

Clinical Manifestation

Isolated injury to the long thoracic nerve is usually manifested as winging of the scapula. Velpeau first described injury to the long thoracic nerve causing paralysis of the serratus anterior in 1837.[196] However, winging of the scapula has many possible causes, with multidirectional instability probably being the most common cause of mild winging. Spinal accessory nerve injury can also cause winging, but this injury tends to be milder and results in more of a rotational deformity of the scapula. Some patients have volitional control over the scapula and can demonstrate significant winging at will.

Nonoperative Treatment

In our opinion, observation should be the standard therapy in idiopathic or nonpenetrating trauma cases. Other than continued use of the shoulder as tolerated, no specific physical therapy protocol has been found to be especially helpful. Braces have been advocated to help hold the scapula against the chest wall[120]; however, although these can be somewhat effective, they are usually found to be awkward and are not well tolerated by patients. Most patients with a nontraumatic or idiopathic cause tend to recover from the paralysis and regain serratus anterior function within 6 months to 1 year.[76]

Operative Treatment

There are potential surgical options available for treating injury to the long thoracic nerve in the early stages. Some surgeons have favored neurolysis of the nerve with decompression at the level of the scalenus medius.[52] However, because it is difficult to be certain where the lesion resides, or if compression (rather than inflammation, for example) is responsible for the dysfunction, we do not recommend this approach for most patients. In cases where there has been no spontaneous recovery, another strategy is to perform neurotization (or nerve transfer) using one or two intercostal nerves or the thoracodorsal nerve (M.B. Wood, personal communication, 2002).[135,204] Because it is not usually clear where the damaged section is, the nerve can be connected with the donor nerve close to the motor end plate. This technique has been helpful in a small number of reported cases.[135,155,192] Many patients with atraumatic lesions recover spontaneously, so we do not routinely recommend surgery for most patients before 6 or 9 months after the nerve deficit develops.

If a patient does not recover serratus anterior function and use of the shoulder is compromised, a number of reconstructive options are available (Fig. 18-10).[9,35,44,81,91,93,121,148,153,154,190,194,199] Scapulothoracic fusion has been performed when the scapula is fixed to the underlying ribs. Although this technique can eliminate winging of the scapula, it will reduce shoulder girdle motion by at least 30%, with mostly forward elevation and extension affected.[27] Pneumothorax is a risk with this technique, and the pseudarthrosis rate is not insignificant. For these reasons, scapulothoracic fusion should be reserved for the salvage situation or for patients with symptomatic facioscapulohumeral dystrophy.

Tendon Transfer

Tendon transfers provide dynamic control of a winging scapula and are now our preferred method in patients with a neurologic deficit that has lasted for 1 year or more. Tubby described transfer of the pectoralis major to the serratus anterior in 1904.[190] Although this transfer might offer initial relief of the winging, the paralyzed serratus anterior tends to stretch out with time, and this procedure is not recommended today. Other techniques described include transfer of the pectoralis minor, rhomboids, or levator scapulae.[35,91,175]

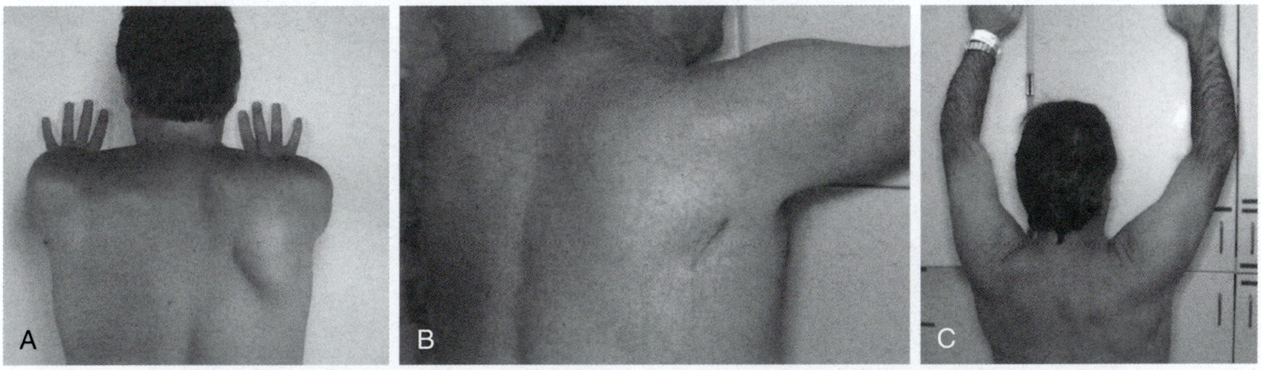

FIGURE 18-10: Long thoracic nerve palsy. A complete long thoracic nerve paralysis from Parsonage-Turner syndrome developed in this 36-year-old man. His winged scapula did not improve after 3 years. He had persistent pain in his shoulder and disability when performing overhead maneuvers. **A,** Prominent right scapula winging is noted preoperatively. **B,** Postoperatively, the winging has disappeared after pectoralis major transfer. The posterior incision has healed well. **C,** Postoperatively, his shoulder arc of motion has improved as well.

Pectoralis Major Transfer

The technique that seems to give the most consistent result is transfer of the pectoralis major to the scapula with tendon graft augmentation. Durman, Ober, and Marmor[56,121,138] each described successful transfer of the pectoralis major with a fascial extension graft in a few cases. More recent studies have demonstrated the excellent ability of this tendon transfer procedure to control winging of the scapula.[44,93,148,153,177,200] The pectoralis major is ideally suited as a transfer to substitute for the paralyzed serratus anterior. The direction of pull of the pectoralis major is similar to the path of the serratus anterior, and the bulk of the pectoralis major provides enough strength to resist winging of the scapula. The technique has been used with transfer of the entire pectoralis major or with only the sternal head (Fig. 18-11); equally good results have been reported with both procedures. However, the sternal head of the pectoralis major is much more in line with the direction of pull of the serratus anterior than is the clavicular head, and it also provides for a less bulky transfer. Furthermore, the sternal head is more substantial than the clavicular head and provides a stronger tendon transfer. Potential concerns of cosmesis or visible deformity of the anterior chest wall should be minimal. In most instances regardless of whether the entire pectoralis major or only the sternal head is transferred, there is little change in the normal contour of the anterior chest.

This procedure can be performed with a single large incision across the axilla or through two separate incisions. The two-incision technique is not technically harder than a single incision and is somewhat more cosmetic and is the preferred procedure. The choice of tissue for augmentation of the transferred pectoralis major tendon depends on the surgeon's preference. The most common choice has been a large portion of fascia lata rolled into a tube. Other graft options include semitendinosus or gracilis autograft or allograft.[178] Fascia lata can be rolled into a spiral tube and draped around the pectoralis major muscle and tendon to provide very strong proximal fixation.

More recently, Elhassan and Wagner reported on the outcome of direct transfer of the sternal head of the pectoralis major with its bony insertion to the scapula for patients with symptomatic scapula winging as result of chronic long thoracic nerve palsy.[64]

Technique

Pectoralis transfer to the scapula augmented with fascia lata is performed with the patient positioned in the lateral decubitus position for easy access to the anterior and posterior aspects of the shoulder and the lateral aspect of the ipsilateral thigh. The anterior approach is usually performed while a second surgical team is simultaneously harvesting the fascia lata. This approach is made somewhat easier by the lateral position. The anterior incision (4 to 6 cm long) is made almost entirely in the axillary crease and is extended only a centimeter superiorly. This technique results in a well-hidden, cosmetic incision. The sternal head of the pectoralis major is easily identified at the inferior margin of the muscle. It wraps posteriorly under the clavicular head and inserts more medial and superior to it. The sternal head is detached directly off the humerus, with care taken to avoid damage to the biceps tendon. The sternal head is then freed up medially onto the chest wall to allow greater excursion of the muscle. The harvested fascia lata graft should measure approximately 14 × 5 cm. The fascia lata is rolled into a spiral tube, draped around the pectoralis major tendon and muscle, and secured with multiple sutures. A heavy running locking suture is then placed through the fascia lata graft and tagged for transfer.

The posterior incision should be made at the junction of the middle and distal lateral edges of the scapula. It is important that an assistant manually pushes the scapula as far anteriorly and laterally as possible. When this

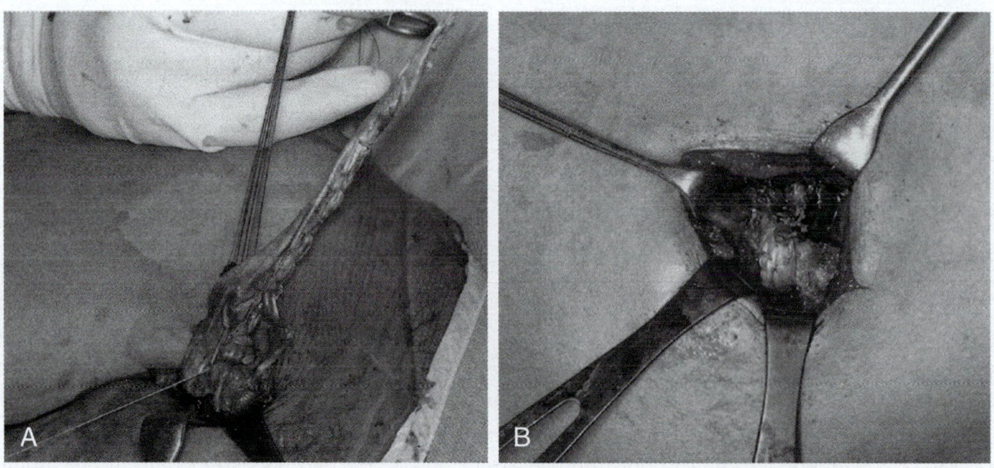

FIGURE 18-11: Operative images of long thoracic nerve palsy. **A,** Axillary exposure showing the sternal portion of the pectoralis tendon reinforced with a fascia lata graft before its transfer posteriorly to the scapula. **B,** The posterior approach shows the tendon secured to the scapula.

position is achieved, a 4-cm incision is made over the lateral edge of the scapula, and the muscles are cleared off the bone and retracted. An 8- to 10-mm hole is created in the scapula with a bur, just medial to the thick lateral mass of the scapula, to ensure a strong bony bridge during the healing period. A large bone hook is helpful at this stage to secure the scapula. Using a large, blunt clamp, a subcutaneous path is created from the anterior incision along the chest wall to the posterior incision. Much of this dissection can be performed with digital palpation. This plane is safe because the brachial plexus is more superior and abducted with the arm.

Once a clear path has been created for the pectoralis major and graft, the traction suture is passed posteriorly and the graft is pulled through the scapular fenestration in an anterior-to-posterior direction. The graft is then pulled tight, attempting to abut the native pectoralis major tendon to the scapula. The tendon is then folded back and sutured to itself. It is important for the scapula to be held as far anterior on the chest wall as possible while these sutures are secured. No reports of overtight pectoralis major transfers have appeared in the literature. Any excess graft after suture fixation is excised. Drains are not usually needed at closure, and the arm is placed into a sling.

Direct transfer of the bony insertion of the sternal head of the pectoralis major to the scapula is also performed in the lateral position, but the thigh does not need to be included in the surgical field as there is no need for tendon graft. A small anterior incision is performed from the axillary fold proximally for 5 cm. Exposure of the pectoralis and the separation of the sternal head from the clavicular head are similar to the technique described above. However, when the sternal head is ready to be detached, electrocautery is used to define the bony insertion of the sternal head of the pectoralis major. Before performing the bony detachment, the surgeon can either retract the clavicular head and leave it attached to the humerus, or detach it and reinsert it later at the site of the bony defect created at the site of the bony harvesting of the sternal head of the pectoralis major. We prefer the latter because it makes the freeing of the sternal head of the pectoralis major and obtaining full excursion easier. We use a combination of electrical saw and small osteotomes to perform the bony detachment of the insertion of the sternal head of the pectoralis major. Once the tendon is detached with its bony insertion, the tendon is tagged with a nonabsorbable suture to facilitate its mobilization and transfer (Fig. 18-12). The rest of the steps are very similar to those in the description above, except for the attachment of the tendon. The lower scapula is detached and the lateral distal aspect of it is debrided to obtain bleeding bone (Fig. 18-13). The detached tendon is passed from the anterior to posterior using a grasping instrument (Fig. 18-14), and then multiple (at least five) No. 2 nonabsorbable sutures are placed in transosseous fashion to be used for the repair. Then, bone-on-bone repair is performed using the sutures as cerclage sutures. If the clavicular head was detached, it is reattached at this time to the proximal humerus at the level of the bone defect that is created from bone harvesting. The technique of attachment is very similar to that for biceps repair.

Postoperative Management

Postoperatively, the patient is told to use the sling full time and to avoid any abduction of the shoulder. At 6

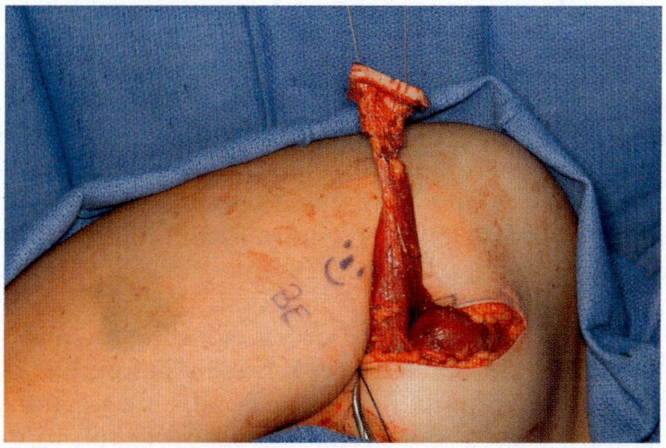

FIGURE 18-12: Sternal head of the pectoralis major detached with its bony insertion and dissected to prepare it for the transfer to the scapula.

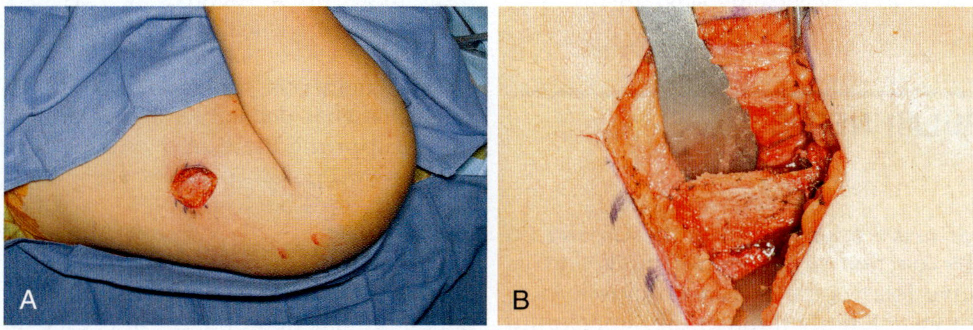

FIGURE 18-13: **A,** Incision placed just distal and lateral to the palpable distal aspect of the scapula. **B,** Preparation of the distal corner of the scapula to have bleeding fresh bone in preparation for the bony transfer.

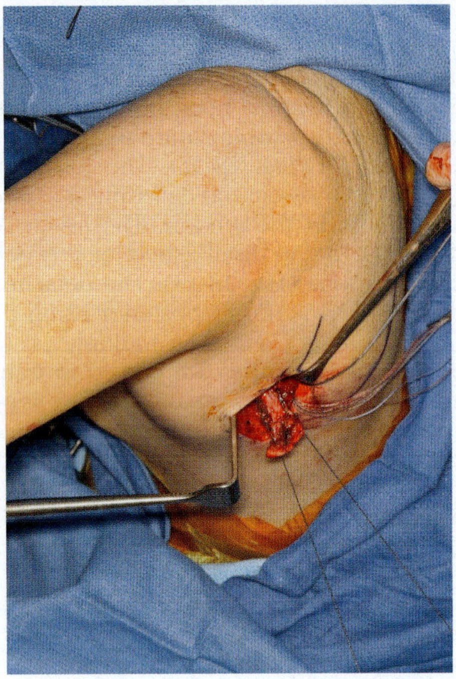

FIGURE 18-14: The sternal head of the pectoralis major is passed from the anterior to the posterior wound and is now ready to be repaired to the distal aspect of the scapula.

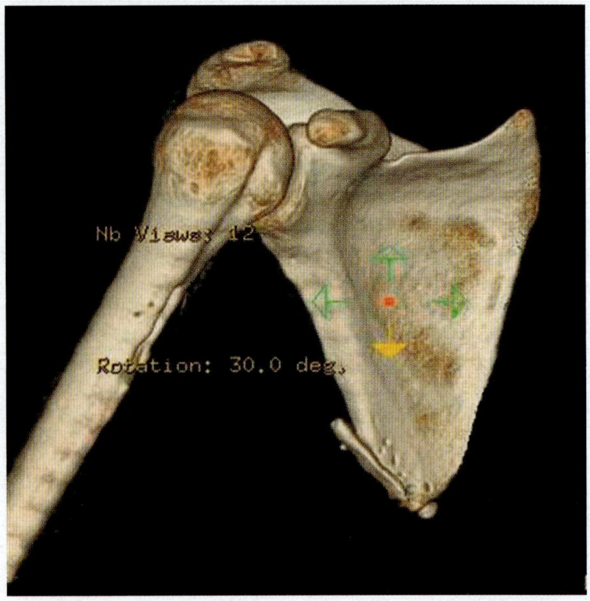

FIGURE 18-15: Three-dimensional computed tomography scan of the scapula showing the healed bony attachment of the sternal head of the pectoralis major to the distal aspect of the scapula.

weeks after surgery, the sling may be discarded and the patient allowed to resume all normal daily activities with the arm, although lifting of objects heavier than 1 kg is not permitted. A formal physical therapy program is not usually necessary. Patients tend to regain a normal range of motion quite readily. It is assumed that healing takes place during the initial 3- to 6-month period, and therefore return to manual labor or sporting activities is allowed after 6 months. However, early failure has occasionally been reported after pectoralis major transfer, apparently related to a premature return to full function before complete healing.[44,93] If a patient, especially an athlete, who has undergone direct transfer of the bony insertion of the sternal head of the pectoralis major wishes to return early to sports activities, a CT scan of the scapula is obtained and the patient is allowed to return much more quickly to full sports activities if it shows adequate bone-to-bone healing (Fig. 18-15).

SUPRASCAPULAR NERVE

Anatomy

The suprascapular nerve originates from the C5 and C6 nerve roots at the junction of the upper trunk and its divisions. The nerve follows the omohyoid muscle posteriorly and then runs inferiorly through the suprascapular notch—a region where it is relatively fixed in position—bridged by the superior transverse scapular ligament. The suprascapular artery and vein typically pass superior to the ligament. After exiting the suprascapular notch, the nerve gives off branches that innervate the supraspinatus. It then continues medial to the superior edge of the glenoid and enters the spinoglenoid notch at the lateral margin of the scapular spine.

As the nerve travels posteriorly, it may be less than 20 mm from the glenoid edge.[19] In the spinoglenoid notch, the spinoglenoid ligament can potentially impinge on the nerve. A spinoglenoid ligament however is not present in all patients.[97] After exiting the spinoglenoid notch, the nerve divides into two to four branches that enter the infraspinatus. Near the suprascapular notch, the suprascapular nerve also supplies articular branches to the shoulder joints. These fibers might explain the pain experienced by patients with suprascapular nerve lesions at the transverse scapular ligament. In contrast, more distal lesions, such as at the spinoglenoid notch, characteristically produce painless atrophy of the infraspinatus.

The cutaneous supply of the suprascapular nerve is still somewhat debatable. Some have described sensory fibers supplying the skin over the posterior of the shoulder; however, few patients are noted to have loss of sensation after nerve injury.

Etiology

Suprascapular neuropathy can occur due to a variety of causes.[195] Direct blunt trauma to the shoulder or sudden twisting of the shoulder can acutely injure the nerve. A

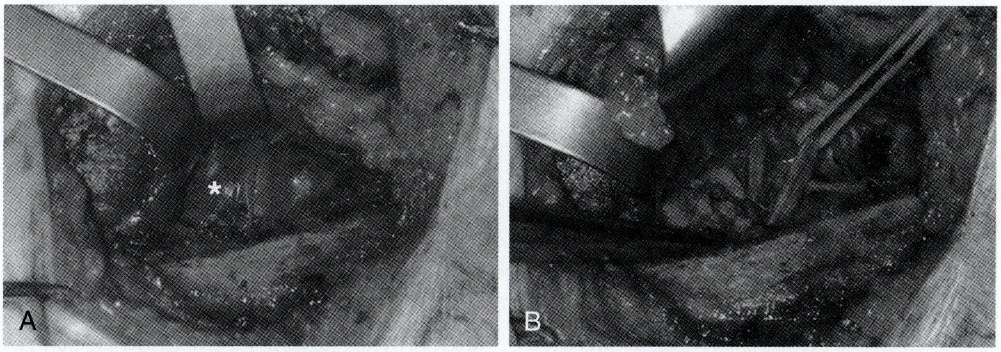

FIGURE 18-16: Suprascapular nerve compression. This 50-year-old man had left shoulder weakness over 6 months and was found to have moderate supraspinatus and infraspinatus weakness (grade 3/5) and atrophy. Electromyography showed denervation changes in the supraspinatus and infraspinatus muscles. Magnetic resonance imaging demonstrated a large ganglion cyst near the suprascapular notch. **A,** At surgery, when the supraspinatus was retracted anteriorly, a large ganglion cyst (*asterisk*) was observed compressing the suprascapular nerve near the suprascapular notch. The nerve was splayed over the top of the cyst and flattened in appearance. **B,** The cyst was resected and the nerve decompressed.

compressive injury can develop at the suprascapular or spinoglenoid notch.

A common cause of nerve compression in this region is a ganglion cyst (Fig. 18-16).[6,7,21,69,128,158] The origin of a cyst in this region is presumed to be from the glenohumeral joint, and it is very often associated with degenerative tears of the glenoid labrum.[7,170] A rare type of cyst, an intraneural ganglion cyst, can affect the suprascapular nerve. With this lesion, mucin is contained within the epineurium of the peripheral nerve. Suprascapular intraneural ganglion cysts have been shown to originate from the glenohumeral joint and to track along the articular branch into the parent nerve as far as the neck (Fig. 18-17). They have also been associated with superior labrum anterior and posterior tears.[174]

Repetitive rotatory motion of the shoulder, such as occurs during many sporting activities, can cause a chronic traction injury of the nerve. Neuropathy of the suprascapular nerve has been noted in participants of baseball, volleyball, tennis, and weightlifting.[1,6,21,25,41,46,59,167] Parsonage-Turner syndrome (acute brachial neuritis) can also result in an idiopathic etiology of suprascapular neuropathy. In rare instances a fracture of the scapula that enters the suprascapular notch can damage the nerve.[23,57,171]

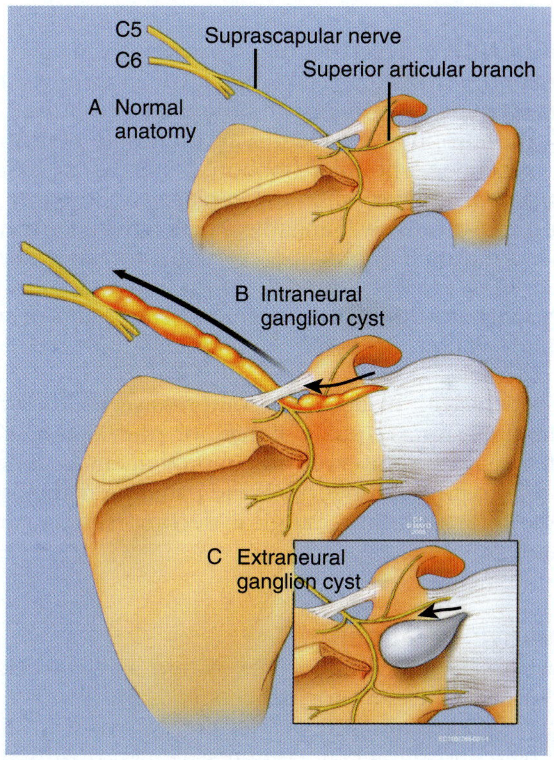

FIGURE 18-17: **A,** Normal anatomy of the suprascapular nerve in the vicinity of the shoulder. **B,** Proximal propagation of a suprascapular intraneural ganglion cyst from the glenohumeral joint along an articular branch into the parent nerve. **C,** An extraneural ganglion cyst originating from the glenohumeral joint may extrinsically compress the neighboring suprascapular nerve. (From Spinner RJ, Amrami KK, Kliot M, et al. Suprascapular intraneural ganglia and glenohumeral joint connections. *J Neurosurg.* 2006;104:551-557.)

Clinical Manifestation and Diagnosis

Patients with a suprascapular nerve injury at the suprascapular notch commonly complain of pain over the posterior and lateral aspects of the shoulder. Pain on deep palpation over the suprascapular notch itself might also be present. In addition, patients might have weakness of abduction, external rotation, or both and may be noted to have atrophy of the supraspinatus and infraspinatus. In many individuals the supraspinatus is difficult to visualize because a well-developed trapezius covers the supraspinatus and makes it difficult to see muscle wasting. Loss of muscle bulk in the infraspinatus however is fairly easy to see on clinical examination. Some patients do not demonstrate any atrophy on examination; shoulder pain and mild weakness of abduction may be the only findings, making a correct diagnosis difficult.

An appropriate clinical examination with EMG/NCS often detects suprascapular neuropathy. The diagnosis can easily be made if conduction velocity is delayed (in comparison to the contralateral side) and fibrillation potentials are noted in the supraspinatus or infraspinatus. In some patients EMG/NCS shows only mild involvement. These patients should be examined carefully for other shoulder pathology that could have been missed during the clinical examination. Surgical treatment tends not to be as beneficial in these patients as in those with substantial changes on EMG/NCS.[7]

Shoulder pain can be caused by several conditions, and thus cervical disk disease, rotator cuff tear, impingement syndrome, and acromioclavicular joint degeneration should all be excluded in these patients, especially those with only mild EMG/NCS findings.

Nonoperative Treatment

Treatment of a patient with suprascapular neuropathy is based on the type of injury and the duration of disability, pain, and atrophy. A patient with a chronic neuropathy from repetitive shoulder motion, such as a baseball or volleyball player, should be placed in therapy and treated conservatively. Similarly, a patient with Parsonage-Turner syndrome should be observed for an extended period. Both groups, if monitored for 2 to 3 months, tend to demonstrate clinical improvement. The results of surgical intervention in these two groups are somewhat unpredictable.[7]

A patient with evidence of compressive neuropathy at either the suprascapular notch or the spinoglenoid notch should be observed for improvement in function over a 3- to 4-month period. If the patient remains symptomatic after that time, surgical decompression can be performed.

Operative Treatment

Early surgical intervention (i.e., within a few weeks) is rarely needed, except for patients with an obvious ganglion cyst noted on MRI or the rare patient with intractable pain and significant compressive neuropathy noted on EMG/NCS. Patients with Parsonage-Turner syndrome experience considerable pain for the first few weeks of the neuropathy, but typically, they do not require operative intervention because their symptoms tend to improve spontaneously over time.

The suprascapular nerve can be approached from an anterior, superior, or posterior direction. The anterior approach demands exposure of at least a portion of the brachial plexus and does not allow exposure of the spinoglenoid notch.[169] A direct superior approach performed by splitting the trapezius in line with its fibers has commonly been recommended. This technique however results in a deep surgical wound in which the suprascapular notch and superior transverse scapular ligament can be visualized, but only a small distance of the suprascapular nerve itself can be exposed.

The posterior approach detaches the trapezius from the spine of the scapula 6 to 8 cm medial to the lateral edge of the acromion. The supraspinatus is then retracted posteriorly to visualize the suprascapular nerve and the notch. Careful exposure should be performed while in the area of the suprascapular notch because the artery and vein travel above this, and occasionally, a branch of the nerve may be positioned above rather than below the superior transverse scapular ligament. If greater exposure of the nerve is needed with this approach, two additional steps can be performed: the trapezius can be detached laterally and anteriorly onto the acromioclavicular joint to allow wide exposure of the nerve. However, at closure, the trapezius will need to be accurately repaired back to the acromion.

If the suprascapular nerve needs to be explored into the spinoglenoid notch, the posterior deltoid can be detached from the spine of the scapula, and exposure of the nerve from the infraspinatus to the suprascapular notch can then be achieved.

In cases involving a ganglion at the spinoglenoid notch, arthroscopic debridement of the cyst is an excellent technique. Arthroscopy also allows visualization of the joint and the opportunity to debride any associated labral tears. Most of these posterosuperior labral tears are not amenable to surgical reattachment. Recently, arthroscopic and endoscopic approaches to decompress the suprascapular nerve at the suprascapular and spinoglenoid notches have been described.[17,92,152]

Outcomes

For patients with suprascapular neuropathy, good or better surgical results have been achieved in the recovery of supraspinatus function. Infraspinatus recovery is more variable. The best results are seen in patients with nerve lesions from masses; the worst are in patients with neuropathy caused by fractures or severe trauma.

THORACIC OUTLET SYNDROME

Thoracic outlet syndrome is a difficult condition to accurately diagnose because of the lack of a gold standard for confirming the diagnosis. Some clinicians believe that it is overdiagnosed, whereas others think that it should be treated more commonly. The correct diagnosis is made more difficult because of the preponderance of subjective symptoms with few objective tests. Both radiographic (including MR neurography) and electrodiagnostic tests have been used to support the diagnosis, but no test is specific for thoracic outlet syndrome. The diagnosis remains primarily one of exclusion and is based on a patient's history and symptoms.

Clinical Manifestation

Despite any controversy about the prevalence of thoracic outlet syndrome, shoulder surgeons will undoubtedly encounter many patients with thoracic outlet symptoms (disputed thoracic outlet syndrome). These patients might complain of pain in the shoulder or neck region with radiation to the forearm or hand. Paresthesias might radiate along the upper part of the arm to the hand. Often, patients perceive loss of sensation along the small and ring fingers. Bilateral symptoms are relatively common, with symptoms greater on the dominant side.

A patient's pain typically begins gradually without a history of trauma. Trauma and impending lawsuits frequently becloud the clinical scenario. Patients often complain of difficulty working overhead. Arm traction, such as carrying a heavy bag or luggage, can increase the symptoms. Although the patient might complain of hand weakness and loss of sensation, the results of motor examination are typically normal.

True neurogenic thoracic outlet syndrome can result from a variant relationship of the neurologic structures to a cervical rib or to fibrous bands and the like, and it typically produces lower trunk compression. These patients might have subtle ulnar-sided lumbrical weakness, or they may display a Gilliatt-Sumner hand (more severe weakness in the intrinsic musculature of the hand beyond the ulnar nerve distribution).[186] In addition, neurovascular compression can result from a reduced costoclavicular space (Figs. 18-18 to 18-20). A vascular disorder (venous or arterial) is occasionally responsible for the symptoms, although this type of vascular thoracic outlet syndrome is less common. In such cases patients often display objective findings, such as a change in the color of their hands or a chronically reduced pulse. Noninvasive vascular studies or an angiogram might demonstrate a compressed area in the vascular system of the upper extremity.

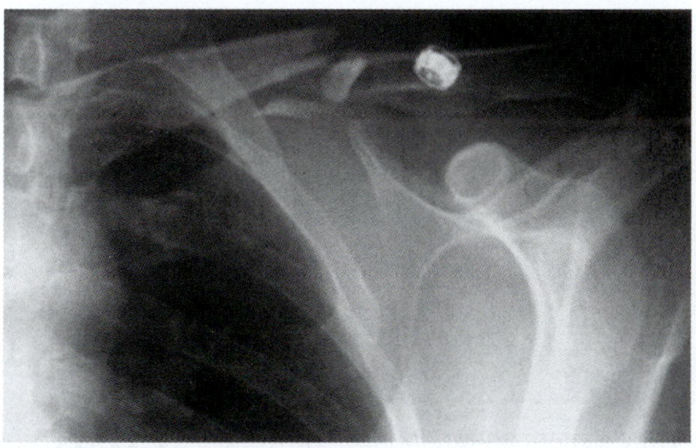

FIGURE 18-18: Clavicle fracture and upper trunk neurapraxia. This 48-year-old man sustained a midshaft clavicle fracture after a fall while snowboarding. Shortly after the injury he noted severe weakness in abduction and mild weakness in elbow flexion. An upper trunk lesion was diagnosed. Plain radiographs demonstrate mild apical angulation of the clavicle fracture. The distal fragment was displaced 8 mm inferiorly. Small butterfly fragments were adjacent to the fracture. This neurologic deficit improved after 4 months.

Diagnosis

Several provocative tests have been described for thoracic outlet syndrome, most of which were originally proposed for vascular conditions.

The Adson test has been described for compression of the subclavian artery. The seated patient turns the head to the affected side while inspiring deeply. The patient's radial artery is palpated and checked for loss of pulse. However, loss of pulse does not by itself indicate thoracic outlet syndrome because a large percentage of the population demonstrates a variation in pulse during different upper extremity maneuvers.

The Wright test involves hyperabduction of the shoulders, with the elbows flexed more than 45 degrees.

The Roos test involves elevation of the arm to 90 degrees of shoulder abduction and external rotation with 90 degree of elbow flexion accompanied by rapid opening and closing of the hands for up to 3 minutes. A modification of the Roos test is the elevated arm stress test, in which the hands are repetitively opened and closed, with the shoulders elevated 180 degrees and the elbows extended. The test is considered positive when the patient reports a reproduction of the symptoms within 30 to 60 seconds.

Percussion of the brachial plexus in the supraclavicular fossa may produce radiating paresthesias.

None of these tests are universally accepted as a gold standard for thoracic outlet syndrome. It is not uncommon to obtain a false-positive result when several of these tests are performed in an asymptomatic patient. The finding of a cervical rib on chest films must also be cautiously interpreted because it is a variation found in 1% of the population.

Treatment

Thoracic outlet syndrome remains a diagnosis of exclusion because no diagnostic tests can accurately pinpoint the condition. In making the diagnosis all aspects of the history and physical examination should be considered carefully. Conservative measures are usually effective and should be the primary treatment. Surgical treatment may offer some benefit in selected patients; however, the techniques are demanding and the potential for complications is high.

If a patient is believed to have thoracic outlet syndrome, conservative management is the usual initial treatment. The patients are taught to avoid activities that aggravate their symptoms. Poor posture is corrected and physical conditioning is improved. An aerobic exercise plan will strengthen the accessory muscles of inspiration, help correct muscle imbalance, and lead to weight loss. Usually, patients follow a conservative management program for at least 9 to 12 months before operative options are considered.

If the patient remains sufficiently symptomatic or disabled, decompression of the brachial plexus with or

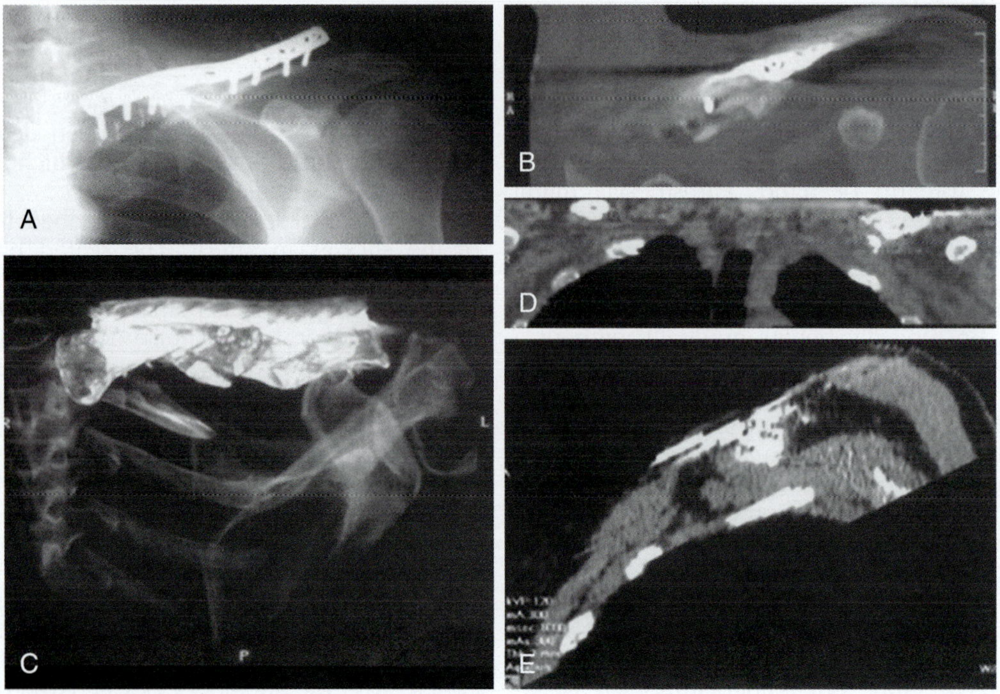

FIGURE 18-19: Brachial plexopathy caused by clavicle malunion. The clavicle fracture in this patient (shown in Fig. 18-18) progressed to nonunion. He also experienced pain near his acromioclavicular joint. He underwent a takedown of the nonunion, bone grafting, and internal fixation with a dynamic compression plate along with distal clavicle resection. The week after surgery he noted ulnar-sided hand paresthesias and then weakness in the hand. Over the next month, severe but incomplete lesions affecting the posterior cord, medial cord, and lateral contribution to the medial cord developed. There is always the potential for iatrogenic compression of the brachial plexus in the thoracic inlet for surgeons operating in or around the clavicle. **A,** Plain radiographs showed the plate fixation and the inferior callus. **B** and **C,** Computed tomographic scans with reconstruction better characterized the inferior callus and showed the reduced costoclavicular space. **D** and **E,** On the left side, the shortest distance between the undersurface of the clavicle callus and the first rib was 10 to 11 mm, versus 13 to 15 mm on the right in the coronal and sagittal planes (**E**). In addition, a well-defined fat plane beneath the clavicle seen on the right side was effaced by a soft tissue density on the left (**D**).

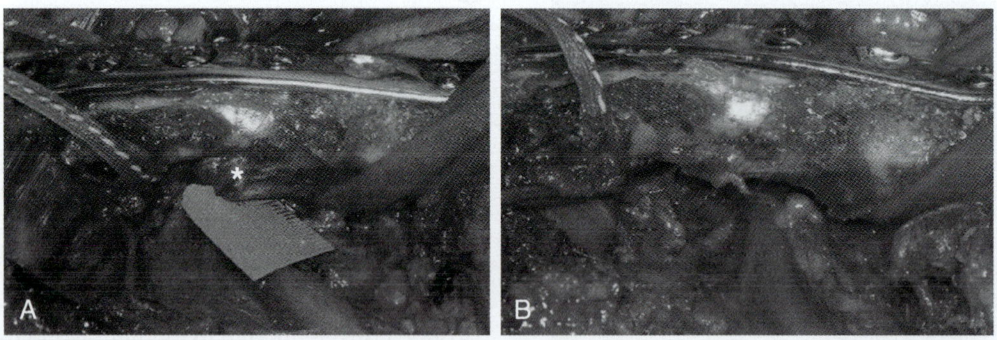

FIGURE 18-20: Brachial plexopathy caused by clavicle malunion (the same patient shown in Figs. 18-18 and 18-19). **A,** Surgery was performed in view of the worsening deficit. A large hypertrophic portion of callus (*asterisk*) was seen compressing the lateral cord. **B,** The bony prominence was resected. Ample room was restored for the underlying neural elements. Passive range of motion did not alter the space, and a first rib resection was not deemed necessary. In the recovery room the patient's hand strength had improved one full grade. He made a full recovery by 3 months. Restoration of a normal costoclavicular space has been associated with favorable recovery of neural function in these types of cases.

without rib resection may be considered. The most common surgical approaches are transaxillary,[159] supraclavicular, or a combination of these. These procedures have advantages and disadvantages, and each has its advocates and critics. However, in general, the results of these techniques have been similar. Leffert and Perlmutter reported a high percentage of excellent results with the transaxillary approach, and Sanders and colleagues reported similar results with a supraclavicular approach.[111,166] Sheth and Campbell reported better symptomatic relief with transaxillary resection of the first rib as compared to supraclavicular neuroplasty of the brachial plexus without rib resection in a randomized trial that compared these two techniques.[168] Surgery should be performed earlier in patients with neurogenic thoracic outlet syndrome.

PARSONAGE-TURNER SYNDROME (BRACHIAL PLEXUS NEUROPATHY)

Brachial plexus neuropathy is also known as *idiopathic brachial plexitis, brachial neuritis, neuralgic amyotrophy, brachial plexus neuropathy, serum neuritis,* and *shoulder-girdle neuritis* among other terms. It also is known as *Parsonage-Turner syndrome* after the two physicians who presented the first large series of patients in 1943.[143] The description dates back to 1887 when Dreschfeld[55] reported two siblings with nontraumatic brachial plexopathy and to 1897 when Feinberg[70] described a case of plexitis after influenza. It is a relatively uncommon condition overall, with an annual incidence rate of one or two cases per 100,000 population.[14] Nevertheless, it is encountered several times per year by those treating shoulder or brachial plexus disorders.

ETIOLOGY

The etiology of this nontraumatic condition remains unclear. It is thought to be immune mediated or inflammatory in nature. Its onset can follow a viral illness or other infection, immunization, pregnancy, trauma, extreme exercise, and surgery.[96,117,127,194] In some ways it is thought to be similar to Bell's palsy affecting the facial nerve. Several pathologic specimens of affected brachial plexus elements have revealed inflammatory changes.[179] A familial component exists as well (hereditary neuralgic amyotrophy)[146,151]; these patients can experience recurrent episodes and are affected at an earlier age than is typical.

Clinical Manifestation

Patients typically have an acute onset of periscapular pain that lasts several days to weeks. Motor weakness in the shoulder and arm associated with sensory loss ensues, usually when the pain is resolving. This triad of pain and motor and sensory disturbance is not always present, and painless neuropathy occurs occasionally. Certain peripheral nerves seem to be preferentially affected, including the long thoracic,[68,142] axillary, suprascapular, anterior interosseous, and radial nerves. The process often involves various components of the brachial plexus diffusely[67] and occurs bilaterally in more than 10% of cases. Other nonbrachial plexus nerves, such as the phrenic nerve, or cranial nerves, such as the spinal accessory nerve, may be involved. The process can also affect a single nerve, such as the anterior interosseous nerve. Men are affected slightly more often than women, generally between the third and sixth decades of life.[160] The disorder is typically monophasic, but recurrent attacks rarely occur.

Diagnosis

The diagnosis of Parsonage-Turner syndrome can often be established by a good history and physical examination, with the exclusion of other disorders. Electrodiagnostic studies typically reveal a patchy, multifocal neurologic process that supports the diagnosis. Other serologic studies and cerebrospinal fluid tests are usually normal. Imaging studies reveal nonspecific changes (such as a high signal intensity in affected muscles on T2-weighted MRI from denervation) but help eliminate other more common diagnoses of the neck and shoulder.

Parsonage-Turner syndrome is often misdiagnosed and is a great masquerader of other diseases. It should be considered when establishing the differential diagnosis of shoulder pain or muscle weakness in the upper limb. It can mimic orthopedic conditions, especially shoulder problems, such as rotator cuff disease, impingement syndrome, adhesive capsulitis, bursitis, and others. Neurologic disorders, including cervical radiculopathy, should be excluded, as should other peripheral nerve conditions, such as mononeuritis multiplex, chronic inflammatory demyelinating polyneuropathy or entrapment syndromes, and transverse myelitis. Anterior interosseous nerve paralysis and long thoracic neuropathy are examples of nerve lesions that are not uncommonly classified as entrapment because of their spontaneous onset that more accurately represents Parsonage-Turner syndrome. In such cases surgeons may take false credit for improving the clinical course by decompressing a nerve that might have recovered anyway based on its own natural history.

Treatment

Treatment is usually supportive and directed at decreasing pain with antiinflammatory agents and other analgesics. Some physicians have tried steroids or intravenous immunoglobulin, although their efficacy has not been established. Maintaining range of motion and performing strengthening exercises are important, and a course of physical therapy is helpful. Residual deformities may be helped in certain cases with tendon transfers, which can provide improved stability or function and pain relief.

Prognosis

Overall, the prognosis is generally favorable, although recovery can take several years. However, not all patients recover, and many experience residual deficits, such as mild scapular winging. It is unknown whether these deficits predispose patients to other shoulder pathology in the long term because of faulty shoulder mechanics. Although this condition has been perceived as one that produces mainly reversible deficits, one series with late follow-up has demonstrated that patients can experience significant disability, limitations in activities of daily living, persistent pain, and difficulty with returning to their original work.[79]

BRACHIAL PLEXUS INJURIES

Brachial plexus lesions (Fig. 18-21) can lead to significant physical disability, psychologic duress, and financial hardship. Complete loss of the use of the limb or a partial loss, such as the limb not allowing the positioning of a working hand in space, results in significant impairment with devastating consequences. Traumatic lesions typically affect young men and often result from automobile or motorcycle accidents. Other mechanisms may be responsible for brachial plexus lesions, including obstetric birth palsy (occurring in approximately 1 in 2000 live births), penetrating injuries, radiation, compression (such as by a mass effect) (Fig. 18-22), tumors, entrapment, iatrogenic causes (such as after first rib resection or shoulder surgery), and inflammation.

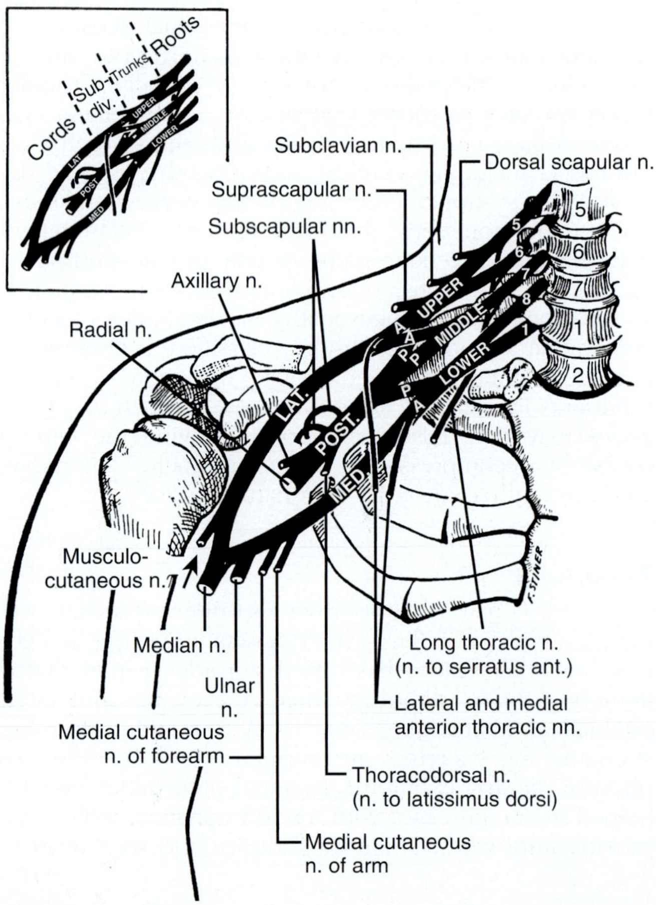

FIGURE 18-21: The brachial plexus. (From Haymaker W, Woodhall B. *Peripheral Nerve Injuries.* Philadelphia: WB Saunders; 1953:210.)

Types

Closed brachial plexus injuries are traction injuries. They result from distraction of the forequarter from the body. Narakas summarized the potential disrupting forces well: "The motorcyclist thrown in the air will have multiple impacts: the car, the roof, the road, each of which will have their own natural history and possible injury."[132] These forces can lead to supraclavicular, retroclavicular, infraclavicular, or combined patterns of injury that affect the brachial plexus from the rootlets to the terminal branches.

Supraclavicular injuries are the most common and the most severe; they are typically related to high-speed injuries. Such injuries most commonly lead to complete lesions (panplexal injuries). Upper-pattern lesions are the second most common (C5, C6, ± C7); lower element (C8, T1) injuries are very rare. Downward traction on the arm or forcible widening of the shoulder-neck angle produces upper trunk injuries, whereas lower trunk injuries are produced by forcible upward traction of the arm. Depending on the duration and the amount of force, stretch injuries can result in neuroma, rupture, or avulsion. Stretch lesions are often longitudinal injuries. Nerve lesions that are in continuity have the best prognosis for recovery but still often need surgical intervention; rupture and avulsion have the poorest prognosis and require surgical intervention. Preganglionic injuries can lead to avulsion from the spinal cord (central avulsion) or rupture just distal to the spinal cord (intradural rupture). Preganglionic injuries can affect the ventral or dorsal root or, more commonly, both of these. Avulsion is more common in the lower elements because of anatomic restraints in the upper levels. The upper elements have proximal branches (e.g., to the phrenic or serratus anterior) and transverse radicular ligaments that may be protective, whereas the lower elements are without these branches or ligaments.

Infraclavicular injuries usually develop after a lower energy impact and are often due to compression rather than traction. Many are incomplete lesions and recover spontaneously without surgery.[109] However, complete lesions do occur, sometimes with rupture and even avulsion. Infraclavicular lesions usually affect the cords and terminal branches and, occasionally, the roots. Injury to one or more terminal branches may occur either as a primary or as a secondary site of injury, together with a supraclavicular or infraclavicular injury. These terminal branch injuries seem to occur at sites where the nerves are relatively fixed. For example, the musculocutaneous nerve may be predisposed to injury at several sites: where it penetrates the coracobrachialis; the suprascapular nerve, at the scapular notch; and the axillary nerve, at the quadrilateral space. Associated vascular injuries

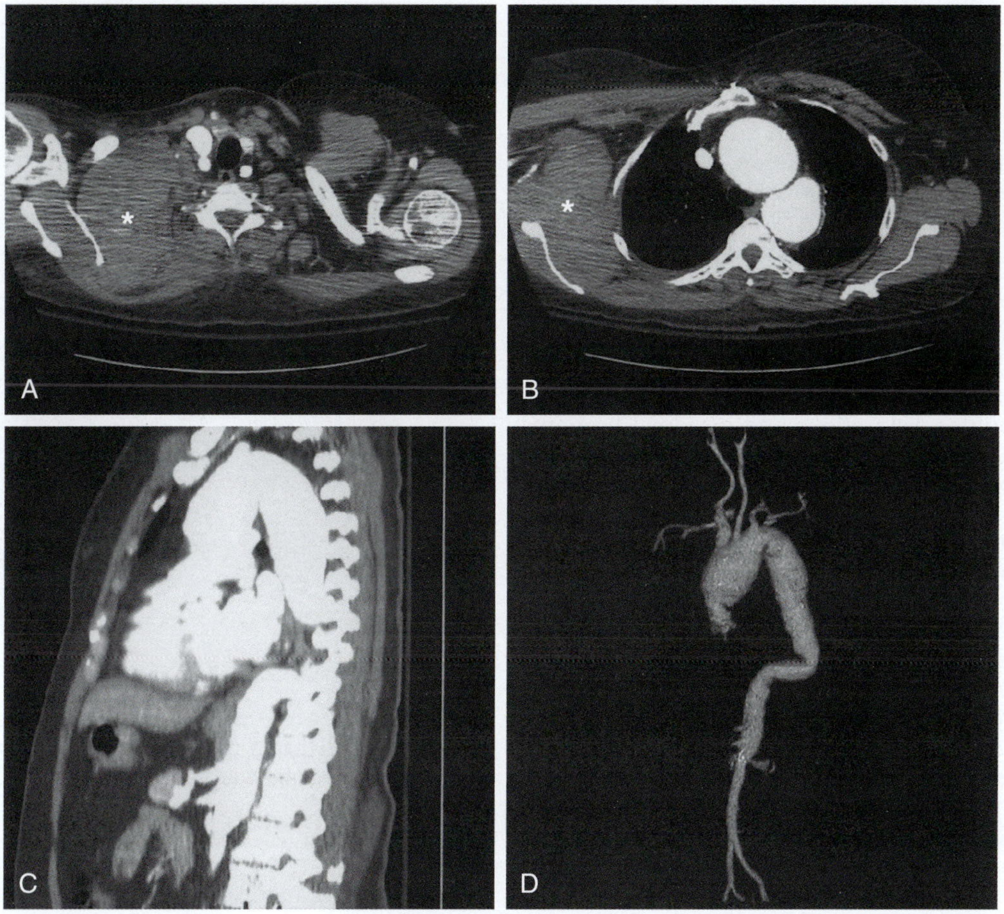

FIGURE 18-22: Brachial plexus compression by a large hematoma. A 55-year-old woman had a history of a previous ascending aortic aneurysm replacement with a composite graft. She was receiving chronic anticoagulation with warfarin (Coumadin) for her aortic valve replacement. She fell from a horse and sustained a tibial plateau fracture. She used crutches clumsily, and a neck hematoma developed "spontaneously"; painful paralysis developed in the right upper limb 1 week later. **A** and **B,** A large (12 × 9 cm) hematoma (*asterisk*), spanning from the supraclavicular portion to the scapula, is compressing the brachial plexus. **C** and **D,** Three-dimensional reconstruction showing a 7-cm aortic aneurysm (also seen in **B**). The aneurysm was an incidental finding, and the hematoma was the result of crutch use and not from a ruptured aneurysm.

occur in 10% to 20% of infraclavicular brachial plexus cases. Coexisting bony injuries (such as clavicle, scapula, or humerus fractures or dislocations) can contribute to the neural injury acutely or in a delayed fashion (e.g., with clavicle nonunion or malunion). Operative dissection of the infraclavicular brachial plexus may be extremely difficult because of the dense fibrosis, which may be especially apparent in cases of previous vascular reconstruction.

Diagnosis

The diagnosis of brachial plexus injuries is often elusive, and the resultant delay can have a negative impact on timely referral for specialized treatment. The diagnosis can be suspected from a good history supported by physical examination and confirmed by electrodiagnostic or imaging studies. The mechanism of the injury—in particular, the position of the neck and arm in relation to the body during trauma—needs to be evaluated. A thorough primary and secondary assessment should be included to identify concomitant injuries to the head, chest, vessels, long bones, pelvis, and spine (associated symptoms and signs of myelopathy should also be sought). Multitrauma is common, and often more critical injuries receive attention, with other (not necessarily minor) injuries potentially being missed. Detailed neurologic testing reveals deficits that affect a discrete pattern.

Ideally, the diagnosis of an injury to the brachial plexus is made in the emergency department. Additional information helpful for the diagnosis includes whether the injury is complete or incomplete, whether it involves the supraclavicular or infraclavicular region (or there is more than one injury), and whether it is a preganglionic or postganglionic injury. These localizations are helpful in planning treatment and predicting the prognosis.

Other diagnostic studies complement the physical examination. Plain radiographs of the chest might reveal an elevated diaphragm from a phrenic nerve injury. Radiographs of the cervical spine and other bones might demonstrate fractures. Angiography should be performed if vascular injury is suspected, especially when an acute brachial plexus injury is present in conjunction with an expanding hematoma, first-rib fracture, widened mediastinum, or upper limb pulse abnormality. Electrodiagnostic studies are most useful about 3 weeks after the injury; these can further localize the lesion and assess the degree of neural involvement. Computed tomography (CT)-myelography[129] should be performed when a supraclavicular lesion has been diagnosed and a preganglionic injury is being considered. We have used shoulder MRI to assess patients with nerve injuries, particularly those associated with shoulder dislocations and proximal humerus fractures to ensure rotator cuff integrity, as well as in isolated suprascapular nerve lesions to identify ganglia. MRI of the brachial plexus is rapidly improving, but we have not yet found this imaging modality to be as helpful as CT-myelography in identifying root avulsions.

A number of features that can be gleaned from a careful history, physical examination, and electrodiagnostic and imaging studies can suggest a preganglionic injury. Such features include deafferentation pain; the finding of Horner syndrome (miosis, ptosis, anhidrosis, and enophthalmos), weak rhomboids or serratus anterior muscles, or the absence of Tinel's sign in the neck on physical examination; electrical studies showing fibrillations in the paraspinal muscles or rhomboids or preserved sensory nerve action potentials in an anesthetic hand with absent motor nerve action potentials; and an elevated hemidiaphragm or associated cervical fractures on radiographs and pseudomeningoceles (Fig. 18-23) or absent nerve rootlets on myelography.

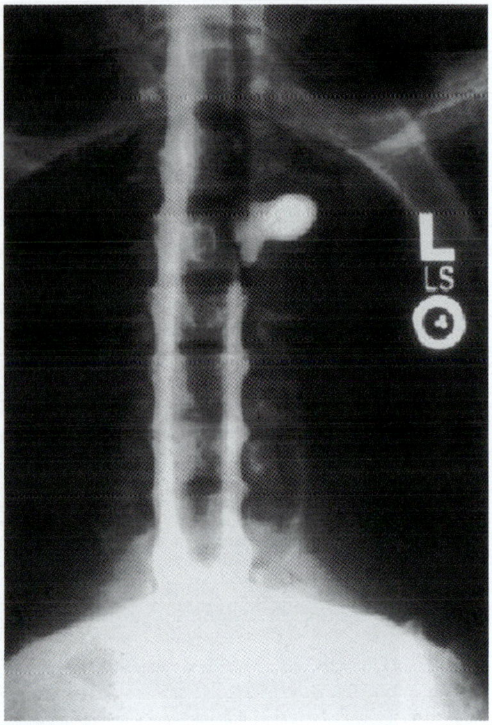

FIGURE 18-23: Large posttraumatic pseudomeningocele suggestive of a preganglionic lesion.

The timely diagnosis of a brachial plexus injury has therapeutic implications. For closed injuries, patients are typically observed for spontaneous improvement over the first several months. It is important to obtain a baseline examination and then monitor clinical and electrophysiologic examinations serially for improvement. Patients who demonstrate improvement within this time frame have sustained a neurapraxic injury. However, it is difficult to preoperatively determine which axonotmetic lesions (those of Sunderland grades II to IV) will recover spontaneously despite their differing prognoses. Grade II is associated with good spontaneous recovery, but grade IV has a poor prognosis.

Patients should receive physical therapy for range of motion to prevent soft tissue contractures and to strengthen working muscles. Neuropathic pain should be managed by a specialist, especially when it is refractory to first-line medications, as is often the case with deafferentation pain.

Nonoperative Treatment

Treating neuropathic pain remains as difficult and challenging an issue as treating loss of function and can also require long-term patient follow-up. Neuropathic pain is best treated by a multidisciplinary approach within a pain clinic setting. Patients can be managed with a combination of various medications titrated to effect by experts in the field under close observation. Other modalities, including psychologic support and physical therapy, should be admixed. Pain can improve over time, especially as reinnervation occurs. Primary nerve-related surgery can help relieve neuropathic pain, either with neurolysis or the resection of neuromas, or with nerve transfers. Patients with refractory pain from a root avulsion can also be treated by creating lesions at the dorsal root entry zone (DREZ lesions)[133] or by spinal cord or motor cortex stimulation.[162]

Operative Treatment

Indications

The decision to operate is complex. Surgery must balance the risks and benefits of waiting for potential spontaneous recovery with the realization that the window of opportunity for nerve recovery is finite. The timing of surgery is critical. Surgery is indicated for closed injuries when sequential examinations have not established objective recovery by 3 to 6 months. Clinical recovery, especially in the proximal muscles, is a favorable sign; however, caution should be taken to avoid undue optimism as there is potential for overinterpretation of an advancing Tinel's sign, a positive squeeze test, or nascent potentials on EMG without additional signs of clinical recovery. If avulsion injury is suspected, surgery may be performed even earlier.

Nerve injuries from sharp objects, such as knives, should be explored early (within several days). Patients with an increasing deficit under observation should undergo early exploration. An increasing deficit often indicates a vascular injury, such as from a pseudoaneurysm or an expanding hematoma. Nerve injuries associated with blunt or contusive lacerations should be explored after several weeks when the nerve ends have demarcated; nerve ends that might have been identified at the time of immediate vascular repair should be tacked down under tension, with definitive treatment performed several weeks later.

Nerve injuries associated with gunshot wounds should generally be treated nonoperatively; the majority of these are not associated with disruption of elements,[99] are neurapraxic, and improve spontaneously. Fortunately, our experience with civilian injuries is limited, and we base our current approach on our vast experience from war injuries. Patients initially evaluated at a late stage (after 9 or 12 months) are better treated with reconstruction (e.g., functional free muscle transfer, tendon transfers, or joint fusion) than with standard nerve surgery (i.e., grafting). Patients in whom distal nerve transfers, such as the Oberlin transfer, can be performed might still benefit from such reconstruction up to 15 months after injury.

Planning

Before surgery, the surgical team should formulate a preoperative plan based on a careful review of all existing clinical and electrophysiologic examinations and studies. Surgeons need to consider a range of factors and tabulate a list of what is and is not working, what is available for transfer, and what is needed. Surgeons must balance realistic goals (e.g., based on injury patterns or the timing of surgery) and expectations of the patient, the family, and themselves. Contingency plans should be established.

General Technique

The brachial plexus is exposed through a supraclavicular or infraclavicular approach, or both, depending on the level or levels of suspected injury. We favor exploration of both regions because we have been surprised by the frequency of double-level injuries. We use a transverse supraclavicular incision rather than a zigzag incision and a separate deltopectoral approach (with detachment of the pectoralis minor). Clavicular osteotomy is seldom necessary except in rare cases with predominantly retroclavicular pathology. If osteotomy is deemed necessary, predrilling and preplating should be performed with a low-contour compression plate (Fig. 18-24). Occasionally, a separate posterior approach to the shoulder or arm is necessary to expose more distal segments of the suprascapular, axillary, and radial nerves.

Exposure of the brachial plexus permits us to perform intraoperative electrophysiologic monitoring. It is well known that direct visualization or palpation of the external surface of a nerve does not accurately predict the nerve's histologic appearance or potential for recovery. We believe that a combination of intraoperative techniques is the most useful way to obtain additional data, define the nerve pathology, and establish the prognosis.

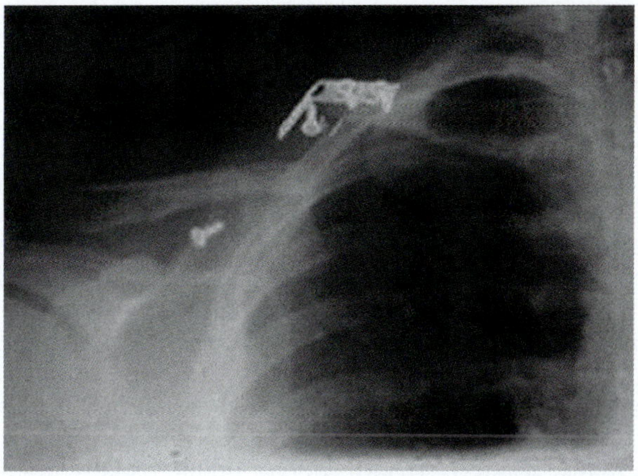

FIGURE 18-24: If clavicular osteotomy is necessary, it should be performed by a surgeon skilled in fixation. This case illustrates inadequate fixation of the clavicular osteotomy with a semitubular plate.

NAPs[100,101,188] can help distinguish preganglionic and postganglionic injuries and can differentiate between grades of axonotmetic injury. Somatosensory evoked potentials (SSEPs) may also be used to determine the presence or absence of nerve root avulsion. Although SSEPs test the sensory pathway per se, in most (but not all) cases, inferences can be drawn about the status of the ventral roots. Another shortcoming of SSEPs is that a positive response can be obtained with as few as 100 to 200 intact nerve fibers.[207] For example, avulsion may be diagnosed with an absent SSEP and a preganglionic NAP. A recovering neuroma will show a regenerative NAP (indicating that the axons are viable). A neuroma that does not conduct an NAP will exhibit flat tracing and will not result in clinical recovery. Motor evoked potentials with transcranial electrical stimulation are becoming more widely used and allow the theoretical advantage of testing the integrity of motor root function.[29,191]

All techniques require experience in interpretation. These types of recordings are better suited for detecting early regeneration in brachial plexus lesions than are compound muscle action potential recordings. Given the distance to the end-organ, it would not be expected that nerve reinnervation has reached the target muscle. However, in partial lesions compound muscle action potentials might also be helpful in determining the severity of the lesion (i.e., the number of functioning axons).

We do not perform hemilaminectomy[33] or histochemical analysis with choline acetyltransferase[89] to identify avulsions, although we recognize the appeal afforded by these techniques.

Nerve Repair

Nerve repair is seldom possible except in instances of acute, sharp injury treated urgently. Standard approaches to brachial plexus surgery include neurolysis of a recovering neuroma that shows a regenerative NAP and grafting of an advanced lesion that does not conduct an NAP or of a rupture; direct repair is not generally practical.[125]

Nerve stumps are sectioned back until good fascicular structure has been identified. Proximal dissection to a foraminal level is sometimes necessary to locate a fascicle of adequate quality in the proximal stump. Plexoplexal grafting is then accomplished by interfascicular repair with microsurgical techniques. Interpositional grafts are placed to ensure adequate coverage of the proximal and distal faces of the nerve ends. Grafts should be sutured in place without tension. Typically, the repairs are performed with the arm abducted and externally rotated. Donor nerve grafts usually include the sural nerve (unilaterally or bilaterally), but other cutaneous nerves in the forearm or arm can also be used. We place several 9-0 sutures to coapt the nerve ends and then reinforce the repair with fibrin glue. Grafts can be sutured in place individually or in cables (after being glued together).

After the repair is completed, the limb is gently mobilized through an arc of motion to test the tension. Unlike some other groups,[119] we do not use intraoperative histology to identify the fascicular structure. The limb is maintained in a shoulder immobilizer for 3 weeks to protect the suture lines. Thereafter, pendulum exercises are initiated and passive and active motion instituted. Therapists provide resting splints for immobile joints. Some groups prescribe electrical stimulation, although this technique has not been validated clinically. Patients are examined every 3 to 4 months for clinical signs of recovery.

Nerve Transfer

Avulsions or preganglionic injuries can be treated by nerve transfer. Nerve transfer (neurotization) exchanges a nonfunctioning nerve with a dispensable or redundant working nerve, nerve branch, or fascicle. Nerve transfers are useful to treat avulsions, to achieve more rapid or predictable recovery of a distal target (i.e., as an alternative to nerve grafting), and to power a free functioning muscle transfer. Nerve transfers provide a source of axons that permits surgeons to reconstruct additional targets with the intent of improving outcomes (Fig. 18-25). This should consist of a large number of pure motor or sensory axons, depending on the type of nerve transfer being performed, and preferably should be synergistic. Patients should be able to relearn the new function independently, although induction exercises and reeducation are necessary components of the postoperative program. Most importantly, when considering any nerve transfer, the cost/benefit ratio as well as the advantages and potential disadvantages of using a specific donor should be considered.

Popular nerve transfers include those of the intercostals,[54,126,130] distal spinal accessory, cervical plexus, thoracodorsal, and pectoral branches.[24] With some of the more aggressive nerve transfers, such as phrenic[84,182,206] or contralateral C7,[85,173] potential risks should be carefully considered. Use of the phrenic nerve and contralateral C7 increases the number of donor nerves available and may allow designing reconstructive strategies that permit more distal reinnervation. Preliminary experience with the hypoglossal nerve[71,118] has been disappointing however. The transfer of ulnar[183] or median[181] nerve

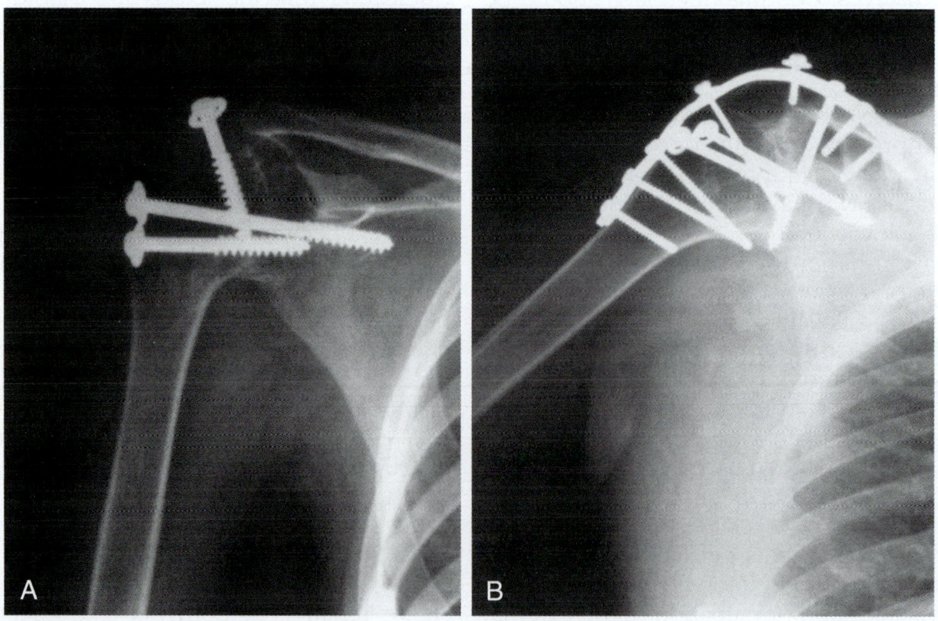

FIGURE 18-25: Shoulder fusion after brachial plexus injury. Two different techniques for shoulder fusion are illustrated. **A,** Large cancellous screws. **B,** A combination of plate and screw fixation.

fascicles to the biceps motor branch or transfer of triceps branches to the axillary nerve[106,108] significantly shortens the time for reinnervation. Several large series have reported minimal morbidity from these techniques.[107,108] Various combinations of nerve transfers are being used as a part of brachial plexus reconstruction.

Historically, the goals for a complete brachial plexus injury were limited. Surgery followed different paths, including "peek and shriek," above-elbow amputation with shoulder fusion, and elbow flexion with biceps neurotization with or without shoulder fusion. The main priorities of brachial reconstruction included restoration of elbow flexion, shoulder abduction, and stability; hand sensibility could only be achieved in some cases. More distal motor function was considered unobtainable because of the length of regeneration needed.

By adding other combinations of nerve transfers, brachial plexus surgeons have recently become more successful in achieving these major goals of restoring elbow flexion, shoulder abduction and stability, and hand sensibility. In the cases with complete avulsion, conventional nerve transfers can include the accessory nerve to the suprascapular nerve, motor intercostals to the biceps, and perhaps sensory intercostals to the median nerve to achieve these goals as part of the primary procedure.

With the emergence of newer techniques, some successful restoration of hand function (grasp and release) has been achieved, even in patients with a flail limb. These results however necessitate a more aggressive approach to reconstruction. Multiple nerve transfers for muscle and sensory function may be performed by themselves or together with free muscle transfer. For example, a single case of panplexus avulsion can be treated with a strategy of multiple neurotization, which might include the phrenic to the suprascapular nerve, the spinal accessory (via a sural nerve graft) to the musculocutaneous nerve, the contralateral C7 to the median nerve with a vascularized ulnar nerve graft, and the intercostals to the radial nerve and the long thoracic nerve.

Another example of brachial plexus reconstruction in evolution can be seen with a typical C5-C6 pattern of functional loss (Erb palsy) as a result of avulsions. Such patients would show an absence of shoulder abduction and external rotation and absence of elbow flexion. A common strategy to improve shoulder abduction is to transfer the spinal accessory nerve to the suprascapular nerve. Improved results can be obtained with double-reinnervation strategies that use this nerve transfer in combination with the transfer of the triceps branch to the axillary nerve.[16,106,108] A further modification is to perform a posterior approach to the accessory-suprascapular nerve transfer (thereby shortening reinnervation time)[12] and to incorporate this posterior approach into a dual-reinnervation strategy.[115]

In the past the most common procedure for elbow reinnervation was the transfer of two or three intercostal nerves. Studies have shown that direct transfer without a bridging nerve graft, performed before 6 months, offers the best results.[39,77,98,161] Others have used the spinal accessory nerve with an intervening sural nerve graft with similar outcomes.[3,163,165] Other nerve transfers that could be performed involved the medial pectoral, thoracodorsal,[47] phrenic, contralateral C7, and even the ipsilateral C7.[85] In the past decade the Oberlin transfer (the transfer of an ulnar nerve fascicle) has been used with great success. Currently, this technique as originally described,[139,185] or as modified, has become extremely popular and widespread. This distal nerve transfer has been performed via an end-to-side technique as well,[75] and some have transferred a median nerve fascicle to an elbow flexor.[181] Superior results have been achieved by transferring fascicles of the ulnar nerve and median nerve to both the biceps and the brachialis muscles.[114,116]

The same clinical pattern of C5 and C6 loss can become more controversial if the surgeon finds C5 and C6 neuromas or ruptures rather than C5 and C6 avulsions. Should a nerve graft from C5, C6, or both be performed if proximal stumps are available, or would nerve transfer(s) or a combination of nerve grafting and nerve transfer be better? Which of these techniques will produce better outcomes? If nerve transfers are to be performed, which ones would provide the best results?

Nerve Reimplantation

Carlstedt and colleagues[31] and other groups[15,74] have attempted the reimplantation of avulsed spinal nerves into the spinal cord. Although regeneration across the central-peripheral nerve interface has been demonstrated in experimental animals and in humans, early experience with this technique in humans has been inferior to other more standard reconstructive procedures. Reimplantation is being performed only at a small number of centers around the world, and its use in humans is still experimental.[187] It remains an exciting possibility for the future.

It is probably best not to treat patients who are initially examined late after injury (after 9 months or 1 year) with nerve grafting. Distal nerve transfers can extend the time interval for reinnervation attempts. A combination of procedures may be considered, including muscle or tendon transfers, free muscle transfer, and bone procedures (shoulder fusion and other augmenting techniques). Options may be limited because of the lack of available donors of sufficient strength.

Muscle Transfer

Free muscle transfer can also be incorporated into the early reconstruction.

Single-muscle transfer is used most commonly to restore elbow flexion and can be accomplished with reliable results. Transfer of the gracilis muscle has been popular, with minimal morbidity of the harvest. Typically, the gracilis muscle origin is secured to the clavicle through drill holes, and the spinal accessory nerve and the gracilis motor nerve can be repaired under the clavicle. Alternatively, two or three intercostal nerves or, when available, a fascicle of the ulnar nerve[88] can be used in place of the spinal accessory nerve. The results of contralateral C7 neurotization of a free muscle have not been as successful.[39] The donor vessels are repaired to the vessels from the thoracoacromial trunk. The tendon of the gracilis is then attached to the biceps tendon. Studies have shown improvement in elbow flexion strength, with 80% of patients achieving MRC grade 3 function or better.[2,37] Free gracilis transfer allows early reinnervation of the free muscle by 3 to 6 months and maximal strength by 18 months.

This free muscle technique can be modified to provide a combined elbow flexion and wrist extension or finger flexion by weaving the tendon beneath the mobile wad into the extensor carpi radialis brevis or the finger flexors. For example, in one series more than half the patients obtained MRC grade M3 function or greater for wrist extension, that is, a full range of motion against gravity.[2] In our experience, elbow flexion is slightly weakened when the free muscle is used for dual transfer rather than just a single function.[13]

Double free muscle transfer for patients with four or five root avulsions has been successfully performed by Doi and colleagues.[53] The lofty goals of these two technically demanding procedures include independent voluntary elbow flexion and extension, independent voluntary finger flexion and extension, and protective sensation in the hand. Stage 1 of the procedure includes exploration of the brachial plexus and free gracilis transfer with spinal accessory neurotization for elbow flexion and finger extension. Stage 2, performed several weeks later, consists of intercostal neurotization of another free gracilis muscle for finger flexion, combined with intercostal motor neurotization of the triceps and sensory neurotization of the median nerve. The gracilis muscle is attached to the second rib and secured into the tendons of the finger and thumb flexors. The donor vessels are repaired to the thoracodorsal vessels. Additional nerve transfers can also be added to provide shoulder function and stabilization using other available donors, such as the phrenic nerve or contralateral C7. In Doi's report 25 of 26 patients obtained good or excellent elbow flexion, and slightly more than half obtained satisfactory prehension (more than 30 degrees of total active motion of the fingers) and could position the hand in space.

Outcomes

Patients with brachial plexus surgery need careful and thoughtful long-term follow-up evaluation. Those who have made insufficient recovery from a primary nerve reconstruction can benefit greatly from a secondary (soft tissue or bone) procedure. Indeed, the surgeon should consider leaving behind some potential donor nerves in case a salvage procedure should be needed. In addition, relatively minor operative procedures, such as flexor-to-extensor tendon transfers, can markedly improve function.

Despite the excitement and improved outcomes brought by these new techniques, the overall results are still sobering when the magnitude of the problem is considered. There is great difficulty with the analysis of outcomes, all too often based on insufficient data from a single surgeon using the same technique at the same time in the same matched set of patients, without long-term follow-up. The definition of a good result or even a uniform classification has not been universally adopted. In the end the study of operative outcomes is a matter of comparing apples, oranges, and lemons.

However, some generalizations can be made regarding outcomes. Ultimate recovery depends on many factors, including the extent and pattern of injury, the age of the patient, the patient's cooperation and rehabilitation, the surgeon's experience, and the time interval between injury and surgery. Outcomes are best for incomplete lesions or neuromas that conduct an NAP. Injuries to the upper plexal elements fare better than those to the lower elements, such as the lower trunk and medial cord; these latter elements do quite poorly with nerve surgery. Infraclavicular lesions and terminal branch injuries do better than supraclavicular injuries (the more distal, the better). The best results can be achieved in those operated on before 6 months and in younger patients. Short grafts do better than long grafts.

Nerve transfers offer the opportunity of speeding up the recovery process. The best results are seen when nerve transfers can be coapted directly without an interpositional graft. Standard nerve transfers to improve the median, ulnar, and distal radial nerve function have not generally fared well. Double innervation of a joint is probably preferable to single innervation.[124] Nerve reconstruction, when achievable, seems to be more functional than tendon transfer or joint fusion.

There have been great strides in brachial plexus reconstruction in recent decades. Outcomes have improved because of increased awareness and improved surgical techniques. In the past, few options were available other than amputation or benign neglect. Brachial plexus injuries have a lifelong impact on the quality of life of affected patients. Most patients still have significant residual loss of function and many experience severe neuropathic pain and become dependent on narcotics.[36] Only about half of these patients return to work. Continued advancement in the basic science, the development of new techniques, and the refinement of described procedures will ultimately improve outcomes and, it is to be hoped, allow many more patients to return to the workforce.

Amputation

Brachial plexus surgery is evolving. Transhumeral amputation, although not widely practiced due to patients' poor compliance with the use of a conventional artificial limb and the lack of pain resolution, has undergone recent developments. The reinnervation of shoulder targets can improve control of not only a stump but also a myoelectric prosthesis.[92] New prostheses using advanced technologies are being designed.

Shoulder Reconstruction Options in Adult Patients With Brachial Plexus Injury

If shoulder function is not restored, at least partially, in adult patients with brachial plexus injury (BPI), their upper extremity function remains substantially limited even when elbow function is restored through nerve repair or transfer or through muscle transfer.[66] The shoulder dysfunction in BPI often manifests as painful inferior subluxation of the shoulder associated with a lack of shoulder external rotation, abduction and flexion. Shoulder internal rotation, manifested by hand on belly position, is usually maintained.

Although shoulder fusion is a potential option for patients with BPI, it is irreversible and requires normal scapulothoracic function, which is usually lacking in many of these patients (Fig. 18-26). Atlan and colleagues reported fair outcomes after shoulder fusion in patients with BPI, but with a 24% rate of nonunion that required reoperation.[10] Cofield and Briggs reported a high complication rate in patients who underwent shoulder fusion, with the worst outcomes in patients with BPI.[43]

Our preference is to attempt tendon transfer whenever it is feasible, and we defer shoulder fusion only as a salvage procedure when there are no muscle transfer options available.

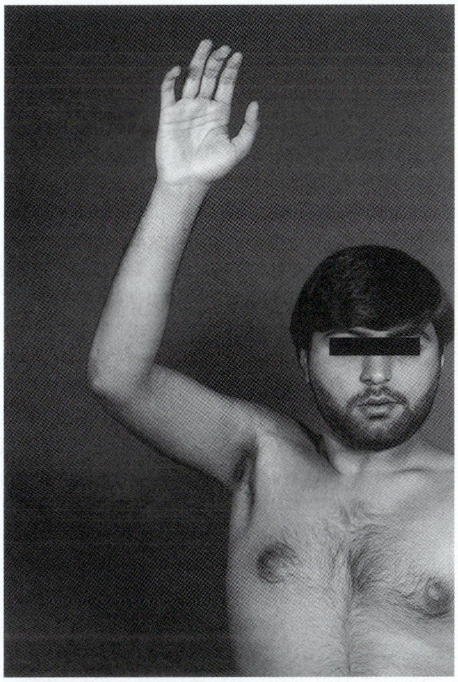

FIGURE 18-26: Brachial plexus reconstruction: nerve transfers for shoulder abduction. This 17-year-old male was in a high-speed motor vehicle accident 6 months previously. He suffered a spinal cord injury that was treated successfully with evacuation of a cervical epidural hematoma acutely. Initially he had a C5-C7 lesion but noted recovery in C6 and C7. Six months after injury, he had a flail shoulder, including weak rhomboids. Electromyography (EMG) showed fibrillations in the midcervical paraspinals. Myelography demonstrated a pseudomeningocele at C5. At surgery, nerve action potentials and somatosensory evoked potentials confirmed a preganglionic injury. He underwent nerve transfers involving the spinal accessory nerve to the suprascapular nerve and a triceps branch to the axillary nerve. By 1 year postoperatively, he had already regained more than 90 degrees of abduction and 45 degrees of external rotation. EMG confirmed nascent potentials in both the infraspinatus and the deltoid muscles.

After restoration of elbow function, patients—especially those who are overweight and women with large breasts—tend to move their elbow while rubbing their hand on their abdomen because of the lack of external rotation. When we ask these patients which single shoulder motion (external/internal rotation, abduction, or flexion) they would prefer if we could only restore one of these for them, more than 90% request shoulder external rotation. For this reason, the reduction of inferior shoulder subluxation and restoration of external rotation are our priorities in the shoulder reconstruction algorithm that we follow in patients with BPI.

Tendon Transfer Options to Restore Shoulder External Rotation in Patients With BPI

The potential tendon transfer options for restoring shoulder external rotation in patients with BPI are: ipsilateral lower trapezius transfer, contralateral lower trapezius transfer, and latissimus major and teres major transfers. Biomechanical comparison of these transfers to the proximal humerus to restore shoulder external rotation showed significant differences, with the best moment arm of external rotation provided by the lower trapezius followed by the teres major and the latissimus dorsi.[87]

With deltoid paralysis, latissimus transfer becomes contraindicated.[80] In addition, except in patients with upper plexus injury, most patients with subtotal or complete BPI do not have normal latissimus or teres major function.

For these reasons, lower trapezius transfer is the "to go" tendon transfer that we recommend for restoring shoulder external rotation in patients with BPI.[61-63] When we have performed lower trapezius transfer, in isolation or as part of multiple tendon transfers, it has reliably stabilized and improved or restored shoulder external rotation in most of our patients.

When the ipsilateral trapezius is paralyzed because the spinal accessory nerve has been used for nerve transfer, the contralateral trapezius becomes the only possible tendon transfer option to restore shoulder external rotation. One of the authors (B.E.) demonstrated in a prior anatomic study the feasibility of transfer of the contralateral lower trapezius origin to the ipsilateral shoulder.[66] We have performed this transfer on 17 patients with very promising results, and for this reason it is now our preferred transfer when the ipsilateral trapezius is not available.

Technique of Lower Trapezius Transfer to the Infraspinatus to Restore Shoulder External Rotation

The patient is placed in the lateral position and the type of incision depends on whether the lower trapezius is to be transferred in isolation or combined with other transfers.

For isolated lower trapezius transfer, double incisions are performed, with one just medial to the spine of the scapula through which the lower trapezius is harvested.

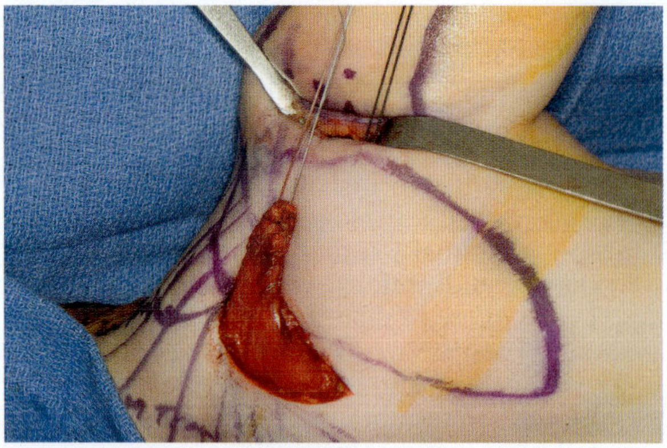

FIGURE 18-27: Harvesting and preparation of the lower trapezius for transfer to the infraspinatus tendon.

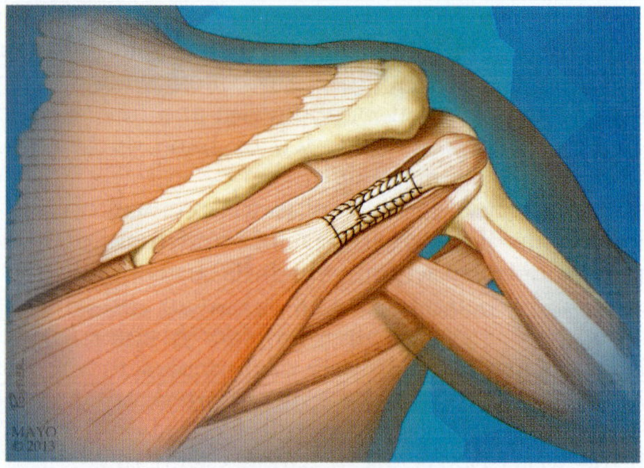

FIGURE 18-28: The direct transfer of the lower trapezius to the infraspinatus. Note the line of pull of the lower trapezius muscle fibers that replicate those of the infraspinatus muscle. (Courtesy Mayo Foundation for Medical Education and Research.)

The most important step in the harvesting of the lower trapezius is to identify its lateral border as it heads toward insertion on the medial spine of the scapula. This portion of the lower trapezius is dissected, elevated, and followed to the insertion on the medial 2 to 3 cm of the spine of the scapula. The tendon is detached and tagged with a suture, and then dissection is performed between the lower and middle trapezius. At this level, the spinal accessory is located on the undersurface of the muscle; thus superficial dissection should be safe. Once sufficient excursion is obtained, the muscle is ready to be transferred (Fig. 18-27).

Exposure of the infraspinatus is accomplished through another incision, an inverted "L," which is placed laterally, with the vertical incision at the level of the joint and the horizontal incision just distal to the spine of the scapula. The posterior half of the deltoid is detached to achieve full exposure of the infraspinatus. As the infraspinatus tendon is almost always intact in patients with BPI, direct transfer of the lower trapezius to the infraspinatus tendon is performed without the need for tendon graft augmentation. The infraspinatus tendon is tagged with a nonabsorbable No. 2 suture in Krakow fashion that will be used for the transfer. The shoulder is placed in maximum external rotation, and a tunnel is created between the medial and lateral wound; the lower trapezius is transferred and repaired to the infraspinatus (Fig. 18-28). We wrap the transferred tendon with TenoGlide (Integra) to reduce the risk of adhesions.

When inferior shoulder subluxation is a major complaint of the patient, we recommend transfer of the upper/middle trapezius to the proximal humerus to stabilize the shoulder at the same time as the transfer of the lower trapezius to restore shoulder external rotation. Although we hope for additional improvement of shoulder abduction with this transfer, we have reported previously that such transfer leads to minimal improvement of shoulder abduction (average, 40 degrees).[62]

Technique of Upper/Middle Trapezius Transfer

With the patient in the lateral position, an inverted U-shaped incision is placed starting medial to the scapula, extending the incision proximally, laterally, and then distally towards the mid-deltoid.

Skin flaps are developed and full exposure of the posterosuperior shoulder and scapulothoracic articulation is achieved.

The lower trapezius harvesting and transfer is then performed as described above.

The middle and lower trapezius are detached from the spine of the scapula, acromion, and lateral clavicle, and an Achilles' tendon allograft is used to augment this part of the muscle. We use the thin part of the tendon graft to wrap the musculotendinous portions of the upper/middle trapezius. We keep the bony attachment of the Achilles tendon attached and use it as part of the transfer to achieve bone-to-bone healing.

After the lower trapezius transfer is complete, additional abduction of the shoulder is performed while keeping the shoulder in external rotation. We aim to abduct to around 90 degrees unless the patient has prior intercostal nerve transfer, in which case we abduct to around 60 degrees to avoid traction injury to the intercostal nerve transfers. TenoGlide is placed on the acromion to reduce the risk of adhesions between the transferred trapezius and the top part of the acromion, and the trapezius prolonged with the Achilles tendon allograft is transferred on top of the acromion to the deltoid insertion (Fig. 18-29). The bone is debrided to have a bleeding surface at the level of insertion, and the bony attachment of the Achilles tendon is internally fixed with two or three screws (3.5 or 4.5 depending on the size of the bone).

Technique of Contralateral Lower Trapezius Origin Transfer to the Infraspinatus Tendon to Restore Shoulder External Rotation

With the patient in the prone position, the thoracic spinous processes are palpated and the T12 level, which

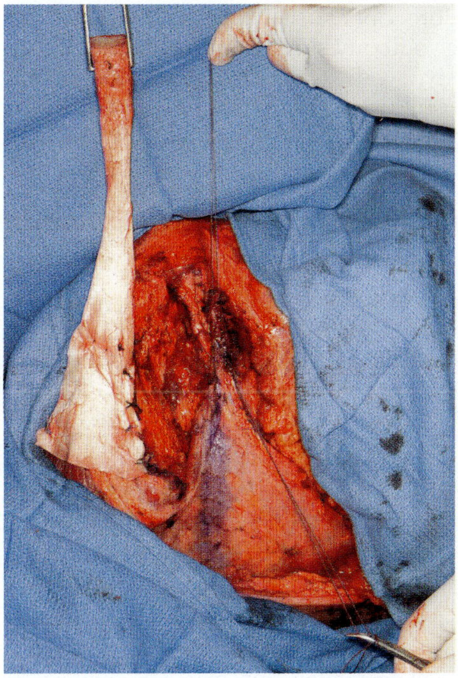

FIGURE 18-29: Intraoperative picture showing the lower trapezius being transferred to the infraspinatus, and the upper/middle trapezius augmented with Achilles' tendon allograft ready for transfer on top of the acromion to the level of the deltoid insertion.

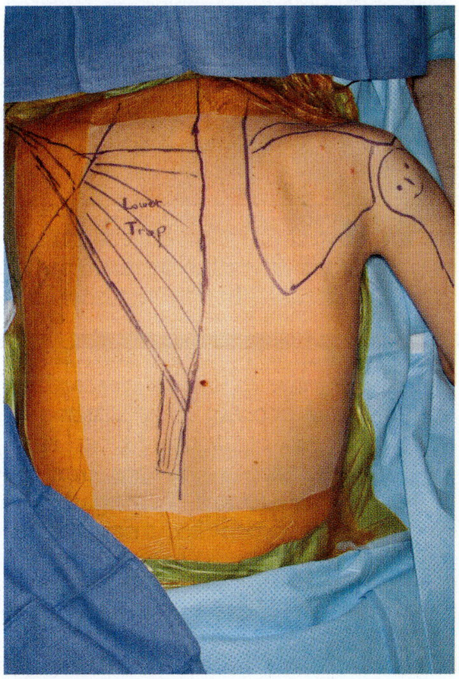

FIGURE 18-30: Marking of the lower trapezius anatomy before surgical harvesting.

is the distal origin of the lower trapezius, is marked (Fig. 18-30). An incision is placed around 2 cm lateral to the level of T12 and extended proximally and distally for around 7 cm. The lower trapezius origin is detached and prolonged with a 5 to 7 cm strip of lumbar fascia.

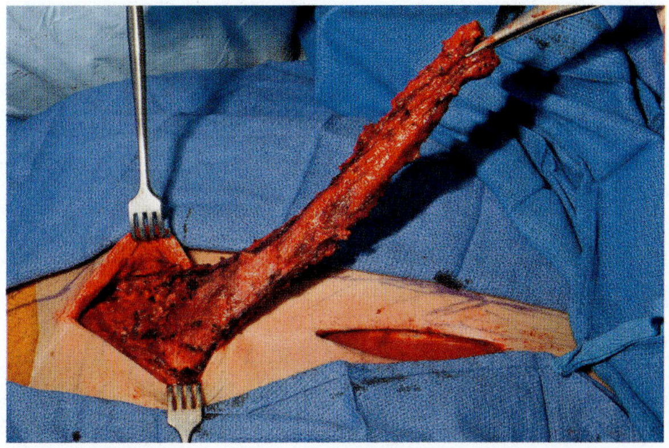

FIGURE 18-31: Harvesting of the lower trapezius origin through double incisions.

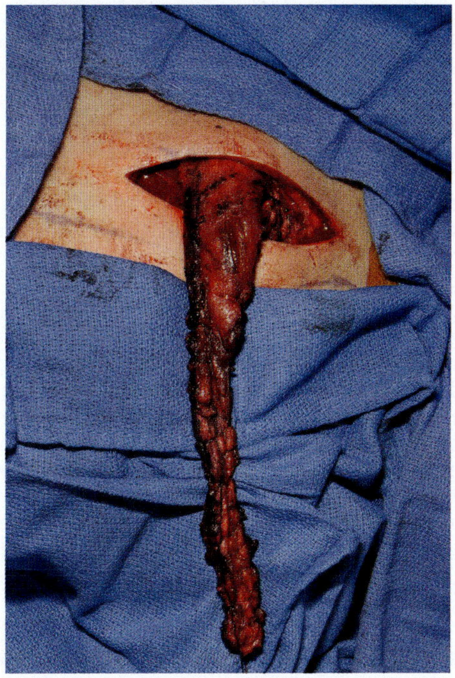

FIGURE 18-32: Note the long reach of the contralateral lower trapezius origin to the ipsilateral shoulder.

Proximal detachment of the lower trapezius is continued through this incision as much as possible and then an additional incision is placed lateral to the thoracic spine, at the level of the spine of the scapula; this is extended distally for around 5 to 7 cm. The detachment is continued using these two incisions, and the lower trapezius is pulled out of the proximal wound (Figs. 18-31 and 18-32). Exposure of the infraspinatus is achieved as described above for the lower trapezius transfer. A tunnel is then created between the paraspinal proximal incision and the lateral incision, and with the shoulder placed in maximal external rotation, the prolonged tendinous aspect of lower trapezius origin is transferred and repaired to the infraspinatus tendon. TenoGlide is used to wrap the transferred muscle to reduce the risk of adhesions.

If latissimus and/or pectoralis major muscles are available for transfer, we add them to the transfers to help restore shoulder flexion. These transfers are much more powerful for restoring the function of the anterior deltoid; we have performed these transfers in 25 patients and achieved an average flexion of 90 degrees.

One more option that we have attempted with very promising outcomes is to perform a reverse shoulder arthroplasty, with transfer of the lower trapezius to restore shoulder external rotation and pedicled pectoralis major or pedicled latissimus dorsi transfer to restore shoulder flexion.

EDITOR COMMENTARY

Samuel Antuña

The authors have brilliantly summarized the approach to the most common neurologic disorders affecting the shoulder.

Shoulder surgeons will face nerve issues in three different situations. First, some patients will present with shoulder pain or dysfunction secondary to nerve compression or paralysis without any significant previous trauma or surgical intervention. This is the case for suprascapular nerve compression or long thoracic nerve paralysis. These clinical scenarios are sometimes difficult to identify and a high degree of suspicion is necessary. Suprascapular neuropathy may need surgical intervention if there is an obvious compression and if neurologic conduction studies are positive; otherwise, it may be a temporary problem that will resolve with time. It is relevant to point out that suprascapular nerve release is not a necessary surgical gesture accompanying massive rotator cuff repair. Several clinical and electrodiagnostic studies have demonstrated that nerve release does not improve patients' pain or clinical outcome.

A second scenario includes patients with previous trauma or surgical intervention who develop neurologic deficit as a complication. This may be a complicated situation both for the patient and for the surgeon. In the traumatic situation it is very important to consider the neurologic status of the patient before any operation is performed. Fortunately, the great majority of patients with nerve palsies after proximal humerus fractures and dislocations recover over time. However, some may not recover completely or may take a long time to do so. Iatrogenic injuries to the axillary and musculocutaneous nerves and to the brachial plexus do occur. In order to minimize their incidence, surgeons must pay full attention to patient positioning and surgical techniques. Some situations may present with higher risk: the implantation of an arthroplasty in a very stiff shoulder may put the brachial plexus at risk for stretching; musculocutaneous nerve injuries have been reported after a Latarjet procedure; and axillary nerve palsies may be seen in difficult shoulder revision arthroplasties or posttraumatic cases.

Finally, patients may present in our clinic asking for reconstructive surgery after permanent nerve injuries that led to shoulder dysfunction, with axillary nerve injuries or brachial plexus palsies being the two most common. Such clinical cases are very demanding and should probably be treated by shoulder surgeons with a very specific interest in nerve reconstruction or tendon transfers. The authors have presented their promising experience with several novel tendon transfers for deltoid paralysis or scapular winging that seem to improve patients' autonomy a great deal. More research in this area is likely in the near future.

In conclusion, this editor believes nerve issues around the shoulder are probably more common than reported in the literature. Exquisite clinical examination is mandatory in any acute shoulder trauma or in patients for whom a revision procedure will be performed. Very stiff shoulders, revision surgery, or nonanatomic repairs represent a risk for iatrogenic nerve injury, and the paralytic shoulder is a challenging problem. Tendon transfers can greatly improve the quality of life of these patients, but these demanding procedures should probably be undertaken by specialized surgeons.

SENIOR EDITOR COMMENTARY

Frederick A. Matsen III

The authors of this chapter are true experts and provide a masterful view of all the major nerve problems and their management. There is little to add, except possibly a simple plan for examination based on the two dimensions of the innervation of the upper extremity. The first dimension is dermatome/myotome based and is the key to evaluating for cervical and upper plexus lesions. C5 provides sensation to the lateral arm, C6 to the lateral forearm and thumb, C7 to the long finger, C8 to the little finger, and T1 to the medial arm. Motorwise, C5 innervates abduction and external rotation, C6 elbow flexion, C7 elbow extension, C8 finger flexion and extension, and T1 intrinsic function of the hand. The second dimension is peripheral nerve based and is the key to evaluating distal plexus and peripheral nerve function. Muscle function is evaluated by looking for atrophy and by actually palpating the muscle for contraction, rather than looking for its action (which can be misleading as different muscles may have similar action). The deltoid is palpated while the arm is extended, abducted, and flexed, checking the axillary nerve. The infraspinatus is palpated while the arm is externally rotated, checking the suprascapular nerve. The biceps is palpated while the arm is flexed, checking the musculocutaneous nerve. The opponens pollicis is palpated while the thumb is opposed, checking the median nerve. The first dorsal interosseous is palpated while the index finger is abducted, checking the ulnar nerve. The extensor pollicis longus is palpated while the thumb is extended, checking the radial nerve. The trapezius is palpated while the shoulder is shrugged, checking the spinal accessory nerve. Because the serratus anterior is difficult to palpate, we check the function of the long thoracic nerve by ensuring the patient can stabilize the scapula to the chest wall when the examiner exerts downward pressure on the arm held horizontally in front of the patient. This whole examination can be completed in much less time than it took to write this paragraph!

CHAPTER 19

The Stiff Shoulder

Matthew F. Dilisio, Bassem T. Elhassan, Laurence D. Higgins, Jon J.P. Warner

The shoulder is a complex articulation consisting of the glenohumeral joint, scapulothoracic joint, and acromioclavicular joint. During normal shoulder elevation, there is a balance of motion between these articulations driven by the shoulder musculature; this provides tremendous mobility, allowing the arm to be placed anywhere in space. Shoulder stiffness, which has numerous etiologies, can be a debilitating and painful problem that disrupts this delicate balance. Recent research has advanced our understanding of the pathogenesis and treatment of the stiff shoulder.

Stiffness about the shoulder was described clinically more than a century ago. It remains a common and frustrating problem seen in orthopedic practice today. A number of clinical scenarios manifest with loss of motion in the shoulder, and the terminology can be confusing. Despite ongoing basic science and clinical research, the mechanisms that lead to the development of a stiff shoulder are not fully understood, and there is still no consensus on the optimal method of treatment.

DEFINITION AND CLASSIFICATION

Classification

Numerous schemes for classifying the stiff shoulder have been proposed over the years. In most a history of some sort of traumatic event is considered a distinguishing factor, but no system has yet been universally accepted.

We prefer to classify the stiff shoulder into two general categories: idiopathic and acquired. The hallmark of both is a significant loss of both active and passive shoulder motion. In the former there is no known intrinsic shoulder disorder, although there may be associated systemic conditions, such as diabetes mellitus. In the latter there is some sort of predisposing condition affecting the shoulder (e.g., surgery or trauma) that is felt to be the initiating factor in the process.

In this chapter we use the term frozen shoulder to describe the idiopathic condition. This group includes patients with diabetes mellitus. All other conditions fall under the category of acquired stiffness. Acquired stiffness can be subdivided to indicate the mechanism associated with the condition (e.g., posttraumatic or postsurgical) (Fig. 19-1).

Primary, Idiopathic Frozen Shoulder

Shoulder stiffness is a general term that encompasses a spectrum of pathology. It was first described as a clinical entity in the late nineteenth century by both Duplay[98] in France and Putnam[274] in the United States. The original term for the condition was *scapulohumeral periarthritis,* which encompassed a number of painful afflictions of the shoulder resulting in stiffness. As knowledge has developed about the specific conditions that can cause a stiff shoulder, this term has fallen out of favor.

In 1934 Codman described a clinical pattern of muscle spasms and glenohumeral stiffness, which he termed the *frozen shoulder.*[69] He stated that this condition was "difficult to define, difficult to treat, and difficult to explain from the point of view of pathology." In many respects this is still true today.

A decade after Codman, Neviaser described a similar condition, a "chronic inflammatory process involving the capsule of the shoulder causing a thickening and contracture of this structure which secondarily becomes adherent to the humeral head." He called it *adhesive capsulitis,* a term he believed better represented the underlying pathology.[238] The term *adhesive capsulitis,* however, has sometimes been used indiscriminately to describe both the idiopathic frozen shoulder and shoulder stiffness related to other causes. Because these are now considered separate entities, it is probably no longer appropriate to use the same term for both.

At a symposium sponsored by the American Academy of Orthopaedic Surgeons in 1992, a workshop committee defined *frozen shoulder* as "a condition of uncertain etiology characterized by significant restriction of both active and passive shoulder motion that occurs in the absence of a known intrinsic shoulder disorder."[365]

In an attempt to obtain a consensus definition and classification of frozen shoulder/adhesive capsulitis from

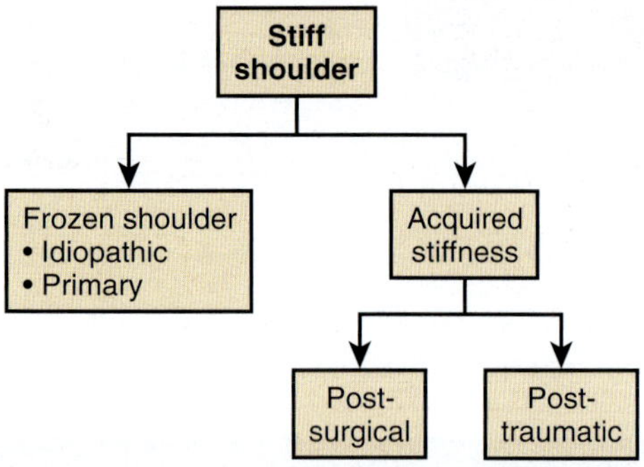

FIGURE 19-1: Classification of shoulder stiffness.

190 shoulder experts from around the world, Zuckerman proposed the definition of frozen shoulder to be "a condition characterized by functional restriction of both active and passive shoulder motion for which radiographs of the glenohumeral joint are essentially unremarkable except for the possible presence of osteopenia or calcific tendonitis." He also classified the condition as primary or secondary based on whether an etiology or associated condition could be identified. He subclassified secondary frozen shoulder as intrinsic (due to rotator cuff or biceps disorders), extrinsic (due to an abnormality remote to the shoulder), or systemic (occurring with associated conditions, such as diabetes mellitus, hyperthyroidism, hypothyroidism, or hypoadrenalism).[366] However, only 66% of the shoulder surgeons agreed with this subclassification of secondary frozen shoulder. We find it optimal to differentiate primary, idiopathic frozen shoulder from secondary frozen shoulder due to surgery, trauma, or other causes (see Fig. 19-1). We do not consider shoulder stiffness associated with a systemic disease, such as diabetes, to be a secondary frozen shoulder.

Secondary Frozen Shoulder

The earliest description of shoulder stiffness following trauma was recorded by Malgaigne in 1859. He wrote with regard to minor nondisplaced, extracapsular fractures about the shoulder[98]:

> There remains long afterward a stiffness, and a difficulty in moving the shoulder; and however great care may be taken, the motion of elevation of the arm will always remain limited; at least I have in no case seen it perfectly restored, even after the lapse of 11 to 15 months.

There is less controversy and confusion surrounding the nomenclature of this clinical entity. Other commonly used terms for the same condition include *posttraumatic stiff shoulder* and *secondary stiffness*. It is unclear whether acquired stiffness can recover without intervention; this is difficult to study because of the heterogeneity of this patient population.

Some degree of shoulder stiffness is typical after bone or soft tissue injuries around the shoulder. Restriction in shoulder motion has been reported after simple contusions, subluxations, dislocations, acromioclavicular joint injuries, clavicle and scapula fractures, and particularly after proximal humerus fractures in the elderly.[75,128]

Especially after repetitive, low-level trauma, localized contractures can develop and can cause motion loss in specific patterns. Isolated posterior capsular contracture is the most commonly described. Neer discussed the impingement syndrome and encouraged therapeutic stretching in forward elevation, internal rotation, and cross-body adduction.[235] Thomas and colleagues[325] and Ticker and colleagues[326] made similar recommendations. In a review of 30 patients from a prospective study of refractory shoulder stiffness, 11 experienced isolated restriction in motion that was attributed to posterior capsular contracture.[145] In each of these patients an associated pathologic process was identified, with a partial-thickness rotator cuff tear being the pathology in seven cases.

Surgical procedures are widely recognized to be a cause of shoulder stiffness. Anterior or posterior capsulorrhaphy, inferior capsular shift, and rotator cuff surgery can all result in limitation of motion, often by design. Tauro found a relatively high incidence of stiffness in patients who underwent surgery for a rotator cuff tear. Patients with more pronounced stiffness often experienced difficulty in regaining normal motion after surgery.[322]

DIAGNOSTIC CRITERIA

Idiopathic frozen shoulder implies a global glenohumeral capsular contracture that occurs in the absence of a definable traumatic event. Acquired stiffness is an extrinsic process related to some other, often traumatic, cause. These conditions might not be mutually exclusive. On rare occasions, inflammation and adhesions have been identified in the subacromial bursa in association with idiopathic frozen shoulder.[142] Although acquired stiffness is generally the result of an extracapsular process, subsequent capsular contracture can develop.

Idiopathic Frozen Shoulder

The lack of consensus regarding nomenclature and classification for frozen shoulder has partly originated from the confusion surrounding necessary and sufficient diagnostic criteria. Many authors, however, have proposed diagnostic criteria for frozen shoulder. Considerations include patient history, relative loss of motion in various planes, motion loss compared with the contralateral shoulder, and radiographic findings.

We do not subscribe to a specific, published set of criteria, but we do consider certain characteristics to be key components in the diagnosis of a frozen shoulder. These include a lack of history of major trauma or surgery about the shoulder, significantly limited passive and active range of motion (ROM) in all planes compared with the contralateral shoulder, and normal radiographs or other advanced imaging studies.

NORMAL MOTION AND PATHOMECHANICS

Understanding the altered mechanics associated with a stiff shoulder requires an understanding of normal shoulder mechanics. Normal shoulder motion involves several interfaces: the articulation between the humeral head and the glenoid (glenohumeral motion), the gliding surface between the proximal humerus and the coracoacromial arch (the subacromial-subdeltoid plane), the articulation between the scapula and the thorax (scapulothoracic motion), and motion through the acromioclavicular joint. Adhesions or contractures at any one of these interfaces can lead to stiff shoulder development.

Glenohumeral Articulation

Under normal circumstances, the shoulder is a remarkably mobile joint. The normal ratio of glenohumeral motion to scapulothoracic motion is 2:1.[114,167,273] The normal surface area of the capsule is nearly twice that of the humeral head[77] and the capsule is inherently loose. In cadaveric tests, Harryman and colleagues measured torsional resistance of the glenohumeral joint with an intact capsule and showed that the capsule remained essentially free of tension until a terminal degree of motion was reached (Fig. 19-2).[146] Most motions during work and activities of daily living are performed in mid-range positions.[149,265] As the end of a ROM is approached, increased tension is seen in the static restraints, notably in the capsule and its associated ligaments: the superior, middle, and inferior glenohumeral ligaments. The humeral head does not simply rotate within the glenoid cavity like a ball and socket joint, but translates over its surface. These ligaments act as restraints to both rotation and translation at the extremes of motion.[219]

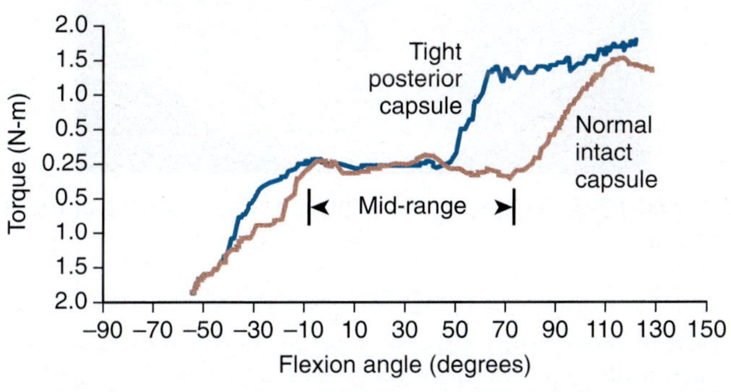

FIGURE 19-2: Under normal circumstances, the static restraints (capsule and ligaments) are under minimal tension in mid range of motion (ROM). These structures become tight at the end of ROMs. In cases of a tight posterior capsule, torsional loads are increased in the mid to high range. (Modified from Harryman DT II, Lazarus MD, Sidles JA, Matsen FA III. Pathophysiology of shoulder instability. In: McGinty JB, Capari RB, Jackson RW, Poehling GG, eds. *Operative Arthroscopy.* 2nd ed. Philadelphia: Lippincott-Raven; 1996:679.)

The anterosuperior capsule in the region of the rotator interval contains the coracohumeral and superior glenohumeral ligaments. It assumes tension with increasing external rotation with the arm in 0 degrees of abduction.[111,147,340] The middle glenohumeral ligament and the anterior band of the inferior glenohumeral ligament become taut with maximal external rotation at 45 degrees and 90 degrees of abduction, respectively.[323,328] The inferior region of the capsule becomes tighter with increasing abduction. The posterior capsule becomes tight in internal rotation with the arm at the side. With increasing angles of elevation, tension is shifted inferiorly.[146,324]

Isolated contractures in specific capsular regions have been described.[118,142,145,237,249,258,326] These have often been created intentionally during procedures for instability.[1] A contracted capsule reduces glenohumeral motion.[146] In a cadaveric study posterior capsular plication was applied to eight shoulders, resulting in limitation of forward elevation, internal rotation, and horizontal adduction. External rotation was unaffected. Tightening of the capsule also increased the torque required to achieve an elevated position (see Fig. 19-2).[146]

Asymmetric tightness of the capsule can cause an obligate translation of the humeral head.[324,148] Normally, the glenohumeral joint displays ball-and-socket mechanics, and the humeral head remains centered within the glenoid fossa except at the extremes of ROM.[273,148] In a cadaveric study when the posterior capsule was surgically tightened, forward flexion caused consistent anterosuperior translation of the humeral head.[146] Clinically, such translation can lead to impingement of the rotator cuff against the coracoacromial arch. This has been described in throwing athletes who develop isolated posterior capsular contractures. Known as *glenohumeral internal rotation deficit,* it can lead to significant pain and disability, especially in overhead athletes.[58] Glenohumeral internal rotation deficit has been associated with partial articular-sided rotator cuff tears, labral tears, and even ulnar collateral ligament tears of the elbow.[15,72,157] Usually, conservative management of this subtle shoulder stiffness can restore physiologic posterior capsular laxity and eliminate the patient's symptoms.

A similar phenomenon can occur with overtightening of the anterior structures, such as with nonanatomic repairs for anterior instability (the Putti-Platt procedure). A chronic contracture of the anterior aspect of the shoulder is almost always associated with a deficit in external rotation compared with the contralateral shoulder. This scenario can result in greater joint reaction forces directed toward the posterior portion of the glenoid and can cause excessive posterior glenoid articular cartilage wear, posterior bony erosion, and osteoarthrosis.[152] Matsen and colleagues have called this process *capsulorrhaphy arthropathy* (Fig. 19-3).[324]

To eliminate pathologic restrictions in motion, a number of techniques, both nonoperative and operative, have been described for capsular release. Although the techniques have evolved, the basic concept of releasing localized or general contractures to improve ROM remains the same.[185,217,237,247,324] The technical details and results of these procedures are discussed in depth later.

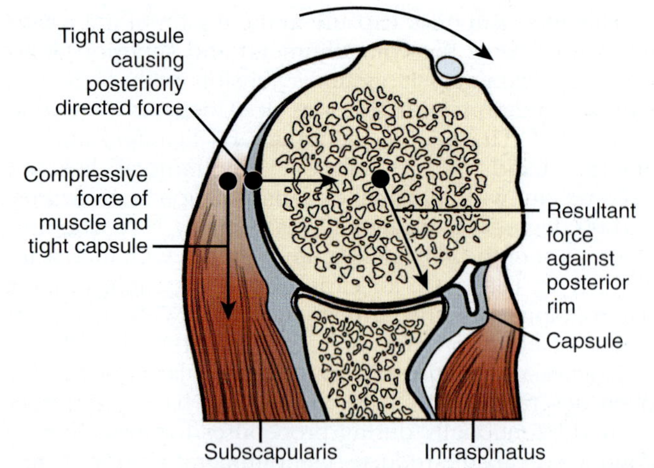

FIGURE 19-3: An asymmetrically tight anterior capsule, such as after a Putti-Platt procedure, causes a loading force against the posterior glenoid rim, which can lead to arthrosis (capsulorrhaphy arthropathy). (From Harryman DT II, Lazarus MD, Sidles JA, Matsen FA III. Pathophysiology of shoulder instability. In: McGinty JB, Capari RB, Jackson RW, Poehling GG, eds. *Operative Arthroscopy.* 2nd ed. Philadelphia: Lippincott-Raven; 1996:686.)

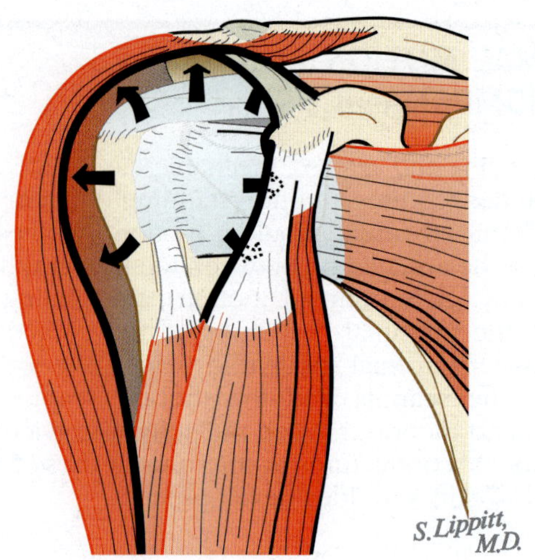

FIGURE 19-4: The humeroscapular motion interface is an important continuum of interfascial sliding surfaces (arrows), including the deep sides of the deltoid, the acromion, the coracoid process and its tendons, the superficial side of the humerus, the rotator cuff, and the long head of the biceps tendon and its sheath. (Modified from Matsen, FA III, Lippitt SB, Sidles JA, Harryman DT II. *Practical Evaluation and Management of the Shoulder.* Philadelphia: Saunders; 1994.)

Subacromial-Subdeltoid Plane

In 1934 Codman stated, "The subacromial bursa itself is the largest in the body and is the most complicated in structure and in its component parts. It is in fact a secondary scapulohumeral joint, although no part of its surface is cartilage."[69]

Matsen and Romeo defined the subacromial-subdeltoid plane interface as a sliding surface between the deep side of the deltoid, the acromion, the coracoid process and its tendons, and the superficial side of the humerus and rotator cuff (Fig. 19-4).[292,324] Normal biceps glide is also necessary for full glenohumeral ROM. If synovitis is present within the glenohumeral joint or biceps tendon sheath, adhesions can spot-weld the long head of the biceps tendon to the capsule or bicipital groove (Fig. 19-5).[142,145,249] Pasteur, in 1932, described peritendinous adhesions within the bicipital groove in patients with frozen shoulder. This finding has also been described since by other authors.[86,159,204,238,262]

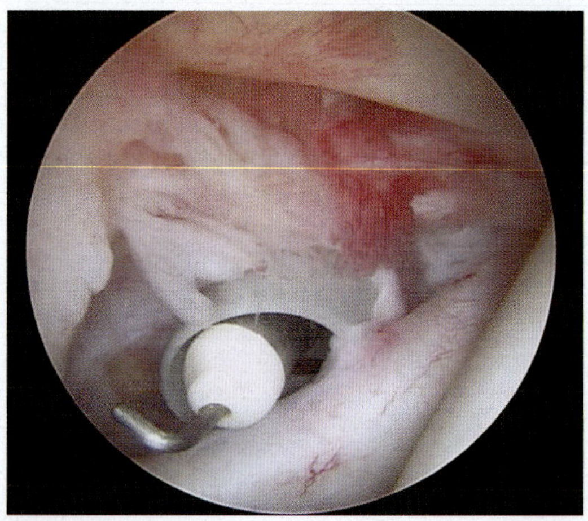

FIGURE 19-5: Biceps tendon adhesions in the setting of frozen shoulder.

Adhesions in this area, which would usually be secondary to trauma or surgery, can substantially limit shoulder motion. Many orthopedic surgeons also struggle with the rehabilitation protocol after shoulder trauma, specifically with proximal humerus fractures. Immobilization can reduce the risk of fracture displacement; however, prolonged immobilization risks stiffness, which can be debilitating even if the fracture has healed in a satisfactory position.

Scapulothoracic Motion

Scapulothoracic mechanics are another important component of shoulder motion. Investigators in the past have determined that scapulothoracic motion is responsible for approximately one third of total shoulder elevation.[114,167] Scapulothoracic motion has been studied in detail by Harryman[147] and McClure.[215] Loss of glenohumeral ROM (e.g., after arthrodesis) can result in an accommodative increase in scapulothoracic ROM.[142] Although it is challenging to clinically measure scapulothoracic motion with accuracy, Nicholson recorded excessive scapular upward rotation (elevation) during active attempts at humeral elevation in patients with frozen shoulder.[245] Lin and colleagues showed increased EMG activity in the upper trapezius, with relatively lower activity in the lower trapezius. These findings have potential implications in the rehabilitation of patients with frozen shoulder.[203]

PATHOPHYSIOLOGY

Although many plausible mechanisms for stiff shoulder development have been proposed, the etiology remains elusive.[154] Advances in basic science research, however, have improved our understanding of the condition. Current efforts are focused on determining both an immunologic basis and the role of cell signaling and inflammatory mediators in its development.

Although recent research has advanced our knowledge of the pathophysiology of the idiopathic frozen shoulder, the exact etiology and mechanism have not yet been established. Our understanding of the disease process is that it is primarily a capsular pathology with signs of inflammation, fibroblast proliferation, and neovascularization. There may be an immunologic component, but there are no reliable laboratory tests or inflammatory markers to diagnose frozen shoulder. There is a clear association of diabetes mellitus and Dupuytren's contracture with frozen shoulder, but the exact pathophysiologic process is mostly speculative. Current research is focused on defining the role of matrix metalloproteinases (MMPs), tissue inhibitors of metalloproteinases (TIMPs), other cytokines, and cytogenetics and their potential role in affecting the natural history of the disease in clinical practice.

Original Theories, Anatomic and Histologic Analysis

In 1896 Duplay's original view of stiff shoulders was that they arose in the subdeltoid region.[98] Riedel subsequently hypothesized that shoulder stiffness may be related to the joint capsule itself.[284] In 1945 Neviaser postulated that idiopathic shoulder stiffness was a capsular pathology. He correlated the surgical, arthrographic, and histologic findings regarding the synovium and capsule of patients with painful shoulder stiffness.[238] Histologically, he identified perivascular infiltration and capsular fibrosis; the synovial layer itself appeared normal. He proposed that shoulder stiffness was due to a tight glenohumeral joint capsule that adhered to itself and the humeral neck, coining the term "adhesive capsulitis." Neer subsequently proposed that coracohumeral ligament contracture also led to shoulder stiffness.[237,258]

Others surgeons continued to histologically analyze the synovium and capsule. Lundberg, too, did not observe any pathologic changes in the synovium. Instead, he found increased collagen density within the capsule and a pattern of glycosaminoglycan distribution that resembled a reparative process.[210] McLaughlin found inflammation in the synovium and biceps sheath in only 10% of his cases.[217] He posited that "acute synovitis represents one phase in the life cycle of this condition."

Hannafin and colleagues attempted to correlate the three histopathologic phases of fibroplasia detected in biopsy samples of patients with frozen shoulder, as described by Neviaser, with findings from clinical examination and arthroscopy. The authors hypothesized that hypervascular synovitis provokes a progressive fibroblastic response in the adjacent capsule, resulting in diffuse capsular fibroplasia and contracture.[140] Based on immunohistochemical and histologic findings, they proposed a cellular pathway that eventually results in the clinical scenario of a frozen shoulder.

Immunologic Analysis

Macnab analyzed biopsy samples obtained during open capsular release and identified round and lymphoid cell infiltrates within the tissue. He hypothesized that this was the result of an autoimmune response directed toward degenerative collagen particles from a hypovascular supraspinatus tendon.[214] Bulgen and colleagues found that patients with a frozen shoulder initially had increased levels of circulating immune complex and C-reactive protein and decreased lymphocyte transformation.[49] The same group subsequently analyzed serum immunoglobulin levels in 25 patients with frozen shoulder and found serum immunoglobulin A levels to be significantly reduced, with this reduction persisting even after clinical recovery.[51,53] Lymphocyte transformation in response to phytohemagglutinin was also significantly depressed in the majority of patients. These early findings suggested an immunologic basis for the disease; however, subsequent reports have failed to support the findings or to identify immunologic tests useful in diagnosis, treatment, or predicting outcome.[361]

Other investigators have attempted to identify factors that predispose patients to shoulder stiffness by using immunologic markers. Initial research was focused on the presence of certain histocompatibility antigens. The presence of human leukocyte antigen (HLA)-B27 was reported as being more common in patients with frozen shoulder (42%) than in controls (10%).[52] This finding, however, was later refuted by the same authors.[51] As of yet, no definite immunologic markers have been defined for patients with frozen shoulder.

A proliferative pathologic repair process initiated by active fibroblasts may occur in response to the inflammatory infiltration of connective tissue by mononuclear cells that produce polypeptide growth factors. Mullett and colleagues[232] examined the response of human fibroblasts to joint aspirates from patients with frozen shoulder and a control group; significantly increased fibroblast proliferation was seen in the patients with frozen shoulder.[232] In another study biopsy samples were taken from the rotator interval in 22 patients undergoing arthroscopic capsular release. Histologic and immunocytochemical analysis revealed the presence of fibroblasts, proliferating fibroblasts, and chronic inflammatory cells (predominantly mast cells). T-cells, B-cells, and macrophages were also present.[138]

Association With Dupuytren Contracture

Many authors dating back to 1936 have reported an association between frozen shoulder and Dupuytren contracture of the hand, with the rate of association ranging from 18% to as high as 52%.[312] More recent investigators have identified similarities in the fibroblastic histologic changes seen in the glenohumeral joint capsule to those seen in Dupuytren contracture.[54,140]

Bunker and Anthony performed manipulation and open excisional biopsy of the coracohumeral ligament and rotator interval capsule in patients who failed to improve with nonoperative treatment of frozen shoulder.[54] The tissue specimens revealed active fibroblast proliferation amidst thick nodular bands of collagen, accompanied by some transformation to a smooth muscle phenotype (myofibroblasts). These histologic features, with neither inflammation nor synovial involvement, are very similar to those seen in Dupuytren contracture. Fibrosis is most evident in later phases of the inflammatory response, and collagen and matrix synthesis takes place after chemotactic and cellular responses. These findings may therefore reflect a later phase of the disease, perhaps following an earlier inflammatory phase.[217] Uhthoff and Boileau confirmed the presence of vimentin, a cytocontractile protein known to be present in Dupuytren contracture, in histologic sections of only the anterior capsular structures in patients with frozen shoulder. This protein was not seen in specimens of the posterior capsule, although type I and type III collagens were. The authors hypothesized that contracture selectively involves only the anterior capsule, whereas fibroplasia involves the entire capsule.[331]

Association With Diabetes Mellitus

The association between idiopathic frozen shoulder and diabetes mellitus is well documented.* However, the exact pathophysiology is still not completely understood. In the 1980s Brownlee and colleagues hypothesized that hyperglycemia leads to faster glycosylation and cross-linking of collagen within the glenohumeral capsule.[43,42] Even though many studies have subsequently demonstrated the association between diabetes and frozen shoulder, there has been little published research since then that has advanced our understanding of the biochemical effect of diabetes on shoulder stiffness.

Cytokinetic, Genetic, and Enzymatic Analysis

The elevation of multiple inflammatory cytokines has recently been linked to idiopathic frozen shoulder. Rodeo and colleagues compared capsular tissue samples from patients undergoing arthroscopy who had frozen shoulder, nonspecific synovitis, or a normal capsule.[291] Their results indicated that cytokines, such as transforming growth factor (TGF-β), platelet-derived growth factor (PDGF), and hepatocyte growth factor are involved in the early inflammatory stages of frozen shoulder. PDGF is a mitogenic agent that causes fibroblastic cell proliferation, and TGF-β increases extracellular matrix production. Suzuki and colleagues further demonstrated that specific growth factors stimulate capsular fibroblasts in a canine model. They found that PDGF-AB, hepatocyte growth factor, and insulin-like growth factor type I all stimulated the migration of fibroblasts from three different parts of a canine shoulder model: the upper and lower parts of the middle glenohumeral ligament and the posterior capsule.[318] Ryu and colleagues found increased vascular endothelial growth factor expression in the synovial tissue of a group of diabetic patients with frozen shoulder; however, its exact role remains undetermined.[299] Elevated levels of inflammatory cytokines interleukin-6 and vascular endothelial growth factor have been found in the synovium of patients with a frozen shoulder, in addition to elevated serum levels of TGF-β.[176,177,209]

MMPs, a family of naturally occurring proteinases that control collagen matrix remodeling, have also been implicated as a contributing factor in the pathogenesis of frozen shoulder.[56,165] Hutchinson and colleagues reported the onset of frozen shoulder in 12 patients with gastric carcinoma after treatment with the synthetic MMP inhibitor, marimastat.[165] This report suggested that the inhibition of MMPs may be associated with frozen shoulder. Bunker and colleagues examined capsular tissue from patients with frozen shoulder.[56] The tissue was analyzed for various factors, including MMPs and their inhibitors.[56] When compared with a normal capsule, the capsule of patients with frozen shoulder demonstrated an increase in messenger RNA for MMPs as well as MMP inhibitors, suggesting that abnormalities in MMP expression are a factor in frozen shoulder. Lubis and colleagues found that the serum MMP-1 and MMP-2 levels were significantly lower in frozen shoulder patients than in patients without a frozen shoulder, while their inhibitors' (TIMP-1 and TIMP-2) levels were significantly higher.[209] Other investigators have found similar MMP abnormalities in synovial tissue.[176,177]

EPIDEMIOLOGY

Studies employing stringent diagnostic criteria for frozen shoulder have defined the incidence in the general population as ranging from 2% to 5%.[77,308] Nearly 70% of patients presenting with frozen shoulder are women, and 20% to 30% develop stiffness in the contralateral shoulder.[139] A recent study demonstrated that 11% of all patients referred to musculoskeletal specialists for a shoulder disorder were ultimately diagnosed with idiopathic frozen shoulder.[174] Recurrence in the same shoulder is quite unusual.[25,59] An accurate incidence of acquired stiffness has yet to be determined, partly because of the variability in this patient population.

PREDISPOSING FACTORS

Age

The majority of patients who seek care for a stiff shoulder, regardless of etiology, are between 40 and 60 years of

*References 13, 17, 38, 112, 200, 206, 210, 231, 259, 260, 293, 302, 336, 357.

age.[45,139,141,233,280,324] It is unusual for an idiopathic frozen shoulder to develop in patients younger than 40 years, with the exception of those who have had insulin-dependent diabetes since childhood. In a large study Lundberg noted that the mean age at the time of presentation was slightly higher in men than in women.[210] However, differences in age relative to sex or type of stiffness were not evident in Harryman and colleagues' series of 126 patients with refractory shoulder stiffness.[144]

Diabetes Mellitus

Patients with diabetes mellitus are clearly at much greater risk for developing limited joint motion[336] not only in the shoulder but also in other joints.[293] Most studies have shown a 10% to 20% incidence of frozen shoulder in these patients, but some have indicated that the rate of incidence may be as high as 35%.[17,38,112,200,210,231,259,260,302,357] The longer a patient has been taking insulin, the greater the risk of developing shoulder stiffness[231] and the greater the resistance to all treatment modalities.[112,302] Patients with childhood-onset diabetes tend to develop stiffness at an earlier age, but in those with adult-onset diabetics the age of presenting with shoulder stiffness is similar to that of the general population. It has been presumed that the severity of diabetes is associated with greater risk of developing a frozen shoulder. However, Yian and colleagues found no association between hemoglobin A1C levels and the prevalence of frozen shoulder in a population of diabetic patients, although the risk increased if patients were taking any medications for diabetes or had developed neurologic manifestations of diabetes.[360]

Insulin-dependent diabetics with joint stiffness in the hands and other major articulations are categorized as having *limited joint motion syndrome*.[293] Diabetics who have cheiroarthropathy (a waxy thickening and induration of the skin associated with flexion contractures of the fingers) as well as a frozen shoulder have higher incidences of retinopathy and bilateral shoulder involvement (77%).[112]

Shoulder stiffness may be the initial manifestation in a patient with diabetes.[304] Lequesne and colleagues discovered 17 patients with glucose intolerance out of 60 new patients with idiopathic frozen shoulder.[200] A diabetes workup should be considered in any patient with newly diagnosed frozen shoulder. Because of the refractory nature of shoulder stiffness in long-term insulin-dependent diabetics, early intervention has been considered appropriate to prevent progressive disability.[112,249,302]

Diabetes not only can put patients at risk for developing a frozen shoulder but also can affect their ultimate outcome. Mehta and colleagues prospectively compared the results of arthroscopic release for frozen shoulder in 42 patients with and without diabetes. The patients in both groups significantly improved, but the Constant score at 6 months was significantly worse in the diabetic patients, with a tendency towards persistent stiffness 2 years postoperatively.[225] Cinar and colleagues also demonstrated that patients with diabetes did worse in terms of pain and motion compared with patients without diabetes after an arthroscopic capsular release.[66]

Non-Shoulder Surgery

Stiffness can also occur after surgery that does not involve the shoulder. Common examples include axillary node dissection and neck dissection, especially when these procedures are combined with radiation therapy.[263,311] Cardiac catheterization in the axilla, coronary artery bypass grafting, and thoracotomy can also restrict shoulder range due to the severe pain after the procedure.[269] In addition, stiffness may be triggered by interventional cardiology procedures, such as cardiac catheterization through the brachial artery[246] or placement of an ipsilateral subpectoral cardiac defibrillator.[57] The incidence of frozen shoulder in a population of male patients who underwent cardiothoracic surgery has been estimated at 3.3%.[329] Frozen shoulder has been described following rehabilitation after breast cancer surgery.[65]

Immobility

In adults immobilization of the shoulder puts it at risk of becoming stiff.[134,172,240,310] A significant number of referrals for shoulder stiffness occur after a period of rest, which has often been recommended by the referring physician. In a review of patients referred to Binder and colleagues, 75% had initially been told to rest the shoulder rather than to perform gentle exercises.[25]

Cervical Disk Disease

Degenerative disk disease between C5-6 and C6-7 has been noted to be more common in patients with shoulder stiffness than in a similar age-matched control group.[358] This association has been supported in other studies.[128,210,217] Patients with symptomatic cervical radiculopathy and a painful shoulder, with or without loss of motion, experienced less pain and were more likely to regain pain-free motion when cervical traction was added to the prescribed exercise regimen.[67]

Thyroid Disorders

Bilateral frozen shoulders are rare but have been reported in the setting of both hyperthyroidism and hypothyroidism.[35,228,316,357] Wohlgethan considered hyperthyroidism, frozen shoulder, and shoulder-hand syndrome to be linked disorders.[355] Resolution of shoulder stiffness has been shown to occur after thyroidectomy and the stabilization of thyroid hormone levels.[255,355]

Cardiac Disease

The association between atherosclerotic coronary vascular disease and shoulder stiffness is well documented.[11,36,105,216,357] In a review of 133 consecutive cases of myocardial infarction, Ernstene and Kinell found 17 patients who complained of unrelenting pain in the shoulder region.[105] Shoulder-hand syndrome, an autonomic dystrophy, may be a sequela of myocardial infarction in 10% to 30% of cases.[229]

Bunker identified raised serum lipid levels in a group of patients with primary frozen shoulder when compared with a group of age- and sex-matched controls,[55] a finding supported by other investigators.[206] However, Austin and colleagues did not find an increased use of lipid-lowering medication in a frozen shoulder cohort compared with the general population.[13]

Pulmonary Disorders

In 1959 Johnson reported that the incidence of frozen shoulder was 3.2% in a population of sanatorium patients with tuberculosis.[172] Saha reported that frozen shoulder occurred more frequently in patients with emphysema and chronic bronchitis, but found no correlation with either the severity or the duration of illness.[301]

Malignancy

Bronchogenic carcinoma and Pancoast tumors of the lung can cause severe shoulder pain that can mimic the early phase of frozen shoulder.[104,156] Other occult neoplastic tumors can be masked by symptoms attributed to a frozen shoulder; these include chest wall tumors, sarcomas, and metastatic disease.[216,239,290,344] Gheita and colleagues found a 15% prevalence of frozen shoulder in 60 patients who had been diagnosed with a malignancy.[119] Malignancy should therefore always be considered in the differential diagnosis when a patient presents with a painful, stiff shoulder that is refractory to initial conservative modalities.

Neurologic Conditions

Shoulder stiffness has been associated with a variety of neurologic disorders. The incidence of frozen shoulder in patients with Parkinson disease is significantly higher than in age-matched controls.[186,285] In 8% of Parkinson disease patients the first symptom was shoulder stiffness, which can occur up to 2 years before the onset of generalized symptoms.[285] Patients with cerebral hemorrhage and cerebral tumors are also at increased risk for frozen shoulder.[45,357]

At least 30% of patients with hemiplegia have shoulder pain and are susceptible to the development of shoulder stiffness.[31,130] Wanklyn and colleagues also found that patients who required transfer assistance were more likely to suffer from shoulder pain.[337] Bruckner and Nye reported a 25% incidence of frozen shoulder in patients who had suffered subarachnoid hemorrhage.[45] They found that the development of stiffness was associated with impaired consciousness, hemiparesis, intravenous (IV) infusion, older age, and depression. In patients with hemiparesis the clinician may find it difficult to distinguish between shoulder stiffness caused by capsular contracture and muscular spasticity.[337] Shoulder-hand syndrome occurs in as many as 30% to 40% of stroke patients and can be terribly disabling. Conversely, Kang and colleagues found that the development of idiopathic frozen shoulder was associated with increased risk of stroke.[178]

Brachial neuritis, a painful neuritis condition also known as Parsonage-Turner syndrome, has been associated with frozen shoulder.[24] Thoracic outlet syndrome, suprascapular neuropathy, and spinal accessory nerve palsy have also been linked to the onset of frozen shoulder.[40,189,263]

Personality Disorders

Some authors have argued that individuals with certain personality characteristics are more likely to develop frozen shoulder. This was first proposed by Codman in 1934 who described four patients with frozen shoulder who "were a little run-down without anything particular the matter."[69] Coventry coined the term *periarthritic personality* and found treatment more challenging in this group.[76] Fleming and colleagues profiled the personality type of 56 patients with a frozen shoulder by using the Middlesex Hospital Questionnaire and found that women with frozen shoulder had significantly greater anxiety levels than did controls.[113] Tyber found the prevalence of depression to be relatively high in a group of 55 patients with painful shoulder syndromes. He included lithium and amitriptyline in his treatment of these patients.[330]

The notion of a characteristic personality disorder is controversial. Wright and Haq found no evidence of this when using the Maudsley Personality Inventory to test 186 patients with a frozen shoulder.[357] Matsen and Harryman reviewed the mental health scores on the Short Form-36 (SF-36) health status questionnaire of 295 patients with either frozen shoulder or acquired stiffness.[144] They found that patients with frozen shoulder and patients with acquired stiffness scored within 95% and 88%, respectively, of the mean score for normal age-matched controls. Debeer and colleagues prospectively evaluated 118 frozen shoulder patients and found no significant difference in personality traits between these patients and controls.[83]

Reaction to Medication

Reports suggest that frozen shoulder can develop after treatment with certain medications. Grasland and colleagues described eight cases of frozen shoulder that developed after the treatment of human immunodeficiency virus (HIV) infection with protease inhibitors.[127] All of these patients received the drug indinavir as part of their regimen and had no other risk factors for frozen shoulder. This association has been confirmed by other investigators.[87,199,268,363] Other medications that have been linked to the onset of frozen shoulder include barbiturates,[223] fluoroquinolones,[115] nelfinavir,[88] and isoniazid.[18,123] The development of a frozen shoulder has also been recently reported after intramuscular vaccination administration.[30,85]

Genetics

A heritability of 42% for frozen shoulder has been reported, although no specific gene has been identified.[136] Wang found over a four times greater risk of developing an idiopathic frozen shoulder in patients with a first degree relative who had developed the disease.[336]

Hypertension

A recent study by Austin and colleagues found an association between idiopathic frozen shoulder and hypertension. In a cohort of patients with the diagnosis of frozen shoulder, the authors found a 50% greater prevalence of antihypertensive medications in these patients than the national average. The authors hypothesized that hypertension is a proinflammatory condition and part of the metabolic syndrome, which can increase the risk of frozen shoulder. However, further research is required to substantiate this.

NATURAL HISTORY

The natural history of frozen shoulder continues to be debated. Many consider primary idiopathic frozen shoulder to be a self-limited disease.[69,280,346] Codman originally stated that "recovery is always sure and can be confidently expected." However, it is not uncommon for patients to continue to have some discomfort and restriction of motion even after the resolution of the thawing phase.[25,129,280,306] Some patients show absolutely no improvement over time or show only mild improvement followed by plateauing.

Meulengracht and Schwartz monitored 65 frozen shoulder patients for 3 years and found 23% developed persistent pain and limitation of shoulder motion.[228] Reeves monitored 41 patients for more than 4 years and identified residual stiffness in more than 60%, with 12% displaying severe restriction in motion.[278] Interestingly, subjective and objective measures of function can differ. At a 3.5-year follow-up, Binder and colleagues found objective motion restriction in 16 of 40 patients, yet only a few complained of significant functional impairment.[25] This result was quite different from the findings of Shaffer and colleagues, who monitored 68 patients with frozen shoulder for approximately 7 years. By objective criteria, 30% of these patients had shoulders that were restricted when compared with the opposite unaffected side, yet 50% complained of persistent pain or stiffness.[306]

Wolf and Green analyzed the influence of several comorbidities on the self-reported functional status of patients with frozen shoulder. They found that increasing numbers of comorbidities were associated with worsening scores on the Disabilities of the Arm, Shoulder, and Hand (DASH) survey, the Simple Shoulder Test (SST), and the SF-36 health status survey.[356]

Involvement of the dominant arm appears to be a good prognostic sign, whereas occupation, ability to work, duration of stiffness, associated injuries, and the treatment program used did not achieve significance when analyzed against other outcome measures.[25,68,145] Patients with insulin-dependent diabetes for more than 10 years tended to have a poorer outcome.[112,168,231]

Hand and colleagues have reported the long-term outcomes of 269 frozen shoulders in 223 patients after a mean follow-up of 4.4 years (range, 2 to 20 years). Of these patients, 59% had normal or near normal shoulders; the remaining 41% reported some ongoing symptoms, but in 94% of the patients, these persistent symptoms were mild. The patients with the most severe symptoms at the onset had the worst long-term prognosis.[139] At a mean follow-up of 9 years (range, 2 to 27 years), Vastamäki and colleagues found that in 94% of the patients the shoulder had improved to near normal with benign neglect. In these patients the duration of symptoms lasted a mean of 15 months.[332]

EVALUATION

In general, a high index of suspicion is necessary to make a definitive diagnosis for primary idiopathic frozen shoulder because other pathologic entities can manifest with shoulder stiffness. A careful history and physical examination are essential. Radiographic and laboratory studies may be helpful in certain instances.

History

As there is no reliable laboratory test or imaging modality for the condition, primary idiopathic frozen shoulder is ultimately a clinical diagnosis. Usually the patient's history and examination provide the only information required to diagnose frozen shoulder. The diagnosis should be considered in patients that present with some degree of pain associated with the corresponding loss of both passive and active ROM. Patients with glenohumeral arthritis often present with similar symptoms, but usually the onset of pain and stiffness occurs over years for arthritis instead of weeks to months as with frozen shoulder. A single true anteroposterior radiograph of the shoulder can easily differentiate idiopathic frozen shoulder from glenohumeral arthritis.

When considering the diagnosis of idiopathic frozen shoulder, it is essential to consider the patient's age, gender, and additional risk factors as outlined in the previous section. Of these, the most relevant are age between 40 and 60 years, female sex, and having diabetes. This pattern can be so reliable that the Chinese refer to idiopathic frozen shoulder as *wishi jian*, which means "fifties shoulder." If a patient lacks these three risk factors, then other diagnoses should strongly be considered.

Stages

Frozen shoulder is classically characterized by three stages: freezing, frozen, and thawing (Fig. 19-6).[144,154,233]

Stage 1: Freezing

This initial stage is characterized by pain. Symptoms have usually been present for several months or less. Typically,

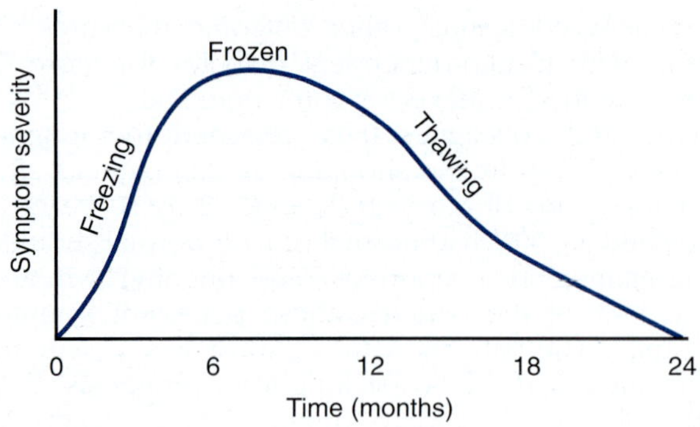

FIGURE 19-6: The traditional stages of primary, idiopathic frozen shoulder with symptom progression and resolution.

patients have what is often described as achy discomfort at rest and severe pain with attempted movements, especially sudden movements. Difficulty with sleeping is an almost universal complaint. Generally, patients limit their use of the affected extremity as discomfort worsens, resulting in loss of function. At this point many patients seek medical attention and the diagnosis can easily be missed. Indeed, many patients are encouraged to immobilize their shoulders, which exacerbates the problem. Reeves wrote that this phase generally lasts between 2 and 9 months.[280]

Stage 2: Frozen

During the frozen phase, the pain tends to abate, but motion becomes severely limited in all planes. Even simple tasks, such as turning off the light and washing hair, become chores. Sleeping is usually problematic. A frozen shoulder is diagnosed in most patients when they enter this stage. Although it can last between 3 and 12 months, the frozen stage can become refractory and last longer.[142,145,249,338]

Stage 3: Thawing

In the final stage ROM slowly returns. As motion improves, residual discomfort generally resolves. Return of flexibility can take months to years.[68,306] Motion restrictions often persist.[25,154] Generally, these restrictions are mild and do not cause significant impairment, but patients should be counseled about this at an early stage.

Differentiating Primary From Secondary Frozen Shoulder

Secondary frozen shoulder does not follow a predictable course like idiopathic frozen shoulder. There are, however, predictable patterns of motion loss after certain injuries. A rotator cuff strain typically causes restricted forward elevation, internal rotation, and cross-body adduction.[142,324,326] This is thought to be related to contracture of the posterior capsule.[146] Articular-sided partial rotator cuff tears are also associated with posterior capsular contractures.[145] Nonanatomic instability repairs result in diminished external rotation. Immobilization after proximal humerus fractures tends to cause a global loss of motion as adhesions form in the subacromial-subdeltoid plane.

Physical Examination

The hallmark of a frozen shoulder is the corresponding loss of both passive and active ROM. A major reason why practitioners that are not experienced with shoulder pathology miss the diagnosis is that they do not test ROM. Instead, the examiner often moves directly to more provocative maneuvers to assess the rotator cuff, which are often positive in frozen shoulder patients. This simple step of testing ROM in the initial evaluation is paramount to avoid subsequent testing and treating being misdirected instead of focusing on the stiffness.

Along with a detailed history, a careful and complete shoulder examination is the key to diagnosing a frozen shoulder. A complete cervical examination should be performed, including neurologic testing of the extremities. The shoulder should be inspected for signs of trauma or previous surgery, which may provide clues for the diagnosis of acquired stiffness. Important landmarks, such as the acromioclavicular joint and bicipital groove, are palpated for tenderness.

ROM, both active and passive, should be tested in all planes and recorded as objectively as possible. This should be repeated in the contralateral shoulder. These measurements are important not only for diagnostic purposes but also to monitor the response to treatment. It is also essential to differentiate glenohumeral motion from humeroscapular motion as many patients with glenohumeral stiffness can compensate with scapulothoracic motion. This is best done by examining the patient in the supine position with the arm free so that the scapula is being compressed against the chest wall through gravity. Alternatively, the examiner can stabilize the scapula with one hand while passively moving the arm with the other. The same measurements should be made at every visit (ideally by the same examiner) and concisely documented until the patient has demonstrated satisfactory improvement. Strength testing of the rotator cuff is performed using standard manual motor testing as well as special tests (belly press, lift-off, lag signs, hornblower's sign). Provocative tests for impingement, acromioclavicular joint pathology, labral tears, instability, and biceps pathology may also be indicated depending on the history and clinical suspicion.

Laboratory Studies

A patient with routine shoulder stiffness does not need laboratory studies for diagnosis or management.[29,287] A complete blood count, C-reactive protein, and erythrocyte sedimentation rate (ESR) may be indicated if there is concern about infection. Decreasing ESR has been observed in patients with successful treatment.[25,228,277,296] In more recent studies, however, ESR has not proved to be reliable or useful when evaluating the patient or monitoring the response to medication.[182,361] A fasting glucose level may be ordered if undiagnosed diabetes mellitus is a concern.[13,200,206,360,336] There are other biochemical mediators associated with frozen shoulder, such as MMPs, TIMPs, TGF-β, and interleukin-6,[176,177,209] but their current role in clinical practice is only experimental.

Imaging

Radiographs

Radiographs are routinely performed for any patient with a stiff shoulder.[324] Specific conditions to be ruled out include fracture, malunion, arthrosis, osteonecrosis, and chronic dislocation. The specific views that are obtained vary depending on the clinical scenario, but a minimum of two orthogonal views is mandatory, including anteroposterior and axillary lateral views. Additional films, such as cervical spine radiographs, may be warranted depending on the clinical suspicion. Radiographs are essential as it can often be difficult to differentiate primary, idiopathic frozen shoulder from glenohumeral arthritis based on history and examination alone.

Routine shoulder radiographs in patients with shoulder stiffness and no history of trauma or surgery are typically normal.[25] Osteopenia of the humeral head may be seen and is probably related to disuse of the extremity.[25,211,282] In approximately 50% of 74 cases of frozen shoulder, Lundberg and Nilsson reported bone loss within a short period.[211] They considered this to be the result of an inflammatory process and not due to disuse alone.

Arthrography

In 1957 Kernwein and colleagues performed arthrographic studies in 12 patients with frozen shoulder.[181] At open biopsy, they found that the capsule and coracohumeral ligament were very contracted, thickened, and inelastic. They also noted the presence of subacute inflammation. Later, Neviaser described the arthrographic findings of adhesive capsulitis, which included decreased joint capacity, obliteration of the reflected axillary fold, and variable filling of the bicipital tendon sheath.[239] No correlation between arthrographic findings and treatment outcome has been found.[25,208] In routine practice today, arthrography is rarely used.

Nuclear Imaging

A bone scan is rarely indicated in the evaluation of a frozen shoulder because these have not proved to be useful in diagnosis, management, or prognosis. Positive bone scans have been reported in as many as 96% of frozen shoulder patients.[334] However, no association has been demonstrated between bone scan activity and the severity of disease, duration of symptoms, arthrographic findings, or ultimate outcome. A bone scan should be ordered only if there is suspicion of a neoplastic process.[25]

Magnetic Resonance Imaging

As techniques and access have improved, magnetic resonance imaging (MRI) has become widely used for evaluating shoulder disorders, including stiffness.[193] Emig and colleagues reported on the MRI characteristics of 10 patients with a frozen shoulder compared with patients without a frozen shoulder.[102] They found the joint capsule and synovium in the frozen shoulder patients to have a combined thickness greater than 4 mm, but they did not observe any significant differences in the volume of intra-articular fluid seen on the MRI scan or in the thickness of the rotator cuff and rotator interval capsule. In a similar study Sofka and colleagues evaluated 46 shoulders with the clinical diagnosis of idiopathic frozen shoulder and attempted to correlate the clinical stage with the MRI characteristics.[313] They found a mean thickness of the axillary pouch of 7.5 mm; this was significantly greater than the axillary pouch measurements in other stages, with means of less than 5.5 mm. Normal capsular and synovial thickness has been found to be less than 3 mm.[218] Abnormalities within the rotator interval are also common. Mengiardi, Gerber, and colleagues described the "subcoracoid triangle sign" as obliteration of the normal-appearing fat between the coracoid process and the coracohumeral ligament on the sagittal oblique images.[227]

The use of IV gadolinium can improve the diagnostic capability of MRI in patients with frozen shoulders. Connell and colleagues noted soft tissue density showing variable enhancement in the rotator interval and partially encasing the biceps anchor on MRI after gadolinium administration.[70] They also noted thickening and gadolinium enhancement of the axillary pouch. Carrillon and colleagues performed IV gadolinium administration followed by MRI and demonstrated enhancement of the synovial lining in patients with frozen shoulder.[61] Tamai and Yamato found enhancement of the joint capsule, which was not seen in patients with subacromial impingement.[321] However, a study that compared findings on MR arthrography in patients with and without frozen shoulder did not identify any specific diagnostic findings for frozen shoulder.[218]

Despite interest shown in it, MRI has not proved to be essential in the diagnosis or management of patients with stiff shoulders, and its routine use in this setting is not supported. Specific indications include concern for underlying rotator cuff integrity and the possibility of a soft tissue or bone neoplasm.

Ultrasound

Several investigators have reported on the use of ultrasound in the evaluation of frozen shoulder.[110,300] Ryu and colleagues noted that the main sonographic feature of frozen shoulder was a constant limitation of the sliding movement of the supraspinatus tendon against the scapula.[300] They reported sensitivity of 91%, specificity of 100%, and accuracy of 92% when comparing ultrasound with arthrography as the gold standard for diagnosis. As with MRI, ultrasound is not a required diagnostic study and is usually indicated only for evaluating the rotator cuff in patients whose physical examination suggests the possibility of a rotator cuff tear coexisting with shoulder stiffness. With the use of ultrasound, Homsi and colleagues found that coracohumeral ligament thickness was greater in idiopathic frozen shoulder patients than in controls.[162]

Arthroscopy

Before performing arthroscopy, the diagnosis of stiffness should already have been made and perhaps confirmed by examination under anesthesia. Arthroscopy allows evaluation and possible treatment of additional pathology, such as rotator cuff tears, impingement, biceps disease, and articular cartilage lesions.

Neviaser described four arthroscopic stages of adhesive capsulitis and proposed that these stages could be used to guide treatment planning[241]:

- A mild erythematous synovitis
- Acute synovitis with adhesions in the dependent folds of the synovial lining
- Maturation of adhesions with less reactive synovitis
- Chronic adhesions without synovitis

Arthroscopic treatment of shoulder stiffness is discussed in detail later in this chapter.

TREATMENT

Frozen shoulder can be a disabling problem for many patients due to the functional limitations and associated pain. Although the literature indicates that most will improve without treatment, many patients are not willing to accept that it may take 2 years for significant resolution of their symptoms[280] (see Fig. 19-6). Most patients present to their physician expecting not only a diagnosis but also a treatment plan to expedite recovery. As with most orthopedic pathology, initial treatment is usually conservative, consisting of activity modification, antiinflammatory medications, and physical therapy. If these treatments fail, there are several more aggressive options, such as manipulation under anesthesia, open surgical release, and arthroscopic release. Many recent publications have focused on the efficacy of arthroscopic procedures to treat frozen shoulder, with promising results.

Understandably, patients become frustrated by continued pain and impaired function. Many are unable to work for some period of time. It is often difficult for patients to understand the condition and accept the uncertainty of resolution. Although there is no consensus on optimal treatment, there appears to be a consensus that some form of treatment, nonoperative or operative, is indicated in any patient with a stiff shoulder.

Nonoperative treatment is the initial approach in almost all patients. This can include oral medications, physical therapy, injections, or other modalities. When patients fail to respond to nonoperative treatment, operative intervention may be indicated. This includes manipulation under anesthesia, surgical release (open or arthroscopic), or some combination of these two treatments.

Nonoperative Treatment

Medication

Various types of analgesics and nonsteroidal antiinflammatory drugs (NSAIDs) have been used as supportive measures to manage the pain and inflammatory component of the stiff shoulder. Their effectiveness in alleviating the pain component has been well established.[26,34,44,97,107,124,164,244,287] Some authors have reported greater improvement in pain in patients who were managed with nonsalicylate analgesics than in those administered NSAIDs.[26] Others have reported that oral steroids produce significantly better improvement in ROM, function, and pain relief in patients with frozen shoulder, but these benefits were not maintained beyond 6 weeks.[47,48] Greater improvement can be expected in patients who combine the intake of such medications with a regular exercise program.[194] Some physicians prescribe short-term, low-dose oral steroids for frozen shoulder, as these can act as a powerful antiinflammatory. Although risks associated with prescribing these medications are small, physicians should still discuss them with patients.[92] We do not routinely prescribe oral steroids for patients as intra-articular steroid injections have been shown to be superior.[207]

Physical Therapy

Physical therapy is a mainstay of initial treatment for shoulder stiffness that has been present for less than 3 to 6 months or in patients who have had no previous treatment.[179] Patients are usually started with active-assisted ROM and gentle passive stretching exercises. Most exercises are easier in the sitting or supine position. Repetition is probably more important than doing one long session. We recommend short sessions of 5 to 10 minutes repeated several times per day, with the goal of trying to push the affected shoulder just slightly past the point of pain during each session. Sometimes it is helpful to have a daily progression chart that the patient can follow. Generally, improvement is seen in small increments. As a result, patients sometimes do not acknowledge their improvement and can become discouraged and frustrated. Patients are encouraged to take NSAIDs and apply heat to the affected shoulder before exercise and to apply ice after exercise. This regimen can help reduce discomfort and improve compliance with the exercises.

Other modalities, such as microwaves, short waves, and heat lamps are sometimes considered as additional measures in the rehabilitation process, although they have not proved to be particularly beneficial in any specific phase of shoulder stiffness.[197] Similarly, adding ultrasound to the physical therapy exercises has not shown any additional benefit to therapy alone.[95,277] Other modalities, such as electrophysiotherapy, massage, or more atypical modalities, such as hyperbaric oxygen and magnetotherapy have been used, but no additional benefit from these could be proved, and none of these treatments fits into a standard shoulder rehabilitation algorithm.[9,33,84,132]

Adding stimuli to distract the mind of the patient from painful sensations has been shown to be helpful during physical therapy exercises. In one study, using audio analgesia as an adjunct to mobilization exercises in patients with chronic frozen shoulder resulted in significant improvement in the recovery of motion and a reduction in the number of treatments necessary for recovery.[99] Using the same rationale, transcutaneous nerve stimulation has been used in patients with frozen shoulder undergoing physical therapy. Rizk and colleagues used transcutaneous nerve stimulation on a group of 28 patients to control their pain during the application of progressive abduction traction.[287] Jurgel and colleagues reported on 10 patients with frozen shoulder who were treated with 4 weeks of rehabilitation that combined exercises with massage and electrical therapy and were able to demonstrate that this protocol improved shoulder ROM in all directions except rotation.[175] They compared this group to a group of 28 patients treated with heat and therapeutic exercises and observed that the increase in ROM was significantly greater in the former group. This may be explained by the strong attachments between collagen fibers, which show high resistance to suddenly applied tension but which also tends to creep when prolonged tension is applied.

Exercises should be performed gently. Forceful stretching maneuvers are contraindicated, especially in the early phases of frozen shoulder. All forms of light resistance strengthening should be postponed until the patient has recovered ROM.[328]

For patients to see improvement from therapy, they must assume primary responsibility for their condition. They should understand and participate actively in the prescribed exercises and be prepared to tolerate some amount of discomfort.[25,76,196,208,238,324,346] Although it can take several months, a closely supervised physical therapy program will lead to improvement in pain and ROM in up to 90% of patients with chronic frozen shoulder.[261] In addition, physical therapy has been shown to improve health-related quality of life.[90]

Nicholson reported on the therapeutic advantage of performing passive stretching in abduction in addition to active ROM exercises.[245] Watson-Jones recommended 3 minutes of active stretching each hour and demonstrated that of 226 frozen shoulders treated with this stretching exercise program alone, only 5% failed to regain satisfactory ROM within 6 months.[346] In another study, 90% of 75 patients who completed a nonoperative program for frozen shoulder achieved satisfactory results, with only 7 patients requiring more aggressive intervention.[131] Russell and colleagues found that a hospital-based group physical therapy program was more effective for restoring ROM and functional scores than individual therapy or a home-based program.[297]

Dudkiewicz and colleagues reported long-term follow-up (mean, 9.2 years; range, 5.5 to 16 years) on 54 frozen shoulder patients who were managed conservatively with physical therapy and NSAIDs.[96] Good long-term outcomes were reported with significantly improved motion in all the measured directions.

Occasionally, physical therapy does not help to improve symptoms in patients with frozen shoulder and at times can even exacerbate them. In one report only 60% of patients who received physical therapy, along with other modalities, achieved the ability to sleep pain-free after 5 months of treatment.[287] Hazelman reported on a group of patients who received physical therapy alone; one third of them experienced an increase in pain, and only half of this group experienced significant improvement with exercises.[153] Diercks and Steven conducted a prospective study on 77 patients with frozen shoulder to compare the effect of intensive physical therapy and manual stretching versus home exercises within the pain limits ("supervised neglect").[91] At 24 months' follow-up, 89% of patients treated with supervised neglect had normal or near-normal painless shoulder function with a Constant score greater than 80. However, only 63% of patients in the group that received intensive physical therapy reached a Constant score of 80 or higher.

Lin and colleagues demonstrated the existence of trapezius muscle imbalance with overactivity of the upper compared with the lower trapezius muscle in patients with frozen shoulder.[202] They concluded that this imbalance in the trapezius muscle might contribute to scapular substitution in compensation for impaired glenohumeral motion and thus rehabilitation of the trapezius should be included in the therapy protocol for patients with frozen shoulder.

Injections

Several different types of injections have been described for treating shoulder stiffness. The simplest types include intra-articular and subacromial injections. Most of the reports on intra-articular injections involve patients with frozen shoulder and not those with acquired stiffness.[50,73,125,160,210,353] Intra-articular injections can be administered along with distention arthrography (brisement), combining chemical and mechanical modalities of treatment.[191,278] Other types of injections include periarticular (trigger point) injections[315,327] and nerve blockade injections (of the suprascapular and upper and lower subscapular nerves).[173]

Intra-Articular Injections

It has been proposed that shoulder stiffness begins with an inflammatory phase followed by scar formation. The theoretical rationale for an intra-articular steroid injection is therefore to inhibit this inflammatory phase, reduce pain, and prevent further development of stiffness. The reported effectiveness of intra-articular steroid injections varies widely.[46,89,276,325]

In most instances intra-articular injections are administered in combination with a physical therapy protocol. For this reason, it is difficult to determine the efficacy of this treatment as an isolated modality. Some investigators have suggested that intra-articular corticosteroid injections provide little or no benefit in the management of shoulder stiffness.[10,46,195,276] Conversely, other investigators have shown beneficial effects from intra-articular steroid injections, mainly of improvement in pain but not in ROM.[276,296,349] When an injection and exercise regimen was compared with analgesics alone, greater improvement was observed with the former.[78]

Widiastuti and Sianturi compared oral triamcinolone intake versus intra-articular triamcinolone injection and concluded that intra-articular steroid administration provided significantly faster improvement when compared with the oral route.[351] Lorbach and colleagues demonstrated similar findings.[207] Williams and colleagues compared exercises and repetitive intra-articular injections of hydrocortisone acetate to serial stellate ganglion blocks, but they were unable to demonstrate significant differences between the treatment groups.[353]

Others have demonstrated intra-articular steroid injections to be more advantageous than trigger point injections. In one study 25% of patients with frozen shoulder benefited from an intra-articular injection, whereas none of the patients who received trigger point injections experienced significant relief.[160] In a study by Carette and colleagues corticosteroid injection plus exercise led to significantly greater improvement than exercise alone or placebo treatment.[60] However, according to Thomas's group this improvement may be related to a decrease in pain rather than a real improvement in ROM.[325] Ryans and colleagues demonstrated in a randomized, blinded, placebo-controlled study that an intra-articular steroid injection was effective in improving shoulder-related disability, which, in combination with home exercise therapy, led to improvement in shoulder external rotation 6 weeks after treatment.[298]

Subacromial injections might also have a role. A prospective, randomized, observer-blind study comparing subacromial steroid injection and physiotherapy demonstrated that injections were as effective as physical therapy alone or in combination.[79] Some investigators have suggested the administration of a combination of injections into both the joint and the subacromial space. However, in comparative studies, no significant differences in pain relief and shoulder ROM at follow-up examination were demonstrated after combined injections.[50,283] This is not unexpected because in frozen shoulder and many cases of acquired stiffness, much of the pathology is intra-articular. Oh and colleagues demonstrated no significant difference in pain, Constant score, or ROM between intra-articular and subacromial injections at more than 6 weeks after injection. These authors concluded that subacromial injections are a reasonable alternative to glenohumeral injections.[252] We routinely perform fluoroscopic glenohumeral injections for all idiopathic frozen shoulder patients because we believe that much of the acute pain associated with the condition may be from glenohumeral synovitis, which is clearly evident in our arthroscopic experience.

In our practice we believe that during the early phase of frozen shoulder, patients might not be able to tolerate physical therapy exercises because of pain. In such cases an intra-articular steroid injection might provide enough relief for the patient to begin an exercise program. We agree with the approach of Weiss and Ting[349] and recommend that all intra-articular injections be performed under radiologic guidance to confirm intra-articular placement. In one study physicians were monitored during the intra-articular injection of radiopaque dye, and the majority of them were unsuccessful in delivering the fluid into the shoulder joint.[283]

When recommending an intra-articular steroid injection, it should be kept in mind that this treatment is not completely benign and complications have been reported. The deleterious effects of intra-articular steroids on tendon metabolism and articular cartilage have been shown in numerous studies.[70,180,319] A case of fatal clostridial myonecrosis after an intra-articular injection of steroids in the shoulder has also been reported.[305] Harryman and Lazarus reported on six cases of chronic sepsis after shoulder arthrography and steroid injections.[143] Shoulder fusion was performed in some of these cases.

Other types of intra-articular injections have garnered interest.[294,320] Tamai and colleagues demonstrated that intra-articular injection of hyaluronate led to the suppression of synovitis, suggesting it has an antiinflammatory property.[320] In a randomized study intra-articular injection of sodium hyaluronate plus steroid was compared with steroid alone for the treatment of frozen shoulder, and both groups improved substantially.[294] Rovetta and colleagues showed that an intra-articular injection of sodium hyaluronate was not as effective in improving ROM in the first 3 months after administration as an intra-articular injection of steroid or physical therapy.[295] In another study intra-articular hyaluronic acid was injected into painful shoulders due either to frozen shoulder or to osteoarthritis.[192] In a short-term follow-up both groups improved substantially in joint comfort and mobility.[192]

Intra-articular injection of enzymatic proteases, such as α-chymotrypsin and hyalase have been used to break up glenohumeral capsular fibrosis.[14,192,294] A few studies have reported the results of intra-articular injection of α-chymotrypsin and hyalase combined with physiotherapy,[14,22] but beneficial effects of this treatment modality were not conclusive. These enzymes are rarely used in current practice.

Capsular Distention

Payr first reported *capsular distention,* also known as *distention arthrography* or *brisement,* in 1931.[264] This is a technique that relies on rupturing the glenohumeral capsule by fluid injection.[6,73,137,191,210,230,254,264,278,307] By injecting progressively higher volumes of fluid into the glenohumeral joint, the pressure eventually builds up until it is high enough for the capsule to be disrupted. This is evident when the pressure of the injection decreases significantly. When capsular disruption occurs, it usually involves the weakest point in the capsule, the biceps tendon sheath, or the subcoracoid bursa.[278]

During the initial injection phase, an arthrogram is often obtained to confirm that the fluid is being injected inside the joint. Some surgeons inject 60 to 100 mL before manipulation in order to produce hydrostatic distention of the joint capsule.[73] More fluid is then injected until the intra-articular pressure increases progressively from 800 mmHg up to a maximum of 1500 mmHg.[133,150,278] Variations of this technique include the injection of saline with local anesthesia and arthroscopic distention.[108,120,163,208,254,280]

Capsular distention has received wide attention because it can be performed in a radiology suite or in an office setting and carries low risk. Several authors have claimed that it is a simple procedure to perform and that it is an effective mechanism for achieving lasting symptomatic relief in patients with frozen shoulder.[106,288,307,310] However, a review of the literature reveals that the results of this modality are variable, as with all other methods of treatment of frozen shoulder.[2,116,254] In addition, steroid injections or manipulations are often performed in conjunction with distention arthrography, which makes comparison between reports and the evaluation of its effectiveness very difficult.

Most cases of distention arthrography reported in the literature have been performed for frozen shoulder. In one study the outcomes of distention arthrography for frozen shoulder and acquired stiffness were compared, with better rates of recovery after 6 months observed in the frozen shoulder group.[279]

In a double-blind prospective study involving 45 patients with frozen shoulder, a comparison was made between distention and nondistention arthrography combined with intra-articular steroid injection.[74] A significant improvement in nocturnal pain was demonstrated in both groups during the first 3 months following the procedure, but no significant difference in ROM and degree of pain relief could be demonstrated between the two groups after 3 months. Rizk and Pinals performed brisement on 16 patients by injecting 30 mL of fluid that contained 20 mL of contrast material, 2 mL of steroid, and 8 mL of lidocaine. This led to capsular rupture in all patients, as evidenced by dye extravasation into the subscapular recess or subacromial space.[289] Thirteen patients experienced immediate relief of pain, with this improvement maintained for 6 months. In two patients who did not experience pain relief, the rupture of the capsule occurred at the level of the distal bicipital sheath. A more recent study by Amoretti and colleagues showed similar results.[3] In addition, Khan and colleagues demonstrated that distention arthrography with intra-articular steroid administration and physical therapy was superior to physical therapy alone.[184]

The patients who experience good results after brisement are those with less severe restriction of ROM and a moderate joint distention before rupture.[6] Improvement in ROM is expected after repeated injections. In a study by Piotte and colleagues the efficacy of repeated distention arthrographies performed at 3-week intervals was evaluated.[270] They showed that two distention arthrographies with steroid, combined with a home exercise program, significantly improved shoulder impairments and disability. However, they were not able to demonstrate a benefit from a third brisement.

When brisement is compared with manipulation under anesthesia (MUA), the reports are variable.[278,279,307] One study by Sharma and colleagues demonstrated significantly better results after distention arthrography.[307] However, other studies have shown that distention arthrography compares unfavorably with MUA.[278,279]

Periarticular Trigger Point Injection and Nerve Blockade

Trigger points are well-localized painful areas around the subscapularis tendon and the periscapular muscles. It is believed that the tenderness of these points is secondary to fibrositis or myofascial inflammation.[169,327] In a study by Steinbrocker and Argyros that included 45 patients with no control group, 95% of patients restored 85% of their function after multiple injections into the joint capsule, bicipital tendon, supraspinatus tendon, and subdeltoid bursa.[315] Other studies have shown that injections into sites other than those mentioned by Steinbrocker and Argyros, including the periarticular region, did not provide long-term benefit or pain relief.[160,234]

The idea of performing nerve blockade to improve the pain component of frozen shoulder started with Wertheim and Rovenstine[350] and later Kopell and Thompson[189] who realized that the suprascapular nerve innervates the joint capsule and could be the main pain generator in patients with frozen shoulder. They demonstrated that suprascapular nerve blockade performed on 20 patients led to substantial pain relief within 24 hours in most of the patients.

For the same reasons, other authors have recommended a suprascapular block with a local anesthetic and steroid to relieve pain.[62,81,125] In a randomized case-control study patients with a diagnosis of frozen shoulder were randomized into either a suprascapular nerve blockade group or a placebo cohort.[80] Significant improvement in pain was demonstrated in the treated patients at 1 month after injection. Another study compared suprascapular nerve blockade to intra-articular corticosteroid injection and found improved pain relief and function in the nerve block group.[173] Repeated suprascapular nerve blockade has also been shown to improve patients' tolerance to deep pressure on the shoulder and to improve passive ROM in frozen shoulder associated with reflex sympathetic dystrophy.[342]

Jankovic and van Zundert studied five patients with frozen shoulder who did not respond to conventional treatment. All these patients underwent a combination of subscapularis nerve blockade along with infiltration of trigger points and all experienced significant pain relief.[169] The authors concluded that the combination of nerve block and trigger point infiltration of the subscapularis muscle might have both therapeutic and diagnostic value for the treatment of frozen shoulder.

Other Modalities

Acupuncture

In a study by Sun and colleagues patients were randomized into two groups to receive physical therapy alone or therapy plus acupuncture, with significant improvement seen in the Constant scores of the patients in the acupuncture group.[317] In another study by Lin and colleagues 150 patients were randomized into three groups and treated with regional nerve blocks, electroacupuncture, or a combination of both treatments.[202] The combination of both treatments resulted in significantly better ROM and longer-lasting pain relief than either treatment alone. Another study showed that undergoing six acupuncture sessions led to complete recovery in patients with frozen shoulder who had experienced limited success with conventional physical therapy.[103]

Calcitonin

The injection of subcutaneous calcitonin and mobilization therapy has been studied prospectively in 50 patients with shoulder stiffness secondary to a number of different etiologies.[334] A significant effect on pain reduction was observed in patients with posttraumatic shoulder stiffness when compared with stiffness from other causes. Other investigators using this modality have documented similar improvement in patients with frozen shoulder and other inflammatory conditions.[8]

Radiation Therapy

Coventry surmised in 1953 that radiation therapy did not bring much benefit in the treatment of chronic frozen shoulder.[76] In a study by Quin radiation therapy was compared with heat and ultrasound but no treatment advantage was found.[277] In another prospective study of 233 patients improvement was found in only 26% of patients.[151] However, in other large series radiation therapy was shown to improve pain in up to 70% of patients with shoulder stiffness, although the long-term risks were not evaluated.[7,32,39,151,364] Radiation therapy might have a role as a treatment option in patients with stiff shoulder-related heterotopic ossification to prevent recurrence after excision. Otherwise, the use of radiation in the United States for the treatment of idiopathic frozen shoulder has been abandoned.

Operative Treatment

Patients who do not regain satisfactory ROM or fail to demonstrate progress after 3 to 6 months of nonoperative care may be candidates for operative intervention. Around 5% to 20% of patients who continue to have significant loss of shoulder motion will remain functionally disabled.[25,68,280,309] Management options include MUA (with or without arthroscopy) or surgical release (open or arthros copic).[142,145,196,216,249,272,303,338] Patients should understand that any form of operative intervention will usually be followed by intensive physical therapy. The decision to proceed with surgical treatment is controversial as some surgeons consider frozen shoulder to be a self-limited process. However, many patients are not willing to accept the prolonged pain and stiffness associated with the natural history of the disease, and so one of the main premises of operative intervention is to expedite the recovery process even if long-term outcomes may be equivalent.

Manipulation Under Anesthesia

Historically, closed MUA has often been recommended as the next step after the failure of nonoperative treatment in patients with stiff shoulder.[98,243,274] However, cases of acquired stiffness in which extra-articular adhesions have developed, as well as changes to the articular anatomy, might not respond well to manipulation.[152,212,213,272,362] Manipulation might be attempted in the acute phase of motion loss when therapy has failed to result in regained motion.

Patients with worsening symptoms after at least 3 months of an appropriate nonoperative exercise program are candidates for MUA.[142,145,183,210] Most reports of MUA have been for patients with frozen shoulder, and the results of this intervention are varied.[63,86,134,135,155,226,354] In one study a greater degree of improvement was achieved in patients who were symptomatic for more than 6 months before manipulation compared with those with a shorter duration of symptoms.[183] This is probably related to the timing of the intervention in relation to the inflammatory phase of frozen shoulder. This phase is usually painful, and as pointed out by Neviaser and Neviaser, any operative intervention in this stage is likely to exacerbate the patient's symptoms and motion loss because of increasing capsular injury.[243] Manipulation should be postponed until pain is experienced only at the extremes of motion, which indicates resolution of the inflammatory phase.

In reports by Neviaser and DePalma the immediate effects of manipulation on structures about the shoulder were observed with arthroscopic and open surgery.[86,243] Tears were seen in the subscapularis muscle and tendon, the anterior and inferior capsule, the supraspinatus tendon, and the long head of the biceps tendon.[143] In addition, because many patients with frozen shoulders have osteopenia of the proximal humerus, fractures may occur with manipulation.[253] Harryman reported on a referred patient with a complete brachial plexus palsy after MUA that resulted in anteroinferior dislocation.[143] The reported cumulative risk of an adverse event after MUA is less than 1%.[63,135,275]

Although complications can arise, other authors have contended that manipulation is a safe and reliable treatment if performed appropriately. Atoun and colleagues manipulated 32 shoulders and showed that manipulation was not associated with rotator cuff tears, fractures, dislocations, or nerve palsies in their cohort.[12]

As with patients with severe osteopenia, MUA is not recommended for patients with long-term diabetes mellitus (lasting longer than 20 years) because these patients are extremely resistant to this method of treatment.[142,145,168] In two studies with short follow-up of approximately 6 months, recurrent stiffness was reported to be between 5% and 20%.[325,354] However, in a study with a longer follow-up of patients with long-term, insulin-dependent diabetes, Janda and Hawkins reported an unacceptably high rate of recurrent stiffness after MUA.[168]

Manipulation can be performed under either regional or general anesthesia, although anesthesia with local injection combined with hydrostatic distention has also been reported.[73] It is essential during the manipulation that complete muscle paralysis be achieved. A regional block is advantageous because the patient can witness the improved ROM immediately after surgery. The immediate postoperative pain is also eliminated, which allows immediate participation in ROM exercises. The block can be administered as a single injection or with placement of an indwelling interscalene catheter.[41,125] A single block of 0.5% bupivacaine provides anesthesia for approximately 12 hours and can be repeated on postoperative days 1 and 2 for continued analgesic effect. If an interscalene block is used, the patient can be maintained on a continuous drip of bupivacaine that provides continuous pain relief during the patient's hospital stay and substantially improves the patient's ability to comply with the intensive physical therapy exercises postoperatively. The addition of systemic steroids has not been shown to have any lasting benefit.[20,205,228]

Codman and Neviaser both described attaching the arm to the bed in a position of abduction and external rotation in order to maintain the motion obtained by the manipulation.[69,240] This maneuver can require significant narcotic analgesia and primarily stretches the anteroinferior portion of the capsule, with the remaining sections of capsule left in a position that can lead to recurrence of the contracture. Other authors have recommended traction to stretch residual contractures and improve motion.[240,242]

To perform the manipulation, the patient is placed supine on the operating room table. Complete muscular paralysis facilitates the procedure and minimizes the risk of fracture. The axillary border of the scapula is stabilized, allowing isolated glenohumeral movement. A constant controlled force is applied to the proximal end of the humerus while the scapula is kept stable; any sudden force increases the risk of fracture or injury to shoulder soft tissues.[155] Gradual traction and flexion are carried out first until an audible and palpable release is heard and felt, indicating rupture of the inferior capsule. The arm is then manipulated into adduction across the patient's chest to stretch or rupture the posterior capsule and restore internal rotation. We perform these manipulations first in order to minimize the theoretical risk of fracture due to the increased torque produced with the rotational movements that follow. The arm is then moved to the side of the body and is held at the supracondylar level while the forearm is rotated very gently into external rotation, taking care not to exert an excessive force that would risk elbow ligament injury. Abduction in the scapular plane is performed with additional internal and external rotation to further release the anterior and posterior capsule. Some steps may be gently repeated until ROM similar to that of the contralateral shoulder is achieved.

Charnley warned against beginning the manipulation with an abduction force because he believed that external rotation had to be achieved first to prevent dislocation.[63] Nevertheless, many authors recommend starting with an initial abduction force.[135,141] A good prognostic sign is the production of crepitus followed by immediate full ROM.[141,183,275] If crepitus does not occur, increased force should not be applied.[142,210] Repeat manipulation may be indicated if the recovered motion is not symmetrical to the opposite side or if motion loss recurs within a short period postoperatively.[134,141] Some authors have reported good results with translational rather than rotational manipulative forces and recommend their application to lessen the chance of fracture.[271]

Although its use has not been proved to enhance the outcome in patients with stiff shoulders, many authors recommended corticosteroid injections after MUA to reduce pain, diminish local inflammation, and decrease the chances of early healing of the disrupted capsule.[135,142,155] In a study of more than 100 patients who underwent MUA, codeine was the only medication required to control pain in the immediate postmanipulation period.[275] In a study by Weiser in which MUA was performed under a local anesthetic, there was full recovery in 60% of patients with three to five treatment sessions.[348] In another study by Thomas and colleagues, 30 patients with frozen shoulders were randomly allocated to one of two groups, one with manipulation and intra-articular steroid injection and the other with intra-articular steroids alone.[325] Of the patients managed with MUA and steroid injection, 80% had decreased pain at follow-up; 40% achieved good ROM, whereas only 47% of patients who received steroid alone had decreased pain, and only 13% achieved good ROM.

The reported outcomes of MUA with or without steroid injection have been highly variable. Good results have been reported in most reviews, except with the long-term diabetic population that is resistant to this treatment and is at a high risk of developing recurrences.[134,143] Haines and Hargadon reported on 78 patients with a mean preoperative duration of symptoms of 2 to 6 months who underwent MUA and steroid injection.[135] At a mean follow-up of 12 weeks, 83% of the patients regained 80% of their glenohumeral motion. Hill and Bogumill reported on 14 frozen shoulder patients with a mean preoperative duration of symptoms of 5.4 months, who underwent MUA and steroid injection.[158] At a mean follow-up of 22 weeks, 75% of the patients were pain-free. Kivimaki and Pohjolainen reported on 24 patients who underwent either MUA alone or MUA with steroid injection and found same results in both groups at 4 months' follow-up.[187]

Weber and colleagues reported on 43 patients with frozen shoulder and a mean preoperative duration of symptoms of 6 months who underwent MUA along with inpatient physiotherapy.[347] At a mean follow-up of 4.7 years, 73% of the patients had gained full recovery of function. Harmon reported on MUA in three separate follow-up studies 2 to 3 years after manipulation, in which 64% to 94% of patients achieved painless motion.[141] Dodenhoff and colleagues reported on 37 patients with a mean preoperative duration of symptoms of 8 months who underwent MUA. They found that 94% patients were satisfied with their result, but 12.8% retained significant persistent disability.[94]

Othman and Taylor reported on 74 patients who underwent MUA and found that significant improvement in range and comfort occurred as early as 3 weeks postoperatively.[257] Sharma and colleagues reported on 32 patients who underwent either MUA or distention with local anesthesia and found significantly better results in the distention group.[307] In a study by Reichmister and Friedman 97% good results were reported in patients who underwent MUA, but 8% of their patients required a second manipulation.[281] Melzer and colleagues reported on 110 patients, comparing those who underwent physiotherapy with medication, as needed, with those who underwent MUA; they concluded that physiotherapy was better than MUA.[226] In a study by Farrell and colleagues MUA was performed on 25 patients with frozen shoulder. The authors reported significant improvement in pain and function, which was maintained for 15 years postoperatively.[109]

Ekelund and Rydell reported on 22 patients who underwent distention arthrography with local anesthetic and steroid followed by MUA and found that 91% of patients had no or slight pain and 83% had almost normal ROM.[100] Similar studies have been performed with local intra-articular anesthesia and manipulation, with the authors claiming successful pain relief and recovery of motion in almost two thirds of patients, with a greater percentage of patients relieved of discomfort alone.[120,208] Lundberg noted that MUA did not affect the natural history or the time course of the disease.[210]

Manipulation and Arthroscopy

MUA usually produces capsular rupture, leading to improved motion, but does not affect intra-articular synovitis. Synovitis may be a major precipitating factor in the development of shoulder stiffness and a contributing factor leading to the recurrence of contracture. In a study by Pollock and colleagues 83% of patients with frozen shoulder who were treated with MUA and arthroscopic debridement achieved a successful result, although patients who were recalcitrant to treatment underwent additional release of the coracohumeral ligament.[272] In a study by Andersen and colleagues 79% of patients who had MUA followed by arthroscopic debridement were pain-free, and 75% had normal ROM at 12 months of follow-up.[4] In a recent study Rill and colleagues demonstrated that frozen shoulder patients with pain and stiffness refractory to conservative means did well following manipulation and arthroscopic release.[286]

Open Surgical Release

Patients who have acquired stiffness resulting from contracture of the extra-articular soft tissues, such as after a Putti-Platt procedure, are unlikely to benefit from MUA. They might not be good candidates for arthroscopic release because the contracture involves both the subscapularis tendon and the capsule.[142,185,237] Open surgical excision of the scar and release of extra-articular adhesions, with or without Z-plasty of the capsule and subscapularis tendon, may be the treatment of choice in this population.

Historically, Codman described open lysis of adhesions in the subacromial and subdeltoid bursae.[69] In patients who experience recurrent stiffness after MUA, Neviaser found it necessary to perform an arthrotomy through an anterior axillary approach, releasing periarticular adhesions and the contracted articular capsule from the humeral head.[238,240] Leffert recommended targeting the structures responsible for restricted motion with a surgical release when patients failed to improve after 6 months of a nonoperative treatment regimen.[196] Lippman suggested the open release of adhesions around the long head of the biceps tendon to liberate the shoulder from stiffness.[204] Simmonds proposed complete excision of the long head of the biceps tendon in cases of severe frozen shoulder.[309] He noted no intra-articular adhesions between the surface of the joint and the articular capsule when he performed these procedures; however, the operative management that he described did not lead to improvements in ROM. Matsen and Kirby recommended open surgical release of the capsule in patients with shoulder stiffness if they failed to improve after 6 months of home exercise therapy.[221] They found this approach to be safer than MUA for patients with osteoporosis and recalcitrant stiffness.

Harmon performed soft tissue release of contracted tissues about the joint in eight patients who failed to improve after gentle manipulation and found the outcome to be similar to that in patients who underwent closed manipulation alone, except two patients who had intractable stiffness.[141] He also treated 30 cases of stiffness with acromioclavicular joint and acromial excision and was able to restore active abduction to around 160 degrees by the third postoperative month.

Kernwein and colleagues performed open release of the capsule and coracohumeral ligament in 4 of 12 patients with frozen shoulder.[181] Tissues were found to be markedly thickened and inelastic. In a study by Ozaki and colleagues the authors reported their findings during the surgical release of 17 patients who had recalcitrant shoulder stiffness.[258] They found that the contracted coracohumeral ligament in the rotator interval was the major tether restricting glenohumeral motion, and they noted that the long head of the biceps tendon was inflamed and stenosed beneath this contracted structure. Nobuhara and colleagues, who performed rotator interval capsular release on 21 shoulders and obtained remarkable improvement in ROM, also appreciated the role of the rotator interval in stiff shoulders.[248]

In one study 25 of 75 patients who failed therapy and MUA underwent open surgical release.[256] At surgery, the coracohumeral ligament was found to be fibrotic and contracted and was excised. Of these 25 patients, 20 achieved good or excellent results; outcomes were worse in patients with long-term diabetes.

As an alternative to the open release of contracted tissues, Baumann described denervation of the ventral aspect of the shoulder capsule, reporting that this method caused a progressive decrease in or total elimination of shoulder pain in 85% of 20 shoulders treated in this fashion.[19] However, this is the only report about this particular technique.

Another population who develops internal rotation contracture is that of patients who had a stroke; as a result, their internal rotator muscles, including the pectoralis major and the subscapularis muscles, spasm and eventually shorten and contract. Braun and colleagues incised the pectoralis major muscle, excised the subscapularis tendon, and preserved the anterior capsule in 13 patients who had this problem.[37] Ten of these 13 patients regained complete pain relief, 20 degrees of external rotation, and 90 degrees of abduction.

When we perform an open surgical release, our preference is to place the patient in the beach chair position.

An interscalene nerve block is performed usually along with general anesthesia. Patients are admitted postoperatively for 48 hours and undergo supervised physical therapy exercises.

We favor the deltopectoral approach unless a prior incision dictates another approach. Layered dissection is performed to excise scar in all tissue planes. The shoulder is placed in abduction and slight flexion to relax the deltoid. Adhesions in the subdeltoid plane are released, taking special care not to injure the axillary nerve, which can be palpated in the substance of the deltoid 3 to 5 centimeters distal to the lateral aspect of the acromion. Once all adhesions have been removed from the subdeltoid region, the humerus may rotate freely beneath the deltoid and the dissection is extended medially to release the adhesions from the subacromial space.

Next, the interval between the conjoined tendon and subscapularis muscle is addressed. The axillary nerve is identified and protected throughout the procedure to allow thorough releases to be performed safely. Adhesions are released by a combination of blunt and sharp dissection. The subscapularis tendon is identified and the rotator interval is released from the humerus to the coracoid.[236,279]

The shoulder is examined at this point to evaluate the effectiveness of the release. In patients with severe internal contractures the subscapularis tendon as well as the anterior capsule is usually shortened and scarred. In such a case, the subscapularis tendon and capsule can be released in the coronal plane using Z-plasty. With this method, the superficial half of the tendon remains attached to the muscle, and the deep half remains attached to the lesser tuberosity. Stay sutures may be placed in the superficial tendon and are used to pull on the muscle, aiding the dissection and the excision of scars tethering the subscapularis muscle to the surrounding tissues. This often requires identification of the axillary nerve and placement of a vessel loop around it to protect it. However, we rarely now perform this procedure to lengthen the tendon. Instead, a complete release of the subscapularis from the anterior glenoid neck and subcoracoid space as well as anteriorly, after identifying the axillary nerve, can achieve sufficient excursion of the tendon to restore physiologic external rotation.

The posterior and inferior capsules are released further if abduction and internal rotation are still limited. A humeral head retractor is placed to retract the head posteriorly to expose the posterior capsule, which is then released from inferior to superior. The shoulder is then placed in maximal external rotation with the arm at the side of the body, and the subscapularis is repaired in a lengthened position using large nonabsorbable braided sutures.

Once the repair is completed, the shoulder is reexamined and the safe zone of early passive ROM is determined. This information is relayed to the physical therapist who will be performing the passive ROM exercises on the patient. In postoperative rehabilitation early, passive rather than active ROM is started until soft tissue healing is substantial at around 4 weeks.

Disadvantages of open surgical release include postoperative pain and the need to protect a repaired or lengthened subscapularis tendon, which explains the less predictable results reported using this technique in patients with acquired stiffness.[117,118,121,339,341] Many of these patients have a concomitant injury to the joint or more extensive soft tissue damage that can limit motion recovery. Successful outcomes are determined by the quality of the surrounding tissue envelope and the status of the articular surfaces.[152,185,212,213]

Arthroscopic Capsular Release

History

Conti, from France, performed the first arthroscopic partial release of a stiff shoulder capsule in 1979.[71] He used a trocar and forceps to release the rotator interval, and he injected intra-articular steroid and performed gentle manipulation. He reported on 18 patients on whom he performed this technique; 16 of them recovered fully within 3 weeks and the other two recovered within 3 to 6 months.

In 1980 Wiley and Older reported on a new arthroscopic technique that they had performed in 10 patients with stiff shoulders.[352] In this technique they performed an arthroscopic examination of the glenohumeral joint, combined with joint distention to stretch the tight capsular constraints and then performed a manipulation. All 10 patients were relieved of their symptoms after the procedure.

In 1986 Ogilvie-Harris and Wiley used blunt instruments and lacerated the anterior capsule to release a tight glenohumeral joint in patients with recalcitrant stiffness secondary to frozen shoulder.[251] They reported satisfactory results in most of the 81 patients on whom they performed this technique. Their results were less satisfactory in patients who had diabetes.

In 1994 Pollock and colleagues reported on 30 shoulders treated with manipulation under interscalene block, followed by diagnostic arthroscopy, debridement of the glenohumeral joint and subacromial space, and sectioning of the coracohumeral ligament.[272] Twenty-five (83%) of the patients had satisfactory results, but only 64% of the patients with diabetes had satisfactory results.

Warner introduced the modern technique of arthroscopic capsular release for primary, idiopathic frozen shoulder in 23 patients in 1997. He performed a complete rotator interval release in addition to complete sectioning of the anterior capsule, middle glenohumeral ligament, and anteroinferior glenohumeral ligament. Significant gains in motion were immediately achieved at the time of surgery, and these were sustained at follow-up of a minimum of 2 years.[339] The technique has evolved to include release of the posterior capsule.[21,145,188,267,338] Chen and colleagues found that extending the release posteriorly beyond the anteroinferior glenohumeral ligament to the posteroinferior glenohumeral ligament improved short-term ROM, but there was no significant difference at 6 months.[64] We routinely extend the capsular release posteriorly to include posteroinferior glenohumeral ligament in order to relieve any internal rotation deficit, which, in our experience, is present in nearly all patients with significant idiopathic adhesive capsulitis.

The morbidity associated with complete arthroscopic capsular release is minimal when compared with open release, with similar rates of recurrent stiffness and earlier pain relief. Complications reported include complete axillary nerve palsy,[145] anterior dislocation occurring immediately postoperatively,[338] and contracture recurrence, which can occur in up to as many as 11% of patients.[345]

Clinical Outcomes

Harryman and colleagues demonstrated a remarkable improvement in six of nine health status scores on the SF-36 general health survey and excellent recovery of function as shown by results of SST after arthroscopic capsular release.[145] They did not observe any significant differences between diabetic and nondiabetic patients, although refractory stiffness developed in three patients with insulin-dependent diabetes. Warner and colleagues reported similar results, with a mean increase of 48 points in Constant score.[338] Similar improvement in Constant scores have been reported by Gerber and colleagues,[117] Jerosch,[170] Bennett,[23] and Massoud and colleagues.[220]

Nicholson reported the results of arthroscopic capsular release in 68 patients with shoulder stiffness secondary to five different etiologies[246]:

1. Idiopathic
2. Postsurgical
3. Posttraumatic
4. Diabetic
5. Impingement syndrome with secondary stiffness

He was able to demonstrate that arthroscopic capsular release was equally effective in relieving pain and restoring function and motion across the five groups of patients.

Gerber and colleagues demonstrated improvement in ROM, pain scores, and Constant scores in 45 shoulders that underwent arthroscopic capsular release for frozen shoulder.[117] They observed that patients with idiopathic frozen shoulder did better after arthroscopic capsular release than the posttraumatic and postsurgical patients. Similarly, Holloway and colleagues reported on 50 patients who underwent arthroscopic capsular release for frozen shoulder with excellent postoperative outcomes.[161] However, patients with shoulder stiffness secondary to a postsurgical etiology achieved less improvement in pain, subjective function, ROM, and overall satisfaction.

Most investigators have reported successful and durable results of arthroscopic capsular release for frozen shoulder. However, more than 50% of patients reported by Segmuller and colleagues were found to have persistent stiffness in internal rotation at a mean follow-up of 13.5 months after arthroscopic inferior capsulotomy performed with cutting diathermy.[303] Despite this residual limitation of function, 88% of the patients were satisfied with their outcome, and 87% had good to excellent results according to their Constant scores.

Better results, with up to 95% of patients achieving complete, painless ROM, were reported in a study by Yamaguchi and colleagues when capsulotomy was combined with the placement of an intra-articular pain pump containing 0.5% bupivacaine.[359] However, recent evidence of the chondrotoxic effect of intra-articular bupivacaine has led many surgeons to refrain from the use of these pumps.[5,16,122,222,314]

Many recent studies have also demonstrated good results. Elhassan, Higgins, Warner, and colleagues demonstrated that arthroscopic release was an effective procedure for shoulder stiffness regardless of the etiology, but patients with postsurgical stiffness did not fare as well as patients with idiopathic or posttraumatic frozen shoulder.[101] Jerosch and colleagues concluded that arthroscopic capsular release is effective for treating both primary and secondary frozen shoulder, according to their findings at a mean follow-up of 3 years.[171] Le Lievre and colleagues found that arthroscopic capsular release is a durable procedure, with pain relief and motion maintained at a mean follow-up of 7 years, with motion essentially equivalent to that of the contralateral shoulder.[198] Waszczykowski and colleagues found that there was no significant decrease in strength in patients followed up a minimum of 2 years after an arthroscopic capsular release.[343]

Subscapularis Release

After its initial description by McLaughlin, subscapularis tendon release has been reported by several authors as part of a complete capsular release.[93,166,217,266,267] Ide and colleagues reported on 42 patients with shoulder stiffness secondary to various etiologies. All the patients underwent complete capsular release with release of the intra-articular subscapularis tendon if the patient had loss of external rotation.[166] The results at 7.5 years follow-up were 84% excellent, 7% good, and 9% poor. No complications were reported. Pearsall and colleagues reported on 35 patients who underwent capsular and subscapularis release; only one of these patients had possible subscapularis insufficiency postoperatively.[266,267]

Similarly, Diwan and colleagues presented a case-controlled cohort study of 40 patients divided into two cohorts.[93] The first cohort of 18 patients underwent a standard arthroscopic anteroinferior release of the capsule. The second cohort of 22 patients underwent the same release along with an extended posterior release and release of a portion of the intra-articular part of the subscapularis tendon as well as a modified physical therapy program. Both groups showed significant reduction of pain by 1 week postoperatively, but improved ROM was seen in the second group. No instability or subscapularis weakness, as determined by the lift-off test, was seen in either group.

Liem and colleagues demonstrated that concomitant release of the intra-articular portion of the subscapularis in addition to an arthroscopic capsular release demonstrated good clinical results without a resultant internal rotation deficit.[201] However, despite the results of this study, we do not recommend routine subscapularis release for frozen shoulder because a thorough and safe arthroscopic release usually restores adequate motion without the need to transect the subscapularis.

Cost-Effectiveness and Value

In the current political and socioeconomic climate of the United States, demonstrating clinical utility alone is no longer sufficient to support the effectiveness of a procedure. A greater emphasis is being placed on value, which takes into account not only patient outcomes but also cost.[27,28] Maund and colleagues have contended that the poor quality of the data precludes a definitive cost-effectiveness analysis among the various treatments of frozen shoulder.[224] Steroid injection and physical therapy was the only treatment that demonstrated a statistically significant clinical benefit in the short term. In response Dattani and colleagues evaluated the cost and outcomes of treating 100 patients with an arthroscopic capsular release, concluding that arthroscopic treatment was a cost-effective procedure that can restore health-related quality of life in most patients within 6 months of surgery.[82] Currently, there is insufficient evidence available to make a compelling determination of the most cost-effective way to manage frozen shoulder.

Comparative Analysis

In a prospective study by Hsu and Chan of 75 patients in 1991, shoulder arthroscopy with distention or manipulation led to better outcomes than physical therapy alone. They favored arthroscopic distention over manipulation because it provided valuable insight into the intra-articular pathology and was more controllable.[163]

In another study comparing manipulation with arthroscopic release in patients with resistant frozen shoulder, Ogilvie-Harris and colleagues also showed significantly better results with arthroscopic release at 2 to 5 years of follow-up.[249] Their arthroscopic release technique included synovectomy in the rotator interval, division of the anterior capsule and the superior glenohumeral ligament, and division of the subscapularis tendon and the inferior capsule. Patients with diabetes initially did worse, but the final outcome for these patients was similar to that for patients without diabetes. The authors concluded that despite the worse outcomes initially reported in diabetic patients with frozen shoulder, these patients still do well after arthroscopic release if they undergo early intervention. Ogilvie-Harris and Myerthall demonstrated no pain and symmetrical motion in 13 of 17 diabetic patients with frozen shoulder who had undergone arthroscopic release.[250]

There have been several recent publications evaluating the efficacy of arthroscopic capsular release for frozen shoulder, and the trend appears to be shifting towards shoulder surgeons performing arthroscopic releases rather than manipulations for recalcitrant frozen shoulder. However, Grant and colleagues were unable to demonstrate any significant difference when comparing arthroscopic releases to closed manipulation. They noted that the quality of evidence was low, and that high-quality studies are needed to definitively compare the procedures.[126] Walther and colleagues retrospectively reviewed the results of 54 patients treated with arthroscopic subacromial decompression and manipulation, arthroscopic subacromial and glenohumeral release, or selective glenohumeral releases only, and found no significant difference between the surgical strategies.[335] Currently, there is insufficient definitive evidence to recommend a single treatment strategy over another.

AUTHORS' PREFERED TREATMENT

Nonoperative Treatment

We advocate a nonoperative protocol using the Jackins (University of Washington) exercise program[143] once the following criteria are satisfied: there has been a comprehensive history and physical examination, comorbid treatable conditions have been managed, the inflammatory plane has been resolved, and analgesics or NSAIDs have been initiated with titration to the patient tolerance.

The Jackins program is performed 5 times daily (with each exercise repeated 8 to 10 times) after the application of heat to the shoulder to improve flexibility. Pain is ideally managed with oral analgesics or a nonsteroidal medication, or both. Although we prefer not to prescribe narcotics, administration is considered on a case-by-case basis, often before therapy or to facilitate sleep. Intra-articular injection with a long-acting anesthetic (bupivacaine 0.5%) and steroid (dexamethasone or methylprednisolone) may be helpful, especially in the acute inflammatory phase. In addition, if the patient is in the more acute inflammatory stage, and it is made more painful by physical therapy, a short hiatus in therapy may be beneficial. We recommend the resumption of therapy with less intensity once the flare resolves.

Of particular importance is the strict avoidance of strengthening exercises during this stretching phase. We believe the premature use of a strengthening program might serve to inflame the affected shoulder. Even isometric exercises should be avoided until the patient's motion closely approximates normal.

The role of the therapist has several facets. Many of the Jackins exercises are suitable for a home-based program, but we find that early supervision is particularly helpful to ensure that patients are stretching appropriately. The introduction of joint mobilization exercises, particularly for internal rotation, can restore motion in a more timely fashion. Finally, the therapist may be able to more accurately chart progress and provide encouragement during the lengthy recuperative process. We encourage patients to see a physical therapist on a biweekly basis once the patient is comfortable with the home exercise program.

Manipulation Under Anesthesia

Indications and Contraindications

Indications for MUA include failure to progress in motion gains despite 4 to 6 months of regular Jackins exercises or failure to obtain pain relief or increased ROM despite intra-articular steroid injection and 3 months of Jackins exercises. The current role of manipulation in our practice is limited and has been superseded by arthroscopic release.

Contraindications include the inflammatory phase of frozen shoulder, failed previous MUA, concomitant rotator cuff tear, severe osteopenia with a significant risk of fracture if MUA is performed, neurologic injury, secondary stiffness as a result of previous surgery (especially rotator cuff repair), posttraumatic stiffness, and chronic insulin-dependent diabetes mellitus.

Technique

The stepwise approach to MUA is critical to ensure that the glenohumeral capsule is ruptured anteriorly, anteroinferiorly, inferiorly, posteroinferiorly, and posteriorly. We prefer to rupture the inferior capsule first because this minimizes glenohumeral torque and therefore potentiates less fracture risk than rotation.

The use of two-finger force is a suitable and appropriate guideline, particularly for rotational movements, to help avoid fracture or other injury. If the capsule cannot be ruptured with this quantity of force, conversion to arthroscopic release may be indicated. To facilitate conversion, manipulations may be performed in a beach chair position to allow scapular stabilization and easy conversion to arthroscopic or open techniques as necessary.

During manipulation, palpable and audible confirmation of capsular and/or adhesion rupture is routinely encountered. If this release does not occur, or if, despite release, motion is incompletely restored, we recommend proceeding with arthroscopic or open release. We routinely employ interscalene block anesthesia with an indwelling catheter if possible, which provides significant perioperative analgesia and allows the patient to engage in physical therapy on the day of surgery and twice daily afterward. It is customary for patients to be admitted for 48 hours while the indwelling catheter is in place to facilitate early ROM in a painless fashion, which we believe is extremely beneficial to restoring motion and showing the patient what the potential improvement in motion will be.

Strategy

Sagittal manipulation into forward flexion with force applied as proximal on the arm as possible to minimize torque (by reducing the lever arm) should rupture the inferior capsule. Coronal manipulation into abduction with scapular stabilization by exerting a downward pressure on the scapula (at approximately 90 to 100 degrees) completes the inferior capsular rupture. Combined abduction and external rotation (at 90 degrees), along with gentle manipulation using the two-finger approach, ruptures the anteroinferior capsule. Midrange abduction (at 45 degrees) and external rotation ruptures the middle glenohumeral ligament and capsule. Adduction with external rotation ruptures the anterior capsule and superior glenohumeral ligament. Cross-body adduction with the arm at 90 degrees, bringing the humerus under the chin, ruptures the posterior capsule. Combined internal rotation and abduction in the coronal plane further releases the posterior capsule.

Provided that the contralateral extremity has a full physiologic ROM, we use this as a guide to ensure completeness of MUA. Although some surgeons advocate the injection of intra-articular steroids at the end of the procedure, we do not do this routinely. The addition of a short course of oral steroids (methylprednisolone) might play a role if it is clinically indicated for patients with significant pain in the absence of contraindications for steroid use (i.e., diabetes).

Postoperative Management

We consider it extremely important to initiate physical therapy on the day of the manipulation. A physical therapist demonstrates motion restoration to the patient and reinforces the benefits of sustained stretching at numerous intervals. We encourage patients to follow Jackins' recommendation regarding the frequency of stretching.

In contrast to the home-based program described by Jackins, we believe that outpatient physical therapy is of significant benefit. We routinely recommend supervised therapy for 5 days per week for the first 2 weeks, then 4 days a week for 2 weeks, and finally 3 days a week. After MUA, patients might experience pain that inhibits an independent program, and having a skilled therapist who performs joint mobilization and edema control and monitors progress is of great benefit for the first 4 postoperative weeks. Thereafter, as the pain subsides, patients are transitioned to a home exercise program. Full motion is typically restored within 3 months after manipulation, although it is not uncommon for subtle motion loss to be present.

Operative Treatment

Arthroscopic Capsular Release

In our experience surgical treatment for idiopathic frozen shoulder is necessary for less than 5% of those seeking care. For patients in whom a concerted conservative approach has failed and who experience recalcitrant shoulder stiffness, arthroscopic release of these contractures is offered. The main objective is to perform a systematic release, as indicated, for the rotator interval, the superior glenohumeral ligament, the coracohumeral ligament, the anterior capsule, the middle glenohumeral ligament, the inferior glenohumeral ligament (anterior and posterior bands), the inferior capsule, and the posterior capsule.

There are several benefits to an arthroscopic release, many of which are simply benefits of arthroscopic surgery over similar open procedures. One particular advantage of the arthroscopic approach is the enhanced visualization that this approach affords the surgeon. The pathologic capsule can be visualized directly and can be released accordingly. Comorbid conditions can be addressed in a relatively atraumatic fashion. Specifically, biceps tendon disease may be addressed simultaneously with a tenotomy or tenodesis with little to no effect on the capsular release or subsequent physical therapy. Concomitant synovitis, which appears to be ubiquitous, may be addressed throughout the joint. The evaluation of the subacromial space and the need for soft tissue or bony decompression is easily achieved. Finally, aggressive physical therapy is immediately acceptable.

Technique

The procedure is performed in a beach chair position with a pneumatic arm holder (Spyder Arm Holder, Tenet Medical) to aid in positioning the extremity. A standard posterior portal is placed approximately 1 cm medial to the edge of the posterolateral acromion and 2 cm inferior to the acromion. Routine arthroscopic equipment is employed and a radiofrequency device for tissue ablation and coagulation is mandatory. We prefer not to manipulate the joint before arthroscopy because this creates a substantial hemarthrosis and allows fluid extravasation from the joint from the start of the arthroscopy. We record a detailed assessment of the passive ROM for forward flexion, abduction, external rotation in adduction and abduction, and internal rotation prior to entering with arthroscopic instruments.

A standard anterior superior portal is created with an outside-in technique, using an 18-gauge spinal needle to localize the incision. A standard 5.5-mm cannula is inserted, often over a metal trocar, because the tissue in the rotator interval as well as the anterior capsule may be hypertrophic. We attempt a diagnostic arthroscopy, but if the glenohumeral joint is too tight to safely visualize structures without risking chondral damage, comprehensive visualization is completed after the release. Synovitis is addressed and the biceps is thoroughly evaluated. The biceps is aggressively treated with tenotomy or tenodesis if there are signs of significant tendinopathy, partial tearing, tenosynovitis, or subluxation or if the excursion of the biceps in the intertubercular groove is restricted. A systematic capsular release follows.

Rotator Interval and Anterior Capsular Release

We start our capsular release from the glenohumeral joint,[333] even though other authors have described good results with debridement of the interval from an extra-articular arthroscopic approach.[190] Starting above the superior glenohumeral ligament, a hook-tipped radiofrequency device is used to divide the superior glenohumeral ligament and the anterior capsule to the superior border of the intra-articular subscapularis. During this release, the rotator interval, which is generally contracted, is released and the humeral head translates inferiorly and laterally, allowing the arthroscope to be advanced and markedly facilitating visualization. The middle glenohumeral ligament is released as it crosses posterior to the subscapularis. The anterior capsule is released inferiorly past the anterior band of the inferior glenohumeral ligament. From this position, the axillary nerve is in close proximity and attention is directed to the posterior capsule.

Posterior Capsular Release

For patients with a restricted internal rotation, a posterior capsular release follows. A switching stick is placed to maintain the position of the posterior portal, and the arthroscope is placed in the anterior portal. Once anterior visualization is confirmed, a 5.5-mm cannula is placed over the switching stick and advanced intra-articularly. The hook-tipped radiofrequency device is placed through the posterior cannula and the cannula is gently moved to lie just outside of the joint. This allows the radiofrequency device to release the capsule just adjacent to the glenoid. In this region the capsule overlies the muscular component of the posterior rotator cuff, and this allows confirmation of a complete posterior capsular release. The release extends inferiorly through the posterior band of the inferior glenohumeral ligament. The radiofrequency device is then used to carefully work inferiorly, keeping in mind that the axillary nerve is in close proximity to the capsule. The inferior capsule is carefully released, layer by layer, until the posterior and anterior capsulotomies are connected. Figures 19-7 to 19-10 illustrate the sequence of arthroscopic capsular release.

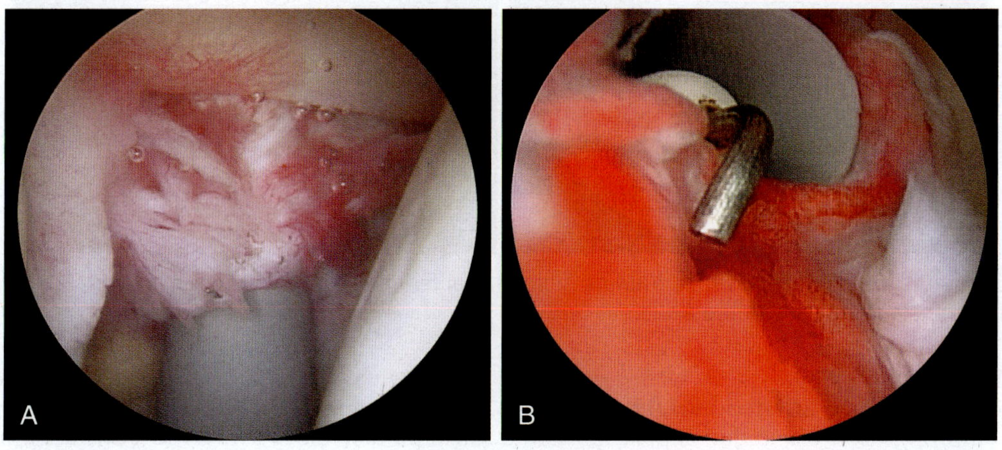

FIGURE 19-7: Right shoulder, viewing from the posterior portal. **A,** Thick scar in the rotator interval. Biceps tendon on top, humeral head on the left. **B,** Typical appearance of synovitis intra-articularly.

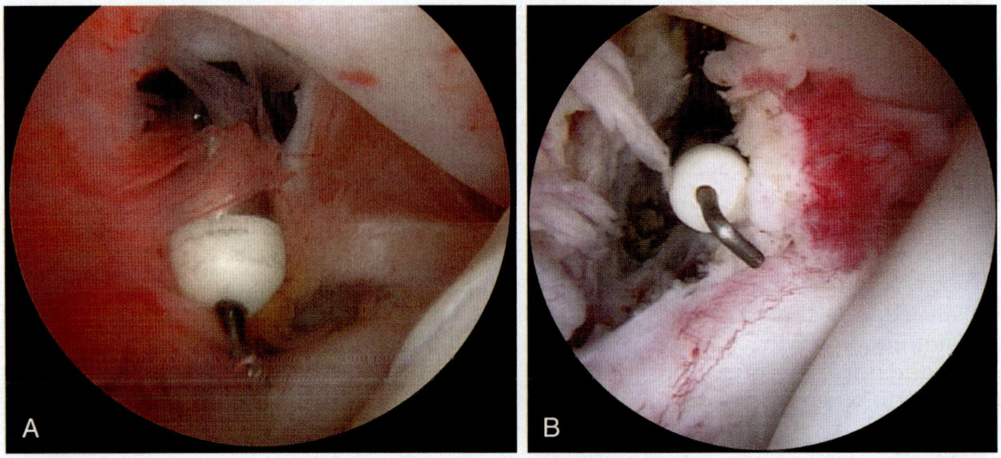

FIGURE 19-8: **A,** Anterior rotator interval release. Note the hook-tipped electrode, which facilitates the release. **B,** Completion of rotator interval release.

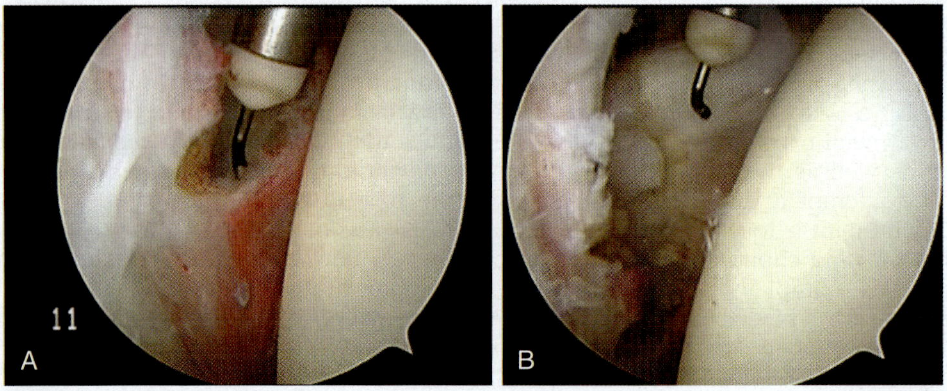

FIGURE 19-9: Release of the middle glenohumeral ligament and inferior glenohumeral ligament. **A,** The intra-articular subscapularis is left intact as the middle glenohumeral ligament is released. **B,** Completion of release through the inferior glenohumeral ligament. Note the muscle fibers of the subscapularis.

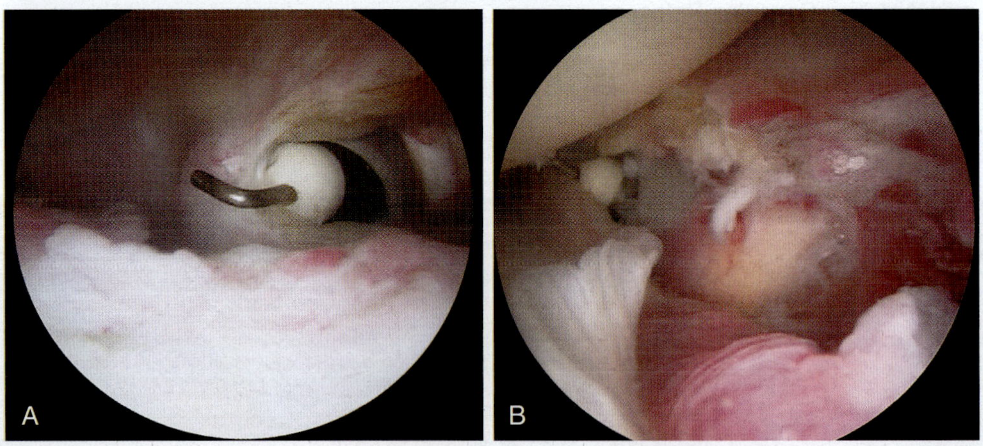

FIGURE 19-10: Posterior capsular release. **A,** Viewing from the anterior portal; the release begins 1 cm from the labrum. **B,** Completion of the posterior release to the axilla.

Subacromial Lysis of Adhesions

The arthroscope may now be inserted into the subacromial space, and thorough soft tissue decompression may be performed. In cases of primary frozen shoulder there are rarely thick adhesions in this region. Posttraumatic or postsurgical cases often have thick, dense subacromial adhesions, and the radiofrequency device is used to meticulously peel away the adhesions and rotator cuff from the acromion. Hasty debridement or manipulation can damage the rotator cuff. The coracoacromial arch is not violated unless there is a significant acromial spur that necessitates bony decompression. Meticulous hemostasis in the subacromial space and the glenohumeral joint is confirmed. At this juncture, the arm may be removed from the arm holder and ROM assessed. A gentle manipulation is performed as described earlier. If loss of motion persists even after complete capsular release and subacromial debridement, then an open release may be needed to address extracapsular scarring or to permit tendon mobilization or Z-plasty lengthening for the treatment of any residual loss of external rotation. The shoulder's motion in all planes is recorded, and this is conveyed to the physical therapist.

Postoperative Management

Passive ROM exercises begin immediately with the therapist, based on the knowledge of ROM obtained after release and manipulation. We do not use continuous passive ROM machines for the shoulder because we believe that there is not only substantial scapulothoracic movement with these devices but also that these machines do not adequately manipulate into the end ROM, which is critical for maintaining and optimizing recovery. The hospital course is typically 48 hours, with therapy twice daily. The patient is instructed to initiate outpatient physical therapy 5 days a week for the first 2 weeks and is then reassessed to determine the adequacy of treatment and the frequency of therapy thereafter.

Open Surgical Release

With the advances in extra-articular arthroscopy and the accomplishment of accurate dissection without open release, the relative indications for and frequency of open surgical release have decreased. However, the arthroscopic application of release has several shortcomings. Dense scar, which may be adherent to neurovascular structures, is difficult to manage arthroscopically. Arthroscopic release does not practically allow lengthening of the subscapularis, which may be necessary to improve ROM. Occasionally, the shoulder is so stiff that it is difficult to introduce the arthroscope and instruments without risking damage to articular cartilage.

In certain cases, arthroscopic release may be combined with open release. Releases of the rotator interval and the posterior, inferior, and anterior capsular regions may be performed arthroscopically followed by open release of extra-articular adhesions. This may be especially relevant in the setting of previous open anterior surgery, stiffness after fracture, stiffness following rotator cuff surgery, and stiffness after shoulder arthroplasty.

Technique

Careful examination, with accurate ROM measurement under anesthesia compared with that of the normal contralateral shoulder, will define planes of restricted motion and focus the nature of the release. Subdeltoid adhesions, in contrast to intra-articular capsular contracture, rarely respond to MUA. In fact, the potential to create injury, including fractures of the humerus and rotator cuff tears (particularly subscapularis rupture), has been the basis for our strong recommendation to not perform an MUA when a subdeltoid release is indicated.

The surgical release should be systematic and precise. Even if other incisions (such as saber type) are present, a deltopectoral incision should be used because its extensile nature will maximize exposure. For dense adhesions in the subdeltoid space, two approaches are recommended. The first involves dissection distal to the rotator cuff musculature beginning just proximal to the deltoid insertion. The distal aspect of an extended deltopectoral incision is rarely involved with dense scar, and dissection along the shaft of the humerus is safe in this zone. Careful dissection proximally follows and facilitates identification of the plane between the rotator cuff and deltoid. Movement of the arm, particularly rotation, further exposes this interface and allows dissection up into the subacromial space. The second approach is to the subacromial space, ensuring the coracoacromial ligament is preserved if possible. After the rotator cuff is identified, hypertrophic bursa and scar may be excised.

Although dense scar can occur in the subdeltoid plane, dissection here is typically straightforward and does not require dissection of neurovascular structures. The axillary nerve does not require exposure, and the plane for mobility is often clearly visualized with humeral motion, in contrast to the plane between the conjoined tendon and the underlying subscapularis. At times, external rotation can ease dissection, but it can also close the interval, and forward flexion with internal rotation might improve visualization. The axillary and musculocutaneous nerves, as well as the remainder of the brachial plexus, are in close proximity and may be damaged not only by dissection but also during retraction.

If adequate motion is obtained and scar still exists within this plane, we take a more conservative approach that stops short of complete resection of scar anterior to the subscapularis. There are data suggesting that fatty infiltration of the subscapularis may be related to aggressive dissection and injury to the small motor branches to the subscapularis; this has tempered our previous enthusiasm for a more extensive dissection. These small motor nerves are difficult to dissect and may be unwittingly damaged during dissection.

If full motion is not obtained, a more aggressive dissection is mandated, with isolation or identification of the axillary nerve and unfettered access to the entire subdeltoid space. This extra-articular release is completed with an intra-articular subscapularis release, constituting a 360-degree release of the subscapularis. After complete extra-articular mobilization, if external rotation is not at least 40 degrees, a formal lengthening of the rotator cuff is necessary. Although there are several options to accomplish this, it is our strong preference to avoid it if at all possible.

Subscapularis Lengthening

Lengthening of the subscapularis is an undesirable but potentially necessary adjunct to obtain ROM, primarily external rotation. The association between loss of external rotation after instability procedures and the onset of early osteoarthrosis has been clearly defined. We therefore attempt to obtain at least 40 degrees of external rotation; however, there are no data defining this as the necessary arc of motion to obtain. There are three commonly employed techniques to lengthen the subscapularis, described in order of preference. The coracohumeral ligament should be released in each of these scenarios.

The choice of technique for subscapularis lengthening is predicated on several criteria. If the subscapularis has previously been repaired, or if a previous surgical approach has been made through the subscapularis, it is critical to assess the quality and thickness of the tendon. If the tendon is robust, a 360-degree release and capsular release may be all that is needed. For thick tendons, a Z-lengthening is possible, but this is a poor option if the tendon is thin and atrophic. Medialization of the tendon, our preferred option, is effective for all tendon thicknesses, although it is clear that the healing potential of any technique is affected by subscapularis quality.

Our preferred approach is a subscapularis slide, which involves medialization of the tendon insertion on the lesser tuberosity. As the lesser tuberosity is only slightly more than 1 cm, the gains with this approach are more modest. Typically, 1 cm of medialization of the tendon increases external rotation by 15 to 20 degrees with the benefit of a lower risk of subscapularis rupture.

For a subscapularis slide, the arm is placed in neutral to external rotation. By placing a freer elevator in the joint through the rotator interval, the attachment of the subscapularis can clearly be identified. The subscapularis and capsule are meticulously and sharply dissected off the humerus as a single unit until the muscular portion of the subscapularis is encountered (bottom third of the subscapularis). At this point, the muscle fibers are left intact and only the capsule is divided along the articular edge of the humerus. During this mobilization, it may be beneficial both to tag the subscapularis and to progressively externally rotate the humerus to keep the structures under tension to facilitate the release. Maintaining the inferior subscapularis attachment and remaining entirely within the joint protects the axillary nerve. Once the intra-articular release is completed, the subscapularis tendon is reattached to the humerus. This is accomplished by placing large (No. 2 or 5) nonabsorbable sutures through the tendon in a modified Mason-Allen configuration and placing sutures in a transosseous configuration at the articular margin. This effectively lengthens the subscapularis by medializing its attachment.

Alternatively, in thick tendon a Neer Z-lengthening of the subscapularis may be performed. With careful dissection, the anterior half of the subscapularis tendon is divided just at the margin of the lesser tuberosity, leaving the posterior half of the tendon attached. Tagging sutures are placed in the tendon, and the anterior half of the tendon is dissected medially to the level of the anterior glenoid. The anterior capsule is then divided at this level just lateral to the anterior glenoid rim. By entering the joint, the inferior capsule may be preserved while the axillary nerve is protected. Closure of the anterior flap lateral edge to the posterior (or deep) flap medial edge effectively lengthens the subscapularis by approximately 2 cm, with a corresponding gain of 40 degrees of external rotation.

Any surgery to the subscapularis results in weakening of the tendon, and particular care should be given to ensure healing of the construct. External rotation stretching must be judicious in the first 2 months, and resisted internal rotation must be restricted for at least 3 months. In addition, the motion safely obtained intraoperatively should be conveyed directly to the therapist caring for the patient. A lack of communication can lead to subscapularis rupture and its sequelae.

Postoperative Management

Patients are admitted for a 2-day hospital stay with a continuous interscalene catheter infusion for pain management. The intraoperative measurement of safe motion is initiated immediately in a passive fashion. Daily physical therapy complements a home-based program of motion every 2 hours within safe zones. We do not use shoulder continuous passive motion devices for the reasons stated previously. The entire process focuses upon ROM for the first 6 weeks, with absolute avoidance of strengthening exercises during this period. Isometric strengthening commences when near-symmetric ROM is achieved.

SUMMARY

Our knowledge about the stiff shoulder continues to broaden. Definitions have become clearer and the classification system has become more precise. Accordingly, treatment algorithms have become more streamlined and clinical studies have become more specific in terms of individual patient populations. Although the pathogenesis is still elusive, ongoing basic science research has given us more insight into the cellular and biochemical pathways that result in shoulder stiffness.

Above all, the diagnosis of a stiff shoulder depends on awareness of the problem. The history and physical examination are paramount, and ancillary studies may also be helpful in certain circumstances. It is important to understand the natural history so that patients are well informed and can actively participate in decision-making.

No treatment has proved to be definitive. In fact, the literature supports many forms of treatment, both operative and nonoperative. All of these treatments have potential advantages and disadvantages, and therefore the treatment approach should be tailored to each individual patient to ensure the best possible outcome. In the future we can expect scientific breakthroughs to lead to the development of new treatment modalities and ultimately to improved clinical outcomes.

Acknowledgments

We acknowledge the contributions of Douglas T. Harryman II, MD, Mark D. Lazarus, MD, and Nathan K. Endres, MD to this chapter in earlier versions of this textbook.

INTERNATIONAL EXPERT COMMENTARY

I.A. Trail

The authors are to be congratulated on producing an excellent and thorough review on what can be one of the most perplexing problems confronting shoulder surgeons. As they point out, much of this confusion stems from inconsistencies within various classifications and, as such, the difficulty in comparing outcomes of the various treatments. The terms "idiopathic frozen shoulder" and "adhesive capsulitis" have been used for over 100 years and describe a particular clinical entity. Most clinicians recognize a history of spontaneous shoulder pain that often disturbs sleep and requires strong analgesics. Occasionally, the pain can be preceded by a minor traumatic event. If symptoms persist, however, active and passive shoulder movements often diminish. Generally, the disease process can last 12 to 18 months, and if untreated while the pain subsides, shoulders can be left with significant stiffness. This often occurs in the absence of any obvious etiology and with normal investigations, particularly radiologic assessment. On occasion, however, the condition can be associated with certain debilitating illnesses and indeed with injury to the ipsilateral limb. The condition is also seen more often in patients who have diabetes or hypothyroidism.

Currently, the diagnosis is made purely on the basis of history and examination, as there is no specific diagnostic test. The absence of such a test can obviously make any scientific study difficult. The definition derived by the American Academy of Orthopaedic Surgeons in 1992 although undoubtedly includes classical cases of frozen shoulder, it unfortunately leaves the door open for the potential inclusion of other causes of stiffness.

The picture is further complicated by the use of the terms "primary" and "secondary" as first used by Zuckerman in 2011. Secondary frozen shoulder was further subclassified into intrinsic, extrinsic, and systemic. In all these, however, stiffness is predominantly a symptom of an alternative disease process (such as rotator cuff impingement or glenohumeral arthritis).

Finally, there is also a group of patients who predominantly present with stiffness, not falling into any recognized clinical pattern and for whom no obvious etiology can be identified. Often these patients are the subject of a medicolegal case involving compensation as a consequence of an accident. Diagnosis in this group is established by exclusion. Often these patients do not respond well to recognized treatment modalities.

As stated previously, the diagnosis for "primary frozen shoulder/adhesive capsulitis" is made principally based on the history. The overriding feature, at least at initial presentation, is severe pain. Examination will reveal a significant loss of movement in all planes. Typical features include the loss of passive and active internal and external rotation with the arm in neutral. This, in the presence of a normal plain radiograph, is usually enough to make the diagnosis. Otherwise, there are no definitive investigations, particularly blood tests. Other investigations, including ultrasound, MRI and MR arthrogram, while often demonstrating typical features, are not sufficient in isolation to make the diagnosis, although they can of course be helpful in excluding other pathology. For the so-called "secondary frozen shoulder," history and examination will lead the clinician to a specific diagnosis that should be confirmed by investigation. As stated previously, stiffness can simply be one symptom of this disease process.

With regard to management, although exact details relating to the natural history remain unclear, as the authors have described, it is generally held that over a period of 12 to 18 months the initial severe pain subsides and movements return. In many instances patients, even if untreated, can regain a satisfactory ROM. Undoubtedly, however, older patients can be left with significant loss of movement. Given the severity and the prolonged nature of the pain, most patients nowadays seek medical advice. Once the diagnosis is made, the primary and most important facet of treatment is pain control. This is usually achieved by a combination of oral analgesics and antiinflammatories, along with the pain-relieving modalities of physiotherapy. On occasion the pain is particularly refractory and nerve blocks can be of value. Once pain relief has been obtained, attempts can be made to regain motion. In the first instance this would again take the form of physical therapy. Indeed, this can be used either in isolation or in combination with other treatment modalities. Adequate pain relief and physical therapy would in the first instance form the basis of treatment for the majority of patients. Although it is not clear as to how often this is successful, it is assumed that the majority of patients recover.

With regard to alternative management, the authors have pointed out a particular problem when comparing treatments for frozen shoulder: many treatments are sequential; that is, they are not directly comparable. For example, most patients would only consider some form of intervention, particularly surgery, once conservative treatment has failed. In the first instance this will take the form of an injection of local anesthetic and steroid into the glenohumeral joint. As the authors have discussed, this is often the first intervention preferred by orthopedic surgeons, and again it is successful in a large number of refractory cases. The use of alternative materials, such as hyaluronic acid, does not appear to be widespread. Should these fail and the patient continues to experience severe pain and stiffness, many surgeons would offer more radical intervention. In the first instance this would take the form of MUA with either a general anesthetic or a regional block. This is often accompanied by an intra-articular injection of local anesthetic and steroid along with a further course of intense physiotherapy. In our unit patients are only considered for this if recovery of movement plateaus during the initial phase of physical therapy. Again, manipulations are often successful, although technique is important and care should be taken, particularly when attempting to restore internal/external rotation; there have been reported instances of humerus fractures with the latter. Experience has shown the effectiveness of manipulation, although it is less effective in patients who suffer from diabetes. Consideration should also be given to the timing of surgery. Traditionally and following the work of Neviaser, it has been held that manipulation should only be undertaken once the pain begins to subside. That is, manipulation too early in the disease process can result in an exacerbation of symptoms. Although this view is generally held by a majority of orthopedic surgeons, scientific proof remains aloof. It is clear, however, that for many

Continued

INTERNATIONAL EXPERT COMMENTARY—cont'd

patients who do undergo a manipulation under anesthesia, recovery can be dramatic.

With the advent of arthroscopy, many clinicians have replaced manipulation or combined it with arthroscopic examination and capsular release of the shoulder joint. This certainly has the advantages of resulting in a more controlled release and mobilization. It is particularly helpful if there is a marked restriction of internal/external rotation. It also has the advantage of excluding any additional intra-articular pathology. Plainly, however, it does involve a more prolonged anesthetic with associated cost implications. It may be that this should only be reserved for the most severe and resistant cases.

One other treatment modality described by the authors is ultrasound-guided capsular or hydrostatic capsular distention. This is often undertaken by a radiologist as an outpatient procedure. As the authors stated, it carries low risk and is simple to perform. Personal experience does indicate that a number of patients gain significant and almost immediate symptomatic relief. It should be noted, however, that these patients often receive an intra-articular injection of local anesthetic and steroid followed by a course of physical therapy.

To conclude therefore the authors have produced a chapter that not only describes the typical features of frozen shoulder/adhesive capsulitis but also the difficulties incumbent with various classifications. The problem is compounded by the fact that for "primary frozen shoulder" there is no specific diagnostic test. For the so-called "secondary frozen shoulder," stiffness should be regarded as a symptom of a particular pathology. As such it is not clear why this definition is required. Added to that, treatment is often sequential with only a small minority of patients actually requiring definitive intervention. As such, and as the authors point out, this makes any comparison difficult and indeed a review of literature reveals that most studies are at best level four/five evidence. Despite this, however, "primary frozen shoulder/adhesive capsulitis" remains a common diagnosis and certainly one from which the majority of patients should make a complete recovery.

EDITOR COMMENTARY

Edward V. Fehringer

I commend the current (and prior) authors for assimilating and presenting a vast amount of work about a simple and common process. Shoulder stiffness is like many conditions in medicine: when we understand it and how to diagnose even subtle cases, the more we see and diagnose. Although the etiology often may elude us, as with the case of so many etiologies that are multifactorial, hopefully the scientific methods that we employ will help eliminate the "idiopathic" adjective. Meanwhile, we diligently observe and diagnose as we can, humbly keeping in mind that, as the authors note, many physicians have achieved success with different forms of nonoperative and operative treatment.

History, examination, and plain radiographs constitute the majority of stiff shoulder workups. As have many others, I have successfully used the Jackins home exercise program as well as formal physical therapy with results that depended on severity, length of disease, coexisting diabetes, and, seemingly most important, patient compliance.

Despite the trend toward arthroscopic release, I have found outpatient manipulation to be useful under a one-shot interscalene block with an intravenous propofol adjunct, with formal physical therapy beginning immediately. I have also found this approach to be reasonable in some patients with non-insulin-dependent diabetes if they have passive elevation greater than roughly 120 degrees. In those with insulin-dependent diabetes I have found arthroscopic release works well with the lowest risk of recurrence.

For patients with prior surgical intervention or fracture, I have found that humeroscapular motion interface scar release is paramount. If prior surgery was performed in open fashion, I have found an open approach to be more helpful in this plane due to scar density. Furthermore, I have found a concomitant capsular release to be often unnecessary in these shoulders if open release and manipulation is planned and a combined arthroscopic capsular release and arthroscopic/open release in the humeroscapular interface to be of value, particularly in patients with diabetes and prior surgical intervention and/or a prior fracture. For the open portion, I have used deltopectoral approaches but have found a deltoid split (a skin incision in skin lines) to be very useful in accomplishing a comprehensive interface release.

Regarding subscapularis lengthening and bony decompressions, I do not perform these. I have found subscapularis insufficiency to be a particularly troublesome entity to deal with. I have therefore maintained it in cases of shoulder stiffness, with anecdotal success. With respect to bony decompressions of the subacromial space, I have found the release of contracted soft tissues almost always to be adequate for motion restoration. Furthermore, I am concerned about the bleeding bone surface on the undersurface of the coracoacromial arch and its potential contribution to additional scarring in the humeroscapular motion interface following release, especially in shoulders with a high propensity for recurrent stiffness.

CHAPTER 20

The Shoulder in Athletes

Neal S. ElAttrache, Justin L. Hodgins, Guillem Gonzalez-Lomas, Christopher S. Ahmad

Repetitive overhead movements and contact sports exert great stress on the shoulder, often at extreme ranges of motion. As a result, the shoulder is a common site of pathology and disability in athletes. Each athlete presents unique diagnostic and therapeutic challenges, and an understanding of sport-specific biomechanics and pathology is essential. Throwing athletes, for example, repeatedly accelerate and decelerate their shoulder over a wide arc of rotation, causing repetitive microtrauma to the static and dynamic stabilizers of the glenohumeral and scapulothoracic joints. In contrast, collision athletes are prone to sudden macrotrauma to the stabilizing static and dynamic elements of the shoulder. This chapter provides a comprehensive overview of the pathophysiology, evaluation, and management of shoulder injuries specific to repetitive overhead and collision athletes.

SPORTS-SPECIFIC BIOMECHANICS

The Kinetic Chain

The kinetic chain of motion can be described as the sequential activation of all body areas through a link segment, progressing from the lower extremity through the trunk to the rapidly accelerating upper extremity.[255] Overhead athletes must efficiently preserve the transmission of force from their legs and trunk to the force-delivery mechanism of their arm in a coordinated cascade of movements. The legs and trunk generate rotational and linear momentum, producing a significant proportion of the energy in the overhead motion. In tennis the legs and trunk are responsible for 50% to 55% of the total force generation required for a power serve.[212] A variety of studies have demonstrated that poor flexibility or muscle imbalances throughout the kinetic chain are common in patients with shoulder injuries, such as shoulder impingement,[220,333,342] rotator cuff tears,[252,342] and instability.[252,346] In one study that examined physical features in 64 throwers with labral tears, 46 (72%) showed infraspinatus and teres minor weakness on resisted external rotation, 31 (48%) demonstrated lower back inflexibility, 28 (44%) showed trunk and hip core musculature weakness by failing a Trendelenburg test, and 25 (39%) had asymmetrically decreased internal rotation of the nondominant hip.[55] Injuries to the foot and ankle, tightness of the muscles crossing the hip and knee joints, weakness of hip abductors and trunk stabilizers, and conditions that alter spinal alignment can all influence kinetic chain energy transmission.

In the baseball pitcher, improper conditioning of the core and trunk can influence the positioning of the throwing arm and may result in excessive force transmission across the stabilizing structures of shoulder; this can compromise performance and predispose the athlete to injury.[319] The "slow arm position"[58,104] describes the disengaged transmission of force with compensatory increases in lumbar lordosis during the acceleration phase, which places the arm behind the body and the scapular plane.[58,104] The shoulder is forced to assume a hyperabducted, externally rotated position that moves the arm out of the safe zone of glenohumeral angulation described by Jobe and colleagues.[265] This position creates a violent acceleration out of the late cocking position, increasing compression loads and shear and traction on the rotator cuff, glenoid, and capsulolabral complex. The resultant forces can injure the posterior capsule, tear and peel the labrum off the glenoid, tear and delaminate the rotator cuff, and injure or stretch the anterior capsular restraints.

THROWING ATHLETES

Athletes who perform repetitive overhead motions exert abnormal stresses on the shoulder that vary in magnitude and anatomic location depending on the sport. Repetitive throwing motions can result in overuse-type injuries with the potential for acute injuries superimposed on chronic changes, a combination that can present therapeutic challenges.

Baseball Pitching

The baseball pitch has been studied extensively and is often used to extrapolate implications for other overhead sports.[109] The predicament of the pitcher's shoulder, the

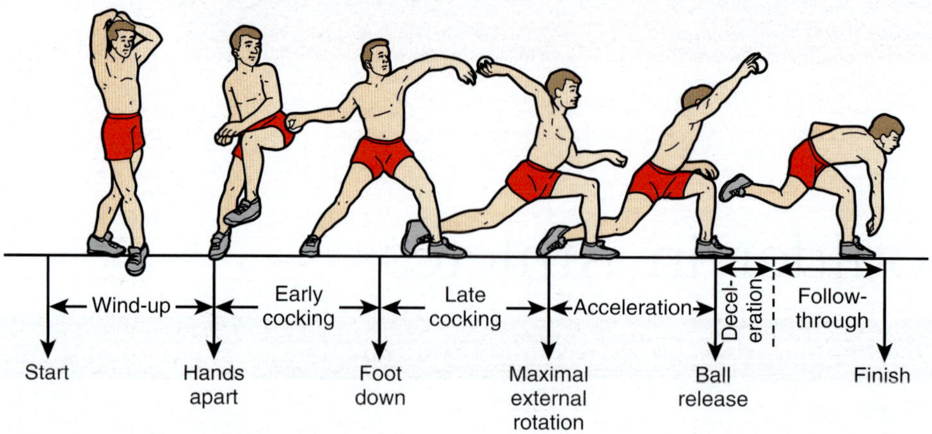

FIGURE 20-1: The baseball pitch has been divided into six phases: (1) wind-up, (2) early cocking, (3) late cocking, (4) acceleration, (5) deceleration, and (6) follow-through.

thrower's paradox,[355] describes the delicate balance of sufficient mobility to foster extreme rotations while maintaining adequate stability to prevent subluxation of the humeral head. In addition, the shoulder must withstand substantial repetitive forces during a pitching motion. Professional pitchers generate up to 92 N-m of humeral rotation torque, which is greater than the torsional failure limit in human cadaveric shoulders.[290] Glenohumeral compressive loads as high as 860 N can be created with concomitant humeral angular velocities as high as 7000 degrees per second.[328] To counteract these forces and keep the humeral head centered in the glenoid, there is significant eccentric contraction of the posterior rotator cuff (the supraspinatus, infraspinatus, and teres minor).

The six phases of the baseball pitch have been extensively examined (Fig. 20-1). Most pitchers incorporate their own style into pitches, particularly during the wind-up and follow-through phases. Regardless of the appearance of the pitch during these phases, correct fundamental pitch mechanics are paramount throughout the entire motion for effective throwing and injury prevention. Improper mechanics at any stage during this energy transfer can lead to injury and affect performance. An experienced coach educated in throwing mechanics is invaluable to the young athlete in preventing and recovering from injury through detecting and correcting subtle abnormalities in form. High-speed video evaluation is a useful tool that provides pitchers and their coaches with visual feedback about technique. The following sections provide a detailed account of the correct mechanics at each pitching phase and resultant pathology associated with poor form.

Wind-up

The wind-up (Fig. 20-2) sets the tone for the rest of the pitch, and poor mechanics during this phase can propagate through the remaining pitch phases. The feet are positioned parallel to one another and perpendicular to the rubber on the mound as the pitcher faces the batter. The right-handed pitcher then places the right foot parallel to the rubber stopper on the pitching mound. As the left leg is elevated, the pitcher keeps the hips level to the ground and points them toward home plate while maintaining balance. The hips then begin driving forward toward home plate and the right hand with the ball exits the left hand glove (Fig. 20-3A). Inexperienced throwers often have flawed form with poor trunk tilt and less hip advancement toward home plate (Fig. 20-3B).

During the wind-up phase, the pitcher should be balanced when the leading leg reaches its highest point. If the pitcher begins to fall forward prematurely as a result of poor balance, the delivery will be rushed and pitch velocity lessened. If the hips fail to point toward home plate, the leading leg will land in an incorrect direction during subsequent pitch phases.

Early Cocking

The hand comes out of the glove while maintaining a position on top of the ball and the shoulder remains internally rotated (see Fig. 20-2B). As the hand brings the ball back and laterally, the shoulder is elevated in the scapular plane past 90 degrees and externally rotated to approximately 45 degrees. The hips are driven toward home plate but the pelvis does not rotate. The phase ends with the left foot landing on the mound, which decelerates the driving lower extremity and trunk.

Two common errors that should be avoided in this phase are "pie throwing" and "opening up" too soon. First, if the hand is rotated under the ball (the "pie-throwing" position seen in Fig. 20-4B) instead of remaining on top (Fig. 20-4A), the humerus externally rotates and places the humeral head in a vulnerable position for anterior subluxation and instability. Second, the lead foot should land pointing toward home plate (Fig. 20-5A). Flaws observed in inexperienced pitchers include abduction of the lead leg when landing on it. For example, a right-handed pitcher with poor form would place the lead left foot on the first-base side of the mound (Fig. 20-5B). This premature opening causes early pelvis rotation with a consequent loss of velocity and increased anterior shoulder strain.[108,109] Movement of the lower extremity and trunk with their substantial

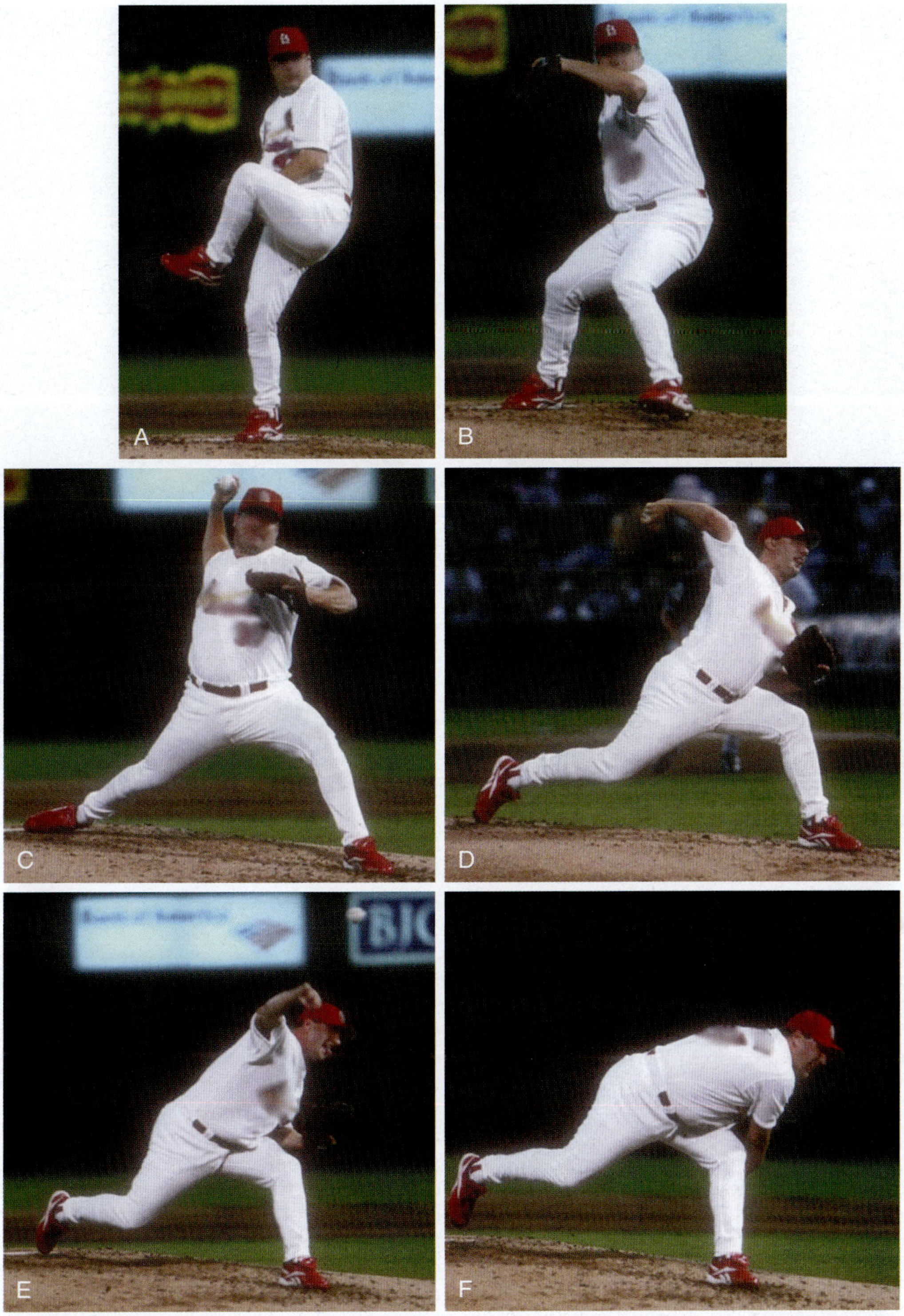

FIGURE 20-2: **A,** Wind-up: the leading leg is elevated while the hips are kept level and pointing toward home plate. **B,** Early cocking: the throwing hand (not seen) must remain on top of the ball, keeping the shoulder internally rotated to minimize the anterior subluxation that can occur if the shoulder is externally rotated during this phase. **C,** Late cocking: a rapid arc of humeral external rotation from 45 degrees to 170 degrees occurs in the scapular plane. **D,** Acceleration: the propulsive force during acceleration begins in the lower extremities, and the kinetic energy is transferred through the trunk and into the shoulder, elbow, and wrist. **E,** Deceleration: the periscapular muscles contract eccentrically to dissipate excess kinetic energy. **F,** Follow-through: eccentric contraction by the scapular rotator muscles continues to decelerate the arm, and the posterior capsule experiences tension as the arm adducts. During the follow-through, the shoulder should internally rotate and horizontally adduct across the body.

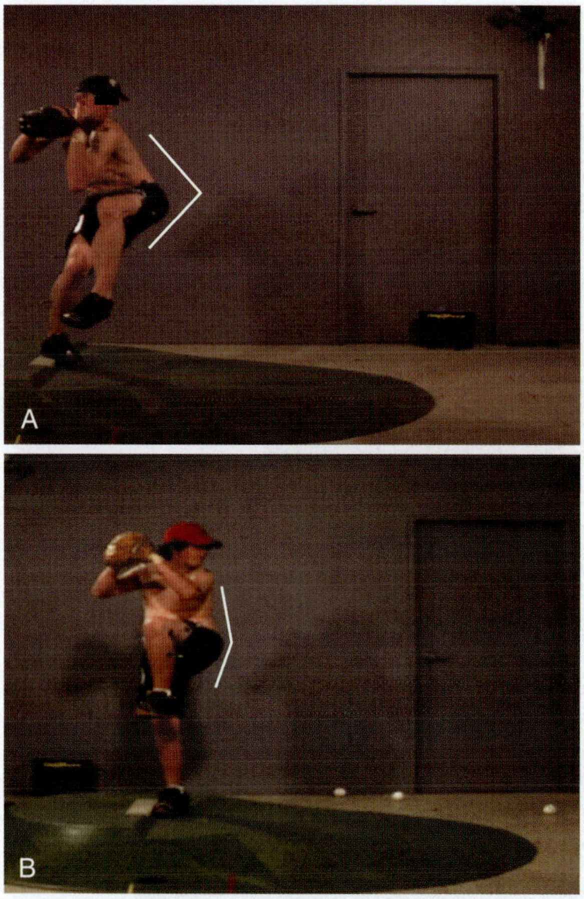

FIGURE 20-3: **A,** The mature thrower leads with his hip toward home plate. **B,** The immature player fails to lead with his hip.

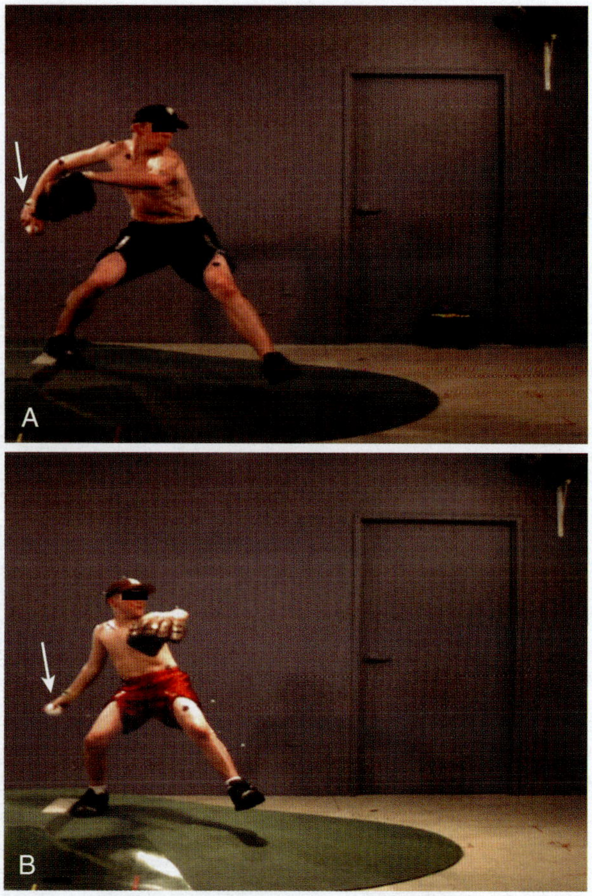

FIGURE 20-4: **A,** The mature player keeps his hand on top of the ball during early cocking. **B,** The immature player brings his hand under the ball during early cocking.

mass creates maximal energy in the lower body that is transferred to the upper extremity and finally to the ball. This requires timed and delayed upper body rotation that allows the energy to develop in the lower extremity and trunk.

Late Cocking

The left foot hits the ground pointing in the direction of home plate, leaving the legs stretched apart (see Fig. 20-2C). The weight of the body is evenly distributed on both legs, and the torso balances in an upright position between the legs. Trunk rotation is delayed as long as possible while the right humerus externally rotates from approximately 45 degrees to 170 degrees in its position in the scapular plane. At this time, the periscapular muscles, including the trapezius, rhomboids, levator scapulae, and serratus anterior, keep the scapula stabilized, and the biceps brachii keeps the elbow flexed at slightly more than 90 degrees. Eccentric contraction of the subscapularis muscle decelerates the externally rotating humerus.

Most injured pitchers experience pain during the late cocking phase. During this phase, at maximal external rotation (nearing 170 degrees), the arm should be abducted 90 to 100 degrees. Throwing with reduced external rotation at the time the foot makes contact with the ground may be associated with increased strain on the anterior shoulder during acceleration and ball release.

Periscapular muscular weakness may also predispose to injury during the late cocking phase. The serratus anterior is significantly less active in pitchers with shoulder instability than in those with normal shoulders.[117] To compensate for diminished serratus anterior strength, the thrower might drop the elbow thus decreasing the degree of scapular rotation and the elevation needed. If this pathologic process continues, the player might attempt to compensate further by moving the humerus behind the scapular plane. If symptoms arise, the player reduces the amount of external rotation to protect against shoulder pain and arches the back into hyperlordosis to compensate for the decreased humeral external rotation. Early recognition of muscle imbalances in the thrower allows the surgeon to institute an early, focused physical therapy program to strengthen the affected structures and protect against the vicious cycle of compensatory pathologic throwing.

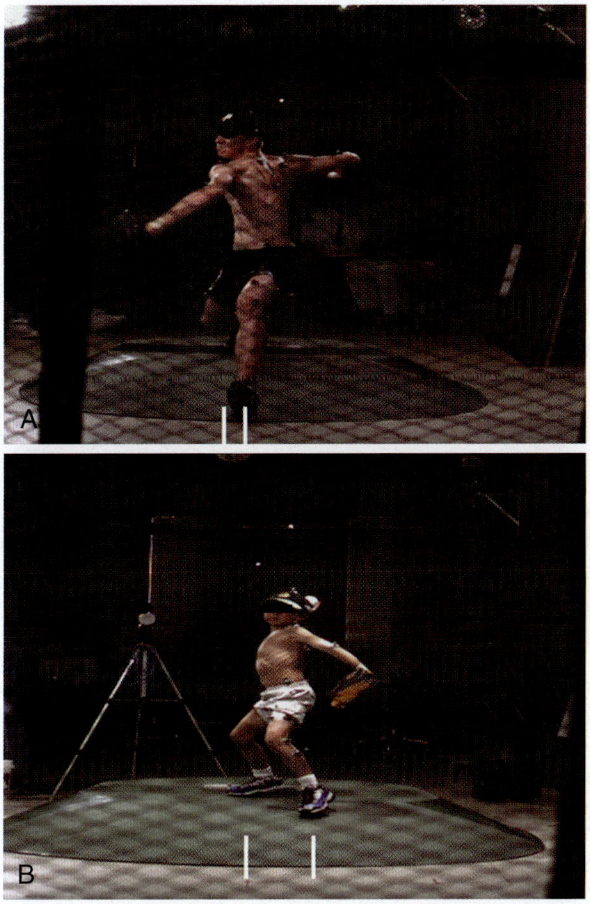

FIGURE 20-5: **A,** The mature player keeps his hips closed, and his lead foot is directed toward home plate. **B,** The immature player opens his pelvis, and his lead foot is directed inside of home plate.

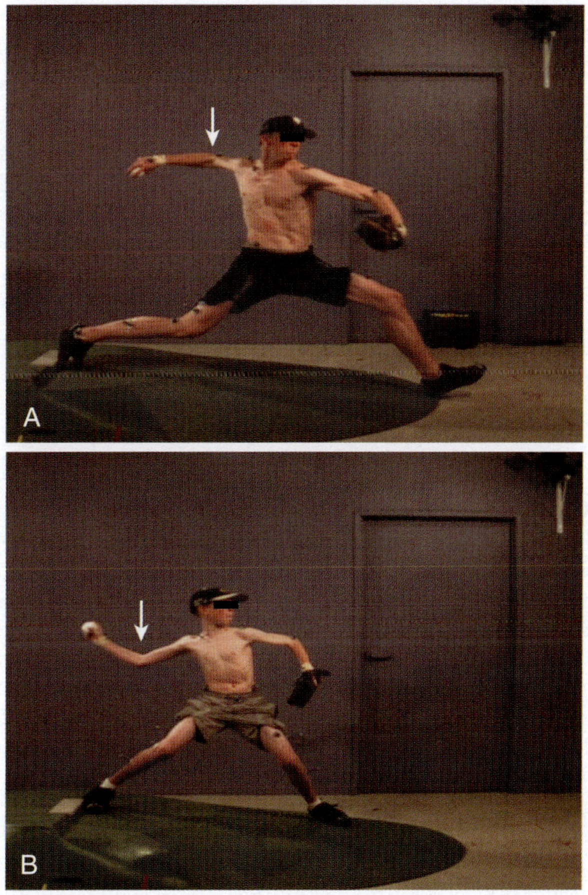

FIGURE 20-6: **A,** The mature player keeps his throwing elbow high (arrow). **B,** The immature player drops his throwing elbow (arrow).

The elbow should reach its highest point in late cocking (Fig. 20-6A); inexperienced throwers often have their elbows in a suboptimal lower position (Fig. 20-6B).

Acceleration

Once the humerus reaches maximal external rotation, the hand carrying the ball accelerates in a rapid arc of internal rotation (see Fig. 20-2D). The energy of the lower extremity and trunk is transferred through the shoulder to the elbow and wrist as the body falls forward. Immediately prior to the release of the ball, the arm internally rotates 80 degrees, reaching peak angular velocities near 7000 degrees per second. Within 0.05 seconds, the ball is released with speeds exceeding 90 mph.[93]

A pitcher with a painful shoulder may lead with the elbow during the acceleration phase, or reduce horizontal abduction while increasing elbow flexion to bring the ball closer to the shoulder. Although this maladaptive position reduces the load on the shoulder, it increases the load on the medial elbow, predisposing it to injury.[109] If the thrower opens up too quickly, positioning the elbow behind the plane of the scapula, the glenohumeral joint hyperangulates, resulting in more pronounced internal impingement (Fig. 20-7).

Deceleration

After the ball release, the right hip rises up and over the left leg. The right foot lifts off the mound and the pitcher performs a controlled fall forward (see Fig. 20-2E). In this phase the teres minor, infraspinatus, and scapular rotator muscles contract eccentrically to dissipate the kinetic energy that was not transferred to the ball. The glenohumeral distraction forces at this time can reach 1 to 1.5 times body weight; these forces are absorbed by the shoulder capsule and posterior rotator cuff.[58]

Follow-through

The arm continues to descend, and the right leg lands on the ground in a controlled fashion (see Fig. 20-2F). Eccentric contraction by the scapular rotator muscles continues to decelerate the arm, and the posterior capsule experiences tension as the arm adducts. During the follow-through, the shoulder should internally rotate and horizontally adduct across the body. If the arm instead finishes facing home plate, excessive stresses are transferred to the shoulder.

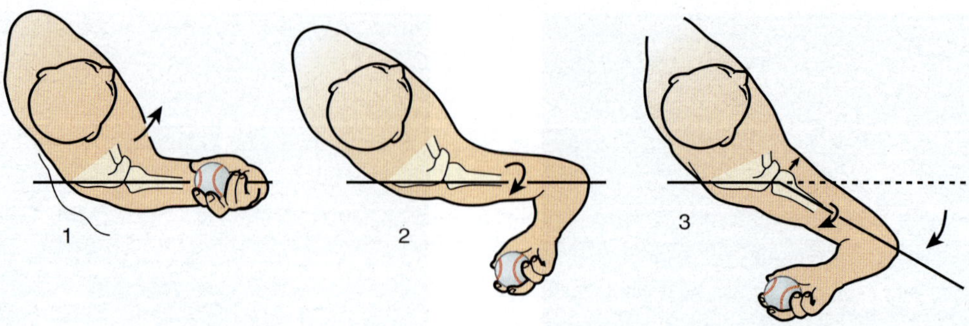

FIGURE 20-7: When the elbow moves posterior to the plane of the scapula, the shoulder is hyperabducted, increasing the risk of internal impingement.

Football Throwing

Although similar in some respects, the overhead throwing motion in football has fundamental differences in shoulder position and stresses compared with the overhead throwing motion in baseball. This is largely attributable to the greater weight of the football (0.42 kg versus 0.14 kg for the baseball).[111,221] The observed injury patterns also differ, with predilection towards overuse disorders, such as biceps tendonitis and rotator cuff injury, as well as traumatic conditions, including rupture of the pectoralis major (PM) muscle.[31,228]

Electromyographic analysis demonstrates four distinct phases in football throwing.[159] Early cocking is initiated at rear foot plant and continued to maximal shoulder abduction and internal rotation. Late cocking starts at maximal shoulder abduction and internal rotation and ends with maximal shoulder external rotation. Acceleration begins with maximal shoulder external rotation and completes with release of the ball. Finally, the follow-through phase is the period from ball release to maximal horizontal adduction.

The kinematics and kinetics of the baseball pitch and football pass have been compared; pitchers produce significantly greater forces and torques in the shoulder during arm deceleration.[111] Quarterbacks demonstrate less motion in their legs, pelvis, and torso, which limits the force transmission compared with that experienced in pitchers. When combined with a lower throwing frequency, fewer games in a season, and greater rest periods between games, quarterbacks are also less prone to many of the overuse injuries characteristic of pitchers.[111]

NONTHROWING OVERHEAD ATHLETES

Tennis

The tennis serve has been likened to an overhead pitch, with similar biomechanical forces responsible for injury. As in throwing, the shoulder is driven through a highly dynamic arc of motion, often exceeding the biomechanical constraints of the joint. Within this context, the shoulder has to maintain a balance between flexibility and instability. As with pitching, optimal kinetic chain energy transfer, proper scapular movement, and rotator cuff function are prerequisites to mitigating shoulder injury. However, there are several key differences.[110] In the tennis serve, the racquet provides an added source of kinetic energy in addition to the human kinetic chain to generate ball velocity. Instead of releasing the ball as in the pitching motion, the tennis player repetitively strikes the ball in a fashion that makes the shoulder susceptible to overuse injury. Tennis players typically have stronger internal rotator muscles than the external rotator muscles, and this imbalance can predispose to injury during arm deceleration.[69]

The tennis serve has five distinct phases (Fig. 20-8), similar to the baseball pitch: wind-up (the knees are flexed and the trunk is rotated), early cocking, late cocking (where the shoulder is maximally abducted and externally rotated), acceleration, and follow-through.

Swimming

The demands on the shoulders of competitive swimmers are immense, and the number of strokes exceeds 500,000 per arm per year.[14] The freestyle swimming stroke has been subdivided into five distinct phases: hand entry, catch, in-sweep, finish, and recovery (Fig. 20-9). Swimming strokes repetitively place the shoulder in the impingement position described by Neer and Welsh.[240] Consequently, shoulder pain and dysfunction in swimmers have traditionally been equated with subacromial impingement and rotator cuff tendinitis.

Biomechanical analyses of shoulder function have found that swimmers suffer from a variety of problems common to all overhead athletes.[214] Impressive shoulder laxity is observed in swimmers, placing them in the spectrum of multidirectional instability; this is a consequence of tremendous forces on soft tissue stabilizers and extreme motion requirements, combined with swimmers' propensity for baseline ligamentous laxity. Associated muscle imbalances therefore can contribute to pathologic instability processes in these shoulders. As in throwing, the swimmer's shoulder must maintain the narrow margin

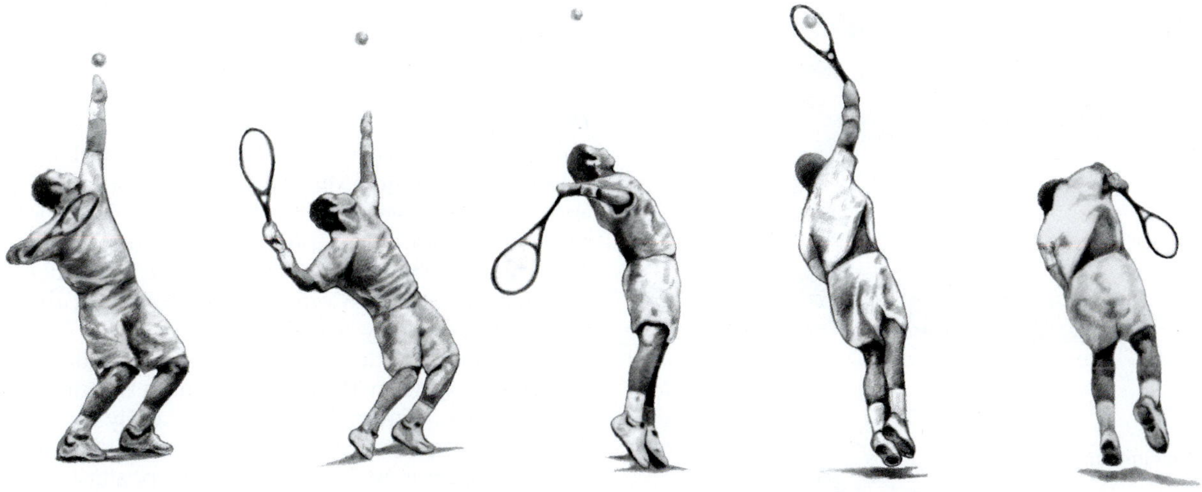

FIGURE 20-8: The tennis serve has been divided into five phases, akin to those of the baseball pitch. These include the wind-up, early cocking, late cocking, acceleration, and follow-through. The shoulder kinematics resemble those of the overhead throw. (Courtesy Nicholas Frankfurt.)

between having enough flexibility to generate body propulsion and developing pathologic instability. Proper strength and coordination of the dynamic scapular stabilizers (the levator scapulae, rhomboids, and trapezius) and glenohumeral stabilizers (the rotator cuff) are critical in preventing symptomatic instability.

Phases of Freestyle Swimming

Hand Entry

In the initial catch, the swimmer's hand enters the water with the shoulder in internal rotation. Swimmers are trained to completely elevate the shoulder at this time while flexing the elbow in order to catch the water. The hand then extends under the water as the palm turns to face down. The lift provided by the water upon hand entry generates a large force on the glenohumeral joint, particularly when the swimmer's arm nears full extension. This force forward elevates the shoulder, placing it in the classic impingement position.

Yanai and Hay have recommended four changes in the technique to reduce impingement during this phase. The first three—streamlining hand entry, strengthening muscles that resist forcible elevation (the latissimus dorsi, PM, teres major, and biceps brachii), and bending the elbow to decrease moment arm length—all reduce the forcible moment arm. The fourth involves externally rotating the scapula on hand entry to reduce the angle subtended by the axis of the humerus and the superior border of scapula, lessening subacromial impingement.[366,367]

Catch

The hand entry foreshadows the next phase of the stroke, called the catch. As soon as maximal arm extension in the water is reached, the pulling arm begins an S-shaped pull, which coincides with the opposite hand's emergence from the water. The elbow flexes as the hand begins to pull the body over itself, generating the highly propulsive phase of the stroke. As the hand continues to push back, it moves in a downward and outward direction. At the mid pull-through point, the humerus is aligned perpendicular to the swimmer's torso, with the hand still cranial to the shoulder.

During the catch phase, the shoulder is adducted and internally rotated. A common technical error during this phase is the dropped elbow. Counsilman and colleagues demonstrated that the dropped-elbow stroke combines external rotation and adduction at the shoulder, whereas the correct, high-elbow technique combines internal rotation with abduction.[85] Richardson found that the increased glenohumeral external rotation placed the muscles of propulsion (the latissimus dorsi and triceps) at a mechanical disadvantage.[278]

The correct high-elbow technique provides a mechanical advantage, but it also increases the percentage of the stroke during which the shoulder is left in the impingement position.[367] Swimmers might adopt the faulty dropped-elbow technique at the onset of incipient impingement in an attempt to curtail pain during the stroke (or secondary to fatigue). Accordingly, biomechanical studies have measured decreased activity in the anterior and middle deltoids when the elbow is dropped, suggesting that the faulty technique uses less energy.[299]

In-Sweep

As the hand reaches the deepest point, the downward motion shifts to an upward, inward, and backward motion, and the hand pushes toward the midline of the body and toward the swimmer's chest. Problems in this phase relate to the stabilizing periscapular muscles, particularly the serratus anterior in the overhead motion. In the swimmer with a painful shoulder, the serratus anterior muscle activity drops considerably.[299] This is likely

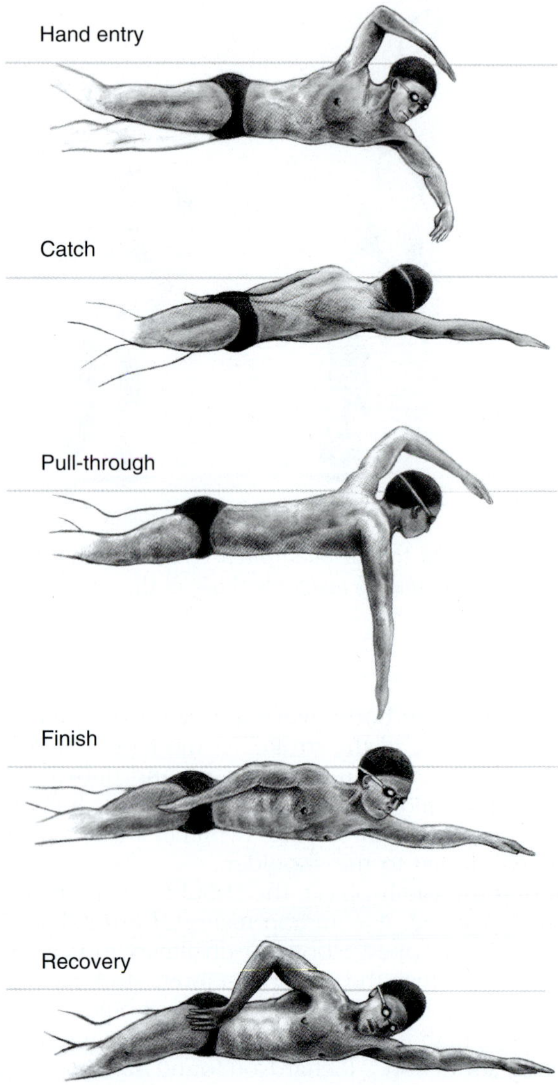

FIGURE 20-9: The swimming stroke is divided into five phases: hand entry, catch, in-sweep, finish, and recovery. (Courtesy Nicholas Frankfurt.)

to be secondary to fatigue due to constant splinting of the painful shoulder. The rhomboids attempt to stabilize the scapula, but because they are antagonists of the serratus anterior, normal synchronous scapular rotation is disrupted.

Finish

The finish is the culmination of the S-shaped pull. The hand turns outward and backward as it is pushed from underneath the body. The humerus must internally rotate significantly to help the hand move in this direction. The hand then flexes upward toward the water surface while still moving backward. The phase ends as the hand breaks the surface of the water. During the finish, the swimmer with impingement might excessively roll the body in an attempt to reduce the amount of internal rotation (painful in impingement) the shoulder has to produce to have the hand exit the water. This is manifested by a noticeably early hand exit.

Recovery

The recovery phase begins with the hand exiting the water. As the hand exits the water, the shoulder abducts and externally rotates as it is brought forward for the next arm entry. Shoulder impingement occurs during a large part of this phase, particularly if the shoulder is kept internally rotated.[367] Codman first described the prerequisite of externally rotating the shoulder in order to achieve full abduction.[74] Otherwise, the greater tuberosity comes in contact with the acromion at about 90 degrees of abduction. Externally rotating as early as possible in the recovery phase reduces the amount of time that the shoulder spends in an impingement position.[366,367]

Instability in Swimmers

The biomechanics of swimming favors swimmers with higher degrees of shoulder laxity.[216] As a result of this self-selection, elite swimmers tend to be hyperlax at baseline and are more at risk for related shoulder pathology.[219] Fine-wire electromyography (EMG) studies have demonstrated that swimming strokes require the shoulder adductors and internal rotators to produce the majority of the propulsive force, and they minimally tax the external rotators.[29,217,218,245,261] Therefore like throwers, swimmers and water polo players significantly increase their internal rotator and adductor/external rotator and abductor strength ratio.[217,218] Whereas a normal shoulder might be able to compensate for these muscle imbalances, a shoulder with excessive laxity might not. As a result, the glenohumeral joint can have subluxation episodes, leading to other painful chronic injuries, such as labral tears, subacromial impingement, and bicipital tendinitis.[131,216]

During the swimming stroke, the force applied to the hand by the water results in an anteriorly directed vector thrust at the shoulder.[216] In a lax shoulder, this force can shift the humeral head excessively, injuring the labrum or the joint surface itself. The external rotators attempt to restrain the humeral head from anterior translation, becoming fatigued and prone to develop tendinitis. Some authors have cited overworked external rotators as a cause of the posterior shoulder pain commonly seen in swimmers with anterior instability.[216] The mainstay of treatment is a rehabilitation program aimed at maintaining normal rotator cuff strength ratios and periscapular muscle strengthening; this has been effective in ameliorating pain and dysfunction.[215] Open and arthroscopic surgical stabilization treatments for elite swimmers with symptomatic instability have not been as successful as for other athletes, with only an estimated 20% returning to their preinjury level of performance.[233]

Impingement in Swimmers

Swimmer adaptations to this provocative shoulder arc of motion can affect pathology and convalescence. For example, unilateral breathing increases impingement on the shoulder ipsilateral to the breathing side.[366] Having the swimmer switch to bilateral breathing can reduce the risk of developing clinical symptoms. Maintaining a high elbow on recovery, avoiding an extended position of the arm before hand entry, and increasing body roll all reduce the percentage of the stroke that the shoulder is in the impingement position. Other conservative measures, such as rest (during which a kickboard can be used), ice, nonsteroidal antiinflammatory drugs (NSAIDs), and a structured rehabilitation program, usually yield successful results. Supraspinatus tendinopathy induced by high-volume swimming should also be considered as a source of shoulder pain as its incidence in elite swimmers has been underestimated.[302] Refractory cases might respond to subacromial decompression, although this is not conducted routinely.[282,288]

Golf

Chronic shoulder overuse injuries can affect golfers, especially because elite-level and some recreational players perform up to 2000 swings per week.[149] Ninety percent of shoulder problems in golfers involve the lead arm (the left arm in a right-handed golfer).[202,264]

The golf swing is divided into five phases (Fig. 20-10): the takeaway (from address until the club is horizontal), the backswing (from horizontal to the top of the backswing), the downswing (from the top of the backswing until the club is horizontal), acceleration (from horizontal club to impact), and follow-through (from ball contact until the end of the swing).[172]

Each phase of the golf swing can cause specific pathology. During the backswing, the lead shoulder moves into internal rotation, forward flexion, and cross-body adduction. This position can cause subacromial impingement and acromioclavicular joint pathology. Posterior pain during the top of the backswing, with the arm fully adducted across the body, can indicate posterior glenohumeral instability. Symptoms during the follow-through, with the lead shoulder abducted and externally rotated, are consistent with anterior instability or biceps tendinitis.

Repetitive swinging of the golf club can eventually overwhelm normal shoulder restraints, especially when performed incorrectly or erratically. Fine-wire EMG studies have demonstrated that whereas professional golfers consistently activate the same sequence of muscles with every swing, recreational golfers tend to produce different muscle-activation patterns and do not duplicate their swing with each shot.[151,264] Similarly, higher handicap players typically experience injuries that result from improper swing mechanics, whereas lower handicap and professional players are susceptible to overuse injuries.[20] The following section presents the most typical golf injuries that affect the shoulder.

Subacromial Impingement and Rotator Cuff Injury

The golfer's lead shoulder is placed in the position of impingement at the extremes of motion: the top of the backswing and the end of the follow-through. Furthermore, a patient with preexisting rotator cuff disease may have a weak takeaway, which can exacerbate poor swing mechanics and worsen impingement. During the backswing, the lead shoulder can be subjected to subacromial impingement, acromioclavicular compression, and, less commonly, coracoid impingement. During the downswing, impact, and follow-through, the trailing shoulder is subject to stress on the superior labrum, coracoid impingement, and humeral head chondral injury.

Several reports have examined impingement in golfers. Studies have found that 26%[203] to 93%[148] of patients with golf-related shoulder symptoms have rotator cuff or subacromial disease. Golfers may be more amenable to successful surgical treatment compared with other overhead athletes, such as throwers, because of the relatively lighter demands placed on their shoulders. Vives and colleagues found that of 29 recreational golfers with subacromial disease and rotator cuff tears, acromioplasty and mini-open repair returned all but three to playing with their previous handicaps and driving distances within 3 years.[337] A case report has described successful arthroscopic subacromial decompression for impingement in a professional golfer that allowed him to return to competitive play.[149]

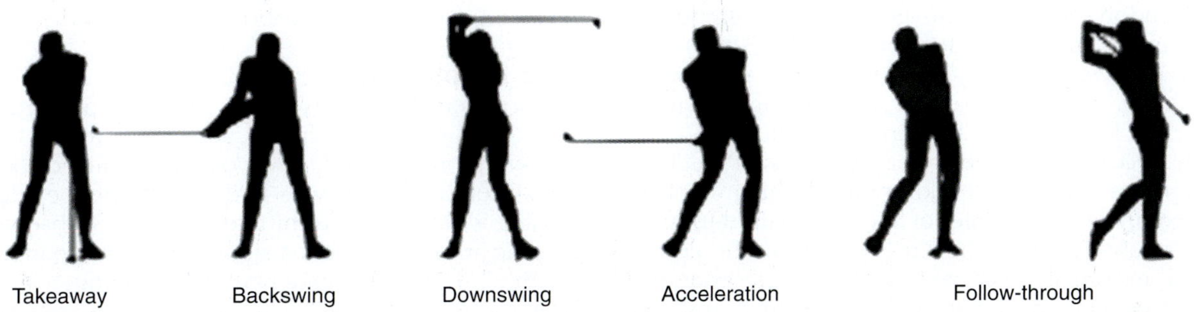

FIGURE 20-10: The golf swing is divided into five phases: the takeaway (from address until the club is horizontal), the backswing (from horizontal to the top of the backswing), the downswing (from the top of the backswing until the club is horizontal), acceleration (from the horizontal to ball impact), and follow-through (from ball contact to the end of the swing). (From Kim DH, Millett PJ, Warner JJ, Jobe FW. Shoulder injuries in golf. *Am J Sports Med.* 2004;32[5]:1324-1330.)

Acromioclavicular Joint Disease

Acromioclavicular joint disease is also prevalent in golfers. Those who complain of symptoms often cite the top of the backswing as problematic, when the lead arm assumes a cross-body adduction position and compresses the acromioclavicular joint. In a study of 35 elite golfers, of whom about half had acromioclavicular joint arthritis, all but one returned to competitive play after treatment.[203] Treatment consisted of physical therapy, swing modification, or, in refractory cases, distal clavicle excision.

Glenohumeral Instability

Golfers can be susceptible to glenohumeral instability, especially because generating a powerful swing requires maximizing the shoulder turn relative to the hip turn.[47] Posterior instability has been described as occurring in up to 12% of golfers with shoulder pain. Some authors have hypothesized that in patients with posterior instability, the subscapularis is relatively stronger than the rest of the rotator cuff, rendering the glenohumeral joint susceptible to posterior forces, which are exacerbated by fatigue to the serratus anterior.[134] Symptoms of pain and instability appear in the lead arm at the top of the backswing when it is placed in maximal adduction.

Physical examination findings in these patients demonstrate posterior instability on load and shift and posterior apprehension with loading in internal rotation and adduction. Small case series have described the successful treatment of posterior instability with therapy, posterior capsulorrhaphy, and subacromial decompression, if indicated.[134] A posterior labral (reverse Bankart) lesion has been successfully treated with arthroscopic repair.[103] Although the patient did not demonstrate signs of posterior instability, he did report pain on posterior load and shift and posterior apprehension tests. Golfers may also experience anterior instability, particularly with the lead arm in the follow-through phase of the swing, when it is in maximal abduction and external rotation. This is often successfully treated in golfers with physical therapy consisting of rotator cuff and scapular stabilizer strengthening,[149,202] with surgical treatment reserved for refractory cases.[149]

Superior Labrum and Biceps Disease

Superior labrum anterior and posterior (SLAP) lesions and biceps tendon disorders in golfers are infrequently reported in the literature.[172] Patients with SLAP tears complain of pain in the lead shoulder at the end of the backswing or beginning of the downswing when the shoulder is loaded and the arm is adducted across the body. Occasionally, the golfer complains of mechanical symptoms, such as clicking or catching. Isolated biceps tendinitis causes anterior shoulder pain during the end of follow-through when the lead arm shoulder is extended, maximally abducted, and externally rotated.

Initial treatment with rest, physical therapy, and anti-inflammatories is usually successful. Persistent symptoms can be addressed arthroscopically with SLAP repair or debridement as needed. Reports of treatment for SLAP tears or biceps lesions in golfers remain limited and the outcomes largely unknown. Older patients with SLAP lesions may be best treated with biceps tenodesis.

Glenohumeral Arthritis

Up to 25% of golfers in the United States are 65 years or older, and thus glenohumeral arthritis is a common condition in the golfer population. Total shoulder arthroplasty has been successful in returning golfers to their sport. One study found that 23 of 24 patients were able to resume playing golf at an average of 4.5 months after surgery, the majority actually improving their scores at an average of 53 months of follow-up, without component loosening.[142] These findings have been reproduced in the literature with return to play rates ranging from 77%[210] to 100%,[297] with modest improvements in both handicap and driving distance.[254]

A typical postoperative rehabilitation program is as follows: putting may be started 6 to 8 weeks after surgery, with light chipping and pitching drills allowed at 10 to 12 weeks. At 3 months, once the subscapularis is well-healed, midiron shots may be incorporated. Long irons and woods may be used at 4 months, and a full round of golf may be played at 5 to 6 months, barring any symptoms at any point during the rehabilitation.

ASYMPTOMATIC THROWING SHOULDER ADAPTATION

Overall Motion

The dominant shoulder of a thrower exhibits adaptive changes. It is well documented in throwers that with the shoulder abducted to 90 degrees, external rotation significantly increases by as much as 10 degrees compared with that of the contralateral arm, and internal rotation is diminished; this is known as glenohumeral internal rotation deficit (GIRD).[26,45,114,144,147,152,351,354] The gain in external rotation is often associated with an equal loss in internal rotation. In asymptomatic throwers therefore the total arc of shoulder motion is maintained, but it is shifted in external rotation by 10 degrees.[223,272,305] There is controversy regarding the anatomic changes responsible for the observed glenohumeral rotation changes, with studies examining soft tissue and bone adaptations.

Bone Adaptations

Developmental changes in the proximal humerus occur in young throwers. Mair and colleagues found that 55% of asymptomatic and 62% of symptomatic skeletally immature baseball players had radiographic evidence of physeal widening.[201] Krahl and colleagues observed that pitching arms underwent a significant increase in humeral length.[178] The developmental bone changes in young throwers also include increased humeral retroversion, which shifts the shoulder arc of motion, with the greatest change occurring in those aged 13 to 14 years.[223] These early changes lead to permanent change in the proximal humerus anatomy. Crockett and colleagues[86] showed that professional pitchers' dominant shoulders have 17 degrees greater humeral retroversion compared with their nondominant shoulders and that there may also be adaptive changes in retroversion within the glenoid.[42] Wyland and colleagues further suggested that concurrent increases in dominant shoulder humeral retroversion and glenoid retroversion are coupled during skeletal development; these were observed as a 2:1 "thrower's ratio" in 32 professional pitchers.[362]

As the normal humeral retroversion angle decreases from 78 degrees to 30 degrees during development, Yamamoto and colleagues[365] hypothesized that repetitive throwing did not increase retroversion in dominant shoulders but rather restricted the physiologic de-rotation of the humeral head during growth.[90,97,98] Humeral osseous adaptation may therefore explain the decrease in internal rotation and most of the increase in external rotation in asymptomatic throwers.

Capsuloligamentous Changes

Soft tissue adaptations are also thought to occur. The anterior capsule and glenohumeral ligaments become more lax in throwing shoulders, and the posterior capsule and glenohumeral ligaments become stiffer. The etiology of these changes remains a controversial subject. Two major theories exist, each proposing different inciting capsular adaptations to repetitive throwing. One argues that throwers initially develop a posterior capsular contracture; the other proposes that they develop an adaptive anterior capsular laxity.

Posterior Capsular Contracture Theory

Burkhart and colleagues proposed that a fundamental adaptation in throwers is a posterior capsular contracture that, although initially asymptomatic, can eventually have significant pathologic implications. They reasoned that in the overhead thrower, the posterior capsule must withstand tensile forces of up to 750 N during the deceleration and follow-through phases.[56] These posterior tensile forces are resisted by the eccentric contraction of the rotator cuff, primarily the infraspinatus, and by the posteroinferior capsule (the posterior band of the inferior glenohumeral ligament) (Fig. 20-11). With repetitive infraspinatus eccentric contraction during deceleration and follow-through, the muscle belly loses active tension, gains passive muscle tension, and develops disturbed proprioception.[274] As a result, higher loads are imposed on the posteroinferior capsule, which then becomes hypertrophied and stiffer.

The theory proposes that this posterior contracture shifts the center of rotation of the shoulder to a more posterosuperior location, creating posterosuperior instability and functional consequences for the shoulder in abduction and external rotation. Grossman and colleagues[120] created a posterior capsular contracture in a cadaveric model and found that the shoulder center of rotation did in fact shift posterosuperiorly in abduction and external rotation, allowing increased clearance of the greater tuberosity over the posterior glenoid rim. The humeral head could consequently externally hyperrotate, producing increased shear in the rotator cuff tendon and internal impingement that is more pronounced.

The rationale for this hypothesis is based on O'Brien's concept of the inferior glenohumeral ligament complex (Fig. 20-12) acting as a hammock to support the humeral head with the arm in abduction.[246] In abduction and external rotation, the posterior band of the inferior glenohumeral ligament is shifted under the humeral head.

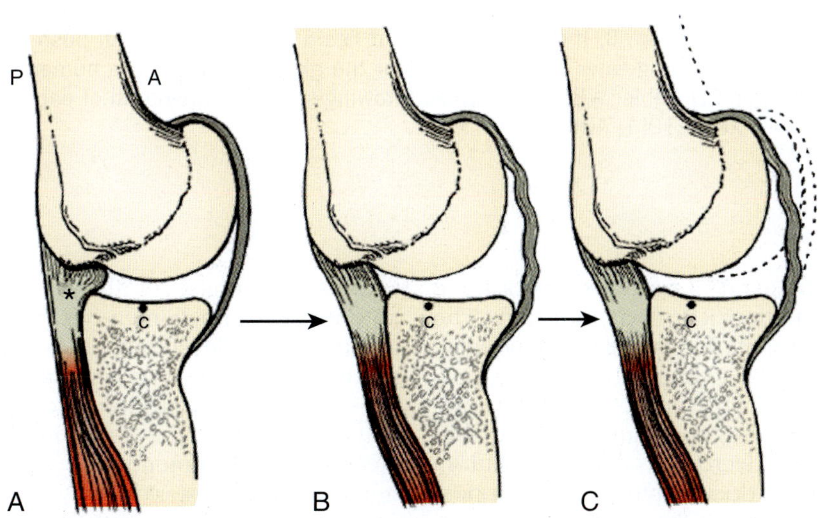

FIGURE 20-11: The posterior capsule and posterior rotator cuff are stressed by tensile forces during the follow-through and deceleration phases of throwing. Repetitive throwing can instigate a focal fibroblastic response in the posterior capsule, and the capsule reacts by becoming hypertrophied and stiff. If the capsule becomes stiff, the center of rotation of the shoulder is shifted to a more posterosuperior location. **A,** The figure shows the original center of rotation of the humeral head (c). **B,** The center of rotation is shifted posterosuperiorly. **C,** A further shift posterosuperiorly as the posterior capsule becomes hypertrophied and stiff. *A,* Anterior; *P,* posterior.

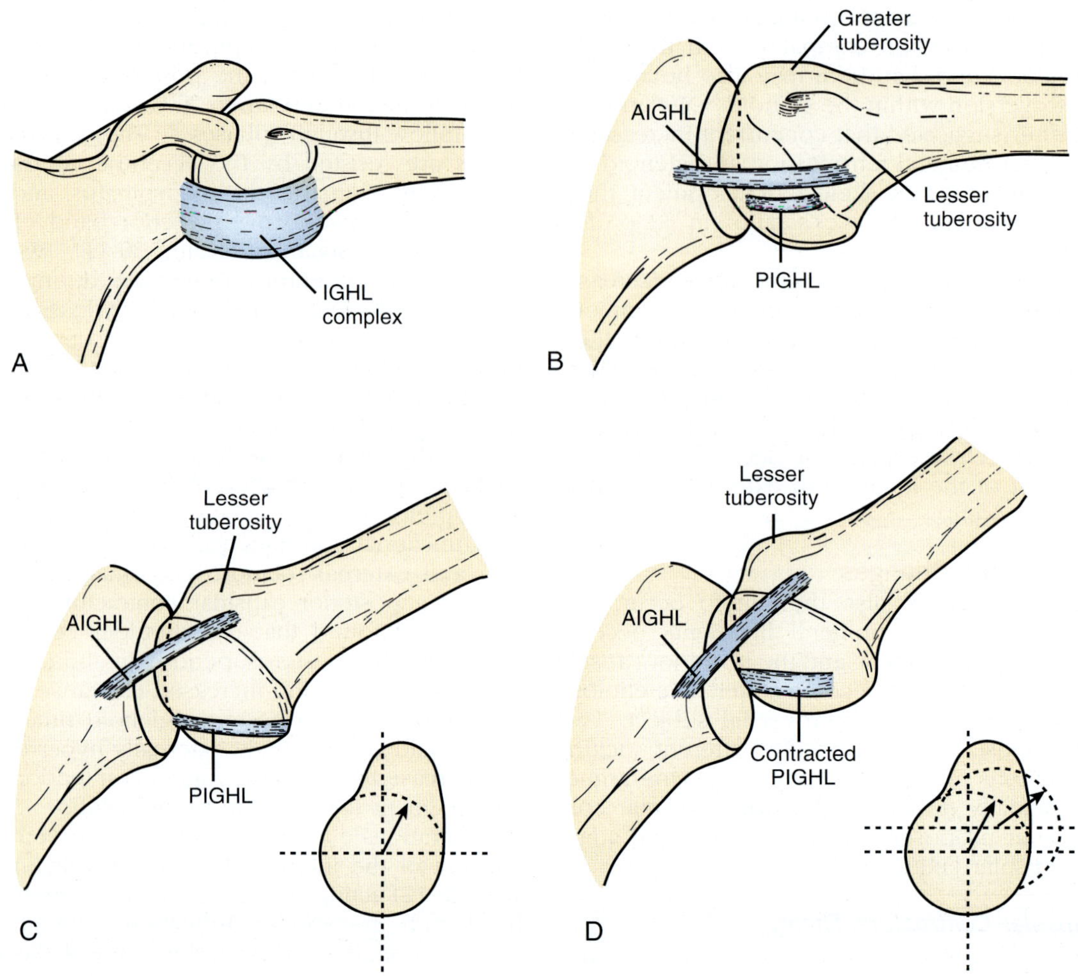

FIGURE 20-12: A model of the inferior glenohumeral ligament (IGHL) adaptation complex helps explain glenohumeral internal rotation deficit and hyperexternal rotation in the throwing athlete. **A,** The IGHL complex. **B,** The complex can be simplified into two bands: the anterior IGHL (AIGHL) and the posterior IGHL (PIGHL). In abduction and external rotation, the posterior band of IGHL is shifted under the humeral head. **C,** If the posterior band has a contracture, it will push the humeral head in a posterosuperior direction. **D,** This allows the greater tuberosity to clear the glenoid rim and the humerus to externally rotate more easily. (From Burkhart SS, Morgan CD, Kibler WB. The disabled throwing shoulder: Spectrum of pathology. Part I: Pathoanatomy and biomechanics. *Arthroscopy.* 2003;19[4]:404-420.)

Posterior band contracture exerts a posterosuperior force on the humeral head, shifting it in that direction. The shift creates a relative anteroinferior capsular redundancy. The net effect of the capsular changes (contracted posterior capsule and relative lengthening of the anteroinferior capsule) and the posterosuperior humeral head shift is increased external and decreased internal rotation. However, other studies have documented significant posterior laxity instead of tightness in throwers,[42,86,226,305] supporting the idea that GIRD likely arises from both ligamentous and osseous adaptations.[86]

Adaptive Capsular Laxity Theory

Other authors have proposed that repetitive shoulder microtrauma to the anterior capsule, particularly during the cocking phase of throwing, can lead to stretched anterior capsuloligamentous structures. The stretched anterior capsule allows the greater external rotation routinely seen in overhead throwers; it can also lead to symptomatic anterior microinstability.[114,144,147] These authors attribute the loss of internal rotation to two factors: the aforementioned osseous adaptation of the humerus and posterior muscle tightness resulting from eccentric posterior muscle contraction during the deceleration phase of throwing.[86]

Several studies have quantified capsular laxity in the context of throwing. Sethi and colleagues found an increased anteroposterior glenohumeral translation of more than 3 mm in pitchers' dominant shoulders compared with the nondominant arm.[305] Borsa and colleagues

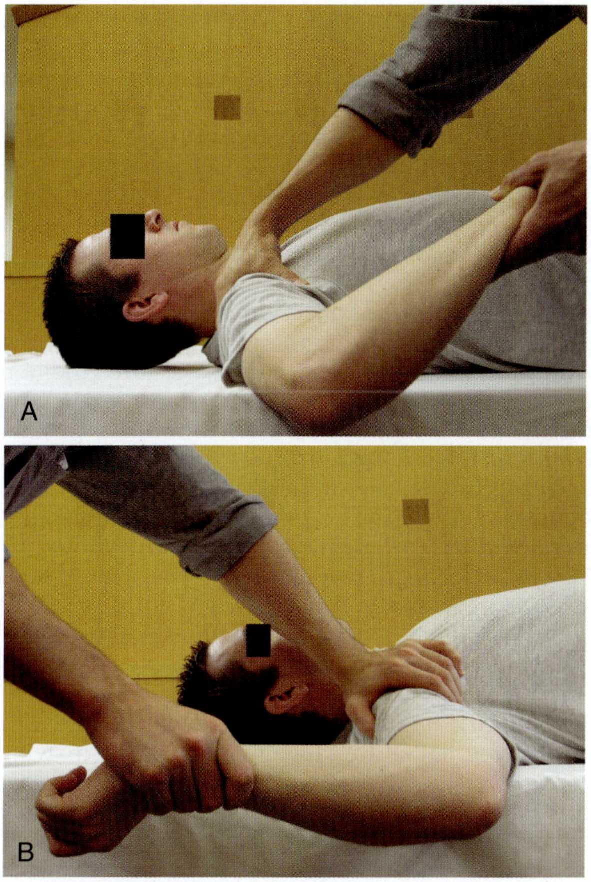

FIGURE 20-16: **A,** At rest, the biceps tendon does not transmit torsional forces. **B,** In humeral external rotation and abduction, the long head of the biceps tendon transmits a torsional force to the posterior labrum, peeling it back.

tears and labral fraying in 73.3% of non-overhead athletes as evidence that internal impingement may not be a phenomenon unique to throwers.[46]

Posterior Capsular Contracture

The theory describing adaptive changes to the posterior capsule has been outlined earlier. In the context of throwing pathology, the contracture of the posterior capsule initiates a cascade that some authors believe explains most overhead arm pathology. Once there is posterosuperior instability and the humeral head is shifted posterosuperiorly, kinetic chain dynamics are affected. The arm loses even more internal rotation and arm acceleration, and therefore ball velocity is lost. Over time, posterior SLAP tears can occur from posterosuperior contact of the labrum and the greater tuberosity. The posterior cuff undersurface begins to fail, and the picture of internal impingement arises. In a small cohort of mainly older patients, attenuation of the anterior capsule occurred with continued throwing, leading to eventual permanent deformation and anterior microinstability.[236]

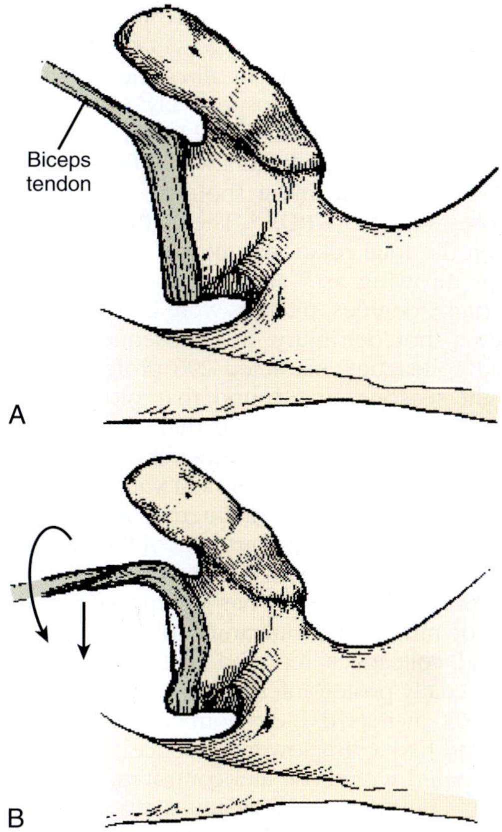

FIGURE 20-17: Measurement of internal **(A)** and external **(B)** rotation with the arm at 90 degrees of abduction and the scapula stabilized in the supine position.

Glenohumeral Internal Rotation Deficit

As described earlier in the discussion on shoulder adaptations to throwing, over time the throwing shoulder develops increased external rotation and disproportionately decreased internal rotation (GIRD). By convention, glenohumeral rotation is measured with the patient either supine or sitting and with the shoulder abducted 90 degrees in the plane of the body. The scapula must be stabilized either against the examination table, if the patient is supine, or by the examiner's hand, if the patient is sitting. Glenohumeral rotation is then measured up to the point that the scapula begins to move on the posterior chest wall or provides resistance (Fig. 20-17). Failure to stabilize the scapula incorporates scapulothoracic motion into the total rotational arc, leading to confounding measurements.

GIRD resulting in a loss of total rotational arc of greater than 20 degrees compared with the contralateral side puts the shoulder at risk for injury.[56,164] Indeed, severe GIRD is more prevalent in symptomatic shoulders. Verna studied 39 professional pitchers with GIRD greater than 35 degrees (with 25 degrees or less of total internal rotation) during a baseball season.[336] He found that 60% of them developed shoulder problems that required them to stop pitching. In a case series of overhead athletes with arthroscopically proven type II SLAP lesions, Kibler found that severe GIRD (average, 33 degrees; range, 26 to 58 degrees) was present in all of them.[56]

Wilk and colleagues prospectively evaluated passive ROM and shoulder injuries in 122 professional baseball pitchers and found that pitchers with GIRD were at almost twice the risk of sustaining shoulder injuries compared with those without GIRD.[353] The authors further noted that when the total rotational motion deficit between the dominant throwing arm and the nonthrowing arm was greater than 5 degrees, pitchers were 2.5 times more likely to sustain a shoulder injury. In a subsequent investigation Wilk and colleagues examined 296 professional pitchers over eight seasons, and found that pitchers with total rotational motion deficits more than 5 degrees in their throwing shoulders were 2.6 times more likely to suffer an elbow injury. This was consistent with previous studies that suggested that a loss of internal rotation increased the load on the medial compartment of the elbow, leading to potential ulnar collateral ligament injury.[95,113]

Symptomatic GIRD likely has a component of posterior capsular or muscular contracture. In a prospective study Kibler and colleagues reported that tennis players who performed daily posteroinferior capsular stretching to minimize GIRD increased their dominant shoulder internal rotation and had a 38% lower incidence of shoulder problems compared with those in a control group who did not stretch.[163,165] Burkhart and colleagues reported that 90% of throwers with symptomatic GIRD (>25 degrees), and almost all young collegiate or high school athletes, responded well to a posteroinferior capsular stretching program (over as little as 2 weeks) that reduced GIRD to an acceptable level (defined as either <20 degrees or <10% of the total rotation in the nonthrowing shoulder).[56]

Alternatively, various developmental adaptations seen in the glenohumeral joint of the overhead throwing athlete have also been suggested as possible reasons for losses in internal rotation, with osseous adaptations (retroversion)[86,272] and muscular adaptations[42,354] both being implicated. In a study of adolescent baseball players by Hibberd and colleagues, age-related increases in GIRD were primarily attributed to humeral retrotorsion rather than to soft tissue tightness.[129] When the GIRD measurements of players of various age groups were adjusted for retrotorsion, no differences in GIRD were detected. Noonan and colleagues further investigated the relationship between GIRD and humeral retrotorsion in 222 professional baseball pitchers.[243] Pitchers with GIRD displayed significantly less humeral torsion (i.e., greater retrotorsion) in their dominant arm compared with those without GIRD as well as greater side-to-side difference in humeral torsion. These authors suggested that greater humeral retrotorsion may place greater stress on the posterior shoulder, resulting in motion deficits and may predispose these pitchers to shoulder injury.

SICK Scapula and Scapular Dyskinesis

The scapula has three main functions during throwing that maximize force transmission from the trunk and torso to the humerus while avoiding risk of labral and rotator cuff injury.[10] First, the scapula must optimize the position of the glenoid with respect to the rapidly rotating humeral head. Second, it must fluidly retract and protract around the thoracic wall as the arm moves through the phases of throwing, maintaining glenohumeral angulation within a safe zone. Third, it must act as a stable base for the origin of the extrinsic and intrinsic shoulder muscles that provide glenohumeral compression and regulate arm motion. These functions require optimal strength and coordination of the periscapular muscles. Weakness, inflexibility, or an imbalance of the periscapular and posterior rotator cuff muscles disturbs the normal anatomic static and dynamic relationships of the scapula. Burkhart and colleagues called the abnormally positioned thrower's scapula a *SICK scapula* (scapular malposition, inferior medial border prominence, coracoid pain, and dyskinesis of scapular movement).[58] Aberrant scapulothoracic motion has been called *scapular dyskinesis.*[164,166]

The SICK scapula is an extreme form of scapular dyskinesis. Morgan also used the term "SICK scapula" to specifically define the static asymmetrical position of the thrower's scapula, in contrast to "scapular dyskinesis," which describes abnormal scapular motion.[236] The hallmark of the SICK scapula is an asymmetrically drooping throwing shoulder and medial scapular winging (Fig. 20-18). The scapular malposition is a combination of four changes in position: upward tilting, protraction, forward tilting in the sagittal plane, and inferior translation. Burkhart and colleagues have described three different subtypes of this syndrome depending on the structures fatigued. The first two are associated with posterosuperior labral tears and internal impingement, and the third is associated with rotator cuff tears. Type I stems from weak lower trapezius and serratus anterior muscles and inflexibility of pectoralis major and minor. This causes inferomedial scapular winging at rest and greater winging on cocking. Type II is predominantly caused by upper and lower trapezius and rhomboid weakness and does not have a large inflexibility component.[58] It is identified by complete medial winging at rest, which worsens with cocking. Type III is associated with impingement lesions and involves superomedial winging of the scapula.

The SICK scapula predisposes the shoulder to labral and rotator cuff tears because the scapula sits in a more protracted and upwardly tilted orientation, positioning the glenoid so it faces more anteriorly and superiorly. This position leads to three developments: anterior tension, posterior compression, and increased glenohumeral angulation. First, with glenoid protraction, the anterior band of the inferior glenohumeral ligament tightens, limiting anterior translation of the humeral head; over time, the ligament becomes susceptible to chronic strain.[346] Second, simultaneously, the posterior edge of the glenoid is brought toward the humerus, placing the posterosuperior labrum and rotator cuff at risk of injury. Finally, excessive protraction increases glenohumeral angulation, which in a thrower will result in the arm lagging behind the body.

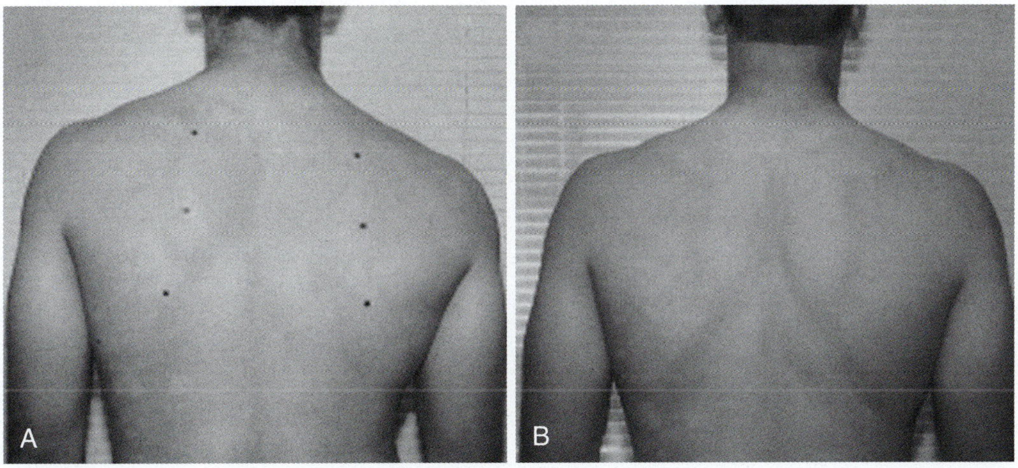

FIGURE 20-18: **A,** A patient with a SICK scapula (scapular malposition, inferior medial border prominence, coracoid pain, and scapular dyskinesis) demonstrates scapular asymmetry with inferior medial border prominence. **B,** After a therapy regimen consisting of scapular stabilizer muscle strengthening and reeducation, the scapulae are symmetrical. (From Burkhart SS, Morgan CD, Kibler WB. The disabled throwing shoulder: Spectrum of pathology. Part III: The SICK scapula, scapular dyskinesis, the kinetic chain, and rehabilitation. *Arthroscopy.* 2003;19[6]:641-661.)

Excessive external rotation in this setting has two deleterious consequences: it exacerbates the aforementioned biceps peel-back effect,[58] and with preexisting scapular protraction, external rotation and abduction can result in posterosuperior glenoid impingement.[164,167] One study examined throwers with proven posterosuperior labral tears and found that a total of 60 out of 64 (94%) showed patterns of dynamic scapular dyskinesis.[55]

Morgan has described a cascade of events that explains many pathologies associated with the SICK scapula: coracoid pain due to pectoralis minor traction tendinopathy, superior medial angle scapular pain from levator scapulae insertional tendinopathy, subacromial origin pain from acromial malposition and decreased subacromial space from upward tilting, acromioclavicular joint pain caused by anterior joint incongruity, sternoclavicular pain, thoracic outlet syndrome radicular pain, and subclavian vascular problems, such as arterial pseudoaneurysm or venous thrombosis.[236]

Treatment for SICK scapula consists of scapular stabilizer muscular strengthening and reeducation.[58,165,168,235,236] The kinetic chain is incorporated into the rehabilitation. The involved side is addressed first using closed-chain exercises followed by open-chain exercises. Scapular rehabilitation has been successful in returning patients with SICK scapula to their previous level of competitive play (Fig. 20-19).

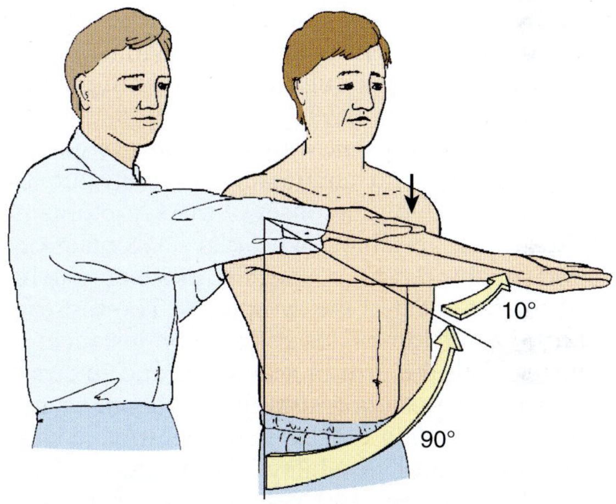

FIGURE 20-19: In the active compression test, the patient's arm is forward-flexed to 90 degrees, adducted 10 to 15 degrees, and maximally internally rotated. The patient resists as the examiner applies a uniform downward force. The patient then maximally supinates the arm and the maneuver is repeated. (Modified from O'Brien SJ, Pagnani MJ, Fealy S, et al. The active compression test: A new and effective test for diagnosing labral tears and acromioclavicular joint abnormality. *Am J Sports Med.* 1998;26[5]:610-613.)

EVALUATION OF THE OVERHEAD ATHLETE

The evaluation of the overhead athlete can be a diagnostic challenge that requires the close integration of history and physical examination findings while utilizing a systematic approach. Many of the traditional examination tests of the shoulder have not been validated or critically evaluated to a significant extent and should therefore be used only as an adjunct to a wider global assessment. In addition, the precise pathophysiology of many shoulder conditions remains unknown, leaving the interpretation of some examination maneuvers uncertain.

History

A sport-specific approach should be used when evaluating the shoulder in an athlete. It can be helpful to observe the athlete in a situation specific to their sport, but often this is not practical for the clinician. Alternatively, coaches and athletic trainers can provide invaluable insight into the athlete's practice or performance-related complaints.

In throwers a detailed history with the chronology of symptoms is essential. In many cases the athlete only describes vague discomfort associated with throwing and a decrease in performance. Pitchers commonly complain of loss of pitch control and loss of velocity and also describe symptoms distant from the shoulder joint. A preseason examination is also critical to document baseline shoulder stability, strength, and ROM, which can be used as a reference when evaluating a mid-season injury. Instability often exists in these patients, but they do not present with symptoms of frank subluxation or dislocation. The throwing phase in which the pain occurs gives direct clues to the underlying pathoanatomy. For example, pain during cocking is often a result of instability or internal impingement with a type II SLAP lesion, whereas pain during follow-through arises from rotator cuff or posterior capsular problems.

Swimmers will often complain of pain during the catch or the recovery, when the shoulder is more often in the provocative impingement position. In swimmers instability is often the principal culprit, exacerbating symptoms of impingement.

Athletes can also present with symptoms of gross instability. As traumatic and atraumatic instability are treated differently, determining the onset of the symptoms is critical. For example, an athlete who plays a contact or collision sport might report a specific incident (such as a dislocation) that initiated the symptoms. The history often suggests the direction of instability. For instance, symptoms elicited with the arm in adduction and internal rotation may suggest posterior instability, whereas symptoms reproduced by holding objects with the arms at the sides often indicate inferior instability. The location of pain or instability, its duration, and response to prior treatment should be noted for all athletes.

Physical Examination

As outlined in the biomechanics section, pathology related to overuse injuries is a continuum and the result of a highly coordinated cascade of movements. Therefore when investigating shoulder complaints, the clinician should also perform a global assessment of related joints, including the spine, elbow, hips, and core area.

Inspection

Both upper extremities should be exposed. The examination begins with inspection of the shoulders for symmetry, with special attention to the acromioclavicular joints, scapular asymmetry, and hypertrophy of the muscles of the dominant arm. Muscle atrophy, particularly the infraspinatus in baseball players, and scapular winging should be noted, as should any surgical incisions.

Range of Motion

Both active and passive ranges of motion (ROM) of the glenohumeral and scapulothoracic joints are measured. Forward elevation in the plane of the scapula, external rotation, and internal rotation in both 0 degrees and 90 degrees of abduction should be documented (in 0 degrees of abduction this is the highest spinal level the patient can reach with the thumb behind the back). During forward elevation with the arm at the side, the 2:1 glenohumeral/scapular motion ratio should be maintained. (The first half of the motion is primarily glenohumeral, and the second half of the elevation arc should move in a 1:1 glenohumeral/scapulothoracic ratio.) As noted previously, the dominant arm in many overhead athletes may demonstrate an increase in external rotation and a concomitant loss in internal rotation. These rotational values should be compared with those of the contralateral limb, and the total arc of motion for both shoulders recorded.

Examination of the scapula should include observing the cervical and thoracic posture, scapular symmetry at rest and with ascending and descending arm motion in both flexion and abduction, and active scapular retraction and elevation.

Palpation

Several structures can be easily palpated, including the glenohumeral joint lines, the acromioclavicular joint, the long head of the biceps (LHB) tendon, and the coracoid process. Tenderness over the acromioclavicular joint is suggestive of acromioclavicular joint pathology. Tenderness over the LHB tendon may indicate tendinitis or a SLAP tear. Coracoid process tenderness suggests pectoralis minor tendinitis or tightness, which has been correlated with scapular protraction and dyskinesis.[58]

Strength

Manual muscle strength testing should aim to isolate the muscle being tested, comparing the injured with the uninjured side. The supraspinatus can be isolated in the empty can position. The subscapularis is best assessed either by the lift-off test described by Gerber and Krushell[116] or by the internal rotation lag sign, which is more sensitive.[128]

Internal Impingement

Apprehension Relocation

The patient is positioned supine on a table. The shoulder is brought into the classic position of internal impingement (≥90 degrees of external rotation, ≥90 degrees of abduction). An anteriorly directed force applied on the posterior aspect of the shoulder will elicit pain but not apprehension. The pain is then relieved with the examiner's hand applying a posteriorly directed force on the anterior aspect of the shoulder.

Active Compression Test

The active compression test, also known as the *O'Brien test* (see Fig. 20-19), evaluates pathology of the biceps and superior labrum complex. The shoulder is brought to 90 degrees of forward flexion and 15 degrees of adduction. Resisted forward elevation is then performed with the thumb pointing down (internal rotation) and pointing up (external rotation). Deep pain during internal rotation but not during external rotation indicates a biceps-labrum complex problem. Pain on top of the shoulder is likely to be due to acromioclavicular joint pathology.

Impingement

Neer Impingement Sign

The shoulder is forcibly elevated while stabilizing the scapula. If there is impingement, pain is classically reproduced at about 90 degrees of forward elevation.

Hawkins Impingement Sign

The shoulder is placed in 90 degrees of forward elevation and 30 degrees of forward flexion and is forcibly internally rotated. Pain evoked in this position is considered a further evidence of impingement.

Acromioclavicular Joint

Acromioclavicular joint pathology is a clinical diagnosis. Pain in the acromioclavicular joint with cross-body adduction and tenderness over the acromioclavicular joint are relatively sensitive and specific. Pain in the acromioclavicular joint area during the active compression test can also denote acromioclavicular joint pathology.

Scapular Provocative Maneuvers

Scapular Assistance Test

Scapular upward rotation is assisted by manually stabilizing the upper medial scapular border and rotating the inferomedial border as the arm is abducted. A positive test relieves symptoms of impingement, clicking, or rotator cuff weakness that are present without the manual assistance.

Scapular Retraction Test

The entire medial border of the scapula is manually stabilized. In patients with apparent rotator cuff weakness and a protracted scapula, if the manual stabilization increases strength, this is positive for scapular dyskinesis. In patients with a positive apprehension relocation test, if the stabilization reduces the pain of impingement during the test, this also suggests that the scapula should be included in the rehabilitation protocol.

Imaging

Standard radiographs and magnetic resonance imaging (MRI) are a critical part of the diagnostic armamentarium for treating athletes' shoulders. Imaging interpretation and diagnoses are discussed in detail in another chapter.

TREATMENT

Posterior Capsule Contracture

Nonoperative Treatment

Nonoperative management has proven successful in managing excessive GIRD (greater than 20 degrees).[96] Some authors have described a series of exercises that theoretically improve posterior capsular contracture and reduce GIRD with some reliability. These include sleeper stretches (Fig. 20-20), in which the athlete lies on one side with the shoulder in 90 degrees of flexion, in neutral rotation, with the elbow in 90 degrees of flexion as well. The shoulder is then passively internally rotated by pushing the forearm toward the table around the fixed point of the elbow.[58]

Others have recommended stretches to improve posterior shoulder flexibility, although they have cited posterior muscle contracture rather than capsule tightness as the component that requires stretching.[354] These stretches include the internal rotation stretch and the horizontal adduction stretch. In the internal rotation stretch, the arm is placed in the throwing (cocked) position and then internally rotated to stretch the posterior rotator cuff. In the horizontal adduction stretch, the arm is horizontally adducted while the scapula is stabilized. The pectoralis minor should also be stretched. This can be effected by placing a rolled towel between the supine athlete's shoulder blades and steadily pushing posteriorly on the shoulders. In addition to the aforementioned stretches, the trapezius muscle and the periscapular retractor and protractor muscles should be strengthened.

Operative Management

The rate of failure of conservative measures, such as sleeper stretches, is exceedingly low, and operative management should only be pursued after aggressive physiotherapy. A thorough examination under anesthesia should be performed prior to diagnostic arthroscopy, documenting bilateral shoulder ranges of motion at 0 and 90 degrees of abduction to confirm the presence of a posterior capsule contracture. The procedure consists of an arthroscopic posteroinferior quadrant capsulotomy, from the 6 o'clock position to the 3 o'clock or 9 o'clock position. The capsule should be incised until the muscle belly of the external rotators can be visualized. Morgan found an average of 62 degrees (range, 55 to 68 degrees) of increase in internal rotation after the capsulotomy.[236] Yoneda and colleagues[371] performed posterior capsular releases on 16 patients and reported that 11, including all four who had no other concomitant lesions, returned to their preinjury level of performance.

SLAP Lesions

Variations in Normal Superior Labrum Anatomy

Appreciating the normal anatomic variants of the superior labrum and biceps insertion is critical to recognizing abnormal pathology. First, the labrum inferior to the glenoid equator is consistently a rounded, fibrous structure continuous with the articular cartilage, whereas the superior labrum has a high degree of normal variation, typically either rounded (Fig. 20-21A) or meniscoid (see Fig. 20-21B), with the meniscal component overlying but not attached to the glenoid articular surface. In one series 49 of 191 patients demonstrated a mobile meniscoid type of superior labrum at arthroscopy and were treated with

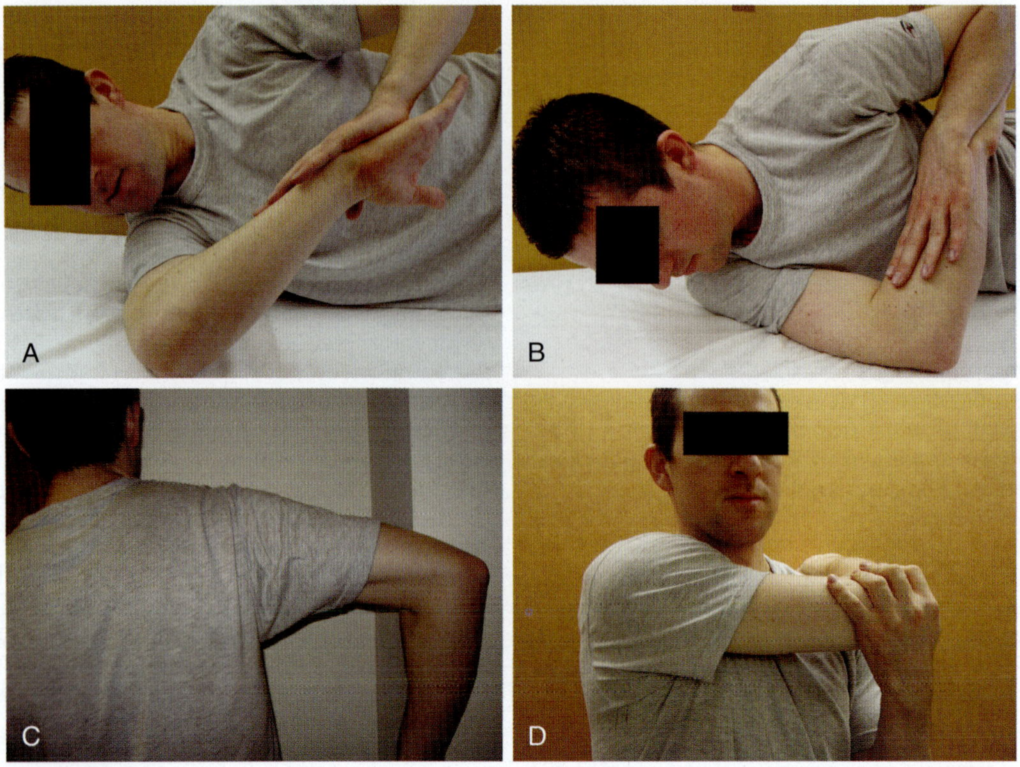

FIGURE 20-20: **A,** The sleeper stretch stretches the posterior capsule. The patient lies on one side with the shoulder neutrally rotated and in 90 degrees of flexion. The elbow is held in 90 degrees of flexion. The forearm is pushed down toward the table to stretch the posterior capsule. **B,** The rollover sleeper stretch in which the patient is lying on the stomach, thereby adducting the arm. As with the sleeper stretch, the forearm is pushed toward the table to stretch the posterior capsule. **C,** In the doorway stretch, the patient stands in a doorway with the shoulder abducted 90 degrees and maximally internally rotated. The door frame is used to apply leverage to the forearm to further internally rotate the shoulder and stretch the posterior capsule. **D,** The cross-arm adduction stretch stretches the posterior rotator cuff and the posterior capsule.

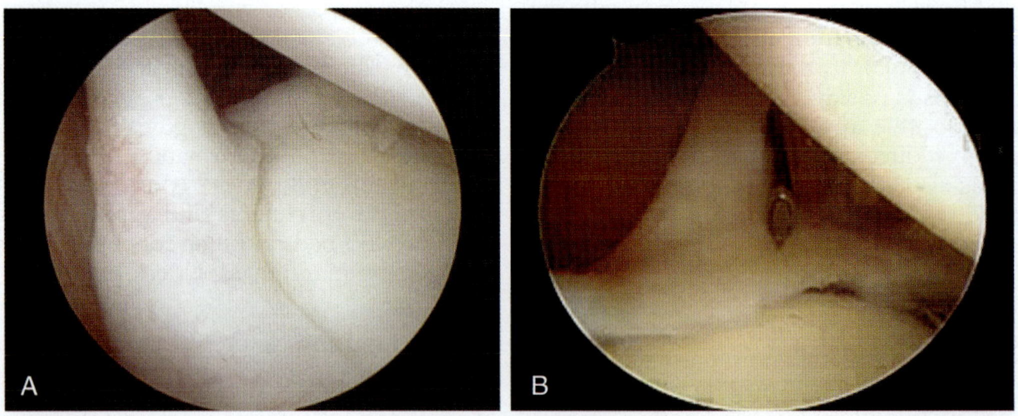

FIGURE 20-21: **A,** Round morphology of the superior labrum. **B,** Meniscoid morphology of the superior labrum.

observation alone. Only one of these patients became clinically symptomatic, which highlights the nonpathologic nature of this anatomic variant.[88]

Second, there are three predominant labral variations that occur in over 10% of the population as reported by Rao and colleagues.[271] The sublabral recess represents a small potential space under the biceps anchor and the anterosuperior labrum and is often present at the 12 o'clock position. The Buford complex is a normal variant that consists of a cordlike middle glenohumeral ligament that originates directly from the superior labrum at the base of the biceps tendon. As a result, there is an absence of anterosuperior labral tissue (Fig. 20-22). The sublabral foramen also involves a cordlike middle glenohumeral

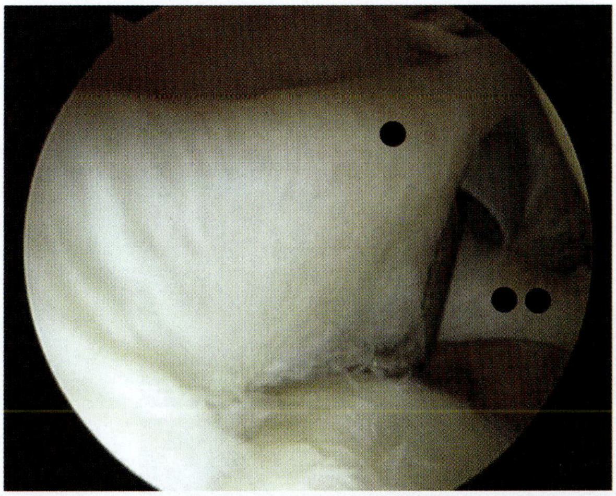

FIGURE 20-22: Example of a Buford complex with a cord-like middle glenohumeral ligament (double dots) underneath the probe attaching to the anterior biceps (single dot) and a sublabral foramen inferior to the middle glenohumeral ligament.

ligament that attaches directly to the anterosuperior labrum, creating a hole between the ligament and the glenoid. Inappropriate surgical attachment of this cordlike middle glenohumeral ligament to this void on the anterosuperior glenoid results in painful restriction of external rotation and elevation. The incidence of the cordlike middle glenohumeral ligament in isolation (18%) is more common than that in combination with the Buford complex (1% to 2%).[136,356]

Superior Labrum-Biceps Complex and Stability

The labrum adds stability to the glenohumeral joint by providing depth and surface area to the glenoid.[135,314] The function of the LHB tendon in glenohumeral stability remains controversial. For example, studies using EMG suggest that the biceps muscle is active with elbow function only.[191,364] Other biomechanical studies however suggest that the biceps tendon might act as an anterior and inferior dynamic stabilizer of the glenohumeral joint.[139,283] One study found that isolated lesions of the anterosuperior portion of the labrum that do not involve LHB had no significant effect on anteroposterior or superoinferior glenohumeral translation. In contrast, complete lesions of the superior labrum and biceps insertion resulted in significant increases in glenohumeral translation.[249] Biomechanical studies have demonstrated that repair of type II SLAP lesions restores glenohumeral stability in both anterior-posterior and inferior translations.[48,49,253]

Classification

Snyder originally described four types of SLAP lesions[312]:

- *Type I lesions* consist of fraying and degeneration of the superior labrum without instability of LHB attachment (Fig. 20-23A).
- *Type II lesions* consist of detachment of the biceps tendon anchor from the superior glenoid tubercle (Fig. 20-23B). Morgan and colleagues later subclassified type II SLAP lesions into anterior, posterior, and combined anterior-posterior lesions.[237]
- *Type III lesions* consist of a bucket-handle tear of a meniscoid superior labrum with an intact biceps tendon anchor (Fig. 20-23C).
- *Type IV lesions* consist of a superior labral tear that extends into the biceps tendon (Fig. 20-23D).

Historically, the incidence of each type of lesion has been reported as 74% type I, 21% type II, 0.7% type III, and 4% type IV. In addition, most SLAP lesions (123 of 139, 88%) can be associated with other intra-articular lesions.[174] Different SLAP types may also coexist as complex lesions; typically, type III or IV lesions manifest in conjunction with a significantly detached biceps anchor (a type II lesion).

Several modifications have been made to the original Snyder classification. Maffet and colleagues[199] expanded the criteria to include three additional subtypes: type V lesions where an anteroinferior Bankart labral lesion exists in continuity with a SLAP tear, type VI lesions with biceps tendon separation and an unstable flap tear of the labrum, and type VII lesions with separation of the biceps tendon–superior labrum complex that extends anteriorly to the middle glenohumeral ligament. Powell and colleagues[267] added three further types: type VIII lesions, where a type II tear has a posterior extension to the 6 o'clock position; type IX lesions, representing a more extensive tear with circumferential involvement of the labrum; and type X lesions, where a superior labral tear is combined with a posteroinferior labral tear (a reverse Bankart lesion).

SLAP Lesions and Throwing

Andrews and colleagues[9] first observed anterosuperior glenoid labrum tears in throwers and postulated that these resulted from traction injuries that occurred in the follow-through phase of throwing, with the biceps eccentrically decelerating the rapidly extending elbow. Burkhart and Morgan described the "peel-back" phenomenon occurring during late cocking, reproducible during an arthroscopic examination, consisting of a torsional force applied to the biceps anchor.[54] Torsional forces in the biceps-labral complex increase as the arm moves into abduction and hyperexternal rotation. The biceps tendon changes from a relative horizontal to a vertical position, producing a twist at the base and thus transmitting the torsional forces to the posterosuperior labrum.

Biomechanical studies have further improved our understanding of the various mechanisms by which SLAP lesions are created. Bey and colleagues[25] found that traction on the biceps tendon can reproducibly create type II SLAP lesions if the glenohumeral joint is inferiorly subluxated. Clavert and colleagues[67] simulated falls on an outstretched hand and found that falling forward on an outstretched hand reliably produced type II SLAP lesions. They postulated that shearing forces were critical to the pathogenesis of these lesions. Kuhn and colleagues[182] studied the throwing motion and found SLAP lesions

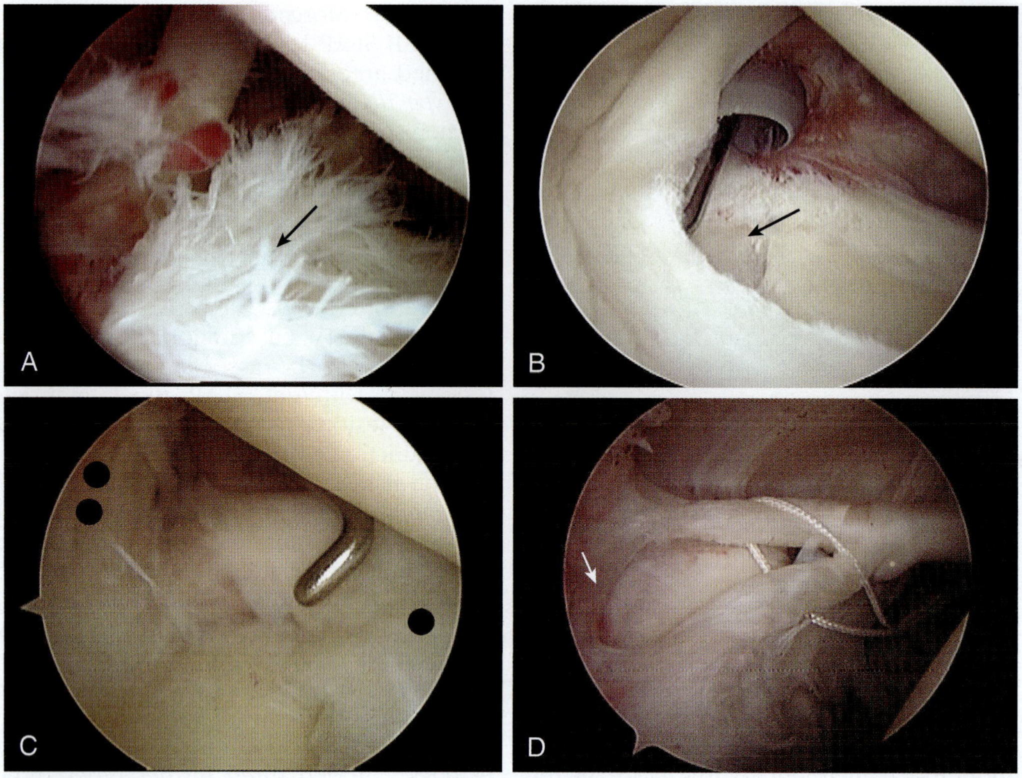

FIGURE 20-23: **A,** Type I SLAP (scapular malposition, inferior medial border prominence, coracoid pain, and scapular dyskinesis) lesion. Fraying (arrow) of the superior labrum without degeneration of the biceps anchor. **B,** Type II SLAP lesion. Detachment (arrow) of the biceps tendon anchor from the superior glenoid tubercle. **C,** Type III SLAP lesion. Bucket-handle tear of a meniscoid labrum (single dot) with an intact biceps tendon anchor (double dots). **D,** Type IV SLAP lesion. A superior labral tear that extends into biceps tendon. The arrow points to superior labral detachment extending into the split biceps.

occurred more commonly in the late cocking position than in the early deceleration position, further supporting the "peel-back" mechanism of injury.

Diagnosis

History

The clinical presentation of the SLAP tear varies; it may be the result of a single traumatic event or it can be more subtle as seen in the overhead athletes. Anterior shoulder pain is the most common complaint, but throwing athletes may present with impaired performance or a loss of velocity and control. Anterosuperior or posterosuperior shoulder pain may be exacerbated by overhead activities, and mechanical symptoms, including popping, locking, and snapping, can occur with unstable tears. Frank instability symptoms are rare, but may be present if the tear extends into the anterior ligament and labrum, resulting in a Bankart lesion.

Anterior traction injuries result from sports, such as water skiing, where the shoulder is pulled forward. Superior traction injuries result from attempting to break a fall from a height. Inferior traction injuries result from a sudden inferior pull.[199,312] Compression of the glenohumeral joint as a result of a fall onto an outstretched hand in forward flexion and abduction or a direct blow to the glenohumeral joint causes an impaction injury of the humeral head against the superior labrum and the biceps anchor.[107,311,312] A type II lesion results when the biceps tendon is avulsed from the superior glenoid as it is tensioned over the humeral head. If a meniscoid-type superior labrum is present, a type III or IV lesion can result with the formation of a bucket-handle fragment.

Physical Examination

The clinical diagnosis of superior labral lesions is challenging, and numerous examination maneuvers have been described for them. Most of these tests are relatively sensitive, but often lack specificity. They include the active compression, compression-rotation,[318] Speed,[107,311] and apprehension-relocation tests. For the active compression test,[247] the arm is positioned in 15 degrees of adduction and 90 degrees of forward elevation. The examiner applies a downward force on the forearm while the hand is pronated and supinated and compares the resulting pain and weakness. A positive test occurs when the patient reports pain that is worse in the pronated position.

Many other tests have been described, including the biceps load test II,[169] the anterior slide test,[162] and the pain provocation test,[229] but their utility has been questioned. Meserve and colleagues[224] performed a meta-analysis that evaluated the sensitivity and specificity of physical exam maneuvers for SLAP lesions. They suggested that the active compression test is the most sensitive and also the most predictive for ruling out SLAP tears. Furthermore, Cook and colleagues[80] conducted a prospective case-control study testing the diagnostic accuracy of five unique tests (the active compression, Speed, biceps load II, dynamic labral shear, and labral tension tests) and concluded that each of these provided little or no value for the diagnosis of SLAP tears.

Imaging

Radiographic evaluation includes anteroposterior, axillary, and outlet views of the shoulder. No specific radiographic abnormalities are pathognomonic for SLAP tears, but concomitant bony lesions including posterior labral ossification, outlet impingement, and acromioclavicular joint disease can be detected. MRI-enhanced arthrography is superior to plain MRI for diagnosing SLAP lesions as the intra-articular contrast medium provides a clearer delamination of the normal anatomic variants of the superior labrum.[22] The diagnostic feature of the MR arthrogram is contrast between the superior labrum and the glenoid that extends around and under the biceps anchor on the coronal oblique image (Fig. 20-24). The axial views visualize possible extension into the anterior and or posterior labrum. MR arthrography is also helpful in identifying the presence of a spinoglenoid cyst and provides the best differentiation between a type II SLAP tear and a normal sublabral recess.[143] Bencardino and colleagues[22] demonstrated a sensitivity of 89%, specificity of 91%, and accuracy of 90% for detecting labral lesions using MR arthrography.

However, despite excellent sensitivity in identifying SLAP lesions, not all abnormalities are clinically significant, and thus careful correlation with physical examination and clinical history is warranted. There can be a high incidence of clinically false-positive MRI findings in the dominant shoulder of the overhead athlete, including partial- or full-thickness rotator cuff tears, labral ossification, and partial tears of the anteroinferior or superior glenoid labrum.[176]

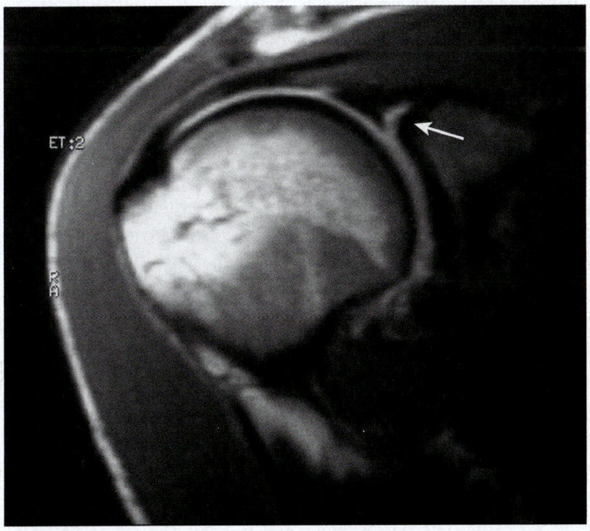

FIGURE 20-24: Coronal image of a magnetic resonance arthrogram demonstrating a superior labral tear (arrow).

Arthroscopic Evaluation

Although the history, physical examination, and MRI can provide useful information in the diagnosis of SLAP lesions, diagnostic arthroscopy remains the gold standard.[227] It is essential to view the joint from both the anterior and posterior portals to thoroughly assess the degree of involvement. Diagnosis of type II lesions can be challenging as the normal superior labrum often has a small cleft between it and the glenoid, especially in the setting of a meniscoid labrum. The stability of the biceps anchor is determined by probing and attempting to elevate the labrum and biceps. The glenoid articular cartilage usually extends medially over the superior corner of the glenoid. An absence of cartilage in this region indicates labral detachment. Traction on the biceps tendon is indicative of a loss of integrity at the superior labral attachment. Burkhart and Morgan[54] have described an arthroscopic examination for "peel back." The arm is placed in a throwing position with humeral external rotation, and the labrum peels away from the posterosuperior glenoid.

Treatment

Nonoperative Management

The role of nonoperative management of unstable SLAP lesions remains controversial. Snyder has argued that nonoperative treatment generally yields poor results, although few studies have focused on the natural history of nonsurgical SLAP tears. In one study patients were treated with an extended trial of activity modification, rehabilitation exercises, corticosteroid injections, and NSAIDs without any significant relief of their symptoms.[251] In contrast, Edwards and colleagues demonstrated that 10 (67%) of 15 overhead throwing athletes treated with a nonoperative regimen were able to return to the same or improved level of play compared with preinjury.[99]

For patients with an acute injury, initial treatment should be directed at eliminating pain, restoring motion, correcting strength deficits, and restoring normal synchronous muscle activity. This includes rest from provocative activities, antiinflammatory medication, and therapeutic modalities. Strengthening is initiated once the pain is resolved. For throwing athletes, a gradual return to throwing may begin as muscle balance and ROM are restored. Treatment may be directed toward surgical intervention if there is failure of the nonoperative program, early suspicion of significant mechanical dysfunction, or a seasonal timing issue.

In throwing athletes, SLAP lesions may coexist with articular-sided tears of the rotator cuff and posterior capsular contractures. Classic subacromial bursitis symptoms and external impingement might also be present. Kibler and colleagues[167] found a high incidence of scapular dyskinesis associated with SLAP lesions. Nonoperative management should therefore include stretching maneuvers for the posterior capsule and rotator cuff as well as exercises for balance and for restoring scapular dynamic stability. Symptoms of subacromial bursitis may be treated with NSAIDs or subacromial corticosteroid injection. Rotator cuff strengthening may proceed only after the restoration of proper capsular elasticity and scapular dynamics. This process can require 6 to 12 weeks before throwing can be initiated. Treatment may be directed toward earlier surgical intervention if there is failure of the nonoperative program, persistent pain, mechanical symptoms and dysfunction, or seasonal timing issues.

Operative Management

The surgical management of SLAP lesions continues to evolve. Treatment options include debridement, labral repair, biceps tenodesis, and combinations of these. Labral repair is performed using suture anchors with either traditional knots or knotless techniques.

Type I SLAP lesions are typically treated with debridement alone. Type II SLAP lesions can be debrided or repaired back to the glenoid rim with suture anchors. For type III SLAP lesions, if the unstable bucket-handle fragment is small, simple resection suffices, but repair is preferable if the unstable fragment is large. Type IV SLAP lesions are treated similarly to type III lesions, and the tendon split is managed with tenotomy, tenodesis, or repair. Management options for the biceps tendon depend on the age and activity level of the patient and on the condition of the remainder of the tendon. Superior labral tears should not be repaired in the face of adhesive capsulitis and should be repaired with caution in patients with significant glenohumeral chondromalacia. Further tightening these shoulders with labral repair can significantly aggravate pain, further compromise their ROM, and accelerate the development of glenohumeral arthrosis.

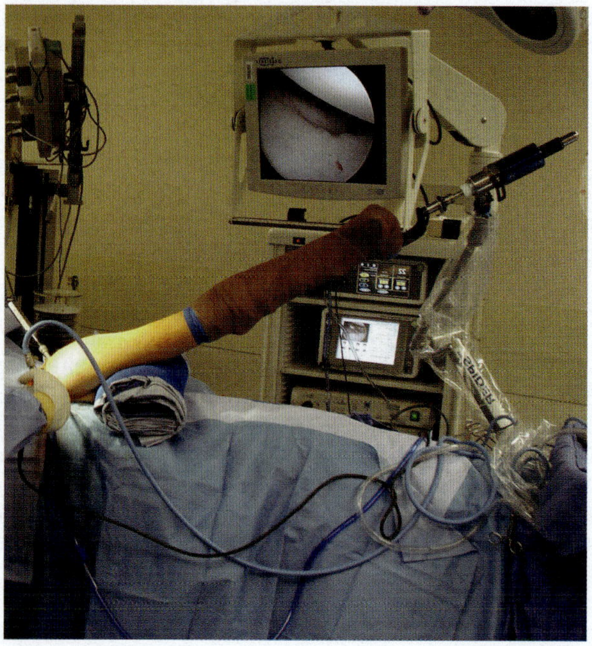

FIGURE 20-25: The patient is placed in the lateral decubitus position to facilitate visualization of the anterior and posterior labrum.

Surgical Repair Technique

Although labral repairs may be performed in either the beach chair or the lateral decubitus position, we prefer the lateral decubitus position with traction to improve superior visualization and provide better access to the posterior labrum (Fig. 20-25). The patient is positioned in approximately 20 degrees of reverse Trendelenburg position and tilted slightly posteriorly to bring the glenoid parallel to the floor. Typically, 10 lb of traction is applied to the arm with a modular joint distractor or a limb positioner, with care taken to avoid overdistraction in order to prevent brachial plexus injury.

Diagnostic arthroscopy is used to confirm the diagnosis of a SLAP lesion. The superior labrum is probed to test the integrity of the biceps-labral attachment to the glenoid. True avulsion of the superior labrum is indicated by fraying and irregularity of the labral undersurface as well as visible chondromalacia of the normally smooth hyaline cartilage of the underlying superior glenoid rim. Arthroscopic examination should include placing the shoulder in the late cocking position of throwing and examining the posterosuperior labrum for possible peel back. During this test, pathologic hypermobility of the posterosuperior labrum and traction of the posterior capsule causes the biceps-labral complex to be pulled medially off the articular edge of the glenoid. The articular surface of the rotator cuff is also examined in this position for delamination and tears. The stability of the entire circumference of the labrum as well as that of anterior and posterior capsule is examined.

Degenerative tissue is debrided from the labrum, biceps, and articular surface of the rotator cuff. This facilitates visualization of damaged tissue that might require repair. In cases of extensive labral tearing or concomitant rotator cuff pathology, our preferred order of repair is as follows: the anteroinferior labrum, proceeding superiorly along the anterior glenoid to the glenoid sulcus; the posteroinferior labrum, proceeding from inferior to superior; the anterosuperior labrum; and finally the rotator cuff.

Care should be taken not to overtighten the tissue or over-constrain the biceps anchor. Placement of anchors anterior to the biceps tendon should be avoided to prevent inadvertent tightening of the middle glenohumeral ligament or closure of a sublabral forearm, which can cause loss of external rotation.[371] Sutures should be placed so as to include the labrum and just enough of the capsular reflection to ensure tissue integrity. Likewise, anchors and sutures should not be placed directly at the biceps-labral base in order to preserve maximal biceps excursion with external and internal rotation.

For a reparable superior labral lesion, the anterior and posterior extent of the labral avulsion is determined. An anterior portal high within the rotator interval provides

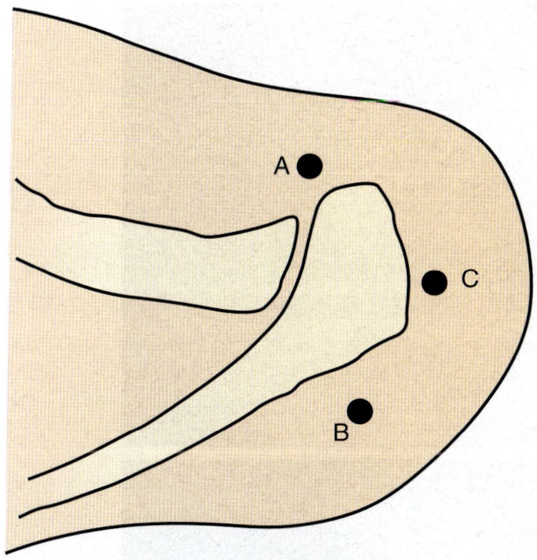

FIGURE 20-26: Portals used for labral repair include anterior **(A)**, posterior **(B)**, and the portal of Wilmington **(C)**.

the best angle of inclination for placing anchors in the anterosuperior glenoid rim (Fig. 20-26). Prior to anchor insertion, the bony surface should be debrided to enhance healing. A motorized shaver is introduced through the anterior working portal to prepare the superior neck of the glenoid beneath the detached labrum. Preferably, percutaneous techniques that minimize morbidity to the supraspinatus tendon should be used. A spinal needle is used to find a position at the desired angle on the glenoid at the location of the Wilmington portal, posterior to the biceps. A small stab incision allows introduction of the drill guide, which penetrates the supraspinatus tendon (Fig. 20-27). The anchor is placed adjacent to the biceps tendon at the glenoid articular margin. The suture anchor must be visualized and confirmed to be in bone, and it must be tested with tension to confirm its security. Suture passage through the labrum is next; we prefer the suture-shuttling technique as the instruments have low profiles and are less traumatic to the labral tissue. In this technique the suture limb facing the labrum is retrieved from the anterior portal. The suture-passing device is passed through the labrum, and the suture shuttle is retrieved through the anterior portal (Fig. 20-27D). The suture is then shuttled through the labrum and out the posterior cannula. If a vertical mattress stitch is elected for a meniscoid labrum, the second suture limb is passed through the labrum. Both suture limbs are then retrieved through the anterior cannula, with the cannula placed posterior to the biceps to facilitate knot tying. Knot tying should aim to ensure the knots are kept away from the glenohumeral articulation. A probe is used to assess the stability and tension of the repair. The process of anchor placement, suture passing, and knot tying is repeated anteriorly and posteriorly as needed (Fig. 20-27F).

Knotless fixation devices have the advantages of eliminating the need for knot-tying and reducing potential chondral irritation from the knots themselves (Fig. 20-28). The results of SLAP repairs have not been as consistent in throwing athletes as in other patient populations. Dines and ElAttrache[94] have suggested that the limited glenohumeral joint space combined with the bulky knots used to secure the labrum to the anchor may be a cause of discomfort. They prefer a horizontal mattress-knotless anchor technique that better recreates the normal meniscoid appearance of the superior labrum.

Rehabilitation

Postoperatively, the shoulder should be protected in a sling for 3 weeks to prevent undue stress on the biceps tendon. The patient begins elbow, wrist, and hand exercises immediately postoperatively and gentle pendulum exercises in 1 week. Strengthening exercises for the rotator cuff, scapular stabilizers, and deltoid are initiated with the goal of restoring full ROM at 6 weeks. Biceps strengthening is initiated 8 weeks postoperatively. Vigorous or strenuous lifting activities are implemented after 3 months, and at 4 months, throwing athletes can begin an interval throwing program on a level surface. They continue a stretching and strengthening program, with particular emphasis on posteroinferior capsular stretching. At 6 months, pitchers may begin throwing full speed, and at 7 months they are allowed maximal effort throwing from the mound.

Outcomes

Historically, simple debridement yielded poor results for unstable SLAP lesions.[83] As fixation techniques evolved, outcomes of surgical repair have improved. Stapling[369] and absorbable tack devices[251,292,301] initially yielded good outcomes compared with debridement alone, but these were later abandoned due to implant-related complications, including synovitis, foreign body reaction, adhesive capsulitis, and breakage.[50,251,355]

Suture anchors have emerged as the gold standard for repair, achieving more reliable results compared with previous devices.[158,170,237,368] Kim and colleagues[170] reported 94% satisfactory results after repair with suture anchors in 34 patients with isolated SLAP lesions; 91% regained their preinjury level of shoulder function. Similarly, 87% of throwing athletes in a study by Morgan and colleagues[237] were able to return to preinjury levels of throwing after suture anchor repair. However, although these studies demonstrated a high level of success following repair, more recent investigations indicate that returning overhead athletes to their preinjury level of performance may be more difficult than previously thought. Yung and colleagues[373] reported that elite overhead athletes may take longer to rehabilitate before returning to sport. Of the 13 patients involved in overhead sports in their cohort, 4 took more than 11 months to return and 1 never returned to competitive play. Sayde and colleagues[293] published a systematic review involving 506 patients with type II SLAP tears from 14 studies. Although "good to excellent" satisfaction was reported for the patient population as a whole, only 63% of overhead athletes were able to return to their previous level of play. The authors did note that there may also be a high incidence of concomitant pathology (such as rotator cuff tears or instability), especially in the throwing athletes, which

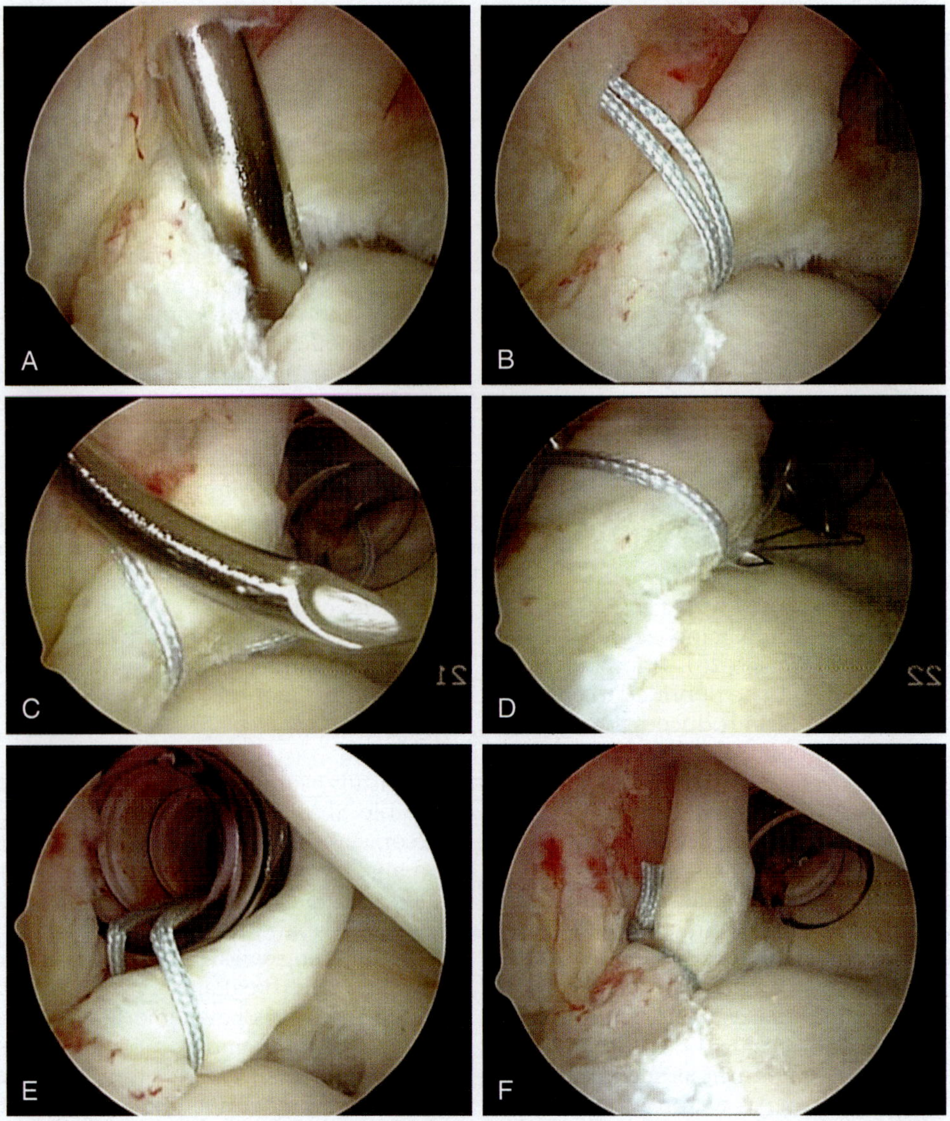

FIGURE 20-27: Percutaneous SLAP (scapular malposition, inferior medial border prominence, coracoid pain, and scapular dyskinesis) lesion repair technique. **A,** Anchor guide in position on the glenoid. **B,** Anchor placed. **C,** Suture passer introduced percutaneously. **D,** Suture passing. **E,** Knot tying with the anterior cannula placed posterior to the biceps tendon. **F,** First anchor complete.

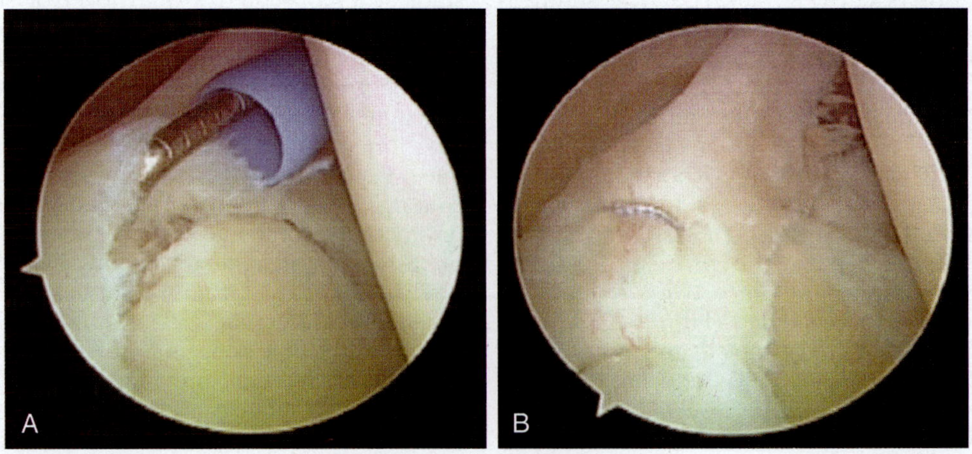

FIGURE 20-28: Knotless SLAP (scapular malposition, inferior medial border prominence, coracoid pain, and scapular dyskinesis) lesion repair. **A,** Probe demonstrating tear. **B,** Two knotless vertical mattress sutures have been placed.

may have affected the final outcomes. Furthermore, most studies included a mixed population of young competitive athletes with older recreational athletes and reported outcomes as an initial "return to sport" rather than full return to the prior level of performance. In an investigation of SLAP repairs in elite overhead athletes, Neri and colleagues[241] showed a return to preinjury level of competition in only 57% of the patients. Inability to return to competition was correlated with the presence of partial-thickness rotator cuff tears.

Other studies have implicated age as a risk factor for SLAP repair failure. Provencher and colleagues[269] prospectively evaluated 179 patients with type II SLAP tears and demonstrated a 37% repair failure rate with 28% of patients requiring revision surgery. Age over 36 years was cited as an independent risk factor for failure. Despite these recent reports, SLAP repairs in this subset of patients continue to increase.[344,376]

Biceps Tenodesis

Tenodesis of LHB for lesions associated with rotator cuff tears has yielded satisfactory results.[33,35,36] As the reported results of SLAP repairs in overhead athletes have been inconsistent, some authors have suggested biceps tenodesis as an alternative to reinsertion (labral repair).[39] There has been speculation over the rationale for why some overhead athletes have difficulty returning to sport following SLAP repair. Alpantaki and colleagues[8] showed that LHB is innervated by a dense network of sensory sympathetic fibers, and these fibers may serve as a source of residual pain following arthroscopic SLAP repair. Rigid fixation of the superior labrum using suture anchors may also restrict the physiologic excursion of the biceps anchor during shoulder elevation, abduction, and rotation, generating pain in throwing movements.[141] Studies have also demonstrated reduced vascularity in the superior osseous glenoid and the superior labral complex.[82] A biceps tenodesis can be advantageous in this environment as it eliminates the pull of the biceps on the repair site and does not require healing in the relatively avascular superior glenoid.[119]

A biceps tenodesis attempts to circumvent potential sources of residual biceps pain in the athlete and can be performed using an all-arthroscopic suprapectoral or an open subpectoral technique. The optimal surgical approach, tenodesis location, and choice of fixation have been the subject of considerable research, but there is a lack of consensus over these in the orthopedic community.

Arthroscopic Biceps Tenodesis Technique

Our preferred technique places the tenodesis location distal to the bicipital groove and is performed according to the method previously described by Lutton and colleagues[197] (Fig. 20-29). The procedure is completed in the modified beach chair position using regional (interscalene) anesthesia. The surgical arm is positioned and adjusted with the use of a limb positioner. Standard arthroscopic portals including a posterior viewing and anterior working portal through the rotator interval are utilized. LHB is released from its superior labral attachment using arthroscopic scissors and the remaining stump and superior labrum are debrided. A tagging suture is not routinely placed in LHB prior to tenotomy. The arthroscope is inserted into the subacromial space and a lateral portal is created using an outside-in technique. Bursectomy of the subdeltoid space is completed to facilitate visualization.

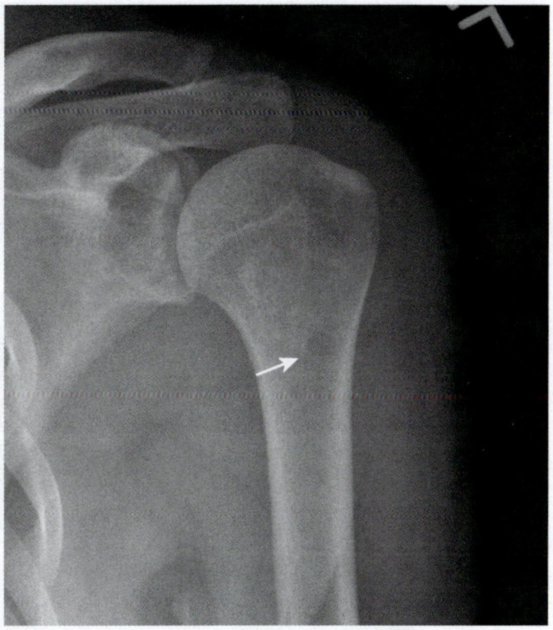

FIGURE 20-29: Postoperative radiograph showing the typical appearance of the bone tunnel for all-arthroscopic suprapectoral biceps tenodesis below the bicipital groove.

The 30-degree arthroscope is redirected into the anterolateral portal and the arm positioned to 60 degrees of forward elevation, 30 degrees of external rotation, and 30 degrees of abduction to aid identification of LHB within the bicipital groove (Fig. 20-30A). Electrocautery is used to release the biceps sheath posterior at the distal groove region, and the LHB tendon is identified. The transverse humeral ligament is left intact covering the groove. The upper border of the PM tendon is isolated and identified with electrocautery (Fig. 20-30B). An accessory anteroinferior "biceps portal" is then established after localization with an 18-gauge spinal needle for the appropriate orthogonal angle to the intended bony tenodesis site, which is below the groove and just proximal to the PM tendon. The location of the site is based on anatomic landmarks and the need to maintain the appropriate length-tension relationship; it is marked on the humerus.[91] LHB is retrieved through the biceps portal with a Kelly clamp and secured with a No. 2 high-tensile suture passed in a whipstitch configuration, ending approximately 25 to 30 mm from the tenotomized end. The diseased portion of the proximal tendon is excised (Fig. 20-30C) and LHB is sized to determine the diameter of the humeral socket.

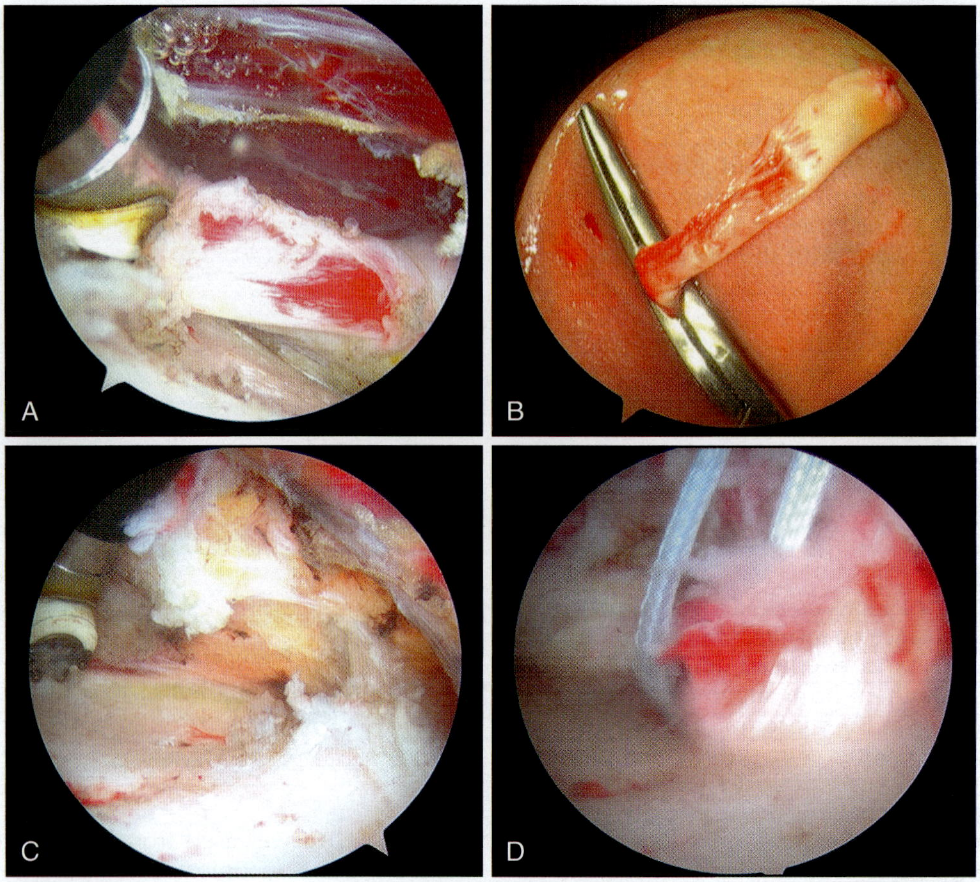

FIGURE 20-30: All-arthroscopic biceps tenodesis technique. **A,** Biceps tendon within the bicipital groove. **B,** Identification of the pectoralis major tendon at the inferior bicipital groove. **C,** Diseased biceps tendon brought outside of skin through the biceps portal. **D,** Fixation of the biceps tendon into the humerus with an interference screw.

The LHB tendon is pulled out through the "biceps portal" and controlled with sutures. The tenodesis site is then once again confirmed arthroscopically to be just proximal to the upper border of the PM tendon and below the groove in a bony site that is no longer grossly concave nor bound by the transverse humeral ligament. A terminally threaded guide pin is inserted through the biceps portal unicortically into the desired tenodesis location and the near cortex is overreamed by 0 to 0.5 mm to the anticipated screw diameter using a cannulated reamer. The appropriate-sized cannulated biotenodesis screw (6.25 to 8 mm × 15 mm) is loaded and secured to the distal end of LHB with an additional No. 2 suture running through a cannulated tenodesis screw (Arthrex Inc.). The tendon is inserted into the depth of the humeral socket and the tenodesis screw advanced 1 mm proud of the cortical surface at the tenodesis site (Fig. 20-30D). The No. 2 suture is then passed through the screw and tied to the No. 2 whipstitched suture to create a suture anchor-type construct to reinforce the interference screw tenodesis.

Outcomes

Early reports of biceps tenodesis for SLAP lesions have shown promising results, but most were limited to older recreational athletes. Boileau and colleagues[39] prospectively evaluated SLAP repair with suture anchor fixation versus arthroscopic biceps tenodesis in two cohorts of patients with type II SLAP tears, of whom 60% were overhead athletes. Following biceps tenodesis, 13 patients (87%) were able to return to their previous level of sports participation, compared with only 20% after SLAP repair. However, treatment allocation in this study was not randomized and the decision regarding repair versus tenodesis was made according to surgeon preference, with tenodesis reserved for patients older than 30 years. Gottschalk and colleagues[119] retrospectively reported on 33 patients (mean age, 46 years) who underwent open subpectoral biceps tenodesis for type II and type IV SLAP tears. Eighty-nine percent of patients were able to return to their preinjury level of activities, including softball, weightlifting, golf, skiing, racket ball, and boxing. The authors concluded that biceps tenodesis was a safe, effective treatment alternative for primary SLAP repair.

Although exceedingly rare, complications of subpectoral biceps tenodesis have been reported.[34,242] These include tenodesis failure, wound infections, musculocutaneous neuropathy, and humerus fractures.[273,300] Postoperative fractures have been attributed to malpositioned tenodesis tunnels, but the stress riser associated with a humeral bone tunnel for tenodesis is an important consideration in the athlete, particular when performing movements as aggressive as throwing. It is preferable in the throwing athlete to use a smaller size interference screw and to position the tenodesis tunnel more proximally in the humerus where the diameter is larger.

Rotator Cuff Tears

Rotator cuff injury is a common source of pain and dysfunction in overhead athletes due to the tremendous stresses imparted to the dynamic stabilizers of the shoulder by repetitive acceleration, deceleration, and overhead motion during throwing and other overhead sports. For the young elite throwing athlete, reports of full-thickness rotator cuff tears are rare and are primarily limited to contact athletes, resulting from a single traumatic event.

Partial-Thickness Rotator Cuff Tears

Partial-thickness rotator cuff tears can be bursal-sided, intrasubstance, or articular-sided. In athletes, articular-sided tears predominate; these are referred to as PASTA (partial articular-sided supraspinatus tendon avulsion) lesions, a term coined by Snyder.[310] Up to 40% of professional pitchers have completely asymptomatic PASTA lesions.[78] When symptoms arise, their onset is usually insidious. The thrower complains of anterosuperior pain with throwing and loss of velocity. The tear typically arises at the articular side of the supraspinatus-infraspinatus interval, posterior to the location of the full-thickness tears commonly seen in the older population. Within the continuum of throwing shoulder pathology, PASTA lesions often occur in combination with other pathologic entities, such as GIRD, posteroinferior capsular contracture, scapular dyskinesis, and SLAP tears, including posterosuperior labral injury and detachment and anterior capsular attenuation.[57]

Several theories exist regarding the causes of partial-thickness rotator cuff tears in the overhead throwing athlete. Andrews and colleagues[9] theorized that articular-sided tears resulted from repetitive eccentric traction forces to the supraspinatus and infraspinatus tendons during the deceleration through release phases of throwing. Davidson and colleagues[87] hypothesized that these tears arose as a result of internal impingement in the cocking position. In this position repetitive contact between the articular side of the rotator cuff and the posterosuperior glenoid generates microtrauma on the cuff side. This pathology is aggravated by anterior subluxation and instability, particularly if the dynamic stabilizers become fatigued. Burkhart and colleagues[57] noted the association between articular-sided rotator cuff tears and posterior type II SLAP lesions via the peel-back mechanism and postulated that the primary etiology of PASTA lesions was posterior capsular contracture leading to posterosuperior migration of the humeral head.

Nonoperative Treatment

Nonoperative treatment for partial-thickness rotator cuff tears includes stretching of the posterior capsular tissues to address loss of internal rotation, rotator cuff strengthening programs (including eccentric and plyometric exercises), periscapular muscle strengthening, trunk and lower extremity strengthening exercises, restoration of proper throwing mechanics, NSAIDs, and corticosteroid injections.

Operative Treatment

Thorough diagnostic arthroscopy is required to identify other causative pathology that may be responsible for the patient's symptoms, especially in the throwing athlete. Surgical options for PASTA lesions include debridement of the rotator cuff tear, subacromial decompression, arthroscopic in situ repair, or completion of the tear followed by open, miniopen, or all-arthroscopic repair. Tears can be classified according to the percentage thickness of the tear, the number of tendons involved, or whether the tear involves the bursal or articular side. Weber found that repairs to tears with more than 50% of the tendon-insertion width in a medial to lateral direction were more successful.[343] Mazzocca and colleagues[209] found in a cadaver model that when articular-sided partial tears reached 50% of depth or greater, this surpassed a critical limit and significantly increased strain in the remaining intact bursal tendon fibers.[209]

The surgical treatment of partial-thickness rotator cuff tears remains controversial, especially in throwing athletes. We have generated several guidelines based on the percentage of tendon torn. The normal footprint of the supraspinatus insertion ranges from approximately 12 to 21 mm in width, and therefore the involved percentage of tendon torn can be calculated. If 25% of the cuff is torn, rotator cuff debridement and subacromial debridement are performed. If 50% of the cuff is torn, an in situ all-arthroscopic repair to the footprint is performed without completing the tear. If more than 75% of the cuff is torn, the tear is completed and an all-arthroscopic rotator cuff repair is performed. Bursal-sided tears show superior results when an acromioplasty is concurrently performed. Intratendinous repair is performed for intratendinous laminar tears. In younger throwing athletes intratendinous repairs are preferable, and acromioplasty should be avoided if there is no evidence of bursal-sided damage.

It is important to recognize the normal bare area that exists between the articular margin and the posterior rotator cuff insertion (Fig. 20-31A). In throwing athletes repairs must be avoided in this area as the humeral head undergoes normal contact with the posterosuperior glenoid, and there is a risk of limiting rotation essential for throwing movements. Occasionally, anterior rotator cuff detachments are repaired to bone in the farthest anterior aspect of the rotator cuff footprint because this area has less normal internal impingement contact in throwing athletes (Fig. 20-31B).

Tear Completion Technique

When we perform tear completion, we prefer an all-arthroscopic over a mini-open rotator cuff repair. In addition to allowing concomitant pathology to be

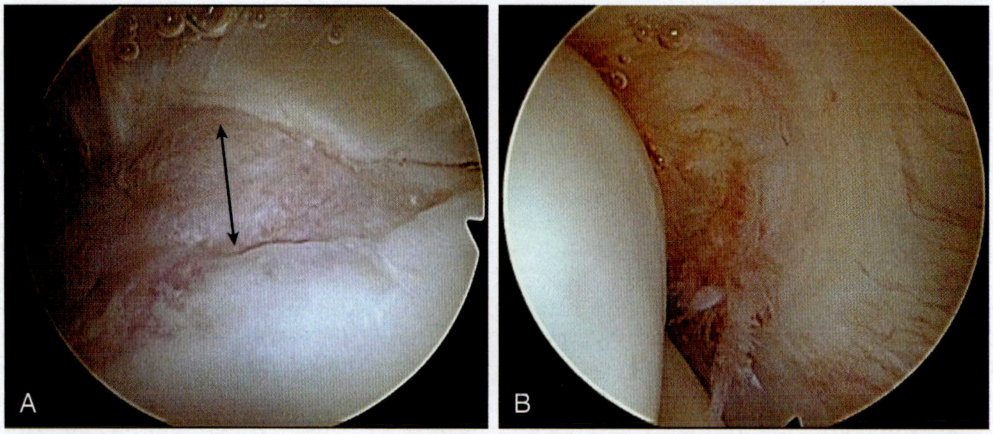

FIGURE 20-31: **A,** Posterior rotator cuff attached laterally with a bare area (arrow) between the attachment and cartilage surface. **B,** Anterior rotator cuff attached adjacent to articular cartilage.

addressed and avoiding the long recovery of deltoid detachment, current techniques for arthroscopic rotator cuff repair result in adequate strength of fixation and restore the cuff insertional footprint. Suture bridge techniques have been shown to biomechanically replicate transosseous tunnel repair techniques, creating tissue compression against the tuberosity to enhance healing.[257]

Research studies have demonstrated that transosseous tunnel repair techniques provide improved footprint coverage,[12] pressurized contact area at the footprint,[256] and reduced motion at the footprint tendon-bone interface compared with standard double-row fixation.[4] It is believed that improved contact characteristics help maximize the healing potential between the repaired tendons and the greater tuberosity.

In Situ Transtendon Technique

The in situ transtendon technique is indicated for the noncompetitive thrower with a 50% PASTA lesion. Glenohumeral arthroscopy is performed, revealing a typically frayed and degenerated undersurface of the supraspinatus and infraspinatus. Debridement exposes the medial aspect of the rotator cuff footprint (Fig. 20-32A).

Before the tear is repaired, the subacromial space is inspected and a bursectomy is performed. Performing a bursectomy prior to placing anchors in a transtendon fashion is essential as prolific subacromial bursa can obscure the suture limbs making retrieval and tying difficult. A suture marker can be placed to allow correlation of the articular surface tear to its general location on the bursal side of the rotator cuff. If the residual portion of the lateral rotator cuff is thin or if a concomitant bursal surface tear is present, the tear is completed, and a standard rotator cuff repair is performed. However, if a significant amount of robust tendon remains attached to the footprint of the rotator cuff, a transtendon arthroscopic repair is indicated.

The arthroscope is reintroduced into the glenohumeral joint. Anchors can be placed through the posterior viewing portal after switching the scope to view from the anterior portal. The shoulder is rotated to obtain the correct angle and location for anchor placement on the tuberosity. If necessary, anchors can be placed percutaneously through the remaining bursal lamina of the tendon. If repairing the avulsed tendon back to bone, care should be taken to leave several millimeters of bone between the articular margin of the humeral head and the tendon repair site. Only the anterior supraspinatus attaches adjacent to the articular margin. The more posterior supraspinatus and infraspinatus attach several millimeters from the margin. Elimination of this bare area results in contact of the tendon against the posterosuperior glenoid with abduction and external rotation; motion restriction ensues, and the site will probably fail to heal.

After anchors are placed, suture passing is performed (Fig. 20-32B). Several devices may be used to accomplish this, but we prefer a shuttling technique with an 18-gauge spinal needle to minimize the trauma to the intact rotator cuff that larger suture-passing devices may create. One suture limb is retrieved through one of the working cannulas. A spinal needle is used to penetrate the first intact bursal cuff and then the articular-sided tear lamina (Fig. 20-32C). A monofilament suture is run through the needle and used to shuttle the anchor suture from the anterior cannula through the tear. This is repeated for all sutures, and typically a double-loaded suture anchor is employed (Fig. 20-32D). If the tear extends farther anteriorly, additional anchors may be placed and the steps repeated. The arthroscope is introduced in the subacromial space and the sutures are tied (Fig. 20-32E). Finally, the glenohumeral joint is visualized once more to inspect the restoration of the rotator cuff footprint (Fig. 20-32F).

Rehabilitation

The postoperative rehabilitation protocol after transtendon rotator cuff repair is similar to that for the standard arthroscopic rotator cuff repair. After the procedure, the treated arm is placed at the side in a sling with a small pillow. The sling is worn continuously for 6 weeks, except

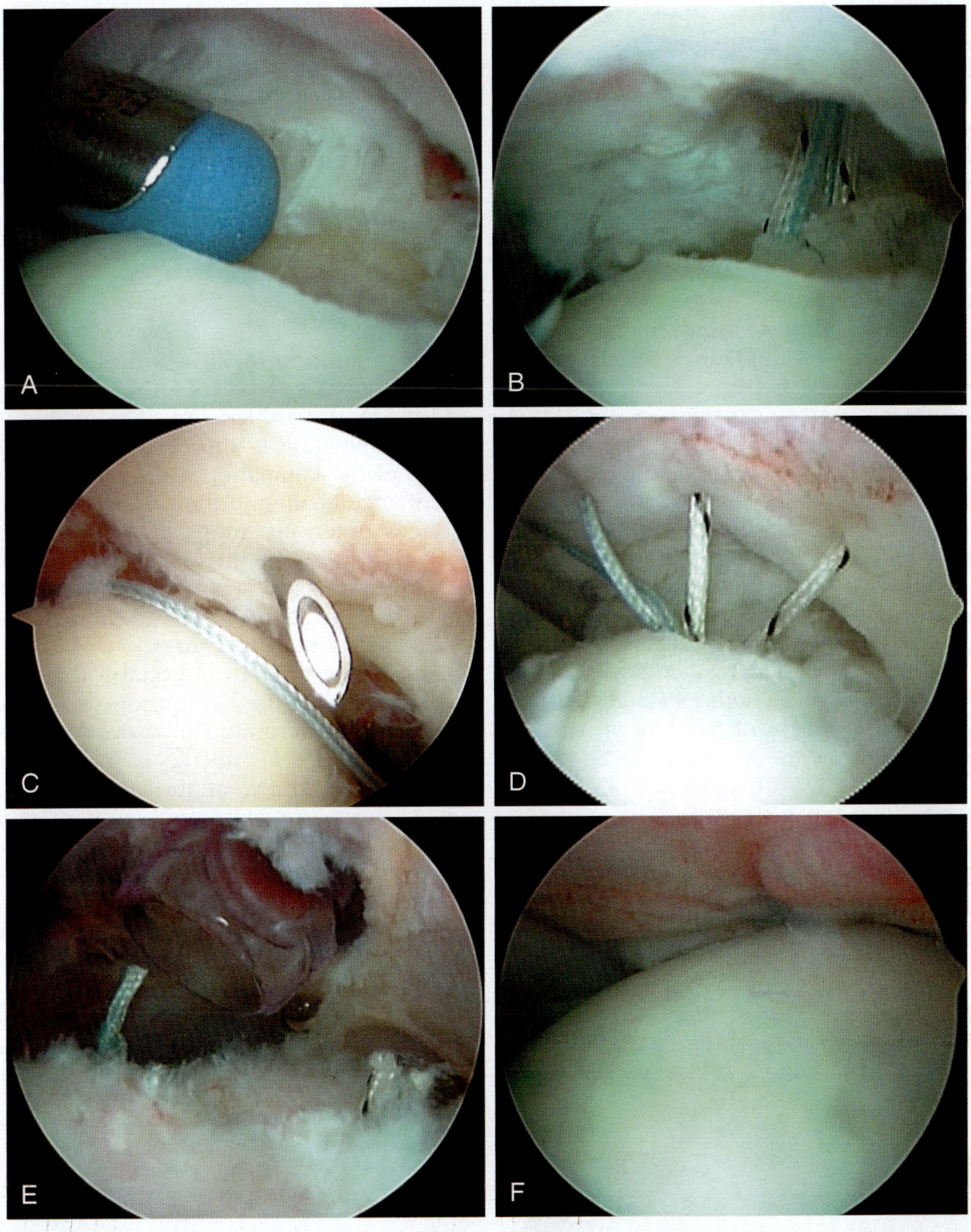

FIGURE 20-32: PASTA repair (partial articular-sided supraspinatus tendon avulsion) technique. **A,** Debridement of a frayed tendon in an area of a partial articular surface tear and debridement of the rotator cuff footprint on the tuberosity using the shaver introduced through the anterior cannula. **B,** A suture anchor passed percutaneously through the tendon and anchored just lateral to the articular margin. **C,** A spinal needle is used to shuttle anchor sutures through the articular-sided tear lamina. **D,** All suture limbs passed. **E,** Knots tied in the subacromial space. **F,** The repair visualized intra-articularly.

during bathing and exercises. Active elbow flexion and extension are encouraged. Patients may begin passive external rotation exercises immediately postoperatively, but overhead stretching is avoided until after 6 weeks in order to avoid stressing the repair. At 6 weeks, the sling is discontinued, and overhead stretches with a rope and pulley and internal rotation stretches are commenced. Isotonic strengthening is not initiated until 10 to 12 weeks after surgery, at which point we begin rehabilitation of the rotator cuff, deltoid, and scapular stabilizers. Progressive activities are incorporated as the patient's strength allows, and unrestricted activities are usually resumed 6 to 12 months following surgery.

Outcomes

The management of rotator cuff injuries in the overhead athlete remains challenging as the orthopedic literature lacks sufficient outcome reports to guide the operative management for this unique subset of patients. Lo and colleagues[193] reported satisfaction with results in all 25 patients who had a minimum of 1-year follow-up evaluation following arthroscopic transtendon rotator cuff repair. The mean UCLA shoulder score for these patients increased from 15 preoperatively to 32 postoperatively. Ide and colleagues reported results of arthroscopic transtendon repair in patients with larger than 6-mm partial-thickness articular-side tears of the supraspinatus tendon and found good or excellent results in 16 of 17 patients.[137] Of six overhead throwing athletes, two returned to their previous sports at the same level, three returned to a lower level, and one was unable to return. The authors concluded that arthroscopic transtendon repair is a safe, reliable procedure in patients with grade 3 (>50%) partial-thickness articular-sided tears.

Liem and colleagues[192] retrospectively reported on 21 amateur and recreational overhead athletes playing six different sports. Arthroscopic repair techniques led to good clinical results, with all the patients returning to sport after an average of 6 months at a self-reported performance level of 91% of their noninjured condition. However, 5 patients (24%) experienced subsequent retearing within 2 years. Similarly, a systematic review performed by Strauss and colleagues[320] reported outcomes on the arthroscopic management of partial-thickness rotator cuff tears. These authors suggested that most tears involving 50% or less of the tendon can be treated with debridement without acromioplasty with good results, although there was an incidence of progression to full-thickness tears in 6.5% to 34% of patients. Repair was indicated for tears greater than 50% of the tendon, and there was no evidence to suggest that tear completion and repair produced superior outcomes over transtendon repair techniques.

PAINT Lesions

PAINT (partial articular-sided intrasubstance tear) lesions were originally described by Conway[79] as a specific type of partial articular-sided rotator cuff tear common in throwers, which involves the intratendinous aspect of the posterior rotator cuff. Conway observed that in throwers, tears often extend into the middle layers of the infraspinatus tendon (Fig. 20-33). Sonnabend and colleagues[313] observed that a synovial lining can form in the laminated aspects of the tear, which compromises intrinsic healing potential. The goal of surgical repair is to obtain side-to-side healing while avoiding repair to the greater tuberosity footprint.

Technique

The technique to repair a PAINT lesion resembles an in situ transtendon repair with respect to portal placement and diagnostic arthroscopy. The magnitude and mobility of the lamination is appreciated using a grasper, and the inside of the lamination is abraded with a shaver or rasp to enhance healing. If the tear is retracted posteriorly and reduces anteriorly more anatomically, the sutures are passed first through the posterior aspect and then through the anterior aspect of the lamina, using the anterior cannula (Figs. 20-34 to 20-36). Mattress sutures are then placed from outside (bursal surface) to inside using a spinal needle and No. 2 nonabsorbable sutures.

A spinal needle is introduced percutaneously just lateral to the acromion in order to penetrate the intact bursal lamina. The needle is maneuvered to penetrate the articular lamina at the desired location. A needle meniscal repair device with a wire shuttle is used to retrieve the suture (Fig. 20-37). Alternatively, a monofilament suture is passed and retrieved through the anterior cannula and tied to the No. 2 nonabsorbable suture.

The spinal needle is reintroduced, penetrating both laminae, and a monofilament suture is introduced and brought out through the anterior cannula and tied to the previous braided suture. It is then shuttled through the rotator cuff to create a mattress suture. These steps are repeated to create the required number of mattress

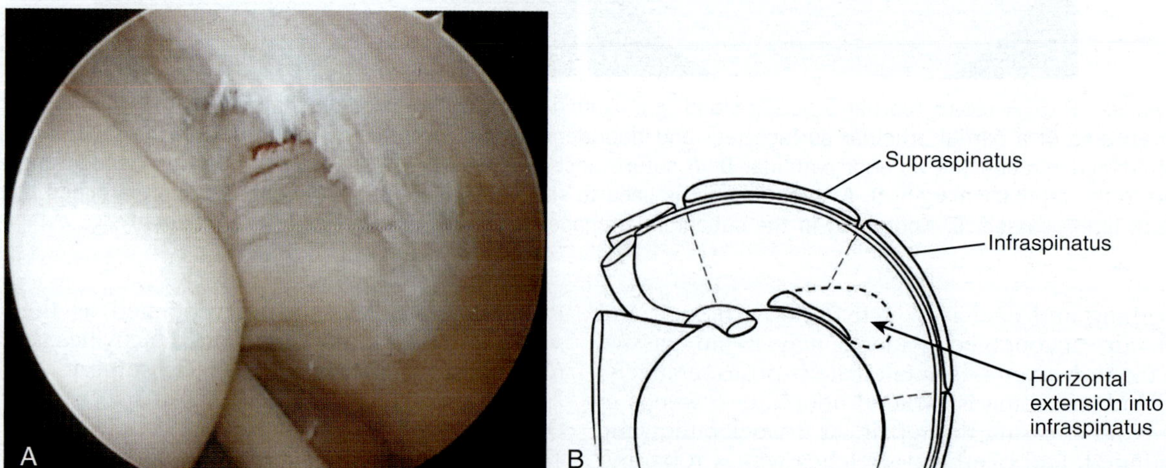

FIGURE 20-33: Intraoperative image **(A)** and schematic **(B)** of a large intratendinous partial-thickness rotator cuff tear at the junction of the supraspinatus and infraspinatus. (**B,** From Conway JE. Arthroscopic repair of partial-thickness rotator cuff tears and SLAP lesions in professional baseball players. *Orthop Clin North Am.* 2001;32[3]:443-456.)

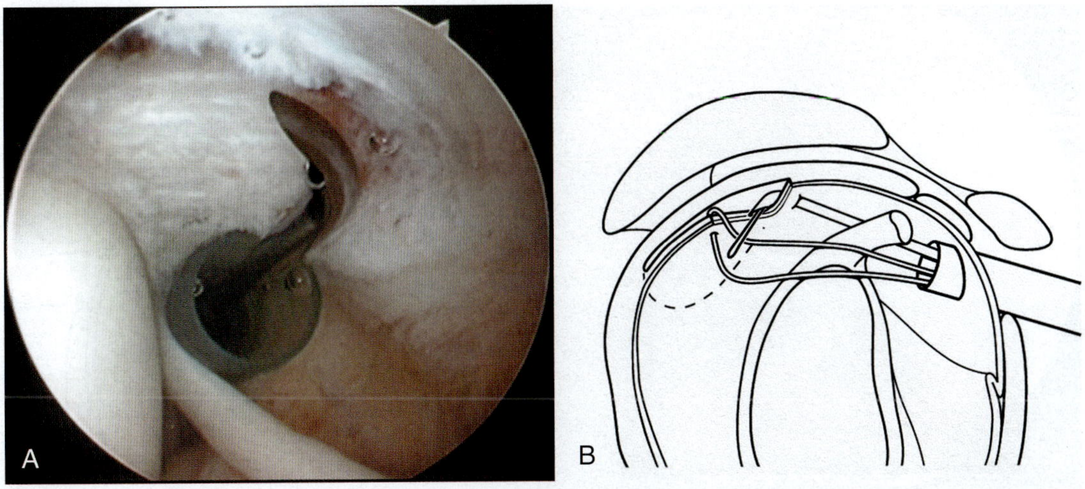

FIGURE 20-34: Intraoperative image **(A)** and schematic **(B)** of a suture lasso introduced and used to pass a No. 2 braided suture through the anterior and posterior aspects of the leading edge of the intratendinous tear. (**B,** From Conway JE. Arthroscopic repair of partial-thickness rotator cuff tears and SLAP lesions in professional baseball players. *Orthop Clin North Am.* 2001;32[3]:443-456.)

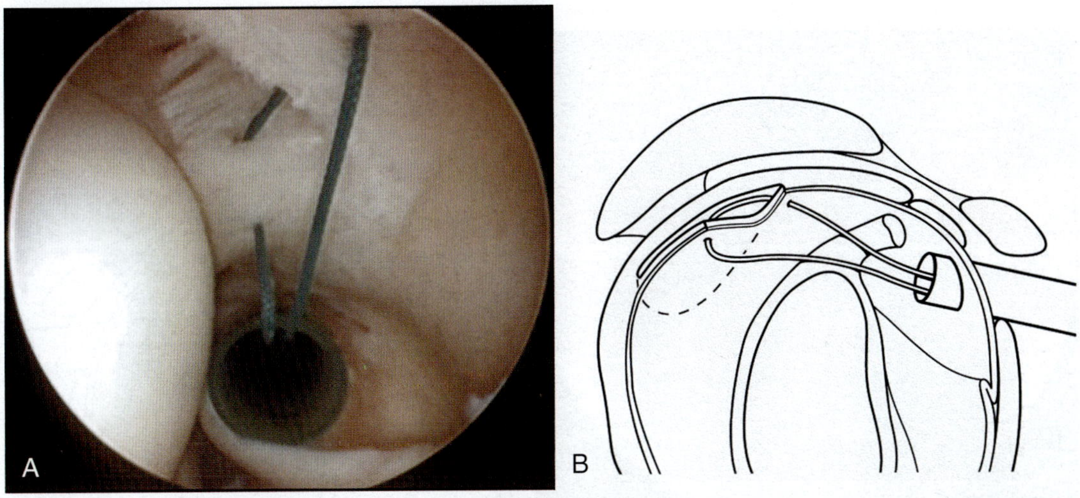

FIGURE 20-35: Intraoperative image **(A)** and schematic **(B)** after the first suture is passed. (**B,** From Conway JE. Arthroscopic repair of partial-thickness rotator cuff tears and SLAP lesions in professional baseball players. *Orthop Clin North Am.* 2001;32[3]:443-456.)

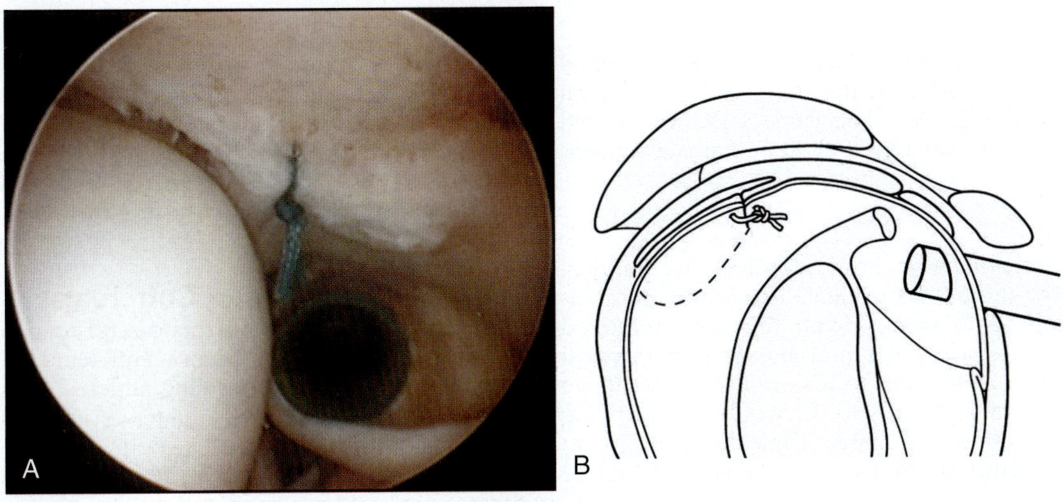

FIGURE 20-36: Intraoperative image **(A)** and schematic **(B)** of the suture limbs being tied intra-articularly, stabilizing the intratendinous tear. (**B,** From Conway JE: Arthroscopic repair of partial-thickness rotator cuff tears and SLAP lesions in professional baseball players. *Orthop Clin North Am.* 32[3]:443-456, 2001.)

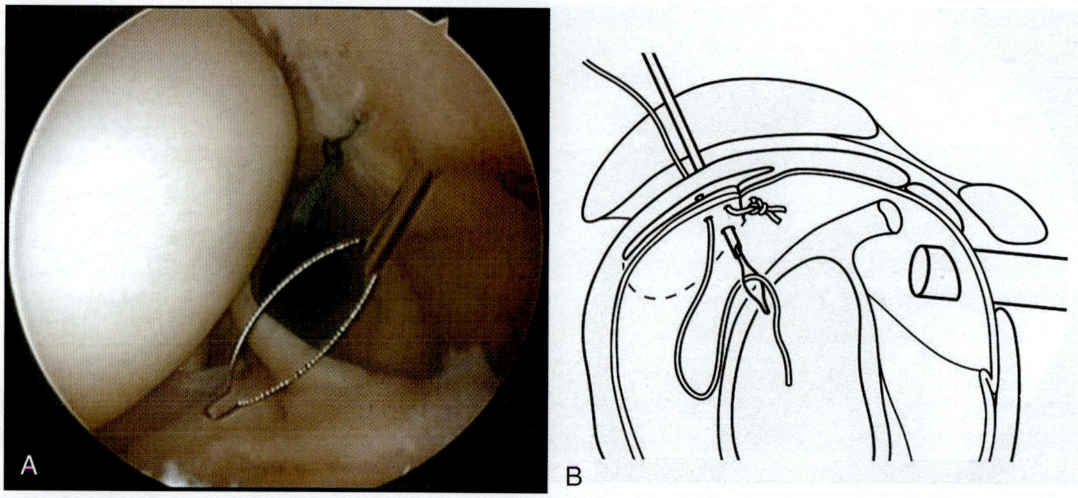

FIGURE 20-37: Intraoperative image **(A)** and schematic **(B)** of a meniscal suturing device used to shuttle suture limbs through the intralaminar component of the tear. (**B,** From Conway JE. Arthroscopic repair of partial-thickness rotator cuff tears and SLAP lesions in professional baseball players. *Orthop Clin North Am.* 2001;32[3]:443-456.)

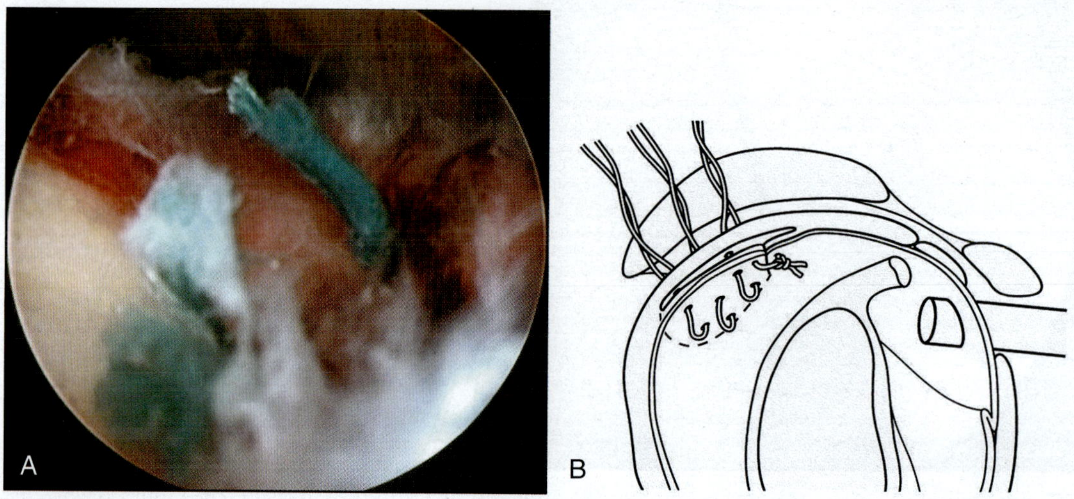

FIGURE 20-38: Intraoperative image **(A)** and schematic **(B)** of the suture limbs being shuttled out through the subacromial space and tied. (**B,** From Conway JE. Arthroscopic repair of partial-thickness rotator cuff tears and SLAP lesions in professional baseball players. Orthop Clin North Am. 2001;32[3]:443-456.)

sutures. The camera is then placed in the subacromial space and the sutures are tied through a standard lateral working portal (Fig. 20-38). The camera is then placed back in the glenohumeral joint and the repair is evaluated (Fig. 20-39).

Rehabilitation

The goals of rehabilitation are to protect the surgical repair and allow the tissues to heal. The arm is immobilized in a sling for 6 weeks, with the sling removed several times a day for passive motion exercises. Physical therapy is initiated at 3 weeks to restore ROM, and active strengthening is initiated at 8 to 12 weeks. A throwing program is initiated at 4 months. Typically, a return to competitive throwing can be expected between 6 and 12 months.

Outcomes

Conway[79] found that of 14 baseball players (mean age, 16 years) who underwent repairs of intratendinous rotator cuff tears and concurrent pathology (including labral and SLAP tears), 89% were able to return to baseball at the preinjury level or higher at 16-month follow-up.

Full-Thickness Rotator Cuff Tears

Although partial-thickness rotator cuff tears are relatively common, full-thickness rotator cuff tears are much less prevalent in overhead throwing athletes. The few reports of complete tears in elite athletes typically involve traumatic dislocations in contact sports such as rugby.[118] In general full-thickness tears carry a poor prognosis in professional athletes, particularly elite throwers.

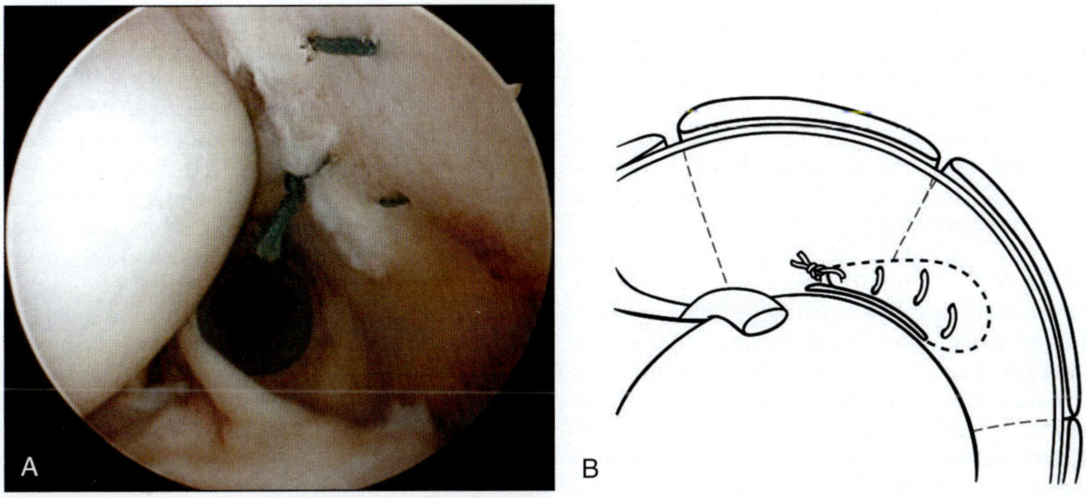

FIGURE 20-39: Intraoperative image **(A)** and schematic **(B)** of the completed repair approximating the leaves of the intralaminar tear. (**B,** From Conway JE. Arthroscopic repair of partial-thickness rotator cuff tears and SLAP lesions in professional baseball players. *Orthop Clin North Am.* 2001;32[3]:443-456.)

Mazoue and Andrews[313] reported the results after mini-open repair of full-thickness rotator cuff tears in 16 professional baseball players. At a mean follow-up of 66.6 months for the pitchers, only 1 player (8%) was able to return to a high competitive level of baseball with no significant shoulder dysfunction. The authors concluded that it is difficult for a professional baseball pitcher to return to a competitive level of pitching after a full-thickness rotator cuff repair with a mini-open approach. Tibone and colleagues[326] studied 45 athletes who underwent repair of either a partial (30 patients) or complete (15 patients) rotator cuff tear with anterior acromioplasty. Although 87% of the patients felt improved from their preoperative status, only six (32%) of the 22 pitchers and throwers who played at either professional or collegiate level returned to their preinjury level of competition.

Posterior Ossification of the Shoulder (Thrower's Exostosis)

First described in 1941, the Bennett lesion (or "thrower's exostosis") is a mineralization of the posteroinferior glenoid observed in overhead throwing athletes.[23] The etiology of the reactive bone formation is related to the capsular traction associated with the repetitive stresses involved in throwing.[18,195] The lesion is found in the area of the attachment of the posterior band of the inferior glenohumeral ligament complex.[195] These lesions have been associated with posterior shoulder pain during the late cocking, acceleration, or follow-through phases of the throwing motion.[222] However, Wright and Palleta[361] studied 55 asymptomatic major league pitchers with routine preseason radiographs and found 22% to have a Bennett lesion. They concluded that concomitant pathology should be suspected when evaluating throwers with posterior shoulder pain as well as this lesion.

Bennett originally recommended excision of the exostosis.[23] Lombardo and colleagues have described a series of athletes with a successful return to throwing following open excision of the lesion.[195] Ferrari and colleagues[105] reviewed seven pitchers with Bennett lesions; all had complained of posterior shoulder pain at some point and all had posteroinferior glenoid tenderness to palpation. They underwent arthroscopic surgery on their shoulders. Posterior labral tears were noted in six of the seven pitchers and were debrided arthroscopically. In addition, these six players demonstrated posterior rotator cuff damage. Six of the seven pitchers returned to pitching at or above their preinjury level.

Meister and colleagues reported on 22 throwers with posterior glenoid osteophytes and posterior shoulder pain that underwent arthroscopic treatment.[222] Of these, 21 demonstrated undersurface rotator cuff tears, and 15 had posterior labral tears. The rotator cuff and labral tears were debrided. In 11 of the patients the posterior glenoid osteophyte was debrided arthroscopically; the indication for debridement was posterior shoulder pain, posterior glenoid rim and capsule tenderness, and a large osteophyte easily accessible by a small capsular incision at the glenoid rim. Eighteen of the players were available for long-term follow-up (at a mean of 6.3 years); 10 of the 18 players were able to return to their preinjury level of sports participation. A trend toward a poor result was noted when the area of the exostosis exceeded 100 mm^2, but the results showed no differences in outcome related to player position, size of the rotator cuff tear, labral damage, or exostosis debridement. The authors concluded that the exostosis should be excised if it is prominent and easily accessible and if it is associated with posterior shoulder pain and tenderness.

Yoneda and colleagues[370] reported on 16 baseball players who underwent the arthroscopic removal of symptomatic Bennett lesions. None of the players had an isolated Bennett lesion: biceps and labral complex injuries were detected and treated in 4 patients, articular-sided partial-thickness rotator cuff tears were debrided in 6 patients, posteroinferior labral injuries were repaired in 4 patients, and a Bankart or an anterosuperior labral injury was repaired in 2. At a minimum of 1 year of follow-up, 11 of the 16 patients had returned to their previous level of competition.

In summary, the approach to treating this lesion is based on the overall shoulder pathology. We recommend a trial of nonoperative treatment that includes rest, posterior capsular stretching, strengthening, and then a throwing program. If nonoperative treatment fails, arthroscopy is indicated and the management of concomitant lesions is addressed. The arthroscopic technique to address a Bennett lesion depends on the integrity of the posterior labrum. When a tear is present, the surgeon can displace the labrum, working through the tear to resect the ossification, and later repair the posterior labrum. When a tear is absent, a capsular window is created to resect the osteophyte (Fig. 20-40). The posterior capsule is left open to relieve the traction etiology of the lesion and address capsular contracture.

Anterior Shoulder Instability in Athletes

Anterior shoulder dislocations are common among contact athletes. Hovelius[133] reported that 40% of dislocations occurred in patients 22 years of age or younger. Baker and colleagues[16] noted that 75% of all shoulder dislocations occur in the position of external rotation and abduction during athletic activities. The pathoanatomy resulting from traumatic anterior instability varies. Rowe and colleagues[287] found the anterior labral tears, as described by Bankart, were the essential lesion of instability in 70% of cases of traumatic instability that required surgery. Superior labral lesions have also been associated with anterior instability as well as plastic deformation of the inferior glenohumeral ligament complex. Bigliani and colleagues[83] showed that an intrasubstance ligament injury occurs before labral avulsion. In addition, bony lesions caused by a compression fracture at the posterolateral margin of the humeral head, termed the *Hill-Sachs lesions,* have been reported in more than 80% of cases of traumatic instability and have been suggested as a risk factor for recurrence.

The concern over initial traumatic shoulder dislocations in athletes stems from the high reported rates of recurrence after nonoperative management. Simonet and Cofield[309] reported that young athletes had an 82% rate of recurrence compared with 30% in nonathletes. This association between recurrence and being an athlete however has been challenged by other authors who did not find such a correlation.[132,324] Rowe and colleagues[284] found a 100% redislocation rate in patients younger than 10 years, 94% between the ages of 10 and 20 years, and 79% between the ages of 20 and 30 years. The type of sport can also influence recurrence with nonoperative treatment. Taylor

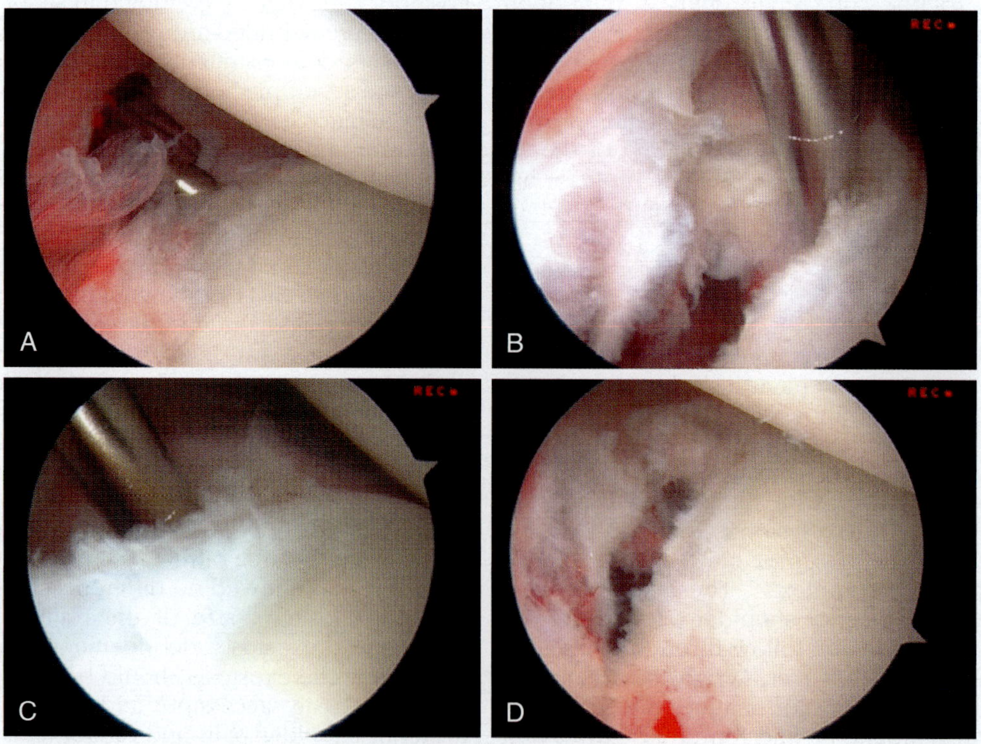

FIGURE 20-40: A, Bennett lesion of the posterior glenoid viewed from the anterosuperior portal. **B,** Posterior capsulectomy performed with a mechanical shaver. **C,** Osteophyte resection using a mechanical shaver. **D,** Completed resection with the posterior capsule left open.

and Arciero[322] reported a 90% rate of redislocation in athletic military cadets involved in collision sports. Athletes in collision sports, such as football, hockey, and rugby, are particularly prone to recurrence because of the high-impact nature of their sport. In 29 athletes who underwent arthroscopic stabilization, Rhee and colleagues[276] found that 28% of the collision athletes redislocated compared with 6.7% of the noncollision athletes.

Nonoperative Treatment

The overall recurrence rate following nonoperative management of traumatic anterior shoulder dislocations ranges from 33% to 67%.[275] Despite these relatively high incidences of recurrence, nonsurgical management continues to be the initial treatment of choice for first-time dislocators. Multiple risk factors for recurrent instability have been identified, including young age, athletic activity, male sex, and the presence of an anterior bone deficiency.[40,65]

Traditionally, immobilization in internal rotation had been implemented, but the suggested duration and position of immobilization continues to evolve. For instance, Simonet and Cofield[309] suggested 6 weeks in internal rotation. In contrast, Buss and colleagues[59] used no immobilization but instead initiated immediate rotator cuff and periscapular strengthening for in-season athletes; however, these authors reported an in-season recurrence rate of 41%. Bottoni and colleagues[43] employed a protocol that advocated immobilizing the shoulder for 4 weeks followed by a rehabilitation program; they found that 75% of nonoperatively treated patients experienced dislocation recurrences. McCarty and colleagues[211] suggested that patients should meet the following six criteria before being allowed to return to their sport:

1. Little or no pain
2. Patient's subjective impression of stability
3. Near-normal ROM
4. Near-normal strength
5. Normal functional ability
6. Normal sport-specific skills

These authors also recommended that the patient should wear a brace to prevent external rotation and abduction while playing.

Itoi and colleagues[140] performed an MRI study showing greater anatomic reduction in the anterior labrum with the humerus in external rotation rather than in the internal rotation position in which most patients are immobilized. They then compared 3 weeks of immobilization in internal rotation versus external rotation and found that the 15.5-month average follow-up recurrence rate was 30% for those in internal rotation versus zero for those in external rotation.[138] However, these results have not been reproduced by others, and the suggested duration and position of immobilization remains an area of controversy.[259]

Operative Treatment

Surgical treatment should be considered for patients identified as being at high risk of recurrent instability or failing nonoperative measures. In the athletic population, decision-making regarding the type of procedure and surgical timing can be challenging. In-season athletes may be managed initially nonoperatively and undergo rehabilitation with return to sport when the previously listed criteria are met and may subsequently undergo stabilization after their season is complete. Others involved in high-risk activities, such as football, white-water kayaking, and rock climbing, should be considered for early stabilization.[321]

Both open and arthroscopic surgical procedures are commonly utilized in the treatment of anterior shoulder instability, and the optimal approach is the subject of considerable scrutiny. Clinical results in the literature for arthroscopic stabilization now rival traditional open approaches to shoulder instability.[77,115,171,173,205,206,316,323,357] Initial poor results of arthroscopic instability surgery have been attributed to inadequate techniques to correct all the necessary pathologic components of glenohumeral instability, including labral tears and capsular laxity.[75,76,156,157,315,317] Arthroscopic results have improved through a combination of better understanding and recognition of these pathologic elements along with improved surgical techniques, including the use of multiple working portals, better anchor and suture-passing instrumentation, more accurate anchor placement, and more precise capsulorrhaphy.[77,84,115,171,173,189,206,289,303,316,323,357,] Suggested advantages to arthroscopic treatment include improved diagnostic capabilities to identify and treat specific pathology, less iatrogenic damage to local tissues (the subscapularis tendon), reduced postoperative pain, and improved cosmesis.[208,291] Others have argued that the open procedures have superior outcomes with lower recurrence in specific patient populations. Ultimately, the preferred surgical technique depends on a variety of patient characteristics, bony and capsulolabral pathoanatomy, and surgeon comfort level.

Some authors have suggested that a patient's participation in a collision sport necessitates open reconstruction. Rhee and colleagues,[276] for example, found that in a study group of 48 shoulders (of 46 collision athletes) there was a 25% recurrence rate of postoperative instability in those who underwent an arthroscopic repair versus a 12.5% recurrence rate in the open group. However, these athletes had all experienced multiple (>17) preoperative episodes of dislocation. Uhorchak and colleagues[334] found that of 66 collision or contact athletes they treated with open modified Bankart repair and anterior capsulorrhaphy, only two experienced recurrent dislocations after surgery, although 13 patients had post-surgical subluxation. Pagnani and Dome[250] found that 55 of 58 football players achieved a good or excellent result after open anterior stabilization. However, arthroscopic techniques have improved over time, and successful stabilization in contact and collision athletes has been reported.[208] Other indications that previously required an open approach but have now become arthroscopically manageable include an attenuated capsule, HAGL (humeral avulsion of glenohumeral ligament) lesions, and revision surgery cases.

Risk Factors for Failure of Arthroscopic Stabilization

In recent years arthroscopic stabilizations have become more common, and there has been an abundance of studies reporting clinical outcomes and recurrence rates. In a prospective evaluation of arthroscopic Bankart repairs, Voos and colleagues[338] suggested that the risk factors for failure are age less than 25, ligamentous laxity, and the presence of a Hill-Sachs lesion measuring more than 250 mm^3. Calvo and colleagues[65] prospectively evaluated 61 patients treated arthroscopically for anterior instability and identified age less than 28 years, diffuse ligamentous laxity, glenoid bone loss greater than 15%, and resumption of contact sports as independent risk factors for failure of repair. Similarly, Porcellini and colleagues[266] retrospectively reported on 625 patients that underwent arthroscopic Bankart repair and found age at the time of the first dislocation, male sex, and the time from the first dislocation until surgery to be significant risk factors for recurrence.

Using a prospective case-control study of 131 patients, Boileau and colleagues[17] developed the instability severity index score (ISIS) as a simple tool for predicting the risk of failure after arthroscopic stabilization. The strongest risk factors for failure included patient age less than 20 years, involvement in competitive or contact sports or those involving forced overhead activity, shoulder hyperlaxity, a Hill-Sachs lesion on an anteroposterior radiograph, and/or loss of the sclerotic inferior glenoid contour. The recurrence rate was also significantly higher in competitive athletes (50%) than in those participating in recreational sports (14.9%).

Bone Deficiencies and Anterior Instability

Hill-Sachs lesions have been reported to occur in 32% to 51% of initial anterior dislocations,[63,133] and anteroinferior glenoid deficiencies (bony Bankart lesions) have been reported in 22% of primary dislocations.[285] Concurrent glenoid and humeral head bone defects exist in nearly 100% of cases of recurrent shoulder dislocators.[52,63] In cases of bony defects higher rates of recurrent instability have been reported after traditional Bankart repair.[52,287,341] Burkhart and DeBeer[52] compared recurrence rates after arthroscopic stabilization and found that 67% of patients with significant bone defects of either the glenoid or humeral head redislocated compared with 4% of those without such defects. For contact athletes with bony deficiencies, the dislocation recurrence rate after arthroscopic management was 89%.

Glenoid Bone Loss

In collision athletes significant glenoid bone loss, classically termed the *inverted-pear glenoid*, remains a relative contraindication for arthroscopic management.[52] In normal circumstances the anteroinferior rim of the glenoid should be readily visible on both the anteroposterior and axillary radiographs, with the loss of the normal contour suggesting glenoid bone loss, especially in the setting of recurrent instability. Advanced imaging with axial CT scans and three-dimensional rendering is preferred for evaluation of glenoid morphology and osseous defects (Fig. 20-41).[33] Many authors have attempted to quantify the critical amount of isolated anterior glenoid bone loss that results in anterior instability, and most agree that glenoid lesions greater than 20% to 25% of the articular surface require a bone grafting procedure (Fig. 20-42).[140,194] This threshold may be lower in the setting of combined defects, such as an engaging Hill-Sachs impaction fracture, the so-called "bipolar" shoulder lesions. However, with improved techniques, encouraging results have been achieved with arthroscopic management in the setting of bony defects. Mologne and colleagues[232] reported no redislocations in 11 patients with 20% to 30% bony glenoid loss and a bone fragment, who were followed up at an average of 34 months after arthroscopic stabilization. Two of 10 patients with a

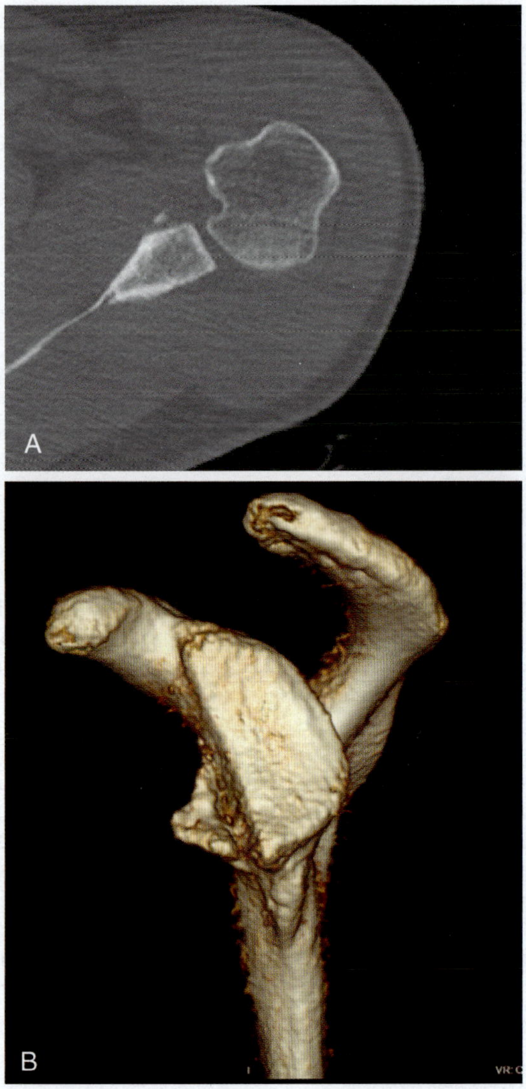

FIGURE 20-41: **A,** Axial computed tomographic (CT) scan through the inferior aspect of the glenoid, demonstrating anterior glenoid deficiency. **B,** Three-dimensional CT reconstruction of the scapula with humeral subtraction.

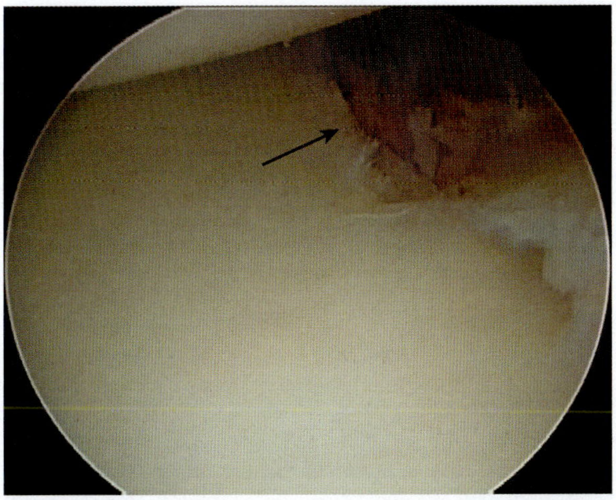

FIGURE 20-42: Arthroscopic view from the anterior portal demonstrating an inverted pear glenoid (arrow), which denotes significant anteroinferior bony deficiency.

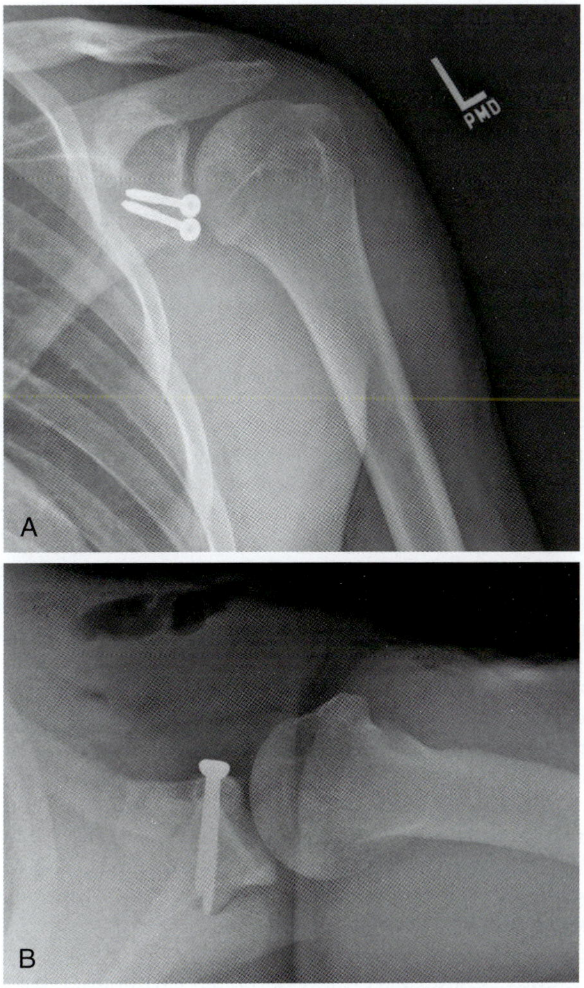

FIGURE 20-43: **A,** Postoperative anteroposterior radiograph after coracoid transfer. **B,** Postoperative axial radiograph after coracoid transfer.

glenoid defect but no visible bone fragment had subluxation symptoms, and another patient experienced redislocation and required revision open surgery.

The most commonly performed bone grafting operation for anterior glenoid bone loss is the open Latarjet procedure. The native coracoid process is osteotomized from its base and transferred with the attached conjoin tendon so that its longitudinal axis is oriented parallel to the face of the glenoid.[321] The fragment is secured with rigid screw fixation (Fig. 20-43A, B). The operation can also be performed arthroscopically; this can be technically challenging, requires specialized equipment, and is associated with a long learning curve.[37,184] Excellent outcomes with very low recurrence rates at long-term follow-up have been reported for the Latarjet procedure. Burkhart and colleagues[53] noted a recurrence rate of 4.9% in 47 modified Latarjet reconstructions; similarly, Schmid and colleagues[296] reported no recurrences in 49 consecutive patients in their series, and the best outcomes were associated with optimal graft placement. Other authors have even suggested the Latarjet as a primary stabilization procedure for contact athletes in the absence of significant anterior glenoid bone loss.[155] Alternatively, high satisfaction and low recurrence rates have been reported with other bone grafting techniques, including autogenous tricortical iliac crest graft and distal tibial allograft.[77,232,268]

Humeral Head Bone Loss

Previously, the presence of a large engaging Hill-Sachs lesion has been a relative contraindication for arthroscopic stabilization.[52] An "engaging" lesion is one that engages the rim of the glenoid when the shoulder is physiologically abducted and externally rotated (Fig. 20-44).[341] When patients with these lesions are treated with arthroscopic Bankart repair alone, recurrence rates can be unacceptably high, especially in the contact athlete.[341] Hill-Sachs lesions may represent 12.5% to 20% or more of the humeral head diameter, although preoperatively

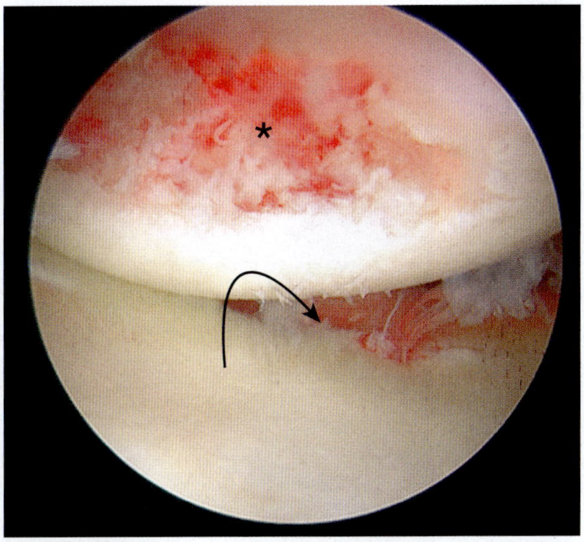

FIGURE 20-44: Arthroscopic image demonstrating a Hill-Sachs lesion (asterisk) engaging over the anterior glenoid rim (arrow) when the arm is brought into abduction and external rotation.

determining the extent of the lesions can be challenging (Fig. 20-45).[304] A CT scan with three-dimensional rendering can help quantify the size and depth of the lesion as well as identify any glenoid deficiencies (Fig. 20-46).

Several procedures to address large humeral head defects have been introduced, including humeral head osteotomy, anterior capsular plication, osteochondral allograft, humeroplasty, and limiting resurfacing arthroplasty.[13,70,180,345,363] Although good clinical results may be achieved, these procedures require an open approach, with its associated morbidity, and may be associated with complications, such as nonunion and glenohumeral osteoarthritis.[61] Wolf and colleagues[359] recently described an arthroscopic technique known as the Hill-Sachs remplissage, which consists of advancing the infraspinatus muscle and posterior capsule into the osseous defects of the Hill-Sachs lesion using suture anchors (Fig. 20-47). This technique was later modified by Koo and colleagues[177] such that the sutures are tied over the tendon rather than the muscle. The infraspinatus tenodesis serves as a checkrein against anterior translation of the humeral head and effectively converts an intra-articular lesion to an extra-articular one.[61] A theoretical disadvantage of the procedure is the loss of external rotation from the nonanatomic advancement of the tendon.

In a recent systematic review, Ahmad and colleagues[61] evaluated outcomes of arthroscopic Hill-Sachs remplissage. Most authors performed the procedure on patients where a Hill-Sachs lesion was identified on preoperative imaging and the humeral head defect engaged on the anterior aspect of the glenoid during dynamic arthroscopic assessment. In almost all the patients there was no "substantial" anterior glenoid bone loss, with most authors frequently citing less than 25% as candidates for the procedure. The overall recurrence rate was reported as 5.4% in 167 shoulders and the change in external rotation was from a mean of only 57.2 degrees preoperatively to a mean of 54.6 degrees postoperatively. Similarly, Boileau

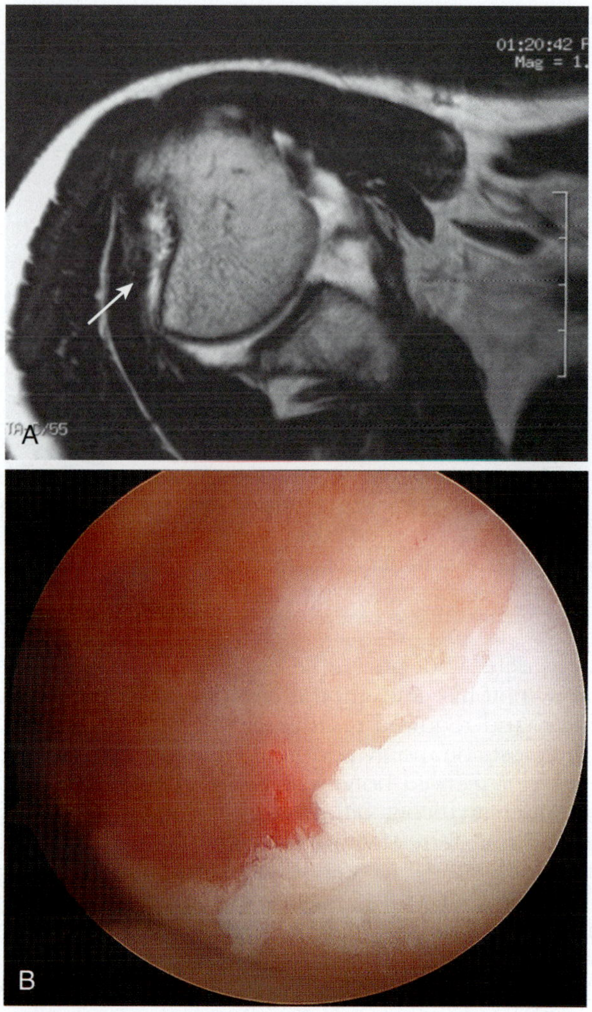

FIGURE 20-45: A significant Hill-Sachs lesion leading to persistent instability. **A,** Magnetic resonance axial image. **B,** Arthroscopic view from the posterior portal.

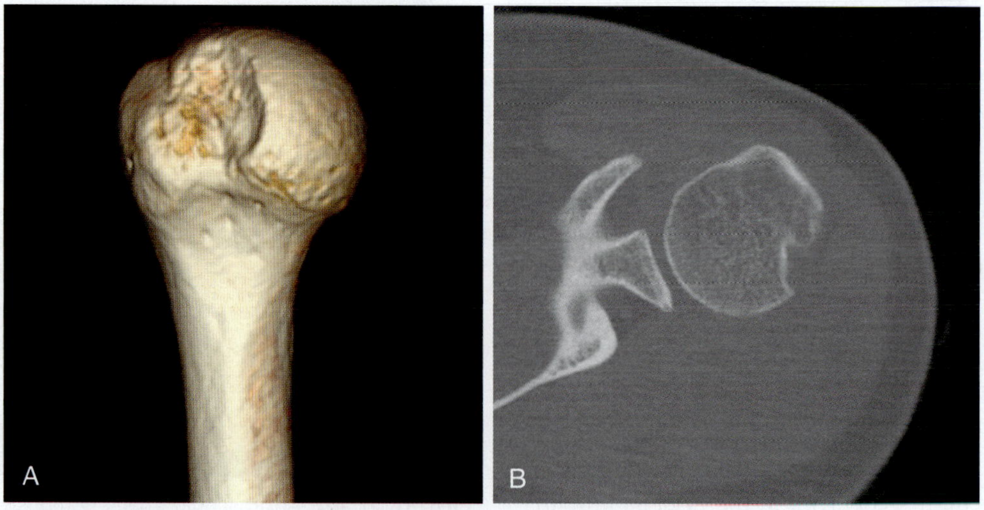

FIGURE 20-46: **A,** Three-dimensional computed tomographic (CT) scan showing a large Hill-Sachs lesion. **B,** Axial CT scan through the superior aspect of the humeral head demonstrating a deep Hill-Sachs defect.

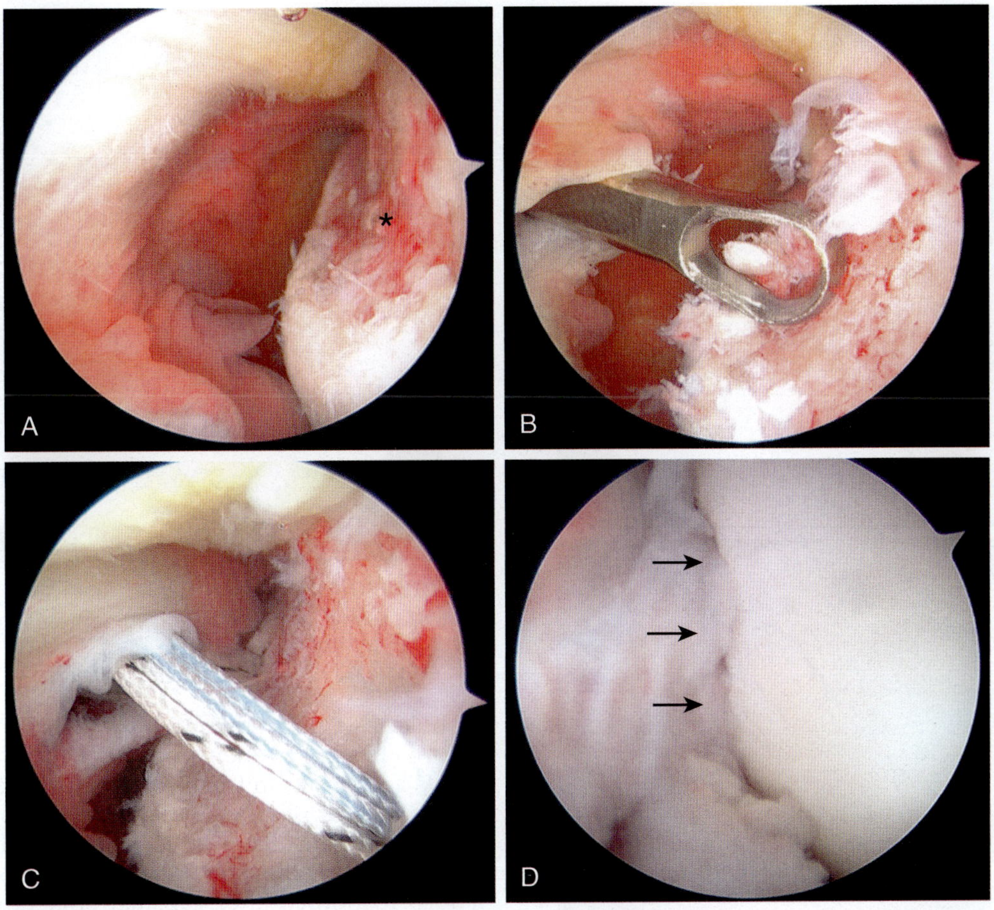

FIGURE 20-47: Arthroscopic Hill-Sachs remplissage technique. **A,** An identified Hill-Sachs defect (asterisk). **B,** Preparation of the humeral defect to create a bleeding surface. **C,** Two suture anchors are introduced into the humeral defect. **D,** Limbs from suture anchors are tied over the infraspinatus tendon and the Hill-Sachs defect is filled with the posterior capsule and infraspinatus tendon.

and colleagues[38] noted an approximate loss of 8 degrees of external rotation in 47 patients; however, 90% were able to return to playing sports, with 68% at their preinjury level of competition. The authors concluded that the loss of rotation was not clinically significant.

Arthroscopic Bankart Repair Surgical Technique

Examination under anesthesia is performed after the induction of either regional or general anesthesia in the supine position. The degree of anterior, posterior, and inferior instability is assessed. Similar to SLAP lesion management, we prefer the lateral decubitus position (see Fig. 20-25) with the table and arm position as previously described.

A standard posterior viewing portal is created 2 cm inferior to the posterolateral edge of the acromion. Diagnostic arthroscopy is performed, and the anterior and superior labrum as well as the undersurface of the rotator cuff is examined. A spinal needle is introduced anteriorly and used to probe the superior labrum as well as the anterior labrum before committing to the location of the anterior superior portal. Proper anterior portal placement is critical, especially when addressing multiple areas of a detached labrum. A cannula is introduced high in the rotator interval adjacent to the biceps tendon, and a probe is used to test the stability of the biceps anchor and labrum attachments to the superior and anterior glenoid.

A second cannula is placed in the rotator interval immediately adjacent to the edge of the subscapularis tendon (Fig. 20-48). This portal provides appropriate access and an angle for anchor placement from the inferior pole of the glenoid to the superior sulcus. The arthroscope is then switched to the anterior portal for better assessment of the posterior labrum, evaluation of the anterior glenoid for bony deficiency, and identification of anterior labral periosteal sleeve avulsion (ALPSA) lesions (Fig. 20-49).

In cases of combined labral pathology (such as posterior labral detachment or posterior instability and multidirectional instability), all posterior work is performed while viewing from the high anterior portal. Posterior anchor placement is performed through an accessory posterior portal placed more laterally and with a higher

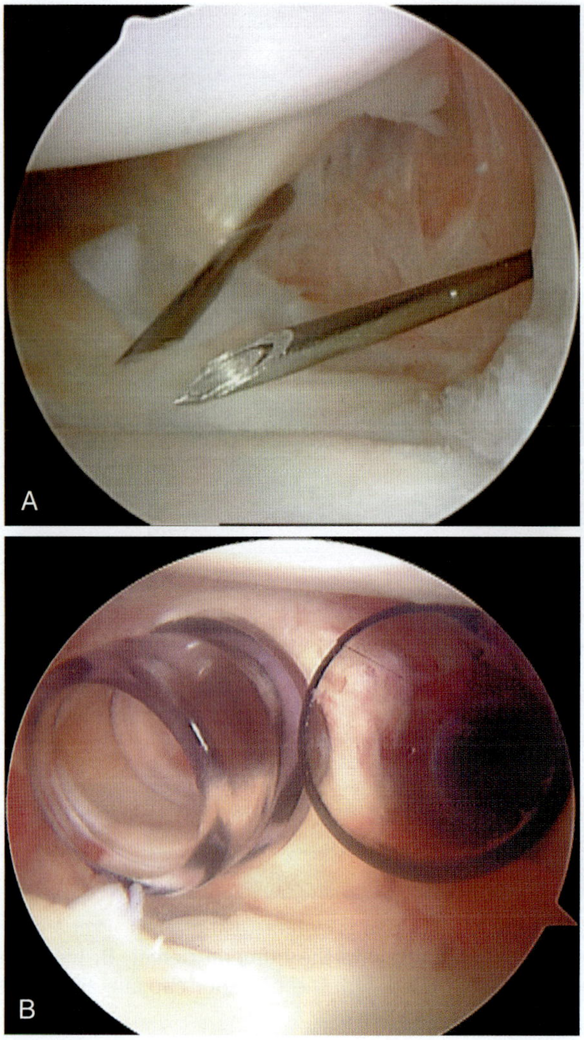

FIGURE 20-48: **A,** Spinal needles introduced adjacent to the biceps tendon and the superior edge of the subscapularis tendon. **B,** Two cannulas placed.

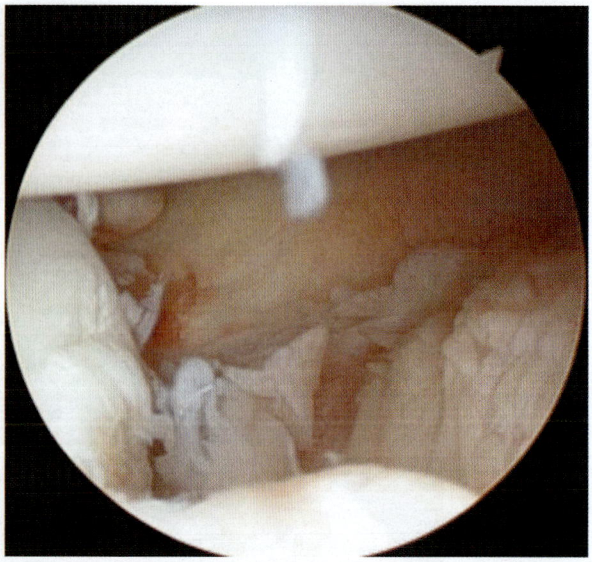

FIGURE 20-49: Anterior labral periosteal sleeve avulsion (ALPSA) lesion visualized from the anterosuperior portal.

angle of inclination to the glenoid than the standard posterior viewing portal. In the event of labral pathology in multiple locations, all labral tissue is mobilized, and all glenoid surfaces are prepared for healing by abrading the bone (Fig. 20-50).

The sequence of repair is then as follows:

1. Place the anterior suture anchors, pass the suture, and tie a knot.
2. Place the posterior suture anchors, pass the suture, and tie a knot.
3. Place the SLAP lesion anchor, pass the suture, and tie a knot.

Knot tying may be completed through the same anterior portal. Anchors should be placed 4 to 5 mm apart until the labrum is secured. The typical anterior instability repair requires a minimum of three anterior anchors.

Alternatively, a percutaneous technique has been developed to further enhance the management of all pathology. This technique allows more precise anchor placement and maneuvering of suture-passing instruments and results in less rotator cuff and capsule morbidity.[175] Capsular plication can also be combined with labral repair, including 1 cm of capsule in each suture anchor stitch; this has been shown to return glenohumeral translations to normal after capsular stretching was induced in a cadaver model.[5] Arthroscopic anteroinferior plication effectively reduces anterior translation and external rotation. Capsulolabral buildup might help limit anterior translation without affecting rotation. Plication results in a shift of the glenohumeral center of rotation posteriorly and inferiorly. Caution should be taken to avoid overtightening the capsule in a throwing athlete.

Posterior Shoulder Instability in Athletes

Posterior shoulder instability is less common than anterior instability, with a reported incidence of 2% to 12% of all cases of shoulder instability.[11] Recurrent posterior subluxation however has become increasingly recognized as a cause of shoulder disability in athletes.[3,230,325,329,357,358] These patients have been shown to have greater glenoid retroversion and more chondral and labral injuries when compared with the nonathlete patients.[44] No single essential lesion occurs in all cases of posterior shoulder instability, and posterior shoulder subluxation is often accompanied by various pathologic lesions and can be associated with multidirectional instability.[130,329] Despite increased awareness of this condition, the diagnosis, classification, and treatment of recurrent posterior instability remain challenging.

Many operative procedures have been described for the treatment of posterior shoulder instability. Overall, outcomes have been less consistent than those of anterior instability, but arthroscopic stabilization has been shown

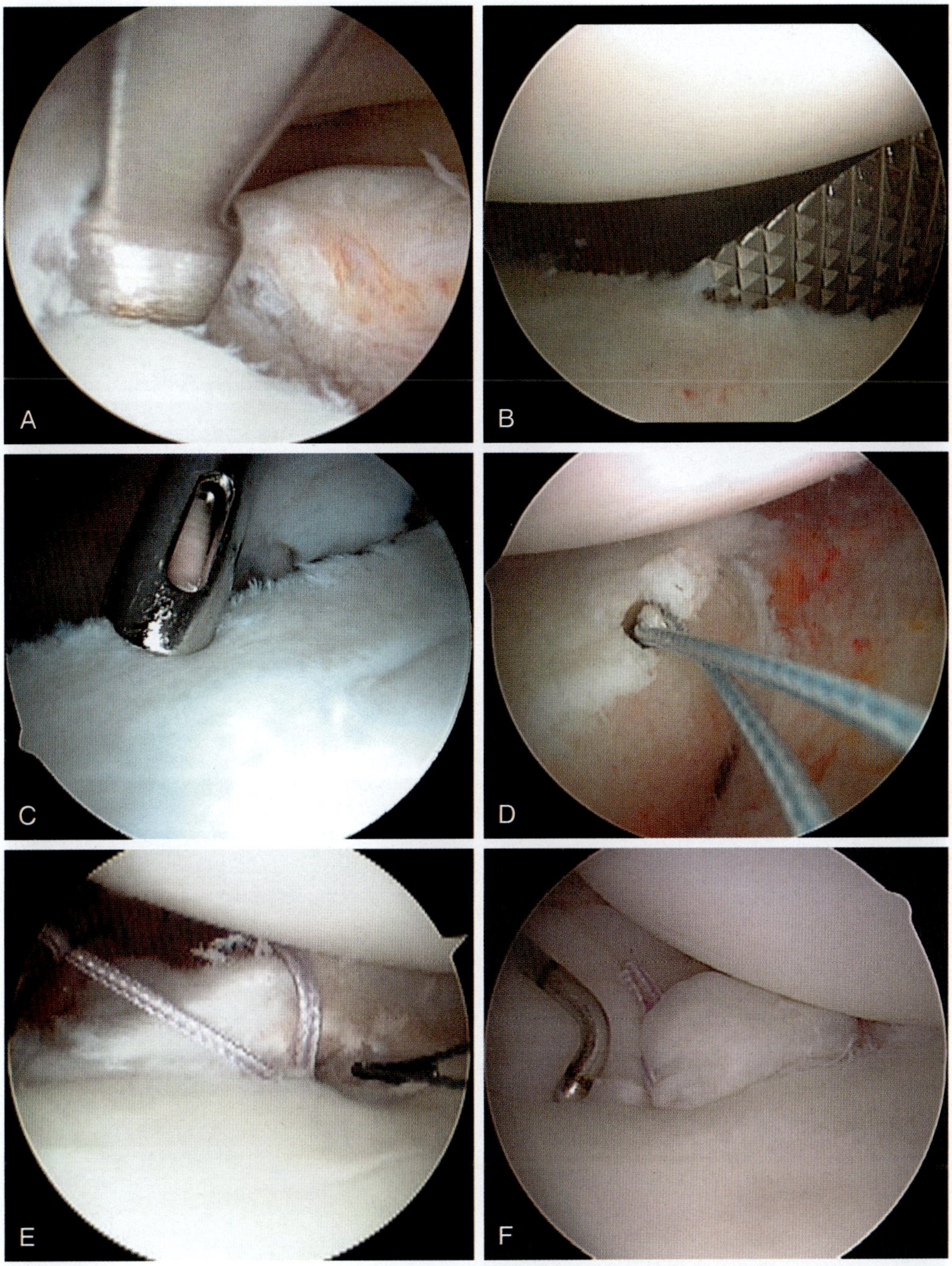

FIGURE 20-50: A, Elevator used to mobilize capsulolabral tissue. **B,** Rasp used to abrade the anterior glenoid. **C,** Anchor drill guide on the face of the glenoid. **D,** Anchor position on the glenoid face as viewed from the superior portal. **E,** Suture passer through the capsulolabral tissue. **F,** Completed repair.

to be an effective and reliable treatment for unidirectional posterior instability.[130] Arthroscopy allows improved identification of the intra-articular pathology associated with posterior instability, such as posterior capsular laxity, posterior capsular tears, or detachment of the posterior capsulolabral complex.[357]

Posterior Labral Repair Surgical Technique

We prefer the lateral decubitus position for improved access to the posterior labrum. The technique is detailed in Figure 20-51. After full visualization of the extent of the labral tear from both portals, the arthroscope is placed in the high anterior portal, and the posterior portal is used for instrumentation. An accessory posterior portal more lateral and distal to the standard posterior portal allows better access to the working area. The torn labrum is mobilized from the glenoid rim with an arthroscopic elevator, and a rasp is used to abrade the capsule. A motorized synovial shaver is used to debride the glenoid rim to a bleeding surface.

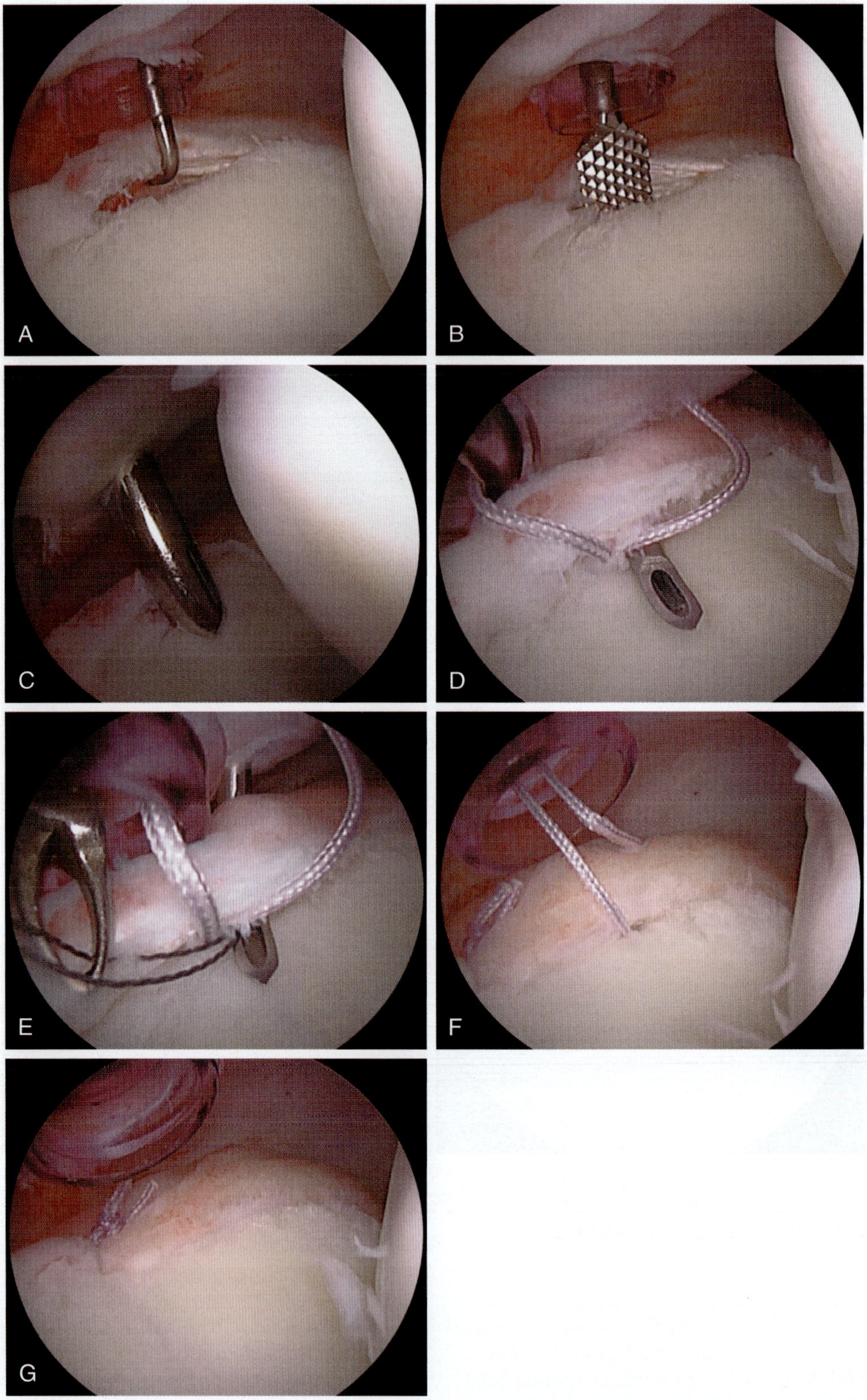

FIGURE 20-51: **A,** Posterior labral tear probed. **B,** Rasp to stimulate healing. **C,** Anchor placed. **D,** Suture passer penetrating the capsulolabral tissue. **E,** Wire used to shuttle the suture. **F,** Sutures retrieved out of the posterior cannula for knot tying. **G,** Completed repair.

Suture anchors are inserted at the articular margin of the glenoid rim. The number of suture anchors used is tailored to the size of the labral tear. Once all of the suture anchors have been inserted, a suture passer is delivered through the capsule and torn labrum and advanced superiorly, reentering the joint at the edge of the glenoid articular cartilage. This technique reintroduces tension into the posterior band of the inferior glenohumeral ligament to help achieve posterior stability. The degree of capsular advancement is tailored to the specific injury pattern. Patients with acute traumatic injuries with minimal capsular stretching undergo minimal capsular advancement, whereas patients with chronic capsular stretching require greater advancement. The anchor suture is shuttled through the capsulolabral complex and then tied. Additional plication sutures are placed if capsular laxity is not sufficiently addressed with the initial capsulolabral plication with suture anchors. Percutaneous anchor insertion and suture passing may also be employed.

Rehabilitation

Immediately following surgery, the shoulder is immobilized in a sling in 30 degrees of external rotation for 4 to 6 weeks, depending on the amount of capsular laxity seen at the time of surgery, with greater laxity requiring longer immobilization. Active elevation of the arm should not be permitted until the fourth week.

Following the immobilization, gentle passive ROM exercises are initiated at 4 to 6 weeks, and gentle, pain-free internal rotation is allowed. Active assisted ROM exercises and isometric internal and external rotation exercises are also initiated. By 2 to 3 months after surgery, ROM is progressed to achieve the full passive and active ROM. At this time, strengthening exercises are also instituted, with emphasis on the rotator cuff and posterior deltoid. Active internal rotation with surgical tubing is also incorporated.

At approximately 6 months postoperatively, a sport-specific rehabilitation protocol is initiated. In general, the athletes must achieve full, painless ROM, full strength, and endurance comparable with that of the contralateral side before they return to full competition. Most patients return to full competition by 6 months after surgery.

Throwing athletes require special consideration, and they should follow a specific protocol in which throwing distance and speed is closely monitored and slowly advanced over 2 to 3 months. Once the throwing athlete is able to perform full-speed throwing for 2 consecutive weeks without symptoms, he or she can be allowed to return to full competition.

Outcomes

Wolf and Eakin[358] examined 14 patients who underwent an arthroscopic capsular plication for unidirectional posterior instability. Preoperatively, all 14 had excessive posteroinferior capsular laxity, with 12 of them having concurrent posterior labral pathologic conditions. At a mean of 33 months of follow-up, 12 patients had achieved good to excellent results and 13 had a resolution of instability. Kim and colleagues[171] prospectively studied 27 athletes with traumatic unidirectional recurrent posterior subluxation who were treated with arthroscopic posterior labral repair and capsular shift. Incomplete labral lesions were converted to complete detachments and repaired back to the glenoid with suture anchors. Postoperatively, all the patients had significantly improved shoulder function and shoulder instrument scores. Shoulder stability was restored in all but one patient, and all but one were able to return to their prior sports activities with few or no limitations.

Bradley and colleagues[44] prospectively studied 100 patients who underwent arthroscopic posterior capsulolabral reconstruction. A subset of 51 shoulders in contact athletes were compared with the entire group of 100 shoulders. At a mean of 27 months postoperatively, the mean American Shoulder and Elbow Surgeons score improved from 50.36 to 85.66 ($P < .001$). There were significant improvements in stability, pain, and function based on standardized subjective scales. However, there were no significant differences for any outcome measure when the contact athletes were compared with the entire cohort. The authors concluded that arthroscopic capsulolabral reconstruction is an effective, reliable treatment for symptomatic unidirectional recurrent posterior glenohumeral instability in an athletic population. Overall, 89% of patients were able to return to their sport, with 67% able to return to their preinjury level.

In a recent systematic review and meta-analysis of posterior instability of the shoulder, DeLong and colleagues[89] reported that patients treated with arthroscopic procedures have superior outcomes compared with those with open procedures with respect to recurrence rate, patient satisfaction, return to sport, and return to the previous level of sport. Despite similar results in outcomes measures with the overall athletic population, overhead athletes were less likely to return to their preinjury level of sports performance compared with contact athletes. The authors also noted that arthroscopic stabilization procedures utilizing suture anchor techniques showed lower rates of recurrence than anchorless repairs in highly active young adults.

NEUROVASCULAR INJURIES

In cases of suspected neurologic injuries in athletes, a thorough and detailed history and physical examination are paramount for differentiating between neurovascular injury and shoulder pathology. In general, reports of acute-onset neck and arm pain or paresthesias should herald the possibility of a neurologic injury.

Burner (Stinger) Syndrome

The burner (or stinger) syndrome occurs in athletes in contact and collision sports. The incidence in collegiate football players has been reported to be from 49% to 65%, and recurrence rates have been reported to be as high as 87%.[190] The injury results from traction or compression of the upper trunk of the brachial plexus at or near Erb's point. Possible predisposing factors include cervical stenosis.[225] Burners affect mostly younger athletes. Older athletes tend to develop cervical root injuries instead, related to degenerative disk changes and spinal stenosis.

History

Typically, the symptoms are incited by lateral neck flexion with contralateral shoulder depression, placing the brachial plexus under traction, although compression mechanisms can also generate burners. The symptoms include an immediate, sharp burning pain that radiates down the arm, with or without paresthesias and weakness. Immediate motor examination may be normal, although strength can deteriorate over hours to days after injury.[126]

Physical Examination

The patient should be examined for upper extremity strength and sensation in all nerve root distributions, particularly those involved in the upper trunk (the shoulder external rotators, deltoid, and biceps). Evaluations should be repeated at the following game and every week for the first 2 weeks to monitor any late onset of weakness or paresthesias. Cervical radiographs should be obtained if the athlete reports neck pain, neck stiffness, or pain with neck motion. Bilateral arm involvement could suggest cervical cord injury. If cervical spine or cord injury is suspected, the athlete should be immobilized on the field on a spine board. Helmet and shoulder pads should be left in place and the athlete should quickly be extracted to a better-equipped facility for further management.

EMG is recommended if weakness persists 3 weeks after injury. It should be noted however that 80% of patients demonstrate abnormal EMG findings up to 53 months after injury.[127] Computed tomography or MRI is indicated if disk or spine injury is suspected or if EMG demonstrates a nerve root lesion.[6]

Treatment

The decision on when the athlete can return to sports is purely clinical. Generally accepted criteria for return to play include the following: full, painless neck and arm ranges of motion; resolution of any paresthesias; negative Spurling's test, brachial plexus stretch, and axial compression tests; and normal manually tested motor strength. Abnormal EMG readings are not an absolute contraindication to return to play.[127] Neck and shoulder muscle strengthening rehabilitation programs as well as built-up collars have been shown to be somewhat effective in reducing recurrence.[127] If the athlete has cervical foraminal stenosis, he or she should be advised to discontinue playing contact sports.[66]

Quadrilateral Space Syndrome

The quadrilateral space is bounded by the teres major and minor muscles, the proximal humerus, and the long head of the triceps. Compression of the axillary nerve and posterior circumflex humeral artery within this space by abnormal fibrous bands or muscle hypertrophy is termed the *quadrilateral space syndrome*.[62] Other causes of compression in this space include extreme abduction and external rotation, such as in the late cocking phase of throwing and space-occupying cysts.[62]

History and Physical Examination

Patients are typically athletes between 20 and 40 years of age. Although the presentation is variable, patients often report nondermatomal pain, including night pain, paresthesias to the lateral arm, weakness in forward elevation and abduction, and easy fatigability in overhead positions. Physical examination should incorporate 1 to 2 minutes of shoulder elevation and abduction, which often reproduces the symptoms. Deltoid atrophy can be apparent.

Diagnosis

Diagnostic studies should include plain radiographs. EMG studies in cases of quadrilateral space syndrome are usually normal.[62] Subclavian arteriography, performed using Seldinger's technique (dye injected first with the arm at the side and then with the humerus in abduction and external rotation), is considered diagnostic when positive (i.e., if the posterior humeral circumflex artery fills when the arm is at the side but not when it is in abduction and external rotation).[62] MR angiography has a significant false-positive rate and has little value in diagnosing this condition.[231]

Treatment

Initial treatment should be conservative. Patients who do not improve after 3 to 6 months should be evaluated for surgery. Open surgical decompression can be performed using a posterior approach. The deltoid is reflected laterally and the teres minor insertion is detached to decompress the space and provide visualization of the fibrous bands, which are released. Cahill and Palmer found that of 18 patients who underwent this procedure, 8 experienced complete relief of symptoms, 8 experienced moderate relief, and 2 experienced no relief.[62]

Suprascapular Nerve Entrapment

The suprascapular nerve is a mixed motor and sensory nerve with consistent contributions from C5 and C6 that branches off the upper trunk of the brachial plexus at Erb's point. It passes under the transverse scapular ligament (the suprascapular artery courses superiorly) and through the suprascapular notch to provide motor function to the supraspinatus. At this point, it also sends sensory branches to the posterosuperior glenohumeral joint, the acromioclavicular joint, and the coracoacromial ligament. The nerve continues around the spine of the scapula toward the spinoglenoid notch, where it dives down to innervate the infraspinatus muscle.

The nerve can be injured by compression or traction. The two most common sites of entrapment are the suprascapular notch and the spinoglenoid notch. Possible causes of compression include a hypertrophied transverse scapular ligament, a narrow suprascapular notch, ganglion or labral cysts, or a lipoma. Traction injuries can occur due to scapular depression and retraction, hyperabduction, and cross-arm adduction with forward flexion. Ferretti and colleagues[106] reported that of 96 asymptomatic volleyball players, 12 had an isolated suprascapular neuropathy with infraspinatus atrophy confirmed by EMG as well as decreased external rotation power. The authors reasoned that the cocked position of serving in volleyball, coupled with forceful external rotation, trapped the nerve in the spinoglenoid notch. Ringel and colleagues[280] have also demonstrated suprascapular neuropathy in pitchers due to repetitive throwing.

Diagnosis

Patients present with vague, deep aching pain over the lateral and posterior shoulder. The pain can radiate down the arm and into the neck. Tenderness may be elicited from the suprascapular notch and the acromioclavicular joint (from the sensory branches). Initially, weakness in arm elevation, abduction, and external rotation may be seen. Atrophy of the supraspinatus and infraspinatus is only seen months after injury.

Standard imaging should be obtained but is usually negative. MRI can show ganglion cysts, muscle atrophy, or associated SLAP tears (Fig. 20-52).[106] Electrodiagnostic tests might show signs of denervation. Successful pain relief with a lidocaine injection into the suprascapular notch is diagnostic.

Treatment

Initial treatment is nonsurgical management with activity modification. Antiinflammatories and a strengthening program typically yield positive results. Martin and colleagues[207] found that 12 of 15 patients achieved good or excellent results with nonoperative treatment. Indications for surgical decompression include persistent pain and limitation after 6 months of nonsurgical care and cases with clear evidence of a compressing structure, such as a ganglion cyst. In all patients with preoperative and postoperative MRI, complete resolution of the cyst was documented.

To decompress the nerve at the suprascapular notch, a superior approach, elevating or splitting the trapezius, with care to avoid injury to the suprascapular artery and vein, followed by resection of the suprascapular ligament, has proven successful.[64] To decompress the nerve at the spinoglenoid notch, a posterior approach, retracting the posterior deltoid and elevating the infraspinatus, may be used. The suprascapular nerve usually lies just posterior to the notch in fibroadipose tissue and must be carefully dissected.

Spinoglenoid cysts are most often associated with a type II SLAP lesion.[68,73,161,277,331,332] Several studies have demonstrated good results with arthroscopic treatment that includes cyst decompression and labral repair.[2,19,71,263] Our preference is therefore to decompress the cyst arthroscopically as part of the labral repair preparation followed by labral repair as previously described in the labral repair section of this chapter.

Youm and colleagues studied the outcome of labral repair with intraoperative cyst decompression.[372] Ten patients with spinoglenoid cysts and associated superior labral tears, demonstrated on preoperative MRI, underwent surgical repair of the labral tear; this was performed without formal cyst aspiration, debridement, or excision. At a mean of 10.2 months after surgical repair, all eight patients who underwent postoperative MRIs showed complete resolution of the cyst, along with labral healing. Four patients with suprascapular neuropathy based on preoperative EMG studies recovered strength and demonstrated normal nerve conduction studies postoperatively. All the patients were able to return to work with no restrictions on activities, and all were satisfied with their outcomes.

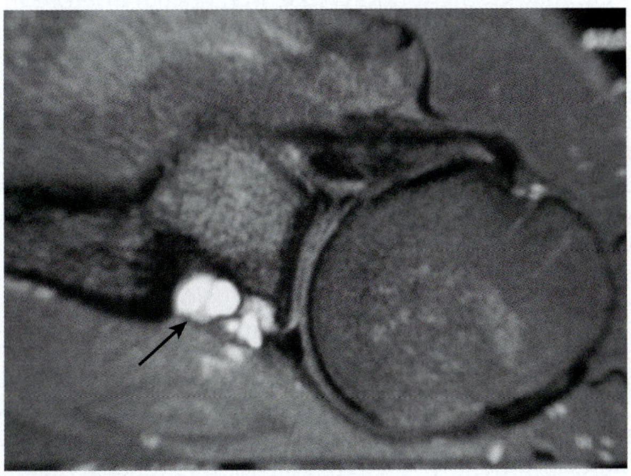

FIGURE 20-52: Axial magnetic resonance images demonstrating a spinoglenoid cyst (*arrow*) and the adjacent posterior superior labral tear.

Thoracic Outlet Syndrome

Thoracic outlet syndrome represents signs and symptoms of compression of neurovascular structures as they exit the thoracic cavity toward the upper extremities. It occurs more commonly in women than men at a ratio of 3.5 : 1.[187] Athletes with thoracic outlet syndrome complain of neck and shoulder pain and tingling or numbness in the upper extremities. Typically, the sensory disturbance is on the ulnar aspect of the hand and forearm. Venous compression can cause unilateral arm swelling.

Physical Examination

During the physical examination, the examiner should look closely for signs of muscle atrophy or weakness, which indicate neuropathy. Several diagnostic tests (the Adson, Wright, and costoclavicular tests) have been devised, with variable diagnostic utility.[187] The hallmark of each test is both pulse diminution during a provocative maneuver and the reproduction of the presenting symptoms.

To perform Adson's test, the radial pulse is checked first with the arm at the side. The patient takes a deep breath, hyperextends the arm, and turns the head toward the involved extremity. The pulse is checked in this position. A diminished pulse is only diagnostic if symptoms are recreated. A positive test indicates compression within the scalene triangle.

Wright's test involves comparing the pulse at rest with the pulse after the patient inhales deeply and abducts and externally rotates the arm. A positive test (a diminished pulse) indicates compression in the subcoracoid region, specifically under the pectoralis minor.

The costoclavicular test is performed by having the patient thrust the shoulders backward and downward to reduce the space between the clavicle and the first rib.

Other helpful diagnostic adjuncts include electromyographic and somatosensory evoked potentials, MR angiograms, and arteriograms.[102,339] Other diagnoses, such as a Pancoast tumor, should be ruled out.

Treatment

Initially, conservative measures, including physical therapy, should be started. Obesity, worker's compensation, and associated distant compression neuropathies have been shown to adversely affect nonoperative outcomes.[244] In refractory cases, surgical options consist of first rib resection, pectoralis minor tenotomy, claviculectomy, or scalene muscle release.[187]

Effort Thrombosis

Spontaneous venous thrombosis of the upper extremity, also known as *Paget-Schroetter syndrome,* occurs without underlying etiologic factors and is associated with repetitive upper extremity activities.[183] It has been described in young, athletic patients in a variety of sports, including swimming, weightlifting, and tennis and may be related to repetitive venous compression.[92] Compression of the subclavian vein has been observed in the cocking position of throwing (abduction with external rotation).

History and Diagnosis

Athletes present with a gradual onset of swelling that occurs over 1 to 7 days, arm ache, mottling of the skin, and tiredness of the arm. Venography confirms the diagnosis. Hypercoagulable states should be ruled out.

Treatment

Nonoperative treatment consisting of bed rest, elevation of the extremity, and anticoagulation therapy has led to high rates of recurrence and disability. In response to the failure of traditional conservative management, Machleder proposed that maintaining the patency of the subclavian vein was the key to long-term symptom relief.[198] To achieve reliable venous patency, he outlined the following protocol: transluminal thrombolytic therapy followed by 3 months of anticoagulation therapy with warfarin, with subsequent transaxillary first rib resection and thoracic outlet decompression. Urschel and Razzuk[335] reported excellent results in 211 patients using a similar regimen. Following this treatment, athletes have returned to their previous level of activity within 1 year of injury.[92]

MUSCLE RUPTURES AFFECTING THE SHOULDER GIRDLE

Rupture of the Pectoralis Major Tendon

Historical Review

Rupture of the PM tendon has been steadily increasing in incidence, particularly over the last decade. This has been attributed to the widespread increase in athletic activities in the general population and to weight training with the recreational use of anabolic steroids.[101] The problem has been reported almost exclusively in male patients, and most PM ruptures occur in individuals aged between 20 and 40 years. Rupture of PM follows extreme muscle tension or direct trauma, or a combination of both. The great majority of cases occur as a result of bench pressing, although other strenuous activities have been reported as causative including rugby, wrestling, snowboarding, skiing, and boxing.[124,179,213,270,295,375] Another common mechanism of injury is when a person attempts to break a fall, resulting in a severe force being applied to a maximally contracted PM muscle.

Wolfe and colleagues[360] provided an explanation, supported by cadaver and clinical studies, for the high rate of injury with bench pressing. Their patients described the rupture as occurring when the bar was at its lowest point with the shoulders extended to 30 degrees, during the eccentric phase of contraction. At this point, the fibers of the lowest portion of the sternal head become disproportionately stretched. Elliot and colleagues[100] showed by electromyographic studies that the PM muscle is maximally activated at the initiation of the lift with the humerus in the extended position. Wolfe and colleagues[360] proposed that the application of a maximal load to inferior fibers that are stretched to an extreme mechanical disadvantage results in rupture of these fibers. Continued loading then increases the tension on the remaining fibers of the sternal head, which fail. This explanation might account for the increased incidence of rupture of the sternal head during weightlifting.

Anatomy

PM arises in a broad sheet as two distinct heads—an upper clavicular head and a lower sternocostal head—that spread to a complex trilaminar insertion along the lateral edge of the intertubercular sulcus. A portion of the sternocostal head spirals on itself to produce the round appearance of the anterior axillary fold, with the result that the lowermost fibers are inserted most proximally on the humerus and in a crescent into the capsule of the shoulder joint. The two laminae of the tendons fuse immediately before insertion on the humerus. In a recent cadaver study both the anterior and posterior layers of the full tendon averaged a mean length of 5.4 cm.[112]

Classification

The traditional classification of PM tendon ruptures was described by Tietjen according to the extent and site of the rupture.[330]

Type 1 injuries consist of a contusion or sprain.
Type 2 injuries represent partial ruptures.
Type 3 injuries are complete ruptures.

Type 3 is further subdivided according to the location of the rupture, including the muscle belly, the musculotendinous junction, or avulsion of the tendon insertion from the humerus. A more comprehensive classification devised by ElMaraghy and Devereaux[101] includes the

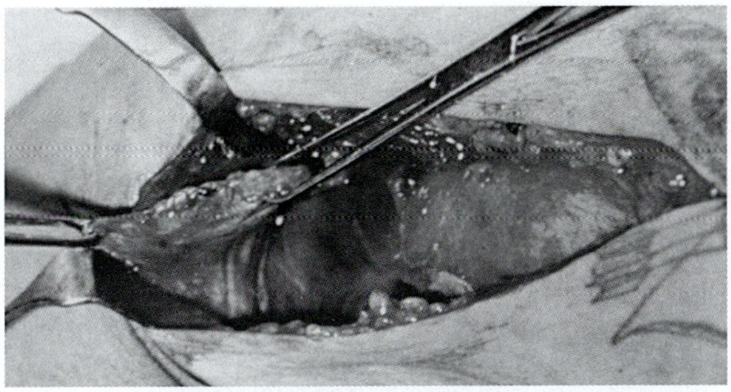

FIGURE 20-53: Intraoperative findings of the pectoralis major tendon avulsed from its humeral origin.

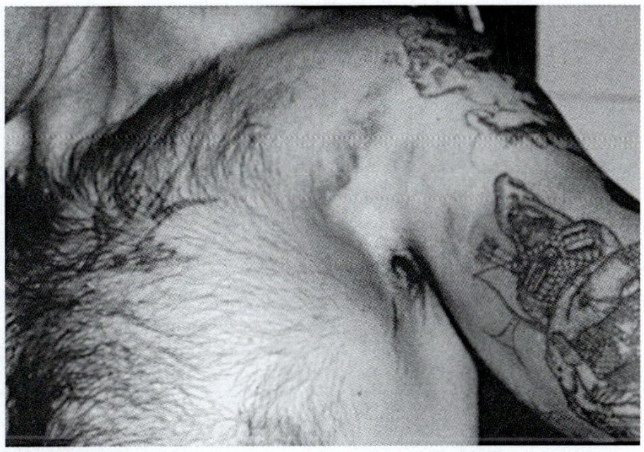

FIGURE 20-54: Rupture of the pectoralis major in a 30-year-old weightlifter. (Courtesy J.J. Brownles, MD.)

chronicity, location, thickness, and width of the tear, each of which potentially affect clinical decision-making and treatment.

Partial tears are more common than complete tears. They usually occur at the musculotendinous junction, whereas complete tears primarily occur at the tendon-bone interface.[213] Most case series report the predominant lesion as an avulsion of the tendon from the humerus (Fig. 20-53). In a series of 78 reported cases, tearing at the musculotendinous junction occurred in 17 cases, tendinous ruptures accounted for three cases, and only two cases involved rupture of the muscle itself.[213]

Clinical Findings

A history of excessive muscle stress, a direct blow, or a crush injury in the shoulder region is often reported. Symptoms include severe, sharp, and often burning pain; a tearing sensation; and possibly an audible "pop" heard by the patient. The injury can be accompanied by significant swelling and ecchymosis. Immediate shoulder dysfunction is apparent.

The physical findings depend on the site of rupture. If the muscle is injured in its proximal portion, the swelling and ecchymosis are usually noted on the anterior part of the chest wall on the involved side. The muscle belly retracts medially toward the axillary fold, resulting in an asymmetric muscle outline and a prominent bulge. Rupture in the distal portion can cause swelling and ecchymosis in both the arm and the chest; the body of the muscle bulges on the chest, and this bulging causes the axillary fold to become thin (Fig. 20-54). The shoulder is tender at the site of rupture, and a visible or palpable defect is usually present, but can be partially obscured acutely as a result of soft tissue swelling.

Resisted adduction and internal rotation of the arm may be weak and accompanied by accentuation of the defect and pain. In chronic cases weakness is the predominant finding, with the palpable defect being confirmatory.

Imaging Evaluation

Radiographs generally fail to reveal any bone abnormality, and the loss of the normal PM shadow is an inconsistent sign of rupture. MRI is the imaging modality of choice for assessment of PM injury and can be very useful in tear characterization and surgical planning.[77A] MRI can also distinguish partial from complete tears and distinguish acute from chronic injuries.[77A] Acute tears demonstrate hemorrhage and edema on MRI (Fig. 20-55), whereas chronic tears demonstrate fibrosis and scarring.[77A] However, a standard shoulder MRI does not contain sufficient sequences extending caudally to identify a PM tear at the tendinous insertion, and dedicated chest sequences extending superiorly from the quadrilateral space and inferiorly to the deltoid tuberosity are required.[186] MRI may be used to monitor interval healing when patients are treated conservatively and to evaluate muscle quality before returning to competitive sports.

Nonoperative Treatment

Nonoperative treatment of PM ruptures is generally reserved for low-demand and elderly patients or those with medical comorbidities that preclude surgical repair. Partial PM ruptures or lesions of the muscle belly often respond to conservative treatment. The early application of cryotherapy for swelling control and a program of shoulder-mobilizing exercises (both passive and active assisted) help restore shoulder function. Passive stretching exercises should begin immediately in the rehabilitation program, followed by active assisted and active exercises during a 6-week period. Resistance exercises and strengthening may begin 2 to 3 months after the injury.[262]

Tears that occur at the musculotendinous junction require special attention. Many surgeons opt to treat these injuries nonoperatively due to technical challenges in obtaining adequate fixation medially within the muscle belly to perform surgical repair; nevertheless, successful direct repair to the tendon stump has been reported.[279]

Surgical Treatment

Various repair techniques for anatomic reattachment of the tendon to its insertion on the humeral cortex have been described in the literature. Preferred fixation methods include transosseous sutures, suture anchors, and cortical button fixation. Sherman and colleagues[307]

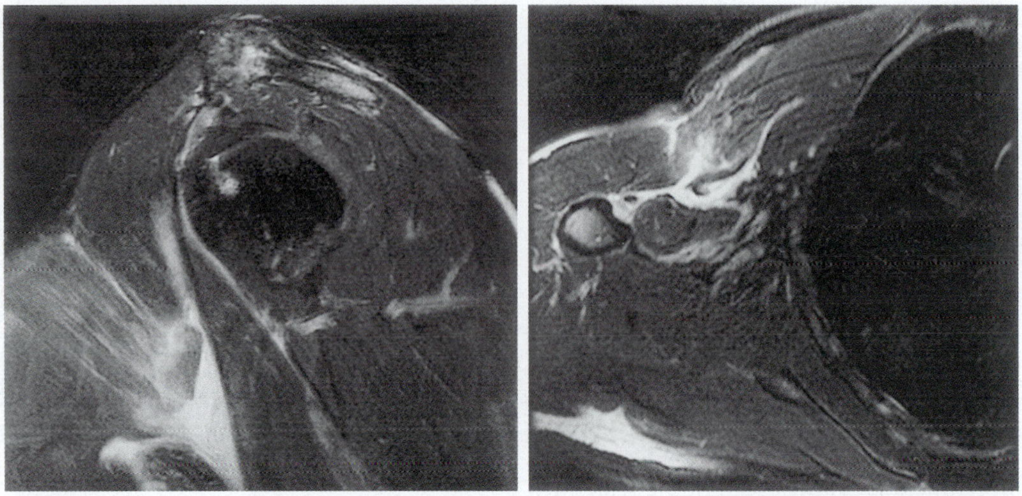

FIGURE 20-55: Sagittal and axial magnetic resonance image demonstrating an avulsion of the pectoralis major tendon from its origin on the humerus.

directly compared these three fixation methods but did not identify any significant differences between them in mechanical loading or failure properties.[307] For situations in which some tendon remains attached to the humerus, Orava and colleagues[248] described an effective method of treatment by end-to-end repair of the tendons, reinforcing the repair with retention sutures into bone.

Tears of the musculotendinous junction can be sutured directly; however, the shredding of tissue structure associated with muscle substance tears offers poor substance for repair, and only imperfect results can be anticipated with this injury. The chronicity of a tear can also impact the surgical technique; reconstruction options, including the use of Achilles tendon allograft,[154] fascia lata allograft,[308] and bone–patellar tendon autograft[258] have been described.

Outcomes

The literature overwhelmingly supports surgical treatment for active individuals with only infrequent reports of high demand patients being successfully managed nonoperatively.[1,185,262,294,295]

Hanna and colleagues[124] examined 22 patients with complete tears of PM by objective strength and subjective functional outcome measures. Injuries sustained in athletic activities were the mechanism in 19 of the 22 cases: 10 patients treated by surgical repair were compared with 12 patients treated nonoperatively. In the group treated surgically the injured arm regained an average of 99% and 97% of the strength of the uninjured arm as assessed by dynamometer testing of peak torque and work, respectively, whereas patients treated nonsurgically regained only 56% of the strength of the uninjured arm. Only one patient who did not undergo repair returned to full function.

Schepsis and colleagues[295] reported on 17 patients with PM injuries; four were treated nonoperatively and 13 with surgery in two groups according to injury type. The authors found an overall satisfaction rating of 96% in the acute injury surgical group, 93% in the chronic injury surgical group, and 51% in the nonoperative group. Isokinetic testing showed adduction strength to be 102% that of the unaffected side in the acute injury surgical group, 94% in the chronic injury surgical group, and 71% in the nonoperative group. The authors concluded that there were no significant differences in outcome between patients treated operatively for acute or chronic injuries but that surgically treated patients fared significantly better than patients treated nonoperatively.

In a meta-analysis of 112 cases of PM rupture, Bak and colleagues[15] found 88% excellent or good results for patients treated surgically versus 27% for patients treated conservatively. They also found that significantly more patients achieved an excellent outcome when surgery was performed within 8 weeks of the injury than when surgery was delayed. They concluded that surgical treatment, preferably within the first 8 weeks after the injury, has a significantly better outcome than conservative treatment or delayed repair.

Good outcomes can still be achieved for chronic tears and so chronicity should not preclude surgical management as a treatment option, even years after the original injury.[60] The precise definition of a chronic tear varies in the literature, but most authors agree that tendon retraction can occur as early as 3 weeks following injury. Additional medial fascial releases may be required for tendon mobilization and a reconstruction rather than a primary repair may be indicated if sufficient mobilization of the tendon is not possible. When attempting to repair a chronic tear, allograft and autograft options should be considered. Autograft techniques include hamstring, fascia lata, and bone–patellar tendon–bone autografts.[60,258] Good reported outcomes have been achieved with allograft reconstruction, which has the advantages of avoiding the morbidity associated with autograft harvest and tailored physical dimensions.[154,308,374]

CONCLUSION

Shoulder injuries in athletes are highly prevalent and potentially debilitating conditions. The treating orthopedic surgeon must pay special attention to the acuity and severity of the symptoms, with particular focus on sport-specific biomechanics. New understanding of the pathophysiology of shoulder injuries in various sports, as well as their management, has improved clinical results. Nonoperative rehabilitation and arthroscopic and open techniques, applied judiciously, can improve shoulder outcomes and return the athlete to the sports arena as quickly and as wholly as possible.

EDITOR COMMENTARY

Edward V. Fehringer

Dr. ElAttrache and colleagues have again done a remarkable job of consolidating and updating the terrific work that has gone into the diagnosis and treatment of shoulder injuries in athletes as well as the acute and chronic conditions that plague these shoulders. Many forms of diagnosis and treatment have evolved since the previous edition of this text. Arthroscopic techniques have continued to be increasingly utilized in the treatment of most shoulder disorders in athletes, except for PM tears and possibly traumatic anterior instability cases in collision athletes and/or those with significant bone loss on the glenoid and/or humeral side(s).

Considerable controversy persists regarding many forms of treatment of the athlete's shoulder. Probably none have been more extensively studied than the throwing shoulder, particularly in baseball pitching. It would seem more comprehensive approaches are in order to identify inefficient joints, muscles, and movement patterns prior to the development of symptoms for which only rest or surgery is the answer. Clearly, due to a number of variables, the overuse or stress conditions that we most often see in our clinics would be markedly reduced if we could identify their root causes. A focus on the "prehab" aspect of throwing seems essential for us to address throwing injuries in athletes before they happen.

We often have inadequate acumen from which to draw to address shoulder and arm pain in throwers. Often without practical methods or reliable resources that can be used before injuries require surgery, we generally recommend rest and/or volume reduction. Yet, if the causes of symptoms are inefficient movement patterns, the symptoms will return if the inefficiencies are not eliminated once throwing has resumed. Models such as the Texas Baseball Ranch in Montgomery, Texas, and the Florida Baseball Ranch in Plant City, Florida, use several disciplines and modalities to identify potential movement pattern causes of pain. Their groups provide practical methods to retrain the body to throw in a more "connected" fashion in an effort to throw more safely and durably. Pain, very simply, is used as information. That information helps them design "prehab" programs designed specifically for individuals, as no two people are alike. Ron and Jill Wolforth of the Texas Baseball Ranch and Randy Sullivan of the Florida Baseball Ranch use this "hyperpersonalization" approach aimed at harnessing the athletic ability present in each individual and avoiding patterns that cause pain. Perhaps approaches such as theirs will help us more commonly identify injuries before they require sutures and grafts.

SENIOR EDITOR COMMENTARY

Frederick Matsen III

The athlete with a shoulder problem presents a particularly difficult management challenge. The surgeon is faced with a highly motivated patient who was once able to perform almost superhuman feats with his or her arm, but whose sport has led to failure of the shoulder to perform at the desired level. The patient is desperate to regain his or her prowess, and the surgeon is desperate to help. Modern diagnostic tools, such as MRI and arthroscopy, reveal a wide range of "findings," but it is nontrivial to relate these findings, such as partial-thickness articular-sided cuff tears or labral fraying, to the patient's functional difficulties. It is even more challenging to decide if placing sutures in a damaged labrum or rotator cuff will make it more resistant to failure than before it was injured. Sometimes these attempts at repair create new problems, such as refractory shoulder stiffness. These issues are particularly problematic for the athlete who is getting older, yet longs for a youthful body. For these reasons, the prospect of operating on the shoulder of an athlete requires judgment based on personal experience, with the outcomes of such surgeries coupled with humility regarding the patient's chances of regaining the desired level of function.

A particularly confusing element of the athlete's shoulder is the use of the term "impingement." The ICD-9-CM Diagnosis Code 726.10 used to refer to "impingement syndrome" is described as "Disorders of bursae and tendons in shoulder region, unspecified." With the current knowledge of the pathogenesis of "disorders of bursae and tendons in the shoulder region" and with diagnostic tools such as MRI, we can reliably differentiate tendinitis, partial-thickness cuff tears, and full-thickness cuff tears. We recognize that pain and limitation of internal rotation of the elevated arm is likely to be due to posterior capsular tightness rather than to acromial pathology. We can now safely retire the term, "impingement syndrome" and avoid treating individuals with a "positive Hawkins impingement test" by performing an acromioplasty.

The authors of this chapter have brought a mature view of the athlete's shoulder. Their combined wealth of experience has emphasized the importance of solid mechanics, good coaching, and overall conditioning in the prevention and treatment of shoulder disorders. Finally, they have provided a realistic and appropriately humble assessment of our ability to "fix" the shoulder of an athlete who has lost the speed of his fast ball or who can no longer place her serve where she wants it or who is no longer able to execute a half-million swimming strokes per year.

CHAPTER 21

Occupational Shoulder Disorders

Manny Halpern, Brent Mollon, Joseph D. Zuckerman

Musculoskeletal disorders can be characterized as "work-related diseases." The World Health Organization (WHO) has described these diseases as multifactorial, with work contributing significantly, although not exclusively, to their causation.[146] The term "disorder" is more appropriate when some of the outcomes of these conditions are of uncertain pathogenesis and may consist of symptoms without obvious clinical signs.[138] The term "work-related musculoskeletal disorders" (WMSDs) has come to replace "repetitive strain injuries" or "cumulative trauma disorders." The National Safety Council Standards Committee, accredited by the American National Standards Institute, has combined the etiologic notions implied in these terms to define a musculoskeletal disorder (MSD) as a disturbance in the regular or normal function of muscle, tendon, tendon sheath, nerve, bursa, blood vessel, bone, joint, or ligament that results in altered structure or impaired motor or sensory function. Accordingly, WMSDs are MSDs that may be caused, aggravated, or precipitated by intense, repeated, or sustained work activities with insufficient recovery. WMSDs generally develop over a period of weeks, months, or years.[103] It follows that MSDs can be partially caused by adverse work conditions, can be exacerbated by workplace exposure, and can impair work capacity. The National Research Council adopted a similar definition but emphasized that none of the common MSDs are uniquely caused by work exposure and that physical and social aspects of life outside work need to be considered.[102] In this respect MSDs would be more accurately defined as activity-related conditions rather than work-related ones. Nevertheless, this chapter will focus on the impact of occupational factors.

MSDs of the upper extremities are diffuse neuromuscular illnesses with significant proximal upper body findings that affect distal function.[108] The boundaries of the shoulder region are not clearly defined because the neck, shoulder, and upper part of the arm operate as a functional unit. A further complication is that most of the musculoskeletal problems of this region are nonspecific and without well-defined diagnoses. Apart from variable location, the current definitions of MSDs lack criteria for the intensity, frequency, and duration of the symptoms that would be indicative of a "case." Case status is currently based on symptoms that have occurred within a specific time frame (such as 1 week), at a specific frequency (such as three episodes in the past year), for a given duration (such as a single episode lasting more than 5 days), or for a combination of frequency and severity.[14]

In this chapter occupational shoulder disorders (OSDs) are defined as work- or activity-related MSDs of the shoulder region. Diagnoses include trapezius and parascapular myalgia, rotator cuff and bicipital tendinitis, impingement syndrome, and subacromial/subdeltoid bursitis. Tension neck and cervical syndrome may be considered as being alternative terms for trapezius myalgia. This chapter will cover primarily the myalgias, as the other conditions have been covered elsewhere in this textbook.

The chapter excludes several other clinical diagnoses. Primary frozen shoulder is idiopathic, and secondary frozen shoulder is usually due to the progression of one of the aforementioned conditions or is a consequence of systemic disease. Frozen shoulder therefore does not conform to the definition of an MSD. Thoracic outlet syndrome (TOS) has been defined as an essentially vascular phenomenon that can be objectively documented. Neurogenic TOS however is a controversial diagnosis that may often rely on physical findings when laboratory tests are often negative. Pascarelli and Hsu[108] encountered neurogenic TOS in 70% of shoulder and upper extremity patients, mostly computer operators and musicians, and postulated that the condition is related to postural derangement. Although thoracic outlet decompression has been advocated in the past to treat a presumed compressive etiology, recent literature has suggested that workers with a diagnosis of TOS who underwent surgery were more likely to be disabled at 1 year and were 21% more likely to describe new neurologic findings when compared with workers that did not undergo surgery.[41] Some state workers' compensation boards now require objective evidence of brachial plexus involvement prior to authorizing decompression for TOS; this has resulted in denial of the vast majority of procedures proposed in recent years.[42,137] We cannot comment therefore on the etiologic relationship of TOS to work-related disability, and we do not consider this condition to be an OSD at this time.

The chapter reviews the epidemiology, etiology, and suggested treatment of OSDs. It also explores the relationship of acromioclavicular and glenohumeral arthritis to occupational factors and provides general information on the primary and secondary prevention of MSDs in occupational settings. The workers' compensation system has been implicated as a contributing factor in the reporting of MSDs. Therefore the influence of workers' compensation on the outcome of treatment is examined. Finally, the chapter reviews the current disability compensation systems.

OCCUPATIONAL SHOULDER DISORDERS

This chapter uses the descriptive term *occupational shoulder disorder* (OSD) to denote WMSDs of the shoulder.[8] The alternative term *occupational cervicobrachial disorders* appeared mainly in the Japanese, Australian, and Scandinavian literature in the 1970s and 1980s but has not been adopted in the United States. Another term *work-related upper extremity musculoskeletal disorders* has also been used, but it includes the elbow, forearm, wrist, and hand.[91] Similarly, the Cochran Collaboration review coined the term *complaints of the arms, neck, and shoulders* (CANS),[9] defined as "musculoskeletal complaints of arm, neck and/or shoulder not caused by acute trauma or by any systemic disease."[134] The factor "Work-relatedness" is not mentioned in the CANS model. Ergonomic workloads, such as repetitive and forceful motion, work organizational factors, and psychosocial work factors have definitely been implicated as causes of CANS but these risk factors are activity-related rather than work-related. A well-known clinical problem concerning musculoskeletal disorders of the shoulder, such as tendonitis and bursitis, is that they are difficult to differentiate but can be identified as a group. Consensus was therefore reached to use the term *subacromial impingement syndrome* in CANS for a disorder that includes the rotator cuff syndrome; tendonitis of the infraspinatus, supraspinatus and subscapularis muscles; and bursitis in the shoulder area. Specific complaints included under CANS are cervical disk hernia, frozen shoulder, and subacromial impingement syndrome (tendinitis and bursitis of the shoulder and rotator cuff syndrome).[68]

The term OSD refers to a symptom complex that is characterized by vague pain about the shoulder girdle, including the paracervical, parascapular, and glenohumeral musculature.[8,44,55,89,136] It may also be associated with pain that radiates into the region of the upper part of the arm.[7] OSDs are thought to be the result of cumulative trauma associated with the performance of certain activities and tasks.[13,139,141]

Epidemiology

The variable definitions of the disorders make it difficult to estimate the burden of OSDs in the general population. The National Health Interview Survey for 1995 showed a 1.74% prevalence of impairment from upper extremity or shoulder MSDs. However, estimates of incidence in the *general* population, as opposed to the *working* population, are unreliable because more than 80% of the adult population in the United States is in the workforce.[102]

The annual survey of occupational injuries and illnesses conducted by the Bureau of Labor Statistics (BLS) is the most frequently referenced source of information on WMSDs in the United States. The U.S. Department of Labor defines an MSD as an injury or disorder of the muscles, nerves, tendons, joints, cartilage, or spinal discs. MSDs do not include disorders caused by slips, trips, falls, motor vehicle accidents, or similar accidents. In 2013 there were 307,640 cases of MSDs, accounting for 33% of the injuries and illnesses that involved days away from work—similar to previous years. Shoulder injuries amounted to 86,690 or 7.5% of all nonfatal injuries and 23% of all WMSD. The incidence of shoulder injuries was 8.2 per 10,000 full-time employees, with the highest incidence (12.9 per 10,000) in local government. The median time away from work due to an occupational shoulder injury was 24 days; this was longer than the median time for all MSDs combined. Sprains and strains accounted for 63% of the shoulder injuries, followed by soreness (22%). The incidence rate for males was higher than that for females (9.1 vs. 7.0 per 10,000 full-time workers), with the highest rate (10.4 per 10,000) found among those aged 45 to 54 years.[24,131]

Courtney and Webster[31] cross-tabulated the BLS data and found that the most frequent shoulder injuries were sprains, strains, and tears caused by overexertion; these ranked second to overexertion back injuries. In half the cases these injuries resulted in 6 days' absence from work. The most severe shoulder injuries however were those with "general symptoms" resulting from bodily reaction and overexertion, with a median of 128 days away from work.

The Safety & Health Assessment & Research for Prevention program of the Washington State Department of Labor and Industries used Washington State Fund-accepted claims data to estimate the burden of workers' compensation claims for rotator cuff syndrome [International Classification of Diseases (ICD-9-CM) codes 726.1, 726.11, and 840.4; Current Procedural Terminology codes 23410, 23412, 23415, and 23420] and shoulder WMSDs.[117] Men accounted for about two thirds of the claims, and the median age of the claimants was in the mid-30s. Of all WMSDs of the upper extremity, rotator cuff syndrome incurred the highest median cost per compensable claim: the cost increased from $3,570 in 1987 to $9,410 in 1992 and then decreased to $6,462 in 1995. The median cost of shoulder WMSDs in that period was $350. For both rotator cuff syndrome and shoulder WMSDs, the mean burden was much higher than the median because of skewed distributions; mean costs were $15,790 per case of rotator cuff syndrome and $7,980 per shoulder WMSD. The mean time lost per claim was 263 days (median, 97) for rotator cuff syndrome and 213 (median, 41) for shoulder WMSDs. The data for Washington State are likely to be representative of other states, as the data for WMSDs of the upper extremity collected by Liberty Mutual across the United States (covering 10% of the private workers' compensation market) were similarly skewed.[59]

Most of what is known about the etiology of MSDs comes from epidemiologic studies.[102] However, the published prevalence and incidence data should be viewed critically. As discussed earlier, there is a lack of agreement on case definitions, which has resulted in epidemiologic studies reporting widely different estimates for the burden associated with these disorders. In the literature reporting on neck and shoulder WMSDs, results from contrasting definitions have produced differences in prevalence (55% vs. 20% to take the most extreme), overall disability (14.6% vs. 23.2%), difficulty at work (8% vs. 15.5%), and the proportion of patients reporting that pain interfered with work (27.3% vs. 16.2%).[108] Studies using different case definitions therefore lack comparability.[108] Furthermore, this literature demonstrates that MSDs are not unique to any specific occupational group, with reported occupations ranging from meat processors to apparel workers or assemblers in the manufacturing industries to office-based data entry operators. Etiologically therefore MSDs may be activity-related rather than work-related, and further discussion will focus on the roles of type, intensity, and duration of activity as they relate to OSD.

The common trait of the occupational groups for which high OSD rates are reported is intense exposure to specific activities or work attributes. The attributes associated with an increased probability of MSDs are considered to be risk factors. It is plausible that individuals who engage in light static occupations would be more likely to suffer from trapezius myalgia, whereas those involved in heavy labor would be more susceptible to rotator cuff disease. However, this hypothesis still needs to be fully verified. Nonetheless, attempts have been made to improve understanding of the relationships between activity and OSD. In 1997 the National Institute of Occupational Safety and Health (NIOSH) studied the epidemiologic evidence for the work-relatedness of neck, shoulder, and upper extremity disorders.[17] The focus of the review was to assess the evidence for relationships between MSDs and workplace exposure to the following factors: (1) repetitive exertion, (2) awkward posture, (3) forceful exertion, and (4) hand-arm vibration. The review included studies relevant to shoulder disorders defined by a combination of symptoms and physical examination findings or by symptoms alone, but not specifically defined as tendinitis. NIOSH also included studies for which the health outcome combined neck and shoulder disorders (tension neck, cervical syndrome, TOS, frozen shoulder, tendinitis, and acromioclavicular syndrome), but in which the exposure was likely to have been specific to the shoulder. Diagnoses of shoulder disorders were based on symptoms determined by interview and physical examination. Shoulder tendinitis included supraspinatus, infraspinatus, and bicipital tendinitis.

The review used five criteria for assessing the evidence: strength of association, temporal relationship, consistency of association, coherence of evidence, and the exposure-response relationship.[17] The included studies generally compared workers in jobs that involved higher levels of exposure with workers who had lower levels of exposure, with the degree of exposure determined by observation or measurement of job characteristics. The resulting epidemiologic evidence for the risk factors of upper extremity MSDs is summarized in Table 21-1. In the following we focus on risk factors that could be associated with OSDs.

The review found evidence of a positive association between highly repetitive work (factor 1 in the above list) and OSDs. Of the seven studies that met at least one of the specified criteria, five reported significant associations (with odds ratios [OR] ranging from 1.6 to 5.0). However, the evidence has important limitations. Only three studies specifically addressed the health outcome

TABLE 21-1 Evidence for Causal Relationship Between Physical Work Factors and Musculoskeletal Disorders (MSDs) of the Upper Extremities

		Risk Factors				
MSD Location or Diagnosis	**No. of Studies**	**Force**	**Static or Extreme Postures**	**Repetition**	**Vibration (Segmental)**	**Combination**
Neck and neck/shoulder	>40	++	+++	++	+/0	–
Shoulder	>20	+/0	++	++	+/0	–
Elbow	>20	++	+/0	+/0	–	+++
Carpal tunnel	>30	++	+/0	++	++	+++
Hand/wrist tendinitis	8	++	++	++	–	+++
Hand-arm vibration	20	–	–	–	+++	–

+++, strong evidence; ++, evidence; +0, insufficient evidence; –, evidence of no effect.
Modified from Bernard BP, ed. Musculoskeletal Disorders and Workplace Factors: A Critical Review of Epidemiologic Evidence for Work-Related Musculoskeletal Disorders of the Neck, Upper Extremity and Low Back. *Washington, DC: DHHS (NIOSH), Publication No. 97-141; 1997.*

of shoulder tendinitis, and these studies involved exposure to repetitive activities combined with awkward shoulder postures or static shoulder loads. The other six studies with significant positive associations dealt primarily with symptoms.

The NIOSH review also found evidence of a relationship between OSDs and repeated or sustained shoulder postures with greater than 60 degrees of flexion or abduction (factor 2). Of 13 studies examined, seven reported significant risk estimates (OR, 2.3 to 10.6). There was evidence for both shoulder tendinitis and nonspecific shoulder pain. The evidence for risk involved in maintaining specific shoulder postures was strongest in those with combined exposure to several physical risk factors, such as holding a tool while working overhead. The association was positive and consistent in the six studies that used diagnosed cases of shoulder tendinitis or a constellation of symptoms and physical findings compatible with tendinitis as the health outcome. Only one of the 13 studies failed to find a positive association between exposure and symptoms or a specific shoulder disorder. This result was consistent with evidence in the biomechanical, physiologic, and psychosocial literature.

The NIOSH 1997 report found *insufficient evidence* for a positive association between shoulder MSDs and either force (factor 3) or exposure to segmental vibration (factor 4).

When assessing combinations of the aforementioned factors, the NIOSH review found the strongest associations with WMSDs of the lower part of the back. For the upper extremities, NIOSH needed to combine risk factors (such as force exertion and exposure to hand-arm vibration while operating powered hand tools) to estimate some risk indicators for pathology. Few independent studies at that time had attempted to investigate combined effects on OSDs. The combined effect of forceful movement and vibrating machinery was later empirically demonstrated by Armstrong and colleagues,[11] but a true appreciation of the effect of multiple factors remains poorly investigated.

An additional confounding variable on the risk of a given job-related activity may be the environment in which the activity is performed. Hildebrandt and colleagues[64] reviewed 27 studies that related climatic (i.e., damp, wind, or cold) or seasonal (i.e., summer, winter) factors to MSDs, although none of these studies specifically addressed the subject. Additionally, they distributed a questionnaire to 2,030 workers in 24 different occupations and found that a third of the workers-related symptoms at the lower back and neck-shoulder region could be attributed to climatic conditions, perceiving that these conditions either caused or aggravated their symptoms. Sick leave as a result of neck-shoulder symptoms was associated with climatic factors, particularly draughts and wind. The authors concluded that researchers, workers, and patients consider such a relationship plausible; however, the epidemiologic evidence is still weak.

OSDs are multifactorial in origin and may be associated with both occupational and nonoccupational factors. The relative contributions of these covariates may be specific to particular disorders. For example, the confounders for nonspecific shoulder pain may differ from those for shoulder tendinitis. Two of the most important confounders or effect modifiers for shoulder tendinitis appear to be age and sport activities. Subjects who have been extremely active in sports seem to have an increased risk for shoulder tendinitis and acromioclavicular osteoarthrosis, with those who have been extremely active in sports and also report high exposure to load lifting during work at even greater risk.[120] In other words, sports activities add to the workload on the shoulder and increase the risk for OSDs. Most of the shoulder studies considered the effects of age in their analysis. However, the NIOSH review concluded that it is unlikely that the majority of the positive associations between physical exposure and OSDs are due to the effects of non-work-related confounders, of which age represents the most significant confounder.[17]

Etiology

The etiology of OSDs, in particular trapezius myalgia, is uncertain. Two theories have been proposed: the *organic* or *physiologic theory* and the *psychosocial theory*.[89]

The *organic* or *physiologic theory* is based on the premise that shoulder pain is secondary to statically sustained contraction of the trapezius. Sustained contractions result in increased intramuscular pressure and decreased blood flow. Ischemic conditions occur when intramuscular pressure exceeds the capillary closing pressure at about 30 mm Hg. The increased metabolic demands of the working muscle and the relative ischemia caused by increased intramuscular pressure may contribute to derangements in the balance of intracellular pH/lactic acid, calcium, and potassium.

In a study of 20 assembly line workers with neck and shoulder pain, Bjelle and colleagues found significantly high levels of muscle enzymes, including creatinine phosphokinase and aldolase, in eight workers without any underlying pathology.[18,19] The elevated muscle enzyme levels were found to diminish after 2 to 8 weeks of sick leave. In addition, elevated serum creatinine kinase levels have been observed in welders, cash register operators, and assembly line workers[52] but not in control groups consisting of controllers and forklift drivers. The sustained load necessary for light, static work has been theorized to cause severe adenosine triphosphate depletion, increased permeability, and the resultant release of muscle enzymes.[54]

The level of activity at which a static, isometric contraction of shoulder muscles causes injury is unknown.[132] Several researchers have attempted to identify an endurance limit, defined as the highest force that can be maintain for an "unlimited" period. Jonsson and colleagues suggested that the static load level should always be below 5% of the maximal voluntary contraction (MVC).[76-78] In support of this suggestion Sjogaard and colleagues have shown that muscle fatigue occurs at 5% of MVC after 1 hour of sustained contraction.[118] This endurance was subsequently confirmed by Frey Law and Avin specifically for the shoulder muscles; these authors also provided data to suggest that shoulder muscles were more fatigable than the trunk muscles, which could endure this exertion level for approximately 5 hours.[43] Furthermore, multiple electromyography (EMG) studies have suggested that myalgia patients have abnormally elevated muscle tension. Findings among these patients include (1) higher muscle tension in symptomatic patients,[38,116] (2) higher muscle tension during sleep,[97] (3) higher muscle tension at the painful site,[38] (4) pain even when static muscle contraction is as low as 2% to 5% of MVC,[29] (5) faster fatigue on the painful side,[51] and (6) shorter muscle endurance.[75] EMG findings that showed decrements in the generation of muscle force during repetitive use have provided evidence of either transient motor unit fatigue or permanent skeletal fiber damage.

One theory for decreased fatigue resistance and force generation in myalgia patients is the "Cinderella hypothesis."[102] This hypothesis suggests that muscle damage may be mediated by mechanisms related to muscle recruitment. According to this theory, relatively small, low-threshold, type I motor units are persistently activated and loaded. These are the first motor units recruited for low-force, repetitive endurance work. They remain in action throughout low-level contractions. Because they carry a disproportionate burden, they are referred to as "Cinderella" fibers. Sustained contraction and activation of these motor units causes pain and fatigue and may eventually lead to permanent injury. Muscle fiber damage may ultimately result in interstitial myofibrositis with a persistent reduction in blood flow.[82] Larsson and colleagues performed bilateral open biopsies of the trapezius muscle in 17 patients with chronic myalgia related to static loads during repetitive assembly work and concluded that there was an association between clinical myalgia and the presence of pathologic muscle fibers on histology.[39,83,84] Additional muscle biopsy studies have demonstrated degenerated mitochondria and increased glycogen deposits.[20] Fiber structural damage is also accompanied by products of cell inflammation and necrosis, edema, and leakage of intrafiber proteins and enzymes.[102]

With dropout of some of the muscle fibers, the overall resistance of the motor unit to fatigue is reduced. Clinically, localized fatigue, muscle strain, and pain can occur with very low level contractions, such as those needed to hold the arms in an elevated posture. The trapezius muscle has been found to be affected by jobs that require static muscle overload.[29,47,50,56,70,77,78,142,143] For example, a high prevalence of OSDs has been reported among dental care workers; some were 5.4 times more likely to experience symptoms than a control group of pharmacists.[90] This increased risk is considered to be secondary to maintaining an unsupported awkward working posture with cervical flexion of 45 to 90 degrees and shoulder flexion and abduction of more than 30 degrees for extended periods (Fig. 21-1). Excessive scapular elevation as a result of mental stress or workstation design may also contribute to the increased trapezius load.[53,106]

In contrast to the *organic/physiologic* theory, the *psychosocial theory*[15,16,66,67,127,140] maintains that emotional stress is an etiologic factor in the development of OSDs. The proponents of this theory contend that OSDs occur in jobs that do not involve excessive muscle strain and consequently are not related to overuse but are more a result of psychosocial factors.[87,88,129] In a study of 607 metal industry workers, depression and distress symptoms were found to be predictors of low back pain, neck-shoulder pain, and other musculoskeletal complaints.[126] Workers may fear that if they ignore their symptoms, the symptoms will progress and become permanently disabling. The workers' compensation system can contribute to this problem by awarding benefits based on the recognition that cumulative trauma can cause significant disability. In a study of 201 patients with chronic pain, Tait and colleagues found that patients with litigation claims reported pain of significantly longer duration and had significantly greater disability than nonlitigating patients.[126] Bongers and colleagues found that monotonous work, a high-perceived workload, and time pressures were causally related to musculoskeletal symptoms.[21]

In an attempt to address the complex, multifactorial nature of OSDs, Armstrong and colleagues proposed a model that incorporates both the organic and the psychosocial theories.[10] In this model *exposure* refers to external factors, such as work requirements. The external exposure produces an internal *dose,* which in turn disturbs the internal state of the individual. Such disturbances may be mechanical, physiologic, or psychologic and in turn evoke a certain *response,* mechanical and/or metabolic changes, that occurs at the tissue level. Finally,

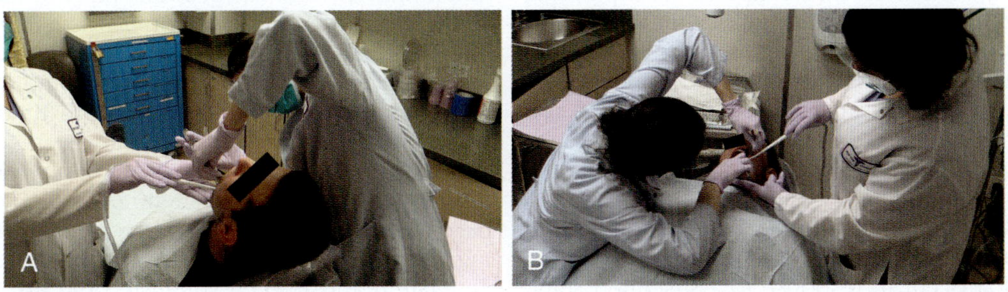

FIGURE 21-1: The exceptionally high rate of occupational cervicobrachial disorder among dentists is thought to result from maintaining an awkward posture for extended periods.

capacity, which can be either physical or psychologic, refers to the ability of the individual to resist destabilization after various doses of exposure. This model provides a framework to explain the relationship between work exposure factors and the different responses that occur, both psychologic and physiologic. A similar model was adopted by the panel of the National Research Council.[102]

Management

Evaluation of a patient with a suspected OSD involves a thorough history and physical examination. The hallmark of OSDs is musculoskeletal pain or discomfort that occurs on the job. Symptoms will vary based on the patient's specific diagnosis. Usually, the underlying diagnosis will fall into one of the following categories: myalgia, tendinitis, or bursitis. In a prospective study of 204 workers with occupationally related upper limb or neck pain, Sikorski and colleagues found that a discrete MSD existed in 58% of cases.[116]

A large proportion of patients diagnosed with an OSD will have signs and symptoms consistent with trapezius myalgia. Symptoms of trapezius myalgia typically include muscle fatigue and stiffness accompanied by subjective pain or headaches. On examination, patients may demonstrate muscle tightness, increased tone, and multiple "trigger points." Occasionally, subtle decreases in range of motion will be seen. Risk factors for myalgia are unvarying stationary positioning of the shoulder and neck, along with prolonged static loading.

Neurologic and vascular conditions such as cervical radiculopathy, TOS, and Raynaud phenomenon could also be associated with OSDs. Congenital or developmental deformities of the shoulder or cervical spine can predispose a worker to OSDs and may need to be addressed. Musculoskeletal neoplasms, both benign (such as osteochondroma) and malignant, can be found about the shoulder girdle and should be considered. Referred sources of pain from other organ systems, including the cardiac, pulmonary, and gastrointestinal systems, should be ruled out.

Several classifications of OSDs have been proposed, and such systems have been used for the development of treatment protocols. A five-grade classification system was developed by the OCD committee of the Japanese Association of Industrial Health (Box 21-1). This system includes tendinitis as well as several neurologic and vascular symptoms that often accompany occupational shoulder pain. A simplified three-stage system was developed by the Occupational Repetition Strain Advisory Committee in Australia. This system is based on the persistence of the symptoms and interference with work (Box 21-2).

Luck and Andersson[89] proposed a pathophysiologic grading system that is a modification of the Australian classification (Box 21-3). This focuses on myogenic pain. The pathophysiologic basis for pain in grade I is metabolic changes that occur in response to a sustained static load. Progression to grade II involves pain that does not resolve overnight and is secondary to muscle inflammation and early interstitial fibrosis. Grade III is characterized by progression to severe myopathy with interstitial fibrosis. It has been proposed that the more advanced the grade, the longer and more aggressive the treatment must be in terms of both time off work and involvement of a multidisciplinary team.[89]

Successful management of the patient requires a multidisciplinary approach. Treatment of physical disorders, psychosocial evaluation, and an appropriate understanding of the work demands are all equally important. Feuerstein and Hickey suggested the use of a multidisciplinary approach that focuses on physical, ergonomic, and psychologic factors.[40] They noted that patients treated

BOX 21-1. Japanese Grading System

Grade I
Subjective complaints without clinical findings

Grade II
Subjective complaints with induration and tenderness of the neck, shoulder, and arm muscles

Grade III
Includes grade II and any of the following:

1. Increased tenderness or enlargement of affected muscles
2. Positive neurologic tests
3. Paresthesia
4. Decrease in muscle strength
5. Tenderness of spinous processes of the vertebrae
6. Tenderness of the paravertebral muscles
7. Tenderness of the nerve plexus
8. Tremor of the hand or eyelid
9. Kinesalgia of the neck, shoulder, and upper extremity
10. Functional disturbance of the peripheral circulation
11. Severe pain or subjective complaints of the neck, shoulder, or upper extremity

Grade IV
Type 1
Severe type of grade III
Type 2
Direct development from grade II without passing through grade III, but having specific findings as follows:

1. Orthopedic diagnosis of the neck-shoulder-arm syndrome
2. Organic disturbances such as tendinitis or tenosynovitis
3. Autonomic nervous disturbances such as Raynaud phenomenon, passive hyperemia, or disequilibrium
4. Mental disturbances, such as anxiety, sleeplessness, thinking dysfunction, hysteria, or depression

Grade V
Disturbances not only at work but also in daily life

BOX 21-2. Australian Staging System

Stage I
Aching and tiredness of the affected limb that occurs during the work shift but subsides overnight and during days off work. There is no significant reduction in work performance, and there are no physical signs. This condition can persist for months and is reversible.

Stage II
Symptoms fail to settle overnight, cause a sleep disturbance, and are associated with a reduced capacity for repetitive work. Physical signs may be present. The condition usually persists for months.

Stage III
Symptoms persist at rest. Sleep is disturbed, and pain occurs with nonrepetitive movement. The person is unable to perform light duties and has difficulty with nonoccupational tasks. Physical signs are present. The condition may persist for months to years.

BOX 21-3. Pathophysiologic Grading System

Grade I (Mild)
Shoulder girdle muscle pain that occurs during work or similar activities and resolves a few hours later; no findings on physical examination.

Grade II (Moderate)
Shoulder girdle muscle pain that persists for several days after work; muscle belly and insertional tenderness on examination.

Grade III (Severe)
Shoulder girdle muscle pain that is constant for weeks or longer; multiple tender areas; palpable induration indicative of muscle fibrosis; muscle belly contracture; reduced range of motion of myogenic origin.

with a multidisciplinary approach had a significantly higher rate of return to work than did those treated with usual care. Johansson and colleagues reported a significant decrease in sick leave, pain intensity, and analgesic use in patients treated with a cognitive-behavioral pain management program. The treatment team included a clinical psychologist, physical therapist, occupational therapist, physical education teacher, vocational counselor, physician, and nurse.[74]

The medical/surgical management of rotator cuff disease, biceps tendonitis, bursitis, and adhesive capsulitis has been covered elsewhere in this textbook. The management of myalgia consists of modalities, such as the application of ice and heat. Range of motion exercises together with strengthening exercises should also be instituted. Antiinflammatory agents may be used in moderate cases, supplemented with low doses of tricyclic antidepressants in more refractory cases. A recent evidence-based systematic review provided evidence for the efficacy of conservative treatments in the management of rotator cuff tendonitis, biceps tendonitis, and trapezius myalgia.[32]

Changes in the workplace can also be beneficial. Introducing more frequent rest breaks and altering the posture and exertion of force at work can help prevent or alleviate OSDs. For example, Hallman and colleagues reported that workers who sat for approximately 9 hours a shift were almost 3 times more likely to report high neck and shoulder pain intensity than those who sat for more moderate durations (about 7 hours).[57] Mekhora and colleagues showed that simple ergonomic interventions, such as adjusting monitor height, seat height, and keyboard height could help reduce symptoms in patients suffering from trapezius myalgia.[94] This, in turn, resulted in less lost work time and higher productivity.[94]

Finally, the psychosocial element of OSDs should not be underestimated. High job demands predict future neck/shoulder pain. It has been suggested that high job demands may increase strain and subsequently increase muscle tension or other physiologic reactions that put individuals at a greater risk for developing neck/shoulder pain.[122] Most theoretical models that describe the relationship between occupational factors and musculoskeletal problems, such as the dose-response or biopsychosocial models, assume that psychosocial stressors at work lead to MSD by eliciting physiologic responses (e.g., by increasing the individual's muscle tension). Thus the psychologic state resulting from the experienced occupational stressors initiates a bodily response that over time may manifest in the form of health problems.[81] Eijckelhof and colleagues found some support for this view: applying simulated workplace stressors (cognitive/emotional stress, work pace, and precision) resulted in increased neck-shoulder and forearm muscle activity; decreased control was not a significant predictor.[35] These elements at work require work organizational changes. In addition to medical management, more aggressive approaches to improve sense of control over symptoms and functional loss, avoidance of unnecessary surgery, assistance to patients in managing residual pain and stress, and attention to employer-employee conflicts are all important in preventing prolonged work disability secondary to upper extremity disorders.[65]

DEGENERATIVE JOINT DISEASE

Although the relationship between cumulative trauma and injury to soft tissues about the shoulder girdle has been delineated, the association of glenohumeral arthritis with occupational factors is less clear.[6,27,86,128,140,147] Unlike the hip and knee, the shoulder is not a weight-bearing joint, and thus symptomatic degenerative arthritis of the glenohumeral joint is less common.

A few studies have investigated the association of glenohumeral arthritis with various occupations. Although some of these studies have reported a relationship between certain occupations and osteoarthritis of the shoulder, a direct association has not been found. Kellgren and Lawrence[80] and later Lawrence[85] found that the prevalence of glenohumeral arthritis in men was influenced by occupation. Waldron and Cox studied the skeletons of 367 workers buried in London between 1729 and 1869 and found no significant relationship between occupation and osteoarthritis of the shoulder.[135] Similarly, in a study that included 151 shoulder dissections, Petersson did not find any convincing evidence to support the notion that occupation is a factor in the development of osteoarthritis of the glenohumeral joint.[111]

As with OSDs, sustained loading may be associated with the development of glenohumeral arthritis. Dentists seem to be susceptible as a result of sustained static loads while maintaining the shoulder in a position of flexion and abduction with elevation of the scapula. In a Finnish study that included 40 dentists, Katevuo and colleagues found that 46% had radiographic evidence of osteoarthritis and 44% had bilateral disease.[79] In contrast, only 13% in the control group—82 farmers presumably unexposed to static load—had findings consistent with osteoarthritis.

It has been speculated that pneumatic drilling may predispose workers to degenerative arthritis. To examine the effect of vibration exposure on the shoulder, Bovenzi and colleagues compared 67 foundry workers who used vibratory tools with 46 heavy manual laborers.[22] They found no significant difference between the two groups in the prevalence of radiographic changes in the shoulder. In general, it has been difficult to differentiate degenerative changes caused by vibration from those that can simply be attributed to heavy manual work.

Degeneration of the acromioclavicular joint is more common than glenohumeral arthritis. As with glenohumeral arthritis, there is little evidence for a relationship with specific occupations. In a radiographic study of bricklayers and blasters, Stenlund and colleagues[121] found that OR for degeneration of the acromioclavicular joint increased with the level of lifetime weight handled on the job. When adjusted for age, construction workers had more than a two times greater risk for osteoarthritis of the acromioclavicular joint than their supervisors. The authors found that construction workers who engaged in sports activity as well were more susceptible to acromioclavicular osteoarthritis. Unlike tendinitis, the risk for those with high workloads did not show job-specific trends: even though most of the loading at work seemed to have been on the left side, the risk for the left shoulder was no greater than that for the right shoulder.[120] It is possible though that OR for the left side in these studies may have been underestimated.[17]

Other studies have reported contrary findings. In a cadaver study De Palma found degenerative changes in almost all subjects older than 50 years.[34] Petersson identified degeneration often in 30- to 50-year-old individuals and regularly in those older than 60 years.[110] Because degeneration occurred with equal frequency in men and women and was of the same severity in the right and left shoulders, occupation may not have been a contributing factor. In a retrospective study that included 83 patients who underwent distal clavicular resection for arthritis, Worcester and Green found no relationship with occupation.[144]

Although a few studies have suggested that the risk factors for OSDs may apply to arthritis, the insidious onset of degenerative disorders makes them more difficult to attribute to work. In summary, there is little evidence that glenohumeral and acromioclavicular osteoarthritis are work related.

PREVENTION

"Ergonomics" is the study of work—the tasks, the technology, and the environment—in relation to human capabilities. In practice, ergonomics is a process of problem solving. This process requires answers to several questions:

1. *Where is the problem?* The jobs or positions targeted for intervention
2. *What is the problem?* The specific risk factors for MSD present on the job, their magnitude, and the body parts at risk
3. *Why is there a problem?* The possible ergonomic root causes of the risk factors, specifically, design hazards that may exacerbate MSDs, such as the design of the workstation, tools, and products that need to be handled, as well as the way that work is organized or the techniques that are used by the individual
4. *What should be done?* Prioritizing hazard control measures

The first two of these points require a surveillance of job hazards. Prevention of WMSDs requires methods that focus on the assessment of risk factors, characterizing the stresses that act on the worker. The assessment should establish the circumstances under which people are affected and the severity of the problems. The physical stresses associated with OSDs rely on the findings of epidemiologic studies. The epidemiologic evidence suggests that several physical stressors play a role in the etiology, either separately or jointly, although the strength of their association with OSDs varies. Therefore the following Occupational data should be collected:

1. Excessive or sustained exertion of force
2. Awkward postures, mainly shoulder flexion/extension or abduction
3. Repetitive motions of the shoulder and neck*
4. Contact with vibrating power tools
5. Low ambient temperature

**Studies usually define repetitive work for the shoulder as activities that involve cyclic flexion, extension, abduction, or rotation of the shoulder joint. The studies operationalize repetitiveness in four ways: (1) the observed frequency of movements past predefined angles of shoulder flexion or abduction; (2) the number of pieces handled per time unit; (3) the duration of short cycle time/repeated tasks within the cycle; and (4) a descriptive characterization of repetitive work or repetitive arm movements.*

Knowledge of the dimensions of the exposure—magnitude, duration, and repetitiveness (frequency)—is necessary to assess the risk. The choice of method is a tradeoff between time, resources, and the level of detail desired. The most cursory task analysis involves a description of the sequence of functions or actions with the use of terms, such as transportation, operation, inspection, or storage. The activities of the upper extremities often require a more detailed analysis, with methods ranging from indirect measures, such as self-reports in interviews or questionnaires, through observations, to direct instrumented measures, such as electrogoniometry, heart rate monitoring, or EMG. These measurements serve to quantify the exposure to risk factors. Muscular stress can be quantified by EMG signals expressed as percent of maximal voluntary contraction or some other reference value. It is not possible to use the arm/hand without stabilizing the rotator cuff girdle and the glenohumeral joint, and therefore work tasks that demand continuous arm movements generate load patterns with a static load component at the shoulder level.[100] The static load of the shoulder muscles may not be high but, as discussed earlier, the low fatigue tolerance of these muscles may cause pain sooner (within about 1 hour of static contraction).

Exposure to external force can be estimated through biomechanical models. Such models for the shoulder are usually based on anthropometric data describing the length of the body segments (hand, forearm, and upper arm), the weight and center of mass of these segments, and their angular configurations with respect to the trunk. The models then calculate the torques acting around the shoulder. Most biomechanical models of shoulder stress underestimate the actual loads. Inertial forces associated with acceleration and deceleration of the body and work object increase the load, and additional loads may also result from antagonistic muscle forces. In addition to the effect on muscle workload, certain shoulder angles produce pressure on internal and surrounding soft tissues. In fact although the required muscle loads actually decrease as the arm-torso angle exceeds 90 degrees, the pressure on soft tissues continues to increase, an effect that is lost in a simple biomechanical assessment.[9]

In summary, the multifactorial nature of WMSDs implies that several categories of ergonomic hazard induce a variety of stressors. It follows that there are often several possible solutions. Exposure to physical stressors can be reduced by modifying the design of the workstation or the tools, redesigning the work objects, reorganizing the sequence of tasks, or implementing any combination of these solutions. The ideal solution would effectively control all or most of the stressors identified on the job. Dealing with multiple risk factors, numerous root causes, and a variety of possible solutions requires the development of professional and administrative strategies.

The strategies adopted to prevent WMSDs can be classified as *primary* and *secondary*. Primary prevention addresses the clinical manifestation of a disease before it occurs. Secondary prevention measures attempt to arrest the development of a disease while it is still in the early symptomatic stage.[112] The first aims at groups of workers, whereas the second focuses on the individual.

By following established practices for controlling exposure to hazardous materials, NIOSH[101] lists four areas of strategy to control and prevent musculoskeletal injuries:

1. Engineering controls to redesign tools, tasks, and workstations.
2. Administrative controls, including:
   A. Work practices (job rotation or enrichment, limited overtime, and rest breaks)
   B. Safe work practice training, including body mechanics
   C. Worker placement evaluation (employee selection)
3. Personal protective equipment, such as gloves, padding, and wrist rests and armrests; NIOSH and the Occupational Safety and Health Administration (OSHA) consider braces to be medical devices rather than personal protective equipment.
4. Medical management to minimize the impact of the health problems.

The goal of NIOSH intervention strategy is to eliminate, reduce, or control the presence of ergonomic hazards. These interventions can be used in both primary and secondary prevention and will be discussed in more detail under secondary prevention.

Primary Prevention

For primary prevention, NIOSH has recommended a tiered hierarchy of controls in which engineering changes are viewed as the first preference, administrative changes are a second preference, and personal protective equipment is the last choice.

The increase in reported cases of MSD and the increase in workers' compensation costs in the United States have prompted some regulatory efforts. Until 1991, attempts to standardize or control exposure to MSD risk factors were limited to specific tasks or situations, such as working with video display terminals or exposure to vibration. After high-profile citations, OSHA issued guidelines in 1993 for managing ergonomics programs.[104] These guidelines were limited to the meatpacking industry, an industry targeted because of a high incidence and severity of MSDs of the upper extremities. OSHA further emphasized that these guidelines were not a standard or regulation. OSHA's approach focused on ergonomics as a process. The guidelines consisted of the following: a discussion of the importance of management commitment and employee involvement, recommended program elements, and detailed guidance and examples for these elements. NIOSH incorporated most of these program elements in its guidelines for setting up an ergonomic program.[99]

OSHA published its Ergonomics Program Standards in the Federal Register (65: 68282-68870) November 14, 2000, but it was rescinded by Congress and President in February 2001. In 2002 OSHA declared its intention to address ergonomics in the work environment in a multi-tiered plan that was to include a combination of enforcement measures, workplace outreach, research, compliance assistance activities, and industry-targeted voluntary guidelines. To date, OSHA has issued guidelines for meat and poultry processing, foundries, shipyards, nursing homes, and retail grocery stores (see https://www.osha.gov/SLTC/ergonomics). The plan is designed to reduce musculoskeletal injuries and focuses on prevention. Rather than deploy specific ergonomic regulations, the enforcement relies still on the General Duty Clause, OSHA Act of 1970, Section 5(a)(1), that states that the employer is to furnish each of his or her employees a place of employment that is free of recognized hazards that are causing or likely to cause death or serious physical harm to employees.

In the absence of federal regulations regarding the prevention of WMSDs, some local initiatives attempted to fill the gap, with varying degrees of success. For example, the states of California and Washington introduced their own ergonomic regulations, although those of Washington were withdrawn in 2003.

Unlike the *program* standards, the American Conference of Governmental Industrial Hygienists chose to develop a *performance* standard for hand activity by using an expert consensus process (Physical and Biological Hazards of the Workplace). Although acceptable work design standards for preventing OSD have not yet been established, recommendations may be made regarding the prevention of localized fatigue. While prevention of fatigue is desirable in its own right, it may be a precursor of MSD. Recommended acceptable exposure limits are 10% of MVC for continuous work and 17% for intermittent work.[9] However, as noted earlier, such guidelines do not take into account the specific tolerance of the shoulder muscles.

Secondary Prevention

In order to estimate the biomechanical load on the body, it is important to know the locations of the manual controls and where materials, parts, and tools are stored and used, as well as the forces required to handle the work objects. Whether estimated as forces through biomechanical models or as muscle tension by EMG measurements, the workload needs to be compared with the individual's strength. Anthropometric tables provide some information on the strength of joints and hands by age and occupation. The analyst may either select a value from the literature that corresponds to the population of interest or use data provided by functional evaluation of a specific individual.

In secondary prevention the control strategies focus on individual patients. Ergonomic accommodations for employees with MSDs fall under the category of secondary prevention. Accommodations are interventions intended to reduce exposure to factors that limit the activities of an individual with impairment. More detailed knowledge is required about the residual abilities and limitations of the individual. Design for an individual requires a functional assessment that specifies that person's strength limits. The clinical evaluator should work closely with the designer during and after design implementation to ascertain that the job can be performed without risk of injury or reinjury.

Three principal means of accommodating impaired or disabled employees may be implemented: client matching, job restructuring, and job modifications.

Client matching, a form of employee selection, is the simplest and most effective way to return a person with a disability to work. It involves ensuring that the job requirements are consistent with the present abilities of the employee. If an employee cannot return to the previous job, an alternative job is found that can be performed without risk of reinjury. This strategy does not attempt to fit the job to the worker because it requires hardly any modifications to the job.

Job restructuring is an administrative control for reducing exposure to a risk factor. Two techniques have been proposed for reducing static load on the shoulder: the introduction of rest breaks and job rotation.

Many studies have attempted to find the optimal rest break frequency, duration, and content to prevent shoulder disorders caused by static, repetitive work. Many of the studies have focused on work at video display terminals (VDT). NIOSH has recommended a 15-minute rest break after 1 to 2 hours of VDT work. Similarly, the Swedish National Board of Occupational Safety and Health has recommended an upper limit of 1 to 2 hours of continuous video display terminal work.[125] The optimal frequency and length of breaks will depend mainly on the type of work that is being performed, the length of time that it can be sustained, and the posture or load that is held. Breaks can be active, with static load being relieved by dynamic muscle work. Short exercise and stretch periods are active breaks and they seem to be more effective than those that involve complete rest.[100]

Static loading of the shoulders can be avoided by rotating from one job to another. This technique requires careful assessment of task demands to ensure that the shoulders will be relieved occasionally. Although this technique is common in manufacturing industries, it is difficult to introduce in office work, which involves fewer tasks with sufficient variability. Workers may however arrange their tasks so that the tasks will periodically take them away from their workstation; for example, they may interrupt typing activities with photocopying, filing, or other duties. This technique can be viewed as a form of active break rather than formal job rotation.

In secondary prevention, job restructuring entails assigning the impaired employee to restricted duties. For example, restructuring the job by assigning heavy lifting tasks to another person would enable a worker with an OSD or low back pain to work while recovering from the injury.

Job modifications and redesign usually involve the use of assistive technology to enable individuals to perform the required tasks. Other employees may also benefit from similar devices. Occasionally, some tasks can be eliminated during the process of introducing new technology.

Case Examples

The following are examples of two cases involving the secondary prevention of OSDs. The first outlines the medical management of a clerical worker with an OSD, and the second demonstrates the application of the ergonomic solving process in secondary prevention.

Case 1

A 41-year-old, right-hand-dominant secretary at a large investment banking corporation had a chief complaint of right shoulder pain. She described a gradual onset of pain that began approximately 1 year before evaluation. She reported diffuse, poorly localized pain about the right side of her neck and right shoulder region. Her pain was intermittent and varied in terms of severity. In general however her pain worsened with work and was alleviated with rest. Specific work activities that exacerbated her symptoms included typing on a keyboard and writing. She spent approximately 9 hours a day in front of a VDT. Initially, her pain occurred solely during work and seemed to resolve at night.

Over the few months prior to the evaluation however her pain lingered into the evening and occasionally persisted into the initial part of the weekend. She had been evaluated previously by several physicians and underwent a rheumatologic workup for inflammatory disease, for which the result was negative. She also underwent electrophysiologic studies, again with negative results. Her physical examination was negative other than the finding of diffuse tenderness of the right trapezius muscle belly. The results of radiographs of the cervical spine and shoulder were negative.

An OSD was diagnosed, and she started on a course of physical therapy that included shoulder and neck range of motion and stretching exercises. She was instructed in muscle relaxation techniques and counseled with regard to limiting the number of hours spent at the computer keyboard, as well as to the value of rest breaks during her workday.

Her workstation was evaluated by an ergonomist, and several modifications were implemented. These modifications included the procurement of a chair with height adjustment, a wider computer keyboard, and an adjustable stand for holding hard copy being transcribed.

After 6 months her symptoms were much improved, and by 1 year she experienced only minor discomfort, which occurred exclusively during her workday and responded to basic stretching maneuvers.

Case 2

A 43-year-old woman complained of pain in her right shoulder, elbow, and index finger. She was living in a suburban area, divorced without children. She had been experiencing the symptoms for about 6 months, since a few weeks after starting working on the assembly line of a plant that produced electric engines for adjusting car seats. At first, the symptoms appeared during the second part of her shift work and usually disappeared on the weekend. When a new engine was introduced, production quotas increased. The symptoms became more severe and frequent, and she sought medical care. OSD and lateral epicondylitis were diagnosed. She was on leave for 1 week but as she was being paid by the piece (i.e., by the number of engines she worked on), she preferred to return to work part time. She experienced difficulty with shopping, dressing, and washing. OSHA had cited the plant for various violations, including underreporting of WMSDs. A review of the recordable cases revealed that the incidence rate of WMSDs at the plant was 13 times higher than the national rate for the manufacturing sector.

As part of medical management of the case, an ergonomic assessment of the workstations on the assembly line was conducted. The patient was observed at her position while she inserted an element into the assembled fixture with a magnetic clip inserter. The results of the assessment are summarized in Box 21-4. Detailed analysis revealed that the task required six operations with the right hand, one of which entailed an awkward posture, exertion of force, and repetitive motion. While using the clip inserter, the right shoulder had to be elevated; the arm was abducted more than 45 degrees and stabilized to enable the transmission of force to the hand tool through the forearm and wrist. The hand tool could not be grasped in a power grip and needed to be steered with the index finger. The operation also required leaning forward while flexing the neck to see the insertion.

Job rotation was not deemed an advisable accommodation because other positions on the assembly line had similar risk factors. Various engineering solutions were proposed, with a focus on a new hand tool and better gloves as first priority.

OUTCOMES OF TREATMENT

Few studies have examined nonoperative treatment outcomes for upper extremity MSDs, and fewer still have focused on OSDs. The outcome measure in occupational health for assessing success in the management of work-related injuries has been return to work. However, besides medical intervention, factors such as age, gender, wages, education, and job characteristics contribute to this outcome.[65] Cheng and colleagues[28] investigated the relationship among employer, provider, and patient outcome measures and how these relate to occupational and clinical factors in a New England workplace physical therapy clinic. They found that 42 patients with OSDs demonstrated significant improvement in self-assessed physical functioning and body pain scores after an average of about seven visits during a 30-day period of physical therapy. Employer and provider outcomes were moderately correlated: full-time workers were more likely to remain on or return to their jobs and so were patients who achieved the physical therapist's goals. Although 77% of the patients remained on or returned to their preinjury jobs, pain scores on discharge were still higher than expected, suggesting that the treatment outcome may not be considered successful from the patient's perspective.

BOX 21-4. Summary of an Ergonomic Assessment of a Case With OSD

Job title: magnetic clip inserter
Number of task elements: right hand 6, left hand 5
Total cycle time: 7 seconds
Date:

Where Is the Problem?
Task element #5 for the right hand: use magnetic clip inserter

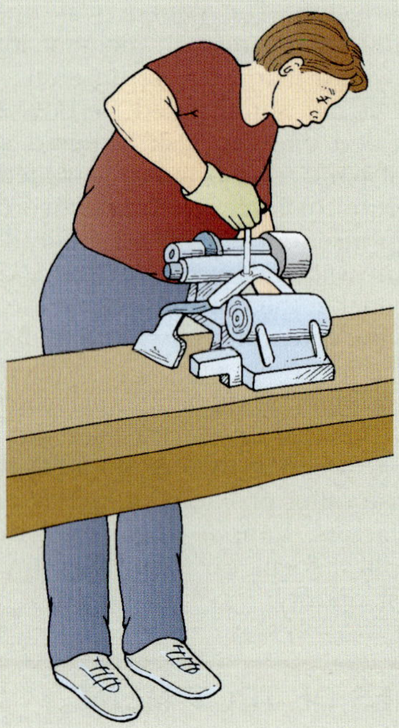

What Is the Problem?
Posture:
Shoulder asymmetry
Right arm abduction >45 degrees
Right forearm pronation

Repetitiveness:
Wrist radial deviation and dorsal flexion

Force:
Right elbow
Right wrist
Right hand palm contact pressure
Right hand fingers 3 and 4 for guiding hand tool

Why Is There a Problem?
Tool Design:
T-handle of magnetic clip inserter

Product Design:
Location of insertion on the fixture

What To Do?
Priority 1:
Change handle of inserter to a power grip
Looser glove with palm padding

Priority 2:
Antifatigue mats
Foot railing

Priority 3:
Change location of clip insertion on the fixture
Tilt the conveyor belt toward the operator

Conclusion
High-risk job for the right shoulder and right elbow

OSD, Occupational shoulder disorder.

Although conflicting results and opinions have been reported in the literature, most studies have found that patients receiving workers' compensation do not respond to surgery with the same success as other patients do.[12,45,60,61,113,114] As an example, Misamore and colleagues reported a comparison of results in two populations of patients undergoing primary repair of the rotator cuff.[96] Twenty-four patients were receiving workers' compensation and 79 were not. The two groups were comparable with regard to age, sex, size of the tear, preoperative strength, pain, and active range of motion. At a mean follow-up of 45 months, only 54% of the compensation group was rated as good or excellent versus 92% of the other patients. Similarly, 42% of the compensation group returned to full activity compared with 94% of their counterparts in the study. No significant differences were noted between the two groups with regard to the amount of time required to return to work, although fewer of the compensation patients returned to full activity. The average return to work time in this study was 6 months. The authors also noted that most of the unsatisfactory results were due to subjective criteria, such as pain, function, and strength. Although both groups had similar active range of motion, fewer than half the patients who were receiving compensation returned to full work activity.

A systematic review and meta-analysis of the surgical international literature shows a strong association between compensation status and poor outcome after surgery.[58] In many studies compensation status was the most significant predictor of outcome when compared with all other diagnostic and demographic variables or treatment variables. Because of the association between compensation and injury, most studies included in the review covered orthopedic, plastic, and spinal surgery. ORs were similar for the five most common procedures (shoulder acromioplasty, carpal tunnel release, lumbar discectomy, lumbar spine fusion, and lumbar intradiscal injection of chymopapain); OR for shoulder acromioplasty was 4.48 against a positive outcome in compensation cases.[58]

Confounding the above discussion is the potential for workers' compensation and legal suits to occur in tandem. Medicolegal factors play an important role in returning to work after an illness or injury, with the potential for secondary gain believed to complicate the recovery of many of these patients.[48,49] For example, one study examined the effect of litigation and workers' compensation claims on the outcome of anterior acromioplasty for chronic inflammation of the supraspinatus tendon due to impingement syndrome.[45] A comparison of three groups (workers' compensation patients, litigation patients, and those with no apparent financial gain) found a significantly longer time to return to work in those receiving workers' compensation (an average of 14.2 weeks compared with 4.7 weeks and 2.5 weeks, respectively). However, these results were confounded by the fact that workers' compensation patients were more often involved in heavy manual labor jobs and therefore may have required a more complete return of shoulder endurance prior to returning. The study found that overall satisfactory pain relief plus return to preinjury work activities was achieved, with 91% of employed patients returning to full employment despite the potential for secondary gain.[45]

EVALUATION OF UPPER EXTREMITY DISABILITY AND IMPAIRMENT

BLS, the National Center for Health Statistics, and Workers' Compensation Awards are primary sources of estimates for occupational illness and injury data. Statistics on disabilities are collected by National Center for Health Statistics through the National Health Interview Survey; the U.S. Census Bureau collects data as part of the Current Population Survey and the Survey of Income and Program Participation. Each agency and instrument for data collection uses a different definition of disability. At the present time, the United States does not have any comprehensive national system to keep track of work-related illness, injury, impairment, or disability. The Survey of Income and Program Participation 2010 reported that 51.4 million working-age people (or 21.3% of the population aged 15 to 64 years) had a *disability*; in about 30.5% of these people the disability was not severe. Approximately 19.9 million people aged 16 to 54 years and older had difficulty with physical tasks relating to upper body functioning, including difficulty with lifting and grasping.[23]

The U.S. Census Bureau reported that in 2008, 10.3 million people (22.1% of the working-age population aged 16 to 64 years) had a disability that prevented or limited work.[130] About a third had a nonsevere work disability. According to the National Health Interview Survey, 16.2 million working-age people had a work limitation (10.5% of the population aged 18 to 64 years).[69]

Disability Versus Impairment

In 2000 the WHO introduced a new framework of reference for classifying the consequences of disease or dysfunction that complemented ICD. The *International Classification of Functioning, Disability, and Health* (ICF) is a classification of health and health-related domains that describe body functions and structures, activities, and participation.[145] The domains are classified with regard to body, individual, and societal perspectives. Because an individual's functioning and disability occur in a context, ICF also includes a list of environmental factors that describe contexts in which individuals live. Having a problem may mean an impairment, limitation, restriction, or barrier, depending on the construct. The WHO moved away from a classification of "impairments" to a classification of problems with body structure and function. Similarly, "disability" is now viewed as limitations in activities, and "handicap" is defined as restrictions in participation.

The classification can be applied to document the impact of shoulder impairment. For example, symptoms of pain in the shoulder would be classified under sensory and pain body functions; changes in range of motion or stability of the joint would be coded under neuromusculoskeletal and movement-related body functions. The location of the disorder may be coded under shoulder structures related to movement (bones, joints, muscles, etc.). Activities related to mobility may be affected, such as lifting or carrying objects, or self-care tasks such as dressing. A disability may ensue if the individual is limited in the performance of these activities. If these limitations cannot be accommodated through assistive technology or social and medical support, this may restrict participation at work and the individual would be considered to be handicapped.

The extent of the problems encountered by an individual may be further expressed according to scales called "qualifiers." For example, the extent of impairment may be rated (qualified) on a scale of 0 for "no impairment" to 4 for "complete impairment." Impairments in body structure use qualifiers of the nature of the change and location that range from 0 for "no change in structure" to 7 for "qualitative changes in structure, including accumulation of fluid." Although the system itself does not provide a link between the scores of clinical assessment tools and these qualifiers, Cieza and colleagues[30] found a high level of agreement between two health care professionals regarding the ICF constructs and eight common health status measurements (e.g., Short Form-36, Pain Disability Index, and Sickness Impact Profile).

The clinical utility of ICF as well as its usefulness for policy making and planning health services is currently under investigation throughout the world. Thus the International Paris Task Force on Back Pain has adopted ICF as a framework for its recommendations.[1] In 2001 the National Committee on Vital and Health Statistics of the Centers for Disease Control and Prevention recommended that the U.S. Department of Health adopt ICF in national studies.[98]

For rehabilitation physicians, ICF has two notable limitations regarding its practicality. One limitation is that it does not yet relate consequences to specific diagnoses thus limiting its use in clinical practice and in planning services. In 2002 the WHO began to select core sets of constructs that may be useful for addressing specific disorders or groups of disorders, such as low back pain.[124] Future efforts may address shoulder disorders. A second limitation lies in the scope of ICF, which covers consequences in areas, such as sexual activity, recreation, home management, self-care, family membership, and social integration. None of these are the domain of government regulation in the United States; compensation systems, such as the Social Security Administration (SSA) and workers' compensation are limited to participation in work and employment. Thus only a limited set of the ICF taxonomy may be useful for establishing work disability.

In 1994 the SSA acknowledged that its disability determination process lacked a conceptually coherent framework.[119] The agency considered the precursor of ICF as a model,[93] but it has not formally adopted a framework yet. The SSA and other agencies involved in the determination of disability maintain the medical model that focuses on impairment, although they do allow considerations regarding limitation of activities, age, work experience, and others in the process. The next section describes the process implemented by these agencies.

Disability Determination

Determination of disability is an administrative process in which the orthopedist plays a key role in the evaluation of impairment.[25] When a disability-determining agency requests that a form be filled out or that an examination be performed, this is usually because an assessment of impairment is being sought. Determination of the impact of an individual's impairment on their functioning in society or, more specifically, on employment is usually performed by the determining agency. The complicated infrastructure of disability determination is based not only on medical impairment but also on an interplay of educational level, work experience, available job opportunities, psychologic factors, age, and socioeconomic background. Judgments based on such a wide range of factors are open to some degree of variation and subjectivity.[2,25,33,107,115,133] A major source of difficulty in the determination of disability is that decisions regarding work capacity rely on medical evaluations. Such evaluations may very well be performed in the absence of an actual assessment of work-related functional capacity.

Medical impairment encompasses both physical and mental entities, with the orthopedic surgeon evaluating anatomic or physiologic defects that interfere with an individual's ability to perform certain functions in a standard fashion. Upper extremity impairments are usually expressed in terms of physical signs, such as joint range of motion or diminution in the generation of force.[2] Several agencies request that impairment be expressed as a percentage in relation to the whole body. Compensation agencies frequently ask the orthopedist to determine work restrictions based on the medical evaluation so they can match abilities and disabilities to specific jobs.

The orthopedist is frequently called on to provide an objective medical evaluation of the impairment during the process of determination of disability. This specialist may be asked to play different roles, such as advisor, objective third-party examiner, patient advocate, or adjudicator, depending on different agencies' needs within the various disability programs. In addition, the orthopedist may be asked to determine and document medical restrictions based on a worker's illness or injury. It is therefore essential that there be a clear understanding of exactly what information the requesting agency needs. It should be recognized that in a "gatekeeper" role, the doctor-patient relationship might be directly affected.

The orthopedist should be knowledgeable and have current information regarding federal and state regulations, as well as employers' work rules. Knowledge of the workplace is an essential component when evaluating a person's disability and return to work. The orthopedist should have a clear understanding of the factors leading to work-related injuries and disorders. A review of work tasks is essential when determining work-relatedness as well as any contributing factors from previous work experience. A comprehensive assessment should include information about non–work-related activities as well, such as spare time and sports activities.

One of the most challenging tasks is to ascertain whether the illness or injury is work related. This undertaking can be complex because not only can there be variations in diagnostic criteria and definitions but also the same disorder may also be considered work-related in one case and not in another. The orthopedist usually has little formal training specific to the workplace. The Quebec Research Institute on Occupational Health and Safety created referral resources on WMSDs, including those of the upper extremity. (One such resource is a guide and tools for modified work, which includes a modified work proposal form for workers with neck or shoulder problems. A second resource is a guide to the diagnosis of work-related shoulder tendonitis.)

Guidelines for Degree of Impairment

The following sources are helpful references that the orthopedist can use to evaluate impairment.

The American Academy of Orthopaedic Surgeons' publication *The Clinical Measurement of Joint Motion*[3] provides a standardized, reproducible, and efficient method for assessment of joint motion. Considerable emphasis is placed on range of motion when evaluating shoulder impairment. Thus when the various agencies request an assessment of impairment, the orthopedist can accurately base the assessment of shoulder impairment on range of joint motion on the unaffected side or can refer to the normal comparative data provided in this publication. Normal joint kinesiology, the range of normal joint motion, and the change in joint motion with age are also discussed.

The American Academy of Orthopaedic Surgeons has published a *Manual for Orthopaedic Surgeons in Evaluating Permanent Physical Impairment.*[4] This publication was an attempt to address the problem of inconsistencies that the orthopedist might face when formulating an opinion on impairment in relation to workers' compensation and personal injury litigation. It proposes a scoring system for the shoulder that can be used as a guide in calculating the percentage of permanent impairment and loss of function in relation to the whole arm.

The American Medical Association has updated their *Guides to the Evaluation of Permanent Impairment*; it is currently in sixth edition.[5] The *Guides* represents a consensus of experts concerning the best practice for evaluation. A format is specified in which data are acquired to analyze, record, and report information about the impairment. The medical evaluation is based on three components. First, the nature of the impairment and its consequences are documented. Second, protocols are provided to evaluate specific organ systems. The musculoskeletal section contains a protocol that can be used to systematically evaluate upper extremity impairment. Third, tables are provided that relate to the evaluation protocols. For the upper extremity, the range of active motion is rounded to the nearest 10 degrees, and a table is provided to calculate the relationship of impairment of the upper extremity to impairment of the whole person. It should be noted that the validity of these measures for the determination of disability has not been adequately studied. The degree to which the procedures predict work disability as a result of soft tissue musculoskeletal impairment has been questioned.[92]

The Minnesota Medical Association has developed a *Revised Temporary Disability Duration Guide*[95] to evaluate a disability that lasts for less than 52 weeks. Determination of impairment is based primarily on the diagnosis and is supported by the medical history, physical findings, and diagnostics.

CURRENT DISABILITY COMPENSATION SYSTEMS

The Americans With Disabilities Act

On July 26, 1990, Congress enacted Public Law 336, the Americans with Disabilities Act (ADA) (http://www.usdoj.gov/crt/ada/adahom1.htm). The act prohibits discrimination and ensures equal opportunity for persons with disabilities in employment, state and local government services, public accommodations, commercial facilities, and transportation. Employment issues are covered by Title I, and the Equal Employment Opportunity Commission (EEOC) is the federal agency that interprets employment discrimination laws and enforces Title I of the ADA. People already in the workforce who incur an MSD have tried to use coverage of the ADA to seek solution to their grievances; these cases have been handled by the EEOC. An idea of the impact of the ADA on OSDs may be obtained from the Job Accommodation Network. In the first quarter of 2002, 12% of the cases handled involved the upper extremities and 13% were related to the back. The total caseload since 1984 has exceeded 305,000.[72] This number is much lower than the burden expected from population surveys. Assuming that only a third of the upper extremity cases were related to the shoulder, the ADA may have affected about 12,000 people with shoulder disabilities.[72]

The intention behind ADA was to protect qualified individuals with disabilities from employment discrimination. To understand who is protected by the ADA, it is necessary to understand the definition of an "individual with a disability" and then to determine whether the individual meets the definition of a "qualified individual with a disability." An individual is protected by the ADA only if both definitions are met.

The ADA defines an *individual with disability* as a person who meets one of the following criteria:

- has a physical or mental impairment that *substantially limits* one or more major life activities
- has a *record of* a statutory disability
- is *regarded as* being disabled

Neck and shoulder MSDs are a "physical impairment" in the ADA sense because they are a "physiologic disorder" and not a physical trait or characteristic. To qualify as an individual with disability, the impairment has to limit major life activities, such as sitting, standing, lifting, and reaching. A limitation has to be described by its *severity*, *duration* (how long it is expected to last), and *impact* (permanent or long term). The diagnosis does not determine disability, only the impact of the impairment. Individuals with shoulder MSDs have encountered the same treatment by the courts as those with low back impairments. The courts have given various interpretations regarding limitations on lifting or reaching as qualifying for disability. To qualify as "substantial," the limitation is expected to affect activities outside work as well as work activities. Limitations on housework, gardening, or child care may not be sufficient. Limitations on performing manual material handling tasks have been rejected on the ground that the limitation has to affect performance in a class of jobs or a broad range of jobs.*

**See Burgard v. Super Value Holdings, Inc., or 1997 U.S. App. Lexis 12228 (10th Cir. 1997) regarding the lower part of the back and Sherrod v. American Airlines, Case No. 97-10011 (5th Cir, January 28, 1998), or McKay v. Toyota Motor Manufacturing, 110 F.3d 369 (1997), regarding neck impairments.*

Even a "30% service-connected" limitation as a result of shoulder impairment may not be sufficient if it is not shown that a major life activity is affected.*

A *qualified individual with disability* is an individual "...who meets the skill, experience, education, and other job-related requirements of a position held or desired and who, with or without reasonable accommodation, can perform the essential functions of a job."

It is sometimes necessary to identify the "essential functions" of a job to know whether an individual with a disability is qualified to do the job. Written job descriptions provide one form of evidence when determining whether a function is essential. Job or task analyses that focus on the results or outcomes of a function are considered more helpful than those focused on the way work is performed.[37] These analyses are particularly important when the function can be performed in only a limited way. As industry attempts to increase efficiency through developing more flexible systems of labor specification, each employee may be asked to perform a wide variety of tasks and functions. The lack of detail in these new forms of job description may make it easier to qualify for a job, but it may also make it more difficult to define the essential functions.

Practices covered by the ADA include, among others, testing, evaluation, medical examination, compensation, and leave. The ADA does not eliminate preplacement medical examination as a selection tool. It mandates that medical screening criteria be job related and consistent with business necessity. The latter may require that the individual pose no direct threat to the health and safety of others. The EEOC[36] interprets "direct threat" to include threat to the health and safety of the applicant, but the EEOC interpretation was rejected by a federal district court in Illinois.† For a physician examiner to make the required assessment, the specific requirements of the job must be determined, including which duties are essential and which are not. The decision-making can be greatly facilitated if job descriptions address the physical requirements of the job and any environmental hazards associated with the work.[26] The ADA limits assessment of an individual's physical capacity if it is unknown what functional abilities are required or what environmental hazards are present.

The EEOC[36] has attempted to clarify some of the issues related to medical examination and testing. In general, tests that measure an applicant's physiologic response (such as heart rate or maximal oxygen uptake) to a physical task (such as running) renders the test a medical examination. As a rule, these tests are interpreted by a health professional. They can be administered after a conditional offer of employment, provided that all candidates are subjected to the same examination regardless of disability [42 U.S.C. §12112(d)(3)]. Strength tests depend on the context in which the test is given. If it is used to determine the capability of performing a specific task (such as lifting a 30-lb box and carrying it for 20 feet), the test is not "medical" and could be administered preoffer. The test measures the weight of the object handled and the distance carried, not the person's physiologic response. The distinction is subtle but legally significant.

**Bailey v. Runyon, Postmaster General, U.S. Postal Service.*

†Kohnke v. Delta Airlines, Inc., 8 NDLR§221 (N.D. Ill. 1966) (No. 93 C 7096).

Workers' Compensation

Workers' compensation is a no-fault insurance system for work-related accidental injury and occupational disease for federal and state workers. Federal government employees receive benefits under the Federal Employees' Compensation Act, and state employees are provided for by separate legislation in state workers' compensation laws enacted by each state. Workers' compensation laws share many characteristics but also have important differences in the federal and state systems. To further complicate the issue of what is compensable under workers' compensation, compensable conditions vary from one state to the next, as well as benefit amounts, processing of claims, and settlement of disputes.[63] It is important that orthopedists understand the requirements of the state workers' compensation system. Under workers' compensation, employers must provide medical treatment and compensation benefits to employees for work-related illness or injury. Employers must demonstrate their ability to pay for workers' compensation costs by obtaining insurance coverage through a state fund or private carrier or by self-insurance. Four categories of compensable disabilities may be provided for under state workers' compensation: temporary total disability, temporary partial disability, permanent total disability, and permanent partial disability. The greatest number of workers' compensation cases is for temporary disability, which accounts for about three fourths of compensable claims. In addition to paying medical expenses and compensating workers for lost wages, state workers' compensation provides for survivors' benefits and vocational rehabilitation. In a study conducted by the Minnesota Blue Cross, workers' compensation costs were found to be almost twice the cost for similar conditions when compared with general liability claims.[95]

To qualify for an award, a worker has to demonstrate that the injury occurred as a result of and in the course of employment. Satisfying the criteria for a compensation claim is not an issue in the case of injuries induced by overt external force; however, in the absence of trauma, assertions of work-relatedness may be more difficult to establish. Most states require that injured employees be unable to perform their level of work or to obtain employment that is suitable to their qualifications and training.

The American Medical Association's *Guides to the Evaluation of Permanent Impairment* provides a standard framework and method of analysis through which physicians can evaluate, report on, and communicate information about shoulder impairment.[5,46] It is either recommended or mandated by law in workers' compensation cases in 38 states and two territories in the United States. The most current edition should be used.

Under workers' compensation, impairment is a medical issue and is defined as an alteration in an individual's health status that interferes with activities of daily living. Using the American Medical Association's guidelines, the orthopedist can represent the degree to which an individual's capacity to carry out daily activities has been diminished. Permanent impairment is defined as impairment that has become static or stabilized during a period sufficient to allow optimal tissue repair and that is unlikely to change despite further medical or surgical therapy.

Under workers' compensation, the evaluation or rating of a disability is a nonmedical assessment. Disability is defined as a decrease or loss or absence of the capacity of an individual to meet personal, social, or occupational demands or to meet statutory or regulatory requirements because of an impairment. A disability refers to a task that an individual cannot do; it arises out of the interaction between impairment and external requirements, with an emphasis on the person's occupation. It logically follows that individuals with impairment are not necessarily "disabled" with regard to their occupation. Individuals with impairment are considered handicapped if there are obstacles to them accomplishing basic activities that can be overcome by compensating in some way for the effects of the impairment. The most common cause of a dispute over compensation claims is determination of the extent of the disability. A physician's expert opinion is then requested, and a hearing is held before the workers' compensation agency.

Railroad and Maritime Workers' Compensation

The Federal Employer's Liability Act (FELA) supersedes state compensation laws and provides for a comprehensive injury compensation system for railroad workers. Unlike state compensation laws, there are no limits on awards, and consequently the system is expensive. Although the physician determines the magnitude of an injured worker's impairment, under FELA a jury decides the degree of disability. The Jones Act provides compensation for maritime workers, with the same rights and remedies as FELA.

Social Security

Two disability compensation programs are administered by the SSA. Workers with a recent work history in employment covered by Social Security are eligible for the Social Security Disability Insurance program. Individuals who have no recent work history but who meet a financial needs test receive benefits under the disability portion of the Supplemental Security Income Program. Both programs use the same definition of disability and the same regulations for determining disability. Disability under the Social Security Program is defined in economic terms and in terms of the individual's ability to work. Individuals are considered disabled if the impairment is of such severity that they are unable to do the work previously performed and are not able to be engaged in any other kind of substantial gainful work as a result of their age, education, and occupational experience. To be considered for benefits, a worker must be unable to work for at least 6 months. This definition of disability is more restrictive than that of other agencies in that the medically determined physical or mental impairment is expected to result in death or to persist for at least 12 months. The impairment must have demonstrable anatomic, physiologic, or psychologic abnormalities demonstrated by medically accepted clinical and laboratory diagnostic techniques. The Social Security Program has established medical criteria, referred to as the "listing of impairments" that define disorders and the level of severity that supposedly prevents a person from working. Unlike workers' compensation, recipients of Social Security are subject to periodic review to determine continued eligibility.

Approximately two thirds of the initial disability claims are denied by Social Security. A claimant's eligibility is determined by a team of examiners based on a review of the records. If a person is denied benefits, there is an appeal process whereby the case is reconsidered by a different team of examiners. If benefits are still denied, the claimant is seen in person by a decision maker, and the claim may go to the Appeals Council of the SSA and ultimately to the federal courts.

The orthopedist is required to furnish sufficient medical evidence to Social Security, including the individual's medical history, clinical findings, laboratory findings, diagnosis based on signs and symptoms, prescribed treatment and prognosis, and a medical source statement describing what work-related activities (such as sitting, walking, lifting, or carrying) the patient can do despite the impairment.

Private Insurance Companies

Individual disability income policies pay a fixed monetary amount of coverage and may be integrated with other public disability programs. They are provided on both an individual and a group basis. In general, benefits may be provided either for a stated period or until the attainment of a specific age. Most policies require that the beneficiary be reexamined by a physician designated by the insurance company to ensure continuation of benefits. Disability is defined in various ways, and the requirements of coverage are determined by each company individually.

Private agencies may request that the orthopedic surgeon determine either short-term or permanent ability to work. The calculation of time off work is often determined by the orthopedist's experience with previous patients having similar diagnoses. Good communication and candor among the orthopedist, the patient, and the insurance company are necessary to achieve the desired goal of return to work.

CONCLUSION

Occupational *shoulder disorders* refer to a symptom complex characterized by vague pain about the shoulder girdle, including the paracervical, parascapular, and glenohumeral musculature. Tendinitis and nerve impingement syndromes are also included under OSDs, but this chapter did not address these. Although not clearly defined, epidemiologic evidence has shown a relationship between mechanical stress, such as static or awkward posture and repetitive motions, and health outcomes classified as OSDs.

Several hypotheses have been postulated to explain the injury mechanism triggered by exposure to the mechanical stressors. Decrements in the generation of muscle force have been demonstrated in EMG studies, as well as by physical and laboratory findings. Damage to contractile structure and reduced blood flow secondary to increased intramuscular pressure have also been reported. In addition, there is evidence for a muscle recruitment mechanism whereby the slow-twitch fibers characteristic of small motor units are recruited first for force and for repetitive, endurance work and remain in action throughout low-level contractions. These motor units of larger muscles, such as the trapezius, are therefore vulnerable to fatigue and damage manifested as myalgia.

Several classifications of OSDs have been proposed, and such systems have been used for the development of treatment protocols. Management consists of modalities such as the application of ice and heat. Range of motion exercises along with strengthening exercises should also be used, and antiinflammatory agents may be helpful. Ergonomic modifications can reduce the exposure to mechanical stress. These modifications are used in primary and secondary prevention of OSDs. The intervention starts with an assessment of the risk factors present in occupational and recreational activities. Engineering modifications are the preferred strategy because they remove the risk at the source, although administrative measures that reduce the exposure are often the first line of action.

Nonoperative treatment can achieve satisfactory outcomes such as reduction of pain and a return to the preinjury activity level. Litigation and workers' compensation claims complicate the recovery, particularly in cases treated surgically.

The WHO has approved an international classification of functioning that can serve to distinguish between disability and impairment. According to this, OSDs are structural and functional body impairments; a disability arises when various activities are limited. Many estimates of impairment from OSDs and disability have been made in the United States, and they depend on the case definition and the method used to collect the data. About 3 million people with disability have a nonsevere condition, whereas about 16 million people of working age have some work limitation. However, determination of disability is largely an administrative process in which the orthopedist plays a key role in evaluation of the impairment. The American Academy of Orthopaedic Surgeons and the American Medical Association have issued the guidelines most commonly used to grade impairments. The most challenging task is to ascertain whether the illness or injury is work related.

The decision regarding public assistance in the case of disability caused by OSDs is framed by the current compensation systems. The most common venue for covering medical costs is private insurance. Workers' compensation is a more common venue for indemnity as well as the treatment costs involved in managing OSDs. However, in the absence of trauma, assertions of work-relatedness may be difficult to establish. The ADA provides a mechanism for accommodations, but it is questionable whether the impact of OSDs will qualify individuals for it. The railroad and maritime workers' Compensation and Social Security are probably the less common systems that provide OSD compensation for workers who meet set criteria.

EDITOR COMMENTARY

Jason E. Hsu

Occupational shoulder disorders are one of the most common musculoskeletal complaints among adults in the workforce. They are associated with substantial lost time off work, and with direct and indirect costs that place a substantial burden on society and our public health systems. The authors of this chapter provide a valuable summary of the definitions, epidemiology, etiology, management, and prevention of these disorders, as well as an excellent overview of the current disability compensation systems in the United States.

This chapter presents physiologic and psychosocial theories for the development of occupational shoulder disorders, and both theories have merit. Work-related shoulder disorders, more so than those in the general population, deserve special consideration with regards to the psychosocial factors. In our practice we have found that patients with work-related claims have significantly inferior clinical outcomes after shoulder arthroplasty, even after accounting for other factors, such as sex, medical comorbidities, etiology, and severity of disease. This is consistent with many other studies that have investigated outcomes in other upper extremity disorders and have noted the same finding. Such results emphasize the difficulty in diagnosing and treating these patients. Management for these patients can be challenged by the fact that physiologic and psychosocial disturbances can be difficult to differentiate, and secondary gain can often cloud the ability of the physician to determine whether the patient's clinical symptoms are a result of structural pathology addressable with surgical intervention.

Our general treatment algorithm for occupational shoulder disorders, from a physical standpoint, includes recommendations for an appropriate exercise regimen. As with our patients in the general population, we often stress the therapeutic and preventative role of general daily exercise, because the physiologic response to cardiorespiratory fitness exercises includes improved systemic circulatory capacity and is likely to induce an elevation in pain thresholds. With

EDITOR COMMENTARY—cont'd

regards to shoulder-specific exercises, the physician, with or without the help of a therapist, must first ensure that shoulder stiffness is not present. If present, an appropriate stretching protocol should be instituted before starting any deltoid or rotator cuff strengthening. The physician or therapist must ensure that the patient can obtain smooth, painless shoulder range of motion prior to starting strengthening. Because myalgias, particularly of the upper trapezius, are extremely common in this population, special attention to the posterior scapular stabilizers through postural exercises and reducing tightness of the pectoralis musculature should be a focus to normalize scapulothoracic kinematics and reduce strain of the upper trapezius. Concurrently, workplace interventions need to be considered for potential kinematic and muscular adaptation changes to eliminate muscular fatigue during specific work tasks.

As important, if not more important, to the physical component of neck and shoulder pain is the psychosocial factors of the patient's overall health. Appropriate social support and job satisfaction must be emphasized and are instrumental to reducing symptoms related to the neck and shoulder. As pointed out by the authors, a multidisciplinary approach involving practitioners focusing on factors beyond the patients' musculoskeletal care is needed for optimal results.

The authors do a fantastic job of appropriately reviewing the nonoperative medical management and workplace modifications for these work-related injuries. They also highlight the fact that workers' compensation patients do not respond to surgery with the same success as the general population. Although this chapter focuses on myalgias, bursitis, and tendonitis, specific note should be made that radiographic findings of acromioclavicular joint degeneration, superior labral tears, and partial thickness rotator cuff tears, among others, are often incidental findings for which surgical intervention is unnecessary. In addition, although used by many agencies to define a constellation of nonspecific inflammatory shoulder symptoms, "impingement syndrome" is a term that we have moved away from using, and the use of anterior acromioplasty in our practice is rare. In our experience, the liberal use of anterior acromioplasty, distal clavicle excision, and biceps tenodesis in patients with occupational disorders often leads to the patients returning to the surgeon or obtaining a second opinion for unresolved shoulder pain and inability to return to work. Similarly, arthroscopic superior labral repair for MRI-documented "SLAP tears" can lead to persistent shoulder stiffness and pain in patients undergoing repair. These failures are not generally the result of a poorly performed surgery, but reflect the difficulty in correctly identifying the pain generators in these patients' shoulders. We rarely perform an acromioplasty and believe that impingement of the anterior acromion onto the rotator cuff is uncommon. Similarly, we are very conservative with indicating superior labral repairs in this patient population, as superior labral tears are often an incidental finding on MRI and distinguishing between a nonpathologic sublabral foramen and a true SLAP tear can be difficult. Repairing these "SLAP tears" often leads to the loss of external rotation and persistent pain.

In conclusion, patients with occupational shoulder disorders merit special consideration regarding nonspecific and nonanatomic shoulder pain, and attention to psychosocial factors is as important as attempting to address physical factors. As the authors point out well, these occupational shoulder disorders can often respond best to nonsurgical treatment, workplace prevention, and workplace modifications. Surgeons should be careful about indicating surgery for nonspecific shoulder pain on the basis of often incidental radiographic findings.

SENIOR EDITOR COMMENTARY

Frederick A. Matsen III

This chapter nicely points out some of the many challenges faced when evaluating and managing shoulder disorders attributed to the patient's employment. One concerning aspect of many occupational disorders is the grab bag of imprecise terms that have been applied to them, such as "complaints of the arms, neck, and shoulders (CANS)," "work-related upper extremity musculoskeletal disorders (WRUEMSDS)," "occupational shoulder disorders (OSDS)," "repetitive motion disorder (RMD)," and "impingement syndrome"; these are conditions that have neither robust diagnostic criteria nor specific treatment for a defined anatomic entity. They leave shoulder surgeons in a very subjective and imprecise position. A well-respected shoulder surgeon once told me that he always gets MRIs on patients with work-related claims "to prove there's nothing wrong." The problem is that we rarely see a normal MRI reading on anyone over the age of 25—everyone has some "findings." As a result, we often see injured workers that have had acromioplasties, acromioclavicular resections, biceps tenodeses, SLAP repairs, and Bankart repairs performed in the absence of supporting evidence from the history and physical exam. The results are predictable.

Occupational disorders usually share some important features. They are thought to be a result of the patient's job. They keep the patient from doing his or her job properly and result in health care costs and loss of earnings for the patient. Furthermore, they raise the question of the patient's entitlement to reimbursement and compensation. For these reasons, occupational disorders create an undeniable conflict between (1) the desire of the patient to emphasize the magnitude of the shoulder disability in order to maximize the support they receive from the employer's insurance and (2) the desire of the employer and the employer's insurance to minimize their coverage for time off work, medical expenses, and long-term disability. The shoulder surgeon is often placed in middle of this conflict and asked to make time-consuming, imponderable, nonmedical determinations, such as the "percent of permanent partial impairment" or defining when the patient is "fixed and stable" or what percentage of the problem was "preexisting" or whether the problem would have arisen in the "absence of the patient's employment." The physician is

Continued

SENIOR EDITOR COMMENTARY—cont'd

rarely an expert in making these determinations, but each decision carries a major impact for the patient and the employer. Patients may feel threatened that the doctor will "cut them off," resulting in a termination of the disability payments that they depend on for family support. This may drive patients to undergo surgical procedures as a demonstration of the severity of the problem. Employers often want the injured worker back only if there are "no restrictions," which is usually a challenge in that we can rarely restore an injured shoulder to normal. Physicians are asked to "approve" various job modifications without detailed knowledge of what the modified job really entails.

In terms of the outcome of treatment, it has been repeatedly demonstrated that workers' compensation is an important comorbidity. Patients insured for on-the-job injuries have poorer outcomes than patients with other types of insurance coverage. Another fact must be recognized: if a patient is out of work for 1 year, the chances of going back to work are slim.

All of these considerations may disincline surgeons from taking on injured workers, but these individuals deserve the same thoughtful care we strive to deliver to all our patients. Our practice is to split the issues into (a) the job and (b) the shoulder. We are up front that no cuff surgery is likely to get a dockworker or carpenter back to 100%. Before considering any surgery, we make sure that the Labor and Industries or Worker's Compensation insurance is formally notified that the injury is likely to prevent full resumption of the preinjury job—without or with treatment. We encourage the parties to begin the process of vocational rehabilitation, again before any interventional treatment. Once the vocational issues are resolved ("this individual will not be able to return to work that requires overhead use of the arm"), we can devote our attention to defining expectations of treatment and trying our best to match these expectations with a realistic presentation of the outcomes we have achieved for patients with similar pathology.

Patients and surgeons faced with job-related injuries face challenges that are not encountered in the management of conditions unrelated to work. These differences need to be carefully considered in planning the evaluation and management.

CHAPTER 22

Tumors and Related Conditions

Robert H. Quinn, Ernest U. Conrad III

Musculoskeletal tumors represent approximately 10% of all orthopedic diagnoses and may present a formidable clinical challenge because of their varying presentations and biologic behavior. They may come to clinical attention either through incidental discovery or because of the resulting symptoms.

This chapter places emphasis on the initial assessment and evaluation along with a review of the salient radiographic and clinical features of the more common lesions, although without an in-depth discussion of any particular lesion. Also discussed are the principles of biopsy and surgical resection, the definition and significance of surgical margins, and the classification of resections and reconstructions.

Tumors involving the shoulder girdle are distinguished by the complex functional anatomy, which poses a challenge both to tumor resection and to the preservation of satisfactory function.

HISTORICAL REVIEW

The term *sarcoma* was used by Abernethy in the nineteenth century to describe tumors that have a firm and fleshy feel. *Sarcoma* refers to malignancies of mesenchymal or connective tissue origin. In the early period sarcomas were lesions of the extremities and were confused with osteomyelitis and other conditions. Even the most accomplished professors of surgery demonstrated little interest in recognizing sarcomas as malignancies distinct from carcinomas, and consequently little work involving classification or treatment was conducted.

An exception was Samuel W. Gross (1837-1884), a well-known surgeon, pathologist, and anatomist at the Jefferson Medical College in Philadelphia, who authored one of the first works that attempted to deal with the classification of various sarcomas, their salient features, indications for treatment, and prognosis. Gross was one of the first to identify sarcomas as a group of tumors distinctly different from carcinomas.[95] With the discovery and development of radiographs (in 1893), various lesions of bone were beginning to attract attention. Gross was one of the first to appropriately identify sarcomas as locally invasive extremity tumors, with frequent metastases to the lungs and that infrequently demonstrated lymphatic or hepatic metastases. In half the cases these unusual lesions were associated with a history of trauma and, according to Gross, they required radical amputation or resection. In retrospect his description of these first cases is remarkable for its clinical accuracy.

The scientific and technical developments in radiology, surgery, and medicine in the early twentieth century resulted in significant advances in orthopedics, which were reflected in improvements in the care of fractures, infections, and tumors. At that time, pathologists and surgeons, such as John Ewing (New York), Ernest A. Codman (Boston), and James Bloodgood (Baltimore), became interested in various tumors of bone.[122] The treatment of sarcomas varied greatly during those early years, but management of these unusual and difficult tumors gradually became more uniform as lesions were recognized histologically and radiographically as distinct entities. The same process of classifying sarcomas into histologic subtypes based on molecular subtype continues today.

Surgical treatment also improved with the developments in pathology and radiology. Aggressive ablative surgery was first recommended by Gross in his classic article on sarcomas[3] and was followed by various innovative surgical techniques.[97,120] Syme of Edinburgh popularized scapulectomy for malignant tumors in 1856.[231] Boris Linberg's classic article in 1928 regarding interscapulothoracic resections for malignancies of the shoulder joint reported on aggressive surgery for skeletal tumors with limb salvage.[124] Since these early reports, dramatic advances in imaging, chemotherapy, pathology, and surgical technique have resulted in improved survival and have allowed more limb-sparing surgery.

In the twentieth century Dallas B. Phemister (1882-1951) of the University of Chicago was one of the first surgeons in North America to demonstrate a special interest in limb-sparing surgery, or "limb salvage" as we know it today.[176] Phemister reviewed the American College of Surgeons' records for osteosarcoma in 1938 and found that only four of 86 extremity cases (4.6%) were treated with a limb-sparing resection.[176] Other reports of limb-sparing surgery at that time described variable results in terms of morbidity and mortality.[157,176] The popularity of limb-salvage surgery reached its zenith in the 1970s and 1980s with an emphasis on the need for appropriate tumor resection and good functional results.

The specialty of musculoskeletal oncology has crystallized from improvements in radiographic staging studies, chemotherapy, pathology, and surgery. One of the most significant developments involved the evolution of a histologic grading system for sarcomas of bone and soft tissue that allows assessment of a patient's prognosis according to the stage of the tumor and the proposed treatment.[39,72,96] This is one of the only systems that appropriately reflects a patient's prognosis based on the most significant determinants of that prognosis: the tumor's mitotic index, histologic subtype, and histologic pleomorphism. This system has demonstrated greater predictability than the previous grading systems. New complementary DNA (cDNA) genotyping of tumors has allowed improved histologic subtyping and the ability to identify molecular defects.[159]

Limb-sparing procedures, when properly executed, involve innovative reconstructive techniques to achieve reasonably functional results. This chapter briefly discusses the indications for, and assessment of, these procedures in terms of functional results and tumor recurrence.

Sarcomas are unusual tumors that require complex treatment. Their rarity and heterogeneity have been major reasons for their haphazard treatment in the past. The difficulties associated with assigning specific subtypes to sarcomas are evidenced by the fact that even among expert pathologists, the agreement rate for subtype is only 61% to 75%,[3,35] with the level of agreement varying by subtype. Recent advances in the molecular phenotyping of these tumors and their corresponding grade and molecular imaging[100] have allowed greater accuracy in tumor subtyping and have facilitated treatment decisions.

ANATOMY

In the shoulder girdle, anatomic considerations are amplified by the proximity of the brachial plexus and major vessels of the upper extremity to the humerus, scapula, and chest wall. It has also been suggested that the shoulder is more prone to intra-articular or pericapsular invasion by sarcomas than are other joints.[168] This may be due to the relatively small joint size or the thin synovial lining of the shoulder or because the biceps tendon provides a direct route into the joint.

Although an evaluation of musculoskeletal tumors frequently refers to the various anatomic compartments of the region involved, the exact anatomy of the compartments of the shoulder remains poorly defined. These compartments include the deltoid compartment, the posterior scapular compartment (supraspinatus, infraspinatus, teres minor, and teres major), the subscapular compartment (subscapularis), the anterior pectoral compartment (pectoralis minor and major), the anterior humeral compartment (biceps and coracobrachialis), the lateral humeral compartment (brachialis), the posterior humeral compartment (medial, lateral, and long head of the triceps), and the intra-articular compartment of the glenohumeral joint (Fig. 22-1). Little work has been done on the true containment or integrity of these compartments, and their boundaries are theoretical.

In skeletally immature patients, the physis often behaves as a barrier to tumor penetration. It is thought that the avascular environment of the physis as well as the presence of antiangiogenic factors inhibit tumor spread.[31,183] Although the vast majority of lesions do not cross the physis, there are a few notable exceptions. These include aneurysmal bone cyst, chondroblastoma, osteogenic sarcoma, and osteomyelitis.

Many anatomic clues are helpful in making the initial diagnosis in patients with an unknown musculoskeletal lesion. For instance, Ewing sarcoma typically develops in the shaft or diaphysis of the humerus; it occurs less frequently in the metaphysis of a long bone. On the other hand, the epicenter of an osteogenic sarcoma is rarely located in the shaft and is usually found in the metaphysis. Primary intra-articular tumors are rare, and an intra-articular lesion is more likely to represent a degenerative, traumatic, or other nonneoplastic diagnosis. Secondary involvement of a joint by an intraosseous malignancy is usually a late phenomenon associated with a longer diagnostic delay or a more aggressive lesion and a worse prognosis (see "Staging and Classification of Tumors" in this chapter).[72,216] Intra-articular malignancies require more complex extra-articular resections.

Particularly difficult locations for neoplasms in the shoulder girdle include those of the brachial plexus or lesions that involve the axillary or brachial vessels. Both the plexus and the axillary vessels are contained within their own sheaths, which can eventually be penetrated or infiltrated by an aggressive lesion. Primary tumors of the brachial plexus (malignant peripheral nerve sheath tumors) usually manifest on clinical examination as a brachial plexus nerve deficit. Any patient with distinct peripheral nerve symptoms associated with a shoulder mass should be assumed to have nerve involvement until it is demonstrated otherwise. Lesions involving the axillary or brachial vessels require magnetic resonance imaging (MRI) to define the precise extent of involvement.

To function normally, the shoulder depends on a well-innervated deltoid and rotator cuff in addition to adequate glenohumeral stability. The deltoid, like most muscle compartments, has anatomic subdivisions (acromial, clavicular, and scapular), but grossly it is a well-defined muscle that is easily resectable, although extremely difficult to reconstruct functionally after proximal humeral resections for bone tumors.

Perhaps the most important anatomic consideration involved in the treatment of shoulder tumors is the anatomy of the axillary nerve and its relationship to the deltoid and surgical exposure. Injuries to the axillary nerve during tumor resection or biopsy can result in partial or complete loss of deltoid function. Thus the

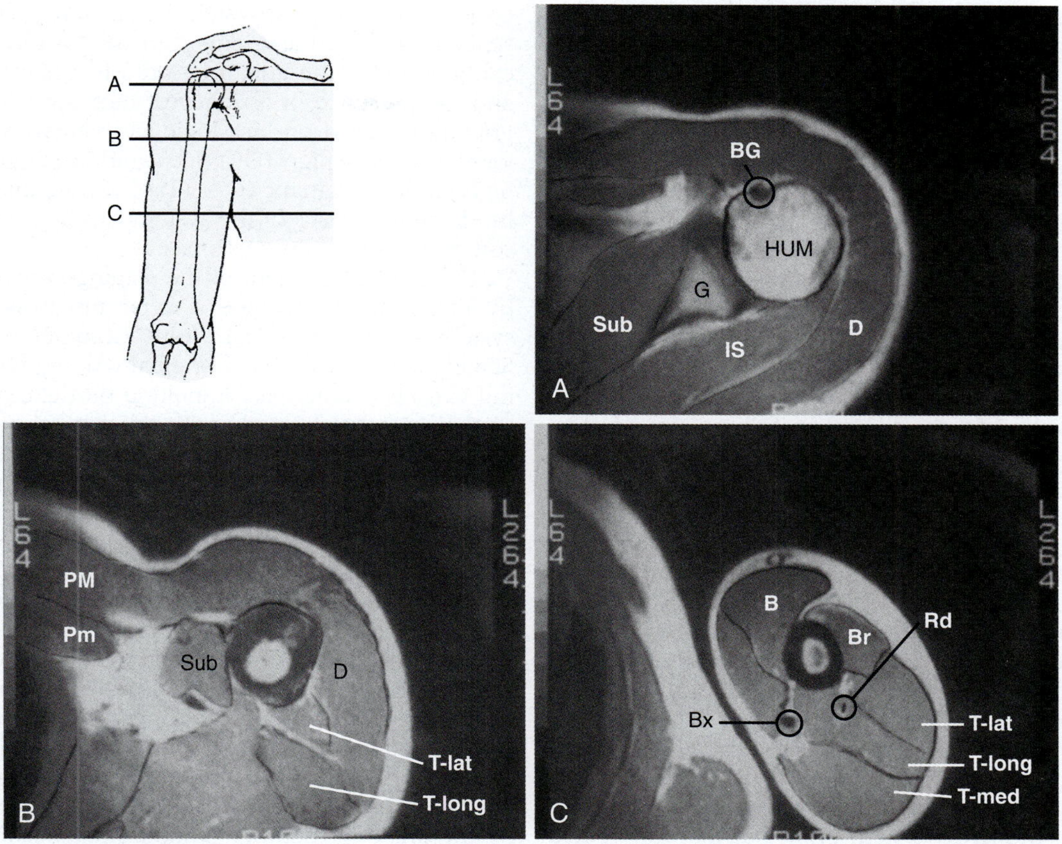

FIGURE 22-1: Shoulder anatomy on axial magnetic resonance imaging. **A,** Transverse image at the level of the glenoid. **B,** Transverse image at the level of the proximal humerus. **C,** Transverse image at the level of the midhumerus. B, biceps brachii; BG, bicipital groove; Br, brachialis; Bx, brachial vessels; D, deltoid; G, glenoid; IS, infraspinatus; Hum, humeral head; PM, pectoralis major; Pm, pectoralis minor; Rd, radial nerve; Sub, subscapularis; T-lat, triceps (lateral head); T-med, triceps (medial head); T-long, triceps (long head).

location of the axillary nerve at the time of biopsy and during resection has great significance. In general, the functional prognosis for tumors of the shoulder girdle is much better if the axillary nerve, deltoid, and rotator cuff are preserved. Glenohumeral joint mechanics can be replaced by shoulder arthroplasty, whereas reconstruction of the deltoid or rotator cuff is significantly more difficult.

STAGING AND CLASSIFICATION OF TUMORS

The early classification system for musculoskeletal tumors was popularized by Lichtenstein, who classified tumors according to basic histologic categories.[121] This descriptive histologic system was useful in identifying general trends in diagnosis and prognosis, but it had limited significance for determining adjuvant treatment (such as chemotherapy or radiation therapy) and prognosis. Today, most staging systems attempt to describe the anatomic extent of the disease as well as the presence or absence of metastases. They allow clinicians to compare clinical information in a clear and consistent manner, and the stage of the tumor enables the physician to provide prognostic information to the patient.

Benign Tumors of Bone

One system that stages benign tumors relies on the radiographic findings and uses an Arabic numeral system (as opposed to the Roman numeral system used for staging malignant disease). Benign disease is denoted as stage 1, 2, or 3, depending on whether the tumor is latent, active, or aggressive. A latent benign lesion does not show active growth and is confined to bone, with minimal or no cortical involvement. A classic example is a nonossifying fibroma. An active lesion shows active growth but is confined within the compartment defined by the surrounding natural boundaries. There may be extensive cortical damage. Aneurysmal bone cysts and chondroblastomas are typically considered to be active lesions. An aggressive lesion has the potential to penetrate or violate natural boundaries, such as cortical bone or periosteum, and to remain locally aggressive without metastasizing. A giant cell tumor of bone is an ideal example. Campanacci has applied this staging system specifically to giant cell tumors in an effort to guide treatment.[26]

Theoretically, only malignant tumors (by definition) can metastasize; however, a counterexample to this is presented by the ability of some histologically "benign" giant cell tumors to "metastasize" to the lung in a few cases.[213] Other aggressive benign tumors (chondroblastoma) have also demonstrated lung metastases in a small number of cases. Stage 2 and 3 lesions account for the vast majority of cases seen in clinical practice.

Although this staging system allows clinicians to characterize typical benign bone lesions, interobserver disagreement diminishes the clinical usefulness of the system in everyday practice.

Malignant Soft Tissue and Bone Tumors

The most commonly cited staging systems for soft tissue sarcomas are the Memorial Sloan-Kettering Cancer Center (MSK) system, the American Joint Committee on Cancer Staging System (AJCC), and the system of Enneking and colleagues.[72] The MSK and AJCC systems both take into account histologic grade, size, location, and the presence of metastases, but they are organized differently.[93,251] The highest category in both of these systems denotes the presence of metastases and therefore the worst prognosis. Critics of the AJCC system point out that the system has not been subjected to multiinstitution scrutiny and is based on an inordinate number of nonextremity tumors.[173]

One of the greatest contributions to today's improved treatment of sarcomas has been the development of a staging system that assists in the selection of treatment, assessment of prognosis, and evaluation of results. Such a classification system was introduced by Enneking in 1980,[72] adopted by the Musculoskeletal Tumor Society, and subsequently accepted, with modifications, by the National Institutes of Health Sarcoma Consensus Study Group as the staging system for all sarcomas.[39] It represents a combined assessment of the histologic, or surgical, grade (G), the anatomic site of primary disease (T), and the presence or absence of metastases (M). Surgical grading is based on histologic assessment, with a lesion identified as benign (G0), low-grade malignant (G1), or high-grade malignant (G2) (Tables 22-1 and 22-2). The fundamental basics of the system can be applied to both soft tissue and bone sarcomas.

The original concept of the staging system as devised by Enneking represented a departure from the staging system of the American Joint Committee for Cancer Staging and End Results,[4] originally designed for evaluating various carcinomas. Enneking thought that the AJCC system correlated poorly with the natural history of sarcomas. He described the salient features of sarcomas with reference to their distinction from carcinomas and the significance of those features regarding staging.[4,9,39]

In contrast to carcinomas, most sarcomas were described as having a similar natural history, one of progressive local invasion and eventual hematogenous pulmonary metastasis. The surgical treatment of sarcomas of the extremities is significantly different from that of lesions of the head and neck, retroperitoneum, trunk, and abdomen. Appropriate surgery with or without adjuvant radiation and chemotherapy remains the definitive treatment of the primary disease for most sarcomas.

The extent of disease in the Enneking system is defined by the anatomic setting. Compartmentalization, or compartmental escape, is an important characteristic of sarcomas, in contrast to previous classification systems and other tumors (carcinomas). A tumor is considered intracompartmental if it is limited by natural boundaries, such as fascia, bone, periosteum, or synovial tissue. A tumor is considered extracompartmental if it penetrates beyond its natural boundaries. It was postulated that the anatomic site (T) was the greatest factor in prognosis because it represented a composite of anatomic site, rate of growth, and delay in diagnosis. The primary extent of disease is initially limited by the natural boundaries of the anatomic

TABLE 22-1 Surgical Staging System: Bone Tumors

Stage	Tumor	Nodes	Metastasis	Grade	Stage Grouping
IA	T1	N0	M0	G1,2	Low grade
IB	T2	N0	M0	G1,2	Low grade
IIA	T1	N0	M0	G3,4	High grade
IIB	T2	N0	M0	G3,4	High grade
III	T3	N0	M0	Any G	—
IVA	Any T	N0	M1a	Any G	—
IVB	Any T	N1	Any M	Any G	—
IVB	Any T	Any N	M1b	Any G	—

Modified from Greene FL, Page DL, Fleming ID, Fritz A. AJCC Cancer Staging Manual. *New York: Springer-Verlag; 2002. Used with the permission of the American Joint Committee on Cancer.*

TABLE 22-2 Surgical Staging System: Soft Tissue Tumors

Stage	Tumor	Node	Metastasis	Grade	Grade	Stage Grouping
I	T1a	N0	M0	G1-2	G1	Low
I	T1b	N0	M0	G1-2	G1	Low
I	T2a	N0	M0	G1-2	G1	Low
I	T2b	N0	M0	G1-2	G1	Low
II	T1A	N0	M0	G3-4	G2-3	High
II	T1b	N0	M0	G3-4	G2-3	High
II	T2a	N0	M0	G3-4	G2-3	High
III	T2b	N0	M0	G3-4	G2-3	High
IV	Any T	N1	M0	Any G	Any G	High or low
IV	Any T	N0	M1	Any G	Any G	High or low

Modified from Greene FL, Page DL, Fleming ID, Fritz A. AJCC Cancer Staging Manual. *New York: Springer-Verlag; 2002. Used with the permission of the American Joint Committee on Cancer.*

compartment in which the lesion is located. Lesions that develop in poorly compartmentalized anatomic sites (such as the groin, popliteal fossa, or perivascular space) are, by the nature of that site, usually associated with a worse prognosis.

The histologic grading system proposed for sarcomas by the Enneking system was simplified to a two-grade system, of high-grade versus low-grade histology. There was no allowance for intermediate-grade histology because there was no intermediate surgical treatment. This system required the pathologist to classify all sarcomas as either high-grade or low-grade lesions, in contradiction to most classic sarcoma grading systems, which typically describe histology as high, low, or intermediate grade. Grading still remains a topic of controversy, especially for soft tissue sarcomas, which do occur as intermediate-grade lesions in certain cases.[52] Tumor grading should not be based on the histologic type alone. The theory that some histologic diagnoses always represent high-grade lesions and a worse prognosis, regardless of their histologic grade, is not generally accepted.

In the original Enneking staging system, the prognosis for a patient with regional lymph node involvement was believed to be as poor as that for a patient with pulmonary metastasis. Therefore lymph node metastasis and pulmonary metastasis were represented by stage III disease. Malignant bone tumors rarely metastasize to lymph nodes. The same holds true for soft tissue sarcomas with a few exceptions: epithelioid sarcoma, clear cell sarcoma, synovial sarcoma, and rhabdomyosarcoma.

Simplicity is both the strength and weakness of the Enneking staging system. By emphasizing high-grade versus low-grade histology and by limiting the number of tumor stages (to IA, IB, IIA, IIB, and III), this system is simple enough to be used by a wide group of specialists and allows a variety of treatments. Thus an IA lesion is malignant, low grade, and intracompartmental. A IIA lesion is high grade and intracompartmental, and IIB is high grade and extracompartmental. Critics of the Enneking system cite the major weaknesses as being the overly simplistic nature of a two-grade system, the fact that subcutaneous sarcomas are difficult to define, and the lack of statistical validation of the system.[173]

In the AJCC system, malignant tumors are denoted as stage I, II, III, or IV (see Table 22-1),[93] depending on the histologic grade (G), primary tumor extent (T), regional nodes (N), and the presence of metastases (M). Grade IV lesions are metastatic, regardless of the grade or anatomic site of the lesion. The system is somewhat different for soft tissue (see Table 22-2).[94]

The anatomic or surgical site classification (T) defines the primary lesion in relation to its position in the anatomic compartment of origin. Tumors are described as encapsulated (T0), intracompartmental (T1), or extracompartmental (T2). This designation is based on the Enneking compartmental theory, in which an anatomic compartment is described as a space or potential space defined by natural boundaries.[72] Tumors contained within an anatomic compartment can violate the boundaries of the compartment with growth—usually a sign of an aggressive benign or malignant tumor. Active benign tumors are typically well encapsulated (T0) and intracompartmental, whereas aggressive benign lesions may be poorly encapsulated but remain intracompartmental (T1). Low-grade malignant lesions are typically intracompartmental (T1), whereas extracompartmental lesions (T2) usually represent high-grade malignancies. Extracompartmental tumors can extend from one compartment into another or from one compartment into a surrounding extrafascial plane, or they can arise within a poorly compartmentalized, extracompartmental space. Poorly compartmentalized anatomic spaces include perivascular areas, such as the subsartorial space of the common femoral artery; the popliteal fossa; the antecubital fossa; or the midhand, midfoot, axilla, or groin.

The stage of the lesion and the surgical margin achieved by a procedure are associated with a certain local recurrence rate as described in the work of Enneking (see the "Surgical Margin" section and Table 22-5). These recurrence rates are based on an extensive retrospective review of the literature and reflect the risk of local recurrence after surgical resection without the use of adjuvant treatment. A benign aggressive (stage 3) lesion treated with a wide margin has a recurrence rate of 10% or less. High-grade malignant tumors (IIB), such as a typical osteosarcoma, require a wide surgical margin that includes a surrounding cuff of normal tissue to prevent a local recurrence.

After careful anatomic staging of the tumor, the appropriate surgical procedure can be predicted by considering the grade of the lesion and the extent of involvement at the primary site (the stage). The difficulty of that resection will also become apparent from this evaluation. A patient's prognosis and the risk of local recurrence can similarly be assessed by considering the grade of the tumor and the surgical margin achieved at the time of the surgical procedure. This *articulation*, or correlation of the tumor stage and the surgical margin, allows an assessment of the risk of local recurrence as a result of the procedure and margin achieved.

Thorough initial evaluation and staging, before treatment, remain the crucial ingredients for a successful outcome. A universally accepted staging classification system is important for directing patient care and for the adequate assessment of clinical results regarding disease-free status. Unfortunately, widespread intraobserver and interobserver disagreement continue to limit the clinical utility of musculoskeletal staging systems.

The staging evaluation involves an assessment by various radiographic studies to determine the precise anatomic extent of the primary disease, as well as whether regional or distant metastases have occurred. Typical staging studies include plain radiographs, along with technetium bone scan, computed tomography (CT), MRI, and other studies that better define a lesion's location. A total body bone scan is the best study to assess the extent of the primary bone lesion and the possibility of bony metastatic disease.[102,218,220] CT scans are excellent for visualizing cortical geography and bone involvement at the primary site on a two-dimensional plane.[72] CT scanning of the lung is routinely performed to assess possible pulmonary metastasis, and it is a more sensitive method than plain radiographs.

MRI is indicated for evaluating soft tissue disease, intramedullary bony disease, and spinal or pelvic lesions.[229] However, MRI does image the peripheral inflammatory reactive zone with a bright signal that might or might not contain a tumor. Similarly, the radiologist can overread soft tissue margins when interpreting malignancies, such as osteosarcoma and Ewing sarcoma[229] because of the inability to distinguish inflammation from tumor on MRI.

Imaging is especially important for tumors in the shoulder area because of the increased complexity of proximal humeral and shoulder girdle tumors.

Although MRI is clearly the optimal imaging modality for demonstrating anatomic detail and the extent of tumor involvement in both bone and soft tissue malignancies, positron emission tomography (PET), using fluorodeoxyglucose, is the preferred dynamic modality for assessing a tumor's degree of malignancy and response to chemotherapy (Fig. 22-2A to C). PET scans have the benefit of being quantifiable; that is, the technique can be validated to yield a specific numerical value, typically referred to as the *standard uptake value* (SUV), which gives an indication of the tumor's degree of malignancy and activity.[38] This assessment is valuable for the initial grading of tumors, evaluating the response to treatment, assessing heterogeneity, and assessing local recurrences.[207] Although PET scans for sarcoma applications are relatively early in their development, there is no doubt that they are valuable for assessing tumor grade, response to treatment, and the possibility of recurrence.

Molecular Biology

The staging systems described thus far use grade, anatomic location, size, and tumor extent to predict tumor behavior and, accordingly, patient survival. In the future it is likely that the greatest improvement in predicting the clinical outcome of musculoskeletal tumors will be made with regard to advances in molecular biology. Sarcomas pose a significant challenge because they comprise a rather diverse and heterogeneous group of neoplasms; additionally, chromosomal translocations are often rather complex and inconclusive.

Despite these inherent challenges, some useful information has been gathered that can help improve the understanding of tumor behavior. For example, overexpression of ErbB-2 or the multidrug resistance gene (*MDR-1*) has been associated with a poor prognosis for patients with osteosarcoma.[10,165] A number of translocations are associated with certain types of sarcomas (Table 22-3). The characteristic t(11;22)(q24;q12) chromosomal translocation resulting in the EWS-FLI1 transcription factor in Ewing sarcoma has been shown to be a positive predictor of survival independent of tumor site, stage, and size.[48] A gene expression signature has been identified in leiomyosarcomas that can predict the development of metastases.[115] High levels of an apoptosis

TABLE 22-3 Chromosomal Translocations

Tumor	Translocation
Ewing sarcoma	t(11;22)(q24;q12)
Synovial sarcoma	t(x;18)(p11;q11)
Extraskeletal myxoid	t(9;22)(q22;q12)
Chondrosarcoma	t(9;17)(q22;q11.2)
Clear cell sarcoma	t(12;22)(q13;q12)
Myxoid liposarcoma	t(12;16)(q13;p11)

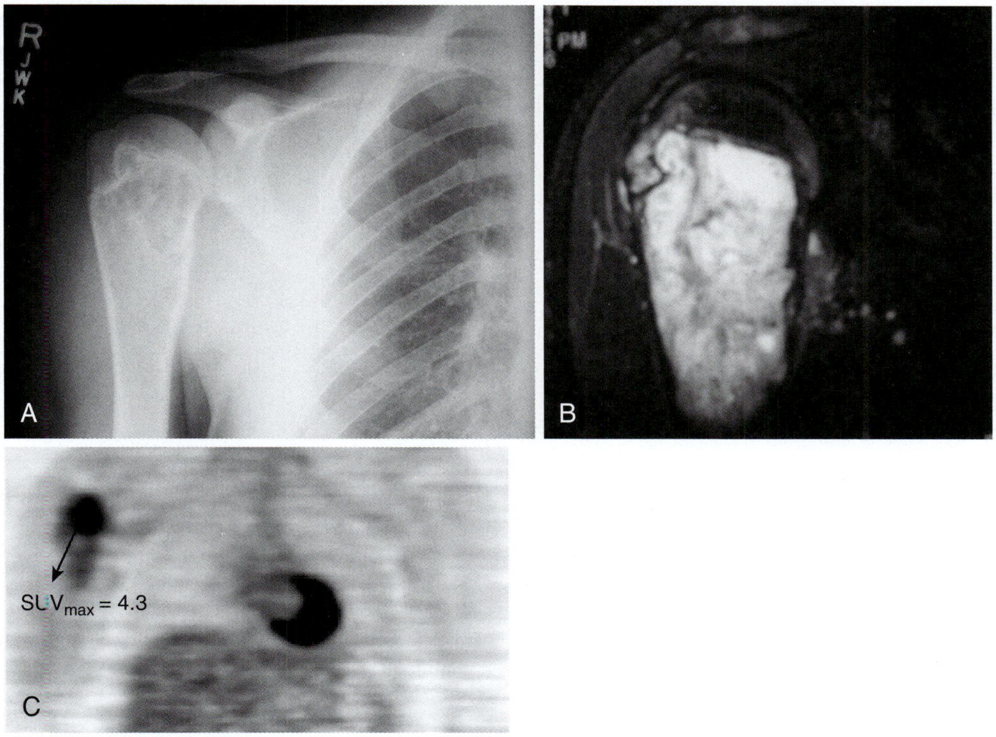

FIGURE 22-2: Pretreatment, preresection imaging of a 16-year-old boy with an osteogenic sarcoma of the proximal aspect of the right humerus. **A,** Plain radiograph. **B,** Magnetic resonance imaging. **C,** Positron emission tomography scan showing a maximum standard uptake value (SUV_{max}) of 4.3 (*arrow*).

inhibitor gene, survivin, can portend a poor prognosis for osteosarcoma patients.[167] Findings such as these might allow the clinician to tailor therapy based on the anticipated outcome of the disease.

Classification of Tumors

Although the histologic classification of tumors has limitations in predicting the prognosis and directing treatment,[100] it does serve a purpose in identifying tumor subtypes and their general tendencies. The most common lesions of bone, cartilage, and soft tissue are described with their general histologic, radiographic, and clinical characteristics. Clinical features, such as patient age, type of radiographic abnormality, and type of tissue involvement can, in many cases, lead to a significant and limited differential diagnosis.

Benign Osseous Lesions

Osteoid Osteoma

Benign osseous lesions of the shoulder are uncommon. Only 10% to 15% of cases of osteoid osteoma and osteoblastoma occur in the shoulder, and when they do occur, they favor the proximal end of the humerus or glenoid.[66,105] Osteoid osteoma typically displays the classic symptom of night pain, which is relieved by salicylates. Radiographically, it is characterized by a large area of reactive bone surrounding a small, subcentimeter radiolucent nidus. On technetium bone scan, osteoid osteoma has impressive increased activity, and the central nidus can be visualized as a distinct cortical hole on CT scanning or tomography. Plain x-ray tomography can also be an effective diagnostic tool for localizing many osteoid osteomas. The differential diagnosis consists of osteoblastoma, osteomyelitis (Brodie abscess), intraosseous ganglion, stress fracture, and bone island. Histologically, this lucent nidus is a well-demarcated, small area of immature and very active osteoblastic tissue. Preoperative localization is an extremely important strategy to prevent intraoperative difficulty in locating these lesions and thus in minimizing local recurrences.

Treatment of an osteoid osteoma may be nonoperative or operative. These tumors will spontaneously involute over time and often can be successfully managed with nonsteroidal antiinflammatory drugs. In reality, however, involution can take many years and few patients are willing (or able) to tolerate such long-term use of nonsteroidal antiinflammatory drugs. CT-guided percutaneous radiofrequency ablation has been popularized as a successful, minimally invasive method of treating osteoid osteomas.[224] Curettage with bone grafting remains the gold standard and recurrence is rare with proper removal of the tumor; however, surgical localization can prove challenging in many anatomic locations.

Osteoblastoma

Some clinicians regard osteoblastoma as a larger version of osteoid osteoma (i.e., giant osteoid osteoma), and it is typified by a large lucent area (>2 cm in diameter) of osteoblastic tissue surrounded by a thin, sclerotic reactive rim of bone.[66] Radiographically, osteoblastoma is generally seen as a lucent lesion that has expanded the overlying cortex into a thin rim. The most common locations include the spine, femur, and tibia. As with osteoid osteoma, osteoblastoma may be difficult to localize radiographically and requires careful preoperative imaging to prevent recurrence. Osteoblastoma, unlike osteoid osteoma, also occurs in an aggressive (stage 3) form that is less well defined radiographically, has a high recurrence rate, and can have a histologic appearance that is difficult to distinguish from low-grade osteosarcoma. Technetium bone scanning and CT scans are good imaging techniques for examining both of these lesions.

BOX 22-1. Signs and Symptoms of Sarcoma

Bone
Bone pain
Night pain
Pain unrelated to joint motion
Tender soft tissue mass

Soft Tissue
Firm mass
Nontender mass
Large (>5 cm) or enlarging
Deep or subfascial

Myositis Ossificans

Myositis ossificans is a benign, reactive, bone-forming process that develops intramuscularly or in the areolar tissues (the tendon, ligament, capsule, and fascia) adjacent to bone. It can occur with or without a history of trauma; without trauma, it may be referred to as *pseudomalignant myositis ossificans* of the soft parts.[162] The pseudomalignant form is typically seen as a symptomatic enlarging soft tissue mass that develops in the second decade of life, and it occurs in the shoulder in 15% of cases.

The typical radiographic appearance is an osseous density in soft tissue that demonstrates peripheral radiographic maturity or margination of the mass, separated from adjacent cortical bone by a narrow zone of uninvolved soft tissue. This characteristic histologic margination or zonation phenomenon (peripheral maturity) is a reflection of the more active (immature) osteoblastic tissue being located centrally in the lesion; this is in contrast to osteosarcoma, which demonstrates the most active histologic area peripherally. Isotope scans of myositis ossificans demonstrate high uptake peripherally that can continue for 8 to 12 weeks or until spontaneous maturation occurs. Before excision, a mature lamellar pattern should be seen radiographically; surgery before that time is associated with a high recurrence rate.

In some patients myositis ossificans may be confused with osteosarcoma or a soft tissue sarcoma, but these tumors do not demonstrate the same zonation or peripheral margination phenomenon, nor do they have the same radiographic characteristics. When the proper diagnosis is uncertain, optimal management includes a complete radiographic evaluation and careful clinical observation rather than a hasty or premature excision or biopsy (which can be difficult to interpret).[42] The radiographic differential diagnosis for myositis ossificans includes extraosseous or parosteal osteosarcoma, synovial sarcoma, vascular lesions, and calcification of soft tissue secondary to necrosis, inflammation, or infection.

Malignant Osseous Lesions

Osteosarcoma

Osteosarcoma is the most common malignant primary bone tumor after myeloma. It is the most common primary sarcoma occurring in the shoulder, followed by Ewing sarcoma and chondrosarcoma. Osteosarcoma demonstrates a bimodal age distribution, with the highest peak occurring in the teenage years (representing primary tumors) and a second peak in the seventh decade (largely representing secondary tumors).

Classic osteosarcoma is a high-grade, aggressive tumor that develops in metaphyseal bone, typically as a stage IIB lesion and usually with an extraosseous soft tissue component present at initial evaluation.[66,106,121] The typical patient experiences intrinsic bone pain at night that is typically unrelated to activity (Box 22-1). The average duration of symptoms at initial assessment is 3 to 6 months, reflecting the subtle nature of the preliminary symptoms and the need for early recognition of intraosseous pain and night pain as warning symptoms.[65,244]

Approximately 10% to 15% of all osteosarcomas occur in the proximal part of the humerus, whereas 1% to 2% develop in the scapula or clavicle.[41,74,106,121] The typical radiograph for osteosarcoma has a sunburst or osteoblastic pattern, with penetration of the adjacent cortex (Fig. 22-3A). Differential diagnosis includes aneurysmal bone cyst, Ewing sarcoma, osteoblastoma, giant cell tumor, and metastatic disease. Osteosarcomas usually have increased activity on bone scan (Fig. 22-3B), and a hemorrhagic soft tissue mass is seen on CT scan (Fig. 22-3C) and MRI (Fig. 22-3D). Arteriography is no longer the technique of choice for evaluating soft tissue involvement, but it may be performed to evaluate major vessel involvement or the response to intraarterial chemotherapy (Fig. 22-3E).[40] In addition to the classic type, variants of osteosarcoma include telangiectatic (vascular) osteosarcoma,[145] secondary osteosarcoma (Paget disease or radiation induced), and various low-grade lesions, such as periosteal and parosteal osteosarcoma.[74,236,237] The basic histologic criterion for the diagnosis of osteosarcoma includes a malignant spindle cell stroma that directly produces neoplastic osteoid.[41,106,121] The overall survival rate at 5 years for patients with osteosarcoma is approximately 70% with appropriate chemotherapy and surgery.[160] Prognostic factors for survival include age, the stage at presentation, and the degree of histologic necrosis at resection (following neoadjuvant chemotherapy).[47]

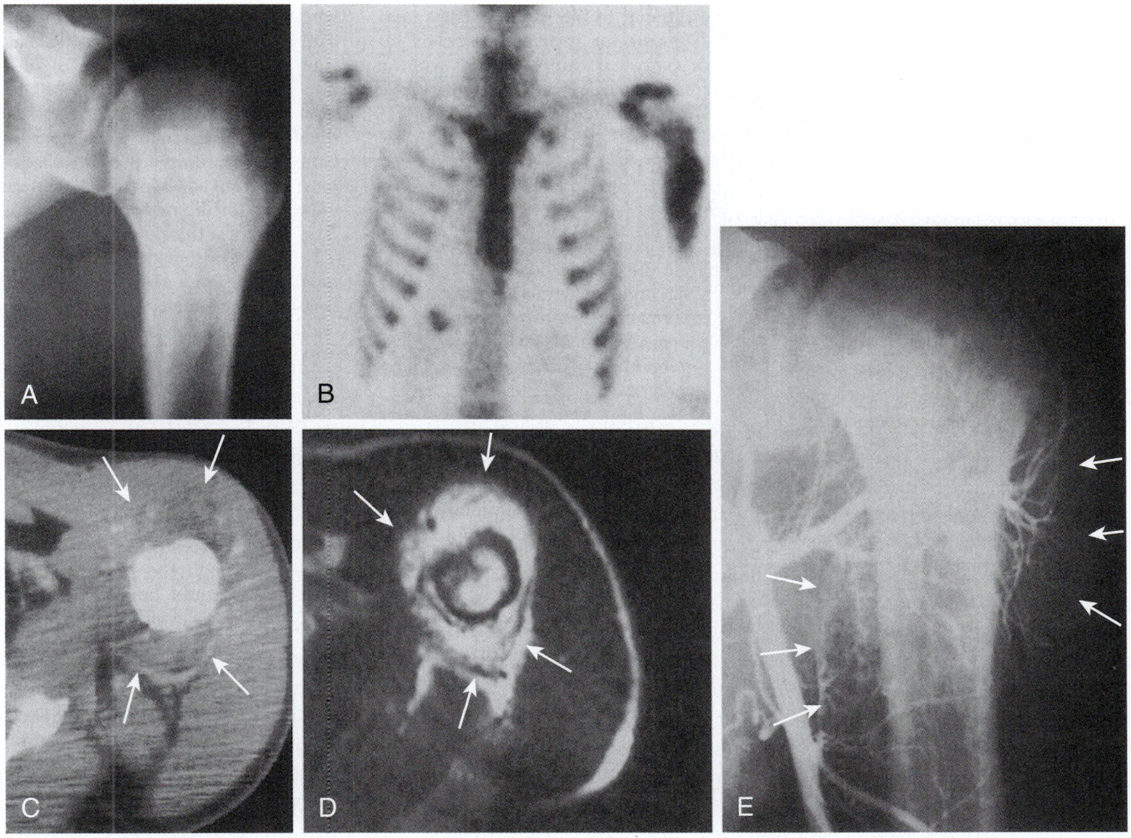

FIGURE 22-3: A, Plain radiograph of an osteosarcoma of the proximal end of the humerus, suggesting minimal soft tissue involvement by tumor. **B,** Bone scan of the same lesion, demonstrating significant extension proximally and distally in the humerus. **C,** A computed tomography scan of the same patient does not demonstrate the extent of soft tissue extension (*arrows*). **D,** Magnetic resonance imaging through the same area of the humerus demonstrating circumferential soft tissue involvement (*arrows*), with much better visualization than was achieved using computed tomography scan. **E,** Arteriogram obtained for intraarterial chemotherapy that demonstrates some soft tissue disease (*arrows*) but with less sensitivity than magnetic resonance imaging.

Benign Cartilaginous Lesions

Osteochondroma

The incidence of cartilaginous tumors in the shoulder is second only to those occurring about the pelvis.[59] Solitary osteochondroma is the most common benign tumor of the shoulder; approximately one fourth of all osteochondromas occur in the proximal part of the humerus. Osteochondromas actually represent a developmental abnormality arising from the peripheral growth plate and are typically active, benign (stage 2) lesions during skeletal growth. The plain radiograph is usually diagnostic in demonstrating a smooth excrescence of metaphyseal cancellous bone that is confluent and continuous with normal metaphyseal bone (Fig. 22-4).

Osteochondromas can appear as pedunculated, stalk-like lesions or as flat, sessile lesions. These tumors are typically diagnosed in the skeletally immature individual. Treatment of a solitary osteochondroma involves excision through the base of the lesion. In the sessile form care should be taken to excise the cartilaginous cap to prevent a recurrence. The most common complication of excision is iatrogenic injury to the adjacent growth plate or neurovascular structures at the time of excision. Adequate

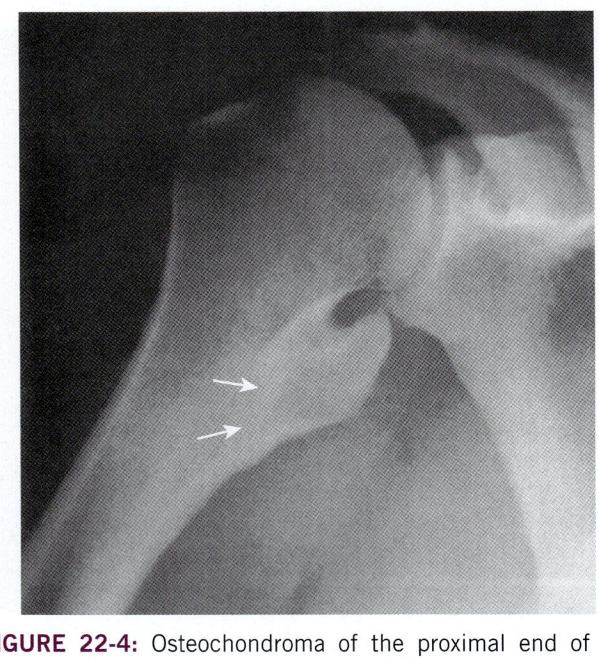

FIGURE 22-4: Osteochondroma of the proximal end of the humerus demonstrating confluence of normal metaphyseal bone and the lesion (*arrows*).

surgical exposure should be emphasized, especially for proximal humeral lesions, which are usually large and adjacent to the major neurovascular bundle.

Concern regarding a possible secondary chondrosarcoma can arise in adult patients with pain, an enlarging soft tissue mass, a thickened cartilaginous cap (>1 to 2 cm), or intraosseous bony erosions. Dedifferentiation is rare and associated with a poor prognosis.[226] The risk of a secondary chondrosarcoma arising out of an osteochondroma is approximately 1% per lesion, although rates as high as 10% to 30% have been reported regarding secondary malignancy in patients with multiple hereditary exostoses.[206]

Chondroblastoma

Chondroblastoma, or Codman tumor, is an unusual benign cartilaginous tumor that occurs in the skeletally immature in the proximal humeral epiphysis (in 25% of cases) as a round or oval lesion containing fine calcifications surrounded by a reactive bony margin.[44,103,114,184] Histologically it consists of aneurysmal tissue, chicken-wire calcifications, and immature paving-stone chondroblasts. Chondroblastoma occurs as an active, benign stage 2 lesion, although it also has a more aggressive stage 3 form. In very rare cases metastasis to the lungs has been demonstrated.

Treatment usually involves extensive intralesional curettage, which results in a large subchondral defect of the humeral head that requires bone graft to prevent subchondral and cartilaginous collapse. An adjuvant agent, such as hydrogen peroxide or cryotherapy, can help reduce local recurrence rates.[239] The radiographic appearance of this epiphyseal lesion is usually typical (Fig. 22-5A and B). The differential diagnosis is dependent on age and includes other benign bone tumors in children and giant cell tumor, chondrosarcoma, or metastatic adenocarcinoma in adults.

Periosteal Chondroma

Periosteal chondroma is another benign cartilaginous lesion of the proximal end of the humerus that is usually located just proximal to the deltoid insertion of the lateral humeral shaft. It typically manifests as a minimally symptomatic or asymptomatic mass that is radiographically evident as a sessile lesion with a distinct, well-defined margin of reactive cortex underlying the radiolucent cartilaginous mass.[118] Marginal excision results in a cortical defect of the humerus that might or might not require bone grafting. There may be recurrence following simple curettage. The differential diagnosis includes periosteal osteosarcoma, which does not have the well-defined underlying sclerotic cortex. Periosteal osteosarcoma is a more aggressive intracortical lesion that can extend into the medullary canal in a small percentage of cases.

Enchondroma

Enchondroma is a benign, central cartilaginous lesion that is most commonly found in the small tubular bones of the hand but which also occurs in the proximal end of the humerus in 10% to 15% of cases.[13,59,107] Enchondromas are usually solitary, but multiple, typically unilateral lesions with extensive deformity that can be seen in Ollier disease (enchondromatosis) (Fig. 22-6) or Maffucci syndrome (enchondromatosis with multiple hemangiomas of skin or viscera, or both).

Treatment of an enchondroma is based on a thorough assessment of the presence of pain and the risk of

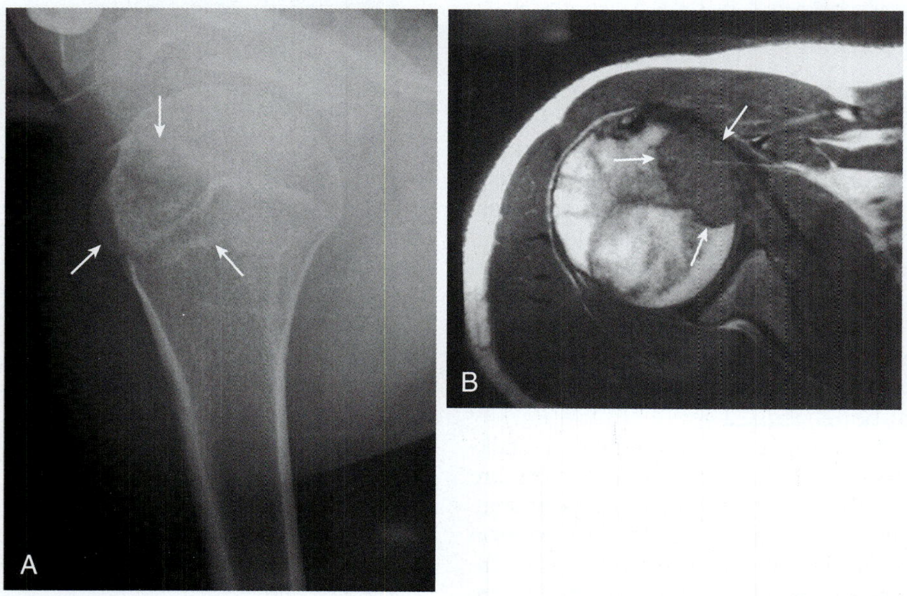

FIGURE 22-5: A, Plain radiograph of a chondroblastoma of the proximal humerus in a 13-year-old boy. Note the typical appearance of the tumor as it crosses the physis. **B,** Axial magnetic resonance imaging demonstrating the extent of bone involvement of this round lesion (*arrow*).

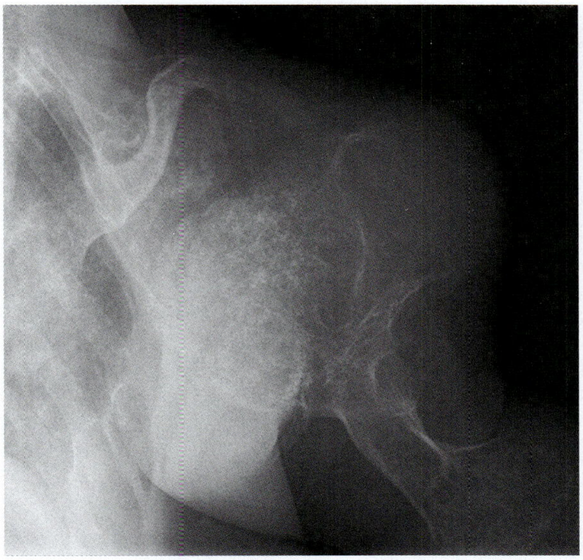

FIGURE 22-6: Plain radiograph of the humerus of an 8-year-old girl with Ollier disease showing the dramatic extent of deformity seen in association with an enchondroma.

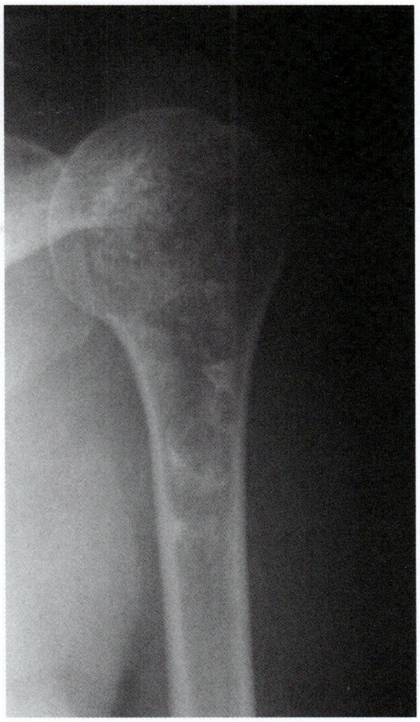

FIGURE 22-7: Plain radiograph of a 45-year-old woman with rotator cuff symptoms and an incidental benign enchondroma. There was no involvement or erosion of the endosteal cortical surface.

fracture. Lesions that are painless can be observed with serial radiographs. If a patient develops pain, or there is evidence of radiographic progression, then reevaluation is essential. The risk of malignant transformation of solitary lesions is extremely small. By contrast, the risk of malignant transformation is 25% to 30% in Ollier disease and even higher in Maffucci syndrome. Malignant degeneration is usually heralded by increased or new pain or by a sharp increase in tumor size.

It is common for enchondromas of the proximal humerus to be encountered incidentally during a work-up for shoulder pain. Unexplained shoulder pain in the presence of an enchondroma can provide a diagnostic dilemma. As enchondromas are rarely symptomatic, every effort should be made to rule out other sources of pain prior to treating the enchondroma. When an enchondroma occurs adjacent to a joint that is symptomatic for degenerative reasons, clinical assessment of bone pain related to the enchondroma may be difficult. This scenario is not uncommon, and it makes the initial evaluation of intraosseous cartilage tumors difficult. The typical radiographic appearance of a benign enchondroma is that of a central lucent lesion with a well-defined bony margin and intrinsic calcifications. Figure 22-7 shows such a lesion in a 45-year-old woman with rotator cuff symptoms and a calcified benign cartilage lesion.

Malignant Cartilaginous Lesions

Chondrosarcoma

Low-grade chondrosarcomas may be difficult to distinguish from enchondromas. Clinical and radiographic clues include pain, large size, increasing size, and full-thickness cortical penetration, particularly with periosteal reaction and/or a soft tissue mass (Fig. 22-8A and B). Technetium bone scans are typically moderately hot for both enchondroma and low-grade chondrosarcoma and are not helpful in distinguishing one from the other. The histologic differentiation between enchondroma and low-grade chondrosarcoma is difficult and requires radiographic correlation.

Microscopic evaluation of low grade cartilage lesions is not diagnostic in a large percentage of cases. Histologic characteristics that suggest malignancy include cellularity, pleomorphism, and evidence of mitotic activity, such as double-nucleated lacunae. These findings are subtle, and the histologic evidence for low-grade chondrosarcoma versus enchondroma is often incomplete and inconclusive.[65,112] This confusion has led to the use of the term "grade one-half" chondrosarcoma to describe cartilage tumors that are histologically borderline between low-grade chondrosarcoma and benign enchondroma.

Primary chondrosarcoma is more commonly seen in the middle to later decades of life, and its incidence in the shoulder is second to that in the pelvis or hip joint.[19,59,87,131,182] It is the most common primary bone malignancy to arise in the coracoid process.[163] These tumors typically manifest as intraosseous lesions with poorly defined margins and faint intrinsic calcifications. The differential diagnosis includes enchondroma, osteosarcoma, and metastases. Less commonly, a primary chondrosarcoma arises from the surface of a bone or joint. Its clinical and radiographic appearance is very subtle, and a diagnostic delay of 6 to 12 months is not uncommon.

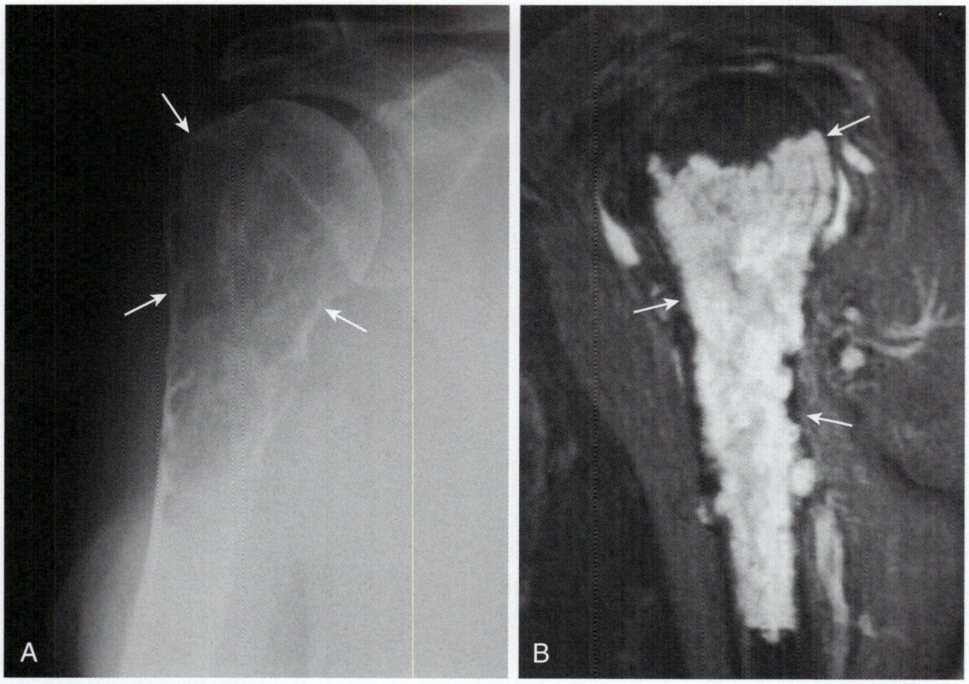

FIGURE 22-8: **A,** Plain radiograph of a 55-year-old man with intrinsic intraosseous pain. The distinct endosteal cortical erosions (*arrows*) suggest a low-grade chondrosarcoma. **B,** Sagittal magnetic resonance imaging of the proximal end of the humerus, demonstrating high signal intensity of cartilage and the extent of intraosseous involvement (*arrows*) by this low-grade chondrosarcoma.

Secondary chondrosarcoma accounts for approximately 25% of all chondrosarcomas, and may be found in patients with a preexisting enchondroma, osteochondroma, multiple enchondromatosis (Ollier disease),[112,114,210] or hereditary multiple osteocartilaginous exostoses.[82]

High-grade lesions are more invasive, have a higher metastatic rate, and usually occur in long-standing lesions as a dedifferentiated chondrosarcoma.[28,42,80,141]

Low-grade chondrosarcomas may be treated surgically with extended curettage utilizing adjuvant and grafting or cementation. High-grade tumors are treated with wide surgical resection. Most chondrosarcomas are considered to be relatively resistant to chemotherapy and radiation therapy, and as a result, uncontaminated surgical resections are an essential part of their treatment.

Synovial Dysplasias

Cartilaginous loose bodies typically arise out of a proliferative synovium in a reactive metaplastic process known as *synovial chondromatosis* (or osteochondromatosis).[150] This process most commonly affects large joints (the knee, elbow, shoulder, and hip) in young adults and results in multiple small, cartilaginous, intra-articular loose bodies as the process matures. In the few cases in which the nodules form a compact mass of cartilage, this may be confused with a low-grade, periarticular or juxta-articular chondrosarcoma. An intra-articular location favors the benign diagnosis of synovial chondromatosis; consequently, sometimes one of the preoperative goals is to determine whether the location is intra-articular or extra-articular. In such cases MRI or CT scan with or without arthrography might pinpoint the exact site of involvement. Synovial chondromatosis is typically a slowly progressive, degenerative disease that ultimately leads to joint destruction. It requires aggressive total synovectomy to prevent persistence or recurrence, and in older patients with degenerative disease, it is well treated with joint excision and replacement. A few reports have associated malignant transformation with long-standing synovial chondromatosis.[156,200]

Another disease associated with proliferating synovium is pigmented villonodular synovitis.[185] It is generally associated with a boggy, inflammatory synovitis, with or without bony erosions, in adolescents or young adults. Histologically, it is an aggressive synovial-histiocytic process that defies description as inflammatory or neoplastic. Treatment for the diffuse form of the disease requires aggressive complete synovectomy. Various forms of radiation therapy have been used in some centers, with acceptable early clinical results.[222] Occasionally, joint degeneration is severe and arthroplasty is recommended.[233]

Miscellaneous Intraosseous Tumors

Simple Bone Cyst

Simple bone cysts, or unicameral bone cysts, occur most commonly in children between the ages of 4 and 12 years. Figure 22-9A shows a simple cyst with a healing pathologic fracture in the humerus of an 8-year-old. The patient remained symptomatic after fracture healing and underwent percutaneous aspiration and injection of autogenous

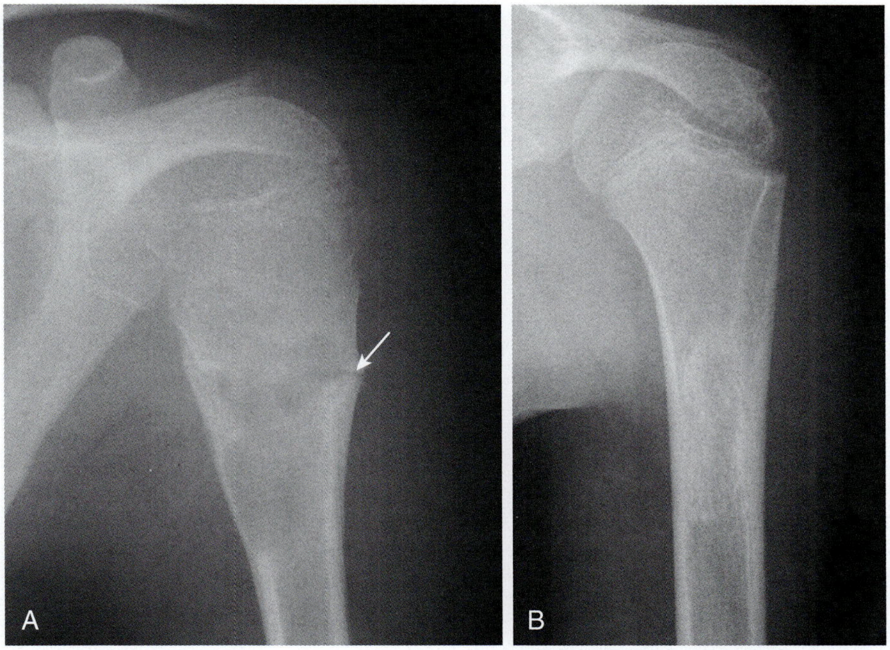

FIGURE 22-9: A, Anteroposterior radiograph of a simple cyst in an 8-year-old boy with a healing pathologic fracture (*arrow*). Note the thin and expanded cortical bone. **B,** At 2-year follow-up, the bone has completely remodeled.

bone marrow and demineralized bone matrix, resulting in complete resolution of the cyst (Fig. 22-9B). Simple bone cysts are well-defined, central radiolucent lesions arising in the metaphysis adjacent to the physis (active) and, with maturation, migrate distally into the diaphysis (latent). Occasionally, a fragment of the cyst wall breaks off and floats into the fluid-filled cyst cavity. Radiographically, this appearance is known as the *fallen-leaf sign*. Simple bone cysts typically involve the proximal part of the humerus (in 50% of cases) and contain straw-colored fluid; they may be confused with an aneurysmal bone cyst or, less often, with fibrous dysplasia.[63,94,129,157,166,203]

The treatments of choice for symptomatic lesions consist of pressure measurement of the cyst, aspiration, and either intraosseous steroid injection or injection of demineralized bone matrix with autogenous bone marrow.[109,194,203] The result is complete healing of the cystic area in approximately 50% of cases and partial healing in 45%.[194] Complete repair after injection is most common in more inactive cysts with lower pressure. Varying results in more recent reports have cast some doubt on the efficacy of steroid injections for simple bone cysts, especially when associated with a venogram at the time of the injection of dye into the lesion.[94] A comparison of injection of steroids versus autologous bone marrow versus allogeneic bone graft has yielded similar success rates; however, multiple steroid injections are often necessary to achieve healing.[32,166]

Recurrence or persistence of the cyst after surgical curettage and bone grafting occurs in approximately 30% of cases. Some diagnostic overlap occurs between aneurysmal and simple cysts in children because some simple cysts can have hemorrhagic fluid and yet do not contain aneurysmal tissue. In general, if a cyst fractures, it is advisable to allow sufficient time for fracture healing before initiating treatment. This can abrogate the need for internal fixation.

Aneurysmal Bone Cyst

Aneurysmal bone cysts are not uncommon in the proximal end of the humerus, but because of their widespread occurrence as a secondary lesion engrafted on other tumors (simple cysts, giant cell tumors, chondroblastomas, or osteoblastomas), the true incidence is unknown. The molecular biology of aneurysmal bone cysts has been elucidated and appears to involve upregulation of oncogenes.[164] The radiographic hallmark is that of a lucent, expansile metaphyseal lesion. MRI shows the presence of fluid-fluid levels (Fig. 22-10). Treatment includes curettage plus bone grafting,[14,64,148] which is associated with a recurrence rate of 20% to 30%. Open growth plates and young age are associated with a higher recurrence risk.[86] Aneurysmal bone cysts can have an aggressive appearance, and a careful biopsy should be performed before curettage to exclude the possibility of telangiectatic osteosarcoma. It may be extremely difficult to distinguish these two entities on frozen section alone. In such cases definitive treatment should be delayed until a final diagnosis is rendered.

Fibrous Dysplasia

Fibrous dysplasia is a congenital dysplasia of bone that often surfaces as a painful lesion secondary to pathologic fracture, microfracture, or the subtle, intrinsic, diaphyseal weakness resulting from pathologic bone. The typical plain radiograph demonstrates a ground-glass density with cortical thickening. Figure 22-11A and B show the plain radiograph and CT scan, respectively, of the humerus of a 20-year-old woman with severe polyostotic fibrous dysplasia. She had a history of chronic pseudarthroses (see Fig. 22-11A) that had persisted despite bracing. When associated with symptoms or pathologic fracture, diaphyseal involvement usually requires intramedullary fixation rather than bone grafting because cancellous bone graft is consistently consumed by the dysplastic process and is ineffective in resolving the weakened dysplastic bone. There may be a role for medical therapy, namely bisphosphonates, in alleviating pain; however, randomized clinical studies are lacking.[29] Histologically, fibrous dysplasia demonstrates a furnace of dysplastic bone activity with similar, impressive increased activity on bone scan.[99,101,108,123,227] Immature islands of bone are seen in a fibrous stroma without osteoblastic rimming.

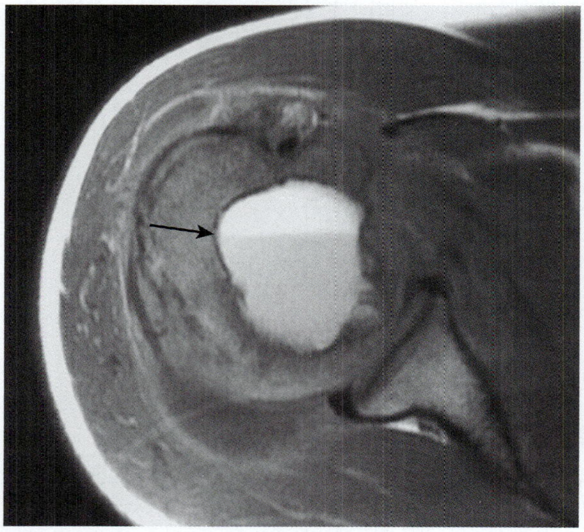

FIGURE 22-10: Axial magnetic resonance imaging of an aneurysmal bone cyst of the humeral head shows the presence of a fluid-fluid level (*arrow*).

Nonossifying Fibroma

Nonossifying fibroma is a benign fibrous lesion that appears radiographically as an eccentric, well-defined, lucent lesion with a scalloped border abutting the adjacent cortex (Fig. 22-12). It is found more commonly in the lower than the upper extremity. When the lesion is smaller than 4 cm, it may be referred to as a *fibrous cortical defect*. When longer than 5 cm or occupying more than half the transverse diameter of the bone, these lesions are at risk for pathologic fracture. The majority of nonossifying fibromas heal spontaneously and require no treatment. Treatment is reserved for lesions with atypical radiographs (which require biopsy) or for symptomatic or larger lesions that require treatment to prevent a pathologic fracture.[5]

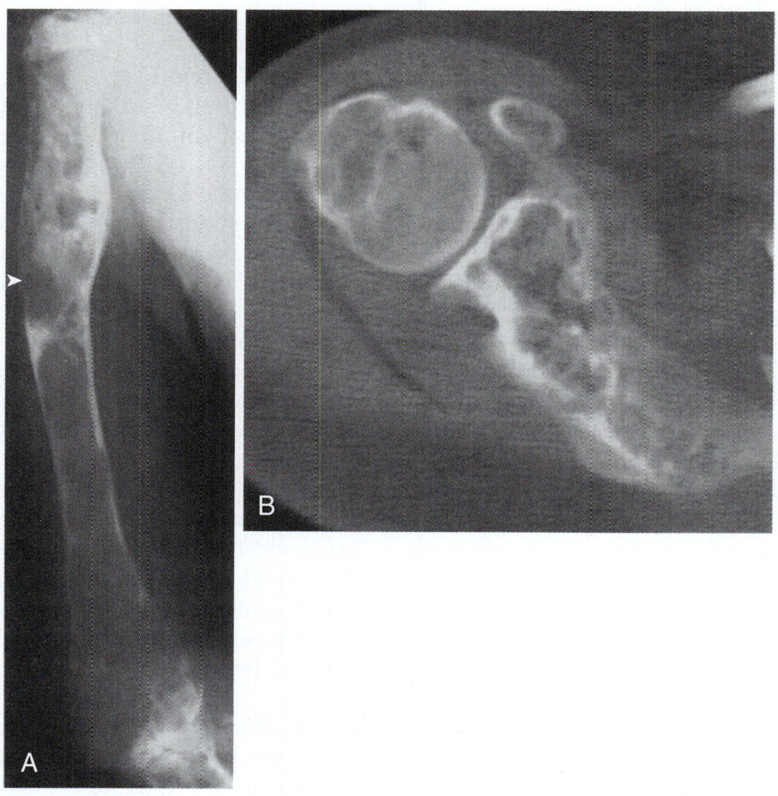

FIGURE 22-11: A, A 20-year-old woman with fibrous dysplasia of the humerus and a chronic pseudarthrosis (*arrow*) resistant to bracing. **B,** Computed tomography scan of the proximal part of the humerus and scapula in the same patient, demonstrating part of her extensive polyostotic disease involving the humerus and scapula, which spared the glenohumeral joint.

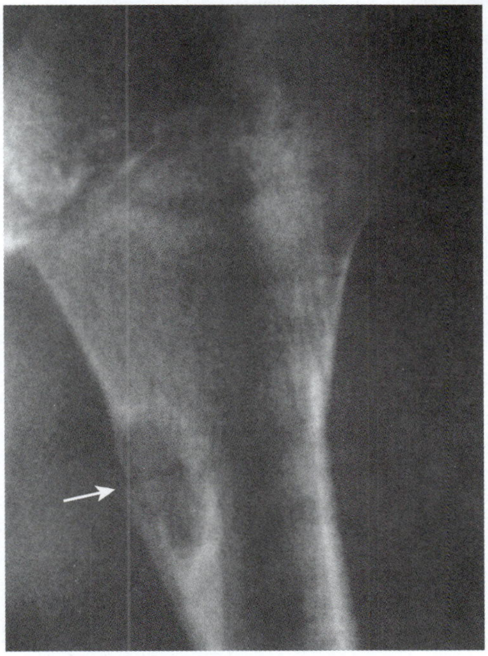

FIGURE 22-12: A small eccentric, juxtacortical nonossifying fibroma manifested as a pathologic fracture (*arrow*).

Giant Cell Tumor

Giant cell tumor (GCT) of bone is a benign, locally aggressive lesion. Although classically considered a benign tumor, in less than 3% of cases GCT of bone has the potential for metastatic pulmonary spread.[37,90,128,138,140,142,174,175] GCT of bone is a common lesion in people between 20 and 40 years of age and develops primarily in the distal end of the femur or proximal part of the tibia (in 60% to 70% of cases). It can also occur in the proximal end of the humerus in 5% to 10% of cases.

GCT is a radiolucent, epiphyseal-metaphyseal tumor that most commonly has a distinct bony margin and is often associated with extensive subchondral bone erosion.[234] There can be bony expansion, cortical destruction, or frank extension of the tumor mass into the soft tissues. Periosteal reaction is uncommon unless there has been a prior pathologic fracture. Although most cases involve solitary lesions, the rare diagnosis of multifocal GCT of bone is usually associated with hand lesions and a slightly younger population. The radiographic differential diagnosis in an adult includes aneurysmal bone cyst, brown tumor of hyperparathyroidism, metastatic adenocarcinoma, lymphoma, chondrosarcoma, intraosseous ganglion, and osteomyelitis.

GCT is typically a Campanacci stage 2 active lesion (in 60% of cases) but is also found as a more aggressive stage 3 tumor in 20% of cases. Treatment of GCT includes curettage with margin extension. The local recurrence rate after curettage alone is 20% to 30% for active lesions versus 5% after extended margin curettage.[26,37,43,89,147]

Margin extension may be achieved mechanically (through burring), or with the use of an adjuvant, such as phenol, bone cement (cementation), or liquid nitrogen (cryotherapy).

Reticuloendothelial Tumors

Tumors of reticuloendothelial origin include a category of intraosseous lesions that arise from marrow stem cells and lesions of similar histology. They are also referred to as round cell or small, blue cell tumors. This category of tumors or abnormalities includes diagnoses, such as leukemia, lymphoma,[230] neuroblastoma, histiocytosis, rhabdomyosarcoma, Ewing sarcoma, infection, and, in adults, multiple myeloma and metastatic adenocarcinoma.

Multiple Myeloma

Multiple myeloma is the most common primary malignancy of bone and typically occurs in the middle decades of life; the shoulder girdle is involved in 5% to 10% of cases.[54,90] The most common site of involvement is the axial skeleton, but multiple distinct lesions develop in the extremities in a significant number of patients and can require surgical stabilization to prevent impending fracture if medical treatment has failed. In patients with a solitary intraosseous myeloma or plasmacytoma of the shoulder at initial evaluation, biopsy is indicated for diagnostic reasons. Multiple myeloma may occur initially in the humerus, scapula, or glenoid as an innocent-appearing bone cyst in a mature adult.

Elevated serum calcium levels, anemia, serum protein electrophoresis, or a distinctly cold bone scan can suggest the diagnosis of myeloma before biopsy in a patient with a solitary lesion or unknown diagnosis. The overall prognosis is poor; however, newer treatments involving aggressive chemotherapy and plasma cell antibodies offer hope for the future. The development of new classes of bisphosphonates has had a positive effect in reducing skeletal events and bone pain.[15]

Figure 22-13A shows the plain radiograph of a 42-year-old man in apparent good health but experiencing shoulder pain. Coronal (Fig. 22-13B) and transverse (Fig. 22-13C) MRI views demonstrate a suprascapular soft tissue lesion that extends anteriorly and posteriorly to the scapula. Open biopsy was diagnostic for multiple myeloma with extensive bone disease. The patient died suddenly 1 week after the biopsy, with an undocumented serum calcium level. All patients with the diagnosis of myeloma need to undergo careful evaluation of their serum electrolytes for the possibility of hypercalcemia, which is usually heralded by altered mental status, fatigue, weakness, or nausea.

Ewing Sarcoma

The second most common intraosseous malignancy in adolescence is Ewing sarcoma, an aggressive marrow cell tumor that appears as a permeative diaphyseal tumor that is poorly marginated and typically associated with a large soft tissue mass.[9,67] Differential diagnosis consists of osteomyelitis, osteosarcoma, lymphoma, eosinophilic granuloma, other round cell tumors, and neuroblastoma, especially in children younger than 2 years.

Figure 22-14A shows such a permeative lesion in the humeral diaphysis of a 16-year-old with a typically hot bone scan (Fig. 22-14B) and an associated soft tissue mass (Fig. 22-14C). Although plain radiography is useful

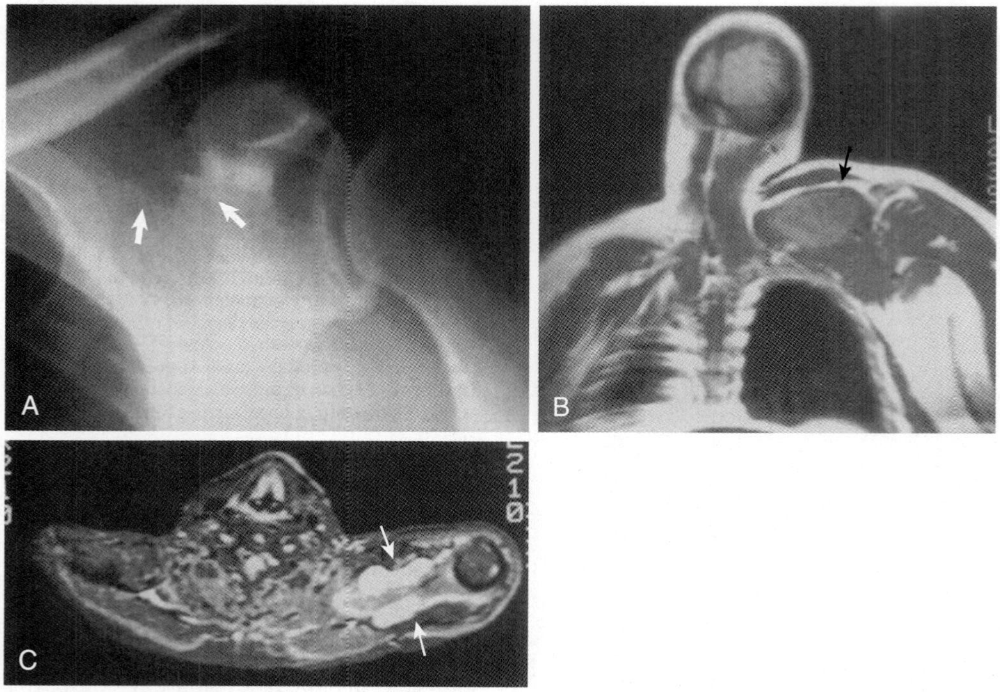

FIGURE 22-13: A, A 42-year-old man with left shoulder pain and a lytic scapular lesion (*arrows*). **B,** Coronal MRI in the same patient demonstrates a suprascapular soft tissue mass (*arrows*). **C,** An axial MRI view of the same patient shows a lesion wrapped anteriorly and posteriorly over the scapula (*arrow*).

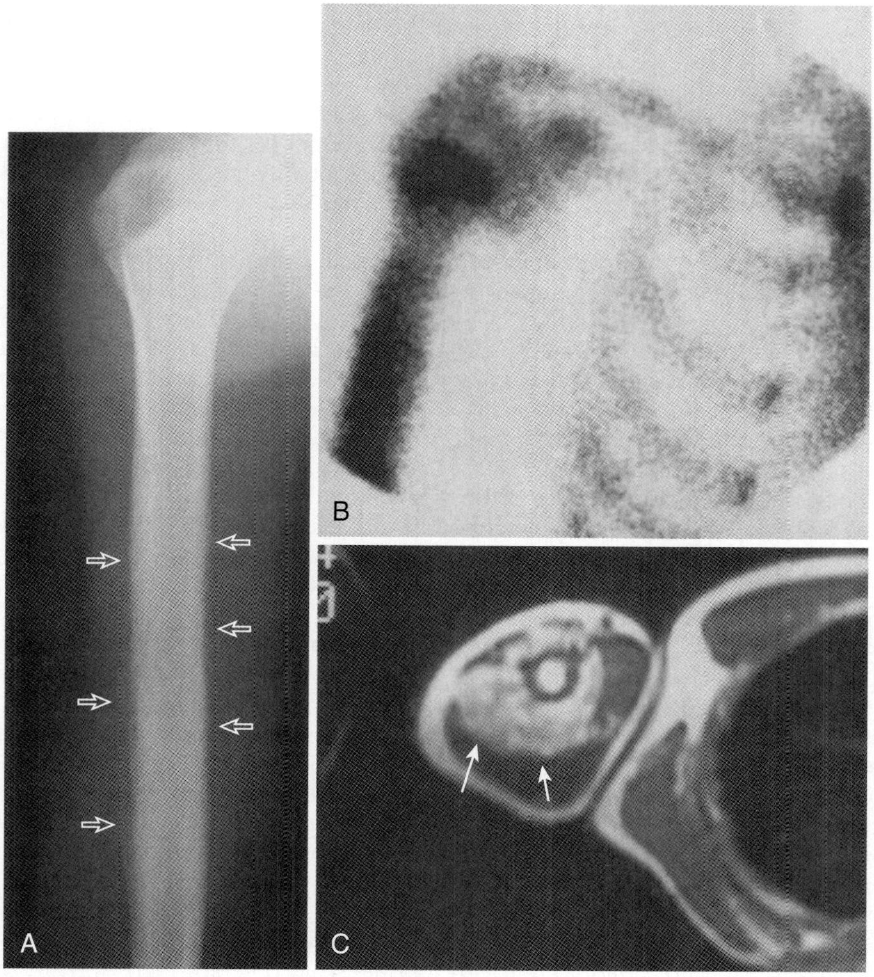

FIGURE 22-14: A, Permeative diaphyseal lesion demonstrating periosteal reaction in a 16-year-old boy (*arrows*). The open biopsy was consistent with Ewing sarcoma. **B,** A bone scan of the same lesion demonstrates significant activity in the humerus. **C,** Axial magnetic reosnance imaging demonstrates a circumferential soft tissue mass (*arrows*) typical of Ewing sarcoma.

for diagnostic purposes, it is not reliable for determining the extent of intramedullary disease. For this reason, an MRI is mandatory before surgery to accurately determine the resection margins. Ewing sarcoma today is primarily treated with aggressive chemotherapy and surgical resection or radiation therapy, depending on the size and location of the primary lesion.

Miscellaneous Dysplasias

Gaucher Disease

Gaucher disease is an uncommon metabolic disorder of the reticuloendothelial system and glucocerebroside-glycolipid metabolism that affects the liver, spleen, and bone marrow.[88] The disease has a higher incidence in the Jewish population and presents most commonly in the first three decades of life, with equal incidence in both sexes. Patients typically present with cytopenia, hepatosplenomegaly, and bone pain.[153] The bone pain is secondary to vascular thrombosis and most commonly occurs in the femoral head, with a high degree of bilaterality.

The disease in many ways represents a form of avascular necrosis of the bone. The humeral head is the second most common site of involvement, and radiographic changes include osteopenia, diaphyseal or medullary expansion, and cortical erosions. The differential diagnosis includes osteomyelitis in the acute setting and round cell tumors in the nonacute setting. Surgical treatment involves internal fixation for fracture prophylaxis or treatment of deformity, joint replacement in adults when indicated, and appropriate management of femoral head necrosis in children. Enzyme replacement is the mainstay of systemic therapy and has been shown to greatly reduce skeletal morbidity.[30]

Paget Disease

Paget disease (also known as osteitis deformans or osteoporosis circumscripta) occurs after the fourth decade and has a slight preponderance in men.[110] It is the second most common metabolic bone disorder in people older than 50 years. Geographically, it appears to have a higher incidence in Great Britain, Western Europe, Australia, and the United States, whereas it is relatively rare in India, Asia, and Africa. Paget disease develops most commonly in the pelvis, skull, lumbosacral spine, femur, and humerus. It can occur in a polyostotic or a monostotic form and is usually evident at the time of initial evaluation. The typical radiographic picture shows cortical thickening, bony enlargement, increased but purposeful trabeculation, and mixed areas of lysis and sclerosis. This is followed by pathologic microfracture and diaphyseal bowing. The differential diagnosis in an adult includes metastatic adenocarcinoma, osteosarcoma, and osteomyelitis. Patients should be assessed by evaluation of serum alkaline phosphatase and urinary hydroxyproline levels, a total body bone scan, and a CT scan or MRI.

Most patients with Paget disease do not require surgical management. The minority of patients who do require surgery usually have musculoskeletal complaints related to deformity, facture, or altered joint mechanics. Patients with Paget disease undergoing orthopedic surgery should, in general, be pretreated to reduce bleeding associated with the hypervascularity of the bone. Paget disease itself is best managed medically with bisphosphonates or calcitonin.[221] Zoledronic acid (approved by the FDA in 2007) is the most recent bisphosphonate to be used for treatment of this condition.

Sarcoma arising out of Paget disease is characterized by a history of progressive pain and a bony lytic lesion with a soft tissue mass (Fig. 22-15A and B). Radiographically, Paget sarcoma of the scapulohumeral area is characterized by predominantly lytic changes in the humerus and purely sclerotic changes in the scapula.[211] Pagetoid sarcoma is a rare variant of osteosarcoma with a very poor prognosis regardless of its site or stage at presentation.[51,135,181] Paget sarcoma is best managed by ensuring a radical surgical margin because of the diffuse nature of the process of Paget disease and the difficulty of assessing the extent of sarcomatous changes.

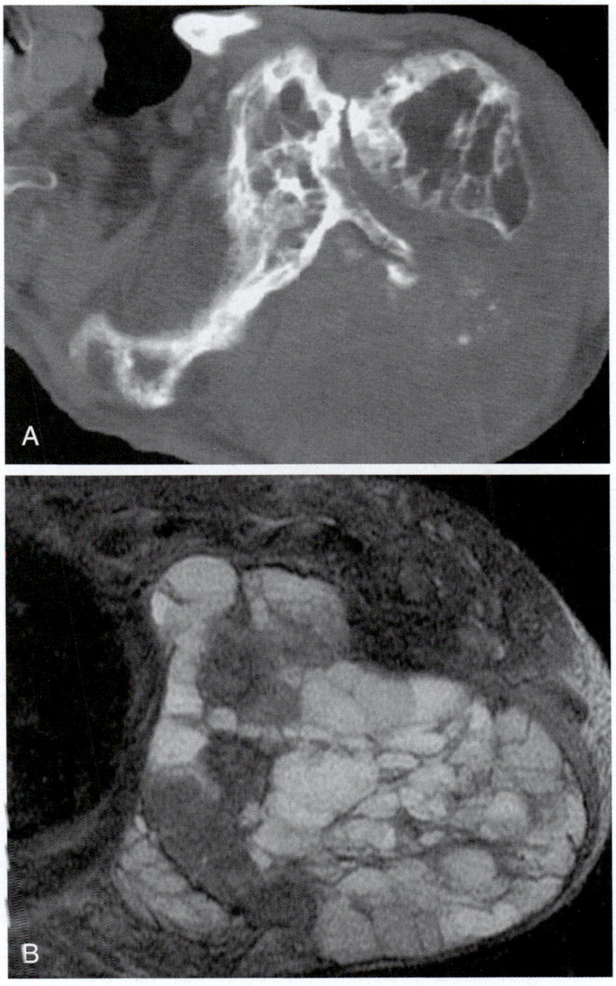

FIGURE 22-15: A, Computed tomography scan of the scapula in a patient with Paget disease shows osteolysis, cortical thickening, and a soft tissue mass. **B,** Axial magnetic resonance imaging demonstrates a soft tissue mass that confirms the suspicion of Paget sarcoma.

Figure 22-16A and B present early and late radiographs of Paget disease in the proximal end of the humerus. The lytic lesion, combined with a history of increasing arm pain, served notice of an early secondary osteosarcoma that showed up 3 months later with a more impressive lytic lesion in the proximal part of the humerus (Fig. 22-16C). Paget disease affected the full humerus, and the bone scan (Fig. 22-16D) was of little help in demarcating bony margins or osseous involvement by this secondary, or pagetoid, osteosarcoma.[121] MRI and CT scans again demonstrate the soft tissue and bony extent of disease in the proximal part of the humerus (Fig. 22-16E and F).

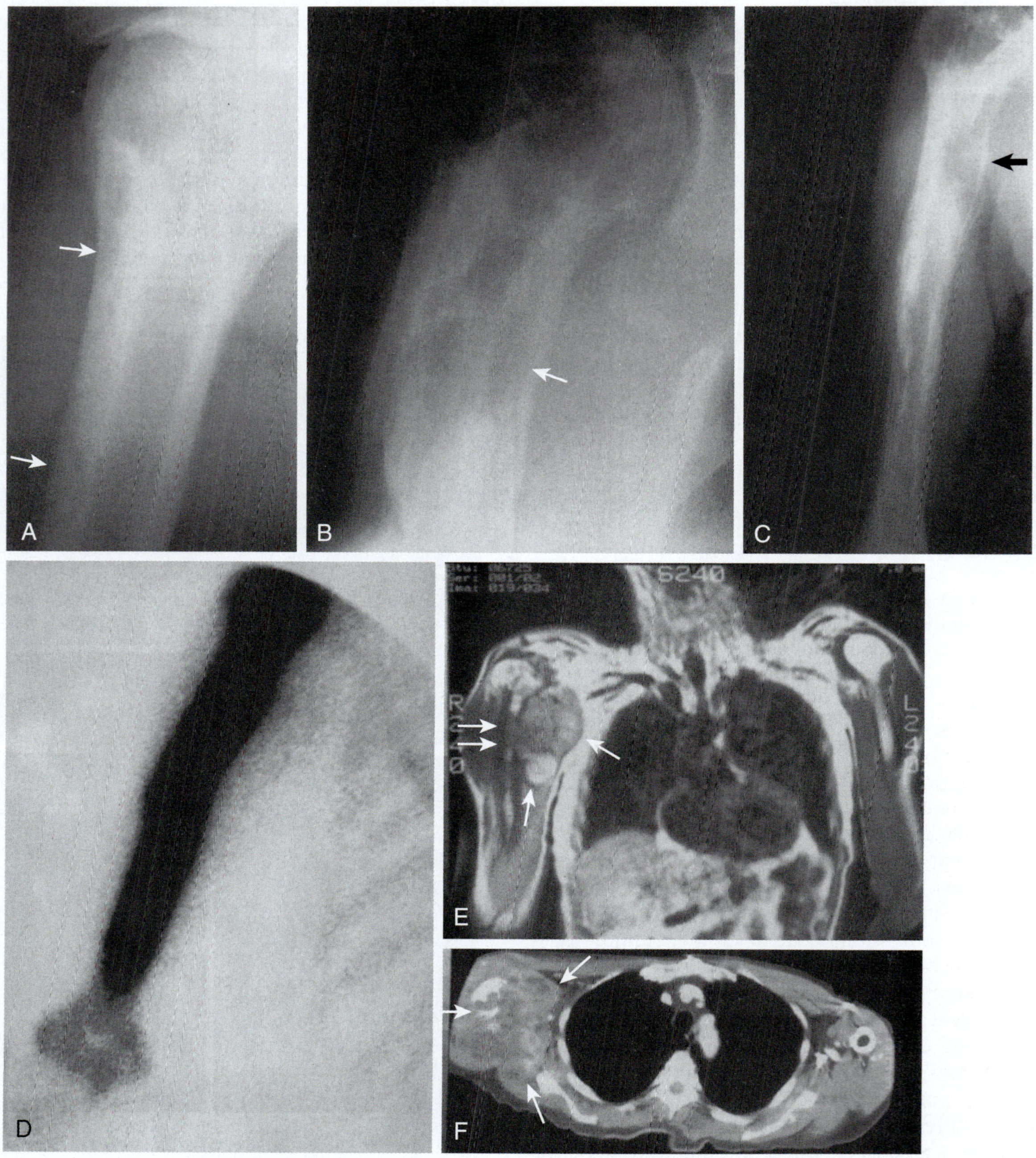

FIGURE 22-16: A, Early Paget disease of the proximal part of the humerus, demonstrating cortical thickening and rarefaction (*arrows*). **B,** The same patient was evaluated years later for shoulder pain and a lytic lesion of the humerus (*arrow*) consistent with a secondary osteosarcoma. **C,** Several months later, this lytic process had become larger (*arrow*) and was associated with a large soft tissue mass (sarcoma). **D,** Bone scanning demonstrates intense humeral activity without distinguishing involvement by Paget disease from sarcomatous changes. **E,** Coronal magnetic resonance imaging shows a large soft tissue mass arising out of the proximal end of the humerus (*double arrows*) and extending into the axilla. **F,** Computed tomography also shows this secondary osteosarcoma with gross destruction of the proximal end of the humerus (*arrows*).

Benign Soft Tissue Tumors

Ganglion

A ganglion is a common soft tissue tumor often confused with other cystic lesions. Ganglia have a thin lining but no true synovial capsule. They are filled with a characteristic gelatinous material. In the shoulder they are often associated with degenerative conditions or a labral tear. MRI is the study of choice for evaluating these lesions and for determining their precise anatomic location. Typically, the MRI shows a rounded or lobular fluid signal mass with low signal on T1-weighted images and high signal on T2-weighted images. When located in the spinoglenoid notch, a ganglion may produce suprascapular nerve palsy secondary to nerve entrapment.[177]

Lipoma

Lipomas can occur intramuscularly or within normal fat planes of the axilla or in the subscapular or other perivascular spaces. They often appear in the anterior deltoid as a large, soft, and nontender intramuscular mass.[62] A few lipomas are tender or firm, and a few have an equivocal history of a change in size. On MRI or CT scan, a benign lipoma usually has a uniform, fatty consistency (Fig. 22-17). Clinically, a liposarcoma has a firmer, denser consistency than that of a lipoma. If a lipoma feels very dense or firm clinically, MRI should be performed for further evaluation. If MRI demonstrates areas of distinctly different density, a biopsy should precede marginal excision to exclude the possibility of a liposarcoma.

Hemangioma

Hemangiomas typically appear as enlarging intramuscular lesions in a child or young adult. They are best visualized by MRI and typically have a serpiginous configuration of vessels. If they are intimately involved with a major vessel, they should also be evaluated with an arteriogram. These lesions do not usually pose diagnostic or surgical problems, with the exception of large hemangiomas or hemangiomatosis of skeletal muscle. These are aggressive, congenital lesions that are often unresectable because of extensive neurovascular and soft tissue involvement.[2,69] Many of these extensive lesions result in amputations because of painful, dysvascular, or infected extremities. Most of these lesions are best diagnosed by open biopsy after MRI, CT scan with contrast, or arteriography. Well-localized lesions are more easily resected than the more extensive congenital lesions. Embolization and interferon treatment have had mixed results in halting the progression of disease.

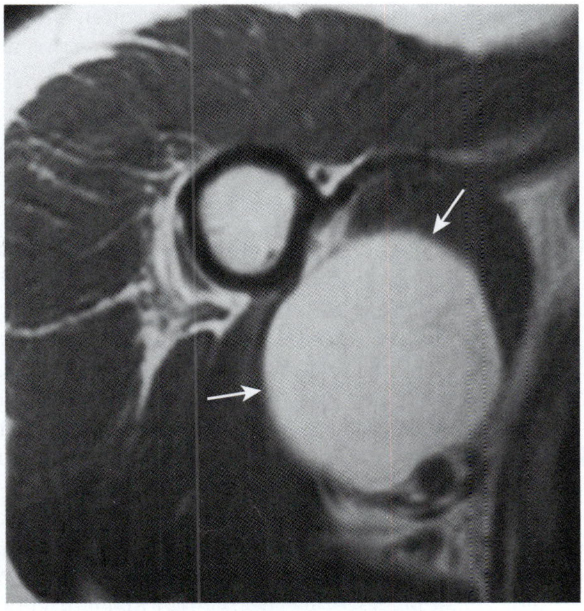

FIGURE 22-17: Axial magnetic resonance imaging of a lipoma (*arrows*) adjacent to the shaft of the proximal humerus. Note the homogeneous fatty signal characteristic of this lesion.

Fibromatosis

Fibromatosis (desmoid tumor) is a locally aggressive (stage 2 or 3) lesion found in young children, teenagers, and young adults. These lesions have a firm consistency on clinical examination and may be associated with osseous erosions or invasion of a neurovascular bundle. Many of these lesions recur locally because of inadequate preoperative staging, underestimation of their potential for local recurrence, and an inadequate surgical margin. Considerable confusion and contradiction is found in the literature regarding the natural history of fibromatosis. Spontaneous regression as described in some publications is unusual except in some congenital forms, and the natural history of lesions in adolescents is progressive growth and recurrence after marginal resection. These lesions rarely demonstrate pulmonary metastasis, and chemotherapy is not usually efficacious, although indications for chemotherapy do exist.[60,75,76,189]

The congenital form of the disease is referred to as *congenital fibrosarcoma*, primarily because of its very impressive histologic cellularity. The adolescent version is best referred to as *aggressive fibromatosis* and behaves as an active aggressive lesion. Preoperative and postoperative MRI studies are mandatory in these patients to fully assess the soft tissue involvement. Bone scans should also be carried out if there is any doubt about secondary bone involvement.

Soft Tissue Sarcomas

Soft tissue sarcomas occur in the upper extremity in approximately one third of all cases. Delays in diagnosis and referral to a specialist are common.[22,33] Moreover, soft tissue sarcomas are often misdiagnosed as benign and patients undergo a contaminated marginal resection of these lesions before definitive biopsy. Soft tissue sarcomas are characterized by four fairly typical clinical characteristics. They generally have a firm consistency and are deep to the superficial muscular fascia, larger than 5 cm, and nontender (Box 22-1). Adequate staging before biopsy is important for soft tissue sarcomas, just as it is for bone sarcomas (Fig. 22-18). In these lesions open biopsy is often, but not always, preferred to needle biopsy for diagnosing both the histologic type and grade of the lesion.

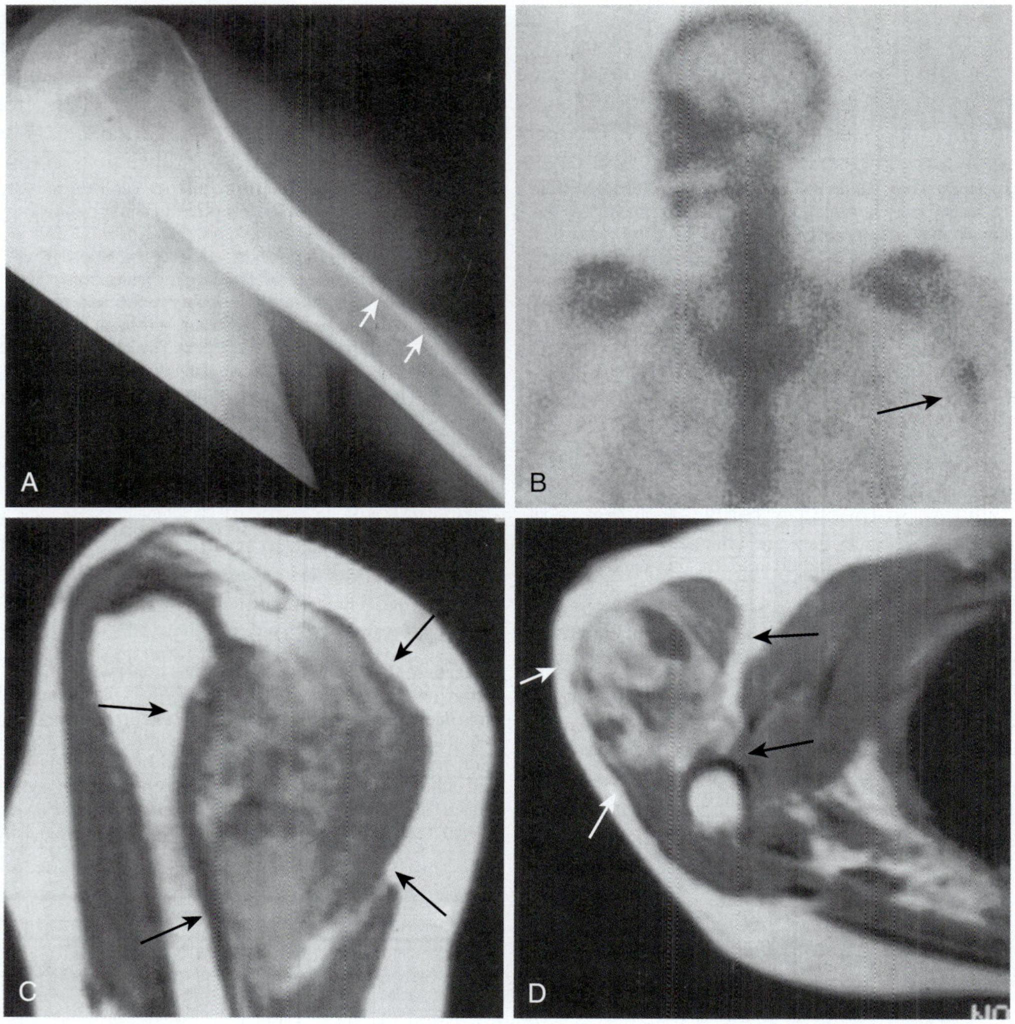

FIGURE 22-18: **A,** Plain radiograph of a 55-year-old woman with a large soft tissue sarcoma at the deltoid. The cortical irregularity at the deltoid insertion (*arrows*) suggests bone invasion. **B,** A bone scan demonstrates distinct bone involvement at the deltoid tubercle with increased uptake (*arrow*). **C,** Sagittal magnetic resonance imaging (MRI) shows a large mass (*arrows*) abutting the proximal part of the humerus. **D,** Axial MRI also suggests posterior humeral cortical invasion by a large deltoid malignant fibrous histiocytoma (*arrows*).

The most common soft tissue sarcoma in adults is malignant fibrous histiocytoma (currently termed myxofibrosarcoma), which occurs most often in older adults (aged 50 to 70 years).[27,75,243] Liposarcoma typically occurs in the lower extremities in young adults as a large lesion with a histology ranging from low grade to high grade or pleomorphic.[27,75,243] Synovial sarcoma[250] is a less common lesion associated with faint soft tissue calcifications, a juxta-articular location, and a high metastatic rate. Fibrosarcoma, rhabdomyosarcoma,[146] leiomyosarcoma, clear cell sarcoma, and epithelioid lesions are other, less common soft tissue malignancies.[77]

Soft tumor sarcomas arising out of a peripheral nerve (peripheral nerve sheath tumors) may occur adjacent to the brachial plexus and present surgical treatment challenges with respect to the brachial plexus, brachial vessels, and the preservation of extremity function. Regardless of the tissue type, the grade of the lesion and the anatomic location of the primary tumor are the most significant factors determining prognosis and treatment. Soft tissue sarcomas of intermediate-grade histology are problematic to treat because of their variable prognosis and response to chemotherapy. There has been some early experience with flow cytometry in identifying more active (aneuploid) tumors, and this knowledge may prove helpful in the future in subclassifying or grading intermediate-grade tumors. Synovial sarcoma, epithelioid sarcoma, and rhabdomyosarcoma are characterized as soft tissue sarcomas with a high incidence (10% to 20%) of regional lymph node metastasis and a poor prognosis,[56,73,125,192,193,219,228] but survival is generally recognized as being closely related to an individual tumor's histologic grade and size.[199]

INCIDENCE OF NEOPLASMS

Malignant tumors arising within the musculoskeletal system are rare and account for 0.5% to 0.7% of all malignancies.[238] They are relatively more common in children, in whom they represent 6.5% of all cancers. Although the incidence of soft tissue sarcomas has little apparent sexual or racial predilection, osteosarcoma and Ewing sarcoma have demonstrated a slight male preference (1.3 : 1.0).[41,104]

The American Cancer Society estimated that in 2015 there would be 11,930 new soft tissue cancers and 2,970 new cancers involving the bone and joints in the United States annually. These were expected to cause an estimated 4,870 deaths from soft tissue cancers and 1,490 from cancers with a bone or joint origin. Various sources have estimated that 1000 to 2000 new cases of osteosarcoma occur annually in the United States.[41,197,238] The true incidence of most of these tumors remains somewhat speculative, largely due to the methods of reporting.

The most common malignancy of the adult musculoskeletal system is metastatic adenocarcinoma, most often from the kidney, lung, breast, or prostate.[65] The most common primary malignancy of bone is multiple myeloma, a plasma cell malignancy usually diagnosed by the medical oncologist rather than the orthopedic surgeon.[90] Multiple myeloma has an incidence that is approximately twice that of osteosarcoma. Excluding multiple myeloma, the most common primary malignant tumor of bone is osteosarcoma. If both benign and malignant primary lesions of the musculoskeletal system are included, cartilaginous tumors are the most common primary lesion (both benign and malignant) of the skeletal system.[41]

Age is a highly important characteristic in the occurrence and distribution of tumors. The overall distribution of tumors by age in decades (Figs. 22-19 and 22-20) demonstrates a preponderance of benign tumors in the skeletons of growing children, with 58% of all benign lesions occurring in the second and third decades. Malignant tumors of the skeleton have a peak incidence in adolescents and middle-aged adults.[41,65,197] Osteosarcoma and Ewing sarcoma are the most common malignant bone tumors in adolescents. In adults osteosarcoma and chondrosarcoma occur with an incidence second only to multiple myeloma and metastatic adenocarcinoma. Osteosarcoma accounts for approximately 40% of all primary malignancies of bone, chondrosarcoma for 20%, and Ewing sarcoma for 12.5%.[41,65,197]

The incidence of tumors by anatomic location is best estimated by a review of the works of Enneking[63] and Dahlin.[41] The overall incidence of primary sarcomas in the shoulder is approximately 15%.[44,63] The shoulder is the third most common overall site for sarcomas, behind the hip-pelvis (first) and the distal femoral and proximal tibial areas of the knee (second). In general, one third of all sarcomas affect the upper extremity.[191] Most shoulder tumors (68.6% to 71.5%) develop in the proximal part of the humerus (Fig. 22-21). Tumors of the shoulder girdle occur in the clavicle (6% to 10% of all cases) and in the scapula (18% to 24%).[41,65]

CLINICAL FEATURES

Despite refinements and developments in the field of musculoskeletal oncology, patients with musculoskeletal

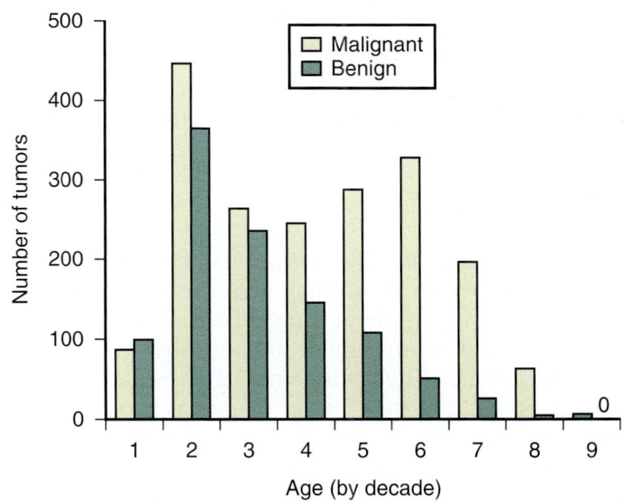

FIGURE 22-19: Distribution of musculoskeletal tumors by age.

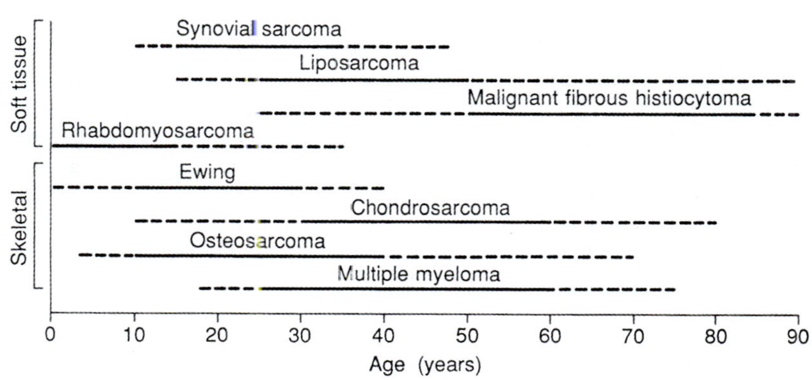

FIGURE 22-20: Sarcomas by age. (Modified from Enzinger FM, Weiss SW. *Soft Tissue Tumors.* St Louis: CV Mosby; 1983.)

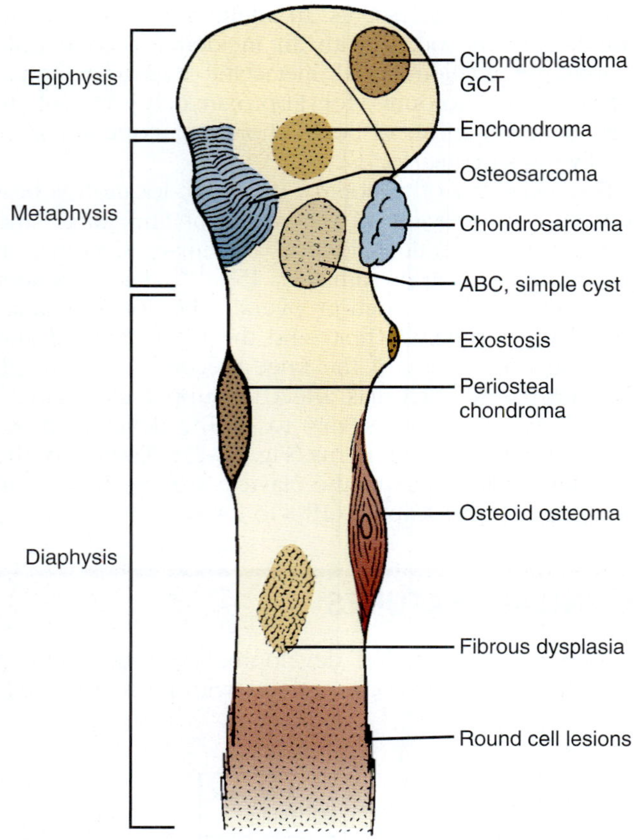

FIGURE 22-21: Common tumors of the proximal end of the humerus. ABC, aneurysmal bone cyst; GCT, giant cell tumor.

malignancies generally experience a 3- to 6-month history of symptoms before an accurate diagnosis is made.[22] The challenge for the general practitioner is to make the diagnosis based on the initial history, physical examination, and plain radiographs. Most of these lesions have a subtle onset, and their initial diagnosis requires attention to certain details and an understanding of a few hallmark signs. The patient's initial assessment remains a crucial step to a successful evaluation and treatment plan. In 70% to 80% of cases it is possible to correctly diagnose and recognize most malignancies based on the initial history, physical examination, and plain radiographs.[65]

Patients with an intraosseous malignancy almost always have pain. The challenge to the physician is to distinguish between the pain of malignancy and the other more common types of musculoskeletal pain. The hallmark symptom of an intraosseous malignancy is pain at night or pain at rest (Box 22-1). Any patient who experiences a symptom of significant pain at night should be carefully assessed radiographically at the time of the first evaluation. As night pain can be a prominent complaint of patients with rotator cuff pathology, evaluation of shoulder symptoms may prove challenging in the presence of an underlying bone lesion. Rarely, a patient presents with a frozen shoulder when the underlying cause is a neoplastic process.[187]

Other pertinent findings in the history that may be helpful include a strong family history of malignancy (adenocarcinoma or sarcoma) or a history in the patient of a previous malignancy that now has metastasized to the skeleton. Weight loss and general malaise may be significant symptoms for metastatic disease, and the physician should initiate a work-up to further evaluate the patient's general health. It is unusual, however, for a patient to have generalized symptoms or metastatic disease as the initial symptom of a sarcoma.

Musculoskeletal neoplasms present a clinical challenge to the orthopedist in determining whether a patient has intraosseous pain or intra-articular pain. This distinction is not readily apparent in the early diagnosis of most intraosseous tumors. A careful physical examination can sometimes elicit findings consistent with joint tenderness, impingement, or weakness, suggesting some sort of intra-articular process. It is unusual for sarcomas to extend into a joint, and the presence of joint findings or symptoms is more consistent with trauma, degenerative disease, or some other nonneoplastic process. In general, intra-articular processes are exacerbated by physical activities and joint motion (see the section on physical examination). Similarly, some patients have referred pain that can lead to an erroneous diagnosis of shoulder pain that actually originated from the cervical spine.

Every adult patient who is evaluated specifically for a possible neoplasm should have a careful general examination of the head and neck, cardiopulmonary status, abdomen, spine, breasts (in women), and prostate (in men), as well as an examination for lymphadenopathy. This sort of general examination is most appropriate for adults older than 35 to 40 years, who are more likely to have metastatic adenocarcinoma. In addition to a specific examination to evaluate patients for a possible neoplasm, all patients should have a complete general musculoskeletal examination to evaluate for joint range of motion, strength, and stability. Regional adenopathy should be routinely sought on examination and will be found with many tumors. It is usually an inflammatory phenomenon, reactive to the tumor. However, lymph node adenopathy larger than 1 cm should be evaluated further by MRI, and biopsy should be performed before a definitive resection of the primary tumor is attempted.

Patients with an aggressive intraosseous malignancy usually have bone tenderness and a mass. The primary site may be deep and well covered by muscle and may be difficult to palpate. Usually, careful palpation will demonstrate the presence or absence of any soft tissue mass. However, low-grade intraosseous lesions might not involve the soft tissues. Extension of an intraosseous malignancy medially toward the major neurovascular bundle, which is close to the humerus, can preclude limb-sparing surgery and is associated with a worse prognosis.

Clinical involvement of the soft tissues can yield important information for directing the MRI scan and other studies. In general, the soft tissue mass produced by an intraosseous malignancy is relatively subtle as an early clinical finding and requires some attention on examination. Soft tissue sarcomas most commonly have a history of a mass. Most soft tissue sarcomas, in contradistinction to intraosseous malignancies, are not painful. All soft tissue lesions should be carefully evaluated for the four characteristics of a soft tissue sarcoma: nontender mass, firm consistency, deep or subfascial location, and a size greater than 5 cm (Box 22-1). Exceptions occur, but as a general rule, these guidelines are very reliable in the initial evaluation of various soft tissue lesions.

The most reliable clinical sign for a soft tissue sarcoma is the consistency or density of the lesion. For instance, the most common soft tissue tumor in an adult is a lipoma, which may be large, deep in location, and nontender; however, its consistency usually indicates whether it is malignant. Lipomas are typically very soft, with the consistency of normal fat, whereas liposarcomas are usually firm. The ability to distinguish the consistency of a soft tissue mass can be a somewhat subtle, but important finding. Anything with a consistency more dense than normal fat should be evaluated carefully. Lipomas that feel firmer than normal fat or are larger than 10 cm should be evaluated by MRI. If a soft tissue mass is thought to be cystic, it is reasonable and advisable to attempt careful aspiration in the clinic to determine whether the lesion contains fluid. Repeated or multiple aspirations are not advised and lead only to contamination of a possible soft tissue sarcoma.

Routine clinical follow-up for a patient with a malignancy is important for detecting progressive disease at an early stage. After the immediate postoperative evaluation, patients with high-grade sarcomas are generally monitored every 3 months for 2 years, every 6 months for another 2 years, and annually thereafter. Intraosseous lesions that appear benign on plain radiographs, or lesions that are discovered incidentally, can be monitored if the plain radiographs are well demarcated and the lesions are obviously benign. If the initial plain radiographs are equivocal, a bone scan and CT or MRI are indicated to determine whether the lesion is active and requires a biopsy or whether it can be monitored clinically. For instance, most low-grade, calcified, or cartilaginous intraosseous lesions can be safely monitored at 6-month intervals.

RADIOGRAPHIC AND LABORATORY EVALUATION

The interpretation of the initial plain radiographs is an important step in the early diagnosis of most musculoskeletal tumors. When dealing with skeletal lesions, the orthopedist should have a system for evaluating the initial plain radiographs and formulating the initial diagnosis. Every bone lesion has a characteristic location, margin, and density that typify it radiographically. These three radiographic characteristics are important in describing a lesion's growth rate and intrinsic density.[63] These concepts originated in a different format from that of Jaffe,[108] who, when evaluating radiographs, first posed the questions "What is the lesion's density?", "What is it doing to bone?", "What is the bone doing to it?", and "What is its location?" This approach helps focus attention on the lesion's growth rate and degree of activity and thus on its malignant potential. With these three characteristics in mind, the initial plain radiographs can be interpreted with the correct diagnosis in most cases.

Location

Where is the lesion located? Is it in the epiphysis, metaphysis, or diaphysis? Are there multiple metastatic sites or one primary site of involvement? For example, an aggressive metaphyseal tumor in an adolescent is very likely to be an osteosarcoma, whereas a diaphyseal lesion is much more likely to be Ewing sarcoma. Whether the lesion is central or eccentric within the bone is also important information. Nonossifying fibroma is almost always eccentric, whereas cartilaginous lesions (enchondromas) are usually centrally located.

Margin

The margin of the lesion on plain radiographs is the best reflection of that lesion's growth rate at the time of the initial evaluation. It refers to the margin or interface between the lesion and surrounding normal bone. If a tumor is slow growing, it will have a distinct or sclerotic margin that demonstrates the ability of the surrounding normal bone to react to it, thus marginating, or walling off, that lesion. A sclerotic or distinct peripheral bony margin indicates a slow-growing or benign lesion and is not generally seen with malignant or aggressive benign tumors. This type of margin reflects the ability of bone to respond to a slowly growing tumor.

At the other end of the spectrum is a lesion that is not well marginated and does not have a sclerotic rim of reactive bone around it. This pattern reflects a more rapidly growing tumor that enlarges at a rate faster than normal bone can react to it. The best examples of an aggressive lesion that infiltrates or percolates through bone are the permeative lesion of Ewing sarcoma or any intramedullary round cell tumor or small blue cell tumor of bone.

Density

The intrinsic density of a lesion within bone or soft tissue is another piece of information contributing to the initial diagnosis. Is the lesion made of bone, cartilage (calcifications), fibrous dysplasia (ground-glass density), or soft tissue (clear)? A truly cystic (or fluid-filled) lesion is most likely to be a benign or infectious lesion in bone or soft tissue, and this cystic nature may be determined clinically or demonstrated by imaging studies.

Evaluation

Complete assessment of a patient with a musculoskeletal lesion involves a careful evaluation of both the clinical and radiographic findings. The complex anatomy and the frequency of referred pain make many diagnoses in the shoulder a challenge.

Appropriate initial radiographs for evaluating most patients include a well-exposed, properly positioned film. It is essential that a well-exposed radiograph of the shoulder be obtained in all patients, especially those with persistent symptoms who may be failing conservative treatment for what is believed to be an intra-articular glenohumeral problem.

For abnormalities noted on plain radiographs, a bone scan is often helpful in determining the activity of the lesion. A whole body bone scan can also determine the presence of other bony lesions.

A CT scan is a valuable procedure for investigating bony detail. This modality is useful for evaluating the characteristics of bony lesions and the extent of cortical involvement from intraosseous or soft tissue lesions adjacent to the cortex. It is also useful for the analysis of a fracture, with a suspicion of it being pathologic in nature. CT scan of the chest (along with plain radiographs) is used to evaluate the presence of metastases, which is important for a newly diagnosed or suspected malignancy. CT scan of the chest, abdomen, and pelvis is an excellent screening tool for an unknown primary tumor when a bone lesion is suspicious for metastatic disease.

MRI provides the greatest detail of soft tissue and bone marrow involvement. It also allows a detailed analysis of a tumor or related abnormality (such as an abscess or hematoma), particularly when used with intravenous gadolinium contrast. MRI is also useful for analyzing exact anatomic location and relationship to other important anatomic structures.

Diagnostic strategies for evaluation of possible skeletal metastases have been reviewed.[195]

Possible tumor involvement of the neurovascular bundle and brachial plexus is best assessed on MRI, whereas arteriography is now reserved specifically for lesions located adjacent to a major vessel. Gallium scans have been used for assessing the extent of soft tissue sarcomas, but they have generally been considered to have inferior resolution quality compared with that of MRI.

Metabolic imaging using radioisotopes, such as fluorodeoxyglucose and others, has received greater attention over the past several years. Such studies are potentially useful in grading tumors (high grade vs. low grade), assessing the response to chemotherapy, and evaluating patients for residual minimal disease.[38,207]

Laboratory

In general, laboratory studies for sarcomas are not of great assistance in making the initial diagnosis. The most common exception is serum alkaline phosphatase, which is often elevated in osteosarcoma or Paget disease.[116] Urinalysis (microscopic hematuria) and the measurement of serum acid phosphatase or prostate-specific antigen levels are helpful in the evaluation of possible malignancies of the prostate or kidney.[172] A hematocrit is useful in evaluating for anemia (which is frequently present in multiple myeloma). White blood cell count, erythrocyte sedimentation rate, and C-reactive protein are often helpful in the diagnosis of infection, although all may be normal in the types of subacute infections that are likely to be confused with neoplasms. Any patient who has multiple myeloma as the differential diagnosis should get serum calcium checked preoperatively to detect hypercalcemia. In addition, these patients should undergo a serum and urine protein electrophoresis study to evaluate their immunoglobulin profile.[108] Lactate dehydrogenase may have prognostic value for osteosarcoma.[8] Abnormalities in electrolytes, blood urea nitrogen, creatinine, and liver function tests may provide clues to the possibility of underlying systemic diseases, some of which can manifest with bone and soft tissue abnormalities.

COMPLICATIONS OF TUMORS

One of the most significant complications of a musculoskeletal tumor is pathologic fracture; the majority of these fractures are secondary to metastatic adenocarcinoma. Approximately one third of all diagnosed cases of breast, pulmonary, thyroid, renal, and prostatic carcinoma involve skeletal metastases.[16,78,98,242] Although the most common site for metastasis is the axial skeleton, approximately 25% of all metastases are located in the shoulder girdle.

Surgery may be indicated to obtain a primary diagnosis by open biopsy or to achieve internal fixation for fracture prophylaxis. Patients with an established tumor diagnosis and lytic lesions that represent bone metastases should, in general, be treated first with chemotherapy and radiation therapy if the evidence indicates that the particular lesion is likely to respond to such treatment. Metastatic lesions that are generally considered to be resistant to radiation therapy or chemotherapy (such as renal cell carcinoma) and lesions that have failed similar previous treatment should be treated surgically. Surgical stabilization or internal fixation is indicated in any patient with an impending or completed pathologic fracture who can tolerate a general anesthetic and who has a life expectancy of at least 1 month. Closed management, usually with a coaptation splint or Sarmiento brace, is relatively poor at relieving fracture symptoms in the humerus because of persistent rotational instability. Healing is generally unpredictable and pain relief is inadequate.

Figure 22-22 shows a pathologic fracture of the proximal part of the humerus in a 65-year-old patient with extensive metastatic disease. His pain was unrelieved with coaptation bracing, and he was treated surgically with methyl methacrylate and short Ender rods placed through the fracture site. His poor medical status and limited life expectancy (several months) dictated this more conservative surgical procedure rather than the usual treatment of hemiarthroplasty. Even patients with widespread metastatic disease can benefit greatly from a careful, but aggressive approach to the management of pathologic fractures versus impending fractures.

The intraosseous sarcomas that result in a pathologic fracture represent less than 10% of all sarcomas, and

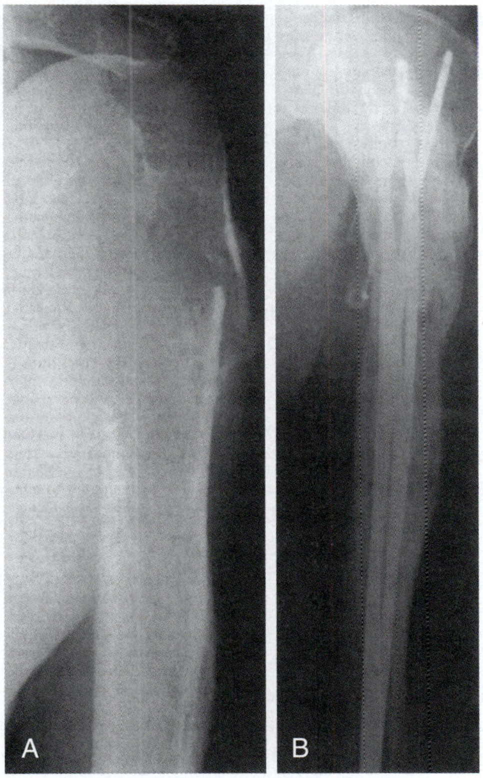

FIGURE 22-22: A, Metastatic adenocarcinoma of the lung in a 65-year-old man with extensive metastatic disease and a pathologic fracture. **B,** Conservative surgical stabilization in this patient involved cementation and placement of a rod through the fracture site.

although they present a challenge, they are no longer considered to be an absolute indication for immediate amputation.[208] Another problem is that of fractures occurring after a poorly designed biopsy, thus emphasizing the need for careful biopsy procedures.

An additional problem arises in patients with Ewing sarcoma in whom a late fracture can develop in a diaphyseal lesion that has been previously irradiated. Such lesions should be stabilized prophylactically with an intramedullary rod to prevent possible fracture if there is any evidence of an impending fracture. Fractures through irradiated bone are unlikely to heal and should be internally fixed or resected as soon as possible.

Fibrous dysplasia is another example of pathologic bone that can require intramedullary fixation to prevent repeated fractures and progressive deformity. Intramedullary fixation is the method of choice because of its biomechanical superiority. Plating with screws is vastly inferior to intramedullary fixation of impending or completed pathologic diaphyseal lesions.

DIFFERENTIAL DIAGNOSIS

The shoulder girdle is an area that presents a challenge to the diagnosis of many different conditions. Its close relationship with the cervical spine and brachial plexus can present a formidable challenge in differentiating cervical spine problems from shoulder problems. The complexity of the soft tissue anatomy of the glenohumeral joint and the difficulty of distinguishing intra- from extraarticular diagnoses are significant, even for the most skilled orthopedist. The confusion that may arise can delay the diagnosis of various musculoskeletal tumors for a significant period.

The differential diagnosis for various musculoskeletal lesions includes the lesions identified in Box 22-2. Although the categories of trauma, tumor, infection, and inflammatory or degenerative disease include the diagnosis in most cases, various dysplastic, hematologic, and metabolic problems are important and require a more extensive evaluation. Certainly, the process of separating out difficult problems starts with an accurate and thorough history and physical examination.

BOX 22-2. Differential Diagnosis of Musculoskeletal Lesions

- Trauma (subtle, bony, acute, chronic)
- Tumor (benign or malignant, primary or metastatic)
- Infection (bacterial, viral, fungal, venereal)
- Inflammatory disease (rheumatoid arthritis, gouty arthropathy, collagen vascular disease, pigmented villonodular synovitis)
- Degenerative disease (osteoarthritis)
- Dysplasias (fibrous dysplasia, Paget disease, multiple hereditary exostoses, neurofibromatosis)
- Hematologic disorders (hemophilia, histiocytosis, myeloproliferative disorder)
- Metabolic disorders (osteomalacia, rickets, hyperparathyroidism, renal osteodystrophy)

Trauma as the cause of lesions of the musculoskeletal system obviously often involves a history of an injury, but incidental trauma is also commonly associated with sarcomas, although no causal relationship has been demonstrated. Chronic injuries or stress fractures are often a more subtle and challenging diagnosis but are less common in the shoulder than in the lower extremity.

Infections are a common problem in healthy young children who suffer from acute hematogenous osteomyelitis or septic arthritis. In fact, the differential diagnosis for any lesion in a child should always include infection as a possible cause. Acute hematogenous osteomyelitis is an unusual problem in adults because osteomyelitis usually develops as a result of traumatic wounds, surgical complications, or chronic decubitus ulcers in adults. Tuberculous or fungal infections are an even greater diagnostic and treatment challenge, and a culture should be performed in all patients with suspected infections. In general, tuberculous infections have an unimpressive amount of reactive bone on radiographs and a chronic history. Whenever an infectious problem is being considered, a biopsy specimen should be sent along with abundant, appropriate material for culture. Some necrotic

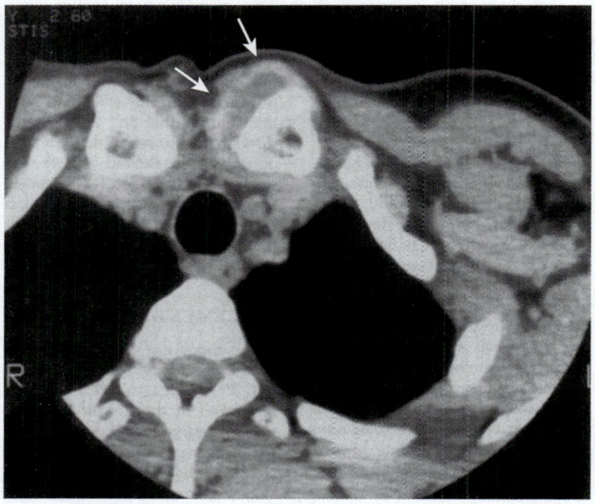

FIGURE 22-23: Computed tomography scan of the sternoclavicular joint in a patient with degenerative joint disease, an effusion, and a soft tissue mass consisting of redundant synovium (*arrow*). This area is difficult to image and could be misinterpreted as a neoplasm.

soft tissue tumors contain pus and strongly resemble a soft tissue abscess. The old adage "always biopsy an infection and culture a tumor" remains good advice as a general rule in the evaluation of any lesion.

Inflammatory and degenerative diseases are usually associated with typical findings on plain radiographs, such as joint space narrowing, subchondral sclerosis, and cyst formation. Clinically, it can be very difficult to distinguish inflammatory or degenerative disease from a subtle neoplasm. The differential diagnosis can also be difficult in children, in whom pauciarticular juvenile rheumatoid arthritis in its initial manifestation can be very difficult to distinguish from septic arthritis and other soft tissue tumors. Figure 22-23 shows a degenerative condition of the sternoclavicular joint in an area that does not easily lend itself to imaging techniques; this degenerative lesion with an apparent soft tissue mass could be misinterpreted as a possible neoplasm of the proximal part of the clavicle. An understanding of the pathology of the sternoclavicular joint is of great assistance in interpreting diagnostic studies of this area.

The most common dysplasias of bone masquerading as neoplasms include fibrous dysplasia in children and Paget disease in adults. These are usually polyostotic "tumors" that actually represent dysplasia of bone. Fibrous dysplasia and Paget disease can often be diagnosed by evaluating plain radiographs and bone scans, as can many of the polyostotic syndromes. Both fibrous dysplasia and Paget disease can require intramedullary fixation to treat chronic, pathologic, painful, and weak long bones. Secondary malignancies are unusual, and are associated with increasing pain and obvious radiographic changes. Other dysplasias include multiple hereditary exostoses and enchondromatoses.

Hematologic disorders (excluding myeloma) that can masquerade as tumors occur most commonly in children or young adults with the various histiocytoses, hemophilia, and other blood dyscrasias. The least aggressive form of histiocytosis is eosinophilic granuloma, which is truly the great imitator in children because it can masquerade as a tumor. Eosinophilic granuloma occurs in the diaphysis and is usually seen as a solitary lesion in a healthy child. However, it can occur as multiple lesions, and when diagnosed in a young child (2 years or younger), there is always the concern that the initial lesion signals the presence of other lesions in the more severe form of the syndrome, such as Hand-Schüller-Christian disease (older children) or Letterer-Siwe disease (infants). Similarly, classic hemophilia or factor VIII deficiency, although uncommon, can show up initially as a solitary knee effusion (septic knee). It is therefore important to obtain an accurate history, and questions should be asked specifically about previous bleeding problems in family members in order to make the diagnosis.

Metabolic disorders in adults can also be difficult diagnoses to make. Adult patients with osteomalacia can have a stress fracture, a hot bone scan, equivocal staging studies, and a risk factor in their history (such as of renal disease or gastrointestinal malabsorption). The syndromes of renal osteodystrophy, osteomalacia, and osteoporosis are unlikely to present as a problem of the upper extremity, but they remain an important part of any complete differential diagnosis. Patients with osteomalacia often have diffuse manifestations of their disease (such as vertebral fractures or osteopenia) and can require a full metabolic work-up that includes serum calcium, PO_4, serum and urinary hydroxyproline, vitamin D, parathyroid hormone levels, bone scan, densitometry, and a tetracycline-labeled iliac crest biopsy.

SURGERY

Biopsy

The management and treatment of any malignancy begins with a sound histologic diagnosis. Biopsy is recommended for all suspicious abnormalities of bone and soft tissue, although, as previously discussed, biopsy of low-grade cartilage and fatty tumors is not usually indicated. Although every institution has its own experiences and prejudices regarding biopsy for sarcomas, open or incisional biopsy is nevertheless regarded by most as the standard method.[216] Incisional biopsy is an operative technique that involves incising a small wedge-shaped piece of tissue from the tumor for histologic evaluation. Its primary advantage over a closed, or needle, biopsy is the acquisition of a larger, more adequate specimen, which is especially important in the challenging diagnosis of sarcoma.

However, open or incisional biopsies do carry a risk of tumor contamination from postoperative hemorrhage. It is important that the surgical principles of incisional biopsy be strictly observed in the shoulder, just as in any other anatomic site. A dissecting hematoma after any biopsy can easily contaminate otherwise normal tissue and expand the required margin for resection, or it can contaminate nearby major neurovascular structures, such as the brachial plexus or brachial vessels, and thus preclude the possibility of a limb-salvage type of resection. In many medical centers with an established sarcoma program, needle biopsies have become the preferred technique for the biopsy of bone and soft tissue lesions.

Mankin and colleagues, under the auspices of the Musculoskeletal Tumor Society,[136] carried out a retrospective evaluation of 329 cases of sarcoma on which biopsies were performed, comparing the biopsies in a referring (primary or secondary) hospital with those performed in a setting with experience in the biopsy of sarcomas. The study concluded that biopsy-related problems were three to five times more common in the outside referring hospital than in the treatment center. The referring hospitals without sarcoma experience had a higher incidence of major diagnostic errors, nonrepresentative biopsies, wound complications, treatment alterations, changes in results, and changes in final results. The incidence of unnecessary amputations was 4.5% of all the cases. This sort of study may be prejudiced in favor of the tertiary institutions due to most of the patients being difficult cases that had been referred for treatment, but the study highlighted a high complication rate for biopsies and the need for careful planning and execution. Higher complication rates and a greater number of diagnostic errors do occur in less experienced centers because of the complexity of the diagnosis and treatment of sarcomas. The best management for all patients with sarcomas is to have the biopsy carried out in an experienced center where the definitive treatment will be rendered.[70]

The best surgical approach for a biopsy of the proximal part of the humerus has traditionally been through the anterior substance of the deltoid (Fig. 22-24). The deltopectoral groove should be avoided because any hematoma after the biopsy might enter the groove, spread proximally into the axilla, and lead to considerable proximal contamination. The joint should not be violated. Although approaching malignant lesions through the anterior deltoid requires resection of that portion of the deltoid with the definitive procedure, it minimizes the risk of contamination. Tumor contamination after the biopsy is a significant problem even in experienced hands, and the following principles of technique should be observed.[136,208]

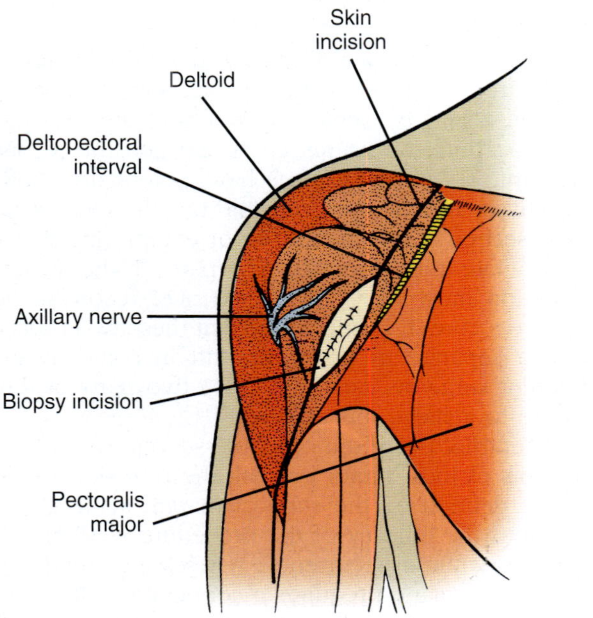

FIGURE 22-24: Biopsy of the proximal end of the humerus.

Placement of the Incision

When performing the biopsy of lesions in the extremities, the surgeon should use a longitudinal (not transverse) incision, usually 4 to 5 cm long (Fig. 22-24). The incision should be placed in the line of the proposed future definitive resection. Around the scapula or clavicle, as in the pelvic girdle, an oblique or transverse incision is appropriate.

Contamination by Tumor Hematoma

If possible, the biopsy of a tumor should always be performed at its most superficial and accessible site. An incisional biopsy technique should involve as little soft tissue dissection as possible. No flaps should be elevated. A lesion biopsy should always be performed away from a major neurovascular bundle or joint to avoid contaminating these structures and thus precluding limb-sparing surgery. This precaution is especially important in the proximal part of the humerus and shoulder because of the proximity of the brachial vessels and brachial plexus.

Before wound closure, strict hemostasis should be carefully accomplished. The use of a tourniquet is not possible in the shoulder, and even in areas where one is used, it should be released before wound closure to achieve hemostasis. Hemostasis may prove to be a challenge in highly vascular malignant lesions in the shoulder, such as angiosarcoma, myeloma, hypernephroma, or Ewing sarcoma. In these situations packing the wound with various coagulant materials in addition to a pressure dressing can prove helpful in enhancing hemostasis. The use of surgical drains or the practice of leaving the wound open after an open biopsy is associated with a higher incidence of wound contamination or infection and is not an accepted method of management.

After achieving hemostasis, the surgeon should meticulously close the biopsy wound and carefully close the deep and superficial layers to prevent late wound dehiscence. The skin is best closed with a subcuticular closure to minimize skin contamination and enable a smaller ellipse of skin to be excised with the main tumor specimen at the time of definitive resection.

Adequacy of the Specimen

Before awakening the patient, it is important to wait for the pathologist to confirm the adequacy of the specimen by frozen section under the microscope. Although it might not be possible to make a definitive diagnosis by frozen section in every case, it is possible to determine whether the specimen contains diagnostic or lesional tissue and thus whether it is an adequate specimen. Bacterial and fungal cultures should be obtained routinely, in addition to sending tissue for special stains, electron microscopy, flow cytometry,[132] or immunohistochemistry. If there is any doubt about the location of a biopsy site in the extremity, pelvis, or spine, an intraoperative radiograph with an appropriate marker should be taken before the biopsy. In many cases of osteogenic sarcoma with a soft tissue mass, it is not necessary to perform a biopsy of the bone to obtain adequate tissue. The biopsy specimen of a bone lesion can often be obtained from its soft tissue extension, thus avoiding fenestration of the bone and the potential complications of postoperative fracture and further contamination from osseous bleeding.

Open Versus Closed Biopsy

The alternatives to an incisional, or open, biopsy include a marginal, or excisional, biopsy or a closed needle biopsy. Excisional biopsy is an acceptable biopsy technique only when used to excise a small lesion (<3 cm) or to excise a lesion that is obviously benign, such as lipoma. Marginal excisional biopsy of a small lesion produces little more contamination than an incisional biopsy and is therefore an adequate technique for that size of lesion. Marginal excision of a tumor, however, is best indicated for benign lesions. Small (≤5 cm) soft tissue sarcomas do develop in the upper extremity, and if there is concern or confusion about a lesion, consultation with a specialist before the biopsy is the appropriate approach.[68]

Needle biopsy can be an appropriate alternative to open biopsy.[21,53,155,204] The disadvantage is the small size of the specimen and the difficulty of assessing whether a lesion is high grade or low grade.[12,21] The attraction of needle biopsy is that it avoids the operative setting, minimizes cost, and is achievable in the clinic, resulting in a quick diagnosis that may be useful in initiating preoperative chemotherapy if a lesion is obviously high grade. The disadvantage of sampling error remains, which has been reported in approximately 25% to 30% of cases.[216]

Needle biopsy is the preferred method for the biopsy of osteosarcoma when the radiographs are typical and only a tissue diagnosis (malignant stroma or osteoid) is required. It has the advantage of a small bone fenestration, thus minimizing both the potential for postbiopsy hemorrhage and the risk of pathologic fracture.

One important indication for needle biopsy is to achieve a "tissue and grade" diagnosis: metastasis, recurrence, or confirmation of an otherwise classic manifestation. In experienced medical centers needle biopsy has now become a relatively reliable method for grading soft tissue sarcomas. The other important indication is the presence of cystic lesions or abscesses. Cystic lesions are not usually malignancies, and in children needle biopsy is a good way to quickly rule out possible infections. It is the preferred method of diagnosing and treating many cystic lesions. If purulent drainage is not obvious, beware of soft tissue sarcomas with central necrosis.

Needle biopsy of soft tissue sarcomas typically involves the use of a trocar cutting needle that delivers a small strip of tissue. Larger trephine or bone marrow needles (3 to 5 mm in diameter) are used for bone lesions. The skinny-needle technique for soft tissue tumors uses a 22-gauge needle for a cytologic smear; this smear requires interpretation by an experienced cytopathologist.

Proceeding immediately with definitive resection after an open biopsy is a treatment alternative that offers the advantage of minimizing the risk of postbiopsy hematoma and contamination. It requires appropriate intraoperative precautions between the biopsy and the definitive resection, such as a change in gowns, gloves, instruments, and operative drapes. Whether it is prudent to proceed with a definitive surgical resection immediately after the frozen section histologic diagnosis depends on the lesion involved and the level of confidence of the pathologist giving the diagnosis. This course of action requires careful planning and a confident, well-informed pathologist at the time of the frozen section biopsy. It is not a reasonable alternative for patients who are candidates for preoperative adjuvant therapy or when the differential diagnosis includes radiation-sensitive tumors, such as lymphomas, which are not treated by resection. When there is doubt regarding whether a lesion is malignant or benign, high grade or low grade, treatment should be delayed until a definitive diagnosis is reached.

Biopsies are a challenging aspect of sarcoma management because of the rarity and complexity of diagnosing and treating these lesions. Although biopsy appears to be a technically small operative procedure, it represents a significant hurdle to achieving an appropriate and successful treatment plan. The complexity of the diagnosis of most sarcomas requires that this significant initial step in the treatment be carried out at a center experienced in the management of sarcomas.[70,136]

Surgical Resections About the Shoulder Girdle

Surgical Margin

Appropriate surgery remains the definitive treatment for most sarcomas at their primary site. Surgical treatment is best described by separately defining the two parts of the procedure: tumor resection part and the reconstructive part. These two aspects have potentially conflicting objectives, and great care should be taken to ensure that the resection is not minimized or compromised in order to facilitate the reconstructive part of the procedure. Resection must take precedence over reconstruction to achieve a cure. It is imperative that these two procedures remain separate in principle, and in some institutions different surgeons carry out these two parts of the procedure to achieve this goal.

When discussing the probable success of a procedure in terms of local tumor control, the resection procedure is best defined by the surgical margin achieved, which describes the efficacy of the procedure in terms of possible future tumor recurrence.[111] Assessing and describing the surgical margin requires a cooperative effort by both the surgeon and the pathologist, who must immediately review the surgical specimen. The four fundamental

TABLE 22-4 Surgical Margins

Surgical Margin	Surgical Procedure	Result
Intralesional	Piecemeal debulking or curettage	Leaves macroscopic tumor
Marginal	Excision of tumor and pseudocapsule through the reactive zone	Leaves microscopic tumor
Wide	Excision of tumor, pseudocapsule, reactive zone, and a cuff of normal tissue	Risk of leaving microscopic tumor
Radical	Extracompartmental procedure removes tumor, pseudocapsule, reactive zone, and the entire compartment	Minimal risk of residual microscopic tumor

From Enneking WF, Spanier SS, Goodman MA. A system for the surgical staging of musculoskeletal sarcoma. Clin Orthop Relat Res. *1980;153:105-120.*

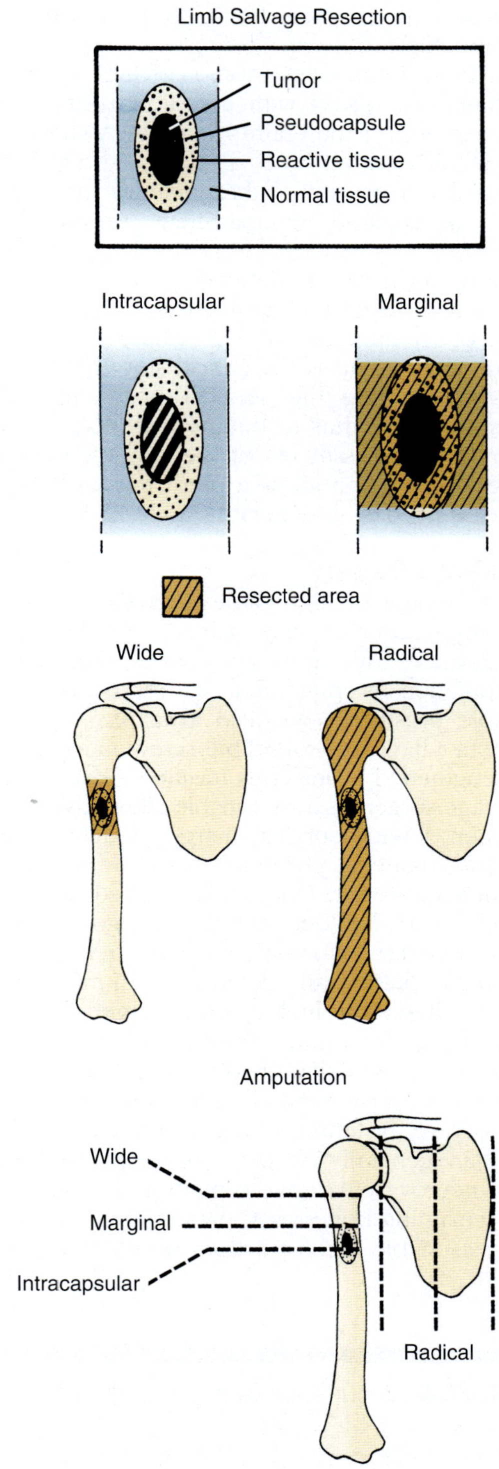

FIGURE 22-25: Surgical margins.

types of margins are intracapsular, marginal, wide, and radical (Table 22-4 and Fig. 22-25).

An intracapsular, or intralesional, surgical margin carries the risk of leaving behind foci of gross tumor. However, this is an acceptable margin when removing benign tumors with low risk of local recurrence, such as nonossifying fibroma or enchondroma.

A marginal surgical margin (Fig. 22-25) involves a plane of dissection through the *reactive zone* located between the tumor and normal tissue. The *reactive zone* refers to tissue surrounding the tumor that is compressed and inflamed by tumor invasion and enlargement. Although this is located outside a tumor's pseudocapsule, it potentially contains foci of microscopic tumor, and thus dissection through this plane risks the possibility of leaving residual microscopic disease. This is an acceptable margin for latent benign bone tumors, such as aneurysmal bone cyst or osteoblastoma, and for most benign soft tissue tumors, such as lipoma and myxoma. However, it is associated with a high recurrence rate in high-grade malignant tumors. This reactive or inflammatory zone usually demonstrates a significant decrease in activity with appropriate chemotherapy.

A wide margin (Fig. 22-25) involves excising the tumor, its pseudocapsule, the surrounding reactive zone, and a cuff of normal tissue. The dissection remains outside the zone of reactive tissue, and thus the tumor specimen contains a cuff of normal tissue around its entire circumference. No specifications or requirements have been determined for the thickness of this cuff of normal tissue. According to this system, however, it is generally believed that a wide margin extends at least 1 to 2 cm. This is the preferred margin of resection for most malignant tumors.

A radical margin (Fig. 22-25) involves an en bloc excision of the tumor, its pseudocapsule, the reactive zone, and the entire compartment within which it is contained.

Radical resections are indicated in the presence of malignancy with skip lesions.

A malignant intraosseous tumor of the proximal end of the humerus treated with a radical surgical margin requires excision of the entire humerus. A similar lesion of the deltoid treated with a radical surgical margin would involve a procedure that includes the total excision of the deltoid compartment from origin to insertion.

The surgical margin is defined by its closest margin. Each particular surgical margin may be achieved by local resection or by amputation (Fig. 22-25). Determination of the surgical margin is the critical step that allows the surgeon to integrate the surgical treatment with the staging system and thus to outline treatment and assess clinical results. Assessments of the surgical margin and the stage of the lesion allow a prediction of local recurrence based on past experience (Table 22-5).

Limb Salvage Surgery

Surgical treatment of high-grade sarcomas of bone can involve amputation or limb salvage. In the skeletally immature patient with significant growth potential remaining, amputation is preferable to resection, although expandable prostheses are also available. These metal arthroplasties have an extendible screw mechanism that can be lengthened at intervals to allow skeletal growth. Limb salvage surgery is a reasonable alternative to amputation when a wide surgical margin is achievable and enough soft tissue is preserved to allow a reasonably good functional result. One study showed limb salvage for tumors of the shoulder girdle to have good intermediate results (average follow-up, 5.3 years) in terms of pain, emotional acceptance, and dexterity.[161] In most cases the functional criteria for limb-sparing surgery are stricter than the criteria for tumor control. Sufficient functional muscle mass is required to obtain a reasonable functional result and to avoid wound complications.[217]

Limb salvage, or limb-sparing, resections of the shoulder girdle are generally indicated for neoplasms that have no major neurovascular involvement and where there is enough remaining bone stock proximally and distally to allow a reasonable reconstruction. In addition adequate soft tissue coverage and deltoid function are required to prevent wound complications and to achieve sufficient functional results.[1,39,57,58,61,127,176] The most common restrictions for effective limb salvage include nerve involvement or the adequacy of soft tissue coverage.

Patients with soft tissue sarcomas or bony sarcomas of the proximal part of the humerus with considerable soft tissue extension are challenging limb salvage candidates. The brachial neurovascular structures and glenohumeral joint are not infrequently involved by the tumor, and careful preoperative staging is essential before deciding on a surgical plan or attempting limb salvage procedures. High-grade malignant tumors of the proximal end of the humerus are typically extracompartmental lesions (grade IIB) that require a wide surgical resection to achieve a cure.

Preoperative staging studies help determine appropriate surgical candidates and the feasibility of a wide surgical resection. The amount of soft tissue involvement and the proximity of the medial neurovascular bundle present a preoperative challenge to determining candidates for limb salvage.

Another preoperative challenge for high-grade sarcomas is assessment of the extent of bone disease and whether this extends into the glenohumeral joint. If the joint is involved, an extracapsular or extra-articular resection is indicated, with resection of the glenoid en bloc with the capsule of the glenohumeral joint and the remainder of the proximal end of the humerus. Preoperative tasks include assessing for distant metastatic disease and determining the extent of bone and soft tissue margins with the planned resection.[39]

The primary site of a tumor to some extent predicts certain resection and reconstruction tendencies. High-grade sarcomas of the proximal part of the humerus are likely to have a close relationship to the medial neurovascular bundle (brachial plexus or brachial artery or vein), axillary nerve, deltoid, or glenohumeral joint. Chest wall involvement with these tumors is less common and usually occurs as a late finding after involvement of the medial neurovascular structures. Obviously, the best limb salvage candidates are those with primary bone tumors that have minimal extraosseous extension. Soft tissue

TABLE 22-5 Recurrence Rate by Surgical Margin Versus Stage

	Recurrence Rate (%)						
	Benign			Malignant			
Surgical Margin	**1**	**2**	**3**	**IA**	**IB**	**IIA**	**IIB**
Intracapsular	0	30	50	90	90	100	100
Marginal	0	0	50	70	70	90	90
Wide	0	0	10	10	30	50	70
Radical	0	0	0	0	0	10	20

Modified from Enneking WF. Musculoskeletal Tumor Surgery. *New York: Churchill-Livingstone; 1983:99.*

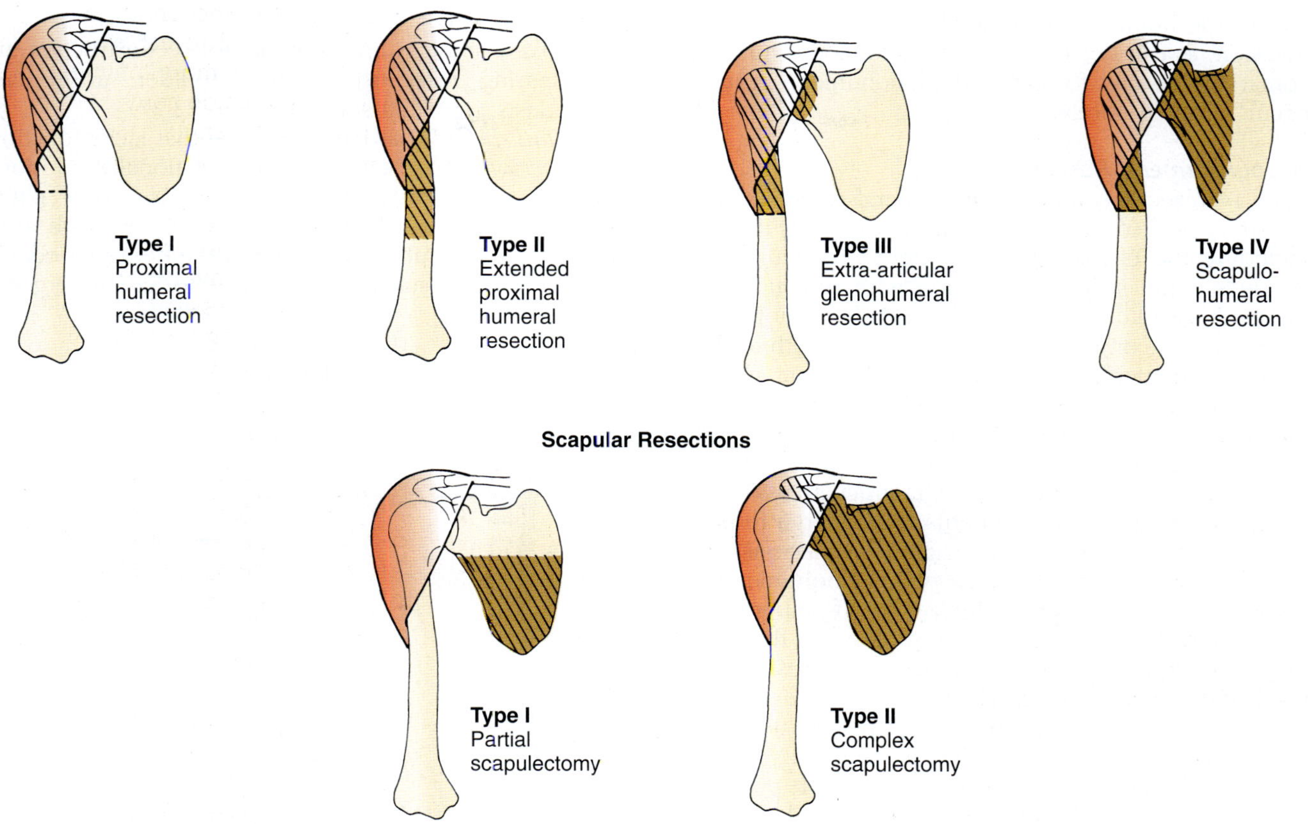

FIGURE 22-26: Classification of shoulder resections. Each type of resection can be subtyped A or B based on the preservation or removal, respectively, of the deltoid.

sarcomas of the shoulder region are easily resected when located in the deltoid, but deltoid resection precludes arthroplasty as a reasonable alternative because of the subsequent loss of active abduction. The following classification system is useful for describing these different resections and the various reconstructive principles (Fig. 22-26).

Short Proximal Humeral Resection

Type I resections, or short proximal humeral resections, are proximal to the deltoid insertion of the humerus (Fig. 22-26). These resections are intra-articular; that is, the bone resection includes the humeral head, and the proximal plane of resection passes through the glenohumeral joint. These resections might or might not involve an en bloc resection of the abductor mechanism. The abductor mechanism includes the rotator cuff, the deltoid muscle, and the deltoid's (axillary) innervation. The sacrifice of any part of this composite results in significantly weakened abduction and a significant change in the expectation of postoperative function (see "Reconstructive Procedures," later). Axillary nerve injury or resection is a common consideration because of the location at the inferior and posterior aspect of the humeral neck.

Proximal humeral resections that include a part of the abductor mechanism are referred to in this classification system as *type IB humeral resections* (Fig. 22-26). Resections of the humerus that do not sacrifice a part of the abductor mechanism are referred to as *type IA resections.* This subclassification into A (preservation of an active abductor mechanism) and B (resection or sacrifice of a part of the abductor mechanism) is also used to classify the other resection types as described.

Long Proximal Humeral Resections

Type II resections (Fig. 22-26) are proximal humeral resections in which the distal osteotomy is made distal to the deltoid insertion. This type usually includes proximal humeral resections longer than 12 cm. They are referred to as type IIA or IIB, depending on whether they spare or include (respectively) the abductor mechanism with the resection. Type II, or long humeral, resections have a longer rehabilitation period and a greater overall incidence of complications or more limited functional results because of the long bone reconstruction and the need to reattach the deltoid.

Glenohumeral Resections

Type III resections of the proximal end of the humerus extend to the glenoid side of the glenohumeral joint in an extra-articular or extracapsular fashion (Fig. 22-26). The proximal bone resection is through the base of the glenoid or scapular neck. Type III resections are typically carried out for high-grade malignancies of the proximal part of the humerus or humeral head with intra-articular invasion, as can occur with osteosarcoma or chondrosarcoma. Indications for type III glenohumeral resections occur relatively rarely.

Scapulohumeral Resections

Type IV resections are scapulohumeral resections of the proximal end of the humerus and scapula (Fig. 22-26), including the classic Tikhoff-Linberg procedure, which involves a full scapular resection with resection of the humeral head.[18,79,124,139] An extended Tikhoff-Linberg resection is a complete scapular resection with a lengthy proximal humeral resection. The resection might or might not include a portion of the deltoid or abductor mechanism (A or B). Modifications of the original Tikhoff-Linberg procedure involve a subtotal scapular resection en bloc along with extra-articular resection of the proximal end of the humerus. These large resections are typically carried out for high-grade lesions of the proximal part of the humerus with glenohumeral joint involvement. One criterion for a Tikhoff-Linberg procedure, as with any limb-sparing surgery, is the lack of involvement of the neurovascular structures (the brachial artery, vein, and brachial plexus). The procedure entails a large scapular resection that is usually left without reconstruction.

Scapulohumeral resections are examples of limb-sparing procedures that result in very limited postoperative function, but they are certainly better compared with forequarter amputation. These resections are accepted well by the patient when the functional limitations are fully discussed before surgery. Postoperatively, patients typically have varying degrees of proximal humeral stability and a well-innervated, functional hand and elbow. Elbow motion depends on the degree of postoperative humeral stability. In this setting where the surgical alternative is an amputation, many patients are satisfied with this limited degree of function.[18,79,124,139,240]

Scapular Resections

Scapular resections may be classified as partial (type I) or complex (type II) resections, depending on whether they include the glenoid (complex) or not (partial) (Fig. 22-26). Partial resections of the scapula are associated with relatively high functional results postoperatively compared with the more restricted functional performance after complex or complete resections of the scapula.[25,143,235]

This classification system does not include other, less common resections about the shoulder, such as various partial or intercalary resections of the humerus that might or might not involve reconstruction. These resections are associated with excellent function postoperatively when the surrounding neurovascular structures and the abductor mechanism are preserved. Partial resection of the humerus may be undertaken for less aggressive benign lesions, such as periosteal chondroma or chondroblastoma. Partial resection of the scapula and clavicle is also unusual and may be undertaken for malignant or benign lesions.[203,204]

Reconstructive Procedures

Three basic choices are available for reconstruction after limb-sparing resection of the shoulder: arthroplasty, arthrodesis, or a flail shoulder (Fig. 22-27).

A *flail shoulder* is defined as one that lacks functional motor power and stability. It is functionally inferior to arthroplasty or arthrodesis but superior to a painful arthroplasty or arthrodesis. A flail shoulder, such as the shoulder that results after a Tikhoff-Linberg procedure is an acceptable result for a patient who has undergone a

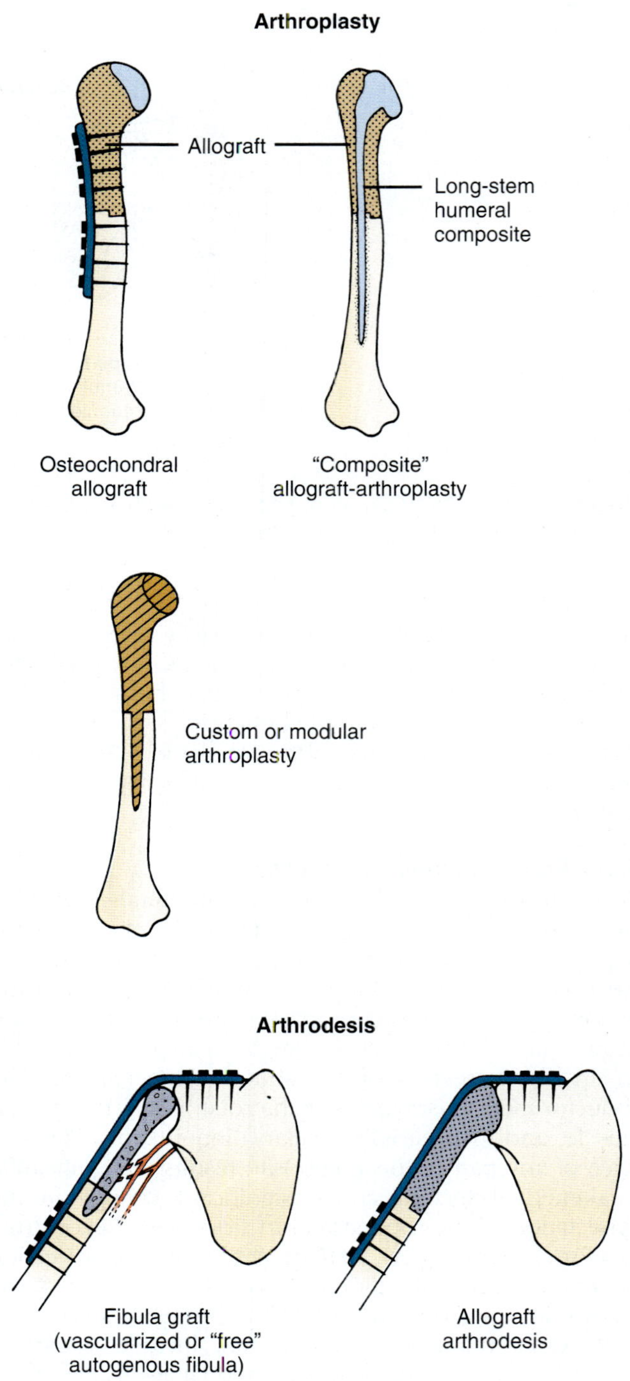

FIGURE 22-27: Reconstruction alternatives.

large scapulohumeral resection for an aggressive tumor. Numerous techniques have been attempted in the past to stabilize the remaining humerus to the chest wall. The original technique of using an intramedullary rod sutured to a proximal rib was discontinued because of the rod migrating into the wound flaps.[25] In addition, suspension of the mid-humerus to the remaining clavicle to achieve some degree of stability has also been attempted. The best method of stabilization involves the reattachment of any remaining proximal musculature to the proximal end of the humerus. A flail shoulder remains a viable alternative after large resections and for the complications of a painful, infected, or failed arthroplasty or arthrodesis. However, a flail joint is unstable, in the true sense of the word, and an attempt should be made to limit instability by soft tissue reconstruction whenever possible.[18,79,124,139,169]

The choice of arthroplasty versus arthrodesis after shoulder resection should be considered carefully with the patient before surgery. The patient's age, personality, vocation, lifestyle, and handedness all affect the decision and should be taken into account. An arthrodesis is more durable than an arthroplasty and may be preferred in young, active patients.

In general, an arthroplasty requires active abduction and glenohumeral stability, both of which call for a competent, functional abductor mechanism. However, what constitutes a functionally competent abductor mechanism is a source of some debate. The abductor mechanism has three basic anatomic components: the deltoid muscle, the rotator cuff muscles (supraspinatus, infraspinatus, and teres minor), and their respective blood supply (circumflex and suprascapular vessels) and innervation (axillary and suprascapular nerves). Resection or injury of the axillary nerve after resection or biopsy of the humerus is not uncommon, and the loss of deltoid function has significant functional consequences. A well-innervated deltoid is the minimal requirement for a functional, stable arthroplasty.

Loss of rotator cuff function has, in the past, required a constrained or semiconstrained arthroplasty, which is associated with greater complications and may have served as an indication for arthrodesis.[179] Newer reconstructive procedures have achieved functional arthroplasties with various unconstrained prostheses using oversized humeral components instead of constrained glenohumeral designs (F.A. Matsen, personal communication, 1988). Press-fit stems and improved screw and washer constructs that better reconstruct the rotator cuff–prosthesis attachment can offer improved results compared with earlier methods.[126] A reverse prosthesis may be especially useful in tumor resections of the shoulder necessitating sacrifice of the rotator cuff, although experience of this is limited.[50] These techniques and others have significantly improved results compared with the high failure rates (50%) in earlier series, but they lack long-term follow-up.[11,92,158,178]

Currently, arthroplasty techniques involve the use of metal, ceramic, or osteochondral allograft implants. The increasing use of allograft transplantation[133,134,171] has had two major effects on the reconstruction of humeral resections. First, it has increased the length of the proximal part of the humerus that can be reconstructed, thereby expanding the indications for limb salvage procedures. Previously, resections were limited to those that could be reconstructed with an autogenous fibular graft or a customized long-stemmed humeral component. It is now possible to replace resections within 8 cm of the distal end of the humerus. Second, allograft reconstructions may be a more reasonable reconstructive alternative in a younger patient because of their potential as a biologic structure. An allograft reconstruction offers the advantages of enhanced soft tissue attachment to the graft, bone union to the remaining humerus, and the potential for transplantation of viable cartilage.

Arthroplasty reconstructions after tumor resection involve the choice of an allograft,[178] a metal[20] or ceramic[20,201,209,214] prosthesis, or a combination of an allograft and a prosthesis, referred to as a *composite reconstruction* (Fig. 22-28).[188] The composite reconstruction involves an allograft or "alloprosthetic" reconstruction that is fixed with a long-stemmed humeral component through the graft and cemented into the remaining humeral bone stock. Composite proximal humeral allografts are the preferred type of allograft reconstruction because of the relatively high failure rate (50%) with osteochondral grafts; they can be cemented or press-fitted into the allograft or the remaining humerus. With this type of reconstruction, reattachment of the deltoid or rotator cuff to the allograft has a distinct advantage over reattachment to metal prostheses.

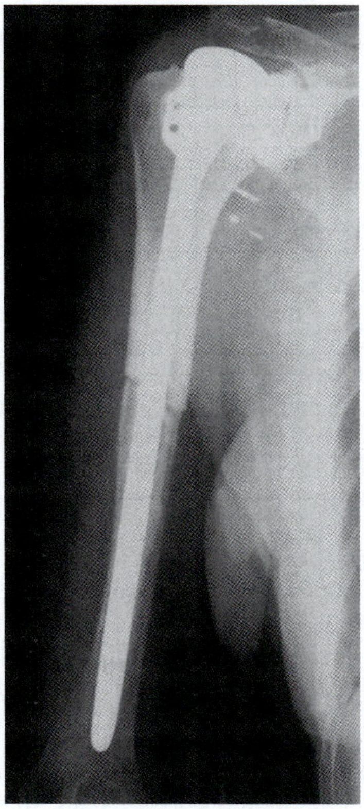

FIGURE 22-28: Composite reconstruction of the proximal part of the humerus.

The greatest challenge after a proximal humeral hemiarthroplasty reconstruction with an allograft is reconstruction of the surrounding soft tissues. Great care has to be taken in reconstructing the glenohumeral joint capsule, the rotator cuff, and the deltoid insertion at the time of transplantation. The processes of bone ingrowth and remodeling, soft tissue attachment, graft fixation, revascularization, and cartilage survival remain areas of active research and clinical investigation. Graft fracture, infection, rejection, and poor function are still serious potential issues that occur in a significant number of patients.[85,133,134,171]

The reconstructive alternative to allograft transplantation is a prosthetic implant of an acceptable metal or ceramic. Prosthetic implants offer the advantage of strength and custom fit, and they are an excellent alternative, especially in older patients. To date, the functional results of arthroplasties in the proximal end of the humerus have been excellent for both composite reconstructions and metal implants.[20,113,188,209,212] In the pediatric population in whom there is an anticipated limb-length discrepancy, an extensible endoprosthesis of the proximal humerus results in good arm function as well as reliable equalization of limb length.[6] As yet, no studies have described comparative differences in function, infection, and revision surgery for these procedures. Newer modular prosthetic designs provide the attractive alternative of a readily available implant that can be customized to the resection defect intraoperatively without delay. These prostheses are newer designs with as yet little clinical follow-up, but they appear to have considerable application in reconstructing the humerus after tumor resection.[188]

Complications following proximal humeral resection and implant hemiarthroplasty reconstructions include instability of the glenohumeral joint, poor rotator cuff function, and aseptic loosening of the implant's humeral stem.

An arthrodesis after tumor resection may be achieved with various bone graft materials, including free or vascularized autogenous fibular grafts or allograft transplantation.[34,36,82,196,241] Resections of up to 5 to 6 cm may be reconstructed with autogenous cancellous grafts from the iliac crest, with or without some shortening of the humerus itself.[23,24,223,225] The remaining humerus should be buttressed against the acromion and might or might not be offset from the glenoid with autogenous grafts. Resections of the humerus up to 20 cm in length may be reconstructed with a vascularized autogenous fibular graft. Free (nonvascularized) autogenous fibular grafts may be used for defects less than 12 cm.[83,205] Nonvascularized fibular grafts longer than 12 cm are associated with a high incidence of graft fracture.[23]

Frozen allograft is a reasonable alternative graft material for shoulder arthrodesis, although achieving bony union can prove challenging.[245] The use of postoperative radiation therapy or chemotherapy has deleterious effects on the bone union of any reconstruction.

Internal fixation of an arthrodesis is best achieved with the use of a long-angled custom plate that enables the patient to avoid prolonged postoperative immobilization and permits enhanced fixation and positioning of the fusion. Such long-angled plates are required for long humeral resections, whereas shorter, more conventional plates may be used for shorter humeral resections.[36] When a long-angled plate is used, at least eight cortices are required for adequate distal humeral fixation. Likewise, scapular fixation requires four or five good scapula screws to prevent a failure of fixation proximally. Careful positioning of the plate at the acromion is necessary to avoid prominence and wound complications. Spica cast immobilization is not required postoperatively if adequate fixation is achieved.[36] Postoperatively, the patient may use a sling with a soft bolster under the elbow. Exercises to improve rhomboid and periscapular strength can begin 6 weeks after surgery and the patient may carefully begin abduction exercises at 8 weeks.[36]

The greatest functional disadvantage of an arthrodesis is the restriction of rotation inherent in the procedure. Most patients are happy with the functional results and obtain adequate abduction (70 to 80 degrees) postoperatively. Limited abduction after arthrodesis usually reflects prolonged immobilization, poor rehabilitation, or a persistent or painful nonunion. The abduction that does occur after arthrodesis is at the scapulothoracic interval and is powered by the rhomboids and other scapular muscles. Patients who are not candidates for an arthroplasty are often good candidates for an arthrodesis because their alternative reconstructive option is usually a flail shoulder.[34,36,84,196] Overall, functional results of arthrodesis are good despite a high complication rate.[81]

Scapular resections are unusual procedures that can involve partial or complex resections.[25,49,143,170,198,202,235] Complex scapular resections in this classification system (see Fig. 22-26) involve a portion of the glenoid. Some experience has been gained in prosthetic replacement of the scapula after total scapulectomy.[55,249] Reconstruction with a scapular prosthesis requires the humeral head replacement to articulate with the prosthetic glenoid. The ideal indication for such a prosthesis is a partial scapulectomy.[55] Eckardt and colleagues[55] reported a series of eight patients treated by endoprosthetic replacement of the scapula for various malignant or benign aggressive lesions. The follow-up on these patients was limited (mean, 20 months), but 50% achieved acceptable (good to excellent) functional results. Likewise, Wittig and colleagues reported a series of three patients who underwent constrained total scapular reconstruction.[249] All of these patients had a stable, painless shoulder with good functional results.[249]

As yet, scapular prosthetic replacement remains a somewhat experimental procedure for which only early, short-term clinical results have been reported. The use of allograft for reconstruction after scapular resection is relatively uncommon, but it can result in good function and stability provided that the rotator cuff mechanism is maintained.[154] Figure 22-29 illustrates the case of a 42-year-old woman with a grade 2 chondrosarcoma of her scapula who underwent resection and reconstruction with a size-matched cadaveric scapular allograft.

Despite the developments and enthusiasm for new techniques of scapular reconstruction, partial and

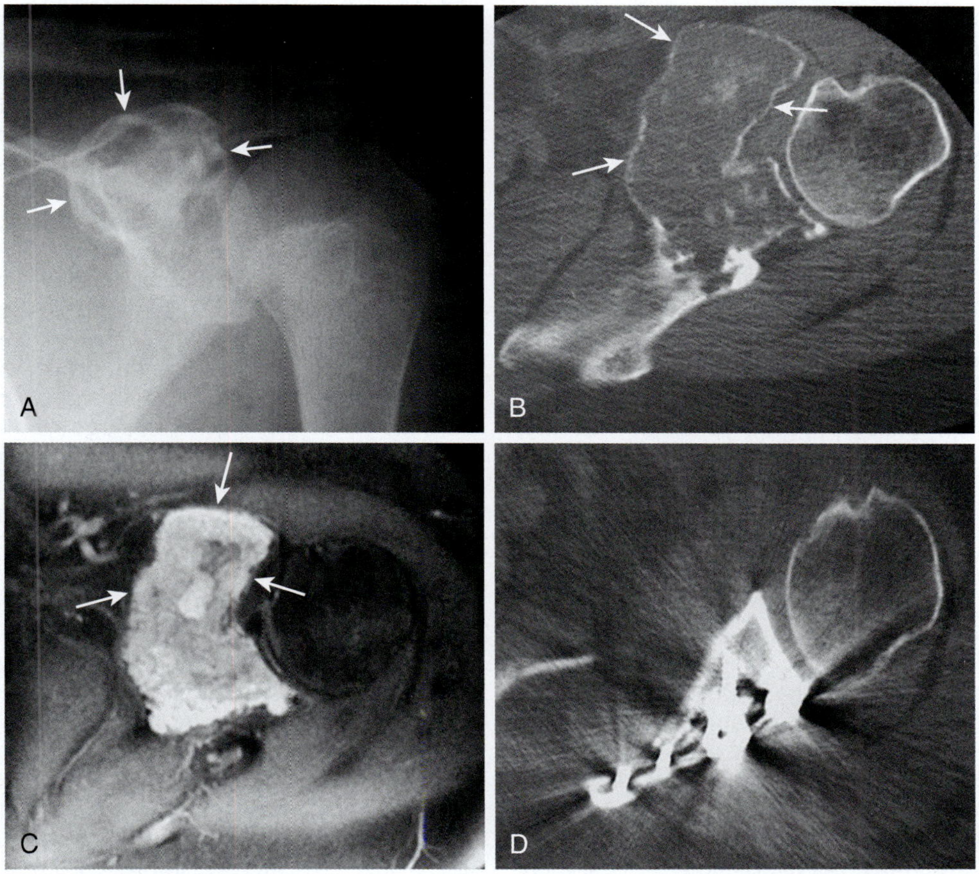

FIGURE 22-29: **A,** Plain film of an expansile scapular grade 2 chondrosarcoma in a 42-year-old woman (*arrows*). **B,** Computed tomography scan showing thinning of the cortical surfaces of the coracoid process and glenoid as well as the presence of calcifications in the lesion. **C,** Magnetic resonance imaging demonstrates the presence of typical high signal intensity from a cartilaginous neoplasm (*arrows*). **D,** Postoperative plain film shows concentric alignment of the patient's native humeral head against a scapular cadaveric allograft.

complete scapulectomies can achieve remarkably good functional results without reconstructive procedures beyond soft tissue closure.

Management of Specific Lesions

Aggressive Benign Bone Tumors

The surgical treatment of active or aggressive benign bone tumors presents a greater challenge when the tumor occurs adjacent to a significant structure, such as a major nerve or vessel, a joint or joint surface, or an active growth plate. Aggressive benign lesions of bone with significant subchondral bone loss often present the greatest challenge in preserving a functional joint.

Aggressive and active benign tumors are typified in the adult by benign giant cell tumor of bone, which occurs in the proximal part of the humerus in 15% to 20% of cases. The choice of treatment for such a lesion includes resection versus intralesional curettage. The latter is usually associated with the use of a local adjuvant to reduce the risk of local recurrence. Various local adjuvants that have been used include the application of liquid nitrogen (cryosurgery) or phenol (phenolization), placement of methylmethacrylate (cementation), mechanical burring, and various forms of cauterization. Wide surgical resection offers the lowest risk of tumor recurrence but represents aggressive treatment for a benign tumor and should be reserved for tumors involving extensive destruction or for those which exhibit multiple recurrences. Experience with curettage and cryosurgery has demonstrated a lower recurrence rate (10%) than with other forms of local adjuvant treatment.[37,90]

Aggressive benign soft tissue tumors are best exemplified by aggressive fibromatosis in young adults; these lesions also require a wide surgical margin to minimize the risk of recurrence. Lesions that are juxtaposed to a major neurovascular structure may be treated with a marginal surgical resection in addition to radiation therapy. Radiation therapy appears to be efficacious in minimizing the recurrence rate after marginal resection, and new chemotherapy agents exist for controlling multiply recurrent desmoid tumors.

Chondrosarcoma of Bone

Chondrosarcoma is the most common primary adult malignancy of bone. It commonly occurs in the proximal part of the humerus. The treatment of low-grade chondrosarcoma typically involves aggressive curettage with local adjuvant treatment (generally employing the same agents used in the treatment of giant cell tumor) and reconstruction with polymethylmethacrylate or allogeneic bone grafting. Chemotherapy and radiotherapy bring no added benefit in the treatment of an intermediate- or low-grade chondrosarcoma. Patients in whom local recurrence develops after surgery can also be treated surgically for this; however, a more aggressive surgical resection is indicated for multiple recurrences.

Intermediate- or high-grade chondrosarcomas are less common and require a wide surgical margin. These higher-grade malignancies cannot reasonably be treated by intralesional procedures because of an increased risk of local recurrence and metastatic disease. These tumors are generally poorly responsive to radiation and chemotherapy.

High-Grade Malignancies of Bone

Osteosarcoma

High-grade osteosarcoma is best treated by preoperative ("neoadjuvant") chemotherapy, reassessment of the response to chemotherapy (restaging), wide margin surgical resection, and postoperative chemotherapy.[47,160,190,215] The reconstruction options previously discussed are commonly employed at the time of resection. Long-term follow-up of limb-sparing surgery for osteosarcoma of the proximal humerus has suggested that prosthetic survival is excellent and function is satisfactory.[247] Postoperative chemotherapy is tailored or adjusted depending on the degree of necrosis in the surgical tumor specimen. This type of treatment was first developed in the Sloan-Kettering T10 methotrexate protocol, with subsequent modifications of pediatric chemotherapy guidelines via the Children's Oncology Group.[47,190,217]

Studies have shown a significant survival correlation with histologic necrosis following chemotherapy, exceeding 90% necrosis on pathologic review of postresection specimens. That degree of necrosis occurs in approximately 50% of pediatric patients.[47]

Patients with metastatic disease provide a significant survival challenge, but up to 25% to 30% can demonstrate long-term survival with chemotherapy and aggressive surgery.

Ewing Sarcoma

Current treatment of Ewing sarcoma is similar to the treatment of osteosarcoma in that preoperative induction chemotherapy is delivered after a histologic diagnosis is obtained with an appropriate biopsy.[91,152,191,225,246] Although treatment of Ewing sarcoma 10 years ago involved a combination of chemotherapy and radiation therapy, several studies that documented a high local recurrence rate, especially with large tumors (greater than 10 cm), led to the preferential use of wide resection surgery for local control.[191] The morbidity may be significant after radiation treatment of lower extremity lesions in young children with Ewing sarcoma.[119,152,225,246] In addition, these patients have one of the highest risks for secondary sarcomas, such as radiation-induced osteosarcoma arising from the radiation field.[130,160]

A wide surgical margin should be the goal of surgical resection, but surgical margins are more difficult to assess with Ewing sarcoma. If the surgical resection is marginal, postoperative radiation therapy is indicated. Patients with Ewing sarcoma typically have a large soft tissue mass that usually demonstrates impressive shrinkage with a reasonable response to chemotherapy.[191,232] The total treatment protocol for Ewing sarcoma usually involves approximately 10 to 12 months of chemotherapy.

Amputations for patients with Ewing or osteosarcoma are now relatively uncommon procedures reserved for young patients (<10 years) with significant growth issues or patients of any age with large or recurrent tumors. Limb salvage patients with unresolved neurovascular or wound complications may also require amputation for the resolution of postoperative complications.

Adult Soft Tissue Sarcomas

Soft tissue sarcomas can occur as high-, low-, or intermediate-grade neoplasms. The goal of surgery is to obtain a tumor-free margin; positive margins increase the risk of tumor recurrence. Soft tissue sarcomas with adequate surgical margins are best treated with the addition of adjuvant radiation therapy. Sarcomas that were initially misdiagnosed as benign and which undergo a contaminated marginal resection should be reexcised with adequate margins. It has been demonstrated that this aggressive two-surgery approach improves survival.[117] Radiation therapy has been shown to improve the local disease-free survival in the shoulder girdle when used to treat large tumors (>5 cm).[149]

Significant controversy exists regarding the use of adjuvant radiation therapy preoperatively versus postoperatively. Proponents of preoperative radiation therapy have argued that the smaller field is a distinct advantage despite a higher incidence of postoperative wound complications. Both approaches are valid.

High-grade soft tissue sarcomas have been treated with preoperative radiation therapy followed by surgical resection and chemotherapy.[7] Local recurrence has not been a significant problem (<10%), whereas pulmonary metastases have posed a problem (10% to 30%). Chemotherapy has demonstrated limited survival advantage in many studies, and its use therefore remains controversial. Many neoadjuvant chemotherapy trials continue to assess early response rates and survival outcomes for the many adult soft tissue sarcoma subtypes. Treatment recommendation and staging assessment guidelines have been established and published by the National Comprehensive Cancer Network.

Metastatic Disease

In the adult population metastatic bone disease is the most common cause of bone destruction in the shoulder. Most lesions in the scapula can be treated with external beam radiation unless there is a pathologic fracture with intra-articular involvement. For the humerus, radiation can be used to treat most small and asymptomatic lesions.

There is ongoing debate regarding the radiographic changes that need to be present to put a long bone at the risk of pathologic fracture. Although the Mirels classification attempts to predict fracture risk in long bones by assigning a score based on anatomic, radiographic, and clinical features, it is nonspecific, and strict adherence to it can result in surgical overtreatment.[46,151] Nevertheless, it is generally agreed that greater than 50% cortical bone destruction in the diaphyseal region puts a patient at risk of pathologic fracture. In this situation surgical treatment is warranted with either plate fixation or an intramedullary device. For lesions involving the humeral head or proximal metaphyseal region, a humeral endoprosthesis is a good option because rigid fixation is difficult to achieve.

Regardless of the surgical procedure, the goal is immediate rigid fixation that provides pain relief and rapid postoperative use of the shoulder and extremity.[17] If the humerus has already fractured from metastatic disease, the same principles of aggressive surgical fixation apply. Palliative forequarter amputation for metastases to the shoulder girdle region should be reserved only for tumors that have major neurovascular or chest wall extension or for severe intractable pain with the loss of limb function.[248]

AUTHORS' PREFERRED METHODS OF TREATMENT

Biopsy

Biopsy of musculoskeletal tumors is always the initial and probably one of the most important steps in evaluating and treating these challenging lesions. The biopsy site should always be placed in the line of a possible future resection and should not be performed before completing an adequate clinical evaluation as well as diagnostic radiographic staging studies. When the staging studies and the clinical findings of the patient suggest a particular lesion, a needle biopsy is our preferred method.

Most classic osteosarcomas have fairly typical radiographic findings and can easily be diagnosed with a needle biopsy. However, when a lesion's diagnosis is still uncertain, even after initial staging studies, an open biopsy provides the best diagnosis. The more generous the biopsy specimen, the easier it is to make the correct diagnosis. In many cases cytogenetic studies are needed to fully analyze the specimen. In general, at least a gram of tissue is required, much more than would be obtainable using needle or core biopsy techniques. Providing enough of a biopsy specimen without contaminating the extremity remains a challenge even for an experienced oncology surgeon. In general, the biopsy should be performed by the surgeon who will carry out the definitive resection.[136]

Surgical Choices

In terms of treatment choices, three different categories of lesions remain a challenge in today's setting: aggressive benign lesions such as giant cell tumor, low-grade malignant lesions such as chondrosarcoma, and high-grade malignant lesions such as osteosarcoma or Ewing sarcoma.

Giant cell tumor, in many cases, is a difficult lesion to treat because it is locally aggressive, causes substantial subchondral bone destruction, and has a high rate of recurrence. It is a difficult tumor to grade histologically and radiographically. Our preferred treatment is curettage along with some method of local "adjuvant" (phenol, burring, cryosurgery, or polymethylmethacrylate). Wide resection should be reserved for tumors associated with substantial bone destruction or multiple recurrences. The experience with curettage and liquid nitrogen has been good regarding tumor control and function of the extremity,[37,90] but this requires careful intraoperative monitoring of the patient for both nitrogen embolic precautions and the protection of soft tissues and neurovascular structures. Denosumab, a RANKL inhibitor, has recently shown significant promise in the systemic treatment of giant cell tumor. Because the long-term effectiveness remains unknown, denosumab treatment should be reserved for multiply recurrent or inoperable tumors.

Low-grade malignancies are typified by low-grade chondrosarcomas, which are difficult lesions to define histologically. Microscopically, a low-grade chondrosarcoma is defined by increased cellularity, binucleated lacunae, and microscopic bone resorption, in addition to the radiographic picture of endosteal cortical resorption and bone destruction. Most of these low-grade lesions are located at the metaphyseal-diaphyseal junction in intramedullary or cancellous bone. Biopsy is unreliable as a diagnostic procedure for this problem. When the diagnosis (enchondroma vs. low-grade chondrosarcoma) is uncertain, we monitor the patient carefully with repeat radiographs every 3 to 6 months and a repeat CT scan or MRI. Treatment of a low-grade malignancy (chondrosarcoma) is similar to that of an aggressive benign lesion (giant cell tumor) with curettage and margin extension. Curettage alone is associated with a very high recurrence rate (70% to 80%) for low-grade malignancies, although recurrence can take 5 to 10 years to appear.

High-Grade Tumors and Preoperative Chemotherapy

High-grade malignancies in the shoulder have a distribution similar to those in other sites, with the most common bone lesions being osteosarcoma and Ewing sarcoma. Most patients with a high-grade malignancy of bone are treated with chemotherapy before surgical resection to minimize local recurrence and to attempt to evaluate tumor response.

Preoperative Adriamycin-based chemotherapy has been effective in improving both overall survival and local recurrence for most pediatric sarcomas. The 5-year survival rates have improved from 25% to 30% previously to a current rate of approximately 60% to 70%. Other improvements in treatment (such as in radiology, pathology, and surgery) have also contributed to this improved survival rate. The chemotherapy protocols are complex and demand a multidisciplinary setting with frequent communication between the chemotherapist and the surgeon.

We also use neoadjuvant chemotherapy for Ewing sarcoma. Although the chemotherapeutic agents are different, the improvement in survival has been similar. Surgical resection is our preferred modality for local control. Adjuvant radiation therapy is often used additionally in the presence of close surgical margins. We rarely use radiation therapy preferentially in the place of surgical resection, except in inoperable tumors, in a palliative setting, or when surgical resection will result in an unacceptable functional outcome.

Soft tissue sarcomas are best treated with surgery and radiation, except in the rare circumstances (generally involving small tumors) where a substantially wide surgical margin can be achieved that precludes the need for radiation therapy. The theoretical benefit of preoperative chemotherapy for soft tissue sarcomas is the early systemic treatment of a systemic disease, minimization of local recurrences, and the opportunity to evaluate the tumor specimen for its response to chemotherapy. However, the survival benefit of chemotherapy remains controversial.

Multiple neoadjuvant chemotherapy trials for adult soft tissue sarcoma have demonstrated an early positive response in soft tissue malignancies using PET imaging that assists with evaluating each patient's response to chemotherapy. National Comprehensive Cancer Network guidelines recommend chemotherapy for high-grade adult soft tissue sarcomas.

Limb-sparing procedures have become quite sophisticated and the functional outcomes are generally good.[71,180] Conversely, there have also been substantial advances in limb prosthetics for amputees. When appropriately performed, limb-sparing procedures do not increase a patient's risk for local recurrence or diminish the patient's chance for survival.[217] Limb salvage surgery should result in a functional outcome at least equivalent to if not greater than what would be obtained with an amputation and appropriate prosthesis. Final decisions regarding limb salvage versus amputation for most patients will depend on the risk, reconstructive risks, and the ability of the patient to tolerate any risk or complications. These decisions are especially compelling when a tumor involves the upper extremity. Communications regarding these decisions are critical.

Musculoskeletal oncology is truly a multidisciplinary specialty centered around the treatment of rare and unusual disorders. Outcomes are best when these patients are treated by an experienced team.

INTERNATIONAL EXPERT COMMENTARY

Simon Carter

The shoulder girdle is the third most common site of primary bone tumors; therefore recognition of the possibility of tumors has to remain in the differential diagnosis of a patient complaining of pain.

Typically the pain complained of is a constant nonmechanical pain that often disturbs sleep. The presence of a mass should also raise concerns. Patients sometimes present with referred pain.

Failure of treatment for a presumed diagnosis should also raise the possibility of a neoplastic condition. The maxim "The correct treatment for the correct diagnosis should result in an improvement" particularly applies to the shoulder. Many patients present late, prejudicing the outcome because of repeated inappropriate treatment for presumed frozen shoulder.

A patient with a suspected tumor of the shoulder should ideally be investigated with targeted imaging, including radiographs and MRI. The diagnosis of a bone tumor can often be made from the plain radiographs, as most tumors have a characteristic appearance; the MRI scan helps in determining the exact site and extent of the lesion.

The differential diagnosis is influenced by the age of the patient; teenagers are the most common age group for osteosarcoma and Ewing sarcoma, whereas middle-aged and elderly most commonly have chondrosarcoma.

The more elderly the patient, the greater is the possibility of plasmacytoma/myeloma and metastatic disease. Myeloma is the most common tumor to arise in bone, with an incidence in the United Kingdom of eight cases per 100,000 compared with an incidence of osteosarcoma of 0.25 cases per 100,000. If metastatic disease is suspected, a thorough history and examination need to be obtained.

Bone scanning is of use in identifying the presence of other sites of bony disease. A request must be made for a whole-body bone scan as often the distal extremities are not imaged. CT of the chest, abdomen, and pelvis are used to identify visceral and chest metastases or the site of the primary disease if the lesion is metastatic.

The presence of a solitary lesion should raise strong suspicion of a primary lesion, and no treatment should be initiated until a definitive diagnosis is obtained, even when there is a pathologic fracture.

After completing the staging studies, a biopsy should be obtained, ideally in the unit that is to treat the patient to avoid contamination of uninvolved tissue compartments and give access to specialty pathologists and techniques. The type of biopsy (such as needle or open) should be determined by the pathologists because the whole purpose of the biopsy is to provide sufficient lesional tissue for diagnosis. Targeted biopsy is important in tumors that have necrotic areas because viable tissue is needed for analysis.

Cartilage tumors represent a difficult diagnostic challenge. Contrast-enhanced MRI scanning helps identify areas of higher metabolic activity, which are more likely to yield diagnostic material. This should be utilized in cases of chondroid lesions that are larger than 5 cm or are painful; that have radiologic features of concern, endosteal scalloping, or peritumoral edema; or are increasing in size on serial radiographs. The use of frozen section has, in the United Kingdom at least, not been popular.

The treatment of the primary tumor depends on the diagnosis and stage of the lesion. Neoadjuvant chemotherapy is used for osteosarcoma and Ewing sarcoma. Chemotherapy is given in a neoadjuvant setting for many reasons, including

INTERNATIONAL EXPERT COMMENTARY—cont'd

an attempt to destroy any metastases that may be present, with the chemonecrosis of the primary tumor being assessed following resection as a surrogate for the response of the metastases. It therefore has a prognostic consequence. The use of neoadjuvant chemotherapy may allow the tumor to decrease in size and/or the margins to become more distinct to allow planning of the definitive resection and, hopefully, better margins of excision.

Inadequate tumor necrosis may require a change in the chemotherapy to alter the outcome, although the evidence supporting such a change in chemotherapy is poor. For Ewing sarcoma, radiotherapy may be used postoperatively if the margins are close and/or there is poor necrosis.

Recent work from our unit has suggested that any viable tumor in the resected specimen indicates that postoperative radiotherapy should be administered to reduce the risk of local recurrence.

Chondrosarcomas are, of course, chemotherapy and radiotherapy resistant and are purely a surgical disease. The principle surgical treatment is resection with reconstruction using a proximal humeral replacement with the shoulder joint stabilized using a mesh or tube. The functional results depend on the extent of bone and soft tissue resection. The function is better if the deltoid insertion is preserved. Benign bone tumors are usually treated using curative biopsy or "curopsy."[186] This simple technique results in about 80% cure in a single stage procedure without the use of adjuvants. Giant cell tumor, if extensive, can be treated medically with the use of denosumab, which allows the lesion to consolidate, and then curettage if there is residual disease. Small chondroid lesions (such as chondroblastomas <2 cm in diameter) can be treated by radiofrequency ablation, avoiding more invasive procedures.

Fibromatosis or desmoid tumors should only be excised if the patient is symptomatic, and resection would not result in a functional deficit. The outcome of treatment is not compromised by delaying surgery and observing the patient. Interestingly, the local recurrence rate is not influenced by the margin of excision, with a reported recurrence rate at primary surgery of about 30%. The decision about treatment must be taken with the expectation of a high rate of recurrence even in expert hands. It must be remembered that fibromatosis does not need to be excised. Indeed, in long-term follow-up it is a self-limiting condition that resolves spontaneously (Figs. 22-30 and 22-31).[45]

The management of metastatic disease depends, of course, on the nature of the primary disease, the presence of other metastases, the disease-free interval and adjuvant treatment, and the prognosis for the patient.

A patient with limited life expectancy could have a "trauma" reconstruction for palliative purposes. If a patient's life expectancy is greater than 6 months, then a resection and reconstruction is appropriate as plating and intramedullary nailing may fail during the life of the patient, and revision sugery may be required. If the metastasis is solitary, there may be an advantage with respect to life expectancy, particularly with breast and renal carcinomas.

Soft tissue sarcomas should be suspected if any of the following features are present: pain, a mass larger than 5 cm in diameter, a mass that is increasing in size, and masses deep to the deep fascia. The chance of malignancy increases with an increasing number of these features.

There is debate about the use of preoperative or postoperative radiotherapy in high-grade soft tissue sarcoma to reduce the risk of local recurrence (although the benefit on survival is not clear). Chemotherapy is reserved usually for patients who present with metastatic disease.

In conclusion, there are many modalities for succesful treatment of tumors around the shoulder, but the clinicians should be wary of unusual symptoms or a failure to respond to treatment; a patient with a tumor may also have a rotator cuff lesion coincidentally. The efficacy of treatment is compromised by delayed presentation. Rapid involvement of a tumor service at an early stage should be encouraged. If there is any doubt, the patient should be investigated quickly; if there is any delay, then rapid referral to a tumor service should be considered.

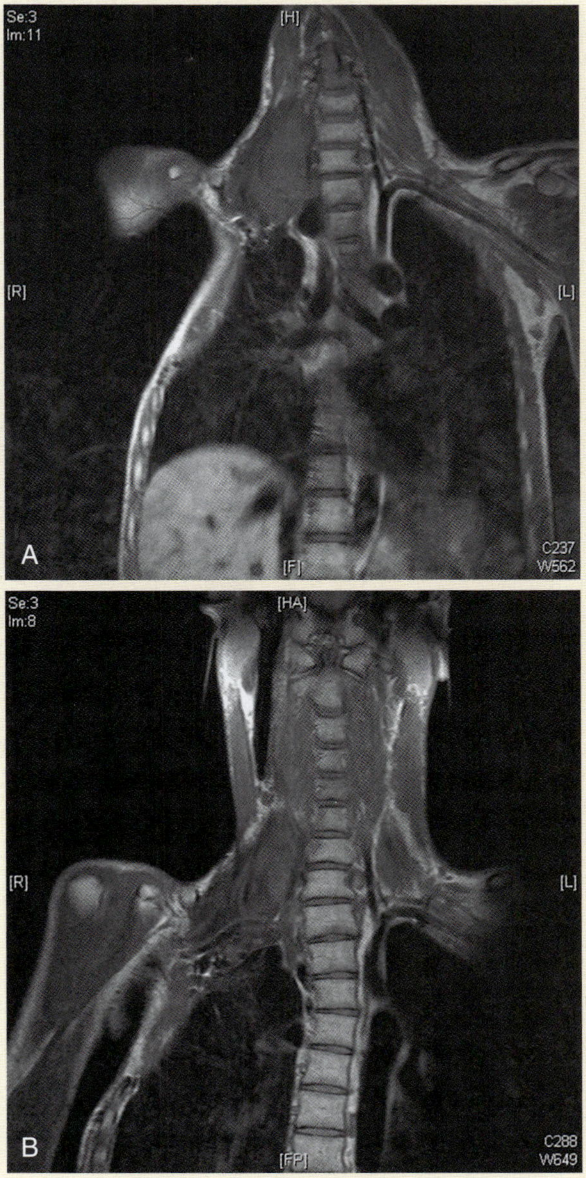

FIGURE 22-30: **A** and **B,** Spontaneous resolution of a desmoid tumor of the base of the neck over a 1-year period.

Continued

INTERNATIONAL EXPERT COMMENTARY—cont'd

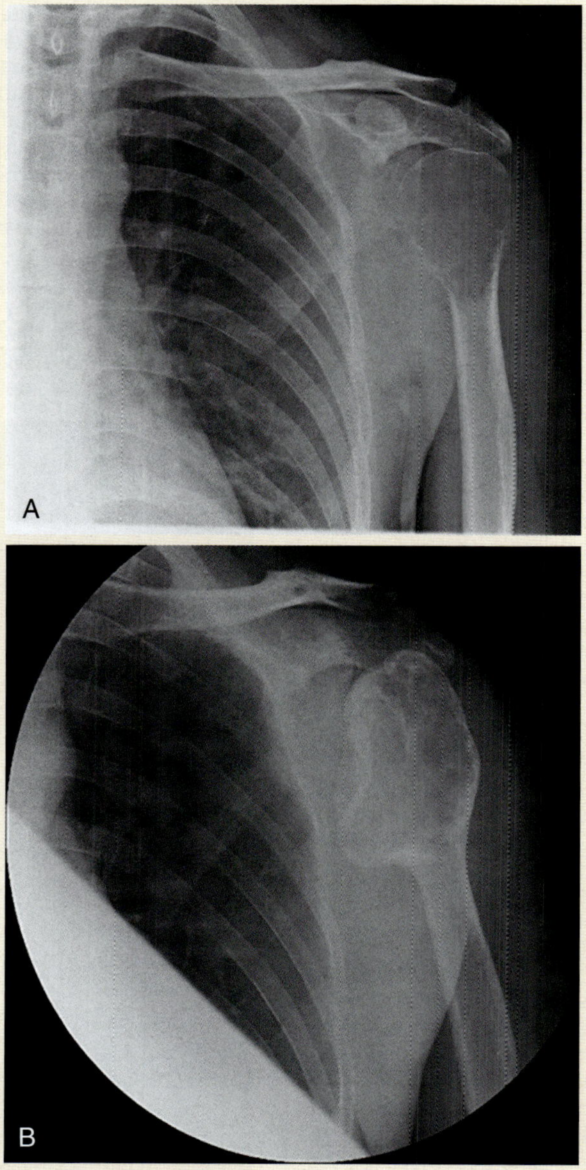

FIGURE 22-31: **A** and **B,** Before and after radiographs of denosumab treatment for giant cell tumor of the humerus after 6 months.

EDITOR COMMENTARY

Steven B. Lippitt

This chapter on shoulder girdle tumors is very well outlined by the authors and logically begins with the complex shoulder anatomy as it relates to tumor biologic behavior and the risks of malignant invasiveness. Relative to other body anatomic regions, the compartments of the shoulder are poorly defined secondary to the traversing brachial plexus and major vessels and the unique biceps long head tendon that provides direct passage to the intra-articular glenohumeral joint. This poses a great challenge in achieving adequate malignant tumor resection while preserving satisfactory shoulder function.

Next, the authors provide the staging and classification for benign and malignant soft tissue and bone tumors. The distinguishing clinical and radiographic features of each lesion are well described with attentive illustrations. Musculoskeletal tumors of the shoulder girdle can have varying presentations. Patients with bone tumors often present with complaint of shoulder pain, including night pain, which can mimic common shoulder disorders, such as rotator cuff disease, arthritis, and frozen shoulder. Patients with soft tissue tumor are often without pain, with a mass discovered incidentally during clinical evaluation. Needless to say, a careful history and physical examination increase the likelihood of early detection of these rare tumors. The male patient should remove his shirt and the female patient should be gowned appropriately to allow full visual inspection and palpation of the shoulder girdle and to allow comparison with the other side to detect subtle asymmetry. In most cases standard orthogonal anteroposterior, scapular lateral, and axillary radiographs will allow accurate detection and even diagnosis of a specific bone tumor. The general practicing shoulder orthopedist must avoid the trap of cursory review of radiographs, inspecting them only for common features, such as acromial spurring, subacromial calcification, and glenohumeral joint space narrowing. The cortical margins and marrow spaces of all bony structures on the radiographs should be systemically followed in a consistent, routine manner to minimize missing subtle, suspicious findings of cortical lucency or irregularity and intramedullary abnormal matrix or calcified lesions. Elderly patients with shoulder pain should especially be considered for differential diagnosis of myeloma or metastatic disease.

Once a bone or soft tissue abnormality is suspected, the appropriate workup should, of course, ensue. This chapter has described the recommended laboratory and special imaging requirements, the principles of biopsy and surgical intervention, the definition and importance of surgical margins, the types of tumor resection, and general concepts regarding subsequent reconstruction. The role of the general orthopedist or shoulder specialist in this process must be carefully considered. All patients with suspected aggressive benign or malignant lesions should be referred to an orthopedic oncologist as part of a multidisciplinary team that includes an interventional radiologist and a musculoskeletal cytopathologist. The tumor biopsy should be very carefully directed as an inappropriate biopsy technique can lead to increased local tumor recurrence or, at worst, can ruin an opportunity for limb salvage, thus requiring amputation. Successful percutaneous needle biopsy typically requires radiographic guidance to obtain adequate viable, representative tissue for specialized histologic exam. An open biopsy of the proximal humerus should be performed through the anterior deltoid and should avoid the standard anterior deltopectoral interval because of the risk of tumor contamination of the adjacent pectoralis major muscle, brachial plexus, and vessels, which makes limb salvage resection often ill-advised. Comparisons of such risks of treatment between an inexperienced center and an experienced cancer center team are well documented.[136,137] Cultures should be obtained routinely with the biopsy regardless of the suspected diagnosis, because infection may simulate any malignancy.

The definitive tumor resection should again reside with the expertise of the specialty trained orthopedic oncologist. The magnitude of the surgical resection will depend on the tumor grade and its anatomic invasiveness, with the final decision about the extent of needed resection often being made at the time of surgery. In limb salvage procedures a functional elbow is highly dependent on the preserved musculocutaneous nerve, while shoulder functional elevation is dependent on the extent of violated rotator cuff, deltoid muscle, or axillary innervation.

The type of shoulder reconstruction plays a secondary role to the adequate wide or radical margin tumor resection. The shoulder specialist's experience in soft tissue repair and arthroplasty techniques may, of course, contribute significantly to the orthopedic oncologist's plan for shoulder reconstruction. Because the planned extent of resection may evolve during surgery, various options of shoulder reconstruction would need to be available.

We are indebted to these authors for the important information in this chapter guiding us with the identification of and appropriate planning for soft tissue and bone lesions, both primary and metastatic. The international perspective on these matters by Dr. Simon Carter, Orthopaedic Oncologist at Royal Orthopaedic Hospital, Birmingham, United Kingdom, is also greatly appreciated. Remember, in our day-to-day shoulder practice, "stay alert!"

Index

Page numbers followed by "*f*" indicate figures, "*t*" indicate tables, "*b*" indicate boxes, and "*e*" indicate online content.

B

C

D

E

F

J

K

L

Q

R

T

U

V

W

Y

Z